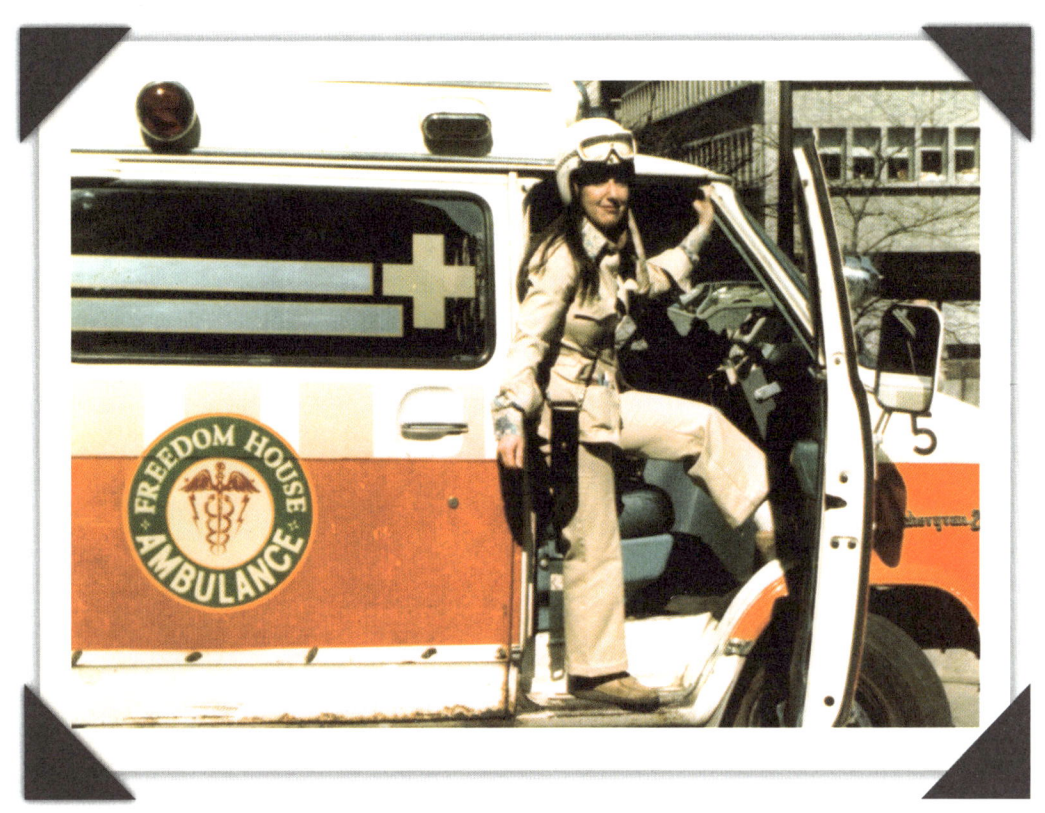

Dedicated to:

Nancy L. Caroline, MD

"The Mother of Paramedics"

1944–2002

AAOS

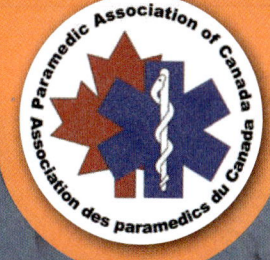

Nancy Caroline's
Emergency
Care in the Streets

Sixth Edition

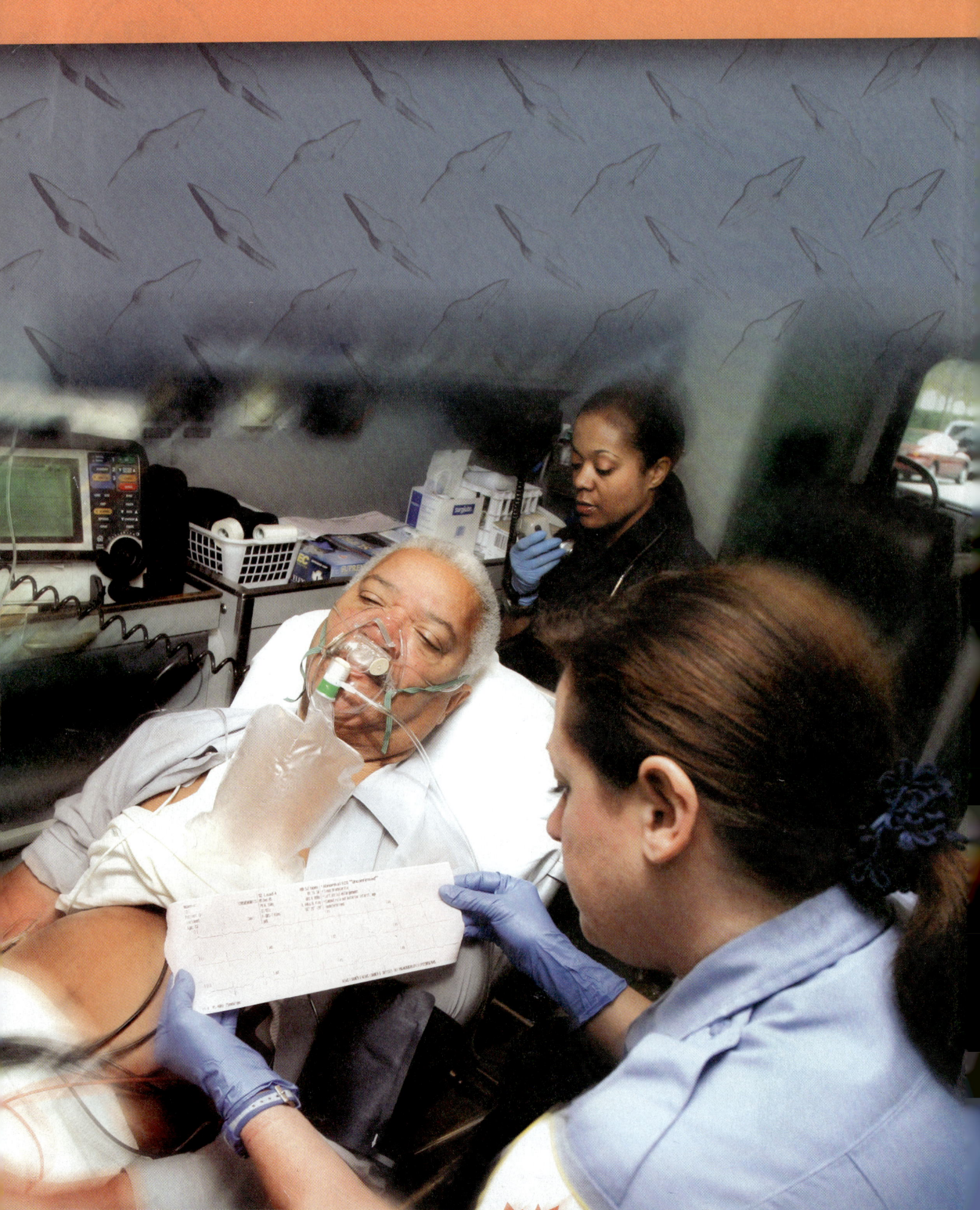

AAOS

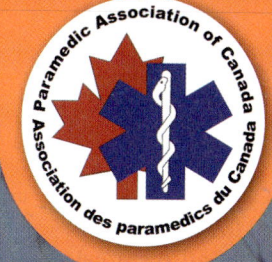

Nancy Caroline's
Emergency
Care in the Streets

Sixth Edition

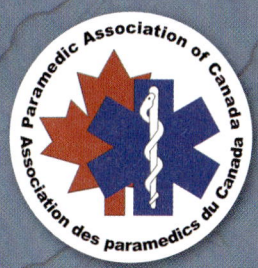

Author:

Nancy L. Caroline, MD

Series Editor:

Andrew N. Pollak, MD, FAAOS

Editors:

Russell D. MacDonald, MD, MPH, FRCPC   Robert J. Burgess, BHSc, ACP, AEMCA, CQIA

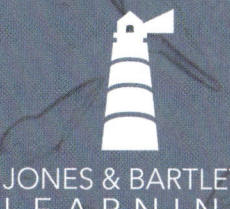

JONES & BARTLETT
LEARNING

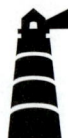

Jones and Bartlett Learning

World Headquarters
Jones & Bartlett Learning
5 Wall Street
Burlington, MA 01803
978-443-5000
info@jblearning.com
www.EMSzone.com

Jones and Bartlett's books and products are available through most bookstores and online booksellers. To contact Jones and Bartlett Publishers directly, call 800-832-0034, fax 978-443-8000, or visit our website, www.jbpub.com.

Substantial discounts on bulk quantities of Jones and Bartlett's publications are available to corporations, professional associations, and other qualified organizations. For details and specific discount information, contact the special sales department at Jones and Bartlett via the above contact information or send an email to specialsales@jbpub.com.

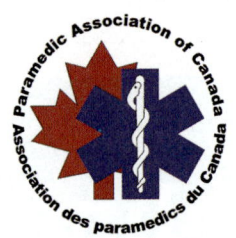

Paramedic Association of Canada
Association des paramédics du Canada
300 March Road, Fourth Floor
Ottawa, Ontario K2K 2E2
613-836-6581
info@paramedic.ca
www.paramedic.ca

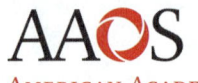

AMERICAN ACADEMY OF ORTHOPAEDIC SURGEONS

Editorial Credits
Chief Executive Officer: Mark W. Wieting
Director, Department of Publications: Marilyn L. Fox, PhD
Managing Editor: Barbara A. Scotese
Associate Senior Editor: Gayle B. Murray

Production Credits

Chief Executive Officer: Clayton Jones
Chief Operating Officer: Donald W. Jones, Jr.
President, Higher Education and Professional Publishing: Robert Holland
Sr., V.P., Sales and Marketing: James Homer
V.P., Production and Design: Anne Spencer
V.P., Manufacturing and Inventory Control: Therese Connell
Publisher, Public Safety: Kimberly Brophy
Director of Marketing: Alisha Weisman
Acquisitions Editor, EMS: Christine Emerton

Editor: Jennifer S. Kling
Associate Managing Editor: Amanda Green
Editorial Assistant: Laura Burns
Senior Production Editor: Susan Schultz
Associate Production Editor: Sarah Bayle
Production Assistant: Tina Chen
Photo Research Manager/Photographer: Kimberly Potvin
Director of Sales and Marketing, Canada: Robert Rosenitsch
Interior Design: Anne Spencer and Kristin E. Parker

Cover Design: Kristin E. Parker
Cartoons: Nick Bertozzi
Composition: diacriTech
Text Printing and Binding: Courier Companies
Cover Printing: Courier Companies
Cover Photograph: Jones and Bartlett Publishers, Courtesy of MIEMSS
Back cover photograph: Photo by Bachrach, all rights reserved
Photos of Nancy L. Caroline provided in loving memory by her mother, Zelda Caroline.

The procedures and protocols in this book are based on the most current recommendations of responsible medical sources. The Paramedic Association of Canada, the American Academy of Orthopaedic Surgeons, and the publisher, however, make no guarantee as to, and assume no responsibility for, the correctness, sufficiency, or completeness of such information or recommendations. Other or additional safety measures may be required under particular circumstances.

This textbook is intended solely as a guide to the appropriate procedures to be employed when rendering emergency care to the sick and injured. It is not intended as a statement of the standards of care required in any particular situation, because circumstances and the patient's physical condition can vary widely from one emergency to another. Nor is it intended that this textbook shall in any way advise emergency personnel concerning legal authority to perform the activities or procedures discussed. Such local determinations should be made only with the aid of legal counsel.

Some images in this book feature models. These models do not necessarily endorse, represent, or participate in the activities represented in the images.

Notice: The patients described in "You are the Paramedic," "Assessment in Action," and "Points to Ponder" throughout this text are fictitious.

ISBN-13: 978-1-284-05103-2

Library of Congress Cataloging-in-Publication Data
Elling, Bob.
  Nancy Caroline's emergency care in the streets. — 6th ed. / Bob Elling,
Michael G. Smith, Andrew N. Pollak.
     p. ; cm.
  Rev. ed. of: Emergency care in the streets / Nancy L. Caroline. 5th ed. c1995.
  Includes bibliographical references and index.
Adapted for use in Canada.
  ISBN-13: 978-0-7637-7399-1 (hardcover)
1. Medical emergencies. 2. Emergency medical technicians. I. Smith, Mike
(Michael Gordon), 1952- II. Pollak, Andrew N. III. Caroline, Nancy L.
Emergency care in the streets. IV. Title. V. Title: Emergency care in the
streets.
  [DNLM: 1. Emergency Treatment. 2. Emergency Medical Services. 3.
Emergency Medical Technicians. WB 105 E46n 2007]
  RC86.7.C38 2007
  616.02'5—dc22   2006103366
6048

Printed in the United States of America
13   10 9 8 7 6 5 4 3 2

Additional illustration and photo credits appear on pages CR.1 and CR.2, which constitute a continuation of the copyright page.

Brief Contents

Contents

SECTION 3 Patient Assessment 12.3

Chapter 12 Patient History 12.4

Paramedic Skill Drills

Resource Preview

CAROLINE'S BACK!

The textbook that is synonymous with paramedic education is back! In the United States, this textbook has been central to paramedic training since the 1970s. Its reputation travelled to Canada where *Emergency Care in the Streets* was adopted by frontline paramedics. Much loved and greatly respected, this textbook is still unrivalled in its ability to speak directly to the paramedic through humour and wisdom. Now, for the first time, this groundbreaking textbook has been adapted by a team of Canadian EMS experts specifically for Canadian paramedics, using the National Occupational Competency Profiles. The Paramedic Association of Canada and the American Academy of Orthopaedic Surgeons are proud to continue Dr. Caroline's legacy. As last, Canadian paramedics have the text they deserve.

Join us in welcoming back Dr. Caroline's legacy, *Emergency Care in the Streets*! The *Sixth Edition* honours Dr. Caroline's work with a clear, empathetic, and understandable writing style full of the humour for which she was known.

Chapter Resources

A multitude of innovative, dynamic features have been incorporated to make learning more engaging, in the spirit of Dr. Caroline's approach. The following pages show you the features to help you learn—from case studies to skill drills to an interactive website. On Dr. Caroline's behalf, the Paramedic Association of Canada and the American Academy of Orthopaedic Surgeons wishes you a successful and rewarding paramedic career!

NOCP Objectives

National Occupational Competency Profiles (NOCP) for paramedic practitioners are provided for each chapter. Appendix C cross-references the NOCP to the entire textbook.

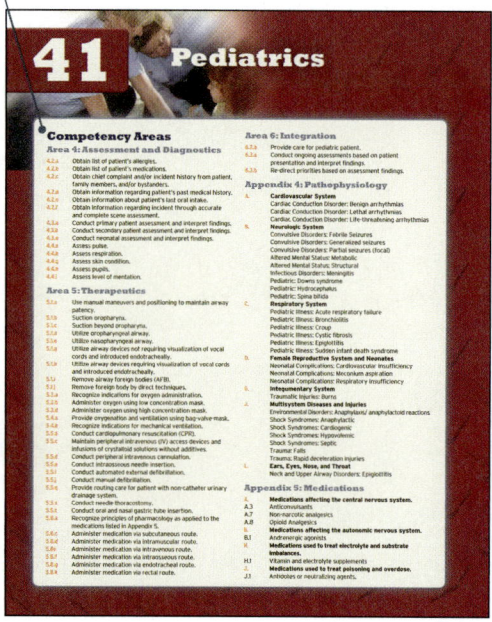

You are the Paramedic

Each chapter contains a progressive case study to start students thinking about what they would do if they encounter a similar case. This feature is a valuable learning tool that encourages critical thinking skills.

The case study introduces patients and follows their progress from dispatch to delivery at the emergency department. The case becomes gradually more detailed as new medical information is presented.

A summary of the case study concludes the chapter.

Notes from Nancy

Provide words of wisdom from Dr. Nancy Caroline.

Special Considerations

Discuss the specific needs and emergency care of special populations, including pediatric patients, geriatric patients, and special needs patients.

Skill Drills

Provide written step-by-step explanations and visual summaries of important skills and procedures.

Documentation and Communication

Provide advice on how to document patient care and tips on how to communicate with other health care professionals.

At the Scene

Discuss practical applications of material for use at the scene.

Controversies

Highlight issues that may be under debate in the prehospital community.

Vital Vocabulary

Terms are easily identified and defined within the text. A comprehensive vocabulary list follows each chapter.

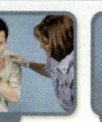
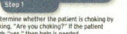
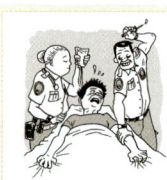
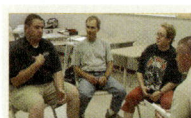

Prep Kit

End-of-chapter activities reinforce important concepts and improve students' comprehension.

Ready for Review

Summarize chapter content in a comprehensive bulleted list.

Assessment in Action

Promote critical thinking with case studies and provide discussion points for classroom presentation.

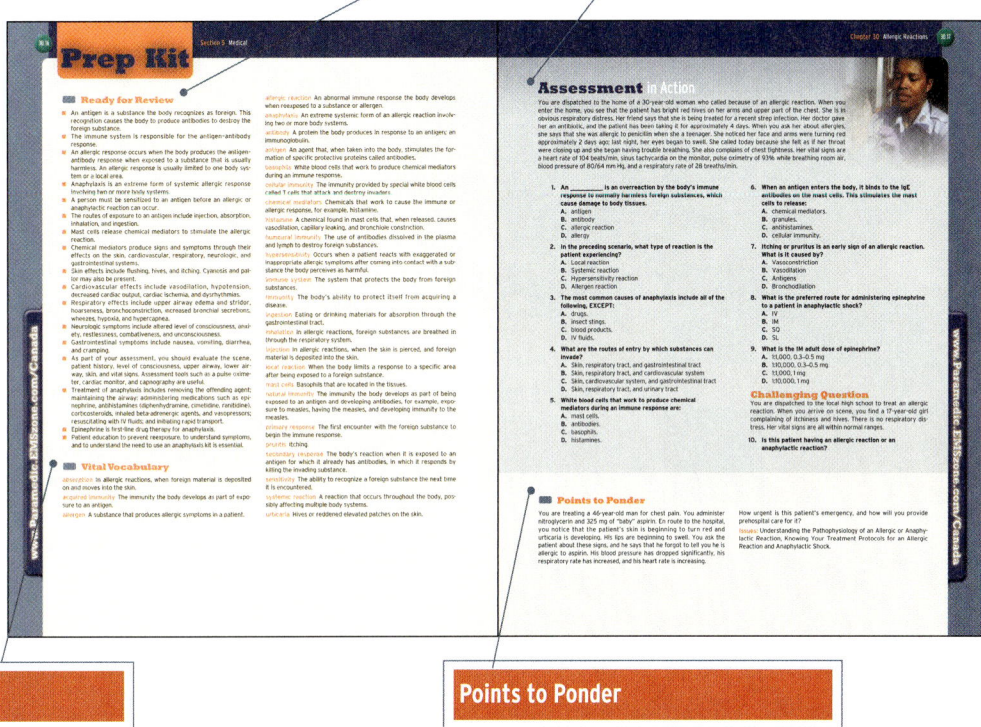

Vital Vocabulary

Provide key terms and definitions from the chapter.

Points to Ponder

Tackle cultural, ethical, and legal issues through case studies.

Technology Resources

www.Paramedic.EMSzone.com/Canada

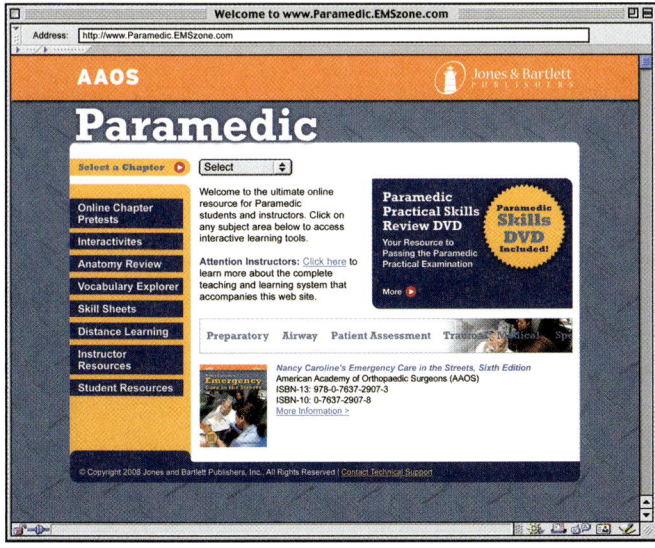

This site has been specifically designed to complement *Nancy Caroline's Emergency Care in the Streets, Sixth Edition* with interactivities and simulations to help students become great paramedics. The following are just some of the resources provided:

- **Chapter pretests** prepare students for training. Each chapter has a pretest and provides instant results and feedback on incorrect answers.
- **Interactivities** allow your students to experiment with the most important skills and procedures in the safety of a virtual environment.
- **Anatomy review** provides interactive anatomical figure-labelling exercises to reinforce students' knowledge of human anatomy.
- **Vocabulary explorer** is a virtual dictionary. Here, students can review key terms, test their knowledge of key terms through flashcards, and complete exercises.

Instructor Resources

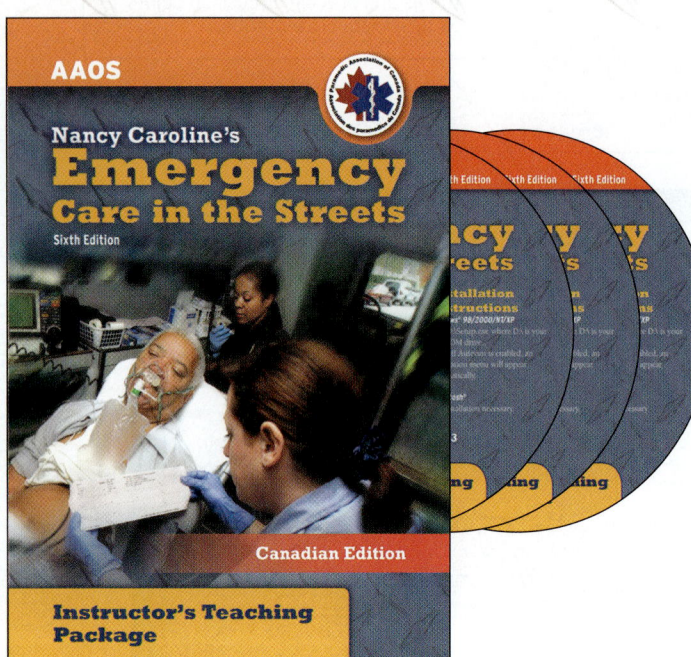

ISBN-13: 978-0-7637-7941-2

This robust package contains everything needed to instruct a dynamic paramedic programme. The CD-ROMs in the package contain:

- **PowerPoint presentations**, providing you with educational and engaging presentations. Following the content of the chapter, the slides also contain case studies and images throughout. The presentations can be modified and edited to meet your needs.
- **Lecture outlines**, providing you with complete, ready-to-use lesson plans that outline all of the topics covered in the chapter. The lesson plans can be modified and edited to fit your course.
- **Image and table bank**, providing you with many of the images and tables found in the text. You can use them to incorporate more images into the PowerPoint presentations, make handouts, or enlarge a specific image for further discussion.
- **Test bank**, providing you with multiple-choice general knowledge and critical thinking questions. With the test bank, you can originate tailor-made classroom exams and quizzes quickly and easily by selecting, editing, organizing, and printing an exam along with an answer key, that includes page references to the text.

The resources found in the Instructor's Package have been formatted so that you can seamlessly integrate them into the most popular course administration tools. Please contact Jones and Bartlett Publishers technical support at www.jbpub.com at any time with questions.

Acknowledgments

Editorial Board

Russell D. MacDonald, MD, MPH, FRCPC
Medical Director, Research Program
Ornge Transport Medicine
Assistant Professor and Co-Director
Emergency Medicine Fellowship Programs
University of Toronto
Toronto, Ontario

Robert J. Burgess, BHSc, ACP, AEMCA, CQIA
Director, Program Operations and Administration
Sunnybrook-Osler Centre for Prehospital Care
Toronto, Ontario

Editors and Authors

SECTION 1

Section Editor: Jan L. Jensen, BSc, ACP
Emergency Health Services
Dalhousie University Division of EMS
Halifax, Nova Scotia

Authors

Chapter 1: Robert J. Burgess, BHSc, ACP, AEMCA, CQIA
Director, Program Operations and Administration
Sunnybrook-Osler Centre for Prehospital Care
Toronto, Ontario

Chapter 1: Bruce K. Farr
Chief and General Manager
Toronto Emergency Medical Services
Toronto, Ontario

Chapter 2: Douglas Andrusiek, MSc, PCP
Director of Research
British Columbia Ambulance Service
Emergency and Health Services Commission
Vancouver, British Columbia

Chapter 2: Carolyn C. Rosenczweig, BA, MD, CCFP, FRCPC
Emergency Physician
Department of Emergency Medicine
Surrey Memorial Hospital
Surrey, British Columbia

Chapter 3: Jan L. Jensen, BSc, ACP
Emergency Health Services
Dalhousie University Division of EMS
Halifax, Nova Scotia

Chapter 3: Russell D. MacDonald, MD, MPH, FRCPC
Medical Director, Research Program
Ornge Transport Medicine
Assistant Professor and Co-Director
Emergency Medicine Fellowship Programs
University of Toronto
Toronto, Ontario

Chapter 4: Wil Bartel, BSc, ACP
Emergency Medical Services Branch
Manitoba Health & Healthy Living
Winnipeg, Manitoba

Chapter 5: Laura Hawryluck, MSc, MD, FRCPC
Associate Professor
Critical Care Medicine
University Health Network
Toronto, Ontario

Chapter 6: Erik N. Vu, ACP, MD, FRPCP, DAvMed
Paramedic and Flight Physician
British Columbia Ambulance Service
Provincial AirEvac and Critical Care Transport Program
Emergency Physician, Vancouver General Hospital
Clinical Instructor, Faculty of Medicine
Department of Emergency Medicine
University of British Columbia
Vancouver, British Columbia

Chapter 7: Vito Sanci, PhD, CCP
Faculty of Medicine
University of Ottawa
Ornge Transport Medicine
Toronto EMS
Toronto, Ontario

Chapter 7: Vincent Teo, BScPhm
Sunnybrook Health Sciences Centre
Toronto, Ontario

Chapter 8: Cathal O'Donnell, MB, FCEM
Consultant in Emergency Medicine
Mid-Western Regional Hospital
Limerick, Ireland

Chapter 9: Doug Fenton, CCP
British Columbia Ambulance Service
Kamloops, British Columbia

Chapter 10: Brad McArthur, CCP(F)
Ornge Transport Medicine
London, Ontario

Chapter 10: Dugg Steary, CCP(F)
Ornge Transport Medicine
London, Ontario

SECTION 2

Section Editor: Jonathon E. Morgan, MD, CCFP(EM), FCFP
Medical Director Northern Region
Ornge Transport Medicine
Sioux Lookout, Ontario

Authors

Chapter 11: Russell D. MacDonald, MD, MPH, FRCPC
Medical Director, Research Program
Ornge Transport Medicine

Assistant Professor and Co-Director
Emergency Medicine Fellowship Programs
University of Toronto
Toronto, Ontario

Chapter 11: Robert J. Burgess, BHSc, ACP, AEMCA, CQIA
Director, Program Operations and Administration
Sunnybrook-Osler Centre for Prehospital Care
Toronto, Ontario

SECTION 3

Section Editor: Graham G. Munro, MHSM, BHSc, CCP
Faculty
School of Biomedical Sciences
Charles Sturt University
New South Wales, Australia

Authors

Chapter 12: Graham G. Munro, MHSM, BHSc, CCP
Faculty
School of Biomedical Sciences
Charles Sturt University
New South Wales, Australia

Chapter 13: Ryan D. Velthuizen, EMTP
Alberta Health Services
Edmonton Zone EMS
St. Albert, Alberta

Chapter 14: Graham G. Munro, MHSM, BHSc, CCP
Faculty
School of Biomedical Sciences
Charles Sturt University
New South Wales, Australia

Chapter 15: Karen Wanger, MDCM, FRCPC, FACEP
Regional Medical Director, Lower Mainland
British Columbia Ambulance Service
Clinical Associate Professor
Faculty of Medicine
University of British Columbia
Vancouver, British Columbia

Chapter 16: Sandra Chad, BA, ACP, EMD
Ajax, Ontario

SECTION 4

Section Editor: Fergal McCourt, MD, MSc, FACEM
EMS Fellow, Division of Emergency Medcine
University of Toronto
Toronto, Ontario

Authors

Chapter 17: Douglas Chisholm, MD, FRCPC
Ornge Transport Medicine
St. Michael's Hospital
University of Toronto
Toronto, Ontario

Chapter 18: Fergal McCourt, MD, MSc, FACEM
EMS Fellow, Division of Emergency Medcine
University of Toronto
Toronto, Ontario

Chapter 19: Rob Ritchie, EMT-P, ACP
Alberta Health Services EMS
Medicine Hat, Aiberta

Chapter 20: Sunil Sookram, MD, FRCPC
Alberta Health Services, Edmonton Zone EMS Medical Director
Alberta Provincial Air Ambulance Medical Director
Associate Clinical Professor, University of Alberta
Edmonton, Alberta

Chapter 21: Sunil Sookram, MD, FRCPC
Alberta Health Services, Edmonton Zone EMS Medical Director
Alberta Provincial Air Ambulance Medical Director
Associate Clinical Professor, University of Alberta
Edmonton, Alberta

Chapter 22: Joseph Ip, MD, MSc, FRCPC
Medical Director
Paramedic Academy
Justice Institute of British Columbia
New Westminster, British Columbia

Chapter 23: Keith Donovan, MD, FRCPC
Associate Professor
Department of Medicine
Division of Emergency Medicine
University of Western Ontario
London, Ontario

Chapter 24: Eli Segal, MD, FRCP, CSPQ
Urgences-santé
SMBD-Jewish General Hospital
McGill University
Montreal, Quebec

Chapter 25: Hal B. Canham, MD, CCFP(EM)
Provincial EMS Medical Director
Alberta Health and Wellness
Edmonton, Alberta

SECTION 5

Section Editor: Jeffrey M. Singh, MD, MSc, FRCPC
Ornge Transport Medicine
Critical Care Medicine
University Health Network
Toronto, Ontario

Section Editor: Randy S. Wax, MD, MEd, FRCPC
Transport Physician
Ornge Transport Medicine
Medical Director
Program for Resuscitation Education and Patient Safety
Mount Sinai Hospital
Assistant Professor and Clinician-Educator
Critical Care
Department of Medicine
University of Toronto
Toronto, Ontario

Authors

Chapter 26: Sean W. Moore, MDCM, FRCPC, FACEP
Transport Physician
Ornge Transport Medicine
Toronto, Ontario

Chapter 27: Michelle Welsford, BSc, MD, ABEM, FACEP, FRCPC
Medical Director
Hamilton Health Sciences Paramedic Base Hospital Program
Associate Professor
McMaster University
Hamilton, Ontario

SECTION 5, continued

Chapter 28: David A. Petrie, MD, FRCP
Associate Professor
Dalhousie University
Halifax, Nova Scotia

Chapter 29: Jeffrey M. Singh, MD, MSc, FRCPC
Ornge Transport Medicine
Critical Care Medicine
University Health Network
Toronto, Ontario

Chapter 29: Randy S. Wax, MD, MEd, FRCPC
Transport Physician
Ornge Transport Medicine
Medical Director
Program for Resuscitation Education and Patient Safety
Mount Sinai Hospital
Assistant Professor and Clinician-Educator
Critical Care
Department of Medicine
University of Toronto
Toronto, Ontario

Chapter 30: Jane Lukins, MBBS, FACEM
Eastern Health
Box Hill, Victoria
Australia

Chapter 31: Michael Feldman, PhD, MD, FRCPC, A-EMCA
Medical Director
Sunnybrook-Osler Centre for Prehospital Care
Assistant Professor
Department of Medicine
University of Toronto
Toronto, Ontario

Chapter 32: William Bradley Snodgrass, EMT–P
Paramedic Program
Medicine Hat College
Medicine Hat, Alberta

Chapter 33: Margaret Thompson, MD, FRCPC, FACMT
Staff Emergency Physician
St. Michael's Hospital
Assistant Professor
Department of Medicine
University of Toronto
Medical Director
Ontario Poison Control Centre
Toronto, Ontario

Chapter 34: Russell D. MacDonald, MD, MPH, FRCPC
Medical Director, Research Program
Ornge Transport Medicine
Assistant Professor and Co-Director
Emergency Medicine Fellowship Programs
University of Toronto
Toronto, Ontario

Chapter 35: Darrell J. Bardua, ACP
Capital District Health Authority
Emergency Health Services
Halifax Regional Municipality
Halifax, Nova Scotia

Chapter 35: Jan L. Jensen, BSc, ACP
Emergency Health Services
Dalhousie University Division of EMS
Halifax, Nova Scotia

Chapter 35: Mark Walker, ACP
Clinical Learning Coordinator
Emergency Health Services
Dartmouth, Nova Scotia

Chapter 36: Valerie Krym, MD, MPH, CCFP(EM)
Senior Medical Consultant
Infectious Diseases Branch
Public Health Division
Ministry of Health and Long-Term Care
Government of Ontario
Assistant Professor
Division of Emergency Medicine
Department of Family and Community Medicine
Faculty of Medicine
University of Toronto
Toronto, Ontario

Chapter 36: Russell D. MacDonald, MD, MPH, FRCPC
Medical Director, Research Program
Ornge Transport Medicine
Assistant Professor and Co-Director
Emergency Medicine Fellowship Programs
University of Toronto
Toronto, Ontario

Chapter 37: Rob Grierson, BSc, BSc(Med), MD, FRCPC
Medical Director
Winnipeg Fire Paramedic Service
Assistant Professor
Department of Emergency Medicine
University of Manitoba
Winnipeg, Manitoba

Chapter 37: Erin R. Weldon, BSc, MD, FRCPC
Associate Medical Director
Winnipeg Fire Paramedic Service
Assistant Professor
Research Director
Department of Emergency Medicine
University of Manitoba
Winnipeg, Manitoba

Chapter 38: Leah Watson, MD, FRCPC
EMS Fellow
University of Toronto
Toronto, Ontario

Chapter 39: Yen Chow, MD, CCFP
Emergency Physician
Thunder Bay Regional Health Sciences Centre
Regional Medical Director
Ornge Transport Medicine
Thunder Bay, Ontario

SECTION 6

Section Editor: Cory Brulotte, MD
Chief Resident
Department of Emergency Medicine
University of Ottawa and the Ottawa Hospital
Ottawa, Ontario

Authors

Chapter 40: Hilary E. A. Whyte, MB, MSc, FRCPC, FRCPI
Associate Professor Paediatrics
University of Toronto
Paediatric Medical Director
Ornge Transport Medicine
Toronto, Ontario

Chapter 41: D. Anna Jarvis, MB, BS, FRCPC, FAAP
Associate Dean, Health Professions Student Affairs
Professor, Department of Paediatrics
Division of Emergency Medicine
The Hospital for Sick Children
University of Toronto
Toronto, Ontario

Chapter 42: Scott Mullin, ACP
Paramedic Program
Medicine Hat College
Medicine Hat, Alberta

Chapter 43: Robin Mason, PhD
Women's College Research Institute
Women's College Hospital
University of Toronto
Toronto, Ontario

Chapter 44: Mary Osinga, BSc, CCP(F)
Ornge Transport Medicine
Paramedic Faculty
Sir Sandford Fleming College
Toronto, Ontario

Chapter 45: Natalie Lavergne, CCP(F)
Ornge Transport Medicine
Ottawa, Ontario

SECTION 7

Section Editor: Steve Darling, BHSc, CCP(F)
York Region EMS
Newmarket, Ontario

Authors

Chapter 46: Steve Darling, BHSc, CCP(F)
York Region EMS
Newmarket, Ontario

Chapter 46: Russell D. MacDonald, MD, MPH, FRCPC
Medical Director, Research Program
Ornge Transport Medicine
Assistant Professor and Co-Director
Emergency Medicine Fellowship Programs
University of Toronto
Toronto, Ontario

Chapter 47: Brian Schwartz, MD, CCFP(EM), FCFP
Senior Director
Sunnybrook-Osler Centre for Prehospital Care
Director, Emergency Management Support
Ontario Agency for Health Protection and Promotion
Toronto, Ontario

Chapter 48: Patrick Auger, BHSc, MEmMTg, CCP(F)
Ornge Transport Medicine
Ottawa, Ontario

Chapter 49: Dean Popov, ACP
Sunnybrook-Osler Centre for Prehospital Care
Toronto, Ontario

Chapter 50: Michael Feldman, PhD, MD, FRCPC, A-EMCA
Medical Director
Sunnybrook-Osler Centre for Prehospital Care
Assistant Professor
Department of Medicine
University of Toronto
Toronto, Ontario

Chapter 51: Saleh Fares, MBBS, FRCPC
EMS Fellow
Division of Emergency Medicine
University of Toronto
Toronto, Ontario

Chapter 51: Abel Wakai, MD, FRCSI, FCEM
Consultant in Emergency Medicine
St. James's Hospital
Dublin, Ireland

APPENDICES

Appendix A: Russell D. MacDonald, MD, MPH, FRCPC
Medical Director, Research Program
Ornge Transport Medicine
Assistant Professor and Co-Director
Emergency Medicine Fellowship Programs
University of Toronto
Toronto, Ontario

Appendix B: Kent Brown
Superintendent EMS
Winnipeg Fire Paramedic Service
Winnipeg, Manitoba

Contributors

Maud Huiskamp, ACP
Lead Educator
Sunnybrook-Osler Centre for Prehospital Care
Toronto, Ontario

Severo Rodriguez, BA, MSc, NR-LP, AEMCA
Program Manager
Southwest Ontario Regional Base Hospital and RTC Programs
London Health Sciences Centre
London, Ontario

Gary Ross, ACP
Educator/Supervisor
Toronto Emergency Medical Services
Toronto, Ontario

Reviewers

Robert O. Brunet
La Cité Collégiale
Ottawa, Ontario

Vlad Chiriac
Durham College
Oshawa, Ontario

Corene Debreuil, PCP, ESI
Regional Health Authority Central Manitoba
Southport, Manitoba

Doug Fenton, CCP
Coordinator, Advanced Programs
Paramedic Academy
Justice Institute of British Columbia
Celista, British Columbia

Dwayne Forsman
Red River College
Winnipeg, Manitoba

Kevin Griffin, MA, BSc, ACP
Durham College
Oshawa, Ontario

John Hein, EMT-P
Staff Development
Emergency Medical Services
The City of Calgary
Calgary, Alberta

Tim Hillier
M.D. Ambulance Care
Saskatoon, Saskatchewan

Ralph Hofmann, MA, BSc, ACP
Associate Dean
School of Health and Community Services
Durham College
Oshawa, Ontario

Jason Hudson, ACP
PCP Instructor
Atlantic Paramedic Academy
Jacksonville, New Brunswick

Mark Hunter, AEMCA, RN, BSCN
Professor
Coordinator, Paramedic Programs
Fanshawe College
London, Ontario

Kevin Keen, AEMCA, AEd
Training Division
Hamilton Emergency Services
Hamilton, Ontario

Shawn Knight, BEd, EMT-P
NAIT
Alberta Health and Wellness
Office of Environmental Health and Safety
Edmonton, Alberta

Doug Kunihiro, BBM, ACP, Dip CS
Faculty, Paramedic Program
Centennial College
Toronto, Ontario

Declan Lawlor, BSc, ACP
Academy of Emergency Training
Burnaby, British Columbia

Derek J. LeBlanc, PCP, BA, MA
Atlantic Health Training and Simulation Centre
Halifax, Nova Scotia

Kent MacDonald, PA
Paramedicine Learning Manager
Holland College
Charlottetown, Prince Edward Island

Alexander (Sandy) MacQuarrie, BSc, MBA, CCP(F)
Atlantic Paramedic Academy
Moncton, New Brunswick

Bill Maser, BEd, MET
School of Health Care
Justice Institute of British Columbia
New Westminster, British Columbia

Terry Price, CCP(F)
Paramedic Program Coordinator
Northern College of Applied Arts and Technology
Timmins, Ontario

Carolyn Ross, PCP
Paramedic Program Coordinator
St. Clair College, Thames Campus
Chatham, Ontario

Lynne Thibeault, RN, ENC, BScN, MEd, NP-PHC
Confederation College
Thunder Bay, Ontario

Dean Vokey, BEd, ACP
Operations Supervisor
Emergency Medical Care, Inc.
Yarmouth, Nova Scotia

The Paramedic Association of Canada, the American Academy of Orthopaedic Surgeons, and Jones and Bartlett Publishers would like to thank the editors, contributors, and reviewers of the US Edition of *Nancy Caroline's Emergency Care in the Streets, Sixth Edition*.

Editorial Board for the US Edition

Bob Elling, MPA, NREMT-P
Andrew N. Pollak, MD, FAAOS
Stephen J. Rahm, NREMT-P
Mike Smith, BS, MICP

Editors and Authors

SECTION 1

Section Editor: David Gurchiek, MS, NREMT-P

Authors

Chapter 1: Don Kimlicka, NREMT-P, CCEMT-P

Chapter 2: Anne Austin, EMT-P, AAS

Chapter 2: Thom Dick, NREMT-B

Chapter 3: Keith Griffiths

Chapter 4: W. Ann Maggiore, JD, NREMT-P

Chapter 5: W. Ann Maggiore, JD, NREMT-P

Chapter 6: Jeffrey Morse, MD

Chapter 7: Geoffrey T. Miller, EMT-P

Chapter 7: Shaun Froshour, NREMT-P

Chapter 8: David Gurchiek, MS, NREMT-P

Chapter 8: Stephen J. Rahm, NREMT-P

Chapter 9: Howard E. Huth, III, BA, EMT-P

Chapter 10: Thom Dick, NREMT-B

Chapter 10: Charles R. Jones, BA, CC-EMTP/TA, CAS, CHS-III

SECTION 2

Section Editor: Stephen J. Rahm, NREMT-P

Author

Chapter 11: Stephen J. Rahm, NREMT-P

SECTION 3

Section Editor: Mike Smith, BS, MICP

Authors

Chapter 12: Mike Smith, BS, MICP

Chapter 13: John F. Elder, EMT-P, CCEMT-P

Chapter 13: Jonathan S. Halpert, MD, FACEP, REMT-P

Chapter 14: Mike Smith, BS, MICP

Chapter 15: Mike Smith, BS, MICP

Chapter 16: Melissa M. Doak, NREMT-P

SECTION 4

Section Editor: Bob Elling, MPA, NREMT-P
Section Editor: Connie J. Mattera, RN, MS, TNS, EMT-P

Authors

Chapter 17: Samuel A. Getz Jr, BS, NREMT-P

Chapter 17: Edward K. Rodriguez, MD-PhD

Chapter 18: Bob Elling, MPA, NREMT-P

Chapter 19: Chad E. Brocato, DHSc, REMT-P

Chapter 20: Charles Bortle, MEd, NREMT-P, RRT

Chapter 20: Jennifer McCarthy, MAs, MICP

Chapter 20: Mark A. Merlin, DO, EMT-P, FACEP

Chapter 21: Stephen J. Rahm, NREMT-P

Chapter 22: Debra Lee, MD

Chapter 23: John Freese, MD

Chapter 24: Samuel A. Getz Jr, BS, NREMT-P

Chapter 24: Robert S. Levy, MD

Chapter 24: Mark A. Merlin, DO, EMT-P, FACEP

Chapter 25: Matthew J. Belan, MD, MBA

Chapter 25: Michael D. Panté, NREMT-P

SECTION 5

Section Editor: Bob Elling, MPA, NREMT-P

Authors

Chapter 26: Charles Bortle, MEd, NREMT-P, RRT

Chapter 27: Bruce Butterfras, MS-Ed, LP

Chapter 27: Deborah J. McCoy-Freeman, BS, RN, NREMT-P

Chapter 28: Charles W. Sowerbrower, MEd, NREMT-P, NCEMSE

Chapter 29: Don Kimlicka, NREMT-P, CCEMT-P

Chapter 29: J. Michael Morrow, MICP, CICP

Chapter 30: Ann Bellows, RN, NREMT-P, EdD

Chapter 31: Charles W. Sowerbrower, MEd, NREMT-P, NCEMSE

Chapter 32: George E. Perry, EdD, NREMT-P

Chapter 33: Mike Smith, BS, MICP

Chapter 34: Don Kimlicka, NREMT-P, CCEMT-P

Chapter 35: Frederick "Fritz" Fuller, REMT-P, PA-C, BS

Chapter 36: Katherine H. West, BSN, MSEd, CIC

Chapter 37: Chris Stratford, RN, BS, EMT-I

Chapter 38: Charles R. Jones, BA, CC-EMT-P/TA, CAS, CHS-III

Chapter 39: Charles R. Jones, BA, CC-EMT-P/TA, CAS, CHS-III

SECTION 6

Authors

Chapter 40: Patricia Chess, MD

Chapter 40: Nirupama Laroia, MD

Chapter 40: Yogangi Malhotra, MD

Chapter 41: Dena Brownstein, MD, FAAP

Chapter 41: Kimberly P. Stone, MD, MS, MA

Chapter 42: Samuel A. Getz Jr, BS, NREMT-P

Chapter 42: Michael D. Panté, NREMT-P

Chapter 42: Jim Upchurch, MD, MA, NREMT-P

Chapter 43: Daniel Doherty, NREMT-P

Chapter 44: Lori L. Bisping, NREMT-P

Chapter 44: Annmary E. Thomas, MEd, NREMT-P

Chapter 45: Deborah Kufs, MS, RN, NREMT-P

SECTION 7

Section Editor: David L. Seabrook, MPA, EMT-P

Authors

Chapter 46: Anne Austin, EMT-P, AAS

Chapter 47: Doyle Dennis, NREMT-P

Chapter 48: Donell Harvin, MPA, NREMT-P

Chapter 49: Norm Rooker, EMT-P

Chapter 49: Hank R. Christen, Jr, MPA

Chapter 50: David L. Seabrook, MPA, EMT-P

Chapter 51: Dennis R. Krebs, NREMT-P

APPENDICES

Appendix A&B: Bob Elling, MPA, NREMT-P

Contributors

Trisha Appelhans

Vicki Bacidore, RN, MSN, ACNP-BC

Darrin M. Batty, AEMT-P

Jeffery L. Beinke, MBA-HCM, BS, REMT-P

Garry Briese

Tom Carpenter, NREMT-P, CCEMT-P

Julie Chase, BS, NREMT-P

Kathleen E. Curran, MICP

Mike Dymes, NREMT-P

Mickey Eisenberg, MD, PhD

Jill E. Hobbs, Editor

Susan M. Hohenhaus, MA, RN, FAEN

Jay Keefauver

Rick Kimball, NREMT-P

Gregg C. Lord, BA, NREMT-P

Patricia Maher, MPA, EMT-P

Brittany Ann Martinelli, MHSc, BSRT,

Scott F. McConnell, FP-C, NREMT-P, MICP, CCEMT-P

Lynette S. McCullough, MPH, EMT-P

David McEvoy, MS, NREMT-P

Eugene Nagel

Deborah L. Petty, BS, EMT-P, I/C

Randy Price, A/As, NREMT-P

Sabra Raulston, NREMT-P

Bernadette A. Royce, BA, FF/EMT-P

Joan Scheffer, EMT-B/WEMT, CRNFA

Jeffrey J. Spencer, BS, EMT-P

Ron Stewart

Barbara O. Ward, BA, MA

Biography

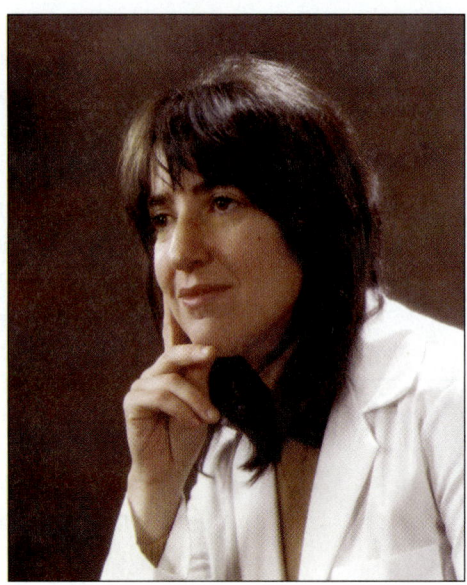

Nancy L. Caroline, MD

Nancy L. Caroline, MD, was only 58 when she died of multiple myeloma in 2002, but her spirit will never leave Emergency Medical Services. She has often been rightly called the Mother of Paramedics because of her dedication to paramedic education.

No physician can be more revered, yet Nancy never used the academic titles to which she was most entitled—everyone from a first year Paramedic to a distinguished leader called Dr. Caroline, simply, "Nancy."

Nancy Lee Caroline was born in the United States in a Boston suburb to Leo and Zelda Caroline in 1944. Nancy had a strong social conscience, and devoted her life to medicine, teaching, and her patients.

Nancy's medical career began at the age of 15 in the pathology laboratory of the famous Benjamin Castleman, MD, at Massachusetts General Hospital. However, Dr. Castleman was unable to pay her for her services, because she was not of legal age to be working for money. Nancy went on to do actual medical research in Dr. Castleman's laboratory, long before she entered college.

Nancy chose to major in linguistics at Radcliffe College. Not surprisingly, it continued to be a point of pride for her to develop a knowledge of the languages in whatever country she was working. She went on to receive her MD from Case Western Reserve University in 1977.

After finishing her residency in Cleveland, Nancy took a fellowship in Critical Care Medicine at the University of Pittsburgh. Beginning in 1974, the late Peter Safar, MD, was overseeing a US Department of Transportation grant to create a curriculum for paramedics. Much of Safar's work began to be delegated to (or, perhaps, seized upon by) the young Dr. Caroline. Because of this work, Nancy served as an advisor to President Gerald Ford on EMS.

Dr. Safar offered Nancy an opportunity, as medical director of Freedom House Enterprises Ambulance Service, to train paramedics chosen from a group of African-American men who did not have a chance to complete their high school educations. Nancy was extremely successful—so successful that she was asked to write a curriculum for paramedic training, a curriculum that was published as *Emergency Care in the Streets*.

Nancy, proud of her Jewish heritage, took an opportunity to emmigrate to Israel as the first medical director of Magen David Adom, Israel's Red Cross society. During her first months in the country, Nancy rose early to attend the extensive Hebrew lessons required of new immigrants, then spent her late afternoons and evenings training the first Israeli paramedics. She would then take a bus home, where she would spend a few precious hours working on the first edition of *Emergency Care in the Streets*.

After her tenure at Magen David Adom came to an end in 1981, Nancy relocated to Nairobi, Kenya, to become Senior Medical Officer of the African Medical and Research Foundation

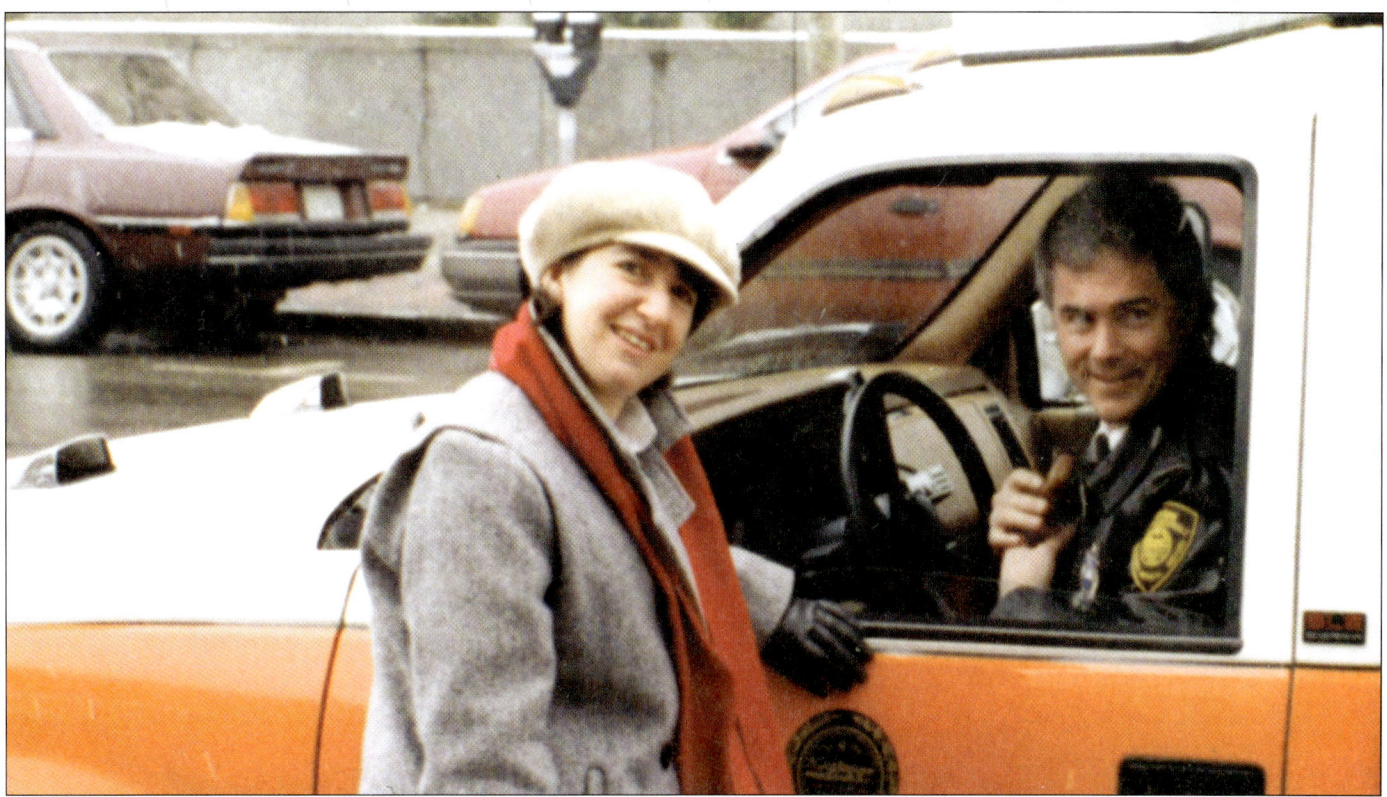

(AMREF), the foundation that oversees the famous Flying Doctor service.

One of Nancy's many duties at AMREF was writing a health advice column for the local newspaper, called "Ask Dr. AMREF." Nancy's famous sense of humor made the column a "must" read in Nairobi. Nancy reported that one reader had all the males on the AMREF staff quite concerned when he began: "Everyone knows that a normal male can go six times in an evening."

No one who ever met her will ever forget her sense of humor, nowhere more evident than in her publications:

Nancy made the editors of a proper Bostonian publishing firm gasp when she wore a hardhat with a revolving red light when she came to call.

Nancy won permission to publish the first cartoon on the cover of the *Journal of the American Medical Association* for her article on the curative power of chicken soup. The cartoonist, her brother Peter, said he was sure it would be the last.

Nancy lost an argument with her editors to have a series of case studies for paramedics called *The Pulseless Man in the Topless Bar*. The case book became *Ambulance Calls* instead—to her undisguised loathing.

During much of her life, Nancy would return to the United States to visit her mother Zelda and her brother Peter. But, on her trips home, Nancy always found time to ride with working paramedics in several cities, to listen to their ups and downs, and to determine what real paramedics needed in the updates of *Emergency Care in the Streets*.

When she became aware of the awful famine that overtook Ethiopia in the early 1980s, Nancy became a consultant for the League of Red Cross Societies, writing a handbook on basic life support and running classes on first aid for African nations.

Nancy worked with the Ethiopian Orthodox Church to provide better nourishment and health care to children in over 600 orphanages, setting up small-scale agricultural projects to feed Africans. In addition, Nancy served as director of medical programs for the American Joint Distribution Committee in Addis Ababa.

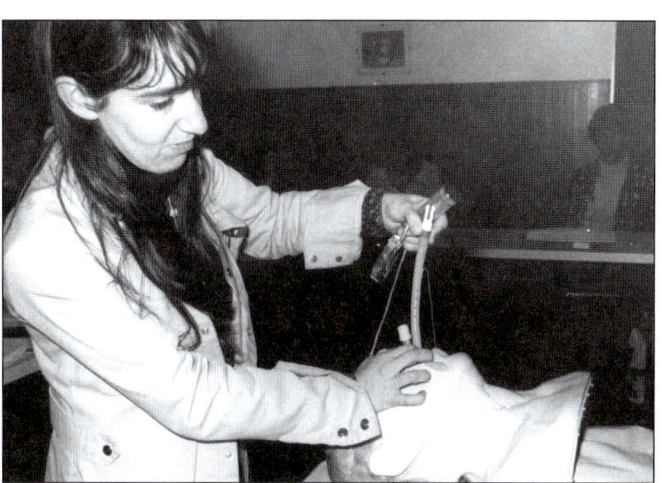

During Nancy's time in Ethiopia, she had to return to the United States for a family emergency. Nancy discovered the only way she could get a plane to the United States was with a substantial cash payment for a ticket. The Christian Bishop of the Ethiopian Orthodox Church, to whom Nancy reported on the orphanages, personally got Nancy on a plane to Boston in short order.

Returning to Israel in 1987, she served as medical consultant for the Center for Educational Technology and for AMREF, developing training materials in emergency medicine and writing correspondence courses for rural health workers in Africa. She also served as an adjunct professor at the University of Pittsburgh's medical school, and, while volunteering in the Department of Oncology in Tel Hashomer, Nancy collaborated with Alexander Waller, MD, on a *Handbook of Palliative Care in Cancer*.

Nancy settled in Metulla, Israel. She realized there was a need for special care in north Israel for people with advanced cancer. In 1995, she founded the Hospice of the Upper Galilee (HUG). In 2002, she married geneticist and molecular biologist Lazarus Astrachan.

Nancy left the world too soon, but few people have done more to leave the world a better place. Despite all her accomplishments, however, the compliment that meant the most to her was to be called the "Mother of Paramedics." Nancy was, no doubt, the best mother paramedics could have.

Foreword

Paramedicine in Canada has finally come of age. The Paramedic Association of Canada (PAC) and its provincial chapters have grown significantly in the past decade, emerging as a strong national voice for paramedics. We also have seen the birth of the EMS Chiefs of Canada (EMSCC) and their role as leaders in the profession, and establishment of Canada's first Provincial College of Paramedicine. Finally, the National Occupational Competency Profiles (NOCPs) have emerged as the national scope of practice for the profession, with education accreditation using the NOCPs as a national standard. Paramedicine now plays an important role in the health care system that is a fundamental part of Canadian society.

This textbook represents another milestone in the coming of age of paramedicine in Canada. It was designed for our paramedics from the ground up, with the NOCPs in mind. We were fortunate to take a wonderful book with an established pedigree, and rewrite it to suit our needs. This is not a mere modification, but a complete transformation that truly meets our needs.

Nancy Caroline was a visionary in EMS education, and wrote her textbook with a style all her own. I am pleased that the first Canadian edition of the textbook that bears her name remains true to her style. For those of you new to *Caroline*, I hope you enjoy her legacy. For those who have come back to *Caroline*, I hope our efforts reflect well on how you remember her.

It is ironic that my EMS career began where Nancy left her mark on EMS education. Although I never had the privilege of meeting her, I worked with many who knew her well. In fact, the EMS providers pictured on the cover of an older edition of *Caroline* were the same paramedics who shared their streetsmarts with me over a decade ago. This first Canadian edition of Nancy's textbook is a tribute to her and those who followed in her footsteps, teaching people like me a thing or two about EMS.

The project to bring the first EMS textbook to paramedics in Canada began almost 10 years ago, just before I left Boston. I thank Dr. Lawrence Mottley and Dr. Peter Moyer for their superb mentorship early in my EMS career and for planting the seeds from which this textbook grew.

It has been my privilege to work with a talented group of over 100 authors, reviewers, section editors, and others who made this landmark textbook possible. This group represents the very best in Canadian EMS leadership, education, and medical direction. The result is a textbook that will serve us well for years to come. I would like to thank each of you for giving your time and sharing your expertise.

This project was endorsed by the PAC and the EMSCC because they recognize education as a key component to growth in this profession. I thank both organizations for their support, and Pierre Poirier and Bruce Farr for their personal support of this project.

I am truly grateful to Jones and Bartlett for believing in this project, offering us the opportunity to bring *Caroline* to Canada, and allowing us to make it truly Canadian. It has been my pleasure to work with the J&B staff.

Last but not least, thank you to Robert Burgess, co-editor on this project, for believing it was possible and playing a major role in helping make it happen.

Russell D. MacDonald
Toronto, Canada
June 2009

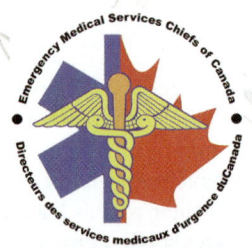

Dear Paramedic,

The EMS Chiefs of Canada (EMSCC) are committed to fostering the growth and development of paramedicine in Canada. In the interest of advancing and aligning EMS leadership in Canada, our White Paper, *The Future of EMS in Canada—Defining the Road Ahead,* details the below noted strategies for the future. The EMSCC recognize that education is a key component to promote this growth.

Specifically;

- A clear core identity,
- Stable funding,
- Systematic improvement,
- Personnel development,
- Leadership support, and
- Mobilized health care

One of the missing pieces has been an EMS textbook written for Canadian paramedics. The first Canadian Edition of *Nancy Caroline's Emergency Care in the Streets* is the long-awaited textbook that meets this need. The author group who wrote and reviewed this textbook includes many well-respected leaders in Canadian EMS education and medical direction. The textbook is the ideal complement to the National Occupational Competency Profiles and will help paramedic educators in Canada deliver truly Canadian-based content for the first time.

We thank Russell and Rob for their expertise, hard work, and dedication to this project. We also thank Jones and Bartlett for supporting paramedicine in Canada and publishing this landmark textbook. This textbook will be a cornerstone in the growth and development of our profession for many years.

On behalf of the EMS Chiefs of Canada, I thank you for your commitment to advancing and aligning EMS in Canada.

Bruce K. Farr
Chief and General Manager
Toronto Emergency Medical Services
President, EMS Chiefs of Canada

ASSOCIATION
MÉDICALE
CANADIENNE

CANADIAN
MEDICAL
ASSOCIATION

CONJOINT
ACCREDITATION SERVICES

Accreditation of
educational programs in:

SERVICES DE L'AGREMENT

L'agrément des
programmes de formation
en :

Cardiology technology/
Technologie de
cardiologie

Cardiovascular perfusion/
Perfusion cardiovasculaire

Clinical genetics/
Génétique clinique

Cytotechnology/
Cytotechnologie

Diagnostic ultrasound
technology/Technologie
d'ultrasonographie

Magnetic resonance
imaging/Imagerie par
résonance magnétique

Medical laboratory
assistant/Adjoint de
laboratoire médical

Medical laboratory
technology/Technologie
de laboratoire médical

Nuclear medicine
technology/Technologie
de la médecine nucléaire

Ophthalmic medical
assisting technology/
Assistance médicale en
ophtalmologie

Orthoptics/Orthoptique

Paramedicine/
Technologie médicale
d'urgence

Physician assistant/
Adjoint au médecin

Radiation therapy
technology/Technologie
de la radiothérapie

Radiological technology/
Technologie radiologique

On behalf of the Canadian Medical Association (CMA), I am pleased to congratulate all those involved in producing the Canadian edition of Caroline's *Emergency Care in the Streets*. This first-ever Canadian textbook in Emergency Medical Services (EMS) is a notable achievement, and marks the continued evolution of EMS education in Canada.

The CMA has long recognized the important roles of all health professions in the continuum of patient care in Canada. The CMA is proud to play a part in the education of EMS providers by providing corporate leadership for the conjoint accreditation process, in an effort to maintain national standards for paramedic programs throughout Canada. Through the collaboration of emergency physicians, paramedics and paramedic educators, paramedic programs are reviewed regularly against national competency requirements to ensure that these programs continue to prepare safe and effective EMS practitioners.

The new Canadian EMS textbook will enhance the ability of paramedic programs to provide an educational experience that is relevant to current EMS practice in Canada. This is truly a milestone in the history of EMS education, and signals the maturity of EMS practice in Canada.

Congratulations on this achievement!

Yours sincerely,

S. Briane Scharfstein, MD, CCFP, MBA
Associate Secretary General, Professional Affairs

A healthy population and a vibrant medical profession • Une population en santé et une profession médicale dynamique

1867, prom. Alta Vista Dr., Ottawa ON K1G 5W8 • cma.ca/accredit / amc.ca/agrement • 613 731-9331 • 800 267-9703

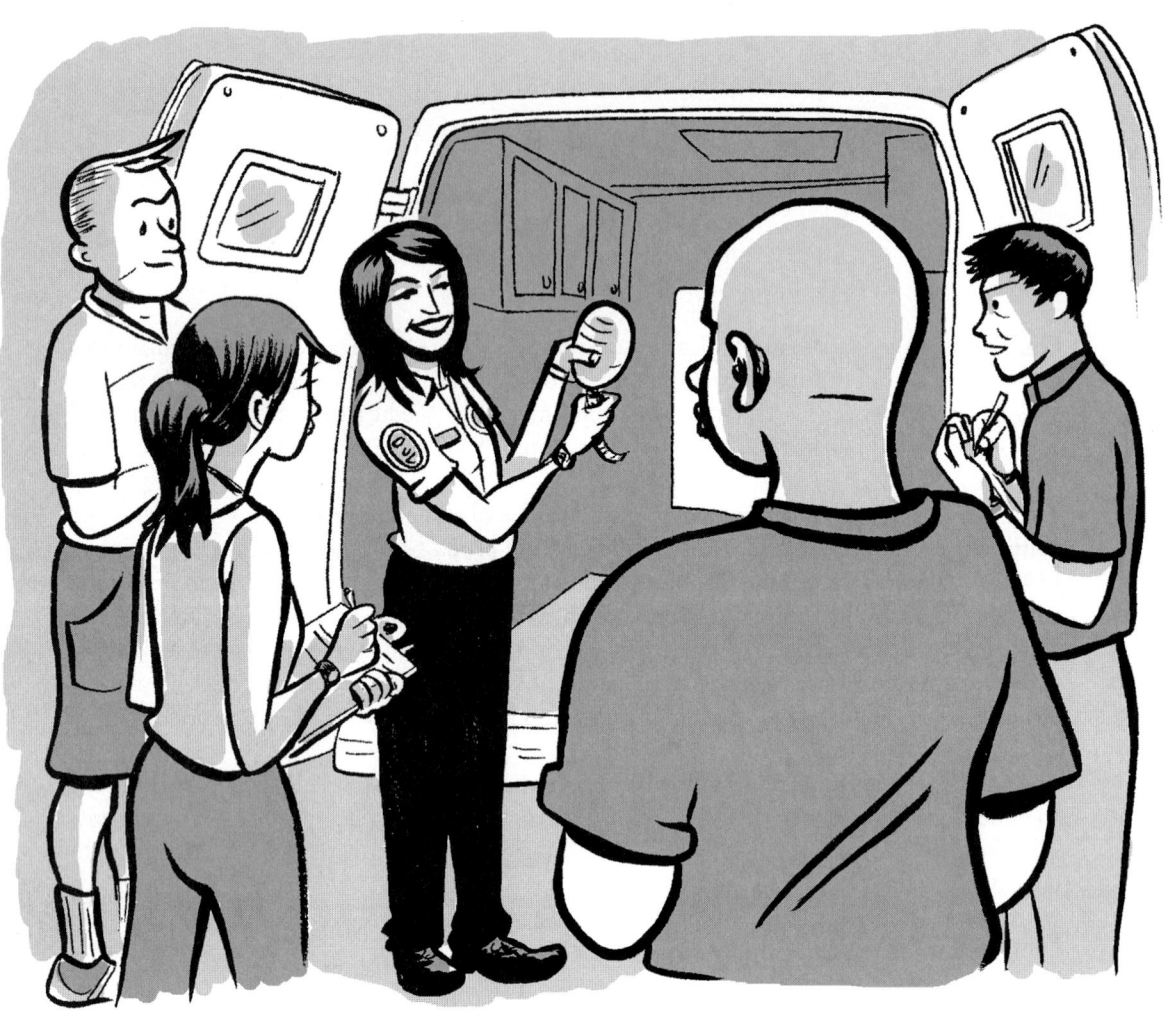

"

If they really want to be paramedics, then we can teach them."

—Eugene Nagel, MD

Preparatory

Section Editor: : Jan L. Jensen, BSc, ACP

EMS Systems, Roles, and Responsibilities

Competency Areas

Area 1: Professional Responsibilities

1.1.a Maintain patient dignity.

1.1.b Reflect professionalism through use of appropriate language.

1.1.c Dress appropriately and maintain personal hygiene

1.1.d Maintain appropriate personal interaction with patients.

1.1.e Maintain patient confidentiality.

1.1.f Participate in quality assurance and enhancement programs.

1.1.h Promote awareness of emergency medical system and profession.

1.1.i Participate in professional association.

1.1.j Behave ethically.

1.1.k Function as patient advocate.

1.2.a Develop personal plan for continuing professional development.

1.2.b Self-evaluate and set goals for improvement, as related to professional practice.

1.2.c Interpret evidence in medical literature and assess relevance to practice.

1.3.a Comply with scope of practice.

1.3.b Recognize "patient rights" and the implications on the role of the provider.

1.4.a Function within relevant legislation, policies, and procedures.

1.5.a Work collaboratively with a partner.

1.5.b Accept and deliver constructive feedback.

1.5.c Work collaboratively with other emergency response agencies.

1.5.d Work collaboratively with other members of the health care team.

1.6.a Exhibit reasonable and prudent judgement.

1.6.b Practice effective problem-solving.

1.6.c Delegate tasks appropriately.

Area 2: Communication

2.1.b Deliver an organized, accurate, and relevant verbal report.

2.1.c Deliver an organized, accurate, and relevant patient history.

2.1.d Provide information to patient about their situation and how they will be treated.

2.1.e Interact effectively with the patient, relatives, and bystanders who are in stressful situations.

2.1.f Speak in language appropriate to the listener.

2.1.g Use appropriate terminology.

2.3.b Practice active listening techniques.

2.4.a Treat others with respect.

2.4.b Exhibit empathy and compassion while providing care.

2.4.d Act in a confident manner.

2.4.e Act assertively as required.

2.4.g Exhibit diplomacy, tact, and discretion.

Area 3: Health and Safety

3.3.a Assess scene for safety.

3.3.b Address potential occupational hazards.

Introduction

Early in the emergency medical services (EMS) system development, the role of a responder was to identify an individual who was ill or injured and rapidly transport the person to a facility, often called "scoop and swoop." Today that has changed dramatically because of the expectations of communities and findings in research. As a paramedic you will encounter many different situations, from life threatening to simply lending an ear to a person just needing a listener. People you meet in the prehospital setting may evaluate you on what they see on television, read in published articles, or your treatment of a loved one. Remember that once you have completed your paramedic training and are certified or licensed, you must not lose recognition that being a certified or licensed paramedic gives you the privilege, not the right, to treat someone who is perhaps experiencing one of the worse moments of their life. Along with that privilege comes a responsibility to maintain your certification and continually upgrade your knowledge and skills. Paramedicine involves life-long learning.

EMS System Development

Pre-20th Century

The modern-day EMS system is a relatively new profession when compared with many other professions Figure 1-1 ▶. Way back in the Babylon of 1700 BC, the medical care professional went to the patient's home, and the Code of Hammurabi (the king who invented rule by law) spelled out protocols and reimbursements for medical care—including punishment for malpractice Figure 1-2 ▶.

Sending the care provider to the patient was the way it was done until Napoleon's time. In the 1790s Jean Larrey, a physician, developed *ambulances volantes,* or flying ambulances. Care was brought to patients in the field as quickly as possible.

The 20th Century and Modern Technology

World Wars I and II saw the development of ambulance corps to rapidly provide prehospital care for and remove injured persons from the battlefields to take them to hospitals far from the front. But, during the 1950s and the Korean War, military medical researchers recognized that bringing the hospital closer to the battlefield would give patients a better chance of surviving Figure 1-3 ▶. Helicopters, another new technology, brought patients to Mobile Army Surgical Hospitals (M*A*S*H units) that helped thousands survive.

In the late 1950s and early 1960s, however, the focus moved back to bringing the hospital to the patient in Northern Ireland, Germany, and Eastern European countries. Mobile intensive care units (MICUs) were staffed by specially trained physicians riding these units. The concept quickly spread to North America, but physicians were in short supply, and those

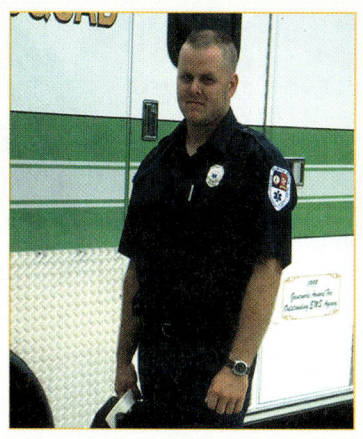

Figure 1-1 Today's paramedics are professionals who are highly trained to provide a wide variety of medical services to the public.

You are the Paramedic Part 1

You are dispatched to an episode of syncope at a local church. En route to the scene, the dispatcher informs you that your patient is an older woman who was reported by family members to have fainted during a church ceremony. She is now conscious and complaining of shortness of breath and light-headedness. Because the location of this call is 15 minutes from your station, additional responders who are closer to the scene have also been dispatched.

First responders quickly arrive on the scene to find a 70-year-old woman surrounded by members of her family, including her grandchildren, the eldest of whom was getting married. Her family members believe she is "just worn out," and think that she should go home and rest. In a brief radio report, the first responders provide you with this updated information. Shortly after arriving at the scene, you introduce yourself to the patient and perform an intial assessment.

Initial Assessment	Recording Time: 0 Minutes
Appearance	Noticeably diaphoretic and pale
Level of consciousness	Conscious but confused
Airway	Patent
Breathing	Increased respirations; adequate depth
Circulation	Very weak radial pulse

1. How is prehospital care initiated for this or any call?
2. What role do dispatchers play in prehospital care?

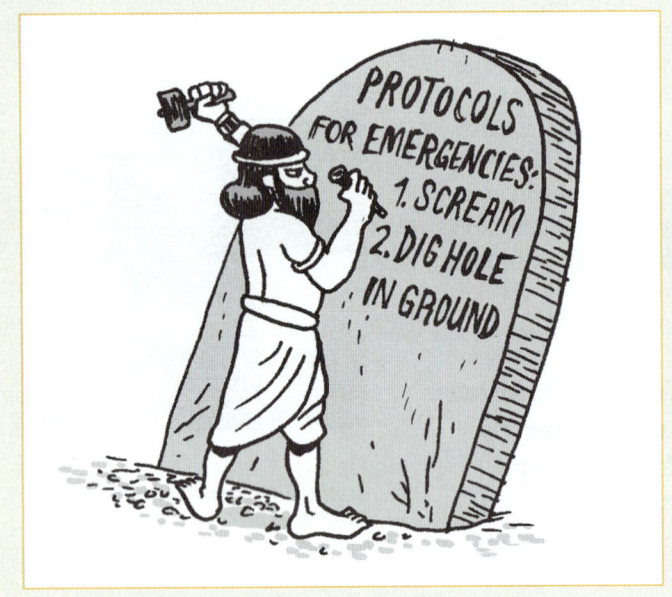

Figure 1-2

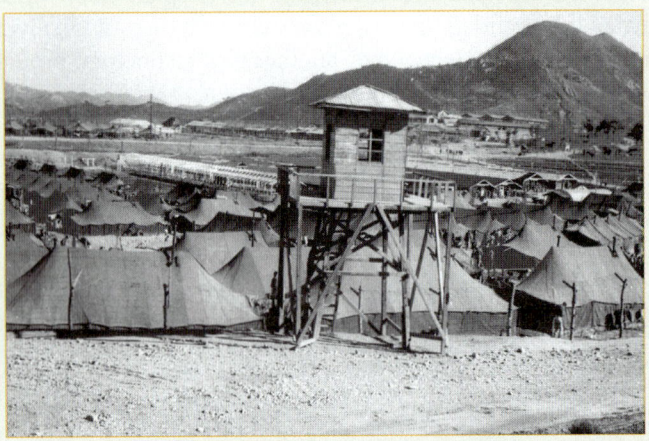

Figure 1-3 Temporary hospitals, such as this one in use during the Korean War, were set up to provide more rapid care for the injured.

Table 1-1	Critical Points

- Develop collaborative strategies to identify and address community health and safety issues.
- Align the financial incentives of EMS and other health care providers and payers.
- Participate in community-based prevention efforts.
- Develop and pursue a national EMS research agenda.
- Pass EMS legislation in each province to support innovation and integration.
- Allocate adequate resources for medical direction.
- Develop information systems that link EMS across its continuum.
- Determine the costs and benefits of EMS to the community.
- Ensure nationwide availability of 9-1-1 as the emergency telephone number.
- Ensure that all calls for emergency help are automatically accompanied by location-identifying information.

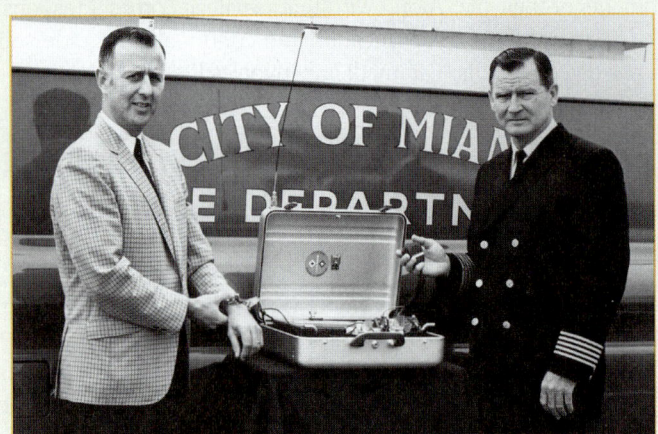

Figure 1-4 Dr. Eugene Nagel, widely considered the father of paramedicine, provided much-needed leadership. Here he is shown (at left) in 1967 with Chief Larry Kenney of the Miami Fire Department, with the first telemetry package to be used by paramedics.

physicians who were interested had minimal expertise to venture into the prehospital area. So a question was asked "Can a nonphysician be trained to perform advanced medical skills?" The answer was "Yes."

In 1966 in the United States, the National Academy of Science and the National Research Council released a "White Paper" entitled "Accidental Death and Disability: The Neglected Disease of Modern Society," in which they outlined 10 critical points (Table 1-1 ▶). From these points the National Highway Safety Act was instituted in 1966. In this act the US Department of Transportation (US DOT) was created, providing authority and financial support for the development of basic and advanced life support programs. The first EMT textbook in the United States, *Emergency Care and Transporta-*

tion of the Sick and Injured, was published by the American Academy of Orthopaedic Surgeons (AAOS) in 1971.

In 1969, the same year the basic training course for EMTs was released, Dr. Eugene Nagel, then of Miami, Florida, began training firefighters from the Miami Fire Department with advanced emergency skills (Figure 1-4 ▲). Dr. Nagel took the use of advanced emergency treatment one step further. He developed a telemetry system that enabled firefighters to transmit a patient's electrocardiogram to physicians at Jackson Memorial Hospital and to receive radio instructions from the physicians regarding what measures to take. Dr. Nagel is often called the "Father of Paramedicine" in the United States.

Many cities set up individual advanced EMS training, and regions added their own spin to what they thought was the essential standard of prehospital care, but it wasn't until 1977 that the first National Standard Curriculum for paramedics was developed by the US DOT. This first paramedic curriculum was based on the work of Dr. Nancy Caroline.

Canadian EMS has similar roots. The need for well-trained paramedics was initially identified in growing urban centres across the country. In Toronto, for instance, the first organized ambulance service hit the streets in 1832, mainly to transport victims of the cholera outbreak that had swept the city of York (as Toronto was then known).

Ambulance services in Canada were a combination of private, publicly funded, and volunteer services. The emphasis on formalizing EMS in Canada was tied to similar activities occurring in the United States. In British Columbia, an organized ambulance service was created in 1974 following government recommendations. Some provinces have only recently moved to organized ambulance services within the last few years. Nova Scotia relied mainly on the Canadian military to provide ambulance services until the creation of a provincial program in 1994. One of the first Canadian air ambulance programs was launched in Saskatchewan in 1946 following the success of the "Royal Flying Doctor" programs in the United Kingdom.

In Canada, the paramedic professional has evolved from the earliest days when ambulance drivers simply transported patients to the hospital to today's professionals who provide a cache of medications and therapies to aid those who need early and immediate interventions. The early 1990s saw paramedic teaching programs included in the Canadian Medical Association's accreditation process. In 2001, the Paramedic Association of Canada issued the National Occupational Competency Profiles (NOCPs) for paramedics. This landmark document was the first to describe the core competencies that paramedics are required to master to practice in Canada. This has led to the development of educational blueprints that have helped begin the process of standardization in this country.

With services provided and coordinated from such a broad base of sources, in the past the challenge has frequently been one of finding common ground for coordinated activities. Factionalized EMS provider groups have been challenged to work together without viewing one another as the competition and

to provide a credible national voice for EMS to be heard across the country, at all levels of government.

The Emergency Medical Services Chiefs of Canada (EMSCC) was incorporated in 2002 as a national forum for information gathering, policy development, and coordinated action by the leadership of Canada's EMS systems. Its membership is drawn from all types of EMS systems across the country, with voting membership open to those who actually operate EMS systems, large and small, and associate membership is available to those who operate within EMS systems in a supervisory or managerial capacity but who are not the senior officers of their respective services. The EMSCC envisions Canadian EMS as a mobile health care service, existing at the centre of the community, reaching into many aspects of community life and community services.

The EMSCC, in its white paper "The Future of EMS in Canada: Defining the New Road Ahead (2006)," has defined a national strategy for EMS, which embraces six key strategic directions:

- **Clear core identity:** Define who and what EMS is, clearly and consistently.
- **Stable funding:** Ensure the consistent availability of those community resources that are required to provide high-quality EMS services.
- **Systematic improvement:** The EMS system must be open to change and directly accountable for performance in a complex and ever-changing environment. It is not enough to say that EMS is doing a good job; EMS must be prepared to prove this, regularly, consistently, and transparently.
- **Personnel development:** Paramedics are one of those rare and wonderful groups for whom learning never stops. EMS must ensure that both education and training of staff are sufficiently robust to enable both personal and professional growth for paramedics, as well as the highest quality of prehospital care, embracing all new and

You are the Paramedic Part 2

As you perform a focused history and physical examination, your partner takes the patient's vital signs. Her pulse rate and blood pressure concern you, and you apply the cardiac monitor. As you question the patient and her family about her medical history and events that have occurred during today's festivities, you immediately note an arrhythmia.

Vital Signs	Recording Time: 5 Minutes
Level of consciousness	Conscious but confused
Skin	Diaphoretic, pale, and cool
Pulse	180 beats/min, regular and weak
Blood pressure	80/42 mm Hg
Respirations	24 breaths/min; adequate depth
SpO_2	95% on 15 l/min using a nonrebreathing mask
ECG	Ventricular tachycardia

3. What prehospital care can PCPs provide for this patient?

appropriate technologies in order to provide the maximum medical benefit to each patient.

- **Leadership support:** Even as we no longer put just anyone in the back of an ambulance, we must also ensure that those responsible for the day-to-day operations and planning of each EMS system have the specific knowledge and skill sets necessary to operate an EMS system at maximum performance.
- **Mobilized health care:** As health care in Canada changes and evolves, EMS must change and evolve along with it. EMS is no longer simply a medical transportation service. There are increasing numbers of places in the world where both the role and the scope of practice of paramedics have evolved to provide definitive primary care outside of traditional clinical venues. Paramedic practitioners have the knowledge and skills required to provide such care.

This collective approach to the fostering of high-quality EMS in Canada has already met with considerable success. A national forum for EMS has been created, along with a highly credible national voice of EMS, which is beginning to influence all levels of government in ways that merely a decade ago would have been regarded as daydreaming. For more information on the EMS Chiefs of Canada organization, be sure to visit their website at *www.emscc.ca.*

Controversies

Many communities initially fought against ambulance drivers "playing doctor," or in other words, becoming paramedics. Now, even the smallest communities expect access to advanced life support (ALS)-trained personnel.

The EMS System

The modern-day EMS system is a complex network of coordinated services providing various levels of prehospital care to a community. These services work in unison to meet both the growing and standing needs of the citizens in the community in which they reside. You, as a paramedic, are part of this network; therefore, you must stay active in your community to be able to meet the ever-changing needs.

The EMS network begins with citizen involvement in the complex EMS system. The public needs to be taught how to recognize that an emergency exists, how to activate the EMS system, and how basic care can be provided before EMS arrives

Figure 1-5 ▶. Remember that the public's idea of an emergency may be drastically different from yours.

At the Scene

A patient may only experience once what a paramedic may experience hundreds of times. Understand the patient's anxiety.

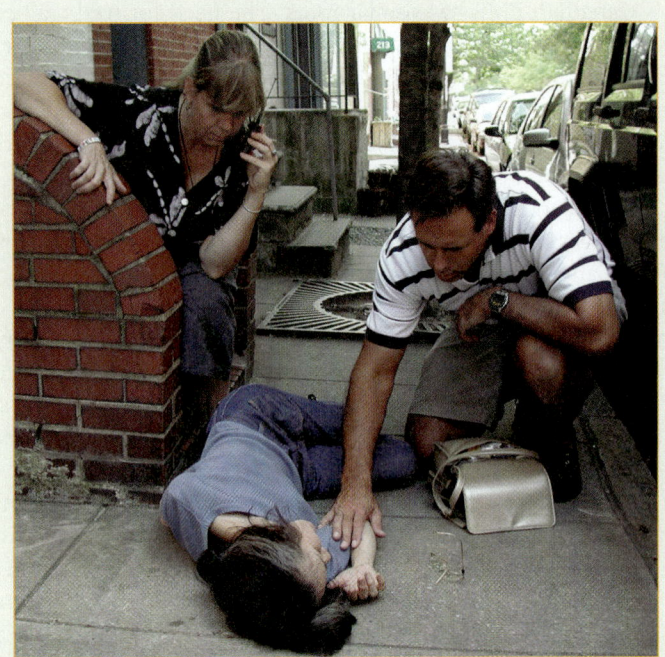

Figure 1-5 One of your roles as a paramedic is educating the public about how to first respond to an emergency, before medical help has arrived.

When you are called to a "sick person" at 02:00 hours who only has a common cold and can't sleep, there is no reason to become angry at the patient, your career, or your EMS system. Instead, use this time to educate the public by offering sympathy and insight on cold treatment, and, perhaps tactfully discuss why a cold is not an emergency. Remember, a paramedic is a public servant. You will often respond to non-emergent calls.

When the public activates the EMS system, their first contact is usually a dispatcher. Requirements for dispatcher training vary greatly from province to province. Dispatchers are limited in their ability to interpret an emergency and in extracting appropriate information from a stressed caller. Once on scene, you have to determine what is really going on, which in many cases is a far cry from what dispatch told you. Despite this or limited information, you, as a paramedic, will develop your prehospital care plan for the patient and decide on the appropriate transport method and receiving facility for your patient.

Being active in your community will keep you on top of the best local resources. When you are drawing up a potential prehospital care plan, you will ask yourself, "Does the receiving facility have the resources needed for this patient?" When you are active in your community, you will know the answer. If the answer is no, the next question, "Is there an appropriate facility within a reasonable distance?" will also be a part of your community knowledge.

There are currently several levels of providers in the EMS system. Each level has a scope of practice, as outlined by the NOCPs. The scope of practice is reevaluated from time to time and may change as a result. Canada's paramedic training programs have an international reputation for producing practitioners who are not only highly skilled, but who also possess a significant level of clinical acumen and critical-thinking ability. Let's take a look at these various levels.

Special Considerations

EMS systems must be capable of handling many different situations including obstetric, pediatric, and geriatric emergencies. Proper procedures, drug dosages, and even assessment techniques are often different in children, adults, and older people.

The Dispatcher

The dispatcher plays a key role in an EMS call. He or she must receive and enter all information on the call, interpret the information, and in turn, relay it to the appropriate resources **Figure 1-6 ▶**. In some locations the dispatcher may be trained as an emergency medical dispatcher (EMD), which charges these individuals with the added task of giving simple medical direction (ie, CPR, bleeding control, etc) to a caller in hopes that this care may benefit the patient until paramedics are on scene.

The Emergency Responder

Not all provinces and territories have this as a certification, and for those that do, there can be considerable variability in requirements. In the generic use of the term, a first responder is usually a person trained in CPR and/or first aid. As a paramedic, one of your jobs will be to familiarize yourself with the level of training of first responders in your EMS system.

The Primary Care Paramedic (PCP)

In most Canadian regions, the primary care paramedic (PCP) is the backbone and primary provider level in many EMS systems. PCPs provide care and transport for the entire spectrum of patients encountered by any EMS system. In addition to oxygen, wound care, splinting, and other basic treatment modalities, PCPs in most of Canada can administer a select number of medications for the treatment of common symptoms, such as ischemic chest pain and shortness of breath. PCPs can also defibrillate unstable cardiac rhythms using AEDs and, in some cases, provide advanced airway procedures using single-lumen airways such as the Combitube or the King airway. Additionally, some PCPs can initiate or maintain intravenous lines and provide certain types of fluid therapy.

The Advanced Care Paramedic (ACP)

The advanced care paramedic (ACP) builds on the knowledge and skills of the PCP. In Canada, ACPs provide what is traditionally considered "advanced life support." ACPs can provide

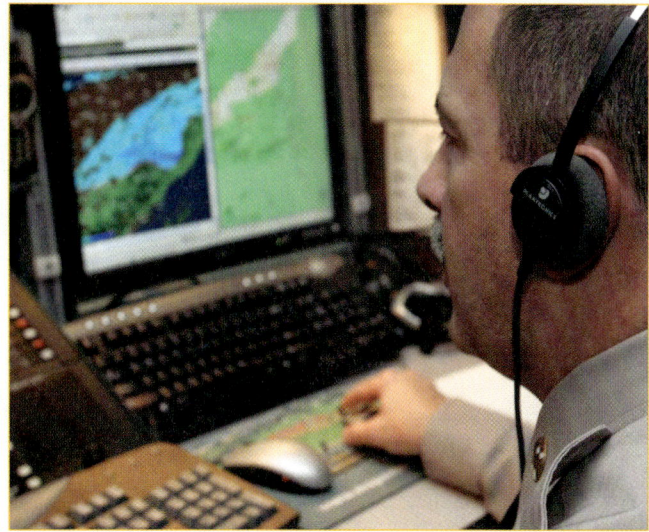

Figure 1-6 The dispatcher coordinates the entire rescue effort. He or she interprets a caller's information and then sends appropriate personnel and resources to the scene.

specific airway measures, including intubation, cricothyrotomy, and needle decompression. The ACP medication list includes a variety of drugs to manage cardiac, respiratory, neurologic, and endocrine emergencies.

The Critical Care Paramedic (CCP)

Critical care paramedics (CCPs) are a unique group of medical practitioners who work primarily in the delivery of air ambulance or land-based critical care interfacility transfer services. Many of the patients managed by these highly trained professionals are complex in nature, often requiring multiple medications, blood products, and mechanical ventilation. Although CCPs participate in emergency responses to accident scenes, their primary role is to move sick patients between facilities.

Paramedic Education

Initial Education

Education may vary from province to province, but in most cases provinces and territories base their paramedic education programs on the NOCPs. Most PCPs receive their initial training at a community college or similar academic institution. This typically, but not always, occurs before the paramedic student is hired by an EMS service. Program lengths vary from less than 1 year in British Columbia to programs, like some in Quebec, that can run longer than 3 years. ACPs are also trained at the community college level; however, many ACPs are already employed as PCPs when they enter training; service-based training programs are not uncommon. ACP programs tend to range from 1 to 2 years in length. There are very few accredited critical care paramedic programs in Canada, and they are almost entirely operated through air ambulance programs. Regardless of program length or paramedic type, the key measure for any educational program is quality. In Canada, paramedic training programs are accredited by the Canadian Medical Association (CMA) after demonstrating that the program meets minimum standards based on the NOCPs.

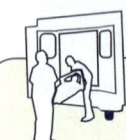

At the Scene

The number of calls you go on isn't the deciding factor on how much more training you need.

Continuing Education

Most provinces require that paramedics show proof of hours spent in continuing education programs. Such programs keep you up-to-date on new research findings and new techniques and skills, and they knock the rust off of skills you seldom use Figure 1-7 ▶. Continuing education can also showcase current issues in your province that impact you and your system's ability to provide quality emergency medical care. Continuing education can be enjoyable and it should be. Whenever possible, you should attend conferences and seminars, ideally with some of them being out of your region and/or province, which helps broaden your knowledge base. It is certainly worth attending conferences that may not be designed for paramedics. Another way to broaden your knowledge base is to read EMS and emergency medicine journals or to attend a journal club. Finally, another great resource for paramedics is the growing number of Internet-

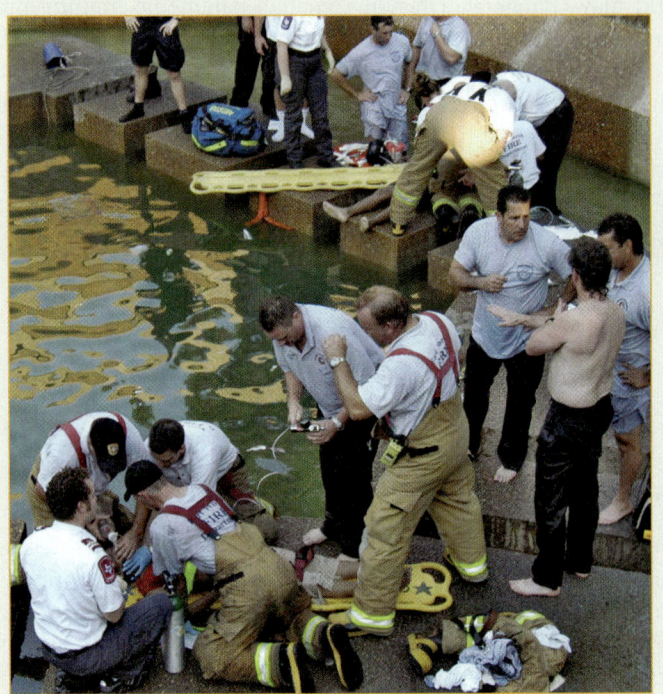

Figure 1-7 Continuing education can keep you up-to-date on technological improvements that are continually made available to paramedics.

based continuing education providers; however, be sure that these programs meet your provincial requirements. Get everyone on your service involved in postcall reviews—they can be very beneficial in identifying problem areas in your practice.

No matter what requirements are mandated by your provincial regulators, responsibility for continuing medical

You are the Paramedic **Part 3**

Your paramedic partner asks the patient whether she has any allergies to medication and then administers an appropriate dose of Versed for sedation. You simultaneously prepare your equipment for synchronized cardioversion and explain to the patient what you must do and what she should expect. You advise the other responders to be prepared for deterioration of the patient's condition and to notify the receiving facility of her condition and the treatment she has received. Having successfully converted your patient's heart rhythm, you take another set of vital signs.

Reassessment	Recording Time: 10 Minutes
Level of consciousness	A (Alert to person, place, and day)
Skin	Pink, warm, and dry
Pulse	88 beats/min, regular and strong
Blood pressure	130/60 mm Hg
Respirations	16 breaths/min and unlaboured
SpO$_2$	99% on 15 l/min using a nonrebreathing mask
ECG	Sinus rhythm

4. What are the advantages of having a paramedic partner?

5. Is there one team member who is more important than another?

education ultimately rests with each individual paramedic. You are the only person who knows which subjects have become alarmingly foggy in your memory and which procedures leave you feeling as if you have ten thumbs. And you are the person who will have to live with the questions and doubts that inevitably arise after something goes wrong in the prehospital environment. Continuing medical education is a way to help make sure that things *don't* go wrong.

National EMS Group Involvement

Many national and provincial organizations exist, and many invite paramedic membership. These organizations do have an impact on the future direction of EMS, so it is very important for you to become involved in them. You will also be able to access many valuable resources to help you develop yourself and your service area and to improve your problem-solving skills. One of the common goals of many national organizations is to promote uniformity of EMS standards and practice throughout the nation. Some of these organizations are listed in   Table 1-2 ▾ .

Licensure, Certification, and Registration

Upon completing a paramedic training program, you will be required to be registered, licensed, and/or certified to practice your profession. Performing functions as a paramedic prior to this is unlawful, or to be more specific, considered practicing medicine without a license. Provincial and local guidelines determine your status when you complete your paramedic training. There are subtle differences between licensure, registration, and certification, which are discussed in Chapter 4. For all intents and purposes, these are essentially the same. Throughout this chapter, to avoid repetition, when we talk about being certified it means the same as holding a license.

Table 1-2	National EMS Organizations

Canada
- The Paramedic Association of Canada (PAC)
- The EMS Chiefs of Canada
- Canadian Association of Emergency Physicians (CAEP)
- Heart and Stroke Foundation

United States
- National Association of Emergency Medical Service Physicians (NAEMSP) Canadian Relations Committee
- National Association of EMS Educators (NAEMSE)
- National Registry of EMTs (NREMT)
- National Association of EMTs (NAEMT)
- Emergency Medical Services for Children (EMS-C)
- American College of Emergency Physicians (ACEP)

Although being certified or registered shows that you have successfully completed a training program and met the provincial requirements to achieve such license, it does not mean that you can perform as a paramedic without the supervision of your service's physician medical director. Agencies (provincial, local, and national) still require that paramedics receive medical direction. The concept and principles of direct medical control will be discussed later in the chapter.

Finally, you may be required to be registered as well as licensed. Registration means that records of your training, local licensure, and recertification will be held by a recognized board of registration and implies that you have successfully completed required provincial testing.

Additionally, some provinces require that paramedic graduates come from an accredited paramedic program. The CMA is the only national accrediting agency for paramedic training programs in Canada.

Reciprocity

Be aware that each province has different registration, certification, and licensing requirements and procedures. Granting recognition to a paramedic from another province or agency is known as reciprocity. This process differs from province to province; in some cases you simply need to be in good standing in your current province to qualify, whereas some provinces require you to challenge their requirements. In other words, you may be required to go through that province's written and/or practical evaluations prior to reciprocity being granted. Others may request your training program transcript and continuing education hours.

Professionalism

During your paramedic education and training process, you learn a vast amount of information designed to make you a health care professional, practicing at the paramedic level. A profession is a field of endeavor that requires a specialized set of knowledge, skills, and expertise, often gained after lengthy training.

As a paramedic, you will be trained at length for certification with standards, competencies, and continuing education requirements.

A paramedic is considered a health care professional. The attributes of a health care professional are that he or she:
- Conforms to the same standards of other health care professions.
- Provides quality patient care.
- Instills pride in the profession.
- Strives continuously for high standards.
- Earns respect from others in the profession.
- Meets societal expectations of the profession whether on or off duty.

As a paramedic, you will be trained for certification using standards, competencies, and continuing education requirements.

The paramedic profession has expected standards and performance parameters as well as a code of ethics. Collectively, these are the standards by which you will be measured as a paramedic.

As a paramedic you must remind yourself that you are in a highly visible role in your community **Figure 1-8 ▾** . Professional image and behaviour must be a top priority. You are a representative of the agency, city, county, district, region, or province you work in. Sometimes, people will make a negative judgment within the first 10 seconds of meeting you. As a paramedic you will be meeting new people as an everyday part of your career. To provide the best possible prehospital care, you must establish and maintain credibility and instill confidence. As you walk into a situation, never forget that a big part of your job is to continually show that you are truly concerned for the well-being of your patients and their families. Your appearance is also of utmost importance—it has more impact than you may think. It is not appropriate to arrive at a call in dirty clothes, with dirty hands, and smelling offensively. You must look and act like a professional at all times.

Other attributes of professionalism as a paramedic include:

- **Integrity.** The single most important attribute. Be open, honest, and truthful with your patients.
- **Empathy.** Show your patients, their families, and other health care professionals that you identified and understand their feelings.
- **Self-motivation.** You should have an internal drive for excellence, which is often a driving force to ensure that you always behave in a professional manner. You will need to continuously educate yourself, accept constructive feedback, and perform with minimal supervision.

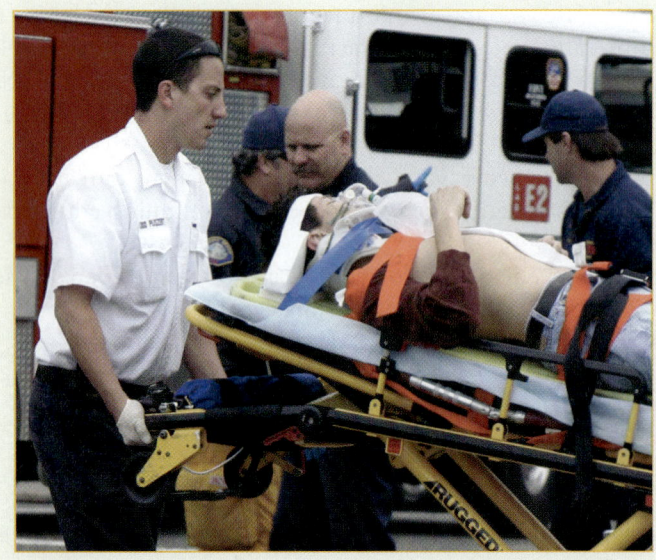

Figure 1-8 Adopting a professional attitude and appearance is a critical part of working with the public and earning their trust.

Notes from Nancy

The role of paramedic entails new prestige, but it also imposes new responsibilities. Paramedics are entrusted with the lives of other human beings, and there is no more awesome or sacred responsibility than that. Your education as a paramedic must not stop with this text. You must continue to read and study and ask questions, to refine your knowledge and skills, so that you may give to each patient the best of which you are capable. You must learn to conduct yourself with humility, to accept criticism, to learn from mistakes as well as from triumphs, and to demand of yourself and your colleagues nothing less than the best. For only then will the title of paramedic signify what it is meant to signify: a commitment to other human beings.

- **Communication.** You must be able to express and exchange your ideas, thoughts, and findings with other professional colleagues. Make conscious reminders to yourself when interacting with patients and their families to listen well and speak directly, without using confusing medical terms **Figure 1-9 ▸** .
- **Teamwork and respect.** Teamwork is required in EMS. On every call, everyone involved must work together to achieve a common goal—to provide the best possible prehospital care to ensure the overall well-being of your patient. Most often in the prehospital setting the paramedic is the team leader. A team leader will not undermine his or her team, but instead will help guide and support the team, remaining flexible and open for change at any moment and communicating at an appropriate place and time with other members of the team to resolve problems. You must always be as respectful of others as you would expect them to be with you.
- **Patient advocate.** You must always act in the best interest of the patient while respecting his or her wishes and beliefs, regardless of your own. This includes patients with special needs or those with different lifestyles, values, and cultures from your own. Never allow your personal feelings about a patient to have an impact on the prehospital care you provide. Respect those you serve. While you need to communicate to do your job, be sure that you maintain a high level of confidentiality. Whatever details you have about your patient, do your best not to talk in front of anyone who is not on your team. When you talk to members of your team, do so quietly and with appropriate respect. Your role in patient advocacy means you should always be on the lookout for spousal or child maltreatment and elder neglect. Make sure you communicate your findings to the appropriate authorities.

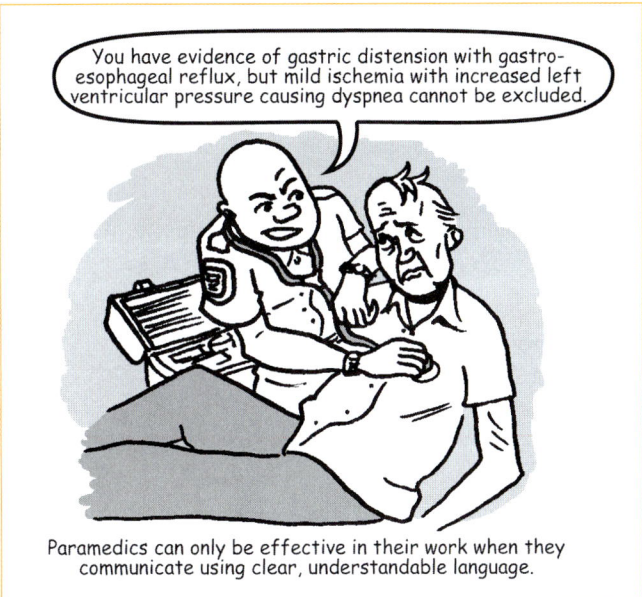

You have evidence of gastric distension with gastro-esophageal reflux, but mild ischemia with increased left ventricular pressure causing dyspnea cannot be excluded.

Paramedics can only be effective in their work when they communicate using clear, understandable language.

Figure 1-9

- **Injury prevention.** A paramedic is in the unique position of seeing the patient's surroundings prior to transport. If you can spot a potential hazard (such as a loose rug at the top of the stairs), use your diplomatic skills and talk about your findings to the patient or a family member. You may prevent a potential injury. Discuss the importance of using bike helmets, safety belts, and child car seats whenever you can. It is another way of preventing injuries.
- **Careful delivery of service.** A paramedic must deliver the highest quality prehospital care. Pay careful attention to detail and continuously evaluate and reevaluate your performance. Use other medical professionals as resources, not adversaries. Follow policies, protocols, and procedures as well as the orders of your superiors.

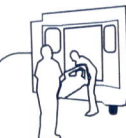

At the Scene

For safety, avoid wearing long necklaces, dangling earrings, or other jewelry that could interfere with your work.

Roles and Responsibilities

So what does it actually mean to be a paramedic? What are my roles? What am I responsible for? These are questions that you should ask yourself throughout your career. The EMS system continues to grow and mature, and with those changes will come new roles and additional responsibilities. Some of the primary responsibilities are shown in **Figure 1-10 ▶** and include:

- **Preparation.** Be prepared physically, mentally, and emotionally. Keep up your knowledge and skill abilities. Be sure you have the appropriate equipment for your call and that it is in good working order.
- **Response.** Responding to the event in a timely, safe manner is very important. High speed—running "hot" without due regard to the safety of you, your partner, your patient, and persons on the highway (even if they should get out of your way but don't)—is not acceptable.
- **Scene management.** Ensuring your own safety and the safety of your team is the first priority. You must also ensure the patient's safety and the safety of any bystanders. Part of your preparation before you reach the scene should include assessing the situation; the nature of the call will give valuable information. Preparing for scene safety starts with the use of personnel protective equipment such as gloves and goggles. The paramedic often sets the example for safety to the members of the EMS team who might believe that running hot is running safe.
- **Patient assessment and prehospital care.** An appropriate organized assessment based on the principles you will learn in this book should be performed on all patients. You will need to recognize and prioritize the patient's needs on the basis of the injuries he or she has sustained or the illness that most urgently needs treatment.
- **Management and disposition.** A paramedic must follow protocols signed off by the medical director. Sometimes, however, when you are in the prehospital environment, you will discover that the protocols might not cover the situation you are in. This is the time that you must radio your medical director or direct medical control for orders. Having a good working relationship with your medical director and direct medical control is critical. You are the eyes, ears, and touch of the medical director. Situations that require a variance of protocol or a decision outside of

You are the Paramedic Part 4

Your patient's pulse has decreased, blood pressure has increased, and she no longer feels short of breath or light-headed. Her skin signs are much improved, with colour returning to her cheeks. Your paramedic partner administers lidocaine, 1 mg/kg of body weight, as well as a maintenance infusion of 2 mg/min. Your patient and her entire family thank you and your partner in the emergency department for your help. You feel gratified to know that all of your hard work has paid off.

6. Why is it important to keep skills and knowledge current?
7. Why is it important to practice these skills as a team?

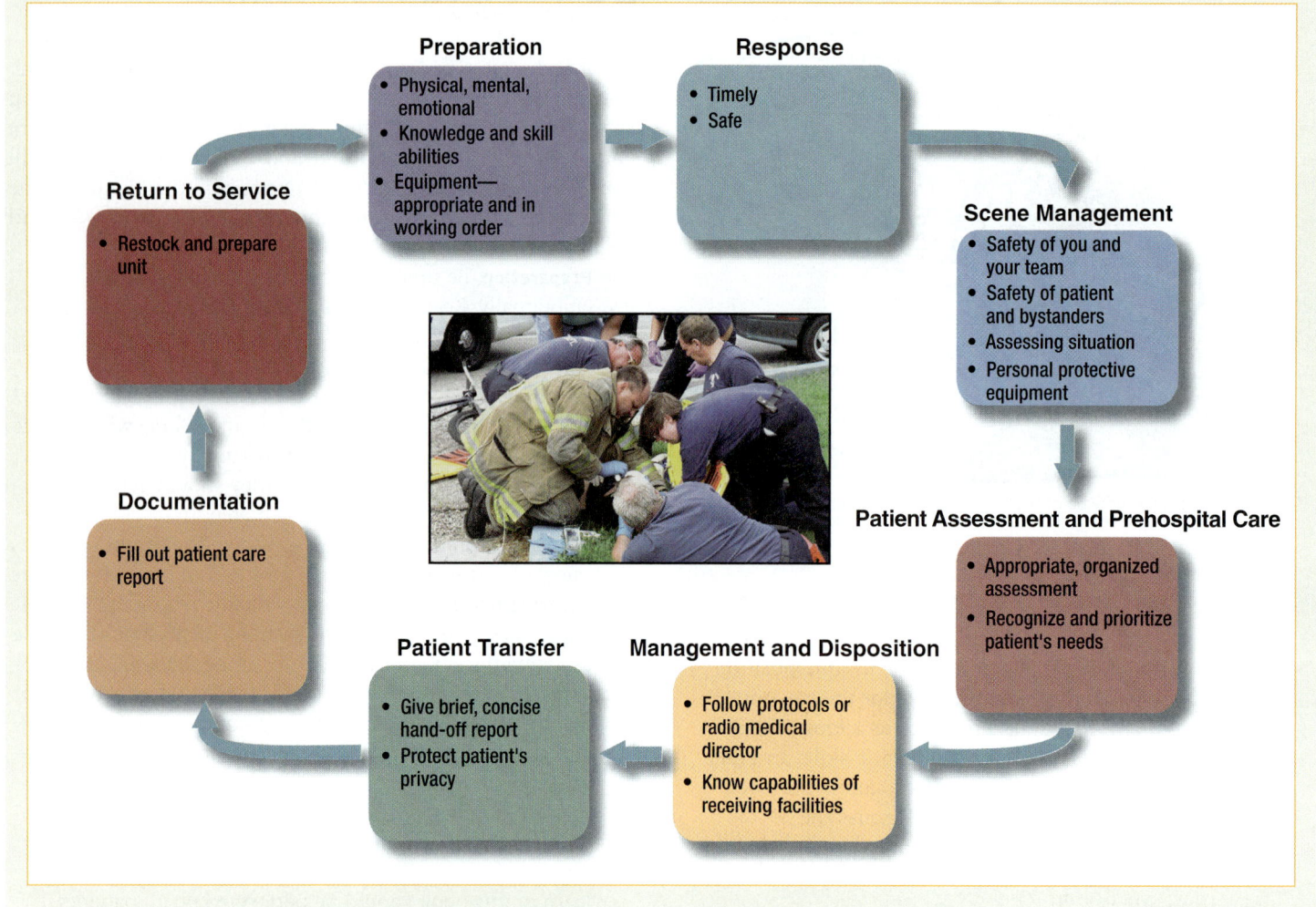

Figure 1-10 Paramedics follow an important sequence of procedures for each emergency call.

your scope of practice need to be communicated with your medical director. You must also make the appropriate transport and destination decisions, often with the cooperation of other medical professionals. Know the capabilities of all receiving facilities with which you may interact; this will assist you in making the right decisions for your patient.

- **Patient transfer.** Once you arrive at the receiving facility, continue to act as a patient advocate and give the appropriate facility staff a brief, concise hand-off report. Once again, use discretion so that you protect your patient's privacy.
- **Documentation.** After you transfer the patient, it is extremely important that a patient care report be filled out immediately. The report serves as a legal record of what you did in the prehospital environment. Physicians must document their care of patients—so must you. Guidelines for documentation will be covered later in this text.
- **Return to service.** Every person on the EMS team is responsible for restocking and preparing the unit as quickly as possible for the next call. Failure to do so can

bring about nasty legal consequences if another call comes in and the unit is not fully restocked and ready to respond.

You are looked upon as a health care professional, so take advantage. Educate the public about what you do and its importance. Get involved with prevention, community, and leadership activities whenever possible **Figure 1-11 ▶**. Never miss an opportunity to teach the community about prevention of injury and illness. Explain to people how to appropriately use your services. For those areas where trained paramedics are few and far between, use your abilities to promote programs that get the public involved in CPR, one of the major determinants of whether a person in cardiac arrest will live or die.

In some regions, paramedics have other health care responsibilities such as working in community clinics, freestanding emergency facilities, and hospitals. Home visits by paramedics under direct medical control are also occurring in many parts of the country.

Paramedics of all EMS levels need to be advocates for prehospital health care, which often means setting out a well thought-out campaign for EMS. Research your community, look at the strengths and weaknesses of the system, and develop

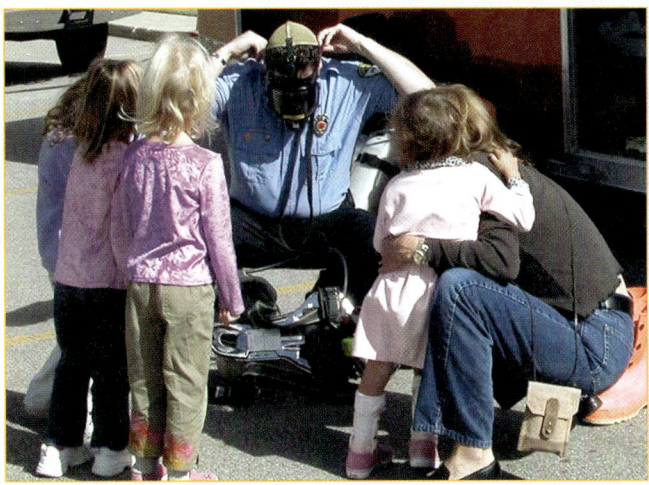

Figure 1-11 Part of your role as a public servant is to interact with and educate the public.

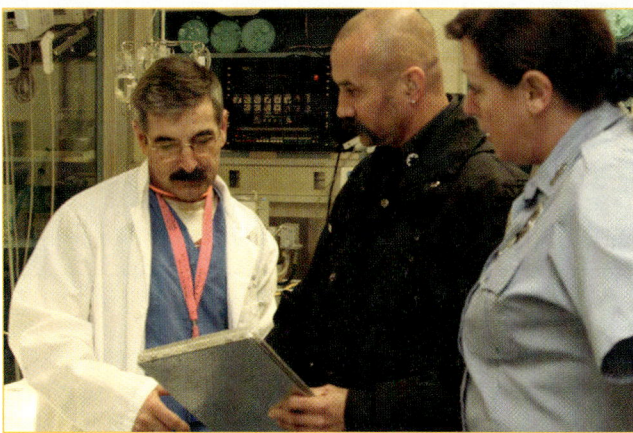

Figure 1-12 Physicians work closely with paramedics through all stages of a patient call. Here, paramedics hand off the patient report to the attending emergency department physician.

Documentation and Communication

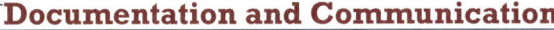

Documentation of equipment repairs and checks is nearly as important as documenting patient prehospital care.

plans for initiatives to improve the system. Many people lack the understanding of what EMS does and recognition of how vital your job can be when a loved one is unexpectedly taken ill. Many programs on television today give the public only a very small insight into the true world of EMS. Some of these programs use unrealistic events or show unrealistic outcomes or inappropriate behaviour on the part of paramedics. By involving yourself in your communities, you can both educate and advocate. It is up to all of us to educate the media and public of the truths in "our world." We must all strive to stay at the top of our profession. Continue your education, become a mentor for new paramedics, and conduct research activities.

Medical Direction

The quickest distinction in the differences among levels of EMS training is that the paramedic carries out invasive procedures—procedures that otherwise are performed only by physicians or other advanced practitioners. The law, however may not give the paramedic independent authority to act. Physicians who are educated about the levels and the extent of the training of paramedics play a vital role in supporting your practice Figure 1-12 ▸ . The role of an EMS medical director includes:

- Educating and training personnel.
- Participating in the selection of new personnel.
- Participating in equipment selection.
- Developing clinical protocols in cooperation with other paramedics who are considered experts in the field.
- Developing and assisting in a quality improvement program.
- Providing input into prehospital care.
- Interfacing between EMS systems and other health care agencies.
- Serving as an EMS advocate to the community.
- Serving as the "medical conscience" of the EMS system.

The medical director also provides direct (either by radio or by electronic communication) and indirect medical control. The benefit to direct medical control is that it provides immediate and specific patient care resources, allows telemetry transmission, allows for continuous quality improvement, and can render on-scene assistance. Indirect medical control allows for the development of protocols, standing orders, procedures, and training. A protocol is a treatment plan for a specific illness or injury. A standing order is a type of protocol that is a written document signed by the EMS system's medical director that outlines specific directions, permissions, and sometimes prohibitions regarding prehospital care that is rendered prior to contacting direct medical control (for example, defibrillation). Protocols are usually developed in conjunction with national standards. For example, EMS personnel use the Heart and Stroke Foundation of Canada advanced cardiac life support algorithms as a protocol for cardiac patients (discussed in detail in Chapter 27). Protocols also dictate what type of equipment and supplies are approved and needed as well as minimum expectations of personnel. The medical director also plays a role after the ambulance call. Medical directors help with patient care report review or even personally perform such reviews to ensure continuous quality improvement.

In some cases you may encounter a physician on scene. If the physician is familiar with EMS protocols or happens to be your medical director, it can be a great help. But you may be caught between what the physician on the scene wants and the protocols that your medical director has given your service. Remember that you work with your physician medical director and you must adhere to the local protocols and standing orders.

You must not lose your cool should the physician on the scene demand direct medical control of the situation.

Politely explain that all your actions must be in accordance with your EMS medical director's protocols. Point out that you can only transfer care of the patient to an onsite physician if that physician is now taking full responsibility for the patient and he or she will be present during transport, riding with the patient in your ambulance to the emergency department. EMS systems have a protocol to address a physician on scene who is not the medical director. Paramedics should consult their local or regional protocols and know how to manage this situation to ensure appropriate prehospital care.

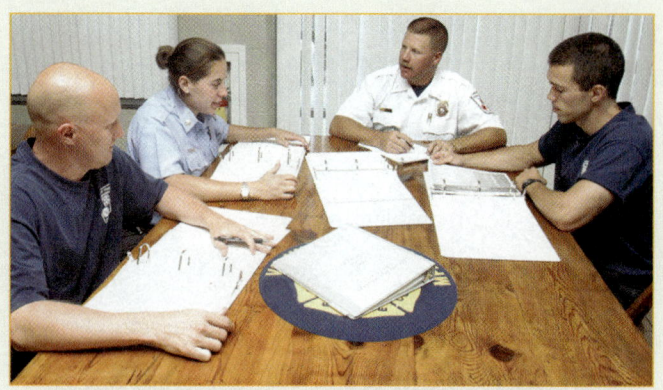

Figure 1-13 Peer reviews should be seen as a constructive part of paramedic practice.

Improving System Quality

Making a good thing better should always be part of your paramedic career. A tool often used to continually evaluate your prehospital care is called continuous quality improvement (CQI). Quality assurance is another process that evaluates problems and finds solutions. CQI is a process of assessing for ongoing improvement without waiting for a problem to arise first. When properly developed and followed, a CQI program can help you and your service.

The process of CQI is dynamic, and your EMS system should develop a structure before a CQI assessment program is started. A good CQI process should include the following:

- Identify any system-wide problem(s).
- Conduct an in-depth review of the problem(s).
- Aid the problem(s) and develop a remedy(ies).
- Develop an action plan for correction of problems.
- Enforce the plan of action.
- Reexamine the problem.
- Identify excellence in patient care.
- Look for modifications that need to be made to protocols and standing orders.
- Identify situations that are currently not addressed by protocols and standing orders.

Although it may not be feasible, all ambulance calls should be reviewed. First and foremost the focus of CQI needs to be on improving patient care.

Some services will choose to do quality assurance as *peer review* Figure 1-13 ▶. Peer review can be a good learning experience if the people doing the reviewing have good guidelines to follow and you keep an open mind. No matter how good your education and training, you will still make mistakes and miss things from time to time. When a peer reviewer finds things you can improve, you should look at it as an educational tool. In an ideal system, the members of the peer review team rotate on and off, meaning that you at some point in time will also serve as a reviewer yourself. Caution: never use this process as a tool to demean or belittle a fellow paramedic. Nor should you discuss your findings with anyone who is not identified as part of the review process. Be professional.

A comprehensive CQI program can help to prevent problems from arising by evaluating day-to-day operations and identifying possible stress points in these operations. These may include:

- Medical direction issues.
- Training.
- Communications.
- Prehospital treatment.
- Transportation issues.
- Financial issues.
- Receiving facility review.
- Dispatch.
- Public information and education.
- Disaster planning.
- Mutual aid.

EMS Research

In the early years of EMS, many standards relating to professionalism, protocols, training, and equipment were developed from "great ideas" or direct experience. The standards for EMS research are now similar to those in any other medical profession. The public of today expects that you, as a paramedic, will do what is medically proven to work in research findings.

Quality EMS research has many benefits for the future. In all health care fields, research determines the effectiveness of treatment—what works and what doesn't. Because funding for

EMS continues to be a problem, it is important that paramedics initiate research and prove that emergency services are necessary.

When you begin your research project, use some form of research ethics board (REB). In 1978, the Medical Research Council of Canada (MRC) outlined the requirements of reviews that would make them acceptable. The first part of research is to identify a specific problem or question. Even if the topic of your project has been researched before, this does not mean you can't revisit it. Sometimes research findings can be flawed and your process may identify flaws or enhance previous research findings. The next step is to decide on what style of research you wish to perform, which may include:

- **Descriptive research.** Research that is basically observation only, where no attempt to change or alter an event occurs.
- **Experimental research.** When a skill, new product, or general idea is used in a trial phase, and the effects are evaluated.
- **Prospective research.** Research that defines a clear problem or question prior to gathering data.
- **Retrospective research.** Research that is based on currently available data.
- **Cross-sectional research.** Research that is based on a group of individuals over an outlined time frame.

Your next step is to outline the group or groups of individuals necessary for the research **Figure 1-14 ▾**. Once the group(s) is identified you may wish to refine the group further, such as giving a specific age bracket, medical condition, or gender. As an example, you may wish to study men between the ages of 20 and 30 who have asthma. Once the list of eligible subjects is identified you should randomly assign patients to each arm of the research. There are many different ways you can achieve this. You may wish to have the computer generate a list of subjects or groups (systematic sampling) or you can set time frame parameters (alternative time sampling). Finally, the least preferred or accurate would be to assign subjects to a specific person or crew (convenience sampling). Even in the best cases, sampling errors can occur. Not everyone will be included in the study, or there may be individuals in the study who meet criteria but still aren't the best representation.

Parameters should be identified in research. They outline the type of individuals who are appropriate for the study. One other tool to use is "blinding," in which subjects are not told the specifics of the project. There are single-, double-, and triple-blinded studies where one, two, or all parties are blinded, respectively. When participants of the research project are advised of all aspects of the project, it is known as an unblinded study.

As your research continues, data will be acquired. You can utilize statistics either in a descriptive or inferential format. Descriptive statistics can also be performed in either a qualitative or quantitative style. The qualitative method does not use numerical information and is the least accurate **Figure 1-15 ▾**. The quantitative approach adds several other possible variables to the research: mean, median, and mode. For example, the mean age of study participants in a study on asthma in men who are between 20 and 30 years old is the average age of the subjects, the median is the midpoint age of the subjects, and the mode is the most frequent age of the subjects. Finally, standard deviation outlines how much those scores in each set will differ from the mean.

As in many aspects of a profession, there are ethical items to consider. When you decide on a research project you must ensure that the risks will not outweigh the benefits. You must acquire consent from the subject(s) and be certain their rights and welfare are adequately protected **Figure 1-16 ▸**. More information on consent will be covered later in this text.

All research projects have the following format:

- **Introduction.** Outlines a brief background of the research, including previous studies, reasons for the study, and a hypothesis of the project.

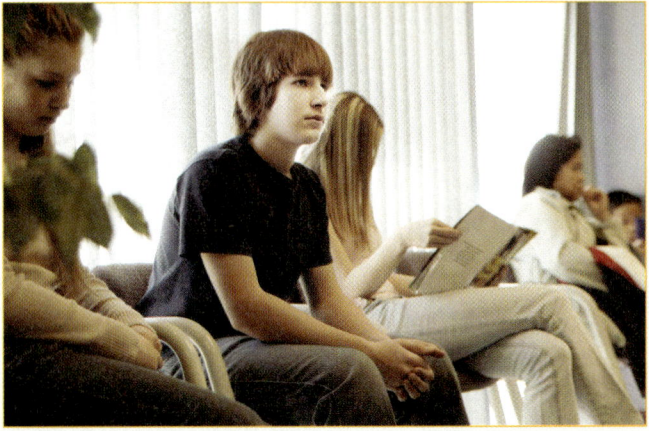

Figure 1-14 Often, medical subjects are paid to participate in research projects. The greater the number of participants, the more reliable the findings.

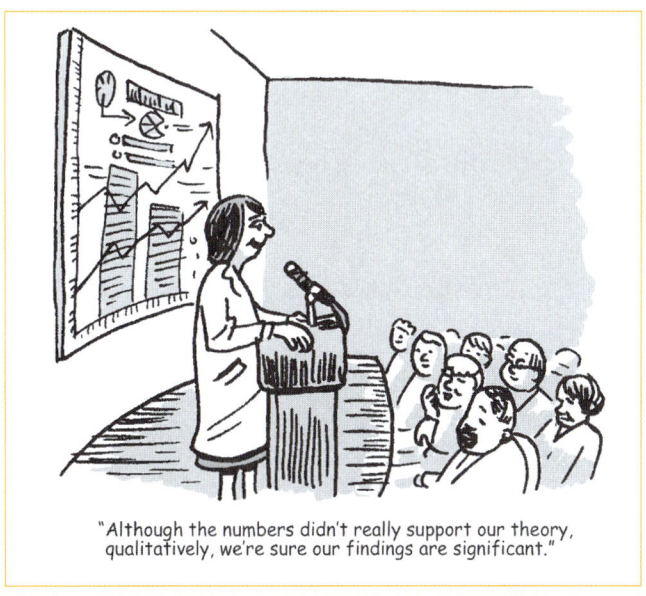

"Although the numbers didn't really support our theory, qualitatively, we're sure our findings are significant."

Figure 1-15

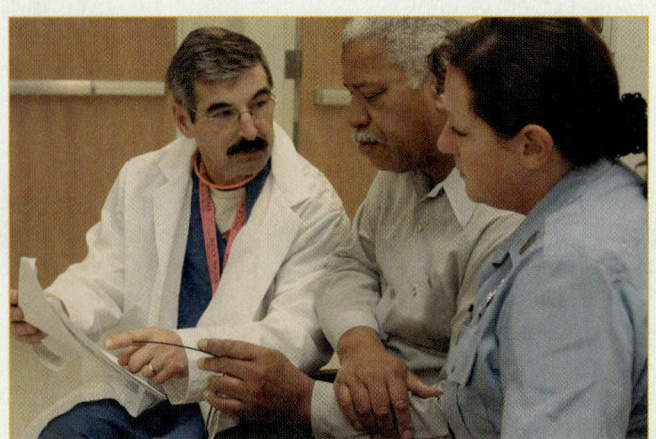

Figure 1-16 Any individual who participates in a research study should be well informed of the goals and parameters of the project.

Table 1-3	Ten Steps to Conducting a Research Project

1. Prepare a question.
2. Write a hypothesis.
3. Decide what you will measure and the best method to use.
4. Outline the population you will use.
5. Identify expected study limitations.
6. Acquire approval of the study by a research ethics board.
7. Obtain needed consent from the population(s) used.
8. Gather data.
9. Analyze your data.
10. Decide what you will do with your final research product.

- **Methods.** Includes a specific description of the project so it can be replicated. This part will outline inclusion and exclusion criteria.
- **Results.** Describes the findings of the project.
- **Discussion.** Details the results of your findings along with the limitations placed on the project and gives ideas you may have that could improve the project next time.
- **Conclusion.** Provides a final summary of information you have outlined in the introduction, methods, results, and discussion sections.

Table 1-3 ▶ lists the steps for conducting a research project. **Table 1-4 ▶** lists questions to answer when evaluating and interpreting research.

Table 1-4	Fifteen Questions to Answer When Evaluating and Interpreting Research

1. Was the research peer reviewed?
2. What was the research hypothesis?
3. Was the study approved by a research ethics board and conducted ethically?
4. What was the population being studied?
5. What were the inclusion and exclusion criteria?
6. What method was used to acquire a sample of patients?
7. How many groups were the patients divided into?
8. How were the patients assigned to the groups?
9. What type of data was gathered?
10. Did the study have enough patients involved?
11. Are there any confounding variables unaccounted for?
12. Were the data analyzed correctly?
13. Is your conclusion logically based from the data?
14. Will it apply in local EMS systems?
15. Were the patients similar to those in your local EMS system?

You are the Paramedic Summary

1. How is patient prehospital care initiated for this or any call?

Prehospital care most often comes with a phone call to 9-1-1, or if the 9-1-1 system does not exist in your service area, with a call to the police or fire department. Educational programs provided by local fire and EMS agencies are vital in guiding the public in how to recognize an emergency, how to access emergency services, and how to provide basic first aid, including cardiopulmonary resuscitation (CPR) and automated external defibrillator (AED) use. If your community has not yet asked for outreach programs, you should initiate them.

2. What role do dispatchers play in prehospital care?

Without dispatchers, appropriate medical, fire, and police resources would not be allocated properly. Dispatchers are highly skilled individuals who are able to calm callers, gather pertinent information regarding the location and nature of the incident, and in some cases provide instruction in basic first aid over the phone. All of these actions are essential in providing prehospital care to the sick and injured.

3. What prehospital care can PCPs provide for this patient?

PCPs can provide essential lifesaving prehospital care by administering oxygen, splinting, controlling bleeding, providing CPR, and using AEDs. Some PCPs have expanded scopes of practice that allow a broader range of skills, depending on local protocols or regulations.

4. What are the advantages of having a paramedic partner?

Some systems provide two paramedics on ALS units, while others do not. Having a paramedic partner is especially helpful when you first begin your career. Some days you will notice that finding a vein for an IV line and opening an airway for an endotracheal tube are more difficult, even for the most seasoned paramedic. Having a partner there to help you is especially advantageous, and your partner can also serve as a sounding board for your ideas and concerns. It is important to note that not all systems run an ambulance with two paramedics; instead, your team may include one paramedic and one other-level paramedic, such as a PCP, so you must be prepared to function as the only paramedic.

5. Is there one team member who is more important than another?

No team member is any more important than another. It is very important to treat all team members with respect—they are all essential in providing quality prehospital care. You, as a paramedic, might be the most highly trained person on the scene, but you must remember your professional demeanour, which includes good manners. Providing quality prehospital care is a team effort, and it serves us well to remember that our purpose is to provide the best prehospital care possible. In the end, if we don't get our act together, only one person pays the true price—the patient we are committed to serve.

6. Why is it important to keep skills and knowledge current?

One of the challenging aspects of being a paramedic is that it is an ever-changing field. Medical research projects track positive and negative impacts of prehospital care. As technology changes and as more information is assessed about using medications and applying patient care techniques, your treatment in the prehospital environment will continue to change and improve.

7. Why is it important to practice these skills as a team?

Because teamwork is an essential element of emergency medicine, it is extremely important to practice working as a team. As each member knows what is expected to meet patient needs, the more effective and efficient prehospital care becomes. An efficient team working together will boost the image of the service in the opinion of the patient, the patient's family members, and the public.

Prep Kit

Ready for Review

- World Wars I and II saw the development of ambulance corps to rapidly care for and remove those injured from the battlefields.
- During the Korean and Vietnam Wars, wounded soldiers could be saved by using helicopters to rapidly remove them from the battlefields to a medical unit.
- In 2001, the Paramedic Association of Canada released the National Occupational Competency Profiles (NOCPs).
- In 2002, the EMS Chiefs of Canada (EMSCC) was incorporated as a national voice and lobby for EMS in Canada.
- In 2007, the EMSCC released its white paper "The Future of EMS in Canada: Defining the New Road Ahead" as a national strategy to direct the growth of EMS in Canada.
- The public needs to be taught how to recognize that an emergency exists, how to activate the EMS system, and how to perform basic prehospital care until EMS arrives.
- The highest level of EMS training is the critical care paramedic.
- Continuing education programs expose paramedics to new research findings and refresh their skills and knowledge.
- Paramedics are required to be licensed and/or certified.
- The paramedic profession contains expected standards and performance parameters as well as a code of ethics.
- Some of the paramedic responsibilities include:
  - Preparation
  - Response
  - Scene management
  - Patient assessment and prehospital care
  - Management and disposition
  - Patient transfer
  - Documentation
  - Return to service
- The medical director provides direct and indirect medical control.
- Research helps bring together the findings of many professionals involved in EMS and brings forth a consensus of what paramedics should or should not do.
- Quality assurance and continuous quality improvement are tools paramedics use to evaluate the care they provide to patients.

Vital Vocabulary

alternative time sampling Time parameters that are set during a research project.

blinding The method of not giving the specifics of a project to the individuals participating in a research or study.

certified A title given when a person has shown that he or she has met requirements based on knowledge of certain facts.

convenience sampling A type of research in which subjects are manually assigned to a specific person or crew, rather than being randomly assigned; the least-preferred component of research.

cross-sectional research A type of research in which information is gathered from a group of individuals over a specific time frame.

descriptive research A type of research in which an observation of an event is made, but without attempts to alter or change it.

direct medical control Medical direction given in real time to an EMS service or paramedic.

emergency medical services (EMS) A health care system designed to bring immediate on-scene prehospital care to those in need along with transport to a definitive medical care facility.

ethical A behaviour expected by an individual or group following a set of rules.

experimental research Describes a new product, skill, or idea that is undergoing research and will be trialed, with the effects evaluated.

health care professional A person who follows specific professional attributes that are outlined in this profession.

indirect medical control Medical direction given through a set of protocols, policies, and/or standards.

inferential A research format that uses a hypothesis to prove one finding from another.

licensed Similar to certified, a person who has shown a degree of competency in a specific occupation and is granted ability to function through a governmental body.

mean The average number in a given research project.

median The midpoint number in a given research project.

medical direction Direction given to an EMS service or paramedic by a physician.

mobile intensive care units (MICUs) An early title given to an ambulance-style unit.

mode The most common number in any given research project.

parameters Outlined measures that may be difficult to obtain in a research project.

profession A specialized set of knowledge, skills, and/or expertise.

professional A person who follows expected standards and performance parameters in a specific profession.

prospective research Specific reason a task or research will be performed before it is started.

protocol A treatment plan developed for a specific illness or injury.

qualitative A type of descriptive statistic in research that does not use numerical information.

quantitative A type of measurement in research that uses a mean, median, and mode.

randomly A way of choosing subjects for a research project without specific reasons.

reciprocity The process of granting licensing or certification to a paramedic from another province or agency.

registration Giving information that will be stored in some form of record book.

research ethics board (REB) A group or institution that follows a set of requirements for ethical review of a research protocol or project, initially devised by Medical Research Council of Canada.

retrospective research Research performed from current available information.

sampling errors Expected errors that occur in the sampling phase of research.

standard deviation In research this outlines how much change from the mean is expected.

standing order A type of protocol that is a written document signed by the EMS system's medical director that outlines specific directions, permissions, and sometimes prohibitions regarding prehospital care that is rendered prior to contacting direct medical control.

systematic sampling A computer-generated list of subjects or groups for research.

unblinded study A type of study in which the subjects are advised of all aspects of the study.

Assessment in Action

You are approximately three fourths of the way through your advanced care paramedic training course. You are not yet certified as an ACP, but you do ride with a local rescue squad as a PCP and "advanced care paramedic resident."

You come upon a motor vehicle collision near your home. No rescue personnel or police are on scene yet. You have your own personal "jump bag" with rescue supplies in your car, including advanced life support supplies you would use as a paramedic. There are two patients, both with significant injuries. They were both unrestrained in the vehicle. One patient is having noticeable trouble breathing.

1. **Even though you are not "on duty," what should you do first in this situation, assuming a bystander has already called for help?**
   A. Call 9-1-1.
   B. Put on gloves and any other personal protective equipment you may need.
   C. Call direct medical control and get permission to treat the patient.
   D. Assess the ABCs.

2. **Which of the following are you *allowed* to do based on the training you already have?**
   A. Provide C-spine stabilization, pressure to stop bleeding, and talk to victims to calm them and let them know what to expect.
   B. Put a c-collar in place, bandage bleeding wounds, and use a Combitube if necessary to help the patient who is having trouble breathing.
   C. Help stop bleeding, and intubate if necessary.
   D. Call direct medical control and ask for permission to treat patients as necessary, including intubation.

3. **If a physician arrives and offers to help, is it appropriate to turn over care to that physician?**
   A. Yes, a physician is a higher authority than you are.
   B. Yes, but only if the physician is willing to take responsibility for the patients, including riding with them to the hospital and signing paperwork.
   C. No, you are not authorized to turn over care until an ALS unit arrives.
   D. It is the option of the EMS crew that arrives on scene.

4. **When EMS arrives on scene, it is your responsibility to:**
   A. explain quickly and accurately your assessments and any treatment or intervention you have administered.
   B. help prepare the patient(s) for transport in any way you can under the direction of the paramedic on scene.
   C. maintain patient care unless the person on scene has the same authority as you or higher.
   D. all of the above.

5. **Are you legally allowed to perform ANY paramedic treatments in this situation?**
   A. Yes
   B. No

6. **Because you are not on duty, is it appropriate to tell the patient "everything will be fine," or do anything else you would not be allowed to do in uniform while working with your agency?**
   A. Yes, you're not on duty, so those sets of rules do not apply. You are acting as a Good Samaritan.
   B. No, you are a health professional whether on duty or off duty, which means being professional at all times.

Challenging Questions

7. **Being a paramedic is not just a job you work during a shift. You are always a paramedic, being a role model for the public at all times. With the increase in television shows that do not always accurately depict the roles of health care providers, do you feel it is your responsibility to educate the public in every situation possible as to what the EMS field is truly like, correct misconceptions, and give an accurate portrayal of what you are responsible for and capable of as a paramedic?**

8. **You are called to the scene of a two-car collision with serious injuries to the drivers and passengers of both vehicles. You call for additional assistance, but know it will be several minutes until more help arrives. Someone stops, and offers his assistance. He does seem to be knowledgeable in what needs to be done for the victims of the accident. Should you enlist his help in stabilizing your patients? Why or why not?**

▬ Points to Ponder

You and your crew are called to a scene in which a car has hit a power pole. Active power lines are down around the vehicle, and the driver seems to be unconscious.

Is your first priority the injured patient, or the safety of yourself and your crew?

Issues: Scene Safety, Patient Care, Patient Access.

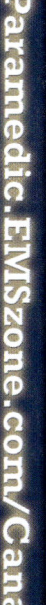

www.Paramedic.EMSzone.com/Canada

The Well-Being of the Paramedic

Competency Areas

Area 1: Professional Responsibilities

1.1.a	Maintain patient dignity.
1.1.b	Reflect professionalism through use of appropriate language.
1.1.c	Dress appropriately and maintain personal hygiene.
1.1.d	Maintain appropriate personal interaction with patients.
1.1.e	Maintain patient confidentiality.
1.1.g	Utilize community support agencies as appropriate.
1.1.j	Behave ethically.
1.1.k	Function as patient advocate.
1.2.b	Self-evaluate and set goals for improvement, as related to professional practice.

Area 2: Communication

2.1.d	Provide information to patient about their situation and how they will be treated.
2.1.e	Interact effectively with the patient, relatives, and bystanders who are in stressful situations.
2.3.a	Exhibit effective non-verbal behaviour.
2.3.b	Practice active listening techniques.
2.3.c	Establish trust and rapport with patients and colleagues.
2.3.d	Recognize and react appropriately to non-verbal behaviours.
2.4.a	Treat others with respect.
2.4.b	Exhibit empathy and compassion while providing care.
2.4.c	Recognize and react appropriately to individuals and groups manifesting coping mechanisms.
2.4.d	Act in a confident manner.
2.4.e	Act assertively as required.
2.4.f	Manage and provide support to patients, bystanders, and relatives manifesting emotional reactions.
2.4.g	Exhibit diplomacy, tact, and discretion.
2.4.h	Exhibit conflict resolution skills.

Area 3: Health and Safety

3.1.a	Maintain balance in personal lifestyle.
3.1.b	Develop and maintain an appropriate support system.
3.1.c	Manage personal stress.
3.1.d	Practice effective strategies to improve physical and mental health related to shift work.
3.1.e	Exhibit physical strength and fitness consistent with the requirements of professional practice.
3.3.a	Assess scene for safety.
3.3.b	Address potential occupational hazards.
3.3.d	Exhibit defusing and self-protection behaviours appropriate for use with patients and bystanders.
3.3.e	Conduct procedures and operations consistent with Workplace Hazardous Materials Information System (WHMIS) and hazardous materials management requirements.
3.3.f	Practice infection control techniques.
3.3.g	Clean and disinfect equipment.
3.3.h	Clean and disinfect an emergency vehicle.

Area 6: Integration

6.1.m	Provide care to patient experiencing terminal illness.

Area 7: Transportation

7.2.a	Utilize defensive driving techniques.
7.2.b	Utilize safe emergency driving techniques.
7.2.c	Drive in a manner that ensures patient comfort and a safe environment for all passengers.

Appendix 4: Pathophysiology

K. **Psychiatric Disorders**
Anxiety Disorders: Acute stress disorder
Anxiety Disorders: Generalized anxiety disorder
Anxiety Disorders: Panic disorder
Anxiety Disorders: Post-traumatic stress disorder
Anxiety Disorders: Situational disturbances

Introduction

Jake Owens is a veteran paramedic who has been in EMS for more than 25 years. Jake has arthritis in his knees and hips, and his back is chronically stiff and sore. He avoids most kinds of exercise because everything he has tried hurts.

When Jake ran his first EMS call, few people thought about paramedic wellness. The slogan of the times was "the patient always comes first." Every third day, Jake was assigned to 24-hour shifts that were so busy, few staffers bothered to cook. Jake and most of his colleagues resorted to fast food while they were on duty, often putting off eating until their last late-night call when they were ravenous. They ate large portions and gulped down large soft drinks and great volumes of coffee to get them through their nights.

Ambulance stretchers typically had to be lifted into and out of ambulances, with or without patients. Two paramedics managed that job by themselves, because there were no first responders. The only way a paramedic could load or unload one of those stretchers was by lifting from the side. To avoid straining his or her back, a paramedic would try to stand very close to the stretcher, spreading his or her thighs widely and lifting with the hands between the knees, about 46 cm apart. The whole procedure put a lot of stress on the lifter's knees and hips.

Between calls, most crews sat and waited—or slept, bracing themselves for repeated wake-up calls. Many smoked more than a pack of cigarettes a day. Paramedics were generally young (usually in their early 20s) with no plans to stay in medical caregiving. Like most people their age, they gave little thought to the long-term consequences of their on-duty lifestyle. But many of them developed life-altering injuries.

Even an expert in human occupational health care could not have devised a more torturous test of human mind or body. Thirty years ago no research project tracked the injuries or the impact of sleep loss and bad eating and exercise habits on ambulance crews. The research about the impact of stress on all health care providers has blossomed in 30 years, culminating in a better understanding of (and hopefully the prevention of) the damage to the physical and mental health of the dedicated professionals on either side of the emergency department door.

Paramedics need to know how to ensure their own well-being and to share what they have learned with other professionals and the public.

Components of Well-Being

Wellness is a baseline state of adjustment to the rigors of life that makes us happy and pain-free most of the time, often brings us joy, and generally produces interactions with others that are

You are the Paramedic Part 1

You are the "newbie" of your crew. Your supervisor has paired you with a veteran paramedic, who is knowledgeable but somewhat cranky. You and your partner have had a long day. Just as you sit down to eat dinner, you are dispatched to a nonemergency transport from a local nursing care facility. As you get up from the table, your partner lets out a big sigh and mumbles something under his breath.

When you arrive, you are greeted by one of the care centre's registered nurses. She tells you this patient is being transported for evaluation by his physician and, as she begins to tell you about the patient's recent history of illness, your partner says, "That's OK. We've got it. Do you have the guy's chart?" She quickly hands you the patient's medical file, and you enter the room to find a morbidly obese 55-year-old man. You estimate his weight to be about 181 kg. You take an initial set of vital signs.

As your partner is readying the stretcher, you ask him if it would be a good idea to call for additional help. He tells you, "No, let's just get this over with."

Initial Assessment	Recording Time: 0 Minutes
Appearance	Eyes open, no apparent distress
Level of consciousness	A (Alert to person, place, and day)
Airway	Open
Breathing	Adequate rate and tidal volume
Circulation	Radial pulse present
Vital Signs	
Skin	Warm, pink, and dry
Pulse	90 beats/min, regular and strong
Blood pressure	160/94 mm Hg
Respirations	22 breaths/min
SpO_2	94% on 2 l/min nasal cannula

1. What is your main concern at the moment?
2. What concerns do you have, if any, regarding your partner's behaviour?
3. Does your partner's attitude have any effect on patient care?

mutually supportive and fulfilling **Figure 2-1** ▾. Wellness has at least three dimensions: the physical, the mental, and the emotional. Many people believe that a fourth dimension, the spiritual, is also essential.

Physical Well-Being

Health care providers have known for years that they are less likely to get hurt if they show up in shape for the work. Your muscle strength, the flexibility of your joints, your cardiac endurance, your emotional equilibrium, your posture (both sitting and standing), your state of hydration, the quality of the foods you eat, and even the amount of sleep you get affect your quality of life. And each of these factors directly impacts the likelihood that you will get through a shift without injury and be able to deal with the mental stress inherent in the job. Let's take a closer look at these factors.

Nutrition

Supervisors and schedule planners understand a lot more about scheduling for good nutrition and hydration today than they did 30 years ago. Even food and drink containers have improved (along with the interiors of vehicles, which now provide space for them). Researchers learned a lot about the consequences of poor nutrition—cardiac illness, type 2 diabetes, obesity, and possibly even Alzheimer's disease. But many paramedics still work 24-hour shifts,

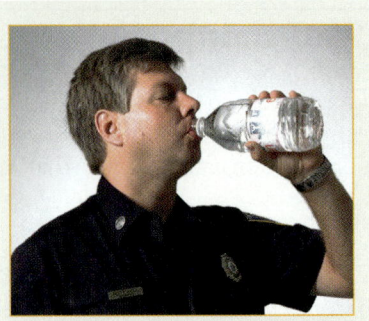

Figure 2-1 Because of the special demands of their job, paramedics must be continually focused on staying both physically and emotionally healthy.

sometimes without scheduled meal breaks. The EMS system is clearly challenged.

Canada's Food Guide is designed to help Canadians make healthy food choices by integrating the science of nutrition and health into a practical pattern of eating. Consuming the amount and type of food recommended and following the tips included in *Canada's Food Guide* will help you to:

- Meet your needs for vitamins, minerals, and other nutrients
- Reduce your risk of obesity, type 2 diabetes, heart disease, certain types of cancer, and osteoporosis
- Contribute to your overall health and vitality

The food guide servings chart shows how much food you need from each of the four food groups every day **Figure 2-2** ▾. It is important for an individual to balance his or her calorie intake with his or her energy needs. A sedentary individual will not need the same quantities of food as the person who is physically active. For instance, a man between the ages of 19 and 30 years with a sedentary lifestyle should consume 2,500 calories a day. If he is active, the intake rises to 3,000 calories a day. *Canada's Food Guide* recommends the following minimum servings from each of the following food groups for a 35-year-old man:

- 8 to 10 vegetables and fruit
- Eight grain products
- Two milk and alternatives
- Three meat and alternatives
- 30 to 45 ml of unsaturated oils and fats

So, what is the best way for a paramedic to sustain energy? Perhaps the best answer to nutrition is to plan your meals before you report for duty. You can keep yourself better hydrated by carrying bottled water instead of buying soft drinks, and minimizing your intake of caffeine. You can stay better nourished and more alert by carrying numerous small snacks (like raisins, nuts, and fruits) you can eat slowly. Taking these steps will also save you lots of money. This is better than speed-eating big, expensive, high-fat meals.

Weight Control

The prehospital environment requires active people who can quickly and accurately observe, assess, access, cope with, and control chaotic situations. Staying fit is a necessity in public service. Patterns of living you develop in your youth are hard to modify in later life—and impose lasting effects on your overall health.

Being active every day is a step toward better

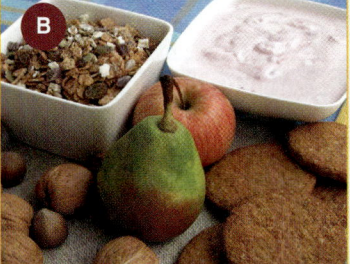

Figure 2-2 *Canada's Food Guide* **(A)** emphasizes a healthy balance of vegetables and fruit, grain products, milk and alternatives, and meat and alternatives, and **(B)** health bars, smoothies, and energy drinks provide a quick, healthy alternative to fast foods.

Source: Eating Well with Canada's Food Guide (2007). www.hc-sc.gc.ca/fn-an/food-guide-aliment/index-eng.php, Health Canada. Reproduced with the permission of the Minister of Public Works and Government Services Canada, 2009.

health and a healthy body weight. *Canada's Physical Activity Guide* recommends building 30 to 60 minutes of moderate physical activity into daily life. You do not have to do it all at once. Add your exercise up in periods of at least 10 minutes at a time. Start slowly and build up.

However, gradual weight reduction, like an exercise program, requires you to plan your meals and your breaks. Rather than taking coffee breaks, some paramedics take breaks by walking or doing other forms of aerobic activity. These paramedics often split a meal between two people when they eat in a restaurant, and they are hearty eaters of salad, vegetables, and fresh-caught broiled fish. You too can do this, with some planning. If you have to eat out, you could order oatmeal or cold cereal for breakfast, a salad (with dressing on the side) and soup for lunch, and roast turkey for dinner.

Exercise

Regular vigorous exercise is closely linked to your body weight, nutritional status, and hydration, and has been shown to improve your sleep, sex life, mental capacity, ability to cope with stress, and overall long-term health. The best exercise program for you depends on your personal preferences. It should be something you enjoy and should be targeted at maintaining, or improving, three areas: your cardiovascular endurance, your flexibility, and your physical strength. More specifically, it should involve enough moderate to vigorous daily physical activity to keep you from gaining weight.

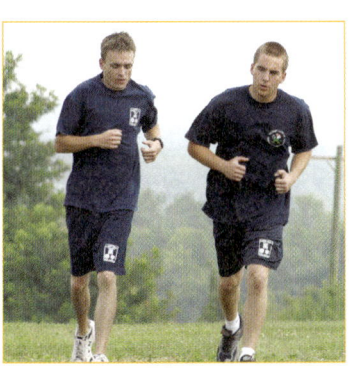

Figure 2-3 Regular exercise—apart from the work you do on calls—should be part of your daily or weekly routine.

It is recommended that adults engage in at least 30 minutes of moderate to vigorous physical activity most days of the week to help build optimal cardiovascular endurance. Working in a busy unit, you probably feel that you get that workout on every call. Back at the station, it is very tempting to prop your feet up and vegetate until the next call. But to stay in good physical condition, you need to find a healthy balance between full-out physical activity (when you are "running hot") and no activity at all **Figure 2-3 ▲**. Most employers realize this and provide their employees with workout equipment to use on each shift.

You should know your target heart rate and attempt to reach this goal every time you exercise. To find your target heart rate, calculate the following:

1. Measure your resting heart rate.
2. Subtract your age from 220. This total is your estimated maximum heart rate.

3. Subtract your resting heart rate from your maximum heart rate. Multiply that figure by 0.7.
4. Add this figure to your resting heart rate.

For example, a 40-year-old man has a resting heart rate of 70 beats/min. Calculations would be as follows:

1. **Resting heart rate.**
   70 beats/min
2. **Maximum heart rate.**
   $220 - 40 = 180$ beats/min
3. **Maximum heart rate minus resting heart rate multiplied by 0.7.**
   $180 - 70 = 110 \times 0.7 = 77$
4. **Target heart rate.**
   $77 + 70 = 147$ beats/min

 At the Scene

Being a paramedic in the prehospital environment is physically and mentally demanding. Following simple guidelines for nutrition, exercise, and mental health will greatly enhance and prolong your career. Recruiting others you work with to join a health maintenance plan that includes these elements will foster teamwork as well as help maintain a balance between your career and your health.

Smoking

If you don't already, *please* don't start! If you do, *please* stop! Not only does this habit fly in the face of everything EMS is about, it also produces many of the most terrible cardiovascular and pulmonary disasters that caregivers in our field confront during the span of our careers. In addition, it sets an awful example for the public—especially to people who have breathing disorders such as asthma. And it makes us look and smell (*Yes, smell!*) like anything but professional caregivers.

Are you a smoker who is trying to quit? Several strategies can help you. First, try to cultivate a relationship with a mentor who was once truly addicted to smoking but who has successfully quit. Use that person as a support,

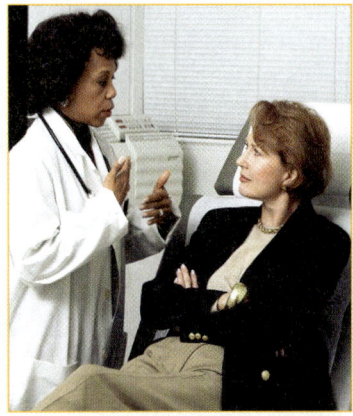

Figure 2-4 Both traditional and alternative health care providers offer a variety of ways to help smokers deal with nicotine addiction.

and draw on his or her advice and encouragement. There are also programs that attack a smoker's psychological dependency. These programs may include instructions and audiotapes, and provide ongoing support. Other options include psychotherapy, hypnotism, and acupuncture.

Talk to your primary care physician. Your doctor should be familiar with more techniques Figure 2-4 ◂ . All of these solutions are cheaper than cigarettes and their attendant health risks.

Circadian Rhythms and Shift Work

EMS imposes schedules on paramedics that conflict with the body's circadian rhythms, or natural timing system. These rhythms are controlled by special areas of the brain, called the suprachiasmatic nuclei, which govern our "internal clocks." Ignoring our circadian rhythms can cause some of us to experience consistent difficulty with sleep, higher thought functions, physical coordination, and even with social functions. You can have trouble focusing during some times of the day or night (so that you simply cannot function as a paramedic) if you don't know what your natural rhythms are, try hard to understand them, and determine a schedule that is best for you. Research on circadian rhythms is only beginning to appear in medical journals, suggesting that some day we might be able to alter our internal clock.

Some tips for dealing with shift work:
- Avoid caffeine.
- Eat healthy meals and try to eat at the same times every day.
- Keep a regular sleep schedule.

The most important point for all paramedics is: don't overlook the need for rest, whatever your rhythms Figure 2-5 ▸ . Many paramedics depend on overtime as part of their normal income. But a paramedic who has been awake and working for 18 to 20 hours straight is only human, and needs rest. You cannot continue to operate an emergency vehicle or administer medications without necessary sleep.

Periodic Health Risk Assessments

Besides sleep, diet, exercise, hydration, and all the other things that make up a healthy lifestyle, you need to be aware of your hereditary factors. Consider what you might know about your immediate family's and your ancestors' health. Alzheimer's disease, chemical addiction, cancer, cardiac illness, hypertension, migraine, mental illness, and stroke all feature prominent hereditary factors. The most common of all heredity health risk factors are heart disease and cancer.

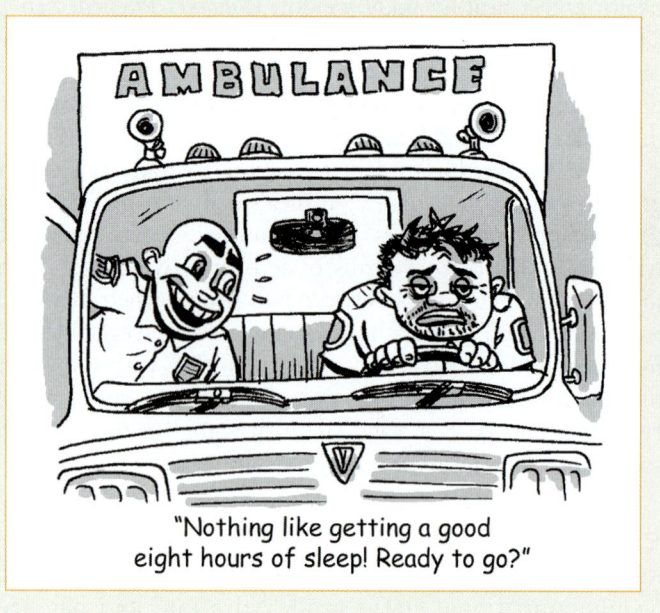

"Nothing like getting a good eight hours of sleep! Ready to go?"

Figure 2-5

Share this information with your personal physician. Your physician is bound by the same oath of confidentiality that you are. Work with him or her to set up a schedule for health assessments, building them into your routine physical checkups. Your physician should be your ally in screening for these diseases and in assessing your lifestyle as well as your heredity.

Body Mechanics

A professional weight lifter typically performs a 30-minute warm-up routine before he or she lifts his or her personal maximum weight. Obviously, that's not an option in any emergency service. But there are a number of habits you can develop that are sure to reduce your exposure to damage from lifting your maximum weight. They include the following:
- *Minimize the number of total body-lifts you have to perform.* When patients need to be lifted, they need to be lifted. But remember that you risk an injury every time you do it. A patient with an arm laceration can stand for a moment while someone rolls the stretcher behind him or her and then helps the patient sit down. Another thing: you can cut your total number of lifts from ground level by

You are the Paramedic Part 2

As you pull the patient across to the stretcher, you feel a slight twinge in your lower back. You hope it's nothing, and prepare to lift your end of the stretcher. As you lift, although you are using proper lifting techniques, you feel a sharp pain in the area of your lumbar spine. You are fairly certain you've just hurt yourself. You tell your partner, who replies, "OK. Well, let's just get this guy to his appointment, and then we'll call the shift captain." Reservedly, you agree, but you must still load the patient in the ambulance.

4. Is this the best course of action?
5. What is the best way to handle this situation?
6. What factors could affect your decisions?

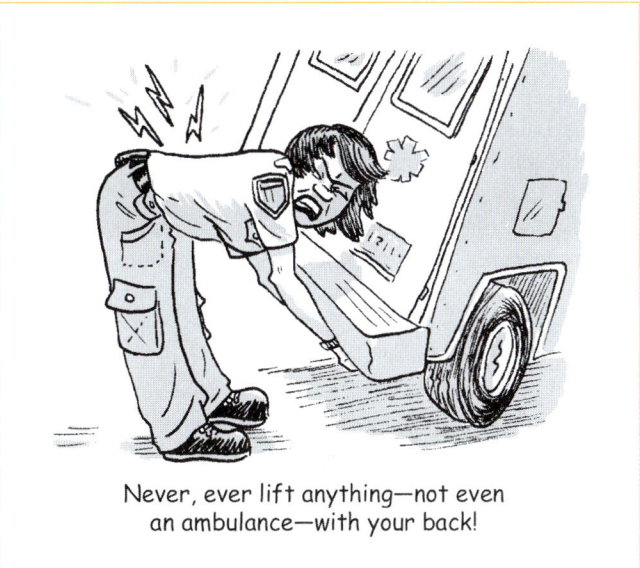

Never, ever lift anything—not even
an ambulance—with your back!

Figure 2-6

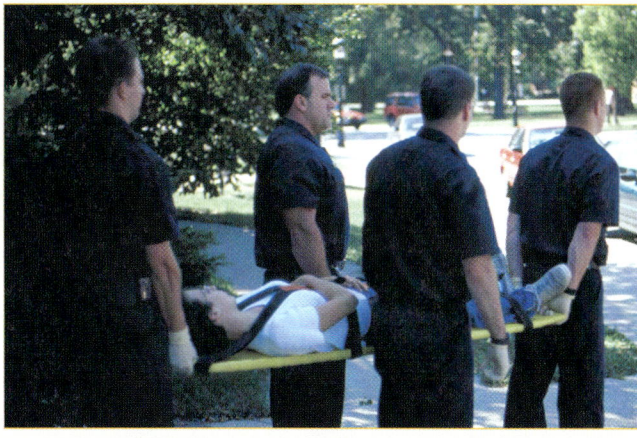

Figure 2-7 Never hesitate to ask for help from your colleagues,
or to provide it when you are asked.

having the stretcher ready in a hands-height position—
never fully lowered. That way, you bend down only
once—to lift the patient on a backboard or accessory
stretcher (scoop/basket). Then, stand where you are and
ask a bystander to roll the cot underneath the backboard
or accessory stretcher. (Don't forget, anytime you walk,
you are balancing on only one foot at a time.)

- *Coordinate every lift in advance.* Make sure that every
member of the team knows what you expect him or her to
do. Just as important, make sure the patient knows it as
well. The last thing you want is for him or her to panic in
midlift and grab someone around the neck, throwing
everyone off balance.
- *Minimize the total amount of weight you have to lift.* If you
have access to a second person who can help lift and load
at the foot end of the stretcher, why not ask for his or her
help? Additionally, consider taking unnecessary equipment
off the stretcher prior to loading or unloading it.
- *Never lift with your back,* not ever. Anyone who has spent a
few years in EMS has made this mistake at least a few
times, citing the pressure of the moment. That pressure
can be a career-ender, unless you're lucky. You cannot trust
luck. The human back is a great weight bearer, but it's a
terrible lifter. To protect your back, follow these
precautions Figure 2-6 ▲ :
  - Always keep your back in a straight, upright position
  and lift without twisting.
  - When lifting, spread your legs about shoulder-width
  apart and place your feet so that your centre of gravity
  is properly balanced.
  - Hold your back upright as you bring your upper body
  down by bending your legs.
  - Lift by raising your upper body and arms and by
  straightening your legs until you are standing.
  - Always lift with your legs, not with your back!
- *Don't carry what you can put on wheels.* Get the ambulance,
and the stretcher, as close to the patient as you can. Use a
stair chair if you have to.
- *Ask for help any time,* without embarrassment or
hesitation—and offer it liberally to others. Anytime you
need to move a patient who cannot or should not walk,
consider the possibility of asking an extra person to help
you Figure 2-7 ▲ . That's not laziness. It's good sense,
and it almost always enhances your body mechanics.

Mental Well-Being

EMS can be a challenging and demanding profession because
paramedics are no less vulnerable to diseases and injuries than
their patients. Paramedics, like the loved ones of their patients,
can be frazzled by the stress of addressing the immediate and
inflexible needs of others.

Mild stress can be a good thing, because it can enhance
your mental acuity. But overwhelming stress can push us
into fight-or-flight syndrome, a physiologic response to a
profound stressor, featuring increased sympathetic tone and
resulting in dilation of the pupils, increased heart rate, dilation of the bronchi, mobilization of glucose, shunting of
blood away from the gastrointestinal tract, and increasing
blood flow to the cerebrum and skeletal muscles. It helps
you deal with the situation right now, but can lead to crushing physical and mental strain if you do not learn appropriate coping skills.

Let's say you need to get away from a marauding grizzly
bear. Your body quickly modifies its performance to enable
you to run from the bear. It borrows blood from your gastrointestinal tract and cerebrum, and shunts the blood to
your skeletal muscles, your adrenal glands, your lungs, and

your reptilian brain (your cerebellum and medulla). Your pupils dilate, enhancing your night vision. You become a running machine—at least for a short time. But you do that at the expense of your higher mental faculties. Your speech becomes clumsy. With those big pupils, you forfeit your depth perception and visual acuity. Your skeletal muscles perform well but, for the time being, you don't feel most kinds of pain such as muscle strain. You lose your fine motor control, so you might have trouble performing motions that require manual dexterity, for example loading a gun or threading a bow and arrow as defence against the bear! You might experience a case of the jitters. And all of that would occur in less than 20 seconds. Your body is preparing you for trouble. You need coping strategies for behaviour that would be most effective in dealing with the situation.

A paramedic needs to be a great observer and a sharp thinker with a two-fisted grip on his or her emotions. Is there a way to control your reactions? It can be difficult, because some events are simply overwhelming. But there are some immediate and long-term techniques that you can use. Remember, the most important thing you can do in modelling your behaviour is to plan for it. Try any or all of these techniques long before you feel yourself melting down at the scene.

You can look and act the part of a professional; take pride in what you do. Caring for people is an ancient pursuit, perhaps the oldest in history. Remind yourself that the world is full of caregivers who do what they do without support, rewards, or recognition from anyone—much less payment. Accept that you are a caregiver with a trust from the public you serve. Because the public elects the officials who certify you, you are responsible to that public in the same way as any other health care professional.

And remember, EMS is a lot bigger than your job, but your life is much bigger than EMS. Keep your lifelong perspective as broad as possible by cultivating relationships with people who are not part of EMS.

Emotional Well-Being

Any professional caregiver needs to have a natural interest in and liking for people. The key to remaining happy in the lifelong practice of critical care medicine is making a deliberate effort to create a healthy balance between life at work and life away. Although many practitioners become very involved in EMS and very dedicated to it, EMS should never be a paramedic's whole life.

EMS does satisfy some of its practitioners' deeply felt needs—especially the need for self-esteem. But, as a popular saying goes, "Don't love something that can't love you back." In fact, many paramedics will say that the more energy you pour into EMS, the more energy it will require to deal with the stress of its importance to you. Why? Because, as another popular saying goes, "Nobody gets out of here alive." Patients can die, regardless of how good their paramedics, nurses, or trauma surgeons are. And you need to recognize that patient death is not your fault, unless you allow your skills, education, or professionalism to decay.

One practical way caregivers manage their balance is by allowing the misfortunes of patients and their families to remind them, year after year, how fortunate they are. Another technique is to faithfully keep a scrapbook. Every thank-you note from a patient or family member goes into that scrapbook and later serves as a reminder that most people appreciate what their prehospital providers do for them.

Develop and nourish your realization that the same situational awareness that you develop in yourself shift after shift as a paramedic can help you to see and appreciate many kinds of beauty in the world around you.

Good health care providers are sensitive people **Figure 2-8 ▸**. They have to be. But part of the price of that trait is that they tend to get their feelings hurt, maybe a little more easily than the average person. They can also be needy, fussy, emotional, and demanding of their leaders. Those are all traits to watch for in colleagues who need to be reminded from

You are the Paramedic Part 3

Because you are on probation, you are afraid to contradict your partner. You assist him in loading the patient into the ambulance, and you are now in great pain. It is all you can do to focus on caring for your patient. He is stable and in a position of comfort. You wish the same statement held true for you. After reading his medical chart, you notify the receiving facility of the incoming patient, pertinent information, and estimated time of your arrival.

Vital Signs	Recording Time: 15 Minutes
Skin	Warm, pink, and dry
Pulse	90 beats/min, regular and strong
Blood pressure	162/94 mm Hg
Respirations	22 breaths/min
SpO_2	95% on 2 l/min nasal cannula

7. What decisions could you have made to prevent this situation?

8. Has prehospital patient care been affected?

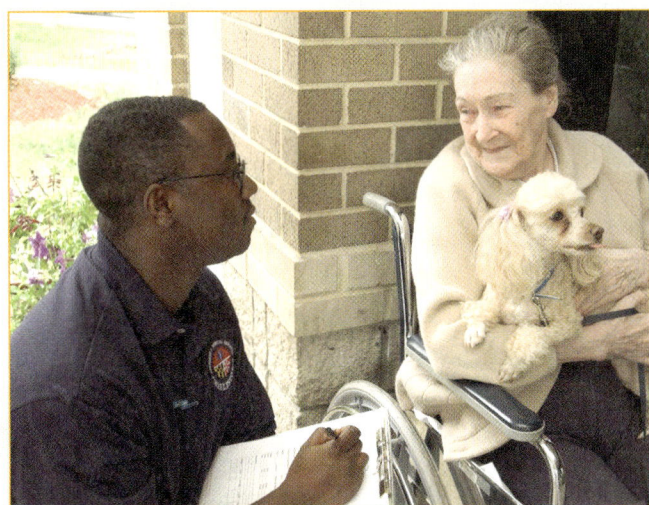

Figure 2-8 One thing that draws people to work as a paramedic is the pleasure of interacting closely with people.

time to time that they're valuable and that what they do matters. You need to remember that too. You should also speak up when you notice that colleagues are not taking care of themselves. You may feel uncomfortable about broaching the subject, but letting them know that you are worried about them can make a difference.

Spiritual Well-Being

Human spirituality is an unseen dimension of human experience. Some people address it with formal religion, but those who do not may still recognize the existence of supernatural power and even of one or more divine entities. Few experienced emergency medical workers deny the possibility of a plane of life beyond our understanding. This possibility may have been reinforced from witnessing the effectiveness of the portable defibrillator, which seems to interrupt the death process, giving paramedics credible and consistent stories from patients.

Medical care supports the dignity and value of life, and the sacredness of individuals. It is essential for you to respect the beliefs of others—those you work with, and patients and their families—to whom those beliefs can be all-important. Your respect for patients' beliefs will also help you in managing effective prehospital patient care. Many paramedics describe a rich sense of their own spirituality that keeps their lives in good perspective.

▮ Stress

All of us have experienced the effects of stress at one time or another. In fact, virtually every human activity involves some degree of stress—sometimes pleasant, sometimes unpleasant, sometimes mild, sometimes intense. And virtually all living creatures are equipped with some sort of inborn stress reaction that enables them to deal effectively with their environment. Hans Selye, MD, PhD, considered the "father of stress theory,"

has defined biological stress as the "nonspecific response of the body to any demand made upon it."

So, stress is a reaction of the body to any agent or situation (stressor) that requires the individual to adapt. Adaptation of one sort or another is necessary all the time, for growth, for development, or just for meeting the demands of everyday life. By itself, then, stress is neither a good thing nor a bad thing, nor should all stress be avoided. After all, self-preservation, one of the most basic requirements of life,

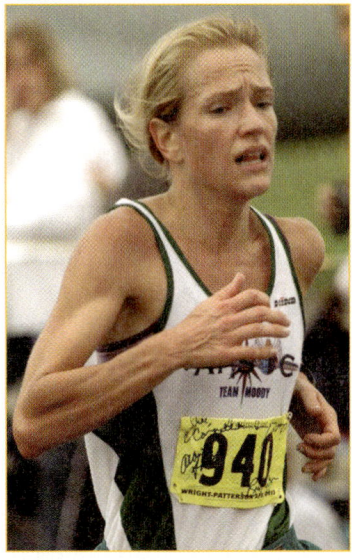

Figure 2-9 Some types of stress, called eustress, are positive and help push us to greater achievements.

would be impossible without a stress-alarm mechanism. Think about that grizzly we talked about earlier. That mechanism also serves you in other ways, for example, motivating you to study for examinations!

It is important to distinguish between injurious and noninjurious stress responses. Selye, for that reason, has classified stress into two categories: eustress (positive stress), the kind of stress that motivates an individual to achieve; and distress (negative or injurious stress), the stress that a person finds overwhelming and debilitating ◖ **Figure 2-9** ▴ ◗. In the rest of this chapter, the kind of stress referred to will be the negative kind of stress.

◖ Documentation and Communication

People from certain cultures and some older patients may believe that showing emotion is a sign of weakness. They may not show the emotions you may readily see in other people in the same situations. Do not assume because they don't indicate stress in the usual ways that they are not distressed. Try to read their body language and hear what they are saying. Also make sure they understand you.

What Triggers Stress

The stress response often begins with events that are perceived as threatening or demanding, but the specific events that trigger the reaction vary enormously from individual to individual. One person may go into a cold sweat even at the *thought* of air travel, while another de-stresses among the clouds piloting an airplane. Learned attitudes strongly affect the situations people find stressful.

The following factors trigger stress in the vast majority of people:

- Loss of a loved one (death of a spouse or family member or going through a divorce) or of a valued possession
- Personal injury or illness
- Major life event (starting or finishing school, marriage, pregnancy, or having children leave home)
- Job-related stress (conflicts with others, excessive responsibility, the possibility of losing your job, or changing a job)

To deal effectively with stress, each of us needs to make a personal appraisal of the stress triggers in his or her life and take action to minimize their effects.

The Physiology of Acute Stress

One of the fundamental models for stress evolved from studies of how humans and other animals responded to threats. It was observed that when a person or a laboratory animal was confronted with a situation that he or she perceived as threatening, a standard series of physiologic reactions was triggered, whatever the threat (this is why Selye referred to stress as a nonspecific response).

Typically, these physiologic reactions prepare the animal for fight-or-flight syndrome by activating the sympathetic nervous system. We will discuss the sympathetic nervous system in Chapter 22. The sympathetic nervous system is the part of the autonomic, or involuntary, nervous system that prepares the body to deal with an emergency.

Generally, the first stage of the stress response is an alarm reaction, which occurs within a fraction of a second after being confronted with a strong stimulus—for instance, a sudden loud noise. The alarm reaction begins with a quick alert response, in which you immediately stop whatever you are doing and focus on the source of the stimulus Figure 2-10 ▾ .

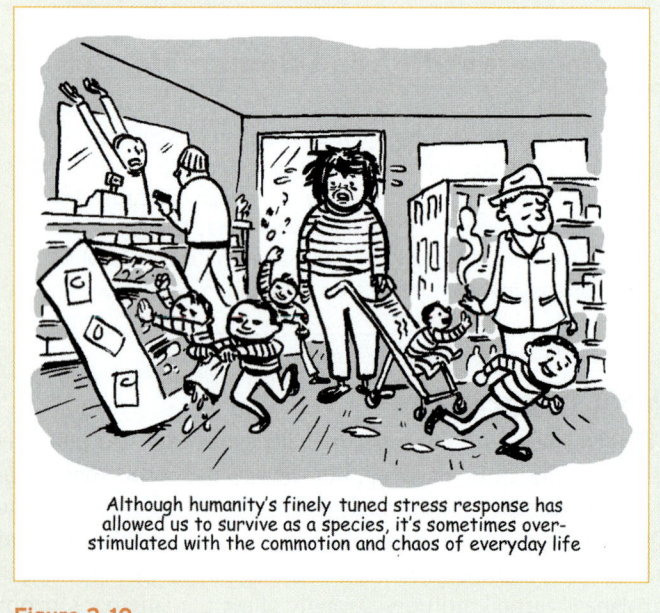

Although humanity's finely tuned stress response has allowed us to survive as a species, it's sometimes overstimulated with the commotion and chaos of everyday life

Figure 2-10

Anyone who has ever startled a grazing deer remembers how the deer exhibited an alert response: it stopped grazing, looked toward the sound that had startled it, and stood absolutely still. Along with the alert response, there is sudden stimulation of the sympathetic nervous system, producing constricted blood vessels, increased heart rate, dilated pupils, erect hair follicles, increased perspiration, and a variety of other physiologic effects. Indeed, we often describe our reactions to a stressful experience in terms of the sympathetic nervous system: "My heart was pounding in my chest." "I broke out in a cold sweat." These are all part of the body's fight-or-flight response to a perceived threat.

For most animals, the fight-or-flight response is a very useful and adaptive mechanism, mobilizing them either to defend themselves (fight) or to run away (flight) in the face of possible danger. Taking either of these steps dissipates the stress, and the animal then goes through a stage of relaxation ("I breathed a sigh of relief when it was over.") and finally returns to its original internal balance. In the modern world, however, the automatic fight-or-flight response to stressful circumstances is probably not as useful as it was in an earlier stage of evolution. Most of the stressors that humans face today are not best solved by fighting or running away.

When a loved one dies or when you lose a job, there is no fight-or-flight outlet for the stress. Under such circumstances, stress becomes chronic, placing our bodies in a continuous, unrelieved state of alert, possibly leading eventually to exhaustion and ill health.

It's important to point out that the stress response is normal. Many people misunderstand the normal physiologic reactions to stressors and interpret the body's preparations for fight or flight as signs of disease, which only serves to increase the level of anxiety. It's essential for paramedics to learn to recognize the symptoms of the stress response, because chronic stress can exact a high toll when it goes unrecognized and unrelieved.

Coping With Your Own Stress

Some early warning signs of your own stress include heart palpitations, rapid breathing, chest tightness, and sweating. Learn to feel yourself entering your fight-or-flight mode. You may notice rapid breathing and breathlessness, unnecessary shouting, and use of curse words that you would not normally use. You may also feel yourself perspiring despite the weather. It is important to the prehospital care of your patients that you try keeping calm to help control the fight-or-flight mechanism in emergencies. Take appropriate action. Initial management techniques include the following steps:

1. **Controlled breathing.** On emergency calls, controlled breathing or taking deep breaths in through the nose and out through the mouth may be the least obvious way to control your anxiety.
2. **Reframing.** Reframing is using your head to look at the situation from a different viewpoint. Instead of thinking "I can't do this," reframe your thoughts to "I trust my training, I can do this."

3. **Progressive relaxation.** After the call, you may find yourself still stressed. Progressive relaxation is a strategy in which you tighten and then relax specific muscle groups to initiate muscle relaxation throughout the body.

Other coping strategies include focusing on the immediate situation while on duty. Off duty, remind yourself (even aloud, although not within the hearing of a patient or his or her loved ones), "I will do my very best, but what I can do to help may not be enough" **Figure 2-11 ▼** .

Coffee is not your friend in avoiding stress reactions. Avoid excessive amounts of stimulants such as caffeine. Faithfully get enough rest, and avoid alcohol during the 24 hours before a duty day. Exercise vigorously and regularly, especially during the 12 hours preceding a shift. Find plenty of things to laugh and joke about, and find compatible partners at work.

A sense of skepticism is valuable to a paramedic, but don't let yourself become cynical and judgmental. Don't spend too long in environments where people don't care about EMS, and avoid prolonged or frequent assignments with cynical people. Study routinely, and keep your certifications and continuing education up-to-date. The social element of continuing education is invaluable in managing stress.

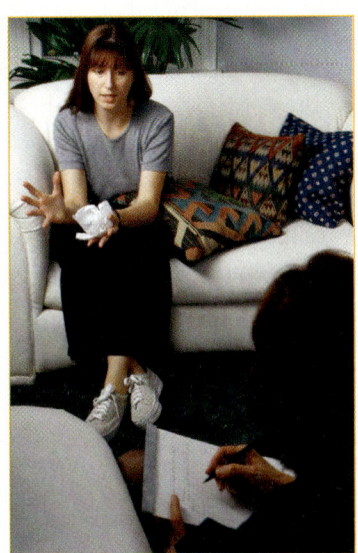

Figure 2-11 Consulting with a professional counselor or therapist can be an important part of dealing with stress and maintaining your emotional well-being.

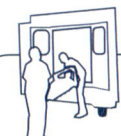

At the Scene

Learn to look for signs of stress in your colleagues and patients. Early discovery can often prevent the situation from worsening.

How People React to Stressful Situations

Anyone—the patient, the family, bystanders, or health care professionals—who confronts critical illness or injury responds in some way to the stresses of each emergency.

Responses of Patients to Illness and Injury

Patients' responses to emergencies are determined by their personal methods of adapting to stress. It will help you as a paramedic to recognize certain common patterns of coping. If the emergency is a medical illness, most people first become aware

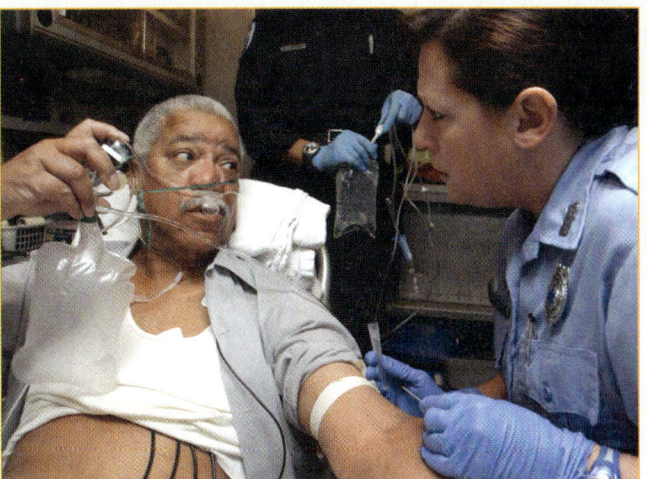

Figure 2-12 The sudden loss of control a patient feels when being treated during an emergency can lead to surprising and sometimes extreme reactions.

of some painful or unpleasant sensations and perhaps a decrease in energy and strength as well. The common response to that awareness is anxiety. Some people exhibit their anxiety by denying it; others become irritable or angry. Once the patient accepts that he or she is ill or injured, any of several common reactions may occur:

- **Fear.** Patients in these situations have realistic fears, such as fear of pain, disability, or death (or fear of their economic effects).

- **Anxiety.** Patients can also experience diffuse anxiety, often stemming from a feeling of helplessness. People who find themselves transformed into patients experience a loss of control. They must place themselves in the hands of a stranger who they must depend on completely and whose competence they cannot really evaluate. People whose self-esteem depends on being active, independent, and aggressive are particularly vulnerable to anxiety when they become ill or injured.

- **Depression.** Depression is a natural response to loss. The patient with a critical illness or injury has lost some bodily function as well as some control. The patient who has had a stroke, for example, may have lost the ability to move an arm or leg on one side of the body and even the ability to speak. It is only natural to feel depressed under such circumstances.

- **Anger.** Anger is one of the most difficult problems for many caregivers to deal with. Suppose a paramedic arrives at the scene of a collision and starts tending immediately to the patient, but the patient becomes hostile and abusive **Figure 2-12 ▲** . The paramedic's natural tendency, under the circumstances, is to think, "Here I am trying to save this guy's life, and he's dumping all over me. Well, he can just go straight to blazes." It is crucial, therefore, to understand that often people respond to discomfort or limitation of function by becoming resentful and suspicious of those around them. A patient who feels angry may vent anger on the rescuer by becoming impatient and irritable or excessively demanding, simply because the rescuer is the most convenient target. A *professional* caregiver realizes in these circumstances that the patient's anger stems from fear and discomfort, and is not really directed at the rescue team.

- **Confusion.** Confusion is especially common among older patients, in whom illness or injury may precipitate disorientation. Such confusion is furthered by the presence of unfamiliar people and equipment, which may seem overwhelming. When a patient appears confused, therefore, it is very important to explain carefully at the outset who you are and what your mission is; thereafter, you should keep up a running commentary on what you are doing to help orient the patient to your role.

In addition to experiencing the reactions just described, most people who have a sudden illness or injury will mobilize one or more psychologic <u>defence mechanisms</u>. Patients and paramedics usually employ these defence mechanisms automatically and subconsciously as a way of relieving personal stress. Here are some examples:

- **Denial.** Many patients tend to ignore or diminish the seriousness of their medical emergencies, because of the anxiety they cause. Denial is often evident in a tendency to dismiss all symptoms with words such as *only* or *a little* (for example, the middle-aged man with chest pain who says, "I'm fine, I'm fine. It's only a little indigestion."). When a patient tries to minimize his or her symptoms in that way, it may be necessary to find a reliable informant among the patient's family or friends so you can obtain more details.

- **Regression.** Regression is a return to an earlier age level of behaviour or emotional adjustment. Regression is often evident in children under stress; for instance, a 10-year-old who sailed through his toilet-training years earlier may suddenly start wetting the bed at night after a stressful experience. Adults too can revert to more childish behaviours under stress. Indeed, when people are injured or become ill, their roles as patients *force* them into a state of dependency, very much like children.

- **Projection.** Projection is attributing your own (sometimes unacceptable) feelings, motives, desires, or behaviour to others. Patients who express vehement indignation or anger at the behaviour of others can unconsciously be denying their own "bad" behaviour by attributing it to other people.

- **Displacement.** Displacement occurs when someone redirects an emotion from the original cause of the emotion (like a cardiac problem) to a more immediate substitute (like a paramedic). Displacement is often the operative mechanism when patients express anger at the paramedic. In reality, patients are angry at someone else—themselves, a family member, fate, God—but they unconsciously redirect their anger toward the stranger who comes to provide medical care. A professional caregiver recognizes that, and accepts it without complaint.

As noted, most of the psychological stress responses are not under your patients' conscious control. Injured patients who respond with anger toward the paramedic often have no perspective on their unpleasant behaviour. The reaction is automatic for the stressed patient.

Just as patients have their own ways of reacting to stress, you have subconscious expectations of how the patient *should* behave when stressed. You might expect a child to cry or to reach out to someone for comfort. But do you allow or tolerate that same reaction in adults?

Often, reactions to illness or injury are rooted in the patient's culture. We live in a multicultural society. Some cultures may openly exhibit their anxieties in what might be termed inappropriate behaviour in another culture. You will not be able to manage prehospital patient care well if you do not respect the culture of your patient.

For example, many patients may react to a situation in what you may think of as quite an emotional way. They may take comfort in having many family members around them for support. This can be quite overwhelming if you come from a cultural background where people are often rather stoic.

Many Canadians place great emphasis on making eye contact, having a firm handshake, and respecting personal space. Some patients may not make eye contact with you because, in their culture, lowered eyes show deference to your authority and uniform. Many people are not comfortable with physical contact (even with their own health care provider) until they have developed a rapport. Obtain permission, if possible, before any hands-on encounters. It is difficult to learn about another culture in an emergency situation, but we need to recognize cultural differences. Learn the cultural differences of the populations you serve, realizing that the reactions you see are only different, not wrong or abnormal **Figure 2-13 ▾** .

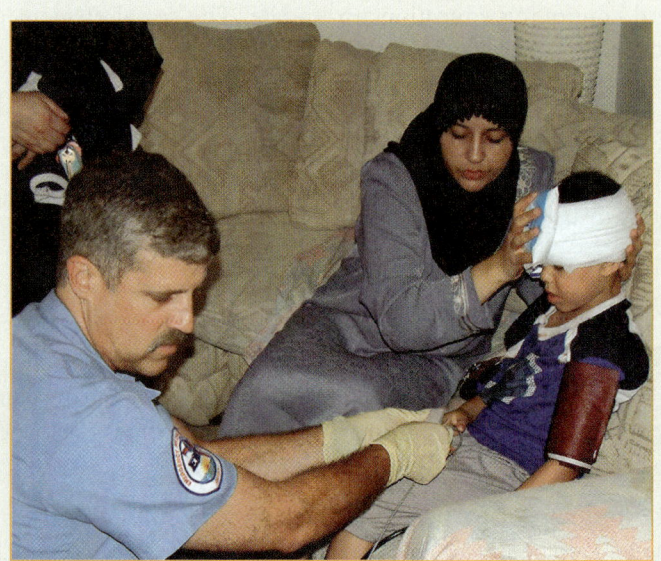

Figure 2-13 Particularly when serving people whose backgrounds are different from your own, you must always maintain an open, nonjudgmental attitude.

Responses of Family, Friends, and Bystanders

Bystanders and family members can exhibit many of the responses that patients exhibit. Family members can be anxious, panicky, or—especially if they are struggling with guilt—angry. Suppose you are called to care for a 4-year-old child who has been struck by a car. The parents of the child are at the scene. Consciously or unconsciously, they feel guilty for what has happened; they may believe, deep down, that if they had kept a closer eye on the child, he or she would not have run out into the street. But, using the mechanisms of projection and displacement, the parents express their guilty feelings as aggression and/or anger toward the rescuers.

They may demand instant action or put pressure on you to move immediately to the hospital. Especially galling may be their implications that you are not competent to handle the situation ("Hurry up and get her to the hospital so that she can be seen by a *doctor!*"). The paramedic needs to recognize that the patient's family and friends have concerns too and that their behaviour, however irritating, arises from distress. Step back emotionally from the situation for a moment. Keep your cool. Calmly explain to the bystanders that there are a few crucial things that the paramedics must get done before attempting move the patient. If necessary, the paramedics have quick radio access to their physician for guidance. Whether dealing with the behaviour of the patient or of those around him or her, the paramedic must constantly remain aware of the distress that lies behind the behaviour. When you are summoned to an emergency, it will never be a festive party. You are entering a situation in which *everyone is under stress,* and you cannot guarantee that people are going to behave appropriately. People who are ordinarily calm and polite in everyday life may not be calm and polite in an emergency. But if *you* can stay calm and polite, no matter what is going on around you, you can improve the behaviour of everyone else at the scene, including your own.

Notes from Nancy

Remember, in emergency situations, everyone is under stress.

Special Considerations

When children are seriously ill or injured, family members and other people at the scene may become frantic. You need to remain calm and confident in your skills, as this may be all that is needed to provide reassurance to everyone at the scene. Remind yourself (and, if you can, the anxious people around you) that scientific studies indicate that paramedic prehospital care and stabilization will improve the patient's chances of a positive outcome.

Responses in Multiple-Casualty Incidents

In a situation involving multiple casualties, such as a train derailment, building collapse, or natural disaster (such as a tornado, flood, or earthquake), both victims and bystanders may react by becoming dazed, disorganized, or overwhelmed. The American Psychiatric Association has identified five categories of reactions in such circumstances. In general, people with these reactions should be removed from the scene.

- **Anxiety.** The normal reactions to such incidents are signs of extreme anxiety, including sweating, trembling, weakness, nausea, and sometimes vomiting. People experiencing this response can recover fully within a few minutes and provide useful assistance if properly directed. Paramedics are not immune to this type of reaction. If you see one of your crew looking a little shaky, the best remedy is to give him or her a specific task ("Get this IV started.").
- **Blind panic.** A more worrisome reaction is blind panic, in which the individual's judgment seems to disappear entirely. Blind panic is particularly dangerous because it is "catchy," and it may precipitate mass panic among others present. For this reason, a panicky bystander needs to be separated quickly from others and, if at all possible, placed under the supervision of a calmer person.
- **Depression.** Depression is seen in the individual who sits or stands in a numbed, dazed state. The depressed bystander needs to be brought back to reality and removed from the scene.
- **Overreaction.** People who overreact tend to talk compulsively, joke inappropriately, become overly active, and race from one task to another without accomplishing anything useful. The person who is overreacting needs to be removed from the area where casualties are being treated.
- **Conversion hysteria.** In conversion hysteria, the patient subconsciously converts anxiety into a bodily dysfunction; he or she may be unable to see or hear or may become paralyzed in an extremity.

We shall go into more detail on how to cope with bystanders in Chapter 48 where we discuss mass-casualty incidents.

Responses of the Paramedic

Health care professionals are not immune to the stresses of emergency situations, and it is to be expected that those dealing with the critically ill and injured will experience a multitude of feelings, not all of them pleasant. The paramedic may feel angry at the demands of the family or the patient, anxious in the face of life-threatening injuries, defensive at inferences he or she is not competent to handle the situation, sad in response to the death of a patient, or any number of these sensations at the same time. These feelings are all perfectly natural, but it is preferable to keep them to yourself during an emergency. An attitude of outward calm and confidence on your part will do much to relieve the anxieties of others at the scene—and that too is part of the paramedic's therapeutic role.

One reaction that is common among health care professionals is a feeling of irritation at the patient who does not appear to be particularly ill. That reaction is especially prevalent among emergency personnel, who are psychologically geared to deal with life-threatening and catastrophic cases and who therefore tend to regard an apparently minor complaint as a burdensome annoyance. Try hard to remember that people define their own emergencies. Also, consider the possibility that people who call 9-1-1 with seemingly minor complaints are not calling for something minor at all—like the woman who called 9-1-1 because she couldn't get to sleep. Her problem was that it was her first night back home after the funeral of her husband. She was scared to death of her first night alone in that bed, thousands of kilometres away from the body of her husband, and she had no one else to call. Anyone who has ever been truly alone knows what an emergency that can be. These victims are not abusing us. They're precisely the ones we're here for.

At the Scene

Do not assume that seemingly nonemergency complaints are not a sign of something wrong. Tunnel vision can cause many mistakes in patient assessments and ultimately in their outcomes.

Burnout

What's this? We've scarcely started the paramedic course, and already we're talking about burnout! Why should we start worrying now about something that may (or may not) happen 10 years down the line?

We need to consider burnout now—at the earliest stage of paramedic training—because now is the time to start developing attitudes and habits that will help prevent burnout, whether 1 year or 20 years down the line.

The dictionary defines <u>burnout</u> as the exhaustion of physical or emotional strength. Burnout is, in fact, a consequence of chronic, unrelieved stress. The paramedic's job, by its very nature, is full of potential stresses. There are the obvious stresses imposed by having to deal, day after day, with mutilating trauma or catastrophic illness. There are, as well, more subtle stresses associated with interpersonal relations, pay, prestige, fringe benefits, and other issues. These complaints and stresses are, no doubt, legitimate. But burnout does not occur solely because of stress. Burnout develops because of the way a person *reacts* to stress.

One person's eustress may be another's distress
Figure 2-14 ▶. The reason is that distress is a *learned* reaction, based on the way an individual perceives and interprets the world around him or her. In other words, distress is nearly always the result of what a person *believes*. Some beliefs are more likely than others to produce stress. Here are some beliefs that are common among paramedics:

- I have to be perfect all the time.
- My safety depends on being able to anticipate every possible danger.
- I am totally responsible for what happens to patients; if they die, it is wholly my fault.
- If there's something I don't know, people will think less of me.
- A good paramedic never makes mistakes.

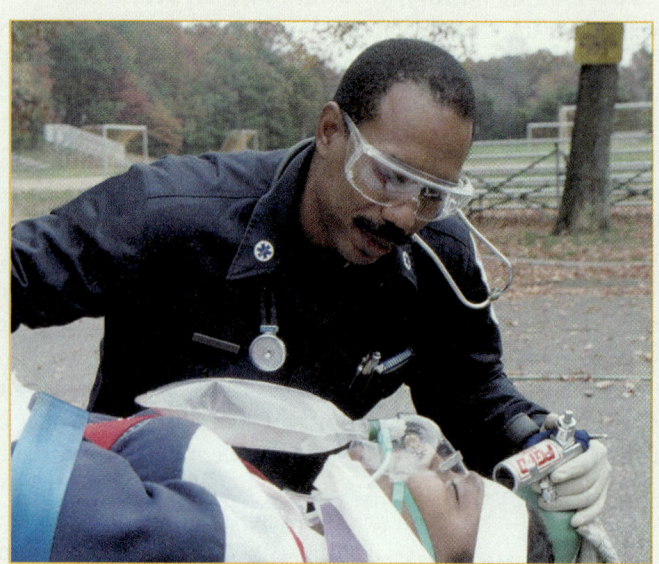

Figure 2-14 Dealing with stress as a paramedic requires the ability to emotionally distance yourself from the situation, and accepting the limits of what you can personally do.

These perfectionist beliefs are very likely to produce stress. They are also false beliefs. Prevention and relief of stress among paramedics begin with the recognition that such beliefs are unrealistic and invalid.

Like many of the conditions we will study in this textbook, burnout is also a sort of illness. And like any other illness, it has signs and symptoms. Learn to look for the symptoms of burnout in yourself and in your colleagues. These symptoms are warning signals, telling you to stop and reexamine your beliefs and your ways of responding to stress. Symptoms of impending burnout include:

- Chronic fatigue and irritability
- Cynical, negative attitudes
- Lack of desire to report to work
- Emotional instability (crying easily, flying off the handle without provocation, laughing inappropriately)
- Changes in sleep patterns (insomnia or sleeping more than usual), and waking without feeling refreshed
- Feelings of being overwhelmed or being helpless or hopeless
- Loss of interest in hobbies
- Decreased ability to concentrate
- Declining health—having lots of colds, stomach upsets, and muscle aches and pains (especially headaches or backaches)
- Constant tightness in your muscles
- Overeating, smoking, or abusing drugs or alcohol

It is preferable, of course, not to wait until symptoms of burnout develop. There are paramedics who have been in the field for 20 years and show no signs whatsoever of burnout, who still report to work every day with the same enthusiasm they did as rookies. What is their secret? In general, the paramedics who do not suffer burnout are those who have learned to respect and value *themselves*. That is not as easy as it sounds. The type of person who chooses to become a paramedic is usually altruistic—someone who puts the needs of others ahead of his or her own needs. In theory, that is very laudable. But in fact, no one can give their best to others for very long if they ignore their own personal needs.

Practically speaking, what does it mean to respect and value yourself? How can you translate that attitude into concrete action? Some of the steps you can take to protect yourself from burnout are summarized in **Table 2-1 ▶**.

Coping With Death and Dying

We all deal with death (remember the quote, "Nobody gets out of here alive"?). What do you say to people who know they're dying? What do you say to a bereaved parent or spouse? How do you deal with your own feelings when a patient has died while under your care? These are all questions we need to be able to answer for ourselves eventually, and it can take a lifetime to sort them out.

Death in the Western hemisphere is generally regarded as a very traumatic experience, something to be feared and postponed as long as possible. It's not that way everywhere in the world. It may help you to know that many seasoned paramedics reveal in candid discussion that they are not afraid to die. Think about it. The average person's only experience with death has been the death of a loved one. It was a rare event. Chances are it was surprising, it was frightening, and it was painful for the survivor.

As a paramedic, you will be there when a lot of people are born and you will be there when a lot of them die. Every one of these encounters is an honour—a most private moment in someone's life, to which you and a small number of your colleagues are invited. Why an honour? Because, in many cultures, these moments are a holy time. These encounters allow you the privilege of meeting someone for the very first time in his or her life—or seeing him or her alive for the very last time. Many of the latter group will exhibit great dignity with their passing, and perhaps show you how to die well someday.

You don't need to experience great frustration because you tried to resuscitate someone and he or she died anyway. For you to resuscitate someone, everything has to go just right. As a paramedic, you will have the opportunity to help a great many people, but you will not be involved in many successful resuscitations, even in the course of a long career. Accept your profession as a calling, and be fulfilled by it. Keep a good grip on your ego, and you will find that "losing" someone will rarely be an issue for you.

What follows here are some general guidelines and techniques for dealing with the dying, their families, and your own stress.

Stages of the Grieving Process

In her classic study, *On Death and Dying*, Elisabeth Kubler-Ross, MD, defined five stages through which grieving people—usually the dying, but sometimes their survivors—often proceed

TABLE 2-1	Nancy's Guidelines for Preventing Burnout

1. Paramedic heal thyself! Take care of your own health.
   - Get enough rest.
   - Eat a balanced diet.
   - Get regular physical exercise—at least 30 minutes of aerobic activity (walking, running, or swimming) three to four times a week.
   - Don't abuse your body. Smoking, overindulgence in alcohol, taking recreational drugs, or self-prescribing any other drugs are all forms of self-abuse.
2. Give yourself some "me" time every day. Some of the most stress-resistant paramedics are those who have learned the techniques of meditation and can thereby escape now and then to a quiet place within themselves. Try different methods of meditation or relaxation and see which one works best for you.
3. Learn how to relax **Figure 2-15 ▼**.
   - Take time for hobbies.
   - Engage in social activities with people not involved in EMS.
   - Leave your job behind when your shift is over.
4. Do not make unreasonable demands on yourself.
   - Forget the idea that you have to be perfect. No one is perfect. If you do the best job you can, that is good enough.
   - You don't have to be right all the time. Accept the fact that now and then you will make a mistake—and that the world will not come to an end on account of it.
5. Do not make unreasonable demands on others.
6. Stay in touch with your feelings.
   - Find someone you can talk to. Share the stress.
   - Cry when you need to. There's no shame in being sad sometimes.
7. Learn techniques for shedding stress while on duty. Don't let stress accumulate.
8. Debrief after tough calls.

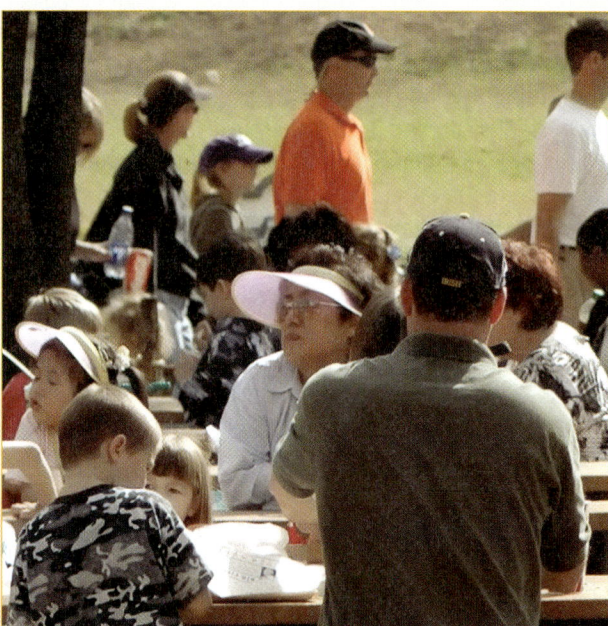

Figure 2-15 One of the best ways of dealing with the stress of working as a paramedic is to invest in relationships and activities outside of work that are meaningful to you.

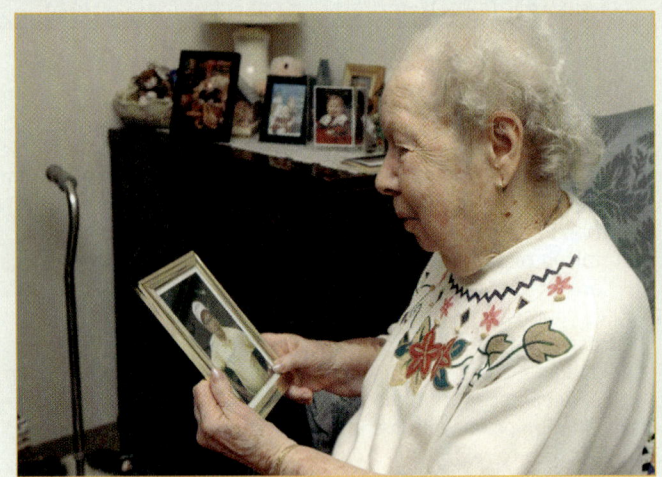

Figure 2-16 People usually go through a lengthy process of grieving before fully accepting the death of a loved one.

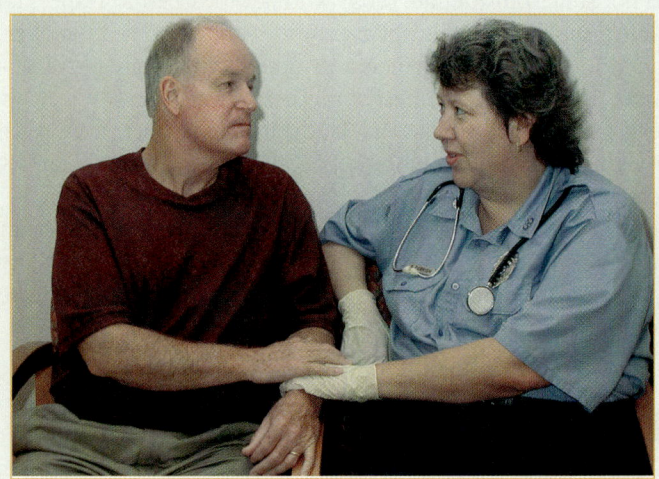

Figure 2-17 Be aware that each patient will have different ways of dealing with his or her immediate situation. Some may be relieved to talk openly about how they feel, while others may have a greater sense of privacy or stoicism.

Figure 2-16 ▲ . Each of these stages in some way helps the dying or their family members adapt to their own reality. It helps to be aware of these stages, and to consider the behaviour of dying patients or their families in the context of the grieving process.

- **Stage 1: Denial.** We have already mentioned denial as a mechanism by which people attempt to ignore a problem or pretend it does not exist. Denial is a way of buffering bad news until we can mobilize the resources to deal with that news more effectively.
- **Stage 2: Anger.** When people can no longer deny the reality of a situation, anger over the loss replaces denial. They may ask, "Why me?" and displace their anger randomly to those around them. As we mentioned earlier, such anger may be very difficult for health care personnel to deal with, and it is necessary again and again to remind yourself, "This patient (or this family member) is not really angry at me. She is angry at the hand life has just dealt her."
- **Stage 3: Bargaining.** When anger does not change the painful reality of a situation, people may resort to bargaining, that is, trying to make some sort of deal in hopes of postponing the inevitable ("If I can just live long enough to see my daughter's wedding, then I'll die in peace.").
- **Stage 4: Depression.** When bargaining fails to change the reality of a loss and people must come to terms with dying, there is suddenly an enormous sense of loss. They may become very quiet. Other people may make the mistake of trying to "cheer them up" at this point. But the people who have experienced the loss typically do not *want* to be cheered up. They want permission to express their sorrow—in words, in tears, or in what Kubler-Ross calls "the silence that goes beyond words." Acknowledge their loss and sadness, and if they act like they want to cry, offer some tissues or a towel and encourage them to "let it out." If they seem to want a hug, offer it. If they seem to just

want to be quiet by themselves, do what you can to accommodate that as well. But try hard not to steer their behaviours in any way unless their behaviour is harmful.
- **Stage 5: Acceptance.** In the final stage of grief, people who are dying prepare to disengage from the world around them. They shed their fears and most of their other feelings as well and begin to loosen the ties that bind them to the living. When the dying enter this acceptance stage, it is often the family that is in need of the most help.

Dealing With the Dying Patient

People who are dying generally know, at the very least, that their situation is serious; they may, in fact, be well aware that they are dying and may want to talk about it. Many health care professionals are reluctant to discuss death with patients, mostly because of their own anxiety about the subject. So they try to maintain an attitude of cheery reassurance ("Everything is going to be all right."), when they both know that everything will *not* be all right. The message patients get is that the subject of dying is taboo and that they'd better keep their feelings about dying to themselves. In fact, perhaps the most important thing you can do for dying patients is to let them know that it's OK to talk about it. There are many ways of doing so. You don't need to come right out and ask, "Do you want to talk about dying?" It's enough to say, "If there's anything worrying you, I'd be glad to listen."

Having made the offer to listen, be prepared to do so. Let patients talk as much as they wish Figure 2-17 ▲ . Make some physical contact. Hold their hand, put a hand on their shoulder, or make some other unmistakable gesture of empathy.

What if patients come straight out and ask you, "Am I going to die?" There is no simple answer as to how to reply to that question, but the answer should acknowledge the seriousness of their condition without taking away all hope. For example, you might say, "You seem to have had a severe heart attack. We're going to give you the best care available, but the situation *is* serious." For patients who know they are dying, it may be a great relief to have someone else acknowledge the fact and thereby give them permission to talk about it.

Dying patients also need to feel that they still have some control over their life. When people lose all control over their life, they may lose a large measure of their dignity and self-respect. As much as possible, explain to them what you are doing and allow them to participate in the treatment. Ask them if there is anyone they would like you to contact or if they have any special instructions they want conveyed to someone. If they *do* ask you to convey a message, *write it down* word-for-word as they state it to you.

Experience tells us that people who know they're going to die usually don't *ask* you if they are going to die. They look you in the eye and *tell* you, "I think I'm going to die." People who ask tend to be fairly stable, but that doesn't mean they're not scared to death. If they appear to be doing OK, let them know that, and tell them not to be afraid, that you've "got them."

Dealing With a Grieving Family

Suppose you are called to the scene where a child has been run over by a truck. You can see at a glance that the child is dead and beyond hope of resuscitation—his skull has been smashed open and his brains are all over the street. Two police officers are restraining the child's mother, who is crying hysterically.

The fact that there is nothing you can do for the child does *not* mean that the call is over. There is another "patient" at the scene—the child's mother—and the call is not over until you have done all you can for her **Figure 2-18 ▾** .

What kinds of things *can* you do for a grieving family? How can you help them begin the process of dealing with their loss? Here are a few guidelines:

- Do *not* try to hide the body of the deceased from the family, even if the body has been badly mutilated. (*Do* hide

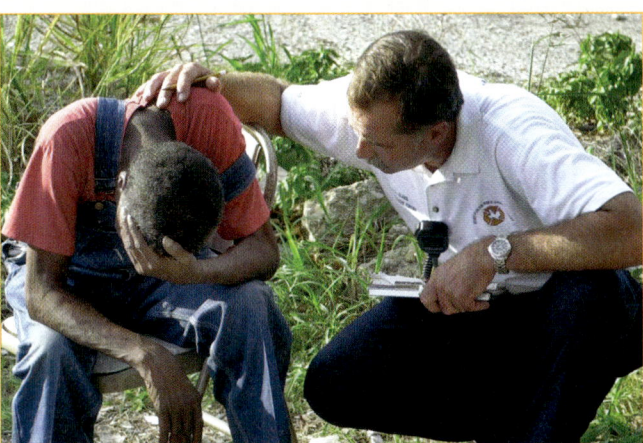

Figure 2-18 While on the scene, one of your responsibilities is to help family members through the initial period after the death of a loved one.

it from the general public, however.) People who are prevented from seeing the body of a loved one may later have enormous difficulty working through their grief, for they may not be able to get beyond their denial.

- For similar reasons, do not use euphemisms for death, such as "expired" or "passed away." The family needs to hear the word "dead."
- Do not be in a hurry to clear away all your resuscitation equipment. Let the family see the equipment before you start tidying up and packing away your gear, so that they will know that everything possible was done to try to save the patient.
- Give the family some time with the remains, especially when the victim is a child. If the death occurred in a public place—as in the hypothetical motor vehicle collision described—move the remains into the ambulance and let the family be alone with the body there. Give them a chance to say goodbye in their own way.
- Try to arrange for further support. Recruit a neighbour to come over, or offer to call the family's clergy.
- Accept the family's right to experience a variety of feelings—guilt, shock, denial, or anger. And when family members do respond with anger, remind yourself yet again, "They aren't really angry at *me.*"

Dealing With a Grieving Child

You need to be particularly sensitive to the emotional needs of children and how they differ depending on their age group. Children up to 3 years of age will be aware that something has happened and people are sad. Family members should be advised to try to maintain the child's routine. They should also watch for irritability and monitor the child's eating and sleeping patterns. Children 3 to 6 years of age believe that death is temporary and may continually ask when the person will return. Family members should be informed that the child may feel responsible for the death and may worry that everyone else they love may also die. The family should emphasize to the child that he or she was not responsible for the death and also that it's OK to cry when you are sad.

Children 6 to 9 years of age may mask their feelings in an effort to not look babyish. Family members should discuss the normal feelings of grieving with the child. Also, they should not hesitate to cry in front of the child. This will convey to the child that crying is acceptable behaviour after the loss of a loved one.

Children 9 to 12 years of age may want to know details surrounding the incident. Family members should encourage the sharing of feelings and memories to facilitate the grieving process.

After the Call Is Over

Some kinds of calls can be real shockers, like the Oklahoma City bombing or the World Trade Center attack in the United States. In those cases, everyone involved in the call is likely to experience some heavy-duty feelings. If these feelings stay bottled up, there may be all sorts of problems later. Every ambulance service, therefore, needs to develop routine procedures for debriefing after any call that involved the death of a patient. All those who participated in the call need a chance to sit down together, in an atmosphere of confidentiality, and air their feelings about what happened.

By definition, a critical incident is one that overwhelms the ability of a paramedic or an EMS system to cope with the experience, either at the scene or later. Some Canadian EMS services deploy specially trained teams to conduct critical incident stress debriefings (CISDs) with emergency personnel who have been involved in particularly traumatic calls or other painful incidents. A CISD is usually held within 24 to 72 hours of the incident. Although public safety organizations have used CISDs for more than 20 years, there is no evidence that they are effective, or that their effects are not actually harmful. The sorts of incidents that are apt to require debriefing include:

- Serious injury or death of a fellow worker in the line of duty
- Suicide of a fellow worker
- Multiple-casualty incidents, such as an airliner crash or train wreck
- Serious injury or death of a child
- Intense media attention to an incident

It is impossible to predict how any given person will react to a particular incident. A call that may be very disturbing to one paramedic may not bother his or her partner at all. People should be offered opportunities to debrief, but debriefings should never be forced upon them.

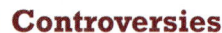

Controversies

There are definitely two sides of the fence on the effectiveness of CISD. Psychology professionals and EMS professionals alike have debated this issue for some time now. Take part in a debriefing whenever you can. Be open-minded about the experience and then draw your own conclusion as to which side of the fence you are on.

Posttraumatic Stress Disorder

Most calls should not disrupt your normal life functions. But, depending on a number of variables, some especially traumatic calls can preoccupy even well-adjusted providers for weeks or even months afterward. This is called posttraumatic stress disorder (PTSD). Most paramedics never experience it, but it's what CISDs were developed to prevent. Let your superiors know if you experience one or more of the following signs of PTSD:

- You have trouble getting an incident out of your thoughts.
- You keep having flashbacks of an incident.
- You have nightmares or other sleep disturbances after an incident.
- Your appetite is not the same after an incident.
- After an incident, you laugh or cry for no good reason.
- You find yourself withdrawing from colleagues and family members after an incident.

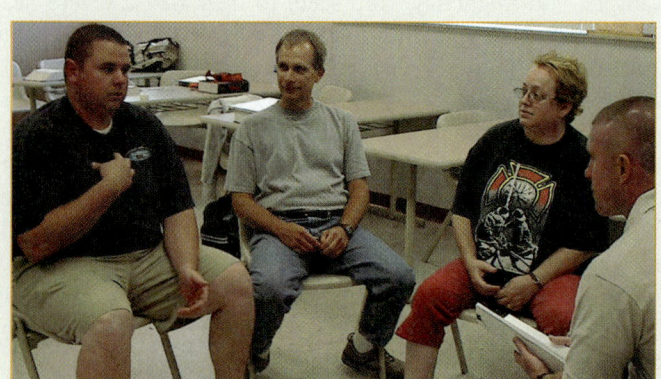

Figure 2-19 A debriefing with colleagues after an especially traumatic or difficult call can help everyone voice their feelings.

The purpose of a CISD is to accelerate the normal recovery process and to help paramedics realize that they are normal people having normal reactions to *ab*normal events **Figure 2-19 ▲** . As mentioned, many EMS systems have CISD management teams to provide support after a traumatic call—and sometimes even during the incident itself. The intervention may take the form of a brief (usually about 30 minutes) defusing session right after the call, in which all who were involved in the incident are offered an opportunity to express their feelings about what happened. As the name implies, a defusing session is intended to remove the explosive potential from a situation and thereby prevent more serious psychological consequences later on.

A formal debriefing is usually coordinated by one or more professional counselors 24 to 72 hours after an incident, when it becomes clear that the incident has had a serious impact and is causing persistent symptoms among the crew. A debriefing usually takes about 3 hours, and is conducted away from the workplace and in a confidential atmosphere so participants can feel free to say what's on their minds.

■ Emergency Vehicle Operations

An emergency vehicle is a four-sided billboard that communicates to the public all the time, whether we realize it or not. It communicates our respect for—or lack of respect for—the safety of others. It communicates our courtesy—or complete lack of it. And it communicates our concern for the comfort and safety of that patient and caregiver in the compartment—or our complete lack of it.

A paramedic's first job is to come home safe to loved ones. There are plenty of paramedics (some whose careers span 20 or 30 years) who have never been involved in an ambulance collision, and not by dumb luck. They understand that safety is deliberate. They understand that operating an ambulance is a public trust. And they never forget that driving an ambulance is dangerous.

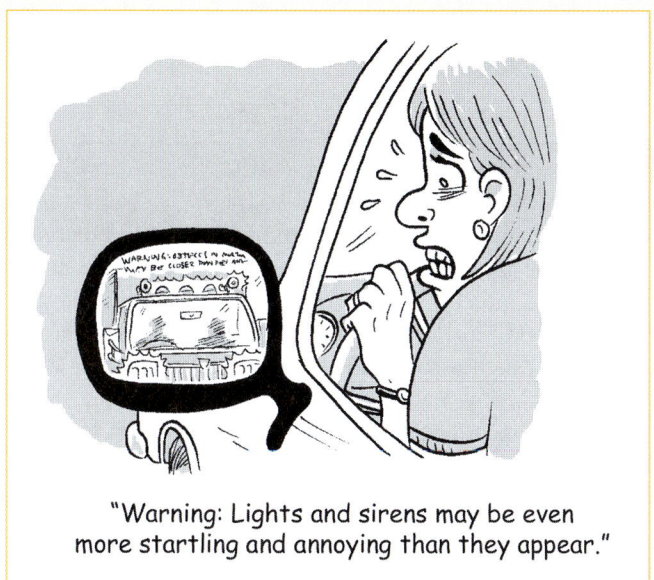

"Warning: Lights and sirens may be even more startling and annoying than they appear."

Figure 2-20

Here are some proven safety tips you can use in your daily driving:

1. Think of your warning equipment as tools you can use to *ask for* (never demand) the right of way.
2. Always allow for the incompetence of other drivers.
3. Come to a full and complete stop when you encounter an opposing signal. Proceed only after you have given other drivers time and cause to anticipate your intentions.
4. Expect some drivers to panic (**Figure 2-20** ▲). If that happens, turn off your siren, switch on the personal address system, and politely say, "Please pull to the right and stop. Thank you." Repeat it in case they don't understand you the first time.
5. Remember, other drivers may not immediately hear your siren when you are travelling at freeway speed. Stay far enough behind other drivers so they can see your lights in their rearview mirrors. Anticipate that, when they notice you, their first instinct will be to slam on their brakes.
6. As frustrating as it may be, control your emotions when it appears that a driver is refusing to yield. Avoid reacting to the situation, which will cause you to lose your cool and potentially worsen it.

Documentation and Communication

When considering transporting a patient with lights and siren on, ask yourself, "Can I justify the potential risk to my safety, my patient's safety, and the safety of others to save a few minutes?" Make sure you can legitimately justify why you transported emergently and document the need to do so.

Besides the general use of lights and the siren, some additional aspects of operating an emergency vehicle deserve special mention.

Using Escorts

When you find yourself responding in tandem with an escort vehicle, remember that the average driver is not likely to understand that one vehicle is escorting another. Most drivers have not had a course in emergency driving. Typically, drivers on a street or highway hear one siren and, especially in their rearview mirrors, will see only the first vehicle in a convoy. Deliberately using an escort is not only a bit pompous, but also dangerous. Do yourself a favor. Minimize the number of times you use any warning equipment and the number of vehicles on a given response. You'll live longer, and so will the public.

Adverse Environmental Conditions

Most of us have enough trouble keeping ourselves visible and trying to predict other drivers' behaviour on clear, sunny days. Add a little bad weather, fog, blowing dust, or slippery asphalt and the average driver can be overwhelmed. Try to be as careful, alert, and predictable for other drivers as you can under the circumstances. When you lose even the slightest visibility, be super observant and expect the worst decision-making from your fellow travellers. In fact, don't even trust yourself under these conditions. Drive slowly, carefully, and remember to sign up for emergency driving classes long before winter, the hurricane season, the wildfire season, or whatever weather torments the paramedics in your region.

Parking at Emergency Scenes

Many of us were taught years ago that when we park in traffic, we should shield ourselves with our equipment and aim the front wheels into traffic. That works fine if you're in law

You are the Paramedic Part 4

Your partner drives to the ambulance entrance of the hospital. It takes every ounce of your concentration to aid your partner in unloading the patient. You tell yourself that you can finish the call but, as you and your partner lower the stretcher to the height of the hospital bed, you are unable to hold up your end. It drops to the floor, and the patient drops with it. Although he appears to be uninjured, the patient screams loudly and immediately threatens to sue you. Your partner now seems to be injured, and the hospital staff members appear to be horrified at what has just transpired.

9. What parts of this situation were preventable?
10. Beyond the physical injuries, what other damage has occurred?

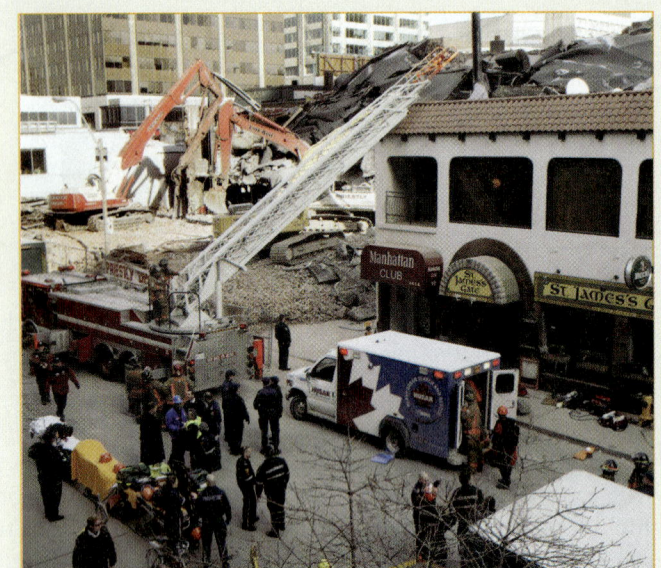

Figure 2-21 Place your vehicle where it can be seen, out of traffic, and where the patient can be easily transported into and out of the vehicle.

enforcement and you need the illumination from your head-lamps anyway, or if you're doing fire suppression and you have access to a front-facing water outlet. But it does you no good at all if you're going to end up loading an ambulance, because ambulances load from the rear. Protect your back; park in the best position for loading **Figure 2-21 ▲**.

There is an exception, and that's if the ambulance happens to be the first equipment on the scene. Just remember: it will need to be moved later on. (Chapter 46 provides a more detailed discussion of this situation.)

Due Regard for the Safety of Others

Everything that makes us paramedics belongs to the public. Our certificates do. Our equipment does. So do the radio frequencies we use every day, and the roads we travel. And so does our occasional prerogative to override certain traffic laws in order to do our jobs. Anyone who operates an emergency vehicle needs to have profound respect for the pain ambulance drivers can inflict on the public by driving too fast, or by insisting on the right-of-way.

People who have abused this privilege tell us that no teacher can possibly describe the horror they felt on the morning after causing a fatality (especially the death of a colleague). These events are always horrible, and they can usually be traced to something that took no more than a couple of seconds to occur. There is no "undo" button in EMS driving, and no amount of shock or grief can ever give us those seconds back.

Although speed is sometimes perceived as the essence of EMS, rest secure in this advice: knowledge is the essence of the

professional paramedic. As you become a paramedic, you will have the most training and the most experience of any EMS provider. Be professional.

Protecting Yourself

Much has changed in EMS since the early 1990s. For one, we have become more aware of the fact that we can be hurt not just by flying bullets, but also by bacteria and viruses found in a patient's body fluids. The use of personal protective equipment (PPE) was not common in the early years. It was a status symbol to see how messy a person could get during the shift because that meant you could "take it" and keep on ticking. Surgeons in the 1800s took similar pride in their messy operating aprons, but they were transmitting infectious diseases by the score. Paramedics in the 2000s take pride in not endangering themselves or their patients.

Face it, there are some nasty germs out there nowadays. Thanks to the research and reporting done by Health Canada, we are now more aware that biohazards are an integral part of our profession and can have long-term effects on the health care worker if certain precautions are not adhered to. Paramedics use routine precautions and appropriate personal protective equipment (PPE) to prevent biohazards and acquiring an infectious or communicable disease.

Use the personal tools that are at your disposal that are designed not only to protect you from your sick patients but to protect them from you! In addition to these tools, consider adopting a practice that doesn't necessarily involve tools, but has proven its worth over the years. Wash your hands!

Personal Protective Equipment and Practices

At a minimum, each ambulance should be equipped with certain PPE because it is an important part of safety for yourself. At a minimum, you should have access to gloves, facial protection (masks and eyewear), gowns, and N95 respirators. The following paragraphs explain the importance of using infection control practices.

Wear Gloves

Gloves are absolutely essential on any EMS call, and some patient encounters warrant more than one set of gloves for a caregiver, depending on the procedure, the patient's history, and the environment **Figure 2-22 ▶**. Anytime you intubate or start an IV, consider following that with a new set of gloves before loading the patient and jumping aboard that ambulance. Gloves are a good idea anytime you sanitize the ambulance too or even handle the cleaning rags. Sterile gloves should be reserved for clean or sterile patient care procedures; they're substantially more expensive than examination gloves. And whatever you've been doing with them, take off your gloves before you drive.

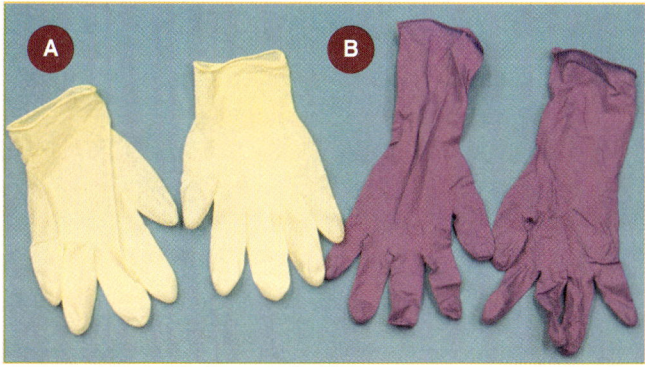

Figure 2-22 Two commonly used types of gloves are (**A**) latex and (**B**) nitrile.

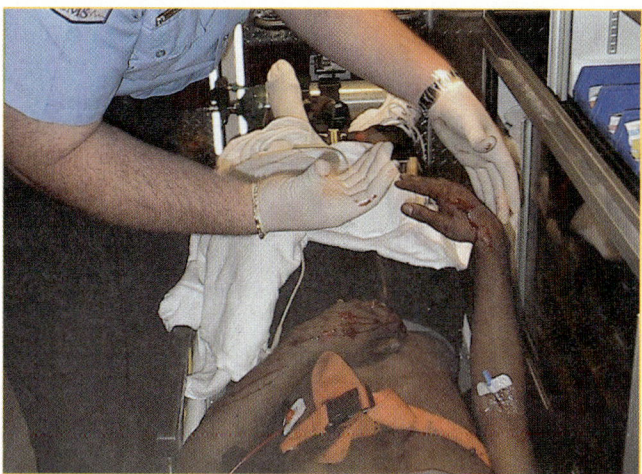

Figure 2-23 Paramedics always need to protect themselves from contact with any type of body fluids.

At the Scene

Get used to washing your hands before and after using the bathroom, before ingesting anything by mouth, before getting into your personal car, and before and after any physical contact between you and a patient or an instrument.

Any advanced medical text on infection control starts with "wash your hands" and ends with it, too.

When you do wash your hands, wash them vigorously with antibacterial soap for at least 30 seconds before rinsing with clean water. If you don't have access to soap and water, carry waterless hand cleaner wipes in your ambulance and use them instead. Isopropyl alcohol, the active ingredient they contain, is a very effective bactericide.

Whatever else you do, wash your hands.

Wash Your Hands

Wash your hands, routinely and often. Long before it was common practice for prehospital caregivers (or any clinical workers) to wear gloves during nonsterile procedures, we learned to wash our hands—sometimes more than 30 times a day, depending on our caseloads. Turn that into a habit. Habits are reliable, even when we're stressed.

Use Lotion

To replenish the natural oils you wash off your skin, and to keep the skin on your hands from cracking, use hand lotion several times a day both on and off duty. For you guys, it's not sissy stuff; it's good sense. Your skin is a very effective barrier to pathogens, as long as it hasn't been breached by the drying effects of frequent washing. And the job of a professional caregiver warrants frequent washing.

Use Eye Protection

Many seasoned paramedics make it their standard practice to wear antisplash eyewear throughout any patient contact. That's a good idea. It's an absolute necessity during suctioning or

intubation procedures. In fact, during intubation, it may be a good idea to use a face shield instead.

Consider Wearing a Mask

Have a cold? Wear a mask—not only to protect your patients and your colleagues from you, but to protect you from additional infections while you are in a weakened state. Have a bad cold? Stay home.

Protect Your Body

Masks and gowns are appropriate whenever you deal with a patient who is extremely messy or bloody 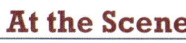 . A large trash bag can be used as a two-armed glove to slide a patient from a couch or bed onto a stretcher if the patient is covered with feces, urine, or blood. Once the patient has been moved, the crew can simply turn the bag inside-out, squeeze the air out of it, tie a knot in its open end, and place it in a hazardous materials bag.

Incontinence barriers should be laid out on a surface when the patient is leaking any type of fluid or has skin lesions.

N95 Respirators

Read some of the recent statistics regarding tuberculosis (TB) and you will realize that this is one of the most common diseases contracted by breathing in germs. The world public health associations estimate that 1.7 *billion* people are affected with TB worldwide, with 3 million deaths a year. The chance of getting the TB bacillus makes it that much more important to wear the N95 respirator **Figure 2-24 ▶** and not just a simple surgical mask.

Clean Your Ambulance and Equipment

Sanitize your patient compartment surfaces frequently, but especially the stretcher, the bench seat, the grab rails, the deck and deck hardware, and the interior and exterior areas around the door handles. These surfaces should be cleaned daily and after every call. The same is true for the door hardware inside (and outside) the cab, the steering wheel and gear-shift lever, the

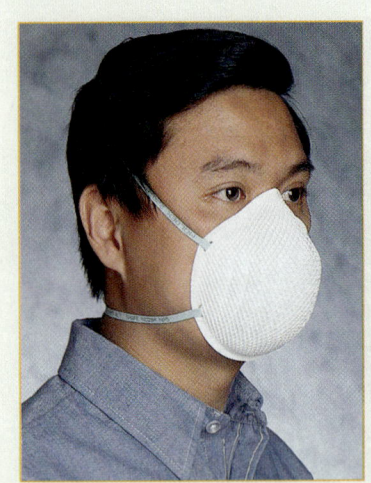

Figure 2-24 Specially designed respirator masks, such as the N95 respirator, protect against infection from tuberculosis bacteria.

emergency brake release, and anything else that you or your colleagues may have handled while wearing contaminated gloves. Remove the stretcher mounts at least once a week to get rid of the dried blood and vomit that tends to accumulate there. It produces an odour that can make some people sick, and it attracts insects such as flies. Clean this area more often if you have had messy calls. Sanitize the phones and microphones as a matter of routine—especially the ones in the patient compartment, which you surely handle while wearing contaminated gloves.

Sanitize or replace your pen often. You typically handle it several times during every call, with your gloves on. Then, you handle it after the call, after you've washed your hands. Likewise, sanitize your stethoscope with alcohol after every call.

Decontamination of equipment and supplies that have been exposed to body substances requires a different cleansing routine than just soap and water. First, any piece of equipment that is intended for single use should be discarded in an appropriate hazardous materials bag. Second, use a commercial disinfecting agent on any piece of equipment that has had direct contact with the patient's skin. Bleach diluted in water (1:10) can also be used as a disinfecting agent. Disinfecting kills many of the microorganisms on the surface of your equipment.

To kill all microorganisms, sterilization by using a commercial sterilizing chemical or pressurized steam is needed. Tools, such as a laryngoscope blade, that come in direct contact with the interior of a patient's body must be sterilized after use.

Properly Dispose of Sharps

Disposal containers (large for the ambulance and small for carry-in gear) for sharps, such as needles and blades, are essential to protect crews against needle sticks or cuts **Figure 2-25 ▸**.

Consider Wearing Body Armour

Body armour can be bulky, expensive, and uncomfortable. It's not nearly as protective against bullets or knives as are self-protective avoidance strategies. But it can protect the wearer from many kinds of chest and abdominal trauma such as those that occur during extrications and in emergency vehicle collisions.

Management of an Exposure

In the event that you have been exposed to a patient's blood or body fluids, follow your local EMS guidelines. Generally, any

paramedic who has been exposed should do the following:

- Wash the affected area immediately with soap and water.
- Comply with all reporting requirements.
- Get a medical evaluation.
- Obtain proper immunization boosters.
- Document the incident, including the actions taken to reduce chances of infection.

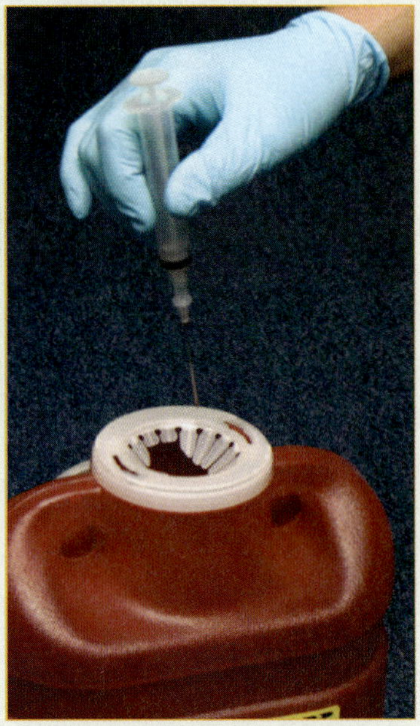

Hostile Situations

Until very recently, paramedics were routinely thrust without assistance into situations involving hostile patients who needed to be restrained, treated, and transported against their will. There is no more dangerous prospect than confronting someone like that without special equipment and plenty of help. A position statement by the National Association of EMS Physicians in December 2003 outlined for the first time an official endorsement of the rights to safety not only of patients but also of their prehospital caregivers. In addition, most modern jurisdictions ask their paramedics to stand back until police have defused these situations (using electric stun devices if necessary).

But paramedics are also exposed to other kinds of hostile situations. If the element of hostility is known or can be anticipated in advance, EMS crews and their first responders should never be allowed to arrive on scene first. Discipline yourself to scrutinize all information that comes to you from others, and remain alert any time you are on duty. Specifically, beware any call dispatched as a fight, stabbing, shooting, domestic disturbance, "person down," or "unknown medical aid." Every one of these calls is suspicious and warrants an initial response by police **Figure 2-26 ▸**. In addition, you should have the prerogative to ask for a police response to any call that your intuition says is violent. Whether or not you ask for police backup may depend on your knowledge of the response area and your analysis of the information you receive from your communications centre.

Do not be afraid of being less than a good caregiver if you ask for police to go in first. You will not be able to treat your patient if you are hurt.

You will surely find that your intuition is a reliable tool that warrants your trust; and it will become more and more sensitive as you gain experience and additional training. Every paramedic should read a book called *The Gift of Fear:*

Figure 2-25 Any needles or blades must be disposed of in special containers.

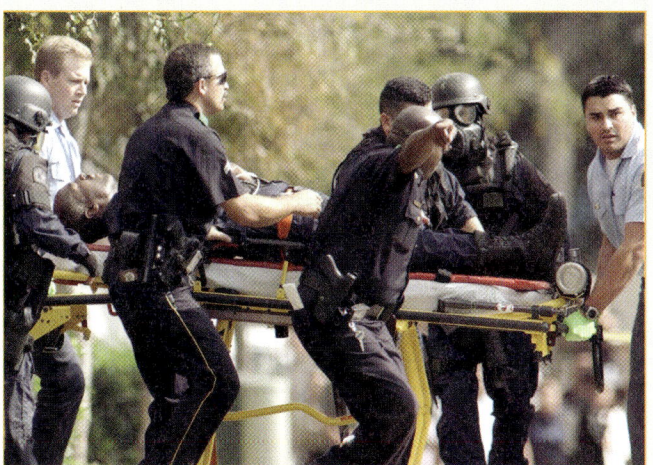

Figure 2-26 Do not hesitate to call for law enforcement if anyone's safety is in question.

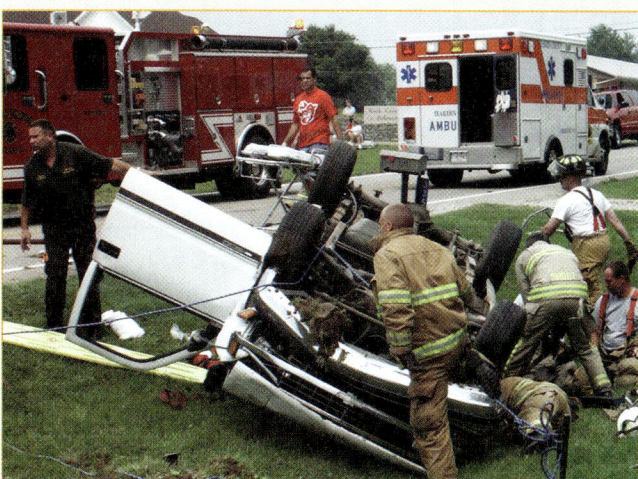

Figure 2-27 At a busy accident scene, it is important to place your vehicle in a safe, visible location, and to minimize the risk of any additional accidents.

At the Scene

Some of the most dangerous calls are those that are not obviously dangerous. The most worrisome calls are those with limited or vague information from the caller. If someone refuses to give information to a dispatcher, it may be because of something they are trying to hide.

Survival Signals That Protect Us From Violence, by Gavin De Becker. It explains how your intuition picks up on small details that your rational side discounts. Intuition is often not the product of your imagination, but of your ability to process small details almost outside of your awareness.

Once you are in contact with a hostile patient, try hard to listen a lot more than you talk. Avoid arguing. Concentrate on de-escalating his or her emotions, because people who are upset don't listen well and they don't reason well either. (Remember fight-or-flight?) Many hostile patients who started out willing to go to the hospital became unwilling because a crew member couldn't resist a "witty" comment.

Learn and use verbal judo. You can learn more about verbal judo by reading *Verbal Judo: Redirecting Behavior With Words,* by George J. Thompson. Verbal judo is a discipline for communication and negotiation that parallels the characteristics of judo, the martial art. As you may know, there are hard forms and soft forms of the martial arts. Judo is a soft form. It's designed to deflect energy or simply move out of its way, rather than inflict it yourself.

Remember that anytime you're on someone else's turf, they have a clear advantage. You can expect them to know everything about their environment while you know nothing (including locations of weapons). Volatile patients in their home environment are much more dangerous there than anywhere else—especially in poor lighting.

Finally, some situations get out of hand due to the paramedic's inability to communicate effectively and build a rapport. Show empathy and understanding on the scene, and you will

develop the trust of your patients. Knowledge of diverse cultures plays a major role in effective communication. "Know your audience" is not just a catch phrase for entertainers. The more you know about the people you serve, the more likely you will know their customs and expectations. You must also be diligent in your pursuit of treating all patients with respect and dignity. Put your personal prejudices aside every time you step on the scene.

Traffic Scenes

The most dangerous kinds of calls you will respond to are the everyday ones, because you naturally get comfortable with them. But regardless of where you are, vehicles move at high speeds, may carry hazardous substances, and may crash into one another in locations that are both dangerous for you and sure to attract spectators. It is important to stay aware of your surroundings, even the familiar ones that you see day in and day out.

Like any scene, your approach to traffic scenes always begins with your familiarity with the response area and your awareness of what the system's other public servants have been doing for the past few hours (because we know you've been paying attention to their frequencies!). This is critical information, because it lets you know your best routing and who might be available to help you with traffic control, air support, hazardous materials, terrain issues, and potential destinations.

Traffic may be only one of the many hazards at the scene of a motor vehicle collision **Figure 2-27 ▲**. The undercarriage of our units are quite hot, especially after travelling 5 to 10 minutes to get to a scene. Parking a hot, running unit on the side of the road in dry grass is just inviting a grass fire. Watch where you park, and the type of material you park over. If you arrive at a scene in the early morning hours, before the sun starts heating up, and park over a liquid spill long enough, it may trigger combustion of the liquid. Sometimes we create our own hazards by carelessly throwing equipment and its packaging all around us at the scene. Not only can people trip over them but we often lose pieces because they get kicked under the vehicles.

At the Scene

If you are the first unit arriving on the scene, do a scene assessment and notify other responding units of any actual or potential hazards that may be present. Your first job is to ensure the safety of the EMS crew—including yourself.

Remember that your primary concern at any scene is safety; safety for yourself as well as for those around you. Identify as many hazards as you can before even leaving your unit. Reviewing the scene before leaving your vehicle goes a long way toward identifying hazards such as fire, unstable vehicles or buildings, unruly crowds, or hazardous materials.

Begin making physical observations a mile or so before you approach the scene. Watch the traffic, pay attention to the wind direction, look for smoke, and begin planning for approaching darkness and for weather-related issues. As you get closer, note the kinds of vehicles and obstacles involved. Make an educated guess about what may have happened. If someone is not yet handling traffic, decide how to control the flow of traffic initially (sometimes it can be a lot more important than medicine at first).

How big an incident do you have, both in size and scope? Are you dealing with commercial carriers of industrial products? What resources will you need immediately? What is the topography? Where will fluids drain naturally? Remember that if you do not have fire on the scene now, it could start quickly as some kinds of fuel begin leaking on hot metal exhaust systems or as a result of electrical arcing.

Where do you eventually want to park? What will your working space be? These are all important considerations, and they will be covered in more detail in Section 7. For now, concentrate more on seeing and protecting the whole scene and not so much on what's wrong with individual patients.

You are the Paramedic Summary

1. What is your main concern at the moment?

Your main concern should be the safety of yourself, your partner, and, finally, your patient. Lifting patients of this size should be performed by an adequate number of responders (no less than four). Your patient is stable, so there is no need for immediate action.

2. What concerns do you have, if any, regarding your partner's behaviour?

It's possible that your partner is having a bad day, is generally disagreeable, or is suffering from burnout. Because you do not know him well yet, it is hard to determine definitively. Employee assistance programs are in existence to aid responders when they are overwhelmed and in need of help.

3. Does your partner's attitude have any effect on prehospital patient care?

He dropped the ball on obtaining essential information regarding this patient's medical history and, most likely, his attitude has affected his patient care on other calls. People suffering from burnout can be more likely to cut corners, make mistakes, and experience problems with colleagues, other medical professionals, and patients. Depending on their condition, these responders may also have difficulty in their personal lives as well.

4. Is this the best course of action?

The best course of action was your first reaction, to call for additional resources. This is appropriate whenever you feel that the number of ambulances, supplies, equipment, or personnel that you have on the scene is inadequate.

5. What is the best way to handle this situation?

Although you might experience grumbling and resistance from your partner, you should tell him that you feel it is unsafe for you and your partner to lift this patient without additional personnel. If you stress the issue of safety, he will likely cooperate with your suggestion.

6. What factors could affect your decisions?

When you are newly hired, no matter how supportive the agency is that you work for, you will be under pressure to perform well. Most agencies have a probationary period for new members during which you can be fired for any reason, or for no reason at all. Obviously, this is a source of stress. No matter how much you are concerned about your employee evaluation, you must put safety first.

7. What decisions could you have made to prevent this situation?

You could have called for additional resources despite the complaints of your partner. You could have requested aid from other employees within the nursing facility. Certified nursing assistants are familiar with appropriate lifting techniques, and with some communication, could aid you in safely moving and lifting the patient. Some departments forbid any nondepartmental personnel from engaging in activities such as this, so always follow local standard operating guidelines.

8. Has prehospital patient care been affected?

Obviously, you must obtain information regarding this patient's medical history and reason for transport. To do otherwise could place the patient at risk. Because the patient's condition was stable, patient care was not jeopardized a great deal. However, if the patient's condition changed rapidly and you were not able to care for the patient because of your own pain, patient care could very well have been compromised.

9. What parts of this situation were preventable?

This situation was entirely avoidable. Don't hesitate to protect yourself. In the end, it was your responsibility to speak up regardless of whether or not it would create an uncomfortable situation with your partner.

10. Beyond the physical injuries, what other damage has occurred?

Because you chose to be agreeable rather than use your common sense and instincts, you not only hurt yourself but also your partner and possibly the patient. Beyond the physical injuries and their associated costs (treatment, rehabilitation, and lost work hours and the resultant overtime), you have damaged the image of your department. This last type of injury is very difficult to fix. The patient will remember what happened, and may choose to sue you, your partner, the department, the city, and the hospital. Depending on what transpires, word of this story could travel to outside parties, including local or national newspapers and/or websites.

Prep Kit

Ready for Review

- Paramedics need to know how to ensure their own well-being.
- Wellness has at least three dimensions: physical, mental, and emotional. It is important to keep all three dimensions healthy and balanced.
- Nutrition plays a key role in maintaining day-to-day energy and maintaining a healthy body for life.
- Practice proper lifting techniques to protect your body and lengthen your career.
  - Minimize the number of total body-lifts you have to perform.
  - Coordinate every lift in advance.
  - Minimize the total amount of weight you have to lift.
  - Never lift with your back.
  - Don't carry what you can put on wheels.
  - Ask for help anytime, without embarrassment or hesitation, and offer it liberally to others.
- Learn how to effectively control stress so that it does not affect your wellness. Take appropriate action. Initial management techniques include:
  - Controlled breathing
  - Reframing
  - Progressive relaxation
- A patient's reaction to stress may include fear, anxiety, depression, anger, confusion, denial, regression, projection, and displacement. Most of these reactions are not under the patient's conscious control. Remember, under emergency situations, everyone is under stress.
- Health care professionals are not immune to the stresses of emergency situations and experience a multitude of feelings, not all of them pleasant. These feelings are normal, but it is better to keep them to yourself during an emergency.
- Burnout is a consequence of chronic, unrelieved stress. Perfectionist beliefs are likely to produce stress.
- As a paramedic, you will be present when a lot of people are born and you will be there when a lot of people die. Every one of these encounters is an honour.
- The patient who is dying may be aware of that fact, and may want to talk about it. One of the most important things you can do for a dying patient is to let him or her know that it is OK to talk about it. Be prepared to listen and provide empathy.
- Critical incident stress debriefings (CISDs) are provided to emergency personnel who have been involved in traumatic calls or other painful incidents.
- An emergency vehicle is an instrument that can either earn its crew a living or kill them. It deserves respect and it warrants understanding.
- Protect yourself by washing your hands; using hand lotion; wearing gloves, eye protection, and a mask and gown (when necessary); cleaning your ambulance and equipment; and properly disposing of sharps.
- Decontamination of equipment and supplies that have been potentially exposed to body substances requires a different cleansing routine than just soap and water; sterilization may be required.
- Keep yourself on "yellow alert" while you are on duty. Do not be afraid to ask for the police to enter a scene first. You will not be able to treat a patient if you or your partner is hurt.
- The most dangerous calls are your everyday ones because you become comfortable with them and let down your guard.
- Your primary concern at any scene is safety—safety for yourself as well as those around you.

Vital Vocabulary

alarm reaction The body's first, "startle" response to a stressor.

alert response The first reaction in the alarm reaction, in which you immediately stop whatever you are doing and focus on the source of the stimulus.

blind panic A fear reaction in which a person's judgment seems to disappear entirely; it is particularly dangerous because it may precipitate mass panic among others.

burnout The exhaustion of physical or emotional strength.

conversion hysteria A reaction in which a person subconsciously transforms his or her anxiety into a bodily dysfunction; the person may be unable to see or hear or may become partially paralyzed.

critical incident An event that overwhelms the ability to cope with the experience, either at the scene or later.

critical incident stress debriefings (CISDs) A confidential peer group discussion in which specially trained teams work with emergency personnel who have been involved in traumatic calls or other painful incidents; CISDs usually occur within 24 to 72 hours of the incident.

defence mechanisms Psychological ways to relieve stress; they are usually automatic or subconscious. Defence mechanisms include denial, regression, projection, and displacement.

denial An early response to a serious medical emergency, in which the severity of the emergency is diminished or minimized. Denial is the first coping mechanism for people who believe they are going to die.

displacement Redirection of an emotion from yourself to another person.

distress A type of stress that a person finds overwhelming and debilitating.

eustress A type of stress that motivates an individual to achieve.

fight-or-flight syndrome A physiologic response to a profound stressor that helps one deal with the situation at hand; features increased sympathetic tone and resulting in dilation of the pupils, increased heart rate, dilation of the bronchi, mobilization of glucose, shunting of blood away from the gastrointestinal tract and cerebrum, and increased blood flow to the skeletal muscles.

posttraumatic stress disorder (PTSD) A delayed stress reaction before an incident, often the result of one or more unresolved issues concerning the incident.

projection Blaming unacceptable feelings, motives, or desires on others.

regression A return to more childish behaviour while under stress.

routine precautions Protective measures for dealing with objects, blood, body fluids, or other potential exposure risks of communicable disease.

stress A nonspecific response of the body to any demand made upon it.

stressor Any agent or situation that causes stress.

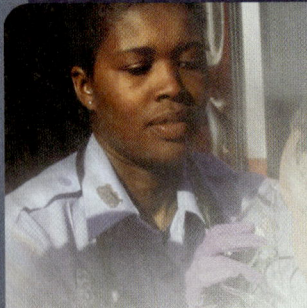

Assessment in Action

On duty, paramedics are expected to be able to perform all the functions of their job. This includes lifting, handling stress, prioritizing patient care, assessing the situation quickly and accurately, keeping themselves and their crew safe, controlling chaotic situations, and dealing with grieving family members. In order to do all of these things, paramedics must take care of themselves outside of the job. They need to keep physically fit, know safe lifting techniques, maintain flexibility, eat right, and much more, as suggested in this book. The following questions pertain to taking care of yourself in order to perform your job at the highest level you can.

1. **Wellness has how many defined dimensions?**
   A. Two—physical and mental
   B. Three—physical, mental, emotional
   C. Three—physical, mental, and spiritual
   D. Four—physical, mental, emotional, and spiritual

2. **Which of these is NOT recommended for paramedics to help themselves stay fit and prepared for their job duties?**
   A. Carrying bottled water instead of buying soft drinks during shifts
   B. Making sure to take vitamins daily
   C. Eating several small, nutritious snacks
   D. Minimizing intake of caffeine

3. **During any given shift you go on approximately seven calls that involve moving quickly, lifting patients, and other related movement. Does this meet the criteria for "regular vigorous exercise"?**
   A. Yes. It gets your heart rate up and exercises various muscles several times during shifts.
   B. No. Regular vigorous exercise means approximately 30 minutes of cardiovascular exercise involving various muscle groups four to five times a week.

4. **What is the suggested exercise program for paramedics?**
   A. Muscle size improvement, cardiovascular endurance, and lifting capabilities
   B. Cardiovascular endurance, flexibility, and physical strength
   C. Flexibility, increasing amounts of weight able to be lifted, and cardiovascular endurance
   D. Physical strength, cardiovascular strength, and concentration on developing muscles most frequently injured in EMS

5. **True or false? Fight-or-flight syndrome can always help in EMS by giving you the energy boost you need to handle a crisis situation.**
   A. True
   B. False

6. **True or false? There is good stress (eustress) and bad stress (distress).**
   A. True
   B. False

7. **Which one of the following is NOT a reaction identified as occurring in multiple-casualty incidents?**
   A. Overreaction—talking or joking inappropriately or racing from one task to another without accomplishing anything
   B. Blind panic—person's judgment seems to disappear entirely
   C. Coping—finding small ways to cope with a situation
   D. Conversion hysteria—patient or bystander subconsciously converts own anxiety into a bodily dysfunction

8. **A patient with serious internal injuries asks you point blank, "Am I going to die?" What would be the best response to this question?**
   A. Be honest, and say that the outlook is not good.
   B. Reassure her that things will be fine.
   C. Be honest but reserved. Assure her that you and all other medical personnel will do your very best to take care of her, but that the situation is serious.
   D. Avoid the question by explaining each procedure you perform on the way to the hospital.

9. **Which of the following is NOT a suggested guideline for helping a grieving family cope with their loved one's death?**
   A. Do not try to hide the body of their loved one from them; give them time alone with the body if requested.
   B. Do not be in a hurry to clear away all resuscitation equipment that was used. Let them see everything possible was done to save their loved one.
   C. Use softer words to present the information, such as "he passed away" or "he's expired."
   D. Accept any feelings the family may go through in your presence, including anger directed toward you.

Challenging Questions

10. **If you cannot easily stay up late at night, be alert during the night, or get up early, can you still successfully work in EMS?**

11. **List some activities and approaches that will help you keep a positive perspective while working in a stressful field.**

12. **A common reaction among paramedics is irritation at being called to help a patient who does not seem particularly ill. When you receive this kind of call, what should you consider?**

Points to Ponder

You are called to the home of a frequent caller for the general complaint of "not feeling well." This person usually calls when she is depressed and lonely, and does not usually have any medical conditions that you can treat. Sometimes, after talking, she says she feels better and refuses transport. Your partner is familiar with her as well. Because of past situations, your partner says you should take your time getting to the scene, neither of you should waste a pair of gloves going in because she is never ill or injured, and the two of you should get through the call as quickly as possible so that you can respond to those who actually need help.

Should you listen to your partner? Should you wear gloves?

Issues: Treating Each Patient, Serving as a Role Model for Scene Safety, Empathy, Working With Other Paramedics.

3 Illness and Injury Prevention

Competency Areas

Area 1: Professional Responsibilities

1.1.g   Utilize community support agencies as appropriate.

1.1.h   Promote awareness of emergency medical system and profession.

1.1.k   Function as patient advocate.

1.2.b   Self-evaluate and set goals for improvement, as related to professional practice.

▌Injury Prevention and EMS

Several years ago, San Diego paramedic Paul Maxwell went on a drowning call. A 2-year-old boy had wandered away from a day care facility and fallen into a neighbour's backyard pool. Despite everyone's best efforts, he could not be resuscitated. The mother was inconsolable, and her cries haunted the paramedic. Maxwell wondered how such tragedies could be prevented—if he could help it, he never wanted to go on another call like that again. Doing a little investigation, and looking up incidents on his EMS system's database, he discovered a pattern of increased drownings in his region. Maxwell made the decision to get involved. In cooperation with his EMS agency, he contacted other groups in his community with an interest in child safety. Using his system's data and motivated by his firsthand knowledge of the suffering that such a death inflicts, Maxwell began a coordinated and successful effort to reduce backyard pool drownings in his community, through both legislation and education. Although the reduction in drownings was incentive enough for Maxwell, he was recognized with a special award by the state of California.

More than a few paramedics have been motivated by their experiences to work actively on prevention. Throughout Canada, paramedics are taking the lead or providing support in a wide variety of interventions—specific prevention measures or activities designed to increase positive health and safety outcomes ▶ **Figure 3-1 ▶** . From beginnings such as these, EMS has emerged as a strong advocate—and practitioner—of injury prevention. Few paramedics see the scene of an injury as a whole: the physical situation, the design flaws in home or highway, and the tragic stress of trauma.

Paramedics, of course, participate in illness prevention such as flu inoculation programs or blood pressure monitoring. However, illness prevention programs are often well-focused by physicians and public health officials. This chapter focuses on injury because of your unique perspective on injuries. Few providers in a hospital or a physician's office are conscious of the physical situation of an accident site for example, or the number of times an incident has occurred at that site. You are uniquely aware. The principles and techniques for illness prevention are not substantially different from those for injury prevention. If you discover a need for a prevention program—perhaps some of your elderly patients might not be getting their influenza or pneumococcal vaccines—by all means, apply the principles.

Common Roots

Injury prevention shares the common root of EMS: the historic National Academy of Sciences/National Research Council 1966 study, "Accidental Death and Disability: The Neglected Disease of Modern Society." The commission noted that just as EMS could help with trauma after an event, injury prevention initiatives could help before an accident happened.

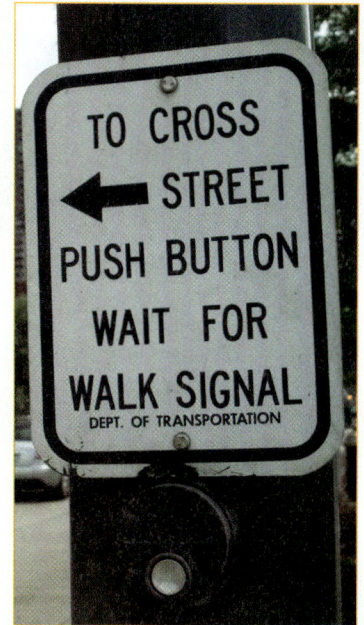

Figure 3-1 Many rules of public safety exist because of the persistent efforts of medical professionals and other involved citizens.

Strengthening this link, the broader definition of injury prevention has always included EMS. Primary injury prevention is defined as keeping an injury from ever occurring. EMS traditionally has focused on secondary injury prevention, reducing the effects of an injury that has already happened. (For the inquiring mind, a third area, tertiary prevention, is defined as the effort to rehabilitate a person who has survived an injury.)

In 1996, the *Consensus Statement on the EMS Role in Primary Injury Prevention* was published. Representing every imaginable EMS constituency, the authors of the statement made clear that primary injury prevention is an "essential" activity "that must

You are the Paramedic Part 1

For the third time in as many months you respond to a call in the same stretch of highway—a winding road along the top of a river gorge. Too many times, the patient is a drunk driver who couldn't negotiate the curve and plunged over the side, unimpeded by guardrails. More often than not, the driver is not wearing a seatbelt. The tragic scenario plays itself out: the driver is thrown from the vehicle, and he or she is severely injured. Your team has a long and treacherous extrication, working on a steep hillside. Everyone on the team knows it will be dangerous. No one has to say it, but you know that the whole team is tempted to think: "Stupid drunks."

This time the driver is a man in his mid-20s. He will live, but appears to have suffered severe head and neck injuries and may never walk again. Later you find out he has a wife and two children, and was coming home after having a few beers at a local tavern after work. By all accounts he is a loving father and husband. He made a mistake, you think, but did he deserve this? After paramedic training, you now wonder, what can I do to prevent another tragedy like this?

1. Why should you consider getting involved in preventing these injuries?
2. What are the risk factors associated with the injuries described here?

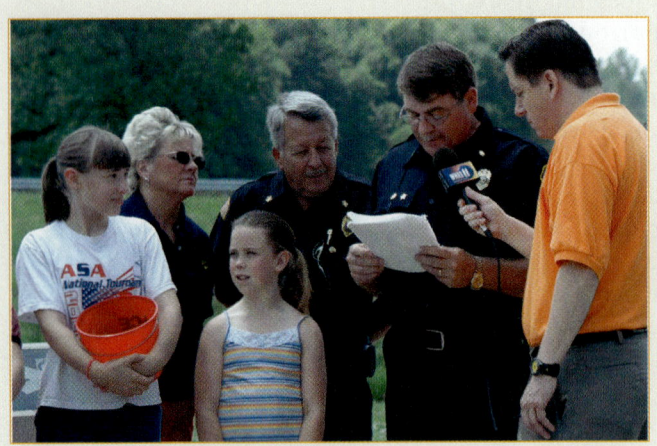

Figure 3-2 Embracing the full role of a paramedic means being involved in the concerns of your community.

Why EMS Should Be Involved

Leaders in both EMS and the prevention field offer the following rationale:

- Paramedics are widely distributed in the population.
- Paramedics reflect the composition of the community they serve.
- In many rural communities, the paramedic might be the most medically sophisticated person.
- If properly coordinated, EMS would provide a formidable resource in the effort to reduce the overall injury burden.
- Paramedics are high-profile role models.
- Paramedics are perceived as champions of their patients.
- Paramedics are welcome in schools and other environments conducive to delivering the prevention message.
- Because they face the results of injuries every day, EMS providers are perceived as authorities on injury and prevention. (A paramedic talking to a city council about drowning prevention legislation, relating a true story about the suffering he or she witnessed, can be an extremely effective teacher.)

be undertaken by the leaders, decision-makers, and providers of every EMS system." The Paramedic Association of Canada and EMS Chiefs of Canada are now advocating that community paramedicine and injury prevention be included in upcoming revisions of the National Occupational Competency Profiles.

Of course, the number one priority for paramedics is to be prepared to respond and treat the injuries that will inevitably occur in their communities. And all paramedics in particularly busy systems will find that time for prevention initiatives will be limited. However, there is a role for every paramedic, at some level, in primary injury prevention **Figure 3-2 ▲**. This includes, first and foremost, teaching others in the health care system and the public *why* you see an injury recurring at the same place.

Injuries as Public Health Threat

Injuries, according to the US National Center for Injury Prevention and Control, part of the Centers for Disease Control and Prevention (CDC), are "the intentional or unintentional damage to the person resulting from acute exposure to thermal, mechanical, electrical, or chemical energy or from the absence of such essentials as heat or oxygen." Historically, injuries were not grouped together. Instead, they were reported under distinct umbrellas, which made it difficult to let the lay population see just how widespread injuries truly are **Figure 3-3 ▶**. Grouping injuries as a common health problem makes it possible to consider the breadth and depth of the problem. It has enabled public health officials and other care providers to call attention to important problems and target more effective interventions.

Intentional injuries, such as assaults or suicide, are included in the definition. EMS can often play a supporting role here too, but can usually have a greater impact in preventing unintentional injuries.

How big a problem are injuries in Canada? To many health experts, it is the largest public health problem facing the country today. According to data collected by the

Notes from Nancy

In addition to being a health care provider, the paramedic—like any other health professional—must also be a health *educator*. Teaching helps the paramedic keep his or her own skills sharp; at the same time, teaching *identifies* the paramedic as a resource person in the community.

Documentation and Communication

Do not forget special population groups in your safety and prevention programs. For instance, there may be different illness and injury patterns related to ethnicity and you can present these topics through your programs. Have printed materials available in all languages spoken throughout your community. Do not neglect people with physical and developmental challenges. Do your best to get the word out in every way possible.

Special Considerations

With a growing geriatric population, a good fall prevention program may be one of the keys to preventing an overload of the health care system. Evaluate all community options available to the older population in your area and bridge any gaps with programs to meet their needs and prevent injuries related to falls.

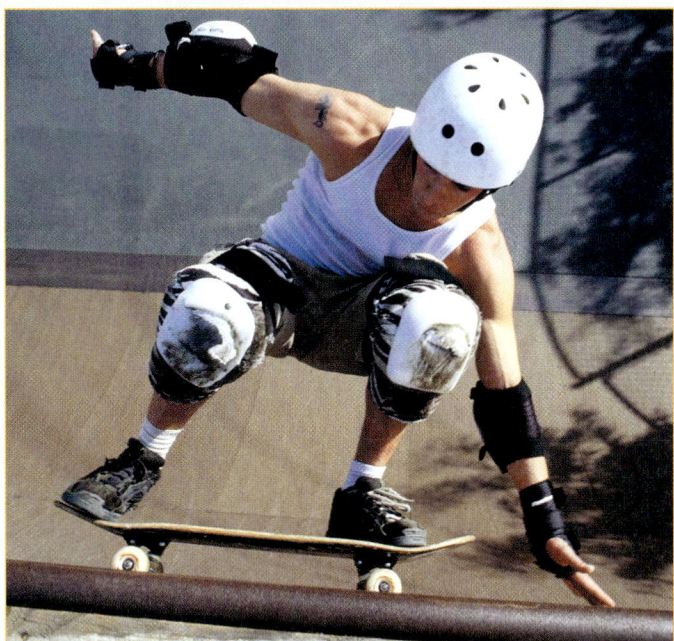

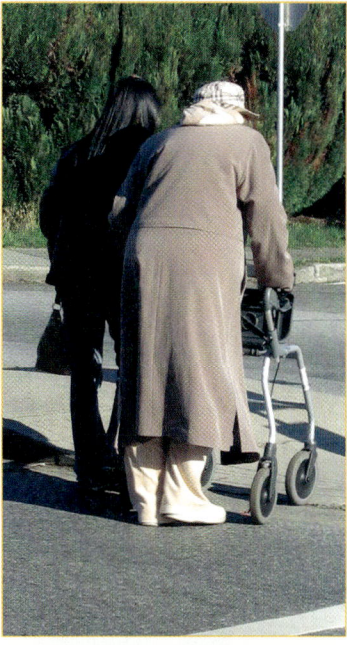

Figure 3-3 Injuries affect people of all age groups and physical abilities. For each potential injury, there are appropriate preventive measures that can and should be taken.

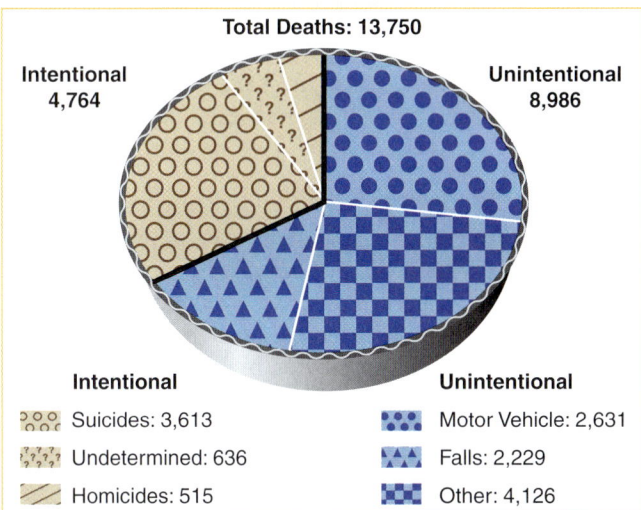

Total Deaths: 13,750

Intentional 4,764   Unintentional 8,986

Intentional
- Suicides: 3,613
- Undetermined: 636
- Homicides: 515

Unintentional
- Motor Vehicle: 2,631
- Falls: 2,229
- Other: 4,126

Figure 3-4 The vast majority of injuries that occur are unintentional—particularly accidents related to driving.

- There were a total of 227,281 hospitalizations due to injury with 111,489 related to falls and 19,783 related to motor vehicle traffic collisions.

Table 3-1 ▸ shows the top 10 causes of death in Canada in 2004. This information is extremely important in understanding how injury impacts different age groups. From ages 1 to 34 years, unintentional injuries are the leading killer. For all ages combined, unintentional injuries are the sixth leading killer.

How much do these injuries cost society, above and beyond the tremendous personal suffering? It is estimated unintentional injuries account for more than $8.7 billion. There is another concept that researchers are using to measure the cost to society: years of potential life lost. It works like this: assume a productive work life until age 65, and deduct the year of death from that age. Thus, an 18-year-old who dies in a car crash has lost 47 years of potential productive work life, whereas someone who dies of a stroke at age 63 years has lost 2 years. Because injuries are a leading cause of death in the young, it quickly adds up **Figure 3-5 ▸**. This method allows a comparison of the years of productive work life lost, disease by disease. This method can measure how many years of usefulness to society a child killed in an accident could have had, comparing those years to those of an older person who, for example, had a myocardial infarction. The value of the comparison is to teach members of your community that the prevention of a childhood accident is of great importance to the community.

It's easier to measure death rates than to measure nonfatal (morbidity) injury rates, because visits to clinics, emergency departments, doctors' offices, and other places for treatment

Public Health Agency of Canada, in 2004 (the latest available year for figures) **Figure 3-4 ▴** :
- In total, 13,750 people died as a result of injury.
- Of those, 8,986 died of unintentional injuries (2,631 motor vehicle traffic collisions and 2,229 falls) and 4,764 died of intentional injuries (3,613 suicides, 636 deaths, and 515 homicides were undetermined).

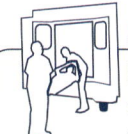

At the Scene

Unintentional falls are the second leading cause of unintentional death behind motor vehicle collisions.

Table 3-1	Top 10 Causes of Death in 2004

1. Circulatory system diseases
2. Cancer
3. Respiratory system diseases
4. Nervous system diseases
5. Endocrine, nutrition, and metabolic diseases
6. Unintentional injuries
7. Digestive system diseases
8. Mental disorders
9. Genitourinary diseases
10. Infectious and parasitic diseases

Source: Leading Causes of Death and Hospitalization in Canada', Table 1: Leading causes of death, males and females combined, www.phac-aspc.gc.ca/publicat/lcd-pcd97/index-eng.php, Public Health Agency of Canada, 2004. Reproduced with the permission of the Minister of Public Works and Government Services Canada, 2009.

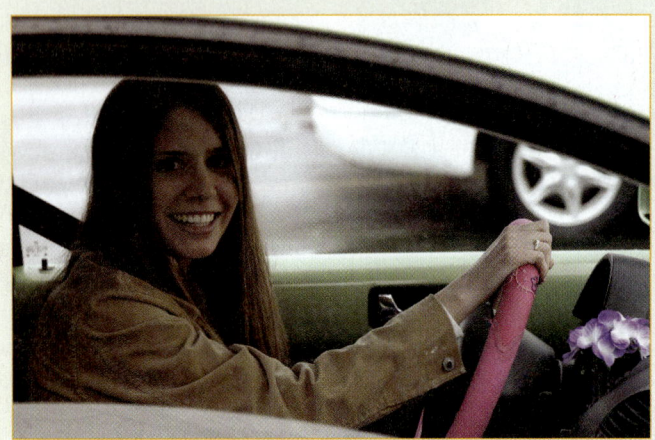

Figure 3-5 The regular use of a seatbelt can have a dramatic effect on the number of years of potential life lost—particularly in younger age groups.

are scattered in a number of agencies and professional groups. In 2004, more than 200,000 Canadians were hospitalized due to unintentional injuries.

▌Principles of Injury Prevention

The 4 Es of Prevention

An injury risk is a potentially hazardous situation in which the well-being of people can be harmed. Interventions need to combine *education* with three other types of interventions: *enforcement, engineering/environment,* and *economic incentives.* These are commonly referred to as the 4 Es of injury prevention [**Figure 3-6 ▸**]. The most effective injury prevention efforts reflect a combination of these interventions.

Education

Most paramedics know that people can behave in ways that cause them to become injured or put others at risk. Many people do not know and therefore cannot assess the risk of doing something—"I didn't know it was unsafe to put my baby's seat in the front passenger seat." Or people know the risk—"I won't wear seatbelts, they are too uncomfortable"—and disregard it anyway. Through education we can often inform people about potential dangers and then act to persuade them to change risky behaviour. Show moms and dads how to use an infant car seat. Tell people about the horrors of being thrown from a vehicle.

To be effective, messages need to be tailored to very specific groups and reinforced with meaningful rewards. Educational techniques that seem to be particularly promising include the use of contracts or participant commitment, incentives, behavioural feedback, and modelling.

However, despite your best efforts, some members of your community may know about a risk but their behaviour will not necessarily change. There are even some paramedics who refuse to wear seatbelts on their rigs! A crucial advantage of any educational effort is that it can pave the way to legislative and environmental/technological changes.

Enforcement

Behaviour can be forced to change by law (that is why it is called law enforcement). Legislation/regulation formulates rules that require individuals, manufacturers, and governments to comply with certain safety practices. Legislation is made by elected government bodies enacting laws that require safe practices. Regulations are made by bureaucracies or agencies that set policies and establish procedures that control the manufacture, sale, and/or use of products. Litigation sets policy when lawsuits are brought against manufacturers or distributors of dangerous products. For example, product liability litigation can encourage manufacturers to remove dangerous products from the market or make them safer. All these measures have been shown to be helpful in enforcement of safety regulations.

You are the Paramedic **Part 2**

You decide your best course of action is to enlist the help of law enforcement officers. They know vehicle collision prevention and detect patterns in highway death and injury. You decide to call your local law enforcement agencies to begin your quest to minimize death and disability resulting from motor vehicle collisions at this particular stretch of road.

3. Which law enforcement agencies could you contact?

4. Who else might be able to help you in assessing road conditions?

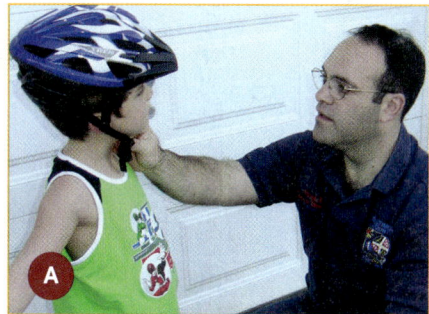
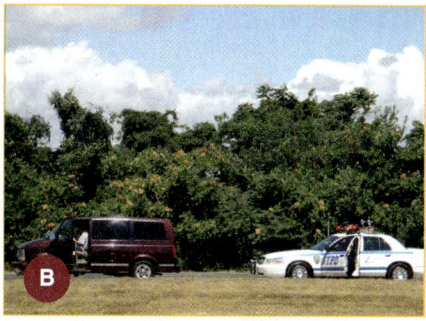
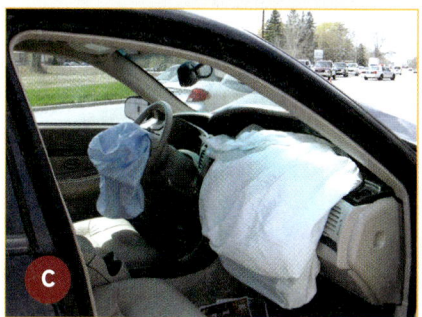
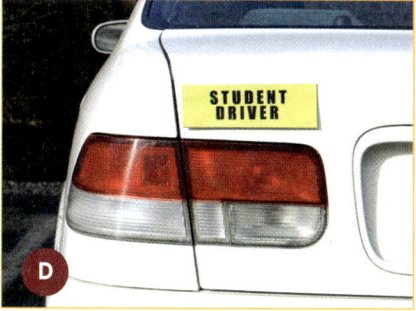

Figure 3-6 A. The four Es of injury prevention start with education. **B.** and **C.** Enforcement and engineering/environment contribute as well. **D.** Economic incentives, such as lower insurance rates for young drivers who have taken approved driver education programs, complete the picture.

Engineering/Environment

Most paramedics know spots where adding guardrails or smoothing out dangerous curves in a road could prevent collisions. Changing the design of products or spaces such as roads can offer automatic protection from injury, often without any conscious change of behaviour by the individual. These are called passive interventions.

For example, making child-resistant bottles is a passive intervention that reduces poisonings, and can be more effective than trying to keep the bottle out of children's reach. Strategies to change the environment can include social, legal, political, and cultural approaches. Environmental modifications, which are often expensive, usually happen when the community's awareness of the problem is raised, causing that community to accept responsibility for change.

At the Scene

The less the personal effort required, the greater the chance that the interventions will be successful.

Economic Incentives

Economic self-interest—saving money on health care costs or insurance rate reduction for careful drivers—provides monetary incentives to reinforce safe behaviour. The threat of lawsuits (and significant monetary damages) often causes manufacturers to improve the safety of consumer products—an economic loss that serves as an incentive to change behaviour. Organizations also recognize the value of offering free or subsidized safety products (bike helmets, fire extinguishers, safety locks) to encourage use.

The Value of Automatic Protections

Passive interventions—those that do not require a conscious decision to act—are often the most successful of all interventions. This approach is also referred to as automatic protection. Examples include the use of sprinkler systems in commercial buildings, air bags in vehicles, or the use of softer, yielding materials for playground surfaces. These measures provide 24-hour protection without requiring a conscious action or decision on the part of the user.

Consider the following injury prevention strategies, comparing education to automatic protection, in the case of head and chest injuries of drivers in motor vehicle collisions:

- **Option 1.** Educate people to buckle up every time they drive.
- **Option 2.** Require that car manufacturers install automatic seatbelts and air bags.

The automatic protection offered by option 2 is more likely to reduce injuries because people do not have to do anything to protect themselves each time they are at risk. Again, however, a combination of approaches—education, enforcement, engineering/environmental modifications, and economic incentives—will result in the most effective strategy. Note that education is still an important aspect of the above examples. Motor vehicle passengers need to know that air bags do not replace the need for seatbelts.

Models for Injury Prevention

A variety of visual models have been created to describe a health problem and how to approach it. The public health model identifies and seeks to control three factors: the host, the agent, and the environment. The public health model triumphed in the prevention and control of diseases such as malaria and polio, sometimes by attacking only two parts of the model. For example, to prevent malaria, you might develop a vaccine, spray pesticides to kill mosquitoes, and/or drain swamps to keep mosquitoes from breeding. These approaches target the host (people), the agent (mosquitoes), and the environment (swamps).

The public health model has been applied to a variety of injury problems. If you add the 4 Es of injury prevention, you can think through appropriate strategies for each part of the model (the host, the agent, and the environment). **Figure 3-7 ▸** sets out the three parts of the public health model using the example of bicycle-vehicle collisions.

The Haddon Matrix

William Haddon, Jr, MD, the US National Highway Traffic Safety Administration's first director, had a mandate to find ways to prevent people from being killed and injured on US highways. Haddon created a matrix that identified several principles of injury prevention. The matrix proved so successful in helping researchers think about injuries, that it was named after Haddon: the Haddon matrix.

Haddon added the factor of *time* to the previous models used to address the causes of injury. The host, agent, and environment are seen as factors that interact over time to cause injury. These factors correspond to three phases of the event: pre-event, event, and post-event. The matrix uses nine separate components to analyze the injury. The Haddon matrix encourages creative thinking in understanding the causes of and potential interventions for injury. **Table 3-2 ▸** shows a Haddon matrix for the example of bicycle-vehicle collisions.

Most paramedics are trained to respond to the post-event—the period of time after an injury has already occurred. The 9-1-1 call is received by the emergency medical dispatcher who sends a service unit to the scene. There, the team members administer emergency prehospital care, a form of secondary intervention that can change the outcome, severity, or result of the event.

You can use the Haddon matrix to trigger your fellow paramedics and others in the community to think about and plan for strategies before the 9-1-1 call comes through. The pre-event phase can get everyone brainstorming about everything that can be done to prevent an injury from occurring. The event phase can get all people involved thinking about interventions to minimize an injury at the time of the event. The post-event phase can address ways to lessen the severity of the injury once it has occurred.

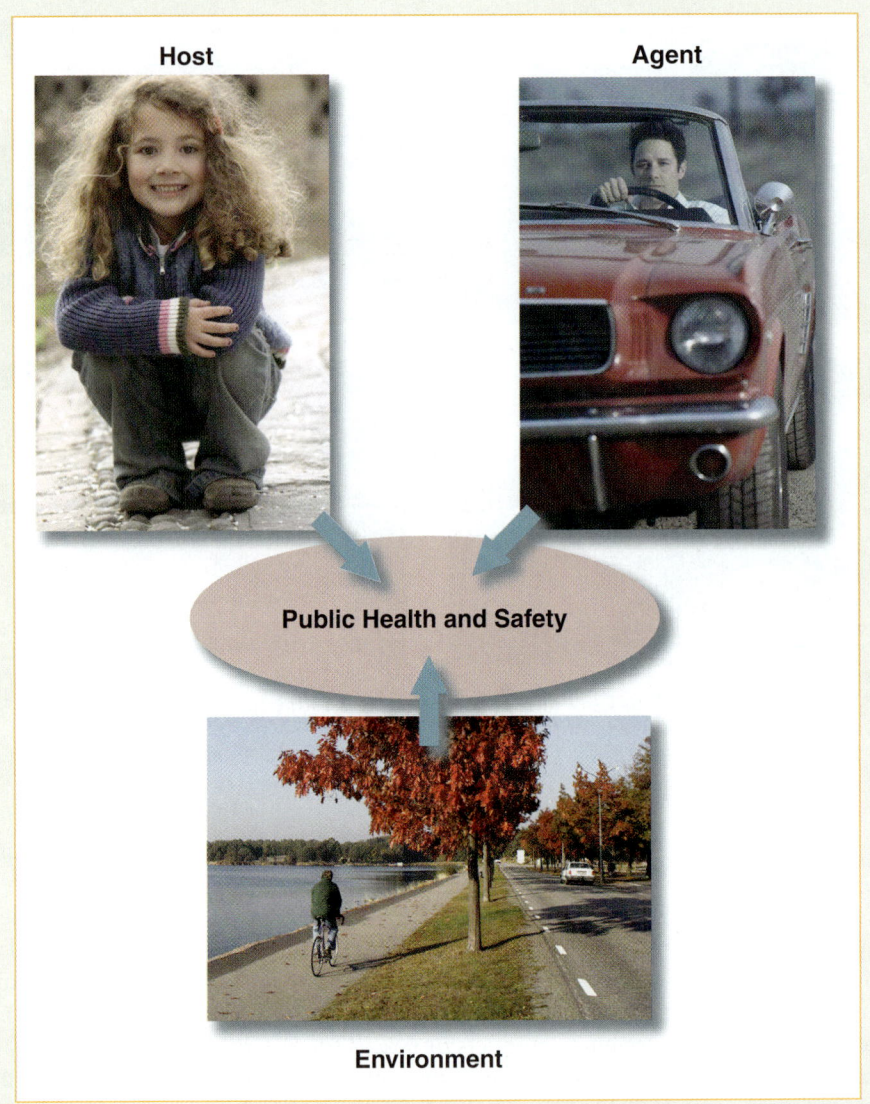

Host

Agent

Public Health and Safety

Environment

Figure 3-7 For bicycle-vehicle collisions, the public health model suggests the need to educate the child (*host*) and driver (*agent*) about safety, minimize the danger of serious injury through the required use of helmets, and perhaps create independent bike paths to separate children from traffic (*environment*).

Injury prevention requires broad and innovative thinking to be most successful. The Haddon matrix helps you to think through which interventions can be effective at certain points in time. Addressing injury prevention within the context of a timeline—pre-event, event, and post-event—can expand our problem-solving capabilities beyond the answer of more education. Blaming the parent for lack of supervision or the driver for going too fast does not generate solutions to the problem of childhood injury. You can generate solutions with physical and measurable attributes using the Haddon matrix as a guide.

Table 3-2	Childhood Motor Vehicle Occupant Injuries Using the Haddon Matrix		
	Host (Human)	**Agent (Car Seat/Vehicle)**	**Environment**
Pre-event	• Wear seatbelt and use car seat at all times. • Make sure babysitter, day care, and extended family members use car seat. • Drive defensively. • Reduce driving during high-risk times, such as rush hour, holiday weekends, or high-speed long-distance travel.	• Maintain up-to-date recall information on car seats. • Manufacture easy-to-use car seats. • Provide 3-point seatbelts in rear seating positions. • Regulate good maintenance and safety features of vehicle.	• Enforce seatbelt and car seat laws. • Encourage safer roads with lower speeds, breakaway poles, and medians. • Encourage low-cost car seat programs. • Conduct media and education campaigns about seatbelts, car seats, drunk driving, and enforcement.
Event	• Driver maintains control of vehicle. • Driver is belted. • Child is restrained.	• Seatbelts and correctly used car seats restrain and protect. • Vehicle design provides collision protection.	• Breakaway signs and light poles are in place. • Guardrails and medians are in place.
Post-event	• Bystanders are trained in first response. • Paramedics are expertly trained in treating pediatric injuries as well as car seat and seatbelt extrications.	• Ambulances are outfitted with up-to-date supplies and equipment designed for children.	• Roadside call boxes are in place. • 9-1-1 and emergency medical dispatch systems are in place. • Adequate road shoulders for emergency use are in place. • There is quality paramedic response and transport. • A trauma centre is nearby.

Injury Surveillance

Surveillance in injury prevention does *not* mean watching over a criminal suspect! In injury prevention, it means watching over society by collecting and analyzing injury data. Injury surveillance is the ongoing, systematic collection, analysis, and interpretation of injury data essential to the planning, implementation, and evaluation of public health practice Figure 3-8 ▶ . These data are collected and then carefully disseminated to individuals or organizations who can use the data to affect change. The final link in the surveillance chain is the application of these data to interventions aimed at preventing injuries.

A strong surveillance system is fundamental to creating an effective injury prevention program. To do the most good, you need to know who is being injured, where, and by what mechanism. The news media may focus on a dramatic incident

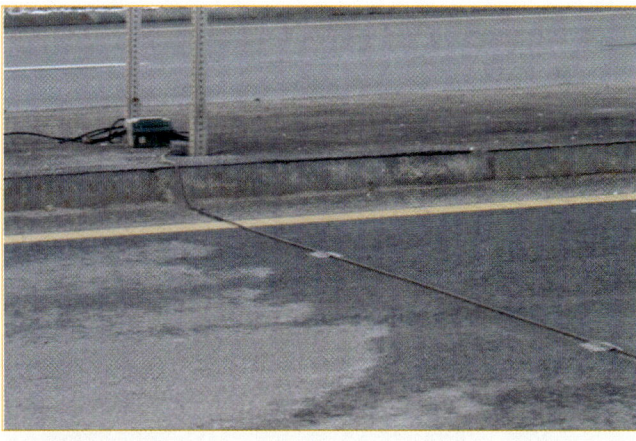

Figure 3-8 One type of surveillance that is familiar to anyone who drives is the use of technology that can tally the number of cars using a particular roadway.

where a dozen people are severely injured, but surveillance data might show that a commonplace, but less newsworthy injury (such as falls among older people) is a greater threat to the community and more easily remedied. As part of the health system, paramedics need to focus on injury prevention. Do not let the headlines be your guide.

Controversies

There is a theory that says if people keep falling off a mountain you should put a fence around the mountain to keep people from climbing it. Another theory says that you should tear down the mountain so that people can't fall off it. Yet another theory says that if you educate people on safe climbing you can prevent them from falling. Finally, there are some who believe an ambulance should be parked at the base of the mountain to save the people who keep falling. So goes the controversy of injury and potential interventions.

Getting Started in Your Community

An abundance of problems faces every community. Each community requires the assessment of the problems that are impairing the health of the largest number of people. Otherwise, you may be overwhelmed with the enormity of the task.

📻 Documentation and Communication

Good documentation on prehospital care reports allows for more consistencies in data gathering, surveillance, and predictions of injury trends.

There is a good chance that, eventually, you can roll up your sleeves and dig in to remedy even the problems that arise from the social conditions causing some injuries. But it will give you and your community a good feeling to address a problem that will have the maximum impact on the community's well-being.

Recognizing Injury Patterns in Your Community

To be effective in prevention, you need to understand the patterns of injuries that occur in your community and learn the characteristics of its population and environment and the types of risks that are present. Your regional or provincial EMS department or public health office will have the most data about injury statistics and is a good starting place to gather information. Many provinces have this information on the Internet. A wide variety of other resources are readily available online, including detailed information about specific problems, case studies, and expert assistance.

Intentional Injuries

Intentional injuries include suicides and suicide attempts, homicides, nonfatal batterings, violent assaults on women (including rapes and spousal abuse), and child and elder maltreatment **Figure 3-9 ▾** .

In 2004 there were 515 homicides and 3,613 suicides. It is estimated that nearly 5,000 intentional injuries are inflicted each year. Researchers are studying the causes of intentional violence in Canada. Certain factors emerge as numerically connected with intentional violence: being male, access to firearms, alcohol abuse, history of childhood maltreatment, mental illness, and poverty. These are all risk factors—characteristics that increase the chances of disease or injury.

It is often overwhelming to consider solutions when the challenges are linked to deeply rooted social ills. How can EMS personnel prevent intentional violence when it is clear that the scope of the problem is a wide one?

One way paramedics have played important supporting roles in programs that seek to reduce suicide, domestic violence, and child maltreatment is by carefully reporting data and noting risk factors while on the scene. Also, paramedics can be taught to identify injuries and risk factors associated with domestic violence or child maltreatment, and report them to the proper channels.

Remember, you are about to become a paramedic. What you do, your expectations of yourself, and your role will filter down to the other members of your crew. Being a conscientious observer will set an example.

Unintentional Injuries

Unintentional injuries have no premeditation; we often call them accidents. **Table 3-3 ▾** shows the top 6 causes of deaths from injury in 2004. Motor vehicle incidents account for the most unintentional deaths, followed by falls, poisonings, suffocations, drowning, and fires and burns. Almost all motor vehicle deaths are classified as unintentional.

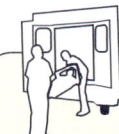

🚑 At the Scene

Remember, you are also a member of "the public" so practice a safe lifestyle on and off the job. Wear seatbelts, safety helmets, and observe safety laws in everything you do.

Figure 3-9 Intentional injuries include all cases of domestic and child maltreatment. As citizens and medical professionals, we are obligated to report all incidents of maltreatment or potentially abusive situations.

Table 3-3	Top 6 Causes of Death From Injury in 2004
1. Motor vehicle collisions	
2. Falls	
3. Poisoning	
4. Suffocation	
5. Drowning	
6. Fire and flame	

Source: Adapted from Public Health Agency of Canada, 2004.

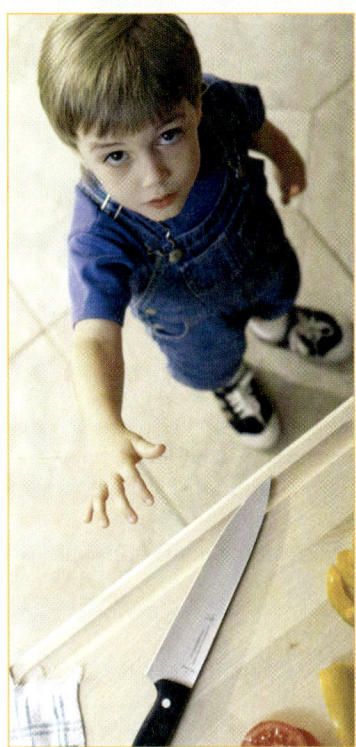

Figure 3-10 Children are at higher risk of sustaining serious injuries from an accident. Parents should always be aware of the potential dangers in reach of a child.

Unintentional Injuries in Children

Many prevention programs have been strongly linked to children, for good reason. Each year 20% to 25% of *all* children sustain an injury sufficiently severe to require medical attention, miss school, and/or require bed rest. Their developing bodies, including a larger head in proportion to the body, thinner skin, and a smaller airway, put them at higher risk of injury and of being more seriously affected by the injury than adults. Each year more than 30,000 injured children require medical treatment **Figure 3-10** ◂ .

Grants, partners, and commercial sponsors support car seat inspections or donations of bike helmets for children because communities recognize that children are at risk. An additional reason to focus on children's issues is the "pass-along effect." Other family members benefit from the message too, such as when a third-grader insists that Daddy buckle up too.

The Safe Kids Canada Campaign is part of a worldwide organization that raises public awareness and is dedicated to reducing childhood injuries. It has an excellent Web site, which can easily be found by looking up the name in a search engine.

Risk Factors for Children

Children at greatest risk of injury are of lower socioeconomic status. The patterns of injury will differ from community to community, but just as the poorest children statistically are at risk of contracting a disease, they are also at risk of injury.

The US CDC reports that home injuries of children occur most frequently where there is/are:

- Water, such as in the kitchen or bathroom, or a backyard swimming pool.
- Intense heat, such as in the kitchen or a backyard barbecue.
- Toxic agents, such as in the kitchen, bathroom, garage, or in a purse.
- High potential "energy," such as in stairwells or loaded firearms.

Many community members have a common belief that schools have become more violent and that intentional injuries are an increasing threat to students. However, *unintentional* injuries—accidents—still represent a much greater threat to health. School injuries occur most frequently during sports activities, industrial arts classes, and on playgrounds.

With the wide variety of injuries affecting children, how do we prioritize prevention efforts? Experts in public health suggest focusing on injuries that have high mortality (death) rates or hospitalization rates, that have a high long-term disability rate, or that have effective countermeasures. The highest priorities are assigned to those types of injuries that are common, severe, and readily preventable.

Community Organizing

Those in EMS who have created successful prevention programs give the following advice for building a team and creating an implementation plan:

- Identify a lead person to coordinate the effort.
- Build as broad a base of support as possible.
- Create a realistic time line for any project, keeping in mind that most must be ongoing to be effective.
- Gather data and facts that pinpoint who is being injured where, with what, and how frequently.
- Choose goals and objectives that are SMART—Simple, Measurable, Accurate, Reportable, and Trackable; build consensus in the community on the need for action.
- Make sure you understand the religious, ethnic, cultural, and language challenges that you may face in implementing an intervention.
- Don't reinvent the wheel—seek out others who have had success with similar interventions or who have expertise in public health.
- Anticipate opposition and expect some losses; turf battles are common but not inevitable.

You are the Paramedic **Part 3**

You have enlisted the help of many different organizations who are now as determined as you are to minimize the recurrence of collisions in this stretch of road. They aid you in performing assessments of the area and making plans to prevent crashes.

5. What groups are potential partners to enlist in a prevention program in this situation?

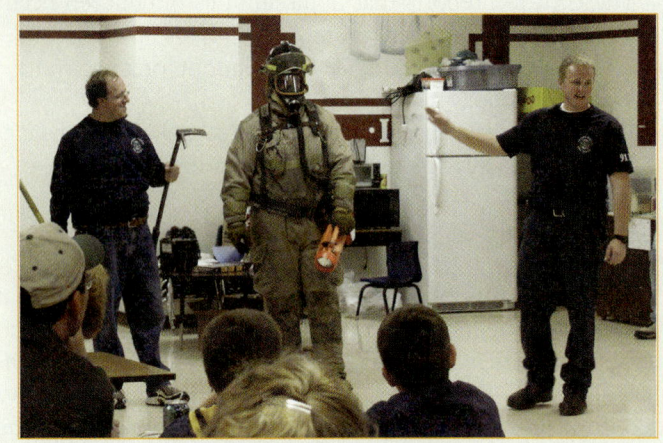

Figure 3-11 An example of an injury prevention program is training to avoid injury in the event of a fire in the home.

- As you lobby to legislators, be brief in phone calls, visits, and testimony.
- Set up your program so that you can measure results and make changes as needed.
- Establish self-sustaining funding sources.
- Keep a sense of humour and persist—change doesn't happen overnight.

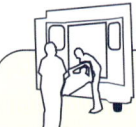

At the Scene

For your first project, start small with realistic goals.

The Five Steps to Developing a Prevention Program

This step-by-step approach to establishing an injury prevention program emphasizes the need to carefully establish goals and objectives with measurable outcomes. (Although the following discusses childhood prevention programs, the methods can be applied to other age groups and their problems.)

1. Conduct a Community Assessment

Bring individuals and groups together to assess what is already being accomplished in your region and to establish what resources (expertise, time, money) are potentially available. Make sure to invite people who represent the community at large, in all its diversity, including survivors of injuries and their families Figure 3-11 ▲ . Potential partners include:

- EMS groups (private and public ground and air ambulance services, fire departments and fire fighter unions, volunteer services, rescue squads, lifeguards)
- Law enforcement (police departments and police officers, unions, sheriff's office, highway patrol, training academies)
- School groups (parent-teacher associations, student clubs, school boards, faculty)
- The media (management, editorial board members, staff reporters)
- Public health officials and health care providers (groups representing emergency physicians and nurses, pediatricians, hospitals, clinics)
- Members of the business community (including those related to insurance, cars, sports, home improvements, safety equipment, local chambers of commerce)
- Religious organizations, civic groups, and service clubs (such as the Kiwanis and the Boy Scouts and Girl Scouts)
- Sports-related organizations (such as Little Leagues or YMCAs)
- Local chapters of nonprofit groups (such as SAFE KIDS Coalitions, Mothers Against Drunk Driving [MADD], the Canadian Red Cross, the Canadian Alzheimer Society)
- Local and national celebrities, community leaders, and elected officials
- Research groups (such as those at universities, private colleges, community colleges)

2. Define the Injury Problem

On the basis of the community assessment and the data you've been able to gather, define the problem in specific quantifiable terms. For example, you should be able to answer the following questions for your community:

- What are the most frequent causes of fatal and nonfatal childhood injuries?
- What populations (by age, location, and other characteristics) are at highest risk of these injuries? When and where are they occurring?
- Using the Haddon matrix, what other factors are associated with these causes?
- What, if anything, is already being done to prevent these injuries?
- Is there an effective intervention available? What resources do you have in order to develop, implement, and evaluate different interventions?

3. Set Goals and Objectives

Goals Make this a broad, general statement about the long-term changes the prevention initiatives are designed to make. (For example, a goal can be to decrease preventable injuries to children on the community's roadways.)

Objectives Make these specific, time-limited, and quantifiable. There are two types: process objectives (1,000 child safety seats will be distributed to low-income families within the next 18 months) and outcome (impact) objectives (the bicycle safety program will increase the rate of helmet use by children younger than 18 years from 30% to 50% within the next 18 months).

4. Plan and Test Interventions

Interventions are the actions you take to accomplish your goals and objectives. Using the 4 Es of prevention and the Haddon matrix, brainstorm options. Consider the resources you have available to commit, and make sure you have thoroughly reviewed what others have already done. You may find communities have had success with similar interventions in similar populations. In that case, you can reliably duplicate their efforts as a process objective. (For example, other groups have shown that bike helmets reduce head injuries; you then need only to demonstrate increased usage of helmets in your targeted population.) Experienced prevention specialists also suggest that you be keenly aware of timing and cultural considerations as you plan your intervention. Getting a sample group together and testing the intervention before actually rolling out the entire program usually helps to improve your chances of success.

5. Implement and Evaluate Interventions

To be credible, your intervention needs to be established so that the results can be measured quantitatively; that is, a formal evaluation will definitely tell you whether you met your goals and objectives. One EMS group knew from previous surveys that the seatbelt usage rate in their community was well below the national average. They established an objective of improving seatbelt usage in their community by 50%. Working with the department of public health in their province, they enacted a series of prevention programs. To measure the effectiveness of different interventions, they put volunteers at selected intersections around the city. They physically counted with a clicker every belted and nonbelted motorist who stopped in front of them. This is extremely important so that your experience can be shared with others. You want to spend your time and resources on efforts you can *show* make a difference. There is a science to planning, implementing, and evaluating an intervention. Seek out others who have knowledge and experience in this facet of injury prevention; it will make for a better program.

Finally, be aware that many, if not most, interventions demand ongoing attention to be effective. Those paramedics who had initial success in reducing backyard drownings saw the numbers go back up a few years after the initial burst of publicity and after enthusiasm for the interventions began to wane. Legislation to fence pools worked well but did not eliminate the problem. They had to gear back up to reestablish the educational interventions that had worked so well originally. Consider building long-term maintenance into any plan to continue the momentum of your program.

Funding a Prevention Program

Ideally, emergency services should have the resources and motivation to include primary prevention activities in their normal operating budget. As a relatively new expansion of the EMS mission, this likely will take time. But motivated services and individuals have found a variety of innovative ways to secure resources including:

- Partnering with the local media to create prevention messages, especially related to seasonal injuries or hazards.
- Seeking grants from regional, provincial, or national organizations. (A good place to start is to contact your provincial EMS office about grant programs.)

- Seeking sponsorships from local nonprofit service organizations or commercial firms, including fire, EMS, and Kiwanis organizations, and car dealerships **Figure 3-12 ▶**.

Networking with other organizations interested in prevention often provides greater leverage in seeking grants or sponsorships. Perhaps the paramedic donates the time of volunteers and is a credible voice in the community, whereas the partner provides organizational resources and knowledge about establishing a scientifically credible injury intervention.

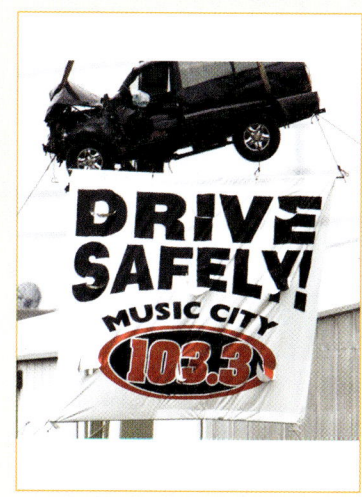

Figure 3-12 Like any successful ad campaign, a public safety program needs to continually remind the public of its message.

How Every Paramedic Can Be Involved

Taking care of patients is the number one job of paramedics. Some won't have the time or inclination to get involved in every aspect of the primary injury prevention measures discussed here. However, there are certain things paramedics can and should do, starting with preventing their own injuries.

Primary injury prevention begins at home, so to speak, by taking care of yourself and at the same time presenting a role model for others in your service and for the community in general. Do you always wear seatbelts, on and off duty? Do you drive safely? Have you prepared yourself physically for the rigors of the job? Do you practice safe lifting techniques? Do you always wear appropriate protective equipment? Do you always maintain scene safety? Your employer will have policies regarding many of these safety issues, but it's up to you to implement them and to take seriously the risks you face everyday on and off the job. Refer back to Chapter 2 to review the appropriate use of personal protective equipment and practices.

Responding to the Call

Perhaps the most ironic, if not most tragic, of all injuries are those caused when an ambulance collides with another vehicle while speeding to a scene, only to find out later the original call was not serious or even one requiring transport. Studies have shown that very few calls demand the use of siren and lights, and many departments now require all ambulances to stop at every stop sign or red light *on every call,* and to maintain strict speed control **Figure 3-13 ▶**. Prioritized dispatch systems

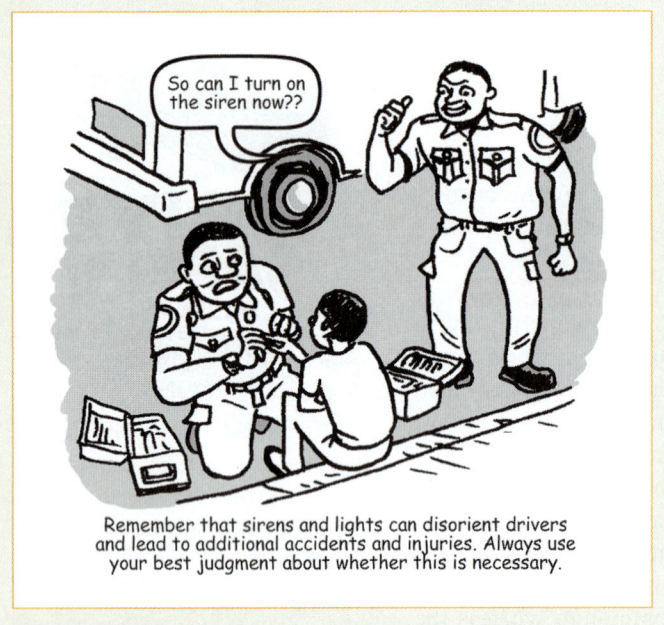

Remember that sirens and lights can disorient drivers and lead to additional accidents and injuries. Always use your best judgment about whether this is necessary.

Figure 3-13

using certified emergency medical dispatchers (EMDs) can provide sophisticated assessments of the need for different levels of response and can improve scene safety while reducing the need for unnecessary responses.

You can provide leadership within your own department for primary injury prevention by advocating policies or equipment that provide a safer environment or initiatives such as a paramedic wellness program. At the same time, you can be a role model by how you personally approach the multitude of decisions you face each day regarding the risks of injury. It is impossible to be a credible advocate for injury prevention if you don't practice what you preach.

Education for Paramedics

Every paramedic should understand the fundamentals of injury prevention. This can easily be the focus of a continuing education program. Some provinces sponsor injury prevention workshops geared specifically to paramedics. Contact your provincial EMS office to see if a workshop can be scheduled for your area, or contact your local public health office to see

what training resources it might have available. There are also excellent self-paced courses and additional information available online.

The "Teachable Moment"

You're on the scene at the site of a collision between two vehicles. The injuries aren't serious, and you notice one of the passengers wasn't wearing a seatbelt. As you prepare him for transport, you look him in the eye and say, "You were very lucky this time . . . the other vehicle didn't hit you square. I've seen plenty of very bad injuries from collisions less serious than this. You really need to wear your seatbelt *every* time you get in the car. It'll save your life."

This was a teachable moment. Educators tell us that there are times when we are more receptive to accepting advice than others. A near-miss like this makes people realize their vulnerability and the true risk of their behaviour—and the lesson is more likely to stick. The paramedic is in the perfect position to articulate and reinforce this message. However, you must use good judgment and be sensitive to the situation. Lecturing a parent immediately after a child has been seriously injured is not going to be effective. What makes a teachable moment?

- The injuries are such that the parents, companions, or the patients themselves will be receptive to the message; you're aware of how ethnic and religious differences must temper the message.
- The scene is conducive to delivering such a message in a nonthreatening, nonjudgmental way. You're not intruding inappropriately or causing embarrassment that could lead to the opposite reaction.
- There is a definitive prevention measure that could have helped, such as using a seatbelt, correct installation of a car seat, wearing a helmet, or keeping firearms locked and safe. Vague advice is less likely to have a lasting effect.

Collection and Analysis of Data

In the opening paragraph of this chapter, we referred to data about backyard drownings. The importance of collecting data in measuring trends, validating interventions, assessing resources, and ultimately persuading others to act cannot be overestimated. For the paramedic, this process starts with the prehospital care report, which is often approached as a

You are the Paramedic Part 4

Much to your disappointment, you are dispatched to the same familiar stretch of road for another motor vehicle collision. Because of your hard work and successful changes to local protocol, members of the flight crew are simultaneously dispatched, and will land in the designated landing zone unless you cancel their response. You arrive to find one male patient who has suffered head injuries and has an altered level of consciousness. You successfully extricate the patient, take spinal precautions, and successfully initiate IVs as well as endotracheal intubation. Just as you finish securing the endotracheal tube, the flight team arrives and now assumes prehospital patient care efforts. The patient is flown to a nearby trauma centre where his head injuries are successfully treated. He makes a full recovery.

6. What other common types of injuries can be easily avoided?
7. Some might question your obligation to this issue. What is your response?

At the Scene

The best teachable moments are those that convey positive reinforcement. If people are wearing seatbelts properly and survive a collision with little or no injuries, tell them, "It's a good thing you had your seatbelts on." You will notice smiles on their faces and they will remember your statement forever.

necessary evil. Standardized coding of incidents is required to collect useful data from far-flung sources. By accurately (and legibly) describing the details of the scene, the external mechanism of injury, the nature of the injury, and the use or absence of protective devices, paramedics can supply important evidence of the scope of a problem and help in monitoring trends.

As a prevention advocate, assess your current prehospital care report to see if it can be modified to be a better tool. Are there ways for the information to be gathered more quickly? Can the information put into a computerized database be promptly updated, easily accessed, and searched? Get involved in local, provincial, or national database systems. Often, much information is being gathered, but agencies aren't consistent or timely in the process, aren't sharing data, or don't have it on a common database. For the injury prevention field, the accurate and timely collection of data is critically important. In EMS, our goal is to put resources into those prevention interventions that can do the most good. This requires documenting injuries and monitoring trends that can be tied to the effects of interventions.

Conclusion

Injury prevention is a complex but rewarding field. Many veteran paramedics have embraced a leadership role in primary prevention after witnessing too many episodes of needless suffering. These leaders recognize their unique role and use their positions to support interventions that make a difference. In their own lives and in their workplace, every paramedic should be proactive in primary injury prevention, whether reducing the odds of a back injury by keeping fit, using proper lifting techniques and protective gear, or taking advantage of a teachable moment with a patient.

Many extend this interest further, reaching out in their communities to become involved as leaders or supporters of a wide variety of prevention programs. They find personal satisfaction and professional fulfillment in the challenge of learning a new field, interacting with a new set of colleagues, and reducing the suffering of those they serve.

You are the Paramedic Summary

1. Why should you consider getting involved in preventing these injuries?

Paramedics should be patient advocates. If you can aid the general public in the prevention of foreseeable injuries, it is your duty to intervene.

2. What are the risk factors associated with the injuries described here?

Risk factors include driving under the influence, failure to use seatbelts, and the age and sex of the driver (as young men typically drive faster and more aggressively than their female and older male counterparts).

3. Which law enforcement agencies could you contact?

Local law enforcement agencies are all appropriate to contact. They will likely have prevention programs and vehicle accident experts on staff who may assist you in minimizing motor vehicle collisions on this stretch of road.

4. Who else might be able to help you in assessing road conditions?

The Department of Transportation is an appropriate agency to contact.

5. What groups are potential partners to enlist in a prevention program in this situation?

You might also consider contacting other service groups in your community who have a desire to combat drunk driving such as MADD and other organizations.

6. What other common types of injuries can be easily avoided?

Injuries involving children, including vehicle collisions and bicycle-related trauma, are also common. There are many programs already designed to target these audiences (for example, dispensing free car seats to new parents and donating bike helmets to children, for those who cannot afford to buy them).

7. Some might question your obligation to this issue. What is your response?

Most people become involved in emergency services because they have a strong desire to help others. As a paramedic, you are responsible to your patients and your community. You should serve as an advocate for those people who cannot care for themselves. This is just another way to perform this service and to have a positive impact on the citizens you serve.

Prep Kit

Ready for Review

- Many paramedics have been motivated by their experience to work actively on injury prevention.
- The 1966 National Academy of Sciences/National Research Council study, "Accidental Death and Disability: The Neglected Disease of Modern Society," noted that EMS could help with trauma after an event, and injury prevention could help prevent an accident before it happens.
- The 1996 *Consensus Statement on the EMS Role in Primary Injury Prevention* emphasized that primary injury prevention is an essential activity of EMS.
- EMS can play a supporting role in preventing intentional injuries and can have an even larger impact in preventing unintentional injuries.
- The years of potential life lost concept is another way to measure the cost of unintentional injury to society. It assumes that an average productive work life continues for 65 years. The age of death is deducted from 65, leaving the years of potential life lost.
- The 4 Es of injury prevention are:
  - Education
  - Enforcement
  - Engineering/environment
  - Economic incentives
- Automatic protections do not include a conscious decision to act and include air bags in vehicles.
- The Haddon matrix uses nine separate components to analyze injury. It encourages creative thinking in understanding the causes and potential interventions for injury.
- Injury surveillance is the ongoing systematic collection, analysis, and interpretation of injury data essential to the planning, implementation, and evaluation of public health practice.
- Paramedics need to focus on injury prevention—do not let the headlines be your guide.
- The five steps to developing a prevention program are:
  - Conduct a community assessment.
  - Define the injury problem.
  - Set goals and objectives.
  - Plan and test interventions.
  - Implement and evaluate interventions.
- Primary injury prevention begins at home by taking care of yourself and presenting a role model for others in your service and in the community.
- The best teachable moments are those that convey positive reinforcement.
- The importance of collecting data in measuring trends, validating interventions, assessing resources, and ultimately persuading others to act cannot be overestimated.

Vital Vocabulary

evaluation Collection of the methods, skills, and activities necessary to determine whether a service or program is needed, likely to be used, conducted as planned, and actually helps people.

goals The end points toward which intervention efforts are directed. A statement of changes sought in an injury problem, stated in broad terms.

Haddon matrix A framework developed by William Haddon, Jr, MD as a method to generate ideas about injury prevention that address the host, agent, and environment and their impact in the pre-event, event, and post-event phases of the injury process.

implementation plan A strategy for carrying out an intervention. Includes goals, objectives, activities, evaluation measures, resource assessment, and time line.

injuries Any unintentional or intentional damage to the body resulting from acute exposure to thermal, mechanical, electrical, or chemical energy or from the absence of such essentials as heat or oxygen.

injury risk A potentially hazardous situation that puts people in a position in which they could be harmed.

injury surveillance The ongoing systematic collection, analysis, and interpretation of injury data essential to the planning, implementation, and evaluation of public health practice.

intentional injuries Injuries that are purposefully inflicted by a person on himself or herself or on another person. Examples include suicide or attempted suicide, homicide, rape, assault, domestic maltreatment, elder maltreatment, and child maltreatment.

interventions Specific prevention measures or activities designed to meet a program objective. Categories include education/behaviour change, enforcement/legislation, engineering/technology, and economic incentives.

morbidity Number of nonfatally injured or disabled people. Usually expressed as a rate, meaning the number of nonfatal injuries in a certain population in a given time period divided by the size of the population.

mortality Deaths caused by injury and disease. Usually expressed as a rate, meaning the number of deaths in a certain population in a given time period divided by the size of the population.

objectives Specific, time-limited, and quantifiable statements that summarize an expected result of an intervention.

outcome (impact) objectives State the intended effect of the program on participants or on the community in such terms as the participants' increased knowledge, changed behaviours or attitudes, or decreased injury rates.

passive interventions Something that offers automatic protection from injury, often without requiring any conscious change of behaviour by the individual; child-resistant bottles and air bags are some examples.

primary injury prevention Keeping an injury from occurring.

process objectives State how a program will be implemented, describing the service to be provided, the nature of the service, and to whom it will be directed.

risk factors Characteristics of people, behaviours, or environments that increase the chances of disease or injury. Some examples are alcohol use, poverty, or gender.

secondary injury prevention Reducing the effects of an injury that has already happened.

unintentional injuries Injuries that occur without intent to harm (commonly called accidents). Some examples are motor vehicle collisions, poisonings, drownings, falls, and most burns.

years of potential life lost A way of measuring and comparing the overall impact of deaths resulting from different causes. It is calculated based on a fixed age minus the age at death. Usually the fixed age is 65 or 70 or the life expectancy of the group in question.

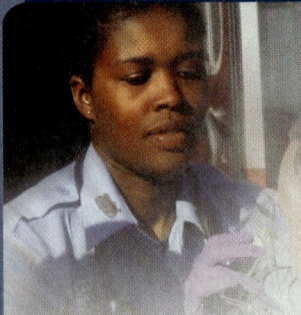

Assessment in Action

There are several things, besides treating injuries, that the paramedic can do to cut down on the number of injuries sustained each year. There is also information about injuries that is important for all paramedics to know. The following questions concern the information that is important to know, and what things paramedics and other health care professionals can do to cut down on the number of injuries sustained each year.

1. **Paramedics are responsible for many duties. However, what is the number one priority of paramedics in their community?**
   A. To be ready to stop and help, whether off duty or on duty
   B. To be prepared to respond and treat injuries that will inevitably occur in their community
   C. To make sure their skills are always up-to-date
   D. To make sure they are good role models in their community

2. **Injuries are defined by the US National Center for Injury Prevention and Control as:**
   A. intentional or unintentional.
   B. resulting from exposure to thermal, mechanical, electrical, or chemical energy.
   C. resulting from the absence of essentials such as heat or oxygen.
   D. all of the above.

3. **One way to measure the cost of injuries to society and the full impact of injury and disease is by using the concept of years of potential life lost. This means:**
   A. assume a productive life until age 65 years for all people, then deduct the year of age at death.
   B. estimate how long that person would have lived given his or her socioeconomic background and genetic makeup, then subtract that number from his or her age at death.
   C. factor in all the patient's health issues at the time of death and estimate how long he or she may have lived based on that information.
   D. compare the cost to society of injuries versus other diseases.

4. **The most successful interventions need to combine education with three other factors. What are they?**
   A. Enforcement, persuasion, modelling of safe behaviour
   B. Legislation, litigation, regulation
   C. Regulatory change, behavioural feedback, economic incentives
   D. Enforcement, engineering/environment, economic incentives

5. **The public health model identifies three influences that cause a health problem. What are they?**
   A. Disease, heredity, lifestyle
   B. Host, agent, environment
   C. Accidents, homicides, suicides
   D. Noneducation, bad lifestyle choices, not using safety measures such as seatbelts

6. **A doctor developed a method to help find ways to prevent people from being killed on highways. He identified several principles of injury prevention and summarized them in a matrix. The host, agent, and environment are seen as factors that interact over time to cause injury. The factors correspond to three phases of the event: pre-event, event, post-event. The matrix discusses nine separate components that contribute to injury. This matrix encourages creative thinking in understanding injury causes and potential interventions. Who was this person, and what is the matrix called?**
   A. William Haddon, Jr, MD; the Haddon matrix
   B. Paul Maxwell; the Maxwell matrix
   C. Ricardo Martinez, MD; the Martinez matrix
   D. Frank Holden; the Holden matrix

7. **Passive interventions in preventing injuries are things such as:**
   A. making seatbelt use a law and adding guardrails to certain roads.
   B. putting safety caps on medicine bottles and putting air bags in cars.
   C. offering monetary discounts for safe driving records.
   D. offering educational classes such as CPR and safe babysitting classes often.

Challenging Questions

8. **You are given the statistics for accidental falls in your town and asked to develop a plan that may reduce the number of falls, given your experience as a paramedic. What are some ideas you can come up with to help reduce the number of falls in your area in the upcoming year?**

9. **What could you and other health care professionals do to decrease the number of people in your area who contract diseases such as chickenpox, tuberculosis (TB), hepatitis, and influenza?**

Points to Ponder

For the fourth time in 3 weeks, you are called to a specific place on a winding highway for a one-car accident. There are no streetlights on this highway, no reflectors to help drivers see how winding it is, and the speed limit is 70 km/h.

What can you do to try to prevent further accidents on this particular stretch of highway?

Issues: Personal Commitment to Prevention, Valuing Personal Safety and Wellness, Teaching Prevention in Your Community.

4 Medical and Legal Issues

Competency Areas

Area 1: Professional Responsibilities

1.1.e	Maintain patient confidentiality.
1.1.j	Behave ethically.
1.3.a	Comply with scope of practice.
1.3.b	Recognize "patient rights" and the implications on the role of the provider.
1.3.c	Include all pertinent and required information on ambulance call report forms.
1.4.a	Function within relevant legislation, policies, and procedures.

Introduction

All medical providers provide care under laws—like many human activities in a democracy. When you become a paramedic, you, too, will be governed by a set of laws affecting how you must treat patients. Your ethical responsibilities, which will be discussed in Chapter 5, differ from legal obligations. Ethics are principles, personal or societal, that determine what is right and wrong. One of the major differences between law and ethics is that laws have sanctions for violation that are enforceable Figure 4-1 ▾ . Laws define our obligations and protect our rights and the rights of others. A paramedic responding to an emergency works within a framework of several types of laws that are set down by either (or both) the federal government or the provincial government:

- Motor vehicle laws for the operation of an emergency vehicle
- EMS legislation
- Medical licensing statutes and regulations
- Civil and criminal statutes about touching, treating, transporting, and possibly injuring another person

It is essential, therefore, that the paramedic have a basic understanding of laws applicable to prehospital emergency care. Failing to perform the job within the law can result in civil liability (as evidenced by an increase in malpractice suits against paramedics) or even criminal liability. It may also result in regulatory action within your province—a disciplinary hearing, for example—or action by your agency and medical director.

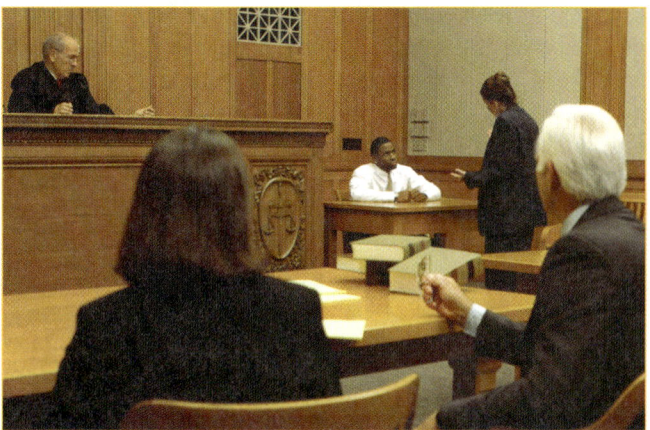

Figure 4-1 Unlike ethics, laws are enforceable rules that all citizens are obliged to follow. Paramedics are sometimes called into court to testify and provide evidence regarding cases under investigation or that are being litigated.

At the Scene

Without question, the best legal protection is to provide a careful, detailed patient assessment and appropriate prehospital medical care, followed by complete and accurate documentation.

In this chapter, we shall review the more important legal concepts affecting the paramedic. However, this text is only a framework to help your understanding. It cannot substitute for competent legal advice because many laws and legal obligations will differ from province to province. Contact an attorney who specializes in the representation of medical professionals if you need legal advice related to your practice. Your supervisor may be able to help you with this or your EMS service may have legal council it uses regularly.

You are the Paramedic Part 1

You are dispatched to an unknown medical problem at a nearby private residence. As you arrive, the patient's wife greets you at the door. She tells you that her husband is a diabetic and that "his sugar must be low." She tells you that he is in the basement and refuses to come upstairs to have something to eat.

As you walk down the basement stairs, you see a 45-year-old man with his back toward you. You call out his name and tell him you are here because his wife is worried that his blood sugar is low. He doesn't acknowledge you. As you attempt to walk in front of him to get eye contact, he takes a swing at you. Unfortunately, you are forced to defend yourself by attempting to restrain the patient. Your partner tries to assist you while simultaneously calling for law enforcement.

Initial Assessment	Recording Time: 0 Minutes
Appearance	Back to you, shoulders raised, fists clenched
Level of consciousness	Conscious
Airway	Open
Breathing	Rapid and deep
Circulation	Unable to assess; patient is combative

1. List the clues that were available to tip you off as to the potential for this patient to become violent.
2. What would be the best course of action at this point?

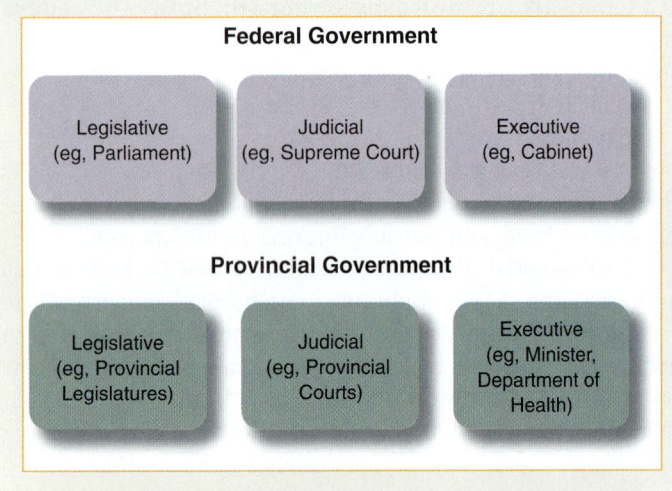

Figure 4-2 Both federal and provincial governments enact and review legislation that is specific to paramedics and their practice.

At the Scene

Many provincial EMS offices have websites with information on laws that affect medical first responders and paramedics. It is a good idea to review the laws of the province in which you are working.

The Legal System in Canada

Although many of our laws are derived from English common law, (or in Quebec, from the French civil code) we have both federal (the big people in Ottawa) and state governments (the folks in your provincial capital) who make, administer, and interpret laws that affect paramedics.

There are three branches of government at each level: the executive, the legislative, and the judicial **Figure 4-2 ▲** . The executive power in Canada is vested in the Queen. In our democratic society, this is only a constitutional convention, because the real executive power rests with the Cabinet. The Cabinet, at the federal level, consists of the Prime Minister and Ministers who are answerable to Parliament for government activities. As well, Ministers are responsible for government departments, such as the Department of Finance and the Department of Justice. When we say "the government" in a general way, we are usually referring to the executive branch.

The legislative branch is Parliament, which consists of the House of Commons, the Senate, and the Monarch or her representative, the Governor General. Most laws in Canada are first examined and discussed by the Cabinet, then presented for debate and approval by members of the House of Commons and the Senate. Before a bill becomes a law, the Queen, or her representative in Canada, the Governor General, must also approve or "assent" to it. This requirement of royal assent is largely ceremonial, because by constitutional convention the Monarch always follows the advice of the government.

The role of the judiciary branch is to interpret and apply the law and the Constitution, and to give impartial judgments in all cases, whether they involve public law, such as a criminal case, or private (civil) law, such as a dispute over a contract. The judiciary also contributes to the common law through the interpretation of previous decisions or setting of new precedents.

Courts have a number of levels as well, including trial court and appellate courts. Departments and agencies reporting to the executive branch often use regulations to specify how things should be done. Agencies, such as Transport Canada at the federal level and the Department of Health at the provincial level, are examples of parts of the administrative branch.

Under Canada's federal system of government, the authority, or "jurisdiction," to make laws is divided between the Parliament of Canada and the provincial and territorial legislatures. Parliament can make laws for all of Canada, but only about matters assigned to it by the Constitution. A provincial or territorial legislature, likewise, can make laws only about matters over which it has been assigned jurisdiction. This means that these laws apply only within the province's borders. The federal parliament deals, for the most part, with issues concerning Canada as a whole, such as trade between provinces, national defence, criminal law, money, patents, and the postal service. The provinces have the authority to make laws concerning education, property, civil rights, the administration of justice, hospitals, municipalities, and other matters of local or private nature within the provinces. Federal law allows territories to elect council with powers similar to those of the provincial legislatures, and citizens of the territories thus govern themselves.

In Canada, generally only provincial governments enact and review legislation that is specific to paramedics and their practice. This is because in most provinces paramedic jurisdiction falls under the Department of Health, which is a provincial responsibility.

Many provinces now have legislation that sets out the framework for regulation of the EMS system. In addition, administrative regulations may be set forth by provincial or municipal governments that regulate the practice of paramedics. In some Canadian provinces, EMS is provided directly by employees of the government department responsible for EMS or through a contractual arrangement with a single agency on a provincewide basis. In these cases, the operational policies of the government department or the contract arrangements may take the place of specific EMS legislation or regulations. It is vital for paramedics to know and understand the laws and administrative regulations that affect practice in their home province. Further, some provinces have enacted legislation to authorize paramedic colleges to oversee the profession. This has been in place in Alberta for some time and is currently underway in Nova Scotia.

Types of Law

Two kinds of law govern paramedics in court: civil law, under which a patient can sue you for a perceived injury, and criminal law, in which the province or federal government will prosecute for breaking a legal statute. Malpractice suits are tried under civil law; misuses of drugs by a paramedic may be tried under criminal law.

A substantial part of civil law is concerned with establishing liability, or responsibility. When a person experiences an injury and seeks redress for that injury, the judicial process must determine who was responsible. A tort is the civil law term for a wrongful act that gives rise to a civil suit. For example, a patient or (if the patient died) the survivor of a patient may be dissatisfied with the prehospital medical care the patient received. The patient or survivor may feel that inadequate prehospital care led to a bad outcome. People have a constitutional right to take legal action against the doctor, nurse, paramedic, or other involved parties. However, the person who is suing must prove that the medical providers he or she is suing caused harm by failing to provide medical care that met the accepted standards. A bad outcome alone does not necessarily mean the medical provider was negligent; however, the patient or survivor has to prove all of the elements of negligence before a lawsuit will be successful.

A legal action of that sort is called a civil suit—that is, an action instituted by a private individual or corporation (the plaintiff) against another private individual or corporation (the defendant)—and the wrongful act that gives rise to a civil suit is called a tort. The objective of a civil suit is usually some sort of compensation (damages) for the injury the plaintiff sustained.

In medical liability cases, the plaintiff usually seeks monetary compensation for physical suffering, mental anguish, medical bills, and sometimes loss of earnings or earning capacity. To succeed in a civil suit, the plaintiff may only need to show that the majority of the reliable evidence favors his or her position.

Few formal records are kept in Canada regarding what behaviours or actions by paramedics pose the greatest risk of lawsuits. However, it is widely believed that two broad areas involve the greatest risk or the greatest number of legal cases. The first is related to calls that result in no transport, including cases where the patient is not transported and their condition subsequently deteriorates and issues related to the dispatch of ambulances where a response is delayed. The second broad, high-risk liability area in EMS is related to the quality of prehospital care provided by paramedics. This includes clinical errors, such as omission to perform a treatment and commission of an unnecessary, harmful intervention.

Vehicle collisions resulting from imprudent operation of emergency vehicles, including during an actual emergency response, are all too common. Each year, these accidents cause serious harm to patients, bystanders, and EMS personnel and result in expensive property damage. Paramedics must be aware that civil suits may occur as a result of these accidents. In some provinces, "no fault" insurance programs are available, which have likely reduced litigation. Canadian precedent, established at least in part through various provincial "no fault" insurance programs, makes such suits less common.

Sometimes the same allegedly wrongful or harmful act that gave rise to a civil suit may also elicit criminal prosecution. A criminal prosecution or provincial statute prosecution is an action taken by the government against a person the prosecutors feel has violated laws. In a criminal or statute case, the government must prove guilt beyond all reasonable doubt: If it does so, the defendant can be fined or imprisoned or both.

The criminal or statute prosecutions that are most likely to apply to prehospital care are assault, battery, false imprisonment, and various provincial traffic laws related to the operation of the ambulance. All of these may arise from complaints about a paramedic's behaviour such as using improper restraining methods, not asking a patient if you may touch him or her before making physical contact, or transporting a patient without his or her consent **Figure 4-3 ▾** .

Assault, battery, and false imprisonment may also be grounds for a civil suit, although suits of this nature against paramedics are rare. But you should know that assault is said to occur when a person (the paramedic) instills the fear of immediate bodily harm or breach of bodily security to another (the patient)—whether or not the threat of harm is actually carried out. Battery occurs when the defendant (the paramedic) touches another person (the patient) without his or her consent. Here are rough working definitions of the difference: saying "I'm going to kick your teeth in" is assault; actually kicking the person's teeth in is battery. Clearly just about any act of medical treatment performed without consent may be considered assault or battery or both, for such acts constitute a threat to the patient's bodily security ("Now I'm going to stick you with this needle. . . .") and an unsanctioned contact with the patient's body.

False imprisonment occurs when a person is intentionally and unjustifiably detained against his or her will. In prehospital care, charges of false imprisonment may arise if a paramedic transports a patient without the patient's consent or uses restraints in a wrongful manner. As we shall see later in this chapter, a paramedic's best protection against these charges is to obtain informed consent for almost everything you do. All medical care providers need to get informed consent, but you will need some guidelines and tips (which come later in this chapter) that most hospital-based personnel don't need to think about.

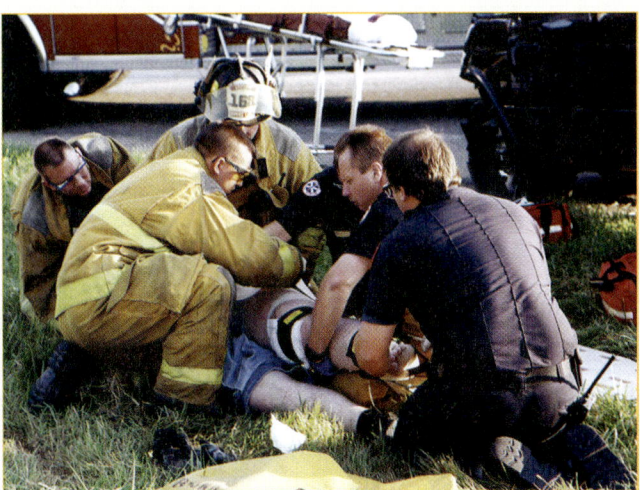

Figure 4-3 Your best prevention against any legal action is to keep the needs of your patient as your top priority and by being an effective and open communicator.

Paramedics may also be sued for <u>defamation</u>, which is intentionally making a false statement through written or verbal communication that injures a person's good name or reputation. <u>Libel</u> is making a false statement in the written form that injures a person's good name. When you write your patient care report, avoid using terms that may be considered insulting or offensive, such as "the patient appears to be drunk." Whatever your personal views, think about the way in which your patient care report would read in court. Don't let any thoughtless comments become evidence against you.

<u>Slander</u> is verbally making a false statement that injures a person's good name. Once again, avoid using terms that could be considered offensive to the patient when passing along prehospital care information to emergency department personnel. Keep in mind always that your patient is very likely a son or daughter, a husband or wife, a brother or sister, or even a father or mother. How would you like information about members of your own family to be treated when information is relayed to the hospital?

How Laws Affect the Paramedic

EMS, as we know it, has been in existence for about 30 years. However, over the last 10 years, the media and public education have made the public aware of what to expect from the local EMS system. If citizens perceive your response as delayed or your efforts as incompetent, they may file lawsuits seeking compensation for injuries they believe were caused by the inadequate EMS response. If you do not explain to your patients why you were delayed, or why a procedure is difficult, you leave yourself open to unasked questions. In the case of health care providers, that silent criticism can lead to the courtroom.

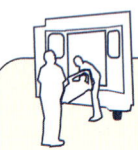

At the Scene

Being courteous, honest, and professional will prevent most patients from complaining or filing lawsuits.

The Legal Process: Anatomy of a Lawsuit

A civil suit begins when a dissatisfied patient contacts an attorney, who then files a document for a lawsuit (called a statement of claim) on behalf of the patient with a local court. The statement of claim will contain the general allegations against the paramedic (let's say it's you) and the EMS system, but may not contain very much specific information about what the patient thinks went wrong. The patient's attorney (or his or her staff) must hand deliver or serve a copy of the statement of claim, and a notice called a summons, to all persons or agencies named in the lawsuit, notifying them of the complaint and the need to respond. From start to finish, a lawsuit may take several years. Because the lawsuit may not begin until several years after the paramedic sees the patient, good documentation after every ambulance call (especially nontransports) is essential to defending a lawsuit.

The response, or statement of claim, will be filed by your EMS service or lawyer. Once the complaint is filed and you (through your lawyer) have answered, a period known as the discovery period begins. The discovery period can last anywhere from a few months to more than 2 years **Figure 4-4 ▾** . During the discovery period, the attorneys on both sides seek to find out as much about the case as possible. They will exchange written questions that must be answered by the parties under oath, and they will also exchange documents, such as the patient's medical record, and take depositions, or statements taken under oath. You should stay in touch with your lawyer during this time and ask for a full explanation of everything that is happening. Your lawyer will also prepare you for a deposition, with instructions on where to go, what to wear, and how to respond to certain types of questions.

Attorneys may also file motions, which are requests for the court to take an action, and argue them before the judge. Your attorney will seek to have the lawsuit dismissed by filing motions. The plaintiff's attorney may ask the court to rule on certain portions of the claim by filing other motions. Either side may file motions asking the court to compel the other side to produce documents or information that is being withheld.

Most civil cases are resolved during a settlement process because it is very expensive and time-consuming to take a case through trial. Settlement processes involve the parties and their lawyers in mediation, which is a conference set up to see if the parties can agree on a dollar amount that will resolve the case, or an arbitration, which is a minitrial in which a single arbitrator or a panel of arbitrators will make a decision based on the evidence presented by both sides. The decision made by the arbitrators is final.

If the case does not resolve itself during a settlement process, it will proceed to trial. Most civil cases in Canada are tried by judges without a jury. However, some civil cases can also be tried

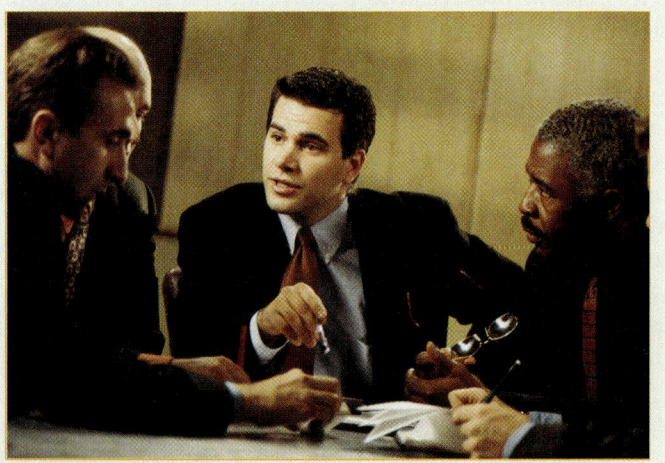

Figure 4-4 The process of a lawsuit can take years, and because of expenses associated with a trial, can result in out-of-court settlements.

by judge and jury. A jury in a civil case is slightly different than in a criminal trial. It has, for example, only six jurors, and the decision does not have to be unanimous, as long as five of the six agree on the verdict.

Notes from Nancy

Probably the most important law affecting paramedics is one that doesn't appear in any of the statute books; it is the *law of doing what is best for the patient.*

Documentation and Communication

If you must deviate from your protocols because of unusual circumstances, consult with direct medical control and make sure you document it well on your patient care report.

Legal Accountability of the Paramedic

A variety of laws and ordinances, many of which differ considerably from province to province, regulate the actions of the public, including paramedics. However, the most important premise for paramedics to remember when working is simply doing what is best for the patient and using common sense. Paramedics are trained in emergency medical care, not law. Every decision regarding prehospital patient care that a paramedic makes, therefore, should be based on the standards of good medical care—*not* on the possible legal consequences. When you do what is best for the patient, it is unlikely you will run afoul of the law—and even if you do get sued, your defence will be greatly enhanced if you have always kept the patient's best interest in mind.

Paramedics always have the responsibility to act in a reasonable and prudent manner and to provide appropriate prehospital care and transportation consistent with their education and training, their medical transport, and other operational protocols of their EMS system.

The Paramedic and the Medical Director

The relationship between the paramedic and the medical director is complex and often not well understood. Ultimately, the paramedic has three lines of authority to answer to: the medical director, the licensing agency, and the employer. Although there is some overlap, it is important to keep these distinctions in mind. Provincial EMS legislation usually requires that the paramedic perform certain advanced life-support procedures and skills only under the supervision of a physician. Legislation may also require the EMS system to have a medical director. It is widely accepted in Canada that the medical director is in a supervisory relationship with the paramedic. Legally speaking, the status of the paramedic as an agent of the physician may vary between provinces, as does the scope of independent practice of paramedics.

The following excerpt from the position statement of the College of Physicians and Surgeons of Manitoba may serve as an example of the relationship. Other provinces may vary.

Delegation of Function

When a physician delegates to another individual any functions which form a part of the practice of medicine, that individual must have the training and qualifications to carry out the duties for which he/she are assigned. Such persons must remain responsible for these duties to the specific delegating medical practitioner.

Transfer of Function

Transfer of function is the performance of a medical function by an individual independent of a qualified physician. Transfer of function can only be considered to a member of a group which is certified as being capable to perform the procedure as a result of education, training, and examination. Transfer of function cannot extend to independent provision of primary care.

Principles of Delegation

The following principles apply to delegation of function:

- The physician remains at all times accountable to the patient for the quality of the patient management program.
- The physician must be aware of what is included in the scope of the delegated function regarding relative liabilities.
- Other individuals may assume responsibility for performing specific functions within the management program when:
  - The physician has ensured that the individual is appropriately trained to do so.
  - The patient accepts care from the individual to whom delegation has been made.
  - The individual accepts the responsibility and acknowledges the supervisory role of a specific physician.

The acts of the paramedic, therefore, may not be held to be the actions of the physician, and the paramedic will be held accountable for his or her own actions. However, the medical director can be held legally accountable and may be named in a civil lawsuit against a paramedic for failing to supervise the paramedic closely enough, or failing to take action when the paramedic's performance is not up to standard. The medical director may restrict the paramedic's practice, or even withdraw supervision entirely from a paramedic if he or she does not believe the paramedic is performing as he or she should. The medical director may also require certain remedial training if the paramedic is weak in some areas of practice. Although the medical director's remedial requirements may ultimately result in employment actions, medical directors are generally not held legally responsible for disciplinary actions taken by employers.

Many of the paramedic's activities require an order from a licensed physician. Orders may be given by radio (direct medical control) or instead may be defined by protocols, or standing orders (indirect medical control), but, in any case, the paramedic is not at liberty to disregard or reverse a physician's order unless, for some reason, the paramedic truly believes that carrying out the order will harm the patient. That fact may give rise to difficult situations, such as instances where paramedics find themselves at the scene of an emergency together with a physician who may not be knowledgeable in prehospital emergency care. Under those circumstances, the paramedics may feel that the orders of the on-scene physician are inappropriate. However, paramedics are on shaky legal ground if they choose to disregard a physician's orders, assuming the physician is licensed in that province and the order is appropriate. To avoid conflicts in such situations, it is best to ask the service medical director to develop protocols ahead of time defining the paramedic's relationship with the medical director of the service and with other physicians in the community, including physician bystanders. A physician bystander should be requested to ride in with EMS if he or she has performed procedures outside the protocols of the paramedics, or has otherwise assumed responsibility for prehospital patient care. Always be sure that the physician is licensed in your province, and document the physician's name and contact information, before allowing him or her to provide prehospital patient care. When conflicts do arise between paramedics and physician bystanders in the field, direct medical control (if available), not the paramedic, should resolve them.

EMS-Enabling Legislation

Most provinces now have what is called EMS-enabling legislation, defining how EMS is structured and designating responsibilities to government agencies. These laws also provide the province's framework for the paramedic's actual practice—what you are permitted to do in the field. For example, EMS legislation may define the need for a medical director, and may also define the scope of practice for the different levels of EMS personnel. The paramedic must be familiar with the EMS legislation in his or her province and any regulations that flow from those statutes.

Administrative Regulations

Administrative regulations—set forth by provincial government departments—also affect and define the specific rules under which paramedics practice. For example, regulations may set out the precise skills and medications to be used by each level of EMS provider. Regulations—usually developed by the province's Department of Health—may further define the paramedic's role in emergency medical care of patients. Regulations may also define the requirements for licensure or certification, renewal requirements, continuing education requirements, and a list of behaviours that may subject paramedics to suspension or revocation of their license or certification.

If a paramedic provides less than adequate prehospital care, or fails to meet the requirements for recertification, the administrative agency may also take action against that paramedic's license. A license is not a right, but rather a privilege, granted by a government agency, allowing the paramedic to provide prehospital care to its citizens. Failure to abide by the regulations can have serious consequences.

Scope of Practice

The scope of practice for paramedics may be spelled out in that province's EMS legislation or regulations. The scope of practice is care that a paramedic is permitted to perform according to the province under its license or certification; however, a local medical director may not permit a paramedic to perform all of the skills or give all of the medications for which he or she is licensed or certified. Some provinces reverse this concept by defining a "scope of independent practice" and allowing the paramedic to add additional scope through transfer or delegation of medical functions from his or her medical director.

A paramedic carrying out procedures for which he or she is not authorized under the enabling legislation is practicing outside his or her scope of practice, which may be considered negligence or, in some provinces, even a criminal offence. The scope of practice should not be confused with the standard of care, which is what a reasonable paramedic in a similar situation would do. This is discussed later in this chapter.

Medical Practice Act

In some provinces physicians and other health care practitioners are enabled to function through the provisions of a Medical Practice Act. This act usually defines the minimum qualifications of those who may perform various health services, defines the skills that each type of practitioner is legally permitted to use, and establishes a means of certification for different categories of health care professionals. Other provinces maintain separate legislation for each category of health care professional. The paramedic should become familiar with the terms of the Medical Practice Act in his or her region.

Privacy of Health Information Acts

The vast majority of health care providers have learned about the principles of Health Information Privacy legislation, which contains stringent privacy requirements for protecting patient information. The Privacy of Health Information Act varies by province and provides for criminal sanctions as well as civil penalties for releasing a patient's private medical information in an unauthorized manner. Generally, medical information can be disclosed only if it is necessary for a patient's treatment or for payment or medical/billing operations, with the specific authorization of the patients. In some cases, research studies will receive approval from research ethics boards to obtain patient information, but certain safeguards are usually required, such as the use of an aggregated form designed specifically for the study (containing only the minimal information required and personal identifiers removed). Typically, health privacy legislation requires each EMS agency to have a privacy officer responsible

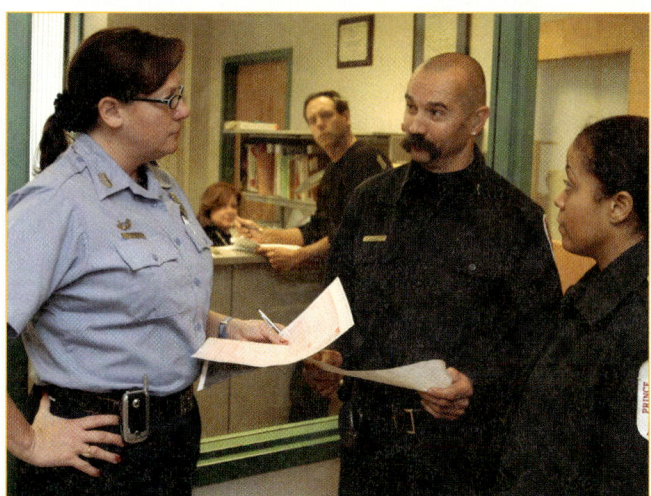

Figure 4-5 Remember that personal health information laws guarantee a patient's confidentiality at all times. Be careful never to discuss a patient's condition in public.

for ensuring that all personal health information (PHI) that the service deals with, in either written or electronic form, not be released in an unauthorized manner. The bottom line is that paramedics must be diligent in following their EMS service's procedures for completing and submitting patient care reports. It is essential they are not lost. As well, paramedics must be careful with the information they disclose by word-of-mouth. Do not casually discuss a patient or a case where anyone might overhear—like an elevator **Figure 4-5 ▲** .

It is not acceptable for EMS patient care reports to be placed in an unsecure location in the ambulance or the EMS station. The only people who should have access to the report are the medical staff the paramedics transferred care to and authorized personnel within the EMS service (for billing and data collection purposes). It is also unacceptable to discuss a patient's PHI in a public forum without that patient's consent. Be aware of sharing "war stories" in a public place, like out for coffee with colleagues or friends. Similarly, paramedics must use caution if a member of the media or the public comes out for a ride-along with your service. Paramedics must make themselves aware of their service's policies in regards to who is permitted to ride-along and how much access they are able to have to the patient. All subpoenas for patient PHI should be directed to the EMS service's Privacy Officer before the information is released. The actual release of the medical record,

even with legal advice, should be delegated only to the senior management of the EMS organization.

Regulations Overseeing Interfacility Patient Transfers

Many patients arrive at smaller community or rural hospitals that do not have the resources to provide all the treatments a patient may require. Patients may be transferred to tertiary health centres for diagnostic procedures or to access specialized health care. In Canada, national standards establishing hospital responsibility for the patient during interfacility transfers do not exist. However, most provinces have policies that establish a referring hospital's responsibility for the care of a patient until that patient is accepted at a receiving hospital.

Paramedics should be certain never to transfer a patient who needs care that falls outside their scope of practice and ensure that the patient is stable enough to transfer. Should a patient need a higher level of care than the paramedics are qualified to provide, it is the responsibility of the transferring hospital to provide someone to accompany the patient, such as a nurse, respiratory therapist, or even a physician. Even when the patient is not going to require interventions that are outside of the paramedic scope of practice, the EMS crew should assess if the care of the patient requires more than one provider in the back. For example, a patient who is intubated and needs to be ventilation en route would likely require more than one provider, if medications need to be given. On these types of critical transfers, anticipate the worst-case scenario and plan accordingly.

It is always wise to discuss all concerns with the sending physician before leaving. Paramedics should also be certain to receive all appropriate paperwork before setting out on a patient transfer, including all pertinent medical records, lab results, x-rays, and other documents. Upon arrival at the receiving hospital, the hospital should have a bed ready for the patient, after agreeing to accept the patient.

Emergency Vehicle Laws

Most provinces have specific statutes that define an emergency vehicle and what traffic should do when one approaches. Although these laws vary somewhat from province to province, it is important to remember that these statutes still require emergency vehicles to be operated in a safe and prudent manner. This includes if it is necessary to have the siren on at all times when the lights are, on how emergency vehicles are to proceed through red

You are the Paramedic Part 2

You feel that for the safety of yourself and your partner you must leave the home. With only two of you, you are not able to safely restrain this patient, who continues to attempt to punch, bite, and kick. Because the patient is combative, you are unable to obtain vital signs.

3. Could your actions be considered abandonment?

4. What other courses of action, if any, could be taken?

lights and intersections, and how other vehicles are to pull over and out of the way. Laws governing emergency vehicle operation do not authorize driving the vehicle in an unsafe manner. If a collision occurs, EMS providers may be found at fault in civil cases brought against the drivers. Worse, if you are the driver, you might also be charged criminally for such situations. This may be likely if the ambulance responding with lights and sirens does not come to a stop at a red light at an intersection to be sure that opposing traffic is stopping, and if excessive speed is used and the ambulance is not able to stop in time to avoid a collision. Some EMS services have implemented vehicle safety programs that monitor each paramedic's driving and cap the speed at which ambulances can travel. Although it is important for paramedics to know the laws of their province about emergency vehicle operation, it is also important to remember that the blue star of life on the side of your vehicle and flashing red lights on top do not exempt you from defensive driving and common courtesy. Drive responsibly.

Immunity: Good Samaritan Legislation

Only four Canadian provinces have some form of Good Samaritan law. These laws are designed to provide a degree of immunity from liability for health care or emergency service providers who stop and help at the scene on an emergency. Unlike the United States, where the laws were initially passed to encourage the public to help at emergency scenes, Canadian Good Samaritan legislation was designed specifically to provide some protection for health care personnel who are off duty and assist at an emergency. The following quotation from the Ontario Good Samaritan law of 2001 is fairly representative of such acts:

Protection from Liability

Despite the rules of common law, a person described in subsection (2) who voluntarily and without reasonable expectation of compensation or rewards provides the services described in that subsection is not liable for damages that result from the person's negligence in acting or failing to act while providing the services, unless it is established that the damages were caused by the gross negligence of the person. 2001, c.2,s.2(1).

Persons Covered

(2) Subsection (1) applies to:

(a) a health care professional who provides emergency health care services or first aid assistance to a person who is ill, injured, or unconscious as a result of an accident or other emergency, if the health care professional does not provide the services or assistance at a hospital or other place having appropriate health care facilities and equipment for that purpose; and

(b) an individual, other than a health care professional described in clause (a), who provides emergency first aid assistance to a person who is ill, injured, or unconscious as a result of an accident or other emergency, if the individual provides the assistance at the immediate scene of the accident or emergency. 2001,c.2,s.2(2).

Note that not all Good Samaritan laws in Canada specifically cover individuals other than health care professionals. According to Ontario's Regulated Health Professions Act, at present paramedics are not considered health care professionals. Therefore, while off duty, paramedics would only be covered under Section 2, Subsection 2b of the Good Samaritan law.

The Ontario Good Samaritan law (and the laws of other provinces) limit the legal protection provided. The emergency care must be given *free of charge* (gratuitously) and does not protect against gross negligence. *Gross negligence* can be defined as any action or omission in reckless disregard of the consequences to the safety or property of another. Sometimes referred to as *very great negligence*, it is more than just neglect of ordinary care toward others or just inadvertence. An example might be a paramedic performing an intervention as a Good Samaritan that the paramedic is not trained or certified to do.

A medical first responder or paramedic providing emergency care while on duty is not, therefore, protected under Good Samaritan laws. As a general rule, if a paramedic has a legal duty to a patient (created by responding in the course of employment), the Good Samaritan law does not apply. Paramedics should be familiar with the applicable legislation in their jurisdiction to determine the protection that applies to them when they are not on duty.

Other Kinds of Immunity
Governmental Immunity

An abiding principal of English law is that you cannot sue the queen (or king) because "the queen can do no wrong." Although the concept of sovereign immunity may limit the liability of paramedics working in government agencies, such as fire departments in the United States, in Canada this concept has been limited through legal precedent in a case known as the *Just decision*. In *Canadian Tort Law, Fifth Edition*, Justice Allen Linden summarized the *Just decision* by saying, "the government must be entitled to govern free from tortious liability. It cannot be a tort for government to govern. However, when a government is supplying services, that is, doing things for its people other than governing, it should be subject to ordinary negligence principles."

Vicarious Liability

It may seem that Canadian paramedics have little if any protection against the financial impact of a civil lawsuit. In reality, the common law in Canada has responded pragmatically to the social needs of employees who may commit a tort in the course of their duties.

An employer may be personally at fault for a tort committed by an employee. For example, the employer may knowingly assign an employee to perform a dangerous task for which he or she is not trained, and thus be liable for injury to others. Although it may not logically follow that the employer should be liable when he or she is not him/herself at fault, and may even have done his best to train the employee to avoid anything that might constitute a tort, the common law has evolved a basis for making the employer liable for the acts of an employee that arise during the course of that employment. Employees generally have limited assets available for redress of the potential harm they can cause. Accordingly, the courts have developed the principle of vicarious liability, whereby employers are held liable to compensate persons for the harm caused by their employees in the course of their employment. The employee remains personally liable for his or her torts, but the best chance of recovery usually lies with the employer.

A consequence of the development of vicarious liability has been that employers generally insure themselves against such losses, and it is unusual for the employee to suffer a financial loss as a direct consequence of a civil judgment. In some provinces, regulations governing the operation of EMS systems may even stipulate a mandatory minimum liability insurance that an employer must carry.

Negligence and Protection Against Negligence Claims

Unless there is some type of immunity, nothing can protect the paramedic from liability for gross negligence, a serious charge. Negligence occurs when a series of events happen:

- The paramedic—or, in some cases, the EMS system—had a legal duty to the patient. For example, a paramedic hired to serve a community has a legal duty to the citizens of that community.
- There was a breach of duty; that is, the person accused of negligence failed to act as another person with similar training would have acted under the same or similar circumstances. Breach of duty may involve doing *less* than one was trained to do (an error of omission—for example, a paramedic who fails to splint an injured extremity) or doing *more* than one was trained to do (an error of commission—for example, an emergency medical responder who sutures a laceration).
- The failure to act appropriately was the proximate cause (the first event in a chain of events) that caused the plaintiff's injury.
- Harm resulted.

Paramedics and the EMS systems in which they work are protected from liability as long as they perform according to the standards expected of paramedics and EMS systems. The paramedic's best protection is to behave in all circumstances according to established procedures and standards set by provincial standards and licensing bodies and national standards such as Canada's National Occupational Competency Profiles (NOCP). Although not all standards are law, they can be introduced as evidence in litigation and may affect the outcome of a suit. It is therefore in your best interest to make sure that your ambulance is maintained in optimal condition and equipped according to prevailing standards and that you follow all protocols as approved by your agency or provincial standard.

A big part of negligence is whether or not there is "foreseeability." This concept implies that the injury, or harm, could have been predicted, or known in advance, and therefore could have been avoided if the proper precautions had been taken. It is foreseeable that giving an incorrect dosage of a drug will result in harm to a patient just as it is foreseeable that running a red light while en route to a call may result in a collision.

Elements of Negligence
Duty

Duty is prescribed by the law: it is what we must do (as paramedics) and how we must do it. Without question, our first duty as paramedics is to do no further harm to a patient. As the Latin phrase (which is thought to have originated with Hippocrates) states: *Primum non nocere* (First, do no harm).

The first element of negligence a patient must prove for a lawsuit to be successful is that of duty. The definitive *Black's Law Dictionary* defines duty, as it is understood in medical negligence, as "an obligation, to which law will give recognition and effect, to conform to a particular standard of conduct towards another." *Black's Law Dictionary* goes on to say that if one fails to perform according to that standard "he becomes subject to liability to the person to whom the duty is owed for any injury sustained by that person of which the conduct is the legal cause."

A great deal of confusion surrounds the concept of legal duty in EMS. For example, many paramedics think that they have a legal obligation to stop at roadside collisions simply because they are paramedics. However, in all but a few provinces, this is not the case. Although a paramedic may feel an ethical or moral obligation to stop and assist, the law in most provinces does not require it. When the paramedic is working a shift, however, or signed up for a particular shift on an "on-call" squad, he or she is obligated to respond to calls during that period.

Popular EMS folklore also says that if you put a sticker that says "paramedic" on your vehicle, this somehow invokes a legal responsibility to stop at all emergencies. But once again, this is not the case **Figure 4-6 ▾** . However, if the paramedic does stop to assist, he or she has a legal duty to perform within the standard of care. If you do stop, there is a further legal duty not to abandon the patient once treatment has begun. Once the

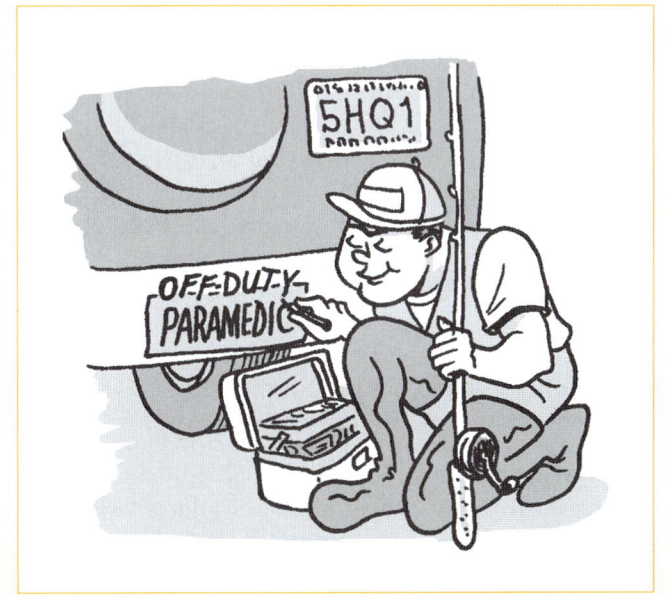

Figure 4-6

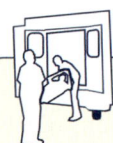

At the Scene

The common law provinces, all provinces except for Quebec, have no laws making it obligatory for people to help someone in need.

Quebec is unique in Canada in imposing a duty on everyone to help a person in peril. The duty to take action stems from the Quebec Charter of Human Rights and Freedoms, enacted in 1975, and the Civil Code.

The Charter contains a provision that imposes an obligation to render aid if it can be accomplished without serious risk to the Good Samaritan or a third person. There is still little jurisprudence interpreting these provisions.

Under the Civil Code, every person is obligated to act as a bon pere de famille, broadly defined as a reasonably prudent person. Failure to do so would amount to fault and lead to legal wrong.

on-duty paramedics arrive on the scene, you may give a report of what you saw and did and then leave the scene.

The concept of duty extends to the paramedic's duties to himself or herself as well. Each of you has an obligation to keep up your licensure or certification, to attend continuing education courses, and to maintain your skills. In addition, you have a duty to maintain your health and psychological well-being so that you will be both mentally and physically prepared for the rigors of your job in prehospital patient care. Further, you have a duty to check your equipment at the beginning of each shift and to take action to ensure that all equipment is functioning properly. Finally, you have a duty to honour your patient's rights to privacy, and their rights to refuse or limit the prehospital care you provide.

In addition, not just individual paramedics but EMS agencies—and even entire EMS systems—can be held to a legal duty. EMS agencies have a duty to respond to calls for aid and to use mutual aid resources appropriately if their own call volume is too heavy to allow response within an appropriate time frame. Some EMS agencies may operate with contracts that specify legal duties, such as minimum response times.

Legal duty is a concept in the law that tells us what our standards of practice are. It is an unpredictable legal concept, often defined in the context of a case tried in a court of law. But the concept of legal duty is used by attorneys defending EMS providers. For example, in a lawsuit against an off-duty paramedic who stopped at an accident to render aid, the paramedic's attorney may attempt to show that the paramedic had no duty to the patient, but instead provided assistance he or she was not required by law to provide.

Breach of Duty

The second element a patient must prove for a lawsuit to be successful is that the paramedic failed to perform within the standard of care. The standard of care is what a reasonable paramedic, in the same or similar situation, would have done. In a lawsuit, a jury will listen to the testimony of expert witnesses on both sides and ultimately decide whether the paramedic's care in the prehospital setting was reasonable or not. These expert witnesses will provide a number of sources on which to base their testimony about whether the paramedic's prehospital care was reasonable. Those sources will include their own training and experience; the paramedic's prehospital training, experience, and continuing education; textbooks; protocols; national standards; standard operating procedures; and the patient care report. (Good documentation will go a long way to prove your high standards of care.)

In Canada, laws typically differentiate between ordinary negligence and gross negligence. How high a standard of care a paramedic will be held to varies from one province to another and depends largely on local precedent.

In those provinces that have Good Samaritan legislation, it typically does not protect against gross negligence. In this case, a lawsuit against a paramedic acting as a Good Samaritan will not be successful unless that paramedic has seriously departed from the accepted standards. Actions are grossly negligent if they are found to be willful or wanton under the law. This is a very difficult standard for a plaintiff to meet. Usually, either intentional conduct or recklessness is essential to a finding of willful or wanton conduct. Gross negligence has been defined as "reckless disregard," "utter indifference," or "conscious disregard" for the safety of others. Usually, if the paramedic can convince the jury that he or she acted in good faith, this will be a defence to a claim of gross negligence.

In other cases, for example, a lawsuit against a paramedic related to a tort while in the course of employment, a plaintiff will only have to show ordinary negligence. This can be a failure to act or a simple mistake that causes harm to a patient. It is much easier for a plaintiff to prove negligence under the ordinary negligence standard.

Proximate Cause

Even in cases where the paramedic had a legal duty to the patient, and the paramedic breached the standard of care, a plaintiff must still link the act that fell below the standard of care directly to his or her injury by showing that the act (or failure to act) proximately caused the harm. *Black's Law Dictionary* defines proximate cause as "that which, in a natural and continuous sequence, unbroken by any intervening cause, produces injury, and without which the result would not have occurred." Simply stated, a plaintiff will have to prove that the paramedic's improper action, or failure to act, was the cause of his or her injury.

Failure to secure a patient on a backboard can be the proximate cause of severing the spinal cord. Demonstrating that an act, or a failure to act, proximately caused an injury is the most difficult part of a lawsuit to prove. It is also the part that defence attorneys spend a great deal of their time on. For example, if paramedics are treating a patient from a motor vehicle collision who has a spinal cord injury and, during patient care, they drop the stretcher, the patient may try to show that his or her injury resulted from the dropped stretcher and not from the collision itself. Careful documentation of the patient's neurologic status at the time you first encounter him or her will be essential to your defence.

Harm

The final element plaintiffs must prove in a negligence lawsuit is that they were harmed. Although physical injury is usually part of any lawsuit for medical negligence, patients also may claim damages for emotional distress, loss of income, loss of enjoyment of life, loss of spousal consortium, loss of household services, and loss of future earning capacity. They will have to show that the paramedic's actions proximately caused each of these kinds of damage.

Abandonment

Abandonment is a form of negligence that involves the termination of care without the patient's informed consent. The term also implies that the patient had a continuing need for medical treatment and that the abrupt termination of treatment was the cause of subsequent injury, illness, or death. Therefore, once you have responded to an emergency, you may not leave a patient in need of medical treatment until another competent health care professional with an equal or higher level of training has taken responsibility for that patient's care. Shocking as it may seem, on more than one occasion, a critically ill or injured patient was left in a busy emergency department by paramedics, and the patient died before emergency department personnel took note of the patient. It is the responsibility of the paramedic to stay with the patient until proper transfer of care has taken place.

Proper transfer of care means transfer of care to another health care professional, not to a stretcher or a clerk! Thus, if you arrive at a busy emergency department with a seriously ill patient, you may have to remain with the patient until emergency department personnel are free to attend to him or her.

Busy emergency departments may direct you to leave your patient in a triage station or waiting area after having been seen by a triage nurse and registered as an emergency department patient. Paramedics should not leave patients in any area of the hospital where they have not or will not be attended to and assessed by medical personnel. You must never leave a patient without giving a full report to a physician, physician assistant, or nurse. If, after the report has been given, the paramedics and the receiving staff person agree that the acuity of the patient is low enough for them to wait in the waiting area, and the emergency staff fully acknowledge the patient is now their responsibility, this is a fine course of action. It becomes an unacceptable course of action when the patient is placed in the waiting room without acknowledgment from the receiving facility.

It is also very important that you leave a copy of your EMS patient care report with the emergency department physician or nurse who is taking over care of your patient. Although many busy services complain that this is difficult to accomplish, it is essential to leave your written report so that the emergency department physician and staff have a written record of your findings of the scene, what prehospital interventions were administered to the patient, and the results of your assessment.

Remember, paramedics are the only health care provider to have first-hand knowledge of the scene. This is valuable information that needs to be passed on, both in verbal and written reports.

It is important to remember that situations in which paramedics attend to a patient but do not transport are a source of legal risk. However, in some situations not transporting a patient does not constitute abandonment. For example, calls are made for ambulances for patients who may not really need treatment or transportation. These calls often arise as a result of a misunderstanding of the EMS system or family, friends, and bystanders being cautious about a medical situation they do not fully understand. Your local medical director should provide protocols for these situations.

In addition, some EMS systems, particular in rural areas, may have mixed personnel (providers of various levels) and may not have a full staff of paramedics at all times. In those areas, even if an advanced care paramedic makes the initial response, if only basic care is required the advanced care paramedic may not need to be part of the transport crew for a situation where the patient does not need advanced care. This is best decided by relaying direct medical control, protocols, or standing orders. If direct medical control is available, a physician should be consulted to confirm that the advanced care paramedic will not be needed for transport. It is the kind of decision that always benefits from the proverbial "two heads are better than one."

Many EMS systems provide a tiered response, with basic life support (BLS) providers reaching the patient quickly, followed by advanced life support (ALS). If a BLS crew responds and makes an improper determination that a patient does not need ALS care, the system may be exposed to liability. Your service needs to work with every provider involved to set up protocols that provide guidance for the situations in which a BLS crew may cancel an incoming ALS crew.

Advance Directives

An advance directive is a written document that expresses the wants, needs, and desires of a patient in reference to his or her future medical care. Advance directives state what medical care the patient wants or doesn't want when the patient is unable to express his or her wishes and generally must be signed by the patient while he or she is capable of doing so. Living wills and organ donation orders are all advance directives.

A do not resuscitate (DNR) order states what life-sustaining emergency procedures should be performed on the patient in situations when the patient's heart has stopped or respirations have ceased. A DNR order is not a "do not care for the patient" order.

For patients who have been identified as organ donors and are critically ill or injured, you may be required to perform some procedures before potential organ procurement, after the patient is deceased. If your EMS system does not already have a protocol for organ donation, assist it in developing protocols to keep organs viable. It is your responsibility to contact your direct medical control for consultation and direction on local prehospital organ procurement procedures.

Whether or not EMS personnel are bound by advance directives is a function of provincial law, and specific provisions vary by province. In Canada, DNR orders generally would not be considered an advance directive, because the patient may not have initiated the document. DNR orders are often limited to terminal patients in a nursing home, hospital, or hospice care and are usually written by the patient's physician, often in consultation with a patient's family or legal designate after the patient becomes unable to make informed decisions about his or her care. These orders remain valid only while the patient is under the direct care of the physician or while in the facility providing care when these orders were written.

One area that may cause conflict for the paramedic is the situation where a patient who has had a DNR order written is sent home with the expectation that he or she will die at home. When death is imminent, the family may become apprehensive and call an ambulance in spite of the plans that may have been made with their physician. Because the patient at home is no longer under the direct care of the facility, you may be required to treat. You must learn what the laws are in your province and follow them.

The ethics of advance directives and organ procurement will be discussed in detail in Chapter 5.

Licensure and Certification

The terms licensure and certification are often confused because, in some provinces, paramedics are considered licensed but in others certified. Some provinces consider paramedics to be both licensed and certified. Certification generally means only evidence of a certain level of training, such as a certificate of completion from a course or school. It is really simply evidence that an individual has a certain level of credentials based on hours of training and examination. It does not address anything more than minimum competency. Licensure, in contrast, is the privilege to practice at a carefully defined level, usually granted by a provincial government agency or self-governing professional authority, such as a College of Paramedics sanctioned by the provincial government. Often, these agencies themselves give licensing examinations.

It is important to remember that, although certain rights do come with a license, a license itself is a privilege granted by a governing authority only on certain conditions, and the paramedic must comply with the authority's requirements for professional behaviour, continuing education, and licensure

renewal, or risk losing that privilege. Those rights may not be conferred in provinces that certify, rather than license, paramedics.

Discipline and Due Process

The rights that come with a license (and with some certificates as well) include what is known as a property interest in your license, because paramedics earn their living by working under their license. However, if a paramedic commits an infraction that jeopardizes that license, he or she may be subjected to a licensure action. The agency that granted the license may seek to restrict, suspend, or even revoke the privilege to practice.

Although legislative provisions vary from province to province, when an administrative agency proposes a licensing action in a province that licenses paramedics, the paramedic generally has a right to due process. Due process is a right to a fair procedure for the action the agency proposes to take. Due process has two components: *Notice* and the *Opportunity to be Heard*. Notice means that the agency must notify the paramedic of the actions that allegedly constitute the infraction. This usually happens by way of a certified letter containing a *Notice of Contemplated Action*. The letter will inform the paramedic of the proposed action to be taken and the sections of the regulations the agency is alleging he or she has violated. The letter will also inform the paramedic of a right to a hearing and the procedure for requesting a hearing. The hearing provides an opportunity for the paramedic to tell his or her side of the story. If the licensing agency still believes that it has grounds for the licensure action after the hearing, it will send a *Notice of Final Action*. The paramedic may also have appeal rights if a final action is taken against his or her license.

Paramedic–Patient Relationships

Confidentiality

The paramedic has an ongoing duty to maintain the confidentiality of the private information shared by the patient **Figure 4-7 ▸** . It is important not to disclose any of the patient's medical information to anyone who does not have a need to know it. As mentioned previously, most provinces have laws pertaining to patient confidentiality; a breach of that confidentiality may provide a means for patients to sue for unauthorized release of their medical information.

You are the Paramedic Part 3

You exit the house, and wait in the locked ambulance for arrival of law enforcement personnel. The patient's wife runs from the home and pleads with you to return inside as her husband is punching through a glass cabinet in the basement. You explain to her that she should wait with you outside until police officers arrive.

5. Was any part of this situation avoidable?

6. What would be helpful in handling this situation?

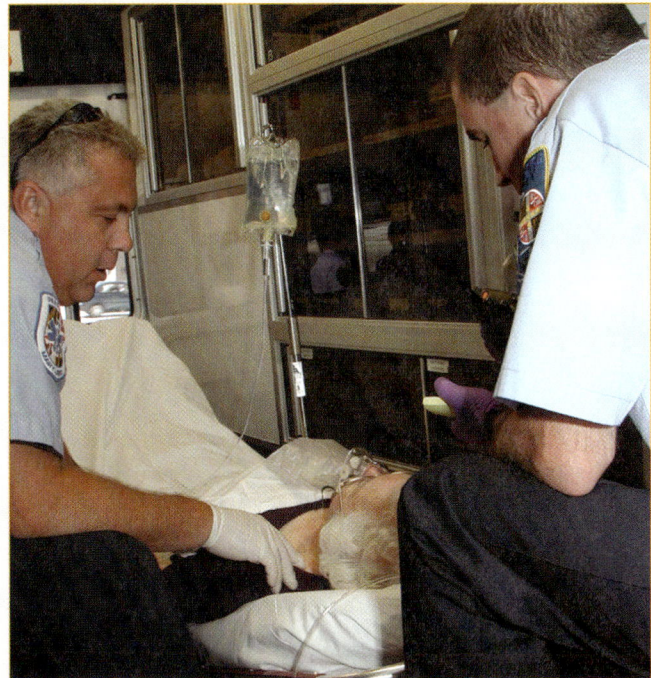

Figure 4-7 When communicating with a patient, be sensitive to his or her point of view, and the environment in which you choose to communicate.

Be careful *where* you talk about patients, too. You must do your best, even at the scene of a collision or in the halls or elevators of hospitals, not to confer in front of bystanders.

As a paramedic, you should become familiar with the laws in your province that are applicable to your EMS operations.

Consent and Refusal

The concepts of consent and refusal can be traced back to the Magna Carta and are clearly embodied in Canadian common law. Canadian common law gives a high degree of protection to an individual's personal security and bodily integrity. It is a basic principle of the common law that every person has the right to be free from unwanted interference or touching, including medical treatment, and no one may administer treatment contrary to the person's wish, even when it may be necessary to preserve that person's life or health. This right is so fundamental that it is entrenched in the Constitution Act of 1982. At common law there are four prerequisites to a valid consent:

1. It must be voluntary;
2. The patient must have legal and mental capacity;
3. It must be specific to both the treatment and the person administering it; and
4. It must be informed.

Common law also permits treatment to be provided without a patient's consent in an emergency, where the health care provider is not aware of any contrary wish having been expressed by the patient when he or she was capable of refus-

ing consent. Adults are presumed to be competent to grant or refuse consent, and in various provinces this presumption has been extended by statute to apply to anyone over the age of 16. With respect to children under the age of 16, the common law has developed the "mature minor rule," which provides that a minor who has a full appreciation of the nature and consequences of medical treatment may consent to (or refuse) that medical treatment.

Common law specifies that only a court-appointed guardian or the court itself, under its *parens patriae* jurisdiction, can consent to or refuse treatment on behalf of an incapable adult patient.

Prior to providing emergency medical care, you must obtain the patient's consent. Any touching of a patient's body without his or her consent may give rise to charges of assault and battery. The concept of consent is predicated on patients who are of legal age and who possess the capacity to make medical care decisions that are appropriate for themselves. This is called decision-making capacity. Patients with decision-making capacity have the right to refuse all or part of the emergency medical care offered to them. There are two types of consent that the paramedic must be familiar with: informed consent and implied consent.

Informed consent must be obtained from every adult patient who has decision-making capacity. Informed consent has two elements.

First, you must tell patients what it is you are proposing to do to them. Before you touch patients, and particularly before you perform any invasive procedure, you must ensure that the patients understand what it is you propose to do to them, and what potential risks the procedure carries. There are a number of things that can get in the way of giving patients the information they need to make their decision, such as language barriers, their emotional state, and their mental abilities. It is usually best to get patients somewhere quiet (such as the back of your EMS unit), where you can calm them down and explain, in a manner they can understand, the nature and extent of the procedure to be performed and the possible risks involved.

Second, patients must give you permission to touch them in the manner you have proposed. This may be done verbally, or by actions such as rolling up a sleeve so that you can take their blood pressure. It is very important that you document how you obtained informed consent in case legal issues arise later. Expressed consent is a type of informed consent that occurs when the patient does something, either by telling you or by taking some sort of action, that demonstrates giving you permission to provide prehospital care.

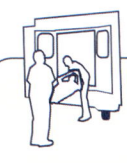

At the Scene

Never *tell* patients that you are going to do a procedure. Instead, *ask* them if you can perform the procedure, even simple procedures, such as taking a blood pressure, and explain to them why they need it.

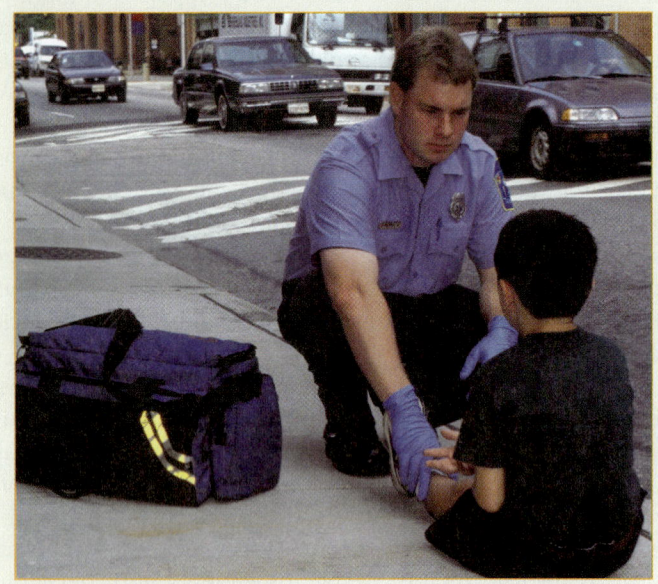

Figure 4-8 Whenever you are dealing with a young child, explain to him or her the need for treatment, and consult his or her parent or guardian.

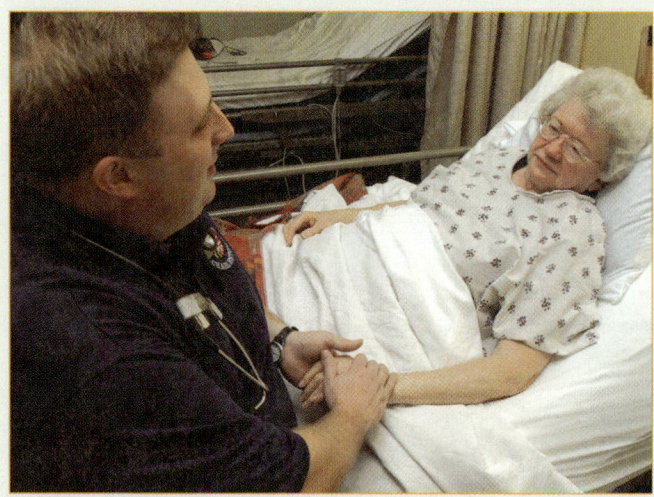

Figure 4-9 When a conscious patient with decision-making capability makes a decision, you must respect that decision.

The other kind of consent is implied consent. In unconscious adults, or in adults who are too ill or injured to consent to emergency lifesaving treatment, their consent is implied. In those cases, the paramedic assumes that the patients would want prehospital care because of the severity of their condition. Generally, when you encounter patients who are seriously injured or extremely ill, they will not have decision-making capacity and their consent to treatment may be implied.

There is nothing in law called *involuntary consent*. Some EMS personnel have been taught the concept of involuntary consent, a term that has been incorrectly applied to describe the permission granted by law enforcement or a legal guardian to treat someone who is under arrest (or otherwise in custody), incapacitated, a minor, or for other reasons. This term is an oxymoron, because consent can *never* be involuntary.

Minors present special issues for the paramedic. Because minors have no legal status, they cannot either consent to or refuse medical care, except in certain cases. Some provinces have enacted legislation that explicitly extends the rights of consent and refusal to children age 16 and older, or, more generally, to children who have the "apparent maturity" to have a full appreciation of the nature and consequences of the proposed medical treatment. In the case of children and adults who have legal guardians, consent must be obtained, if possible, from a parent or legal guardian of the patient. If the parent or guardian is not available, emergency treatment to sustain life may be undertaken without consent under the doctrine of implied consent.

Overall, obtaining consent for adults and children may be somewhat difficult for the new paramedic **Figure 4-8 ▲**. A patient or a guardian of a child may not want you to assess and treat for a variety of reasons. However, as a patient advocate

you will need to be aware of potential problems for obtaining permission and be prepared to discuss the need for care.

Decision-Making Capacity: The Prerequisite for Consent and Refusal

Refusals, like consent, must be informed refusals, and all the same prerequisites apply. Patients must have decision-making capacity in order to be able to refuse care. Decision-making capacity is the ability of patients to understand the information you are providing to them, coupled with the ability to process that information and make a choice regarding medical care that is appropriate for them. Paramedics have a number of tools to use in evaluating patients' decision-making capacity, but the best one is their ability to talk to patients to find out whether patients understand what is happening to them. In addition, if pulse oximetry and blood glucose measurements are outside normal ranges, they can provide measurable information regarding patients' ability to understand and communicate. Detailed documentation of decision-making capacity is important to show that patients were able to understand your proposed plan of prehospital care.

If a conscious patient with decision-making capacity refuses to consent to treatment, that person may not be treated without a court order **Figure 4-9 ▲**. In such instances, the paramedic should consult with direct medical control for instructions. The most prudent approach is for the paramedic to inform the person in a calm and sympathetic manner of the possible consequences of refusing treatment. Bear in mind that many people who refuse medical treatment do so out of fear and emotional distress, and the patient's distress needs to be recognized and dealt with in an understanding way.

It is *not* appropriate nor is it in your interest as an advocate to consider the person who refuses treatment a "bad patient" and to behave in a hostile or aggressive manner toward him or her. Remember, you are at the scene to help the patient, so try to find out what is bothering the patient and why he or she is rejecting help, and always respect their rights.

Bear in mind that some patients refuse treatment as a way of denying that they have a problem—such as the middle-aged man who appears very stoic with chest pain who refuses treatment in order to deny the possibility that he may be experiencing a heart attack. A sympathetic ear and a little reassurance will often convert the problem patient into someone you can help. It is important to inform your patients of the risks of not being assessed by a physician in an emergency department. For this example, the paramedic should inform the man with chest pain that the EMS system has limited diagnostic capabilities, and that he may indeed be having a heart attack (even if it is not showing on the 12-lead ECG). A heart attack that goes undiagnosed is very serious and can lead to more heart damage or possible death.

Sometimes having patients talk by radio or telephone with direct medical control may be helpful. If, however, after your best efforts to talk with patients about their situation and to explain the possible consequences of refusing treatment, they still decline prehospital care, there is little more that you can do. Even at that point, though, do not close any doors. Let patients know that, should they change their mind, you will be willing and ready to help them because that is your job.

Maintain a courteous, concerned attitude. Let patients know that your chief concern is their well-being. Let patients know that it is all right to change their mind. Urge patients to seek further medical evaluation by the doctor of their choice. Help them make concrete plans for follow-up. Sometimes patients will consent to transport but not consent to treatment; others may consent to treatment but refuse transport. If patients refuse transport, try to make sure that someone will be with them after you leave and always advise them to call back for help if needed.

Once again, documentation of patient refusals is critically important should litigation arise in which the patient claims the paramedic abandoned him or her. Document carefully, including the patient's history, all findings of your physical examination and mental status examination, the patient's stated reasons for refusing prehospital care, and all advice given to the patient, including explanations of the risks of refusing such care. It is also important to note how much time you spent attempting to provide prehospital care. The report should be signed by the patient and, preferably, by an impartial observer (for example, a police officer, if present). The purpose of a witness/observer is to *hear* the exchange of the information, not just to sign a piece of paper with his or her name. Soliciting for signatures from others on the scene who may not have been paying attention to your conversation or the information exchanged with the patient may pose legal issues. Soliciting for a signature just to fill in your report is not useful and could be harmful.

It is essential for paramedics to attempt the process of obtaining informed consent to treat the patient (or informed consent to refuse). Just because a patient has signed a refusal form does not mean that the patient has given you an informed refusal. You must have informed the patient of what you propose to do to care for him or her, and the potential risks of refusing that care, in a manner he or she is capable of understanding.

Notes from Nancy

If you place the welfare of the patient ahead of all other considerations, you will rarely if ever commit an unethical act in medical care.

It is often frustrating and difficult for the paramedic, like any other health care provider, to accept the fact that a patient may refuse all or part of prehospital care. However, it is important to respect a patient's rights, regardless of whether it is contrary to your beliefs or what you think you should be doing. Courts have upheld patient refusals when paramedics carefully documented a patient's decision-making capacity, and their explanation of the possible consequences of refusing prehospital care.

A problem sometimes arises in determining whether a person who refuses prehospital care or transport to a hospital has decision-making capacity. Suppose, for example, you are called to help a patient who has had a seizure in a downtown store. By the time you arrive, the seizure is over, and the patient is conscious. She says she is all right, and she refuses to go to the hospital. You smell alcohol on her breath. Does that patient possess the decision-making capacity to refuse treatment? To make that determination, you need to spend a little time evaluating the patient. You should explain to her, "I can't let you go until I've checked you over and until you talk to me enough to convince me that you're OK and that you understand your situation."

In general, any patient with altered mental status or unstable vital signs probably cannot be considered able to refuse transport to the hospital. The paramedic must become proficient in establishing whether a patient has decision-making capacity in a very short time frame, and with minimal information. The criteria for determining mental competence should be spelled out in detail in the protocols of every ambulance service. As a rule, such criteria will include the following:

At the Scene

The potential legal consequences of using reasonable force to bring a patient to the hospital (false imprisonment) are far less serious than the consequences—legal and medical—of a bad outcome (wrongful death or malpractice) if a patient in need of further care is released at the scene. It is always preferable to err on the side of transporting a patient but, in all cases confer first with direct medical control. Depending on the province, police may be empowered to transport a patient for medical evaluation when the patient appears incapable of providing informed consent or refusal. If this is the case, police should always be contacted before attempting to restrain any patient for transport.

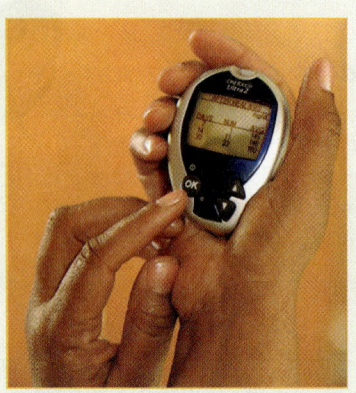

Figure 4-10 Remember that a patient's decision-making ability can be affected by the intake of alcohol or drugs, and by abnormal blood glucose or oxygen saturation levels.

- The patient is oriented to person, place, and day.
- The patient responds to questions appropriately.
- There is no significant mental impairment from alcohol, drugs, head injury, or other organic illness. (Ask family members, if present, whether the patient is behaving the way he or she normally does.) What constitutes significant mental impairment is a judgment call that is very subjective.
- The patient demonstrates to you that he or she understands the nature of his or her condition and the risks of not going to the hospital for immediate care. This can only be done after a thorough explanation of the patient's condition, and the risks of refusal.
- The patient can describe a reasonable plan for follow-up care.
- Oxygen saturation levels are within normal limits.
- Blood glucose levels are within normal limits **Figure 4-10 ▲** .

When patients have a potentially life-threatening illness or injury and there is any doubt as to their decision-making capacity, it is always preferable to transport them to the hospital even if it is against their will. The decision to allow a potentially impaired patient to refuse treatment is a *medical* decision, requiring judgment and experience. That decision is best made by a doctor in the hospital, not by a paramedic on the street.

Psychiatric emergencies present particularly vexing problems of consent. When a person's life is not in danger, a police officer is generally the only individual given the authority to restrain and transport that person against his or her will. An EMS system should not do so except at the express request of the police. Notably, neither a physician nor the patient's family may, in most regions, authorize such transport; they may authorize involuntary *commitment*, but their authority does not extend to the forcible transport of a patient against his or her will. Therefore, it is essential for every EMS service to establish protocols, based on local laws, for dealing with the mentally disturbed patient who refuses transport. In many instances, the participation of the police will be required, and the role of each agency involved should be clearly defined beforehand.

Use of Force: Violent Patients and Using Restraints

The use of force by paramedics against patients has been the cause of numerous lawsuits in recent years. However, in the reality of today's EMS practice, the paramedic will encounter violent

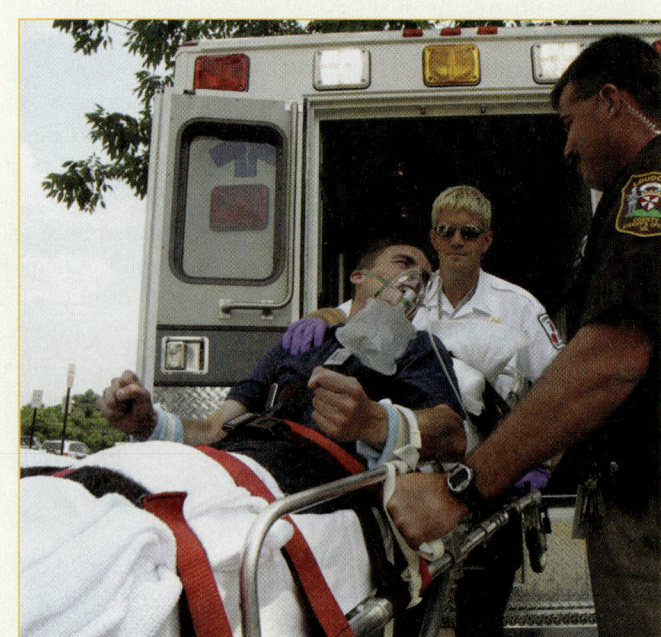

Figure 4-11 Use restraint only when absolutely necessary to ensure your own safety and that of the patient. Remember that it takes several strong people to fully restrain a patient, ideally.

patients who must be restrained in order to protect the patients themselves and to protect those who are trying to care for them.

Under the law, paramedics can use force only in response to a patient's use of force against them. If the paramedic is attacked, he or she may defend himself or herself against the attack. The amount of force that is allowed under the law is either equal to or slightly greater than the force offered by the patient, and must be in response to the patient's actions. Violence against paramedics is on the rise. It is always acceptable—nay, almost obligatory—for paramedics to refuse to enter a dangerous and unsecured situation, or for paramedics to leave a situation that becomes violent, until law enforcement can secure the scene and make it safe for paramedics to enter.

In situations requiring patient restraint for medical reasons, it is important to understand that a paramedic may only restrain patients when they are a danger to themselves or to others **Figure 4-11 ▲** . Violence can be the result of hypoxia, hypoglycemia, mental illness, brain injury, drug abuse or overdose, alcohol, or a variety of other underlying medical and psychiatric causes. Specific medical protocols should cover what is considered appropriate in your EMS system for restraining patients, and should spell out what medications or devices are allowed for use in restraining patients. Many EMS systems now use medications, such as benzodiazepines or antipsychotics, to calm patients who are violent and need transportation to a hospital to discover the underlying medical or psychiatric cause of their outbursts.

Transportation

Patients should be transported to the hospital of their choice when possible and reasonable; however, most EMS systems have protocols that direct paramedics to transport certain types of patients to particular hospitals. The capability of each hospital to care for particular kinds of patients should guide the EMS system in developing transport protocols. Transportation of patients to a facility that does not have the ability to care for their particular illness or injury can result in liability for the paramedic.

Crime Scene and Emergency Scene Responsibilities

When handling a situation involving a death, or any potential crime scene, remember that it may take law enforcement officials some time to figure out whether the scene involved a suicide, homicide, or some other form of criminal activity. It is important for paramedics to use extreme caution and not disturb or destroy potential evidence.

If the scene is a vehicle collision, don't move anything unless you have to—including broken glass, pieces of metal, or even a beer can. Leave dead bodies where they are until a coroner or medical examiner arrives to investigate.

If the incident scene is indoors, don't touch anything you don't have to touch, such as telephones or doorknobs, because of the risk of eliminating fingerprints. Carefully document any statements made by witnesses and get their contact information. Limit the number of EMS personnel who enter the scene, as each person who enters further contaminates what may later turn out to be a crime scene.

Remember that in rape cases the victim may carry vital pieces of evidence, such as fibre or hair, on his or her body—take care to protect this evidence.

If the scene involves a death, stay with the body until the police arrive, and protect the scene from contamination by bystanders, family members, media, or additional EMS personnel.

In most jurisdictions, a paramedic is not legally authorized to pronounce a patient dead. If you have any doubt about the possibility of saving the patient, initiate resuscitation. You can contact direct medical control, if available, for further direction or transport him or her to the hospital. Consult your local or regional protocols to determine what to do in this situation.

Documentation

Importance of Documentation

Even the most skilled and conscientious health care professional may eventually have to go to court as a witness or defendant in a civil or criminal action. The paramedic's best protection in court is a *thorough and accurate medical record*. This cannot be overstressed. The information recorded should contain only a record of the facts of what your findings and patient treatment entailed. Remember, you are at the scene and the emergency department physician is not; therefore, you can assist greatly by painting a picture of what you experienced at the scene. Whenever a paramedic cares for a patient, a careful, detailed record should be made of at least the following information, which are the characteristics of an effective patient care report:

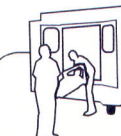

At the Scene

Be aware that at crime scenes the perpetrator may still be at or near the scene and could be a factor in when and how you care for your patient.

You are the Paramedic Part 4

Law enforcement arrives at the scene and successfully restrains your patient, who now has multiple lacerations on his face, arms, and torso. You are able to control major bleeding, initiate an IV, and provide dextrose to raise his blood glucose level. You transport him to the nearest appropriate hospital for further treatment of his injuries. Just as you transfer his care to emergency department staff, the patient's wife bursts through the emergency department doors, screaming at you and your partner and threatening to file a lawsuit. She says, "You abandoned my husband! Now look at him! This is all your fault!"

Reassessment	Recording Time: 20 Minutes
Level of consciousness	A (Alert to person, place, and day)
Skin	Warm, pink, and moist
Pulse	100 beats/min; strong and regular
Blood pressure	112/64 mm Hg
Respirations	24 breaths/min; adequate depth
SpO$_2$	98% on oxygen at 6 l/min via nasal cannula
Blood glucose	6.7 mmol/l

7. Can she prove negligence?

8. Can she file a lawsuit?

- **Date and times.** The time the call was received, the time of your arrival at the scene, the time of your departure from the scene, and the time of your arrival at the hospital.
- **History.** Information elicited from the patient and bystanders. If you are quoting patients or bystanders directly, identify them and put their statements in quotation marks.
- **Observations.** Observations of the scene, particularly if they suggest how the injury took place.
- **Physical examination.** Give a detailed description of your assessments. Include all pertinent negatives, for example, any part of the body you examine and find to be normal.
- **Treatment.** Be precise! Do not write, for example, "IV therapy was given." Write "Medical control was contacted and orders received from Dr. Smith. An 18-gauge Protect-cath IV was initiated in the left forearm; 1 litre bag of normal saline at a to keep vein open rate."
- **Changes.** Note any changes in the patient's status while under your care.

Documentation and Communication

For syncope, pertinent negatives include (but are not limited to) the patient denying that he or she has had recent diarrhea, vomiting, or tarry or bloody stools.

Patient Care Report

The following is an example of a thorough patient care report:

EXAMPLE **PATIENT CARE REPORT**

BLS 7 responded to a 911 dispatch for a patient with chest pain @ a private residence. Arrived @ 3235 1st avenue @ 12:55 to find a 73 y/o female complaining that her grandson "is causing her to have a heart attack." Next-door neighbour, crew from engine 6, & grandson are on scene. Neighbour called 911-dispatch centre.

Subjective
Chief Complaint: Chest Pain
Pt states sudden onset while arguing c̄ grandson. She feels this may have triggered the pain because she was quite upset. She has taken 2 of her own NTG in the last 15 minutes s̄ relief. Describes chest pain as crushing to the left side of her chest radiating to her jaw & left arm. Rates it a 9 on 1-10 scale & states it began 1 hour ago. She also complains of some sweating & SOB. States she has Ø allergies to meds, has medical history of chest pain & takes NTG for relief. States while having lunch, she got into an argument c̄ grandson & started having chest pain. Denies any nausea, vomiting, or dizziness. Grandson stated, "She fell in the kitchen." Pt repeatedly denies falling. Ø evidence of trauma noted on assessment.

Objective
Arrived to find pt sitting on front steps of home, c̄ O2 by NRB 15 lpm being administered by fire fighters. Pt appears to be in moderate distress, anxious, holding her hand to her chest & unable to sit still. Airway—clear. Breathing—lungs clear equal

---

EXAMPLE **PATIENT CARE REPORT**

bilaterally, c̄ good tidal volume, equal rise/fall of chest & Ø noted accessory muscle use. Circulation—strong/regular radial pulse, skin pale/cool/clammy. Disability—alert, able to speak full/clear sentences.
Head—3″ laceration below left eye c̄ swelling & redness left side of face, Ø other trauma noted. Pupils—equal and reactive, Chest—intact, Ø noted change to chest pain c̄ palpation or inspiration. Abd—soft non-tender, Extremities— +PMS in all extremities c̄ equal hand grips. Posterior Body— spinal assessment reveals spinal area non-tender, Ø numbness/tingling/weakness or loss of sensation in any extremity. Baseline Vitals: BP-128/80, P-88, R-20. Refer to vital signs data boxes for times and reassessment.

Analysis
Possible: Cardiac Chest Pain
Rule out: Head / C-Spine Injury

Plan
12:55— Arrive, initial assessment, spinal immobilization equipment applied with no change to PMS post immobilization, vitals assessed, continue O2 at 15 lpm/NRM. Pt states oxygen is not helping her chest pain. Pt agrees to treatment & transport.

13:04— Confirm that NTG is pts, was prescribed by her physician, & she has taken 2 c̄ last one being > 5 minutes ago. Dressed wound with 4×4.

13:06— Paramedic Jones assisted pt in administration of 1 sublingual 0.4 mg NTG tab.

13:10— Moved pt to ambulance, en route to hospital.

13:15— Reassess, pt states the pain is now a "3" on 1-10 scale, she states "SOB is now gone." Skin colour is improved, pt appears more relaxed.

13:17— Vitals reassessed with no change. Pt removed O2 mask stated "I don't need or want this anymore." Explained to pt significant importance of O2 with chest pain and potential for condition to worsen if oxygen is discontinued. Pt still refused NRM or nasal cannula.

13:20— Arrive ED, pt care transferred & report given to RN Turner.

Complete your records as soon as possible after the call. Even a few hours later, the details may become vague in your memory. Write legibly in ink. If your system uses electronic patient care reports, be sure to read your report over for typing errors before printing or transmitting the record. Be as precise and detailed as possible. Document everything you did, and everything about your examination and reassessment of the patient. Remember, *if you don't document it, you can't prove you did it.* Your patient care report becomes a permanent part of the patient's record. It is also a legal document and reflects on its author.

Neatness counts! A sloppy, incomplete record suggests to the reader (and to the court!) that the prehospital care of the patient may also have been sloppy and incomplete

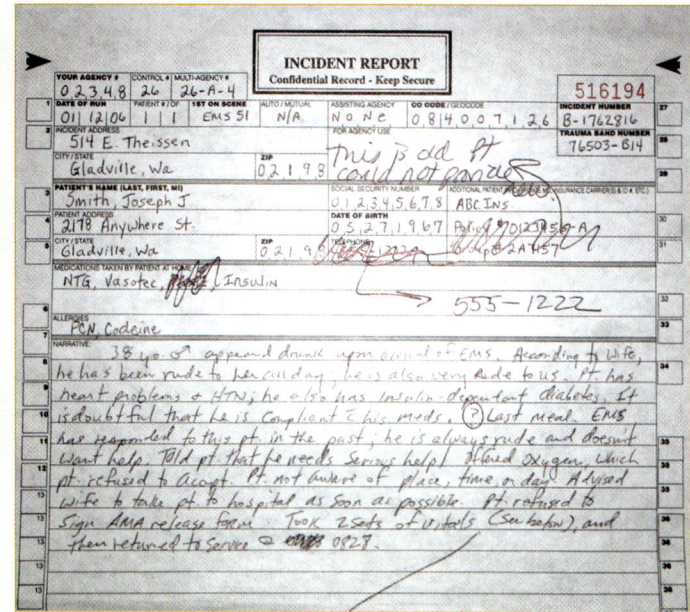

Figure 4-12 Filing a patient care report is a critical part of your responsibilities as a paramedic. **A.** Proper documentation **B.** Improper documentation. Particularly if you sense that there might be legal complications with a patient, take extra time and care to submit a thorough report.

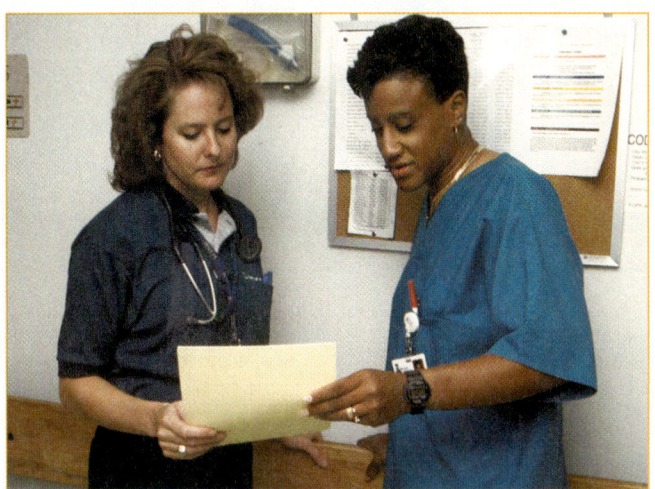

Figure 4-13 Part of ensuring competent and continuous care for each patient is making sure that the patient's report is handed over to appropriate medical personnel at the hospital.

Figure 4-12 ▲ . Such records are red flags to plaintiff's attorneys who consider them an invitation to file suit. Take the time to make your records accurate and thorough. Document any unusual events, including equipment failures, interference by bystanders, getting lost, or other problems you encounter either on the way to or at the scene. These problems should be documented factually and objectively. All crew members—not just the one writing the report—should sign the report legibly, and denote their crew numbers.

There are some things a paramedic should never do in a medical record. It is not the place for creative writing. The medical record is not the place for flippant or derogatory remarks about a patient. Do not use the medical record to blame another medical provider for an adverse event. Find another outlet for your opinions, medical or otherwise. The medical record is the worst possible place to voice frustrations with the administration of the EMS system. You will only hurt, not help, any systems issues that may arise in the course of a lawsuit.

Your Report Becomes Part of the Medical Record

Always leave a copy of your written report at the emergency department. It is critical for you to leave a written record of your prehospital treatment of the patient to ensure continuity of care in the emergency department **Figure 4-13 ◀** . The emergency department staff needs to know how you encountered the patient, what treatment you rendered, and any changes in the patient's condition resulting from your care. Failure to leave a copy of the report can result in duplication of treatment, or a lack of understanding of what precipitated the emergency call. That copy of your report will become a part of the patient's permanent medical record. Paramedics in busy services who race out the door without leaving a record of their care leave themselves open for problems with the legal system and the hospital. Remember, many hospitals caution all health care providers against only giving verbal orders and reports.

Retention of Medical Records

Your call reports should be maintained for a period generally described by provincial law. Providers should never keep personal copies of patient care reports because of the confidential nature of the information contained.

Reportable Cases

Each province has its own requirements regarding categories of cases that must be reported to the appropriate authorities. These cases include some of the most difficult a paramedic will see.

Virtually every province has laws requiring paramedics to report suspected child maltreatment. It is essential for you to be familiar with the reporting requirements of your own province.

The obligation to report is most frequently applied to the following categories of cases:

- Neglect or maltreatment of children
- Neglect or maltreatment of elderly people
- Domestic violence
- Injury sustained during the commission of a felony, or specific injuries considered to be of suspicious origin (such as gunshot wounds or stab wounds)
- Drug-related injuries
- Childbirth occurring outside a licensed medical facility
- Rape
- Animal bites
- Certain communicable diseases

In recent years, increasing emphasis in Canada on privacy related to health information may also restrict the paramedic's ability to report some of these same items. As noted, reporting requirements vary widely from province to province. Learn the laws of your province and observe the reporting obligations that apply to you.

Coroner and Medical Examiner Cases

Every EMS system should have a list of procedures for coroner-medical examiner cases Figure 4-14 ▾ . Although the coroner's law varies somewhat from province to province, generally you should notify the coroner-medical examines service of all deaths, including:

1. Obvious or suspected homicide
2. Obvious or suspected suicide
3. Any other violent or sudden, unexpected death
4. Death of a prison inmate
5. Any sudden or unexpected death occurring outside a health care facility

Special Considerations

Elder maltreatment is as prevalent as child maltreatment in our society. Do not forget to be observant and report any suspicious signs or symptoms to the proper authorities.

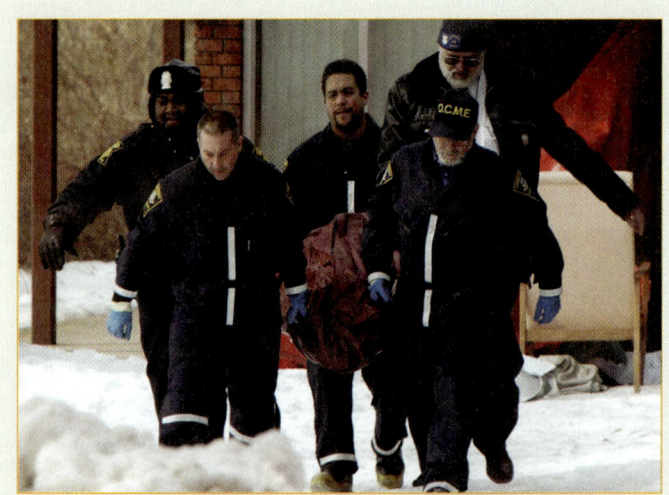

Figure 4-14 In any situation involving the death of an individual, paramedics should contact the coroner-medical examiner service with pertinent details depending on local protocols.

You are the Paramedic Summary

1. What clues, if any, were available to tip you off as to the potential for this patient to become violent?

Most often, body language is a bigger indicator of potential violence than words that patients use. This patient had his back to you with his shoulders raised and fists clenched. These are all indications of impending violence. If you have no indication that the scene is unsafe, and you find yourself in a situation such as this one, maintain a safe distance, never allow the patient to come between you and your exit, call for law enforcement, and immediately leave the scene if you feel you or your partner are in danger.

2. What would be the best course of action at this point?

Your best course of action is to leave the immediate area. It takes, at minimum, four trained personnel to safely restrain a patient (one for each limb). Because you do not have these resources immediately available, you are not able to safely restrain this patient. Unfortunately, violence can erupt very quickly, and it is imperative not to enter a scene you believe is unsafe or to put yourself or your partner in harm's way.

3. Could your actions be considered abandonment?

Technically, you left the patient after you had initiated contact. However, you were unable to render required medical care because of the patient's combative behaviour. You remained ready to provide necessary treatment as soon as the patient had been properly restrained. It could be argued that you should have responded with an adequate number of staff and/or law enforcement because the details of the call were unknown. This could be construed as a grey area, depending on the interpreter.

4. What other courses of action, if any, could be taken?

When you are unsure as to the intent of the patient, or suspect that the patient could become violent, you should avoid any physical movement or verbal statements that may induce anger. It would have been more prudent to slowly initiate contact rather than immediately attempting to gain eye contact.

5. Was any part of this situation avoidable?

As part of your training, you will learn that the brain is very sensitive to lowered levels of blood glucose and blood oxygen. Hypoglycemic and hypoxic states can cause significant deterioration in mental status, sometimes accompanied by bizarre or combative behaviour. Be on the lookout for these things when dealing with known diabetics who have apparent low blood glucose levels.

6. What would be helpful in handling this situation?

The more information that can be obtained regarding the details of the incident prior to your arrival, the greater chance you have of avoiding a situation such as this one. However, for reasons stated earlier, this may not be possible. Be prepared for the unexpected.

7. Can she prove negligence?

If it could be proved that you should have known that the patient was likely to become violent, then negligence could be proven. For instance, if this patient had a history of becoming violent and you did not immediately request appropriate additional resources, then there could be a legitimate claim of negligence.

8. Can she file a lawsuit?

Yes. People can and do file lawsuits for many reasons. The best method of protection is to always follow local protocols, document each call thoroughly, and act in the patient's best interest. Doing these things will minimize chances of a successful lawsuit against you. This does not, however, prevent a lawsuit from occurring.

Prep Kit

◼ Ready for Review

- Paramedics operate in a community that exposes them to professional liability. Failing to perform their job as expected within the medical community, the legal community, and the regulations of the jurisdiction in which they function will expose them to civil and/or criminal liability.
- The foundation of our legal system is our federal government. There are three branches of government: executive, judicial, and legislative.
- There are two types of law: civil and criminal.
  - Civil cases result in monetary damages.
  - Criminal cases result in incarceration of an individual.
- Paramedics are particularly susceptible to charges of assault and battery. Assault is when you instill the fear of bodily harm. Battery is when you (as a paramedic) unlawfully touch another without his or her consent.
- False imprisonment can occur when a paramedic restrains a patient against his or her will. Protection against this charge can exist only if appropriate documentation and policy exist regarding the specific call.
- Defamation, slander, and libel present risks to paramedics when they make statements, either verbal or written, that injure a person's good name. Saying a patient looks drunk is inappropriate. Paramedics should describe the behaviour that reflects their concerns.
- Lawsuits follow a general process that starts with a complaint or notice of complaint, a response or answer by the defendant, discovery, settlement discussions, and trial process.
- Paramedics are subject to multiple legal jurisdictions, including provincial law, provincial regulations, local medical protocol, and departmental policy.
- Medical directors have a supervisory relationship over paramedics.
- Your activities function as an extension of a series of medical directions from the medical director that are either direct or indirect. These directives are binding on paramedics unless they believe that they will cause harm to the patient.
- Provincial legislation enables paramedics to practice in their province. It is the responsibility of paramedics to understand the statutes of the province in which they practice.
- Provincial laws define scope of practice for the paramedic, which specifies the limits of practice allowed under the Medical Practice Act.
- Personal health information laws have been enacted to protect patient information from unlawful and unnecessary dissemination.
- Emergency vehicle operations must be done in a manner that protects the public from further injury. No call can justify driving in a manner that endangers the public.
- You may provide prehospital care when off duty and in some provinces be protected under Good Samaritan laws. Paramedics must remember that they are only protected if they perform within their training and education and if they do not receive any compensation.
- Negligence occurs only when four processes have occurred:
  - Duty to act. The paramedic must have had a duty to act.
  - Breach of duty. The paramedic did not fulfill that duty.
  - Proximate cause. The paramedic's breach of duty caused the plaintiff's injury.
  - Injury resulted. An injury occurred as a result of the above.

- As the highest level of prehospital care providers, paramedics must ensure that they do not abandon their patients. Abandonment can occur anytime paramedics turn over their patients inappropriately or to a level of care lesser than themselves or if they leave a patient without ensuring that the patient had the mental capacity to refuse treatment or transport.
  - Documentation is the best method to prevent the appearance of abandonment.
- Patients have the right to determine their own care. Paramedics must understand their legal limitations based on any advance directives issued by the patient.
- Do not resuscitate (DNR) orders are a specific form of legal directive that generally defines the end-of-life care plan developed by a patient's physician (usually in consultation with a patient or their family). A DNR order is *not* a "do-not-care-for-the-patient" order.
- Provincial jurisdictions issue paramedics either licenses, certificates, or both. Paramedics must understand that the licensure or certification is a privilege extended by the governing authority that allows paramedics to practice within the enacting legislation.
- All patients of sound mind have the legal right under the Canadian Constitution to privacy, consent, and refusal. Paramedics cannot infringe on these inalienable rights unless they believe that patients are not of sound mind and pose a detriment to themselves or others.
- You must obtain informed consent from patients prior to any medical process including examination.
- You must get expressed consent from patients before initiating treatment.
- Implied consent is said to exist when patients are unable to answer for themselves and paramedics deem that treatment is required.
- Minors pose challenges that local jurisdictions must address before a call occurs. In general, if the patient is a minor, the minor may have neither the right to consent to care nor the right to refuse it. Paramedics must always take responsibility for minors.
- Documentation is the lifeblood of a paramedic. All calls should have documentation that reflects what occurred. The documentation must include any and all demographics, times, history of events, physical examinations, treatment processes, and changes.
- Documentation is a legal form that will be used against you if you are part of a legal action.
- Patient refusals and no-transport calls pose a large potential legal liability to paramedics. The only protection against a civil suit over a refusal will be the documentation that the paramedic produces at the time of the incident.
  - A refusal signature without narrative and evidence of a physical examination is worthless.
- Paramedics must plan to protect themselves and their colleagues from violence. Understanding local law enforcement protocols and having medical protocols for the restraint of patients by both physical and chemical methods are necessary.
- Crime scenes present the intersection between EMS and law enforcement. Paramedics have an obligation to assist the law enforcement community in preservation of evidence and documentation of scenes or actions that may later be introduced on behalf of a criminal prosecution.

Vital Vocabulary

abandonment Abrupt termination of contact with the patient without giving the patient sufficient opportunity to find another suitable health care professional to take over his or her medical treatment.

advance directive A written document that expresses the wants, needs, and desires of a patient in reference to future medical care; examples include living wills and organ donation.

assault To create in another person a fear of immediate bodily harm or invasion of bodily security.

battery Any act of touching another person without that person's consent.

certification Evidence of a certain level of training, such as a certificate of completion from a course or school.

civil suit An action instituted by a private individual or corporation against another private individual or corporation.

consent Agreement by the patient to accept a medical intervention.

criminal prosecution An action instituted by the government against a private individual for violation of criminal law.

damages Compensation for injury awarded by a court.

decision-making capacity The patient's ability to understand and process the information you give him or her about your proposed plan of prehospital care.

defamation Intentionally making a false statement, through written or verbal communication, which injures a person's good name or reputation.

defendant In a civil suit, the individual against whom a legal action is brought.

do not resuscitate (DNR) order A physician-initiated set of end-of-life treatment orders developed in consultation with a patient's family or legal designate in the event that the patient is not able to express his or her own wishes and has not left an advance directive.

due process A right to a fair procedure for a legal action against a person or agency; has two components: *Notice* and *Opportunity to be Heard*.

duty Legal obligation of public and certain other ambulance services to respond to a call for help in their jurisdiction.

ethics A set of values in society that differentiates right from wrong.

expressed consent A type of informed consent that occurs when the patient does something, either through words or by taking some sort of action, that demonstrates permission to provide care.

false imprisonment The intentional and unjustified detention of a person against his or her will.

Good Samaritan law A statute providing limited immunity from liability to persons responding voluntarily and in good faith to the aid of an injured person outside the hospital.

gross negligence Negligence that is willful, wanton, intentional, or reckless; a serious departure from the accepted standards.

immunity Legal protection from penalties that could normally be incurred under the law.

implied consent Assumption on behalf of a person unable to give consent that he or she would have done so.

informed consent A patient's voluntary agreement to be treated after being told about the nature of the disease, the risks and benefits of the proposed treatment, alternative treatments, or the choice of no treatment at all.

liability A finding in civil cases that the preponderance of the evidence shows the defendant was responsible for the plaintiff's injuries.

libel Making a false statement in written form that injures a person's good name.

licensure The privilege to practice at a carefully defined level, usually granted by a provincial government agency or self-governing professional body.

Medical Practice Act An act that usually defines the minimum qualifications of those who may perform various health services, defines the skills that each type of practitioner is legally permitted to use, and establishes a means of certification for different categories of health care professionals.

negligence Professional action or inaction on the part of the health care worker that does not meet the standard of ordinary care expected of similarly trained and prudent health care practitioners and that results in injury to the patient.

ordinary negligence Negligence that is a failure to act, or a simple mistake that causes harm to a patient.

plaintiff In a civil suit, the individual who brings a legal action against another individual.

proximate cause The specific reason that an injury occurred; one of the items that must be proven in order for a paramedic to be held liable for negligence.

scope of practice What a province permits a paramedic practicing under its license or certification to do.

slander Verbally making a false statement that injures a person's good name.

standard of care What a reasonable paramedic with training would do in the same or a similar situation.

tort A wrongful act that gives rise to a civil suit.

vicarious liability Protection whereby the employer is held liable to compensate persons for the harm caused by their employees in the course of their employment.

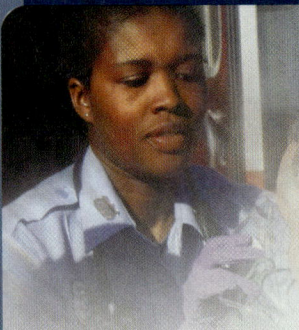

Assessment in Action

You are called to a scene in which a man with altered mental status is bleeding heavily from an open cut on his forehead. The neighbours called 9-1-1 after seeing him in his yard where he was having trouble walking and attempting to mow the lawn in the pouring rain. When you arrive, the man is angry that someone called 9-1-1. He insists that he's fine. He has no memory of how he may have cut his head, isn't making sense, and seems confused. He refuses to let you examine him, refuses to answer any questions, and refuses transport. What would be the appropriate response to the following questions?

1. **Can treating this patient without his consent be considered assault and/or battery?**
   A. Yes
   B. No

2. **What is the difference between *assault* and *battery*?**
   A. Assault is physical contact in a harmful way; battery is severe injury.
   B. Assault is verbal or other threats that instill fear in someone; battery is actually touching someone without their consent.
   C. Assault is verbal threats actually carried out; battery is physically harming someone without any kind of warning to that person.
   D. Assault is physical only; battery is verbal only.

3. **True or false? The scope of practice for a paramedic may vary significantly from province to province.**
   A. True
   B. False

4. **True or false? The medical director has the authority to prevent a paramedic from performing certain skills that he or she is licensed or certified to perform if he or she feels like doing so for some reason.**
   A. True
   B. False

5. **You cannot discuss anything regarding the man in the scenario because of your province's PHI law, which:**
   A. protects the privacy of medical information, insurance information, and any other privacy issues affecting the patient within the health care system.
   B. requires criminal sanctions against anyone who releases private health care information regarding a patient.
   C. requires civil penalties for anyone who uses protected health information in an unauthorized manner.
   D. requires that no personal patient information be released over the radio.

6. **True or false? If your agency is part of a government agency, you cannot be sued for wrongdoing as a paramedic working for that agency.**
   A. True
   B. False

7. **The elements that must be proven for a negligence lawsuit to be successful are:**
   A. duty; breach of duty; proximate cause; and harm.
   B. duty; breach of duty; harm; and abandonment.
   C. breach of duty; harm; abandonment; and proximate cause.
   D. abandonment and breach of duty.

8. **You must obtain consent—either implied or informed (except in some cases)—to do which of the following?**
   A. Touch a patient, treat a patient, transport a patient
   B. Transport a patient
   C. Treat and transport a patient
   D. None of the above

9. **True or false? A patient with some, or all, of the following, is not able to refuse prehospital care.**
   - Patient is not oriented to person, place, and time.
   - Patient demonstrates that he or she does not understand his or her condition or the need for medical attention.
   - It is obvious that the patient is impaired as a result of alcohol or drugs.
   - The patient has an obvious head injury and is not answering questions appropriately.
   A. True
   B. False

10. **What is the paramedic's BEST protection in court, no matter what the charge or case against him or her?**
    A. A good attitude and proper maintenance of skills
    B. His or her reputation, professionally and personally
    C. A thorough and accurate medical record on all patients treated
    D. An exceptional memory of all calls and patients treated

Challenging Questions

11. **You and your crew have transported a patient with minor injuries from a motor vehicle collision. The emergency department is very busy. Your rescue squad is understaffed. It is a rainy night. You pull aside a nurse and give your report. The nurse says he'll get to her as soon as possible. You leave a copy of the call report at the nurses station and leave the patient on the stretcher. What are you doing wrong that you could be sued for later?**

12. **You are called to a scene of domestic violence. The man who attacked his wife has been taken into custody by local police, who are still on the scene. However, the man has injuries that you know require stitches. He is refusing prehospital care. The officers tell you that you can treat and transport him (in their presence) based on the concept of involuntary consent. Why is this not acceptable reasoning? (There is more than one reason.)**

Points to Ponder

You and your partner are dispatched to a dying patient who has a valid advance directive per your EMS system. In this advance directive the patient requests that no resuscitative measures be taken. The only care requested is comfort care.

A hospice volunteer is on scene and has requested transport to the hospital. The patient's daughter, who is the medical power of attorney, is also on scene. She was unaware that the volunteer phoned EMS and is refusing to let you and your partner transport the patient to the hospital. The family members are very upset and becoming angry, repeating over and over "she just wanted to die in the bed her husband died in 40 years ago." They state, "This is difficult enough without you here," and they want you to leave.

Did the volunteer have the right to call EMS without speaking to the family first, in particular the medical power of attorney? Does the medical power of attorney have the right to refuse transporting the patient to the hospital? How do you and your partner resolve these issues?

Issues: Defending the Patient's Right to Die With Dignity, Defending the Value of Advance Directives.

Ethical Issues

Competency Areas

Area 1: Professional Responsibilities

1.1.a	Maintain patient dignity.
1.1.b	Reflect professionalism through use of appropriate language.
1.1.e	Maintain patient confidentiality.
1.1.j	Behave ethically.
1.1.k	Function as patient advocate.
1.2.c	Interpret evidence in medical literature and assess relevance to practice.
1.3.b	Recognize "patient rights" and the implications on the role of the provider.
1.4.a	Function within relevant legislation, policies, and procedures.
1.6.a	Exhibit reasonable and prudent judgment.
1.6.b	Practice effective problem-solving.

Area 2: Communication

2.1.d	Provide information to patient about their situation and how they will be treated.
2.1.e	Interact effectively with the patient, relatives, and bystanders who are in stressful situations.
2.1.g	Use appropriate terminology.
2.3.c	Establish trust and rapport with patients and colleagues.
2.4.a	Treat others with respect.
2.4.b	Exhibit empathy and compassion while providing care.
2.4.g	Exhibit diplomacy, tact, and discretion.

Medical Ethics

Ethics is the philosophy of right and wrong, of moral duties, of responsibilities, and of ideal professional behaviour. Morality is a code of conduct defined by society, religion, culture, or another person that affects one's character, conduct, and conscience.

Ethical dilemmas can be some of the most challenging problems that paramedics and other health care providers face in clinical practice. A number of different ethical theories and frameworks—deontological, utilitarian, virtue, care, relativism, egalitarian, libertarian, and feminism among others—have been developed to guide professional behaviour when faced with these difficult situations. No one theory, however, is able to answer all of the ethical dilemmas that may arise. Similarly, a single theory cannot uniformly guide decision making and professional conduct.

In 1979, Beauchamp and Childress described *principlism*, the theory that four equally important principles are present in all ethical theories: autonomy, beneficence, nonmalfeasance, and justice:

- *Autonomy* reflects the need to respect other people as individuals who have the right to make capable and informed decisions regarding their health care.
- *Beneficence* means doing what is best for the patient.
- *Nonmalfeasance* points to the fundamental medical creed of *premium non nocere*, or "first, do no harm."
- *Justice* reflects the need for fairness and to "treat equal cases equally and unequal cases unequally." The principle of justice incorporates consideration of the distribution of health care resources in patient care.

Today, these four principles are often used in the analysis of ethical dilemmas in an effort to best resolve them. Yet problems remain because these principles may conflict with each other; respect for individual principles may, in fact, suggest a markedly different course of action. For these reasons, the principles do not always provide an answer to a particular situation. Still, they offer an invaluable framework to begin to unpack the issues, to analyze them from different perspectives, and to devise ways to resolve them that will guide conduct and ultimately improve the quality of care provided.

Paramedics need to be open to discussions of ethical issues and be aware of their own moral standards, beliefs, and biases that affect their daily work. Everyone has different beliefs, values, cultural and/or religious backgrounds, personal and professional experiences, and goals that influence their thoughts and actions in daily life. Self-knowledge and awareness of these factors and their potential influence on professional practice is crucial in order to fulfill your professional role and fiduciary duty as a paramedic. The assumption that your patients share your moral standards may frequently be false. Your moral standards may even conflict with your patients' wishes or your patients' best interests. It is important that you put your patient's interests before your own **Figure 5-1 ▾**.

Medical ethics (sometimes called *bioethics*) is a discipline within ethics that discusses and debates dilemmas that arise in caring for patients. Ethical principles have been incorporated into codes of ethics that are meant to guide the conduct and

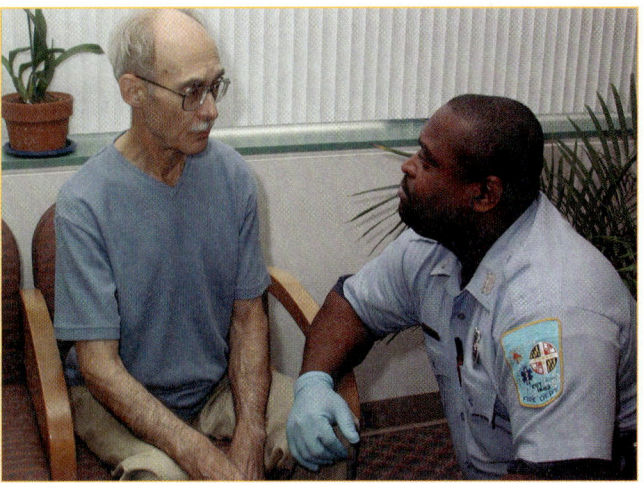

Figure 5-1 As a paramedic serving a diverse public, you will frequently work with people who have cultural backgrounds that are different from your own. Work to set aside your own personal beliefs when making decisions on the patient's behalf.

You are the Paramedic Part 1

You are dispatched to 1625 Lance Lane for a 50-year-old man with an unknown medical problem. En route to the scene, the dispatcher informs you, "CPR is in progress." Your estimated time of arrival to the scene is approximately 15 minutes, but you feel confident this patient has a good chance for survival because your primary service area has a tiered response system.

In a brief radio report, an on-scene emergency medical responder crew advises you that this was a witnessed cardiac arrest. The patient complained of chest pain just prior to collapse, and CPR was started immediately by a family member. No other information is provided. When you ask whether electrical therapy with the AED has been administered, no one replies. You find this odd, and wonder if something is wrong.

1. Are emergency medical responders and volunteer primary care paramedics held to the same standards of prehospital care as staff paramedics?
2. If sensitive information needs to be relayed regarding prehospital care, what other communication options should be available to paramedics?

describe a standard of professionalism for health care providers **Figure 5-2 ▶** . Throughout the ages, there have been many published codes of ethics. The Oath of Geneva, drafted by the World Medical Association in 1948, provides a good example; it is the oath taken by many medical students on completion of their studies, at the time of being admitted to the medical profession:

> I solemnly pledge myself to consecrate my life to the service of humanity; I will give to my teachers the respect and gratitude which is their due; I will practice my profession with conscience and dignity; the health of my patient will be my first consideration; I will respect the secrets which are confided in me; I will maintain by all the means in my power the honor and noble traditions of the medical profession; my colleagues will be my brothers; I will not permit considerations of religion, nationality, race, party politics, or social standing to intervene between my duty and my patient; I will maintain the utmost respect for human life from the time of conception; even under threat, I will not make use of my medical knowledge contrary to the laws of humanity. I make these promises solemnly, freely and upon my honor.

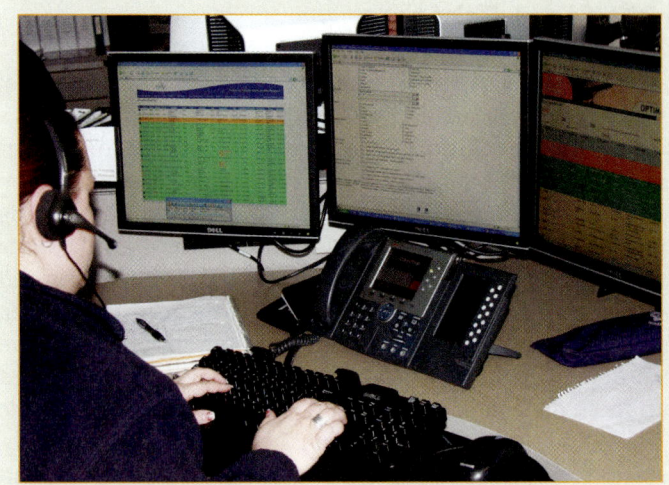

Figure 5-2 When people call 9-1-1, they trust you not only with providing proper medical care, but also with using sound ethical judgment—including the safeguarding of their personal possessions.

You are the Paramedic Part 2

When you arrive, you learn that the AED could not be used because the battery failed. The first emergency medical responders were from a volunteer agency, and no one had been assigned that weekend to check the equipment because it was a holiday and everyone was gone. They ask you not to tell anyone, and promise it will never happen again.

You don't have time to become involved in a detailed discussion, but gather information pertinent to caring for your patient. As you proceed to the hospital, the patient's wife identifies herself, tells you that she is a registered nurse, and asks if she can ride with you to the hospital. En route to the receiving facility, she asks you why the AED failed to operate.

Initial Assessment	Recording Time: 25 Minutes
Level of consciousness	Unresponsive
Airway	Patent
Breathing	Bag-valve-mask ventilations
Circulation	Carotid pulse detected with compressions
Vital Signs	
Skin	Cool, pale/mottled with blue mucosa and moist
Blood pressure	None
Spo$_2$	Unable to read
ECG	Asystole in three leads
Pupils	Fixed and dilated
Treatment	
ETT	8.0 mm/21 cm at the teeth
Oxygen	High-flow via bag-valve-mask device
IV	Normal saline, #1 left antecubital vein, 18-gauge; #2 right antecubital vein, 18-gauge; 1,000 ml normal saline infusing
Medications	Epinephrine, 1:10,000 3 mg IV Atropine, 2 mg IV

3. Is it ever appropriate to conceal information regarding prehospital care?
4. How should you answer the wife's question?
5. How and when should you address her concerns?

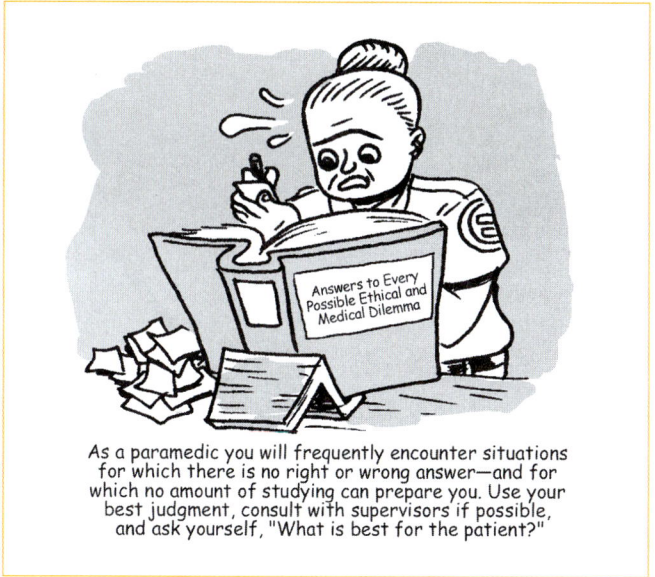

As a paramedic you will frequently encounter situations for which there is no right or wrong answer—and for which no amount of studying can prepare you. Use your best judgment, consult with supervisors if possible, and ask yourself, "What is best for the patient?"

Figure 5-3

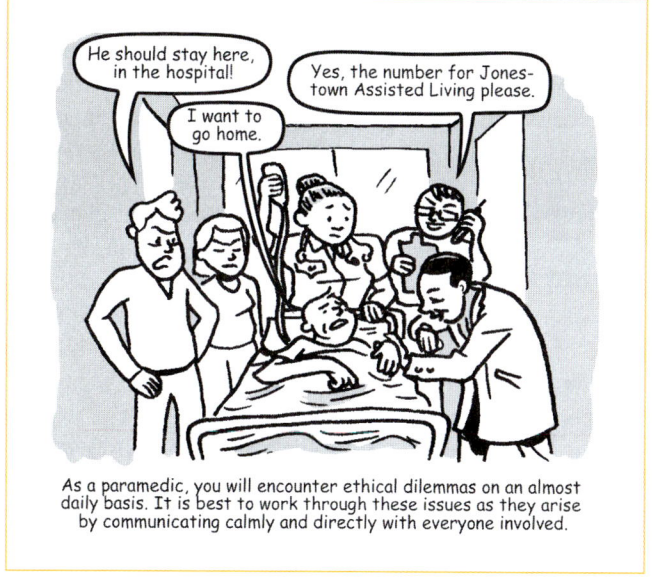

As a paramedic, you will encounter ethical dilemmas on an almost daily basis. It is best to work through these issues as they arise by communicating calmly and directly with everyone involved.

Figure 5-4

The Canadian National Occupational Competency Profiles (NOCPs) include ethical behaviour as one of the first professional behaviours that must be understood, valued, and integrated into paramedic practice. A paramedic's first priority is concern for the welfare of others. All of the various codes of right and wrong must ultimately arise from that concern, and it is a safe generalization that *if you place the welfare of the patient ahead of all other considerations, you will rarely if ever commit an unethical act in medical care* **Figure 5-3 ▲**. It would be impossible to enumerate here all of the ethical dilemmas that you may face in your work as a paramedic. However, if each time you are confronted with a dilemma of right and wrong you ask yourself, "What is in the best interest of the patient?" you will be on firm footing.

Ethics has become the subject of many teaching sessions, because paramedics find themselves in the unique position of being accountable to more systems than the average health care provider in trying to respect the wishes of the patient **Figure 5-4 ▶**. The EMS system, your medical director, the EMS service you work for, and your community's standard of care can compete with the wishes of the patient. These competing interests can create an ethical conflict that you will want to resolve. How can you do this? Communicate, communicate, communicate.

Autonomy

As you learned in the previous chapter, patients have the right to direct their own care, including how they want their end-of-life medical care provided to them. This right, known as patient autonomy, has come to the forefront of medical ethics.

Respect for autonomy promotes the recognition that each patient is a unique person with deeply held values and beliefs and with distinctive past experiences upon which they base important life and health care decisions. This recognition is crucial so that the patient is viewed as a person, not just another "case of x." Moreover, demonstrating respect for autonomy builds trust in the health care team and reveals the caring, empathy, and compassion of high-quality care, often at times when people need it the most.

Capacity

The expression of autonomy in health care decision making is dependent on patients having the capacity to express their wishes with regard to the treatment in question. You should always presume that patients are capable; that is, they are presumed to have the ability to (1) understand information regarding their state of health and treatment options and (2) appreciate the consequences of a given decision or lack of decision. A capable patient has the well-recognized right to autonomy to determine what happens to his or her own body, to accept or refuse medical treatment according to, or even against, the advice of the health care provider. This right to self-determination also extends the right of capable patients to refuse effective treatment options and even life-sustaining ones.

Capacity may vary over time, depending on the patient's state of health (physical, psychological, or emotional) and medications (prescriptions, over-the-counter remedies, or illicit/street drugs). A patient may be capable with respect to consenting to one treatment, yet be incapable with respect to another, especially if the latter is more complicated and more difficult to understand. Some patients may understand the proposed treatment but for a variety of reasons fail to appreciate the consequences of their decisions. Capacity assessments are crucial whenever health care providers initiate a patient care relationship. Repeat assessments are important to monitor possible changes in the patient's condition. Illness, medications, intoxication, and drug use/addictions can alter a patient's capacity temporarily or permanently. As soon as a patient recovers his or her capacity, the patient reassumes control over all of his or her health care decisions and treatment plans.

Consent to Treatment

In the case of an emergency situation where a patient is not capable of consenting to treatment, consent is generally presumed and paramedics are to "err on the side of life" and initiate all required resuscitative treatments. Consent to continue treatment must be obtained at the earliest opportunity from the patient (if capacity is restored) or his or her substitute decision-maker. In all other nonemergency situations, consent to treatment is required—even for treatment by paramedics—before treatment can be initiated.

For consent to be valid, three ethical concepts must be met:

1. The patient must be capable or consent must be given by the patient's legal substitute decision-maker in the event of incapacity.
2. The consent must be informed.
3. The consent must be given voluntarily, without coercion or manipulation.

To be informed, health care providers must provide patients and/or their substitute decision-makers enough information. What constitutes "enough" is the information that would be expected by a reasonable person in the patient's circumstances. The patient must also be given the opportunity and time to ask questions **Figure 5-5 ▶**. Therefore, in order for consent to be informed, the following must be explained:

- A description of why treatment is needed, the recommended treatment, and alternative options
- The expected benefits and the likelihood that these could be obtained
- The material risks of the treatment and the likelihood of their occurrence
- The material side effects of the treatment and the likelihood of their occurrence
- If any of the material risks or side effects were to occur, what other treatment would be required
- The likely consequences of not having the treatment
- An explanation of the health care provider's recommendation in view of the treatment options
- Any questions the patient or his or her substitute decision-maker may have or any information requested

In legal terms, consent can be expressed (orally or in writing) or implied (ie, the patient sticks out his arm for an intravenous start).

A common situation for paramedics is the necessity of treating patients against their wishes. Usually, these patients do not have decision-making capacity, the situation is an emergency, and treatment is given "erring on the side of life." If your patient is the proverbial "guy who doesn't want to admit he's having a

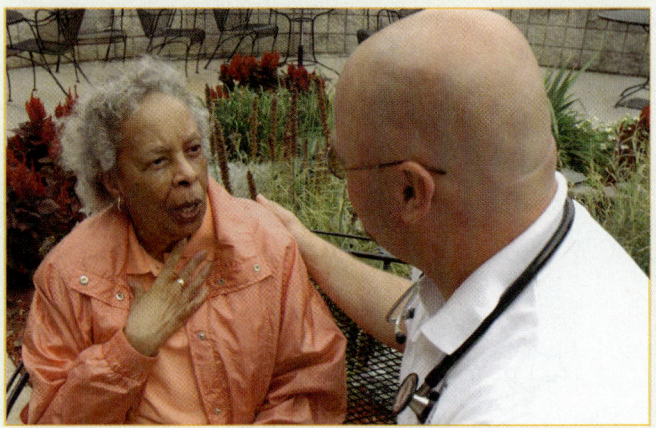

Figure 5-5 Remember that the decision to accept medical treatment is a difficult one. Give the patient time to think and to consider what feels right. Often, this is the first time the patient has had to face the reality of his or her medical condition.

heart attack," you must use your best diplomatic negotiating skills to persuade him to come with you to the hospital. Persuasion (ie, "I really feel you should come to the hospital. We are concerned about you. Your family is concerned about you. We all want to make sure you receive treatment if you need it.") is deemed ethical practice, whereas coercion (ie, "If you don't come to the hospital we will never respond to your 9-1-1 call again.") and manipulation (ie, "If you don't come to the hospital, chances are great that you will die in the next 5 minutes.") are not. The ends do not justify the means, and it does not matter if you are just trying to act in your patient's best interests.

Ideally, these situations should be covered in protocols and discussed in detail regularly with your medical director and paramedic colleagues. Often, paramedics will have "rounds" where difficult cases—both clinically and ethically—are discussed. Learning from others' experiences and debating the issues is the optimal way for all paramedics to improve their practice.

At the Scene

Many provinces and territories have legislation that allows for power of attorney for personal care, advance directives, and living wills. These documents provide paramedics with direction about patient wishes and who can speak for the patient when they are unable to do so. Paramedics should be familiar with legislation and regulations in their jurisdiction and how to respond to the patient's wishes when the patient is unable to express these wishes.

Advance Care Planning

If a patient becomes or is incapable of making decisions, he or she still has a right to be respected and to have a voice in his or her health care and treatment choices. In the event that the patient loses his or her capacity to make such decisions, respect for a patient's autonomy can be achieved through following either: (1) a previously expressed (ie, at a time that the patient was capable) oral or written advance directive or (2) through the appointment of a substitute decision-maker.

The expression of oral and/or written advance directives by capable patients in anticipation of their wishes regarding future health care choices and expected quality of life is sometimes referred to as advance care planning. The wishes themselves, either orally or in writing, are called advance directives. These advance directives only come into effect when a patient becomes incapable of making decisions. However, they do not replace the need to obtain informed consent at the time treatment is actually needed.

The process of obtaining consent to a given treatment at the time of need—even if this entails discussions with a substitute decision-maker and not the patient—allows the review of wishes, values, and beliefs; the revision of goals in context of the patient's situation; and the correction of any misconceptions and misinformation (regarding treatments and/or expected outcomes) that may have influenced previous decisions and advance directives.

Because the patient's wishes may change over time, it is crucial to ensure that they are current before using them to form the basis of important decisions. Patients have the right to change their advance directives at any time, if they are capable. These changes are legally valid and must be considered in any future decisions regarding treatment options, whether the newly expressed advance directive is spoken or written down. In other words, it does not matter if the advance directive is written, what matters is that it is the most current expression of the patient's wishes—of his or her autonomy—that must be respected.

Advance directives often fail to anticipate situations that may arise in a patient's life. For these reasons, their language is vague and subject to interpretation. Rarely do they spell out exactly what kind of treatment a patient wishes to be given, under what circumstances should he or she become incapacitated. At times, they may even be impossible to carry out in view of the patient's condition at the time they come into effect. Furthermore, the diagnosis and prognosis of illness often is not crystal clear, and decision-making regarding initiating, continuing, withholding, and withdrawing treatments can be difficult, even when advance directives have been expressed.

At the Scene

Do not be confused. An advance directive is not the same as a do not resuscitate (DNR) order. The advance directive allows for consent to decisions regarding DNR orders if a patient becomes incapacitated or is unable to make his or her own decisions—assuming a DNR order would reflect the patient's values, beliefs, and treatment goals.

Power of Attorney for Personal Care

A power of attorney for personal care is a formal legal document that may include advance directives; it may also desig-

nate another person to make health care decisions for the patient at any time the patient is unable to make those decisions himself or herself. This appointed person is known as the attorney for personal care and/or the substitute decision-maker. The person designated to make decisions does not have to be the patient's relative; it may be someone close to the patient who understands his or her wishes   Figure 5-6 ▾ .

A patient may also have completed a will appointing an executer of his or her estate and/or a power of attorney for financial matters, designating someone to deal with any financial issues in the event of his or her future incapacity. Neither the attorney for financial matters nor the executer of the estate is automatically able to assume decision-making power regarding health care treatments.

Incapacity and Substitute Decision Making

A substitute decision-maker can be: (1) designated by the patient either orally or in writing; (2) appointed in a legal power of attorney for personal care document; or, (3) depending on jurisdiction, by default according to a preset hierarchy of family members, starting with the patient's spouse or partner   Figure 5-7 ▸ . Health care providers have a duty to explain all treatment choices, their benefits and risks, and recommended course of action to the substitute decision-maker as though they would for the patient.

It is hoped that the substitute decision-maker will have discussed issues of goals, values, and beliefs, especially with regard to health care and perceptions of what gives life quality and meaning, with the patient. Unfortunately, this often is not the case, and substitute decision-makers can be left floundering. Furthermore, substitute decision-makers often have no clear idea of their role and responsibilities and need to be educated by health care providers regarding their obligations when making decisions.

In general terms, substitute decision-makers are bound to make decisions according to previously expressed wishes of the patient that apply to the treatment and current circumstances or, if such wishes do not exist, according to the patient's best

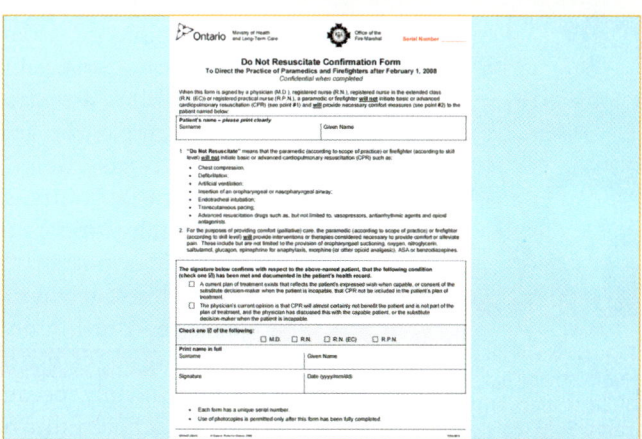

Figure 5-6 An advance directive describing the type of care a person wishes to receive under conditions of a terminal illness or irreversible coma.

Do not Resuscitate Confirmation Form © Queen's Printer for Ontario, 2007. Reproduced with permission.

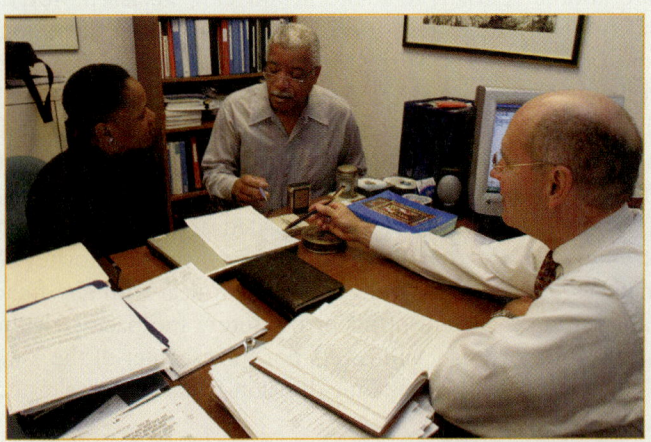

Figure 5-7 A substitute decision-maker (often a child over a certain age or other close relative) is frequently designated when a person draws up a power of attorney for personal care.

interests. Best interests are not an arbitrary concept that the health care provider can judge based on his or her personal belief system or moral code. Best interests are intended to reflect the uniqueness of each patient by mandating consideration of: (1) other values, beliefs, or goals that would have influenced his or her decision making; (2) whether the recommended treatment would improve the patient's condition or quality of life and/or slow, reduce the rate of, or prevent deterioration in health and quality of life; (3) whether the benefits of the recommended treatment would outweigh its risks; and (4) whether the same outcomes could be achieved by a less intrusive treatment plan.

Acting as a substitute decision-maker is not an easy task. Frequently, complex decisions must be made quickly during times of emotional and psychological distress. Open and clear communication, repeated discussions, empathy, and caring are needed to facilitate the process and support the substitute decision-maker and/or family members.

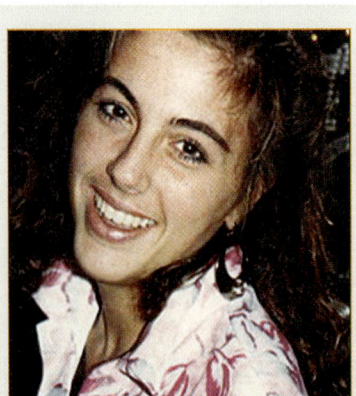

Figure 5-8 Because she did not leave any directive about the type of care she wanted to receive, Terry Schiavo's case became a battleground between family members who held different viewpoints about care of the terminally ill.

As medical technology has made the line between life and death more imprecise, a number of cases have gained the public's attention. For example, the Terry Schiavo case demonstrated that courts will ultimately support the right of a patient, or their closest relative, to make end-of-life decisions **Figure 5-8 ◄**. Unfortunately, because Terry Schiavo did not leave a written advance directive, her husband's decision making was challenged by the family, which ultimately put the case in the courts' hands.

Patients' decisions may not be accepted by other members of the public or other members of the patient's family, but it is important for the paramedic to remember that legally, each person has the right to make decisions about his or her own medical care. Patients may make decisions, such as refusal of treatment, that the paramedic does not agree with, but the paramedic must respect that patient's wishes, assuming the patient has decision-making capacity.

End-of-Life Decision

Paramedics will often deal with patients at the very end of their lives. It is a unique trust in EMS, and these patients, as well as their families, should be treated with the utmost respect and empathy. Paramedics should never think: "Why did they bother to call 9-1-1 if they don't want us to do anything?" That line of thinking is an example of the individual paramedic's own moral code getting in the way of the paramedic's medical ethics. Instead, you must understand that the family of a dying patient, even one under hospice or palliative care, may not know how to check a pulse, and may not understand that difficult, agonal respirations may continue for hours before a patient actually dies. Many people have never been with someone at the moment of death. You have; therefore, you can provide the family with guidance and comfort during such a difficult time. If information and support is partly what they called you for, be sure they receive it—it is part of your job.

Many people will call EMS when a loved one is dying and the death is expected. Whether advance care directives or treatment plans outlining palliative treatments, as opposed to resuscitative ones, can be legally respected by paramedics in these situations varies by jurisdiction. As a paramedic, you need to familiarize yourself with the law and how it operates in your jurisdiction.

DNR Orders

During the last decade, DNR orders were finally recognized in the prehospital setting in some, but not all, jurisdictions. Ethically, all paramedics are part of the medical community and act in ways that other health care professionals do, recognizing that patients have the same rights to direct their care, and to refuse care, outside the hospital that they do inside the hospital.

The legal framework is not always as clear, however, and resuscitation in the field may be mandated even in the face of clearly expressed wishes to the contrary. Some jurisdictions will allow the discontinuing of resuscitative treatments on the authority of the base hospital physician. Paramedics should contact direct medical control in confusing situations involving resuscitation questions and make sure they understand their EMS services' protocols on this before starting work.

■ Withholding or Withdrawing Resuscitation

Modern bioethical guidelines rely on the patient's wishes, values, goals, and best interests and reasonable medical professional judgment (standard of care) in deciding when to stop

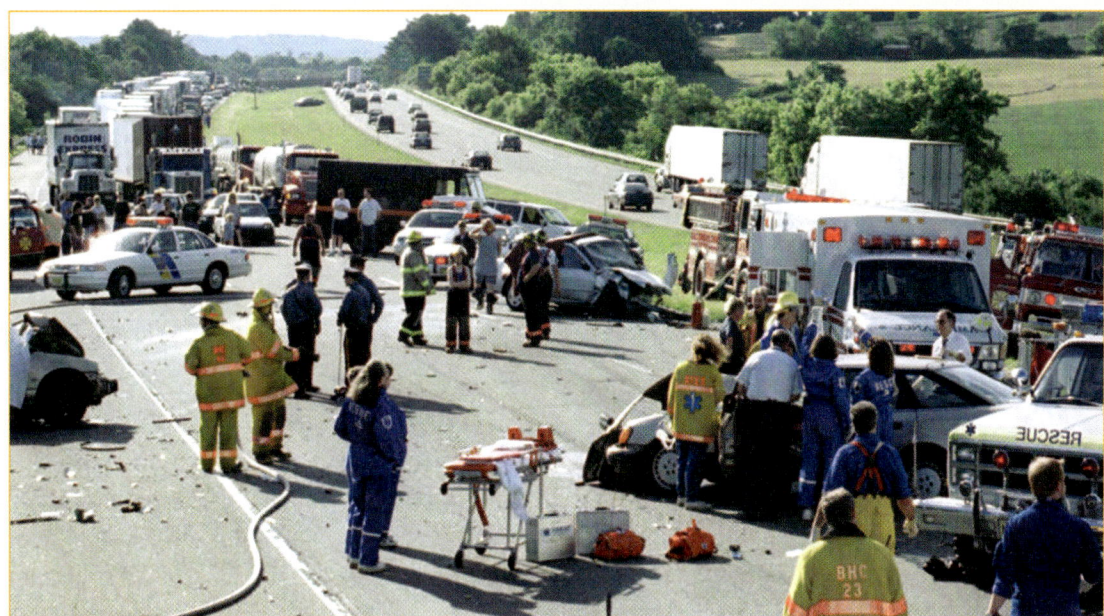

Figure 5-9 Although our instincts are always to try to sustain life at whatever cost, sometimes it is clear that resuscitation efforts will be futile, and should be withheld per local protocols.

For these reasons, the concept of futility can best be thought of through a very narrow definition: A treatment is futile if it would not work. Decisions can also be made to withhold or withdraw treatment if: (1) the patient or his or her substitute decision-maker requests it; (2) the treatment has not attained the preset goals; (3) the treatment is not working, (4) the burdens exceed the benefits and the patient or substitute decision-maker consents to its withholding or withdrawal; or (5) the treatment falls outside a well-recognized and accepted standard of prehospital care. In situations of doubt, paramedics should contact their medical oversight physician for orders and advice.

CPR and resuscitation efforts, as well as when it is appropriate for health care professionals to decline to initiate them at all. Numerous medical studies have shown that resuscitation of medical, as well as trauma patients, is sometimes a futile intervention at the onset or may become futile at some point. Futile resuscitation efforts—interventions that studies have shown do not benefit patients—are not medically, ethically, or legally indicated **Figure 5-9 ▲**.

Problems arise, however, in the use of the concept of futility. Over the years, many definitions of futility have been proposed, yet there is still a lack of clarity and consensus within the medical field. Concerns arise over using the definition of futility in practice, especially in discussions with patients and/or families, because it conveys the notion that patients are not worth the effort. Moreover, through its use and the power it gives them not to initiate or to stop treatment, health care providers may impose their own values and beliefs regarding what constitutes "futility" and "benefit" on others.

Health care providers' perceptions of futility may also give rise to "slow codes" or "Hollywood codes," during which resuscitation efforts are performed deliberately slowly and inadequately and often for show in front of family members. Such practices are completely unethical and should never occur. A patient is either resuscitated to the best of your professional ability or resuscitation efforts are not initiated or stopped in consultation with direct medical control.

Paramedics, especially those working in rural and wilderness situations, will need to carefully consider the time it will take for a patient to reach definitive care at the hospital. The base hospital physician should be contacted for advice and orders. Err on the side of initiating resuscitation in situations of doubt.

Given that EMS resources are not infinite, you will need to consider issues of resource allocation, including your time and putting your unit out-of-service to make a long drive. Use EMS

You are the Paramedic Part 3

After you arrive at the hospital, your patient is pronounced dead. At this point, there is no way for you to know whether the patient could have been saved with the prompt use of the AED. You contact your shift supervisor, notify him of this issue, and contact your medical program director to report the incident to her. You then carefully document all of the pertinent patient care information in the medical incident report.

6. Beyond the documentation required to complete the medical incident report, what else should you document and how?

7. Why is it important to completely and concisely document a call, especially a call such as this one?

8. What is the purpose of quality assurance and quality improvement?

resources in a way that will respond to those in the greatest need first and that will do the most good for the most people in the community. EMS resources should always be used in a manner that provides for the most coverage at all times. These situation should ideally be covered in protocols and discussed regularly and in detail with your medical director.

Each jurisdiction has its own laws that may define the role of the paramedic in resuscitation issues. In some jurisdictions, a paramedic may be able to "pronounce" death, while in others only a medical investigatory or physician may do so. Each paramedic should be aware of requirements for pronouncing death, including how to contact direct medical control if this is required.

> ### At the Scene
>
> It is always a good idea to discuss when to start and when to stop CPR with your partner and other paramedics to ensure that everyone understands the direction of the resuscitation.

In addition to the scenarios described so far, there are some calls where it is appropriate for paramedics not to begin even the most basic life support on a patient in cardiac arrest. Although local protocols will ultimately guide your practice, it may be appropriate to not start resuscitation interventions in situations where the patient is obviously dead, such as when rigor mortis, dependent lividity, cold core body temperature in a warm environment, or injuries incompatible with life have been sustained. Blunt trauma arrest, prolonged response times, and lengthy medical resuscitation efforts may be indications for withdrawal of resuscitative efforts in the field.

These decisions are particularly difficult and emotional when dealing with pediatric patients, although, again, modern medical guidelines weigh against prolonged resuscitation efforts. Studies have shown that paramedics feel particularly uncomfortable about terminating resuscitation in children. "Working a code" simply because the patient is a child who has experienced sudden infant death syndrome (SIDS) may not be legally or ethically appropriate and may actually cause a family additional suffering when they are led to believe that the child may have a chance of survival.

Paramedics tend to be action-oriented people who feel that they must do something (remember, this is *your* moral code). However, there are some situations in which a paramedic can do more for the grieving family than for the patient who has died and, ethically, you should be prepared to support the family. It can be the hardest part of the job.

Training, a review of the available literature, and open discussions about what is medically appropriate in a given EMS system should provide guidance and ease concerns about these difficult situations. Once again, continuing education on the topic of appropriate resuscitation could help paramedics look at this particularly difficult issue from many sides.

> ### Documentation and Communication
>
> Imagine what it would be like to have a family emergency while visiting another country. How difficult would it be for you to trust their medical system knowing it is different than what you are used to?

Do not try to judge whether interventions are futile totally by yourself. Communicate, communicate, and communicate. Ultimately, medical interventions and life-saving attempts may also prolong suffering or fail to return a patient to a meaningful life. In such instances, you need guidance from direct medical control. In order to judge whether a cardiac arrest is the natural end of a life or a reversible response to a treatable medical event requires a thorough understanding of all the consequences of a particular intervention. You are considering the treatment benefit to your patient, who might be beyond your help. Again, communicate.

Conflicts in Professional Integrity and Roles

Paramedics may find themselves in conflict with other health care providers' decisions, such as their paramedic partners, their medical director, or other workers. For example, occasionally a physician will give an order that the paramedic may feel is detrimental

You are the Paramedic Part 4

An internal investigation was initiated by your medical director to determine the appropriate course of action regarding this call. You learn that evidence normally gathered by this agency's AED, including an audio recording of the event, as well as a cardiac strip, are now missing. Without these pieces to the puzzle, the investigation comes to a halt.

You receive a call from one of the paramedics who responded, and he tells you that he witnessed one of the other paramedics destroying the evidence. Even more unnerving, he tells you this has happened before. He is a fairly new paramedic and is afraid that he will be kicked out of the agency if anyone learns that he called you.

9. What should you do?

10. Can individuals as well as departments be sued?

to the patient's best interests. It is important for the paramedic to discuss immediately why he or she feels that way with the physician. Remember, you are often in a better position to see what is going on with the patient, and a big part of your job is to communicate fully with the physician. A paramedic should never perform a procedure or administer a medication that he or she believes will be detrimental to the patient. If a physician, for example, mistakenly orders that a drug be administered via an endotracheal tube when the paramedic has been trained never to use that particular drug by that route, it is important for the paramedic to ask the physician to revisit that order.

However, if the dispute is not resolved, you need to be the patient's advocate and act in his or her best interest. If the doctor is insistent about the orders, there are several ways to handle the problem: (1) tell the doctor that your standing orders are never to administer the drug by endotracheal tube and ask if he or she can suggest other ways of administration and (2) if you are not working with your medical director, tell the doctor that you can only administer the medication if your medical director approves. None of these are even half as good as having a good, trusting relationship with the staff of the emergency department. Communicate!

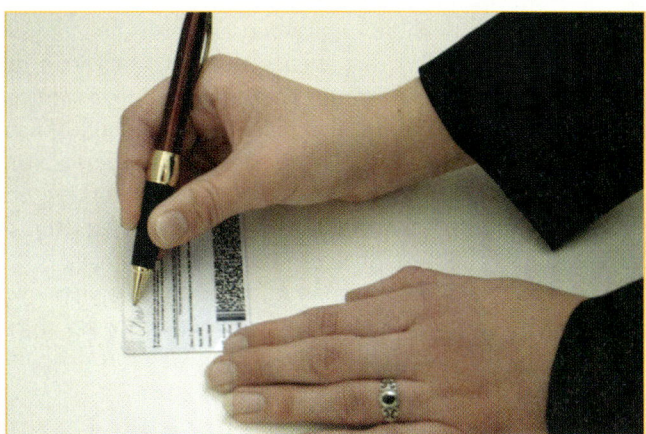

Figure 5-10 Most provinces have an organ donation form on the reverse side of the driver's license.

Organ Donation

A major issue in medical ethics is that of the potential for patients with lethal brain injuries to donate organs. Organ and tissue donation can offer a second chance at life for many people in dire need. It is a gift and an act of kindness that may also comfort the bereaved family. Efforts to increase organ and tissue donation are ongoing worldwide. Many patients with a variety of illnesses may wait years for an organ and ultimately die on the organ recipient list, never having received a chance to live life to the fullest.

Until recently, neurological death (brain death) had to have been declared before a patient could be considered a potential organ donor and before his or her family could be approached and the option of organ donation explained. Although a patient may have a signed donor card, the actual consent to donate or not is a choice that is presented to the family **Figure 5-10 ▶**. If the family refuses consent, their wishes are respected, even when the patient has a signed organ and tissue donor card expressing his or her wish to donate. This practice, although seemingly a violation of the patient's wishes, is performed out of respect for the surviving family members.

Currently, programs that offer the option of donation after cardiac death—usually after a decision has been made to withdraw life support in the Intensive Care unit—are becoming increasingly available. Controversially, some programs are also exploring whether a patient should be kept alive on life support when they have progressed to neurological death (such as in major illness or massive neurological injury). This may allow for a decision to be made about donating organs and tissue after the subsequent cardiac death occurs.

EMS systems should have clear guidelines on any organ or tissue donation process that the service is part of. Generally, you should not be expected to make decisions on whether organs are viable for transplantation. Some EMS services have protocols where you simply notify the next of kin that organ or tissue donation is an option, give them information on a card, and then inform the medical examiner or tissue donation service that the conversation has been initiated. This only occurs if resuscitation is terminated in the field or was not attempted. Several criteria must be met for such a protocol to be initiated (such as assessing the patient's age, comorbidities, time of death, etc.). You should only enter into these conversations if your service has a protocol or guideline for doing so, and you should never put pressure on family members. You are simply providing information.

Ethics and EMS Research

EMS practices have largely emerged on an ad hoc basis based on paramedics' experiences in the prehospital environment. Little research has been performed to confirm the effectiveness of the procedures used in the prehospital setting. Properly randomized, controlled studies in EMS are not common, but they are emerging. Paramedics must remember that the first principle of medical practice is to do no harm and continue to seek further education about the effectiveness of EMS practice. Some aspects of prehospital care are still rooted in anecdotal experience, unsupported by research. Some EMS procedures, however well-intentioned, have been shown to not be helpful to patients. Evidence from research can produce outcomes that are dissimilar from what is expected logically. As a result, paramedics and medical directors need to work together to make sure that their service's protocols are based on the latest evidence.

EMS studies on the critically ill or injured patients without informed consent is a true ethical dilemma—many of the patients paramedics care for are critically ill or injured. These patients are usually unable to give consent, and their physical state is so compromised that even if they are conscious they may not be able to absorb information to give *informed* consent. It is essential for critical interventions for highly acute conditions to be based on evidence, not just on expert opinion or anecdotal evidence. EMS research experts are working hard to develop the best ways to do such research in an ethically sound manner. This text does not cover the many aspects of EMS research, but it is an important topic that impacts every paramedic's practice. Continue to make yourself aware of how researchers are handling this issue and other ethical debates concerning patients in research.

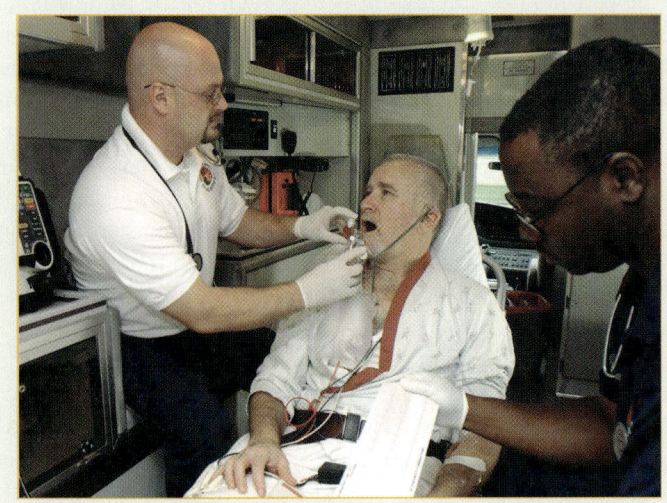

Figure 5-11 One of the best ways to hone your skills as a paramedic is to find a good mentor whose work ethic and attitude you admire.

Ethics in the EMS Workplace: Accountability

Paramedics must be accountable for their actions at all times—accountable to the patient, to the EMS medical director, and to the EMS system as a whole. The paramedic is obligated to consistently meet the expectations of the community, which includes displaying highly ethical behaviour. How a paramedic handles teamwork, his or her attitude on the job, justice and respect for patient autonomy, and his or her patients' cultural and lifestyle diversity will ultimately shape that paramedic's career. Each paramedic must consider what type of a paramedic he or she wants to become **Figure 5-11 ▶**. New paramedics may want to find a mentor whose style and professionalism they strive to emulate.

Professional ethics are extremely important as EMS continues to struggle to be recognized and funded in the same manner as the other medical professions. Immature, unprofessional behaviour and criminal acts, such as sexual misconduct, substance abuse, patient abuse, and harassment of colleagues, have no place in an emerging profession. Off-duty misconduct will affect a paramedic's reputation, and potentially his or her employment. News stories that depict paramedics engaged in immature or illegal activities serve to lessen the public's confidence in EMS. Illegal drug use, selling of drugs, inappropriate

use of emergency vehicles, inappropriate visitors entertained at the emergency base station, or use of alcohol while on duty are strictly forbidden.

The paramedic also cannot stand by silently and watch as other paramedics engage in misbehaviour. The paramedic is ethically required to disclose such activities. Misconduct should be promptly reported to the appropriate chain of command. Similarly, the paramedic is obligated to report medical errors he or she makes or witnesses to the medical direction as soon as possible.

Paramedics who choose to become patient advocates, who participate in and actively seek out the very best in training and professional development, and who put the good of the team above their own personal aspirations will ultimately succeed and be rewarded with a fulfilling EMS career. Human beings seem to perform best when they share themselves and work toward an end much greater than themselves. You probably would not be reading this text if you were not that kind of person. But, you must remember, EMS is an evolving specialty, and the future of it lies in your hands.

You are the Paramedic Summary

Like every profession, not everyone involved in EMS is of high moral character. During the course of your career, you will most likely run across events or situations that require your immediate action. Individuals who are willing to cut corners, conceal their wrongdoings, or engage in otherwise unethical or illegal acts bring the entire emergency medical services profession down. If you choose to look the other way, you become party to their choices. Doing the right thing can sometimes result in personal consequences such as the loss of a job, obtaining a "whistle-blower" reputation, or other negative impacts, but it is your duty to act in the best interests of your patients, your community, and your profession.

1. Are emergency medical responders and volunteer primary care paramedics held to the same standards of prehospital care as staff paramedics?

Ideally, they should be held to the same response and patient prehospital care standards, but sometimes they are not. This is unfortunate, because the patient and the patient's family are unaware of who gets paid and who doesn't. They want a professional—someone who looks and acts the part of a lifesaving team member. Professionalism includes all facets of response and preparation for response. Here are a few examples that encompass the duties of a professional EMS provider:

- Knowing where your equipment is and how to use it.
- Ensuring that all equipment is clean and ready prior to a call.
- Ensuring that adequate amounts of equipment and supplies are available.
- Presenting a professional image by arriving in a clean uniform, clean ambulance, and behaving in a manner consistent with a professional paramedic.

2. If sensitive information needs to be relayed regarding prehospital care, what other communication options should be available to paramedics?

It is never appropriate to ignore an incoming paramedic's radio questions regarding prehospital care or other pertinent information. We've all been in situations where we feel that information needs to be communicated in a discreet manner—information about minors, sexual assaults, child abuse, or other sensitive situations. Use a landline or cellular phone in such instances, even if it is only to let the provider know you need to relay information face-to-face. Failure to communicate with the paramedics will cause them to wonder whether the radio system is malfunctioning, you are ignoring them, or something else is wrong.

3. Is it ever appropriate to conceal information regarding prehospital care?

No. It is never acceptable to cover up mistakes or omissions in patient care. To do so could jeopardize the patient's life. We are all human, and we all make mistakes. Ideally, no mistakes should be made in the prehospital environment, but they can and do happen. If you should find yourself in this situation, immediately report any mistakes or other concerns to the appropriate medical authority.

4. How should you answer the wife's question?

Don't lie. Give her factual information, and stick to what you know. If you are unsure, tell her you don't know, but that you will look into the matter to ensure she receives accurate information.

5. How and when should you address her concerns?

Because you are actively caring for her husband, now is not the time to discuss what has occurred during the call. Ideally, a physician should explain any patient care procedures or complications regarding her husband's care in an environment that is quiet, private, and much less stressful. Adhere to your local standard operating guidelines and other protocols for interacting with a patient's family members. If none are in place regarding a specific issue, use common sense and sensitivity.

6. Beyond the documentation required to complete the medical incident report, what else should you document and how?

You should also fill out an addendum or memo that will not be directly attached to the medical incident report. This type of formal note should include all related information not appropriate to include in a medical document. Include information such as comments from providers, conditions, or items you noticed at the scene or other important information that you believe is pertinent to the call and could likely be forgotten at a later date. Ensure that this is a typed document that includes names, dates, times, witnesses, and references to other appropriate documents. Remember, stick to the facts, and write this as though it could also be subpoenaed at a later time.

7. Why is it important to accurately, concisely, and completely document a call, especially a call such as this one?

All your documentations should reflect a professional image. Misspellings, illegible handwriting, and major omissions all point to one thing—you are not a professional. It can be argued that if your documentation is poor, so is your patient care. Always document with the anticipation that one day a lawyer might have your medical incident report enlarged for a jury to inspect. More important, however, should be your strong desire to provide complete verbal and written reports to ensure your patient has exceptional continuity of care.

8. What is the purpose of quality assurance and quality improvement?

Quality assurance and quality improvement exist to keep paramedics on the right track. These programs should involve an informal and formal method for evaluating all calls and flagging those that need to be reviewed. Paramedics work under the license of a physician. That physician ensures that we adhere to guidelines established by the latest in patient care research. As paramedics, we all benefit from reviewing calls and learning what we did right and what we can improve upon. EMS is an ever-changing field. It is our responsibility to ensure that all that we do is within the guidelines of national accepted standards and the local protocols as set forth by the oversight physician.

9. What should you do?

Obviously, you must keep this individual's name private. His concern regarding a backlash is a valid one. However, you must report this information immediately to your supervisor and medical program director so that corrective action can be taken. Explain to the paramedic what course of action you must take, but tell him that you will protect his identity.

10. Can individuals as well as departments be sued?

Yes! Absolutely! Both can be sued in civil and criminal courts. Don't assume that your EMS service has an insurance policy that will cover your legal fees and other court costs should you be sued as an individual provider. They may or may not. You should be sure to know the content and extent of what your service provides you in terms of legal and liability coverage. Regardless, if you are found to be negligent, your employer may not pay all of your legal expenses. Some paramedics opt to have an insurance policy separate from their employer. Although this is at the paramedic's discretion, it provides the paramedic with additional resources in the event of litigation.

Prep Kit

Ready for Review

- Paramedics who maintain a good, well-rounded general ethical code in their daily lives will be able to carry that through to their profession.
- Paramedics who are concerned for the welfare of others will rarely commit an unethical act in their professional career.
- Paramedics need to keep in mind that all patients have the right to make their own decisions regarding their medical care, regardless of the paramedic's personal or professional views.
- Empathy and compassion are part of a paramedic's job.
- Patients often decide on medical care and treatment issues prior to an emergency. Paramedics need to be familiar with advance directives, DNR orders, powers of attorney for personal care, substitute decision-making guidelines, and organ donation protocols. They need to know how these are operationalized and respected in their practice jurisdiction.
- Futile resuscitation efforts need to be addressed and considered prior to an emergency event. Weighing various ethical issues prior to their occurrence can help prevent and reduce suffering in our patient population.
- Paramedics who strive to become an advocate for their communities and carry a high sense of accountability will not only have a rewarding career, but will also be able to make the right ethical decisions regardless if they are encountered in the prehospital environment, with colleagues, or in their daily lives.

Vital Vocabulary

advance care planning Expression of oral and/or written advance directives by capable patients in anticipation of their wishes regarding future health care choices and expected quality of life.

advance directive A directive from the patient while capable, either orally or in writing, describing his or her wishes for future medical treatment in the event that he or she becomes incapable of making health care decisions.

do not resuscitate (DNR) order A legally binding, written order for health care providers not to provide life-saving measures during cardiac or respiratory arrest; may be created by the physician, the patient, or the patient's substitute decision-maker.

ethics The philosophy of right and wrong.

futile intervention A medical intervention that will not work or will not benefit the patient in any way.

morality Code of conduct defined by society, religion, culture, or another person that affects one's character, conduct, and conscience.

patient autonomy The right to direct one's own care.

power of attorney for personal care A legal document that contains advance directives and appoints another person to make health care decisions, including withdrawal or withholding of care, for the patient in the event that he or she becomes incapable of making such decisions.

substitute decision-maker A person designated by a patient (or by default depending on law in a given practice jurisdiction) to make health care decisions for that person when he or she is unable to do so.

Assessment in Action

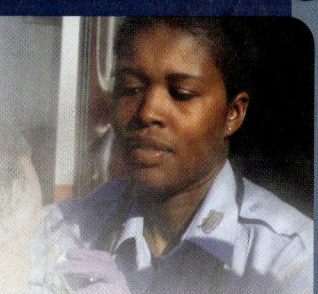

You are dispatched to a messy scene—a two-car, one-motorcycle collision in the pouring rain. When you arrive, you see that the motorcycle driver was not wearing a helmet. The passengers in one of the vehicles were not wearing seatbelts, and the inside of the vehicle smells strongly of alcohol.

1. When you check on the motorcycle driver, he is not breathing and has a partially crushed skull. You are not sure how long he has not been breathing. The head injury may mean that if you revive him, he will be brain damaged. Do you initiate CPR?
   A. Yes
   B. No

2. You recognize that one of the cars has teenagers from a class you recently gave a lecture to on the importance of not drinking and driving and the need to wear seatbelts. They are conscious and alert, but most of them have some kind of injury, and the car smells like alcohol. How do you handle this situation?
   A. As you would any other trauma call, but less gently. Give them the biggest IV needle you can, comment on how careless they were every chance you can, and lecture them on how they could have prevented this if they had listened to your recent lecture and used common sense.
   B. Take care of them last. They were obviously the reason the collision happened in the first place, and they're not hurt badly.
   C. Make them feel as guilty as you can. Tell them the motorcycle driver is most likely dead, and the people in the other car have been hurt by their carelessness and lack of concern for themselves and others.
   D. Assume nothing, and treat all the patients as you would in any trauma call—gently, compassionately, and quickly.

3. You and a colleague disagree on how to treat one victim of the collision. You are the higher-trained paramedic. Your colleague is disagreeing with you very loudly in front of the patient and bystanders. This is making the already injured patient panic and wonder if he is in competent hands. What do you do?
   A. Remind your colleague that you are the highest-trained paramedic on the scene, and therefore the one in charge, so what you say goes, period.
   B. Take the colleague aside quickly, and professionally (and quietly) explain that the scene is not a place to have loud disagreements, you are in command of the scene, you are accepting responsibility, and that differences can be discussed after the call.
   C. Explain to the patient that you are the more experienced paramedic, that you are in charge, and that your colleague has an inferiority complex and has trouble letting someone else be in charge. Then give the colleague a mundane task to do with a different patient to get him out of your way.
   D. Tell the colleague to shut up, and ignore him as you take care of the patient in the way you feel is appropriate.

4. The medical director gives you an order to give one of the patients 2 mg of morphine for pain. However, your patient says that he is not in that much pain and that although he is not allergic to narcotics he doesn't like the effect they have on him. Should you follow the medical director's order as it stands?
   A. Give the medical director the information the patient has shared with you, and ask that he reconsider his order.
   B. Tell the patient that the medical director is your boss, and what he says is to be done without question.
   C. Tell the medical director you will administer the morphine, but don't actually administer it to the patient, making them both happy.
   D. Tell the patient that he may not be in much pain yet, but he will, and the medical director knows what is best.

5. The couple in the car that was hit is older and speaking a foreign language. One of your colleagues says you should treat them last, because they will be difficult to communicate with. How do you handle it?
   A. Agree with him. Your own countrymen come first in your book.
   B. It should make no difference in their treatment. In EMS, all people are equal and are to be treated that way, regardless of ethnicity, insurance status, or religious beliefs.
   C. Take a vote among your colleagues to see who thinks their treatment should come last.
   D. Flip a coin to see who should be treated first.

6. On an off-duty Friday night, some friends call and ask you to a party. You don't have a designated driver, and you can't stay out too late because you have a shift in the morning. What do you do?
   A. Go out and have a good time, life is short. You can drive slowly on the way home and be very careful, it's not too far from your house.
   B. If you go, don't drink. You have a reputation to uphold.
   C. Go, but drink very little, so you're only driving under the influence a little, not a lot.
   D. Just make sure you're completely sober before hitting the road home.

7. **The older woman in the second vehicle tells you she has a terminal illness. When she begins having chest pains, she requests that you do nothing to save her if she should go into cardiac arrest. She does not have any written DNR order documentation with her, however. She is relatively calm and seems to be of sound mind in making her decision. She does not even want the ECG put on her. What do you do?**
    A. Comply with her wishes if she is competent to make the decision.
    B. You cannot comply with her request unless she has a written DNR order with her.
    C. Tell her that you must hook up the ECG machine and treat her until she is at the hospital, where she and a doctor can decide what is best.
    D. Call direct medical control, explain the situation, and ask for advice.

8. **You find out that the motorcycle driver is an organ donor. Direct medical control told you a few seconds ago *not* to initiate CPR based on his severe head injury and lack of breathing. What do you do?**
    A. Call direct medical control and ask about keeping his body alive until his organs can be donated.
    B. Comply with the instructions from direct medical control, ensuring that direct medical control understands the situation, the patient's wishes, and local policies and procedures.
    C. Find out from a close family member what his wishes were, if possible, and follow his wishes if they were known.
    D. He obviously won't need the organs anymore—keep his body alive so they can be given to someone who needs them. The fact that his driver's license says that he is an organ donor is enough to cover any liability.

Challenging Questions

You and your team of three other men are called to the scene of a two-car collision involving several teenage girls. They all claim to be injured only slightly. One of the members of your team jokingly reminds the rest of you that in any trauma the rule is to "strip them" and check them thoroughly. You know they should have a complete physical examination—many patients don't feel other injuries until the adrenaline of the situation has worn off. However, you also know that at least one person on your team is hinting at taking advantage of the situation.

9. **Do you do what is best and give them a thorough examination, while also giving your colleagues a cheap thrill? After all, you're just following the rules.**

10. **Do you point out to your colleagues that what they are doing is unethical and unprofessional, and has no place in the field of EMS?**

11. **Do you report what you saw and heard to the chain of command after the incident is taken care of?**

Points to Ponder

The more time you spend with a new colleague, the more you think he may have a substance abuse problem that is getting worse. He is having trouble remembering things and making quick decisions on the job, which is a "have to" in EMS. You see him taking pills often, but nothing you recognize. When you question him even subtly, he gets defensive and angry. His actions may cause a mistake in the field or put someone in danger. You like him, and he's a good colleague when he isn't affected by whatever he is taking, and you don't want to get him in trouble. What do you do?

Issues: Working With Other Providers, Accountability to the EMS System and the Patient, Maintaining and Encouraging the Standard of Care.

This chapter on pathophysiology has been adapted from *Paramedic: Pathophysiology* (Bob Elling, Mikel A. Rothenberg, MD, and Kirsten M. Elling, 2006, Jones and Bartlett Publishers). It is dedicated to the late Dr. Rothenberg, who, like Dr. Caroline, spent his life helping health care providers understand the complexity of the human body in crisis and injury.

Competency Areas

Appendix 4: Pathophysiology

A. Cardiovascular System
Vascular Disease: Arteriosclerosis
Vascular Disease: Hypertension
Vascular Disease: Thoracic Aortic Dissection
Inflammatory Disorders: Pericarditis
Valvular Disease: Prolapsed Mitral Valve
Valvular Disease: Regurgitation
Valvular Disease: Stenosis
Acute Coronary Syndrome: Infarction
Heart Failure: Cardiomyopathies
Heart Failure: Left-sided
Heart Failure: Pericardial Tamponade
Heart Failure: Right-sided
Cardiac Conduction Disorders: Benign Arrhythmias
Cardiac Conduction Disorders: Lethal Arrhythmias
Cardiac Conduction Disorders: Life-threatening Arrhythmias
Congenital Abnormalities: Ventricular Septal Defect
Traumatic Injuries: Myocardial Contusion

B. Neurologic System
Headache and Facial Pain: Infection
Altered Mental Status: Metabolic
Altered Mental Status: Structural
Chronic Neurologic Disorders: Alzheimer's
Chronic Neurologic Disorders: Multiple Sclerosis
Chronic Neurologic Disorders: Muscular Dystrophy
Chronic Neurologic Disorders: Parkinson's Disease

C. Respiratory System
Medical Illness: Chronic Obstructive Pulmonary Disorder
Medical Illness: Pneumonia/Bronchitis
Medical Illness: Pulmonary Edema
Medical Illness: Pulmonary Embolism
Medical Illness: Reactive Airways Disease/Asthma
Pediatric Illness: Cystic Fibrosis

E. Gastrointestinal System
Esophagus/Stomach: Peptic Ulcer Disease
Liver/Gall Bladder: Cholecystitis/Biliary Colic
Liver/Gall Bladder: Hepatitis

G. Integumentary System
Infectious and Inflammatory Illness: Allergy/Urticaria

H. Musculoskeletal System
Inflammatory Disorders: Arthritis
Inflammatory Disorders: Gout

I. Endocrine System
Acid-Base Disturbances
Diabetes Mellitus
Electrolyte Imbalances
Thyroid Disease

J. Multisystem Diseases and Injuries
Cancer: Malignancy
Hematologic Disorders: Anemia
Hematologic Disorders: Sickle Cell Disease
Infectious Diseases: Acquired Immune Deficiency Syndrome
Infectious Diseases: Influenza Virus
Infectious Diseases: Meningococcemia/Bacteremia
Infectious Diseases: Tetanus
Toxicologic Illness: Prescription Medication
Toxicologic Illness: Non-Prescription Medication
Toxicologic Illness: Recreational
Toxicologic Illness: Poisons (absorption, inhalation, ingestion)
Environmental Disorders: Near Drowning and Drowning
Immunologic Disorders: Autoimmune Disorders
Shock Syndromes: Anaphylactic
Shock Syndromes: Cardiogenic
Shock Syndromes: Hypovolemic
Shock Syndromes: Neurogenic
Shock Syndromes: Obstructive
Shock Syndromes: Septic

K. Psychiatric Disorders
Affective Disorders: Bipolar Disease
Affective Disorders: Depressive Disorders

L. Ears, Eyes, Nose, and Throat
Nasal and Sinus Disorders: Sinusitis
Neck and Upper Airway Disorders: Tonsillitis

Introduction

The human body is made up of cells, tissues, and organs, which function in a constantly changing microenvironment. The study of living organisms with regard to their origin, growth, structure, behaviour, and reproduction is known as biology. Pathophysiology refers to the study (*logos*) of the functioning of the organism (*physiology*) in the presence of suffering/disease (*pathos*). When the normal condition or functioning of the cellular systems breaks down in response to stressors, and the systems can no longer maintain homeostasis, disease may result. Determining the etiology (cause) of this disease process often helps the paramedic identify a reasonable approach to both evaluation and initial treatment of the patient.

To understand how disease may alter cellular function, it is first necessary to understand normal cellular structure and function. This chapter begins by reviewing the structure and function of the cellular system and environment. Following that review is a discussion of how alterations of the environment and its normal homeostasis may result in the state of disease. Next, the impact of genetics on the development of disease states, the role of immunity and self-defence mechanisms in protecting the organism from disease, the states of inflammation and shock, and the role of stress on the development of disease are described and discussed in detail.

Review of the Basic Cellular Systems

Cells

The cell is the basic self-sustaining unit of the human body. As cells grow and mature, they become specialized (eg, kidney cells) through the process of differentiation. Groups of cells form tissues, various types of tissues make up organs, and groups of organs constitute organ systems.

Nearly all cells of higher organisms, except mature red blood cells and platelets, have three main components: the cell membrane, the cytoplasm containing the internal components or organelles, and a nucleus.

The cell membrane consists of fat and protein. It surrounds the cell and protects the internal components within the cytoplasm.

At the Scene

Chemically, fatty compounds—like those in the cell membrane—are neutral (uncharged), whereas electrolytes (sodium and potassium) are water-based (charged). Fats are soluble in oil but not in water. Thus, for a charged molecule to enter through a cell membrane, it has to travel through a special pathway. These transport channels—the so-called ion channels—consist of protein-lined pores that are specifically sized for each substance (calcium and potassium). Local anesthetics (eg, lidocaine) and antiarrhythmic drugs (eg, amiodarone) exert their effects by blocking ion channels.

The organelles, which are found within the cell's cytoplasm (fluid), operate in a cooperative and organized fashion to maintain the life of the cell. They include the following components **Figure 6-1 ▶**:

Ribosomes contain RNA and protein. They interact with RNA from other parts of the cell, joining amino acid chains together to form proteins. When ribosomes attach to endoplasmic reticulum, they create rough endoplasmic reticulum.

You are the Paramedic Part 1

You are complaining to your partner about how taking a pathophysiology review class has nothing at all to do with being a paramedic when you are called to a local dialysis centre for an unknown medical emergency. You are met by a patient care technician who takes you to a 67-year-old woman who appears to be in moderate distress. The nurse caring for the patient states that 30 minutes into dialysis, the patient's blood pressure dropped to 86/44 and she became short of breath. They immediately stopped therapy and called 9-1-1. This occurred approximately 15 minutes prior to your arrival. The nurse further mentions that the patient has a fever of 39.1°C. When questioned, the patient tells you that she missed her last two dialysis sessions because she was not feeling well. She admits to having malaise and a fever for 3 days. She further complains of pain in her right forearm at the site of the dialysis shunt and slight shortness of breath. The patient denies experiencing chest pain, nausea, vomiting, abdominal pain, or dizziness.

Initial Assessment	Recording Time: 0 Minutes
Appearance	Awake and anxious
Level of consciousness	A (Alert to person, place, and day)
Airway	Open
Breathing	Slightly elevated rate with accessory muscle use noted
Circulation	Weak radial pulses with pale, warm, moist skin

1. What are some of the potential complications that can occur from missing dialysis?
2. Does renal disease affect other organ systems?

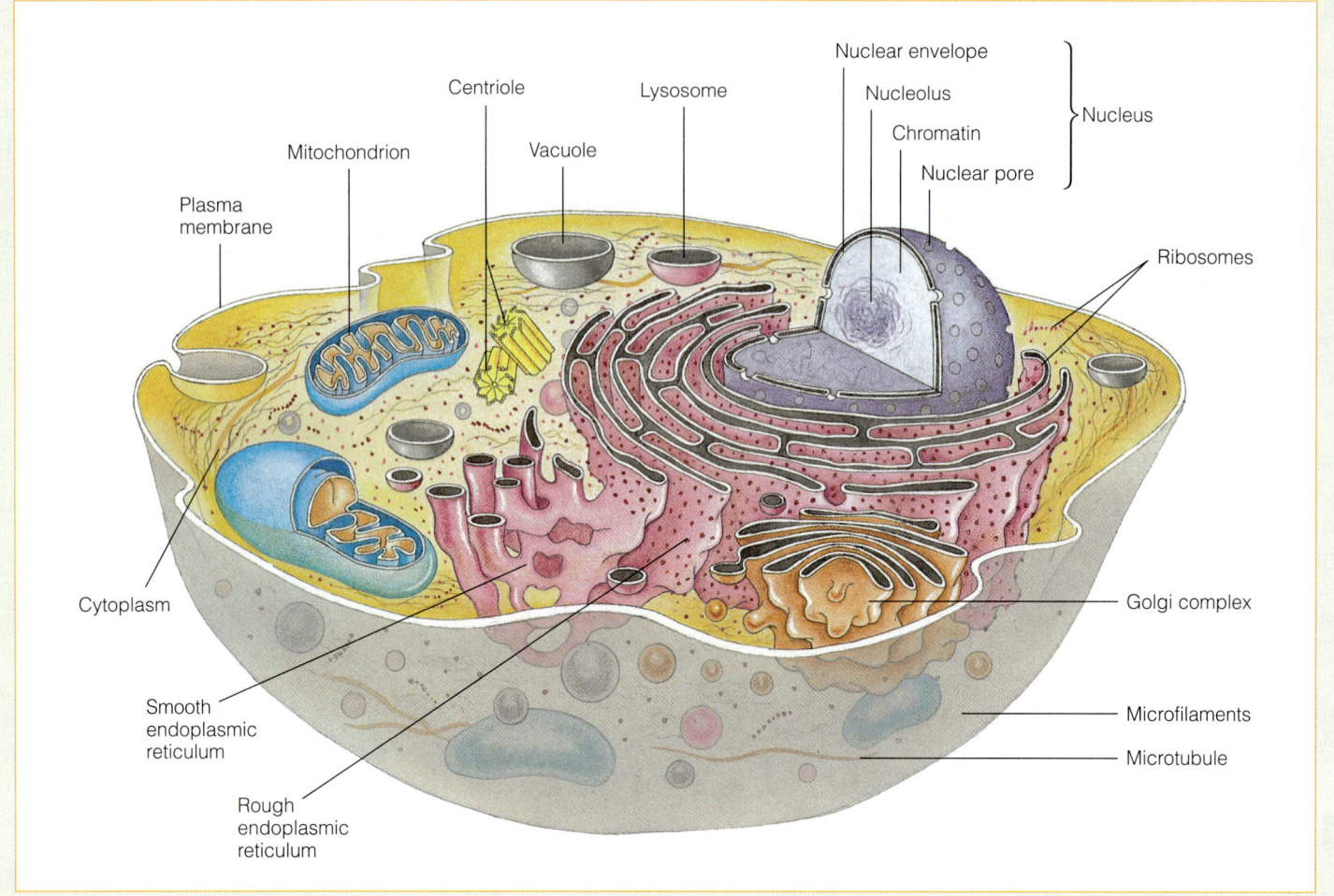

Figure 6-1 The structure of a cell. The cell is divided into nuclear and cytoplasmic compartments. The cytoplasm is packed with organelles, the structures in which the cell carries out many functions.

The *endoplasmic reticulum* is a network of tubules, vesicles, and sacs. Rough endoplasmic reticulum is involved in building proteins. Smooth endoplasmic reticulum is involved in building lipids (fats), such as those found in the cell membranes and those found in carbohydrates.

The *Golgi complex* is located near the nucleus of the cell. It is involved in the synthesis and packaging of various carbohydrates (sugar) and complex protein molecules such as enzymes.

Lysosomes are membrane-bound vesicles that contain digestive enzymes. These enzymes function as an intracellular digestive system, breaking down bacteria and organic debris that have been taken into the cell.

Similar to lysosomes, *peroxisomes* are found in high concentrations in the liver and neutralize toxins such as alcohol.

Mitochondria are small, rod-like organelles that function as the metabolic centre of the cell. They produce adenosine triphosphate (ATP), which is the major energy source for the body.

The nucleus contains the genetic material, called chromatin, and the nucleoli, which are rounded, dense structures that contain ribonucleic acid (RNA). The RNA is responsible for controlling the cellular activities. The nucleus is surrounded by a membrane called the nuclear envelope; the nucleus itself is embedded in the cytoplasm.

Tissues

Tissues are composed of groups of similar cells that work together for a common function. There are four types of tissues: epithelial, connective, muscle, and nerve tissue.

Epithelium covers the external surfaces of the body. Epithelial tissue also lines hollow organs within the body, such as the intestines, blood vessels, and bronchial tubes. In addition to providing a protective barrier, epithelial tissues play roles in the absorption of nutrients in the intestines and the secretion of various body substances. For example, the sweat glands in the dermis layer of the skin—specifically, the stratified squamous epithelial cells—produce a solution containing urea and salt. In contrast, the simple columnar epithelium lines the small intestine and absorbs nutrients from the foods we eat. The epithelial cells that line the inside of blood vessels are called endothelial cells; they regulate the flow of blood through the vessel as well as clotting of the blood (coagulation).

Connective tissue binds the other types of tissue together. Extracellular matrix is a nonliving substance consisting of protein fibres, nonfibrous protein, and fluid that separates connective tissue cells from one another. Collagen is the major protein within the extracellular matrix. At least 12 types of collagen exist, with types I, II, and III being the most abundant. Alterations in collagen structure resulting from abnormal genes or abnormal processing of collagen proteins result in numerous diseases (eg, scurvy). Bone and cartilage are subtypes of connective tissue. Adipose tissue is a special type of connective tissue that contains large amounts of lipids (fat).

Muscle tissue is characterized by its ability to contract. It is enclosed by fascia, which is the layer of fibrous connective tissue that separates individual muscles. Muscles overlie the framework of the skeleton and are classified in terms of both their structure and their function. Structurally, muscle tissue is either striated (ie, microscopic bands or striations can be seen) or nonstriated (also called smooth). Functionally, muscle is either voluntary (consciously controlled) or involuntary (not normally under conscious control).

The three types of muscle are skeletal muscle (striated voluntary), cardiac muscle (striated involuntary), and smooth muscle (nonstriated involuntary). Most of the muscles used voluntarily in day-to-day activities are skeletal muscles. The heart consists of cardiac muscle and has the ability to both contract and generate impulses. Smooth muscle lines most glands, digestive organs, lower airways, and vessels. When a patient's brain senses the need to respond to an environmental stimulus by vasoconstriction, the vessels in the periphery react. For example, the smooth muscle in the bronchioles may vasoconstrict during an asthma attack, leading to wheezing and difficulty moving air out of the lungs. Smooth muscle is also responsible for constriction and dilation of the pupil of the eye when it is exposed to changes in light levels.

Nerve tissue is characterized by its ability to transmit nerve impulses. The central nervous system (CNS) consists of the brain and the spinal cord. Peripheral nerves extend from the brain and spinal cord, exiting from between the vertebrae to various parts of the body.

Neurons are the main conducting cells of nerve tissue, and the cell body of the neuron is the site of most cellular functions. Dendrites receive electrical impulses from the axons of other nerve cells and conduct them toward the cell body, whereas axons typically conduct electrical impulses away from the cell body. Each neuron has only one axon, but it may have several dendrites. Nerve cells are separated by a gap called the synapse. Electrical impulses travel down the nerve and trigger the release of neurotransmitters, which carry the impulse from axon to dendrite.

Homeostasis

Adaptive responses to various stimuli allow the cells and tissues to respond and function in stressful environments, in a constant effort to preserve a degree of stability or equilibrium.

This adaptation process is known as homeostasis (from the Greek words for "same" and "steady"); it is also called the *dynamic steady state.*

Homeostasis is maintained in the body because normal regulatory systems are counterbalanced by counter-regulatory systems. Thus, for every cell, tissue, or organ that performs one function, there is always at least one component that performs the opposing function. For example, the autonomic nervous system consists of the sympathetic and parasympathetic components, which act to speed up or slow down the activity of target organs. Other homeostatic mechanisms include the body's control of its internal temperature despite fluctuations in the external temperature, the regulation of pH and acid–base balance in the body, and the balance of water or hydration in the cells and body of the organism.

Regulatory systems communicate within the body mainly at the cellular level. Cells communicate electrochemically through a process called cell signaling, in which they release molecules (such as hormones) that bind to proteins called receptors, located on the surface of the receiving cells. This signaling triggers chemical reactions in the receiving cells that lead to a biological action. When the action is completed, the opposing system "turns off" the action through a process called feedback inhibition or negative feedback **Figure 6-2 ▸** .

The thermostat mechanism in a home is a good example of a feedback mechanism. In the middle of the winter, heat is constantly being lost through the house's windows, doors, and any poorly insulated areas. The thermostat detects this decrease in temperature and signals the furnace to produce heat to rewarm the house. Once the temperature rises to a certain point, the thermostat gives negative feedback to the furnace, causing it to shut down to prevent overheating. This feedback process keeps the house temperature within a selected range **Figure 6-3 ▸** . Similarly, the body is constantly generating heat through its cellular processes. Five primary mechanisms help the body eliminate excess temperature or heat: convection, conduction, radiation, evaporation, and respiration. In short, the body's thermostat works to balance the generation of heat with the processes of heat elimination.

The human body maintains homeostasis by balancing what it takes in with what it puts out. For example, the body takes in chemicals and electrolytes, food, and water. It utilizes the nutrients, proteins, sugars, and oxygen and then eliminates the unnecessary chemicals and byproducts through respiration (carbon dioxide), urine and sweat (excess liquids), and feces (solid waste). **Figure 6-4 ▸** illustrates this normal balance.

When normal cell signaling is interrupted, disease occurs. The normal counterbalances within the body are rendered ineffective, such that normal regulatory systems begin to operate autonomously. The system stops providing critical negative feedback; instead, it gives unopposed positive feedback.

Excessive output can rapidly upset homeostasis (eg, severe diarrhea kills millions of children each year in some nations, and severe perspiration can cause excessive water loss and dehydration). Likewise, changes in input can alter homeostasis

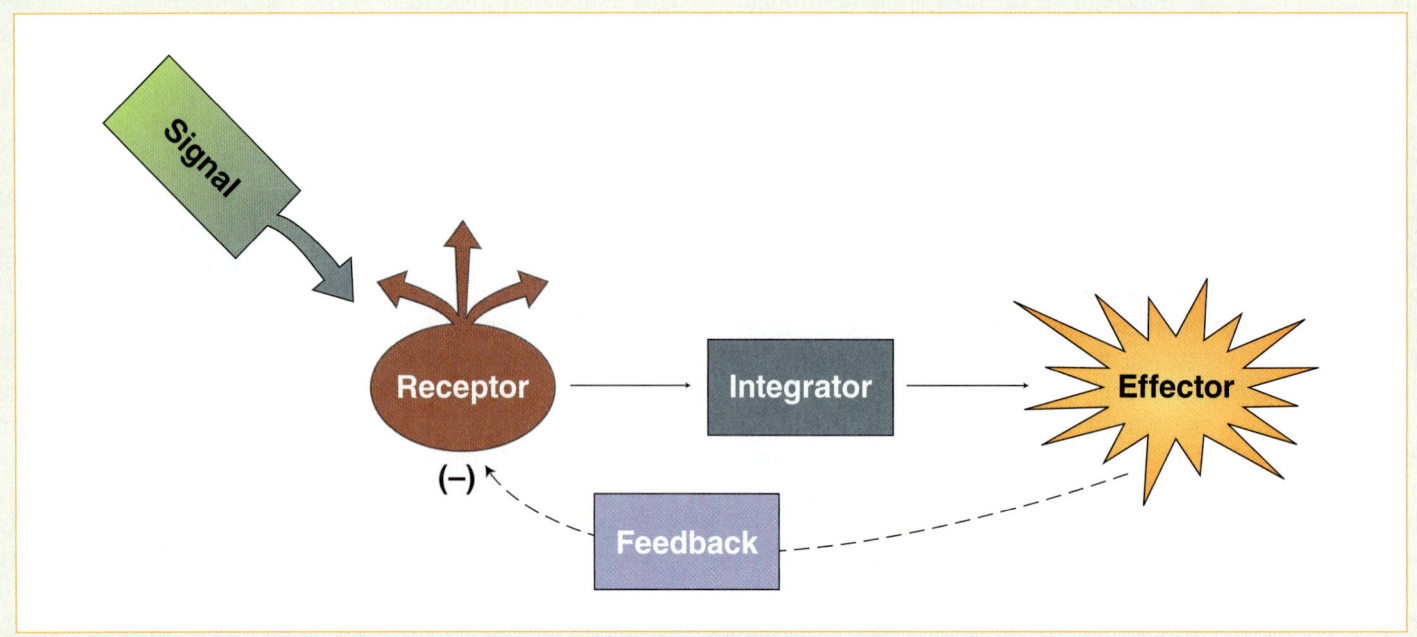

Figure 6-2 Most cellular communication includes a component of negative feedback in which the product of a reaction feeds back information about its own "assembly line," thereby stopping its own production.

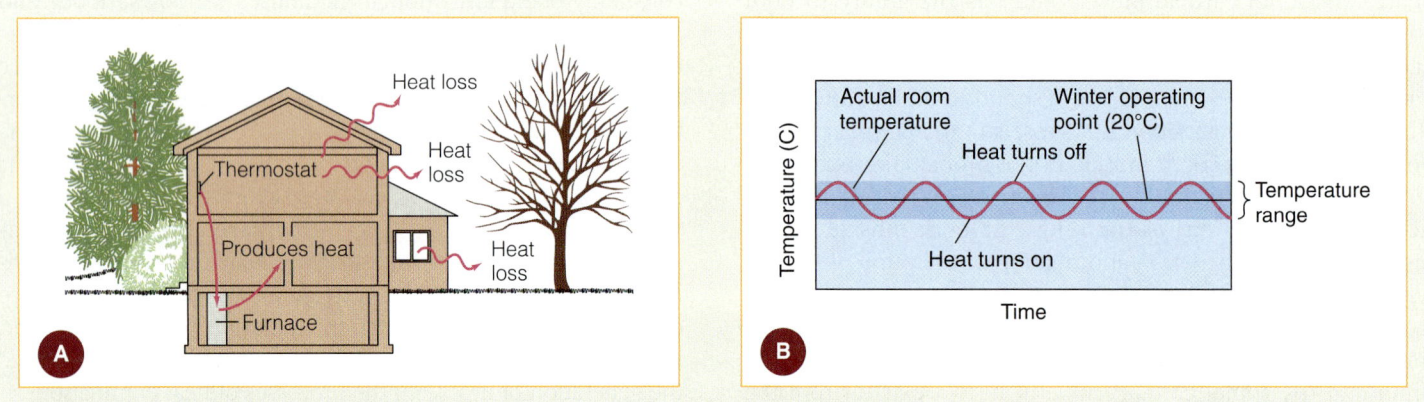

Figure 6-3 Homeostasis and the house. **A.** Heat is maintained in a house by a furnace, which compensates for heat loss. The thermostat monitors the internal temperature and switches the furnace on and off in response to temperature changes. **B.** A hypothetical temperature graph showing temperature fluctuation around the set point.

(eg, going without water for 3 or more days can be life-threatening, and excess salt intake can cause hypertension) **Figure 6-5 ▶**.

The degree of fluid imbalance required to alter homeostasis and result in illness depends on the patient's size, age, and underlying medical conditions. In healthy adults, loss of more than 30% of total body fluid is required, but a loss of only 10% to 15% of total body fluid in a small child could easily result in symptoms. For this reason, fluid therapy is part of the basics of resuscitation.

Ligands

Ligands are molecules that are either produced by the body (endogenous) or given as a drug (exogenous), and that bind any receptor, anywhere, leading to any reaction. In addition to medications, common ligands include hormones, neurotransmitters, and electrolytes.

Hormones are substances that are formed in very small amounts in one specialized organ or group of cells and then carried to another organ or group of cells in the same organism to perform regulatory functions. Endocrine hormones

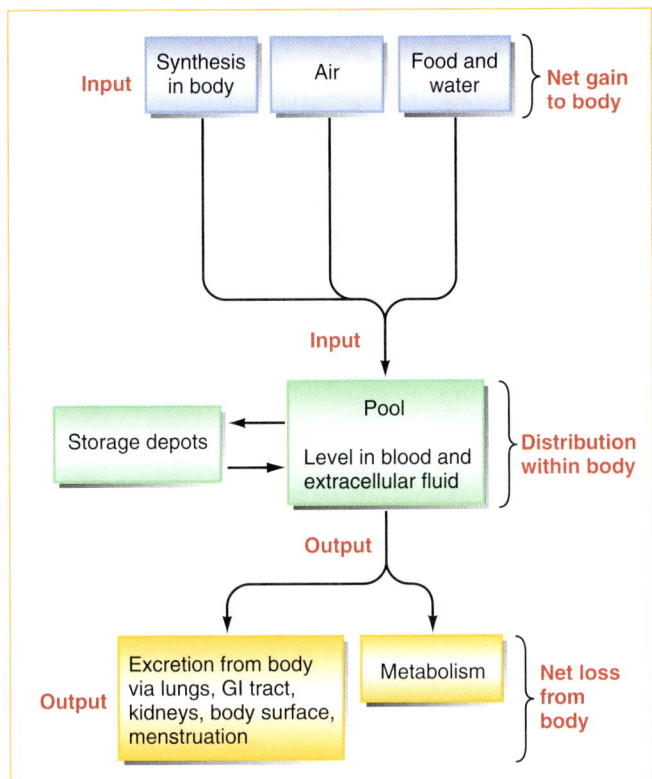

Figure 6-4 Generalized view of the homeostatic system. Inputs and outputs are balanced to maintain more or less constant levels of chemical and physical parameters.

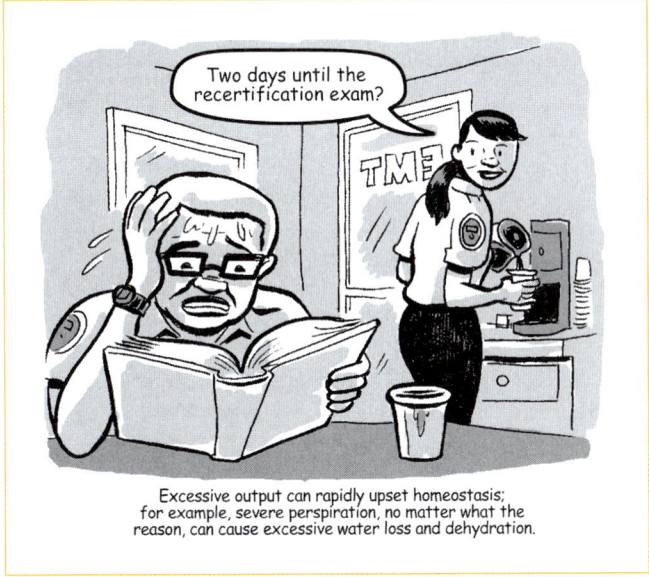

Figure 6-5

(eg, thyroid hormones, adrenal steroids) are carried to their target organ or cell group in the blood. Exocrine hormones reach their target via a specific duct that opens into an organ; examples of exocrine secretions include stomach acids and perspiration. Paracrine hormones (eg, histamine, the hormone released

during allergic and inflammatory reactions) diffuse through intracellular spaces to reach their target. If the hormone acts on the cell that secreted it, it is called an autocrine hormone.

Neurotransmitters are proteins that affect signals between cells of the nervous system. For example, acetylcholine, which aids in the movement of nerve impulses from neuron to neuron, is a neurotransmitter.

Electrolytes play an important role in cell signaling as well as generating the nervous system's action potential. Examples of electrolytes commonly found in the body include sodium, potassium, calcium, and chloride.

Adaptations in Cells and Tissues

When cells are exposed to adverse conditions, they go through a process of adaptation in an attempt to protect themselves from injury. In some situations, the cells change permanently; in others, they change their structure and function only temporarily.

Atrophy is a decrease in cell size due to a loss of subcellular components, which in turn leads to a decrease in the size of the tissue and organ. The actual number of cells remains unchanged. The decreased size represents an attempt to cope with a new steady state with less-than-favourable conditions or a lack of use. For example, a casted, immobilized limb will shrink in size due to disuse atrophy.

Hypertrophy is an increase in the size of the cells due to synthesis of more subcellular components, which in turn leads to an increase in tissue and organ size. For example, the left ventricle in the heart may hypertrophy owing to chronic high resistance pressures from hypertension (elevated blood pressure).

Hyperplasia is an increase in the actual number of cells in an organ or tissue, usually resulting in an increase in the size of the organ or tissue. For example, a callous represents hyperplasia of the keratinized layer of the epidermis of the foot in response to increased friction or trauma.

Dysplasia is an alteration in the size, shape, and organization of cells. It is most often found in epithelial cells that have undergone irregular, atypical changes in response to chronic irritation or inflammation. For example, dysplasia is strongly associated with the development of cancer in the cervix of women who are exposed to human papillomavirus and in the respiratory tracts of smokers.

Metaplasia refers to the reversible, cellular adaptation in which one adult cell type is replaced by another adult cell type. For example, the ciliated and secretory epithelium in the airways of smokers may be replaced by squamous metaplasia.

The Cellular Environment

Distribution of Body Fluids

The cellular environment refers to the distribution of cells, molecules, and fluids throughout the body. This environment changes with aging, exercise, pregnancy, medications, disease,

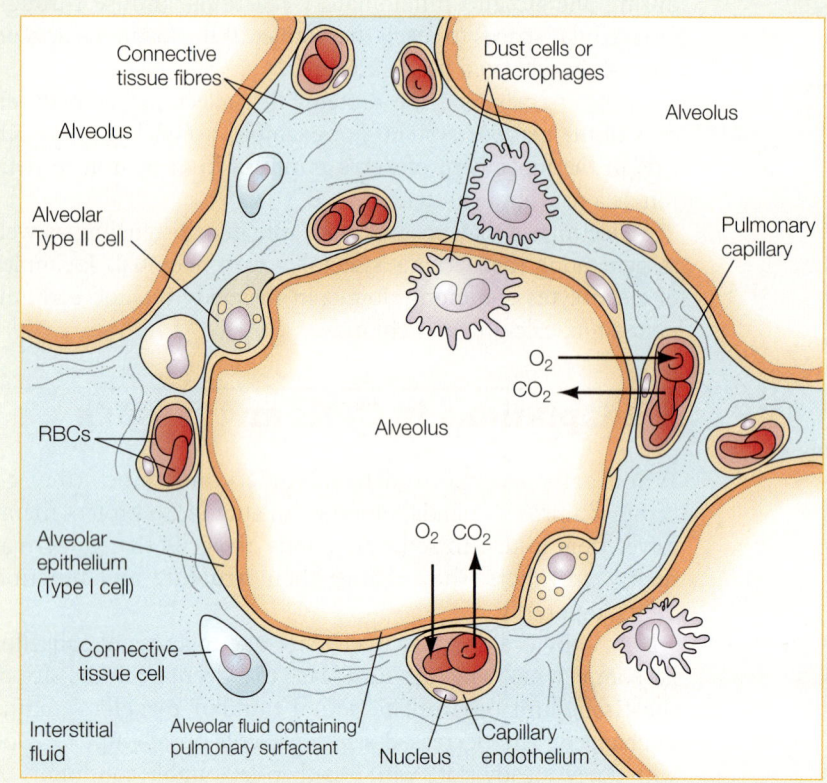

Figure 6-6 Close-up of the alveolus. Oxygen diffuses out of the alveolus and into the capillary. Carbon dioxide diffuses in the opposite direction, entering the alveolar air that is expelled during exhalation. Note the location of the interstitial fluid.

Fluid and Water Balance

The average adult takes in about 2,500 ml of water per day. Sixty percent of this fluid intake occurs by drinking. Another 30% comes from the water in foods, such as fruits. The remaining 10% is a byproduct of cellular metabolism. Most water (60%) is lost in the form of urine; 28% is lost through the skin and lungs; 6% is lost in the feces; and 6% is lost through sweat. The amount of water lost through sweating is highly variable—for example, in hot environmental conditions or during periods of rigorous exercise, it is possible to lose large amounts of fluid.

Water (solvent) and dissolved particles (solutes) move between cells as well as between blood vessels and connective tissues. The two general methods of movement are passive transport and active transport Table 6-1 ▾ .

Water moves between intracellular and extracellular fluid by osmosis. Osmosis is the movement of water down its concentration gradient and across a membrane. Osmotic pressure develops when two solutions of different concentrations are separated by a semipermeable membrane. Water moves from the region of low osmotic pressure to the region of higher osmotic pressure Figure 6-7 ▸ . When you compare the two solutions, the solution with a higher solute

and injury. Body fluids contain water, sodium, chloride, potassium, calcium, phosphorous, and magnesium.

Approximately 50% to 70% of the total body weight is fluid (a component also known as the total body water). The average male is 60% fluid; the average female is 50% fluid. Body fluid is classified into two main types: intracellular fluid (45% of body weight) and extracellular fluid (15% of body weight). (In terms of the total body water volume—as compared to body weight—approximately 75% of the body's fluid is intracellular, and the remaining 25% is extracellular.) The extracellular fluid can be further classified into interstitial fluid (10.5% of body weight; see Figure 6-6 ▴), which surrounds tissue cells and includes cerebrospinal fluid and synovial fluid, and intravascular fluid (4.5% of body weight), which is found within the blood vessels but outside the cells themselves.

Special Considerations

Total body water changes throughout a person's lifetime. At birth, a healthy, full-term infant will have approximately 80% total body water; in older people, total body water may constitute only 45% of body weight. For this reason, dehydration can be a serious concern in geriatric patients.

Table 6-1	Movement of Molecules
Method	**Movement**
Passive transport diffusion	Movement of a substance from an area of higher concentration to an area of lower concentration.
Facilitated diffusion	A transport molecule ("helper" molecule) within the membrane helps the movement of a substance from areas of higher concentration to areas of lower concentration.
Osmosis	The movement of a solvent, such as water, from an area of low solute concentration to one of high concentration through a selectively permeable membrane to equalize concentrations of a solute on both sides of the membrane.
Filtration	The movement of water and a dissolved substance from an area of high pressure to an area of low pressure.
Active transport	Movement via "pumps" or transport molecules that require energy and move substances from an area of low concentration to an area of high concentration.

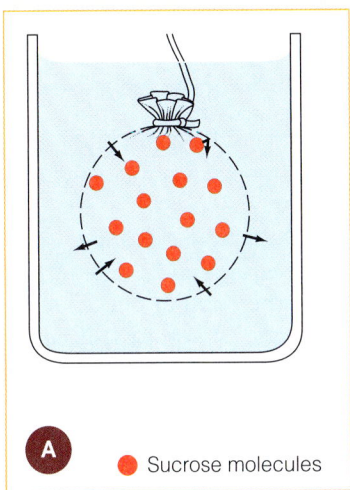

● Sucrose molecules

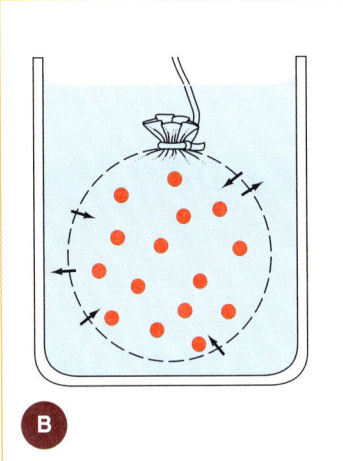

Figure 6-7 Osmosis is the diffusion of water molecules from a region of higher water concentration (or low solute concentration) to one of lower water concentration (or high solute concentration) across a selectively permeable membrane. **A.** To demonstrate the process, immerse a bag of sugar water in a solution of pure water. **B.** Water diffuses into the bag (toward the lower water concentration).

concentration has a higher osmotic pressure and is referred to as a hypertonic solution. The solution with a lower solute concentration has a lower osmotic pressure and is referred to as a hypotonic solution. Solutions with equal solute concentrations are called isotonic solutions (ie, 0.9% NaCl or lactated Ringer's solution).

Intracellular fluid volume is controlled in two ways: by the proteins and organic compounds that cannot escape through the cell membrane and by the sodium–potassium (Na$^+$/K$^+$) membrane pump. Most intracellular substances are negatively charged and so attract positively charged ions, including potassium. Because all of these substances are osmotically active, they can pull water into the cell—even until the cell ruptures. The Na$^+$/K$^+$ pump is responsible for keeping this situation in check and maintaining the cell's electrical potential by continuously removing three Na$^+$ ions from the cell for every two K$^+$ ions that are moved back into the cell. If this pump is impaired due to insufficient potassium in the body, sodium accumulates and causes the cells to swell.

Plasma

Plasma, which makes up about 55% of the blood, is composed of 91% water and 9% plasma proteins. Plasma proteins include albumin, which maintains osmotic pressure; globulin; fibrinogen; and prothrombin, which assists with clotting. Water moves between plasma and interstitial fluid based on conditions known as Starling's forces. Under normal conditions, the amount of fluid filtering outward through the arterial ends of the capillaries equals the amount of fluid that is returned to the circulation by reabsorption at the venous ends of the capillaries.

The equilibrium between the capillary and the interstitial space is controlled by four forces: capillary hydrostatic pressure, capillary colloidal osmotic pressure, tissue hydrostatic pressure, and tissue colloidal osmotic pressure. Capillary hydrostatic pressure pushes water out of the capillary into the interstitial space. Because the pressure is higher on the arterial end than the venous end, more water is pushed out of the capillary on the arterial end and more water is reabsorbed on the venous end. Capillary colloidal osmotic pressure is generated by dissolved proteins in the plasma that are too large to penetrate the capillary membrane. Tissue hydrostatic pressure opposes the pushing of fluids from the capillary into the interstitial space. Tissue colloidal osmotic pressure pulls fluid into the interstitial space.

Capillary and membrane permeability plays an important role in the movement of fluid and the emergence of edema in the surrounding tissues. If permeability increases, capillaries and membranes are more likely to leak. If permeability decreases, capillaries and membranes are less likely to leak.

Alterations in Water Movement: Edema

Edema occurs when excess fluid builds up in the interstitial space. Peripheral edema (eg, in the ankles and feet) is the most common form. Severe edema may be caused by long-standing lymphatic obstruction. If the patient is bedridden, edema may occur in the sacral area (sacral edema). Ascites is the abnormal accumulation of fluid in the peritoneal cavity.

Edema may have any of several causes:

Notes from Nancy

The cardinal sign of overhydration is edema.

- Increased capillary pressure—arteriolar dilation (eg, allergic reactions, inflammation), venous obstruction (eg, hepatic obstruction, heart failure, thrombophlebitis), increased vascular volume (eg, heart failure), increased levels of adrenocortical hormones, premenstrual sodium retention, pregnancy, environmental heat stress, or the effects of gravity from prolonged standing.
- Decreased colloidal osmotic pressure in the capillaries—decreased production of plasma proteins (eg, liver disease, starvation, severe protein deficiency) or increased loss of plasma proteins (eg, protein-losing kidney diseases, extensive burns).

At the Scene

The clinical manifestations of edema may be either local or generalized. Patients may have pulmonary edema for cardiac reasons, or edema may present following near-drowning (submersion) or a narcotic overdose. Excess fluid in the lungs (eg, acute pulmonary edema) impairs the diffusion of oxygen into pulmonary capillaries, making the patient hypoxic. Patients can literally drown in their own fluids if they do not receive proper care.

- Lymphatic vessel obstruction due to infection; disease of the lymphatic structures or their removal (eg, mastectomy and removal of lymph nodes may lead to edema in the upper extremity). In this case, the amount of fluid leaving the arterial end of capillaries does not equal the amount of fluid that returns in the venous side of the capillaries. Hence, more fluid leaves the arterial sides, where the mean forces favouring outward movement are slightly higher, and the additional fluid is picked up by the lymphatic system.

Fluid and Electrolyte Balance

Water balance in the body is maintained through a variety of factors, of which the thirst mechanism and release of anti-diuretic hormone (ADH) are the most important. The renin-angiotensin-aldosterone system also plays a role in water homeostasis. The body's state of hydration is monitored continuously by three types of receptors:

- *Osmoreceptors* monitor extracellular fluid osmolarity. Sensors for these receptors are located primarily in the hypothalamus. When the extracellular fluid osmolarity is too high, they stimulate the production of ADH.
- *Volume-sensitive receptors* are located in the atria. When the intravascular fluid volume increases, the atria are stretched, leading to the release of natriuretic proteins.
- *Baroreceptors* are found primarily in the carotid artery, aorta, and kidneys. They are sensitive to changes in blood pressure.

The most potent stimulation for the release of ADH is an increase in blood osmolarity. When osmolarity increases, the pituitary gland releases ADH, also known as vasopressin. ADH stimulates the kidneys to resorb water, decreasing the blood's osmolarity.

Sodium and Chloride Balance

Sodium is the most common cation (ie, positively charged ion) in the body. The average adult has 60 mEq of sodium for each kilogram of body weight. Most of the body's sodium is found in the extracellular fluid, but a small amount is found in the intracellular fluid. Intracellular sodium is transported out of the cell by the sodium–potassium pump because a resting cell membrane is relatively impermeable to sodium. Sodium also plays an important role in the regulation of the body's acid–base balance (sodium bicarbonate buffer system).

Sodium is taken in with foods. As little as 500 mg per day meets the body's needs.

Sodium is regulated primarily by the renin-angiotensin-aldosterone system (RAAS) and by natriuretic proteins. The RAAS is a complex feedback mechanism responsible for the kidney's regulation of sodium in the body. When sodium is present in excess, it is excreted into the urine; when the body sodium levels are low, the kidneys resorb sodium.

Renin is a protein that is released by the kidneys into the bloodstream in response to changes in blood pressure, blood flow, the amount of sodium in the tubular fluid, and the glomerular filtration rate. When renin is released, it converts the plasma protein angiotensinogen to angiotensin I. In the lungs, angiotensin I is converted rapidly to angiotensin II by angiotensin-converting enzyme (ACE). Angiotensin II, in turn, stimulates sodium resorption by the renal tubules. It also constricts the renal blood vessels, slowing kidney blood flow and decreasing the glomerular filtration rate. As a result, less sodium is filtered into the urine and more sodium is resorbed in the blood. **Figure 6-8 ▶** illustrates the role of the kidneys in the regulation of blood pressure and blood volume.

Angiotensin II is also responsible for stimulating the secretion of the adrenal hormone aldosterone. Aldosterone acts on the kidneys to increase the reabsorption of sodium into the blood and enhance the elimination of potassium in the urine. In addition to the stimulation by angiotensin II, aldosterone release is stimulated by increased extracellular potassium levels, decreased extracellular sodium levels, and release of adrenocorticotropic hormone (ACTH) from the pituitary gland.

Whereas activation of the RAAS leads to retention of sodium and water, production of natriuretic proteins increases when there is too much sodium and water in the body. Natriuretic proteins inhibit ADH and promote excretion of sodium and water by the kidneys.

Chloride is an important anion, or negatively charged ion, that when combined with sodium makes ordinary table salt. When placed in water, the compound will separate into its original ionic form. It assists in regulating the acid–base balance, especially the pH of the stomach, and is involved in the osmotic pressure of the extracellular fluid. Table salt, milk, eggs, and meats all contain chloride. It is often the case that where sodium goes, chloride follows.

Alterations in Sodium, Chloride, and Water Balance

Changes in water content can cause a cell to either shrink or swell. Tonicity refers to the tension exerted on a cell due to

Notes from Nancy

When you eat a bag of potato chips, you ingest a very large quantity of salt. Acutely, the body responds by holding on to water (hence urine output temporarily declines). In normal individuals, the kidneys and other regulatory mechanisms soon straighten things out.

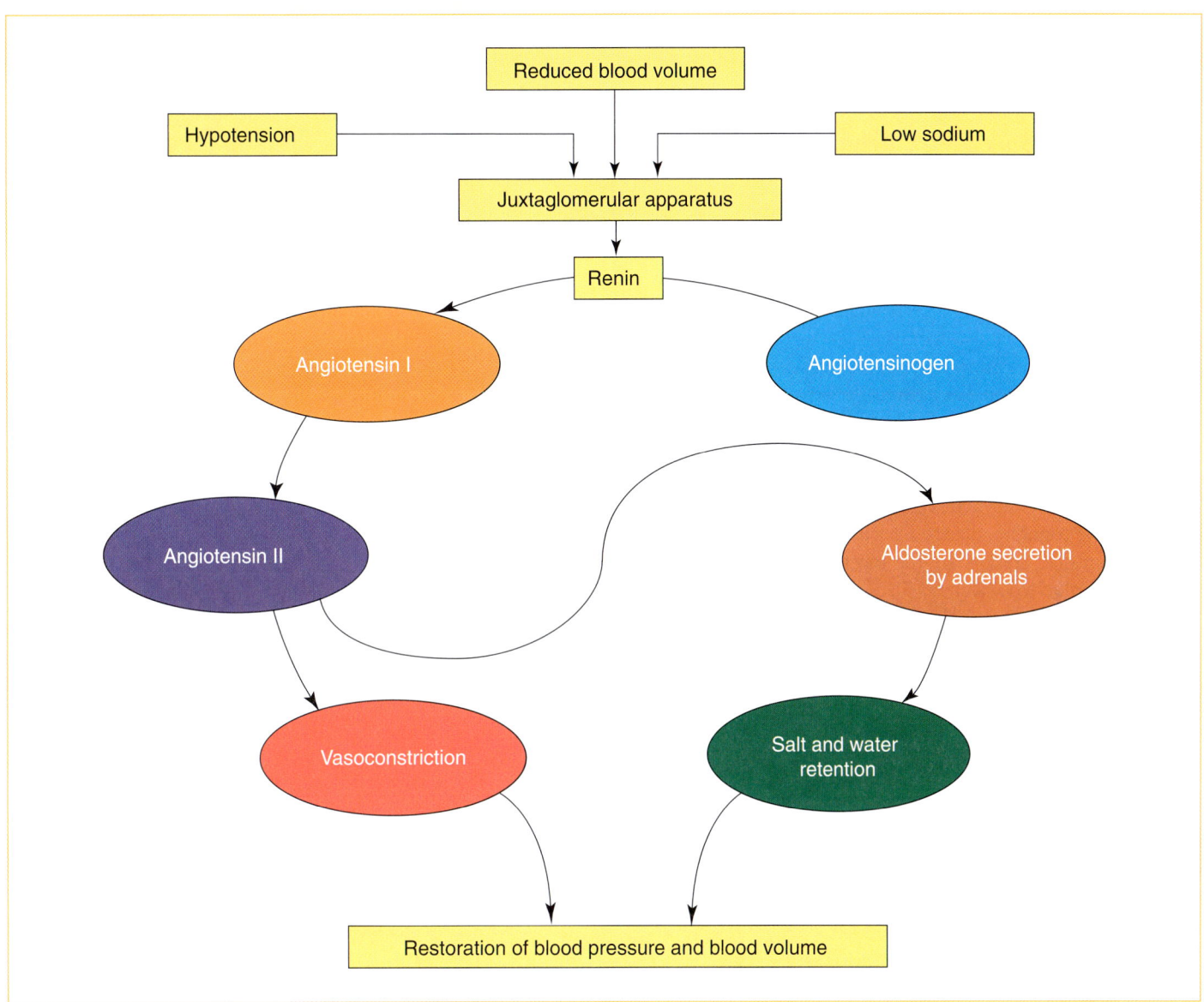

Figure 6-8 Role of the kidneys in regulation of blood pressure and blood volume.

water movement across the cell membrane. When cells are placed in an isotonic solution (ie, one with the same osmolarity as intracellular fluid—280 mOsm/l), they neither shrink nor swell. When cells are placed in a hypertonic solution, water is pulled out of the cells and they shrink. When cells are placed in a hypotonic solution, they swell.

An isotonic fluid deficit is a decrease in extracellular fluid with proportionate losses of sodium and water. An isotonic fluid excess is a proportionate increase in both sodium and water in the extracellular fluid compartment; common causes include kidney, heart, and liver failure. Manifestations of these problems depend on the serum sodium level. When dehydration exists, orthostatic hypotension and decreased urine output (oliguria) are common. Hyperthermia, delirium, and coma may be seen with very high sodium levels (> 160 mmol/l).

A hypertonic fluid deficit is caused by excess body water loss without a proportionate sodium loss (a relative water loss exists). The result is hypernatremia, which is clinically defined as a serum sodium level greater than 148 mmol/l and a serum osmolarity greater than 295 mOsm/kg. A hypotonic fluid deficit is caused by excessive sodium loss with less water loss (a relative water excess exists). This results in hyponatremia, which is characterized by a serum sodium level less than 135 mmol/l and a serum osmolarity less than 280 mOsm/kg.

Causes of hypernatremia and hyponatremia may include excess sweating from hot environmental conditions or exercise as well as gastrointestinal losses through vomiting, diarrhea, inappropriate intravenous fluids, or diuretics. Some patients have nausea and headaches, and others go on to develop seizures and coma. Clinical findings typically depend not only on the absolute sodium level, but also on the time period over which the abnormality developed. Patients who become hyponatremic over a period of days tend to have fewer symptoms than individuals who develop the abnormality acutely.

Alterations in Potassium, Calcium, Phosphate, and Magnesium Balance

Potassium

Potassium (K^+), as the major intracellular cation, is critical to many functions of the cell. Potassium is necessary for neuromuscular control, regulation of the three types of muscles (skeletal, smooth, and cardiac), acid–base balance, intracellular enzyme reactions, and maintenance of intracellular osmolarity. The normal serum level of potassium is in the range of 3.5 to 5.0 mmol/l.

Hypokalemia is defined as a decreased serum potassium level. Common causes include decreased potassium intake, potassium shifts into the cells (eg, insulin, alkalosis, beta-adrenergic stimulation such as with epinephrine), renal potassium losses (eg, increased aldosterone activity, diuretics), and extrarenal potassium losses (eg, vomiting, diarrhea, laxatives). Muscular weakness, fatigue, and muscle cramps are the most frequent complaints in mild to moderate hypokalemia. Flaccid paralysis, hyporeflexia, and tetany may occur with very low levels of potassium (< 2.5 mmol/l). The ECG shows decreased amplitude and broadening of T waves, prominent U waves, premature ventricular contractions and other arrhythmias (eg, torsade de pointes), and depressed ST segments. Although acute hypokalemia can be treated with IV potassium supplementation, this therapy is rarely undertaken in the prehospital setting.

Hyperkalemia is an elevated serum potassium level. Common causes include spurious causes (repeated fist-clenching during phlebotomy, with release of potassium from forearm muscles; specimen drawn from an arm with a potassium infusion), decreased excretion (renal failure, drugs that inhibit potassium excretion [spironolactone, ACE inhibitors, nonsteroidal anti-inflammatory drugs (NSAIDs)]), shifts of potassium from within the cell (eg, burns, metabolic acidosis, insulin deficiency), and excessive intake of potassium. The elevated potassium level interferes with normal neuromuscular function, leading to muscle weakness and, rarely, flaccid paralysis. ECG changes occur in fewer than half of patients with a serum potassium level greater than 6.5 mmol/l and include peaked T waves, widening of the QRS complex, and arrhythmias (eg, ventricular tachycardia).

Hyperkalemia can be life-threatening due to its cardiac manifestations; therefore, it should be treated in the prehospital setting. Calcium administered intravenously immediately antagonizes cardiac conduction abnormalities. Bicarbonate, insulin, and salbutamol shift potassium into the cells during a 15- to 30-minute period.

Calcium

The majority (98%) of the body's calcium is found in the bone and teeth. This element provides strength and stability for the collagen and ground substance that forms the matrix of the skeletal system. Calcium enters the body through the gastro-intestinal tract and is absorbed from the intestine in a process that depends on the presence of vitamin D **Figure 6-9**. Vitamin D is largely obtained through exposure to sunlight, stored in the bone, and ultimately excreted by the kidney. The normal serum calcium level is 2.2 to 2.6 mmol/l.

Hypocalcemia is defined as a decreased serum calcium level. Causes of hypocalcemia include decreased intake or absorption (eg, malabsorption, vitamin D deficit), increased loss (eg, alcoholism, diuretic therapy), and endocrine disease (eg, hypoparathyroidism, sepsis). Symptoms reflect the increased excitation of the neuromuscular and cardiovascular systems. Spasm of skeletal muscle causes cramps and tetany. Laryngospasm with stridor can obstruct the airway. Convulsions can occur as well as abnormal sensations (paresthesias) of the lips and extremities. Prolongation of the QT interval predisposes to the development of ventricular arrhythmias.

Hypercalcemia is an increased serum calcium level. Causes include increased intake or absorption (eg, excess antacid ingestion), endocrine disorders (eg, primary hyperparathyroidism, adrenal insufficiency), neoplasms (eg, cancers), and miscellaneous causes (eg, diuretics, sarcoidosis). Symptoms include constipation and frequent urination (polyuria). Stupor, coma, and renal failure may develop in severe cases. Treatment of the underlying cause is the mainstay of dealing with hypercalcemia. On an acute basis, volume replacement with boluses of 0.45% or 0.9% normal saline may be helpful.

At the Scene

In the presence of tetany, arrhythmias, or seizures, 10% IV calcium gluconate (10 to 20 ml) administered over 10 to 15 minutes is indicated. Oral calcium and vitamin D preparations are appropriate in moderate or asymptomatic cases.

Phosphate

Phosphate is primarily an intracellular anion and is essential to many body functions.

Hypophosphatemia is characterized by a decrease in serum phosphate levels. Causes include decreased supply or absorption (eg, starvation, malabsorption, blocked absorption [aluminum-containing antacids]), excessive loss of phosphate ion (eg, diuretics, hyperparathyroidism, hyperthyroidism, alcoholism), intracellular shift of phosphorous (eg, administration of glucose, anabolic steroids, oral contraceptives, respiratory alkalosis, salicylate poisoning), electrolyte abnormalities (eg, hypercalcemia, hypomagnesemia, metabolic acidosis), and abnormal losses followed by inadequate repletion (eg, diabetic ketoacidosis, chronic alcoholism). Symptoms include muscle weakness, decreased deep tendon reflexes, mental obtundation, and confusion. Weakness is common. Acute, severe hypophosphatemia can lead to acute hemolytic anemia and increased susceptibility to infection. Muscle death (rhabdomyolysis) may also occur. Treatment involves oral replenishment

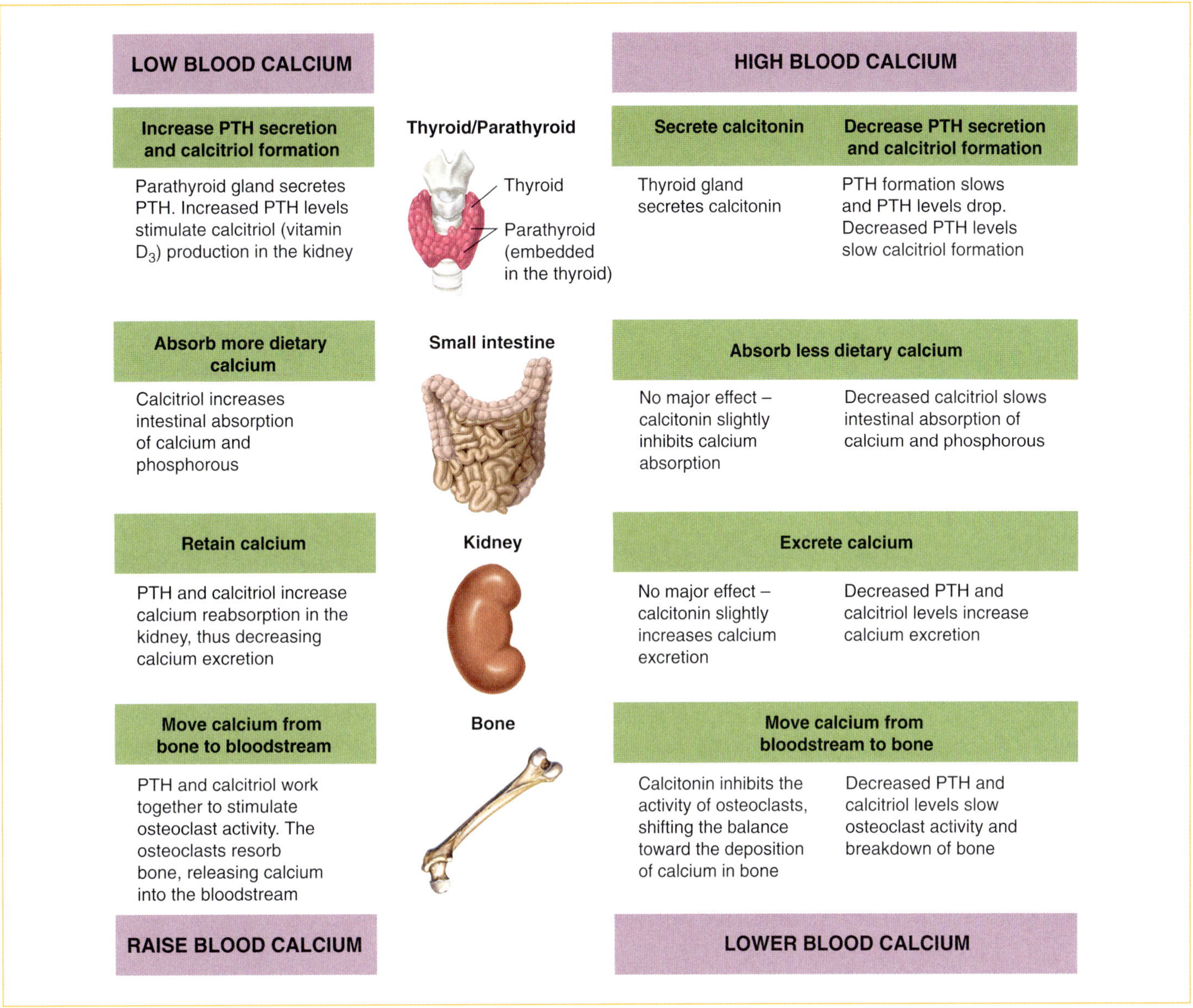

LOW BLOOD CALCIUM		HIGH BLOOD CALCIUM	
Increase PTH secretion and calcitriol formation	Thyroid/Parathyroid	**Secrete calcitonin**	**Decrease PTH secretion and calcitriol formation**
Parathyroid gland secretes PTH. Increased PTH levels stimulate calcitriol (vitamin D_3) production in the kidney	Thyroid / Parathyroid (embedded in the thyroid)	Thyroid gland secretes calcitonin	PTH formation slows and PTH levels drop. Decreased PTH levels slow calcitriol formation
Absorb more dietary calcium	Small intestine	**Absorb less dietary calcium**	
Calcitriol increases intestinal absorption of calcium and phosphorous		No major effect – calcitonin slightly inhibits calcium absorption	Decreased calcitriol slows intestinal absorption of calcium and phosphorous
Retain calcium	Kidney	**Excrete calcium**	
PTH and calcitriol increase calcium reabsorption in the kidney, thus decreasing calcium excretion		No major effect – calcitonin slightly increases calcium excretion	Decreased PTH and calcitriol levels increase calcium excretion
Move calcium from bone to bloodstream	Bone	**Move calcium from bloodstream to bone**	
PTH and calcitriol work together to stimulate osteoclast activity. The osteoclasts resorb bone, releasing calcium into the bloodstream		Calcitonin inhibits the activity of osteoclasts, shifting the balance toward the deposition of calcium in bone	Decreased PTH and calcitriol levels slow osteoclast activity and breakdown of bone
RAISE BLOOD CALCIUM		**LOWER BLOOD CALCIUM**	

Figure 6-9 Regulation of blood calcium levels. Calcitonin has only a weak effect on calcium ion concentration. It is fast-acting, but any decrease in calcium ion concentration triggers the release of parathyroid hormone (PTH), which almost completely overrides the calcitonin effect. In prolonged calcium excess or deficiency, the parathyroid mechanism is the most powerful hormonal mechanism for maintaining normal blood calcium levels.

in mild to moderate cases. Severe cases and symptomatic patients require IV phosphate replacement.

Hyperphosphatemia is defined as an increased serum phosphate level. Causes include massive loading of phosphate into the extracellular fluid (eg, excess vitamin D, laxatives or enemas containing phosphate, IV phosphate supplements, chemotherapy, metabolic acidosis) and decreased excretion into the urine (eg, renal failure, hypoparathyroidism, excessive growth hormone [acromegaly]). Symptoms vary widely, but may include tremor, paresthesia, hyporeflexia, confusion, seizures, muscle weakness, stupor, coma, hypotension, heart failure, and prolonged QT interval. Treatment of the underly-

ing cause and of any accompanying hypocalcemia is the most common therapeutic approach. Saline boluses (forced diuresis) are often helpful.

Magnesium

Magnesium is the second most abundant intracellular cation, after potassium. About 50% of the body's magnesium is stored in the bones, 49% in the body cells, and the remaining 1% in the extracellular fluid. Normal serum levels are 0.8 to 1.2 mmol/l.

Hypomagnesemia is defined as a decreased serum magnesium level. Causes include diminished absorption or intake (eg, malabsorption, chronic diarrhea, laxative abuse, malnutrition), increased renal loss (eg, diuretics, hyperaldosteronism, hypercalcemia, volume expansion), and miscellaneous causes (eg, diabetes, respiratory alkalosis, pregnancy). Common symptoms are weakness, muscle cramps, and tremor. Patients develop marked neuromuscular and central nervous system hyperirritability with tremors and jerking. There may be hypertension, tachycardia, and ventricular arrhythmias. In some patients, confusion and disorientation are prominent features. Treatment consists of IV fluids containing magnesium.

Hypermagnesemia is an increased serum magnesium level. It is almost always the result of kidney insufficiency and the inability to excrete the amount of magnesium taken in from food or drugs, especially antacids and laxatives. Symptoms include muscle weakness, decreased deep tendon reflexes, mental obtundation, and confusion. Weakness is common, and respiratory muscle paralysis or cardiac arrest is possible.

Acid–Base Balance

The measurement of hydrogen ion concentration of a solution is called pH. Normal body functions depend on an acid–base balance that remains within the normal physiologic pH range of 7.35 to 7.45. The mathematical formula for calculating pH is pH = –log [H$^+$], where "log" refers to the base-10 logarithm and [H$^+$] refers to the hydrogen ion concentration. Changes in the pH are exponential, not linear. For example, a change in the pH from 7.40 to 7.20 results in a 10^2 (ie, 100-fold) change in the acid concentration.

To maintain the delicate acid–base balance, the body relies on its buffer systems. Buffers are molecules that modulate changes in pH. In the absence of buffers, the addition of acid to a solution will cause a sharp change in pH. In the presence of a buffer, the pH change will be moderated or may even be unnoticeable in the same situation. Because acid production is the major challenge to pH homeostasis, most physiologic buffers combine with H$^+$.

Buffer systems include proteins, phosphate ions, and bicarbonate (HCO$_3^-$). The large amounts of bicarbonate produced from the carbon dioxide (CO$_2$) made during metabolism create the body's most important extracellular buffer system. Hydrogen and bicarbonate ions combine to form carbonic acid, which readily dissociates into water and carbon dioxide:

$$H^+ + HCO_3^- \Leftrightarrow H_2CO_3 \Leftrightarrow H_2O + CO_2$$

In the bicarbonate buffer system, excess acid (H$^+$) combines with bicarbonate (HCO$_3^-$), forming H$_2$CO$_3$. This compound rapidly dissociates into water and CO$_2$, which is then exhaled. Because the acid is eliminated as water and CO$_2$, the total pH does not change significantly. A similar process occurs with the production of metabolic base (bicarbonate).

Acidosis Versus Alkalosis

When the buffering capacity of the body is exceeded, acid–base imbalances occur. A blood pH greater than 7.45 is called alkalosis; a blood pH less than 7.35 is called acidosis.

If the pH is too low (acidosis), neurons become less excitable and CNS depression results. Patients become confused and disoriented. If CNS depression progresses, the respiratory centres cease to function, leading to the person's death.

If pH is too high (alkalosis), neurons become hyperexcitable, firing action potentials at the slightest signal. This condition first manifests as sensory changes, such as numbness or tingling, then as muscle twitches. If alkalosis is severe, muscle twitches turn into sustained contractions (tetanus) that paralyze respiratory muscles.

Disturbances of acid–base balance are associated with disturbances in potassium balance, in part because of the kidney transport system that moves H$^+$ and K$^+$ in opposite directions. In acidosis, the kidneys excrete H$^+$ and resorb K$^+$. Conversely, when the body goes into a state of alkalosis, the kidneys resorb H$^+$ and excrete K$^+$. A potassium imbalance usually shows up as disturbances in excitable tissues, especially the heart.

Metabolic Versus Respiratory Acid–Base Imbalances

Acid–base disturbances are classified into two general categories: metabolic and respiratory. Each is then broken down into acidosis and alkalosis.

Metabolic acidosis is an accumulation of abnormal acids in the blood for any of several reasons (eg, sepsis, diabetic ketoacidosis, salicylate poisoning). Initially, the Pa$_{CO_2}$ (partial pressure of carbon dioxide) is not affected, but the pH is decreased. Later, the body compensates for the metabolic abnormality by hyperventilating, leading to excretion of CO$_2$ and compensatory respiratory alkalosis. For example, patients with diabetic ketoacidosis often experience *Kussmaul respirations* (deep, rapid, sighing ventilations), in which they hyperventilate to "blow off" CO$_2$ and decrease the acidosis.

Metabolic alkalosis is rarely seen in an acute condition, but is very common in chronically ill patients, especially those undergoing nasogastric suction. It involves either a buildup of excess metabolic base (eg, chronic antacid ingestion) or a loss of normal acid (eg, through vomiting or nasogastric

At the Scene

Respiratory compensation for metabolic problems (acidosis or alkalosis) occurs rapidly and is relatively predictable. Metabolic compensation for respiratory problems (acidosis or alkalosis), if it occurs at all, takes hours to days. Compensation returns the pH toward normal. Acutely, compensation is never complete. Chronic compensation, as in chronic obstructive pulmonary disease (COPD), often does result in a completely normal pH.

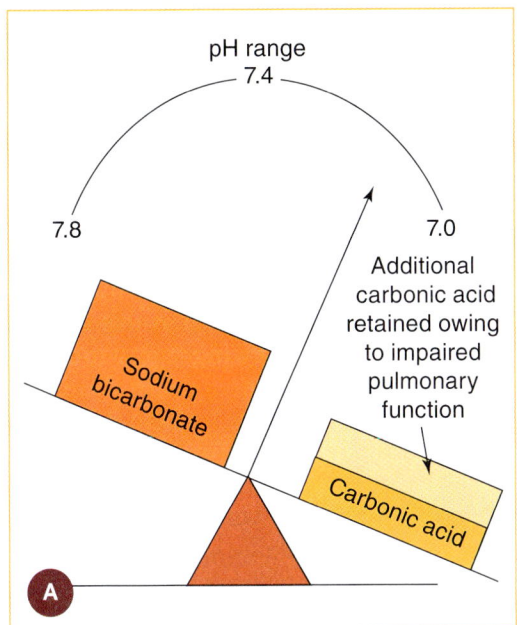

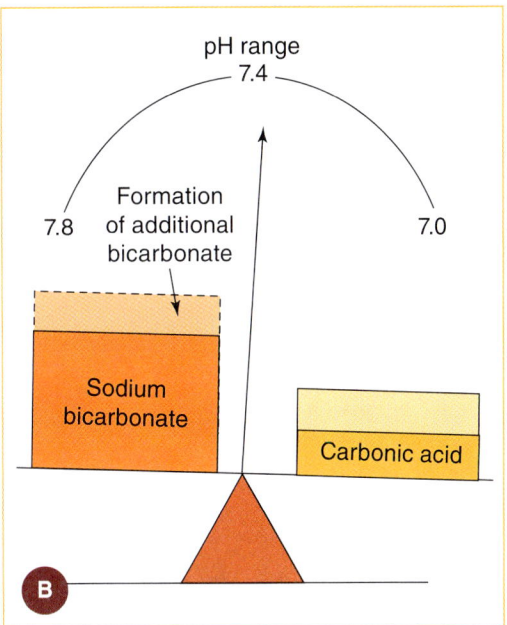

Figure 6-10 A. Derangement of acid–base balance in respiratory acidosis. **B.** Compensation by formation of additional bicarbonate.

Figure 6-11 ▸ . This damage often results in a change in cell shape and function. Functional changes may include an inability to use oxygen appropriately, development of intracellular acidosis, accumulation of toxic waste products, and an inability to metabolize nutrients.

Damage and functional changes in individual cells often have an impact on the entire organism. In some cases, only minor systemic abnormalities are noted, such as fever. At other times, entire organ systems fail and the patient's situation becomes critical (eg, kidney failure). Because all body systems are connected in some manner, dysfunction in one system inevitably affects other systems. When the homeostatic balance in the body is upset, the "scales" can shift in an unfavourable direction.

Cell injury may, up to a point, be repaired with proper treatment. Irreversible injury occurs once cells have passed the "point of no return," after which no treatment will help. Cell death is followed by necrosis, a process in which the cell breaks down. The cell membrane becomes abnormally permeable, leading to an influx of electrolytes and fluids. The cell and its organelles swell. Lysosomes also release enzymes that destroy intracellular components. These processes occur both during and after actual cell death.

suctioning). The pH is high and the Pa_{CO_2} unchanged initially. On a chronic basis, the body compensates by slowing ventilation and increasing the Pa_{CO_2}, thereby creating a compensatory respiratory acidosis.

Respiratory acidosis occurs when CO_2 retention leads to increased Pa_{CO_2} levels. It also occurs in situations of hypoventilation (eg, heroin overdose) or intrinsic lung diseases (eg, asthma or COPD) **Figure 6-10 ▲** .

Excessive "blowing off" of CO_2 with a resulting decrease in the Pa_{CO_2} causes respiratory alkalosis. Although often called hyperventilation, many potentially serious diseases (eg, pulmonary embolism, acute myocardial infarction, severe infection, diabetic ketoacidosis) may be responsible for increased ventilatory levels.

Cell Injury

Cellular injury may result from various causes, such as hypoxia (lack of oxygen), ischemia (hypoxia due to lack of blood supply), chemical injury, infectious injury, immunologic (hypersensitivity) injury, physical damage (mechanical injury), and inflammatory injury. The manifestations of cell injury and death depend on how many and which types of cells are damaged.

Manifestations of cellular injury occur at both the microscopic (structural) and the functional levels. Common microscopic abnormalities (eg, those observed in the cardiac cell undergoing necrosis from hypoxemia for an extended period of time) include cell swelling, rupture of cell membranes or nuclear membranes, and breakdown of nuclear material (chromosomes)

Hypoxic Injury

Hypoxic injury is a common—and often deadly—cause of cellular injury. It may result from decreased amounts of oxygen in the air or loss of hemoglobin function (eg, carbon monoxide poisoning), a decreased number of red blood cells (eg, bleeding), disease of the respiratory or cardiovascular system (eg, COPD), or loss of cytochromes (mitochondrial proteins that convert oxygen to ATP, like that seen in cyanide poisoning).

Although hypoxia by itself has deleterious effects on cells, the damage does not stop there. Cells that are hypoxic for more than a few seconds produce mediators (substances) that may damage other local or distant body locations. The result is a positive feedback cycle in which mediators lead to more cell damage, which leads to more hypoxia, which leads to further mediator production, and so forth.

The earliest and most dangerous mediators produced by cells in response to hypoxia are free radicals. These molecules are missing one electron in their outer shell. The presence of an odd, unpaired electron results in chemical instability

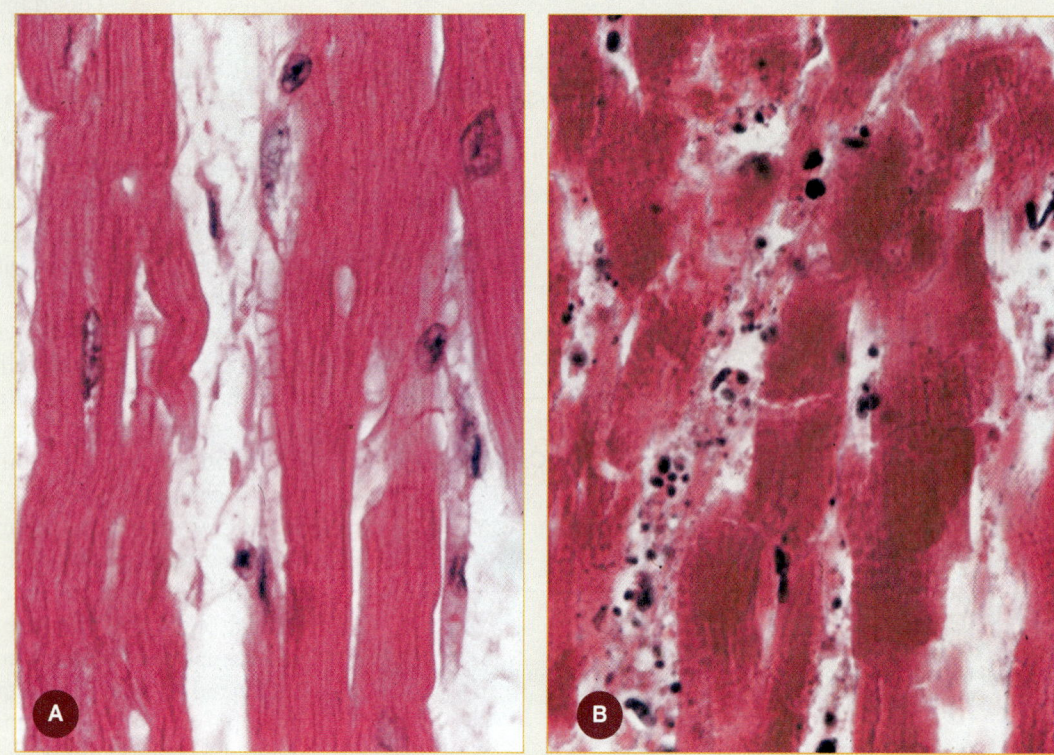

Figure 6-11 Comparison of cardiac muscle fibres. **A.** With necrotic fibres. **B.** Note fragmentation of fibres, loss of nuclear staining, and fragmented bits of nuclear debris. When the cell is injured it swells, resulting in nuclear membrane rupture and breakdown of the nuclear material (original magnification, ×400).

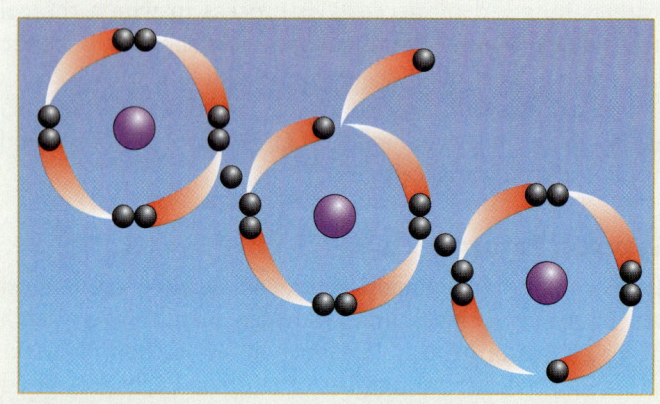

Figure 6-12 Free radicals are missing one electron in their outside orbit. This molecular structure results in chemical instability. Each black dot represents an electron in the outer shell.

Figure 6-12 ▲ . Free radicals randomly attack cells and membranes in an attempt to "steal back" the missing electron. The result is widespread and potentially deadly tissue damage.

Chemical Injury

A variety of chemicals may injure and ultimately destroy cells, including poisons, lead, carbon monoxide, ethanol, and pharmacologic agents. Common poisons include cyanide and pesti-

cides. Cyanide induces cell hypoxia by blocking oxidative phosphorylation in the mitochondria and preventing the metabolism of oxygen. Pesticides block an enzyme, acetylcholinesterase, thereby preventing proper transmission of nerve impulses.

Chronic ingestion of lead, such as that caused by chewing on windowsills painted with lead-based paint, leads to brain injury and neurologic dysfunction. Although all of lead's toxic effects cannot be tied together neatly by pointing to a single unifying mechanism, its ability to substitute for calcium (molecules of lead and calcium are a similar size) is a common factor in many of its toxic actions. Mostly likely lead is "mistaken" for calcium in vital biochemical reactions, leading to abnormal results and dysfunction.

Carbon monoxide binds to hemoglobin, preventing adequate oxygenation of the tissues. Low levels cause nausea, vomiting, and headache. Higher levels result in death.

In lower doses, ethanol causes the well-known effects of inebriation. Higher doses result in severe CNS depression, hypoventilation, and cardiovascular collapse.

Some pharmacologic agents produce toxic products when they are metabolized in the body, especially in "overdose conditions." Acetaminophen (Tylenol), in doses of more than 140 mg/kg in an adult, results in acute overdose, causing the accumulation of toxic intermediates that poison the liver and may lead to death.

Infectious Injury

Infectious injury to cells occurs as a result of an invasion of either bacteria or viruses. Bacteria may cause injury either by direct action on cells or by the production of toxins. Viruses often initiate an inflammatory response that leads to cell damage and patient symptoms.

Virulence measures the disease-causing ability of a microorganism. The pathogenicity of any particular microorganism is a function of its ability to reproduce and cause disease within the human body. In particular, the growth and survival of bacteria in the body depend on the effectiveness of the body's own defence mechanisms and the bacteria's ability to resist those mechanisms. A depressed immune system is less able to fight off microorganisms that the body perceives as harmful; populations with weaker immune systems may include newborn infants, elderly patients, diabetics, and people with cancer or other chronic diseases.

Bacteria

Many bacteria possess a capsule that protects them from ingestion and destruction by phagocytes—cells (eg, white blood cells) that engulf and consume foreign material such as microorganisms and cellular debris Figure 6-13 ▼. Not all bacteria are encapsulated, however. *Mycobacterium tuberculosis,* for example, lacks a capsule, yet stubbornly resists destruction; it can be transported by phagocytes throughout the body. Gram-positive bacteria are distinguished by very thick cell walls composed of many layers of peptidoglycan (amino acids and sugar); conversely, the cell walls of gram-negative bacteria consist largely of lipids. The pathogenic qualities of gram-negative bacteria, which include the microorganism that causes bubonic plague, make them especially problematic for humans.

Bacteria also produce exotoxins or endotoxins—substances such as enzymes or toxins—that can injure or destroy cells. Staphylococci, streptococci, and *Clostridium tetani,* for example, secrete exotoxins into the medium surrounding the cell. Endotoxins are lipopolysaccharides that are part of the cell walls of gram-negative bacteria. When large amounts of endotoxins are present in the body, a person may develop septic shock.

When cells are injured, circulating white blood cells are attracted to the site of injury. White blood cells release endogenous pyrogens, which then cause a fever to develop. Indeed, the body's most common reaction to the presence of bacteria is inflammation. Some bacteria have the ability to produce hypersensitivity reactions. The proliferation of microorganisms in the blood is called bacteremia or sepsis.

Viruses

Viruses are intracellular parasites that take over the metabolic processes of the host cell and then use the cell to help them replicate. A virus consists of a nucleic acid core of either RNA or DNA. Surrounding the viral core is a layer of protein known as the capsid, which protects the virus from phagocytosis. Some viruses have an additional protective coat known as the envelope.

The replication of a virus occurs inside the host cell because viruses do not contain any of their own organelles. Viral infection of a host cell leads to a decreased synthesis of macromolecules that are vital to the host cell. Unlike bacteria, however, viruses do not produce exotoxins or endotoxins.

There may be a symbiotic relationship between a virus and normal cells that results in a persistent unapparent infection. Viruses have been known to evoke a strong immune response and can rapidly produce an irreversible, lethal injury in highly susceptible cells, as is the case with acquired immunodeficiency syndrome (AIDS).

Immunologic and Inflammatory Injury

Inflammation is a protective response that can occur even without bacterial invasion. Infection is characterized by an invasion of microorganisms that causes cell or tissue injury, which leads to the inflammatory response. The immune system protects the body by providing defences to attack and remove foreign organisms such as bacteria or viruses.

Cellular membranes may be injured when they come in direct contact with the cellular and chemical components of the immune or inflammatory process, such as phagocytes (neutrophils and macrophages), histamine, antibodies, and lymphokines. In such a case, potassium leaks out of the damaged cell and water flows inward, causing the cell to swell. The nuclear envelope, organelle membranes, and cell membrane may all rupture, leading to cell death. The degree of swelling and chance of membrane rupture depend on the severity of the immune and inflammatory responses.

Other Injurious Factors

Genetic factors that may damage cells include chromosomal disorders, premature development of atherosclerosis, and obesity (in some cases). There are two ways an abnormal gene may develop in an individual: by mutation of the gene during meiosis, which affects the newly formed fetus, or by heredity. In trisomy 21 (Down syndrome), the child is born with an extra chromosome, usually number 21.

Good nutrition is required to maintain good health and assist the cells in fighting off disease. Nutritional disorders that can injure cells and the organism as a whole include obesity, malnutrition, vitamin excess or deficiency, and mineral excess or deficiency. These conditions can lead to alterations in physical growth, mental and intellectual retardation, and even death in some circumstances.

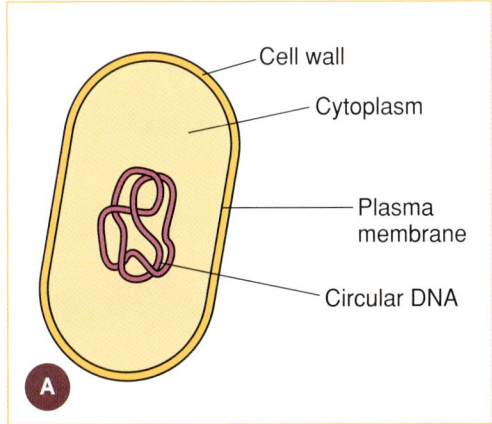

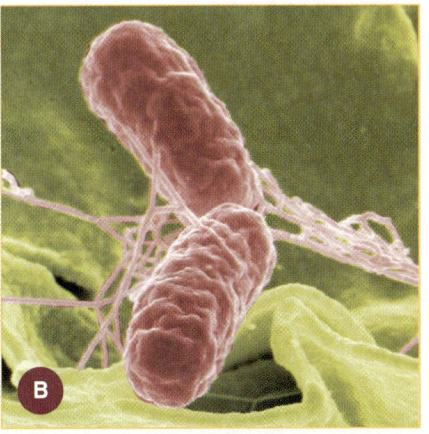

Figure 6-13 General structure of a bacterium. **A.** Bacteria come in many shapes and sizes, but all have a circular strand of DNA, cytoplasm, and a plasma membrane. A cell wall surrounds the membrane in many bacteria. **B.** An electron micrograph of salmonella bacteria. Many bacteria have a capsule that protects them from ingestion and destruction by phagocytes.

Physical agents, such as heat, cold, and radiation, may also cause cell injury—for example, burns, frostbite, radiation sickness, and tumours. The degree of cell injury that results is determined by both the strength of the agent and the length of exposure.

Apoptosis

Apoptosis is normal cell death. It is unique in that it is genetically programmed into the cell as a part of normal development, organogenesis, immune function, and tissue growth. It plays a normal role in aging, early development, menses, lactating breast tissue, thymus involution, and red blood cell turnover.

During apoptosis, cells exhibit characteristic nuclear changes, and they typically die in well-defined clusters rather than in a random fashion. The molecular mechanism underlying apoptosis involves the activation of genes that code for proteins known as caspases. These proteins are essentially cellular "cyanide"—in essence, their production leads to cell suicide. Unlike in the case of cell death from disease processes, proteins and DNA undergo controlled degradation that allows their remnants to be taken up and reused by neighbouring cells. In this way, apoptosis allows the body to eliminate a cell but still "recycle" many of its components. Pathologically, areas that have undergone apoptotic death do not show any evidence of inflammation. In contrast, an inflammatory response is typically observed when cells undergo necrosis from hypoxia or cellular toxins.

Apoptosis can be activated prematurely by pathologic factors such as cell injury. This sort of premature stimulation results in early cell death, which occurs in some forms of heart failure. Another example of pathologic apoptosis is the death of hepatocytes (liver cells) in patients with viral hepatitis. The dying cells form

lumps of chromatin known as Councilman's bodies. Factors that inhibit the normal course of apoptosis result in unwanted cellular proliferation, as in cancer and rheumatoid arthritis (uncontrolled synovial tissue proliferation). **Figure 6-14 ▾** illustrates the process by which cancerous cells develop from normal cells.

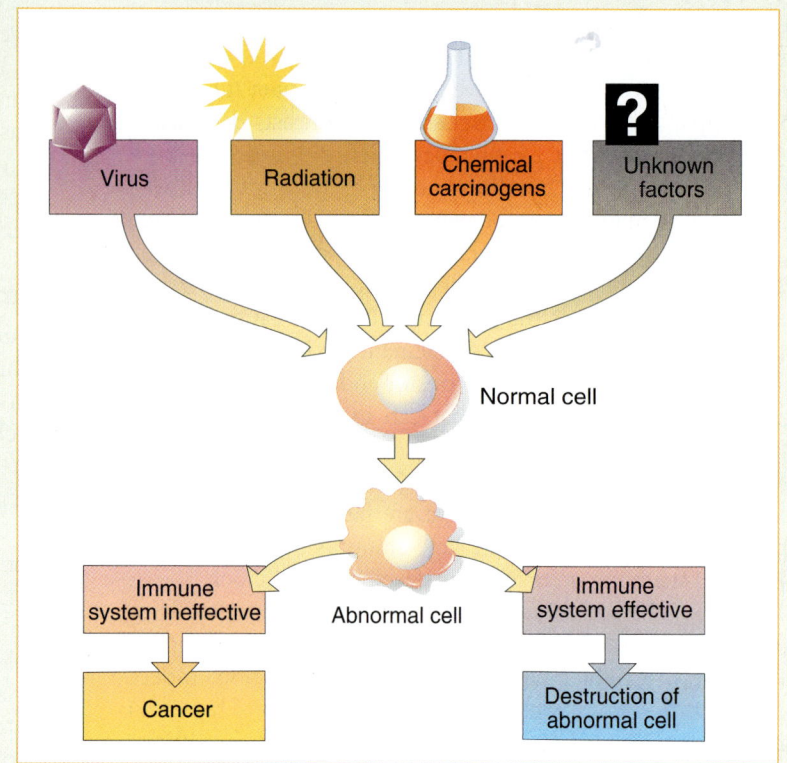

Figure 6-14 The onset of cancer. Viruses and other factors induce a normal cell to become abnormal. When the immune system is working effectively, it destroys the abnormal cells, so no cancer develops. When abnormal cells evade the immune system, they form a tumour and then may become a spreading cancer.

You are the Paramedic Part 2

You ask your partner to place the patient on 100% oxygen via a nonrebreathing mask and get a set of baseline vital signs while you begin to question her regarding her current illness and past medical history. The patient tells you that she has end-stage renal disease and requires dialysis every other day. She was unable to make it to her last appointment because she did not feel well and had no way to get there. She did not call her physician, stating that she thought she could "shake off this bug." She had been taking acetaminophen (Tylenol) every 4 hours for the fever and the pain in her forearm. Her past medical history is significant for hypertension, a myocardial infarction in 2003, and congestive heart failure. Daily medications include Captopril, aspirin, and nitroglycerin as needed.

Vital Signs	Recording Time: 5 Minutes
Skin	Pale, warm, and moist
Pulse	140 beats/min, regular; weak radial
Blood pressure	86/50 mm Hg
Respirations	28 breaths/min, accessory muscle use, rales auscultated half way up the back bilaterally
Spo₂	93% on nonrebreathing mask at 15 l/min of supplemental oxygen

3. What should you monitor your patient for?
4. Which interventions should you consider at this point, if any?

Abnormal Cell Death

If the injury leading to cell degeneration is of sufficient intensity and duration, irreversible cell injury will lead to cell death. Necrosis is the result of the morphologic changes that occur following cell death in living tissues. It may be either simple necrosis (coagulation) or derived necrosis.

Simple necrosis refers to areas of necrosis where the gross and microscopic tissue and some of the cells are recognizable. It may be caused by acute ischemia, acute toxicity (eg, from heavy metals), or direct physical injury (eg, from caustic chemicals and burns).

Derived necrosis includes caseation necrosis, dry gangrene, fat necrosis, and liquefaction necrosis. Caseation necrosis is manifested by the loss of all features of the tissue and cells, so that they come to resemble cheese when viewed through a microscope. Dry gangrene results from invasion and putrefaction of necrotic tissue, after the blood supply is compromised to the tissue and the tissue undergoes coagulation necrosis. Fat necrosis results from the destruction of fat cells, usually by enzymes (ie, pancreatic proteases and lipases). Liquefaction necrosis results from coagulation necrosis followed by liquefaction necrosis of tissues and invasion by putrefying bacteria that grow rapidly in a warm moist environment; the bacteria then produce lytic enzymes and gas.

Genetics and Familial Disease

Factors Causing Disease

Genetic, environmental, age-related, and sex-associated factors can all cause disease. Genetic factors are present at birth and are passed on through a person's genes to future generations. Environmental factors include microorganisms, immunologic and toxic exposures, personal habits and lifestyle, exposures to chemicals, the physical environment, and the psychosocial environment.

Age and sex-associated factors interact with a combination of genetic and environmental factors, lifestyle, and anatomical or hormonal differences. The risk of a particular disease often depends on the patient's age. For example, newborns are at greater risk of certain diseases because their immune systems are not fully developed (see Chapter 41). Teenagers are at high risk of other diseases due to trauma, drugs, and alcohol. The older we become, the greater the risk of cancer, heart disease, stroke, and Alzheimer's disease (see Chapter 42). Some diseases are more prevalent in men, such as lung cancer, gout, and Parkinson's disease. Women are more likely to have osteoporosis, rheumatoid arthritis, and breast cancer.

Some uncontrollable factors (eg, genetics) influence a disease process, but many other factors can be controlled. For example, behaviours such as smoking, drinking alcohol, poor nutrition (eg, excessive fat, salt, and sugar intake; insufficient intake of protein, fruits, vegetables, and fibre), lack of exercise, and stress can all be modified.

Analyzing Disease Risk

Analyzing disease risk involves consideration of disease rates and disease risk factors (both causal and noncausal). All studies of a disease should consider the incidence, prevalence, and mortality of the disease. The incidence is the frequency of disease occurrence (eg, one in four patients has this disease). The prevalence is the number of cases in a particular population over time (eg, last year, more than 100,000 patients had this disease). The mortality is the number of deaths from a disease in a given population (eg, 1 in 50 affected individuals in Canada with this disease will die).

Risk factors, age, and sex differences often interact. For example, suppose a person has a genetic tendency toward coronary artery disease; the risk of myocardial infarction or sudden death is higher in this individual even if he or she exercises regularly and has no other risk factors. A person who smokes heavily but has no other risk factors may have a similarly elevated risk.

Common Familial Diseases and Associated Risk Factors

The terms *genetic risk* and *familial tendency* are often used interchangeably. A true genetic risk is one that is passed through generations by inheritance of a gene. In contrast, with a familial tendency, diseases may "cluster" in family groups despite lack of evidence for heritable gene-associated abnormalities.

Table 6-2 ▸ lists some of the traits and diseases carried on human chromosomes. Autosomal recessive is a pattern of inheritance that involves genes located on autosomes (any chromosome other than sex chromosomes). A person needs to inherit two copies of a particular form of such a gene to show that trait. A parent who carries the gene for an autosomal recessive trait but does not display the trait has a 25% chance of passing the inherited condition to his or her child if the other parent is also a carrier for the trait. If both parents actually have the inherited condition, then all of their children will have the condition. Hemochromatosis, which causes people to accumulate too much iron in their bodies, shows an autosomal recessive pattern of inheritance—a person must inherit a copy of the hemochromatosis gene from each parent to develop the disease.

In autosomal dominant inheritance, a person needs to inherit only one copy of a particular form of a gene to show that trait; it does not matter which form of the gene is inherited from the other parent. A parent has at least a 50% chance of passing on an autosomal dominant inherited condition to his or her child. Familial adenomatous polyposis, which places people at extremely high risk of developing colon cancer, shows an autosomal dominant pattern of inheritance.

Immunologic Disorders

Immunologic diseases are caused by either hyperactivity or hypoactivity of the immune system. Most immunologic diseases that exhibit familial tendencies involve an overactive immune system—for example, allergies, asthma, and rheumatic fever. Often there is significant overlap between causative factors, including the patient's environment. [Table 6-3 ▾] lists common respiratory diseases that may be caused by environmental pollutants, viruses, or bacteria.

Allergies are acquired following initial exposure to a stimulant, known as an allergen. Repeated exposures cause the immune system to react to the allergen [Figure 6-15 ▸]. Although the clinical presentation varies, it usually includes swelling and itching, runny nose, coughing, sneezing, wheezing, and nasal congestion. A person who has an allergic tendency is said to be atopic. Environmental conditions may also increase a person's susceptibility toward an allergic reaction.

Asthma is a chronic inflammatory condition resulting in intermittent wheezing and excess mucus production. Nearly 60% of attacks are precipitated by viral infections. Allergies account for another 20% of asthma attacks, with stress and emotions causing the remainder. In addition to the familial component, chromosomal differences in certain individuals may enhance their susceptibility to asthma.

Rheumatic fever is an inflammatory disease that occurs primarily in children. This disease results from a delayed reaction to an untreated streptococcal infection of the upper respiratory tract (eg, strep throat). Symptoms, which appear several weeks after the acute infection, may include fever, abdominal pain, vomiting, arthritis, palpitations, and chest pain. Recurrent episodes of rheumatic fever may cause permanent myocardial damage, especially to the cardiac valves. A family history of acute rheumatic fever may predispose an individual to the disease.

Cancer

Cancer includes a large number of malignant growths (neoplasms). The prognosis often depends on the extent of its spread (metastasis) and the effectiveness of treatment.

Table 6-2	Traits and Diseases Carried on Human Chromosomes
Autosomal recessive	
Albinism	Lack of pigment in eyes, skin, and hair
Cystic fibrosis	Pancreatic failure, mucus buildup in lungs
Sickle cell anemia	Abnormal hemoglobin leading to sickle-shaped red blood cells that obstruct vital capillaries
Tay-Sachs disease	Improper metabolism of gangliosides in nerve cells, resulting in early death
Phenylketonuria	Accumulation of phenylalanine in blood; results in mental retardation
Attached earlobe	Earlobe attached to skin of the neck
Hyperextendable thumb	Thumb bends past 45° angle
Autosomal dominant	
Achondroplasia	Dwarfism resulting from a defect in epiphyseal plates of forming long bones
Marfan's syndrome	Defect manifest in connective tissue, resulting in excessive growth and aortic rupture
Widow's peak	Hairline coming to a point on forehead
Huntington's disease	Progressive deterioration of the nervous system beginning in late 20s or early 30s; results in mental deterioration and early death
Brachydactyly	Disfiguration of hands, shortened fingers
Freckles	Permanent aggregations of melanin in the skin

Table 6-3	Common Respiratory Diseases		
Disease	**Pathology/Symptoms**	**Cause**	**Treatment**
Emphysema	Breakdown of alveoli; shortness of breath	Smoking and air pollution	Administer oxygen to relieve symptoms; quit smoking; avoid polluted air. No known cure.
Chronic bronchitis	Coughing, shortness of breath	Smoking and air pollution	Quit smoking; move out of polluted area; if possible, move to warmer, drier climate.
Acute bronchitis	Inflammation of the bronchi; yellowy mucus coughed up; shortness of breath	Many viruses and bacteria	If bacterial, take antibiotics, cough medicine; use vapourizer.
Sinusitis	Inflammation of the sinuses; mucus discharge; blockage of nasal passageways; headache	Many viruses and bacteria	If bacterial, take antibiotics and decongestant tablets; use vapourizer.
Laryngitis	Inflammation of larynx and vocal cords; sore throat; hoarseness; mucus buildup and cough	Many viruses and bacteria	If bacterial, take antibiotics, cough medicine; avoid irritants, such as smoke; avoid talking.
Pneumonia	Inflammation of the lungs ranging from mild to severe; cough and fever; shortness of breath at rest; chills; sweating; chest pains; blood in mucus	Bacteria, viruses, or inhalation of irritating gases	Consult physician immediately; go to bed; take antibiotics, cough medicine; stay warm.
Asthma	Constriction of bronchioles; mucus buildup in bronchioles; periodic wheezing; difficulty breathing	Allergy to pollen, some foods, food additives; dandruff from dogs and cats; exercise	Use inhalants to open passageways; avoid irritants.

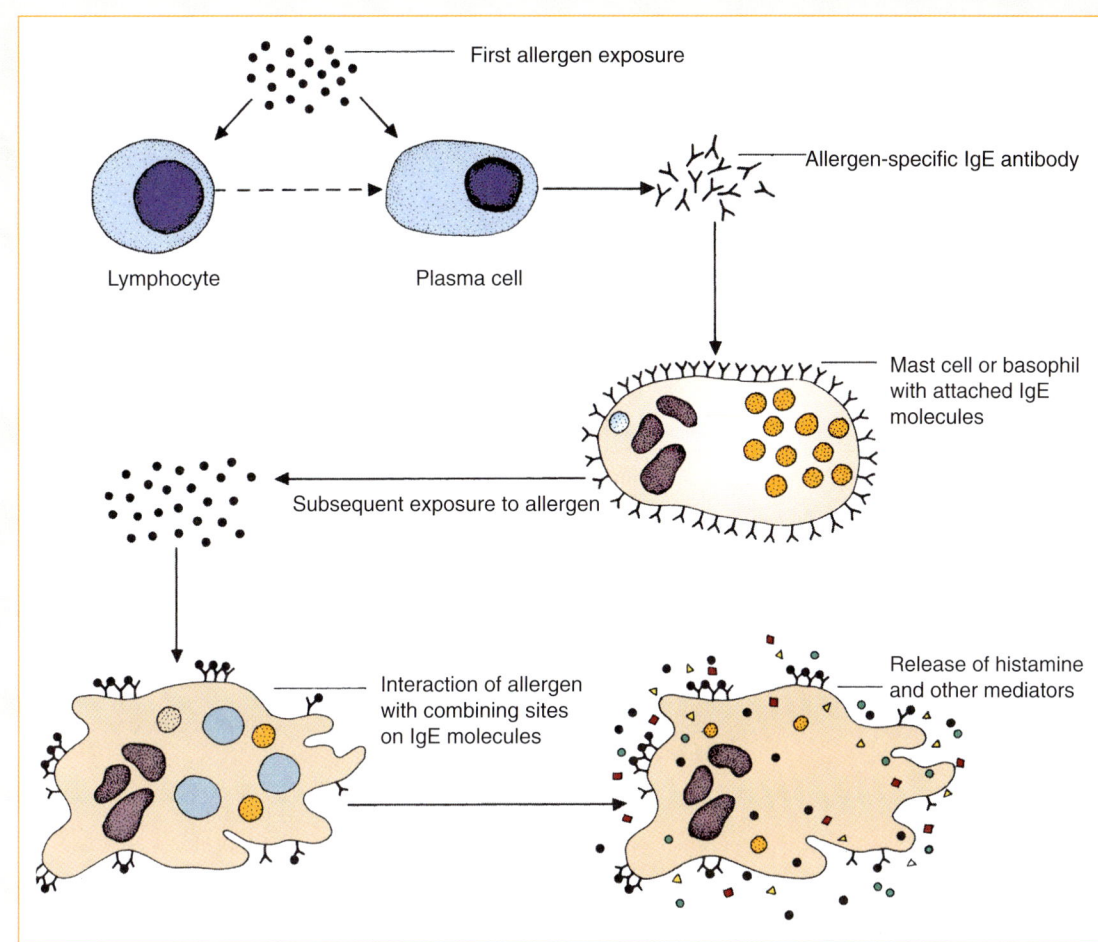

Figure 6-15 Pathogenesis of allergy. First, exposure to an allergen induces formation of specific IgE antibodies in susceptible individuals, which then bind to mast cells and basophils by the nonantigen receptor end of the molecule. Subsequent exposure to the same allergen leads to antigen-antibody interaction, liberating histamine and other mediators from mast cells and basophils. These mediators induce allergic manifestations.

Labels in figure:
First allergen exposure
Lymphocyte
Plasma cell
Allergen-specific IgE antibody
Mast cell or basophil with attached IgE molecules
Subsequent exposure to allergen
Interaction of allergen with combining sites on IgE molecules
Release of histamine and other mediators

is transmitted from generation to generation. The susceptibility may be inherited through either the mother's or the father's side of the family.

Early symptoms of breast cancer are usually detected by the woman during breast self-examination and include a small, painless lump, thick or dimpled skin, or a change in the nipple **Figure 6-16** ▸. Later symptoms include nipple discharge, pain, and swollen lymph glands in the axilla. Treatment depends on the location, size, and metastasis of the tumour.

Colorectal cancer is the third most common type of cancer in both males and females, accounting for a combined 21,500 newly diagnosed cases and 8,900 deaths in Canada each year. Relatives of people who have had colorectal cancer are more likely to develop the disease themselves, and parents can pass on to their children changes in certain genes that can lead to colorectal cancer. Symptoms may be minimal, consisting only of small amounts of blood in the stool. Treatment involves surgery and sometimes chemotherapy. Periodic rectal examinations and colonoscopy are recommended for adults older than 40 years to detect the disease at an early stage.

Lung cancer is the leading cause of death due to cancer in Canada. The major risk factor is cigarette smoking. Research has identified eight alterations in the genetic material of lung cancers that suggest a genetic tendency to develop the disease. Other predisposing factors include exposure to asbestos, coal products, and other industrial and chemical products. Symptoms include cough, difficulty breathing, blood-tinged sputum, and repeated infections. Treatment depends on the type, site, and extent of the cancer and may include surgery, chemotherapy, and/or radiotherapy.

Breast cancer is the most common type of cancer occurring among women and accounts for as many as 22,400 newly diagnosed cases and 5,300 deaths each year in Canada. Women whose first-degree relatives (ie, parent, sister, or daughter) have breast cancer are 2.1 times more likely to develop the disease. Risk varies with the age at which the affected relative was diagnosed; the younger the age at occurrence, the greater the risk posed to relatives. Approximately 5% to 10% of patients with breast cancer demonstrate a pattern of autosomal dominant inheritance, in which cancer predisposition

Endocrine Disorders

Diabetes mellitus is one of the most significant endocrine diseases. This chronic disorder of metabolism is associated with either partial insulin secretion or total lack of insulin secretion by the pancreas, which in turn affects the patient's ability to utilize glucose. Symptoms include excessive thirst and urination, weight abnormalities, and presence of excessive sugar in the urine and the blood.

Ketoacidosis-prone (type 1) diabetes is also known as insulin-dependent diabetes mellitus because patients need exogenous insulin to survive. Nonketoacidosis-prone (type 2) diabetes is called non–insulin-dependent diabetes, even though many type 2 diabetics require exogenous insulin injections. Both forms have a hereditary predisposition. There is no cure

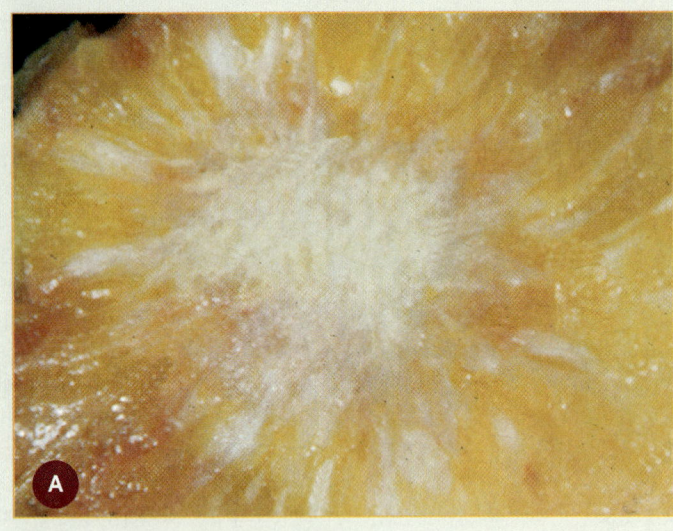

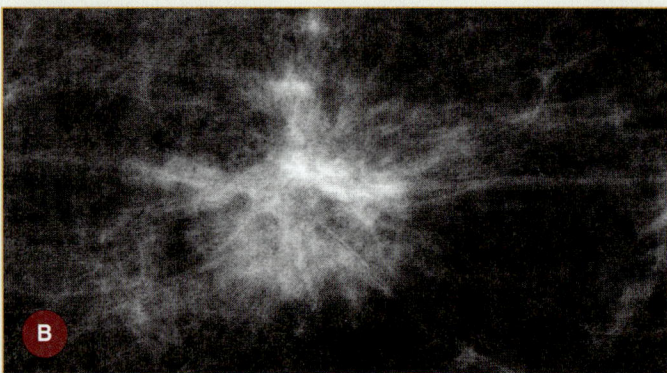

Figure 6-16 Breast carcinoma. **A.** Cross-section of breast biopsy specimen. The tumour appears as a firm, poorly circumscribed mass that infiltrates the surrounding fatty breast tissue. **B.** Appearance of breast carcinoma in a mammogram. The tumour appears as a white area with infiltrating margins.

for type 1 diabetes (other than pancreas transplantation) at the present time; type 2 diabetes can occasionally be brought under control with weight loss.

Hematologic Disorders

Hemolytic anemia is characterized by increased destruction of red blood cells. This disorder has a number of causes, such as an Rh factor blood transfusion reaction, a disorder of the immune system, or exposure to chemicals (eg, benzene and bacterial toxins). **Figure 6-17 ▶** depicts how the body handles iron. Hemolytic anemia following aspirin overdose or penicillin treatment is rare; it is much more common, albeit still rare, with sulfa drugs used to treat urinary tract infection (eg, Septra or Bactrim [trimethoprim-sulfamethoxazole]). An inherited enzyme deficiency (glucose-6-phosphatase dehydrogenase deficiency) markedly increases a person's susceptibility to sulfa drug-induced hemolytic anemia.

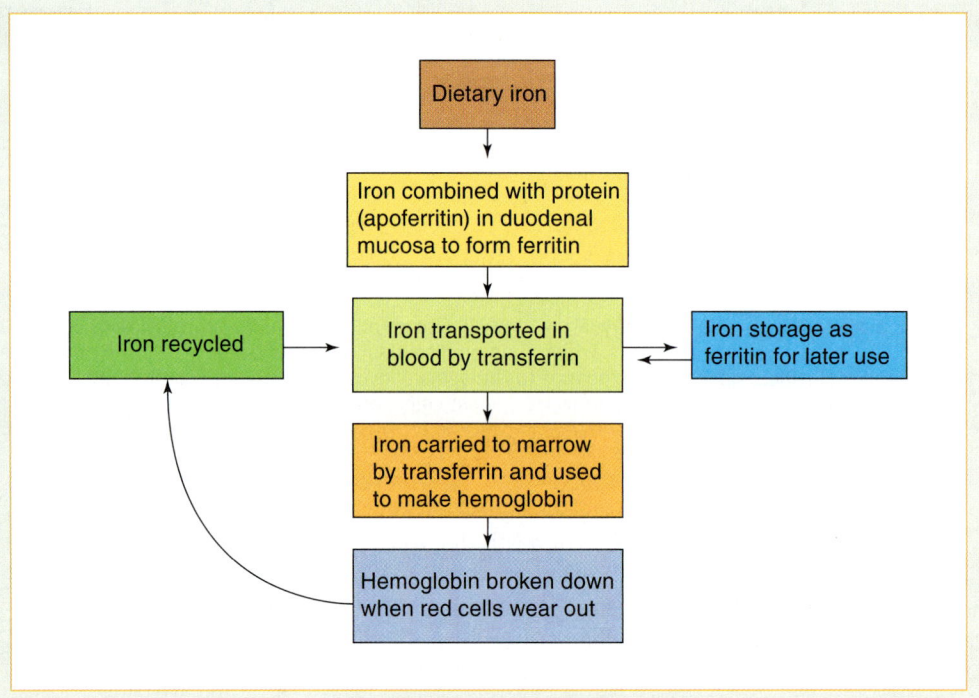

Figure 6-17 Iron uptake, transport, storage, and utilization for hemoglobin synthesis. Most of the iron used for hemoglobin synthesis is recycled from worn-out red cells. Chronic blood loss removes iron-containing cells from the circulation, and the iron contained in the red cells can no longer be recycled to make hemoglobin; this leads to iron deficiency anemia.

Hemophilia is an inherited disorder characterized by excessive bleeding. It is a sex-linked condition, occurring only in males, and is passed from asymptomatic mothers to sons. In this disorder, one of the blood-clotting proteins (usually factor VIII) necessary for normal blood coagulation is missing or is present in abnormally low amounts. Patients experience greater than usual blood loss in dental extractions and following simple injuries. They may also bleed into joints and, rarely, into the brain. Treatment consists of administration of missing blood-clotting factors.

Hemochromatosis is an inherited (autosomal recessive) disease in which the body absorbs more iron than it needs. The excess iron is stored in various organs, including the liver, kidney, and pancreas. Hemochromatosis can lead to diabetes, heart disease, liver disease, arthritis, impotence, and a bronzed skin colour. These symptoms can be avoided by regularly drawing blood (phlebotomy).

Cardiovascular Disorders

Several cardiovascular disorders are known to follow specific patterns of inheritance. Still others have strong familial tendencies (eg, coronary heart disease).

Long QT syndrome is a cardiac conduction system abnormality that results in a prolongation of the QT interval on the ECG. Because most long QT syndromes are inherited in an autosomal dominant manner, all first-degree relatives must also be screened. Sometimes these syndromes are associated with congenital hearing loss, hypertrophic cardiomyopathy, or mitral valve prolapse. Patients are at risk for palpitations and ventricular arrhythmias, especially torsade de pointes. Many patients are asymptomatic until they have an arrhythmia, causing either syncope or sudden death. Always consider syncope under the following conditions to be due to a life-threatening arrhythmia until proven otherwise:

- Exercise-induced syncope
- Syncope associated with chest pain
- A history of syncope in a close family member (ie, parent, sibling, or child)
- Syncope associated with startle (eg, loud noises such as phones or alarm clocks)

Cardiomyopathy is a general term for diseases of the myocardium (heart muscle) that ultimately progress to heart failure, acute myocardial infarction, or death. These diseases cause the heart muscle to become thin, flabby, dilated, or enlarged. One variant, hypertrophic cardiomyopathy, is autosomal-dominant hereditary. The main feature of hypertrophic cardiomyopathy is an excessive thickening of the heart muscle (hypertrophy means to thicken or grow excessively); see **Figure 6-18 ▲**. In addition, microscopic examination of the heart muscle shows that it is abnormal. Patients may have shortness of breath, chest pains, palpitations, or syncope; sudden cardiac death is also possible. Beta blockers are effective treatment in some patients. Others require surgery or an automatic implantable cardiac defibrillator designed to deliver a shock to the heart.

Mitral valve prolapse (MVP; also referred to as a floppy mitral valve) is relatively common, affecting 2.5% of males and 7.6% of females. There is a familial tendency toward MVP, albeit

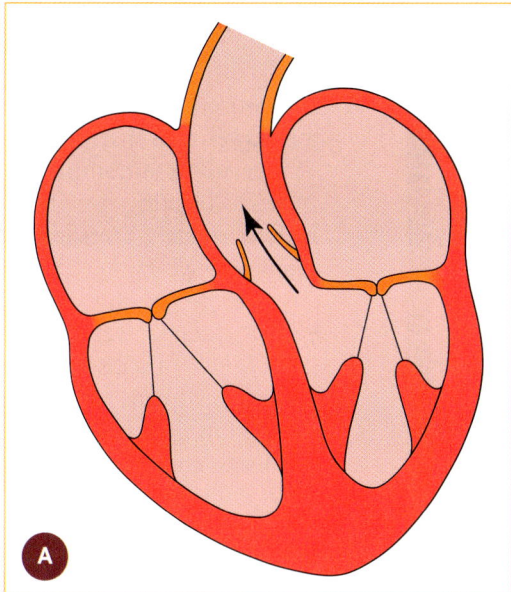
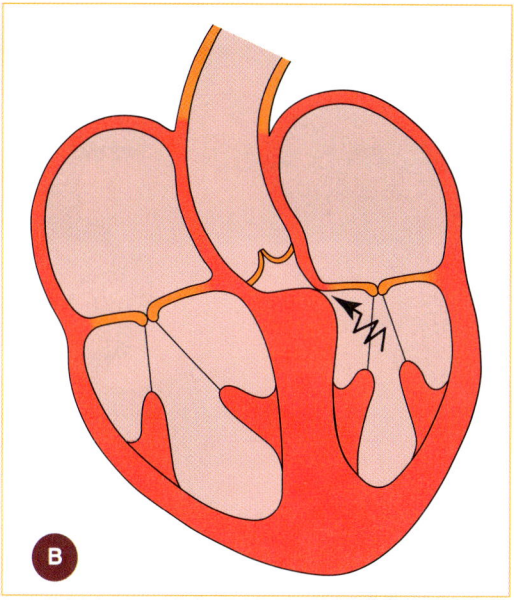

Figure 6-18 Comparison of normal cardiac function with malfunction characteristic of hypertrophic cardiomyopathy. **A.** Normal heart, illustrating unobstructed flow of blood from left ventricle into aorta during ventricular systole. **B.** Hypertrophic cardiomyopathy, illustrating obstruction to outflow of blood from left ventricle by hypertrophied septum, which impinges on the anterior leaflet of mitral valve.

usually in association with other cardiovascular conditions. The mitral valve leaflets balloon into the left atrium during systole. MVP is often a benign, symptomless condition but may be symptomatic (eg, chest pain, fatigue, dizziness, dyspnea, or palpitations). Generally, the only physical finding is a "clicking" sound heard during cardiac auscultation. Cardiac arrhythmias develop in a small number of patients.

Sometimes MVP leads to mitral regurgitation (also called mitral insufficiency), in which a large amount of blood leaks backward through the defective valve. Mitral regurgitation can lead to thickening or enlargement of the heart wall, caused by the extra pumping the heart must do to make up for the backflow of blood. It sometimes causes people to feel tired or short of breath. Mitral regurgitation usually can be treated with medication, but some people need surgery to repair or replace the defective valve.

Coronary heart disease, often called coronary artery disease, is caused by impaired circulation to the heart. Typically, patients have occluded coronary arteries from atherosclerotic plaque buildup. The effects can range from ischemia to infarction and necrosis (death) of the myocardium. Almost half of all cardiovascular deaths result from coronary heart disease. This condition has a familial tendency; significant risk factors for coronary artery disease development include having a father who had an acute myocardial infarction or died suddenly before 55 years of age and having a mother who died before 65 years of age. Other risk factors include hypercholesterolemia, cigarette smoking, hypertension (high blood pressure), age, and diabetes.

Hypercholesterolemia is an elevation of the blood cholesterol level. The blood cholesterol level is further divided into

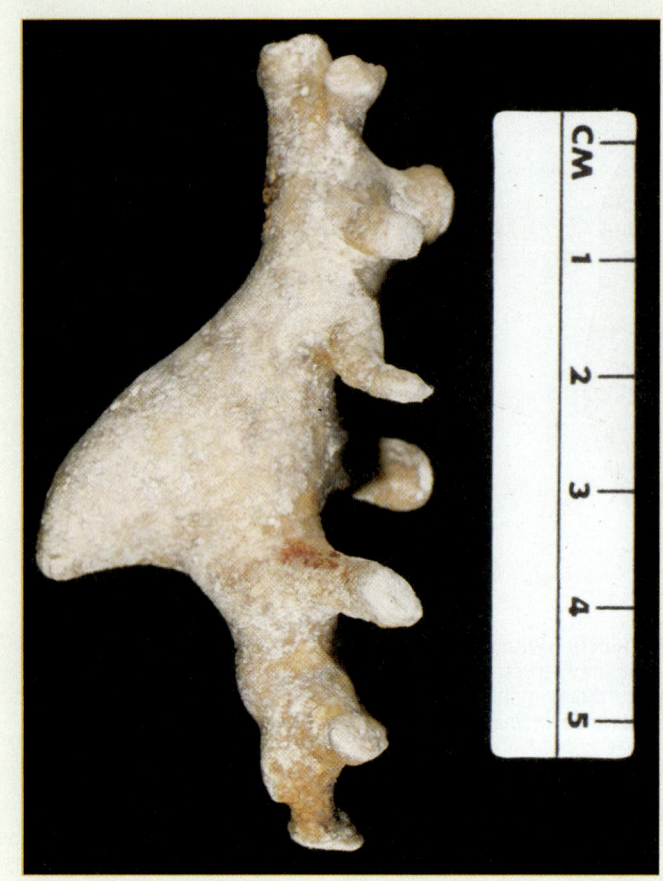

Figure 6-19 Large staghorn-shaped kidney stone.

high-density lipoproteins (HDL; "good cholesterol") and low-density lipoproteins (LDL; "bad cholesterol"). Despite having a normal total cholesterol level, persons with abnormally low levels of HDL and/or elevations of LDL are at an increased risk of coronary heart disease.

Renal Disorders

Gout is an abnormal accumulation of uric acid due to a defect in metabolism. As a result of this defect, uric acid accumulates in the blood and joints, causing pain and swelling of the joints, especially the big toe. Often, the patient has fever and chills. Gout is more common among men than women and usually has a genetic basis. If left untreated, it causes destructive tissue changes in the joints and kidneys. Treatment includes diet and drugs to reduce inflammation and to increase the excretion of uric acid or decrease its formation.

Kidney stones are small masses of uric acid or calcium salts that form in any part of the urinary system (eg, kidney, ureter, or bladder). Often—although not always—stones cause severe pain, nausea, and vomiting when the body attempts to pass them. Although most stones are small, occasionally they become large enough to adopt the internal contours of the kidney **Figure 6-19 ▲** . Researchers have found a gene that causes the intestines to absorb too much calcium, which can lead to the formation of kidney stones. Uric acid stones also often have a genetic basis. Some are small enough to pass in the urine, with or without pain; others must be removed surgically.

Gastrointestinal Disorders

Malabsorption disorders result from defects in the function of the bowel wall that prevent normal absorption of nutrients. The result is a complex of symptoms, including loss of appetite, bloating, weight loss, muscle pain, and stools with high fat content. Diarrhea, which may be bloody, may also be a prominent symptom.

Lactose intolerance is a defect or deficiency of the enzyme lactase, resulting in an inability to digest lactose (milk sugar). Lactase deficiency, which appears to be due to an abnormal gene, affects nearly three-fourths of the world's population. Symptoms include bloating, flatulence, abdominal discomfort, nausea, and diarrhea on ingestion of milk and milk products.

Ulcerative colitis is a serious chronic inflammatory disease of the large intestine and rectum. This disease, which shows a familial tendency, is characterized by recurrent episodes of abdominal pain, fever, chills, and profuse diarrhea, with stools containing pus, blood, and mucus. Treatment consists of anti-inflammatory agents, including corticosteroids. Severe cases may require surgery with removal of parts of the intestinal tract. Patients are at increased risk for developing cancer of the colon.

Crohn's disease is a chronic inflammatory condition affecting the colon and/or terminal part of the small intestine. It is believed to be associated with as-yet-undetermined gene abnormalities. Symptoms include frequent episodes of non-bloody diarrhea, abdominal pain, nausea, fever, weakness, and weight loss. Treatment is by anti-inflammatory agents, antibiotics, and proper nutrition.

Peptic ulcer disease is characterized by circumscribed erosions (ulcerations) in the mucous membrane lining of the gastrointestinal tract—specifically, in the esophagus, stomach, duodenum, or jejunum. Peptic ulcers may result from excess acid production or from a breakdown in the normal mechanisms protecting the mucous membranes. Although this disease appears to have a genetic component, a major contributor to its development is infection with the bacterium *Helicobacter pylori*—the observed familial patterns appear to be due to shared infections with *H pylori*. Symptoms include gnawing pain, which is often worse when the stomach is empty, after the person eats certain foods, or when the patient is under stress. Treatment includes avoidance of irritants (eg, tobacco, alcohol, irritating foods), antibiotics, and drugs to decrease acidity. In refractory cases, surgery may be necessary.

Gallstones (cholethiasis) are stone-like masses in the gallbladder or its ducts caused by precipitation of substances contained in bile (eg, cholesterol, bilirubin). Factors that contribute to their formation include abnormalities in the composition of bile, stasis of bile, and inflammation of the gallbladder with many gallstones. Gallstones may be asymptomatic, but cause symptoms when they obstruct the flow of bile. Small stones that are able to pass into the common duct produce indigestion and biliary colic. Biliary colic pain is sudden in onset and increases steadily to its maximum in approximately 1 hour. The pain is located in the upper right quadrant or the epigastric area and may be referred to the back. Larger stones may cause jaundice (yellow skin and sclerae). Although genetic factors are responsible for at least 30% of symptomatic gallstone disease, heredity probably plays an even larger role in gallstone pathogenesis, because data based on symptomatic gallbladder disease underestimate the true prevalence in the population.

Obesity is an unhealthy accumulation of body fat that has many deleterious side effects, both medical and social. Health risks associated with obesity include hypertension, hyperlipidemia, cardiovascular disease, glucose intolerance, insulin resistance, diabetes, gallbladder disease, infertility, and cancer of the endometrium, breast, prostate, and colon. Although some people likely have a genetic predisposition to obesity, the roles of specific genes in its development have yet to be determined.

Neuromuscular Disorders

Although environmental contributions are highly likely, certain neuromuscular disorders have a familial and genetic basis. Huntington's disease (also called Huntington's chorea), for example, is a hereditary condition (autosomal dominant) characterized by progressive chorea (involuntary rapid, jerky motions) and mental deterioration, leading to dementia. Symptoms usually first appear in the third or fourth decade of life and progress to death, often within 15 years.

Muscular dystrophy is a generic term for a group of hereditary diseases of the muscular system characterized by weakness and wasting of groups of skeletal muscles, leading to increasing disability. The various forms differ in age of onset, rate of progression, and mode of genetic transmission. Duchenne's muscular dystrophy is a sex-linked recessive disease (affecting only males); symptoms first appear around the age of 4 years. Progressive wasting of leg and pelvic muscles produces a waddling gait and abnormal curvature of the spine, progressing to inability to walk and confinement to a wheelchair, usually by age 12 years. There is no specific treatment, and death, usually from heart disorders, often results by age 20 years.

Multiple sclerosis is a progressive disease in which nerve fibres of the brain and spinal cord lose their myelin cover. Although it is not directly inherited, there is a familial predisposition in some cases, suggesting a genetic influence on susceptibility. The disease usually begins in early adulthood and progresses slowly, with periods of remission and exacerbation. Early symptoms include abnormal sensations in the face or extremities, weakness, and visual disturbances (such as double vision), which progress to ataxia (lack of coordination), abnormal reflexes, tremors, difficulty in urination, and difficulty in walking. Depression is also common. There is no specific treatment or cure, but corticosteroids and other drugs are used to treat symptoms.

Alzheimer's disease affects 300,000 Canadians over the age of 65. Although its cause is unknown, the disease results in cortical atrophy and loss of neurons in the frontal and temporal lobes of the brain; in addition, ventricular enlargement occurs due to the loss of brain tissue. Histologic changes in the brain of an Alzheimer's patient include neurofibrillary tangles and senile plaques ◖ **Figure 6-20** ▶ . Studies of the genetics of inherited early-onset Alzheimer's have been linked to mutations on three genes.

Clinical manifestations of Alzheimer's disease occur in three distinct stages. Stage 1 is characterized by memory loss, lack of spontaneity, subtle personality changes, and disorientation to time and date. Stage 2 features impaired cognition and

You are the Paramedic Part 3

You perform a physical examination on the patient while your partner prepares an IV setup. Your physical examination is significant for the following findings: positive jugular vein distention; use of accessory muscles in the neck and shoulders to assist respirations; pitting edema of both lower extremities; and an area surrounding the shunt site on the right arm approximately 10 cm in diameter that is red, swollen, and hot to the touch. As you are completing your assessment, the patient begins to complain of feeling lightheaded. You lower the head of the dialysis chair to a 60° angle, initiate an IV using a 18-gauge catheter in the left antecubital, and begin a fluid bolus of 200 ml.

Reassessment	Recording Time: 10 Minutes
Skin	Pale, warm, and moist
Pulse	140 beats/min, regular; weak radial
ECG	Narrow complex tachycardia with tall T waves
Blood pressure	78/44 mm Hg
Respirations	28 breaths/min laboured
Spo$_2$	93% on nonrebreathing mask at 15 l/min of supplemental oxygen
Pupils	Equal and reactive to light

5. Is the patient going into shock? If so, what type?

6. Why is a fluid bolus appropriate in this setting?

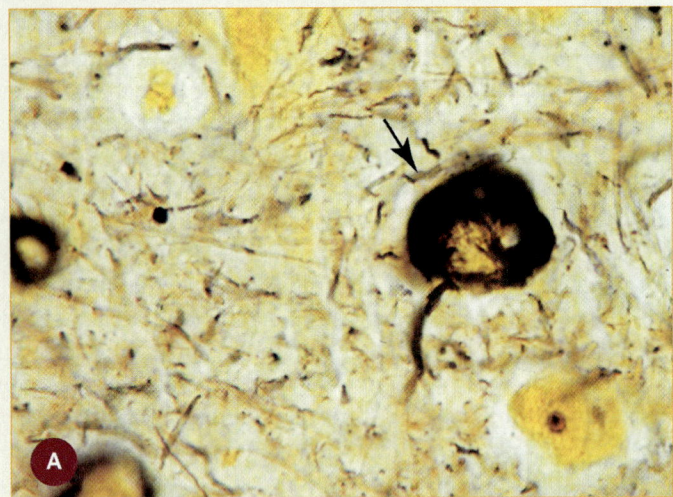 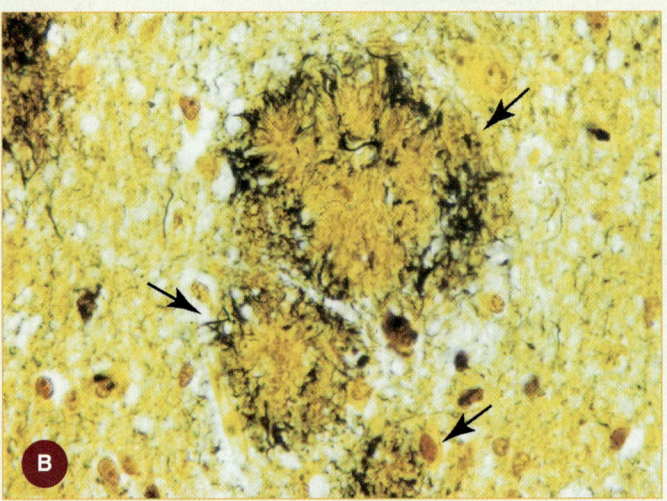

Figure 6-20 Alzheimer's disease. **A.** Thickened neurofilaments encircle and obscure the nuclei of nerve cells (arrow), forming a neurofibrillary tangle (original magnification, × 400). **B.** Three senile plaques (arrows) composed of broken masses of thickened neurofilaments (original magnification, × 100).

Special Considerations

Never assume that new or worsening confusion in a geriatric patient is due purely to Alzheimer's disease, without first considering potentially correctable causes such as new medications, infections, or myocardial infarction. An "apparent" emotional, psychological, or behavioural problem may have an organic cause, especially in the geriatric population.

abstract thinking, restlessness and agitation, wandering, inability to carry out activities of daily living, impaired judgment, and inappropriate social behaviour. Stage 3 involves indifference to food, inability to communicate, urinary and fecal incontinence, and seizures.

Psychiatric Disorders

Some common psychiatric disorders appear to have a familial, and perhaps even genetic, component. For example, schizophrenia comprises a group of mental disorders characterized by gross distortions of reality (psychoses), withdrawal from social contacts, and disturbances of thought, language, perception, and emotional response. Its symptoms are highly varied but may include apathy, catatonia or excessive activity, bizarre actions, hallucinations, delusions, and rambling speech. Although the cause of schizophrenia has not been identified, a combination of hereditary or genetic predisposing factors is likely in most cases.

Manic-depressive disorder (also known as bipolar disorder or manic-depressive psychosis) is a mental disorder characterized by episodes of mania and depression. One or the other phase may be dominant at a given time, and the phases may alternate or aspects of both phases may be present at the same time. The higher rates of bipolar disorder among relatives, identical twins, and biological parents versus adoptive parents have been cited as evidence of the role of genetics in this disorder; the risk within the general population as a whole is approximately 1%. Treatment consists of psychotherapy plus antidepressants and tranquilizers.

Hypoperfusion

Perfusion is defined as delivery of oxygen and nutrients and removal of wastes from the cells, organs, and tissues by the circulatory system. Evaluation of a patient's level of organ perfusion is important in emergency care, especially in diagnosing shock. Hypoperfusion occurs when the level of tissue perfusion decreases below normal.

When the body senses tissue hypoperfusion, it sets compensatory mechanisms into motion. In some cases, this action is sufficient to stabilize the patient. In other cases, the hypoperfusion overwhelms the normal compensatory mechanisms and the patient's condition progressively deteriorates **Table 6-4 ▸**.

In response to hypoperfusion, the body releases catecholamines (ie, epinephrine and norepinephrine), which

Documentation and Communication

The terms *shock* and *hypoperfusion* are usually synonymous, at least when they are applied to multiple body systems. Localized hypoperfusion, such as from arterial occlusion, is *not* shock.

Table 6-4	Signs and Symptoms in the Phases of Hypoperfusion
Compensated	**Decompensated**
■ Agitation, anxiety, restlessness	■ Altered mental status (verbal to unresponsive)
■ Sense of impending doom	■ Hypotension
■ Weak, rapid (thready) pulse	■ Laboured or irregular breathing
■ Clammy (cool, moist) skin	■ Thready or absent peripheral pulses
■ Pallor with cyanotic lips	
■ Shortness of breath	■ Ashen, mottled, or cyanotic skin
■ Nausea, vomiting	■ Dilated pupils
■ Delayed capillary refill in infants and children	■ Diminished urine output (oliguria)
■ Thirst	■ Impending cardiac arrest
■ Normal blood pressure	

produce vasoconstriction (increased systemic vascular resistance). In addition, the RAAS is activated and antidiuretic hormone is released from the pituitary gland. Together these actions trigger salt and water retention as well as peripheral vasoconstriction, thereby increasing blood pressure and cardiac output. Depending on the severity of the insult, variable amounts of fluid will shift from the interstitial tissues into the vascular compartment. The spleen also releases some red blood cells that are normally sequestered there, to augment the oxygen-carrying capacity of the blood. The overall response of the initial compensatory mechanisms is to increase the preload (venous return), stroke volume, and heart rate. The result is usually an increase in cardiac output and myocardial oxygen demand.

As hypoperfusion persists, the myocardial oxygen demand continues to increase. Eventually, the above-normal compensatory mechanisms can no longer keep up with the demand. Myocardial function worsens, with decreased cardiac output and ejection fraction. Tissue perfusion decreases, leading to impaired cell metabolism. Often, the blood pressure decreases, especially in progressive hypoperfusion. Fluid may leak from the blood vessels, causing systemic and pulmonary edema. At this point, other signs of hypoperfusion may be present, such as dusky skin, oliguria, and impaired mentation.

Types of Shock

Shock is an abnormal state associated with inadequate oxygen and nutrient delivery to the metabolic apparatus of the cell, resulting in impairment of cell metabolism and inadequate perfusion of vital organs (see Chapter 18). Once a certain level of tissue hypoperfusion is reached, cell damage proceeds in a similar manner regardless of the type of initial insult. Impairment of cellular metabolism prevents the body from properly using oxygen and glucose at the cellular level. Cells revert to anaerobic metabolism, which causes increased lactic acid production and metabolic acidosis, decreased oxygen affinity for hemoglobin,

decreased ATP production, changes in cellular electrolytes, cellular edema, and release of lysosomal enzymes. Glucose impairment leads to elevated blood glucose levels due to release of catecholamines and cortisol. In addition, fat breakdown (lipolysis) with ketone formation may occur.

Shock can occur due to inadequacy of the central circulation (eg, the heart and the great vessels) or of the peripheral circulation (the remaining vessels, including the microscopic circulation [eg, arterioles, venules, and capillaries, as illustrated in ⟨Figure 6-21 ▸⟩]). From a mechanistic approach, two types of shock are distinguished: central and peripheral. Central shock consists of cardiogenic shock and obstructive shock. Peripheral shock includes hypovolemic shock and distributive shock.

Cardiogenic shock occurs when the heart cannot circulate enough blood to maintain adequate peripheral oxygen delivery. In the case of ischemic heart disease, this requires loss of 40% or more of functioning myocardium. The most common cause of cardiogenic shock is myocardial infarction, either as a single event or by cumulative damage. Other forms of cardiac dysfunction may also result in cardiogenic shock (ie, large ventricular septal defect or hemodynamic significant arrhythmias) (see Chapter 27).

Obstructive shock occurs when blood flow becomes blocked in the heart or great vessels. In pericardial tamponade ⟨Figure 6-22 ▸⟩, diastolic filling of the right ventricle is impaired due to significant amounts of fluid in the pericardial sac surrounding the heart, leading to a decrease in the cardiac output. Aortic dissection leads to a false lumen (aortic opening), with loss of normal blood flow ⟨Figure 6-23 ▸⟩. A left atrial tumour may obstruct flow between the atrium and ventricle and decrease cardiac output. Obstruction of either the superior or inferior vena cava (vena cava syndrome) decreases cardiac output by decreasing venous return. A large pulmonary embolus (blood clot in the lung) or a tension pneumothorax (lung collapse) may prevent adequate blood flow to the lungs, resulting in inadequate venous return to the left side of the heart.

In hypovolemic shock, the circulating blood volume is unable to deliver adequate oxygen and nutrients to the body. Two types of hypovolemic shock—exogenous and endogenous—are possible, depending on where the fluid loss occurs. The most common type of exogenous hypovolemic shock is external bleeding (eg, from an open wound); it may also result from loss of plasma volume caused by diarrhea or vomiting. Endogenous hypovolemic shock occurs when the fluid loss is contained within the body.

Distributive shock occurs when there is widespread dilation of the resistance vessels (small arterioles), the capacitance vessels (small venules), or both. The circulating blood

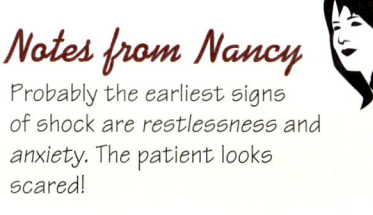

Notes from Nancy
Probably the earliest signs of shock are restlessness and anxiety. The patient looks scared!

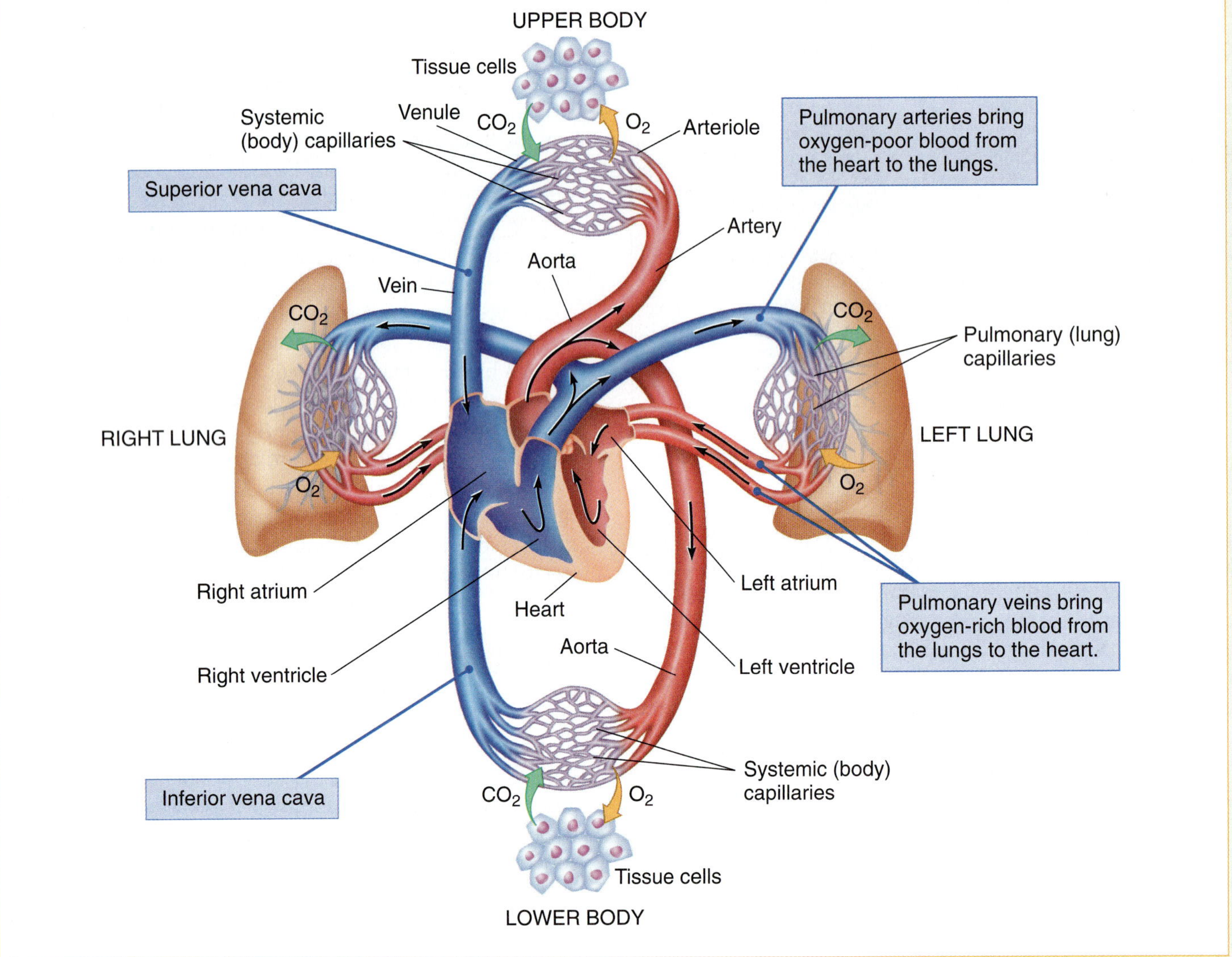

UPPER BODY

Tissue cells

Systemic (body) capillaries

Venule

CO_2

O_2

Arteriole

Pulmonary arteries bring oxygen-poor blood from the heart to the lungs.

Superior vena cava

Artery

Aorta

Vein

CO_2

CO_2

Pulmonary (lung) capillaries

RIGHT LUNG

LEFT LUNG

O_2

O_2

Right atrium

Left atrium

Heart

Right ventricle

Aorta

Pulmonary veins bring oxygen-rich blood from the lungs to the heart.

Left ventricle

Inferior vena cava

CO_2

O_2

Systemic (body) capillaries

Tissue cells

LOWER BODY

Figure 6-21 The circulatory system includes the heart, arteries, veins, and interconnecting capillaries. The capillaries—the smallest vessels—connect with venules and arterioles. At the centre of the system, and providing its driving force, is the heart.

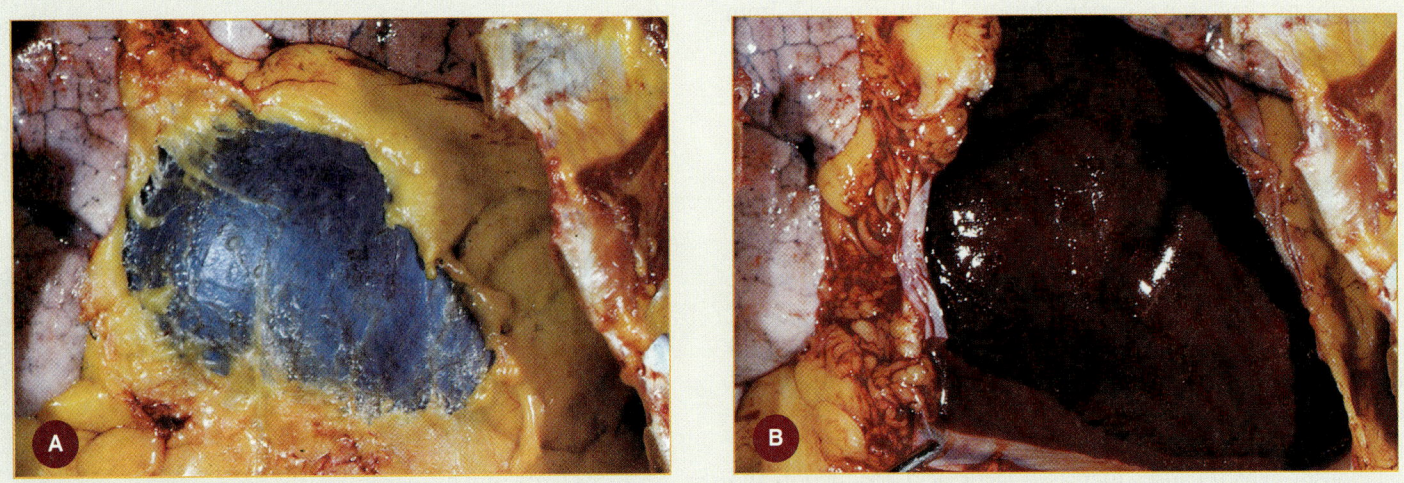

Figure 6-22 Cardiac tamponade secondary to myocardial rupture. **A.** Distended pericardial sac. **B.** Pericardial sac opened, showing clotted blood surrounding the heart, which compressed the heart and prevented filling of the right ventricle in diastole.

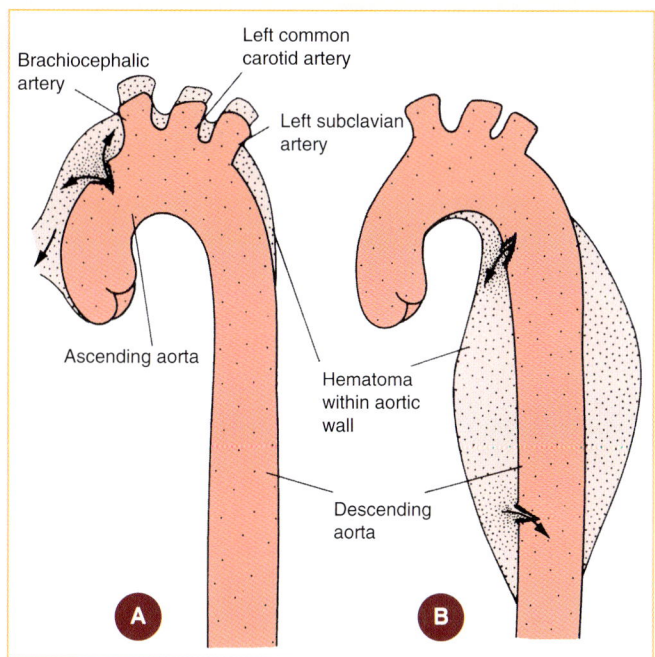

Figure 6-23 Sites of thoracic aortic dissection. **A.** A tear in the ascending aorta causes both proximal and distal dissection. **B.** A tear in the descending aorta may cause extensive distal dissection.

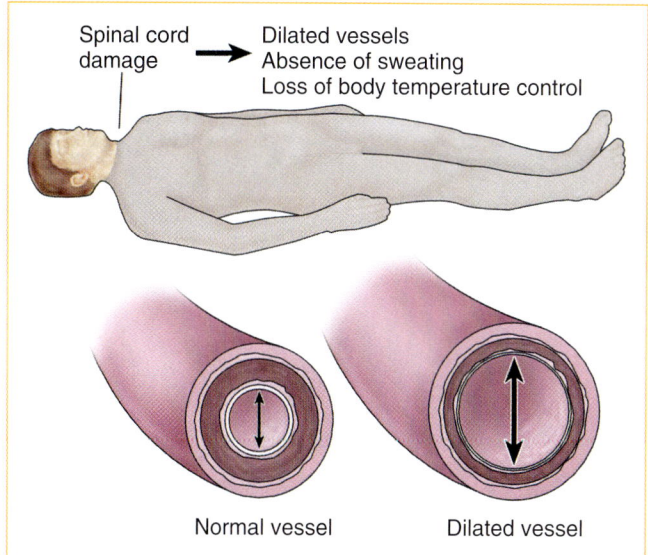

Figure 6-24 Damage to the spinal cord can cause significant injury to the part of the nervous system that controls the size and muscle tone of blood vessels. If the muscles in the blood vessels are cut off from their impulses to contract, then the vessels dilate widely, increasing the size and capacity of the vascular system. The blood in the body can no longer fill the enlarged vessels, resulting in inadequate perfusion and neurogenic shock.

volume then "pools" in the expanded vascular beds, and tissue perfusion decreases. The three most common types of distributive shock are anaphylactic shock, septic shock, and neurogenic shock **Figure 6-24 ▸**.

In anaphylactic shock, histamine and other vasodilator proteins are released upon exposure to an allergen. Anaphylaxis is also accompanied by wheezing and urticaria (hives). The result is widespread vasodilation that causes distributive shock and blood vessels that continue to leak. Fluid leaks out of the blood vessels into the interstitial spaces, resulting in intravascular hypovolemia.

Septic shock occurs as a result of widespread infection, usually bacterial. Complex interactions occur between the bacterial invader and the body's defence systems. Initially, the body's own defence mechanisms may keep the infection at bay. If the normal immune mechanisms become overwhelmed, the body produces a multitude of substances that cause vasodilation and decreased

At the Scene

In anaphylaxis, interstitial fluid may cause significant swelling. In some cases, this swelling may occlude the upper airway, resulting in a life-threatening condition. Recurrent large areas of subcutaneous edema of sudden onset, usually disappearing within 24 hours, are called angioedema. This condition is seen mainly in young women, frequently as a result of allergy to food or drugs.

cardiac output. If left untreated, the result is multiple organ dysfunction syndrome and often death.

Neurogenic shock usually results from spinal cord injury. The effect is loss of normal sympathetic nervous system tone and vasodilation. Often patients have fluid-refractory hypotension due to the degree of vasodilation.

Management of Shock

All types of shock are characterized by reduced cardiac output, circulatory insufficiency, and rapid heartbeat. Although low blood pressure is classically associated with shock, it is a late sign, especially in children. In compensated shock, the systolic blood pressure is within the normal range; in decompensated shock, the systolic blood pressure is less than the fifth percentile for the age.

Clinically, determining the presence or absence of shock requires the evaluation of the presence and volume of the peripheral pulses, and assessment of end-organ perfusion and function. Strength of the peripheral pulses is related to both stroke volume of the heart and pulse pressures. Peripheral pulses should be readily palpable if the person is not in shock, although cold environments or obesity may compromise the presence or strength of these pulses. Skin perfusion in the normal individual results in warm, dry, and pink extremities, fingers, and toes, whereas shock may result in slow, delayed, or prolonged capillary refill time. To test the capillary refill time, briefly squeeze the toe or finger, then look for return of pink colour. A normal capillary refill time is less than 2 seconds

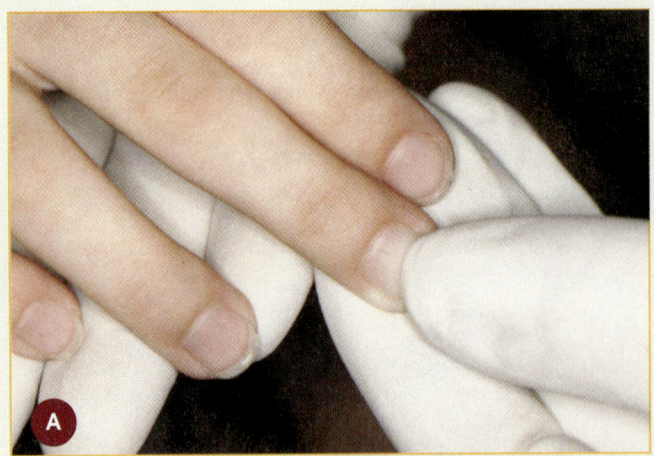

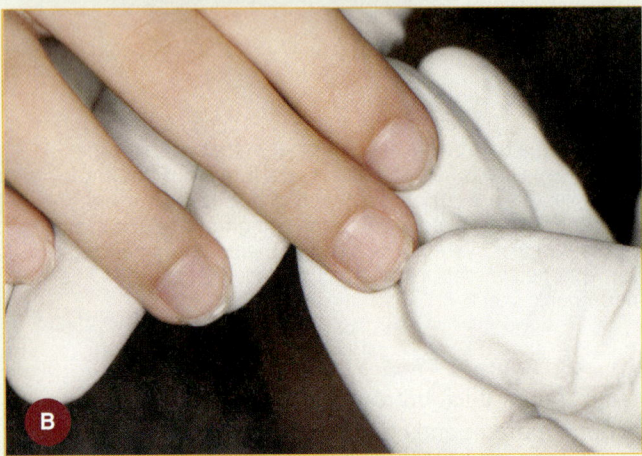

Figure 6-25 Testing capillary refill time. **A.** To test capillary refill, gently compress the fingertip until it blanches. **B.** Release the fingertip and count until it returns to its normal pink colour.

At the Scene

A possible exception to the rule of IV fluid therapy is hypovolemic shock caused by ongoing bleeding. Some studies suggest that fluid therapy to maintain the systolic blood pressure at approximately 80 mm Hg may be safer for the patient than attempting restoration of normotension, which may aggravate ongoing bleeding. As always, follow your local protocols.

after blanching of the toe or finger, whereas a person in shock may have a capillary refill time of more than 2 seconds **Figure 6-25 ▲**. Mottling, pallor, peripheral or central cyanosis, and delayed capillary refill may signal the presence of shock, whereas altered mental status is an indication of inadequate brain tissue perfusion.

Treatment primarily addresses the underlying condition (see Chapter 18).

Multiple Organ Dysfunction Syndrome

Multiple organ dysfunction syndrome (MODS) is a progressive condition usually characterized by concurrent failure of several organs, such as the lungs, liver, and kidneys, along with some clotting mechanisms, which occurs after severe illness or injury. First described in 1975, MODS is associated with a mortality rate of 60% to 90%, and is the major cause of death following sepsis, trauma, and burn injuries.

Primary MODS is a direct result of an insult, such as a pulmonary contusion from striking the chest on the steering wheel during a collision. Secondary MODS is organ dysfunction that occurs as an integral component to the patient's response (eg, renal failure following trauma).

MODS occurs when injury or infection (eg, septic shock) triggers a massive systemic immune, inflammatory, and coagulation response with release of inflammatory mediators. Overactivation of the complement system further increases inflammation and damage to the cells. Overactivation of the coagulation system due to endothelial damage causes uncontrolled coagulation in the microscopic venules and arterioles, which in turn results in microvascular thrombus formation and tissue ischemia. MODS also activates the kallikrein/kinin system, resulting in the release of bradykinin, a potent vasodilator. Vasodilation leads to tissue hypoperfusion and may also contribute to hypotension.

The net outcome of the activation of these systems is maldistribution of systemic and organ blood flow. Often tissues attempt to compensate for this problem by accelerating their metabolism. The result is an oxygen supply and demand imbalance with tissue hypoxia, including tissue hypoperfusion, exhaustion of the cells' fuel supply (ATP), metabolic failure, lysosome breakdown, anaerobic metabolism, and acidosis and impaired cellular function.

MODS typically develops hours to days following resuscitation. Its signs and symptoms include hypotension, insufficient tissue perfusion, uncontrollable bleeding (coagulopathy), and multisystem organ failure. Patients may develop a low-grade fever from the inflammatory response, tachycardia, and dyspnea. They may also be difficult to oxygenate due to the presence of acute lung injury and adult respiratory distress syndrome. During a 14- to 21-day period, renal and liver failure can develop in these patients, along with collapse of the gastrointestinal and immune systems. Cardiovascular collapse and death typically occur within days to weeks of the initial insult.

■ The Body's Self-defence Mechanisms

The immune system includes all structures and processes associated with the body's defence against foreign substances and disease-causing agents. The body has three lines of defence: anatomical barriers, the inflammatory response, and the immune response.

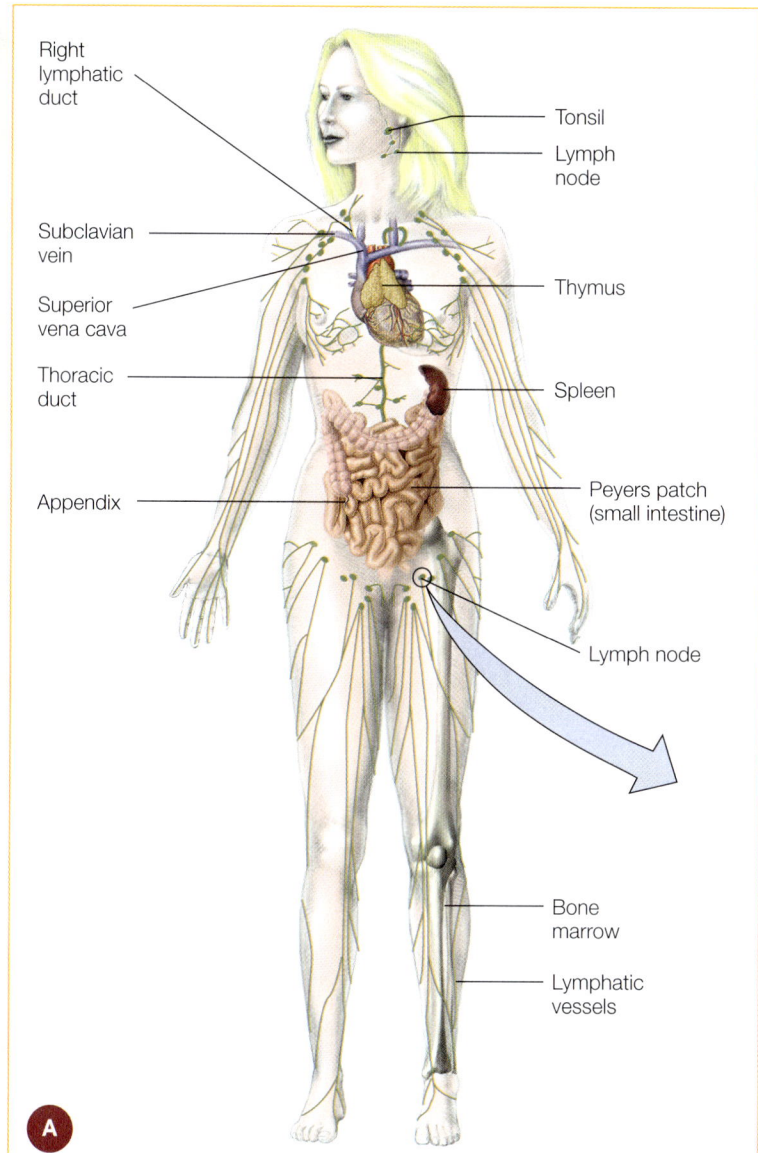

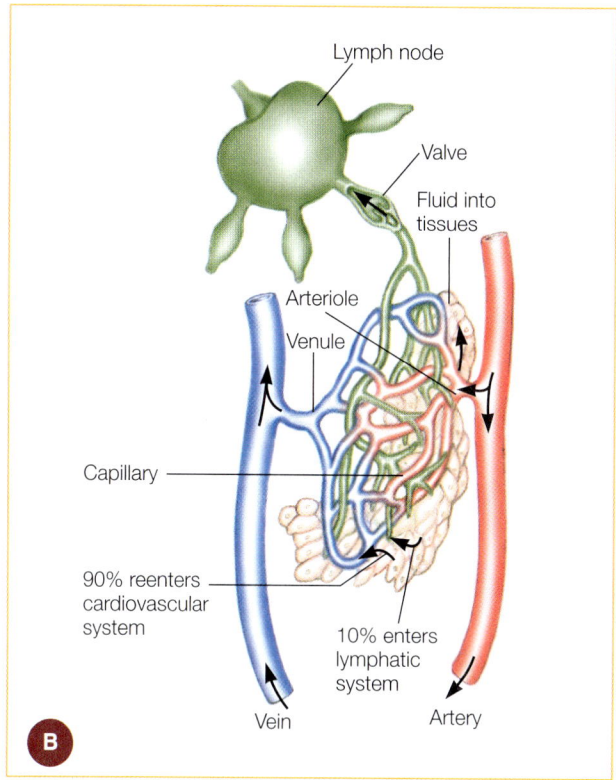

Figure 6-26 The lymphatic system. **A.** The lymphatic system consists of vessels that transport lymph and excess tissue fluid back to the circulatory system. **B.** Lymph is picked up by lymphatic capillaries that drain into larger vessels. Like the veins, the lymphatic vessels contain valves that prohibit backflow. Lymph nodes are interspersed along the vessels and filter the lymph.

Several anatomical barriers decrease the chances of bodily invasion by foreign substances. The skin serves as a major deterrent. Hairs in the upper respiratory tract (the nose) and the lining of the lower respiratory tract (cilia-covered epithelial cells) help repel foreign matter, especially small particles and some bacteria. Acid in the stomach prevents many infectious agents from entering the body via the gastrointestinal tract.

The inflammatory response is a response of the tissues of the body to irritation or injury characterized by pain, swelling, redness, and heat. White blood cells of various types are a major component of this response.

The immune response is the body's defence reaction to any substance that is recognized as foreign. Often, this response is directed toward invading microbes, such as bacteria or viruses. It is also triggered by foreign bodies (eg, a splinter) and even abnormal growths in the cells (eg, a tumour). The immune response involves only one type of white blood cells, namely lymphocytes.

The inflammatory reaction and the immune response are independent processes, although they often occur simultaneously. Inflammation can be present without activation of the immune response, and vice versa.

Not all invaders can be destroyed by the body's immune system. In some cases, the best compromise the body can reach is to control the damage and keep the invader from spreading. Often, the immune system succeeds in preventing severe disease following infection. When the normal systems become overwhelmed or fail, serious disease occurs.

Anatomy of the Immune System

The lymphatic system is a network of capillaries, vessels, ducts, nodes, and organs that helps maintain the fluid environment of the body by producing lymph and conveying it through the body **Figure 6-26 ▲**. The immune system has two anatomical components: the lymphoid tissues and the cells that are responsible for the immune response.

Lymphoid tissues are distributed throughout the body. The two primary lymphoid tissues are bone marrow and the thymus gland. Bone marrow is specialized soft tissue found within bone. Red bone marrow, which is widespread in the bones of children and is found in some adult bones (eg, sternum and ribs), is essential for formation of mature blood cells; it produces B lymphocytes. T lymphocytes originate from precursor cells in the bone marrow, leave the bone marrow, and mature in the thymus gland. This bilobed gland—located below the thyroid gland and behind the sternum—is prominent at birth, increases in size until the body reaches puberty, and then shrinks and decreases in functional activity during adulthood.

In secondary lymphoid tissues (ie, encapsulated and unencapsulated diffuse lymphoid tissues), mature immune cells interact with invaders and initiate a response. Encapsulated lymphoid tissues consist of the lymph nodes and the spleen. Lymph nodes (lymph glands) are small structures that filter lymph and store lymphocytes; they are concentrated in areas of the body such as the axillae, groin, and neck. The spleen is located on the left side of the body, posterior and lateral to the stomach (left upper quadrant); it monitors the blood, destroys worn-out red blood cells, and traps foreign invaders. The diffuse lymphoid tissues are scattered throughout the body.

Lymph is a thin, watery fluid that bathes the tissues of the body; it circulates through lymph vessels and is filtered in lymph nodes. Lymphatic capillaries unite to form the lymph vessels, which eventually coalesce and empty their contents into the central venous circulation (Figure 6-27 ▸). Most lymph empties into the superior vena cava via the thoracic duct, located on the left side of the thorax. The remaining lymph enters the right subclavian vein via three or four lymphatic ducts.

Clusters of lymphoid tissue are associated with the skin and the respiratory, urinary, gastrointestinal, and reproductive tracts. These tissues, which are collectively termed mucosal-associated lymphoid tissue (MALT), contain immune cells that are in a position to intercept pathogens before they reach the general circulation. The tonsils are perhaps the best-known type of MALT. Unencapsulated lymphoid tissue is particularly prominent in the gastrointestinal tract. Called the gut-associated lymphoid tissue (GALT), this tissue lies just under the inner lining of the esophagus and intestines.

The primary cells of the immune system are the white blood cells, or leukocytes. There are five general types (Table 6-5 ▸):

- Basophils contain histamine granules and other substances that are released during inflammatory and allergic responses. They account for less than 1% of the leukocytes but are essential to the nonspecific immune response to inflammation because they release histamine and other chemicals that dilate blood vessels.
- Eosinophils release substances that damage or kill parasitic invaders. They also play a major role in mediating the

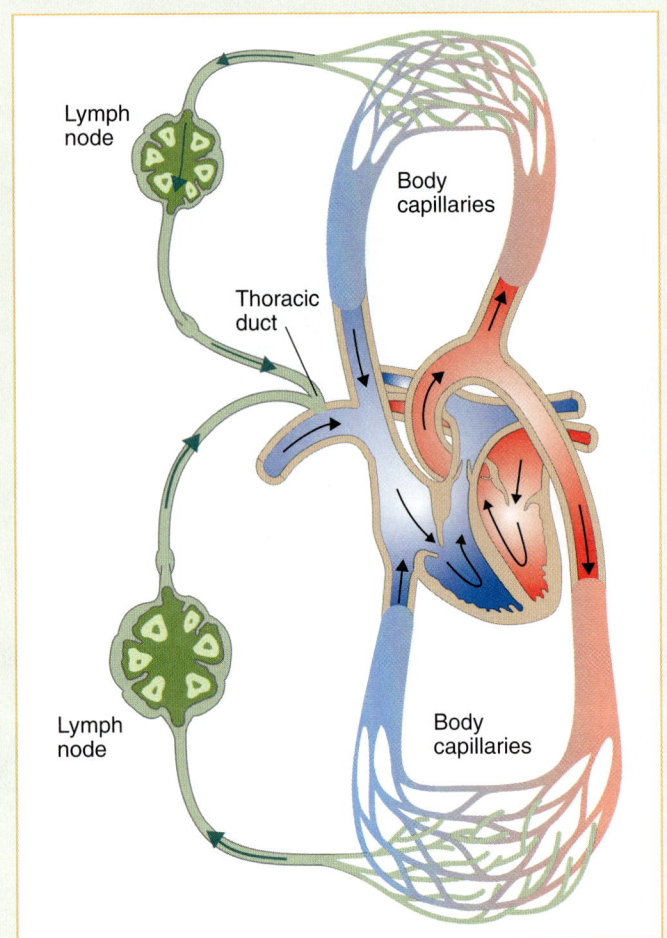

Figure 6-27 The interrelationship of the lymphatic system and the circulatory system. Blood fluid passes out of the arteries in the upper and lower parts of the body, and then enters a system of lymphatic ducts that arise in the tissues. The fluid, called lymph, passes through lymph nodes and on the right side makes its way back to the general circulation via the thoracic duct. Lymph vessels from the left upper quadrant join the thoracic duct and empty into the left subclavian vein. Lymph vessels from the right upper quadrant join together to form the right lymphatic duct, which empties into the right subclavian vein.

allergic response. These white blood cells, which account for 1% to 3% of the leukocytes, release chemoactive substances that can result in severe bronchospasm.

- Neutrophils are the most abundant white blood cells, accounting for 55% to 70% of the leukocytes. They have a segmented nucleus and are often called polymorphonuclear leukocytes ("polys"). Neutrophils are largely responsible for protecting the body against infection and are key components of the first response to foreign body invasion. They are readily attracted by foreign antigens, which they destroy by engulfing and digesting the antigens (phagocytosis).
- Monocytes mature in the blood during their first 24 hours and then travel to the tissues, where they differentiate into macrophages. Macrophages function primarily as

		Table 6-5	Types of White Blood Cells		

Name	Description	Concentration (number of cells/mm³)	Life Span	Function
Neutrophil	Approximately twice the size of red blood cells; multilobed nucleus; clear-staining cytoplasm	3,000–7,000	6 hours to a few days	Phagocytizes bacteria
Eosinophil	Approximately same size as neutrophil; large pink-stained granules; bilobed nucleus	100–400	8-12 days	Phagocytizes antigen-antibody complex; attacks parasites
Basophil	Slightly smaller than neutrophil; contains large, purple cytoplasmic granules; bilobed nucleus	20–50	A few hours to a few days	Releases histamine during inflammation
Monocyte	Larger than neutrophil; cytoplasm greyish-blue; no cytoplasmic granules; U- or kidney-shaped nucleus	100–700	Lasts many months	Phagocytizes bacteria, dead cells, and cellular debris
Lymphocyte	Slightly smaller than neutrophil; large, relatively round nucleus that fills the cell	1,500–3,000	Can persist many years	Involved in immune protection, either attacking cells directly or producing antibodies

scavengers for the tissues. Monocytes and macrophages represent one of the first lines of defence in the inflammatory process.

- Lymphocytes and their derivatives mediate the acquired immune response. Although most lymphocytes are found in the lymphoid tissues, many are found in circulating lymph and blood as well. There are two basic types: B lymphocytes and T lymphocytes.

Mast cells resemble basophils but do not circulate in the blood. They are found in the connective tissues, beneath the skin, in the gastrointestinal mucosa, and in the mucosal membranes of the respiratory system. Mast cells play a role in allergic reactions, immunity, and wound healing.

Characteristics of the Immune Response

The native and acquired immune responses protect the body from potentially infectious agents (eg, viruses, bacteria) and foreign substances that have gained access to the body through the skin or the lining of internal organs.

Native immunity (also called natural or innate immunity) is a nonspecific cellular and humoural (antibody) response that operates as the first line of defence against pathogens. Most native immunity is associated with the initial inflammatory response.

Acquired immunity (also called adaptive immunity) is a highly specific, inducible, discriminatory, and unforgetting method by which armies of cells respond to an immune stimulant. It arises when the body is exposed to a foreign substance or disease and produces antibodies to that invader. Passive acquired immunity is the receipt of preformed antibodies to fight or prevent an infection. Typically passive acquired immunity lasts for a much shorter period of time than active acquired immunity. Examples include transplacental and colostrum (the mother's initial milk to her infant, which is loaded with antibodies); transmission of maternal antibodies, which protect newborn infants until their own immune system matures sufficiently to take over; and injection of immunoglobulin (a concentrated form of antibodies obtained from donors).

The primary (initial) immune response takes place during the first exposure to an antigen (a foreign substance). It may or may not result in clinical symptoms. Sometimes, the initial response of the body is to produce an antibody that causes symptoms on subsequent exposures. The secondary (amnestic) immune response occurs upon repeat exposure to a foreign substance. The body has already developed a "memory" for that substance, so a reaction occurs upon reexposure to it.

The beginning (induction) phase of the immune response occurs when a part of the immune system recognizes an antigen. Antigens may be either immunogenic (ie, elicit an immune response) or nonimmunogenic (do not elicit an immune response). An antibody binds a specific antigen so that the complex can attach itself to specialized immune cells that either ingest the complex to destroy it or release biological mediators such as histamine to induce an allergic/inflammatory response. The specific features of the antigen–antibody interaction depend on the foreign substance involved (Figure 6-28 ▸).

An immunogen is an antigen that activates immune cells to generate an immune response against itself. Thus, an immunogen is an antigen, but an antigen is not necessarily an immunogen. A hapten is a substance that normally does not stimulate an immune response but that can be combined with an antigen and, at a later time, initiate a specific antibody response on its own.

Humoural Immune Response

In humoural immunity, B-cell lymphocytes produce antibodies, which then react with a specific antigen, as shown in (Figure 6-29 ▸).

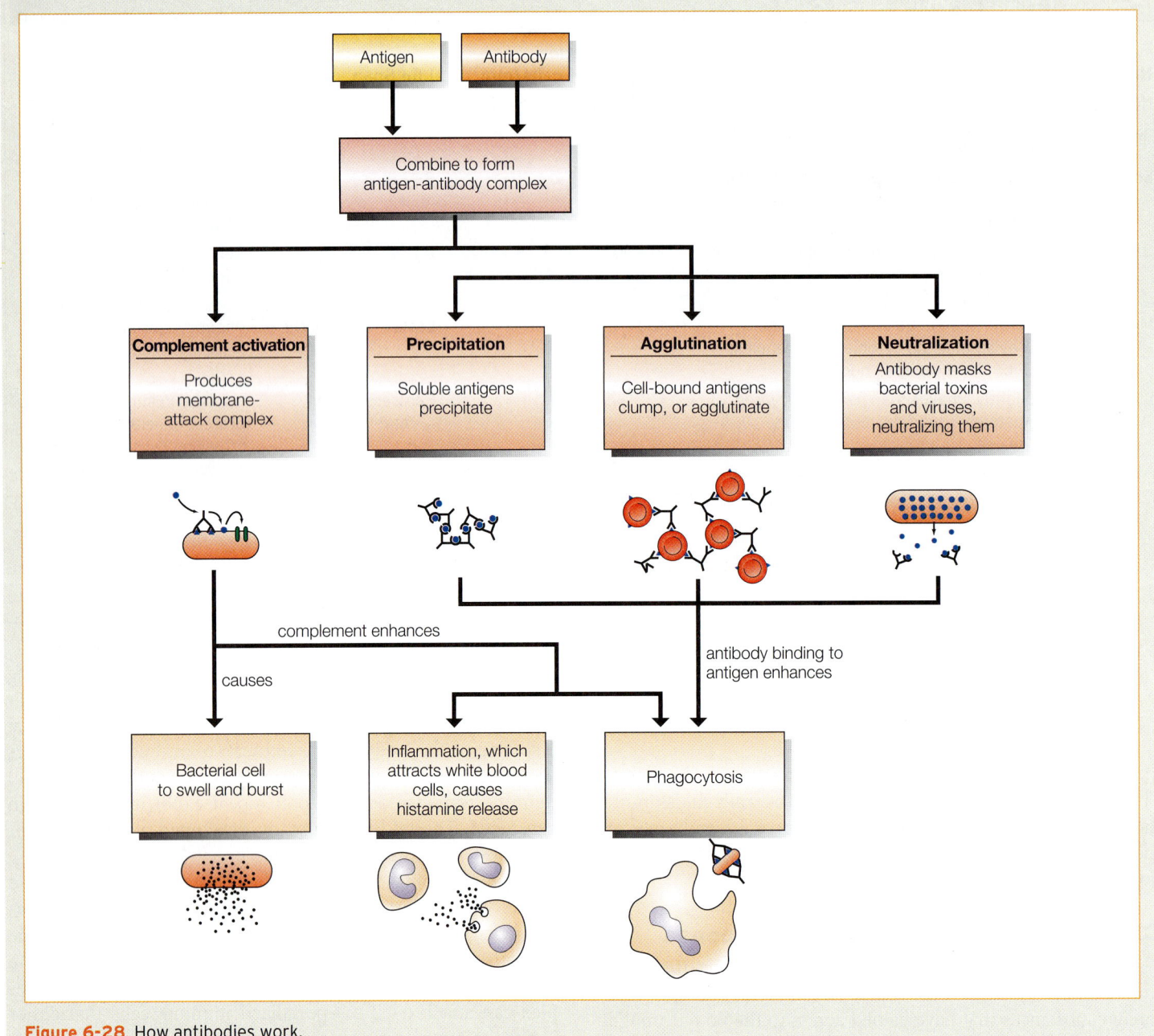

Figure 6-28 How antibodies work.

B Lymphocytes

Like all blood cells, B cells are born in the bone marrow, where they are descended from stem cells. The clonal selection theory holds that each B cell makes antibodies that have only one type of antigen-binding region and, therefore, are specific for a particular antigen, known as the cognate antigen. Antibodies are found on the surface of B cells, where they are able to recognize the presence of their cognate antigens. When a B cell recognizes the cognate antigen, it proliferates to make more identical B cells in an exponential fashion, each of which can make antibodies that recognize the same antigen.

For B cells to produce antibodies, they must first be activated. The most common way this occurs is via helper T cells:

1. A macrophage engulfs the antigen via phagocytosis. It digests the antigen, pushing the discarded particles to the cell surface. These remnants interact with the B cell and a helper T cell.

2. The antigen binds to both the B cell and the helper T cell, activating both.

3. The activated helper T cell secretes a lymphokine, a substance that stimulates the B cells to produce a clone. A clone is a group of identical cells formed from the same parent cell. The clone comprises two types of identical cells that have different functions: plasma cells, which make the antibodies, and memory cells, which "remember" the initial encounter with the antigen.

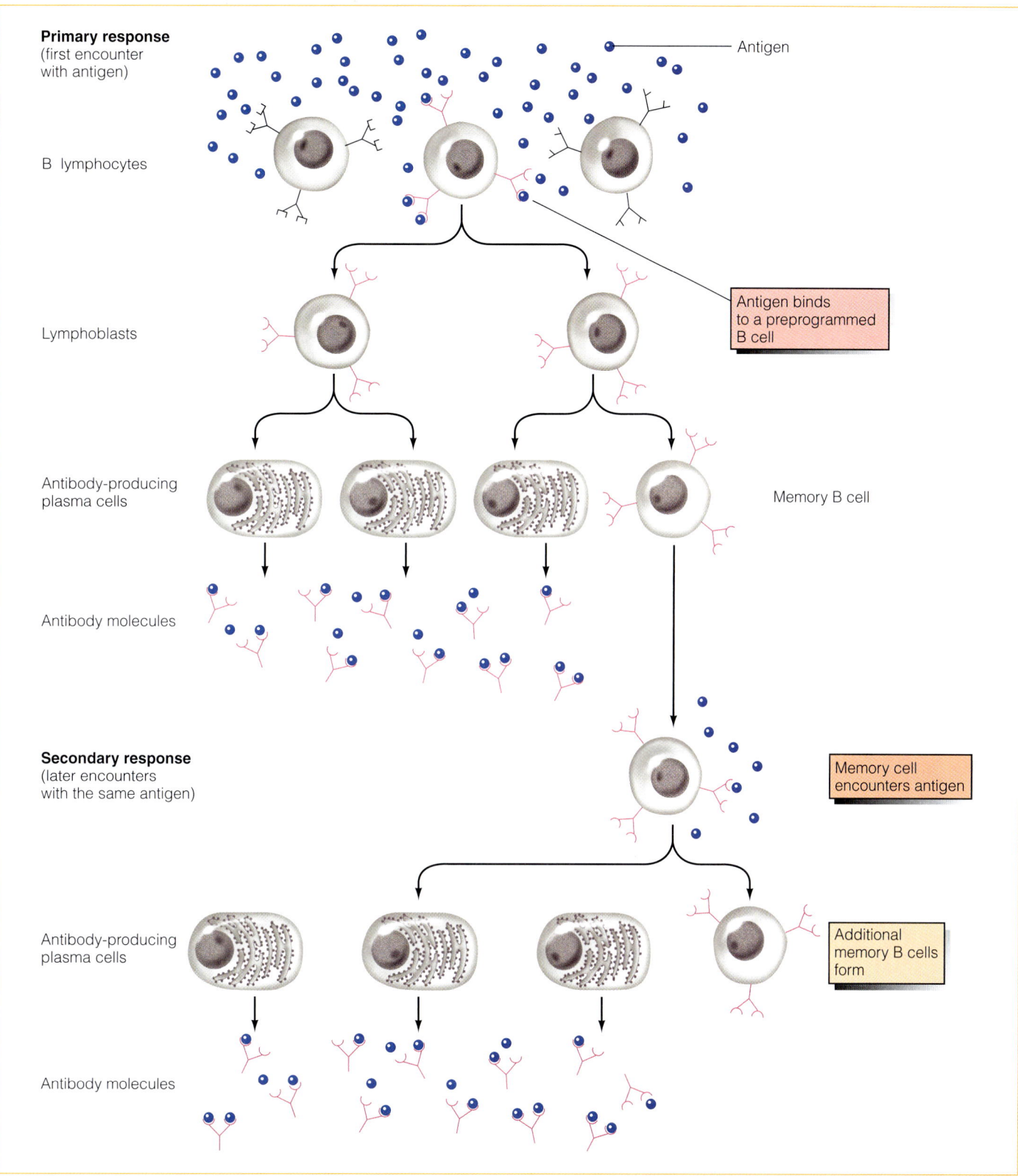

Primary response
(first encounter
with antigen)

B lymphocytes

Antigen

Antigen binds
to a preprogrammed
B cell

Lymphoblasts

Antibody-producing
plasma cells

Memory B cell

Antibody molecules

Secondary response
(later encounters
with the same antigen)

Memory cell
encounters antigen

Antibody-producing
plasma cells

Additional
memory B cells
form

Antibody molecules

Figure 6-29 B-cell activation. Immunocompetent B cells are stimulated by the presence of an antigen, producing an intermediate cell, the lymphoblast. The lymphoblasts divide, producing plasma cells and some memory B cells. Memory B cells respond to subsequent antigen encroachment, yielding a rapid secondary response.

The human body distinguishes between foreign substances and its own cells and tissues by means of the major histocompatibility complex (MHC). A group of genes located on a single chromosome, the MHC permits an individual who is capable of generating an immune response to distinguish *self* from *non-self* (ie, what is foreign). The human leukocyte antigen (HLA) gene complex is the human MHC and is present in all nucleated human cells. It codes for numerous antigens that are unique to an individual. When the immune system "sees" these particular antigens, it recognizes them as "self" and no immune response occurs.

Immunoglobulins

The antibodies secreted by B cells are called immunoglobulins (this text uses use the terms *immunoglobulins* and *antibodies* interchangeably, unless otherwise stated). These Y-shaped proteins consist of a crystallizable fragment (Fc) portion and two antigen-binding fragment (Fab) regions that bind only a specific antigen. The basic antibody molecule has four chains linked into a Y-shape. Each side of the Y is identical, with one light chain attached to one heavy chain

Figure 6-30 ▾. The two arms, or Fab regions, contain antigen-binding sites. The stem, or Fc region, determines to which of the five immunoglobin classes an antibody belongs **Figure 6-31 ▸**.

Most antibodies are found in the plasma, where they make up about 20% of the plasma proteins in a healthy individual.

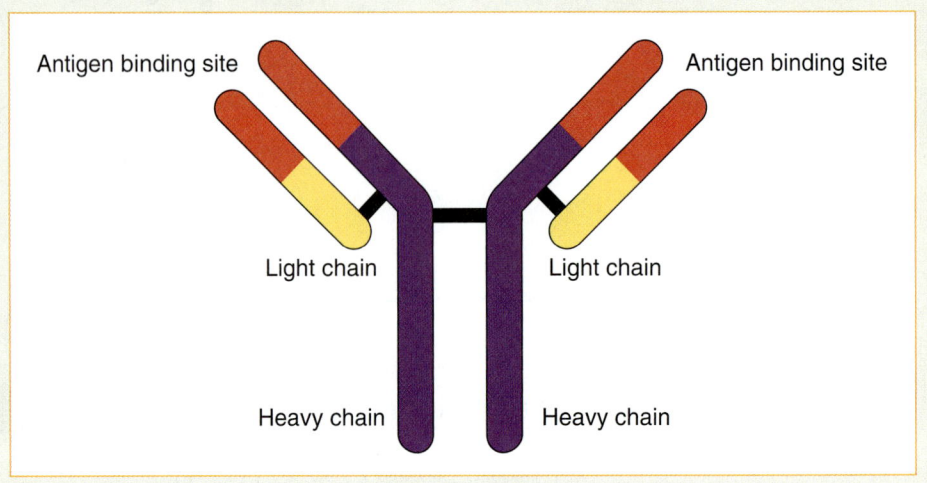

Figure 6-30 Structure of an immunoglobulin molecule.

You are the Paramedic Part 4

You prepare the patient for transport, noting that her breathing is still laboured. She tells you that she is less lightheaded after the first 100 ml of saline has been administered; however, she still complains of being "short-winded." You contact the hospital for further orders, advising an estimated time of arrival of 8 minutes. The emergency department physician has no further orders at this time.

Upon your arrival at the emergency department, you notice that the dialysis nurse is already preparing for Mrs. Jensen. The emergency room physician explains to you that the physical findings are compatible with the beginning of septic shock due to an infection at the shunt site in addition to being volume-overloaded secondary to missed dialysis. He also suspects that Mrs. Jensen's potassium level will be high because of the tall T waves present on the ECG.

When you return to the emergency department that evening with another patient, you check up on Mrs. Jensen. She's resting comfortably in the medical intensive care unit, where she is being treated for sepsis, congestive heart failure, and hyperkalemia (her level was 6.7 mmol/l). After the day's experience, you decide that studying pathophysiology is beneficial after all!

Reassessment	Recording Time: 15 Minutes
Skin	Pale, warm, and moist
Pulse	150 beats/min, regular; weak radial
ECG	Narrow complex tachycardia with tall T waves
Blood pressure	84/56 mm Hg
Respirations	26 breaths/min laboured
Spo$_2$	93% on nonrebreathing mask at 15 l/min of supplemental oxygen
Pupils	Equal and reactive to light

7. How did the inflammatory process manifest itself in this patient?

8. What are other signs and symptoms of hyperkalemia?

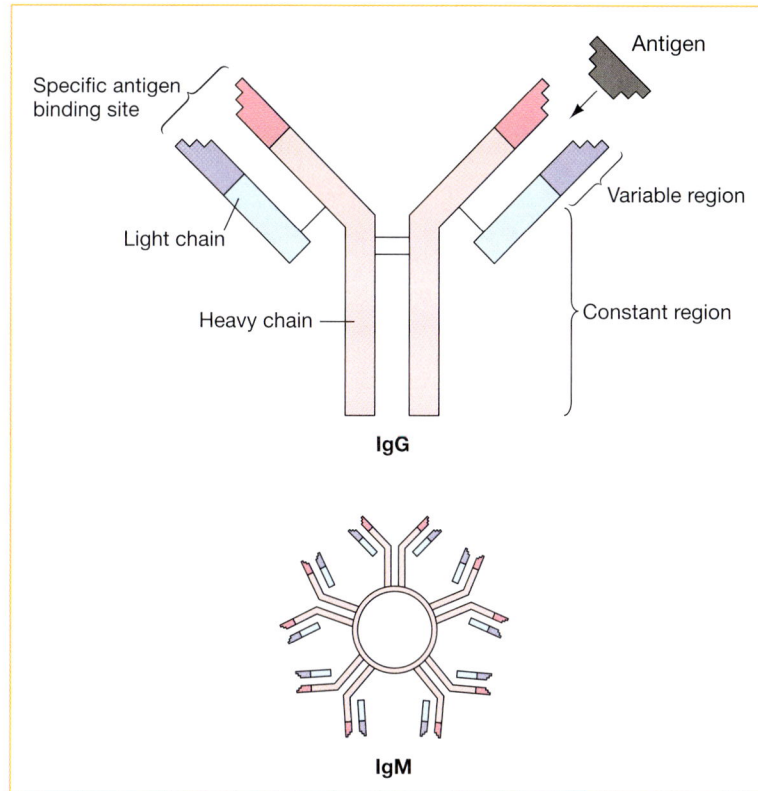

Figure 6-31 General structure of an antibody.

Antibodies make antigens more visible to the immune system in three ways:

- Antibodies act as opsonins. In opsoninization, an antibody coats an antigen to facilitate its recognition by immune cells. Antibodies are not toxic by themselves, but they label antigens so that other immune cells will attack them.
- Antibodies cause antigens to clump for easier phagocytosis (precipitation, also known as agglutination).
- Antibodies bind to and inactivate some toxins produced by bacteria. Macrophages can then ingest and destroy the inactivated toxins.

Antibodies are divided into five general classes of immunoglobulins [Table 6-6 ▶]. Fetal immunity is a passive acquired immunity that is derived primarily from maternal IgG and IgM antibodies. Following delivery, these antibodies persist until the neonate's own B cells take over. A substantial number of antibodies are also transferred through breast milk, which is one of many reasons why experts favour breastfeeding.

Cell-Mediated Immune Response

In cell-mediated immunity, T-cell lymphocytes recognize antigens and contribute to the immune response in two major ways: (1) by secreting cytokines that attract other cells or (2) by becoming cytotoxic and killing infected or abnormal cells. There are four subgroups of T cells:

- *Killer T cells* (also called cytotoxic T cells) destroy the antigen. Cytotoxic T cells help rid the body of cells that

have been infected by viruses as well as cells that have been transformed by cancer. They are also responsible for the rejection of tissue and organ grafts.

- *Helper T cells* activate many immune cells, including B cells and other T cells (also called T4 or CD4+ cells).
- *Suppressor T cells* (also called T8 or CD8+ cells) suppress the activity of other lymphocytes so they do not destroy normal tissue.
- *Memory T cells* remember the reaction for the next time it is needed.

During the cell-mediated response, macrophages ingest pathogens. When a macrophage digests a pathogen, it releases small particles of antigen. This antigen pushes its way to the macrophage surface, where it is recognized by specific T cells. Other T cells, such as helper T cells and killer T cells, bind to the antigen and macrophage, destroying the invader.

Cellular Interactions in the Immune Response

There are remarkable similarities in how the body responds to different kinds of immune challenges. Although the details depend on the particular challenge, the basic pattern is the same—the innate response starts first and is then reinforced by the more specific acquired response. These two pathways are interconnected.

Consider what happens when bacteria enter the body. If the bacteria are not encapsulated, macrophages begin to ingest them immediately. If the bacteria are encapsulated, antibodies

Table 6-6	General Classes of Immunoglobulins
IgG	The most common immunoglobulin. Accounts for 75% of the antibodies in the blood. Found in lymph, synovial fluid, peritoneal fluid, cerebrospinal fluid, and breast milk. IgG is the only immunoglobulin that crosses the placenta, giving infants immunity in the first few months of life.
IgA	Accounts for 15% of the antibodies in the blood. Also found in tears, saliva, respiratory tract secretions, and the stomach. IgA combines with a protein in the mucosa and defends body surfaces against invading microorganisms.
IgM	Accounts for 5% to 10% of the antibodies in the blood and is the dominant antibody in ABO (blood type) incompatibilities. IgM is the initial antibody formed in most infections.
IgE	Accounts for less than 1% of the antibodies in the blood and is associated with allergic reactions. When mast cell receptors combine with IgE and antigen, the mast cells degranulate and release chemical mediators such as histamine.
IgD	Accounts for less than 1% of the antibodies in the blood. The physiologic role of IgD is unclear.

(opsonins) must coat the capsule before they can be ingested by phagocytes.

Components of the cell wall then activate the complement system. Some components of the activated complement system, termed chemotaxins, attract leukocytes from the circulation to help fight the infection. The complement cascade ends with the formation of a set of proteins called the membrane attack complex (MAC). These molecules insert themselves into the bacterial membrane, weakening those areas in the membrane. Ions and water enter the cell through the weakened areas, leading to lysis of the bacterium (a chemical process that does not involve immune cells).

If antibodies to the bacteria are already in the body, they will help the innate response by acting as opsonins and neutralizing bacterial toxins. Although it often takes several days, memory B cells attracted to the infection site will be activated if they encounter an antigen they recognize. If the infection is new to the body (preexisting antibodies are not present), B cells will be activated. Combined with helper T cells and cytokine release, antibodies are produced and memory B and T cells are formed.

T-cell and B-cell function is deficient in older patients. Depressed lymphocyte function is accompanied by a decrease in macrophage activity. Therefore, older people are more prone to experience infections and recover slowly. In addition, older people have increased levels of autoantibodies (antibodies directed against the patient), which partly explains why older people are prone to autoimmune disease.

Acute and Chronic Inflammation

Inflammation is a dynamic process that, once initiated, triggers a complex cascade of events involving both local and systemic events. The two most common causes of inflammation are infection (eg, bacterial or viral) and injury.

The acute inflammatory response involves both vascular and cellular components. After transient arteriolar constriction, the arterioles dilate, allowing an influx of blood under increased pressure. This active hyperemia (increased intravascular pressure) causes the blood vessel to expand; as in a balloon that is being inflated, the vessel walls become thinner. The higher pressure combined with increased vessel wall permeability causes fluid to leak into the interstitial spaces (edema). When enough fluid has escaped into the surrounding area and the intravascular pressure has been released, the vessel wall contracts and the outflow slows, leading to stasis of blood in the capillaries.

A variety of blood cells participate in tissue inflammatory reactions: white blood cells (leukocytes), platelets, mast cells, and plasma cells (B lymphocytes that create antibodies). Specific cell types include neutrophils, monocytes, lymphocytes, eosinophils, basophils, and activated platelets. Chemical mediators, primarily produced by the mast cells, account for the vascular and cellular events that occur during the acute inflam-

At the Scene

Corticosteroids can decrease the initial inflammatory response, which is a necessary part of wound healing. They also increase the risk of wound infection owing to their immunosuppressive activity. This consideration is important in diabetic patients because of their propensity to develop wound infections.

matory response. Cell-derived mediators include histamine, arachidonic acid derivatives, and cytokines (eg, interleukins, tumour necrosis factor).

Mast Cells

Mast cells play a major role in inflammation. During inflammation, they degranulate and release a variety of substances. The major stimuli for the degranulation of mast cells during the inflammatory response are physical injury (eg, trauma), chemical agents (eg, bacterial toxins), and immunologic substances (eg, interaction of an antigen and an IgE antibody).

Following their degranulation, mast cells release vasoactive amines. The most important of these substances, histamine and serotonin, increase vascular permeability, cause vasodilation, and can cause bronchoconstriction, nausea, and vomiting. Because histamine is a preformed vasodepressor amine that is stored in mast cells, it can be released quickly, so its actions are seen early in the inflammatory response. Mast cells also synthesize chemotactic factors that attract neutrophils (neutrophil chemotactic factor) and eosinophils (eosinophilic chemotactic factor).

Mast cells also synthesize leukotrienes. Leukotrienes—also known as slow-reacting substances of anaphylaxis (SRS-A)—are a family of biologically active compounds derived from arachidonic acid. The clinically important leukotrienes participate in host defence reactions and pathophysiologic conditions that paramedics commonly see at the scene, such as immediate hypersensitivity and inflammation. Leukotrienes have potent actions on many parts of the body, including the cardiovascular, pulmonary, immune, and central nervous systems, and the gastrointestinal tract.

Leukotrienes are primarily endogenous mediators of inflammation. They contribute to the signs and symptoms seen in acute inflammatory responses, including responses resulting from the interaction of allergens with IgE antibodies on mast cells. Certain leukotrienes are bronchoconstrictors, stimulate airway mucus secretion, and are very potent at increasing the permeability of postcapillary venules (including those in the bronchial circulation), thereby causing plasma protein exudation (oozing out of the tissue) and edema. Certain leukotrienes may also promote eosinophil migration into the airways of animals and asthmatic patients, and they may also increase bronchial hyperresponsiveness through an action on sensory nerves.

Finally, mast cells synthesize prostaglandins. These substances, which are derived from arachidonic acid, comprise a group of about 20 lipids that are modified fatty acids attached to a five-member ring. Prostaglandins are found in many vertebrate tissues, where they act as messengers involved in reproduction, the inflammatory response to infection, and pain. Aspirin and NSAIDs inhibit prostaglandin synthesis, leading to reduced inflammation and pain.

Plasma Protein Systems

The plasma-derived mediators that modulate the inflammatory process are called plasma protein systems. They include the complement system, the coagulation (clotting) system, and the kinin system. The interaction of these systems is vital to a normal inflammatory response. Each system consists of a cascade of biochemical reactions such that as one compound is produced, it catalyzes the formation of the next compound—much like knocking over a line of dominos.

Complement System

The complement system is a group of plasma proteins that attract white blood cells to sites of inflammation, activate white blood cells, and directly destroy cells. The central compound in this complement cascade is called C3. C3 is produced by one of the two "complement pathways": the classic pathway or the alternate pathway. The classic pathway starts when an antigen–antibody complex binds to a complement component (C1); activation of this pathway is dependent on the presence of antibodies. The alternate pathway can be triggered by bacterial toxins and does not need antibodies to be activated.

Regardless of which pathway is taken, the main products are the same: C3b, anaphylatoxins, and the MAC. C3b coats bacteria, making it easier for macrophages to engulf them. Anaphylatoxins (C3a, C4a, and C5a) stimulate smooth-muscle contraction and increase vascular permeability by stimulating the release of histamine from mast cells and platelets. The MAC is a set of complement proteins (C5b, C6, C7, C8, and C9) that bind to form a hollow tube, much like a short straw, that can puncture into the plasma membrane of a cell. In this way, transmembrane channels are formed that allow ions, water, and other small molecules to pass through, resulting in loss of cellular osmolarity and death of the cell.

Coagulation System

The coagulation system plays a vital role in the formation of blood clots in the body and facilitates repairs to the vascular tree. Inflammation triggers the coagulation cascade, initiating a complex series of reactions that result in the formation of fibrin. Fibrin is the protein that polymerizes (bonds) to form the fibrous component of a blood clot. The various coagulation factors are counterbalanced by a variety of inhibitors, so that the coagulation is restricted to one area. Simultaneously, the fibrinolysis cascade is activated to dissolve the fibrin and create fibrin split products (ie, fragments of the dissolving clot).

Kinin System

The kinin system leads to the formation of the vasoactive protein bradykinin from kallikrein. Kallikrein is an enzyme that is normally found in blood plasma, urine, and body tissue in an inactive state. When it becomes activated, it can dilate blood vessels, influence blood pressure, modulate salt and water excretion by the kidneys, and influence cardiac remodelling after acute myocardial infarction. Bradykinin increases vascular permeability, dilates blood vessels, contracts smooth muscle, and causes pain when injected into the skin.

The kinin system is spurred into action by the activation of Hageman factor (coagulation factor XII). (Table 6-7 ▶ lists the various coagulation factors.) In addition to its role in the kinin system, Hageman factor participates in the clotting, fibrinolytic, and complement cascades. Its activators include bacterial lipopolysaccharides and endotoxin. Activated factor XII triggers the intrinsic clotting cascade, which occurs when blood is exposed to collagen or other substances. For example, when a blood vessel is cut, the skin cells are damaged and the blood comes in contact with collagen. The extrinsic clotting cascade is activated by substances released from injured cells when tissue damage occurs.

Cellular Components of Inflammation

The goal of the cellular component of acute inflammatory response is for inflammatory cells—namely, polymorphonuclear neutrophils (PMNs)—to arrive at the sites within tissue where they are needed. This process involves two major stages: an intravascular phase and an extravascular phase. During the intravascular phase, leukocytes move to the sides of blood vessels and attach to the endothelial cells. During the extravascular phase, leukocytes travel to the site of inflammation and kill organisms. The cellular event sequence is as follows:

1. **Margination.** Loss of fluid from the blood vessels into the inflamed or infected tissue causes the blood left in the vessels to have increased viscosity, which slows the flow of blood and produces stasis. PMNs, which usually travel toward the centre of the vessel, settle toward the sides of the vessel as the blood flow slows down. As stasis develops, leukocytes also move (marginate) toward the sides of blood vessels, where they bump into the endothelial cells and bind to them. Stress can lead to demargination of some white blood cells, which stimulates the bone marrow to produce more white blood cells, which in turn increases the white blood cell count.

2. **Activation.** Mediators of inflammation trigger the appearance of selectins and integrins on the surfaces of endothelial cells and PMNs, respectively.

3. **Adhesion.** PMNs attach to endothelial cells, as mediated by selectins and integrins.

4. **Transmigration (diapedesis).** The PMNs permeate through the vessel wall, moving into the interstitial space.

5. **Chemotaxis.** PMNs move toward the site of inflammation in response to chemotactic factors that are released by

Table 6-7	Coagulation Factors	
Factor Number	**Name**	**Functions**
I	Fibrinogen	Protein synthesized in liver; converted into fibrin in stage 3
II	Prothrombin	Protein synthesized in liver (requires vitamin K); converted into thrombin in stage 2
III	Tissue thromboplastin	Released from damaged tissue; required in extrinsic stage 1
IV	Calcium ions	Required throughout entire clotting sequence
V	Proaccelerin (labile factor)	Protein synthesized in liver; required to form prothrombin activator in both intrinsic and extrinsic stage 1
VII	Serum prothrombin conversion accelerator (stable factor, proconvertin)	Protein synthesized in liver (requires vitamin K); functions in extrinsic stage 1
VIII	Antihemophilic factor (antihemophilic globulin)	Protein synthesized in liver; required for intrinsic stage 1
IX	Plasma thromboplastin component	Protein synthesized in liver (requires vitamin K); required for intrinsic stage 1
X	Stuart factor (Stuart-Prower factor)	Protein synthesized in liver (requires vitamin K); required to form prothrombin activator in both intrinsic and extrinsic stage 1
XI	Plasma thromboplastin antecedent	Protein synthesized in liver; required for intrinsic stage 1
XII	Hageman factor	Protein required for intrinsic stage 1
XIII	Fibrin-stabilizing factor	Protein required to stabilize the fibrin strands in stage 3

bacteria or formed from activated complement, chemokines, or arachidonic acid derivatives (eg, leukotrienes) in response to cell injury.

Figure 6-32 ▶ illustrates the inflammatory response.

Cellular Products of Inflammation

Cytokines are products of cells that affect the function of other cells. Monocytes release monokines, and lymphocytes release lymphokines.

Interleukins include IL-1 (interleukin-1) and IL-2 (interleukin-2), which attract white blood cells to the sites of injury and bacterial invasion. Interferon is a protein produced by cells when they are invaded by viruses. This cytokine is released into the bloodstream or intercellular fluid to induce healthy cells to manufacture an enzyme that counters the infection.

Lymphokines stimulate leukocytes. Macrophage-activating factor stimulates macrophages to help engulf and destroy foreign substances. Migration inhibitory factor keeps white blood cells at the site of infection or injury until they can perform their designated task.

Injury Resolution and Repair

Normal wound healing involves four steps—repair of damaged tissue, removal of inflammatory debris, restoration of tissues to a normal state, and regeneration of cells. Healing after tissue injury or loss caused by inflammation depends on the type of cells that make up the affected organ. Labile cells divide continuously, so organs derived from these cells (eg, skin or intestinal mucosa) heal completely. Stable cells are replaced by regeneration from remaining cells, which are stimulated to enter mitosis. These cells are found in the liver and kidney. Permanent cells, such as nerve cells and cardiac myocytes, cannot be replaced; scar tissue is laid down instead.

Wounds may heal by either primary or secondary intention. Healing by primary intention occurs in clean wounds with opposed margins (eg, a clean surgical wound). First, blood fills the defect and coagulates, forming a scab, which is a mesh-like structure composed of fibrin and fibronectin. If the inflammatory process was severe, tissue may be destroyed and require repair. Next, macrophages remove cellular debris and secrete growth factors. These growth factors stimulate angiogenesis and growth of fibroblasts, leading to the formation of granulation tissue. The epithelium then regenerates, covering the surface defect. Deposition of collagen results in fibrous union. By the end of the first week, 10% of the preoperative strength is regained. Scar maturation occurs as collagen cross-linking takes place. By the end of 3 months, 80% of the normal tensile strength of the tissue has been restored.

Healing by secondary intention occurs in large gaping or infected wounds. Wounds that heal by secondary intention have a more pronounced and prolonged inflammatory phase, causing the neutrophils to persist for days. They also have more abundant granulation tissue. Wound contraction is mediated by myofibroblasts, which help to draw the margins of the wound closer to each other as time passes.

Factors that can lead to dysfunctional wound healing may be either local or systemic. Local factors include infection (when the body's healing efforts are diverted to fight off the cause of the infection); an inadequate blood supply (as in diabetes) that produces tissue hypoxia, which slows wound

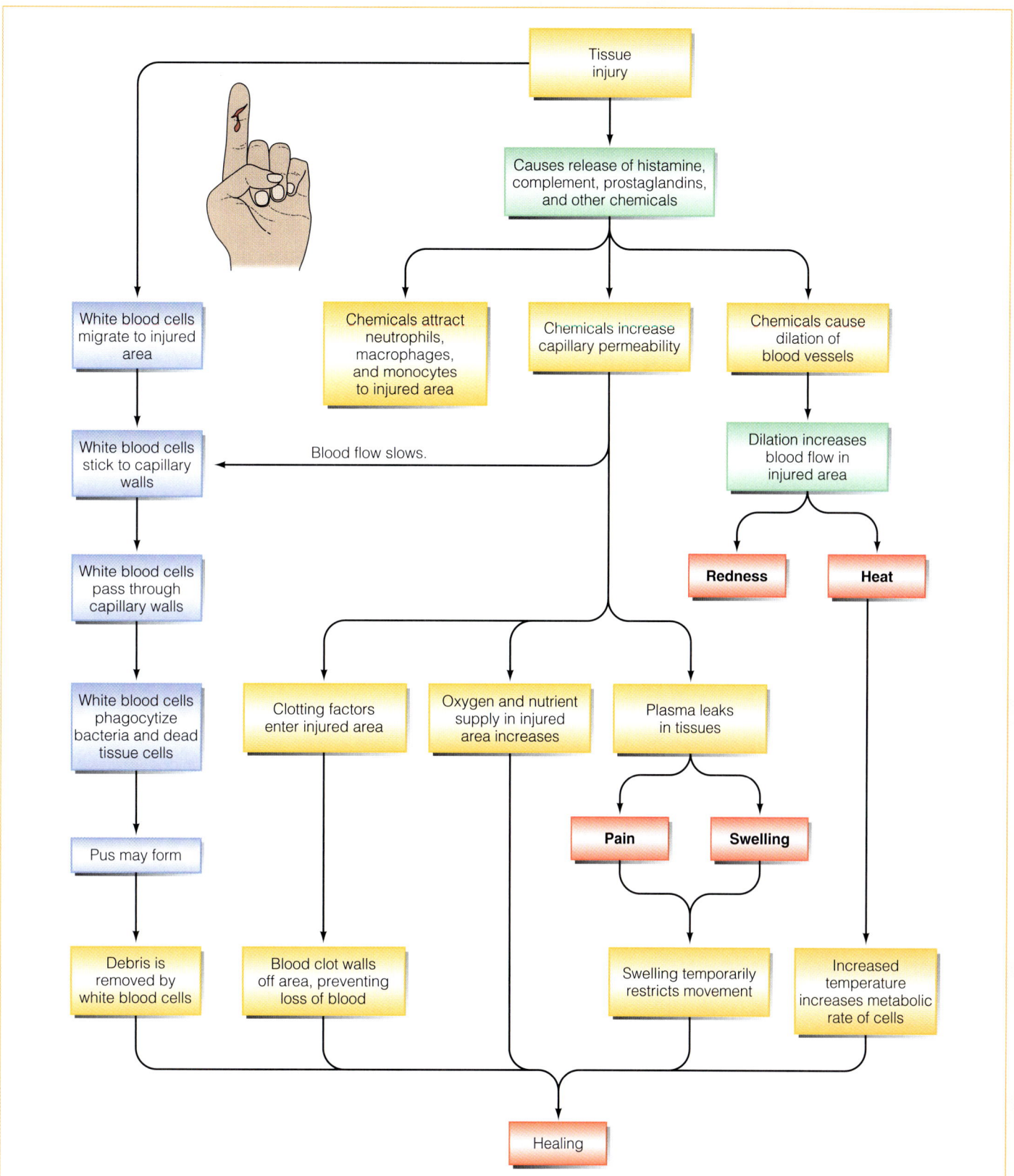

Figure 6-32 The inflammatory response.

healing and may promote infection; and foreign bodies (when present in a wound, they stimulate acute and chronic inflammation, both of which interfere with wound healing).

Systemic factors that influence the healing of a patient's wounds include poor nutritional intake, which leads to poor scar formation and suppression of the immune system, and hematologic abnormalities (proper wound healing requires the presence of adequate numbers of white blood cells). Patients who have impaired bone marrow stores of white blood cells are susceptible to infection and often heal more slowly. Both diabetes and AIDS affect the cells of the immune system, which plays a direct role in wound healing, and increase the likelihood of wound infection. Corticosteroids suppress the initial inflammatory response required for the proper formation of scar tissue and increase the risk of wound infection by slowing the immune system response.

Chronic Inflammation Responses

Chronic inflammation responses are usually caused by an unsuccessful acute inflammatory response due to a foreign body, persistent infection, or antigen. They are associated with an infiltrate containing monocytes and lymphocytes, and usually involve tissue destruction and repair (or scar formation). The vascular events are similar to those that take place in acute inflammation but also include the growth of new blood vessels (a process known as angiogenesis).

Age and the Inflammatory Response

Both newborns and geriatric patients often exhibit relative impairment of their immune systems, potentially slowing their inflammatory response. As a consequence, signs of inflammation may be more subtle in these populations. In addition, wound healing often takes longer, especially in the geriatric patient. The immune system is not fully developed until the child is between 2 and 3 years of age. Therefore, investigation of a fever in younger children must be aggressive and thorough. Many experts recommend hospital admission for a temperature greater than 38°C in a child younger than 3 months.

Variances in Immunity and Inflammation

Hypersensitivity

Hypersensitivity is any bodily response to any substance to which a patient has increased sensitivity. It is a generic term for a variety of reactions. Allergy is a hypersensitivity reaction to the presence of an agent (allergen). Autoimmunity is the production of antibodies or T cells that work against the tissues of one's own body, producing hypersensitivity reactions or autoimmune disease (as in systemic lupus). Isoimmunity is the formation of T cells or antibodies directed against the antigens on another person's cells (typically after the transplantation of an organ or tissues). A blood transfusion reaction is an example

of an isoimmune reaction to another person's red blood cells. The destruction of cells by antibodies or T cells may be either an autoimmune or an isoimmune reaction.

Mechanisms of Hypersensitivity

A hypersensitivity reaction may be immediate, occurring within seconds to minutes, or delayed, occurring hours to days after exposure to an antigen. The speed of symptom evolution depends on the antigen and the type of response the body mounts against it. Hypersensitivity reactions are typically classified into four types: I, II, III, and IV.

Type I Hypersensitivity Reactions

A type I hypersensitivity reaction is an acute reaction that occurs in response to a stimulus (eg, bee sting, penicillin, shellfish). The mechanism involves interaction between the stimulus (antigen) and a preformed antibody of the IgE type. At first exposure to a specific antigen, specific IgE antibodies bind to mast cells via the nonspecific region (Fc) portion. Upon secondary exposure to the same antigen, these bound antibodies are cross-linked by the antigen, resulting in degranulation of the mast cell, and release of histamine and other mediators ► **Figure 6-33** ◄. The released histamine feeds back on both mast cells and eosinophils, leading to the release of additional histamine and other mediators. The severity of the symptoms that a particular patient develops depends on the extent of mediator release.

The degree of severity of hypersensitivity reactions varies from very severe and life-threatening reactions, such as anaphylaxis, to less severe reactions, such as allergic rhinitis (edema and irritation of the nasal mucosa), bronchial asthma (bronchial constriction, mucus production, and airway inflammation), wheal and flare (ie, insect bite leading to vasodilation and swelling), and mild food allergy (leading to diarrhea, gastrointestinal distress, and vomiting). A propensity to type I reactions may be diagnosed through skin tests (eg, patch test, scratch test) and other laboratory procedures (measurement of specific IgE antibody levels). Treatment is avoidance of the antigen, but desensitizing injections may be helpful in severe cases.

Nevertheless, it is impossible to predict how severe any given reaction will be. If a person has had a severe reaction in the past, he or she is at an increased risk for another one with subsequent antigen exposures. You should always assume that an IgE-mediated reaction could rapidly transition into a life-threatening event. These reactions need to be treated quickly, and most prehospital providers are trained to administer epinephrine by using an EpiPen auto-injector or by giving a subcutaneous injection.

Type II Hypersensitivity Reactions

Type II hypersensitivity reactions are cytotoxic (cell destructive) and classically involve the combination of IgG or IgM antibodies with antigens on the cell membrane. Cells are lysed (destroyed), either by complement fixation or by other antibodies. This process also destroys many of the body's healthy cells. Histamine release from mast cells is not involved, and IgG-mediated allergic responses occur within a few hours of

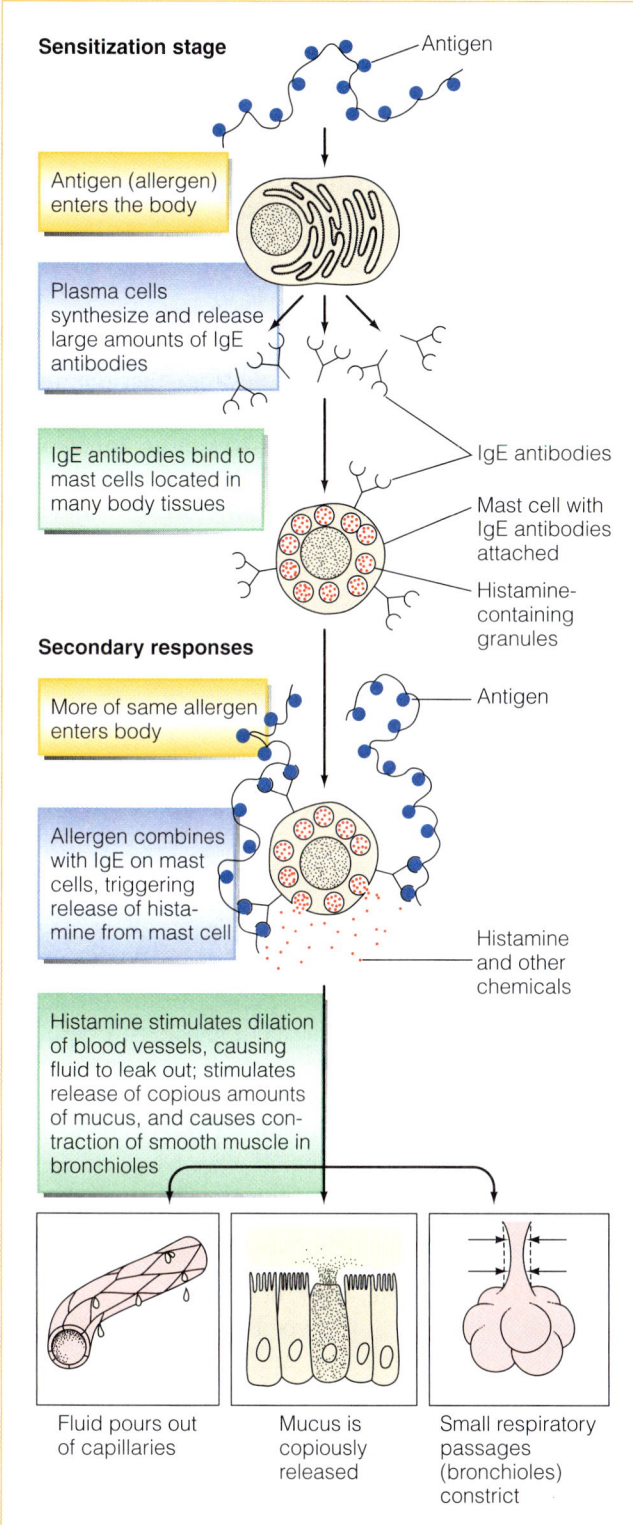

Sensitization stage

Antigen

Antigen (allergen) enters the body

Plasma cells synthesize and release large amounts of IgE antibodies

IgE antibodies bind to mast cells located in many body tissues

IgE antibodies

Mast cell with IgE antibodies attached

Histamine-containing granules

Secondary responses

More of same allergen enters body

Antigen

Allergen combines with IgE on mast cells, triggering release of histamine from mast cell

Histamine and other chemicals

Histamine stimulates dilation of blood vessels, causing fluid to leak out; stimulates release of copious amounts of mucus, and causes contraction of smooth muscle in bronchioles

Fluid pours out of capillaries

Mucus is copiously released

Small respiratory passages (bronchioles) constrict

Figure 6-33 Type I allergic reaction. The antigen stimulates the production of massive amounts of IgE, a type of antibody produced by plasma cells; the IgE, in turn, attaches to mast cells. This is a sensitization stage. When the antigen enters again, it binds to the IgE antibodies on the mast cells, triggering a massive release of histamine and other chemicals. Histamine causes blood vessels to dilate and become leaky, and it promotes increased production of mucus in the respiratory tract. Mast cell degranulation may also cause bronchospasm in some people.

antigen exposure. Examples of IgG-mediated responses include transfusion reactions and newborn hemolytic disease.

Type III Hypersensitivity Reactions

Type III hypersensitivity responses involve primarily IgG antibodies that form immune complexes with antigen to recruit phagocytic cells, such as neutrophils, to a site where they can release inflammatory cytokines. Since histamine release from mast cells is not involved, IgG-mediated allergic responses occur within a few hours of antigen exposure. Reactions may be systemic or localized.

The systemic form is called serum sickness and results from a large, single exposure to an antigen, such as horse antibody serum. Antigen–antibody complexes formed in the bloodstream are then deposited in sites around the body, most notably in the kidney, with resultant inflammatory reactions (eg, serum sickness from penicillin). Signs and symptoms of serum sickness may include fever, malaise, rashes, joint aches, lymphademopathy, and splenomegaly.

The localized form of type III response is called an Arthus reaction. Arthus reactions consist of a circumscribed area of vascular inflammation (vasculitis). An example of an Arthus reaction is farmer's lung (a hypersensitivity pneumonitis), which is a local hypersensitivity reaction in the lung to moulds that grow on hay.

Type IV Hypersensitivity Reactions

Type IV allergic responses, also known as cell-mediated hypersensitivity, are primarily mediated by soluble molecules that are released by specifically activated T cells. These reactions are classified into two subtypes: delayed hypersensitivity and cell-mediated cytotoxicity.

Delayed hypersensitivity involves lymphocytes and macrophages. T cells respond to an antigen and activate CD4 (a helper T cell) lymphocytes. These lymphocytes release mediators that are designed to destroy the foreign substance. Examples include contact hypersensitivity to poison ivy, or the local induration due to mononuclear cell infiltrates from a PPD (tuberculin) skin test.

Cell-mediated cytotoxicity involves only sensitized T cells (CD8 lymphocytes or T killer cells). These cells kill the antigen-bearing target cells rather than activating the CD4 lymphocyte to do so. Examples include the body's response to viral infections, tumour immune surveillance, and the mechanism by which transplant rejection occurs.

Targets of Hypersensitivity

The immune system targets different molecules, depending on the type of hypersensitivity reaction. In allergic reactions, the target is an antigen or allergen. Allergens are substances that cause a hypersensitivity reaction, such as those listed in **Table 6-8 ▶**.

In autoimmune reactions, the target is a person's own tissues. For reasons that are unclear, normal tolerance of "self" tissues breaks down and the immune system treats the body's own tissues as foreign.

Graves' disease is an autoimmune disease caused by thyroid-stimulating or thyroid-growth immunoglobulins.

Table 6-8	Allergens That Can Cause Hypersensitivity Reactions
Type	**Examples**
Inhalants	Pollen, dust, smoke, fungi, plastic, odours
Foods	Eggs, milk, wheat, chocolate, strawberries
Drugs	Aspirin, antibiotics, serums, codeine
Infectious agents	Bacteria, viruses, fungi, animal parasites
Contactants	Animals, plants, metals, chemicals
Physical agents	Light, pressure, radiation, heat and cold

These antibodies activate receptors for thyroid-stimulating hormone, causing increased activity by the thyroid gland. In addition to hyperthyroidism, Graves' disease is associated with characteristic eye changes—lid retraction, stare, and exophthalmus (protrusion of the eyes)—and skin changes (pretibial myxedema—localized edematous skin in the pretibial area).

Type 1 diabetes mellitus is also considered an autoimmune disease. Although the exact insult is unknown (but is suspected to be a viral infection), some agent stimulates the body to produce autoantibodies against beta cells in the pancreas that produce insulin. The result is a deficiency of insulin, and diabetes.

Rheumatoid arthritis is a chronic systemic disease that affects the entire body. One of the most common forms of arthritis, it is characterized by inflammation of the synovium (the connective tissue membrane lining the joint) with resulting pain, stiffness, warmth, redness, and swelling. Inflammatory cells release enzymes that cause damage to bone and cartilage. The involved joint can lose its shape and alignment, resulting in pain and loss of movement. Rheumatoid arthritis is associated with the formation of rheumatoid factor—that is, IgM antibodies to tissue IgG. In the joints, the synovial membrane is thickened due to infiltration of inflammatory cells (lymphocytes).

Myasthenia gravis is an acquired autoimmune disease that is characterized by autoimmune attack on the nerve–muscle junction. The circulating autoantibodies cause abnormal muscle fatigability and typically involve the smallest motor units first, such as the extraocular muscles. This produces ptosis (droopy eyelid) and diplopia (double vision). Other muscles may be involved, causing problems with swallowing (dysphagia). Characteristically, repeated contraction of the affected muscles makes the symptoms worse. Two thirds of patients with myasthenia gravis have thymic abnormalities, with the most common being thymic hyperplasia. A minority of patients have a tumour of the thymus, called a thymoma.

Immune thrombocytopenia purpura (ITP) is a blood disorder in which the patient forms antibodies to blood platelets that cause their destruction. Thrombocytopenia describes a decrease in blood platelets; purpura are purplish areas of the skin and mucous membranes (such as the lining of the mouth)

where bleeding has occurred as a result of decreased or ineffective platelets. Some cases of ITP are caused by drugs, whereas others are associated with infection, pregnancy, or immune disorders such as systemic lupus erythematosus. About half of all cases are classified as "idiopathic" (ie, the cause is unknown).

Bleeding is the main symptom of ITP and can include bruising and tiny red dots on the skin or mucous membranes. In some instances, bleeding from the nose, gums, and digestive or urinary tracts may occur. Rarely, the patient has bleeding within the brain.

Treatment of idiopathic ITP is based on the severity of the symptoms and the patient's platelet count. In some cases, no therapy is needed. In most cases, drugs that alter the immune system's attack on the platelets are prescribed, such as corticosteroids (eg, prednisone) and IV infusions of immunoglobulin. Another treatment that usually results in an increased number of platelets is removal of the spleen, the organ that destroys antibody-coated platelets.

Systemic lupus erythematosus (SLE) is a chronic autoimmune disease with many manifestations. In this disease, the body's own immune system is directed against the body's own tissues. The etiology of SLE is not known. Although this disease is more common in young women, it can occur in either sex at any age. The production of autoantibodies leads to immune complex formation. These immune complexes can then be deposited in glomeruli, skin, lungs, synovium, and mesothelium, among other places. Symptoms include arthritis, a red rash over the nose and cheeks, fatigue, weakness, fever, and photosensitivity. Glomerulonephritis (kidney disease), pericarditis, anemia, and neuritis may develop. In addition, many SLE patients develop renal complications.

Rh factor is an antigen that is present in the erythrocytes (red blood cells) of about 85% of the population. Erythrocytes contain antigens on their surface, which are proteins recognized by the immune system. Within the plasma are antibodies, which are proteins that react with antigens. Individuals are classified as having one of four blood types based on the presence or absence of these specific antigens. This process of classification is referred to as blood typing, or determining the ABO blood group.

Type A blood contains erythrocytes with type A surface antigens and plasma containing type B antibodies; type B blood contains type B surface antigens and plasma containing type A antibodies. Type AB blood contains both types of antigens but the plasma contains no ABO antibodies. Type O contains neither A nor B antigens but contains both A and B plasma antibodies. A person's blood type determines which type of blood he or she may receive in a blood transfusion.

Rh blood groups involve a complex of antigens first discovered in rhesus monkeys. The presence of any of the 18 separate Rh antigens makes an individual's blood Rh positive. If an individual with Rh negative blood were to be exposed to Rh positive blood, antibodies to the antigens could be produced.

Persons who have the factor are designated Rh-positive; those who lack the factor are termed Rh-negative. Blood for transfusions must be classified in terms of its Rh factor, as well as the ABO blood group, to prevent possible incompatibility reactions. If an Rh-negative person receives Rh-positive blood, for example, hemolysis and anemia can result. A similar reaction can occur if an Rh-negative mother exposes her Rh-positive fetus to antibodies to the factor.

Immune and Inflammation Deficiencies

Immunodeficiency is an abnormal condition in which some part of the body's immune system is inadequate, and consequently resistance to infectious disease is decreased. It may be congenital or acquired.

Congenital Immunodeficiencies

Patients with severe combined immunodeficiency disease have defects that involve lymphoid stem cells. As a consequence, both T cells (cellular immunity) and B cells (humoural immunity) are affected. Patients are at risk for infection with all types of organisms (eg, bacteria, mycobacteria, fungi, viruses, parasites). There are two forms of this disease, both of which are inherited.

X-linked agammaglobulinemia is one of the most common forms of primary immunodeficiency. This disease, which affects male infants, is caused by a defect in the differentiation of pre-B cells into B cells. The result is markedly decreased levels of all immunoglobulins and of mature B lymphocytes. T lymphocytes, however, function normally. Patients develop recurrent pyrogenic infections, but have no problems with fungal and viral infections because their cell-mediated immunity is unaffected. These infections first emerge in affected infants at about 6 months of age when maternal immunoglobulin levels have decreased.

Isolated deficiency of IgA is probably the most common form of immunodeficiency. This disease results from a block in the terminal differentiation of B lymphocytes. Most patients are asymptomatic, but some may develop chronic sinus infections. Patients also have an increased incidence of autoimmune disease.

Acquired Immunodeficiencies

Any nutritional deficiency can hamper normal immune function and the inflammatory response. Nutritional deficiencies may depress bone marrow function and diminish white blood cell development **Figure 6-34 ▶**. A lack of protein in the diet, for example, decreases the liver's ability to manufacture inflammatory mediators and plasma proteins.

The stress of trauma can also cause immunodeficiency. Other contributors to this condition may include hypoperfusion or shock, mediator production, damage to vital organs, and the decreased nutrition occurring during trauma states.

Iatrogenic (treatment-induced) immunodeficiency is most frequently caused by drugs. Corticosteroids, whether taken orally or inhaled, suppress the immune system. Often, this results in therapeutic benefit to the patient. In a small number of patients, however, the resulting immunosuppression leads to other diseases (eg, tuberculosis). Usually physicians are very careful about the prescribed duration of this therapy because of

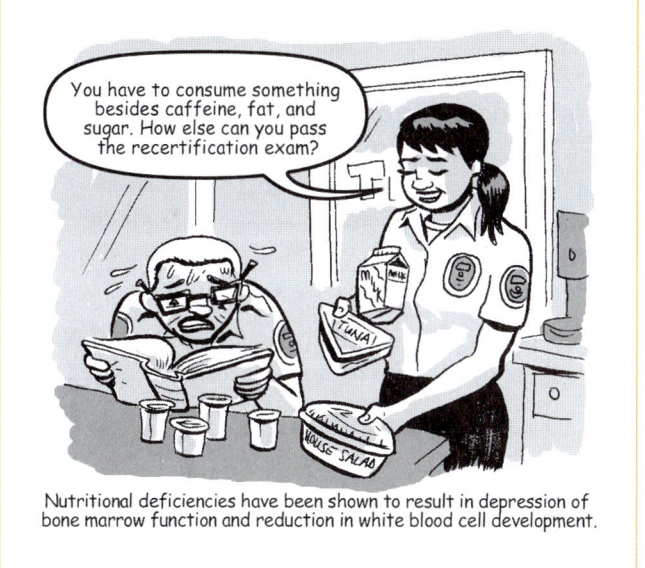

Nutritional deficiencies have been shown to result in depression of bone marrow function and reduction in white blood cell development.

Figure 6-34

its potential for adverse effects. In addition, idiosyncratic reactions to antibiotics may result in bone marrow suppression, as is the case with chemotherapeutic drugs for cancer. Many cases of bone marrow suppression in cancer are direct and predictable side effects of chemotherapy, and not true idiosyncratic, "out of the blue" reactions.

Physical or mental stress has been shown to decrease white blood cell and lymphocyte function. It may also lead to decreased production of various antibodies.

AIDS is an immunodeficiency disease that is caused by the RNA retrovirus HIV (human immunodeficiency virus). HIV binds to the CD4 surface protein of helper T cells, infects these cells, and kills them. Their destruction causes decreased humoural and cell-mediated reactions.

Treatment of Immunodeficiencies

Replacement therapy is available for some types of immunodeficiencies (eg, common variable immunodeficiency). Intravenous gamma globulin has been used in the therapy of a number of immunologic disorders of the nervous system, especially myasthenia gravis and inflammatory neuropathies, with considerable success. Bone marrow transplantation may restore immune competence in persons with acquired causes of immunodeficiency, such as following chemotherapy for cancer. In the future, gene therapy may be useful for treatment of both congenital and acquired causes of immunodeficiency.

Stress and Disease

Stress is the medical term for a wide range of strong external stimuli, both physiologic and psychological, that can cause a physiologic response. Usually, the response to stress is appropriate and beneficial. However, an unchecked stress response can result in deleterious outcomes, including chemical dependency, heart attack, stroke, depression, headache, and abdominal pain.

General Adaptation Syndrome

The general adaptation syndrome, a term introduced by Hans Selye in the 1920s, characterizes a three-stage reaction to stressors, both physical (eg, injury) and emotional (eg, loss of a loved one).

Stage 1: Alarm

The body reacts to stress first by releasing catecholamines, chemical compounds derived from the amino acid tyrosine that act as hormones or neurotransmitters. They are produced mainly from the adrenal medulla and the postganglionic fibres of the sympathetic nervous system. Catecholamines are soluble, so they circulate dissolved in blood. The most abundant catecholamines are epinephrine (adrenaline), norepinephrine (noradrenaline), and dopamine. Adrenaline acts as a neurotransmitter in the CNS and as a hormone in the blood. Noradrenaline is primarily a neurotransmitter of the peripheral sympathetic nervous system but is also present in the blood (mostly through "spillover" from the synapses of the sympathetic system).

Normally, the "fight-or-flight" response that occurs in the alarm reaction prepares the body to deal with stress, but it can also weaken the immune system, leading to infection.

Stage 2: Resistance

Stage 2, the resistance stage, is the body's way of adapting to stressors. It does so primarily by stimulating the adrenal gland to secrete two types of corticosteroid hormones that increase the blood glucose level and maintain blood pressure: glucocorticoids and mineralocorticoids. The most significant glucocorticoid in the body is cortisol, which controls carbohydrate, fat, and protein metabolism. Cortisol also has potent anti-inflammatory actions. Mineralocorticoids (predominantly aldosterone) control electrolyte and water levels in the body, mainly by promoting sodium retention by the kidney.

Continuation of stress and accompanying corticosteroid release eventually leads to fatigue, lapses in concentration, irritability, and lethargy.

Stage 3: Exhaustion

After a long period of stress, the person enters the exhaustion stage. The adrenal glands become depleted, leading to decreased blood glucose levels. The result is decreased stress tolerance, progressive mental and physical exhaustion, illness, and collapse. At this point, the body's immune system is compromised, significantly reducing a person's ability to resist disease. Heart attack, high blood pressure, or severe infection may result.

Effects of Chronic Stress

The hypothalamic-pituitary-adrenal axis (HPA axis) is a major part of the neuroendocrine system that controls reactions to stress. The HPA axis triggers a set of interactions among the glands, hormones, and parts of the midbrain that mediate the general adaptation syndrome. Continued stress, however, leads to loss of these normal control mechanisms. As a result, the adrenals continue to produce cortisol, which exhausts the stress mechanism and leads to fatigue and depression. Cortisol also interferes with serotonin activity, furthering the depressive effect.

Consistently high cortisol levels lead to suppression of the immune system through increased production of interleukin-6, an immune system messenger. Not surprisingly, then, research indicates that stress and depression have a negative effect on the immune system. Reduced immunity renders the body more susceptible to everything from colds and flu to cancer. For example, the incidence of serious illness, including cancer, is significantly higher among people who have suffered the death of a spouse in the previous year. Although severe, prolonged stress does not cause death directly, it does cause the body to lose its ability to fight disease in its effort to manage the stress. Stress also causes the body to release fat and cholesterol into the bloodstream, which in turn leads to clogging of the arteries and may eventually result in heart attack or stroke.

Many people start drinking alcohol to excess to combat their stress. Other manifestations of chronic stress include depression, headaches, insomnia, ulcers, and asthma. Fortunately, this immune suppression process can be corrected with psychotherapy, medication, or any number of other positive influences that restore hope and a feeling of self-esteem. The ability of human beings to recover from adversity is remarkable.

You are the Paramedic Summary

1. What are some of the potential complications that can occur from missing dialysis?

Patients who have end-stage renal disease depend on dialysis to take on the workload of the kidneys, such as being a filter for toxins and maintaining proper fluid balance and electrolyte balance. An interruption in these vital functions can lead to the development of problems such as congestive heart failure, myocardial infarction, pulmonary edema, arrhythmias, electrolyte imbalances, and medication toxicity.

2. Does renal disease affect other organ systems?

Yes; all organ systems are affected by renal failure. Patients can develop problems similar to those experienced by diabetics and patients with hypertension. For example, patients with renal disease often develop problems with peripheral neuropathy, gastrointestinal disturbances, and anemia.

3. What should you monitor your patient for?

The patient is presenting with a number of issues, any of which could potentially lead to problems. First and foremost, she is hypotensive and in respiratory distress. You need to keep a watchful eye on her blood pressure and respiratory status, being prepared to intubate if necessary. The tall T waves on the ECG are characteristic of hyperkalemia. The heart does not play nice in an environment in which the potassium is out of line. Frequently check the monitor for the development of ventricular arrhythmias such as premature ventricular contractions, ventricular tachycardia, and ventricular fibrillation.

4. Which interventions should you consider at this point, if any?

At this point, Mrs. Jensen is receiving high-flow supplemental oxygen. The patient definitely requires cardiac monitoring and intravenous access for possible fluid and medication administration.

5. Is the patient going into shock? If so, what type?

Yes; the patient is going into shock, but which type can be a little tricky. We know from her clinical presentation that septic shock is a possibility due to the signs of infection at the shunt site. With a history of a past myocardial infarction and congestive heart failure, cardiogenic shock cannot be ruled out as a possible cause.

6. Why is a fluid bolus appropriate in this setting?

Hypotension is a common side effect of dialysis that can result from the change in fluid and/or electrolyte distribution. Most patients will respond favourably to a small fluid bolus (200 to 250 ml) returning fluid back to the blood vessels. This small amount of fluid should not have a negative effect in the respiratory status of your patient.

7. How did the inflammatory process manifest itself in this patient?

The inflammatory process manifested itself in both local and systemic effects. Local effects include the development of redness, swelling, tenderness, and heat at the shunt site. Systemic involvement of the inflammatory process is seen in the presence of fever.

8. What are other signs and symptoms of hyperkalemia?

Patient's who have hyperkalemia may also present with irritability, abdominal distention, nausea, diarrhea, oliguria, weakness, or paralysis. Good history taking will help you clue into this serious electrolyte imbalance and initiate therapy!

Prep Kit

■ Ready for Review

- All cells except red blood cells and platelets have three main components: a nucleus, cytoplasm, and a cell membrane.
- There are four major tissue types: epithelial tissue; connective tissue, muscle tissue, and nervous tissue.
- When cells are exposed to adverse conditions, they go through a process of adaptation (which can be temporary or permanent) to protect themselves from injury. Examples of adaptations include atrophy, hypertrophy, hyperplasia, dysplasia, and metaplasia.
- The cellular environment refers to the distribution of cells, molecules, and fluids throughout the body. It changes with aging, exercise, pregnancy, medications, disease, and injury. Body fluids contain water, sodium, chloride, potassium, calcium, phosphorous, and magnesium.
- pH is a measurement of hydrogen ion concentration. Normal body functions depend on an acid–base balance that remains within the normal physiologic pH range of 7.35 to 7.45.
- Cellular injury results from causes such as chemical exposure, infectious agents, immunologic responses, inflammatory responses, prolonged periods of hypoxia, genetic factors, nutritional imbalances, and physical agents.
- Age- and sex-associated factors interact with a combination of genetic and environmental factors, lifestyle, and anatomical or hormonal differences to cause disease.
- Analyzing disease risk involves consideration of disease rates (incidence, prevalence, mortality) and disease risk factors (causal and noncausal). These risk factors, age, and sex differences interact to influence an individual's level of risk.
- A true genetic risk is passed through generations on a gene. In contrast, a familial tendency may "cluster" in family groups despite lack of evidence for heritable gene-associated abnormalities. In autosomal dominant inheritance, a person needs to inherit only one copy of a particular form of a gene to show that trait. In autosomal recessive inheritance, the person must inherit two copies of a particular form of a gene to show the trait.
- Immunologic diseases occur because of hyperactivity or hypoactivity of the immune system. Allergies are acquired following initial exposure to a stimulant, known as an allergen. Repeated exposures cause a reaction by the immune system to the allergen.
- Perfusion is the delivery of oxygen and nutrients to cells, organs, and tissues through the circulatory system. Hypoperfusion occurs when the level of tissue perfusion falls below normal.
- Shock is an abnormal state associated with inadequate oxygen and nutrient delivery to the metabolic apparatus of the cell, resulting in an impairment of cell metabolism.
- Multiple organ dysfunction syndrome (MODS) is a progressive condition usually characterized by combined failure of several organs, such as the lungs, liver, and kidney, along with some clotting mechanisms. It occurs after severe illness or injury.
- The immune system includes all of the structures and processes that mount a defence against foreign substances and disease-causing agents. The body has three lines of defence: anatomical barriers, the inflammatory response, and the immune response.
- The immune system has two anatomical components: the lymphoid tissues of the body and the cells that are responsible for the immune response.
- The primary cells of the immune system are the white blood cells, or leukocytes.
- There are two general types of immune response: native and acquired.
- Immunity may be either humoural or cell-mediated.
- The antibodies secreted by B cells are called immunoglobulins. Antibodies make antigens more visible to the immune system in three ways: by acting as opsonins, by making antigens clump, and by inactivating bacterial toxins.
- The inflammatory response is a reaction of the tissues of the body, triggered by cellular injury, to irritation or injury that is characterized by pain, swelling, redness, and heat.
- The two most common causes of inflammation are infection and physical agents.
- Cytokines are products of cells that affect the functioning of other cells; they include interleukins, lymphokines, and interferon.
- Chronic inflammatory responses are usually caused by an unsuccessful acute inflammatory response after the invasion of a foreign body, persistent infection, or antigen.
- Normal wound healing involves four steps: repair of damaged tissue, removal of inflammatory debris, restoration of tissues to a normal state, and regeneration of cells.
- Wounds may heal by either primary or secondary intention.
- Hypersensitivity is an increased bodily response to any substance to which the person is abnormally sensitive. A hypersensitivity reaction may be immediate, occurring within seconds to minutes, or delayed, occurring hours to days after exposure to the antigen.
- Immunodeficiency may be congenital or acquired.
- Stress does not cause death directly, but it can permit diseases that ultimately lead to the patient's death to flourish.
- The general adaptation syndrome describes the body's short-term and long-term reactions to stress.

■ Vital Vocabulary

acidosis A blood pH of less than 7.35.

acquired immunity A highly specific, inducible, discriminatory, and permanent method by which literally armies of cells respond to an immune stimulant.

activation Mediators of inflammation trigger the appearance of molecules known as selectins and integrins on the surfaces of endothelial cells and PMNs, respectively.

active hyperemia The dilation of arterioles after transient arteriolar constriction, which allows influx of blood under increased pressure.

adhesion The attachment of PMNs to endothelial cells, mediated by selectins and integrins.

adipose tissue A connective tissue containing large amounts of lipids.

alkalosis A blood pH of greater than 7.45.

allergen Any substance that causes a hypersensitivity reaction.

allergy Hypersensitivity reaction to the presence of an agent (allergen) that is intrinsically harmless.

anaphylactic shock A severe hypersensitivity reaction that involves bronchoconstriction and cardiovascular collapse.

angiogenesis The growth of new blood vessels.

antibodies Proteins secreted by certain immune cells that bind antigens to make them more visible to the immune system.

antigen A foreign substance recognized by the immune system.

apoptosis Normal, genetically programmed cell death.

Arthus reaction A localized reaction involving vascular inflammation in response to an IgG-mediated allergic response.

asthma A chronic inflammatory lower airway condition resulting in intermittent wheezing and excess mucus production.

atopic The medical term for having an allergic tendency.

atrophy A decrease in cell size due to a loss of subcellular components.

autoantibodies Antibodies directed against the patient.

autocrine hormone A hormone that acts on the cell that has secreted it.

autoimmunity The production of antibodies or T cells that work against the tissues of a person's own body, producing autoimmune disease or a hypersensitivity reaction.

autosomal dominant A pattern of inheritance that involves genes that are located on autosomes or the nonsex chromosomes. You only need to inherit a single copy of a particular form of a gene to show the trait.

autosomal recessive A pattern of inheritance that involves genes located on autosomes or the nonsex chromosomes. You must inherit two copies of a particular form of a gene to show the trait.

axon Part of the neuron that conducts the impulses away from the cell body.

basophils Approximately 1% of the leukocytes, they are essential to nonspecific immune response to inflammation due to their role in releasing histamine and other chemicals that dilate blood vessels.

bone marrow Specialized tissue found within bone.

buffers Molecules that modulate changes in pH to keep it in the physiologic range.

capillary refill time A test done on the fingers or toes by briefly squeezing the toe or finger, then evaluating the time it takes for the pink colour to return.

cardiogenic shock A condition caused by loss of 40% or more of the functioning myocardium; the heart is no longer able to circulate sufficient blood to maintain adequate oxygen delivery.

cell-mediated immunity Immune process by which T-cell lymphocytes recognize antigens and then secrete cytokines (specifically lymphokines) that attract other cells or stimulate the production of cytotoxic cells that kill the infected cells.

cell signaling The process by which cells communicate with one another.

central shock A term that describes shock secondary to central pump failure, it includes both cardiogenic shock and obstructive shock.

chemotaxins Components of the activated complement system that attract leukocytes from the circulation to help fight infections.

chemotaxis The movement of additional white blood cells to an area of inflammation in response to the release of chemical mediators, such as neutrophils, injured tissue, and monocytes.

coagulation system The system that forms blood clots in the body and facilitates repairs to the vascular tree.

complement system A group of plasma proteins whose function is to do one of three things: attract leukocytes to sites of inflammation, activate leukocytes, and directly destroy cells.

connective tissue Tissue that serves to bind various tissue types together.

cytokines Products of cells that affect the function of other cells.

dendrites Part of the neuron that receives impulses from the axon and contains vesicles for release of neurotransmitters.

distributive shock Occurs when there is widespread dilation of the resistance vessels (small arterioles), the capacitance vessels (small venules), or both.

dysplasia An alteration in the size, shape, and organization of cells.

endocrine hormones Hormones that are carried to their target or cell group in the bloodstream.

endothelial cells Specific types of epithelial cells that serve the function of lining the blood vessels.

eosinophils Cells that make up approximately 1% to 3% of the leukocytes, which play a major role in allergic reactions and bronchoconstriction in an asthma attack.

epithelium Type of tissue that covers all external surfaces of the body.

etiology The cause of a disease process.

exocrine hormones Hormones that are secreted through ducts into an organ or onto epithelial surfaces.

feedback inhibition Negative feedback resulting in the decrease of an action in the body.

fibrin A whitish, filamentous protein formed by the action of thrombin on fibrinogen. Fibrin is the protein that polymerizes (bonds) to form the fibrous component of a blood clot.

fibrinolysis cascade The breakdown of fibrin in blood clots, and the prevention of the polymerization of fibrin into new clots.

free radicals Molecules that are missing one electron in their outer shell.

general adaptation syndrome A three-stage description of the body's short-term and long-term reactions to stress.

gut-associated lymphoid tissue (GALT) The lymphoid tissue that lies under the inner lining of the esophagus and intestines.

hapten A substance that normally does not stimulate an immune response but can be combined with an antigen and at a later point initiate an antibody response.

helper T cells A type of T lymphocyte that is involved in both cell-mediated and antibody-mediated immune responses. It secretes cytokines that stimulate the B cells and other T cells.

hemochromatosis An inherited disease in which the body absorbs more iron than it needs and stores it in the liver, kidneys, and pancreas.

hemolytic anemia A disease characterized by increased destruction of the red blood cells. It can occur from an Rh factor reaction, exposure to chemicals, or a disorder of the immune system.

hemophilia An inherited sex-linked disorder characterized by excessive bleeding.

histamine A vasoactive amine that increases vascular permeability and causes vasodilation.

homeostasis is a term derived from the Greek words for "same" and "steady." All organisms constantly adjust their physiologic processes in an effort to maintain an internal balance.

hormones Proteins formed in specialized organs or glands and carried to another organ or group of cells in the same organism. Hormones regulate many body functions, including metabolism, growth, and temperature.

humoural immunity The immunity that utilizes antibodies made by B-cell lymphocytes.

hypercalcemia A condition in which calcium levels are elevated.

hypercholesterolemia An elevated blood cholesterol level.

hyperkalemia An elevated blood serum potassium level.

hypermagnesemia An increased serum magnesium level.

hypernatremia A blood serum sodium level greater than 148 mmol/l and a serum osmolarity greater than 295 mOsm/kg.

hyperphosphatemia An elevated blood serum phosphate level.

hyperplasia An increase in the actual number of cells in an organ or tissue, usually resulting in an increase in size of the organ or tissue.

hypersensitivity A generic term for bodily responses to a substance to which a patient is abnormally sensitive.

hypertonic solution A solution with an osmolarity greater than intracellular fluid.

hypertrophy An increase in the size of the cells due to synthesis of more subcellular components, leading to an increase in tissue and organ size.

hypocalcemia A decreased serum calcium level.

hypokalemia A decreased blood serum potassium.

hypomagnesemia A decreased serum magnesium level.

hyponatremia A blood serum sodium level that is less than 135 mmol/l and a serum osmolarity that is less than 280 mOsm/kg.

hypoperfusion A condition that occurs when the level of tissue perfusion decreases below that needed to maintain normal cellular functions.

hypophosphatemia A decreased blood serum phosphate level.

hypothalamic-pituitary-adrenal (HPA) axis A major part of the neuroendocrine system that controls reactions to stress. It is the mechanism for a set of interactions among glands, hormones, and parts of the midbrain that mediate the general adaptation syndrome.

hypotonic solution A solution with an osmolarity lower than intracellular fluid.

hypovolemic shock A condition that occurs when the circulating blood volume is inadequate to deliver adequate oxygen and nutrients to the body.

immune response The body's defence reaction to any substance that is recognized as foreign.

immune system The body system that includes all of the structures and processes designed to mount a defence against foreign substances and disease-causing agents.

immunodeficiency An abnormal condition in which some part of the body's immune system is inadequate, and consequently resistance to infectious disease is decreased.

immunogen An antigen that activates immune cells to generate an immune response against itself.

immunoglobulins Antibodies secreted by the B cells.

incidence The frequency with which a disease occurs.

inflammatory response A reaction by tissues of the body to irritation or injury, characterized by pain, swelling, redness, and heat.

interferon Protein produced by cells in response to viral invasion. Interferon is released into the bloodstream or intercellular fluid to induce healthy cells to manufacture an enzyme that counters the infection.

interleukins Chemical substances that attract white blood cells to the sites of injury and bacterial invasion.

isoimmunity Formation of antibodies or T cells that are directed against antigens or another person's cells.

isotonic solution A solution with the same osmolarity as intracellular fluid (280 mOsm/l).

kinin system A general term for a group of polypeptides that mediate inflammatory responses by stimulating visceral smooth muscle and relaxing vascular smooth muscle to produce vasodilation.

leukocytes The white blood cells responsible for fighting off infection.

leukotrienes Arachidonic acid metabolites that function as chemical mediators of inflammation. Also known as slow-reacting substances of anaphylaxis (SRS-A).

ligand Any molecule that binds a receptor leading to a reaction.

lymph A thin, watery fluid that bathes the tissues of the body.

lymphatic system A network of capillaries, vessels, ducts, nodes, and organs that helps to maintain the fluid environment of the body by producing lymph and transporting it through the body.

lymphocytes The white blood cells responsible for a large part of the body's immune protection.

lymphokines Cytokines released by lymphocytes, including many of the interleukins, gamma interferon, tumour necrosis factor beta, and chemokines.

macrophages Cells that developed from the monocytes that provide the body's first line of defence in the inflammatory process.

margination Loss of fluid from the blood vessels into the tissue, causing the blood left in the vessels to have an increased viscosity, which in turn slows the flow of blood and produces stasis.

mast cells The cells that resemble basophils but do not circulate in the blood. Mast cells play a role in allergic reactions, immunity, and wound healing.

membrane attack complex (MAC) Molecules that insert themselves into the bacterial membrane, leading to weakened areas in the membrane.

metaplasia A reversible, cellular adaptation in which one adult cell type is replaced by another adult cell type.

mitochondria The metabolic centre or powerhouse of the cell. They are small and rod-shaped organelles.

monocytes Mononuclear phagocytic white blood cells derived from myeloid stem cells. They circulate in the bloodstream for about 24 hours and then move into tissues to mature into macrophages.

mortality The number of deaths from a disease in a given population.

mucosal-associated lymphoid tissue (MALT) The lymphoid tissue associated with the skin and the respiratory, urinary, and reproductive traits as well as the tonsils.

multiple organ dysfunction syndrome (MODS) A progressive condition usually characterized by combined failure of several organs, such as the lungs, liver, and kidney, along with some clotting mechanisms, which occurs after severe illness or injury.

native immunity A nonspecific cellular and humoural response that operates as the body's first line of defence against pathogens.

negative feedback The concept that once the desired effect of a process has been achieved, further action is inhibited until it is needed again; also called feedback inhibition.

neurogenic shock This condition usually results from spinal cord injury. The effect is loss of normal sympathetic nervous system tone and vasodilation.

neurotransmitters Proteins that transmit signals between cells of the nervous system.

neutrophils Cells that make up approximately 55% to 70% of the leukocytes responsible in large part for the body's protection against infection. They are readily attracted by foreign antigens and destroy them by phagocytosis.

nucleus A cellular organelle that contains the genetic information. The nucleus controls the function and structure of a cell.

obstructive shock This occurs when there is a block to blood flow in the heart or great vessels.

oliguria Decreased urine output.

opsoninization Occurs when an antibody coats an antigen to facilitate its recognition by immune cells.

organelles Internal cellular structures that carry out specific functions for the cell.

osmosis The movement of water down its concentration gradient across a membrane.

paracrine hormones Hormones that diffuse through intracellular spaces to their target.

pathophysiology The study of how normal physiologic processes are affected by disease.

perfusion The delivery of oxygen and nutrients to the cells, organs, and tissues of the body. Also involves the removal of wastes.

pericardial tamponade Impairment of diastolic filling of the right ventricle due to significant amounts of fluid in the pericardial sac surrounding the heart, leading to a decrease in the cardiac output.

peripheral nerves All of the nerves of the body extending from the brain and spinal cord.

peripheral shock A term that describes shock secondary to peripheral circulatory abnormalities—includes both hypovolemic shock and distributive shock.

pH The measure of acidity or alkalinity of a solution.

phagocyte A kind of cell that engulfs and consumes foreign material such as microorganisms and debris.

phagocytosis Process in which one cell eats or engulfs a foreign substance to destroy it.

polymorphonuclear neutrophils (PMNs) A type of white blood cell formed by bone marrow tissue that possesses a nucleus consisting of several parts or lobes connected by fine strands; a variety of leukocyte.

polyuria Frequent and plentiful urination.

prevalence The number of cases of a disease in a specific population over time.

prostaglandins A group of lipids that act as chemical messengers.

pyrogens Chemicals or proteins that travel to the brain and affect the hypothalamus, and stimulate a rise in the body's core temperature.

renin-angiotensin-aldosterone system (RAAS) A complex feedback mechanism responsible for the kidney's regulation of sodium in the body.

Rh factor An antigen present in the erythrocytes (red blood cells) of about 85% of people.

ribonucleic acid (RNA) Nucleic acid associated with controlling cellular activities.

septic shock This occurs as a result of widespread infection, usually bacterial. Untreated, the result is multiple organ dysfunction syndrome (MODS) and often death.

serotonin A vasoactive amine that increases vascular permeability to cause vasodilation.

serum sickness A condition in which antigen antibody complexes formed in the bloodstream deposit in sites around the body, most notably in the kidney, with resultant inflammatory reactions.

slow-reacting substances of anaphylaxis (SRS-A) Biologically active compounds derived from arachidonic acid called leukotrienes.

T killer cells Cells released during a type IV allergic reaction that kill antigen-bearing target cells.

tonicity Tension exerted on a cell due to water movement across the cell membrane.

transmigration (diapedesis) The PMNs permeate through the vessel wall, moving into the interstitial space.

urticaria Multiple small, raised areas on the skin that may be one of the warning signs of impending anaphylaxis. Also known as hives.

vasculitis An inflammation of the blood vessels.

vasoactive amines Substances such as histamine and serotonin that increase vascular permeability.

virulence A measure of the disease-causing ability of a microorganism.

Points to Ponder

You have a new partner for the day and you respond to a "difficulty breathing" call. Once there, your patient advises that he has an "autoimmune disease." Your partner leans over to you and says quietly, "Oh no, this guy has AIDS and we're going to get it."

How are you going to explain this patient's medical condition to your partner without doing so in front of your patient?

Issues: Bloodborne Pathogens, Autoimmune Diseases, Universal Precautions.

Assessment in Action

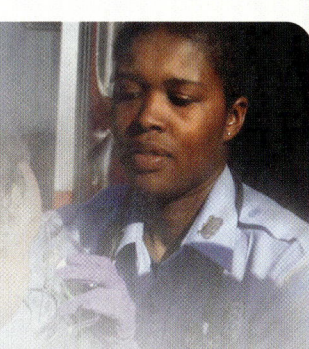

You have responded to a 40-year-old male patient who crashed on his motorcycle. The patient is wearing a helmet and is conscious but agitated and restless. You notice a large amount of blood on the ground around the patient's lower body. As you complete your assessment, you find the patient has an unstable pelvis and an open femur fracture. Your initial vital signs are blood pressure, 136/70 mm Hg; pulse, 100 beats/min; and respiration, 16 breaths/min. You know your patient has lost a considerable amount of blood and are concerned the patient may start exhibiting signs of shock.

1. **What are the two types of shock?**
   A. Arterial and venous
   B. Central and peripheral
   C. Hypovolemic and systemic
   D. Peripheral and distributive

2. **What type of shock involves fluid loss?**
   A. Anaphylactic
   B. Cardiogenic
   C. Hypovolemic
   D. Septic

3. **What are the two types of hypovolemic shock and which one is exhibited by this patient?**
   A. Exogenous and endogenous
   B. Aerobic and anaerobic
   C. Kallikrein and kinin
   D. Angiotensin and aldosterone

4. **Based on your assessment of this patient, his agitation, anxiety, and restlessness may be a sign of:**
   A. decompensated shock.
   B. compensated shock.
   C. neurogenic shock.
   D. distributive shock.

5. **Which adult blood pressure reading would represent decompensated shock?**
   A. The systolic blood pressure is greater than 5% for the age range.
   B. The systolic blood pressure is less than 5% for the age range.
   C. The diastolic blood pressure is greater than 5% for the age range.
   D. The diastolic blood pressure is less than 5% for the age range.

6. **A normal capillary refill time should be:**
   A. more than 4 seconds.
   B. 3 to 4 seconds.
   C. greater than 2 seconds.
   D. less than 2 seconds.

Challenging Question

7. **Your unit has a pair of MAST (military antishock trousers) in the inventory. Since your patient has an obvious pelvic injury and a decompensated blood pressure, should you use them?**

7 Pharmacology

Competency Areas

Area 4: Assessment and Diagnostics

4.2.a   Obtain list of patient's allergies.
4.2.b   Obtain list of patient's medications.

Area 5: Therapeutics

5.8.a   Recognize principles of pharmacology as applied to the medications listed in Appendix 5.
5.8.b   Follow safe process for responsible medication administration.

Appendix 5: Medications

A.   **Medications affecting the central nervous system.**
A.1   Opioid Antagonists
A.2   Anaesthetics
A.3   Anticonvulsants
A.5   Anxiolytics, Hypnotics, and Antagonists
A.7   Non-narcotic Analgesics
A.8   Opioid Analgesics
A.9   Paralytics

B.   **Medications affecting the autonomic nervous system.**
B.1   Adrenergic Agonists
B.2   Adrenergic Antagonists
B.3   Cholinergic Agonists
B.4   Cholinergic Antagonists

C.   **Medications affecting the respiratory system.**
C.1   Bronchodilators

D.   **Medications affecting the cardiovascular system.**
D.1   Antihypertensive Agents
D.2   Cardiac Glycosides
D.3   Diuretics
D.4   Class 1 Antidysrhythmics
D.5   Class 2 Antidysrhythmics
D.6   Class 3 Antidysrhythmics
D.7   Class 4 Antidysrhythmics
D.8   Antianginal Agents

E.   **Medications affecting blood clotting mechanisms.**
E.1   Anticoagulants
E.2   Thrombolytics
E.3   Platelet Inhibitors

F.   **Medications affecting the gastrointestinal system.**
F.1   Antiemetics

G.   **Medications affecting labour, delivery, and postpartum hemorrhage.**
G.1   Uterotonics
G.2   Tocolytics

H.   **Medications used to treat electrolyte and substrate imbalances.**
H.1   Vitamin and Electrolyte Supplements
H.2   Antihypoglycemic Agents

I.   **Medications used to treat/prevent inflammatory responses and infections.**
I.1   Corticosteroids
I.2   NSAIDs
I.3   Antibiotics
I.4   Immunizations

J.   **Medications used to treat poisoning and overdose.**
J.1   Antidotes or Neutralizing Agents

Introduction

The word *pharmacology* comes from the Greek words *pharmakon* (meaning "drug" or "poison") and *logos* (meaning "word" or "discourse"). The goal of emergency pharmacology in the prehospital setting is to use medications to reverse, prevent, or control various diseases and illnesses, chronic and acute. To achieve this goal, prehospital providers must be able to interpret a patient's history and physical findings, formulate a management plan, and incorporate appropriate treatment modalities, including pharmacology and medication administration. Medication errors are the leading cause of patient safety errors in health care. For this reason, medications must always be delivered according to the *six rights:* the Right patient, the Right medication, the Right dose, the Right route, the Right time, and the Right patient care report (PCR) documentation (Table 7-1 ▶). This chapter will aid you in understanding the medications used to treat specific medical problems, how they are administered to achieve therapeutic and nontoxic levels, and their actions, absorption, and elimination, while keeping in mind the six rights of medication administration.

All medications are poisons if they are given to the wrong patient or in toxic quantities. For this reason, paramedics and health care personnel must have a strong understanding of pharmacology and use great caution when administering medications to patients. In this chapter, the drugs and doses mentioned comply with nationally accepted guidelines. Paramedics must become familiar with the specific medications, uses, and doses that are used in their systems as approved by the medical director. The medications discussed in this chapter may not be administered without authorization of medical direction through approved standing orders or by direct verbal communication with an authorized direct medical control physician.

Historical Trends in Pharmacology

The use of chemical compounds to treat illnesses is an ancient practice. Records of medication use date back thousands of years from the use of plants and minerals to today's modern and ever-changing methods of synthetic and laboratory-engineered medications. The study of medications and their effect or actions on the body is called pharmacology.

Ancient Health Care

Ancient Egyptian health care was heavily influenced by spiritual beliefs. It did, however, incorporate basic first-aid techniques to treat obvious external injuries. Ancient doctors also used chemical compounds to treat certain ailments. In fact, documents have been found containing formularies for more than 700 medications.

The Pre-Renaissance and Post-Renaissance Periods

During the medieval period, doctors had no concept of viruses or bacteria or their infectious properties. It was believed that sickness represented punishment for one's sins. Attempts to treat ailments centered on approaches intended to counteract the presenting symptoms. Presenting symptoms were categorized based on their moisture and temperature: Blood was hot and wet, phlegm was cold and wet, black bile was cold and dry, and yellow bile was hot and dry. According to the prevailing theory of the time, based on the ancient four humours theory of the Greek physician Hippocrates (460–370 BC), when a person became sick, one of these four items was out of balance. Phlegm, for example, needed to be counteracted by its opposite, yellow bile. Therefore, the patient would need to take a

You are the Paramedic Part 1

You and your partner are on your way back to the station when you are called to an assisted-living facility for an unknown medical. Upon arrival, you are met in the lobby by the patient's son, who brings you back to the apartment. The door to the apartment is open when you get there, and you see an older man sitting on a recliner in the living room. As you approach him and introduce yourself, you note that he is pale and slightly diaphoretic. He tells you that he has been feeling "skips in his chest" for the past couple of hours and that he becomes extremely lightheaded when he stands. He also says he feels "a little winded" and states that his vision "is off." He denies having any chest pain, headaches, or any other symptoms. He states that he takes heart medications but cannot recall what they are. His son recalls that his father keeps a list of his medications and medical history on an index card in his wallet.

Initial Assessment	Recording Time: 0 Minutes
Appearance	Awake and ill-appearing
Level of consciousness	A (Alert to person, place and day)
Airway	Open and clear
Breathing	Slightly elevated rate with adequate chest rise and volume
Circulation	Weak, irregular radial pulses with pale, cool, moist skin

1. What are some potential differential diagnoses?
2. What types of medications might your patient be taking?

Table 7-1	**The Six Rights of Medication Administration**

1. Right patient

Although you will typically treat one patient at a time, sometimes you may have to manage multiple patients. It is critical to confirm the identity of a patient before administering any medication—especially when patients are unconscious or are unable to communicate (because of extremes of age, altered consciousness, or other factors). Always make an attempt to have the patient confirm his or her identity verbally, or confirm the identity of the patient yourself through identification devices (bracelets, ID cards). A critical issue, as identified in your SAMPLE history, is to ensure that the patient does not have allergies to the medication(s) you intend to give **Figure 7-1 ▶** .

2. Right medication

Administration of the wrong medication is the most common medication-related error. Several factors may lead to "wrong medication" errors, including similar labelling and packaging, similar names and storage practices, and poor communication. Always repeat back (echo) the medication order, and confirm that the packaging matches the intended order. Avoid using abbreviations, verify the route of administration, and always recheck the order before administration.

3. Right dose

Dosages of nearly every medication depend on patient-specific factors (such as medical condition, weight, age); the actual dosage called for is often not equal to the amount supplied in an ampoule or prefilled syringe in the prehospital setting. Therefore, you will have to calculate the patient's specific dose from the supplied medication, and determine how to dilute, mix, or reconstitute it properly prior to administration. When calculating the correct dose, always recheck your math and, if possible, have your partner recheck and verify the final dose.

4. Right route

Many medications can be administered by a variety of routes; the optimal route depends on the patient's condition and the speed with which the medication needs to take effect. Errors can occur when medication doses and routes are confused. For example, intravenous (IV) drip doses can be different concentrations than the same medication injected into an IV as a bolus. Another important route-related issue is the patient's condition. If a patient is in profound shock, you must consider how well the medication will be absorbed and distributed to target tissues. Choosing the right route makes a big difference in allowing the medication to have the correct effect.

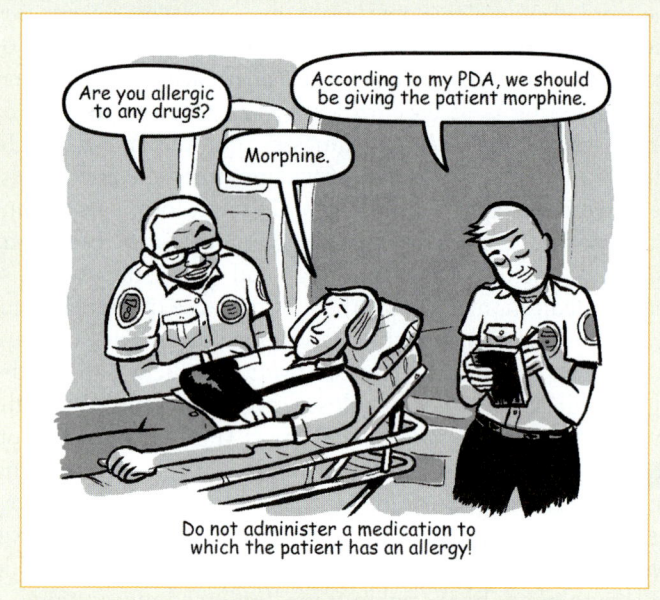

Do not administer a medication to which the patient has an allergy!

Figure 7-1

5. Right time

Because all medications take a certain amount of time to take effect and may have the potential to interfere with other medications, you must always follow the recommended guidelines for the proper frequency of medication administration. Evaluate the patient's condition and vital signs before and after you administer any medication, and document any noted response or change in the patient's condition. Also remember that some medications require a specific administration frequency to maintain a therapeutic level.

6. Right documentation and reporting

Because paramedics frequently transfer care of a patient to other health care providers, it is critical to document in writing the medications administered, specifically, the dose, including route and time when they were administered, and what kinds of changes the patient has experienced, if any. Whenever possible, communicate this information in writing, on the PCR, and in a verbal report to the next level of care.

---

prescription made from plants and animals that were hot and dry and likely contained a fair amount of bile. After the Renaissance, medication use took on a slightly more scientific approach. Through the process of observation, early health care providers began to recognize—albeit to a limited extent—that certain compounds (such as plants and minerals) were effective for treating some ailments and ineffective for others. For example, opium, the raw substance collected from certain poppies (*Papaver somniferum*) was known to reduce pain and induce sleep. In 1805, the German chemist Friedrich Sertürner isolated morphine as the active ingredient from the raw substance.

Modern Health Care

The modern pharmaceutical industry began in the 19th century with the discovery of highly active medicinal compounds that could be manufactured most efficiently on a large scale. Today, pharmaceuticals form the basis of a billion dollar industry. Thanks to the thousands of <u>drugs</u> currently in use and the new drugs approved on a daily basis, health care has made tremendous strides in our ability to care for sick and injured people. Although not every condition has a cure, virtually all diseases can be treated to some degree with medications.

Pharmaceuticals can be expected to continue to make great strides in all aspects of disease treatment. As cancer rates continue to rise, treatments and cures for this set of diseases are the focus of much research. Remarkable progress continues to be made in the prevention and treatment of heart disease and stroke. The pharmaceutical industry is likely to continue expanding into biotechnology, including the use of compounds to target specific proteins or DNA. Ideally, work on the molecular level will lead to the eradication of some of the leading killers of today.

Medication Names

A medication is a drug that has been approved by the government agency that regulates pharmaceuticals. In Canada, that agency is the Health Products and Food Branch (HPFB). The Food and Drugs Act (FDA) is the applicable legislation that ensures public safety with regard to medications. A *drug*, as defined by Health Canada, is any substance or mixture of substances manufactured, sold, or represented for use in (a) the diagnosis, treatment, mitigation, or prevention of a disease, disorder, or abnormal physical state or its symptoms, in human beings or animals; (b) restoring, correcting, or modifying organic functions in human beings or animals; or (c) disinfection in premises in which food is manufactured, prepared, or kept.

Medications may be available either with or without a prescription. Prescription-only medicines (POM) are available at a pharmacy and may be purchased only with a prescription from a physician or other health care professional with the ability to prescribe, such as a dentist or nurse practitioner. In contrast, over-the-counter (OTC) medications do not require a prescription and are available in many places—pharmacies, convenience stores, and grocery stores, for example—without special restrictions. Prescription-only medicines can be given OTC status only if they are considered safe enough that most people will not hurt themselves accidentally by taking the medication as instructed.

Pharmaceutical companies invest billions of dollars each year in research and development. Not surprisingly, they are eager to protect their investments by obtaining patents on their new drugs. A patent gives its holder exclusive rights to produce and sell the drug until the patent expires. After it loses its patent, the medication may then be available as a generic drug (nonpatented) from multiple sources.

Because thousands of medications are already on the market and more emerge every year (hundreds are approved each year in Canada alone), a systematic way of naming them is essential. All medications are assigned three names: chemical, generic, and trade.

- The chemical name describes the drug's chemical makeup—that is, its composition and molecular structure.
- The generic name (or nonproprietary name) is a general name for a drug. Although it is not manufacturer-specific, the generic name is usually created by the company that first manufactures the chemical. The generic name is generally derived from the chemical name but is shorter and simpler. In the 1950s, the World Health Organization

(WHO) initiated the International Nonproprietary Name (INN) Program to standardize generic drug names. Health Canada provides final approval of drug names eligible to be used in Canada.

- The trade name (or brand name) is the unique name under which the original manufacturer registers the new drug with the HPFB. Use of the "registered" symbol (®) in the upper-right corner of the trade name indicates that it has been registered as a trademark; a trade name may also be identified by capitalizing the name. If a given drug is marketed by a number of manufacturers, it may have several trade names. Some familiar trade names include Lipitor (a cholesterol-lowering medication), Reactine (used to treat common allergies), and Xanax (used to treat anxiety disorders).

To see how this naming system works, consider the names given to amiodarone, an important antidysrhythmic carried by paramedics:

- Chemical name: 2-butyl-3-benzofuranyl 4-[2-(diethylamino)-ethoxy]-3,5-diiodophenyl ketone hydrochloride
- Generic name: amiodarone
- Trade names: Cordarone

In this text, we will refer to drugs by their generic names. When a drug is widely known by its trade name, the trade name will be capitalized and placed in parentheses in this text after the generic name—for example, diazepam (Valium), norepinephrine (Levophed), furosemide (Lasix), naloxone (Narcan), and oxytocin (Pitocin).

Sources of Drugs

The drugs we use are derived from four principal sources: animal, plant, mineral, and synthetic compounds Figure 7-2 ▸ . Plant sources of drugs include a variety of roots, leaves, flowers, and seeds. For example, digitalis, which is used in the treatment of heart failure, is prepared from the dried leaves of a wildflower called purple foxglove. In contrast, insulin, a medication taken by diabetics, is usually prepared from the pancreas of animals (primarily pigs). Armour, a thyroid medication, is derived from desiccated pig thyroid. Minerals used in the treatment of medical problems include calcium, iron, and magnesium. Drugs that are manufactured synthetically include synthetic forms of vitamins, steroids, narcotics, and many others.

Sources of Drug Information

In addition to standard continuing education, you should stay abreast of newly approved medications and current research. Drug information may be obtained from many sources, many of which are available in print and electronic formats. Table 7-2 ▸ discusses some of the most up-to-date and reliable resources.

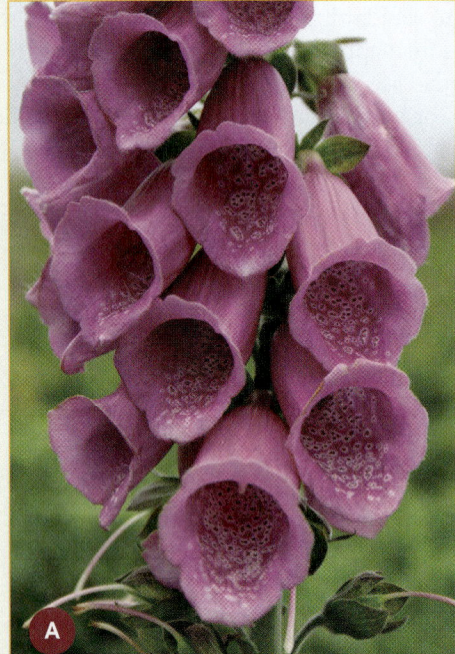
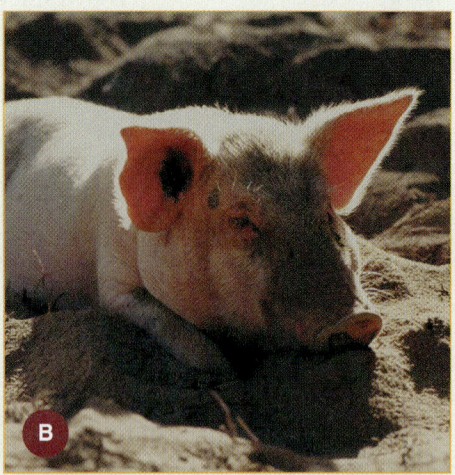
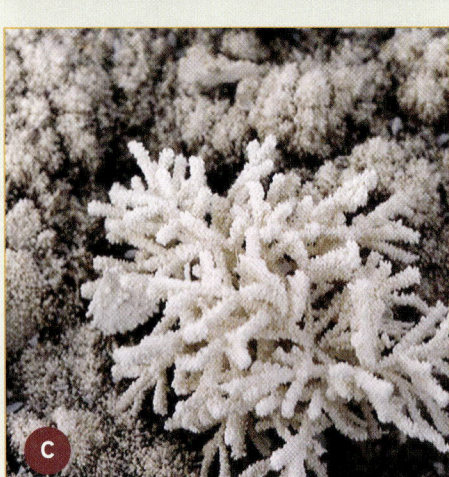
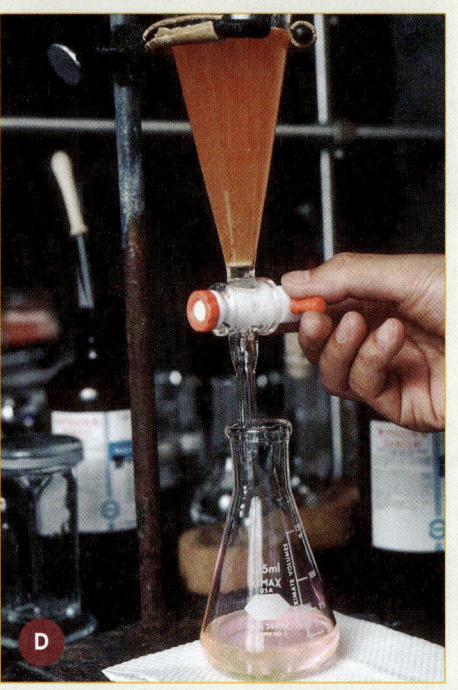

Figure 7-2 Drug sources and examples. **A.** Plant source. **B.** Animal source. **C.** Mineral source. **D.** Laboratory source.

information. The most accurate sites are updated and then revised in your download site (for example, your PDA) on a regular basis.

Canadian Regulation of Pharmaceuticals

The manufacture of pharmaceuticals in Canada and most other countries is subject to a variety of laws and regulations. The goal of these laws and regulations is to protect consumers. In particular, they prohibit manufacturers from making false claims about their drugs' benefits or advising patients to administer the drugs incorrectly. They also seek to protect patients from drugs that might cause harm and require drug manufacturers to publish information about side effects and known potential harmful effects of their products.

Laws and regulations also outline standards for drug manufacture to ensure that drugs produced by different manufacturers are of uniform strength and purity. In Canada, the HPFB ensures that manufacturers produce drugs that meet government standards.

Drug-Related Legislation

The Food and Drugs Act, first passed in 1920, and most recently revised in 1985, aims to protect the public from mislabelled, poisonous, or otherwise harmful foods and medications. It applies to all food, drugs, natural health products, and medical devices sold in Canada and governs the sale, advertisement, and labelling of products to ensure consumer safety and prevent deception.

The *Controlled Drugs and Substances Act* (1996) replaces the *Narcotic Control Act*, which was passed in 1961. It governs the production, registration, distribution, and possession of narcotic and controlled substances. The drugs are organized into eight schedules, each associated with varying control measures, depending on their dependence and abuse potential and their usefulness in medical therapy. Schedules I to V list different controlled substances, schedule VI lists precursors to "designer drugs" or other controlled substances, and schedules VII and VIII specify amounts of substances in schedule II associated

In recent years, the Internet has emerged as an invaluable resource for drug information. Familiarize yourself with reputable and reliable Internet resources. Software versions of some of these resources, such as Epocrates, are available for notebook computers, personal digital assistants (PDAs), and pocket personal computers. No matter which format you use, be sure to research the resource's accuracy before relying on the

Table 7-2	Sources of Drug Information
Source	**Description**
Health Canada HPFB–Therapeutic Products Directorate (TPD)	Ensures that safe and efficacious drugs are available in Canada; aims to balance potential health benefits with risks and patient safety posed by drugs.
Compendium of Pharmaceuticals and Specialties (CPS)	Compiles data on most medications available in Canada; uses the information on file with the HPFB; includes all of the necessary information on indications, dosages, contraindications, and adverse reactions. The book's size makes it difficult for use on an ambulance, but CD-ROM and online versions make it more accessible in the prehospital environment.
Hospital formulary	A list of drugs, dosage forms, package sizes, and drug strengths stocked by hospitals and pharmacies; published as a quick reference to assist the physician and nursing staffs; divided into four general sections: introduction, therapeutic index, drug monographs, and general reference.
Drug inserts	Printed document included in the packaging provided by the drug's manufacturer; generally the same information submitted and approved by the HPFB; when available, serves as a valuable reference; should not be confused with the information provided by a pharmacy when a patient receives a prescription, which is useful in obtaining information pertaining to a drug but is not necessarily all inclusive.
*United States Pharmacopeia Drug Information (USP DI)**	A compendium that provides another source of useful and miscellaneous drug information for pharmacists and medical practitioners; includes generic and trade names; information may not be limited to drugs approved for use by the FDA in the United States.

*Note: This is a US reference, and some drug names may differ in Canada.

- **Schedule I** includes narcotics such as opium, heroin, morphine, and cocaine.
- **Schedule II** includes cannabis and cannabis resin.
- **Schedule III** includes stimulants, such as amphetamines, and hallucinogens, such as LSD.
- **Schedule IV** includes substances such as anabolic steroids, barbiturates, and benzodiazepines.
- **Schedule V** includes phenylpropanolamine.
- **Schedule VI** includes precursors that can be converted or used to produce "designer drugs" or other controlled substances.
- **Schedule VII** defines limits associated with application of cannabis-related penalties, cannabis (3 kg), and cannabis resin (3 kg).
- **Schedule VIII** defines limits associated with application of cannabis-related penalties, cannabis (30 g), and cannabis resin (1 g).

At the Scene

It is important for you to become familiar with "street" names of these commonly used and abused drugs. Most users will not tell you they took methylenedioxymethamphetamine; most likely you will hear terms like ecstasy or XTC. Research or look up these common street terms.

with lesser penalties. It is illegal to import, export, traffic, or possess substances in schedules I, II, and III. The offences in schedule IV are similar to those for I, II, and III, except that there is no offence for simple possession. It is illegal to import, export, or possess for trafficking substances in schedules V and VI.

Manufacturing-Related Regulations

Legislation also focuses on guaranteeing standardization of doses. Standardization assures patients that when they take a medication with a stated amount of the active ingredient, they will, in fact, receive that amount of the drug. Clearly, no one would want to be prescribed a certain dose of a drug and find that the actual medication contained twice (or half) the amount of active ingredient stated on the drug's label. The amount of active ingredients must be within 95% to 105% of that stated on the label. For example, if the label says "300 mg of amiodarone," the medication must contain between 285 mg and 315 mg of the drug.

The pharmaceutical manufacturers and the HPFB use two techniques to analyze the content of a drug: assays and bioassays. An assay is an analysis of the drug itself to evaluate its potency. A bioassay is a procedure for determining the concentration, purity, and/or biological activity of a substance by measuring its effect on an organism, tissue, cell, or enzyme.

Government Agencies That Regulate Drugs

Today, regulation of drugs in Canada falls under the jurisdiction of several agencies.

- The HPFB is Canada's federal authority responsible for the regulation of health products and food, through enforcement of the Food and Drugs Act. It also oversees the safety and efficacy of veterinary drugs sold in Canada. Furthermore, the HPFB is responsible for the promotion of health and well-being of Canadians. Within the HPFB, there are three directorates:
  - The Therapeutic Products Directorate (TPD) reviews the safety and efficacy of pharmaceuticals and medical devices and authorizes their use in Canada.
  - The National Health Products Directorate (NHPD) regulates natural health products, such as vitamin or herbal supplements.
  - The Biologics and Genetic Therapies Directorate (BGTD) regulates biological (eg, vaccines) and radiopharmaceutical drugs.
- The Office of Controlled Substances (OCS) ensures that controlled substances and drugs are not diverted for illegal use. It develops legislation, regulations, policies, and operations to support the control of illicit drug use.
- The Pharmaceutical Advertising Advisory Board (PAAB) and Advertising Standards Canada (ASC) independently review pharmaceutical advertisements to determine compliance with the Food and Drugs Act. Note that in Canada only limited direct-to-consumer advertising is permitted for prescription drugs (drug name only).
- The Marketed Health Products Directorate (MHPD) is responsible for post-marketing surveillance of adverse events secondary to marketed drugs. In the event that a product's quality or safety comes into question, it can work with other Health Canada directorates to remove the product from market or provide safety information.

The Drug-Approval Process

New drugs are constantly being developed. The commercialization process, however, takes years—the average time for a drug to be developed, tested, and approved is about 9 years. In some cases, manufacturers spend most of those 9 years developing a drug only to find out that the drug does not work as envisioned or is too dangerous for human consumption.

All new drugs must go through animal studies and clinical trials in humans before they are approved for distribution.

Animal Studies

Animal studies are designed to identify tissues and organs sensitive to the drug's actions and to elucidate the drug's pharmacodynamic and pharmacokinetic properties. Testing in at least two animal species is required by law. After successful completion of animal studies, an investigational new drug may enter clinical trials in humans.

Clinical Trials

Clinical trials proceed in four phases:

- **Phase I.** The new drug is tested in healthy volunteers to compare human data with those in animals, to determine safe doses of the drug, and to assess its safety.
- **Phase II.** These trials are performed in homogenous populations of patients (50 to 300 patients). In double-blind studies, one group receives the drug and the other group receives a placebo. These studies are designed to evaluate the drug's efficacy and safety and to establish which form is the most effective dose.
- **Phase III.** In these clinical trials, the drug is made available to a larger group of patients (several thousand). These studies, which usually last several years, evaluate the drug's efficacy and monitor the nature and incidence of side effects.
- **Phase IV.** After successful completion of Phase III clinical trials, the drug company can submit a New Drug Submission (NDS) to the HPFB for approval to market the drug. Phase IV trials compare the new drug with others on the market and examine the drug's long-term efficacy and cost-effectiveness.

Newly Approved Drugs

If the TPD of Health Canada approves the drug company's NDS and is satisfied that its manufacturing process follows the Food and Drugs Act, it will issue the drug a Notice of Compliance (NOC). This indicates that the drug has been reviewed and is authorized for marketing in Canada. All drugs are also issued a Drug Identification Number (DIN), which is a unique identifier for the drug. With the increasing number of naturopathic medicines appearing on the market, Health Canada now assigns Natural Product Numbers (NPN) to natural products that meet safety and proper labelling standards for OTC natural products.

Health Canada does allow practitioners access to drugs currently not available on the Canadian market (eg, investigational drugs) through the Special Access Program (SAP) for treating patients with serious conditions for which conventional therapies have failed.

Special Considerations in Drug Therapy

Pregnant Patients

Administration of any medication to a pregnant woman poses two pharmacologic challenges: It can alter the mother's anatomy and physiologic functions, and it has the potential to directly harm the fetus. For this reason, you must be familiar with how a particular medication might affect the fetus before you consider giving it to a pregnant patient. The US Food and Drug Administration (FDA) has developed a rating scale regarding the risk to the mother and fetus for medications; categories include A, B, C, D, and X. (An explanation of these ratings can be found in the medication reference materials mentioned earlier.) Health care providers in Canada also use this rating scale and categories. The MOTHERISK program at Toronto's Hospital for Sick Children has gathered the largest database of drugs used in pregnancy and maternal risk information in the world. This database is publically accessible and a useful resource to health care professionals. In the prehospital environment, you must be able to quickly evaluate the risks versus the benefits of the drug's administration. Does the potential benefit to the mother outweigh the risk to the fetus? If the drug is the only option for saving the mother's life, then that consideration would be paramount. When in doubt, contact direct medical control to discuss the situation.

To see how the twin concerns of mother and fetus play into your decision to administer a particular medication, let's examine the profile for amiodarone:

- **Drug:** Amiodarone (Cordarone). An antiarrhythmic
- **Category:** D, crosses placenta. There are no adequate human studies of effects on the mother or fetus. Congenital hypothyroidism has been described in the second trimester (the drug is 38% iodine by weight). Fetal bradycardia.
- **Breastfeeding:** Excretion into breast milk is significant. Elimination half-life is 58 days. The American Academy of Pediatrics has classified amiodarone as a drug "for which the effect on nursing infants is unknown but may be of concern."
- **Neonatal side effects:** May accumulate in infant with breastfeeding. Possible hypothyroidism.

Pediatric Patients

Medications have much different effects in adults than they do in children—whether the pediatric patient is a newborn, a neonate, an infant, or a toddler. In particular, infants do not achieve the same level of hepatic function as adults until they reach about 6 months of age; as a consequence, babies have a sharply reduced metabolic capacity. Similarly, the products of metabolism in children can vary from those seen in adults, which may sometimes result in unexpected responses. At the same time, children can metabolize some medications much more quickly than adults do, so they may require relatively higher doses or more frequent administration of some medications. The incomplete development of the gastrointestinal tract in young infants slows absorption of oral medications and delays elimination, so the same medication would be more potent in an infant than in an adult.

Geriatric Patients

The changes in pharmacokinetics in geriatric patients are comparable to those observed in young children. In elderly people, hepatic functions and gastrointestinal activity slow, which in turn delays absorption and elimination. In addition, geriatric patients are often taking several medications; these concomitant therapies may interact and modify one another's effects.

You are the Paramedic Part 2

You ask your partner to place the patient on 100% oxygen via nonrebreathing mask and obtain a set of vital signs while you begin to question the patient further about his current illness and past medical history. The patient's son explains that his father was discharged from the hospital last week for problems associated with his heart. He hands you an index card that contains his father's medical history and list of medications. You note that the patient has a history of atrial fibrillation, congestive heart failure, and stable angina. Daily medications include digoxin, 0.125 mg every morning; warfarin (Coumadin), 3 mg every morning; furosemide (Lasix), 60 mg with breakfast and 60 mg at bedtime; diltiazem CD (Cardizem CD), 240 mg every morning; and nitroglycerin as required for chest pain. As you are looking over the list, the son pulls you over to side of the room and quietly expresses his concern about his father's medication compliance, as he has noticed that his father can be forgetful and may be taking his medication more often than it is prescribed.

Vital Signs	Recording Time: 5 Minutes
Skin	Pale, cool, and moist
Pulse	45 beats/min, irregular; weak radial
Blood pressure	72/50 mm Hg
Respirations	24 breaths/min, rales auscultated at bases
Sp_{O_2}	96% on nonrebreathing mask at 15 l/min of supplemental oxygen

3. What type of drug is diltiazem and how does it work?

Special Considerations

Pediatric and geriatric patients often have slower absorption and elimination times, necessitating modification of the doses administered. Pregnant patients are limited in the medications they can take because of risk to the fetus.

Furthermore, because they may have a large number of medications to be taken and alterations in their normal mental status, geriatric patients may unintentionally overdose on a particular drug or forget to take it.

The Scope of Management

Safe and Effective Drug Administration

One of the principal areas in which your activities differ from those of an MFR is in the administration of a long list of pharmacologic agents. Such agents have lifesaving and life-endangering potential, depending on how they are used. The wrong drug or the wrong dose of the right drug can kill a patient as effectively as a lethal weapon. For this reason, you must be intimately familiar with the pharmacologic agents used in the prehospital environment—their indications and contraindications, their side effects, and their dangers. Nowhere in emergency care can ignorance or carelessness on the part of paramedics do so much harm as in the administration of drugs. As a paramedic, you will be responsible for ensuring that administration of medications in the prehospital environment is safe, therapeutic, and effective.

Legal, Moral, and Ethical Responsibilities

When administering medications to a patient, you are legally responsible for the appropriate use and documentation of that therapy. Even if another paramedic prepares the medication and hands a syringe to you to administer, you are still the person responsible. Always have a clear understanding of which medication you are administering and why you are administering it.

Put yourself in the shoes of your patient. How much confidence would you have in the person providing your care if he or she did not have a complete understanding of each drug, when to use it, and how it works? In addition to the obvious legal responsibility, we have a moral and ethical responsibility to ensure that we administer drugs safely.

The following guidelines will help you fulfill your responsibilities.

- Make certain you understand the precautions and contraindications associated with each medication. In addition, consider the precautions and contraindications as they relate to this case.
- Practice proper administration techniques. The manner in which you administer the medication will directly affect how the drug works and may prevent complications such as infection.
- Know the side effects associated with the particular medication, and understand how to observe for, and document, side effects experienced by your patient. Being familiar with the medication's classification will assist you in understanding its side effects.
- Understand the pharmacokinetics and pharmacodynamics of the medications.

As health care has evolved in the prehospital setting, the list of medications administered by paramedics has expanded in tandem. Keeping abreast of all the information is a challenge that you will face throughout your entire career. Do not hesitate to use references to refresh your memory. Having appropriate material readily available will prove beneficial, especially when you need to make important decisions.

Try to obtain concise yet thorough information about the patient's medication use. It is essential to get an accurate list of the patient's current prescribed medications because this list may

Notes from Nancy

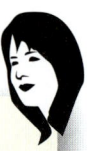

Do not trust your memory in an emergency!

At the Scene

The ever-growing variety of medications available makes it impossible for you to know everything about each drug. Do not hesitate to contact medical direction or consult a reference guide when faced with a medication you are not intimately familiar with.

Notes from Nancy

There are, in fact, tens of thousands of possible drug interactions, particularly in a society like ours, in which people take a lot of pills. The books on drug interactions are often the size of the Toronto or Vancouver telephone directories, and no human brain could be expected to absorb all that information.

reveal clues about the patient's medical history. It is also necessary for deciding appropriate drug therapy so that you may avoid potentially dangerous drug interactions. Determine what, if any, OTC medications the patient may have taken. Find out if the patient is taking any recreational drugs, vitamins, herbal remedies, or alternative medicines. All of these substances can have significant interactions with the medications used in emergency settings—and they may even be the culprit causing the patient's current condition.

Finally, remember that the patient has the right to refuse treatment. Be sure to fully inform your patient about the care that you are giving, including any medications that may be administered and the potential effects and side effects that the patient may experience.

Pharmacology and the Nervous System

Medications administered as part of the care provided in the prehospital setting exert their effects largely by acting on the nervous system. For this reason, it is critical that you understand the functioning of the nervous system as it relates to pharmacology.

Anatomically, the nervous system is made up of the central nervous system (CNS; the brain and spinal cord) and various types of peripheral nerves. The two major types of peripheral nerves are the afferent nerves (Latin: *ad,* "to" + *ferre,* "to bear"), which carry sensory impulses from all parts of the body to the brain, and the efferent nerves (Latin: *efferns,* "to bring out"), which carry messages from the brain to the muscles and all other organs of the body.

Functionally, the nervous system is divided into two primary components (**Figure 7-3 ▲**): the CNS and the peripheral nervous system (PNS).

At the Scene

At the Scene

Virtually all medications used in the prehospital setting may interact with other medications, including those taken by the patient on a daily basis. A concise list of the patient's medications will help ensure safe and accurate drug administration.

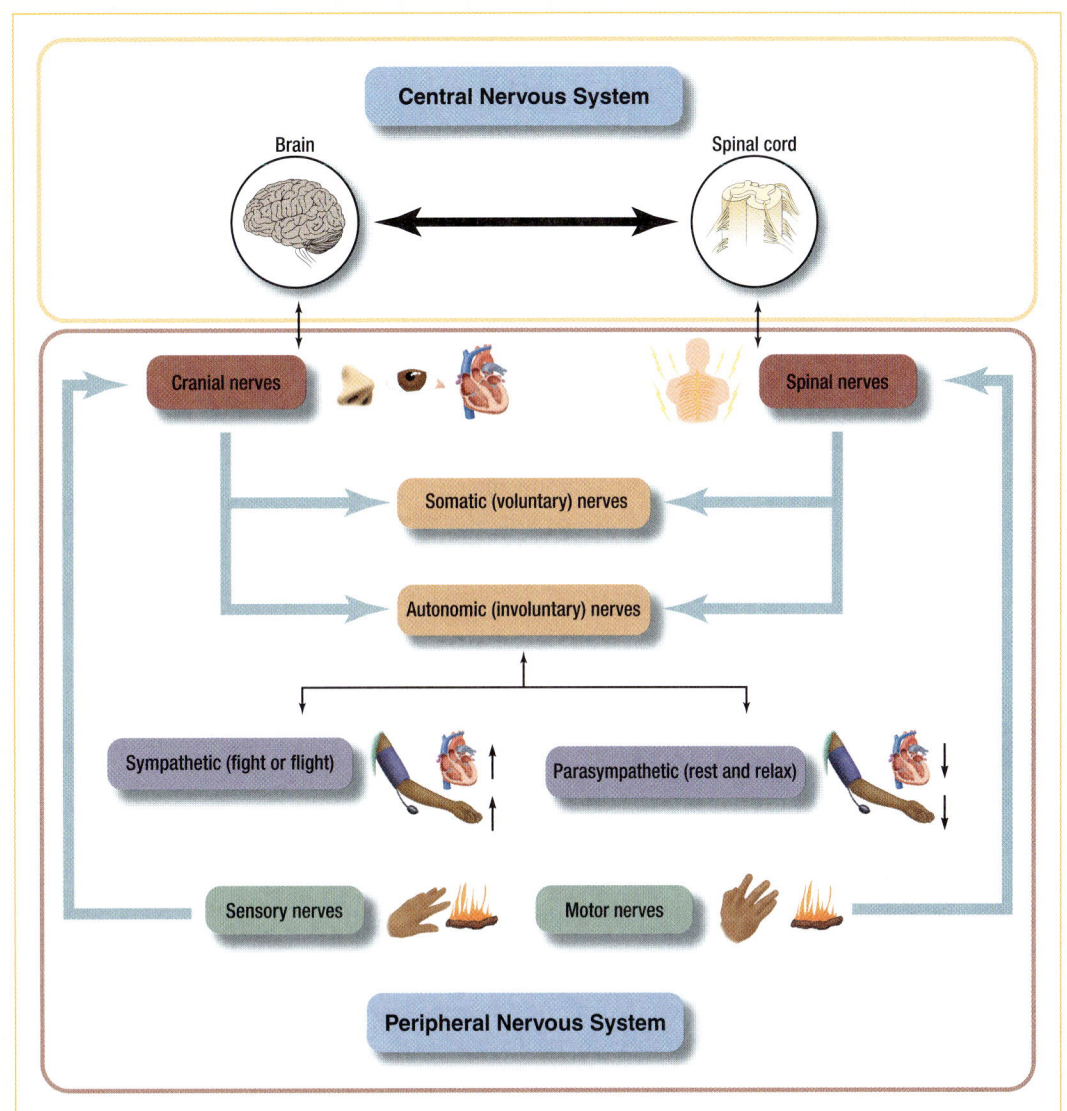

Figure 7-3 Organization of the nervous system.

Central Nervous System

The CNS functions as the control centre for all other nervous system functions. One can easily think of the CNS like the CPU (central processing unit) in a home computer. The CPU in a computer carries out all calculations, coordinating a wide array of incoming and outgoing information from the many cables and connections of the computer. The CNS receives input from many receptors throughout the body, interprets the stimulus received via these sensory neurons, and makes decisions and directs actions to be carried out at target sites and organs throughout the body. These messages are then sent back out to the body via motor neurons or effectors, which carry out the desired action in various muscles and glands throughout the body. Computers work in a similar manner—the CPU interprets data from the keyboard, mouse, disk drives, and so forth and makes decisions and produces output actions such as printing. The whole system is connected by cables that function like the efferent and afferent nerves, sending and receiving information back and forth between the various components.

Peripheral Nervous System

The peripheral nervous system (PNS) consists of all nervous tissue outside of the brain and spinal cord and is separated into two divisions: the somatic nervous system and the autonomic nervous system (ANS). The ANS is particularly vulnerable to the administration of prehospital medications. It is considered to be "automatic" or involuntary because we cannot control its functioning or force functions under its control to happen or not happen.

The autonomic nervous system (ANS) sends sensory impulses from internal structures (such as blood vessels, the heart, and organs of the chest, abdomen, and pelvis) through afferent autonomic nerves to the brain. Afferent neurons are an essential element in reflex regulation of the ANS. The responses to these stimuli sent by afferent neurons are carried back to the organ systems by efferent autonomic nerves, which cause appropriate responses from the organs of the body to change the way they are functioning or behaving. The ANS transmits nerve impulses from the CNS to effector organs through two types of neurons: preganglionic and postganglionic. The preganglionic neurons originate in the CNS, emerge through the brain stem or spinal cord, and make connections at ganglia (groupings of nerve cell bodies located in the PNS). Ganglia act as relay stations through which a ganglionic transmitter relays the impulse to the postganglionic neurons. The postganglionic neurons terminate and stimulate the effector organs (such as smooth muscle, glands, and cardiac muscle) **Figure 7-4 ▶** .

To see how this system works, consider what happens when specialized sensory organs in the carotid sinus and aortic arch detect the pressure within each of these areas. This stimulus is signalled to the CNS via afferent neurons, causing the efferent branch of the system to respond and effecting pressure changes within the system.

The ANS is divided into two further subsystems: the sympathetic nervous system and the parasympathetic nervous system. These two systems have opposing effects on the body.

Sympathetic Nervous System

The sympathetic nervous system, responsible for the fight-or-flight response, is the dominant system during periods of stress

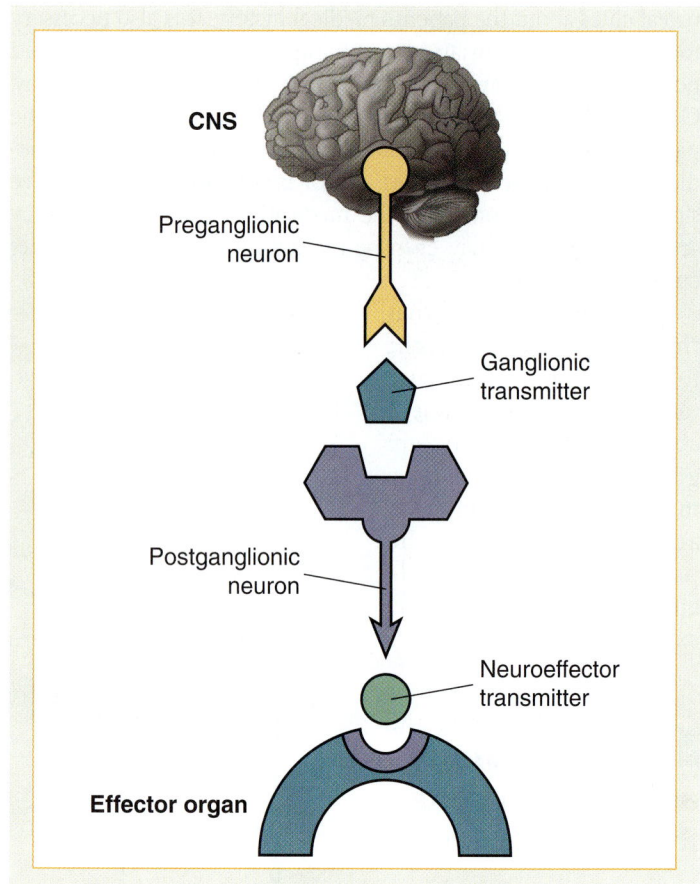

Figure 7-4 Efferent neurons of the ANS.

and activity. It is also a key player in the regulation of hypoglycemia, hypothermia, and trauma.

The sympathetic nerves have their origins in the thoracic and lumbar sections of the spinal cord. They exit the spinal cord through the spinal nerves, which then extend to two types of ganglia: sympathetic chain ganglia and collateral ganglia. Working through these ganglia, the sympathetic nervous system increases heart rate and blood pressure, the release of energy stores throughout the body, and blood flow to the skeletal muscles and heart by diverting flow from the skin and other internal organs. Sympathetic stimulation also results in dilation of the pupils and bronchioles of the respiratory system. The net goal of sympathetic stimulation is to provide the body with energy, oxygen, and the ability to react to stressful situations. The primary chemical messengers of the sympathetic nervous system are norepinephrine and epinephrine. The nerve fibres that release norepinephrine are referred to as adrenergic nerve fibres.

To better understand how sympathetic influences are working, let's look at the heart. The heart rate and force of contraction in response to stress are primarily under the control of the sympathetic nervous system. Sympathetic nerve fibres stimulate all parts of the atria and ventricles. Stimulation of the sympathetic nervous system releases epinephrine, a primary chemical messenger that activates a specific type of receptor in

Sympathetic nervous system terminology:

- **Adrenergic.** Relating to nerve fibres that release norepinephrine or epinephrine
- **Sympathomimetic.** Effects resembling those caused by stimulation of the sympathetic nervous system, such as the effects seen after an injection of epinephrine
- **Sympatholytic.** Interfering with or inhibiting the effect of the impulses from the sympathetic nervous system

An easy way to remember these two terms is:

- When you *mimic* something, you imitate it (sympatho*mimetic*).
- When you *lyse* it, you break it down (sympatho*lytic*).

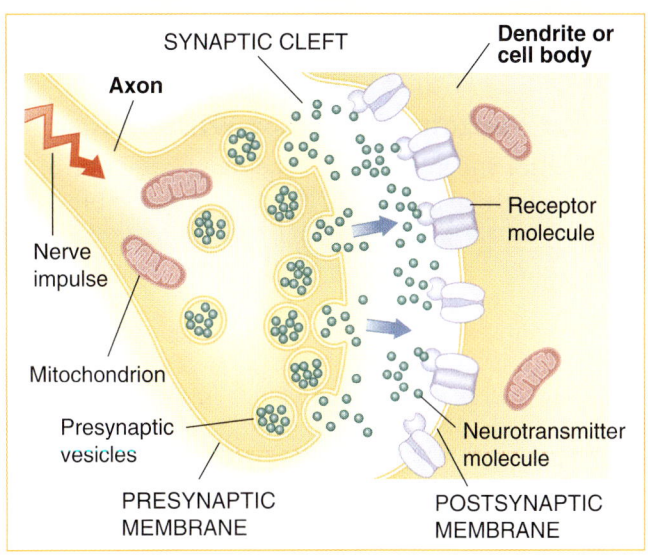

Figure 7-5 A synaptic cleft.

the heart known as the beta-1 adrenergic receptor. Epinephrine affects the heart by increasing the rate of contraction, the conduction velocity, and the force of contraction in the ventricular muscle. The result: increased systemic heart rate and blood pressure. The same actions occur when you administer an injection of epinephrine; this effect is referred to as a *sympathomimetic* response.

Parasympathetic Nervous System

The parasympathetic nervous system is the dominant system during periods of rest and relaxation. It sometimes is referred to as the rest-and-digest system. The nerves associated with the parasympathetic system have their origins in the brain stem and sacral segments of the spinal cord. The nerves from the brain stem pass through four of the cranial nerves: oculomotor (III), facial (VII), pharyngeal (IX), and vagus (X). These nerves innervate most of the body, including the eyes, salivary glands, ears, lungs, and abdominal organs. The sacral segments innervate the kidneys, urinary bladder, sexual organs, and the terminal large intestine.

To see how the sympathetic and parasympathetic nervous systems work in conjunction, consider the effect of these two systems on the heart. The heart, like most major organs and glands, receives sympathetic and parasympathetic stimuli. The sympathetic stimulus increases the heart rate and contractility of the muscle; the parasympathetic impulses decrease the rate and contractility. The constant tug-of-war between these two sets of stimuli determines the final heart rate and contractility status.

Neurochemical Transmission

Neurotransmission is the process of chemical signalling between cells. This process involves several steps. Let's look at a cholinergic neuron to describe the process. A cholinergic neuron is one that releases the chemical acetylcholine (ACh).

The first step involves the synthesis of ACh. Here choline is taken from extracellular fluid, along with sodium, into the neuron where it is turned into ACh. Second, the ACh is stored in vesicles in the nerve terminal. The third step involves the release of ACh from the nerve ending. This occurs when an action potential arrives at the nerve ending, stimulating the voltage-sensitive channels to open and release ACh into the synaptic gap (the space between the cell membrane of an axon terminal and of the target cell with which it synapses, also called the *synaptic cleft*) **Figure 7-5 ▲**. The fourth step involves binding of released ACh to a receptor. Once ACh is released from the synaptic vesicles, it diffuses across the synaptic space and binds to receptors on the next, or target, cell. The binding of ACh to the receptor causes a response within the cell, and a new nerve impulse is initiated.

Receptors are unique molecular structures or sites on the surface or interior of a cell that bind with substances such as hormones, drugs, and neurotransmitters. Receptors are highly specialized and, in most cases, respond only to a particular substance. It is easy to think of the receptor-neurotransmitter relationship like a lock and key. If every neurotransmitter stimulated every receptor, there would be tremendous competition and confusion within the body's cells.

The fifth step involves the degradation of ACh. Once the new nerve impulse is initiated, an enzyme called acetylcholinesterase (AChE) is released, which breaks ACh into choline and acetate. The sixth and final step is the recycling of choline by the neurons so that it can be made into ACh for a subsequent action or transmission.

Other Receptors

In addition to neurotransmission, other methods of chemical signalling occur through local mediators and the secretion of hormones. Most cells in the body secrete chemicals that may act at the local area and stimulate changes in their immediate environment. Nearly all of these locally released chemicals are destroyed or removed by the cells and do not enter blood circulation and create changes throughout the entire body. A good example of a local mediator is histamine.

Hormones are secreted by specialized cells into the bloodstream. Hormones are transported throughout the entire body and have a broad range of effects at various target tissues.

Altering Neurotransmission With Drugs

In some cases and conditions, it becomes necessary to alter normal neurotransmission. This can be accomplished by using drugs that mimic or inhibit neurotransmission. Some medications inhibit the release of neurotransmitters, and others block the receptor sites along the neural pathway. For example, contamination involving organophosphates (pesticides) alters neural transmissions. In this case, the ACh released by the organophosphate binds to the AChE, making it ineffective. The final result is overstimulation of the nerves due to an excess of ACh in the synaptic cleft. In this case, a medication is needed to break the bond between the organophosphate and AChE so that AChE can break down the ACh and terminate the nerve stimulation. The drug of choice is 2 PAM chloride, which is effective at cleaving the organophosphate from AChE and allowing it to break down the excess ACh, terminating nerve stimulation and returning it to a normal state. There are many medications that can alter normal neurotransmission.

Selective Drug Action: Nicotinic and Muscarinic Receptors

Nicotinic receptors are present in many tissues in the body, including the CNS and the PNS. These receptors function at the neuromuscular junctions of somatic muscles, and stimulation causes muscular contraction. Nicotinic receptors are triggered by the neurotransmitter ACh, but they are also opened by nicotine. Nicotinic effects are those of sympathetic overactivity and neuromuscular dysfunction and include tachycardia, hypertension, dilated pupils, muscle fasciculation (involuntary contractions or twitching of groups of muscle fibres), and muscle weakness.

Muscarinic receptors are found throughout the body as subcomponents of the CNS and ANS **Figure 7-6 ▸**. The primary neurotransmitters for muscarinic receptors are ACh and muscarine. Muscarinic effects result in parasympathetic overactivity and include bradycardia, miosis (pinpoint pupils), sweating, blurred vision, excessive lacrimation (tearing), excessive bronchial secretions, wheezing, shortness of breath, coughing, vomiting, abdominal cramping, diarrhea, and urinary and fecal incontinence. Atropine is a common medication that is given in the prehospital setting to reverse the effects of muscarinic overstimulation.

General Properties of Medications

Drugs adjust or influence the body's existing functions; they usually do not provide the body with functions it does not already have. To exert their effects, they must interact with various cells and tissues in the body, and they typically work through several mechanisms of action rather than relying on a single action. In most cases, medications may bind to a receptor site and trigger a stimulus; in some cases, they change the chemical properties of cells and tissues. They may also combine with other chemicals within cells or organ systems to aid in elimination or bind to receptors to alter the normal metabolic functions of cells and tissues.

Receptors are specialized target molecules that are present on the surface of cells or within the cell. They bind a medication and mediate its pharmacologic effect. Medications may interact with a variety of receptor sites—for example, enzymes, nucleic acids, and membranous receptors. Once the medication and the receptor site bind, a biological response follows. The magnitude of this response is directly proportional to the number of these drug-receptor sites.

The attraction between a medication and its receptors is referred to as affinity. The stronger the affinity between the two, the stronger the resulting bond. In some cases, different medications have affinity for the same receptor site; however, it is unlikely that both will bind with the same strength, which means that one medication inevitably takes priority.

A medication that stimulates a response in a receptor site is called an agonist. The strength of its effect depends on the concentration of the agonist at the receptor site, which is in

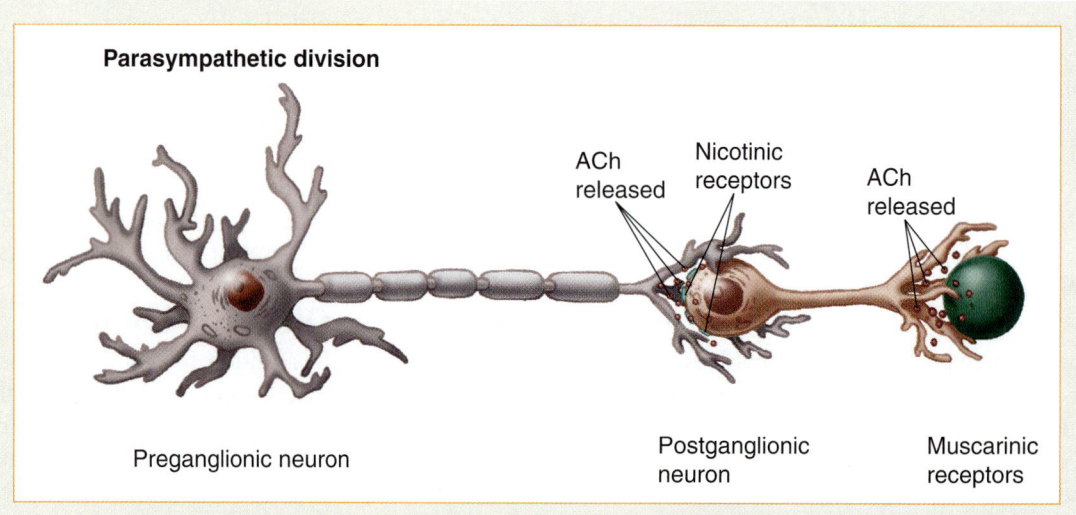

Parasympathetic division

ACh released

Nicotinic receptors

ACh released

Preganglionic neuron

Postganglionic neuron

Muscarinic receptors

Figure 7-6 Muscarinic receptors are present on some sympathetic and all parasympathetic target tissues.

turn determined by the dose administered and the drug's rate of absorption, distribution, and metabolism.

Drug Forms

Drugs come in many forms, solid and liquid, each of which has special properties. In the prehospital environment, you will use only a limited subset of the drug forms described herein.

Liquid Drug Forms

- **Solution.** A liquid containing one or more chemical substances entirely dissolved, usually in water, for example, normal saline solution (The majority of medications used by paramedics are solutions.)
- **Suspension.** Preparation of a finely divided drug intended to be (or already) incorporated in a suitable liquid, for example, amoxicillin, supplied as a powder requiring the addition of water (Note: All bottles containing suspensions must be shaken thoroughly before use because their ingredients tend to separate on standing.)
- **Fluid extract.** Concentrated form of a drug prepared by dissolving the crude drug in the fluid in which it is most readily soluble; standardized such that 1 milliliter (ml) contains 1 gram (g) of the drug, for example, many herbal supplements and remedies, such as saw palmetto
- **Tincture.** Dilute alcoholic extract of a drug such as tincture of iodine, used as a skin antiseptic
- **Spirits.** Preparation of a volatile substance dissolved in alcohol, such as spirits of ammonia, formerly used to rouse people from fainting through its noxious odour
- **Syrup.** Drug suspended in sugar and water to improve its taste, such as cough syrup and syrup of ipecac
- **Elixir.** Solution with alcohol and flavouring added, such as cough medicines, particularly those formulated for children
- **Milk.** Aqueous suspension of an insoluble drug, such as milk of magnesia
- **Emulsion.** Preparation of one liquid (usually an oil) distributed in small globules in another liquid (usually water), for example, some preparations of diazepam (Valium); often used as lubricants
- **Liniments** and **lotions.** Preparations of drugs for external use, usually to relieve discomfort such as pain or itching or to protect the skin, for example, calamine lotion

Solid Drug Forms

- **Extract.** A concentrated preparation of a drug made by putting the drug into solution (in alcohol or water) and evaporating the excess solvent until the concentration reaches a prescribed standard, for example, liver extract, which has been used in the treatment of anemia, prepared by dissolving ground mammalian liver and allowing the solvent to evaporate; extract is then incorporated into a tablet or capsule

- **Powder.** A drug that has been ground into pulverized form, for example, mixtures of powdered sodium bicarbonate and calcium carbonate, used as an antacid in the treatment of ulcers; example in prehospital care: activated charcoal powder
- **Capsule.** A cylindrical gelatin container enclosing a dose of medication, for example, many over-the-counter pain medications, such as ibuprofen (Advil). These are available as hard gelatin (often containing dry powder medication) or soft gelatin (often containing liquid medication) capsules.
- **Pulvule.** Resembles a capsule, but it is not made of gelatin and does not separate; usually are proprietary forms of a drug, such as propoxyphene hydrochloride (Darvon)
- **Tablet.** A powdered drug that has been moulded or compressed into a small disk, such as aspirin tablets; example in prehospital care: nitroglycerin tablets. This is the most commonly used solid dosage form. Many variations of tablets are available to optimize their intended effect, such as enteric-coated, rapid-dissolve, chewable, or effervescent tablets.
- **Suppository.** A drug mixed in a firm base that melts at body temperature and is shaped to fit the rectum, urethra, or vagina; may be used for local action (for example, glycerin suppositories to promote evacuation of the rectum) or for systemic effect (for example, diazepam [Valium] suppositories to treat seizure disorders and status epilepticus in children)
- **Ointment.** A semisolid preparation for external application to the body, usually containing a medicinal substance, for example, neomycin ointment, a topical antibiotic
- **Patch.** A medication impregnated into a membrane or adhesive that is applied onto the surface of the skin, for example, nitroglycerin patch **Figure 7-7** ▾

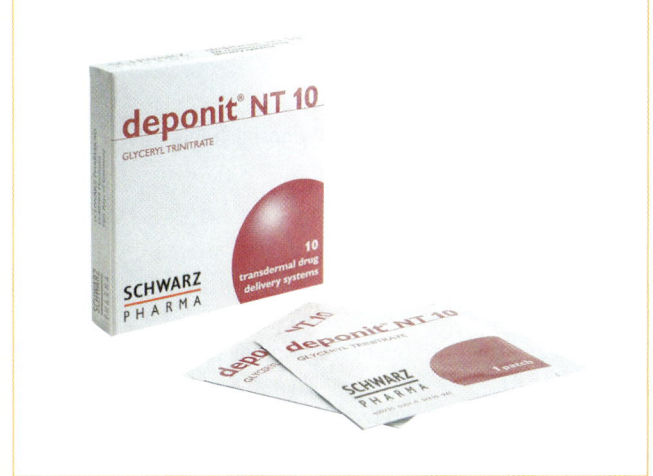

Figure 7-7 Nitroglycerin patch.

Gaseous Drug Forms

Medications may also come in the form of a vapour. Gaseous medications are primarily used in operating suite anesthesia. To create the gas, a medication in liquid form is placed into a machine that promotes vapourization. The vapours are inhaled by the patient to induce anesthesia. An example of a medication administered as a vapour is sevoflurane (Ultane).

■ Overview of the Routes of Drug Administration

Rates of Drug Absorption

How you choose to administer a drug—that is, the mode of administration—affects the rate at which the body absorbs the drug and, ultimately, the onset of its therapeutic effects. The action of a drug, especially the speed with which it works, is also influenced by the way it enters the body—that is, the route of administration. Obviously, drugs injected directly into the circulation, such as IV or intraosseous (IO) injections, enter the bloodstream the most rapidly. Nearly as fast is the absorption across the respiratory mucosa when drugs are sprayed down an endotracheal tube or breathed in from an inhaler. Other mucosal surfaces, such as those found in the rectum, provide for rapid absorption as well, albeit at an unpredictable rate. Intramuscular (IM) injection is slower because the drug must be picked up from the muscles by the circulating blood; the same is true of subcutaneous (SC) injections, which are absorbed more slowly than IM injections. Near the slowest end of the scale are drugs administered orally (PO). The slowest absorption of all is across intact skin.

Table 7-3 ▾ summarizes the rates of absorption. Note that the route of administration that is appropriate for one drug

Table 7-3	Rates of Absorption by Different Routes
Route of Administration	**Time Until Drug Takes Effect***
Topical	Hours to days
Oral	30–90 min
Rectal	5–30 min (unpredictable)
SC injection	15–30 min
IM injection	10–20 min
Sublingual tablet	3–5 min
Sublingual injection	3 min
Inhalation	3 min
Endotracheal	Unknown; unpredictable
IO	60 s (considered best alternate route if no IV access)
IV	30–60 s
Intracardiac	15 s (no longer recommended in cardiac arrest)
*In a healthy person with normal perfusion.	

may be unsuitable for another drug, so for any given drug it is essential to know the routes by which it may be given.

Local or Systemic Effects

Drugs may produce their effects locally, systemically, or both. Local effects result from the direct application of a drug to a tissue—for example, when you apply a lotion to the skin to relieve itching. Systemic effects occur after the drug is absorbed by any route and distributed by the bloodstream; they almost invariably involve more than one organ, although the response of one or another organ may predominate.

The action of a drug is rarely a completely fixed property of the medication. Instead, the effect of any given drug typically varies depending on the patient, the dose, the route by which the drug is given, and the drug's metabolic rate.

■ Routes of Drug Administration

The routes of administration are classified into three categories based on how the medication is absorbed and distributed: percutaneous, enteral, and parenteral. Medications given via the percutaneous routes are applied to and absorbed through the skin or mucous membranes. Enteral medications are administered and absorbed somewhere along the gastrointestinal tract, most commonly orally. Any route of administration that does not cause the drug to be absorbed through the skin, mucous membranes, or gastrointestinal tract is considered parenteral. The actual route of administration you select in the prehospital environment is dependent on the medication and the intended effect.

Percutaneous Routes

Percutaneous routes of medication administration are those for any medication that is absorbed through the skin or through a mucous membrane. Drugs may be applied topically—that is, on the surface of the body. Ordinarily, the intact skin is an effective barrier to absorption of drugs, but some drugs have been specially prepared to cross the barrier at a very slow rate, so the route is useful for sustained release of drugs for a long period. Thus, some patients take nitroglycerin in the form of a cream rubbed into the skin or a patch pasted onto the skin. Estrogens (female hormones) are also sometimes given in the form of a patch.

Administration via the transdermal route is generally performed by placing medication directly onto the patient's skin. It is also easily controlled by simply removing and wiping the medication from the skin, which causes the effect to quickly subside. Although the rate of absorption is consistent, steady, and predictable, it can be affected by the thickness of the skin and the presence of scar tissue at the site of administration. It can also be affected by the amount of peripheral circulation. Conditions that decrease peripheral circulation, such as hypothermia and hypotension, will lead to a slower rate of absorption. In a febrile patient, the rate of absorption would be much quicker than anticipated.

Administering medications through mucous membranes is becoming increasingly popular in the prehospital setting. This route allows for the medication to be absorbed at a moderate to rapid rate. Sublingual (SL) administration refers to giving a medication—nitroglycerin, for example—under the tongue. Drugs given sublingually are usually rapidly absorbed, with effects becoming apparent within a few minutes. The buccal route (between the cheeks and gums) may be used to give glucose gel to a hypoglycemic diabetic patient. The nasal route is an increasingly popular way to aerosolize and administer medications. Naloxone given intranasally, for example, is quickly absorbed into the blood vasculature in the nasopharynx. Although this route of administration is less commonly used in the prehospital setting, drops may be placed in the eye to be absorbed in the conjunctival sac or in the ear (aurally) to fight infection or minimize pain.

The pulmonary route of drug administration is used to deliver medications directly to the pulmonary system through inhalation or injection. In the inhalation route, the drug is placed in a nebulizer that reduces it to a mist, which the patient then breathes in. In the lungs, the drug is absorbed into the bronchioles and alveolar sacs. Paramedics can also administer medications through an endotracheal tube, placing it in liquid form into the bronchioles and alveolar sacs to be absorbed. Only certain medications are suitable to be given via the endotracheal tube. NAVEL is a handy mnemonic that will help you recall which drugs can be delivered in this way: Naloxone, Atropine, Vasopressin, Epinephrine, and Lidocaine. If medications are given via the endotracheal route, the dose must be doubled to achieve the same effects as if given intravenously. Currently, the endotracheal tube route is not recommended in cardiac arrest because the effectiveness of medication absorption is questionable at best. The IV and IO routes are preferred in these cases. Specific routes and the steps of administration are discussed further in Chapter 8.

Enteral Routes

Medications that are given via one of the enteral routes are absorbed somewhere along the gastrointestinal tract. Most patients take their daily medications at home by the oral route (per os, or PO) because that route is painless, convenient, and economical. Drugs taken by mouth are absorbed at an unpredictable but generally slow rate from the stomach and intestines—usually somewhere between 30 and 90 minutes. Because absorption is slow and unpredictable, drugs are rarely given by the oral route in emergency situations. The

one exception is aspirin for patients suspected of having acute coronary syndrome (ACS); its administration requires an adequate level of consciousness to prevent aspiration, however. In some cases, you may need to administer medications via a gastric tube, which allows for access directly to the gastrointestinal system.

Drugs may be administered rectally for their local effect; they may also be given rectally because they are irritating if given orally or because the patient cannot take an oral medication (for example, if vomiting). In the prehospital setting, the rectal route can be considered if quick IV access is impractical. The extreme vascularity of the rectum promotes rapid but sometimes unpredictable absorption. Medications administered rectally (per rectum, or PR) generally do not pass through the liver and, therefore, are not subjected to hepatic alterations.

Parenteral Routes

Parenteral routes include those in which medications are administered via any route other than the alimentary canal (digestive tract), skin, and mucous membranes. They are generally administered via syringes and needles. In most cases, parenteral routes allow for the fastest absorption rate.

The IV route is the most rapidly effective—but also the most dangerous route of administration. Drugs given intravenously go directly into the bloodstream and to the target organs, without any appreciable delay in absorption. Thus, IV injection enables you to deliver a known quantity of drug over a known period; that is, it allows the most accurate control of dosage. It is a dangerous route, however, precisely because the entire dose of the drug is delivered in one blast, so a toxic reaction is much more likely. Absorption of an IV drug usually takes about 30 to 60 seconds. The absorption rate will be slowed in heart failure (because of the longer circulation time). In cardiac arrest with CPR in progress, an IV drug will take 3 to 4 times longer than usual to reach its target organ because the cardiac output is only one third of the normal rate. As a consequence, it will take at least 1 or 2 minutes after giving an emergency drug during CPR to ensure that the drug has circulated adequately. Always prepare to administer a medication in cardiac arrest by drawing it up ahead of time. Administer drugs during compression cycles to enhance distribution whenever possible, and never interrupt compressions to administer a medication during cardiac arrest. In general, IV drugs should be given *slowly,* unless you receive contrary orders. In the prehospital environment, it is unacceptable to administer a medication by direct venipuncture because this technique may result in infiltration of the drug. Infiltration is the escape of fluid into the surrounding tissue, which causes a localized area of edema, and is discussed in more detail in Chapter 8.

The intraosseous (IO) route is becoming increasingly popular in the prehospital setting. This route has long been used for pediatric patients, but with the advent of convenient devices for adult use, it is quickly becoming a standard when quick IV access is not practical. Any medication that can be given intravenously can be given intraosseously. The rate of absorption and time of onset have been shown to be identical if not better because the medicine enters a noncollapsible channel with rapid flow into the central circulation.

Drugs given by the intramuscular (IM) route take longer to act than those given intravenously because they must first be absorbed from the muscle into the bloodstream. By the same token, IM medications have a longer duration of action than IV drugs because they are absorbed gradually during a period of minutes to hours. Obviously, absorption of medications given by the IM or SC route depends on adequate blood flow to muscles and peripheral tissues, which is not the case in shock or cardiac arrest. Therefore, IM injections should be given only to patients with adequate perfusion.

An IM injection usually involves volumes of about 1 to 5 ml and is given into the deltoid muscle of the upper arm (the preferred site for prehospital applications) or into the upper outer quadrant of the gluteus muscle of the buttocks. (The technique for IM injection is described later in this chapter.) The use of the deltoid muscle of the arm has the advantage that the rate of drug absorption can be slowed in case of an adverse reaction. Should dyspnea, dizziness, itching, edema, urticaria,

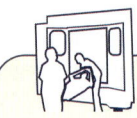

At the Scene

Do not give IM or SC injections to patients with impaired peripheral perfusion.

wheezing, or any other sign of an allergic reaction develop following an IM (or SC) injection in the arm, you should immediately fasten a tourniquet proximal to the injection site and then manage the patient as described in Chapter 30.

With the subcutaneous (SC or SQ) route, a small amount (usually less than 2 ml) of drug is injected into the fat or connective tissue beneath the skin. Medications administered by this route are absorbed more slowly and over a more prolonged period than when they are given intravenously; the peak drug effect usually occurs within about 30 minutes. The SC route is used to administer epinephrine in asthmatic attacks of mild to moderate severity. These injections are usually given under the skin of the upper outer arm, anterior thigh, or abdomen.

▌ Pharmacokinetics

Every medication has varying effects on the body. Pharmacokinetics is the study of the metabolism and action of medications within the body, with particular emphasis on the time required for absorption, duration of action, distribution in the body, and method of excretion.

Absorption

Absorption of medications refers to the transfer of a medication from its site of administration into the body to specific target organs

You are the Paramedic Part 3

You perform a physical examination on the patient while your partner prepares an IV set up. You document the following findings: positive JVD; rales auscultated at the bases; slight swelling around the ankles; and a slow, irregular, weak pulse. You ask the patient to describe his vision problems. He explains that for the past 2 days his sight has been blurry and objects have had a yellow-green circle around them. He jokingly tells you that this blurriness interferes with him being able to complete the morning crossword puzzle and watch his game shows at night.

You establish an 18-gauge IV in the right AC and begin to administer a 200-ml fluid bolus. Before leaving for the hospital you perform a 12-lead ECG, which shows atrial fibrillation at a rate in the 40s with frequent PVCs. Recalling the information on cardiac medication from a recent in-service you know that both digoxin and diltiazem CD can lower the heart rate. You also know that the patient is symptomatic from the low heart rate and PVCs. Unsure of how to proceed with treatment, you decide to contact direct medical control for guidance.

Reassessment	Recording Time: 10 Minutes
Skin	Pale, cool, and moist
Pulse	42 beats/min, irregular; weak radial
ECG	Atrial fibrillation with a slow ventricular response and frequent PVCs
Blood pressure	78/44 mm Hg
Respirations	24 breaths/min, slight increase work of breathing
Spo_2	96% on nonrebreathing mask at 15 l/min of supplemental oxygen
Pupils	Equal and reactive to light

4. Does the patient present with signs and symptoms of possible drug toxicity? If so, which medications are in question?

5. What treatment will increase the patient's blood pressure?

and tissues. The ultimate goal is for the medication to reach a therapeutic concentration in the bloodstream. Achieving this therapeutic concentration depends partially on the rate and extent to which the drug is absorbed. The rate and extent are, in turn, dependent on the ability of the medication to cross the cell membrane.

Mechanisms of Medication Absorption

A medication may cross the cell's membrane by one of two mechanisms: active transport or passive diffusion (discussed in Chapter 8). In active transport, specialized proteins that span the membrane of a cell facilitate the movement of the medication inside target tissues and cells. This energy-dependent process uses a carrier-mediated mechanism to assist the medication into the cell and can move the drug across the concentration gradient (from an area of lower concentration to an area of higher concentration). In contrast, passive diffusion (also known as absorption) of a medication does not use energy or carrier-mediated mechanisms. Instead, medications move from an area of high concentration to an area of low concentration. Lipid-soluble medications move easily across most cell membranes, as do water-soluble drugs via aqueous channels.

Blood Flow and Medication Absorption

A properly functioning circulatory system greatly enhances the rate of medication absorption. If the body area to which a medication is applied (for example, transdermal route) or injected (for example, IM route) has a good vascular system and a rich blood supply, the rate of absorption is enhanced. In contrast, areas of the body with poor blood supply or particular routes of administration (for example, SC route) may be associated with a delay in the rate of absorption. As mentioned earlier, medications administered via the IV route are immediately passed throughout the circulatory system, absorbed, and delivered to target tissues and organs. In patients in profound states of shock or circulatory compromise, absorption may be delayed with any of the administration methods.

Surface Areas and Medication Absorption

All medications must pass through nontarget cells to reach their intended receptor target; these nontarget cells may include the skin, mucosa, and intestinal tissue. The larger the surface area that is available to the medication as a "launching pad," the greater the amount of absorption and the more quickly the medication can reach its target and take effect.

Another factor affecting the absorption rate is the nature of the cells that the medication is trying to pass through. Single layers of cells, like the tissue of the intestines, readily transport medications. In contrast, multilayer tissues like the skin require more time for absorption.

Medication Concentration and Absorption

The concentration of the medication administered affects its absorption as well. Pharmaceutical manufacturers use this fact to their advantage—for example, by altering a medication's coating to tweak the ultimate rate of absorption. Medications that are administered in high doses are generally absorbed more quickly than medications that are administered at lower doses.

When medications are administered to a patient, they eventually become distributed throughout the entire body. Thus, the higher the concentration in the body, the greater the absorption. For this reason, giving very high concentrations or doses to speed absorption is not a good idea. Once a medication is administered, it will continue to circulate in the body and affect its target receptors until the drug is eliminated. Typically, when continued doses are required, two approaches to administration are used. First a loading dose—a large dose of the same concentration that temporarily exceeds the body's ability to eliminate the medication—is given to quickly reach a therapeutic level. It is followed by a maintenance dose—a smaller dose administered over time and intended to maintain a therapeutic level of the medication at the receptor site. Loading doses are typically based on the volume of distribution, which takes into account the patient's weight; maintenance doses are selected based on the body's ability to eliminate the medication.

Environmental pH and Medication Absorption

Most medications are weak acids or weak bases. Once in solution, they become ionized (electrically charged). Most medications reach a state of equilibrium between their ionized and nonionized forms, facilitating their absorption. The pH of a medication affects its ability to ionize. Medications that are weak acids are able to ionize much better in an alkaline environment, whereas medications that are weak bases are able to ionize more completely in an acidic environment.

Medications administered by any route inevitably undergo side reactions—that is, reactions with nontarget cells and tissues—before they reach their intended destination. A critical consideration for the effectiveness of any drug is how much of it is still active by the time it reaches its target organ. This property, called the drug's bioavailability, must be taken into account when selecting the dose to ensure that enough medication is being absorbed at the target organ to achieve the desired effect.

Distribution

Medication distribution is the process by which a medication moves throughout the body. Blood is the primary distribution vehicle. Factors that change the way blood flows through the body will change the way medications are transported to the target tissue. If the patient's overall cardiac output is diminished, the medication will not move as quickly. Along the same lines, if blood is not moving efficiently to a particular part of the body, the distribution may be slowed. For example, if the patient is cold, the blood is shunted away from the skin and peripheral extremities. In such a case, an antibiotic intended to fight an infection in the foot will not arrive at that area as quickly as intended.

The only way a medication molecule can actually be used by the body is if it is not bound with anything else—that is, it must be "free drug." Because of this, the extent to which the medication binds with nontarget cells affects its intensity and duration of action. Not all of the medication molecules are floating around the blood at the same time. Medications have a tendency to collect in certain areas of the body that act as storage sites. Typically, drugs will become bound to fat, muscle tissue, and bone, thereby limiting the amount of medication that is free in the bloodstream. In particular, lipid-soluble medications have a high affinity for adipose (fat) tissue. As a consequence, low blood flow may allow for their extended retention in the adipose tissue. Still other medications have an unusual affinity for bone tissue. Molecules of these drugs will accumulate after the drug is absorbed onto the bone crystal surface.

In contrast, while roaming around the body in the bloodstream, the medication may become bound to plasma proteins. Such a drug–protein complex cannot be used by the body, so its formation lowers the therapeutic concentration of the drug. The amount of free drug is always proportional to the amount of bound drug. Thus, as the free drug is used and eliminated, the drug–protein complexes break down and release more free drug to replace what has been used.

In particular, molecules of a medication may become bound to the plasma protein known as albumin. Albumin, which is too large to diffuse out of the bloodstream, essentially kidnaps drug molecules, making them ineffective. Albumin is not in endless supply, however. Furthermore, other medications may be competing to bind to the same albumin. As such, the amount of free drug is influenced by the amount of available albumin. Some conditions may cause a decrease in the albumin levels, particularly those that involve decreased liver functions. Even if the albumin levels are normal, the amount of affinity for albumin that one medication has compared with another can affect free-drug levels (think of it like magnets and a metal screw for the albumin, with one magnet being stronger than the other).

Other aspects of the body may also prevent medication molecules from being distributed to certain tissue. The blood-brain barrier is a single layer of capillary endothelial cells. It allows only lipid-soluble medications to enter the brain and cerebrospinal fluid. In a pregnant patient, the placental barrier consists of membrane layers separating blood vessels of the mother and the fetus. Much like the blood-brain barrier, the placental barrier does not permit most non–lipid-soluble medications to pass to the fetus. This is not an impregnable barrier, however; some non–lipid-soluble medications can cross the placental barrier, so you must understand which medications can be given to a pregnant patient and in which situations.

Biotransformation

The manner in which the body metabolizes medications is referred to as biotransformation. It occurs in one of two ways: by transforming the medication into a metabolite or by making the medication more water soluble. Only medication molecules that are in a free-drug form are able to be biotransformed.

Drug manufacturers use this fact to their advantage when creating medications, known as prodrugs, that become active only *after* they undergo biotransformation. Most of the biotransformation takes place in the liver. The endoplasmic reticulum of hepatocytes contains the enzymes primarily responsible for biotransformation.

The biotransformation of a medication directly affects the route chosen to deliver a medication. All blood that comes from the gastrointestinal tract must pass through the liver before moving on to the rest of the body. This gives the liver the opportunity to partially or completely inactivate drugs long before they reach the intended target tissue, a scenario known as the first-pass effect. Because of the first-pass effect, some medications can be given only parenterally. For example, insulin must always be given subcutaneously—never orally. The liver would completely inactivate insulin if it were to undergo the first-pass effect, making it useless. Even medications that are not completely inactivated by the first-pass effect sometimes require a higher dose when given orally to ensure that enough of the drug survives to have a therapeutic effect.

Liver enzymes can act on a drug in two ways, or phases. In phase 1, the enzymes may oxidize the drug or bind it with oxygen molecules. The enzymes may also hydrolyze the medication, decomposing it by a reaction with water. In either case, the medication becomes more soluble with water. In phase 2, the medication molecules combine with a chemical found in the body; this interaction is known as a conjugation reaction. Phase 1 and phase 2 allow the drug to move to the next stage, excretion.

Excretion

In excretion, the body eliminates the remnants of the drug, which could be toxic or inactive metabolites. (Recall that the liver may have inactivated at least some of the drug through biotransformation.) Excretion occurs primarily through the kidneys via three mechanisms:

- **Glomerular filtration.** A passive process in which blood flows through the glomeruli of the kidneys. These structures are bundles of capillaries within a capsule. A differential in pressure forces wastes away from the blood into the capsule where it is transported for excretion via the urine.
- **Tubular secretion.** An active transport process in which medications are bound to specific transporters aiding in their elimination.
- **Partial reabsorption.** This occurs when some amount of the drug is reabsorbed after being filtered.

The same factors that affect absorption can also affect excretion, particularly the environmental pH—in this case, the pH of the urine. In this case, if the medication is acidic in an alkaline urine, the medication will more readily move into the urine for excretion. Conversely, an alkaline medication in an acidic urine environment will also readily move to the urine. The closer the pH, the slower the medication will be excreted.

Pharmacodynamics

Pharmacodynamics is the way in which a medication produces the response we intended, also known as the mechanism of action. It also encompasses the factors that may alter the intended response and any side effects or unexpected effects.

Theories of Drug Action

Medications cause their action on the body by four mechanisms:

- They may bind to a receptor site.
- They may change the physical properties of cells—typically, by changing the osmotic balance.
- They may chemically combine with other chemicals (such as with the goal of turning the substance into a nonproblematic chemical).
- They may alter a normal metabolic pathway (such as by interrupting the normal growth process of cells).

Medications that bind to a receptor site are the most prevalent, particularly in the prehospital setting. Receptor sites are specialized proteins on a cell that receive chemical mediator messages to stimulate a particular response. For example, when ACh attaches to receptor sites in the heart, it causes the heart rate to slow. Cellular responses can be wide ranging depending on the chemical mediator and the cells being stimulated. A medication molecule will have one of two effects when it attaches to a receptor site: It may stimulate the receptor site to cause the response it normally does (agonist), or it may block the receptor site from being stimulated by other chemical mediators and inhibit the normal response (antagonist). Some medications can also act as agonist-antagonists, or partial agonists, by performing both roles. In any event, the medication molecule must compete with the naturally occurring chemical mediator. To win this battle, the medication molecule must have a higher affinity for the receptor than the chemical mediator does. In addition, more than one medication may vie for the same receptor.

Once the medication is bound to the receptor site, it initiates a chemical change that produces the expected effect. In some cases, this chemical change *is* the intended effect. In other cases, the initial chemical change releases a second compound (known as a second messenger) that actually causes the intended effect. Cyclic adenosine monophosphate (cAMP) is the most common second-messenger chemical related to pharmacology. Once cAMP enters the cell, it triggers the release of still other enzymes, which then carry out their own functions.

The number of available receptors is inconsistent and can be affected by the actual number of sites present, the number already occupied by another chemical mediator, and the number occupied by another medication. As medication molecules bind to the receptor sites, the number of receptors decreases, a process known as down-regulation. However, some medications can actually increase the number of available receptor sites, a process known as up-regulation.

Drug-Response Relationship

Once the medication finds the target tissue, it needs to accumulate to a sufficient concentration to produce its desired effect. The drug-response relationship correlates the amount of medication given and the response it causes. Most of this information comes from the plasma-level profiles, which describe the length of onset, duration, and termination of action. They also allow pharmacologists to determine the minimum level of medications to be effective and how much it would take to become toxic to the patient. When administering a medication, we need to know how long it will take for the concentration of the medication at the target tissue to reach the minimum effective level—that is, the onset of action. We also need to know how long the medication can be expected to remain above that minimum level to provide the intended action—that is, the duration of action. The termination of action is the amount of time after the concentration level falls below the minimum level to the time it is eliminated from the body. All of these factors affect the therapeutic index—the ratio of a drug's lethal dose for 50% of the population (LD_{50}) to its effective dose for 50% of the population (ED_{50}). In other words, the therapeutic index gives an indication of a medication's margin of safety. The plasma profile also provides information about the medication's biological half-life—that is, the time it takes the body to eliminate half of the drug.

Factors Affecting Drug Responses

A chief variable affecting the action of a drug is patient characteristics. Patients differ from one another in several ways with respect to how they react to medications:

- **Age.** Patients of different ages may have very different responses to the same drug. Older people, for example, tend to be much more sensitive to the effects of drugs and often require smaller doses than younger patients. It is not, however, solely a matter of dose. Some drugs actually have different effects altogether in different age groups. Barbiturates, for example, act as sedatives in most adults, but in older patients, they may produce excitement or agitation.
- **Weight.** Many drugs are formulated for an average adult, usually considered to be a 70-kg person. Clearly, however, the ultimate concentration in the body of a given dose of a drug will be quite different if the same drug is taken by a 48-kg person and a 136-kg person. To correct for differences in weight between patients, when specifying drug doses for emergency care, we usually give the dose in milligrams of the drug per kilogram of the patient's body weight (mg/kg).

- **Sex.** Although most sex differences in how a medication reacts are based on general differences in body mass, some medications can have varying effects in the different sexes, particularly when they are based on hormones.
- **Environment.** The environmental milieu can influence a medication's reaction because of the psychologic and physiologic stresses imposed on the patient. In addition, a particular reaction to an environmental factor, such as seasonal allergies, can alter response to a medication.
- **Time of administration.** The time at which a patient is given a medication relative to other events may affect the reaction. If a patient takes an oral medication immediately after eating, the time of onset is likely to be slowed compared with taking the same drug on an empty stomach or during physical activity such as exercise.
- **Condition of the patient.** The patient's overall state of health will also affect the response to many drugs. If the kidneys are not working properly, for example, medications may not be excreted efficiently, so the concentration of a drug may build up inside the body until it reaches toxic levels. If the patient is in shock and, therefore, by definition, the peripheral tissues are not normally perfused, it may take hours before the patient will absorb a drug that has been given by injection. Medications may also not be effective in a hypothermic patient until the person warms up.
- **Genetic factors.** In some cases, a patient's genetics may alter body systems and affect the reaction to a certain medication. If a patient lacks necessary enzymes or has a lower metabolism, for example, the response to a medication might be significantly delayed.
- **Psychologic factors.** In several research studies, patients given a false medication were found to exhibit the effects of the real medication. These patients believed they were taking the real medication and tricked their bodies into having the same response, known as the placebo effect.

Predictable Responses

Because of the extensive research that goes into developing and testing a medication before it is approved, we generally have a good idea of what a particular drug will do to the patient. Obviously, we expect to see the desired response after giving the medication. At the same time, we should anticipate responses beyond the desired effect. Side effects are reactions that can manifest as signs or symptoms that are not what we wanted to happen but nevertheless are expected based on how the medication works. Every medication has some side effects—even oxygen. The trick is to be able to evaluate the benefits compared with the risks associated with the side effects. If the patient's condition will improve more so than deteriorate from side effects, we are likely to give the medication. Conversely, if the side effects overburden or even hurt the patient more so than provide benefit, we would withhold the drug. This trade-off is known as the risk-benefit ratio.

Iatrogenic Responses

An iatrogenic response is an adverse condition inadvertently induced in a patient by the treatment given. An example of this would be the patient who develops a urinary tract infection after insertion of an indwelling (for example, Foley) catheter. When administration of drugs leads to symptoms that mimic naturally occurring disease states, it is known as an iatrogenic drug response.

Unpredictable Responses

Even though the doses of medications are carefully tested and designed for specific conditions, some patients have adverse effects that are not anticipated. The most common unpredictable response encountered in the prehospital setting is an allergic reaction. An allergic reaction occurs when the patient is extremely sensitive, or hypersensitive, to the medication or one of its ingredients. Because the patient is hypersensitive, the drug activates the immune system. Allergic reactions are unpredictable—unless the patient has had an allergic reaction to the same drug in the past—and may lead to life-threatening anaphylaxis. The paramedic should remain alert for an allergic reaction after administering *any* drug.

In rare cases, the patient may experience a completely unique response that is specific to that person; it is not seen in other patients. This situation is known as an idiosyncrasy.

Patients who take a particular medication for an extended period can build up tolerance to it. In these cases, the patient will have a decreased response to the same amount of medication, often requiring higher doses than normal. Along the same lines, a patient could develop a tolerance as a result of prolonged administration of a separate medication. Known as cross-tolerance, this phenomenon is often seen in patients who take many pain medications. When taking a medication such as oxycodone, the patient becomes tolerant to opiate-based medications. If you administer morphine for pain, the patient may not have the same response as other patients because of cross-tolerance. Tachyphylaxis is a condition in which the patient rapidly becomes tolerant to a medication. It can occur with just a couple of doses and is most often seen with sympathomimetic agents.

Any medication needs to reach a minimum concentration in the target tissue before it becomes effective; that concentration is reached by providing a specific dose. If several doses are given in a relatively short time, the patient may experience a cumulative effect. A cumulative effect is the increased effect when a medication is given in several successive doses, which might result in therapeutic or nontherapeutic effects.

With prolonged administration of a medication, a patient can become drug-dependent. In this case, the person will have significant symptoms if he or she stops using the medication.

Many patients take multiple medications at one time. It is possible for the effects of one medication to alter the response of another medication, a phenomenon known as a drug interaction. The interaction may not always be one we can anticipate. Just because two medications are sympathomimetics, for example, it does not necessarily mean the patient will experience a more dramatic sympathetic response. It is possible to see the opposite response or a completely unrelated response. When the patient is taking more then one medication, one medication could block the body's response to another medication. We can also use this fact as an advantage. For example, if the patient has taken an opiate-based drug such as morphine, we have the ability to administer another medication, naloxone, to block the response to the morphine.

A summation effect is an additive effect—that is, two drugs given to the patient have the same effect that doubles the response exhibited by the patient. When the patient receives two drugs that have the same effect but produces a response greater than the sum of their individual responses, the result is known as synergism. At times, the interaction between two medications can cause one drug to enhance the effect of another, known as potentiation. For example, acetaminophen (Tylenol) and alcohol interact. In this case, it is well known that high doses of acetaminophen are damaging to the liver. When alcohol is ingested along with acetaminophen, more of the medication is taken up into the liver and may result in acute liver failure. This phenomenon is referred to as the alcohol-acetaminophen syndrome. Some potentiation effects are known and can be exploited to achieve a desired effect; in other cases, potentiation may occur unexpectedly. A direct biochemical interaction that takes place between two drugs is referred to as interference.

Drug Storage

Many medications can be altered by extremes of temperature, exposure to direct sunlight, or excessive humidity. In most cases, the potency of the medication is decreased and, in some cases, the actual molecular components can be degraded and made inactive. Each manufacturer must provide guidance on the proper storage for each medication that is approved by the HPFD. In general, medications should be kept out of direct sunlight and stored in temperatures between approximately 15°C and 30°C. You should be conscious of these general guidelines, use your best judgment, and ensure that medications are stored in areas that are not routinely or constantly exposed to poor climate conditions. Every department should have a written protocol or procedure for the specific handling of every medication, fluid, or diluent on the vehicle or in the station to guide you on how best to store and handle medications used in daily practice.

Security of Controlled Medications

Nearly every medication used in the prehospital setting is a prescription medication; however, some are controlled substances and have more stringent control guidelines. Minimum requirements for the storage of controlled substances include a securely locked, substantially constructed cabinet with no sign or any other indication that the cabinet is used for the storage of controlled substances. Cabinets constructed of materials that are fragile and/or allow visualization, such as glass or plastic, are considered inappropriate for this purpose. A controlled substance

disposition record must be maintained, and thorough documentation must be completed for any use of a controlled substance. This includes the disposal of any leftover waste medication that was not administered during patient care. Any expired controlled substances must be returned to the agency or departmental officer in charge of maintenance and dispersal of controlled substances and must also be documented in the disposition record(s). Note that these are general guidelines. Every department must have a written protocol and procedure for the use, storage, disposition, and documentation of controlled substances.

Components of a Drug Profile

According to federal law, every medication must include a drug profile in the packaging when it is distributed from the manufacturer. The drug profile is a document that contains all of the information pertaining to the medication. Understanding this profile will aid you in selecting the most appropriate medication for your patient.

Drug Names

The drug profile includes the generic and trade names of the medication. It is also common to find the chemical name and a graphic representation of the drug molecule.

Classification

Each medication falls into a specific classification based on its effect on the patient and its mechanism of action. Having an understanding of the properties of each classification and knowing which medications fall within each classification will simplify the inherent memorization process involved with learning the drugs.

Mechanisms of Action

The mechanism of action describes how the medication causes its intended effect: by binding to a receptor site, by changing the physical properties of cells, by chemically combining with other chemicals, or by altering a normal metabolic pathway.

Indications

A medication's indications are the reasons or conditions for which the medication is given. The indications are selected based on what the medication was designed to accomplish and what has been approved by the HPFD.

Pharmacokinetics

The pharmacokinetics section describes how the medication is absorbed, distributed, and eliminated from the body. This is useful information when deciding which of the available routes of administration are most appropriate for the patient's condition. This section will also typically quantify the medication's expected time of onset and its duration of action.

Side and Adverse Effects

This section lists the undesired effects from the medication that were found during development of the drug. You should discuss these side effects with your patients so they can make an informed decision about their care and know what to expect.

Routes of Administration

Drugs may be given through a variety of routes—orally, subcutaneously, intravenously, and so forth. A drug that is therapeutic when given by one route may be lethal when given by another.

Drug Forms

Medications can come in several forms. This section of the drug profile lists available forms and their concentrations. The forms may include tablets, ampules, or vials, to name a few. Concentrations are always listed as how much medication comes diluted in how much fluid.

Dosages

The dose is the amount of the medication that should be administered for a particular condition. It is important to consider the patient's age and weight and the form in which the drug usually supplied.

Contraindications

There will almost always be conditions under which it is inappropriate to administer a particular medication. Those conditions are listed in the contraindications section of the drug profile. If a medication is given when a contraindication is present, it will most likely harm the patient.

Special Considerations

The special considerations section contains all the information necessary to safely and effectively administer the medication to pediatric patients, geriatric patients, pregnant patients, and any other special groups defined for the drug. It will also include other important information that did not appear elsewhere in the drug profile.

▌Drugs by Classifications

Classifications of drugs are based on the effect the drugs will have on a particular part of the body or on a specific condition. Antiemetic medications, for example, suppress the sensation of nausea. Many medications fall into more than one classification. For example, promethazine (Phenergan) is an antiemetic and an antihistamine. This section discusses the many classifications of drugs and their subcategories.

Analgesics and Antagonists

Analgesics include medications that relieve pain—that is, induce analgesia. Analgesia is the absence of the sensation of pain. (It is different from anesthesia, which will be discussed shortly.) Sometimes the analgesic itself is not sufficient to relieve pain, in which case an adjunct medication may be given to enhance the effects of the analgesic.

The most common class of medications used for analgesia in the prehospital setting comprises the opioid agonists. Opioid agonists, which are similar to or derived from the opium plant, bind to opiate receptors. By blocking these receptors, they prevent the neurons from sending pain signals. These medications are also CNS depressants. Fentanyl (Sublimaze) is a popular opioid agonist because it is rapid-acting, is very potent, and has a relatively short duration of action. The patient will experience analgesia within about 90 seconds, and the drug's effective duration lasts approximately 30 minutes.

Morphine has long been a popular option for the prehospital induction of analgesia. In addition to analgesia, morphine has a tendency to cause a euphoric feeling. Morphine has direct applications in cardiac emergencies because it decreases the workload on the heart (that is, cardiac preload and afterload) and, thereby, decreases the heart's consumption of oxygen.

Several nonopioid analgesics exist, many of which are available as OTC drugs. Many of these nonopioid analgesics have antipyretic properties as well, meaning they can reduce the patient's fever. All of them alter the production of prostaglandins and cyclooxygenase (Cox) to produce their effects. Three forms of nonopioid analgesics are particularly popular: salicylates (such as aspirin); nonsteroidal anti-inflammatory drugs (NSAIDs), such as ibuprofen; and para-aminophenol derivatives (such as acetaminophen [Tylenol]).

Documentation and Communication

> When treating a patient's pain, assess the patient's pain on a scale of 0 to 10 before and after treatment, and clearly document your assessment on the PCR.

Opioid antagonists reverse the effects of opioid drugs. They work by competitively binding with the opiate receptors in an antagonistic manner, meaning they do not stimulate the receptor to initiate its action. As a result of this binding, the opioid molecules cannot get to the receptor. The most common opioid antagonist used in the prehospital setting is naloxone (Narcan).

Opioid agonist-antagonists have agonistic and antagonistic properties. They are often preferred because they can decrease pain but do not diminish the function of the respiratory system or lead to dependence or addiction, unlike some other analgesics.

Anesthetics

Anesthetic medications are intended to induce a loss of sensation to touch or pain. Anesthesia can be achieved systemically, regionally, or locally. Systemic anesthesia, also known as general anesthesia, is often done through the inhalation of volatile vapourized liquids and is predominantly reserved for operating room use. Regional anesthesia focuses on a particular portion of the body, such as the legs or the arms. Local anesthesia causes a loss of sensation to touch or pain at a specific isolated spot on the body where a procedure is to take place. Regional and local anesthesia are achieved through the injection of a medication into particular locations to block nerve impulses. In other cases, the patient is given an anesthetic via inhalation, using a mask and anesthesia machine to deliver the medication.

Anesthetics are commonly grouped based on their onset of action and the duration of their effects. Ultra–short-acting agents such as thiopental sodium (Pentothal), hexobarbital, and methohexital have an onset of less than 45 seconds and generally last for 15 minutes to 3 hours. Short-acting agents such as secobarbital and pentobarbital have an onset of 10 to 15 minutes and last for 2 to 4 hours. Intermediate agents such as amobarbital and butabarbital have an onset of 15 to 30 minutes and a duration of 4 to 6 hours. Long-acting agents such as phenobarbital and barbital have an onset of 30 to 60 minutes and a duration of 6 to 8 hours.

Anesthetics have some drawbacks. In particular, they can slow the functioning of the respiratory system, CNS, and cardiovascular system.

In the prehospital setting, anesthesia (sedation) is desired before invasive procedures such as endotracheal intubation or cardioversion. In the prehospital environment, we typically administer benzodiazepines, opioids, or nonbarbiturate hypnotics to achieve a level of anesthesia.

Antianxiety, Sedative, and Hypnotic Drugs

Not surprisingly, few people would want to be awake and alert during an invasive procedure. To counteract the anxiety before such a procedure takes place, patients may take drugs that produce sedation. To ensure that they sleep through the event, they receive drugs that produce hypnosis. Drugs that create sedation and hypnosis include benzodiazepines, barbiturates, opioid agonists, and nonbarbiturate hypnotics.

Benzodiazepines are the sedatives most commonly used to prepare patients for invasive procedures. Although their exact mechanism of action is not fully understood, these drugs are believed to affect the inhibitory neurotransmitter gamma-aminobutyrate acid (GABA) in the brain. Benzodiazepine molecules bind to a receptor near GABA binding sites, which is thought to enhance their affinity for GABA. This increased affinity causes brain activity to slow. Midazolam (Versed) is a popular benzodiazepine that is relatively short acting; it has a 30- to 60-minute duration of action. In addition, midazolam has a potent amnesic effect, meaning that it inhibits the patient's ability to recall the procedure; its onset of action is approximately 1 to 3 minutes. Diazepam (Valium) is a moderately long-acting benzodiazepine with a 30- to 90-minute duration of action but a slower onset, approximately 5 minutes.

Barbiturates are believed to work very similarly to benzodiazepines by increasing the affinity between receptor sites and the inhibitory neurotransmitter GABA. Thiopental (Pentothal) is a short-acting barbiturate that has an onset of action of approximately 10 to 20 seconds and a duration of action of

5 to 10 minutes. It has limited use in the prehospital setting, however, because it is associated with significant side effects.

The nonbarbiturate hypnotics have almost identical properties to benzodiazepines and barbiturates in terms of how they affect GABA receptors. The difference is that nonbarbiturate hypnotics tend to have comparatively fewer side effects, particularly in terms of cardiovascular compromise. Etomidate (Amidate) is a common choice when a nonbarbiturate hypnotic is required. This ultra–short-acting medication has an onset of action of 5 to 15 seconds and maintains its effects for approximately 3 to 5 minutes. Etomidate has minimal effects on hemodynamic stability and decreases intracranial pressure and cerebral oxygen metabolism, making it a good choice for use in the prehospital setting.

Propofol (Diprivan), another nonbarbiturate hypnotic, has an extremely rapid time of onset, typically exerting its effects within 10 to 20 seconds. The effects are short-lived, however, and last only 10 to 15 minutes.

Anticonvulsants

A seizure, in general terms, is a state of neurologic hyperactivity. Active seizures generally require treatment in the prehospital setting because of the complications associated with them. Although the exact mechanism behind anticonvulsant medications is not completely clear, these drugs are believed to work by inhibiting the influx of sodium into cells. This halt of sodium transport decreases the cells' ability to depolarize and propagate the seizures. Several other types of drugs are used as anticonvulsants, including benzodiazepines, barbiturates, hydantoins, and valproic acids.

CNS Stimulants

Stimulation of the CNS can be accomplished one of two ways: by increasing excitatory neurotransmitters or by decreasing inhibitory neurotransmitters. Amphetamines, prescription and illicit, are examples of CNS stimulants. They increase the release of dopamine and norepinephrine to increase wakefulness and awareness. They also increase tachycardia and hypertension and can cause seizures and psychosis. Methylphenidate (Ritalin) works in similar manner but is intended to allow patients to better focus and avoid distraction.

Psychotherapeutic Drugs

Most psychotherapeutic drugs work by blocking dopamine receptors in the brain. Patients may occasionally have ill effects from their use or overuse. Schizophrenia is often treated with medications that fit into the phenothiazine and butyrophenone classifications. These medications are associated with a host of side effects, which may include extrapyramidal symptoms, orthostatic hypotension, and sedation. They also have a tendency to cause sexual dysfunction. Extrapyramidal symptoms include a wide array of symptoms such as involuntary movements, tremors, rigidity, muscle contractions, restlessness, and changes in breathing and heart rate. One of the more common involuntary movements noted is associated with the mouth, lips, and tongue. For example, the patient may have facial tics, roll the tongue, and lick the lips.

Depression is a common disorder for which many treatments are available. In particular, it is often treated with selective serotonin reuptake inhibitors (SSRIs) and monoamine oxidase inhibitors (MAOIs), which block the metabolism of monoamines in the brain. Although their popularity is waning, tricyclic antidepressants (TCAs) are still occasionally used as antidepressants. The TCAs have powerful inhibitory effects:

- They block the neurotransmitters norepinephrine and serotonin from being reabsorbed in the brain.
- They block ACh from reaching its receptors, which may lead to tachycardia.
- They block alpha-1 receptors, which may produce orthostatic hypotension.

Drugs for Specific CNS and PNS Dysfunctions

The central nervous system (CNS) agents are a class of drugs that produce physiologic and psychologic effects through a variety of mechanisms. These agents can be divided into two groups: specific agents, which bring about an identifiable mechanism with unique receptors for the agent, and nonspecific agents, which produce effects on different cells through a variety of mechanisms. The nonspecific agents are generally classified by the focus of action or specific therapeutic use, for example, antiobesity agents.

Another common group of CNS agents is stimulants, which exert their action by excitation of the CNS. Some of the specific drugs included in this group are caffeine, cocaine, and various amphetamines. All of these drugs are used to enhance alertness and reduce drowsiness and fatigue. However, high doses of these agents can cause increased nervousness, irritability, tremors, and headache. Some people may also experience withdrawal symptoms when they stop taking stimulants.

In other cases, patients may be prescribed CNS depressants. These agents are used to slow brain activity. They may be prescribed to treat anxiety, muscle tension, pain, insomnia, stress, panic attacks, and, in some cases, seizures. Some other CNS depressants are used as anesthetics. Examples of CNS depressants include lorazepam (Ativan), triazolam (Halcion), chlordiazepoxide (Librium), diazepam (Valium), alprazolam (Xanax), and opiclone (Imovane).

Drugs Affecting the Parasympathetic Nervous System

Stimulation of the parasympathetic nervous system produces myriad effects. For example, it causes the pupils to constrict and produces bronchoconstriction. It has cardiac effects, too—it causes the heart to slow and reduces its contractile force. In the digestive system, increased activity of the parasympathetic nervous system stimulates secretions from digestive glands and enhances the activity of the smooth muscles found along the digestive tract.

Cholinergic Medications

All preganglionic and postganglionic parasympathetic nerves use ACh as the neurotransmitter. Acetylcholine, which has a short life span, is deactivated by AChE. Two types of ACh receptors, collectively known as cholinergic receptors, are found in the parasympathetic system: nicotinic receptors and muscarinic receptors. The nicotinic receptors are found in all autonomic ganglia and at the neuromuscular junctions. The muscarinic receptors, which are widespread throughout the body, enable the parasympathetic nervous system to respond to stimulation. Cholinergic medications (also known as parasympathomimetics) stimulate the cholinergic receptors. Anticholinergic medications (also known as parasympatholytics) block the cholinergic receptors.

Cholinergic medications may act directly or indirectly on cholinergic receptors. A drug that has direct action binds with these receptors, thereby blocking ACh from exerting its effects. A drug that has indirect action interacts with AChE, thereby allowing ACh to avoid deactivation. If excessive cholinergics are present, the patient may exhibit the SLUDGE phenomena: increased Salivation/sweating, Lacrimation, Urination, Defecation/drooling/diarrhea, Gastric upset/cramps, and Emesis. Patients exposed to certain fertilizers, insecticides, VX (a nerve agent), and sarin gas exhibit SLUDGE symptoms because all of these substances have cholinergic properties. Weapons of mass destruction are covered in Chapter 48.

Anticholinergic Medications

Anticholinergic medications work in opposition to the parasympathetic nervous system by blocking the muscarinic and nicotinic receptors:

- **Muscarinic cholinergic antagonists** block ACh exclusively at the muscarinic receptors. Atropine, for example, is a muscarinic cholinergic antagonist; it decreases secretions, increases heart rate, dilates the pupils, and decreases gastrointestinal system activity.
- **Nicotinic cholinergic antagonists** block ACh exclusively at the nicotinic receptors. This inhibition effectively disables the ANS, so it is virtually never used.

Neuromuscular blocking agents affect the somatic (motor) nervous system by inducing paralysis. Two classes of paralytics are used to induce paralysis in the prehospital setting: depolarizing neuromuscular blocking agents and nondepolarizing neuromuscular blocking agents. All neuromuscular blocking agents bind to the somatic ACh receptors at the neuromuscular junction. Depolarizing medications stimulate depolarization of the muscle cells, which manifests as fasciculations—that is, muscle twitches. The medication then produces continuous stimulation of the muscle cell, which does not allow it to return to its resting (repolarized) state. In contrast, nondepolarizing agents bind in a competitive but nonstimulatory manner to part of the ACh receptor. As a result, these drugs do not cause fasciculations. The lack of fasciculations, coupled with the availability of reversal agents, might suggest that nondepolarizing neuromuscular blocking agents would be preferred over depolarizing agents. In reality, nondepolarizing agents tend to have a long onset and duration of action, which significantly reduces their desirability in prehospital care.

Succinylcholine is a depolarizing neuromuscular blocking agent that is the paralytic of choice for prehospital airway management. Despite its promotion of depolarization, it is favored because of its rapid onset of action (less than 45 seconds) and its short duration of action (4 to 5 minutes).

Some newer versions of nondepolarizing neuromuscular blocking agents offer shorter onset times relative to succinylcholine, but little progress has been made in shortening their duration of action. The extended duration of action is a problem because if an endotracheal intubation attempt is unsuccessful, the patient is left without spontaneous respiration for more than 30 minutes. Vecuronium is a newer nondepolarizing neuromuscular blocker that produces paralysis in as little as 30 seconds but has an intermediate duration of action of approximately 30 minutes.

Rocuronium works similarly to vecuronium. It also has a fairly rapid onset of 45 seconds, but its duration of action can be as long as 45 minutes. Rocuronium may be substituted for succinylcholine if the extended recovery time is acceptable, such as following successful endotracheal intubation.

Pancuronium is another neuromuscular blocking agent that may be used in the prehospital setting. It is important to keep in mind that acceptable conditions for endotracheal intubation generally take 90 to 120 seconds after administration of the drug, and ventilation and oxygenation must be ensured during the interval. In addition, the paralysis can last anywhere from 45 to 90 minutes. Some consider this unfavourable in situations calling for paralyzing the patient for airway management, which are time critical situations. The 90-plus-second onset time, especially compared with other shorter acting paralytics, does not make this drug the best choice. Furthermore, the duration of 45 to 90 minutes means that if the intubation attempt were unsuccessful, we would have a completely paralyzed patient for upwards of an hour without appropriate means of ventilation.

Drugs Affecting the Sympathetic Nervous System

Medications may be given to a patient in an effort to stimulate the sympathetic nervous system (sympathomimetics) or inhibit the sympathetic nervous system (sympatholytics). These medications can be selective or nonselective in terms of the receptors they affect.

Sympathomimetics stimulate the adrenal medulla so that it releases norepinephrine and epinephrine, the major neurotransmitters in the sympathetic nervous system. Norepinephrine and epinephrine, in turn, stimulate one of two types of sympathetic receptors: dopaminergic receptors and adrenergic receptors.

Stimulation of dopaminergic receptors produces dilation of the renal, coronary, and cerebral arteries. As yet, no medications have been marketed that specifically target these receptors.

Four types of adrenergic receptors are distinguished, based on their effects when stimulated:

- **Alpha-1 receptors.** Produce peripheral vasoconstriction, are associated with mild bronchoconstriction, and speed metabolism
- **Alpha-2 receptors.** Control the release of norepinephrine
- **Beta-1 receptors.** Increase the heart rate, cause cardiac muscle to contract, strengthen cardiac contraction, produce automaticity, and trigger cardiac electrical conduction
- **Beta-2 receptors.** Stimulate vasodilation and bronchodilation

A medication that agonizes (stimulates) the alpha-1 receptors increases blood pressure by increasing cardiac preload and afterload. When these receptors are antagonized (suppressed), the blood pressure is lowered by preventing vasoconstriction. This tends to cause feedback responses as the body attempts to compensate for the decreased blood pressure. Most notably, the heart rate increases and the body attempts to increase blood volume by reabsorbing sodium and water in the kidneys.

In the prehospital setting, we often agonize the beta-1 receptors in an attempt to treat cardiac arrest and hypotension. Stimulation of these receptors increases myocardial contractility (also known as inotropy). In contrast, antagonizing the beta-1 receptors lowers the blood pressure by limiting the myocardial contractility and the heart rate (chronotropy). It also decreases impulse generation in the heart and slows the conduction at the atrioventricular node, thereby treating tachycardia.

Stimulation of the beta-2 receptors allows us to treat asthma and other diseases that cause excessive narrowing of the bronchioles. Keep in mind that when using beta-2 agonists, the patient may exhibit some beta-1 effects as well. Beta-2 antagonism serves no clinical purpose; there are no circumstances in which we want to reduce the amount of air getting to the lungs via bronchoconstriction.

Skeletal Muscle Relaxants

Overstimulation of the nicotinic cholinergic transmission process can cause skeletal muscle spasms, which are very uncomfortable at best and painful at worst. Three types of skeletal muscle relaxants may provide relief: central acting, direct acting, and neuromuscular blocking. Central-acting medications work by producing CNS depression in the brain. Direct-acting medications target the muscles themselves to produce relaxation. Neuromuscular blockers produce complete paralysis.

Drugs Affecting the Cardiovascular System

The walls of the heart are composed of many interconnected cells. These cells are specialized to serve particular functions: Some conduct electrical impulses; others cause the heart to contract. Medications targeting the cardiovascular system are classified according to their effects on these specialized cells.

Medications that affect the heart rate are said to have a chronotropic effect. Inotropic effects are changes in the force of contraction. When a drug alters the velocity of the conduction of electricity through the heart, it is said to have a dromotropic effect. All three types of effects can be positive or negative. In other words, if there is a positive chronotropic effect, the heart rate has increased. If there is a negative inotropic effect, the heart is not squeezing as forcefully.

Cardiac glycosides are a class of medications that are derived from plants. These drugs block certain ionic pumps in the heart cells' membranes, which indirectly increases calcium concentrations. Digoxin, for example, may have positive inotropic effects or a combination of modest negative chronotropic and more dramatic negative dromotropic effects. Cardiac glycosides in general have a small therapeutic index (margin of safety), however, and are associated with numerous side effects.

Antiarrhythmic medications have long been used in the prehospital setting to treat and prevent cardiac rhythm disorders. These medications can have direct and indirect effects on cardiac tissue. Antiarrythmics are further classified into four groups according to their fundamental mode of action on the heart:

- **Sodium channel blockers** slow the conduction through the heart; in other words, they have a negative dromotropic effect.
- **Beta blockers** reduce the adrenergic stimulation of the beta receptors.
- **Potassium channel blockers** increase the heart's contractility (positive inotropy) and work against the reentry of blocked impulses.
- **Calcium channel blockers** block the inflow of calcium into the cardiac cells, thereby decreasing the force of contraction and automaticity. They may also decrease the conduction velocity (negative dromotropic effect).

Antihypertensive Medications

Over 5 million Canadians have hypertension. Medications administered to treat hypertension, known as antihypertensives, have the following treatment goals: keep blood pressure within normal limits, maintain or improve blood flow, and reduce the stress placed on the heart. Because these drugs are often administered for many years (even on a lifelong basis), the agent selected for a particular patient should not produce tolerance or have unbearable side effects.

Diuretic medications cause the kidneys to remove excess amounts of salt and water in the body. By lowering the total fluid volume, they reduce the level of stress placed on the cardiovascular system. In particular, they lower the preload on the heart and decrease the stroke volume. Thiazides, a type of diuretic medication often given with other antihypertensive medications, specifically control the sodium and water quantities excreted by the kidneys. Loop diuretics lower the concentration of sodium and calcium ions in the body; unfortunately, their use may also lead to excessively low levels of potassium.

Vasodilator medications act on the smooth muscles of the arterioles and veins. This property explains why nitroglycerin, a vasodilator, is so beneficial in treating myocardial ischemia. Unfortunately, the dilation of these vessels prompts a response from the sympathetic nervous system. As a consequence, when vasodilators are used to lower blood pressure, the patient must also take medications that inhibit the sympathetic nervous system.

Sympathetic blocking agents include beta blockers and adrenergic inhibitors. Beta blockers compete with epinephrine to bind with available receptor sites, thereby diminishing the effects of beta stimulation. The exact mechanism of action of adrenergic inhibitors has not been clearly elucidated but, like beta blockers, these medications decrease cardiac output and diminish the production of renin. Renin is one component of the renin-angiotensin-aldosterone system, which partially controls blood pressure.

Angiotensin-converting enzyme (ACE) inhibitors also target the renin-angiotensin-aldosterone system. ACE inhibitors suppress the conversion of angiotensin I to angiotensin II.

In contrast, angiotensin II receptor antagonists block angiotensin II from binding to its receptor sites. These drugs have been used to treat congestive heart failure and vascular diseases.

Calcium channel blockers have antiarrhythmic and antihypertensive properties. By causing the dilation of coronary arteries, they enable more oxygen to reach the heart via coronary artery dilation. In addition, they prevent the contraction of smooth vascular muscle, which reduces resistance in the peripheral vascular system.

Anticoagulants, Fibrinolytics, and Blood Components

Platelets repair damage in the blood vessels. This function is critical because defects in blood vessels can cause blood flow to slow, sometimes enough to result in the formation of a blood clot (also known as a thrombus). Abnormal thrombi may cause a life-threatening crisis such as ACS or stroke. A variety of medications are used to prevent or minimize the detrimental effects of thrombi.

Antiplatelet agents interfere with the aggregation, or collection, of platelets. They do not break down aggregated platelets but simply prevent further buildup of these blood cells. Notably, salicylic acid (aspirin) has significant antiplatelet properties and has proved important in the prehospital setting thanks to its ability to minimize the damage to the myocardium in ACS.

Anticoagulant drugs, as their name suggests, work against coagulation, thereby preventing thrombi from forming. Some patients can be prescribed anticoagulants on a long-term basis as a preventive measure, thereby avoiding the formation of thrombi associated with surgeries and certain cardiovascular conditions. You need to be aware of anticoagulant use, particularly when patients are involved in some sort of traumatic injury. Just as anticoagulants prevent blood coagulation in the vascular system, they can also prevent the life-saving coagulation needed to prevent blood loss.

Once a blood clot has formed, a <u>fibrinolytic agent</u> may be administered to dissolve the thrombus and prevent it from breaking off and entering the bloodstream, where it might do further damage. Fibrinolytic agents actually promote the digestion of fibrin. The use of fibrinolytic medications in the prehospital setting remains controversial and, in some circumstances, other forms of reperfusion therapy may be indicated.

Antihyperlipidemic Medications

Although the significance of high cholesterol as an indicator for heart disease remains a topic of discussion, many doctors prefer to treat hyperlipidemia (high cholesterol) in an effort to stave off future problems for their patients. Several types of medications are available to control cholesterol levels. HMG (3-hydroxy-3-methylglutaryl) coenzyme A reductase inhibitors—commonly referred to as statins—are especially popular choices. These medications disrupt the cholesterol production pathway in the body.

Mucokinetic and Bronchodilator Drugs

Serious respiratory emergencies often arise from severe narrowing of any portion of the respiratory tract. The respiratory tract is lined by smooth muscle fibres that influence the diameter of the airway. Control of the smooth muscles is maintained by the ANS. Namely, the parasympathetic nervous system stimulates the airway to constrict, whereas the sympathetic nervous system causes the airway diameter to dilate. Sympathetic stimulation is a result of epinephrine stimulation of the beta-2 receptors.

Many respiratory emergency treatments attempt to expand the respiratory tract by using sympathomimetic medications. These medications are classified according to their effects on the receptors. Some medications are nonselective: They affect alpha, beta-1, and beta-2 receptors alike. Stimulation of alpha receptors reduces vasoconstriction, which in turn reduces mucosal edema. Stimulation of beta-1 receptors increases the patient's heart rate and the force of myocardial contraction. Most beneficial to patients with respiratory issues, stimulation of the beta-2 receptors produces bronchodilation and vasodilation.

Complications arise when patients with respiratory emergencies eventually experience decreased amounts of oxygen to the vital organs, including the heart. As nonselective sympathomimetics begin exerting their effects, the increased heart rate and greater force of contraction lead to a higher demand for oxygen—but, of course, oxygen is already in short supply in a respiratory emergency. For this reason, it is preferable to treat respiratory emergencies with medications specific to beta-2 receptors. Such drugs produce smaller increases in heart rate and force of contraction and, thereby, dramatically decreases the body's rate of oxygen consumption.

A second-line treatment in a respiratory emergency is the class of drugs known as <u>xanthines</u>. These drugs relieve airway constriction by relaxing the smooth muscles of the bronchioles and stimulating cardiac muscles to work harder, thereby increasing blood flow. They also stimulate the CNS—in fact, one notable xanthine is the well-known CNS stimulant, caffeine.

Other respiratory medications suppress the inflammatory response that typically causes acute distress for patients with restrictive airway diseases. In the acute care setting, steroids—including methylprednisolone (Solu-Medrol) and dexamethasone (Decadron)—can be administered for this purpose.

Oxygen and Miscellaneous Respiratory Drugs

Oxygen is the most commonly used medication in the prehospital setting. And it is, in fact, a medication—which means it has appropriate and inappropriate uses and some side effects. Supplementary oxygen therapy is covered in depth in Chapter 11.

Patients may be taking a gamut of medications to treat respiratory problems, depending on their symptoms. Especially during the cold and influenza seasons, use of OTC decongestant medications is common. Try to find out what medications your patient is taking, and know the effects that these drugs may have on other medications and the signs and symptoms they can produce. Although each decongestant varies slightly in terms of its mechanism of action, all such medications seek to reduce tissue edema, facilitate drainage, and maintain the patency of the sinuses. For example, pseudoephedrine, a sympathomimetic, can cause the expected responses associated with medications in this class.

Unfortunately, the fact that these and other medications are readily available sometimes leads to their illicit use. People looking for a high have been known to overdose on decongestants and cold products—particularly pseudoephedrine, dextromethorphan, and diphenhydramine.

Drugs Affecting the Gastrointestinal System

Several classes of medications that target the gastrointestinal system are available; the exact choice of drug depends on the specific complaint. Patients experiencing nausea and vomiting may be treated in the prehospital setting with antiemetic medications. Promethazine, which is technically classified as an antihistamine and a sedative, has significant antiemetic effects and may sometimes be administered to relieve a patient's nausea. Like other antihistamines, this drug works as a competitive antagonist, blocking histamines from binding to H-1 receptors. **Table 7-4 ▸** lists other gastrointestinal agents.

Eye Medications

Ophthalmic (eye) medications are virtually always administered in the form of drops directly to the eye. The exact treatment depends on the patient's particular condition but often includes anti-infective agents and drugs intended to reduce swelling (such as NSAIDs and steroids). Ophthalmic administration of medications in the prehospital setting is generally limited to anesthetic purposes to relieve isolated irritation or to ease flushing of the eye. Tetracaine (Pontocaine) is a topical anesthetic used with a Morgan lens to flush debris or contamination from the eye. Tetracaine reduces the pain and discomfort that may be associated with these injuries.

Table 7-4	Gastrointestinal Agents
Agent(s)	**Action**
Antacids	Neutralize stomach acid, used to relieve acid indigestion, upset stomach, "sour stomach," and heartburn; typically are OTC preparations, for example, Mylanta, Tums, Maalox, and milk of magnesia
Antiflatulents	Prevent or are used to treat excessive gas in the intestinal tract, for example, simethicone (Gas-X, Ovol)
Digestants	Used to aid in or stimulate the digestive process; for example, lactase, used by people who are intolerant to dairy products
Antiemetics	Prevent or arrest vomiting, for example, include promethazine (Phenergan), prochlorperazine (Stemetil), metoclopramide (Maxeran), and ondansetron (Zofran)
Cannabinoids	Provide relief to people whose chemotherapy drug causes *minimal* nausea and vomiting; believed to work in an area of the brain thought to be partly responsible for causing nausea and vomiting; mild drowsiness, dizziness, and euphoria are common side effects
Emetics	Used to promote or cause vomiting, for example, syrup of ipecac
Cytoprotective agents	Predominantly used to treat peptic ulcer disease; provide protection to the lining of the stomach and the duodenum to allow ulcers to heal, for example, misoprostol (Cytotec)
H₂-receptor antagonists and proton pump inhibitors	Reduce acid production in the stomach; act by blocking the receptors or proton pumps of acid-producing cells in the stomach, for example, include ranitidine (Zantac) and omeprazole (Losec)
Laxatives	Stimulate loosening, relaxation, or evacuation of the bowels; sometimes maltreated by patients with eating disorders and can lead to profound dehydration if taken improperly; often used for in-hospital management of ACS patients to avoid vagal stimulation during bowel movements
Antidiarrheals	Used to prevent or treat diarrhea and frequently found as OTC preparations, such as loperamide (Imodium)

Patients may be prescribed antiglaucoma drugs that are used to treat glaucoma, an eye disease characterized by abnormally high intraocular fluid pressure, damaged optic disc, hardening of the eyeball, and partial to complete loss of vision. Common examples include timolol (Timoptic), brimonidine (Alphagan), and latanoprost (Xalatan). All of these agents are prepared as eye solutions or ointments in some cases. Other agents include mydriatic and cycloplegic agents. Mydriatic agents are used to dilate the pupils, and cycloplegics are used in the treatment and evaluation of eye problems and include tropicamide (Mydriacyl), cyclopentolate (Cyclogyl), and topical atropine. Several other medications used in the prehospital setting are contraindicated in the presence of glaucoma, so having an idea of which medications the patient may be taking for this condition will assist you in making appropriate decisions about your patient's care.

Ear Medications

Much like ophthalmic medications, medications affecting the ear (otic) are generally administered in the form of drops directly to the ear. The exception occurs in the rare case of a significant infection of the ear, which may require systemic antimicrobial medications. Most otic medications have anti-infective and anti-inflammatory effects. Prehospital administration of otic medications is not indicated.

Drugs Affecting the Pituitary Gland

Although not used in the prehospital setting, medications are available to treat pituitary disorders. These drugs may be administered to shrink or eradicate pituitary tumours. They can also block the pituitary gland from making too much hormone.

Drugs Affecting the Parathyroid and Thyroid Glands

Thyroid disorders are not an uncommon finding in patients treated by paramedics. There are two medical options for treating thyroid disorders: Medications suppress the activity of the thyroid (used in hyperthyroidism) or replace missing thyroid hormones (used in hypothyroidism). Levothyroxine (Synthroid) is a popular medication used to replace the hormones missing in hypothyroidism.

Drugs Affecting the Adrenal Cortex

Most of the treatment for disorders of the adrenal cortex involves the use of corticosteroids. Corticosteroids have anti-inflammatory properties and can have profound metabolic effects.

Drugs Affecting the Pancreas

A variety of medications are available to affect the pancreas. Still others may not act on the pancreas directly, but rather alter the way insulin (produced by the pancreas) is utilized by the body.

To directly affect the pancreas, sulfonylureas increase insulin secretion from the pancreatic beta cells. This medication is effective only if patients have residual beta cell function. Insulin sensitivity is increased by thiazolidinediones and biguanides, which are oral antidiabetic agents.

Drugs for Labour and Delivery

The use of medications for women in labour is generally limited to situations in which the delivery is abnormal or complicated, which is relatively rare. Of course, if the labour were normal, you probably would not be there. The medications administered in this situation have one of two effects: precipitating labour or inhibiting labour. Currently, only one HPB-approved medication to facilitate labour is available, oxytocin (Pitocin). Oxytocin is a naturally occurring hormone that has multiple reproductive functions. Boosting the levels of oxytocin increases the force and frequency of contractions. This drug is also used to reduce postpartum hemorrhage.

If labour begins before the baby is fully developed or if the labour is causing danger to the mother or baby, medications with tocolytic properties can be used. Tocolytic medications suppress the force and frequency of uterine contractions. Magnesium sulfate is the medication most commonly used for this purpose. It relaxes the smooth muscles, including those located in the uterus. Terbutaline is a beta agonist that has also been used as a tocolytic agent.

Drugs Affecting the Reproductive System
Medications and the Male Reproductive System

With the exception of antibiotics and antivirals for specific infections, a majority of the medications prescribed to affect the male reproductive system are intended to treat erectile dysfunction. Although you will not need to be involved in the treatment of erectile dysfunction, you need to be aware of whether the patient is being treated because of the complications that can arise in prehospital care. Phosphodiesterase inhibitors—for example, sildenafil (Viagra), vardenafil (Levitra), and tadalafil (Cialis)—are commonly prescribed to relax the smooth muscles of the corpora cavernosa and induce vasodilation. Using other vasodilatory medications, particularly nitroglycerin, within 24 to 48 hours of having taken a phosphodiesterase inhibitor can have serious implications for the patient's blood pressure. Always ask patients if they have used erectile dysfunction medications before administering nitroglycerin to avoid profound hypotension **Figure 7-8 ▶**.

Medications and the Female Reproductive System

Female reproductive medications perform a variety of functions, from contraception to promoting conception. Most of the medications carry out their functions by altering the reproductive hormones. Contraceptive medications contain synthetic hormones that trick the body into believing the ovary has already released an ovum, which in turn prevents an ovum from being released for fertilization. Antibiotics and antifungal medications may be used for specific conditions. Involvement of paramedics in administering medications affecting the female reproductive system is not indicated.

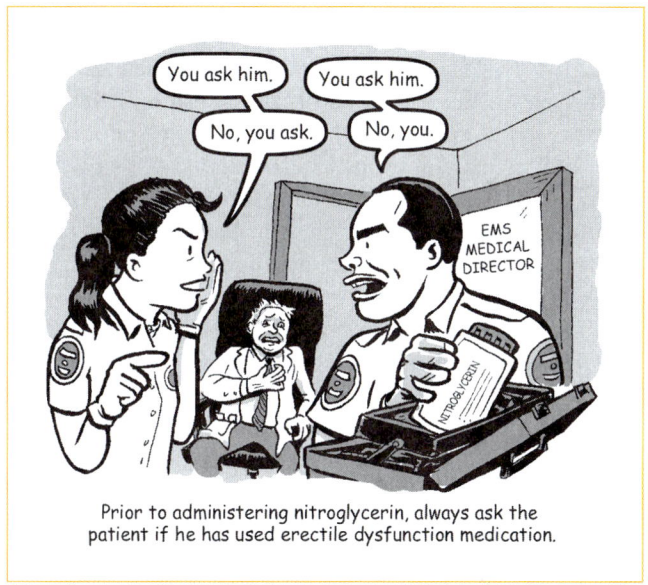

Prior to administering nitroglycerin, always ask the patient if he has used erectile dysfunction medication.

Figure 7-8

You are the Paramedic Part 4

You make contact with direct medical control, where the physician advises you to administer 500 mg of calcium chloride IV and closely monitor the patient's vital signs. Upon safe transfer of the patient at the hospital the physician explains that the patient is likely experiencing the effects of digitalis and calcium channel blocker toxicity.

Reassessment	Recording Time: 15 Minutes
Skin	Pink, warm, and dry
Pulse	74 beats/min, irregular; strong radial
ECG	Atrial fibrillation
Blood pressure	118/84 mm Hg
Respirations	22 breaths/min
Spo₂	98% on nonrebreathing mask at 15 l/min of supplemental oxygen
Pupils	Equal and reactive to light

6. What does it mean when a medication has a low therapeutic index?

7. What occurs when one drug potentiates a second drug?

Antineoplastic Drugs

Antineoplastic medications are designed to combat cancer. Most chemotherapy medications are antineoplastic drugs that work by targeting the DNA within the cancerous cells. As yet, these medications do not have the ability to single out cancerous cells, so their systemic side effects are typically significant. As paramedics, we are called to care for cancer patients from time to time; an understanding of their condition and treatments will assist you in treating them effectively.

Drugs Used in Infectious Diseases and Inflammation

Drugs Used to Treat HIV Infection

There are a number of drugs used for treating HIV infection. The first group of drugs used to treat HIV infection, called nucleoside reverse transcriptase inhibitors, interrupts the virus during an early stage of replication (that is, when the virus is making copies of itself). These drugs may slow the spread of HIV in the body and delay the acquisition of opportunistic infections. This class of drugs is also referred to as nucleoside analogs. Examples include the drugs zidovudine (AZT) and lamivudine (3TC). A second class of drugs, non-nucleoside reverse transcriptase inhibitors, also inhibits early stage viral replication. An example includes efavirenz.

A third class of drugs for treating HIV infection, called protease inhibitors, interrupts the virus during replication at a later step in its life cycle; for example, ritonavir.

A new class of drugs, known as fusion inhibitors, has also been approved by the HPFB as a treatment for HIV infection. Enfuvirtide (Fuzeon, or T-20), for example, prevents the HIV-1 virus from entering immune cells by blocking the merger of the virus with the cell membranes. This drug is designed for use in combination with other anti-HIV treatment. It reduces the level of HIV infection in the blood and may be active against HIV that has become resistant to current antiviral treatment schedules.

Antibiotics

Antibiotic medications are actually a subclassification of antimicrobial medications. Antibiotics are themselves classified into several categories based on their composition and the types of bacteria they target. Not all antibiotics affect all types of infections. Antibiotics generally work by killing the bacteria (bactericidal) or by preventing multiplication of the bacteria (bacteriostatic) and thereby allowing the body's immune system to overcome the infectious invaders. Many patients are allergic to certain antibiotics. Thus, although we do not administer antibiotics in the prehospital setting, we should ascertain specific medication allergies of our patients.

Antifungal, Antiviral, and Antiparasitic Medications

Treating fungal infections in humans, particularly systemic infections, can be much more difficult than treating bacterial or viral infections. The basic cellular structure is nearly identical between humans and fungi. Because antimicrobial medications target a specific structure within the infective organism, it is a challenge to identify a medication that will not harm human cells as well. One difference between human and fungal cells is that fungal cells use ergosterol instead of cholesterol as part of the cellular wall. Polyene medications cause the fungal cells' contents to leak out, causing them to die. Two other classes of antifungal medications, the imidazoles and the triazoles, work by inhibiting certain enzymes, thereby blocking fungal cell wall synthesis.

Antiviral medications work by a variety of mechanisms. Some antiviral medications inhibit the replication of RNA and DNA in the virus. Others inhibit the penetration and uncoating of the virus in the host cell. Still others can act as prodrugs, boosting the effectiveness of other antiviral medications given concurrently.

Antiparasitic medications target parasites (organisms that live in or on the living tissue of a host organism at the expense of that host). For example, mebendazole (Vermox) is an antiparasitic medication used to treat pinworm (enterobiasis). Pinworm infection is one of the most common parasitic infections in Canada and the United States. **Table 7-5 ▼** lists types of antifungal, antiviral, and antiparasitic agents.

Nonsteroidal Anti-inflammatory Drugs

The NSAIDs are designed to reduce pain, inflammation, and fever. They work by inhibiting the cyclooxygenase (COX) enzymes, which produce the chemical prostaglandin; prostaglandin, in turn, promotes pain, inflammation, and fever.

Table 7-5	Antifungal, Antiviral, and Antiparasitic Agents
Agent(s)	**Action**
Antimalarial	Any drug used to prevent or treat malaria: chloroquine, an antimalarial drug used to treat malaria and amebic dysentery; mefloquine hydrochloride (Larium and Mephaquin), an antimalarial drug effective in cases that do not respond to chloroquine and said to produce harmful neuropsychiatric effects in some people; primaquine and quinine, bitter alkaloids extracted from cinchona bark
Antiviral	A group of medications used to treat viral diseases; includes acyclovir
Antituberculous	A group of medications used in the treatment of tuberculosis, including isoniazid, rifampicin, pyrazinamide, and ethambutol
Antiamebiasis	Medications used to treat amebas in the body
Anthelmintics	Medications used to treat parasitic intestinal worms
Antifungal	A group of medications used to treat both local (mycotic) and systemic fungal infections; includes fluconazole and clotrimazole (Canesten)
Leprostatic	A group of medications used in the treatment and management of leprosy

There are two COX enzymes, known as COX-1 and COX-2. Some NSAIDs can be nonselective or semiselective in targeting only the COX-2 enzymes. It has been shown that COX-2 medications are associated with a lower incidence of bleeding and ulcers.

Aspirin differs slightly from other NSAIDs in that it targets the COX-1 enzymes to reduce platelet aggregation, which provides great benefit in patients who are suspected of having a myocardial infarction. This selectivity also explains why you cannot substitute another NSAID such as ibuprofen, which targets COX-2 to a much greater extent, for aspirin in this situation.

Uricosuric Drugs

Uric acid is found in the blood and is excreted by the kidneys. If uric acid levels are too high, this chemical can be deposited in the form of solid crystals in the joints—a condition known as gout. Uricosuric medications are designed to lower the uric acid levels in the blood by increasing its excretion by the kidneys into the urine.

Serums, Vaccines, and Other Immunizing Agents

Serums, vaccines, and other immunizing agents all fall into the immunobiological medications category. Immunizations can consist of antigens (vaccines, toxoids) or antibodies (immune globulins, antitoxins). A toxoid is a modified bacterial toxin that has been made nontoxic but retains the ability to stimulate the formation of antibodies. A vaccine, a suspension of whole (live or inactivated) or fractionated bacteria or viruses that have been made nonpathogenic, is given to induce an immune response and prevent disease.

Drugs Affecting the Immunologic System

Patients who undergo organ transplantation or have an autoimmune disease are often prescribed immunosuppressant medications. Immunosuppressants are intended to inhibit the body's ability to attack the "foreign" organ or, in the case of autoimmune diseases, the medications inhibit the body's attack on itself. These drugs are generally derived from fungi or bacteria and tend to have a complicated mechanism of action. Put succinctly, they inhibit lymphocytes and T cells from carrying out their immune functions.

Dermatologic Drugs

A wide variety of afflictions can affect a patient's skin, from infections to cancer. The specific medication used will be determined by the condition itself. Although several systemic medications can be used to treat dermatologic disorders, a majority of the drugs used will be applied topically. In addition, medications used to affect other areas of the body can be given through the skin (that is, transdermally). Nitroglycerin for patients with chest pain and fentanyl for pain management, for example, are commonly encountered medications that are administered transdermally.

Vitamins and Minerals

Vitamins and minerals are necessary substances that allow for normal metabolism, growth and development, and cellular function. Patients may be taking vitamin and mineral supplements to replace deficient items or as a preventive measure. Vitamins affect a wide variety of functions, but one particular we focus on in the prehospital setting is thiamine (vitamin B_1). Thiamine aids in converting carbohydrates into energy. People with alcoholism, among others, have a propensity to be deficient in this vitamin. It is sometimes appropriate to give thiamine intravenously to patients with risk factors for thiamine deficiency before administering dextrose in an attempt to facilitate effective metabolism.

Fluids and Electrolytes

Several types of IV fluids may be administered to patients. Crystalloid solutions are typically used in the prehospital setting and can be isotonic, hypotonic, or hypertonic. Isotonic solutions provide a stable medium for the administration of medication and provide effective fluid and electrolyte replacement. Hypertonic solutions help provide nutrition. Hypotonic solutions are beneficial in dehydration situations but not in hypovolemic cases. In addition to crystalloids, you may administer colloid solutions to your patients. IV fluids are discussed in detail in Chapter 8.

Antidotes and Overdoses

The management of overdose reflects the agent that the patient has consumed. Antidotes can function antagonistically by blocking receptor sites that would otherwise be stimulated by the agent. They can transform the agent into an inert, nonhazardous form to facilitate excretion. Alternatively, they may bind to the agent to prohibit its absorption into the bloodstream. Overdoses and their antidotes are discussed in depth in Chapter 33.

▌ Tying It All Together

As you review the various classifications of medications on the preceding pages, you will probably ask yourself why you need to know all of these because you don't administer them in the prehospital setting. And that is a very good question.

The answer is that there is a tremendous amount of information that can be obtained about your patient's current condition and medical history based on the medications taken. Having an understanding of which types of medications have specific functions allows you to more effectively assess your patient's condition(s). If your patient is unresponsive and you find a spilled bottle of nitroglycerin tablets, what will you suspect? Knowing what nitroglycerin is used for and the effects it has on the body allows you to significantly narrow down the possible conditions your patient might have.

In addition to the assessment of the current condition, you can also gather significant information about the patient's medical history. Again, a general understanding of the uses and effects of different medications provides the clues you need to obtain a large portion of the patient's medical history even when the patient is unable to answer. Furthermore, it is common for patients to forget about a medical condition or not consider it a medical *problem*. For example, a patient may tell you that you he does not have high blood pressure, but when you review his prescription medications, you find labetalol. Because you know that labetalol is often used to treat hypertension, you question him again. He may respond this way: "I don't have high blood pressure because that medication lowers it." This proves to be very useful information that you might have missed had you not understood the classifications of medications.

In addition, a patient's medications may alter the clinical presentation of some conditions. As you probably already know, a patient who is in hypovolemic shock will have an increased pulse rate followed by a decrease in blood pressure. What do you think you will see in a patient with hypovolemic shock but who is taking a prescription medication intended to block beta adrenergic receptors?

Once you have an idea of the condition the patient has and know the medical history, you can begin to develop your pharmacologic treatment plan. Understanding the classifications of medications has a role in this situation as well. You need to develop a treatment plan that will treat the patient's condition while considering the negative effects and interactions with the patient's other medications.

You are the Paramedic Summary

1. What are some potential differential diagnoses?

Your patient presents with a combination of symptoms: palpitations, mild shortness of breath and visual disturbances. Looking at this trio of symptoms, cardiac problems such as a silent MI, high blood pressure, and abnormal heart rate or rhythm are good possibilities. The mention that he has a history of "heart problems" also helps to tip the scale in this direction.

2. What types of medications might your patient be taking?

There are a variety of different types of medications that he could be taking for heart problems—including a diuretic, a beta blocker, a calcium channel blocker, or an ACE inhibitor.

3. What type of drug is diltiazem (Cardizem) and how does it work?

Diltiazem is a calcium channel blocker. This drug lowers blood pressure by decreasing peripheral vascular resistance. It helps decrease the work load of the heart by diminishing myocardial and smooth muscle contraction. Calcium channel blockers are also effective in the management of fast cardiac rhythm disturbances because of their ability to decrease the conduction of electrical impulses through the heart.

4. Does the patient present with signs and symptoms of possible drug toxicity? If so, which medications are in question?

Yes, drug toxicity, specifically digoxin and diltiazem, is a possibility. When taken in excess, either medication can cause a significant drop in a patient's hemodynamic status, which explains the problems with the heart rate and blood pressure, but what about the vision disturbances? One of the other side effects of digoxin toxicity is visual disturbances, including the presence of a yellow-green halo around objects and blurred vision.

5. What treatment will increase the patient's blood pressure?

In this case the best treatment is to reverse the effects of the calcium channel blocker, diltiazem, by administering calcium chloride.

6. What does it mean when a medication has a low therapeutic index?

The therapeutic index measures the safety of the drug. It is calculated by dividing the lethal dose 50 (LD_{50}) by the effective dose 50 (ED_{50}). The closer the answer is to 1, the more harmful the drug is. Since the therapeutic index for digoxin is close to one, the amount of medication between a normal dose and a toxic dose is very small, making it easy for toxic levels to develop. Because of this, patients who take digoxin frequently have their blood levels checked to make sure that they are within the therapeutic range.

7. What occurs when one drug potentiates a second drug?

When potentiation occurs, the effect of one drug increases the effect of another. In your patient, the administration of diltiazem increased the amount of digoxin in the blood, leading to the increased effects of digoxin and an increased chance of toxicity.

Prep Kit

Ready for Review

- In the prehospital setting, the goal of emergency pharmacology is to use medications to reverse, prevent, or control various diseases and illnesses, chronic and acute.
- Medications must always be delivered according to the *six rights:* the Right patient, the Right medication, the Right dose, the Right route, the Right time, and Right documentation on your PCR.
- A medication is a drug that has been approved by the government agency that regulates pharmaceuticals.
- The manufacture of pharmaceuticals in Canada is subject to a variety of laws and regulations that aim to prohibit manufacturers from making false claims about their drugs' benefits and advising patients to administer the drugs incorrectly.
- Drugs are derived from four principal sources: animal, plant, mineral, and synthetic compounds.
- Special considerations exist when administering medications to pregnant women, children, and older people.
- Paramedics are legally responsible for the appropriate use of medications and documentation of medication therapy. Always have a clear understanding of which medication you are administering and why you are administering it.
- Medications administered as part of the care provided in the prehospital setting exert their effects largely by acting on the nervous system.
- The peripheral nervous system is separated into two divisions: the somatic nervous system and the ANS. The ANS is particularly vulnerable to the administration of prehospital medications. It is considered to be "automatic" or involuntary because we cannot control its functioning or force functions under its control to happen or not happen. The sympathetic nervous system, which gives the fight-or-flight response, is the dominant system during periods of stress and activity. The parasympathetic nervous system is the dominant system during periods of rest and relaxation.
- Neurotransmission is the process of chemical signalling between cells.
- Receptors are unique molecular structures or sites on the surface or interior of a cell that bind with substances such as hormones, drugs, and neurotransmitters. Receptors are highly specialized and, in most cases, respond only to a particular substance, much like a lock and key.
- Normal neurotransmission can be altered by using drugs that mimic or inhibit neurotransmission. Some medications inhibit the release of neurotransmitters, and others work by blocking the receptor sites along the neural pathway.
- Drugs adjust or influence the body's existing functions by interacting with various cells and tissues in the body, and they typically work through several mechanisms of action rather than relying on a single action. In most cases, medications may bind to a receptor site and trigger a stimulus; in some cases, they change the chemical properties of cells and tissues. They may also combine with other chemicals within cells or organ systems to aid in elimination or bind to receptors to alter the normal metabolic functions of cells and tissues.
- Drugs are available in a wide array of forms, including liquids, solids, and vapours. In the prehospital environment, you use only a limited subset of drug forms.
- The mode of administration affects the rate at which the body absorbs the drug, and the route of administration affects the speed with which a drug works.
- Local effects result from the direct application of a drug to a tissue. Systemic effects occur after the drug is absorbed by any route and distributed by the bloodstream.

- The routes of administration are classified into three categories based on how the medication is absorbed and distributed: percutaneous (applied to and absorbed through the skin), enteral (absorbed somewhere along the gastrointestinal tract), and parenteral (any route of administration that does not cause the drug to be absorbed through the skin, mucous membranes, or gastrointestinal tract).
- Every medication has varying effects on the body. The study of the metabolism and action of medications within the body is called pharmacokinetics, which focuses particularly on the time required for absorption, duration of action, distribution in the body, and method of excretion.
- A medication's ability to reach a therapeutic concentration in the bloodstream depends partially on the rate and extent to which the drug is absorbed. Rate and extent are dependent on the ability of the medication to cross the cell membrane, which occurs by active transport or passive diffusion.
- Blood is the primary distribution vehicle for medications. Factors that change the way blood flows through the body will change the way medications are transported to the target tissue.
- Biotransformation, or the way in which the body metabolizes medications, occurs by transforming the medication into a metabolite or by making the medication more water-soluble.
- Excretion occurs primarily through the kidneys via glomerular filtration, tubular secretion, and partial reabsorption.
- Medications cause their action on the body by binding to a receptor site, changing the physical properties of cells, chemically combining with other chemicals, or altering a normal metabolic pathway.
- The drug-response relationship correlates the amount of medication given and the response it causes.
- Factors affecting how patients react to medications include age, weight, sex, environment, time of administration, condition of the patient (overall state of health), genetic factors, and psychologic factors.
- Every medication has some side effects that are known and anticipated, although occasionally unanticipated adverse reactions (iatrogenic responses) are seen.
- Extremes of temperature, exposure to direct sunlight, or excessive humidity may decrease the potency of some medications or degrade the actual molecular components and make the medication inactive.
- Understanding drug profiles will help you select the most appropriate medication for your patients.
- Classifications of drugs are based on the effect the drugs will have on a particular part of the body or on a specific condition.

Vital Vocabulary

absorption The process by which a medication's molecules are moved from the site of entry or administration into the body and into systemic circulation.

adrenal medulla The inner portion of the adrenal glands that synthesizes, stores, and eventually releases epinephrine and norepinephrine.

adrenergic Pertaining to nerves that release the neurotransmitter norepinephrine or noradrenaline (such as adrenergic nerves, adrenergic response). The term also pertains to the receptors acted on by norepinephrine, that is, the adrenergic receptors.

afferent nerves The nerves that carry sensory impulses from all parts of the body to the brain.

affinity The force attraction between medications and receptors causing them to bind together.

agonist A substance that mimics the actions of a specific neurotransmitter or hormone by binding to the specific receptor of the naturally occurring substance.

analgesia The absence of the sensation of pain.

analgesics A classification for medications that relieve pain, or induce analgesia.

anesthetic A type of medication intended to induce a loss of sensation to touch or pain.

angiotensin converting enzyme (ACE) inhibitors Medications that suppress the conversion of angiotensin I to angiotensin II.

angiotensin II receptor antagonists Medications that are similar to ACE inhibitors but work by selectively blocking angiotensin II at their receptor sites.

antagonist A molecule that blocks the ability of a given chemical to bind to its receptor, preventing a biological response.

antiarrhythmic medications The medications used to treat and prevent cardiac rhythm disorders.

antibiotic medications The medications that fight bacterial infection by killing the bacteria or by preventing multiplication of the bacteria to allow the body's immune system to overcome them.

anticholinergic Of or pertaining to the blocking of acetylcholine receptors, resulting in inhibition of transmission of parasympathetic nerve impulses.

anticoagulant drugs The medications used to prevent intravascular thrombosis by preventing blood coagulation in the vascular system.

anticonvulsant medications The medications used to treat seizures, which are believed to work by inhibiting the influx of sodium into cells.

antihypertensives The medications used to control blood pressure.

antineoplastic medications The medications designed to combat cancer.

antiplatelet agents The medications that interfere with the collection of platelets.

autonomic nervous system (ANS) The component of the peripheral nervous system that sends sensory impulses from internal structures (such as blood vessels, the heart, and organs of the chest, abdomen, and pelvis) through afferent autonomic nerves to the brain.

barbiturates Any medications of a group of barbituric acid derivatives that act as central nervous system depressants and are used as sedatives or hypnotics.

benzodiazepines Any medications of a group of psychotropic agents used as antianxiety, muscle relaxants, sedatives, or hypnotics.

bioavailability The amount of a medication that is still active once it reaches its target tissue.

biological half-life The time it takes the body to eliminate half of the drug.

biotransformation A process by which a medication is chemically converted to a different compound or metabolite.

buccal route A medication route in which medication is administered between the cheeks and gums.

calcium channel blockers The medications that suppress arrhythmias, provide more oxygen to the heart via coronary artery dilation, and reduce peripheral vascular resistance.

capsule A cylindrical gelatin container enclosing a dose of medication.

cardiac glycosides A classification of medications that naturally occur in plant substances and that block certain ionic pumps in the heart cells' membranes, which indirectly increases calcium concentrations; an example is digoxin.

chemical name A description of the drug's chemical composition and molecular structure.

cholinergic Fibres in the parasympathetic nervous system that release a chemical called acetylcholine.

chronotropic Affecting the rate of rhythmic movements, such as the heartbeat. A positive chronotropic effect would result in increasing the heart rate.

CNS stimulants Any medications or agents that increase brain activity.

contraindications In health care, conditions or factors that increase the risk involved in using a particular drug, carrying out a medical procedure, or engaging in a particular activity.

cross-tolerance A form of drug tolerance in which patients who take a particular medication for an extended period can build up a tolerance to other medications in the same class.

cumulative effect An effect that occurs when several successive doses of a medication are administered or when absorption of a medication occurs faster than excretion or metabolism.

depolarizing neuromuscular blocking agents Medications designed to keep muscles in a contracted state.

distribution The movement and transportation of a medication throughout the bloodstream to tissues and cells of the body and, ultimately, to its target receptor.

diuretic medications The medications designed to promote elimination of excess salt and water by the kidneys.

dopaminergic receptors The receptors believed to cause dilation of the renal, coronary, and cerebral arteries.

dromotropic Relating to or influencing the conductivity of nerve fibres or cardiac muscle fibres.

drugs Any substance or mixture of substances manufactured, sold, or represented for use in the diagnosis, treatment, mitigation, or prevention of a disease, disorder, or abnormal physical state or its symptoms, in human beings or animals.

duration of action How long the medication concentration can be expected to remain above the minimum level needed to provide the intended action.

efferent nerves The nerves that carry messages from the brain to the muscles and all other organs of the body.

elixir A solution with alcohol and flavouring added.

emulsion A preparation of one liquid (usually an oil) distributed in small globules in another liquid (usually water).

enteral routes The medication administration routes in which medications are absorbed somewhere along the gastrointestinal tract.

excretion The elimination of toxic or inactive metabolites from the body. This is primarily done by the kidneys, intestines, lungs, and assorted glands.

extract A concentrated preparation of a drug made by putting the drug into solution (in alcohol or water) and evaporating off the excess solvent to a prescribed standard.

fibrinolytic agents The only medications available to dissolve blood clots after they have already formed; the drugs promote the digestion of fibrin.

fluid extract A concentrated form of a drug prepared by dissolving the crude drug in the fluid in which it is most readily soluble.

ganglia Groupings of nerve cell bodies located in the peripheral nervous system.

generic drug A medication that is not patented.

generic name A general name for a drug that is not manufacturer-specific; usually the name given to the drug by the company that first manufactures it.

hypnosis Altered consciousness often caused by hypnotic drugs, which are used to induce sleep.

iatrogenic response An adverse condition inadvertently induced in a patient by the treatment given.

idiosyncrasy An abnormal (and usually unexplained) reaction by a person to a medication, to which most other people do not react.

immunobiological medications The medications that include serums, vaccines, and other immunizing agents.

immunosuppressant medications The medications intended to inhibit the body's ability to attack the "foreign" organ or, in the case of autoimmune diseases, the medications that inhibit the body's attack on itself.

indications The reasons or conditions for which the medication is given.

inotropic Affecting the contractility of muscle tissue, especially cardiac muscle.

interference A direct biochemical interaction between two drugs.

intramuscular (IM) route A method of delivering a medication into the muscle of the body. This is accomplished by placing a needle into a muscle space and injecting the medication into the tissue.

intraosseous (IO) route A method of delivering a medication into the marrow cavity of a bone. This is accomplished by placing a rigid needle into the marrow cavity and flushing a medication into the space.

liniments Liquid preparations of drugs for external use, usually to relieve some discomfort (such as pain, itching) or to protect the skin.

local anesthesia A type of anesthesia that causes a loss of sensation to touch or pain at a specific isolated spot on the body where a procedure is to take place.

local effects The effects that result from the direct application of a drug to a tissue, for example when lotions are applied to the skin to relieve itching.

loop diuretics Medications that inhibit the reabsorption of sodium and calcium ions and that can cause an excessive loss of potassium.

mechanism of action The way in which a medication produces the intended response.

medication A licensed drug taken to cure or reduce symptoms of an illness or medical condition or as an aid in the diagnosis, treatment, or prevention of a disease or other abnormal condition.

milk In the context of pharmacology, an aqueous suspension of an insoluble drug.

muscarinic cholinergic antagonists Medications that block acetylcholine exclusively at the muscarinic receptors; an example is atropine.

neuromuscular blocking agents Medications that affect the parasympathetic nervous system by inducing paralysis.

neurotransmission The process of chemical signalling between cells.

nicotinic cholinergic antagonists Medications that block the acetylcholine only at nicotinic receptors.

nonbarbiturate hypnotics Medications designed to sedate without the side effects of a barbiturate.

nondepolarizing neuromuscular blocking agents Medications designed to cause temporary paralysis by binding in a competitive but nonstimulatory manner to part of the ACh receptor. Do not cause fasciculations.

nonopioid analgesics Medications designed to relieve pain without the side effects of opioids.

nonspecific agents Medications that produce effects on different cells through a variety of mechanisms. Generally classified by the focus of action or specific therapeutic use.

nonsteroidal anti-inflammatory drugs (NSAIDs) Medications with analgesic and fever-reducing properties.

ointment A semisolid preparation for external application to the body, usually containing a medicinal substance.

onset of action The time needed for the concentration of the medication at the target tissue to reach the minimum effective level.

opioid agonist-antagonists Medications designed to relieve pain without the side effects of opioids.

opioid agonists Chemicals that are similar to or derived from the opium plant.

opioid antagonists A classification of medications that reverses the effects of opioid drugs.

para-aminophenol derivatives Medications designed to reduce fevers and relieve pain.

parenteral routes Medication routes in which medications are administered via any route other than the alimentary canal (digestive tract), skin, or mucous membranes.

patch A solid medication impregnated into a membrane or adhesive that is applied to the surface of the skin.

percutaneous routes The medication routes of any medication absorbed through the skin or a mucous membrane.

peripheral nervous system (PNS) Consists of all nervous tissue outside of the brain and spinal cord and is subdivided into two divisions, the *somatic* and *autonomic* nervous systems.

pharmacodynamics The branch of pharmacology that studies reactions between medications and living structures, including the processes of body responses to pharmacologic, biochemical, physiologic, and therapeutic effects.

pharmacokinetics The study of the metabolism and action of medications with particular emphasis on the time required for absorption, duration of action, distribution in the body, and method of excretion.

pharmacology The branch of medicine dealing with the actions of drugs in the body—therapeutic and toxic effects—and development and testing of new drugs and new uses of existing ones.

potentiation In health care, the effect of increasing the potency or effectiveness of a drug or other treatment; may occur by administering two medications concurrently, and one increases the effect of the other.

powder A drug that has been ground into pulverized form.

pulmonary route A medication route in which medication is administered directly to the pulmonary system through inhalation or injection.

pulvule A solid medication form that resembles a capsule but it is not made of gelatin and does not separate.

regional anesthesia A type of anesthesia that focuses on a particular portion of the body, such as the legs or the arms.

sedation An effect in which the patient experiences decreased anxiety and inhibition.

side effects Reactions that can manifest as signs or symptoms that are not desired but are expected based on how the medication works.

skeletal muscle relaxants Medications that provide relief of skeletal muscle spasms.

sodium channel blockers Antiarrhythmic medications that slow conduction through the heart.

solution A liquid containing one or more chemical substances entirely dissolved, usually in water.

specific agents Medications that bring about an identifiable mechanism with unique receptors for the agent.

spirits A preparation of a volatile substance dissolved in alcohol.

stimulants An agent that increases the level of body activity.

subcutaneous (SC or SQ) route A medication route in which injections are given beneath the skin into the fat or connective tissue immediately underlying it.

sublingual (SL) A medication route in which medication is administered under the tongue.

summation effect The process whereby multiple medications can produce a response that the individual medications alone do not produce.

suppository A drug mixed in a firm base that melts at body temperature and is shaped to fit the rectum, urethra, or vagina.

suspension A preparation of a finely divided drug intended to be (or already) incorporated in a suitable liquid.

sympathetic blocking agent An antihypertensive medication that decreases cardiac output and rennin secretions.

sympathomimetics The medications administered to stimulate the sympathetic nervous system.

synergism An interaction of two or more medications that results in an effect that is greater than the sum of their effects if taken independently.

syrup A drug suspended in sugar and water to improve its taste.

systemic anesthesia A type of anesthesia often done through the inhalation of volatile vapourized liquids and predominantly reserved for operating room use; also called general anesthesia.

systemic effects The effects that occur after the drug is absorbed by any route and distributed by the bloodstream; almost invariably involve more than one organ.

tablet A powdered drug that has been moulded or compressed into a small disk.

tachyphylaxis A condition in which the patient rapidly becomes tolerant to a medication.

termination of action The amount of time after the medication's concentration falls below the minimum effective level until it is eliminated from the body.

therapeutic The desired or intended action of a medication.

therapeutic index The ratio of a drug's lethal dose for 50% (LD_{50}) of the population to its effective dose for 50% (ED_{50}) of the population; a medication's margin of safety.

thiazides A type of diuretic medication that specifically controls the sodium and water quantities excreted by the kidneys.

tincture A dilute alcoholic extract of a drug.

tolerance A physiologic response that requires a patient to take an increased medication dose to produce the same effect that formerly was produced by the lower dose.

toxoid A modified bacterial toxin that has been made nontoxic but retains the ability to stimulate the formation of antibodies.

trade name The brand name registered to a specific manufacturer or owner; also called proprietary name.

transdermal route A medication route generally performed by placing medication directly onto the patient's skin.

uricosuric medications The medications designed to lower the uric acid level in the blood by increasing the excretion by the kidneys into the urine.

vaccine A suspension of whole (live or inactivated) or fractionated bacteria or viruses that have been made nonpathogenic; given to induce an immune response and prevent disease.

vapour A gaseous medication form primarily used in operating room anesthesia.

vasodilator medications The medications that work on the smooth muscles of the arterioles and/or the veins.

xanthines A classification of medications that affect the respiratory smooth muscle and that relax bronchiole smooth muscles, stimulate cardiac muscle, and stimulate the central nervous system.

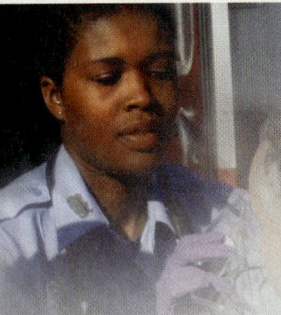

Assessment in Action

You and your partner have responded to a call for chest pain. The patient is a 68-year-old man who describes the pain as being a 20 on a 1-to-10 scale with 10 being the worst pain ever. As your partner connects the patient to the monitor, you start gathering your patient's history. The patient has had a previous cardiac event and has been prescribed a "beta blocker."

1. **What is the primary action of a beta blocker?**
   A. It reduces the adrenergic stimulation of the beta receptors in the heart.
   B. It increases the adrenergic stimulation of the beta receptors in the heart.
   C. It reduces the cholinergic stimulation of the beta receptors in the heart.
   D. It increases the cholinergic stimulation of the beta receptors in the heart.

2. **You decided to give your patient salicylic acid once you determine that he is not allergic to it. Salicylic acid is a(n):**
   A. calcium channel blocker.
   B. sympathomimetic.
   C. antiplatelet agent.
   D. antihypertensive.

3. **Your patient has not taken any of his own nitroglycerin, so you decide to give him a dose of yours. How are you going to deliver the medication?**
   A. IV push
   B. Sublingual
   C. Intramuscular
   D. Subcutaneous

4. **How long should it take for the nitroglycerin to take effect through this route of administration?**
   A. 15 to 20 minutes
   B. 10 to 15 minutes
   C. 5 to 10 minutes
   D. Less than 5 minutes

5. **Your patient is still having substantial chest pain after the nitroglycerin, and you decide that he will benefit greatly from analgesia. Which medication is an analgesic?**
   A. Morphine
   B. Naloxone (Narcan)
   C. Oxygen
   D. Salbutamol

6. **What is a specific cardiac action of the analgesic mentioned in question 5 that should benefit this patient?**
   A. It has a chronotropic action that slows the heart rate.
   B. It decreases the workload on the heart.
   C. It increases the workload on the heart.
   D. It decreases ectopic beats.

Challenging Question

7. **If this patient had taken three doses of his own nitroglycerin, would you still give him three doses of yours?**

▬ Points to Ponder

You respond to a mutual aid request from a neighbouring jurisdiction for a cardiac arrest. When you arrive on the scene, you find that the local fire service arrived ahead of you. The fire crew has a paramedic on board and has secured the airway and inserted an IV line. You introduce yourself and your MFR partner to the crew and assume responsibility for administering the medications. You ask your partner to hand you some epinephrine. Your partner pulls the unfamiliar drug box over and starts rummaging through looking for a particular colour of label, which he cannot find. All of the medications are unboxed and stored in elastic loops in a soft-sided pack. You look back at your partner to see what the hold-up is and you see the medication pack.

Are all medication boxes standardized by the colour of the box? Who has the responsibility to select the correct medication?

Issues: Working With Other Responders, Properly Administering Medication.

8 Vascular Access and Medication Administration

Introduction

Vascular access is often needed in emergency medicine for patients in hemodynamically unstable condition and in need of intravenous (IV) fluids, various medications, or both. A number of techniques are used to gain vascular access in the prehospital setting, including cannulation of a peripheral extremity vein, external jugular vein cannulation, and intraosseous access for infusion. In critically ill or injured patients, survival often depends on your ability to obtain vascular access quickly and effectively. Because these procedures are invasive, you must be proficient, yet cautious. Significant harm to the patient can result from improper technique and/or insufficient knowledge of the medication(s) being administered.

This chapter begins with an overview of fluids and electrolytes—balanced and imbalanced—and the processes of osmosis and diffusion. Next, it discusses the various types of IV solutions used in the prehospital setting and the techniques of IV therapy and intraosseous infusion. Finally, it describes the mathematical principles used in pharmacology, calculating medication doses (bolus and maintenance infusion), and the various routes for administering medications.

Fluids and Electrolytes

The human body is composed mostly of water, which provides the environment in which the chemical reactions necessary to life take place. Water also serves as a transport medium for nutrients, hormones, and waste materials. The total body water (TBW) constitutes 60% of the weight of an adult and is distributed among the following compartments Figure 8-1 ▶ :

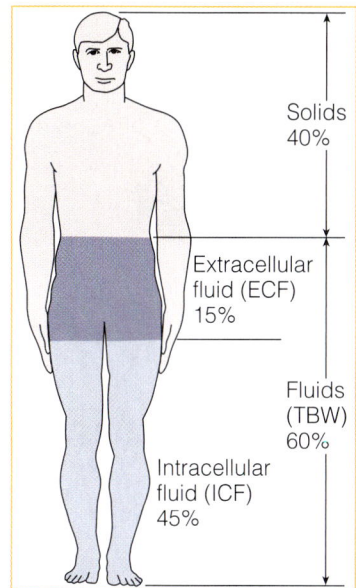

Figure 8-1 Distribution of water throughout the body.

- Intracellular fluid (ICF) is the water contained inside the cells; it normally accounts for 45% of body weight.
- Extracellular fluid (ECF), the water outside the cells, accounts for 15% of body weight and is further divided into two types of fluids:
  - Interstitial fluid, the water bathing the cells, accounts for about 10.5% of body weight. The interstitial fluid also includes special fluid collections, such as cerebrospinal fluid and intraocular fluid.
  - Intravascular fluid (plasma), the water within the blood vessels, carries red blood cells, white blood cells, and vital nutrients. Intravascular fluid normally accounts for about 4.5% of body weight.

You are the Paramedic Part 1

You are dispatched to the home of a 70-year-old woman who has diabetes. A neighbour found her lying on a couch in her living room. The neighbour tells you she tried to wake up the patient, but was unable to do so. The patient appears to be unconscious; she is pale and noticeably diaphoretic. She is breathing, but her respirations are rapid and shallow.

Your general impression of the patient and her environment reveals no signs of injury. After carefully moving the patient to the floor, you perform an initial assessment. Your partner opens the jump kit in preparation for treatment.

Initial Assessment	Recording Time: 0 Minutes
Level of consciousness	U (Unresponsive)
Airway	Patent; airway is clear of secretions
Breathing	Respirations, rapid and shallow
Circulation	Radial pulses, rapid and weak; skin, pale and diaphoretic; no gross bleeding

1. Is this a medical patient or a trauma patient?
2. What are your initial priorities of prehospital care?
3. What is the most appropriate initial airway management for this patient?
4. Does this patient require immediate medication therapy?

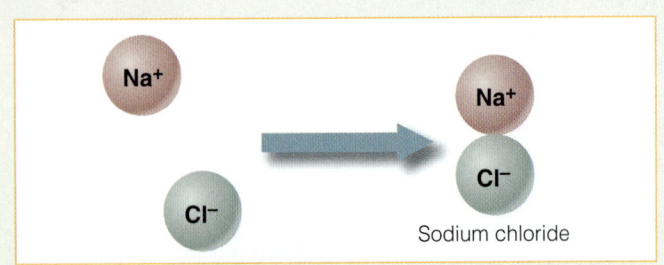

Figure 8-2 When sodium (Na⁺) and chloride (Cl⁻) unite, they form salt (sodium chloride [NaCl]).

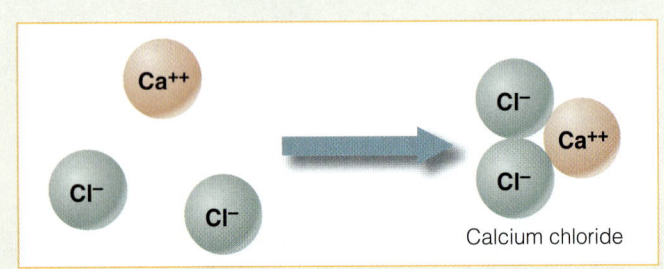

Figure 8-3 A doubly charged (bivalent) cation such as calcium (Ca⁺⁺) needs two anions.

The fluids in the body are composed of dissolved elements and water, a combination known as a solution. A solution is a mixture of two things:

- Solvent. The fluid that does the dissolving, or the solution that contains the dissolved components
- Solute. The dissolved particles contained in the solvent

Water in the body serves as the universal solvent, dissolving a variety of solutes. These solutes can be classified as electrolytes or nonelectrolytes.

Electrolytes

Atoms carry charges—some positive, some negative. Two or more atoms that bond together form a molecule. When atoms bond together, they share and disperse their charges throughout the molecule. Organic molecules contain carbon atoms—for example, table sugar ($C_6H_{12}O_6$). By contrast, inorganic molecules do not contain carbon—for example, table salt (NaCl). Inorganic molecules give rise to electrolytes (so called because of their ability to conduct electricity) when they dissociate in water into their charged components.

Electrolytes, also called ions, are reactive and dangerous if left to circulate in the body. The body, however, uses the energy stored in these charged particles. Electrolytes help to regulate everything from water levels to cardiac function and muscle contractions. Water in the body stabilizes the electrolyte charges so that the electrolytes can aid in the metabolic functions that are necessary for life.

Each electrolyte has a unique property or value to the body. If the electrolyte has an overall *positive* charge, it is called a cation; if it has an overall *negative* charge, it is called an anion. The major cations of the body include sodium, potassium, calcium, and magnesium; bicarbonate, chloride, and phosphorous are the major anions.

The internationally accepted unit of measurement for electrolytes is the millimole (mmol). One millimole of any cation is able to react completely with 1 mmol of any anion. For example, sodium (Na⁺) is a singly charged (monovalent) cation, and chloride (Cl⁻) is a singly charged anion. Thus 1 mmol of Na⁺ will react with 1 mmol of Cl⁻ to form NaCl—ordinary table salt **Figure 8-2 ◂**. Calcium (Ca⁺⁺) has two positive charges (bivalent) and reacts completely with two singly charged anions **Figure 8-3 ◂**.

Sodium

Sodium (Na⁺) is the principal extracellular cation needed to regulate the distribution of water throughout the body in the intravascular and interstitial fluid compartments. Its role in maintaining adequate cellular perfusion gives rise to the saying, "Where sodium goes, water follows."

Potassium

About 98% of all the body's potassium (K⁺) is found inside the cells of the body, making it the principal intracellular cation. Potassium plays a major role in neuromuscular function and in the conversion of glucose into glycogen. Cellular potassium levels are regulated by insulin. The sodium-potassium (Na+-K+) pump is helped by the presence of insulin and epinephrine. Low potassium levels—hypokalemia—in the serum (blood plasma) can lead to decreased skeletal muscle function, gastrointestinal disturbances, and alterations in cardiac function. High potassium levels in the serum—hyperkalemia—can lead to hyperstimulation of neural cell transmission, resulting in cardiac arrest.

Calcium

Calcium (Ca⁺⁺) is the principal cation needed for bone growth. It also plays an important part in the functioning of heart muscle, nerves, and cell membranes and is necessary for proper blood clotting.

Low serum calcium levels—hypocalcemia—can lead to overstimulation of nerve cells. Signs and symptoms of hypocalcemia include skeletal muscle cramps, abdominal cramps, carpopedal spasms, hypotension, and vasoconstriction.

High serum calcium levels—hypercalcemia—can lead to decreased stimulation of nerve cells. Signs and symptoms of hypercalcemia include skeletal muscle weakness, lethargy, ataxia, vasodilation, and hot, flushed skin.

Magnesium

Magnesium (Mg⁺⁺) has an important role as a coenzyme in the metabolism of proteins and carbohydrates. In addition, it acts in a manner similar to calcium in controlling neuromuscular irritability.

Bicarbonate

Bicarbonate (HCO_3^-) levels are the determining factor between acidosis and alkalosis in the body. Bicarbonate is the primary buffer used in all circulating body fluids.

Chloride

Chloride concentration is a primary determinant of stomach pH. It also regulates extracellular fluid levels.

Phosphorous

Phosphorous (P) is an important component in adenosine triphosphate (ATP), the body's powerful energy source.

Nonelectrolytes

The body also contains solutes that have no electrical charge. These nonelectrolytes include glucose and urea. The normal concentration of glucose in the blood, for example, is 4 to 8 mmol/l.

Fluid and Electrolyte Movement

Water and electrolytes move among the body's fluid compartments according to some basic chemical and biological tenets. One governing principle is that unequal concentrations on different sides of a cell membrane will move to balance themselves equally on both sides of the membrane. Balance across a cell membrane has two components:

- Balance of compounds (for example, water and electrolytes) on either side of the cell membrane
- Balance of charges [the positive ($^+$) or negative ($^-$) charges carried on the atoms] on either side of the cell membrane

When concentrations of charges or compounds are greater on one side of the cell membrane than on the other side, a gradient is created. The natural tendency for materials is to flow from an area of higher concentration to one of lower concentration, establishing a concentration gradient. Gradients are categorized according to the type of material that flows down them: Chemical compounds flow down chemical gradients; electrical currents flow down electrical gradients. The process of flowing down a gradient depends on whether the cell membrane will allow the material to pass through it. Certain compounds can travel freely across the cell membrane (a kinetically favourable situation that requires little energy), whereas others require active transport across the membrane because of the size of the compound or because of an incompatible charge.

Diffusion

When compounds or charges concentrated on one side of a cell membrane move across it to an area of lower concentration, the process is called diffusion. To visualize this situation, imagine that too many people show up for a theatre performance. The management decides to open another seating area to accommodate the crowd. Patrons (charges or compounds) are concentrated in a small area (the cell) outside the door (the cell membrane) leading to the new seating area. When the theatre manager opens the door, patrons can move through it (selective cell membrane permeability) from the congested area (down a concentration gradient). The patrons spread themselves out evenly (diffuse) throughout the total area, with some choosing to stay behind in the original seating area as others move into the new area, until all have an equal amount of room.

Filtration

Filtration, another type of diffusion, is commonly used by the kidneys to clean blood. Water carries dissolved compounds across the cell membranes of the tubules of the kidney. The tubule membrane traps these dissolved compounds but lets the water pass through in much the same way that a coffee filter traps the grounds as water passes through it. This cleans the blood of wastes and removes the trapped compounds from circulation so they can be flushed out of the body. The antidiuretic hormone (ADH) prevents the loss of water from the kidneys by causing its reabsorption into the tubules.

Active Transport

Often, the cell must maintain an imbalance of compounds across its membrane to achieve some metabolic purpose. For example, in the sodium-potassium pump, the cell uses sodium outside the cell and potassium inside the cell for depolarization. To maintain this imbalance, the cell must use energy in the form of ATP and actively transport compounds across its membrane. Even though active transport demands a high-energy expenditure, its benefits outweigh the initial use of ATP. Pumping sodium out of the cell and potassium into the cell has the added benefit of moving glucose into the cell at the same time.

Osmosis

As noted earlier, fluid compartments in the body are separated from one another by membranes, such as the cell membranes and the membranes lining blood vessels. The concentration of fluid in those compartments—that is, the number of solute particles—is chiefly influenced by the process called osmosis. If two solutions are separated by a semipermeable membrane (eg, a cell membrane), water will flow across the membrane *from* the solution of *lower* solute concentration *to* the solution of *higher* solute concentration. The net effect is to equalize the solute concentrations on both sides of the membrane.

The effects of osmotic pressure on a cell constitute the tonicity of the solution **Figure 8-4 ▸**. Tonicity reflects the concentration of sodium in a solution and the movement of water in relation to the sodium levels inside and outside the cell.

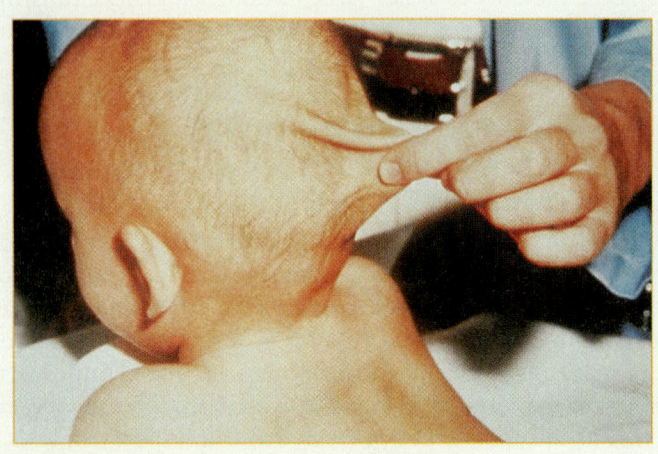

Figure 8-4 Tonicity.

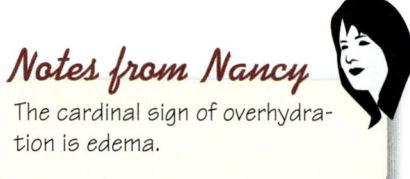

Figure 8-5 Skin tenting is a sign of dehydration.

Abnormal States of Fluid and Electrolyte Balance

The healthy body maintains a delicate balance between intake and output of fluids and electrolytes, ensuring that the internal environment remains fairly constant. The internal environment's resistance to change is called homeostasis. The ill or injured body, however, may be unable to maintain homeostasis, and excesses or deficits of fluids and electrolytes may occur. You need to know when IV fluids are indicated, what kinds of fluids are required in different situations, and when IV fluids can be dangerous. Although verbal orders or protocols will largely govern the use of IV fluids in the prehospital environment, you must still use your judgment when administering IV fluids.

A healthy person loses approximately 2 to 2.5 l of fluid daily through urine output and through the lungs (exhalation) and skin. These losses are replaced by intake of fluids and by nutrients that are partially converted to water in their metabolism. In illness, abnormal states of hydration may occur in which intake and output are no longer in balance.

Dehydration

Dehydration is defined as inadequate total systemic fluid volume Figure 8-5 ◂ . It is usually a chronic condition of elderly or very young people and may take days to manifest. As fluid is lost from the vascular compartment, the body reacts by shifting interstitial fluid into the vascular area; fluid also shifts from the intracellular to the extracellular compartments. As a consequence, a total systemic fluid deficit occurs.

Signs and symptoms of dehydration include decreased level of consciousness, postural hypotension, tachypnea, dry mucous membranes, tachycardia, poor skin turgor, and flushed, dry skin. Causes of dehydration include diarrhea, vomiting, gastrointestinal drainage, hemorrhage, and insufficient fluid or food intake.

Notes from Nancy

The cardinal sign of overhydration is edema.

Overhydration

When the body's total systemic fluid volume increases, overhydration occurs. Fluid fills the vascular compartment, filters into the interstitial compartment, and is forced from the engorged interstitial compartment into the intracellular compartment. This fluid backup can lead to death Figure 8-6 ▸ .

Signs and symptoms of overhydration include shortness of breath, puffy eyelids, edema, polyuria, moist crackles (rales), and acute weight gain. Causes of overhydration include unmonitored IVs, kidney failure, and prolonged hypoventilation.

IV Fluid Composition

The use of IV fluids can significantly alter the patient's condition and facilitate patient treatment. Each bag of IV solution must be sterile and safe; therefore, each bag of IV solution is individually sterilized Figure 8-7 ▸ . The compounds and ions dissolved in the solutions are identical to the ones found in the body.

Sodium is used as the benchmark to calculate a solution's tonicity. The concentration of sodium in the cells of the body is approximately 0.9%. Altering the concentration of sodium in the IV solution, therefore, can move the water into or out of any fluid compartment in the body.

Types of IV Solutions

There are five basic types of IV solutions: isotonic, hypotonic, hypertonic, crystalloid, and colloid. IV fluids use combinations of these solutions to create the desired effects inside the body.

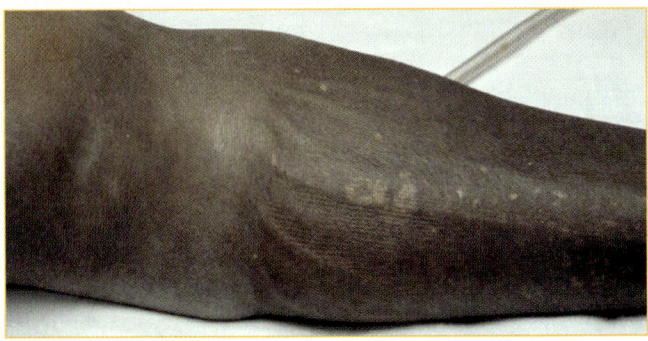

Figure 8-6 In an overhydrated patient, fluid backup occurs.

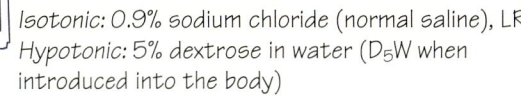

At the Scene

Isotonic: 0.9% sodium chloride (normal saline), LR
Hypotonic: 5% dextrose in water (D₅W when
introduced into the body)
Hypertonic: 3.0% saline, blood products, albumin, pentaspan

contents of the intravascular compartment without shifting fluid to or from other compartments, or changing cell shape—an important consideration when dealing with hypotensive or hypovolemic patients. When administering isotonic solutions, you must be careful to avoid fluid overloading. Patients with hypertension and congestive heart failure are at greatest risk of this problem. The extra fluid increases preload, which in turn increases the workload of the heart, creating fluid backup in the lungs.

Lactated Ringer's (LR) solution is generally used in the prehospital environment for patients who have lost large amounts of blood. It contains lactate, which is metabolized in the liver to form bicarbonate—the key buffer that combats the intracellular acidosis associated with severe blood loss. LR solution should not be given to patients with liver problems because they cannot metabolize the lactate.

D_5W, 5% dextrose in water, is a unique type of isotonic solution. As long as it remains in the bag, it is considered an isotonic solution. Once it is administered, however, the dextrose is quickly metabolized, and the solution becomes hypotonic.

Hypotonic Solutions

A hypotonic solution has an osmolarity less than that of serum. When this fluid is placed in the vascular compartment, it begins diluting the serum. Soon the serum osmolarity is less than that of the interstitial fluid; water is pulled from the vascular compartment into the interstitial fluid compartment, causing cells to swell and possibly burst from the increased intracellular osmotic pressure.

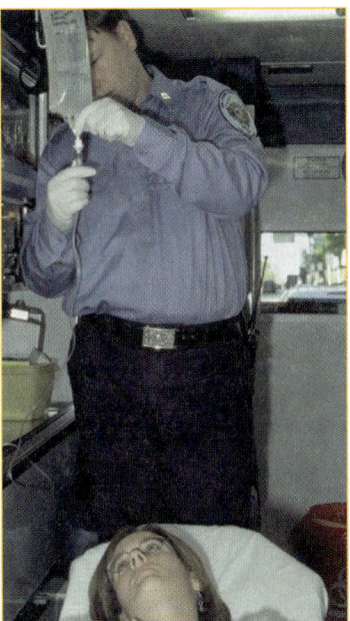

Figure 8-7 Each bag of IV solution must be sterile and safe.

Fluid movement across a cell membrane resulting from hypertonic, isotonic, and hypotonic solutions is illustrated in **Figure 8-8 ▾**. IV fluids introduced into the circulatory system can affect the tonicity of the extracellular fluid, resulting in dire consequences unless care is used.

Isotonic Solutions

Isotonic solutions such as normal saline (0.9% sodium chloride) have almost the same osmolarity (concentration of solute) as serum and other body fluids. As a consequence, isotonic solutions expand the

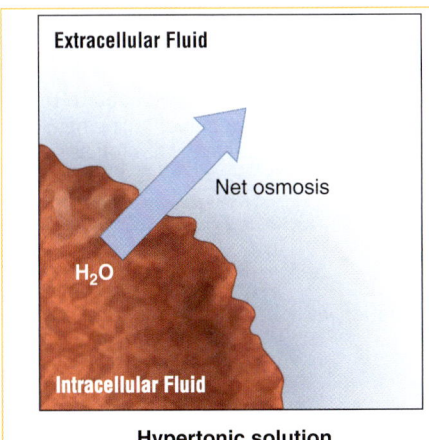 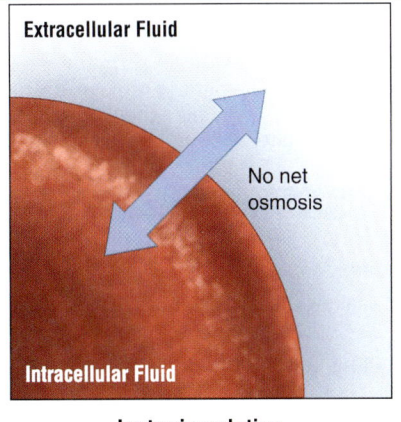 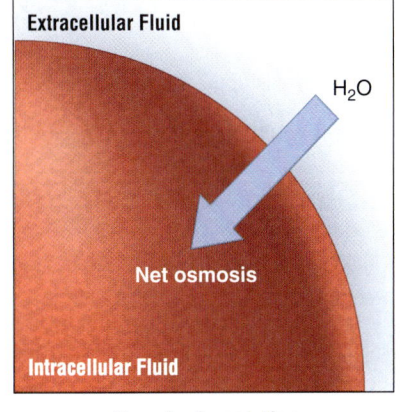

Figure 8-8 Fluid movement with hypertonic, isotonic, and hypotonic solutions.

Hypotonic solutions hydrate the cells while depleting the vascular compartment. They may be needed for a patient who is receiving dialysis because dialysis therapy dehydrates the cells.

Hypotonic solutions can cause a sudden fluid shift from the intravascular space to the cells, leading to cardiovascular collapse and increased intracranial pressure from shifting fluid into the brain cells. For example, giving D_5W for an extended period can increase intracranial pressure. This makes hypotonic solutions dangerous for patients with stroke or any head trauma. Administering these solutions to patients with burns, trauma, malnutrition, or liver disease is also hazardous because these patients are at risk for developing third spacing, an abnormal fluid shift into the interstitial compartment.

Hypertonic Solutions

A hypertonic solution has an osmolarity higher than that of serum, meaning that the solution has more ionic concentration than serum and pulls fluid and electrolytes from the intracellular and interstitial compartments into the intravascular compartment. The danger is that the cells may collapse from the increased extracellular osmotic pressure. Hypertonic solutions shift body fluids into the vascular spaces and help stabilize blood pressure, increase urine output, and reduce edema. These fluids are rarely, if ever, used in the prehospital setting.

Often the term "hypertonic" is used to refer to solutions that contain high concentrations of proteins. These proteins have the same effect on fluid as sodium. Careful monitoring is needed to guard against fluid overloading when using hypertonic fluids, especially with patients with impaired heart or kidney function. Also, hypertonic solutions should not be given to patients with diabetic ketoacidosis or others at risk of cellular dehydration.

Crystalloid Solutions

Crystalloid solutions are dissolved crystals (eg, salts or sugars) in water. The ability of these fluids to cross membranes and alter fluid levels makes them the best choice for prehospital care of injured patients who need body fluid replacement. When you use an isotonic crystalloid for fluid replacement to support blood pressure after blood loss, remember the 3-to-1 replacement rule: *3 ml of isotonic crystalloid solution is needed to replace 1 ml of patient blood.* This amount is needed because approximately two thirds of the infused isotonic crystalloid solution will leave the vascular spaces in about 1 hour.

When you replace lost volume, it is imperative to remember that crystalloid solutions cannot carry oxygen. Boluses of 20 ml/kg should be given to maintain perfusion (ie, radial pulses, adequate mental status) but not to raise blood pressure to the patient's normal level. Increasing blood pressure too much with IV solutions not only dilutes remaining blood volume, thereby decreasing the proportion of hemoglobin, but also may increase internal bleeding by interfering with hemostasis—the body's internal blood-clotting mechanism.

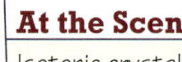

At the Scene

Isotonic crystalloid solutions—normal saline and LR—replace lost volume but do not carry oxygen. Replace lost volume to maintain perfusion, but recognize the need for rapid transport.

Colloid Solutions

Colloid solutions contain molecules (usually proteins) that are too large to pass out of the capillary membranes and, therefore, remain in the vascular compartment. These very large protein molecules give colloid solutions a very high osmolarity. As a result, they draw fluid from the interstitial and intracellular compartments into the vascular compartments. Colloid solutions work very well in reducing edema (eg, in pulmonary or cerebral edema)

You are the Paramedic Part 2

Your partner is appropriately managing the patient's airway. The patient remains unconscious and unresponsive. Your rapid head-to-toe assessment reveals no gross injury or bleeding. The patient is wearing a medic-alert bracelet that identifies her as a diabetic. The neighbour tells you that she just spoke with the patient approximately 1 hour earlier and she was fine. Baseline vital signs reveal the following:

Vital Signs	Recording Time: 5 Minutes
Blood pressure	100/60 mm Hg
Pulse	120 beats/min, weak and regular
Respirations	30 breaths/min and shallow (baseline); your partner is assisting ventilation with a bag-valve-mask device and 100% oxygen
Sao₂	99% (with assisted ventilation and 15 l/min of oxygen)
Skin	Cool, pale, and moist

5. Given the patient's history, what additional assessment should you perform?

6. When starting an IV for this patient, what solution should you use?

while expanding the vascular compartment. They could cause dramatic fluid shifts and place the patient in considerable danger if they are not administered in a controlled setting. For this reason, colloids are rarely used in the prehospital setting. Examples of colloids are albumin, dextran, and pentaspan.

Oxygen-Carrying Solutions

Obviously, the best fluid to replace lost blood is whole blood. Unlike the crystalloid and colloid solutions, whole blood contains hemoglobin, which carries oxygen to the body's cells. On occasion (eg, aeromedical transports, mass-casualty incidents), O-negative blood—a universally compatible blood type—may be used outside a hospital setting. However, because of the refrigeration requirements and other storage issues, general use of whole blood is impractical in the prehospital setting.

Synthetic blood substitutes, which do have the ability to carry oxygen, are being researched and, in some places, tested. They show great potential for improving the way you treat patients who have lost large amounts of blood. Not only would these synthetic blood substitutes expand circulating volume, but they also would carry and deliver oxygen to the part of the body that needs it the most—the cell.

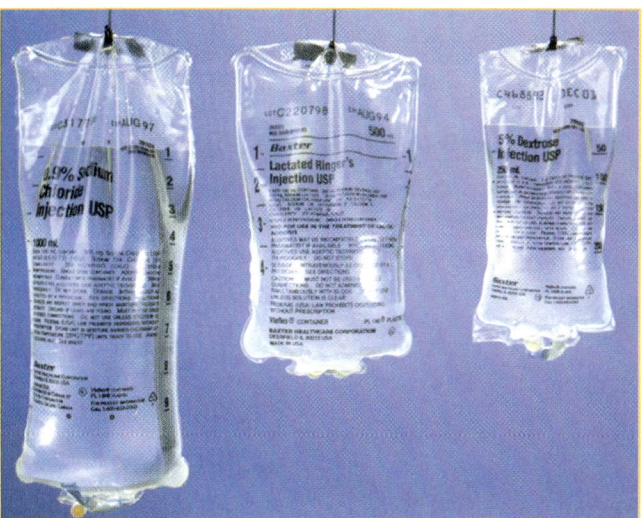

Figure 8-9 IV solution bags come in different fluid volumes.

▎IV Techniques and Administration

Intravenous means "within a vein." Intravenous (IV) therapy involves cannulation of a vein with a cannula to access the patient's vascular system. It is one of the most invasive techniques you will perform as a paramedic. Peripheral vein cannulation involves cannulating veins of the periphery—that is, veins that can be seen and/or palpated (eg, veins of the hand, arm, or lower extremity and the external jugular vein).

The most important point to remember about IV therapy is to keep the IV equipment sterile. Forethought and attention to detail will help prevent mental and procedural errors while starting the IV. One way to ensure proper technique is to develop a routine to follow as you assemble the appropriate equipment.

Assembling Your Equipment

To avoid delays and IV site contamination, gather and prepare all your equipment before you attempt to start an IV. In some cases, the patient's condition may make full preparation difficult, so working as a team becomes critical. The members of your own crew, by anticipating your needs, often make the assembly of IV equipment possible.

Choosing an IV Solution

When choosing the most appropriate IV solution, you must identify the needs of your patient. Ask yourself these questions:
- Is the patient's condition critical?
- Is the patient's condition stable?
- Does the patient need fluid replacement?
- Will the patient need medications?

In the prehospital setting, the choice of IV solution is usually limited to two isotonic crystalloids, normal saline and LR solution. D_5W is often reserved for administering medication because the presence of dextrose has the potential to alter fluid and electrolyte levels in the body.

Each IV solution bag is wrapped in a protective sterile plastic bag and is guaranteed to remain sterile until the posted expiry date. Once the protective wrap is torn and removed, however, the IV solution must be used within 24 hours. The bottom of each IV bag has two ports: an injection port for medication and an access port for connecting the administration set. A removable pigtail protects the sterile access port. Once this pigtail is removed, the bag must be used immediately or discarded.

IV solution bags come in different fluid volumes **Figure 8-9 ▲**. Volumes commonly used in hospitals are 1,000 ml, 500 ml, 250 ml, 100 ml, and 50 ml; the more common prehospital volumes are 1,000 ml and 500 ml. The smaller volumes (250 ml and 100 ml) typically contain D_5W or saline and are used for mixing and administering maintenance medication infusions.

Choosing an Administration Set

An administration set moves fluid from the IV bag into the patient's vascular system. IV administration sets are sterile as long as they remain in their protective packaging. Each set has a piercing spike protected by a plastic cover. Once this spike is exposed and the seal surrounding the cap is broken, the set must be used immediately or discarded.

On most drip sets, a number on the package indicates the number of drops it takes for a millilitre of fluid to pass through the orifice and into the drip chamber **Figure 8-10 ▶**. Administration sets come in two primary sizes: microdrip and macrodrip. Microdrip sets allow 60 gtt (drops) per millilitre (ml)

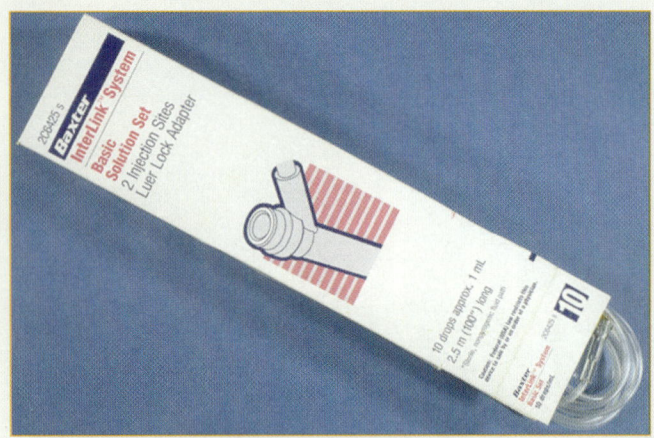

Figure 8-10 The number visible on the drip set refers to the number of drops it takes for a millilitre of fluid to pass through the orifice and into the drip chamber.

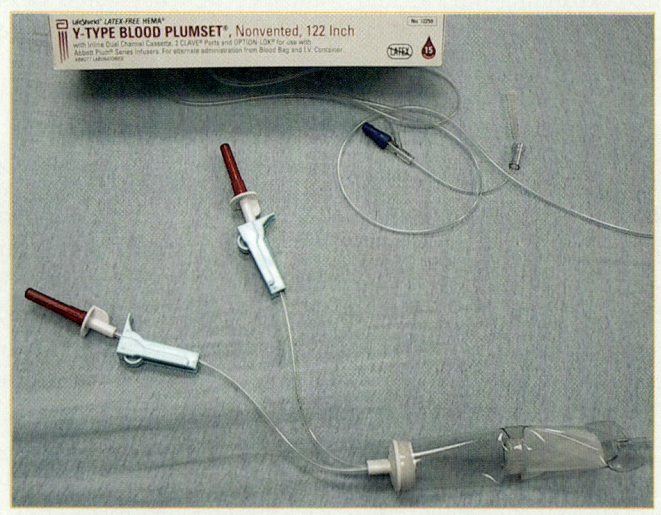

Figure 8-11 Most blood sets have dual piercing spikes that allow two bags of fluid to be used at once for the same patient.

through the needlelike orifice inside the drip chamber. They are ideal for medication administration or pediatric fluid delivery because it is easy to control their fluid flow. Macrodrip sets allow 10 or 15 gtt/ml through a large opening between the piercing spike and the drip chamber. They are best used for rapid fluid replacement.

Preparing an Administration Set

After choosing the IV administration set and the IV solution bag, verify the expiry date of the solution and check for solution clarity. Prepare to spike the bag with the administration set. The steps for this procedure are shown here and illustrated in ▶ **Skill Drill 8-1** ▶ :

1. Remove the rubber pigtail found on the end of the IV bag by pulling on it. The bag is still sealed and will not leak until the piercing spike punctures this port. Remove the protective cover from the piercing spike. (Remember, this spike is sterile!) **Step 1** .

2. Slide the spike into the IV bag port until you see fluid enter the drip chamber. Squeeze or compress the drip chamber until it is approximately half full **Step 2** .

3. Allow the solution to run freely through the drip chamber and into the tubing to prime the line and flush the air out of the tubing **Step 3** .

4. Twist the protective cover on the opposite end of the IV tubing to allow air to escape. Do not remove this cover yet, because the cover keeps the tubing end sterile until it is needed. Let the fluid flow until air bubbles are removed from the line before turning the roller clamp wheel to stop the flow **Step 4** .

5. Go back and check the drip chamber; it should be only half-filled. The fluid level must be visible to calculate drip rates. If the fluid level is too low, squeeze the chamber until it fills; if the chamber is too full, invert the bag and the chamber and squeeze the chamber to empty the fluid back into the bag **Step 5** . Hang the bag in an appropriate location with the end of the IV tubing easily accessible.

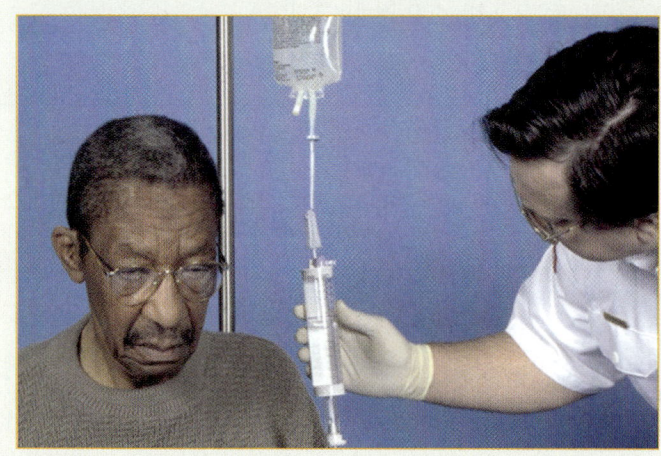

Figure 8-12 Volutrol administration set.

Other Administration Sets

Blood tubing is a macrodrip administration set that is designed to facilitate rapid fluid replacement by manual infusion of multiple IV bags or IV and blood replacement combinations. Most blood tubing administration sets have dual piercing spikes that allow two bags of fluid to be used simultaneously for the same patient **Figure 8-11 ▲** . The central drip chamber has a special filter designed to filter the blood during transfusions.

Fluid control for pediatric patients and certain geriatric patients is very important. A microdrip set called a Volutrol (or Buretrol) allows you to fill a 100- or 200-ml calibrated drip chamber with a specific amount of fluid and administer only that amount to avoid inadvertent fluid overload **Figure 8-12 ▲** . These are commonly used in pediatric patients. A proximal roller clamp enables you to shut off the Volutrol drip chamber from the IV bag. If the patient needs additional fluids, simply open the proximal roller clamp and fill the Volutrol with more fluid.

Skill Drill 8-1: Spiking the Bag

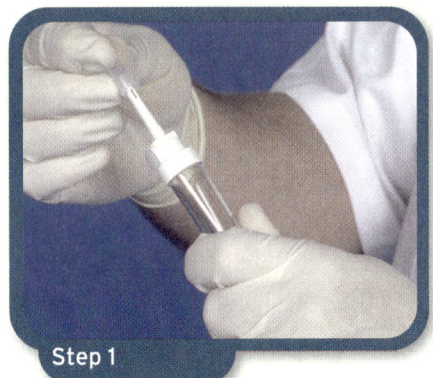

Step 1

Pull on the rubber pigtail on the end of the IV bag to remove it. Remove the protective cover from the piercing spike.

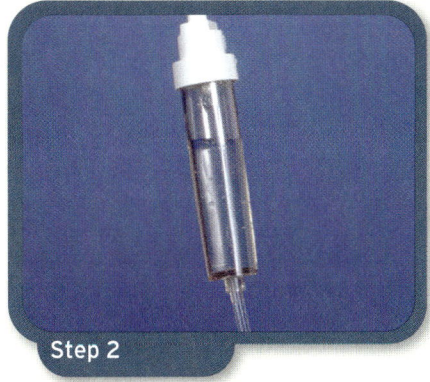

Step 2

Slide the spike into the IV bag until you see fluid enter the drip chamber. Squeeze or compress the drip chamber until it is approximately half full.

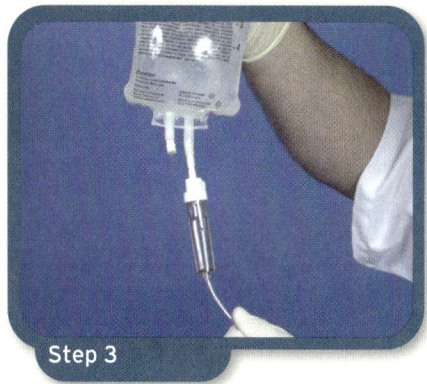

Step 3

Allow the solution to run freely through the drip chamber and into the tubing to prime the line and flush the air out of the tubing.

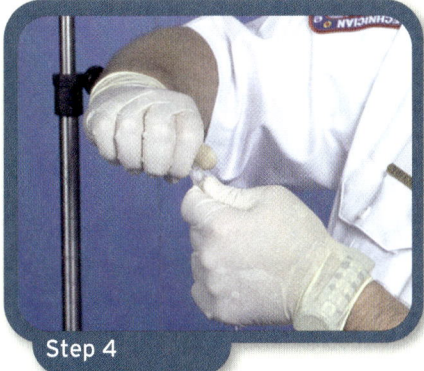

Step 4

Twist the protective cover of the opposite end of the IV tubing to allow air to escape. Do not remove this cover yet. Let the fluid flow until air bubbles are removed from the line before turning the roller clamp wheel to stop the flow.

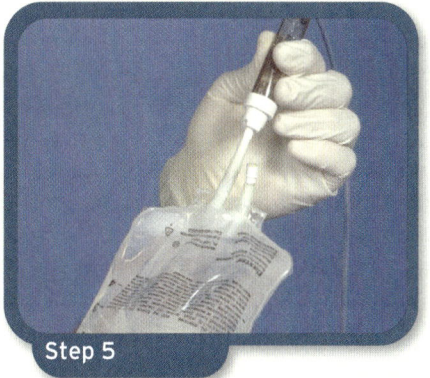

Step 5

Check the drip chamber; it should be only half-filled. If the fluid level is too low, squeeze the chamber until it fills; if the chamber is too full, invert the bag and the chamber and squeeze the chamber to empty the fluid back into the bag. Hang the bag in an appropriate location.

Choosing an IV Site

It is important to select the most appropriate vein for IV cannula insertion. Avoid areas of the vein that contain valves because a cannula will not pass through these areas easily and the needle may cause damage. Valves can be recognized as small bumps located in the vein. Use the following criteria to select a vein:

- Locate the vein section with the straightest appearance **Figure 8-13 ▶**.
- Choose a vein that has a firm, round appearance or is springy when palpated.
- Avoid areas where the vein crosses over joints.
- Avoid edematous extremities and any extremity with a dialysis fistula or on the side a mastectomy was done.

If IV therapy is being given for a life-threatening illness or injury, this choice is often limited to the areas that remain open during hypoperfusion. Otherwise, limit IV access to the more distal areas of the extremities: *Start distally, work proximally.* If the most distal site ruptures or infiltrates, you can move up the extremity to the next appropriate site. Because failed cannulation brings the possibility of leakage into the surrounding tissues, any fluid introduced immediately below an

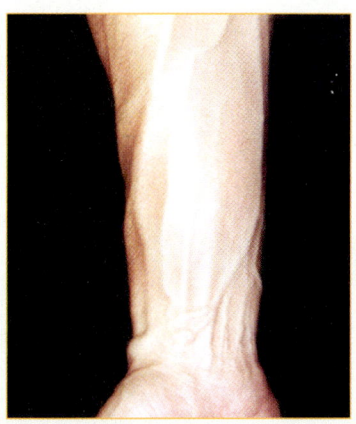

Figure 8-13 Look for veins that are relatively straight and spring back when palpated.

open wound has the potential to enter the tissue and cause damage.

Large protruding arm veins can be deceiving in terms of their ease of cannulation. Often these bulging veins can roll from side to side during a cannulation attempt, causing you to miss the vein. A remedy is to apply manual traction to the vein to lock it into position. Traction techniques differ depending on the location chosen for cannulation. Hold hand veins in place by pulling the skin over the vein taut with the thumb of your free hand as you flex the patient's hand Figure 8-14 ▾ . Stabilize wrist veins by flexing the wrist and pulling the skin taut over the vein. Applying lateral traction to the vein with your free hand can stabilize veins in the forearm and antecubital areas. Stabilizing and cannulating the external jugular vein requires a different approach (discussed later in this chapter).

The patient's opinion should also be considered when selecting an IV site because he or she may know an IV location that has worked in the past. Avoid attempts to insert an IV in an extremity if it shows signs of trauma, injury, or infection; if it has an arteriovenous shunt for renal dialysis; or if it is on the same side a mastectomy was done. Also, pay careful attention to areas of the vein that have track marks; they are usually a sign of sclerosis caused by frequent cannulation or puncture of the vein, for example from IV drug abuse.

Some protocols allow IV cannulation of leg veins. Use caution when cannulating veins in these areas because they can place the patient at greater risk of venous thrombosis and subsequent pulmonary embolism.

Choosing an IV Cannula

Cannula selection should reflect the purpose of the IV, the age of the patient, and the location for the IV. The most common types used in the prehospital setting are over-the-needle cannulas and butterfly cannulas. An over-the-needle cannula

Figure 8-15 ▾ is a Teflon cannula inserted *over* a hollow needle. A butterfly cannula is a hollow, stainless steel needle with two plastic wings to facilitate its handling Figure 8-16 ▾ . Through-the-needle cannulas are plastic cannulas inserted *through* a hollow needle; these cannulas are rarely used in the prehospital setting.

Table 8-1 ▸ lists the advantages and disadvantages of over-the-needle cannulas. These cannulas are preferred for use in the prehospital setting for infusing IV fluids or medications in adults and children. They are more readily secured, are less cumbersome than the butterfly cannula, and allow for greater patient movement without the need to immobilize the entire limb.

Table 8-2 ▸ lists the advantages and disadvantages of butterfly cannulas.

Over-the-needle cannulas come in different gauges and lengths Figure 8-17 ▸ . The smaller the gauge of the cannula, the larger the diameter. Thus a 14-gauge cannula is of larger diameter than a 22-gauge cannula; 14 gauge is the largest, 27 gauge is the smallest. The larger the diameter, the more fluid that can be delivered through it. The most common lengths are 1¼" and 2¼".

Select the largest-diameter cannula that will fit the vein you have chosen or that will be the most appropriate and comfortable for the patient. An 18- or 20-gauge cannula is usually a good size for adults who do not need fluid replacement. Metacarpal veins of the hand can usually accommodate 18- or

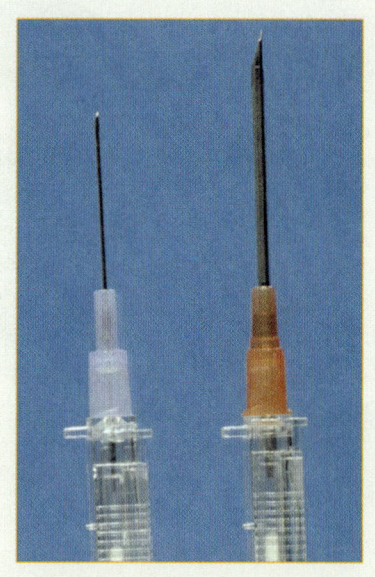

Figure 8-15 Over-the-needle cannulas.

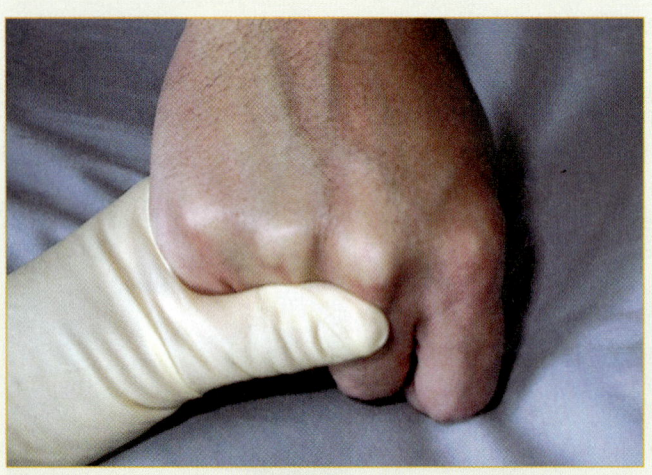

Figure 8-14 Hold hand veins in place by pulling the skin over the vein taut with the thumb of your free hand as you flex the patient's hand.

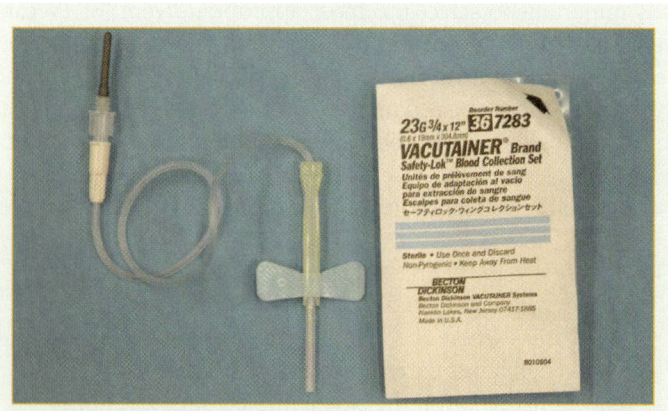

Figure 8-16 Butterfly cannula.

At the Scene

As a general rule, you should start distally and work your way up the patient's extremity when starting an IV. For patients who need rapid fluid replacement, are in cardiac arrest, or are otherwise hemodynamically unstable, however, you should use the antecubital vein. Unlike other extremity veins (eg, hand, forearm), this vein is usually visible and easier to palpate. A neck vein or an adult IO are other options.

Special Considerations

If you are using an over-the-needle cannula to start an IV in a pediatric patient, choose among the 20-, 22-, 24-, or 26-gauge cannulas, depending on the child's age. Butterfly cannulas can be placed in the same locations as over-the-needle cannulas and in visible scalp veins in pediatric patients. Scalp veins are best used in young infants.

20-gauge cannulas. A 14- or 16-gauge cannula should be used when the patient requires fluid replacement (eg, for hypovolemic shock). You should be able to insert a 14- or 16-gauge cannula into an antecubital vein or external jugular vein in the average adult.

In recent years, an attempt has been made to create over-the-needle cannulas that minimize the risk of a contaminated stick—when a paramedic punctures his or her skin with the same cannula that was used to cannulate the vein of a patient. For example, some of these newer cannulas offer automatic needle retraction after insertion, usually accomplished with a locking slide mechanism or a spring-loaded slide mechanism.

Inserting the IV Cannula

Each paramedic has a unique technique to insert an IV, and you should observe many different techniques to determine what works best for you. Two considerations, however, apply to *any* technique: (1) Keep the beveled side of the cannula up when inserting the needle in a vein **Figure 8-18 ▾**, and (2) maintain adequate traction on the vein during cannulation.

Apply a tourniquet above the site you have chosen for the insertion to allow blood to fill the veins. This creates additional vascular pressure to engorge the veins with blood below the band. It should be snug enough to significantly diminish venous flow but should not hamper arterial flow. The tourniquet should be left in place only long enough to complete the IV insertion, obtain blood samples (if needed), and attach the

Table 8-1	Advantages and Disadvantages of Over-the-Needle Cannulas	
Advantages	**Disadvantages**	
■ Less likely to puncture the vein than a butterfly cannula	■ Risk of sticking the paramedic with contaminated needle as it is withdrawn	
■ More comfortable once in position	■ More difficult to insert than other devices	
■ Radiopaque for easy identification during x-ray	■ Possibility of cannula shear	

Table 8-2	Advantages and Disadvantages of Butterfly Cannulas	
Advantages	**Disadvantages**	
■ Easiest venipuncture device to insert	■ May easily cause infiltration	
■ Useful for scalp veins in infants and in small, difficult veins in geriatric patients for obtaining blood samples	■ Possible blood cell damage when drawing blood through the butterfly cannula	
■ Small, short needles	■ Small-gauge needles limit fluid flow	

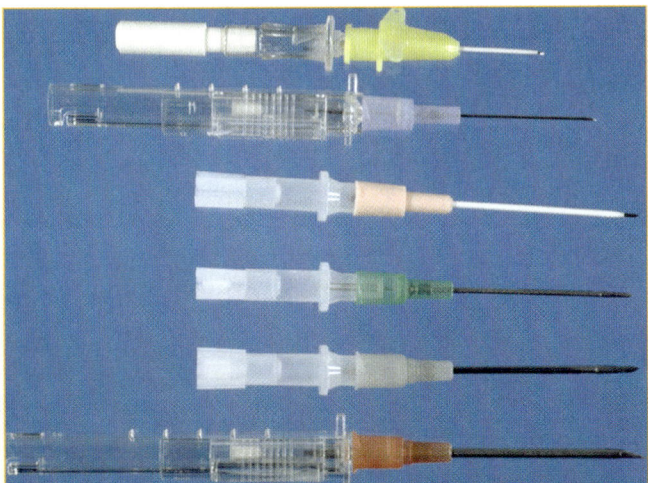

Figure 8-17 Note the difference in the lengths and diameters of over-the-needle cannulas.

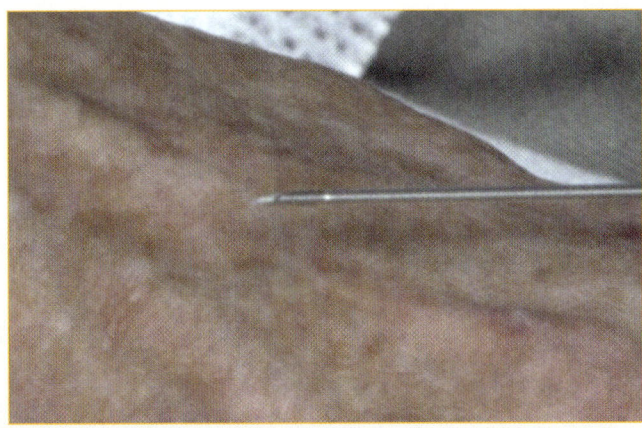

Figure 8-18 Keep the beveled side of the cannula up when inserting the needle into a vein.

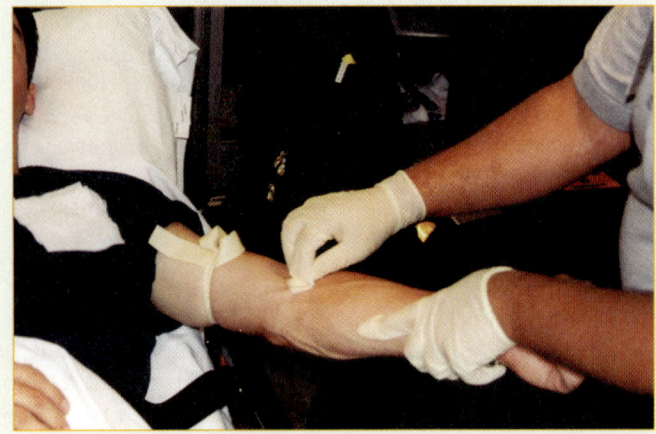

Figure 8-19 When cleansing the site for IV cannulation, use the first alcohol pad or iodine swab to clean in a circular motion from the inside out, then use the second to wipe straight down the centre of the vein.

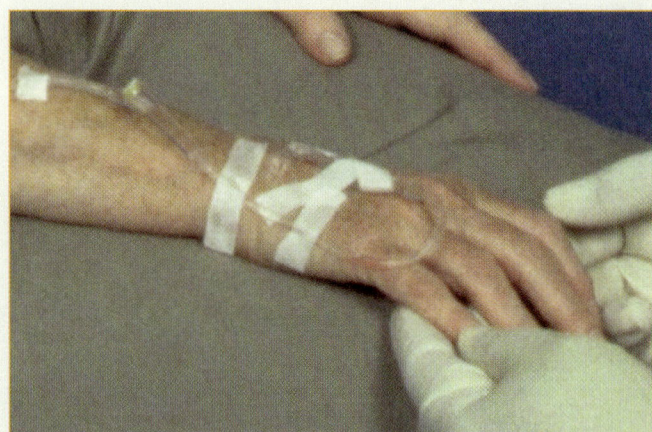

Figure 8-20 Tape the area so that the cannula and tubing are securely anchored.

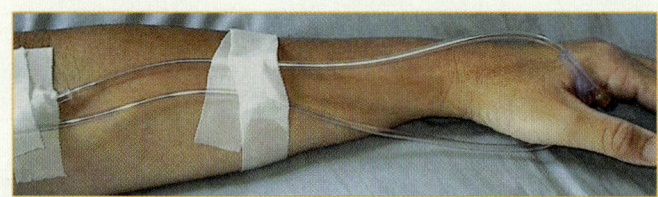

Figure 8-21 Loosely wrap the IV line around the patient's thumb and secure it to the forearm.

line. *Do not leave the tourniquet in place while you assemble IV equipment.*

Tourniquets can be difficult to manage, especially if you are wearing gloves. You should develop a technique that will allow you to release the tourniquet with a small tug on one end. Items that can be used as tourniquets include a Penrose drain, a blood pressure cuff, or in a pinch, surgical hose.

Once you have selected an insertion site, prep it with an alcohol or iodine swab **Figure 8-19 ▲**. Apply gentle downward or lateral traction on the vein with your free hand while holding the cannula, bevel side up, in your dominant hand. Take care as you apply traction to avoid collapsing the vein. Begin by establishing an insertion angle of about 45°. Advance the cannula through the skin until the vein is pierced (you should see a flash of blood in the cannula flash chamber); then immediately drop the angle down to about 15° and advance the cannula a few more centimetres to ensure the cannula sheath is in the vein. Slide the sheath off the needle and into the vein; do not advance the needle too far because it can lacerate the vein. After the cannula is fully advanced, apply pressure to the vein just proximal to the end of the indwelling cannula, remove the needle, and dispose of it in a sharps container, or in the case of other style cannulas, trigger the shielding device.

Securing the Line

Once the cannula is in position and the contents of the IV bag are flowing properly, you must secure the IV. Tape the area so that the cannula and tubing are securely anchored in case of a sudden pull on the line **Figure 8-20 ▶**. Tear the tape before you start the IV, because you will need one hand to stabilize the site while you tape the IV. Double back the tubing to create a loop that will act as a shock absorber if

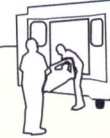

At the Scene

Iodine helps to make veins more visible in dark-skinned people. As with any patient, make sure the patient is not allergic to iodine.

the line is pulled accidentally. Cover the insertion site with sterile gauze, and secure it with tape or use a commercially manufactured device. Avoid circumferential taping around any extremity, as it may impair circulation.

The steps for establishing vascular access are as follows **Skill Drill 8-2 ▶**:

1. Choose the appropriate fluid, and examine the bag for clarity and expiry date.

   Make sure that no particles are floating in the fluid and that the fluid is appropriate for the patient's condition.

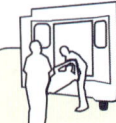

At the Scene

To further stabilize the IV line, loosely wrap it around the patient's thumb and secure it to the forearm **Figure 8-21 ▲**. This will prevent disruption of the IV if the line is pulled.

2. Choose the appropriate drip set, and attach it to the fluid. A macrodrip set (eg, 10 gtt/ml) should be used for a patient who needs volume replacement; a microdrip set (eg, 60 gtt/ml) should be used for a patient who needs a medication route.

3. Fill the drip chamber by squeezing it (Step 1).

4. Flush or "bleed" the tubing to remove any air bubbles by opening the roller clamp (Step 2). Make sure no errant bubbles are floating in the tubing.

5. Tear the tape before venipuncture, or have a commercial device available (Step 3).

6. Apply gloves before making contact with the patient. Palpate a suitable vein (Step 4). Veins should be "springy" when palpated. Stay away from areas that are hard when palpated.

7. Apply the tourniquet above the intended IV site (Step 5). It should be placed approximately 15 to 25 cm above the intended site.

8. Clean the area using aseptic technique. Use an alcohol pad to cleanse in a circular motion from the inside out. Use a second alcohol pad to wipe straight down the centre (Step 6).

9. Choose the appropriately sized cannula, twist the cannula to break the seal. Do not advance the cannula upward, as this may cause the needle to shear the cannula. Examine the cannula and discard it if you discover any imperfections (Step 7). Occasionally you will find "burrs" on the edge of the cannula.

10. Insert the cannula at an angle of approximately 45° with the bevel up while applying distal traction with the other hand (Step 8). This traction will stabilize the vein and help to keep it from "rolling" as you stick.

11. Observe for "flashback" as blood enters the cannula (Step 9). The clear chamber at the top of the cannula should fill with blood when the cannula enters the vein. If you note only a drop or two, you should gently advance the cannula farther into the vein.

12. Occlude the cannula to prevent blood leaking while removing the stylet (Step 10). Place the thumb of the hand not holding the cannula over the end of the cannula that is currently situated inside the vein to prevent blood running out when you remove the needle. With practice, you will be able to feel the cannula.

13. Immediately dispose of all sharps in the proper container (Step 11).

14. Attach the prepared IV line (Step 12).

15. Remove the tourniquet (Step 13).

16. Open the IV line to ensure fluid is flowing and the IV is patent. Observe for any swelling or infiltration around the IV site (Step 14). If the fluid does not flow, check whether the tourniquet has been released. If infiltration is noted, immediately stop the infusion and remove the cannula while holding pressure over the site to prevent bleeding.

17. Secure the cannula with tape or a commercial device (Step 15).

18. Secure IV tubing and adjust the flow rate while monitoring the patient (Step 16).

Documentation and Communication

To document an IV, you need to include four things:
- The gauge of the needle
- The site (for example, left forearm, left external jugular)
- The type of fluid you are administering
- The rate at which the fluid is running

For example, if you initiated an IV in the left antecubital fossa with an 18-gauge cannula and are infusing normal saline at a rate of 120 ml per hour, the documentation should appear as follows:

18g IV left antecubital fossa NS @ 120 ml/h

At the Scene

Helpful IV Hints
- Allow the arm to hang off the stretcher.
- Pat or rub the area.
- Apply chemical heat packs for about 60 seconds.
- If you meet resistance from a valve, elevate the extremity.
- After two misses, let your partner try (Figure 8-22 ▶).
- Try sticking without a tourniquet if the IV keeps infiltrating.
- Never pull the cannula back over the needle.
- The more IVs you perform, the more proficient you will become.

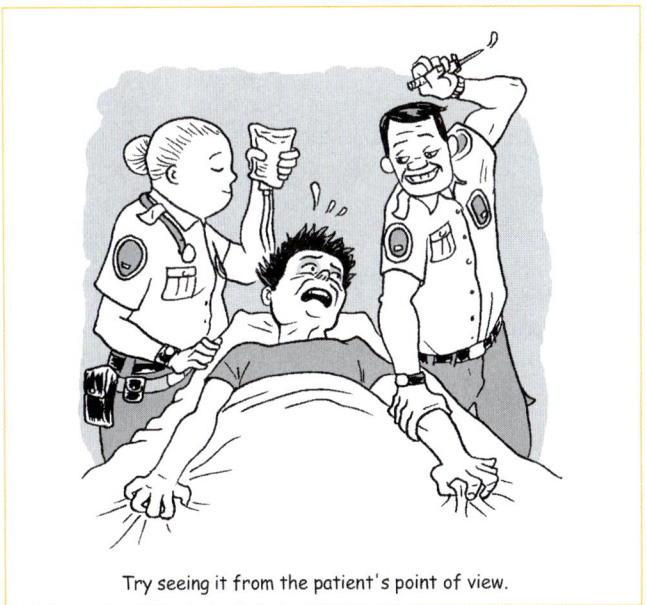

Try seeing it from the patient's point of view.

Figure 8-22

Skill Drill 8-2: Obtaining Vascular Access

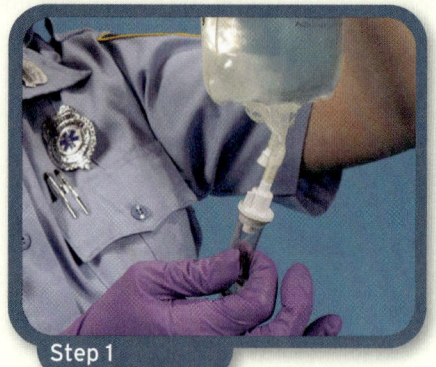

Step 1

Fill the drip chamber by squeezing it.

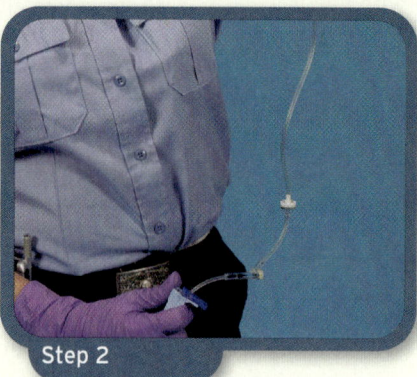

Step 2

Flush or "bleed" the tubing to remove any air bubbles by opening the roller clamp.

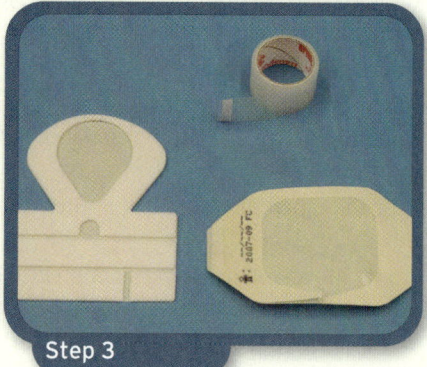

Step 3

Tear the tape before venipuncture, or have a commercial device available.

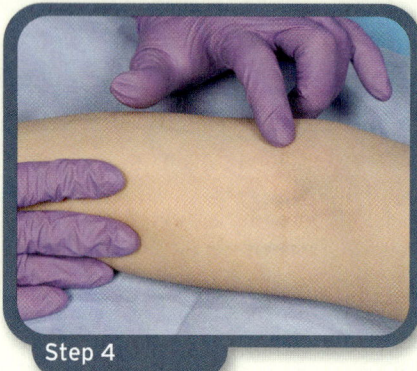

Step 4

Apply gloves before making contact with the patient. Palpate a suitable vein.

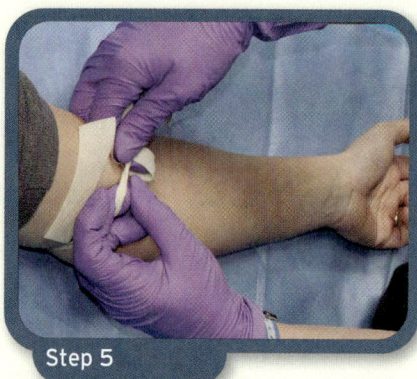

Step 5

Apply the tourniquet above the intended IV site.

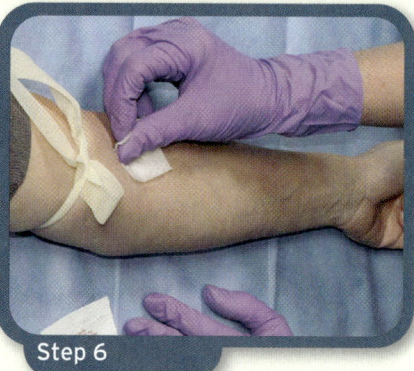

Step 6

Clean the area using aseptic technique. Use an alcohol pad to cleanse in a circular motion from the inside out. Use a second alcohol pad to wipe straight down the centre.

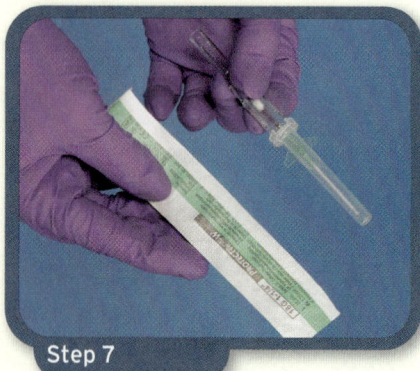

Step 7

Choose the appropriately sized cannula, and examine it for any imperfections.

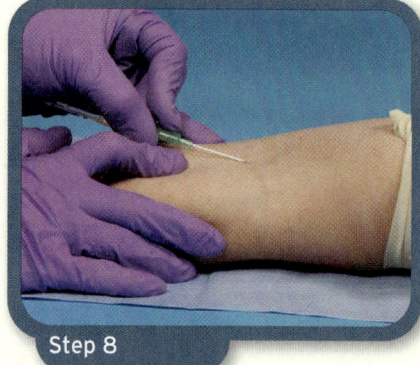

Step 8

Insert the cannula at an angle of approximately 45° with the bevel up while applying distal traction with the other hand.

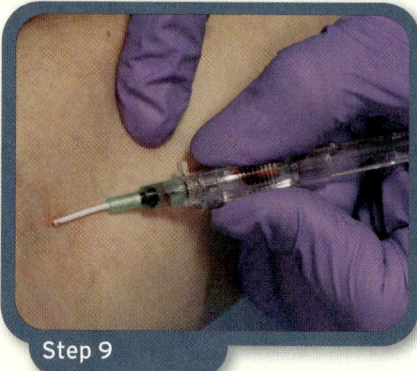

Step 9

Observe for "flashback" as blood enters the cannula.

Skill Drill 8-2: Obtaining Vascular Access (*continued*)

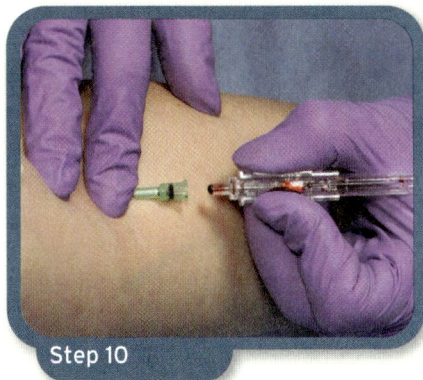

Step 10

Occlude the cannula to prevent blood leaking while removing the stylet.

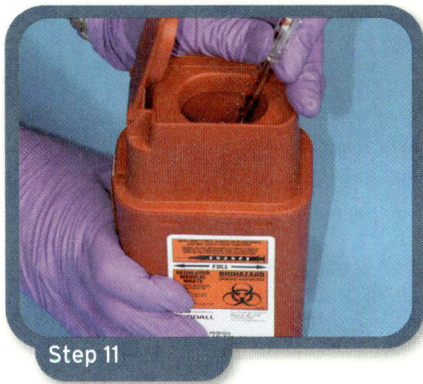

Step 11

Immediately dispose of all sharps in the proper container.

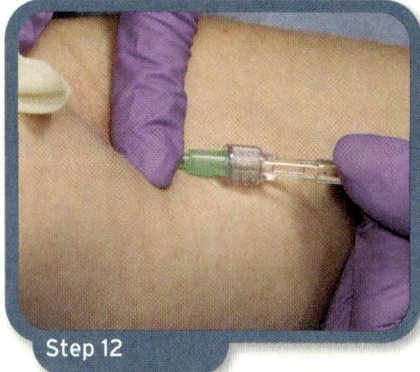

Step 12

Attach the prepared IV line.

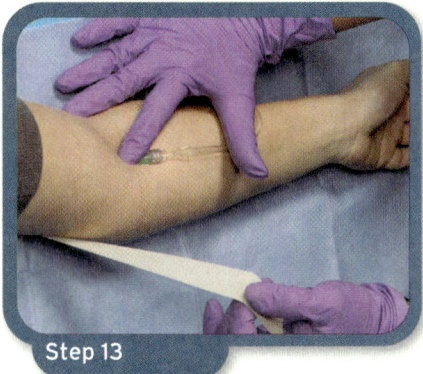

Step 13

Remove the tourniquet.

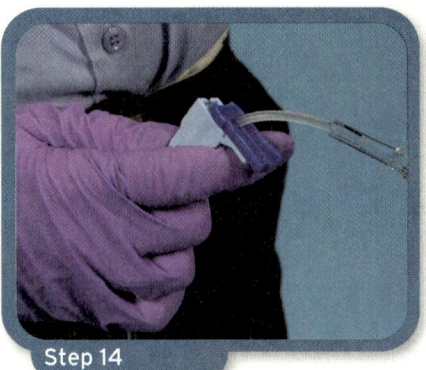

Step 14

Open the IV line to ensure fluid is flowing and the IV is patent. Observe for swelling or infiltration around the IV site.

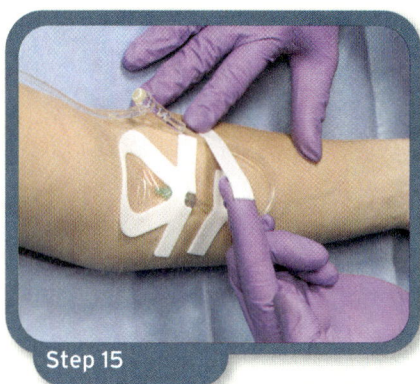

Step 15

Secure the cannula with tape or a commercial device.

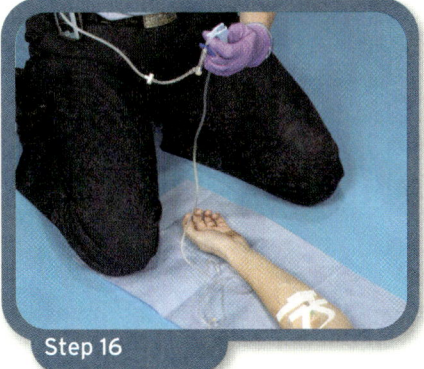

Step 16

Secure the IV tubing and adjust the flow rate while monitoring the patient.

At the Scene

Saline locks (buff caps) are a way to maintain an active IV site without running fluids through the vein. These access ports are used primarily for patients who do not need additional fluids but who may need rapid medication delivery (eg, in case of congestive heart failure or pulmonary edema). A saline lock is attached to the end of an IV cannula and filled with approximately 2 ml of normal saline to keep blood from clotting at the end of the cannula **Figure 8-23 ▾** . Because this is a sealed-access site, the saline remains in the port without entering the vein, preventing clotting. These devices are also known as intermittent (INT) sites because they eliminate the need to reestablish an IV each time the patient needs medication or fluid.

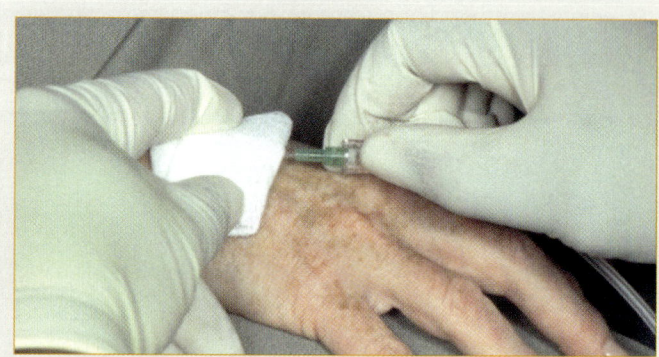

Figure 8-24 When removing a cannula and IV line, pull gently and apply pressure to control bleeding.

Changing an IV Bag

You may have to change the IV bag for some patients, particularly those who require larger volumes of IV fluid (ie, for hypovolemic shock). Do not allow an IV fluid bag to become *completely* depleted of fluid. Change the bag when about 25 ml of fluid is left.

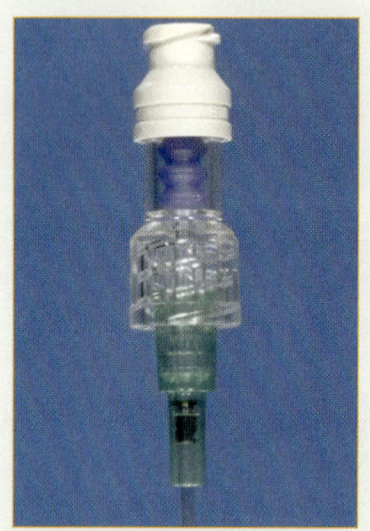

Figure 8-23 A saline lock is attached to the end of an IV cannula and filled with approximately 2 ml of normal saline to keep blood from clotting at the end of the cannula.

There are two important points to remember when changing an IV bag. First, like the initial setup of the IV bag and administration set (see Skill Drill 8-1), replacing the IV bag is a sterile process. If the equipment becomes contaminated, replace it and use new equipment. Second, never allow the administration set to become depleted of fluid; always ensure that some fluid remains in the drip chamber and tubing of the set. This simple action will prevent air from entering the patient's vein.

The steps for changing an IV fluid bag are as follows:

1. Stop the flow of fluid from the depleted bag by closing the roller clamp.
2. Prepare the new IV bag by removing the pigtail from the piercing spike port. Inspect the new bag of IV fluid for clarity and discolouration and to ensure that the expiry date has not passed.
3. Remove the piercing spike from the depleted bag and insert it into the port on the new bag. *Do not touch the piercing spike of the administration set.*
4. Ensure that the drip chamber is appropriately filled, and then open the roller clamp and adjust the fluid rate accordingly.

Discontinuing the IV Line

To discontinue the IV line, shut off the flow from the IV with the roller clamp. Gently peel the tape back toward the IV site. As you get closer to the site and the cannula, stabilize the cannula while you loosen the remaining tape holding the cannula in place. Do not remove the IV tubing from the hub of the cannula. Fold a 10 × 10 cm piece of gauze and place it over the site, holding it down while you pull back on the hub of the cannula. Gently pull the cannula and the IV line from the patient's vein while applying pressure to control bleeding **Figure 8-24 ▴** .

External Jugular Vein Cannulation

The external jugular (EJ) vein **Figure 8-25 ▸** runs downward and obliquely backward behind the angle of the jaw until it pierces the deep fascia of the neck just above the middle of the clavicle. It ends in the subclavian vein, where valves retard backflow of blood. The EJ vein is fairly large and usually easy to cannulate; however, because the vein lies so near the surface of the skin, it rolls if the vein is not appropriately anchored during cannulation. It is also very near other vessels (such as the carotid artery) that may be damaged during cannulation.

You should exhaust all other means of cannulating a peripheral vein (ie, in the arm or hand) before attempting cannulation of the EJ vein. Although it is a "peripheral" vein, more risks are associated with cannulation of this vein—namely, inadvertent puncture of the carotid artery, a *rapidly* expanding hematoma if infiltration occurs, and air embolism.

Follow these steps to cannulate the external jugular vein:

1. Place the patient in a supine, head-down position to fill the jugular vein. Turn the patient's head to the side opposite the intended venipuncture site. *Always feel carefully for a pulse before cannulating an external jugular vein. It is imperative not to pierce the carotid artery.*
2. Appropriately cleanse the venipuncture site.
3. Occlude the jugular vein with your finger, distal to the cannula insertion site, to facilitate backflow of blood; this will allow the vein to become more visible.

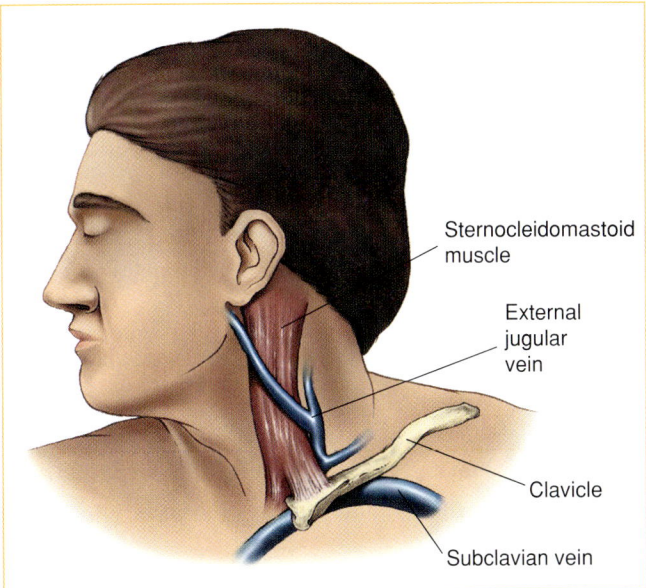

Figure 8-25 Anatomy of the external jugular vein.

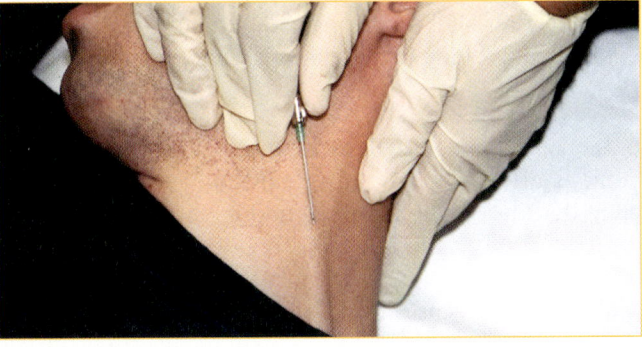

Figure 8-26 The external jugular vein requires a specific insertion site midway between the angle of the jaw and the midclavicular line with the cannula pointed toward the shoulder on the same side as the venipuncture.

4. Align the cannula in the direction of the vein, with the point aimed toward the shoulder on the side of the venipuncture (**Figure 8-26 ▲**).
5. Make the puncture midway between the angle of the jaw and the midclavicular line. Stabilize the vein by placing a finger lightly on top of it just above the clavicle.
6. Proceed as described for cannulation of a peripheral vein. *Do not let air enter the cannula once it is in the vein.*
7. Tape the line securely but do *not* put circumferential dressings around the neck.

Factors Affecting IV Flow Rates

Several factors can influence the flow rate of an IV. For example, if the IV bag is not hung high enough, the flow rate will

not be sufficient. Perform the following checks after completing IV administration and whenever a flow problem occurs:

- *Check the IV fluid.* Thick, viscous fluids such as blood products and colloid solutions infuse slowly and may be diluted to help speed delivery. Cold fluids run more slowly than warm fluids. If possible, warm IV fluids before administering them in a cold environment.
- *Check the administration set.* Macrodrips are used for rapid fluid delivery; microdrips deliver a more controlled flow.
- *Check the height of the IV bag.* The IV bag must be hung high enough to overcome gravity. Hang it as high as possible.
- *Check the type of cannula used.* The larger the diameter of the cannula (the smaller the number—for example a 14-gauge is of larger diameter than a 20-gauge), the more fluid can be delivered.
- *Check the tourniquet.* Do not leave the tourniquet on the patient's arm after completing the IV.

Potential Complications of IV Therapy

Problems associated with IVs can be categorized as local or systemic reactions. Local reactions include problems such as infiltration and thrombophlebitis. Systemic complications include allergic reactions and circulatory overload.

Local IV Site Reactions

Most local reactions require that you discontinue the IV and reestablish the IV in the opposite extremity. Examples of local reactions include infiltration; thrombophlebitis; occlusion; vein irritation; hematoma; nerve, tendon, or ligament damage; and arterial puncture.

Infiltration

Infiltration is the escape of fluid into the surrounding tissue, which causes a localized area of edema. Causes of infiltration include the following problems:

- The IV passes completely through the vein and out the other side.
- The patient moves excessively.
- The tape used to secure the IV becomes loose or dislodged.
- The cannula is inserted at too shallow an angle and enters only the fascia surrounding the vein (this problem is more common with IVs in larger veins, such as those in the upper arm and neck).

Signs and symptoms of infiltration include edema at the cannula site, continued IV flow after occlusion of the vein above the insertion site, and patient complaints of tightness and pain around the IV site.

If infiltration occurs, discontinue the IV and reestablish it in the opposite extremity or in a more proximal location on the same extremity. Apply direct pressure over the swollen area to reduce further swelling or bleeding into the tissue. Avoid wrapping tape around the extremity, as it could create a tourniquet.

Thrombophlebitis

Infection and thrombophlebitis (inflammation of the vein and the presence of a clot) may occur in association with venous cannulation; both conditions are most frequently caused by lapses in aseptic technique. Thrombophlebitis is commonly encountered in patients who abuse drugs as well as in patients who are receiving long-term IV therapy in a hospital or hospice setting or with vein-irritating solutions (eg, dextrose solutions, which have a very low pH, or hypertonic solutions of any sort). It can also be produced by mechanical factors, such as excessive motion of the IV needle or cannula after it has been placed.

Thrombophlebitis is usually manifested by pain and tenderness along the vein and redness and edema at the venipuncture site. These signs generally do not appear until after several hours of IV therapy, so you are unlikely to see a case of thrombophlebitis in the prehospital setting unless you are doing an interhospital transport of a patient with an established IV. In such a case, stop the infusion and discontinue the IV at that site. Warm compresses applied to the site may provide some relief.

It is far better to prevent thrombophlebitis or infection than to treat it afterward. To prevent thrombophlebitis, take the following measures:

- Use a povidone-iodine preparation to scrub and disinfect the skin over the venipuncture site; then do a final wipe with an alcohol swab. Make certain the site is dry before initiating the venipuncture.
- Always wear gloves when doing a venipuncture.
- After inserting the cannula, cover the puncture site with a sterile dressing.
- Anchor the cannula and tubing securely to prevent motion of the cannula within the vein.

Occlusion

Occlusion is the physical blockage of a vein or cannula. If the flow rate is not sufficient to keep fluid moving out of the cannula tip such that blood enters the cannula, a clot may form and occlude the flow. The first sign of an occlusion is a decreasing drip rate or the presence of blood in the IV tubing. With a positional IV site, fluid flows at different rates depending on the position of the cannula within the vein; these differences can produce occlusions. Positional IVs may be necessary because of proximity to a valve or because of patient movement that allows the line to become physically blocked, such as resting on the line or crossing arms. Occlusion may also develop if the IV bag nears empty and the patient's blood pressure overcomes the flow, causing fluid backup in the line.

If occlusion occurs, follow the steps shown in **Skill Drill 8-3 ▶** to determine whether the IV should be reestablished:

1. Select and assemble a sterile 10-ml syringe and large-gauge needle. If your service uses needleless IV systems, a needle is not required (**Step 1**).
2. Select an injection port closest to the IV site, and swab it with an alcohol wipe.

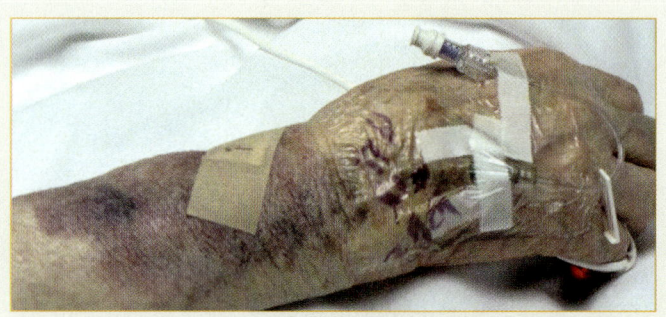

Figure 8-27 Hematomas can be caused by the improper removal of a cannula, resulting in pooling of blood around the IV site, leading to tenderness and pain.

3. Insert the needle into the injection port. If your service uses needleless IV systems, connect the syringe to the injection port (**Step 2**).
4. Pinch the line in between the injection port and IV bag.
5. Gently pull back on the plunger to disrupt the occlusion and reestablish flow.
6. If flow is reestablished, ensure that the rate is sufficient.
7. If you are unable to reestablish flow, discontinue the IV and reestablish it in the opposite extremity or at a proximal location in the same extremity (**Step 3**).

Vein Irritation

Occasionally, a patient will experience vein irritation from the IV fluid. Patients who have this problem often complain immediately that the solution is bothering them (ie, tingling, stinging, itching, and burning). In such cases, observe the patient closely in case an allergic reaction to the fluid develops.

Vein irritation is usually caused by a too-rapid infusion rate. If redness develops at the IV site—a sign suggesting thrombophlebitis—discontinue the IV and save the equipment for later analysis. Reestablish the IV in the other extremity with new equipment in case the old equipment contained unseen contaminants.

Hematoma

A hematoma is an accumulation of blood in the tissues surrounding an IV site, often resulting from vein perforation or improper cannula removal. Blood can be seen rapidly pooling around the IV site, leading to tenderness and pain **Figure 8-27 ▲** . Patients with a history of vascular diseases (including diabetes) and patients taking certain medications (eg, corticosteroids or a blood thinner like Coumadin) can have a predisposition to vein rupture or to hematoma development with IV insertion.

If a hematoma develops while you are attempting to insert a cannula, stop and apply direct pressure to help minimize bleeding. If a hematoma develops after a successful cannula insertion, evaluate the IV flow and the hematoma. If the hematoma appears to be controlled and the flow is not affected, monitor the IV site and leave the line in place. If the hematoma develops as a result of discontinuing the IV, apply direct pressure with a 10 cm × 10 cm gauze pad to the site.

Skill Drill 8-3: Determining Whether an IV Is Viable

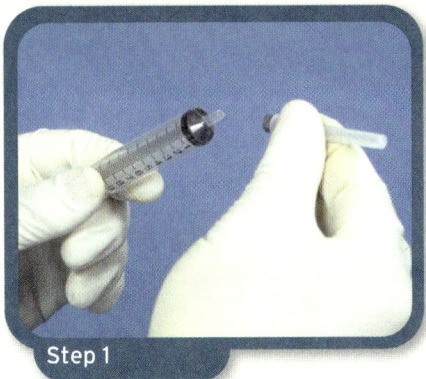

Step 1

Select and assemble a sterile 10-ml syringe and large-gauge needle. If using a needleless system, a needle is not required.

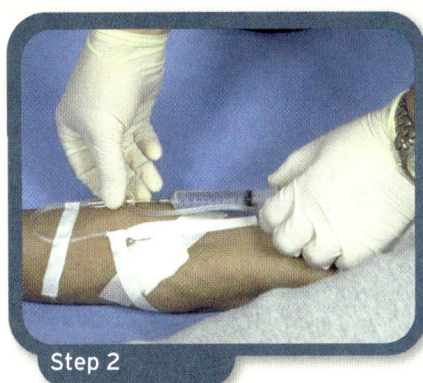

Step 2

Select an injection port near the IV site, and swab it with an alcohol wipe.

Insert the needle into the injection port. If using a needleless system, connect the syringe to the injection port.

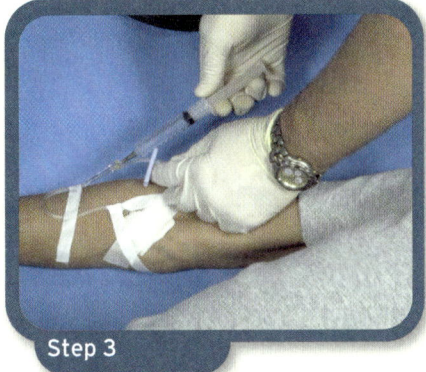

Step 3

Pinch the line in between the injection port and IV bag.

Gently pull back on the plunger to disrupt the occlusion and reestablish flow. If flow is reestablished, ensure that the rate is sufficient.

If the occlusion does not dislodge, discontinue the IV and reestablish it in the opposite extremity or at a proximal location on the same extremity.

Nerve, Tendon, or Ligament Damage

Improper identification of anatomical structures around the IV site can lead to perforation of tendons, ligaments, and nerves. Selecting an IV site located near joints increases the risk for perforation of these structures. When this type of injury occurs, patients will experience sudden and severe shooting pain. Numbness or tingling in the extremity after the incident is common. Immediately remove the cannula and select another IV site.

Arterial Puncture

You may accidentally puncture the wrong blood vessel if the vein selected for cannulation lies near an artery. *The risk of arterial*

puncture is especially high when cannulating an external jugular vein—be careful! If you insert a cannula into an artery by mistake, bright red blood will spurt back through the cannula. The blood's colour and its flow characteristics will alert you to your error. *Immediately withdraw the cannula, and apply direct pressure over the puncture site for at least 5 minutes or until bleeding stops.*

To avoid cannulating an artery, always check for a pulse in any vessel you intend to cannulate. Under normal circumstances, veins are near the skin surface and arteries lie much deeper. On occasion, an anatomical anomaly occurs and the vessels become transpositioned, resulting in an artery being very superficial.

Systemic Complications

Systemic complications can evolve from reactions or complications associated with IV insertion. They usually involve other body systems and can be life-threatening. If the IV line is established and patent in such a patient, do not remove it because it may be needed for treatment. Potential systemic complications include allergic reactions, pyrogenic reactions, circulatory overload, air embolus, vasovagal reactions, and cannula shear.

Allergic Reactions

Often, allergic reactions associated with IV therapy are minor. However, anaphylaxis—a potentially life-threatening condition—is possible and must be treated aggressively. Allergic reactions can result from a person's unexpected sensitivity to an IV fluid or medication. Such sensitivity could be unknown to the patient, so you must maintain vigilance with any IV for a possible allergic reaction.

The patient presentation depends on the extent of the reaction. Common signs and symptoms of an allergic reaction include itching (pruritus), shortness of breath, edema of face and hands, urticaria (hives), bronchospasm, and wheezing.

If an allergic reaction occurs, discontinue the IV and remove the solution. Leave the cannula in place as an emergency medication route. Attach a saline lock, if available.

Notify direct medical control immediately, and maintain an open airway. Monitor the patient's ABCs and vital signs. Keep the solution or medication for evaluation by the hospital (Chapter 30 covers allergic reactions and anaphylaxis in more detail).

Pyrogenic Reactions

Pyrogens are foreign proteins capable of producing fever. Their presence in the infusion solution or administration set may induce a pyrogenic reaction, which is characterized by an abrupt temperature elevation (as high as 41.1°C) with severe chills, backache, headache, weakness, nausea, and vomiting. Occasionally vascular collapse occurs, with all the signs and symptoms of shock. The reaction usually begins within 30 minutes after the IV infusion has been started.

If you observe *any* signs of such a reaction—for example, if the patient complains of a headache or backache after you have started running fluids—*stop the infusion immediately!* Start a new IV in the other arm with a *fresh infusion solution,* and remove the first IV. If the patient is showing signs of shock, treat as any other case of shock.

Pyrogenic reactions can be largely avoided by inspecting the IV bag carefully before use. If the bag has any leaks or if the fluid looks cloudy or discoloured, select another bag.

Circulatory Overload

Healthy adults can handle as much as 2 to 3 extra litres of fluid without compromise. Problems occur, however, when the patient has cardiac, pulmonary, or renal dysfunction; these types of dysfunction do not tolerate any additional demands from increased circulatory volume. The most common cause of circulatory overload in the prehospital setting is failure to readjust the drip rate after flushing an IV line immediately after insertion. Always monitor the IV to ensure the proper drip rate. If available, consider using a Volutrol (Buretrol) administration set for patients who are at risk for circulatory overload.

Signs and symptoms of circulatory overload include dyspnea, jugular vein distention, and hypertension. Crackles (rales) are often heard when evaluating breath sounds. Acute peripheral edema can also be an indication of circulatory overload.

To treat a patient with circulatory overload, slow the IV rate to keep the vein open and raise the patient's head to ease respiratory distress. Administer high-flow oxygen, and monitor vital signs and breathing adequacy. Some EMS systems will have standing orders and others will prompt the paramedic to contact direct medical control immediately, because certain drugs can be given to reduce the circulatory volume.

Air Embolus

For patients who are already ill or injured, however, *any* air introduced into the IV line can present a problem. Properly flushing an IV line will help eliminate the likelihood of air embolus. Although IV bags are designed to collapse as they empty to help prevent this problem, this collapse does not always occur. Be sure to replace empty IV bags with full ones.

> ### Special Considerations
> It is easy to overload older patients who need large amounts of IV fluids. Administer small boluses of fluid (200 to 300 ml), and check breath sounds before and after each bolus to ensure that the lungs remain "dry."

If your patient begins developing respiratory distress with unequal breath sounds, consider the possibility of an air embolus. Other associated signs and symptoms include cyanosis (even in the presence of high-flow oxygen), signs and symptoms of shock, loss of consciousness, and respiratory arrest.

Treat a patient with a suspected air embolus by placing the patient on his or her left side with the head down to trap any air inside the right atrium or right ventricle, administering 100% oxygen, and rapidly transporting to the closest appropriate facility. Be prepared to assist ventilation if the patient experiences inadequate breathing.

Vasovagal Reactions

Some patients have anxiety concerning needles or the sight of blood. Such anxiety may cause vasculature dilation, leading to a drop in blood pressure and patient collapse. Patients can present with anxiety, diaphoresis, nausea, and syncopal episodes.

Treatment for patients with vasovagal reactions centres on treating them for shock:

1. Place patient in shock position.
2. Apply high-flow oxygen.
3. Monitor vital signs.
4. Establish an IV in case fluid resuscitation is needed.

Cannula Shear

Cannula shear occurs when part of the cannula is pinched against the needle, and the needle slices through the cannula, creating a free-floating segment. The cannula segment can then travel through the circulatory system and possibly end up in the pulmonary circulation, causing a pulmonary embolus. Treatment involves surgical removal of the sheared tip. If you suspect a cannula shear, place the patient in a left lateral recumbent position with his legs down and his head up to try to keep the cannula remnant out of the pulmonary circulation.

Cannula hubs are radiopaque (ie, they appear white in an x-ray) to aid in diagnosing this type of problem. Never rethread a cannula. Dispose of the used one and select a new cannula.

Patients who have experienced cannula shear with pulmonary artery occlusion present with sudden dyspnea, shortness of breath, and possibly diminished breath

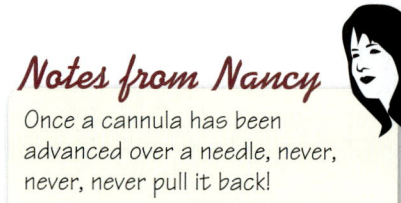

Notes from Nancy

Once a cannula has been advanced over a needle, never, never, never pull it back!

sounds. Their symptoms mimic the presentation of an air embolus and can be treated the same way. Such patients need continued IV access, and you must try to obtain an IV site in the other extremity.

Obtaining Blood Samples

If blood samples are needed, you should obtain them at the same time you start the IV. Evidence suggests that obtaining blood through equipment designed to start an IV access line is prone to hemolysis. In the prehospital setting, the goal should first be on starting the IV and then looking for a phlebotomy site on the other extremity or distal to the IV fluid site. If you have difficulty drawing blood, however, stop and finish the IV.

To obtain blood samples when starting an IV, you will need the following equipment:

- 15- or 20-ml syringe
- 18- or 20-gauge needle
- Self-sealing blood tubes

The blood-tube tops usually come in red, blue, green, and lavender, and should be filled in that order. Use the following mnemonic to help remember the order for filling the tubes: Red Blood Gives Life. The *red*-topped tube contains no additives and is intended to clot if blood typing is needed. The *blue*-topped tube contains the preservative EDTA and is used to help determine a patient's prothrombin time and partial thromboplastin time (values that are used to calculate the patient's blood clotting time). The *green*-topped tube is filled with heparin to prevent clotting and is used to evaluate the patient's electrolyte and glucose levels. *Lavender*-topped tubes are filled with sodium citrate and are often used for a complete blood count, including hematocrit and hemoglobin values.

After the IV cannula is in place, occlude the cannula and remove the tourniquet. Attach a 15- or 20-ml syringe to the hub of the IV cannula and draw the necessary amount of blood. *Do not leave the tourniquet on while drawing blood with the syringe; doing so may cause waste products to build up in the blood and could skew laboratory test results.* Detach the syringe after the required amount of blood has been obtained, attach the IV tubing, and begin the infusion. Attach an 18- or 20-gauge needle to the syringe, fill the blood tubes with the necessary amount of blood, and immediately dispose of the syringe and needle in a puncture-proof sharps container. *Exercise extreme caution when filling blood tubes with this technique; you are handling a "live" needle!*

If IV therapy is not indicated but blood samples are required, you can obtain them by using a cylindrical device that attaches to an 18- or 20-gauge sampling needle (a Vacutainer). The blood tubes are inserted into the Vacutainer after the needle it is attached to has entered the vein. To obtain blood using a Vacutainer, follow these steps:

1. Apply a tourniquet, and locate a suitable vein—typically, the antecubital vein. Follow PPE and routine precautions.

2. Prep the vein as you would when starting an IV—use an alcohol prep or iodine swab, and cleanse the area in a

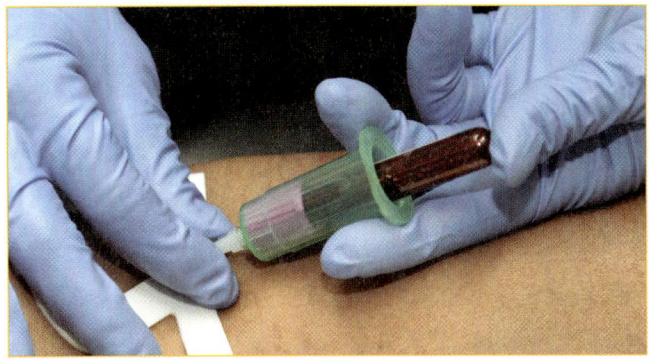

Figure 8-28 Obtaining blood samples with a Vacutainer.

circular motion, starting from the inside and working your way out.

3. Insert the needle (already attached to the Vacutainer) into the vein.

4. Remove the tourniquet, and insert blood tubes into the Vacutainer to obtain the necessary amount of blood **Figure 8-28 ▲**.

5. Remove the needle from the vein, and apply direct pressure.

6. Dispose of the needle in a puncture-proof sharps container.

7. Label all the tubes with patient's name, the date, the time, and your name as soon as possible to avoid mixing tubes with those of another patient.

Once the blood tubes are filled, gently turn them back and forth several times to mix the anticoagulant and blood evenly. The exception is the red-topped tube, which is intended to separate the serum from the other blood components. Avoid shaking this tube after the blood has clotted, because the motion may destroy the sample.

For blood tubes to be viable for testing, they must be at least three fourths full. Follow local protocols for the types of blood tubes to fill. All blood samples need to be labelled immediately with the patient's name, the time, and the site from which the blood draw was drawn; this should also be documented in your final chart. Remember to alert the receiving hospital staff that you have drawn blood, because they may want to affix their own labels and send the samples to the lab.

Intraosseous Infusion

Intraosseous means "within the bone." Intraosseous (IO) infusion is a technique of administering fluids, blood and blood products, and medications into the intraosseous space of a long bone, usually the proximal tibia.

Long bones consist of a shaft (diaphysis), the ends (epiphyses), and the growth plate (epiphyseal plate) **Figure 8-29 ▶**.

The intraosseous (IO) space collectively comprises the spongy cancellous bone of the epiphyses and the medullary cavity of the diaphysis. Its vasculature drains into the central circulation by a network of venous sinuses and canals.

When a patient is in shock, cardiac arrest, or an otherwise hemodynamically compromised condition, peripheral veins

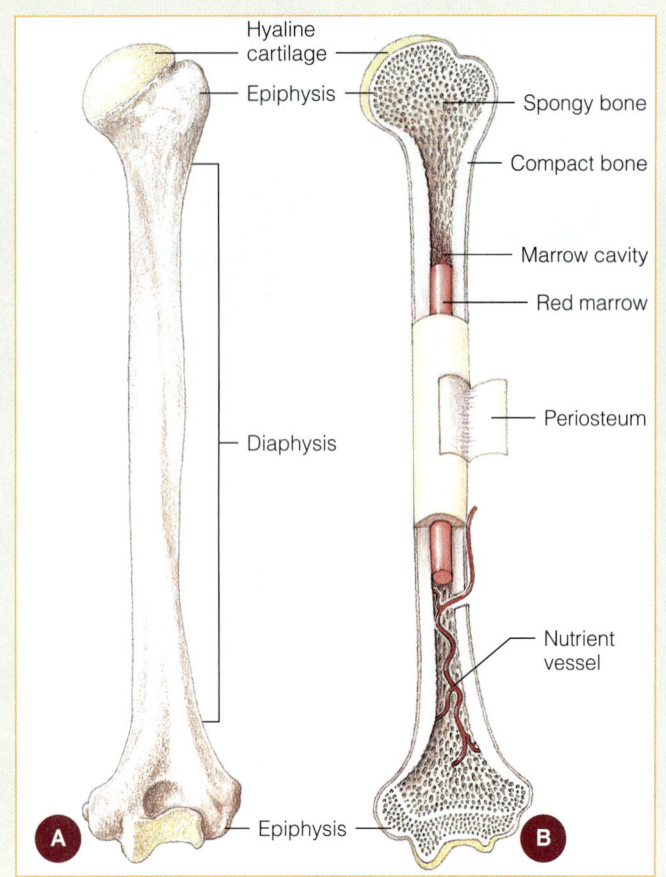

Figure 8-29 The components of a long bone. **A.** The humerus. Note the long shaft and dilated ends. **B.** Longitudinal section of the humerus showing compact bone, cancellous (spongy) bone, and marrow.

Labels for Figure 8-29:
- Hyaline cartilage
- Epiphysis
- Diaphysis
- Epiphysis
- Spongy bone
- Compact bone
- Marrow cavity
- Red marrow
- Periosteum
- Nutrient vessel

often collapse, making IV access extremely difficult, if not impossible. However, the IO space remains patent, unless the patient has suffered trauma to its bony structure (eg, a fracture). For this reason, the IO space is commonly referred to as a "noncollapsible vein." It quickly absorbs IV fluids and medications and rapidly gets them to the central circulation—as rapidly as is possible with the IV route. Anything that can be given via the IV route—crystalloids, medications, and blood and blood products—can be given via the IO route.

IO infusion is indicated when you are unable to obtain IV access in a critically ill or injured patient (eg, in profound shock, cardiac arrest, or status epilepticus). Historically, IO infusion was reserved for children younger than 6 years when IV access could not be obtained within 3 attempts or 90 seconds. Although this still holds true, IO infusion is an alternative means of establishing vascular access in critically ill or injured adults.

Equipment for IO Infusion

Several products are used for placing an IO needle into the IO space: manually inserted IO needles, the *FAST1®*, the EZ-IO, and the Bone Injection Gun (BIG). Use of these devices requires specialized training and thorough familiarity with each

device's features, functionality, and clinical application. If your EMS system uses any of these devices, follow local protocols regarding their application.

Manually inserted IO needles (ie, Jamshedi needle, Cook cannula) were the original devices used for establishing IO access in children and are still widely used in the prehospital setting. They consist of a solid boring needle (trocar) inserted through a sharpened hollow needle **Figure 8-30 ▾**. The IO needle is pushed into the bone with a screwing, twisting action. Once the needle pops through the bone, the solid needle is removed, leaving the hollow steel needle in place. The IV tubing is attached to this cannula.

Because manually inserted IO needles are long, rest at a 90° angle to the bone, and are easily dislodged, they require full and careful immobilization. Stabilization is critical for these lines to maintain adequate flow. Stabilize the IO needle in the same manner that you would any impaled object.

The *FAST1®* (First Access for Shock and Trauma) was the first IO device approved for use in adults; *it is not used in children.* Four design elements allow for this device's IO placement in the sternum: an infusion tube and subcutaneous portal, an introducer, a target/strain relief patch, and a protective dome **Figure 8-31 ▾**. The company that developed this device chose sternum placement based on the ease of locating the manubrium and the easier penetration than other bones.

The EZ-IO features a sealed, hand held, lithium battery powered medical drill to which a special IO needle is attached **Figure 8-32 ▸**. This device is used to insert an IO needle into the proximal humerus, proximal tibia, or distal tibia of adults and children when immediate vascular access is needed

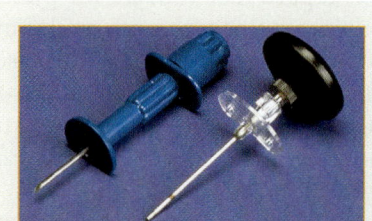

Figure 8-30 Manually inserted IO needles.

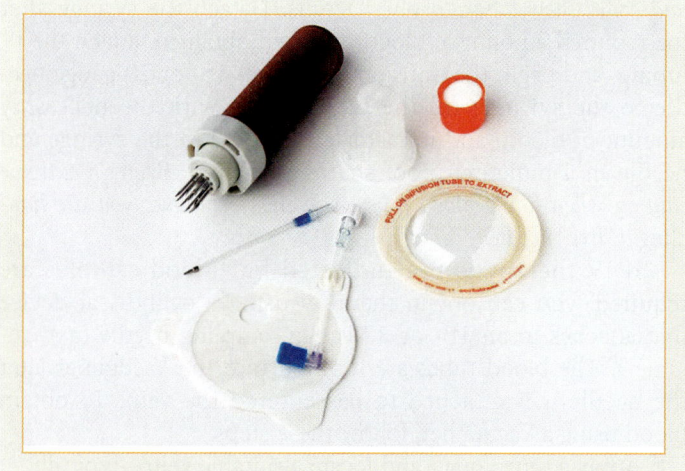

Figure 8-31 *FAST1®* sternal IO device.

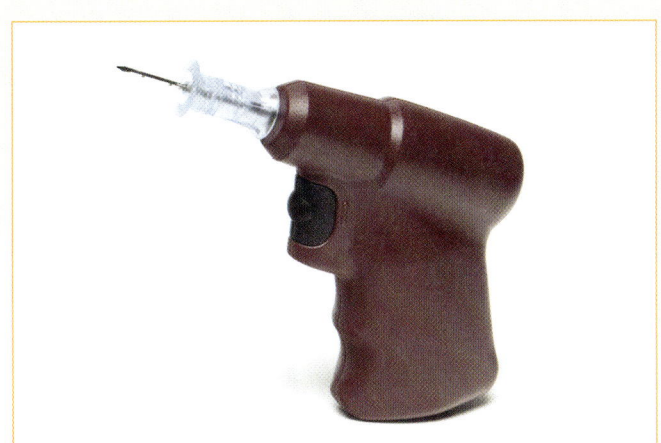

Figure 8-32 EZ-IO.

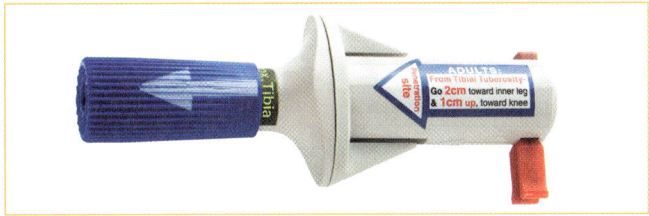

Figure 8-33 Adult BIG.

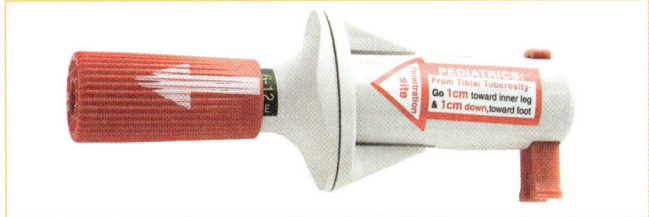

Figure 8-34 Pediatric BIG.

in acute situations. The EZ-IO driver (medical drill) is universal, but three different weight-based, single-use needle sets are available for adults, children, and patients with excessive tissue over the insertion site.

The Bone Injection Gun (BIG) is a spring-loaded device that is used to insert an IO needle into the proximal tibia of adult and pediatric patients. It comes in an adult size **Figure 8-33 ▲** and a pediatric size **Figure 8-34 ▲**, though both versions offer the same operational features.

Performing IO Infusion

The technique for performing IO infusion requires proper anatomical landmark identification. The flat bone of the proximal tibia—the most commonly used site—is located medial to the tibial tuberosity, the bony protuberance just below the knee.

Follow these steps to perform IO infusion using a manually inserted IO needle **Skill Drill 8-4 ▶**.

1. Check the selected IV fluid for proper fluid, clarity, and expiry date. Look for discolouration and for particles floating in the fluid. If found, discard the bag and choose another bag of fluid.

2. Select the appropriate equipment, including an IO needle, syringe, saline, and extension set **Step 1**. A three-way stopcock may also be used to facilitate easier fluid administration.

3. Select the proper administration set. Connect the administration set to the bag.
   Prepare the administration set. Fill the drip chamber and flush the tubing. Make sure all air bubbles are removed from the tubing.

4. Prepare the syringe and extension tubing.

5. Cut or tear the tape. This can be done at any time before IO puncture.

6. Take PPE and routine precautions **Step 2**. *This must be done before IO puncture.*

7. Identify the proper anatomical site for IO puncture **Step 3**. When using the BIG in an adult, go 2 cm from the tibial tuberosity toward the inner leg, and then 1 cm up toward the knee. When using the EZ-IO, go down 2 cm from the patella to the tibial tuberosity, then 1 cm toward the inner leg. It is important to avoid penetrating the epiphyseal (growth) plate in children. When using the BIG in a child, go 1 to 2 cm from the tibial tuberosity toward the inner leg, and then 1 cm down toward the foot.

8. Cleanse the site appropriately. Follow aseptic technique by cleansing in a circular manner from the inside out.

9. Perform the IO puncture, by first stabilizing the tibia, then placing a folded towel under the knee, and finally holding in a manner to keep your fingers away from the site of puncture.

10. Insert the needle at a 90° angle to the leg. Advance the needle with a twisting motion until a "pop" is felt **Step 4**. Unscrew the cap, and remove the stylet from the needle **Step 5**.

11. Attach the syringe and extension set to the IO needle. Pull back on the syringe to aspirate blood and particles of bone marrow to ensure proper placement.

12. Slowly inject saline to ensure proper placement of the needle. Watch for extravasation, and stop the infusion immediately if it is noted. It is possible to fracture the bone during insertion of the IO. If this happens, you should remove the IO and switch to the other leg.

13. Connect the administration set and adjust the flow rate as appropriate **Step 6**. Fluid does not flow as rapidly through an IO cannula as through an IV line; therefore, crystalloid boluses should be given with a syringe in children and a pressure infuser device in adults.

14. Secure the needle with tape, and support it with a bulky dressing. Stabilize in place in the same manner that an

Skill Drill 8-4: IO Infusion

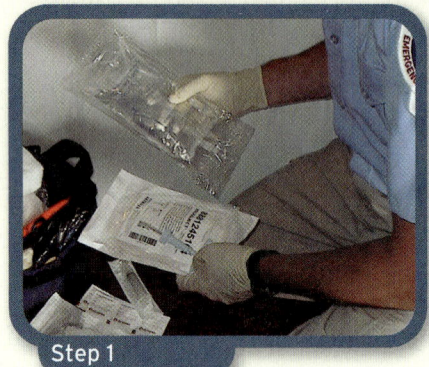

Step 1

Check selected IV fluid for proper fluid, clarity, and expiry date.

Select the appropriate equipment, including an IO needle, syringe, saline, and extension tubing.

Select the proper administration set. Connect the administration set to the bag. Prepare the administration set, syringe, and extension tubing.

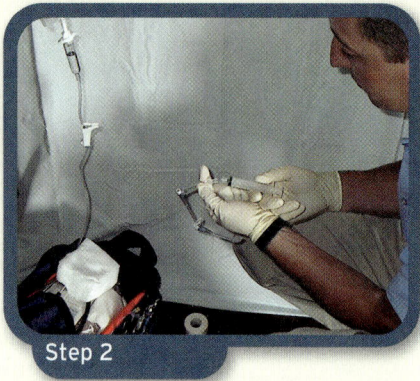

Step 2

Take PPE and routine precautions.

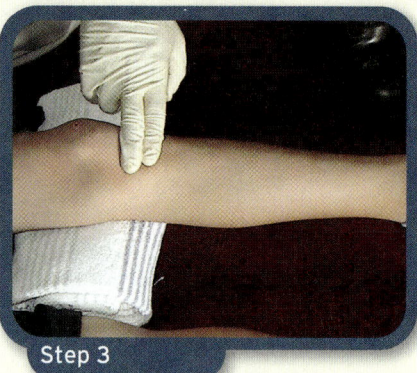

Step 3

Identify the proper anatomical site for IO puncture.

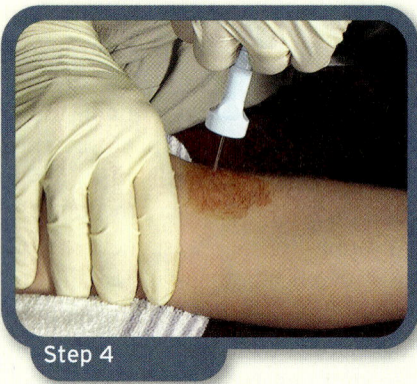

Step 4

Cleanse the site appropriately.

Stabilize the tibia, and insert the needle at a 90° angle, advancing it with a twisting motion until a "pop" is felt.

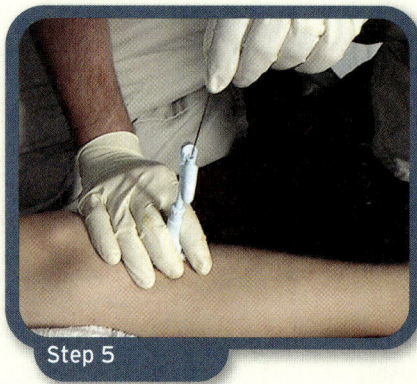

Step 5

Unscrew the cap, and remove the stylet from the needle.

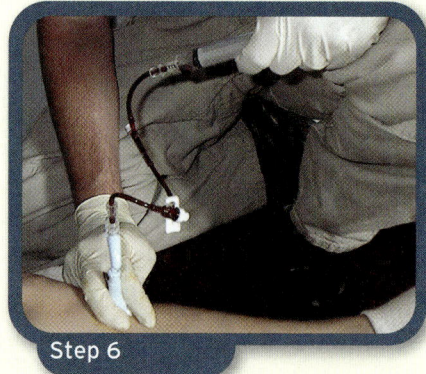

Step 6

Attach the syringe and extension set to the IO needle.

Pull back on the syringe to aspirate blood and particles of bone marrow to ensure proper placement.

Slowly inject saline to ensure proper placement of the needle.

Watch for extravasation, and stop the infusion immediately if it is noted.

Connect the administration set, and adjust the flow rate as appropriate.

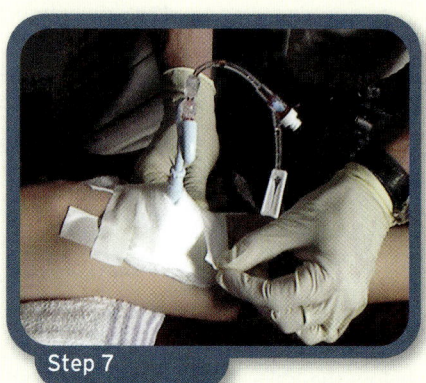

Step 7

Secure the needle with tape, and support it with bulky dressing.

impaled object is stabilized. Use bulky dressings around the cannula, and tape securely in place. Be careful not to tape around the entire circumference of the leg, as this could impair circulation and potentially result in compartment syndrome (Step 7).

15. Dispose of the needle in the proper container.

Potential Complications of IO Infusion

If proper technique is used (ie, proper anatomical landmark identification, aseptic technique), IO infusion is associated with a relatively low complication rate. The same potential complications associated with IV therapy—thrombophlebitis, local irritation, allergic reaction, circulatory overload, and air embolism—can occur with IO infusion, as well as several others unique to this method of infusion.

Extravasation occurs when the IO needle does not rest in the IO space, but rather rests outside the bone (because the bone was missed completely or is fractured). In such a case, IV fluid will collect in the soft tissues. The risk of extravasation can be reduced significantly by using the proper insertion technique: *Insert the IO needle at a 90° angle to the bone.* Extravasation should be suspected if the infusion does not run freely or if the site—especially the posterior aspect of the leg—rapidly becomes edematous. If this occurs, discontinue the infusion immediately and reattempt insertion in the opposite leg. Undetected extravasation could result in compartment syndrome.

Osteomyelitis is inflammation of the bone and muscle caused by an infection. According to several studies, osteomyelitis occurs in fewer than 0.6% of IO insertions.

Failure to identify the proper anatomical landmark can damage the growth plate, potentially resulting in long-term bone growth abnormalities in children.

If your insertion technique is too forceful, or if you use an IO needle that is too large for the patient's age or size, fractures can occur.

Through-and-through insertion occurs when the IO needle passes through *both* sides of the bone. To avoid this, stop inserting the needle when you feel a pop. If you feel a "pop, pop," you have likely passed the needle through both sides of the bone. Remove the needle and attempt insertion on the opposite extremity.

A pulmonary embolism (PE) can occur if particles of bone, fat, or marrow find their way into the systemic circulation and lodge in a pulmonary artery. Suspect a PE if the patient experiences acute shortness of breath, pleuritic chest pain, and cyanosis.

Contraindications to IO Infusion

Cannulation of a peripheral vein remains the preferred route for administering IV fluids and medications. If a functional IV line is available—in a pediatric patient or an adult—IO cannulation is *not* indicated. Other contraindications to IO cannulation and infusion include fracture of the bone intended for IO cannulation, infection of skin overlying the bone intended

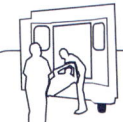

At the Scene

With the exception of the FAST1 sternal IO device, all IO devices—manual, spring-loaded, and battery-powered—are primarily used to insert an IO needle into the IO space of the proximal tibia. However, other anatomical locations, such as the distal tibia and distal femur, may also be acceptable locations for IO needle insertion.

for IO cannulation, osteoporosis, osteogenesis imperfecta (a congenital disease resulting in fragile bones), and bilateral knee replacements (obviously more relevant in adults).

Calculating Fluid Infusion Rates

Once the IV or IO cannula is in place, you need to adjust the flow rate according to the patient's clinical condition or as dictated by direct medical control. To do so, you must know the following information:

- The volume to be infused
- The period over which it is to be infused
- The properties of the administration set you are using— that is, how many drops per millilitre (gtt/ml) it delivers

Documentation and Communication

When you start an IV for the purpose of administering a medication, you should set the flow rate just slow enough to keep the vein patent. This slow flow rate can be documented using the acronym TKVO which stands for *To Keep Vein Open*.

By knowing in advance the volume to be infused, the period over which it will be infused, and the properties of the administration set, you can easily calculate the flow rate:

$$\text{gtt/min} = \frac{\text{volume to be infused} \times \text{gtt/ml of administration set}}{\text{total time of infusion } in\ minutes}$$

For example, suppose the physician orders an infusion of 1 l (1,000 ml) of normal saline to be infused in 4 hours, and the macrodrip administration set provides 10 gtt/ml:

Total volume to be infused = 1,000 ml
gtt/ml of the administration set = 10
Time of infusion (in minutes) = 240

$$gtt/min = \frac{1,000 \ ml \times 10 \ gtt/ml}{240 \ minutes} = approximately \ 42 \ gtt/min$$

At the Scene

If the physician orders a specific number of millilitres to be administered per hour (ml/h), a quick and easy way to calculate the number of drops per minute (gtt/min) is to divide the number of millilitres per hour:

- By 6, if using a macrodrip that provides 10 gtt/ml
- By 4, if using a macrodrip that provides 15 gtt/ml
- By 1, if using a microdrip set that provides 60 gtt/ml

Medication Administration

Before administering any medication to a patient, you must have a thorough understanding of how the medication will affect the human body—negatively and positively. This includes familiarity with the medication's mechanism of action, indications, contraindications, side effects, routes of administration, pediatric and adult doses, and antidotes (if available) for adverse reactions (see Chapter 7).

The first rule of medicine is *primum non nocere,* "The first thing (is) to do no harm." For example, administering the drug atropine to a patient with asymptomatic bradycardia could result in undesirable tachycardia and potential hemodynamic compromise. As a result, you have caused harm to the patient who otherwise did not need the drug. It is, therefore, paramount to ensure that a particular drug is clearly indicated to treat the patient's condition.

You must also have an understanding of basic math for pharmacology to calculate the appropriate medication dose. This section begins with a review of basic mathematical principles as they apply to pharmacology and concludes with the various methods of medication administration.

Drug doses and flow rate calculations are often sources of confusion for many prehospital personnel, yet they are skills you will need to utilize frequently in the prehospital setting and during your initial training while practicing at skill stations. As a paramedic, you must learn to quickly and accurately calculate medication doses to maximize the chance for a positive patient outcome. Disastrous results, including death, may be the outcome if you administer an inappropriate drug or dose, give it by the wrong route, or give the medication too rapidly or too slowly.

Mathematical Principles Used in Pharmacology

The Metric System

The metric system is a decimal system based on multiples of ten (Figure 8-35 ▾). In this system, the basic unit of length is the metre (m), the basic unit of volume is the litre (l), and the basic unit of weight is the gram (g). Prefixes indicate the fraction of the base being used. Commonly used prefixes, from smallest to largest, include *micro-* (0.000001), *milli-* (0.001), *centi-* (0.01), and *kilo-* (1,000).

Drugs are supplied in a variety of weights and volumes, and you will be required to convert those weights to volume to administer the appropriate dose of a medication to your patient. (Table 8-3 ▸) lists the symbols of weight and volume, with their respective abbreviations, that are used in the metric system. (Table 8-4 ▸) lists the metric units of weight and volume and their equivalents.

Weight and Volume Conversion

To administer the appropriate dose of a medication to a patient, you must be able to convert larger units of weight to smaller ones (for example, g to mg) and larger units of volume to smaller ones (for example, l to ml). Conversely, you must be able to convert smaller units of weight to larger ones (for example, mg to g) and smaller units of volume to larger ones (for example, ml to l).

Drugs are packaged in different units of weight and volume. However, the weight (for example, μg, mg, g) and volume (for example, ml) of the drug to be administered usually comprise only a fraction of the total amount of its packaged form. For example, you may need to administer 50 mg of a drug to a patient, but the drug is packaged in grams. Therefore, you must be able to convert grams to milligrams and then determine how much volume is required to achieve the desired dose.

Weight Conversion

Converting weight is simply a matter of multiplying or dividing by 1,000 *or* moving the decimal point three places to the right or left.

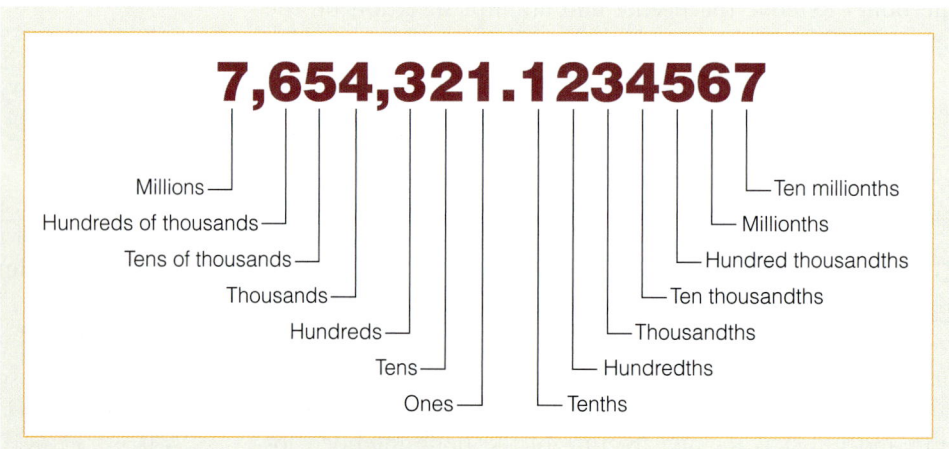

7,654,321.1234567

Millions
Hundreds of thousands
Tens of thousands
Thousands
Hundreds
Tens
Ones
Tenths
Hundredths
Thousandths
Ten thousandths
Hundred thousandths
Millionths
Ten millionths

Figure 8-35 Decimal scale.

Table 8-3	Symbols Used in the Metric System

Symbols of weight (smallest to largest)

- microgram = µg (or mcg)
- milligram = mg
- gram = g (or gm)
- kilogram = kg

Symbols of volume (smallest to largest)

- millilitre = ml
- decilitre = dl
- litre = l

Table 8-4	Metric Units and Their Equivalents

Units of weight (smallest to largest)

- 1 µg = 0.001 mg
- 1 mg = 1,000 µg
- 1 g = 1,000 mg
- 1 kg = 1,000 g

Units of volume (smallest to largest)

- 1 ml = 1 cc*
- 100 ml = 1 dl
- 1,000 ml = 1 l

*One millilitre (ml) of water weighs 1 g and occupies 1 cubic centimetre (cc) of volume. Thus a ml and a cc both express one one-thousandth of a litre and are, therefore, equivalent expressions.

To convert a larger unit of weight to a smaller one, *multiply* the larger unit of weight by 1,000 *or* move the decimal point three places to the *right:*

EXAMPLE

Converting 2 g to mg (2 g = X mg)

2 g × 1,000 = 2,000 mg *or* 2.000 g = 2,000 mg
$\longrightarrow$

To convert a smaller unit of weight to a larger one, *divide* the smaller unit of weight by 1,000 *or* move the decimal point three places to the *left:*

EXAMPLE

Converting 200 µg to mg (200 µg = X mg)

200 µg ÷ 1,000 = 0.2 mg *or* 200.0 µg = 0.2 mg
$\longleftarrow$

Volume Conversion

In the prehospital setting, you will usually deal with only two measurements of volume: millilitres and litres. The formula is the same as for converting units of weight: Divide or multiply by 1,000 *or* move the decimal point three places to the left or right.

When converting a smaller unit of volume to a larger one, *divide* the smaller unit of volume by 1,000 *or* move the decimal point three places to the *left:*

EXAMPLE

Converting 100 ml to l (100 ml = X l)

100 ml ÷ 1,000 = 0.1 l *or* 100.0 ml = 0.1 l
$\longleftarrow$

To convert a larger unit of volume to a smaller one, *multiply* the larger unit of volume by 1,000 *or* move the decimal point three places to the *right:*

EXAMPLE

Converting 1.5 l to ml (1.5 l = X ml)

1.5 l × 1,000 = 1,500 ml *or* 1.500 l = 1,500 ml
$\longrightarrow$

Converting Pounds to Kilograms

The only apothecary-to-metric conversion that you will likely make in the prehospital setting is from pounds (apothecary) to kilograms (metric).

Although many of the drugs given in emergency medicine are administered in a standard dose (eg, 1 mg of epinephrine), others are administered based on the patient's weight in kilograms (eg, 1 to 1.5 mg/kg of lidocaine). In addition, most drugs administered to pediatric patients are based on their weight in kilograms.

Two formulas can be used to convert pounds to kilograms. Use whichever one is easiest for you to remember.

Formula 1: Divide the patient's weight in pounds by 2.2
(1 kg = 2.2 lb)

For example, when converting a 170-lb man's weight to kilograms, the formula would be as follows:

---

170 lb ÷ 2.2 = 77.27 kg

Because the value following the decimal point in this example is less than 0.5, you may round the patient's weight in kilograms to 77. If the value after the decimal point had been greater than 0.5, you would round the weight in kilograms to 78. Although this may seem negligible, it is good practice to administer the *most* appropriate amount of the drug to the patient.

> Formula 2: Divide the patient's weight in pounds by 2 and subtract 10% of that number

For example, when converting a 120-lb woman's weight to kilograms, the formula would be as follows:

> Step 1: 120 lb ÷ 2 = 60
> Step 2: 60 × 10% = 6
> Step 3: 60 − 6 = 54 kg
> NOTE: This formula provides an approximate weight and is not exact.

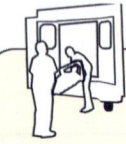

At the Scene

Carry a calculator or EMS guide to assist you in converting pounds to kilograms or when calculating a drug dosage.

Other Systems of Measurement

The apothecary system was formerly used by physicians and pharmacists but has been largely replaced by the metric system. It is based on 480 grains (gr) to 1 oz and 16 oz to 1 lb. The grain (gr) is the basic unit of weight and is approximately the weight of a drop of water. The minim is the unit of volume and is approximately the volume of a drop of water. Additional units of volume are the pint (pt), quart (qt), and gallon (gal). Fractions are used in the apothecary system.

You may also encounter the household system, which consists of measurements such as drops, teaspoons, tablespoons, and cups. This system is rarely, if ever, used for drug dosage calculation or administration in the prehospital setting.

The Fahrenheit and Celsius (or centigrade) temperature scales are commonly used to measure temperature. On the Celsius scale, water freezes at 0° and boils at 100°. On the Fahrenheit scale, water freezes at 32° and boils at 212°. Normal body temperature is 98.6° Fahrenheit and 37° Celsius. Values on each of these scales can easily be interconverted by using the following equations:

- To convert Fahrenheit to Celsius: Subtract 32, then multiply by 0.555 (5/9)

> 98.6°F − 32 × 0.555 = 36.9 (37°C)

- To convert Celsius to Fahrenheit: Multiply by 1.8 (9/5), then add 32

> 37°C × 1.8 + 32 = 98.6°F

Calculating Medication Doses

There are multiple formulas for calculating medication doses. This chapter focuses on those formulas that most students find easy to understand. For other calculation formulas, you are encouraged to consult with your instructor. The method of drug dose calculation demonstrated in this chapter is based on the following three factors:

- Desired dose
- Concentration of the drug available (dose on hand)
- Volume to be administered

Desired Dose

The desired dose (ie, the drug order) is the amount of a drug that the physician orders or is indicated in your local standing order protocols for you to give to a patient. It may be expressed as a standard dose (eg, 5 mg of diazepam [Valium], 25 g of 50% dextrose) or as a specific number of micrograms, milligrams, or grams per kilogram of body weight (eg, 1 to 1.5 mg/kg of lidocaine).

Drug Concentrations

After receiving a drug order (desired dose), you must determine how much of the drug that you have available. In other words, you must know its concentration—the total weight (μg, mg, or g) of the drug contained in a specific amount of volume (ml or l). Sometimes this information is printed on the label of the drug container (eg, Drug X at a concentration of 5 mg/ml); other containers may list the total weight and total volume of the drug separately (eg, 50 mg of drug Y in 10 ml). The following are examples of common prepackaged drug concentrations:

- Lidocaine, 100 mg/10 ml
- Epinephrine, 1 mg/10 ml
- Furosemide, 40 mg/4 ml
- Adenosine, 6 mg/2 ml
- 50% dextrose, 25 g/50 ml

In the preceding examples, notice that the drugs are contained in different volumes of solution. *To administer a drug, you must know the weight of the drug that is present in 1 ml.* This information will tell you the concentration of the drug that you have on hand. The formula for calculating this is as follows:

> Total weight of the drug ÷ total volume in millilitres
> = weight per millilitre

By using this formula, you can easily calculate how much of the drug is contained in each millilitre.

> **EXAMPLE**
>
> Lidocaine, 100 mg/10 ml
>
> 100 mg (total weight) ÷ 10 ml (total volume) = 10 mg/ml

Things become a bit trickier when the label of the drug lists the drug concentration as a percentage—for example, "1% lidocaine." What *percentage* means in terms of drug concentration is the number of *grams present in 100 ml*. Thus 1% lidocaine contains 1 g of drug in every 100 ml (1 dl). By dividing the numerator and denominator by 100, we arrive at a concentration of 10 mg/ml:

$$\frac{1\,g}{100\,ml} = \frac{1{,}000\,mg}{100\,ml} = 10\,mg/ml$$

Documentation and Communication

To prevent errors when documenting decimals, write 0.2 mg or 2 mg instead of .2 mg or 2.0 mg, which could easily be mistaken for 2 mg or 20 mg, respectively.

Volume To Be Administered

After determining the concentration of the drug present in each millilitre, you must calculate how much volume is needed to give the amount of the drug ordered (desired dose). Use the following formula to calculate the volume to be administered:

Desired dose (mg) ÷ concentration of drug on hand (mg/ml)
= volume to be administered

EXAMPLE 1

Direct medical control orders you to administer 5 mg of diazepam (Valium) to your patient for sedation. You have a vial of diazepam, which contains 10 mg in 2 ml. How many millilitres of diazepam must you give to achieve the ordered dose of 5 mg?

Step 1: Determine the concentration (in mg/ml).

10 mg ÷ 2 ml = 5 mg/ml (concentration)

Step 2: Determine how much volume to administer.

5 mg (desired dose) ÷ 5 mg/ml (concentration) = **1 ml**

EXAMPLE 2

You are ordered to administer 12.5 g of dextrose to a hypoglycemic patient. You have a prefilled syringe of 50% dextrose containing 25 g in 50 ml. How many millilitres of dextrose will you give?

Step 1: Determine the concentration (in g/ml).

25 g ÷ 50 ml = 0.5 g/ml (concentration)

Step 2: Determine how much volume to administer.

12.5 g (desired dose) ÷ 0.5 g (500 mg)/ml (concentration) = **25 ml**

Weight-Based Drug Doses

As mentioned earlier, some medication doses are based on the patient's weight in kilograms. Determining the appropriate dose for the patient requires simply adding one step to the formula we just discussed—conversion of the patient's weight in pounds to kilograms. Remember, 1 kg = 2.2 lb.

EXAMPLE

A 7-year-old girl requires 0.02 mg/kg of atropine to treat symptomatic bradycardia. You have a prefilled syringe of atropine containing 1 mg in 10 ml. The child's mother tells you that she weighs 60 lb. How many milligrams will you give to this child (that is, what is the desired dose)? How much volume will you give to achieve the required dose?

Step 1: Convert the child's weight in pounds to kilograms.

Formula 1: 35 lb ÷ 2.2 = 15.9 kg (round to 16 kg)

Formula 2: 35 lb ÷ 2 − 10% = 15.75 kg (round to 16 kg)

Step 2: Determine the desired dose.

0.02 mg × 16 kg = 0.32 mg (round to 0.3 mg [desired dose])

Step 3: Determine the concentration.

1 mg ÷ 10 ml = 0.1 mg/ml (concentration)

Step 4: Determine how much volume to administer.

0.3 mg (desired dose) ÷ 0.1 mg/ml (concentration) = **3 ml**

Calculating the Dose and Rate for a Medication Infusion

Non–Weight-Based Medication Infusions

Following the administration of certain drugs, you may need to begin a continuous infusion to maintain a therapeutic blood level of the drug to prevent a recurrence of the condition. Medication infusions are usually ordered to be administered over a specified period, usually per minute.

To calculate a continuous medication infusion that is not weight-based, you must know the following information in advance:

- The desired dose (μg/min or mg/min)
- The properties of the administration set you are using (eg, microdrip [60 gtt/ml])

You will use the same formula to calculate a drug dose as previously discussed. Then, however, you will calculate the desired dose to be administered continuously—usually a certain number of micrograms (μg) or milligrams (mg) per minute.

For example, suppose you have just administered 75 mg of lidocaine to your patient in cardiac arrest, after which time the cardiac rhythm converts to a perfusing rhythm. Direct medical control then orders you to begin a continuous lidocaine infusion at 2 mg/min. You must determine at how many drops per minute (gtt/min) to set the IV drip rate to deliver the 2 mg/min desired dose. To do so, you will add a certain amount of lidocaine into a bag of IV fluid. For demonstrative purposes, we will add 2 g (2,000 mg) of lidocaine to a 500-ml bag of normal saline, a common combination. The formula to calculate the continuous infusion rate is as follows:

Step 1: Determine the concentration.

2 g (2,000 mg) of lidocaine ÷ 500 ml of normal saline
= 4 mg/ml (concentration)

Step 2: Determine the amount of volume to infuse per minute (ml/min).

For this calculation, you must recall the desired dose—in this case, 2 mg/min. To determine the number of ml/min, you perform the following calculation:

2 mg (desired dose) ÷ 4 mg/ml (concentration) = 0.5 ml/min

Step 3: Determine how many drops per minute (gtt/min) at which to set the IV flow rate.

For this calculation, you must know the number of drops per millilitre (gtt/ml) that your IV administration set delivers—a microdrip (60 gtt/ml) or a macrodrip (10 or 15 gtt/ml). For a microdrip administration set (typically used when administering a continuous medication infusion), the number of drops per minute for the IV flow rate would be calculated as follows:

0.5 ml/min × 60 gtt/ml ÷ total time in minutes (1) = 30 gtt/min

Weight-Based Medication Infusions

Some continuous medication infusions are based on the patient's weight in kilograms. Dopamine, for example, is typically administered in a range of 5 to 20 µg/kg/min. By using the previously discussed formula and factoring in the patient's weight in kilograms to determine the desired dose, we will calculate the IV drip rate for a 70-kg patient who requires a continuous dopamine infusion at 5 µg/kg/min. For demonstrative purposes, we will add 800 mg of dopamine to a 500-ml bag of normal saline, a common combination.

Step 1: Determine the desired dose.

5 µg/kg/min × 70 kg = 350 µg/min (desired dose)

Step 2: Determine the concentration.

800 mg (800,000 µg) of dopamine ÷ 500 ml of normal saline = 1.6 mg/ml (concentration)

The caveat here is that dopamine is administered in *micrograms*, not milligrams. Therefore, we must convert the 1.6 mg/ml concentration to µg/ml. Recall that to convert a larger unit of weight to a smaller one, you must multiply by 1,000 *or* move the decimal point three places to the *right;* in other words, 1.6 mg is equal to *1,600 µg.*

Step 3: Determine the amount of volume to infuse per minute (ml/min).

Again, you must recall the desired dose—in this case, 350 µg/min. To determine the number of ml/min, the calculation continues as follows:

350 µg (desired dose) ÷ 1,600 µg/ml (concentration) = 0.22 ml/min

Step 4: Determine how many drops per minute (gtt/min) at which to set the IV flow rate.

Again, you must know the properties of the administration set you are using. In this example, we will use the microdrip (60 gtt/ml). The number of drops per minute for the IV flow rate would be calculated as follows:

0.22 ml/min × 60 gtt/ml ÷ total time in minutes (1) = 13.2 gtt/min (round to 13 gtt/min)

Pediatric Drug Doses

There are numerous methods for determining the appropriate dose of medication for a pediatric patient. Many paramedics use length-based resuscitation tape measures **Figure 8-36 ▾**; others carry an EMS field guide with tables or charts specific to pediatric patients. Most drugs used in pediatric emergency medicine are based on the child's weight in kilograms. With the exception of the obviously smaller doses and volumes, the calculations for pediatric drug dosing and medication infusions are the same as they are for adults.

Medical Direction

Medication administration is governed by your local protocols, the best evidence within the literature, and/or direct medical direction. The medical director for your service may allow the administration of certain medications as long as the patient meets certain criteria.

For example, for an unconscious diabetic patient with a confirmed blood glucose reading of 2 mmol/l, the paramedic may be allowed by written protocols (standing orders) to administer 50% dextrose ($D_{50}W$). Standing orders are a form

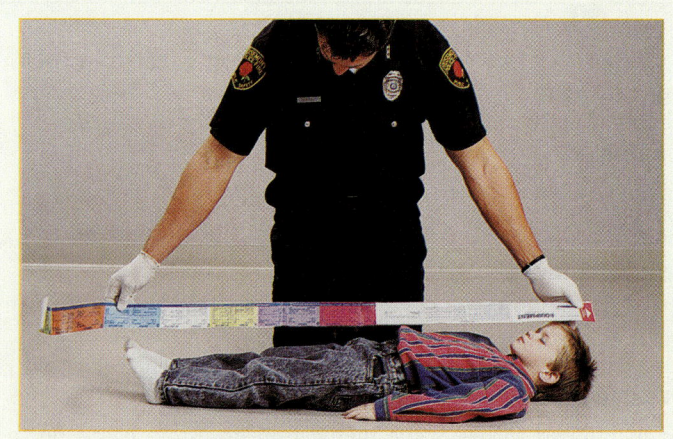

Figure 8-36 Use of a length-based resuscitation tape measure is one method of calculating pediatric drug doses. The tape measure estimates the child's weight (up to 34 kg) based on his or her length.

of indirect medical control, in which the paramedic performs certain predefined procedures without any consultation.

Some EMS system medical directors may not allow paramedics to perform certain procedures (for example, administering medications) before making contact with him or her. This is referred to as direct medical control.

Local policies and procedures are designed to guide you in specific situations. When questions or unusual situations arise—even if you function primarily by standing orders—contacting direct medical control for consultation is recommended in EMS systems that have this as an option.

Paramedic's Responsibility Associated With Drug Orders

The danger of something going wrong when administering a drug—for example, administering the wrong drug or the wrong dose of a drug—can be minimized by following a set procedure that incorporates a number of safety precautions. In EMS systems that require an online physician consultation:

1. Make sure the base physician understands the situation. The decision to order the administration of any given drug is complex, involving such considerations as the patient's age, weight, clinical status, allergy history, concomitant medical problems, and other drugs he or she may be taking. Thus, it is critical that you obtain and communicate complete and accurate information about the patient to enable the physician to make prudent and correct decisions about drug administration.

2. Make sure you understand the physician's orders clearly. If the orders are unclear or seem—on the basis of your knowledge—to be in error (for example, dosage more than the usual range, an unusual route of administration), *ask the physician to repeat the order.* Do not assume that the doctor is infallible, especially at 3:00 AM.

3. Always repeat any orders, word for word, back to the physician before administering a medication, to confirm that you received and understood the order accurately. In the repetition, state the *name of the drug,* the *dose,* and the *route* by which it is to be given. As a paramedic, you are just as responsible for the administration of the drug and its possible consequences as the physician giving the order, so be absolutely certain which drug is to be administered, in what dose, and by which route. If your partner does not hear the exchange of information, you should repeat the order to him or her as an additional safety measure.

4. If the patient is conscious, or if there is another reliable source of information, confirm that the patient is not allergic to the drug that has been ordered.

5. Read the label carefully as you take the vial or syringe from its box and again before you give the drug. Note the *drug concentration* printed on the label and the drug's *date of expiry.*

6. Check for defects in the vial, preloaded syringe, or ampule, and make sure that the fluid inside is not cloudy, discoloured, or precipitated. Check whether the container itself appears to be cracked or damaged. If the medication looks suspicious in any way, do *not* use it.

7. If you have orders to administer more than one drug, make sure that the drugs are compatible. Some drugs will not mix with others. For example, if sodium bicarbonate ($NaHCO_3$) is mixed with calcium chloride ($CaCl$), an insoluble precipitate, calcium carbonate ($CaCO_3$), will form in the solution. Should any cloudiness occur after a drug has been injected into IV tubing, *clamp the tubing immediately* and replace it with a new administration set.

8. Notify the physician when the medication has been administered.

9. Monitor the patient for possible adverse side effects.

10. Dispose of the syringe and needle safely. Do *not* try to recap the needle, for the likelihood is quite high of sticking yourself in the process; rather, dispose of the needle and syringe in a sharps container.

Notes from Nancy
Never guess what the physician has ordered. When in doubt, ask.

The "Six Rights" of Drug Administration

If given inappropriately, some medications can have lethal effects. Paramedics are dedicated to helping others, not harming them. Before giving *any* drug, review the "six rights" of medication administration:

- Right patient
- Right drug
- Right dose
- Right route
- Right time
- Right documentation

Verify that this is indeed the *right patient.* In multipatient situations, reconfirm the patient's name and compare it with the wrist band or triage tag.

Read the drug label at least three times before administration to ensure that you have the *right drug:*

1. When it is still in the drug box it came in
2. When you prepare the drug for administration
3. Before actually administering the drug to the patient

You are responsible for knowing the appropriate doses for the medications you carry on your ambulance. You are also responsible for accurately calculating the appropriate dose of the drug. Always recheck your drug calculations before administration to ensure that you are administering the *right dose.*

It is imperative that you know the *right route* for the drug or drugs that you are about to administer. A drug given by an inappropriate route—even if it is the right drug—could have disastrous and possibly fatal consequences.

Knowledge of the indications, contraindications, therapeutic effects, side effects, and appropriate doses for each of the drugs that you carry on your ambulance is critical to safe patient care.

Based on the patient's clinical presentation, you must know the *right time* to administer a medication (that is, when the medication is indicated). Of equal if not greater importance is knowing when *not* to administer a medication (that is, when the medication is contraindicated). Furthermore, some of the medications you carry on the ambulance have specific intervals for repeated doses; you must be aware of these drugs and the appropriate intervals at which they are administered.

Recall the adage, "If you did not document it, you did not do it." Always document the following information on the patient care report after administering a medication:

- Name of the drug
- Dose of the drug
- Time you administered the drug
- Route of administration
- Your name or the paramedic who administered the drug
- Patient's response to the medication, whether positive or negative

Documentation and Communication

If you administer a controlled substance to your patient (eg, morphine, midazolam [Versed], fentanyl), document the amount of medication that you gave to the patient and the amount of medication that you wasted (did not give to the patient). EMS systems are held to the standards of a governing body (such as Health Canada) in terms of how controlled substances are documented. In general, amounts administered and wasted are documented and require a cosignature, along with general medication counts every 12 to 24 hours to track the accuracy of the drug's usage and supporting documentation.

Local Drug Distribution System

Before responding to an EMS call, you must ensure that all equipment on the ambulance is fully functional; this verification is made during your check of the ambulance at the beginning of your shift. All medications must be checked to ensure that they are not expired or damaged and that they are readily available in the right quantity. You must be thoroughly familiar with the system used to exchange and replace outdated or damaged drugs in your EMS system.

You are also responsible for the documentation and security of all controlled substances carried on your ambulance, including accounting for all controlled substances that were wasted (ie, residual medication that was not administered to the patient). Follow the specific policies and procedures of your local drug distribution, security, and accountability system.

Medical Asepsis

Medical asepsis is the practice of preventing contamination of the patient by using aseptic technique. This method of

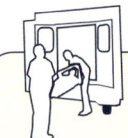

At the Scene

In addition to ensuring that medications have not expired or become contaminated, you must ensure that the medications are kept at the recommended temperatures while stored in your ambulance. Refer to the package insert for the medication for this information.

You are the Paramedic Part 3

Your partner obtains a blood glucose reading of 2 mmol/l. You initiate an IV line of normal saline with an 18-gauge cannula and set the rate to keep vein open (TKVO). A police officer arrives at the scene and obtains additional information from the neighbour. You quickly reassess the patient.

Reassessment	Recording Time: 9 Minutes
Level of consciousness	Unresponsive
Airway and breathing	Airway remains patent; ventilation is assisted by bag-valve-mask device and 100% oxygen
Blood pressure	104/64 mm Hg
Pulse	118 beats/min, weak and regular
Sao$_2$	99% (with assisted ventilation)
Blood glucose	2 mmol/l

The patient requires 50% dextrose (D$_{50}$W) to treat her hypoglycemia. You open the box, remove the drug, and prepare to administer it.

7. What does the "%" in 50% dextrose mean?

8. What is the concentration of D$_{50}$W that you have on hand?

9. What are the "six rights" of medication administration?

cleansing is intended to prevent contamination of a site when performing an invasive procedure such as starting an IV or administering a medication. Medical asepsis may be accomplished through the use of sterilization of equipment, antiseptics, or disinfectants.

Clean Technique Versus Sterile Technique

Some of the equipment you will use in the prehospital environment has been sterilized for patient safety. For example, some medications have been packaged using sterile technique. Sterile technique refers to the destruction of all living organisms and is achieved by using heat, gas, or chemicals.

Because it is almost impossible to maintain a sterile environment in the prehospital environment, you must practice medical asepsis to reduce the risk of contamination and infection. Examples of medical asepsis include handwashing, wearing gloves, and keeping equipment as clean as possible. For example, the site on a patient's hand that has been cleaned with iodine and alcohol before starting an IV is said to be "medically clean."

If you open an IV cannula package and the IV cannula inadvertently falls to the ground or otherwise comes in contact with a contaminated surface, discard it and use a new IV cannula. If you have already cleaned the injection port on the IV tubing where you intend to inject a medication and you inadvertently touch the cleaned injection port, recleanse the port before injecting the medication. You must always make a *conscious* effort to prevent contamination—whether handling equipment, supplies, or the patient. This is the cornerstone of maintaining a medically clean environment.

Antiseptics and Disinfectants

Antiseptics are used to cleanse an area before performing an invasive procedure such as IV therapy or medication administration. Even though antiseptics are capable of destroying pathogens, they are not toxic to living tissues. Isopropyl alcohol (rubbing alcohol) and iodine are the two most common antiseptics you will use in the prehospital environment.

Disinfectants, by contrast, are toxic to living tissues; therefore, you should never use them on a patient. Use disinfectants only on nonliving objects such as the inside of the ambulance, laryngoscope blades, and other nondisposable equipment. Examples of common disinfectants include Virex, Cidex, and Microcide.

Routine Precautions and Contaminated Equipment Disposal

Personal Protective Equipment

Treat any body fluid as being potentially infectious. Many patients who harbor infectious diseases may be asymptomatic and/or unaware that they are infected. As a paramedic, you owe it to yourself to protect yourself by taking the proper precautions when starting an IV or administering a medication. Minimum personal protective equipment (PPE) for these procedures include wearing gloves and protective eyewear (ie, goggles, face shield). If blood splattering is possible, full facial protection is indicated.

Handwashing is the *most* effective way to prevent the spread of disease. It should be a routine practice for you, between all patients. Note, however, that handwashing alone will not prevent you from being infected; use the appropriate precautions as dictated by the situation.

Disposal of Contaminated Equipment

After an IV cannula or needle has penetrated a patient's skin, it is contaminated. Considering the fact that accidental needlesticks are the most common route for disease transmission in the health care setting, you must always handle contaminated equipment carefully and dispose of it immediately and properly. Sharps are any contaminated item that can cause injury. Sharps include IV needles and cannulas, broken ampules or vials, and anything else that can penetrate or lacerate the skin.

Immediately dispose of all sharps in a puncture-proof sharps container that bears a biohazard logo **Figure 8-37 ▶**. Sharps containers should be readily accessible; place at least two in the back of the ambulance so that your handling of needles, cannulas, and other sharps is kept to a minimum amount of time. In addition, you should have a smaller sharps container in your jump kit for immediate disposal of sharps while not in the ambulance. **Table 8-5 ▶** lists some safe practices that will minimize your risk of an inadvertent needlestick. As always, follow your agency's exposure control plan.

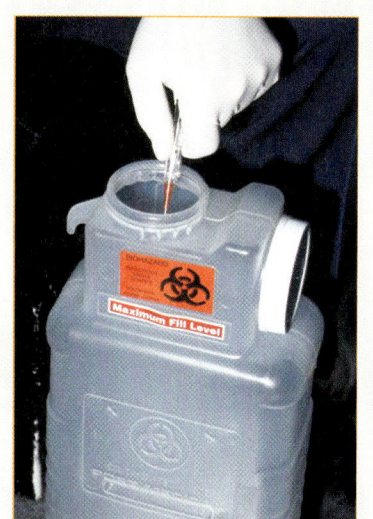

Figure 8-37 Always dispose of sharp objects or blood-filled items in a puncture-proof sharps container.

Enteral Medication Administration

The enteral route refers to any route in which medication is absorbed through some portion of the gastrointestinal tract. Enteral medication routes include the oral, gastric tube, and rectal administration routes.

Table 8-5	Minimizing Your Risk of a Needlestick

- *Immediately* dispose of all sharps in a puncture-proof sharps container. *Do not* drop the sharps on the floor for later disposal, and *do not* attempt to recap a needle and syringe before placing it in the sharps container.
- When possible, perform all invasive procedures at the scene. If your patient's condition warrants starting an IV or administering a medication en route to the hospital, *use extreme caution* as it is extremely dangerous and not recommended. Although most paramedics become proficient at starting IVs in the back of a moving ambulance, it may be necessary to have your partner briefly stop the ambulance, especially if you are travelling over rough terrain.
- Recap needles *only* as an absolute last resort. If you must recap a needle, use the one-handed technique. Place the needle cover on a stationary surface, then slide the needle—with one hand—into the needle cap.

Oral Medication Administration

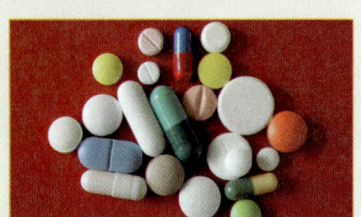

Figure 8-38 Tablets and capsules, oral medications typically taken by mouth, enter the bloodstream through the digestive system.

Most patients take their daily medications at home by the oral route (PO [per os]). Forms of solid and liquid oral medications include capsules, timed-release capsules, lozenges, pills, tablets, elixirs, emulsions, suspensions, and syrups **Figure 8-38 ▲** (see Chapter 7).

Drugs taken by mouth are absorbed at a slow rate from the stomach and intestines—usually somewhere between 30 and 90 minutes. Because absorption is slow, drugs are rarely given by the oral route in the prehospital setting.

To give oral medications, you may use a small medicine cup, a medicine dropper, a teaspoon, an oral syringe, or a nipple. Gather the appropriate equipment for the form of medication you are administering. Check for indications, contraindications, precautions, and review the six rights before administering any medication.

Follow these steps when administering an oral medication **Figure 8-39 ▶**.

1. Take routine precautions.
2. Determine the need for the medication based on patient presentation.
3. Obtain a focused history and physical examination, including any drug allergies.
4. Follow standing orders, or contact direct medical control for permission.
5. Check the medication to be sure it is the right medication, it is not cloudy or discoloured, and its expiry date has not passed.
6. Determine the appropriate dose. If using a liquid medication, pour the desired amount into a calibrated cup.

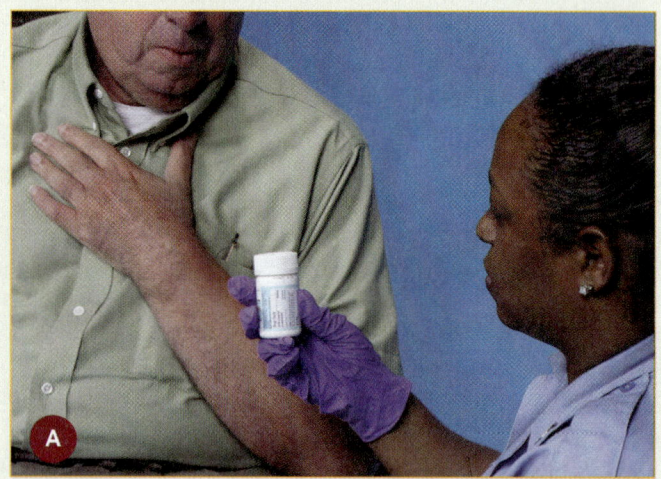

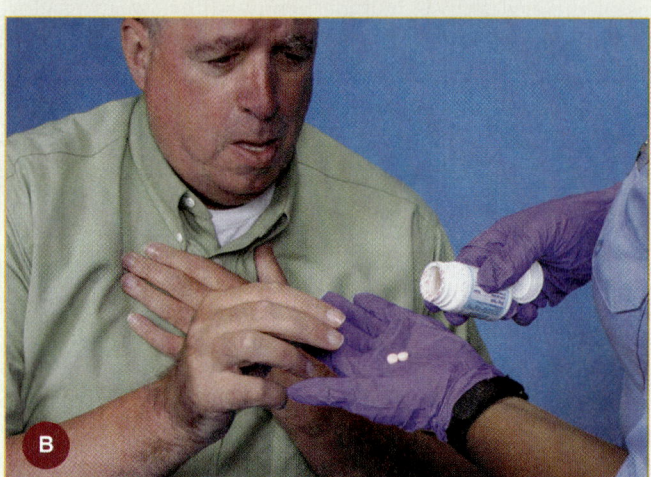

Figure 8-39 Administering an oral medication. **A.** Check the medication and its expiry date. **B.** Have the patient take the medication. Provide a glass or cup of water if necessary.

7. Instruct the patient to swallow the medication with water, if administering a pill or tablet.
8. Monitor the patient's condition, and document the medication given, route, time of administration, and response of the patient.

Gastric Tube Medication Administration

Gastric tubes (orogastric or nasogastric) are occasionally inserted in the prehospital setting to decompress the stomach. However, gastric tube placement also provides a route for enteral medication administration. Although most medications given via the gastric tube are administered in a hospital setting, activated charcoal for certain toxic ingestions—particularly in patients with a depressed swallowing mechanism or decreased level of consciousness—is the most likely scenario in which a gastric tube would be used as a medication route in the prehospital setting. Chapter 11 describes insertion of orogastric and nasogastric tubes. Follow these steps to administer

Skill Drill 8-5: Administering Medication via the Gastric Tube

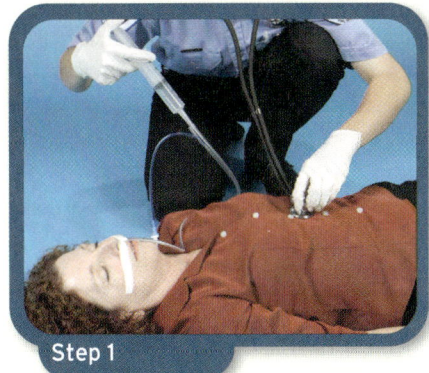

Step 1

Attach a 60-ml syringe to the proximal end of the gastric tube, and slowly inject air into the tube while auscultating over the epigastrium to confirm proper placement.

For further confirmation of correct tube placement, aspirate with the syringe and observe for gastric contents.

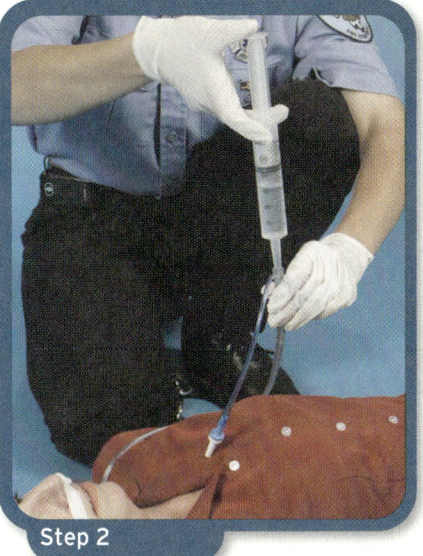

Step 2

Inject 30 to 60 ml of normal saline into the gastric tube to irrigate the tube.

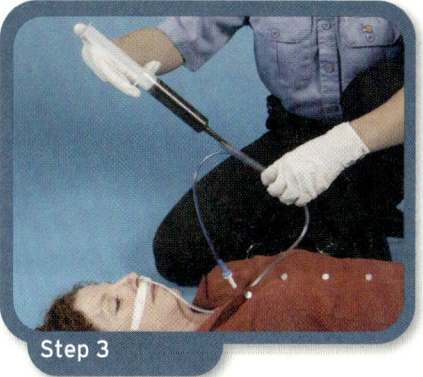

Step 3

Inject the appropriate amount of medication into the gastric tube.

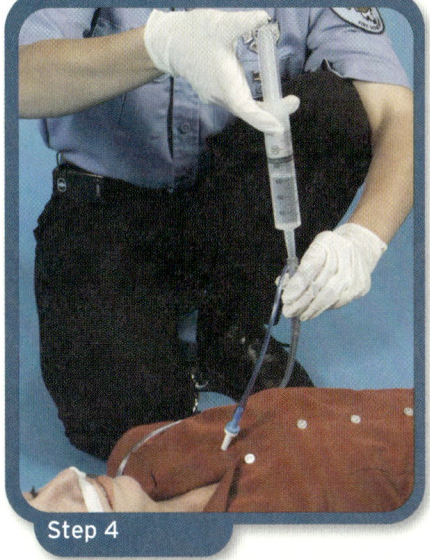

Step 4

Flush the gastric tube with 30 to 60 ml of normal saline to ensure dispersal of the drug into the stomach.

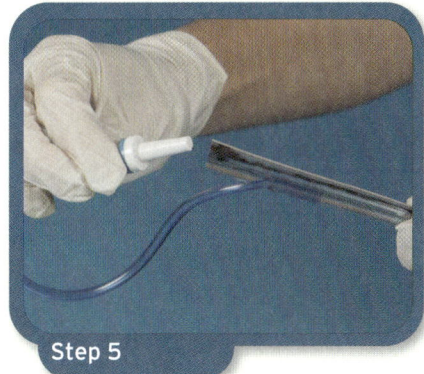

Step 5

Clamp off the proximal end of the gastric tube; do not reattach the tube to suction.

Monitor the patient for adverse reactions, and repeat the medication dose if indicated.

medications via the gastric tube after the tube has been inserted **Skill Drill 8-5 ▲**.

1. Take routine precautions.
2. Confirm proper gastric tube placement. Attach a 60-ml cone-tipped syringe to the gastric tube and slowly inject air as you or your partner auscultates over the epigastrium **Step 1**.

   To further confirm proper placement, withdraw on the plunger of the syringe and observe for the return of gastric contents in the tube. Leave the gastric tube open to air.

3. Draw up 30 to 60 ml of normal saline into the syringe, and irrigate the gastric tube **Step 2**. If you meet resistance, ensure that the tube is not kinked.
4. Draw up the appropriate amount of medication, and slowly inject it into the gastric tube **Step 3**.
5. Inject 30 to 60 ml of normal saline into the gastric tube following administration of the medication **Step 4**. This will ensure that the tube is flushed and that the patient has received the entire dose of the medication.

6. Clamp off the proximal end of the gastric tube (Step 5). Do not attach the gastric tube to suction because this will result in removal of the medication from the stomach. Monitor the patient for adverse reactions. Repeat the medication dose if indicated.

Rectal Medication Administration

Certain drugs may be administered rectally if you are unable to establish IV or IO access. In the prehospital environment, diazepam (Valium) can be administered rectally in pediatric patients because IV access can be challenging enough under normal circumstances, and even more so when the child is having a seizure. Because the rectal mucosa is highly vascular, medication absorption is rapid and predictable (Figure 8-40 ▾). Certain antiemetic medications are available in suppository form, and under certain circumstances, you might be asked to administer them. A suppository is a drug mixed in a firm base that melts at body temperature and is shaped to fit the rectum.

Follow these steps to administer a drug via the rectal route:

1. Take routine precautions and use appropriate PPE.

2. Determine the need for the medication based on patient presentation.

3. Obtain a focused history and physical examination, including any drug allergies.

4. Follow standing orders, or contact direct medical control for permission.

5. Determine the appropriate dose, and check that the medication is the right medication, there is no cloudiness or discolouration, and the expiry date has not passed.

6. When inserting a suppository, use a water-soluble gel for lubrication. Insert the suppository into the rectum approximately 2.5 to 3.8 cm while instructing the patient to relax and not to bear down.

7. For medications in liquid form, some modifications are needed. You may use a nasopharyngeal airway, a small endotracheal tube, the plastic sheath of an IV cannula, or a well-lubricated, 1-ml syringe as your delivery device. Determine the best option based on the size of your patient.

- Lubricate the end of the device you have choosen with a water-soluble gel, and gently insert it approximately 2.5 to 3.8 cm into the rectum (Figure 8-41 ▾).
- Instruct the patient to relax and not to bear down.
- With a *needleless* syringe, gently push the medication through the tube.
- Once the medication has been delivered, remove and dispose of the tube or syringe in an appropriate container.

8. Monitor the patient's condition, and document the medication given, route, time of administration, and response of the patient.

▌Parenteral Medication Administration

The parenteral route refers to any route other than the gastrointestinal tract. Parenteral routes for medication administration

> ### At the Scene
>
> Diazepam (Valium) is available in a specially designed container, for rectal adminstration.
> The distal end of the container is tapered, which facilitates insertion into the rectum. This feature eliminates the need for syringes or other methods of injecting the medication into the rectum.

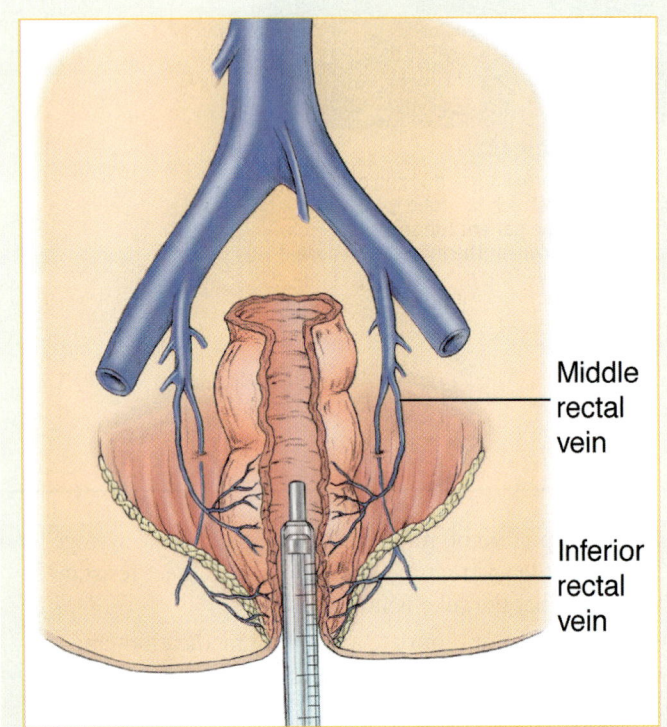

Figure 8-40 The rectal mucosa is highly vascular. It rapidly and predictably absorbs medications.

Middle rectal vein

Inferior rectal vein

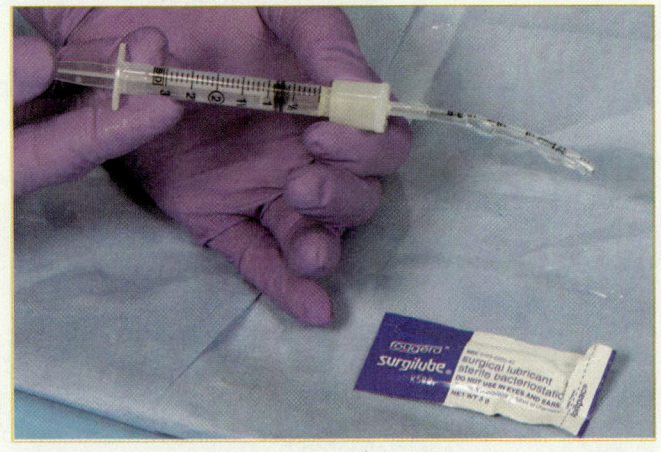

Figure 8-41 Syringe attached to an endotracheal tube.

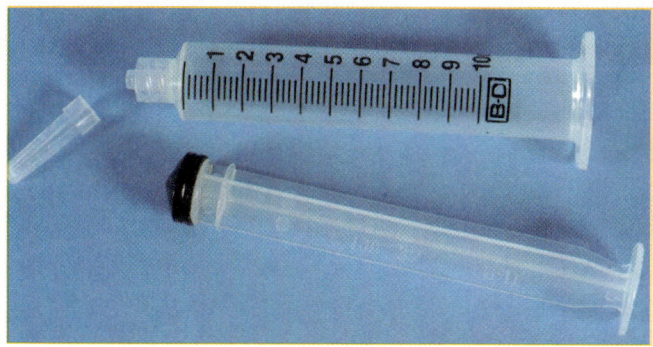

Figure 8-42 A syringe consists of a plunger, body or barrel, flange, and tip.

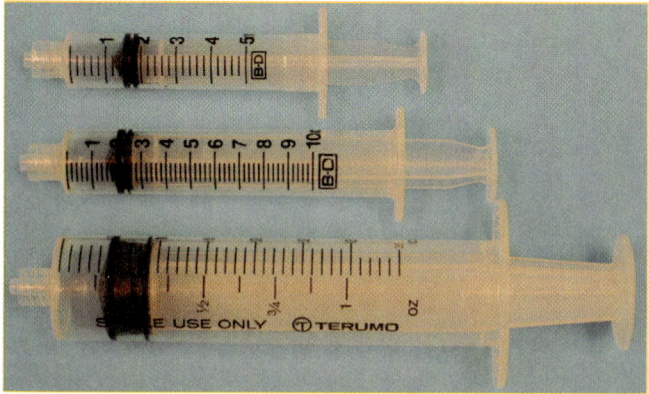

Figure 8-43 Syringes come in a variety of sizes. Some come with needles already attached, others without needles attached.

include the intradermal, subcutaneous, intramuscular, intravenous, intraosseous, and percutaneous routes. Compared with enterally administered medications (eg, oral, gastric tube), parenterally administered medications are absorbed into the central circulation more quickly and at a more predictable rate, thus achieving their therapeutic effects faster. Of the parenteral drug routes, IV administration is the route most commonly used in the prehospital setting and generally is the quickest route for getting medication into the central circulation.

Syringes and Needles

A variety of needles and syringes are used for administering parenteral medications. Most syringes come prepackaged in colour-coded packs with a needle already attached. The needles and syringes may also be packaged separately. Syringes consist of a plunger, body or barrel, flange, and tip Figure 8-42 ▲ . Most syringes are marked with 10 calibrations per millilitre on one side of the barrel, where each small line represents 0.1 ml; the other side of the barrel is marked in minims. Syringes vary from 1 ml to 60 ml; the 3-ml syringe is the one most commonly used for injections. Syringe selection is based on the volume of medication that you will administer Figure 8-43 ▲ .

Hypodermic needle lengths vary from 1 to 5 cm for standard injections. As with IV cannulas, the gauge of the

needle refers to the diameter: The smaller the number, the larger the diameter. Common needle gauges range from 18 to 26. The needle gauge used depends on the route of parenteral medication administration. Smaller-gauge needles, for example, are used for subcutaneous injections, whereas larger-gauge needles are used for intramuscular and IV injections.

The proximal end of the needle, or hub, attaches to the standard fitting on the syringe. The distal end of the needle is beveled.

Packaging of Parenteral Medications
Ampules

Ampules are breakable sterile glass containers that are designed to carry a single dose of medication Figure 8-44 ▶ . They may contain as little as 1 ml or as much as 10 ml, depending on the medication.

When drawing a medication from an ampule, follow the steps in Skill Drill 8-6 ▶ .

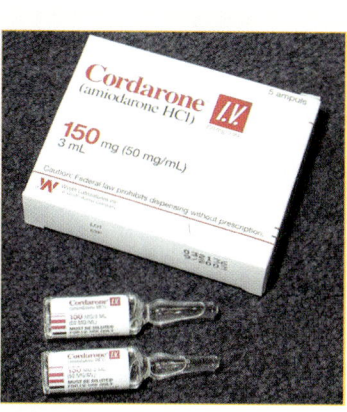

Figure 8-44 Ampules.

1. Check the medication to be sure that the expiry date has not passed and that it is the correct drug and concentration.
2. Shake the medication into the base of the ampule. If some of the drug is stuck in the neck, gently thump or tap the stem Step 1 .
3. Using a 10 × 10 cm gauze pad or an alcohol prep, grip the neck of the ampule and snap it off. Drop the stem in the sharps container Step 2 .
4. Insert the needle into the ampule without touching the outer sides of the ampule. Draw the solution into the syringe, and dispose of the ampule in the sharps container Step 3 .
5. Hold the syringe with the needle pointing up, and gently tap the barrel to loosen air trapped inside and cause it to rise Step 4 . Press gently on the plunger to dispel any air bubbles Step 5 .
6. Recap the needle using the one-handed method.

Vials

Vials are small glass or plastic bottles with a rubber-stopper top; they may contain single or multiple doses of a medication Figure 8-45 ▶ . When using a vial of medication, you must first determine how much of the drug you will need and how many doses are in the vial.

For a single-dose vial, you will draw up the entire amount in the vial. For multiple-dose vials, you should draw up only the amount needed. Remember that once you remove

Skill Drill 8-6: Drawing Medication From an Ampule

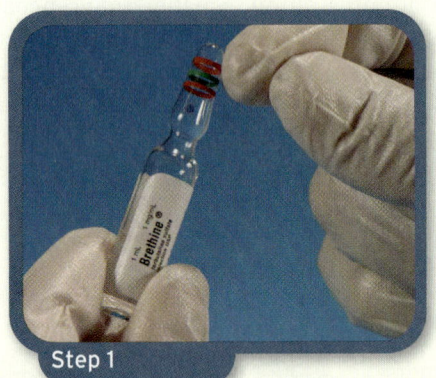

Step 1

Gently tap the stem of the ampule to shake medication into the base.

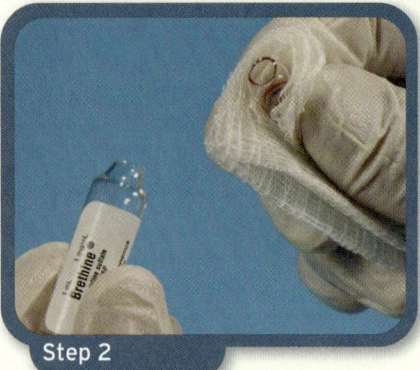

Step 2

Grip the neck of the ampule using a 10 × 10 cm gauze pad, and snap the neck off.

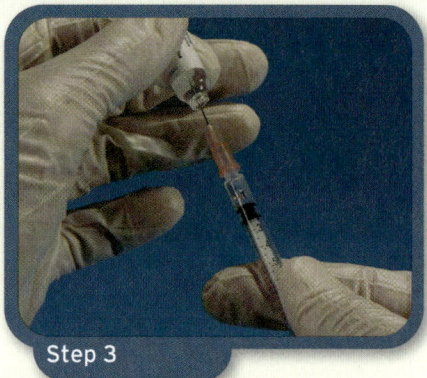

Step 3

Without touching the outer sides of the ampule, insert the needle into the medication in the ampule, and draw the solution into the syringe.

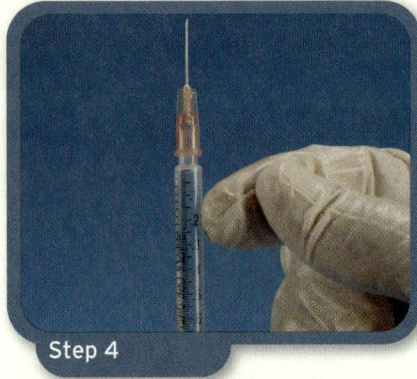

Step 4

Holding the syringe with the needle pointing up, gently tap the barrel to loosen air trapped inside.

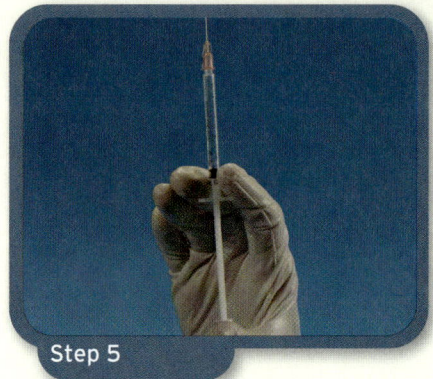

Step 5

Gently press on the plunger to dispel any air bubbles, and recap the needle using the one-handed method.

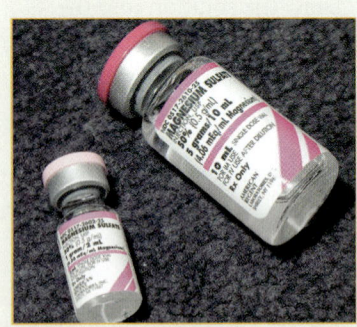

Figure 8-45 Vials (single-dose and multidose).

the cover from a vial, it is no longer sterile. If you need a second dose, clean the top of the vial with alcohol before withdrawing the medication.

Some medications that are stored in vials may need to be reconstituted, such as methylprednisolone sodium succinate (Solu-Medrol) and glucagon. Glucagon is stored in two vials, one with the powdered form of the drug and the other with sterile water. Drug reconstitution involves injecting the sterile water (or provided diluent) from one vial into the vial that contains the powder, thereby making a solution for injection. To reconstitute the contents of two vials, draw the fluid out of the first vial and inject it into the vial that contains the powder. Shake the vial vigorously to mix the medication before drawing out the contents for administration.

Solu-Medrol is stored in a Mix-o-Vial, a single vial divided into two compartments by a rubber stopper **Figure 8-46 ▶**. To reconstitute a drug that is

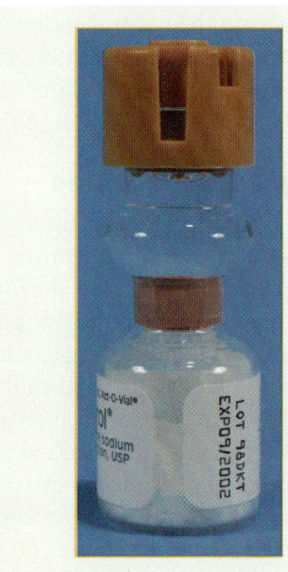

Figure 8-46 A Mix-o-Vial.

Skill Drill 8-7: Drawing Medication From a Vial

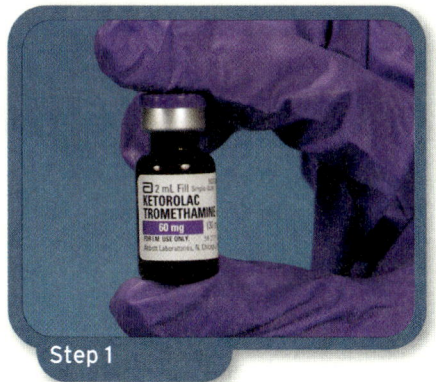

Step 1

Check the medication and its expiry date.

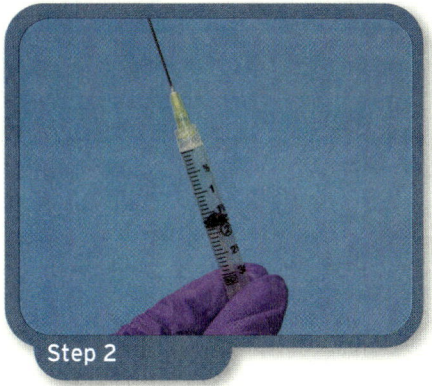

Step 2

Determine the amount of medication needed, and draw that amount of air into the syringe.

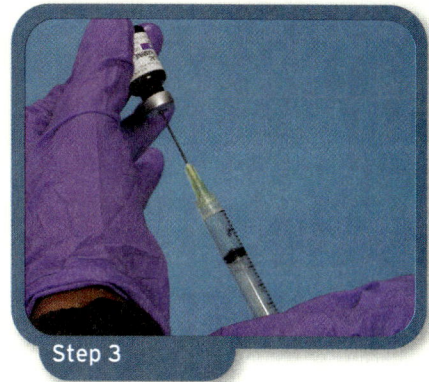

Step 3

Invert the vial, and insert the needle through the rubber stopper. Expel the air in the syringe into the vial, and then withdraw the amount of medication needed.

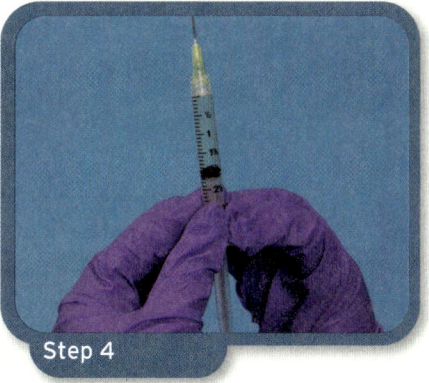

Step 4

Withdraw the needle, and expel any air in the syringe.

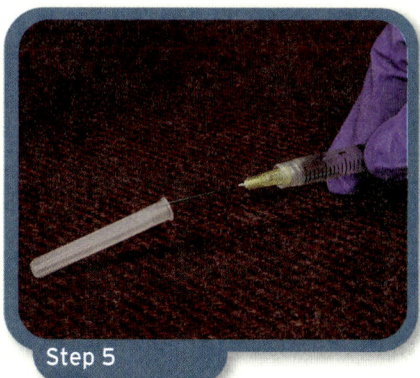

Step 5

Recap the needle using the one-handed method.

---

contained in a Mix-o-Vial, squeeze the two vials together, which releases the centre stopper and allows the contents to mix. Shake vigorously to mix the contents before drawing out the medication.

When drawing medication from a vial, follow the steps in **Skill Drill 8-7 ▲**.

1. Check the medication to be sure that the expiry date has not passed and that it is the correct drug and concentration (Step 1).

2. Remove the sterile cover, or clean the top with alcohol if the vial was previously opened.

3. Determine the amount of medication that you will need, and draw that amount of air into the syringe (Step 2). Allow a little extra room to expel some air while removing air bubbles.

4. Invert the vial, and insert the needle through the rubber stopper into the medication. Expel the air in the syringe into the vial and then withdraw the amount of medication needed (Step 3).

5. Once you have the correct amount of medication in the syringe, withdraw the needle from the vial and expel any air in the syringe (Step 4).

6. Recap the needle using the one-handed method (Step 5).

Prefilled Syringes

Prefilled syringes are packaged in tamper-proof boxes. Two types of prefilled syringes exist: those that are separated into a glass drug cartridge and a syringe, **Figure 8-47 ▸**, and pre-assembled prefilled syringes **Figure 8-48 ▸**. These syringes are designed for ease of use. After all, it is much easier and quicker to use a prefilled syringe when you are treating a patient in cardiac arrest than it is to draw up each individual dose.

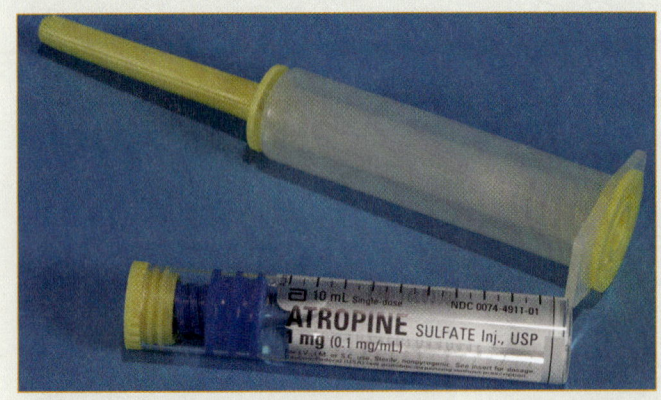

Figure 8-47 Two-part prefilled syringes are separated into a glass drug cartridge and a syringe.

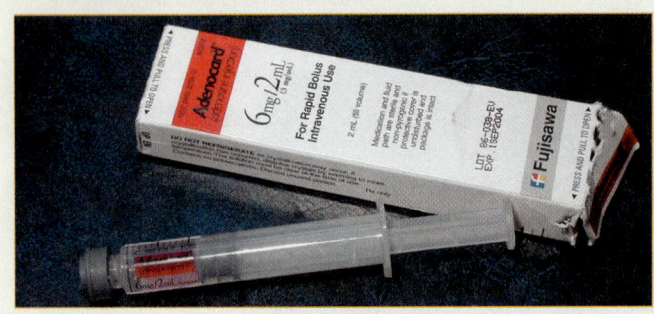

Figure 8-48 Preassembled prefilled syringe.

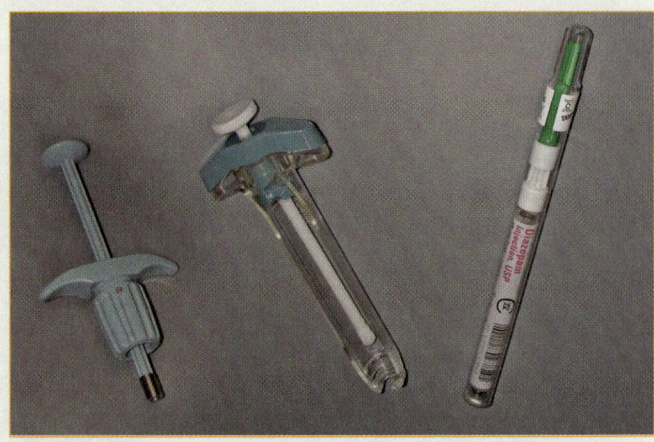

Figure 8-49 Reusable syringes (left). Disposable medication cartridge (right).

At the Scene

Whenever you use a needle to draw up medication from an ampule or vial, hold the syringe against your palm with the needle pointing up and draw the ampule or vial down onto the needle using the thumb and forefinger of the palm the syringe is braced against to avoid sticking yourself. This especially applies if you are in a moving ambulance.

To assemble the two-part prefilled syringe, pop the caps off of the syringe and the drug cartridge, insert the drug cartridge into the barrel of the syringe, and screw them together. Remove the needle cover, and expel air in the manner previously described. Follow the steps for the route the medication is to be given.

Single-dose disposable medication cartridges that are inserted into a reusable syringe are also available. These syringes are commonly referred to as Tubex, Aboject, and Carpuject syringes **Figure 8-49**.

Intradermal Medication Administration

Intradermal injections involve administering a small amount of medication—typically less than 1 ml—into the dermal layer, just beneath the epidermis. The technique involves the use of a 1-ml syringe (for example, a tuberculin syringe) and a 25- to 27-gauge, 1- to 2.5-cm needle.

When selecting a site for an intradermal injection, you should avoid areas that contain superficial blood vessels to minimize the risk of systemic medication absorption. Because of their high visibility and relative lack of hair, the most common anatomical locations for intradermal injections are the anterior forearm and upper back.

Medications administered intradermally have a very slow rate of absorption; there is minimal to no systemic distribution. The medication remains locally collected at the site of the injection. Unless you are anesthetizing the skin before establishing an IV, you will rarely use the intradermal route to administer medications in the prehospital setting. Instead, these injections are typically given in a physician's office or in the hospital to test a patient for allergies or to perform a PPD (purified protein derivative)—a skin test for tuberculosis.

Follow these steps to administer a medication via the intradermal route:

1. Take routine precautions.
2. Determine the need for the medication based on patient presentation.
3. Obtain a focused history and physical examination, including any drug allergies and vital signs.
4. Follow standing orders, or contact direct medical control for permission.
5. Check the medication to ensure that it is the correct one, that it is not cloudy or discoloured, and that the expiry date has not passed, and determine the appropriate amount to give for the correct dose.
6. Advise the patient of potential discomfort while explaining the procedure.
7. Assemble and check equipment needed: alcohol preps and a 1-ml syringe with a 25- to 27-gauge, 1-cm or 2.5-cm needle. Draw up the correct dose of medication.

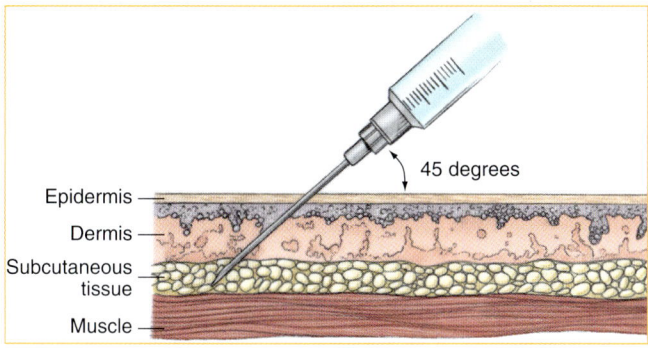

Figure 8-50 A subcutaneous injection is below the dermis and above the muscle.

8. Cleanse the area for administration using aseptic technique.
9. Pull the skin taut with your nondominant hand.
10. Insert the needle at a 10° to 15° angle with the bevel up.
11. Slowly inject the medication while observing for the formation of a wheal, or small bump, which indicates that the medication is collecting in the intradermal tissue.
12. Remove the needle. Immediately dispose of the needle and syringe in the sharps container.
13. Monitor the patient's condition, and document the medication given, route, administration time, and response of the patient.

Subcutaneous Medication Administration

Subcutaneous (SC) injections are given into the loose connective tissue between the dermis and the muscle layer **Figure 8-50 ▲**. Volumes of a drug administered subcutaneously are usually 1 ml or less. The injection is performed using a 24- to 26-gauge 1.27- to 2.5-cm needle. Common sites for SC injections—in both adults and children—include the upper arms, anterior thighs, and the abdomen **Figure 8-51 ▶**. Patients who take insulin injections usually vary the sites owing to the multiple (usually daily) injections they require.

Follow the steps in **Skill Drill 8-8 ▶** to administer a medication via the subcutaneous route:

1. Take routine precautions.
2. Determine the need for the medication based on patient presentation.
3. Obtain a focused history and physical examination, including any drug allergies and vital signs.
4. Follow standing orders, or contact direct medical control for permission.
5. Check the medication to ensure that it is the correct one, that it is not cloudy or discoloured, and that the expiry date has not passed, and determine the appropriate amount and concentration for the correct dose **Step 1**.
6. Advise the patient of potential discomfort while explaining the procedure.

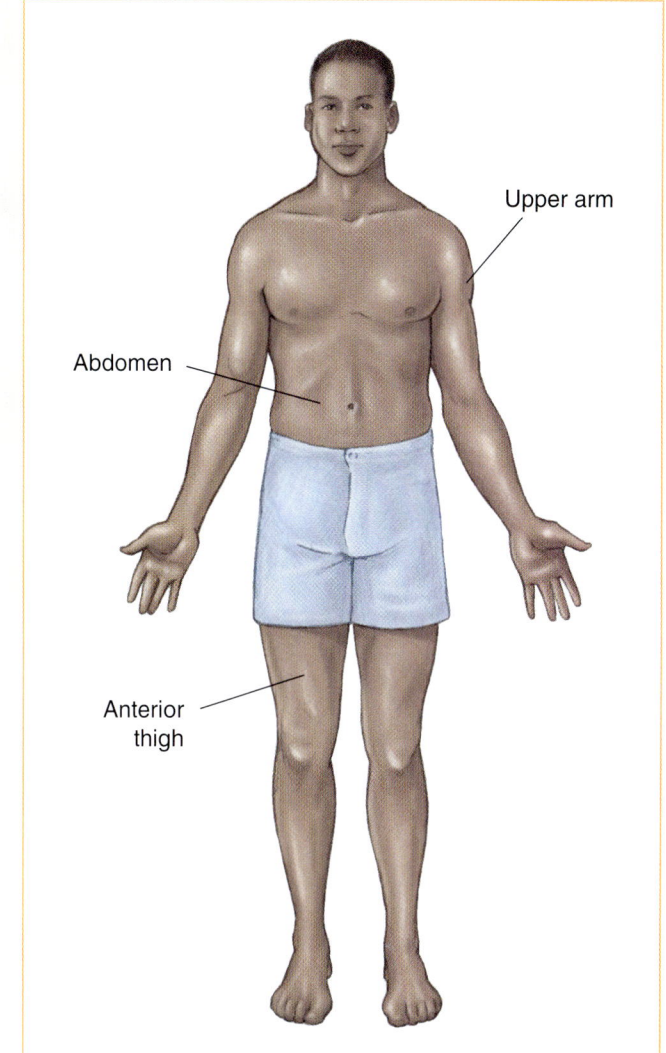

Figure 8-51 Common sites for subcutaneous injections.

7. Assemble and check equipment needed: alcohol preps and a 3-ml syringe with a 24- to 26-gauge needle. Draw up the correct dose of medication **Step 2**.
8. Cleanse the area for the administration (usually the upper arm or thigh) using aseptic technique **Step 3**.
9. *Pinch the skin* surrounding the area, advise the patient of a stick, and insert the needle at a *45° angle*.
10. Pull back on the plunger to aspirate for blood. The presence of blood in the syringe indicates you may have entered a blood vessel. In such a case, remove the needle, and hold pressure over the site. Discard the syringe and needle in the sharps container. Prepare a new syringe and needle, and select another site.
11. If there is no blood in the syringe, inject the medication and remove the needle. Immediately dispose of the needle and syringe in the sharps container **Step 4**.

Skill Drill 8-8: Administering Medication via the Subcutaneous Route

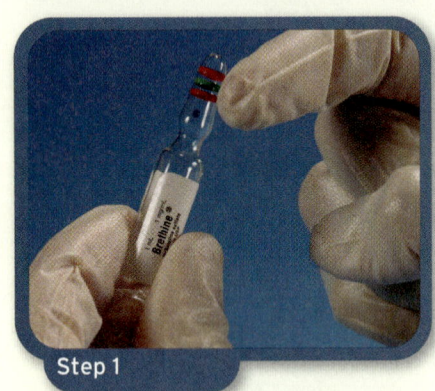

Step 1

Check the medication to ensure that it is the correct one, that it is not discoloured, and that the expiry date has not passed.

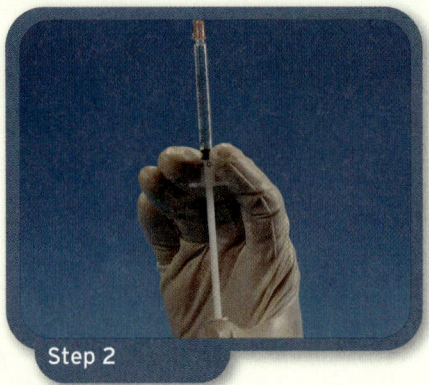

Step 2

Assemble and check the equipment. Draw up the correct dose of medication.

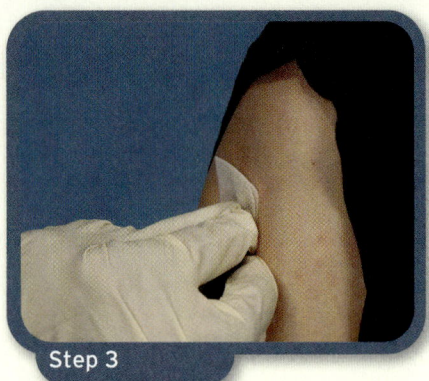

Step 3

Using aseptic technique, cleanse the injection area.

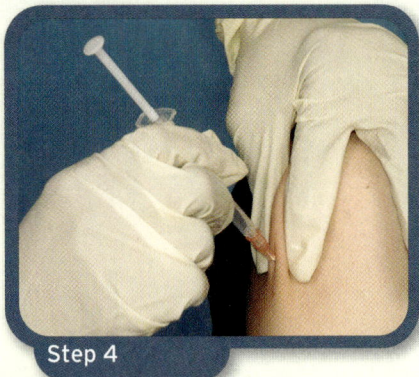

Step 4

Pinch the skin surrounding the area, and insert the needle at a 45° angle. Pull back on the plunger to aspirate for blood. If there is no blood, inject the medication, remove the needle, and hold pressure over the area. Immediately dispose of the needle and syringe in the sharps container.

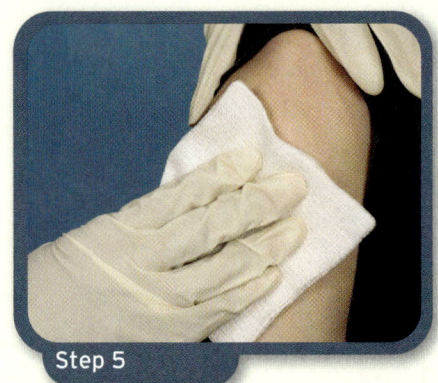

Step 5

To disperse the medication, rub the area in a circular motion. Monitor the patient's condition.

12. To disperse the medication through the tissue, rub the area in a circular motion with your gloved hand.
13. Properly store any unused medication.
14. Monitor the patient's condition, and document the medication given, route, administration time, and response of the patient (**Step 5**).

Intramuscular Medication Administration

Intramuscular (IM) injections are given by penetrating a needle through the dermis and subcutaneous tissue and into the muscle layer (**Figure 8-52** ▶). This technique allows administration of a larger volume of medication (up to 5 ml) than the subcutaneous route. Because there is also the potential for damage to nerves due to the depth of the injection, it is important to choose the appropriate site. Common anatomical sites for IM injections for adults and children include the following:

- **Vastus lateralis muscle**—the large muscle on the lateral side of the thigh.
- **Rectus femoris muscle**—the large muscle on the anterior side of the thigh.
- **Gluteal area**—the buttocks, specifically the upper lateral aspect of either side.
- **Deltoid muscle**—the muscle of the upper arm that covers the prominence of the shoulder. The site for injection is approximately 4 to 5 cm below the acromion process on the lateral side (**Figure 8-53** ▶).

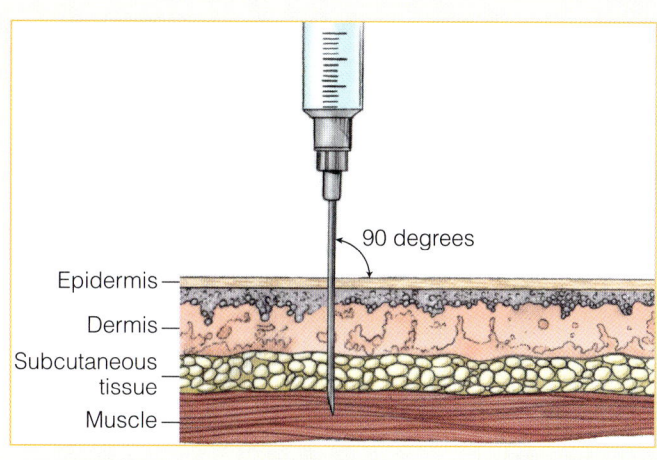

Figure 8-52 An intramuscular injection is below the dermis and subcutaneous layer and into the muscle.

4. Follow standing orders, or contact direct medical control for permission.
5. Check the medication to ensure that it is the correct one, that it is not cloudy or discoloured, and that the expiry date has not passed, and determine the appropriate amount and concentration for the correct dose (**Step 1**).
6. Advise the patient of potential discomfort while explaining the procedure.
7. Assemble and check equipment needed: alcohol preps and a 3- to 5-ml syringe with a 21- or 22-gauge, 2.5- or 5-cm needle. Draw up the correct dose of medication (**Step 2**).
8. Cleanse the area for administration (usually the upper arm or the hip) using aseptic technique (**Step 3**).
9. *Stretch the skin* over the cleansed area, advise the patient of a stick, and insert the needle at a *90° angle.*
10. Pull back on the plunger to aspirate for blood. The presence of blood in the syringe indicates you may have entered a blood vessel. In such a case, remove the needle, and hold pressure over the site. Discard the syringe and needle in the sharps container. Prepare a new syringe and needle, and select another site.
11. If there is no blood in the syringe, inject the medication and remove the needle. Immediately dispose of the needle and syringe in the sharps container (**Step 4**).
12. To disperse the medication through the tissue, rub the area in a circular motion with your gloved hand (**Step 5**).
13. Store any unused medication properly.
14. Monitor the patient's condition, and document the medication given, route, administration time, and response of the patient.

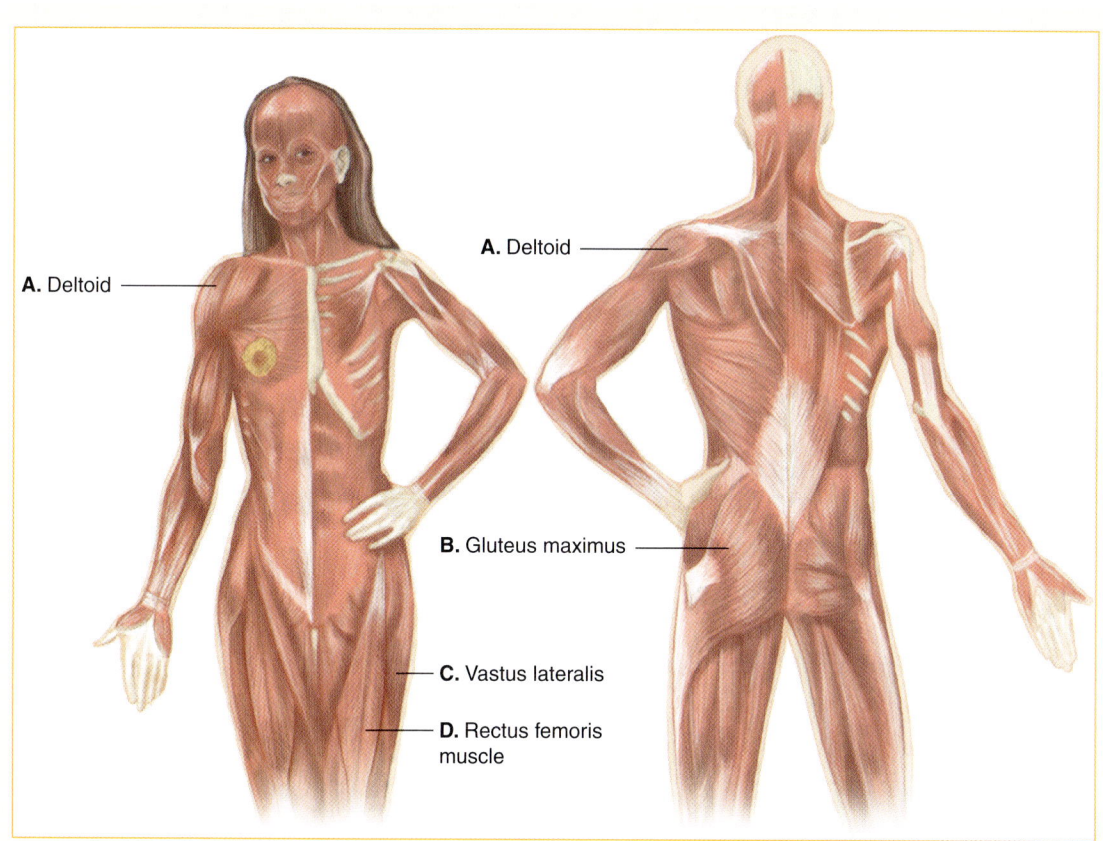

Figure 8-53 Common sites for intramuscular injections. **A.** Deltoid muscle. **B.** Gluteal area. **C.** Vastus lateralis muscle. **D.** Rectus femoris muscle.

Follow the steps in (**Skill Drill 8-9** ▸) to administer a medication via the intramuscular route:

1. Take routine precautions.
2. Determine the need for the medication based on patient presentation.
3. Obtain a focused history and physical examination, including any drug allergies and vital signs.

IV Bolus Medication Administration

The IV route places the drug directly into the circulatory system. It is the fastest route of medication administration because it bypasses most barriers to drug absorption. As a result, *there is no room for error with IV administration.* (See "Potential Complications of IV

Skill Drill 8-9: Administering Medication via the Intramuscular Route

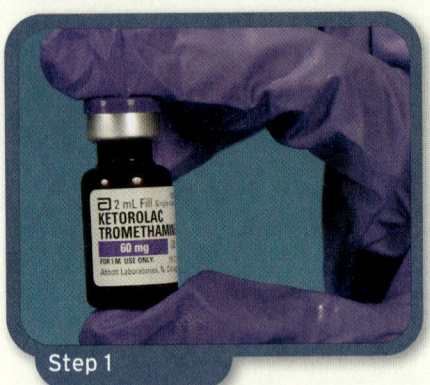

Step 1

Check the medication to ensure that it is the correct one, that it is not discoloured, and that its expiry date has not passed.

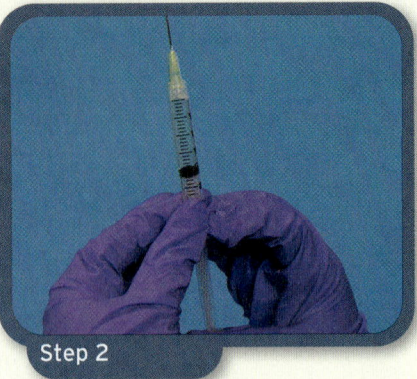

Step 2

Assemble and check the equipment. Draw up the correct dose of medication.

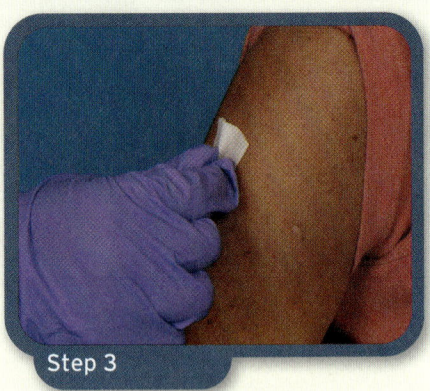

Step 3

Using aseptic technique, cleanse the injection area.

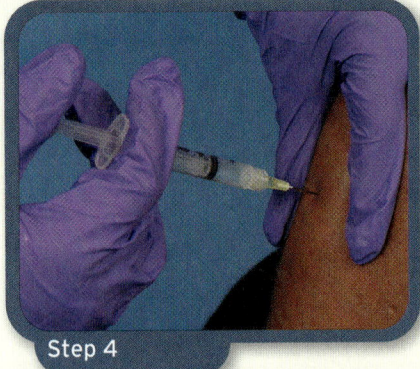

Step 4

Stretch the skin over the area, and insert the needle at a 90° angle. Pull back on the plunger to aspirate for blood. If there is no blood, inject the medication and remove the needle. Immediately dispose of the needle and syringe in the sharps container.

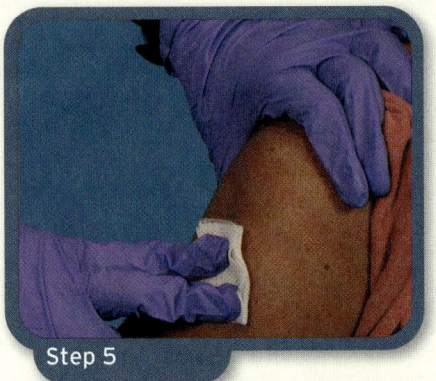

Step 5

To disperse the medication, rub the area in a circular motion. Monitor the patient's condition.

At the Scene

Effective absorption of medications administered by the subcutaneous and intramuscular routes requires adequate peripheral perfusion. This is clearly not the case in patients in profound shock or cardiac arrest. Therefore, subcutaneous and intramuscular injections should not be given to patients with inadequate perfusion.

Therapy" earlier in this chapter for details on what can go wrong.) Drugs are administered by direct injection with a needle and syringe into an established peripheral IV line. Many services now use needleless systems to provide protection against needlesticks.

When using a needleless system, the syringe simply screws into the injection port of the administration set (IV tubing).

A bolus is a single dose, usually given by the IV route. When given in one mass, it may consist of a small or large quantity of a drug and can be given rapidly or slowly, depending on the drug. Some medications, such as lidocaine and amiodarone, require an initial bolus and then may require a continuous IV infusion to maintain a therapeutic level of the drug.

Follow the steps in **Skill Drill 8-10 ▶** when administering a medication via the IV bolus route:

1. Take routine precautions.
2. Determine the need for the medication based on patient presentation.
3. Obtain a focused history and physical examination, including any drug allergies and vital signs.

4. Follow standing orders, or contact direct medical control for permission.

5. Check the medication to ensure that it is the correct one, that it is not cloudy or discoloured, and that the expiry date has not passed, and determine the appropriate amount and concentration for the correct dose.

6. Explain the procedure to the patient and the need for the medication.

7. Assemble needed equipment, and draw up medication. Expel any air in the syringe. Draw up 20 ml of normal saline to use as a flush for the medication.

8. Cleanse the injection port with alcohol, or remove the protective cap if using the needleless system (**Step 1**).

9. Insert the needle into the port, and pinch off the IV tubing proximal to the administration port. Failure to shut off the line will result in the medication taking the pathway of least resistance and flowing into the bag instead of into the patient.

10. Administer the correct dose of the medication at the appropriate rate. Some medications must be administered very quickly, while others must be pushed slowly to prevent adverse effects (**Step 2**).

11. Place the needle and syringe into the sharps container.

Skill Drill 8-10: Administering Medication via the Intravenous Bolus Route

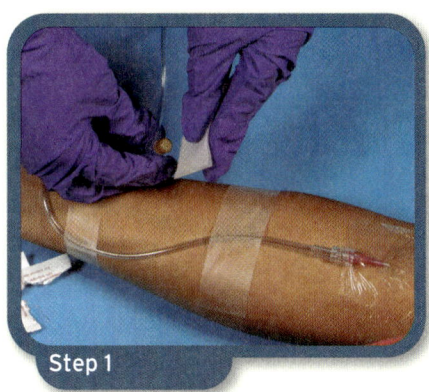

Step 1

Assemble and check the equipment. Cleanse the injection port, or remove the protective cap if using the needleless system.

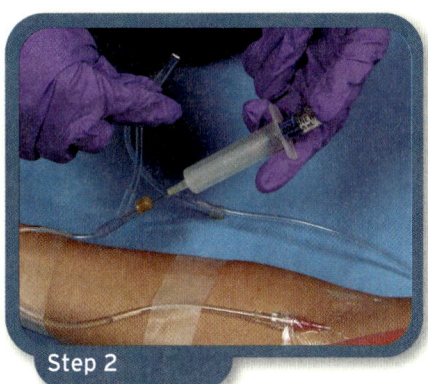

Step 2

Insert the needle into the port, and pinch off the IV tubing proximal to the administration port. Administer the correct dose at the appropriate rate.

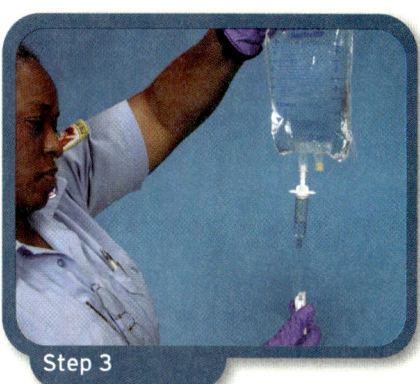

Step 3

Unclamp the IV line to flush the medication into the vein, allowing it to run briefly wide open, or flush with a 20-ml bolus of normal saline. Readjust the IV flow rate to the original setting, and monitor the patient's condition.

You are the Paramedic Part 4

After administering 50 ml of 50% dextrose, the patient's level of consciousness rapidly improves. She pushes the bag and mask away from her face but will tolerate a nonrebreathing mask. She is obviously confused about what happened, but consents to EMS transport to the hospital. You apprise her of the events that transpired and reassess her. Your partner retrieves the stretcher from the ambulance.

Reassessment	Recording Time: 12 Minutes
Level of consciousness	A (Alert to person, place, and day)
Airway and breathing	Airway remains patent; respirations, 18 breaths/min with adequate depth
Blood pressure	112/70 mm Hg
Pulse	88 beats/min, strong and regular
Sao$_2$	99% (with 100% oxygen)
Blood glucose	4 mmol/l

10. Does this patient require an additional dose of 50% dextrose?

11. Does this patient require an IV bolus of normal saline?

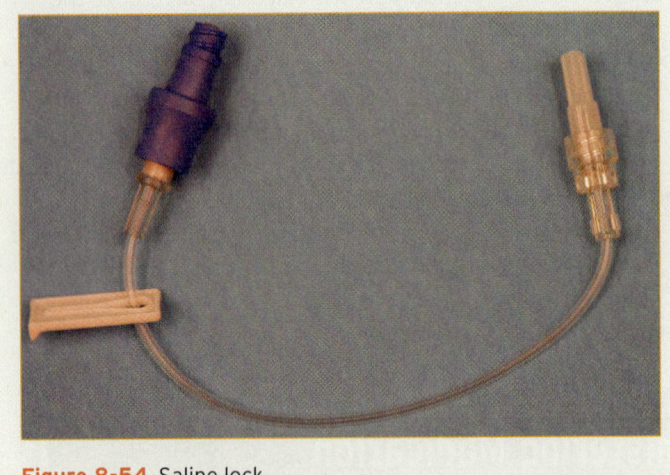

Figure 8-54 Saline lock.

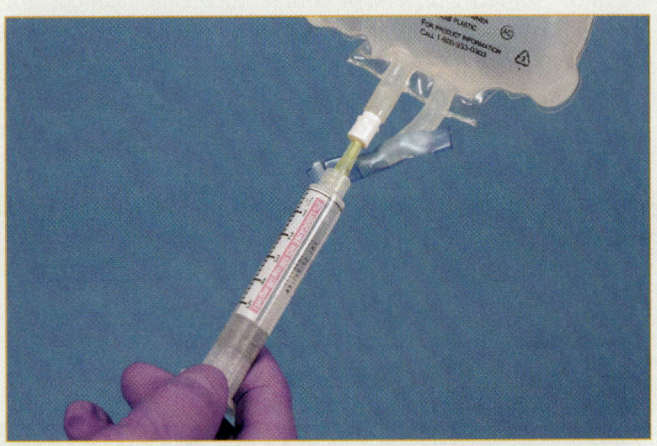

Figure 8-55 Adding medication to an IV bag.

12. Unclamp the IV line to flush the medication into the vein. Allow it to run briefly wide open, or flush with a 20-ml bolus of normal saline.
13. Readjust the IV flow rate to the original setting (Step 3).
14. Properly store and label any unused medication.
15. Monitor the patient's condition, and document the medication given, route, time of administration, and response of the patient.

As discussed earlier in this chapter, saline locks are used for patients who are not in need of IV fluid boluses but may need medication therapy. Follow these steps to administer a medication through a saline lock (Figure 8-54 ▲):

1. Take routine precautions.
2. Determine the need for the medication based on patient presentation.
3. Obtain a focused history and physical examination, including any drug allergies and vital signs.
4. Follow standing orders, or contact direct medical control for permission.
5. Check the medication to ensure that it is the correct one, that it is not cloudy or discoloured, and that the expiry date has not passed, and determine the appropriate amount and concentration for the correct dose.
6. Explain the procedure to the patient and the need for the medication.
7. Assemble needed equipment, and draw up the medication. Draw up 20 ml of normal saline to use as a flush for the medication.
8. Cleanse the injection port with alcohol, or remove the protective cap if using the needleless system.
9. Insert the needle into the port while holding it carefully, or screw the syringe onto the port.
10. Pull back slightly on the syringe plunger, and observe for blood return. If blood appears, slowly inject the medication, watching for infiltration. If resistance is felt, or if the patient complains of any discomfort, discontinue

administration immediately. A new site will need to be established.
11. Place the needle and syringe into the sharps container.
12. Clean the port, and insert the needle with the syringe containing the flush.
13. Flush the saline lock, and place the needle in the sharps container.
14. Store any unused medication properly.
15. Monitor the patient's condition, and document the medication given, route, time of administration, and response of the patient.

Adding Medication to an IV Bag

Certain medications are added to the IV solution itself to be administered as a maintenance infusion—for example, dopamine, lidocaine, and epinephrine. All of these medications require careful titration to achieve the desired effect.

The steps for adding medication to an IV bag are as follows:

1. Check the fluid in the IV bag for clarity or discolouration, and ensure that the expiry date has not passed.
2. Check the *drug name* on the ampule, vial, or prefilled syringe. Check the *concentration of the drug* it contains (for example, µg/ml or mg/ml).
3. *Compute the volume* of the drug to be added to the IV bag. Draw up that amount in a syringe (if a prefilled syringe is used, note the proportion of the volume of the syringe required).
4. Cleanse the medication injection port on the IV bag with an alcohol swab.
5. Inject the desired volume of medication into the IV bag by puncturing the rubber stopper on the medication injection port (Figure 8-55 ▲).
6. Withdraw the needle, and dispose of the needle and syringe in the sharps container. Agitate the IV bag gently to ensure that the added drug is well mixed in the solution.
7. *Label the IV bag* with the name of the medication added, the amount added, the concentration of medication in the

At the Scene

Medications that are used for maintenance infusions (for example, lidocaine and dopamine) are commonly premixed and prepackaged, which eliminates the need to calculate and draw up the appropriate amount of medication to add to the bag. However, you must still be aware of the concentration (for example, µg/ml or mg/ml) of drug in the premixed solution and the appropriate maintenance infusion rate.

IV bag (for example, µg/ml or mg/ml), the date and time, and your name.

8. Attach the IV administration set, and prepare the IV bag as discussed earlier in this chapter.

Electromechanical Infusion Pumps

When administering a medication maintenance infusion, you should use an electromechanical infusion pump, if available. The infusion pump can also be used to deliver IV fluid maintenance infusions in children and elderly patients to minimize the risk of a "runaway IV" and subsequent circulatory overload.

Most infusion pumps allow you to set the parameters of medication administration—drug concentration and volume to be infused—and will then calculate the appropriate infusion rate. This feature allows for precise medication dosing, minimizing the risk of delivering too little or too much medication.

Electromechanical infusion pumps deliver fluids or medications via positive pressure. Although medications delivered in this manner can result in infiltration of a vein, most infusion pumps are equipped with an alarm that indicates a change in the flow pressure. Other common safety features include alarms that alert you to the presence of occlusion (eg, air in the tubing) or depletion of the medication. Some infusion pumps are designed to accommodate the IV tubing to regulate the flow of IV fluids or medications **Figure 8-56 ▼**, whereas others are designed to accommodate a needleless syringe **Figure 8-57 ▶**.

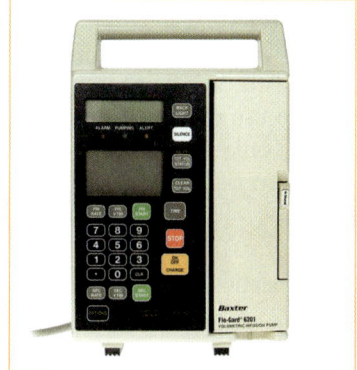

Figure 8-56 Infusion pump that accommodates IV tubing.

IO Medication Administration

The IO route is used for critically ill or injured children and adults when IV access is difficult or impossible to obtain. Any fluid or medication that may be given through an IV line—bolus or maintenance infusion—can be given by the IO route. Shock, status epilepticus, and cardiac arrest are but a few of the reasons for establishing IO access. Unlike with an IV line, fluid does not flow well into the bone because of resistance; therefore, it is necessary to use a large syringe to infuse the fluid. A pressure infuser device—a sleeve placed around the IV bag and inflated to force fluid from the IV bag—should be used when infusing fluids in adults.

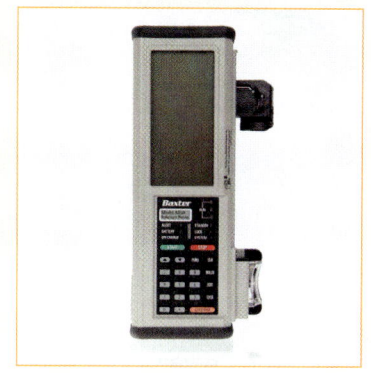

Figure 8-57 Syringe-type infusion pump.

Complications of using the IO route are similar to those of the IV route. Along with the complications discussed earlier in this chapter, there is also the potential for compartment syndrome if fluid leaks outside the bone and into the osteofascial compartment.

Follow the steps in **Skill Drill 8-11 ▶** to administer a medication via the IO route:

1. Take routine precautions.
2. Determine the need for the medication based on patient presentation.
3. Obtain a focused history and physical examination, including any drug allergies and vital signs.
4. Follow standing orders, or contact direct medical control for permission.
5. Check the medication to ensure that it is the correct one, that it is not cloudy or discoloured, and that the expiry date has not passed, and determine the appropriate amount and concentration for the correct dose.
6. Explain the procedure to the patient and/or parent and the need for the medication.
7. Assemble needed equipment, and draw up the medication. Also draw up 20 ml of normal saline for a flush **Step 1**.
8. Cleanse the injection port of the extension tubing with alcohol, or remove the protective cap if using the needleless system **Step 2**.
9. Insert the needle into the port, and clamp off the IV tubing proximal to the administration port. This is usually managed with a three-way stopcock. Failure to shut off the line will result in the medication taking the pathway of least resistance and flowing into the bag instead of into the patient.
10. Administer the correct dose of the medication at the proper push rate. Some medications must be administered very quickly, while others must be pushed slowly to prevent adverse effects **Step 3**.
11. Place the needle and syringe into the sharps container.

Skill Drill 8-11: Administering Medication via the IO Route

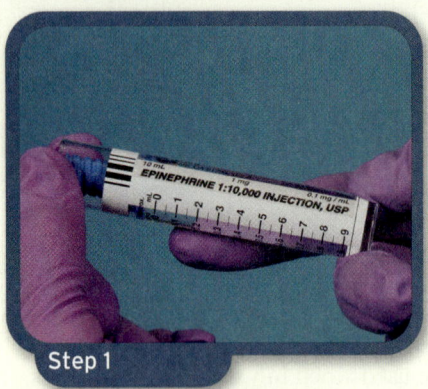

Step 1

Check the medication to ensure that it is the correct one, that it is not discoloured, and that the expiry date has not passed.

Assemble the equipment, and draw up the medication. Draw up 20 ml of normal saline for a flush.

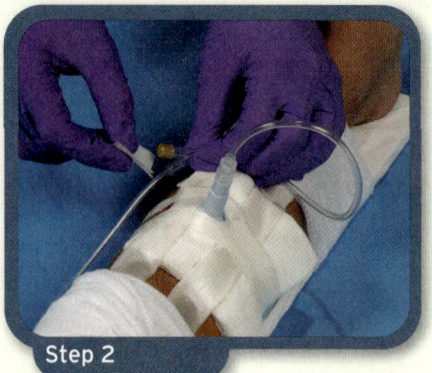

Step 2

Cleanse the injection port, or remove the protective cap if using the needleless system.

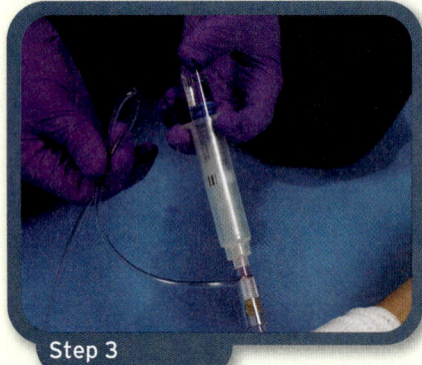

Step 3

Insert the needle into the port, and pinch off the IV tubing proximal to the administration port. Administer the correct dose at the proper push rate.

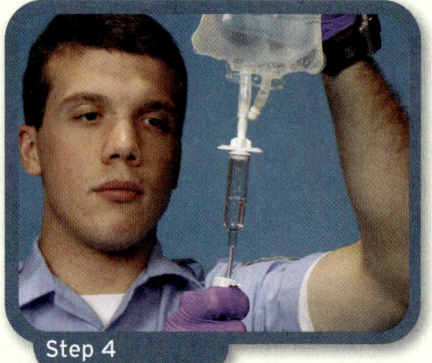

Step 4

Unclamp the IV line to flush the medication into the vein, allowing it to run briefly wide open, or flush with a 20-ml bolus of normal saline.

Readjust the IV flow rate to the original setting, and monitor the patient's condition.

12. Unclamp the IV line to flush the medication into the vein. Flush with at least a 20-ml bolus of normal saline.

13. Readjust the IV flow rate to the original setting.

14. Store any unused medication properly.

15. Monitor the patient's condition, and document the medication given, route, time of administration, and response of the patient (**Step 4**).

Percutaneous Medication Administration

With percutaneous routes of administration, medications are applied to and absorbed through the skin and mucous membranes. Because percutaneously administered medications

bypass the gastrointestinal tract, their absorption is more predictable. Percutaneous routes of medication administration include the transdermal, sublingual, buccal, ocular, aural, and nasal routes.

Transdermal Medication Administration

Transdermal medications are applied topically—that is, on the surface of the body. Ordinarily, intact skin is an effective barrier to absorption of drugs. However, some drugs have been specially prepared to cross that barrier at a very slow steady rate, so the transdermal route is useful for the sustained release of certain medications.

Nitroglycerin, estrogen, nicotine, and analgesic patches, for example, are applied to the skin and release medications over a specified period. Creams, lotions, and pastes (eg, nitroglycerin paste, corticosteroid cream) are also transdermally administered medications.

Factors that can increase the speed of transdermal absorption include administration of too much of the medication (ie, inadvertent or intentional overdose) and thin or nonintact skin. Decreased speed of transdermal absorption can be caused by factors such as thick skin, scar tissue in the area to which the medication is applied, and peripheral vascular disease.

Other than assisting a patient with his or her transdermal medication, there is rarely a need to use this route of administration in the prehospital setting. Should a situation arise that requires you to administer a transdermal medication patch or paste, follow these steps:

1. Take routine precautions.

2. Determine the need for the medication based on patient presentation.

3. Obtain a focused history and physical examination, including any drug allergies and vital signs.

4. Follow standing orders, or contact direct medical control for permission.

5. Check the medication patch or cream to ensure that it is the correct one and that the expiry date has not passed, and determine the appropriate amount for the correct dose.

6. Explain the procedure to the patient and the need for the medication.

7. Clean and dry the area of the skin where the medication will be applied.

8. Apply the medication to the area in accordance with the manufacturer's specifications.

9. Monitor the patient's condition, and document the medication given, route, time of administration, and response of the patient.

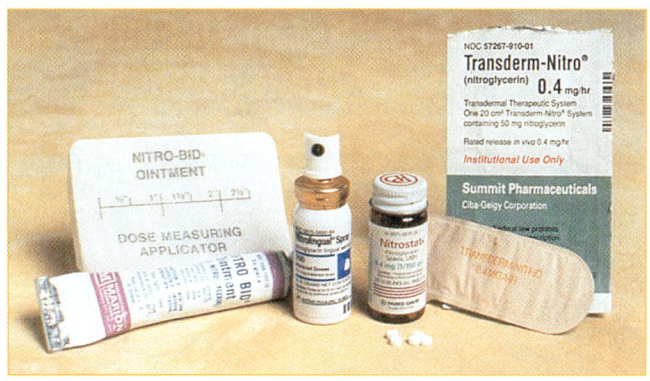

Figure 8-58 Nitroglycerin is often given sublingually as a spray or a tablet. It is also available as a transdermal patch or paste and can be administered as an IV drip as well.

At the Scene

During assessment of your patient, look for transdermal medication patches, especially narcotic and nitroglycerin patches, which can result in hypotension. If the patient is already in a hemodynamically unstable condition, narcotics and nitroglycerin may complicate the clinical picture.

Sublingual Medication Administration

The sublingual (under the tongue) region is highly vascular, so medications given via the sublingual route are rapidly absorbed. Sublingually administered medications, relative to enterally administered medications, get into the circulation much faster. Nitroglycerin—spray or tablet—is a drug that is most commonly administered via the sublingual route **Figure 8-58 ▶** .

Drugs may also be *injected* into the network of veins (venous plexus) under the tongue (strictly speaking, that is another form of intravenous injection). This technique is especially useful for giving narcotic antagonists to patients who have overdosed on heroin because finding a suitable vein in such patients may be nearly impossible.

To administer a sublingual medication, follow these steps **Skill Drill 8-12 ▶** .

1. Take routine precautions.

2. Determine the need for the medication based on patient presentation.

3. Obtain a focused history and physical examination, including any drug allergies and vital signs.

4. Follow standing orders, or contact direct medical control for permission.

5. Check the medication to ensure that it is the correct one and that its expiry date has not passed, and determine the appropriate amount for the correct dose.

6. Ask the patient to rinse his or her mouth with a little water if the mucous membranes are dry **Step 1** .

7. Explain the procedure, and ask the patient to lift his or her tongue. Place the tablet or spray the dose under the tongue, or ask the patient to do so.

8. Advise the patient not to chew or swallow the tablet, but to let it dissolve slowly.

9. Monitor the patient's condition, and document the medication given, route, administration time, and response of the patient **Step 2** .

Buccal Medication Administration

The buccal region, which is also highly vascular, lies in between the cheek and gums. Most medications administered via the buccal route are in the form of tablets. It is becoming a popular route to consider in prehospital medicine and is often seen in the special needs pediatric setting.

To administer a medication via the buccal route, follow these steps:

1. Take routine precautions.

2. Determine the need for the medication based on patient presentation.

3. Obtain a focused history and physical examination, including any drug allergies and vital signs.

4. Follow standing orders, or contact direct medical control for permission.

5. Check the medication to ensure that it is the correct one and that its expiry date has not passed, and determine the appropriate amount for the correct dose.

6. Explain the procedure to the patient and the need for the medication.

7. Place the medication in between the patient's cheek and gum, or ask the patient to do so.

8. Advise the patient not to chew or swallow the tablet, but to let it dissolve slowly.

9. Monitor the patient's condition, and document the medication given, route, administration time, and response of the patient.

Skill Drill 8-12: Administering Medication via the Sublingual Route

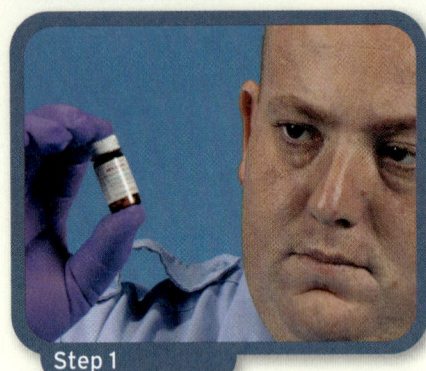

Step 1

Check the medication for drug type and its expiry date, and determine the appropriate amount for the correct dose.

Have the patient rinse his or her mouth with a little water if the mucous membranes are dry.

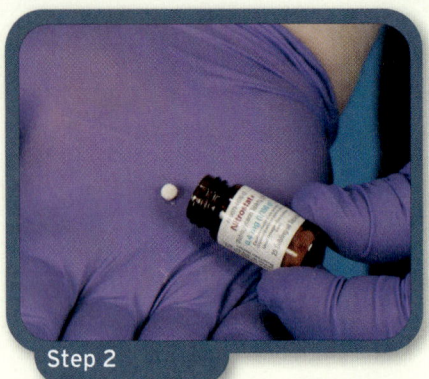

Step 2

Explain the procedure to the patient, and ask the patient to lift his or her tongue. Place the tablet or spray the dose underneath the tongue, or have the patient do so.

Advise the patient not to chew or swallow the tablet, but to let it dissolve slowly.

Monitor the patient, and document the medication given, the route, administration time, and the response of the patient.

At the Scene

Wear gloves when administering nitroglycerin. Otherwise, the medication can be absorbed through your skin.

Ocular Medication Administration

Drops or ointments are commonly administered via the ocular route. Ocular medications are typically administered for pain relief, allergies, drying of the eyes, or infections. Other than assisting a patient with his or her ocular medication or irrigating a patient's eyes following a toxic exposure, none of the medications used in the prehospital setting are administered via the ocular route.

If a patient asks you to assist him or her with ocular medication administration, follow these steps:

1. Take routine precautions.
2. Confirm that the medication is prescribed to the patient.
3. Place the patient in a supine position, or have the patient place his or her head back and look up.
4. *Without touching the eyeball,* expose the conjunctiva by gently pulling down on the lower eyelid.
5. Administer the required amount of medication on the conjunctival sac by using an eye dropper. Do not apply the medication directly on the eyeball.
6. Advise the patient to close his or her eyes for 1 to 2 minutes.
7. Document the medication name, dose, and administration time.

Aural Medication Administration

Certain medications—mainly antibiotics, analgesics, and earwax removal preparations—are administered via the mucous membranes of the aural (ear) canal. As with ocular medications, the aural route is rarely, if ever, used in the prehospital setting.

If you are asked by the patient to assist in administering his or her aural medication, follow these steps:

1. Take routine precautions.
2. Confirm that the medication is prescribed to the patient.
3. Place the patient on his or her side with the affected ear facing up.
4. Expose the ear canal by pulling the ear up and back (adults) or down and back (infants and children).
5. Administer the medication in the appropriate dose with a medicine dropper.
6. Document the medication name, dose, and administration time.

Intranasal Medication Administration

Intranasal (within the nose) medications include nasal spray for congestion or solutions to moisten the nasal mucosa. In recent years, this route of medication administration has become increasingly more popular in the prehospital setting. Intranasally administered medications are rapidly absorbed, providing a more rapid onset of action than IM injections. Administration of emergency medications via the intranasal route is performed with a mucosal atomizer device (MAD) **Figure 8-59 ▶**. The MAD attaches to a syringe and allows you to spray (atomize) select medications into the nasal mucosa.

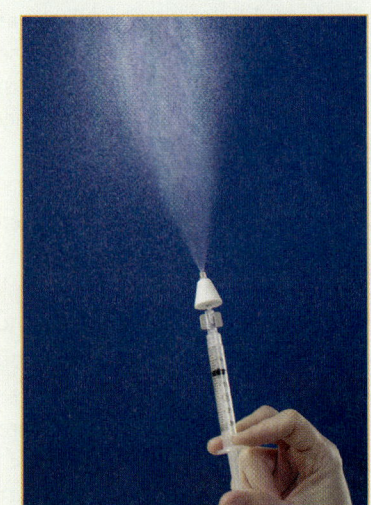

Figure 8-59 Mucosal atomizer device (MAD).

Owing to the molecular structure of drugs, only a few emergency medications can be given intranasally, including naloxone and midazolam. Follow local protocol, or consult with direct medical control about the appropriate doses of these medications and any other medications that may be administered intranasally.

To administer a drug via the intranasal route, follow these steps:

1. Take routine precautions and use appropriate PPE.
2. Determine the need for the medication based on patient presentation.
3. Obtain a focused history and physical examination, including any drug allergies and vital signs.
4. Follow standing orders, or contact direct medical control for permission.
5. Check the medication to ensure that it is the correct one, that it is not cloudy or discoloured, and that the expiry date has not passed.
6. Draw up the appropriate dose of medication in the syringe.
7. Attach the mucosal atomizer device to the syringe.
8. Explain the procedure to the patient (or to a relative if the patient is unconscious) and the need for the medication.
9. Spray *half* of the medication dose into each nostril.
10. Dispose of the atomizer device and syringe in the appropriate container.
11. Monitor the patient's condition, and document the medication given, route, time of administration, and response of the patient.

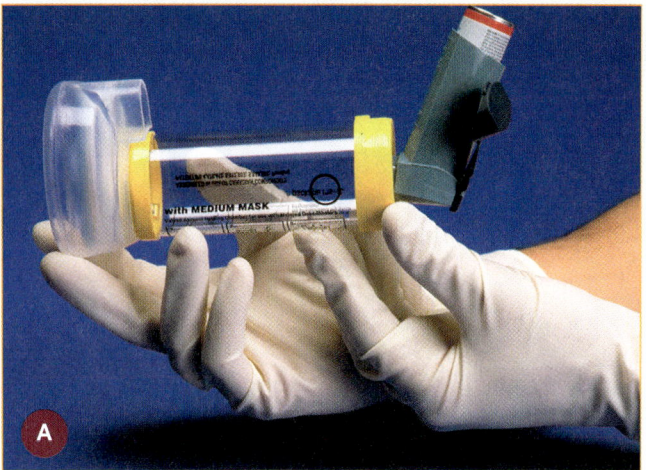

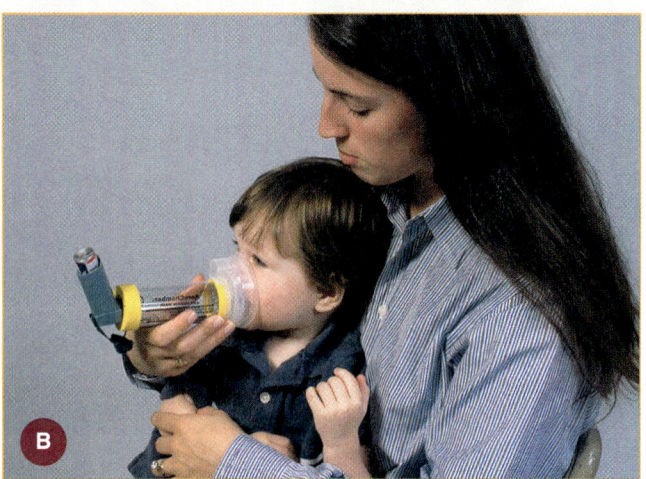

Figure 8-61 A. In children, an MDI and spacer can be used with or without a mask. **B.** Children as young as 6 months can use a mask and spacer device.

Medications Administered by the Inhalation Route

Nebulizer and Metered-Dose Inhaler

Many medications used in the treatment of respiratory emergencies are administered via the inhalation route. The most common inhaled medication is oxygen. Beta$_2$ agonist bronchodilators (eg, salbutamol) are often administered in the prehospital setting for patients experiencing respiratory distress caused by certain obstructive airway diseases, such as asthma, bronchitis, and emphysema. Other medications, such as ipratropium bromide—an anticholinergic bronchodilator—are also administered via the

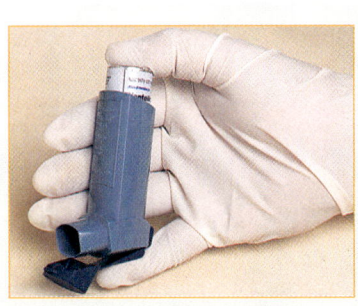

Figure 8-60 Some medications are inhaled into the lungs with an MDI so that they can be absorbed quickly into the bloodstream.

inhalation route. Check your drug reference guide or the package insert for the indications, contraindications, and precautions before giving any of these medications.

A patient with a history of respiratory problems will usually have a metered-dose inhaler (MDI) to use on a regular basis or as needed **Figure 8-60 ◀**. Medications administered by the MDI can be delivered through a mouthpiece held by the patient or by a mask—with or without a spacer device—for young children and patients who are unable to hold the mouthpiece **Figure 8-61 ▲**. The paramedic should check the MDI device to determine if it needs to be shaken before drug delivery to ensure that the device delivers the appropriate drug dose.

For more severe problems, liquid bronchodilators may be aerosolized in a nebulizer for inhalation. Small-volume nebulizers (also called updraft or hand-held nebulizers) are the most commonly used method of administration of inhaled medications in the prehospital setting **Figure 8-62 ▶**. Oxygen or a compressed air source is connected to the nebulizer to produce the aerosolized mist.

Follow the steps in **Skill Drill 8-13 ▶** to administer a medication via a small-volume nebulizer:

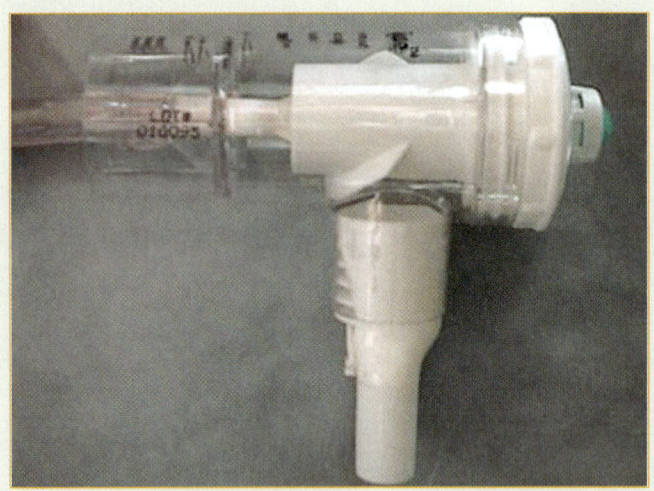

Figure 8-62 A small-volume nebulizer is used to deliver medications via aerosolized mist.

to breathe. Have the patient breathe as deeply as possible and hold his or her breath for 3 to 5 seconds before exhaling. Continue to coach the patient as needed.

10. Monitor the patient's condition, and document the medication given, route, time of administration, and response of the patient to the medication (Step 4).

11. Cardiac monitoring is essential when administering a beta agonist. If cardiac dysrhythmias are noted, stop the administration of the medication, administer high-flow oxygen, and contact direct medical control.

Some patients with respiratory emergencies may be breathing inadequately (ie, inadequate tidal volume, fast or slow respiratory rate) and will not be able to effectively inhale beta-agonist medications into the lungs via a nebulizer or an MDI. In this case, assist with bag-valve-mask ventilation and attach a small-volume nebulizer to the ventilation device. Place a short piece of corrugated tubing—separated by a T piece to connect the nebulizer to—between the bag and mask or endotracheal tube if the patient is intubated.

1. Take routine precautions.

2. Determine the need for an inhaled bronchodilator based on patient presentation.

3. Obtain a focused history and physical examination, including any drug allergies and vital signs.

4. Follow standing orders, or contact direct medical control for permission.

5. Check the medication and its expiry date. Make sure that you have the right medication and that it is not cloudy or discoloured (Step 1).

6. If the medication is in a premixed package, add it to the bowl of the nebulizer. If it is not premixed, add the medication to the bowl and mix it with the specified amount of normal saline, usually 3 ml (Step 2).

7. Connect the T piece with the mouthpiece to the top of the bowl, or the mask to the bowl, and connect it to the oxygen tubing.

8. Set the flowmeter at 6 l/min to produce a steady mist (Step 3).

9. With the MDI or hand-held nebulizer in position, instruct the patient on the proper way

Skill Drill 8-13: Administering a Medication via a Small-Volume Nebulizer

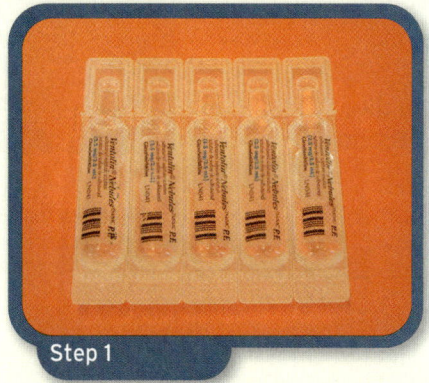

Step 1

Check the medication and the expiry date.

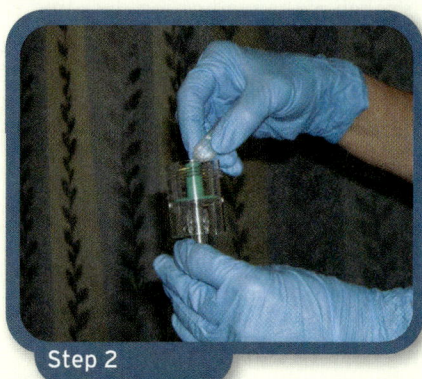

Step 2

Add premixed medication to the bowl of the nebulizer.

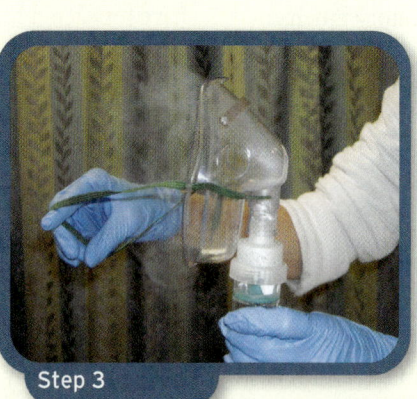

Step 3

Connect the T piece with the mouthpiece to the top of the bowl, connect it to the oxygen tubing, and set the flowmeter at 6 l/min.

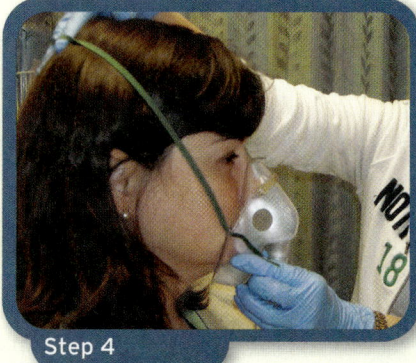

Step 4

Instruct the patient to breathe as deeply as possible and hold his or her breath for 3 to 5 seconds before exhaling. Monitor the patient for effects.

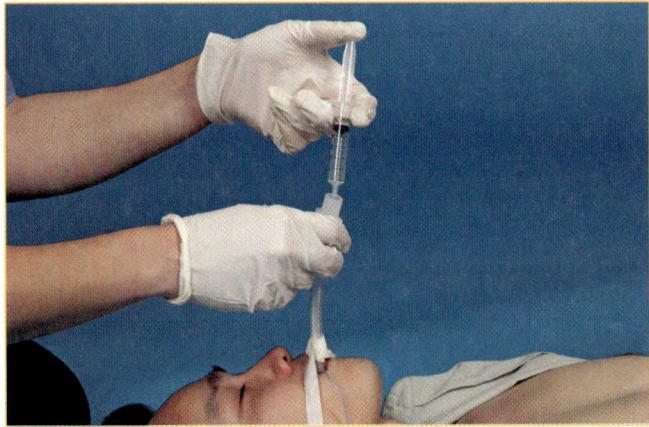

Figure 8-63 Administering medication via the ET tube.

Endotracheal Medication Administration

The 2005 International Liaison Committee on Resuscitation guidelines no longer advocate administration of drugs by the endotracheal route. If IV access is not possible, the guidelines now recommend establishing access using the IO route. New devices make this easy in resuscitation settings. If IV or IO access is unavailable, certain resuscitative medications can be administered down the endotracheal (ET) tube, as a last resort. For the medication to be adequately dispersed throughout the tracheobronchial tree, you must administer 2 to 2.5 times the standard IV dose. *Only* four medications should be given down the ET tube; they can easily be remembered by the mnemonic LEAN: Lidocaine, Epinephrine, Atropine, Naloxone.

To administer medications via the ET tube, follow these steps:

1. Draw up the appropriate dose of the medication to be administered as your partner ventilates the patient. Dilute the appropriate dose of the medication in 10 ml of normal saline.
2. Disconnect the bag-valve-mask device from the ET tube, and rapidly instill the medication down the ET tube **Figure 8-63** .
3. Immediately reconnect the bag-valve-mask device to the ET tube, and ventilate the patient briskly to facilitate passage of the drug down the trachea and into the lungs.

Rates of Medication Absorption

The speed at which a drug is absorbed is directly related to the route by which it is given. Obviously, drugs injected directly into the bloodstream (ie, as IV or IO injections) gain access to the central circulation the fastest. Oral medications take longer to achieve their therapeutic effects, because they must be absorbed through the gastrointestinal tract first. **Table 8-6** summarizes the various medication routes and their rates of absorption.

Table 8-6	Medication Routes and Rates of Absorption
Route of Administration	**Onset of Action***
Intraosseous	30–60 s
Intravenous	30–60 s
Endotracheal	2–3 min†
Inhalation	2–3 min
Sublingual	3–5 min
Intramuscular injection	10–20 min
Subcutaneous injection	15–30 min
Rectal	5–30 min
Oral	30–90 min
Topical	Minutes to hours

*In a healthy person with adequate perfusion.

†Recent data suggest that ET drug administration may be less effective than previously thought, especially in poor perfusion states.

You are the Paramedic Summary

1. Is this a medical patient or a trauma patient?

You have not obtained enough information to be able to establish whether this is a medical patient or a trauma patient. Your index of suspicion should increase for the potential for trauma in this case, especially because no one witnessed the events preceding the patient's condition. Further assessment of the patient and her surroundings is required. If there is *any* potential for trauma, then treat her accordingly (ie, spinal motion restriction precautions). Paramedics should not be too hasty to "label" a patient as being a medical or trauma patient; this requires a careful assessment. Some patients have *both* medical and traumatic elements to their condition.

2. What are your initial priorities of care?

Immediate care for this patient involves carefully moving her to the floor (with spinal precautions if trauma is suspected) and performing an initial assessment. This is the most important aspect of initial patient care. You *must* be able to *rapidly identify and correct* immediate threats to life. This patient is unresponsive; clearly, her condition requires immediate treatment.

3. What is the most appropriate initial airway management for this patient?

The patient is unconscious and unresponsive, so you must immediately ensure that her airway is open and clear of secretions. Furthermore, her respirations are rapid and shallow (reduced tidal volume). Initial airway management should include inserting an oral or nasal airway adjunct and assisting ventilation with bag-valve-mask ventilation and 100% oxygen. Rapid, shallow respirations will result in decreased minute volume. If this is not *immediately* treated, significant hypoxia and acidosis will develop.

4. Does this patient require immediate medication therapy?

Other than 100% oxygen, which you have already administered, further assessment is required before determining whether medication therapy is indicated. Although the patient's history of diabetes and clinical presentation are highly suggestive of hypoglycemia, they are not conclusive. In some diabetic patients, it may be difficult to differentiate between hypoglycemia and hyperglycemia, especially if the patient is unconscious.

5. Given the patient's history, what additional assessment should you perform?

Obviously, you should test the blood glucose level of any unconscious patient—with or without a history of diabetes. This is especially true if you observe signs suggesting hypoglycemia. Adequate glucose to the brain is just as critical as oxygen; without it, permanent brain damage or death can occur. Because hypoglycemia is an easily correctable condition, rapid blood glucose testing should be performed and, if needed, treated immediately.

6. When starting an IV for this patient, what solution should you use?

An isotonic crystalloid (most often normal saline) is the fluid of choice for the vast majority of patients that you will treat in the prehospital setting. A D_5W solution (or any glucose-containing solution) should not be used in patients with diabetes. D_5W is a more appropriate choice when mixing a medication to deliver in a maintenance infusion. Patients with diabetic ketoacidosis, for example, are typically dehydrated from the osmotic diuresis caused by excess blood glucose levels. Isotonic crystalloids, because they remain in the vascular space for longer periods, are needed for rehydration and maintenance of adequate perfusion.

7. What does the "%" in 50% dextrose mean?

In terms of medication concentration, *percent* refers to the number of grams present in 100 ml (1 dl) of volume. Therefore, 50% dextrose contains a concentration of 50 g (50,000 mg) of dextrose in 100 ml of volume. Because 50% dextrose is dispensed in a 50 ml volume, there are 25 g of medication in the container.

8. What is the concentration of $D_{50}W$ that you have on hand?

The concentration on hand represents the total amount of weight (μg, mg, or g) present in 1 ml. $D_{50}W$ represents 50 g of dextrose in 100 ml of volume. However, because $D_{50}W$ is contained in only 50 ml, you have only 25 g of dextrose in one pre-filled syringe. To determine the concentration on hand, divide the total number of milligrams (25 g = 25,000 mg) by the total volume (50 ml): 25,000 mg ÷ 50 ml = 500 mg/ml.

9. What are the "six rights" of medication administration?

Before administering any medication, you must review the six rights to ensure that safe and effective patient care is given: (1) right patient, (2) right drug, (3) right dose, (4) right route, (5) right time, and (6) right documentation. You can cause further harm to the patient if a drug—even if it's the right drug—is given at the wrong time, by an inappropriate route, or in the wrong dose.

10. Does this patient require an additional dose of 50% dextrose?

Based on a post-$D_{50}W$ glucose reading of 4 mmol/l and the patient's obvious clinical improvement, additional doses of $D_{50}W$ are not indicated. However, the question remains as to why her blood glucose level dropped initially. Ask further questions to explore this issue, such as when she last ate, what she ate (if she ate), if she took her insulin and how much, and if she has any other medical problems. During transport, continue to monitor the patient's level of consciousness and reassess her blood glucose level as needed.

11. Does this patient require an IV bolus of normal saline?

The IV line can remain at a TKVO rate; there is no need for fluid boluses. At present, the patient's vital signs indicate hemodynamic stability. Her heart rate, which was 120 beats/min initially, was likely due to a sympathetic nervous system discharge in response to hypoglycemia, not hypovolemia. Following administration of the $D_{50}W$, the patient's heart rate promptly recovered. No mechanism for volume loss has been identified (eg, vomiting, diarrhea).

Prep Kit

Ready for Review

- The cellular environment contains charged ions, called electrolytes, that are used by the cell for different purposes. These electrolytes include sodium, potassium, calcium, bicarbonate, chloride, and phosphorous. Their electrical charges must remain in balance on either side of the cell membrane.
- There must be a balance of compounds on either side of the cell membrane. If an imbalance occurs, the cell can move chemicals or charges across its membrane by various methods, including osmosis, diffusion, active transport, and filtration.
- Understanding the workings of the intracellular and extracellular chemicals and charges will provide you with a better foundation for understanding why different types of IV solutions are administered for different conditions.
- Techniques for gaining vascular access include cannulation of a peripheral extremity vein, cannulation of the external jugular vein, and cannulation of the IO space. Although the ultimate goal of vascular access is to be able to administer fluids and medications, each of these techniques requires a different approach and must be practiced frequently for initial and ongoing proficiency.
- Several different IV administration sets exist, and you must know which one is most appropriate for a given patient condition. Microdrip sets (60 gtt/ml) are commonly used for medication infusions. Macrodrip sets (10 or 15 gtt/ml) are used when the patient requires IV fluid boluses to treat dehydration, hypovolemic shock, and other states of hemodynamic instability.
- You must consider two factors when choosing an IV cannula: gauge and length. The larger the gauge (the smaller the number), and the shorter the length, the more fluid that can be infused through it. Over-the-needle cannulas are the most commonly used IV cannulas in the prehospital setting.
- Cannulation of a peripheral extremity vein is the preferred initial means of establishing vascular access. If it is unsuccessful and the patient is critically ill or injured, proceed with IO cannulation without delay. External jugular vein cannulation is usually attempted only after all other techniques of gaining vascular access have failed.
- IO cannulation and infusion are no longer reserved for children only; they can also be used to establish emergency vascular access in adults. The IO space, which acts like a sponge, quickly absorbs fluids and medications and rapidly transports them to the central circulation.
- Although peripheral veins often collapse when a patient is in shock or cardiac arrest, the IO space tends to remain patent. Thus IO cannulation and infusion—in children and adults—may be lifesaving measures if peripheral venous access is not possible. Any fluid or medication that can be administered via the IV route can be administered via the IO route and can travel to the central circulation just as rapidly.
- You must be thoroughly familiar with the equipment you are using when performing IO cannulation. Follow local protocols and attend in-service training regarding the specific equipment used for IO cannulation in your EMS system.
- Use aseptic technique when performing any invasive procedure to minimize the risk of patient contamination. Always use PPE and routine precautions when performing an invasive procedure to maximize your own safety.
- Along with the dispensing of medications comes the responsibility to be thoroughly familiar with each medication carried on your ambulance. Carry an EMS guide or other reference to look up unfamiliar drugs or to confirm the doses and routes of drugs that you are familiar with. Remember: *First, do no harm.*
- Good math skills and a thorough understanding of the metric system are imperative to providing the right dose of a drug to your patient. The six rights of medication are right patient, right drug, right dose, right route, right time, and right documentation. Administering the wrong drug, using the wrong route, or giving the wrong dose can have disastrous effects.
- All equipment used in the administration of medications must be kept sterile to prevent contamination of the patient. Use PPE and routine precautions to protect yourself. Needleless systems have made older needle systems increasingly obsolete, as the former systems decrease the incidence of needlesticks.
- As a paramedic, you must be familiar with the various routes of medication administration, including the proper use of equipment and proper anatomical locations for administration via each route.
- Enteral medication administration includes the administration of all drugs that may be given through any portion of the gastrointestinal tract. The parenteral route includes any method of drug administration that does not pass through the gastrointestinal tract.
- The IV and IO routes are the fastest routes of medication administration; the oral and transdermal (topical) routes are the slowest.
- When in doubt, always follow local protocols or contact direct medical control as needed for direction when administering a medication. *Never make a hasty critical decision before consulting with a physician!*

Vital Vocabulary

access port A sealed hub on an administration set designed for sterile access to the IV fluid.

acidosis A pathologic condition resulting from the accumulation of acids in the body.

administration set Tubing that connects to the IV bag access port and the cannula to deliver IV fluid.

alkalosis A pathologic condition resulting from the accumulation of bases in the body.

ampules Small glass containers that are sealed and the contents sterilized.

anion An ion that contains an overall negative charge.

antecubital The anterior aspect of the elbow.

anticoagulant A substance that prevents blood from clotting.

antidiuretic hormone (ADH) A hormone produced by the pituitary gland that signals the kidneys to prevent excretion of water.

antiseptics Chemicals used to cleanse an area before performing an invasive procedure, such as starting an IV; not toxic to living tissues; examples include isopropyl alcohol and iodine.

aseptic technique A method of cleansing used to prevent contamination of a site when performing an invasive procedure, such as starting an IV.

ataxia A staggered walk or gait.

aural Pertaining to the ear.

bivalent An ion that contains two charges.

blood tubing A special type of macrodrip administration set designed to facilitate rapid fluid replacement by manual infusion of multiple IV bags or IV-blood replacement combinations.

bolus A term used to describe "in one mass"; in medication administration, a single dose given by the IV or IO route; may be a small or large quantity of the drug.

Bone Injection Gun (BIG) A spring-loaded device that is used for inserting an IO needle into the proximal tibia in adult and pediatric patients.

buccal Between the cheek and gums.

butterfly cannula A rigid, hollow, venous cannulation device identified by its plastic "wings" that act as anchoring points for securing the cannula.

cannula shear Occurs when a needle is reinserted into the cannula, and it slices through the cannula, creating a free-floating segment.

cannulation The insertion of a cannula, such as into a vein to allow for fluid flow.

carpopedal spasms Hand or foot spasms; usually the result of hyperventilation or hypocalcemia.

cation An ion that contains an overall positive charge.

Celsius scale A scale for measuring temperature in which water freezes at 0° and boils at 100°.

colloid solutions Solutions that contain molecules (usually proteins) that are too large to pass out of the capillary membranes and, therefore, remain in the vascular compartment.

concentration The total weight of a drug contained in a specific volume of liquid.

concentration gradient The natural tendency for substances to flow from an area of higher concentration to an area of lower concentration, within or outside the cell.

contaminated stick The puncturing of an emergency care provider's skin with a needle or cannula that was used on a patient.

crystalloid solutions Solutions of dissolved crystals (for example, salts or sugars) in water; contain compounds that quickly dissociate in solution.

D_5W An intravenous solution made up of 5% dextrose in water.

dehydration Depletion of the body's systemic fluid volume.

depolarization The rapid movement of electrolytes across a cell membrane that changes the cell's overall charge. This rapid shifting of electrolytes and cellular charges is the main catalyst for muscle contractions and neural transmissions.

desired dose The amount of a drug that the physician orders for a patient; the drug order.

diaphysis The shaft of a long bone.

diffusion A process in which molecules move from an area of higher concentration to an area of lower concentration.

diluent A solution (usually water or normal saline) used for diluting a medication.

direct medical control Type of medical control in which the paramedic is in direct contact with a physician, usually via two-way radio or telephone.

disinfectants Chemicals used on nonliving objects to kill organisms; toxic to living tissues; examples include Virex, Cidex, and Microcide.

drip chamber The area of the administration set where fluid accumulates so that the tubing remains filled with fluid.

drug reconstitution Injecting sterile water or saline from one vial into another vial containing a powdered form of the drug.

electrolytes Charged atoms or compounds that result from the loss or gain of an electron. These are ions that the body uses to perform certain critical metabolic functions.

enteral route A route of medication administration that involves the medication passing through a portion of the gastrointestinal tract.

epiphyseal plate The growth plate of a bone; a major site of bone development during childhood.

epiphyses The ends of a long bone.

external jugular (EJ) vein Large neck vein that is lateral to the carotid artery.

extracellular fluid (ECF) The water outside the cells; accounts for 15% of body weight.

EZ-IO A hand-held, battery-powered driver to which a special IO needle is attached; used for insertion of the IO needle into the proximal tibia of children and adults.

Fahrenheit scale A scale for measuring temperature in which water freezes at 32° and boils at 212°.

fascia The fibrelike connective tissue that covers arteries, veins, tendons, and ligaments.

FAST1® A sternal IO device used in adults; stands for First Access for Shock and Trauma.

flash chamber The area of an IV cannula that fills with blood to help indicate when a vein is cannulated.

gastric tubes Tubes that are commonly inserted in patients in the prehospital setting to decompress the stomach; can also be used to administer certain enteral medications.

gauge The internal diameter of an IV cannula or needle.

gtt A unit of measure that indicates drops.

hematoma An accumulation of blood in the tissues beneath the skin; a potential complication of IV therapy.

hemostasis The body's natural blood-clotting mechanism.

homeostasis The balance of all body systems of the body; also known as homeostatic balance.

hypercalcemia A high serum calcium level.

hyperkalemia A high serum potassium level.

hypertonic solution A solution that has a greater concentration of sodium than does the cell; the increased osmotic pressure can draw water out of the cell and cause it to collapse.

hypocalcemia A low serum calcium level.

hypokalemia A low serum potassium level.

hypotonic solution A solution that has a lower concentration of sodium than does the cell; the increased osmotic pressure lets water flow into the cell, causing it to swell and possibly burst.

infiltration The escape of fluid into the surrounding tissue; the result of vein perforation during IV cannulation.

inhalation Breathing into the lungs; a medication delivery route.

interstitial fluid The water bathing the cells; accounts for about 10.5% of body weight; includes special fluid collections, such as cerebrospinal fluid and intraocular fluid.

intracellular fluid (ICF) The water contained inside the cells; normally accounts for 45% of body weight.

intradermal the layer of the dermis, just beneath the epidermis; a medication delivery route.

intramuscular (IM) Into a muscle; a medication delivery route.

intranasal Within the nose.

intraosseous Within the bone.

intraosseous (IO) infusion A technique of administering fluids, blood and blood products, and medications into the intraosseous space of a long bone, usually the proximal tibia.

intraosseous (IO) space The spongy cancellous bone of the epiphyses and the medullary cavity of the diaphysis, collectively.

intravascular fluid Plasma; the water within the blood vessels, which carries red blood cells, white blood cells, and vital nutrients; normally accounts for about 4.5% of body weight.

intravenous Within a vein.

intravenous (IV) therapy Cannulation of a vein with an IV cannula to access the patient's vascular system.

ionic concentration The amount of charged particles found in a particular area.

ions Charged atoms or compounds that results from the loss or gain of an electron.

isotonic crystalloids Intravenous solutions that do not cause a fluid shift into or out of the cell; examples include normal saline and lactated Ringer's solutions.

isotonic solution A solution that has the same concentration of sodium as does the cell. In this case, water does not shift, and no change in cell shape occurs.

lactated Ringer's (LR) solution A sterile isotonic crystalloid IV solution of specified amounts of calcium chloride, potassium chloride, sodium chloride, and sodium lactate in water.

local reactions Reactions that occur in a localized area; a potential complication of IV therapy.

macrodrip sets Administration sets named for the large orifice between the piercing spike and the drip chamber; allow for rapid fluid flow into the vascular system; allow 10 or 15 gtt/ml, depending on the manufacturer.

medical asepsis A term applied to the practice of preventing contamination of the patient by using aseptic technique.

metabolic Pertaining to the breakdown of ingested foodstuffs into smaller and smaller molecules and atoms that are used as energy sources for cellular function.

metered-dose inhaler (MDI) A pressurized canister that delivers a specific dose of a medication; commonly used for beta-agonist bronchodilators.

metric system A decimal system based on tens for the measurement of length, weight, and volume.

microdrip sets Administration sets named for the small needlelike orifice between the piercing spike and the drip chamber; allow for carefully controlled fluid flow and are ideally suited for medication administration; allow for 60 gtt/ml.

milliequivalent (mEq) Unit of measure for electrolytes.

Mix-o-Vial A single vial divided into two compartments by a rubber stopper; Solu-Medrol is stored this way.

monovalent An ion that contains one charge.

mucosal atomizer device (MAD) A device that attaches to the end of a syringe that is used to spray (atomize) certain medications via the intranasal route.

nebulizer A device for producing a fine spray or mist that is used to deliver inhaled medications.

nonelectrolytes Solutes that have no electrical charge; include glucose and urea; measured in milligrams (mg).

normal saline A solution of 0.9% sodium chloride; an isotonic crystalloid.

occlusion Blockage, usually of a tubular structure such as a blood vessel or IV cannula.

ocular Pertaining to the eye.

osmolarity The ability to influence the movement of water across a semipermeable membrane.

osmosis The movement of water across a semipermeable membrane (for example, the cell wall) from an area of lower to higher concentration of solute molecules.

osteogenesis imperfecta A congenital bone disease that results in fragile bones.

osteomyelitis Inflammation of the bone and muscle caused by infection.

overhydration An increase in the body's systemic fluid volume.

over-the-needle cannula A Teflon (plastic) cannula inserted over a hollow needle.

parenteral route A route of medication administration that involves any route other than the gastrointestinal tract.

Penrose drain A type of surgical drain often used as a tourniquet.

percutaneous Through the skin or mucous membrane.

peripheral vein cannulation Cannulating veins of the periphery, that is, those that can be seen and/or palpated. Examples of peripheral veins include those of the hand, arm, and lower extremity and the external jugular vein.

piercing spike The hard, sharpened plastic spike on the end of the administration set designed to pierce the sterile membrane of the IV bag.

postural hypotension Symptomatic drop in blood pressure related to the patient's body position; detected by measuring pulse and blood pressure while the patient is lying supine, sitting up, and standing. An increase in pulse rate and a decrease in blood pressure in any one of these positions is considered a positive sign for this condition.

prefilled syringes Medication syringes that are prepackaged and prepared with a specific concentration.

pressure infuser device A sleeve that is placed around the IV bag and inflated to force fluid to flow from the IV bag and into the tubing.

pulmonary embolism A blood clot or foreign matter trapped within the pulmonary circulation.

pyrogenic reaction A reaction characterized by an abrupt temperature elevation (as high as 41° C) with severe chills, backache, headache, weakness, nausea, and vomiting; a potential complication of IV or IO therapy.

radiopaque Feature of an IV cannula (or any other object) that allows it to appear on an x-ray.

saline locks Special types of IV devices that eliminate the need to hang a bag of IV fluid; also called a buff cap or INT (intermittent); commonly used for patients who do not require fluid boluses but may require medication therapy.

self-sealing blood tubes Glass tubes with self-sealing rubber caps; used to obtain blood samples for laboratory analysis.

sharps Any contaminated item that can cause injury; includes IV needles and cannulas, broken ampules or vials, or anything else that can penetrate or lacerate the skin.

sodium-potassium (Na+-K+) pump The mechanism by which the cell brings in two potassium (K+) ions and releases three sodium (Na+) ions.

solute The dissolved particles contained in the solvent.

solution Combination of dissolved elements (solutes) and water (solvent).

solvent The fluid that does the dissolving, or the solution that contains the dissolved components.

standing orders A form of indirect medical control, in which the paramedic performs certain predefined procedures before contacting the physician.

sterile The destruction of all living organisms; achieved by using heat, gas, or chemicals.

subcutaneous (SC) Into the tissue between the skin and muscle; a medication delivery route.

sublingual Under the tongue; a medication delivery route.

syncopal episodes Fainting; brief losses of consciousness caused by transiently inadequate blood flow to the brain.

systemic complications Reactions that affect systems of the body.

third spacing The shifting of fluid into the tissues, creating edema.

thrombophlebitis Inflammation of a vein.

through-the-needle cannulas Plastic cannulas inserted through a hollow needle; referred to as Intracaths.

www.Paramedic.EMSzone.com/Canada

tonicity The osmotic pressure of a solution, based on the relationship between sodium and water inside and outside the cell, that takes advantage of their chemical and osmotic properties to move water to areas of higher sodium concentration.

total body water (TBW) Total amount of water in the human body; accounts for approximately 60% of the weight of an average man; divided into various compartments.

track marks The visible scars from repeated cannulation of a vein; commonly associated with illicit drug use.

transdermal Across the skin; a medication delivery route.

tubules Sections of the kidney where the filtration of wastes, electrolytes, and water is controlled.

Vacutainer A cylindrical device that attaches to an 18- or 20-gauge sampling needle; accommodates self-sealing blood tubes when obtaining blood samples.

venous thrombosis The development of a stationary blood clot in the venous circulation.

vials Small glass or plastic bottles that contain medication; may contain single or multiple doses.

Volutrol A special type of microdrip set that features a 100- or 200-ml calibrated drip chamber; used for fluid regulation in patients prone to circulatory overload, such as pediatric and elderly patients; also called a Buretrol.

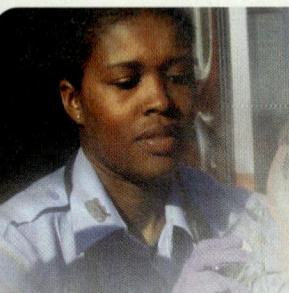

Assessment in Action

You and your partner are dispatched to an apartment complex because of a possible overdose. Law enforcement personnel are already present and radio you that the scene is secure. When you enter the apartment, you find the patient, a 30-year-old man, unconscious on the couch. With the assistance of law enforcement personnel, you and your partner quickly move the patient to the floor and perform an initial assessment. The patient has sonorous respirations and a slow, weak radial pulse. There is no gross bleeding or evidence of trauma.

1. **How will you treat this patient initially?**
   A. Apply oxygen via nonrebreathing mask.
   B. Suction his oropharynx for 15 seconds.
   C. Provide bag-valve-mask ventilation and 100% oxygen.
   D. Manually open his airway and insert an airway adjunct.

2. **Your partner assesses the patient's respirations and notes that they are slow and shallow. What should you direct him to do?**
   A. Apply a nonrebreathing mask set at 15 l/min.
   B. Provide bag-valve-mask ventilation and 100% oxygen.
   C. Assess the patient's oxygen saturation with a pulse oximeter.
   D. Help you prepare to perform immediate endotracheal intubation.

3. **Following additional assessment of the patient, you suspect a narcotic overdose. While your partner continues to manage the patient's airway, you prepare to establish vascular access. Which of the following statements regarding vascular access is MOST correct?**
   A. You should immediately insert an IO cannula into the patient's proximal tibia.
   B. External jugular vein cannulation is preferred when patients are deeply unconscious.
   C. 5% dextrose in water (D_5W) is the fluid of choice for patients who may require volume expansion.
   D. The antecubital vein is the preferred vein to use when starting an IV on a critically ill or injured patient.

4. **Which of the following IV cannulas will allow you to deliver the greatest amount of volume in the *shortest* period?**
   A. 14-gauge, 3.2-cm cannula
   B. 14-gauge, 5.7-cm cannula
   C. 16-gauge, 3.8-cm cannula
   D. 18-gauge, 5.7-cm cannula

5. **Vascular access has been obtained. Your protocols call for the administration of naloxone (Narcan) in a dose of 2 mg. You have a prefilled syringe of naloxone that contains 10 mg in 5 ml. How many millilitres of naloxone will you administer to achieve the desired dose of 2 mg?**
   A. 1 ml
   B. 2 ml
   C. 3 ml
   D. 4 ml

6. **Compared with medications administered via the enteral route, parenteral medications:**
   A. must be instilled through a gastric tube.
   B. can be delivered only by the IV route.
   C. do not pass through the gastrointestinal tract.
   D. reach the central circulation at a much slower rate.

7. **Which of the following medication routes has the *slowest* rate of absorption?**
   A. Intravenous
   B. Transdermal
   C. Subcutaneous
   D. Intramuscular

www.Paramedic.EMSzone.com/Canada

8. Shortly after administering naloxone to your patient, the IV line infiltrates. You obtain a blood glucose reading of 2.2 mmol/l and must administer glucagon via the IM route. However, glucagon must be reconstituted before being administered. What does drug reconstitution involve?

A. Administration of the drug during a period of at least 5 seconds

B. Delivering the medication in the form of a maintenance infusion

C. Diluting the drug with at least 5 ml of normal saline or sterile water

D. Adding diluent to the powdered form of the drug to make a solution

Challenging Questions

A 54-year-old male is found unconscious in his home by a close friend. The patient is unresponsive, breathing slowly and shallowly, and is bradycardic. As your partner begins ventilation assistance with a bag-valve-mask device and 100% oxygen, you find a bottle of hydrocodone—a potent narcotic analgesic—on an adjacent table. The prescription was filled 2 days prior and is now empty. According to the friend, the patient recently had bilateral knee replacements, and was prescribed the medication for pain relief. He further states that the patient has "emotional problems." Recognizing that the patient will require naloxone (Narcan), you attempt to establish a peripheral IV line, but are unsuccessful after several attempts. Your partner reports that she is not having difficulty with bag-valve-mask ventilation.

9. Should you intubate this patient?

10. What alternate medication routes are available to administer the naloxone?

Points to Ponder

You and your partner are treating a 35-year-old man with a headache. The patient is conscious and alert and denies chest pain or shortness of breath. His blood pressure is 130/84 mm Hg, heart rate is 44 beats/min and regular, and respirations are 16 breaths/min and unlaboured. Further assessment reveals that the patient's skin is pink, warm, and dry, and his lungs are clear to auscultation bilaterally. The cardiac monitor reveals sinus bradycardia at 40 beats/min.

An IV line is established and set at a to keep vein open (TKVO) rate. As you are obtaining the patient's medical history, your paramedic partner administers 1 mg of atropine sulfate to the patient. Following administration of the atropine, the patient experiences tachycardia at a rate of 130 beats/min and becomes anxious and nauseous. However, his symptoms have resolved by the time you arrive at the hospital.

Analyze this situation and explain what happened.

Issues: Recognizing a Patient in Stable Versus Unstable Condition, Understanding the Need to Verify the "Six Rights" of Medication Administration, Documenting and Reporting a Medication Error.

9 Human Development

Competency Areas

Area 2: Communication

2.1.d Provide information to patient about their situation and how they will be treated.
2.1.f Speak in language appropriate to the listener.
2.1.g Use appropriate terminology.
2.3.a Exhibit effective non-verbal behaviour.
2.3.b Practice active listening techniques.
2.3.c Establish trust and rapport with patients and colleagues.
2.3.d Recognize and react appropriately to non-verbal behaviours.

Area 4: Assessment and Diagnostics

4.3.o Conduct neonatal assessment and interpret findings.

Area 5: Therapeutics

5.4.a Provide oxygenation and ventilation using bag-valve-mask.

Area 6: Integration

6.2.a Provide care for neonatal patient.
6.2.b Provide care for pediatric patient.
6.2.c Provide care for geriatric patient.

Appendix 4: Pathophysiology

A. Cardiovascular System
Congenital Abnormalities: Atrial septal defect
Congenital Abnormalities: Patent ductus arteriosus
Congenital Abnormalities: Transposition
Congenital Abnormalities: Ventricular septal defect

Introduction

One of the most interesting things about humans is that we evolve—not just as a species, but also as people over our life span. Paramedics must be aware of both the obvious and subtle changes that a person undergoes physically and mentally at various stages of life and understand how these changes might alter the approach to patient care.

Infants

As any parent can attest, infants (1 month to 1 year) develop at a startling rate ▶Figure 9-1▶. Neonates (birth to 1 month) are covered in detail in Chapter 40: *Neonatology*.

Physical Changes

Vital Signs

▶Table 9-1▶ lists the normal ranges of vital signs for various age groups. The younger the person, the faster the pulse rate and respirations. At birth, a pulse rate of 90 to 180 beats/min and a respiratory rate of 30 to 60 breaths/min are considered normal. After about a half hour, an infant's heart rate often drops to around 120 beats/min and the respiratory rate adjusts to between 30 to 40 breaths/min. Tidal volume in infants starts at 6 to 8 ml/kg. By age 1 year, the volume increases to 10 to 15 ml/kg.

Blood pressure directly corresponds to the patient's weight, so it typically increases with age. At birth, the average systolic blood pressure of an infant is 50 to 70 mm Hg. By 1 year of age, it is in the range of 70 to 95 mm Hg.

Weight

An infant usually weighs 3 to 3.5 kg at birth. After birth, infants usually lose 5% to 10% of their birth weight due to the loss of fluid in the first week. Then they normally gain weight in their second week of life. From here on, infants grow at a rate of about 30 g per day, doubling their weight by 4 to 6 months and tripling it by age 1 year.

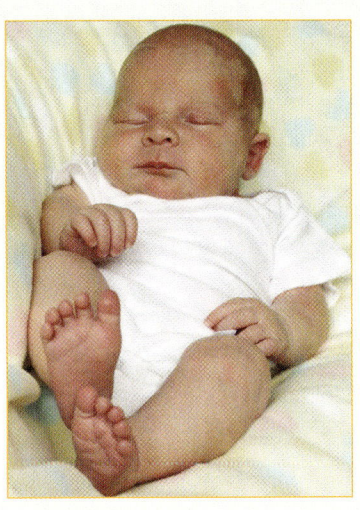

Figure 9-1 An infant.

Cardiovascular System

Prior to birth, fetal circulation occurs through the placenta, which is connected to the ductus venosus and ductus arteriosus. Just after birth, the ductus venosus constricts and closes.

> **At the Scene**
>
> Infants often land head first when they fall because their heads account for 25% of their total body weight. Also, most infants cannot stretch out their arms in time to cushion or slow their fall. Keep this point in mind when considering spinal immobilization on an infant.

You are the Paramedic Part 1

You and your partner have just finished checking your rig when you hear the dispatcher: "Ambulance 5281, respond to 788 Elm Street for a 16-year-old female complaining of abdominal pain."

When you arrive at the residence, you are greeted by an anxious man who introduces himself as the patient's father. While holding his terrified and screaming 2-year-old son, he cries, "My daughter's upstairs in her bedroom with her mom. I think her appendix burst!" Upon entering the patient's bedroom, you introduce yourself and see the patient curled in a fetal position on the floor, writhing in pain and complaining of nausea. She moans, "My stomach hurts, please help me!" You begin your initial assessment of the patient as her parents watch intently over your shoulder.

Initial Assessment	Recording Time: 0 Minutes
Appearance	Fetal position, obvious distress
Level of consciousness	A (Alert to person, place, and day)
Airway	Open
Breathing	24 breaths/min and adequate
Circulation	Strong radial pulses at 118 beats/min, no external bleeding

1. What are your differential diagnoses given the information provided?
2. How would you approach your patient interview?
3. What could explain the slightly elevated patient respirations and pulse?

Table 9-1	Vital Signs at Various Ages			
Age	Pulse Rate (beats/min)	Respirations (breaths/min)	Blood Pressure (mm Hg)	Temperature (°C)
Newborn (0 to 1 month)	90 to 180	30 to 60	50 to 70	36.7 to 37.8
Infant (1 month to 1 year)	100 to 160	25 to 50	70 to 95	36 to 37.6
Toddler (1 to 3 years)	90 to 150	20 to 30	80 to 100	36 to 37.6
Preschool age (3 to 6 years)	80 to 140	20 to 25	80 to 100	36
School age (6 to 12 years)	70 to 120	15 to 20	80 to 110	36
Adolescent (12 to 18 years)	60 to 100	12 to 16	90 to 110	36
Early adult (19 to 40 years)	70	12 to 20	90 to 140	36
Middle adult (41 to 60 years)	70	12 to 20	90 to 140	36
Late adult (61 and older)	Depends on health	Depends on health	Depends on health	36

As a consequence, the infant's blood pressure changes, and the foramen ovale, an opening in the septum of the heart, closes. The ductus arteriosus also constricts and closes, resulting in circulation through the pulmonary system and the veins and arteries (rather than through the placenta) as well as increased vascular resistance and decreased pulmonary resistance **Figure 9-2 ▶**. Transposition of the great arteries is a very rare congenital abnormality where the aorta and pulmonary artery positions on the heart are reversed. It requires surgery since it results in hypoxemia.

Pulmonary System

Prior to an infant's first breath, the lungs have never been inflated. An infant's first breath is therefore forceful—it has to be!

Infants are primarily "nose breathers" for the first month of their lives. Infants younger than 6 months are particularly prone to nasal congestion, which can cause viral upper respiratory infections. If you receive a call for a baby choking, always make sure the infant's nasal passages are clear and unobstructed by mucus.

The rib cages of infants are less rigid than those of older humans, and the ribs sit horizontally. This explains the diaphragmatic breathing ("belly breathing") in infants.

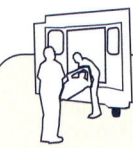

At the Scene

When you are counting respirations in an infant, count the number of times the abdomen rises instead of concentrating solely on the chest rise.

Two other important anatomical points related to an infant's airway, when compared with an adult's, are the proportionally large size of the tongue and the proportionally shorter and narrower airway. As a result of these factors, infants can much more easily occlude their airway than older children or adults can.

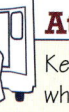

At the Scene

Keep the infant's unique airway anatomy in mind when you are selecting an appropriate upper airway adjunct, the proper advanced airway, and the most appropriate sized endotracheal tube.

When providing bag-valve-mask ventilations to an infant, you need to be aware that an infant's lungs are fragile. Ventilations that are too forceful can result in trauma from pressure, or barotrauma.

Renal System

Infants can become easily dehydrated because their kidneys usually cannot produce concentrated urine. An infant's urine consists mainly of water, which can cause the child to develop electrolyte imbalances.

Immune System

While in the womb, infants collect antibodies from the maternal blood. For the first year of life, the infant maintains some of the mother's immunities, so he or she has naturally acquired passive immunities. Infants can also receive antibodies via breastfeeding, further bolstering their immune system.

Nervous System

Although the infant's nervous system is developed at birth, its evolution continues after birth. For example, the newborn lacks the ability to localize and isolate a particular response to sensation. Motor and sensory development are most developed in the cranial nerves, which control blinking, sucking, and gag reflexes.

An infant is born with certain reflexes. The moro reflex (startle reflex) happens when an infant is caught off guard by something or someone; the infant opens his or her arms wide, spreads the fingers, and seems to grab at things. A palmar grasp occurs when an object is placed into the infant's palm. The rooting reflex takes place when something touches an infant's cheek; the infant will instinctively turn his or her head toward the touch. In conjunction with the sucking reflex, which occurs when an infant's lips are stroked, these reflexes are often tested when feeding.

An infant's fontanelles allow the head to be moulded **Figure 9-3 ▶**—for example, when the newborn passes through the birth canal. These three or four bones of the skull eventually bind together and form suture joints within 18 months of birth. If the anterior fontanelle is sunken, the infant is most likely dehydrated.

Perhaps the neurologic development that is of most interest to parents is the development of a sleep pattern. Some

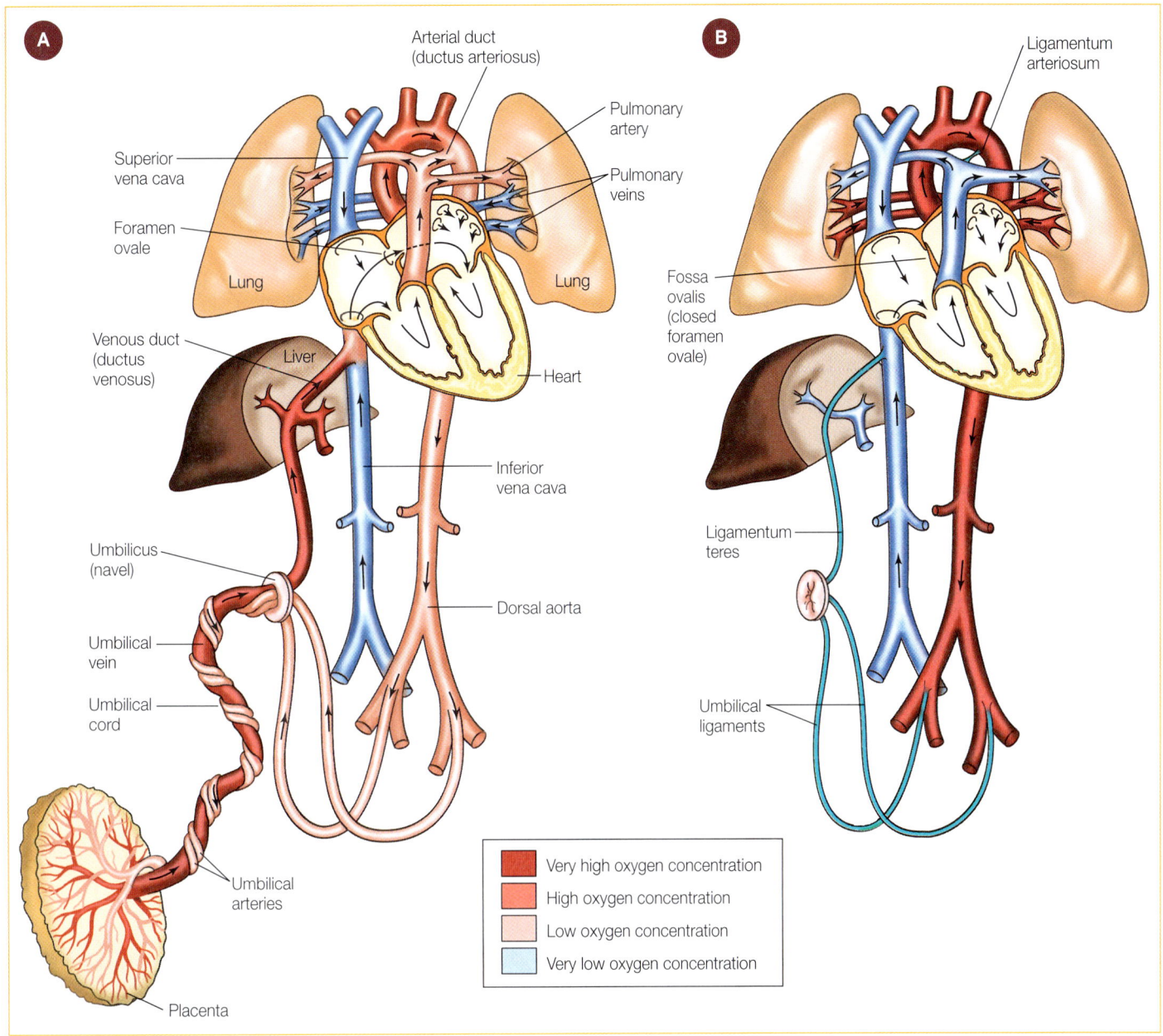

Figure 9-2 Fetal circulation before birth (**A**) and after birth (**B**).

physicians suggest that parents wake infants every few hours for both feeding and safety (eg, to guard against sudden infant death syndrome [SIDS]). Others suggest that infants should be left to sleep so that they can adjust to family life and develop a circadian rhythm, ideally within 4 months after birth. (For more information on SIDS, see Chapter 41.)

Musculoskeletal System

Growth plates, located on either end of an infant's bone, aid in lengthening a child's bones. Epiphyseal plates, or secondary bone-growing plates, are also present. Bones grow in thickness

by building on themselves. In contrast, an infant's muscles account for approximately 25% of his or her total weight.

Psychosocial Changes

An infant's psychosocial development begins at birth and continues to evolve as the infant interacts with and reacts to the environment. Parents often obsess about whether their child is developing within the socially accepted norms. **Table 9-2 ▶** outlines typical ages at which major psychosocial changes are noticed.

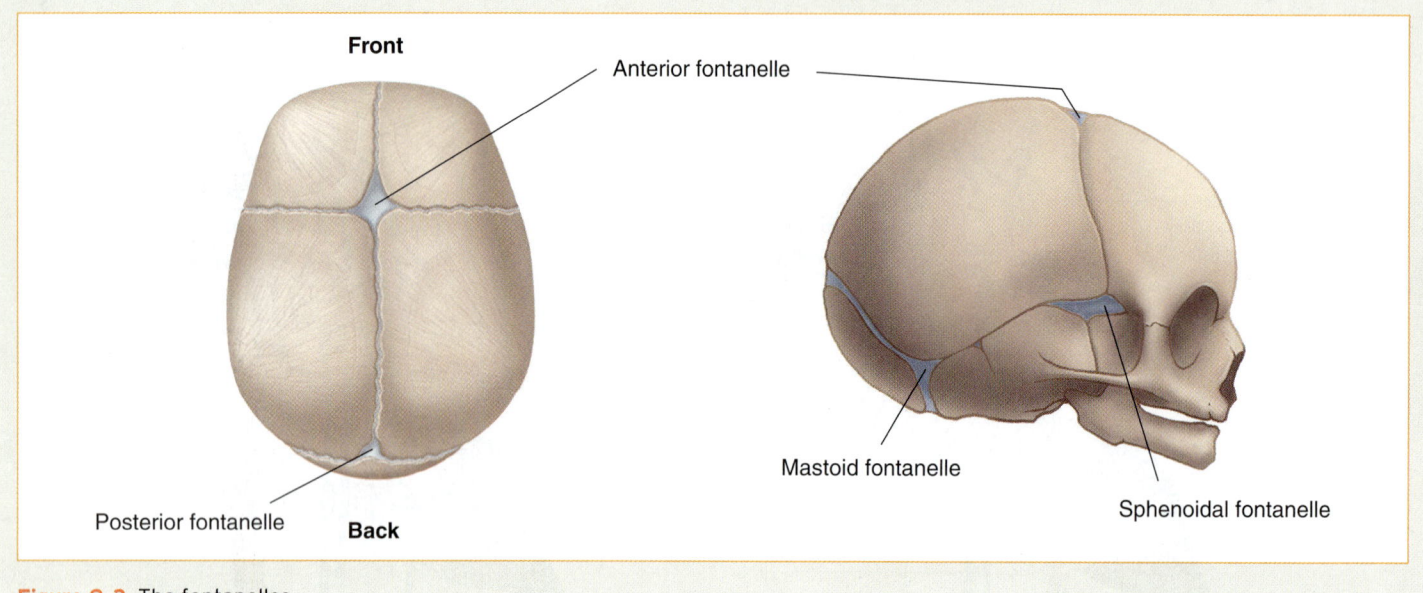

Figure 9-3 The fontanelles.

Table 9-2	Noticeable Characteristics at Various Ages
Age	**Characteristic**
2 months	Can recognize familiar faces; able to track objects with the eyes
3 months	Can bring objects to the mouth; can smile and frown
4 months	Reaches out to people; drools
5 months	Sleeps through the night; can tell family from strangers
6 months	Teething begins, sits upright in a chair, one-syllable words spoken
7 months	Afraid of strangers, mood swings
8 months	Responds to "no"; can sit alone; plays peek-a-boo
9 months	Pulls himself or herself up; places objects in mouth to explore them
10 months	Responds to his or her name; crawls efficiently
11 months	Starts to walk without help; frustrated with restrictions
12 months	Knows his or her name; can walk

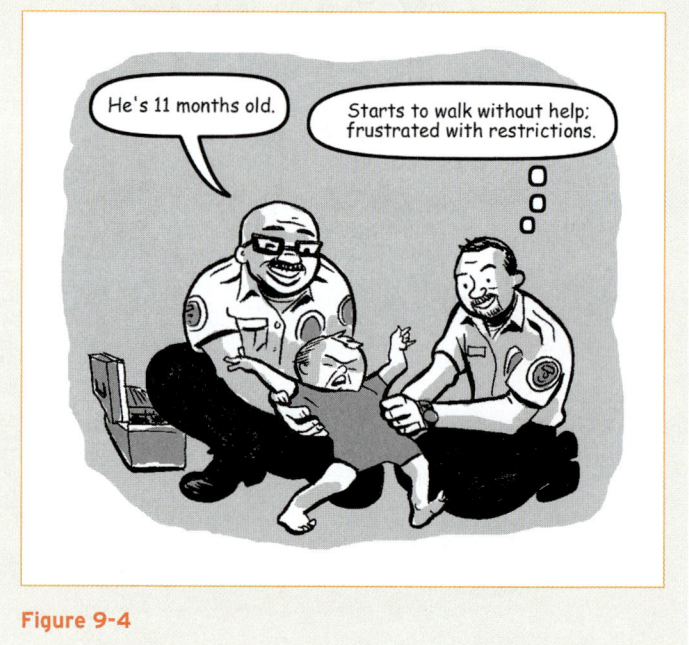

Figure 9-4

In most infants, the primary method of communicating distress is through crying **Figure 9-4 ▸** . Parents can often tell what is upsetting their child simply by listening to the tone of the child's crying—that is, they know the difference between tears for anger, frustration, pain, fear, hunger, discomfort, and sleepiness. Infants occasionally make another distinct cry—an alarming distressed cry. This cry may be heard when an unexpected event occurs, causing a situational crisis for the infant.

The key to having a happy, healthy infant is spending time with the child. Nevertheless, infants often have their own timetable as to when they will become attached to their parents and other family members. Bonding, or the formation of a close, personal relationship, is usually based on a secure attachment. A secure attachment occurs when an infant understands that parents or caregivers will be responsive to his or her needs. This realization encourages a child to reach out and explore, knowing that his or her parents will provide a "safety net."

Another type of attachment, referred to as anxious avoidant attachment, is observed in infants who are repeatedly rejected. These children develop an isolated lifestyle where they do not have to depend on the support and care of others.

Trust and mistrust refers to a stage of development from birth to about 18 months of age. Most infants desire that their world be planned, organized, and routine. When their caregivers and parents provide this environment for them, the infant gains trust in those individuals. The opposite also holds true Figure 9-5 ▶ .

A toddler's cardiovascular system isn't dramatically different from that of an adult. A toddler's lungs continue to develop more bronchioles and alveoli. Although toddlers and preschoolers have more lung tissue, they do not have well-developed lung musculature. This anomaly prevents them from sustaining deep or rapid respirations for an extended period of time.

The loss of passive immunity in the immune system is possibly the most obvious development at this stage of human life. "Colds" often develop that may manifest as gastrointestinal distress or upper respiratory tract infections. As toddlers spend

Toddlers and Preschoolers

Physical Changes

In toddlers (ages 1 to 3 years Figure 9-6 ▶) and preschoolers (ages 3 to 6 years Figure 9-7 ▶), the heart rate and respiratory rate are slower than the corresponding vital signs in infants, whereas the systolic blood pressure is higher (approximately 100 mm Hg). At the same time, weight gain should level off.

At the Scene

When dealing with patients who are very young, try to keep their routine the same by keeping family and familiar items nearby.

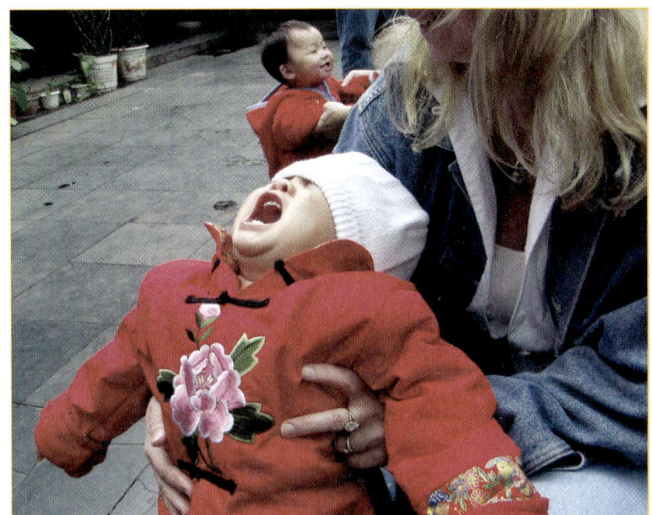

Figure 9-5 If an infant perceives that his or her parents or caregivers will not provide an organized, routine environment, the infant can develop behavioural problems.

You are the Paramedic Part 2

You apply supplemental high-flow oxygen to your patient, place her in a position of comfort, and begin your focused assessment and history. Your assessment reveals right-sided lower abdominal pain rated as 9 on a 10-point scale, with radiation to the back and groin. You continue to ask your patient questions about her history. Her father provides answers about her prior knee surgery a few years ago, and the fact that she takes fexofenadine and salbutamol for her allergies and asthma.

When you ask the patient about her last menstrual period, you discover that she is taking extended-cycle birth control pills for regulation of her menstrual cycle and that her last period was a little less than 2 months ago. Per her medication schedule, her next menstrual period is due in about a month and a half. When you ask the patient whether there is any chance she may be pregnant, she adamantly denies the possibility, and her father is insulted that you would ask such a question.

Assessment	Recording Time: 10 Minutes
Skin	Pale, warm, and moist
Pulse	118 beats/min
Blood pressure	130/88 mm Hg
Respirations	24 breaths/min
Spo2	100% on 15 l/min nonrebreathing mask on supplemental oxygen

4. What are your differential diagnoses now?

5. What is your next step in treatment of this patient?

6. Do you allow the parent to ride in the compartment of the ambulance along with the patient?

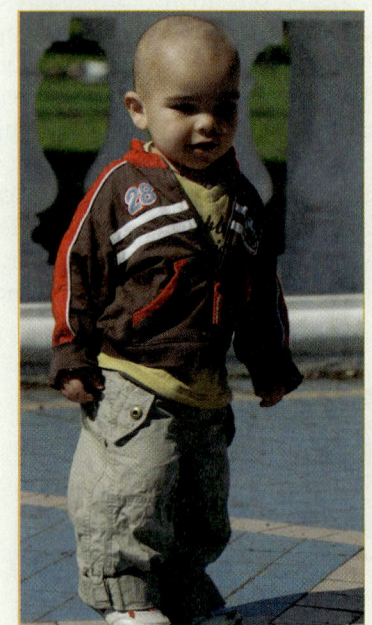

Figure 9-6 A toddler.

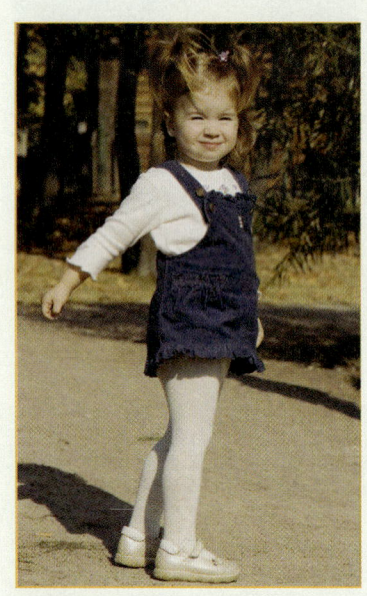

Figure 9-7 A preschooler.

more time around playmates and classmates, they acquire their own immunity as the body is exposed to various viruses and germs.

Neuromuscular growth also makes considerable progress at this age. Toddlers and preschoolers spend a great deal of time finding out exactly how to use their expansive nervous system and the muscles it controls by walking, running, jumping, and playing catch **Figure 9-8 ▶**. This stage also includes the continued development of the renal system and of elimination patterns (ie, toilet training).

Other developments that occur during this time frame include the emergence of "baby" teeth. Teething (ie, "breaking teeth" through the gums) can be painful and accompanied by fever. In addition, parents and toddlers are enthralled with sensory development—for example, tickling.

Psychosocial Changes

This period of development is often exciting for parents. The toddler or preschooler is learning to speak and express himself or herself, thereby taking a major step toward independence. By the age of 3 or 4 years,

At the Scene

With toddlers and preschoolers, you might try to "break the ice" by giving them a teddy bear and explaining what you are going to do by showing them on the teddy bear. Such children may be able to understand by show-and-tell more clearly than using only a verbal description.

most children can use and understand full sentences. As they progress through this stage of their life, they will go from using language to communicate what they want, to using language creatively and playfully.

This is also the time when toddlers begin to interact with other playmates and start to play games. Playing games teaches control, following of rules, and even competitiveness. A lot of learning and development takes place by the child watching his or

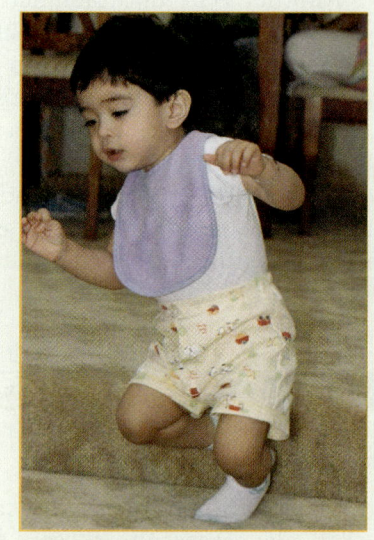

Figure 9-8 Toddlers learn to walk, one of the major milestones in life.

her peers during group outings, such as "play dates" with other children. Of course, behaviour observed on television and computers can also be learned, which is why some parents limit their children's viewing choices or the amount of time they devote to these activities. During this phase of development, children also learn to recognize sexual differences by observing their role models.

School-Age Children

Physical Changes

From ages 6 to 12 years, a school-age child's vital signs and body gradually approach those observed in adulthood **Figure 9-9 ▶**. Obvious physical traits and body function changes become apparent as most children grow about 2 kg and 6 cm each year. Their permanent teeth also come in during this period.

Psychosocial Changes

Children are engaged in a lot of psychosocial growing up during the school years. Parents as a whole do not devote as much time to their

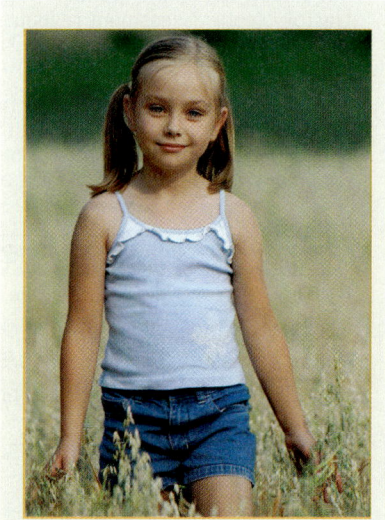

Figure 9-9 A school-age child.

children during this phase. Nevertheless, it is at this critical time in human development that children learn various types of reasoning. In preconventional reasoning, children act almost purely to avoid punishment and to get what they want. In conventional reasoning, they look for approval from their peers and society. In postconventional reasoning, children make decisions guided by their conscience.

During this stage, children begin to develop their self-concept and self-esteem. Self-concept is our perception of ourselves; self-esteem is how we feel about ourselves and how we "fit in" with our peers.

Adolescents (Teenagers)

Physical Changes

The vital signs of adolescents (ages 12 to 18 years Figure 9-10 ▾) begin to level off within the adult ranges, with a systolic blood pressure generally between 90 and 110 mm Hg, a pulse rate between 60 and 100 beats/min, and respirations in the range of 12 to 16 breaths/min. Adolescence is also the time of life when humans experience a growth spurt (ie, an increase in muscle and bone growth) and blood changes. As a whole, boys experience this stage of development later in life than girls do. When this period of growth has finished, however, boys are generally taller and stronger than girls.

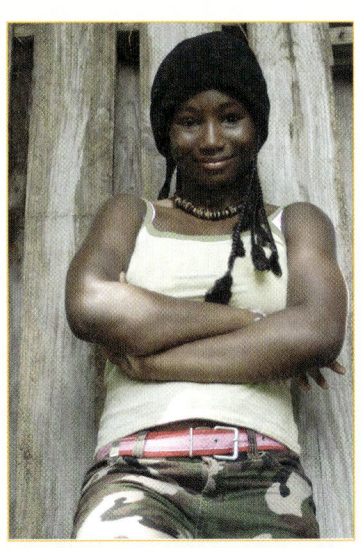

Figure 9-10 An adolescent.

One of the more subtle changes during this phase of life is the maturation of the human reproductive system. Secondary sexual development begins, along with enlargement of the external sex organs. Pubic hair and axillary hair begin to appear. Voices start to change in range and depth. In females, the breasts and thighs increase in size as adipose tissue is deposited there. Menstruation begins during this time; menarche is starting to occur at increasingly younger ages, however, so it is not uncommon to begin menstruation prior to becoming a teenager. Another key development in female teenagers is the release of follicle-stimulating hormone and luteinizing hormone, both of which increase estrogen and progesterone production. In contrast, the hormone gonadotropin is secreted in males and results in the production of testosterone. Acne can occur due to hormonal changes.

Psychosocial Changes

Adolescents and their families often deal with conflict as teenagers try to gain control of their lives from their parents. Privacy becomes an issue among adolescents, their siblings, and their parents. Adolescents may struggle to create their own identity—to define who they are Figure 9-11 ▾ . They may also show greater interest in sexual relations. Many adolescents

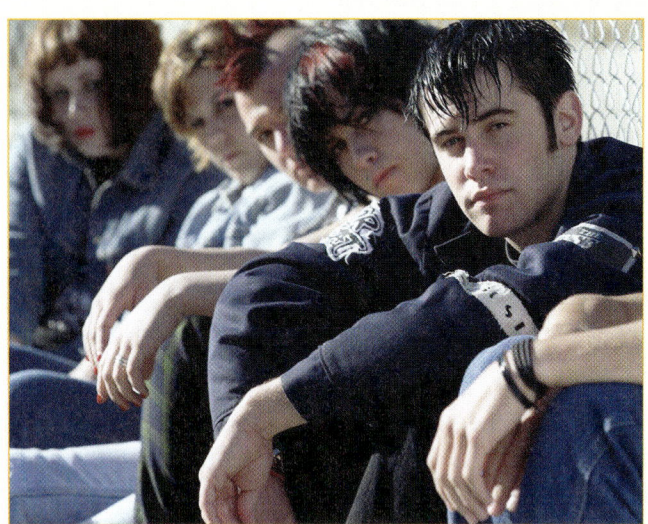

Figure 9-11 Adolescents want to fit in and may struggle to create an identity.

You are the Paramedic Part 3

You and your partner load your frightened patient into the back of your ambulance and begin the 20-minute transport to the local hospital. You asked the father to ride in the cab of the ambulance, telling him that he'd be safer there.

Once you are in the back of the ambulance, you ask the patient again about her sexual activity and the possibility of pregnancy, reminding her that it is important to her health that you know the truth. She confides in you that she is sexually active and that she missed taking a couple of her birth control pills in the past few months. She says, "I'm freaking out. I think I'm pregnant and my dad's going to kill me!" You try to calm the patient and continue to provide prehospital care, including the initiation of an IV line. At the hospital, you give your report to the emergency department nurse and your partner shows the patient's father to the waiting area.

7. What is your primary differential diagnosis now?

8. Did this diagnosis alter your care?

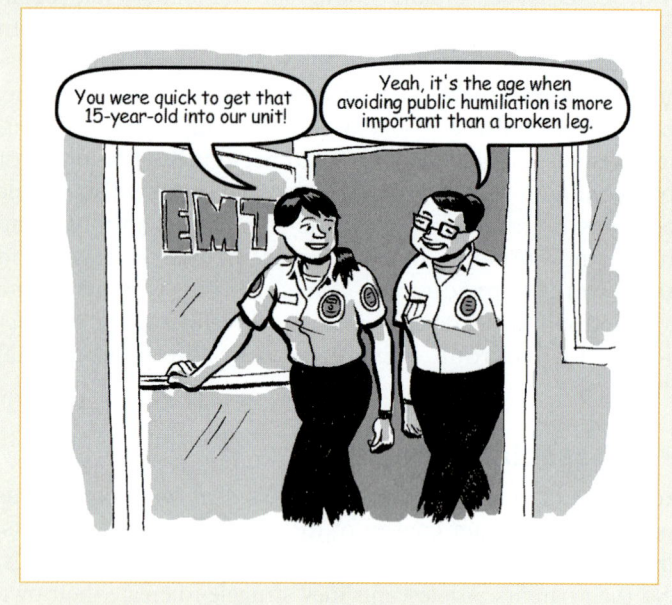

Figure 9-12

At the Scene

When you interview adolescents in the presence of their family, they may not tell you the complete truth so as to protect their privacy or image. It is best to ask these patients certain questions in total privacy, where they feel they can answer without constraint.

are fixated on their public image and are terrified of being embarrassed **Figure 9-12 ▲** . At this age, a code of personal ethics is developed, based partly on parents' ethics and values and partly on the influence of the teenager's environment. At this tumultuous time, teenagers are at a higher risk than other populations for suicide and depression.

Early Adults

Physical Changes

Early adults range in age from 19 to 40 years **Figure 9-13 ▶** . Their vital signs do not vary greatly from those seen throughout adulthood. Ideally, the human heart rate will stay around 70 beats/min, the respiratory rate will stay in the range of 12 to 20 breaths/min, and the systolic blood pressure will be approximately 120/80 mm Hg.

From age 19 years to just a little after 25 years, the human body should be functioning at its optimal level. After this point, the disks in the spine begin to settle, and height can sometimes be affected, causing a "shrinking." Fatty tissue increases, which leads to weight gain. Muscle strength

decreases, and the reflexes slow. For all these reasons, accidents are common causes of death in this age group.

Psychosocial Changes

Three words best describe a human's world during this stage of life: work, family, stress. During this period, humans strive to create a place for themselves in the world, and many do everything they can to "settle down." Along with this natural tendency to settle comes

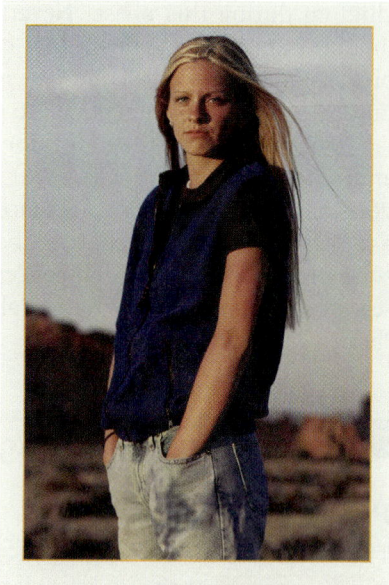

Figure 9-13 An early adult.

love and childbirth. Despite all of this stress and change, this age group enjoys one of the more stable periods of life.

Middle Adults

Physical Changes

Middle adults are ages 41 to 60 years **Figure 9-14 ▼** . This group is vulnerable to vision and hearing loss. Cardiovascular health also becomes an issue in many of these individuals, as does the greater incidence of cancer. In women, menopause— the cessation of menstruation—begins in the late 40s or early 50s.

Psychosocial Changes

Middle adults tend to focus on achieving their life's goals, as they realize that they are approaching the halfway point in human life expectancy. At this point, many parents must cope with becoming a married couple

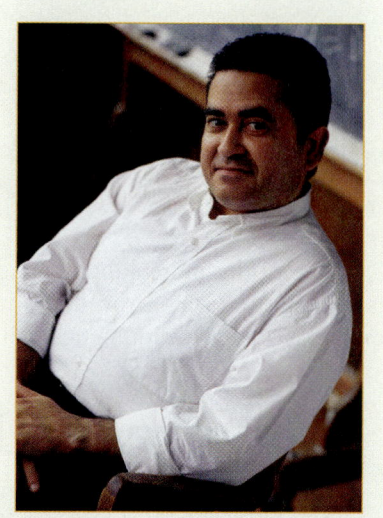

Figure 9-14 A middle adult.

again and reprioritize their lives as their children leave the home, creating "empty nest" syndrome. Finances may become a worrisome issue, as people look forward to retirement and experience small crisis moments. The term *mid-life crisis* describes a person who makes a dramatic gesture in a bid to

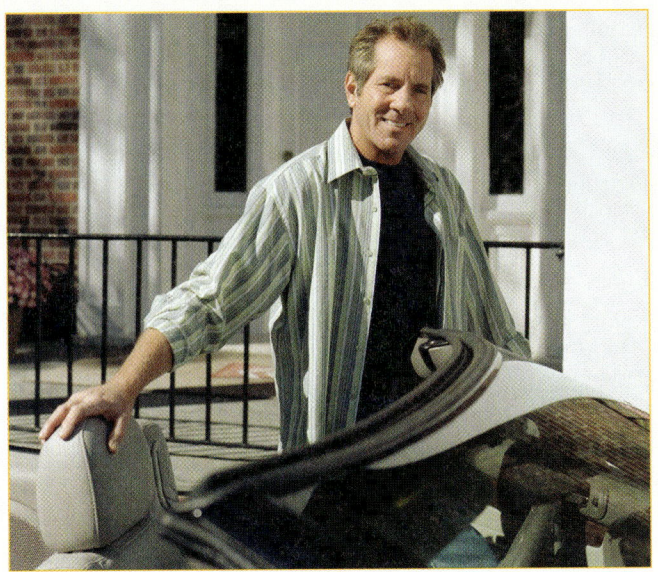

Figure 9-15 The classic example of the mid-life crisis is the middle-age man who buys a fancy, expensive sports car!

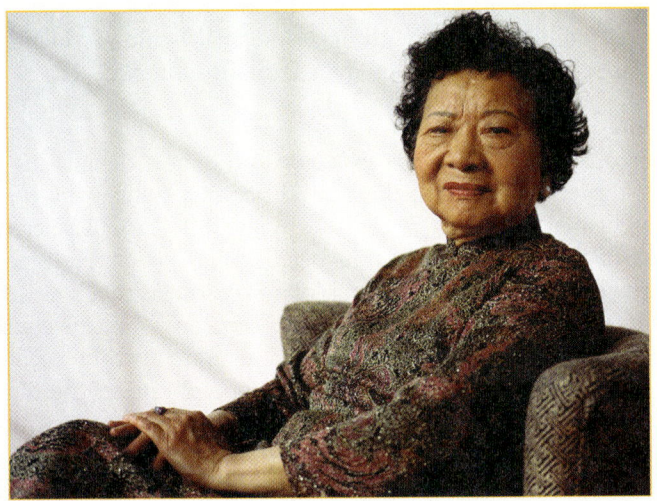

Figure 9-16 A late adult.

reclaim his or her youth. The classic example is the 45-year-old father of three who buys a bright red, two-seat convertible sports car Figure 9-15 ▲ .

Late Adults

Physical Changes

Late adults include those ages 61 and older Figure 9-16 ▲ . Life expectancy is constantly changing. When the first edition of this text was printed in 1979, life expectancy was about 75 years. It is approximately 80 years at this time, with maximum life expectancy estimated at 120 years.

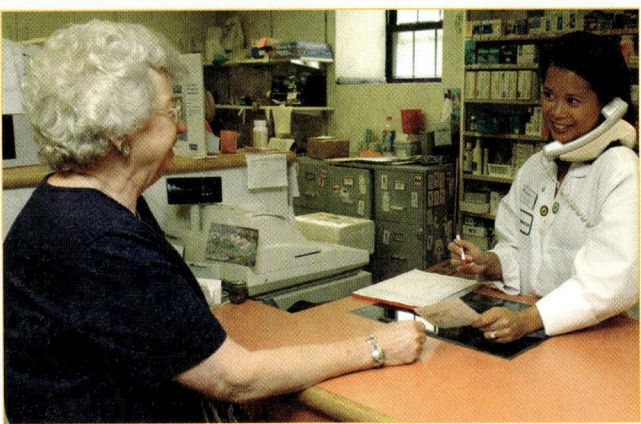

Figure 9-17 Older people are often on multiple medications to help them stay active.

Later in life, the vital signs depend on the patient's overall health, medical conditions, and medications taken. Today's late adults are staying active longer than their ancestors. Thanks to medical advances, they are often able to overcome numerous medical problems, but may need multiple medications to do so Figure 9-17 ▲ .

Cardiovascular System

Cardiac function declines with age consequent to anatomical and physiologic changes that are largely related to atherosclerosis. In this disorder, which most commonly affects coronary vessels, cholesterol and calcium build up inside the walls of blood vessels, forming plaque. The accumulation of plaque eventually leads to partial or complete blockage of blood flow. Atherosclerosis can also contribute to development of an aneurysm, or weakening and bulging of the blood vessel wall; an aneurysm may potentially rupture if it is subjected to high stretching forces. More than 60% of people older than age 65 have atherosclerotic disease.

Other age-related changes typically include a decrease in heart rate, a decline in cardiac output (the amount of blood circulated each minute), and the inability to elevate cardiac output to match the demands of the body. The vascular system also becomes stiff. For example, the pressure of systole increases with age. The left ventricle must then work harder, so it becomes thicker, losing its elasticity in this process. The thickening and stiffening of this muscle hinders filling in the ventricle, thereby decreasing cardiac output. Similar stiffening occurs in the heart valves, which may impede normal blood flow into and out of the heart. As the blood passes through these stiffened valves, a heart murmur may be heard, even in the absence of disease. Decreases in elastin and collagen in blood vessel walls, in turn, reduce the elasticity of the peripheral vessels by as much as 70%. Compensation for blood pressure changes will be hampered because these vessels are less able to distend and contract.

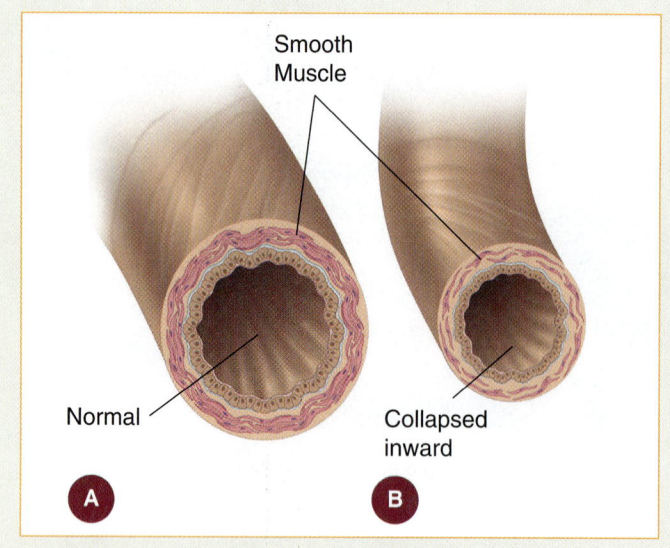

Figure 9-18 **A.** Healthy muscle in a younger patient's airway helps maintain the open airway during the pressures of inhalation. **B.** Muscle weakening with age can lead to airway collapse that may produce wheezing.

Respiratory System

In late adults, the size of the airway increases and the surface area of the alveoli decreases. The natural elasticity of the lungs also decreases, forcing them to use their intercostal muscles more to breathe. In addition, the chest becomes more rigid because of calcification of the ribs to the sternum, which adds to the difficulty of breathing.

The loss of the mechanisms that protect the upper airway can include a decreased ability to clear secretions as well as decreased cough and gag reflexes. The cilia that line the airways diminish with age, while the innervation of the structures in the airway provides increasingly less sensation. Without the ability to maintain the upper airway, aspiration and obstruction become more likely.

When a younger patient inhales, the airway maintains its shape, allowing air to enter. As the smooth muscles of the lower airway weaken with age, strong inhalation can make the walls of the airway collapse inward and cause inspiratory wheezing Figure 9-18 ▲. The collapsing airways result in low flow rates, because less air can move through the smaller airways, and air trapping, because air does not completely exit the alveoli (incomplete expiration).

By age 75 years, the vital capacity (the volume of air moved during the deepest inspiration and expiration) may amount to only 50% of the vital capacity noted in young adulthood. Factors contributing to this decline include loss of respiratory muscle mass, increased stiffness of the thoracic cage, and decreased surface area available for the exchange of air.

Physiologically, vital capacity decreases and residual volume (the amount of air left in the lungs after expiration of the maximum possible amount of air) increases with age. As a consequence, stagnant air remains in the alveoli and hampers gas exchange. This effect can produce hypercarbia (increased carbon dioxide in the bloodstream) and acidosis, even when the person is at rest.

Renal and Gastric Systems

In the kidneys, both structural and functional changes occur in the late adult. The filtration function of these organs, for example, declines by 50% between the ages of 20 and 90 years. Kidney mass decreases by 20% over the same span. The number of nephrons—the basic filtering units in the kidneys—also declines between the ages of 30 and 80 years. Aging kidneys respond less efficiently to hemodynamic stress (ie, stress relating to the circulation of blood) and to fluid and electrolyte imbalances.

Changes in gastric and intestinal function may inhibit nutritional intake and utilization in older adults. For example, taste bud sensitivity to salty and sweet sensations decreases. Saliva secretion decreases, which reduces the body's ability to process complex carbohydrates. Gastric motility slows with age because of the loss of intestinal tract neurons, which can lead older adults to feel constipated or not hungry. Likewise, gastric acid secretion diminishes. Blood flow in the mesenteries (membranes that connect organs to the abdominal wall) may drop by as much as 50%, decreasing the ability of the intestines to extract nutrients from digested food. Gallstones become increasingly common with age, and anal sphincter changes reduce elasticity and can produce fecal incontinence.

Nervous System

Nervous system changes can result in the most debilitating of age-related ailments. In the central nervous system, the brain weight may shrink 10% to 20% by age 80 years. A selective loss of 5% to 50% of neurons occurs, and the surviving neurons shrink in size. The frontal lobe may lose as much as 20% of its synapses (the junctions between neurons) over the course of a person's life. Motor and sensory neural networks become slower and less responsive. The metabolic rate in the older brain does not change, however, and oxygen consumption remains constant throughout life.

The brain, which is surrounded by the meninges, takes up almost all of the space in the skull. Cerebrospinal fluid protects the brain inside these membranes. Unfortunately, age-related shrinkage creates a void between the brain and the outermost layer of the meninges, which provides room for the brain to move when stressed. This shrinkage also stretches the bridging veins that return blood from inside the brain to the dura mater. If trauma moves the brain forcibly, the bridging veins can tear and bleed Figure 9-19 ▶. Bleeding can empty into this void, resulting in a subdural hematoma, which may go unnoticed for some time. Increased intracranial pressure is required for signs of head trauma to be present; the intracranial pressure will not rise—and, therefore, its signs will not be present—until the void has been filled and pressurized. (For more information, see Chapter 21.)

Functioning of the peripheral nervous system also slows with age. Sensation becomes diminished and misinterpreted. The resulting slowdown in reflexes may contribute to the incidence of trauma. Nerve endings deteriorate, and the ability of

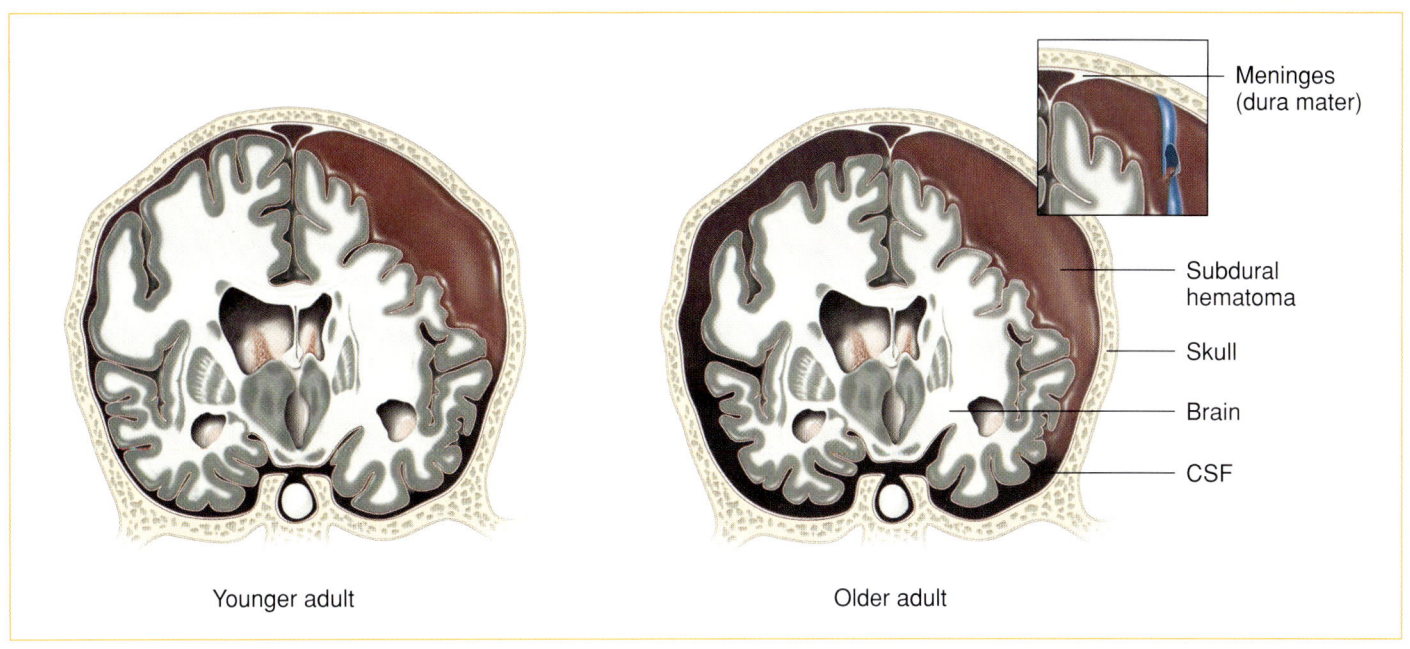

Younger adult   Older adult

Meninges
(dura mater)

Subdural
hematoma

Skull

Brain

CSF

Figure 9-19 Brain atrophy with age can make tearing of the bridging veins more likely with trauma. It may also create a space into which bleeding can occur without producing immediate signs of increased intracranial pressure.

the skin to sense the surroundings becomes hindered. Hot, cold, sharp, and wet items can all create dangerous situations because the body cannot sense them quickly enough.

Sensory Changes

Pupillary reaction and ocular movements become more restricted with age. The pupils are generally smaller in older patients, and the opacity of the eye's lens diminishes visual acuity and makes the pupils sluggish when responding to light. Visual distortions are also common in older people. Thickening of the lens makes it harder for the eye to focus, especially at close range. Peripheral fields of vision become narrower, and a greater sensitivity to glare constricts the visual field.

Hearing loss is about four times more common than loss of vision in late adults. Changes in several hearing-related structures may lead to a loss of high-frequency hearing, or even deafness.

Psychosocial Changes

Paramedics should treasure their opportunities to spend time with and communicate with late adults. Many of them have amazing stories and experiences to share with us, yet we often take them for granted. Our elderly share with us a great amount of wisdom, and we need to remind them of their self-worth. Indeed, until about 5 years before death, most late-stage adults retain high brain function. In the 5 years preceding death, however, mental function is presumed to decline, a theory referred to as the terminal drop hypothesis.

As the elderly population continues to grow, we have the responsibility to seek out unique ways to accommodate their needs during their last 20 to 40 years of life. While many older adults refuse to give up the independence of having their own home, the number of assisted-living communities is growing.

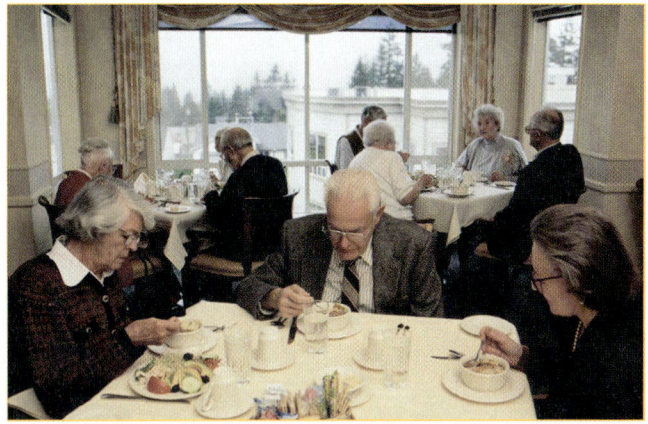

Figure 9-20 Many older adults live in assisted-living facilities.

These facilities allow older adults to live in campus-based communities with people in their own age group, while enjoying the privacy of their own apartment and the security of nursing care, maintenance, and food preparation, if desired **Figure 9-20 ▲**. Unfortunately, these facilities can be expensive.

Most people need to deal with financial issues throughout their lives. Few things in life produce more worry and stress than money problems. Late adults, in particular, may constantly worry about rising costs of health care and are often forced to make decisions such as whether to pay for groceries or their medication. Modern families often take less responsibility for their elderly family members than earlier generations did. Today, more than 50% of all single women in Canada who are 65 years of age or older are living at or below the poverty level. This problem remains to be resolved.

You are the Paramedic Summary

1. What are your differential diagnoses given the information provided?

Differential diagnoses should include, but are not limited to, ovarian cysts, influenza, gastroenteritis, appendicitis, pregnancy, ectopic pregnancy, hernia, menstrual cramps, abdominal aortic aneurysm, psychological emergency, and nephritis.

2. How would you approach your patient interview?

In approaching this patient, you need to remember that she is very much capable of being a woman in physical terms, but may still be a teenage girl at a social and emotional level. Treat her with respect and privacy.

3. What could explain the slightly elevated patient respirations and pulse?

A response to pain and/or anxiety can increase the pulse, blood pressure, and respirations.

4. What are your differential diagnoses now?

At this point, you cannot rule out any differential diagnosis. Nevertheless, you should maintain a high index of suspicion for ectopic pregnancy.

5. What is your next step in treatment of this patient?

The paramedic should initiate IV access and draw blood samples while keeping the patient in the best position for comfort and repeated reassessment of her condition.

6. Do you allow the parent to ride in the compartment of the ambulance along with the patient?

The parent should ride in the front seat of the ambulance on the way to the hospital for two very important reasons:

- The parent is safer when wearing a seatbelt in the passenger seat in the cab.
- With the parent in the front of the ambulance, he or she can still be near the child without being in range of the paramedic's voice. The paramedic can then ask the patient questions and ensure patient privacy while promoting forthright answers.

7. What is your primary differential diagnosis now?

Your primary diagnosis at this point should be to rule out ectopic pregnancy.

8. Did this diagnosis alter your prehospital care?

The possibility of ectopic pregnancy shouldn't alter your prehospital care, but it will better prepare you for transition of patient care at the hospital. You will also be able to provide better comfort for your extremely anxious patient.

Prep Kit

Ready for Review

- While each developmental stage is marked by different changes and characteristics, infants (1 month to 1 year) develop at a startling rate.
- The vital signs of toddlers (ages 1 to 3 years) and preschoolers (ages 3 to 6 years) differ somewhat from those of an infant.
- From ages 6 to 12 years, the school-age child's vital signs and body gradually approach those observed in adulthood.
- The vital signs of adolescents (ages 12 to 18 years) begin to level off within the adult ranges.
- Early adults are those who are age 19 to 40 years.
- Middle adults are those who are age 41 to 60 years.
- Late adults are those who are age 61 years and older.
- Vital signs do not vary greatly through adulthood.

Vital Vocabulary

adolescents Persons who are 12 to 18 years of age.

aneurysm A swelling or enlargement of part of a blood vessel, resulting from weakening of the vessel wall.

anxious avoidant attachment A bond between an infant and his or her parent or caregiver in which the infant is repeatedly rejected and develops an isolated lifestyle that does not depend upon the support and care of others.

atherosclerosis A disorder in which cholesterol and calcium build up inside the walls of the blood vessels, forming plaque, which eventually leads to partial or complete blockage of blood flow.

barotrauma Injury resulting from pressure disequilibrium across body surfaces, for example from too much pressure in the lungs.

bonding The formation of a close, personal relationship.

conventional reasoning A type of reasoning in which a child looks for approval from peers and society.

ductus arteriosus A duct that is present before birth that connects the pulmonary artery to the aorta in order to move unoxygenated blood back to the placenta.

ductus venosus A duct that is present before birth that connects the placenta to the heart in order to move oxygenated blood to the fetus.

early adults Persons who are 19 to 40 years of age.

fontanelles Areas where the infant's skull has not fused together; usually disappear at approximately 18 months of age.

foramen ovale An opening in the septum of the heart before birth, and which closes after birth.

growth plates Structures located on either end of an infant's bone, which aid in lengthening bones as the child grows.

hypercarbia Increased carbon dioxide levels in the bloodstream.

infants Persons who are from 1 month to 1 year of age.

late adults Persons who are 61 years old or older.

life expectancy The average amount of years a person can be expected to live.

mesenteries The membranes that connect organs to the abdominal wall.

middle adults Persons who are 41 to 60 years of age.

moro reflex An infant reflex in which, when an infant is caught off guard, the infant opens his or her arms wide, spreads the fingers, and seems to grab at things.

nephrons The basic filtering units in the kidneys.

palmar grasp An infant reflex that occurs when something is placed in the infant's palm; the infant grasps the object.

postconventional reasoning A type of reasoning in which a child bases decisions upon his or her conscience.

preconventional reasoning A type of reasoning in which a child acts almost purely to avoid punishment to get what he or she wants.

preschoolers Persons who are 3 to 6 years of age.

rooting reflex An infant reflex that occurs when something touches an infant's cheek, and the infant instinctively turns his or her head toward the touch.

school age A person who is 6 to 12 years of age.

secure attachment A bond between an infant and his or her parent or caregiver, in which the infant understands that the parents or caregivers will be responsive to his or her needs and take care of him or her when help is needed.

sucking reflex An infant reflex in which the infant starts sucking when his or her lips are stroked.

terminal drop hypothesis The theory that a person's mental function declines in the last 5 years of life.

toddlers Persons who are 1 to 3 years of age.

transposition Congenital abnormality where the aorta and pulmonary artery positions on the heart are reversed.

trust and mistrust A phrase that refers to a stage of development from birth to approximately 18 months of age, during which infants gain trust of their parents or caregivers if their world is planned, organized, and routine.

www.Paramedic.EMSzone.com/Canada

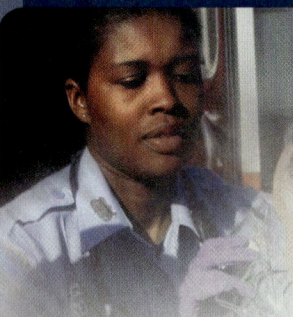

Assessment in Action

Your unit has arrived on the scene of a motor vehicle collision in which a minivan has rear-ended another vehicle at a fairly low speed. The minivan's airbag did not deploy. Inside the minivan you have four patients. The driver of the vehicle is a 38-year-old woman who was wearing a seatbelt. In the passenger seat is a 70-year-old woman who was also wearing a seatbelt. In the back seat are an infant who is restrained in a car seat and a toddler who has freed himself from his car booster seat.

1. **Which of your patients will be most prone to having airway occlusion problems?**
   A. Infant
   B. Adolescent
   C. Early adult
   D. Late adult

2. **When you assess the infant's vital signs, what should a normal respiratory rate be?**
   A. 12 to 20 breaths/min
   B. 18 to 24 breaths/min
   C. 30 to 60 breaths/min
   D. 26 to 40 breaths/min

3. **When you assess the infant's respiratory rate, you notice that the infant's chest is not moving but his abdomen is moving with his respirations. Is this a normal finding?**
   A. No, there is obviously an injury to the infant's chest.
   B. No, loosen the car seat straps and see if that makes a difference.
   C. No, remove the infant from the car seat immediately.
   D. Yes, infants are normally "belly breathers."

4. **The toddler in the vehicle is withdrawing from your attempts at a hands-on assessment. How will you continue to assess this toddler?**
   A. Reason with him.
   B. Explain what you want to do.
   C. Show the child what you are going to do using a prop.
   D. Let a family member continue the assessment.

5. **When doing your assessment on the 70-year-old patient, you attempt to check the pulse, motor function, and sensation on her lower extremities. The pulse is very hard to locate, and sensation appears to be nonexistent. You see no signs of trauma to the patient's lower extremities. To what source can you attribute this loss of sensation?**
   A. Peripheral nerve function slows with aging.
   B. You must be missing a traumatic injury.
   C. There is no change to nerve function but there is with circulation.
   D. The patient is cold and does not adjust well.

6. **The female patient in the driver's seat is approximately 38 years old. What would you expect her normal vital signs to be if she had not been involved in this accident?**
   A. P = 70, R = 30, BP = 180/90
   B. P = 70, R = 16, BP = 120/80
   C. P = 100, R = 30, BP = 180/90
   D. P = 100, R = 16, BP = 120/80

Challenging Question

You have notified your dispatcher that you will need a second ambulance to respond to this location due to the number of patients. All of the patients appear to have nonemergent injuries, which allows you to choose which patients will travel together.

7. **How will you use your knowledge of human development to make this decision?**

Points to Ponder

You are about to transport a toddler to the hospital for a minor laceration that will need a few stitches. The toddler will not lie down on the stretcher and fights your attempts to calm him down. The mother of the child is willing to ride with you to the hospital.

Where will you have her ride—in the front passenger seat or in the treatment compartment in visual contact with the child?

Issues: Physical and Psychological Changes in Human Development, Stranger Anxiety.

10 Patient Communication

Competency Areas

Area 1: Professional Responsibilities

1.1.b Reflect professionalism through use of appropriate language.

1.1.d Maintain appropriate personal interaction with patients.

1.1.e Maintain patient confidentiality.

1.1.j Behave ethically.

1.1.k Function as patient advocate.

1.3.b Recognize "patient rights" and the implications on the role of the provider.

Area 2: Communication

2.1.d Provide information to patient about their situation and how they will be treated.

2.1.e Interact effectively with the patient, relatives, and bystanders who are in stressful situations.

2.1.f Speak in language appropriate to the listener.

2.1.g Use appropriate terminology.

2.3.a Exhibit effective non-verbal behaviour.

2.3.b Practice active listening techniques.

2.3.c Establish trust and rapport with patients and colleagues.

2.3.d Recognize and react appropriately to non-verbal behaviours.

2.4.a Treat others with respect.

2.4.b Exhibit empathy and compassion while providing care.

2.4.c Recognize and react appropriately to individuals and groups manifesting coping mechanisms.

2.4.d Act in a confident manner.

2.4.e Act assertively as required.

2.4.f Manage and provide support to patients, bystanders, and relatives manifesting emotional reactions.

2.4.g Exhibit diplomacy, tact, and discretion.

2.4.h Exhibit conflict resolution skills.

Introduction

The scenario with the Kellars in *You are the Paramedic Part 1* illustrates the importance of something we all need to remember throughout our careers. However well-intentioned we may be, some paramedics see people not as people, but as their medical problems. That's a shallow approach to emergency medicine in the prehospital environment. It always begins with something else that's hard to teach, and which most of us never hear much about. The following pages are intended to guide you through the art and skills of communicating with people on the worst days of their lives.

People are not just medical puzzles for you to solve, and they're certainly not just nuisances or interruptions. They're the reason paramedics exist. And they deserve your best efforts at service—what that "S" in EMS stands for.

Being a good paramedic requires a major talent for multi-tasking. When you're kneeling in front of Mr. Kellar, who is sitting there on his couch and denying his symptoms, you should also be aware that Mrs. Kellar, seated right there next to him, is scared to death that she could lose him. More than that, you have to *feel* something for both of them. These are abilities you would not expect to find, and probably wouldn't need, in most other jobs. These abilities are the gifts of caregivers.

Internal Factors for Effective Communication

You need to be able to *naturally like people* (which is difficult for some people). You don't have to like them all, and you don't have to like them every day. But liking them has to be real for you, and it has to come easily. Why? Because when they defecate in your ambulance, vomit on your shoes, or bleed all over your clean uniform, you have to be able to tolerate that

without so much as a syllable of protest. These events are all part of a paramedic's job.

This chapter is based on the presumption that you like people, you care about them, and you honestly want to serve them. You'd better. Because if you don't, they will pick up your true feelings and poor attitude in the blink of an eye—and so will their families. And if you don't like people, you're pretty much guaranteed to hate doing what paramedics do every day: serving people, in their own time and on their own terms. As a paramedic you may see people looking their worst. They may smell like urine, vomit, digested blood, stale perspiration, feces, or worse. But that's how real people really are, especially when they're sick. If you expect anything else, the mistake will be all yours and your patients will pay for it in the marginal prehospital care they may get from you. And you'll pay for it by having a really short career.

At least half of the calls you will run as a paramedic will take you into people's homes, day and night and in the most private moments of their lives. Try to see every invitation into the home of someone else as a personal honour in a time and place where no one else would be welcome **Figure 10-1 ▶**. You will be there when a lot of people are born, and you will be there when a lot of people die. In many cultures, people believe that God is present in times like these. Whether you subscribe to that belief or not, try hard to sense the privilege of being invited. It can make your career a lasting and fulfilling experience, instead of a source of drudgery.

External Factors for Effective Communication

A paramedic who looks the part of a professional inspires a lot more confidence in patients, in family members, and in the public than one who pays no attention to his or her appearance

You are the Paramedic Part 1

Mary and Bill Kellar have been married for 44 years. Their four children have all moved away, and the two of them share a quiet suburban home in Ontario. Late one evening while watching TV, Mary notices that one side of her husband's face appears flaccid. When she asks him if he is all right, he says he's fine, but his words are slurred and difficult to understand. She waits only a few more minutes before announcing that she is going to call for help, and she dials 9-1-1 despite his protests. The paramedics who arrive a few minutes later are obviously tired from previous calls.

Initial Assessment	Recording Time: 0 Minutes
Appearance	Flaccid and weak muscles on left side of patient's face
Level of consciousness	A (Alert to person, place, and day)
Airway	Open
Breathing	Normal rate; adequate depth
Circulation	Radial pulse present

1. What communication difficulties do you immediately anticipate in this scenario?

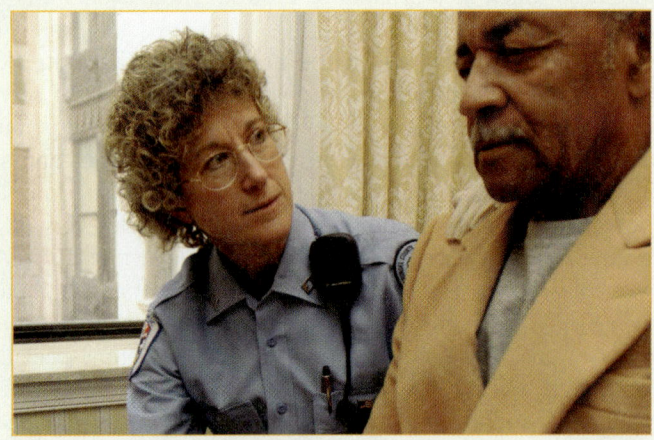

Figure 10-1 Think of it as an honour to be asked into a patient's home. Be respectful, and always be kind.

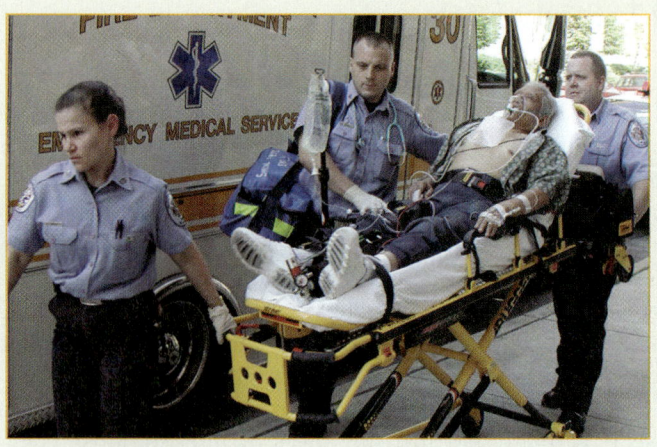

Figure 10-2 One way to comfort patients is to look as though you can help them, to look in charge. Be sure that your uniform is clean and that your shoes are clean, in good shape, and polished.

Figure 10-2 ▶ . You've heard this in other chapters but listen to this advice once again: polish your leather shoes and iron your shirt before you show up for work. Make it easy for others to read your first name and at least your last initial, as well as your level of certification. Learn the principles of professional etiquette, and make sure your overall behaviour inspires respect in people you don't know. That's more than making nice; it's what a professional does.

At the Scene

Patients will pick up on how you treat or are treated by other paramedics at the scene. If you are treated with respect, and if you treat the other paramedics with respect, the patient will see this and have more confidence in you as well.

If you want people to tell you about their problems, convince them you want to hear what they have to say. Communication is the act of transmitting information to another person—and, for paramedics, it can be verbal or through body language. Give patients your undivided attention; don't treat them like nuisances. There's nothing worse than talking about someone in his or her presence, as though he or she is an inanimate object—or worse, as though the person doesn't even exist. And it's unforgivable to ask someone a question you're just going to repeat later because you didn't pay attention to the answer the first time. Jot it down. When it's time to communicate, *communicate*. That means listen, don't just talk. Listening is part of communicating too, because it transmits information as well.

An excellent way to convince someone that you're really listening to him or her is a technique called "active listening." Almost all professional interviewers use it routinely. Active listening is repeating the key parts of a patient's responses to

You are the Paramedic Part 2

Mary gets the impression from the paramedics' demeanour that they would prefer to be somewhere else. Twice she asks them what they think is happening to Bill, but they don't reply. Instead, they focus on applying oxygen, starting an IV, attaching electrodes, and performing various other skills and assessments. They don't talk to the patient except to ask questions, and they don't seem to appreciate or address the fact that Mary is terrified.

Vital Signs	Recording Time: 3 Minutes
Skin	Pale and cool; perspiring
Pulse	88 beats/min, irregular
Blood pressure	184/94 mm Hg
Respirations	18 breaths/min
SpO_2	97% on 15 l/min via nonrebreathing mask

2. Describe what the phrase "total patient care" means to you.

questions. Especially when you're taking notes at the same time, it helps you to convince patients that you really want to hear what they're saying. Active listening also helps confirm the information patients are providing. This ensures there is no misunderstanding between you and your patients.

Some specific expressions that are helpful are:

- When patients thank you, say, "You're very welcome!" (not "No problem." "No problem" implies, "That's OK; you aren't too much of a nuisance." It's definitely not as nice as saying, "You're welcome.")
- When patients apologize to you because they're incontinent or vomiting or because you have to carry them down a flight of stairs, tell them something like, "It's OK; you don't need to be sorry. This is what we do, *and we're here because we want to be.*"

If you like serving people, these kinds of expressions will feel natural to you, and no doubt you will find your colleagues imitating you after only a short time.

Try hard not to shout. Some scenes are very noisy. But even so, when you shout, so does everyone else. And when people are shouting, they tend to get excited. If you're answering a call in a noisy place such as a bar, ask the bartender to help by turning off the music, turning up the lights, and keeping an eye on the other patrons. (In this type of situation, get your patient out of there as soon as you can.) Move the patient to your "office"—the back of the ambulance. If you must use a compressor or run a noisy diesel on the scene, shut it off as soon as you can to cut down on the noise level. Meanwhile, try to talk close to your patient's ears in a calm voice. It lets him or her know that you have your emotions under control, which helps him or her stay calm as well. Try managing your history-taking all at one time. Taking the patient's medical and health history helps you stay organized and encourages people to take your questions seriously.

If you want reliable answers to personal questions, try to manage your scene so you can ask these kinds of questions quietly and in private. Even if you do earn a patient's trust, there are things people just don't want to talk about in front of others. Don't forget to ask a few payoff questions—questions that don't fall under the category of routine medical history but that, time after time, will net you information that's critical to a presumptive diagnosis. Some payoff questions are listed and explained later in this chapter.

Some scenes are easy to manage. But paramedics very often work in bizarre, noisy, chaotic, and sometimes dangerous environments that are challenging at best **Figure 10-3 ▶**. Under these circumstances, communicating with patients (and their family members) is especially critical to the skills of assessment and the art of bringing about calm (and therefore healing).

Developing Rapport

When you find yourself standing at someone's bedside in the middle of the night, if you really don't want to be there, if you

Special Considerations

Do not assume that all elderly patients are hard of hearing. You will be put in your place if you begin by talking loudly or too slowly to an older patient only to be told by the patient, "I'm not deaf."

really don't care how he or she feels, and if you just want to get back to bed, he or she will get the message, *whether you intended to send it or not*. Nothing you pretend, say, or do will fool your patient. If you really *do* want to be there, you really *do* care, and you really *don't* mind being awakened, your patient will get that message too.

People in crisis are highly perceptive, and there is no greater crisis than being scared to death that you're about to lose someone you love more than anyone in the whole world.

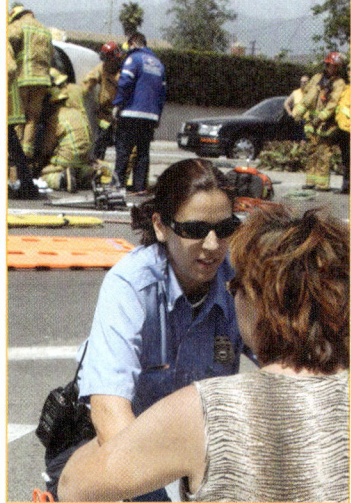

Figure 10-3 Even in the most chaotic conditions, try to create a safe zone for your patient. Shut out everything else the best you can, and focus on helping this one person.

Your most essential challenge as a therapeutic communicator is to convey calm, unmistakable, genuine concern for someone you've never met. People in crisis do much better if someone like you can relieve their fear and help them to harness their own internal healing power.

Watch Your Inflection

Your voice is just as important in communication as your words. You know what someone's voice sounds like when he or she is really concerned for you. Think about how the voice of someone who cares for you sounds when you are hurt or upset. Use that calm and steady tone of reassurance to reinforce your interest in and concern for the patient.

Respond to the Patient

There is probably nothing as insulting to a patient as asking or telling a caregiver something and receiving no response at all. Regardless of what the patient says, acknowledge what he or she said. If you are not comfortable responding, simply nod or restate what the patient said, without providing a definitive answer right away. If you later figure out how you can give more information, you may tell the patient at that point.

Tell People Who You Are

Once you break that initial ice with someone, tell him or her who you are. That's just common courtesy, but it is often overlooked by medical professionals. Tell them something more too. Tell them you're a paramedic. Remember, they're about to entrust their privacy and their medical well-being to someone they didn't know a moment ago. They deserve to know what you know (and what you don't). By introducing yourself, you are also saying, "You are, no matter what the indignities of treatment, in charge of your health care, and you can communicate with me as an equal."

Use the Patient's Name

Most of us use the same few words to greet our patients, both in the prehospital environment and in the hospital: "Hi. What's the problem?" That's OK for an amateur, but it doesn't say much for a professional. Why? Because people's names are important to them and to their families. Your name is the first thing you receive after birth, and it's the only thing you keep when you die (think about every gravestone you've ever seen). As a caregiver, use the importance of a person's name like a tool.

Don't just start your patient contact with a question about the medical problem. Introduce yourself, and then ask patients their name. That simple practice tells them their discomfort is important, but it also opens a window through which you can quickly assess a lot. Think about that for a few moments.

When you address patients with an expression like, "Hi. My name is Lee Jones and I'm a paramedic. What's your name?" what do they have to be able to do in order to answer appropriately? They have to go through a very specific sequence of physical and mental processes, which amounts to a mini-mental status examination. Consider the following:

- They have to hear your words.
- They have to locate the source of your voice and meet your gaze.
- They have to process the meaning of your words (in your common language).
- They have to formulate a meaningful, accurate response from memory.
- They have to put their response into coherent speech.
- They have to be able to do all of that within about 1 second.

During that second, if you're close enough to see the size of their pupils, you can assess their mental state and the function of at least six pairs of cranial nerves. That's a fair amount of assessment.

In addition, you've communicated something very important to the patient and his or her family just by asking that question—your respect. Part of your respectful behaviour is to introduce yourself with your full name and your profession. You've told him or her (and family members), "Mr. or Mrs. Edwards, you may be about to lose your dignity and possibly your shorts, but you're going to be able to keep your name." Finally, using the names of people is good for us and for our colleagues. It reminds us that we're not just dealing with broken brains and broken livers and broken hearts day after day. Instead, we're dealing with *people*. It also lets the patient establish the level of formality they are comfortable with. If they say, "You can call me Joey," then do so, but if they say, "I am Mr. Jones," do not call them Joey, Buddy, or any other pet name.

Anticipate and Deal With Fear

Usually, after a few weeks of ambulance calls, you will be impressed with the fact that most patients are scared to death of the situation. If the patient isn't afraid, consider that one or more of his or her loved ones may be absolutely terrified Figure 10-4 ▶ . Reassurance may be one of the most important treatments you can provide.

You are the Paramedic Part 3

As the paramedics assess Mr. Kellar, his wife hears them casually discussing the likelihood of stroke. This is her worst nightmare, because their physician had warned Bill about the risks of his high blood pressure and high cholesterol. After repeated attempts to communicate with the paramedics have failed, she becomes so frustrated that she screams, "Why do you keep ignoring me?"

Reassessment	Recording Time: 7 Minutes
Level of consciousness	A (Alert to person, place, and day)
Skin	Pale and cool; perspiring
Pulse	88 beats/min, irregular
Blood pressure	184/98 mm Hg
Respirations	18 breaths/min
SpO_2	96% on 15 l/min via nonrebreathing mask
ECG	Atrial fibrillation

3. Although the paramedics in this scenario are attending to the patient's medical needs, could the wife have a valid complaint regarding their caregiving?

4. How can your introductions (or lack thereof) and general demeanour affect your ability to communicate with your patients as well as with their friends and family members?

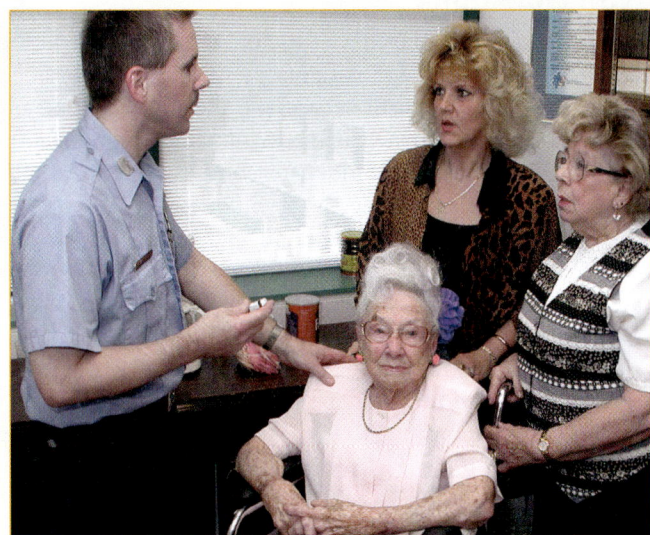

Figure 10-4 As soon as possible, you or your partner should explain to the patient's family members what is happening and what they can do. This information can help them deal with their fear and worry.

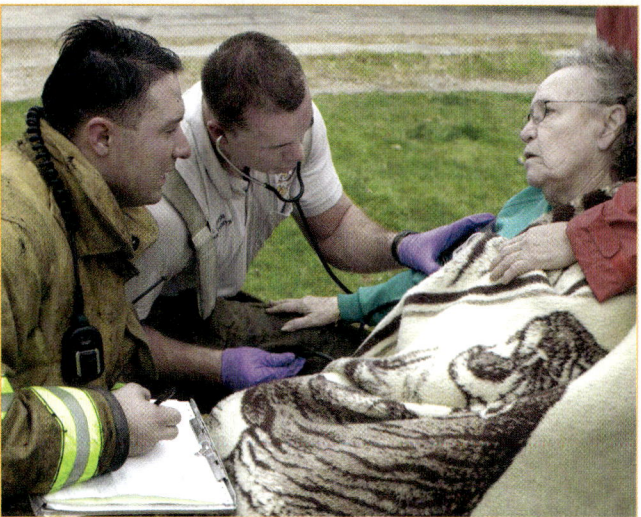

Figure 10-5 Show your patient the same respect you'd want others to show your father or brother or your mother or sister. Protect modesty with a blanket or towel.

How do you control fear? First, by your own sense of competence and professional calm. Second, by honestly caring about someone (a fact that, like kindness, patients and family members alike can easily detect). Third, by giving people information. When someone wakes up in the middle of the night with a dull, crushing chest pain, that person doesn't want to be treated like a child or someone who cannot understand what is happening. Tell your patients what you think is happening. Show patients what their ECG reveals, tell them their blood pressure, explain how you're planning to make them better, and let them know how they're doing. There is no better way to harness a patient's own power to self-heal, nor is there a better way to harness the healing power of loved ones, while at the same time stabilizing their emotions.

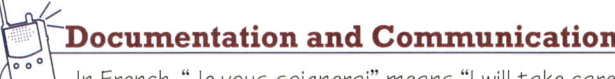

Documentation and Communication

In French, "Je vous soignerai" means "I will take care of you."

Respect the Importance of Pain

When someone tells you he or she is in pain, let that person know you grasp and appreciate the situation, and then do something about it. One of the most grievous offenses by caregivers (in and out of hospitals) is ignoring pain. People deserve to have their pain relieved as completely as possible, then and there—with a medical consultation if necessary. Don't make them wait. You wouldn't want your loved ones to wait for pain relief. A patient should never have to be patient about any pain you can alleviate, whether in the prehospital environment or in the hospital.

Respect and Protect People's Modesty

Modesty matters—no matter how acute the medical condition. It's especially important to the very old, adolescents, and sometimes, the very young. If the patient is not personally sensitive to modesty (because of an impaired mental state, for example), family members most certainly are **Figure 10-5 ▲**.

Help, Don't Judge

When you become a paramedic, you will need to know a person's medical history in order to help him or her. For example, you will need to use naloxone to treat an opiate addict. Sadly, drug and alcohol addicts support their addictions by lying. Few addicts will admit to drinking more than two beers, let alone to taking an opiate. Here's where your own moral code has to take a backseat to professional ethics. Try to avoid judging patients because the causes of addiction can be very complex. We can't pretend to know why people make the choices they make; we, as health care providers, see only the results of these choices.

When you ask someone an uncomplicated question using plain, simple language, and he or she responds with an unnecessarily complicated or inappropriate response, one of the things you should probably consider is the possibility that the patient is lying. Of course, that's not always true. Also, one of the most common strategies people develop to cope with stress is lying. Plenty of people who are not addicted lie, too. Patients may also be mentally impaired (by chemicals, hypoxia, psychiatric disorders, or other causes of disorganized thinking). But lying does happen often enough, so you should anticipate it.

Whatever you do, don't appoint yourself judge. Instead, merely consider this individual a poor historian and move on with your interview. One of the things that can happen to you over time if you allow yourself to judge people is that you can become cynical. Professional skepticism is a useful tool; it facilitates sound, clinical decision-making. But cynicism is skepticism gone wild and is unproductive to you and your patients.

Conducting the Interview

The reason we question people is to find out how they're feeling, what happened that may have made them sick or hurt them, and what their lives have been like. But to quote the old expression about computers: "Garbage in, garbage out." If we're not careful about what questions we ask, we may not obtain the information we need. Following are three techniques that can make your questioning more productive.

Open-Ended Questions

When you need to know how someone feels, first try asking a question that makes the patient do the thinking. This is an open-ended question—a question that does not have a yes or no answer, and which does not give the patient specific options to choose from. For instance, if you ask patients to describe their own chest pain, don't suggest qualities like sharpness, dullness, or pressure. Instead, let them think of a word that describes how the pain feels; their own words will probably more accurately describe what they are feeling. Some examples of open-ended questions are:

- How have you been feeling lately?
- Do you have an idea of what is causing this?
- Do you have any other concerns about your health?
- Is there anything else you would like to discuss?

Closed-Ended Questions

Sometimes (for example, when you're trying to find out about a patient's medical history) you need answers to specific questions. In these cases, try a direct, or closed-ended question. In fact, it's a good idea to develop a standard set of questions concerning medical history that you ask almost all patients. Avoid talking down to them (that's insulting), but avoid using medical terms. Instead, try using words that people without medical training can understand. Your standard questions may include the following:

- Have you ever had any heart problems?
- Any lung problems?
- Any high or low blood pressure?
- Diabetes?
- Seizures?
- Fainting spells?
- Any prior head injury?
- Do you have both lungs and both kidneys?

If the patient is female and of childbearing age (generally, 12 to 50 years old), be sure to ask about her history of pregnancies, deliveries, and abortions, when her last menstrual period was and if it was normal, and if she has had any gynecologic surgeries.

Payoff Questions

Most seasoned paramedics have developed their own repertoire of additional questions for patients in specific circumstances. We call them payoff questions because they're like icebergs—tiny questions that can reveal huge subsurface issues. Sometimes these issues are the hidden reason we've been called to help someone. Some examples of payoff questions are:

- Have you ever felt like this before?
- Have you been upset about anything lately?
- Are you afraid of someone? (Save this one for the privacy of the ambulance.)
- Have you been thinking about hurting yourself?
- What happened the last time you felt this way?

Strategies to Elicit Useful Responses to Questions

To get the right answers, it's not always enough just to ask the right questions. Why? Because when people are in crisis, some of them are terrible communicators. It can be almost impossible to think and organize your thoughts when you are terrified. Fortunately, good interviewers also have the following tools to use to get answers.

Facilitate the Response

If patients hesitate to answer questions completely, encourage them to provide you with more information. One useful expression is simply, "Please say more." Another is, "Please feel welcome to tell me about that."

Be Quiet

If you sense that patients are trying to put something into words but are having trouble expressing themselves, try this famous tip "Never miss a good opportunity to shut up." Be patient. Don't say anything at all for a few seconds. Let them talk.

Documentation and Communication

If you must stop patients from talking to get an urgent task done, explain to them why they need to be quiet and that they will be able to talk to you when you finish your task.

Clarify the Response

If you don't understand what patients have told you, ask them to explain what they mean. This communicates that you are listening and taking their comments seriously. It may also help you understand what they are trying to tell you.

Redirect the Response

Sometimes patients will mention something in passing or will avoid answering a specific question. You can politely redirect their attention to that question (several times, if necessary) until you get them to answer it.

Interpret the Response

If you've tried clarification and you're still not sure what patients are trying to tell you, sometimes it helps to vocalise what you think they've said and invite them to correct you.

Simplify and Summarize the Response

Some patients have a hard time speaking plainly, no matter how hard they try. It can be difficult to communicate with people who have psychiatric problems, who fabricate their diseases, and who are afraid or upset. If patients give you a confusing or disorganized response, try putting their comments into simpler terms and see if they agree with your synopsis. It can help them focus their thoughts and help you as an interviewer.

■ Common Interviewing Errors

None of us is perfect, and all of us have made errors in the course of questioning patients. Learn to improve your interviewing skills by observing what other paramedics have done:

Assume Nothing!

Most mistakes caregivers make have happened as the result of assuming things. Assuming that a patient is faking unconsciousness or seizures, assuming that a companion is a spouse, assuming that a fight victim is a member of a gang, or assuming that a patient is inebriated are very common mistakes. Try hard to become a careful observer and to keep your mind open to a wide range of possibilities. Remember that when we assume, sometimes it makes an "ass" out of "u" and "me."

Giving Medical Advice

Patients and their families often ask their paramedics for medical advice, in much the same way as they would consult a physician. That's an honour, because it conveys their trust. Patients may even ask you to comment on a decision by their physician. Don't fall for that one (however well-intentioned the question may be). Instead, suggest they obtain their medical advice from a doctor.

Providing False Hope

Try not to overencourage patients or their family members if a patient is very ill. You can't possibly see in advance what's going to happen to someone. But remember that the question, "Am I going to die?" is a lot different than the statement, "I think I'm going to die." Lots of patients whose status seems very stable will ask you if they're going to die. A good answer to that one is, "Some day—but you look pretty good to us today." Another option is "I don't know, but I sure hope not. What do you think?" As for the latter case, patients who look you right in the eye and tell you they feel they're going to die are probably right. People in cardiogenic shock or who have end-stage chronic obstructive pulmonary disease do that with uncanny regularity. Invite their family members to give them a kiss before taking them to the emergency department. It may be their last opportunity, and they will treasure that memory forever.

If the patient or a family member asks you if the patient is going to die, and the patient is not in stable condition, you could say, "We think he (or she) is very sick, but we're doing everything we possibly can to help."

Assuming Excessive Authority

Just as we're not qualified to judge people, it's important to remember that we're not police officers either. Adopting the no-nonsense demeanour of a law officer can frighten your patient, and make your job of caring for that patient nearly impossible. (How do *you* feel when you are pulled over, even for expired tags, by a law officer?)

You are the Paramedic Part 4

Upon seeing his wife so distraught, Mr. Kellar becomes upset as well. He tries to explain that she has recently had a heart attack, but his words are garbled and the paramedics are unable to understand him, in spite of his best efforts, so his message goes undelivered.

Reassessment	Recording Time: 10 Minutes
Level of consciousness	A (Alert to person, place, and day)
Skin	Pale, cool, and moist
Pulse	98 beats/min, irregular
Blood pressure	190/104 mm Hg
Respirations	18 breaths/min
Spo$_2$	96% on 15 l/min via nonrebreathing mask
ECG	Atrial fibrillation
Blood glucose	5.5 mmol/l

5. How has this crew's lack of people skills affected this call?

6. Can this situation be mended?

Sidestepping the Truth

Patients deserve to know what their blood pressure is and what their ECG reveals about them. Their blood sugar (blood glucose level) isn't a secret you need to keep from them, nor is your presumptive diagnosis. When patients ask you what you think is wrong, remember that you're serving them. Remind them that you don't have definitive answers and that you're not a physician, but tell them what you think may be going on. Be honest and sincere about what you're telling them, but never harsh.

Distancing Yourself From Patients as People

Another Western medical technique for maintaining the relationship between physicians and patients is professional distancing—that is, avoiding contact with patients as people. This can take the form of using lots of big, complicated medical words you hope they won't understand, and answering patients' questions with half-truths. No matter who uses these techniques, do not adopt them as your own. They will not serve your own or your patients' well-being in the long run.

Nonverbal Skills

People in crisis are still people, and you can use many of the same methods that other professional interviewers use to get them to tell you things. Following are a few of those skills or tools.

Eye Contact

Direct eye contact is something you avoid with animals; they perceive it as a sign of aggression. But people expect brief, frequent, direct eye contact, especially when they need reassurance. "Seeing eye-to-eye" with people generally communicates honesty and concern and is considered a baseline necessity of sincere communication of any kind Figure 10-6 . Think about that when you start to interview a patient with your mirrored sunglasses on.

You won't always have time to simply visit with some patients, especially if they're very sick. But try to remember that when a patient's status is subacute, your busy hands may correlate to you engaging in less (or no) eye contact. If the patient needs someone to talk to, take the time to listen when you can.

Touch

Some people don't like to be touched at all; to others, it's a valuable assurance that someone cares about them. You should try gently touching patients on a neutral part of the body, such as a shoulder or arm, especially when you're trying to reassure them or mitigate their fear Figure 10-7 . But watch how they react. If they pull away from you, chances are that touch in this instance won't be a valuable strategy. If they react positively (for instance, by leaning toward you or seeming to relax), then touch as a form of reassurance will work with them.

Gentleness

Being gentle is actually a quality of touch (mentioned above). You can use it even with a patient who prefers not to be

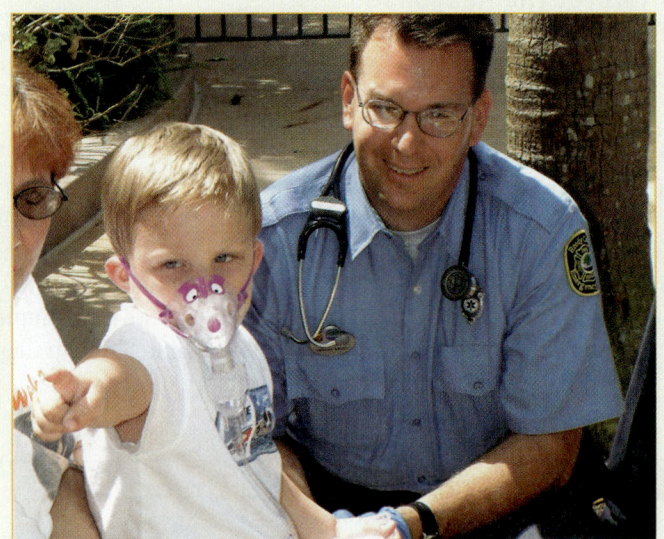

Figure 10-6 Whenever possible, put yourself at eye level with your patient. This is especially important when you're treating a child or an adult who is bedridden or wheelchair bound.

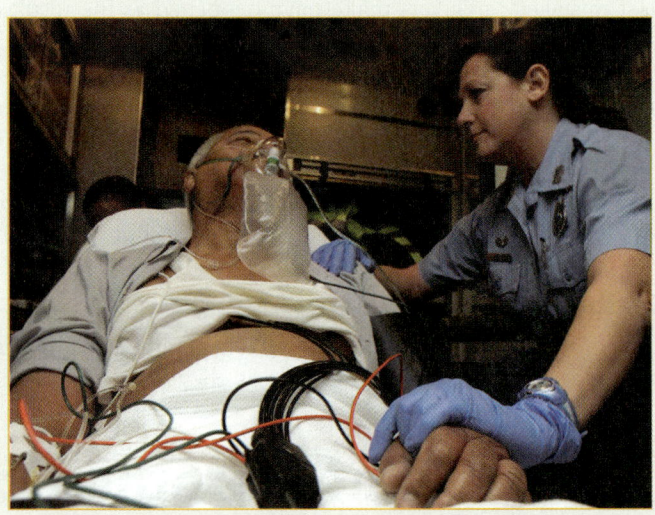

Figure 10-7 A gentle touch on the hand, arm, or shoulder can comfort someone who is sick or hurt and very scared.

touched. Gentleness can be the easy way you place the head of your stethoscope against the patient's chest or the way you apply a blood pressure cuff or blanket.

Posture

When you're dealing with patients who are terrified, don't stand in front of them with your arms folded across your chest. That conveys confrontation, not concern. Instead, try to position yourself at the same level as (or below the level of) their eyes. Sit or kneel at an angle that would not encroach on their personal space. For instance, lots of paramedics squat on the floor or ground in front of people who are seated in a car or on a bus bench or couch. Some choose to sit on the drug box.

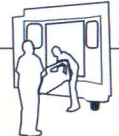

At the Scene

Avoid whispering, laughing, or snickering with your partner or other responders in front of or within hearing distance of the patient. It is unprofessional. Even if it is not about them, they will feel as if it is.

Demeanour

A pleasant demeanour comes easily to people who like people. To others, it doesn't come at all; and it's one of the reasons we emphasized liking people earlier in this chapter. It's absolutely necessary when you're dealing with people in crisis, because they need to see you as someone who is safe to be with, who does not pose a threat, and who honestly cares. With that comes the belief that you are going to handle the crisis.

Therapeutic Smile

Anyone who has dealt with even a few scared people can tell you that a smile can greatly help relieve stress. Think back to a time when you were troubled by something and someone's smile told you that everything was going to be OK. Your ability to smile can be just as valuable when you're dealing with people in crisis.

Assessing Mental Status

Excellent communication is vital in assessing how alert and oriented your patients are. There are many useful techniques for assessing mental status, and most of them are simple and based on plain old common sense. We have already discussed the most versatile first step ever invented: asking a patient for his or her name. Beyond that, consider the patient's ability to express himself or herself in the following ways.

Appropriate Humour

The highest form of mental function is the spontaneous expression of appropriate humour. To generate that degree of mental status, a person has to possess a high degree of cognitive function and an intact memory. People who aren't thinking clearly don't have the neuronal function to invest in spontaneous humour.

Timing of Responses to Questions

Assess how long it takes a patient to respond appropriately to your questions. A patient who is thinking clearly should be able to answer simple questions that make sense within 1 second.

Memory (Person, Place, Day, and Event)

Patients should be able to tell you quickly and accurately who they are and who you are, where they are, what day of the week it is, and what happened that necessitated your being called. Incorrect responses to any of these constitute a memory dysfunction and therefore decreased blood flow to the brain.

Ability to Obey Simple Commands

Any disruption in a patient's ability to comply with requests in the preceding steps indicates a brain dysfunction in the cerebrum or possibly the cerebellum. The dysfunction may be acute and could even be preexisting.

Special Interview Situations

There are situations in paramedic practice that may require special communication techniques. Some of these may include uncommunicative patients, hostile patients, very old or very young patients, and patients with special needs. Stereotyping any of these groups of patients, however, will only work

You are the Paramedic Part 5

The paramedics attempt to calm Mrs. Kellar and apologize to her. She is now crying uncontrollably, and says she's experiencing chest pain and shortness of breath. She sits down next to her husband and self-administers a nitroglycerin tablet under her tongue. An IV of normal saline has been established at a to keep vein open rate.

Reassessment	Recording Time: 15 Minutes
Level of consciousness	A (Alert to person, place, and day)
Skin	Pale and cool; perspiring
Pulse	118 beats/min, irregular
Blood pressure	188/102 mm Hg
Respirations	18 breaths/min
Spo$_2$	98% on 15 l/min via nonrebreathing mask
ECG	Atrial fibrillation

7. What would be the best course of action in this situation?
8. What are the different forms of communication and how do they impact patient prehospital care?

against effective communication. A good paramedic is never judgmental about his or her patients. No one calls you to judge them or their circumstances; they call for your medical care! But you can and should try the following techniques when you find yourself *not* communicating well with some patients.

People Who Are Unmotivated to Talk

There's nothing wrong with a little quiet; in fact, people who talk too much can be fairly irritating. When patients refuse to talk and you're not seeing signs of decreased mental status, there's no need to force the issue. Instead, make lots of eye contact, express your concern in every way possible, explain everything you are doing, invite them repeatedly to answer questions, and let them know it's all right if they don't wish to talk. This strategy of accepting them as they are can be very effective at breaking down barriers.

People Who Are Hostile

You are guaranteed to receive some unpleasant insults from people who are in crisis, and the insults will probably happen quite frequently. It's especially predictable when you're dealing with people who are chemically impaired. Discipline yourself never to respond in kind. Nothing escalates a situation faster than trading insults. Very often, when it involves a patient or bystanders, there are plenty of witnesses. It makes no sense and it can be very dangerous, especially when you're on their turf (about which you know nothing and they know everything). Remember, you're a helper. Remember, just as you can't fix everybody medically, you can't fix everybody emotionally either. Consider the possibility that you may not be able to defuse someone's anger. If the situation gets out of control, you may have to defer to police.

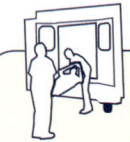

At the Scene

Learn to look for aggressive body language that signals increased anger and a possible attack such as clenched fists, intense staring directed at you, and breathing heavily through clenched teeth.

People Who Are Very Old or Very Young

Try not to presume that older people are any harder to communicate with than anyone else just because they're older. Their illnesses may tend to be more complex than the illnesses of younger people because they may have more than one disease or disorder and they may be taking more kinds of medicines concurrently. You may note individual differences among the geriatric population related to hearing, eyesight, mental status, and mobility; you need to adapt to them. The fact remains, older people are individuals and their differences are individual.

Children can be difficult patients because they pose communication challenges, even to the best paramedic. They tend to protest pain vigorously, they may be afraid of strangers (like

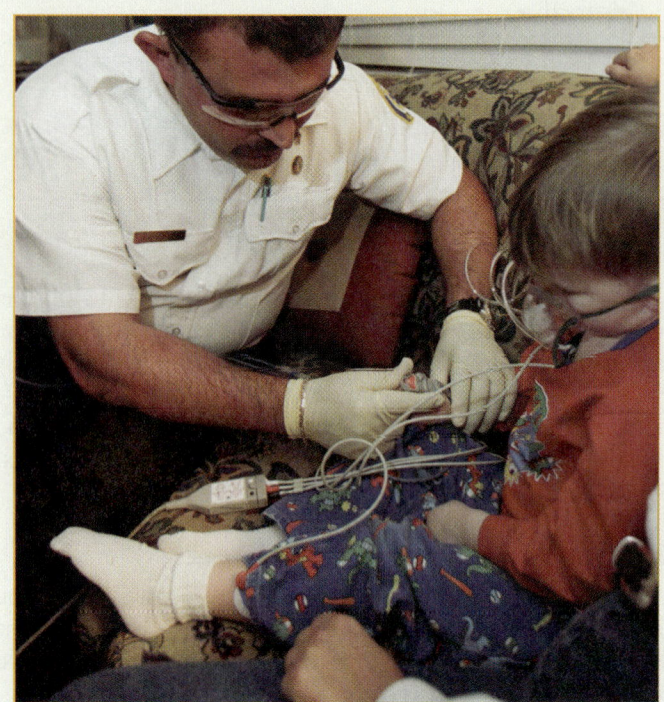

Figure 10-8 When you're examining a very young child, involve the parents. Have the father hold the child on his lap, or ask the mother to keep the toddler occupied while you work.

you), they may panic when separated from their parents, and their bodies may not be as familiar to many of us as are the bodies of adults. With a little practice, we can become comfortable treating them too.

Equipment (such as stethoscopes or needles) is not as important early in our contact with children as are friendly eye contact, smiles, and calm, subdued explanations, geared to match each child's age. Discipline yourself to minimize your movements, lower your voice, and touch as gently as you can. Try placing yourself at or below the child's eye level, for instance by sitting on the floor and placing the child on the stretcher or on a parent's lap **Figure 10-8 ▲**. If possible, involve a parent in the hands-on prehospital care of a conscious small child (for instance, by holding an extremity while you insert an IV). This is much less helpful when treating older children but is more important with infants and toddlers.

When parents are not available, toys are very useful for bridging the emotional gap between paramedics and some kids. Many crews stock their ambulances with teddy bears for toddlers. Short of those, you can make a serviceable chicken out of an examination glove by inflating the glove and marking its eyes with a felt marker **Figure 10-9 ▶**. You are more likely to connect with the child if you do this right in front of the child rather than if you ask someone else to do it.

Adolescents (beginning at about age 12) may not want their parents present at all during questioning or examination. In fact, an adult who insists on monitoring your conversation

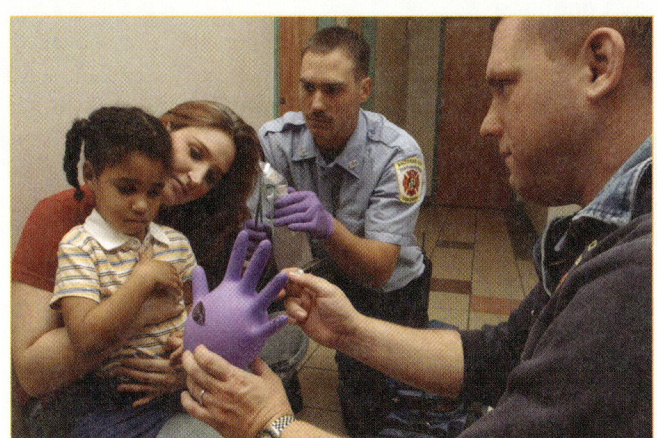

Figure 10-9 An examination-glove chicken can put a youngster at ease.

with an adolescent should raise questions in your mind. Don't refuse the prerogative of a parent, but be sure you communicate the situation to the emergency department physician, and chart it accurately. Generally, it's a good idea to deal with adolescents as adults. You gain better cooperation from them by offering them options and honouring their choices. (Hint: Never offer an option you know you can't honour.) Make special efforts to protect the modesty of adolescents in particular. They are, for the most part, obsessed with their image and what others think of them.

People Who Live With Special Challenges

It would be a mistake to overlook the needs of people who have speech, hearing, sight, or other kinds of communication disorders. Many caregivers enroll in sign-language or lip-reading classes to facilitate communication with these patients.

When you encounter a patient who has trouble communicating, remember that family members or primary caregivers who know these patients well can facilitate your efforts. Just as importantly, they can also help you to alleviate fear.

Many caregivers find that touch and eye contact are helpful bridging mechanisms when dealing with these patients. For example, a light touch on a patient's shoulder can convey kindness, while a firm grasp can express reassurance. Some patients respond well to brief, one-armed hugging. In still other situations, you can grasp a patient's face between your hands and use your eyes to convey concern or to calm him or her down.

Documentation and Communication

Many hospitals and 9-1-1 emergency communications centres have interpreter capabilities and are a good resource for communicating with patients who speak a language that is different from yours. Know what resources are available for patients who use sign language as a means of communication as well.

Cross-Cultural Communication

To effectively communicate to save lives, you must strive to understand the differences inherent in all peoples, then you can adjust your efforts to accommodate and overcome cultural barriers. The most common barriers to communication include the barriers of race, ethnicity, age, gender, language, education, religion, geography, and even economic status. The combination of all these groups can be defined as "culture." No matter who we are, or where we come from, or how open-minded we think ourselves to be, we *all* have some level of prejudice we must be conscious of. You cannot treat your patients effectively if you use your own culture as your only reference—it is much like imposing your own morality on patients. While understanding other cultures is not necessarily an ethical issue, it still is best not to have preconceived ideas about how you should communicate when you care for a patient.

Cultural sensitivity and cultural diversity have become important buzzwords in business today. There are literally thousands of classes and seminars on how to deal with cultural differences of both employees and business contacts. What do all these classes and seminars actually teach? In a word, "respect."

Sounds simple enough in theory, but in practice? Many people fall short of giving even basic respect in everyday interactions, let alone in a health care environment. In Canada, emphasis falls on getting the job done, and many people seem to be too hurried and busy, and too self-absorbed, to be really concerned about how we are viewed. We can offend with the abruptness of our behaviour. In other cultures, appearance and manners mean everything and lack of respect is unforgivable.

While the social practices, mannerisms, etiquette, and idiosyncrasies of all cultures are too numerous to list in one book, let alone in a chapter, it is highly important that you be open to educating yourself. It is the responsibility of the individual paramedic to research what cultural groups, ethnic groups, or religious groups are prevalent in his or her area of practice and learn how to deal with each culture accordingly. You may not get everything right when you encounter a representative from one of these groups, but your efforts at communicating will translate the idea of respect and that makes all the difference in the world.

Manners

Manners are also important. Canadian culture has come to a place where many young people no longer have even a rudimentary understanding of good manners. Pop culture has destroyed many concepts of appropriateness in dress and behaviour. Take for instance, the ubiquitous baseball cap. Not too long ago, it was considered rude for a man to wear a hat indoors, when a woman walked by, or even in a bar. Today we wear baseball caps with our paramedic uniforms. We wear them inside, outside, backwards, and sideways. Some people wear them with remarks or pictures on them that are designed to shock. While wearing a baseball cap has become accepted practice in some places in Canada, many people are offended if they see a hat worn indoors. However, in another culture, covering your head by wearing a hat at all times is considered a demonstration of your faithfulness to God. It is important for the paramedic to know the difference.

Additionally, many of the polite forms of address have fallen by the wayside. Patients have been referred to as "dude," "mac," "man," and even "bubba." Responses to patient's questions have included "naw," "yep," "yeah," and "nuh uh." This is slang, it is lazy, and it is not professional. Get used to saying "Yes sir," "No ma'am," "Thank you," and "Please." You would be amazed at how far such niceties go in instilling confidence and establishing a professional relationship with your patient.

"Would you . . . ," "Could you . . . ," and "May I . . ." are equally important. Most people like to give permission before being touched. Lack of address and assumption of permission is particularly demeaning to an elderly person in a nursing home. You are nonverbally communicating, "You are not important enough or mentally competent enough to be asked for permission."

Manners are also important in the area of involuntary bodily functions, which often have the embarrassing tendency to erupt while performing a patient examination. Simply say, "Excuse me," and the embarrassment should be temporary.

Hand Gestures

Another Canadian usage that may be looked upon with disfavour is our use of hand gestures. The thumbs-up sign that Canadians use to indicate "everything is OK" or "ready to go" is actually the equivalent of an extended middle finger in many Arabic and some Latin countries.

The OK sign, made with thumb and index finger circled, and the other three fingers extended, is standard Canadian for "good to go." In Latin countries, it is a reference to a circular orifice located posteriorly. It also has this meaning in Germany, Italy, and Russia. In France, the gesture means zero and can be used to indicate something is worthless. In other cultures, it represents the evil eye. In Japan, it indicates that money is needed, or that coins are preferred.

The extended middle finger is probably the rudest gesture in the Canadian gesture catalog. In Japan, the middle digit is used as the index finger and has the same significance as pointing. Please remember this fact when providing prehospital care to a Japanese family, and they seem to "flip you off" when you ask to be shown where it hurts.

Body Language

Body language and gestures are common the world over, but an innocent gesture in one country may be a serious insult in another. Perhaps the most cross-cultural gesture, and the easiest to remember, is the simple smile. A smile is readily received by most every culture on earth and has the tendency to convey good will and acceptance. Practice it often when dealing with patients.

Every culture in the world has its own peculiarities and social and religious practices that are unique. The list below is by no means all-inclusive, but illustrates some of the differences you may see when providing cross-cultural prehospital care:

- **Bowing.** Shows rank and status in Japan. The deeper the bow, the more respect is communicated.
- **Touching the head.** Many Asians do not touch the head. The head is considered the most sacred part of the body and is the residence of the soul. Touching the head may put the soul in jeopardy.
- **Touching with the left hand.** Islamic and Hindu cultures avoid touching with the left hand, as traditionally this hand was used for unclean functions. It is considered rude and offensive to offer the left hand in greeting.
- **Feet.** Showing the bottom of the feet is considered offensive in Muslim nations, as well as most of Thailand. To point the soles of your shoes or the soles of your feet at someone is to say "you are beneath my feet" or "you are worth less than dirt."
- **Slouching.** Considered rude in Japan and in Northern European areas.
- **Hands in pockets.** A gesture of disrespect in Turkey.
- **Sitting with legs crossed.** Disrespectful in Turkey and Ghana.
- **Hands on hips.** Sign of hostility in Mexico and Argentina.
- **Eye contact.** Avoid direct eye contact to show respect in most Asian, African, Latin American, and Caribbean cultures (Somalian and Brazilian cultures are exceptions). Prolonged eye contact is acceptable in Arab, Somalian, and Brazilian cultures; in these cultures, it is believed prolonged eye contact communicates honesty and interest in the recipient.
- **Nodding.** Indian and Arabic people may signal agreement by moving the head from side-to-side (the Western "no" gesture). They may indicate no by tipping the head back, and clicking the tongue against the roof of the mouth.

You are the Paramedic Summary

Your ability to communicate compassion, care, and understanding can be just as important as your ability to start IVs and perform other advanced life-support skills. If you rebel against acquiring the emotional intelligence that will help you communicate effectively, you will likely experience a bumpy road as a paramedic. Possessing a high emotional intelligence quotient will positively affect your relationships with subordinates, peers, and superiors, as well as with your patients. Possessing an understanding of the human side of EMS is essential to becoming an outstanding paramedic.

1. **What communication difficulties do you immediately anticipate in this scenario?**

Patients experiencing a stroke can have difficulties understanding and communicating language. You should immediately be concerned with communication when you suspect your patient is experiencing a stroke. As you can imagine, it would be very frustrating and frightening to understand speech but be unable to respond (or vice versa). If normal methods of communication fail, think outside the box to effectively communicate with your patient.

2. **Describe what the phrase "total patient care" means to you.**

Total patient care involves caring for all of the patient's needs, including his or her physical, mental, and emotional needs. To ignore any of these is not caring for the entire patient and is therefore considered incomplete prehospital care. To ignore a patient's pain, for instance, is not only poor patient prehospital care but can also be considered grounds for a lawsuit if you have the ability to medicate or otherwise ease the patient's pain and fail to do so.

3. **Although the paramedics in this scenario are attending to the patient's medical needs, could the wife have a valid complaint regarding their caregiving?**

Yes! Although the paramedics are tired, they should not ignore questions from the wife, nor should they treat the patient as though he is a manikin. It's important to remember that paramedics exist to care for life-threatening conditions. Your prehospital care needs to include an education and communication component. If you choose not to work on your people skills or to learn the qualities needed for emotional intelligence, you will likely experience difficulties in communicating and caring for your patients.

4. **How can your introductions (or lack thereof) and general demeanour affect your ability to communicate with your patients as well as with their friends and family members?**

Failing to establish a connection with your patients will likely cause problems with your patients right from the start. You need to quickly establish a bond of trust between yourself and your patient. It can be difficult if you are tired, hungry, or otherwise having a bad day, but failing to do so will translate these feelings to your patients who may respond negatively to them.

5. **How has this crew's lack of people skills affected this call?**

Their failure to address the softer aspects of patient prehospital care really made this call more difficult than it needed to be. Total patient care should also encompass the needs of family members or other loved ones. Failure to address their questions or concerns can directly and negatively affect patient prehospital care and, in some instances, can exacerbate a patient's medical condition. If you don't have time to address every issue, at minimum, acknowledge questions and explain that you will address their questions after you have finished with the task at hand.

6. **Can this situation be mended?**

It is very difficult to undo a situation such as this one. One bad PR move can cost an EMS or fire agency and its personnel in many ways. It is very important to keep and maintain the public's trust, and one incident can destroy years of good relations between members of the public and an EMS agency.

7. **What would be the best course of action in this situation?**

Calling an additional crew to diffuse the situation (as well as to transport Mrs. Kellar to the hospital for her chest pain) would be the best course of action. Consider the possibilities of what would happen if her condition suddenly worsened (for example, if she had an acute myocardial infarction and had a cardiac arrest). Obviously, offering a sincere apology is ideal, although it may not be enough in this situation. Requesting an additional crew to interject new faces may be required to calm both patients as well as to provide the required medical care they both need.

8. **What are the different forms of communication and how do they impact patient prehospital care?**

Much of how we communicate as people is done without the use of words. Body language is very powerful and can send a very different message than what is being communicated through words. Be mindful of your facial expressions, stance, and tone of voice as these will communicate your true intention or message beyond your words. Sometimes it's not what you say but how you say it that has the biggest impact on what is communicated between you and your patient.

Prep Kit

Ready for Review

- People are not just medical puzzles for us to solve; they are the reason we as paramedics exist.
- Most of the people you will meet during responses will be in crisis, and having the worst days of their lives.
- At least half of the calls you will run as a paramedic will take you into people's homes, day and night, and in the most private moments of their lives. Try to see every invitation into the home of someone else as a personal honour in a time and place where no one else would be welcome.
- If you want people to tell you about their problems, convince them you want to hear what they have to say. Give them your undivided attention.
- Active listening is repeating the key parts of a patient's responses to questions. It helps confirm the information the patient is providing. This ensures there is no misunderstanding.
- Your most essential challenge as a therapeutic communicator is to convey calm, unmistakable, genuine concern for someone you've never met.
- When you first meet your patients, introduce yourself and ask them for their name. By doing so, you communicate your respect for them.
- Even if you're not convinced that patients are in real trouble, consider the possibility that they're scared to death.
- When patients tell you they're in pain, let them know you grasp and appreciate their situation, and then do something about it.
- Modesty matters, no matter how acute the medical condition. If the patient is not personally sensitive to it, family members most certainly are.
- When you need to know how patients feel, try asking open-ended questions—questions that do not have a yes or no answer, and which do not give them specific options to choose from.
- When you're trying to find out about facts (for example, a medical history), use closed-ended, or direct, questions.
- If you sense that patients are trying to put something into words, but are having trouble, be patient. Don't say anything at all for a few seconds. Let them talk.
- Never assume. Try hard to become a careful observer and to keep your mind open to a wide range of possibilities.
- Nonverbal communication can be as powerful as words.
- Direct eye contact generally communicates honesty and concern.
- Posture is important. Try to position your eyes at the same level or below the level of the patient's eyes.

- A smile can greatly help relieve a stressful situation. Your ability to smile can be valuable when you're dealing with people in crisis.
- The highest form of mental function is the spontaneous expression of appropriate humour.
- Assess how long it takes for a patient to respond appropriately to your questions. Patients who are thinking clearly should be able to answer simple questions within 1 second.
- Patients should be able to tell you accurately who they are and who you are, where they are, what time of day it is, and what happened that necessitated your being called.
- When you ask patients to perform a simple task, they should be able to do the task correctly within about 1 second.
- When a patient refuses to talk and you're not seeing signs of decreased mental status, there's no need to force the issue. Instead, make lots of eye contact, express your concern in every way possible, explain everything you are doing, invite them repeatedly to answer questions, and let them know it's all right if they don't wish to talk.
- Try not to presume that older people are any harder to communicate with than anyone else, just because they're older.
- Children can pose treatment and communication challenges even to the best of us. Minimize your movements, lower your voice, and touch them as gently as you can—possibly without gloves at first. Try keeping your eye level at or below the child's, by sitting on the floor and placing the child on the stretcher or on a parent's lap.
- When you encounter a patient who has trouble communicating, remember that family members or primary caregivers who know these patients well can facilitate your efforts. Just as importantly, they can also help you alleviate fear.
- Dealing with people of cultures different from your own can be challenging. It's always considered a mark of your respect if you make an effort to learn about their language and culture.

Vital Vocabulary

closed-ended question A question that is specific and focused, either demanding a yes or no answer, or an answer chosen from specific options.

communication The transmission of information to another person—whether it be verbal or through body language.

open-ended question A question that does not have a yes or no answer, and which does not give the patient specific options to choose from.

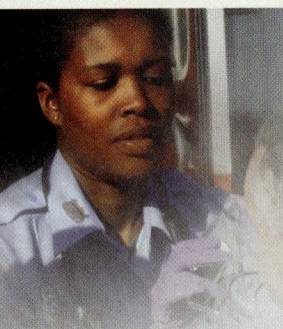

Assessment in Action

Your crew gets a call to the home of an older couple. The man has been sick with a cough and fever and is now vomiting. His wife is extremely concerned. She is also lonely and happy for the chance to talk to anyone at all. When you arrive, she takes her time telling you how his illness started, how he is doing now, and then starts talking about how long they've been married, their children, and so on. In this situation, how would you answer the following questions?

1. The act of communicating involves:
   A. talking as much as listening.
   B. listening as much as talking.
   C. listening only.
   D. talking only.

2. If the man or woman in this scenario was hard of hearing, how would you handle it?
   A. Scream at him or her at the top of your lungs.
   B. Get closer to him or her, but try not to be exceptionally loud.
   C. Tell him or her to turn up his or her hearing aid.
   D. Do whatever it takes to get the information you need, including talking loudly or writing notes.

3. If the woman in this scenario was a person who calls paramedics for every ache and pain and, as much as you like people, she drives you crazy, how would you react?
   A. Let your impatience show, hoping she will get to the point of the visit so you can do your job.
   B. Ignore her and concentrate on talking to her ill husband since he is the patient.
   C. Be patient and redirect her when she gets off track, without letting your impatience show.
   D. Listen to her whole story, picking out what's needed, and thinking about what job you'd like to switch to when you're done with that shift.

4. Just in case your patient has chest pain or cardiac issues, you need to ask if he's taking any erectile dysfunction medication. Since this couple is older, how would you go about this?
   A. Explain that you need to know some personal information in case of any cardiac issues, and explain the possible interaction with nitroglycerin or other cardiac medications.
   B. Ask her directly, making a joke out of it to make her more comfortable.
   C. Ask him instead, elbowing him jokingly and referring to "keeping her happy."
   D. Ask them both very professionally, and see who answers.

5. With this older couple, would you call them by their first names or use their last names with Mr. and Mrs.?
   A. Call them whatever you want, you are in charge and they are the patients.
   B. Call them by their first name to let them know you remember who they are and are on a very personal level with them.
   C. Call them pet names like "honey" and "sugar."
   D. Call them by their last names preceded by Mr. and Mrs. unless they say otherwise.

6. What if the woman in this scenario was so scared for her husband that she was having trouble staying calm and answering questions?
   A. Tell her to calm down and that she's doing him no good acting like that.
   B. Keep your voice calm and even. Get close enough to him so that you can do some assessments while you try to calm her down with your own calm demeanour.
   C. Have your partner take her out of the room so she isn't a distraction, and try to get the information that you need from her husband.
   D. Let your partner try to talk to her about her family while you try to talk with the patient.

7. After examining the man in this scenario, you have no idea what may be wrong with him, or if taking him to the hospital will make any difference. His wife asks you what you think. What is your best option?
   A. Tell her the truth; you have no idea, he's just sick.
   B. Talk in big medical terms she won't understand, and get busy transporting him so she can't ask for clarification.
   C. Tell her that she must face that they're both getting old and they will be more and more ill as time goes on, she should just get used to it.
   D. Tell her that you have some ideas, but it's best to let the doctor check him out. He'll be taken care of by you and the hospital staff.

Challenging Questions

An older woman fell in the shower and hurt her hip badly. You are told she has a history of osteoporosis. When you arrive, she is still lying in the bathtub with a towel covering her; her family didn't want to move her. You can see and sense that she is very modest and doesn't want that towel moved so that you can assess her injury.

8. What is the best way to handle this situation?

You have been called to the home of a 14-year-old girl who has severe cramps and heavy vaginal bleeding. You need to ask her about her sexual activity, and if there is any chance that she may be pregnant. Her parents are standing right there.

9. What should you do?

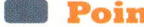 ## Points to Ponder

You are called to the scene of a vehicle collision in which the driver of one car has significant leg injuries. He is conscious and alert, and is also deaf.

How would you best communicate with this patient?

Issues: Communicating With Patients in Special Situations, Alternative Strategies for Communication.

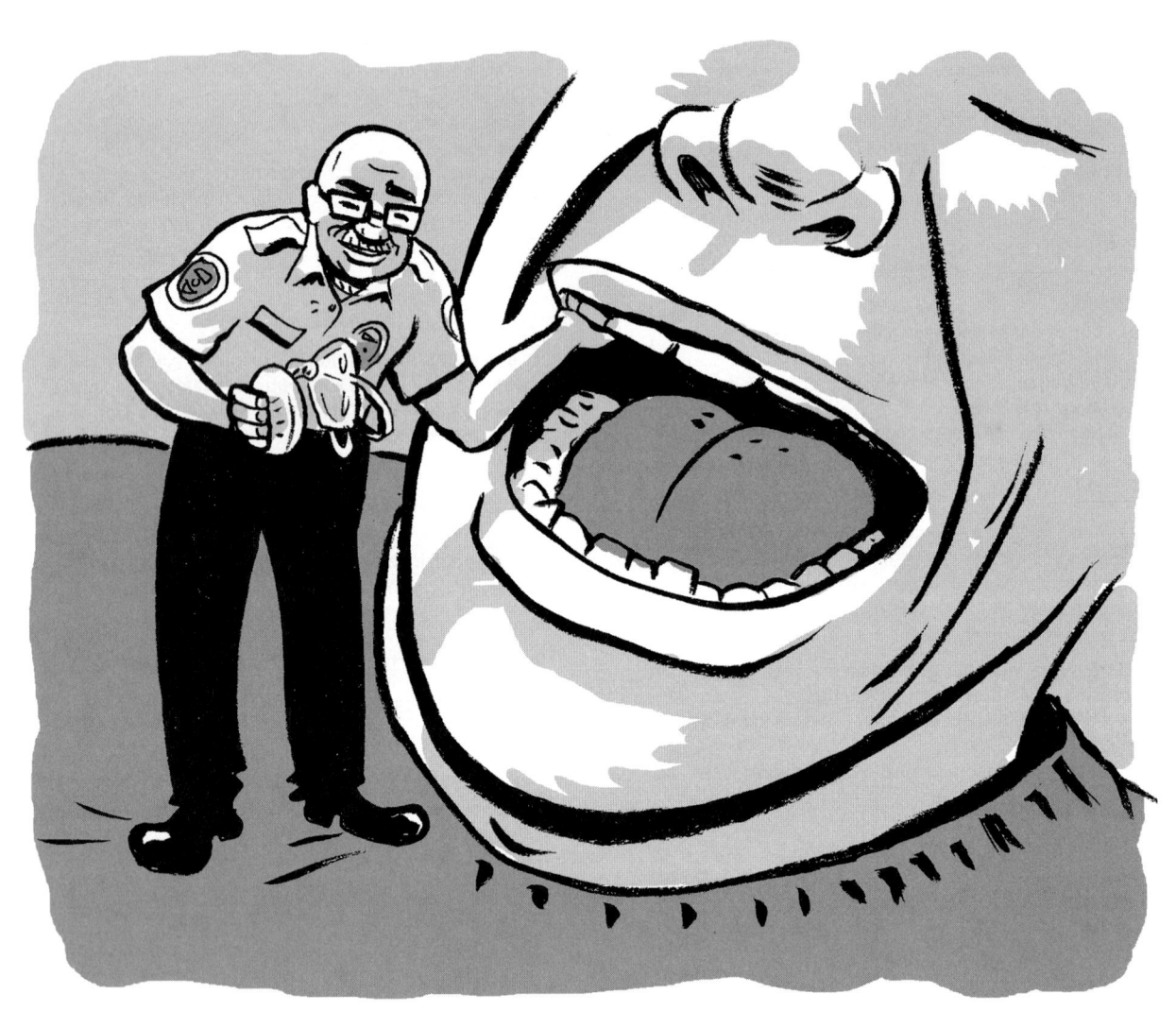

My five rules of airway management are pretty simple. 1. Blue is bad. 2. Oxygen is good. 3. Air should go in and out. 4. Noisy breathing is obstructed breathing. 5. Bare the chest!"

—Ronald D. Stewart, OC, MD, FRCPC, DSc

Airway

Section 2

Section Editor: Jonathon E. Morgan, MD, CCFP(EM), FCFP

 11 | **Airway Management and Ventilation** 11.4
Russell D. MacDonald, MD, MPH, FCFP, FRCPC,
Robert J. Burgess, BHSc, ACP, AEMCA, CQIA

11

Airway Management and Ventilation

Competency Areas

Area 1: Professional Responsibilities

1.3.a	Comply with scope of practice.
1.5.a	Work collaboratively with a partner.
1.6.a	Exhibit reasonable and prudent judgement.
1.6.c	Delegate tasks appropriately.

Area 2: Communication

2.4.d	Act in a confident manner.
2.4.e	Act assertively as required.

Area 3: Health and Safety

3.3.a	Assess scene for safety.
3.3.b	Address potential occupational hazards.
3.3.f	Practice infection control techniques.
3.3.g	Clean and disinfect equipment.

Area 4: Assessment and Diagnostics

4.2.a	Obtain list of patient's allergies.
4.2.b	Obtain list of patient's medications.
4.2.c	Obtain chief complaint and/or incident history from patient, family members, and/or bystanders.
4.2.d	Obtain information regarding patient's past medical history.
4.2.f	Obtain information regarding incident through accurate and complete scene assessment.
4.3.a	Conduct primary patient assessment and interpret findings.
4.3.b	Conduct secondary patient assessment and interpret findings.
4.3.e	Conduct respiratory system assessment and interpret findings.
4.4.a	Assess pulse.
4.4.b	Assess respiration.
4.4.d	Measure blood pressure by auscultation.
4.4.g	Assess skin condition.
4.4.i	Assess level of mentation.

Area 5: Therapeutics

5.1.a	Use manual maneuvers and positioning to maintain airway patency.
5.1.b	Suction oropharynx.
5.1.c	Suction beyond oropharynx.
5.1.d	Utilize oropharyngeal airway.
5.1.e	Utilize nasopharyngeal airway.
5.1.f	Utilize airway devices not requiring visualization of vocal cords and not introduced endotracheally.
5.1.g	Utilize airway devices not requiring visualization of vocal cords and introduced endotracheally.
5.1.h	Utilize airway devices requiring visualization of vocal cords and introduced endotracheally.
5.1.i	Remove airway foreign bodies (AFB).
5.1.j	Remove foreign body by direct techniques.
5.1.k	Conduct percutaneous cricothyroidotomy.
5.1.l	Conduct signal cricothyroidotomy.
5.2.a	Recognize indications for oxygen administration.
5.2.b	Take appropriate safety precautions.
5.2.c	Ensure adequacy of oxygen supply.
5.2.d	Recognize different types of oxygen delivery systems.
5.2.e	Utilize portable oxygen delivery systems.
5.3.a	Administer oxygen using nasal catheter.
5.3.b	Administer oxygen using low concentration mask.
5.3.c	Administer oxygen using controlled concentration mask.
5.3.d	Administer oxygen using high concentration mask.
5.3.e	Administer oxygen using pocket mask.
5.4.a	Provide oxygenation and ventilation using bag-valve-mask.
5.4.b	Recognize indications for mechanical ventilation.
5.4.c	Prepare mechanical ventilation equipment.
5.4.d	Provide mechanical ventilation.
5.8.a	Recognize principles of pharmacology as applied to the medications listed in Appendix 5.
5.8.e	Administer medication via intravenous route.

Area 6: Integration

6.1.c	Provide care to patient experiencing illness or injury primarily involving respiratory system.
6.1.j	Provide care to patient experiencing illness or injury primarily involving eyes, ears, nose, or throat.

Appendix 4: Pathophysiology

C.	**Respiratory System**
	Medical Illness: Aspiration
	Traumatic Injuries: Aspirated foreign body
	Traumatic Injuries: Tracheobronchial disruption
L.	**Ears, Eyes, Nose, and Throat**
	Neck and Upper Airway Disorders: Epiglottitis
	Neck and Upper Airway Disorders: Obstruction
	Neck and Upper Airway Disorders: Tracheostomies
	Neck and Upper Airway Disorders: Trauma injury– blunt/penetrating

Appendix 5: Medications

A.	**Medications affecting the central nervous system.**
A.5	Anxiolytics, Hypnotics, and Antagonists
A.8	Opioid Analgesics
A.9	Paralytics
D.	**Medications affecting the cardiovascular system.**
D.4	Class 1 Antidysrhythmics
J.	**Medications used to treat poisoning and overdose.**
J.1	Antidotes or Neutralizing Agents

Maintaining a Patent Airway: A Critical Concern

Establishing and maintaining a patent (open) airway and ensuring effective oxygenation and ventilation are vital aspects of effective patient prehospital care. Attempting to stabilize a patient whose airway is compromised is futile. No airway, no patient—it's that simple! The human body needs a constant supply of oxygen to carry out the physiologic processes necessary to sustain life; the airway is where it all begins. Few situations will cause such acute deterioration and death more rapidly than airway and ventilation compromise. Therefore, the patient's airway must remain patent at all times.

The function of the respiratory system is quite simple: It brings in oxygen and eliminates carbon dioxide (the primary waste product of aerobic metabolism). If this process is interrupted, vital organs of the body will not function properly. For example, the brain can survive for only 6 minutes or so without oxygen before permanent brain damage is virtually assured.

Failure to manage the airway or inappropriate management of the airway is a major cause of preventable death in the prehospital setting. Unfortunately, basic techniques to secure a patent airway are commonly neglected or performed improperly in the rush to proceed to advanced interventions. Poor technique (eg, improper mask size, improper bag-valve-mask seal, improper airway positioning) and failure to reassess the patient's condition merely serve to increase mortality and morbidity.

Health care providers must understand the importance of early detection of airway problems, rapid and effective intervention, and continual reassessment of a patient with airway or breathing compromise.

This chapter examines the airway in detail, beginning with a review of the anatomy and physiology of the respiratory system. It follows a "basic-to-advanced" approach, just as airway management should be performed in the prehospital environment. The chapter describes the various techniques of opening and maintaining a patent airway, recognizing and treating airway obstructions, assessing a patient's ventilation status, administering supplemental oxygen, and providing ventilatory assistance. Advanced techniques, including advanced airway devices and procedures, are then discussed in detail.

Anatomy of the Upper Airway

The upper airway consists of all anatomical airway structures above the level of the vocal cords. Its major functions are to warm, filter, and humidify air as it enters the body through the nose and mouth. The first portion of the upper airway, the pharynx (throat), is a muscular tube that extends from the nose and mouth to the level of the esophagus and trachea. The pharynx is composed of the nasopharynx, oropharynx, and laryngopharynx (also called the hypopharynx). The laryngopharynx is the lowest portion of the pharynx; it opens into the larynx anteriorly and the esophagus posteriorly **Figure 11-1 ▾** .

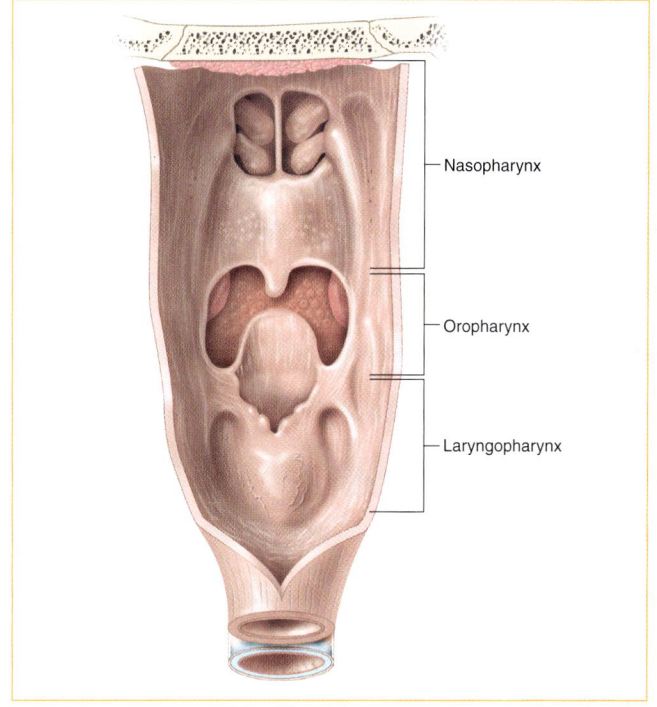

Figure 11-1 The pharynx.

You are the Paramedic Part 1

You are dispatched to a grocery store for a 50-year-old man with difficulty breathing. You and your paramedic partner reach the scene in approximately 5 minutes. Upon arrival, you find the patient sitting on a bench in front of the store. He is conscious, alert, and in mild respiratory distress. He tells you, in complete sentences, that he suddenly began having trouble breathing while inside the store.

1. Is this patient's airway patent?
2. How will you proceed with your assessment of this patient?

Nasopharynx

On inhalation, air normally enters the body through the nose and passes into the nasopharynx, which is formed by the union of the facial bones.

The entire nasal cavity is lined with a ciliated mucous membrane that keeps contaminants such as dust and other small particles out of the respiratory tract. In illness, the body produces additional mucus to trap potentially infectious agents. This mucous membrane is extremely delicate and has a rich blood supply. Any trauma to the nasal passages, such as improper or overly aggressive placement of airway devices, may result in profuse bleeding from the posterior nasal cavity. Bleeding from this area cannot be controlled by direct pressure. Extrinsic factors (eg, cocaine use) can also damage the delicate nasal passages or the septum, which separates the two nares.

Three bony shelves, called turbinates, protrude from the lateral walls of the nasal cavity and extend into the nasal passageway, parallel to the nasal floor. The turbinates serve to increase the surface area of the nasal mucosa, thereby improving the processes of warming, filtering, and humidification of inhaled air.

The nasopharynx is divided into two passages by the nasal septum, a rigid partition composed of bone and cartilage. Normally, the nasal septum is in the midline of the nose. In some people the septum may be deviated to one side or the other—a condition that becomes important when contemplating insertion of a nasal airway.

The sinuses are cavities formed by the cranial bones. Fractures of these bones may cause cerebrospinal fluid (CSF) to leak from the nose (cerebrospinal rhinorrhea) or the ears (cerebrospinal otorrhea). The sinuses prevent contaminants from entering the respiratory tract and act as tributaries for fluid to and from the eustachian tubes and tear ducts.

Oropharynx

The oropharynx forms the posterior portion of the oral cavity, which is bordered superiorly by the hard and soft palates, laterally by the cheeks, and inferiorly by the tongue **Figure 11-2 ▾**. The 32 adult teeth are embedded in the gums in such a manner that significant force is required to dislodge them. However, trauma of lesser severity may result in fracture or avulsion of the teeth, potentially obstructing the upper airway or causing aspiration of tooth fragments into the lungs.

The tongue is a large muscle attached to the mandible and the hyoid bone—a small, horseshoe-shaped bone to which the jaw, epiglottis, and thyroid cartilage attach as well. From an airway perspective, the most important anatomical consideration regarding the tongue is its tendency to fall back and occlude the posterior pharynx when the mandible relaxes. In fact, the tongue is the most common cause of anatomical upper airway obstruction, especially in patients with a decreased level of consciousness.

The palate forms the roof of the mouth and separates the oropharynx and nasopharynx. Its anterior portion, which is formed by the maxilla and palatine bones, is called the hard palate. The soft palate is posterior to the hard palate.

The adenoids, which are located on the posterior nasopharyngeal wall, are lymphatic tissue that filters bacteria. The tonsils, which are also made of lymphatic tissue, are located in posterior pharynx; they help to trap bacteria. The adenoids and

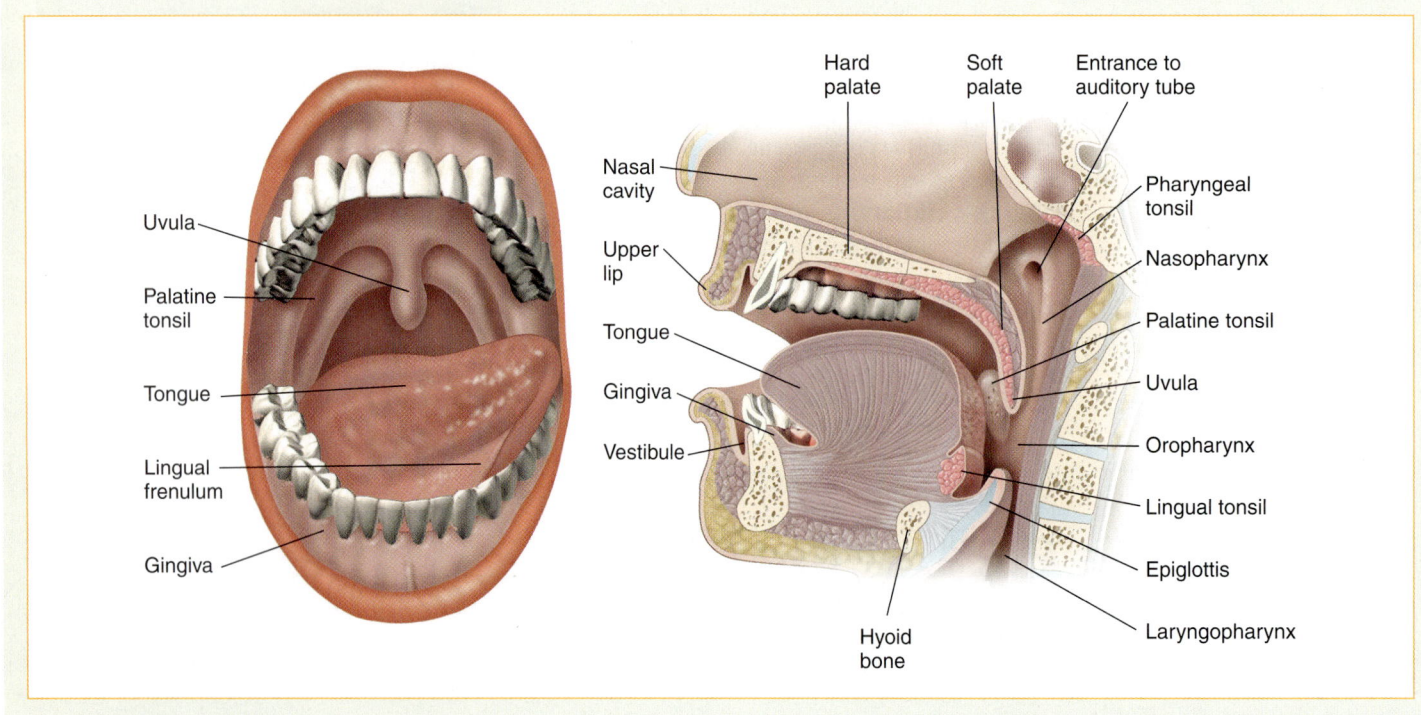

Figure 11-2 The oral cavity.

tonsils often become swollen and infected. Severe swelling of the tonsils can potentially cause obstruction of the upper airway.

The uvula, a soft-tissue structure that resembles a punching bag, is located in the posterior aspect of the oral cavity, at the base of the tongue.

The superior border of the glottic opening is the epiglottis. This leaf-shaped cartilaginous flap prevents food and liquid from entering the larynx during swallowing.

The vallecula is an anatomical space, or "pocket," located between the base of the tongue and the epiglottis. It is an important landmark for endotracheal intubation.

Larynx

The larynx is a complex structure formed by many independent cartilaginous structures (Figure 11-3 ▾). It marks where the upper airway ends and the lower airway begins.

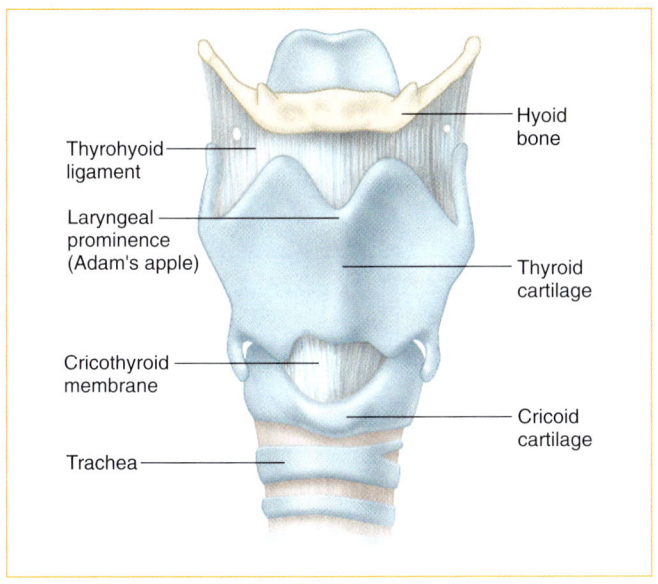

Figure 11-3 The larynx.

The thyroid cartilage is a shield-shaped structure formed by two plates that join in a "V" shape anteriorly to form the laryngeal prominence known as the Adam's apple. The thyroid cartilage is suspended in place by the thyroid ligament and is directly anterior to the glottic opening.

The cricoid cartilage, or cricoid ring, lies inferiorly to the thyroid cartilage; it forms the lowest portion of the larynx. The cricoid cartilage is the first ring of the trachea and the only upper airway structure that forms a complete ring.

Between the thyroid and cricoid cartilages is the cricothyroid membrane, which is a site for emergency surgical and nonsurgical access to the airway (cricothyrotomy). Because it is bordered laterally and inferiorly by the highly vascular thyroid gland, paramedics must locate the anatomical landmarks carefully when accessing the airway via this site.

The glottis, also called the glottic opening, is the space in between the vocal cords and the narrowest portion of the adult's airway (Figure 11-4 ▸). Airway patency in this area is heavily dependent on adequate muscle tone. The lateral borders of the glottis are the vocal cords. At rest, these white bands of tough tissue are partially separated (ie, the glottis is partially open). During forceful inhalation, the vocal cords open widely to provide minimum resistance to air flow.

The arytenoid cartilages are pyramid-like cartilaginous structures that form the posterior attachment of the vocal cords; they are valuable guides for endotracheal intubation. As the arytenoid cartilages pivot, the vocal cords open and close, which regulates the passage of air through the larynx and controls the production of sound; hence, the larynx is sometimes called the "voice box."

The pyriform fossae are two pockets of tissue on the lateral borders of the larynx. Airway devices are occasionally inadvertently inserted into these pockets, resulting in a tenting of the skin under the jaw.

When the airway is stimulated (eg, during aspiration of foreign material or submersion incident), defensive reflexes cause a laryngospasm—spasmodic closure of the vocal cords, which causes a partial of complete airway obstruction.

You are the Paramedic Part 2

Closer examination of the patient reveals that he has mild accessory muscle use and intercostal retractions. As your partner opens the equipment bag, you perform an initial assessment and note the following:

Initial Assessment	Recording Time: 0 Minutes
Appearance	Obvious respiratory distress; anxious; pale
Level of consciousness	A (Alert to person, place, and day)
Airway	Open and clear
Breathing	Increased respiratory rate, laboured breathing with adequate tidal volume
Circulation	Skin, pale and diaphoretic; radial pulse, rapid and bounding

3. What immediate management is indicated for this patient?
4. What questions would be pertinent to ask this patient?

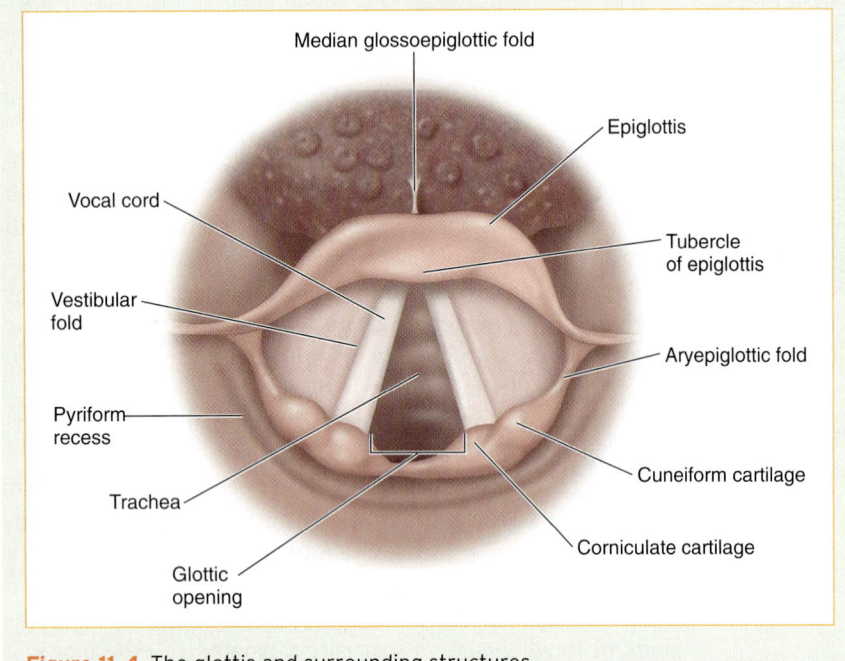

Figure 11-4 The glottis and surrounding structures.

Labels in Figure 11-4:
- Median glossoepiglottic fold
- Epiglottis
- Vocal cord
- Tubercle of epiglottis
- Vestibular fold
- Aryepiglottic fold
- Pyriform recess
- Cuneiform cartilage
- Trachea
- Corniculate cartilage
- Glottic opening

This reflex normally lasts a few seconds. Persistent laryngospasm can threaten the airway by preventing ventilation altogether.

Anatomy of the Lower Airway

The function of the lower airway is to exchange oxygen and carbon dioxide. Externally, it extends from the fourth cervical vertebra to the xiphoid process. Internally, it spans the glottis to the pulmonary capillary membrane.

The trachea, or windpipe, is the conduit for air entry into the lungs. This tubular structure is approximately 10 to 12 cm in length and consists of a series of C-shaped cartilaginous rings. The trachea begins immediately below the cricoid cartilage and descends anteriorly down the midline of the neck and chest to the level of the fifth or sixth thoracic vertebra. It divides into the right and left mainstem bronchi at the level of the carina. These bronchi are lined with mucus-producing cells and beta-2 receptors that, when stimulated, result in bronchodilation.

The right bronchus is somewhat shorter and straighter than the left bronchus. Thus an endotracheal tube that is inserted too far will often come to lie in the right mainstem bronchus.

All of the blood vessels and the bronchi enter each lung at the hilum. The lungs consist of the entire mass of tissue that includes the smaller bronchi, bronchioles, and alveoli **Figure 11-5 ▶** . In total, the adult lungs can hold approximately 6 l of air.

The right lung has three lobes and the left lung has two lobes, which are covered with a thin, slippery outer lining called the visceral pleura. The parietal pleura lines the inside of the thoracic cavity. A small amount of fluid is found between the pleurae, which decreases friction during breathing.

Upon entering the lungs, each bronchus divides into increasingly smaller bronchi, which in turn subdivide into bronchioles. The bronchioles, which are made of smooth muscle, dilate or constrict in response to various stimuli. The smaller bronchioles branch into alveolar ducts that end at the alveolar sacs.

The balloon-like clusters of single-layer air sacs known as alveoli are the functional site for the exchange of oxygen and carbon dioxide. This exchange occurs by simple diffusion between the alveoli and the pulmonary capillaries.

The alveoli are lined with a proteinaceous substance called surfactant, which decreases surface tension on the alveolar walls and keeps them expanded. If the amount of pulmonary surfactant is decreased or the alveoli are not inflated, they will collapse—a condition called atelectasis.

Lung and Respiratory Volumes

The total lung capacity in the average adult male is approximately 6 l, but only a fraction of this capacity is used during normal breathing. While a small amount of gas exchange occurs in the alveolar ducts and terminal bronchioles, most of the gas exchange occurs in the alveoli.

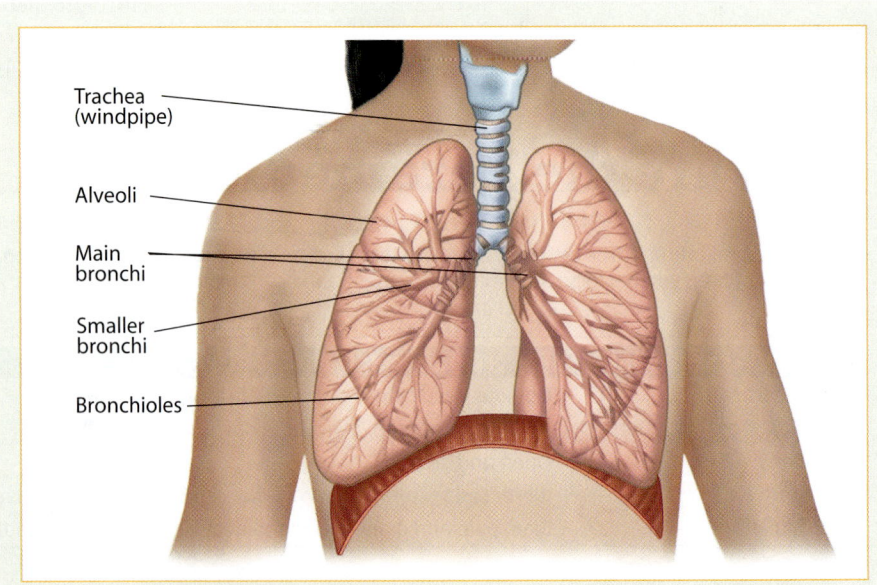

Labels in Figure 11-5:
- Trachea (windpipe)
- Alveoli
- Main bronchi
- Smaller bronchi
- Bronchioles

Figure 11-5 The trachea and the lungs (lower airway structures).

Special Considerations

Although the maneuvers, techniques, and indications for airway management are essentially the same in children as they are in adults, several anatomical differences in the child make mastery of these techniques critical.

Infants and small children have a proportionately larger occiput, which causes the head to flex when the child lies supine; this position itself can cause an airway obstruction. When positioning the airway of an infant or child, you should place a folded towel under his or her shoulders to maintain a neutral position of the head.

Compared to adults, children have a proportionately smaller mandible and a proportionately larger tongue **Figure 11-6 ▶** . Both factors increase the incidence of airway obstruction in children.

The child's epiglottis is more floppy and omega-shaped than an adult's. As a consequence, it must be lifted out of the way to visualize the vocal cords for intubation **Figure 11-7 ▶** .

In general, the infant's and child's airway is smaller and narrower at all levels. The larynx lies more superior and anterior than in an adult—an important consideration when visualizing the vocal cords for intubation. The larynx is also funnel-shaped due to the narrow, underdeveloped cricoid cartilage. In children younger than 10 years, the narrowest portion of the airway is at the cricoid ring. Further narrowing of the child's inherently narrow airway, such as that caused by soft-tissue swelling or foreign body aspiration, can result in a major decrease in airway resistance and breathing inadequacy.

Children do not have well-developed chest musculature, and their ribs and cartilage are softer and more pliable than an adult's. As a result, the thoracic cavity cannot optimally contribute to lung expansion. Children rely heavily on their diaphragm for breathing, which moves their abdomen in and out. For this reason, infants and children are commonly referred to as "belly breathers."

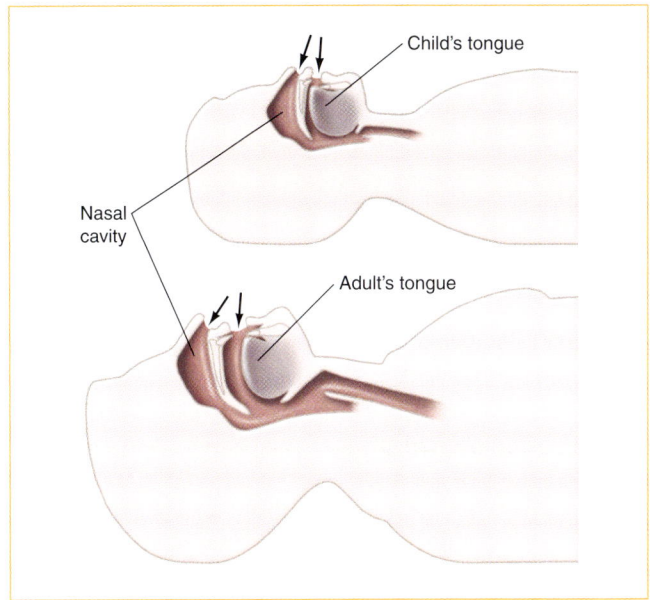

Figure 11-6 In children, the mandible is proportionately smaller and the tongue is proportionately larger than in an adult.

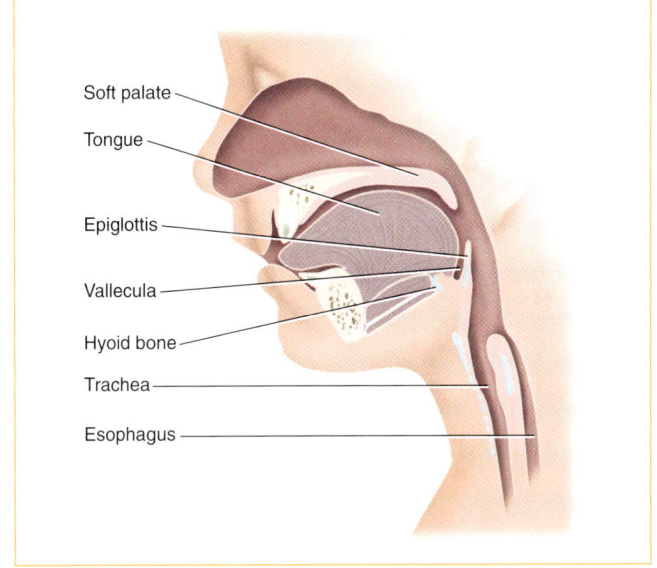

Figure 11-7 The child's epiglottis and surrounding structures.

Tidal volume (V_T), a measure of the depth of breathing, is the volume of air that is inhaled or exhaled during a single respiratory cycle. Normal tidal volume in the average adult male is 5 to 7 ml/kg (approximately 500 ml). In infants and children, normal tidal volume is approximately 6 to 8 ml/kg. Inspiratory reserve volume is the amount of air that can be inhaled in addition to the normal tidal volume; it is normally about 3,000 ml.

In the adult, about 30% of the normal tidal volume remains in the upper airway passages; this so-called dead space volume (V_D) is approximately 150 ml. Dead space is any portion of the airway where air lingers, but does not participate in gas exchange. The anatomical dead space includes the trachea and larger bronchi, where residual gas may remain at the end of inhalation. Certain respiratory diseases increase dead space by creating intrapulmonary obstructions or atelectasis; these areas are called physiologic dead space.

The remaining volume of inhaled air, which does reach the alveoli and therefore does participate in gas exchange, is called alveolar volume. Alveolar volume is equal to tidal volume minus dead space volume; it is approximately 350 ml in the average adult male.

It is important to understand the concepts of minute volume (V_M) and minute alveolar volume (V_A). Minute volume is simply the amount of air that moves in and out of the respiratory tract per minute; it is determined by multiplying the tidal volume by the respiratory rate ($V_M = V_T \times RR$). Minute alveolar volume (V_A) is the amount of air that actually reaches the alveoli per minute and participates in gas exchange; it is determined by multiplying the tidal volume (minus dead space volume) by the respiratory rate. For example:

$$(500 \text{ ml } [V_T] - 150 \text{ ml } [V_D]) \times 16 \text{ breaths/min} = 5{,}600 \text{ ml } (V_A)$$

Minute volume will increase if the tidal volume, respiratory rate, or both, increases. Conversely, minute volume will decrease if the tidal volume, respiratory rate, or both, decreases. As the respirations become faster, however, they typically become more shallow (reduced tidal volume). When respirations are too rapid *and* too shallow, the inhaled air may reach only the anatomical dead space before it is promptly exhaled, resulting in decreased minute alveolar volume.

Table 11-1 ▶ demonstrates how tidal volume and respiratory rate can influence a patient's minute alveolar volume and, therefore, overall breathing adequacy. This information will prove useful for assessing a patient's breathing adequacy and identifying patients who require assisted ventilation.

Following an optimal inspiration, the amount of air that can be forced from the lungs in a single exhalation is called the functional residual capacity. The amount of air that you can exhale following normal (relaxed) exhalation is called the expiratory reserve volume; this amount is about 1,200 ml. Even if you exhale forcefully, however, you cannot completely empty your lungs of air. Residual volume is the air that remains in the

Table 11-1	How Tidal Volume and Respiratory Rate Affect Minute Alveolar Volume
Example 1: Normal tidal volume and respiratory rate	
(500 ml [V_T] - 150 ml [V_D]) × 16 breaths/min = **5,600 ml (V_A)** *Good!*	
Example 2: Reduced tidal volume and a normal respiratory rate	
(250 ml [V_T] - 150 ml [V_D]) × 14 breaths/min = **1,400 ml (V_A)** *Not good!*	
Example 3: Reduced tidal volume and a slow respiratory rate	
(350 ml [V_T] - 150 ml [V_D]) × 6 breaths/min = **1,200 ml (V_A)** *Not good!*	
Example 4: Reduced tidal volume and a fast respiratory rate	
(200 ml [V_T] - 150 ml [V_D]) × 40 breaths/min = **2,000 ml (V_A)** *Not good!*	

lungs after maximal expiration; it is also about 1,200 ml in the average adult male.

The fraction of inspired oxygen (F_{IO_2}) is the percentage of oxygen in inhaled air. F_{IO_2} increases when supplemental oxygen is given to a patient and is commonly documented as a decimal point.

Ventilation

Ventilation is the process of moving air into and out of the lungs. If a patient is not breathing or is breathing inadequately, he or she no longer has an effective mechanism to intake oxygen and eliminate carbon dioxide. Therefore, in addition to oxygenation, ensuring adequate ventilation is one of the highest priorities in treating any patient.

Ventilation consists of two phases:

- **Inspiration** (inhalation) is the process of moving air into the lungs.
- **Expiration** (exhalation) is the process of moving air out of the lungs.

Documentation and Communication

A person breathing room air, which contains 21% oxygen, would be documented as having an F_{IO_2} of 0.21. A nonrebreathing mask, which delivers about 90% oxygen, would be documented as delivering an F_{IO_2} of 0.90 to an adequately breathing patient.

You are the Paramedic Part 3

Your partner applies a nonrebreathing mask on the patient and sets the flow rate at 15 l/min as you perform a focused history and physical examination. The patient tells you that he has congestive heart failure. The following baseline vital signs are obtained:

Vital Signs	Recording Time: 2 Minutes
Respirations	28 breaths/min, laboured, adequate depth
Pulse	120 beats/min, regular and bounding
Skin	Pale and diaphoretic
Blood pressure	144/94 mm Hg
Spo$_2$	95% while receiving 100% oxygen via nonrebreathing mask

5. Is this patient breathing adequately? Why or why not?
6. What are the signs of inadequate ventilation?

One ventilation cycle consists of one inspiration, which occupies approximately one third of the ventilation cycle, and one expiration, which occupies the remaining two thirds.

Regulation of Ventilation

The body's need for oxygen is dynamic; it is constantly changing. The respiratory system must be able to accommodate those changes in oxygen demand by altering the rate and depth of ventilation. These changes are regulated primarily by the pH of the CSF, which is directly related to the amount of carbon dioxide dissolved in the plasma portion of the blood (Pa_{CO_2}). The regulation of ventilation involves a complex series of receptors and feedback loops that sense gas concentrations in the body fluids and send messages to the respiratory centre in the brain to adjust the rate and depth of ventilation accordingly.

Neural Control of Ventilation

Neural (nervous system) control of breathing can be traced to the medulla. The involuntary control of breathing originates in the brain stem—specifically, in the pons and the medulla. The impulses for automatic breathing descend through the spinal cord and can be overridden (to a point) by voluntary control, such as when you talk or hold your breath.

Two types of motor nerves affect breathing. The phrenic nerves innervate the diaphragm. The intercostal nerves innervate the external intercostal muscles between the ribs.

The respiratory centre in the medulla is divided into three regions: the respiratory rhythmicity centre, the apneustic centre, and the pneumotaxic centre. The respiratory rhythmicity centre sets the respiratory rate. During normal, quiet breathing, it gradually increases the stimulation for inhalation over 2 seconds and then relaxes for 3 seconds, allowing passive exhalation, and then repeats the cycle. This results in a resting respiratory rate.

As the chest expands, mechanical (stretch) receptors in the chest wall and bronchioles send a signal to the apneustic centre via the vagus nerve to inhibit the inspiratory centre, and expiration occurs. This feedback loop, which combines neural and mechanical control, is called the Hering-Breuer reflex. It is a protective mechanism that terminates inhalation, thus preventing overexpansion of the lungs.

The apneustic centre influences the respiratory rate by increasing the number of inspirations per minute. Its activity is countered by the functioning of the pneumotaxic centre, which inhibits inspiration. In times of increased demand, the pneumotaxic centre decreases its influence, thereby increasing the respiratory rate.

Chemical Control of Ventilation

The respiratory system must keep the blood's concentrations of oxygen and carbon dioxide and its acid-base balance within a very narrow range. The body has a number of chemoreceptors that monitor the levels of O_2, CO_2, and the pH of the CSF and provide feedback to the respiratory centres to modify the rate and depth of breathing based on the body's needs at any given time Figure 11-8 ▶.

The chemoreceptors that monitor the carbon dioxide content in arterial blood are located in the carotid bodies and the

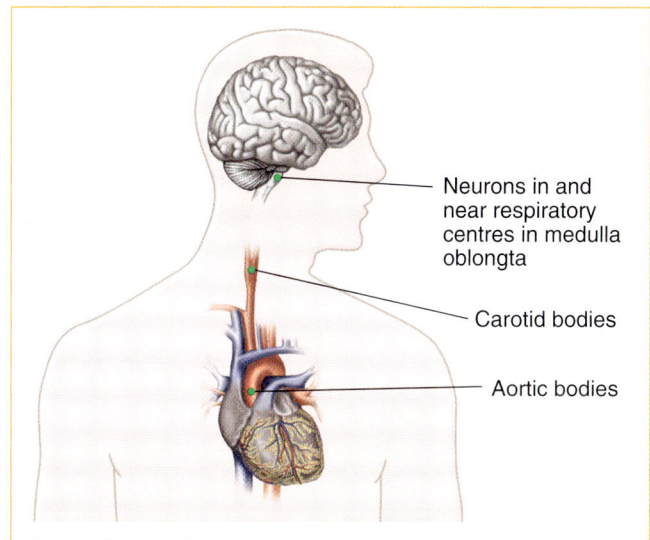

Figure 11-8 Chemoreceptors (locations).

- Neurons in and near respiratory centres in medulla oblongta
- Carotid bodies
- Aortic bodies

aortic arch. These receptors sense minute changes in the Pa_{CO_2} and send signals to the respiratory centres via the glossopharyngeal nerve (ninth cranial nerve) and the vagus nerve (tenth cranial nerve).

Central chemoreceptors, which monitor the pH of the CSF, are located adjacent to the respiratory centres in the medulla. An increase in the acidity (decreased pH) of the CSF triggers these chemoreceptors to increase the rate and depth of breathing. These receptors are very sensitive to small changes in pH and provide for "fine-tuning" of the body's acid-base balance.

Under normal circumstances, fluctuations in Pa_{CO_2} and pH of the CSF are the dominant influence on respiration, and the primary respiratory drive derives from the body's attempt to regulate the Pa_{CO_2} within normal limits. However, some patients with chronic respiratory diseases are unable to take in O_2 and eliminate CO_2 effectively, so their respiratory centres have gradually accommodated to high Pa_{CO_2} levels.

In such cases, the body uses a "backup system" to control breathing. Although the primary control of breathing is based on the Pa_{CO_2} and the pH of the CSF, the chemoreceptors in the carotid bodies and aortic arch also respond to decreased levels of oxygen dissolved in the plasma (Pa_{O_2}). In this scenario, the chemoreceptors send messages to the respiratory centre to increase the rate and depth of breathing. This secondary control of breathing is called the hypoxic drive. Usually only end-stage COPD patients are on hypoxic drive.

Control of Ventilation by Other Factors

Numerous factors other than changes in the pH and Pa_{CO_2} can influence ventilation. As the body temperature rises (ie, in the case of fever), respirations increase in response to the increased metabolic activity. Certain medications cause respirations to increase or decrease, depending on their physiologic action. For example, amphetamines produce a sympathomimetic effect and would cause an increase in respirations,

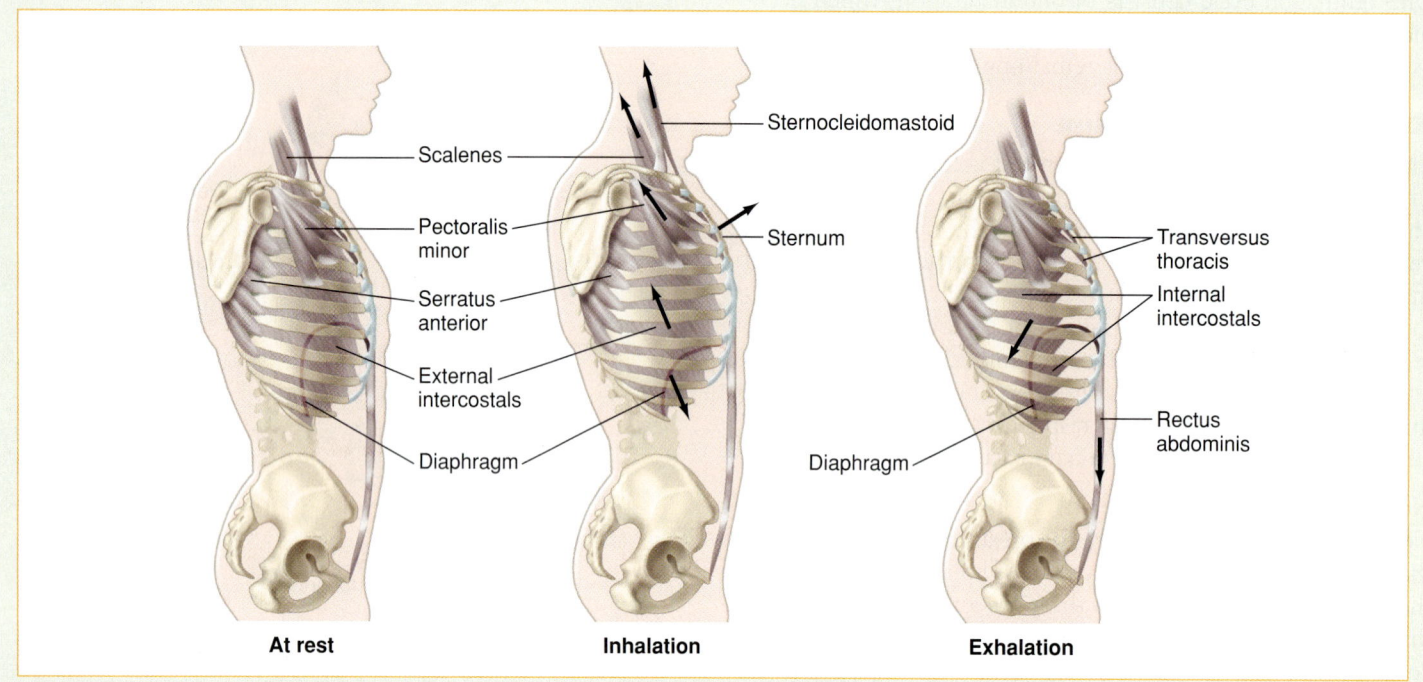

Figure 11-9 The mechanics of breathing.

whereas narcotic analgesics (eg, morphine, fentanyl) would cause a decrease in respirations due to their central nervous system depressant effects. Pain and strong emotions can also increase respirations.

Hypoxia is a powerful stimulus to breathe, and would result in increased respirations in an effort to bring more oxygen into the body. Conversely, acidosis increases respirations as a compensatory response to promote the elimination of excess carbon dioxide produced by the body.

A person's metabolic rate also influences the rate of breathing. When the metabolic rate is high (eg, during exercise), respirations increase to eliminate the excess carbon dioxide produced. Conversely, when the metabolic rate is low (eg, during sleep), respirations slow.

The Mechanics of Ventilation

Ventilation is accomplished through pressure changes in the lungs, which in turn are brought about by contraction and relaxation of the intercostal muscles and diaphragm. The diaphragm is the major muscle of breathing. It separates the thoracic cavity and the abdominal cavity.

Inhalation is an active process that is initiated by contraction of the respiratory muscles. As the diaphragm contracts after receiving impulses from the phrenic nerves it flattens out, increasing the vertical dimensions of the thorax. At the same time, the intercostal muscles contract after receiving impulses from the intercostal nerves, causing the ribs and sternum to move upward and outward, increasing the horizontal dimensions of the chest cavity. The net effect is to increase the volume of the chest. The lungs, being highly elastic and "glued" via the

visceral pleura to the chest wall, undergo a comparable increase in volume. The air in the lungs now suddenly occupies a larger space, so the pressure within the lungs drops rapidly. As the air pressure inside the chest falls below that of the outside atmosphere, air begins to flow from the region of higher pressure (outside the body) to the region of lower pressure (the lungs)—a process called negative-pressure ventilation. When the pressures inside and outside the lungs are equalized, inhalation stops. Oxygen and carbon dioxide then diffuse across the alveolar-capillary membrane in the lungs.

In contrast to inhalation, exhalation is a passive process. At the end of inhalation, the respiratory muscles relax. The natural elasticity (recoil) of the lungs passively exhales the air. **Figure 11-9 ▲** illustrates the processes of inhalation and exhalation.

At the Scene

Normal breathing involves negative intrathoracic pressure and the pulling of air into the lungs.

With ineffective chest movement (eg, reduced tidal volume) or no chest movement (eg, apnea), negative intrathoracic pressure cannot be created. The only way to move air into the lungs is then by positive-pressure ventilation, the forcing of air into the lungs. Positive pressure can be created with a bag-valve-mask device, pocket face mask, or a mechanical ventilation device.

Respiration

Every living cell in the body requires an uninterrupted supply of oxygen to carry out its metabolic processes. The cells of the brain and heart, for example, can tolerate only very short periods of oxygen deprivation—usually less than about 6 minutes—after which they will die. Once brain cells or myocardial (heart muscle) cells have died, they can never be replaced.

The same metabolic processes that consume oxygen produce carbon dioxide as a waste product. This carbon dioxide must be carried away from the cell and disposed of, or it may accumulate to toxic levels. Therefore, the body needs a mechanism to eliminate the carbon dioxide produced by metabolism.

As it happens, the body very economically uses the same mechanism—respiration—to ensure a constant oxygen supply and to remove the excess carbon dioxide. Two types of respiration occur in the human body: external and internal. External respiration (pulmonary respiration) is the exchange of gases between the lungs and the blood cells in the pulmonary capillaries. Internal respiration (cellular respiration) is the exchange of gases between the blood cells and the tissues **Figure 11-10 ▶**.

Gas exchange in the body occurs by diffusion, a process in which a gas moves from an area of higher concentration to an area of lower concentration. Both oxygen and carbon dioxide pass through the alveolar membrane by diffusion.

Dissolved oxygen crosses the pulmonary capillary membrane and binds to the hemoglobin molecule of the red blood cell. Without hemoglobin, oxygen transport is not possible. Consequently, replacing large amounts of lost blood with isotonic crystalloid solutions (eg, normal saline, lactated Ringer's), which lack hemoglobin, will be not be as effective as replacing lost blood with whole blood or packed red blood cells.

Approximately 97% of the body's total oxygen is bound to hemoglobin; the remainder is dissolved in the plasma portion of the blood. A pulse oximeter reads the percentage of hemoglobin that is saturated with oxygen (SpO_2), which is normally greater than 95%. The remaining oxygen that is dissolved in the plasma makes up the partial pressure of oxygen (PaO_2 or PO_2).

The majority of carbon dioxide is transported in the blood in the form of bicarbonate ions, with about 33% being bound to the hemoglobin. As O_2 crosses from the alveoli into the blood, CO_2 diffuses from the blood into the alveoli. The carbon dioxide dissolved in the plasma makes up the partial pressure of CO_2 ($PaCO_2$ or PCO_2).

Causes of Decreased Oxygen Concentrations in the Blood

Numerous conditions can result in decreased blood-oxygen concentrations. A lower partial pressure of atmospheric oxygen, such as an environment rich in carbon monoxide (CO), decreases the available amount of oxygen. CO has a much greater affinity for hemoglobin than oxygen (250 times more). Severe bleeding decreases the hemoglobin levels in the blood,

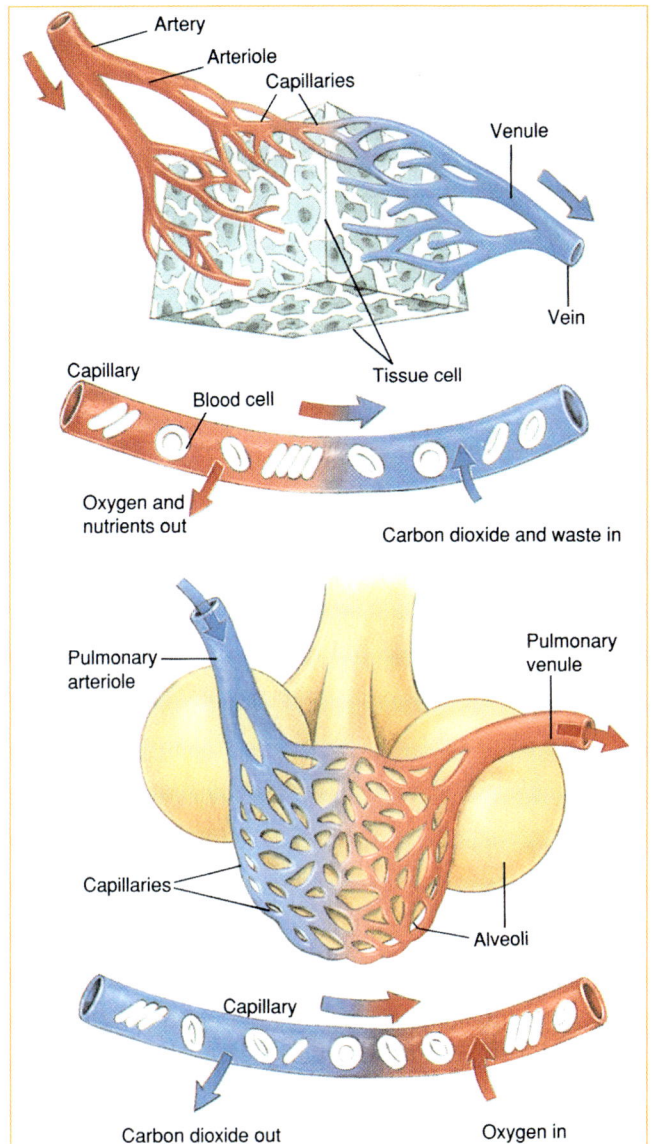

Figure 11-10 Internal and external respiration.

thereby decreasing the oxygen-carrying capability of the blood and, in turn, decreasing the amount of oxygen available to the cells. Anemia, a deficiency of red blood cells, results in a chronically decreased ability of the blood to carry oxygen. Without sufficient circulating red blood cells, there is nothing for the hemoglobin molecule to unite with.

Conditions that reduce the surface area for gas exchange also decrease the body's available oxygen supply—for example flail chest, diaphragmatic injury, simple or tension pneumothorax, open pneumothorax (sucking chest wound), hemothorax, and hemopneumothorax.

Decreased mechanical effort also decreases the availability of oxygen for respiration. Patients experiencing severe chest pain secondary to trauma or a medical condition tend to breathe as shallowly as possible in an effort to reduce chest wall movement and alleviate the pain; this is called "respiratory splinting." Traumatic asphyxia, an injury caused by severe compression of the chest, and hypoventilation from any cause also result in decreased oxygen levels in the blood.

Medical conditions such as pneumonia, pulmonary edema, and chronic obstructive pulmonary disease (COPD) may also result in decreased blood-oxygen levels. These conditions decrease the surface area of the alveoli either by damaging the alveoli or by leading to an accumulation of fluid in the lungs. Nonfunctional alveoli inhibit the diffusion of oxygen and carbon dioxide. As a result, blood entering the lungs from the right side of the heart will bypass the alveoli and will return to the left side of the heart in an unoxygenated state, a condition called intrapulmonary shunting.

Causes of Abnormal Carbon Dioxide Concentrations in the Blood

The $Paco_2$ in the arterial blood represents a balance between the CO_2 produced in metabolism and the CO_2 eliminated during ventilation. The amount of CO_2 produced normally remains relatively constant. As the metabolic rate goes up (eg, fever), however, more CO_2 is produced. As the metabolic rate falls (eg, hypothermia), the production of CO_2 declines. The type of metabolism also influences CO_2 production, with any metabolic process that results in the formation of acids increasing the amount of CO_2 in the blood. For example, excess lactic acid in the blood (caused by anaerobic metabolism) or excess ketoacids in the blood (caused by fat metabolism due to absent cellular glucose) will increase the circulating levels of CO_2.

If CO_2 production exceeds the body's ability to eliminate it by ventilation, the level of $Paco_2$ rises to produce hypoventilation. Theoretically, hypoventilation can occur in two ways: CO_2 production can exceed the body's ability to eliminate it, or CO_2 elimination can be depressed to the extent that it no longer keeps up with normal metabolism.

At the other extreme is hyperventilation, which occurs when CO_2 elimination exceeds CO_2 production. For example,

Table 11-2	Carbon Dioxide Balance	
	Hypoventilation	Hyperventilation
Minute volume	↓	↑
CO_2 elimination	↓	↑
$Paco_2$	↑ (hypercarbia)	↓ (hypocarbia)

patients experiencing an anxiety attack tend to breathe very deep and very fast (eg, minute volume is increased), so they eliminate CO_2 at a rate faster than their body produces it. The level of CO_2 in their blood then falls below normal and they experience symptoms such as dizziness and numbness/tingling in the face and extremities.

Given a steady rate of CO_2 production and CO_2 elimination, $Paco_2$ is directly proportional to minute volume **Table 11-2 ▲**. Decrease the minute volume, and you decrease CO_2 elimination, so CO_2 builds up in the blood (hypercarbia). Increase the minute volume, and you increase carbon dioxide elimination, so the level of CO_2 in the blood falls (hypocarbia).

The Measurement of Gases

Dalton's law of partial pressure states that the total pressure of a gas is the sum of the partial pressure of the components of that gas, or the pressure exerted by a specific atmospheric gas. The major components of air are nitrogen (78.62%); oxygen (20.84%); CO_2 (0.04%); and water vapour (0.50%).

▌ Airway Evaluation

The importance of carefully assessing a patient's airway and ventilatory status cannot be overemphasized. In the prehospital environment, you will encounter patients with a variety of airway problems—some of these problems are easily corrected, others require aggressive management. *The prehospital care you*

You are the Paramedic Part 4

As you continue with your focused history and physical examination of the patient, you note that his level of consciousness has diminished and that cyanosis is developing around his mouth. You perform an immediate reassessment.

Reassessment	Recording Time: 5 Minutes
Level of consciousness	V (Responsive to verbal stimuli); confused
Respirations	32 breaths/min, shallow
Pulse	130 beats/min, weak and regular
Skin	Pale and diaphoretic, developing perioral cyanosis
Blood pressure	130/78 mm Hg
Spo_2	82% while breathing 100% oxygen via nonrebreathing mask

7. How should you adjust your treatment for this patient? Why?

provide to a patient with an airway or breathing problem is only as good as the assessment you perform.

Essential Parameters

Breathing at rest should appear effortless, not laboured. If you can see or hear a patient breathing, there is usually a problem. Normally, an adult at rest should have a respiratory rate between 12 and 20 breaths/min (Table 11-3 ▾). The respirations should be of adequate depth (tidal volume) and follow a regular pattern of inhalation and exhalation.

Patients experiencing respiratory distress often attempt to compensate with preferential positioning, such as an upright tripod position (elbows out), or a semi-Fowler's (semi-sitting) position. Patients with respiratory distress will avoid a supine position.

Recognition of Airway Problems

A patient who is conscious, alert, and able to speak to you in complete sentences has no immediate airway or breathing problems. Nonetheless, you must still closely monitor a patient's airway and breathing status and be prepared to intervene should his or her condition deteriorate. Changes in respiratory rate, depth, and regularity may be subtle. If these subtleties are overlooked, and the appropriate prehospital care is not provided, the patient's outcome may be less than desirable. In case of inadequate breathing, it is critical to intervene immediately with some form of positive-pressure ventilation and 100% oxygen.

The adult patient with an abnormal respiratory rate must be evaluated for other signs of inadequate ventilation (Table 11-4 ▾). Causes of inadequate ventilation include severe infection (sepsis), trauma, brain stem insult, a noxious or oxygen-poor atmosphere, and renal failure, to name a few. In addition to inadequate ventilation, causes of respiratory distress may include upper and/or lower airway obstructions, impairment of the respiratory muscles (eg, spinal cord injury), or impairment of the nervous system (eg, head injury, drug overdose).

Table 11-3	Normal Respiration Rate Ranges
Adults	12 to 20 breaths/min
Children	15 to 30 breaths/min
Infants	25 to 50 breaths/min

Table 11-4	Signs of Inadequate Breathing

- Slow (< 12 breaths/min) or fast (> 20 breaths/min) respirations
- Shallow breathing (reduced tidal volume)
- Adventitious (abnormal) breath sounds
- Altered mental status
- Cyanosis

Dyspnea is defined as any difficulty in respiratory rate, regularity, or effort. It may result from hypoxemia, a decrease in arterial oxygen levels. If left untreated, hypoxemia will progress to hypoxia, a lack of oxygen to the body's cells and tissues. Untreated hypoxia will lead to anoxia, an absence of oxygen that results in cellular and tissue death.

If a patient's airway is not patent, or if breathing is absent or inadequate, all therapies that you may attempt will prove futile. Proper airway management involves opening the airway, clearing the airway, assessing breathing, and providing the appropriate intervention(s)—in that order.

Evaluation of the airway includes the techniques of look, listen, and feel. Visual techniques should be used at first sight of the patient. The following questions must be answered when assessing the patient with respiratory distress:

- How is the patient positioned?
  - Is he or she in a tripod position?
  - Is the patient experiencing orthopnea (dyspnea while lying down)?
- Is rise and fall of the chest adequate (eg, adequate tidal volume)?
- Is the patient gasping for air (air hunger)?
- What is the skin colour?
- Is there flaring of the nostrils?
- Is the patient breathing through pursed lips?
- Do you note any retractions (skin pulling in between and around the ribs during inhalation):
  - Intercostal?
  - At the suprasternal notch?
  - At the supraclavicular fossa?
  - Subcostal?
- Is the patient using accessory muscles to breathe? (Accessory muscles, which are not normally used during normal breathing, include the sternocleidomastoid muscles of the neck.)
- Is the patient's chest wall moving symmetrically? (Asymmetric chest wall movement, when one side of the chest moves less than the other, indicates that airflow into one lung is decreased.)

Listen for air movement at the patient's nose and mouth. Is the patient taking a series of quick breaths, followed by a prolonged exhalation phase? If so, this is a sign of inadequate ventilation.

Auscultate breath sounds with a stethoscope. Breath sounds should be clear and equal on both sides of the chest (bilateral), anteriorly and posteriorly. Compare each apex (top) of the lung to the opposite apex and each base (bottom) of the lung to the opposite base (Figure 11-11 ▸).

If you are ventilating the patient with a bag-valve-mask device, note any resistance or change in ventilatory compliance. Increased compliance means that air can be forced into the lungs with relative ease; decreased compliance suggests an upper or lower airway obstruction.

Assess for pulsus paradoxus (paradoxical pulse), which occurs when the systolic blood pressure drops more than 10 mm Hg during inhalation. A change in pulse quality, or even the disappearance of a pulse during inhalation, may also be detected. Pulsus paradoxus is typically seen in patients with decompensating COPD, severe pericardial tamponade, or other conditions that increase intrathoracic pressure (eg, tension pneumothorax, severe asthma attack).

A history of the patient's present illness is a vital part of your assessment of the patient with respiratory distress. You should ask questions to determine the evolution of the current problem:

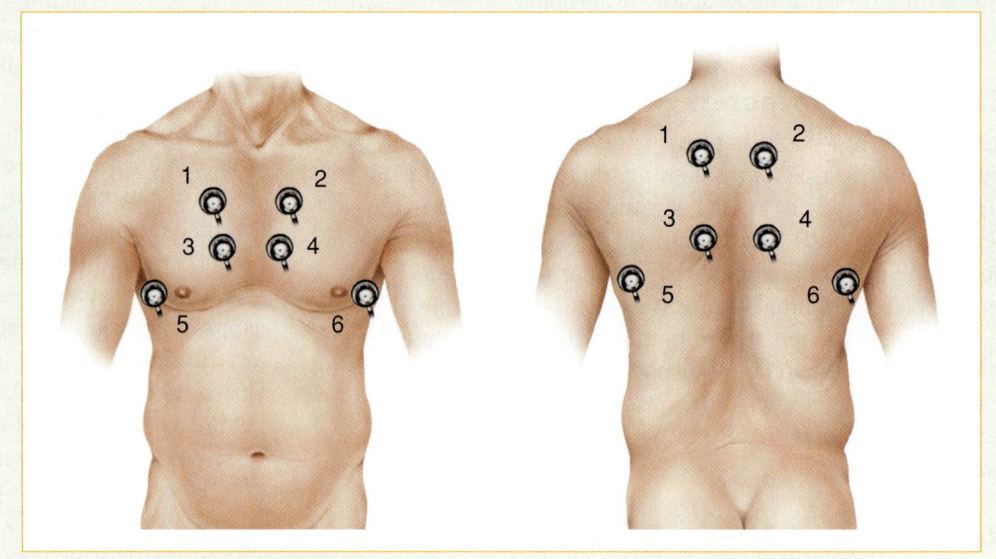

Figure 11-11 Auscultation of breath sounds (1 to 6).

- Was the onset of the problem sudden or gradual over time?
  - Some people may perceive respiratory distress that occurred 2 days prior as arising gradually, when, in fact, the onset was sudden; the patient may have simply waited 2 days before calling for help.
- Is there any known cause or "trigger" of the event?
  - Asthma is commonly exacerbated by stress or cold weather. A foreign body airway obstruction is commonly preceded by a sudden onset of difficulty in breathing during a meal or, in children, while playing with small toys or other objects.
- What is the duration (is it constant or recurrent)?
- Does anything alleviate or exacerbate the problem?
- Are there any other associated symptoms, such as a productive cough, chest pain or pressure, or fever?
- Were any interventions attempted prior to EMS arrival?
- Has the patient been evaluated by a physician or admitted to the hospital for this condition in the past?
  - Determine specifically whether the patient was hospitalized or merely seen in the emergency department and then released. If the patient was hospitalized, ask whether he or she was admitted to an intensive care unit (ICU) or a regular, unmonitored floor. A condition that warranted an ICU admission is clinically significant.
- Is the patient currently taking any medications?
  - Ask whether the patient has had any changes in his or her current prescription, such as a new medication or changes in the prescribing directions of an existing medication.
- Does the patient have any risk factors that could cause or exacerbate his or her condition, such as alcohol or illicit drug use, cigarette smoking, or a poor diet?

Evaluate the patient for any modified forms of respiration. Protective reflexes of the airway include coughing, sneezing, and gagging. Coughing is a forceful exhalation produced with a greater than normal volume of breath. The patient whose

cough mechanism is suppressed—whether by drugs, by pain, by trauma, or by any other cause—is at serious risk of aspirating foreign material.

Sneezing is also a sudden, forceful exhalation, but in this instance air is expelled through the nose rather than through the mouth. Sneezing is usually elicited by irritation of the nose.

Gagging is a forceful muscular contraction of the pharyngeal muscles and the glottis. This reaction is automatic when something touches an area deep in the oral cavity. The gag reflex helps protect the lower airway from aspiration, or entry of fluids or solids into the trachea, bronchi, and lungs.

Sighing is a slow, deep inhalation followed by a prolonged and sometimes quite audible exhalation. Sighing periodically hyperinflates the lungs, thereby reexpanding

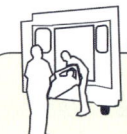

At the Scene

Important questions to ask the patient with respiratory distress are:

- Have you ever been held in the emergency department overnight for the same problem?
- Have you ever been admitted to the hospital for the same problem?
- Have you ever been admitted to an intensive care unit for the same problem?
- Have you ever been intubated for the same problem?

A condition serious enough to warrant admission or intubation requires urgent attention to prevent a repeat occurrence. This information will serve to increase your index of suspicion and prepare you for a potential rapid deterioration in the patient's condition.

Table 11-5	Abnormal Respiratory Patterns
Cheyne-Stokes respirations	Gradually increasing rate and depth of respirations followed by gradual decrease of respirations with intermittent periods of apnea; associated with brain stem insult.
Kussmaul respirations	Deep, gasping respirations; common in diabetic coma (ketoacidosis).
Biot respirations	Irregular pattern, rate, and depth with intermittent periods of apnea; results from increased intracranial pressure.
Agonal respirations	Slow, shallow, irregular respirations or occasional gasps; results from cerebral anoxia; may be seen briefly after the heart has stopped as the brain continues to send signals to the respiratory muscles.

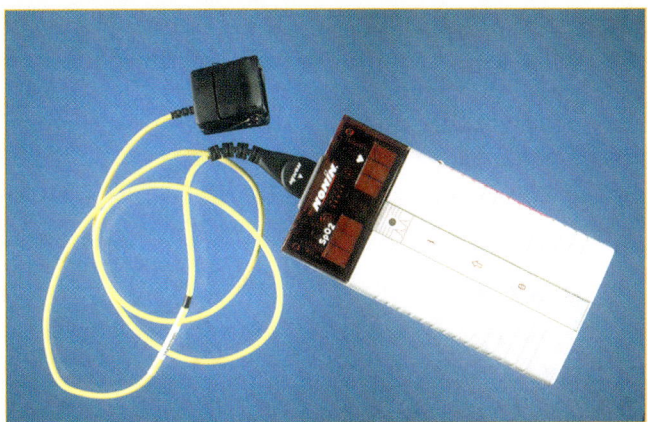

Figure 11-12 A pulse oximeter.

atelectatic (collapsed) alveoli. The average person sighs about once per minute.

Hiccuping is a sudden inhalation, due to spasmodic contraction of the diaphragm, cut short by closure of the glottis. Hiccuping serves no physiologic purpose, although persistent hiccups may be clinically significant.

Patients with serious injuries or illness may present with changes in their respiratory pattern. **Table 11-5 ▲** shows various abnormal respiratory patterns and their causes.

Diagnostic Testing

In addition to your hands-on assessment of the patient with an airway or breathing problem, several methods and devices are used to quantify oxygenation and ventilation. Pulse oximetry is a simple, rapid, safe, and noninvasive method of measuring—minute by minute—how well a person's hemoglobin is saturated.

A pulse oximeter **Figure 11-12 ▶** measures the percentage of hemoglobin in the arterial blood that is saturated. Under normal circumstances, hemoglobin is saturated with oxygen. When carbon monoxide is available, hemoglobin will bind to it rather than oxygen, and can "fool" the oximeter. A sensor probe, clipped to the patient's finger or ear lobe, uses a light-emitting diode (LED) to transmit light through the vascular bed to a light-sensing detector. The amount of light transmitted across the vascular bed depends on the proportion of hemoglobin that is saturated with oxygen. To ensure that the instrument is measuring arterial and not venous oxygen saturation, pulse oximeters are designed to assess only pulsating blood vessels. As a consequence, they also measure the patient's pulse. One way to check the functioning of a pulse oximeter is to compare the pulse reading it provides with your own measurement of the patient's pulse by palpation.

A normally oxygenated, normally perfused person should have an SpO_2 between 95% and 99%. Any reading below 95% indicates respiratory compromise; a reading below 90% signals a need for aggressive oxygen therapy.

Situations in which pulse oximeters may be useful in prehospital emergency care include the following:

- **Monitoring the oxygenation of a patient during an intubation attempt.** The low-saturation alarm on the pulse oximeter can signal that the paramedic should abort the intubation attempt and ventilate the patient.

- **Identifying deterioration in a trauma victim.** In the patient with multiple trauma, the signs of a developing tension pneumothorax, for instance, may not be evident until the problem is quite advanced. A declining SpO_2 level can alert the paramedic that something bad is happening and prompt a search for the cause of the problem.

- **Identifying deterioration in the cardiac patient.** Pulse oximetry may enable early identification of patients who are experiencing congestive heart failure in the wake of a myocardial infarction.

- **Identifying high-risk patients with respiratory problems.** For example, pulse oximetry may identify patients with asthma who are having serious attacks or patients with emphysema who are in severe decompensation.

- **Assessing vascular status in orthopaedic trauma.** Pulse oximetry is useful in assessing a fractured extremity to evaluate the pulse distal to the fracture. Loss of a pulse means that the limb is in jeopardy and may require urgent action in the prehospital setting if transport time is long. A pulse oximeter clipped to a finger or toe on a broken limb might provide critical information about the ongoing circulation to the limb.

The usefulness of a pulse oximeter depends on its ability to provide accurate information. A pulse oximeter that gives a reading of 99% when the patient is actually severely hypoxemic will not be much help to anyone. Be aware of circumstances that might produce erroneous readings:

- **Bright ambient light** may enter the spectrophotometer of the pulse oximeter and create an incorrect reading. Protect the sensor clip by covering it with a towel or aluminum foil.
- **Patient motion** can confuse the pulse oximeter, as it may mistake motion for arterial pulsation and read the oxygen saturation from a vein rather than an artery.
- **Poor perfusion** makes it difficult for the oximeter to sense a pulse and therefore to generate a reading. Poor perfusion occurs in states such as shock, cardiac arrest, and cold exposure. If the patient's limbs are vasoconstricted and cold, it may be necessary to place the pulse oximeter clip on the ear lobe or nose.
- **Nail polish** will prevent the sensor from working properly. Carry disposable acetone (nail polish remover) swabs to quickly remove nail polish.
- **Venous pulsations** may occur in some patients with right-sided heart failure. If a vein is pulsating, the oximeter may regard it as an artery and measure venous oxygen saturation.
- **Abnormal hemoglobin** may produce a falsely high SpO_2. Carboxyhemoglobin, for example, is formed by the attachment of CO to the hemoglobin molecule. Because the pulse oximeter cannot distinguish between oxyhemoglobin (hemoglobin that is occupied by oxygen) and carboxyhemoglobin, it may give a high SpO_2 reading for a patient who is severely hypoxemic from CO poisoning. The results of pulse oximetry should therefore be interpreted cautiously in victims of smoke inhalation or other circumstances likely to have produced CO poisoning.

When in Doubt, Look at the Patient!

Always weigh the information provided by pulse oximetry (or any other device) against clinical observations. If the patient is turning blue and struggling to breathe, you may ignore the pulse oximeter reading that says the patient is adequately oxygenated.

The steps for performing pulse oximetry are listed here and shown in **Skill Drill 11-1 ▶**.

1. Clean the patient's finger. Place the index or middle finger into the pulse oximeter probe. Turn on the pulse oximeter and note reading of the SpO_2 **Step 1**.
2. Palpate the radial pulse to ensure that it correlates with the display on the pulse oximeter **Step 2**.

In patients with certain reactive airway diseases (eg, asthma), bronchoconstriction can be evaluated by measuring the peak rate of a forceful exhalation

with a peak expiratory flow monitor. An increasing peak expiratory flow suggests that the patient is responding to treatment (eg, inhaled bronchodilators). A decreasing peak expiratory flow may be an early indication that the patient's condition is deteriorating.

Peak expiratory flow varies based on sex, height, and age. Normal adults have a peak expiratory flow rate of 350 to 750 ml.

The steps for performing peak expiratory flow measurement are listed here and shown in **Skill Drill 11-2 ▶**.

1. Place the patient in a seated position with the legs dangling. Assemble the flowmeter and make sure that it reads zero **Step 1**.
2. Ask the patient to take a deep breath, place the mouthpiece in his or her mouth, and ask the patient to exhale as forcefully as possible. Make sure no air leaks around the device or comes from the patient's nose **Step 2**.
3. Perform the test three times, and take the best rate of the three readings **Step 3**.

■ Airway Management

A patient who is conscious and is talking, screaming, or crying has a patent airway. In a patient with an altered LOC, however, the airway is often not patent and manual maneuvers will be

---

Skill Drill 11-1:
Performing Pulse Oximetry

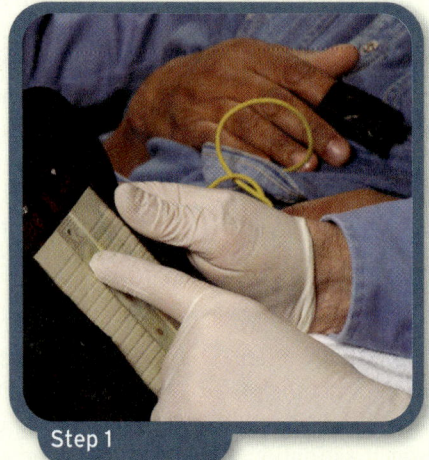

Step 1

Clean the patient's finger and place his or her finger in the pulse oximeter probe. Turn on the pulse oximeter and note the display of the SpO_2.

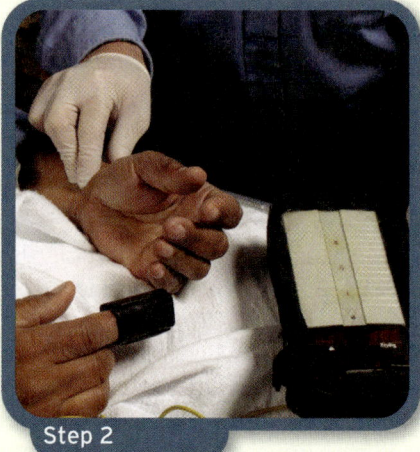

Step 2

Palpate the radial pulse to ensure that it correlates with the display on the pulse oximeter.

Skill Drill 11-2: Peak Expiratory Flow Measurement

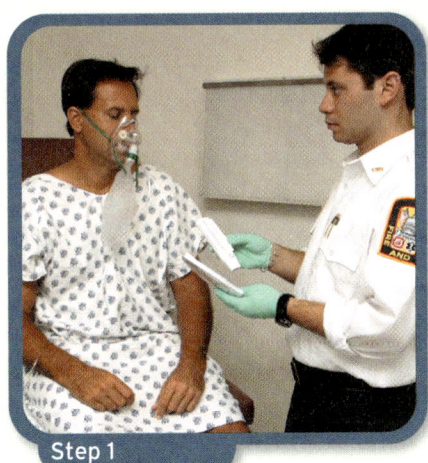

Step 1

Assemble the flowmeter and make sure it reads zero.

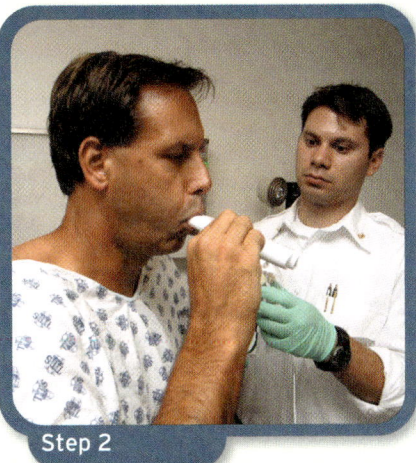

Step 2

Ask the patient to take a deep breath, place the mouthpiece in his or her mouth, and ask the patient to exhale as forcefully as possible. Make sure no air leaks around the device or comes from the patient's nose.

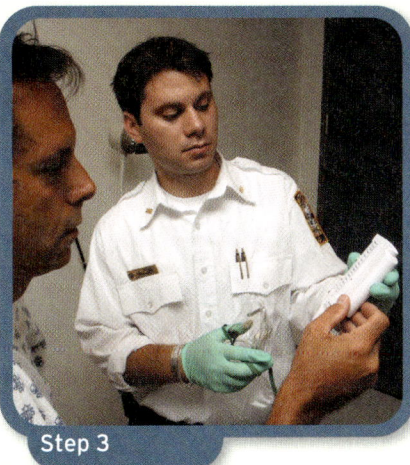

Step 3

Perform the test three times, and take the best rate of the three readings.

---

required to open it. In addition, artificial airway adjuncts may be needed to assist in maintaining the airway

Positioning the Patient

In a perfect world, all patients would present in a supine position, so that you could quickly open the airway, assess breathing, and intervene without moving them. If patients are found unconscious and in a prone position, however, you must position them properly so that you can open the airway, assess respirations, and provide ventilations if needed.

To move a patient to a supine position, log roll the individual as a unit. Once the patient is in a supine position, open his or her airway and assess breathing status. The recovery position, which involves placing the patient in a left lateral recumbent position, can be used in all nontrauma patients who are unconcious or have a decreased LOC who are able to maintain their own airway spontaneously and are breathing adequately **Figure 11-13 ▶**.

Manual Airway Maneuvers

In the unconscious patient or patient with a decreased LOC, the most common cause of airway obstruction is the patient's tongue **Figure 11-14 ▶**. To correct this problem, manually maneuver the patient's head to propel the tongue forward and open the airway. Techniques used to accomplish this include the head tilt–chin lift maneuver and the jaw-thrust maneuver (with or without head tilt).

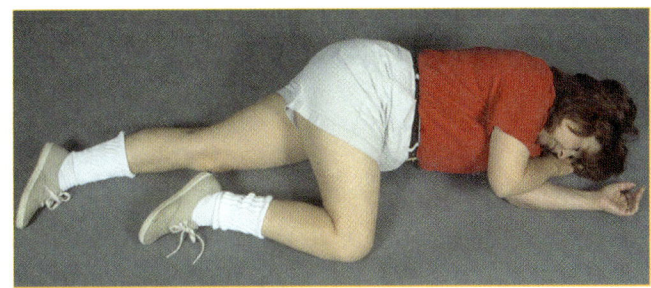

Figure 11-13 The recovery position.

Head Tilt–Chin Lift Maneuver

Opening the airway to relieve an obstruction can often be done quickly and easily by simply tilting the patient's head back and lifting the chin. This head tilt–chin lift maneuver is the preferred technique for opening the airway of a patient who has not sustained trauma. Occasionally, this simple maneuver is all that is required for the patient to resume breathing. Following are some considerations when using the head tilt–chin lift maneuver:

- **Indications.** An unresponsive patient, no mechanism for cervical spine injury, or a patient who is unable to protect his or her own airway.
- **Contraindications.** A responsive patient or a patient with possible cervical spine injury.

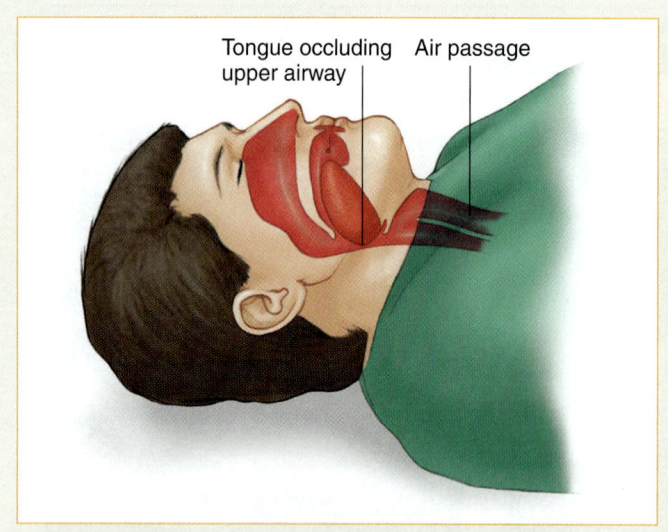

Figure 11-14 When the tongue falls back and occludes the posterior pharynx, it may obstruct the airway.

- **Advantages.** No equipment is required, and the technique is simple, safe, and noninvasive.
- **Disadvantages.** It is thought to be hazardous to patients with spinal injury and does not protect from aspiration. Perform the head tilt–chin lift maneuver in the following manner **Skill Drill 11-3 ▸**.

1. With the patient in a supine position, position yourself beside the patient's head **Step 1**.
2. Place one hand on the patient's forehead, and apply firm backward pressure with your palm to tilt the patient's head back **Step 2**. This extension of the neck will propel the tongue forward, away from the posterior pharynx and clear the airway.

3. Place the tips of your fingers of your other hand under the lower jaw near the bony part of the chin **Step 3**. Do not compress the soft tissue under the chin, as this may block the airway.
4. Lift the chin upward, bringing the entire lower jaw with it, helping to tilt the head back **Step 4**. Do not use your thumb to lift the chin. Lift so that the teeth are nearly brought together, but avoid closing the mouth completely. Continue to hold the forehead to maintain backward tilt of the head.

Jaw-Thrust Maneuver

If you suspect that the patient has experienced a cervical spine injury, open his or her airway with the jaw-thrust maneuver. In this technique, you open the airway by placing your fingers behind the angle of the jaw and lifting the jaw forward. The jaw is displaced forward at the mandibular angle. You can easily seal a mask around the patient's nose and mouth while performing this maneuver. Following are some considerations when using the jaw-thrust maneuver:

- **Indications.** An unresponsive patient, possible cervical spine injury, or a patient who is unable to protect his or her own airway.
- **Contraindications.** A responsive patient with resistance to opening the mouth. The jaw-thrust maneuver may be needed in the responsive patient who has sustained a jaw fracture to keep the tongue away from the back of the throat.
- **Advantages.** May be used in patients with cervical spine injury, may use with cervical collar in place, and does not require special equipment.
- **Disadvantages.** Cannot maintain if patient becomes responsive or combative, difficult to maintain for an extended period of time, very difficult to use in conjunction with bag-valve-mask ventilation, thumb must remain in place to maintain jaw displacement, requires second paramedic for bag-valve-mask ventilation, and does not protect against aspiration.

You are the Paramedic Part 5

You are now assisting the patient's breathing with a bag-valve-mask device and 100% oxygen. You radio the EMD and ask for an engine company to respond for manpower assistance. Your partner quickly reassesses the patient and notes the following:

Reassessment	Recording Time: 8 Minutes
Level of consciousness	P (Responsive to painful stimuli)
Respirations	36 breaths/min, shallow (baseline); you are assisting ventilations with a bag-valve-mask device and 100% oxygen
Pulse	150 beats/min, regular and weak
Skin	Pale and diaphoretic extremities and trunk; facial cyanosis
Blood pressure	118/70 mm Hg
Sp_{O_2}	86% while being ventilated with a bag-valve-mask device and 100% oxygen

8. Why is your patient's condition not improving with assisted ventilation?
9. What must you do to correct the situation?

Skill Drill 11-3:
Head Tilt–Chin Lift Maneuver

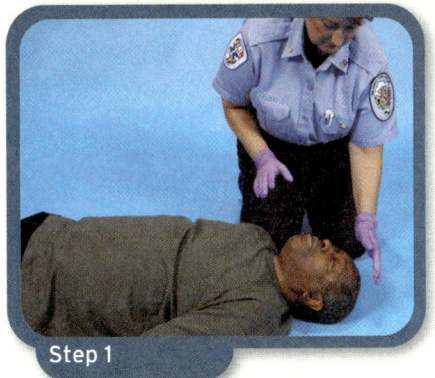

Step 1

Position yourself at the side of the supine patient.

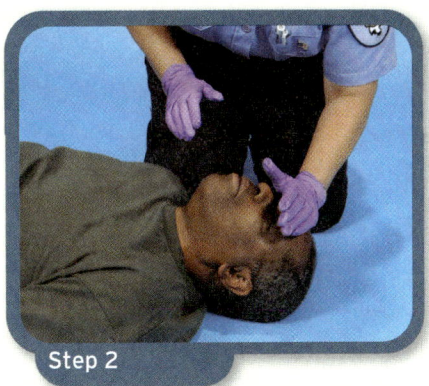

Step 2

Place your hand closest to the patient's head on the forehead.

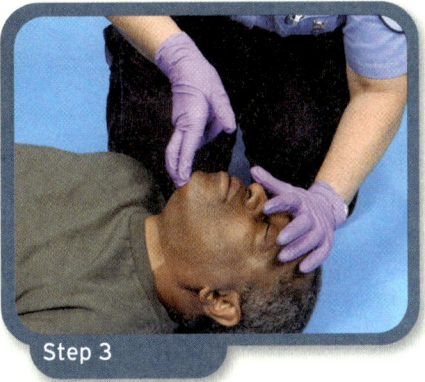

Step 3

With your other hand, place two fingers on the underside of the patient's chin.

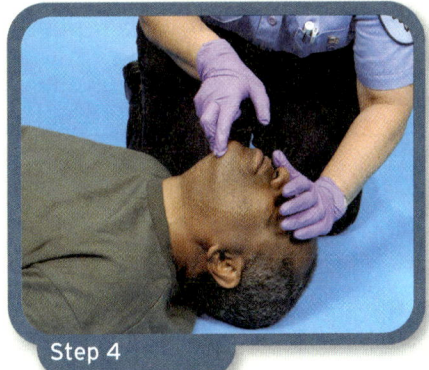

Step 4

Simultaneously apply backward and downward pressure to the patient's forehead and lift the jaw straight up. Do not depress the soft tissue below the chin.

Jaw-Thrust Maneuver With Head Tilt

The jaw-thrust maneuver with head tilt is similar to the head tilt–chin lift maneuver, with a few exceptions. Following are some considerations when using the jaw-thrust maneuver with head tilt:

- **Indications.** An unresponsive patient or a patient unable to protect his or her own airway.
- **Contraindications.** A responsive patient or a patient with a possible cervical spine injury.
- **Advantages.** It is noninvasive and does not require special equipment.
- **Disadvantages.** It is difficult to maintain, requires a second paramedic for bag-valve-mask ventilation, and does not protect against aspiration.

Perform the jaw-thrust maneuver with head tilt in the following manner **Skill Drill 11-5 ▸**.

1. Position yourself at the top of the patient's head **Step 1**.
2. Place the meaty portion of the base of your thumbs on the zygomatic arches, and hook the tips of your index fingers under the angle of the mandible, in the middle indent below the patient's ear **Step 2**.
3. Displace the jaw upward and tilt the head back **Step 3**.

Tongue-Jaw Lift Maneuver

The tongue-jaw lift maneuver is used more commonly to open a patient's airway for the purpose of suctioning or inserting an oropharyngeal airway. It cannot be used to ventilate a patient, because it will not allow for an adequate mask seal on the patient's face. Perform the tongue-jaw lift in the following manner **Skill Drill 11-6 ▸**.

1. Position yourself at the side of the patient **Step 1**.
2. Place the hand closest to the patient's head on the forehead **Step 2**.
3. With the other hand, reach into the patient's mouth and hook your first knuckle under the incisors or gum line. While holding the patient's head and maintaining the hand on the forehead, lift the jaw straight up **Step 3**.

Perform the jaw-thrust maneuver in the following manner **Skill Drill 11-4 ▸**.

1. Position yourself at the top of the supine patient's head **Step 1**.
2. Place the meaty portion of the base of your thumbs on the zygomatic arches and hook the tips of your index fingers under the angle of the mandible, in the indent below each ear **Step 2**.
3. While holding the patient's head in a neutral inline position, displace the jaw upward and open the patient's mouth with the tips of your thumbs **Step 3**.

If you are unable to open the airway with the jaw-thrust maneuver, you should carefully perform the head tilt–chin lift maneuver.

▌ Airway Obstructions

The airway connects the body to the life-giving oxygen in the atmosphere. If it becomes obstructed, this lifeline is cut and

Skill Drill 11-4: Jaw-Thrust Maneuver

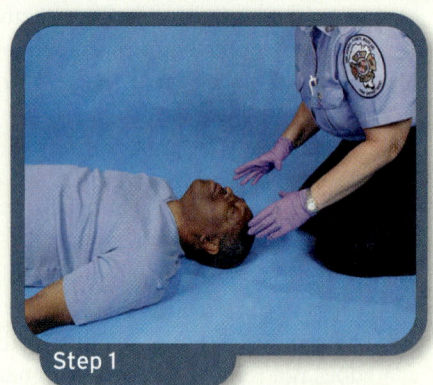

Step 1

Position yourself at the top of the patient's head.

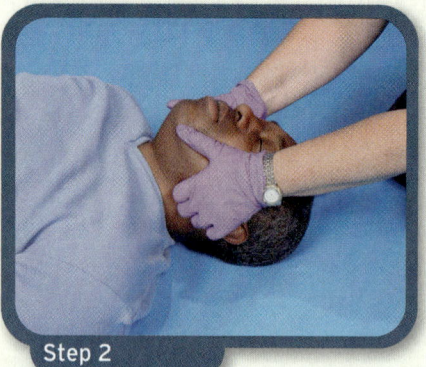

Step 2

Place the meaty portion of the base of your thumbs on the zygomatic arches, and hook the tips of your index fingers under the angle of the mandible, in the indent below each ear.

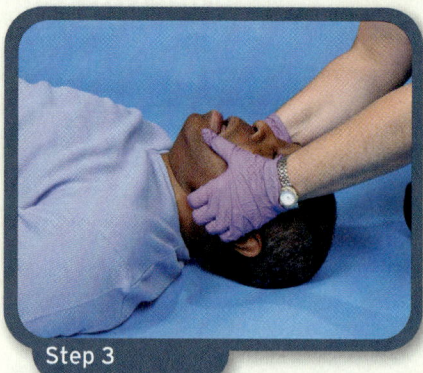

Step 3

While holding the patient's head still, displace the jaw upward and open the patient's mouth with your thumb tips.

Skill Drill 11-5: Jaw-Thrust Maneuver With Head Tilt

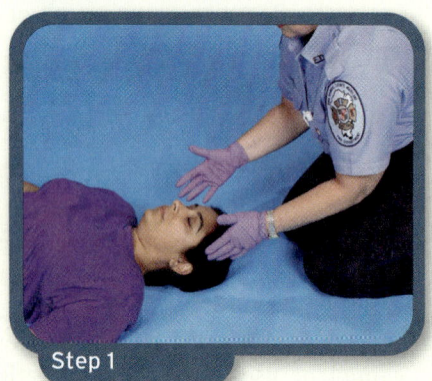

Step 1

Position yourself at the top of the patient's head.

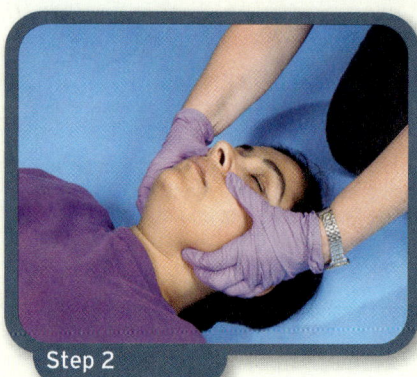

Step 2

Place the meaty portion of the base of your thumbs on the zygomatic arches, and hook the tips of your index fingers under the angle of the mandible, in the middle indent below each ear.

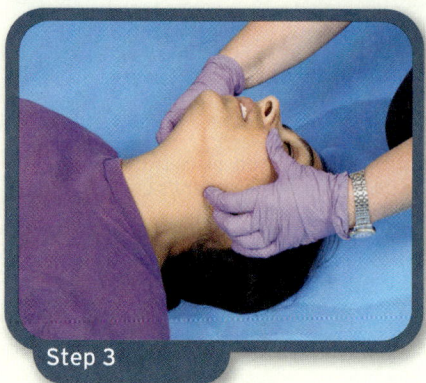

Step 3

Displace the jaw upward and tilt the head back.

the patient dies—often within minutes. The paramedic must recognize the signs of an obstructed airway and immediately take corrective action.

Causes of Airway Obstruction

In an adult, sudden foreign body airway obstruction usually occurs during a meal. In children, it typically occurs while eating or playing with small toys. An otherwise healthy child who presents with a sudden onset of difficulty breathing—especially in the absence of fever—should be suspected of having a foreign body airway obstruction. A multitude of other conditions can cause an airway obstruction, however, including the tongue, laryngeal edema, laryngeal spasm (laryngospasm), trauma, and aspiration.

Skill Drill 11-6: Tongue-Jaw Lift Maneuver

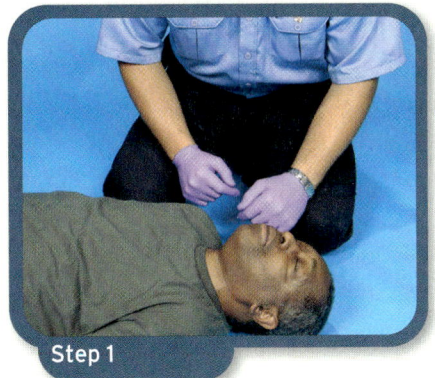

Step 1
Position yourself at the patient's side.

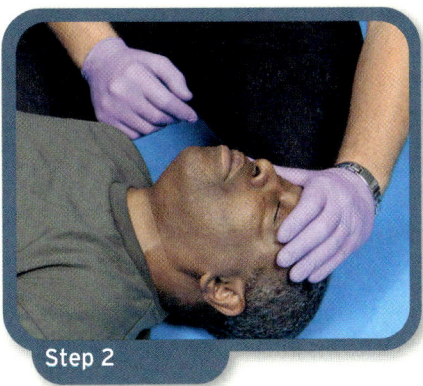

Step 2
Place the hand closest to the patient's head on the forehead.

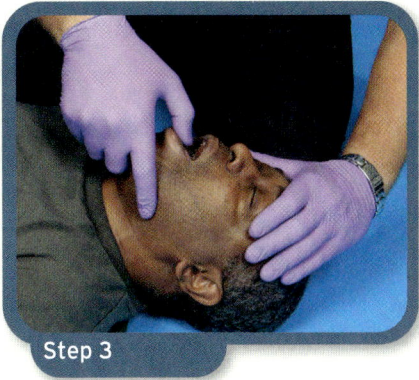

Step 3
With your other hand, reach into the patient's mouth and hook your first knuckle under the incisors or gum line. While holding the patient's head and maintaining the hand on the forehead, lift the jaw straight up.

When the airway is obstructed secondary to an infectious process or a severe allergic reaction, repeated attempts to clear the airway as if it were obstructed by a foreign body will be unsuccessful and potentially harmful. These patients require specific management (discussed in the appropriate chapters of this book) and prompt transport to an appropriate medical facility.

Tongue

In the patient with an altered LOC, the jaw relaxes and the tongue tends to fall back against the posterior wall of the pharynx, closing off the airway. A patient with partial obstruction from the tongue will have snoring respirations; a patient whose airway is completely obstructed will have no respirations. Obstruction of the airway by the tongue is simple to correct using a manual maneuver (eg, head tilt–chin lift, or jaw-thrust).

Foreign Body

A large number of people die from foreign body airway obstructions each year, often as the result of choking on a piece of food. The typical victim is middle-aged or older and wears dentures. He or she has usually had a few alcoholic drinks, which depresses protective reflexes and adversely affects a person's judgment regarding how large a piece of food can be prudently placed in the mouth. Additionally, patients with conditions that decrease their airway reflexes (eg, stroke) are at an increased risk for a foreign body airway obstruction. A foreign body may cause a mild or severe airway obstruction, depending on the size of the object and its location in the airway.

Signs may include choking, gagging, stridor, dyspnea, aphonia (inability to speak), and dysphonia (difficulty speaking). Treatment for the patient depends on whether he or she is effectively moving air. Techniques for foreign body airway obstruction removal will be discussed later in this chapter.

Laryngeal Spasm and Edema

A laryngeal spasm (laryngospasm) results in spasmodic closure of the vocal cords, completely occluding the airway. It is often caused by trauma during an overly aggressive intubation attempt or immediately upon extubation, especially when the patient has an altered LOC.

Laryngeal edema causes the glottic opening to become extremely narrow or totally closed. Conditions that commonly cause this problem include epiglottitis, anaphylaxis, or inhalation injury (eg, burns to the upper airway).

Airway obstructions caused by laryngeal spasm or edema may be relieved by positive-pressure ventilation using a bag-valve-mask or an upward pull of the jaw in an attempt to reposition the airway. In certain cases, muscle relaxant medications may be effective in relieving laryngeal spasm. Do not let your guard down after the laryngospasm has appeared to have resolved; resolution of the crisis does not mean that laryngospasm will not recur. The patient should be transported to the hospital for evaluation.

Fractured Larynx

Airway patency depends on good muscle tone to keep the trachea open. Fracture of the larynx increases airway resistance by decreasing airway size secondary to decreased muscle tone, laryngeal edema, and ventilatory effort. An advanced airway may be required to maintain a patent airway.

Aspiration

Aspiration of blood or other fluid significantly increases mortality. In addition to potentially obstructing the airway, aspiration destroys delicate bronchiolar tissue, introduces pathogens into the lungs, and decreases the patient's ability to ventilate (or be ventilated).

Suction should be readily available for any patient who is unable to maintain his or her own airway. Patients requiring emergency care should always be assumed to have a full stomach.

Recognition of an Airway Obstruction

A foreign body lodged in the upper airway can cause a mild (partial) or severe (complete) airway obstruction. A rapid but careful assessment is required to determine the seriousness of the obstruction, as the differences in managing mild versus severe cases are significant.

A patient with a mild airway obstruction is conscious and able to exchange air, but may show varying degrees of respiratory distress. The patient will usually have noisy respirations and may be coughing. He or she may wheeze between coughs but does not become cyanotic. *Patients with a mild airway obstruction should be left alone! A forceful cough is the most effective means of dislodging the obstruction.* Attempts to manually remove the object could force it farther down into the airway and cause a severe obstruction. Closely monitor the patient's condition and be prepared to intervene if you see signs of severe airway obstruction.

A patient with a severe airway obstruction typically experiences a sudden inability to breathe, talk, or cough—classically during a meal. The patient may grasp at his or her throat (universal sign of choking), begin to turn cyanotic, and make frantic, exaggerated attempts to move air Figure 11-15 ▸ . Patients with a severe airway obstruction have a weak, ineffective, or absent cough and are in marked respiratory distress; weak inspiratory stridor and cyanosis are often present.

Emergency Medical Care for Foreign Body Airway Obstruction

If the patient with a suspected airway obstruction is conscious, ask, "Are you choking?" If the patient nods "yes," begin treatment immediately. If the obstruction is not promptly cleared, the amount of oxygen in the blood will decrease dramatically, resulting in severe hypoxia and death.

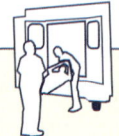

At the Scene

Causes of Airway Obstruction

- Relaxation of the tongue in an unresponsive patient
- Foreign objects—food, small toys, dentures
- Blood clots, broken teeth, or damaged oral tissue following trauma
- Airway tissue swelling—infection, allergic reaction
- Aspirated vomitus (stomach contents)

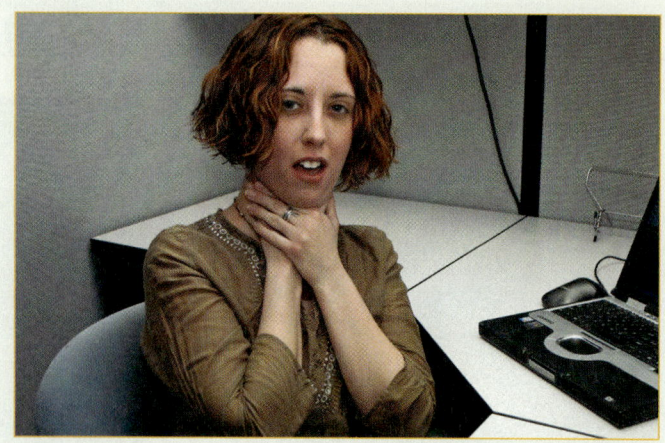

Figure 11-15 The universal sign of choking.

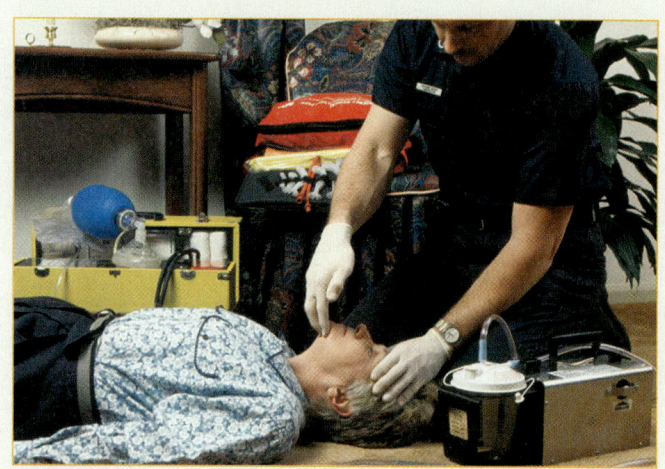

Figure 11-16 Securing and maintaining a patent airway and ensuring adequate ventilation are among the most important steps in caring for an unconscious patient.

Manage any unresponsive person as if he or she has a compromised airway. Open and maintain the airway with the appropriate manual maneuver (eg, head tilt–chin lift for non-trauma patients, jaw-thrust for trauma patients), assess for breathing, and provide artificial ventilation if necessary Figure 11-16 ▲ .

If, after opening the airway, you are unable to ventilate the patient (no chest rise and fall) or you feel resistance when ventilating, reopen the airway and again attempt to ventilate the patient. Lung compliance is the ability of the alveoli to expand when air is drawn into the lungs, either during negative-pressure ventilation or positive-pressure ventilation. Poor lung compliance is characterized by increased resistance during ventilation attempts.

If large pieces of vomitus, mucus, loose dentures, or blood clots are found in the airway, sweep them forward and out of the mouth with your gloved index finger. *Blind finger sweeps of the mouth—regardless of the patient's age—are not recommended and may cause further harm; only attempt to remove foreign bodies that you can see and easily retrieve.* After the patient's airway is open, insert your index finger down along the inside of the patient's cheek and into his or her throat at the base of the tongue, then try to hook the foreign body to dislodge it and maneuver it into the mouth. Take care not to force the foreign body deeper into the airway. Do *not* blindly insert any object into the patient's mouth to remove a foreign body, because anything jammed into the throat can damage the delicate structures of the pharynx and compound the obstruction with hemorrhage. Suctioning should be used to clear the airway of secretions as needed.

Special Considerations

According to current Emergency Cardiovascular Care (ECC) guidelines, a child is defined as a patient from 1 year of age to the onset of puberty (12 to 14 years of age).

The steps for managing a severe airway obstruction in a conscious adult or child are listed here and shown in **Skill Drill 11-7 ▾**.

1. Determine whether the patient is choking by asking, "Are you choking?" If the patient nods "yes," then help is needed **Step 1**.

2. Perform the Heimlich maneuver until the object is expelled or the patient becomes unresponsive **Step 2**.

The steps for managing a severe airway obstruction in an unconscious adult or child are listed here and shown in **Skill Drill 11-8 ▸**.

1. Open the airway with the head tilt–chin lift maneuver and look in the patient's mouth **Step 1**. If you see the object, carefully remove it from the patient's mouth.

2. Attempt to ventilate the patient **Step 2**. If unsuccessful, reopen the airway and again attempt ventilation.

3. Perform chest compressions **Step 3**. Perform 30 chest compressions if you are by yourself or if the patient is an adult; perform 15 chest compressions if two paramedics are present or if the patient is a child. In the child, chest compressions can be performed with one or two hands, depending on the size of the child.

4. Open the airway with the head tilt–chin lift maneuver and look in the patient's mouth **Step 4**. If you see the object, carefully remove it from the patient's mouth. Repeat steps 2 through 4 until successful or until help arrives.

The steps for managing a severe airway obstruction in a conscious infant are listed here and shown in **Skill Drill 11-9 ▸**.

1. Perform five back blows (slaps) **Step 1**.

2. Perform five chest thrusts **Step 2**. Repeat steps 1 and 2 until the object is expelled or the infant becomes unresponsive.

The steps for managing a severe airway obstruction in an unconscious infant are listed here and shown in **Skill Drill 11-10 ▸**.

1. Open the infant's airway with slight extension of the neck and look in the mouth **Step 1**. If you see the object, carefully remove it from the infant's mouth.

2. Attempt to ventilate **Step 2**. If unsuccessful, reopen the airway and again attempt ventilation.

3. Perform chest compressions **Step 3**. Perform 30 chest compressions if you are by yourself; perform 15 chest compressions if two paramedics are present.

4. Open the infant's airway with slight extension of the neck and look in the mouth **Step 4**. If you see the object, carefully remove it from the infant's mouth. Repeat steps 2 through 4 until successful or until help arrives.

Skill Drill 11-7: Managing Severe Airway Obstruction in a Conscious Adult or Child

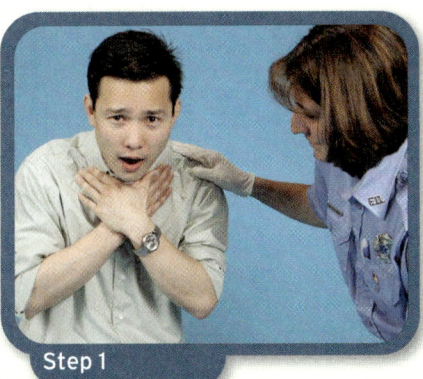

Step 1

Determine whether the patient is choking by asking, "Are you choking?" If the patient nods "yes," then help is needed.

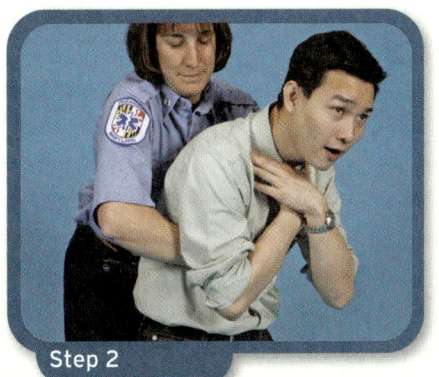

Step 2

Perform the Heimlich maneuver until the object is expelled or the patient becomes unresponsive.

Skill Drill 11-8: Managing Severe Airway Obstruction in an Unconscious Adult or Child

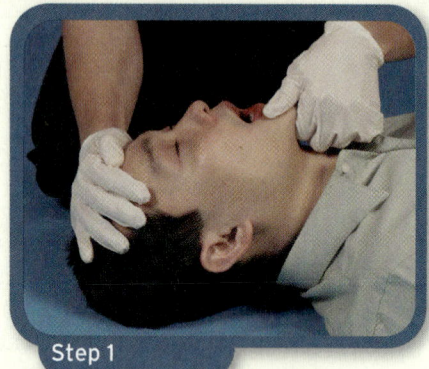

Step 1

Open the airway and look in the mouth. If you see the object, carefully remove it from the patient's mouth.

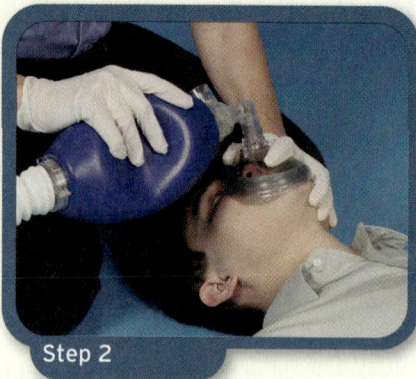

Step 2

Attempt to ventilate the patient. If unsuccessful, reopen the airway and again attempt ventilation.

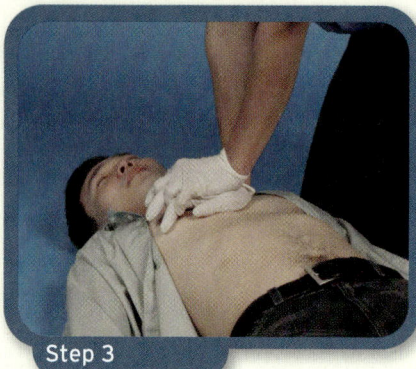

Step 3

Perform chest compressions.

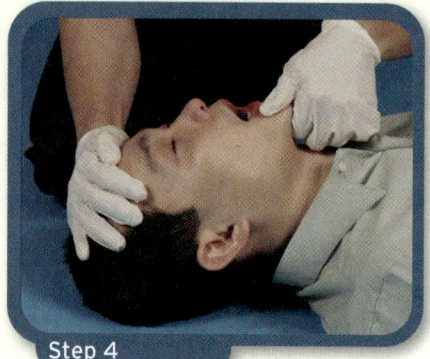

Step 4

Open the airway and look in the mouth. If you see the object, carefully remove it from the patient's mouth. Repeat steps 2 through 4 until successful or until help arrives.

Skill Drill 11-9: Managing Severe Airway Obstruction in a Conscious Infant

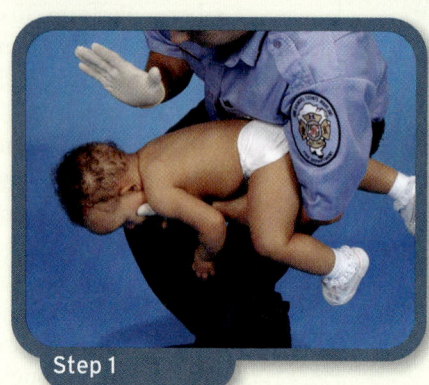

Step 1

Perform five back blows (slaps).

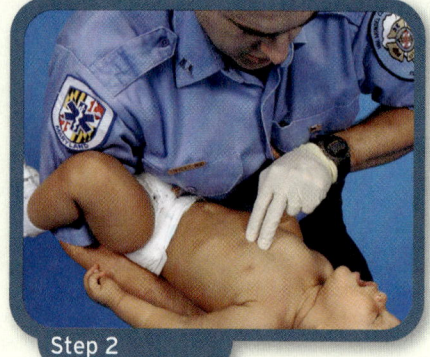

Step 2

Perform five chest thrusts. Repeat steps 1 and 2 until the object is expelled or the infant becomes unresponsive.

The Heimlich maneuver (abdominal thrusts) is the most effective method of dislodging and forcing an object out of the airway. It aims to create an artificial cough by forcing residual air out of the victim's lungs, thereby expelling the object. You should perform the Heimlich maneuver on any conscious child or adult with a severe airway obstruction until the obstructing object is expelled or until the patient becomes unresponsive. If the conscious patient with a severe airway obstruction is in the advanced stages of pregnancy or is morbidly obese, perform chest thrusts instead of abdominal thrusts.

If you are unable to relieve a severe airway obstruction in an unconscious patient with the basic techniques previously discussed, you should proceed with direct laryngoscopy (visualization of the airway with a laryngoscope) for the removal of the foreign body in unresponsive patients. Insert the laryngoscope blade into the patient's mouth. If you see the foreign body, carefully remove it from the upper airway with Magill forceps, a special type of curved forceps **Figure 11-17 ▶**. The steps for removal of an upper airway obstruction with Magill forceps are listed here and shown in **Skill Drill 11-11 ▶**.

1. With the patient's head in the sniffing position, open the patient's mouth and insert the laryngoscope blade **Step 1**.
2. Visualize the obstruction, and retrieve the object with the Magill forceps **Step 2**.
3. Remove the object with the Magill forceps **Step 3**.
4. Attempt to ventilate the patient **Step 4**.

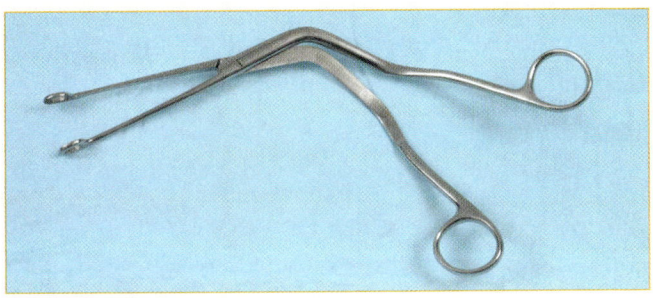

Figure 11-17 Magill forceps.

At the Scene

A patient with a severe upper airway obstruction has very little time before severe hypoxia develops. If several attempts to relieve the obstruction with conventional BLS methods fail, you should proceed with direct laryngoscopy without delay. As you are performing BLS maneuvers, your partner should be preparing the laryngoscope handle and blade.

Suctioning

When the patient's mouth or throat becomes filled with vomitus, blood, or secretions, a suction apparatus enables you to remove the liquid material quickly and efficiently, thereby allowing you to ventilate the patient. Ventilating a patient with secretions in his or her mouth will force material into the lungs, resulting in an upper airway obstruction or aspiration. Therefore, clearing the patient's airway with suction, if needed, is your next priority after opening the patient's airway. *If you hear gurgling, the patient needs suctioning!*

Suctioning Equipment

Ambulances should carry both a fixed suction unit (which operates off a vacuum from the engine manifold) and a portable suction unit (battery operated or hand powered) **Figure 11-18 ▶**. Regardless of your location—in the patient's residence, the middle of a field, or in the back of the ambulance—you must have quick access to suction. It is essential for resuscitation.

Mechanical or vacuum-powered suction units should be capable of generating sufficient vacuum and the amount of suction should be adjustable for

Skill Drill 11-10: Managing Severe Airway Obstruction in an Unconscious Infant

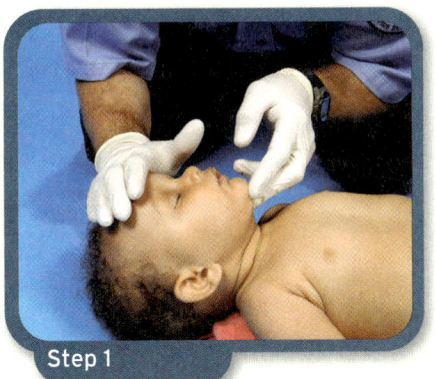

Step 1

Open the infant's airway and look in the mouth. If you see the object, carefully remove it from the infant's mouth.

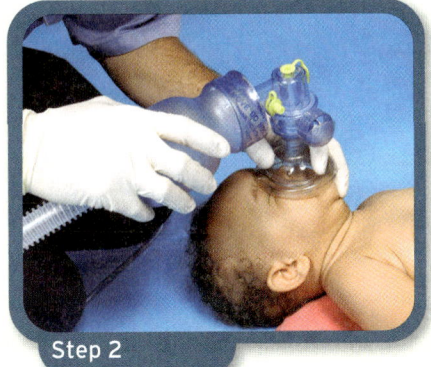

Step 2

Attempt to ventilate. If unsuccessful, reopen the airway and again attempt ventilation.

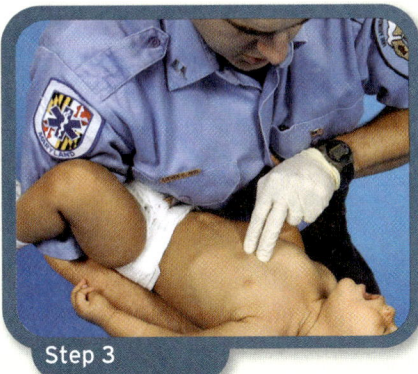

Step 3

Perform chest compressions.

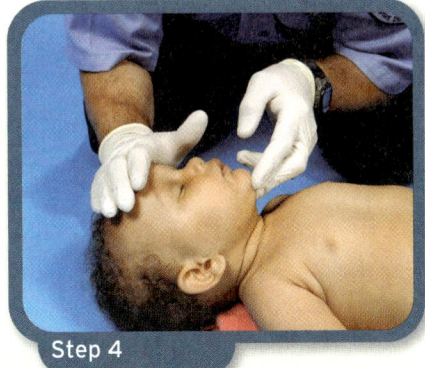

Step 4

Open the infant's airway and look in the mouth. If you see the object, carefully remove it from the infant's mouth. Repeat steps 2 through 4 until successful or until help arrives.

Notes from Nancy

Carry your intubation kit with you whenever you respond to a call in a restaurant.

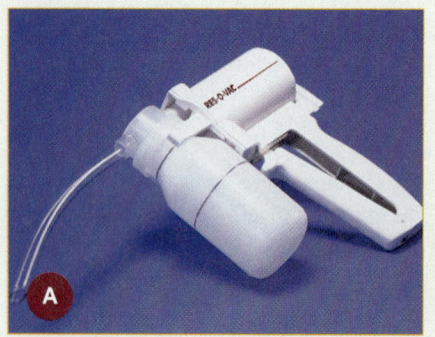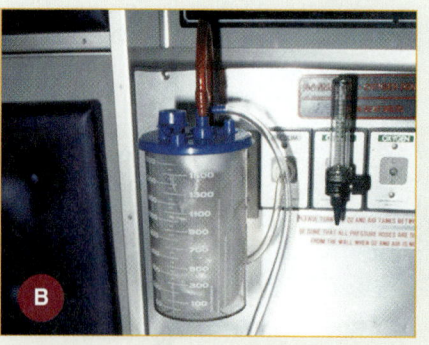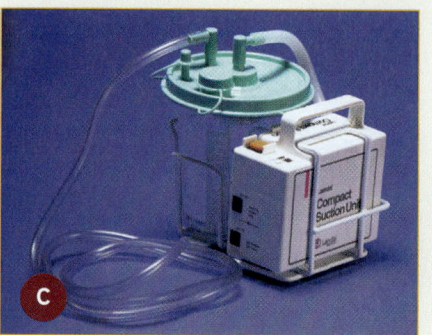

Figure 11-18 Suctioning equipment is essential for good airway management. **A.** Hand-operated device. **B.** Fixed unit. **C.** Portable unit.

Skill Drill 11-11: Removal of an Upper Airway Obstruction With Magill Forceps

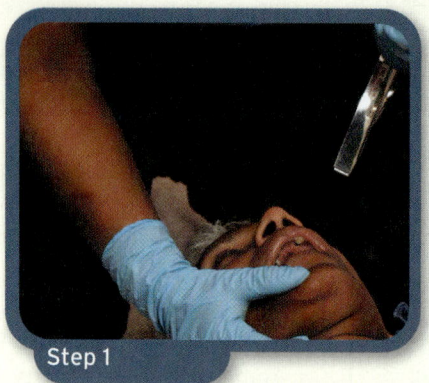

Step 1

With the patient's head in the sniffing position, open the patient's mouth and insert the laryngoscope blade.

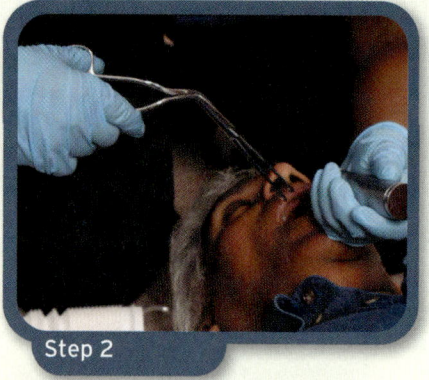

Step 2

Visualize the obstruction, and retrieve the object with the Magill forceps.

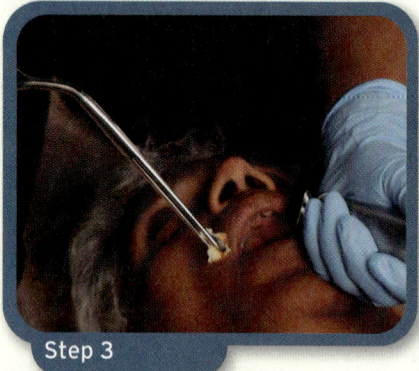

Step 3

Remove the object with the Magill forceps.

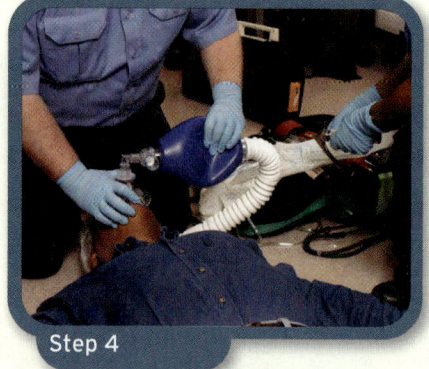

Step 4

Attempt to ventilate the patient.

most common types of suction devices.

Regardless of which type of suction unit you are using, the device must be able to generate enough vacuum pressure to adequately suction the patient's mouth and oropharynx. In addition to the suctioning unit, the following supplies should be readily accessible at the patient's head:

- Wide-bore, thick-walled, nonkinking tubing
- Soft and rigid suction catheters
- A nonbreakable, disposable collection bottle
- A supply of water for rinsing the catheters

A suction catheter is a hollow, cylindrical device that is used to remove fluids and secretions from the patient's airway. A Yankauer catheter (tonsil-tip catheter) is a good option for suctioning the pharynx in adults and the preferred device for infants and children. These plastic-tip catheters have a large diameter and are rigid, so they do not collapse. Rigid catheters are capable of suctioning large volumes of fluid rapidly. Tips with a curved contour allow for easy, rapid placement in the pharynx Figure 11-19 ▸ .

use in children and intubated patients. Check the vacuum on the mechanical suction unit at the beginning of every shift by turning on the device, clamping the tubing, and making sure the pressure gauge registers sufficient vacuum. Ensure that all battery-charged units have fully charged batteries. Table 11-6 ▸ lists the advantages and disadvantages of the

Soft plastic, nonrigid catheters, sometimes called French or whistle-tip catheters, can be placed in the oropharynx or nasopharynx or down an endotracheal (ET) tube. They come in various sizes and have a smaller diameter than hard-tip catheters. Soft catheters are used to suction the nose and liquid secretions in the back of the mouth and in situations in which

Table 11-6	Suction Devices	
Suction Device	**Advantages**	**Disadvantages**
Hand powered	• Lightweight • Portable • Mechanically simple • Inexpensive	• Limited volume • Limited suction • Manually powered • Fluid contact • Components not disposable • Not routinely recommended
Oxygen-powered portable	• Lightweight • Small	• Limited suction power • Uses a lot of oxygen for limited suctioning power
Battery-operated portable	• Lightweight • Portable • Excellent suction power • May "field troubleshoot" most problems with the device	• More complicated mechanics • May lose battery integrity over time • Some fluid contact • Components not disposable
Mounted vacuum powered	• Extremely strong vacuum • Adjustable vacuum power • Components disposable	• Not portable • Fluid contact • Cannot "field service" or substitute power source

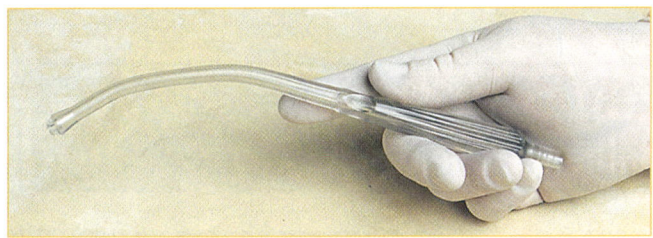

Figure 11-19 Tonsil-tip catheters are a good choice for suctioning the oropharynx because they have wide-diameter tips and are rigid.

you cannot use a rigid catheter, such as for a patient with a stoma ▸ Figure 11-20 ▸ . For example, a rigid catheter could break a tooth in a patient with clenched teeth, whereas a flexible catheter may be worked along the cheeks without causing injury. Suction tubing without the attached catheter facilitates suctioning of large debris in the oropharynx and allows access to the back of the pharynx in a patient with clenched teeth.

Suctioning Techniques

Mortality increases significantly if a patient aspirates; therefore, suctioning the upper airway is critical to prevent aspiration. Suctioning removes not only liquids from the airway, but also oxygen. For that reason, any patient who is to be suctioned should be adequately preoxygenated first; this will provide a small oxygen reserve that can be drawn upon while you are suctioning. Even so, each suctioning attempt must be limited to a maximum of 15 seconds in the adult (less in infants and children). Be careful not to stimulate the back of

You are the Paramedic Part 6

The patient's airway has been cleared appropriately and bag-valve-mask ventilations with 100% oxygen are continued. The engine arrives and two firefighters assist you in loading the patient into the ambulance, where you attach a cardiac monitor, start an IV, and perform a reassessment. The closest appropriate hospital is approximately 40 km away.

Reassessment	Recording Time: 11 Minutes
Level of consciousness	V (Responsive to verbal stimuli)
Respirations	28 breaths/min, shallow (baseline); you are assisting ventilations with a bag-valve-mask device and 100% oxygen
Pulse	120 beats/min, regular and weak
Skin	Remains pale and diaphoretic; facial cyanosis is improving
Blood pressure	114/72 mm Hg
SpO_2	95% while receiving assisted ventilations with a bag-valve-mask device and 100% oxygen

10. What is your most appropriate action at this point?

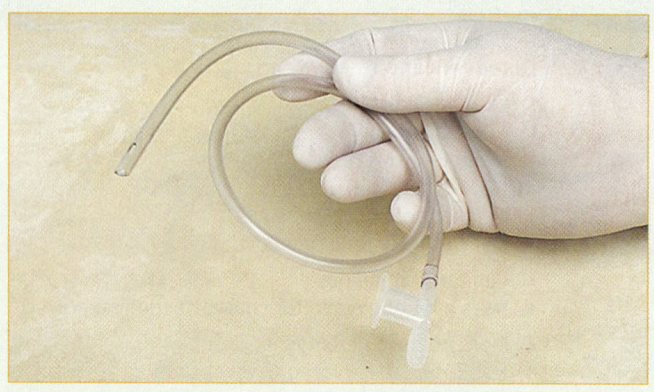

Figure 11-20 French (whistle-tip) cannulas are used in situations in which rigid cannulas cannot be used, such as when a patient has a stoma or if the patient's teeth are clenched.

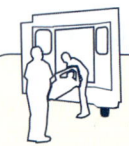

At the Scene

Suctioning Time Limits

Adult	15 seconds
Child	10 seconds
Infant	5 seconds

4. Apply suction in a circular motion as you withdraw the cannula. Do not suction an adult for more than 15 seconds (Step 4).

Airway Adjuncts

The first step in the initial management of an unconscious patient is to open the airway, initially by manual methods (eg, head tilt–chin lift, jaw-thrust). If the patient has an altered LOC, an artificial airway may then be needed to help maintain an open air

the throat of a young child or infant as the vagal stimulus can cause the heart rate to drop. After the patient has been suctioned, continue ventilation and oxygenation.

Soft-tip cannulas must be lubricated when suctioning the nasopharynx and used through an ET tube. The cannula is inserted, and suction is applied during extraction of the cannula to clear the airway. After the patient has been suctioned, reevaluate the patency of his or her airway, and continue to ventilate and oxygenate as needed.

Before inserting any suction cannula into a patient, make sure you measure for the proper size, going from the corner of the mouth to the earlobe. Never insert a cannula past the base of the tongue, as it may cause the patient to gag or vomit.

The steps for properly suctioning a patient's airway are listed here and shown in Skill Drill 11-12 ▶.

1. Turn on the assembled suction unit (Step 1).
2. Measure the cannula from the corner of the mouth to the earlobe (Step 2).
3. Before applying suction, open the patient's mouth by using the crossfinger technique or tongue-jaw lift, and insert the tip of the cannula to the predetermined depth. Do not suction while inserting the cannula (Step 3).

Skill Drill 11-12: Suctioning a Patient's Airway

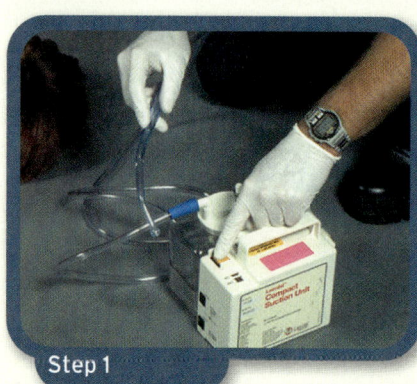

Step 1
Make sure the suctioning unit is properly assembled, and turn on the suction unit.

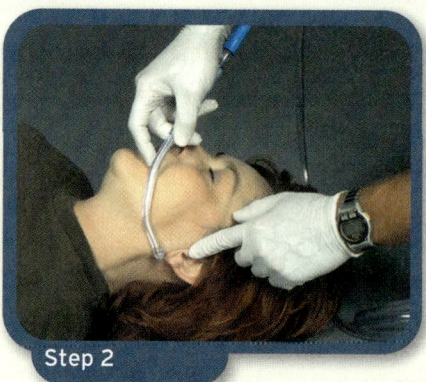

Step 2
Measure the cannula from the corner of the mouth to the earlobe.

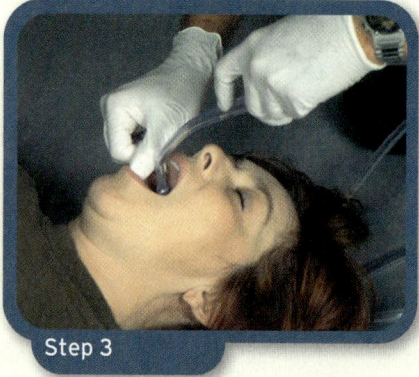

Step 3
Open the patient's mouth, and insert the cannula to the predetermined depth without suctioning.

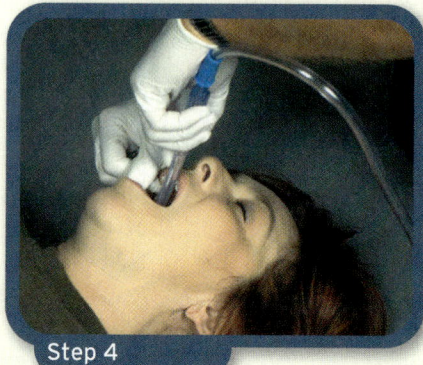

Step 4
Apply suction in a circular motion as you withdraw the cannula. Do not suction an adult for more than 15 seconds.

passage. *An artificial airway is not a substitute for proper head positioning.* Even after an airway adjunct has been inserted, the appropriate manual position of the head must be maintained.

Oropharyngeal Airway

The oropharyngeal (oral) airway is a curved, hard plastic device that fits over the back of the tongue with the tip in the posterior pharynx **Figure 11-21 ▾**. It is designed to hold the tongue away from the posterior pharyngeal wall, and its use makes it much easier to ventilate patients with a bag-valve-mask device. The oral airway can also serve as an effective bite-block, preventing an intubated patient from biting down on the ET tube.

An oral airway should be inserted promptly in unresponsive patients—breathing or not—who have no gag reflex. Because its distal end sits in the back of the throat, this device will stimulate gagging and retching in a patient with an intact gag reflex. For that reason, the oropharyngeal airway should be used only in unconscious, unresponsive patients without a gag reflex. *If the patient gags during insertion of the oral airway, remove the device immediately and be prepared to suction the oropharynx.* Following are some considerations when using an oropharyngeal airway:

- **Indications.** Unconscious patients, absent gag reflex.
- **Contraindications.** Conscious patients, patients with a gag reflex.
- **Advantages.** Noninvasive, easily placed, prevents blockage of the glottis by the tongue.

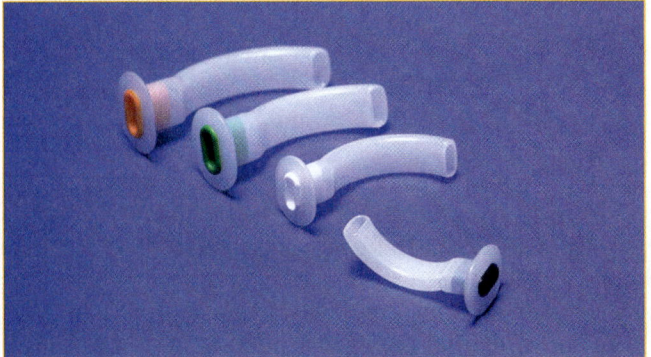

Figure 11-21 An oral airway is used for unconscious patients who have no gag reflex. It helps to keep the tongue from blocking the airway.

- **Disadvantages.** Does not prevent aspiration.
- **Complications.** Unexpected gag may cause vomiting, pharyngeal or dental trauma with poor technique.

If the oral airway is improperly sized or is inserted incorrectly, it could actually push the tongue back into the pharynx, creating an airway obstruction. Rough insertion of the airway can injure the hard palate, resulting in oral bleeding and creating a risk of vomiting or aspiration. Prior to inserting an oral airway, suction the oropharynx as needed to ensure that the mouth is clear of blood or other fluids. If the patient gags while being suctioned, consider using a nasopharyngeal airway instead. The steps for inserting an oral airway are listed here and shown in **Skill Drill 11-13 ▸**.

1. To select the proper size, measure the distance from the patient's earlobe to the corner of the mouth **Step 1**.
2. Open the patient's mouth with the crossfinger technique or tongue-jaw lift. Hold the airway upside down with your other hand. Insert the airway with the tip facing the roof of the mouth **Step 2**.
3. Rotate the airway 180°, flipping it over the tongue. When inserted properly, the airway will rest in the mouth, with the curvature of the airway following the contour of the teeth. The flange should rest against the lips, with the distal end in the posterior pharynx **Step 3**.

If you encounter difficulty while inserting the oral airway, try this alternative technique **Skill Drill 11-14 ▸**.

1. Use a tongue blade to depress the tongue, ensuring that the tongue remains forward **Step 1**.
2. Insert the oral airway sideways from the corner of the mouth, until the flange reaches the lips **Step 2**.
3. Rotate the oral airway 90°, removing the tongue blade as you exert gentle backward pressure on the oral airway, until the flange rests securely in place against the lips **Step 3**.

Skill Drill 11-13: Inserting an Oral Airway

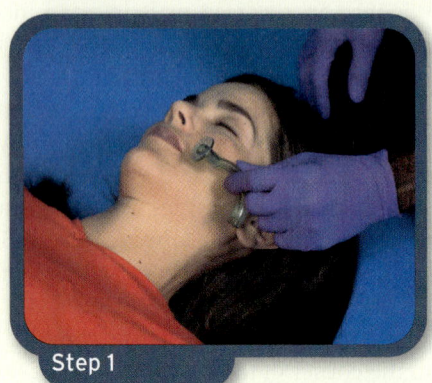

Step 1

Determine the size of the airway by measuring the distance from the patient's earlobe to the corner of the mouth.

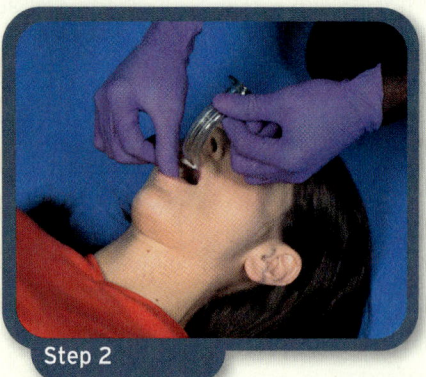

Step 2

Open the patient's mouth with the crossfinger technique or tongue-jaw lift. Hold the airway upside down with your other hand. Insert the airway with the tip facing the roof of the mouth and slide it in until it touches the roof of the mouth.

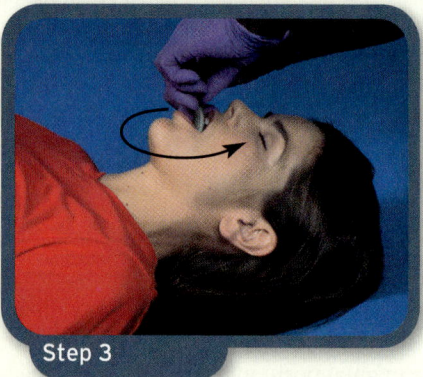

Step 3

Rotate the airway 180°, flipping it over the tongue. Insert the airway until the flange rests on the patient's lips. In this position, the airway will hold the tongue away from the posterior pharynx.

Skill Drill 11-14: Inserting an Oral Airway With a 90° Rotation

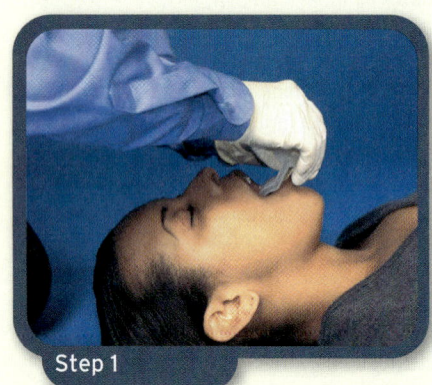

Step 1

Depress the tongue with a tongue blade so the tongue remains forward.

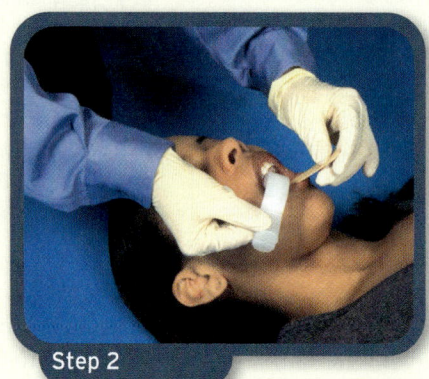

Step 2

Insert the oral airway sideways from the corner of the mouth, until the flange reaches the lips.

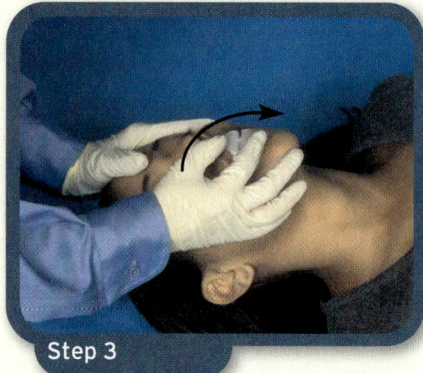

Step 3

Rotate the oral airway 90°, and remove the tongue blade as you exert gentle backward pressure on the oral airway until the flange rests securely in place against the lips.

Nasopharyngeal Airway

The nasopharyngeal (nasal) airway is a 15-cm long, soft, rubber tube that is inserted through the nose into the posterior pharynx behind the tongue, thereby allowing passage of air from the nose to the lower airway. The nasal airway is much better tolerated than an oral airway in patients who have an intact gag reflex yet an altered LOC **Figure 11-22** . Do not use this device when is the patient has experienced trauma to the nose or you have reason to suspect a skull fracture (eg, CSF leakage from the nose). Although unlikely, inserting the airway in such cases may cause it to enter the brain through the hole caused by the fracture.

The nasopharyngeal airway must be inserted gently to avoid precipitating epistaxis (nosebleed). Lubricate the airway generously with a water-soluble jelly, preferably one that contains local anesthetic, and slide it gently, tip downward, into one nostril. *Do not try to force it.* If you meet resistance, try to

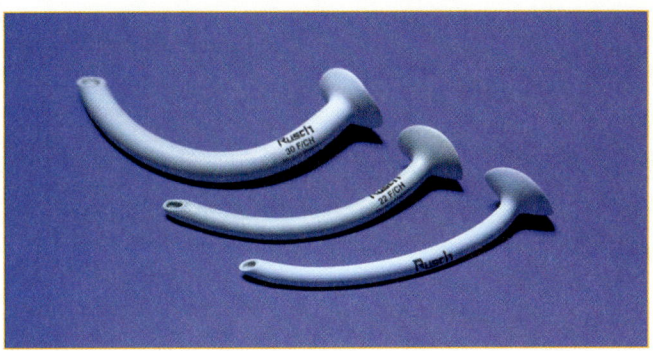

Figure 11-22 A nasal airway is better tolerated by patients who have an intact gag reflex.

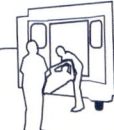
pass the airway down the other nostril. Following are considerations when using a nasopharyngeal airway:

- **Indications.** Unresponsive patients, patients with an altered mental status who have an intact gag reflex.
- **Contraindications.** Patient intolerance, caution in the presence of facial fracture or skull fracture.
- **Advantages.** Can be suctioned through, provides a patent airway, can be tolerated by awake patients, can be safely placed "blindly," does not require the mouth to be open.
- **Disadvantages.** Poor technique may result in severe bleeding (resulting epistaxis may be extremely difficult to control), does not protect from aspiration.

The steps for inserting a nasal airway are listed here and shown in **Skill Drill 11-15 ▶**.

1. Before inserting the airway, make sure you have selected the proper size. Measure the distance from the tip of the nostril to the earlobe. In almost all individuals, one nostril is larger than the other. The diameter should be roughly equal to the patient's little finger **Step 1**.
2. After lubricating the nasal airway with a water-soluble gel, place the airway in the larger nostril, with the curvature of the device

following the curve of the floor of the nose and the bevel facing the septum **Step 2**.

3. Place the bevel toward the septum and insert it gently along the nasal floor, parallel to the mouth. *Do not force the airway* **Step 3**.
4. When completely inserted, the flange should rest against the nostril. The distal end of the airway will open into the posterior pharynx **Step 4**.

As an alternative, the proper size of nasal airway can be determined by measuring from the tip of the nostril to the angle

Skill Drill 11-15:
Inserting a Nasal Airway

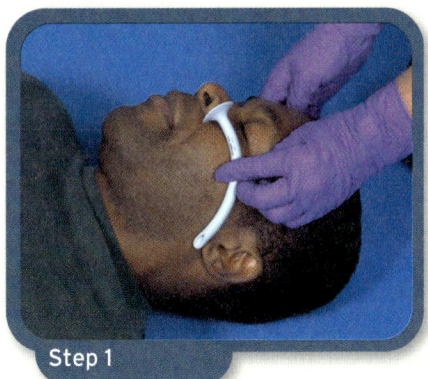

Step 1

Determine the size of the airway by measuring the distance from the tip of the nose to the patient's earlobe. Coat the tip with a water-soluble lubricant.

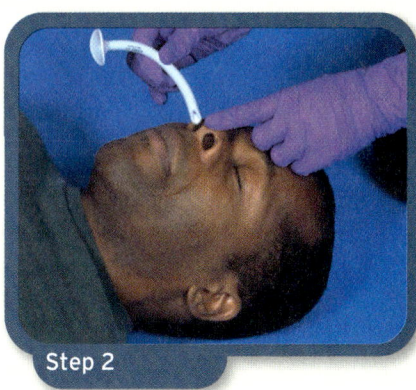

Step 2

Insert the lubricated airway into the larger nostril, with the curvature following the floor of the nose and the bevel facing the septum.

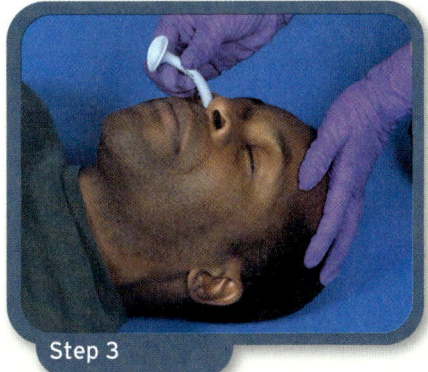

Step 3

Gently advance the airway. If using the left nostril, insert the nasal airway until it meets with resistance, then rotate the airway 180° into position. *This rotation is not required if you are using the right nostril.*

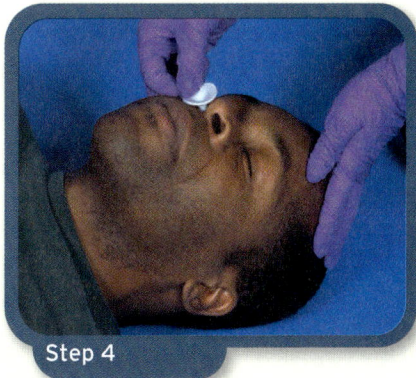

Step 4

Continue until the flange rests against the nostril. If you feel any resistance or obstruction, remove the airway and insert it into the other nostril.

of the jaw rather than the earlobe. If the nasal airway is too long, it may obstruct the patient's airway. If the patient becomes intolerant of the nasal airway, gently remove it from the nasal passage. Although the nasal airway is not as likely to cause vomiting as the oral airway, you should still have suction readily available.

Supplemental Oxygen Therapy

Supplemental oxygen should be administered to any patient with potential hypoxia, regardless of his or her clinical appearance. In some conditions, a part of the patient's body does not receive enough oxygen, *even though the oxygen supply to the body as a whole is entirely adequate.* For example, when a patient experiences an acute myocardial infarction (heart attack), a portion of the myocardium is hypoxic, *even though the rest of the body is well oxygenated.* Increasing the available oxygen supply also enhances the body's compensatory mechanisms during shock and other distressed states.

The oxygen-delivery method must be appropriate for the patient's ventilatory status and should be reassessed frequently and adjusted accordingly based on the patient's clinical condition and breathing adequacy. When a patient needs oxygen, the paramedic's first priority is to provide that oxygen quickly.

Oxygen Sources

Pure (100%) oxygen is stored in seamless steel or aluminum cylinders, whose colours may vary from silver, to chrome, to green, or some combination thereof. Make sure that the cylinder is labeled "medical oxygen." Also, look for letters and numbers stamped on the collar of the cylinder or on the tag attached to the cylinder Figure 11-23 ▶ . Of particular importance are the month and year stamps, which indicate when the cylinder was last hydrostat tested.

Oxygen cylinders are available in various sizes. You will most often use the D cylinder, which contains 350 l of oxygen and is typically carried from the ambulance to the patient, and the M cylinder, which contains 3,450 l of oxygen and remains on board the ambulance as a main supply tank. The E (or super/jumbo) cylinder, another common size, holds 625 l of oxygen.

Oxygen delivery is measured in terms of litres per minute (l/min). As a precaution against running out at an inconvenient moment, you should replace an oxygen cylinder with a full one when the pressure falls to 200 psi or below. That level is called the safe residual pressure, indicating that it is *unsafe* to continue using the oxygen cylinder. On the basis of the pressure in the oxygen cylinder and the flow rate of oxygen delivery, you can calculate how long the supply of oxygen in the cylinder will last—that is, the tank life Table 11-7 ▶ .

Liquid Oxygen

Liquid oxygen is oxygen that is cooled to its aqueous state. It converts to a gaseous state when warmed. Although much larger volumes of gaseous oxygen can be stored in the aqueous state, units for liquid oxygen generally require upright storage

At the Scene

It should be routine procedure at the beginning of every shift to open the main cylinder valve on the vehicle's oxygen supply and check the pressure remaining in the cylinder. Check the pressure gauges on all portable cylinders after every call in which oxygen is used. Replace oxygen cylinders when their pressure reaches or falls below 200 psi. Always carry at least one backup cylinder in the ambulance—you may not have a chance to return to your station for a full cylinder.

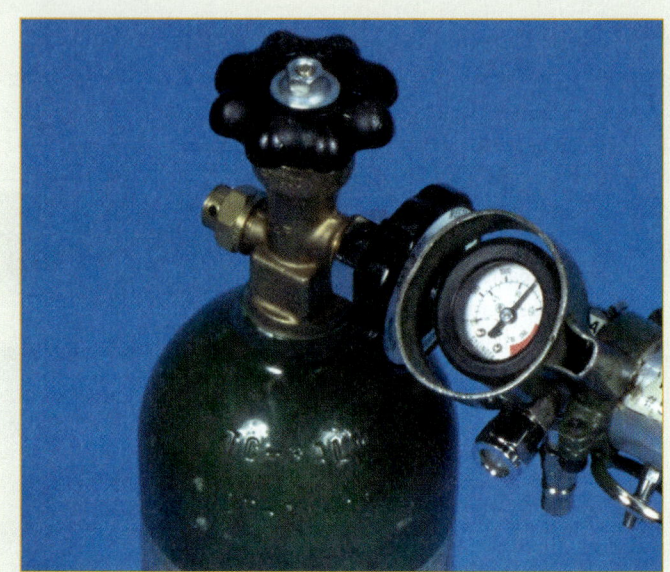

Figure 11-23 Oxygen cylinders for medical use have a series of letters and numbers stamped into the metal on the collar of the cylinder.

Table 11-7	Oxygen Cylinders: Duration of Flow	
Formula		
Tank pressure in psi − 200 psi (the safe residual pressure) × cylinder constant / Flow rate in l/min		= Duration of flow in minutes
Cylinder Constant		
D = 0.16		G = 2.41
E = 0.28		H = 3.14
M = 1.56		K = 3.14
Calculation		
Determine the life of a D cylinder that has a pressure of 2,000 psi and a flow rate of 15 l/min.		
(2,000 [psi] − 200 [safe residual pressure] × 0.16 [cylinder constant]) / 15	=	$\frac{288}{15 \text{ (l/min)}}$ = 19.2 (19) min
Note: psi indicates pounds per square inch.		

The formula shown:

$$\frac{\text{Tank pressure in psi} - 200 \text{ psi (the safe residual pressure)} \times \text{cylinder constant}}{\text{Flow rate in l/min}} = \text{Duration of flow in minutes}$$

$$\frac{(2{,}000\,[\text{psi}] - 200\,[\text{safe residual pressure}] \times 0.16\,[\text{cylinder constant}])}{15} = \frac{288}{15\,(\text{l/min})} = 19.2\,(19)\ \text{min}$$

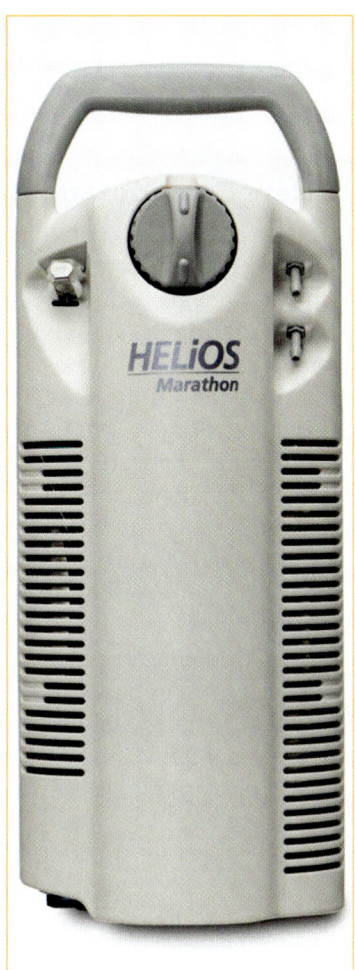

Figure 11-24 Liquid oxygen converts to a gas when warmed. It must be stored upright.

Figure 11-24 ◂. Additionally, there are special requirements for large volume storage and cylinder transfer.

Oxygen Regulators and Flowmeters

High-pressure regulators are attached to the cylinder stem to deliver cylinder gas under high pressure. These regulators are used to transfer cylinder gas from tank to tank, such as when you are refilling a portable oxygen cylinder.

The pressure of gas in a full oxygen cylinder is approximately 2,000 psi. Clearly, this is far too much pressure to deliver directly into a patient's airway. Instead, gas flow from an oxygen cylinder to the patient is controlled by a therapy regulator, which attaches to the stem of the oxygen cylinder and reduces the high pressure of gas to a safe range (about 50 psi).

Flowmeters, which are usually permanently attached to the therapy regulator, allow the oxygen delivered to the patient to be adjusted within a range of 1 to 25 l/min. The two types of flowmeters most commonly used are the pressure-compensated flowmeter and the Bourdon-gauge flowmeter.

A pressure-compensated flowmeter incorporates a float ball within a tapered calibrated tube; this float rises or falls based on the gas flow in the tube. The gas flow is controlled by a needle valve located downstream from the float ball. Because this type of flowmeter is affected by gravity, it must remain in an upright position to obtain an accurate flow reading Figure 11-25 ▸.

By contrast, the Bourdon-gauge flowmeter is not affected by gravity and can be placed in any position. This pressure gauge is calibrated to record the flow rate Figure 11-26 ▸. The major disadvantage of this type of flowmeter is that it does not compensate for backpressure. As a result, it will usually record a higher flow rate when there is any obstruction to gas flow downstream.

Preparing an Oxygen Cylinder for Use

Prior to administering supplemental oxygen to your patient, you must prepare the oxygen cylinder and therapy regulator. To place an oxygen cylinder into service, follow these steps Skill Drill 11-16 ▸.

1. Inspect the cylinder and its markings. Remove the plastic seal covering the valve stem opening (if commercially filled). Inspect the opening to ensure that it is free of dirt or other debris. With the tank facing away from yourself and others, use an oxygen wrench to "crack" the cylinder—quickly opening and closing the valve to ensure that dirt particles and other contaminants do not enter the oxygen flow Step 1.

2. Attach the regulator/flowmeter to the valve stem, ensuring that the pin-index system is correctly aligned. A metal or plastic O-ring is placed around the oxygen port to optimize the airtight seal between the collar of the regulator and the valve stem Step 2.

3. Place the regulator collar over the cylinder valve, with the oxygen port and pin-indexing pins on the side of the

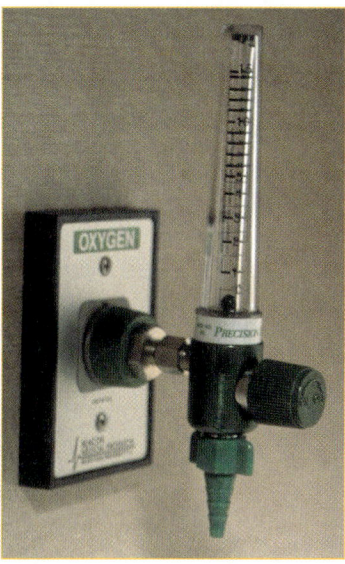

Figure 11-25 Pressure-compensated flowmeters contain a float ball that rises or falls based on the gas flow in the tube. It must remain in an upright position for an accurate flow reading.

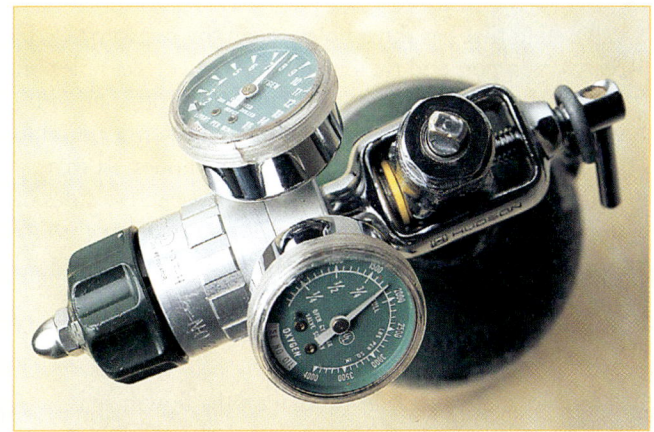

Figure 11-26 The Bourdon-gauge flowmeter is not affected by gravity and can be placed in any position.

Skill Drill 11-16: Placing an Oxygen Cylinder Into Service

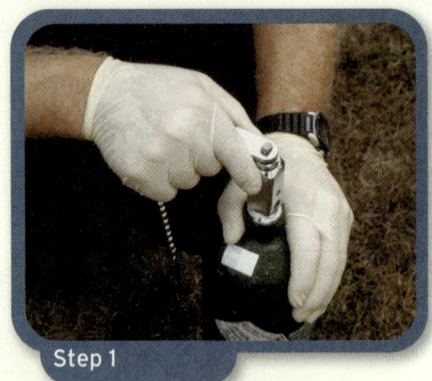

Step 1

Using an oxygen wrench, turn the valve counterclockwise to "crack" the cylinder.

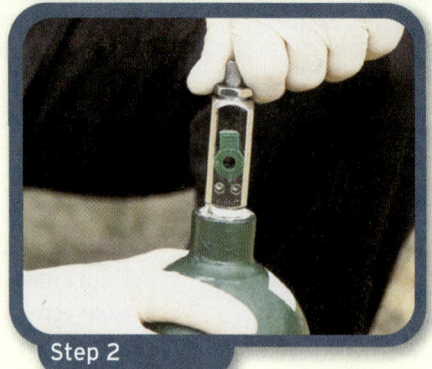

Step 2

Attach the regulator/flowmeter to the valve stem using the two pin-indexing holes, and make sure that the O-ring is in place over the larger hole.

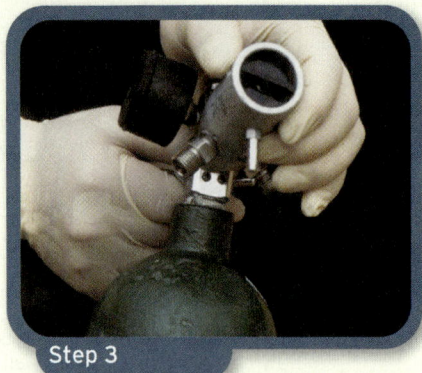

Step 3

Align the regulator so that the pins fit snugly into the correct holes on the valve stem and hand-tighten the regulator.

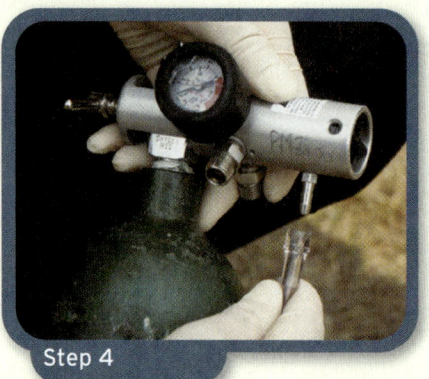

Step 4

Attach the oxygen connective tubing to the flowmeter.

flowmeter and select the oxygen flow rate that is appropriate for your patient's condition **Step 4**.

Safety Considerations

Any cylinder containing compressed gas under high pressure has the potential, under the right conditions (actually, the *wrong* conditions!), to assume the properties of a rocket. Furthermore, oxygen presents the additional hazard of fire, because it supports the combustion process. For these reasons, safety precautions are necessary when you are handling oxygen cylinders:

- Keep combustible materials, such as oil or grease, away from contact with the cylinder itself, the regulators, fittings, valves, or tubing.
- Do not permit smoking in any area where oxygen cylinders are in use or on standby.
- Store oxygen cylinders in a cool, well-ventilated area. Do not subject the cylinders to temperatures above 50°C.
- Use an oxygen cylinder only with a safe, properly fitting regulator valve. Regulator valves for one gas should never be modified for use with another gas.
- Close all valves when the cylinder is not in use, even if the tank is empty.
- Secure cylinders so that they will not topple over. In transit, keep them in a proper carrier or rack, or strap them onto the stretcher with the patient.
- When working with an oxygen cylinder, always position yourself to its side. Never place any part of your body over the cylinder valve! A loosely fitting regulator can be blown off the cylinder with sufficient force to demolish any object in its path.
- Have the cylinder hydrostat tested every 10 years, to make sure it can still sustain the high pressures required. The original test date is stamped onto the cylinder together with its serial number.

valve stem that has three holes. Align the regulator so that the oxygen port and the pins fit into the correct holes on the valve stem; align the screw bolt on the opposite side with the dimpled depression. Tighten the screw bolt until the regulator is firmly attached to the cylinder. At this point, you should not see any space between the sides of the valve stem and the interior walls of the collar **Step 3**.

4. With the regulator firmly attached, open the cylinder and read the pressure level on the regulator gauge. Follow your local protocols regarding minimum cylinder pressures.

5. A second gauge or a selector dial on the flowmeter indicates the oxygen flow rate. Attach the oxygen connective tubing to the "Christmas tree" nipple on the

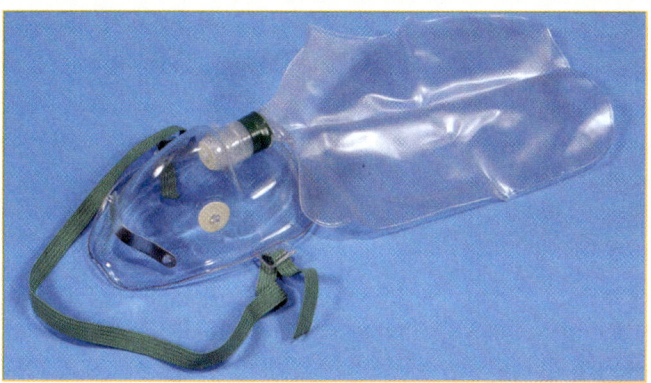

Figure 11-27 Nonrebreathing mask.

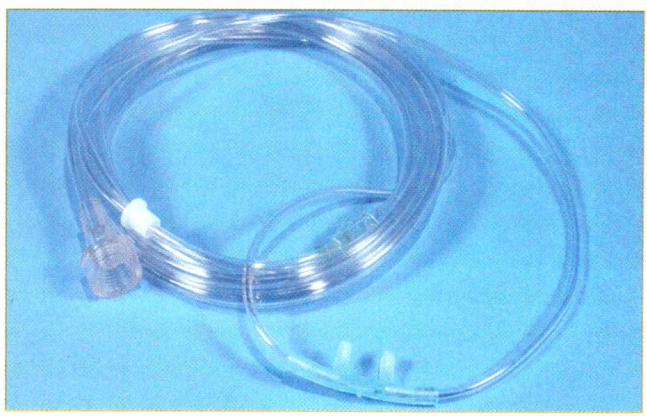

Figure 11-28 Nasal cannula.

Supplemental Oxygen-Delivery Devices

The most common oxygen-delivery devices that you will use in the prehospital setting are the nonrebreathing mask, nasal cannula, and bag-valve-mask device. However, if your EMS system performs interfacility transfers, you may encounter other oxygen-delivery devices, such as the simple face mask, partial rebreathing mask, and Venturi mask. Small-volume nebulizers, which are typically used to deliver aerosolized medications, may also be used to administer supplemental oxygen.

Nonrebreathing Mask

The nonrebreathing mask is the preferred device for delivering supplemental oxygen to spontaneously breathing patients in the prehospital setting. With a good mask-to-face seal and a flow rate of 15 l/min, it is capable of delivering between 90% and 100% inspired oxygen.

The nonrebreathing mask is a combination mask and reservoir bag system. Oxygen fills a reservoir bag that is attached to the mask by a one-way valve. This permits the patient to inhale from the reservoir bag but not to exhale back into it. The only gas that can enter the reservoir, therefore, is 100% oxygen piped in from the oxygen cylinder. Exhaled gas escapes through one-way flapper valves located on the side of the mask Figure 11-27 ▲.

Prior to administering oxygen to a patient with a nonrebreathing mask, you must ensure that the reservoir bag is completely filled. The oxygen flow rate is adjusted from 12 to 15 l/min to prevent collapse of the bag during inhalation. Use a pediatric nonrebreathing mask, which has a smaller reservoir bag, for infants and small children; they inhale smaller volumes of air.

The nonrebreathing mask is indicated for spontaneously breathing patients who require high-flow oxygen concentrations (eg, shock, hypoxia from any cause) and have adequate tidal volume (ie, good chest rise). Contraindications include apnea and poor respiratory effort. Because the nonrebreathing mask delivers oxygen passively, the patient's respirations must be of adequate depth to open the one-way valve and draw air from the reservoir bag into the lungs. A patient with reduced tidal volume (shallow breathing) will benefit very little, if any, from the nonrebreathing mask.

Nasal Cannula

The nasal cannula delivers oxygen via two small prongs that fit into the patient's nostrils Figure 11-28 ▲. With an oxygen flow rate of 1 to 6 l/min, the nasal cannula can deliver an oxygen concentration of 24% to 44%. Higher flow rates will merely irritate the nasal mucosa without increasing the delivered oxygen concentration. An oxygen humidifier should be used when delivering oxygen via nasal cannula for a prolonged period of time, as it will help prevent mucosal drying and irritation.

The nasal cannula provides low to moderate oxygen enrichment and is most beneficial to patients who require long-term oxygen therapy (eg, for COPD). It is ineffective if the patient is apneic, has poor respiratory effort, is severely hypoxic, or is a mouth-breather. In the prehospital setting, the nasal cannula is primarily used when patients who need oxygen cannot tolerate a nonrebreathing mask.

The nasal cannula is generally well tolerated, especially in patients who are claustrophobic and intolerant of an oxygen

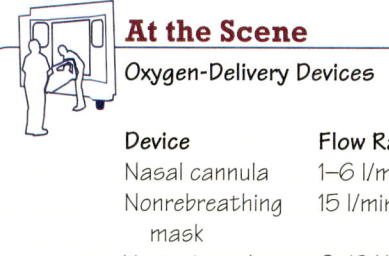

At the Scene

Oxygen-Delivery Devices

Device	Flow Rate	Oxygen Delivered
Nasal cannula	1–6 l/min	24%–44%
Nonrebreathing mask	15 l/min	90%–100%
Venturi mask	6–12 l/min	24%–50%
Bag-valve-mask device with reservoir	15 l/min – flush	Nearly 100%

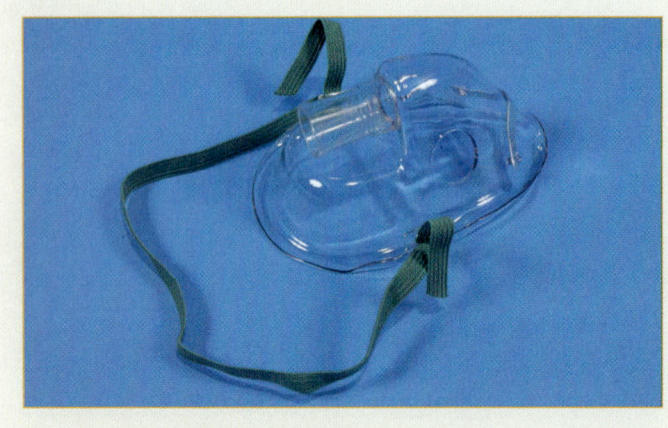

Figure 11-29 Simple face mask.

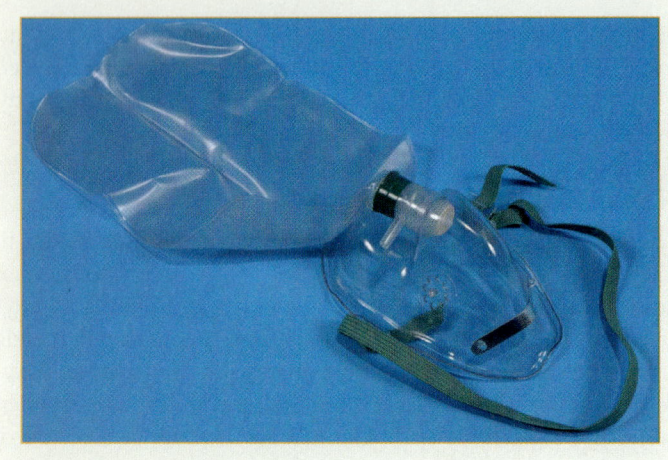

Figure 11-30 Partial rebreathing mask.

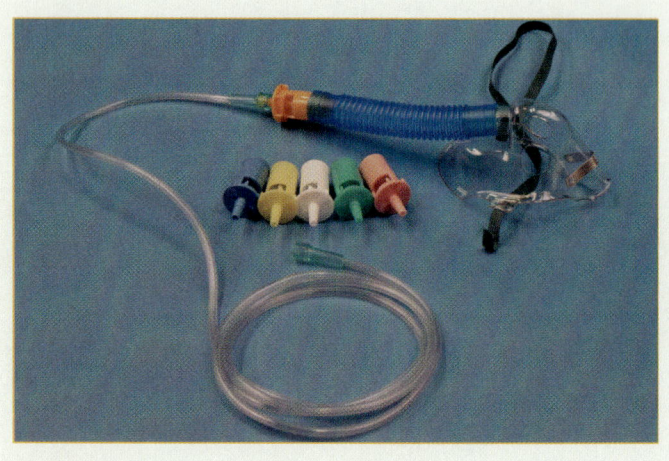

Figure 11-31 Venturi mask.

mask over their face. However, it does not deliver high volumes or concentrations of oxygen.

Simple Face Mask

A simple face mask is a full mask enclosure with open side ports. Room air is drawn in through the side ports on inhalation, diluting the concentration of inspired oxygen Figure 11-29 ▲. Exhaled air is vented through holes on each side of the mask. The simple face mask will deliver between 40% and 60% oxygen at 10 l/min. If there is a leak around the face, however, the amount of inspired oxygen decreases. The simple face mask can deliver oxygen concentrations only slightly higher than those delivered by the nasal cannula. These devices are rarely used in the prehospital environment.

Partial Rebreathing Mask

A partial rebreathing mask is similar to the nonrebreathing mask except that it lacks a one-way valve between the mask and the reservoir Figure 11-30 ▲. Room air is not drawn in with inspiration, but residual expired air is mixed in the mask and rebreathed.

Contraindications are the same as for the nonrebreathing mask—any patient with apnea or inadequate tidal volume. Because inspired gas is not mixed with room air, higher concentrations are attainable—at flow rates of 6 to 10 l/min, an oxygen concentration of 35% to 60% becomes possible. Increasing oxygen flow rate beyond 10 l/min will not enhance the oxygen concentration, and leakage from the mask around the face decreases oxygen concentration. These devices are rarely used in the prehospital environment.

Venturi Mask

The Venturi mask draws room air into the mask along with the oxygen flow, allowing for the administration of highly specific oxygen concentrations Figure 11-31 ▲. Depending on the adapter used, the Venturi mask can deliver 24%, 28%, 35%, 40%, or 50% oxygen. Venturi masks are especially useful in the hospital management of patients with COPD and other chronic respiratory diseases. They offer little advantage in prehospital care, except in the long-range transport of such patients.

Hi-Ox Mask

The Hi-Ox mask is a modification of the nonrebreathing mask. Like the nonrebreathing mask, the patient inhales oxygen from the reservoir bag via a one-way valve. Unlike the nonrebreathing mask, the patient's exhaled breath passes through another one-way valve and then through a high-efficiency filter before exiting the mask. This system provides the spontaneously breathing patient with a high concentration of supplemental oxygen and protects the paramedics from exhaled respiratory secretions and communicable diseases. In many EMS systems, the Hi-Ox mask or other similar device is used routinely for patients with febrile respiratory illness who require supplemental oxygen.

Small-Volume Nebulizer

A nebulizer is used primarily to deliver aerosolized medications. Oxygen enters an aerosol chamber that contains

Table 11-8	Methods of Positive-Pressure Ventilation

- Mouth-to-mask
- Two-person bag-valve-mask device
- Flow-restricted, oxygen-powered ventilation device
- One-person bag-valve-mask device

Note: The methods are listed in order of preference, because research has demonstrated that personnel who ventilate patients infrequently have great difficulty maintaining an adequate seal between the mask and the patient's face.

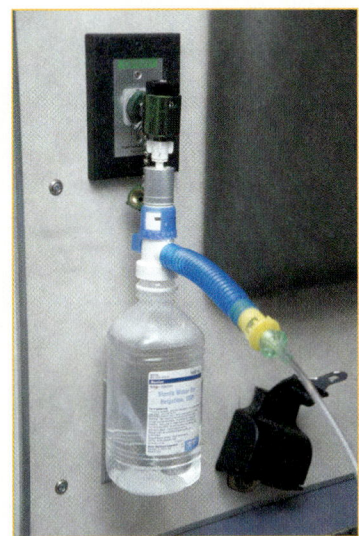

Figure 11-32 Administering humidified oxygen is preferred for long-range transports to avoid drying the patient's mucous membranes.

3 to 5 ml of fluid. The pressurized oxygen in this chamber aerosolizes the oxygen for inhalation. You will learn how to administer bronchodilators in this manner.

Oxygen Humidifier

Oxygen stored in cylinders has zero humidity, and it is not a good idea to deliver dry gases to a patient's airway, especially for long periods of time. In fact, oxygen that is entirely devoid of moisture will rapidly dry the patient's mucous membranes. An oxygen humidifier consists of small bottle of water through which the oxygen leaving the cylinder becomes moisturized before it reaches the patient Figure 11-32 ▲ . Because the humidifier must be kept in an upright position, however, it is practical only for the fixed oxygen unit in the ambulance.

Humidifying oxygen and nebulizers, however, increase the risk of aerosolizing respiratory secretions and spreading communicable diseases. As a result, many EMS agencies do not permit use of humidified oxygen, nebulizers, or related devices. You should consult with your EMS service prior to using humidified oxygen, nebulizers, or related devices.

Assisted and Artificial Ventilation

A patient who is not breathing needs artificial ventilation with 100% oxygen. The same is true of patients who are breathing inadequately, such as those with fast or slow respirations, reduced tidal volume, or an irregular pattern of respirations. These patients need ventilation assistance to improve oxygenation and facilitate CO_2 elimination from the body.

Inadequate negative-pressure ventilation is treated with some form of positive-pressure ventilation, which involves forcing air into the patient's lungs. The techniques used differ only in the power source used to generate the pressures and the airflows required for inflating a patient's lungs Table 11-8 ◄ .

Mouth-to-Mouth and Mouth-to-Nose Ventilation

Consider the following scenario: You are relaxing by the side of a local swimming pool when you see a teenager being fished out of the water, apparently unconscious. You race over to him and tilt his head back to open his airway; then you look, listen, and feel for breathing and determine that he is apneic. What should you do next? Because you don't ordinarily bring resuscitation equipment to the pool, you will have to initiate positive-pressure ventilations with the only equipment immediately available to you—your own mouth and lungs.

Mouth-to-mouth is the most basic form of ventilation. Mouth-to-nose simply involves ventilating through the nose, rather than through the mouth. Indications for this type of ventilation include apnea and when other ventilation devices are not available.

The disadvantages of mouth-to-mouth or nose ventilation include psychological barriers secondary to sanitary and communicable disease issues. There is a potential for exposure to blood and other body fluids through direct contact with the patient's mouth or nose. Although mouth-to-mouth or mouth-to-nose ventilation requires no special equipment, allows you to deliver excellent tidal volume, and provides 16% oxygen to the patient (adequate to sustain life), other methods of providing positive-pressure ventilation are safer for the rescuer.

There are also some potential complications associated with mouth-to-mouth or mouth-to-nose ventilation. Hyperventilation of the patient's lungs may occur, especially if the patient is small and the rescuer is overzealous. Hyperventilation of the

At the Scene

Airway management and ventilation procedures often expose you to blood, vomitus, and oral secretions. While blood is the most potentially infectious body fluid, you should exercise great caution to avoid contact with all body fluids. At a minimum, you should wear gloves for all airway and ventilation procedures and when handling airway equipment that has been contaminated with body fluids. To mitigate the risk of splashing or droplets of body fluid coming in contact with your mouth, nose, and eyes, wear a mask and protective eyewear or a face shield, especially when placing an advanced airway. In cases of significant blood splashing, such as in trauma, you should also wear a protective gown, if possible. You should consult your EMS agency and local regulations regarding the use of personal protective equipment when performing airway maneuvers.

Skill Drill 11-17: Mouth-to-Mask Ventilation

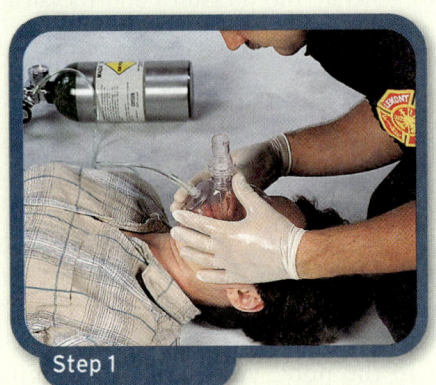

Step 1

Once the patient's head is properly positioned, place the mask on the patient's face. Seal the mask to the face using both hands.

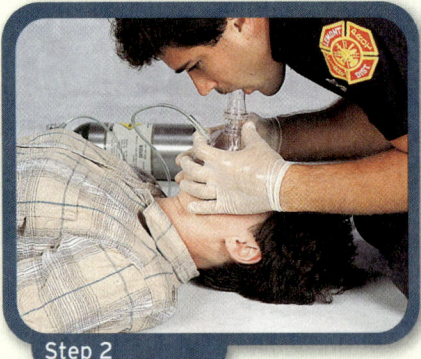

Step 2

Exhale into the open port of the one-way valve for 1 second as you watch for visible chest rise.

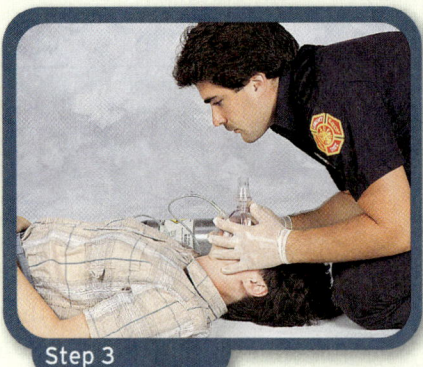

Step 3

Watch for the patient's chest to fall during exhalation.

rescuer is another potential complication. Rapid, deep breathing, especially for prolonged periods of time, decreases carbon dioxide levels in the blood and, in severe cases, could cause the rescuer to lose consciousness. Gastric distension may also occur, increasing the risk of vomiting and aspiration; this clearly would be detrimental to the patient but would also expose the rescuer to the patient's vomitus.

To avoid putting yourself in a position where mouth-to-mouth or mouth-to-nose ventilation is the only option, ensure that you have access to a pocket mask or face shield—or anything with a barrier device—regardless of where you are. The use of mouth-to-mouth or mouth-to-nose ventilation is not recommended for paramedics due to the risk of communicable disease.

Mouth-to-Mask Ventilation

Mouth-to-mask ventilation employs the same readily available power source as mouth-to-mouth or mouth-to-nose (the rescuer's lungs), but eliminates direct contact with the patient's mouth or nose. Use of a one-way valve over the mask's mouthpiece virtually eliminates any possibility of contact with the patient's secretions and diverts the patient's exhaled air away from the paramedic's mouth Figure 11-33 ▶ .

Because you are able to use both hands to hold the mask to the patient's face, it is easier to maintain an effective seal and deliver excellent tidal volume. If the pocket face mask is not equipped with an oxygen inlet valve, then you will deliver 16% oxygen to the patient. When its inlet valve is connected to an oxygen source at a flow rate of 15 l/min, the pocket mask can deliver up to 55% oxygen to the patient.

Complications associated with using a pocket face mask are the same as for mouth-to-mouth or mouth-to-nose ventilation—hyperinflation of the patient's lungs, hyperventilation of the rescuer, and gastric distension.

Figure 11-33 Pocket mask with a one-way valve.

The steps for performing mouth-to-mask ventilations are listed here and shown in Skill Drill 11-17 ▲ .

1. Kneel at the patient's head. Open the airway with the appropriate manual maneuver. Connect the one-way valve to the face mask. Place the mask over the patient's face, ensuring that the top is over the bridge of the nose and the bottom is in the groove between the lower lip and chin. Grasp the patient's lower jaw with the first three fingers on each hand. Place your thumbs on the dome of the mask. Make an airtight seal by applying firm pressure between the thumbs and the fingers. Maintain an upward and forward pull on the lower jaw with your fingers to keep the airway open Step 1 .

2. Take a breath and exhale through the open port of the one-way valve. Breathe into the mask for 1 second, observing visible chest rise Step 2 .

3. Remove your mouth, and watch for the patient's chest to fall during passive exhalation Step 3 .

Skill Drill 11-18: One-Person Bag-Valve-Mask Ventilation

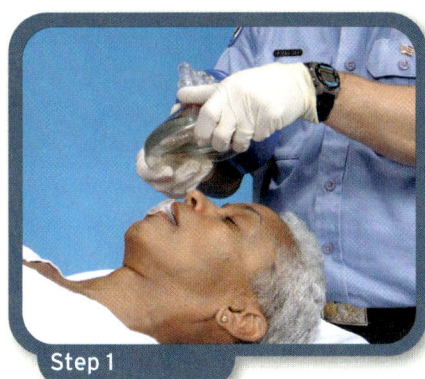

Step 1

Choose the proper mask size to seat the mask from the bridge of the nose to the chin.

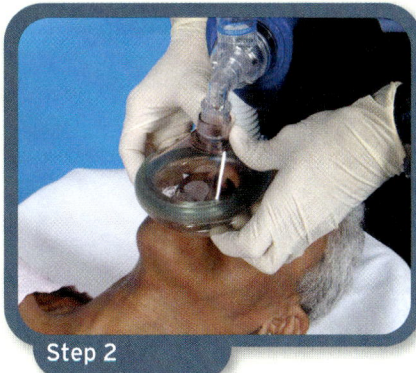

Step 2

Position the mask on the patient's face and ensure an adequate seal.

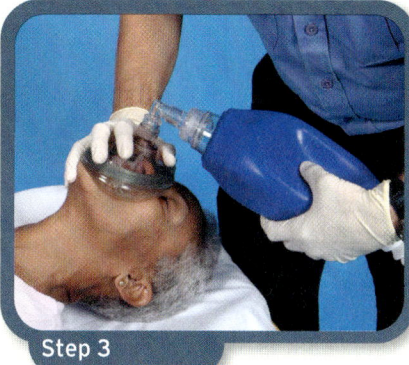

Step 3

Open the patient's airway and hold the mask in place with one hand as you squeeze the bag with the other hand. Allow the bag to reinflate slowly and completely.

Table 11-9	Ventilation Rates

Adult*

- Apneic with a pulse: 10 to 12 breaths/min
  - With *or* without an advanced airway in place (eg, ET tube, LMA)
- Apneic and pulseless: 8 to 10 breaths/min
  - After an advanced airway has been inserted
- Ventilations can be asynchronous with chest compressions

Infant and Child*

- Apneic with a pulse: 12 to 20 breaths/min
  - With *or* without an advanced airway in place (eg, ET tube, LMA)
- Apneic and pulseless: 8 to 10 breaths/min
  - After an advanced airway has been inserted
- Ventilations can be asynchronous with chest compressions

*Avoid hyperventilating any patient. Hyperventilation may lower carbon dioxide levels in the blood, which may be injurious. In addition, hyperventilated lungs will increase intrathoracic pressure and impede venous return, lowering cardiac output. Hyperventilation also increases the risk of regurgitation and aspiration.

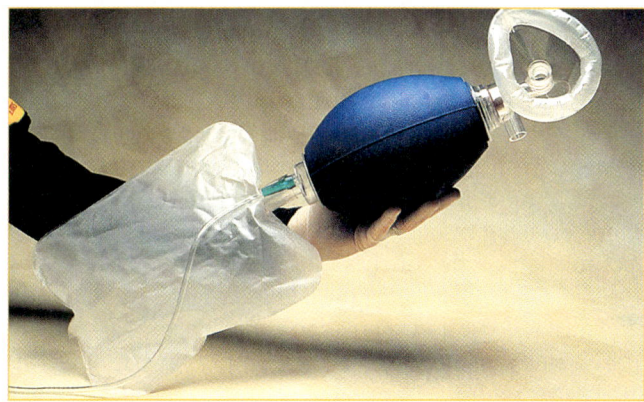

Figure 11-34 Bag-valve-mask device.

Ventilation effectiveness is best determined by watching the patient's chest rise and fall and feeling for resistance of the patient's lungs as they expand. You should also hear and feel air escape as the patient exhales. If the patient is in cardiac arrest, your breaths do not need to be synchronized to chest compressions. Make sure that you provide the correct number of breaths per minute for the patient's age (Table 11-9 ▲).

One-Person Bag-Valve-Mask Ventilation

The bag-valve-mask device is the most common device used to ventilate patients in the prehospital environment (Figure 11-34 ▶). With an oxygen flow rate of 15 l/min and a reservoir attached, the bag-valve-mask device can deliver almost 100% oxygen to the patient. Bag-valve-mask ventilations are indicated for apneic patients and for patients who are breathing inadequately, as long as they can tolerate the device.

This technique provides an excellent barrier from blood and other body fluids and allows the rescuer to ventilate the patient for extended periods of time without fatigue.

A major challenge is maintaining an effective mask-to-face seal. The single person operating a bag-valve-mask device must be able to perform three tasks with only two hands: keeping the airway properly positioned, maintaining a mask seal, and squeezing the bag. Complications associated with the one-person bag-valve-mask ventilation technique are typically related to inadequate tidal volume delivery, which usually occurs secondary to poor technique, inadequate mask-to-face seal, or gastric distension.

The steps for performing the one-person bag-valve-mask ventilation technique are listed here and shown in (Skill Drill 11-18 ▲).

1. Choose the proper mask size to seat the mask from the bridge of the nose to the chin (Step 1).
2. Position the mask on the patient's face and ensure an adequate seal (Step 2).

3. Open the patient's airway and hold the mask in place with one hand. Squeeze the bag completely over 1 second with the other hand and watch for visible chest rise. Allow the bag to reinflate slowly and completely (**Step 3**).

Two-Person Bag-Valve-Mask Ventilation

In contrast to the one-person technique, two-person bag-valve-mask ventilation is a much more efficient means of providing artificial or assisted ventilations. With two paramedics, one can maintain an adequate mask-to-face seal, while the other squeezes the bag. This will facilitate the delivery of excellent tidal volume and high oxygen concentrations. Indications for the two-person bag-valve-mask technique include apnea, inadequate breathing, inability to ventilate the patient with one paramedic, and spinal injury. Contraindications include patients who are intolerant of the device.

The only major disadvantage of the two-person bag-valve-mask technique is that it requires additional personnel, who are not always present on every call. Complications include hyperinflation of the patient's lungs and gastric distension. For these reasons, the patient must be constantly monitored for adequate chest rise and ventilation compliance.

The steps for performing the two-person bag-valve-mask ventilation technique are listed here and are shown in **Skill Drill 11-19** ▲ .

1. The first paramedic maintains a mask seal by the most appropriate method (**Step 1**).
2. The second paramedic squeezes the bag completely with both hands over 1 second, observing for visible chest rise (**Step 2**).

Three-Person Bag-Valve-Mask Ventilation

The one-person, two-person, and three-person bag-valve-mask techniques can be understood in terms of progressive difficulty. If you cannot ventilate a patient effectively with one paramedic, use two. If you cannot ventilate effectively with two, use three. With this approach, there are very few patients that you cannot ventilate.

The three-person bag-valve-mask technique is indicated for apneic patients, patients who are breathing inadequately, patients who cannot be ventilated by one or two paramedics, and patients with a possible spinal injury. It is contraindicated in patients who are intolerant of the device.

The major disadvantage is that this technique requires additional personnel. Furthermore, the area around the

Skill Drill 11-19: Two-Person Bag-Valve-Mask Ventilation

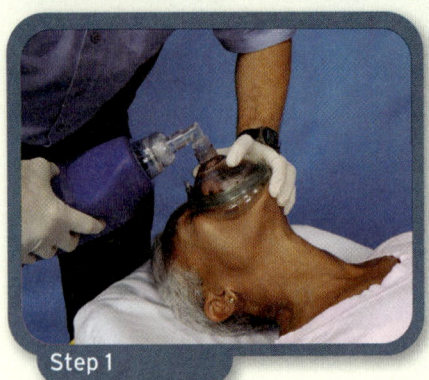

Step 1
The first paramedic maintains the mask seal by the most appropriate method.

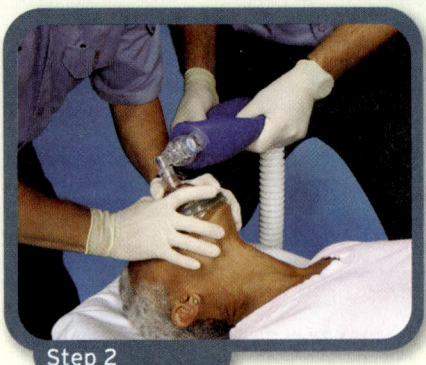

Step 2
The second paramedic squeezes the bag completely over 1 second to provide visible chest rise.

patient's head can become very crowded when he or she is being ventilated by three paramedics.

Complications associated with the three-person bag-valve-mask technique are the same as those for the one-person and two-person techniques—hyperinflation of the patient's lungs and gastric distension. Therefore, the patient must be continually monitored for adequate chest rise and ventilation compliance. If the patient's chest does not rise and fall during ventilations, you may need to reposition the head, insert an airway adjunct, or apply cricoid pressure.

The steps for performing the three-person bag-valve-mask ventilation technique are listed here and shown in **Skill Drill 11-20** ▶ .

1. The first paramedic maintains a mask seal by the most appropriate method (**Step 1**).
2. The second paramedic squeezes the bag completely with both hands over 1 second (**Step 2**).
3. The third paramedic applies cricoid pressure (**Step 3**).

The bag-valve-mask device may also be used in conjunction with an ET tube or with other advanced airway devices such as the Combitube and the laryngeal mask airway (LMA).

Flow-Restricted, Oxygen-Powered Ventilation Device

A third potential source for artificial ventilation is the flow-restricted, oxygen-powered ventilation device (FROPVD), also referred to as a manually triggered ventilator or demand valve **Figure 11-35** ▶ . The FROPVD can be used to ventilate apneic patients or to administer supplemental oxygen to spontaneously breathing patients. Its plastic housing includes a 15/22-mm adapter designed to fit onto standard ventilation masks as well as advanced airways (eg, ET tube, Combitube).

Skill Drill 11-20: Three-Person Bag-Valve-Mask Ventilation

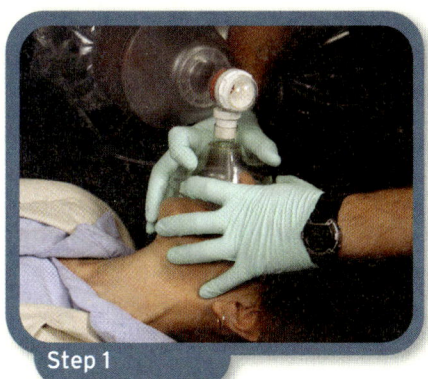

Step 1

The first paramedic maintains a mask seal by the most appropriate method.

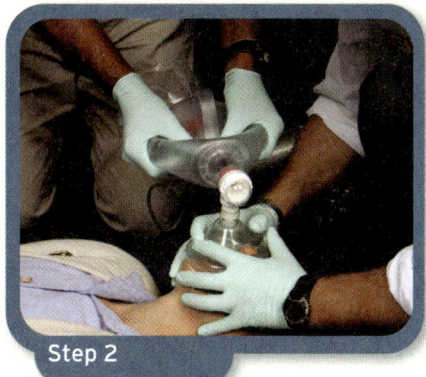

Step 2

The second paramedic squeezes the bag over 1 second to achieve visible chest rise.

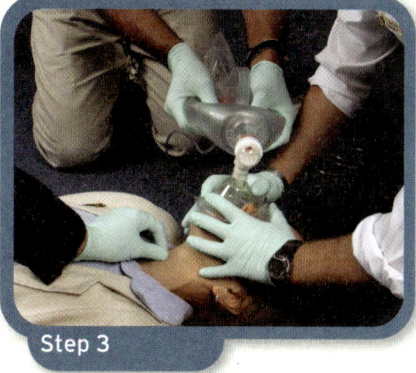

Step 3

The third paramedic applies cricoid pressure.

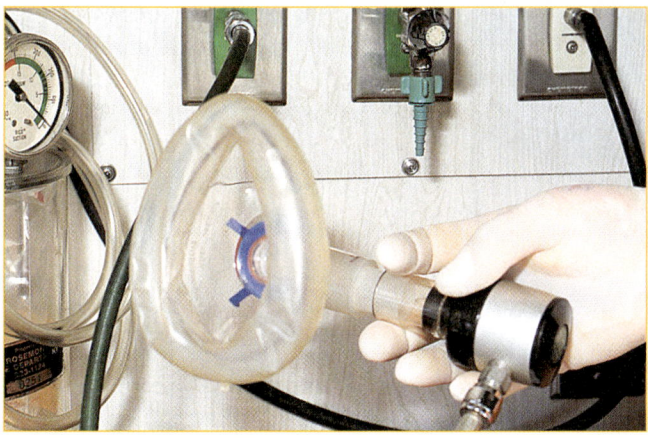

Figure 11-35 Flow-restricted, oxygen-powered ventilation device.

At the Scene

Indications That Artificial Ventilation Is Adequate*

- Adequate and equal chest rise and fall with ventilation
- Ventilations are delivered at the appropriate rate:
  - 10 to 12 breaths/min for adults
  - 12 to 20 breaths/min for infants and children
- Heart rate returns to a normal range

Indications That Artificial Ventilation Is Inadequate

- Minimal or no chest rise and fall
- Ventilations delivered too fast or too slow for patient's age
- Heart rate does not return to a normal range

*In patients who are apneic with a pulse (ie, not in cardiac arrest).

The FROPVD has a demand valve that is triggered by the negative pressure generated during inhalation. This valve automatically delivers 100% oxygen as the spontaneously breathing patient begins to inhale and stops the flow of gas at the end of inhalation. Generally, patients find it most comfortable if they hold the mask to their face themselves. The FROPVD delivers only the volume needed by the patient during inhalation, rather than wasting oxygen by providing a constant flow. Because the FROPVD makes an airtight seal with the patient's face, the patient inhales almost 100% oxygen. If the patient is conscious, he or she must have adequate tidal volume to be able to self-administer oxygen via the FROPVD. Do not use this device if the spontaneously breathing patient has an altered level of consciousness or is intolerant of the FROPVD.

For ventilation of apneic patients, a pushbutton on top of the FROPVD can control the flow of oxygen. When the button is depressed, 100% oxygen streams out at a fixed flow rate of 40 l/min. This flow continues until the operator takes his or her finger off the button or the pop-off valve releases when the device reaches the preset pressure limit of 30 cm H_2O.

The valve opening pressure at the cardiac sphincter (opening into the stomach) is also about 30 cm H_2O. This limited pressure is a disadvantage for certain patients who need greater pressure to overcome increased airway resistance, including those with COPD or an airway obstruction. Therefore, whenever you are ventilating patients with a FROPVD, ensure that they are receiving enough volume by observing the chest for adequate rise.

Unlike a bag-valve-mask device or pocket mask, the FROPVD requires an oxygen source to function—a potential disadvantage. In addition, the operator cannot feel whether the patient is being adequately ventilated with this device. Changes in compliance can be an important early indication of an impending problem. You must closely monitor the patient

Skill Drill 11-21: Flow-Restricted, Oxygen-Powered Ventilation for Apneic Patients

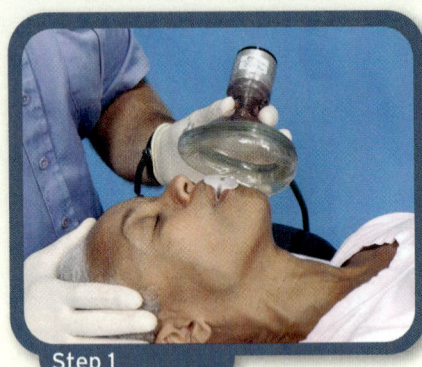

Step 1

Choose the proper mask size to seat the mask from the bridge of the nose to the chin.

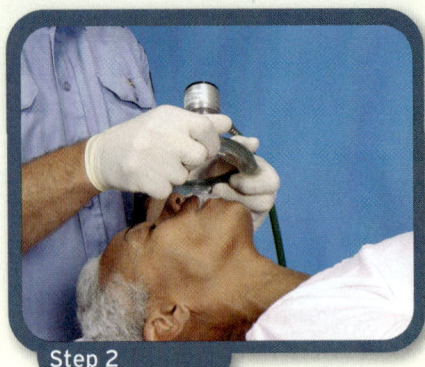

Step 2

Position the mask on the patient's face by the most appropriate method.

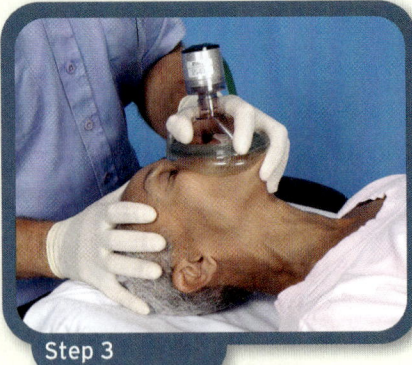

Step 3

Open the patient's airway and hold the mask with one hand.

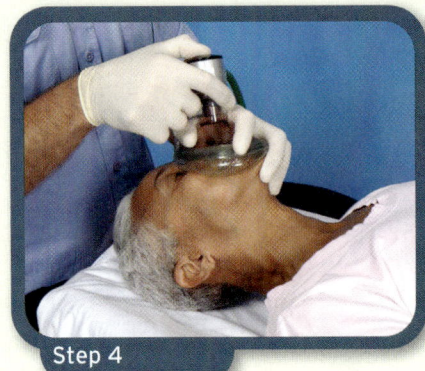

Step 4

Press the ventilation button until you achieve visible chest rise.

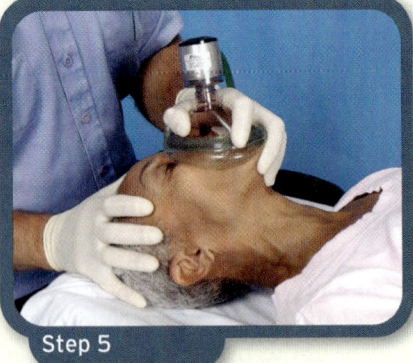

Step 5

Allow the patient to exhale passively.

This device *should not* be used when ventilating infants or children or for patients with possible cervical spine or chest injury. *Cricoid pressure should be maintained whenever FROPVDs are used to ventilate nonintubated patients.* This will help to reduce the incidence of gastric distension.

The steps for ventilating an apneic patient with the FROPVD are listed here and shown in **Skill Drill 11-21 ◂**.

1. Choose the proper mask size to seat the mask from the bridge of the nose to the chin **Step 1**.
2. Position the mask on the patient's face by the most appropriate method **Step 2**.
3. Open the patient's airway and hold the mask in place with one hand, maintaining an adequate mask-to-face seal **Step 3**.
4. Press the ventilation button until you see visible chest rise **Step 4**.
5. Allow the patient to exhale passively **Step 5**.

The steps for administering supplemental oxygen to a spontaneously breathing patient with the FROPVD are listed here and shown in **Skill Drill 11-22 ▸**.

1. Prepare your equipment by attaching the appropriate-sized mask to the FROPVD and ensuring that it is connected to an oxygen source **Step 1**.
2. Whenever possible, have the patient hold the mask to his or her own face to maintain a good seal **Step 2**.
3. When the patient inhales, the negative pressure created will trigger the valve within the FROPVD and deliver 100% oxygen **Step 3**.

being ventilated mechanically and remain vigilant for changes in his or her condition.

The FROPVD has been used in EMS for several years; however, recent findings suggest that they should not be used routinely because of the high incidence of gastric distension and damage to intrathoracic structures caused by barotrauma.

Continuous Positive Airway Pressure

Continuous positive airway pressure (CPAP) delivers positive pressure to the airways of a spontaneously breathing patient

Skill Drill 11-22: Flow-Restricted, Oxygen-Powered Ventilation Device for Conscious, Spontaneously Breathing Patients

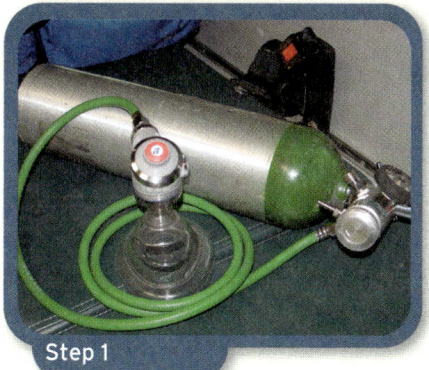

Step 1

Prepare your equipment.

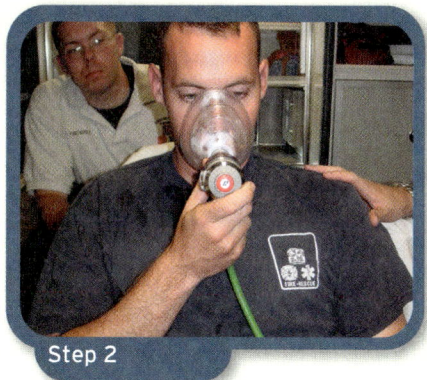

Step 2

Whenever possible, have the patient hold the mask to his or her own face to maintain a good seal.

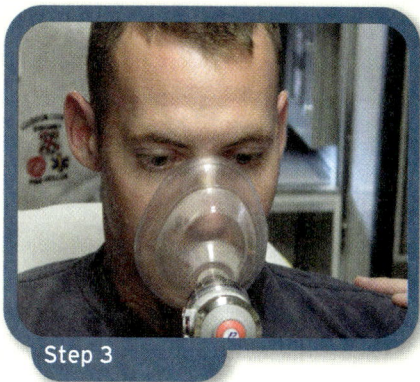

Step 3

When the patient inhales, the negative pressure created will trigger the valve within the FROPVD and deliver 100% oxygen.

At the Scene

A number of EMS agencies provide interfacility transport of mechanically ventilated patients. The discussion of respiratory physiology and mechanical ventilation associated with ventilator-dependent patients is complex. Advanced and critical care paramedics who transport patients using mechanical ventilators require specific training in the management of a mechanically ventilated patient and ventilator-related complications. Paramedics should refer to their protocols and procedures regarding management of ventilator-dependent patients and the operation of the ventilator used in their service.

Special Considerations

Artificial Ventilation of the Pediatric Patient

The flat nasal bridge of the pediatric patient makes achieving an effective mask-to-face seal more difficult in children than in adults. Furthermore, compressing the mask against the face to improve mask seal may result in obstruction. The best mask seal is achieved by the two-person bag-valve-mask ventilation technique with jaw displacement, although current standards support either the one- or two-paramedic technique.

A pediatric bag-valve-mask device with a minimum tidal volume of 450 ml should be used for full-term neonates and infants. In children (1 year of age to the onset of puberty [12 to 14 years of age]), consider the size of the child when determining bag size. An adult bag with a 1,500-ml volume may be used, but a pediatric bag-valve-mask is preferred. Children older than 12 to 14 years of age require the adult-sized bag-valve-mask for adequate ventilation. Choose a size to ensure a proper mask fit. The mask should reach from the bridge of the nose to the cleft of the chin. A length-based resuscitation tape may also be used to determine the most appropriate-sized bag-valve-mask device for pediatric patients who weigh up to 34 kg.

When you are ventilating a pediatric patient, ensure that there is a proper mask seal by using the EC-clamp technique 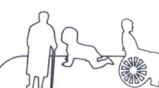 *. Place the mask over the mouth and nose, avoiding compression of the eyes. With one hand, place your thumb on the mask at the apex (over the nose) and your index finger on the mask at the chin to form a "C." With gentle pressure, push down on the mask to establish an adequate seal. Maintain the airway by lifting the bony prominence of the chin with your remaining fingers, forming an "E." Avoid placing pressure on the soft area under the chin, as this may cause an airway obstruction.*

during the respiratory cycle. With CPAP, the patient exhales against positive pressure (positive end-expiratory pressure [PEEP]); this prevents atelectasis, forces fluid from the alveoli, and improves pulmonary gas exchange. CPAP is an effective treatment for patients with cardiogenic pulmonary edema, and has been shown to reduce the need for intubation when used in conjunction with drug therapy.

CPAP is delivered through a tight-fitting face mask that is attached to an oxygen source; the amount of PEEP can be adjusted between 2.5 and 10 cm H_2O. Patient anxiety is common during initial CPAP therapy; coaching and reassurance are often needed to facilitate compliance. After applying the CPAP device, observe for signs of clinical improvement, which include decreased work of breathing, increased ease in speaking, decreases in respiratory and heart rate, and increased SaO_2.

Experts have not determined whether CPAP is useful in the prehospital setting. Initial small EMS studies suggest that CPAP may provide symptom relief for patients with acute respiratory

(continued on next page)

(continued)

Say, "Squeeze," as you compress the bag as a guide for squeezing. Provide just enough volume to initiate chest rise. Do not overinflate. Obtain adequate chest rise with each ventilation. Pause to allow adequate time for exhalation. Begin releasing the bag and say, "Release, release," to allow time for air to escape. Continue ventilations using the "squeeze, release, release" method.

During ventilation, look for adequate chest rise. Listen for bilateral lung sounds at the third intercostal space on the midaxillary line. Also assess the patient for improvement in skin colour and heart rate.

If needed, you may apply cricoid pressure to minimize gastric distension and passive regurgitation. Locate the cricoid ring by palpating the trachea for a prominent horizontal band inferior to the thyroid cartilage and the cricothyroid membrane. Apply gentle downward pressure using one fingertip in infants and the thumb and index finger in children. Avoid excessive pressure, as it may cause tracheal compression and obstruction in infants.

If performed correctly, bag-valve-mask ventilation is a perfectly acceptable method to oxygenate and ventilate a pediatric patient. Indeed, it may actually be more effective and cause less injury to use a bag-valve-mask device to ventilate the pediatric patient and provide prompt transport to the hospital rather than to attempt intubation.

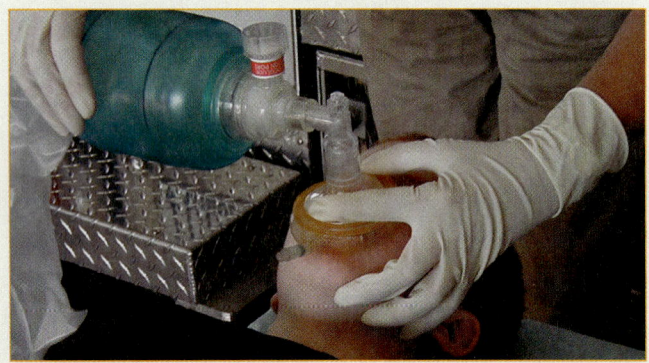

Figure 11-36 The EC-clamp technique will facilitate proper hand placement to maintain a good mask-to-face seal.

failure. Large emergency department and hospital-based studies have demonstrated that noninvasive ventilation methods, such as CPAP, improve respiratory distress symptoms and can avert the need for tracheal intubation, but there is no effect on mortality. Services that carry out interfacility patient transport are equipped to manage patients receiving noninvasive ventilation such as CPAP. These patients are typically more stable than emergency response patients, and noninvasive ventilation is a useful method to support oxygen and ventilation needs in this patient population. Although CPAP is useful in this situation or as a bridge to more definitive airway management, the overall role and benefit of CPAP in the prehospital setting has yet to be determined.

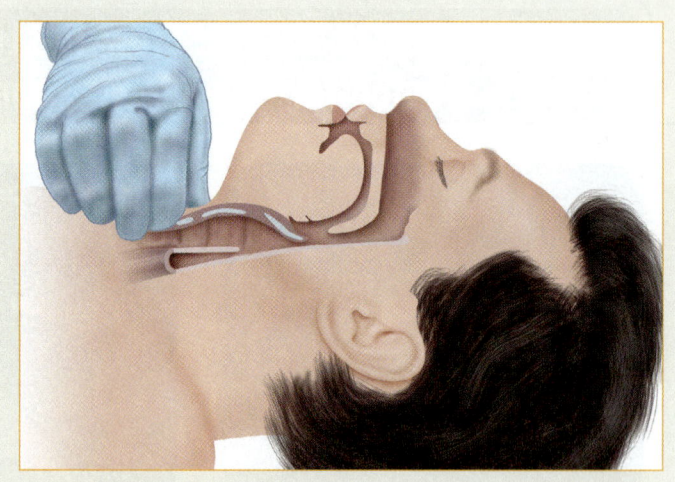

Figure 11-37 Cricoid pressure, or the Sellick maneuver.

Cricoid Pressure (Sellick Maneuver)

When ventilating any patient who is not intubated, you must be alert for gastric distension. This problem can be partially prevented or alleviated by using the <u>Sellick maneuver</u>, also called <u>cricoid pressure</u>. When performed properly, this noninvasive procedure can also help prevent passive regurgitation with aspiration during positive-pressure ventilation.

When you apply posterior pressure to the cricoid cartilage, the esophagus is partially occluded between the cricoid ring and the cervical vertebrae, providing more air delivery into the lungs and less air delivery into the stomach **Figure 11-37 ▲**. Cricoid pressure is indicated only in unconscious patients who cannot protect their own airway and are at imminent risk for vomiting (or if vomiting is occurring). This technique can also be used during endotracheal intubation to move the larynx posteriorly and facilitate an adequate view of the vocal cords.

Disadvantages of this technique include extreme or a large quantity of emesis if pressure is removed; therefore, cricoid pressure should be maintained until the patient is intubated. In addition, the procedure requires two paramedics. If a cervical spine injury is present, cricoid pressure may cause further injury, so this technique is contraindicated in these patients. Potential complications associated with cricoid pressure include trauma to the larynx if excessive force is used, esophageal rupture from unrelieved high gastric pressures, and obstruction of the trachea when the technique is used in small children.

The steps for performing cricoid pressure are listed here and shown in **Skill Drill 11-23 ▶**.

1. Visualize the cricoid cartilage **Step 1**.
2. Palpate the cricoid cartilage to confirm its location—inferior to the thyroid cartilage **Step 2**.
3. Apply firm pressure on the cricoid ring with your thumb and index finger on either side of the midline. Maintain pressure until the patient is intubated **Step 3**.

Skill Drill 11-23: Cricoid Pressure (Sellick Maneuver)

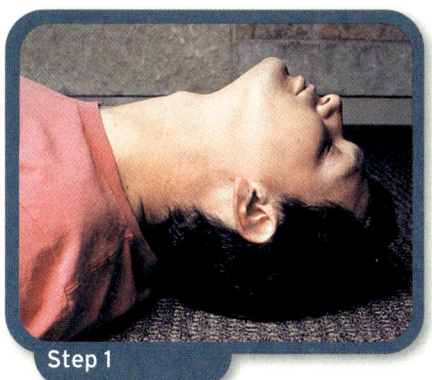

Step 1
Visualize the cricoid cartilage.

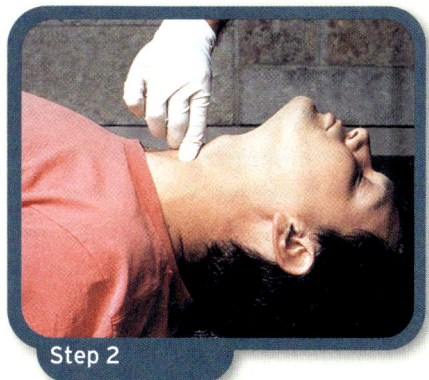

Step 2
Palpate to confirm its location.

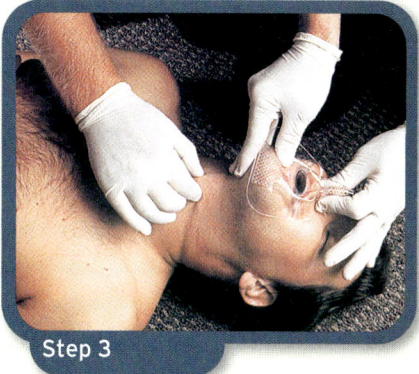

Step 3
Apply firm pressure with your thumb and index finger on either side of the midline.

Gastric Distension

Any form of artificial ventilation that blows air into the patient's mouth—as opposed to blowing air directly into the trachea via an endotracheal tube—may lead to inflation of the patient's stomach with air. Gastric distension is especially likely to occur when excessive pressure is used to inflate the lungs, when ventilations are performed too fast, or when the airway is partially obstructed during ventilation attempts. The pressure in the airway forces open the esophagus, and air flows into the stomach. Gastric distension occurs most often in children but is common in adults as well.

A distended stomach is harmful to the patient for at least two reasons. First, it promotes regurgitation of stomach contents, and vomitus creeping up the back of the throat rapidly finds its way into the patient's lungs (aspiration). Second, a distended stomach pushes the diaphragm upward into the chest, reducing the amount of space in which the lungs can expand.

Signs of gastric distension include an increase in the diameter of the stomach, an increasingly distended abdomen, and increased resistance to bag-valve-mask ventilations. If these signs are noted, you should reassess and reposition the airway as needed, apply cricoid pressure, and observe the chest for adequate rise and fall as you continue ventilating. In addition, limit ventilation times to 1 second or the time needed to produce adequate chest rise.

Invasive Gastric Decompression

Invasive gastric decompression involves inserting a gastric tube into the stomach and then removing the contents with suction. The gastric tube is a very effective tool for removing air and liquid from the stomach, as it decreases the pressure on the diaphragm and virtually eliminates the risk of regurgitation and aspiration.

The gastric tube can be inserted into the stomach through the mouth (orogastric [OG] tube) or through the nose (nasogastric [NG] tube). It should be considered for any patient who will need positive-pressure ventilation for an extended period of time, especially if he or she is not intubated. An NG or OG tube should also be inserted when gastric distension interferes with ventilations—for example, when children are receiving positive-pressure ventilation or have swallowed large volumes of air secondary to increased work of breathing.

NG and OG tubes must be used with extreme caution in any patient with known esophageal disease (eg, tumours or varices). They should never be used in a patient whose esophagus is not patent. After insertion, make sure that the tube has been placed into the stomach. Occasionally it may remain in the esophagus without actually entering the stomach (supragastric placement) or may have been inadvertently placed into the trachea.

As a reminder, paramedics should always take routine precautions and use appropriate PPE when inserting an orogastric or nasogastric tube.

Nasogastric Tube

An NG tube is inserted through the nose, into the nasopharynx, through the esophagus, and into the stomach **Figure 11-38 ▸** . In airway management and ventilation, it decompresses the stomach, thereby decreasing pressure on the diaphragm and limiting the risk of regurgitation. The NG tube is also used to perform gastric lavage—a procedure in which the stomach is decontaminated following a toxic ingestion.

The NG tube is relatively well tolerated, even by patients who are awake. Patients can still talk with an NG tube in place, and, after a few hours, most get used to it. For these reasons, the NG route of insertion is generally preferred for conscious patients.

During the insertion of an NG tube, most patients who are awake will gag and may vomit, even if their gag reflex is suppressed. In a patient with a decreased level of consciousness, vomiting can seriously threaten the airway.

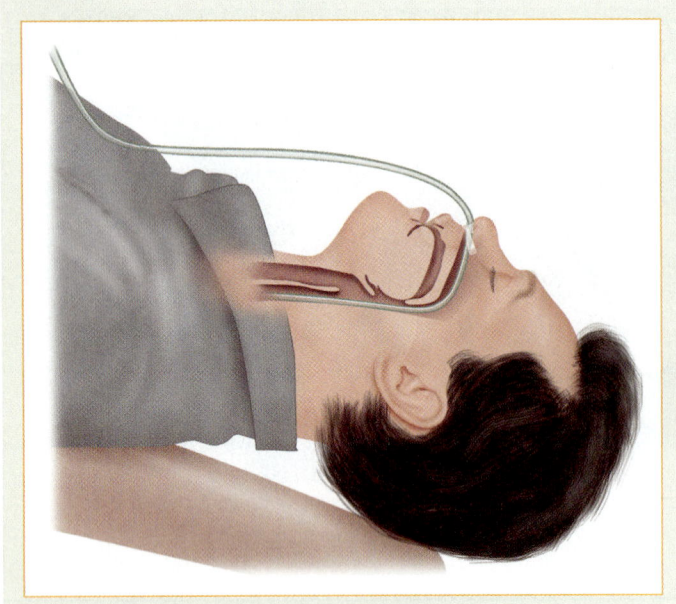

Figure 11-38 Nasogastric tube.

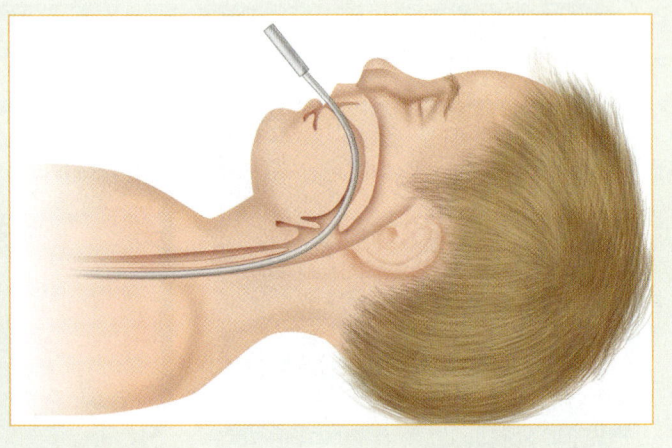

Figure 11-39 Orogastric tube.

8. Confirm proper placement: auscultate over the epigastrium while injecting 30 to 50 ml of air into the tube and/or observe for gastric contents in the tube (Step 8).
9. Apply suction to the tube to aspirate the stomach contents, and secure the tube in place (Step 9).

As a reminder, paramedics should always take routine precautions and use appropriate PPE when inserting an orogastric or nasogastric tube.

Orogastric Tube

An OG tube serves the same purpose as an NG tube but is inserted through the mouth instead of the nose (Figure 11-39 ▲). The advantages and disadvantages of the OG tube are essentially the same as they are for the NG tube. The major differences are that the OG tube carries no risk of nasal bleeding and is safer in patients with severe facial trauma. Additionally, you can use larger tubes, which is helpful if the patient requires aggressive gastric lavage.

The OG tube, however, is less comfortable for conscious patients, causing gagging much more often, and increases the possibility of vomiting. Conscious patients also tend to bite the tube as it is passed orally.

The OG route is generally preferred for patients who are unconscious without a gag reflex. Because these patients need aggressive airway management, the OG tube is almost always inserted *after* the patient's airway is protected with an ET tube; insertion of the OG tube before intubating the patient may obscure your view of the vocal cords.

The steps of OG tube insertion are listed here and shown in (Skill Drill 11-25 ▶).

1. Position the patient's head in a neutral or flexed position (Step 1).
2. Measure the tube for the correct depth of insertion (mouth to ear to xiphoid process) (Step 2).
3. Lubricate the tube with a water-soluble gel (Step 3).
4. Introduce the tube at the midline, and advance it gently into the oropharynx (Step 4).
5. Advance the tube into the stomach (Step 5).

Insertion of an NG tube in patients with severe facial injuries, particularly midface fractures and skull fractures, is contraindicated. In such patients, the NG tube may be inadvertently inserted through the fracture and into the cranial vault. For patients with these conditions, use the OG route of insertion.

Poor technique during NG tube insertion can cause trauma to the nasal passageways, esophagus, or gastric lining; therefore, you must use caution and be gentle when inserting the tube.

Use of the NG tube in patients who are not intubated interferes with the mask seal of the bag-valve-mask device. If you cannot effectively ventilate a patient because of severe gastric distension, however, you must balance the benefit of gastric decompression against the risk of a poor mask seal and determine which has a higher priority. Of course, if the patient is unconscious and requires endotracheal intubation, you can easily pass the ET tube around the NG tube.

The steps of NG tube insertion are listed here and shown in (Skill Drill 11-24 ▶).

1. Explain the procedure to the patient, and oxygenate him or her, if necessary and possible. Ensure that the patient's head is in a neutral position. Suppress the gag reflex with a topical anesthetic spray (Step 1).
2. Constrict the blood vessels in the nares with a topical alpha agonist (Step 2).
3. Measure the tube for the correct depth of insertion (nose to ear to xiphoid process) (Step 3).
4. Lubricate the tube with a water-soluble gel (Step 4).
5. Advance the tube gently along the nasal floor (Step 5).
6. Encourage the patient to swallow or drink to facilitate passage of the tube into the esophagus (Step 6).
7. Advance the tube into the stomach (Step 7).

Skill Drill 11-24: Nasogastric Tube Insertion in a Conscious Patient

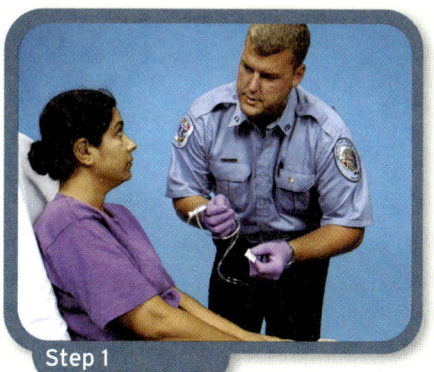

Step 1

Explain the procedure to the patient, and oxygenate the patient if necessary. Ensure that the patient's head is in a neutral position and suppress the gag reflex with a topical anesthetic spray. Use routine precautions and appropriate PPE.

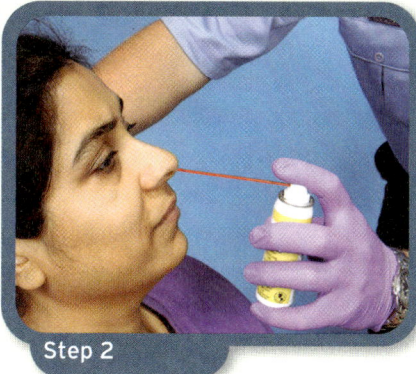

Step 2

Constrict the blood vessels in the nares with a topical alpha agonist.

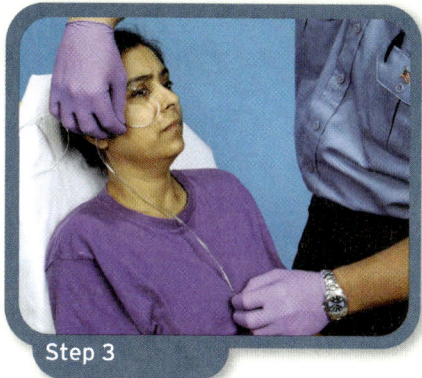

Step 3

Measure the tube for the correct depth of insertion (nose to ear to xiphoid process).

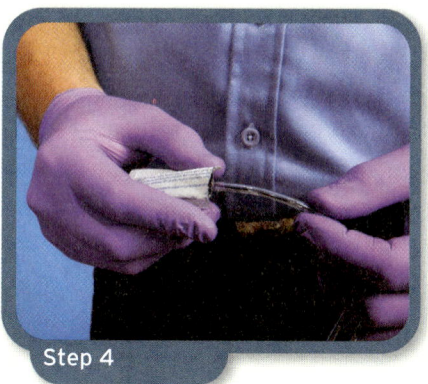

Step 4

Lubricate the tube with a water-soluble gel.

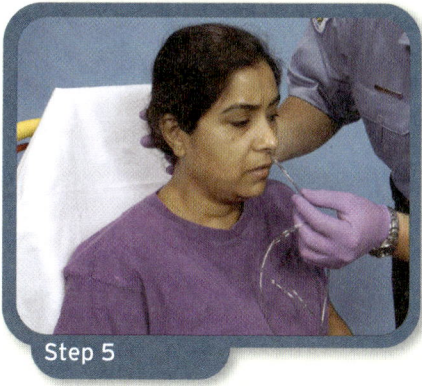

Step 5

Advance the tube gently along the nasal floor.

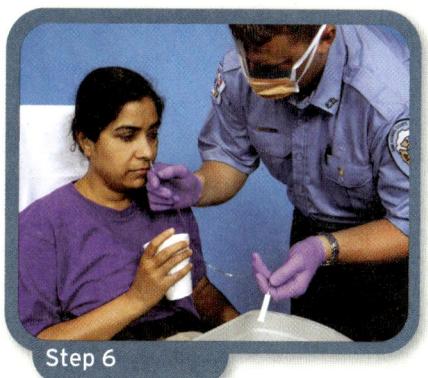

Step 6

Encourage the patient to swallow or drink to facilitate passage of the tube.

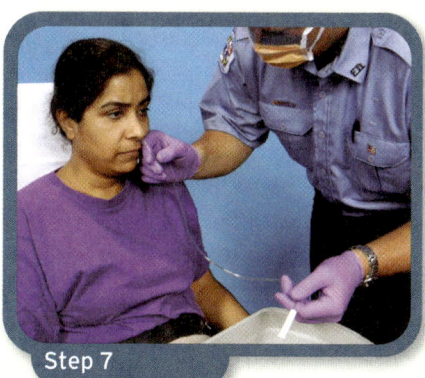

Step 7

Advance the tube into the stomach.

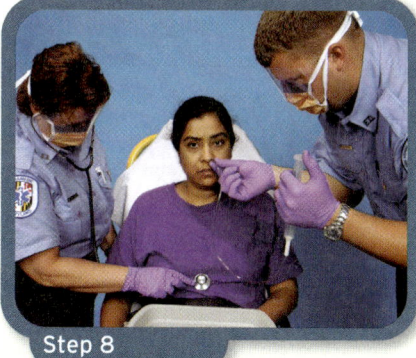

Step 8

Confirm proper placement: auscultate over the epigastrium while injecting 30 to 50 ml of air and/or observe for gastric contents in the tube. There should be no reflux around the tube.

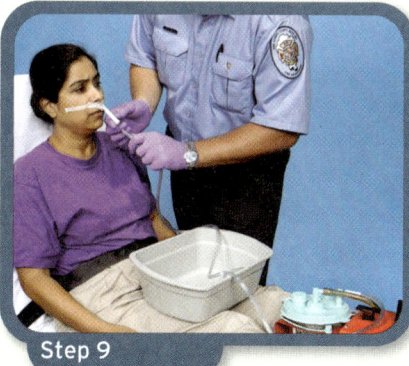

Step 9

Apply suction to the tube to aspirate the gastric contents, and secure the tube in place.

Skill Drill 11-25: Orogastric Tube Insertion

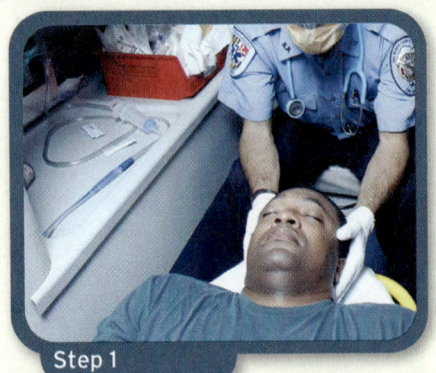

Step 1

Position the patient's head in a neutral or flexed position. Use routine precautions and appropriate PPE.

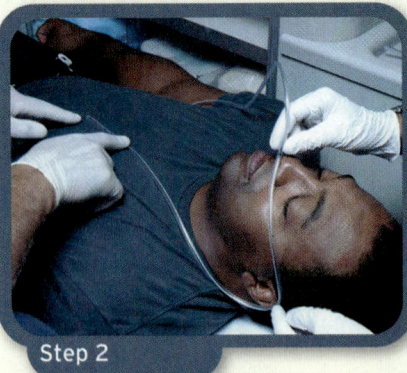

Step 2

Measure the tube for the correct depth of insertion (mouth to ear to xiphoid process).

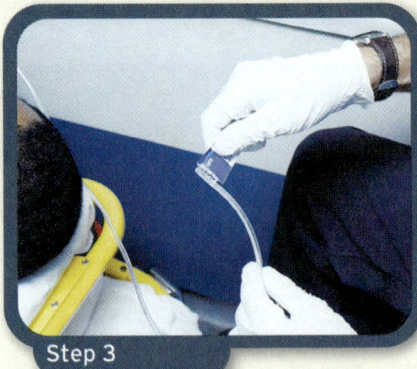

Step 3

Lubricate the tube with a water-soluble gel.

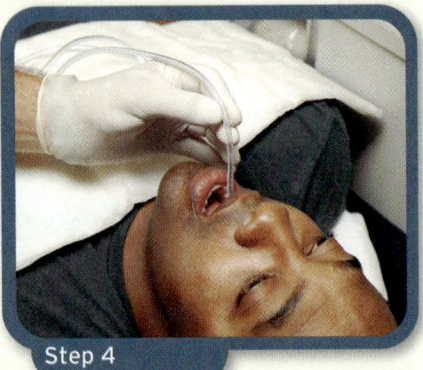

Step 4

Introduce the tube at the midline, and advance it gently into the oropharynx.

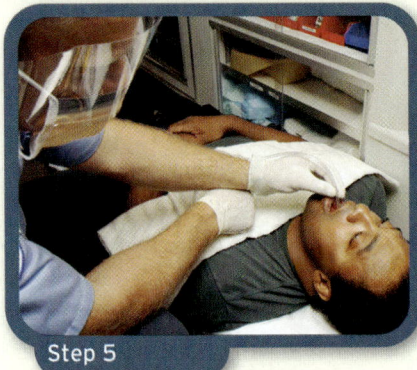

Step 5

Advance the tube into the stomach.

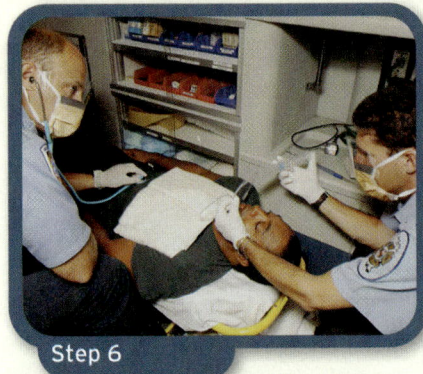

Step 6

Confirm proper placement: auscultate over the epigastrium while injecting 30 to 50 ml of air and/or observe for gastric contents in the tube. There should be no reflux around the tube.

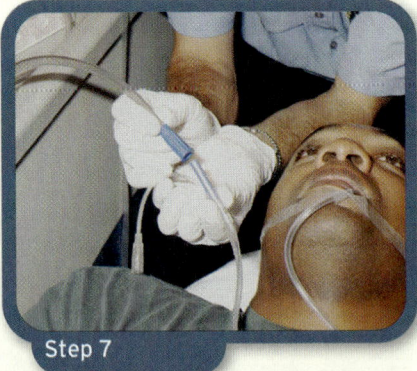

Step 7

Apply suction to the tube to aspirate the stomach contents, and secure the tube in place.

6. Confirm proper placement: Auscultate over the epigastrium while injecting 30 to 50 ml of air and/or observe for gastric contents in the tube. There should be no reflux around the tube Step 6 .

7. Apply suction to the tube to aspirate the stomach contents, and secure the tube in place Step 7 .

Advanced Airway Management

One of the most common mistakes in the situation of respiratory or cardiac arrest is to proceed with advanced airway management too early, forsaking the basic techniques of establishing and maintaining a patent airway in a patient who is already hypoxemic. There is no question that a patient who has arrested requires oxygenation and ventilation, but advanced airway management, such as endotracheal intubation, is not a substitute for basic techniques. *Never abandon the basics of airway management and immediately proceed with advanced techniques simply because you can.*

Another common mistake is failure to identify a potentially difficult airway in a patient who is not in respiratory or cardiac arrest. In certain patients, the paramedic can predict a difficult intubation. Paramedics should always remember that a difficult intubation is something that can be anticipated and prepared for. Two mnemonics can be used to help predict difficulties in airway management.

You can predict difficulties with bag-valve-mask ventilation by remembering MOANS:

M *Mask seal*—problems getting a good seal with the mask

O *Obese*—obese people are difficult to bag-valve-mask ventilate because of their increased body weight

A *Aged*—the elderly tend to be difficult to bag-valve-mask ventilate due to loss of connective tissue and bony structure on their face

N *No teeth*—forming a good seal with the mask is difficult in edentulous patients

S *Stiff lungs*—patients with underlying lung disease require higher pressures to ventilate, and this may be difficult to do with bag-valve-mask ventilation

If you identify a patient with one or more of these features, you should anticipate that bag-valve-mask ventilation may be difficult. Two-person bag-valve-mask ventilation with an airway adjunct may be necessary for effective bag-valve-mask ventilation.

The second mnemonic, LEMON, can predict difficulty with endotracheal intubation:

L *Look*—look externally for obvious anatomical deformities such as obesity, craniofacial abnormalities, neck masses, large tongue, or trauma to the face and neck. Any external deformity or abnormality suggests a difficult intubation.

E *Evaluate the 3-3-2 rule*—the width from the front of the chin to the hyoid bone should be at least three fingerbreadths wide, the width of the patient's mouth opening should be at least three fingerbreadths wide, and the distance from the mandible to the hyoid bones should be at least two fingerbreadths wide. If one or more of these widths or distances do not meet the 3-3-2 rule, you should anticipate a difficult intubation.

M *Mallampati scale*—oral access is assessed using the Mallampati scale Figure 11-40 ▾ . Visibility of the oral pharynx can range from complete visualization (class I) to no visualization at all (class IV). Class III and IV predict difficulty in endotracheal intubation.

O *Obstruction*—you can anticipate a difficult intubation if there is obstruction in the airway, such as epiglottitis, neck injury, tumour in the pharynx, or any other clinical feature to suggest an obstruction (eg, snoring, noisy breathing, abnormal voice).

N *Neck mobility*—if a patient has limited neck mobility due to arthritis, surgery, or cervical spine immobilization, you can anticipate some difficulty with intubation.

If you identify a patient who fails the LEMON assessment, you should prepare an alternative method for oxygenating and ventilating the patient *before* attempting the intubation. Being prepared with all the necessary equipment enables you to proceed to plan B without delay if the first method fails.

Tracheal intubation is a mechanical skill that can be taught to paramedics in a short period of time. The art of airway management, including tracheal intubation, requires a good understanding of anatomy, physiology, and disease processes that affect oxygenation and ventilation. Everyone can agree that the patient who suffers a respiratory or cardiac arrest needs rapid and definitive airway management, whereas the patient with mild shortness of breath due to pneumonia does not need intubation. The challenge to you, as a paramedic, is to sort out the patients between these two extremes, identifying which ones can be managed without intubation and which ones will need intubation. Intubation is an invasive procedure with multiple risks. When considering intubation, you should always remember to first do no harm.

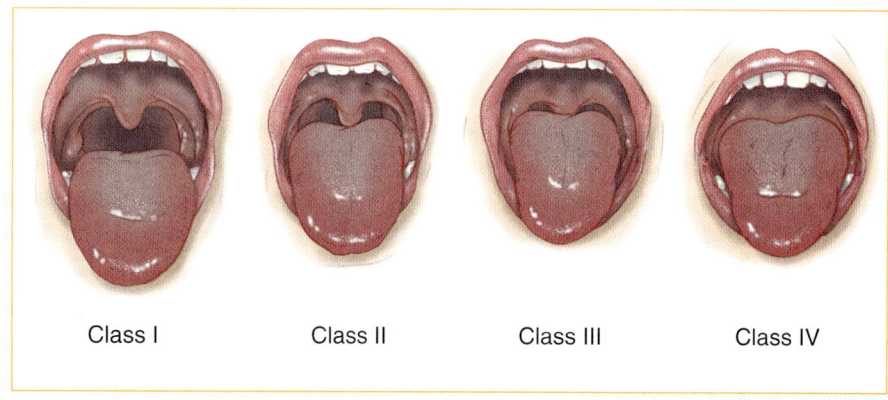

Class I   Class II   Class III   Class IV

Figure 11-40 Mallampati scale.

Endotracheal Intubation

Endotracheal intubation is defined as passing an endotracheal (ET) tube through the glottic opening and sealing the tube with a cuff inflated against the tracheal wall. When the tube is passed into the trachea through the mouth, the procedure is called orotracheal intubation. When the tube is passed into the trachea through the nose, the procedure is called nasotracheal intubation.

Intubation of the trachea is the *most* definitive means of achieving complete control of the airway. A solid understanding of the basics of this technique is needed when making urgent decisions about when to intubate a patient. Following are considerations when performing endotracheal intubation:

- **Indications.** Present or impending respiratory failure, apnea, inability of the patient to protect own airway, control of ventilation for therapeutic reasons (eg, control Pa_{CO_2}).
- **Contraindications.** None in emergency situations. However with inexperienced personnel, other advanced airways (eg, Combitube or LMA) may be easier and equivalent.
- **Advantages.** Provides a secure airway, protects against aspiration, provides an alternate route to IV/IO for certain medications (as a last resort).
- **Disadvantages.** Requires special equipment, bypasses physiologic functions of the upper airway (warming, filtering, humidifying).
- **Complications.** Bleeding, hypoxia, laryngeal swelling, laryngospasm, vocal cord damage, mucosal necrosis, barotrauma, dental injury, inadvertent tube displacement (right mainstem bronchus, esophagus, hypopharynx).

The basic structure of an endotracheal (ET) tube **Figure 11-41 ▶** includes the proximal end, the tube itself, the cuff and pilot balloon, and the distal tip. The proximal end is equipped with a standard 15/22-mm adapter that allows it to be attached to any ventilation device. It also

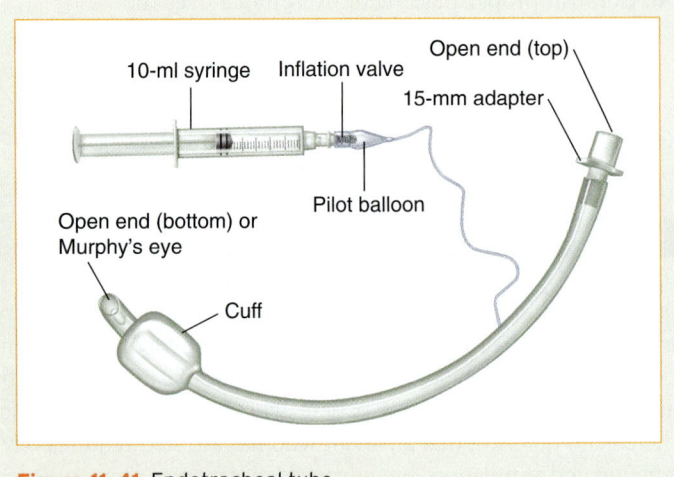

Figure 11-41 Endotracheal tube.

includes an inflation port with a pilot balloon; the distal cuff is inflated with a syringe attached to the inflation port, which has a one-way valve. The pilot balloon indicates whether the distal cuff is inflated or deflated once the tube has been inserted into the mouth.

You are the Paramedic Part 7

One of the firefighters drives your ambulance to the hospital so that your partner can assist you with bag-valve-mask ventilation using 100% oxygen en route to the hospital. You find that you are having difficulty maintaining an adequate mask-to-face seal with the bag-valve-mask device; the patient looks worse. You tell the firefighter to stop the ambulance so that you and your partner can safely assess and treat the problem. Reassessment of the patient reveals the following:

Reassessment	Recording Time: 16 Minutes
Level of consciousness	U (Unresponsive)
Respirations	30 breaths/min and shallow (baseline); you are having difficulty maintaining an adequate mask-to-face seal with the bag-valve-mask device
Pulse	160 beats/min, regular and weak
Skin	Severe facial cyanosis
Blood pressure	98/58 mm Hg
Spo2	83% while receiving assisted ventilations with a bag-valve-mask device and 100% oxygen

11. What are the signs of inadequate artificial ventilation?

12. What management is required to prevent further deterioration of this patient's condition?

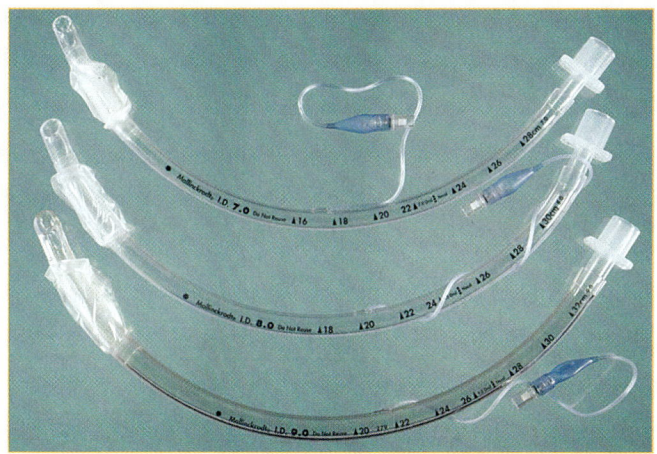

Figure 11-42 Endotracheal tubes are available in a variety of sizes.

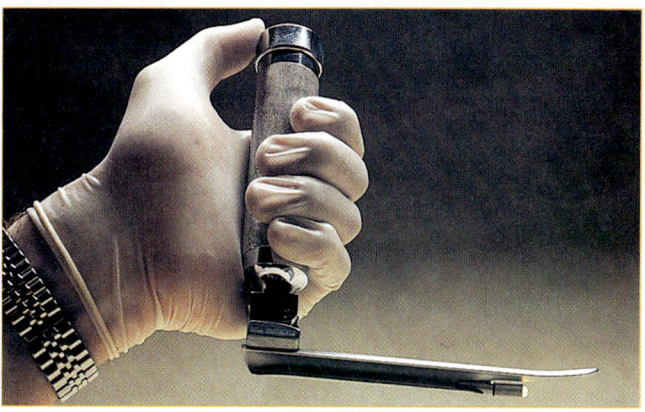

Figure 11-43 A laryngoscope with a straight blade.

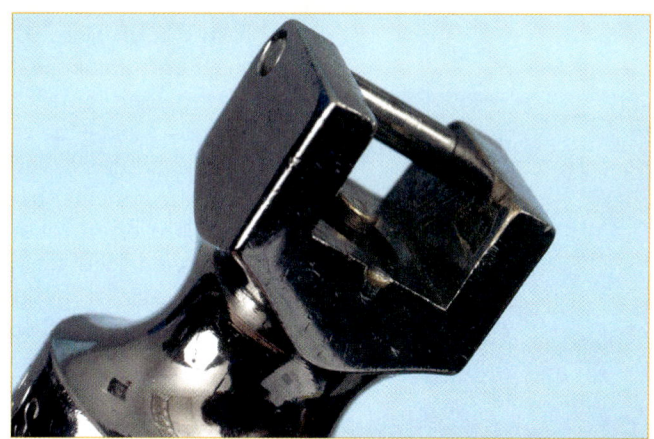

Figure 11-44 The laryngoscope's handle has a bar designed to connect with a notch on the blade.

Centimetre markings along the length of the tube provide a measurement of its depth. The distal end of the tube has a beveled tip to facilitate insertion and an opening on the side called Murphy's eye, which enables ventilation to occur even if the tip becomes occluded by blood, mucus, or the tracheal wall.

Endotracheal tubes range in size from 2.5 to 9.0 mm inside diameter in 0.5-mm increments, and their length ranges from 12 to 32 cm Figure 11-42 ▲ . Sizes ranging from 5.0 to 9.0 mm are equipped with a distal cuff that, when inflated, makes an airtight seal with the tracheal wall. A tube that is too small for the patient will lead to an increased resistance to airflow and difficulty in ventilating. A tube that is too large can be difficult to insert and may cause trauma. Normally, an adult female will require a 7.0- to 8.0-mm tube, while an adult male will require a 7.5- to 8.5-mm tube.

ET tubes ranging from 2.5 to 4.5 mm are used in pediatric patients. In children the funnel-shaped cricoid ring (the narrowest portion of the pediatric airway) forms an anatomical seal with the ET tube, eliminating the need for a distal cuff in most cases. There are limited situations where a cuffed pediatric tube may be used in the hospital setting. The proximal end of the tube still has a 15/22-mm adapter for use with standard ventilation devices, and the distal end has a beveled tip with distal end markings. However, because it lacks a balloon cuff, there is no pilot balloon.

A number of anatomical clues can help determine the proper size of ET tube for adults and children. The internal diameter of the nostril is a good approximation of the diameter of the glottic opening. The diameter of the little finger, nare, or the size of the thumbnail is also a good approximation of airway size. Because all attempts to predict the tube size required for a given patient are estimates, however, you should always have *three* ET tubes ready: one tube of the size you *think* will be appropriate, one a size larger, and one a size smaller.

The laryngoscope and blade are required to perform orotracheal intubation by direct laryngoscopy—a procedure in which the vocal cords are directly visualized for placement of the ET tube. The laryngoscope consists of a handle and interchangeable blades Figure 11-43 ▲ . The handle contains the power source for the light on the laryngoscope blade. Most laryngoscopes run on batteries, but some are rechargeable. The handle has a bar designed to connect with a notch on the blade Figure 11-44 ▲ . When the blade is moved into the perpendicular position, the bright light shines near the tip of the blade.

The two most common types of laryngoscope blades are the straight (Miller) blade and the curved (Macintosh) blade. The straight laryngoscope blade is designed so that its tip will extend beneath the epiglottis and lift it up Figure 11-45 ▶ —a particularly useful feature in infants and small children, who often have a long, floppy epiglottis that is difficult to elevate out of the way with a curved blade. In the adult, use of a straight blade requires great care; if used improperly and levered across the upper jaw, the straight blade is more likely to damage the patient's teeth. The curved laryngoscope blade is less likely to be levered against the teeth by an inexperienced paramedic and is usually preferred by beginners and experienced intubators alike Figure 11-46 ▶ . The direction of the curve conforms to that of the tongue and pharynx, so the

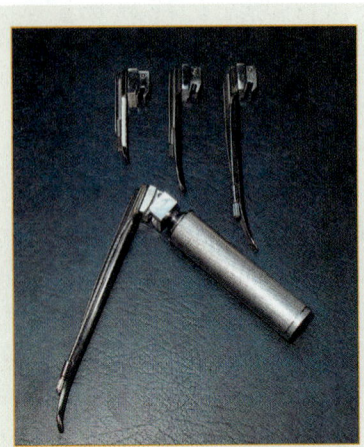

Figure 11-45 A straight (Miller) blade with three additional size blades shown.

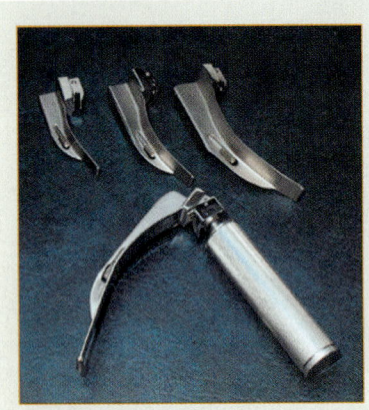

Figure 11-46 A laryngoscope and an assortment of curved (Macintosh) blades.

blade follows the outline of the pharynx with relative ease. The tip of the curved blade is placed in the vallecula (the space between the epiglottis and the base of the tongue) rather than beneath the epiglottis; it indirectly lifts the epiglottis to expose the vocal cords. You should have *both* curved and straight blades readily available during an orotracheal intubation attempt.

Blade sizes range from 0 to 4. Sizes 0, 1, and 2 are appropriate for infants and children, whereas 3 and 4 are considered adult sizes. For pediatric patients, blade sizes are often recommended based on the child's age or height. Most paramedics choose the blade for adults based on experience and the size of the patient (3 for average-sized adults and 4 for larger persons).

It is common, especially in emergency situations, to be unable to obtain a full view of the glottic opening. The stylet, a semirigid wire that is inserted into the ET tube to mould and maintain the shape of the tube, enables you to guide the tip of the tube over the arytenoid cartilage, even if you cannot see the entire glottic opening. This device should be lubricated with a water-soluble gel to facilitate its removal, and its end should be bent to form a gentle "hockey stick" curve. The end of the stylet should rest at least 1.3 cm back from the end of the ET tube;

Controversies

If you cannot obtain vascular access (eg, IV, IO), your protocols may allow you to administer certain resuscitative medications via the ET tube. Epinephrine and atropine are the most commonly administered drugs using the endotracheal route. They are administered by this route as a last resort, during a cardiac arrest where there is no other vascular access. Medications can be administered via the endotracheal route in a dose that is 2 to 2.5 times the standard IV/IO dose.

if the stylet protrudes beyond the end of the tube, it may damage the vocal cords and surrounding structures. Bend the other end of the stylet over the proximal tube connector, so that the stylet cannot slip farther into the tube.

Magill forceps have two uses in the emergency setting. First, they are used to remove airway obstructions under direct visualization, as discussed earlier in this chapter. Second, they are used to guide the tip of the ET tube through the glottic opening if you are unable to get the proper angle with simple manipulation of the tube.

Orotracheal Intubation by Direct Laryngoscopy

Orotracheal intubation by direct laryngoscopy involves inserting an ET tube through the mouth and into the trachea while visualizing the glottic opening with a laryngoscope; it is by far the most common method of performing endotracheal intubation in the emergency setting. Following are some considerations when performing orotracheal intubation by direct laryngoscopy:

- **Indications.** Apnea, hypoxia, poor respiratory effort, suppression or absence of a gag reflex.
- **Contraindications.** Caution in an unsuppressed gag reflex.
- **Advantages.** Direct visualization of anatomy and tube placement, ideal method for confirming placement, may be performed in breathing or apneic patients.
- **Disadvantages.** Requires special equipment.
- **Complications.** Dental trauma, laryngeal trauma, misplacement (right main stem bronchus, esophagus, hypopharynx).

Table 11-10 ▶ summarizes the equipment and preparation required prior to performing orotracheal intubation. Make a copy of this table and tack it to your intubation kit, so that you can check the kit systematically at the beginning of every shift.

Routine Precautions and Personal Protective Equipment

Intubation may expose you to blood or other body fluids, so take proper precautions when performing this procedure. In addition to gloves, wear a mask that covers your *entire* face, which will be relatively close to the patient's mouth and nose, and that will protect you if the patient vomits or coughs during intubation.

Preoxygenation

Adequate preoxygenation with a bag-valve-mask device and 100% oxygen is a critical step prior to intubating a patient. You should preoxygenate the apneic or hypoventilating patient for 2 to 3 minutes. During the intubation attempt, the patient will undergo a period of forced apnea when he or she will not be ventilated. The goal of preoxygenation is to prevent hypoxia from occurring during this time. Unfortunately, you will be unable to perform an extensive preintubation evaluation of the patient, and patients who are intubated in the prehospital setting are usually physiologically unstable.

You should monitor the patient's SpO_2 and achieve as close to 100% saturation as possible during the 2- to 3-minute period of preoxygenation. During the intubation attempt itself, you must continually monitor the SpO_2. Do not let it fall below 95%.

Table 11-10	Preparing Equipment* for Intubation
Equipment	**What to Check, Prepare, and Assemble**
Ventilation equipment	Have an assistant ventilate the patient while you are assembling, checking, and preparing your equipment. Ensure that the patient is being ventilated with 100% oxygen and that the pulse oximeter reading is greater than 95%.
Endotracheal tube	Select the proper size ET tube (7.0- to 8.0-mm for an adult female; 7.5- to 8.5-mm for an adult male). Inject 10 ml of air into the cuff, and ensure that the cuff holds air. Confirm that the 15/22-mm adapter is firmly inserted into the tube. Insert the stylet, and ensure that the tip is proximal to Murphy's eye. Bend the tube/stylet into a "hockey stick" configuration. Increase the angle of the bend if you anticipate a difficult intubation.
Laryngoscope and blades	It is best to have an assortment of blades available because some patients are easier to intubate with one than with another. Confirm the blade that you plan to use is free of any nicks (which could easily cause soft-tissue trauma). Check the bulb to ensure that the light is "bright, white, steady, and tight." The light should be bright enough so that it is uncomfortable to look at directly. It should be white, not yellow or dim. The light should not flicker, especially as the blade is moved on the handle. Most important, the bulb must be tightly screwed into the blade to prevent it from being aspirated into the airway.
Towels	Towels are needed to position the patient's head.
Suction	Suction may be needed to clear the airway of secretions to obtain an adequate laryngoscopic view of the glottic opening.
Magill forceps	Have Magill forceps available should you need to guide the ET tube into the trachea or if you encounter a foreign body obstruction during laryngoscopy.
Confirmation devices	Stethoscope and an end-tidal carbon dioxide ($Etco_2$) detector.
ET tube securing device	Have the appropriate device readily available to secure the tube (eg, tape or a commercial Et tube securing device).

*The paramedic should also prepare backup or rescue equipment in case initial attempts at intubation fail.

At the Scene

Ideally, the patient should have an Spo_2 of 100% (or as close to it as possible) prior to the intubation attempt. If you are attempting to preoxygenate the patient, and the Spo_2 continues to drop despite your best efforts at manual airway management and ventilation, it is best to proceed with intubation without delay.

At the Scene

If the patient has experienced a possible neck injury, his or her head must be placed in a neutral in-line position. Do not use the sniffing position or extend the patient's head in any way. Intubation of the trauma patient is most effectively performed by two paramedics. One paramedic maintains manual in-line stabilization of the patient's head and neck in the neutral position to prevent any further injury, and the second paramedic performs the intubation.

The consequences of even brief periods of hypoxia can be disastrous. Do not rely solely on pulse oximetry to quantify a patient's oxygenation status; it can produce falsely high readings, even if the patient is severely hypoxic. Although some sequelae of hypoxia are dramatic and occur immediately, most are subtle and occur gradually. Clearly, some of the poor neurologic outcomes following aggressive airway management result from intubation-induced hypoxia or inappropriate ventilation-induced hypo- or hypercarbia.

Positioning the Patient

Successful laryngoscopy will be extremely difficult—if not impossible—to perform without proper positioning of the patient's head. The airway has three axes: the mouth, the pharynx, and the larynx. When the head is in a neutral position, these axes are at acute angles, facilitating entry of food into the esophagus rather than into the trachea 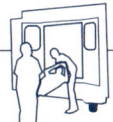 **Figure 11-47A ▶** . Although this positioning is advantageous to the conscious, spontaneously breathing patient, the angles of these axes make laryngoscopy difficult.

To facilitate visualization of the airway, the three axes must be aligned to the greatest extent possible. This is most effectively achieved by placing the patient in the "sniffing" position (the position of the head when intentionally sniffing). The position involves approximately a 20° extension of the atlanto-occipital joint and a 30° flexion of the neck at C6 and C7 for patients with short necks and/or no chins, increasing the angle even further will help improve visualization. The Sellick maneuver further improves the ability to see the vocal cords **Figure 11-47B ▶** .

In most supine patients, the sniffing position can be achieved by extending the head and elevating the occiput 2.5 to 5 cm. Elevate the head and/or neck with folded towels until the ear is at the level of the sternum **Figure 11-48 ▶** . When you are using towels, their thickness can easily be adjusted by changing the number of folds. With obese patients, padding under the head alone may not result in the sniffing position; you may need to add padding under the shoulders and neck as well. To determine whether the patient is in a true sniffing position, view the person from the side to evaluate the adequacy of his or her head position.

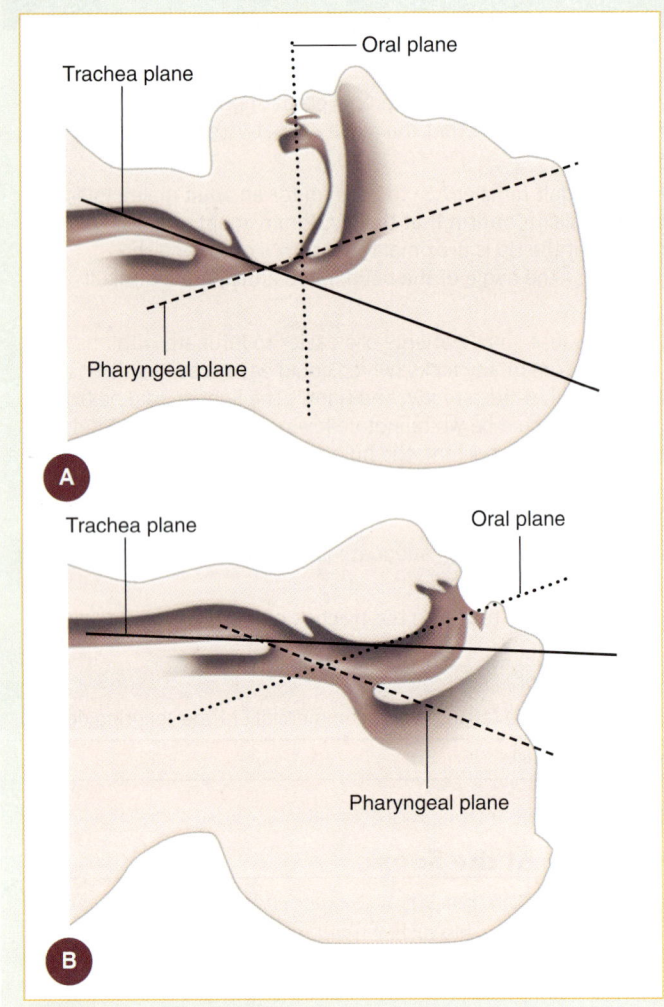

Figure 11-47 Three axes of the airway: oral, pharyngeal, and tracheal. **A.** Neutral position. **B.** Sniffing position.

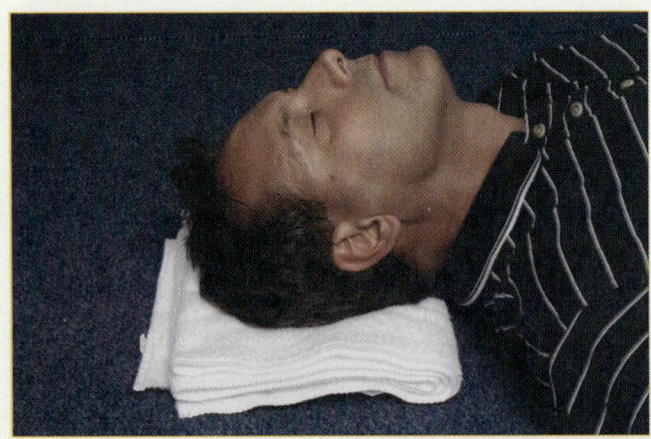

Figure 11-48 Head elevation is best achieved with folded towels positioned under the head.

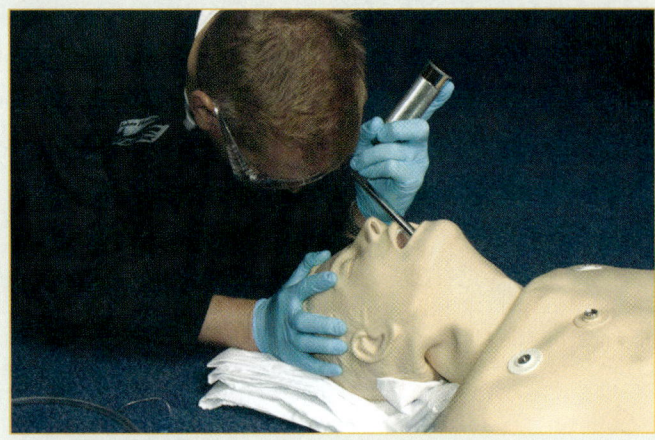

Figure 11-49 If the patient is on the floor or ground, you may need to kneel and lean forward or lie on the floor to get into the proper position.

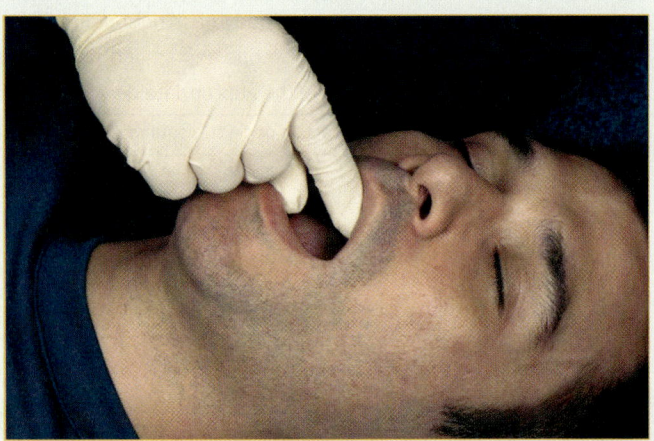

Figure 11-50 Place the side of your right-hand thumb just below the bottom lip and push the mouth open, or scissor your thumb and index finger between the molars.

Blade Insertion

After you have properly positioned the patient's head and provided preoxygenation, direct your partner to stop ventilating. Position yourself at the top of the patient's head. If the patient is on a stretcher, you can squat to put your head at the level of the patient's face. If the patient is on the floor or ground, you may need to kneel and lean forward or lie down to get into the proper position **Figure 11-49 ▲**.

Grasp the laryngoscope with your left hand and hold it as low down on the handle as possible. If the patient's mouth is not open, the easiest technique is to place the patient's head in extension. If the patient has a suspected neck or cervical spine injury, however, you must not reposition the patient's head and neck. Alternatively, you can place the side of your right-hand thumb just below the bottom lip and push the mouth open, or "scissor" your thumb and index finger between the molars **Figure 11-50 ▲**.

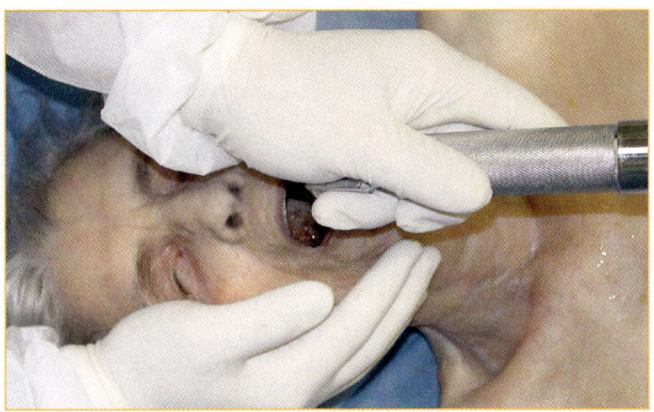

Figure 11-51 The tongue is a sticky, amorphous structure that can be a major hindrance to visualizing the airway. Proper use of the laryngoscope is critical to controlling the tongue.

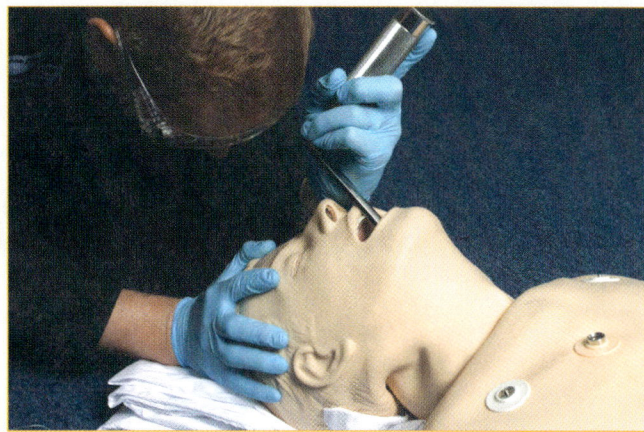

Figure 11-53 Keep your back and your left arm straight as you pull upward. This allows you to use the strength of your shoulders to lift the patient's jaw.

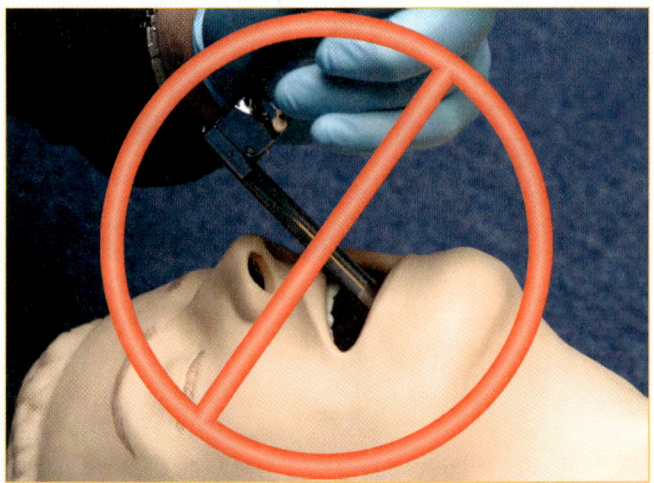

Figure 11-52 Prying against the upper teeth with the laryngoscope can result in breaking and potential aspiration of the teeth. Don't do it!

Insert the blade into the *right* side of the patient's mouth. Use the flange of the blade to sweep the tongue gently to the left side of the mouth while moving the blade into the midline. Take care not to catch the patient's lips between the laryngoscope blade and the teeth. Moving the tongue from right to left is a critical step. If you simply insert the blade in the midline, the tongue will hang over both sides of the blade and all you will see is the tongue   `Figure 11-51 ▲` .

Slowly advance the blade—the curved blade into the vallecula or the straight blade beneath the epiglottis—while sweeping the tongue to the left. Exert *gentle* traction at a 45° angle to the floor as you lift the patient's jaw. *Do not "pry" back on the laryngoscope;* this will cause you to use the patient's upper teeth as a fulcrum, resulting in breaking and potential aspiration of teeth   `Figure 11-52 ▲` . It may also cause you to injure the patient's esophagus if you are using the straight blade. Keeping your back and your left arm straight as you pull upward allows you to use the strength of your shoulders to lift the patient's jaw

and decreases the likelihood of levering the laryngoscope blade against the patient's teeth   `Figure 11-53 ▲` . The correct motion is similar to holding a wine glass and offering a toast.

Visualization of the Glottic Opening

Continue lifting the laryngoscope as you look down the blade. You should see some familiar anatomical landmarks—the epiglottis or the arytenoid cartilage. Identifying these structures enables to you make small adjustments in the position of the blade to aid in visualization of the glottic opening.

With the curved blade, walk the blade down the tongue because you know that the vallecula and the epiglottis lie at the base of the tongue. With the straight blade, insert the blade straight back until the tip touches the posterior pharyngeal wall.

As you continue to work the tip of the blade into position (lifting the epiglottis with the straight blade or the vallecula with the curved blade), the glottic opening should come into full view. The vocal cords are the white fibrous bands that lie

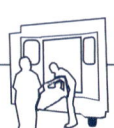

At the Scene

Improving Your Laryngoscopic View: The Sellick Maneuver and the BURP Maneuver

When the angle of the pharynx and the larynx is particularly acute, it is often difficult to see the entire glottic opening. You can do two things to increase the percentage of the glottic opening that you can see: the Sellick maneuver or the BURP maneuver. The Sellick maneuver, which reduces the incidence of gastric distension during positive-pressure ventilation, also moves the larynx more posteriorly. If applied by an assistant during direct laryngoscopy, it reduces the acuity of the angle between the pharynx and larynx and can improve your laryngoscopic view. BURP refers to backward, upward, rightward pressure used in conjunction with the Sellick maneuver to help bring the larynx into better view.

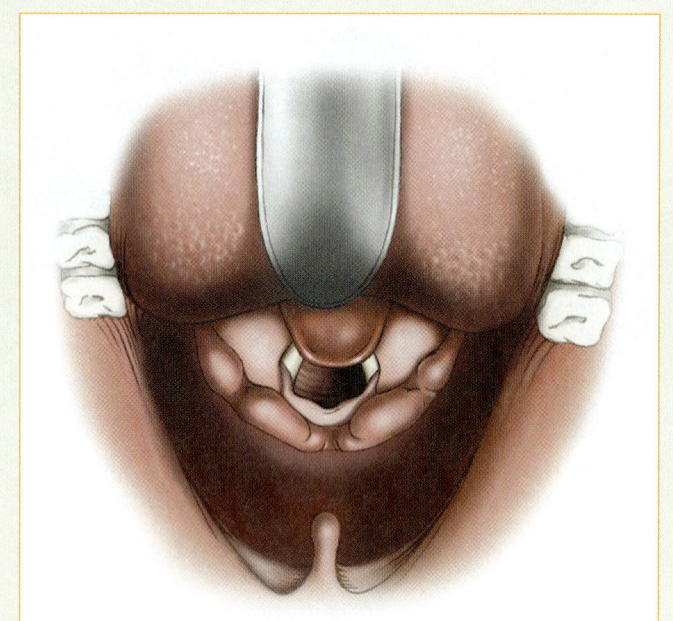

Figure 11-54 Laryngoscopic view of the vocal cords (white fibrous bands).

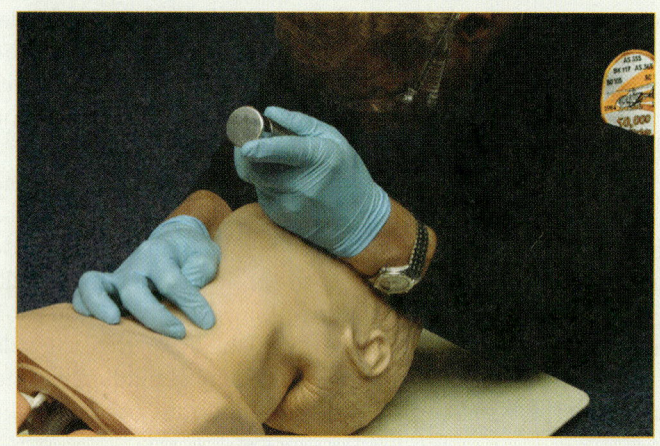

Figure 11-55 BURP maneuver.

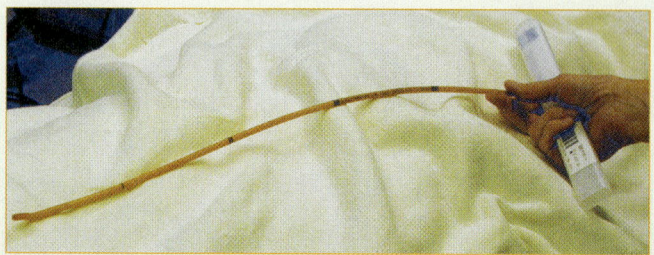

Figure 11-56 The gum elastic bougie device.

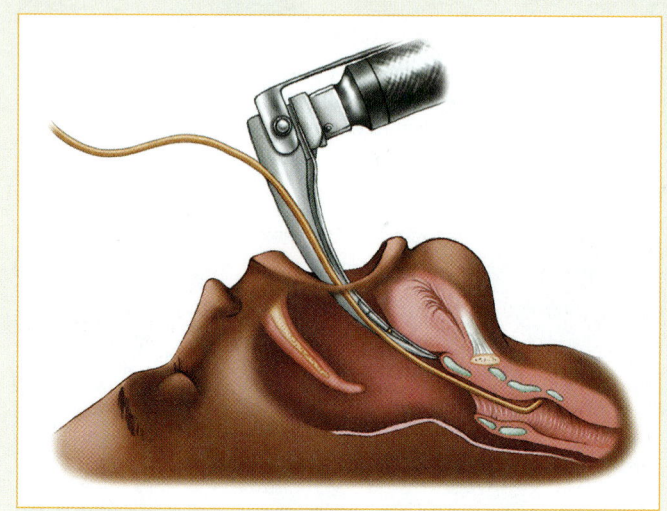

Figure 11-57 The angle at the distal tip of the gum elastic bougie facilitates entry into the glottic opening and enables you to feel the ridges of the tracheal wall.

vertically within the glottic opening; they should be slightly open **Figure 11-54 ▲**.

If you are having difficulty seeing the glottic opening, take your right hand and locate the lower third of the thyroid cartilage. By applying Backward, Upward, and Rightward Pressure (the BURP maneuver), you can often move the larynx into view **Figure 11-55 ▲**. This may be more effective than cricoid pressure alone. Unfortunately, sometimes when you let go to pass the tube with your right hand, you will lose view of the vocal cords. If possible, have an assistant hold the larynx in position as you pass the tube. The BURP maneuver can also be applied to the cricoid ring or the hyoid bone.

The gum elastic bougie, also called the Eschmann stylet, is a flexible device that is approximately 1 cm in diameter and 60 cm long **Figure 11-56 ▶**. It can make intubation possible in some difficult situations, especially when your view of the glottic opening is limited. The gum elastic bougie is rigid enough that it can be easily directed through the glottic opening, yet flexible enough that it does not cause damage to the tracheal walls.

The gum elastic bougie is inserted through the glottic opening under direct laryngoscopy. The angle at its distal tip facilitates entry into the glottic opening and enables you to "feel" the ridges of the tracheal wall **Figure 11-57 ▲**. Once the gum elastic bougie is placed deeply into the trachea, it becomes a guide for the ET tube. Simply slide the tube over the gum elastic bougie and into the trachea. Remove the gum elastic bougie, ventilate, and confirm proper ET tube placement.

Tube Insertion

Once you have visualized the glottic opening, pick up the preselected endotracheal tube in your right hand, holding it near the connector as you would hold a pencil. Under direct vision, insert the tube from the right corner of the patient's mouth through the vocal cords. Continue to insert the tube until the proximal end of the cuff is 1 to 2 cm past the vocal cords. *You must see the tip of the ET tube pass through the vocal cords. If you cannot see the vocal cords, do not insert the tube!* An ET tube shoved blindly down the throat will often come to rest in the esophagus, not in the trachea; the only way to be certain that the tube has

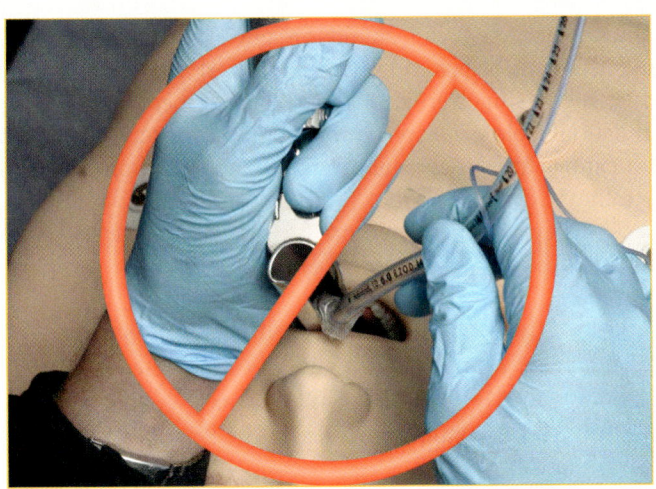

Figure 11-58 Placing a tube down the barrel of the blade obscures your view of the glottic opening.

At the Scene

An intubation attempt should not take more than 30 seconds. If you are unable to intubate the patient within 30 seconds, abort the attempt and reoxygenate the patient for at least 30 seconds to 1 minute with 100% oxygen before attempting intubation again.

Multiple intubation attempts, provided that you perform appropriate oxygenation and ventilation in between attempts, will generally not harm your patient; however, prolonged individual attempts will. During CPR, compressions should not be stopped for more than 10 seconds.

passed through the vocal cords is to *see* it pass through the vocal cords. If you take your eye off the tip of the tube (and the vocal cords), even for a second, you significantly increase the likelihood of allowing the tube to slip into the esophagus.

A common mistake of beginners is to try to pass the tube down the barrel of the laryngoscope blade—especially when using a straight blade. The laryngoscope blade is not designed as a guide for the tube; it is a tool used only to visualize the glottic opening. Placing the tube down the barrel of the blade will obscure your view of the glottic opening **Figure 11-58**.

Ventilation

After you have seen the cuff of the ET tube pass roughly 1.3 cm beyond the vocal cords, gently remove the blade, hold the tube securely in place with your right hand, and remove the stylet from the tube. Inflate the distal cuff with 5 to 10 ml of air and then detach the syringe from the inflation port. If the syringe is not removed immediately following inflation of the distal cuff, air from the cuff may leak back into the syringe, resulting in a loss of an adequate seal between the cuff and the tracheal wall. Avoid inflating the distal cuff with excess pressure as this may cause tissue necrosis of the tracheal wall.

Have your assistant attach the bag-valve-mask device to the ET tube and continue ventilation. As the first ventilations are delivered, look at the patient's chest to ensure that it rises with each ventilation. At the same time, listen with a stethoscope to both the stomach over the epigastrium and then the lungs at both the apices. If the tube is properly positioned, you will hear a quiet epigastrium and equal breath sounds bilaterally. Epigastric sounds may be transmitted to the lungs in obese patients or those with significant gastric distension, however, leading you to believe that you have inadvertently intubated the esophagus.

Confirmation of Tube Placement

Visualizing the ET tube passing in between the vocal cords is your first (and most reliable) method of confirming that the tube has entered the trachea; however, you must continue gathering information to assess the location of the tube. A misplaced tube that goes undetected is a fatal error. You *must* incorporate multiple assessment findings into the determination of where the tube is located.

Auscultation is the first step in confirming proper tube placement. Unequal or absent breath sounds suggest esophageal placement, right mainstem placement, pneumothorax, or bronchial obstruction.

Bilaterally absent breath sounds or gurgling over the epigastrium when auscultating during ventilation indicates that you have intubated the esophagus rather than the trachea. In that case, you must remove the ET tube and be prepared to vigorously suction the patient's airway. If gastric distension is present, the likelihood of emesis is increased. After clearing the airway with suction (if needed), ventilate the patient with 100% oxygen for 30 seconds to 1 minute before you make another attempt at intubation.

Paramedics who are skilled at advanced airway management may opt to leave the esophageal ET tube in place. This makes it easier to identify the esophagus and guide the next ET tube placement attempt or placement of the gum elastic bougie. The decision to remove an esophageally placed ET tube before or after further intubation attempts will depend on your skill as an intubator and your EMS agency.

If breath sounds are heard only on the right side of the chest, the tube has likely been advanced too far and entered the right mainstem bronchus. Follow these steps to reposition the tube:

1. Loosen or remove the tube securing device.
2. Deflate the distal cuff.
3. Place your stethoscope over the left side of the chest.
4. While ventilation continues, *slowly* retract the tube while simultaneously listening for breath sounds over the left side of the chest.
5. Stop as soon as bilaterally equal breath sounds are heard.
6. Note the depth of the tube (in cm) at the patient's teeth.
7. Reinflate the distal cuff.
8. Secure the tube.
9. Resume ventilations.

If the ET tube has been properly positioned in the trachea, the bag-valve-mask device should be easy to compress and you

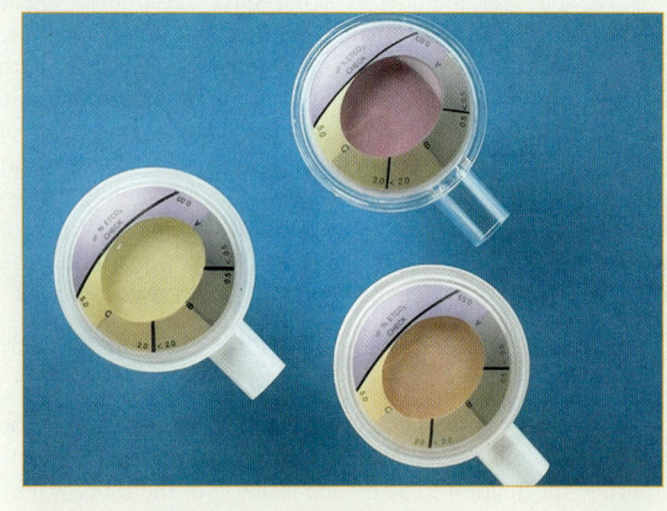

Figure 11-59 Colourimetric capnographers.

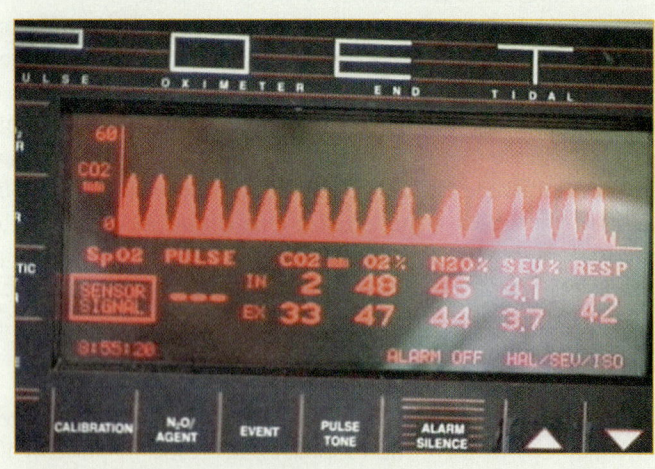

Figure 11-60 A capnometer.

should see corresponding chest expansion. Increased resistance (decreased ventilation compliance) during ventilations may indicate gastric distension, esophageal intubation, or tension pneumothorax. Any of these conditions warrant immediate reassessment and corrective action.

End-tidal carbon dioxide ($ETCO_2$) detectors detect the presence of carbon dioxide in exhaled air. Because carbon dioxide is not present in the esophagus, use of the $ETCO_2$ detector is a very reliable method for confirming proper tube placement and is a *mandatory* method to confirm endotracheal tube placement in the prehospital setting. $ETCO_2$ detectors may be colourimetric, digital, or digital/waveform. A capnographer attaches in between the ET tube and bag-valve-mask device. It contains colourimetric paper, which should turn yellow during exhalation, indicating proper tube placement (**Figure 11-59 ▲**). A capnometer performs the same function and attaches in the same way as a capnographer, but provides a readout of the patient's exhaled carbon dioxide (**Figure 11-60 ▲**). Ongoing assessment with digital capnometry is an excellent indicator of continued correct

placement of the ET tube, especially in the back of a moving ambulance, where breath sounds are often difficult to hear. If the patient's $ETCO_2$ begins to fall, it should alert you that a problem exists, such as inadvertent ET tube displacement or inadequate ventilation. Note that capnography may be inaccurate in patients with cardiac arrest, who are severely acidotic and only eliminating minimal carbon dioxide.

The steps for performing $ETCO_2$ detection are listed here and shown in (**Skill Drill 11-26 ▸**).

1. Detach the ventilation device from the ET tube (**Step 1**).
2. Attach an in-line capnographer or capnometer to the proximal adapter of the ET tube (**Step 2**).
3. Reattach the ventilation device to the ET tube, and resume ventilations (**Step 3**).
4. Monitor the capnographer or capnometer for appropriate reading (appropriate colour change or digital reading) (**Step 4**).

The $ETCO_2$ detector should be in place as soon as the ET tube is inserted to help confirm correct tube placement.

Although $ETCO_2$ detection is useful to confirm tube placement, quantitative measurement of $ETCO_2$ is more useful clinically. Many portable monitor/defibrillators used in the prehospital setting can display a numerical real-time measurement of exhaled $ETCO_2$. This numeric value is clinically relevant. Prehospital studies have shown that inadequate or excessive ventilation of intubated patients can lead to hypercarbia or hypocarbia. The abnormally high or low $ETCO_2$ is potentially harmful. Once a patient is intubated, close monitoring of $ETCO_2$ helps direct the rate of ventilation and tidal volume to prevent hypocapnia and hypercapnia. Failure to properly monitor $ETCO_2$ and maintain it in the appropriate range is known to be harmful and can lead to poor patient outcome. This is particularly true in patients with closed head injuries. Protocols that target prehospital ventilation and prevent hypocapnia and hypercapnia are just as important as providing supplemental oxygen and monitoring oxygen saturation to prevent hypoxia. Monitoring the $ETCO_2$ waveform is now also recommended for intubated patients throughout the periarrest period of a cardiac arrest resuscitation. The waveform helps monitor CPR quality and can detect a return or loss of spontaneous circulation by increases or decreases in $ETCO_2$, respectively. Paramedics performing tracheal intubation should know if their monitor measures quantitative $ETCO_2$ and whether their local or regional protocols have $ETCO_2$ target ranges for patients who are intubated and ventilated.

The esophageal detector device (EDD) is another method of helping confirm proper ET tube placement. The EDD is a bulb or syringe with a 15/22-mm adapter. With the syringe model, the syringe is attached to the end of the ET tube and the plunger is withdrawn, creating negative pressure (**Figure 11-61 ▸**). If the tube is in the trachea (which has rigid, noncollapsible walls), air is easily drawn into the syringe and the plunger does not move when released. Unlike the trachea, however, the esophagus is a flaccid, easily collapsible tube. Thus, if the tube is in the esophagus, a vacuum is created as the EDD's plunger is withdrawn and the plunger moves back toward zero when released.

Skill Drill 11-26: Using Colourimetric Capnography for Carbon Dioxide Detection

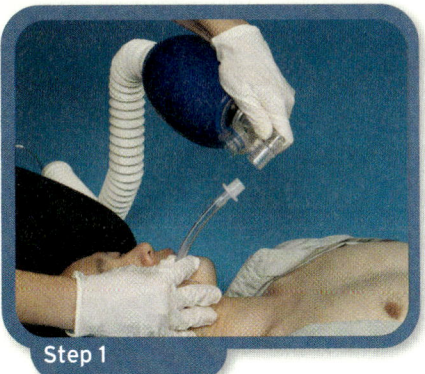

Step 1

Detach the ventilation device from the ET tube.

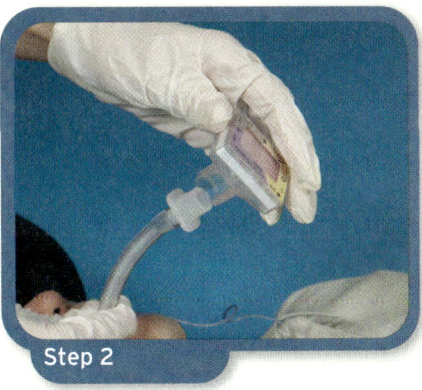

Step 2

Attach an in-line colourimetric capnographer or capnometer to the proximal adapter of the ET tube.

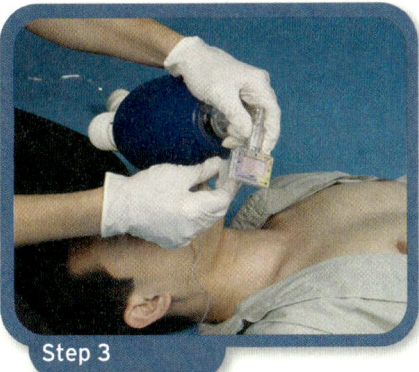

Step 3

Reattach the ventilation device to the ET tube, and resume ventilations.

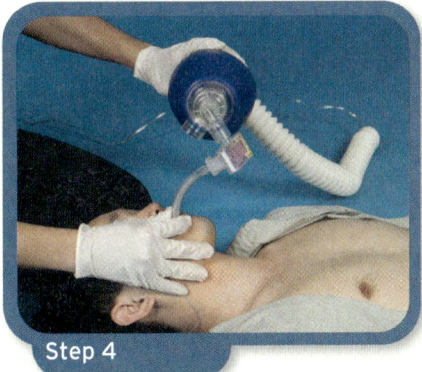

Step 4

Monitor the device for appropriate reading (appropriate colour change or digital reading).

With the bulb model, the bulb is squeezed and then attached to the end of the ET tube. If it remains collapsed or inflates slowly, the esophageal wall has occluded the distal tip of the tube, indicating that esophageal intubation has likely occurred. If the bulb briskly expands, the tube is properly positioned in the trachea **Figure 11-62 ▾**.

The EDD is not a very reliable indicator that the ET tube is in the trachea and should not be used for definitive confirmation of proper tube placement. Remember that multiple methods for confirming proper tube placement must be used.

After confirming proper tube placement, note and mark the ET tube with an ink line or piece of tape at the point where it emerges from the patient's mouth; this will enable medical personnel involved in the subsequent care of the patient to determine whether the tube has slipped in or out. The average depth for adult patients is 21 to 25 cm.

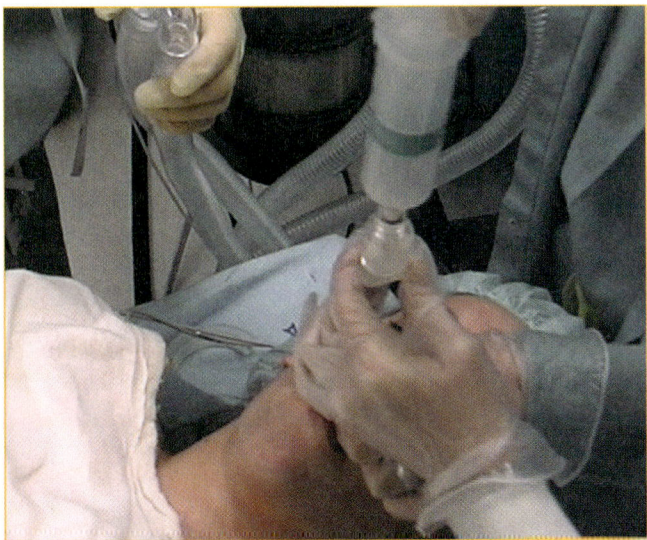

Figure 11-61 With the esophageal detector device syringe, the ability to freely withdraw air indicates placement of the tube in the trachea.

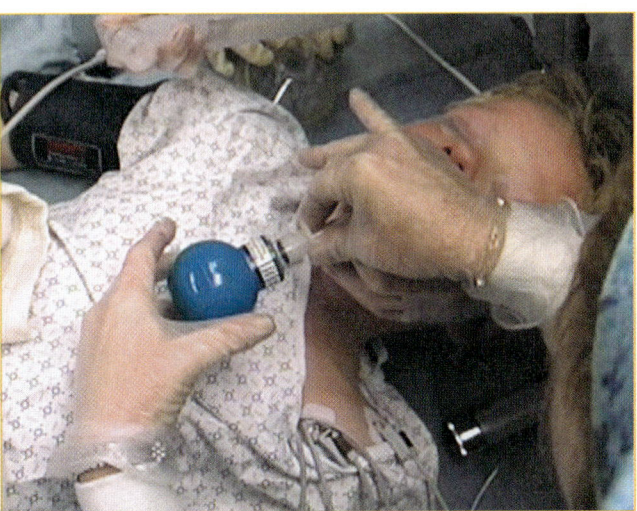

Figure 11-62 If the ET tube is in the trachea, the EDD bulb should briskly fill with air.

Skill Drill 11-27: Securing an Endotracheal Tube With Tape

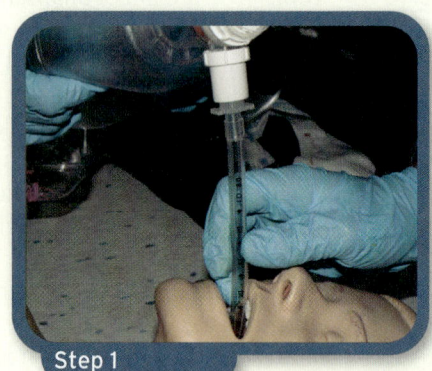

Step 1

Note the centimetre marking on the tube at the level of the patient's teeth.

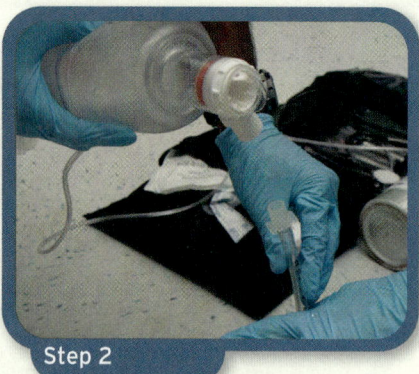

Step 2

Remove the bag-valve-mask device from the ET tube.

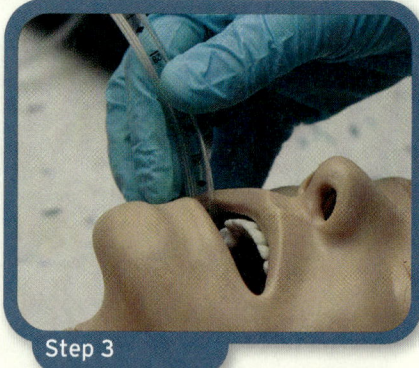

Step 3

Move the ET tube to the corner of the patient's mouth.

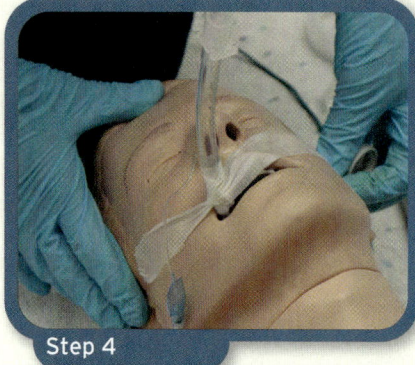

Step 4

Encircle the ET tube with tape, and secure the tape to the patient's maxilla (using tincture of benzoin to facilitate tape adhesion).

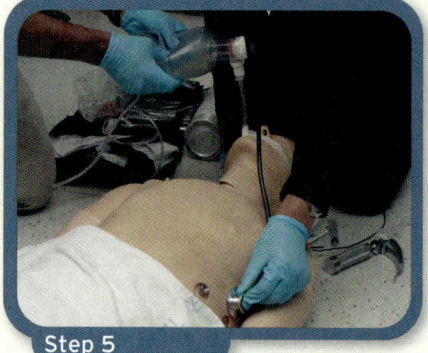

Step 5

Reattach the bag-valve-mask device, and auscultate again over the apices and bases of the lungs and over the epigastrium.

Securing the Tube

The last, and very important step, is to secure the ET tube. Inadvertent extubation caused by the patient or someone else is relatively common and can be very traumatic to the patient. There are few things more discouraging than to accomplish a difficult intubation, only to have the tube slip out of the trachea. Reintubation will almost certainly be even more difficult. *Never take your hand off the ET tube before it has been secured with tape or a commercial device!* Even then, it is a good idea to support the tube manually while you ventilate the patient to avoid a sudden jolt from the bag-valve-mask device that yanks the tube from the trachea.

Many commercial tube-securing devices are available. You should be familiar with the specific device used by your EMS system. Every paramedic should also know how to secure a tube using tape, because it is almost always available. The steps for securing an ET tube with tape are listed here and shown in **Skill Drill 11-27 ▲**.

1. Note the centimetre marking on the tube at the level of the patient's teeth **Step 1**.
2. Remove the bag-valve-mask device from the ET tube **Step 2**.
3. Move the ET tube to the corner of the patient's mouth **Step 3**.
4. Encircle the ET tube with tape, and secure the tape to the patient's maxilla (using tincture of benzoin to facilitate tape adhesion) **Step 4**.
5. Reattach the bag-valve-mask device, and auscultate again over the apices and bases of the lungs and over the epigastrium **Step 5**.

At the Scene

The presence of condensation (vapour mist) in the ET tube during exhalation is not a reliable indicator that the ET tube is in the trachea. Tube misting by itself should not be used for definitive confirmation of proper tube placement. Instead, use multiple methods to confirm proper tube placement.

The steps for securing an ET tube with a commercial device are listed here and shown in **Skill Drill 11-28 ▸**.

1. Note the centimetre marking on the tube at the level of the patient's teeth **Step 1**.
2. Remove the bag-valve-mask device from the ET tube **Step 2**.
3. Position the ET tube in the centre of the patient's mouth **Step 3**.
4. Place the commercial device over the ET tube. Tighten the screw to secure it in place **Step 4**. Fasten the strap.
5. Reattach the bag-valve-mask device, and auscultate again over the apices and bases of the lungs and over the epigastrium **Step 5**.

If the patient bites the tube or experiences a seizure, the ET tube may become occluded; therefore, after properly securing the tube, insert a bite block or oral airway in between the patient's molars. Many commercially manufactured ET tube-securing devices feature a built-in bite block for this purpose.

It is also important to minimize head movement in the intubated patient. With a firmly secured tube, the tip can move as much as 5 cm during head flexion and extension. Consider applying a cervical collar, placing the patient on a backboard, and stabilizing the patient's head with lateral immobilization blocks to reduce the likelihood of tube dislodgement during transport.

The steps for orotracheal intubation by direct laryngoscopy are summarized here and shown in **Skill Drill 11-29 ▸**.

1. Use routine precautions and PPE (gloves and face shield as a minimum) **Step 1**.
2. Preoxygenate the patient for 2 to 3 minutes with a bag-valve-mask device and 100% oxygen **Step 2**.
3. Check, prepare, and assemble your equipment **Step 3**.
4. Place the patient's head in the sniffing position **Step 4**.
5. Insert the blade into the right side of the patient's mouth, and displace the tongue to the left **Step 5**.
6. Gently lift the long axis of the laryngoscope handle until you can visualize the glottic opening and the vocal cords **Step 6**.
7. Insert the ET tube through the right corner of the mouth, and visualize its entry between the vocal cords **Step 7**.

At the Scene

No single test for correct ET tube placement is 100% accurate. Always use at least two methods of tube placement confirmation.

8. Remove the laryngoscope from the patient's mouth **Step 8**.
9. Remove the stylet from the ET tube **Step 9**.
10. Inflate the distal cuff of the ET tube with 5 to 10 ml of air, and detach the syringe from the inflation port **Step 10**.
11. Attach an end-tidal carbon dioxide detector to the ET tube to confirm tube placement **Step 11**.
12. Attach the bag-valve-mask device, ventilate, and auscultate over the epigastrium first and then apices and bases of both lungs **Step 12**.
13. Secure the ET tube **Step 13**.
14. Place a bite block in the patient's mouth **Step 14**.

Nasotracheal Intubation

Nasotracheal intubation is the insertion of a tube into the trachea through the nose. In the prehospital setting, it is usually performed without directly visualizing the vocal cords—hence the term "blind" nasotracheal intubation.

Blind nasotracheal intubation is an excellent technique for establishing control over the airway in situations where it is either difficult or hazardous to perform laryngoscopy. Because the procedure must be performed on patients with spontaneous breathing, it is less likely to result in hypoxia.

Indications and Contraindications

Nasotracheal intubation is indicated for patients who are breathing spontaneously, but require definitive airway management to prevent further deterioration of their condition. Conscious patients or patients with an altered mental status and with an intact gag reflex, who are in respiratory failure secondary to conditions such as COPD, asthma, or pulmonary edema, are excellent candidates for nasotracheal intubation.

Nasotracheal intubation is contraindicated in apneic patients (eg, in respiratory or cardiac arrest); such patients should receive orotracheal intubation. This procedure is also contraindicated in patients with head trauma and possible midface fractures, as evidenced by CSF drainage from the nose following a head injury. In these patients, a nasally inserted ET tube may enter the cranial vault and penetrate the brain. Other contraindications to nasotracheal intubation include anatomical abnormalities, such as in patients with a deviated septum, patients with nasal polyps, or patients who frequently use cocaine. Nasal insertion of an ET tube in these patients may result in severe epistaxis.

Documentation and Communication

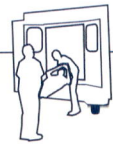

On the patient care report, document the means of assessing placement of the ET tube, such as breath sounds, visualization, and capnography or capnometry findings. The depth of the tube, as noted by the centimetre marking at the patient's teeth, should also be documented. Additionally, indicate when correct placement was confirmed: at the time the ET tube was placed, when the patient was moved into the ambulance, and upon arrival at the hospital.

Skill Drill 11-28: Securing an Endotracheal Tube With a Commercial Device

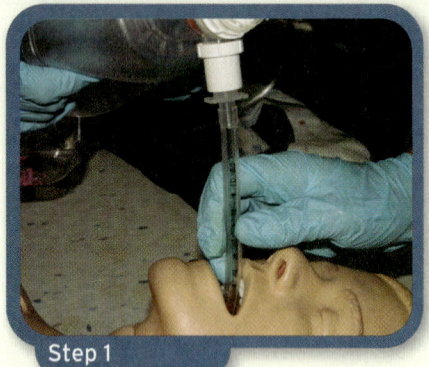

Step 1

Note the centimetre marking on the tube at the level of the patient's teeth.

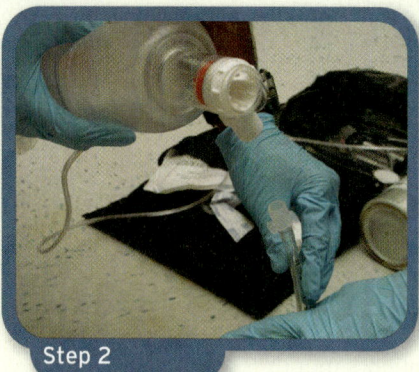

Step 2

Remove the bag-valve-mask device from the ET tube.

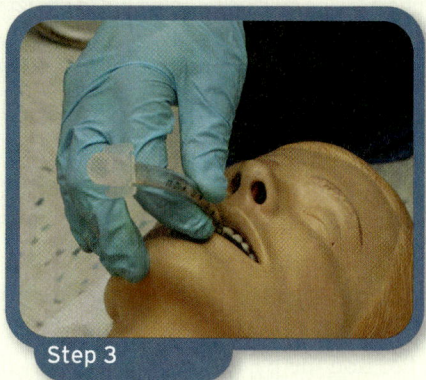

Step 3

Position the ET tube in the centre of the patient's mouth.

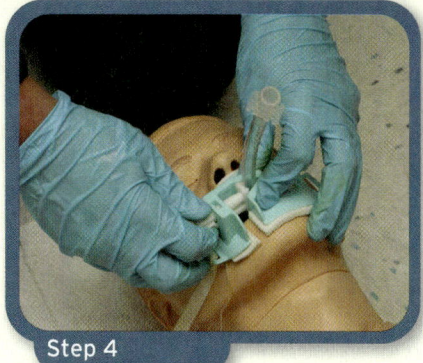

Step 4

Place the commercial device over the ET tube. Tighten the screw and fasten the strap to secure.

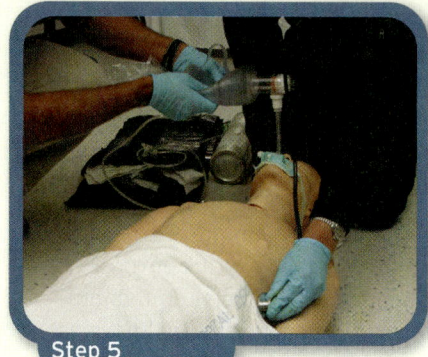

Step 5

Reattach the bag-valve-mask device, and auscultate again over the apices and bases of the lungs and over the epigastrium.

You are the Paramedic Part 8

After definitively securing the patient's airway, you may attach the patient to a transport ventilator and continue transport. En route, you note marked improvement in his condition. Your reassessment reveals the following:

Reassessment	Recording Time: 22 Minutes
Level of consciousness	P (Responsive to painful stimuli); improving, patient is becoming resistant to the ET tube
Respirations	Ventilate with 100% oxygen at a rate of 12 breaths/min
Pulse	118 beats/min, regular and stronger
Skin	Cyanosis is dissipating; skin is cool and dry
Blood pressure	118/70 mm Hg
Spo₂	97% while being ventilated with 100% oxygen

13. Should you extubate this patient? Why or why not?
14. Are any pharmacologic interventions required?

Skill Drill 11-29: Intubation of the Trachea Using Direct Laryngoscopy

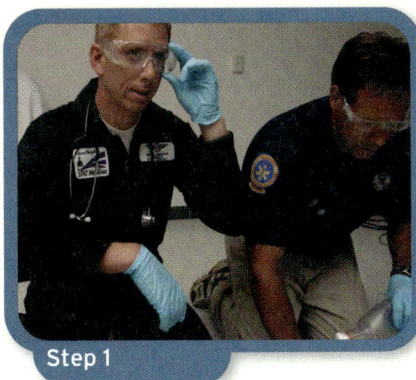

Step 1

Use routine precautions and PPE (gloves and face shield).

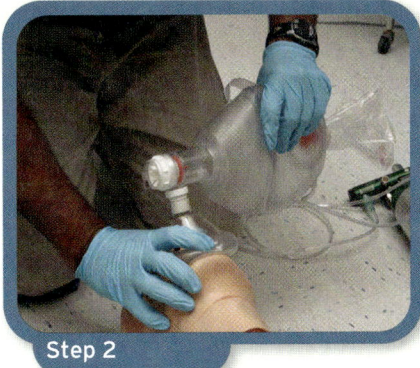

Step 2

Preoxygenate the patient for 2 to 3 minutes with a bag-valve-mask device and 100% oxygen.

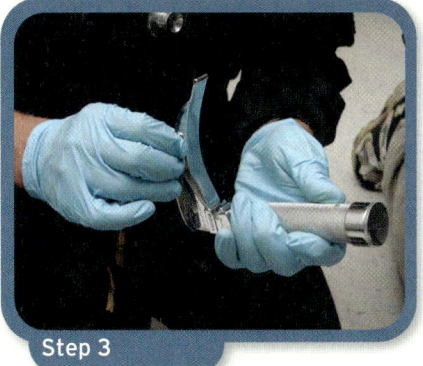

Step 3

Check, prepare, and assemble your equipment.

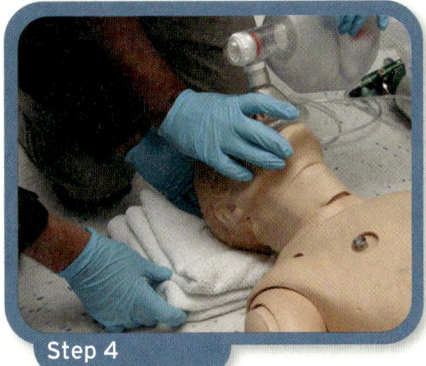

Step 4

Place the patient's head in the sniffing position.

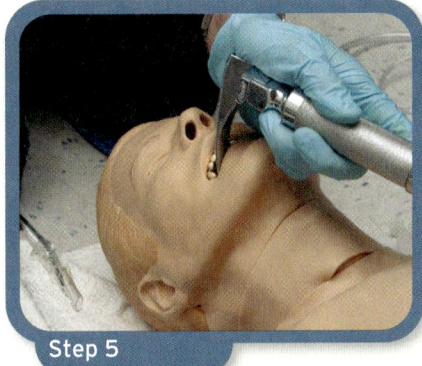

Step 5

Insert the blade into the right side of the patient's mouth, and displace the tongue to the left.

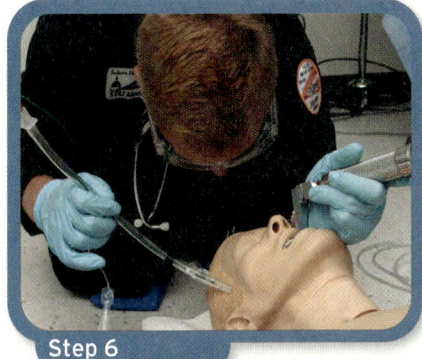

Step 6

Gently lift the long axis of the laryngoscope handle until you can visualize the glottic opening and the vocal cords.

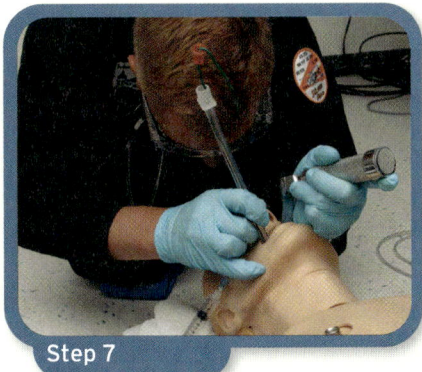

Step 7

Insert the ET tube through the right corner of the mouth, and visualize its entry between the vocal cords.

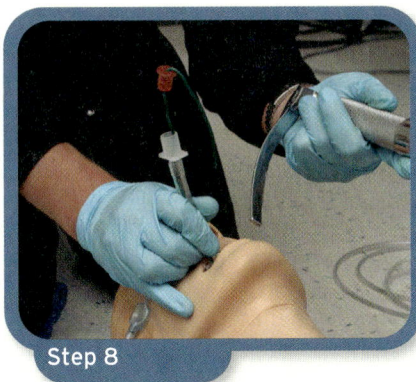

Step 8

Remove the laryngoscope from the patient's mouth.

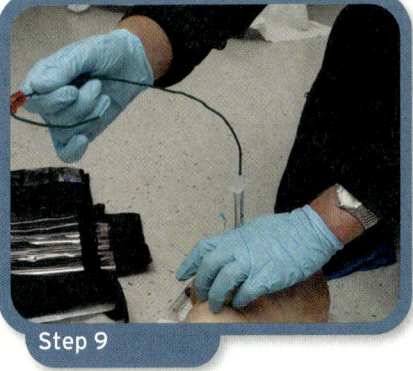

Step 9

Remove the stylet from the ET tube.

Skill Drill 11-29: Intubation of the Trachea Using Direct Laryngoscopy (*continued*)

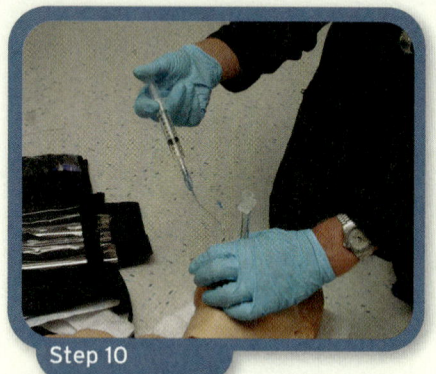

Step 10

Inflate the distal cuff of the ET tube with 5 to 10 ml of air, and detach the syringe from the inflation port.

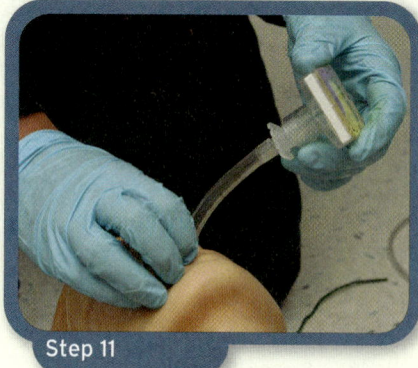

Step 11

Attach the end-tidal carbon dioxide detector to the ET tube and confirm presence of end-tidal carbon dioxide.

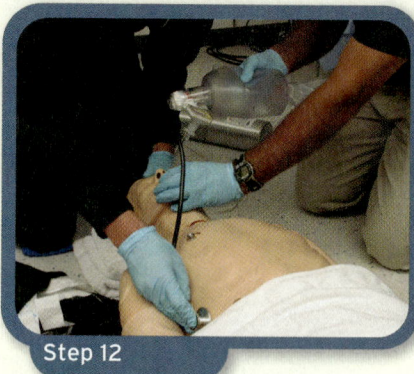

Step 12

Attach the bag-valve-mask device, ventilate, and auscultate over the epigastrium and over the apices and bases of both lungs.

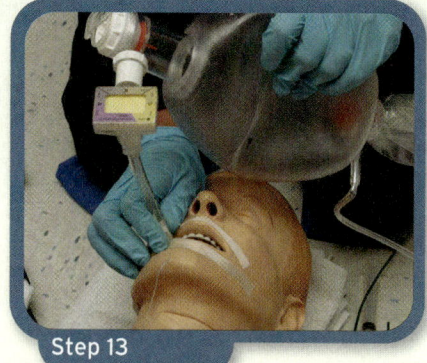

Step 13

Confirm placement and then secure the ET tube.

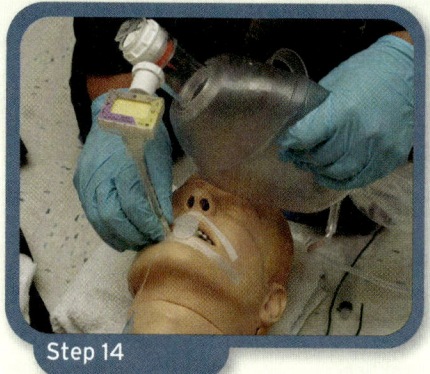

Step 14

Place a bite block in the patient's mouth.

Likewise, you should avoid nasotracheal intubation, if possible, in patients with blood-clotting abnormalities or in those who take anticoagulation medications (eg, Coumadin). These conditions also increase the likelihood and severity of epistaxis following insertion of anything in the nose.

Advantages and Disadvantages

The primary advantage of blind nasotracheal intubation is that it can be performed on patients who are awake and breathing. This procedure does not require that you place anything in the mouth (eg, laryngoscope), so the nasotracheal route is associated with much less retching and a lower risk of vomiting in patients with an intact gag reflex.

Another major advantage of nasotracheal intubation is that there is no need for a laryngoscope, which eliminates the risk of trauma to the teeth or soft tissues of the mouth. Because the patient's mouth does not need to be opened, this technique is better suited to patients with limited temporomandibular joint mobility, such as those with mandibular wiring, mandibular fractures, seizures, or clenched teeth (trismus).

Nasotracheal intubation does not require the patient to be placed in a sniffing position, which makes it an ideal technique for intubating patients with a possible spinal injury, unless a midface fracture is suspected. Finally, because the tube is inserted through the nose, the patient cannot bite the tube. Furthermore, it can be secured more easily than a tube that is inserted orally because the nose generally has fewer secretions than the mouth.

On the downside, because nasotracheal intubation is a blind technique, the paramedic cannot use one of the major tube confirmation methods—visualizing the tube passing through the vocal cords. Confirming proper tube position is important, regardless of which intubation method is employed; however, the paramedic should be even more diligent when confirming tube placement following nasotracheal intubation.

Complications

Bleeding is the most common complication associated with nasotracheal intubation. If intubation is successful, the airway is protected and the risk of aspiration is eliminated. However, severe bleeding can occur, especially with rough technique, posing an additional threat to an already compromised airway as the swallowing of blood greatly increases the likelihood of vomiting and subsequent aspiration.

The incidence of bleeding associated with nasotracheal intubation can be reduced by being very gentle when inserting the tube into the nostril and by lubricating the tip with a water-soluble gel. If available, an anesthetic lubricant containing a vasoconstrictive agent (eg, phenylephrine hydrochloride [Neo-Synephrine]) will reduce the amount of patient discomfort as well as the likelihood and severity of nasal bleeding.

Equipment

The same equipment used for orotracheal intubation—minus the laryngoscope and stylet—is used for blind nasotracheal intubation. Standard ET tubes can be used for both orotracheal and nasotracheal intubation, although they should be 1.0 to 1.5 mm smaller when inserted nasally. When choosing the size of tube, select one that is slightly smaller than the nostril in which it will be inserted.

Some ET tubes have been designed specifically for blind nasotracheal intubation. For example, the Endotrol tube **Figure 11-63** is slightly more flexible than a standard ET tube and is equipped with a "trigger" that is attached to a piece of line, which is itself attached to the tip of the tube. Pulling the trigger moves the tip of the tube anteriorly and increases the tube's overall curvature. This feature replaces the function of the stylet.

The movement of air through the ET tube helps determine proper tube placement following nasotracheal intubation. A number of devices have been developed to allow the paramedic to confirm successful nasotracheal intubation without the need to place his or her face next to the tube and thus risk contact with contaminants in the patient's exhaled breath **Table 11-11** .

Technique for Nasotracheal Intubation

When you perform blind nasotracheal intubation, you use the patient's spontaneous respirations to guide the ET tube into the trachea and confirm proper placement. The tube is advanced as the patient inhales, at which point the vocal cords are open at their widest, which facilitates placement of the tube into the trachea.

Table 11-11	Devices Used to Determine Maximum Airflow Through the Tube During Nasotracheal Intubation
Humid-Vent 1	Device that attaches to the 15/22-mm adapter at the end of the ET tube to prevent secretions from being expelled from the tube.
BAAM® (Beck Airway Airflow Monitor)	A small whistle that attaches to the 15/22-mm adapter and emits a high-pitched sound as air moves in and out of the tube.
Stethoscope with head removed	Stethoscope tubing placed in the proximal 2 to 3 cm of the ET tube enables the paramedic to hear air movement without placing his or her face next to the tube.
IV tubing attached to an earpiece	The tubing in the proximal 2 to 3 cm of the ET tube enables the intubator to hear air movement without placing his or her face next to the tube.

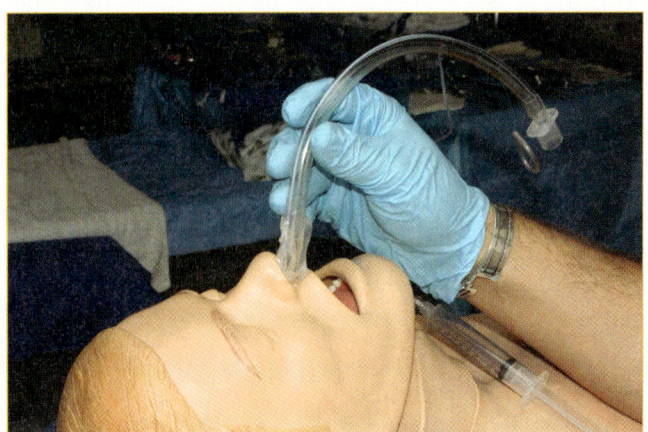

Figure 11-64 Aim the tip of the tube straight back toward the ear.

After preparing your equipment and preoxygenating the patient, insert the tube into the nostril with the bevel facing toward the nasal septum. The right nostril is typically used because the curvature of the tube is in the correct orientation in relation to the bevel. If the right nostril is obstructed or if significant resistance is met, insert the tube into the left nostril, but rotate the tube 180° as its tip enters the nasopharynx.

The angle of insertion is critical when performing nasotracheal intubation. Aim the tip of the tube straight back toward the ear **Figure 11-64** . The goal is to follow the floor of the nasal cavity until the tube enters the nasopharynx. *Do not* insert the tube with the tip aimed upward toward the eye, as this can damage the turbinates and cause significant bleeding.

As the tube is advanced into the nasopharynx, you will begin to hear air rushing in and out of the tube as the patient breathes. Your goal is to position the tube just above the glottic

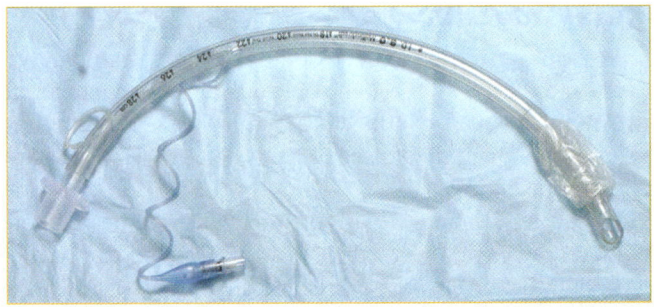

Figure 11-63 The Endotrol tube makes the nasotracheal procedure safer, easier, and more efficient.

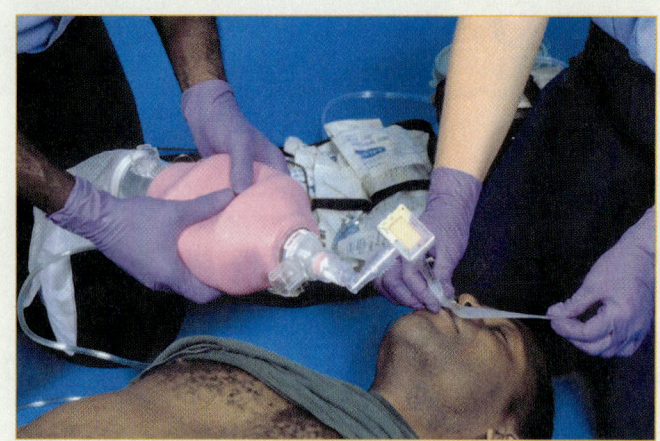

Figure 11-65 Clean up any secretions or excess lubricant and secure the tube with tape.

opening so that the patient will draw the tube into the trachea when he or she inhales deeply. Manipulate the patient's head to control the position of the tip of the tube. Cup your left hand (if the tube is inserted in the right nostril) under the patient's occiput. Move the patient's head until you find the position that offers the maximum amount of air moving through the tube. At this point, the tube should be positioned just above the glottic opening.

As the patient inhales, the negative pressure created by inhalation facilitates movement of the tube through the glottic opening. Instruct the patient to take a deep breath, and *gently* advance the tube with the inhalation. Placement of the tube in the trachea will be evidenced by an increase in air movement through the tube.

If you see a soft-tissue bulge on either side of the airway, the tube has probably been inserted into the pyriform fossa. Hold the patient's head still and slightly withdraw the tube. Once maximum airflow is detected, advance the tube on inhalation. If you do not see a soft-tissue bulge and no air is moving through the tube, the tube has entered the esophagus. Withdraw the tube until you detect airflow, and then extend the head.

Once the tube has been properly positioned, inflate the distal cuff with the minimum amount of air necessary to achieve an airtight seal. Attach a bag-valve-mask device to the tube and ventilate the patient according to his or her clinical condition. Because you do not have the benefit of visualizing the tube passing in between the vocal cords, confirmation (by multiple techniques) and continuous monitoring of proper tube position is more important following blind nasotracheal intubation than with any other intubation technique. Although the movement of air in and out of the tube during breathing is a good indicator that the tube is in the trachea, it is not foolproof. Additional indicators of successful placement include the patient coughing when the tube is passed and the patient is no longer able to talk. In many cases, only the tip of the ET tube has passed through the glottic opening; even slight patient movement may dislodge the tube, potentially unrecognized,

into the esophagus. Movement of the tube can also result in right mainstem placement.

Clean up any secretions or excess lubricant and secure the tube with tape **Figure 11-65 ◀**. Document the depth of insertion at the nostril and monitor it frequently to detect movement of the tube.

The steps for performing blind nasotracheal intubation are listed here and shown in **Skill Drill 11-30 ▶**.

1. Use routine precautions and PPE (gloves and face shield at a minimum) **Step 1**.
2. Preoxygenate the patient whenever possible with a bag-valve-mask device and 100% oxygen **Step 2**.
3. Check, prepare, and assemble your equipment **Step 3**.
4. Place the patient's head in a neutral position **Step 4**.
5. Pre-form the ET tube by bending it in a circle **Step 5**.
6. Lubricate the tip of the tube with a water-soluble gel **Step 6**.
7. Gently insert the ET tube into the most compliant nostril with the bevel facing toward the nasal septum and advance the tube along the nasal floor **Step 7**.
8. Advance the ET tube through the vocal cords as the patient inhales **Step 8**.
9. Inflate the distal cuff with 5 to 10 ml of air and detach the syringe **Step 9**.
10. Attach an end-tidal carbon dioxide detector to the ET tube **Step 10**.
11. Attach the bag-valve-mask device, ventilate, and auscultate over the apices and bases of both lungs and over the epigastrium **Step 11**.
12. Secure the ET tube **Step 12**.

Digital Intubation

Suppose you are in the midst of attempting to intubate your patient and suddenly the light on your laryngoscope sputters out. You must have a contingency plan for these kinds of unexpected events, including a set of fresh batteries and a back-up laryngoscope handle.

Fortunately, there *is* a way to intubate the trachea without a laryngoscope. Digital intubation (also referred to as "blind" or "tactile" intubation) involves directly palpating the glottic structures and elevating the epiglottis with your middle finger while guiding the ET tube into the trachea by feel. Being adept at digital intubation provides you with an option in some extreme

Skill Drill 11-30: Blind Nasotracheal Intubation

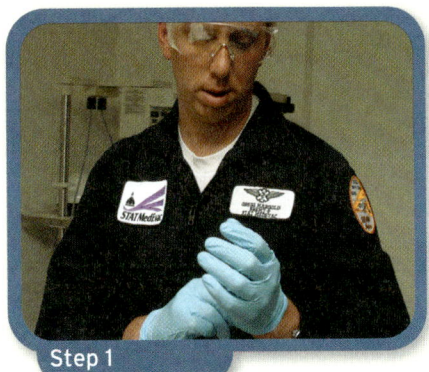

Step 1

Use routine precautions and PPE (gloves and face shield at a minimum).

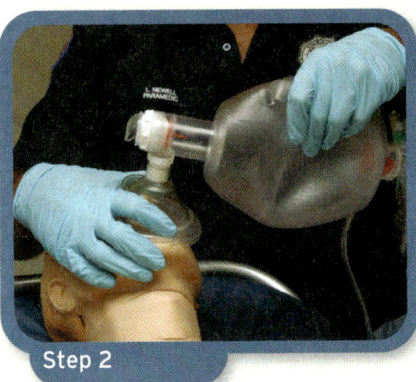

Step 2

Preoxygenate the patient whenever possible with a bag-valve-mask device and 100% oxygen.

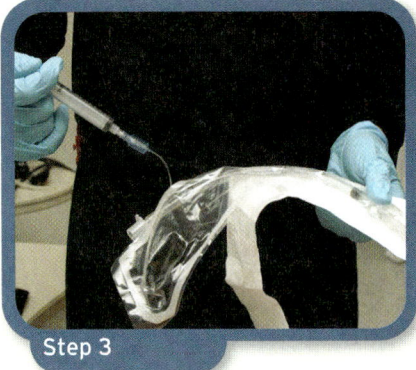

Step 3

Check, prepare, and assemble your equipment.

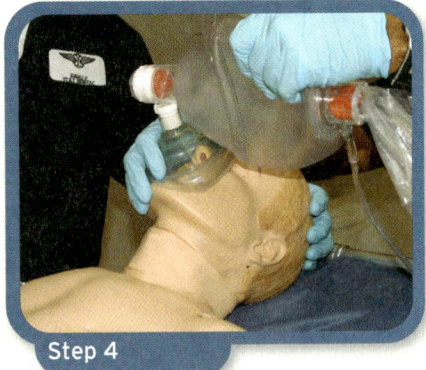

Step 4

Place the patient's head in a neutral position.

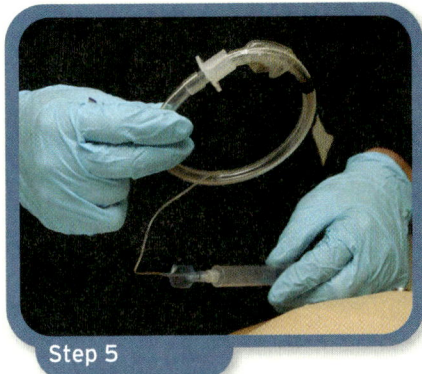

Step 5

Pre-form the ET tube by bending it in a circle.

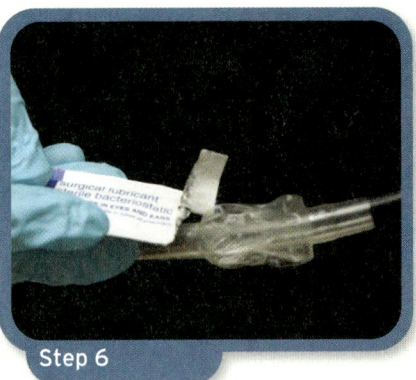

Step 6

Lubricate the tip of the tube with a water-soluble gel.

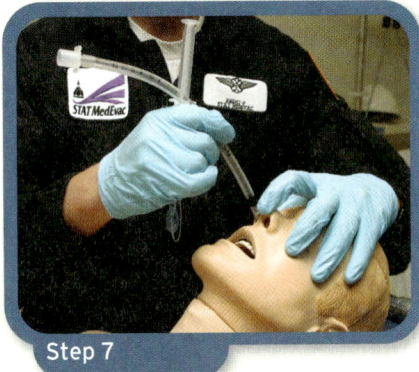

Step 7

Gently insert the ET tube into the most compliant nostril, with the bevel facing toward the nasal septum and advance the tube along the nasal floor.

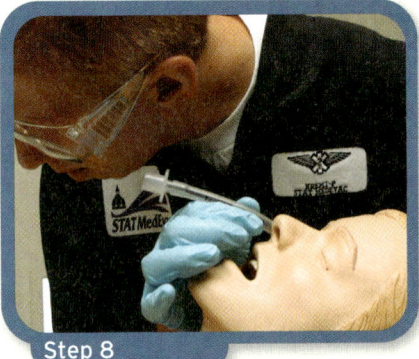

Step 8

Advance the ET tube through the vocal cords as the patient inhales. The BAAM® device can be helpful in this step.

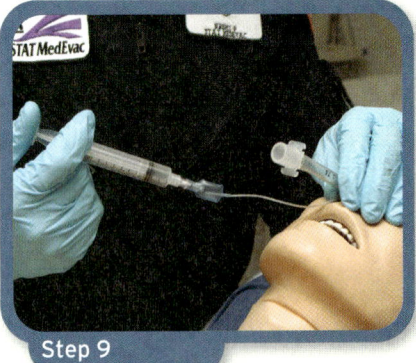

Step 9

Inflate the distal cuff with 5 to 10 ml of air and detach the syringe.

Skill Drill 11-30: Blind Nasotracheal Intubation (*continued*)

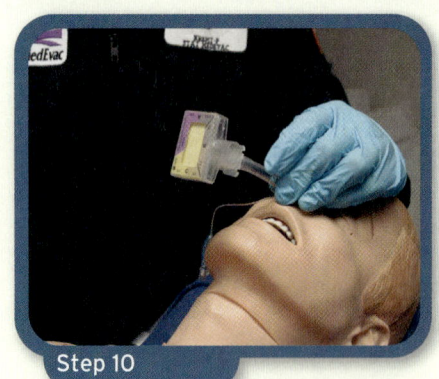

Step 10

Attach an end-tidal carbon dioxide detector to the ET tube.

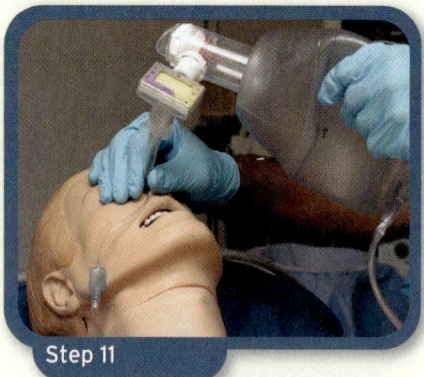

Step 11

Attach the bag-valve-mask device, ventilate, and auscultate over the apices and bases of both lungs and over the epigastrium.

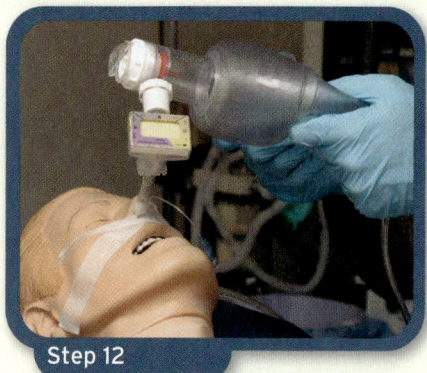

Step 12

Confirm placement and then secure the ET tube.

circumstances, such as equipment failure when attempting to intubate an apneic patient, who, because of his or her apnea, is not a candidate for blind nasotracheal intubation.

Indications and Contraindications

Digital intubation may be used in the following exceptional circumstances:

- A laryngoscope is not available or has malfunctioned.
- Other techniques to intubate the patient have failed.
- The patient is in a confined space.
- The patient is extremely obese or has a short neck.
- Copious secretions obscure your view of the airway.
- The head cannot be moved due to trauma or immobilization equipment interferes with direct laryngoscopy.
- Massive airway trauma has made visualization of the intubation landmarks impossible.

Although digital intubation can be performed in pediatric patients, the size of the paramedic's fingers (it takes two fingers) relative to the size of the child's mouth usually makes the technique impossible. Also, digital intubation is absolutely contraindicated if your patient is breathing, is not unconscious, or has an intact gag reflex.

Advantages and Disadvantages

Because digital intubation does not require a laryngoscope, this technique is most advantageous in the event of equipment failure. It is also ideal in situations in which your view of the vocal cords is obscured by copious, uncontrollable oral secretions. Because digital intubation does not require the patient's head to be in a sniffing position, it can be performed on trauma patients and patients whose heads cannot be placed in a sniffing position (eg, obese or short-necked patients).

The major disadvantage of digital intubation is that it requires you to place your fingers in the patient's mouth, thus

At the Scene

Always check your intubation equipment at the beginning of each shift to ensure that it is fully functional. Failure to do so increases the risk of equipment breakdown when it is needed the most. Digital intubation, although an acceptable technique, is clearly the least desirable option. Having functional equipment when you need it will avoid the need to stick your fingers down the patient's throat to place the ET tube.

posing a risk of being accidentally bitten. Digital intubation should therefore be performed only in patients who are unresponsive and apneic, *and* who have a bite block in their mouth to prevent closure. There is also a potential risk of exposure to an infectious disease. The patient's teeth could easily tear through a paramedic's gloves and cut his or her fingers, especially if the teeth are sharp or broken.

Successful placement of the ET tube via digital intubation depends on frequency of practice, experience, manual dexterity, and the size and length of the paramedic's fingers. Paramedics with short fingers or fingers that are large in diameter will have greater difficulty performing digital intubation.

Digital intubation should only be attempted as a last resort, when there is no other rescue airway device. You should remember that bag-valve-mask ventilation may be a more suitable and safer alternative to digital intubation.

Complications

Misplacement of the ET tube is the major complication of digital intubation. Although the intubation is tactilely guided, it is easy to misdirect the tip of the tube during insertion. Therefore, diligent attention to tube confirmation is absolutely essential with this technique.

Because it does not require the use of a laryngoscope, digital intubation is associated with a much lower incidence of dental trauma; however, the insertion of a bite block or dental prod can cause lip trauma, tooth damage, or both. Additionally, vigorous attempts at insertion or improper technique can cause airway trauma or swelling.

Any intubation attempt, regardless of the technique used, can result in hypoxia. Therefore, you must carefully monitor the patient's clinical condition (eg, pulse oximetry, skin colour, heart rate) during the technique, limit your intubation attempts to 30 seconds, and ventilate the patient appropriately in between attempts.

Equipment

Less equipment is needed for digital intubation. In fact, you will usually attempt the digital technique because you have limited (or malfunctioning) equipment. Except for the laryngoscope, you will essentially use the same equipment required for orotracheal intubation, plus your fingers. That is, you will need traditional intubation equipment and supplies—a stylet, EtCO$_2$ detector or EDD, and an appropriate device to adequately secure the tube.

Technique for Digital Intubation

Today, because of the variety of alternative airway devices available (eg, Combitube, PtL, King airway, LMA), digital intubation is rarely performed. Nonetheless, you should work, through frequent practice, to become just as skilled and competent with digital intubation as you are with more common advanced airway management techniques.

Prepare your equipment for the digital intubation as your assistant is ventilating the patient with a bag-valve-mask device and 100% oxygen. Select an ET tube that is one half to a full size smaller than that used for intubation with direct laryngoscopy. In this technique, the tip of the tube is guided into the trachea while using your index finger as a leverage point. A stylet provides the tube with the rigidity necessary to make the bend in the tube. Two configurations are recommended; you should practice with both to determine which you prefer.

- In an "open J" configuration, the stylet is inserted and a large J shape is made in the distal end of the tube.
- In the "U-handle" configuration, the tube is bent into a U shape and the proximal half of the tube is bent into a 90° handle toward your dominant hand **Figure 11-66 ▶**.

Because a sniffing position is not required to perform digital intubation, the paramedic can be positioned at the patient's left side facing toward the head. This position facilitates digital intubation if the patient is trapped in a seated or standing position **Figure 11-67 ▶**.

Before even considering placing your fingers in the patient's mouth, insert a bite block or the flange of an oral airway, turned sideways, between the patient's molars **Figure 11-68 ▶**. This will prevent complete closure of the patient's mouth, affording protection for your fingers in the event of a sudden change in consciousness or seizure.

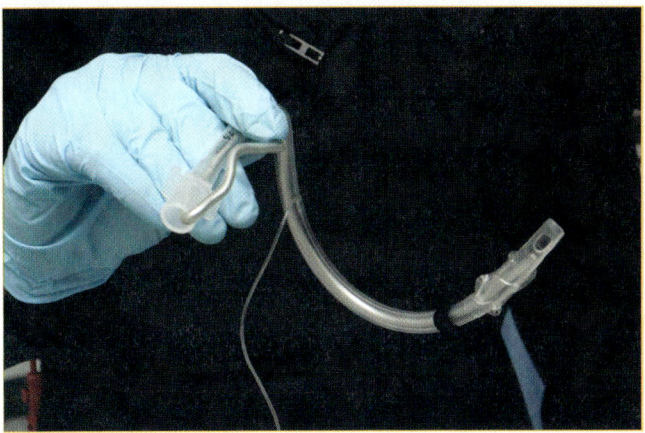

Figure 11-66 The U-handle configuration.

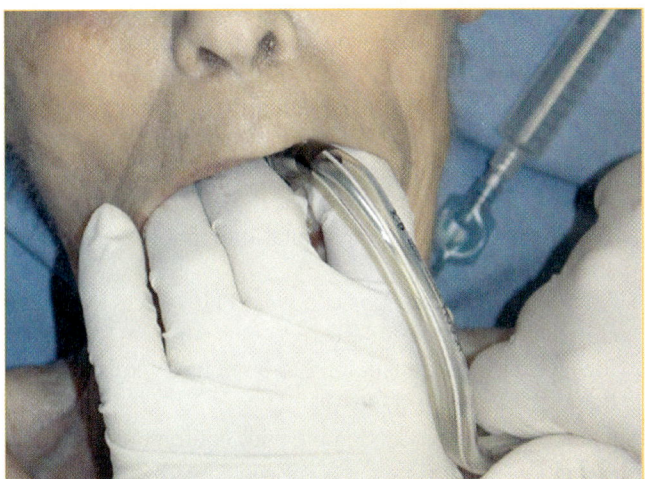

Figure 11-67 If the patient is trapped in a seated or standing position, digital intubation can be performed from a position facing the patient.

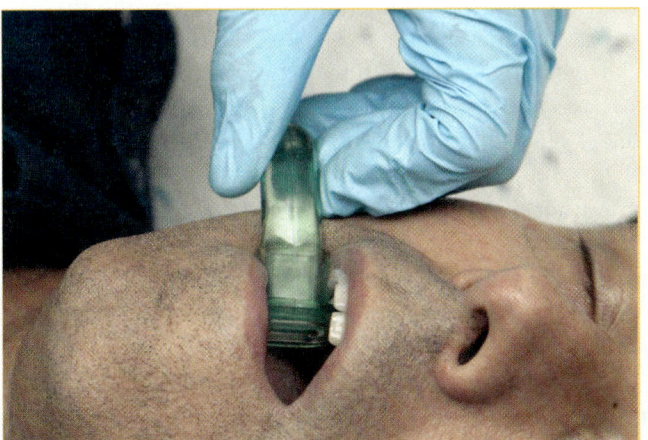

Figure 11-68 The flange of an oral airway can be inserted into the mouth and turned sideways to act as a bite block.

Insert the index and middle fingers of your left hand into the right side of the patient's mouth. Press down against the tongue as you slide your fingers along the midline of the tongue until you can feel the epiglottis. Then pull the epiglottis forward with your middle finger.

Hold the endotracheal tube in your right hand, as you would hold a pencil, and insert it into the left side of the patient's mouth. Advance the tube along the outer surface of your left index finger or between your middle and index fingers, and guide its tip toward the glottis. Once you feel the cuff of the tube pass about 5 cm beyond the tip of your finger, stabilize the tube with your right hand while you gently withdraw your two left fingers from the patient's mouth.

After the tube has been positioned and stabilized manually, carefully remove the stylet and inflate the distal cuff with 5 to 10 ml of air (don't forget to detach the syringe from the inflation port). Attach the bag-valve-mask device to the ET tube—with an EtCO₂ detector between the bag and tube—and ventilate the patient while observing for visible chest rise.

Because digital intubation is truly a blind technique, rigorous tube confirmation protocol must be followed. Auscultate both lungs and over the epigastrium, monitor $EtCO_2$, and properly secure the tube in place. Continue ventilations according to the patient's clinical condition.

The steps for performing digital intubation are listed here and shown in **Skill Drill 11-31** ▶.

1. Take routine precautions and wear PPE (gloves and face shield at a minimum) (Step 1).
2. Preoxygenate the patient for 2 to 3 minutes with a bag-valve-mask device and 100% oxygen (Step 2).
3. Check, prepare, and assemble your equipment (Step 3).
4. Bend the ET tube by placing a slight curve at its distal end (like a hockey stick) (Step 4).
5. Place the patient's head in a neutral position (Step 5).
6. Place a bite block in between the patient's molars to prevent the patient from biting your fingers (Step 6).
7. Insert your left middle and index fingers into the patient's mouth and shift the patient's tongue forward as you advance your fingers toward the patient's larynx (Step 7).
8. Palpate and lift the epiglottis with your left middle finger (Step 8).
9. Advance the tube with your right hand and guide it in between the vocal cords with your index finger (Step 9).
10. Remove the stylet from the ET tube (Step 10).
11. Inflate the distal cuff of the ET tube with 5 to 10 ml of air and detach the syringe (Step 11).
12. Attach the $EtCO_2$ detector to the ET tube (Step 12).
13. Attach the bag-valve-mask device, ventilate, and auscultate over the apices and bases of both lungs and over the epigastrium (Step 13).
14. Secure the ET tube (Step 14).

Tracheobronchial Suctioning

Tracheobronchial suctioning involves passing a suction catheter into the ET tube to remove pulmonary secretions. The first rule to remember about performing tracheobronchial suctioning is this: Don't do it if you don't have to! This kind of suctioning requires strict attention to sterile technique, which is nearly impossible to maintain when you're in a ditch by the side of the road. Suctioning the trachea can also cause cardiac dysrhythmias; cardiac arrest has been reported during tracheobronchial suctioning. For these reasons, you should avoid suctioning through an ET tube *unless secretions are so massive that they interfere with ventilation.* If tracheobronchial suctioning must be performed, use a sterile technique (if possible), and monitor the patient's cardiac rhythm and oxygen saturation during the procedure. Preoxygenation of the patient is essential prior to performing tracheobronchial suctioning. In order to minimize the risk of exposure to respiratory secretions and disease transmission, a closed, in-line suction catheter device should be incorporated into the ventilation circuit. This system makes tracheobronchial suctioning possible without detaching the bag-valve-mask device from the ET tube and potentially exposing the paramedic to any respiratory secretions.

If an in-line suctioning system is not available, you must take care to prevent exposure to respiratory secretions. Prelubricate a soft-tip (whistle-tip) catheter and hyperoxygenate the patient for at least 2 to 3 minutes. It may be necessary to inject 3 to 5 ml of sterile water down the ET tube to loosen thick pulmonary secretions.

Gently insert the suction catheter down the ET tube until resistance is felt. Apply suction as the catheter is extracted, taking care not to exceed 15 seconds in the adult patient. After tracheobronchial suctioning is complete, continue ventilations using the bag-valve-mask device, and reassess the patient.

The steps for performing tracheobronchial suctioning are listed here and shown in **Skill Drill 11-32** ▶.

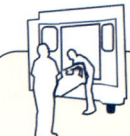

At the Scene

Endotracheal Intubation: Points to Remember

- Never attempt endotracheal intubation before the patient has been adequately preoxygenated.
- Assemble and check all your equipment before you begin.
- Position is everything! Ensure that the patient's head is in the proper position to align the airway axes.
- Don't rush! Work with *deliberate* speed.
- Get it right the first time. The second attempt will likely be more difficult. Remember that a patent BLS airway is acceptable until a more experienced paramedic has time to pass an advanced airway.
- Confirm that the ET tube is in the right place. Take *nothing* for granted.
- Secure the ET tube appropriately. Otherwise, you'll soon be trying to put it back in again.
- Even when the tube is properly secured, stabilize it with your hand as you ventilate the patient.

Skill Drill 11-31: Digital Intubation

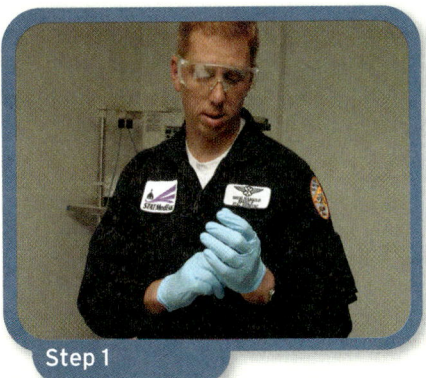

Step 1

Take routine precautions and wear PPE (gloves and face shield at a minimum).

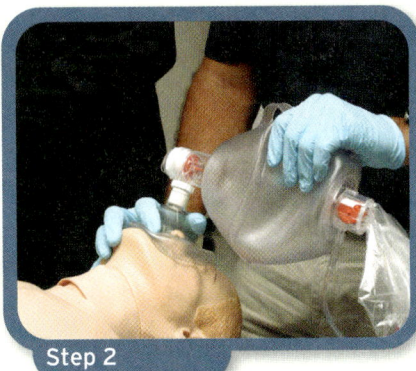

Step 2

Preoxygenate the patient for 2 to 3 minutes with a bag-valve-mask device and 100% oxygen.

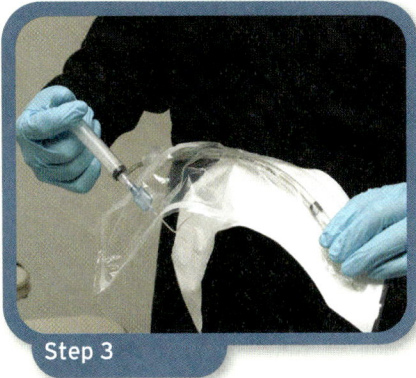

Step 3

Check, prepare, and assemble your equipment.

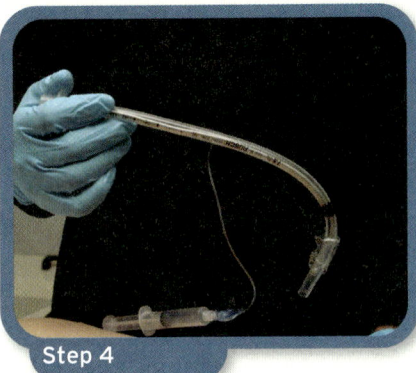

Step 4

Bend the ET tube by placing a slight curve at its distal end (like a hockey stick).

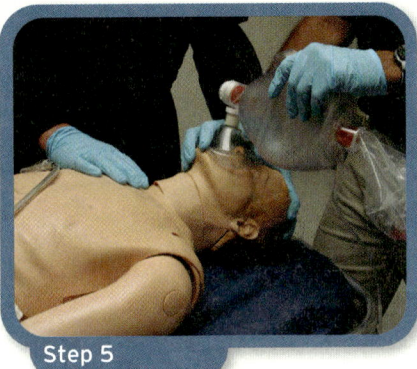

Step 5

Place the patient's head in a neutral position.

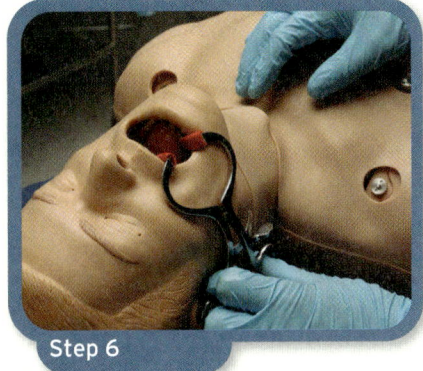

Step 6

Place a bite block in between the patient's molars to prevent the patient from biting your fingers.

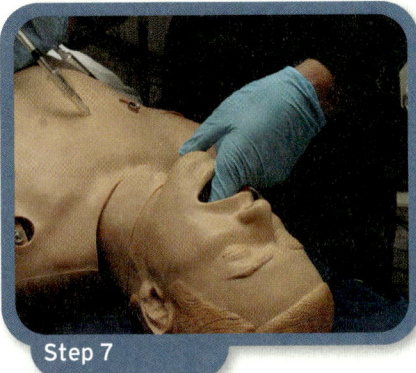

Step 7

Insert your left middle and index fingers into the patient's mouth and shift the patient's tongue forward as you advance your fingers toward the larynx.

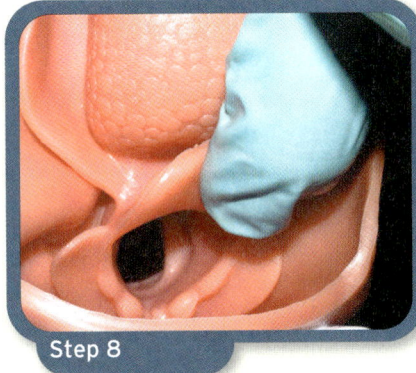

Step 8

Palpate and lift the epiglottis with your left middle finger.

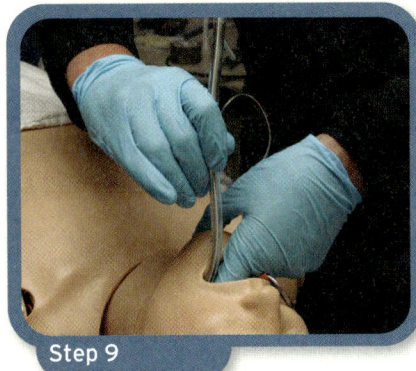

Step 9

Advance the tube with your right hand and guide it in between the vocal cords with your left index finger.

Skill Drill 11-31: Digital Intubation (continued)

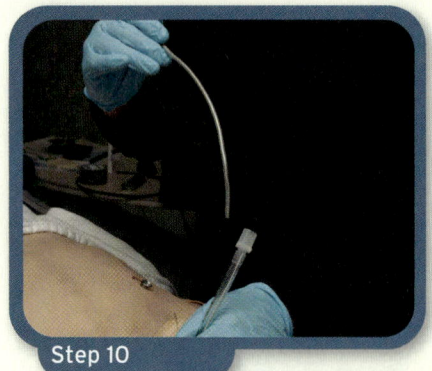

Step 10

Remove the stylet from the ET tube.

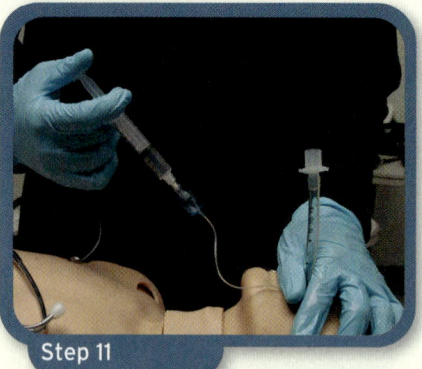

Step 11

Inflate the distal cuff of the ET tube with 5 to 10 ml of air and detach the syringe.

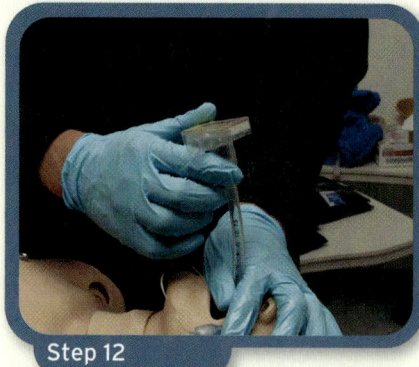

Step 12

Attach the $Etco_2$ detector to the ET tube.

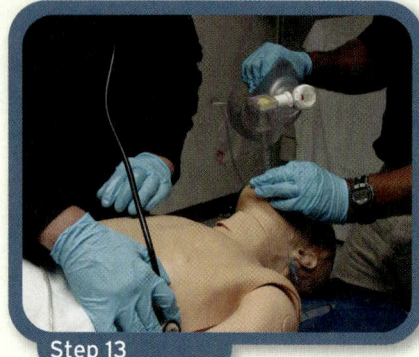

Step 13

Attach the bag-valve-mask device, ventilate, and auscultate over the apices and bases of both lungs and over the epigastrium.

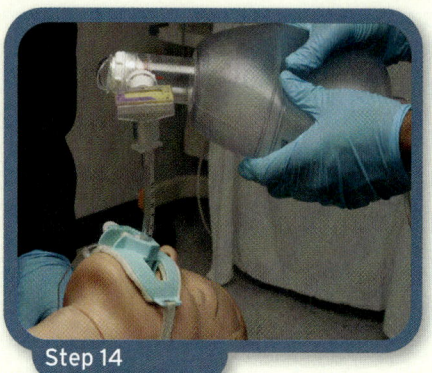

Step 14

Secure the ET tube.

You are the Paramedic Part 9

The patient is now calm and compliant with the ET tube and mechanical ventilations, but you note a decrease in his oxygen saturation and an increase in his heart rate. You immediately reassess breath sounds and epigastric sounds and determine that the ET tube is still correctly placed; the $Etco_2$ detector confirms this.

Reassessment	Recording Time: 27 Minutes
Level of consciousness	Sedated
Respirations	Ventilated with 100% oxygen at a rate of 12 breaths/min; gurgling is heard in the ET tube
Pulse	130 beats/min, strong and regular
Skin	Pink and moist
Blood pressure	122/74 mm Hg
Spo_2	90% while being ventilated with 100% oxygen

15. What has most likely caused this patient's increased heart rate and decreased Spo_2?

16. How will you remedy the situation?

Skill Drill 11-32: Performing Tracheobronchial Suctioning

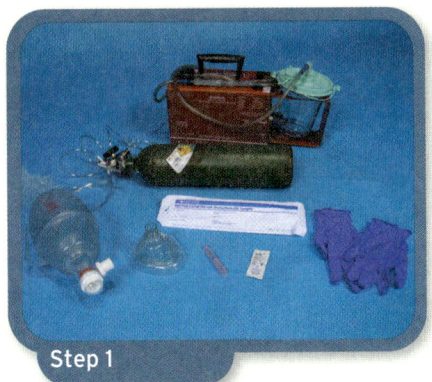

Step 1

Use routine precautions and PPE. Check, prepare, and assemble your equipment.

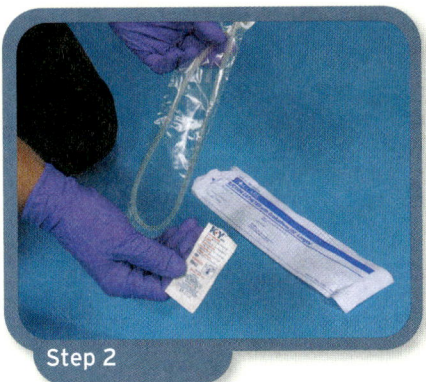

Step 2

Lubricate the suction catheter.

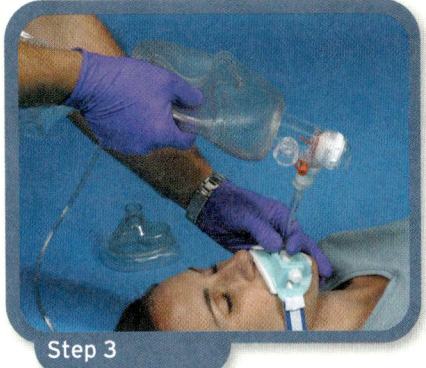

Step 3

Preoxygenate the patient.

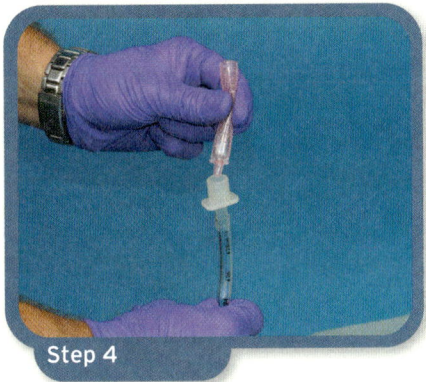

Step 4

Detach the bag-valve-mask device and inject 3 to 5 ml of sterile water down the ET tube.

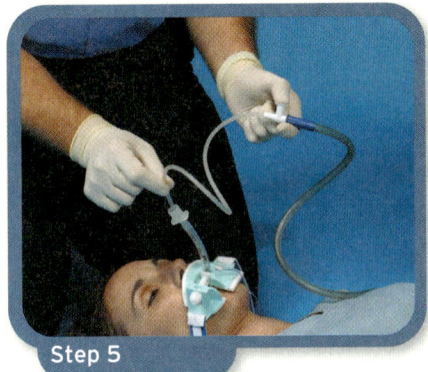

Step 5

Gently insert the catheter into the ET tube until resistance is felt.

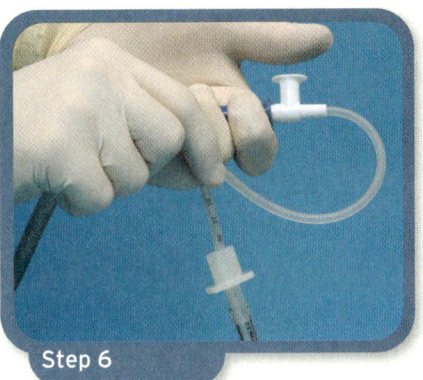

Step 6

Suction in a rotating motion while withdrawing the catheter. Monitor the patient's cardiac rhythm and oxygen saturation during the procedure.

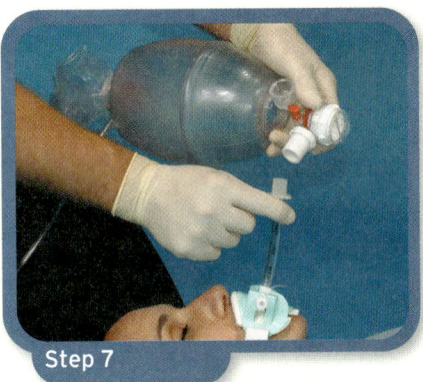

Step 7

Reattach the bag-valve-mask device and resume ventilation and oxygenation.

1. Use routine precautions and PPE. Check, prepare, and assemble your equipment (Step 1).
2. Lubricate the suction catheter (Step 2).
3. Preoxygenate the patient (Step 3).
4. Detach the bag-valve-mask device and inject 3 to 5 ml of sterile water down the ET tube (Step 4).
5. Gently insert the catheter into the ET tube until resistance is felt (Step 5).
6. Suction in a rotating motion while withdrawing the catheter. Monitor the patient's cardiac rhythm and oxygen saturation during the procedure (Step 6).
7. Reattach the bag-valve-mask device and resume ventilation and oxygenation (Step 7).

(**Skill Drill 11-33**) lists the steps for performing tracheobronchial suctioning using an in-line suction device:

1. Use routine precautions and wear PPE.
2. Check, prepare, and assemble your equipment.
3. Connect suction to the in-line suction catheter.
4. Preoxygenate the patient.
5. Gently advance the in-line suction catheter down the ET tube until resistance is felt.
6. Suction in a rotating motion while withdrawing the catheter into the sidearm of the in-line device. Monitor the patient's cardiac rhythm and oxygen saturation during the procedure·
7. Resume ventilation and oxygenation.

Extubation in the Prehospital Environment

Extubation is the process of removing the tube from an intubated patient. Patients are rarely extubated in the prehospital setting. Generally, the only reason to consider performing extubation in the prehospital setting is if the patient is *unreasonably* intolerant of the ET tube (eg, extremely combative, gagging, or retching). In general, it is better to sedate the patient rather than remove the ET tube, but this may not be an option in all EMS systems or in patients who are hemodynamically unstable. Prior to considering extubation, you should contact direct medical control or follow locally established protocols.

The most obvious risk associated with extubation is overestimation of the patient's ability to protect his or her own airway. Additionally, when extubation is performed on conscious patients, there is a high risk of laryngospasm, and most patients experience some degree of upper airway swelling because of the trauma of having the tube in the trachea. These two facts, along with the ever-present potential for vomiting, make successful reintubation challenging, if not impossible. If you are not *absolutely* sure that you can reintubate the patient, do not remove the tube! In most cases, this involves sedating the patient with a benzodiazepine or possibly even using a paralytic agent. Extubation in the prehospital setting is absolutely contraindicated if there is *any* risk of recurrent respiratory failure or if you are uncertain that the patient can maintain his or her own airway spontaneously.

If extubation in the prehospital environment is indicated, first preoxygenate the patient. Discuss the procedure with the patient, and explain what you plan to do. If possible, have the patient sit up or lean slightly forward; this will place him or her in a safe position should vomiting occur after extubation. Assemble and have available all equipment to suction, ventilate, and reintubate, if necessary. After confirming that the patient remains responsive enough to protect his or her own airway, suction the oropharynx to remove any secretions or debris that may threaten the airway once the tube has been removed. Deflate the distal cuff on the ET tube as the patient begins to exhale so that any accumulated secretions proximal to the cuff are not aspirated into the lungs. On the next exhalation, *remove the tube in one steady motion,* following the curvature of the airway. Consider placing a towel or emesis basin in front of the patient's mouth in case vomiting occurs.

The steps for performing extubation are listed here and shown in (**Skill Drill 11-34** ▸)

1. Preoxygenate the patient (Step 1).
2. Ensure that ventilation and suction equipment are immediately available (Step 2).
3. Confirm patient responsiveness (Step 3).
4. Lean the patient forward (Step 4).
5. Suction the oropharynx (Step 5).
6. Deflate the distal cuff of the ET tube (Step 6).
7. Remove the ET tube as the patient coughs or begins to exhale (Step 7).

Pediatric Endotracheal Intubation

Although endotracheal intubation has been considered the means for definitive prehospital airway management in adults, recent studies suggest that effective bag-valve-mask ventilations in the pediatric patient can be as effective as intubation for EMS systems that have short transport times. However, if bag-valve-mask ventilations are not producing adequate ventilation and oxygenation, the infant or child may require intubation. Indications for endotracheal intubation in pediatric patients are the same as those in adults:

- Cardiopulmonary arrest
- Respiratory failure/arrest
- Traumatic brain injury
- Unresponsiveness
- Inability to maintain a patent airway
- Need for prolonged ventilation
- Need for endotracheal administration of resuscitative medications (if no IV or IO)

Certain anatomical differences between children and adults (**Table 11-12** ▸) play a key role in performing a successful intubation, as proper airway positioning is critical.

Laryngoscope and Blades

Although any laryngoscope handle can be used to intubate a child, most paramedics prefer the thinner pediatric handles. Straight blades facilitate lifting of the floppy epiglottis. If a curved blade is used, the tip of the blade is positioned in the

Skill Drill 11-34: Performing Extubation

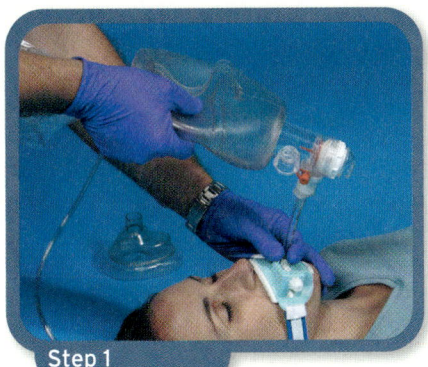

Step 1

Preoxygenate the patient.

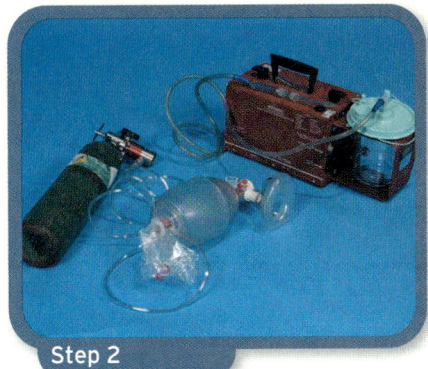

Step 2

Ensure that ventilation and suction equipment are immediately available.

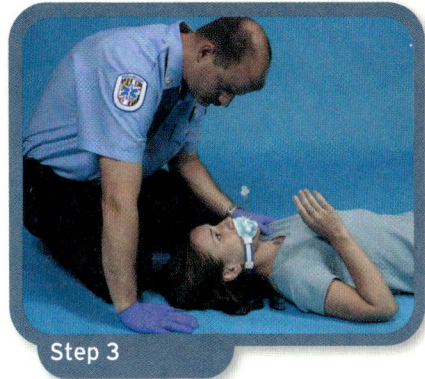

Step 3

Confirm patient responsiveness.

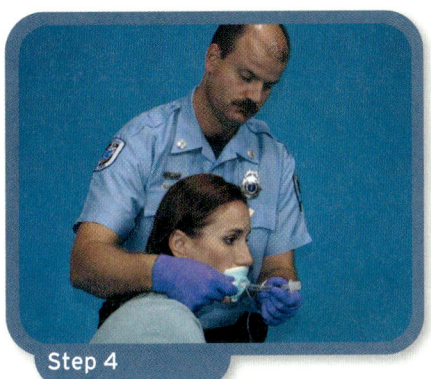

Step 4

Lean the patient forward.

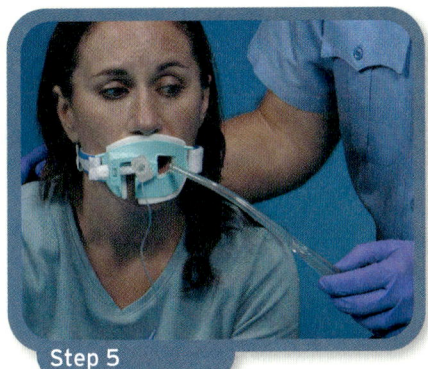

Step 5

Suction the oropharynx.

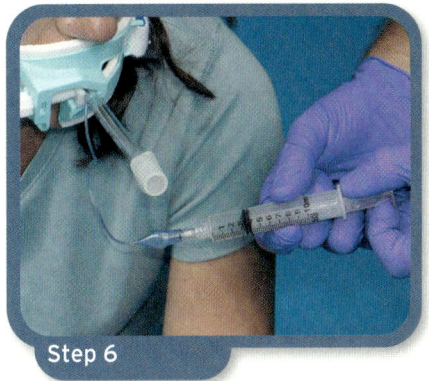

Step 6

Deflate the distal cuff of the ET tube.

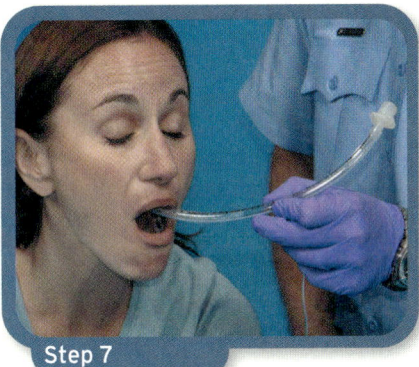

Step 7

Remove the ET tube as the patient coughs or begins to exhale.

Table 11-12   Differences in the Pediatric Airway

- Infants have a larger, rounder occiput, which causes the head of an infant or small child who lies supine to be in a flexed position.
- In children, the tongue is proportionately larger and the mandible is proportionately smaller—differences that increase children's propensity for airway obstruction.
- The epiglottis in a child is more floppy and omega-shaped, so it must be lifted, or positioned, out of the way to visualize the vocal cords.
- The trachea in a child is smaller, shorter, and narrower than an adult's, and it is positioned more anteriorly and superiorly.
- The narrowest portion of the child's airway is the cricoid ring, which is below the vocal cords (subglottic), and the anatomy below the vocal cords is funnel-shaped. This makes a cuff less necessary for occluding the trachea.

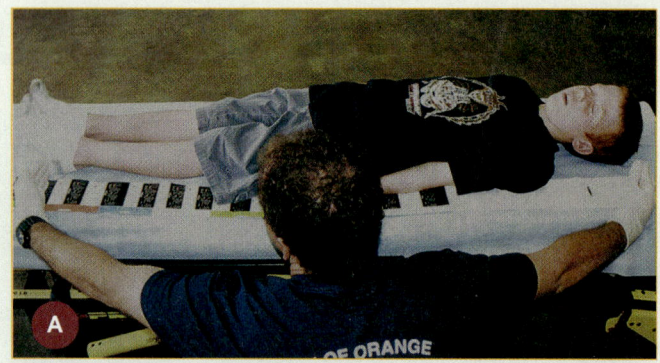

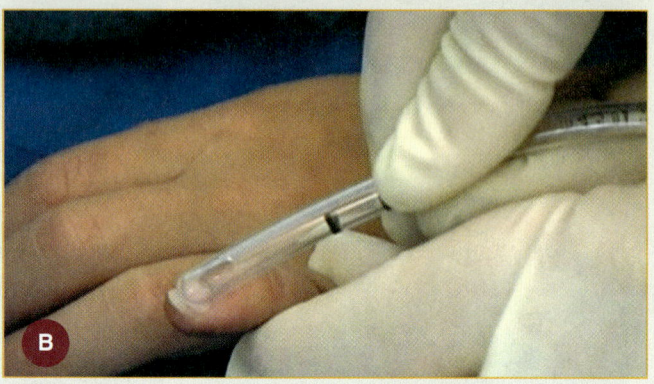

Figure 11-69 A. A length-based resuscitation tape can help estimate a child's ET tube size. **B.** The width of the child's small fingernail can be used to estimate ET tube size.

vallecula to lift the jaw and epiglottis to visualize the vocal cords.

The blade should extend from the child's mouth to the tragus of the ear. Acceptable means of measuring this length include use of a length-based resuscitation tape measure or using the following general guidelines:

- Premature newborn: size 0 straight blade
- Full-term newborn to 1 year of age: size 1 straight blade
- 2 years of age to adolescent: size 2 straight blade
- Adolescent and older: size 3 straight or curved blade

Endotracheal Tubes

ET tube size can be selected by using a length-based resuscitation tape measure **Figure 11-69A ▸**. For children older than 1 year of age, the following formulae can be used:

- Age (in years) ÷ 4 + 4 for an uncuffed tube
- Age (in years) ÷ 4 + 3 for a cuffed tube
  - A 4-year-old child would need a 5.0-mm uncuffed tube (4 [age in years] ÷ 4 + 4 = 5.0) or a 4.0-mm cuffed tube (4 [age in years] ÷ 4 + 3 = 4.0)

Certain anatomical clues, such as the nares or the width of the child's small fingernail **Figure 11-69B ▸** can be used to estimate tube size, or you can follow general guidelines based on the child's age **Table 11-13 ▸**.

Uncuffed ET tubes were long considered necessary until the child reached 8 to 10 years of age, because the narrowest part of the airway was below the cords and would provide a suitable seal against a properly sized ET tube. Uncuffed tubes were also considered necessary to prevent ischemic and damage to the tracheal mucosa. With newer tube and cuff designs, it is no longer necessary to use an uncuffed tube in patients 1 year or older. New guidelines permit the use of a cuffed tube in these children. The advantage of using a cuffed tube is prevention of a large air leak and prevention of aspiration of stomach contents. You must always be cautious to avoid excessive cuff inflation and prevent ischemia and damage to the tracheal mucosa at the level of the cricoid ring. You must remember that a cuffed tube is necessary in pediatric patients once they reach adolescence, typically beyond 8 to 10 years of age.

Table 11-13   Guidelines for Selecting Pediatric Endotracheal Tubes

Age	ET Tube (mm)	Insertion Depth (cm)
Premature infant	2.5–3.0 uncuffed	8.0
Full-term infant	3.0–3.5 uncuffed	8.0–9.5
Infant to 1 year	3.5–4.0 uncuffed	9.5–11.0
Toddler	4.0–5.0 uncuffed or cuffed	11.0–12.5
Preschool	4.5–5.5 uncuffed or cuffed	12.5–14.0
School age	5.5–6.5 uncuffed or cuffed	14.0–20.0
Adolescent	7.0–8.0 cuffed	20.0–23.0

When selecting the appropriate size ET tube, you should have a tube one size smaller as well as one size larger than expected for situations in which there is variability in the child's upper airway diameter.

The appropriate depth of insertion of the ET tube is 2 to 3 cm beyond the vocal cords. After the tube has been inserted, the depth at the corner of the child's mouth should be recorded and monitored. For uncuffed tubes, a black band—the vocal cord guide—often encircles the tube at its distal end. When you see this band at the level of the vocal cords, stop. Cuffed tubes should be inserted until the cuff is just below the level of the vocal cords. Another guideline is to insert the tube to a depth equal to three times the inside diameter (mm) of the ET tube. For example, a 4.0-mm tube should be inserted to a depth of 12.0 cm (12.0 = three times 4 mm).

Pediatric Stylet

The use of a stylet, for the most part, is a matter of personal preference when intubating the pediatric patient. If a stylet is used, insert it into the ET tube, stopping at least 1 cm from the end of the tube. Pediatric stylets will fit into tubes of size 3.0 to 6.0 mm, whereas the adult stylets are used for tubes of size 6.0 mm and larger. After inserting the stylet into the ET tube, bend the tube into a gentle upward curve. In some cases, bending the tube into the shape of a hockey stick is beneficial.

Preoxygenation

Adequate preoxygenation with a bag-valve-mask device and 100% oxygen prior to attempting intubation cannot be overemphasized—airway obstruction and hypoxia are the most common cause of cardiac arrest in the pediatric population. While preoxygenating the child, you must also ensure that the child's head is in the proper position; this is the neutral position for patients with suspected trauma or the sniffing position otherwise. If needed, insert an airway adjunct; in conjunction with proper manual positioning of the head, it will maintain airway patency and facilitate effective ventilation.

Additional Preparation

Stimulation of the parasympathetic nervous system with resultant bradycardia can occur during intubation in children; therefore, you should apply a cardiac monitor. A pulse oximeter should be used throughout the intubation attempt to monitor the child's oxygen saturation. In addition, suction should be readily available to clear oral secretions from the child's airway. Atropine sulfate in a dose of 0.02 mg/kg (minimum dose of 0.1 mg) may be administered to prevent vagal-induced bradycardia secondary to parasympathetic stimulation.

Intubation Technique

With the child's head in a sniffing position, open his or her mouth by applying thumb pressure on the chin. If an oral airway has been inserted, remove it. If needed, suction the child's mouth and pharynx to remove any secretions.

Hold the laryngoscope handle in your left hand, using your thumb, index finger, and middle finger to hold the handle (the "trigger finger" position). Insert the laryngoscope blade in the right side of the child's mouth, sweeping the tongue to the left side and keeping it under the blade. Advance the blade straight along the tongue, while applying gentle traction upward along the axis of the laryngoscope handle at a 45° angle. *Never use the teeth or gums as a fulcrum for the blade.* A child's teeth could easily be loosened or cracked during a traumatic intubation attempt.

When the blade passes the epiglottis, gently lift the epiglottis if you are using a straight blade. If you are using a curved blade, place the tip of the blade in the vallecula, and lift the jaw, tongue, and blade gently at a 45° angle.

Identify the vocal cords and other normal anatomical landmarks. If they are not visible, have your partner gently apply cricoid pressure. Additional gentle suctioning may be needed to facilitate your view of the vocal cords.

Hold the ET tube in your right hand, and insert the tube from the right-side corner of the child's mouth. Do not pass the tube through the channel of the laryngoscope blade, as you will lose sight of the vocal cords. Guide the tube through the vocal cords, and advance the tube until the glottic/vocal cord mark (black band) is positioned just beyond the vocal cords (approximately 2 to 3 cm). Record the depth of the tube as measured at the right-side corner of the child's mouth, and remove the laryngoscope blade.

Carefully remove the stylet if one was used, while holding the tube securely in place. Next, recheck the tube depth to ensure that it did not become displaced during removal of the stylet. If you are using a cuffed ET tube, inflate the cuff until the pilot balloon is full. Suction the tracheal tube if fluid is present. Attach the tube to a bag-valve-mask device and 100% oxygen. Release cricoid pressure, if used.

Confirm proper ET tube placement by using one or more techniques. Observe the patient for bilateral chest rise during ventilation. Auscultate over the epigastrium and the lungs bilaterally at the midaxillary line at the third intercostal space, listening for two breaths in each location. If breath sounds are absent over the lungs or heard over the epigastrium, the tube may not be in the trachea. To correct this, withdraw the tube, bag-valve-mask ventilate, and prepare to reintubate. If breath sounds are decreased on the left side, the tube may be positioned too deep and aimed toward or in the right mainstem bronchus. To correct this problem, listen to the left side of the chest while ventilating and *carefully* withdrawing the tube, until breath sounds are equal on both sides of the chest. Re-record the depth of the tube.

Breath sounds travel easily in a child because of a child's small chest size. Auscultate over the epigastrium to ensure that no bubbling or gurgling sounds are present. These sounds indicate esophageal intubation, mandating immediate removal of the tube, suctioning as needed, and ventilation with a bag-valve-mask device and 100% oxygen prior to reattempting intubation.

Additional clinical methods to confirm proper ET tube placement include improvement in the child's skin colour, pulse rate, and oxygen saturation, as well as use of an $EtCO_2$ detector. When using these devices in children, remember two important points: (1) The adult colourimetric $EtCO_2$ detector cannot be used in children weighing less than 15 kg, use a specifically designed pediatric colourimetric $EtCO_2$ detector; and (2) the esophageal bulb or syringe cannot be used in children weighing less than 20 kg.

After you confirm proper tube placement, hold the ET tube firmly in place and secure it with tape or a commercially available device. Although several methods for securing an ET tube exist, no single method is foolproof. One person should always hold the tube in place while another properly secures it.

It is important to reconfirm tube placement not only after securing the tube but also following any patient movement because tubes can easily become dislodged. To do so, auscultate for epigastric sounds and bilateral breath sounds. Once tube position has been confirmed, resume ventilations with 100% oxygen at the appropriate rate.

If you realize the tube is too large or you cannot identify the vocal cords and glottic landmarks, abort the intubation attempt and ventilate the child with the bag-valve-mask device and 100% oxygen. Modify your equipment selection accordingly, and start the procedure from the beginning. If intubation cannot be accomplished after two attempts, discontinue attempts, and resume bag-valve-mask ventilation for the remainder of the transport.

The steps for performing pediatric endotracheal intubation are listed here and shown in Skill Drill 11-35 ▸.

1. Take routine precautions and wear PPE (gloves and face shield at a minimum) Step 1 .
2. Check, prepare, and assemble your equipment Step 2 .
3. Manually open the child's airway and insert an adjunct if needed Step 3 .
4. Preoxygenate the child with a bag-valve-mask device and 100% oxygen for at least 30 seconds Step 4 .
5. Insert the laryngoscope in the right side of the mouth and sweep the tongue to the left. Lift the tongue with firm, gentle pressure. Avoid using the teeth or gums as a fulcrum Step 5 .
6. Identify the vocal cords. If the cords are not yet visible, instruct your partner to apply cricoid pressure Step 6 .
7. Introduce the ET tube in the right corner of the child's mouth Step 7 .
8. Pass the ET tube through the vocal cords to approximately 2 to 3 cm below the vocal cords. Inflate the cuff if a cuffed tube is used Step 8 .

9. Attach an EtCO₂ detector to confirm tube placement Step 9 .
10. Attach the bag-valve-mask device, and auscultate over the epigastrium to ensure there are no breath sounds and over each lateral chest wall high in the axillae to ensure there are equal breath sounds Step 10 .
11. Secure the ET tube, noting the placement of the distance marker at the child's teeth or gums and reconfirm tube placement Step 11 .

If an intubated child's condition acutely deteriorates, you must take immediate action to identify and correct the underlying problem. The DOPE mnemonic (Displacement, Obstruction, Pneumothorax, and Equipment failure) can be used to recall the common causes of acute deterioration in the intubated child Table 11-14 ▾ .

Complications of Endotracheal Intubation

Complications associated with endotracheal intubation in the pediatric patient are essentially the same as those for adult patients:

- **Unrecognized esophageal intubation.** *Frequently* monitor the position of the tube, especially after *any* major patient move.
- **Induction of emesis and possible aspiration.** *Always* have a suctioning device immediately available.
- **Hypoxia resulting from prolonged intubation attempts.** Limit pediatric intubation attempts to *20 seconds.* Monitor the child's cardiac rhythm and oxygen saturation during intubation.
- **Damage to teeth, soft tissues, and intraoral structures.** Technique, technique, technique!

Table 11-14	Troubleshooting Acute Deterioration With the DOPE Mnemonic in the Intubated Child
Displacement	■ Reauscultate over the epigastrium and lungs for breath sounds.
	■ If breath sounds are absent and you hear epigastric gurgling, immediately remove the ET tube, suction as needed, and ventilate with a bag-valve-mask device and 100% oxygen.
	■ If breath sounds are stronger on the right, slowly withdraw the tube until they are equal bilaterally.
Obstruction	■ If thick pulmonary secretions are interfering with your ability to effectively ventilate the intubated child, perform tracheobronchial suctioning.
	■ Consider tube obstruction if ventilation compliance is decreased (eg, it is hard to squeeze the bag).
Pneumothorax	■ Suspect a pneumothorax if breath sounds are stronger on the *left* and decreased or absent on the right; such findings are not consistent with right mainstem intubation.
	■ Suspect a pneumothorax if breath sounds are stronger on the *right* and decreased or absent on the left and this does not improve with tracheal tube repositioning.
	■ Ventilation compliance may also be decreased in a child with a pneumothorax; suspect a pneumothorax if this occurs despite proper tracheal suctioning, confirming the tracheal tube is patent, and there is no bag-valve-mask or ventilator malfunction.
	■ If trained and certified to do so, prepare to perform needle decompression of the side of the chest suspected to have a pneumothorax.
Equipment failure	■ Ensure that you are delivering 100% oxygen.
	■ Check the reservoir bag on the bag-valve-mask device for tears, ensure that the device is attached to a 100% oxygen source, and check the bag itself for tears.
	■ Immediately replace defective or damaged equipment.

Skill Drill 11-35: Performing Pediatric Endotracheal Intubation

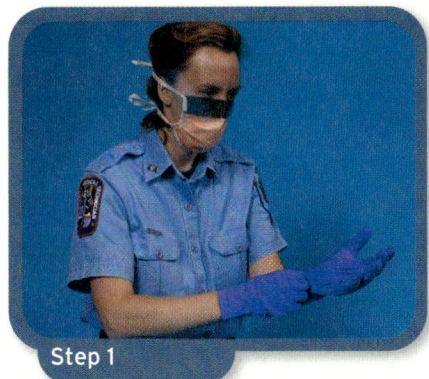

Step 1

Take routine precautions and wear PPE (gloves and face shield at a minimum).

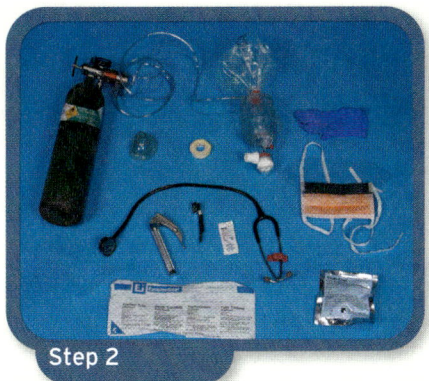

Step 2

Check, prepare, and assemble your equipment.

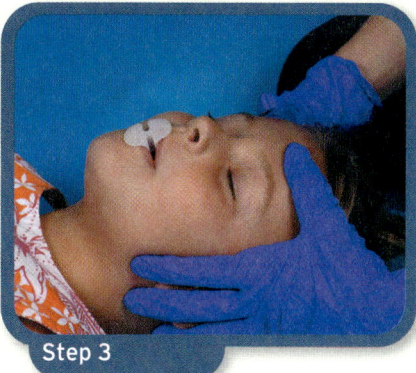

Step 3

Manually open the child's airway and insert an adjunct if needed.

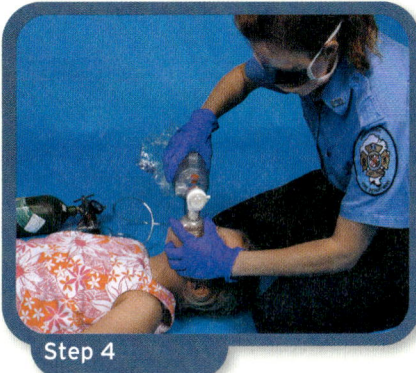

Step 4

Preoxygenate the child with a bag-valve-mask device and 100% oxygen for at least 30 seconds.

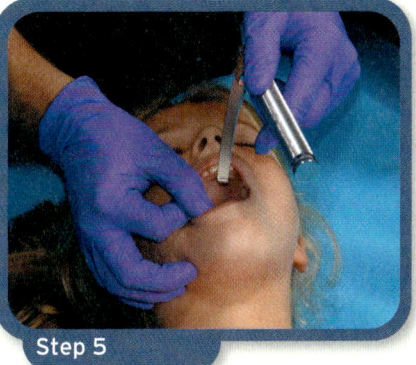

Step 5

Insert the laryngoscope in the right side of the mouth and sweep the tongue to the left. Lift the tongue with firm, gentle pressure. Avoid using the teeth or gums as a fulcrum.

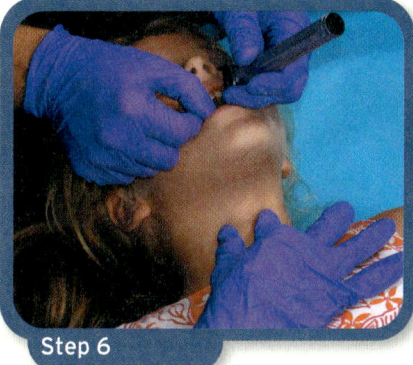

Step 6

Identify the vocal cords. If the cords are not yet visible, instruct your partner to apply cricoid pressure.

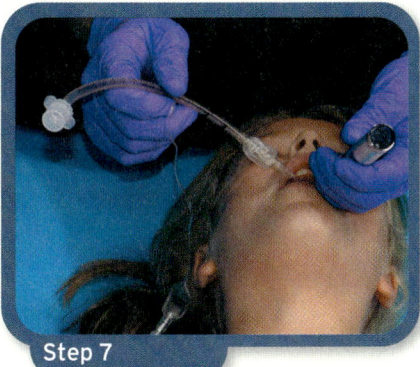

Step 7

Introduce the ET tube in the right corner of the child's mouth.

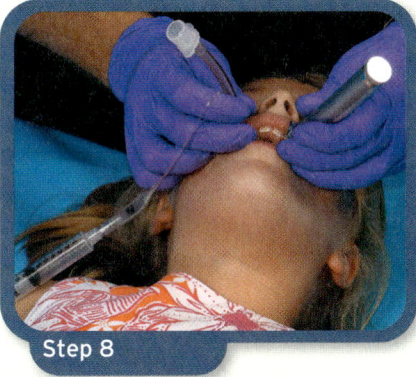

Step 8

Pass the ET tube through the vocal cords to approximately 2 to 3 cm below the vocal cords. Inflate the cuff if a cuffed tube is used.

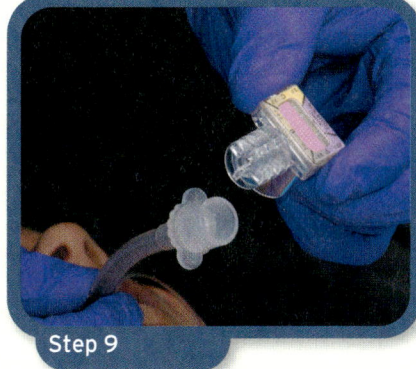

Step 9

Attach an $Etco_2$ detector to confirm tube placement.

Skill Drill 11-35: Performing Pediatric Endotracheal Intubation (*continued*)

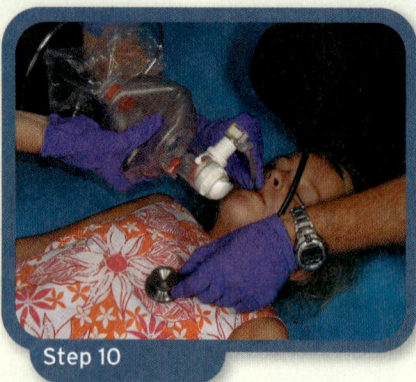

Step 10

Attach the bag-valve-mask device, and auscultate over the epigastrium to ensure there are no breath sounds and over each lateral chest wall high in the axillae to ensure there are equal breath sounds.

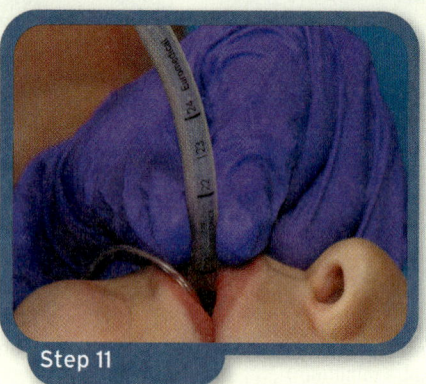

Step 11

Secure the ET tube, noting the placement of the distance marker at the child's teeth or gums and reconfirm tube placement.

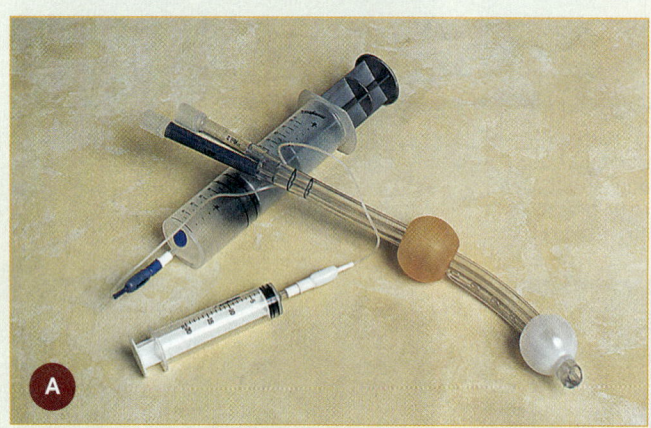

A

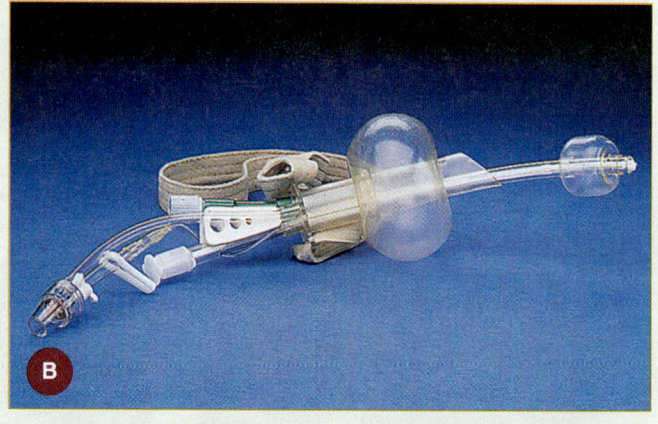

B

Figure 11-70 **A.** Combitube. **B.** Pharyngeotracheal lumen airway.

At the Scene

A single pediatric intubation attempt should not exceed 20 seconds. If intubation cannot be performed within this time frame, abort the attempt and resume bag-valve-mask ventilations with 100% oxygen.

Multilumen Airways

Compared with esophageal airways, the Combitube and the pharyngeotracheal lumen airway (PtL) have shown to provide better airway management and ventilation **Figure 11-70 ▲** .

Both devices have a long tube that is blindly inserted into the airway. This tube can be used for either esophageal obturation or endotracheal intubation; as a result, ventilation is possible regardless of whether the tube is placed into the esophagus or the trachea. The presence of an oropharyngeal balloon also eliminates the need for a mask seal.

These devices have two lumens, each with a 15/22-mm ventilation adapter. The proper port for ventilation depends on where the tube is positioned during insertion. Both types of multilumen airways have a proximal cuff, which is inflated in the oropharynx to eliminate the need for a face mask.

Indications and Contraindications

Multilumen airways are indicated only for use in unresponsive, apneic patients without a gag reflex. If the patient regains consciousness, the device must be removed.

These devices are contraindicated in pediatric patients, and they should be used only for patients between 1.5 and 2.1 m tall. While there is only one size PtL, a smaller version of the Combitube, called the Combitube SA (small adult), can be used on adults taller than 1.2 m. Because the tube is typically inserted into the esophagus, neither the PtL nor the Combitube should be used in patients with esophageal trauma, known esophageal diseases (eg, cancer, varices), or in those who have ingested a caustic substance.

Advantages and Disadvantages

The major advantage of the multilumen airway is that, in effect, it cannot be improperly placed; effective ventilation is possible if the tube enters the esophagus or the trachea. Insertion of the multilumen airway is also technically easier than endotracheal intubation. Furthermore, because insertion of the airway is performed with the patient's head in the neutral position, cervical spine movement is kept to a minimum. Additionally, no mask seal is required to ventilate with the Combitube or PtL.

Multilumen airways also provide some patency to the airway. If the tube is placed in the trachea, it functions exactly like an ET tube, and no upper airway positioning is required. If the tube is placed in the esophagus, the pharyngeal balloon creates an airtight seal in the oropharynx, making the tongue position less of a factor in the maintenance of a patent airway. A jaw-thrust maneuver should easily alleviate any ventilatory difficulty if the epiglottis partially obstructs the airway.

Use of a multilumen airway requires strict attention and good assessment skills because ventilation in the wrong port results in no pulmonary ventilation. These devices are usually considered temporary airways and should be replaced as soon as possible. The pharyngeal balloon mitigates, but does not completely eliminate, the risk of aspiration. Additionally, intubating the trachea via direct laryngoscopy with a multilumen airway in place, although possible, can be extremely challenging.

Complications

The most significant complications associated with the use of multilumen airways are unrecognized displacement of the tube into the esophagus and esophageal trauma. Good assessment skills are essential to properly confirm tube placement, and multiple confirmation techniques should be employed following insertion of the device. Care and proper technique during insertion and transport are essential to minimize trauma to the esophagus.

Laryngospasm, vomiting, and possible hypoventilation may occur during insertion of a multilumen airway.

Ventilation may be difficult if the pharyngeal balloon pushes the epiglottis over the glottic opening. A few cases of difficult ventilation have occurred with multilumen airways. However, in all cases, ventilation became easier when the device was withdrawn 2 to 4 cm.

Equipment

The PtL consists of two tubes and two cuffs. The longer tube passes through the shorter, wider tube. The longer tube is 31 cm long and 8 mm in diameter and usually is inserted into the esophagus. This tube is open at its distal tip and has a balloon at its distal end. A semirigid stylet maintains the curvature and rigidity of the long tube and occludes the tip. The shorter tube is 21 cm long and is designed to come to rest with its distal tip deep in the oropharynx. A large low-pressure cuff is inflated proximal to the tip of the shorter tube. Both cuffs are inflated simultaneously with an in-series valve system that can be inflated with a bag-valve-mask device. The short tube is made of hard plastic to resist damage from biting, and a strap goes around the head to secure the device Figure 11-71 ▾ .

The Combitube consists of a single tube with two lumens, two balloons, and two ventilation ports. One lumen is open at its distal end; the other is closed. The closed lumen has side holes distal to the pharyngeal balloon. The proximal balloon is designed to be inflated with air and provides a pharyngeal seal. The distal balloon is inflated with air and makes an airtight seal with the walls of the trachea (if placed in the trachea) or leads to esophageal obturation (if placed in the esophagus) Figure 11-72 ▸ . You should refer to the manufacturer's instructions on the amount of air used to inflate each balloon.

Technique for Multilumen Airway Insertion

While multilumen airways can be used to ventilate regardless of whether the tube is placed into the esophagus or the trachea, this flexibility makes confirmation of ventilation extremely important. If you use the wrong port, the patient will not receive any pulmonary ventilation. Confirmation of ventilation is, therefore, a critical part of the procedure for using multilumen airways.

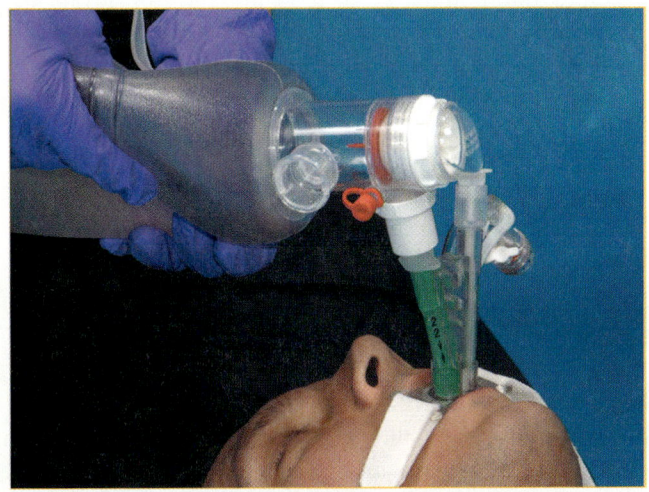

Figure 11-71 Ventilation with a PtL in place.

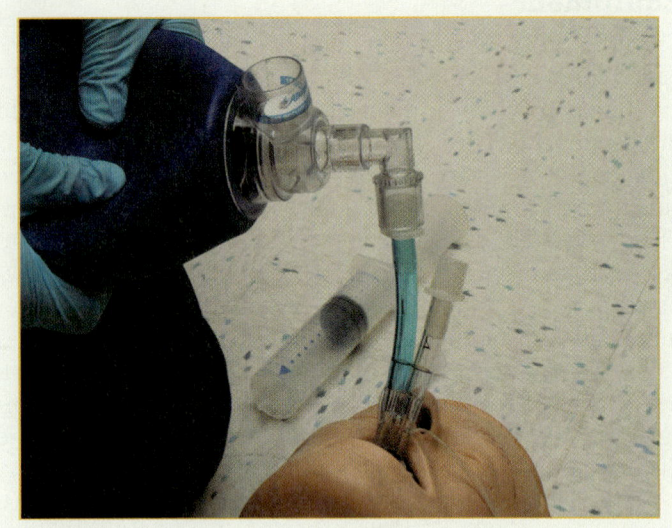

Figure 11-72 Ventilation with a Combitube in place.

Procedures Before and During Insertion

Check and prepare all your equipment. Check both cuffs to ensure that they hold air. The patient should be preoxygenated with a bag-valve-mask device and 100% oxygen before insertion. *Ventilation should not be interrupted for longer than 30 seconds to accomplish airway placement.* For both PtL and Combitube insertion, the patient's head should be placed in a neutral position.

- *Forwardly displace the jaw.* With the patient's head in a neutral position, insert the thumb of your gloved nondominant hand into the patient's mouth and lift the jaw. This action lifts the hyoid bone and pulls the base of the tongue off the posterior pharyngeal wall.
- *Insert the device.* Following the curvature of the tube, insert the device blindly into the posterior pharynx. Insert the Combitube until the incisors are between the two black lines printed on the tube. Insert the PtL until the flange comes to rest on the teeth. Be gentle, and stop advancing the tube if you meet resistance.
- *Inflate the cuffs.* In the PtL, the cuffs inflate together through an in-line valve system. Attach a bag-valve-mask device to the inflation adapter, and inflate the cuffs until the pilot balloon is firm. Close the clamp to prevent air leakage. In the Combitube, two independent inflation valves must be inflated sequentially. The first inflation valve goes to the pharyngeal balloon and is inflated with air. The second inflation valve inflates the distal balloon and is filled with air.

Procedures After Insertion

After you inflate the balloons, begin to ventilate the patient. With the PtL, first ventilate through the short tube (the tube without the stylet); with the Combitube, ventilate through the longer (blue) tube. Confirm adequate chest rise and the presence of breath sounds. If there are no breath sounds and

the chest does not rise during ventilation, switch immediately to the other ventilation port. Be sure to continuously monitor ventilation. Both multilumen airways are generally secure in the airway owing to the large pharyngeal balloons. Nevertheless, the head strap of the PtL should be attached because inadvertent removal of a multilumen airway would be traumatic.

The steps for insertion of a PtL are listed here and shown in **Skill Drill 11-36 ▸**.

1. Take routine precautions and wear PPE (gloves and face shield at a minimum) **Step 1**.
2. Preoxygenate the patient with a bag-valve-mask device and 100% oxygen **Step 2**.
3. Place the patient's head in a neutral position **Step 3**.
4. Open the patient's mouth with the tongue-jaw lift maneuver, and insert the PtL in the midline of the patient's mouth **Step 4**.
5. Inflate the proximal and distal cuffs **Step 5**.
6. Ventilate the patient through the pharyngeal (green) tube first. If the chest rises, continue to ventilate through the green tube **Step 6**.
7. If the chest does not rise, remove the stylet from the clear tube and ventilate through the clear tube **Step 7**.
8. Confirm placement by auscultating for breath sounds over the lungs and gastric sounds over the abdomen **Step 8**.

The steps for insertion of a Combitube are listed here and shown in **Skill Drill 11-37 ▸**.

1. Take routine precautions and wear PPE (gloves and face shield at a minimum) **Step 1**.
2. Preoxygenate the patient with a bag-valve-mask device and 100% oxygen **Step 2**.
3. Gather your equipment **Step 3**.
4. Place the patient's head in a neutral position **Step 4**.
5. Open the patient's mouth with the tongue-jaw lift maneuver, and insert the Combitube in the midline of the patient's mouth. Insert the tube until the incisors lie between the two reference marks **Step 5**.
6. Inflate the pharyngeal cuff with the recommended volume of air **Step 6**.
7. Inflate the distal cuff with the recommended volume of air **Step 7**.
8. Ventilate the patient through the pharyngeal (blue) tube first. Chest rise indicates esophageal placement of distal tip; continue to ventilate **Step 8**.
9. No chest rise indicates tracheal placement; switch ports and ventilate **Step 9**.
10. Confirm placement by auscultating for breath sounds over the lungs and gastric sounds over the abdomen **Step 10**.

▌The King Airway

The King airway is a relatively new airway device that is available in several different versions. It is designed as an alternate to the Combitube or PtL. The King airway is blindly inserted

Skill Drill 11-36: Insertion of the PtL

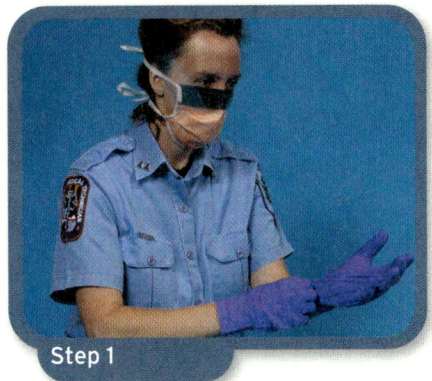

Step 1

Take routine precautions and wear PPE (gloves and face shield at a minimum).

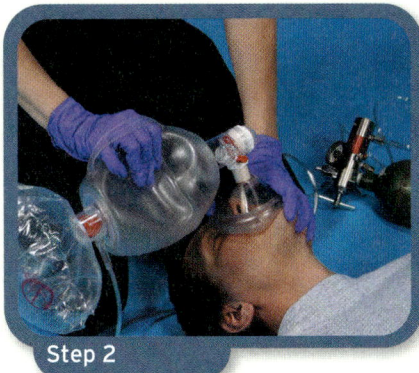

Step 2

Preoxygenate the patient with a bag-valve-mask device and 100% oxygen.

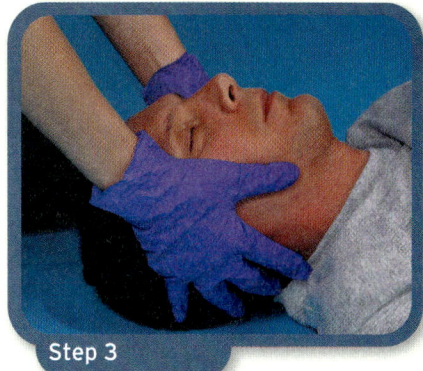

Step 3

Place the patient's head in a neutral position.

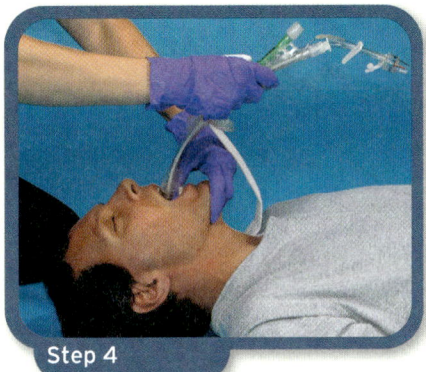

Step 4

Open the patient's mouth with the tongue-jaw lift maneuver, and insert the PtL in the midline of the patient's mouth.

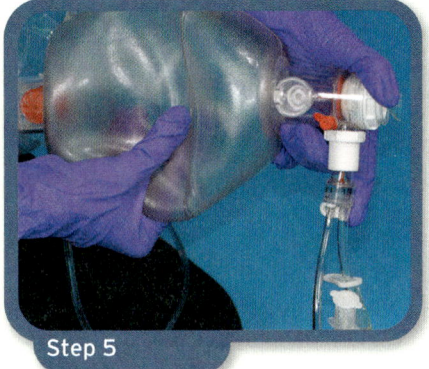

Step 5

Inflate the proximal and distal cuffs.

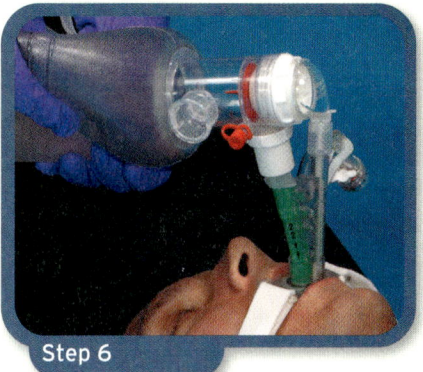

Step 6

Ventilate the patient through the pharyngeal (green) tube first. If the chest rises, continue to ventilate through the green tube.

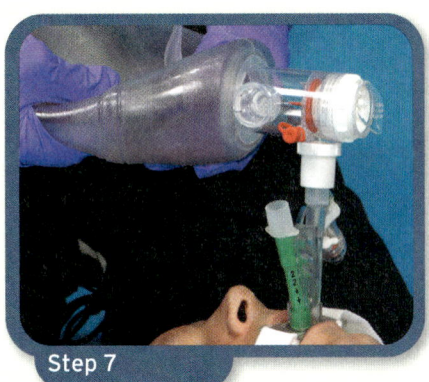

Step 7

If the chest does not rise, remove the stylet from the clear tube and ventilate through the clear tube.

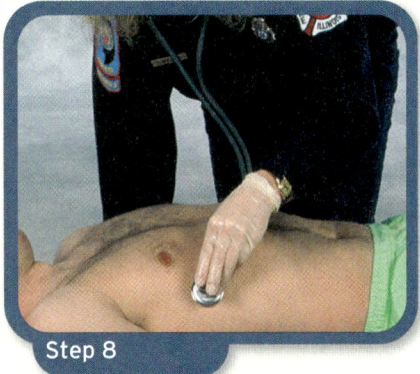

Step 8

Confirm placement by auscultating for breath sounds over the lungs and gastric sounds over the abdomen.

Skill Drill 11-37: Insertion of the Combitube

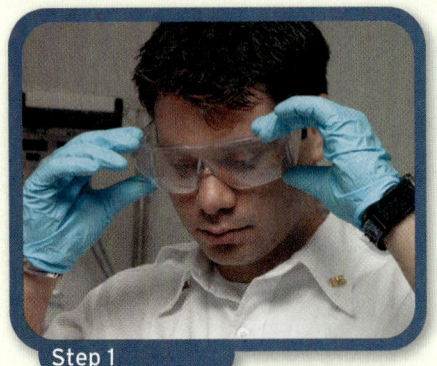

Step 1

Take routine precautions and wear PPE (gloves and face shield at a minimum).

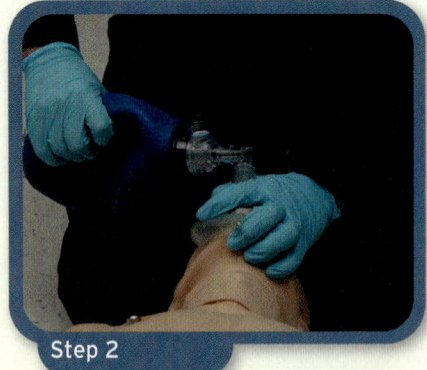

Step 2

Preoxygenate the patient with a bag-valve-mask device and 100% oxygen.

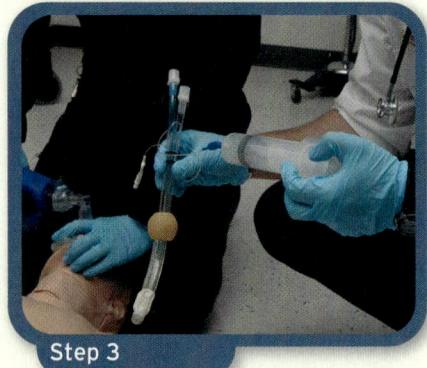

Step 3

Gather your equipment.

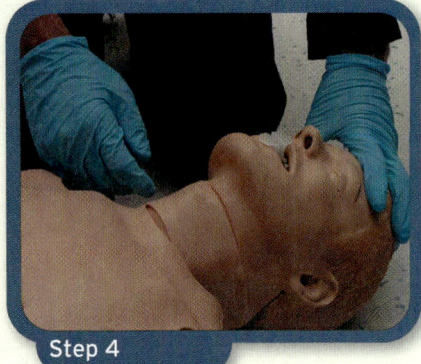

Step 4

Place the patient's head in a neutral position.

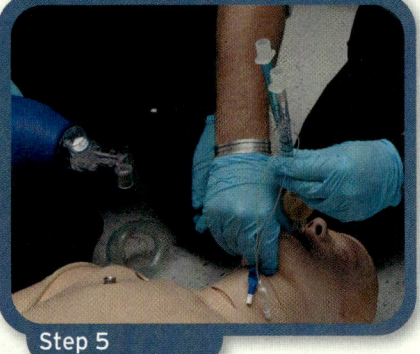

Step 5

Open the patient's mouth with the tongue-jaw lift maneuver, and insert the Combitube in the midline of the patient's mouth. Insert the tube until the incisors lie between the two reference marks.

into the mouth and seats itself in the oropharynx and supraglottic space once the balloon is inflated **Figure 11-73 ▶**. When the position is confirmed, it can adequately oxygenate and ventilate the patient. Studies show the King LT is easier and quicker to place than the Combitube, and can be used successfully as a rescue airway device for failed tracheal intubation attempts.

Indications and Contraindications

The King airway should be considered as a possible alternative to bag-valve-mask ventilation in the place of a Combitube or PtL, or when a rescue device is required for a failed tracheal intubation attempt. It has the same disadvantages, complications, and special considerations as the Combitube and PtL.

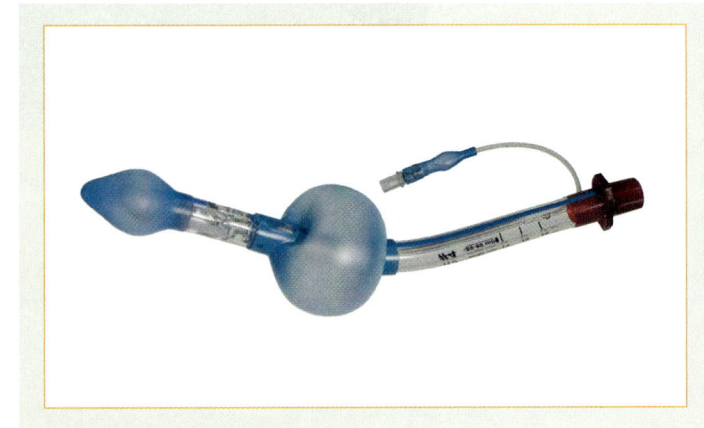

Figure 11-73 King LT airway.

Skill Drill 11-37: Insertion of the Combitube (*continued*)

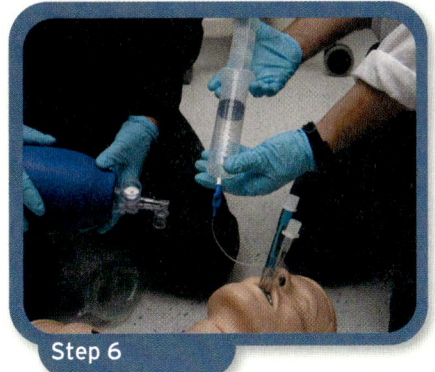

Step 6

Inflate the pharyngeal cuff with the recommended volume of air.

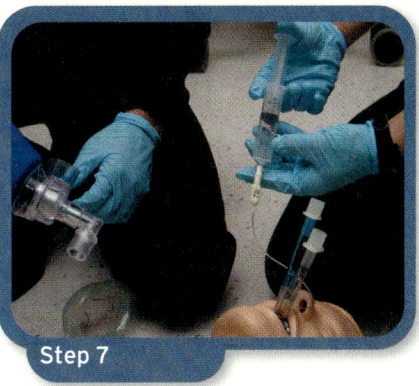

Step 7

Inflate the distal cuff with the recommended volume of air.

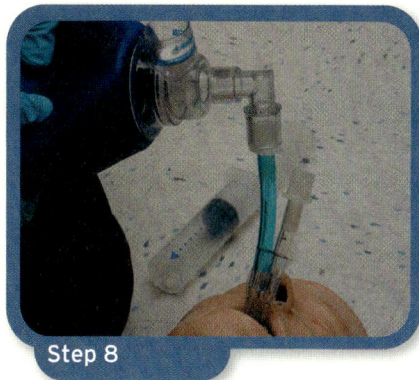

Step 8

Ventilate the patient through the pharyngeal (blue) tube first. Chest rise indicates esophageal placement of distal tip; continue to ventilate.

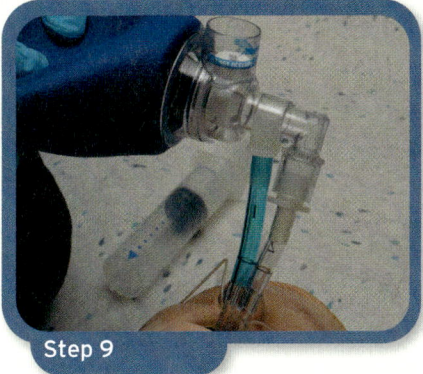

Step 9

No chest rise indicates tracheal placement; switch ports and ventilate.

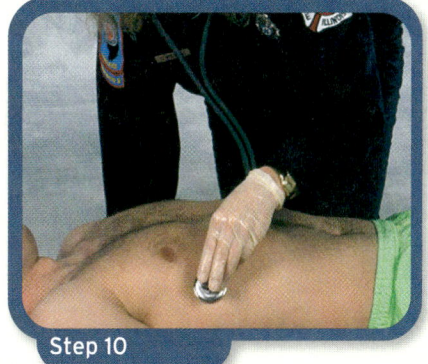

Step 10

Confirm placement by auscultating for breath sounds over the lungs and gastric sounds over the abdomen.

Unlike some multilumen airway devices, the King airway has a single inflation port. You should refer to the manufacturer's instructions on the amount of air required to inflate the balloon and properly seat the device.

Technique for King Airway Insertion

The King airway comes in many sizes; the patient's size and weight determines the size that should be used. The cuff has a one-way valve and, once in position, should be inflated with the amount of air recommended by the manufacturer. Check and prepare all equipment. Check the cuff by inflating it with 50% more air than is required for that size airway. The cuff should then be completely deflated so that no folds appear in the cuff. Preoxygenate the patient with a bag-valve-mask device and 100% oxygen prior to inserting the ing airway. Ventilation should not be interrupted for more than 30 seconds to accomplish placement of the King airway.

- Place the patient's head in a neutral position, unless contraindicated. Hold the King airway at the connector with your dominant hand. Using your other hand, open the patient's jaw, and apply jaw thrust or chin lift unless contraindicated by cervical spine precautions.
- Insert the airway tip into the corner of the mouth, and advance the tip behind the base of the tongue while rotating the tube back to the midline so the blue orientation line faces the patient's chin.
- Continue to advance the tube until the base of the connector is aligned with the patient's teeth or gums.
- Inflate the cuff with the recommended amount of air or to just seal the device.
- Attach the tube to the bag-valve-mask device and confirm tube placement.
- Once placement is confirmed, secure the tube and begin ventilating the patient.

The steps for insertion of a King airway are listed here and shown in **Skill Drill 11-38 ▾**:

1. Take routine precautions and wear PPE (gloves and face shield at a minimum) **Step 1**.
2. Preoxygenate the patient with a bag-valve-mask device and 100% oxygen **Step 2**.
3. Gather your equipment **Step 3**.
4. Place the patient's head in the neutral position.
5. Open the patient's mouth with the jaw-chin lift maneuver, and insert the King airway in the corner of the mouth **Step 4**.

6. Advance the tip behind the base of the tongue while rotating the tube back to midline so that the blue orientation line faces the patient's chin.
7. Advance the tube until base of connector is aligned with teeth or gums. Do not use excessive force.
8. Inflate the cuff with the recommended amount of air or to just seal the device **Step 5**.
9. Attach the tube to the bag-valve-mask device and confirm tube placement **Step 6**.
10. Once placement is confirmed, secure the tube and begin ventilating the patient.

Skill Drill 11-38: Insertion of the King Airway

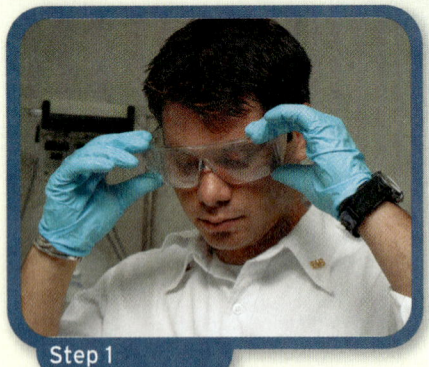

Step 1

Take routine precautions and wear PPE (gloves and face shield at a minimum).

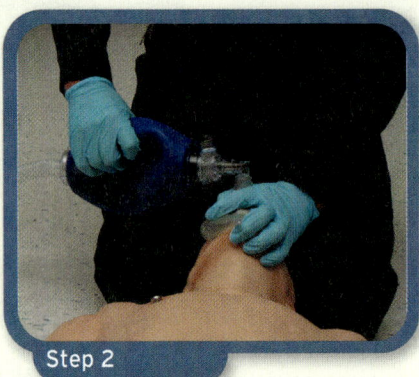

Step 2

Preoxygenate the patient with a bag-valve-mask device and 100% oxygen.

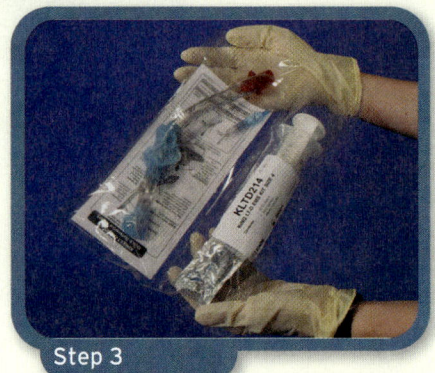

Step 3

Gather your equipment.

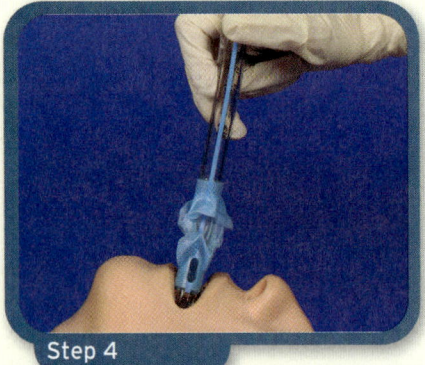

Step 4

Place the patient's head in the neutral position. Open the patient's mouth with the jaw-chin lift maneuver, and insert the King Airway in the corner of the mouth.

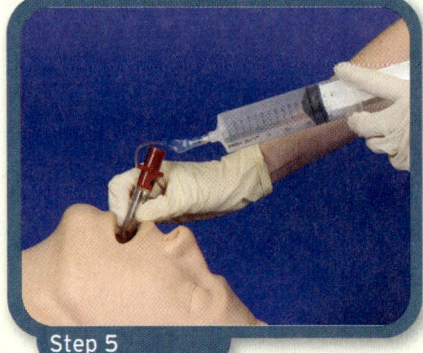

Step 5

Advance the tip behind the base of the tongue while rotating the tube back to midline so that the blue orientation line faces the patient's chin. Advance the tube until base of connector is aligned with teeth or gums. Do not use excessive force. Inflate the cuff with the recommended amount of air or to just seal the device.

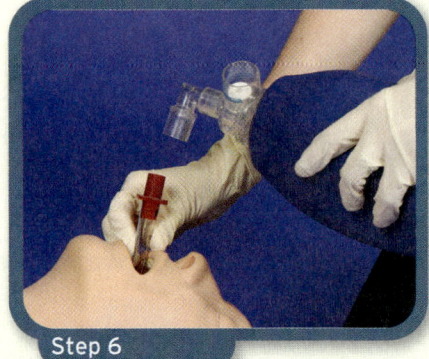

Step 6

Attach the tube to the bag-valve-mask device and confirm tube placement. Once placement is confirmed, secure the tube and begin ventilating the patient.

The Laryngeal Mask Airway

The laryngeal mask airway (LMA) was originally developed for use in the operating room as an alternative to bag-valve-mask ventilation. It is commonly used during short surgical procedures, but can take the place of endotracheal intubation, when longer periods of anesthesia are required Figure 11-74 ▾ . The LMA was not designed for emergency use, and, is not a replacement for endotracheal intubation. It has a role in emergency situations when attempts at intubation have failed, multilumen airways (eg, PtL, Combitube) are not available, and the only viable option is mask ventilation.

The LMA is designed to provide a conduit from the glottic opening to the ventilation device. It surrounds the opening of the larynx with an inflatable silicone cuff positioned in the hypopharynx. When properly inserted, the opening of the LMA is positioned at the glottic opening, and the tip is inserted into the proximal esophagus, the lateral portions in the pyriform fossae, and the upper border at the base of the tongue. The inflatable cuff conforms to the contours of the airway and forms a relatively airtight seal Figure 11-75 ▸ .

Indications and Contraindications

The LMA should be considered as an alternative to bag-valve-mask ventilation when the patient cannot be intubated.

The manufacturers of the LMA indicate that it should be used only in patients who are fasting. Unfortunately, this would eliminate all emergency patients paramedics encounter in the prehospital setting. These patients should always be presumed to have full stomachs. The LMA, however, could be used as a potential alternative to bag-valve-mask ventilation in the prehospital setting when attempts at intubation have failed.

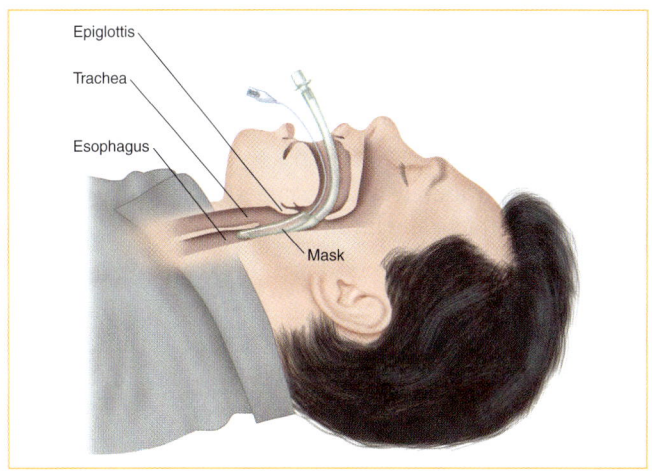

Figure 11-75 The opening of the LMA is positioned at the glottic opening, the tip at the entrance of the esophagus, the lateral portions in the pyriform fossae, and the upper border at the base of the tongue.

The LMA is less effective in obese patients and should not be used in morbidly obese patients. Pregnant patients and patients with a hiatal hernia are at an increased risk for regurgitation and must be evaluated carefully if LMA use is considered. The LMA is ineffective for the ventilation of patients requiring high pulmonary pressures (eg, COPD, congestive heart failure).

Advantages and Disadvantages

The LMA has been shown to provide better oxygenation than bag-valve-mask ventilation with an oral airway. Furthermore, ventilation with the LMA does not require the continual maintenance of a mask seal. Compared to endotracheal intubation, LMA insertion is easier and does not require laryngoscopy. There is also significantly less risk of trauma to soft tissue, vocal cords, the tracheal wall, and teeth. The LMA provides protection from upper airway secretions, and the tip of the LMA wedged into the proximal esophagus may provide some obturation.

The main disadvantage of the LMA, especially in emergencies, is that it does not provide protection against aspiration. In fact, the LMA actually increases the risk of aspiration if the patient regurgitates because his or her stomach contents would most likely be directed into the trachea. During prolonged

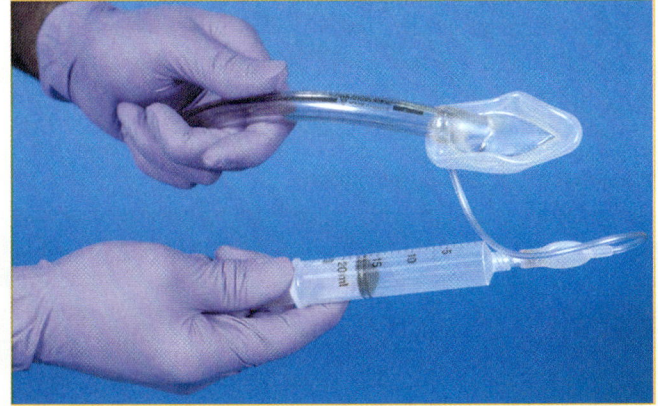

Figure 11-74 The laryngeal mask airway.

Documentation and Communication

If adverse events occur with the use of advanced airway devices, such as bleeding or trauma, be sure to document these occurrences on the patient care report form.

LMA ventilation, some air may be insufflated into the stomach because the seal made in the airway is not airtight. Because of this risk of aspiration, the LMA is unlikely to replace endotracheal intubation in prehospital emergency airway management. *The LMA should not be considered a primary airway device for emergency patients.* It should, however, be considered as a rescue airway in patients who cannot be endotracheally intubated.

Complications

The most significant complications associated with use of the LMA involve regurgitation and subsequent aspiration. The incidence of LMA misplacement in the operating room is relatively low and appears to decrease with experience. Nonetheless, the paramedic should observe the patient for clinical indications of inadequate ventilation (eg, chest rise, breath sounds) during LMA ventilation. Hypoventilation of patients who require high ventilatory pressures can also occur. A few cases of upper airway swelling have been reported.

Equipment

The LMA comes in many sizes, with the size based on the patient's weight. The device consists of an inflatable cuff attached to an obliquely cut tube. The cuff provides a collar that positions the opening of the tube at the glottic opening when inflated. Two vertical bars at the opening of the tube prevent occlusion. The proximal end of the tube is fitted with a standard 15/22-mm adapter that is compatible with any ventilation device. The cuff has a one-way valve assembly and should be inflated with a predetermined volume of air based on the size of the airway **Figure 11-76 ▸** . Note that a common mistake is to select a size that is too small. This results in the inability to ventilate effectively.

Technique for Laryngeal Mask Airway Insertion

Procedures Before and During Insertion

Check and prepare all equipment. Check the cuff of the LMA by inflating it with 50% more air than is required for that size airway. Next, deflate the cuff so that no folds appear near the tip. Deflation is best accomplished by pressing the device, cuff down, on a flat surface **Figure 11-77 ▸** . Lubricate the base of the device.

Preoxygenate the patient with a bag-valve-mask device and 100% oxygen prior to inserting the LMA. Ventilation should not be interrupted for more than 30 seconds to accomplish placement of the LMA. Place the patient's head in a sniffing position, unless there is a suspected neck injury.

- *Insert your finger between the cuff and the tube.* Proper insertion of the LMA depends on holding the device properly. Place the index finger of your dominant hand in the notch between the tube and the cuff. Open the patient's mouth.

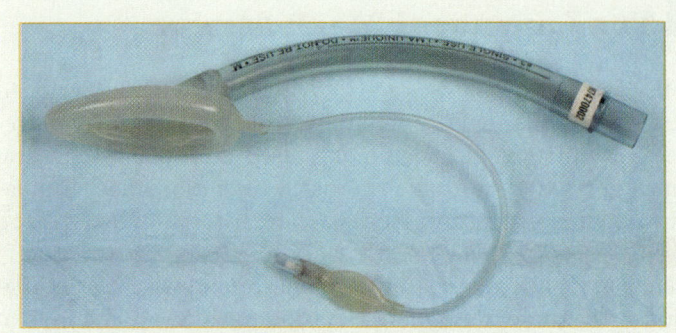

Figure 11-76 The LMA with the cuff inflated.

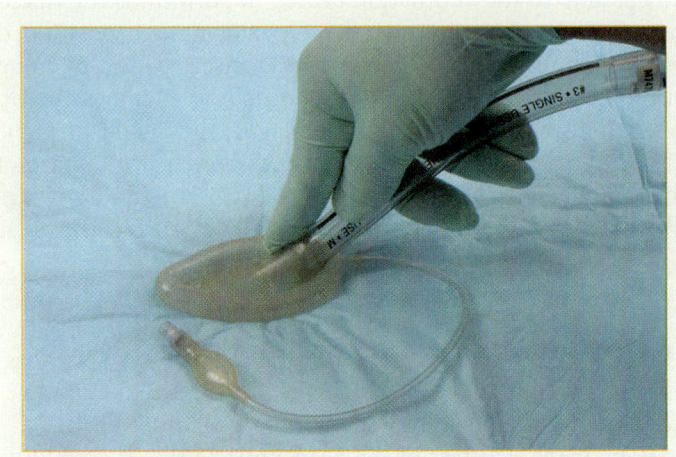

Figure 11-77 Press the LMA, cuff down, against a flat surface to remove all wrinkles from the cuff.

- *Insert the LMA along the roof of the mouth.* The key to proper insertion is to slide the convex surface of the LMA along the roof of the mouth. Use your finger to push the airway against the hard palate. Once it slides past the tongue, the LMA will move easily into position.
- *Inflate the cuff.* Inflate the cuff of the LMA with the amount of air indicated for that size airway. If the LMA is properly positioned, it will move out of the airway slightly (1 to 2 cm) as it seats into position.

Procedures After Insertion

Following inflation of the cuff, attach the bag-valve-mask device and begin to ventilate the patient. Confirm chest rise and the presence of breath sounds. Continuously and closely monitor for regurgitation in the tube. Carefully reassess the airway during any patient movement, and be prepared to ventilate with a bag-valve-mask device and 100% oxygen if the LMA becomes dislodged.

A 6.0-mm ET tube can be passed through a size 3 or 4 LMA, allowing for intubation. The vertical bars are designed to allow a well-lubricated tube to pass straight through, and research in the operating room found a high success rate of endotracheal intubation following this technique. Some LMAs are designed to accept and guide an ET tube into the trachea and may prove to be a viable alternative to direct laryngoscopy Figure 11-78 ▸ .

The steps for inserting an LMA are summarized here and shown in Skill Drill 11-39 ▸ .

1. Take routine precautions and wear PPE (gloves and face shield at a minimum).
2. Check the cuff of the LMA by inflating it with 50% more air than is required for that size airway. Then deflate the cuff completely Step 1 .
3. Lubricate the base of the device Step 2 .
4. Preoxygenate the patient with a bag-valve-mask device and 100% oxygen. Ventilation should not be interrupted for more than 30 seconds to accomplish LMA placement. If the patient is not suspected of having a neck injury, place the patient's head in the sniffing position Step 3 .
5. Insert your finger between the cuff and the tube. Place the index finger of your dominant hand in the notch between the tube and the cuff. Open the patient's mouth Step 4 .
6. Insert the LMA along the roof of the mouth. Use your finger to push the airway against the hard palate Step 5 .
7. Inflate the cuff with the amount of air indicated for that sized airway Step 6 .
8. Attach the bag-valve-mask device and begin to ventilate the patient. Confirm chest rise and the presence of breath sounds. Continuously and closely monitor the patient Step 7 .

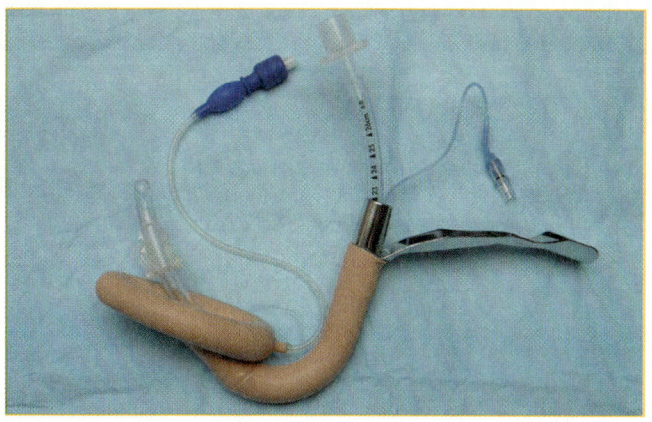

Figure 11-78 The intubating LMA with a 6.0-mm ET tube.

▌Pharmacologic Adjuncts to Airway Management and Ventilation

Pharmacologic agents in airway management are used to decrease the discomfort of intubation, decrease the incidence of complications associated with laryngoscopy and intubation, and make aggressive airway management possible for patients who need it but who are too conscious or combative to cooperate.

Sedation in Emergency Intubation

Sedation is used in airway management to reduce the patient's anxiety, induce amnesia, and to decrease the gag reflex. It is useful for anxious, combative, or agitated patients, as well as for patients who need aggressive airway management but who are too conscious to tolerate intubation. If used properly, and under the correct circumstances, sedation effectively increases patient compliance, thus making definitive airway management easier and safer to perform. If used improperly, however, it can cause further harm.

The complications associated with sedation in airway management are related primarily to undersedation or oversedation. Undersedation can result in poor patient cooperation, the complications of gagging (eg, trauma, tachycardia, hypertension, vomiting, or aspiration), and incomplete amnesia of the event. Oversedation can result in uncontrolled general

You are the Paramedic Part 10

Your patient's condition has now stabilized. He is delivered to the emergency department, where you give your verbal report to the attending physician. The patient is admitted with a diagnosis of acute exacerbation of congestive heart failure.

Reassessment	Recording Time: 35 Minutes
Level of consciousness	Sedated
Respirations	Ventilated with 100% oxygen at a rate of 12 breaths/min
Pulse	100 beats/min, strong and regular
Skin	Pink and moist
Blood pressure	130/80 mm Hg
Spo₂	98% while being ventilated with 100% oxygen

17. What treatment would have been appropriate had this clinically unstable patient been too conscious or combative to intubate?

Skill Drill 11-39: LMA Insertion

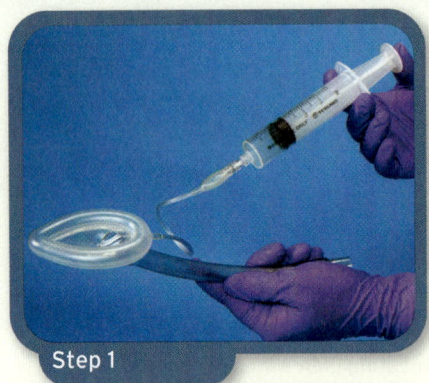

Step 1

Check the cuff of the LMA by inflating it with 50% more air than is required for that size airway. Then deflate the cuff completely.

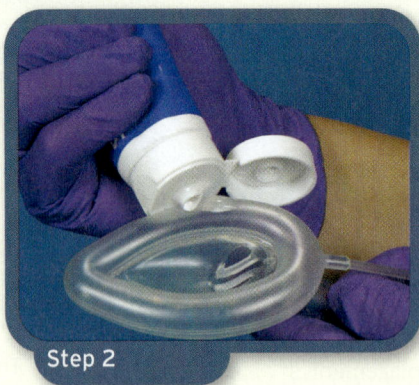

Step 2

Lubricate the base of the device.

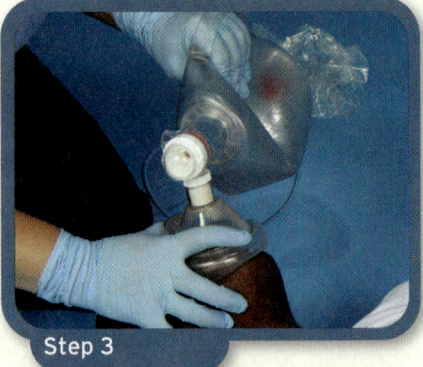

Step 3

Preoxygenate the patient with a bag-valve-mask device and 100% oxygen. Ventilation should not be interrupted for more than 30 seconds to accomplish LMA placement. Place the patient's head in the sniffing position, if neck injury is not suspected.

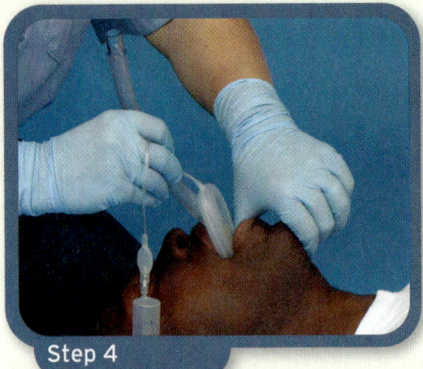

Step 4

Insert your finger between the cuff and the tube. Place the index finger of your dominant hand in the notch between the tube and the cuff. Open the patient's mouth.

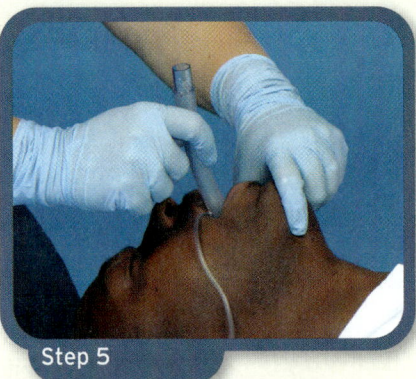

Step 5

Insert the LMA along the roof of the mouth. Use your finger to push the airway against the hard palate.

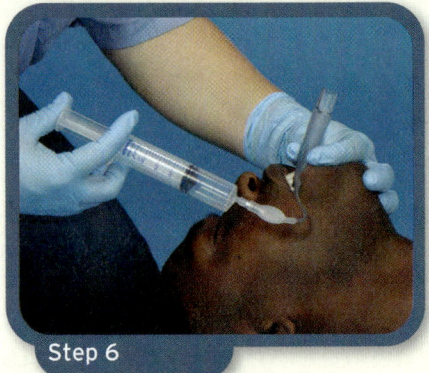

Step 6

Inflate the cuff with the amount of air indicated for that size airway.

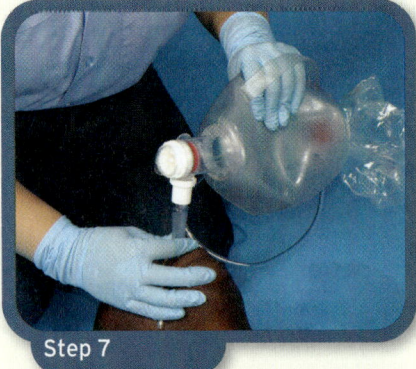

Step 7

Attach the bag-valve-mask device and begin to ventilate the patient. Confirm chest rise and the presence of breath sounds. Continuously and closely monitor the patient.

anesthesia, loss of protective airway reflexes, respiratory depression, complete airway collapse, and hypotension.

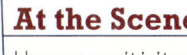

At the Scene

Hypersensitivity to sedative medications is the primary contraindication to the use of these drugs. Obtain an accurate medical history prior to giving any drug to any patient.

The level of sedation desired dictates the amount of the medication administered. The patient's response to sedatives is dose dependent. The paramedic should follow local protocols and medical directives, and may consult with direct medical control regarding the appropriate dose for a given patient.

Two major classes of sedatives are commonly used in airway management: analgesics and sedative-hypnotics **Table 11-15 ▾**. Analgesics decrease the perception of pain. Sedative-hypnotics induce sleep and decrease anxiety; they do not reduce pain.

Butyrophenones

Butyrophenones are potent, effective sedatives. Two of these drugs, haloperidol (Haldol) and droperidol (Inapsine), are frequently used in emergency situations for anxiolysis, the relief of anxiety. These medications are effective for calming agitated patients, trauma patients who are combative, patients who are experiencing alcohol withdrawal, and patients with acute psychoses. They do not produce apnea and have little effect on the cardiovascular system. Droperidol is faster acting than haloperidol and is generally preferred in emergency situations. Butyrophenones are not recommended for induction of anesthesia. Butyrophenones can decrease seizure threshold, increasing the risk of a seizure in a patient at risk for seizures.

Benzodiazepines

Benzodiazepines are sedative-hypnotic drugs. Diazepam (Valium) and midazolam (Versed) provide muscle relaxation and mild

sedation and are used extensively as anxiolytic and anticonvulsant medications. They also provide antegrade amnesia, which is beneficial when you are performing invasive or uncomfortable procedures; the patient will not be able to recall the event.

Midazolam is two to four times as potent as diazepam, is faster acting, and has a shorter duration of action. In doses of 0.2 mg/kg IV, midazolam produces loss of consciousness in 30 to 60 seconds and lasts up to 20 minutes. Midazolam can be used to induce general anesthesia prior to intubation; however, these large doses increase the likelihood of complications. Respiratory depression and hypotension are potential side effects of benzodiazepine administration. Lower doses (0.05 to 0.1 mg/kg) are often used as part of a rapid sequence intubation to avoid some of the adverse side effects, but these doses do not typically result in optimal intubating conditions.

Flumazenil (Romazicon) is a benzodiazepine antagonist that can reverse the effects of diazepam and midazolam.

Barbiturates

Barbiturates are sedative-hypnotic medications that have a long history of use. When administered intravenously, thiopental (Pentothal) and other related barbiturates cross the blood–brain barrier rapidly and act on gamma-aminobutyric acid (GABA) receptors, causing rapid onset of profound CNS depression. A single dose of 3 to 5 mg/kg IV thiopental results in loss of consciousness in 30 seconds and lasts 5 to 8 minutes. Barbiturates can cause significant respiratory depression and a drop in blood pressure of approximately 10% in normovolemic patients. This drop in blood pressure can be profound and potentially irreversible in hypovolemic patients.

Opioids/Narcotics

Opioids are potent analgesics with sedative properties. Narcotics are used in emergency airway management as a premedication, during induction, and in maintenance of sedation/amnesia. The two most commonly used narcotics for airway management are fentanyl (Sublimaze) and morphine. Fentanyl is 70 to 150 times more potent than morphine. It has a short onset of action and a relatively short duration of action.

Opioids can cause profound respiratory and central nervous system depression and produce severe hypotension and bradycardia, especially in hemodynamically unstable patients. These negative effects can be reversed with naloxone (Narcan), a narcotic antagonist.

Etomidate

Etomidate (Amidate) is a nonnarcotic, nonbarbiturate hypnotic-sedative drug. It is a fast-acting agent of short duration. This drug has little effect on heart rate, blood pressure, cerebral blood flow, and intracranial pressure, and does not cause the histamine release and bronchoconstriction that may occur with other agents. However, a high incidence of uncomfortable myoclonic muscle movement is associated with its use. Etomidate is a useful induction agent in patients with coronary artery disease, increased intracranial pressure, or borderline hypotension/hypovolemia. The initial dose of etomidate, as part of a rapid sequence intubation, is 0.3 mg/kg IV. At present, etomidate is

Table 11-15	Sedatives Used in Airway Management
Drug Type	**Examples**
Butyrophenones: sedative	Haloperidol (Haldol) Droperidol (Inapsine)
Benzodiazepines: sedative-hypnotic	Diazepam (Valium) Midazolam (Versed)
Barbiturates: sedative-hypnotic	Thiopental (Pentothal)
Narcotics (opioids): sedative-analgesic	Fentanyl (Sublimaze) Morphine
Other agents	Etomidate (Amidate): sedative-hypnotic Ketamine (Ketalar): sedative-analgesic-hypnotic Propofol (Diprivan): sedative-hypnotic

not widely available because Health Canada has not approved it for general release. It is, however, available in controlled release in some settings, including some EMS agencies. You are advised to refer to your EMS agency's established protocols and medical directives to determine if etomidate is available for advanced airway management in your EMS service.

Ketamine

Ketamine (Ketalar) is a drug with sedative, analgesic, and hypnotic properties. It was created in the laboratory from phencyclidine (PCP). Ketamine has potent sedative, analgesic, and hypnotic properties. Protective airway reflexes are maintained, and there is little respiratory depression following administration. Ketamine is also very hemodynamically stable, making it a useful agent in patients who are hemodynamically unstable. After a dose of 1 to 2 mg/kg IV, it produces loss of consciousness in 30 to 60 seconds and lasts up to 15 minutes.

At the Scene

Combativeness, aggressiveness, and belligerence should be considered signs of cerebral hypoxia until proven otherwise. You must be firm and direct, but still treat your patients with respect and empathy. Keep in mind that they are fighting for their lives, not with you.

Ketamine is not commonly used in emergency situations involving adults because of the incidence of nightmares, referred to as emergence phenomenon. In children, these emergence phenomena are less common; therefore, ketamine is used as a sedative, analgesic, and hypnotic agent in the pediatric population.

There is also conflicting evidence regarding ketamine use in patients with elevated intracranial pressure. It may increase cerebral blood flow, resulting in further increases in intracranial pressure. Although this may lead to further brain injury, this must be balanced against its cardiovascular stability that prevents hypotension, a common side effect of other agents used in rapid sequence intubation.

Ketamine is not frequently used in the prehospital setting for airway management. It does, however, have a specific role in airway management of the patient with severe acute asthma. Its bronchodilator properties and the fact that the patient maintains their protective airway reflexes makes it a suitable induction agent in these patients.

Neuromuscular Blockade in Emergency Intubation

Cerebral hypoxia can make an ordinarily docile person combative, aggressive, belligerent, and uncooperative. This can make for a very difficult and potentially dangerous situation—both for the patient and for the paramedics. The patient with cerebral hypoxia must be treated with aggressive oxygenation and ventilation, but his or her combativeness often makes this a difficult, if not impossible, task to perform. Clenching of the patient's teeth due to spasm of the jaw muscles (trismus) and vocal cords spasm (laryngospasm) can also hamper your efforts to obtain a definitive airway.

In the past, it was common practice to physically restrain the patient to obtain a definitive airway. A safer, more effective approach is to "chemically paralyze" the patient with neuromuscular blocking agents (paralytics). With the patient chemically paralyzed and sedated, his or her protective airway reflexes are lost; you can effectively perform oxygenation and ventilation, and the patient will not gag during insertion of an ET tube.

Neuromuscular Blocking Agents

Although sedatives alone can be used to facilitate intubation, the incidence of complications and side effects are high. In well-trained and skilled hands with the appropriate equipment and the appropriately selected patient, it is much more effective to administer a drug specifically designed to induce paralysis. Paralytic drugs affect all skeletal muscles, including the diaphragm and the intercostal muscles. Within about a minute of receiving an IV dose of a paralytic, a patient will become *totally* paralyzed. That is, the patient will stop breathing; his or her jaw muscles will go slack, and the base of the tongue will flop back against the posterior pharynx and obstruct the airway. Put bluntly, paralytics convert a breathing patient with a marginal airway into an apneic patient with no airway. Before you bring about such a change, you must be *absolutely* sure that you can place an ET tube into the patient's trachea within the next 30 seconds. Once a patient is paralyzed, you are completely responsible for that patient's breathing and well-being. Fortunately, paralytic agents do not affect cardiac or smooth muscle.

A paralyzed patient will *appear* to be asleep or unconscious, but is not! Paralytic agents, unlike sedatives, have no effect on level of consciousness. The patient is fully aware and can hear, feel, and think.

Pharmacology of Neuromuscular Blocking Agents

To understand how medications induce paralysis, recall how skeletal muscles contract. All skeletal (striated) muscles are voluntary and require input from the somatic nervous system to initiate contraction. As an impulse to contract reaches the terminal end of a motor nerve, acetylcholine (ACh) is released into the synaptic cleft (the junction between the nerve cell and the muscle cell). This neurotransmitter diffuses across the short distance of the synaptic cleft and binds to receptor sites on the motor end plate. Acetylcholine occupying the receptor sites triggers changes in electrical properties of the muscle fibre, a process called depolarization. When enough motor end plates have been depolarized, a threshold is reached and the muscle fibre contracts. Depolarization lasts for only a few milliseconds because of the presence of acetylcholinesterase, an enzyme that quickly removes acetylcholine from the synaptic cleft and from the receptors on the motor end plate.

Paralytic medications all function at the neuromuscular junction and relax the muscle by impeding the action of acetylcholine. Collectively, all paralytics are referred to as neuromuscular blocking agents. They are classified into two categories: depolarizing and nondepolarizing agents.

Table 11-16 ▸ lists the standard dosages for these agents used in the prehospital setting.

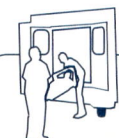

At the Scene

Paralysis Versus Sedation

Imagine what it must be like to be completely paralyzed. You can't blink, talk, move, and, most importantly, breathe! You are completely dependent upon others to keep you alive. Paralytic agents do not induce sedation or amnesia. If you administer only a paralytic agent, the patient will be fully conscious and remember the entire event. Therefore, unless contraindicated, you must sedate a patient who is paralyzed. **Paralysis without sedation is considered a form of patient maltreatment!**

Depolarizing Neuromuscular Blocking Agents

Depolarizing neuromuscular blockers competitively bind with the acetylcholine receptor sites but are not affected as quickly by acetylcholinesterase. Therefore, they cause depolarization of the muscle and prevent future signals for depolarization from having an effect because all of the acetylcholine receptor sites are already occupied.

Succinylcholine chloride (Anectine) is the only depolarizing neuromuscular blocking agent. Because succinylcholine causes depolarization, fasciculations—characterized by brief, uncoordinated twitching of small muscle groups in the face, neck, trunk, and extremities—can be observed during its administration Figure 11-79 ▸ . These fasciculations tend to cause generalized muscle pain at the termination of paralysis (when the succinylcholine wears off).

At the Scene

If you administer only a depolarizing paralytic (eg, succinylcholine) to your patient, you will have to give the medication by continuous infusion or administer a bolus every 5 minutes. This significantly increases the risk of complications. Repeat dosing with a depolarizing agent only is not routine practice to maintain paralysis.

Depolarizing neuromuscular blockers are characterized by a very rapid onset (45 to 90 seconds) of total paralysis and a relatively short duration of action (15 minutes). For this reason, succinylcholine is often used as an initial paralytic. With this drug, if you are unable to secure the patient's airway, you have to support ventilation for only a short period of time before the patient can breathe again on his or her own.

Succinylcholine should be used with caution in patients with burns, crush injuries, and blunt trauma—that is, conditions that can result in hyperkalemia, because succinyl-

Table 11-16	Neuromuscular Blocking Drug Dosages
Drug	**Dosage**
Succinylcholine (depolarizing)	1.5 to 2.0 mg/kg via IV push (initial dose) - Repeat doses can be given based on the patient's response
Vecuronium (nondepolarizing)	0.1 mg/kg via IV push (initial dose for adults and children older than 10 years of age) - 0.01 to 0.015 mg/kg can be given 25 to 40 minutes after initial dose
Pancuronium (nondepolarizing)	0.06 to 0.1 mg/kg via IV push (initial dose for adults and children older than 1 month of age) - Can repeat at 0.01 mg/kg every 20 to 60 minutes as needed
Rocuronium	0.6 to 1.2 mg/kg IV push (initial dose) - 0.1 to 0.3 mg/kg IV push can be given every 20 to 30 minutes for subsequent doses

Table 11-17	Contraindications for Succinylcholine Administration
Condition	**When Not to Administer Succinylcholine**
Burns to > 10% of body surface area	48 hours to 6 months after burn
Abdominal sepsis	3 or more days after onset of sepsis
Crush injuries	3 days to 6 months after crush injury
Illness causing paralysis (including stroke)	3 days to 6 months after illness
Neuromuscular disorders	Do not administer if active
History or family history of malignant hyperthermia	Do not administer

choline may exacerbate the hyperkalemia, resulting in dangerous cardiac arrhythmias. Table 11-17 ▴ lists associated conditions that may result in severe hyperkalemia when succinylcholine is administered. Additionally, because its chemical structure is similar to that of acetylcholine, succinylcholine can cause bradycardia, especially in pediatric patients. Premedication with atropine, which prevents succinylcholine-induced bradycardia, should precede the administration of succinylcholine in

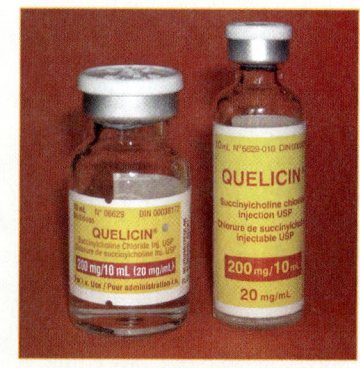

Figure 11-79 Succinylcholine.

pediatric patients. Finally, succinylcholine must be refrigerated in order to prevent it from degrading. When stored at room temperature, such as in your drug box, succinylcholine lasts for as little as two weeks and as long as three months. Succinylcholine must also be protected from light to prevent degrading.

Nondepolarizing Neuromuscular Blocking Agents

Nondepolarizing neuromuscular blockers also bind to acetylcholine receptor sites; however, unlike depolarizing neuromuscular blockers, they do not cause depolarization of the muscle fibre. When given in sufficient quantity, the amount of nondepolarizing medication exceeds the amount of acetylcholine in the synaptic cleft, and the critical threshold of depolarization cannot be achieved. Thus, when nondepolarizing paralytics are administered in small quantities prior to administering a depolarizing paralytic, they prevent fasciculations. The defasciculating dose is typically 10% of the normal dose; it does not induce paralysis, but does cause weakness.

The most commonly used nondepolarizing neuromuscular blockers are vecuronium (Norcuron), pancuronium (Pavulon), and rocuronium (Zemuron). Rocuronium **Figure 11-80 ▸** has the most rapid onset of action (45 to 90 seconds) of the nondepolarizing agents, and an intermediate duration of action (20 to 45 minutes). Vecuronium **Figure 11-81 ▸** has a rapid onset of action (2 minutes), but a longer duration of action (45 minutes). Pancuronium **Figure 11-82 ▸** also has a rapid onset of action (3 to 5 minutes), and a slightly longer duration of action (1 hour).

Nondepolarizing neuromuscular blockers, because of their longer duration of action, are ideal when the patient requires extended periods of paralysis, such as when there is a prolonged transport time or when the patient's airway has been secured and you need to manage other injuries or conditions. However, these agents should be given carefully before the patient's airway has been secured because their duration of action is prolonged when compared to succinyl choline.

The prolonged duration of action may not be a drawback due to recent developments in drug research. There is a new class of drugs, known as modified γ-cyclodextrins, that encapsulate certain nondepolarizing neuromuscular blocking agents, such as rocuronium, and cause the blocking agents to dissociate with the nicotinic receptor. While not a true reversal drug, this encapsulation and dissociation effectively ends the neuromuscular blockage. The new drug is being studied in clinical trials. If the trials are successful, class they could allow those practicing RSI to reverse the effects of nondepolarizing neuromuscular blocking agents in the event of an intubation failure or problem where blockage reversal is required immediately.

Rapid-Sequence Intubation

Rapid-sequence intubation (RSI) represents a culmination and integration of all of your airway, problem-solving, and decision-making skills into one procedure. It includes the safe, smooth, and rapid induction of sedation and paralysis followed immediately by intubation. Although RSI has been successfully performed in the operating room for years, its use in the prehospital setting is relatively new. It is generally used for conscious or combative patients who need to be intubated but who are unable or unwilling to cooperate. It is also used when intubation requires minimal or no physiologic disturbance, such as in patients with increased intracranial pressure.

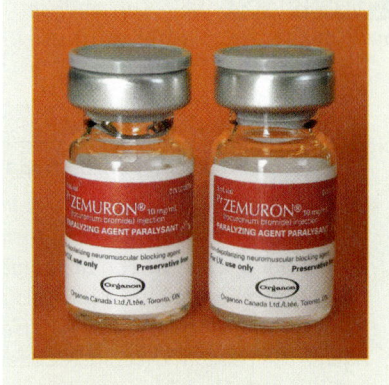

Figure 11-80 Rocuronium.

The general steps for RSI are the same for all patients; however, different protocols are used for normal, stable patients and unstable patients. Prior to proceeding with RSI, or any advanced airway maneuver for that matter, you must properly assess the patient's airway for any anticipated difficulties. If you anticipate any difficulty, you should consider not proceeding with an RSI and instead use some other technique to secure the airway. In all cases, you should be familiar with your local and regional EMS protocols and directives in order to safely secure the airway without endangering the patient's safety and well-being.

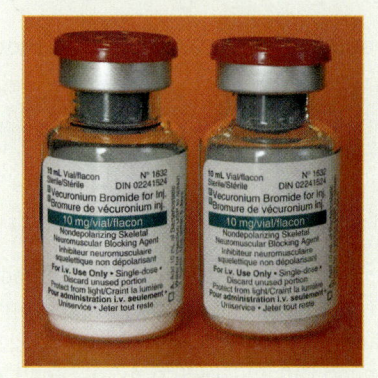

Figure 11-81 Vecuronium.

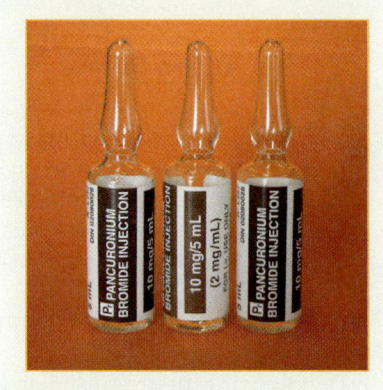

Figure 11-82 Pancuronium.

Preparation of the Patient and Equipment

The experience of being intubated is frightening for patients, so you must explain what you are going to do and reassure the patient that he or she will be asleep during the procedure and will not feel or remember anything. Place the patient on a cardiac monitor and pulse oximeter. Check, prepare, and assemble your equipment and ensure that it is in good working order. In particular, have suction *immediately* available, and the equipment for your backup plan if your first intubation method fails.

Preoxygenation

Adequately preoxygenate the patient with 100% oxygen to ensure that positive-pressure ventilation will not be necessary until the patient has been successfully intubated Figure 11-83 ▸. If the patient is not ventilating adequately, you will need to assist ventilations during the procedure itself.

Premedication

Stimulation of the glottis associated with intubation can cause dysrhythmias and a substantial increase in intracranial pressure (ICP)—a particularly problematic issue for patients with closed head injuries or other conditions associated with increased ICP. If you are performing RSI on a patient with closed head trauma, you may administer 1 to 1.5 mg/kg IV of lidocaine. While the evidence is not conclusive, lidocaine may decrease the risk of dysrhythmias and the spike in ICP associated with stimulation of the upper airway.

As previously discussed, you may also choose to administer a defasciculating dose (typically 10% of a normal dose) of a nondepolarizing paralytic, if time permits. Atropine sulfate should also be administered to decrease the incidence of bradycardia associated with the administration of succinylcholine. The usual dose for the adult is 0.5 mg and 0.02 mg/kg (minimum dose 0.1 mg) for infants and children.

Sedation and Paralysis

As long as the patient is hemodynamically normotensive (systolic BP > 90 mm Hg), administer a sedative agent to induce sedation and amnesia. Immediately thereafter, administer succinylcholine. Paralysis will begin in 30 seconds and will be complete within 2 minutes. Wait for paralysis to take place, ensuring optimal intubating conditions before proceeding with your intubation attempt.

Posterior Cricoid Pressure

Immediately after the patient is sedated and paralyzed, have an assistant apply posterior cricoid pressure Figure 11-84 ▸. As long as the patient's oxygen saturation is maintained, do not provide positive-pressure ventilation, as this will significantly increase the risk of regurgitation and aspiration.

Intubation

Intubate the trachea as carefully as possible Figure 11-85 ▸. If you cannot accomplish the intubation within 30 seconds, stop and ventilate the patient for 30 seconds to 1 minute with a bag-valve-mask device and 100% oxygen before trying again. *If you must ventilate the patient with a bag mask, do so slowly (1 second per breath [enough to produce visible chest rise]) while maintaining cricoid pressure to minimize the risk of regurgitation.* If the patient is inadequately paralyzed, you may give a second dose of succinylcholine.

Once the tube is in the trachea, inflate the cuff, remove the stylet, verify correct position of the ET tube, and release cricoid pressure. Secure the tube in place as normal and continue ventilations at the appropriate rate.

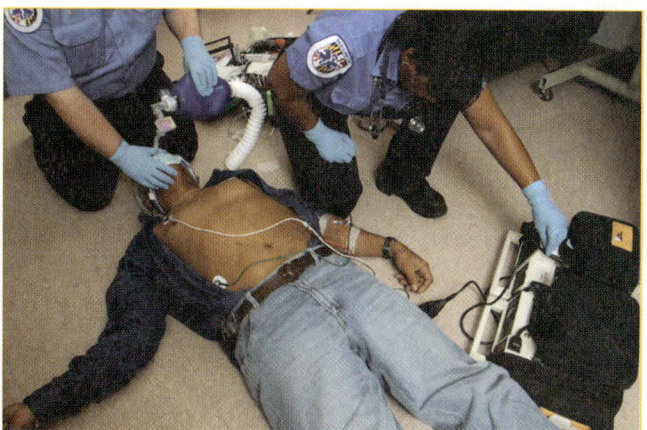

Figure 11-83 Preoxygenate the patient prior to performing rapid-sequence intubation.

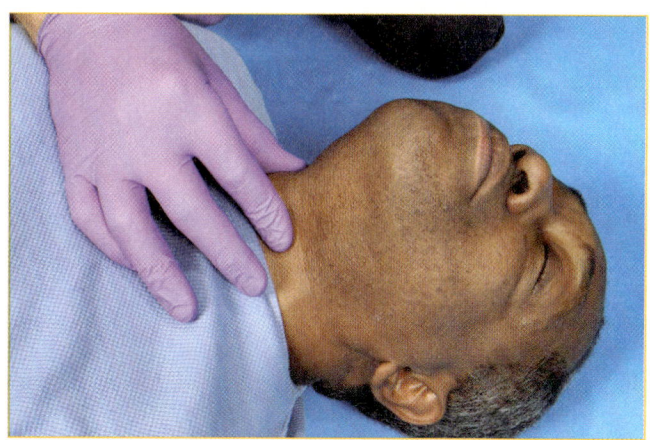

Figure 11-84 A second paramedic should apply posterior cricoid pressure to reduce the risk of regurgitation.

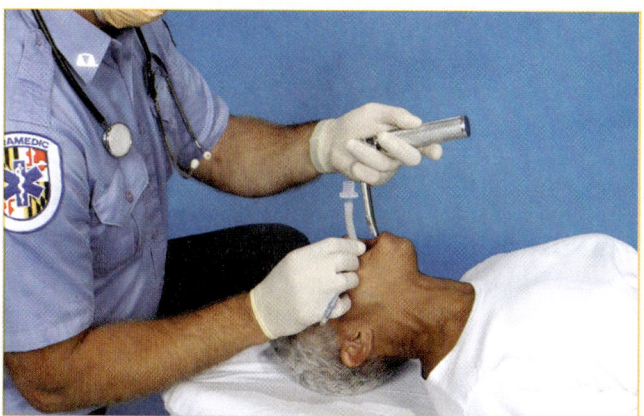

Figure 11-85 Intubate the trachea.

At the Scene

Rapid-sequence intubation should be attempted only if you have confidence that you will be able to intubate and ventilate the patient, or ventilate the patient without intubation, if necessary. Otherwise, a patient who has been sedated and paralyzed will die. Above all else, *do no harm!*

Maintenance of Paralysis and Sedation

When you are *absolutely* sure that you have successfully intubated the trachea, administer a nondepolarizing blocker to maintain long-term paralysis. Continue to administer a sedative if the patient's blood pressure is adequate. Monitor the patient's heart rate and blood pressure to ensure that sedation is not wearing off.

Although the general steps of RSI are the same for all patients, some modification is necessary for unstable patients. If the patient's oxygen saturation drops at any point, you have no choice except to ventilate (just do it slowly). If the patient is hemodynamically unstable, you must judge whether sedation is appropriate or whether the risk of profound hypotension is too great to sedate the patient prior to inducing paralysis. **Table 11-18** lists sample protocols for RSI in hemodynamically normal and unstable patients.

■ Failure to Intubate

No matter how careful, prepared, and skilled you are, some intubations will be unsuccessful or impossible. If the intubation attempt fails, go back to basics—bag-valve-mask ventilation. In most cases, and if done properly, bag-valve-mask ventilation should allow you to oxygenate and ventilate the patient. This gives you time to go to your plan B. A number of options are available to secure an airway in a patient you are unable to intubate, but are still able to ventilate.

Several rescue devices are available that you can use as plan B. The first three are the esophageal obturator airway (EOS), the esophageal gastric tube airway (EGTA), and the laryngeal mask airway (LMA). They were discussed in previous sections of this chapter. Although some EMS agencies use them as the airway device of choice for primary and some advanced paramedics, they should be considered rescue airway devices for advanced and critical care paramedics with advanced airway management skills. As a rescue device, these three devices are temporary measures to secure an airway, oxygenate, and ventilate. They are not definitive airway management tools.

Transillumination Techniques for Intubation

Transillumination intubation, like digital intubation, is rarely considered a first-line technique to definitively secure the airway, but it may prove valuable in some situations. The tissue that overlies the trachea is relatively thin. Therefore, a bright light source placed inside the trachea emits a bright, well-circumscribed light that is visible on the outside of the trachea and the external soft tissue that overlies it.

Table 11-18	Sample Protocols for Rapid-Sequence Intubation

For hemodynamically normal patients

1. Take routine precautions and wear PPE (gloves and face shield at a minimum).
2. Prepare patient and equipment.
3. Preoxygenate with 100% oxygen for at least 2 to 3 minutes.
4. Consider a defasciculating dose of nondepolarizing paralytic, lidocaine, and/or atropine.
5. Sedate.
6. Administer succinylcholine.
7. Apply cricoid pressure.
8. Intubate, verify tube placement, and release cricoid pressure.
9. Administer a nondepolarizing paralytic and maintain adequate sedation.

For hemodynamically unstable patients

1. Take routine precautions and wear PPE (gloves and face shield at a minimum).
2. Prepare patient and equipment.
3. Preoxygenate and ventilate as necessary.
4. Consider sedation.
5. Administer succinylcholine.
6. Apply cricoid pressure.
7. Intubate, verify tube placement, and release cricoid pressure.
8. Administer a nondepolarizing paralytic.

A number of devices can be used to intubate the trachea with the transillumination technique. You should be familiar with your specific equipment and consult the product documentation for instructions in its use. In this section, the term "lighted stylet" will be used generically to describe any malleable stylet with a bright light source at its distal end that can be used to guide intubation.

Indications and Contraindications

Transillumination intubation can be used whenever a patient needs to be intubated, but is usually performed after other intubation techniques have failed. This technique is absolutely contraindicated in patients with an intact gag reflex and in those with an airway obstruction. When determining whether transillumination should be attempted, you should consider the amount of soft tissue overlying the trachea. Obese patients and patients with short, muscular necks may be difficult to transilluminate.

Theoretically, it is possible to perform transillumination in pediatric patients; however, the stylet *must* be able to fit inside the ET tube. Most lighted stylets will not fit in tubes smaller than 6.0 mm.

Advantages and Disadvantages

Because transillumination does not involve the use of a laryngoscope, it largely avoids the problems associated with laryngoscopy (eg, dental trauma, soft-tissue trauma). In contrast to other blind intubation techniques (eg, digital, nasotracheal), transillumination adds a visual parameter—a light at the midline of the neck—which increases the chance for successful tube placement. Furthermore, this technique does not require visualization of the glottic opening, so the tube can be placed through copious secretions. Finally, because the patient's head does not need to be in a sniffing position, transillumination can be safely performed in patients with a possible spinal injury.

The major disadvantages of transillumination are the requirement for special equipment—namely, a bright light source at the tip of the malleable stylet as well as being proficient with its use. As a consequence of this requirement, transillumination can be difficult or impossible to perform in brightly lit areas. If you are inside, you may be able to dim the lights and perform this procedure.

Complications

Although transillumination is not an entirely blind technique, the intubator cannot directly visualize the tube passing between the vocal cords. Therefore, misplacement of the tube in the esophagus is the main complication associated with the technique. Pay strict attention to tube confirmation techniques following transilluminated-guided intubation.

Equipment

Whether specifically designed or modified, the single most important piece of equipment required for transillumination-guided intubation is a device with a rigid stylet and a bright light source at the end. Because the light may not always be aimed directly at the skin surface, it should shine laterally as well as forward. The lighted stylet must be long enough to accommodate a standard-length ET tube, and there should be some method of adequately securing the stylet within the tube.

Technique for Transillumination-Guided Intubation

As with any intubation technique, the patient must be preoxygenated for at least 2 to 3 minutes with a bag-valve-mask device and 100% oxygen. Your assistant can perform this task as you prepare your equipment.

Select the appropriately sized ET tube and check the cuff to ensure that it holds air. Lubricate and insert the lighted stylet so that the light is positioned immediately at (but not beyond) the tip of the tube. Ensure that the stylet is firmly seated into the tube.

Prepare the tube by bending it into the proper shape to facilitate entry of the tube into the trachea as well as to ensure that the light will be visible at the anterior neck. The stylet should be straight, with a sharp 90° angle in the tube/stylet just proximal to the cuff. This bend in the tube must be sharp, as it will act as the pivot point when you direct the stylet into the trachea; it will also place the light in the proper position to illuminate the anterior part of the neck.

Place the patient's head in a neutral or slightly extended position. This position will move the epiglottis off the posterior pharyngeal wall and facilitate entry of the ET tube into the glottic opening. Extension of the patient's head will also provide maximum exposure of the anterior part of the neck, enhancing visualization of the lighted stylet under the soft

tissue as it moves down the airway. The intubator is typically positioned at the patient's head.

While holding the lighted stylet in your dominant hand, displace the patient's jaw forwardly by grasping it with your thumb and forefinger. This step will ensure that the epiglottis is not covering the glottic opening. Turn on the lighted stylet and insert the device in the midline of the patient's mouth, with the tip directed toward the laryngeal prominence. The goal is to lift the epiglottis with the ET tube/stylet combination.

As you continue to insert the tube/stylet, draw your wrist toward you. The light should become visible at the midline of the neck. A tightly circumscribed light slightly below the thyroid cartilage indicates that the tip of the tube has entered the trachea. A faintly glowing light and bulging of the soft tissue above the thyroid cartilage indicates that the tip of the tube is in the vallecular space. If this occurs, withdraw the tube slightly, displace the jaw forward, and re-advance the tube/stylet assembly. A dim, diffuse light at the anterior part of the neck typically indicates esophageal placement. In this case, slightly withdraw the tube/stylet assembly and slightly extend the patient's head. You may also consider increasing the angle of the bend in the tube. These actions should reposition the tube/stylet assembly at the glottic opening. If you continue to encounter difficulty, abort the procedure and ventilate the patient with a bag-valve-mask device and 100% oxygen prior to reattempting insertion of the tube/stylet.

Once a bright, tightly circumscribed light is visible at the midline and just below the thyroid cartilage, hold the stylet in place and advance the tube approximately 2 to 4 cm into the trachea. When the tube is securely in the trachea, manually stabilize it in place with your nondominant hand and carefully withdraw the lighted stylet.

Inflate the distal cuff of the ET tube with 5 to 10 ml of air, detach the syringe from the inflation port, and attach the bag-valve-mask device to the ET tube. Ventilate the patient while auscultating over the apices and bases of both lungs and over the epigastrium. Following subjective and objective confirmation of proper tube placement, secure the tube in place with the appropriate device and continue ventilations according to the patient's clinical condition.

The steps for performing intubation with the transillumination technique are listed here and shown in **Skill Drill 11-40 ▸**.

1. Take routine precautions and wear PPE (gloves and face shield at a minimum) (Step 1).
2. Preoxygenate the patient for 2 to 3 minutes with a bag-valve-mask device and 100% oxygen (Step 2).
3. Check, prepare, and assemble your equipment (Step 3).
4. Insert the lighted stylet into the ET tube (Step 4).
5. Bend the ET tube by placing a slight curve at its distal end (like a hockey stick) and turn on the lighted stylet (Step 5).
6. Lift the patient's tongue and mandible anteriorly (Step 6).
7. Insert the ET tube into the midline of the patient's mouth and slowly advance toward the larynx (Step 7).
8. Observe for a tightly circumscribed light at the midline of the neck and advance the ET tube 2 to 4 cm farther (Step 8).

Skill Drill 11-40: Transillumination Intubation

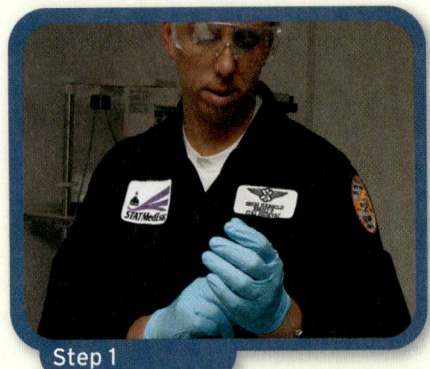

Step 1

Take routine precautions and wear PPE (gloves and face shield at a minimum).

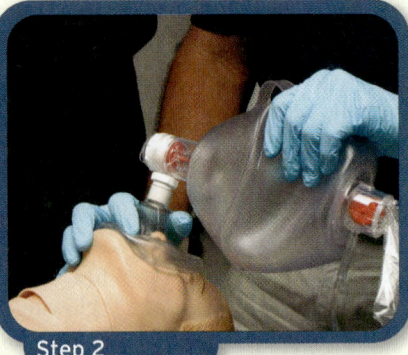

Step 2

Preoxygenate the patient for 2 to 3 minutes with a bag-valve-mask device and 100% oxygen.

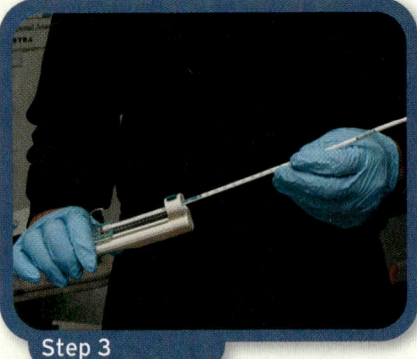

Step 3

Check, prepare, and assemble your equipment.

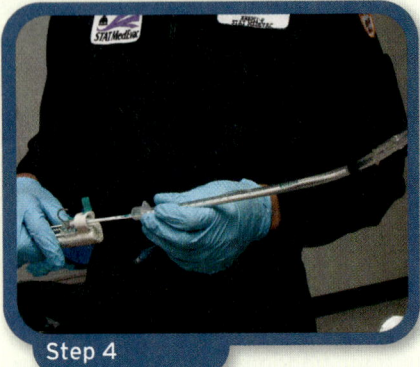

Step 4

Insert the lighted stylet into the ET tube.

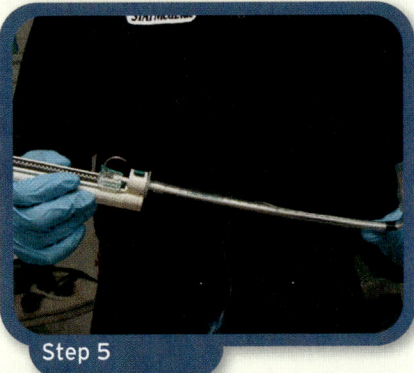

Step 5

Bend the ET tube by placing a slight curve at its distal end (like a hockey stick) and turn on the lighted stylet.

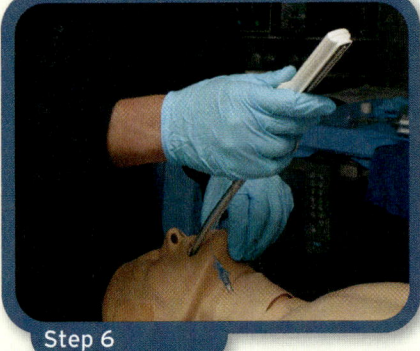

Step 6

Lift the patient's tongue and mandible anteriorly.

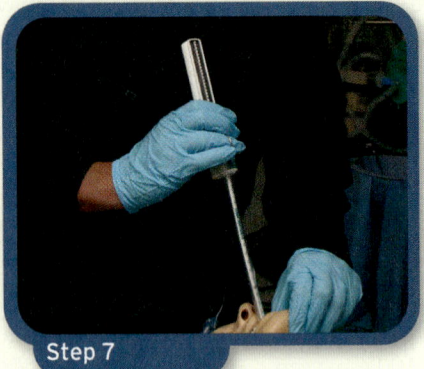

Step 7

Insert the ET tube into the midline of the patient's mouth and slowly advance toward the larynx.

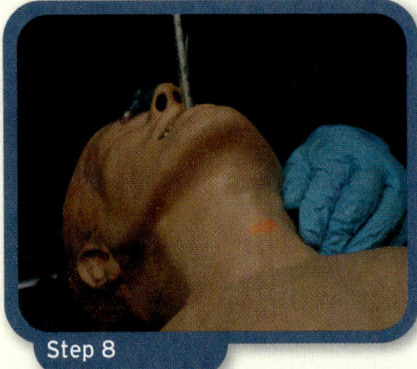

Step 8

Observe for a tightly circumscribed light at the midline of the neck and advance the ET tube 2 to 4 cm farther.

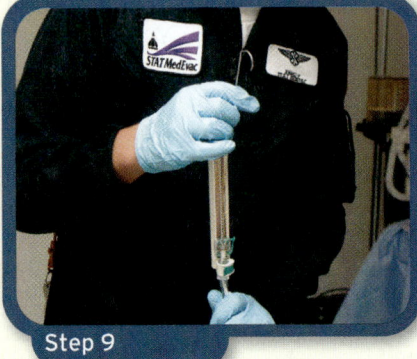

Step 9

Remove the stylet from the ET tube.

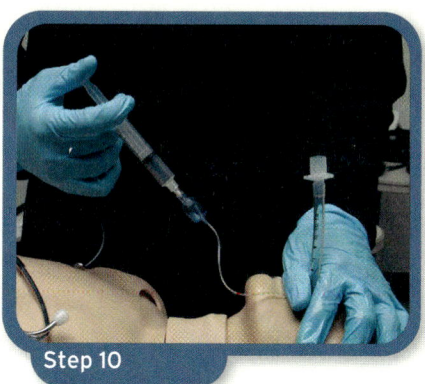

Skill Drill 11-40: Transillumination Intubation (continued)

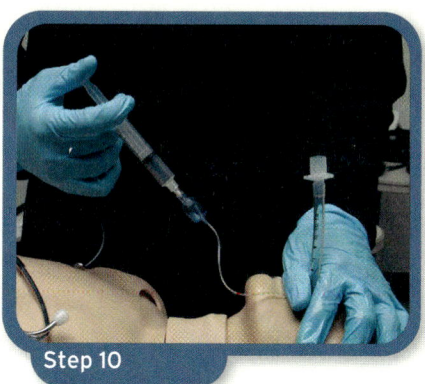

Step 10

Inflate the distal cuff of the ET tube with 5 to 10 ml of air and detach the syringe.

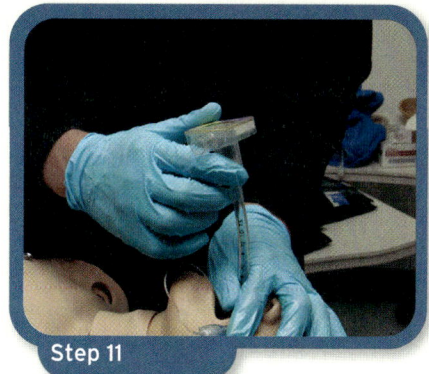

Step 11

Attach the Etco₂ detector to the ET tube.

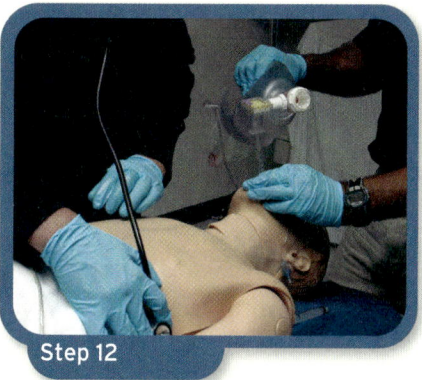

Step 12

Attach the bag-valve-mask device, ventilate, and auscultate over the apices and bases of both lungs and over the epigastrium.

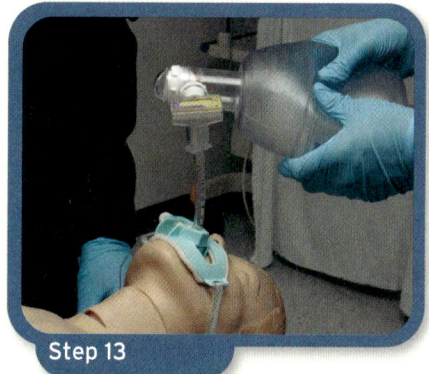

Step 13

Secure the ET tube and recheck breath sounds.

last resort when you are unable to intubate the patient using first-line or rescue devices and are unable to ventilate the patient using bag-valve-mask ventilation. To perform these procedures, you must be familiar with the key anatomical landmarks that lie in the anterior aspect of the neck **Figure 11-86 ▸**.

In addition, you must be familiar with the important blood vessels in this area. The superior cricothyroid vessels run at a transverse angle across the upper third of the cricothyroid membrane. The external jugular veins run vertically and are located lateral to the cricothyroid membrane. If the cricothyroid membrane is incised vertically when performing a cricothyrotomy, the jugular veins can be avoided altogether.

When performing cricothyrotomy, you should expect to encounter some minor bleeding from the subcutaneous and small skin vessels as you incise the cricothyroid membrane. This bleeding should be easily controlled with light pressure after the tube has been inserted into the trachea.

9. Remove the stylet from the ET tube (**Step 9**).
10. Inflate the distal cuff of the ET tube with 5 to 10 ml of air and detach the syringe (**Step 10**).
11. Attach the Etco₂ detector to the ET tube (**Step 11**).
12. Attach the bag-valve-mask device, ventilate, and auscultate over the apices and bases of both lungs and over the epigastrium (**Step 12**).
13. Secure the ET tube (**Step 13**).

Surgical and Nonsurgical Airways

Two methods of securing a patent airway can be used when conventional techniques and methods fail: the open (surgical) cricothyrotomy and translaryngeal cannula ventilation (nonsurgical, or needle cricothyrotomy). These are considered a

Open Cricothyrotomy

Open cricothyrotomy (surgical cricothyrotomy) involves opening the cricothyroid membrane with a scalpel and inserting an endotracheal or tracheostomy tube **Figure 11-87 ▸** directly into the subglottic area (below the vocal cords) of the trachea. The cricothyroid membrane is the ideal site for making a surgical opening into the trachea because no important structures lie between the skin and the airway. The airway at this level lies relatively close to the skin and is easy to enter through the thin cricothyroid membrane. The posterior wall of the airway at this level is formed by the tough cricoid cartilage, which helps prevent accidental perforation through the back of the airway into the esophagus.

Indications and Contraindications

Open cricothyrotomy is indicated only when you are unable to secure a patent airway with more conventional means and are unable to oxygenate and ventilate the patient. *It is not the preferred means of initially securing a patient's airway;*

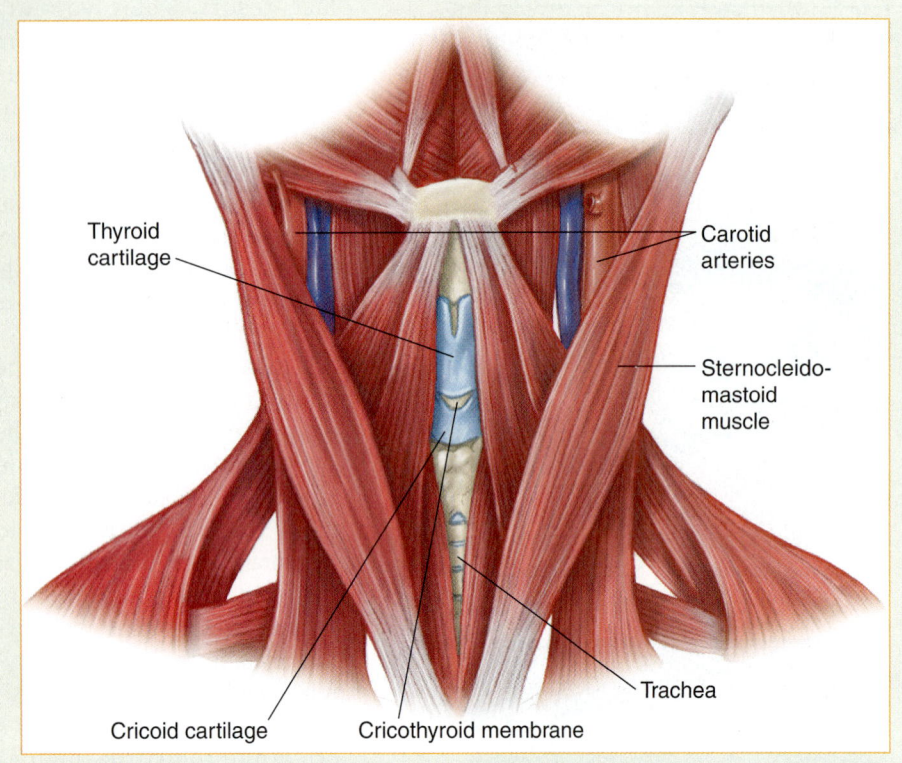

Figure 11-86 Anatomy of the anterior part of the neck.

Thyroid cartilage
Carotid arteries
Sternocleido-mastoid muscle
Cricoid cartilage
Cricothyroid membrane
Trachea

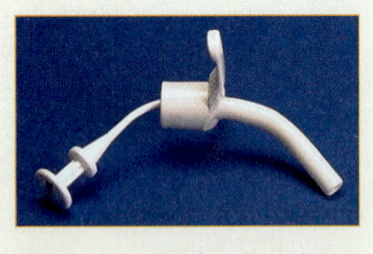

Figure 11-87 Tracheostomy tube.

to identify the correct anatomical landmarks (cricothyroid membrane), crushing injuries to the larynx and tracheal transection, underlying anatomical abnormalities (eg, trauma, tumours, or subglottic stenosis), and age younger than 8 years. The larynx of a small child is generally unable to support a tube large enough to produce effective ventilation without causing damage to the larynx; you would be safer performing a needle cricothyrotomy (discussed later in this chapter) in young children.

In situations where cricothyrotomy is contraindicated, the paramedic must rapidly transport the patient to the closest appropriate facility, where an emergency tracheostomy can be performed.

Advantages and Disadvantages

Open cricothyrotomy can be performed quickly, is technically easier than performing a tracheostomy, and can be performed without manipulating the cervical spine. The latter characteristic is especially advantageous because many cricothyrotomies involve patients with massive facial trauma.

Disadvantages of cricothyrotomy include difficulty in performing the procedure in children (younger than 8 years) and in patients with short, muscular, or fat necks. In contrast to needle cricothyrotomy, an open cricothyrotomy is more difficult to perform; however, inserting a large-bore tube (eg, an ET tube or tracheostomy tube) enables you to achieve greater tidal volume, which facilitates more effective oxygenation and ventilation.

rather it is considered a last resort when all other attempts and methods have failed. For example, if you are unable to intubate a patient but can provide effective bag-valve-mask ventilations, cricothyrotomy would not be appropriate.

It is also an appropriate method to secure a patent airway in the setting of a severe foreign body upper airway obstruction that cannot be extracted with Magill forceps and direct laryngoscopy, airway obstructions from swelling (eg, epiglottitis, anaphylaxis, upper airway burns), massive maxillofacial trauma, and the inability to open the patient's mouth. Patients with massive maxillofacial trauma **Figure 11-88 ▶** often have associated mandibular fractures, which makes it extremely difficult to maintain an effective mask-to-face seal with a bag-valve-mask device. Intubation in these patients would also be extremely difficult due to posterior tongue lacerations with profuse bleeding. In such cases, frequent suctioning to prevent aspiration would delay intubation and increase patient hypoxia.

As noted earlier, the main contraindications for open cricothyrotomy are the ability to secure a patent airway by less invasive means or lack of familiarity and training to perform a cricothyrotomy. Other contraindications include inability

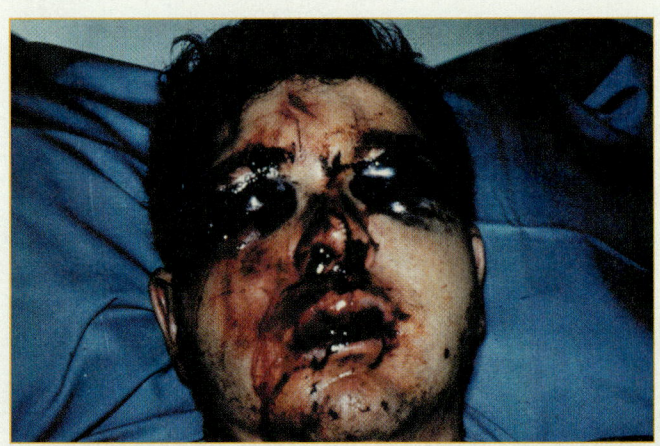

Figure 11-88 Patients with massive maxillofacial trauma often have mandibular fractures or profuse oral bleeding, both of which can make bag-valve-mask ventilations or intubation extremely difficult, if not impossible, to perform.

Complications

You should expect some minor bleeding when performing an open cricothyrotomy. More severe bleeding is usually the result of inadvertent laceration of the external jugular vein. Incising the cricothyroid membrane vertically, instead of horizontally, will minimize this potential complication. It will also minimize the risk of damaging the highly vascular thyroid gland. After the incision has been made, *gently* inserting the tube will minimize the risk of perforating the esophagus or damaging the laryngeal nerves.

An open cricothyrotomy must be performed quickly. Taking too long to complete a cricothyrotomy will result in unnecessary hypoxia to the patient, which may result in cardiac arrhythmias, permanent brain injury, or cardiac arrest.

At the Scene

Frequent practice on a cadaver, if available, or a special cricothyrotomy manikin, will maximize your ability to perform cricothyrotomy quickly. In general, skills that are not frequently performed in the prehospital setting should be routinely practiced to maintain proficiency and competence.

Tube misplacement should be suspected when subcutaneous emphysema is encountered after performing a cricothyrotomy. Subcutaneous emphysema occurs when air infiltrates the subcutaneous (fatty) layers of the skin, and is characterized by a "crackling" sensation when palpated.

Any invasive procedure performed in the prehospital setting carries the risk of infection to the patient. Therefore, you should make all attempts to maintain aseptic technique when performing an open cricothyrotomy.

Equipment

Commercially manufactured cricothyrotomy kits are available **Figure 11-89 ▶**. If such a kit is not available, however, you must prepare the following equipment and supplies:

- Scalpel
- ET tube or tracheostomy tube (6.0 mm minimum)
- Commercial device (or tape) for securing the tube
- Curved hemostats
- Suction apparatus
- Sterile gauze pads for minor bleeding control
- Bag-valve-mask device attached to 100% oxygen

Technique for Performing Open Cricothyrotomy

Once you determine that an open cricothyrotomy is needed, you must proceed rapidly, yet cautiously. Identify the cricothyroid membrane by palpating for the V notch of the thyroid cartilage, which feels like a high, sharp bump. Stabilize the larynx between your thumb and middle fingers while you palpate with your index finger. When you have located the V notch, slide your index finger down into the depression between the thyroid and cricoid cartilage; that is the cricothyroid membrane.

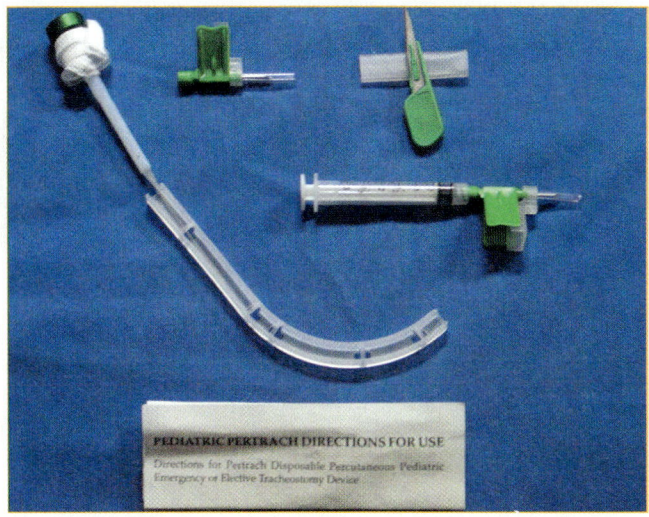

Figure 11-89 Cricothyrotomy kit.

While you are locating and preparing the site, your partner should be preparing your equipment as well as ensuring that the cardiac monitor and pulse oximeter are attached to the patient.

Maintain aseptic technique as you cleanse the area with an antiseptic cleaning solution; avoid touching the area once cleansed. While stabilizing the larynx with one hand, make a 1- to 2-cm vertical incision over the cricothyroid membrane. Some advocate making an additional 1-cm incision horizontally across the membrane to facilitate easier placement of the tube. If you elect to do so, remember that the thyroid gland and external jugular veins are lateral to the area and can be damaged if the horizontal incision is too long. Once the incision has been made, insert the curved hemostats into the opening and spread it apart. Your partner should be readily available to control any bleeding that might occur.

With the trachea exposed, gently insert a 6.0-mm cuffed ET tube or a 6.0 tracheostomy tube and direct it into the trachea. Once the tube is in place, inflate the distal cuff with the appropriate volume of air. Attach the bag-valve-mask device to the standard 15/22-mm adapter on the tube and ventilate the patient while your partner auscultates to ensure the absence of epigastric sounds, as well as the presence of bilaterally clear breath sounds. If epigastric sounds are heard, you have likely perforated and inadvertently inserted the tube into the esophagus.

Additional confirmation of correct tube placement can be accomplished by attaching an $EtCO_2$ detector in between the tube and bag-valve-mask device. After confirming proper tube placement, ensure that any minor bleeding has been controlled, properly secure the tube, continue to ventilate the patient at the appropriate rate, and transport as soon as possible.

The steps for performing an open cricothyrotomy are listed here and shown in **Skill Drill 11-41 ▶**.

1. Take routine precautions and wear PPE (gloves and face shield at a minimum) **Step 1**.
2. Check, assemble, and prepare the equipment **Step 2**.

Skill Drill 11-41: Performing an Open Cricothyrotomy

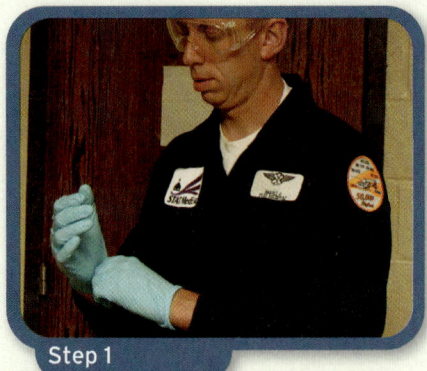

Step 1

Take routine precautions and wear PPE (gloves and face shield at a minimum).

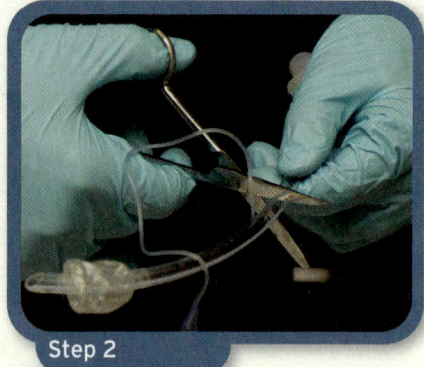

Step 2

Check, assemble, and prepare the equipment.

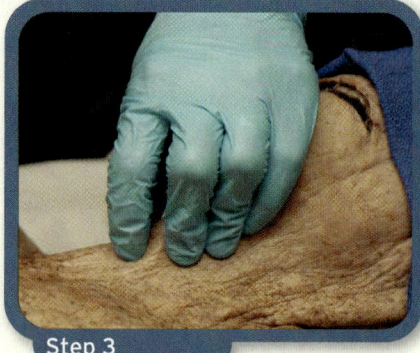

Step 3

With the patient's head in a neutral position, palpate for and locate the cricothyroid membrane.

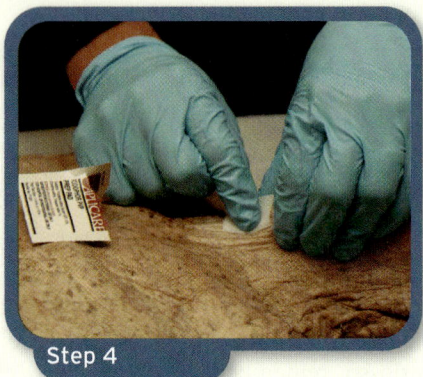

Step 4

Cleanse the area with an antiseptic cleaning solution.

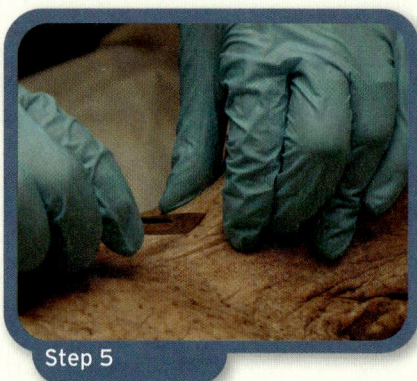

Step 5

Stabilize the larynx and make a 1- to 2-cm vertical incision over the cricothyroid membrane.

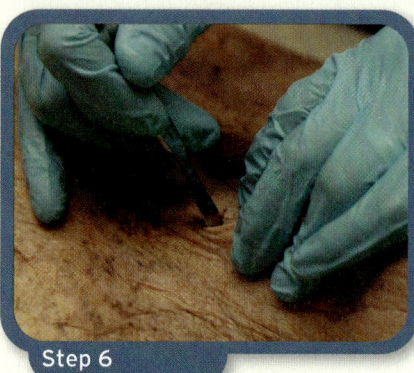

Step 6

Puncture the cricothyroid membrane and make a horizontal cut 1 cm in each direction from the midline.

3. With the patient's head in a neutral position, palpate for and locate the cricothyroid membrane (Step 3).

4. Cleanse the area with an antiseptic cleaning solution (Step 4).

5. Stabilize the larynx and make a 1- to 2-cm vertical incision over the cricothyroid membrane (Step 5).

6. Puncture the cricothyroid membrane and make a horizontal cut 1 cm in each direction from the midline (Step 6).

7. Spread the incision apart with curved hemostats (Step 7).

8. Insert the tube into the trachea (Step 8).

9. Inflate the distal cuff of the tube (Step 9).

10. Attach an $EtCO_2$ detector in between the tube and the bag-valve-mask device (Step 10).

11. Ventilate the patient and confirm correct tube placement by auscultating the apices and bases of both lungs and over the epigastrium (Step 11).

12. Secure the tube with a commercial device or tape. Reconfirm correct tube placement and resume ventilations at the appropriate rate (Step 12). Transport as soon as possible.

Needle Cricothyrotomy

Needle cricothyrotomy also uses the cricothyroid membrane as an entry point into the airway. In this procedure, a 14- to 16-gauge over-the-needle IV catheter (angiocath) is inserted through the cricothyroid membrane and into the trachea. Adequate oxygenation and ventilation are then achieved by attaching a high-pressure jet ventilator Figure 11-90 ▶ to the hub of the catheter. Known as translaryngeal catheter ventilation, this procedure is commonly used as a temporary measure until a more definitive airway can be obtained (eg, via open cricothyrotomy or tracheostomy).

Skill Drill 11-41: Performing an Open Cricothyrotomy (*continued*)

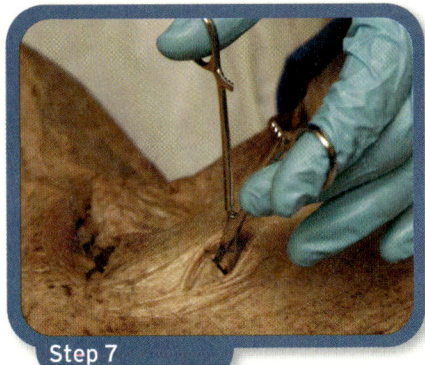

Step 7

Spread the incision apart with curved hemostats.

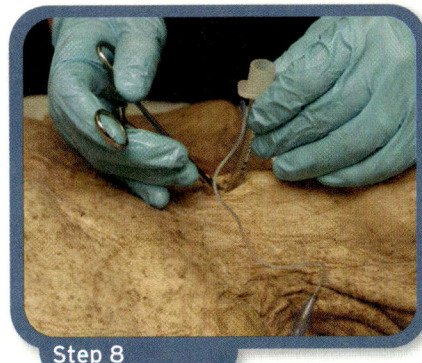

Step 8

Insert the tube into the trachea.

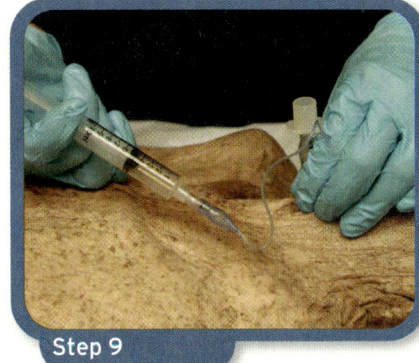

Step 9

Inflate the distal cuff of the tube.

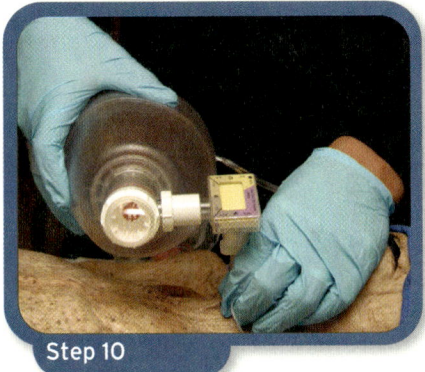

Step 10

Attach an $Etco_2$ detector in between the tube and the bag-valve-mask device.

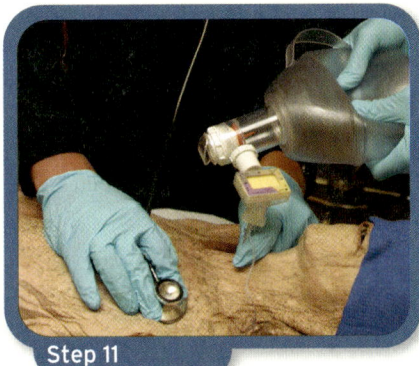

Step 11

Ventilate the patient and confirm correct tube placement by auscultating the apices and bases of both lungs and over the epigastrium.

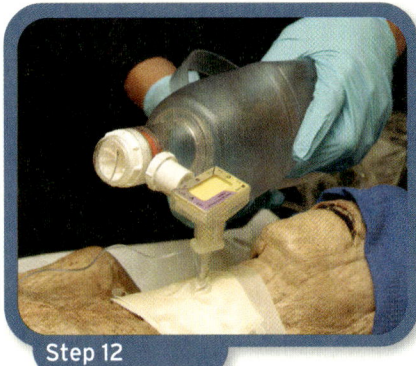

Step 12

Secure the tube with a commercial device or tape. Reconfirm correct tube placement and resume ventilations at the appropriate rate.

Indications and Contraindications

The indications for needle cricothyrotomy and translaryngeal catheter ventilation are the inability to ventilate the patient by other, less invasive techniques such as bag-valve-mask or the LMA. Needle cricothyrotomy is indicated only when you are unable to secure a patent airway with more conventional means and are unable to oxygenate and ventilate the patient. It is not the preferred means of initially securing a patient's airway; it is a last resort when all other attempts and all methods have failed.

It is also an appropriate method to oxygenate the patient in the setting of a complete foreign body upper airway obstruction that cannot be extracted with Magill forceps and direct laryngoscopy, airway obstructions from swelling (eg, epiglottitis, anaphylaxis, upper airway burns), massive maxillofacial trauma, and the inability to open the patient's mouth. In these situations, there is an anatomical cause resulting in an inability to intubate and ventilate. Needle cricothyrotomy is

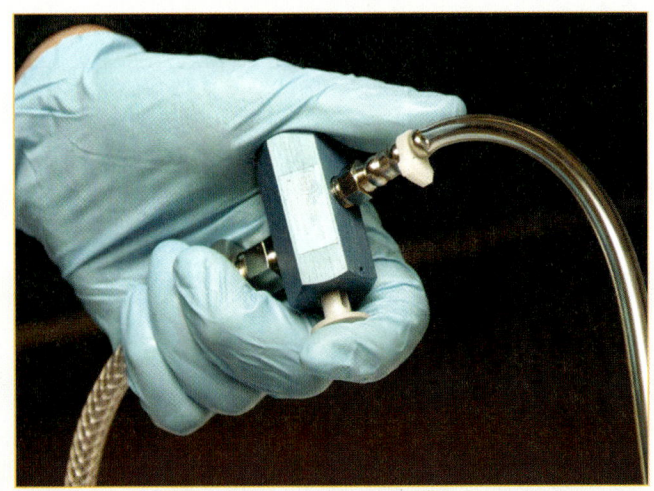

Figure 11-90 High-pressure jet ventilator.

contraindicated in patients who have a complete airway obstruction above the site of catheter insertion.

Unlike all other initial and rescue airway devices, needle cricothyrotomy and transtracheal ventilation only oxygenate the patient (ie, provide adequate oxygenation). These techniques do not adequately ventilate (ie, allow exhalation of carbon dioxide in adequate quantities). As a result, the patient's $PaCO_2$ and end-tidal CO_2 will rise quickly with these forms of ventilation. Therefore, this is strictly a temporary measure, requiring emergent transport to the hospital for a more definitive airway.

In addition, the high-pressure ventilator used with needle cricothyrotomy increases intrathoracic pressure, thus resulting in barotrauma and a potential pneumothorax. Barotrauma can also be caused by overinflation of the lungs with the jet ventilator, so care must be taken to open the release valve only until the patient's chest adequately rises.

If the equipment necessary to perform translaryngeal catheter ventilation is not immediately available, you should opt to perform another rescue airway technique.

Advantages and Disadvantages

Compared with an open cricothyrotomy, needle cricothyrotomy is faster and technically easier to perform. In particular, it is associated with a lower risk of causing damage to adjacent structures because you are puncturing the cricothyroid membrane with an IV catheter—not incising it with a scalpel. Needle cricothyrotomy also allows for subsequent intubation attempts because it uses a small-bore catheter, thus allowing an ET tube to easily pass beside it. This could be particularly beneficial if you do not have the equipment or protocols to perform an open cricothyrotomy. In addition, this procedure does not require manipulation of the patient's cervical spine.

There are, however, some disadvantages to performing a needle cricothyrotomy. Using a smaller-bore tube (angiocath) to ventilate the patient does not provide protection from aspiration as an ET tube or tracheostomy tube. (A larger-bore tube, combined with the distal cuff, would fill the diameter of the trachea, protecting it from esophageal regurgitation.) Also, this

At the Scene

If you do not have a transtracheal jet ventilator available, but have the requisite training and certification to perform needle cricothyrotomy, there is an alternative—albeit less effective—method of ventilating the patient via needle cricothyrotomy. Attach a 7- to 7.5-mm ET tube adapter into the barrel of a 10-ml syringe. Next, connect the syringe to the IV catheter that has been inserted into the cricothyroid membrane. Connect the bag-valve-mask device to the ET tube adapter and begin ventilations. Although you will not be able to deliver nearly the tidal volume as would be possible with a jet ventilator, this approach may be your only alternative to provide some oxygenation and ventilation until a more definitive airway can be achieved at the emergency department.

technique requires a specialized, high-pressure jet ventilator to deliver adequate tidal volume. This jet ventilator will expend high volumes of oxygen very rapidly.

Complications

Improper catheter placement can result in severe bleeding secondary to damage of adjacent structures. Even if the catheter is correctly placed, excessive air leakage around the insertion site can cause subcutaneous emphysema, especially if the patient has undetected laryngeal trauma. If too much air infiltrates into the subcutaneous space, compression of the trachea and subsequent obstruction may occur.

Extreme care must be exercised when ventilating the patient with a jet ventilator. The release valve should be opened just long enough for adequate chest rise to occur. Overinflation of the lungs can result in barotrauma, which carries the risk of pneumothorax. Conversely, opening the release valve for too short a period of time could cause hypoventilation, resulting in inadequate oxygenation and ventilation.

Equipment

The following pieces of equipment are needed to perform needle cricothyrotomy and translaryngeal cannula ventilation:

- Large-bore IV catheter (14 to 16 gauge)
- 10-ml syringe
- 3 ml of sterile water or saline
- Oxygen source (50 psi)
- High-pressure jet ventilator device and oxygen tubing

Technique for Performing Needle Cricothyrotomy

In preparing your equipment, draw up approximately 3 ml of sterile water or saline into a 10-ml syringe and attach the syringe to the IV catheter. Next, place the patient's head in a neutral position and locate the cricothyroid membrane. If time permits, cleanse the area with an antiseptic cleaning solution.

While you are stabilizing the patient's larynx, carefully insert the needle into the midline of the cricothyroid membrane at a 45° angle toward the feet (caudally). You should feel a pop as the needle penetrates the membrane. After the pop is felt, insert the needle approximately 1 cm farther, and then aspirate with the syringe. If the catheter has been correctly placed, you should be able to easily aspirate air and see the saline or water bubbling within the syringe. If blood is aspirated or if you meet resistance, you should reevaluate catheter placement because it is likely outside the trachea.

After confirming correct placement, advance the catheter over the needle until the catheter 0hub is flush with the skin, then withdraw the needle and place it in a puncture-proof biohazard container. Next, attach one end of the oxygen tubing to the catheter and the other end to the jet ventilator.

Begin ventilations by opening the release valve on the jet ventilator and observing for adequate chest rise. Auscultation of breath and epigastric sounds will further confirm correct catheter placement. To prevent overexpansion of the lungs and subsequent barotrauma, turn the release valve off as soon as you see the chest rise. Exhalation will occur passively via the glottis. Ventilate the patient as dictated by his or her clinical condition.

Secure the catheter by placing a folded gauze pad under the catheter and taping it in place. Continue ventilations while frequently reassessing the patient for adequacy of ventilations as well as for potential complications (eg, subcutaneous emphysema from incorrect placement).

The steps for performing needle cricothyrotomy with translaryngeal catheter ventilation are listed here and shown in **Skill Drill 11-42 ▶**.

1. Take routine precautions and wear PPE (gloves and face shield at a minimum) **Step 1**.
2. Attach a 14- to 16-gauge IV catheter to a 10-ml syringe containing approximately 3 ml of sterile saline or water **Step 2**.
3. With the patient's head in a neutral position, palpate for and locate the cricothyroid membrane **Step 3**.
4. Cleanse the area with an antiseptic cleaning solution **Step 4**.
5. Stabilize the larynx and insert the needle into the cricothyroid membrane at a 45° angle toward the feet **Step 5**.
6. Aspirate with the syringe to determine correct catheter placement **Step 6**.
7. Slide the catheter off of the needle until the hub of the catheter is flush with the patient's skin **Step 7**.
8. Place the syringe and needle in a puncture-proof container **Step 8**.
9. Connect one end of the oxygen tubing to the catheter and the other end to the jet ventilator **Step 9**.
10. Open the release valve on the jet ventilator and adjust the pressure accordingly to provide adequate chest rise **Step 10**.
11. Auscultate the apices and bases of both lungs and over the epigastrium to confirm correct catheter placement **Step 11**.
12. Secure the catheter with a gauze pad and tape. Continue ventilations while frequently reassessing for adequate ventilations and any potential complications **Step 12**. Transport as soon as possible.

Special Patient Considerations

Laryngectomy, Tracheostomy, Stoma, and Tracheostomy Tubes

A laryngectomy is a surgical procedure in which the larynx is removed. This procedure is performed by making a tracheostomy (surgical opening into the trachea), thus creating a stoma, an orifice that connects the trachea to the outside air. The tracheal stoma is located in the midline of the anterior part of the neck. Surgical removal of the entire larynx is called total laryngectomy. A person who has had this procedure is a laryngectomee, or "neck breather"—he or she breathes through the hole in his or her neck. Because there is no longer any connection between the patient's pharynx and lower airway, you cannot ventilate such a patient by the mouth-to-mouth or mouth-to-nose technique. The air blown into the mouth or nose can only go down the esophagus into the stomach; it will not reach the lower airway.

A partial laryngectomy entails surgical removal of a portion of the larynx. People who have had this procedure are called "partial neck breathers"—they breathe through *both* the stoma and the nose or mouth. In practice, you may not be able to tell if an apneic laryngectomee is a neck breather or only a partial neck breather until you attempt artificial ventilation.

Suctioning of a Stoma

You may encounter patients who require suctioning of thick secretions from the stoma. Failure to recognize and identify these patients could result in hypoxia. It is not uncommon for a patient's stoma to become occluded with mucous plugs. Patients with laryngectomies possess a less efficient cough; therefore, they will have difficulty spontaneously clearing the stoma by themselves.

Suctioning of the patient's stoma must be performed with extreme care, especially if laryngeal swelling is suspected. Even the slightest irritation of the tracheal wall can result in a violent laryngospasm and complete airway closure. Limit suctioning of the stoma to 10 seconds.

The steps for suctioning a stoma are listed here and shown in **Skill Drill 11-43 ▶**.

1. Take routine precautions and wear PPE (gloves and face shield at a minimum) **Step 1**.
2. Preoxygenate the patient with a bag-valve-mask device and 100% oxygen **Step 2**.
3. Inject 3 ml of sterile saline through the stoma and into the trachea **Step 3**.
4. Instruct the patient to exhale, and insert the catheter (without providing suction) until resistance is felt (no more than 12 cm) **Step 4**.
5. Suction while withdrawing the catheter as you instruct the patient to cough or exhale **Step 5**.
6. Resume oxygenating the patient with a bag-valve-mask device and 100% oxygen **Step 6**.

Ventilation of Stoma Patients

Neither the head tilt–chin lift nor the jaw-thrust maneuver is required for ventilating a patient with a stoma. If the patient has a stoma and no tracheostomy tube in place, ventilations can be performed using the mouth-to-stoma (with a resuscitation mask) technique or with a bag-valve-mask device. Regardless of the technique used, you should use an infant- or child-size mask to make an adequate seal over the stoma. Seal the patient's nose and mouth with one hand to prevent the leakage of air up the trachea. Release the seal of the patient's mouth and nose following each ventilation, allowing exhalation to occur through the upper airway. Two paramedics are needed to perform bag-valve-mask device-to-stoma ventilations: one to seal the nose and mouth and the other to squeeze the bag-valve-mask device. If you are unable to ventilate a patient who has a stoma, try suctioning the stoma and mouth with a French or soft-tip catheter before providing artificial ventilation through the nose and

Skill Drill 11-42: Performing Needle Cricothyrotomy and Translaryngeal Cannula Ventilation

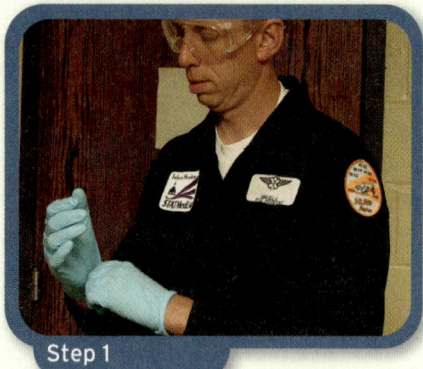

Step 1

Take routine precautions and wear PPE (gloves and face shield at a minimum).

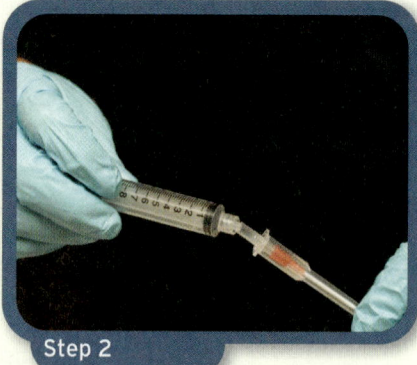

Step 2

Attach a 14- to 16-gauge IV catheter to a 10-ml syringe containing approximately 3 ml of sterile saline or water.

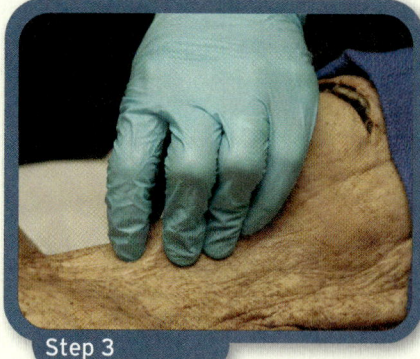

Step 3

With the patient's head in a neutral position, palpate for and locate the cricothyroid membrane.

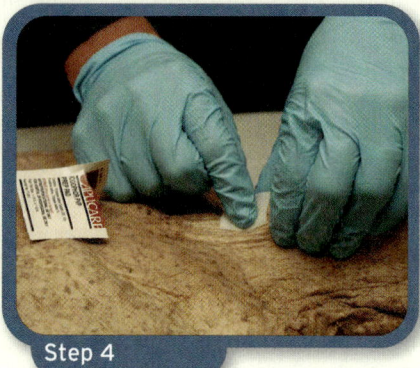

Step 4

Cleanse the area with an antiseptic cleaning solution.

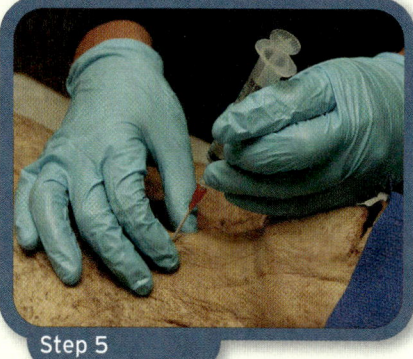

Step 5

Stabilize the larynx and insert the needle into the cricothyroid membrane at a 45° angle toward the feet.

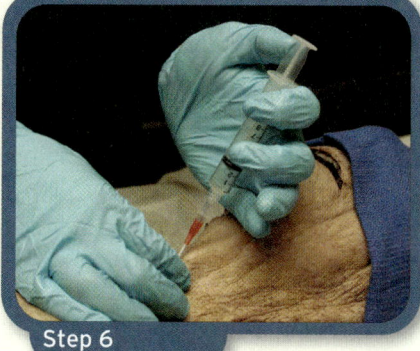

Step 6

Aspirate with the syringe to determine correct catheter placement.

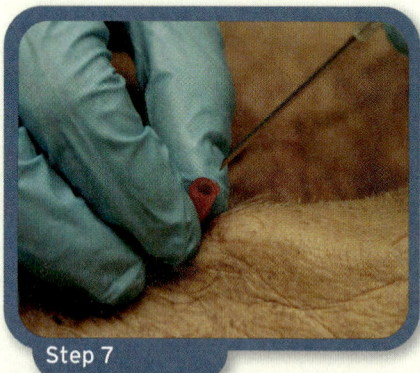

Step 7

Slide the catheter off of the needle until the hub of the catheter is flush with the patient's skin.

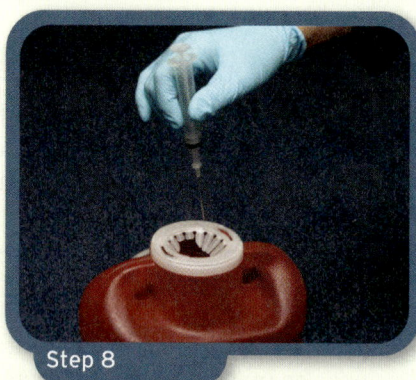

Step 8

Place the syringe and needle in a puncture-proof container.

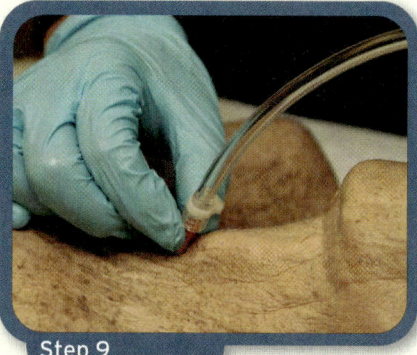

Step 9

Connect one end of the oxygen tubing to the catheter and the other end to the jet ventilator.

Skill Drill 11-42: Performing Needle Cricothyrotomy and Translaryngeal Cannula Ventilation (*continued*)

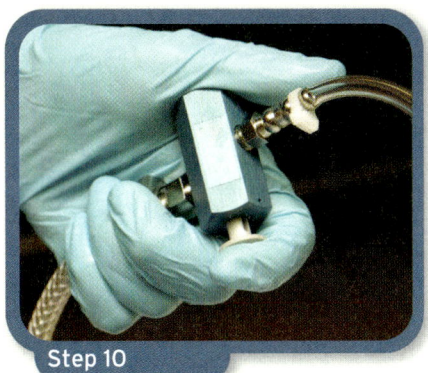

Step 10

Open the release valve on the jet ventilator and adjust the pressure accordingly to provide adequate chest rise.

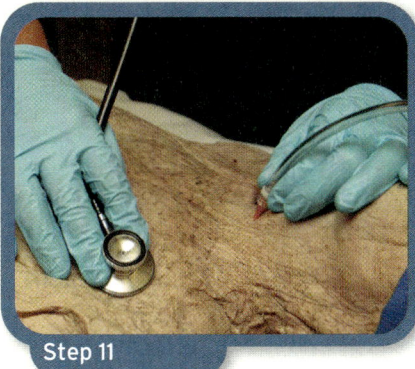

Step 11

Auscultate the apices and bases of both lungs and over the epigastrium to confirm correct catheter placement.

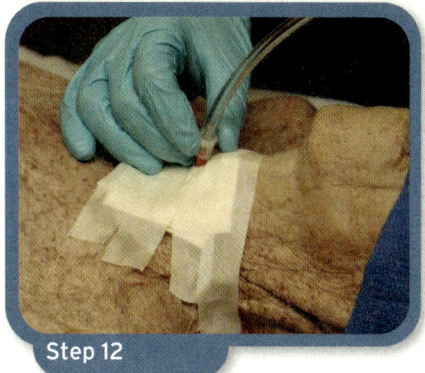

Step 12

Secure the catheter with a gauze pad and tape. Continue ventilations while frequently reassessing for adequate ventilations and any potential complications.

Skill Drill 11-43: Suctioning of a Stoma

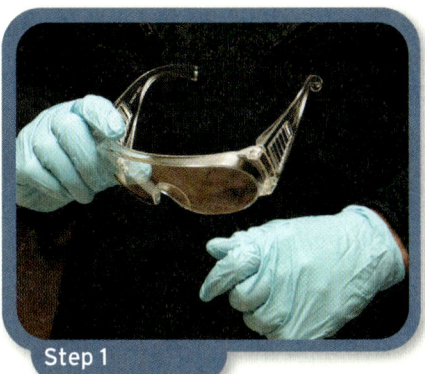

Step 1

Take routine precautions and wear PPE (gloves and face shield at a minimum).

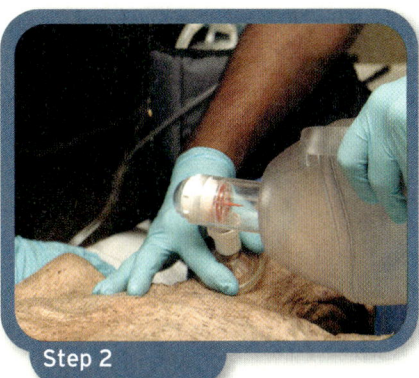

Step 2

Preoxygenate the patient with a bag-valve-mask device and 100% oxygen.

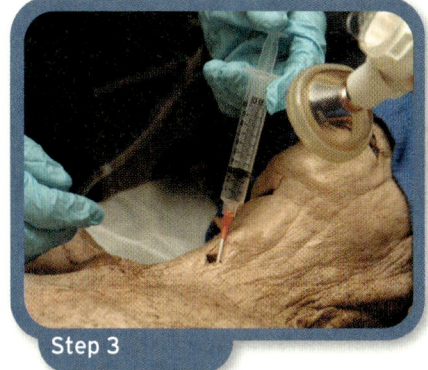

Step 3

Inject 3 ml of saline through the stoma and into the trachea.

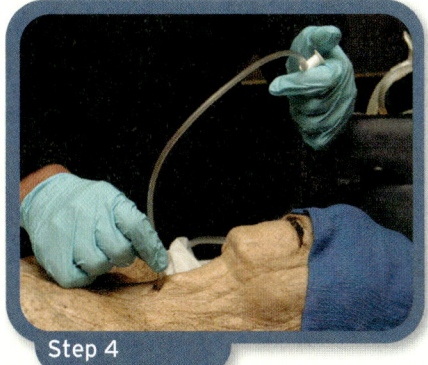

Step 4

Instruct the patient to exhale, and insert the catheter (without providing suction) until resistance is felt (no more than 12 cm).

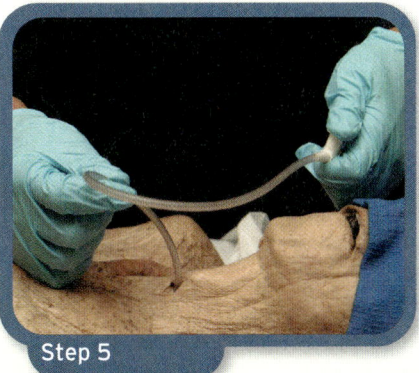

Step 5

Suction while withdrawing the catheter as you instruct the patient to cough or exhale.

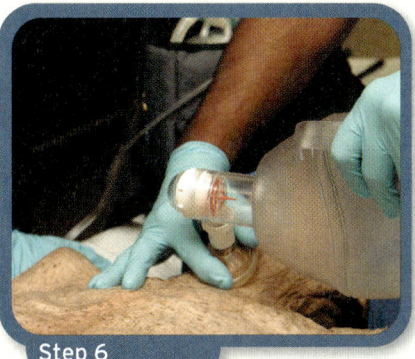

Step 6

Resume oxygenating the patient with a bag-valve-mask device and 100% oxygen.

mouth. If you seal the stoma during ventilation, the ability to artificially ventilate the patient in this way may be improved, or it may help to clear any obstructions.

The steps for performing bag-valve-mask device-to-stoma ventilation are listed here and shown in **Skill Drill 11-44 ▸** .

1. With the patient's head in a neutral position, locate and expose the stoma **Step 1** .

2. Place the bag-valve-mask device over the stoma and ensure an adequate seal **Step 2** .

3. Ventilate the patient by squeezing the bag-valve-mask device, and assess for adequate ventilation by observing chest rise and feeling for air leaks when using a mask. Seal the mouth and nose if an air leak is evident from the upper airway **Step 3** .

4. Auscultate over the lungs to confirm adequate ventilation **Step 4** .

Tracheostomy Tubes

A tracheostomy tube is a plastic tube placed within the tracheostomy site (stoma) **Figure 11-91 ▸** . It requires a 15/22-mm adapter to be compatible with ventilatory devices, such as a mechanical ventilator or bag-valve-mask device. Patients with a tracheostomy tube may receive supplemental oxygen via tubing designed to fit over the tube or by placing an oxygen mask over the tube. Ventilation is accomplished by simply attaching the bag-valve-mask device to the tracheostomy tube.

Patients with a tracheostomy tube who experience sudden dyspnea often have thick secretions in the tube. In this case, perform suctioning through the tracheostomy tube as you would through a stoma.

When a tracheostomy tube becomes dislodged, stenosis (narrowing) of the stoma may occur. Stenosis is potentially life-threatening because soft-tissue swelling decreases the stoma's diameter and impairs the patient's ventilatory ability. In such cases, you may not be able to replace the tracheostomy tube itself and may have to insert an ET tube into the stoma before it becomes totally occluded. Because the patient with the stoma already has a significant medical problem (eg, brain injury, chronic respiratory insufficiency), he or she may be less tolerant of even brief periods of hypoxia.

Skill Drill 11-44: Bag-Valve-Mask Device-to-Stoma Ventilation

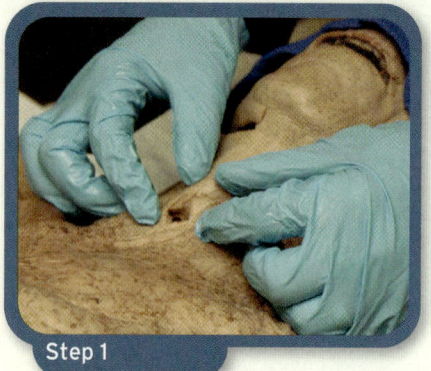
Step 1
With the patient's head in a neutral position, locate and expose the stoma.

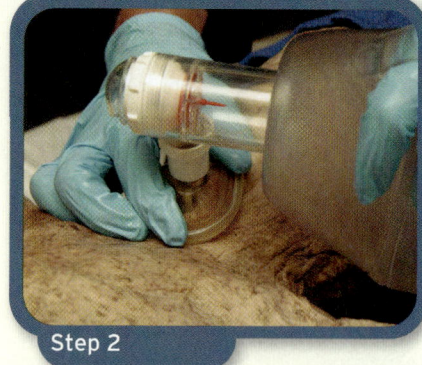
Step 2
Place the bag-valve-mask device over the stoma and ensure an adequate seal.

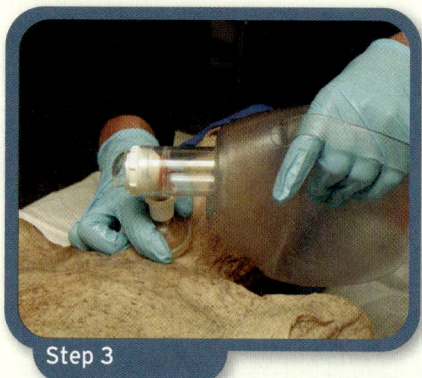
Step 3
Ventilate the patient by squeezing the bag-valve-mask device, and assess for adequate ventilation by observing chest rise.

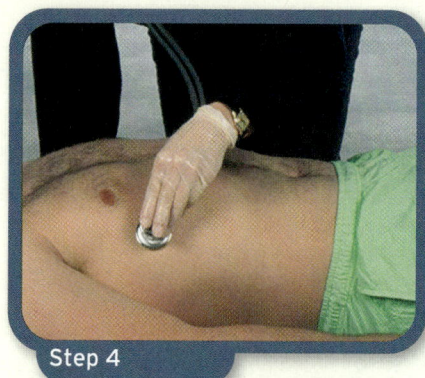
Step 4
Auscultate over the lungs to confirm adequate ventilation.

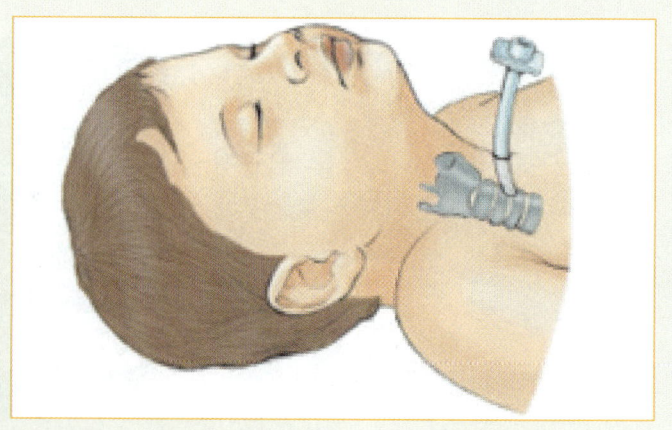
Figure 11-91 A tracheostomy tube.

Skill Drill 11-45: Replacing a Dislodged Tracheostomy Tube

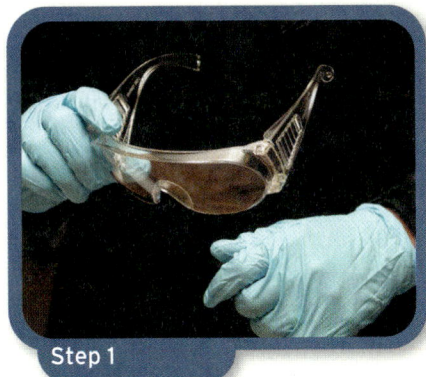

Step 1

Take routine precautions and wear PPE (gloves and face shield at a minimum).

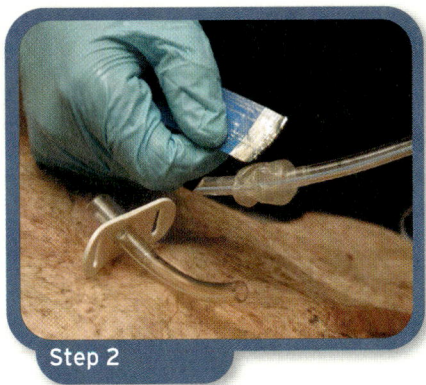

Step 2

Lubricate the same-sized tracheostomy tube or an ET tube (at least 5.0 mm).

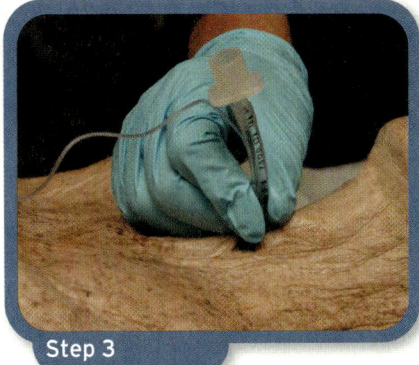

Step 3

Instruct the patient to exhale, and gently insert the tube approximately 1 to 2 cm beyond the balloon cuff.

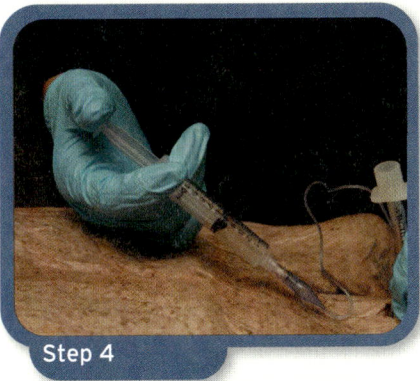

Step 4

Inflate the balloon cuff.

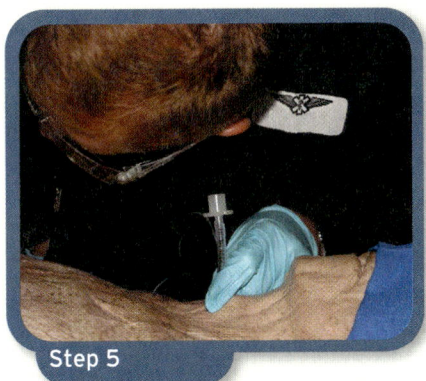

Step 5

Ensure that the patient is comfortable, and confirm patency and proper placement of the tube by listening for air movement from the tube and noting the patient's clinical status. Ensure that a false lumen was not created.

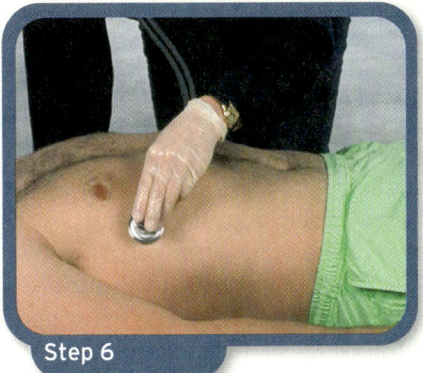

Step 6

Auscultate the lungs to confirm correct tube placement.

The steps for replacing a dislodged tracheostomy tube are listed here and shown in **Skill Drill 11-45 ▲**.

1. Take routine precautions and wear PPE (gloves and face shield at a minimum) **Step 1**.
2. Lubricate the same-sized tracheostomy tube or an ET tube (at least 5.0 mm) **Step 2**.
3. Instruct the patient to exhale, and gently insert the tube approximately 1 to 2 cm beyond the balloon cuff **Step 3**.
4. Inflate the balloon cuff **Step 4**.
5. Ensure that the patient is comfortable, and confirm patency and proper placement of the tube by listening for air movement from the tube and noting the patient's clinical status. Ensure that a false lumen was not created **Step 5**.
6. Auscultate the lungs to confirm correct tube placement **Step 6**.

Dental Appliances

Dental appliances, which are frequently encountered in the elderly population, can take many different forms: dentures (upper, lower, or both), bridges, individual teeth, and braces (in the younger population). When assessing the airway of a patient with a dental appliance, especially one who is semiconscious or unconscious, you must determine whether the appliance is loose or fitting well. If the dental appliance fits well, leave it in place. A well-fitting appliance helps to maintain the face's structure, facilitating an effective mask-to-face seal if the patient requires ventilation via pocket mask or bag-valve-mask device. If the appliance is loose, however, it could easily become an airway obstruction, and should be removed.

If the unconscious patient has an airway obstruction caused by a dental appliance, perform the usual steps in clearing an obstruction, such as chest compressions, direct laryngoscopy, and use of the Magill forceps. Great care must be taken if the obstruction is caused by a bridge; these devices often contain sharp metal ends that can easily lacerate the posterior pharynx or larynx.

Often it is not the dental appliance itself that hinders the paramedic's ability to perform a safe and effective intubation, but rather attempts to identify and remove the device. The paramedic may become overly concerned with the presence of the dental appliance rather than concentrating on performing the intubation. Additionally, the oropharyngeal anatomy may be somewhat distorted by the presence of a dental appliance.

In general, it is best to remove dental appliances before intubating a patient. Once the ET tube is in place and has been secured, removal of the dental appliance will be extremely difficult and dangerous, as it may cause dislodgement of the tube or inflict unnecessary oropharyngeal trauma.

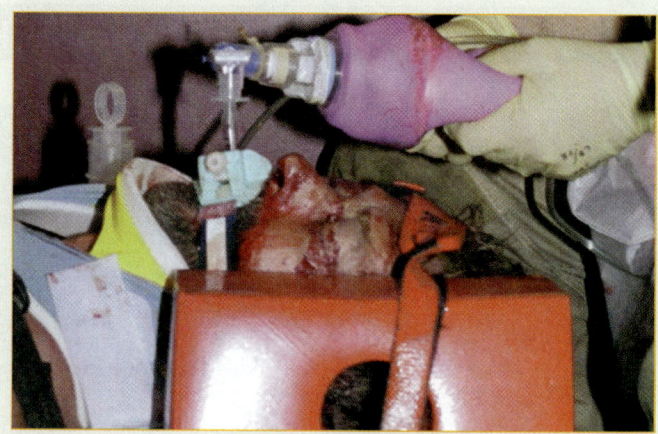

Figure 11-92 Airway management can be especially challenging in patients with facial injuries.

Facial Trauma

It can be especially challenging to effectively manage the airway of a patient with facial injuries **Figure 11-92 ▶**. Because the face is highly vascular, facial trauma can result in severe tissue swelling and bleeding into the airway. Control bleeding with direct pressure and suction the airway as needed. You may encounter a patient with severe facial trauma who is breathing inadequately *and* has severe oropharyngeal bleeding—both problems are life-threatening. This situation is most effectively managed by suctioning the patient's airway for 15 seconds (less in infants and children) and then providing positive-pressure ventilation for 2 minutes. This alternating pattern of suctioning and ventilating should continue until the oral secretions have been cleared or the patient has been intubated.

Facial injuries should also increase your index of suspicion for a cervical spine injury. Therefore, when managing the

airway, use the jaw-thrust maneuver and keep the patient's head in a neutral in-line position. Endotracheal intubation of the trauma patient is most effectively performed by two paramedics—one who maintains neutral in-line stabilization of the patient's head and the other who performs the intubation. An alternative technique, especially if you are the only paramedic managing the patient's airway, is to stabilize the patient's head in a neutral in-line position with your thighs and then perform the intubation.

When ventilating the patient with facial injuries, stay alert for changes in ventilation compliance or sounds that may indicate laryngeal edema (eg, stridor). If you are unable to effectively ventilate or orally intubate the patient with severe facial injuries, perform a cricothyrotomy (surgical or needle).

You are the Paramedic Summary

1. Is this patient's airway patent?

Although the patient is experiencing respiratory distress, he is conscious, alert, and talking in complete sentences. Therefore, his airway appears to be patent *at this time*.

2. How will you proceed with your assessment of this patient?

You have already formed a general impression of the patient as you approached him. You must now perform an initial assessment of the patient to determine if he has any problems with airway, breathing, or circulation that require immediate treatment.

3. What immediate management is indicated for this patient?

Immediate management for this patient includes administering 100% supplemental oxygen via nonrebreathing mask. He is experiencing signs and symptoms of hypoxemia, such as pallor, diaphoresis, tachypnea, and tachycardia. You must closely monitor his respiratory effort and be prepared to assist ventilations if his breathing becomes inadequate (eg, a reduced tidal volume, profoundly laboured breathing).

4. What questions would be pertinent to ask this patient?

During your focused history and physical examination of the patient, you should use the OPQRST mnemonic to question the patient regarding his present illness. Pertinent questions for a patient complaining of dyspnea include the pattern of the problem (acute or chronic), factors that provoke or palliate his respiratory distress (Can he lie flat?), the patient's perception of the severity of his respiratory distress, and the time of onset. Also determine whether the patient has any medical problems that could be causing (or be exacerbated by) his respiratory distress—for example, congestive heart failure, asthma, COPD, or recent pneumonia.

5. Is this patient breathing adequately? Why or why not?

Although his respirations are tachypneic (28 breaths/min) and laboured, his respirations are producing adequate tidal volume at the present time, which suggests that his respiratory effort is adequate. Close monitoring for signs of inadequate breathing is essential, however. You must be prepared to assist ventilations if needed.

6. What are the signs of inadequate ventilation?

Signs of inadequate ventilation include a slow (< 12 breaths/min) or fast (> 20 breaths/min) respiratory rate, reduced tidal volume (shallow breaths), an irregular pattern of inhalation and exhalation, cyanosis, and a decreased mental status.

7. How should you adjust your treatment for this patient? Why?

This patient's respiratory effort is no longer adequate. His level of consciousness has decreased, his heart rate has increased, his respirations have become shallow (reduced tidal volume), and cyanosis is developing around his lips. Additionally, his oxygen saturation is falling despite 100% oxygen via nonrebreathing mask. Therefore, you must begin assisting his ventilations with a bag-valve-mask device and 100% oxygen. Because of his decreased mental status, a nasopharyngeal airway should be inserted to assist in maintaining airway patency.

8. Why is your patient's condition not improving with assisted ventilation?

As evidenced by the patient's gurgling respirations, oral secretions are impairing your ability to effectively ventilate him. Patients with congestive heart failure, especially during periods of exacerbation, frequently cough up pink, frothy sputum. These secretions must be cleared from the airway to allow effective oxygenation and ventilation.

9. What must you do to correct the situation?

When you hear gurgling, think suction! This patient's oropharynx must be suctioned to clear the secretions from his airway, thus improving your ability to effectively oxygenate and ventilate him. This suctioning should not exceed 15 seconds.

If the patient continues to produce oral secretions, you have two problems to manage: aspiration of secretions and inadequate respiratory effort. This is most effectively managed by suctioning the oropharynx for 15 seconds and providing positive-pressure ventilation for 2 minutes. This alternating pattern of suctioning and ventilating should continue until the oral secretions have been removed or the patient's airway has been definitively secured with an ET tube.

10. What is your most appropriate action at this point?

Suctioning the patient's airway has improved his condition (eg, increased Sp_{O_2}, improved mentation, decreased heart rate), but he is still in need of ventilatory assistance and the closest hospital is 40 km away. Immediate transport, with further management en route, is an appropriate intervention. Another option, given this patient's progressive deterioration, would be to proceed with intubation prior to transport rather than trying to manage an unstable airway through a lengthy transport.

11. What are the signs of inadequate artificial ventilation?

Signs of inadequate artificial ventilation include minimal or absent rise of the chest, a heart rate that does not improve, persistent or worsening cyanosis, and a decreasing Sp_{O_2} despite ventilations. Remember, it can be very difficult to ventilate an adult patient with a bag-valve-mask device by yourself, especially if you don't do so on a regular basis. The one-person bag-valve-mask technique takes practice and experience. This is why it is so important to ensure that two paramedics are available to ride in the patient care compartment en route to the hospital for a patient with an unstable airway.

12. What management is required to prevent further deterioration of this patient's condition?

This patient's clinical condition has deteriorated significantly: He is unresponsive, his respirations have slowed, and he is profoundly cyanotic. Your bag-valve-mask ventilations are not effective because of an ineffective mask-to-face seal (a common complication). This patient's airway needs to be definitively secured with an ET tube, before his condition further deteriorates to respiratory or cardiac arrest.

13. Should you extubate this patient? Why or why not?

Absolutely not! The improvement in this patient's clinical condition is the result of your intubation and providing him with 100% oxygen directly into his lungs. There is no guarantee that he will be able to maintain his own airway or you will be able to reintubate him.

14. Are any pharmacologic interventions required?

Instead of extubating a patient and facing the potential risks associated with removal of the tube (eg, laryngospasm, regurgitation with aspiration), it is *safer* and more efficient to sedate the patient. A variety of sedative-hypnotic drugs can be used for this purpose, including midazolam (Versed) and diazepam (Valium). Follow your locally established protocols regarding sedation agents and dosages.

15. What has most likely caused this patient's increased heart rate and decreased Sp_{O_2}?

Acute deterioration in the condition of an intubated patient is usually caused by one of the following: tube dislodgement, obstruction of the tube with secretions, pneumothorax, or equipment failure. Although you hear gurgling in the ET tube, you have already reconfirmed proper placement of the ET tube by auscultation and capnography. The ET tube is probably partially occluded with pulmonary secretions—most likely secondary to the patient's congestive heart failure.

16. How will you remedy the situation?

Occlusion of the ET tube can interfere with effective oxygenation and ventilation of the intubated patient, and must be treated by suctioning the tracheobronchial tree. Preoxygenate the patient for 30 seconds to 1 minute. Inject 3 to 5 ml of sterile saline or water down the ET tube to loosen the secretions, and insert a soft-tip catheter down the ET tube until you meet resistance. Suction in a circular motion while withdrawing the catheter. *Do not exceed 15 seconds during any one suction attempt.* Because suctioning can result in hypoxia, you should closely monitor the patient's cardiac rhythm and oxygen saturation.

17. What treatment would have been appropriate had this clinically unstable patient been too conscious or combative to intubate?

Patients who require intubation, but who are too conscious or combative to tolerate laryngoscopy and tube placement, are candidates for rapid-sequence intubation (RSI), especially if your transport time to the hospital will be lengthy. RSI involves sedating the patient to induce amnesia and suppress the gag reflex. A neuromuscular blocking drug (paralytic) is then given to induce paralysis, facilitating placement of the ET tube. After the patient has been intubated, sedation and paralysis are maintained as needed. RSI is not without risk: You must be absolutely certain that you will be able to intubate the patient once he or she is paralyzed. Follow locally established protocols and/or consult with direct medical control as needed regarding RSI.

Prep Kit

■ Ready for Review

- The upper airway consists of all structures above the vocal cords—the larynx, oropharynx, nasopharynx, and tongue. Its functions include warming, filtering, and humification of inhaled air.

- The lower airway consists of all structures below the vocal cords—the trachea, mainstem bronchi, bronchioles, pulmonary capillaries, and alveoli. Pulmonary gas exchange takes place at the alveolar level in the lungs.

- The diaphragm is the major muscle of breathing; it is innervated by the phrenic nerves. The intercostal muscles, the muscles between the ribs, are innervated by the intercostal nerves. Accessory muscles, which are used during times of respiratory distress, include the sternocleidomastoid muscles of the neck.

- The primary breathing stimulus in a healthy patient is based on increasing arterial carbon dioxide levels. The hypoxic drive—a backup system to breathe—is based on decreasing arterial oxygen levels.

- Ventilation is the movement of air into and out of the lungs. Negative-pressure ventilation is the drawing of air into the lungs due to changes in intrathoracic pressure. Positive-pressure ventilation is the forcing of air into the lungs and is provided via bag-valve-mask device, pocket mask, or mechanical ventilation device to patients who are not breathing (apneic) or are breathing inadequately.

- Manual airway maneuvers include the head tilt–chin lift, jaw-thrust (with and without head tilt), and the tongue-jaw lift.

- Regardless of the patient's condition, his or her airway must remain patent at all times. Clearing the airway means removing obstructing material; maintaining the airway means keeping it open, manually or with adjunctive devices.

- Airway obstruction can be caused by choking on food (or, in children, on toys), epiglottitis, inhalation injuries, airway trauma with swelling, and anaphylaxis. It is critical to differentiate between a mild (partial) airway obstruction and a severe (complete) airway obstruction.

- Chest compressions, finger sweeps (only if the object can be seen and easily retrieved), manual removal of the object, and attempts to ventilate is the recommended sequence of events to attempt to remove a foreign body airway obstruction in the unconscious adult. Abdominal thrusts should be performed continuously in the conscious adult or child with an airway obstruction until the obstruction is relieved or he or she becomes unresponsive.

- Back slaps and chest thrusts are performed to relieve a severe airway obstruction in conscious infants. Chest compressions are performed in unconscious infants with a severe airway obstruction.

- Patients with a mild airway obstruction should be closely monitored and transported. Encourage the patient who is coughing forcefully to continue coughing, as it is the most effective way of clearing the airway.

- If conventional methods of airway obstruction removal fail, perform direct laryngoscopy and attempt to retrieve the object with Magill forceps.

- Basic airway adjuncts include the oropharyngeal (oral) airway and the nasopharyngeal (nasal) airway. The oral airway keeps the tongue off of the posterior pharynx; it is used only in unresponsive patients without a gag reflex. The nasal airway is better tolerated in patients with altered mental status who have an intact gag reflex.

- Oropharyngeal suctioning may be required after opening a patient's airway. Rigid (tonsil-tip) catheters are preferred when suctioning the pharynx. Soft, plastic (whistle-tip) catheters are used to suction secretions from the nose, and can be passed down the endotracheal tube to suction pulmonary secretions.

- Oropharyngeal suction should be limited to 15 seconds in the adult, 10 seconds in the child, and 5 seconds in the infant.

- The recovery position involves placing the patient in a left lateral recumbent position. It is the preferred position to maintain the airway of unconscious patients without traumatic injuries, who are breathing adequately.

- Adequate breathing features a respiratory rate between 12 and 20 breaths/min, adequate depth (tidal volume), a regular pattern of inhalation and exhalation, symmetrical chest rise, and bilaterally clear and equal breath sounds.

- Inadequate breathing features a rate that is too slow (< 12 breaths/min) or too fast (> 20 breaths/min), a shallow depth of breathing (reduced tidal volume), an irregular pattern of inhalation and exhalation, asymmetrical chest movement, adventitious airway sounds, cyanosis, and an altered mental status.

- The nonrebreathing mask is the preferred device for delivering oxygen to adequately breathing patients in the prehospital setting; it can deliver up to 90% oxygen when the flow rate is set at 15 l/min. The nasal catheter should be used if the patient cannot tolerate the nonrebreathing mask; it can deliver oxygen concentrations of 24% to 44% when the flowmeter is set at 1 to 6 l/min. Other types of oxygen delivery devices include the simple face mask, partial rebreathing mask, and Venturi mask.

- The pulse oximeter measures the percentage of blood that is saturated with oxygen (Spo_2). This type of measurement depends on adequate perfusion to the capillary beds and can be inaccurate when the patient is cold, is in shock, or has been exposed to carbon monoxide.

- Peak expiratory flow is a fairly reliable assessment of the severity of a patient's bronchoconstriction. It is also used to gauge the effectiveness of treatment, such as inhaled beta-2 agonists (eg, salbutamol).

- Patients with inadequate breathing require some form of positive-pressure ventilation; patients with adequate breathing who are suspected of being hypoxemic require 100% supplemental oxygen via nonrebreathing mask. Never withhold oxygen from any patient suspected of being hypoxemic.

- Unrecognized inadequate breathing will lead to hypoxia, a dangerous condition in which the body's cells and tissues do not receive adequate oxygen.

- The methods of providing artificial ventilation—in order of preference—include the two-person bag-valve-mask technique; the flow-restricted, oxygen-powered ventilation device (FROPVD); and the one-person bag-valve-mask technique. Use extreme caution with the FROPVD and never use this device in children and those with cervical spine or thoracic injuries.

- Ventilating too forcefully or too fast can cause gastric distension, which can cause regurgitation and aspiration. Delivering ventilations over 1 second and the use of posterior cricoid pressure (Sellick maneuver) will reduce the incidence of gastric distension and the associated risk of regurgitation/aspiration.

- Invasive gastric decompression involves the insertion of a gastric tube into the stomach. A nasogastric (NG) tube is inserted into the stomach via the nose; an orogastric (OG) tube is inserted into the stomach via the mouth.

- Unresponsive patients or patients who cannot maintain their own airway should be considered candidates for endotracheal intubation, the insertion of an endotracheal (ET) tube into the trachea. In orotracheal intubation, the ET tube is inserted into the trachea via the mouth; in nasotracheal intubation (a blind technique), the ET tube is inserted into the trachea via the nose.
- Tracheobronchial suctioning is indicated if the condition of the intubated patient deteriorates due to pulmonary secretions in the ET tube.
- Extubation should not be performed in the prehospital setting unless the patient is unreasonably intolerant of the tube. It is generally best to sedate the intubated patient who is becoming intolerant of the ET tube.
- Alternative airway devices, which may be used if endotracheal intubation is not possible or is unsuccessful, include the Combitube, pharyngeotracheal lumen airway (PtL), and the laryngeal mask airway (LMA), and intubation with the use of a lighted stylet (transillumination).
- Pediatric endotracheal intubation involves the same technique as for adult patients, but with smaller equipment.
- Patients with a tracheal stoma or tracheostomy tube may require ventilation, suctioning, or tube replacement. Ventilation through a tracheostomy tube involves attaching the bag-valve-mask device to the 15/22-mm adapter on the tube; ventilation of the patient with a stoma and no tracheostomy tube can be performed with a pocket mask or bag-valve-mask device. Use pediatric-size masks when ventilating a patient through his or her stoma.
- Open (surgical) cricothyrotomy involves opening the cricothyroid membrane, inserting a tracheostomy tube or ET tube into the trachea, and ventilating the patient with a bag-valve-mask device. Needle cricothyrotomy involves inserting a 14- to 16-gauge over-the-needle catheter through the cricothyroid membrane and ventilating the patient with a high-pressure jet ventilation device.
- Rapid-sequence intubation (RSI) involves using pharmacologic agents to sedate and paralyze the patient to facilitate placement of an ET tube. It should be considered when a conscious or combative patient requires intubation and there are no contraindications.
- Drugs used for RSI include sedatives, hypnotics, and neuromuscular blocking agents (paralytics).
- Check for loose dental appliances in a patient before providing artificial ventilation. Loose dental appliances should be removed to prevent them from obstructing the airway; tight-fitting dental appliances should be left in place during artificial ventilation.
- Dental appliances should be removed before intubating a patient. Removing them after the patient has been intubated may result in inadvertent extubation.
- Patients with massive maxillofacial trauma are at high risk for airway compromise due to oral bleeding. Assist ventilations and provide oral suctioning as needed.

Vital Vocabulary

accessory muscles Muscles not normally used during normal breathing; includes the sternocleidomastoid muscles of the neck.

acetylcholine (ACh) Chemical neurotransmitter of the parasympathetic nervous system.

adenoids Lymphatic tissues located on the posterior nasopharyngeal wall that filter bacteria.

adventitious Abnormal.

agonal respirations Slow, shallow, irregular respirations or occasional gasping breaths; results from cerebral anoxia.

alveolar volume Volume of inhaled air that reaches the alveoli and participates in gas exchange; equal to tidal volume minus dead space volume and is approximately 350 ml in the average adult.

alveoli Balloon-like clusters of single-layer air sacs that are the functional site for the exchange of oxygen and carbon dioxide in the lungs.

anatomical dead space Includes the trachea and larger bronchi. The air remaining in these areas is the result of residual gas in the upper airway at the end of inhalation.

anoxia An absence of oxygen.

antegrade amnesia Inability to remember from this point in time forward.

anxiolysis Relief of anxiety.

aphonia Inability to speak.

apneustic centre Portion of the brain stem that influences the respiratory rate by increasing the number of inspirations per minute.

arytenoid cartilages Pyramid-like cartilaginous structures that form the posterior attachment of the vocal cords.

aspiration Entry of fluids or solids into the trachea, bronchi, and lungs.

asymmetric chest wall movement When one side of the chest moves less than the other; indicates decreased airflow into one lung.

atelectasis Collapsing of the alveoli.

atlanto-occipital joint Joint formed at the articulation of the atlas of the vertebral column and the occipital bone of the skull.

bag-valve-mask device Manual ventilation device that consists of a bag, mask, reservoir, and oxygen inlet; capable of delivering up to 100% oxygen.

barbiturates Sedative-hypnotic medications; includes drugs such as thiopental (Pentothal) and methohexital (Brevital).

barotrauma Trauma resulting from excessive pressure.

benzodiazepines Sedative-hypnotic drugs that provide muscle relaxation and mild sedation; includes drugs such as diazepam (Valium) and midazolam (Versed).

Biot respirations Irregular pattern, rate, and depth with intermittent periods of apnea; results from increased intracranial pressure.

Bourdon-gauge flowmeter An oxygen flowmeter that is commonly used because it is not affected by gravity and can be placed in any position.

bronchioles Subdivision of the smaller bronchi in the lungs; made of smooth muscle and dilate or constrict in response to various stimuli.

BURP maneuver Acronym for Backward, Upward, Rightward Pressure.

butyrophenones Potent, effective sedatives; includes drugs such as haloperidol (Haldol) and droperidol (Inapsine).

capnographer Device that attaches in between the endotracheal tube and bag-valve-mask device; contains colourimetric paper, which should turn yellow during exhalation, indicating proper tube placement.

capnometer Device that attaches in the same way as a capnographer, but provides a light-emitting diode (LED) readout of the patient's exhaled carbon dioxide.

carboxyhemoglobin Abnormal hemoglobin that is formed by the attachment of carbon monoxide to the hemoglobin molecule.

carina Point at which the trachea bifurcates (divides) into the left and right mainstem bronchi.

cerebrospinal otorrhea Cerebrospinal fluid drainage from the ears.

cerebrospinal rhinorrhea Cerebrospinal fluid drainage from the nose.

chemoreceptors Monitor the levels of O_2, CO_2, and the pH of the CSF and then provide feedback to the respiratory centres to modify the rate and depth of breathing based on the body's needs at any given time.

Cheyne-Stokes respirations Gradually increasing rate and depth followed by a gradual decrease with intermittent periods of apnea; associated with brain stem insult.

Combitube Multilumen airway device that consists of a single tube with two lumens, two balloons, and two ventilation ports; an alternative device if endotracheal intubation is not possible or has failed.

continuous positive airway pressure (CPAP) A form of noninvasive ventilation in which the patient exhales against positive-pressure via a tight-fitting face mask; used to treat patients with cardiogenic pulmonary edema.

cricoid cartilage Forms the lowest portion of the larynx; also referred to as the cricoid ring; the first ring of the trachea and is the only upper airway structure that forms a complete ring.

cricoid pressure The application of posterior pressure to the cricoid cartilage to reduce the risk of regurgitation during positive-pressure ventilation; also called the Sellick maneuver.

cricothyroid membrane A thin, superficial membrane located between the thyroid and cricoid cartilages that is relatively avascular and contains few nerves; the site for emergency surgical and nonsurgical access to the airway.

curved laryngoscope blade Also called the Macintosh blade; designed to fit into the vallecula, indirectly lifting the epiglottis and exposing the vocal cords.

cyanosis Blue or purple skin; indicates inadequate oxygen in the blood.

dead space Any portion of the airway that does not contain air and cannot participate in gas exchange.

depolarizing neuromuscular blockers Competitively bind with the acetylcholine receptor sites but are not affected as quickly by acetylcholinesterase; includes drugs such as succinylcholine.

diaphragm The major muscle of breathing. It is the anatomical point of separation between the thoracic cavity and the abdominal cavity.

diffusion Movement of a gas from an area of higher concentration to an area of lower concentration.

digital intubation Method of intubation that involves directly palpating the glottic structures and elevating the epiglottis with your middle finger while guiding the ET tube into the trachea by feel.

direct laryngoscopy Visualization of the airway with a laryngoscope.

dysphonia Difficulty speaking.

dyspnea Any difficulty in respiratory rate, regularity, or effort.

emergence phenomenon Nightmares associated with the use of ketamine.

endotracheal intubation Passing an endotracheal (ET) tube through the glottic opening and sealing the tube with a cuff inflated against the tracheal wall.

endotracheal (ET) tube Tube that is inserted into the trachea; equipped with a distal cuff, proximal inflation port, a 15/22-mm adapter, and cm markings on the side.

end-tidal carbon dioxide ($Etco_2$) detectors Device that detects the presence of carbon dioxide in exhaled air.

epiglottis Leaf-shaped cartilaginous structure that closes over the trachea during swallowing.

esophageal detector device (EDD) Bulb or syringe that is attached to the proximal end of the ET tube; a device used to confirm proper ET tube placement.

etomidate A nonnarcotic, nonbarbiturate hypnotic-sedative drug; also called Amidate.

exhalation Passive movement of air out of the lungs; also called expiration.

expiration Passive movement of air out of the lungs; also called exhalation.

expiratory reserve volume The amount of air that you can exhale following a normal exhalation; average volume is about 1,200 ml.

external respiration The exchange of gases between the lungs and the blood cells in the pulmonary capillaries; also called pulmonary respiration.

extubation The process of removing the tube from an intubated patient.

fasciculations Characterized by brief, uncoordinated twitching of small muscle groups in the face, neck, trunk, and extremities; caused by the administration of depolarizing neuromuscular blocking agents (eg, succinylcholine).

flow-restricted, oxygen-powered ventilation device (FROPVD) Also referred to as a manually triggered ventilator or demand valve. Can be used to ventilate apneic or to administer supplemental oxygen to spontaneously breathing patients.

fraction of inspired oxygen (Fio_2) The percentage of oxygen in inhaled air.

functional residual capacity The amount of air that can be forced from the lungs in a single exhalation.

gag reflex Automatic reaction when something touches an area deep in the oral cavity; helps protect the lower airway from aspiration.

gastric distension Inflation of the patient's stomach with air.

gastric tube A tube that is inserted into the stomach to remove its contents.

glottis The space in between the vocal cords that is the narrowest portion of the adult's airway; also called the glottic opening.

gum elastic bougie Also called the Eschmann stylet; a flexible device that is inserted in between the glottis under direct laryngoscopy. The ET tube is then threaded over the device, facilitating its entry into the trachea.

head tilt–chin lift maneuver Manual airway maneuver that involves tilting the head back while lifting up on the chin; used to open the airway of a semiconscious or unconscious nontrauma patient.

Heimlich maneuver Abdominal thrusts performed to relieve a foreign body airway obstruction.

hemoglobin An iron-containing protein within red blood cells that has the ability to combine with oxygen.

Hering-Breuer reflex A protective mechanism that terminates inhalation, thus preventing overexpansion of the lungs.

Hi-Ox mask A mask that allows the patient to inhale oxygen from a reservoir bag via a one-way valve and exhale breath through another one-way valve through a high-efficiency filter before exiting the mask.

hilum Point of entry of all of the blood vessels and the bronchi into each lung.

hyoid bone A small, horseshoe-shaped bone to which the jaw, tongue, epiglottis, and thyroid cartilage attach.

hypercarbia Increased CO_2 content in arterial blood.

hyperventilation Occurs when CO_2 elimination exceeds CO_2 production.

hypocarbia Decreased CO_2 content in arterial blood.

hypoventilation Occurs when CO_2 production exceeds the body's ability to eliminate it by ventilation.

hypoxemia A decrease in arterial oxygen levels.

hypoxia A lack of oxygen to the body's cells and tissues.

hypoxic drive Secondary control of breathing that stimulates breathing based on decreased PaO_2 levels.

inspiration The active process of moving air into the lungs; also called inhalation.

inspiratory reserve volume The amount of air that can be inhaled after a normal inhalation; the amount of air that can be inhaled in addition to the normal tidal volume.

intercostal nerves Nerves that innervate the external intercostal muscles, the muscles between the ribs.

internal respiration The exchange of gases between the blood cells and the tissues; also called cellular respiration.

intrapulmonary shunting Bypassing of oxygen-poor blood past non-functional alveoli.

jaw-thrust maneuver Manual airway maneuver that involves stabilizing the patient's head and thrusting the jaw forward; the preferred method of opening the airway of a semiconscious or unconscious trauma patient.

jaw-thrust maneuver with head tilt Manual airway maneuver that involves thrusting the jaw forward while tilting back on the head.

ketamine A drug with sedative, analgesic, and hypnotic properties; created in the laboratory from phencyclidine (PCP).

King airway A single-lumen airway device that serves as an alternative to ventilation with a bag-valve-mask or for procedures where tracheal intubation is not possible.

Kussmaul respirations Deep, gasping respirations; common in diabetic coma (ketoacidosis).

laryngeal mask airway (LMA) Device that surrounds the opening of the larynx with an inflatable silicone cuff positioned in the hypopharynx; an alternative device to bag-valve-mask ventilation.

laryngectomy A surgical procedure in which the larynx is removed.

laryngoscope Device that is used in conjunction with a laryngoscope blade in order to perform direct laryngoscopy.

laryngospasm Spasmodic closure of the vocal cords.

larynx A complex structure formed by many independent cartilaginous structures that all work together; where the upper airway ends and the lower airway begins.

lung compliance The ability of the alveoli to expand when air is drawn into the lungs, either during negative-pressure ventilation or positive-pressure ventilation.

Magill forceps A special type of forcep that is curved, thus allowing the paramedic to maneuver it in the airway.

minute alveolar volume The amount of air that actually reaches the alveoli per minute and participates in gas exchange.

minute volume The amount of air that moves in and out of the respiratory tract per minute.

Murphy's eye An opening on the side of an endotracheal tube at its distal tip that enables ventilation to occur even if the tip becomes occluded by blood, mucus, or the tracheal wall.

nasal catheter Delivers oxygen via two small prongs that fit into the patient's nostrils. With an oxygen flow rate of 1 to 6 l/min, the nasal catheter can deliver an oxygen concentration of 24% to 44%.

nasal septum A rigid partition composed of bone and cartilage; divides the nasopharynx into two passages.

nasogastric (NG) tube Gastric tube is inserted into the stomach through the nose.

nasopharyngeal (nasal) airway A soft rubber tube about 15 cm long that is inserted through the nose into the posterior pharynx behind the tongue, thereby allowing passage of air from the nose to the lower airway.

nasopharynx The nasal cavity; formed by the union of the facial bones.

nasotracheal intubation Insertion of an endotracheal tube into the trachea through the nose.

nebulizer Device used primarily to deliver aerosolized medications. Oxygen enters an aerosol chamber that contains 3 to 5 ml of fluid. The pressurized oxygen in this chamber aerosolizes the medication for inhalation.

needle cricothyrotomy Insertion of a 14- to 16-gauge over-the-needle IV catheter (angiocath) through the cricothyroid membrane and into the trachea.

negative-pressure ventilation Drawing of air into the lungs; airflow from a region of higher pressure (outside the body) to a region of lower pressure (the lungs); occurs during normal (unassisted breathing).

nondepolarizing neuromuscular blockers Binds to acetylcholine receptor sites; however, unlike depolarizing neuromuscular blockers, they do not cause depolarization of the muscle fibre; includes drugs such as vecuronium (Norcuron) and pancuronium (Pavulon).

nonrebreathing mask A combination mask and reservoir bag system. Oxygen fills a reservoir bag that is attached to the mask by a one-way valve. This permits the patient to inhale from the reservoir bag but not to exhale back into it. With a good mask-to-face seal and a flow rate of 15 l/min, it is capable of delivering up to 90% inspired oxygen.

open cricothyrotomy Also referred to as a surgical cricothyrotomy; an emergent procedure that involves incising the cricothyroid membrane with a scalpel and inserting an endotracheal or tracheostomy tube directly into the subglottic area of the trachea.

opioids Also called narcotics; potent analgesics with sedative properties; includes drugs such as fentanyl (Sublimaze) and alfentanil (Alfenta).

orogastric (OG) tube Gastric tube inserted into the stomach through the mouth.

oropharyngeal (oral) airway A hard plastic device that is curved in such a way that it fits over the back of the tongue with the tip in the posterior pharynx.

oropharynx Forms the posterior portion of the oral cavity, which is bordered superiorly by the hard and soft palates, laterally by the cheeks, and inferiorly by the tongue.

orotracheal intubation Insertion of an endotracheal tube into the trachea through the mouth.

orthopnea Positional dyspnea.

oxygen humidifier Small bottle of water through which the oxygen leaving the cylinder is moisturized before it reaches the patient.

oxyhemoglobin Hemoglobin that is occupied by oxygen.

palate Forms the roof of the mouth and separates the oropharynx and nasopharynx.

pancuronium A nondepolarizing neuromuscular blocking agent; used to maintain paralysis following succinylcholine-facilitated intubation; also called Pavulon.

paralytics Also called neuromuscular blocking agents; paralyzes skeletal muscles; used in an emergency situation to facilitate intubation.

parietal pleura Thin membrane that lines the chest cavity.

partial laryngectomy Surgical removal of a portion of the larynx.

partial rebreathing mask Similar to the nonrebreathing mask except that there is no one-way valve between the mask and the reservoir. Room air is not entrained with inspiration; however, residual expired air is mixed in the mask and rebreathed.

patent Open.

peak expiratory flow An approximation of the extent of bronchoconstriction; used to determine whether patients are improving with therapy (eg, inhaled bronchodilators).

pharyngeotracheal lumen airway (PtL) Multilumen airway device that consists of two tubes and two cuffs; an alternative device if endotracheal intubation is not possible or has failed.

pharynx Throat.

phrenic nerves Nerves that innervate the diaphragm.

physiologic dead space Additional dead space created by intrapulmonary obstructions or atelectasis.

pneumotaxic centre Area of the brain stem that has an inhibitory influence on inspiration.

positive-pressure ventilation Forcing of air into the lungs.

pressure-compensated flowmeter An oxygen flowmeter that incorporates a float ball within a tapered calibrated tube. The float rises or falls according to the gas flow within the tube. Because this type of flowmeter is affected by gravity, it must remain in an upright position to obtain an accurate flow reading.

primary respiratory drive Normal stimulus to breathe; based on fluctuations in Paco$_2$ and pH of the CSF.

pulse oximeter Device that measures oxygen saturation.

pulsus paradoxus A drop in the systolic BP of 10 mm Hg or more; commonly seen in patients with pericardial tamponade or severe asthma.

pyriform fossae Two pockets of tissue on the lateral borders of the larynx.

rapid-sequence intubation (RSI) A specific set of procedures, combined in rapid succession, to induce sedation and paralysis and intubate a patient quickly.

recovery position Left-lateral recumbent position; used in all semiconscious and unconscious nontrauma patients, who are able to maintain their own airway spontaneously and are breathing adequately.

residual volume The air that remains in the lungs after maximal expiration.

respiration The exchange of gases between a living organism and its environment.

retractions Skin pulling in between and around the ribs during inhalation.

rocuronium A nondepolarizing neuromuscular blocking agent; used to maintain paralysis following succinylcholine-facilitated intubation; also called Zemuron.

safe residual pressure A term that implies that it is *unsafe* to continue using an oxygen cylinder with a pressure of less than 200 psi.

sedation Reduction of a patient's anxiety, induction of amnesia, and suppression of the gag reflex.

Sellick maneuver The application of posterior pressure to the cricoid cartilage to minimize the risk of regurgitation during positive-pressure ventilation; also referred to as cricoid pressure.

simple face mask A full mask enclosure with open side ports. Room air is drawn in through the side ports on inhalation, diluting the concentration of inspired oxygen. Exhaled air is vented through holes on each side of the mask. The simple face mask will deliver between 40% and 60% oxygen at 10 l/min.

sinuses Cavities formed by the cranial bones that trap contaminants from entering the respiratory tract and act as tributaries for fluid to and from the eustachian tubes and tear ducts.

stenosis Narrowing.

stoma The resultant orifice of a tracheostomy that connects the trachea to the outside air; located in the midline of the anterior neck.

straight laryngoscope blade Also called the Miller blade; designed to lift the epiglottis and expose the vocal cords.

stylet A semirigid wire that is inserted into the ET tube to mould and maintain the shape of the tube.

succinylcholine chloride A depolarizing neuromuscular blocker frequently used as the initial paralytic during rapid-sequence intubation; causes muscle fasciculations; also referred to as Anectine.

surfactant A proteinaceous substance that lines the alveoli; decreases alveolar surface tension and keeps the alveoli expanded.

therapy regulator Attaches to the stem of the oxygen cylinder, and reduces the high pressure of gas to a safe range (about 50 psi).

thyroid cartilage The main supporting cartilage of the larynx; a shield-shaped structure formed by two plates that join in a "V" shape anteriorly to form the laryngeal prominence known as the Adam's apple.

tidal volume A measure of the depth of breathing; the volume of air that is inhaled or exhaled during a single respiratory cycle.

tongue-jaw lift maneuver A manual maneuver that involves grasping the tongue and jaw and lifting; commonly used to suction the airway and to place certain airway devices.

tonsils Lymphatic tissues that are located in the posterior pharynx; they help to trap bacteria.

tonsil-tip catheter A hard or rigid suction catheter; also called a Yankauer catheter.

total laryngectomy Surgical removal of the entire larynx.

total lung capacity The total volume of air that the lungs can hold; approximately 6 l in the average adult male.

trachea The conduit for all entry into the lungs; a tubular structure that is approximately 10 to 12 cm in length and is composed of a series of C-shaped cartilaginous rings; also called the windpipe.

tracheobronchial suctioning Passing a suction catheter into the endotracheal tube to remove pulmonary secretions.

tracheostomy Surgical opening into the trachea.

tracheostomy tube Plastic tube placed within the tracheostomy site (stoma).

translaryngeal cannula ventilation Used in conjunction with needle cricothyrotomy to ventilate a patient; requires a high-pressure jet ventilator.

transillumination intubation Method of intubation that uses a lighted stylet to guide the endotracheal tube into the trachea.

trismus Clenched teeth caused by spasms of the jaw muscles.

turbinates Three bony shelves that protrude from the lateral walls of the nasal cavity and extend into the nasal passageway, parallel to the nasal floor; serve to increase the surface area of the nasal mucosa, thereby improving the processes of warming, filtering, and humidification of inhaled air.

upper airway Consists of all anatomical airway structures above the level of the vocal cords.

uvula A soft-tissue structure that resembles a punching bag; located in the posterior aspect of the oral cavity, at the base of the tongue.

vallecula An anatomical space, or "pocket," located between the base of the tongue and the epiglottis; an important anatomical landmark for endotracheal intubation.

vecuronium A nondepolarizing neuromuscular blocking agent; used to maintain paralysis following succinylcholine-facilitated intubation; also called Norcuron.

ventilation The process of moving air into and out of the lungs.

Venturi mask A mask that has a number of interchangeable adapters that draws room air into the mask along with the oxygen flow; allows for the administration of highly specific oxygen concentrations.

visceral pleura Thin membrane that lines the lungs.

vocal cords White bands of tough tissue that are the lateral borders of the glottis.

whistle-tip catheters Soft plastic, nonrigid catheters; also called French catheters.

Assessment in Action

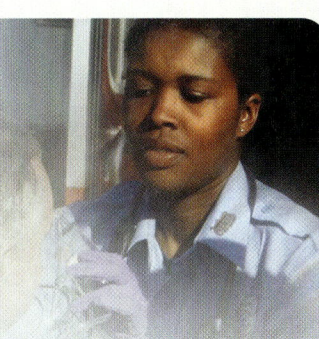

You are dispatched to a residence for an "unconscious male." You arrive at the scene 6 minutes after being dispatched and are met at the door of the residence by a frantic woman.

Your initial assessment reveals that the man is unresponsive. His respirations are slow and shallow, and his pulse is rapid and weak. Further assessment reveals facial cyanosis and vomitus around his mouth. The patient's wife tells you that she thinks her husband has had a stroke. You and your partner begin immediate treatment; a second paramedic unit is dispatched to the scene to provide assistance.

1. **Vomitus that has been aspirated into the lungs will:**
   A. cause a rapid, fatal infection.
   B. impair pulmonary diffusion.
   C. increase ventilation compliance.
   D. require deep tracheal suctioning.

2. **The goal of providing assisted ventilation to a hypoventilating patient is to:**
   A. minimize hypocarbia.
   B. reduce gastric distension.
   C. improve cardiac output.
   D. maintain minute volume.

3. **Signs of adequate ventilation in the adult include:**
   A. pink mucous membranes.
   B. a prolonged exhalation phase.
   C. a shallow depth of breathing.
   D. respirations of 30 breaths/min.

4. **Positive-pressure ventilation is defined as:**
   A. forcing air into the lungs.
   B. drawing air into the lungs.
   C. deep spontaneous breathing.
   D. a reduction in tidal volume.

5. **Which of the following oxygen delivery devices is MOST appropriate for a patient with suspected hypoxemia and adequate tidal volume?**
   A. Nasal catheter
   B. Simple face mask
   C. Nonrebreathing mask
   D. Bag-valve-mask device with reservoir

6. **Negative-pressure ventilation occurs when:**
   A. the diaphragm relaxes and ascends.
   B. pressure within the thoracic cavity decreases.
   C. air is blown into the lungs with a bag-valve-mask device.
   D. a patient is ventilated with a demand valve.

7. **The volume of air moved into and out of the lungs per breath is called:**
   A. tidal volume.
   B. stroke volume.
   C. minute volume.
   D. alveolar volume.

8. **The primary respiratory drive in a healthy individual is based on:**
   A. decreasing Pa_{O_2} levels.
   B. the pH of venous blood.
   C. progressive hypocarbia.
   D. increasing P_{CO_2} levels.

9. **In contrast to hypoxia, hypoxemia is defined as:**
   A. a complete lack of oxygen to the brain.
   B. a deficiency of oxygen in the arterial blood.
   C. decreased oxygen to the body's tissues and cells.
   D. an insufficient supply of oxygen to the myocardium.

10. **What is the MOST commonly encountered problem when ventilating a patient with the one-person bag-valve-mask technique?**
    A. Inability to squeeze the bag
    B. Forgetting to attach the reservoir
    C. Difficulty maintaining a mask seal
    D. Not manually positioning the head

11. **The phrenic nerves innervate the:**
    A. diaphragm.
    B. intercostal muscles.
    C. accessory muscles.
    D. pons and medulla.

12. **Physiologic dead space would increase with:**
    A. atelectatic alveoli.
    B. increased tidal volume.
    C. reduced minute volume.
    D. gastric distension.

13. **Alveolar surface tension would increase with:**
    A. positive-pressure ventilation.
    B. inadvertent esophageal intubation.
    C. increased ventilatory compliance.
    D. a deficiency of pulmonary surfactant.

14. **What is the usual anatomical dead space volume in the average adult male?**
    A. 70 ml
    B. 150 ml
    C. 200 ml
    D. 350 ml

15. **The exchange of gases between a living organism and its environment is called:**
    A. ventilation.
    B. respiration.
    C. expiration.
    D. inhalation.

16. **If performed properly, the Sellick maneuver will minimize the risk of:**
    A. shallow breathing.
    B. excessive tidal volume.
    C. gastric distension.
    D. tracheal intubation.

17. **The volume of air that remains in the lungs after maximal expiration is called:**
    A. residual volume.
    B. expiratory reserve volume.
    C. inspiratory reserve volume.
    D. functional residual capacity.

18. **A patient who has an altered mental status and has shallow respirations should be treated initially with:**
    A. immediate endotracheal intubation.
    B. a nonrebreathing mask at 15 l/min.
    C. insertion of a laryngeal mask airway.
    D. some form of positive-pressure ventilation.

19. **Which of the following MOST accurately describes pulsus paradoxus?**
    A. An increase in the heart rate during inhalation
    B. A decrease in systolic BP during inhalation
    C. An increase in diastolic BP during exhalation
    D. A decrease in the heart rate during exhalation

20. **Which of the following respiratory patterns is characterized by occasional, irregular, shallow breaths?**
    A. Biot breathing
    B. Agonal breathing
    C. Cheyne-Stokes breathing
    D. Kussmaul breathing

21. **Immediately after inserting an endotracheal tube through the vocal cords, the paramedic should:**
    A. begin ventilations.
    B. attach an $Etco_2$ detector.
    C. inflate the distal cuff.
    D. auscultate for breath sounds.

22. **To properly align the three airway axes prior to endotracheal intubation, the patient's head should be placed in what position?**
    A. Sniffing
    B. Flexed
    C. Extended
    D. Neutral

23. **Multilumen airway devices are not intended to be used in patients who:**
    A. are deeply unconscious.
    B. weigh more than 75 kg.
    C. have an esophageal disease.
    D. are in cardiopulmonary arrest.

24. **Following a needle cricothyrotomy, ventilations are MOST effectively performed with which of the following devices?**
    A. Bag-valve-mask device and 100% oxygen
    B. Flow-restricted oxygen-powered device
    C. ET tube adapter and a 10-ml syringe
    D. High-pressure jet ventilation device

25. **Medications used during rapid-sequence intubation (RSI) include which of the following?**
    A. Epinephrine
    B. Succinylcholine
    C. Amiodarone
    D. Furosemide

Challenging Question

You and your partner are caring for a 67-year-old man with congestive heart failure. The patient is extremely restless and agitated, and is labouring to breathe. Your repeated attempts to provide 100% oxygen via nonrebreathing mask have failed; the patient keeps pulling the mask away from his face. He is becoming physically exhausted; however, he is still agitated and noncompliant with your treatment. He has cyanosis to his face, an oxygen saturation of 78%, an end-tidal carbon dioxide reading of 15 mm Hg per capnometry, and a weak pulse at 120 beats/min. The closest appropriate medical facility is 25 km away.

26. **What measures must be taken to prevent this patient from developing cardiac arrest?**

Points to Ponder

Your partner is attempting to perform endotracheal intubation on a middle-aged unconscious, apneic man. The patient is attached to a cardiac monitor, which is displaying a normal sinus rhythm, and a pulse oximeter, which is reading 98%. Approximately 15 seconds into the intubation attempt, you note that the patient's heart rate has dropped approximately 30 beats/min and the pulse oximeter now reads 82%. You immediately advise your partner of the change in the patient's condition, to which he replies, "I still have 15 seconds left." He continues with the intubation attempt, which is successful. As you are in the process of securing the ET tube in place, the patient experiences cardiac arrest. Despite aggressive management and prompt transport to the hospital, the patient dies.

Why did this patient experience cardiac arrest? What could have been done to prevent it?

Issues: Knowing When to Abort an Intubation Attempt, Understanding the Importance of Adequate Oxygenation and Ventilation, Working Effectively as a Team.

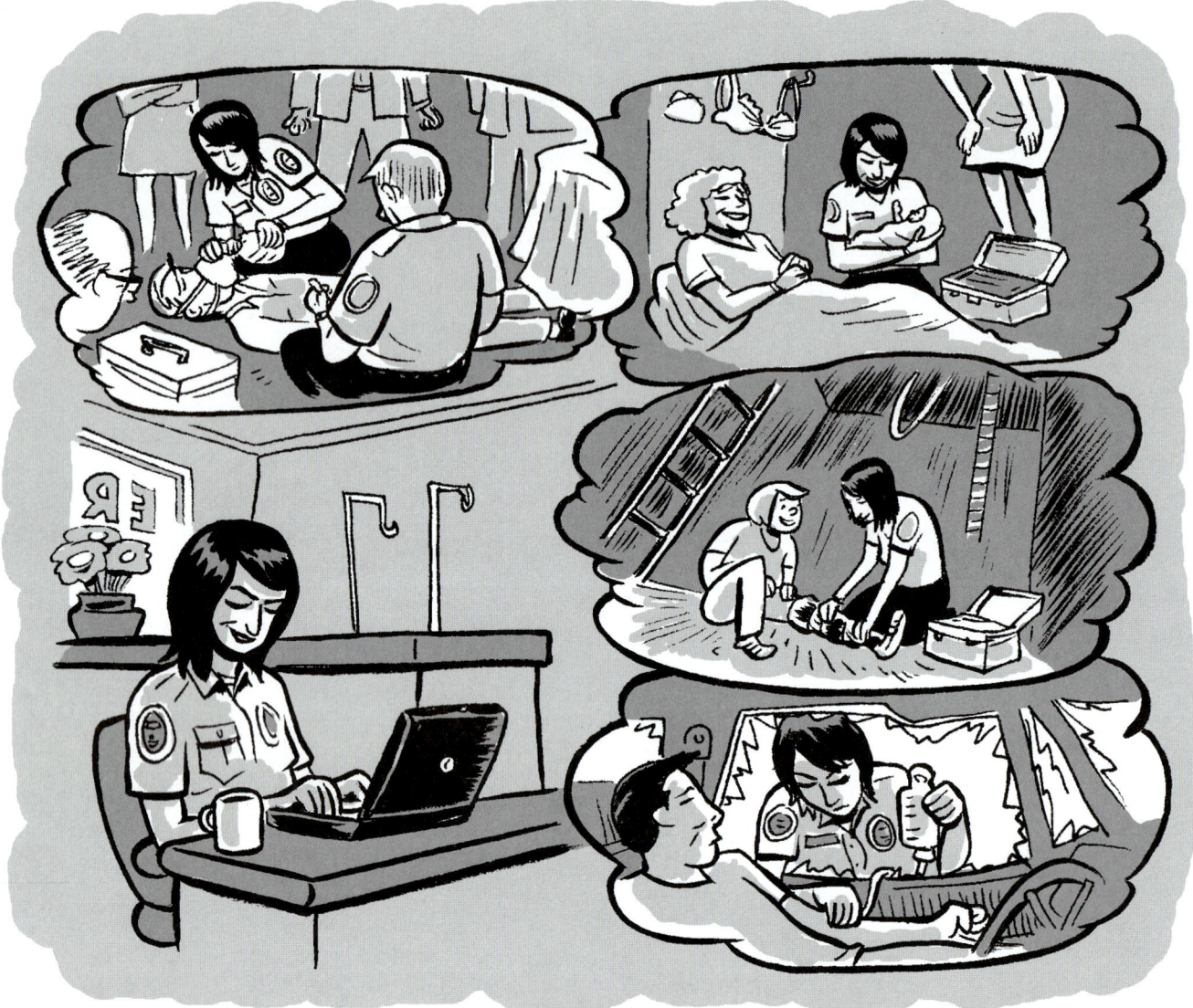

"

I learned the special stresses and constraints of rendering care outside the controlled conditions of a hospital: CPR in a crowded restaurant, childbirth in the lingerie section of a department store, splinting at the bottom of an elevator shaft, intravenous infusions inside a wrecked automobile."

—Nancy L. Caroline, MD

Patient Assessment

Section Editor: Graham G. Munro, MHSM, BHSc, CCP

3

Section

Competency Areas

Area 1: Professional Responsibilities

1.1.b Reflect professionalism through use of appropriate language.

1.1.c Dress appropriately and maintain personal hygiene.

1.1.d Maintain appropriate personal interaction with patients.

1.5.a Work collaboratively with a partner.

Area 2: Communication

2.1.c Deliver an organized, accurate, and relevant patient history.

2.1.d Provide information to patient about their situation and how they will be treated.

2.1.e Interact effectively with the patient, relatives, and bystanders who are in stressful situations.

2.1.f Speak in language appropriate to the listener.

2.1.g Use appropriate terminology.

2.3.a Exhibit effective non-verbal behaviour.

2.3.b Practice active listening techniques.

2.3.c Establish trust and rapport with patients and colleagues.

2.3.d Recognize and react appropriately to non-verbal behaviours.

2.4.c Recognize and react appropriately to individuals and groups manifesting coping mechanisms.

2.4.g Exhibit diplomacy, tact, and discretion.

Area 4: Assessment and Diagnostics

4.2.a Obtain list of patient's allergies.

4.2.b Obtain list of patient's medications.

4.2.c Obtain chief complaint and/or incident history from patient, family members, and/or bystanders.

4.2.d Obtain information regarding patient's past medical history.

4.2.e Obtain information about patient's last oral intake.

Introduction

Most practicing first responders, paramedics, nurses, and physicians quickly learn that patient assessment is one of the most important parts of their job. Assessment combines a number of steps—assessing the environment, getting your patient's chief complaint, taking care of life-threatening problems, taking your patient's medical history, and doing a physical examination. One of the most unique things about your patient assessment skills is that *there is no limit to how good they can be*. With a positive attitude and a commitment to excellence, you will have the opportunity to continue to polish and improve these critical skills throughout your career as a paramedic.

Paramedics often work with seriously ill or injured patients without the input of specialized resources, like clinical laboratories and x-ray departments Figure 12-1 ▶ . However, you can be confident in a good initial diagnosis if you learn excellent history-taking skills. Many physicians say that hospital tests more often than not confirm a diagnosis the physician arrived at *by taking a patient history*.

To the patient, the entire assessment process should appear to be a seamless process. To the paramedic, it is most often a blend of questions and answers with a physical examination. What varies from patient to patient is the number and types of questions that must be asked and to what extent the patient should be examined before an initial diagnosis is reached. Never forget that the entire patient assessment process should be organized and systematic, but, at the same time, be reasonably flexible.

Aside from performing the initial assessment, which focuses on the identification and correction of any life threats to the patient, virtually all of the remaining history-gathering and physical examination components come with a lot of latitude as to when each is sequenced into the patient assessment process. In other words, you can do the majority of your assessment and examination in the order that is in the best interest of patient care, *once the initial assessment and correction of life threats is completed.*

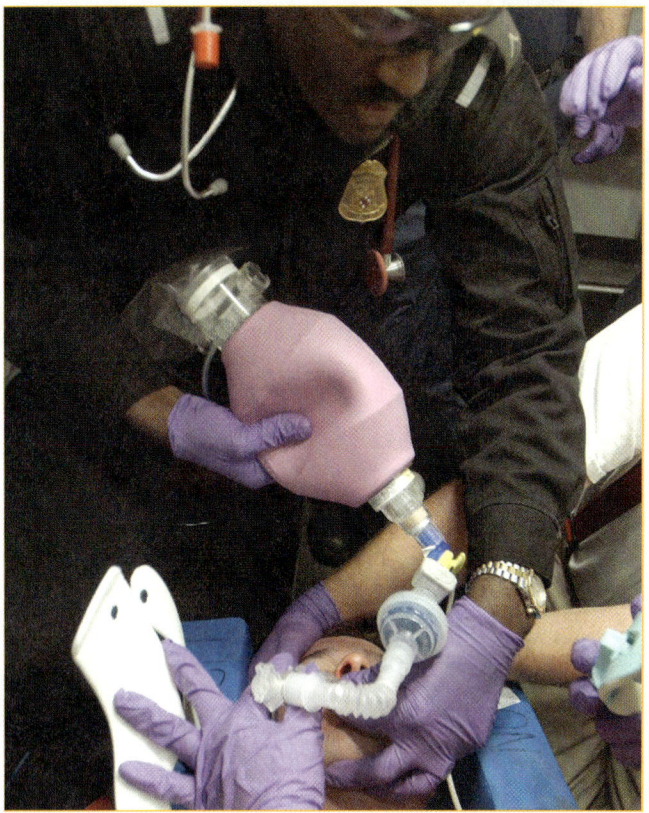

Figure 12-1 As a paramedic, you will work with seriously ill or injured patients.

You are the Paramedic Part 1

You are dispatched to 3401 Webberville Road for a 65-year-old man who has "passed out." En route to the scene, the emergency medical dispatcher informs you that your patient is now conscious and alert and reportedly was stung by a bee.

As you arrive on the scene, someone waves for you from the backyard of the residence. As you approach, you see a man seated at a picnic table surrounded by an obviously concerned group of people. There are a few large bowls of food placed in the middle of the table, and several insects are flying around them. You introduce yourself to the group, and they introduce you to your patient, Lawrence Smith. Your patient's adult daughter tells you that they were all eating dinner when the patient was stung by a bee. He is complaining of itching at the sting site and dizziness.

Initial Assessment	Recording Time: 0 Minutes
Appearance	Eyes open, talking with family members
Level of consciousness	A (Alert to person, place, and day)
Airway	Patent
Breathing	Adequate rate and tidal volume
Circulation	Radial pulse present

1. What are your immediate concerns?
2. At this point, what would you want to know about his medical history?

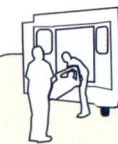

At the Scene

For peak efficiency, communicate your patient assessment findings with your partner(s) and share with them the patient care plan.

Most EMS teams are made up of two people working in tandem to quickly identify and address the patient's needs. The EMS team may be composed of two paramedics, or, it may be a split team, with one advanced care and one primary care paramedic. In either case, with the limited physical resources of a two-person team, working in the dynamic, unstable prehospital environment, providing quality patient care can be quite a challenge.

A key part of making your practice of prehospital care successful is for you to develop and cultivate your own style of assessment and an overall strategy for evaluating and providing care for the patients you will encounter in the unique and varied circumstances in the field setting. You will have to work within the parametres of the published standards of care in your system, adding your own personal touches, for example, what gear you take in on a given call or whether you like to kneel or sit while you interview the patient.

Always remember that your overall job as a paramedic is to quickly identify your patient's problem(s), set your care priorities, develop a patient care plan, and quickly and efficiently execute the patient care plan.

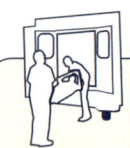

At the Scene

In prehospital emergency care, the priorities of evaluation and treatment are based on the degree of threat to the patient's life.

Sick Versus Not Sick

The most important assessment skill for a paramedic to acquire, and one that comes only from lots of experience, is quickly determining whether the patient is *sick* or *not sick.* This quick visual assessment is based on the chief complaint, respirations, pulse, mental status, and skin signs and colour. For trauma patients, the mechanism of injury and obvious trauma should be factored in as well. These items together reflect the overall performance of the respiratory, cardiovascular, and neurologic systems and can quickly provide you with a sound medical basis for determining whether a patient is in stable or unstable condition. Abnormalities in any of these areas could indicate a life-threatening condition.

If the patient is sick, the next step is to determine "how sick." On one end of the sick scale is a patient with a miserable sinus infection. Is the patient sick? Yes. Is this a life-threatening event? Probably not. On the other end of the scale is a patient who is a dusky grey, struggling to answer your questions, and exhibiting one- or two-word dyspnea (so short of breath that only one- or two-word bursts are possible). Is the patient sick? Yes. Is this a life-threatening event? Unlike the previous scenario, the answer is yes.

Documentation and Communication

One key to getting a good patient history is to develop rapport with your patient—even though you spend only a short time with him or her.

Every time you assess a patient, you have to *qualify* whether your patient is sick or not sick, and then you must *quantify* how sick the patient is. Once this has been accomplished, you are in a position to decide what, if any, care needs to be provided at the scene versus in the ambulance, en route to the hospital.

Making Your Initial Diagnosis

More often than not, you will make your initial diagnosis based on the *patient history* and the *chief complaint.* Your ability to obtain quality information from patients with differing educational, cultural, and ethnic backgrounds; patients with various levels of cognitive ability; and patients impaired by alcohol or drugs is no small challenge. In addition, you still have to ask the right questions to get the information needed to make the best decisions for your patient.

For the most part, being good at patient assessment is a lot like being a good detective. As you interview your patient, you will sift through the information you obtain, and throughout that process, you will continuously glean clues **Figure 12-2 ▾** . On the basis of clues, you will ask more questions to seek information relevant to the patient's chief complaint. You may pursue one line of questioning about current medications that yields nothing important, yet the next line of questioning about medical history is a goldmine.

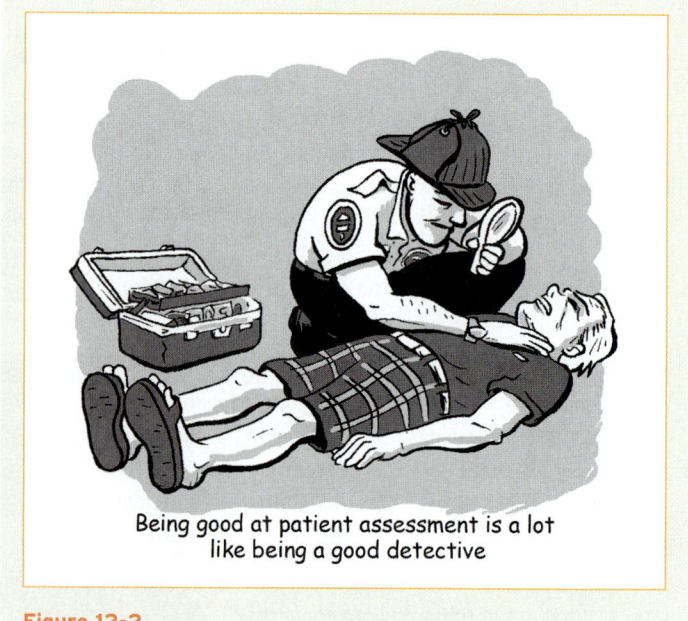

Being good at patient assessment is a lot like being a good detective

Figure 12-2

Controversies

There is much controversy about paramedics making a "diagnosis" in the prehospital environment. However, an "initial diagnosis" must be made to understand which treatment protocol to use.

Just as the veteran detective methodically collects and analyzes clues to ultimately "solve the case," so must you use a similar process to best meet your patient's needs.

In time, every paramedic develops his or her own *style* of patient assessment. As you work at developing this most important job skill, it is critical that you need to think of patient assessment as a "fluid" process. The overall assessment process must be organized and systematic but still flexible enough to allow you to maximize your information gathering. As the patient interview unfolds, you need to be able to change the sequence of your questioning as the situation or patient's condition dictates. You must know when to expand your questioning to elicit more information and when to focus your questioning to ascertain the most relevant facts.

Medical Versus Trauma

Last, keep in mind that there are two basic categories of patient problems: medical and trauma. For patients with medical problems, identifying their chief complaint and sifting carefully through their medical history will allow you to provide the quality care the patients need.

Unlike medical emergencies, trauma calls are generally the result of unexpected events. When trauma is the primary culprit, the patient's medical history often has little or no impact on your care plan. Because of that, trauma cases require a modified approach to assessment. That will be covered in more detail in Chapter 13.

That said, it is important to never forget that medical events can cause trauma; for example, a person with diabetes takes insulin, forgets to eat breakfast, the blood glucose level drops, and, as a result, the person falls down the steps. By comparison, traumatic events can produce medical problems; for example, a person with asthma wrecks a new car and the stress of the event results in an asthma attack. Keep your mind open to the varied patient care scenarios you may encounter in your practice so you are mentally ready to respond to your patient's needs.

Evaluation of the Emergency Scene

Regardless of when and where you respond to an emergency call, the *very first step, before patient care is initiated,* is to *take a look around* and evaluate the overall safety and stability of the emergency scene for any risks to you or any other member of the rescue team, the patient, and any friends, family, and bystanders **Figure 12-3 ▶**.

If you do not take a few moments to evaluate the scene and address safety issues, you may find that you and/or your partner have joined the list of casualties. An injured paramedic simply adds to the list of injured and subtracts from the list of rescue resources, making more work for the rest of the rescue team.

Notes from Nancy

Dead heroes can't save lives. Injured heroes are a nuisance. So check the scene for hazards before you lurch in.

Content of the Patient History

Patient Information

There are a number of components that collectively make up the patient history. On most calls, the two most important pieces of patient history information that you need to obtain are the patient's name and the chief complaint. After that, you can obtain the rest of the patient history in whatever order is most conducive to good patient care and most convenient.

Your first step in approaching your patient is to introduce yourself and to explain that you are a paramedic. Then you can ask your patient his or her name and why he or she asked for your help (the chief complaint). Along with the patient's *name,* you need to ask about the *date, time, location,* and *events* surrounding the current situation. This is important information and gives you the chance to quickly determine if the patient is alert to person, place, time, and events. Your EMS system may require you to collect some additional identifying data such as age, sex, race, address, marital status, and occupation. You will

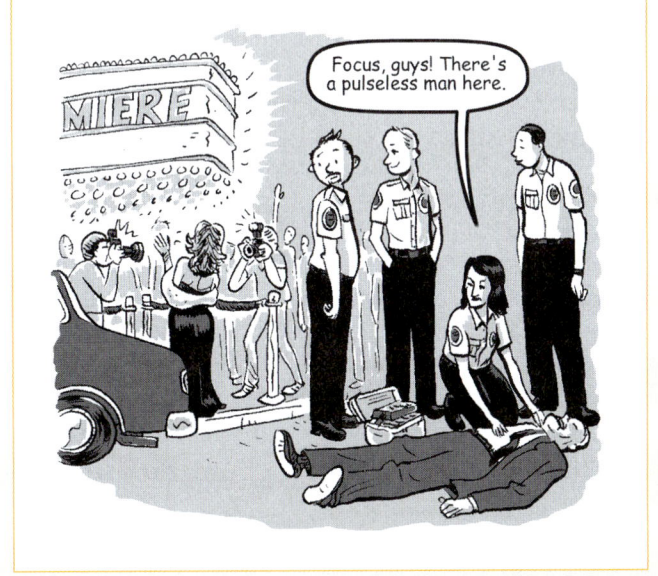

Figure 12-3

also want to know who called 9-1-1; did the patient place the call for help, or was it a friend, family member, or bystander who placed the call?

If first responders are already on the scene, find out the information they have already obtained and the results of any care they provided. This information saves time by avoiding your having to ask the same questions again, which in turn, keeps the patient from getting frustrated. Is bleeding controlled? Was oxygen administered?

Learning About the Present Illness

Once the meet-and-greet phase is over, start gathering information. Again, take a moment to make sure the patient is as comfortable as possible before you start—warm or cool enough, privacy ensured—and that you have gained the patient's confidence and trust.

The history of the present illness starts with one of the most open-ended of all medical questions: "What's going on today that made you call 9-1-1?" An open-ended question cannot be answered with a "yes" or "no." This or a similar question gets the ball rolling. More often than not, the answer you get involves some problem(s) with the person being in pain or discomfort. If your patient's behaviour is inappropriate, you must first eliminate any physiologic causes, such as hypoxia or hypoglycemia, before you consider the possibility that it might be a psychiatric emergency.

Sometimes patients will have multiple complaints. Let's say a 64-year-old man tells you, "I'm really weak, and it feels like there are butterflies in my chest." You will need to figure out whether these symptoms are related. If you believe that they are related, to provide appropriate care, you need to identify the *origin of the problem.* In this case, you may want to ask, "Have you had this problem before?"

On the other hand, let's say your patient is complaining of "being dizzy and having pain in her left ankle." You can ask a couple of questions and may determine, for example, that the two complaints are not related. You must then decide which of the two is your priority.

Once you've established the chief complaint(s), you will want to flesh out the history of the present illness, which should provide you with a clear sequence and chronologic account of the patient's signs and symptoms, that is, *what happened* and *when.*

You need to ask about the patient's *general state of health* and any serious childhood or adult illnesses. Ask about any mental health problems the patient might be having and whether he or she has ever been hospitalized for a mental health problem. Although it is often difficult for patients and families to admit to

Documentation and Communication

The history of present illness should always be documented clearly and accurately. This is often the most important information, medically and legally.

mental health problems, if you are matter-of-fact and dignified in asking the question, you can get a "straight" answer.

You will also need to ask about any accidents or injuries the patient had within the last month or so and about any operations or hospitalizations within the last 6 months or so.

One of the more challenging aspects of the history-taking process is that of pulling together the patient's *current health status,* because it is made up of many unrelated pieces of information. However, it often ties together some of the past history with the history of the current event, so it has definite value to the assessment process. The simple fact of the matter is, you don't need to obtain each and every piece of information on the following list for every patient. It takes time and practice and a certain amount of common sense for you to know the right questions to ask each patient.

Questions that will be most helpful in getting a useful history include the following:

- What prescription medicines are you currently taking? How much and how often? (Patients can and do confuse when and how to take their medications—and if your patient has, you could be witnessing a drug reaction. Also, as you gain paramedic experience, your familiarity with the drugs will give you an idea of the patient's illness. Medications will also give you a clue about mental health problems or dementia without your needlessly antagonizing a reluctant patient.)
- Do you take any over-the-counter medication like aspirin, herbs, or vitamins?
- Are you allergic to any medicines or other substances?
- Do you smoke? How much? Do you drink beer, wine, or cocktails? How often?
- Have you been smoking or taking drugs other than cigarettes? Assure your patient of confidentiality.
- What did you have to eat yesterday and today?
- Ask about screening tests that are appropriate. For example, for difficulty breathing ask: "Have you had a chest x-ray lately?"
- Are your immunizations up-to-date? How about a flu shot or pneumococcal vaccine? Ask about children's immunizations, too.
- Have you been getting a good night's sleep? Look for maladaptive sleep patterns.
- Do you like to exercise? How much?
- What kinds of chemical cleaners do you have in your house? Do you have any strong chemicals where you work? You might need to probe for environmental hazards.
- Does the family use seatbelts and car seats for the children? Do you have any baby gates? Are medicines locked away (if it seems necessary)?
- Do you have a history of any specific diseases in your family?
- Where do you live? What do you like to do at home? Is there anyone in your life that you might be afraid of? You might need to assess a difficult home situation.
- How do you spend your time during the day?

- Do you have anything in your religion that would prevent me from administering treatment?
- Are you an optimistic person? You might feel it important to get your patient's overall outlook on life.

Special Considerations

In some cases, a patient's religious beliefs may be relevant, for example if the beliefs pertain directly to medical care. If your patient indicates that such beliefs are important, this information should be passed along to emergency department staff.

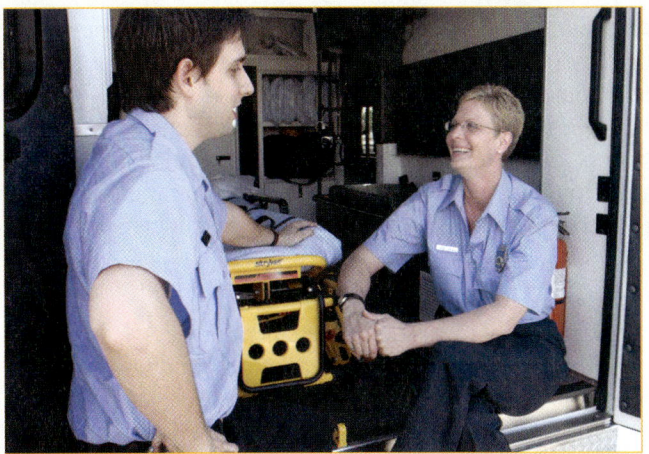

Figure 12-4 Your appearance should be professional and your demeanour positive and friendly.

You have to decide which of the listed items you want to explore and which you do not. For a really sick patient with immediate life threats, you may have no time to explore any of them. For a patient in stable condition who appears to be in no apparent distress, you may have time and decide to explore all relevant topics.

Last, you'll want to do a quick check on the body systems. A great way to gain insight is to ask, "Has your doctor ever told you that you have a heart, lung, or brain problem?" After that, you can ask about things like bowel movements, and so on, which tend to be non–life threatening.

Techniques for History Taking

Setting the Stage for Quality Patient Care

Every time you care for a patient, you must first establish a professional relationship. In most cases, this is a *short-term* relationship, less than 2 hours' duration, until you provide your hand-off report and turn the patient over to the emergency department staff.

Your Demeanour and Appearance

Although time is short, you will want to have a positive patient outcome in the care you provide and the communication you establish with all involved. When you first meet your patient, they should be looking at a clean, neat, health care provider. You should have good personal hygiene and grooming and attire that is professional, clean, and pressed **Figure 12-4 ▶**. If you look professional, your patient will likely develop a good first impression of you.

Along with your appearance, there is the matter of your demeanour. On every call, your attitude is always on display. If you are unhappy, a look of unhappiness is almost certainly on your face. Your facial expression and body language can send powerful messages. If you have come to believe that calls to 9-1-1 need to meet *your* expectations, *you are wrong*. If patients think a problem is serious enough to merit a call to 9-1-1, you have an obligation to treat patients and their complaints accordingly—professionally and to the best of your ability.

Introduce yourself to your patient and tell him or her the name of your service and your certification level. Introduce your partner as well.

Try to interview the patient in a private setting. Don't hesitate to ask any nonessential personnel to leave the room or to at least step back because you will frequently find yourself asking your patients personal or intimate questions. Most people do not want to admit some bad habits (for example, cigarettes) that have a negative impact on their health. But you need to know. If the setting makes the patient uncomfortable, the patient may choose to not answer your questions or to answer inaccurately. Working to ensure the patient's privacy, confidentiality, and comfort level goes a long way toward establishing positive patient rapport and encourages more honest, open communication.

Confidentiality

As discussed in Chapter 4, it is your duty to maintain confidentiality of the patient's information. The Canada Health Act, and the various provincial health information privacy acts govern the gathering and disclosure of patient information. You need to be familiar with the relevant laws. Also, showing the patient that you respect the confidentiality of his or her medical information helps build rapport and contributes to total patient care.

How to Address the Patient

After introducing yourself, ask the patient his or her name and how he or she would like to be addressed. Err on the side of formality, using Mr., Miss, Mrs., or Ms. There is a world of difference in Mr. John Markham (formal), John (more casual), or Johnnie (really casual). Your patient will say, "Call me John" if that is what he prefers. Calling patients by the name of their choosing is professional, but assuming formality will help establish more rapport than being too familiar.

Avoid "catch-all names" or "pet names" like pal, buddy, sport, dude, friend, honey, sweetie, cutie, and darling. You can bog down the process of obtaining a history by demeaning the patient and treating the patient unprofessionally. Using casual nicknames also can be problematic when there are cultural differences. Some terms have negative connotations in some cultures. You need to be familiar with the cultural groups in your area and with issues that could lead to misunderstanding.

Note Taking

As you get ready to start the assessment process, let the patient know that you are going to be asking a number of questions and that while he or she is answering, you or your partner will be taking notes. This lets patients know they aren't being ignored and that the information being provided is important enough to write down **Figure 12-5 ▶**.

Too often, paramedics read off a list of questions to patients to fill in all the blanks on the call report. With this approach comes the problem of making little to no eye contact with the patient. Don't bury your nose in the clipboard! If possible, position yourself at the eye level of your patient.

Reviewing the Medical History and Information Reliability

Frequently, you will obtain information not just from your patient but also from other sources. It is important that you document the source of this information in your record. Family members are commonly involved at emergency scenes, as are friends. Law enforcement personnel and bystanders also can be valuable sources of information.

A large number of the patient contacts in day-to-day EMS are routine patient transfers from assisted living or extended care facilities to the hospital and back. Take a few moments to review the transfer paperwork. You need to know the medical history of the patient so you are prepared to provide care should your planned routine transfer suddenly turn unroutine.

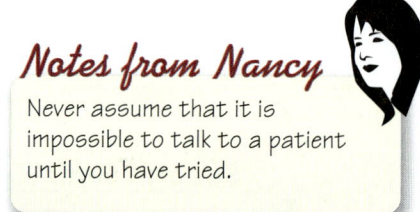

Notes from Nancy

Never assume that it is impossible to talk to a patient until you have tried.

Keep in mind the importance of evaluating your sources of information for reliability. Although the medical records in the transfer packet from an extended care facility should be assumed to be reasonably accurate, individual performances of caregivers vary. When all is said and done, you are responsible for patient care decisions, so make sure you work with information that is as accurate as possible.

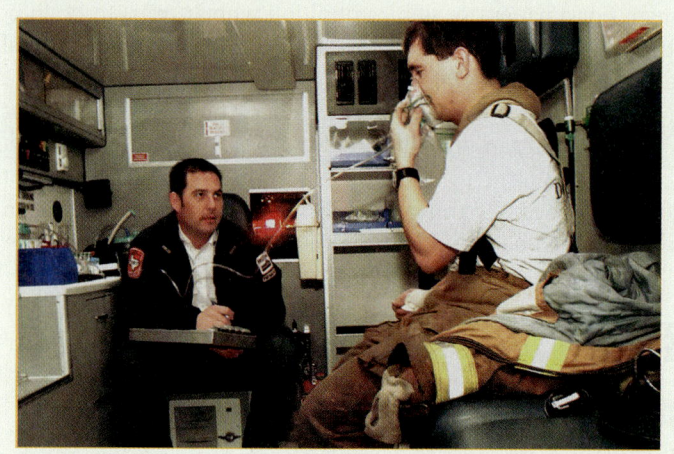

Figure 12-5 You may want to take notes during the patient history.

You are the Paramedic Part 2

After moving the bowls of food out of the immediate area and asking the other members of the family to give you and your patient some privacy, you notice localized swelling and redness at the sting site and a venom sac embedded in his skin. You scrape the stinger away with a tongue depressor, obtain vital signs, give the patient high-flow supplemental oxygen, and insert an 18-gauge intravenous (IV) cannula in the right antecubital vein to give normal saline to keep vein open. The patient denies having shortness of breath and any history of severe allergic reactions. He also denies carrying or using an EpiPen or having taken any antihistamines before your arrival. When you ask about his medical history, he says he has occasional chest pain with exertion and that his only medication is nitroglycerin. He has no allergies to medication. He tells you that currently he has no chest pain.

Vital Signs	Recording Time: 3 Minutes
Skin	Localized redness and swelling at the sting site and hives on the abdomen
Pulse	98 beats/min, regular
Blood pressure	108/58 mm Hg
Respirations	24 breaths/min
Spo$_2$	100% with oxygen at 12 to 15 l/min via nonrebreathing mask

3. What medication(s) would you administer to this patient?
4. What other assessment tools would you like to use?

Communication Techniques

Encourage Dialogue

On the basis of the questions asked and answers received, you will make patient care decisions. A number of approaches and conversation techniques can help to improve the volume and quality of information you obtain during the patient interview.

Facilitation

A dictionary definition of facilitation is to "make easy or easier." Facilitation in communication means using techniques that permit your patient to feel open to giving you some of the most delicate information he or she can share. Patients of all ages are hesitant to share private or embarrassing information. Your job is to make your patients feel so secure with you that they will give you the information you need.

The most important thing you can do to facilitate the information exchange is pay attention. Maintain eye contact if it is culturally appropriate. Some cultures consider constant eye contact to be a sign of aggression and may avoid eye contact for that reason, not because they are not listening. Use phrases that encourage the patient to share more information such as, "That's helpful," "Anything else you can think of?" or "Please go on." Nodding your head and using an appropriately placed, "Okay," every now and then lets the patient know you are getting the message.

> ### Documentation and Communication
> Do not put ideas into the patient's head, such as, "Is the pain in your chest a dull ache that is behind your sternum and radiates into your jaw?"

Another helpful facilitation technique is repeating key information from the patient's answers.

Patient: *"I've been feeling weird since I got up, and my chest just aches bad. It never felt like this before."*
Paramedic: *"Your chest aches?"*
Patient: *"Real bad. I've never had it ache like this."*
Paramedic: *"You've had chest pain before?"*
Patient: *"Yeah, I've been seeing a heart doctor pretty regularly for going on 5 years now. Used to be I would get kind of a squeezing feeling in my chest, I'd take a nitro, and it would go away. Well, this is nothing like that! I took two nitro right away, and I'll bet it's been close to an hour and a half, and nothing has changed."*

In this case, with just two short questions, you greatly expanded what you knew about the patient. You now know that the patient:

- Has a history of heart disease.
- Has been seeing a cardiologist for 5 years.
- Is having pain today that is different from and more serious than pain in the past.
- Is having pain today that is the worst it has ever been.

- Has taken nitroglycerin for symptom relief in the past.
- Took two nitroglycerin doses today that failed to relieve the symptoms.

Reflection

Reflection is the *repetition* of a word or phrase that a patient has used to encourage more detail.

Your patient might say: *"I couldn't catch my breath."*
You could respond: *"You couldn't catch your breath, Mrs. Slocum?"*
Your patient might elaborate: *"I don't know. I recall my heart just all of a sudden seemed to start beating really fast, and then I got scared, and all of a sudden I was breathing superfast but not getting enough air."*

Reflection is a powerful tool for getting a good patient history for two reasons: (1) Reflection usually does not break the flow or your patient's thoughts. It helps you both stay focused. (2) The information you will obtain is not biased by "leading" the patient. You are using the words the patient used, not your own description, which is very important in good histories.

Clarification

Clarification is the technique of asking your patients for more information when some aspect of the history is vague or unclear to you **Figure 12-6 ▾**. The clearer you are about your patient's condition, the more helpful and appropriate your care will be. On the other hand, if you are unsure about your patient's problem, the more likely your care is based on guesswork and happenstance.

Paramedic: *"What's going on today, Mrs. Hendrickson?"*
Patient: *"Oh I don't know. I'm just . . . well I'm just not feeling like myself."*
Paramedic: *"I'm sorry. Could you try to be a little more specific? If you could do that, it will help me figure out what's going on with you today."*
Patient: *"I'm always full of energy first thing in the morning, but I'm so weak right now that I couldn't even take Princess out to do her business."*

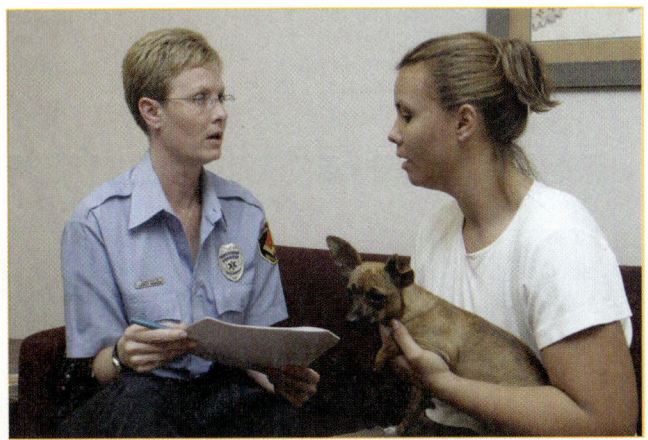

Figure 12-6 Use clarification to gain more information about the patient's chief complaint.

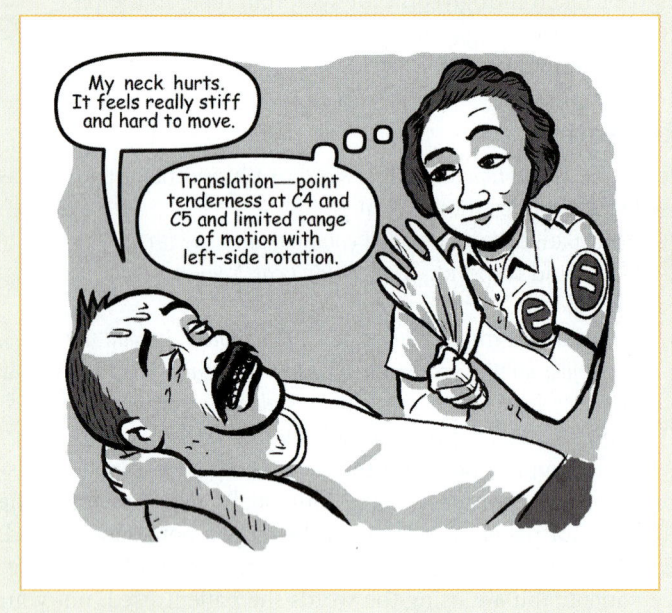

Figure 12-7

Documentation and Communication

Layman's Lingo	EMS Lingo
My sugars	I'm a diabetic
Fell out	Had a syncopal episode
Has the fits	History of seizures
Water pills	Furosemide (Lasix)

With this example, having identified the chief complaint as "weakness" is medically clearer than the complaint of "not feeling like myself."

Clarification is one of the more frequently used interview techniques in EMS. By the nature of your job, you may want to speak and listen to the language of medicine, but the average layperson has a limited medical vocabulary. Patients will generally use nonmedical terms to answer your assessment questions **Figure 12-7** . You will need to clarify what they mean.

Empathetic Response

Empathy is often described as one step further than sympathy; empathy is a psychological gift that allows you to feel what your patient is feeling—putting yourself into his or her shoes. At times, you will hear sad and tragic information from your patients. Do not hesitate to communicate your feelings and address the emotional impact of what has been said **Figure 12-8** .

> Paramedic: *"What is the reason you called for help today, Mr. Ortiz?"*
> Patient: *"I've just been horribly depressed."*
> Paramedic: *"And why is that, Mr. Ortiz?"*
> Patient: *"My wife and two kids were hit and killed by a drunk driver 6 months ago, and I just can't get over it."*
> Paramedic: *"I am so sorry to hear that, Mr. Ortiz. That seems so wrong to me."*

Mr. Ortiz, the man who has lost his entire family, might not have an overt medical problem, but certainly you should consider the possibility that he might be so depressed that some kind of mental health referral is needed.

You are the Paramedic Part 3

With your patient's blood pressure low, his pulse rate elevated, and the presence of hives, you consider epinephrine administration. With his heart history and lack of breathing difficulty, epinephrine should be administered with caution. You decide that the subcutaneous route of 0.3 to 0.5 mg 1:1,000 is appropriate, and your partner begins preparing the equipment and site. You also choose to administer diphenhydramine (Benadryl) IV, but just as you move your patient to the stretcher, you see a small, open pill bottle lying on his chair.

Reassessment	Recording Time: 5 Minutes
Skin	Slightly moist, pale, and warm
Pulse	100 beats/min, regular
Blood pressure	108/58 mm Hg
Respirations	24 breaths/min
Spo$_2$	100% with oxygen at 12 to 15 l/min via nonrebreathing mask
ECG	Sinus rhythm with no ectopy

5. What could be another reason for his low blood pressure and elevated pulse rate?
6. What should you immediately ask your patient?
7. Should you consider rethinking your diagnosis and treatment plans now?

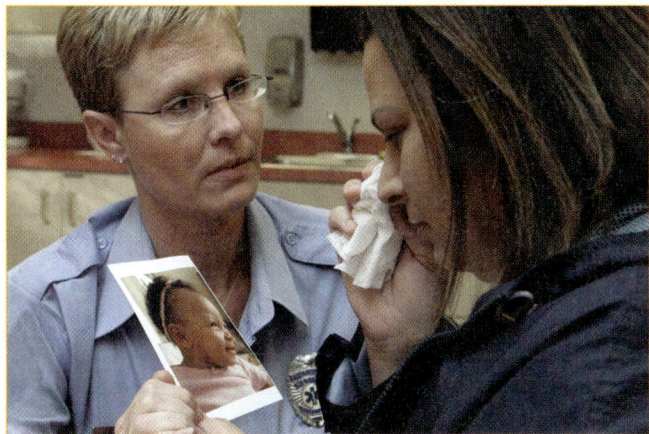

Figure 12-8 Be empathetic when the patient conveys sad or tragic information.

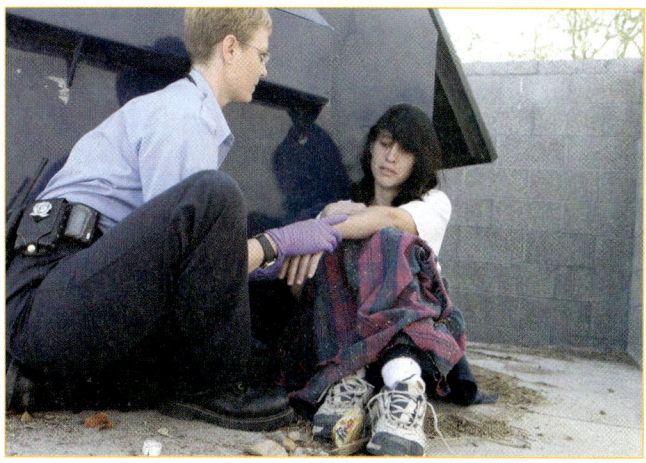

Figure 12-9 Use a nonjudgmental approach when confronting a patient.

Paramedics, unlike most other health care providers, see people when the illness or trauma just occurred. Your patients are uniquely vulnerable and uniquely demanding. Try your best to develop empathy for your patients.

Remember that in earlier chapters we discussed being active in your community to keep yourself aware of other sources of help for your patients. Empathy can help you set your patient on a path to healing—no matter what the diagnosis.

Confrontation

Confrontation is making your patients aware that you perceive something that is not consistent with their behaviour, the actual scene, or the information the patient is giving you. Nevertheless, avoiding confrontations with your patients is a good practice. If you must confront a patient, for example about using illegal drugs or alcohol, a professional approach can help you get medically appropriate information. Sometimes patients want a chance to deal with their problems. The key is to remain professional and nonjudgmental **Figure 12-9 ▶** .

Patient: *"My life just sucks. I don't know why I even go on living."*
Paramedic: *"Are you considering suicide?"*
Patient: *"I'm thinking that might just be the best thing."*
Paramedic: *"Have you made plans on how you are going to do it?"*
Patient: *"I don't know, I haven't given it that much thought."*

This patient's response clearly points toward possible suicide. Use a direct approach and ask the patient about whether he is contemplating suicide and if so, if he has a plan. This information helps you assess how distressed the patient is so that you can decide how to best ensure safe transport of the patient.

Interpretation

If your patient refuses to give you information, you need to infer what could be causing the distress and then ask the patient if you are right. (In the preceding situation, the paramedic, who spoke with a clearly distressed patient used interpretation about whether the patient was suicidal.)

The skill of interpretation demands that paramedics use their best diplomatic skills. One of the best phrases with which to begin an inference is the ever-reliable, "So, if I understand you correctly . . ."

Asking About Feelings

Asking about feelings is one of the most difficult roles of a paramedic. But as part of a good health history, you will need to ask if a patient is tired, depressed, or any number of feelings that are most easily dealt with by denial. (You will even need to ask these questions of a colleague if you see the symptoms.)

Try to keep possible unpleasant sights, sounds, and smells from your patient who is feeling badly. You can also validate feelings. "This is a tough situation." That's empathy in action. Do your best to attend to psychological needs at the scene. It is a tough job, but these needs profoundly affect physical health.

Be effective. Do not ask, "Are you okay?" This is the most tempting of all questions (and it *can* be answered with a yes or no!). Instead, ask for facts first, then follow up. Even with someone you know quite well, you need to establish rapport to ask a question about how he or she is feeling. Most of us would deny that we are exhausted, frazzled, scared, or depressed. Your patients met you only a few minutes ago. Establish that you are a caring health professional during a series of "safe" questions about physical health.

Getting More Information

You've gotten a lot of information from your patient, but in many cases, you need to refine your thinking to come up with a valid diagnosis. Let's say you were exploring a particular symptom such as "abdominal pain" with your patient. (As you will soon learn, abdominal pain can suggest a startlingly large number of diagnoses.) Some possible questions you might ask the patient about the *region* or location of the pain include the following:

- Where exactly does it hurt?
- Does it hurt in one particular spot or in a general area?
- Can you point to where it hurts with one finger?
- Does the pain stay right there, or does it move or radiate anywhere else?
- If your pain does move or radiate, where does it go?

Questions you may ask about the *quality* of the abdominal pain include the following:

- What type of pain is it: a sharp pain or more of a dull ache?
- Does the pain come and go, or is it constant?
- If you wanted me to feel the same feeling that you do, what would you do to me to make me feel that way?

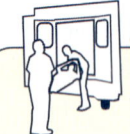
At the Scene

Letting patients describe their pain in their own words will be very helpful for your assessment.

Questions you may ask about the *severity* of the abdominal pain include the following:

- In your opinion, how bad is this pain?
- Is it more of an uncomfortable feeling or a feeling of hurt?
- Would you say the pain is similar to or worse than with previous episodes?
- On a scale of 1 to 10, with 10 being the *worst* pain you've ever felt and 1 being very minor, how would you rate your pain?

The questions in these lists are not exhaustive or all-inclusive. Add and modify questions to the patient interview as you need to. Subtract questions if time is of the essence. Use open-ended questions whenever you can (Figure 12-10 ▾). Pin your patient down

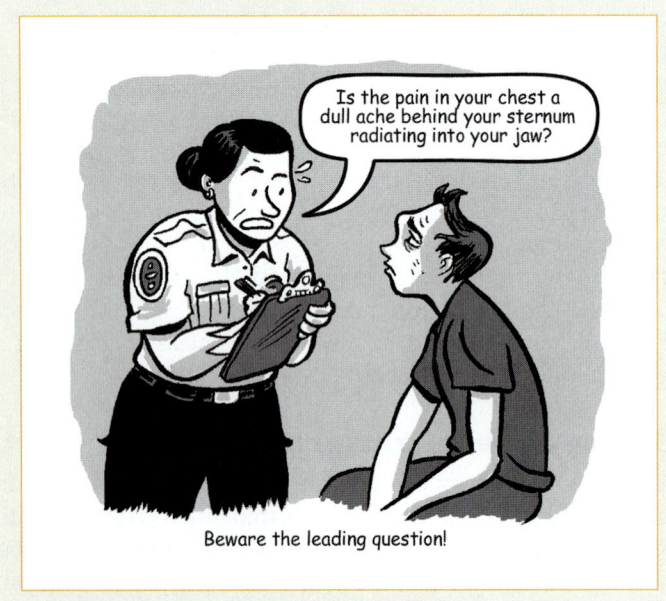

Is the pain in your chest a dull ache behind your sternum radiating into your jaw?

Beware the leading question!

Figure 12-10

with a close-ended question if that's what the situation requires.

Try to be *orderly* and *systematic* in your information gathering and assessment, while at the same time *flexible* in your approach. Being flexible in an emergency is a lot harder than it sounds, but it is attainable with practice—lots and lots of practice.

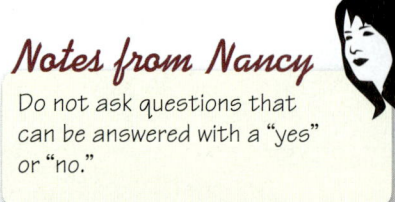
Notes from Nancy

Do not ask questions that can be answered with a "yes" or "no."

You could probably use some help in remembering what to cover. The mnemonic OPQRST offers an easy-to-remember approach to analyzing a patient's chief complaint that is simple and effective.

- **Onset.** When did you start to feel pain?
- **Provocation.** What do you think brought on your pain?
  - Did the pain start all of a sudden or come on over a period of time?
  - Does anything make the pain go away or feel better or feel worse?
- **Quality.** If you were trying to make me feel the way you do, what would you do to me to give me that same feeling?
- **Region/Radiation/Referral.**
  - Can you point to the place where it hurts with one finger?
  - Does the pain stay there, or does it go somewhere else?
- **Severity.** On a scale of 1 to 10, with 1 being very minor and 10 the worst pain you've ever felt, how would you rank this?
- **Time.** How long have you felt this way?

Documentation and Communication

Documenting pain severity ratings is important. Also note how distressed the patient appears: mild, moderate, or severe.

Clinical Reasoning

The results of your questions should expand your thinking about problems and other body systems that are associated with the symptoms your patient has mentioned. In Chapter 15, you will learn the details of critical thinking. Critical thinking consists of (1) concept formation, (2) data interpretation, (3) application of principles (guidelines or algorithms), (4) reflection in action (being willing to change course as you interpret your patient's condition), and (5) reflection on action (doing honest and thorough postcall critiques to benefit learning).

Being able to think and perform well under pressure is a big part of being able to be good paramedic. In many ways, critical thinking and decision making are just two more skills you will need to work on, not just while you are a student, but for the rest of your career as a practicing paramedic.

One of the most important elements of the interview process is for you to be a *great listener,* and a big part of being a great listener is also being a *patient listener.* For a number of reasons, patients can be slow to respond. Maybe they didn't hear your question. Maybe they didn't understand you. Maybe they are afraid to answer. There are many possible explanations. Ask, then wait, and give your patients time to gather their thoughts so they can answer you.

Communicate with your patients by using terminology matched to their knowledge and understanding. For example, a patient who is an emergency department nurse or a retired surgeon will understand medical terminology. On the other hand, a patient who speaks little English needs simple and focused communication.

Throughout the assessment process, look for nonverbal communication, such as changes in facial expression, heavy sighs, or aggressive gestures (finger pointing), any of which can impact your information processing.

Direct Questions

To complete the history, direct questions could be required. Patients might not be giving you easy-to-digest facts about themselves, and if you need a date, time, or other specific information, you should ask for it.

Getting a History on Sensitive Topics

As a paramedic, you will be privileged to care for people who depend on you during some of the worst moments of their lives. You represent hope and comfort no matter how difficult, even horrific, your patient's situation might be.

Some sensitive factors like drug and alcohol abuse can stand in the way of your best efforts for the health of your patients. Here are some ways that can help you be the paramedic you want to be, no matter how sensitive the situation.

Alcohol and Drug Abuse

People who regularly abuse drugs or alcohol become adept at hiding the signs and symptoms from their friends, family, and workplace associates and denying there is a problem. Such denial can go on for years, and the signs and symptoms can be hidden even from people closest to the patient.

If asked how much alcohol or drug has been consumed, the amount is often understated. Some experienced paramedics say the standard answer to the question about how many drinks is "two," when the behaviour indicates many more. Slightly *fewer* than half of all motor vehicle collisions involve alcohol. Just *more* than half of all motor vehicle collisions that result in fatalities involve alcohol **Figure 12-11 ▶** .

It is probable that an alcohol-impaired patient will give an unreliable history. Do not assume that all that you are told is completely accurate. Keep in mind that alcohol can mask any number of signs and symptoms. When a patient who experienced a significant traumatic event denies neck or back pain, if you smell what you believe to be alcohol on the patient's breath or behaviour raises your suspicion of alcohol or drug use, take precautions to restrict spinal motion.

Alcohol is a legal drug. If your patient is using other substances to "get high," using them is most likely illegal. The fear of punishment for illegal use of drugs might lead patients to deny their use. Let your patient know that you are a medical person and anything that he or she tells you will be kept in confidence. Do your best to win your patient's trust because you need the information to provide proper treatment.

Keep your best professional attitude as you work with patients you suspect of using drugs or alcohol. Paramedics should never judge their patients by appearances or behaviour. An unkempt homeless person might be in desperate need of assessment for head trauma, not alcoholism. A suburban executive might have hit his head during a collision, but drinking alcohol might be the cause of the accident.

Physical Abuse and Domestic Violence

As a paramedic, you are required to report a case if you have reason to suspect physical abuse or domestic violence. Although it is inappropriate for you to accuse someone of abuse at the scene, never hesitate to call for law enforcement personnel if you have reason to believe that abuse has occurred. They will help stabilize the scene and provide another set of professional eyes.

A number of clues may lead you to suspect domestic violence. Injuries inconsistent with the information you are being given are common, as are multiple injuries in various stages of healing. Unspoken messages can be given by the family's behaviour. Maybe it's the cowering posture of the woman at the kitchen table as her husband or significant other towers over her and answers your questions for her. If the injured family member does not give you the information but waits for someone else to speak up, that's a clue that the injured family member is being repressed. You can suggest that the significant other who is doing all the talking go to the

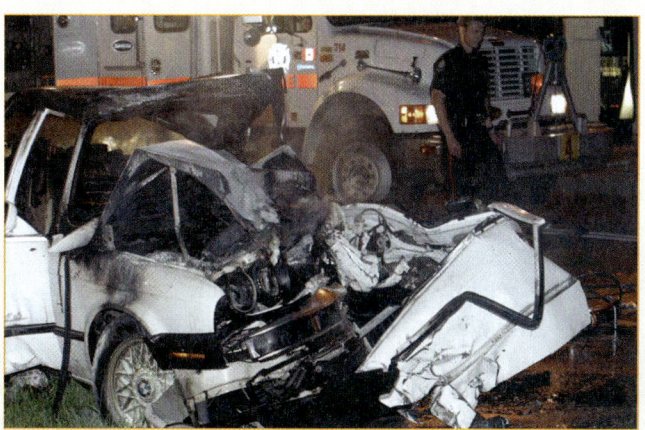

Figure 12-11 Many collisions involve alcohol. In these cases, the patient history may not be reliable.

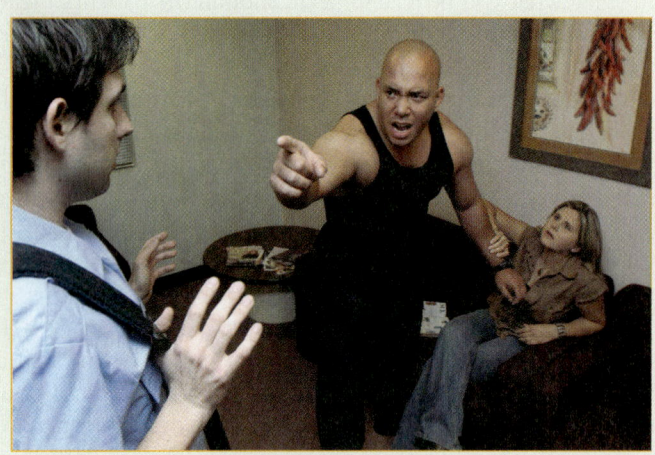

Figure 12-12 Do not handle potentially violent calls alone. Summon law enforcement personnel.

At the Scene

If you find yourself suddenly in a potentially dangerous position and your partners are not aware of it, use a predetermined code word to alert them. One inconspicuous code is to use the trade name of something in your ambulance—"could you get the Ferno stretcher?" Your partners should know that it means there is danger and that they should summon law enforcement personnel.

rig to help with the gurney. The moment the door shuts, you may receive valuable information, such as, "My husband is beating me and I'm scared to death. You've got to get me out of here before he kills me or one of the kids." *Immediately* request law enforcement personnel if this or if anything close to this happens.

Emergency scenes involving domestic violence are some of the most dangerous for EMS and law enforcement professionals alike   **Figure 12-12 ▲** . Don't even think of handling them without law enforcement personnel on hand.

Sexual History

A number of factors may influence a patient about being less than forthcoming about sexual history. Religious upbringing, cultural or societal mores, and exotic or bizarre sexual tastes may inhibit a patient from sharing sexual history because this is truly one of the most private and personal aspects of a person's life. When the topic is someone's sexual history, obtaining the history in as private a setting as possible is essential.

Keep your questions focused and on task. For a female patient complaining of acute abdominal pain, foul smelling vaginal discharge, pain on urination, genital lesions, or similar complaints, you will need to know such things as when your patient last had a period and when she last had sexual intercourse. You will also need to find out if there is vaginal bleeding, whether she has had multiple sex partners, the

Special Considerations

Some younger teens may be confused when asked about sexual issues. Be direct and avoid using questions like, "Are you sexually active?" because they may think active means often.

characteristics of the vaginal discharge, and whether she uses a birth control method.

Male patients with complaints of pain on urination, discharge from the penis, genital lesions, and so forth, need to be asked about their most recent sexual encounter, whether they use condoms, the characteristics of their discharge and lesions, and so forth.

You may need to ask female and male patients if they have ever been tested for HIV, AIDS, or hepatitis. Do not interject any opinions or biases about sexual choices or behaviour. Their choices aren't your choices, just as your choices are not theirs. Every patient you care for deserves to be treated with compassion and respect.

Special Assessment Challenges

Simply put, it is impossible to address every scenario you may encounter in your work as a paramedic, but there are a number of special assessment challenges that occur often enough to be worth talking about.

Silence

When you are on a mission to obtain your patient's history in a timely manner, a period of silence on the part of your patient can make you uneasy. Don't let it. Your patient may be simply trying to gather his or her thoughts, trying to recall possibly distant details relative to the questions(s) you just asked, or trying to decide if he or she trusts you enough to answer your question(s) truthfully or at all. In any case, be patient.

Keep your antenna extended for nonverbal signs of distress. Pain, psychological distress, or fear often register in body movements and facial expression.

As you work in the prehospital environment while you are a student, you will learn how to read the many nonverbal cues that patients give. The paramedics you work with will help, as will working with experienced caregivers in the emergency department and the hospital. Although paramedics work outside the hospital, you will still find help in learning to read nonverbal cues from everyone you work with.

Another pair of essential skills you can learn from these seasoned veterans are how to time your questions and how to be patient. Learn to ask questions and then *wait*. What seems like an eternity to you is but 1 or 2 seconds to your patients, as they think, retrieve facts, or assess your trustworthiness.

Overly Talkative Patients

On the other side of the coin are overly talkative patients. Some people learn to talk endlessly as a way of socializing, but you must consider possible clinical reasons for the chattiness. Recovering from a fight-or-flight situation, consuming a triple espresso 15 minutes ago, or an illegal drug—cocaine, crack, or methamphetamine—might be the reason. Whatever the cause, the first requirement of dealing with a talkative patient is to keep your patience (again). Try giving the patient free reign for the first few minutes. You might not be able to get as comprehensive a history as you would like with such a patient, given the limits on your time.

After a few minutes, try interrupting your patient to ask for clarification of a piece of information. This gives you an opportunity to quickly summarize what you have just heard.

One thing is for sure: you are better off with too much information than with too little or no information.

Patients With Multiple Symptoms

Although your calls would be much simpler if your patients had only a single complaint, that is not reality. Sometimes you will be presented with "linked" complaints such as, "It feels like my heart is just fluttering, and I'm really dizzy." In this case, both symptoms can be tied to the patient having a high pulse rate.

Then again, especially with the older population, it is entirely possible and, in many cases, entirely likely that you are dealing with multiple causes. A patient with diabetes who is having a cardiac crisis may easily forget that he or she has taken insulin and takes it again. One of the classic musts in EMS is to *always check the blood glucose level* on patients who have *altered mentation,* whether they have a history of diabetes or not.

You need to learn to prioritize your patient's complaints. Only when that is accomplished can you develop an appropriate care plan as you decide which of your patient's problems you need to address and in which order you need to address them.

No matter how sure you are about your initial diagnosis, *always* remain open to the possibility that something else is going on with your patient.

Notes from Nancy

If you don't ask, you won't find out.

Anxious Patients

Believe it or not, you are the cause of many of your patients being overly anxious. No matter how much the public loves to watch emergencies on TV, it is frightening to see an ambulance, fire engine, or squad car pull up and stop in front of the house. You should expect your patient to initially be somewhat anxious, but he or she should start to calm down shortly after your arrival. If not, it's time to open your mind up to other

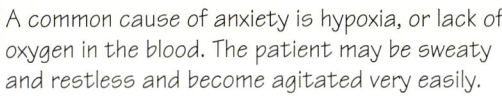

At the Scene

A common cause of anxiety is hypoxia, or lack of oxygen in the blood. The patient may be sweaty and restless and become agitated very easily. Hypoxia is often misinterpreted as panic.

possibilities. High anxiety is a sign of physiologic shock beginning to set in. You will need to be ready to treat immediately. Or your patient could be hiding something, such as physical abuse or the use of illegal drugs.

Whatever the case, be sensitive to verbal and nonverbal clues, always keeping in mind that any information you fail to obtain could be the information you need to treat your patient.

Reassurance

When communicating with patients, paramedics should be poised and confident, with a positive demeanour. With that positive demeanour also comes the temptation to reassure your patients, sometimes inappropriately. Be cautious about what you tell your patients so that you don't make promises you can't deliver.

For example, it can be tempting to reassure a metal worker who caught his wedding ring on a piece of metal that a couple of stitches should make him good as new. However, many circumferential finger cuts can result in an amputation. Imagine how much distress you will cause your patient when he arrives at the hospital and the news is not so cheery.

In addition, if your reassurance is inappropriate, your patient could choose not to share quite as much information as he or she might have under other circumstances, leaving you with less information rather than more.

Anger and Hostility

Frequently you will find yourself the target of patients' and family members' frustrations, which may manifest as anger or outright hostility. Anger and hostility at unfairness and harsh realities are normal. Remember, don't take these situations personally—take them professionally.

The most important skill that you can use is not to get angry yourself. When you are in control of your own anger, you can work to calm the situation. Be attentive to changes in body language, such as threatening gestures or an escalating volume of the conversation or, worse yet, having a heated dialogue melt down into an outright yelling match. When people are angry or hostile, the worst thing you can do is get angry yourself.

As with any call, establishing a safe and secure scene is your first order of business. If you cannot calm the patient or family members, it's time to consider possibly calling for law enforcement personnel. If the patient or a family member is hostile, you might need to tell the person directly that if he or she continues to shout, you will not feel safe enough to do your assessment and will need to call law enforcement personnel. However, if the patient and/or the family members are already angry, telling them that the police are on the way is not going to make them any happier. In worst case scenarios, you may have to withdraw to the safety of your ambulance to wait for the police to arrive.

If the hostile person suddenly leaves the room, especially in the middle of the conversation, you or your partner should follow the person, while working to calm him or her and defuse the situation. What you are also doing is making certain that the person doesn't go back to the bedroom, get a handgun out of the nightstand, and come back and shoot you, your partner, and maybe even the spouse.

Intoxication

When your patient is intoxicated, whether from alcohol or drugs, taking a good medical history becomes very difficult. Intoxication may mask symptoms, such as pain. With intoxication also comes a decrease in patience; while the patient is trying to explain things to you, his or her hostility or anger can escalate faster than if he or she were not intoxicated. A common scenario for this type of situation occurs at minor fender benders, where the intoxicated person wants to get back in the car and continue on his or her way after having run into a stoplight or fire hydrant. The patient's behaviour can become explosive. Your ability to be patient and diplomatic with your communication is paramount.

As frustrating as dealing with intoxicated people can be, do your best to remain objective and nonjudgmental. Remember, one of the keys to being a good paramedic is that *you have to like people,* but that in no way means that you *have to like what people do.*

Crying

Sometimes people cry because they are happy or sad. Although these are certainly common reasons for crying, other possibilities exist.

When the unexpected strikes, it can overwhelm people emotionally. Patients and their family members, along with their friends and neighbours, can suddenly find themselves under extreme levels of stress as a result of the emergency situation at hand. Just as some people react with anger and hostility to a stressful situation, others cry.

Once again, patience goes a long way. You can't expect the crying to immediately stop by yelling, "Quit crying!" Be patient.

Fortunately, the presence of paramedics arriving on the scene often exerts a calming effect. During the course of your career, you will be surprised at how often you hear someone say, usually the very moment you walk in the door, something like, "Thank goodness, the paramedics are here!" Collectively, your calm demeanour and patient approach; appropriate touch, such as a hand on the shoulder; and a quiet, "I'm in control now," tone of voice will help get the crying to stop and allow you to move on to other matters.

Depression

Depression is a common reason for seeking medical attention. If a patient seems sad, hopeless, restless, and irritable; has sleep or eating disruptions; says that he or she feels his or her energy

You are the Paramedic **Part 4**

Your patient admits to taking his nitroglycerin after being stung. He tells you that his doctor told him to "take it when he feels bad." So he did.

Reassessment	Recording Time: 10 Minutes
Skin	Localized redness and swelling at the sting site and hives on the abdomen
Pulse	96 beats/min, regular
Blood pressure	112/64 mm Hg
Respirations	24 breaths/min
Spo$_2$	100% with oxygen at 12 to 15 l/min via nonrebreathing mask
ECG	Sinus rhythm; no ectopy

8. What could have happened if you had continued to treat according to your original diagnosis?

9. What is your updated assessment and treatment plan?

10. What is important to remember when talking with the average person about medications and medical history?

is low; or has pain for which you cannot find a source, consider that your patient might be depressed.

There are two basic types of depression. Situational depression describes a reaction to a stressful event in a patient's life. Chronic depression is ongoing and does not seem to have an apparent cause. Depression is a normal human response. In the case of situational depression, many people accept what has happened and begin to get on with their life again.

However, sometimes this doesn't happen and they fall victim to chronic depression. Both forms of depression can lead to harmful behaviour, including suicide. You must ask about your patient's feelings to assess for risk of suicide. If the patient indicates he or she could do away with himself or herself, you must follow your service's protocol for behavioural or psychiatric emergencies. Remember that depression is caused by a neurochemical imbalance in the brain and cannot be easily "shaken off" or "got over."

Sexually Attractive or Seductive Patients

It is not abnormal for clinicians and patients to be sexually attracted to each other. Although these feelings are normal, it is never appropriate for a clinician to act on them. If a patient becomes seductive or makes sexual advances, frankly but firmly make clear that your relationship is professional, rather than personal. Should this occur, try to keep your partner, a member of the law enforcement community, or a family member in the room with you at all times as a witness to any events that occur and a support person to help the patient recognize that the behaviour is inappropriate.

Make absolutely certain that you don't cross the line that separates personal from professional behaviour, and don't allow the patient to cross that line either.

Confusing Behaviours or Histories

Paramedics sometimes find that the patient's history given at the scene is very different from the history the patient gives to the physician in the hospital emergency department. Sometimes the information is so different that it seems as if this is an entirely different patient. Patients may be too frightened or embarrassed to give particular information to a paramedic but will give a physician the vital information.

Don't forget how many other possibilities can account for confusing behaviour on the part of your patients, such as hypoxia, a toxic environment, a cerebrovascular accident (stroke), or transient ischemic attack. You will need to consider the possibility of mental illness or drug-induced delirium. Last, don't forget to consider some organic cause such as Alzheimer's disease, dementia, or a brain tumour. The human brain is an impressive organ, and there are a number of reasons it may malfunction.

Limited Education or Intelligence

Never, ever presume that you will not be able to get a history from a patient—any patient. Some patients will not have much knowledge of the health care system or its specialized vocabulary. Other patients will be developmentally challenged. Assume that you can get at least some worthwhile history from all patients. Assume that it is your job to keep asking questions in different ways until you get the answers you need.

Don't try to impress patients with medical terminology. Simple phrases will do a much better job. Asking someone, "Do you think you are having an attack of unstable angina?" may get you little more than a blank stare in return. On the other hand, "Are you having chest pain?" may get you just the information you need to proceed with caring for your patient.

Your patient doesn't need a master's degree to provide you with an accurate medical history. You can frequently get adequate information from patients with a limited education or intellectual capabilities. Be alert for partial answers to your questions or omissions. The patient may not know or be able to recall the information you are requesting. For patients who are severely mentally challenged, you may need to get information from family members, friends, or another caregiver.

Language Barriers

The world has many groups of people who do not speak the primary language of the countries in which they live. But when they are sick, you will want to give them the best possible care **Figure 12-13 ▼**.

The first person to look to for help is someone who speaks your language and your patient's language—an interpreter. (If there are large groups of people who speak one language in your service area, it would be wise to learn how to ask for an interpreter in that other language.)

Often, the only person available to interpret will be your patient's child—children absorb a new language quickly in their schools. If you can find someone older and not so intimately attached to your patient, it would be better for getting a

Documentation and Communication

In French, "Parlez-vous Anglais?" means "Do you speak English?"

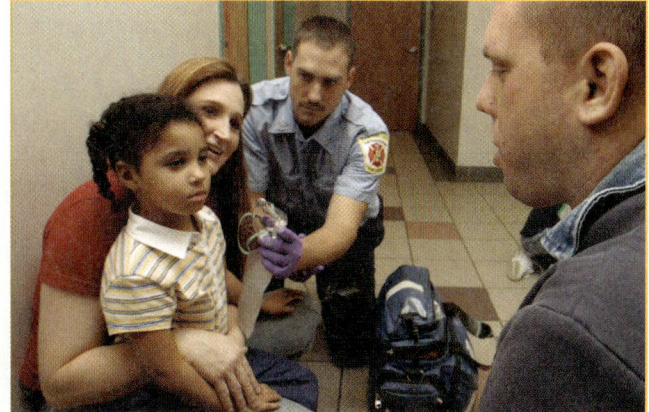

Figure 12-13 You will work with people of other cultures, which may require using an interpreter.

Documentation and Communication

Be aware that medical terms and jargon often do not translate well, such as "ECG leads," "CAT scan," "JAWS," and "stool."

At the Scene

Patients' medication(s), their living quarters, and the name of their doctor can often give clues about medical history. For example, insulin means the patient has diabetes; oxygen tanks and nebulizers in the house probably denote chronic lung disease; and the physician's name can be that of a specialist, like an oncologist or psychiatrist.

good history. Keep your questions as straightforward as possible, and do your very best not to scare a child.

You must not, however, let a few broken words of yours be a substitute for an interpreter. Also understand that simply turning up the volume on your questioning does nothing to overcome a language barrier.

Hearing Problems

Another interesting challenge includes working with patients with hearing problems. Hearing problems can range from a slight impairment to total deafness. For patients such as older people who may only have minimal impairment, speaking slowly and slightly louder may be all that is necessary. For people with a more severe problem, you may want to let them wear your stethoscope as you hold the bell and speak to them. If you do this, make sure to clean the earpieces before you offer them to the patient and before you put them back on.

When addressing patients who are totally deaf but who can read lips, address them face-to-face, slowing your speech slightly so that you are speaking clearly. With medical communications, however, you should find an interpreter who knows American Sign Language (ASL). Writing out medical communications is also a way of getting a patient history. You can resort to writing your questions and have the patients write their answers. In a pinch, it's better than nothing.

On your successful completion of a paramedic program, two of the best investments in continuing education you can make for your future are learning a second language and learning sign language.

Visual Impairment or Blindness

Many patients with varying degrees of visual impairment are self-sufficient and live independent, productive lives. People who are blind have the greatest challenge. First, and foremost, be careful to announce yourself, giving your patient your identity and your reason for being there. Be cautious, and if you pull up a chair to sit next to a blind patient, remember to put it back exactly where you found it. The same is true if furniture has to be moved to provide access or egress for the gurney. Blind people who have their living environments situated the

way they want it can get around with remarkable ease. Make sure you leave things the way you found them.

Once you move the patient to the rig, he or she is in a foreign environment and dependent on the paramedics for transport and assistance with an orderly transition into the emergency department. Be sure to tell the person what you are doing and the location of the transport vehicle at all times (for example, "We'll be at the hospital in about 10 minutes." "We're at the hospital and will be wheeling you off the ambulance and into the emergency department in just a minute."

Family and Friends

Some of your patients might not be able to give you any or much information, and you will need to turn to their family and friends. You need the information to help your patient, but the farther you go from the primary source, the more chance for inaccuracy. Try to obtain accurate data when possible; the more accurate your data, the easier it will be to form an accurate initial diagnosis and provide the best care possible.

Also, you are in a delicate position because you cannot reveal medical information about your patient to the family, so forming your questions will be difficult. Nevertheless, information about your patient is critical, so work with people who can help your patients.

Conclusion

As a paramedic, you can do so much more for your patient than you could as a primary care paramedic. But you must also be aware that being able to do more means that you must know more—not only more about health, disease, and injury, but also more about your patients. A good history, which demands good communications skills and unflagging attention to detail, is an important building block of prehospital care.

You will constantly be reviewing how to do history taking better and better, not only as part of your classes, but also as part of your efforts to maintain and upgrade your prehospital patient care skills.

You are the Paramedic Summary

1. What are your immediate concerns?

Scene safety is your first priority, and with the continued presence of bees, the food should be removed and/or the patient should be removed from the immediate area. The last thing you need is for your patient to be stung again.

2. At this point, what would you want to know about his medical history?

It is vital to know whether your patient has a history of severe allergic reaction, especially associated with bee stings. Should your patient have a history of anaphylaxis, you should be on high alert because the likelihood of recurrence is extremely high.

3. What medication(s) would you administer to this patient?

The standard medications for administration to patients with signs and symptoms of anaphylaxis include epinephrine and diphenhydramine. Patients who have significant hypotension and wheezing should receive 0.3 to 0.5 milligrams of epinephrine, 1:10,000 IV; for other patients who are not experiencing severe hypotension or airway compromise, who have relevant medical histories, or are older, epinephrine, 0.3 to 0.5 milligrams 1:1,000 subcutaneously, will likely be a better choice. You must consider all factors when choosing the route and dose of epinephrine administration. Diphenhydramine is indicated because it will prevent the remaining histamine from entering the cells. But, as for all treatments, you should follow local protocols.

4. What other assessment tools would you like to use?

Obviously with the patient's heart history, the cardiac monitor is an essential assessment tool. Depending on the patient's chief complaint and your impression, you may also decide to obtain a 12-lead ECG.

5. What could be another reason for his low blood pressure and elevated pulse rate?

Nitroglycerin causes blood pressure to drop, and when this occurs, assuming the patient is not also taking a beta-blocker, the pulse rate will increase to compensate.

6. What should you immediately ask your patient?

You should ask if he took his nitro before your arrival. This would also explain his hypotension, increased pulse rate, and lack of shortness of breath associated with expected airway edema in anaphylaxis.

7. Should you consider rethinking your diagnosis and treatment plans now?

Armed with this new, very important information, you decide that diphenhydramine is a good choice, and epinephrine is not needed at this time. After confirming clear lung sounds, a fluid bolus to increase blood pressure rather than the use of alpha- and beta-agonists is indicated. Follow local protocols.

8. What could have happened if you had continued to treat according to your original diagnosis?

Giving epinephrine to a healthy, young patient who does not need it will probably be well tolerated and will not cause harm. However, your patient is older and has a history of angina with exertion; the increased myocardial oxygen demand associated with the faster, more forceful pumping of the heart with epinephrine administration could cause your patient to have a heart attack. Remember, first, do no harm.

9. What is your updated assessment and treatment plan?

Confirm with your patient the absence of chest pain, tightness, heaviness, or squeezing. Reassess the presence of clear and equal breath sounds, obtain a 12-lead ECG, and provide a saline bolus to raise your patient's blood pressure. Follow your local protocols for the management of these patients following administration of epinephrine for anaphylaxis. Administer 25 to 50 mg of diphenhydramine IV as originally planned because he has hives and will benefit from administration of the antihistamine.

10. What is important to remember when talking with the average person about medications and medical history?

It's important to remember that your patients are laypeople who might not know why they are taking various medications. Although in this scenario you asked questions about medications that you know would be appropriate in the treatment of a severe allergic reaction, your patient will probably not know the how's and why's of administering various medications, including the ones taken on a daily basis. It makes sense to you, but it may be confusing to him. Sound your patient out, however. Your patient might be a retired health care worker who would clearly understand what you are doing.

Prep Kit

Ready for Review

- Patient assessment consists of two sets of skills: taking an excellent patient history and doing a good physical assessment.
- Patient history is a primary means of diagnosing the chief complaint in the prehospital environment. Some physicians say that all the sophisticated tests available in a modern hospital only confirm what they learn in taking a patient's history.
- The first part of a patient's history also serves as a good mental status examination: ask for the patient's name; the date, time, and location; the chief complaint, and the events. You will know if there is a cognition problem if your patient cannot put this information together.
- Ask if your patient has had these symptoms before, the general state of his or her health, and any serious illnesses. Inappropriate behaviour should also be noted. Write down a list of medications your patient is taking and allergies to medications.
- The best questions to use in getting a medical history are open-ended questions. Resist the temptation to run through a checklist in which the answers are yes or no.
- The mnemonic OPQRST offers an easy-to-remember template approach to analyzing a patient's chief complaint: Onset, Provocation, Quality, Region/radiation/referral, Severity, and Time.
- Use constructive communications skills as you talk with your patient: facilitation, reflection, clarification, empathy, confrontation, interpretation, and asking directly about feelings.

- When more information is required, remember to be sensitive in using direct questions. A paramedic represents power and authority to a sick person—think about how you feel when your physician asks direct questions of you.
- Remember to work on strategies within your service and with your partner for positive communications with patients who are silent, overly talkative, seductive, having multiple symptoms, anxious, needing reassurance, angry or hostile, intoxicated, crying, or depressed.

Vital Vocabulary

chief complaint The problem for which the patient is seeking help.

history of the present illness Elaboration of the patient's chief complaint.

initial diagnosis A determination of what a paramedic thinks is the patient's current problem, usually based on the patient history and the chief complaint.

patient history Information about the patient's chief complaint, present symptoms, and previous illnesses.

signs Indications of illness or injury that the examiner can see, hear, feel, smell, and so on.

symptoms The pain, discomfort, or other abnormality that the patient feels.

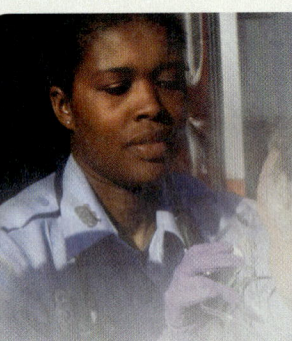

Assessment in Action

It is 3:00 AM, and you respond to a private residence. You have responded to a call dispatched as "unknown medical." On arrival, the scene is safe and you find a 56-year-old man, who is conscious, alert, and oriented. You and your partner introduce yourselves, explaining that you are paramedics from the city ambulance service. The patient is seated on the edge of his bed. He is having obvious difficulty breathing and is anxious and pale. His wife tells you that her husband was awakened from sleep by chest pain and shortness of breath. She is concerned about the current events.

1. **In an effort to establish the chief complaint and history of present illness, you should:**
   A. ask why 9-1-1 was called.
   B. consult the wife to determine the chief complaint. This will keep the patient calm.
   C. request previous medical documentation, which can be reviewed to determine the patient's medical problems.
   D. ask the patient what is wrong tonight and have him describe the symptoms he is having and how long the symptoms have been occurring.

2. **To assist in analyzing the chief complaint, you should use a mnemonic that is easy to remember or a template to help elicit all aspects of the complaint. The most commonly used mnemonic is:**
   A. ABCD.
   B. OPQRST.
   C. MNOP.
   D. RSTUV.

3. **Facilitation eases the flow of information and includes all the following, EXCEPT:**
   A. paying attention.
   B. maintaining good eye contact.
   C. repeating key information.
   D. suggesting symptoms and signs.

4. **The patient says something you do not fully understand. How can you clarify what he said?**
   A. Ask him to clarify—explain unclear complaints in his own words.
   B. Give him examples of how the condition affects most people.
   C. Suggest medical terminology so that you can better define his complaint.
   D. Ask bystanders or family for their impression of the complaint.

5. **You must ask the patient what medication he is taking. This is important because medications can suggest past and present illnesses. To best determine medications that are being taken, you should:**
   A. review his pharmacy receipts.
   B. call his physician.
   C. consult his relatives.
   D. ask him what medications, including prescription, over-the-counter, and herbal supplements he is taking.

6. **The posture of the patient's wife stiffens, and she begins to look angry. She starts yelling at you and your partner, telling you to hurry up and do something. You should:**
   A. have your partner take her aside and calmly explain what you are doing.
   B. call for back up at the first opportunity.
   C. have police stand by during the history taking.
   D. ignore her.

7. **You smell alcohol on the patient's breath. You wonder if he might be intoxicated. Problems encountered with intoxicated patients include which of the following?**
   A. Intoxicated patients may not understand what you are trying to say, making effective communications difficult or impossible.
   B. Intoxication may mask symptoms, making treatment decisions difficult.
   C. Intoxicated patients can present potentially violent situations.
   D. All of the above.

Challenging Questions

8. **You are dispatched to an unknown injury. You and your partner arrive on scene and hear loud noises and yelling from inside the residence. You then hear the sound of glass breaking. What should you do?**

9. **You arrive on scene at the home of a patient with hearing difficulty. What can you do to better enable effective communications?**

▬ Points to Ponder

You respond to a medical call involving a 46-year-old man. On arrival you recognize the patient as a teacher at the local middle school. You ask why you were called today and the patient tells you that he has been experiencing serious anxiety. You inquire about medical history, and your patient tells you that he checked himself into a psychiatric hospital during the summer break to get treatment for paranoia.

After shift, you are eating dinner at a popular restaurant with your partner and two other paramedics from your service. They ask if anything interesting happened today. You begin to tell them about the teacher, and your eyes meet those of your partner. You realize that this is not appropriate.

Why is this not appropriate, and what should you do now?

Issues: Confidentiality, History Taking.

13 Physical Examination

Competency Areas

Area 4: Assessment and Diagnostics

4.3.a   Conduct primary patient assessment and interpret findings.

4.3.b   Conduct secondary patient assessment and interpret findings.

4.3.c   Conduct cardiovascular system assessment and interpret findings.

4.3.d   Conduct neurological system assessment and interpret findings.

4.3.e   Conduct respiratory system assessment and interpret findings.

4.3.g   Conduct gastrointestinal system assessment and interpret findings.

4.3.h   Conduct genitourinary system assessment and interpret findings.

4.3.i   Conduct integumentary system assessment and interpret findings.

4.3.j   Conduct musculoskeletal system assessment and interpret findings.

4.3.m   Conduct assessment of the ears, eyes, nose, and throat and interpret findings.

4.4.a   Assess pulse.

4.4.b   Assess respirations.

4.4.c   Conduct non-invasive temperature monitoring.

4.4.d   Measure blood pressure by auscultation.

4.4.e   Measure blood pressure by palpation.

4.4.g   Assess skin condition.

4.4.h   Assess pupils.

4.4.i   Assess level of mentation.

Appendix 4: Pathophysiology

L.   **Ears, Eyes, Nose, and Throat**
Eyes—Medical Illness: Cataracts

Introduction

Physical examination is the process by which quantifiable, objective (based on fact or observable) information is obtained from a patient about his or her overall state of health. This information is compared with subjective (observed or perceived by the patient), historical information that is obtained from the patient. Armed with these two types of information, you can make a comprehensive assessment of the patient. While performing an assessment, you may see the patient's condition as a clinical manifestation; however, a caring and empathetic approach will yield better results and a more accurate evaluation. Likewise, a professional appearance and demeanour will instill trust and confidence in the abilities of the care provider.

The physical examination consists of two elements—obtaining vital signs that measure overall body function, and performing a head-to-toe survey that evaluates the workings of specific body organ systems. This survey is done in a sequential manner, ensuring that every aspect of the body's function is evaluated. Of course, the conditions in the prehospital setting may determine precisely how the physical examination is performed. Sometimes, the physical examination may be condensed. For example, for an unresponsive medical patient or a trauma patient with a significant mechanism of injury (MOI), a rapid trauma/medical assessment can be performed.

The overall patient assessment is intended to determine whether a problem exists, so that actions can be taken to manage that problem. Before you can appreciate abnormalities on examination, you must understand the wide variety of normal presentations. This is something that can be learned only through direct hands-on experience and interaction with patients. Thus every patient encounter represents an opportunity for you to gain experience about the normal human condition.

Examination Techniques

The techniques of inspection, palpation, percussion, and auscultation allow you to use your physical senses to obtain physical information and to understand the normal (versus abnormal) functions of a patient's body. Inspection involves looking at the patient, either in general or at a specific area (ie, a patient's overall appearance from the doorway versus looking specifically at the chest wall for abnormalities/deformities) **Figure 13-1 ▾**. Palpation is physical touching for the purpose of obtaining information—for example, tenderness (elicited pain), deformity, crepitance, mass effect, pulse quality, and abnormal organ enlargement **Figure 13-2 ▸**.

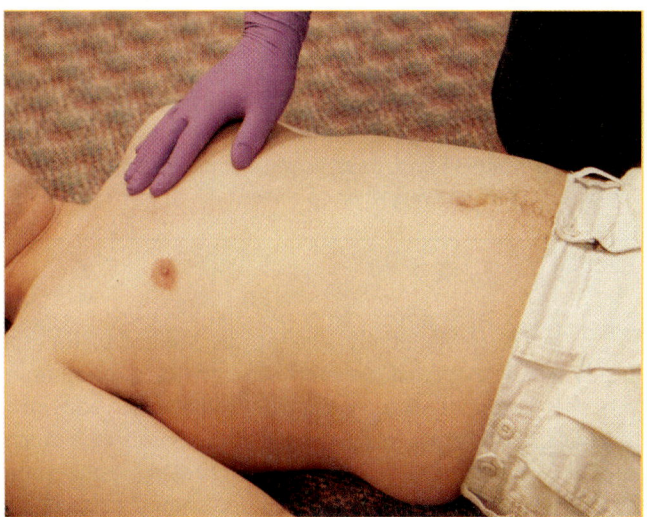

Figure 13-1 Inspection.

You are the Paramedic Part 1

You and your partner brave the harsh winter winds as you leave the protective warmth of the emergency department and race to your truck. It is one of the coldest days of the season and, unfortunately, one of the busiest. Just as you manage to get the truck heated, you and your partner are dispatched to a doctor's office for a patient complaining of shortness of breath. When you arrive, you are immediately brought to an examination room where you find a 75-year-old man in acute respiratory distress.

Initial Assessment	Recording Time: 0 Minutes
Appearance	Patient is leaning forward in tripod position
Level of consciousness	A (Alert to person, place, and day)
Airway	Open
Breathing	Rapid and shallow, visible retractions and audible wheezes, pursed lip breathing
Circulation	Strong radial pulses; pale, warm skin with cyanotic lips and nail beds

1. What is your general impression of the patient? Is he sick or not sick?
2. What do you think is the most valuable assessment tool at your disposal?

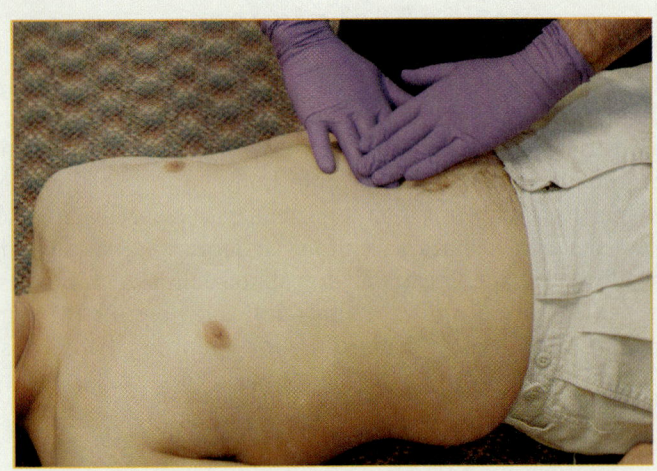

Figure 13-2 Palpation.

At the Scene

When done properly, palpation should never cause harm. Deep palpation requires practice and knowing when to stop.

<u>Percussion</u> entails gently striking the surface of the body, typically where it overlies various body cavities. This technique allows the paramedic to detect changes in the densities of the underlying structures. For example, percussion of a normal lung will yield medium to loud, low-pitched, resonant sounds. Percussion sounds over muscle and bone should be soft, high-pitched, and flat. Percussion sounds over hollow organs such as the intestines are often described as loud, high-pitched, and tympanic (like a drum).

Percussion is a skill that requires a lot of practice to perfect. Follow the steps in ⟨ **Skill Drill 13-1** ⟩:

1. Place your nondominant hand lightly against the surface to be examined ⟨ **Step 1** ⟩.
2. Hyperextend the middle finger and apply firm pressure to the surface to be percussed ⟨ **Step 2** ⟩.
3. Directly strike the middle phalanx of the middle finger with one or two fingertips of the other hand ⟨ **Step 3** ⟩.
4. Apply the same force over each area of the body to accurately compare the sounds produced by percussion.

<u>Auscultation</u> involves listening with a stethoscope ⟨ **Figure 13-3** ▸ ⟩. The body generates a variety of high- and low-frequency sounds—both normal and abnormal—that can be detected via auscultation. Bowel sounds can be assessed via auscultation, as can lung sounds. Appreciating the presence of and differences in auscultated sounds requires keen attention.

Vital Signs

Vital signs consist of a measurement of pulse rate, rhythm, and quality; respiratory rate, rhythm, and quality; blood pressure; temperature; and pulse oximetry. Other than overall patient appearance, vital signs are the most basic objective data for determining

---

At the Scene

There are important differences between the bell and diaphragm of the stethoscope. The bell is cup-shaped and is used to listen for deep and low-pitched sounds (heart sounds). It is placed very lightly on the skin, just enough to make a seal. The diaphragm is flat-shaped and is used to listen for high-pitched sounds (breath, bowel, and normal heart sounds); it is placed firmly on the skin.

Skill Drill 13-1: Percussion

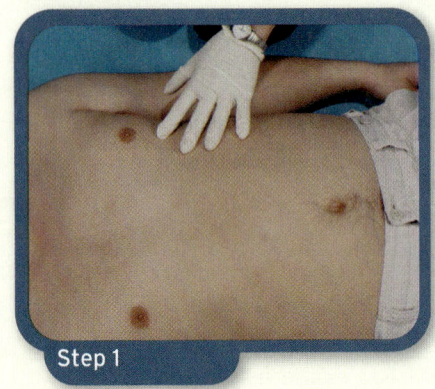

Step 1

Place your hand lightly against the surface to be examined.

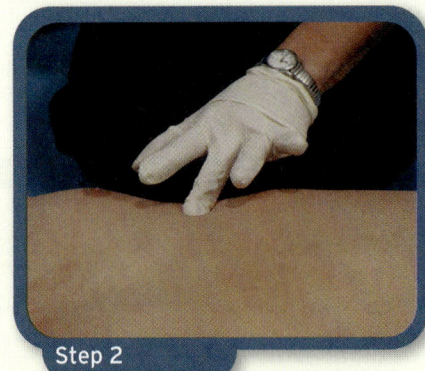

Step 2

Hyperextend the middle finger and apply firm pressure.

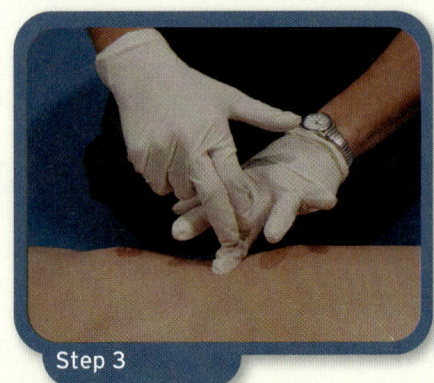

Step 3

Strike the middle finger with one or two fingertips of the other hand.

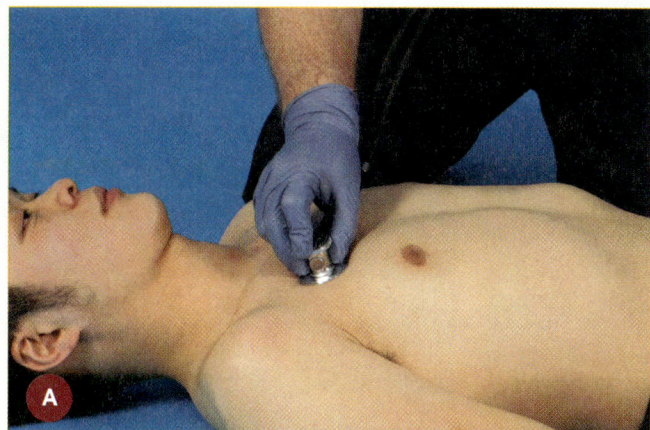

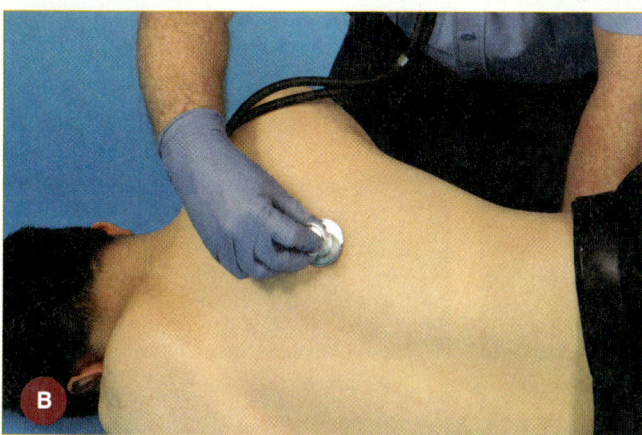

Figure 13-3 Auscultation of the (**A**) anterior chest and the (**B**) posterior chest.

At the Scene

Be aware that the patient's age, underlying physical and mental conditions, and current medications can affect the patient's vital signs. Like any other assessment tool, consider the vital signs but devote your attention to the patient.

patient status. Their measurement requires the paramedic to use the techniques of auscultation, palpation, and inspection.

Vital signs are aptly named; strict attention should be paid to the assessment of these critically important parameters. Normal limits can vary depending on several factors, including age and medication use, and vital signs should be interpreted with those factors in mind. Vital signs should be obtained both accurately and serially to help determine overall stability of the patient. Because vital signs can change dramatically over relatively short time periods, failing to check them frequently, especially in the context of a significantly ill or injured patient, can lead to faulty patient care.

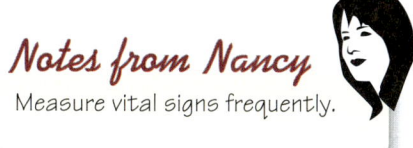

Notes from Nancy
Measure vital signs frequently.

Blood Pressure

Blood pressure is the measurement of the force exerted against the walls of the blood vessels. It is commonly measured in a peripheral artery, although it can be obtained essentially anywhere in the circulatory system. Blood pressure is the product of cardiac output and peripheral vascular resistance, so it includes two components: systolic pressure and diastolic pressure. Systolic pressure is created by the left ventricle while it is contracting (ie, in systole). Diastolic pressure is the result of residual pressure in the system while the left ventricle is relaxing (ie, in diastole). Normally, diastolic pressure should not go to zero, because peripheral vascular resistance in the arteriolar side of the circulatory system should continually provide for a diastolic pressure. The coronary arteries receive blood flow by this mechanism, so lower diastolic pressure means less myocardial perfusion.

At the Scene

Many patients exhibit an increase in blood pressure due to anxiety and the stress of an acute injury or illness. Look at your patient as well as trends in vital signs before concluding that the blood pressure is truly abnormal.

Blood pressure must be measured using a cuff that is appropriate to the patient's size and habitus (physique or body build). Too small or tight a cuff will yield an artificially high pressure; too large or loose a cuff will give inappropriately low results. Although blood pressure ideally will be auscultated, it can be palpated to estimate the systolic pressure. Periodic inspection of the blood pressure cuff's gauge is important, as it can lose accuracy and require recalibration.

Pulse

Pulse measurements should assess the rate, presence, location, quality, and rhythm of the pulses. To palpate the pulse, gently compress an artery against a bony prominence, which allows you to feel the pressure wave generated by the heart's contraction. Pulses can be obtained at several points in the body, including the radial, brachial, femoral, and carotid arteries **Figure 13-4 ▶**. When formally counting the pulse rate, time the pulses for a minimum of 15 seconds and then multiply by 4 to obtain the rate per minute. Palpating a pulse is a basic way to evaluate perfusion and cardiac output. Paramedics should compare proximal and distal pulses during patient evaluations.

Although it is appropriate to check for the presence of a central pulse in an unresponsive patient, the actual pulse rate

At the Scene

Whenever possible, avoid taking a blood pressure on a painful/injured extremity, an arm with an arteriovenous shunt or fistula, or on a post-mastectomy side. This can cause pain and/or result in inaccurate readings. This can also damage a shunt or fistula.

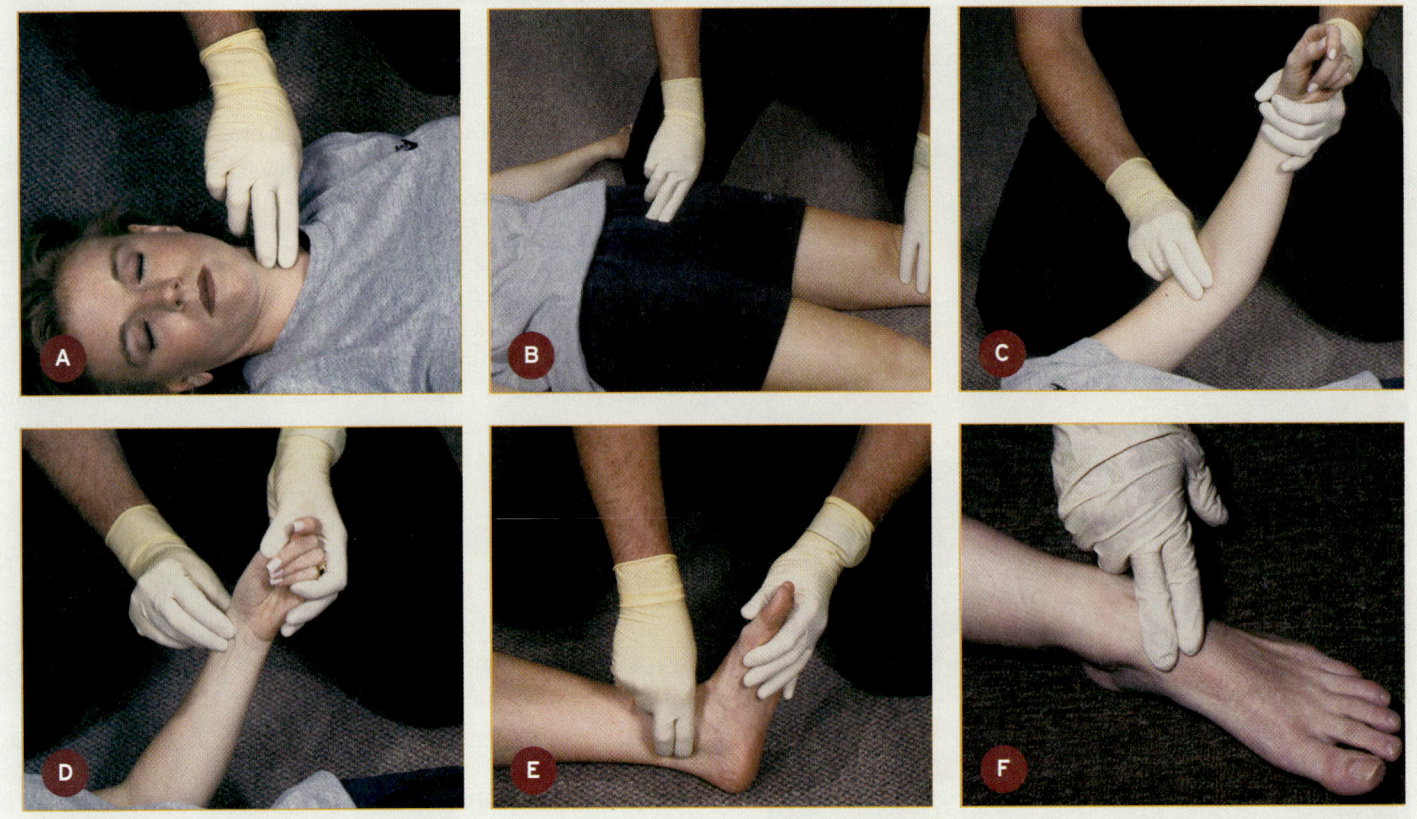

Figure 13-4 Common pulse points. **A.** Carotid pulse. **B.** Femoral pulse. **C.** Brachial pulse. **D.** Radial pulse. **E.** Posterior tibial pulse. **F.** Dorsalis pedis pulse.

Special Considerations

Palpating the pulse in an infant may present a problem. Because an infant's neck is often very short and fat, and its pulse is often quite fast, you may have a hard time finding the carotid pulse. Therefore, in infants younger than 1 year, you should palpate the brachial artery to assess the pulse.

should be counted in the most peripheral location that can be palpated, to aid with rapid estimation of the blood pressure. In the responsive patient, you may want to determine respiratory rate while you appear to be checking the pulse; this may decrease patients' tendency to inadvertently alter their breathing pattern or rate when they become aware of being evaluated.

Respiration

The respiratory rate is typically measured by inspection of the patient's chest, but respiratory movements can also be assessed by visualizing portions of the abdominal wall, neck, face, and overall accessory muscle use. Although the absolute respiratory rate is important, the quality of the respiratory effort should be evaluated as well. In particular, you should learn to recognize pathologic respiratory patterns or rhythms (eg, tachypnea, Kussmaul, Cheyne-Stokes, and Biot breathing). Similarly, you should recognize

breathing difficulties when patients exhibit tripod positioning, accessory muscle use, or retractions. This information is especially helpful in the assessment of pediatric patients. Respiratory rate should be measured for a minimum of 30 seconds, and then multiplied by 2 to obtain the rate per minute.

Temperature

Many methods can be used to evaluate body temperature. If you use a tympanic device for obtaining a patient's body temperature, however, be aware of extrinsic factors that may increase or decrease the temperature reading.

Pulse Oximetry

Arterial oxygen saturation determination made via <u>pulse oximetry</u> has earned a place in emergency health care as part of regular vital signs monitoring (**Figure 13-5 ▸**). Although pulse oximetry is a valuable tool, it should never be used as an

At the Scene

The accuracy of tympanic membrane temperatures has been called into question by some data, especially in patients with severe infections. If your patient looks sick, feels warm, and the tympanic membrane temperature is "normal," consider using a different type of thermometer.

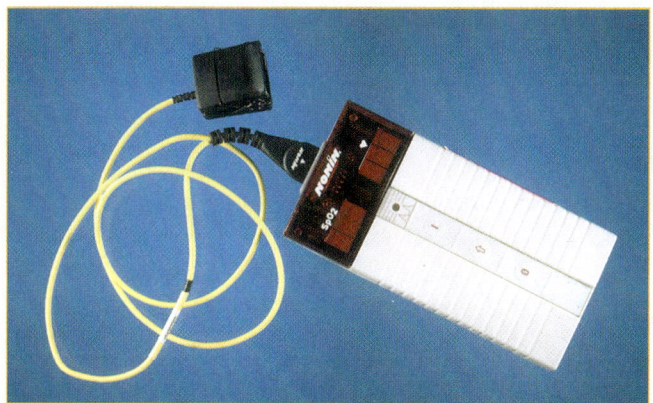

Figure 13-5 A pulse oximeter.

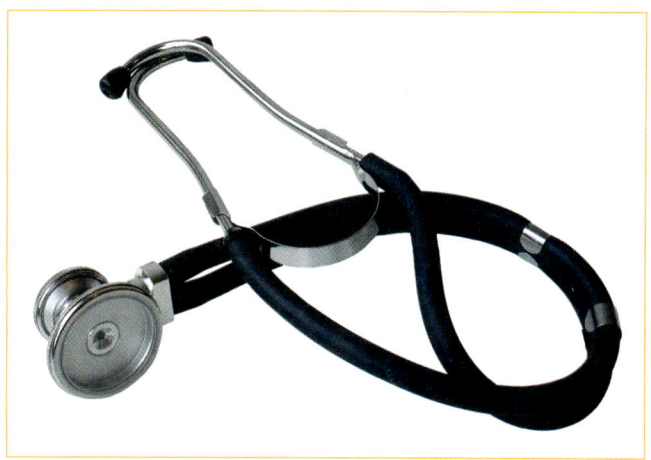

Figure 13-7 Stethoscope.

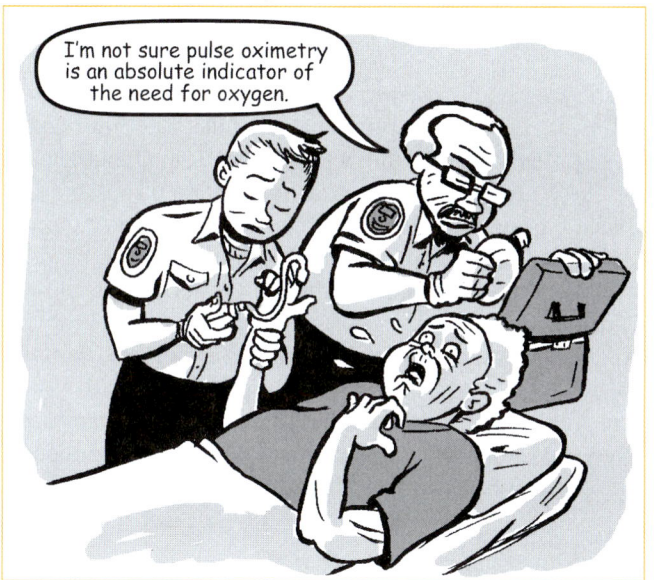

Figure 13-6

absolute indicator of the need for oxygen therapies. Pulse oximetry measures the percentage of hemoglobin saturation and can provide inaccurate information in certain situations. Paramedics need to understand potential complications with pulse oximetry in order to appropriately process the information it provides Figure 13-6 ▲. Inaccurate readings may be obtained for a variety of reasons—a hypotensive or cold patient, carbon monoxide poisoning, abnormal hemoglobin (ie, sickle-cell disease), vascular dyes, patient motion, and incorrect placement.

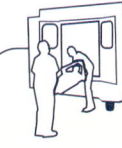

At the Scene

Remember to look at your patient, not the "number." If the patient looks sick, and the pulse oximetry reading is "normal," then the patient is still sick.

Equipment Used in the Physical Examination

Equipment used to perform the physical examination includes a stethoscope, blood pressure cuff (sphygmomanometer), ophthalmoscope, otoscope, scissors, a reliable light source, gloves, and a sheet or blanket.

Stethoscopes Figure 13-7 ▲ are available in two forms: acoustic and electronic. Today's acoustic stethoscope, which is the most commonly seen in the prehospital setting, consists of two earpieces attached to an air-filled tube that connects to a chest piece. The chest piece has two sides—a diaphragm (plastic disk) and a bell (hollow cup)—that can be placed against the patient to sense sounds. The diaphragm is vibrated by the sounds of the body, which are then transmitted up to the stethoscope's earpieces; thus the diaphragm side is used to pick up higher-frequency sounds. The bell, which usually transmits lower-frequency sounds, senses the sounds directly off the skin of the patient.

The acoustic stethoscope doesn't amplify sounds; rather, it simply blocks out ambient noises, allowing the paramedic to hear and appreciate the sounds of the body. In contrast, the electronic stethoscope converts the acoustic sound waves into an electronic signal that is then amplified.

The sphygmomanometer, or blood pressure cuff, is used in the measurement of the patient's blood pressure Figure 13-8 ▶. This device consists of an inflatable cuff, which occludes blood flow, and a manometer (pressure meter), which is used to determine the pressure in the artery at various points in the physical examination. These two components are connected via tubing. In manual cuffs, a separate tube connects to an inflation bulb.

Many sizes of blood pressure cuffs are available, and using the appropriate size for the patient is essential to obtain an accurate reading. The cuff should be one half to two thirds the

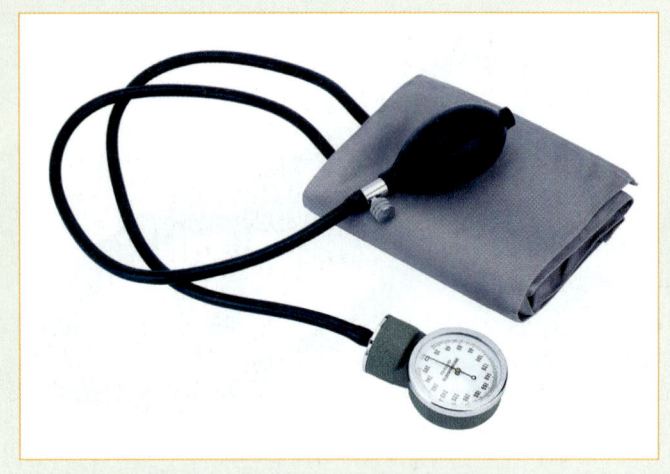

Figure 13-8 Sphygmomanometer.

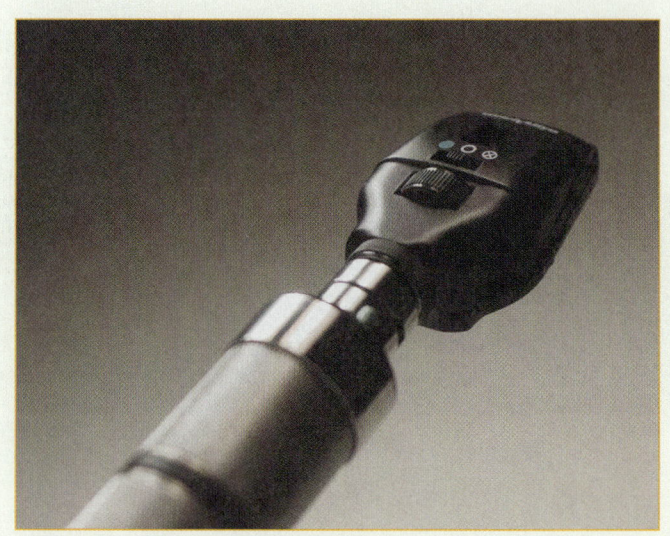

Figure 13-9 Ophthalmoscope.

size of the upper arm. The blood pressure measurement is separated into systolic and diastolic pressures and is reported in millimetres of mercury (mm Hg).

The ophthalmoscope allows you to look into a patient's eyes and view the retina and aqueous fluid. This tool consists of a concave mirror and a battery-powered light, which is usually contained in the device's handle 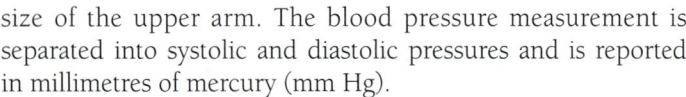. The care provider looks through a monocular eyepiece that is usually equipped with a rotating disk of lenses; selection of a lens allows for adjustment of the depth and magnification. Use of the ophthalmoscope is usually reserved for hospital and physician's office examination, because effective evaluation requires dilation of the patient's pupils with medication.

The otoscope is used to evaluate the ears of a patient. This instrument consists of a head and a handle. The head contains an electric light source and a low-power magnifying lens. The front of the headpiece has an attachment for a disposable plastic earpiece (speculum). The examiner inserts the speculum into the ear and looks through a lens on the rear of the headpiece. Some otoscopes include a sliding rear window that allows for the insertion of an additional instrument (eg, to remove ear wax). Most have an insertion point for a bulb that is used to push air into the ear canal, allowing the examiner to visualize the movement of the tympanic membrane. The batteries are located in the handle unless it is a wall-mounted unit, such as those found in a physician's office.

You are the Paramedic Part 2

Your partner starts to obtain the patient's vital signs and you begin your patient assessment. The medical assistant tells you that the patient made an emergency appointment this morning for increasing shortness of breath that began last night around 10:00 PM. He presented in severe respiratory distress with an increased work of breathing and audible wheezes. He was administered a nebulizer treatment with 0.25 mg of salbutamol (Ventolin) 20 minutes prior to EMS being called. Your examination reveals that the patient is still experiencing severe respiratory distress. He has a barrel-shaped chest with marked intercostal and supraclavicular retractions, pursed lipped breathing, audible inspiratory and expiratory wheezes, and can only speak in one- or two-word sentences. You also observe cyanosis around his mouth and nail beds with clubbing of the fingers. The medical assistant also provides you with the patient's medical history, which is significant for a 60-year smoking habit, emphysema, and hypertension. He is prescribed nebulizer treatments with 2.5 mg of salbutamol (Ventolin)/normal saline four times a day, two puffs of budesonide (Pulmicort) inhaler twice a day, 200 mg of metoprolol-SR (Apo-metoprolol SR) once a day, and home oxygen at 3 l/min. He has an allergy to iodine and penicillin.

Vital Signs	Recording Time: 5 Minutes
Skin	Pale, warm, with cyanotic lips and nail beds
Pulse	130 beats/min, regular; strong radial
Blood pressure	168/82 mm Hg
Respirations	40 breaths/min, laboured, audible wheezes
Spo$_2$	70% on nasal cannula at 4 l/min

3. Which signs and symptoms are acute? Which are chronic?
4. Which interventions should you consider at this point?

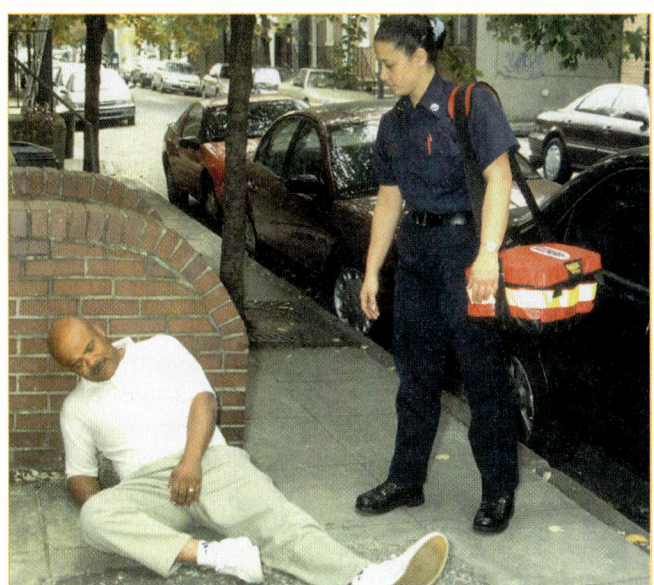

Figure 13-10 Get a general impression of the overall situation as you approach the patient.

The General Impression

The general impression begins as you approach the scene, simultaneously sizing up the situation and the patient's overall presentation **Figure 13-10 ▲** . A quick look at the environment in which the patient is found and the general appearance of the patient provides a substantial amount of information before you ask the first question. An important skill that many paramedics develop is a sense as to when a patient is seriously ill, based primarily on his or her initial appearance. The expression "sick or not sick?" sums up this approach.

Look for signs of significant distress such as mental status changes, anxiousness, laboured breathing, difficulty speaking, diaphoresis, obvious pain, obvious deformity, and guarding or splinting of a painful area. It is not uncommon for persons experiencing substantial and incapacitating pain to present with a quiet and still affect.

Other aspects that may be readily apparent and worth noting as you develop a general impression include dress, hygiene, expression, overall size, posture, untoward odours, and overall state of health. When characterizing the overall state of the patient, be sure to use appropriate terms to describe the degree of distress: no apparent distress, mild (slight or not harsh), moderate (small or average), acute (very great or bad), and severe (dangerous or difficult to endure). Other acceptable terms to describe the general state of a patient's health include chronically ill, frail, feeble, robust, and vigorous.

Perhaps the quickest and most reliable initial way to evaluate a patient's overall degree of distress is to look at the skin. Relatively subtle but serious changes in overall perfusion are usually manifested early on in the skin's appearance. Evaluate the skin's colour, relative moisture, and relative temperature. Note any obvious lesions or deformities.

Pallor is present when red blood cell perfusion to the capillary beds of the skin is poor. You may also be able to detect pallor by looking at the patient's lips or eye conjunctiva. Cyanosis indicates a relative lack of oxygen perfusion, although the number of red blood cells may be adequate to carry any available oxygen. Cyanosis correlates extremely well with low arterial oxygen saturation. It can be visualized generally in the skin, but more specifically in the fingernail beds, face, and lips.

Ecchymosis is localized bruising or blood collection within or under the skin. Evaluate large ecchymoses for the possibility of serious underlying soft-tissue, bony, or organ injury. Serious wounds to the head, neck, and torso should also be noted, as well as any evidence of a potential hemorrhage.

The Physical Examination

The physical examination of a patient in the prehospital setting is the most important skill a health care provider can master. This ability is first developed as a primary care paramedic and should be refined as an advanced practitioner. Starting intravenous access, pushing medications, and performing endotracheal intubation are simply mechanical skills that require only practice to achieve proficiency. The skills of patient assessment and interpreting the findings of a physical examination, by comparison, truly separate the accomplished paramedic from the basic provider. The physical examination consists of a comprehensive review of systems to determine the nature and extent of the patient's illness or injury.

Mental Status

Evaluation of a patient's mental status involves assessing cognitive function (ie, ability to use reasoning or perception). At a minimum, evaluate the patient's degree of alertness. This assessment is accomplished by using the Alert and Oriented (AO) × 4 method, which means the patient is alert to person, place, time, and events leading up to this particular moment. The AVPU scale is a rapid method of assessing the patient's level of consciousness using one of the following four designations:

- **A** *Alert* (oriented to person, place, and day)
- **V** Responds to *Verbal* stimuli
- **P** Responds to *Painful* stimuli
- **U** *Unresponsive*

When classifying the response to stimuli, grade the patient according to the best response you can elicit. For example, a patient passed out on the street who moans in response to a loud shout from the paramedic would score a V on the AVPU scale. Response to tactile stimuli (eg, pinching the nail bed, twisting the skin of the forearm) would earn a P. No response to verbal or tactile stimuli would be classified as U.

Skin, Hair, and Nails
Skin
The skin, which is the largest organ system in the body, serves three major functions: It regulates the temperature of the body, transmits information from the environment to the brain, and protects the body in the environment.

Special Considerations

Mental status may be difficult to evaluate in children. First, determine whether the child is alert. Even infants should be alert to your presence and should follow you with their eyes (a process called "tracking"). Ask the primary caregiver whether the child is behaving normally, particularly in regard to alertness. Most children older than 2 years should know their own name and the names of their parents and siblings. Evaluate mental status in school-age children by asking about holidays, recent school activities, or teachers' names.

The skin is the major organ governing the body's thermoregulation. In a cold environment, constriction of the blood vessels shunts blood away from the skin to decrease the amount of heat radiated from the body surface (observed as pale skin). When the outside environment is hot, the vessels in the skin dilate, the skin becomes flushed or red, and heat radiates from the body surface. Also, in a hot environment, sweat is secreted to the skin surface from the sweat glands. Energy, in the form of body heat, is lost during the evaporation process, which causes body temperature to fall.

Information from the environment is carried to the brain through a rich supply of sensory nerves that originate in the skin. Nerve endings that lie in the skin are adapted to perceive and transmit information about heat, cold, external pressure, pain, and the position of the body in space. In this way, the skin recognizes changes in the environment. It also reacts to pressure, pain, and pleasurable stimuli.

The skin is composed of two layers: the epidermis and the dermis (**Figure 13-11 ▶**). The epidermis, or outermost layer, is the body's first line of defence. It serves as the principal barrier against water, dust, microorganisms, and mechanical stress. Underlying the epidermis is the dermis—a tough, highly elastic layer of connective tissues. This complex material is composed chiefly of collagen fibres, elastic fibres, and a mucopolysaccharide gel. Numerous fibroblasts (cells that secrete collagen, elastin, and ground substance) are found within the dermis as well.

The dermis is subdivided into the papillary dermis and a reticular layer. The vasculature inside the papillary dermis serves two functions—it provides nutrients to the epidermis, and aids in thermoregulation. Dilation of these vessels increases blood flow to the skin, allowing heat to dissipate. Conversely, blood vessel constriction results in retention of heat. The reticular layer consists of dense, irregular connective tissue, which provides both strength and elasticity. With age,

the skin undergoes significant changes, including loss of the collagen connective tissues and diminished capillary supply.

Examination of the skin involves both inspection and palpation. Pay careful attention to the skin colour, moisture, temperature, texture, turgor, and any significant lesions. Look for evidence of diminished perfusion, evaluate for pallor and cyanosis, and be wary of diaphoresis. Reddened or pink skin can be seen in a variety of normal states, but it is also evident in states of relative vasodilation (flushing). Flushed skin is usually apparent in patients with fever, and it may be seen in patients experiencing an allergic process. Reddened skin should also be considered in the context of superficial burns.

Examining the skin for changes in perfusion is usually best accomplished in areas where the epidermis is thinnest, such as the fingernails, lips, and conjunctivae. It is sometimes useful to examine the palms and soles as well. Pale skin is a relatively common finding in the seriously ill patient and may indicate severe vasoconstriction, as seen in profound anemia, acute cardiovascular events, other shock-like states, and hypothermia. Local areas of blanched, cool, white skin are typical of frostbite. Although cyanotic skin is commonly seen in states of oxygen desaturation, it can also be a function of hypothermia, especially in very young patients. Mottling is a typical finding in states of severe protracted hypoperfusion and shock and is readily evident in pediatric patients.

It takes practice to accurately gauge patients' relative perfusion and hydration status. Becoming familiar with the abnormal findings of the skin and mucous membranes is an excellent aid in judging both. Turgor relates directly to hydration. Poor skin turgidity is an expression of poorly hydrated skin, with associated tenting evident in extreme cases, particularly in young children (**Figure 13-12 ▶**). Because of normal changes in elastin and connective tissues with advanced age, skin turgor is an insignificant indicator in geriatric patients, as is skin that is

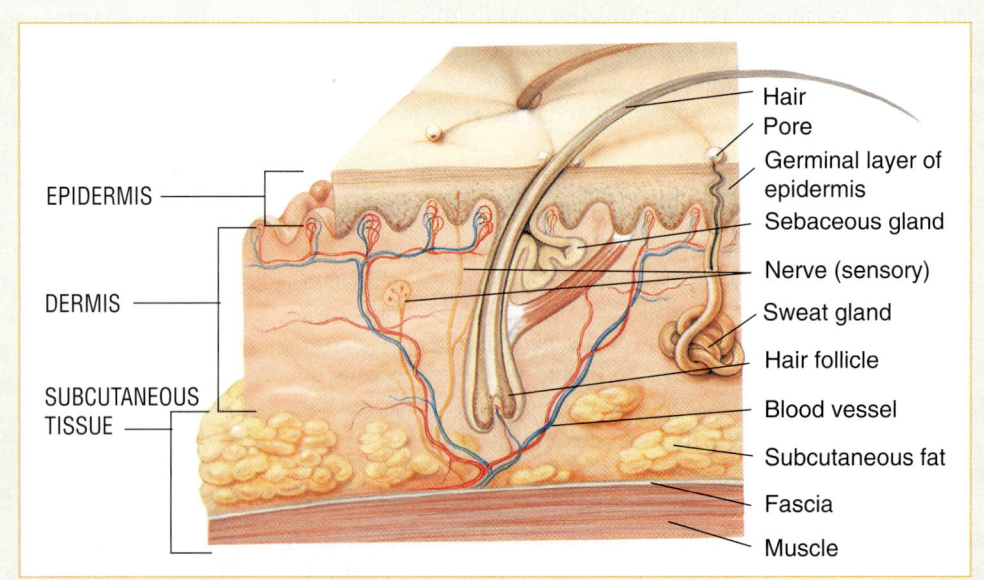

EPIDERMIS

DERMIS

SUBCUTANEOUS TISSUE

- Hair
- Pore
- Germinal layer of epidermis
- Sebaceous gland
- Nerve (sensory)
- Sweat gland
- Hair follicle
- Blood vessel
- Subcutaneous fat
- Fascia
- Muscle

Figure 13-11 The skin is composed of a tough external layer (the epidermis) and a vascular inner layer (the dermis).

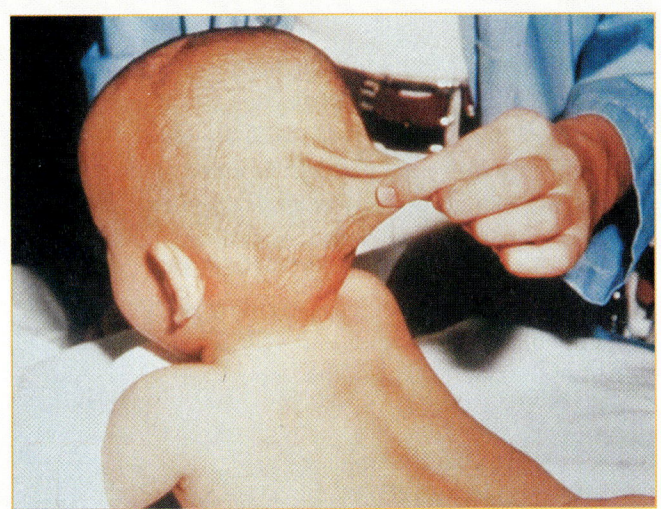

Figure 13-12 Tenting is evident with extreme dehydration.

Special Considerations

When assessing skin turgor in an older patient, use the skin of the upper chest. This is a much more reliable indicator than the extremities.

abnormally dry to the touch. Paying attention to skin temperature can sometimes prove useful when trying to determine the etiologies of different problems (eg, respiratory distress). Sometimes making a clinical distinction between congestive heart failure with pulmonary edema versus pneumonia is a function of the patient's temperature, which may be readily apparent from tactile examination of the skin.

Skin lesions may sometimes be the only external evidence of a serious internal injury. Take note of any large areas of ecchymosis, palpable crepitus (palpable fractures), and open wounds. Devastating internal injuries can result from wounds whose only external signs are relatively benign-appearing penetrations. Be aware of any body areas that are hidden by clothing or by devices such as a backboard and head immobilizer. Always visually inspect and manually palpate the patient's back and expose body parts. Likewise, evaluation for rashes is usually best accomplished by discreetly examining areas of skin otherwise hidden by clothing.

Hair

Examination of the hair is done by inspection and palpation. In this survey, note the quantity, distribution, and texture of the hair. Recent changes in the growth or loss of hair can indicate an underlying endocrine disorder, such as diabetes, or may result from treatment modalities for disease

At the Scene

When inspecting the skin, always be alert for signs of possible abuse or maltreatment. Multiple bruises at different stages of healing or even pressure sores may raise concerns about possible physical abuse and should be reported.

processes (eg, chemotherapy or radiation treatment of cancer). Although the recent loss of hair may be related to a disease process, the thinning and loss of hair can also be a normal finding in the older patient.

Nails

The examination of the fingernails and toenails can reveal many subtle findings **Table 13-1 ▾**. The colour, shape, texture, and presence or absence of lesions should all be assessed. The normal nail should be firm and smooth on palpation. Normal changes to the nails with aging include the development of striations and a change in colour (yellowish tint) related to the reduction in body calcium.

Head, Ears, Eyes, Nose, and Throat

The head, ears, eyes, nose, and throat (HEENT) examination consists of a comprehensive evaluation of the head and related structures. It is crucial because the head contains the brain, numerous important sensory organs, and all of the upper airway anatomy. The eyes are a nervous system structure that involves both motor pathways (lids, extraocular muscles, pupillary constrictors, corneal blink reflex) and sensory pathways. The ears provide for both hearing and balance control. The nose is a sensory organ involved with the senses of smell and taste; it also plays an important role in assisting with breathing. The throat consists of the mouth and posterior pharynx, and all the structures intrinsic to them. This complicated organ simultaneously coordinates many motor and sensory functions, while also coordinating the initial activities of both the respiratory and digestive systems.

Table 13-1	**Abnormal Findings in the Nails**	
Condition	**Findings**	**Possible Cause**
Beau's lines	Transverse depressions in the nail inhibiting growth	Systemic illness, severe infection, or nail injury
Clubbing	The angle between the nail and the nail base approaches or exceeds 180°	Flattening and enlargement of the fingertips is associated with chronic respiratory disease
Psoriasis	Pitting, discolouration, and subungual thickening of the nail	
Splinter hemorrhages	Red or brown linear streaks in the nail bed	Bacterial endocarditis or trichinosis
Terry's nails	Transverse white bands that cover the nail except for the distal tip	Cirrhosis

Head

The head is divided into two parts: the cranium and the face. The cranium, or skull, contains the brain. The brain connects to the spinal cord through the foramen magnum, a large opening at the base of the skull. The most posterior portion of the cranium is the occiput. On each side of the cranium, the lateral portions are called the temples or temporal regions. Between the temporal regions and the occiput lie the parietal regions. The forehead is called the frontal region. Just anterior to the ear, in the temporal region, you can feel the pulse of the superficial temporal artery. A layer of muscle fascia covers the skull. The thick skin covering the cranium, which usually bears hair, is called the scalp.

Within the skull lie the meninges, three distinct layers of tissue that suspend the brain and the spinal cord within the skull and the spinal canal. The dura mater is the tough, fibrous, outer layer that resembles leather. It forms a sac that contains the central nervous system (CNS), with small openings through which the peripheral nerves exit. The inner two layers of the meninges, called the arachnoid and the pia mater, are much thinner than the dura mater. They contain the blood vessels that nourish the brain and spinal cord. Cerebrospinal fluid (CSF) is produced in a chamber inside the brain, called the third ventricle. CSF fills the space between the meninges and acts as shock absorber.

When you are examining the head, you should both feel it and inspect it visually. This step is important in the management of potential trauma patients and with patients who have altered mental status or are unresponsive. If you find evidence of external bleeding, attempt to separate the hair manually and irrigate the clot; this should allow you to identify the source of bleeding. Evaluate the skull for any deformity, step-off, or tenderness. Observe the general shape and contour of the skull.

In children younger than 18 months, routinely palpate the anterior fontanelle (the "soft spot"). Prior to its normal physiologic closure, it can serve as an excellent relative indicator of hydration and intracranial pressure. The fontanelle is usually characterized as open and flat (the normal state), bulging (common while crying, pathologic when observed in a quiet child), and sunken (in severe dehydration).

When you are evaluating the face, observe the colour and moisture of the skin, as well as expression, symmetry, and contour of the face itself. Also pay attention to any swelling or apparent areas of injury, and note any signs of respiratory distress. Use the mnemonic DCAP-BTLS—Deformities, Contusions, Abrasions, Punctures/penetrations, Burns, Tenderness, Lacerations, and Swelling—to assist you during the physical examination. Follow the steps in Skill Drill 13-2 ▶ to assess the head:

Special Considerations

Always inspect the fontanelle in infants.
Bulging = Increased intracranial pressure in a quiet child
Sunken = Dehydration

1. Visually inspect the head, looking for any obvious DCAP-BTLS Step 1 .
2. Palpate the top and back of the head to locate any subtle abnormalities Step 2 . Use a systematic approach, going from front to back, to ensure that nothing is missed.
3. Part the hair in several places to examine the condition of the scalp. Identify any lesions under the hair Step 3 .
4. Note any pain during the process (this examination should not cause the patient any pain).
5. Palpate the structure of the face noting any DCAP-BTLS. Pay attention to the condition of the skin, hair distribution, and shape of the face Step 4 .

At the Scene

Protecting fragile CNS structures from further damage is vital to the patient's prospects for living a normal life. Lean toward caution and overprotection in assessing and treating possible brain and spinal cord injuries.

Eyes

The eyes are a tremendously complex sensory organ Figure 13-13 ▶ . They process light stimuli for the brain, so that the brain is able to decode light impulses presenting to the eyes and form a visual image. The eyes are a critical link to the CNS, and as such they allow the examiner to more precisely assess the functions of the CNS.

Each eye consists of an anterior chamber and a posterior chamber, which are always assessed in a standardized fashion (ie, from "front to back"). The outer aspects of the eye are checked first, with deeper structures subsequently evaluated. General issues to ask about include any pain or redness, loss of vision, diplopia (double vision), photophobia, blurring, discharge, and corrective lens use.

After addressing these general questions, assess for visual acuity (VA)—that is, the ability or inability to see, and how well the patient can see. Check VA by examining each eye in isolation. If corrective lenses are normally worn, check VA with the correction in place. The standard device for checking VA is the Snellen ("E") chart Figure 13-14 ▶ , although it is not an appropriate tool in the prehospital setting. More appropriate tools in this environment include simple tests such as light/dark discrimination and finger counting. Finger counting should be done from a noted distance, typically 2 m, 1 m, and 30 cm. Reporting on VA must include the distance from which finger counting was measured.

The pupil is a circular opening in the centre of the pigmented iris of the eye. The diameter and reactivity of the patient's pupil to light reflect the status of the brain's perfusion, oxygenation, and condition. The pupils are normally round and of approximately equal size; they serve as optical diaphragms, adjusting their size depending on the available light. In normal room light, the pupils appear to be midsized. With less light, they dilate to allow more light to enter the eye, making it possible to

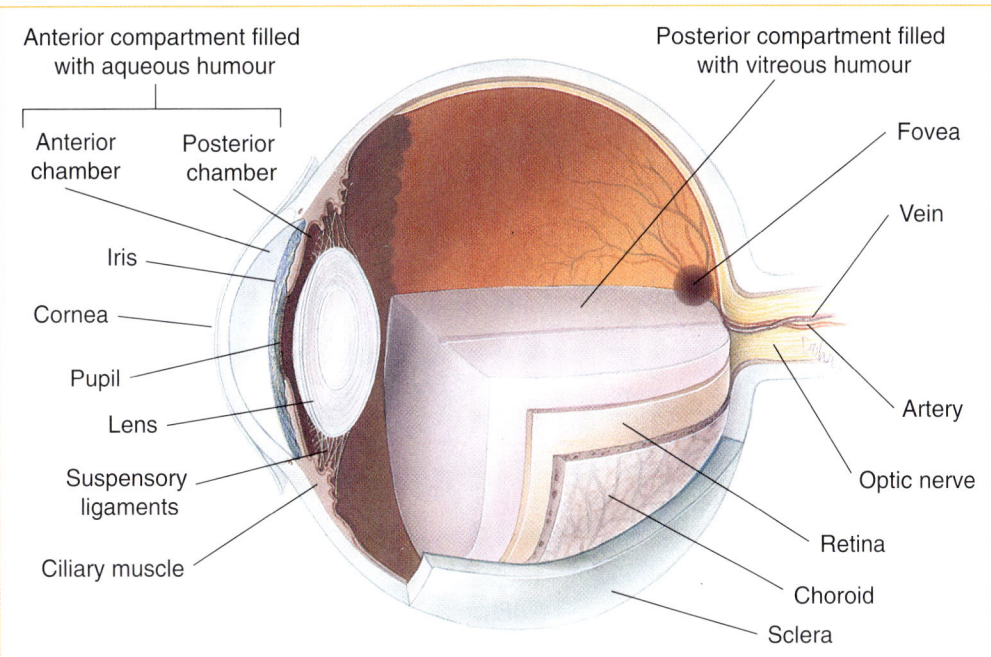

Anterior compartment filled with aqueous humour

Anterior chamber

Posterior chamber

Iris

Cornea

Pupil

Lens

Suspensory ligaments

Ciliary muscle

Posterior compartment filled with vitreous humour

Fovea

Vein

Artery

Optic nerve

Retina

Choroid

Sclera

Figure 13-13 The structure of the eye.

Skill Drill 13-2: Assessing the Head

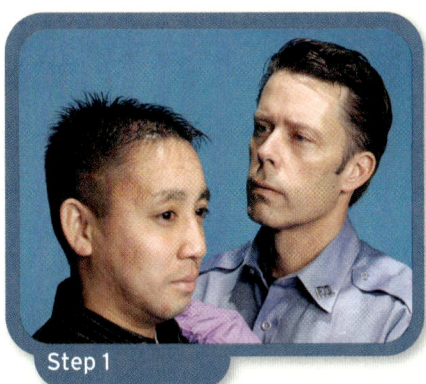

Step 1

Visually inspect the head, looking for any obvious DCAP-BTLS.

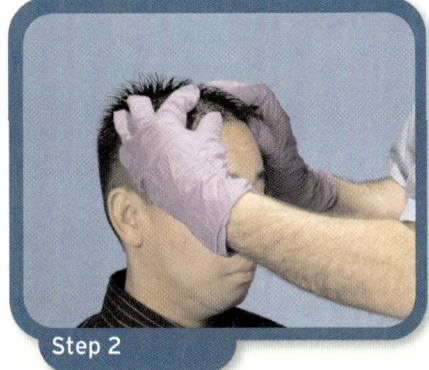

Step 2

Palpate the top and back of the head to locate any subtle abnormalities.

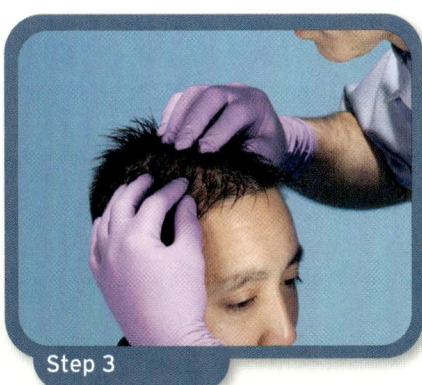

Step 3

Part the hair in several places to examine the condition of the scalp.

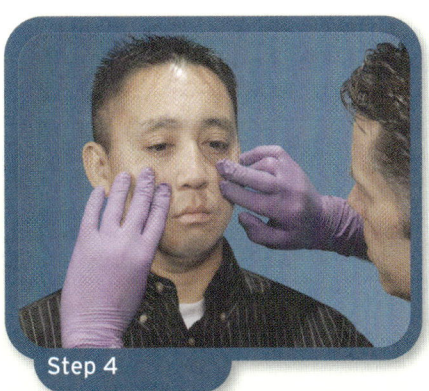

Step 4

Palpate the structure of the face, noting any DCAP-BTLS.

see even in dim light. With high light levels or when a bright light is suddenly introduced, the pupils instantly constrict, allowing less light to enter and protecting the sensitive receptors in the inner eye from damage. When a brighter light is introduced into one eye (or higher levels of light enter one eye only), both pupils should constrict equally to the appropriate size for the pupil receiving the most light.

In the absence of any light, the pupils will become fully relaxed and dilated. When light is introduced, each eye sends sensory signals to the brain, indicating the level of light received. Pupil size is regulated by a series of continuous motor commands that the brain automatically sends through the oculomotor nerves (third cranial nerve) to each eye. Normally, pupil size changes instantly to any change in light level.

When assessing the pupils, check for size (in millimetres), shape, and symmetry. Also check for a reaction to light shined on them, performing this assessment in as darkened an environment as possible. Asymmetric pupils (anisocoria, which can be found in 20% of the population) may indicate significant ocular or neurologic pathology, but must be correlated with the patient's overall presentation **Figure 13-15** ▶. Topical applications of certain medicines and substances can also provoke pupilary changes. The early assessment of the pupils in patients with a decreased level of awareness is important because the pupils reflect any responses or changes to the autonomic nervous system that are in direct response to any illness, injury, or involvement of drugs or toxins. This can aid you in determining a possible cause for your patient's condition.

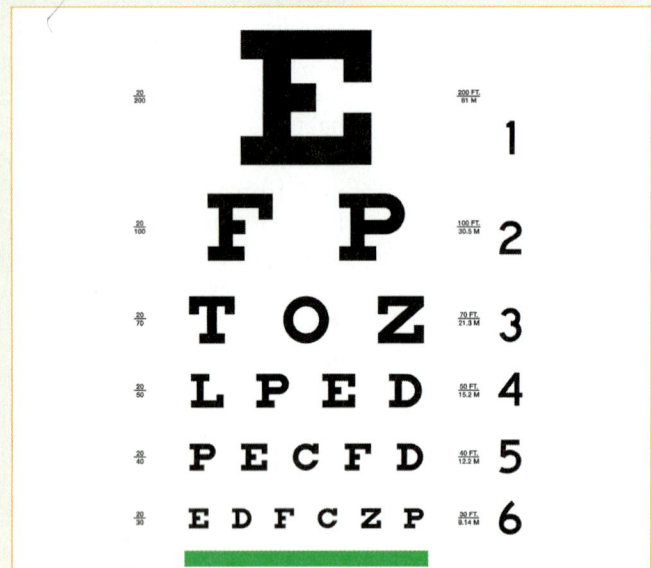

Figure 13-14 Due to its size and complexity, the Snellen chart is not a good prehospital tool.

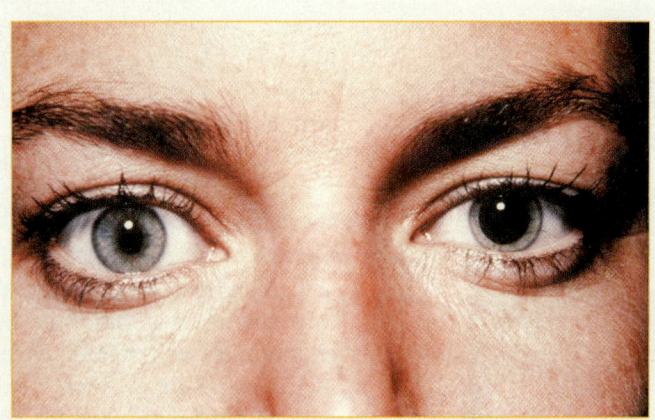

Figure 13-15 Asymmetric pupils may be normal or may signify a severe brain injury.

Muscles are responsible for physically moving the eyes from side to side and up and down, which allows for seamless binocular vision. When asked to follow a finger moved in a "Z" or "H" pattern, the eyes should move smoothly and symmetrically with the finger. Visual field examination assesses the retina's (and therefore the optic nerve's) ability to perceive light. This is done by checking the patient's peripheral vision, examining each eye in isolation.

Following the general eye examination, a more precise pen light examination is typically undertaken Figure 13-16 ▶ . Check the lids, lashes, and tear ducts. Look for foreign bodies, evidence of wounds and trauma, and discharge. Turn up the lids to look for foreign bodies, and inspect the conjunctivae and sclera. The sclera ought to be white, not jaundiced or injected (red). Painless subconjunctival hemorrhage is a common but benign presentation. The conjunctivae ought to be

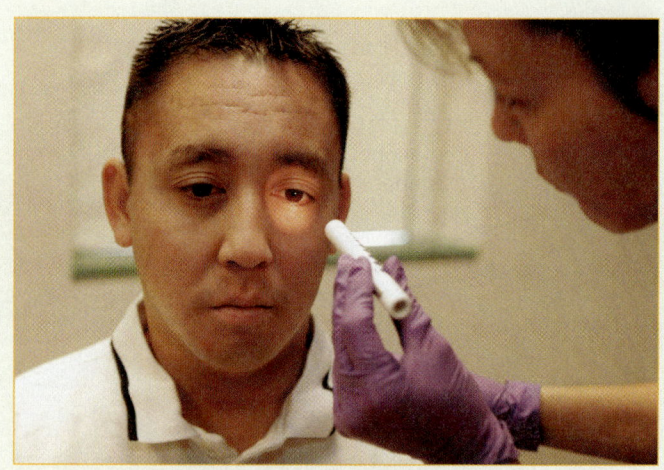

Figure 13-16 Pen light examination of the eye.

pink—not cyanotic, pale, or overly reddened. The cornea and lens will be difficult to examine without additional assessment tools—although in a trauma situation, you should note whether the globe is patent. Next, examine the anterior chamber and iris for clarity, noting any cloudiness or bleeding. Finally, examine the posterior chamber and retina; however, this examination is more useful after chemical dilation of the pupil and appropriate use of an ophthalmoscope. Follow the steps in Skill Drill 13-3 ▶ and Skill Drill 13-4 ▶ :

1. Examine the exterior portion of the eye. Look for any obvious trauma or deformity Step 1 .

2. Ask the patient about any pain, altered vision (eg, blurred or double vision), discharge, or sensitivity to light.

3. Measure visual acuity by having the patient count the number of fingers you are holding up at varying distances (usually 2 m, 1 m, and 30 cm away from the patient). Perform this examination on each eye independently of the other Step 2 .

4. Examine the pupils for size, shape, and symmetry. They should be equal.

5. Test the pupils for their reaction to light. Both pupils should constrict when exposed to light, and they should be equal in their response Step 3 .

6. Test for cranial nerve function by asking the patient to follow your fingers in a "Z" or "H" pattern. Note any abnormal movement of the eyes Step 4 .

7. Inspect the eyelids, lashes, and tear ducts for evidence of trauma, foreign bodies, or discharge Step 5 .

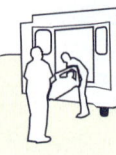 **At the Scene**

You may find that your patient's eye movement is not parallel. Failure to follow in a certain direction indicates weakness of an extraocular muscle or dysfunction of a cranial nerve innervating it.

Skill Drill 13-3: Examining the Eye

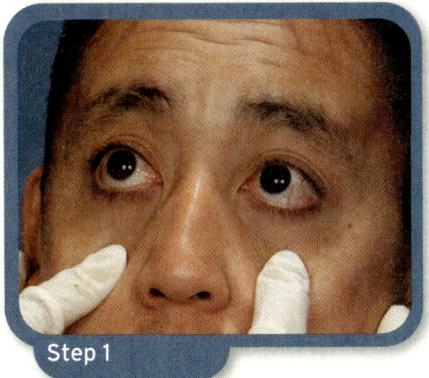

Step 1

Examine the exterior portion of the eye.

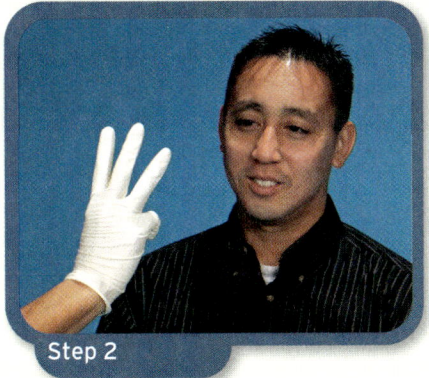

Step 2

Measure visual acuity by having the patient count the number of fingers you are holding up at varying distances.

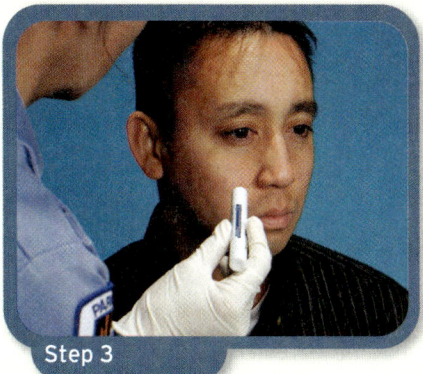

Step 3

Test the pupils for their reaction to light.

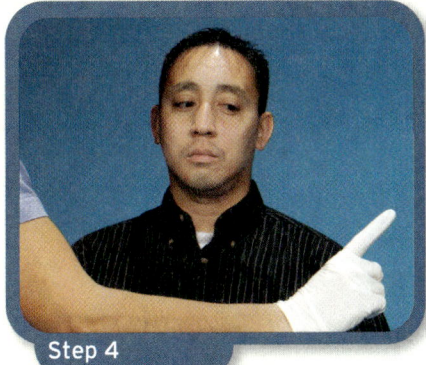

Step 4

Test for cranial nerve function by asking the patient to follow your fingers in a "Z" or "H" pattern.

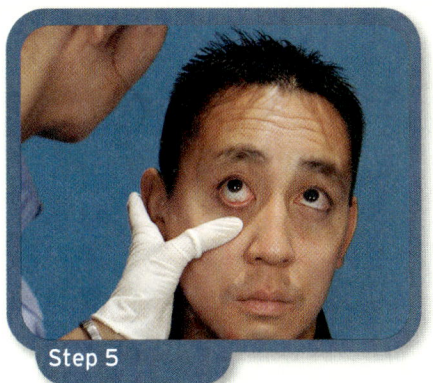

Step 5

Inspect the eyelids, lashes, and tear ducts.

1. Darken the environment as much as possible.
2. Ask the patient to look straight ahead and focus on a distant object (Step 1).
3. Set the light on the ophthalmoscope to a setting no brighter than necessary and the lens to 0 unless another setting works better for your eyes.
4. Use your right hand and eye to examine the patient's right eye; use your left hand and eye to examine the patient's left eye (Step 2).
5. Place the scope to your eye and look into the patient's pupil from 25 to 50 cm away at a 45° angle to the eye. You should see the retina as a "red reflex" or a bright orange glow (Step 3).
6. Slowly move toward the patient to appreciate the structures of the fundus. Adjust the lens as needed to improve the focus. Locate a blood vessel and follow it back to the disk. Use this blood vessel as a point of reference.

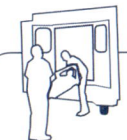 **At the Scene**

Cataracts appear as opaque black areas against the red reflex.

7. Inspect for the size, colour, and clarity of the disk. Note the integrity of the blood vessels and any lesions present on the retina. Move nasally to observe the macula (Step 4).
8. Repeat the process with the other eye.

Ears

The ear is a sensory organ that is chiefly involved with hearing and sound perception but is also intimately involved with balance control. The ear consists of an outer portion, a middle portion, and an inner portion Figure 13-17 ▶ .

The external ear consists of the pinna, or auricle (the part lying outside of the head), and the external auditory

Skill Drill 13-4: Eye Examination With an Ophthalmoscope

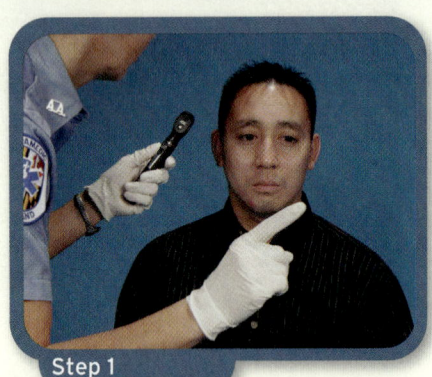

Step 1

Ask the patient to look straight ahead and focus on a distant object.

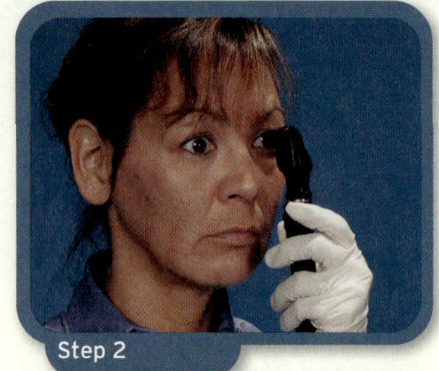

Step 2

Use your right hand and eye to examine the patient's right eye; use your left hand and eye to examine the patient's left eye.

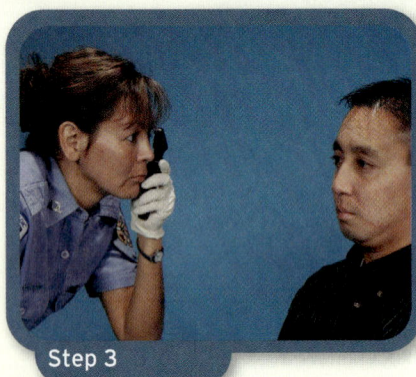

Step 3

Place the scope to your eye and look into the patient's pupil from 25 to 50 cm away at a 45° angle to the eye.

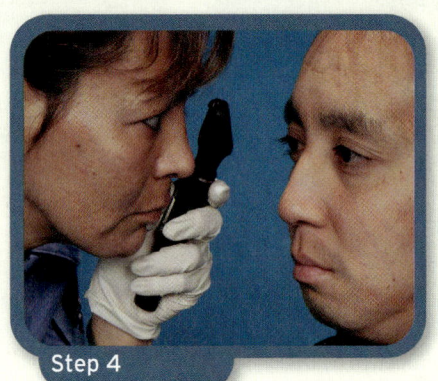

Step 4

Inspect for the size, colour, and clarity of the disk.

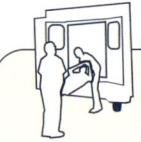

At the Scene

Use of the ophthalmoscope requires frequent practice. It is not routinely used in prehospital care.

canal, which leads in toward the tympanic membrane, or eardrum.

The middle ear contains three small bones (hammer, anvil, and stirrup) that move in response to sound waves hitting the tympanic membrane. This mechanism controls how we hear and differentiate sounds. The middle ear is connected to the nasal cavity by the Eustachian tube, or internal auditory canal. This connection permits equalization of pressure in the middle ear when external atmospheric pressure changes.

The inner ear consists of bony chambers filled with fluid. As the head moves, so does the fluid. In response, fine nerve endings within the fluid send impulses to the brain, indicating the position of the head and the rate of change of position.

Assessing the ears essentially involves checking for new aberrations in hearing perception plus inspecting and palpating for wounds, swelling, or drainage (pus, blood, CSF). Often the mastoid process of the skull, which is palpated immediately posterior to the auricle, is assessed for discolouration and tenderness (Battle's sign). Abnormalities of the external canal and tympanic membrane are visualized by use of an otoscope. Follow the steps in **Skill Drill 13-5 ▸** :

1. Select an appropriately sized speculum. Dim the lights as much as possible.
2. Ensure that the ear is free of foreign bodies.
3. Place your hand firmly against the patient's head and gently grasp the patient's auricle. Move the ear to best visualize the canal, usually upward and back in the adult patient **Step 1** .
4. Instruct the patient not to move during the examination to avoid damaging the ear.
5. Turn on the otoscope and insert the speculum into the ear **Step 2** . Insertion toward the patient's nose usually provides the best view. Don't insert the speculum deeply into the canal.
6. Inspect the canal for any lesions or discharge. A small amount of cerumen (ear wax) is normal **Step 3** .
7. Visualize the tympanic membrane (eardrum), and inspect it for integrity and colour. It should be translucent or a pearly grey colour. Note any signs of inflammation, including swelling or discolouration (pink or redness in the canal or tympanic membrane).

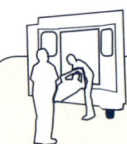

At the Scene

When looking for a foreign body, don't advance an otoscope tip blindly; you may accidentally push the foreign body in further.

Nose

The nose is a sensory organ involved with smell and taste; it is also part of the respiratory system. In assessing injuries involving the nose, it helps to picture the inside of the nose itself **Figure 13-18 ▶**. The nasal cavity is divided into two sections or chambers by the nasal septum, which is made of cartilage. Each nasal chamber contains three layers of bone (the turbinates) that are covered with a moist lining. Both chambers have superior, middle, and inferior turbinates. During nasal breathing, the air moves through the nasal chambers and is humidified as it passes over the turbinates. The turbinates are highly vascular and can cause profuse bleeding if damaged.

When checking the nose, assess it both anteriorly and inferiorly. Look for evidence of asymmetry, deformity, wounds, foreign bodies, discharge or bleeding, and tenderness. Note any evidence of respiratory distress, such as flaring of the nostrils. Inspect the exterior of the nose, looking for colour changes, symmetry, and structural abnormalities. The nose should be firm and the nares clear of obstruction. Examine the column of the nose; it should be midline with the face. Inspect the septum for any deviation from midline. The nares should be symmetrical. Slight deviation or asymmetry of the nares, septum, and column are normal findings; however, gross abnormalities should be noted. Note any drainage or discharge. Small amounts of mucosal discharge are normal, but large amounts of mucus and any blood or CSF fluid are serious findings.

Throat

Assessment of the throat should include an evaluation of the mouth, the pharynx, and sometimes the neck. The throat is a conduit for both respiration and digestion, and it's in close proximity to numerous vital neurovascular structures.

As part of the assessment of overall hydration status, pay close attention to the lips, teeth, oral mucosa, and tongue. In patients who present with markedly altered mental status, you'll need to rapidly determine upper airway

OUTER EAR   **MIDDLE EAR**   **INNER EAR**

Pinna — External auditory canal — Tympanic membrane — Semicircular canals — Oval window — Vestibular nerve — Cochlear nerve — Cochlea — Vestibule — Round window — Eustachian (auditory) tube — Malleus — Incus — Stapes

(Not to scale)

Figure 13-17 The structure of the outer, middle, and inner ear.

Skill Drill 13-5: Examining the Ear With an Otoscope

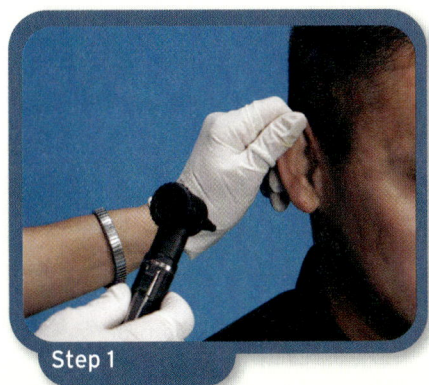

Step 1

Place your hand firmly against the patient's head and gently grasp the patient's auricle.

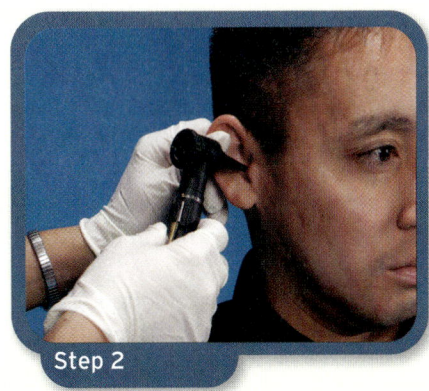

Step 2

Turn on the otoscope and insert the speculum into the ear.

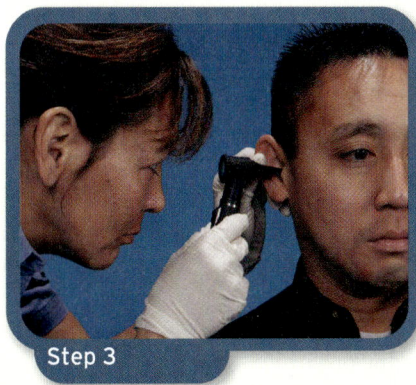

Step 3

Inspect the canal for any lesions or discharge.

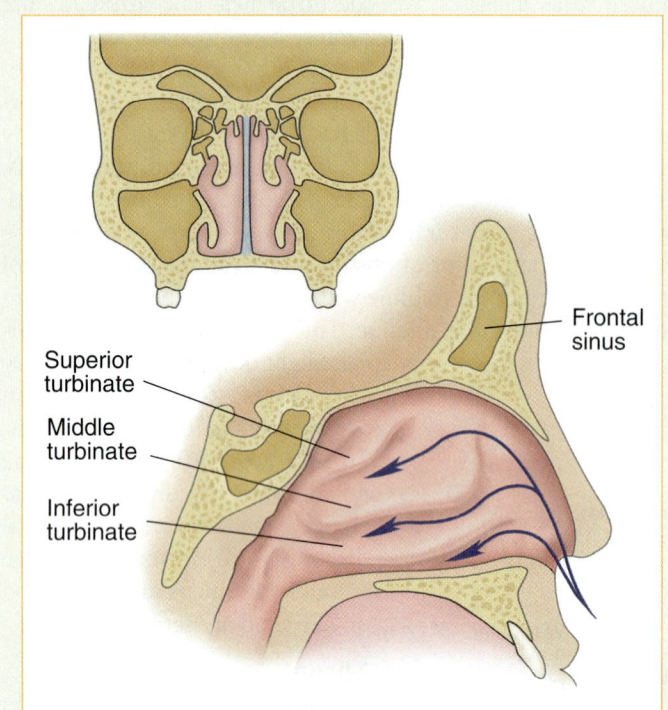

Figure 13-18 The nose has two chambers, divided by the septum. Each chamber is composed of layers of bone called turbinates. Above the nose are the frontal sinuses. On either side of the nose are the orbits of the eyes.

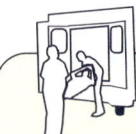

At the Scene

Frank blood or clear, watery drainage (CSF) from the ears or nose following trauma suggests a basilar skull fracture.

status; prompt assessment of the throat and upper airway structures is mandatory. Depending on the situation, assess for the presence of a foreign body or aspiration in either the throat or lower airway structures. Situations requiring removal of foreign bodies, secretions, or blood can manifest in many types of emergency cases. Always be prepared to assist with clearing the pharynx using manual techniques and suction.

The examination of the mouth begins with the lips, which should be pink and free of edema or surface irregularities. Confirm that the mouth is symmetrical. The gums should be pink, with no lesions or edema. Inspect the airway to ensure that it's free of obstructions. Visualize the tongue, noting its colour, size, and moisture. The tongue should be located at midline, without swelling, and moist. Examine the oropharynx, identifying any discolouration or pustules that might indicate an infection. Note any unusual odours on the breath, as they can indicate certain illnesses. Inspect the uvula for edema and redness.

The neck is an extraordinarily muscular region, through which many vital structures pass. External anatomy includes the jaw, cricothyroid membrane, external jugular veins, thyroid

cartilage, suprasternal notch, and cervical spinous processes. When assessing the neck, take the time to look for any abnormalities, including those related to symmetry, masses, and venous distention. When noting venous distention, consider the patient's body position relative to lying flat (0°). Describe how far up the neck the distention tracks (from the base of the neck to the angle of the jaw), using either an approximate or centimetre scale. Palpate the carotid pulses and note relative strength of impulse. Look for any pulsating or expanding mass near the carotid pulse point. Palpate the suprasternal notch in an effort to identify any tracheal deviation. Have the patient open and close the jaws while you palpate over the temporomandibular joint during your examination of the jaw. To examine the neck, follow the steps in **Skill Drill 13-6 ▶**:

1. If trauma is suspected, take precautions to protect the cervical spine **Step 1**.
2. Assess for the usage of accessory muscles during respiration.
3. Palpate the neck to find any structural abnormalities or subcutaneous air, and to ensure the trachea is midline. Do not spend a lot of time doing this, because it can be difficult to assess. Most tracheal deviation is picked up on chest x-ray. Begin at the suprasternal notch and work your way toward the head **Step 2**. Be careful about applying pressure to the area of the carotid arteries, as it may stimulate a vagal response.
4. Assess the lymph nodes and note any swelling, which may indicate infection **Step 3**.
5. Assess the jugular veins for distention; it may indicate a problem with blood returning to the heart **Step 4**.

Cervical Spine

The cervical spine is the pathway by which the spinal cord makes its way out of the brain and into the torso, enabling the spinal nerves to emanate to and innervate the rest of the body **Figure 13-19 ▶**. It is also the point at which the head connects to the body. The spine is supported by a large mass of muscle, as well as multiple tendinous and ligamentous supports. Cervical injury can present in a variety of ways, and the assessment for such injury must be conducted in a careful manner.

Evaluate the patient first for the MOI and then for the presence of pain. Does the patient have an altered mental status, or did a loss of consciousness occur at the time of the event? Is there a significant MOI, or do multiple or serious distracting injuries make assessment of the cervical spine difficult? Is the patient under the influence of any intoxicating substances? Being able to confidently answer all of those questions will allow you to decide which patients may (or may not) require further treatment of a potential cervical spine injury.

When examining the cervical spine, inspect and palpate it, looking for evidence of tenderness and deformity. Midline posterior tenderness involving the bony spinous processes should always raise concerns. Palpable discomfort over the lateral aspects of the neck usually signals a muscular or ligamentous problem, not an injury to the bony spinal column itself. Any manipulations that result in pain, tenderness, or tingling

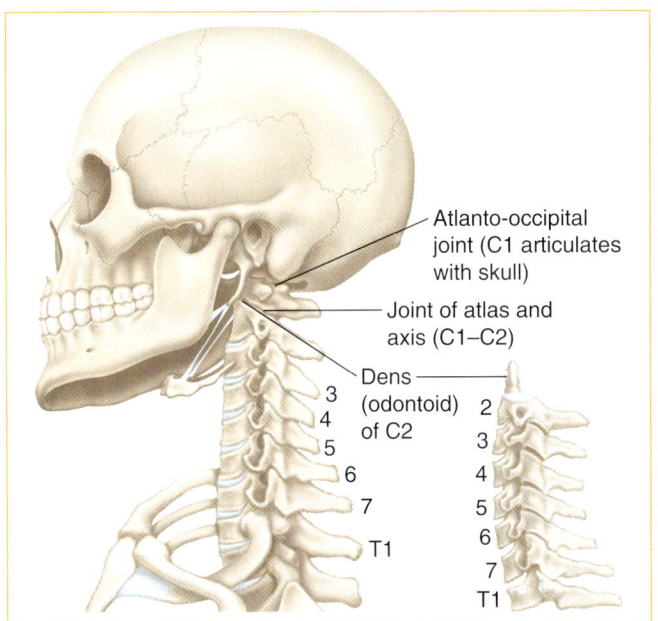

Figure 13-19 The cervical vertebrae.

should prompt you to stop the examination *immediately* and place the patient into a properly sized collar. With any complaints of neck pain in patients who have suffered a significant MOI, immediate stabilization of the head and neck is essential. Continued assessment of a patient's range of motion should take place only when there is no potential for serious injury.

When ranging the neck to assess for an underlying injury, first perform the activity in a passive manner, in which you are in control of the head and neck. Next, conduct the examination actively—that is, with the patient performing the directed maneuvers but being cautioned to stop if he or she experiences any pain or tingling. When checking range of motion, first slowly rotate the head from shoulder to shoulder. Then extend the head back, followed by flexing of the head and neck, touching chin to chest. Any discomfort elicited by these maneuvers should prompt you to terminate the examination immediately and protect the patient's spine.

Chest

The chest (or thorax) consists of the superior aspect of the torso, from the base of the neck to the diaphragm as delineated by the costal arch **Figure 13-20 ▶** . The chest wall is divided into anterior and posterior portions—literally, the patient's front and back. The back of the chest extends down the patient's back, posteriorly, which tends to move up and down with breathing. The chest contains many vital structures, including the lungs and mediastinal elements (heart, great vessels). The chest wall serves as a protective covering for the internal components. It consists of numerous musculoskeletal, vascular, nervous, connective, and lining structures.

Typically, the chest examination proceeds in three phases. The chest wall is checked, a pulmonary evaluation is conducted, and finally the cardiovascular assessment is performed. The chest must be inspected to assess for deformities in wall patency as well as to look for external clues of respiratory distress. Expose the chest and then begin its assessment, using the techniques of inspection, palpation, percussion, and auscultation. The examination of the posterior chest is the

Skill Drill 13-6: Examining the Neck

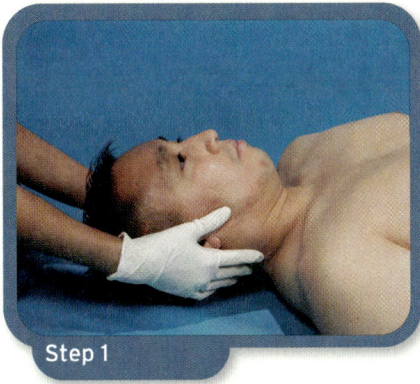

Step 1

If trauma is suspected, take precautions to protect the cervical spine.

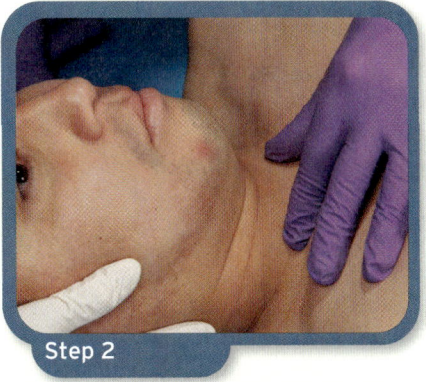

Step 2

Palpate the neck to find any structural abnormalities or subcutaneous air, and to ensure the trachea is midline. Begin at the suprasternal notch and work your way toward the head.

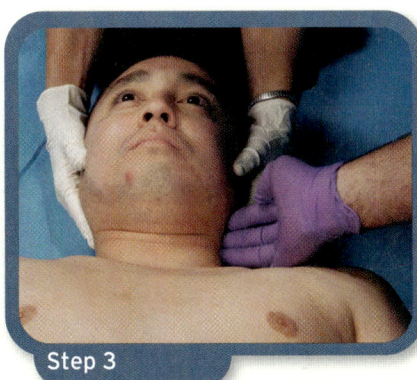

Step 3

Assess the lymph nodes.

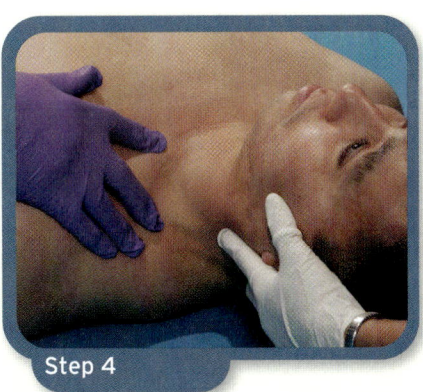

Step 4

Assess the jugular veins for distention.

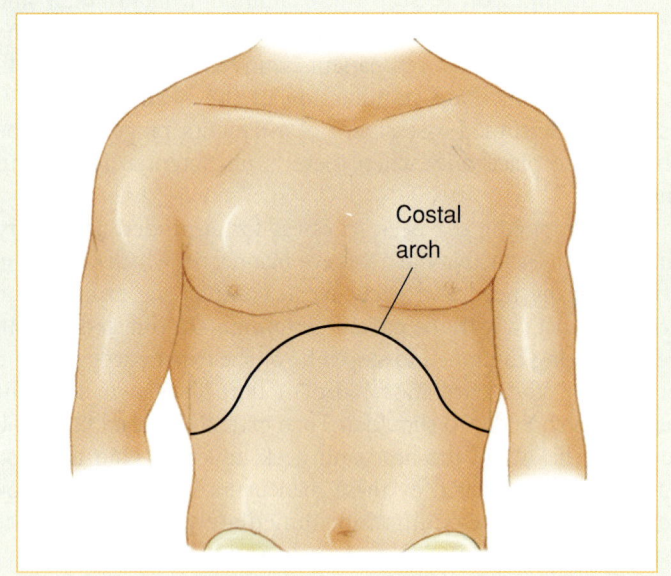

Figure 13-20 The chest (thorax) consists of the superior aspect of the torso, from the base of the neck to the diaphragm as delineated by the costal arch.

Costal arch

chest wall for respiratory effort, and document the respiratory rate, depth, and rhythm. Listen to the patient's breathing, and note the general shape of the chest wall. Pay close attention to any signs of abnormal breathing movements (paradox, accessory muscle use, impaired or diminished breathing movement) and retractions (suprasternal, sternal, intercostal, and subcostal). The presence of retractions is an important indicator of pulmonary issues, especially in children. Note any chest deformities, such as barrel chest (chronic obstructive pulmonary disease [COPD]), flail segments/subcutaneous air (trauma), kyphoscoliosis of the spine (compression fractures, COPD), significant bruising, and any suspicious wounds.

When palpating the chest wall, note any tenderness or crepitance/crepitus. Be sure to palpate areas that were initially noted to be abnormal on inspection. Palpation will also enable you to better appreciate respiratory symmetry and expansion. Although often impractical in the prehospital environment, percussion of the chest wall can allow for enhanced evaluation of the underlying chest cavity by distinguishing either dullness or hyperresonance versus normal resonance.

Auscultate the breath sounds **Figure 13-21 ▶**. The lungs consist of five discrete lobes: The right side contains the right upper, right middle, and right lower lobes; the left side contains the left upper and left lower lobes, as well as the lingual

same as the examination of the anterior chest. Follow the steps in **Skill Drill 13-7 ▶**:

1. Ensure the patient's privacy as best you can.
2. Inspect the chest for any obvious DCAP-BTLS **Step 1**.
3. If you find any open wounds, dress them appropriately.
4. Note the shape of the patient's chest—it can give you clues to many underlying medical conditions (eg, emphysema or bronchitis) **Step 2**.
5. Look for any surgical scars that may be a result of pacer implantation or a midline scar (a "zipper") that indicates previous cardiac surgery. Palpation of the chest may also reveal air under the skin (ie, subcutaneous emphysema).
6. Auscultate the lung fields, noting any abnormal lung sounds **Step 3**.
7. Use percussion to detect any abnormalities **Step 4**.
8. Auscultate for heart tones.
9. Repeat the appropriate portions of the examination for the posterior aspect of the thorax.

Compare the two sides of the chest for symmetry. Observe the

Skill Drill 13-7: Examining the Chest

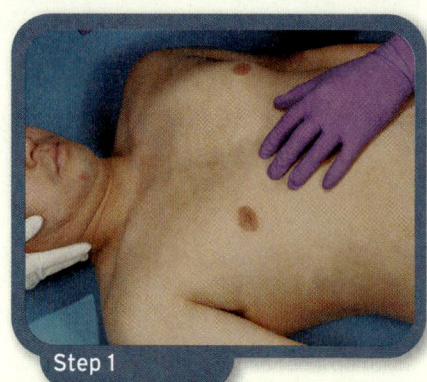

Step 1

Inspect the chest for any obvious DCAP-BTLS.

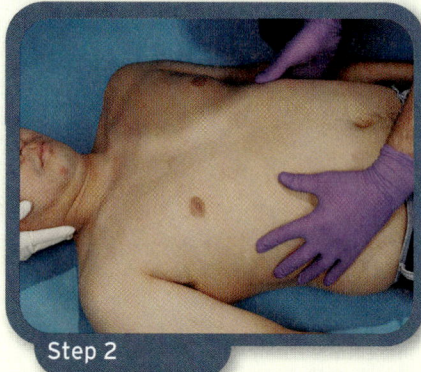

Step 2

Note the shape of the chest.

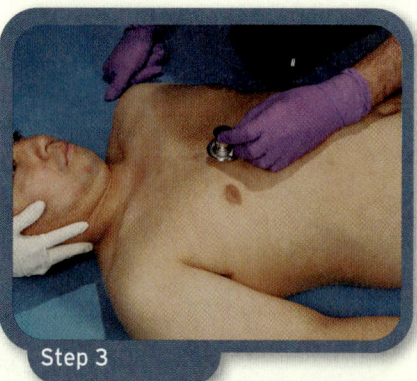

Step 3

Auscultate the lung fields, noting any abnormal lung sounds.

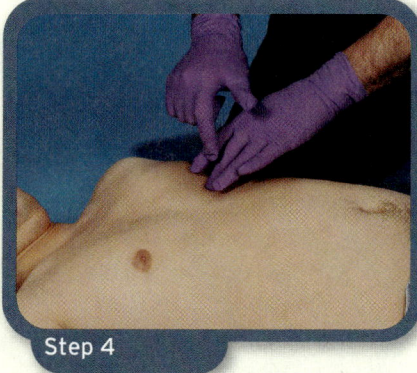

Step 4

Percuss the chest to detect any abnormalities.

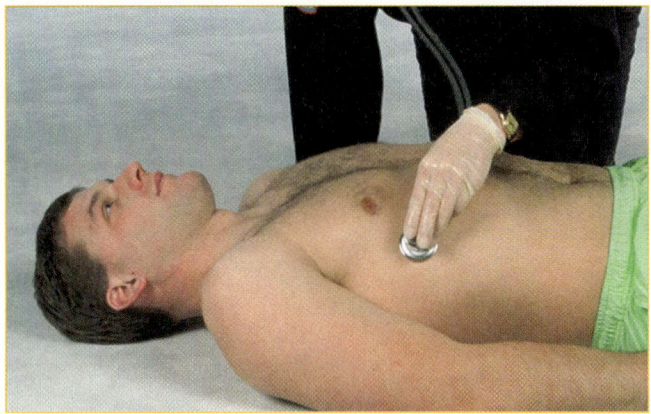

Figure 13-21 Auscultate the breath sounds on both sides of the chest.

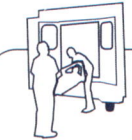

At the Scene

Lungs are hyperinflated with chronic emphysema, resulting in hyperresonance where you would expect cardiac dullness.

Figure 13-22 ▶ . During your examination, listen over each lobe, both anteriorly and posteriorly. Have the patient take as deep a breath as he or she can via an open mouth to facilitate your auscultatory assessment. Listen to as many portions of the lungs as possible, preferably avoiding any bony prominences, attached medical equipment, or clothing. Always use the best stethoscope available.

Normal lung sounds include bronchial, vesicular, and bronchovesicular sounds. They are a function of the particular

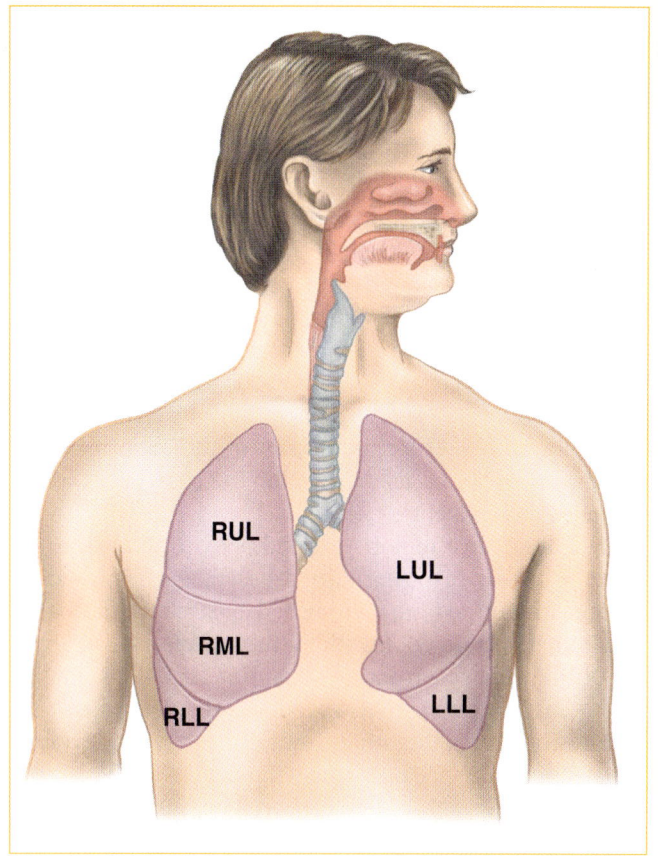

Figure 13-22 The five lobes of the lungs.

pulmonary structure that air is passing through. Pathologic or adventitial breath sounds include wheezes and crackles. They are indications of lung tissue consolidation, atelectasis, edema, mucus collection, and hemorrhage. Stridor is an abnormal

You are the Paramedic Part 3

You administer another nebulizer treatment with 2.5 mg of Ventolin/normal saline via face mask as you prepare him to be moved to the ambulance. Once you have your patient safely in the back you establish an IV of normal saline in his left antecubital vein with an 18-gauge cannula. Upon reassessment of the patient following the breathing treatment, you find that he still has audible inspiratory and expiratory wheezes and increased work of breathing evidenced by intercostal and supraclavicular retractions. The patient states that he does not feel any relief and asks if there is anything else you can do. You administer a second breathing treatment with 2.5 mg of salbutamol (Ventolin)/normal saline and contact direct medical control for additional orders.

Reassessment	Recording Time: 12 Minutes
Skin	Pale, warm, and dry with cyanotic nail beds and lips
Pulse	138 beats/min, regular, strong distal pulses
ECG	Sinus tachycardia
Blood pressure	164/82 mm Hg
Respirations	38 breaths/min, laboured
Spo$_2$	78% on a nebulizer at 8 l/min
Pupils	Equal and reactive to light

5. Would an increased work of breathing be present upon reassessment of the patient if your treatment was effective?

6. How should your patient management progress?

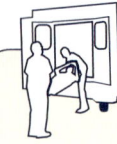

At the Scene

Percussion of the chest produces hyperresonance when the thorax is full of air and hyporesonance, or dullness, when it's full of blood.

respiratory sound of the upper airway that is often apparent on general examination, but can also be auscultated in more subtle presentations. Rubs can be heard emanating from either the lungs or the heart. A rub is produced by a partial loss of intrapleural integrity, when an abnormal collection of fluid has accumulated between a portion of the visceral and parietal pleura, resulting in "pleuritic" pain and a perceived rub on auscultation. Be sure of the location of the abnormal sound, because sounds can be referred within the chest cavity, particu-larly in pediatric patients.

One of the most important—and perhaps most often over-looked—aspects of pulmonary assessment is appreciating when breath sounds are diminished or absent. You can't be aware of this phenomenon without first developing an appreci-ation of the wide spectrum of normal presentations that exist. Before going out into the field, you should spend many hours listening to normal breath sounds, in order to develop an understanding of what constitutes the many variations of nor-mal breathing. After that, you'll spend time listening to patients with respiratory difficulty, preferably alongside an experienced individual who can point out the significant variations in the presenting abnormalities.

Decreased breath sounds can be localized to a portion of one lung, or they can encompass the entire chest. When hypoventilation is suspected, you must take immediate action. Decreased breath sounds typically signal a lack of respiratory excursion or decreased tidal volume. Numerous problems can cause decreased breath sounds, including pneumothorax, hemothorax, pleural effusion, pulmonary edema, atelectasis/consolidation, exacerbated COPD, status asthmati-cus, opiate intoxication, pneumonia, bronchitis, and altered mental status.

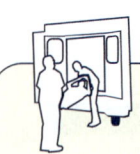

At the Scene

Normal breathing should be quiet and not grossly evident to you. If you can see or hear the patient breathe, there's a problem.

Cardiovascular System

The cardiovascular system circulates blood throughout the body, an activity that maintains perfusion of the body's tissues Figure 13-23 ▶ . The cardiovascular system comprises a pump (the heart), a set of pipes (the blood vessels), and a liq-uid transported within those pipes (blood).

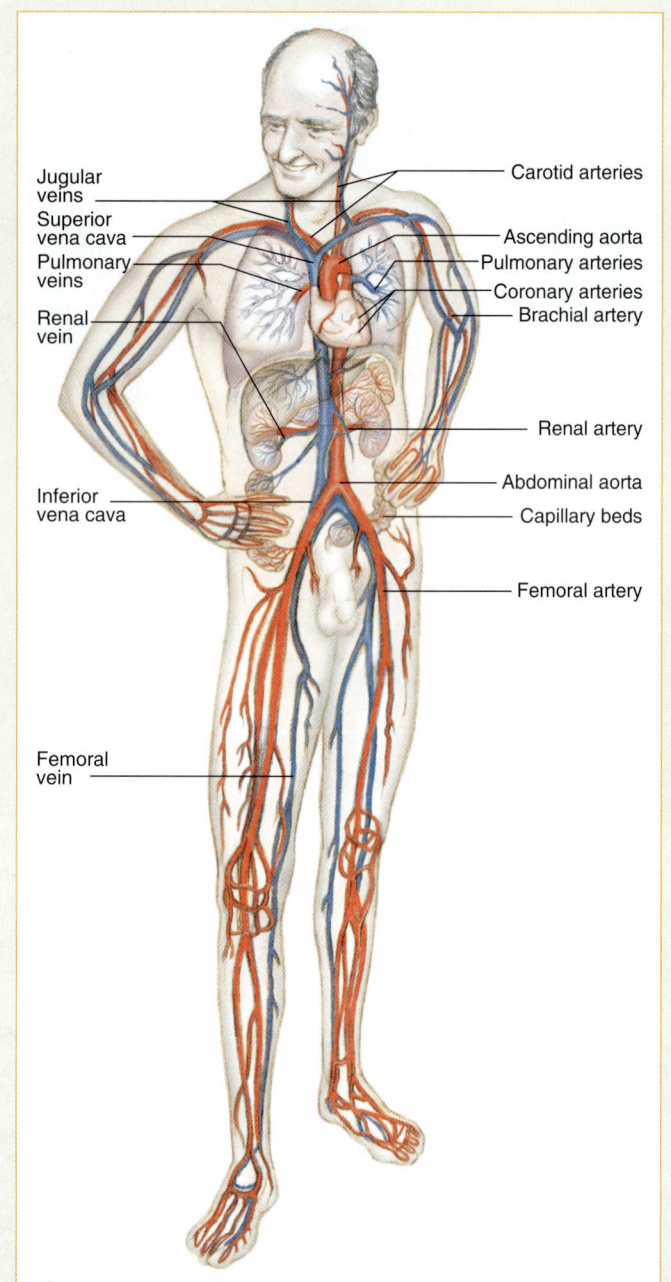

Jugular veins
Superior vena cava
Pulmonary veins
Renal vein
Inferior vena cava
Femoral vein

Carotid arteries
Ascending aorta
Pulmonary arteries
Coronary arteries
Brachial artery
Renal artery
Abdominal aorta
Capillary beds
Femoral artery

Figure 13-23 The cardiovascular system.

Blood consists of plasma, red blood cells, white blood cells, and platelets. Plasma is essentially a mild saline solution, but it also contains blood-clotting factors and particles that play important roles in the body's immune response.

The complex arrangement of connected tubes in the circu-latory system includes the arteries, arterioles, capillaries, venules, and veins. This system is entirely closed, with capillar-ies connecting the arterioles and the venules.

Blood flows through two circuits in this system: the sys-temic circulation in the body and the pulmonary circulation in the lungs. The systemic circulation carries oxygen-rich blood from the left ventricle through the body and back to the right

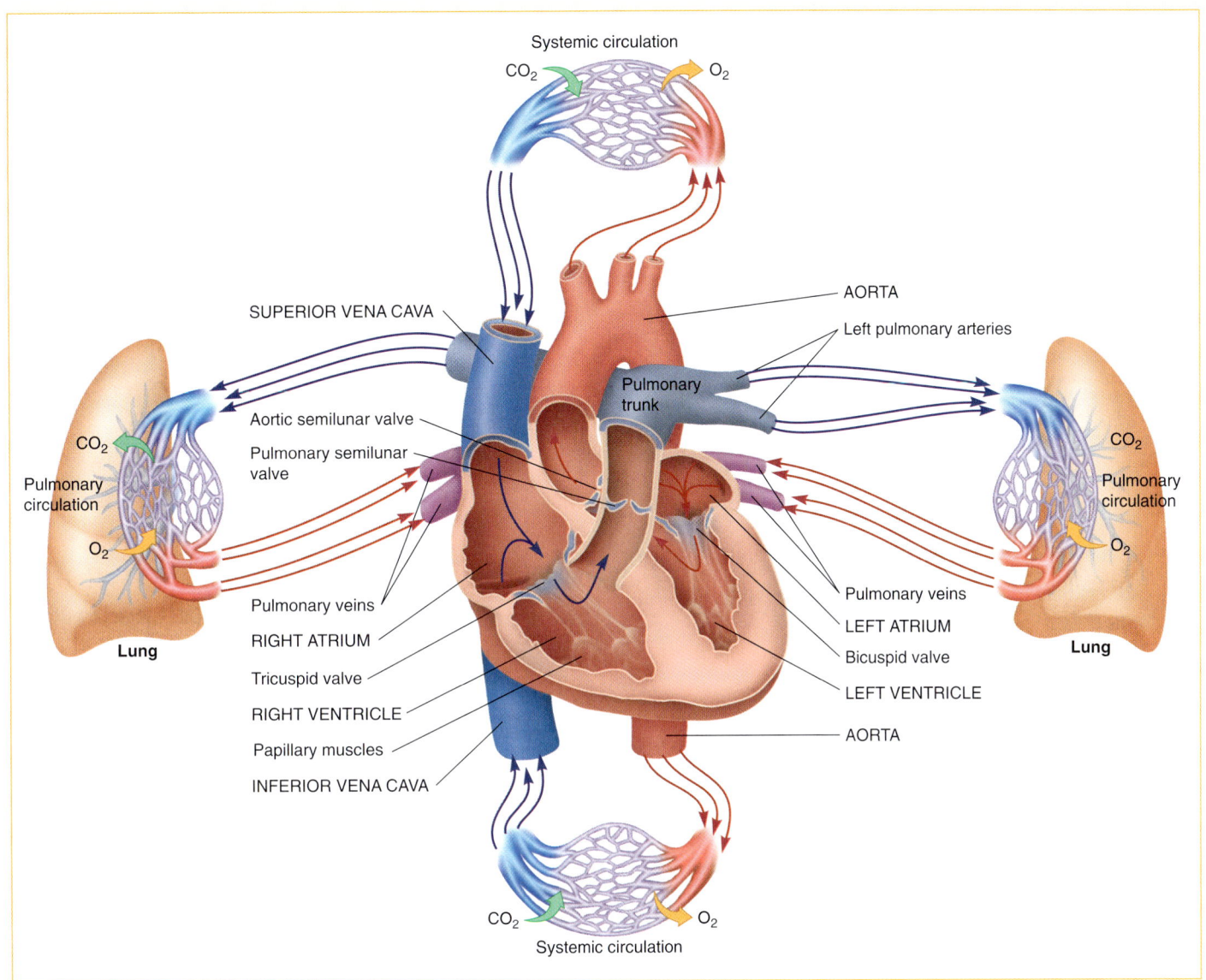

Figure 13-24 Blood flow through the heart and lungs.

atrium. As this blood passes through the tissues and organs, it gives up oxygen and nutrients and absorbs cellular wastes and carbon dioxide. The cellular wastes are, in turn, eliminated as the blood flows through the liver and the kidneys. The pulmonary circulation carries oxygen-poor blood from the right ventricle through the lungs and back into the left atrium.

The cardiac cycle involves the events of cardiac relaxation (diastole), filling, and contraction (systole). These mechanical events are coordinated electrically with the heart's pacing and conduction system. The heart consists of four chambers: two atria (upper chambers) and two ventricles (lower chambers). Each side of the heart contains one atrium and one ventricle. The interatrial septum (membrane) separates the two atria; a thicker wall, the interventricular septum, separates the right and left ventricles. Each atrium receives blood that is returned

to the heart from other parts of the body; each ventricle pumps blood out of the heart. The upper and lower portions of the heart are separated by the atrioventricular valves, which prevent backward flow of blood. The semilunar valves, which are located between the ventricles and the arteries into which they pump blood, serve a similar function Figure 13-24 ▲.

Blood enters the right atrium via the superior and inferior vena cavae and the coronary sinus, which consists of veins that collect blood returning from the walls of the heart. Blood from four pulmonary veins enters the left atrium. Between the right and left atria is the fossa ovalis, a depression that represents the former location of the foramen ovale, an opening between the two atria that is present in the fetus.

The cardiac cycle coordinates the movement of blood between the chambers of the heart. The atria always relax and

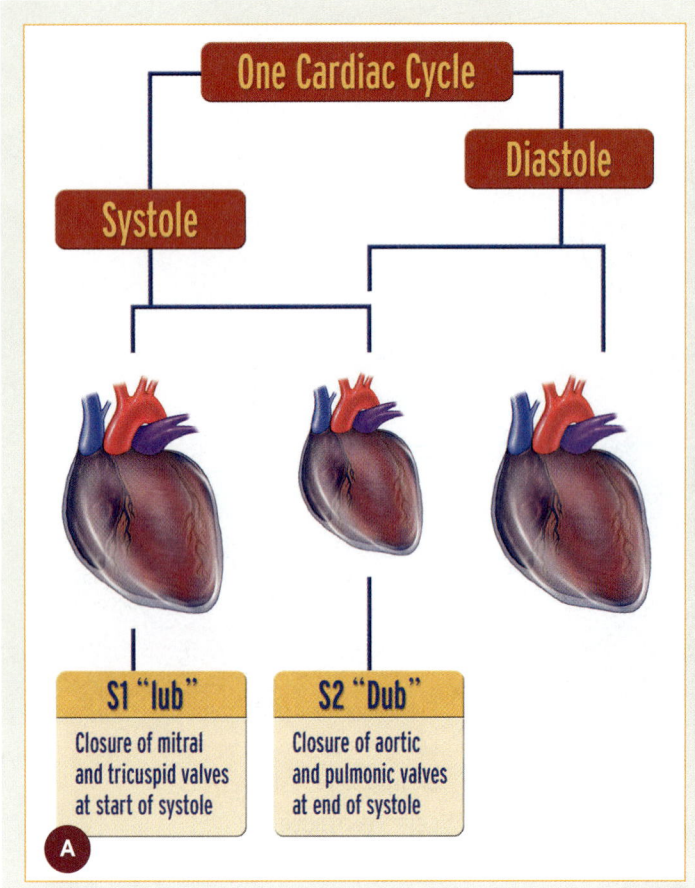

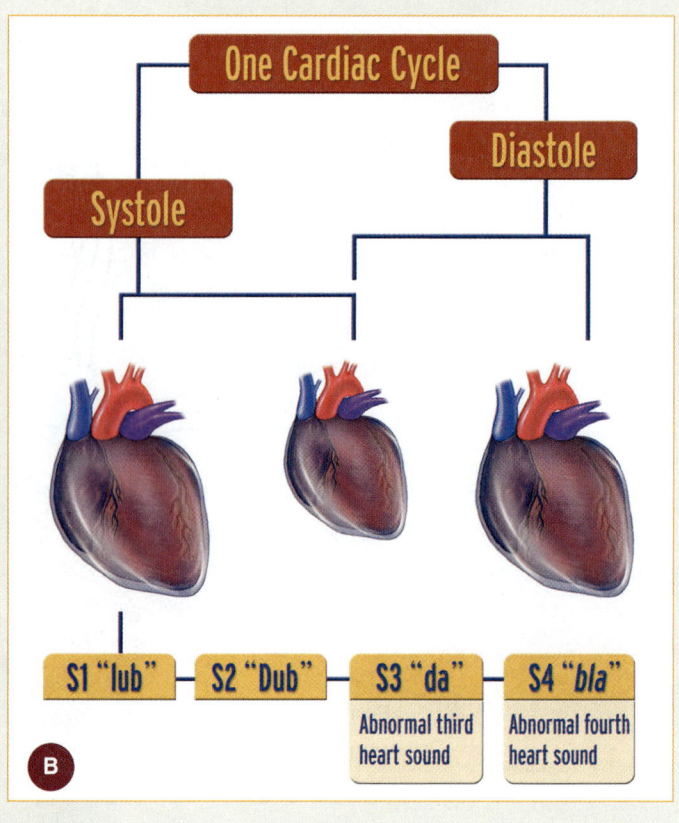

Figure 13-25 Heart sounds. **A.** The normal S_1 and S_2 heart sounds. **B.** The abnormal S_3 and S_4 heart sounds.

contract together, as do the ventricles. While the atria are contracting (and filling the ventricles), the ventricles are relaxing. Conversely, when the ventricles are contracting, the atria are relaxing, being filled by either the vena cava or the pulmonary veins.

The contraction and relaxation of the heart, combined with the flow of blood, generates characteristic heart sounds during auscultation with a stethoscope. The normal pattern sounds much like this: "lub-DUB lub-DUB, lub-DUB . . ." The "lub" is referred to as the first heart sound or S_1, and the "DUB" (emphasized because it is often louder) as the second heart sound or S_2. Pathologic heart sounds include S_3 and S_4 **Figure 13-25 ▲**. The S_3 or third heart sound is a soft, low-pitched heart sound that occurs about one third of the way through diastole. Although S_3 is sometimes present in healthy young people, it most commonly is associated with abnormally increased filling pressures in the atria secondary to moderate to severe heart failure. S_4, which is considered a "gallop" rhythm, is a moderately pitched sound that occurs immediately before the normal S_1 sound; it's always abnormal. The S_4 sound

At the Scene

The S_3 sound is associated with heart failure and is always abnormal in patients over 35 years of age.

represents either decreased stretching (compliance) of the left ventricle or increased pressure in the atria.

Heart sounds can be appreciated by listening to the chest wall in the parasternal areas superiorly and inferiorly as well as in the region superior to the left nipple. Follow the steps in **Skill Drill 13-8 ▶**:

1. Place the patient in one of these positions to bring the heart closer to the left anterior chest wall:
   - Sitting up and leaning slightly forward **Step 1**
   - Supine
   - Left lateral recumbent position
2. Place your stethoscope at the fifth intercostal space over the apex of the heart **Step 2**.
3. To appreciate the S_1 sound, ask the patient to breathe normally and hold the breath on expiration.
4. To appreciate the S_2 sound, ask the patient to breathe normally and hold the breath on inhalation **Step 3**.
5. Auscultate the area above the left nipple to listen for S_3 and S_4 heart sounds.

Korotkoff sounds are detected while listening to a patient's blood pressure. A bruit is an abnormal "whoosh"-like sound that indicates turbulent blood flow moving through a narrowed artery (most significant in the carotid arteries). A murmur is an abnormal whoosh-like sound heard over the heart that indicates turbulent blood flow around a cardiac valve. Murmurs are

Skill Drill 13-8: Auscultation of Heart Sounds

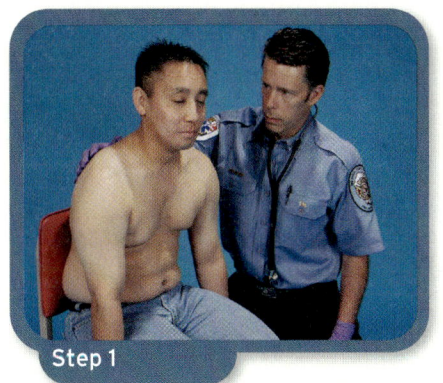

Step 1

Place the patient in a position that will bring the heart closer to the left anterior chest wall, such as sitting up and leaning slightly forward.

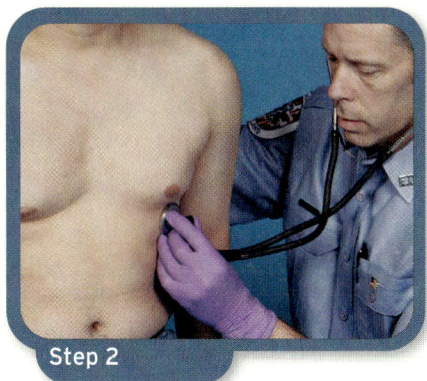

Step 2

Place your stethoscope at the fifth intercostal space over the apex of the heart.

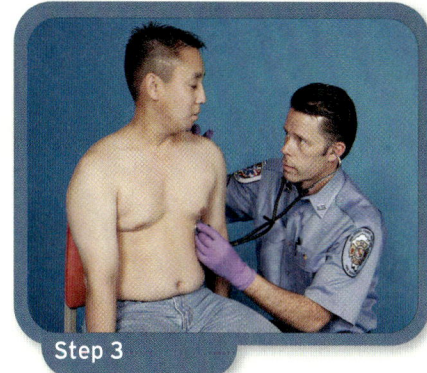

Step 3

Ask the patient to breathe normally and hold the breath on inhalation.

graded as a range of intensity from 1 (softest) to 6 (loudest). Many people have normal, physiologic murmurs. In some patients, they can represent a degree of pathology, depending on the nature of the underlying problem and the specific anatomy of the valve involved. To fully appreciate the nature and quality of normal heart sounds and murmurs, you must thoroughly practice your listening skills using excellent equipment.

Arterial pulses are a physical expression of systolic blood pressure. They are caused when contraction of the left ventricle and ejection of blood into the systemic circulation generate a pressure wave, which then travels throughout the arterial system. Arterial pulses are palpable wherever an artery crosses a bony prominence.

Venous pressure tends to be very low. In fact, in the normal setting, the pressure in the vena cava just before blood is received into the right atrium is close to zero. Veins are relatively nonmuscular, thin-walled vessels that have no effect on systemic vascular resistance and do not assist in promoting systemic blood pressure. Blood flows through the venous system and returns to the heart in part because it is propelled from behind in a continuous fashion, draining the capillary network. Most venous return of blood is a function of the respiratory cycle, generated by negative intrathoracic pressure that is developed at inspiration during normal breathing.

Occasionally, you can estimate the capacity of the venous system by observing a patient's jugular venous pressure, also known as jugular venous distention (JVD). In right-sided heart failure, blood tends not to be readily accepted into the right atrium. Venous capacitance increases in an effort to compensate for this failure, which in turn results in elevated pressures and corresponding JVD. JVD can be most readily observed by

evaluating the anterolateral aspects of the neck; it can also be provoked in a normal person by having the person lie supine and elevate the legs. While examining a patient for JVD, it is important to note how much distention is present, measured in terms of centimetres of distention from the origin of the jugular vein at the base of the neck. Note the angle of the patient relative to 0° (flat) while making the observation.

In situations involving hypotension, there may be no evidence of JVD, even while the patient is supine. Hypotensive patients with JVD must be carefully assessed as to the nature of their condition, however. Depending on the clinical situation, patients with JVD may be experiencing cardiogenic shock or have a ruptured cardiac valve. In the setting of chest trauma, neck vein distention and hypotension may symbolize a tension pneumothorax or pericardial tamponade.

The ability of the circulatory system to constrict and dilate can diminish markedly as a person ages. Although this limitation may vary considerably from patient to patient, an older patient's ability to compensate for cardiovascular insults may be profoundly curtailed by age-related changes, especially arterial atherosclerosis and diabetes. In addition, many medications that older persons routinely use to manage problems such as high blood pressure can negatively affect the body's ability to handle sudden changes in the demand for blood supply. By contrast, children and young adults have an enhanced ability to vasoconstrict and increase the pulse rate to compensate for a vascular insult; this compensation mechanism can fool paramedics into believing that young patients are "less sick" than they actually are.

When you are examining the cardiovascular system, pay attention to arterial pulses, noting their location, rate, rhythm, and quality. Obtain an accurate blood pressure, and repeat this measurement periodically to assess the patient's hemodynamic stability. Examine the jugular veins for distention. While inspecting and palpating the chest, listen for heart sounds. Feel the chest wall to locate the point of maximum impulse (PMI), and then listen over the areas where the cardiac valves are. The aortic valve is found near the second intercostal space, to the right of the sternum. The pulmonic valve lies near the second intercostal space, to the left of the sternum. The tricuspid valve is auscultated over the lower left sternal border. The mitral valve can be appreciated over the cardiac apex, lateral to the lower left sternal border near the midclavicular line. Note the intensity of the heart sounds, and listen for S_1, S_2, and any extra sounds and murmurs.

Abdomen

Because of the large number of organs within the abdomen, the location of organs and their related medical complaints are most easily described by dividing the abdomen into imaginary quadrants. The umbilicus (navel) serves as the central reference point. The diaphragm, the large dome-shaped muscle used for respiration, is at the top of the abdominal cavity, and the pelvis is at the bottom. The quadrants are divided by a set of imaginary perpendicular lines intersecting at the umbilicus **Figure 13-26 ▾**.

The abdomen contains almost all of the organs of digestion, the organs of the urogenital system, and significant neurovascular structures. The abdominal wall is a relatively thick muscular organ that overlies the peritoneum. The peritoneum is itself a well-defined layer of fascia made up of the parietal and visceral peritoneum. Abdominal organs are often characterized as being either intraperitoneal or extraperitoneal, depending on where they reside in relation to this layer. Intraperitoneal organs include the stomach, proximal duodenum of the small intestine, pancreas, jejunum, ileum, appendix, cecum, transverse colon, sigmoid colon, proximal rectum, liver, gallbladder, spleen, omentum, and female internal genitalia. Extraperitoneal organs include the mid- and distal duodenum, abdominal aorta, mid- and lower rectum, kidneys, pancreatic tail, adrenal glands, ureters, renal blood vessels, gonadal blood vessels, ascending colon, descending colon, and urinary bladder.

The abdominal organs can be topographically organized and sequentially assessed by viewing the overlying abdominal wall in a subdivided fashion. This is typically done in quadrants—left upper quadrant (LUQ), right upper quadrant (RUQ), left lower quadrant (LLQ), right lower quadrant (RLQ)—or ninths: right hypochondrial, RH; epigastric, E; left hypochondrial, LH; right lumbar, RL; umbilical, U; left lumbar, LL; right iliac, RI; hypogastric, H; left iliac, LI **Figure 13-27 ▾**.

Abdominal pain and associated concerns are common complaints, but their cause is often difficult to identify. Obtaining any appropriate history relevant to the situation is critical to help elucidate the nature of the problem. Historical information should include the location, quality, and severity of the discomfort; time of onset and duration of symptoms; significant activities at onset of distress; any aggravating or

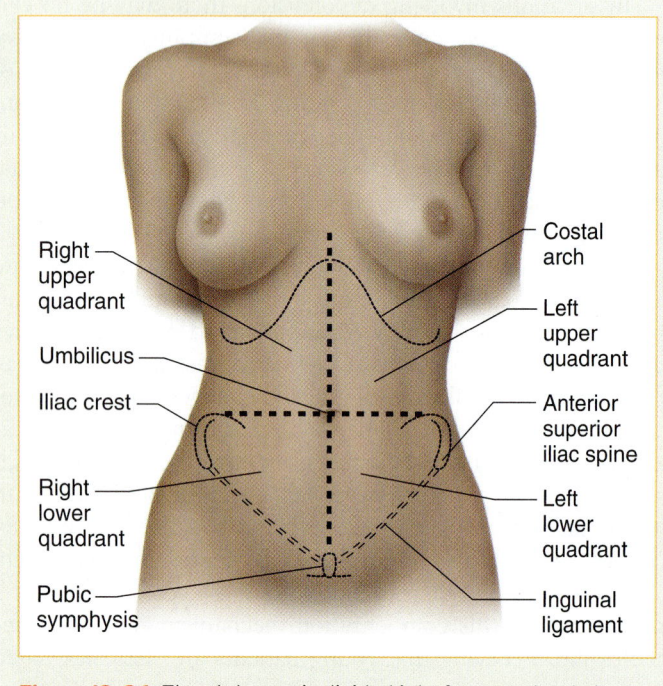

Figure 13-26 The abdomen is divided into four quadrants by imaginary vertical and horizontal lines.

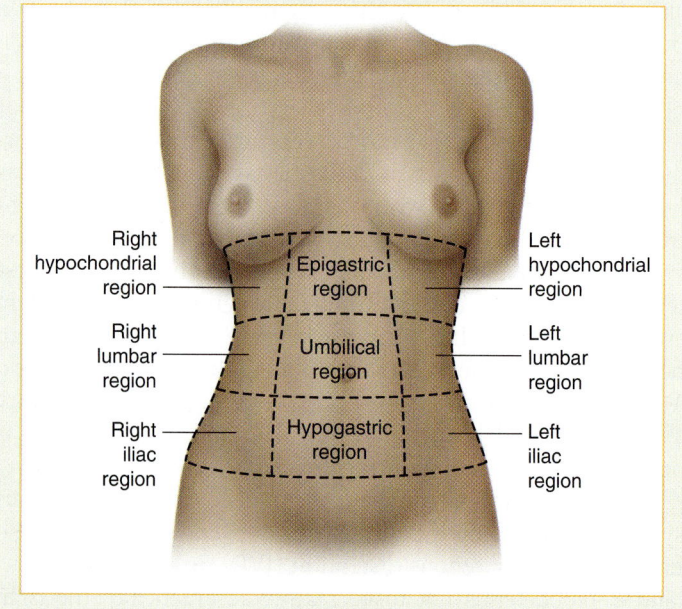

Figure 13-27 The abdomen can also be divided into nine regions.

At the Scene

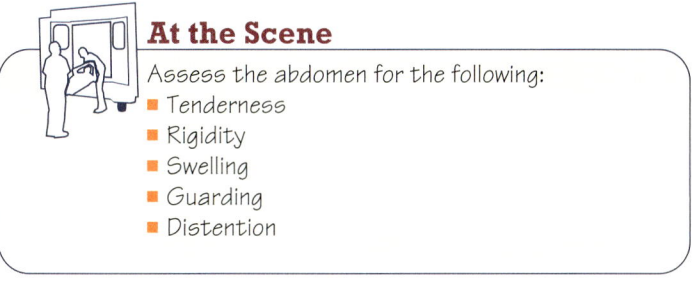

Assess the abdomen for the following:

- Tenderness
- Rigidity
- Swelling
- Guarding
- Distention

alleviating factors; and any associated symptoms, including nausea, vomiting, febrile symptoms, or changes in dietary, bowel, or bladder habits.

When you are examining a patient's abdomen, generally it's best to make the patient as comfortable as possible. Sometimes this requires giving some pain medication first, as the patient may be more cooperative and better able to focus with less discomfort. To assess the abdomen, the patient must be in a supine position. To examine and palpate/percuss over the posterior aspects of the abdomen, however, you should either sit the patient up or log roll him or her at some point.

Prior to palpating the abdomen, have the patient point to the area of greatest discomfort. Avoid touching that area until last. Work slowly and avoid quick movements. When appropriate, speak with the patient about the nature of the illness while palpating the abdomen. Once an area of tenderness has been localized, attempt to visualize which structures may underlie it and think about what might potentially be causing the problem. In situations of penetrating trauma, this step is less of a priority: It is difficult to localize which areas may be damaged with a high-velocity wound by visualizing and palpating the abdominal wall. Always proceed with abdominal assessment in a systematic fashion, routinely performing inspection, auscultation, percussion, and palpation, in that order. Follow the steps in **Skill Drill 13-9 ▶**:

1. Inspect the abdomen for any DCAP-BTLS **Step 1**.
2. Note any surgical scars, as they may be clues to an underlying illness.
3. Look for symmetry and the presence of any distention.
4. Auscultate the abdomen for bowel sounds **Step 2**.

5. Perform percussion.
6. Palpate the four quadrants of the abdomen in a systematic pattern, beginning with the quadrant farthest from the patient's complaint of pain **Step 3**.
7. Note any tenderness or rigidity, and pay special attention to the patient's expressions as they may yield valuable information **Step 4**.

When you are inspecting the abdomen, look at the skin as well as the contour and overall appearance of the abdominal wall. Identify any scars, wounds, striae, dilated veins, bruises, rashes, and discolourations. Note any generalized distension or localized masses.

At the Scene

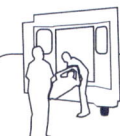

When palpating the abdomen, always begin on the side opposite the site of pain.

Skill Drill 13-9: Examining the Abdomen

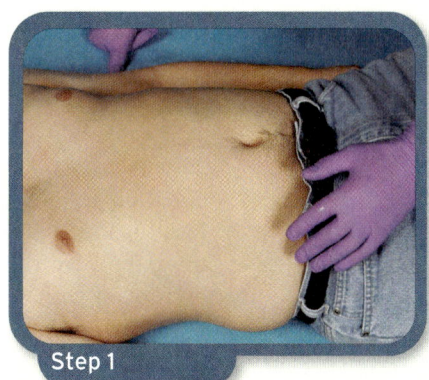

Step 1

Inspect the abdomen for any DCAP-BTLS.

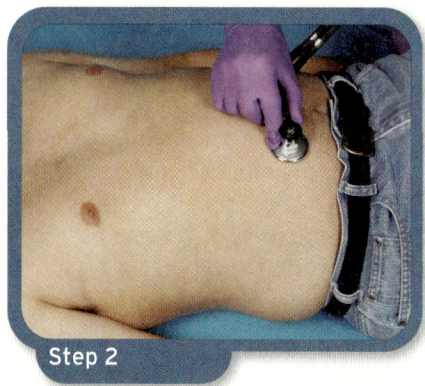

Step 2

Auscultate the abdomen for bowel sounds.

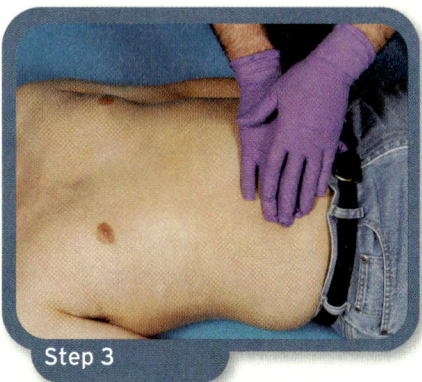

Step 3

Palpate the four quadrants of the abdomen in a systematic pattern, beginning with the quadrant farthest from the patient's complaint.

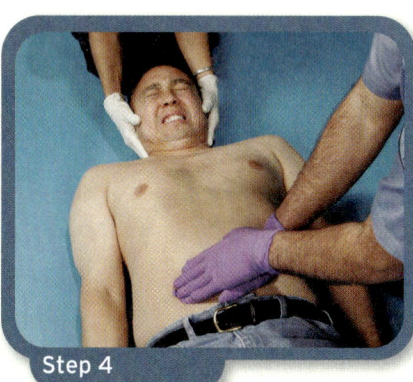

Step 4

Note any tenderness or rigidity.

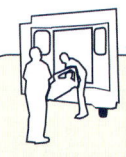

At the Scene

Restlessness and constant repositioning occur with colicky pain of gastroenteritis or bowel obstruction. Absolute stillness, resisting any movement, is demonstrated with the pain of peritonitis. Knees flexed, facial grimacing, and rapid/uneven respirations also indicate signs of pain.

The abdomen can be described as flat, rounded, protuberant (bulging out), scaphoid, or pulsatile. Any abdominal distention needs to be distinguished from obesity. An obese abdomen tends to be more protuberant than distended, and is typically exceptionally pliable. A patient with intra-abdominal pathology who also happens to have significant obesity will present a challenge in this regard.

Some patients may have ascites, a collection of fluid within the peritoneal cavity. Ascites is consistent with an underlying edema, but instead of affecting the interstitial tissues of the legs, it involves the abdomen. The patient's abdomen may appear markedly distended, and a visible or palpable fluid wave may be evident during examination, with shifting dullness noted to percussion. Ascites is most typically seen in patients who suffer from liver disease, but it can also be appreciated with underlying malignancy and, to a certain extent, with renal and cardiac insufficiency.

Auscultation of the abdomen is commonly performed as part of the routine abdominal examination, although it may have limited utility in the prehospital setting. To hear bowel sounds, the setting must be fairly optimal and you should take enough time to ensure an adequate assessment. Differentiating normal from abnormal can sometimes be challenging, so you should practice this skill on many healthy individuals to get a full appreciation for the abnormal situations you are likely to encounter.

When you are assessing bowel sounds, make note of their presence or absence. Sometimes the abnormality is characterized by hyperactivity or hypoactivity, rather than a total lack of sounds. Bowel sounds can also be described as increased, decreased, or absent. In the case of hyperactive sounds, note their frequency and character. With an obstruction, the sounds are often referred to as high-pitched and tinkling.

Palpation yields perhaps the most significant diagnostic information during the abdominal examination—that is, tenderness (elicited pain). You may then be able to correlate historical information related to the patient's current illness or

At the Scene

Hyperactive sounds are loud, high-pitched, rushing, or tinkling sounds that signal increased motility. Hypoactive or absent sounds follow recent abdominal surgery or are a sign of inflammation of the peritoneum.

situation and the findings from the examination, and determine what's wrong.

A patient who contracts his or her abdominal muscles shows the sign called guarding. Guarding can be either a voluntary or involuntary act, and is typically encountered when the patient has peritoneal irritation. Such irritation may arise when an organ underlying the peritoneum becomes inflamed, or when a hollow organ ruptures and empties its contents into the peritoneal cavity. In trauma cases, however, solid-organ bleeding does not always result in peritoneal irritation and guarding. Large-volume bleeding with peritoneal distention will result in this phenomenon, for example. Marked peritoneal irritation and guarding is referred to as abdominal rigidity. This clinically important feature often results in urgent surgical evaluation and intervention. Guarding and rigidity are often encountered in trauma patients, but may also be seen in cases of appendicitis, cholecystitis, hollow-organ perforation, pancreatitis, and diverticulitis.

At the Scene

Pain upon release of pressure confirms rebound tenderness, which is a reliable sign of peritoneal inflammation such as with appendicitis.

Patients with less discrete guarded tenderness to palpation may have a more visceral problem. Although this may represent an early manifestation of a serious condition, it can also be associated with various degrees of bowel obstruction, renal colic, biliary colic, or urinary tract infection. Often the pain is less localized on palpation, and is deep-seated and poorly described by the patient. Cases of colic typically involve a problem with peristalsis, the wave-like contraction motion of a hollow tubular structure (eg, small and large intestine, common bile duct, or ureter). A stone may obstruct the tube, for example, or an adhesion or hernia may prevent proper intestinal peristalsis. Some patients will describe the pain as "wave-like," or waxing and waning in nature. Other lower abdominal sources of pain and tenderness include genitourinary processes.

Vascular sources can cause significant abdominal pain, most notably aortic aneurysm. Occasionally a markedly dilated aorta can be seen pulsating in the upper midline abdomen. Palpation will enable the provider to estimate its diameter. A ruptured aortic aneurysm also tends to be tender to palpation, and care should be taken to minimize manipulation of an aneurysm once it is suspected. The aorta is a retroperitoneal structure, however, so a lack of obvious findings while assessing the anterior abdomen does not rule out this diagnosis in an otherwise proper clinical setting. Other notable palpable abdominal wall masses include hernia, a localized weakening of the abdominal wall musculature. Sometimes hernias are congenital phenomena; oftentimes, they are acquired. They can result in strangulation of the underlying intestine.

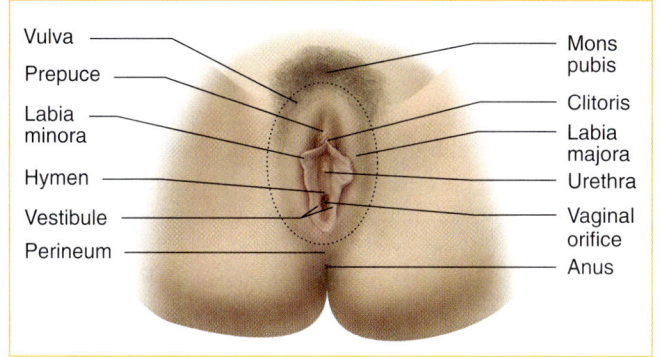

Figure 13-28 The female external genitalia.

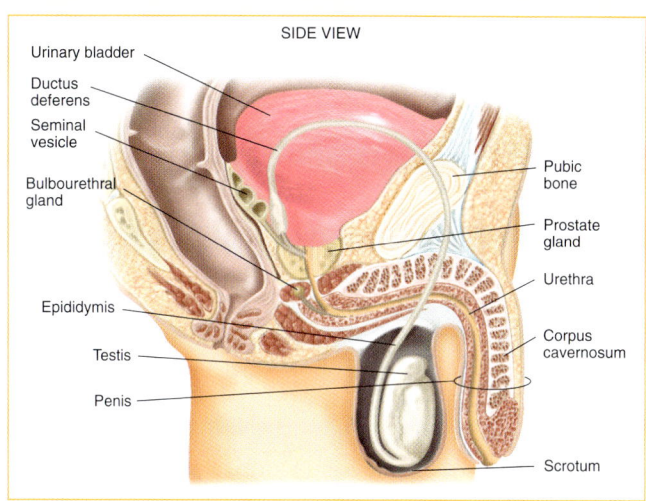

Figure 13-29 The male genitalia.

Female Genitalia

The female genitalia consist of the ovaries, fallopian tubes, uterus, vagina, and external genitalia **Figure 13-28 ▲** . The ovaries lie in the lowermost abdomen, in the inguinal regions, just superior to the inguinal creases. During a woman's reproductive years, the ovaries produce specialized hormones and ova. Hormonal regulation results in the maturation and release of an ovum roughly once a month as part of the menstrual cycle during that time.

After its release by the ovary, the ovum enters the fallopian tube and travels to the uterus. In the nonpregnant state, the uterus is a small structure, which is not palpable on external examination. This hollow, very muscular organ opens via the cervix into the vagina. Its inner lining thickens in response to hormonal stimulation, corresponding with the ripening and release of an ovum from the ovary.

The uterus receives sperm via the vagina and cervix. Pregnancy can result if sperm and ova successfully combine and become implanted in the lining of the uterine wall. If such fertilization does not occur, the uterine lining will slough and pass from the body with the menstrual flow.

In general, assessment of female genitalia is performed in a limited and discreet fashion. Always keep the patient appropriately draped during the course of the examination. Male paramedics should be assisted by a female. Reasons to examine the genitalia include concern over life-threatening hemorrhage or imminent delivery in childbirth.

While assessing the abdomen, palpate both the bilateral inguinal regions and the hypogastric region. If the decision is made to examine the genitalia specifically, limit the examination to inspection only. Pain and tenderness in the fallopian tubes and ovaries can be elicited during patient assessment. Clinically significant causes of this pain include ectopic pregnancy, complications of third-trimester pregnancy, and nonpregnant ovarian problems or pelvic infections. In the trauma patient where pelvic fracture is a concern, genital bleeding is a possibility, albeit an unlikely one. In the case of injury involving intentional trauma, significant bleeding is possible; if you must intervene in this kind of situation, be sure to preserve any garments and give them to the police as soon as possible. In general, make note of the amount and quality of any bleeding, as well as any inflammation, discharge, swelling, or lesions of the genitalia.

Male Genitalia

The male reproductive system consists of the testes, reproductive ducts, prostate, penis, and urethra **Figure 13-29 ▲** . The testes are analogous to the ovaries, in that they are the principal organs of reproduction and are responsible for manufacturing sperm. The testes, which lie outside the torso in a sac called the scrotum, produce hormones, seminal fluid (semen), and reproductive cells (sperm). The sperm and seminal fluid are transported from the testes to the lower abdomen, where they are stored in the seminal vesicles.

During sexual intercourse, semen is ejaculated through the urethra. During its passage through the urethra, the prostate gland adds fluids to the semen. The urethra passes through the penis, which is a highly vascular structure. Reflexive arteriolar dilation within the penis results in penile engorgement and subsequent erection.

When you are examining male genitalia, make certain that your partner is present and perform the examination in a limited and discreet fashion. In the prehospital setting, situations requiring assessment of the male genitalia are limited. Always assess the entire abdomen and note any pertinent findings, as occasionally lower abdominal problems are referred from the genitalia. Situations of testicular torsion or inguinal hernia sometimes present with a complaint of lower abdominal pain but minimal abdominal tenderness. In the case of a trauma patient, assess for the possibility of significant genital bleeding and injury, or underlying fracture. Note any inflammation, discharge, swelling, or lesions.

Anus

The anus—the distal orifice of the alimentary canal—is often evaluated at the same time as the genitalia. It is examined in only a limited number of circumstances, and is always done with the patient appropriately draped and your partner present. Examination usually occurs with the patient lying in a laterally recumbent position, and involves inspection only. Examine the sacrococcygeal and perineal areas, noting obvious bleeding, trauma, lumps, ulcers, inflammation, rash, and abrasions.

Musculoskeletal System

The extremities consist of both soft tissues and bones. Joints are areas where bone ends abut each other and form a kind of hinge, creating a jointed appendage. Joints are filled with shock-absorbing linings and fluid (synovium), and are held together by ligaments. They allow the body to perform mechanical work. Indeed, the mechanical process of motion becomes possible when the joints are flexed and extended by skeletal (or striated) muscles that traverse the joints. Skeletal muscles are anchored to bone via tendons, with each muscle being named according to its location and function.

The principal joints of the upper extremities include the shoulder (acromioclavicular and glenohumeral joints), elbow (olecranon), and wrist (radiocarpal). The principal joints of the lower extremities include the hip (acetabulum), knee (patellar), and ankle (tibiotalar).

As joints age, they become more vulnerable to repetitive motion stress and trauma, and they lose much of their articular abilities due to inflammation and breakdown of the synovium. Disruption of the bones, joints, and soft tissues can take a variety of forms, and discomfort or disability may be a manifestation of an acute problem, a chronic problem, or a combination of the two.

Common types of musculoskeletal and soft-tissue injuries include fractures, sprains, strains, dislocations, contusions, hematomas, and open wounds. Fractures may be characterized in a number of ways. For example, an open fracture is essentially a fracture with direct communication to the exterior surface of the body, or simply an open wound in close proximity to the site of a presumed fracture.

Although fractures always involve a pathologic process, it is important to distinguish a pathologic fracture from a physiologic fracture. A physiologic fracture occurs when abnormal forces are applied to normal bone structures, producing a fracture. A pathologic fracture occurs when normal forces are applied to abnormal bone structures, producing a fracture. Physiologic fractures occur in the setting of high-force injury. Pathologic fractures often occur in settings of decreased bone density, such as osteopenia or occult malignancy.

When you are examining the skeleton and joints, pay attention to both their structure and their function. Consider

how the joint and associated extremity look and how well they work. Does the extremity look normal, and does it move easily? In particular, note any limitation in range of motion, pain with range of motion, or bony crepitance. When assessing the joints and extremities, look for evidence of inflammation or injury, such as swelling, tenderness, increased heat, redness, ecchymosis, or decreased function. Also evaluate the joint or extremity for obvious deformity, diminished strength, atrophy, or asymmetry from one side to the other. The examination of the musculoskeletal system should not cause the patient any pain; if any occurs, it should be considered an abnormal finding. Follow the steps in **Skill Drill 13-10** :

1. Beginning with upper extremities, inspect the skin overlying the muscles, bones, and joints for soft-tissue damage (**Step 1**).
2. Note any deformities or abnormal structure.
3. Check for adequate distal pulse, motor, and sensation to each extremity (**Step 2**).
4. Inspect and palpate the hands and the wrists, noting any DCAP-BTLS.
5. Ask the patient to flex and extend the joints of the fingers, hands, and wrist, noting any abnormalities in the range of motion. If the patient experiences any discomfort, stop that portion of the examination immediately (**Step 3**).
6. Inspect and palpate the elbows, noting any abnormalities. Ask the patient to flex and extend the elbow to determine the range of motion.
7. Ask the patient to turn the hand from the palm-down position to the palm-up position and back again, noting any pain or abnormalities (**Step 4**).
8. Inspect and palpate the shoulders. Ask the patient to shrug the shoulders and raise and extend both arms (**Step 5**).
9. Inspect the skin overlying the lower extremities.
10. Beginning with the feet, inspect and palpate the bony structures, noting any abnormalities (**Step 6**).
11. Ask the patient to point and bend the toes to establish the range of motion (**Step 7**).
12. Ask the patient to rotate the ankle, checking for pain or restricted range of motion (**Step 8**).
13. Inspect and palpate the knee joints and patella. Ask the patient to bend and straighten both to establish the range of motion (**Step 9**).
14. Check for structural integrity of the pelvis by applying gentle pressure to the iliac crests and pushing in and then down (**Step 10**).
15. Ask the patient to lift both legs by bending at the hip and then turning the legs inward and outward. Note any abnormalities (**Step 11**).

Often the diagnosis of a problem involving the shoulders and related structures can be made simply by noting the patient's posture at the time of first contact with paramedics **Figure 13-30** . For example, a glenohumeral joint dislocation may be manifested as the loss of normal contour of the shoulder, with abnormal squaring of the lateral aspect of the

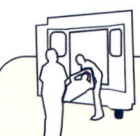

At the Scene

Point tenderness is the most reliable indicator of an underlying closed fracture.

Skill Drill 13-10: Examining the Musculoskeletal System

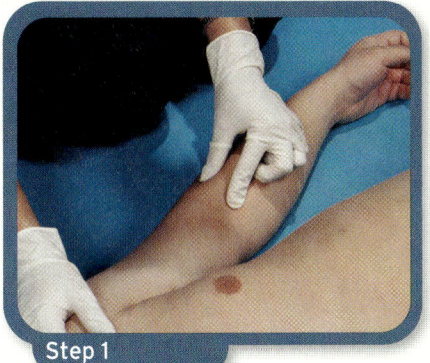

Step 1

Inspect the skin overlying the muscles, bones, and joints for soft-tissue damage.

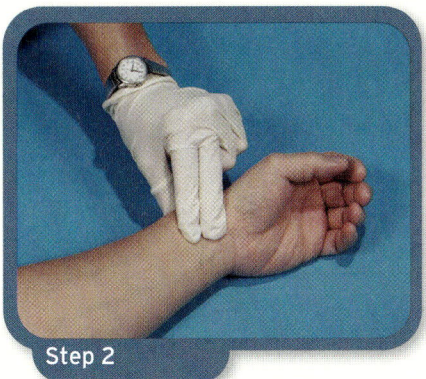

Step 2

Check for adequate distal pulse, motor, and sensation to each extremity.

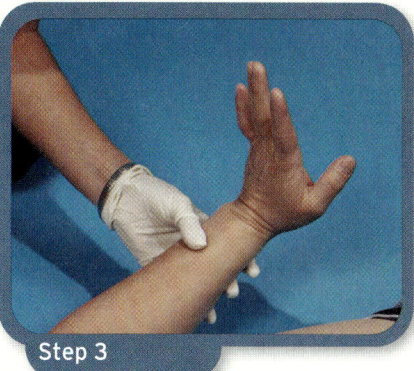

Step 3

Ask the patient to flex and extend the joints of the fingers, hands, and wrist to establish range of motion.

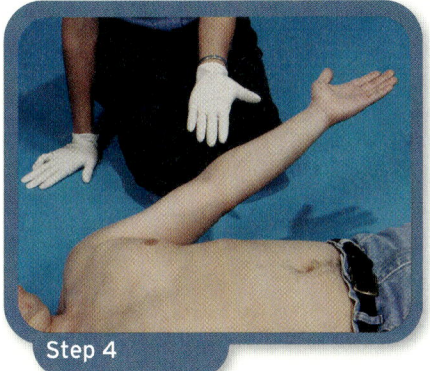

Step 4

Ask the patient to turn the hand from the palm-down position to the palm-up position and back again.

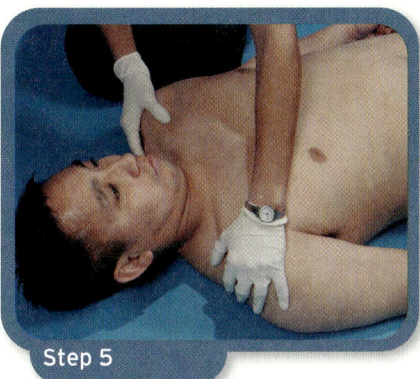

Step 5

Inspect and palpate the shoulders.

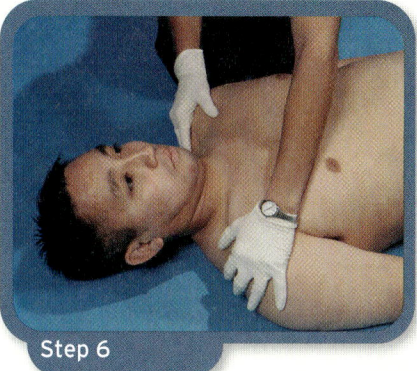

Step 6

Inspect and palpate the bony structures.

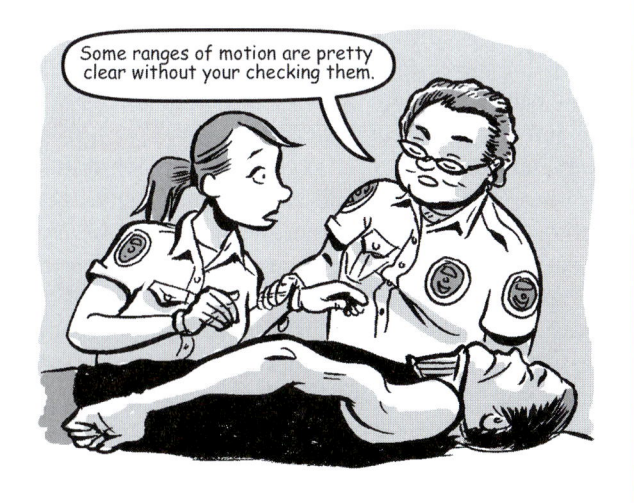

Some ranges of motion are pretty clear without your checking them.

Figure 13-30

shoulder and the humeral head visible and/or palpable in the soft tissues of the chest wall, in the subacromial region Figure 13-31 ▶.

When you are palpating the proximal upper extremity and shoulder, be sure to assess the sternoclavicular joint, acromioclavicular joint, subacromial area, and bicipital groove (origin of the biceps, just distal to the anterior aspect of the humeral head). Note any tenderness, swelling, crepitance, deformity, rotation, or ecchymosis in these areas.

When possible, check the patient's range of motion by asking the patient to raise the arms to the vertical position, above the head. Next, have the patient demonstrate external rotation and abduction by placing both hands behind the neck with the

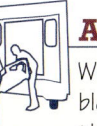

At the Scene

When you are assessing a patient with a possible shoulder dislocation, position yourself behind the patient and compare the shoulders. The dislocated side is usually lower than the uninjured side.

Skill Drill 13-10: Examining the Musculoskeletal System (*continued*)

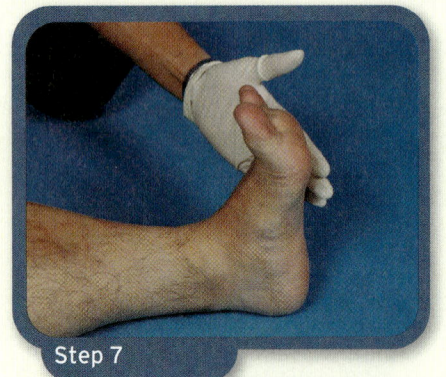

Step 7

Ask the patient to point and bend the toes to establish range of motion.

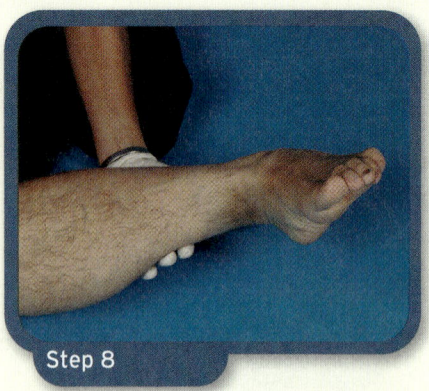

Step 8

Ask the patient to rotate the ankle, checking for pain or restricted range of motion.

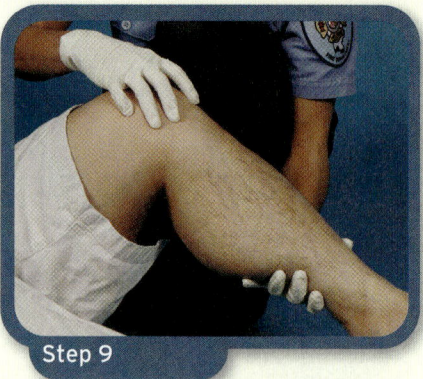

Step 9

Inspect and palpate the knee joints and patella. Ask the patient to bend and straighten both to establish range of motion.

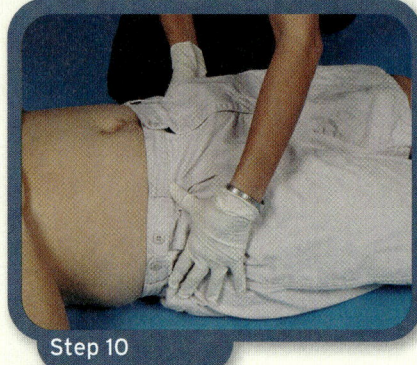

Step 10

Check for structural integrity of the pelvis by applying gentle pressure to the iliac crests and pushing in and then down.

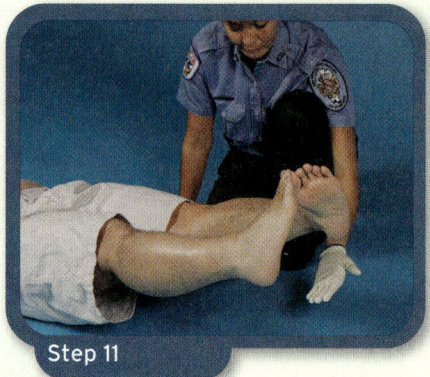

Step 11

Ask the patient to lift both legs, bending at the hip and then turning the legs inward and outward.

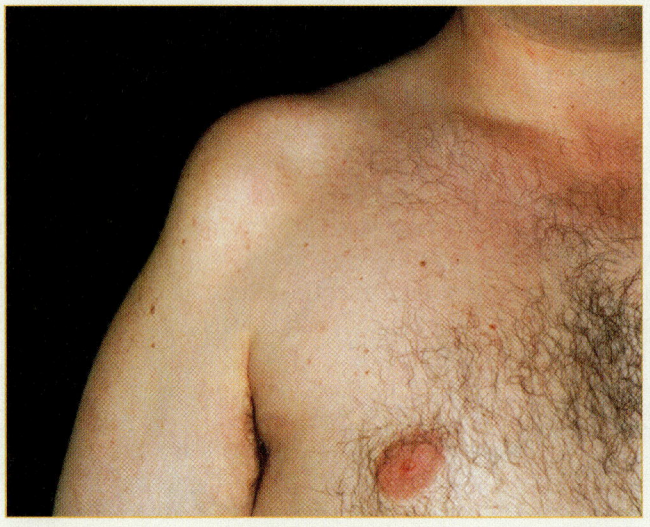

Figure 13-31 Abnormal squaring of the shoulder.

elbows out to the sides. Finally, perform internal rotation by having the patient place both hands behind the low back.

Evaluation of the elbows should start with an overall inspection for gross deformity or abnormal rotation. Palpate the elbow between the epicondyles and olecranon, and palpate the epicondyles and olecranon themselves **Figure 13-32 ▶**. Note any tenderness, crepitance, swelling, or thickening. Range-of-motion testing should be performed last, as suspicion of significant pathology or fracture of the elbow mandates appropriate immobilization as soon as possible. When ranging the elbows, flex and extend them both passively and actively. Then have the patient supinate and pronate the forearms while the elbows are flexed at the patient's sides.

When you are checking the hands and wrists, inspect them for any abnormalities, including swelling, redness, contusions, wounds, nodules, deformities, or atrophy. Palpate the hands, feeling the medial and lateral aspects of each interphalangeal joint on each finger **Figure 13-33 ▶**. Squeeze the hands, compressing the metacarpophalangeal joints. Palpate the carpal bones of the wrists, noting any areas of swelling,

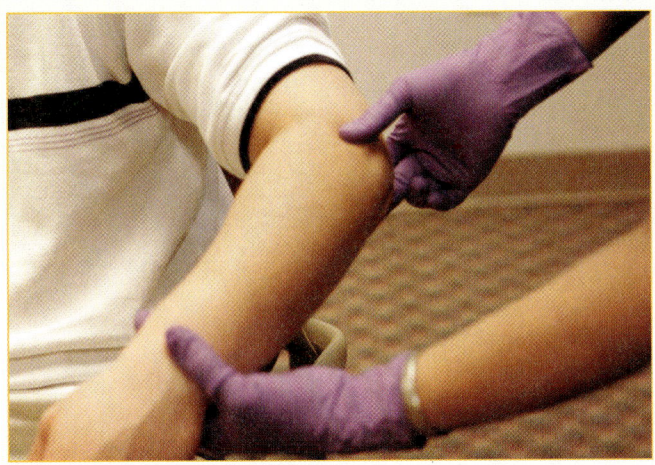

Figure 13-32 Palpate the elbow.

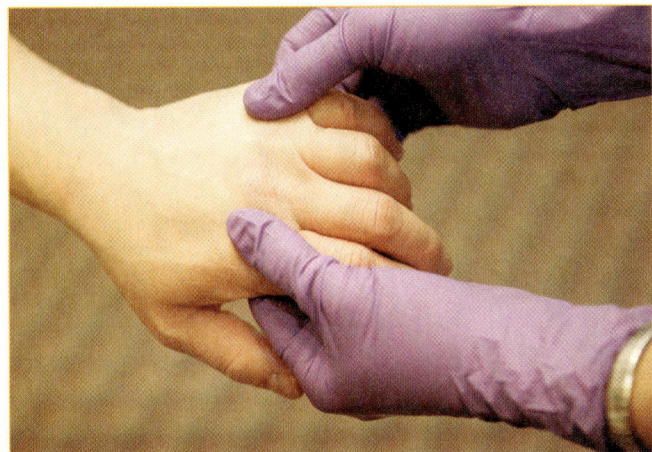

Figure 13-33 Palpate the fingers.

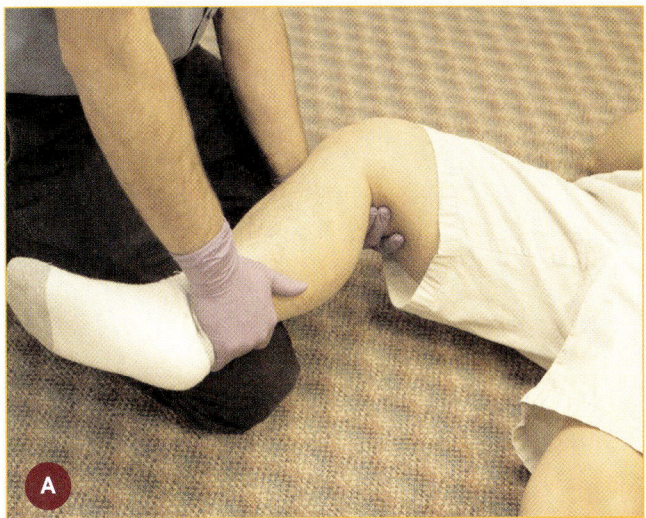

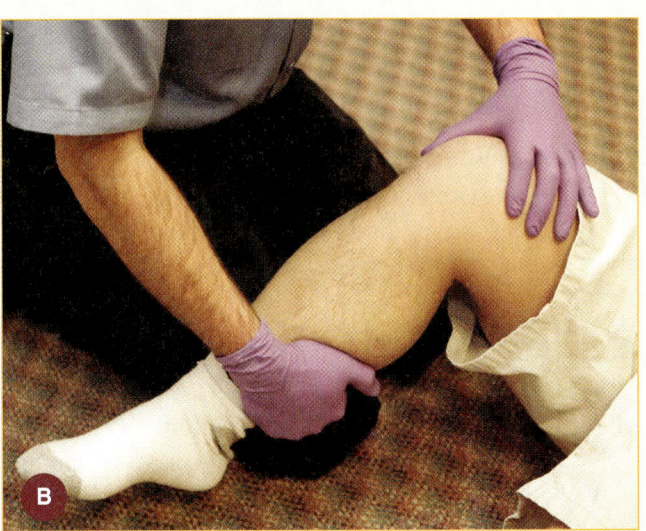

Figure 13-34 Examination of the lower extremities. **A.** Hip. **B.** Knee.

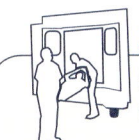

At the Scene

Heberden's and Bouchard's nodules are hard and nontender, and occur with osteoarthritis.

tenderness, or bogginess. Perform range-of-motion evaluations by asking the patient to make fists with both hands, then extend and spread the fingers, then flex and extend the wrists, and finally move the hands laterally and medially with the palms facing down. Check capillary refill, symmetry of radial pulses, and overall limb temperature at this point.

A rapid appreciation of injury or disability involving the lower extremities can be made by evaluating the patient's ability to walk. Of course, this may not be a practical first approach to assessment in many prehospital cases.

Examination of the knees and hips begins with inspection of overall alignment and deformity of the lower extremities Figure 13-34 ▶. Identify any lower extremity shortening and/or rotation, either internal or external; these findings are often evident with an injury to the proximal aspects of the lower extremity. Look for evidence of thickening, swelling, or bruising of the thigh. Note any crepitance or palpable tenderness. If possible, range the knees and hips in an effort to determine the presence of underlying injury to those structures. Ask the patient to bend each knee and raise the bent knee toward the chest. Assess for rotation and abduction of the hips, both passively and actively. Palpate each hip individually—specifically, distal to the inguinal crease and over the anterior, lateral, and posterior aspects. Finally, palpate and compress the pelvis.

When you are examining the ankles and feet, observe all surfaces. Note any wounds, deformities, discolourations, nodules, or swelling. Palpate all aspects of the feet and ankles, noting tenderness, bogginess, swelling, or crepitance. Measure distal pulses over the dorsalis pedis and posterior tibialis, and assess capillary refill and overall limb temperature at this point. Assess range of motion by having the patient plantar flex, dorsiflex, and invert and evert the ankles and feet. Be sure to

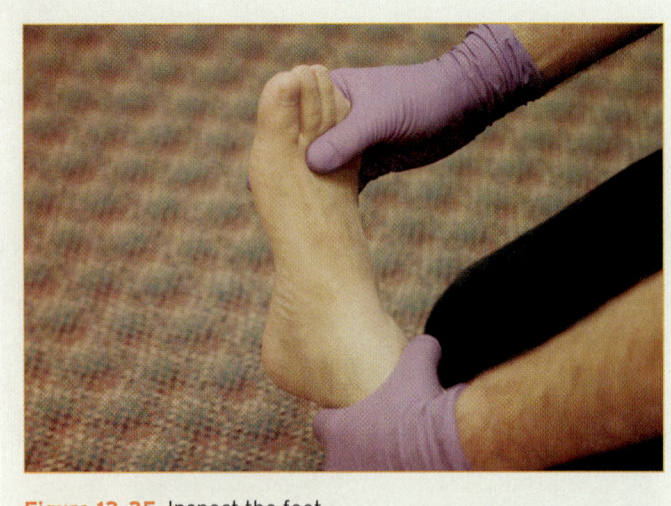

Figure 13-35 Inspect the feet.

check the forefoot and toes by inspection, palpation, and range-of-motion testing (Figure 13-35 ▲).

Peripheral Vascular System

The peripheral vascular system comprises all aspects of the circulatory system, except for the heart, the great vessels immediately involved with the mediastinum, and the coronary circulation. Thus it includes all of the body's arteries, veins, arterioles, venules, capillaries, lymphatics, and the respective fluids that fill these structures.

The lymphatic system is an intricate network of nodes and ducts of various sizes that are dispersed throughout the body (Figure 13-36 ▶). Lymph nodes are larger accumulations of lymphatic tissue, and smaller amounts of lymph are distributed by tissue throughout the body. All lymphatic tissue contains large numbers of immunologically active cells; thus the lymphatics manage a key function in the body's immune system. The ducts contain a fat-rich fluid known as lymph, which transports materials from the lymph tissue into the central venous circulation via the thoracic ducts.

Perfusion occurs in the peripheral circulation via the network of capillary beds. Blood cells and plasma in close proximity to tissue offload substances required by the cells for proper metabolic functioning, and simultaneously pick up metabolic wastes for transport out of the tissues, ultimately for elimination from the body. Impaired functioning of the peripheral vascular system means that the capillary beds can't provide for adequate tissue and organ perfusion—this is a significant source of morbidity and mortality. Diseases of the peripheral vascular system are often seen in patients with other underlying medical conditions, such as diabetes, hypertension, dyslipidemia, obesity, and tobacco use. These disease processes typically target and cause malfunctioning of the smaller-diameter vessels of the peripheral vascular system, resulting in disease states of the tissues and organs that depend on those vessels for proper functioning. With age and the occurrence of these various disease processes, the vasculature becomes less able to rapidly manage changes in perfusion requirements, so it can itself become a source of illness.

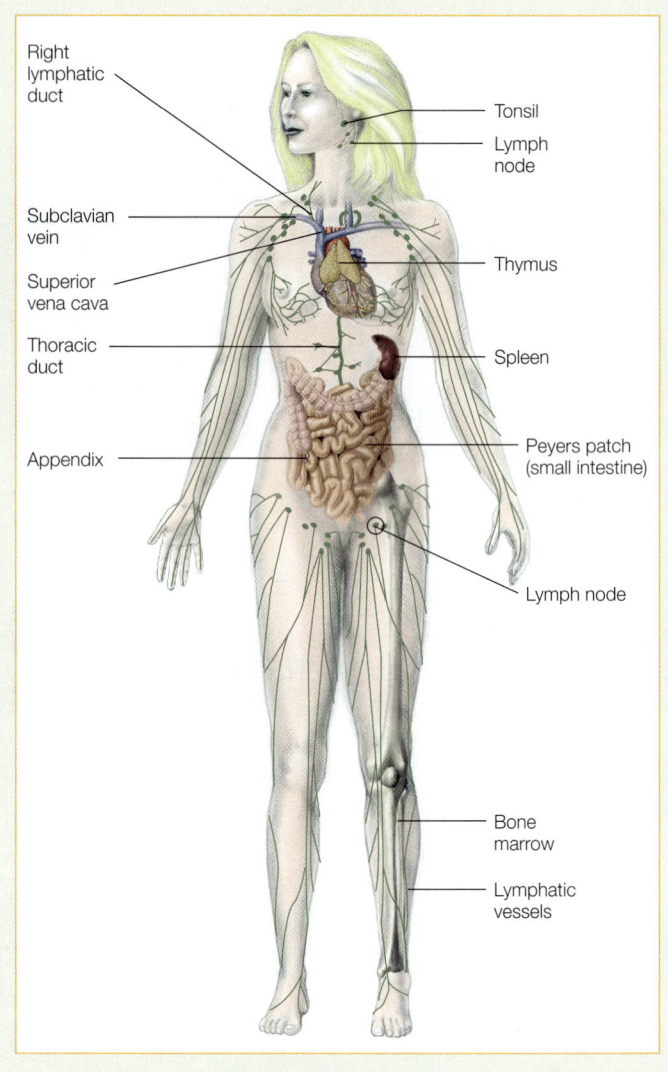

Figure 13-36 Lymphatic system.

When you are assessing the peripheral vascular system, pay attention to both the upper and lower extremities. Look for signs indicative of either acute or chronic vascular problems. A wide range of disorders can affect the peripheral vascular system—from chronic venous stasis and lymphedema to intermittent claudication (cramp-like pain in the lower legs due to poor circulation) and acute arterial occlusion. Peripheral vascular disease can manifest in many forms, depending on the point in the vasculature where the abnormality is located. Carotid artery disease can manifest as a stroke, for example, while arterial embolization involving the mesenteric vessels can result in bowel ischemia and necrosis. In the extremities, involvement of the peripheral vasculature can result in limb ischemia. Follow the steps in Skill Drill 13-11 ▶ :

1. While examining the upper extremities, note any abnormalities in the radial pulse, skin colour, or condition   Step 1 .
2. If abnormalities are noted in the distal pulse, work your way proximally, checking these pulse points and noting your findings   Step 2 .

3. Palpate the epitrochlear and brachial nodes of the lymphatic system, noting any swelling or tenderness (Step 3).

4. Examine the lower extremities, noting any abnormalities in the size and symmetry of the legs (Step 4).

5. Inspect the skin colour and condition, noting any abnormal venous patterns or enlargement (Step 5).

6. Check distal pulses, noting any abnormalities (Step 6).

7. Palpate the inguinal nodes for swelling or tenderness (Step 7).

8. Evaluate the temperature of each leg relative to the rest of the body and to each other.

9. Evaluate for pitting edema in the legs and feet (Step 8).

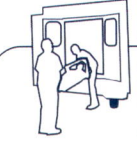

At the Scene

Pitting edema 4-point scale:
+1 = 0–7.5 mm
+2 = 7.5 mm–15 mm
+3 = 15 mm–30 mm
+4 = >30 mm

When you are checking the upper extremities, inspect them from fingertips to shoulders. Note the extremity's relative size, and evaluate it for symmetry by comparing one side to the other. Pay attention to any obvious swelling, unusual venous patterns, the colour and texture of the skin, and the colour of the nail beds. Palpate the radial pulses, and compare each side to the other. In situations of unilaterally absent pulses, check proximally over the brachial pulse sites. When you are evaluating a limb for ischemia, consider the five Ps of acute arterial insufficiency: Pain, Pallor, Parasthesias/Paresis, Poikilothermia (inability to maintain a constant core body temperature independent of ambient temperature), and Pulselessness. The loss of a palpable pulse is probably the worst indicator of such a problem, as it's considered a late finding. If indicated, palpate the epitrochlear and axillary lymph nodes, noting their size, tenderness, overlying redness, and mobility.

Proper evaluation of the vascular status of the lower extremities requires the patient to be lying down and draped appropriately. Remove the patient's socks, stockings, and shoes before proceeding with the examination. Inspect the lower extremities from the groin and buttocks to the feet. Always examine the lower extremities by comparing the right side to the left. Look at the size and symmetry of the legs, noting any localized versus generalized swelling. Pay attention to any remarkable superficial venous patterns or venous enlargement. Observe the skin pigmentation, as well as the skin colour and texture. Rubor, ecchymosis, or pallor may all be encountered in patients who are suffering from significant vascular insufficiency. Also note the presence of any rashes, scars, and ulcers, and determine whether they are shallow or deep.

Palpate pulses in the lower extremities to assess the arterial circulation. In particular, palpate pulses over the dorsalis pedis, the posterior tibialis, and the femoral regions. The popliteal pulse can also occasionally be appreciated. Note the temperature

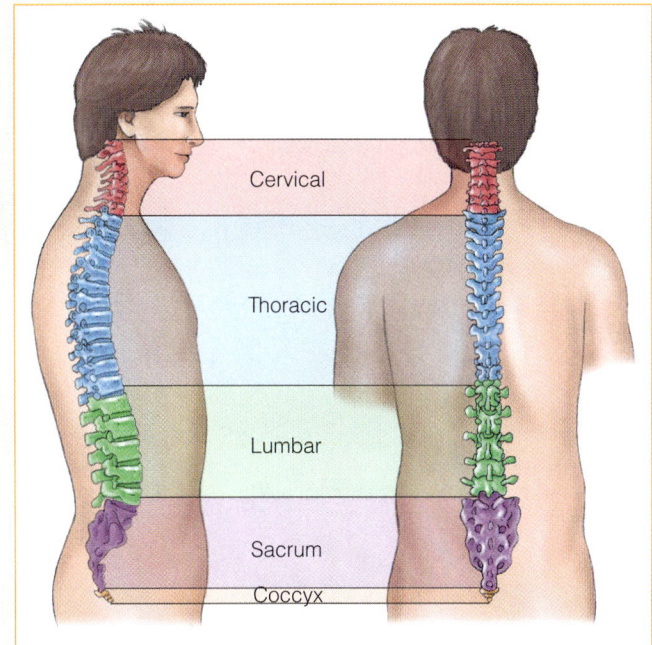

Figure 13-37 The five sections of the spinal column.

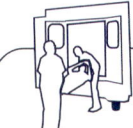

At the Scene

Bilateral, dependent, pitting edema occurs with systemic conditions such as heart failure and hepatic cirrhosis. Unilateral edema occurs with local conditions such as occlusion of a deep vein.

of the feet and legs, and attempt to palpate edema in the legs. To do so, press your thumb over the dorsum of the foot and anteriorly over the tibias, holding the thumb with firm, gentle pressure for at least 5 seconds. If indicated, palpate the superficial inguinal lymph nodes, noting their size, tenderness, any overlying redness, and mobility.

Spine

The spine represents the core of the axillary skeleton. It consists of 33 individual vertebrae, the lower nine of which are fused (Figure 13-37 ▲). The vertebrae are irregularly shaped bones that articulate with each other in a complex fashion. The spine provides anchoring points for the skull, shoulders, ribs, and pelvis. It also protects the spinal cord and provides the passageway through which spinal nerves travel to and from the peripheral nervous system.

When you are assessing the spine, begin by inspecting the back from both the posterior and lateral aspects. The spine features several curves, representing the cervical, thoracic, and lumbar regions. Lordosis refers to the inward curve of the lumbar spine just above the buttocks. An exaggerated form of lordosis results in swayback. Kyphosis refers to the outward curve of the thoracic spine. It is frequently exaggerated in elderly persons due to degenerative joint disease, osteoporosis, and vertebral

Skill Drill 13-11: Examining the Peripheral Vascular System

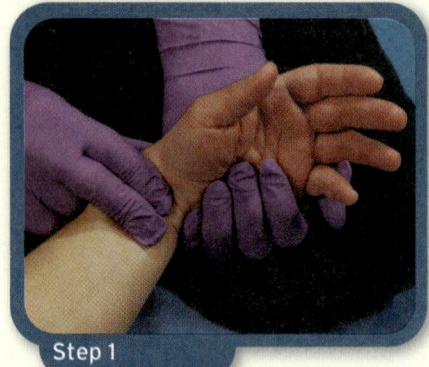

Step 1

Note any abnormalities in the radial pulse, skin colour, or condition.

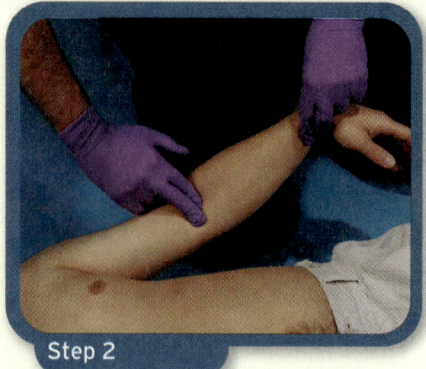

Step 2

If abnormalities are noted in the distal pulse, work your way proximally, checking these pulse points and noting your findings.

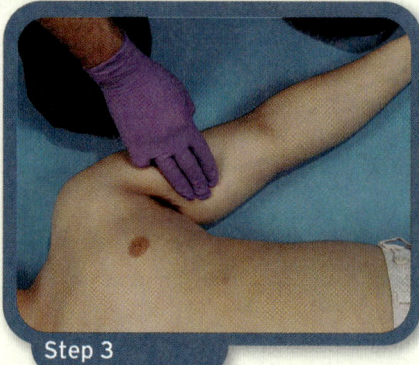

Step 3

Palpate the epitrochlear and brachial nodes of the lymphatic system, noting any swelling or tenderness.

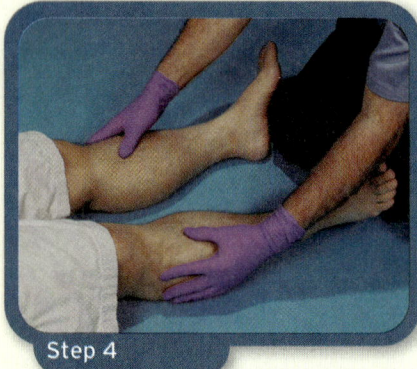

Step 4

Examine the lower extremities, noting any abnormalities in the size and symmetry of the legs.

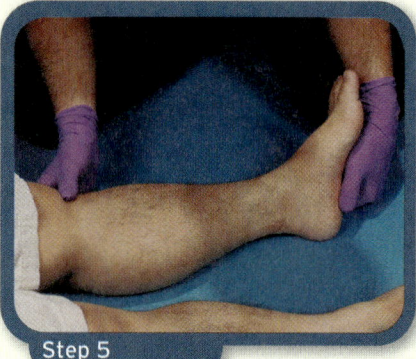

Step 5

Inspect the skin colour and condition, noting any abnormal venous patterns or enlargement.

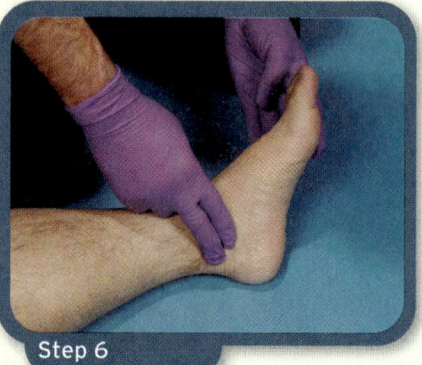

Step 6

Check distal pulses.

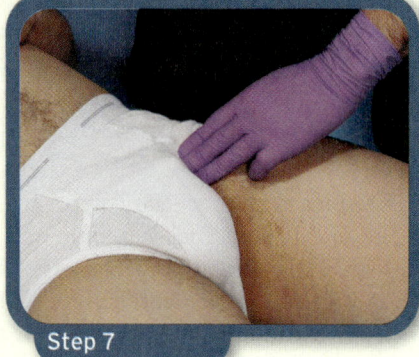

Step 7

Palpate the inguinal nodes for swelling or tenderness.

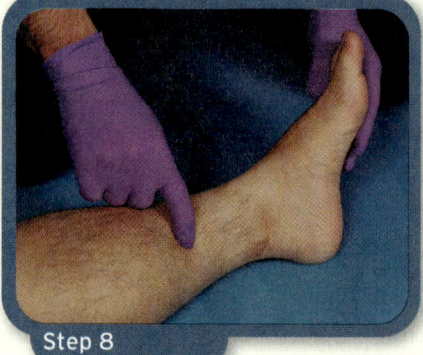

Step 8

Evaluate for pitting edema in the legs and feet.

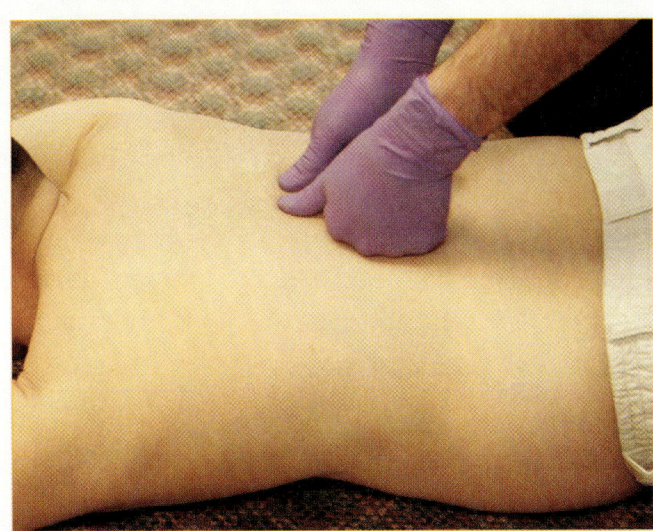

Figure 13-38 When you are palpating the spine, use the thumb to touch each spinous process.

compression fractures. At its worst, kyphosis can become a source of restrictive lung disease, a form of COPD. Scoliosis is a sideways curvature of the spine, and is always abnormal. When you are examining the spine, look for differences in the height of the shoulders as well as differences in the heights of the iliac crests of the pelvis. Be sure to take a moment and look at the entire back at this point, noting any wounds or ecchymosis.

Palpation of the spine is typically done while the patient is supine, often when he or she has been log rolled onto one side to facilitate access to the back and placement of a spinal immobilization device. When you are palpating the spine, use the thumb to touch each spinous process **Figure 13-38 ▲**. This allows you to identify any tenderness, step-off, or crepitance. Identification of an abnormality should prompt you to institute proper splinting and protective measures.

While you are examining the spine, it's also appropriate to check the rest of the back for any other significant findings on palpation. Tap over the costovertebral angles, and palpate the scapulae, paraspinal areas, and base of the neck. Also check the buttocks.

Finally, perform a range-of-motion evaluation. Although this evaluation may be of limited utility in the prehospital setting, in areas that practice selective spinal immobilization, it may prove quite helpful. Range of motion should always be checked passively first, with the paramedic controlling the range. It's then done actively, with the patient controlling the range. If at any time during ranging you elicit pain in the spine or tingling in the extremities, stop that phase of assessment immediately and immobilize the spine. Ranging the cervical spine should require rather limited movements. In contrast, ranging the remainder of the spine may include somewhat exaggerated motions, including flexion and extension, with the patient front- and back-bending. Lateral bending can also be appreciated, as can leftward and rightward rotation. Pay attention to the smoothness and symmetry of the patient's movements,

along with the actual degree of motion elicited. Follow the steps in **Skill Drill 13-12 ▶**:

1. Inspect the cervical, thoracic, and lumbar curves for any abnormalities **Step 1**.
2. Evaluate the heights of the shoulders and the iliac crests **Step 2**. Differences from one side to the other may indicate abnormal curvature of the spine.
3. Palpate the posterior portion of the cervical spine, noting any point tenderness or structural abnormalities **Step 3**.
4. In the nontrauma patient, and in the absence of reported pain, ask the patient to move the head forward, backward, and from side to side **Step 4**.
5. Move down the spine, palpating each vertebra with the thumbs to note any tenderness or instability **Step 5**.
6. In the absence of pain or trauma, ask the patient to bend at the waist in each direction to establish the range of motion **Step 6**.

Nervous System
Structure and Function of the Nervous System

The nervous system is the body's master control system. It constantly receives information about the body's internal and external environments, and it continuously readjusts the body's systems in response to changes in those environments. The nervous system includes two portions: the central nervous system (CNS), which consists of the brain and spinal cord, and the peripheral nervous system (PNS), which includes the remaining motor and sensory nerves.

The brain is an extraordinarily complex structure, with an enormous perfusion requirement. It is constantly active at both conscious and unconscious levels. The brain comprises the cerebrum, cerebellum, and medulla (brain stem). The cerebrum takes charge of all of the brain's conscious processes; it's divided into four discrete lobes (frontal, temporal, parietal, and occipital). The cerebellum is responsible for coordinating balance. The brain stem handles all of the unconscious deeper processes.

With the exception of the cranial nerves, all nerves are ultimately channeled to the brain via the spinal cord. The spinal cord plays the role of a large conduit, passing information back and forth along itself. The peripheral nerves that emanate from the spinal cord, which are known as spinal nerves, have both motor and sensory pathways. Motor nerves control some aspect of motion or movement, whereas sensory nerves receive external signals and send them to the brain for processing and motor response. Motor tracts run from the spinal cord to the body outwardly; sensory nerves run from the body to the cord inwardly.

Skill Drill 13-12: Examining the Spine

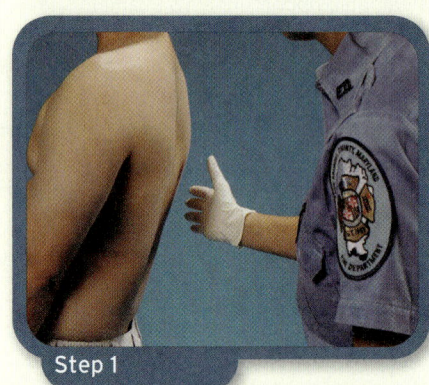

Step 1

Inspect the cervical, thoracic, and lumbar curves for any abnormalities.

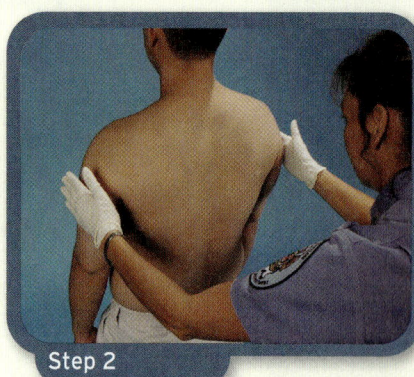

Step 2

Evaluate the heights of the shoulders and the iliac crests.

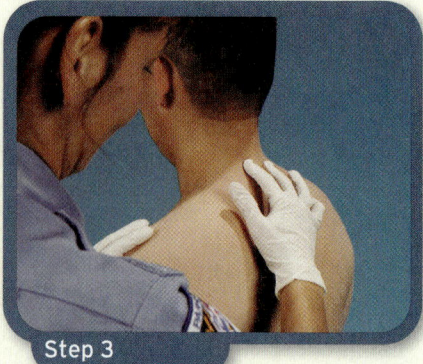

Step 3

Palpate the posterior portion of the cervical spine, noting any point tenderness or structural abnormalities.

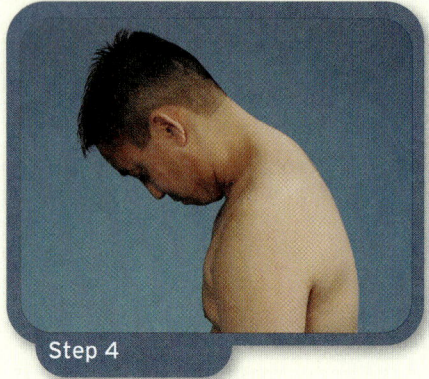

Step 4

In the nontrauma patient, and in the absence of reported pain, ask the patient to move the head forward, backward, and from side to side.

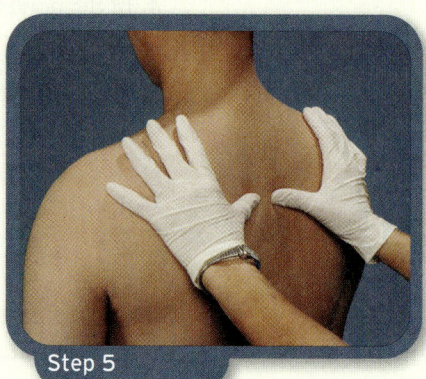

Step 5

Palpate each vertebra with the thumbs.

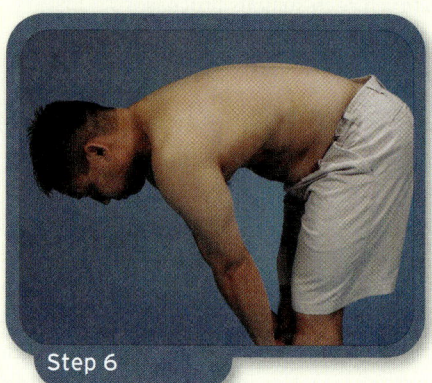

Step 6

In the absence of pain or trauma, ask the patient to bend at the waist in each direction to establish the range of motion.

Cranial nerves are not mediated by the spinal cord but rather go directly to and from the brain, originating at the medulla. They innervate the face, head, and parts of the neck, with the exception of the vagus nerve, which runs down the neck and into the chest and abdomen. There are 12 cranial nerves in total. They play roles in a wide variety of motor and sensory functions **Table 13-2 ▶** that involve both the voluntary and autonomic nervous systems (discussed later in this section).

The peripheral nerves are covered with a sheet-like material called myelin. Myelin promotes rapid transmission of impulses along the nerve. In the newborn, several of the major motor pathways (or long tracts) are not fully myelinated. Over time, however, myelin is completely deposited and the motor pathways become fully functional. Conversely, with advancing age and the occurrence of various disease states, neurologic functions can deteriorate. This failure may take the form of a cognitive problem (eg, dementia), or it may lead to a physical

disability (eg, the problems seen with parkinsonism and cerebrovascular disease).

In addition to the central/peripheral distinctions, the nervous system may be divided into involuntary (autonomic) and voluntary portions, with the autonomic nervous system being further subdivided into the sympathetic and parasympathetic systems. Reflexes are involuntary motor responses to specific sensory stimuli, such as a tap on the knee or stroking the eyelash. The location of what is stimulated determines which muscle will contract to produce a reflexive response. Spinal reflexes occur when sensory input comes from receptors in the muscles, joints, and skin. The motor response to this stimulation occurs entirely within the spinal cord; no brain processing is required. Other reflexes include the deep tendon reflexes and the superficial and brain stem reflexes. Primitive reflexes—including the Babinski, grasping, and sucking signs—are normal findings in infants. In older people, once the long motor pathways of the PNS have become fully myelinated, the primitive reflexes

Table 13-2 Cranial Nerves

Number	Name	Motor vs Sensory	Functions
I	Olfactory	Sensory	Smell
II	Optic	Sensory	Light perception and vision
III	Oculomotor	Motor	Pupil constriction, eye movements
IV	Trochlear	Motor	Eye movements
V	Trigeminal	Motor and sensory	Motor: chewing Sensory: face, sinuses, teeth
VI	Abducens	Motor	Eye movements
VII	Facial	Motor	Facial movements
VIII	Vestibulocochlear	Sensory	Hearing, balance perception
IX	Glossopharyngeal	Motor and sensory	Motor: throat and swallowing, gland secretion Sensory: tongue, throat, ear
X	Vagus	Motor and sensory	Heart, lungs, palate, pharynx, larynx, trachea, bronchi, GI tract, external ear
XI	Spinal accessory	Motor	Shoulder and neck movements
XII	Hypoglossal	Motor	Tongue, throat, and neck movements

At the Scene

A Babinski test may be used to check for neurologic function in an unresponsive patient. This is accomplished by stimulating the sole of the foot by rubbing with your thumb or running a pen or other pointed object along the sole of the foot. Babinski reflex occurs when the great toe flexes and the other toes fan out. The presence of this reflex in adults indicates a neurologic injury. Do NOT perform a Babinski test on a patient who has injuries to the lower extremities. This could cause the patient to pull the leg back, causing pain.

represent abnormal findings, typical of injury or disconnection between the cerebral cortex and the brain stem.

The Neurologic Examination

When you are performing a neurologic examination, you need to focus on several key concepts (Skill Drill 13-12). At a bare minimum, the neurologic examination should determine the patient's baseline mental status (AVPU), cranial nerve function (pupils, eyes, smile, speech, swallow, shoulder shrug), distal motor function (ability to move), and distal sensory function (ability to feel). It may also test the deep tendon reflexes if necessary.

First, assess the patient's overall mental status. Is the patient awake? If so, is the patient alert, and to what degree? If a change in level of consciousness has occurred, what kind of stimulus does it take to get a response, and to what degree does the patient's mental status improve? In the case of an altered mental status, do you observe any unusual postures? Is there any alteration in physical status (eg, is the ability to move successfully and symmetrically preserved)?

The Glasgow Coma Scale was designed as a tool to assist in better assessing subjects with significant alterations in mental status; it was originally intended for use in the trauma setting. It simultaneously scores several parameters, including eye opening, verbal acuity, and motor activity, and attempts to provide a numerical score as a rapid means of defining severity of brain dysfunction and potential prognosis. Follow the steps in **Skill Drill 13-13**:

1. Assess the patient's mental status by using the AVPU mnemonic.
2. Note the patient's posture.
3. Evaluate cranial nerve function **Step 1**.
4. Evaluate the patient's neuromuscular status by checking muscle strength against resistance **Step 2**. Use the grading system described below to grade all extremities.
5. Evaluate the patient's coordination by performing the finger-to-nose test using alternating hands **Step 3**.
6. If appropriate, test the patient's gait and balance by having the patient walk heel-to-toe or perform the heel-to-shin stance **Step 4**.
7. Perform the pronator drift test by asking the patient to close his or her eyes and hold both arms out in front of the body **Step 5**. There should be no difference in movement on either side.
8. Evaluate the patient's sensory function by checking his or her responses to both gross and light touch.
9. If appropriate, check for deep tendon reflexes.

Notes from Nancy
Restlessness is a danger signal!

After assessment of the patient's overall mental status, you should begin the comprehensive neurologic examination. Of course, such an examination is not needed in every case. Its details may vary greatly, depending on the nature of the patient's problem. Also, many portions of the neurologic examination may have been completed earlier, during other aspects of the patient assessment. Keep track of these initial findings so that you can report them, they are not needlessly repeated, and any subsequent changes in status can be noted. Are left- and right-sided motor and sensory findings symmetrical? If not, how do they differ? Does the presenting problem appear to be more of a CNS or a PNS malfunction?

When testing the cranial nerves, a number of simple maneuvers can be employed to determine the presence and degree of disability **Table 13-3**. With practice, the entire cranial nerve examination can be performed in less than 3 minutes.

Adequate evaluation of the motor system involves assessment of several distinct areas. Although motor activity may

Skill Drill 13-13: Examining the Nervous System

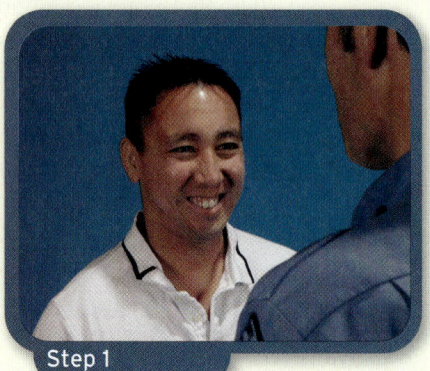

Step 1

Evaluate cranial nerve function.

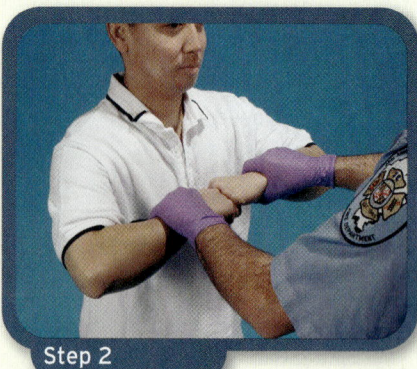

Step 2

Evaluate the patient's neuromuscular status by checking muscle strength against resistance.

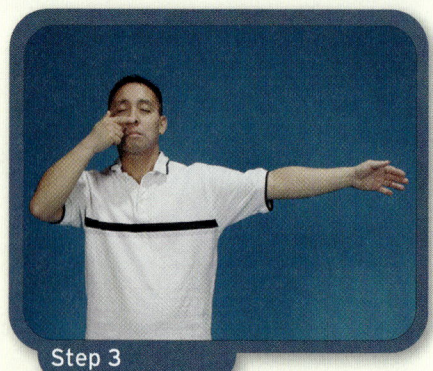

Step 3

Evaluate the patient's coordination by performing the finger-to-nose test using alternating hands.

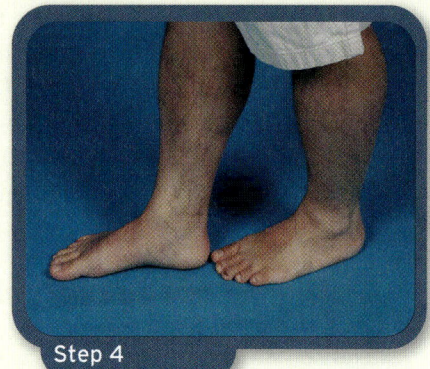

Step 4

If appropriate, test the patient's gait and balance by having the patient walk heel-to-toe or perform the heel-to-shin stance.

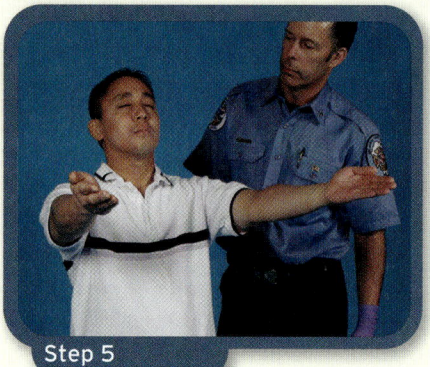

Step 5

Perform the pronator drift test by asking the patient to close his or her eyes and hold both arms out in front of the body.

Table 13-3	Tests for Disability in Cranial Nerves
Cranial Nerve	**Test**
I	Check smell
II	Check visual acuity
III	Check pupil size, shape, symmetry, response to light, eye movements
IV	Check eye movements
V	Check jaw clench; touch both sides of face at forehead, cheeks, and jaw
VI	Check eye movements
VII	Check facial symmetry; look for abnormal movements; raise eyebrows, grin broadly, frown, shut eyes tightly, puff out cheeks; note any asymmetry
VIII	Check hearing and balance
IX, X	Check swallowing; perform general physical examination
XI	Check shoulder shrug; turn head from left to right and back
XII	Check swallowing; turn head from left to right and back

represent the localized workings of the musculoskeletal system, the nervous system has an overriding influence on motor activity. Observe the patient's initial posture and body position **Figure 13-39 ▶** as well as the body position both at rest and with movement, if appropriate. Watch for any apparent involuntary movements, and document their quality, rate, rhythm, and amplitude. Try to determine whether these involuntary movements are related to the patient's posture or activity, and think about whether their presentation

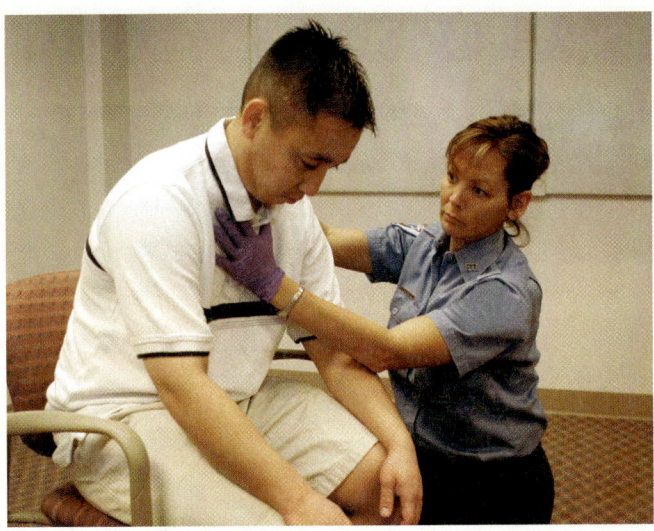

Figure 13-39 Note the patient's posture and body position.

Table 13-4	Scoring of Deep Tendon Reflexes
Grade	**Deep Tendon Reflex Response**
0	No response
1+	Sluggish
2+	Active (expected response)
3+	Slightly hyperactive
4+	Hyperactive

includes a component of fatigue or emotion. Make a general assessment of the bulk of the patient's major muscle groups. Compare these muscles' sizes and contours. Note associated muscle tone by checking for resistance to passive movement.

Probably the single most important part of the motor examination is the evaluation of overall muscle strength. To perform this assessment, have the patient actively move against the examiner's resistance. Strength is graded on a scale of 1 to 5:

1: No muscle contraction or twitch detectable,

2: Only active movement with gravity eliminated,

3: Active movement against gravity obtained,

4: Active movement against some resistance or with fatigue evident,

5: Active movement against full resistance without evident fatigue.

Strength is expressed as a ratio—for example, "strength is 4 over 5 (4/5) in the bilateral upper and lower extremities"; 5/5 is a state of normal muscle tone. When checking strength, and depending on the location of the muscle groups involved, be prepared to test for flexion, extension, grip, abduction, adduction, and opposition.

Checking coordination is an important part of the neurologic examination because it tests a variety of nervous system functions, especially those involving cerebellar functioning. Coordination is assessed by evaluating a patient's ability to perform rapid alternating movements, point-to-point movements (including finger-to-nose and heel-to-shin testing), stance, and gait. Gait and stance should be evaluated only in those subjects whose status allows them to be safely placed in a standing position. Note any upper extremity tremors, flaps, or pronator drift at this point as well.

Just as evaluation of motor function tests the workings of the nervous system from the brain outward to the body, testing sensory function checks the workings of the nervous system from the body inward to the brain. In general, sensory

processes are tested bilaterally, looking for changes in symmetry from one side to the other, as well as comparing proximal to distal processes. When performing the initial assessment on a patient appearing in extremis, a sensory examination is typically the first evaluation done. Initial "shake and shout" maneuvers represent an attempt to find evidence of preserved higher cerebral functioning. Typically these tests look for any response to gross stimuli (eg, a loud shout in the face) or implementation of more noxious forms of stimuli (eg, squeezing the nail bed, twisting the skin of the forearm). As part of a general examination of the sensory system, minimal perception of gross versus light touch should be tested (no equipment is required). More involved sensory evaluation involves checking sharp versus dull perception and two-point discrimination. Sensation is commonly reported in relation to dermatomal location on the body's surface. Dermatomes are distinct areas of skin that correspond to specific spinal or cranial nerve levels where sensory nerves enter the CNS.

Follow the steps in **Skill Drill 13-14 ▸** to evaluate deep tendon reflexes. Scoring of deep tendon reflexes is covered in **Table 13-4 ▲** .

1. Place the patient in the sitting position **Step 1** .

2. Flex the patient's arm to 45° at the elbow. Locate the biceps tendon in the antecubital fossa. Place your thumb over the tendon, with your fingers behind the elbow. Strike your thumb with the reflex hammer, noting the flexion of the elbow **Step 2** .

3. With the patient's arm remaining at a 45° angle, rest the patient's forearm on your arm with the hand slightly pronated. Strike the patient's brachioradial tendon proximal to the wrist, noting the flexion of the elbow **Step 3** .

4. Flex the patient's arm at the elbow 90° and rest his or her hand against the body. Locate and strike the triceps tendon, noting contraction of the triceps or extension of the elbow **Step 4** .

5. Flex the patient's knee to 90°, allowing the leg to dangle. Support the upper leg with your hand, and strike the patellar tendon just below the patella. Note the contraction of the quadriceps and the extension of the lower leg **Step 5** .

6. With the patient's leg in the same position, hold the heel of the patient's foot in your hand. Strike the Achilles tendon, noting the plantar flexion of the foot **Step 6** .

Skill Drill 13-14: Evaluation of Deep Tendon Reflexes

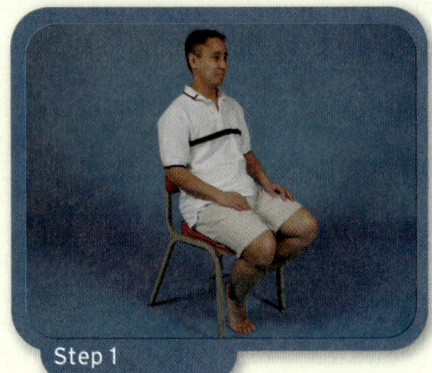

Step 1

Place the patient in the sitting position.

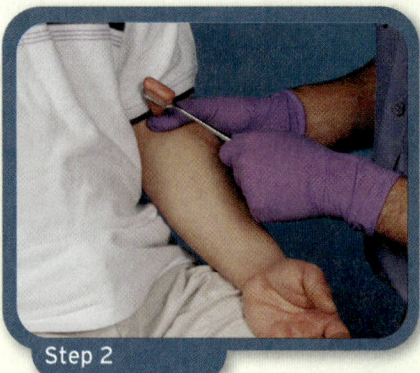

Step 2

Flex the patient's arm to 45° at the elbow. Locate the biceps tendon in the antecubital fossa. Place your thumb over the tendon, with your fingers behind the elbow. Strike your thumb with the reflex hammer, noting the flexion of the elbow.

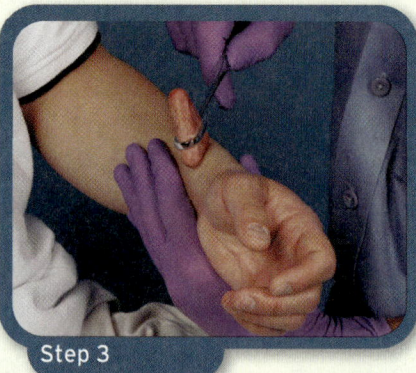

Step 3

With the patient's arm remaining at a 45° angle, rest the patient's forearm on your arm with the hand slightly pronated. Strike the patient's brachioradialis tendon proximal to the wrist, noting the flexion of the elbow.

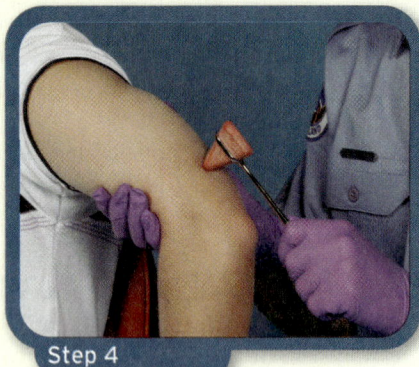

Step 4

Flex the patient's arm at the elbow 90° and rest his or her hand against the body. Locate and strike the triceps tendon, noting contraction of the triceps or extension of the elbow.

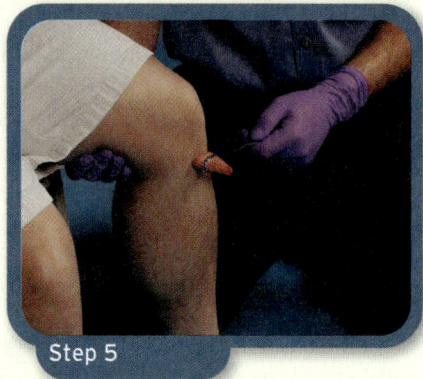

Step 5

Flex the patient's knee to 90°, allowing the leg to dangle. Support the upper leg with your hand, and strike the patellar tendon just below the patella.

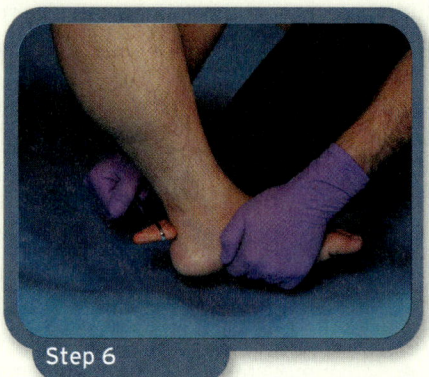

Step 6

With the patient's leg in the same position, hold the heel of the patient's foot in your hand. Strike the Achilles tendon.

Results of the Neurologic Examination

Abnormal findings on the neurologic examination can take a wide variety of forms. Most common are mental status changes that can represent any number of acute and chronic processes, many of which have a nonneurologic origin. Oftentimes, mental status changes represent changes in perfusion or are encountered as a subtle indicator of early sepsis (which is very common in the elderly population).

Distinguishing between delirium and dementia, when dealing with a patient with abnormal mental status, is also important. Delirium is more consistent with an acute sudden change in mental status, secondary to some significant underlying aberration. Dementia is representative of a gradual and pervasive deterioration of cognitive cortical functions, typically secondary to the slow progression of some disease state.

Commonly encountered motor abnormalities include facial and extremity strength asymmetry along with difficulty in speaking (aphasia). These signs are very typical of cerebrovascular disease. Other commonly encountered abnormalities include ataxia, dystonia, seizures, vertigo, visual changes, tinnitus, and tremor. In the setting of trauma, global changes in mental status are more indicative of intracranial mass lesions, whereas decreased extremity motor function may present with proximal versus distal asymmetry and objective parasthesias (tingling or sensory changes), which is more consistent with a spinal lesion.

Physical Examination of Infants and Children

When caring for infants and children, you'll need to alter your approach to patient assessment in general. Because a young child might not be able to speak, your assessment of his or her condition must be based in large part on what you can see and hear yourself.

Examining a child requires understanding that you may have to deal with several sources of information. Families may be helpful in providing vital information about the injury or illness. If possible, and if the patient is of an adequate age and developmental status, you should also attempt to elicit some information from the patient.

In the physical examination, the goals of assessment in children are the same as those for adult patients. If possible, obtain the permission of the parent or guardian before conducting an examination. Explain to the child that you're going to check him or her because you're a paramedic, and that you're here to help. In a situation of acute life-threatening illness or injury, rapidly conduct the initial assessment and manage life-threatening conditions as with an adult patient.

When time permits, consider certain age-related strategies for attempting to facilitate the examination. Overall, children tend to do better being examined from toe to head, as opposed to the reverse method commonly used with adults. This strategy tends to gain trust and decreases the child's fear. Infants are usually not to be overly distressed by being manipulated by adults, so the basic approach to assessment is reasonable with them. Pay close attention to vital signs and physical findings, as the ability to obtain a helpful history is limited.

Children are prone to dehydration and infection (eg, sepsis), and assessment for trauma should always be a consideration as well. Children from 1 to 3 years of age can be challenging to work with, and as a rule will strenuously object to being touched or manipulated by a stranger. The toe-to-head approach is a good strategy in this age group. Decide which aspects of the examination must be performed, set some reasonable ground rules for the examination, and then examine the patient accordingly. Practice ways to safely and adequately hold young patients to facilitate the assessment. If possible, have family members assist with this task.

Children from 4 to 5 years of age are typically much less of a management challenge for the paramedic. They are usually cooperative and helpful with the examination, and the standard head-to-toe approach can usually be employed. School-age children tend to be cooperative as well, and should be actively engaged in the examination process. Be sure to take the time to explain what you're doing while you're examining them.

Adolescent evaluation can be a bit more demanding, as these patients tend to have feelings more directed at preserving their autonomy, and can be concerned about how a given situation may involve either parents or peers. They also tend

You are the Paramedic Part 4

You contact the receiving facility and give a report to the emergency department physician, noting the patient's level of distress and a 20-minute transport time due to weather. The physician asks you to administer 125 mg of methylprednisolone (Solu-Medrol) IV and a third breathing treatment with 2.5 mg of salbutamol (Ventolin)/0.5 mg of ipratropium (Atrovent). She also asks you to be prepared to intubate in case your patient's condition begins to deteriorate.

As ordered, you administer the 125 mg of methylprednisolone (Solu-Medrol) IV, begin a third breathing treatment, and prepare for intubation just in case. Ten minutes away from the hospital the patient grabs you by the arm and whispers that he can't keep breathing any longer and loses consciousness. You ask your partner to contact dispatch and pull over so that you can intubate. Using a size 3 Macintosh blade you are able to visualize the vocal cords and insert an 8.0-mm endotracheal tube. Endotracheal tube placement is further confirmed with bilateral breath sounds, equal and symmetric, chest rise, and a positive end-tidal CO_2 waveform. After confirming tube placement you secure the tube at the 23-cm mark at the lip and transport is resumed.

You arrive at the hospital approximately 12 minutes later. The patient is immediately placed on a ventilator. Three hours later he is admitted to the medical intensive care unit with an exacerbation of his emphysema. He is treated successfully with antibiotics and aggressive respiratory therapy and is discharged home 8 days later.

Reassessment	Recording Time: 25 Minutes
Skin	Pale, warm, and dry, with cyanotic lips and nail beds
Pulse	120 beats/min, regular, with strong distal pulses
ECG	Sinus tachycardia
Blood pressure	148/78 mm Hg
Respirations	12 breaths/min on bag-valve-mask ventilation
SpO_2	86% on bag-valve-mask ventilation at 100% supplemental oxygen
Pupils	Equal and reactive to light

7. Why is it important to reassess your patient after each treatment intervention?

to be very concerned with bodily integrity, so be prepared to reassure them that things are okay if a physical finding is not concerning.

When you are dealing with the assessment of children, some general principles apply. No matter how stressful or disturbing the situation, remain calm, patient, and gentle. Be honest with children; if something is likely to hurt, say so—but without much else in the way of fanfare. If at all possible, attempt to keep children and parents together. Many children normally harbor fears over separation; in the setting of acute illness or injury, these anxieties will only be worsened. Remember that pediatric patients presenting in the prehospital setting are often victims of trauma. Be sure to appropriately assess for injury, and treat appropriately. Don't neglect a child's pain.

Recording Examination Findings

Medical information may be presented in both verbal and written forms. Recording of information should always be done in as orderly and concise a fashion as possible, without omitting important information. The obtained information may then be practically and accurately relayed to the receiving medical staff. In addition, documentation ensures that an accurate historical accounting of the patient's problems prior to entering the hospital will legally exist in the formal medical record. A number of acceptable formats are currently in use. You must use the forms that are recommended by your medical director. Modification of a format is acceptable, so long as it preserves the basic requirements for medical documentation.

A physical examination requires a physical interaction between the patient and the care provider, and it can be successfully performed on a patient who can't communicate. When you are recording examination findings, note objective signs,

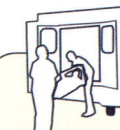

At the Scene

Remember the legal and ethical components to the physical examination:

1. Respect the patient's autonomy in decision making.
2. Be accountable to the patient.
3. Respect the patient's confidentiality and privacy.
4. Obtain consent.
5. Recognize assault and battery.
6. Understand and respect advanced directives.
7. Document facts accurately and nonjudgmentally.

pertinent negatives, and other similar relevant information. Objective information is commonly recorded in a standard format, in the same order as used for the verbal or written report.

Limits of the Physical Examination

The ability to competently perform a physical examination is one of the most valuable skills a paramedic can possess. This examination can, for example, uncover information that the patient is unable or unwilling to share. An accomplished clinician will use this skill in conjunction with the patient interview and other diagnostic tools to form an impression and formulate a treatment plan.

Nevertheless, despite the emphasis placed on a comprehensive physical examination, it has limitations. Even the most experienced physician understands that not everything can be discovered in the examination. In the prehospital setting, it's important to remember that evaluation by a trained physician and laboratory and radiographic studies may be needed for a definitive diagnosis.

You are the Paramedic Summary

1. What is your general impression of the patient? Is he sick or not sick?

You see an elderly man in a tripod position in obvious respiratory distress. His breathing is rapid and shallow. He has retractions and audible wheezes, and cyanosis is present not only in the fingertips but in the lips as well. Your general impression should be "I have a sick patient here!"

2. What do you think is the most valuable assessment tool at your disposal?

Cardiac monitor? No, try again. Blood pressure cuff? Nah! Pulse oximeter? Keep trying! Stethoscope? Good guess, but not quite. You are the most valuable assessment tool that you have! Think about it. You are able to gather information and form the general impression of a patient without using any equipment, right? If the patient is talking to you upon arrival, he or she has a patent airway. Checking a radial pulse will not only tell you the pulse rate, but the quality of pulse and skin temperature as well. You can visualize skin colour, check for symmetric chest rise, retractions, and work of breathing. Abnormal breath sounds such as wheezes, stridor, and rhonchi may be severe enough to be heard without a stethoscope. Don't forget about smell. The nose knows when odours such as ketones, alcohol, and cyanide are present. All of this information can be obtained without the use of any equipment.

3. Which signs and symptoms are acute? Which are chronic?

The chronic signs and symptoms of COPD are clubbing of the fingers, cyanotic nail beds, barrel-shaped chest, and pursed-lipped breathing. Acute signs and symptoms include abnormal breath sounds. A decreased oxygen saturation, shallow breathing, and rapid respiratory rate may be both acute and chronic. This is where you need to ask the patient what is normal for him and move forward from there. For example, your patient's normal oxygen saturation may be 84%, which is definitely decreased; therefore, an oxygen saturation level of 70% indicates an acute condition requiring your attention.

4. Which interventions should you consider at this point, if any?

The focus of treatment needs to be decreasing your patient's work of breathing. Supplemental oxygen can be applied via non-rebreathing mask. (Yes, it is safe to do this provided you keep reassessing your patient to make sure he doesn't become apneic or develop altered mental status!) Pharmacologic treatment is achieved by the administration of a bronchodilator such as salbutamol (Ventolin). Bronchodilators will help by relaxing the muscles surrounding the bronchioles, allowing air to flow more freely into and out of the lungs.

5. Would an increased work of breathing be present upon reassessment of the patient if your treatment was effective?

This is a tough question. It may take a while for the patient's work of breathing to return to what is normal for him. Don't get discouraged if after the first treatment he is still experiencing increased work of breathing. Remember to also reassess breath sounds, pulse rate, and pulse oximetry and be sure to document your findings.

6. How should your patient management progress?

Listen to your patient; he knows his condition better than you! He is telling you that the breathing treatment is not working. Administering additional nebulizer treatments with salbutamol (Ventolin) or a combination of salbutamol (Ventolin) and ipratropium (Atrovent) is appropriate. Depending upon your individual protocols, direct medical control may need to be contacted for further orders including the administration of a corticosteroid such as methylprednisolone (Solu-Medrol) or magnesium sulfate, a smooth-muscle relaxer.

7. Why is it important to reassess your patient after each treatment intervention?

Imagine being put in the middle of an unfamiliar country without a map, compass, or means of communication. How would you find your way out? Without reassessing your patient, how would you get the information necessary to guide further treatment? In your patient, it would be important to note respiratory rate and effort, changes in breath sounds, an improvement in his ability to speak, mental status, pulse rate, and pulse oximetry. Are the breathing treatments working or do you need to consider adding other medications? Can the patient maintain his own airway or do you need to control it via bag-valve-mask ventilation or endotracheal intubation? Remember, your patient can provide you with the clues you need as long as you look for them.

Prep Kit

Ready for Review

- Physical examination is the process by which quantifiable, objective information is obtained from a patient about his or her overall state of health.
- The physical examination consists of two elements: obtaining vital signs that measure overall body function, and performing a head-to-toe survey that evaluates the workings of specific body organ systems. This survey is done in a sequential manner, ensuring that every aspect of the body's function is evaluated.
- The techniques of inspection, palpation, percussion, and auscultation allow you to use your physical senses to obtain physical information and to understand the normal (versus abnormal) functions of a patient's body.
- Vital signs consist of a measurement of blood pressure; pulse rate, rhythm, and quality; respiratory rate, rhythm, and quality; temperature; and pulse oximetry. Other than overall patient appearance, vital signs are the most basic objective data for determining patient status.
- The general impression begins as you approach the scene, simultaneously sizing up the overall situation and the patient's appearance. Review the environment in which the patient is found and the general state of the patient's health.
- The physical examination consists of a comprehensive review of systems to determine the nature and extent of the patient's illness or injury.
- Evaluate the patient's mental status using the AVPU scale.
- When you are examining the head, you should both feel it and inspect it visually. This step is important in the management of potential trauma patients and with patients who have altered mental status or are unresponsive.
- When you are evaluating the face, observe the colour and moisture of the skin, as well as expression, symmetry, and contour of the face itself. Pay attention to any swelling or apparent areas of injury, and note any signs of respiratory distress. Use the mnemonic DCAP-BTLS.
- When you are assessing the pupils, check for size (in millimetres), shape, and symmetry. Also check for a reaction to light shined on them.
- Cervical injury can present in a variety of ways, and the assessment for such injury must be conducted in a careful manner. Evaluate the patient first for the MOI and then for the presence of pain.
- Any manipulations of the spine that result in pain, tenderness, or tingling should prompt you to stop the examination *immediately* and place the patient into a properly sized collar. With any complaints of neck pain in patients who have suffered a significant MOI, immediate stabilization of the head and neck is essential.

- Typically, the chest examination proceeds in three phases: the chest wall is checked, a pulmonary evaluation is conducted, and finally the cardiovascular assessment is performed. Inspect the chest to assess for deformities in wall patency and to look for external clues of respiratory distress.
- Heart sounds can be appreciated by listening to the chest wall in the parasternal areas superiorly and inferiorly as well as in the region superior to the left nipple.
- Because of the large number of organs within the abdomen, the location of organs and their related medical complaints are most easily described by dividing the abdomen into imaginary quadrants.
- When you are inspecting the abdomen, look at the skin as well as the contour and overall appearance of the abdominal wall. Identify any scars, wounds, striae, dilated veins, bruises, rashes, and discolourations. Note any generalized distention or localized masses.
- When you are examining the skeleton and joints, pay attention to both their structure and their function. Consider how the joint and associated extremities look and how well they work.
- When you are assessing the joints and extremities, look for evidence of inflammation or injury, such as swelling, tenderness, increased heat, redness, ecchymosis, or decreased function. Also evaluate the joint or extremity for obvious deformity, diminished strength, atrophy, or asymmetry from one side to the other.
- The examination of the musculoskeletal system should not cause the patient any pain; if any occurs, it should be considered an abnormal finding.
- Palpation of the spine is typically done while the patient is supine, often when he or she has been log rolled onto one side to facilitate access to the back and placement of a spinal immobilization device.
- When you are palpating the spine, use the thumb to touch each spinous process. Identification of an abnormality should prompt you to institute proper splinting and protective measures.
- The neurologic examination should determine the patient's baseline mental status (AVPU), cranial nerve function (pupils, eyes, smile, speech, swallow, shoulder shrug), distal motor function (ability to move), and distal sensory function (ability to feel). It may also test the deep tendon reflexes if necessary.
- You need to alter your approach to patient assessment when dealing with infants and children. Because a young child might not be able to speak, your assessment of his or her condition must be based in large part on what you can see and hear yourself. Family members or caregivers may also be able to provide useful information.
- Medical information may be presented in both verbal and written forms. Recorded information should be orderly, concise, and complete.

Vital Vocabulary

aphasia The impairment of language that affects the production or understanding of speech and the ability to read or write.

ascites Abnormal accumulation of fluid in the peritoneal cavity.

auscultation The method of listening to sounds within the body with a stethoscope.

bruit An abnormal "whoosh"-like sound of turbulent blood flow moving through a narrowed artery.

crepitus Crackling, grating, or grinding that is often felt or heard when two ends of bone rub together.

cyanosis A bluish-grey skin colour that is caused by reduced levels of oxygen in the blood.

delirium Change in mental status that is marked by the inability to focus, think logically, and maintain attention.

dementia The slow onset of progressive disorientation, shortened attention span, and loss of cognitive function.

dermatomes Distinct areas of skin that correspond to specific spinal or cranial nerve levels where sensory nerves enter the CNS.

ecchymosis Localized bruising or blood collection within or under the skin.

foramen magnum A large opening at the base of the skull.

Glasgow Coma Scale Scoring system used to determine level of consciousness.

guarding Contraction of the abdominal muscles in patients.

hernia Protrusion of any organ through an opening into a body cavity where it does not belong.

inspection Looking at the patient, either in general or at a specific area (ie, a patient's overall appearance from the doorway, versus looking specifically at the chest wall for abnormalities/deformities).

Korotkoff sounds Sounds related to blood pressure that are heard by stethoscope.

kyphosis Outward curve of the thoracic spine.

lordosis Inward curve of the lumbar spine just above the buttocks. An exaggerated form of lordosis results in the condition known as swayback.

mottling A blotchy pattern on the skin; a typical finding in states of severe protracted hypoperfusion and shock.

murmur An abnormal "whoosh"-like sound heard over the heart that indicates turbulent blood flow around a cardiac valve.

occiput The most posterior portion of the cranium.

opthalmoscope An instrument used to look into a patient's eyes and view the retina and aqueous fluid; consists of a concave mirror and a battery-powered light that is usually contained in the handle.

otoscope A tool used to the ears of a patient; consists of a head and a handle. The head contains an electric light source and a low-power magnifying lens.

pallor Paleness.

palpation Physical touching for the purpose of obtaining information.

parasthesias Tingling or sensory change.

pathologic fracture A fracture that occurs when normal forces are applied to abnormal bone structures.

percussion Gently striking the surface of the body, typically overlying various body cavities to detect changes in the densities of the underlying structures.

perfusion The circulation of blood within an organ or tissue in adequate amounts to meet the cells' needs.

physical examination The process by which quantifiable, objective information is obtained from a patient about his or her overall state of health.

physiologic fracture A fracture that occurs when abnormal forces are applied to normal bone structures.

primitive reflexes Reflex reactions such as Babinski, grasping, and sucking signs normally found in very young patients.

pulse oximetry An assessment tool that measures oxygen saturation of hemoglobin in the capillary beds.

reflexes Involuntary motor responses to specific sensory stimuli, such as a tap on the knee or stroking the eyelash.

rubor Redness; one of the classic signs of inflammation.

rubs Lung sound produced by a partial loss of intrapleural integrity, when an abnormal collection of fluid has accumulated between a portion of the visceral and parietal pleura, resulting in "pleuritic" pain and a perceived rub on auscultation.

scoliosis Sideways curvature of the spine.

stridor A harsh, high-pitched, crowing inspiratory sound, such as the sound often heard in acute laryngeal obstruction.

tenting A condition in which the skin slowly retracts after being pinched and pulled away slightly from the body; a sign of dehydration.

turgor Loss of elasticity in the skin.

vasoconstriction Narrowing of a blood vessel, such as with hypoperfusion or cold extremities.

vasodilation Widening of a blood vessel.

visual acuity (VA) The ability or inability to see, and how well one can see.

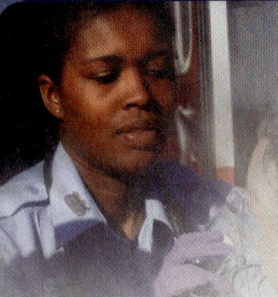

Assessment in Action

You're dispatched to the home of a 24-year-old woman who is complaining of abdominal pain. On your arrival, she is bent over, grasping her abdominal wall, and tells you the pain is very intense. Her vital signs are within normal limits. You begin to ask questions and perform your physical examination.

1. _____ is a rapid method of assessing the patient's level of consciousness.
   A. APU
   B. C&O×3
   C. AVPU
   D. AO×4

2. Inspection involves:
   A. looking at the patient, either in general or at a specific area.
   B. the physical touching for the purpose of obtaining information.
   C. gently striking the surface of the body, typically overlying various body cavities.
   D. listening with a stethoscope.

3. Measuring _____ require(s) the paramedic to utilize the techniques of auscultation, palpation, and inspection.
   A. blood pressure
   B. pulse rate
   C. heart rate
   D. vital signs

4. Blood pressure must be measured with a cuff that's appropriate to the patient's size. If you use a blood pressure cuff that is too small or tight you will yield an(a)_____.
   A. artificially low blood pressure
   B. artificially normal blood pressure
   C. artificially high blood pressure
   D. normal pressure

5. Because of the large number of organs within the abdomen, the _____ serves as a central reference point.
   A. lower rib cage
   B. pelvic girdle
   C. xyphoid process
   D. umbilicus

6. The above patient is complaining of pain near her gallbladder. This would be located in the_____.
   A. RUQ
   B. LUQ
   C. RLQ
   D. LLQ

7. When a patient is contracting his or her abdominal muscles, this is called_____.
   A. rigidity
   B. guarding
   C. soft
   D. nontender

Challenging Question

8. Are there any special considerations you should take into account based on your patient's gender?

Points to Ponder

You are dispatched to the home of a 65-year-old woman who is complaining of a feeling of general malaise that began about 4 days ago. When you arrive on scene, the patient appears to be in no distress. You introduce yourself and begin your physical examination. The patient denies having any chest pain, shortness of breath, nausea, or vomiting. Her vital signs are as follows: respiratory rate, 18 breaths/min; pulse oximetry reading, 99% on room air; blood pressure, 110/70 mm Hg; and pulse rate, 75 beats/min with a normal sinus rhythm on the monitor.

The patient states that she "hasn't felt right" for a few days and she called now because she had no way to get to the doctor.

Where should you begin your examination?

Issues: Understanding the Importance of a Complete Physical Examination, Understanding the Need for a Caring Attitude When Performing a Physical Examination, Understanding the Importance of a Professional Appearance and Demeanour When Performing a Physical Examination.

14 Patient Assessment

Competency Areas

Area 1: Professional Responsibilities

1.5.c Work collaboratively with other emergency response agencies.

Area 2: Communication

2.2.a Record organized, accurate, and relevant patient information.

2.3.a Exhibit effective non-verbal behaviour.

2.3.b Practice active listening techniques.

2.3.c Establish trust and rapport with patients and colleagues.

2.3.d Recognize and react appropriately to non-verbal behaviours.

Area 3: Health and Safety

3.2.b Transfer patient from various positions using applicable equipment and/or techniques.

3.2.c Transfer patient using emergency evacuation techniques.

3.3.a Assess scene for safety.

3.3.b Address potential occupational hazards.

3.3.e Conduct procedures and operations consistent with Workplace Hazardous Materials Information System (WHMIS) and hazardous materials management requirements.

3.3.f Practice infection control techniques.

Area 4: Assessment and Diagnostics

4.1.a Rapidly assess a scene based on the principles of a triage system

4.1.b Assume different roles in a mass casualty incident.

4.1.c Manage a mass casualty incident.

4.2.a Obtain list of patient's allergies.

4.2.b Obtain list of patient's medications.

4.2.c Obtain chief complaint and/or incident history from patient, family members, and/or bystanders.

4.2.d Obtain information regarding patient's past medical history.

4.2.e Obtain information about patient's last oral intake.

4.2.f Obtain information regarding incident through accurate and complete scene assessment.

4.3.a Conduct primary patient assessment and interpret findings.

4.3.b Conduct secondary patient assessment and interpret findings.

4.3.c Conduct cardiovascular system assessment and interpret findings.

4.3.d Conduct neurological system assessment and interpret findings.

4.3.e Conduct respiratory system assessment and interpret findings.

4.3.g Conduct gastrointestinal system assessment and interpret findings.

4.3.h Conduct genitourinary system assessment and interpret findings.

4.3.i Conduct integumentary system assessment and interpret findings.

4.3.j Conduct musculoskeletal assessment and interpret findings.

4.3.m Conduct assessment of the ears, eyes, nose, and throat and interpret findings.

4.3.n Conduct multisystem assessment and interpret findings.

4.3.o Conduct neonatal assessment and interpret findings.

4.3.p Conduct psychiatric assessment and interpret findings.

4.4.a Assess pulse.

4.4.b Assess respiration.

4.4.c Conduct non-invasive temperature monitoring.

4.4.d Measure blood pressure by auscultation.

4.4.e Measure blood pressure by palpation.

4.4.g Assess skin condition.

4.4.h Assess pupils.

4.4.i Assess level of mentation.

4.5.a Conduct oximetry testing and interpret findings.

Area 6: Integration

6.3.a Conduct ongoing assessments based on patient presentation and interpret findings.

6.3.b Re-direct priorities based on assessment findings.

Appendix 4: Pathophysiology

B. **Neurologic System**
Traumatic Injuries: Head Injury

C. **Respiratory System**
Traumatic Injuries: Pneumothorax (simple, tension)

D. **Female Reproductive System and Neonates**
Pregnancy Complications: Ectopic pregnancy

E. **Gastrointestinal System**
Small/Large Bowel: Appendicitis

J. **Multisystem Diseases and Injuries**
Shock Syndromes: Cardiogenic
Trauma: Assault
Trauma: Falls
Trauma: Rapid deceleration injuries

Scene Assessment

Routine Precautions and PPE
Scene Safety
Consider Mechanism of Injury/Nature of Illness
Determine the Number of Patients
Consider Additional Resources
Consider C-Spine Immobilization

Initial Assessment

Approach and Form a Working Diagnosis
Assess Mental Status
Assess the Airway
Assess Breathing
Assess Circulation
Identify Priority Patients and Make Transport
  Decisions

Trauma Patients   **Medical Patients**

Focused History and Physical Examination

Reconsider Mechanism of Injury	
Significant Mechanism of Injury	**No Significant Mechanism of Injury**
Rapid Trauma Assessment	Focused Trauma Assessment Based on Chief Complaint
Baseline Vital Signs	Baseline Vital Signs
SAMPLE History	SAMPLE History
Reevaluate Transport Decision	Reevaluate Transport Decision

Focused History and Physical Examination

Evaluate Responsiveness	
Responsive	**Unresponsive**
History of Illness	Rapid Medical Assessment
SAMPLE History	Baseline Vital Signs
Focused Medical Assessment Based on Chief Complaint	SAMPLE History
Baseline Vital Signs	Reevaluate Transport Decision
Reevaluate Transport Decision	

Detailed Physical Examination

Perform the Detailed Physical Examination
Reassess Vital Signs

Ongoing Assessment

Repeat the Initial Assessment
Reassess and Record Vital Signs
Repeat the Focused Assessment
Check Interventions

Introduction

Patient assessment is the platform upon which quality prehospital care is built and the single most important skill you bring to bear on patient care. Patient assessment is a complex skill made up of two primary components: information gathering and physical examination. In the first component, called history-taking, you try to determine the nature of the patient's problems by asking questions, listening to and analysing answers, and observing the way the patient presents and the setting in which he or she is found. In the second component, called physical assessment, you perform a hands-on evaluation of the patient to further explore the chief complaint(s) and to detect injuries or signs of illness.

This chapter describes the skill of patient assessment, focusing primarily on the *what* aspects of patient assessment (that is, what needs to done as part of an organized, systematic assessment). Chapters 12 and 13 presented the *how* aspects of the patient assessment in more detail. Now you will learn how to pull everything together. Please note that pediatric assessment in covered in detail in Chapter 41: *Pediatrics*.

The information gleaned during the patient assessment process helps you make key prehospital care decisions. The first and most important question during the initial assessment is always "Does my patient have any life-threatening conditions?" If life threats are present, you must quickly decide how to address them. Patient findings obtained early in the assessment process often dictate whether the patient needs to be transported by ground or by air ambulance and to which facility. For these reasons, your patient assessment skills are the single most important tools in your paramedic toolbox. While *some* of your patients may need spinal immobilization and *others* may need a breathing treatment, *all of your patients* need excellent patient assessment.

The fundamental components of your job are to identify problems (the chief complaint, or why someone called 9-1-1), set priorities (rank the problems from most to least serious), develop a prehospital care plan (address the problems), and execute the plan (provide care for the patient). As you gain experience and complete more calls, however, the breadth and depth of your knowledge base should increase and you should see a corresponding increase in your assessment skills. Patient assessment is a skill that you should hone *throughout your entire paramedic career*.

The Elements of Patient Assessment

Several elements make up the skill of patient assessment, with each being used in some way to gather information. The primary source of information during your assessment is usually the patient, but you will also gather information from sources such as the patient's family or friends or eyewitnesses to the emergency event. That information is then added to information gathered from the emergency scene itself, along with the data you obtain from your diagnostic tools and tests (such as cardiac monitor, glucometer, pulse oximetry, and capnography).

Care in the prehospital setting is very similar to the process used in solving a "whodunit" murder mystery. In this case, however, you are the detective, and the mystery is finding out what is wrong with your patient and what you can do about it. To solve the mystery, you gather "clues" about your patient's problem, sift through the clues, and analyze the data. Missed clues resulting from a weak, disorganized, or incomplete patient assessment may keep you from solving the mystery, which in the real world equates with your patient getting less than optimal prehospital care.

You are the Paramedic Part 1

You are dispatched to a local high school football practice for a "player down." Upon arrival, you find a 17-year-old youth lying on the sidelines, unconscious. His teammates tell you that they were participating in a no-contact, warm-up drill when Mike suddenly collapsed. They also state that Mike had no complaints just before the event and seemed to be "just fine."

In your initial assessment, the patient responds only to deep, painful stimuli, and you find no obvious signs of trauma. The team's coach isn't sure if Mike has any medical conditions, and he can't provide any further information.

Initial Assessment	Recording Time: 0 Minutes
Appearance	Wearing full protective gear; supine
Level of consciousness	P (Responsive to painful stimuli)
Airway	Patent
Breathing	Slightly fast but adequate
Circulation	Strong, full radial pulse

1. What is the best method of airway assessment and management for a patient who is wearing a football helmet and shoulder pads?
2. Although other players deny the occurrence of any trauma, should you immobilize this patient?

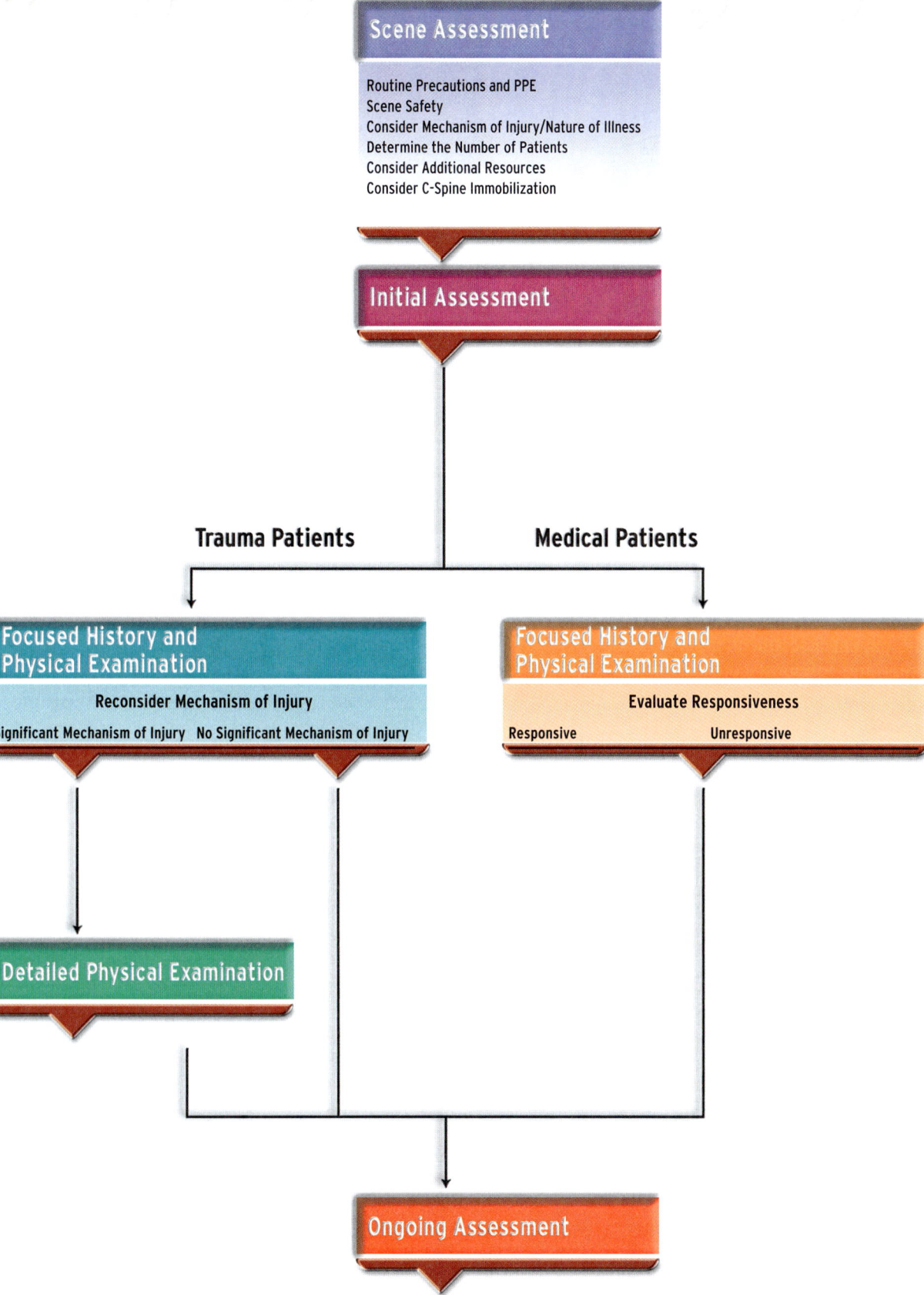

Scene Assessment

Routine Precautions and PPE
Scene Safety
Consider Mechanism of Injury/Nature of Illness
Determine the Number of Patients
Consider Additional Resources
Consider C-Spine Immobilization

Initial Assessment

Trauma Patients

Focused History and Physical Examination

Reconsider Mechanism of Injury

Significant Mechanism of Injury   No Significant Mechanism of Injury

Detailed Physical Examination

Medical Patients

Focused History and Physical Examination

Evaluate Responsiveness

Responsive   Unresponsive

Ongoing Assessment

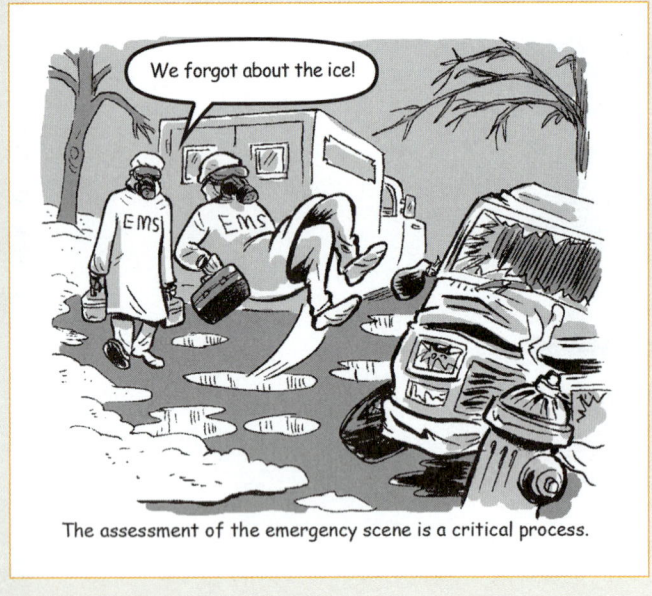

Figure 14-1

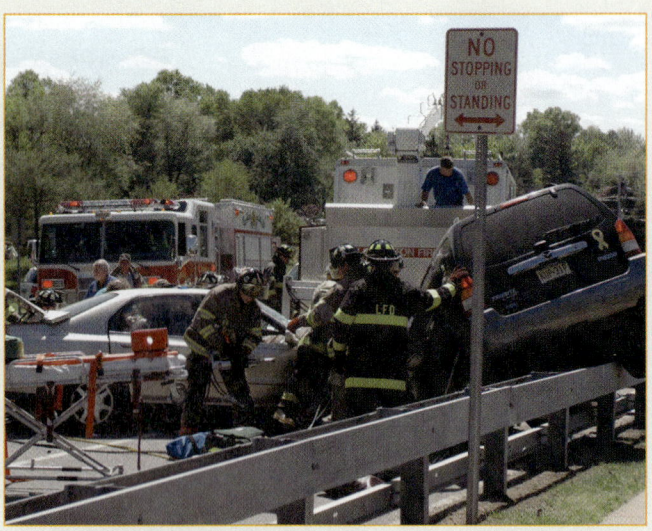

Figure 14-2 Motor vehicle collision scenes have many risks to you, your partners, and the patient.

Scene Assessment and Evaluation

Routine Precautions

The first step of the patient assessment process is the scene assessment. Your first and foremost concern on any call is ensuring your own safety and the safety of the other paramedics 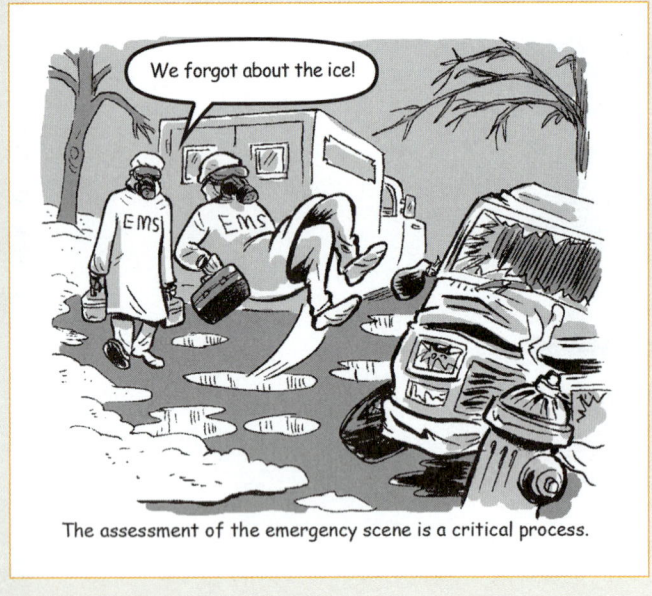. You are of no value to the patient if you get injured and can't provide care. Suppose you get an infectious disease because you neglected to follow personal protective equipment (PPE) procedures; you may then miss time from work because you are sick. In the worst-case scenario, you might contract a career-ending or life-threatening disease, all because you chose to ignore the requirement for use of PPE or did not take routine precautions.

You should wear properly sized gloves on every call. If blood or other fluids could potentially splash or spray, wear eye protection. When inhaled particles are a risk factor, wear a properly sized and fitted mask (HEPA or N95). In rare cases, a gown is also indicated. Always take the steps necessary to protect yourself on calls. When in doubt about the nature of the threat, it's always better to err on the side of caution and protect yourself too much rather than too little. Infection control is covered in depth in Chapters 2 and 36.

Scene Safety

In the assessment and evaluation of the emergency scene, the main focus is to ensure the safety and well-being of the paramedics and any other emergency responders. Ask yourself, "Is it safe for me and my team to enter this scene and to approach the patient?" To answer that question, you need to use a "wide-angle lens" thought process when you assess and evaluate the scene. Some of the issues you might encounter in particular scenes are described next.

Collision and rescue scenes often include multiple risks, such as unstable vehicles, moving traffic, jagged metal and broken glass, fire or explosion hazards, downed power lines, and, possibly, hazardous materials **Figure 14-2 ▲** .

Toxic substances are found at many scenes. From the lawn and garden chemicals found in almost every home to the countless chemicals used in industry and manufacturing, you should always be alert for the presence of toxic substances. You should also be wary of working in toxic environments (that is, the atmosphere itself). Smoke is the by-product of incomplete combustion and can contain many toxins, pathogens, and carcinogens. In these cases, having proper body and respiratory protection is a must before entering the scene and initiating patient care **Figure 14-3 ▶** .

Don't just think of crime scenes in the past tense because there is always the possibility that more violence may occur. Under ideal circumstances, when dispatched to a potential crime scene, law enforcement personnel should enter and secure the scene first. All too frequently, however, the paramedics arrive first

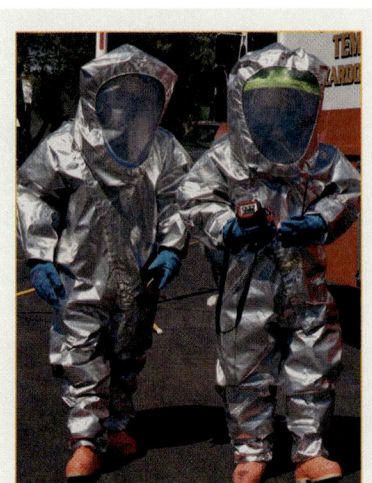

Figure 14-3 Scenes involving toxic substances may require specially trained rescuers with extra protective equipment.

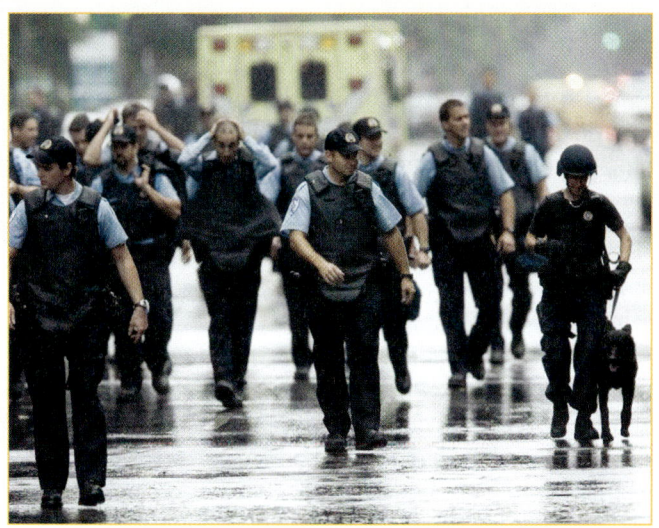

Figure 14-4 If the scene is unsafe, request law enforcement support, and wait in your vehicle at a safe distance.

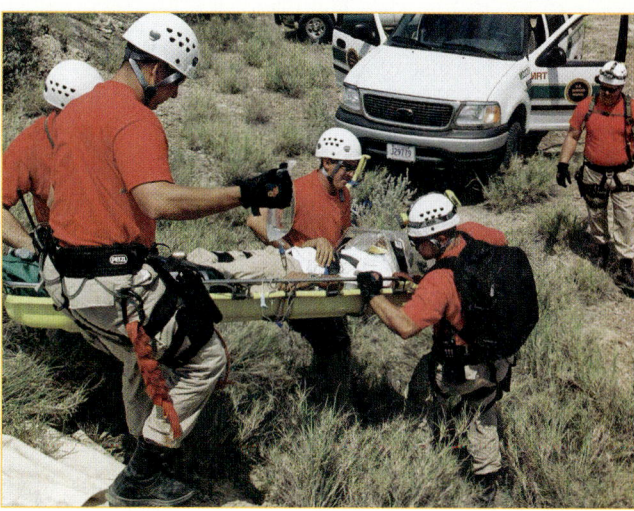

Figure 14-5 At times you may need a team to carry patients out of areas with unstable terrain.

and unknowingly enter a crime scene. For example, the dispatch centre might receive a call for a "man down"; on arrival, the paramedics might discover that the patient has been stabbed three times in the chest. Law enforcement personnel should be requested immediately in such cases because it is nearly impossible for you and your partner to control the scene and provide prehospital care for the patient at the same time **Figure 14-4 ▲** —and because the perpetrator could return with more firepower.

When faced with a currently unstable scene or a scene that begins deteriorating (for example, people become progressively louder or more unruly or make aggressive gestures or threats), consider retreating to the vehicle until the scene is secured and deemed safe. If you believe that you can pull it off safely, remove the patient from the scene with you, but making such an attempt is clearly a judgment call on your part.

Unstable surfaces are everyday occurrences in the prehospital setting. In some parts of Canada, snow- or ice-covered surfaces can persist for 3 or 4 months out of the year. In some parts of the country, it typically rains from November to May. Most of Canada has terrain issues ranging from minor hills to mountains to sandy beaches. Thus, working on unstable surfaces is an inevitable part of prehospital medicine **Figure 14-5 ▶** . Take the time to make all of your patient lifts and moves as safe and controlled as possible. Just making a mental commitment to focus on this aspect of your practice will go a long way toward helping prevent a fall and a possible injury. Also, consider investing in a good pair of boots that will serve to keep your feet comfortable and to provide good traction, which helps to avoid surprise slips.

Behavioural emergencies are common and challenging calls, and they always present with the possibility of some sort of violent outbreak occurring. With the continued increase in the manufacture and abuse of methamphetamine, paramedics are seeing a growing number of patients who are on the tail end of multiple sleepless days fueled by methamphetamine. The people are often paranoid, emotionally unstable, and almost always armed, making them far more a threat than an average patient with a non–drug-induced behavioural emergency. In addition, methamphetamine and crack users are at high risk of experiencing excited or agitated delirium, such that they may present in a blind rage and are almost uncontrollable. In one case, the patient was shot with a TASER device by law enforcement personnel *14 times in fewer than 5 minutes*; despite this barrage, it still took six people to secure the patient in handcuffs and place him on the stretcher. There is a clear message here: Never hesitate to call for law enforcement assistance when managing any patient who has the potential for becoming violent.

While protecting the emergency response team is clearly a priority, so is protecting the patient and bystanders. Establishing a perimeter around an emergency scene may prevent bystanders from entering a dangerous scene and potentially becoming patients themselves. Environmental issues can also influence scene safety and the prehospital care process. The longer a patient is exposed to wind and rain, the more likely hypothermia will become a factor. Of course, leaving a patient lying on a hot asphalt highway as the midday sun beats down is not good medicine either. When the environment is unfriendly, perform the initial assessment, address life threats, and get the patient into the controlled environment of the ambulance as quickly as possible.

Mechanism of Injury/Nature of Illness

Most calls to 9-1-1 will be for a medical emergency or some form of trauma. A generic-sounding call such as a "sick man" in no way guarantees that a sick, hypoglycemic patient didn't also fall and injure himself as a result of a low blood glucose level. Or, a trauma patient may have wrecked her car when she passed out because of an abnormal heart rhythm. Prudent paramedics keep their minds open to multiple possibilities when trying to figure out just what's going on with patients. The mechanism of injury (MOI) is the way in which traumatic injuries occur—the forces that act on the body to cause damage. Assessing and evaluating the MOI can help you predict the likelihood of certain injuries having occurred and estimate their severity. (The patterns of injuries sustained in traumatic events are discussed in detail in Chapter 17.)

On purely medical calls, you should quickly determine from the patient (or family, friends, or bystanders) why paramedics were requested. The nature of illness (NOI) is the general type of illness a patient is experiencing.

At this point, if there is more than one patient or the patient is obese, you can call for additional resources. If multiple patients are present and have similar symptoms or complaints, you might consider carbon monoxide poisoning (or contact with some other noxious agent) or food poisoning as prime candidates. Irrespective of the cause of the problem, the presence of multiple patients means that they must be triaged to determine which additional resources you need and how you will allocate the resources.

Once you have identified the total number of patients and estimated the severity of their injuries, you should request any additional resources—for example, fire, police, rescue, public utilities, or hazardous materials personnel—needed to support the efforts of first responders already on the scene.

The process of scene assessment is completed in a very short time. Once you have digested the dispatch information, evaluated the overall scene and safety, determined the MOI or NOI, and summoned additional help, you are ready to manage prehospital care. By contrast, if the responding crew can manage the situation without further assistance, you should assess the need for spinal motion restriction and continue with patient care. Based on the scene assessment and MOI, paramedics must ensure that spinal motion restriction takes place on reaching the patient. Indications for spinal motion restriction will be covered further in Chapter 22.

At the Scene

Assessing the safety of a scene before entering may be the single most important way in which paramedics can attend to their own well-being. Subtle signs of danger not immediately recognized and neutralized—or avoided—at this point can become more threatening without being noticed once you shift your attention to patient assessment and prehospital care. Initial scene assessment often allows you to distinguish between a manageably safe scene and one that could spin dangerously out of control without further warning.

You are the Paramedic Part 2

As you gain access to the patient's airway, your partner applies a pulse oximeter and obtains vital signs. High-flow supplemental oxygen is applied, venous access is established, and the patient is readied for transport.

Vital Signs	Recording Time: 5 Minutes
Level of consciousness	V (Responsive to verbal stimuli) with a Glasgow Coma Scale score of 7
Skin	Pink, warm, and moist
Pulse	70 beats/min, regular
Blood pressure	104/68 mm Hg
Respirations	24 breaths/min
Spo2	100% while breathing room air

3. Because this patient is a minor, what are some important considerations for treatment and transport?
4. Of all your differential diagnoses, which ones should be considered a diagnosis of exclusion?

Patient Assessment

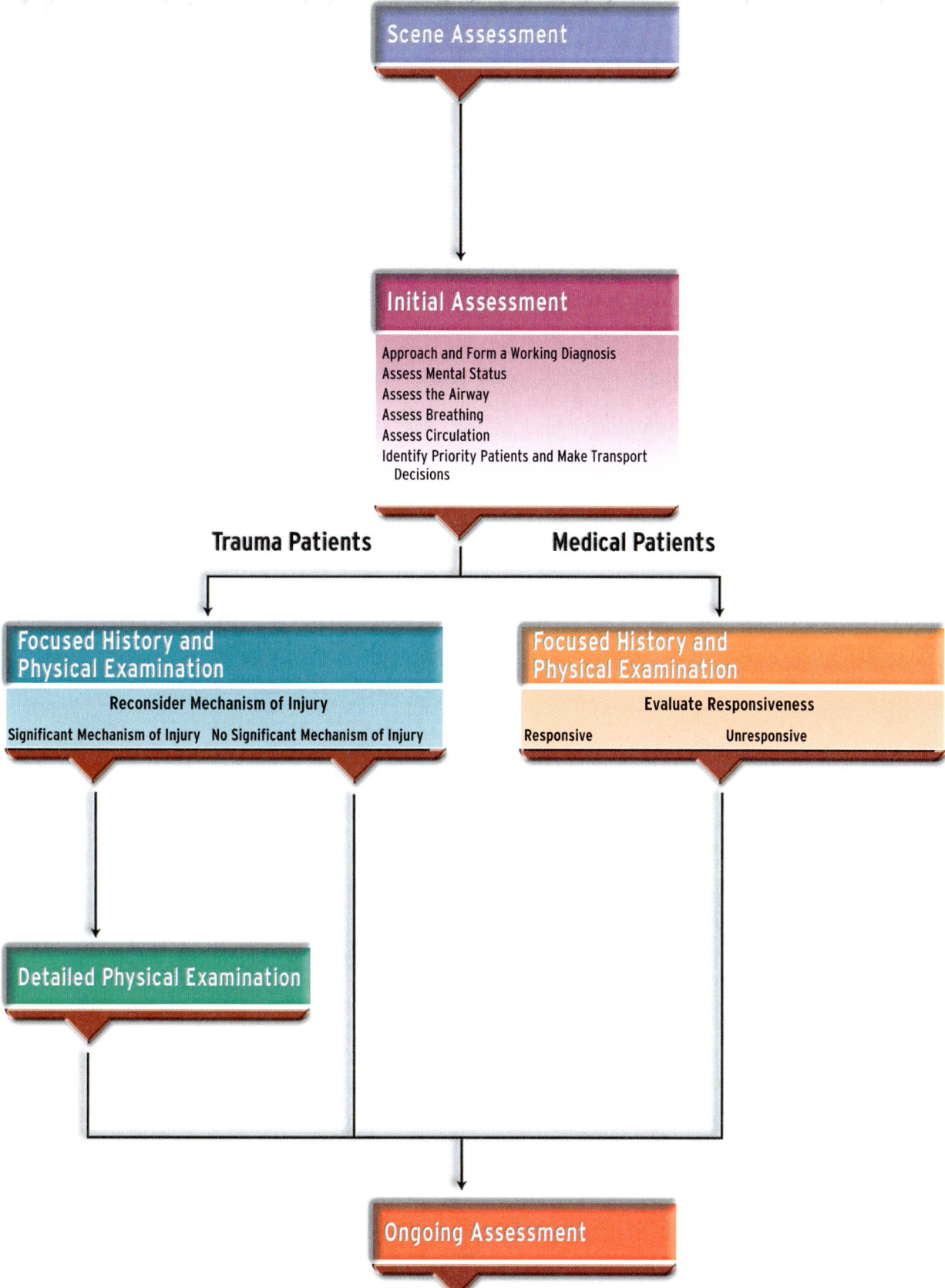

Scene Assessment

Initial Assessment

Approach and Form a Working Diagnosis
Assess Mental Status
Assess the Airway
Assess Breathing
Assess Circulation
Identify Priority Patients and Make Transport
 Decisions

Trauma Patients **Medical Patients**

Focused History and Physical Examination

Reconsider Mechanism of Injury

Significant Mechanism of Injury No Significant Mechanism of Injury

Focused History and Physical Examination

Evaluate Responsiveness

Responsive Unresponsive

Detailed Physical Examination

Ongoing Assessment

The Initial Assessment

The initial assessment is the most time-intensive portion of the assessment process because it focuses on the identification and management of life-threatening problems. In the first 60 to 90 seconds, as you look at, talk with, and touch your patient, you should be able to identify threats to the ABCs. More often than not, you will form a working diagnosis for your patient based almost solely on the initial presentation and chief complaint.

Each of us, without even trying or being conscious of doing so, makes dozens of observations about the appearance of another person during the first few seconds of an encounter—for example, whether the other person is sitting or standing, overweight or thin, smiling or frowning, dressed neatly or sloppily. In assessing a patient, we must make similar observations, but in a much more conscious, objective, and systematic manner, looking for specific clues to give us an immediate sense of the seriousness of the situation. A complaint of "I just can't catch my breath" that comes to you in one- or two-word bursts clearly points to a very sick patient. A patient complaining of "chest pain" after being stabbed in the chest is an even more obvious example of a priority.

You are trying to answer two questions: Is my patient sick? If so, how sick is he or she? In the case of trauma, the questions take a slightly different form: Is my patient hurt? If so, how badly hurt is he or she?

Whether it is medical or trauma, the first question is a qualification and the second is a quantification. "Is my patient sick?" has a yes or no answer, whereas "How sick is my patient?" attempts to rate the event's severity. With time and experience, you should be able to answer both questions in that 60- to 90-second window, forming your working diagnosis.

Once these questions are answered, you can move forward with determining your priorities of prehospital care, developing a care plan, and putting the care plan into action. If the primary problem seems to be a traumatic injury, identify and evaluate the MOI. If the primary problem seems to be medical, identify the NOI. As you mentally move through this process, keep in mind that an injured patient might have a medical component to his or her problem, just as a patient with a medical emergency might have a trauma component to his or her problem.

You will also need to identify the age and sex of your patient because each can change how your patient presents. For example, an older woman having a heart attack may have an atypical presentation (no chest pain) compared with the more traditional presentation seen with an older man with the same condition. Likewise, a girl of middle school age will often be more emotionally mature than a boy of the same age, changing how each answers your questions and reacts to the emergency itself.

The information gleaned from the initial assessment is crucial to the overall outcome for your patient. Treat life threats as you find them, but also decide what additional prehospital care is needed, what needs to be done on scene versus en route,

when to initiate transport, and which facility is most appropriate given your patient's needs.

Assess the Patient's Mental Status and Neurologic Function

The patient's mental status is often one of the prime indicators of how sick the patient really is. Changes in the state of consciousness may provide the first clue to an alteration in the patient's condition, so establish a baseline as soon as you encounter the patient. At the same time you are assessing mental status, if trauma is involved, you need to decide whether you will implement spinal motion restriction procedures.

The quickest and simplest way to assess the patient's mental status or level of consciousness (LOC) is to use the AVPU process:

A *Alert* to person, place, and day
V Responsive to *Verbal* stimuli
P Responsive to *Pain*
U *Unresponsive*

You can further assess mental status by considering whether the patient is alert and oriented (A × O) in four areas: person, place, day, and the event itself. Assessing whether the patient can recall his or her name and the day tests long-term memory, whereas assessing whether the patient knows where he or she is and what happened tests short-term memory.

The most reliable and consistent method of assessing mental status and neurologic function is the Glasgow Coma Scale (GCS), which assigns a point value (score) for eye opening, verbal response, and motor response; these values are totaled for a total score **Table 14-1 ▶**. While it may take slightly longer to perform than the AVPU, the GCS provides much greater insight into the patient's overall neurologic function.

Let's work through a scenario. You encounter an older man who tracks you with his eyes as you enter his room. As you

Table 14-1	Glasgow Coma Scale					
Eye Opening		**Best Verbal Response**		**Best Motor Response**	
Spontaneous	4	Oriented and converses	5	Follows commands	6
To verbal command	3	Disoriented conversation	4	Localizes pain	5
To pain	2	Speaking but nonsensical	3	Withdraws to pain	4
No response	1	Moans or makes unintelligible sounds	2	Decorticate flexion	3
		No response	1	Decerebrate extension	2
				No response	1

Scores:
14–15: Mild dysfunction
11–13: Moderate to severe dysfunction
10 or less: Severe dysfunction (The lowest possible score is 3.)

speak with the man, you note that his verbal response is disoriented, even though he follows your commands. His GCS values would be 4, 4, and 6, for a total score of 14. By comparison, if the patient opened his eyes only to pain, moaned as the only verbal response, and withdrew to pain, he would be assigned GCS values of 2, 2, and 4, for a total score of 8. When reporting a GCS score, it is important to break down the score into its component parts, because two patients with the same GCS can present differently depending on their scores for each category. Clearly, a child or infant will respond differently than an adult. A modified assessment should be used for these patients. This is addressed in Chapter 41.

Assess the Patient's Airway Status

Assessment of the patient's airway status focuses on two questions: Is the airway open and patent? Is it likely to remain so? For air to be drawn into the lungs, the airway has to be properly positioned and not obstructed (open from an anatomical perspective). If you hear sonorous (snoring respirations), think "position problem"—the sounds you are hearing are most likely from the tongue partially obstructing the airway. If you hear gurgling or bubbling sounds, think "suction"—there are most likely fluids such as blood, mucus, or vomit in the mouth or posterior pharynx.

When approaching airway management, think from the simple to the complex. The easiest problem to solve is one of position. Its resolution requires no equipment and can be done quickly. The possibility of a spine injury (or lack thereof) drives the decision of which technique to use to open the airway (head tilt–chin lift or jaw-thrust maneuver). In the case of obstruction, such as by food, BLS procedures to clear the obstruction require no equipment and can be done quickly.

Assessment of a patient's airway is completed in the same way regardless of the patient's age. In responsive patients of any age, talking or crying will give clues about the adequacy of the airway. For all unconscious patients, you must establish responsiveness and look, listen, and feel for breathing. If breathing is ineffective or absent, you must open the airway with a head tilt–chin lift (in nontrauma patients) or jaw thrust (in trauma patients).

When performing the head tilt–chin lift maneuver, remember the anatomical differences in the various age groups and make sure that you do not create an airway obstruction with an improper position of the head. Infants and young children do not have the developed tracheal rings that provide support, which means the trachea is easily collapsed or occluded when the head position changes.

Suctioning takes longer (because of the need to set up and use the equipment) and is a more complicated procedure than positioning. If you suction the patient for too long, you create a new problem: hypoxia. However, you need to suction the airway until it is clear. Concerns about causing hypoxia are minor compared to the need to clear the airway and prevent aspiration.

If a mechanical means is required to keep the airway open and patent, you must choose an airway adjunct. If you opt to place an oropharyngeal or nasopharyngeal airway, you must retrieve the equipment, choose the right size for the specific patient, and then place the airway. This procedure takes considerable time.

If you determine that the patient cannot maintain his or her airway and you cannot maintain it by any other means, you need to use a more invasive technique, such as endotracheal intubation. This invasive procedure involves several pieces of equipment: a laryngoscope handle, a laryngoscope blade, a properly sized endotracheal tube, a syringe, a stylet, an OPA, an end-tidal carbon dioxide detector, a bag-valve-mask device, and a method to secure the tube once it is placed. Obviously, gathering the equipment, preparing the patient, and performing the intubation procedure is more time-intensive than previously mentioned interventions.

Other airway management options include bag-valve-mask ventilation or use of a multilumen airway, laryngeal mask airway, or surgical airway (discussed in Chapter 11).

Assess the Patient's Breathing

Breathing is proportional and related to airway adequacy. The assessment of breathing likewise focuses on two questions: First, is the patient breathing? If not, then you have to breathe for the patient. Second, if the patient is breathing, is breathing adequate?

Recall from Chapter 11 that the respiratory rate multiplied by the tidal volume inspired with each breath equals the minute volume. For example, a patient breathing slowly and deeply at 10 breaths/min and 500 ml/breath has a minute volume of 5,000 ml. By comparison, a patient breathing faster and shallower at a rate of 24 breaths/min and 200 ml/breath would have a minute volume of 4,800 ml. On a per-minute basis, the volumes of the two patients are virtually identical, even though the second patient is breathing more than twice as fast as the first patient. Always keep in mind that the amount of air actually moved in and out of the lungs each minute is the best measure of breathing adequacy. Besides the assessment of tidal volume, note the patient's breathing rate, work of breathing (accessory muscle use), breath sounds, skin colour, and LOC or mental status as part of the breathing assessment.

The techniques used to assess a patient's breathing status are not new: Look, listen, and feel. Look for chest rise and fall, noting symmetry of the chest wall and depth of respirations. Listen for breath sounds by using your sense of hearing or by auscultation with a stethoscope. Note adventitious lung sounds, and treat the patient accordingly. Finally, feel for air movement by placing your cheek or the palm of your hand near the patient's mouth.

Assess the Patient's Circulation

Assessing the pulse gives a rapid check of the patient's cardiovascular status and provides information about the rate, strength, and regularity of the heartbeat. In adults and children, the pulse is best palpated over the radial (responsive) and carotid or femoral (unresponsive) artery by using the tips of your index and middle fingers. In responsive or unresponsive infants, palpate the pulse over the brachial artery. First measure the pulse rate by counting the number of beats during 15 seconds; then multiply by 4. If the pulse is irregular or slow, it is best to count for a full minute.

As you count the pulse rate, note the force of the pulse. A normal pulse feels "full," as if a strong wave has passed beneath your fingertips. When there is severe vasoconstriction or in the case of hypotension with a fast pulse, the pulse may feel weak or "thready." By comparison, a patient who is hypertensive will produce a pulse that is more forceful than usual—a "bounding" pulse.

Finally, note the rhythm of the pulse. A normal rhythm is regular, like the ticking of a clock. If some beats come early or late or are skipped, the pulse is irregular. Although many cardiac dysrhythmias are not life threatening, in the case of heart blocks, an irregular pulse can indicate a serious condition. As such, consider all patients with an irregular pulse at risk until proven otherwise.

Report your findings by describing the rate, force, and rhythm of the pulse. For example, state that "The patient's pulse was 72, full, and regular," or "The pulse was 138, thready, and regular."

As part of this phase of the initial assessment, assess the patient's skin for colour, temperature, and moisture. Collectively, these criteria provide insight into the patient's overall

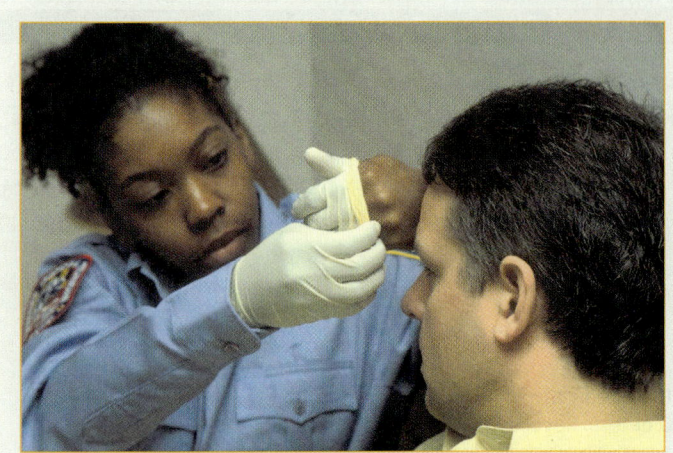

Figure 14-6 Assessing the skin condition. Use the back of the hand to assess the temperature and moisture of the skin.

Table 14-2	Inspection of the Skin	
Skin Colour	**Possible Cause**
Red	Fever Hypertension Allergic reactions Carbon monoxide poisoning (late sign)
White (pallor)	Excessive blood loss Fright
Blue (cyanosis)	Hypoxemia
Mottled	Cardiovascular embarrassment (as in shock)

perfusion. Use the back of your hand to assess the warmth and moisture of the patient's skin because it tends be more sensitive than your palm Figure 14-6 ▲ .

The colour of the skin Table 14-2 ▲ , especially in light-skinned patients, reflects the status of the circulation immediately underlying the skin, including the oxygen saturation of the blood. In people of colour, changes may not be readily evident in the skin but may be assessed by examining the mucous membranes (such as the lips or conjunctivae). When the blood vessels supplying the skin are fully dilated, the skin becomes warm and pink. When the blood vessels supplying the skin constrict or the cardiac output drops, the skin becomes pale or mottled and cool. If the patient does not get enough oxygen, as in the case of a narcotic overdose where the patient is breathing four times per minute, the blood will desaturate as the oxygen level drops; the skin will turn a dusky grey or blue (cyanosis). Pallor occurs if arterial blood flow ceases to part of the body, as in the case of a blood clot or massive bleeding. Hypothermia will also result in pallor as the body shunts blood to the core and away from the extremities.

Skin temperature rises as peripheral blood vessels dilate; it falls as blood vessels constrict. Fever and high environmental temperatures usually stimulate vasodilation, whereas shock

Table 14-3	Palpation of the Skin
Skin Condition	**Possible Cause**
Hot, dry	Excessive body heat (heat stroke)
Hot, wet	Reaction to increased internal or external temperature
Cool, dry	Exposure to cold
Cool, wet	Shock

elicits vasoconstriction. Normal skin is moderately warm and dry. The dryness or moisture of the skin is largely determined by the sympathetic nervous system. Stimulation of the sympathetic nervous system, as in shock or any other severe stress, causes sweating. Depression of the sympathetic nervous system, as in an injury to the thoracic or lumbar spine, can cause the skin in the affected area to become abnormally dry and cool **Table 14-3 ▲** .

Identify Priority Patients

Early in the assessment process, you need to identify priority patients who will benefit from limited time at the scene and rapid transport, as in the case of a patient with internal bleeding from trauma. Such a patient needs to see a surgeon who will surgically repair the injuries and replace the lost blood, neither of which can be accomplished in the prehospital setting except under extreme circumstances.

When you have a priority patient, you need to expedite transport, doing only what is absolutely necessary at the scene and handling everything else en route, including the appropriate focused history and physical examination. Determining a priority patient requires that you think through a variety of possibilities:

- **Poor general impression.** The patient is in obvious distress and does not "look well."
- **Unresponsive patients.** Unresponsiveness is never a good sign and typically points to a patient in serious or critical condition.
- **Responsive but does not or cannot follow commands.** Altered mentation is another bad sign; the question you need to answer is "How bad?"
- **Difficulty breathing.** Breathing problems are one of the most common chief complaints in prehospital care. Patients who have difficulty breathing are in trouble; those who are "working to breathe" are in serious trouble.
- **Hypoperfusion or shock.** Without question, hypoperfusion or shock is an obvious sign of a high-risk patient. Weak or absent peripheral pulse, sustained tachycardia, and pale, cool, wet skin all point to serious consequences.
- **Complicated childbirth.** Anything that presents from the birth canal other than the newborn's head represents a situation not likely to be managed in the out-of-hospital setting.
- **Chest pain with a systolic blood pressure less than 90 mm Hg.** Especially in the context of tachycardia, this sign indicates cardiac compromise and a high-risk patient in unstable condition.
- **Uncontrolled bleeding.** Whether internal or external, such bleeding is a serious life threat.
- **Severe pain anywhere.** Any person with severe pain, especially enough to wake the person up in the middle of the night, should be considered a priority patient.
- **Multiple injuries.** While a patient may have multiple minor injuries that by themselves aren't serious, several small problems can add up to one big problem.

You are the Paramedic Part 3

The patient's mother is contacted at work. She reports that, other than mild scoliosis identified during his freshman year, Mike's health history is unremarkable. She further states that her son has a 4.0 GPA and no history of problems at school. When asked, she denies Mike having any recent history of significant trauma and drug use beyond "sneaking a few beers with friends."

Reassessment	Recording Time: 15 Minutes
Level of consciousness	V (Responsive to verbal stimuli) with a Glasgow Coma Scale score of 7
Skin	Pink, warm, and moist
Pulse	72 beats/min, regular
Blood pressure	106/70 mm Hg
Respirations	24 breaths/min with adequate depth
Spo₂	100% on room air
Temperature	37°C
Pupils	3 mm/PEARRL
Blood glucose	8.5 mmol/l

5. Does this patient need high-flow supplemental oxygen? Why or why not?

6. Should this patient be intubated? Why or why not?

Focused History and Physical Examination

Patient Assessment

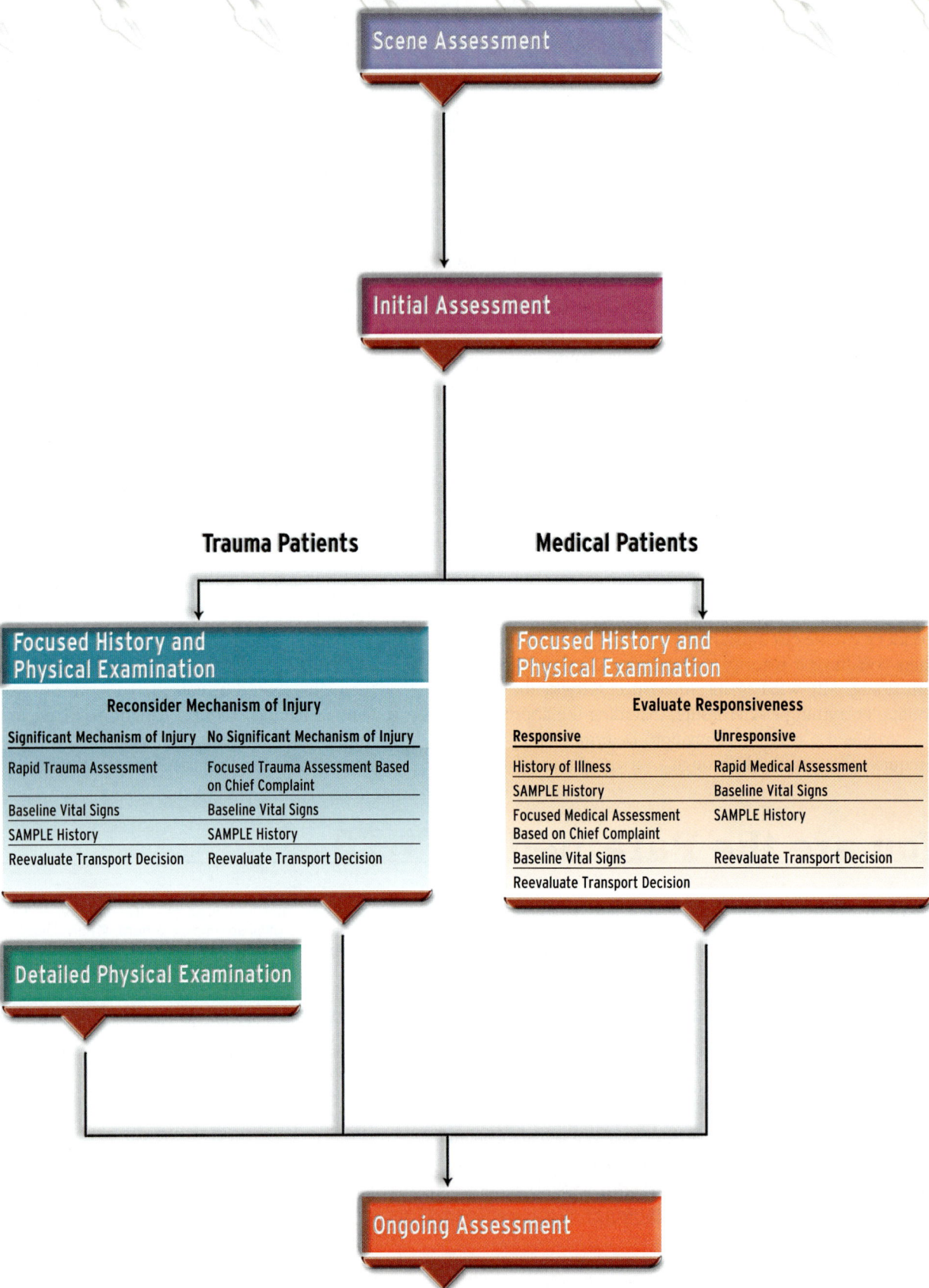

Scene Assessment

Initial Assessment

Trauma Patients   **Medical Patients**

Focused History and Physical Examination

Reconsider Mechanism of Injury

Significant Mechanism of Injury	No Significant Mechanism of Injury
Rapid Trauma Assessment	Focused Trauma Assessment Based on Chief Complaint
Baseline Vital Signs	Baseline Vital Signs
SAMPLE History	SAMPLE History
Reevaluate Transport Decision	Reevaluate Transport Decision

Focused History and Physical Examination

Evaluate Responsiveness

Responsive	Unresponsive
History of Illness	Rapid Medical Assessment
SAMPLE History	Baseline Vital Signs
Focused Medical Assessment Based on Chief Complaint	SAMPLE History
Baseline Vital Signs	Reevaluate Transport Decision
Reevaluate Transport Decision	

Detailed Physical Examination

Ongoing Assessment

The Focused History and Physical Examination

Once the initial assessment is complete and all life threats have been addressed, you can move into the focused history and physical examination phase of patient assessment. Although the problems of many patients—especially older ones—will have medical and traumatic aspects, we will look at medical and trauma patients separately in this section.

Responsive Medical Patients

For a responsive patient with a medical problem, you will usually form your working initial diagnosis based on information gathered during the history-taking process. The focused physical examination and any diagnostic tests you perform after taking the history will help further pinpoint the problem.

With a responsive medical patient, you must first identify the chief complaint. In most cases, some type of pain, discomfort, or body dysfunction (such as hasn't had a bowel movement in 4 days) prompts the call for help. In some cases, the complaint may be vague (such as "I just don't feel right today"). Vague complaints are common in older people. They challenge you to ask the right questions and be a patient listener as you work to obtain the information you need to make good prehospital care decisions Figure 14-7 ▾ .

History of the Present Illness

After determining the chief complaint, you should obtain the history of the present illness. The mnemonic OPQRST provides a helpful template through which to elaborate on the chief complaint: Onset, Provocation, Quality, Region/radiation/referral, Severity, and Timeframe. (The use of OPQRST is explained in detail in Chapter 12.) As part of the focused history and physical examination, the SAMPLE mnemonic can also be useful in the interviewing process: Signs and

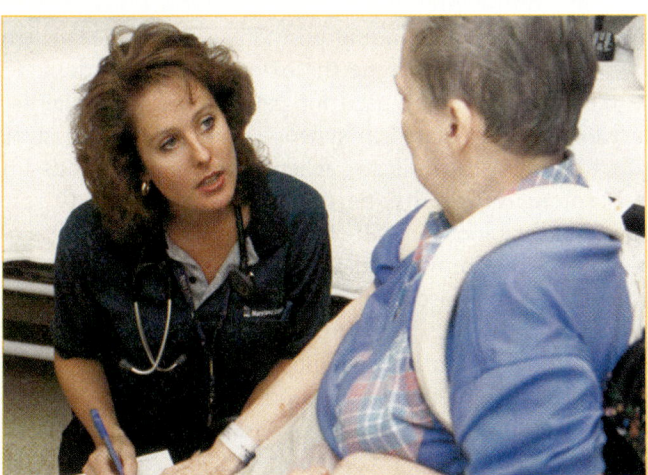

Figure 14-7 Be patient when obtaining information about a vague complaint.

symptoms of current complaint; Allergies; Medications; Pertinent past history; Last oral intake; and Events that led to the current injury or illness.

While taking the history, look for a medical information tag or card. Medical identification devices may take the form of a bracelet, necklace, or wallet card. Such a device is used to identify patients with a history of allergies, certain medical conditions (such as diabetes, cardiac conditions, hypertension, renal disease), and other conditions that may need to be addressed in the treatment of the patient.

Past Medical History

The past medical history is frequently linked to the patient's current problem. For example, people with diabetes who don't manage their blood glucose levels experience progressively worsening problems with their peripheral circulation, eyesight, and kidney function. Also, stable angina frequently transitions into unstable angina; at some point, the patient's condition may worsen and the patient may have a heart attack.

Components of the past medical history include the patient's general state of health, childhood and adult diseases, surgeries and hospitalizations, psychiatric or mental health illness, and traumatic injuries. As you inquire about the patient's past medical history, take the time to explore how some of his or her problems were solved (for example, "It took a couple of breathing treatments before I felt better" or "After my last asthma attack, I had to be intubated and was in the hospital on a ventilator for a week").

Equally important is the case in which the patient presents with a problem he or she has never experienced. An acute presentation of a new problem or condition is best considered serious until proven otherwise.

Current Health Status

The patient's current health status is a composite picture that includes numerous factors in the patient's life. To some degree, each of these items may have contributed to the problem you are confronted with today:

- Dietary habits
- Current medications (including prescription, over-the-counter, herbal, and recreational drugs)
- Allergies (environmental and medication)
- Exercise (or lack thereof)
- Alcohol or tobacco use
- Recreational drug use (if the patient is forthcoming)
- Sleep patterns and disorders
- Immunizations (such as flu shots, tetanus)

Focused Physical Examination

The focused physical examination should be driven by the information you gathered during the initial assessment and the history-taking phase. For a patient who tells you, "I just can't catch my breath," assessment of breath sounds early on is a must. If the patient tells you, "My leg feels numb," assessment of pulse, motor function, and sensation in the affected and unaffected extremities is indicated. You need to exercise good judgment to make the best use of your time. Don't waste time palpating a patient's abdomen or auscultating heart sounds if the person complains of a stiff neck. In general, the out-of-hospital care you provide for a responsive medical patient will be driven by your local protocols in conjunction with your consultation with the base station physician.

The most common complaints from a responsive medical patient will involve the head, heart, lungs, or abdomen, individually or in combination.

For patients with a "head" problem (confusion, headache, altered mentation), you should assess and palpate the head looking for signs of trauma. Check for facial asymmetry, such as facial droop or other signs of a suspected stroke. Dilated or constricted pupils may point to recreational drug use, whereas red conjunctiva may suggest drug or alcohol use. Elevated blood pressure often accompanies a headache, possibly secondary to hypertension.

For a suspected heart problem, assess the pulse for regularity and examine the skin for signs of hypoperfusion (pallor, cool, wet) or oxygen desaturation (cyanosis). Listen to breath sounds—many cardiac problems are associated with respiratory problems (such as rales secondary to pulmonary edema). Obtain baseline vital signs. Serious hypotension with sustained or progressive tachycardia is common in cardiogenic shock; stay alert for this condition because its mortality rate is more than 80%. Check for jugular venous distension (JVD) because it can indicate heart failure or pneumothorax. Examine the extremities for signs of peripheral edema that may result from right-sided heart failure.

For patients with respiratory complaints, assess breath sounds early and often. Possible findings or problems include the following:

- Lung fields with absent breath sounds: pneumothorax
- Silent breath sounds: status asthmaticus
- Lung fields with areas of consolidation: pneumonia
- Wheezing (localized or diffuse): asthma or bronchoconstriction
- Crackles: pulmonary edema, heart failure, toxic inhalation, submersion

For any patient with a respiratory complaint, be alert for the appearance of accessory muscle use or retractions, both of which are signs of increased work of breathing. Also, keep an eye out for the signs of ventilatory fatigue, such as decreased mentation or a tired, worn-out appearance that often precedes ventilatory failure and, frequently, respiratory or cardiac arrest. Watch for the appearance of JVD with respiratory patients because it may point to pneumothorax or heart failure.

One of the most challenging complaints in the out-of-hospital setting is that of abdominal pain because it can result from multiple causes and often presents with little or no external signs. Three basic mechanisms produce abdominal pain:

- *Visceral pain* results when hollow organs are obstructed, thereby stretching the smooth muscle wall, which in turn produces cramping and more diffuse, widespread pain.
- *Inflammation* or irritation of the somatic pain fibres located in the skin, the abdominal wall, and the musculature may produce sharp, localized pain, as in the case of pelvic inflammatory disease or appendicitis. If gastric contents, blood, or urine enters the peritoneum, it will also produce somatic pain, albeit usually much less localized and more diffuse.

- *Referred pain* has its origin in a particular organ but is described by the patient as pain in a different location. Examples include flank pain associated with kidney stones, inner thigh pain from appendicitis or pelvic inflammatory disease, scapular pain from cholecystitis, and groin pain (waves of pain) from renal colic.

Inspection and palpation of the abdomen can provide valuable information, although it is often general. Tightness or guarding can result from internal bleeding, an inflamed organ, and many other causes. With upper left quadrant pain, possible sources include a ruptured spleen from a sickle cell crisis and mononucleosis. Patients with lower left abdominal pain, especially if they have a history of constipation, nausea, vomiting, and fever, should be suspected of having diverticulitis. With lower right abdominal pain, appendicitis is a likely culprit. Generalized abdominal pain in women of childbearing age can be the result of an ectopic pregnancy, a ruptured ovarian cyst, or some other obstetric or gynecologic problem.

During the focused physical examination, along with history taking, obtain a full set of vital signs, including an auscultated blood pressure, accurate pulse and respiratory rates, and the patient's temperature. Use other diagnostic tools as indicated.

Baseline vital signs are an integral part of any focused history and physical examination. Clues provided will help you determine the seriousness of the patient's condition and the function of internal organs. Remember that shock, whether medical or trauma-related, is seen in different stages. Changes in a patient's blood pressure may be the last piece of evidence paramedics see when shock changes from one level to the next. Keep in mind that blood pressure must be sufficient to maintain adequate end-organ perfusion.

Orthostatic vital signs and the tilt test are measurements of a patient's blood pressure and pulse that are taken in the supine and sitting or standing positions. The results of such a test can help you determine the extent of volume depletion. The tilt test is generally used for patients with complaints of nausea, vomiting, diarrhea, syncope, and potential gastrointestinal problems; it indicates whether the patient needs fluid replacement. Normally, baroreceptors in the body sense changes in the blood pressure and volume and stimulate a catecholamine and renin-aldosterone response. This, in turn, causes peripheral vasoconstriction, increased heart rate, and fluid retention, which puts more blood into core circulation and increases volume. In patients who are volume-depleted, there is not enough circulating blood to push into the core circulation, especially when they move from a supine position to sitting or standing.

In some studies, a tilt test or orthostatic change is considered positive when the patient's blood pressure shows a decrease in systolic pressure (up to 20 mm Hg), an increase in

Focused History
and Physical Examination

At the Scene

Many technological devices are available to paramedics to aid in patient assessment. While they are excellent equipment, always remember that you are assessing a patient—not a machine. Take the time to explain what your tools are and why you are using them. This simple action may help lessen patient anxiety.

diastolic pressure of 10 mm Hg (a narrowing pulse pressure), and an increase in heart rate by 20 beats/min. Vital signs should be taken at 1-minute intervals between moving a patient to a new position, and the cuff should be placed on the same arm in the same location. Documentation should include whether the pulse was regular, if the patient is being monitored and there is an attached strip, and whether the patient is experiencing other symptoms. If fluid replacement is given, paramedics should repeat the orthostatic assessment.

An Unresponsive Medical Patient

With an unresponsive medical patient, you start at a disadvantage in your assessment because your most reliable source of information—the patient—can't answer your questions. Owing to this serious limitation, assessment of an unresponsive medical patient looks much like a trauma assessment. You must rely on a thorough head-to-toe physical examination plus the normal diagnostic tools (pulse oximetry, capnography, cardiac monitor, and glucometer) to acquire the information needed to care for your patient. If family or friends are present, they may be able to provide information about the chief complaint, history of the present illness, past medical history, and possibly current health status. Nevertheless, the information they offer is almost never as good as that provided directly by the patient.

After completing the initial assessment, and assuming you have ruled out trauma, position unresponsive medical patients in the recovery position (left lateral recumbent position) to facilitate drainage of vomit, blood, or other fluids and to help prevent aspiration. If trauma is a factor, position the patient in neutral alignment, place a properly sized and fitted rigid cervical collar, and implement spinal motion restriction procedures as per the local protocol.

Perform a thorough assessment of the head, neck, chest, abdomen, pelvis, posterior body, and extremities, looking for signs of illness such as rash or urticaria, fever, unusual or excessive bruising, pulmonary or peripheral edema, and irregular pulse. Follow up your examination with at least two sets of vital signs—one taken now and another taken a few minutes after you've started your initial interventions (such as supplemental oxygen and IV therapy). The first set establishes a baseline (baseline vital signs); the second and additional sets (serial vital signs) provide comparative data to help you evaluate whether the patient's condition is improving, status quo, or worsening. If time allows, additional sets of vital signs add further data, allowing you to map trends (such as a progressively

increasing pulse rate). Make sure the vital signs include an auscultated blood pressure, accurate pulse and respiratory rates, and the patient's temperature. A recheck of breath sounds is always a prudent choice as well.

Unconscious, unresponsive medical patients should always be considered in unstable condition and at high risk, so rapid transport to the appropriate facility is indicated. Throughout transport, perform ongoing assessment, which includes rechecking the ABCs and reassessing anything associated with the patient's chief complaint.

Trauma Patients

Focused History and Physical Examination

Trauma patients may be classified into two major groups: patients with an isolated injury and patients with multisystem trauma. The biggest difference from an assessment perspective is that an isolated injury allows you to immediately focus on the main problem. In contrast, with multisystem trauma, you must first find all (or as many as you can reasonably find) of the various problems (for example, a hematoma on the forehead, a fractured arm, and neck and lower back pain). Then you need to prioritize the injuries by severity and the order in which you plan to address them. During the assessment, you must continually think about how each injury or condition relates to the others. For example, the mortality rate for a patient with a serious traumatic brain injury who has just a single episode of hypotension doubles. In such a case, not recognizing and addressing the hypotension and the lack of adequate perfusion pressure has a huge impact—in some cases, a fatal impact.

Another important consideration is the "high visibility factor" of many injuries, which sometimes creates a visual distraction. A compound fracture of the lower leg and ankle, with the foot twisted sideways and jammed under the brake pedal in a car, is not a pretty sight—but it is not a life-threatening injury. Because of the visual distraction, you might focus on the grossly deformed ankle and miss the early signs and symptoms of shock caused by the internal injuries and bleeding that you can't see.

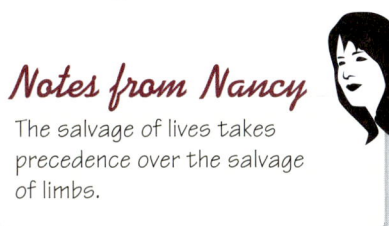

Notes from Nancy

The salvage of lives takes precedence over the salvage of limbs.

As you move into the focused history and physical examination of a trauma patient, quickly revisit all of the information from your initial assessment, including reconsidering the mechanism of injury. Collectively, these data may help you identify patients who need to be priority transports to the trauma centre.

A number of mechanisms have the potential to produce life-threatening injuries **Figure 14-8 ▶**:

- Ejection from *any* vehicle (car, motorcycle, or all-terrain vehicle)
- Death of another patient in the same passenger compartment

Focused History and Physical Examination

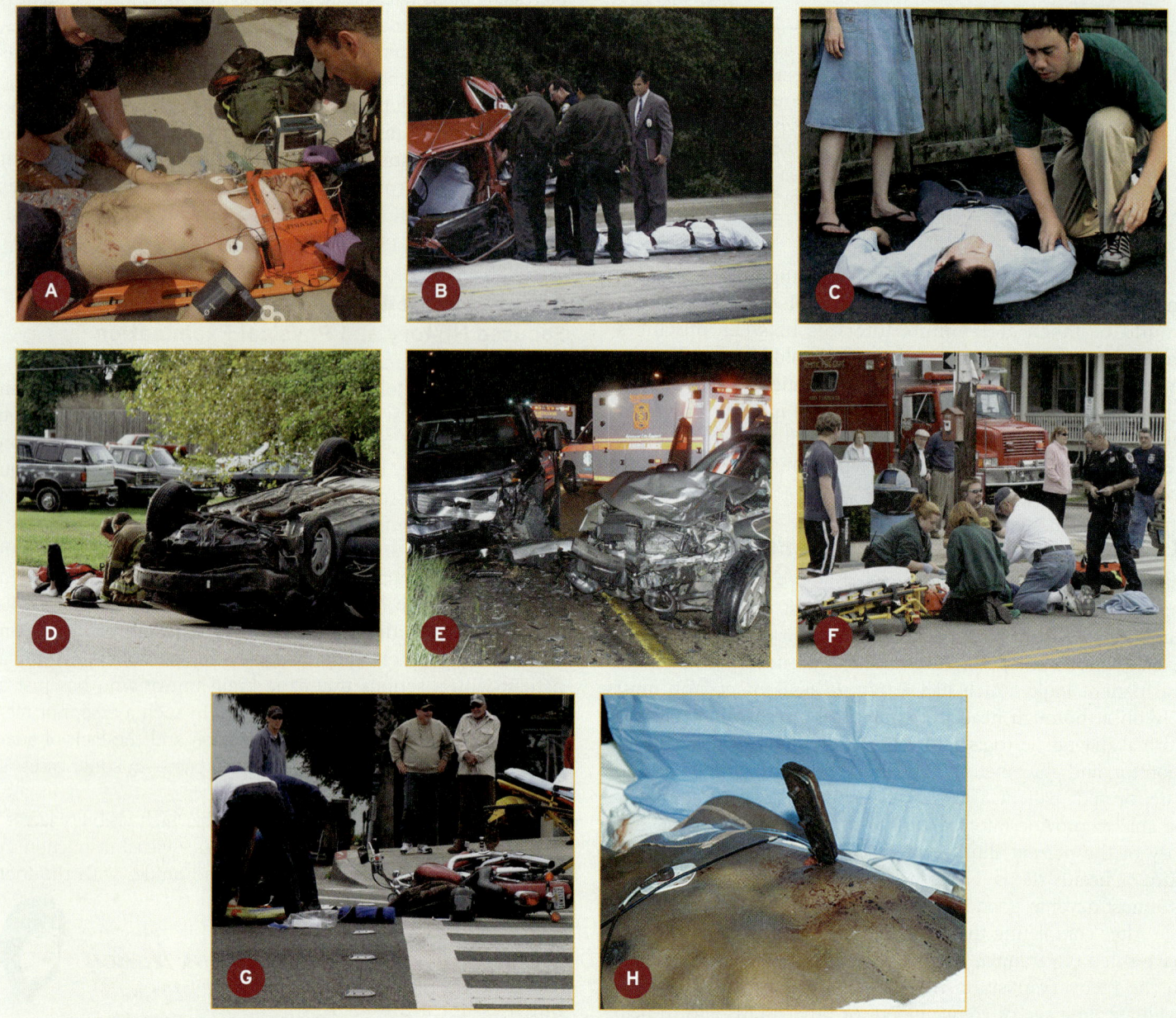

Figure 14-8 Significant mechanisms of injury. **A.** Ejection from *any* vehicle (car, motorcycle, ATV). **B.** Death of another patient in the same passenger compartment. **C.** Falls from more than 7 m. **D.** Vehicle rollover. **E.** High-speed motor vehicle collision. **F.** Vehicle-pedestrian collision. **G.** Motorcycle collisions. **H.** Penetrating wounds to the head, chest, or abdomen.

- Falls from more than 7 m (or three times the patient's height)
- Vehicle rollover (unrestrained occupant)
- High-speed motor vehicle collision
- Vehicle–pedestrian collision
- Motorcycle collision
- Penetrating wounds to the head, chest, or abdomen

If the patient is an infant or a child, mechanisms of injury that would indicate a high-priority patient include falls from more than 3 m, a bicycle collision, or being struck by a vehicle **Figure 14-9 ▶** .

In many cases, multiple mechanisms of injury have come into play—for example, a T-bone collision that leaves the patient with a crushed upper arm and pelvic girdle and also penetrating trauma from the piece of door trim impaled in his chest. A patient with any of the previously mentioned mechanisms should immediately raise your index of suspicion. Two or more mechanisms of injury markedly increase the chance of a patient sustaining a serious or fatal injury.

Several other mechanisms of injury are also worth considering. Seatbelts, even when properly positioned, can cause injuries as the car and its occupants decelerate in a collision.

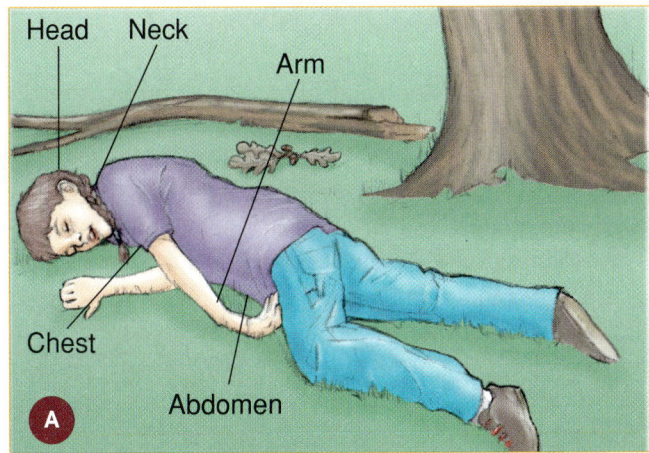

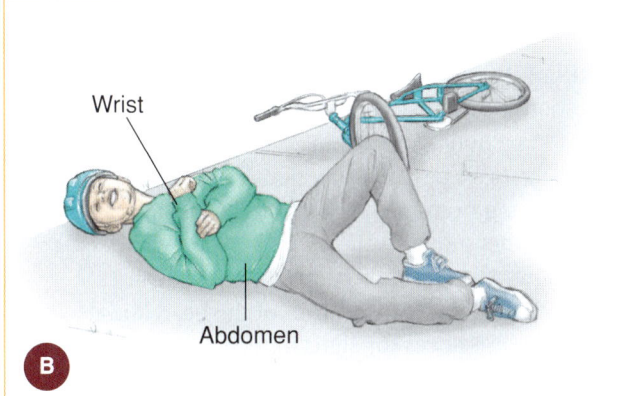

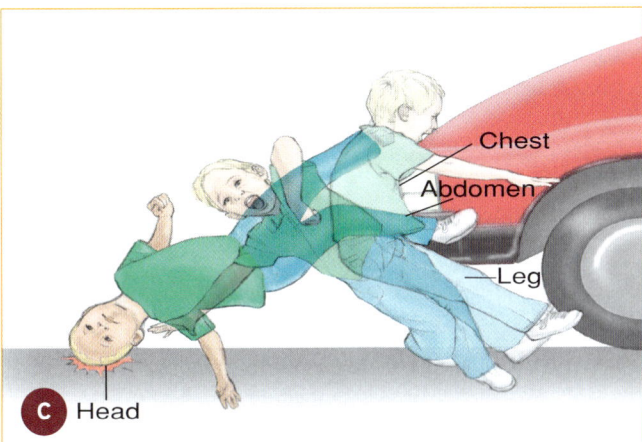

Figure 14-9 Significant mechanisms of injury for an infant or child. **A.** Falls from more than 3 m. **B.** Bicycle collision. **C.** Pedestrian–vehicle collision.

Check the clavicles where the shoulder strap crosses. The clavicles are small bones, and the subclavian vein and arteries run directly underneath them. In shorter patients, the shoulder strap mounted on the B column in a car can ride up across the neck, increasing the risk of soft-tissue and cervical spine injury. Examine the area where the lap belt crosses the pelvic girdle. If the belt is not across the iliac spine but has ridden up over the lower abdomen, the patient has an increased risk of organ damage and thoracic or lumbar spine injury. Passengers who

tuck the shoulder harness under their arms for comfort and are then involved in rollover accidents are at high risk of death from liver injuries caused by the improperly positioned belt.

Airbags have saved countless lives, but many people don't realize that an airbag is a secondary restraint system, designed to work with seatbelts to reduce injuries. When the seatbelt is not used and a collision occurs, the airbag deploys, momentarily catching the patient. As the airbag deflates, it releases the driver or passenger, who continues moving forward and may go down-and-under (into the dashboard) or up-and-over (into the steering wheel and/or windshield). When working any collision with airbag deployment, lift the bag and look underneath for a bent steering wheel—another potential source of life-threatening internal injuries. Be very cautious when accessing patients in the front compartment of a vehicle where the air bag has not deployed even though damage to the vehicle indicates that it should have. Air bags can deploy spontaneously, causing severe injury or death to the patient or rescuer.

Child safety seats have also saved countless lives **Figure 14-10 ▶**. If they are improperly installed or positioned in the vehicle, however, they can be rendered useless as a safety device. If the car seat comes loose during a collision, the risk of face, head, neck, and spine trauma to the child increases markedly. Similarly, if the child is too large or too small for the seat, the seat will not provide the intended level of protection.

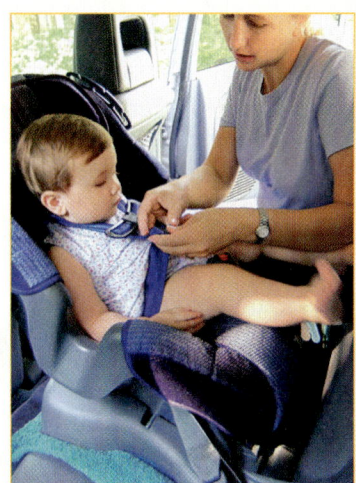

Figure 14-10 A child should be properly positioned in a car seat in the rear seats of the vehicle.

Any trauma patient who is unresponsive or has altered mental status should be considered a high-risk, priority patient and requires immediate transport to a trauma centre. An unconscious, unresponsive patient may have a traumatic brain injury, stroke, hypoglycemia, or alcohol or drug intoxication. All are bad—even potentially lethal—events, with some (such as traumatic brain injury) being devastating injuries.

Rapid Trauma Assessment

The rapid trauma assessment is a specialized tool that is typically sandwiched between the initial assessment and the focused physical examination of a trauma patient. This assessment is usually performed on patients with any significant mechanism of injury. As with any aspect of patient assessment involving inspection, always stay alert for any medical alert bracelets or devices and take note of any scars indicating that the patient has had open heart surgery or had a pacemaker or automated internal cardioverter-defibrillator implanted in the chest wall.

The rapid trauma assessment is usually performed after the initial assessment and all life threats to airway, breathing, and circulation have been identified and addressed. If the patient is responsive, identify the chief complaint(s) and symptoms, and then use this information to guide and direct your assessment. Give the patient who has been involved in any kind of significant traumatic event a quick once-over from head-to-toe by performing a rapid trauma assessment. Keep in mind that the most visible injury you may be looking at (the scalp laceration) or the most painful injury the patient complains about (the fractured and dislocated ankle) may not be nearly as serious as the most lethal injury the patient has (the ruptured spleen). A splenic injury, for example, is less visible and less painful than the other two injuries.

Before you begin the rapid trauma assessment, make sure that the patient's cervical spine is manually immobilized in the neutral position. Quickly reassess the patient's current mental status, comparing it with the baseline you established when you first encountered the patient. Last, revisit your transport decision. If you decide the patient needs immediate transport, you should perform the rapid trauma assessment while the patient is being immobilized and prepared for transport, so that the moment you get the patient loaded, you can head to the hospital.

The model of rapid trauma assessment discussed here is organized and systematic. While it isn't the only way to perform such an assessment, it's a good way to do one. **Skill Drill 14-1 ▶** shows the steps of the rapid trauma assessment, which are also described in the following paragraphs. As you evaluate each region, use the mnemonic, DCAP-BTLS:

1. Start the rapid trauma assessment at the patient's head, inspecting and palpating the skull for any asymmetry (such as knots, depressions) or bleeding (Step 1).

2. Palpate down the posterior cervical spine, feeling for any step-offs or knock-offs and looking for any signs of trauma (Step 2). Be alert for a facial grimace or moan that may be a clue of tenderness on the cervical spine.

3. Quickly look in and behind the patient's ears for blood, cerebrospinal fluid (CSF), or bruising (all signs of a possible skull fracture or traumatic brain injury) (Step 3). Move your head to look; *don't turn the patient's head.*

4. Check the pupils, and quickly palpate the orbits, doing both sides in unison. Feel from the nose out to the lateral edge, including upper and lower ridges (Step 4).

5. Inspect the nose for bleeding and other signs of trauma (Step 5).

6. Assess the mouth for blood or other fluids that may need suctioning (Step 6). Ask a responsive patient to run the tongue around the inside of the teeth to feel whether anything seems to be broken or displaced. If the patient is unresponsive, open the mouth and look for injury or a need for suctioning.

7. Assess the neck for JVD, subcutaneous emphysema (a sign of air leaking from the chest), or tracheal shift (a very late sign of a pneumothorax) (Step 7). Note whether a medical identification tag is present.

8. On completing your inspection of the head and neck, examine your gloves for signs of bleeding, and place a properly sized rigid cervical collar (Step 8).

9. Inspect and palpate the chest. Place your thumbs in the suprasternal notch and follow both clavicles out to the shoulder girdle, keeping the clavicles (commonly fractured bones) between your thumb and finger. This technique

You are the Paramedic Part 4

You are providing supplemental high-flow oxygen at 12 l/min via a nonrebreathing mask and infusing normal saline at 30 ml/h. The patient's heart is in sinus rhythm, and you have not intubated him. The end-tidal carbon dioxide detector reads 34 mm Hg with a normal waveform.

Upon arrival at the hospital, the patient is transferred to the care of the emergency department staff with no change in his status. Blood is drawn, and all laboratory values are unremarkable, including the drug screen, which comes back negative. However, the patient remains unconscious for approximately 2 hours.

Reassessment	Recording Time: 20 Minutes
Level of consciousness	Glasgow Coma Scale score of 7
Skin	Pink, warm, and moist
Pulse	72 beats/min, regular
Blood pressure	104/68 mm Hg
Respirations	24 breaths/min with adequate depth
SpO$_2$	100% on supplemental oxygen
Pupils	3 mm/PEARRL

7. If no initial diagnosis is possible, what should your prehospital care goals be?

8. Under normal circumstances, when an abrupt loss of consciousness occurs, which four primary probabilities should you consider as part of your rule-out diagnosis?

allows you to feel most of the entire length of the bone while maintaining continuous contact (Step 9). At the same time, inspect the chest for symmetrical rise and fall and for any signs of retractions or other excessive "work of breathing."

10. Gently place your palm on the sternum; press down and then side-to-side to check stability as you assess for a flail chest or fractured sternum (Step 10).

11. Barrel-hoop the rib cage under the armpits and then at the costal margin to assess for fractured ribs (commonly broken bones) or a flail chest (Step 11). Be firm but gentle. Fractured ribs are painful enough without undue pressure being placed on them. If you find large bruised areas, make special mental note: You may be looking at a flail segment but one that does not show the classic paradoxical ("seesaw") movement because the body is still "splinting" the segment with muscle spasm.

12. If you log roll the patient to move him or her to a backboard, examine and palpate the thoracic and lumbar spine for step-offs or knock-offs as you also look for puncture wounds or other signs of trauma (Step 12).

13. Inspect and palpate all four quadrants of the abdomen, being alert for rigidity, guarding, bruising, and tenderness (Step 13). While you are palpating the abdomen, be alert for a grimace or moan from the patient, which indicates that you touched something that caused pain or discomfort. Given the number of organs in and adjacent to the abdomen, one or more is likely to be injured in any significant traumatic event. Be quick but thorough with your assessment of the abdomen.

14. Move to the pelvic girdle, and gently but firmly assess flexion and compression by pressing down and then inward on the iliac crest, feeling for any sign (instability or pain) that the pelvic girdle is damaged (Step 14).

15. Gently palpate over the bladder (Step 15). If the groin area is wet or bloody or if the patient complains of pain in the area, quickly examine the groin and the genitalia.

16. Inspect and palpate both lower extremities from hip to ankle, looking for signs of bleeding or swelling (Step 16). Note whether one extremity is shorter than the other or if either or both are rotated abnormally (signs of fracture or dislocation).

17. After you have inspected and palpated both legs, simultaneously assess pedal pulses (Step 17), noting whether they feel similar. A difference in pulse quality (one weaker than the other) points to a potentially serious vascular disruption. Bilateral loss of motor function suggests a spinal cord injury, whereas unilateral loss of function is most likely musculoskeletal in origin, except in the case of a suspected stroke. In a responsive patient, check motor function and sensation of the extremities as well (distal pulse, motor function, and sensation).

18. Check your gloves for blood (Step 18).

19. Inspect and palpate the arms, and assess the pulse, motor function, and sensation (Step 19) just as you did with the legs. Check for a medical identification tag.

20. Check your gloves for blood (Step 20).

21. Assess the back. You can slide your hands under the retroperitoneal area to palpate the bottom of the thoracic spine and some of the lumbar spine. Unless you log roll the patient, however, you won't be able to inspect and palpate the entire back. Inspect and palpate the back to whatever extent you can (Step 21).

22. One last time, check your gloves for blood (Step 22).

When you complete the rapid trauma assessment, obtain a set of baseline vital signs. If you have the resources, have another paramedic take the vital signs while you do your rapid trauma assessment; it is efficient, saves time, and is a good practice.

Also, mentally compile a list of all that you now know about your patient, including the chief complaint, the history of the present event, the medical history, and any information about the patient's current health status. Combine that knowledge with the other information and insights you have gained from your various assessments, along with the information obtained from your diagnostics, and you should have more than enough information to make good clinical choices for your patient.

The rapid trauma assessment will help you find any life threats you may have missed in the initial assessment, but it needs to be done quickly. While it generally follows the pattern of a detailed physical examination, the rapid trauma assessment is much, much quicker. A detailed physical examination can take 15 minutes or more; with practice, you can perform a rapid trauma assessment in 2 or 3 minutes. *But you must understand that it takes lots and lots of practice* (Figure 14-11 ▾).

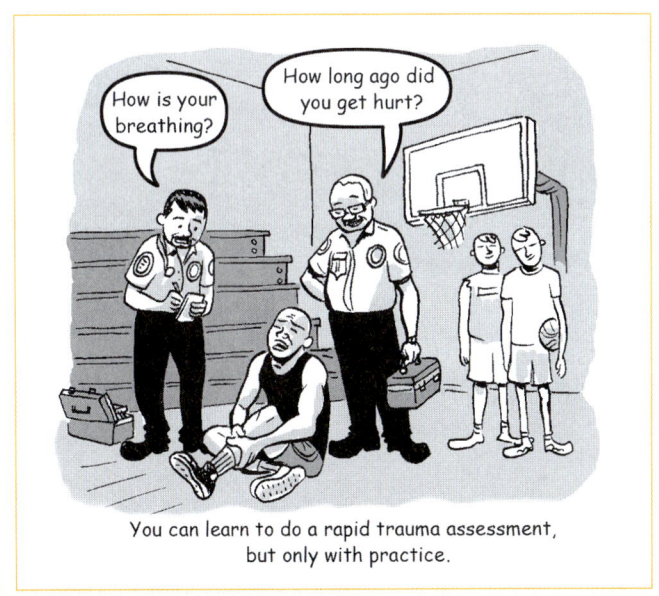

You can learn to do a rapid trauma assessment, but only with practice.

Figure 14-11

Focused History
and Physical Examination

Skill Drill 14-1: The Rapid Trauma Assessment

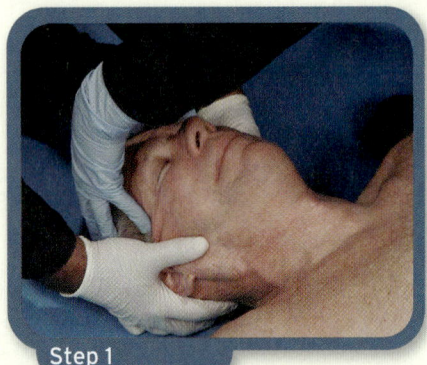

Step 1

Inspect and palpate the skull.

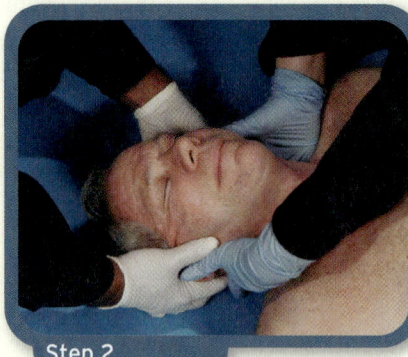

Step 2

Palpate down the posterior cervical spine.

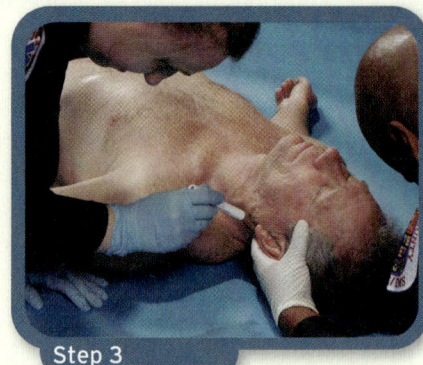

Step 3

Look in and behind the patient's ears.

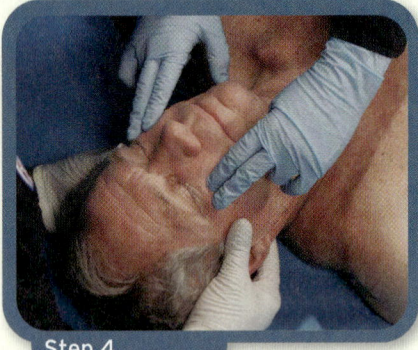

Step 4

Check the pupils, and quickly palpate the orbits.

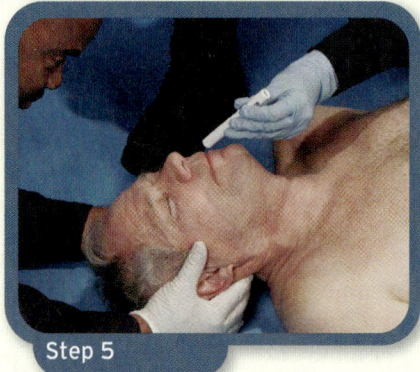

Step 5

Inspect the nose.

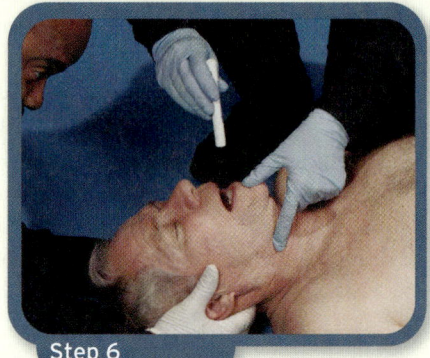

Step 6

Assess the mouth.

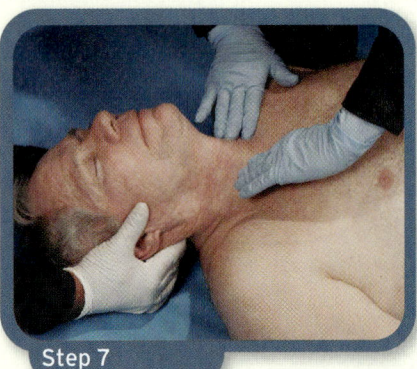

Step 7

Assess the neck.

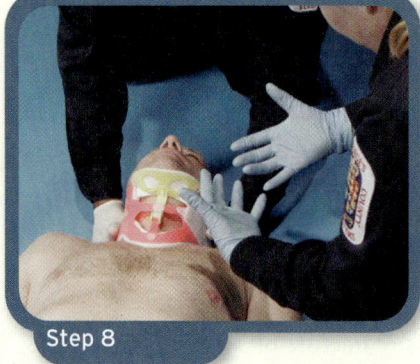

Step 8

Check your gloves for any signs of bleeding. Place a properly sized rigid cervical collar.

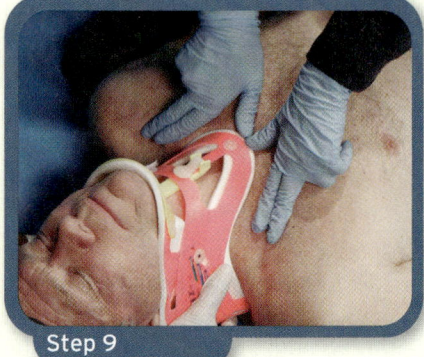

Step 9

Inspect and palpate the chest.

Skill Drill 14-1: The Rapid Trauma Assessment (*continued*)

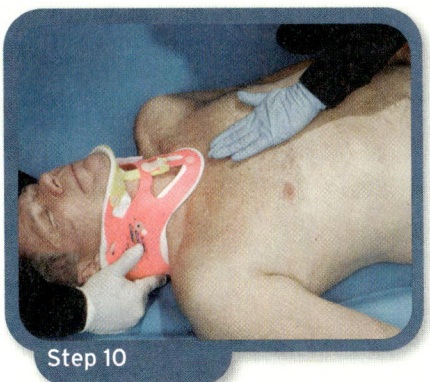

Step 10

Assess for a flail chest or fractured sternum.

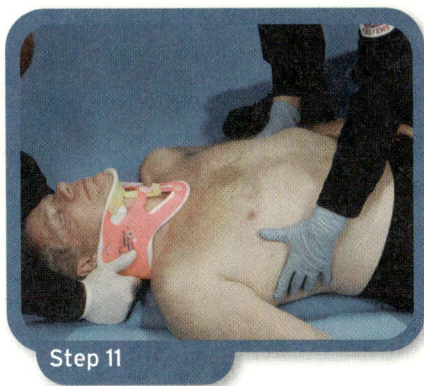

Step 11

Assess for fractured ribs or a flail chest.

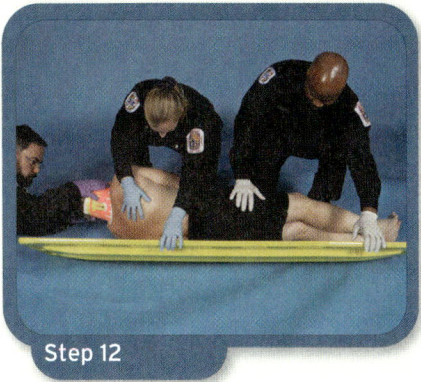

Step 12

If you log roll the patient to a backboard, examine and palpate the thoracic and lumbar spine.

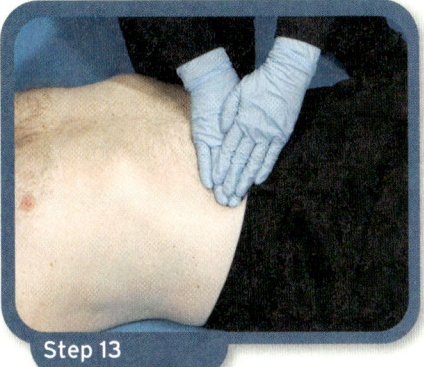

Step 13

Inspect and palpate all four quadrants of the abdomen.

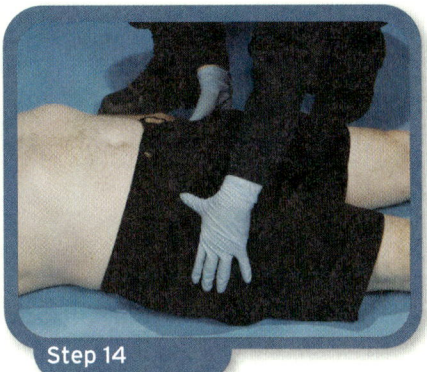

Step 14

Assess the pelvic girdle.

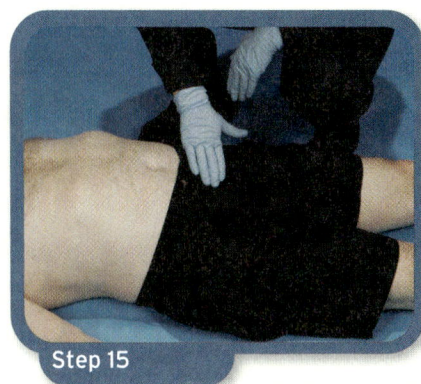

Step 15

Palpate over the bladder.

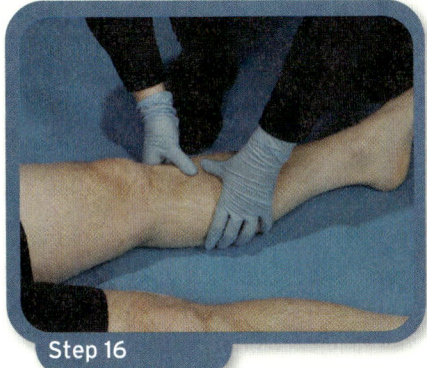

Step 16

Inspect and palpate both lower extremities from hip to ankle.

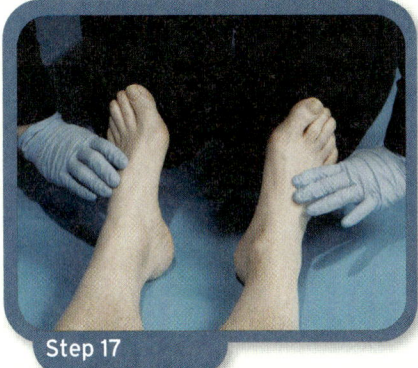

Step 17

Simultaneously assess pedal pulses.

Focused History and Physical Examination

You are the Paramedic Part 5

As the neurosurgeon begins evaluation of the patient, he shakes the patient's big toe and speaks to him. To his surprise, Mike says, "I'm fine, thank you!" On reassessment of his mental status, the patient receives a GCS score of 15 and shows no neurologic deficits. A comprehensive assessment by the neurosurgeon includes a computed tomography scan and magnetic resonance imaging, both with negative results.

The patient was discharged home, allowed to return to school the following day, and cleared for athletic activities 1 week later. No final determination for the transient loss of consciousness was identified.

Skill Drill 14-1: The Rapid Trauma Assessment (*continued*)

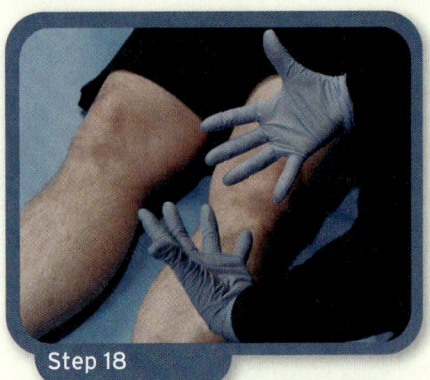

Step 18

Check your gloves for blood.

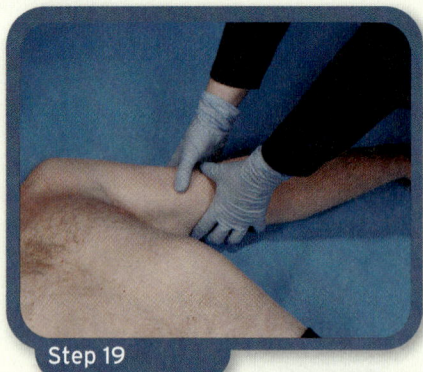

Step 19

Inspect and palpate the arms, and assess pulse, motor function, and sensation.

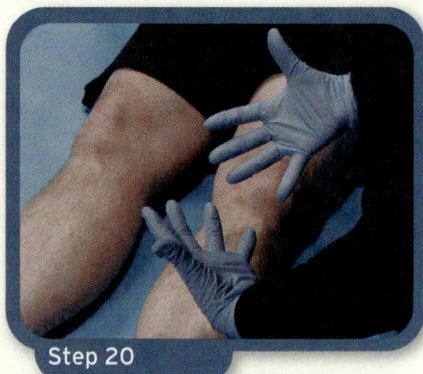

Step 20

Check your gloves for blood.

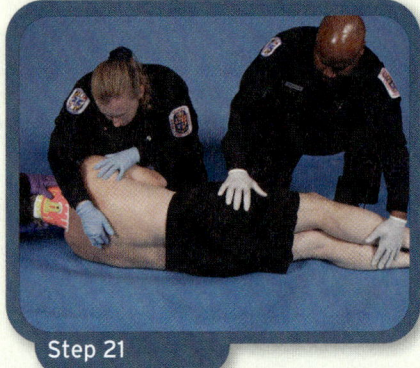

Step 21

Inspect and palpate the back.

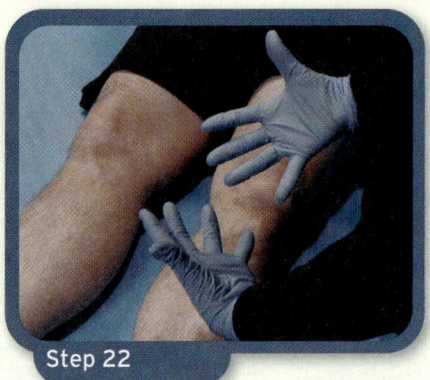

Step 22

Check your gloves for blood.

At the Scene

It may be difficult to assess the stability of a large patient's chest for paradoxical motion. Try fanning out the fingers of both of your hands as wide as possible; then assess the up-and-down motion of the patient's breathing. This will give you a better assessment of equality and movement of the chest with respiration.

Patients With Minor Injuries or No Significant Mechanism of Injury

Most trauma calls involve patients with a single, isolated injury or, on occasion, several minor injuries. In almost all of these cases, the lack of serious or critical injuries is consistent with the lack of a significant mechanism of injury: A collision on the basketball court results in a sprained ankle; a skater crashes and ends up with a Colles fracture; a loose piece of metal spins off a lathe in the machine shop, lacerating the machinist's forearm. Patients should not show any signs of systemic involvement (hypotension). If they do, there is more going on than an isolated injury. You need to continue with your assessment with the goal of finding the more serious problem.

Patient Assessment

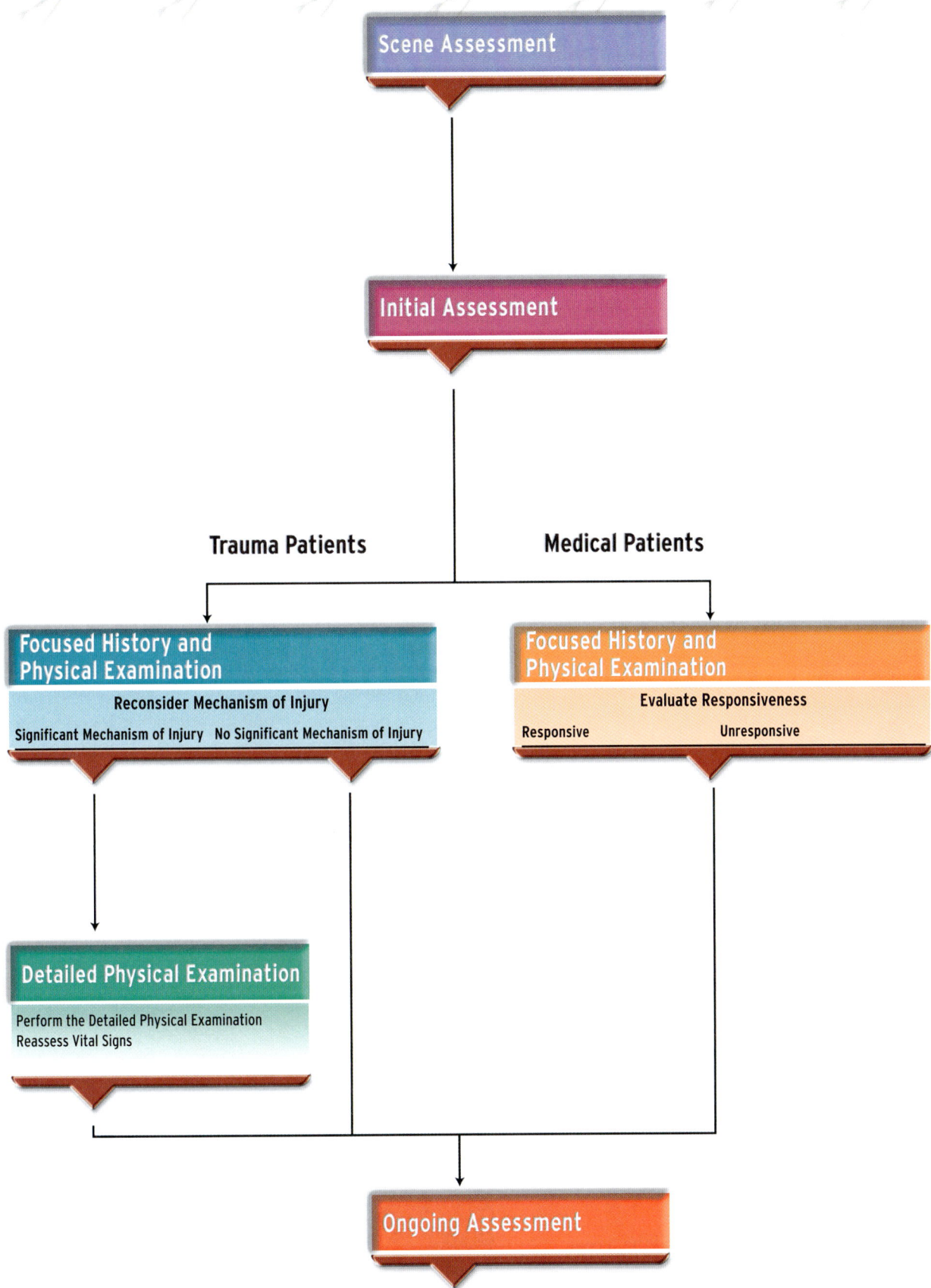

Scene Assessment

Initial Assessment

Trauma Patients

Medical Patients

Focused History and Physical Examination

Reconsider Mechanism of Injury

Significant Mechanism of Injury · No Significant Mechanism of Injury

Focused History and Physical Examination

Evaluate Responsiveness

Responsive · Unresponsive

Detailed Physical Examination

Perform the Detailed Physical Examination
Reassess Vital Signs

Ongoing Assessment

The Detailed Physical Examination

The detailed physical examination is another specialized form of patient assessment. In many cases, you won't need to do this assessment (such as for a finger laceration) or won't have time (such as when you have a patient in serious or critical condition). The detailed physical examination can take 15 minutes or more to gather a more detailed and comprehensive history and perform a detailed and thorough physical examination (such as checking range of motion [ROM]).

In the majority of cases when you perform a detailed physical examination, it will be done on a trauma patient en route when you have extended transport time (usually more than 15 minutes). Frequently, you will find yourself modifying the examination based on the patient's chief complaint. Use this tool as you see fit—or not at all, if you don't think it will provide meaningful information.

The detailed physical examination can be stressful and produce anxiety in patients because you are asking them to divulge personal information to a paramedic they have known for 10 minutes, and they would normally share such information only with their personal physician, whom they may have known for 10 years. Be respectful of patients' privacy, and maintain your most professional demeanor as you perform a detailed physical examination.

As you prepare to perform this examination, you will want to review the patient data gathered when you identified the chief complaint and performed the initial assessment. Add in the history of the present illness, the medical history, and the current health status. Keeping this information in mind will help keep you focused and on task as you delve into your patient's problem(s).

A detailed physical examination seeks to define complaints or problems that were not identified in the focused history and physical examination. During this process, paramedics reevaluate any treatment that is under way, based on new information gathered. New treatments are also started to deal with problems found during the detailed physical examination. In addition, paramedics reevaluate the patient's vital signs and assess trends in any changes.

Begin your detailed physical examination by evaluating the patient's mental status:

- Is the patient's appearance and behaviour appropriate?
- How is the patient's posture and general motor behaviour?
- Evaluate the patient's speech and language by listening to what the patient says and how he or she says it.
- Pay attention to the patient's thought process and perceptions.
- Assess the insights the patient does or does not have, along with the judgments the patient makes. (The patient is really sick but doesn't want to go to the hospital today ". . . but maybe tomorrow.")
- Assess memory and attention in the remote and the recent domains. For example, ask about memorable past birthdays, then about the events of the day.
- Evaluate new learning ability. For example, give the patient a simple phrase to remember (such as "You can't teach an

old dog new tricks" or "Jack and Jill went up the hill") and explain that you plan to ask the patient about the phrase in a little while. Wait 5 minutes and do just that.

After you complete the mental status examination, begin the general survey of the patient. Assess the patient's LOC and compare it with baseline data. Has the LOC changed? If so, how? What is the skin colour? Are there any visible lesions? Look carefully at the patient's facial expression. Does the patient show obvious signs of anxiety or distress, or does the patient look pale and lethargic as if he or she might be in end-stage shock? Assess the patient's apparent state of health and ask yourself that all-important question: "Sick or not sick?" (In the case of trauma, this question becomes "Hurt or not hurt?")

Other considerations covered in the detailed physical examination include the following:

- The patient's height and weight (Are they proportional to the patient's build?)
- Dress, grooming, and personal hygiene
- General posture, gait, and motor activity
- Unusual breath or body odours
- Skin colour, temperature, moisture, and turgor

Head and Face

Start your hands-on assessment at the patient's head. Inspect and feel the entire cranium for signs of deformity or asymmetry, being careful not to palpate any depressions, lest you push bone fragments into the cranial vault or the brain **Figure 14-12 ▾**. Note any warm, wet areas; they usually represent blood, CSF, or a combination of the two.

Carefully inspect and palpate the upper and lower orbits, starting at the nose and working toward the lateral edge. Assess the eyes for shape and symmetry, and check the pupils for size and reactivity (fixed, dilated, sluggish). Evaluate whether the eyes move in harmony (conjugate gaze) and whether they can track in all fields (up, down, left, right, across). Note periorbital ecchymosis (raccoon's eyes).

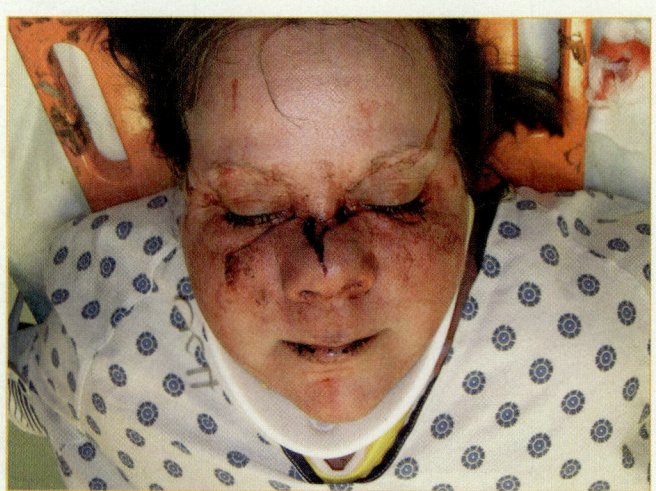

Figure 14-12 Do not palpate any depressions in the skin; you could push bone fragments into the cranial vault or brain.

Inspect and palpate the nose for structural integrity, and look inside for signs of trauma and fluids that may need suctioning. If there is drainage, determine whether it is bloody or clear (in which case, it could be mucus or CSF). Inspect and palpate the maxilla and the mandible, assessing the integrity and symmetry of both structures. Open the mouth, and look for signs of trauma (such as cracked or missing teeth, missing crowns or on-lays). Check the bite for fit. Be alert for any unusual odours on the patient's breath (such as alcohol or ketones). Check the posterior pharynx for fluids that may need to be suctioned.

Check in, around, and behind the ears for fluids or bruising (Battle's sign). Look carefully into the ear canal, and examine the structure of the ear for signs of trauma. Inspect the anterior part of the neck, assessing for JVD, swelling, and other signs of trauma. Assess for midline placement of the trachea.

Chest and Lungs

Before starting the physical examination of the chest, look at the overall symmetry, then assess for equal rise and fall, and finally look for retractions, accessory muscle use, and other signs of increased work of breathing. Remember—flail segments may not have paradoxical movement early on due to the splinting effect of muscle spasms. When you reassess lung sounds later, look for signs of flail segments that may just be presenting.

Inspect and palpate the clavicles from the suprasternal notch out to the shoulder girdles. Assess the ROM of the acromioclavicular joint. Confirm that the sternum is structurally intact. By using the flat surface of your palms, barrel-hoop the rib cage, feeling for asymmetry, deformities, and unstable segments, and evaluate the overall integrity of the chest wall. If the environment is quiet enough, percuss the chest for hyperresonance (pneumothorax, asthma, chronic obstructive pulmonary disease) and hyporesonance (hemothorax). Finally, assess breath sounds in a minimum of six fields.

Cardiovascular System

Check and compare distal pulses. Reassess the skin condition for pallor and diaphoresis (signs of sympathetic discharge). Be alert for patients with sustained bradycardia (which lowers blood pressure and may decrease the patient's mental state) or tachycardia (increases cardiac workload and may lower blood pressure). Run a 3-lead ECG for all patients with a cardiac history. If the patient has a significant heart history and you have the time, acquire a 12-lead ECG. It would be tragic to miss an evolving MI due to hypotension caused by trauma. If the environment is quiet enough, consider auscultating for abnormal heart sounds.

Abdomen

Start your assessment of the abdomen by inspecting the entire area for signs of swelling or bruising. Bluish discolouration in the periumbilical area (Cullen's sign) is indicative of intraperitoneal hemorrhage, with two of the more common causes being ruptured ectopic pregnancy and acute pancreatitis. Look for a rash or other signs of an allergic reaction. Take note of scars from previous trauma or surgeries.

Palpate each quadrant gently but firmly, and recognize that the patient may respond in many ways. A moan, a guarding posture or withdrawing, or a facial grimace all send the same message: You have touched something or somewhere that causes pain or discomfort. That information is worth pursuing with your assessment. Consider any signs or symptoms of abdominal injury as serious and indicative of a high-priority patient in unstable condition.

Rebound tenderness checks are rarely done in the prehospital setting primarily because they can be painful for the patient as you slowly push down and then rapidly release sections of the abdomen. A positive sign (the patient cries out or withdraws) indicates peritoneal irritation.

Genitalia

Unless the patient complains of pain or discomfort or of feeling that he or she is bleeding, there is no reason to examine the genitalia. If you note wetness or bleeding during your examination, you should examine the genitalia because these vascular organs can bleed extensively when injured. Take note of priapism in male patients; a prolonged erection is usually the result of a spinal cord injury.

In cases of sexual assault or rape, handle all clothing per local protocol and bag it with any other evidence (no biodegradable garbage bags). Sexual assault and rape have huge psychological impacts. Be as supportive, caring, and nonjudgmental as possible throughout your prehospital care for the patient. It is almost always helpful to have a paramedic who is the same sex as the patient involved in care. If that is not possible, however, do not delay prehospital care of the patient because of it.

Anus and Rectum

Unless the patient has a history or indication of trauma to the anus or rectum, there is generally no reason to examine this area. With a positive history or signs or symptoms of trauma, examine the area to assess for the need of bleeding control or another intervention (such as treatment for shock, care of eviscerated parts).

Peripheral Vascular System

Moving from the upper extremities to the lower limbs, inspect the extremities for asymmetry and any skin signs, such as bruising, pallor, mottling, or other signs of trauma. Check skin temperature and moisture. When you assess pulses in the extremities, do both sides simultaneously so that you can compare pulse strength, rate, and regularity from side to side. A significant variation in pulse strength in one extremity, especially when associated with pallor or cyanosis, points to vascular compromise.

Detailed Physical Examination

Musculoskeletal System

Start your assessment of the musculoskeletal system by performing a global inspection of the patient. Do all extremities appear to be properly positioned and functioning normally? If the patient is standing or seated, assess his or her posture for signs of scoliosis or the telltale lean of a suspected stroke. Look for redness or inflammation at the joints (signs of arthritis). Stay alert for red, swollen areas on the extremities, especially those that are warm to the touch (signs of a clot or thrombus).

Check the ROM. First, have patients move the extremities by themselves; significantly decreased ROM in this setting may be attributed to joint-related problems. Next, have patients work their extremities through a normal ROM, only this time with you providing resistance against their movements. Decreased or diminished ROM under these circumstances usually points to muscular weakness or atrophy or possibly problems with innervation. Assess for equality of grips.

Nervous System

The check of the nervous system is one of the most time-consuming elements of the detailed physical examination, mainly because it involves five separate miniassessments: mental status, motor response, cranial nerve function, reflexes, and sensory response.

The mental status examination essentially repeats the examination done in the rapid trauma assessment. Think of it as checking "mental vital signs." Assess the patient's LOC, and compare it with your baseline and any other LOC checks during other parts of your assessment. A handy mnemonic to guide you through the mental status examination is the mnemonic COASTMAP:

- **Consciousness.** Along with LOC, note the patient's ability to pay attention and concentrate. Is the patient easily distracted?
- **Orientation.** Ask about the year, season, month, day, and date. Have the patient identify the present location—that is, province, town, and specific location. Can the patient recall and describe the event(s) currently going on?
- **Activity.** Does the patient appear anxious or restless? Is he or she sitting very still, scarcely moving at all? Is he or she making any strange or repetitive motions (possibly because of methamphetamine use)?
- **Speech.** Note the rate, volume, articulation, and intonation of the patient's speech. Does it sound pressured? Does the speech have a flat, monotone delivery consistent with depression? Is the speech garbled or slurred (dysarthria)? Garbled or slurred speech may have many causes,

including alcohol or drug impairment, stroke, and head injury.

- **Thought.** Listen to the patient's story. What's on his or her mind? Is the patient making sense? Is there anything unusual about his or her reasoning? Is the patient expressing apparently false ideas (delusions)? Are voices telling the patient what to do or think (psychotic)? Does the patient report that people are "out to get me" (paranoia)?
- **Memory.** You can usually form an impression of the patient's memory by listening to his or her reconstruction of events. A more precise assessment requires asking a few questions. Ask the patient if you may test his or her memory. If the patient assents, slowly say the names of three unrelated subjects (such as apple, bicycle, sewing machine). Now ask the patient to repeat those words; that will test registration. A few minutes later, ask the patient if he or she can remember the three words you named before; that tests retention and memory.
- **Affect.** The patient's affect (mood) may be most apparent in his or her body language. The patient sitting with shoulders drooping and head bent, for example, conveys depression. Note whether the affect—the expression of inner feelings—seems appropriate to the situation.
- **Perception.** Detecting disorders of perception may be difficult because patients are often hesitant to answer questions about hallucinations. Sometimes it is helpful to ask the patient, "Do you ever hear things that other people can't hear?"

It is also helpful to assess the following:

- **Cranial nerves.** Quickly assess the cranial nerves, as described in Chapter 13.
- **Motor system.** Take an overall look at how the patient moves. Are his or her movements smooth or jerky? Note unusual or repetitive movements. Check for muscle strength by assessing bilateral grips.
- **Reflexes.** By using a reflex hammer, evaluate the patient's deep tendon reflexes in the knees and elbows for diminished or heightened responses. Additional reflex checks are probably not warranted in the prehospital environment.
- **Sensory system.** By using the appropriate tools, test the patient for pain (dull versus sharp), sensation, position, and vibration. Compare distal sensation and proximal sensation and one side with the other as you assess the dermatomes.

After completing this assessment, make certain that all assessment findings have been accurately recorded, take one more set of vital signs, and recheck breath sounds.

Patient Assessment

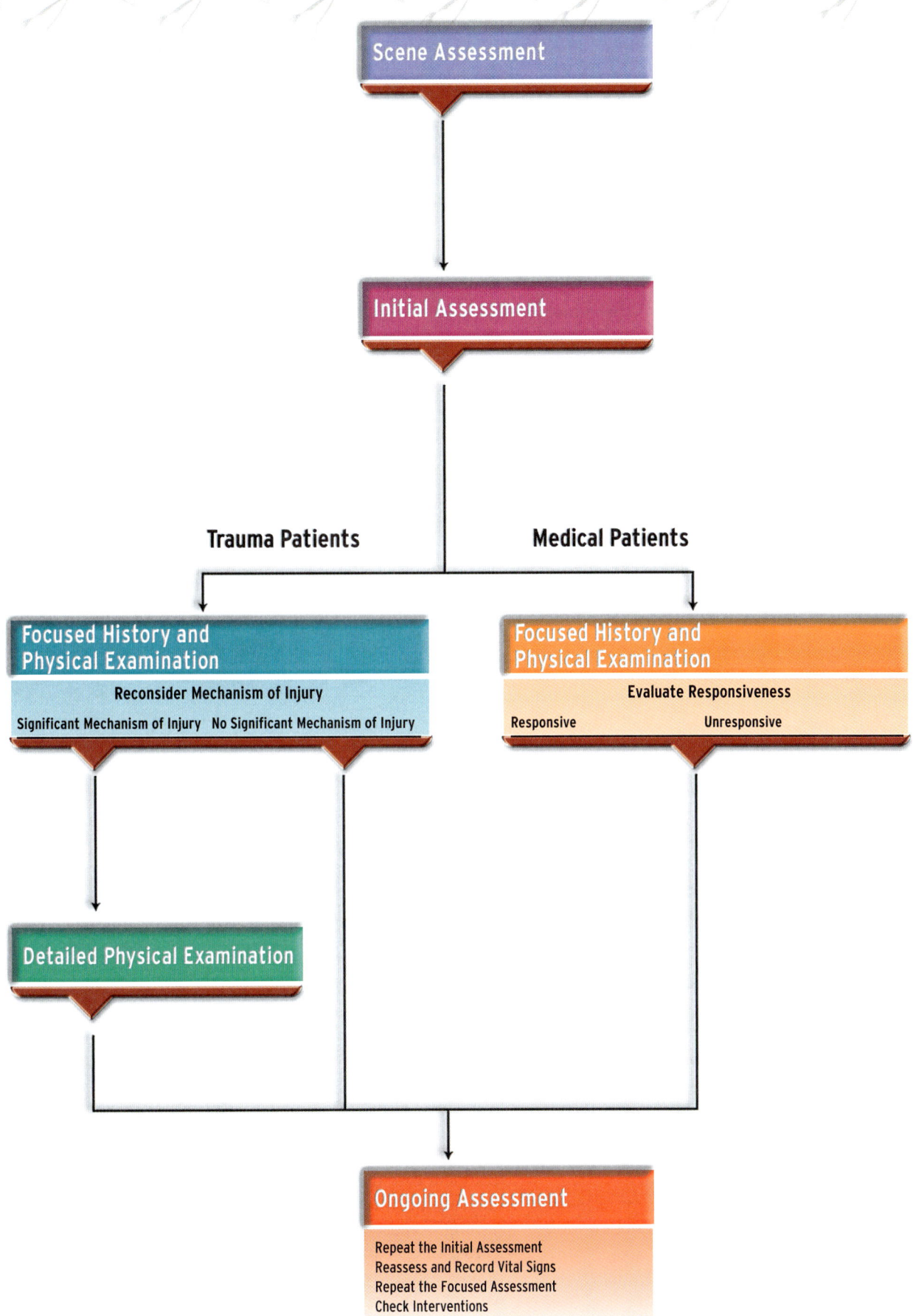

Scene Assessment

Initial Assessment

Trauma Patients

Medical Patients

Focused History and Physical Examination
Reconsider Mechanism of Injury
Significant Mechanism of Injury   No Significant Mechanism of Injury

Focused History and Physical Examination
Evaluate Responsiveness
Responsive   Unresponsive

Detailed Physical Examination

Ongoing Assessment
Repeat the Initial Assessment
Reassess and Record Vital Signs
Repeat the Focused Assessment
Check Interventions

The Ongoing Assessment

After the initial assessment, the ongoing assessment is the single most important assessment process you will perform. It represents a continuous, yet cyclical, process that you perform throughout transport, right up to the time you turn patient prehospital care over to the emergency department staff. For patients in stable condition, you should do an ongoing assessment every 15 minutes or so. For patients in unstable condition, you need to make a concerted effort to repeat the ongoing assessment every 5 minutes.

Reassessment of Mental Status and the ABCs

The ongoing assessment combines repetition of the initial assessment, reassessment of vital signs and breath sounds, and repetition of the focused assessment. During the ongoing assessment, you continue to evaluate and reevaluate the patient's status and any treatments already administered. Trends in the patient's current condition may give clues about the effectiveness of treatments: Have they improved the patient's condition? Are identified problems better or worse? This information indicates which changes have occurred and which critical conditions have been addressed and corrected.

First, compare the patient's LOC with your baseline assessment. Is the LOC changing? If so, how? If mentation is decreasing, can the patient still protect the airway? If you have doubts, consider inserting an advanced airway.

Second, review the patient's airway. Is it patent? Swelling, bleeding, or just a change of position can obstruct the airway in the blink of an eye, so make certain that the airway is properly positioned and dry. Always be prepared to suction, and don't delay if you hear gurgling in the upper airway. It's far better to prevent aspiration than to treat it later. If the airway needs to be secured, *do it immediately,* and intubate the patient. Once intubation is accomplished, recheck lung sounds and perform oximetry and capnography periodically to confirm that the tube is properly placed.

Third, reassess breathing. Is the patient breathing adequately? If not, figure out why and fix the problem. For hypoventilation, assist breathing with oxygen and a bag-valve-mask device. Correct hypoxia with high-concentration oxygen therapy. For patients with diminished or absent breath sounds, JVD, and progressive dyspnea (signs of pneumothorax), decompress the chest.

Stay alert for signs that the patient is experiencing ventilatory fatigue (for example, decreasing pulse oximetry reading, looks increasingly tired). Be especially alert for this possibility in children because it is a classic sign that precedes disaster for the patient. Patients of any age who are going into ventilatory fatigue need to have their airway managed for them.

Finally, reassess the patient's circulation. Assess overall skin colour as an initial measure of cardiovascular function and hemodynamic status. With pale, cool, wet skin, think shock; with cyanosis, think oxygen desaturation; with mottling, think end-stage shock.

Make certain that all bleeding is controlled. If you find blood-soaked dressings, add more fresh dressings to the stack and rebandage in place. Reassess the blood pressure, watching closely for signs that the patient is beginning to decompensate.

Reassess the pulse, including its rate, strength, and regularity. Progressive tachycardia may indicate that the patient is still bleeding, is hypoxic, or is developing cardiogenic shock. In contrast, sustained or progressively worsening bradycardia may reflect rising intracranial pressure (from trauma or a stroke) or end-stage shock.

Reassessment of Prehospital Care and Transport Priorities

After repeating the initial assessment as part of your ongoing assessment, think about your present care plan. Have you addressed all life threats? Based on what you now know, do you need to revise your priority list? If so, make the change and get on with prehospital care. In contrast, if your plan is working well and you've addressed most or all of the patient's complaints, there is no need to revise the care plan.

While you are reevaluating your prehospital care priorities, you should reassess the transport plan as well. Should routine transport be stepped up to priority? Is the patient's condition worsening to the point that you need to consider diverting to a closer facility? Do you need to set up a rendezvous with an air ambulance and fly the patient to the health care facility? If your patient's condition has improved and stabilized, you should step down from priority and transport the patient as a routine case, the clearly safer choice.

Get another complete set of vital signs, and compare them with the expected outcomes from your therapies. For example, if you administered a 500-ml bolus of normal saline to a patient with gastrointestinal bleeding, you usually would expect a rise in blood pressure and a decrease in pulse rate. With any priority patient, you should have, at a minimum, three sets of vital signs—and that would be if you had a short transport. With most priority patients, you will have four or five sets of vital signs. Thus, you can look for trends or patterns such as a slowing pulse, rising blood pressure, and erratic respiratory patterns that represent the Cushing's reflex, a grave sign for patients with head trauma. Alternatively, narrowed pulse pressure, muffled heart tones, and JVD are associated with cardiac tamponade (Beck's triad), usually secondary to penetrating chest trauma.

The last element of the ongoing assessment is to revisit the patient's complaints (from the focused history), along with your interventions. Have any complaints improved or resolved? Has the 9 over 10 chest pain improved with the nitroglycerin you administered? Did the second salbutamol treatment ease the patient's breathing? Which situations remain unresolved? Situations that are worsening are especially concerning because they could mean an unseen problem or ineffective interventions. If you have not reached the receiving facility, get ready to do the ongoing assessment again—that's why it's called the ongoing assessment.

You are the Paramedic Summary

1. What is the best method of airway assessment and management for a patient who is wearing a football helmet and shoulder pads?

The quickest way to access this patient's airway is to remove the helmet's face guard rather than the entire helmet. This technique addresses two issues, airway assessment and management, and keeps the spine in a neutral position should the patient require spinal immobilization. (Spinal immobilization is covered in Chapter 22.)

2. Although the players deny any trauma, should you immobilize this patient?

There is no evidence to suggest that this patient requires spinal precautions. When in doubt, err on the side of caution and immobilize the patient. This will be a determination for you to make in accordance with your local protocols.

3. Because this patient is a minor, what are some important considerations for treatment and transport?

Most high schools require an updated student file that includes current phone numbers for parents in case of an emergency. If the parents are unavailable, this patient would be treated and transported under the rules of implied consent.

4. Of all your differential diagnoses, which ones should be considered a diagnosis of exclusion?

Although at some point during the course of your career you will likely encounter patients who exaggerate signs or falsify symptoms (including feigning unconsciousness), this should be the last thing you suspect, even in patients who have a history of malingering. Consider this possibility only after you've carefully reviewed all other potential causes. Doing otherwise will likely cause a misdiagnosis and/or delay of essential prehospital care and prompt transport.

5. Does this patient need high-flow supplemental oxygen? Why or why not?

The adage, "Never withhold oxygen," is good advice. It is appropriate to apply high-flow oxygen because the patient is unconscious and can benefit from supplemental oxygen therapy. Be ever mindful of what you're doing and why, especially when administering drugs, including oxygen. Note that pulse oximetry is not always accurate, even when it provides a reading. Patients with carbon monoxide poisoning may have an acceptable or even a 100% oximetry reading. Patients who have cold hands or who wear nail polish may initially have a lower pulse oximetry reading but, in fact, are better oxygenated than their carbon monoxide–poisoned counterparts.

6. Should this patient be intubated? Why or why not?

It can be argued that because this patient is unconscious, he cannot maintain his airway and should, therefore, be intubated via rapid-sequence induction (RSI; "Less than 8, intubate!"). If an airway cannot be kept patent with basic techniques, insert an endotracheal tube. Before making this decision, look at the patient's vital signs, oximetry and capnography readings, and other signs. Is the patient ventilating and oxygenating adequately? All information in this scenario would suggest that the answer to this question is "yes." However, there is new research to suggest that effective bag-valve-mask ventilation with an oral airway in place can adequately oxygenate and ventilate a patient without exposing them to the potential risks of intubation. Your local protocols dictate the when, how, why, and where of intubation, and over the course of your career the role of intubation is likely to change. This patient can be managed effectively without taking the risks of RSI.

7. If no initial diagnosis is possible, what should your prehospital care goals be?

As a paramedic, your goals are to assess and treat any life-threatening conditions, monitor ABCs, provide supportive measures, and continue to search for underlying causes of the patient's signs and symptoms.

8. Under normal circumstances, when an abrupt loss of consciousness occurs, which four primary probabilities should you consider as part of your rule-out diagnosis?

Any sudden change in mentation should make you question the presence of underlying illnesses or injuries related to the neurovascular system as well as hypoglycemia, drug toxicity, and cardiac arrhythmias.

Prep Kit

▬ Ready for Review

- Patient assessment is the platform on which quality prehospital care is built and the single most important skill you bring to bear on patient prehospital care.
- Patient assessment is a complex skill made up of two primary components: information gathering and physical examination.
- Several elements make up the skill of patient assessment, with each being used in some way to gather information.
- The first step of the patient assessment process is the scene size-up because your first and foremost concern on any call is ensuring your own safety and the safety of the other EMS team members.
- During the initial assessment, in the first 60 to 90 seconds, as you look at, talk with, and touch your patient, you should be able to identify threats to the ABCs.
- Once the initial assessment is complete and all life threats have been addressed, you can move into the focused history and physical examination phase of patient assessment.
- The detailed physical examination can take 15 minutes or more for a more detailed and comprehensive history and a more detailed and thorough physical examination (such as checking ROM).
- After the initial assessment, the ongoing assessment is the single most important assessment process you will perform.

▬ Vital Vocabulary

alert and oriented (A × O) A determination made when assessing mental status by looking at whether the patient is oriented to four elements: person, place, time, and the event itself. Each element provides information about different aspects of the patient's memory.

AVPU A method of assessing mental status by determining whether a patient is Awake and alert, responsive to Verbal stimuli or Pain, or Unresponsive; used principally in the initial assessment.

Beck's triad The combination of a narrowed pulse pressure, muffled heart tones, and JVD associated with cardiac tamponade; usually resulting from penetrating chest trauma.

current health status A composite picture of a number of factors in a patient's life, such as dietary habits, current medications, allergies, exercise, alcohol or tobacco use, recreational drug use, sleep patterns and disorders, and immunizations.

Cushing's reflex The combination of a slowing pulse, rising blood pressure, and erratic respiratory patterns; a grave sign for patients with head trauma.

detailed physical examination The part of the assessment process in which a detailed area-by-area examination is performed on patients whose problems cannot be readily identified or when more specific information is needed about problems identified in the focused history and physical examination.

focused history and physical examination The part of the assessment process in which the patient's major complaints or any problems that are immediately evident are further and more specifically evaluated.

focused physical examination The examination done on a responsive medical patient, driven by the information gathered during the initial assessment and the history-taking phase.

Glasgow Coma Scale (GCS) An evaluation tool used to determine level of consciousness, which evaluates and assigns point values (scores) for eye opening, verbal response, and motor response, which are then totaled; effective in helping predict patient outcomes.

history of the present illness Information about the chief complaint, obtained using the OPQRST mnemonic.

initial assessment The part of the assessment process that helps you identify immediately or potentially life-threatening conditions so that you can initiate lifesaving prehospital care.

mechanism of injury (MOI) The way in which traumatic injuries occur; the forces that act on the body to cause damage.

nature of illness (NOI) The general type of illness a patient is experiencing.

ongoing assessment The part of the assessment process in which problems are reevaluated and responses to treatment are assessed.

past medical history Information obtained during the patient history, such as the patient's general state of health, childhood and adult diseases, surgeries and hospitalizations, psychiatric and mental illnesses, or traumatic injuries, which may relate to the patient's current problem.

rapid trauma assessment A unique and specialized assessment performed between the initial assessment and the focused physical examination of a trauma patient, usually on patients with a significant mechanism of injury, assessing specific parts of the entire body.

scene assessment A quick assessment of the scene and its surroundings made to provide information about scene safety and the mechanism of injury or nature of illness, before you enter and begin patient prehospital care.

working diagnosis The overall initial impression that determines the priority for patient prehospital care; based on the patient's surroundings, the mechanism of injury, signs and symptoms, and the chief complaint.

Assessment in Action

Your unit has been dispatched to a motor vehicle collision in which a small car has struck a utility pole. Dispatch has advised you that there appears to be one patient in the vehicle. As you arrive on the scene, you notice that the wooden utility pole is leaning at a 45° angle toward the car, and the utility wires are hanging low over the vehicle but not touching it. Without leaving the unit, you see a person sitting in the driver's seat who appears to be leaning over the steering wheel but is not moving. You are not sure, but you believe you see the top of a child's car seat in the rear of the car. No traffic or crowd control has been started, and you do not see a utility crew on the scene.

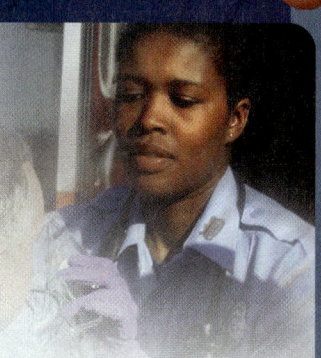

1. **What is the first step in your patient assessment?**
   A. Assess the patient's chief complaint.
   B. Perform a detailed physical examination to determine the extent of the condition.
   C. Perform a scene assessment.
   D. Assess AVPU.

2. **What is the first and foremost concern during your scene assessment?**
   A. The patient's level of consciousness
   B. The patient's breathing
   C. The safety of you and the rest of your team members
   D. The safety of the patient and their family members

3. **What best describes the term mechanism of injury?**
   A. The forces that act on the body to cause damage
   B. The internal forces of the human body
   C. The way an accident happened
   D. The external circumstances that caused an accident to happen

4. **How long should your initial assessment take?**
   A. 10 to 20 seconds
   B. 30 to 40 seconds
   C. 60 to 90 seconds
   D. More than 90 seconds

5. **A rapid trauma assessment be should performed on any trauma patient with a(n):**
   A. fracture.
   B. significant MOI.
   C. significant medical history.
   D. significant NOI.

6. **When should a detailed physical examination be done?**
   A. For every patient encounter
   B. When you have time on scene to complete it
   C. While you are transporting the patient to the hospital
   D. During the scene assessment

Challenging Questions

You arrive at a construction site where a worker fell approximately 10 m from a ladder and landed on his left side. Your initial assessment does not reveal threats to the ABCs. The patient, who is conscious and alert, complains of pain to the left side of his body; he denies having chest pain and shortness of breath and states that he did not lose consciousness. Other than some minor abrasions to the patient's left arm and lateral thigh, the remainder of your examination is unremarkable. Your partner reports the following vital signs: blood pressure, 126/76 mm Hg; pulse rate, 86 beats/min and regular; and respirations, 14 breaths/min and unlaboured.

7. **Does this patient require transport to a trauma centre?**

8. **Could you defend a transport mode of code 3 for this patient?**

Points to Ponder

You and your partner have been dispatched to a call for "chest pain." When the dispatcher provides an update, he states that the patient is a 70-year-old woman who started having chest pain about 2 hours ago. The patient has a cardiac history, but the extent of the history is unclear because of a language barrier. The dispatcher also states that there is an 8-year-old child with the patient.

Upon arrival, you find the patient sitting upright in a chair. She is leaning slightly forward, with her arms folded across her chest. You introduce yourself and ask her for information about her chief complaint. She looks up at you and says, "No English," in a heavy accent that you do not recognize. You have already formed your initial impression of the patient and have determined that she is in considerable distress.

How do you proceed with your physical assessment given that this patient does not speak English and you do not speak her native language? Would you consider using the 8-year-old as an interpreter? How will you address a time delay in your assessment progression?

Issues: Assessing Persons of Differing Cultures, Communications Barriers, Time Delay During Assessment.

Critical Thinking and Clinical Decision Making

Competency Areas

Area 1: Professional Responsibilities

1.6.a Exhibit reasonable and prudent judgement.
1.6.b Practice effective problem-solving.
1.6.c Delegate tasks appropriately.

Area 2: Communication

2.3.a Exhibit effective non-verbal behaviour.
2.3.b Practice active listening techniques.
2.3.c Establish trust and rapport with patients and colleagues.
2.3.d Recognize and react appropriately to non-verbal behaviours.
2.4.a Treat others with respect.
2.4.b Exhibit empathy and compassion while providing care.
2.4.d Act in a confident manner.
2.4.g Exhibit diplomacy, tact, and discretion.

Area 6: Integration

6.1.a Provide care to patient experiencing illness or injury primarily involving cardiovascular system.
6.1.b Provide care to patient experiencing illness or injury primarily involving neurological system.
6.1.c Provide care to patient experiencing illness or injury primarily involving respiratory system.
6.1.d Provide care to patient experiencing illness or injury primarily involving genitourinary/reproductive systems.
6.1.e Provide care to patient experiencing illness or injury primarily involving gastrointestinal system.
6.1.f Provide care to patient experiencing illness or injury primarily involving integumentary system.
6.1.g Provide care to patient experiencing illness or injury primarily involving musculoskeletal system.
6.1.h Provide care to patient experiencing illness primarily involving immune system.
6.1.i Provide care to patient experiencing illness primarily involving endocrine system.
6.1.j Provide care to patient experiencing illness or injury primarily involving eyes, ears, nose, or throat.
6.1.k Provide care to patient experiencing illness or injury due to poisoning or overdose.
6.1.l Provide care to patient experiencing non-urgent medical problem.
6.1.m Provide care to patient experiencing terminal illness.
6.1.n Provide care to patient experiencing illness or injury due to extremes of temperature or adverse environments.
6.1.o Provide care to patient based on understanding of common physiological, anatomical, incident, and patient-specific field trauma criteria that determine appropriate decisions for triage, transport, and destination.
6.1.p Provide care for patient experiencing psychiatric crisis.
6.2.b Provide care for pediatric patient.
6.2.c Provide care for geriatric patient.
6.2.d Provide care for physically-challenged patient.
6.2.e Provide care for mentally-challenged patient.
6.3.a Conduct ongoing assessments based on patient presentation and interpret findings.
6.3.b Re-direct priorities based on assessment findings.

Appendix 4: Pathophysiology

The reader must have knowledge of the areas presented in Appendix 4.

Introduction

The most fundamental description of what a paramedic does on a day-to-day basis is as follows: identify problems, set patient care priorities, develop a prehospital care plan, and, finally, execute that plan. You might think that this sounds like cookbook medicine, and in a way you would be correct. However, effective cookbook medicine requires the paramedic be a *thinking cook*, because patients often do not present exactly as those described in a textbook. To complicate matters further, the prehospital environment is constantly changing, which can affect the stability of any scene Figure 15-1 ▾ . A paramedic is expected to work in this environment and provide *quality* prehospital patient care.

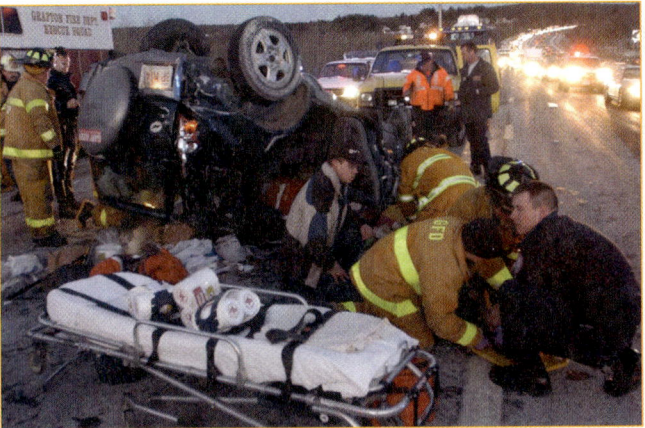

Figure 15-1 Your work as a paramedic will rarely be done in a quiet, stress-free place. You will have to learn the skill of making decisions in a chaotic environment.

This chapter is divided into two parts: first, an explanation of critical thinking, and second, how you can apply critical thinking skills in the streets. Initially, you will learn about *the science of thinking*. Then comes the practical subject matter: how to use this knowledge and *take it to the streets*. To master critical thinking, you will need to know the cornerstone thinking processes and terms.

The Cornerstones of Effective Paramedic Practice

Gathering, Evaluating, and Synthesizing

The first cornerstone of your practice is having the ability to *gather, evaluate,* and *synthesize* information. Every day, call by call, you will find yourself challenged as you try to obtain information from patients of different age groups and educational backgrounds, with varying abilities to communicate. Most patients do not know what information is useful to you and what is not. Your challenge on every call is to gather the information you need in an efficient manner and to not become impatient if the patient seems to digress. Many times, alcohol or other drug use will impair a patient's ability to respond to your questions, which will further complicate your information gathering. The patient's illness or injury may impair his or her ability to relay information clearly.

Once you have gathered the information, you must assess and evaluate it to formulate a prehospital care plan. You must check the validity of the information—often relying on your own judgment and communication skills. For example, let's say you encounter a patient with a minor sprained ankle who immediately asks you for morphine for pain. Your first thought might be that this person is an illicit drug user. Another consideration, however, is that your patient is a health care professional or knowledgeable in medicine and has a low tolerance

You are the Paramedic Part 1

During the past two weeks, the cold and flu season has hit and has affected many members of the community, including some of your colleagues. While checking the unit at the beginning of your shift, you get a call-out.

You are dispatched to 1611 Lynne Lane for a 65-year-old woman complaining of weakness, fatigue, and dizziness. A family member requested no lights or siren. As you arrive on the scene, you are met by the patient's daughter, who called 9-1-1 after speaking to her mother on the phone. She explains that her mom believes "she just has a cold." Her daughter is concerned it might be something more.

Initial Assessment	Recording Time: 0 Minutes
Appearance	Eyes open, flat affect
Level of consciousness	A (Alert to person, place, and day)
Airway	Patent
Breathing	Rapid with adequate tidal volume
Circulation	Radial pulse present, fast

1. When do you begin patient assessment?
2. What are the benefits and the risks of diagnosing based on dispatch?

At the Scene

Remember, your professional ethics demand that you consider all the possibilities when communicating with a patient. You must not judge. You must figure out: what does your patient need?

At the Scene

Hypercarbia means an excess of carbon dioxide (CO_2) in the blood, as indicated by an elevated PCO_2 level.

for pain. If morphine is not the first-line drug for a sprained ankle, you will need to explain this to your patient. The thinking paramedic must consider all possibilities to be as objective as possible in the decision-making process.

Once you have evaluated the information you obtained from the scene, the patient, or a bystander, you need to process—or *synthesize*—this information.

For example, consider a patient, a 64-year-old man having chest pain, who has had type 1 diabetes since childhood, started smoking in high school, and has had chronic obstructive pulmonary disease (COPD) since his 50s. Synthesis requires that you look at each of those three facts about your patient, any of which may or may not be life threatening. Your job is to paint a mental picture of how each fact affects the other **Figure 15-2 ◀**.

In this scenario, we know that diabetes is a metabolic dysfunction that includes a disorder of circulation. Although an extremely low level of blood glucose may kill someone or result in brain damage quickly, a chronic, higher-than-normal blood glucose level takes its toll on every organ and every system. Think about how many long-term diabetics you encounter with vision problems or amputated fingers or toes. The patient's COPD, which is primarily a disease of gas exchange, at some point results in some combination of hypoxia (low levels of oxygen in the blood) and hypercarbia (high levels of carbon dioxide in the blood). You need to assess the new onset of chest pains. One of the possibilities is that coronary artery disease has caused one or more of the vessels of the heart muscle to become blocked, in turn causing a part of the heart to begin to necrose or die. Taking all of the information you have gathered and synthesizing it would basically work something like this: "I have a patient with diseases of

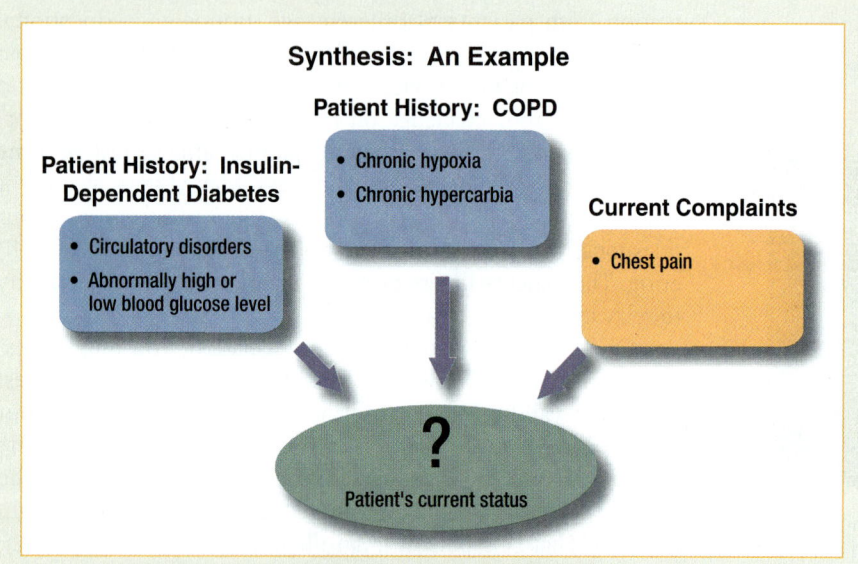

Figure 15-2 When you synthesize patient information you have gathered, you will assess the relative importance of the patient's medical history (blue boxes) and his or her current complaints (yellow box). These factors all affect each other.

You are the Paramedic Part 2

The patient tells you that she's sorry her daughter has bothered you. She tells you that she asked her daughter to bring over some food and cold medicine, not for her to call an ambulance. She says it's true that she hasn't been feeling well since early this morning, but she doesn't think it's anything major. She apologizes to you again and says, "I'm sure you have better things to do."

Vital Signs	Recording Time: 10 Minutes
Skin	Slightly moist, slightly pale, and warm
Pulse	110 beats/min, regular
Blood pressure	130/82 mm Hg
Respirations	36 breaths/min
Spo₂	95% on room air

3. What are pertinent negatives?

4. What information is missing from the above assessment?

both circulation and gas exchange. There is a chance that part of the patient's heart is dying because vessels are unable to deliver oxygenated blood to a portion of the heart muscle." You must treat the combined effect of your patient's disease processes to prevent the unperfused section of heart from dying, which may cause the death of your patient. That is synthesis—taking conditions and assessing their potential for having life-threatening impact. In the end, the patient could be having a heart attack, a life-threatening problem.

Developing and Implementing a Patient Care Plan

The second cornerstone of your practice is the *development and implementation of a patient care plan*. This is actually much simpler than analyzing the validity of the information you've gathered. Once you've determined the patient's primary problem by identifying the chief complaint and establishing an initial diagnosis, your care plan is almost always defined by the patient care protocols or standing orders in the EMS system where you work. Protocols, or standing orders, define the essential standard of care for patients with certain injuries, illnesses, or behavioural conditions. They further specify your performance parameters, which define what you can or cannot do without direct medical control, as well as when you need to contact direct medical control before providing care. Collectively, standing orders and protocols promote both a standard approach and a standard of quality care as defined by regional, provincial, or national standards.

Unfortunately, protocols, standing orders, and patient care algorithms only address classic patient care presentations. They frequently don't address vague patient complaints that don't fit into a neat clinical description—nor do they address patients with multiple disease etiologies (remember synthesis?) and/or those patients who will require multiple treatment modalities as part of the care plan.

So, your next step is to figure out what you should do in your patient's best interest.

Judgment and Independent Decision Making

The third cornerstone is *judgment and making independent decisions* Figure 15-3 ▶ . Let's say that you encounter a machinist who has had an incident in which one of the parts of a machine has seriously gashed the upper part of his leg. You can see significant amounts of blood gushing from the area of his femoral artery with every contraction of his heart. You realize that you do not have time to make radio or cell phone contact with a base station doctor, identify your unit and yourself, present the patient problem, get directions for prehospital patient care, and *then* take action before the patient may die. Even under the best circumstances, your patient would have died long before your "call the doc" process was completed. To save the patient, you recognize the severed artery as an immediate life threat and apply continuous direct pressure, possibly combined with use of a pressure point to control the bleeding.

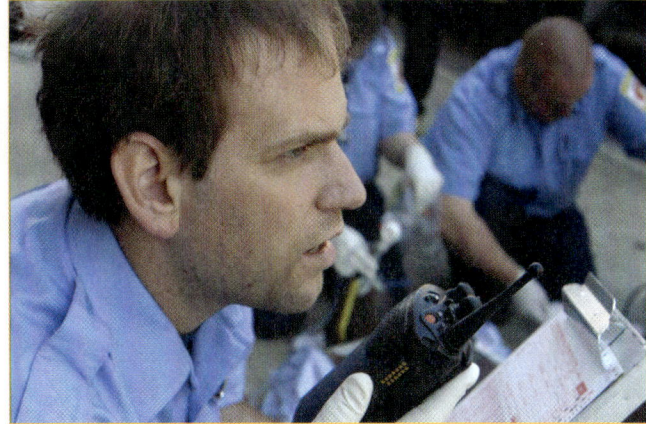

Figure 15-3 Each call that you do will have its own unique circumstances and challenges. Much of your skill rests with the use of careful, nonjudgmental decision making.

The use of tourniquets is becoming more prominent in the prehospital and military settings. There is good evidence to support their use.

Another scenario you may encounter—a patient in cardiac arrest on his or her front porch. With your resource hospital only a few blocks away, you choose to do CPR and shock any shockable rhythm (as you will learn in Chapter 27). After that, you secure the airway, administer oxygen, load the patient, and transport, performing CPR and administering medication en route. Put that same patient in a third-story attic apartment with a small, almost useless stairway access, and you may find yourself dealing with outcomes ranging from the patient being either fully resuscitated and viable or pronounced dead. Because of the restrictive physical requirement, you realize it is impossible to quickly and efficiently get the patient out of the house and en route to the care facility. As such, you manage the patient to one end point or another. Either the resuscitation gets called off, or you get the patient back and stabilized before you attempt to package and transport. As circumstances change, so may your patient care plan. However, that will only happen if you are using your critical thinking and decision-making skills to the best of your abilities.

Documentation and Communication

Documenting difficulties such as darkness, limited access, and unruly crowds that you encounter while caring for a patient will help to justify your decisions made for prehospital patient care.

Thinking Under Pressure

The fourth and final cornerstone of your practice is your ability to *think and work under pressure*. Imagine ringing the doorbell at the address to which you have been dispatched and having the door open, at which point a hysterical mother hands you her cyanotic, apneic 2-year-old who she just dragged out of the bottom of the bathtub. Your critical thinking faculties should tell you to get that child breathing in the next handful of seconds or you will have a full cardiac arrest on your hands, diminishing the likelihood of saving the child's life. Only a combination of excellent knowledge coupled with excellent psychomotor clinical skills will allow you to avert a patient care disaster: the death of a child. To accomplish that, you must be able to work under extreme pressure and be able to perform both quickly and effectively.

The Range of Patient Conditions

One of the key elements of your practice is to be able to quickly determine if your patient is *sick or not sick*. For patients who are sick, you must further be able to quantify *how sick they are*. That will, in turn, allow you to make good choices as to what prehospital care you must provide at the scene and what care you should provide in the back of the ambulance while en route. It is difficult to define *sick*. A patient might think of sick as having a bad cold. Sick to an emergency health care provider means, "Does this patient have an acute life-threatening process?" or "Is this patient unstable?" An experienced paramedic, nurse, or physician can differentiate between sick and not sick, often within seconds, by just looking at the patient. You should consciously make this

Special Considerations

The best way to recognize "sick" infants and small children is to know what "not sick" infants and small children act like according to their age. To improve your ability to recognize this difference, take every opportunity you can to assess children, take every continuing education pediatrics course, and read every article you can.

determination for every patient you see so that over time it becomes an immediate, unconscious, reflex determination.

Clear thinking in a chaotic emergency starts with a triage model. Critical patients need immediate prehospital care to survive. Serious patients need care within the next few minutes to possibly the next half hour (or they become critical patients) to have a positive outcome **Figure 15-4 ▶**. The two groups of patients that are left are the mortally wounded or dead, and those often termed the walking wounded or minimally injured.

Examples of patients with *critical life threats* would include those with:

- Major multisystem trauma
- Devastating single-system trauma
- Airway compromise or an unsecured airway
- Severe hemodynamic instability (eg, from blood loss, sepsis, or arrhythmia)

- Severe burn injury, including facial and airway burn
- Acute presentations of chronic conditions
Examples of patients in *serious condition* would include those with:
- Multisystem trauma with relatively stable vital signs
- Various medical presentations, including pneumonia or COPD with exacerbation and early signs of fatigue (will progress to respiratory failure if not corrected), altered mental status from mild hypoglycemia (will progress to coma and seizure if not corrected)
- Significant burn injury
Examples of patients who are "walking wounded" or have *minimal, non-life-threatening injuries* would include those with:
- Small lacerations
- Minor or longstanding medical complaints with no new changes and stable vital signs
- Partial-thickness burns of an extremity of less than 5% body surface area

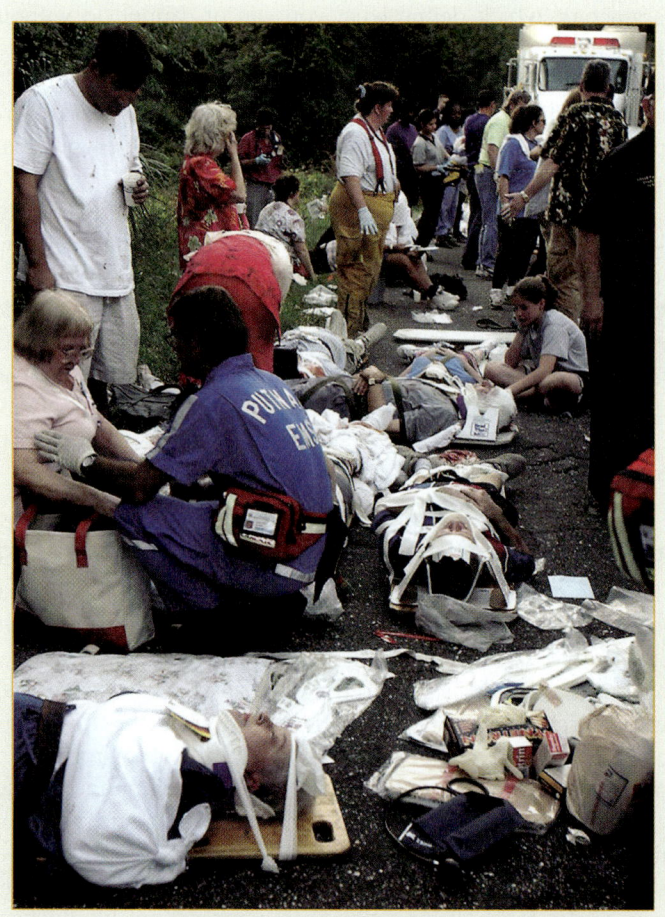

Figure 15-4 With multiple patients, you must quickly assess and prioritize the urgency of each person's condition. After assessing the scene, call for additional help.

Critical Thinking and Clinical Decision Making

It is important for you to have a command of the vocabulary for the process psychologists and philosophers call *thinking* and *decision making*. By having a better understanding of how your thoughts are formed and processed, you can make the best decisions possible in caring for your patients **Figure 15-5 ▾** .

Concept Formation

The first stage of the thought process in prehospital care is that of gathering information—things you see, hear, smell, or feel. This process is concept formation. In EMS, you will form your concepts on several variables, including your initial assessment of your patient's condition, your general impression, including assessment of your patient's affect, the patient's vital signs, and actual measurements from your other diagnostic EMS tools.

The process starts as you arrive at the scene and evaluate it from a safety perspective for both the EMS team and your patient. You need to evaluate the mechanism of injury for trauma, or for medical calls, the nature of the present illness. How does your patient present? Does the patient appear uncomfortable, or frightened, or deathly ill? You need to assess the patient's level of consciousness (LOC), in part to determine whether the person can provide you with reliable information to act on. This initial evaluation of their LOC will also establish a baseline for you to refer to later as the call progresses and the patient's condition changes.

At the Scene

Observe family members for clues also. Do they seem worried or nervous? Does calling 9-1-1 seem "routine" for them? Are they huddled in a corner crying or are they trying to watch television during your assessment? Be alert for situations that are not what they seem to be.

You move further into the information gathering process as you perform your initial assessment, focusing on the identification of any serious threats to your patient's life that you need to immediately address. You continue on as you perform an appropriate physical examination. As you examine your patient, identify the patient's chief complaint, and get a pertinent medical history, including any medications the patient is taking: prescription, over-the-counter, illicit, or possibly herbal.

One of the most important observations you need to judge is your patient's affect—or emotional state reflected in physical behaviour **Figure 15-6 ▾** . The affect might not tally with what patients tell you. For example, suppose you have a patient who presents with the hyper-kind-of-manic behaviour associated with amphetamine abuse, yet denies any drug use. You might even see drug paraphernalia. You must balance the story you are getting with the patient's affect—there should be a match. If there isn't a reasonable match, you need to ask yourself why.

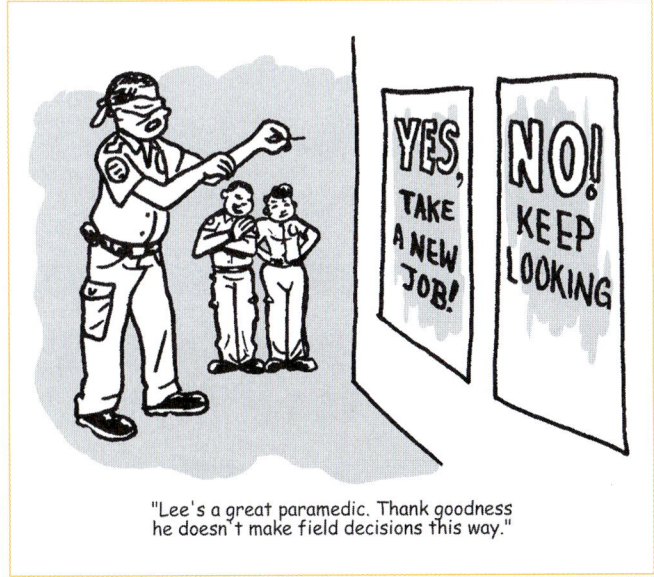

"Lee's a great paramedic. Thank goodness he doesn't make field decisions this way."

Figure 15-5

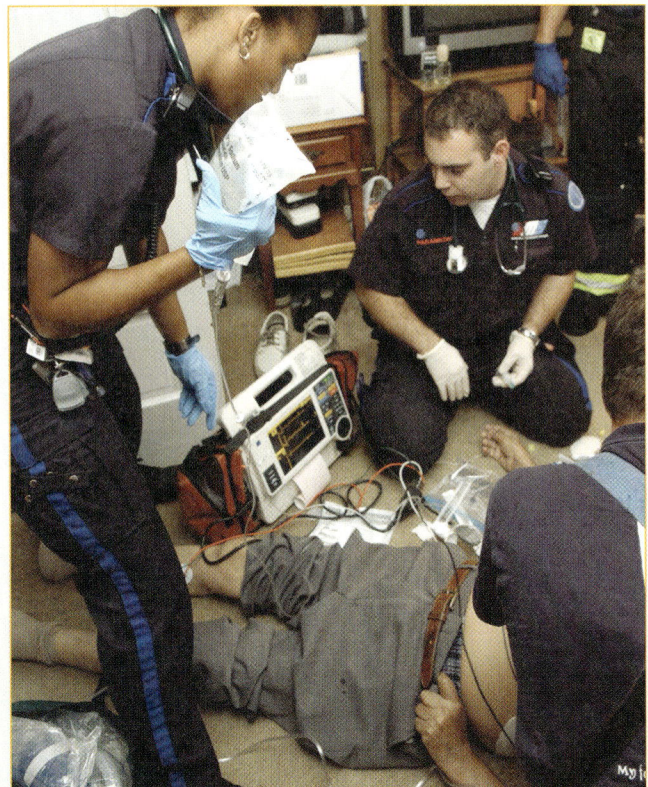

Figure 15-6 Take in clues not only from your patient's status, but also from his or her surroundings. Assess the entire environment to make sure that you fully understand how it may impact your patient's condition.

Also on your information-gathering quest is obtaining the patient's vital signs by using your primary diagnostic tools: the glucometer, pulse oximeter, capnometer, cardiac monitor, blood pressure cuff, and stethoscope.

Data Interpretation

During the second stage of the critical thinking process, you must evaluate all the information that you have gathered, which is called data interpretation. You will need a good background in anatomy and physiology as well as pathophysiology so you understand both how the body works, and when problems arise, how it responds to those problems. Another key element is your experience. If you have come to the advanced care paramedic program with lots of experience as a primary care paramedic, you will have an excellent platform to build on.

How you think and form conclusions is affected not only by the attitudes of patients, but by your attitude as a paramedic. This means, for example, that you should never consider a call a waste of your time or talent. Furthermore, unprofessional comments such as "I can't believe you called us for THIS!" show a lack of compassion and interest in providing the best possible prehospital care   Figure 15-7 ▶ . Every call is an opportunity to hone your communication and medical skills.

Having a negative attitude about any patient or patient care situation will almost guarantee that the care you provide will be suboptimal. To maintain the standards set by your profession, you must provide the best care you can for every patient you encounter. Period.

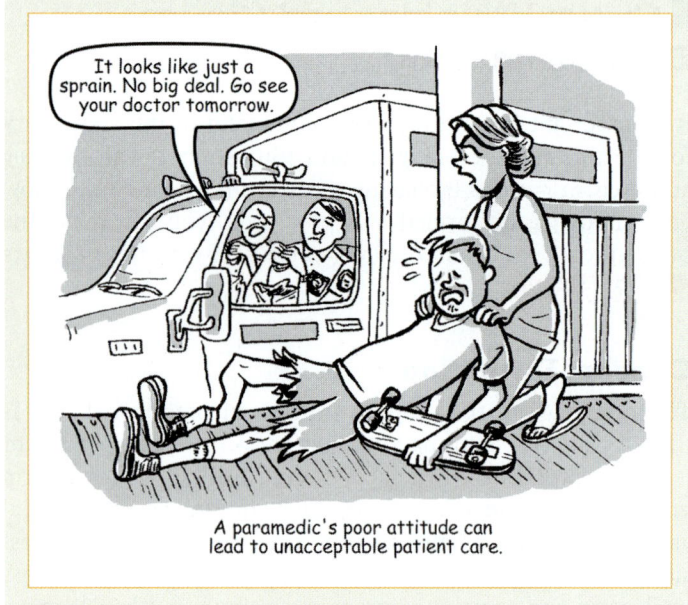

A paramedic's poor attitude can lead to unacceptable patient care.

Figure 15-7

Application of Principle

The next stage of the critical thinking process in EMS comes when you develop your initial diagnosis. Think of it as being "tentative" or "preliminary." It is what you feel is at the root of your patient's problem, and what you will focus your patient care efforts on correcting. In addition to the main initial diagnosis, there are often a number of other possibilities in the back of your mind. This list is the *differential diagnosis*.

You are the Paramedic Part 3

The patient denies having a recent history of productive cough, fever, chills, body aches, nausea, or vomiting, but does admit she's felt quite tired and a bit short of breath since she woke around 6 AM.

Your partner asks her if she wishes to be transported to the hospital, and she asks, "Do I really need to go?" You tell her since her daughter was concerned enough to call 9-1-1 coupled with her feeling of shortness of breath, these are both good reasons to be transported to the hospital for further evaluation. After hearing this explanation, she agrees to treatment and to transport. You place her on oxygen, start an 18-gauge IV of normal saline in her right hand to keep the vein open, and place her on the cardiac monitor.

Reassessment	Recording Time: 15 Minutes
Skin	Slightly moist, pale, and warm
Pulse	102 beats/min, regular
Blood pressure	130/74 mm Hg
Respirations	30 breaths/min
SpO_2	98% on 4 l/min via nasal cannula
Temperature	37°C
ECG	Sinus rhythm

5. How can a patient's opinion affect treatment and transport decisions?
6. Can men and women have different symptoms of acute illness?

Your prehospital care plan is driven by the patient care protocols or standing orders in the system where you work. They represent the standard of care and describe the treatments and interventions you are expected to provide. In addition, they further define what you as a paramedic can do without contacting direct medical control, as well as what therapies or interventions you cannot do without obtaining orders from medical control.

Reflection in Action

You are now actively treating your patient while at the same time monitoring the effects of your interventions. Think of *reflection in action* as simply *thinking while doing.*

Let's say your patient was complaining of having "difficulty breathing." You apply a nonrebreathing mask with oxygen flowing at 15 l/min. After a few minutes you ask, "Is it getting any easier for you to breathe?" Too often, paramedics get caught up in thinking they must do one thing after another, frequently forgetting to periodically check and see whether what they are doing is actually solving the problem and making the patient feel better. If you ask your patient how your treatment is working, you will also be reassessing your patient ▶ Figure 15-8 ▾ . Reassessment is an important and continuous part of your patient care. Reassessment also allows you to monitor the accuracy of your preliminary diagnosis. If the response to treatment is not what you expect, you may need to reconsider that diagnosis and pay more attention to other items on your differential diagnosis.

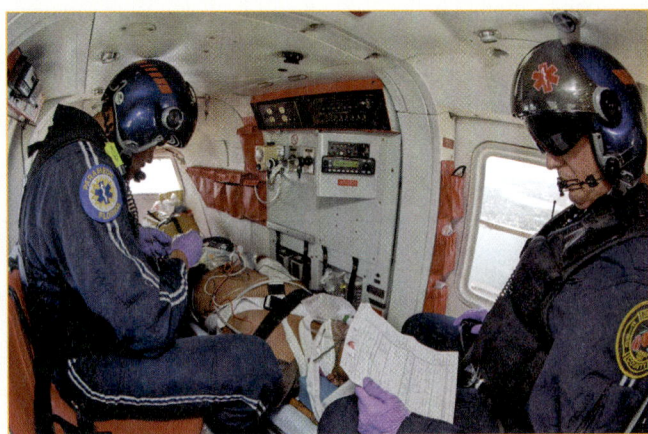

Figure 15-8 A patient's condition can change rapidly—especially if he or she is critically ill or injured. Monitor any changes to a patient's condition.

Documentation and Communication

It is important not only to document procedures done and medications given but also what effect the procedure or medication had, if any.

In another scenario, let's say you are treating a 58-year-old man who experienced chest pain while moving some rocks to landscape his yard. Although he has no previous cardiac history, he is in the right age group for a heart problem to appear. When you ask him if he can pinpoint where the pain seems to be, he points to a spot on his chest directly over his heart. You continue down the same care plan.

Then you ask if anything makes the pain better or worse, and the patient explains that if he holds his left arm still the pain goes away. However, upon movement it hurts terribly in the area over his heart. This information is important, because you know that pain associated with a heart attack is not usually relieved by just keeping one's arm still. You must consider this information along with the responses to other questions about the nature of the pain and associated symptoms. The patient may be having pain from a musculoskeletal injury. You also know that the pain from a heart attack can present in a variety of ways; therefore, you should ask questions designed to differentiate between the two problems. If this seems to be a musculoskeletal injury, you should revise your impression and treatment plan.

Instead of giving the patient aspirin, nitroglycerin, and high-flow oxygen for a possible heart attack, you should begin by providing treatment designed for musculoskeletal pain. If the picture changes with further questioning or physical examination, you may revise your prehospital care plan once more.

One of the key elements of this stage of the critical thinking process is to avoid *tunnel vision* and always keep your mind open to all the possible causes of your patient's current condition. Your patient might be having a heart attack that presents in a way that is not in the textbooks. Reassess constantly.

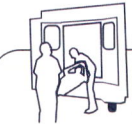

At the Scene

Tunnel vision, ie, seeing little and missing a lot— the demise of many paramedics.

Reflection on Action

The last stage in the critical thinking process occurs after the call is over and is commonly associated with call review or critiques. This is the time when you look back at the total call and reflect on how you processed the signs and symptoms and reached the decisions that you did. One of the most difficult aspects of this stage is learning to say either, "I was wrong" or "I made a mistake." Both are difficult phrases for any health care provider to say, because none of us wants to make an error or ever be wrong. However, there is not a single health care provider who doesn't make a mistake every now and then.

In truth, you will periodically encounter patients with atypical presentations, or, in other words, patients who just don't follow the textbook. For example, you may see a patient with a neck fracture who has no pain. Even though pain is the single best predictor of a possible spine injury, it is not an absolute predictor 100% of the time. To make an accurate diagnosis, you must also

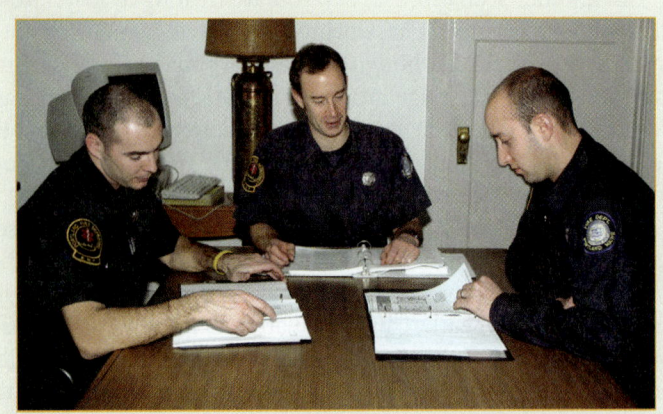

Figure 15-9 A formal review, or audit, of your performance can seem intimidating. However, it is also an opportunity for you to gain important feedback and improve yourself professionally.

bring into play all that you have learned about communication and the ethical treatment of patients—your patient might come from a culture that denies having pain.

Reflection gives you the chance to continuously improve your thinking and decision making, and, in turn, your patient care as you modify your experience base. Always having a "learning attitude" makes every call you go on, every class you take, and every call review you attend an opportunity to improve yourself to provide better prehospital care for your patients **Figure 15-9 ▲** . When your call gets selected for a continuous quality improvement audit, look at it as an opportunity to have an outside reviewer look at your work in hopes that you continue to grow and improve in your practice. See it as a growth opportunity. Growth won't happen if you can't admit to your mistakes or if you are unwilling to learn. Never *ever* forget that the successful completion of the paramedic class is really just the starting point

in your career. To provide the best possible prehospital care requires that you make a commitment to a lifetime of learning. The most important trait for a lifetime career is a true desire to become better and better as a paramedic.

Let's review the fundamental elements of the critical thinking and decision-making process. As you look over each item on the following list, ask yourself, *"Do I have this quality already or do I need to develop it?"*

- Adequate fund of knowledge in anatomy and pathophysiology
- Ability to gather and organize data and form concepts
- Ability to focus on specific and multiple elements of data
- Ability to identify and deal with medical ambiguity— uncertainty regarding the specific cause of the patient's condition; few calls follow the scripts in your protocols
- Ability to differentiate between relevant and irrelevant data
- Ability to analyze and compare similar situations
- Ability to analyze and compare contrary situations
- Ability to construct arguments and articulate your reasoning
- Ability to begin to act when needed while still gathering information

From Theory to Practical Application

A number of factors come into play with every call, making each one unique to a certain degree. Consider the following:

You are dispatched to a "car off the road" involving a single car with four passengers that has spun off into a ditch at an estimated speed of 100 km/hr. Think about how each of the following variables might change the call and how you might manage it:

- None of the passengers had on a seatbelt.
- The car was travelling at 100 km/hr.
- The vehicle flipped over and is on its roof.

You are the Paramedic Part 4

You are writing your patient care report when you hear the emergency department physician say, "Mrs. Jones, it appears that you are having a heart attack." Your heart drops as you realize you hadn't even considered this diagnosis. As the doctor passes by, he tells you the news. This means your call will be brought up in your department's monthly quality assurance/quality improvement review.

Reassessment	Recording Time: 20 Minutes
Skin	Slightly moist, pink, and warm
Pulse	94 beats/min, regular
Blood pressure	130/80 mm Hg
Respirations	30 breaths/min
Temperature	37°C
ECG	Sinus rhythm

7. Do good paramedics make errors like this one?
8. How can a paramedic's attitude affect patient care?
9. What was done right in this call?
10. How could this error have been avoided?

- It's −10°C outside, and the collision was not discovered for at least an hour.

As you can see from the list, each variable change creates dozens of possible "new" outcomes, and as those possibilities increase so does your challenge as a paramedic to manage the call and patient care properly.

Few of the calls you respond to on a day-to-day basis represent true life-threatening emergencies. That doesn't in any way imply that they are less important; just that they are less challenging to your medical expertise. They may be challenging in other ways. Remember that every call, no matter how trivial appearing to you, is important to the patient and can be a learning experience for all involved.

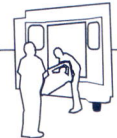

At the Scene

Never be fooled by patients who initially appear uninjured or healthy. Never hesitate to do a thorough evaluation, history, and physical examination.

To focus yourself even further consider this:

- Minor medical and traumatic events require very little critical thinking, and, as such, decision making is relatively easy.
- Patients with obvious life-threats pose limited critical thinking challenges, and again, simple decision making.
- Patients whose conditions fall somewhere around the midpoint on the spectrum between "no-big-deal" minor and "oh-my-gosh" serious pose the greatest critical thinking and decision-making challenges to you as a paramedic.

As we transition into the street application of this material, keep in mind that behind your uniform you are just a person like anybody else, and because of that, you, too, have to deal with the impact of the "fight or flight" response when confronted with extreme cases that push *your* buttons (sensory overload). The hormonal response has both a positive and a negative impact on you. On the positive side, you may have enhanced visual and auditory acuity as well as improved reflexes and muscle strength. On the negative side, you may have impaired critical thinking skills and diminished concentration and assessment abilities. One way to counter these negative effects is to improve your mental conditioning. Practice your skills until you can do them almost instinctively and can perform them on command, almost flawlessly, in the skills lab setting. Once you reach that level, you can draw on these skills in a real-life setting, allowing you to better focus on patient assessment or other decision-making areas.

Facilitate better thinking under pressure by memorizing the following mental checklist for all calls:

1. Take a moment to *scan the situation.*
2. Take another moment to *stop and think.*
3. *Make decisions and act* on behalf of the patient.
4. *Stay calm,* and maintain clear, concise *mental control.*
5. Plan to regularly and continually *reevaluate the patient.*

Taking It to the Streets

Having now looked at the science side of critical thinking, let's transition to the practical side. When you are out on a call, critical thinking can be summed up with the *Six Rs.*

1. Read the Scene

The emergency scene is a relative goldmine of information readily available to you, if you are wise enough to mine it. Equally important to consider is that this information is *only* available at the scene and becomes unavailable once you initiate transport to the hospital. Some of the primary elements involved in reading the scene are: evaluating the overall safety of the situation, the environmental conditions, the immediate surroundings, access and exit issues, and finally evaluating the mechanism of injury **Figure 15-10 ▾**. In particular, when you are looking at the mechanism of injury, take time to evaluate all aspects. For example, with a motor vehicle collision look at the length of the skid marks or note whether there are

Notes from Nancy

If you do not take a few moments to survey the scene . . . , you are very likely to become one of the casualties yourself. And a paramedic who is injured because he or she rocketed out of the ambulance without taking a good look around, will be of no benefit to the patient(s). Indeed, an injured paramedic just increases the number of victims that the remaining rescue personnel have to care for, and that will very likely detract from the prehospital care given to the other patients. The moral is: Dead heroes can't save lives. Injured heroes are a nuisance, so check the scene for hazards before you lurch in.

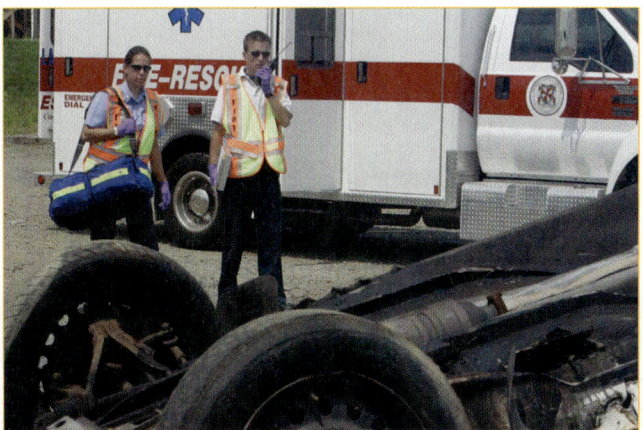

Figure 15-10 Although you need to focus on treating patients as soon as possible, always take a moment to register important information about the scene. What has happened that will help you assess each patient's condition?

none, what the vehicle struck, how much intrusion there is into the passenger compartment, and whether seatbelts were worn. In another example, the case of an elderly patient found unconscious at home, you would look for neatness or disarray in the home and the presence or absence of multiple pill bottles. You would also note exactly where the patient was found (in bed, on the floor, etc.).

Other issues when you "read the scene" include assessing the environment in which the patient was found. Was it hot, cold, wet? Also, are there eyewitnesses or friends or family to provide additional information?

2. Read the Patient

Probably one of the greatest skills you can develop is learning to read a patient quickly. As you approach the patient, does the patient see you and track you with his or her eyes? Offer the patient your hand to shake, and introduce yourself and ask why 9-1-1 was called. If the patient takes your hand and answers you appropriately, you have just determined that the patient has a Glasgow Coma Scale score of 15 (spontaneous eye opening, follows commands, appropriate verbal response). Other components of effectively reading a patient include:

- **Observe** the patient. What's the patient's LOC and level of comfort or discomfort? Skin colour? Position? Work of breathing? Any obvious deformity or asymmetry? **Figure 15-11 ▾**
- **Talk** to the patient. Determine the chief complaint. Is this a new problem or the worsening of a preexisting condition? Obtain the medical history and the history of the present problem.
- **Touch** the patient. What's the skin temperature and moisture level like? Assess the pulse rate, regularity, and strength.
- **Auscultate** lungs sounds. Confirm the adequacy or inadequacy of respirations and reassess the patency of the airway.

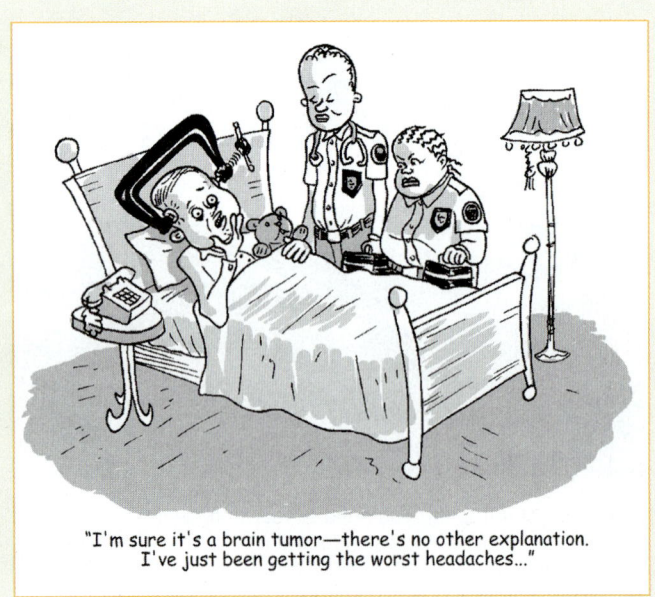

"I'm sure it's a brain tumor—there's no other explanation. I've just been getting the worst headaches..."

Figure 15-11

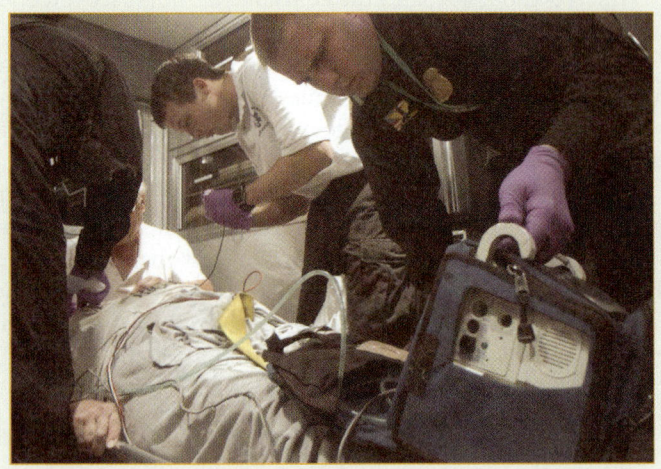

Figure 15-12 The more accurate your patient readings, the more reliable your diagnosis will be. Take the time to collect a set of baseline vital signs on every patient.

- **Identify** life threats. Correct any life threats relative to airway, breathing, and circulation in the order you find them.
- **Obtain** complete and accurate vital signs **Figure 15-12 ▴**. For every patient, even for transfer patients, a baseline set of vital signs is a must. For patients with serious problems, two sets of vital signs provide comparative data. With critical patients, three or more sets of vital signs allow you to assess trends and to reassess whether the patient's condition is stabilizing, getting better, or getting worse. If your patient's condition is getting worse, multiple sets of vital signs provide some indication of how fast the patient's condition is deteriorating. Learn to integrate the taking of vital signs into the timely movement of the patient to the hospital. Determine what you need to do right away and what can wait for later during transport.

3. React

You must begin patient prehospital care by addressing life threats in the order you find them. Next, consider the worst-case scenario that could be causing your patient's symptoms, and either rule it out or rule it in. After that, your primary focus should be to determine the most common and probable cause for the patient's current condition. By addressing the worst-case scenario, you can try to avoid any catastrophes in patient prehospital care and then can take the time to look for less lethal problems.

If, at the end of your assessment, you haven't been able to develop an initial diagnosis, it is acceptable to provide prehospital

Controversies

EMS services have for many years treated patients with prophylactic treatments even when there is no evidence to support the need. Should every trauma patient be immobilized on a backboard? Should every unconscious person be given Narcan?

care based on the presenting signs and symptoms. If your patient is having difficulty breathing, you administer high-flow oxygen and place the patient in a position of comfort. For symptoms of shock, you elevate the feet, provide a cover for warmth, administer high-flow oxygen, and establish a large-bore IV line while you continue to try to search for the cause of the condition. When you put the limited physical and technical resources of the pre-hospital environment up against the number of possible diagnoses a patient might have, you will find that you will regularly be treating patients who cannot be diagnosed until they reach the hospital. In some cases, the diagnosis may elude the doctor as well, so this is nothing to be ashamed of or worried about. It is simply a reality of medicine and has to be dealt with in a professional fashion.

4. Reevaluate

As patient prehospital care is continuing, another key element of good care is to make certain that you follow up on any interventions. See whether the splint you applied has eased the pain in your patient's injured leg. If you are treating frequent PVCs (premature ventricular contractions) with an antidysrhythmic medication, check the monitor to see whether the contractions have resolved. On challenging calls, once paramedics get into the treatment mode, they too often just focus on *doing things* and forget to see whether the *things they are doing* are actually improving the patient's situation.

As you reassess your patient, take the time to add any information you may have gathered from the detailed or focused physical examination and add it to the information you found in the initial assessment. Say you find that your patient has no breath sounds in the upper right lobes secondary to a fractured rib that caused a small pneumothorax. By itself, the small pneumothorax is not an immediate life threat to a relatively healthy individual. But let's say the patient also has bilateral fractured femurs, significant blood loss, and a minor head injury. Under those circumstances, a small pneumothorax may complicate matters far more than if it were the only condition. When you encounter patients, especially trauma patients, with multiple pathophysiologies, it is up to you to add them up as you develop your care plan to make sure nothing is overlooked that can be addressed on the scene.

5. Revise the Plan

As you continue to provide care for your patient, you may get indications that what you once thought was a head injury is a problem secondary to glue sniffing; two very different causes. The thinking paramedic, no matter how sure he or she is of the initial diagnosis, always keeps part of the thought process open to other possibilities **Figure 15-13 ▸**. As other information becomes available as the call unfolds, you should always be prepared to change directions as necessary. By remaining mentally "light on your feet," you position yourself to be receptive to changing presentations or circumstances, which, in turn, helps you avoid tunnel vision.

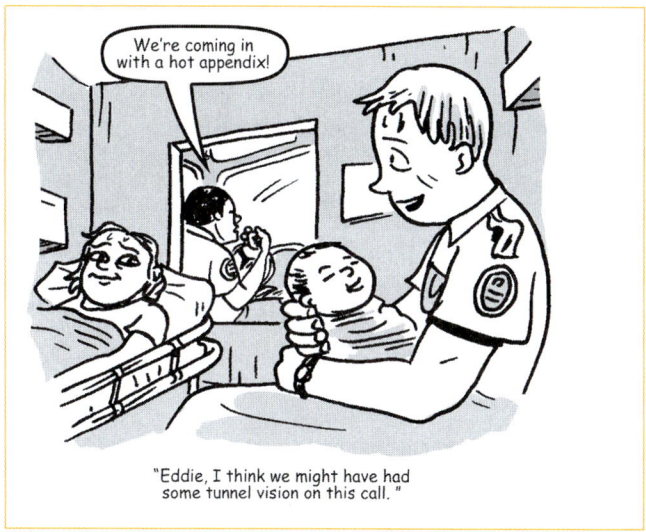

"Eddie, I think we might have had some tunnel vision on this call."

Figure 15-13

6. Review Your Performance

Again, once a call is over, you as a paramedic have the opportunity to look back and reexamine your work **Figure 15-14 ▾**. Whether this review is in the formal setting of a continuous quality improvement (CQI) meeting or just back at the station reviewing the call with your partner, taking the time to critically look at your work allows you real growth opportunities. This is particularly true when an error has occurred. While success is satisfying and certainly feels good, there is little growth opportunity to be had. However, when an error does occur, take the time to analyze the call so that you can identify what circumstances arose to create the error. Was it a system problem? Did you misjudge the call? Errors will only change if you want to find out what they were, and why they recurred. Excellence in prehospital care is the gradual result of you as a paramedic constantly striving to improve your practice, which requires that you *always* have an attitude that is open to learning.

Being a thinking paramedic will only happen if you choose to work on your critical thinking skills throughout your career. As you continue to improve the way you think and make decisions, your patient care will improve as well. Your reward will be excellence in your practice—the ultimate job satisfaction.

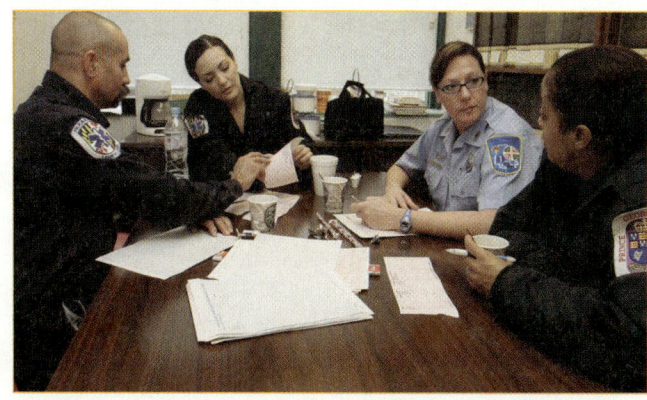

Figure 15-14 You will learn something new with every patient interaction. One of the best ways to review your performance—and to learn—is to talk it over with peers, keeping patient confidentiality in mind.

You are the Paramedic Summary

1. When do you begin patient assessment?

Most people consider patient assessment to begin as early as dispatch, but some would argue there is one step even before the dispatch. Fire departments are well-versed in the aspects of preplanning. They regularly inspect buildings in their response area to identify life, fire, and special hazards related to that structure. Good paramedics know their primary service areas, and can use this information to add even further understanding to information that dispatchers provide regarding their patients. As a good paramedic, your antennae would go up when dispatched to a local orchard for difficulty breathing. Could your patient be suffering from anaphylaxis related to a bee sting or a respiratory emergency related to the inhalation of a pesticide?

2. What are the benefits and the risks of diagnosing based on dispatch?

Dispatchers are adept at gathering and distilling information from 9-1-1 callers. Dispatchers not only gather information, but calm callers, provide instructions, and send appropriate resources to a caller's location. Despite the dispatcher's best efforts, the information gained from callers may or may not be accurate. Oftentimes, this information gives you a good list of possible causes related to a patient's chief complaint, but it is very important to refrain from making a diagnosis. Information provided by the dispatcher should be used to see the big picture, where you can begin to determine whether other resources are likely to be necessary and discuss en route to the scene what role you and the other paramedic will play. The bottom line—generate a list of possible causes, but be flexible!

3. What are pertinent negatives?

Pertinent negatives are findings you would expect to see in a medical condition, but do not. If a paramedic suspects an infection, you would ask questions about the recent history of a productive cough, fever, or chills—all indicators of infection. If your patient denies having any of these signs and symptoms, you are faced with a pertinent negative—it is possible that your patient does not have an infection.

4. What information is missing from the above assessment?

Temperature can yield a wealth of information, particularly in this case. The presence or lack of fever can aid you in narrowing down your list of possible causes. All of your assessment tools aid you in narrowing your list of differential diagnoses.

5. How can a patient's opinion affect treatment and transport decisions?

Patients sometimes self-diagnose, and often only want your reassurance that they don't need to go to the hospital. Don't let a patient talk you into a different diagnosis. Of course, you will respect your patient's feelings and opinions but you must consider them in light of your physical findings.

6. Can men and women have different symptoms of acute illness?

More and more is being learned about the differences of men and women in their response to acute illness. In most classic heart attack scenarios, the patient experiences chest pain, but many of the studies done to describe heart attacks were done using male patients. This symptom is not required to question the presence of a myocardial infarction. Postmenopausal women may have only associated complaints of a sudden onset of generalized weakness, fatigue, dizziness, or shortness of breath. Obtaining an adequate medical history to include all possible risk factors can also provide a wealth of information to aid you in narrowing your list of possible causes.

7. Do good paramedics make errors like this one?

Yes. Like everyone, we all make errors. In our work, mistakes are not welcomed and may result in loss of life. This is why we must assess and reassess our patients and why we must strive to maintain our skills and improve our knowledge. The key is to learn from errors, both your own and those of others.

8. How can a paramedic's attitude affect patient care?

Because we are human, we can allow our personal feelings to affect patient care. This is not always a bad thing, but our personal attitudes should never have a negative impact on patient care. Being tired, hungry, or otherwise distracted is not your patient's concern. Your patient's needs come first, and second only to the safety of yourself and your crew.

9. What was done right in this call?

You erred on the side of the patient. Although you failed to adequately gather data about your patient's condition, you encouraged her to seek evaluation by a physician. Being genuinely concerned for the patient's well-being will oftentimes prevent poor patient care or outcomes. You also provided oxygen, established an IV, and placed her on the cardiac monitor. Your assessment and care, albeit incomplete, did have a positive effect. When reviewing calls, it is important to note what you do right as well as what you can improve on.

10. How could this error have been avoided?

For all calls, you should have a list of possible causes. Always be suspicious for serious, life-threatening conditions. Rule out the worst possible scenario. Don't make assumptions or be complacent or lazy. Every patient deserves a thorough assessment regardless of time of day or if your needs are or aren't being met at the time. It's also important to continue to read the latest in medical research. Medicine is an evolving field, and each year more is learned about the human body and its response to various treatments.

Prep Kit

Ready for Review

- The first cornerstone of your practice as a paramedic is having the ability to *gather*, *evaluate*, and *synthesize* information.
- Once you have gathered information, you must assess and evaluate this information as to its validity and the impact it will have on the patient care plan you are developing.
- Once you have evaluated the information you obtained from the scene, the patient, or any bystanders, then you need to process—or *synthesize*—that information.
- The second cornerstone of your practice is the *development and implementation of patient care plans*.
- Your care plan is almost always defined by the patient care protocols or standing orders in the EMS system where you work.
- The third cornerstone is *judgment and making independent decisions*.
- The fourth and final cornerstone of your practice is your ability to *think and work under pressure*.
- The first stage of the thought process in prehospital care is gathering information—things you see, hear, smell, or feel. This is *concept formation*.
- The second stage of the critical thinking process is data interpretation—evaluating the information you have gathered.
- The last stage in the critical thinking process occurs after the call is over and is commonly associated with call review or critiques. Look back at the total call and reflect on how you processed the signs and symptoms and reached the decisions that you did.

- The *Six Rs* can be used to summarize what must be done on a call:
  - Read the scene
  - Read the patient
  - React
  - Reevaluate
  - Revise the plan
  - Review your performance
- Excellence in prehospital care results from a constant striving to improve your practice, which requires that you ALWAYS have an attitude that is open to learning.

Vital Vocabulary

concept formation Pattern of understanding based on initially obtained information.

cookbook medicine Treatment based on a protocol or algorithm without adequate knowledge of the patient being treated.

data interpretation The process of formulating a conclusion based on comparing the patient's condition with information from your training, education, and past experiences.

medical ambiguity Uncertainty regarding the specific cause of the patient's condition.

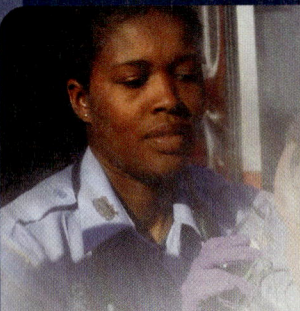

Assessment in Action

You are called to a scene where a 16-year-old male has had a seizure, is vomiting, and isn't making much sense to his family. By the time you get there, he is making a little more sense and is no longer actively vomiting. The family tells you he came home from a party, began vomiting almost immediately, and had a mild seizure that lasted about a minute. He has not answered any of their questions, and they have no idea what he may have eaten or taken at the party.

1. **You introduce yourself to the family and the patient, and ask him how he is feeling. He doesn't answer. You tell him you'd really like to help him feel better, and need for him to answer your questions and be honest. You can see that his pupils are very dilated, he is sweating, and his face is very pale. He doesn't want to answer any of your questions, but does shake his head "no" when you ask if he drank or took any kind of drugs at the party. What do you do?**
   A. Continue with your evaluation as you normally would, in front of his family, despite his denial of having drunk alcohol or taken any drugs.
   B. Tell him you know he's lying based on what his body is telling you, and be confrontational until he tells you what he drank or took.
   C. Try to embarrass him in front of his family so he will tell you the truth.
   D. Continue your evaluation as normal, until you can get him in a private setting so that he may be more inclined to be honest because he is not in front of his family.

2. **In the back of your ambulance, the teen still denies having taken or drank anything. The symptoms he is experiencing tell you otherwise. What do you do?**
   A. Try to scare him by telling him that he will get much worse, and could even die, if he is not honest so you can treat him appropriately.
   B. Call direct medical control, give them all known information, and ask what you should do.
   C. Treat him based on what you *think* he may have taken, without confirmation from the patient himself.
   D. Take him to the hospital and let the doctor deal with him.

3. **In the back of the ambulance, the teenager admits to drinking some beer at the party. He says he is not on any medications, has no known allergies, has never had any type of seizure previously, and has never taken drugs. His pupils are still dilated, he is still somewhat confused, he is sweating and pale, and he is developing stomach cramps. He begins vomiting again, but does not smell like beer at all. He seems to be getting worse. He does not want to go to the hospital, and begs you not to tell his parents about the beer. What do you do?**
   A. Tell his parents you believe he may have a stomach virus, keeping his secret for him. After all, you were a teenager once too and have had your share of partying days.
   B. Tell his parents the truth—that you believe he has taken some kind of drug and that he needs to be taken to the emergency department for treatment, asking their permission to take him against his will for treatment.
   C. Honour the teenager's request to deny treatment, tell him what risks he is facing, and that you will be happy to return and take him to the emergency department if he changes his mind.
   D. Tell his parents nothing except that you are taking him to the hospital for evaluation and that he cannot refuse treatment because he has an altered mental status.

4. **While in the ambulance, your partner suggests the possibility that the teenager, based on his symptoms, is experiencing some kind of blood glucose issue. What do you do?**
   A. Consider this possibility and check the teenager's blood glucose level.
   B. Tell your partner that you are in charge, you've already made up your mind about what is wrong with the teenager, and that is that.
   C. Call direct medical control and ask if you should even consider any possibility of blood glucose issues.
   D. Tell your partner when he has the experience and knowledge that you have, he can make the decision.

5. **The patient's family is impatiently waiting outside your ambulance. His mother begins knocking on the door, then banging on it, insisting she know exactly what is being said and done to her son. She begins yelling and swearing that you are not doing your job right, she doesn't trust you, and she no longer wants you to treat her son. What do you do?**
   A. Send your partner out to calm her down, explaining that you are evaluating her son and doing what is best for him.
   B. Ignore her and continue to evaluate and treat her son.
   C. Explain to her how sick her son is, and that he must be treated based on his altered mental status, with or without her consent.
   D. Let her into the ambulance, apologize, explain what you are doing, what you believe is wrong, what you think will happen if he is not treated at all, and ask that she give her consent.

6. **If the young man mentioned in the above scenario had a rapidly deteriorating mental status (confusion that got worse and worse in a short amount of time) and other signs, such as his breathing rate also deteriorated, how would this affect your evaluation and treatment?**
   A. It would not affect it; you would evaluate and treat him as you would in other questions listed above.
   B. You would panic, tell his parents the outlook was not good, and take him to the emergency department as quickly as possible.
   C. You would tell his parents that their son's condition was his own fault for drinking alcohol while under age or taking drugs, and he should have known better.
   D. You would treat all symptoms as they occurred on your way to the emergency department.

7. **What if the patient in the scenario became combative, stubborn, and mean, and insisted that you give him narcotic pain medication before you do anything else? What if he would not allow you to examine or otherwise treat him unless you did this first? You know he needs to go to the hospital, and that he has more problems than just the pain he is dealing with. What would you do?**
   A. Give him the pain medication to make him more cooperative, and to make your assessment, diagnosis, and treatment easier.
   B. Bribe him—tell him if he's cooperative for the evaluation and treatment, you will give him what he wants (even if you have no intention of doing so).
   C. Tell him that you work under a physician and have certain rules you must follow, which do not allow you to give him the pain medication he wants unless you do a full examination and diagnosis and your medical director allows it.
   D. Tell him that if he does not cooperate and let you do your job, you will tell his parents that you believe he has taken drugs, and may even get the police involved.

Challenging Questions

You are called to the home of an older man whose neighbours saw him walking around his house and yard late in the evening in his underwear, seeming confused. When you arrive, he does not answer his open front door. You walk in, calling his name, and take note of some small insulin syringes lying on the kitchen counter. You find him standing in the backyard, looking confused. When you introduce yourself and question him, he says he has no idea why he's in the backyard and had no idea he wasn't dressed. You note that he is also wearing a medical ID bracelet, but it does not have a condition listed on it. He asks you at least four times who you are, and why you're there. You ask him how he's feeling; he says he's fine. You ask him about his medical history, asking specifically if he is diabetic. He tells you he is not. But you know from neighbours that he lives alone. He is extremely confused and irrational.

8. **Do you listen to your patient's answers and put faith into them, assuming he knows what he is talking about, and try to assess and diagnose him based on that information? Or do you take into account his behaviour and what you have seen (insulin syringes, medical ID bracelet), heard, and observed?**

9. **If the patient in this scenario were naked and began saying inappropriate things to your young female partner, how would you (and your partner) handle it?**

▣ Points to Ponder

You are dispatched to a "two-vehicle collision that occurred at a slow speed; minor or no injuries reported by bystander."

How should you prioritize this call?

Issues: Preparation, Priorities, Response Time to Scene.

www.Paramedic.EMSzone.com/Canada

16

Communications and Documentation

Competency Areas

Area 1: Professional Responsibilities

1.1.a Maintain patient dignity.

1.1.b Reflect professionalism through use of appropriate language.

1.1.c Dress appropriately and maintain personal hygiene

1.1.d Maintain appropriate personal interaction with patients.

1.1.e Maintain patient confidentiality.

1.1.f Participate in quality assurance and enhancement programs.

1.1.g Utilize community support agencies as appropriate.

1.1.h Promote awareness of emergency medical system and profession.

1.1.i Participate in professional association.

Area 2: Communication

2.1.a Deliver an organized, accurate, and relevant report utilizing telecommunication devices.

2.1.b Deliver an organized, accurate, and relevant verbal report.

2.1.c Deliver an organized, accurate, and relevant patient history.

2.1.d Provide information to patient about their situation and how they will be treated.

2.1.e Interact effectively with the patient, relatives, and bystanders who are in stressful situations.

2.1.f Speak in language appropriate to the listener.

2.1.g Use appropriate terminology.

2.2.a Record organized, accurate, and relevant patient information.

2.2.b Prepare professional correspondence.

2.3.a Exhibit effective non-verbal behaviour.

2.3.b Practice active listening techniques.

2.3.c Establish trust and rapport with patients and colleagues.

2.3.d Recognize and react appropriately to non-verbal behaviours.

Introduction

In EMS communication, relaying information from one person to another becomes extremely urgent in the short time that you will have to care for a patient. That information needs to move rapidly, efficiently, and effectively. As a paramedic, you must be able to effectively communicate verbally and in writing with many other people.

You need to know what constitutes an EMS communications system, who needs to be able to talk with whom, what technical resources are available to you to make those conversations possible, and what you can do to make communications as efficient as possible. You also need to understand the crucial role of the emergency medical dispatcher (EMD) in facilitating all phases of EMS communications. You need to know how to organize patient information into a brief, orderly verbal report that can be transmitted by radio or by telephone.

Written communication in the form of reports or documentation is as vital to your patient care as following local medical protocols. Learning to write effectively and accurately with only the absolutely necessary subjective information is an important paramedic skill. Subjective information includes the symptoms patients describe—the degree of pain, for example. Objective information includes the measurable signs that you observe and record, such as blood pressure. You must record subjective *and* objective information and the details of patient care for every call in a written or computer-based report, and in some cases, both. This report needs to be complete, accurate, and legible because it can provide the basis of defence in legal proceedings and is of vital importance to your service or agency for many other reasons as well, including facilitation of quality prehospital care, continuity, and billing insurance. Your written report should "paint a picture" of the entire call that is clear and accurate to the reader.

Phases of Communication

Communication during an emergency call has several phases that are essential to appropriate prehospital care and transportation. You will be exchanging information with many people, including the patient, bystanders with valuable information, the patient's family, direct medical control, the receiving medical facility staff, your dispatch centre, law enforcement officials, and other paramedics. One paramount responsibility in an emergency is communication with your partner. Staying in constant touch will keep each of you on top of your responsibilities and working effectively as a team while providing prehospital care for your patient.

Each phase of the communication process requires using terminology understood by the people you are communicating with. Patients might need you to explain their medical condition in terms they know and understand. When you relay information to the receiving medical facility, you can use the medical terminology you have learned to make your radio report clear. The old saying, "When in Rome, do as the Romans do," applies in EMS. Using medical terminology and avoiding slang terms shows your professionalism and respect for everyone you work with.

Although you might not think of yourself as a "number-crunching" scholar, collecting information and data is essential to EMS. You can help gather the data, analyze it, and determine what changes are necessary by writing clear, accurate, and easy-to-read reports. Although data collection may seem time-consuming, ensure that the information you

You are the Paramedic Part 1

It is a beautiful summer day when you and your partner are dispatched to a bicycle collision at 1277 Cochran Mill Road. On arrival, you are greeted by a bystander who tells you that during his usual afternoon walk he found a woman lying next to the trail. He said he was worried she had been hit by a car or was otherwise injured, so he didn't move her and immediately called 9-1-1.

You find a 45-year-old woman lying on the ground and unresponsive. Her bike is lying on top of her, and she is wearing a helmet, bike shorts, and a T-shirt.

Initial Assessment	Recording Time: 0 Minutes
Appearance	Pale, obviously diaphoretic
Level of consciousness	U (Unresponsive)
Airway	Open; secretions present
Breathing	Noisy breathing present; secretions present
Circulation	Rapid radial pulse present

1. Why did the dispatcher supply very little information for this call?
2. What immediate challenges do you foresee regarding this call?
3. How does the initial information you're given from dispatchers, family, bystanders, or other responders impact your decisions regarding prehospital care?

record and report to your EMS agency is accurate for data collection, billing, and reporting purposes. Even in cases of multiple-casualty incidents (MCIs), collecting data is especially essential for determining patient care totals, severity of injuries, outcomes, and mass care procedures.

Who Needs to Communicate With Whom?

For the EMS system to work, a number of people have to be able to contact a number of other people. Let's follow an emergency call from its inception to its conclusion to see who needs to reach whom.

The first stage of the EMS response is notification, that is, someone has to tell EMS that an emergency exists. Usually notification is carried out by telephone or cellular phone, and the person requesting help communicates with the <u>emergency medical dispatcher (EMD)</u>. A universal emergency telephone number—9-1-1 in most places in Canada—and the availability of telephones and cellular phones in most places has greatly helped notification. Notification may, less frequently, come by radio, when the emergency is detected by a law enforcement or other public vehicle.

The next step is <u>dispatch</u>, communicating from the service headquarters with the responding paramedic team. The person who directs that team to the scene of the emergency is called the dispatcher **Figure 16-1 ▾**. Dispatch may be accomplished by telephone, pager, fax, or two-way radio that may include <u>push-to-talk</u> technology. Push-to-talk devices can include mobile phones or walkie-talkies known as half-duplex devices. These allow the voice to be transmitted when a button is pushed and allow the listener to hear if the button is released. Most telecommunications equipment today uses digital technology rather than direct or analogue transmission and radio tubes. Digital technology offers many advantages in terms of speed, privacy, programmability, and the global positioning system, or GPS. Many dispatch centres use <u>computer-aided dispatch</u> systems, automated computer systems that process

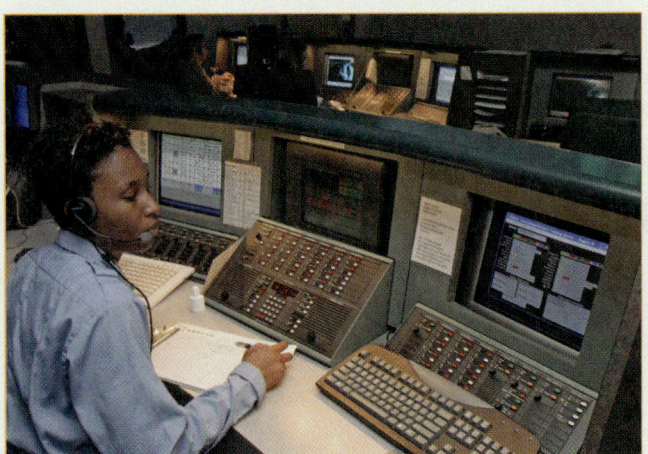

Figure 16-1 The dispatcher receives the call to 9-1-1 and dispatches EMS to the scene.

the information received and assist dispatchers with multiple functions and tasks.

Your dispatcher may have to speak with you en route to give you additional information about the call. You may need to request other resources, such as police, fire, hazardous materials, or another specialty rescue unit. Communications between you and the dispatcher are usually carried out by <u>mobile</u> (in the vehicle) or <u>portable</u> (in your hand) radios. Cellular telephones may also be used for that purpose provided coverage is available.

Your service might require special training in <u>emergency medical dispatch</u> procedures, which means your dispatchers may be able to provide basic medical instructions to callers who are able to provide basic first aid steps while you are on your way. Some dispatch centres have trained paramedics to relay basic medical instructions to callers when needed. Such prearrival instructions give your service what many in EMS call "zero response time," providing immediate aid and assistance, which can be vital in saving a life. Simple but lifesaving acts such as clearing an obstructed airway, performing chest compressions, or reassuring the patient can be carried out by a layperson under the instructions of a good dispatcher. In many cases, these prearrival instructions may bring a sense of emotional support to a caller in a time of great need, reassuring people close to the patient that everything that can be done is being done and actively getting the caller to perform lifesaving tasks.

Your dispatcher can give you prearrival information that will keep you on top of events as they are unfolding, with updates on the situation and your patient while you are en route.

Once you are at the scene, communications among you, the receiving facility, and your medical control are necessary to allow physician orders for invasive procedures to be transmitted and to coordinate the care of your patient. Your direct medical control physician can receive any required telemetry for patient assessment. In the early years, it was a common practice for paramedics to send electrocardiograms (ECGs) to direct medical control. For a time, the transmission of a lead II ECG was discontinued in most communities because of competition for the air waves, and direct medical control physicians let paramedics work under more expanded standing orders. The most recent Heart and Stroke Foundation recommendations support a paramedic acquiring 12-lead ECG and either transmitting it to medical control or interpreting it to identify potential changes due to cardiac ischemia. In some services, a facsimile, or fax, of the ECG is transmitted directly by cellular phone to the coronary catheterization laboratory to help the staff determine the best treatment, preparing for fibrinolytic therapy or a catheterization procedure.

Communication with the physician in charge, whether by voice or telemetry, can require two-way radios, a telephone <u>patch</u> (telephone-to-radio connection), cellular telephones, or facsimile capabilities.

Once your patient is ready to be moved, you must communicate with the receiving facility to let the hospital know what to expect. Once again, most ambulance-to-hospital communications are by radio, but cellular telephones also have an

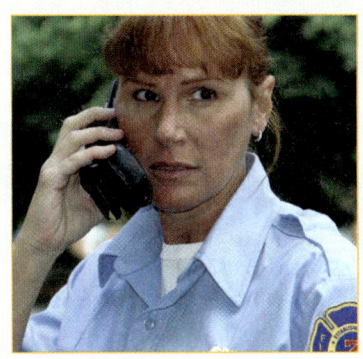

Figure 16-2 Use of cellular phones is becoming more common in EMS communications systems.

increasingly important role Figure 16-2 ◄. Computer-based transmissions are also becoming more widely used. Some services have wireless systems that transmit the data in the prehospital care report (PCR) to the emergency department (ED) as the ambulance is pulling into the hospital's parking lot. Once back at their station, these lucky paramedics transmit the billing and patient profile to the service's computer as the ambulance pulls into the garage. The data is sent to the EMS agency headquarters before the crew actually steps out of the ambulance!

These communications links are essential to ensure an efficient response to an emergency call. However, a complete EMS communications system requires a few other components as well:

- It is highly desirable to link all area hospitals into the communications network. In case of a disaster, multiple casualties may be appropriately distributed and hospitals may be informed of the number of patients they will be receiving. Interhospital communications can be carried out by telephone networks, by radio, or through computer-based programs. Some hospitals now participate in regional programs that allow hospital bed availability to be displayed on a computer screen and shared in case of diversion and overcrowding issues.

- Other agencies that may be involved in an emergency response (police, fire, public utilities, helicopter services, poison centres) should be able to communicate with one another. Cellular technology has made such communications much more accessible, but a backup radio network is still desirable in case telephone lines and frequencies become overloaded during an MCI. Satellite phones, which often work when the cellular system is down, are an additional tool a paramedic may have available to assist in communicating during a disaster. Coordination of such systems should be done well in advance of a disaster and tested periodically to ensure the system will work.

- Finally, it is important, especially in disasters, to be aware of other broadcast systems that may be recruited to assist in communications within the community.

Components of an EMS Communications System

Even though the digital revolution will improve communications, most EMS communications systems today are based on the use of radios, so you need to learn about what radio signals

are and what equipment is available for sending and receiving radio signals.

Radio Communications and Telemetry

Radio transmits signals by electromagnetic waves. Remember, energy can be emitted in the form of waves or particles. When energy is emitted in the form of waves, the energy can be characterized by the length of the waves it produces. Energy of a relatively long wavelength produces audible sound; energy of shorter wavelength is in the infrared light spectrum. Between sound and infrared light are the wavelengths for radio transmission. Radio wavelengths are used for tuning by adjusting your radio to the proper frequency—how frequently the wave recurs in a given time (usually 1 second). Short wavelengths are repeated more often—with higher frequency—than longer wavelengths. Radio frequencies are designated by their cycles per second, or hertz (Hz) (named for the man who first described the propagation of electromagnetic waves). The following abbreviations are commonly used:

- hertz (Hz)—cycles per second
- kilohertz (kHz)—1,000 cycles per second
- megahertz (MHz)—1 million cycles per second
- gigahertz (GHz)—1 billion cycles per second

Radio waves are confined to the part of the electromagnetic frequency spectrum extending from 3 kHz to about 3,000 GHz. A normal voice channel requires a minimum of 3 kHz. Frequency bands are portions of the radio frequency spectrum assigned for specific uses. The most commonly used bands for medical communications are the very high frequency (VHF) band and the ultrahigh frequency (UHF) band. The VHF band extends from roughly 30 to 175 MHz and has been arbitrarily divided into a low band (30 to 50 MHz) and a high band (150 to 175 MHz). The low-band frequencies may have ranges up to 3,200 km but are unpredictable because changes in ionospheric conditions may cause "skip interference," with patchy losses in communication. The high-band frequencies are almost wholly free of skip interference, but at a price—a much shorter transmission range. The most commonly used of the VHF high-band frequencies for emergency medical purposes are in the 150 to 160 MHz range. The UHF band extends from 300 to 3,000 MHz, with most medical communications occurring around 450 to 470 MHz. At these frequencies, communications are entirely free of skip interference and have minimal noise (signal distortion). The UHF band has better penetration in dense metropolitan areas, and UHF reception is usually quite adequate inside buildings. The UHF band, however, has a shorter range than the VHF band, and energy at UHF is more readily absorbed by rain and environmental objects, such as trees and brush.

Radios that operate at 800 MHz are common in EMS systems. This frequency offers excellent penetration of buildings and has minimal interference and reduced channel noise. Because of this, it works quite well in metropolitan areas; 800 MHz also allows for trunking, in which multiple agencies or systems can share frequencies. An 800-MHz radio can also be linked to a computer system to transmit voiceless communications. The use of trunked systems has allowed the dispatcher to reprogram the radios so that agencies that do not routinely talk to each other can easily do so at the scene of a mass-casualty incident, a rescue, a hazardous materials incident, or other special operations.

Agencies within the federal government control the allocation of frequencies in Canada. VHF frequencies have been set aside for general emergency radio communications and UHF band assignments for ambulance-to-hospital telemetry systems, especially where communications from physicians to rescue personnel are needed to consult or direct patient care activities. Those band assignments will be given to you by your EMS system.

Biotelemetry

Biotelemetry (usually called simply telemetry) is the capability of measuring vital life signs and transmitting them to a distant terminal. Biotelemetry started out with ECGs but often is used for other measurements.

The term *biotelemetry* in emergency medical care is usually shortened to *telemetry*. Most often, telemetry is a short way of saying you are transmitting an ECG signal from your patient to a distant receiving station. The standard ECG is composed of low-frequency signals (100 Hz or less), which would be filtered out by a voice communications system. To make sure voice communication doesn't filter the ECG out, the ECG signal must be encoded if it is to be sent over the same radio channels used to transmit voice. The ECG signal is encoded by using a reference audio tone, for example at 1,000 Hz, which is made to vary with the voltage generated by the electric events in the heart. The reference tone, or calibration, of a varying 1,000-Hz tone is used to modulate the frequency of the transmitter to ensure that all signals are being transmitted. When the ECG signal is received at the distant terminal at the receiving hospital or medical control, it is amplified and decoded to produce a voltage that is an exact replica of the original. That voltage is then converted to the graphic plot seen on the oscilloscope or printout.

ECG telemetry over UHF frequencies is confined to one lead of a 12-lead ECG, so it can be used to interpret cardiac rhythms. For a more complete diagnosis of an ECG, such as in the case of examining the ECG of a patient with suspected acute coronary syndrome, one must examine all 12 leads of the ECG. Some EMS systems use facsimile technology to allow transmission of ECGs, including 12-lead ECGs, to receiving hospitals before the arrival of the ambulance at the facility.

Distortion of the ECG signal by extraneous spikes and waves is known as noise and may arise from a variety of sources:

- Muscle tremor
- Loose ECG electrodes
- Sources of 60-cycle alternating current (AC), such as transformers, power lines, and electric equipment
- Attenuation (reduction) of transmitter power, caused by weak batteries or transmission beyond the range of the transmitter

In the past several years, as paramedics have become more and more skilled in dysrhythmia recognition, the trend has been to make less and less use of ECG telemetry; rather, most systems rely solely on the paramedic's assessment of the patient's cardiac rhythm and rarely require confirmation of the assessment by a physician. Just as ECG telemetry seemed headed for the fate of the horse-drawn ambulance, however, two developments occurred to bring about a reassessment of prehospital ECG telemetry. First, conclusive research on the use of fibrinolytic agents indicated that the earlier the agents were given during an acute myocardial infarction, the better the chances of myocardial reperfusion. Second, cellular telephone and facsimile technology made it possible to transmit a 12-lead ECG from a moving ambulance to a hospital and, therefore, to diagnose myocardial infarction before the patient reaches the hospital. At the least, such early diagnosis enables the EMS service to bypass the closest hospital and take the patient to a designated cardiac centre and notify the cardiac intervention lab to prepare for primary angioplasty and stenting of the blocked coronary artery immediately after the patient arrives or, in some EMS systems, even deliver the fibrinolytic therapy in the prehospital setting. Because technology can facilitate assessment and treatment in the prehospital setting, it is probable that telemetry in one form or another will remain a part of emergency care for some time. Information other than ECGs may also be transmitted to the receiving hospital before the patient arrives. Because advancements in technology are occurring rapidly, EMS systems must keep up with the technology that will allow better methods for communication of patient information.

Cellular Telephones

Cellular telephones operate on 3 watts of power or less. Mobile antennas are much closer to the ground than base station antennas, so communications from the unit are typically limited to 16 to 24 km over average terrain. Base station antennas are usually located on high sites to increase the coverage area.

Cellular telephones are becoming more common in EMS communications systems. These telephones are simply low-power portable radios that communicate through a series of interconnected repeater stations called "cells" (hence the name "cellular"). Cells are linked by a sophisticated computer system and connected to the telephone network. Cellular telephones are also popular with other public safety agencies, particularly as more cell sites are constructed in rural areas.

Cell phones have advantages that radio does not: (1) The public is encouraged to make use of the free service for 9-1-1 or other emergency numbers. (2) Cell phone technology incorporates GPS to let emergency responders know where the patient is.

Many cellular systems make equipment and air time available to EMS services at little or no cost as a public service. The public is often able to call 9-1-1 or other emergency numbers on a cellular telephone free of charge. However, this easy access may result in overloading and jamming of cellular systems in MCI and disaster situations, and you should have a backup communications plan in your service to circumvent these overloads.

Most newer cell phones have GPSs built in specifically for emergencies. (It is possible to turn off GPS in a cellular phone but not for EMS). The so-called enhanced 9-1-1 helps the EMS operator know exactly where the cell call is being placed from. In the past, when a cell phone call was made by a patient who drove off the road, rescuers would need to search blindly because many patients became unconscious or did not know their location. Many vehicles also have vehicle locator and navigation systems that notify emergency services when a collision has occurred. These, too, are based on GPS technology. Typically, these cell phone calls for emergency services may go through a routing centre rather than directly to the local dispatch centre. The 9-1-1 cellular calls often go through a regional or provincial system operated by the cellular phone service provider. They have predetermined protocols to determine the caller's location and forward the call to the appropriate public service answering point.

Modes of Radio Operation

Assigned radio frequencies may be used in a variety of systems. In a simplex system, portable units can transmit only in one mode (voice or telemetry) or receive (voice) at any given time. A simplex system requires only a single radio frequency. A network that uses two different frequencies at the same time, to permit simultaneous transmission and reception (like a telephone), is referred to as duplex. Another alternative is to combine, or multiplex, two or more signals—such as the paramedic's voice and the patient's ECG—for simultaneous transmission on one frequency.

Suppose that an ambulance service wanted the possibility of voice communications and continuous telemetry. There are at least four ways to design the communications system to meet those requirements:

- The ambulance could transmit on two frequencies of a UHF-frequency pair (channel) allocated for telemetry (duplex). One frequency would transmit the voice signal and the other, the telemetry signal. Such a system requires that the ambulance have two UHF transmitters (one for voice, one for telemetry) and one receiver (voice).
- The ambulance service could multiplex (combine) telemetry and voice on one frequency of the allocated UHF pair and receive voice communications on the other frequency of the pair. That requires only one UHF transmitter on the vehicle, but the base station must be fitted with demultiplexing equipment to separate the two signals coming in on one frequency.
- The ambulance could transmit telemetry data on one frequency of the allocated telemetry pair and transmit voice data on a VHF frequency. That requires a UHF and a VHF transmitter on the vehicle (two simplex systems).
- As noted, there is an increasing trend toward using cellular telephones for ECG telemetry. Cellular phones have full duplex capability, a multitude of available channels, a very high-quality signal that is unlikely to degrade over distance, and a much lower capital and maintenance cost.

Building Blocks of a Communications System

Although EMS communications systems vary considerably among one another, most systems serving moderate to large populations are constructed of the following components.

You are the Paramedic Part 2

You see that additional assistance will be required to extricate the patient from her bike, and you request it. A crew is dispatched from a nearby fire station. You and your partner err on the side of caution and initiate spinal precautions. Your partner controls the patient's cervical spine while you manage the airway.

Firefighters quickly arrive and extricate the patient and place her on the backboard. You next insert an intravenous (IV) line, and, per local protocol, perform a blood glucose check. No trauma is noted beyond a few minor abrasions to her right arm, shoulder, and leg.

Vital Signs	Recording Time: 5 Minutes
Level of consciousness	Unresponsive, with a Glasgow Coma Scale score of 5
Skin	Pale, cool, and diaphoretic
Pulse	128 beats/min, strong and regular
Blood pressure	132/86 mm Hg
Respirations	22 breaths/min
Spo$_2$	92% ambient air

4. How did this call change from dispatch to arrival?
5. Given her level of consciousness, what concerns do you have regarding her airway?
6. What are your top priorities at the moment?

Base Stations

The base station is a collection of radio equipment consisting, at minimum, of a transmitter, receiver, and antenna. The base station serves as a dispatch and coordination area and ideally should be in contact with all other elements of the system. Base stations generally use relatively high power output (45 to 275 watts).

The base station must be equipped with an antenna sited in suitable terrain, preferably on a hill or high building, close to the base. The antenna system has a vital part in transmission and reception efficiency. A good antenna system can compensate for limits on power output and human-made signal distortion in the area.

Mobile Transmitter/Receivers (Transceivers)

A mobile transmitter/receiver, or mobile transceiver, is a two-way radio mounted in a vehicle. Mobile transmitter/receivers come in a variety of power ranges, and the power output largely determines the distance over which the signal can be effectively transmitted. A transmitter in the 7.5 watt range, for example, will transmit for distances of 16 to 19 km over slightly hilly terrain. Transmission distances are greater over water or flat terrain and reduced in mountainous areas or where there are many tall buildings. Mobile transmitters with higher outputs have proportionally greater transmission ranges. Today, the typical mobile transmitter operates at between 20 and 50 watts.

Portable Transmitter/Receivers

Portable, handheld radios are useful when paramedics must work at a distance from their vehicle but need to stay in communication with the base or with one another Figure 16-3 ▾ . Portable units may also be used by physician consultants when not stationed at the hospital. Portable units usually have power outputs of up to 5 watts and, thus, have limited range by themselves, although the signal of a handheld transmitter can be boosted by retransmission through the vehicle.

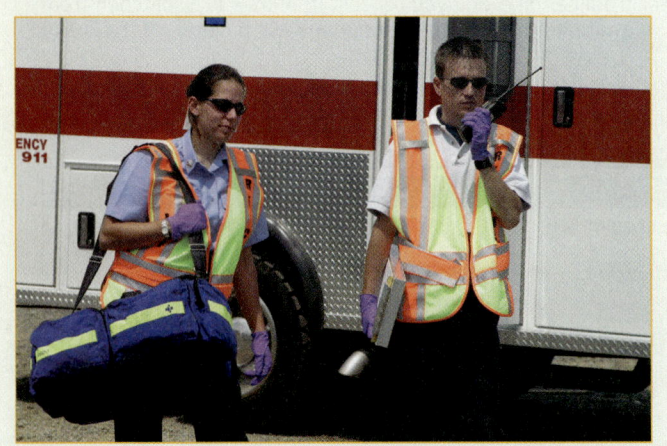

Figure 16-3 A portable radio is essential if you need to communicate with the dispatcher or direct medical control when you are away from the ambulance.

Repeaters

A repeater is a miniature base station used to extend the transmitting and receiving range of a telemetry or voice communications system Figure 16-4 ▾ . Repeaters may be stationary in one location (fixed repeaters) or carried in emergency vehicles (mobile repeaters). A repeater picks up a weak signal and retransmits it at a higher power on another frequency, so it extends the range of low-power portables and allows more members of the system to hear one another. This is how the trooper on the side of the highway can talk to a supervisor on the other end.

Remote Consoles

A remote console, usually located in the ED of a hospital, is a terminal that receives transmissions of telemetry and voice from the out-of-hospital environment and transmits messages back, usually through the base station. Remote consoles are connected to the base station by dedicated telephone lines, microwave, or radio. They contain an amplifier and speaker for incoming voice reception, a decoder for translating the telemetry signal into an oscilloscope tracing or printout, and a microphone for voice transmission.

Backup Communications Systems

In addition to radio communications, most systems use landline (telephone) backup to link various fixed components of the system, such as hospitals, public safety services, and poison control. Telephones may also be patched into radio transmissions through the base station, enabling, for example, communication between paramedics using radios in the prehospital environment and a physician using his or her telephone at home. Finally, as mentioned earlier, cellular telephones are becoming an increasingly important part of EMS communications, overcoming many of the problems of overcrowded EMS radio frequencies. Cellular phones are cheaper than radios and generally give a much clearer signal. Furthermore, they enable a paramedic in the prehospital environment to communicate with anyone who has a telephone—the patient's family physician, an injured child's parent, or an expert in another province who can advise on a hazardous materials situation. The possibilities are as varied as the listings in the telephone directory.

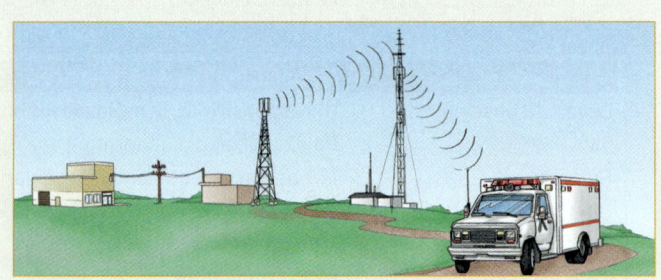

Figure 16-4 A message is sent from the control centre by a landline to the transmitter. The radio carrier wave is picked up by the repeater for rebroadcast to outlying units. Return radio traffic is picked up by the repeater and rebroadcast to the control centre.

Communicating by Radio

The effectiveness of an EMS communications network depends on the technical hardware and on the people who use it. Communicating effectively by radio under emergency conditions requires skill and experience. Some paramedics "freeze" at the microphone, whereas others find themselves acting out their latent ambitions as disk jockeys with unlimited streams of patter. Neither behaviour is appropriate or useful. Effective radio communication in EMS requires knowledge of the rules that govern the communications and an understanding of conventions for transmitting medical information by radio. It is not complicated if you bear in mind that the purpose of talking on the radio is to transmit pertinent information. Keep communications simple, brief, and direct.

Notes from Nancy
The purpose of talking on the radio is to transmit pertinent information.

You should practice effective communications skills and be familiar with all of the various methods of communication that will be required through your radio. As part of your job, you will need to demonstrate how to communicate effectively with your dispatcher for the call, from call receipt to call end. In addition, you must be able to effectively communicate with the receiving medical facility and deliver a precise and direct radio report in an organized and systematic manner.

Government Regulations

As mentioned earlier, the federal government assigns and regulates all radio and television communications in Canada. For radio, the government issues licenses, allocates frequencies, establishes technical standards, and establishes and enforces rules and regulations for the operation of radio equipment. Officials monitor transmissions on various frequencies and conduct spot checks of base stations to ensure that they are properly licensed. Fines can be imposed for failing to follow rules and regulations.

The use of obscenities and the transmission of messages unrelated to provision of medical services are forbidden. When it is necessary to communicate a personal message to a paramedic in the prehospital environment, it is best simply to notify her or him by radio to contact the base by phone. Similarly, a paramedic with a personal request of the dispatcher should use a telephone, not a two-way radio to communicate that message **Figure 16-5 ▶**.

Clarity of Transmission

The basic model of communication, whether by radio, intercom, telephone, or face-to-face involves a *sender,* a clear message, a *receiver,* and a *feedback loop* to ensure that the exact message that was sent is received and interpreted properly by the receiver. The purpose of communications equipment is to

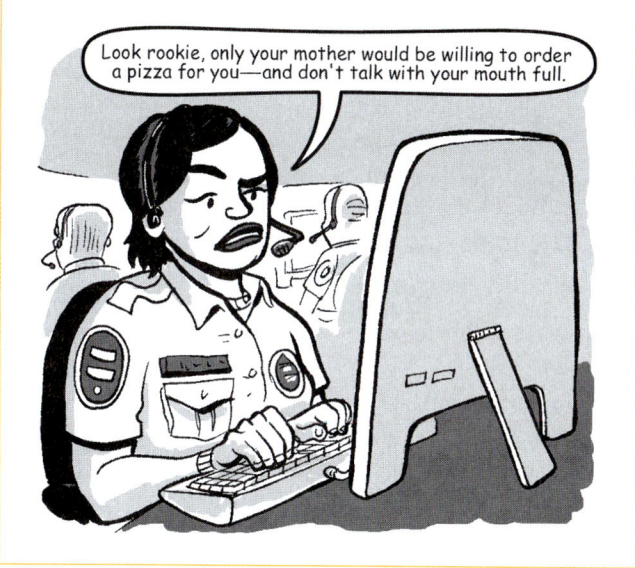

Figure 16-5

permit communication. That sounds obvious, yet it is often forgotten. Simply blurting something into a microphone is not communicating. For communication to occur, someone at the other end of the radio has to be able to hear and understand what you say. The first principle of communicating by radio is clarity.

A number of guidelines can help you improve the clarity of transmissions:

- Before you begin to transmit, listen to make sure the channel is clear. If another radio transmission is in progress, wait until the parties have finished transmitting before you try to get on the air. Cutting in on someone else's transmission will only ensure that neither of you will be adequately heard.
- Once the channel is quiet, press the transmit key for at least 1 second before you start speaking to ensure that the beginning of your message is not lost.
- Start your transmission with the identifying information: give the number or the name of the unit being called first, then your own identification (for example, "Foothills Hospital, this is Medic 3"). That way, the unit being called is alerted immediately and will be listening when you give your own identification, so they can reply at once, "Go ahead, Medic 3." If you do say, for example, "Medic 3 calling Foothills Hospital", the recipients might listen only when you've mentioned their identification and, therefore, will miss your identification. So what inevitably happens then is, "This is Foothills Hospital. What unit is calling?" That extra transmission is a waste of time.
- Keep your mouth close to the microphone, but not too close. About 5 to 8 cm is usually ideal.
- Speak clearly and distinctly, pronouncing each word carefully.

- Don't shout! Shouting distorts the signal. Speak in a normal pitch; very high- and low-pitched sounds do not transmit well. Whispering is not effective for transmitting.
- Don't talk with your mouth full. It muffles transmission.
- Keep calm and keep your voice free from emotion. You don't have to imitate a talking computer; a normal conversational tone is fine. Just keep your voice and mind free of panic, anger, excitement, and other feelings that can distort your transmission and your judgment.

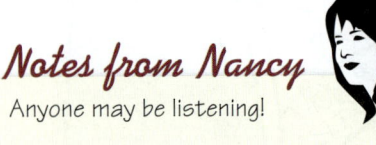

Notes from Nancy
Anyone may be listening!

- Keep your transmissions brief. Air time is precious, and emergency medical frequencies are not the place for long philosophic dialogues. Try having your radio reports taped at some point to critique your own transmissions and perfect your style.
- If you have a long message to transmit, break up the message into 30-second segments, checking at the end of each segment to determine whether it was received and understood.
- Don't waste air time with unnecessary phrases, such as "be advised." Also bear in mind that courtesy is taken for granted; there is no need to use air time for social graces such as "please," "thank you," and "how nice to hear your voice."
- When speaking a word or name that might be misunderstood, spell it out, using the international phonetic alphabet (Table 16-1 ▾) or a similar system. Suppose, for example, you are asking the hospital to notify the patient's family doctor whose name might be mistaken for that of another doctor on the staff; you might say, "Notify Dr. Wilby. That's Dr. WHISKEY-INDIA-LIMA-BRAVO-YANKEE, Wilby."
- When presenting numbers that might be misunderstood, transmit the number as a whole, then digit by digit. For example, if the respirations are 16, you would say, "The respirations are sixteen, that is, one-six."

Content of Transmissions

Radio transmissions for emergency medical services should be brief, to the point, and professional in tone (Figure 16-6 ▾). Here are some guidelines about what should and should not be included in EMS radio communications:

- The first thing to remember when you get "on the air" is that your words are, quite literally, in the air, floating around for anyone to hear. Remember, anyone may be listening (Figure 16-7 ▾).

  The medical staff at the local ED, a patient signing in at the front desk of another ED, a 12-year-old radio buff playing with his scanner at home . . . any of them may be listening with great attention to your transmission. Therefore, it is essential to protect the privacy of the patient at all times. Do not use the patient's name on the air, and do not transmit personal information about the patient. Also, check local laws applicable to your EMS systems. Certain types of cases, such as rape or psychiatric problems, confidential communicable disease history (such as HIV status), are best identified on the

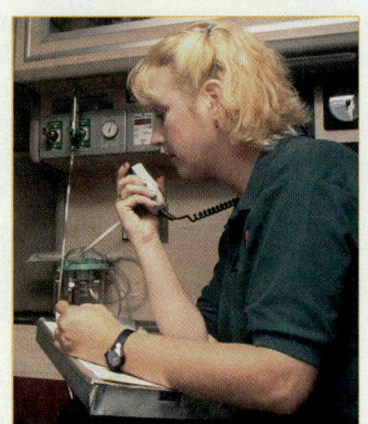

Figure 16-6 The patient report should be given in an objective, accurate, professional manner.

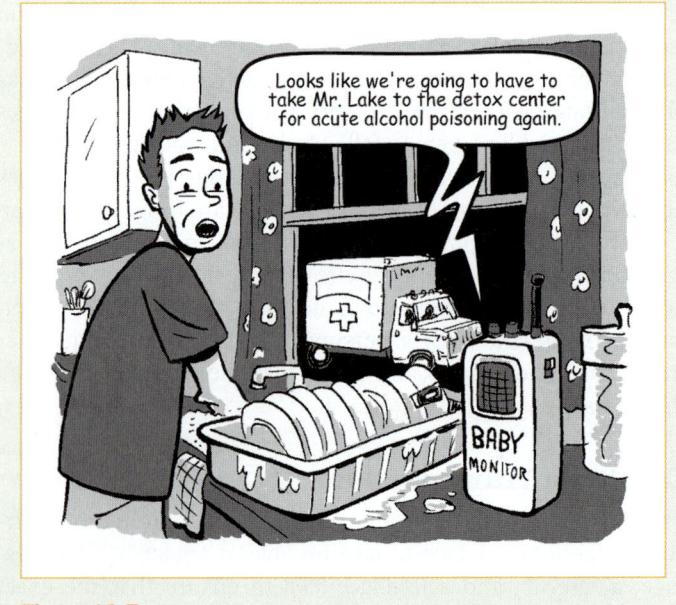

Figure 16-7

Table 16-1	International Phonetic Alphabet	
A Alpha	**J** Juliette	**S** Sierra
B Bravo	**K** Kilo	**T** Tango
C Charlie	**L** Lima	**U** Uniform
D Delta	**M** Mike	**V** Victor
E Echo	**N** November	**W** Whiskey
F Foxtrot	**O** Oscar	**X** X-ray
G Golf	**P** Papa	**Y** Yankee
H Hotel	**Q** Quebec	**Z** Zebra (or Zulu)
I India	**R** Romeo	

air by an established code or given in face-to-face communications when you arrive in the ED.

Don't assume that your cellular telephone offers you protected conversations. There are scanners on the market that can tune into the local cellular frequencies. So don't say anything on the radio or the cellular phone that you don't want everyone in town to hear.

- Be impersonal. Use "we," not "I," to refer to yourself, and use proper names and titles ("Sergeant York," not "Billy") to refer to others when necessary.
- Don't try to be a comedian or a critic. There is no place for unprofessional behaviour, sarcasm, or other poor conduct on emergency medical radio frequencies.
- Don't use profane language on the air. Aside from the reflection on your professional character, the government might issue civil monetary penalties, revoke a license, or deny a renewal application.
- Use professional language, but don't show off. Once again, remember that the object of the exercise is to communicate information, not to stun your listener into awe and admiration. Using proper medical terminology is advisable when done correctly.
- Avoid using words that are difficult to hear. The word "yes," for example, is easily lost in transmission; use "affirmative" instead. Similarly, use "negative" instead of "no."
- Use standard formats agreed on by your EMS service for transmission of information. The patient's history, for example, should always be presented in the same order. When the listeners know what they are listening for, they are less likely to miss parts of the transmission.
- When you finish transmitting, obtain confirmation that the transmission was received. When you receive instructions by radio from the dispatcher or from direct medical control, echo the order back to make certain you have understood it correctly. Thus, for example, if the physician instructs you to administer 75 mg of lidocaine slowly IV, you would respond, "That is lidocaine, 75 milligrams, repeat, 75 milligrams, slowly IV. Is that confirmed?"
- Question any orders you did not hear clearly or did not understand.
- Use EMS frequencies only for emergency medical communications.

Codes

Some ambulance services still use radio codes; most do not. Codes were used for several reasons:

- To maintain security of communication
- To keep air time as brief as possible
- To diminish the likelihood of misunderstanding or noise
- To prevent the patient, family, and bystanders from understanding what is being said

The last-mentioned reason is particularly important when the information you need to convey to the dispatcher or

physician could alarm the patient. Suppose that you want to tell the physician that your patient is probably having an acute myocardial infarction and is in very serious condition. It is preferable that the patient not be privy to that assessment because it could increase anxiety and possibly worsen the patient's condition. In fact, it is best not to be sitting right next to the patient when transmitting your report to the emergency department.

For a code to be of any use, everyone using the radio must know the meaning of the code words. When codes are used, therefore, they should be simple and standardized within a given region, and a copy of the code should be posted at every radio terminal.

The ten-code system, once commonly used, has been phased out in many EMS systems. If codes are still used in your agency, be sure to learn the code system used.

When and if you use codes, remember that one of their main purposes is to shorten air time.

Whenever codes are used, they should be kept simple and reserved for cases in which they are really needed. During MCIs, when personnel unfamiliar with the codes

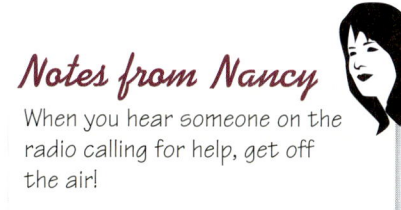

Notes from Nancy

When you hear someone on the radio calling for help, get off the air!

may be staffing radios and when everyone is apt to be anxious, it is usually best to abandon codes and use words that all understand. Most services use standard terms rather than codes for regular day-to-day operations as well.

Relaying Information to Direct Medical Control

Radio communications between paramedics in the prehospital environment and their direct medical control physician need to be concise and accurate. A standard format for communicating patient information over the radio will ensure that significant information is relayed in a consistent manner and that nothing is omitted **Figure 16-8 ▶**.

When relaying medical information in person, such as when a bedside transfer of patient care occurs, be mindful of the information you are supplying, many times in the presence of the patient **Figure 16-9 ▶**. At times, it may be more practical to step outside the patient care room or to speak in a softer tone to provide the history and transferring information to the receiving medical practitioner. In addition, be brief. At this time, additional information should be shared that may not have been given in the radio report to the receiving facility. Ensure you are providing this information in person to a medical practitioner of an equal or a higher level of care to avoid abandonment and confidentiality issues and to ensure continuity of care. In many cases, a copy of the written report will be given to the receiving facility before you leave. Be sure

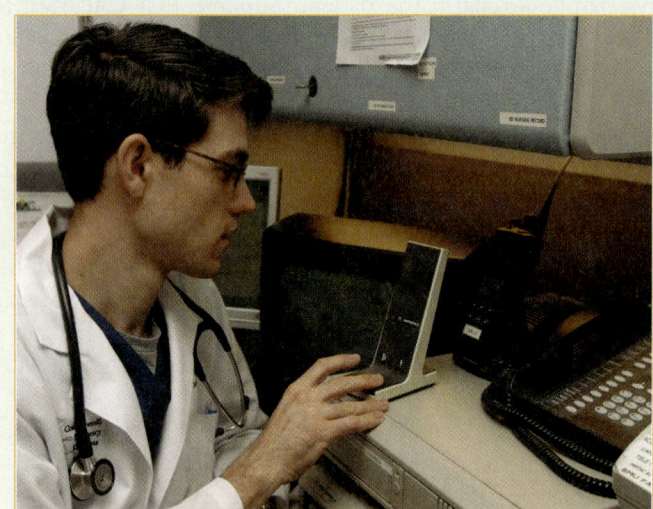

Figure 16-8 Use a standard format for communicating patient information to direct medical control.

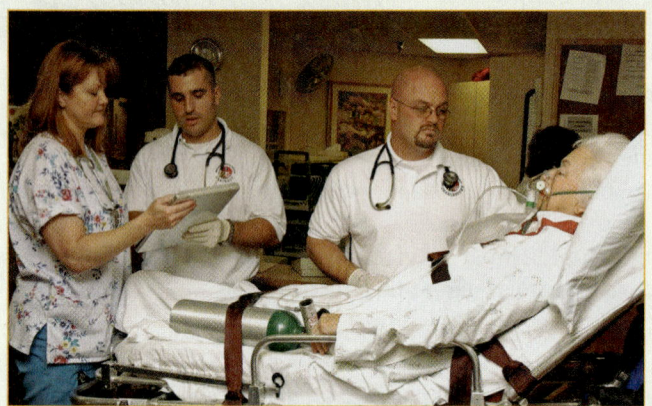

Figure 16-9 Be mindful of how you provide your report when the patient is present.

to follow local or regional protocols on providing patient care reports.

Format for Reporting Medical Information

The following list shows the items that should be included when reporting medical information:

- The patient's age and sex
- The patient's chief complaint
- A brief, pertinent history of the present illness or injury
- Anything the physician needs to know about the patient's other medical history relative to the current situation, including major underlying medical conditions, medications, and important allergies
- The patient's level of consciousness and degree of distress
- The vital signs
- The pertinent physical findings in head-to-toe order
- ECG findings
- Treatment given so far and response to treatment

For example, here is a transmission regarding a patient in congestive heart failure: "We have a 53-year-old man complaining of severe shortness of breath, which wakened him from sleep and is worse when he is lying down. He has a history of hypertension and takes Diuril. He is alert but in significant respiratory distress, with a pulse of 130 and regular, respirations 36 and laboured, and BP 190/120. Physical examination reveals no JVD but crackles and wheezes in both lung fields. He has 2+ pitting ankle edema. We are sending you an ECG."

The preceding transmission can be relayed in less than 30 seconds, and any physician hearing that information will immediately recognize that this is a hypertensive patient in moderately severe left-sided heart failure.

When paramedics call in without a standard reporting format, the physician might have to waste time gleaning the information needed to know what is going on. Consider the following dialogue:

You are the Paramedic Part 3

The glucometer reads "2.2." You immediately tell your partner, who assembles a preloaded syringe containing $D_{50}W$. As you give the dextrose, your patient's level of consciousness begins to improve. The patient no longer needs ventilatory assistance. She remains somewhat confused but can provide her name and states that she has type 2 diabetes. You provide supplemental oxygen at 15 l/min via nonrebreathing mask, and her ECG indicates sinus tachycardia.

Reassessment	Recording Time: 10 Minutes
Level of consciousness	Alert, with a Glasgow Coma Scale score of 14
Skin	Pale, warm, slightly diaphoretic
Pulse	120 beats/min, strong and regular
Blood pressure	128/86 mm Hg
Respirations	20 breaths/min
Spo2	95%
Blood glucose	2.2 mmol/l

7. As your patient's level of consciousness improves, what issues do you foresee?

8. How does your ability to effectively communicate impact patient care?

Paramedic: *We have a patient with a pulse of 130, a blood pressure of 190/120, and respirations of 30. We're sending you a strip.*

Physician: *Fine, but what's his problem?*

Paramedic: *He's short of breath.*

Physician: *How long has this been going on?*

Paramedic: *Just a minute (pause). He says it woke him up from sleep about an hour ago.*

Physician: *Does he have any underlying medical problems?*

Paramedic: *He takes medicine for hypertension.*

Physician: *Is he in any distress?*

Paramedic: *Yeah, he's having a hard time breathing.*

Physician: *What do his lungs sound like?*

Paramedic: *He has crackles and wheezes all over.*

Clearly, disorganized and incomplete communication is not efficient. It is a waste of time and causes frustration. The physician might respond to transport him immediately rather than try to get complete information. To avoid ineffective dialogues, gather your information thoroughly at the scene, organize it clearly in your mind, and only then get on the air to the physician. Because even the best of us can be rattled under pressure, it's a good idea to write the reporting format on a card and affix the card to your handheld transmitter or the dashboard of the ambulance so you may refer to it while reporting in.

Dispatching

The verb "to dispatch" means "to send out on a mission," but the EMD does a lot more than just send ambulances out to emergencies. The EMD functions as a vital part of the paramedic team who obtains as much information as possible about the emergency, then directs the appropriate vehicle to the scene, and provides the caller with whatever advice may be needed to manage the situation until help arrives. The EMD also monitors and coordinates communication with the prehospital environment and maintains written records pertaining to the response to the call.

Let us consider the EMD's tasks in each phase of the call.

Receipt of the Call for Help

Whenever someone telephones for an ambulance, the EMD has to assume that the caller needs help, even if the caller is too upset to be clear about the nature of the problem. The EMD, therefore, has to be able to put himself or herself in the caller's place and understand the caller's distress. That means the EMD must:

- *Answer the telephone promptly*, within two or three rings; each ring may seem like an eternity to a panicky person.
- *Identify himself or herself and the agency*. The caller needs immediate confirmation of having reached the right number.
- *Speak directly into the mouthpiece*, clearly and without mumbling.
- *Observe telephone courtesy*. The EMD must be calm and professional, informing the caller exactly what is being done and how soon assistance can be expected. As mentioned earlier, in some cases, EMDs provide prearrival

instructions such as in the form of emergency medical dispatching—the EMD relays vital first aid information to the caller who can then apply the aid techniques while waiting for the ambulance to arrive.

- *Take charge of the conversation*. Once the EMD has identified the ambulance service, he or she must start asking the caller questions to which immediate answers are needed. Questions pertaining to safety issues are a priority. Additional useful information may also be obtained, such as specific situations the EMS crew might encounter: Is the residence door locked? What pets does the patient have? These nuggets of information are invaluable in the prehospital environment.

Information Gathering

The method used to gather information from a caller is most often a series of short questions asked by the EMD. When a call for EMS comes in, the EMD should elicit the following minimum information:

- The exact location of the patient(s), including the street name and number; the proper geographic designation (such as whether the street is East Maple or West Maple) and the name of the community (adjacent towns may have streets by the same name). If the call comes from a rural area, the dispatcher should try to establish landmarks (such as the nearest cross-street or business establishment, water tower, or antenna).
- The telephone number (call-back number) of the caller, in case the call is disconnected or there is a need to phone the caller back for more information. It is not uncommon for paramedics not to be able to find the address and to ask for help from the original caller. Asking for the caller's telephone number also helps discourage nuisance calls to EMS because prank callers are reluctant to supply their phone numbers. Finally, the caller's telephone exchange may help to pinpoint his or her location if the caller is unfamiliar with the region, as is often the case of a traveller calling from the road. In services equipped with an enhanced 9-1-1 system, a lot of the information mentioned—such as the phone number and location of the caller—is recorded automatically through sophisticated telephone technology, and the EMD need only confirm the information on the screen.
- The caller's perception of the nature of his or her or the patient's problem.
- Specific information concerning the patient's condition that will help evaluate the urgency of the situation and the EMD's need to provide the caller with prearrival instructions by phone. The EMD should ask specifically:
  - Is the patient conscious?
  - If not, is the patient breathing?
  - Is the patient bleeding badly?
- If the emergency is a motor vehicle collision, further important information should be obtained:
  - The kinds of vehicles involved (that is, cars, trucks, motorcycles, buses). If a truck is involved, is there any indication of the cargo it is carrying? A truck carrying

dynamite requires a different approach from one carrying bananas!

- The number of persons injured and an estimate of the extent of injuries. This information will enable the EMD to estimate the magnitude of the problem.
- Apparent hazards at the scene, such as heavy traffic, downed power lines, fire, spilled chemicals, and peculiar odours.

Information about such hazards enables the EMD to contact other agencies that may have to be involved, such as utility workers to take care of downed wires or an engine company to deal with spilled fuel. In most modern dispatch centres, the EMD has visual prompts with the key questions to ask on the computer screen.

Dispatch

At the point when your EMD has obtained the address of the emergency, the telephone number of the caller, and the apparent problem, the EMD should ask the caller to wait on the line. The EMD must then decide, assuming the call is a medical emergency within the service's jurisdiction, which crew(s) and vehicle(s) will be dispatched. That decision will be governed by the nature and location of the call and the availability of various units at the time. The appropriate crew is contacted and informed of the nature of the call and its exact location ("Medic 5, possible heart attack at 573 East Main Street, that's five-seven-three East Main Street with Jones Drive on the cross"). Once the ambulance is dispatched, the EMD may return to the telephone to obtain the rest of the information previously outlined. Further questioning may reveal special conditions that might affect your travel to the scene or your actions at the scene. If so, that information should be relayed to you while you are en route, for two reasons:

- So that you may know if the response requires travel under emergency conditions, using emergency warning devices
- So that while en route you may anticipate and prepare for tasks to be performed at the scene: assembling the equipment to deliver a baby or transmitting cardiac information to the receiving hospital

The EMD might also remind you to buckle up en route to the scene because this is usually the most dangerous part of the call!

Advice to the Caller

After directing you and any rescue crew(s) to the scene and alerting all of you to any special conditions, your EMD should return to the telephone and tell the caller what is being done ("An ambulance is on the way and should be there in about 5 minutes."). If your EMD suspects your patient has a life-threatening emergency, your EMD should also provide instructions to the caller in very simple terms about emergency care techniques (such as airway maintenance, Heimlich maneuver, CPR, hemorrhage control). The caller is likely to be in an agitated state, so instructions must be clear and simple.

Excellent protocols have been developed for giving such instructions by telephone, and all EMDs should undergo training in those procedures.

Ongoing Communications With the Scene

It is important for your EMD to monitor the communications of the ambulance and to be aware of what is occurring at the scene. Your EMD must coordinate communications between the ambulance and direct medical control and contact any other agencies (such as fire and police) whose presence may be required at the scene. The EMD should also receive and record communications from you when you are in the prehospital environment regarding the following:

- The time the ambulance departed for the scene
- The time the ambulance arrived at the scene
- The time the crew made contact with the patient
- The time the ambulance left the scene
- The time the ambulance arrived at the hospital
- The time the ambulance went back in service

Paramedics involved in giving emergency care simply don't have time to keep looking at their watches and recording the moment each of those events occurred. The times cited, along with the time the call was received, must be recorded accurately at the communications centre **Figure 16-10 ▾**. The easiest way to accomplish that is to have paramedics radio in at each time indicated (for example, "En route to hospital") and for the EMD to record the times. Your record of the times permits a gamut of medical, administrative, and academic evaluations. Your supervising medical personnel can evaluate the appropriateness of the time emergency personnel spend with a patient, and managers can assess how long it takes a team to get back in service after a call.

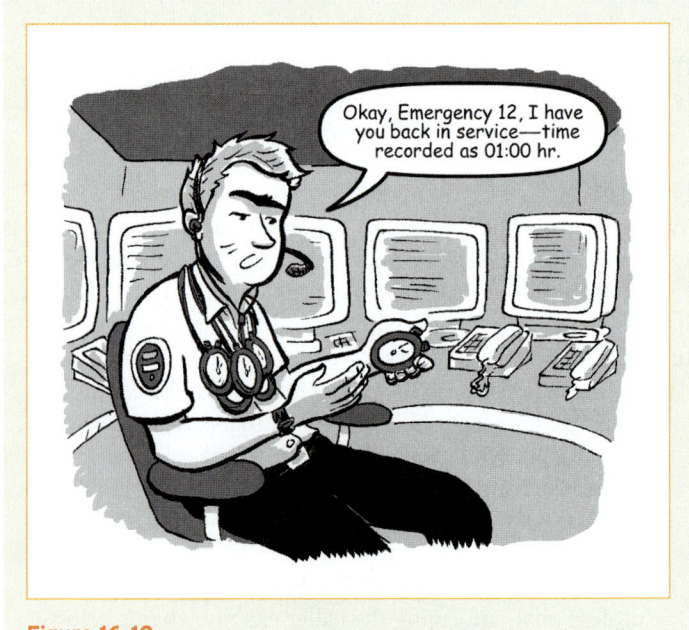

Figure 16-10

Table 16-2	Phases of Dispatch
Information Gathered	**Dispatcher Action**
Address of incident	Answers telephone promptly
Call-back number	Identifies agency
Perceived problem	Dispatches (first) ambulance
Patient's name	
Patient's condition	Gives patient care instructions
For road collision:	by phone if required
Number of vehicles	
Kinds of vehicles	
Number of victims	
Hazards at the scene	Notifies responding ambulances
	of special situations
	Dispatches additional
	ambulances as needed
	Contacts other agencies
	as needed
	Monitors communications
	from the scene

Table 16-3	Military Times		
Regular Time	**Military Time**	**Regular Time**	**Military Time**
Midnight	0000	Noon	1200
1:00 AM	0100	1:00 PM	1300
2:00 AM	0200	2:00 PM	1400
3:00 AM	0300	3:00 PM	1500
4:00 AM	0400	4:00 PM	1600
5:00 AM	0500	5:00 PM	1700
6:00 AM	0600	6:00 PM	1800
7:00 AM	0700	7:00 PM	1900
8:00 AM	0800	8:00 PM	2000
9:00 AM	0900	9:00 PM	2100
10:00 AM	1000	10:00 PM	2200
11:00 AM	1100	11:00 PM	2300

The phases of the EMD's work are summarized in Table 16-2 ▲.

Documenting Times

In general, it is routine practice to use standard military time when documenting times for calls. Most dispatchers use this format when providing times over the radio as well. Table 16-3 ▲ shows how military time relates to standard AM and PM time.

Factors That May Affect Communications

In communication, many things may go wrong, and not all of them are equipment failures. You need to be prepared for such situations. Radio communication is very technical and technology-driven. At times, systems may have problems, such as radio tower issues, computer crashes, and audio problems, and you may have to adapt to necessary changes. Follow your local protocols regarding radio failure.

You have learned how important communication skills are in previous chapters. You can be faced with a number of problems, including patients who do not speak your primary language or patients with communication disorders. Ask "those in the know" about telephone interpreters, people on your service who speak more than one language, and learn what you can do before you see your patients. Review your patient assessment skills for patients with impaired hearing.

Documentation and Communication

Cultural diversity is found in EMS every day. If you are not familiar with the various cultures present in your community, consider a training session in which leaders from various cultural organizations in your community are invited to meet your organization members. This could open up dialogue for both groups and could create an avenue for growth and development to reduce communication barriers in EMS calls. In addition, training members of your EMS organization to speak other languages that are spoken in your area may also be of significant benefit to your community.

Documentation

What do you call the report in your agency or EMS setting? Here is a list of different terms used to describe the written documentation or report for calls for service:

- Patient care report (PCR)
- Prehospital patient report (PPR)
- Ambulance call report (ACR)
- Call report
- Trip sheet
- Run sheet
- Run report
- Ambulance trip sheet

Whatever you call it, do you know and understand the importance of it? The adage, "No job is finished until the paperwork is done" is very true in EMS. Your written report, most commonly referred to as the PCR (prehospital/patient care report), is the only written record of the events that transpired during the call for service. It needs to be one of the most important skills you learn as a paramedic. It will be the legal record for the call and a part of the patient's medical record and the hospital's ED chart. The PCR provides for a continuum of patient care on arrival at the receiving facility. Time will not allow you to relay all of the information obtained through patient assessment and findings in a radio report or the verbal report on arrival. Your verbal report should be a brief summary of the assessment findings and the event, but your written report should be a more detailed account from the very moment the call began until it concluded. The written report should accurately reflect, or paint a picture, of the events of the call.

Although you may include subjective information from the patient, such as statements from him or her about symptoms, no bias or personal opinions (subjectivity) of yours should be contained within your written report. Poorly written, inappropriately documented PCRs could have adverse implications for patient care and for your career. Omissions or errors in your report could lead to further errors in care. Improper and inadequate reports also could result in litigation, loss of job or position, a negative reflection on one's reputation as an EMS professional, and more.

No matter your particular writing style, your report should be complete, well-written, legible, professional, and your sole source of information about the call. Your report may also be used in legal proceedings. In some cases, it may be your only defence against a complaint about a call—if you document what happened, you will have solid evidence of your conduct and what transpired on the call. Your memory may not serve you well 5 years from now, but your written report will remain the same. If it is well written, it will jog your memory and should provide a picture of the events of the call to all who read it. As a health care professional, it is important that you use proper spelling, proper grammar, and accurate terminology in your report. Do not attempt to use medical terms and abbreviations if you do not fully understand their meaning. Never make up your own abbreviations because they will only be meaningful to you and could confuse others. Doing so could result in patient care errors and leave your professional character at stake if the report is called into question.

In addition, you should write every PCR as if your medical director were reading it, such as in a quality assurance review. Your report is the only record (unless your medical director was on the call with you) of why you performed a certain procedure or why you administered a particular medication to a patient. Reports that your medical director and EMS agency can read and understand will help them evaluate your performance accurately.

On occasion, EMS reports may be requested for medical audits and other educational settings. Call reviews, or sessions in which peers and other medical professionals review care reports for adherence to local protocols, quality assurance, and quality monitoring, may occur. Your written and computer-based reports may be used to calculate the number of times you have performed a specific skill, such as medication administration or oral intubation. Always accurately document all skills attempted and performed with patient care.

Billing and administration are significant reasons why PCR writing needs to be accurate and complete. Most EMS agencies now need to bill for services to recover the costs of providing patient care. For complete and accurate revenue recovery, you must ensure that all procedures performed are documented, insurance codes obtained, and the appropriate medical necessity signature obtained (where required). You need to document why a patient may have needed emergency care, especially in the case of private or scheduled transports, to ensure your service's billing information will result in payment from the responsible insurer, agency, or private payer. You will often be trained by your agency and its billing company about what additional forms you need to complete as a part of each EMS response. Paramedics may grumble about these tasks, but you must understand that it is a necessary portion of the call to complete billing paperwork and to supply the most accurate and defensible information to the EMS agency. Just as billing has become necessary in EMS, so has research. Proper documentation done by all paramedics often justifies innovative, lifesaving techniques when data are put together by researchers. Many provinces now require EMS agencies to submit data to their provincial EMS office to verify call volumes and skills used. These data may include the number of calls an agency responds to, the types of calls, care provided, and patient outcomes. Such patient care data collection can lead to improvement of the EMS system as a whole.

Do you know if the procedures you are performing are making a difference in your patient's outcome? Your careful documentation of procedures is the basis of research and evaluation of their effectiveness. Research is very difficult to do without accurate data and information. In many provinces, regional or provincial databases exist or are being developed to capture call and patient care. Their purpose is to enable researchers to examine trends, analyze care processes, and determine ways to improve the provision of prehospital care. The data for these important initiatives come from your written report.

Medical Terminology

Using medical terminology correctly is essential to EMS communications. You should learn the established and accepted medical terms and abbreviations for your EMS operations. Some EMS systems have specific approved lists of medical abbreviations and terms that must be used.

Medical terminology may seem to be a foreign language. Well, it is! Most terminology comes from the ancient Roman language, Latin. In addition, some common words used in EMS such as "packaging a patient for transport" or "bagging the patient during airway management" might be used. Be sure to know acceptable terms and words used in your EMS agency. An ongoing review of the anatomy and physiology chapter can help you become familiar with medical terminology. Let's take a more in-depth look at commonly used medical terms and their meanings.

Medical Abbreviations

Medical abbreviations can be very useful for documentation purposes, but you must be certain the abbreviations you are using are consistent with approved medical abbreviations in your EMS system. Incorrect or inappropriate medical abbreviations can cause confusion and, in the worst cases, could lead to medication and treatment errors. You should learn the approved medical abbreviations for your service area before you use them in a report. Each EMS system should have a list of approved medical abbreviations available for use and documentation purposes. Once again, accuracy, neatness, and completeness reflect a professional writing style. Common medical abbreviations are listed in the student workbook and website for this text. Note that many abbreviations have more than one meaning, so extreme care is needed when using them. Paramedics should contact their service to determine which abbreviations are appropriate or acceptable for use in their jurisdiction.

Documenting Incident Times

Keeping good records of time is essential to all EMS operations. The role of timekeeper falls to dispatchers. You must also keep track of time during your documentation of the incident. You should compare your times with those of the dispatcher to ensure accuracy and proper timekeeping. Several times are absolutely vital to be kept and documented for accurate report writing.

- **Time of call.** The time when the call for help is placed or requested
- **Time of dispatch.** Time when call is toned or alerted for a response
- **Time of arrival at the scene.** Time when EMS unit arrives on scene
- **Time with patient.** Time recorded when patient contact is made (this may not be the same time of arrival, for example, a patient on the 17th floor of a high-rise building; should include the time it takes to physically get to the patient)

- **Time of medication administration.** Time when medications are administered for adherence to protocols
- **Time of departure from scene.** Time recorded when EMS unit leaves the scene
- **Time of arrival at medical facility.** Time when arriving at medical facility (if a patient is transported)
- **Time back in service.** Time when EMS unit and crew are ready for return to service

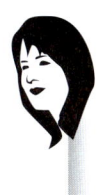

Notes from Nancy

Symptoms belong in the history. Signs belong in the physical examination.

General Documentation Considerations

Paramedics must know and understand that EMS documentation is a required and necessary element of patient care. Paramedics should pride themselves not only on their patient care skills, but also on their documentation skills.

Documentation of the narrative portion of the PCR should be a detailed segment indicating the elements of the call. It should be written in a format accepted by your agency and should be accurate and complete. Simply writing "followed ACLS protocols" may not be sufficient documentation for your agency or medical director. Specifics of the call should be recorded such as "the patient was intubated with a 7.5 ETT and ventilatory assistance provided with supplementary oxygen at 15 l/min. ETT placement was confirmed by breath

You are the Paramedic Part 4

As your patient becomes alert and oriented, she tells you that she was riding her bike home from work when she became shaky. She says that she thought she had some candy in her backpack but was unable to find it. She decided to continue home, and the next thing she remembered she was lying on the ground surrounded by strangers.

Reassessment	Recording Time: 15 Minutes
Level of consciousness	Alert, with a Glasgow Coma Scale score of 15
Skin	Pale, warm, slightly diaphoretic
Pulse	110 beats/min, strong and regular
Blood pressure	126/82 mm Hg
Respirations	18 breaths/min
SpO_2	98%
Blood glucose	6.3 mmol/l

9. How do body language and tone of voice communicate as much or more than words?
10. How does total patient care enter into this scenario?
11. What is the purpose of documentation?
12. Who is your documentation audience?

sounds, chest rise, and a tube check, before securing the ETT at the mark of 26 at the teeth. The end-tidal CO_2 detector and pulse oximeter were placed immediately and their readings were: _____ and _____ [Be sure to clarify which is which.]."

Any direct medical control orders received and medical advice given should be documented in the narrative section. In some EMS systems, items such as consultations, orders requested or received from direct medical control, and any refusal situations in which direct medical control has been consulted should be documented in detail in the narrative section. Simply writing "see refusal on back" is not an effective method of patient care documentation.

Many methods for narrative documentation exist. Your EMS agency or medical director may prefer a specific method to be used when documenting PCRs. Be familiar with the approved methods and all required elements for report writing for your agency. Some examples of narrative writing styles for reports are as follows:

- **Chronological order.** This is telling the narrative in a story format from the time of the initial dispatch until the call was completed. If used regularly, this format allows you to explain the call from start to finish.
- **SOAP method: Subjective, Objective, Assessment, and Plan (for treatment).** Simple and logical method used to document various aspects of the patient care encounter
- **CHARTE method: Chief complaint, History, Assessment, Treatment (Rx), Transport, and Exceptions.** Similar to the SOAP format for report writing but allows you to break the narrative down into logical sections similar to that of your EMS assessment
- **Body systems approach.** Documenting each body system from head to toe. This method of report writing may be difficult to apply in EMS and may be too time-consuming for paramedics.

Regardless of the style of narrative report writing you and your service agree on, be sure to follow it routinely. Switching from one format to another or attempting to change formats during report writing may lead you to forget certain elements or essential details that should have been included. Proper grammar and spelling are essential when writing reports. You might consider carrying a pocket guide, reference, or medical terminology book in your ambulance to avoid spelling errors.

Notes from Nancy

Always report your findings in the same sequence, regardless of the sequence in which they were actually obtained.

Pertinent negatives should be documented when writing your EMS report. This is a record of negative findings that warrant no care or intervention but indicate that a thorough and complete examination and history were performed. For example, "The patient denies any shortness of breath with his chest pain, patient denies any radiation of the chest pain to other parts of the body." This would indicate that you not only

obtained the information about the chest pain, but also inquired about shortness of breath and radiation of the pain.

The use of pertinent spoken accounts made by your patient and others on scene may be essential to the continuum of patient care. If you use any spoken accounts made by the patient or others, be sure to indicate who made the statement and place the exact words in quotations. This may include statements about the patient's behaviour, the mechanism of injury, safety-related information such as the use of weapons, information that may be useful to criminal investigators as a part of their investigation, disposition of valuables, admissions of suicidal intentions made by a patient, or any first aid interventions provided by bystanders before the arrival of EMS.

Other Elements Essential to EMS Report Writing

You should also document the use of mutual aid services such as helicopters, specialized rescue teams, and other agencies called in to assist. Unusual occurrences should be documented as well, including having to secure the patient with restraining devices for safe transport or other situations in which unusual circumstances arise. If you need to summon an additional crew for lifting a heavy patient or if you will have an extended scene time owing to a prolonged extrication, this information should be clearly documented to explain why "something out of the ordinary" occurred.

Elements of a Properly Written Report

Documentation accuracy depends on all information being provided, such as times, narrative information, and checkboxes, and it must be comprehensive and precise. All sections should show that you have completed them, even if a section was not applicable to the call. For example, if your PCR has a section of check boxes for specific information on cardiac arrest calls but the call you are documenting was not a cardiac arrest call, note that on the report in a manner that is approved by your agency. Simply leaving the boxes blank may raise questions about the completeness of the report.

All reports should be legible and written in ink. The colour of ink used may be determined by your EMS agency. Standard ink colours of black and blue are most commonly selected. Handwriting, especially in the narrative portion of the report, needs to be neat and easily read by others. In addition, take great care to not contaminate your written reports with any liquid found in the prehospital environment. Evidence of your own rehydration activities should not appear on your written report! Place all your completed reports in a secure location agreed on by you and your partner that protects the patient's privacy, until they can be secured in the proper place at your EMS agency office or headquarters.

The PCR needs to be timely, even in EMS systems where call volume is high. If you respond to multiple calls without accurately completing PCRs before proceeding to the next call, details may be forgotten and important information left out, or worse, inaccurate information may be written. Your EMS agency should allow you a reasonable amount of time to complete your reports, replenish supplies, and clean and disinfect vehicles *before* returning them to service. Some jurisdictions and services require that copies of written reports be supplied to the receiving facility or hospital within a specific timeframe, such as 24 hours. Know the applicable laws and requirements of your province and EMS system. In some systems, paramedics fax the completed form to the ED because the hospital has a secure fax location that meets confidentiality requirements.

If you encountered any problems responding to or during the call of which your service administration should be aware, follow the documentation policy of your agency. Usually these problems or incidents (ie, an injury on the call, an infectious disease exposure, a delayed response, a conflict at the scene with family or other response agencies, an MCI, etc) will involve filing an agency special incident report. All PCRs should be free of jargon, slang, and opinions of the paramedic. Be certain that your documentation is not libelous. Only true and accurate statements should be documented. If quotes of bystanders or statements made by the patient are used, be sure to indicate who made them and place the exact words in quotations on the report.

All reports should be reviewed by the paramedic who authors them before submitting them to the receiving medical facility and to the paramedic's EMS agency. Reviewing for completeness, accuracy, grammar, spelling, and proper use of medical terminology and abbreviations will help ensure a well-written and well-documented report.

Too often, we ignore the importance of report writing and documentation in EMS. Negative sentiments are often associated with report writing, but you should not let them "get to you." Be positive; report writing reflects on the paramedic who authors the report. When you file a complete, well-documented, legible report, you have done the most important part of the completion of your call.

Documenting Patient Care Refusal

Legal aspects of patient care were discussed in Chapter 4, but here we will discuss the necessary documentation in more depth. Refusal of care is one of the most difficult elements of patient care documentation. Competent adult patients have the right to refuse medical care or to consent to treatment. You must know and understand the rights of your patients. You should also be very familiar with the applicable laws in your province about patient care and who has the right to refuse such care. For a person to refuse care, the decision should be a valid one based on the patient's knowledge of his or her situation.

Your most important job is to ensure that your patient is well informed about the situation at hand. You should have explained and the patient must understand, in great detail, the potential consequences of refusing medical care when it may be warranted, including possible death. Unconscious patients may be treated under implied consent. All paramedics should be familiar with the laws of their province regarding the age of consent, care of minors, emancipated minors, and people with mental or cognitive impairments, such as mental illness or the effects of drug or alcohol use. Above all else, you need to ensure that every reasonable effort has been made for the patient's welfare and best interests.

It is essential that you have a witness to the process involved in making sure your patient has sufficient knowledge of the situation to make an informed choice. If the patient refuses to sign the form for refusing treatment, your witness should also be present. The observations of the witness should be documented, and the name and contact information of the witness should be included.

A complete history and assessment should be performed or attempted when possible and practical. This includes obtaining a full set of baseline vital signs. A patient's refusal to allow such an assessment should be well documented on the PCR. Be sure to evaluate the patient's mental status. Mental status may be considered impaired if the person is not oriented to person, time, or place or makes nonsensical statements. The impairment can be a result of an injury, a medical condition such as electrolyte imbalance or hypoglycemia, mental illness, or drugs or alcohol.

The patient must be fully informed of the situation, the right to receive and refuse medical care, and the consequences of such a refusal of care. This needs to be done in a language that the person understands and documented on the PCR. If the person refusing care has an obvious injury or medical condition that requires immediate medical attention, you should involve direct medical control for further guidance and assistance. If direct medical control is contacted, it should be documented on the PCR, including the events that transpired.

Always politely and tactfully explain to patients that they have the right to change their mind and may recall EMS later. Such an exchange of information should be witnessed and documented with signatures and identifying information such as phone numbers of the witnesses involved, who frequently may be law enforcement personnel or others at the scene.

The PCR should be thoroughly completed and well documented for all patient refusals of care. At times, patients may agree to transport but want to refuse a particular procedure such as intravenous therapy or backboarding procedures. In such cases, refusal of the specific procedure(s) should be handled as if it is a refusal of care, including an explanation of associated risks and complications of refusal, a signature by the patient acknowledging refusal of a portion of care, a witness, and complete and accurate documentation.

Special Considerations in Documentation

In unusual circumstances, you may have to use other means of documentation, such as triage tags in an MCI (covered in Chapter 47). Rather than waiting until an MCI occurs, become familiar the triage tags, learn where they are stored, the information needed on the tags, and situations that may warrant their use in your agency or department.

If your response to a call has been cancelled, be sure to document who cancelled the response, such as law enforcement, on the PCR. In addition, if the patient left the scene before your arrival, document any information known about the patient's departure.

Documentation Revisions, Corrections, and Lost Reports

At times, it may be necessary to write a revision or correct your PCR. Although every attempt should be made to be accurate and legible on the initial report, if a report has to be revised or corrected, you must note the date and time of the revised report and the purpose for writing the revision or making the correction. Never discard or destroy the original PCR.

Only the person who wrote the original report can revise it. Additions or notations added by others after the completion of the report may raise questions about the authenticity of the report and the confidentiality practices of your agency. Routine administrative report handling and reviews are necessary for entering information into computer databases, billing for services, and quality assurance monitoring. At no time should administrative activities involve altering or rewriting the report or portions of it.

When writing your report, if you make an error, place a single line through the error and initial the line and date it; write the corrected information next to it Figure 16-11 ▾. Do not erase information, scribble through errors, use correction fluid, or use correction tape. Remember, the PCR is a legal document.

If you forgot to include important information, you may need to write an addendum to your report. You may also need to write an addendum if you are asked to write statements of events for matters related to quality assurance or risk management and to answer complaints. An addendum added to your

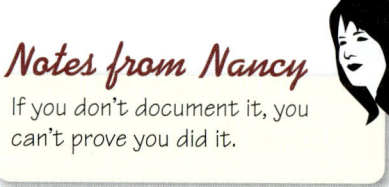

Figure 16-11 If you make a mistake in writing your report, the proper way to correct it is to draw a single horizontal line though the error, initial it, and write the correct information next to it.

original report should be noted as added to the original and the reason for the late entry and should include the date of entry, the time of entry, and signature of the author.

Supplemental narratives also may be needed if additional information becomes available after the original report has been written. Such reports should be documented with the date, time, and the reason for the added information and signed by the author. Some EMS services use a supplemental report to write lengthy information when space on the original report is limited. Follow your service's policies for using supplemental reports and the procedures for writing them. Regardless of when they are added, they should be attached in some way to the original report for record keeping purposes.

You may be required to obtain and document billing information for the EMS service provided. You need to understand the sensitive and confidential nature of such information and the laws and regulations pertaining to billing and documentation security under confidentiality laws. EMS agencies should take care not to add additional information provided by billing clerks or others after the report has been submitted. Doing so might be in violation of local, provincial, or federal laws. If you have additional information to document after handing in the form, follow the policy of your agency regarding whether a supplementary form is needed.

Lost reports pose huge legal implications for paramedics, EMS agencies and departments, and medical directors. All paramedics are responsible to ensure that their reports are completed and turned in as required by policy or procedure. Do not keep copies of your reports—if you need to document numbers of procedures or ages of patients for

Notes from Nancy

If you don't document it, you can't prove you did it.

your paramedic internship, follow the specific policy of your training centre. If lost reports are an ongoing problem for an agency or provider, steps should be taken to correct the problem. Know that attempting to recreate PCRs is irresponsible and possibly illegal. Also, record keeping may be a legal requirement in your province, and there may also be a specified time requirement for submission of reports.

The Effects of Poor Documentation

Documentation directly affects the quality of care provided after you have delivered the patient to the hospital. Inappropriate, inaccurate, and poor documentation can adversely affect the quality of care received by patients after arrival at the hospital. Let's say you administered a medication en route to the hospital but forgot to document the medication and the times you administered it. The patient could be overmedicated because of your failure to document the care you provided. Documenting what the patient or family members tell you and your findings from examining the patient enhances the quality of care. For example, if hospital staff know that a patient has a seizure disorder or that a patient who's had transient ischemic attacks in the past had symptoms of stroke en route to the hospital, proper care can be planned.

In addition there are legal implications of documentation. Poorly written, inaccurate, or illegible reports might lead a judge or jury to decide in favor of the plaintiff. On the other hand, a lawyer may decide not to pursue a case when the documentation reveals a correctly written and well-documented report.

Not only are there potential legal implications for paramedics, but their reputations also are affected by their documentation skills. Poorly written, inappropriate, or inaccurate reports might make others question the care provided, whereas well-written reports show organizational skills, knowledge of patient conditions and needs and proper documentation, and respect for organizational policies and procedures. Part of being a good paramedic is completing the paperwork and reports as required. If writing reports is difficult for you, seek additional classes or study report-writing skills to enhance your abilities. Your agency or service might have an educational program to assist you with such education and training.

Computer-Based Reporting

In this era of computer-based technology, paramedics are faced with technology in the ambulance in many forms. One such form involves electronic reporting devices and electronic reporting means. Electronic reporting may assist you in writing accurate, timely, and legible reports. Many will also link to software-based computer programs that capture the data for research and reporting to enhance the EMS system. Knowing the number of endotracheal tubes inserted by a paramedic or how many times CPR was performed by your agency can help in tailoring continuing education to meet the specific needs of agency paramedics. Most provinces have laws requiring EMS agencies to report certain types of data to the provincial EMS office. The use of computer-based EMS report writing programs helps in this task **Figure 16-12** .

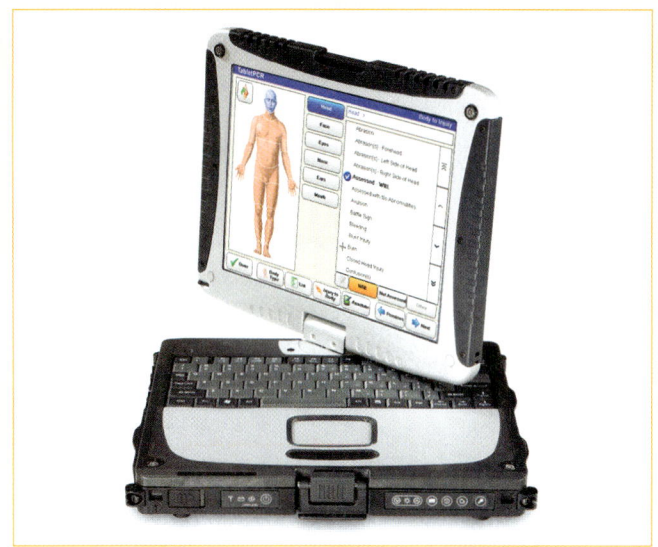

Figure 16-12 A tablet PC-based reporting system.

█ Conclusion

Assume the personal responsibility of writing detailed, accurate EMS reports with an emphasis on good documentation skills. Reports should be concise, accurate, and timely. EMS agencies and departments should have a process to ensure that all reports are well written and a quality assurance program to ensure that what was written in the PCR actually occurred as stated on the call.

Promote quality patient care and set a good example by writing accurate, legible EMS reports. The reports should be complete to the point that people reviewing them, whether your medical director or the administrative office clerk billing for the service provided, can read them and understand exactly what transpired on the EMS call. If your report does not paint a clear picture of what happened, it isn't written well.

Documentation and Communication

To understand how electronic data collection can improve operations, consider the following two methods (paper versus electronic).

Paper

- Citizen calls for assistance.
- Dispatcher hand writes the information.
- Ambulance is dispatched with the information given over radio. Information may need to be reconfirmed two or three times.
- The crew treats the patient and transports to the hospital.
- At the hospital, a handwritten PCR is generated.
- A copy is left at the hospital and the original logged and stored at the station.
- The paperwork is picked up and taken to the headquarters station (sometimes located far away) where it is reviewed, sorted, and coded by the supervisor.
- The paperwork is forwarded to the business office where it is entered into a computer system for billing.
- The supervisor in charge of quality assurance (QA)/ quality improvement (QI) manually sorts through PCRs for review.

Electronic

- Citizen calls for assistance.
- Dispatcher electronically enters information while on the phone with the caller.
- Dispatcher assigns the call to an ambulance in the computer-aided dispatch, immediately pulling up a map on the computer screen showing the exact location of the call.
- Dispatcher pages the crew; crew steps into ambulance.
- If a mobile data terminal is installed in the ambulance, the problem, any hazards associated with the address, and the street address with a location on a computer map are right there.
- EMS arrives on scene and treats the patient. Transport is completed.
- The crew fills out a short paper form with the basics of demographics and treatments given. This form is left with the ED staff.
- The crew syncs its laptop with the server through a Wi-Fi (wireless-fidelity) connection. Information gathered by the dispatcher is downloaded into the patient record.
- En route to the station, the crew uses a touch screen to select information for the PCR, which reduces the narrative required and allows for drawing injuries and complaints on an anatomical model.
- A legible, comprehensive report is synced by Wi-Fi connection to the server at the headquarters station.
- The server faxes the PCR automatically to the receiving ED.
- The QA/QI process is streamlined. The supervisor has direct access to any PCR from any computer terminal to review the report and can search for PCRs that meet certain criteria.
- The billing office staff has immediate access to the record.

You are the Paramedic Summary

1. Why did the dispatcher supply very little information for this call?

Dispatchers do an outstanding job of calming 9-1-1 callers, obtaining information, and providing lifesaving instructions. They accomplish all of this with their voice and their communication skills. However, despite their best efforts, callers sometimes are unable to provide enough information or unknowingly provide inaccurate information. Although you might have an excellent idea about the nature of the call before arrival, it's important to keep these issues in mind en route to the scene.

2. What immediate challenges do you foresee regarding this call?

This incident was unwitnessed. No one can provide information about the nature of her injuries, her downtime, or any medical problems she may have. When dealing with these sorts of unknowns, it's best to err on the side of the worst-case scenario. Although she had protective gear on, it is possible that she could have a spinal injury.

3. How does the initial information you're given from dispatchers, family, bystanders, or other responders impact your decisions regarding patient care?

Sometimes certain portions of information can be stressed too much or omitted entirely. Don't get locked into a line of treatment without first considering other possibilities. Make sure to assess the scene in addition to your patient. Get a good view of the big picture and all its possibilities before narrowing your view.

4. How did this call change from dispatch to arrival?

Originally, this seemed to be a trauma call. As with all trauma patients, it's important to consider the underlying cause of the incident because sometimes the causes are medical. For example, if you are unable to find a cause for someone's involvement in a motor vehicle collision, such as road conditions, animals, or debris in the roadway, stop and think of medical emergencies, such as cerebrovascular accident (stroke), myocardial infarction, and hypoglycemia.

5. Given her level of consciousness, what concerns do you have regarding her airway?

Although you can readily correct her decreased level of consciousness and, therefore, her airway patency issues with the administration of dextrose, it is important to assess and consider the possibility that she aspirated gastric contents, which, if she did, could result in aspiration pneumonia. She should be transported for further evaluation for possible aspiration and of medication dosages and unrecognized trauma.

6. What are your top priorities at the moment?

As always, your top priorities are airway, breathing, and circulation. As prehospital providers, our job is to handle life-threatening emergencies first and then, time permitting, assess and treat other conditions. With all of your patients, you should attempt to ascertain the underlying reason for the physical manifestations such as decreased level of consciousness.

7. As your patient's level of consciousness improves, what issues do you foresee?

Sometimes patients who regain consciousness do not understand why they should be transported to the hospital. Frequently these patients will refuse treatment and/or transport. It is your job to act in their best interests and advise them of their needs and the consequences that could result from their refusal. If they refuse your help, it should be an informed refusal.

8. How does your ability to effectively communicate impact patient care?

If you are a poor communicator, whether in verbal or nonverbal communication, your patient possibly will not get the needed care. If you are unable to establish trust, a patient may be reluctant to provide information or to trust your suggestions.

9. How do body language and tone of voice communicate as much or more than words?

Much of what we communicate is nonverbal. If your words don't match your facial expression, tone of voice, and body language, it's likely that your words won't be heard and your nonverbal cues will. Be aware of what you say with your nonverbal language.

10. How does total patient care enter into this scenario?

Communicating that you care about the patient's well-being is accomplished through your words and actions. Sometimes what patients care about most is not what concerns you the most. Try to put yourself in your patients' shoes and address what's important to them and what they need in terms of medical care.

11. What is the purpose of documentation?

Because we, as prehospital providers, see our patients for such a short period of time, we can forget that we are but one link in the large chain of the continuum of care. It is important to bear this in mind when completing your medical incident reports. Your report will follow your patient as they travel through their hospital care and discharge. The purpose of our documentation is to provide a clear picture for all the health care professionals who were not on the scene of the emergency. Be clear. Be concise. Be complete.

12. Who is your documentation audience?

For the most part, your documentation will be viewed by other health care professionals for the purposes of understanding the nature of the patient's initial (or exacerbated) illness or injury; however, documentation is sometimes also viewed by litigators. Issues such as sloppy penmanship, misspelled words, and incomplete documentation can give the appearance that you are lazy, incompetent, or both. To help keep this in sight, imagine each of your reports being picked over by an attorney and viewed by a judge and jury. Also remember that it may take years for a case to go to trial, and you will likely have forgotten much of the call. Your documentation will aid your memory and provide evidence of your patient care.

Prep Kit

■ Ready for Review

- You must be able to rapidly, efficiently, and effectively communicate when responding to a call to fulfill your role as a paramedic.
- The phases of communication include notification, potential prearrival instructions for the caller, dispatch, communication during on-scene care, and communication with the receiving facility while en route.
- The dispatcher communicates with people who call in an emergency, and sends the EMS unit to the scene. Most of their telecommunication is done through digital technology.
- The dispatcher identifies the exact location of the patient, the telephone number, the nature of the problem, and specific information about the patient's condition and emergency, such as the types of vehicles involved in a car collision or hazards at the scene.
- The dispatcher is also responsible for monitoring communications with the ambulance, coordinating communication with direct medical control and other agencies, and recording the times when the various phases of the call occurred.
- Emergency medical dispatch is special training which teaches dispatchers to provide basic medical instructions to emergency callers over the phone. Updates resulting from this prearrival care can be communicated to the EMS crew as they are en route.
- Radio is one of the main methods of communication in EMS. The most commonly used bands for medical communications are the very high frequency (VHF) band and ultrahigh frequency (UHF) band. The higher the band, the less interference there is, but the shorter the transmission range.
- Trunking is the ability for multiple agencies or systems to share frequencies. This allows the dispatcher to reprogram radios so that agencies which do not normally talk to each other are able to, if necessary, such as in a mass-casualty incident.
- The federal government controls frequency allocation and licensing in Canada. It also establishes technical standards for radio equipment, establishes and enforces rules and regulations for the operation of radio equipment, and monitors transmissions. Communications over frequencies allotted for medical purposes are supposed to be used strictly for that purpose.
- Biotelemetry (often referred to as telemetry) is used to transmit vital life signs to a distant terminal. In EMS it is usually used for transmitting an ECG. This can be useful in diagnosing myocardial infarction and can allow the hospital to prepare to administer fibrinolytic therapy.
- Cellular telephones are becoming more common in EMS communications systems. Many newer cell phones have global positioning systems built in which aid the enhanced 9-1-1 operator to determine exactly where the call is being made.
- Systems used for radio transmission include simplex, duplex, and multiplex. Simplex operates on one frequency and only allows transmission to go one way. Duplex operates on two frequencies and allows simultaneous transmission and reception. Multiplex operates on two or more frequencies and allows for more than one transmission simultaneously.
- An EMS communications system consists of a base station, mobile and portable transmitters or receivers, a repeater, a remote console, and a landline or backup communications system.
- Keep radio communication simple, brief, and direct. One of the main goals is clarity. Use the international phonetic alphabet to aid transmission of spellings.
- Remember that your words can be heard by anyone who is listening. Keep your communications professional at all times. Do not transmit the patient's name or personal information over the radio; this would be in violation of confidentiality laws.

- Most ambulance systems use plain English in radio communications, but some use radio codes. If your agency uses codes, be sure to learn them.
- When reporting medical information, include the patient's age and sex, chief complaint, brief history, level of consciousness, degree of distress, vital signs, physical findings, ECG findings, and treatment.
- Your written report, or patient care report, is the only record of events that transpired during the call and serves as a legal record. It should be complete, well-written, legible, and professional. Proper use of terminology is essential. Learn common medical abbreviations.
- You will need to write a narrative in your patient care report. There are many methods, including chronological order, the SOAP method, the CHARTE method, and the body systems approach. Learn the method used by your system.
- The patient care report needs to be filled out in a timely manner. Be sure to fill it out directly after the call.
- If a patient refuses care, ensure that you have obtained vital signs and a complete history, fully inform the patient of the situation, involve direct medical control if needed, and thoroughly document the situation.
- If you must revise or correct your patient care report, note the date, time, and purpose for the correction. Place a single line through the error, initial it, and write the correct information next to it.
- Inaccurate or poor documentation could lead to subsequent caregivers providing inappropriate care to the patient. It could also work against you in a lawsuit, and negatively affect your reputation.

■ Vital Vocabulary

base station Assembly of radio equipment consisting of at least a transmitter, receiver, and antenna connection at a fixed location.

biotelemetry Transmission of physiologic data, such as an ECG, from the patient to a distant point of reception (commonly referred to in EMS as "telemetry").

cellular telephones Low-power portable radios that communicate through an interconnected series of repeater stations called "cells."

computer-aided dispatch An automated computer system that processes the information received and assists the dispatcher with multiple functions and tasks.

dispatch To send to a specific destination or to send on a task.

duplex Radio system using more than one frequency to permit simultaneous transmission and reception.

emergency medical dispatch First aid instructions given by specially trained dispatchers to callers over the telephone while an ambulance is en route to the call.

emergency medical dispatcher (EMD) A person who receives information and relays that information in an organized manner during the emergency.

encoded A message is put into a code before it is transmitted.

enhanced 9-1-1 system An emergency call-in system in which additional information such as the phone number and location of the caller is recorded automatically through sophisticated telephone technology and the dispatcher need only confirm the information on the screen.

frequency In radio communications, the number of cycles per second of a signal, inversely related to the wavelength.

hertz (Hz) Unit of frequency equal to 1 cycle per second.

landline Communications system linked by wires, usually in reference to a conventional telephone system.

mobile In radio communications, a radio that is affixed to an EMS vehicle, but the vehicle can move around.

multiplex Method by which simultaneous transmission of voice and ECG signals can be achieved over a single radio frequency.

noise In radio communications, interference in a radio signal.

patch A connection between a telephone line and a radio communications system enabling a caller to get "on the air" by dialing into a special telephone.

portable A handheld radio that can be carried on a person and used for communications away from a vehicle.

push-to-talk Commonly abbreviated as PTT, a method for communicating on a half-duplex communications system by pushing a button on the communication device to send and releasing the button to receive.

repeater Miniature transmitter that picks up a radio signal and rebroadcasts it, extending the range of a radio communications system.

simplex Method of radio communication using a single frequency that enables transmission or reception of voice or an ECG signal but is incapable of simultaneous transmission and reception.

ten-code A radio code system using the number 10 plus another number.

transceiver A radio transmitter and receiver housed in a single unit; a two-way radio.

trunking Sharing of radio frequencies by multiple agencies or systems.

ultrahigh frequency (UHF) band The portion of the radio frequency spectrum between 300 and 3,000 mHz.

very high frequency (VHF) band The portion of the radio frequency spectrum between 30 and 150 mHz.

wavelength The distance in a propagating wave from one point to the corresponding point on the next wave.

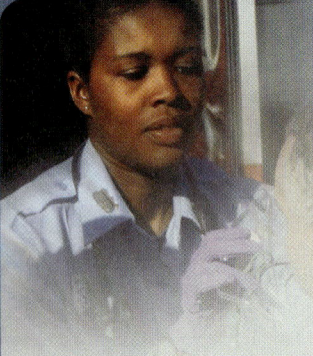

Assessment in Action

You are dispatched to a nursing home for a patient in respiratory distress. When you arrive, you find the patient with agonal respirations, and he is cold to the touch and grossly diaphoretic. His heart rate is 50 beats/min; his rhythm on the monitor is junctional. He has no palpable radial pulses and a palpable systolic blood pressure of 70 mm Hg. The staff stated he was "just fine" 30 minutes before they called 9-1-1. He was found slumped in his chair.

Your treatment for this patient includes an IV of normal saline, open wide for fluid volume, and endotracheal intubation with a 7.5 ET tube. You transport and transfer the patient to the emergency department staff on arrival. You now need to prepare the PCR.

1. **Which of the following statements is true for a PCR?**
   A. It is the only written record of the prehospital events.
   B. Documentation in the PCR is one of the most important skills learned as a paramedic.
   C. It is a legal record and part of the patient's medical record.
   D. All of the above.

2. **When a paramedic intubates a patient, all of the following should be documented, EXCEPT:**
   A. the size of the tube.
   B. the brand of the tube.
   C. who intubated the patient.
   D. the confirmation devices used.

3. **There are several charting "systems" a paramedic can use when documenting. They include all of the following, EXCEPT:**
   A. SOAP.
   B. CHARTE.
   C. body system approach.
   D. SOPE.

4. **How should you document a patient's words?**
   A. Document using quotes on the PCR.
   B. Write down what the patient stated.
   C. Rephrase what the patient said.
   D. Use a special incident report to state what the patient said.

5. **True or false? Pertinent negatives should be documented when writing your PCR.**
   A. True
   B. False

6. **Ensuring that documentation is complete, accurate, and legible is part of the _____ of paramedics.**
   A. standing orders
   B. direct medical control responsibilities
   C. professional responsibilities
   D. department of health requirements

7. **The best time for a paramedic to write the PCR is:**
   A. en route to the hospital.
   B. after a verbal patient report to the receiving hospital.
   C. after returning to headquarters.
   D. while waiting to transfer the patient at the receiving hospital.

8. **When a PCR is inappropriate or care is inadequately documented, it can be presumed that:**
   A. the paramedic had a bad day.
   B. the paramedic was not trained properly.
   C. others may question the care given to the patient.
   D. the paramedic forgot to include something.

9. **The documentation of starting IVs in the prehospital environment should include all of the following, EXCEPT:**
   A. the size of the cannula used.
   B. the site of the IV.
   C. multiple attempts if not successful on the first try.
   D. who adjusted the drip.

Challenging Questions

You are dispatched for a motor vehicle collision. When you arrive, you find a male patient, unknown age, unconscious, and unresponsive in the street. He appears to have a significant head injury; as you examine him, you notice brain matter on the road. His injuries are incompatible with life. The ECG shows asystole in all three leads. You call your direct medical control physician, who pronounces the patient dead. There are two other vehicles involved in this collision with a total of three patients who have minor injuries.

10. **How do you properly document this call?**

11. **Why is accurate documentation important?**

Points to Ponder

You are dispatched to a private residence for a person having a seizure. While responding, you are informed by your dispatcher that the call has been upgraded to a cardiac arrest. You arrive at the home and are unable to gain access. You advise your dispatch centre. The dispatcher uses the call-back number received with the 9-1-1 call. Someone runs from next door and tells you that the call is at another house. You go over, treat the patient, and transport to the hospital. After the call, you find out you received the wrong address—the 9-1-1 call originated at the house you were sent to because the person in need did not have a phone.

What information could have helped you en route to the call? How do you document the delay in patient contact, especially because this was a cardiac arrest and seconds matter?

Issues: Understanding the Role of Your Dispatch Centre, Advocating Among Peers, Completing Documentation, Resolving the Negative Attitude Toward Documentation.

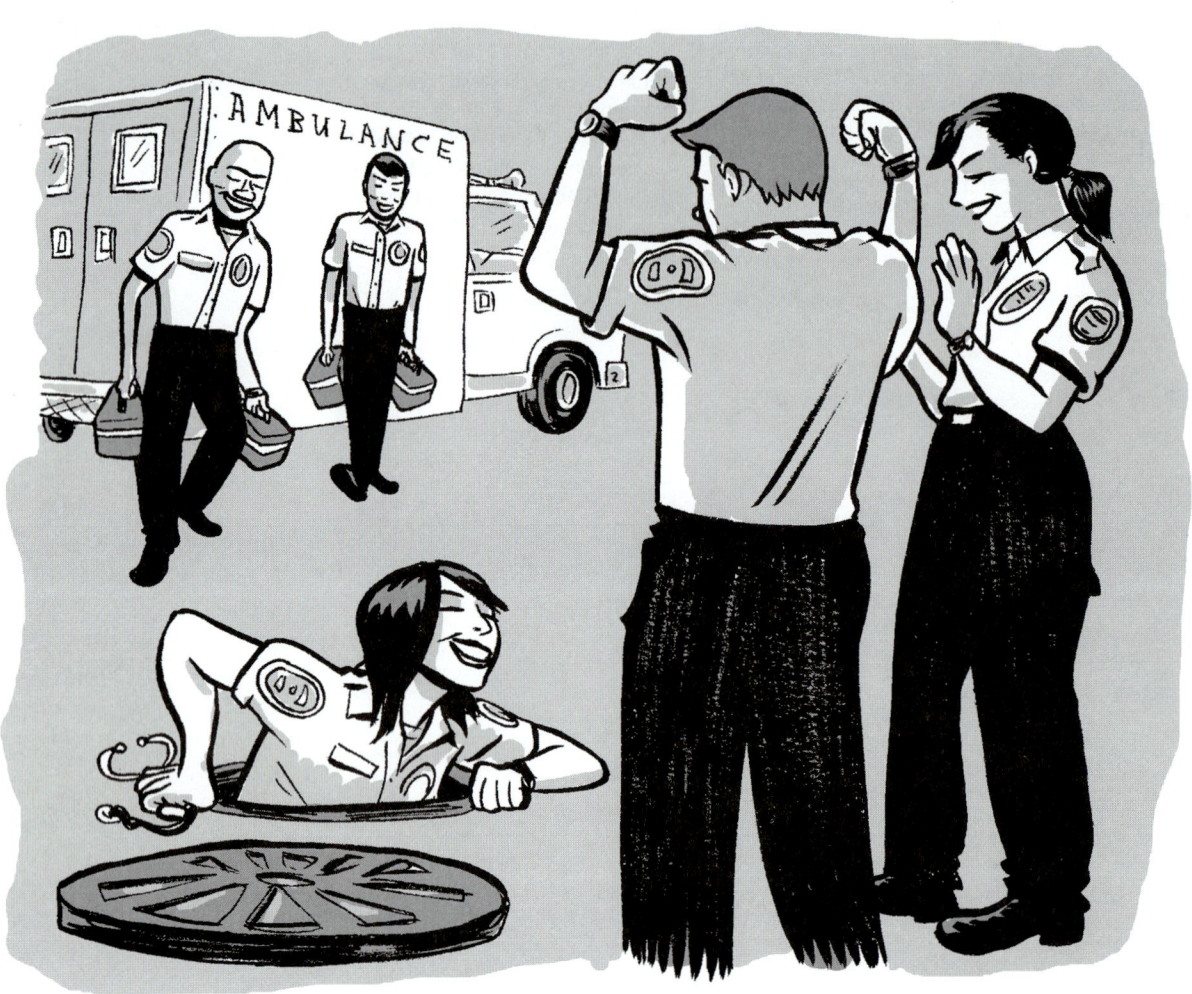

"

The first time I climbed into a sewer to do a resuscitation, I realized there were lots of things they never told me in medical school."

—Nancy L. Caroline, MD

Trauma

4

Section Editor: Fergal McCourt, MD, MSc, FACEM

Competency Areas

Area 1: Professional Responsibilities

1.4.a   Function within relevant legislation, policies, and procedures.

Area 4: Assessment and Diagnostics

4.2.f   Obtain information regarding incident through accurate and complete scene assessment.

4.3.a   Conduct primary patient assessment and interpret findings.

4.3.b   Conduct secondary patient assessment and interpret findings.

4.3.n   Conduct multisystem assessment and interpret findings.

Area 6: Integration

6.1.g   Provide care to patient experiencing illness or injury primarily involving musculoskeletal system.

6.1.o   Provide care to patient based on understanding of common physiological, anatomical, incident, and patient-specific field trauma criteria that determine appropriate decisions for triage, transport, and destination.

6.3.a   Conduct ongoing assessments based on patient presentation and interpret findings.

6.3.b   Re-direct priorities based on assessment findings.

Area 7: Transportation

7.4.b   Recognize the stressors of flight on patient, crew, and equipment, and the implications for patient care.

Appendix 4: Pathophysiology

C.   **Respiratory System**
Traumatic Injuries: Flail chest
Traumatic Injuries: Penetrating injury

E.   **Gastrointestinal System**
Traumatic Injuries: Abdominal injuries—penetrating/blunt

G.   **Integumentary System**
Traumatic Injuries: Lacerations/avulsions/abrasions

H.   **Musculoskeletal System**
Skeletal Fractures: Appendicular
Skeletal Fractures: Axial

J.   **Multisystem Diseases and Injuries**
Trauma: Assault
Trauma: Blast injuries
Trauma: Crush injuries
Trauma: Falls
Trauma: Rapid deceleration injuries

L.   **Ears, Eyes, Nose, and Throat**
External, Middle, and Inner Ear Disorders: Traumatic ear injuries

Introduction

Trauma, defined as a transfer of energy applied clinically, is the leading cause of death in Canadians younger than age 45. With improvements in health care and management of chronic diseases, death rates due to conditions such as heart disease, neoplasms, cerebrovascular events, and respiratory illnesses have decreased significantly in younger age groups. Unintentional trauma, often referred to as the "silent epidemic," represents a major health concern. It has been estimated that 90% of these injuries are preventable. In Canada, trauma accounted for 7,076 deaths and almost 2 million hospital days in 2004.

Basic concepts of the mechanics and biomechanics of trauma will help you analyze and manage your patient's injuries. Analyzing a trauma scene is a vital skill because you are the eyes and ears of the emergency department physicians at the scene of the trauma. Your paramedic-written patient history and verbal reports are the *only* source for physicians and surgeons to understand the events and mechanisms that led to your trauma patient's injuries. Your information is critical as a foundation to visualize and search for injuries that may not be apparent on physical examination.

Trauma, Energy, Biomechanics, and Kinematics

Trauma is the acute physiologic and structural change (injury) that occurs in a patient's body when an external source of

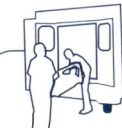

At the Scene

The top five causes of trauma death are motor vehicle collisions, falls, poisonings, burns, and drownings.

energy dissipates faster than the body's ability to sustain and dissipate it **Figure 17-1** ▾.

If your patient's body is in a vehicle that smashes into a wall, the energy delivered by the moving vehicle is released when the car is stopped by the wall. Your patient's body is moving at the same speed as the vehicle, and his or her body does not have bumpers to absorb the energy from stopping. If the energy is not absorbed in other ways, the patient's body absorbs it, often causing bones to break and internal organs to rupture—what you see as traumatic injuries.

Different forms of energy produce different kinds of trauma. These external energy sources can be mechanical, chemical, thermal, electrical, and barometric.

Mechanical energy is energy from motion (kinetic energy ie, a moving vehicle) or energy stored in an object

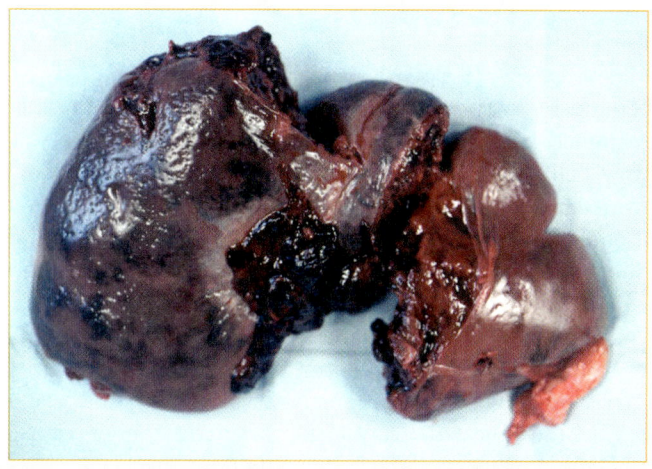

Figure 17-1 Traumatic injury occurs when the body's tissues are exposed to energy levels beyond their tolerance. Some traumatic injuries may not be visible. This photo shows a ruptured spleen.

You are the Paramedic Part 1

You are dispatched to 1601 South Main Street for "man fallen from a roof." This address is located in the business district of your service area. En route to the call, you learn that this man had been running from police and had come from a building in the downtown area. The patient is in police custody, and the scene is considered safe.

You arrive but are unable to assess much because the patient is combative and unwilling to answer your questions. You can see that his skin is slightly moist and a bit pale.

Initial Assessment	Recording Time: 0 Minutes
Appearance	Grimacing, screaming, punching
Level of consciousness	A (Alert to person, place, and day)
Airway	Patent
Breathing	Rapid and deep
Circulation	Unable to assess due to patient combativeness

1. What initial information about the fall gives rise for concern?
2. How does knowing your primary service area impact your understanding of potential patient injuries?
3. Given the location, what other conditions are you worried about?

(potential energy—a concrete bridge abutment). Kinetic energy would be found in two moving vehicles colliding. Potential energy would be present in a fall from a height. In that case, gravity would be the *potential* source of energy that can cause the object to fall. Chemical energy can be found in an explosive or an acid or even from a reaction to an ingested or medically delivered agent or drug. Electrical energy comes in the form of high voltage electrocution or a lightning strike. Barometric energy can result from sudden and radical changes in pressure, often occurring during diving or flying.

Biomechanics is the study of the physiology and mechanics of a living organism using the tools of mechanical engineering. Biomechanics provides a way of analyzing the mechanisms and results of trauma sustained by the human body. Kinetics studies the relationships among speed, mass, direction of the force, and, for paramedics, the physical injury caused by speed, mass, and force. Knowledge of kinetics can help you predict injury patterns found in a patient.

Factors Affecting Types of Injury

The kind of injury resulting after trauma is sustained will be determined by the ability of the patient's body to disperse the energy delivered by the traumatic event. Some patients' bodies can stretch and bend to absorb the energy of the traumatic event. But other patients' bone and tissue cannot absorb the energy. For example, a healthy football player can absorb a "hit" on the playing field better than an older man with diminished bone mass.

External factors that determine types of injury include the amount of *force* and *energy* delivered. The amount of injury (force) your patient sustains varies with the size (or mass) of the object delivering the force and energy, with the change in velocity (how fast your patient or the object is travelling), with acceleration or deceleration (how much the object or your patient speeds up or slows down), and with the body area to which the force is applied. This is a real world application of Newton's second law of motion (force = mass × acceleration). The primary reasons for the extent of trauma your patients sustain are the amount of energy in the object and the mechanism by which the object is delivered to the body. The body receives wider-spread trauma from a cannon ball (more energy inside) than it does from a bullet, although both are often lethal.

Duration and *direction* of the force of application are also important. The *rate of force application* affects trauma because energy that is applied rapidly is not tolerated as well as a similar amount of energy delivered over a longer period. For example, energy delivered rapidly can cause broken wrists, whereas longer-term energy delivery might show up as a repetitive stress injury—even though the amount of force might ultimately be exactly the same. In vehicle collisions, paramedics learn to recognize the directional patterns in injuries from front-end, side, and rear-end collisions.

The larger the area of force dissipation, the more pressure is reduced to a specific spot on the body, often without making a visible cut. Bullet impact is less if the energy in the bullet is dissi-

pated over the ceramic plate inside a bulletproof vest than if all the force of the bullet is applied at a small location on the skin.

In trauma medicine, this spreading of impact is described as *blunt trauma*. Paramedics at all levels quickly learn in the prehospital environment that blunt trauma is difficult to diagnose because there is often little external damage. Paramedics study kinetics to help them diagnose this potentially lethal, but sometimes invisible, form of trauma.

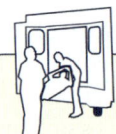

At the Scene

Suspect a spinal injury when you see a cracked windshield, steering wheel or dashboard damage, intrusion into a vehicle, or fractured feet or ankles after a fall. It will make a difference in how you handle the ABCs.

The position of the trauma victim—how he or she is positioned—at the time of the event is an external factor. Seatbelts have done a great deal to effect the reduction in lethal injuries by keeping occupants in positions less likely to cause fatal injuries.

Internal injuries sustained when the break point of an organ is exceeded can be difficult to diagnose. There may be external markers, such as contusions, abrasions, lacerations, and punctures.

The *impact resistance of body parts* will also have a bearing on types of tissue disruption. Impact resistance is often determined by what is inside your patient's organs: gas, liquid, or solid.

Paramedics need to know that organs that have gas inside, such as in the lungs and intestinal tract, will scatter energy more than liquid or solid boundaries. This means that the organ around the gas will be easily compressed, so look for lung and intestinal trauma first. Water-bearing organs include the vascular system, the liver, spleen, and muscle. Water-bearing tissues are less compressible than gas-containing tissues. Solid density interfaces occur mostly in bones such as in the cranium, spine, and long bones.

Because many injuries are not obvious on first presentation, understanding the effects of forces and energy transfer patterns will help in the assessment of the *mechanism of injury* (MOI), which in turn can help predict the most likely type of injuries you will see when you are in the out-of-hospital setting **Figure 17-2 ▶**. Paramedic students need to learn to have a *high index of suspicion* for injuries that otherwise might be undetected for several hours. Anticipate the possibility of specific types of injury: you will help your patient and the trauma team who will need your assessment of the scene.

▍Trauma Centres

Paramedics need a good working knowledge of the hospital resources with a reasonable idea of how long transport will take. Frequently, you will be the decision maker about where

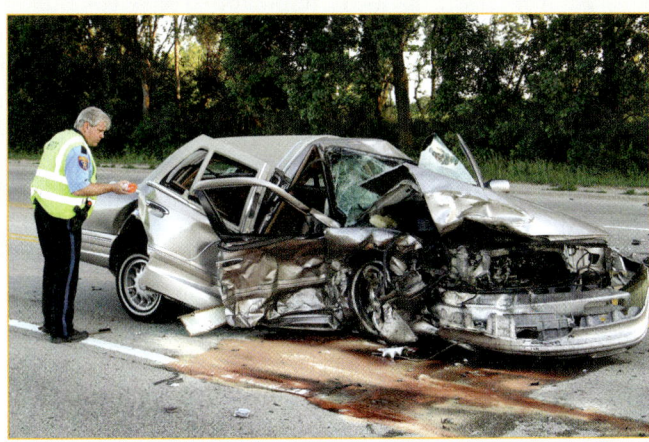

Figure 17-2 The appearance of the car can provide you with critical information about the severity of the collision and the possible injuries to the occupants.

Documentation and Communication

So much emphasis is placed on the MOI because obtaining a complete and accurate history of the incident can help predict as many as 95% of the injuries present. After ensuring your personal safety and maintaining the ABCs, the mechanism of injury is key information to obtain from the trauma scene. You must report the MOIs to the receiving trauma centre or emergency department. You are the eyes and ears of the trauma team at the scene of the injury.

your patient should be transported. Before you even get to the scene, you should know what is available in your area.

The Committee on Trauma (COT) of the American College of Surgeons is the governing body responsible for the designation of trauma centres in the United States. There are four separate categories of verification in the COT's program (Level I, II, III, and IV).

The Trauma Association of Canada (TAC) has developed similar guidelines for the organization and staffing of tertiary, district, and rural centres. Tertiary care centres in Canada are approximately equivalent to a Level I trauma centre as described by the American College of Surgeons.

Tertiary Trauma Centre (Level I)
- Plays the leading role within the regional or community trauma system. It has the capability of providing definitive care for seriously injured patients. The centre assumes the leadership role in the delivery of optimal care to the injured patient, research, teaching, data collection, evaluation, and the injury control and prevention program.
- Serves as a facility for the resuscitation of acutely injured patients, as well as the regional referral centre for severely

injured patients. The centre must have a comprehensive external disaster response plan.
- Participates in research at the clinical and/or basic science level and in the management activities related to trauma care.
- Undertakes educational activities including the teaching of undergraduate and postgraduate physicians, as well as other allied health professionals. Teaching also includes outreach education throughout the region and public educational programs.
- Collects, analyzes, and produces reports on data, and participates in a provincial trauma registry. Participates in epidemiological studies of injury.
- Provides leadership in injury control and prevention programs, including identification of prevention priorities and strategies.
- Identifies the need for new resources.

District Trauma Centre (Level II)
- May be an urban hospital or rural community hospital.
- Is a strategically located centre with resources, human and physical, sufficient to treat single system injuries, some multisystem injuries, and fulfill resuscitation requirements prior to referral to a tertiary care centre.

Primary Trauma Centre (Level III)
- Is a smaller, general practitioner hospital or nursing station that serves as an initial "clearing station" and refers all but minor injuries to either its district trauma centre or to a tertiary trauma centre, following appropriate consultation.

Currently, there are 15 accredited Tertiary Trauma Centres in Canada. In some provinces, "trauma networks" have been established, with a lead trauma hospital providing Level I care.

Criteria for Referral to a Trauma Centre

Paramedics are responsible for determining whether a patient should go to a trauma centre—and at what level. In all provinces, trauma centres have been created in large urban centres and bypass and triage criteria have been established. You may also have to determine whether air transport is required to a tertiary or lead trauma centre. *The criteria for transport to a trauma centre vary from system to system.* Every paramedic should know his or her local and regional protocols for triage and bypass to a trauma centre. In January 2009, the US Centers for Disease Control and Prevention released their Guidelines for Field Triage of Injured Patients, derived from recommendations of a national expert panel. The guidelines state that patients meeting one of the following criteria should be preferentially transported to a designated trauma centre:

1. If one of the following is present, the patient should be referred to a trauma centre:
   - GCS (Glasgow Coma Scale score) < 14
   - RR (respiratory rate) < 10 or > 29
   - SBP (systolic blood pressure) < 90
   - RTS (revised trauma score) < 11
   - PTS (pediatric trauma score) < 9

2. If one of the following is diagnosed in the prehospital environment, the trauma centre is a more appropriate triage endpoint:
   - Flail chest
   - Two or more proximal long bone fractures
   - Amputation proximal to wrist or ankle
   - All penetrating trauma to head, neck, torso, or extremities proximal to elbow or knee
   - Any limb paralysis
   - Pelvic fractures
   - Combination of trauma with burns
   - Open and depressed skull fractures
   - Major burns

3. Evaluate at this point the MOI and examine the trauma scene for evidence of high-energy trauma. If one of the following is present, refer to a trauma centre:
   - Ejection from vehicle
   - Death in same passenger compartment
   - Pedestrian thrown or run over or vehicle–pedestrian injury at > 8 km/h
   - Initial speed > 65 km/h
   - High-speed motor vehicle collision (> 65 km/h)
   - Intrusion into passenger compartment of > 30 cm
   - Major vehicle deformity > 50 cm
   - Extrication time > 20 minutes
   - Falls > 6 m
   - Rollover (unrestrained passenger)
   - Motorcycle collision at > 35 km/h or with separation of rider and bike

4. If none of the above criteria is met, then consider transfer to trauma centre if:
   - Patient of age < 5 or > 55 years
   - Pregnancy > 20 weeks
   - Known immunosuppressed patients

   - Known cardiac disease or respiratory disease comorbidity
   - Type 1 diabetes, cirrhosis, morbid obesity, or coagulopathy

The prehospital assessment of trauma patients is key to their management and transport to the appropriate definitive care facility.

Transport Considerations

When making a decision to transport a patient, several options must be considered. What are the needs of the patient? What is the level of the receiving facility? The patient should be transported to the closest, most appropriate facility to receive optimal care. You must also decide on the mode of transport that will offer the greatest benefit. Should you call for air transport, or is ground transport sufficient?

When making the decision to transport by ground, several factors should be taken into consideration. Can the appropriate facility be reached within a reasonable timeframe by ground? What is the extent of injuries? If in a congested area, can the patient be transported to a more accessible landing zone for air medical transport?

Air transport must be considered in several situations: (1) when there is extended transport time by ground, (2) when there are multiple casualties, (3) when extrication times are prolonged and patients are critically injured, and (4) when there are long distances to an appropriate facility as opposed to the closest emergency department. There also may be other times that air transport is appropriate Figure 17-3 ▾ . If the patient can be transported to definitive care within a reasonable amount of time by ground, there is no need to call for air transport. Take into consideration the time it will take for the aircraft to lift off, travel, and land, just to reach the scene. By weighing the timeframe against transport by ground, you will be able to make an informed decision. Also take into account the terrain. Is there a safe area for landing? If not, how far will the patient need to be transported to reach a secure landing zone? If there is a great distance, ground transport may be a more reasonable option. Once the decision is made to call for

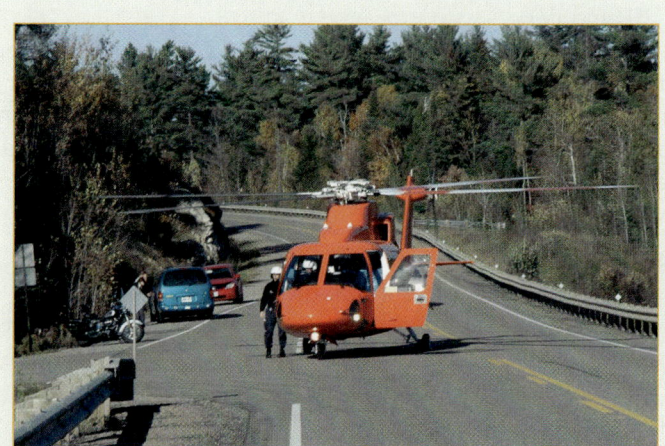

Figure 17-3 A helicopter may be used to transport patients quickly to the proper trauma centre.

air medical transport, contact your dispatcher to request a unit, or follow local protocols regarding contacting air support.

Helicopter Triage Criteria

All levels of prehospital paramedics should recognize the need for and criteria used in making the decision to use aeromedical

At the Scene

The Platinum Ten Minutes refers to the goal of the maximum time spent at a scene for a critical trauma patient. Scene times should be limited as much as possible to get the patient to more definitive care at a trauma centre. Trauma, more often than not, means that onsite stabilization is a questionable paramedic procedure. However, other problems may be better handled by onsite paramedic stabilization. One of your major tasks as a student paramedic is to learn the difference between the two.

transport in their service area. The key to success is recognizing the need for the aeromedical transport of patients and activating the service as early as possible. The trauma triage guidelines in this chapter should be used as a guideline, but providers must know their local and regional criteria for activation of a helicopter EMS response for trauma patients.

■ A Little Physics

Although drivers of motor vehicles might not obey the community's traffic laws, they must—whether they want to or not—obey the laws of physics that govern all objects on our

planet. A little familiarity with these laws will help you understand more about the mechanisms of trauma.

Velocity (V) is the distance an object travels per unit time. The difference between velocity and speed is that velocity is also defined by moving in a specific direction. Acceleration (a) of an object is the rate of change of velocity that an object is subjected to, whether speeding up or slowing down. Gravity (g) is the downward acceleration that is imparted to any object on earth by the effect of the earth's mass. During each second of a fall, the velocity or speed of the falling object increases by 9.8 m/sec^2.

Controversies

Some situations may have contraindications or relative contraindications for aeromedical transport. These situations include traumatic cardiac arrest, inclement weather conditions, extremely combative patients, morbidly obese patients, patients with barotrauma (diving injuries may necessitate lower flying altitudes), and situations in which ground transport and appropriate level of care are available and would permit quicker care.

The kinetic energy (KE) of an object is the energy associated with that object in motion. It reflects the relationship between the weight (mass) of the object and the velocity at which it is travelling and is expressed mathematically as:

$$\text{Kinetic energy} = \frac{\text{Mass}}{2} \times \text{Velocity}^2$$

$$\text{or, KE} = \frac{m}{2} \times v^2$$

You are the Paramedic Part 2

The police officers advise you that the patient was probably under the influence of PCP (phencyclidine hydrochloride), and in his attempts to avoid arrest, he climbed up a fire escape and fell. He landed on his hands and feet, stumbled for a few steps, and continued to try to run away unsuccessfully.

Vital Signs	Recording Time: 5 Minutes
Level of consciousness	V (Responsive to verbal stimuli)
Skin	Slightly moist, slightly pale, and cool
Pulse	Carotid (unable to access radial pulses because patient is being restrained); rapid (142 beats/min)
Blood pressure	168 by palpation
Respirations	60 breaths/min
Sao$_2$	99% while breathing room air

4. Given commonalities of fire escape locations, what other information do you have?
5. How does your patient's condition hinder your assessment techniques?
6. How do you compensate for this hindrance?

Thus, velocity has a much greater effect on KE than weight because it is squared   Figure 17-4 ▾ .

In other words, an object increases its kinetic energy more by increasing its velocity than by increasing its mass. The kinetic energy of an object involved in a collision must be *dissipated* as the object comes to rest. The kinetic energy of a car in motion that stops suddenly must be somewhere   Figure 17-5 ▸ . In a car, kinetic energy can be dissipated by braking, transforming to heat (another form of energy). If all the energy is not transformed into heat, however, the KE is transformed into deformed metal (potential energy), which results in damage to the car and its occupants. The mechanics of dissipation can result in injury. For example, a car travelling at 56 km/h hits a wall, which stops the car, but the driver is still travelling at 56 km/h until stopped by the seatbelts or the air bag, or, if not wearing a seatbelt, the steering wheel, dashboard, or windshield.

Speed kills exponentially: look what happens when velocity increases 10 km/h versus when the person weighs in at 10 kg heavier.

- 70 kg person at 10 km/h = 3,500 KE units
- 70 kg person at 20 km/h = 28,000 KE units
- 70 kg person at 30 km/h = 63,000 KE units
- 70 kg person at 40 km/h = 112,000 KE units
- 80 kg person at 40 km/h = 128,000 KE units
- 70 kg person at 55 km/h = 211,750 KE units
- 70 kg person at 65 km/h = 295,750 KE units

Note that when weight increases by 10 kg but velocity remains the same, there is not much change in the kinetic energy. However, when the velocity increases from 55 to 65 km/h (a difference of only 10 km/h), the KE (remember, that's energy in motion!) increases by 90,000 KE units!

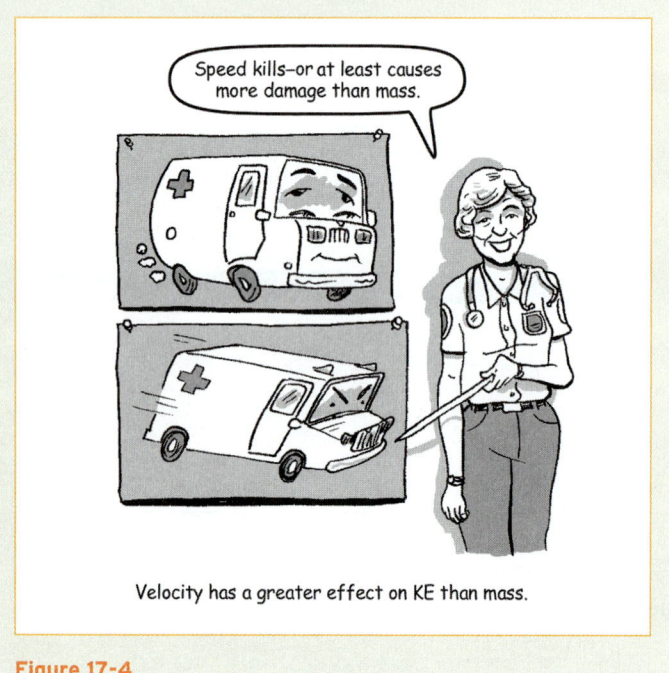

Speed kills—or at least causes more damage than mass.

Velocity has a greater effect on KE than mass.

Figure 17-4

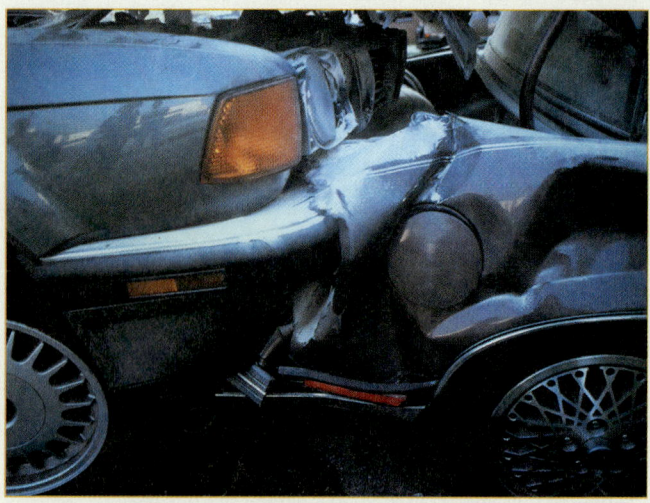

Figure 17-5 The kinetic energy of a speeding car is converted into the work of stopping the car, usually by crushing the car's exterior.

Modern cars are designed to have crumple zones to maximize the amount of energy dissipated by deformation before the passenger compartment is involved. Because the vehicle damage so often shows just how fast the car was going, the amount of damage provides information to help in your decision about transferring your patient to a trauma centre.

In addition to the velocity at which the car (and its passengers) are travelling, the vehicle's angle of impact (front collision versus side impact, or how your patient hit the inside of a vehicle), the differences in the sizes of the two vehicles, and the restraint status and protective gear of the occupants will affect the amount of energy dissipation that affects your patients in a collision.

Remember the laws of physics that no driver can break? Here's a quick review. The law of conservation of energy states that energy can be neither created nor destroyed, it can only change form. Energy generated from a sudden stop or start must be transformed to one of the following energy forms: thermal, electrical, chemical, radiant, or mechanical (as discussed earlier).

Energy dissipation, as you know, is the process by which KE is transformed into one of these forms of mechanical energy. When a car stops slowly, its KE is converted to thermal energy—heat—by friction of the braking action. If the car wrecks, KE is also dissipated into mechanical energy as the car body crumples in a collision. Mechanical energy is further dissipated in the form of injury as the occupants sustain fractures or other bodily harm.

Protective devices such as seatbelts, air bags, and helmets are designed to *manipulate* the way in which energy is dissipated into injury. For example, a seatbelt converts kinetic energy of the occupants into a seatbelt–to-body pressure force rather than into a steering wheel deformation against the torso or a windshield shattering against the head.

Newton's first law of motion states that a body at rest will remain at rest unless acted on by an outside force. Similarly, a body in motion tends to remain in motion at a constant velocity, travelling in a straight line, unless acted on by an outside force. Most bodies in motion (without the assistance of a motor or other propulsion device) tend to eventually stop owing to the action of forces of friction, wind resistance, or other force resulting in deceleration.

Newton's second law of motion states that the force that an object can exert is the product of its mass times its acceleration:

Force = Mass (Weight) × Acceleration (or Deceleration)

The higher an object's mass and acceleration, the higher the *force* that needs to be applied to make a change of course or stop the object. Remember our cartoon? Force equals mass × acceleration or deceleration. Deceleration is slowing to a stop. Rapid deceleration, as may occur in a collision, dissipates tremendous forces and, therefore, major injuries. Deceleration and acceleration can also be measured in numbers of g forces. One g force is the normal acceleration of gravity. A two or three g acceleration or deceleration force is, logically enough, two or three times the force associated with the acceleration of gravity. A two g deceleration would make you feel like you are twice as heavy as you are at rest. Three g acceleration would make you feel three times heavier. High-speed collisions can generate decelerations in *hundreds* of g's. The human limit to deceleration is about 30 g.

In a *head-on collision* with two vehicles travelling in opposite directions along a straight line, transferred energy is represented in part as the sum of both their speeds. If a car strikes an immovable object, forces generated come from the speed of the only moving object. In a *rear impact* of two vehicles travelling along the same line, the energy potential is lessened because it is the difference in speed between them, also known as the *closing speed*.

It is important to have an understanding of these laws of physics because they help define the types and patterns of trauma you will see in the prehospital environment. You are the most important witness the hospital trauma team has—the information you learn from physics will affect the outcome of your patient's life.

Types of Trauma

Injuries are generally described as the consequence of blunt or penetrating trauma. Blunt trauma refers to injuries in which the tissues are not penetrated by an external object **Figure 17-6** . Blunt trauma commonly occurs in motor vehicle collisions, in pedestrians hit by a vehicle, in motorcycle collisions, in falls from heights, in serious sports

injures, and in blasts when no shrapnel is involved and the pressure wave is the primary cause of the injuries.

Penetrating trauma results when tissues are penetrated by single or multiple objects **Figure 17-7** . Penetrating trauma results from gunshot wounds caused by a single or multiple projectiles, stab wounds, and blasts with shrapnel or secondary projectiles. Penetrating trauma may also occur in combination with blunt injuries such as in implement injuries during a motor vehicle collision or a fall out of a tree and onto a fence.

At the Scene

As a general rule, the entrance wound is smaller than the exit wound. Assume that cavitation involves internal structures that are not readily visible on your clinical examination.

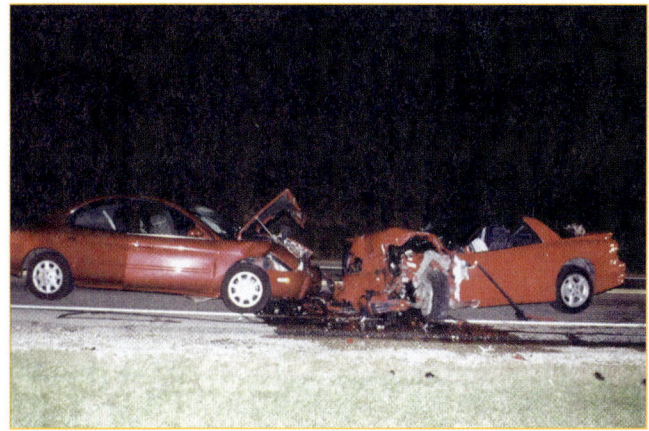

Figure 17-6 Blunt trauma typically occurs in motor vehicle collisions.

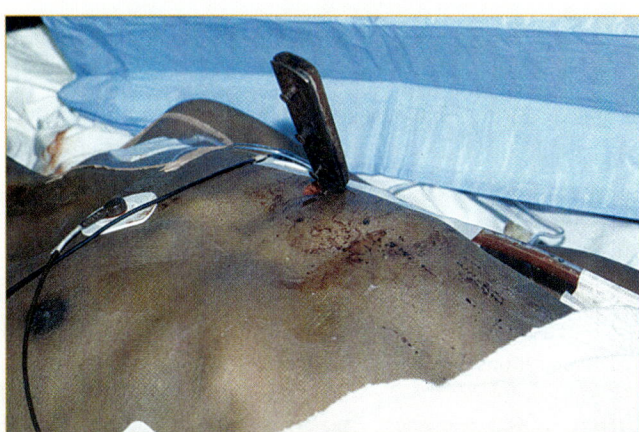

Figure 17-7 Injuries from low-energy penetrations, such as a stab wound, are caused by the sharp edges of the object moving through the body.

Injuries Caused by Deceleration

Abrupt deceleration injuries are produced by a sudden stop of a body's forward motion. Whether from a fall, shaking a baby, or a high-speed vehicle collision, decelerating forces can induce shearing, avulsing, or rupturing of organs and their restraining fascia, vasculature, nerves, and other soft tissues. These injuries are often invisible during examination, so every paramedic needs to understand how such injuries are sustained.

The head is particularly vulnerable to deceleration injuries. The brain is a fairly heavy organ that lies in fluid inside the skull. Any trauma that will jerk the patient's head causes the brain to hit the inside of the skull, causing bleeding, bruising, tearing, and crush injuries. All of these injuries are extremely dangerous and might not show up on a cursory examination. Your paramedic index of suspicion should be on high alert for these injuries.

The chest is vulnerable to aorta injury. The *aorta,* the largest blood vessel in the body, is the most common site of deceleration injury in the chest. The aorta is often torn away from its points of fixation in the body. Shearing of the aorta can result in rapid loss of all the body's blood and immediate death.

Abdominal blunt trauma results as the forward motion of the body stops and internal organs continue their forward motion, resulting in tearing at their points of attachment and shearing injuries. Organs that can be affected include the liver, kidneys, small intestine, large intestine, pancreas, and spleen.

Kidneys are injured as forward motion produces tears to the organ or to points of attachment through the renal arteries. Also, as forward motion is restrained by the large bowel, the small bowel can tear and result in free air in the abdomen. Trauma can also do damage without tearing by causing an insufficient supply of blood to the bowel. The spleen can also be torn, sometimes resulting in left upper quadrant pain and life-threatening internal bleeding.

Injuries Caused by External Forces

Crush and compression injuries are the result of forces applied to the body by things external to the body at the time of impact. Crush and compression injuries occur *at* the time of impact, unlike deceleration injuries, which occur *before* impact. Crush and compression injuries are often caused by dashboards, windshields, the floor, and heavy objects falling on the body.

Compression head injuries, which may result in skull fractures, often are associated with cervical spine injury. The more severe the head injury, the more likely a cervical spine injury has also occurred. Brain tissue does not compress; it swells within the enclosed area of the skull. As the brain swells inside the skull, it is crushed, causing a catastrophic injury.

Compression injuries of the chest may produce *fractured ribs,* which can lead to internal injuries of the lungs and heart. One of the signs of a lung injury is a *flail chest,* a condition in which a section of the chest wall moves paradoxically with respirations (moves opposite of normal). Fractured ribs may also cause blood or air to seep into the chest space, which would require decompression and placement of a chest tube. Blunt cardiac injury can compress the heart against the chest wall, causing arrhythmias and direct injury to the heart muscle. If the lungs are compressed, acute respiratory distress syndrome (ARDS) can require intubation to maintain your patient's breathing.

Almost all abdominal organs can be affected by hitting an external object. Organs often injured are the pancreas, spleen, liver, and kidneys. Compression against the seatbelt may result in *bowel rupture, bladder rupture, diaphragm tearing,* and *spinal injuries.* The aorta continues from the chest down into the abdomen, where it can be involved in vascular injury.

You are the Paramedic Part 3

The police officers restrain the patient so that you can perform your initial assessment and a rapid trauma assessment, while taking spinal precautions. You are able to apply a cervical collar and minimize his movement on a backboard. During your rapid trauma assessment, you find that he has deformity of both legs below the knees. He also has some abrasions to both hands and arms. It appears as though the majority of force was absorbed by the legs during the fall.

Reassessment	Recording Time: 10 Minutes
Level of consciousness	V (Responsive to verbal stimuli)
Skin	Slightly moist, slightly pale, and cool
Pulse	Carotid (unable to access radial pulses as patient is being restrained); rapid
Blood pressure	168 by palpation
Respirations	60 breaths/min
Sao_2	98% while breathing room air; patient noncompliant with nonrebreathing mask

7. Given this information, what other injuries do you suspect?

8. How can a patient who is under the influence of drugs be difficult to manage?

9. In addition to trauma, what other medical emergencies can ensue from the use of PCP?

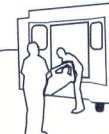

At the Scene

According to Transport Canada:

- 660,000 motor vehicle collisions occurred in 2003.
- Motor vehicle collisions were the cause of 2,766 fatalities in 2003.
- Fatalities and injuries have declined about 15% between 1994 and 2003, despite an increase in the number of registered motor vehicles.
- For the past 10 years, single-vehicle collisions have accounted for about 50% of all fatal collisions.
- Most deadly collisions occur on rural roads; 67% of fatal collisions took place on rural roads in 2003.
- Four out of five serious collisions occur in clear weather.
- The largest number of fatalities occurred in the 25- to 34-year age group. The second most at-risk age group was 65+ years.
- Of fatally injured drivers, 32% had a blood alcohol concentration over the legal limit of 17 mmol/l. In 1987, 47% of fatally injured drivers were legally intoxicated.
- 40% of vehicle occupants who died were not wearing seatbelts. 90% of Canadians regularly use seatbelts.
- Motor vehicle collisions accounted for 26,676 hospitalizations in 2004.
- Motor vehicle collisions accounted for just under one half of major injuries in Canada in 2004.
- 52% of fatalities were drivers.
- 23% of fatalities were passengers.
- 13% of injuries were pedestrians.
- Motorcyclists accounted for 1 in 16 of the total road fatalities in Canada.

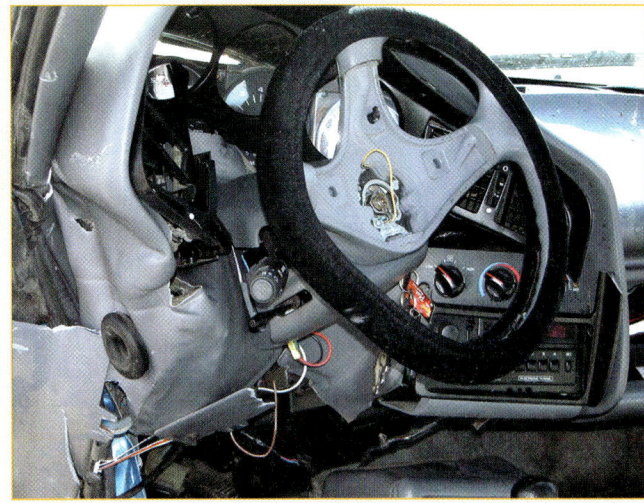

Figure 17-8 Deceleration of the occupant starts during sudden braking and continues during impact and collision. The appearance of the interior of the car can provide you with information about the severity of the patient's injuries.

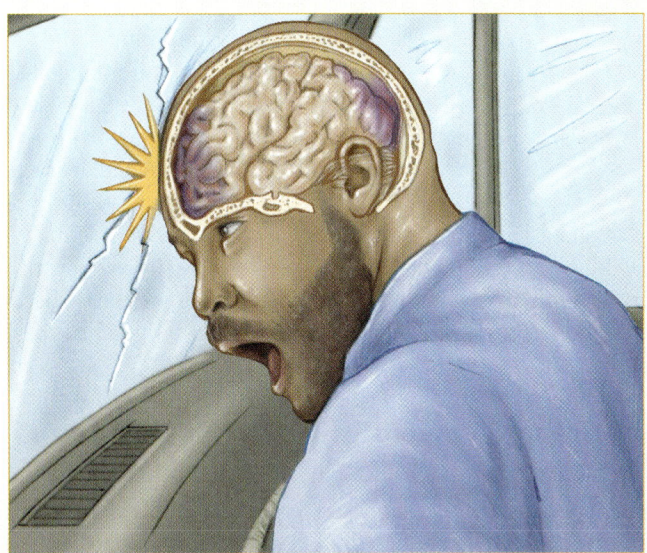

Figure 17-9 Deceleration of internal organs involves the body's supporting structures and movable organs that continue their forward momentum until stopped by anatomical restraints. In this illustration, the brain continues its forward motion and strikes the inside of the skull, resulting in a compression injury to the anterior portion of the brain and stretching of the posterior portion.

Pelvic fractures also result from external compressive trauma, potentially injuring the bladder, vagina, rectum, lumbar plexus, and pelvic floor and leading to severe bleeding from the large arteries near the hip bones.

Motor Vehicle Collisions

When a motor vehicle collides with another object, trauma in the collision is composed of *five phases* tied to the affects of progressive deceleration. The first phase, *deceleration of the vehicle,* occurs when the vehicle strikes another object and is brought to an abrupt stop. The forward motion of the car continues until its KE is dissipated in the form of mechanical deformation and damage to the vehicle and occupant or until the restraining force of the object is removed (for example, sheared off pole, yielding of a guard rail) and the vehicle motion continues until its KE is gently dissipated by drag or continued braking. The second phase is *deceleration of the occupant,* which starts during sudden braking and continues during impact and collision. This results in deceleration, compression, and shear trauma to the occupants **Figure 17-8 ▸** . The effects on vehicle occupants will vary depending on the mass of each occupant, protective mechanisms

in the vehicle such as restraints and air bags, body parts involved, and points of impact. The third phase, *deceleration of internal organs,* involves the body's supporting structures (skull, sternum, ribs, spine, and pelvis) and movable organs (brain, heart, liver, spleen, kidneys, and intestine) that continue their forward momentum until stopped by anatomical restraints **Figure 17-9 ▲** . Energy is dissipated by internal organs as they are injured. Movement of fixed and nonfixed parts may result in tears and shearing injuries. The fourth phase is the result of *secondary collisions,* which occur when a vehicle occupant is hit by objects moving within the vehicle such as packages, animals, or other passengers. These objects may continue to travel at the vehicle's initial speed and then hit a passenger who has come to rest. These types of collisions have been known to cause severe spine and head trauma. The final phase is the result of *additional impacts* that the vehicle may receive, as when it is hit and deflected into another vehicle, tree, or another

At the Scene

Don't forget that the collision of internal organs striking against the body can result in severe damage, though this may not always be obvious.

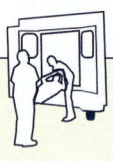

Notes from Nancy

When the windshield is cracked or broken, the front seat occupant has a cervical spine injury until proven otherwise.

object. This may increase the seriousness of original injuries or cause further injury. For example, a frontal collision may cause a posterior hip dislocation and an acetabular fracture via a dashboard mechanism and a subsequent side impact from another vehicle may add a lateral compression pelvic ring injury, resulting in complex pelvic and acetabular trauma. **Table 17-1 ▶** shows the structural clues, body clues, and resulting injuries for different types of collisions.

Predicting Types of Injury by Examining the Scene

Important clues to predict injury types can be obtained by paying attention to the history of the collision and by an examination of the scene. Using your new-found knowledge of the physics of trauma, you can make a good estimate of how injured your patients might be by looking at the amount of damage around the scene. How dented and deformed the vehicle looks is a clear indication of the forces involved and of the degree of deceleration sustained by your patient. Dents and deformities on the inside of the vehicle will show you the point of impact on the patient. Do a quick check for injury types visible on your patient: head injury or seatbelt marks show what parts of the body may have been involved in energy absorption. Tire skid marks at the scene indicate whether significant energy was dissipated by braking before collision. Debris along the course of the collision may indicate multiple collisions and different force vectors acting on the patient along the course of the collision.

There are primarily *five types of impact patterns:* Frontal or head on, lateral or side impact, rear impact, rotational, and rollover. In *frontal and head-on collisions,* the front end of the car distorts as it dissipates kinetic energy and decelerates its forward motion. Passengers decelerate at the same rate as the vehicle. In a 45 km/h collision, the front end of an average car will crush 60 cm at the rough estimate of 1.5 cm of deformity for each 1 km/h. The forces applied to the driver will differ based on car design, materials, and safety features of the vehicle. The interior will also suggest possible injuries by the damage your patient's body has done to the dash, windshield, or steering wheel, for example.

Position at the precise time of impact is very important in determining an occupant's movements and injuries during a collision. Unrestrained occupants usually follow one of two trajectories, a *down-and-under pathway,* or an *up-and-over pathway.*

The down-and-under pathway is travelled by an occupant who slides under the steering column **Figure 17-10 ▶**. As the vehicle is decelerating, the occupant continues to travel downward and forward into the dashboard or steering column, led by the knees. The knees hit the dashboard, transmitting the energy of the deceleration up the femurs to the pelvis. With knees locked in the dash and hips in the seat, force vectors go down the tibia and along the femur. If the feet are not locked by folding floorboards or brake pedals, energy along the tibia will be transferred to the lower leg, with no immediate injury. If the feet are locked in place, midshaft femur fracture can occur. In some cases, the heads of the femurs will dislocate. If the occupant's knees hit the dashboard, look for a fracture-dislocation of the knee or for hip and pelvic fractures or hip dislocation. Your patient's torso can twist in such a way that his or her head hits the steering column. Always look for spinal injuries.

The upper torso continues forward until it impacts the car, be it the steering wheel or the seatbelt and air bag protection system. Look for rib fractures or pulmonary or cardiac injuries caused by internal striking and compressing. When your patient is a child, assume that there will be pulmonary or cardiac injuries—children have more flexible ribs but often sustain compression injuries. Remember how gas-containing organs absorb more of the energy of the collision?

Notes from Nancy

When there is damage to the steering assembly, there is critical injury to the driver until proven otherwise.

In the up-and-over pathway, the lead point is the head. In this sequence, rotation occurs around the ankles with the torso moving in an upward and forward direction. The head takes a higher trajectory, impacting the windshield, roof, mirror, or dashboard, causing compression and deceleration injuries in your patient that can include significant head and cervical spine trauma. The anterior part of the neck may strike the

Table 17-1	MOI: Motor Vehicle Collision	
Structural Clues	**Body Clues**	**Look for These Injuries**
Head-on collision		
Deformed front end Cracked windshield	Bruised or lacerated head or face	• Brain injury • Scalp, facial cuts • Cervical spine injury • Tracheal injury
Deformed steering column	Bruised neck Bruised chest	• Sternal or rib fracture • Flail chest • Myocardial contusion • Pericardial tamponade • Pneumothorax or hemothorax • Exsanguination from aortic tear
Deformed dashboard	Bruised abdomen Bruised knee, misplaced kneecap	• Ruptured spleen, liver, bowel, diaphragm • Fractured patella • Dislocated knee • Femoral fracture • Dislocated hip
Lateral collision		
Deformed side of car	Bruised shoulder	• Clavicular fracture • Fractured humerus • Multiple rib fractures
Door smashed in	Bruised shoulder or pelvis	• Fractured hip • Fractured iliac wing • Fractured clavicle or ribs
"B" pillar deformed	Bruised temple	• Brain injury • Cervical spine fracture
Broken door or window handles	Bruised or deformed arms	• Contusions
Broken window glass	Dicing lacerations	• Multiple lacerations
Rear-end collision		
Posterior deformity of the vehicle	Secondary anterior injuries, especially if the patient was unrestrained	• "Whiplash" injuries • Cervical spine fractures • Deceleration injuries of a head-on collision
Headrest not adjusted		

steering wheel, causing laryngeal fracture, serious lacerations, and other soft-tissue injury.

Ejection is possible if the windshield does not stop the body from projecting through it. This leads to second-impact injuries when the body contacts the ground or objects outside of the car. These injuries can be as severe as initial-impact injuries, and they increase the likelihood of great vessel damage and death. The spine absorbs energy as it is compressed between the stationary head and the moving torso, which leads to injury.

A dangerous lung injury may occur if your patient reflexively takes a deep breath just before impact, hyperinflating the lungs and closing the glottis. The impact of the steering wheel can injure the lungs via generation of pressures beyond the capabilities of lung tissue, like a "paper bag being exploded" (60% to 70% of pneumothoraces may occur this way) **Figure 17-11 ▸**.

The abdomen, pelvis, or upper thigh contacts the lower aspect of the steering wheel or dash, and lower leg fractures could be present. **Table 17-2 ▸** lists the "ring" of chest injuries that can occur from impacting the steering wheel or the dashboard.

Lateral impact, "T"-bone, and *side collisions* impart energy to the near-side occupant almost directly to the pelvis and chest **Figure 17-12 ▸**. Unrestrained occupants will remain almost motionless, literally having the car pushed out from under them. Seatbelts do little to protect these passengers because they are designed to limit forward hinging injuries, not side impacts. As one vehicle makes contact

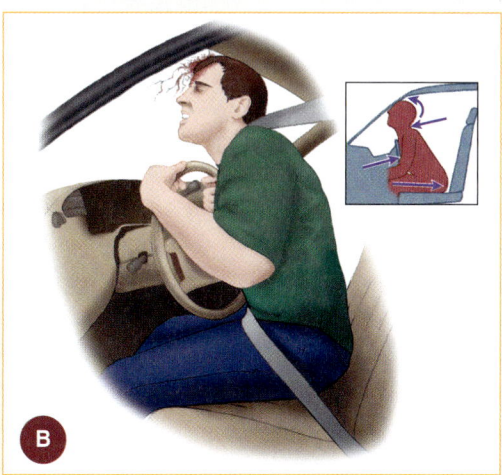

Figure 17-10 A. The down-and-under pathway. **B.** The up-and-over pathway.

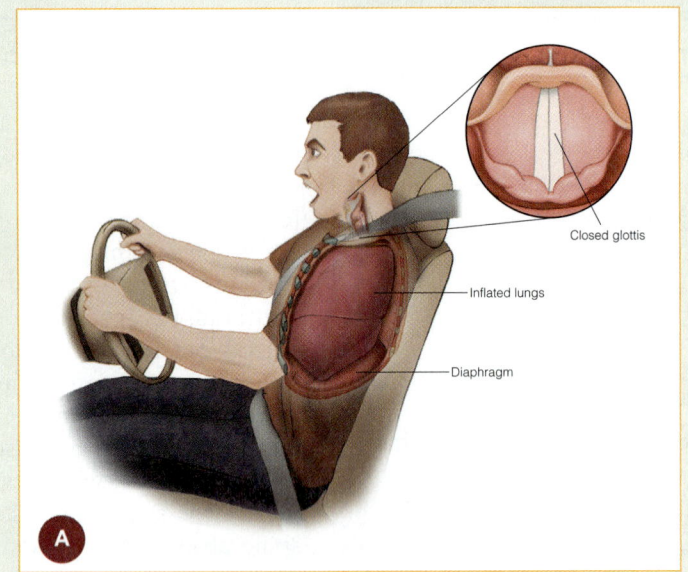

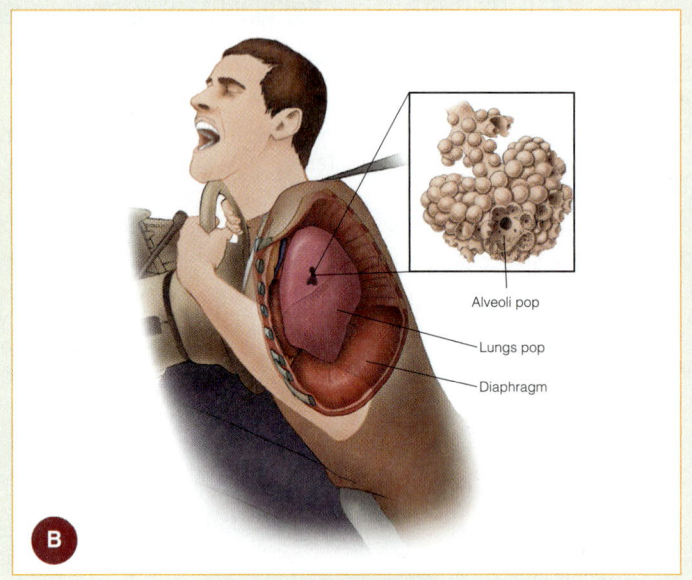

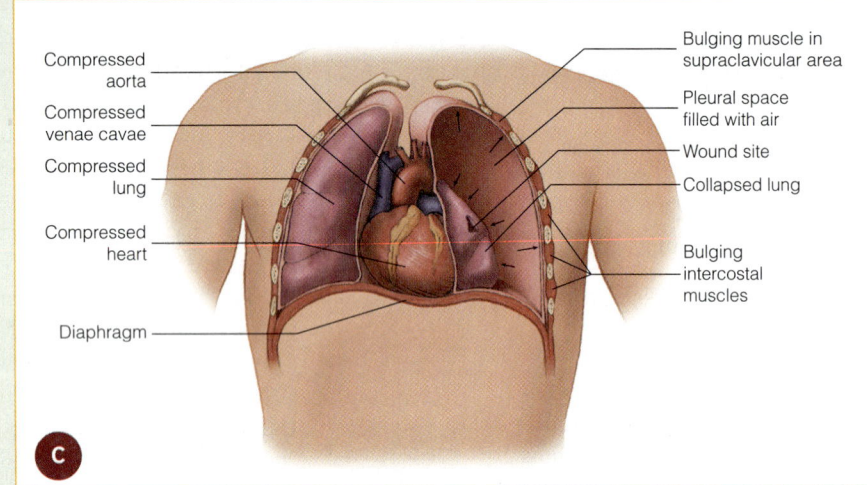

Figure 17-11 The paper-bag syndrome. **A.** The occupant takes a deep breath just before colliding, closing the glottis and filling the lungs with air. **B.** The occupant's chest hits the steering wheel, popping the alveoli in the lungs. **C.** A pneumothorax results.

Table 17-2	"Ring" of Chest Injuries From Impacting the Steering Wheel or Dashboard

- Facial injuries
- Soft-tissue neck trauma
- Larynx and tracheal trauma
- Fractured sternum
- Myocardial contusion
- Pericardial tamponade
- Pulmonary contusion
- Hemothorax, rib fractures
- Flail chest
- Ruptured aorta
- Intra-abdominal injuries

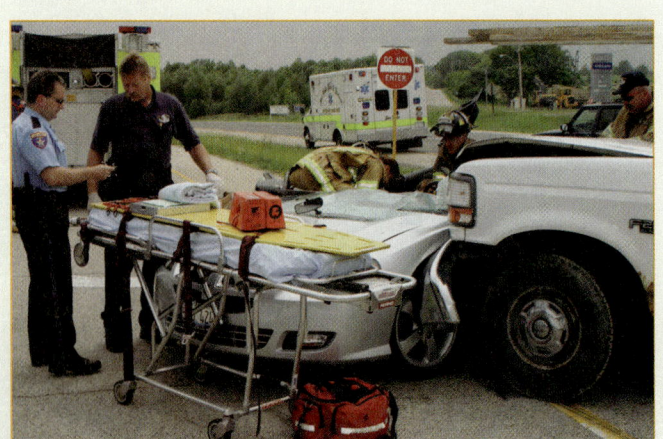

Figure 17-12 In a lateral collision, the car may be struck above its centre of gravity and begins to rock away from the side of impact. This causes a type of lateral whiplash in which the passenger's shoulders and head whip toward the intruding vehicle.

with the side of the other vehicle, the occupant nearest the impact is hit by the door of the car as the passenger compartment begins to deform and collapse. The head can strike the hood of the impacting vehicle or object. Injury results from direct trauma to the affected side and to tension developed on the far side. Older vehicles may not have safety glass on the side windows. Upper extremity trauma depends on the spatial orientation of the arm at impact. The shoulder frequently rotates outward and posteriorly, exposing the chest and ribs to injury. Forces transmitted to the chest cause rib fractures, lateral flail chest, and lung contusions. If the humerus remains between the door and chest, the clavicle may absorb side motion and fracture. As the body of the occupant is pushed in one direction, the head moves toward the impacting object, creating a line of tension along the contralateral side. This may result in ligamentous disruption and dislocation of the spine on the opposite side of the impact. The far-side occupant, if properly restrained, has the advantage of "riding down" with the car, thereby receiving considerably less force. If unrestrained, he or she may move in a direction parallel but opposite to the impact. This passenger receives forces similar to any unrestrained occupant. Furthermore, because both passengers travel in a direction parallel to impact but in opposite directions, they collide with each other, causing additional injury.

In a lateral collision, if the greater trochanter of the femur is impacted and transmits forces to the pelvis, sometimes it may be driven through the acetabulum into the pelvis. If the force reaches the ilium, the pelvis may also fracture. The typical pattern of pelvic injury that occurs in this scenario is a lateral compression injury that trauma surgeons call pelvic ring disruption. Lateral compression injuries are less serious than anterior compression injuries. Death in lateral collisions is usually the result of associated torso or head injuries.

Rear-impact collisions have the most survivors, if the driver and passengers are properly restrained **Figure 17-13 ▾** . If the vehicle coming from the rear is travelling at excessive speed, however, most bets on survivability are off. Most often in this kind of collision, a stationary (or slower moving) vehicle is struck from behind and the impact energy is transmitted as a sudden forward accelerating force. The neck hyperextends as the body moves forward relative to the head. The head does not move forward with the body unless a headrest is in the proper position; if the headrest is not in proper position, the head is snapped back and then forward. Because most seats have some degree of elasticity after the sudden forward acceleration has ended, the stored potential energy in the seat is converted to an energy of forward motion, which can aggravate the hyperextension trauma to the neck and then follow with some rebound forward flexion of the head on the chest resulting in hyperflexion. A third episode of extension may occur as the chest moves forward. This is the so-called whiplash injury.

In a rear-impact collision, energy is imparted to the front vehicle, which accelerates rapidly, while frontal impact energy to the rear driver is reduced because energy is being transferred to the front car. One concern with rear-impact collisions is the frequency with which seat backs collapse, causing unrestrained occupants to be propelled into the back seat. Head restraints developed to prevent the head and torso from moving separately are not always adjusted correctly. Many are placed too low and act as a fulcrum that may actually facilitate the extension injury. They need to be adjusted so they are behind the head and not behind the neck.

A *rotational* or *quarter-panel impact* occurs when the collision is off centre. In this case, rotation occurs as part of the car continues to move and part of the car comes to a stop. The vehicle stops at the point of impact, but the opposite side continues in rotational motion around the impact point. The point of greatest speed loss of the vehicle is the site where the greatest damage to the occupant will occur. The resultant forces act along a vector oblique to the direction of travel. For example, in a ten o'clock impact with twelve o'clock being frontal, the driver would initially move forward and then diagonally as the vehicle rotates, striking the A pillar, the support for the windshield. The front-seat passenger would strike the rearview mirror area. The point of greatest deceleration becomes the location of the most severely injured patients. Occupants tend to receive a combination of frontal and lateral injuries. Because rigid objects may be in line with vector forces, head injuries may result. Three-point belts are effective in preventing injury in angled collisions of up to 45°.

Rollover scenarios have the greatest potential to cause lethal injuries. Injuries will be serious even if seatbelts are worn. However, if your patients did not wear seatbelts, they may be ejected, and they will have been struck hard with each change in direction the car makes with the rollover. Even a restrained occupant's head and neck will change direction with each change in the vehicle's position.

Ejection of the patient from the vehicle increases the chance of death by 25 times **Figure 17-14 ▸** . One of three ejected victims will sustain a cervical-spine fracture. A partial ejection can result in an arm or leg injured by being caught between the vehicle and the ground.

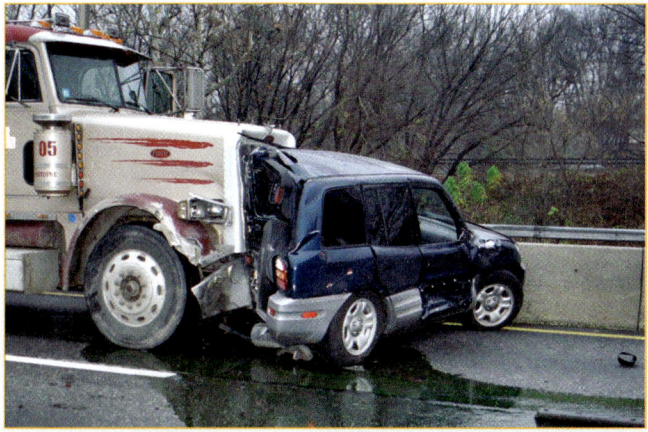

Figure 17-13 Rear-end impacts often cause whiplash-type injuries, particularly when the head and/or neck is not restrained by a headrest.

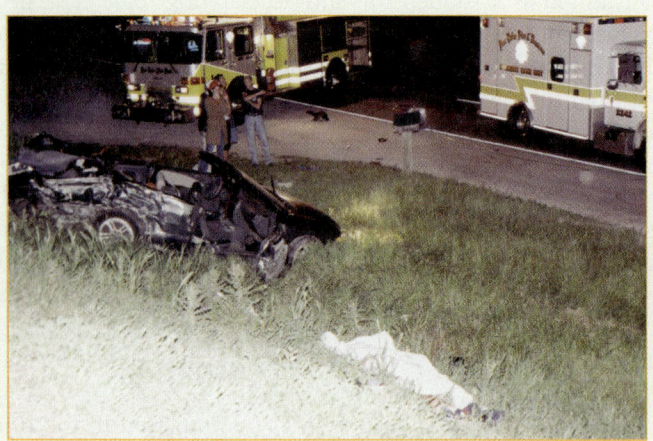

Figure 17-14 Occupants who have been ejected or partially ejected may have struck the interior of the car many times before ejection.

Restrained Versus Unrestrained Occupants

Seatbelts are highly effective because they stop the motion of any vehicle occupant who will otherwise travel at the same speed as the vehicle, until stopped. The seatbelt, although capable of delivering some injury at high speeds, will prevent the serious-to-fatal injuries of being unrestrained in the car and being ejected from the car. One of every 13 victims of ejection sustains major and permanent cervical spine damage. Restrained victims "ride down" the deceleration with belt elasticity and crush time of the car, with a nearly 45% reduction in fatalities. Restraints limit the contact of the occupants with the interior of the vehicle, prevent ejection, distribute deceleration energy over a greater surface, and prevent the occupants from violently contacting each other. As a result, all types of injuries are decreased, including head, facial, spine, thoracic, intra-abdominal, pelvic, and lower extremities, and ejection is also limited.

All arguments against seatbelt use are unfounded. Every unrestrained passenger poses a hazard to themselves and to other occupants in the vehicle, especially for front seat passengers who are at double risk for injury in a front-end collision if the back seat occupants are unrestrained.

Specific injuries associated with seatbelt use include cervical fractures due to flexion stresses and neck sprains due to deceleration and hyperextension. Most serious injuries occur because the patient did not use the seatbelt correctly. If the occupant does not use the lap strap, severe upper body injuries, including spinal injuries and decapitation, can occur. If the seatbelt is placed above the pelvic bone, abdominal injuries and lumbar spine injuries result.

Air bags were another great step up for patient safety. They have reduced deaths in direct frontal collisions by about 30%. Front air bags will not activate in side impact collisions or impacts to the front quarter panel, and without the use of a seatbelt, they are insufficient to prevent ejection. They are self-deflating and function only for a first impact, not the secondary ones. The rapidly inflating bag can also result in secondary injuries from direct

contact with the air bag or from the chemicals used to inflate it. Common injuries include abrasions and burns to the face, chest, and arms; minor corrosive toxic effects, chemical keratitis, conjunctivitis, or corneal abrasion, and inhalation injuries **Figure 17-15 ▼** .

Small children can be severely injured or killed if air bags inflate while they are in the front seat. That is why all paramedics are encouraged to participate in teaching parents how to properly place and secure children's car seats.

Unique Patient Populations

Increased morbidity and mortality, especially chest trauma, is more common in *geriatric patients,* particularly rib and sternal fractures. Fatalities also increase if *child* restraint devices are improperly installed or used. Children who have outgrown a car seat but are too small to be restrained by belts designed for adults are at risk for hyperflexion and abdominal injury.

> **Special Considerations**
>
> The different mechanisms of injury in children and the unique anatomical features of children together produce predictable patterns of injury. Because penetrating injuries are uncommon and because the head (compared with the rest of the body) is larger in childhood, injured children often have blunt injuries primarily involving the head. If the energy impact is severe and involves the entire body, the child may have a pattern involving the head, chest, abdomen, and long bones.

Pregnant women in general wear seatbelts less frequently than do nonpregnant women owing to the unproven concern that the seatbelt may increase damage to the unborn child in the case of a collision. However, no study has reported that seatbelts increase

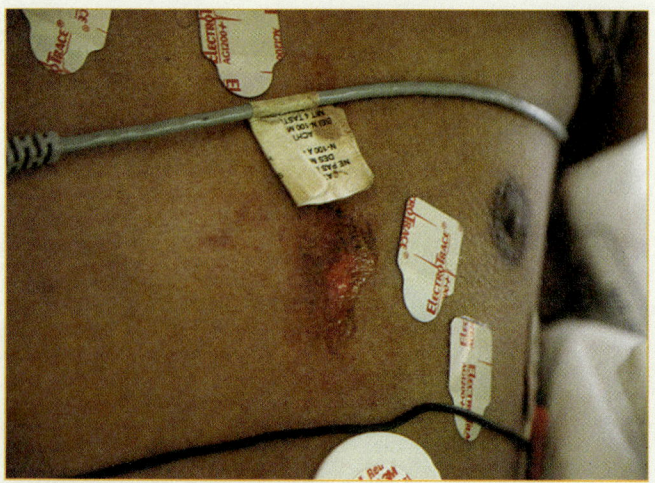

Figure 17-15 Air bags can cause abrasions to the face, chest, and arms.

fetal mortality. If lap belts are worn alone and too high, they allow enough forward flexion and subsequent compression to rupture the uterus because deceleration forces are transmitted directly to the uterus. Lap belts with shoulder harnesses are essential to provide equal distribution of forces and to prevent forward flexion of the mother. Without the shoulder harness, the protuberant uterus will also receive the impact of the steering wheel or dashboard. Steering wheel or dashboard injuries sustained because seatbelts were not worn or worn improperly are associated with a 50% fetal death rate.

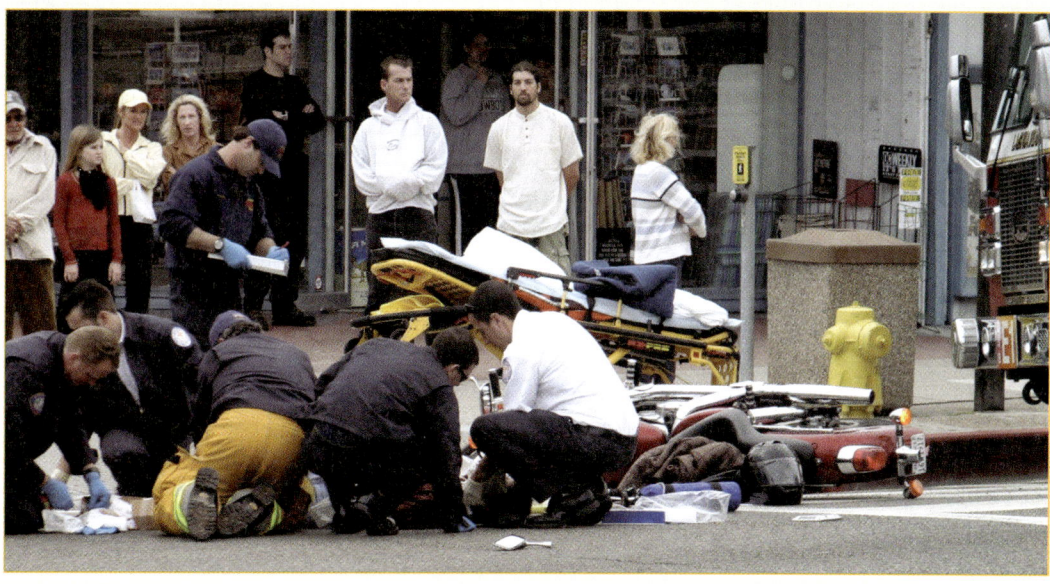

Figure 17-16 At a motorcycle collision scene, attention should be given to the deformity of the motorcycle, the side of most damage, the distance of skid in the road, the deformity of stationary objects or other vehicles, and the extent and location of deformity in the helmet.

Motorcycle Collisions

In 2003, motorcycles made up only 1 of every 51 vehicles on the road. Despite this, motorcycles still accounted for 6.4% (177) of Canada's road user fatalities in 2003. Motorcycling deaths increased significantly in the 45- to 54-year age group from 1994 to 2003 and decreased slightly in most other age groups.

In a motorcycle collision, any structural protection afforded to the victims is not derived from a steel cage, as is the case in a car, but from protective devices worn by the rider, that is, helmet, leather or abrasion-resistant clothing, and boots. While helmets are designed to protect against impact forces to the head, they transmit any impact into the cervical spine, and as such, do not protect against severe cervical injury. Leather and synthetic gear worn over the body was initially designed to protect professional riders in competition, where falls tend to be controlled and result in long sliding mechanisms on hard surfaces rather than multiple collisions against road objects and other vehicles. Leather clothing will protect mostly against road abrasion but offers no protection against blunt trauma from secondary impacts. In a street accident, collisions occur usually against other larger vehicles or stationary objects.

When you are assessing the scene of a motorcycle collision, attention should be given to the deformity of the motorcycle, the side of most damage, the distance of skid in the road, the deformity of stationary objects or other vehicles, and the extent and location of deformity in the helmet Figure 17-16 ▲ . These findings can be helpful in estimating the extent of trauma in a patient.

There are *four types of motorcycle impacts*. In a *head-on collision,* the motorcycle strikes another object and stops its

> **Special Considerations**
> Changes in vision, hearing, posture, and motor ability predispose older people to a greater risk of being struck by a vehicle.

forward motion while the rider and parts of the motorcycle that are broken off continue their forward motion until stopped by an outside force, such as drag from the road or another opposing force from a secondary collision. Because the motorcycle's centre of gravity is above the front axle, there is a forward and upward motion at the point of the collision, causing the rider to go over the handlebars. If the rider's feet remain on the pegs or pedals, the forward and upward motion of the upper torso is restrained by femurs and tibias, producing bilateral femur or tibia fractures and severe foot injuries.

For motorcycles with a low riding seat below the level of the gas tank, such as Japanese racing bikes or Italian transalpine style motorcycles, the tank can act as a wedge on the pelvis during the initial phase of the collision resulting in severe APC (anterior-posterior compression) injuries to the pelvis, often resulting in severe neurovascular compromise. Open pelvic fractures are also common, resulting in severe perineal injuries with loss of the pelvic floor. Mortality associated with open pelvic fractures approaches 50%.

In an *angular collision,* the motorcycle strikes an object or another vehicle at an angle so that the rider sustains direct crushing injuries to the lower extremity between the object and the motorcycle. This usually results in severe open and comminuted lower extremity injuries with severe neurovascular compromise, often requiring surgical amputation.

Traumatic amputations are also common high-speed injuries. After the initial crush injury to the lower extremity, mechanisms such as those described in the head-on collision also apply. Often the rider is propelled over the hood of the colliding vehicle. Because the collision is at an angle, severe thoracoabdominal torsion and lateral bending spine injuries can result, in addition to head injury and pelvic trauma.

An *ejected* rider will travel at high speed until stopped by a stationary object, another vehicle, or by road drag. Severe abrasion injuries (road rash) down to bone can occur with drag. An unpredictable combination of blunt injuries can occur from secondary collisions.

A technique used to separate the rider from the body of the motorcycle and the object to be hit is referred to as *laying the bike down*. It was developed by motorcycle racers and adapted by street bikers as a means of achieving a controlled collision. As a collision approaches, the motorcycle is turned flat and tipped sideways at 90° to the direction of travel so that one leg is dropped to the grass or asphalt. This slows the occupant faster than the motorcycle, allowing for the rider to become separated from the motorcycle. If properly protected with leather or synthetic abrasion-resistant gear, injuries should be limited to those sustained by rolling over the pavement and any secondary collision that may occur. When executed properly, this maneuver prevents the rider from being trapped between the bike and the object. However, a rider unable to clear the bike will continue into the vehicle, often with devastating results.

With any type of collision, the helmet should remain on unless airway management techniques cannot be performed with the helmet in place or the helmet does not fit snuggly to the head. Dents and abrasions must be assumed to have caused c-spine fractures until proven otherwise by an x-ray. Precautions should be taken to remove the helmet, which should be cut if it cannot be removed without introducing further deformation to the neck.

Pedestrian Injuries

In 2003, 379 pedestrians were killed and 13,340 were injured in Canada. Canadian seniors over age 65 accounted for 31.4% of pedestrian fatalities, even though they comprise only 12.8% of the population. Approximately 50% of urban pedestrian fatalities occurred at intersections. In 2003, 44 deaths were a result of bicycles being hit by a vehicle.

More than 85% of pedestrians are struck by the vehicle's front end, sustaining a predictable pattern of injuries starting with those caused by direct impact with the bumper. Adult injuries are generally lateral and posterior because adults tend to turn to the side or away from impact, whereas children will face forward into the oncoming vehicle.

There are *three predominant mechanisms of injury*. When the vehicle strikes an adult body with its bumpers, it creates lower extremity injuries, particularly to the knee and leg. These are in the form of various patterns of tibia-fibula fractures, often open knee dislocations and tibial plateau fractures. Usually the tibia is fractured on the side of impact; the impact potentially fractures the other leg as well. Knee dislocations are common with severe multiligamentous injury.

In the prehospital environment, a dislocated knee should be splinted in the position found if the patient has good distal PMS—pulse, and motor and sensory function. It is key to remember that if the knee reduces spontaneously, you must communicate this to the trauma team verbally and in your report. Spontaneous reduction is an indication of possible vascular injury that can be missed by the trauma team if you do not report the spontaneous reduction.

A *second impact* occurs as the adult is thrown on the hood and/or grille, resulting in head, pelvis, chest, and coup-contrecoup traumatic brain injuries. Lateral compression pelvic fractures are common in this mechanism and can cause open fractures with bony punctures of the vagina in women and in other viscera. A *third impact* occurs when the body strikes the ground or some other object after it has been subjected to a sudden acceleration by the colliding vehicle.

Pediatric patterns of pedestrian injury are different from patterns in adults. Small children are shorter, so the car bumper is more likely to strike them in the pelvis or torso, causing severe injuries from direct impact **Figure 17-17 ▼**. Although they are less likely than adults to fly over the hood of the car, they are more likely to be run over by the vehicle as they are propelled to the ground by the impact. Multiple extremity and pelvic fractures and abdominal and thoracic crush injuries are to be expected. Closed head trauma often kills young patients.

The <u>Waddell triad</u> refers to the pattern of vehicle–pedestrian injuries in children and people of short stature: (1) The bumper hits the pelvis and femur instead of the knees and tibias. (2) The chest and abdomen hit the grille or low on the hood of the car (sternal and rib fractures). (3) The head strikes the vehicle and then the ground (skull and facial fractures, facial abrasions, and closed head injury).

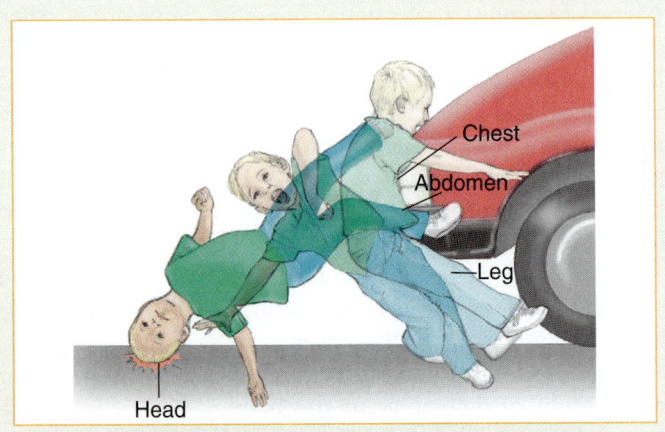

Figure 17-17 In car versus pedestrian collisions, children frequently sustain multisystem injuries involving the head, chest, abdomen, and long bones.

Falls From Heights

High falls most commonly involve children younger than 5 years of age who are left unsupervised near a high window (more than 3 m) or on a porch higher than 3 m with inadequate railings. Adult falls from heights usually occur in the context of criminal activity, attempted suicide, or intoxication such as in alcohol, narcotic, or hallucinogen use, especially PCP.

Remember that a fall produces acceleration downward at 9.8 m/sec^2. On contact with the floor or ground, an instantaneous deceleration occurs that decelerates the victim from whatever velocity had been achieved at the end of the fall to zero velocity. If a person falls for 2 seconds, the speed at impact is nearly 20 m/sec.

The severity of injuries you can expect to find in your patient will depend on a number of factors, all of which will be important in your patient assessment:

- **Height.** The height from which the patient has fallen will determine the *velocity* of the fall. A person falling one storey (3.5 m) onto concrete, for example, will fall at about 9 m/sec and experience an impact force of about 48 g. A person falling from the second storey (8 m) will reach a velocity of 14 m/sec and experience an impact force of 95 g on the same surface. Height plus stopping distance predicts the magnitude of deceleration forces. Assuming an average storey or floor is 3.5 m, a fall of four stories will kill 50% of those who fall. A fall of seven stories will kill 90% of those who fall.
- **Position.** The position or orientation of the body at the moment of impact will also be a determinant of type of injuries sustained and their survivability. Children tend to fall headfirst, owing to the relatively greater mass of a child's head, so head injuries are common in children, as are injuries to the wrists and upper extremities when the child attempts to break his fall with outstretched arms. Adults, on the other hand, usually try, when not intoxicated, to land on their feet, thus controlling their fall. However, they often tilt backward, landing on their buttocks and outstretched hands. The group of potential injuries from a vertical fall to a standing position is commonly referred to as the *Don Juan syndrome* or *lover's leap* pattern of injuries **Figure 17-18 ▶**. Injuries include foot and lower extremity fractures, along with hip, acetabular, and pelvic ring and sacral fractures. Lumbar spine axial loading also results in vertebral compression and burst fractures particularly of T12-L1 and L2. Vertical deceleration forces to organs (liver, spleen, and aorta) and fractures of the forearm and wrist (Colles' fracture) are also common.
- **Area.** The area over which the impact is distributed—the larger the area of contact at the time of impact, the greater the dissipation of the force and the lesser the peak pressures generated.
- **Surface.** The surface onto which the person has fallen and the degree to which that surface can deform (degree of plasticity) under the force of the falling body can help dissipate the forces of sudden deceleration. Deep snow, for example, has a relatively large capacity to deform, whereas concrete has scarcely any plasticity. Also, contrary to what may be expected, water also has very little plasticity at high-speed impacts. The surface of contact may also present hazards in the form of irregularities or protruding structures; it is far more dangerous to fall onto a wrought-iron picket fence, for example, than onto the grass beside it. If the surface does not conform, the unprotected body will.
- **Physical condition.** The physical condition of the patient in the form of preexisting medical conditions may also influence the injuries sustained. Most notably is the case of older patients with osteoporosis, a condition that predisposes to fractures even with minimal falls. Patients with hematologic conditions resulting in an enlarged spleen may also be more prone to a ruptured spleen in a fall. Children younger than 3 years of age have fewer injuries from falls greater than three stories than do older children and adults, most likely because of the more elastic nature of their tissues and less ossification.

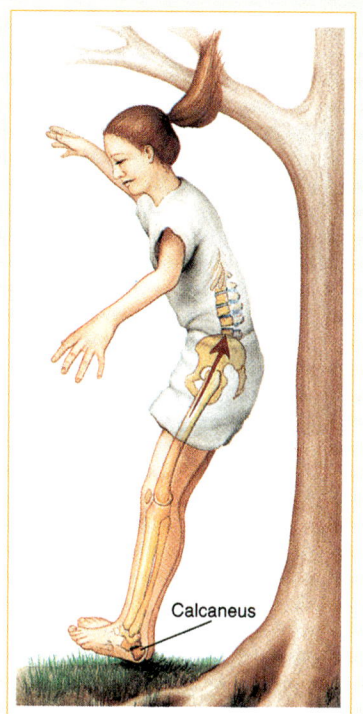

Figure 17-18 When an adult jumps or falls and lands on his or her feet, the energy is transmitted to the spine, sometimes producing a spinal injury in addition to injuries to the legs and pelvis.

Calcaneus

Penetrating Trauma

Unlike blunt trauma, which can involve a large surface area, penetrating trauma involves a disruption of the skin and underlying tissues in a small, focused area. Although a variety of objects may cause penetrating injuries in a variety of settings, penetrating trauma is usually interpreted as being more specific to injuries caused by firearms, knives, and other devices used as a means to cause intentional or accidental harm.

In Canada, the most common sources of penetrating injuries are firearms **Figure 17-19 ▶**. In 2002, 816 Canadians died from gun-related injuries. Deaths from firearms have fallen steadily from 1979 to 2002, mostly because of a decrease in gun-related suicides. In Canada, 80% of gun fatalities are suicides, 15% are homicides, and 4% are unintentional. Homicide deaths involving firearms also fell in Canada, falling from 0.8 deaths per 100,000 in the 1980s to 0.4 deaths per

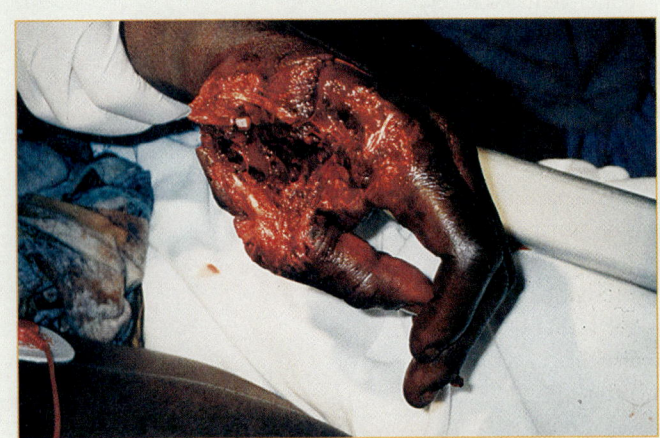

Figure 17-19 Guns are a common cause of penetrating trauma, as shown in this case.

100,000 in 2002. Guns are used in about one third of homicide cases. In 2002, death rates from gun injuries were about the same in all age groups over 15 years.

The risk of dying from a firearms-related injury is significantly higher in the United States than in Canada. In 2000, American males were three times more likely to die from a gun injury than Canadian males. American females were seven times more likely to die from a gun injury. Gun-related deaths are also much higher, per capita, in the Northern territories than in the rest of Canada.

Stab Wounds

The severity of a stab wound depends on the anatomical area involved, depth of penetration, blade length, and angle of penetration. A stab wound may also involve a cutting- or hacking-type force such as in machete wounds, which not only can result in laceration, but also can cause fractures and blunt injury to underlying soft tissues and bone and potentially amputation.

Neck wounds can involve critical anatomical structures such as the carotid arteries, subclavian vessels, apices of the lung, the upper mediastinum, trachea, esophagus, and thoracic duct. Deep neck wounds of sufficient energy can result in spinal cord involvement and cervical fracture.

Lower chest or upper abdominal wounds have the potential of involving the thoracic and abdominal cavities, depending on the location of the diaphragm at the time of injury, that is, whether the person was taking a breath or exhaling.

Be careful when documenting the location, size, and nature of stab wounds, because your records may be used in criminal proceedings. The pattern of stab wounds closely relates to the mechanism of injury. Wounds delivered to the back are generally downward, whereas stab wounds from the front are generally upward, although this may be difficult to determine from inspecting the wound externally.

Gunshot Wounds

Firearms are the primary mechanism resulting in penetrating trauma. The amount of damage a firearm can cause will depend on a number of factors, including the type of firearm (rifle, shotgun, or handgun), velocity of the projectile, physical design of the projectile, the distance to the target from the muzzle of the firearm, and the type of tissue that is struck.

There are hundreds if not thousands of firearm models and designs. However, they can be classified primarily into three types: shotguns, rifles, and handguns.

Shotguns fire round pellets (referred to as "shot"), from about half a dozen to several dozen at a time, depending on the type of load used. The load denominated 00 or 000 "buckshot" is the larger pellets, and smaller shot such as No. 7 is a common fowl hunting shot or "birdshot." At short range, even the smaller shot can cause devastating injuries. Shotgun shells can also be loaded with a single large and heavy projectile called a sabot, which can cause even worse harm. A shotgun typically has a smooth bore, and its numerous projectiles are not stabilized in flight by spin, as is the single projectile fired from a

You are the Paramedic Part 4

After the patient is placed on the backboard, you decide to load the patient into the ambulance where you reattempt splinting of injured extremities, establish vascular access, and administer a 500-ml bolus of normal saline en route to the hospital. You alert the hospital staff of the need for security personnel on your arrival to the emergency department.

Reassessment	Recording Time: 15 Minutes
Level of consciousness	V (Responsive to verbal stimuli)
Skin	Slightly moist, slightly pale, and cool
Pulse	136 beats/min
Blood pressure	160/88 mm Hg
Respirations	34 breaths/min
Sa_{O_2}	98% while breathing room air; patient noncompliant with nonrebreathing mask
ECG	Sinus tachycardia with occasional unifocal premature ventricular contractions

10. What will remain a concern throughout this call?

rifle barrel. The pellets, therefore, leave the barrel and immediately start dispersing so that the shot density (that is, the separation between any two pellets) at the time of impact on a target will be determined by the distance travelled.

At very close range (less than 10 m), a shotgun can induce destructive injuries. Entrance and exit wounds can be very large, with shotgun wadding, bits of clothing, skin, and hair driven into the wound that can cause massive contamination, leading to increased infection potential should the patient survive the initial trauma.

Rifles are firearms firing a single projectile at very high velocity through a grooved barrel that imparts a spin to the projectile that stabilizes the projectile's flight for accuracy.

Handguns are of two types: revolvers and pistols. Revolvers have a cylinder holding from 6 to 10 rounds of ammunition, and pistols have a separate magazine holding as many as 17 rounds of ammunition in some models. Handguns also have rifled barrels to impart spin to a bullet, but their accuracy is more limited than a rifle's because their barrels (and sight radius) are shorter. The ammunition handguns fire is also, in general, less powerful than ammunition fired from rifles, and handguns fire at lower velocities.

The most important factor for the seriousness of a gunshot wound is the *type of tissue* through which the projectile passes. Tissue of high elasticity like muscle, for example, is better able to tolerate stretch (temporary cavitation) than tissue of low elasticity, like the liver. A high-velocity bullet fired through a fleshy part of the leg may do much less damage than a relatively low-velocity bullet that punctures the aorta or the liver. Many bullet wounds of the extremities that are found to have caused no fracture or neurovascular compromise will be treated by the trauma team with splinting and a single dose of antibiotic without a need for wound exploration or bullet retrieval.

An entry wound is characterized by the effects of initial contact and implosion. Skin and subcutaneous tissues are pushed in, cut, or abraded externally as missile fragments pass and heat is transferred to the tissues. At close range, tattoo marks from powder burns can occur. At extremely close ranges, burns can occur from muzzle blast. Heavy wound contamination results from negative pressure generated behind the travelling projectile, which sucks surrounding elements such as clothing into the wound, greatly increasing infection potential.

Deformation and tissue destruction sustained in soft tissues and bone is based on a combination of factors, including density, compressibility, missile velocity, and missile fragmentation. The initial path of tissue destruction is caused by the projectile crushing the tissue during penetration. This creates a permanent cavity that may be a straight line or an irregular pathway as the bullet is deflected into a number of angles after initial penetration. Pathway expansion refers to the tissue displacement that occurs as the result of low-displacement shock waves (sonic pressure waves) that

travel at the speed of sound in tissue (four times the speed of sound in air). These shock waves push tissues in front of and lateral to the projectile and may not necessarily increase the wound size or cause permanent injury, but they result in cavitation (cavity formation). Tissue is compressed and accelerated away, causing injury. The waves of tissue are similar to throwing a rock into a pond. The rock creates a hole in the pond that quickly refills while waves emanate from the penetrating "wound," or hole in the pond.

Bowel, muscle, and lung are relatively elastic, resulting in fewer permanent effects of temporary cavitation. Liver, spleen, and brain are relatively inelastic, and the temporary cavity may become a permanent defect. Missile fragmentation is a major cause of tissue damage as the projectile sends off fragments that create their own separate paths through tissues. Secondary missiles can also be generated by pieces of bone, teeth, buttons, or other objects encountered in the projectile's path as it enters the body. Exit wounds occur when the projectile has sufficient energy that is not entirely dissipated along its trajectory through the body. The projectile then exits the patient and can injure other bystanders as well.

The size of the exit wound depends on the energy dissipated and the degree of cavitation at the point of exit. Exit wounds usually have irregular edges and may be larger than the entry wound **Figure 17-20 ▾**. There may be multiple exit wounds in the case of fragmentation. The number of exit wounds and the extent of tissue damage encountered must be assessed and carefully documented.

At the Scene

Don't assume that a bullet followed a straight path between the entrance and exit sites. It may ricochet inside the body, especially off bones, and travel in many different directions.

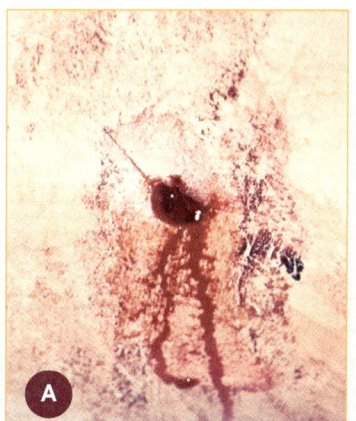 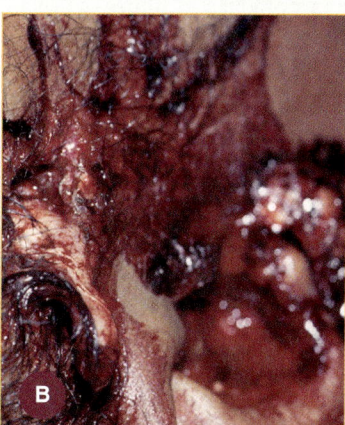

Figure 17-20 A. Entrance wound from a gunshot. **B.** Exit wound from a gunshot.

Shotgun wounds are the result of tissue impacted by numerous projectiles. As described earlier, the greater the distance from the muzzle to the target, the more dispersion the multiple projectiles will have and the more KE that will be lost before impact. Thus, shotguns are most lethal when used as short-range weapons. Also, the velocity of each pellet is less than the velocity of any bullet fired from a rifle.

Wounding potential from an injury sustained from a shotgun depends on the powder charge, the size and number of pellets, and the dispersion of the pellets. Dispersion is in turn determined by the range at which the weapon was fired, the barrel length (shorter barrels have more scatter), and the type of choke at the end of the barrel.

To give the trauma team at the hospital as much information as possible, try to obtain the following information:

- *What kind of weapon* was used (handgun, rifle, or shotgun; type and calibre, if known)?
- At *what range* was it fired?
- *What kind of bullet* was used? (Ideally, see if the police can find an unfired cartridge.)

What to look for:

- Powder residue around the wound
- Entrance and exit wounds (the exit wound is usually larger and more ragged)

In the real world, the assailant is usually gone, along with the weapon, and patient care is the first goal of paramedics, a far more pressing matter than obtaining answers to the previous questions. Be careful, again for legal reasons, when describing entry or exit wounds in your documentation. It may be better to simply describe the location(s) and/or shape(s) of wounds. Leave forensics to the experts.

Blast Injuries

Although most commonly associated with military conflict, blast injuries are also seen in civilian practice in mines, shipyards, chemical plants, and, increasingly, in association with terrorist activities. People who are injured in explosions may be injured by any of four different mechanisms (**Figure 17-21** ▶):

- **Primary blast injuries.** These are due entirely to the blast itself, that is, damage to the body caused by the pressure wave generated by the explosion.
- **Secondary blast injuries.** Damage results from being struck by flying debris, such as shrapnel from the device or from glass or splinters, that have been set in motion by the explosion. Objects are propelled by the force of the blast and strike the victim, causing injury. These objects can travel great distances and be propelled at

tremendous speeds, up to nearly 5,000 km/h for conventional military explosives.

- **Tertiary blast injuries.** These occur when the patient is hurled by the force of the explosion against a stationary object. A "blast wind" also causes the patient's body to be hurled or thrown, causing further injury. In some cases, wind injuries can amputate limbs.
- **Miscellaneous blast injuries.** These include burns from hot gases or fires started by the blast, respiratory injury from inhaling toxic gases, and crush injury from the collapse of buildings, among others.

The vast majority of patients who survive an explosion will have some combination of the four types of injury mentioned. We will confine our discussion here to primary blast injuries because they are the most easily overlooked.

The Physics of an Explosion

When a substance is detonated, a solid or liquid is chemically converted into large volumes of gas under pressure with resultant energy release. Propellants, like gunpowder, are explosives designed to release energy relatively slowly compared with high explosives (for example, trinitrotoluene), which are designed to detonate very quickly. Composition C4 can create initial pressures of more than 27.5 million kilopascals ("4 million pounds per square inch"). This generates a pressure pulse in the shape of a spherical

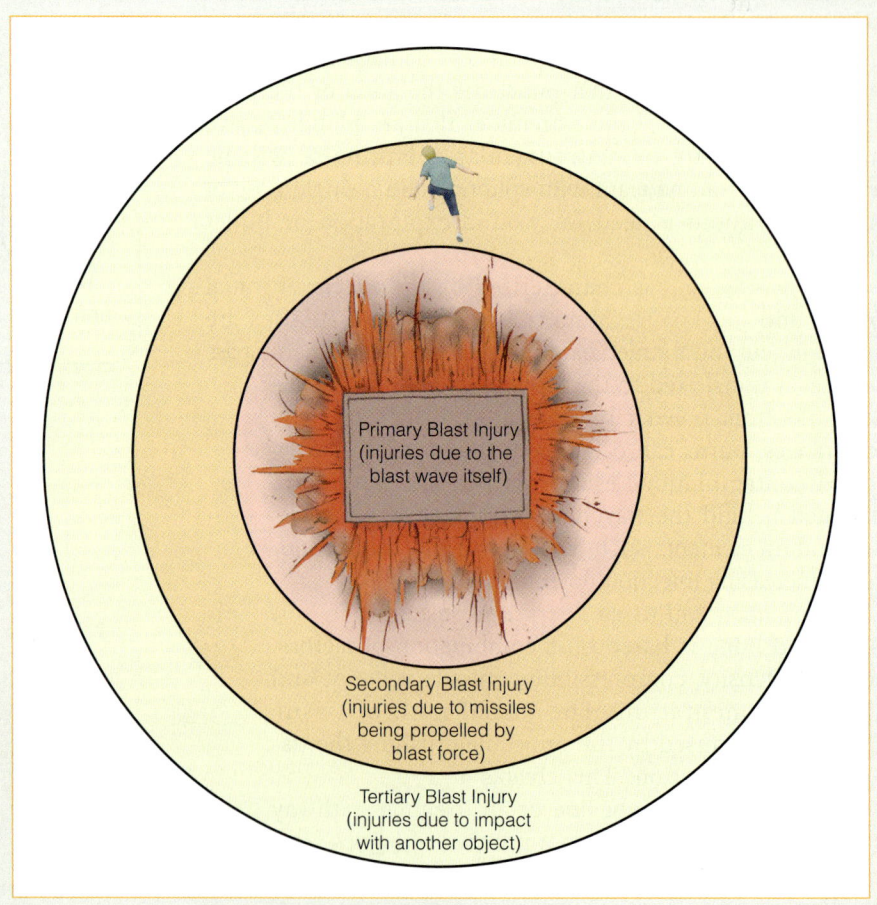

Figure 17-21 The mechanisms of blast injuries.

blast wave that expands in all directions from the point of explosion. Flying debris and high winds commonly cause conventional blunt and penetrating trauma.

Components of Blast Shock Wave

The leading edge of the shock wave is called the blast front. A positive wave pulse refers to the phase of the explosion in which there is a pressure front higher than atmospheric pressure. The peak magnitude of the wave experienced by a patient becomes lessened the farther the person is from the centre of the explosion. The increase in pressure from a blast can be so abrupt that high-explosive blast waves are also referred to as "shock waves." Shock waves possess a characteristic, brisance, that describes the shattering effect of the wave and its ability to cause disruption of tissues as well as structures. Tissue damage is dependent on the magnitude of the pressure spike and the duration of force application. The negative wave pulse refers to the phase in which pressure is less than atmospheric; it may last 10 times as long as the positive wave pulse. It occurs as air displaced by the positive wave pulse returns to fill the space of the explosion. It can lead to massive movements of air resulting in high-velocity winds.

The speed, duration, and pressure of the shock wave are affected by the following:

- The *size* of the explosive charge. The larger the explosion, the faster the shock waves and the longer they will last.
- The nature of the *surrounding medium*. Pressure waves travel much more rapidly in water, for example, and are effective at greater distances in water than in air.
- The *distance* from the explosion. The farther one is from the explosion, the slower the shock wave velocity and the longer its duration.
- The presence or absence of *reflecting surfaces*. If the pressure wave is reflected off a solid object, its pressure may be multiplied several times. For example, a shock wave that might cause minimal injury in the open can cause devastating trauma if the patient is standing beside a wall or similar solid object.

The changes in pressure produced by the shock wave are accompanied by transient *winds,* sometimes of very high velocity, that can accelerate small objects to speeds of greater than 100 metres per second (m/sec). A missile travelling at 15 m/sec can easily penetrate human skin; at 120 m/sec, a missile can enter any of the major body cavities and cause serious internal injury. Blast winds can also send the human body flying against larger, more stationary objects, or as mentioned previously, amputate limbs.

In an *underwater explosion,* a shock wave travels at greater velocity than in open air, thereby making it possible to receive injuries at three times the distance that would normally be required to receive such injuries. This is because positive pressures are higher and there are no negative pressures or high-velocity wind. Blast fragments and gases move shorter distances in water.

An explosion is significantly more damaging in *closed spaces* because of a limited dissipation environment for the forces involved and for the generation of toxic gases and smoke. The blast wave is magnified when it comes into contact with a solid surface such as a wall, causing patients near a wall to be hit with significantly higher pressure, resulting in increased risk of injury and death.

Remember the discussion of the types of tissue and the effect of trauma on tissues that contain air, water, or bone? Blast pressures cause destruction at the interface between tissues of different densities or the interface between tissues and trapped air. When the shock wave passes from a higher to lower density medium, a severe pressure disturbance develops at the interface of the denser medium. The result is fragmentation of the heavier medium, or spalling. When the shock wave contacts small gas bubbles, the bubbles are compressed and high local pressures are created, called implosion. The bubbles can then reexpand and cause further damage. *Acceleration and deceleration* of organs at their fixation points will occur in a manner similar to that in blunt trauma.

Tissues at Risk

Air-containing organs such as the middle ear, lung, and gastrointestinal tract are most susceptible to pressure changes. Junction between tissues of different densities and exposed tissues such as head and neck are prone to injury as well. The ear is the organ system most sensitive to blast injuries. The tympanic membrane evolved to detect minor changes in pressure and will rupture at pressures of 0.35 kg/cm^2 above atmospheric pressure. Thus, the tympanic membranes are a sensitive indicator of the

> **Notes from Nancy**
>
> When there is evidence of ear problems after an explosion, look for serious injury to the lungs.

possible presence of other blast injuries. The patient may complain of ringing in the ears, pain in the ears, or some loss of hearing, and blood may be visible in the ear canal. Dislocation of structural components of the ear, such as the ossicles conforming the inner ear, may occur. Permanent hearing loss is possible.

Primary pulmonary blast injuries occur as contusions and hemorrhages. When the explosion occurs in an open space, the side toward the explosion is usually injured, but the injury can be bilateral when the victim is located in a confined space. The patient may complain of tightness or pain in the chest and may cough up blood and have tachypnea or other signs of respiratory distress. Subcutaneous emphysema (crackling due to the presence of air under the skin) over the chest can be palpated, indicating air in the thorax. Pneumothorax is common and may require emergency decompression (which will be covered in the chapter on pulmonary injuries) in the prehospital environment for your patient to survive. Pulmonary edema may ensue rapidly. If there is *any* reason to suspect lung injury in a blast victim (even just the presence of a ruptured eardrum), administer oxygen. Avoid giving oxygen under positive pressure, however (that is, by demand valve) because that may simply increase the damage to the lung. Be cautious as well with intravenous fluids, which may be poorly tolerated in patients with this lung injury and result in pulmonary edema.

One of the most concerning pulmonary blast injuries is arterial air embolism, which occurs on alveolar disruption with subsequent air embolization into the pulmonary vasculature. Even small air bubbles can enter a coronary artery and cause myocardial injury. Air embolism to the cerebrovascular system can produce disturbances in vision, changes in behaviour, changes in state of consciousness, and a variety of other neurologic signs.

Notes from Nancy

If the victim of a blast injury has any neurologic abnormalities, notify medical control at once!

Solid organs are relatively protected from shock wave injury but may be injured by secondary missiles. Hollow organs, however, may be injured by similar mechanisms as for lung tissue. Perforation or rupture of the bowel and colon is a risk. Underwater explosions result in the most severe abdominal injuries.

Neurologic injuries and *head trauma* are the most common causes of death from blast injuries. Subarachnoid (beneath the arachnoid layer covering the brain) and subdural (beneath the outermost covering of the brain) hematomas are often seen. Permanent or transient neurologic deficits may be secondary to concussion, intracerebral bleeding, or air embolism. Instant but transient unconsciousness, with or without retrograde amnesia, may be initiated not only by head trauma, but also by cardiovascular problems. Bradycardia and hypotension are common after an intense pressure wave from an explosion. This is a vagal nerve–mediated form of cardiogenic shock without compensatory vasoconstriction (for example, vasovagal syncope).

Extremity injuries, including traumatic amputations, are common. Other injuries are often associated with tertiary blasts. Patients with traumatic amputation by postblast wind are likely to sustain fatal injuries secondary to the blast. In present combat, improved body armour has increased the number of survivors of blast injuries from shrapnel wounds to the torso. The number of severe orthopaedic and extremity injuries, however, has increased. In addition, while body armour may limit or prevent shrapnel from entering the body, it also "catches" more energy from the blast wave, possibly resulting in the victim being thrown backward, thus increasing potential spine and spinal cord injury.

Although blast injuries have usually been the domain of military surgeons, they often occur in industrial settings and are, unfortunately, more common today owing to the increased use of explosives as a tool for urban terrorism. Although civilian blast injuries in an industrial or mining setting used to be mostly characterized by blast injuries and burns, terrorist bombs often have shrapnel. Paramedics should be fully educated and aware of what to expect in these scenarios.

You are the Paramedic Summary

1. What initial information about the fall gives rise for concern?

The height of buildings without occupants and drug-related nature of the incident create concern about safety issues for yourself, your partner, the police, and the general public at large.

2. How does knowing your primary service area impact your understanding of potential patient injuries?

Being familiar with various aspects of your response area can aid you in understanding potential hazards or general conditions of an area. In this case, because it is a nonresidential area with buildings much higher than a typical single-family residence, you begin to wonder about the height of the fall and extent of the patient's injuries.

3. Given the location, what other conditions are you worried about?

This is a business location where the ground will be asphalt or concrete. The surface that an individual lands on implies much information about the forces placed on the body. Residential areas have more areas with grass, dirt, or gravel, which can absorb energy as a result of the impact of a fall.

4. Given commonalities of fire escape locations, what other information do you have?

If the fire escape is located in an alley, the patient can become entangled in lines or wires of various uses and can land on objects such as parked cars, dumpsters, or other people.

5. How does your patient's condition hinder your assessment techniques?

Patients under the influence of drugs can be unwilling or unable to provide reliable information about their injuries because their mentation and ability to perceive pain can be greatly diminished. When a patient not under the influence would guard an injury or self-splint a fracture, patients under the influence have lost these safety mechanisms and can fail to provide feedback that could aid you in determining the extent of their injuries.

6. How do you compensate for this hindrance?

You must rely on the information given to you by the mechanism of injury, any available witnesses, and your assessment techniques to determine the location and nature of the patient's injuries. Understanding the forces placed on the body in common traumatic injuries will aid you in treating obvious and not obvious injuries.

7. Given this information, what other injuries do you suspect?

Given the height of the fall and his position upon landing, you would also suspect lumbar spine fractures. The force of landing on pavement will travel up the heels, legs, and into pelvis and spine.

8. How can a patient who is under the influence of drugs be difficult to manage?

These patients will fail to comply with simple commands or treatment, and you may find it extremely difficult to provide necessary treatment. Depending on their reaction to the drugs, they can remove intravenous lines and otherwise fail to remain still despite obvious injuries.

9. What other medical emergencies can ensue from the use of PCP?

Depending on the amount and route of administration, PCP can result in hallucinations, paranoia, psychosis, cardiac arrhythmias, seizures, hyperthermia, kidney failure, and death. Sedation may be required, especially if the patient cannot be restrained by other means. Any patient who requires restraints must be continually monitored, particularly if chemical restraints must be used.

10. What will remain a concern throughout this call?

When dealing with a patient who is under the influence of drugs or alcohol and who exhibits combative behaviour, you must remain diligent regarding scene safety. These patients can be very unpredictable, and law enforcement personnel should accompany you in the ambulance during transport.

Prep Kit

Ready for Review

- Trauma is the primary cause of death and disability in people 1 to 45 years old.
- The amount of force and energy delivered are factors in the extent of trauma sustained. Duration and direction of the force of application are also important.
- Understanding the effects of forces and energy will help in developing a high index of suspicion for the mechanism of injury and the likely types of injuries.
- There are three categories of trauma centres accredited by the Trauma Association of Canada. Tertiary care trauma centres provide the highest level of care and are the equivalent of Level I centres as described by the American College of Surgeons. Your local EMS system may have other designations for trauma referral centres.
- Situations in which there is extended transport time by ground, mass casualties, prolonged extrication times, and critically injured patients, or when there is a long distance to an appropriate facility may warrant transporting a patient via air medical transport.
- Kinetic energy (KE) of an object is the energy associated with that object in motion. It reflects the relationship between the weight (mass) of the object and the velocity at which it is travelling.
- In a motor vehicle collision, the angle of impact, mechanical characteristics of the vehicle, and the occupant's position at the time of impact will determine types of injury.
- The law of conservation of energy states that energy can be neither created nor destroyed, it can only change form.
- Trauma in a collision is composed of five phases representing the effects of progressive deceleration: deceleration of the vehicle, deceleration of the occupant, deceleration of internal organs, secondary collisions, and additional impacts.
- There are five primary types of impacts: frontal or head on, lateral or side, rear, rotational, and rollover.
- The front seat occupants of vehicles during a frontal or head-on collision usually follow one of two trajectories, a down-and-under pathway or an up-and-over pathway.
- Protective devices such as seatbelts, air bags, and helmets are designed to manipulate the way in which energy is dissipated.
- Adult pedestrians involved in a collision experience three predominant mechanisms of injury: lower extremity injuries from the initial hit, second impact injuries from being thrown onto the hood or grille, and third impact injuries when the body strikes the ground or another object.
- The severity of injuries from falls from heights depends on the height, position, and orientation of the body at the moment of impact; the area over which the impact is distributed; the surface onto which the person falls; and the physical condition of the patient.
- The severity of a stab wound depends on the anatomical area involved, depth of penetration, blade length, and angle of penetration. Carefully document the location of stab wounds.
- Firearms are the primary mechanism resulting in penetrating trauma. The magnitude of tissue damage depends on the projectile's velocity, the orientation of the projectile as it entered the body, the distance from which the weapon was fired, the design of the projectile, and the type of tissue through which the projectile passed.
- Blast injuries include primary, secondary, tertiary, and miscellaneous injuries.

Vital Vocabulary

acceleration The rate of change in velocity.

acute respiratory distress syndrome (ARDS) A respiratory syndrome characterized by respiratory insufficiency and hypoxemia.

angle of impact The angle at which an object hits another; this characterizes the force vectors involved and has a bearing on patterns of energy dissipation.

arterial air embolism Air bubbles in the arterial blood vessels.

avulsing A tearing away or forcible separation.

barometric energy The energy that results from sudden changes in pressure as may occur in a diving accident or sudden decompression in an airplane.

biomechanics The study of the physiology and mechanics of a living organism using the tools of mechanical engineering.

blast front The leading edge of the shock wave.

blunt cardiac injury Contusion as the heart is compressed between the sternum and the spine.

blunt trauma An impact on the body by objects that cause injury without penetrating soft tissues or internal organs and cavities.

brisance The shattering effect of a shock wave and its ability to cause disruption of tissues and structures.

cavitation Cavity formation; shock waves that push tissues in front of and lateral to the projectile and may not necessarily increase the wound size or cause permanent injury but can result in cavitation.

chemical energy The energy released as a result of a chemical reaction.

deceleration A negative acceleration, that is, slowing down.

electrical energy The energy delivered in the form of high voltage.

entry wound The point at which a penetrating object enters the body.

exit wound The point at which a penetrating object leaves the body, which may or may not be in a straight line from the entry wound.

gravity The acceleration of a body by the attraction of the earth's gravitational force, normally 9.8 m/sec^2.

implosion A bursting inward.

kinetic energy The energy associated with bodies in motion, expressed mathematically as half the mass times the square of the velocity.

kinetics The study of the relationship among speed, mass, vector direction, and physical injury.

law of conservation of energy The principle that energy can be neither created nor destroyed, it can only change form.

mechanical energy The energy that results from motion (kinetic energy) or that is stored in an object (potential energy).

missile fragmentation A primary mechanism of tissue disruption from certain rifles in which pieces of the projectile break apart, allowing the pieces to create their own separate paths through tissues.

negative wave pulse The phase of an explosion in which pressure from the blast is less than atmospheric pressure.

Newton's first law of motion The principle that a body at rest will remain at rest unless acted on by an outside force.

Newton's second law of motion The principle that the force that an object can exert is the product of its mass times its acceleration.

pathway expansion The tissue displacement that occurs as a result of low-displacement shock waves that travel at the speed of sound in tissue.

penetrating trauma Injury caused by objects that pierce the surface of the body, such as knives and bullets, and damage internal tissues and organs.

permanent cavity The path of crushed tissue produced by a missile traversing part of the body.

positive wave pulse The phase of the explosion in which there is a pressure front with a pressure higher than atmospheric pressure.

potential energy The amount of energy stored in an object, the product of mass, gravity, and height, that is converted into kinetic energy and results in injury, such as from a fall.

pulmonary blast injuries Pulmonary trauma resulting from short-range exposure to the detonation of high explosives.

shearing An applied force or pressure exerted against the surface and layers of the skin as tissues slide in opposite but parallel planes.

spalling Delaminating or breaking off into chips and pieces.

trauma Acute physiologic and structural change that occurs in a victim as a result of the rapid dissipation of energy delivered by an external force.

tympanic membrane The eardrum; a thin, semitransparent membrane in the middle ear that transmits sound vibrations to the internal ear by means of the auditory ossicles.

velocity The speed of an object in a given direction.

Waddell triad A pattern of vehicle–pedestrian injuries in children and people of short stature in which (1) the bumper hits pelvis and femur, (2) the chest and abdomen hit the grille or low hood, and (3) the head strikes the ground.

whiplash An injury to the cervical vertebrae or their supporting ligaments and muscles, usually resulting from sudden acceleration or deceleration.

■ Points to Ponder

You and your partner are dispatched as a second paramedic unit to assist in a two-car motor vehicle collision. You arrive on scene and are directed to a vehicle approximately 100 metres from the initial impact. Witnesses state that this vehicle was struck on the passenger side at a high rate of speed and slid out of control through a metal fence and the driver's side is now resting against a large tree. You are told that the other vehicle involved in the collision drove through a red light, driving approximately 80 km/h. The passenger side has an intrusion of more than 60 cm. There are two women inside the van. They are conscious, alert, and orientated and very upset, crying hysterically. The fire department is extricating the patients from the vehicle.

What is the mechanism(s) of injury to the vehicle? What type of injuries would you suspect the patients may have? What are major concerns and thoughts you must have during your assessment and treatment of these trauma patients? What level trauma hospital would you take these patients to?

Issues: Understanding Kinematics of Trauma, Predicting Injury Patterns, Examining the Scene and Patients, Knowledge of Trauma Centre Levels.

Assessment in Action

You are dispatched for a single motor vehicle collision and encounter a wet, slippery road. The driver of the vehicle is slumped in the driver compartment. Witnesses tell you that she was driving and then suddenly lost control of her vehicle, struck a mail box, and then drove head on into a telephone pole.

1. **What is Newton's first law of motion?**
   A. The force that an object can exert is the product of its mass times its acceleration.
   B. A body at rest will remain at rest and a body in motion will remain in motion unless acted on by an outside force.
   C. Energy cannot be created or destroyed but can be changed in form.
   D. Kinetic energy is a function of an object's weight and speed.

2. **Trauma in a collision is composed of how many phases, which represent the effects of progressive deceleration?**
   A. 2
   B. 3
   C. 4
   D. 5

3. **A patient's ability to dissipate the energy determines the pattern of injury.**
   A. True
   B. False

4. **What type of impact would you suspect in the preceding scenario?**
   A. Lateral
   B. Rear
   C. Frontal
   D. Rotational

5. **Injuries are generally categorized as:**
   A. head and spinal trauma.
   B. extremity and body trauma.
   C. blunt and penetrating trauma.
   D. closed and open trauma.

6. **The role of air bags is to:**
   A. cushion forward movement of the occupant.
   B. protect the occupant from ejection.
   C. accelerate the occupant away from the point of impact.
   D. block the occupant's view of the impact.

Challenging Questions

You are dispatched to a woman who has fallen. On arrival, you find a 38-year-old woman supine on the ground. Initially, she is responsive to deep painful stimuli.

7. **The severity of injuries will depend on a number of factors that will be important in assessing the patient. List these factors.**

18 Bleeding and Shock

Competency Areas

Area 4: Assessment and Diagnostics

4.3.a   Conduct primary patient assessment and interpret findings.

4.3.b   Conduct secondary patient assessment and interpret findings.

4.3.c   Conduct cardiovascular system assessment and interpret findings.

4.3.d   Conduct neurological system assessment and interpret findings.

4.3.e   Conduct respiratory system assessment and interpret findings.

4.3.f   Conduct obstetrical assessment and interpret findings.

4.3.g   Conduct gastrointestinal system assessment and interpret findings.

4.3.h   Conduct genitourinary system assessment and interpret findings.

4.3.i   Conduct integumentary system assessment and interpret findings.

4.3.j   Conduct musculoskeletal assessment and interpret findings.

4.3.k   Conduct assessment of the immune system and interpret findings.

4.3.l   Conduct assessment of the endocrine system and interpret findings.

4.3.m   Conduct assessment of the ears, eyes, nose, and throat and interpret findings.

4.3.n   Conduct multisystem assessment and interpret findings.

4.4.a   Assess pulse.

4.4.b   Assess respiration.

4.4.c   Conduct non-invasive temperature monitoring.

4.4.d   Measure blood pressure by auscultation.

4.4.e   Measure blood pressure by palpation.

4.4.f   Measure blood pressure with non-invasive blood pressure monitor.

4.4.g   Assess skin condition.

4.4.h   Assess pupils.

4.4.i   Assess level of mentation.

4.5.a   Conduct oximetry testing and interpret findings.

4.5.b   Conduct end-tidal carbon dioxide monitoring and interpret findings.

4.5.c   Conduct glucometric testing and interpret findings.

4.5.d   Conduct peripheral venipuncture.

4.5.e   Obtain arterial blood samples via radial artery puncture.

4.5.f   Obtain arterial blood samples via arterial line access.

4.5.g   Conduct invasive core temperature monitoring and interpret findings.

4.5.h   Conduct pulmonary artery catheter monitoring and interpret findings.

4.5.i   Conduct central venous pressure monitoring and interpret findings.

4.5.j   Conduct arterial line monitoring and interpret findings.

4.5.k   Interpret laboratory and radiological data.

4.5.l   Conduct 3-lead electrocardiogram (ECG) and interpret findings.

4.5.m   Obtain 12-lead electrocardiogram and interpret findings.

Appendix 4: Pathophysiology

J.   **Multisystem Diseases and Injuries**
Shock Syndromes: Anaphylactic
Shock Syndromes: Cardiogenic
Shock Syndromes: Hypovolemic
Shock Syndromes: Neurogenic
Shock Syndromes: Obstructive
Shock Syndromes: Septic

Introduction

After managing the airway, recognizing bleeding and understanding how it affects the body are perhaps the most important skills you will learn as a paramedic. Any kind of bleeding is potentially dangerous because it may eventually lead to shock. Uncontrolled bleeding may lead to serious injury and, ultimately, death.

Bleeding is also the most common cause of shock. As used in this chapter, shock describes a state of collapse and failure of the cardiovascular system. Shock is actually a normal compensatory mechanism used by the body to maintain systolic blood pressure (BP) and brain perfusion during times of distress. This response can accompany a broad spectrum of events, ranging from trauma to heart attacks to allergic reactions. If not treated promptly, shock will injure the body's vital organs and ultimately lead to death. Your early and rapid actions can help significantly reduce the morbidity and mortality rates from bleeding and shock.

Anatomy and Physiology of the Cardiovascular System

The cardiovascular system is designed to carry out one crucial job: keep blood flowing via the lungs to the peripheral tissues. In the lungs, blood dumps the gaseous waste products of metabolism—chiefly carbon dioxide—and picks up life-sustaining oxygen. In the peripheral tissues, the process is reversed: Blood unloads oxygen and picks up wastes. If blood flow were to stop or slow significantly, the results would be catastrophic. Oxygen delivery to the heart, brain, and other vital organs would be disrupted. For a few minutes, the cells could switch to an emergency metabolic system—one that does not require oxygen (anaerobic metabolism), but that form of metabolism produces even more acids and toxic wastes. The cells of the organs of the body would have nowhere to eliminate their wastes and would rapidly be affected by the toxic by-products of their own metabolism.

To keep the blood moving continuously through the body, the circulatory system requires three intact components **Figure 18-1** ▶ :

- A functioning pump: the heart
- Adequate fluid volume: the blood and body fluids
- An intact system of tubing capable of reflex adjustments (constriction and dilation) in response to changes in pump output and fluid volume: the blood vessels

All three components must interact effectively to maintain life. If any one becomes damaged or is deficient, the whole system is in jeopardy.

Structures of the Heart

The heart is a muscular, cone-shaped organ whose function is to pump blood throughout the body. Located behind the sternum, the heart is about the size of a closed fist, weighing 280 to 350 g

You are the Paramedic Part 1

You and your partner have just finished dinner on what has been a quiet night shift. Suddenly, chatter erupts on the police scanner and you are called to a shooting at a local gas station/minimarket. The dispatcher alerts you that police on the scene are requesting "a rush on the bus."

As you park in front of the store, you notice a crowd gathering on the sidewalk. Police officers are establishing a perimeter. You grab your initial assessment bag and head inside as your partner pulls out the stretcher with the help of a police officer.

As you enter the store, a detective informs you, "There was a robbery; the clerk was shot and the perpetrator has left the scene." You observe a 22-year-old man sitting on the floor behind the counter and leaning against the wall. He is holding his left upper quadrant with his bloody hand. The patient appears to weigh about 80 kg. Although he is conscious, alert, and in obvious pain, he tells you that the shooting occurred just as the clock struck 23:00. It is now 23:10, and you hit the elapsed time counter on your digital watch as you don your personal protective equipment (PPE). As you begin to talk to the patient, you reach down to palpate his radial pulse but cannot feel it.

Initial Assessment	Recording Time: 0 Minutes
Appearance	Awake and anxious
Level of consciousness	A (Alert to person, place, and day)
Airway	Open and clear
Breathing	Rapid, shallow, and laboured
Circulation	Unpalpable radial pulse

1. Does the lack of significant visible bleeding and the fact that he is alert indicate that this patient is not bleeding seriously?
2. What is the significance of time in this type of incident?

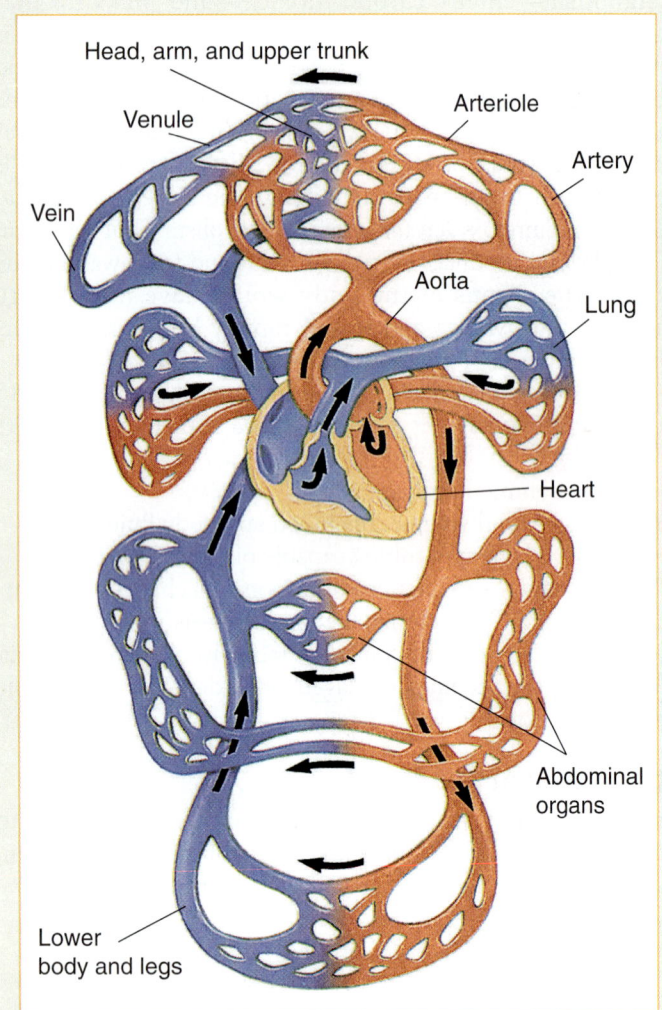

Figure 18-1 The circulatory system requires continuous operation of its three components: the heart, the blood and body fluids, and the blood vessels.

Labels in figure: Head, arm, and upper trunk; Venule; Arteriole; Vein; Artery; Aorta; Lung; Heart; Abdominal organs; Lower body and legs

atrium (Figure 18-2 ▸). Blood from the upper part of the body returns to the heart through the superior vena cava; blood from the lower part of the body returns through the inferior vena cava (the larger of the two veins). From the right atrium, blood passes through the tricuspid valve into the right ventricle. The right ventricle then pumps the blood through the pulmonic valve into the pulmonary artery and then to the lungs.

In the lungs, oxygen is returned to the blood and carbon dioxide and other waste products are removed from it. The freshly oxygenated blood returns to the left atrium through the pulmonary veins. Blood then flows through the mitral valve into the left ventricle, which pumps the oxygenated blood through the aortic valve, into the aorta (the body's largest artery), and then to the entire body.

The Cardiac Cycle

The cardiac cycle is the repetitive pumping process that begins with the onset of cardiac muscle contraction and ends with the beginning of the next contraction. Myocardial contraction results in pressure changes within the cardiac chambers, causing the blood to move from areas of high pressure to areas of low pressure. The valves ensure that blood is pumped in a forward direction.

The pressure in the aorta against which the left ventricle must pump blood is called the afterload. The greater the afterload, the harder it is for the ventricle to eject blood into the aorta. A higher afterload, therefore, reduces the stroke volume, or the amount of blood ejected per contraction.

The amount of blood pumped through the circulatory system in 1 minute is referred to as the cardiac output (CO). CO is expressed in litres per minute (l/min). The cardiac output equals the pulse rate multiplied by the stroke volume:

Cardiac Output = Stroke Volume × Pulse Rate

in men and 225 to 280 g in women. Roughly two thirds of the heart lies in the left part of the mediastinum, the area between the lungs that also contains the great vessels.

The human heart consists of four chambers: two atria (upper chambers) and two ventricles (lower chambers). Each atrium receives blood that is returned to the heart from other parts of the body; each ventricle pumps blood out of the heart. The upper and lower portions of the heart are separated by the atrioventricular valves, which prevent backward flow of blood. The semilunar valves, which serve a similar function, are located between the ventricles and the arteries into which they pump blood.

Blood Flow Within the Heart

Two large veins, the superior vena cava and the inferior vena cava, return deoxygenated blood from the body to the right

Factors that influence the pulse rate, the stroke volume, or both will affect CO and, therefore, oxygen delivery (perfusion) to the tissues.

Increased venous return to the heart stretches the ventricles somewhat, resulting in increased cardiac contractility. This relationship, which was first described by the British physiologist Ernest Henry Starling, is known as the Starling law of the heart. Starling noted that if a muscle is stretched slightly before it is stimulated to contract, it would contract with greater force. Thus, if the heart is stretched, the muscle contracts more forcefully.

Although the amount of blood returning to the right atrium varies somewhat from minute to minute, a normal heart continues to pump the same percentage of blood returned, a measure called the ejection fraction. If more blood returns to the heart, the stretched heart pumps harder rather than allowing the blood to back up into the veins. As a result, more blood

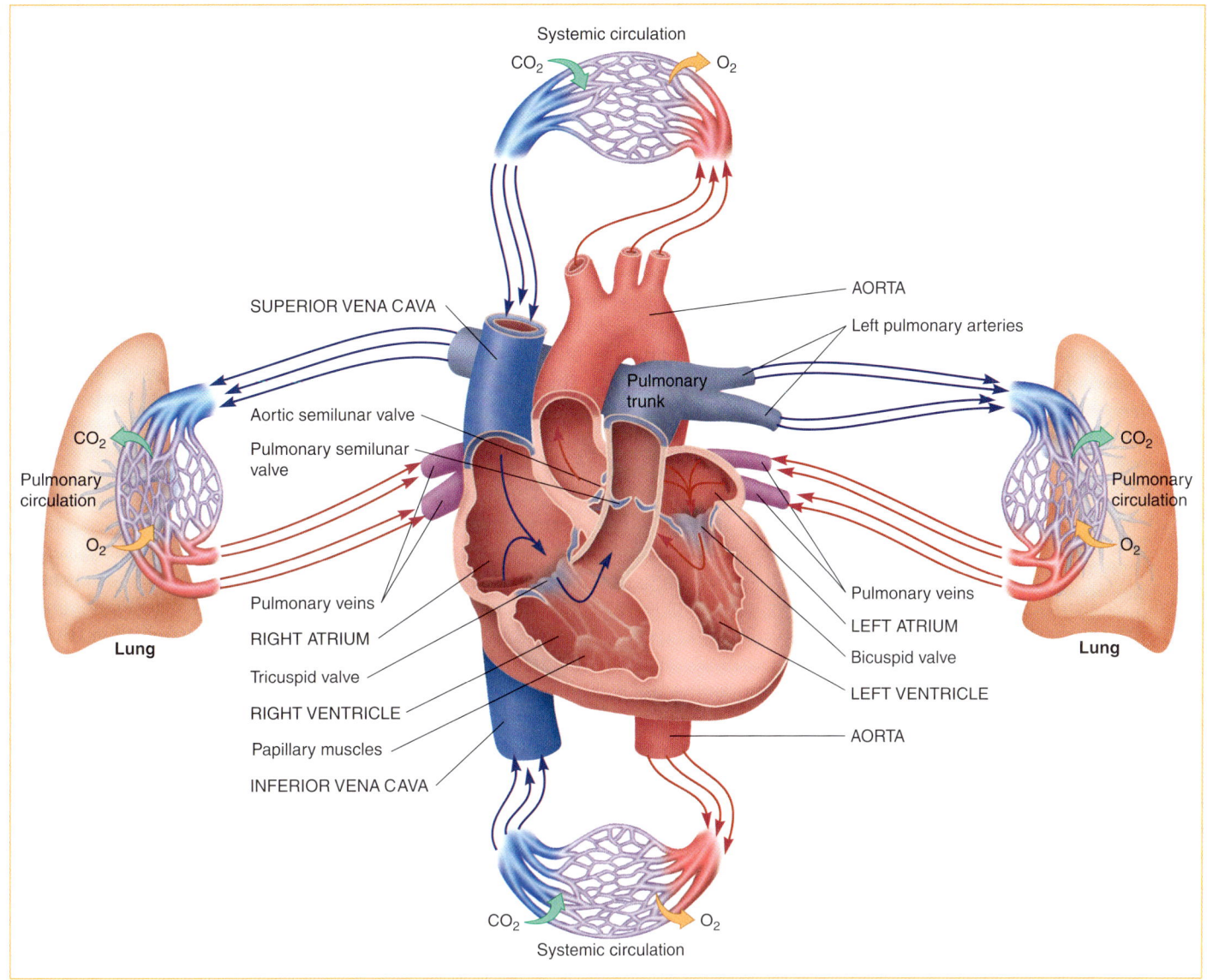

Figure 18-2 Circulation begins in the heart muscle.

is pumped with each contraction, yet the ejection fraction remains unchanged: The amount of blood that is pumped increases, but so does the amount of blood returned. This relationship maintains normal cardiac function when a person changes positions, coughs, breathes, or moves.

Blood and Its Components

Blood consists of plasma and formed elements or cells that are suspended in the plasma. These cells include red blood cells (RBCs), white blood cells (WBCs), and platelets. The purpose of blood is to carry oxygen and nutrients to the tissues and cellular waste products away from the tissues. In addition, the formed elements serve as the mainstay of numerous other body functions, such as fighting infections and controlling bleeding.

Plasma is a watery, straw-coloured fluid that accounts for more than half of the total blood volume. It consists of 92% water and 8% dissolved substances such as chemicals, minerals, and nutrients. Water enters the plasma from the digestive tract, from fluids between cells, and as a by-product of metabolism.

The disk-shaped RBCs (erythrocytes) are the most numerous of the formed elements. Erythrocytes are unable to move on their own; instead, the flowing plasma passively propels them to their destinations. RBCs contain hemoglobin, a protein that gives them their reddish colour. Hemoglobin binds oxygen that is absorbed in the lungs and transports it to the tissues where it is needed.

Several types of WBCs (leukocytes) exist, each of which has a different function. The primary function of all WBCs is to fight infection. Antibodies to fight infection may be produced, or leukocytes may directly attack and kill bacterial invaders.

Platelets are small cells in the blood that are essential for clot formation. The blood clotting (coagulation) process is a complex series of events involving platelets, clotting proteins in the plasma (clotting factors), other proteins, and calcium. During coagulation, platelets aggregate in a clump and form much of the foundation of a blood clot. Clotting proteins produced by the liver solidify the remainder of the clot, which eventually includes red and white blood cells.

Blood Circulation and Perfusion

Arteries are blood vessels that carry blood away from the heart. Veins are blood vessels that transport blood back to the heart. As arteries get farther from the heart, they become smaller. Eventually, they branch into many small arterioles, which themselves divide into even smaller capillaries (microscopic, thin-walled blood vessels). Oxygen and nutrients pass out of the capillaries and into the cells, and carbon dioxide and waste products pass from the cells and into the capillaries by a process called diffusion. To return deoxygenated blood to the heart, groups of capillaries gradually enlarge to form venules. Venules then merge together, forming larger veins that eventually empty into the heart, via the superior and inferior vena cavae.

Perfusion is the circulation of blood within an organ or tissue in adequate amounts to meet the cells' current needs for oxygen, nutrients, and waste removal. Blood must pass through the cardiovascular system at a speed that is fast enough to maintain adequate circulation throughout the body, yet slow enough to allow each cell time to exchange oxygen

and nutrients for carbon dioxide and other waste products. Although some tissues, such as the lungs and kidneys, never rest and require a constant blood supply, most tissues require circulating blood only intermittently, but especially when they are active. Muscles, for example, are at rest and require a minimal blood supply when you sleep. In contrast, during exercise, muscles need a large blood supply. As another example, the gastrointestinal (GI) tract requires a high flow of blood after a meal. After digestion is completed, it can do quite well with a small fraction of that flow.

The autonomic nervous system monitors the body's needs from moment to moment, adjusting the blood flow as required. During emergencies, it automatically redirects blood away from other organs and toward the heart, brain, lungs, and kidneys. Thus, the cardiovascular system is dynamic, constantly adapting to changing conditions. Sometimes, however, it fails to provide sufficient circulation for every body part to perform its function, resulting in hypoperfusion or shock.

The heart requires constant perfusion, or it will not function properly. The brain and spinal cord cannot go for more than 4 to 6 minutes without perfusion, or the nerve cells will be permanently damaged—recall that cells of the central nervous system do not have the capacity to regenerate. The kidneys will be permanently damaged after 45 minutes of inadequate perfusion. Skeletal muscles cannot tolerate more than 2 hours of inadequate perfusion. The GI tract can exist with limited (but not absent) perfusion for several hours. These times are based on a normal body temperature (37.0°C). An organ or tissue that is considerably colder is better able to resist damage from hypoperfusion because of the slowing of the body's metabolism.

You are the Paramedic Part 2

Additional help arrives on the scene as you complete your initial assessment. Your partner has brought in the stretcher and is beginning to administer supplemental oxygen via a nonrebreathing mask at 15 l/min. Police inform you that the robber's weapon may have been a "sawed-off shotgun" that was fired at a fairly close range. The patient tells you a single shot was fired after he told the robber that he would not open the safe.

You give the patient some gauze and tell him to hold it firmly against the wound. When you complete your initial assessment of the patient, you decide to perform the rapid physical examination in the back of the ambulance and the SAMPLE history as you have time, given the higher priorities and need for rapid transport.

Initial Assessment	Recording Time: 3 Minutes
Breathing	Rapid, laboured, but no obstructions to breathing process (flail segment, punctures, or impaled objects). Oxygen has been started.
Circulation	A rapid, weak carotid pulse can be felt, the external bleeding is easily controlled with direct pressure and gauze. The skin is pale, cool, and moist.

3. On the basis of the information you have so far, and remembering that the patient weighs approximately 80 kg, how much blood did he have before the incident? How much could he have lost so far?

4. What phase or stage of shock is this patient in?

5. Which BLS and ALS interventions would be most appropriate for this patient at this time? Should you insert an intravenous (IV) line at the scene?

▌ Pathophysiology of Hemorrhage

Hemorrhage simply means bleeding. Bleeding can range from a "nick" to a capillary while shaving, to a severely spurting artery from a deep slash with a knife, to a ruptured spleen from striking the steering column during a car collision. External bleeding (visible hemorrhage) can usually be easily controlled by using direct pressure or a pressure bandage. Internal bleeding (hemorrhage that is not visible) is usually not controlled until a surgeon locates the source and sutures it closed. Because internal bleeding is not as obvious, you must rely on signs and symptoms to determine the extent and severity of the hemorrhage.

External Hemorrhage

External bleeding is usually due to a break in the skin. Its extent or severity is often a function of the type of wound and the types of blood vessels that have been injured. (Wound types are discussed in detail in Chapter 19.) Bleeding from a capillary usually oozes, bleeding from a vein flows, and bleeding from an artery spurts.

These descriptions are not infallible. For example, considerable oozing from capillaries is possible when a patient gets a very large abrasion (such as the road rash when a cyclist slides along the pavement without protective clothing). Likewise, varicose veins on the leg can produce copious bleeding.

Arteries may spurt initially, but as the patient's BP decreases, often the blood simply flows. In addition, an artery that is incised directly across or in a transverse manner will often recoil and attempt to slow its own bleeding. By contrast, if the artery is cut on a bias, it does not recoil and continues to bleed.

Some injuries that you might expect to be accompanied by considerable external bleeding do not always have serious hemorrhaging. For example, a person who falls off the platform at the train station and is run over by a train may have amputations of one or more extremities, yet experience little bleeding because the wound was cauterized by the heat of the train's wheels on the rail. Conversely, a person who pulled over on the shoulder of the road and was removing the jack from his car's trunk when another motorist slammed into the rear of the car, pinning him between the two vehicles, may have severely crushed legs. In such a case, bleeding may be severe, with the only effective means of bleeding control being two tourniquets.

Internal Hemorrhage

Internal bleeding as a result of trauma may appear in any portion of the body. A fracture of a small bone (such as humerus, ankle, or tibia) produces a somewhat controlled environment in which a relatively small amount of bleeding can occur. By contrast, bleeding into the trunk (that is, thorax, abdomen, or pelvis), because of its much larger space, tends to be severe and uncontrolled. Nontraumatic internal hemorrhage usually occurs in cases of GI bleeding from the upper or lower GI tract, ruptured ectopic pregnancies, ruptured aneurysms, or other conditions.

Any internal bleeding must be treated promptly. The signs of internal hemorrhage (such as hematoma) do not always develop quickly, so you must rely on other signs and symptoms and an evaluation of the mechanism of injury (MOI) to make this diagnosis. Pay close attention to patient complaints of pain or tenderness, development of tachycardia, and pallor. In addition to evaluating the MOI, be alert for the development of shock when you suspect internal bleeding.

Management of a patient with internal hemorrhaging focuses on the treatment of shock, minimizing movement of the injured or bleeding part or region, and rapid transport. The patient will likely need a surgical procedure to stop the bleeding. In recent years, ultrasound has been used to locate bleeding in the emergency department (ED) before moving the patient to the surgical suite for the ultimate resolution of the problem.

Controlled Versus Uncontrolled Hemorrhage

Bleeding that you can control (such as external bleeding that responds to a pressure bandage) and bleeding that you cannot control (such as a bleeding peptic ulcer) are serious emergencies. As a consequence, the initial assessment of the patient includes a search for life-threatening bleeding. If found, the hemorrhage must be controlled; if the hemorrhage cannot be controlled in the prehospital environment, all of your efforts should concentrate on attempting to control the bleeding as you rapidly transport the patient to the ED.

Most external bleeding can be managed with direct pressure, although arterial bleeding may take 5 or more minutes of direct pressure to form a clot. Military experience has shown that the use of pressure points is not as effective as previously thought and is difficult to manage while trying to rapidly evacuate a person from the battlefield. For this reason, most military medical training calls for use of a tourniquet for external bleeding to an extremity that cannot be controlled with direct pressure and a pressure bandage.

Because most cases of internal bleeding are rarely fully controlled in the prehospital setting, a patient with this type of injury needs rapid transport to the ED. Some strategies may be effective in the prehospital environment depending on the cause of the bleeding. For example, the external circumferential pressure of the pneumatic antishock garment/military antishock trousers (PASG/MAST) may help control the massive bleeding that accompanies a pelvic fracture. The paramedic should consult their local or regional protocols regarding use of binders or PASG/MAST.

The Significance of Bleeding

When patients have serious external hemorrhage, it is often difficult to determine the amount of blood loss. Blood looks different on different surfaces, such as when it is absorbed in clothing versus when it has been diluted by being mixed in water. Although you should attempt to determine the amount of external blood loss, the patient's presentation and your assessment will ultimately direct your prehospital care and treatment plan.

Human adult male bodies contain approximately 70 ml of blood per kilogram of body weight, whereas adult female bodies contain approximately 65 ml/kg. The body cannot tolerate an acute blood loss of more than 20% of this total blood volume. If the typical adult loses more than 1 l of blood, significant changes in vital signs will occur, including increasing heart and respiratory rates and decreasing BP. An isolated femur fracture, for example, can easily result in the loss of 1 l or more of blood in the soft tissues of the thigh.

Because infants and children have less blood volume than their adult counterparts, they may experience the same effect with smaller amounts of blood loss. For example, a 1-year-old child has a total blood volume of about 800 ml, so significant symptoms of blood loss may occur after only 100 to 200 ml of blood loss. To put this in perspective, remember that a soft drink can holds roughly 345 ml of liquid **Figure 18-3**.

How well people compensate for blood loss is related to how rapidly they bleed. A healthy adult can comfortably donate one unit (500 ml) of blood in a period of 15 to 20 minutes without having ill effects from this decrease in blood volume. If a similar blood loss occurs in a much shorter period, hypovolemic shock, a condition in which low blood volume results in inadequate perfusion and even death, may rapidly develop.

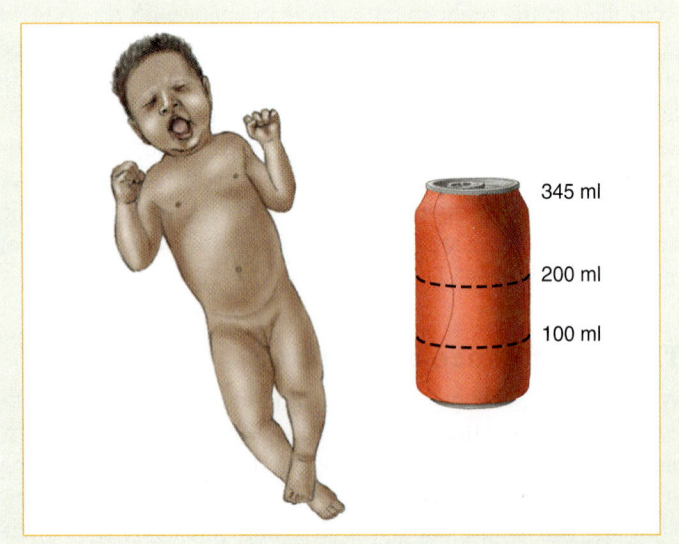

345 ml
200 ml
100 ml

Figure 18-3 A soft drink can holds roughly 345 ml of liquid.

Consider bleeding to be serious if any of the following conditions are present:

- A significant MOI, especially when the MOI suggests that severe forces affected the abdomen or chest
- Poor general appearance of the patient
- Signs and symptoms of shock
- Significant amount of blood loss
- Rapid blood loss
- Uncontrollable bleeding

Physiologic Response to Hemorrhage

Typically, bleeding from an open artery is bright red (because of the high oxygen content) and spurts in time with the pulse. The pressure that causes the blood to spurt also makes this type of bleeding difficult to control. As the amount of blood circulating in the body drops, so does the patient's BP and, eventually, the arterial spurting diminishes.

Blood from an open vein is much darker (low oxygen content) and flows steadily. Because it is under less pressure, most venous blood does not spurt and is easier to manage. Bleeding from damaged capillary vessels is dark red and oozes from a wound steadily but slowly. Venous and capillary bleeding is more likely to clot spontaneously than arterial bleeding.

On its own, bleeding tends to stop rather quickly, within about 10 minutes, in response to internal clotting mechanisms and exposure to air. When vessels are lacerated, blood flows rapidly from the open vessel. The open ends of the vessel then begin to narrow (vasoconstrict), which reduces the amount of bleeding. Platelets aggregate at the site, plugging the hole and sealing the injured portions of the vessel, a process called hemostasis. Bleeding will not stop if a clot does not form. Direct contact with body tissues and fluids or the external environment commonly triggers the blood's clotting factors.

Despite the efficiency of this system, it may fail in certain situations. A number of medications, including anticoagulants such as aspirin and prescription blood thinners, interfere with normal clotting. With a severe injury, the damage to the vessel may be so extensive that a clot cannot completely block the hole. Sometimes, only part of the vessel wall is cut, preventing it from constricting. In these cases, bleeding will continue unless it is stopped by external means. In a case involving acute blood loss, the patient might die before the body's hemostatic defences of vasoconstriction and of clotting can help.

Assessment of a Bleeding Patient

The assessment of any patient begins with a good scene assessment and proceeds to your general impression and initial assessment. Once the scene is deemed safe to enter, you will need to don the appropriate level of personal protective equipment (PPE). Depending on the severity of bleeding and your initial diagnosis, this will entail gloves, mask, eyeshield, and, when the patient is very bloody or blood is spurting, a gown **Figure 18-4**.

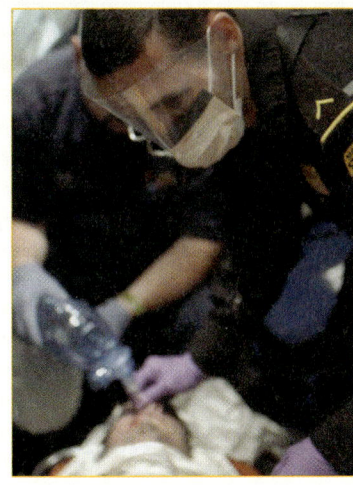

Figure 18-4 Depending on the severity of bleeding and your initial diagnosis, PPE will entail gloves, mask, eyeshield, and, in some cases, a gown.

During the initial assessment, after determining the patient's mental status with AVPU, you must locate and manage immediate threats to life involving the airway, breathing, and circulation. Ensure that the patient has a patent airway. If you observe bleeding from the mouth or facial areas, keep the suction unit within reach.

If the patient has minor external bleeding, you can note it and move on with the initial assessment; management of this problem can wait until the patient has been properly assessed and prioritized. Do not get sidetracked by applying dressings and bandages to a patient who has much more serious problems. If major external bleeding is present, you should deal with it during the initial assessment. If you suspect internal bleeding, begin management by keeping the patient warm and administering supplemental oxygen by a nonrebreathing mask at 15 l/min.

At the Scene

When you are dealing with a bleeding patient, be sure to take necessary precautions to protect yourself from splashing or splattering. Wear appropriate PPE, including gloves, gown, mask, and eye protection. This is especially essential when arterial bleeding is present. Also remember that frequent, thorough handwashing between patients and after every call is a simple yet important protective measure.

Carefully assess the MOI in trauma patients because it may be your best indicator that the patient has sustained an internal injury and may be bleeding. **Table 18-1 ▶** lists some MOIs that can give clues about internal bleeding.

During your focused history, elaborate on the patient's chief complaint using the OPQRST mnemonic, and obtain a history of the present illness using SAMPLE. Are there any

At the Scene

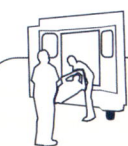
Consider any patient exhibiting signs and symptoms of shock without obvious injury to have probable internal bleeding, usually in the abdominal cavity.

Table 18-1	The MOI: Indicators of Internal Bleeding
Mechanism of Injury	**Potential Internal Bleeding Sources**
Fall from a ladder striking head	Head injury or hematoma
Fall from a ladder striking extremities	Possible fractures; consider chest injury
Child struck by car (Waddell triad)	Head trauma, chest and abdomen injuries, leg fractures
Fall on outstretched arm	Possible broken bone or joint injury
Child thrown or falls from height	Children usually have a head-first impact, causing head injury
Unrestrained driver in head-on collision (up-and-over route)	Head and neck, chest, abdomen injuries
Unrestrained driver in head-on collision (down-and-under route)	Knees, femur, hip, and pelvis injuries
Unrestrained front-seat passenger, side impact collision with intrusion into vehicle	Humerus broken exposing the chest wall (possible flail chest); pelvis and acetabulum injuries
Unrestrained driver crushed against steering column	Chest and abdomen injuries, ruptured spleen, neck trauma
Road bike or mountain bike (over the handlebars)	Fractured clavicle, road rash, head trauma if no helmet
Abrupt motorcycle stop, causing rider to catapult over the handlebars	Fractured femurs, head and neck injuries
Diving into the shallow end of a swimming pool	Head and neck injuries
Assault or fight	Punching or kicking injury to chest and abdomen and the face
Blast or explosion	Injury from direct strike with debris; indirect and pressure wave in enclosed space

signs and symptoms of hypovolemic shock? Ask the patient if they have pain or if he or she experiences any dizziness. Ask the patient about current medications that may thin the blood and about any history of clotting insufficiency. Assess for tenderness, bruising, guarding, or swelling. These signs and symptoms may indicate internal bleeding.

During the physical examination (rapid or focused, depending on the MOI), note the colour of bleeding and try to determine its source. Bright red blood from a wound or the mouth, rectum, or other orifice indicates fresh arterial bleeding. Coffee-ground emesis is a sign of upper GI bleeding; this kind of blood is old and looks like used coffee grounds.

Melena, the passage of dark, tarry stools, indicates lower GI bleeding. Hematochezia, by contrast, is the passage of stools containing bright red blood and may indicate bleeding near the external opening of the colon. Hemorrhoids in the lower colon tend to cause hematochezia. Hematuria (blood in the urine) may suggest serious renal injury or illness. Nonmenstrual vaginal bleeding is always significant as well.

Management of a Bleeding Patient

Always wear appropriate PPE when treating bleeding patients. As with all prehospital care, ensure that the patient has an open airway and is breathing adequately. Provide high-flow supplemental oxygen, and assist ventilation if needed, paying special attention to cervical spine control in trauma patients.

Managing External Hemorrhage

To control external hemorrhaging, follow these steps:
1. Apply direct pressure over the wound.
2. Elevate the injury above the level of the heart if no fracture is suspected.
3. Apply a pressure dressing.

A tourniquet is generally used only as a last resort, when it may be necessary to sacrifice the limb to save the life.

Bleeding From the Nose, Ears, and Mouth

Bleeding from the nose (epistaxis) or bleeding from the ears following a head injury may indicate a skull fracture. In such a case, you should not attempt to stop the blood flow. If you suspect a skull fracture, cover the bleeding site loosely with a sterile gauze pad to collect the blood and help keep contaminants away from the site—there is always a risk of infection to the brain with a skull fracture. Apply light compression by wrapping the dressing loosely around the head. If blood or drainage contains cerebrospinal fluid, there will be a characteristic staining of the dressing that resembles a bull's-eye target.

Bleeding From Other Areas

With bleeding from other areas of the body, control bleeding through use of direct pressure and elevation, if appropriate. Apply pressure dressings, especially at pressure points for the upper and lower extremities. In addition, use splints as necessary, always following your local protocols. Pack large, gaping wounds with sterile dressings. Consider applying the PASG/MAST, if your local protocols permit, but reserve the tourniquet for use as a last resort.

Once bleeding is controlled and a sterile dressing and pressure bandage have been applied, keep the patient warm and in the appropriate position. Allow the patient's condition to dictate the mode of transport.

Special Management Techniques for External Hemorrhage

Much of the bleeding associated with broken bones occurs because the sharp ends of the bones lacerate vessels, muscles, and other tissues. As long as a fracture remains unstable, the bone ends will move and continue to damage tissues and vessels. They may also break up clots that have partially formed, resulting in ongoing bleeding. For these reasons, immobilizing a fracture is a priority in the prompt control of bleeding. Often, simple splints will quickly control the bleeding associated with a fracture. If not, you may need to use another splinting device.

Air Splints

Air splints can control the bleeding associated with severe soft-tissue injuries, such as massive or complex lacerations, or with fractures. They also stabilize the fracture itself. An air splint acts like a pressure dressing applied to an entire extremity rather than to a small, local area.

Once you have applied an air splint, monitor circulation in the distal extremity. Because an air splint is typically inflated to approximately 50 mm Hg (so you can still dent the splint with your fingertips), it would not be appropriate to use on arterial bleeding because the splint would not actually control the bleeding until the patient's systolic BP dropped to the pressure of the splint.

Hemostats

Although hemostats may be helpful when a vessel has been severed, especially if it has retracted into the surrounding tissue, they often cause significant damage to the vessel and surrounding tissue. Be sure to check your local protocols about the use of hemostats in your area.

Tourniquets

The tourniquet is useful if a patient is bleeding severely from a partial or complete amputation and other methods of bleeding control have proved ineffective. The paramedic should realize that its application can cause permanent damage to nerves, muscles, and blood vessels, resulting in the loss of an extremity. The procedure for tourniquet application is shown in Skill Drill 19-2 in Chapter 19. Whenever applying a tourniquet, make sure you observe the following precautions:

- Do not apply a tourniquet directly over any joint. Keep it as close to the injury as possible.
- Use the widest bandage possible. Make sure that it is tightened securely.
- Never use wire, rope, a belt, or any other narrow material as the tourniquet; it could cut into the skin.
- Use wide padding under the tourniquet, if possible, to protect the tissues and help with arterial compression.

- Never cover a tourniquet with a bandage. Leave it open and in full view.
- Do not loosen the tourniquet after you have applied it. Hospital personnel will loosen it once they are prepared to manage the bleeding.

Pneumatic Antishock Garment/Military Antishock Trousers

MAST, also known as PASG, is an inflatable garment that surrounds the legs and abdomen of a patient to provide circumferential pressure. It is by far one of the most controversial pieces of equipment used in the prehospital setting. This device is primarily used for controlling blood loss and is not designed for resuscitation, except with authorization of direct medical control in a few situations of extreme hypotension **Figure 18-5 ▾** .

In the 1980s, researchers began to question whether this device, and IV fluid infusion, were really effective in the treatment of shock. The use of this device remains highly controversial, be sure to check with and adhere to your local protocols **Figure 18-6 ▸** .

By applying uniform pressure to sources of bleeding, the PASG/MAST, when pumped up to the point where the Velcro crackles (60 to 80 mm Hg), seems to control bleeding and promote hemostasis. The circumferential pressure also compresses the tissue and vessels and, ultimately, results in a decrease in the vascular container size under the suit. With this increase in the systemic vascular resistance (SVR), it has been theorized that a small amount of blood (approximately 200 ml) is autotransfused back to the torso and the mean arterial pressure (MAP) increases. These effects increase the patient's CO.

The PASG/MAST raises the BP of a patient in shock. Whether elevating the BP is beneficial has not been proved. Some researchers believe that raising the BP before bleeding has been controlled may have harmful effects, for example by promoting further bleeding. However, raising the patient's BP improves prefusion to vital organs and can be useful to *paramedics,* because veins that were collapsed and invisible may "pop up" after the device has been inflated, making the job of inserting IV lines easier.

The inflated device provides a good splint for a fractured pelvis, but only does a marginal job splinting fractures of the lower extremities. Ideally, fractures of the femur should be traction-splinted in conjunction with the application of the PASG/MAST.

As yet, we do not know whether the PASG/MAST improves the overall outcome for seriously injured patients. Recent research at Baylor College of Medicine suggests that, at least in certain types of injuries, the device does not improve chances of survival and may adversely affect the outcome. Medical directors of local EMS systems should stay abreast of the research in this area and make their decisions regarding deployment of the device accordingly.

In EMS systems that continue to use the PASG/MAST, use is appropriate in patients with shock from blood loss (hemorrhagic shock) in the following circumstances:

- To stabilize suspected pelvic fractures with hypotension
- To begin to control severe hypotension (systolic BP < 50 to 60 mm Hg)
- To begin to control suspected intraperitoneal bleeding with hypotension (solid organs such as the liver and spleen, mesenteric vessels)
- To begin to control retroperitoneal bleeding with hypotension (such as in kidneys, aorta, and vena cavae)

Current contraindications to use of the PASG/MAST include the following:

- Penetrating thoracic trauma
- Splinting of the lower extremities in the absence of hypotension. The PASG/MAST is not a good splint and has been known to cause compartment syndrome of the calf when fractures were present.

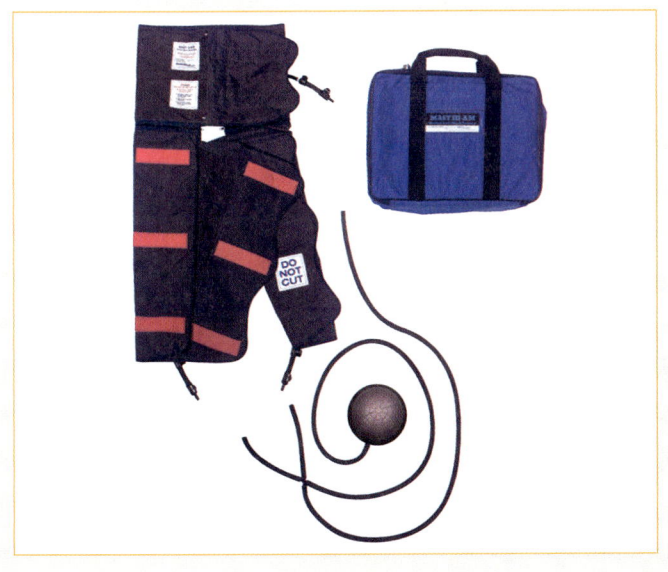

Figure 18-5 PASG/MAST device.

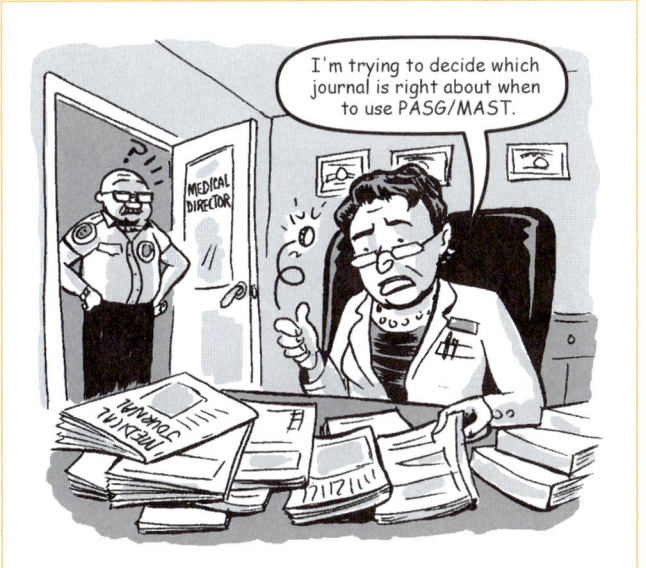

Figure 18-6

- Evisceration of abdominal organs
- Impaled objects of the abdomen
- Pregnancy
- Acute pulmonary edema
- Traumatic cardiac arrest
- Major head injuries

The steps in applying the device are described here and shown in **Skill Drill 18-1 ▾** :

1. Rapidly expose and examine the areas to be covered by the PASG/MAST. Pad any exposed bone ends to prevent puncture of the garment as it is inflated.

2. Apply the garment. If you will immobilize or move the patient on a backboard, lay the device out on the board before rolling the patient onto it. Position the top of the abdominal section of the PASG/MAST below the lowest rib to ensure that it does not compromise chest expansion **Step 1** .

3. Close and fasten both leg compartments and the abdominal compartment **Step 2** .

4. Open the stopcocks (valves) to the compartments you are preparing to inflate, ensuring that the other compartments are closed off.

5. Auscultate breath sounds for pulmonary edema before inflation **Step 3** .

6. Inflate the compartments with the foot pump to 60 to 80 mm Hg (until the Velcro crackles). Turn off compartment valves after inflation to maintain pressure in the garment. When using the device to stabilize a pelvic fracture, apply pressure only until the garment is firm to the touch. Overinflation may cause the bones to shift, creating further injury and bleeding. Higher inflation pressures may cause local tissue damage and/or compartment syndrome **Step 4** .

7. Check the patient's BP. Continue to monitor serial vital signs at least every 5 minutes because a patient who is subjected to this intervention is considered unstable. Remember that the pressure gauges on the device

Skill Drill 18-1: Applying PASG/MAST

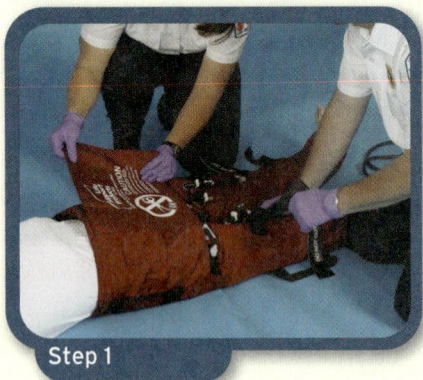

Step 1

Rapidly expose and examine the areas to be covered by the device. Pad any exposed bone ends. Apply the garment so that the top is below the lowest rib.

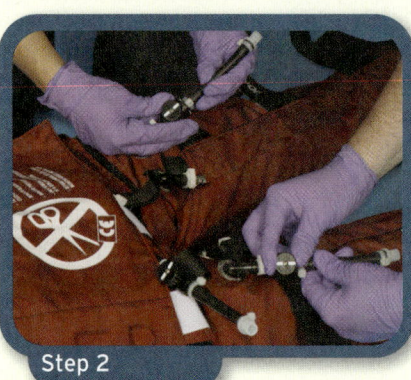

Step 2

Close and fasten both leg compartments and the abdominal compartment.

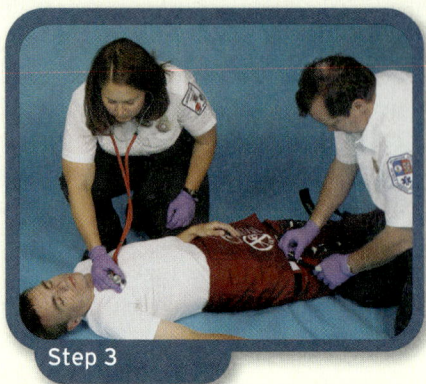

Step 3

Open the three stopcocks (valves). Auscultate breath sounds for pulmonary edema before inflation.

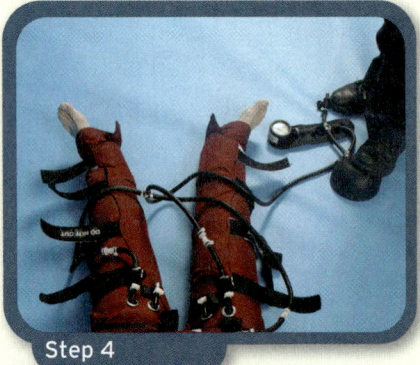

Step 4

Inflate with the foot pump until the Velcro crackles (approximately 60 to 80 mm Hg).

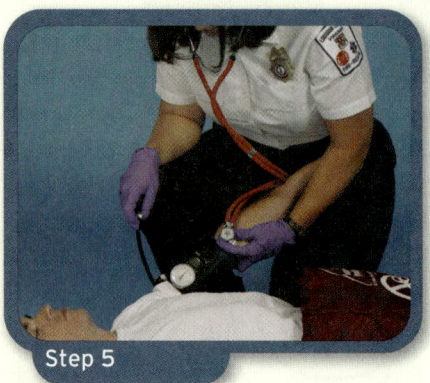

Step 5

Check the patient's BP again, and begin transport if not already in the transport mode.

measure the air pressure in the device—not the patient's BP. Be aware of temperature extremes or external pressure changes that might significantly affect the pressure exerted by the PASG/MAST, thus requiring frequent monitoring and adjustment (Step 5).

The simplest rule to remember regarding deflation of the PASG/MAST is this: Do not deflate the device in the prehospital environment. To the extent that the device supports the BP and provides hemostasis, the effects will be reversed when the PASG/MAST is deflated. An extreme case in which it might be necessary to deflate the device in the prehospital setting—albeit with direct medical control's permission—would be for a suspected ruptured diaphragm (causing abdominal contents to herniate into the chest cavity immediately after inflation of the device). It is desirable, therefore, to have restored at least some of the patient's circulating blood volume before releasing the pressure provided by the PASG/MAST. Remember that the patient's container size will have been decreased and deflation will increase the container, potentially leading to dramatic declines in the SVR, preload (venous return), and CO.

Before the PASG/MAST is deflated in the hospital setting, the patient should have at least two large-bore IV infusions running, with typed and cross-matched blood on standby. If the patient's serial vital signs are relatively stable and the ED physician so instructs, cautious deflation of the PASG/MAST may proceed as follows:

1. Record the patient's pulse and BP.
2. Slowly deflate the abdominal section *only*.
3. Recheck the patient's serial vital signs for 5 to 10 minutes. If the BP drops by 5 mm Hg or more, infuse 100 to 200 ml of fluid until the BP restabilizes.
4. When the patient's vital signs are again stable, slowly deflate one leg section.
5. Recheck the vital signs for 5 to 10 minutes. If there is another BP drop, again infuse volume until the BP comes back up.
6. If vital signs are stable, deflate the other leg section—again slowly, with careful monitoring of BP every few minutes.

In severely injured patients, this deflation procedure, which can take between 20 and 60 minutes, will usually not be feasible. Instead, the patient must be taken straight to the operating room with the PASG/MAST still on and inflated.

Managing Internal Hemorrhage

The definitive management of a patient with internal hemorrhage occurs in the hospital. Prehospital management of suspected internal bleeding involves treating for shock and splinting injured extremities:

1. Keep the patient supine, open the airway, and check breathing and pulse.
2. Administer high-flow supplemental oxygen and assist ventilation if needed.
3. Splint broken bones or joint injuries. If a pelvic fracture is suspected, you may consider use of the PASG/MAST if your local protocols permit.

4. Place blankets under and over the patient to maintain body heat.
5. If no fractures are suspected, elevate the legs 30 cm. While en route to the ED, insert a large-bore (14- or 16-gauge) IV cannula, and administer a fluid challenge of 250 ml (provided the lungs are clear). Insert an IV line at the scene only if transport is delayed (such as if the patient is entrapped). Whenever possible, use warm IV fluids to prevent the patient from becoming chilled.
6. Consider giving pain medication if the vital signs are stable and after consultation with direct medical control.
7. Monitor the serial vital signs, and watch diligently for developing shock.

If the patient shows any signs of shock (hypoperfusion), transport rapidly while providing aggressive management en route. Because a patient in shock is usually emotionally upset, you should provide psychological support as well.

Transportation of Patients With Hemorrhage

In case of hemorrhage, the issue is not whether the patient will be transported, but rather how fast the transport decision should be made and where the patient should be taken for definitive care. There are a few exceptions to this rule—for example, in the case of a minor wound, the decision to transport a patient should take into consideration factors such as the need for stitches, whether the patient has had a tetanus shot in the past 10 years, and whether the patient or his or her companion is reliable and will follow up properly. (Wounds are discussed in more detail in Chapter 19.)

Most patients with internal or external hemorrhage will need to be transported to a hospital for further care. Consideration for the priority of the patient and the availability of a regional trauma centre should be your concerns when making a transport decision in such cases. Patients who have severe internal or external bleeding, especially if uncontrolled, will usually be candidates for surgical interventions and should be transported to a facility with those capabilities. Patients with specific causes of bleeding such as major trauma or specific devastating wounds (such as leg amputation, glove avulsion) should be taken to a facility that is fully prepared to care for the patient. In EMS systems with helicopters available, it may be appropriate to consider this method of transportation for a patient with suspected severe internal or uncontrollable external bleeding.

Pathophysiology of Shock

Hypoperfusion occurs when the level of tissue perfusion decreases below normal. Early decreased tissue perfusion may result in subtle changes, such as altered mental status, before a patient's vital signs (blood pressure, pulse, respiratory rate) appear abnormal. Shock refers to a state of collapse and failure of the cardiovascular system that leads to inadequate circulation, creating inadequate tissue perfusion. Like internal bleeding, shock cannot be seen. It is not a specific disease or injury, but rather a dangerous condition that results in inadequate flow of blood to the body's cells and failure to rid the body of metabolic wastes.

Notes from Nancy

Don't wait until the BP falls before you suspect shock and begin treatment!

When the body senses tissue hypoperfusion, compensatory mechanisms are set into action. In some cases, this is enough to stabilize the patient's condition. In other cases, the severity of disease or injury overwhelms the normal compensatory mechanisms, leading to progressive deterioration in the patient's condition. Evaluation of a patient's level of organ perfusion is important in diagnosing shock. If the conditions causing shock are not promptly addressed, the patient will rapidly deteriorate. Perfusion depends on CO, SVR, and transport of oxygen:

Cardiac Output = Pulse Rate × Stroke Volume

Blood Pressure = Cardiac Output × Systemic Vascular Resistance

Because the heart cannot pump out what is not in its holding chambers, BP varies directly with CO, SVR, and blood volume. Hypoperfusion, therefore, can result from inadequate CO, decreased SVR, or the inability of RBCs to deliver oxygen to tissues.

At the Scene

Remember that BP may be the last measurable factor to change in shock. The body has several automatic mechanisms to compensate for initial blood loss and to help maintain BP. Thus, by the time you detect a drop in BP, shock is well developed. This is particularly true in infants and children, who can maintain their BP until they have lost close to half their blood volume.

Mechanisms of Shock

Recall that normal tissue perfusion requires three intact mechanisms: a pump (heart), fluid volume (blood and body fluids), and tubing capable of reflex adjustments (constriction and dilation) in response to changes in pump output and fluid volume (blood vessels). If any one of those mechanisms is damaged, tissue perfusion may be disrupted, and shock will ensue.

When shock arises because of failure of the heart's ability to pump effectively due to muscle dysfunction, it is called cardiogenic shock (*cardio* = heart + *genic* = causing). Cardiac arrest is the most drastic form of cardiogenic shock, but not the only form. Cardiogenic shock may occur secondary to myocardial infarction, cardiac arrhythmias, pulmonary embolism, severe acidosis, or a variety of other conditions. All of these conditions have one thing in common: They interfere with the heart's ability to pump normally.

Shock may also occur because of a loss of fluid volume; perfusion cannot take place if there isn't enough fluid to propel through the system. When shock comes about because of inadequate volume, it is termed hypovolemic shock (*hypo* = deficient + *vol* = volume + *emia* = in the blood). Volume can be lost as blood (hemorrhagic shock), plasma (as in burns), or electrolyte solution (as in vomiting, diarrhea, sweating). Suspect a hypovolemic component of shock in any patient with unexplained shock, and treat the patient for hypovolemia first.

Failure of vasoconstriction (that is, a decrease in the peripheral vascular resistance [PVR]) may lead to neurogenic shock, so called because the sympathetic nervous system ordinarily controls the dilation and constriction of blood vessels. In a healthy person, the calibre of the blood vessels constantly changes in response to signals from the nervous system, allowing the body to adapt to changes in position, fluid volume, and so forth. When you stand up, for example, blood vessels in your legs reflexively constrict to divert the circulation toward more vital areas, like the brain. Similarly, when you donate a pint of blood or sweat a litre of fluid, your blood vessels constrict to accommodate a smaller fluid volume. In certain situations, nervous system control over the calibre of blood vessels becomes deranged—for example, after spinal cord injury—and the blood vessels lose their tone and dilate. A given blood volume then has to be accommodated quite suddenly in a much larger container. The net effect is a relative hypovolemia (the volume in the container is now inadequate relative to the increased size of the container), which the body experiences as shock.

More than one component of the circulatory system may be affected in case of shock. For example, a patient in shock after a myocardial infarction is likely to have an element of cardiogenic shock, because the damaged heart can no longer pump efficiently, and an element of hypovolemic shock, if the patient has been vomiting, sweating, or too nauseated to take in fluids. Some types of shock always result from combined deficits from both fluid leakage into the interstitial space as well as vasodilatation.

Certain categories of patients are at high risk to develop shock. They include patients known to have had trauma or bleeding, elderly people, patients with massive myocardial infarction, pregnant women, and patients with a possible source for septic shock (such as burned patients and people with diabetes or cancer).

Notes from Nancy

Suspect a hypovolemic component of shock in any patient with unexplained shock, and treat for hypovolemia first.

Compensation for Decreased Perfusion

Central among the homeostatic mechanisms that regulate cardiovascular dynamics are those that maintain BP. When any event results in decreased perfusion (such as in blood loss, myocardial infarction, loss of vasomotor tone, or tension pneumothorax), the body must respond immediately to preserve the vital organs. Baroreceptors located in the aortic arch and carotid sinuses sense the decreased blood flow and activate the vasomotor center, which oversees changes in the diameter of blood vessels, to begin constriction of the vessels.

Stimulation typically occurs when the systolic pressure is between 60 and 80 mm Hg in adults or even lower in children. A decrease in systolic pressure to less than 80 mm Hg stimulates the vasomotor centre to increase arterial pressure by constricting vessels. The drop in arterial pressure decreases the stretching of the arterial walls, thereby decreasing baroreceptor firing, stimulating the vasoconstrictor centre of the medulla. The sympathetic nervous system is also stimulated as the body recognizes a potential catastrophic event.

In response to hypoperfusion, the renin-angiotensin-aldosterone system is activated and antidiuretic hormone is released from the pituitary gland. Together, these mechanisms trigger salt and water retention and peripheral vasoconstriction. The result is an increase in the patient's BP and CO. Depending on the severity of the insult, variable amounts of fluid will shift from the interstitial tissues into the vascular compartment. The spleen also releases some RBCs that are normally sequestered there to augment the blood's oxygen-carrying capacity. The overall response of the initial compensatory mechanisms is to increase the preload, stroke volume, and pulse rate, which usually results in an increase in CO.

As hypoperfusion persists, the myocardial oxygen demand continues to increase. Eventually, the accelerated compensatory mechanisms are no longer able to keep up with the body's demand. Myocardial function then worsens, with decreased CO and ejection fraction. Tissue perfusion decreases, leading to impaired cell metabolism. Often, the systolic BP decreases, especially in progressive hypoperfusion or "decompensated" shock. Fluid may leak from the blood vessels, causing systemic and pulmonary edema. Other signs of hypoperfusion may also be present, such as dusky skin colour, oliguria, and impaired mentation.

The body produces its own "medicines," epinephrine and norepinephrine, in the adrenal glands in response to hypoperfusion. These substances are released by the body as part of the global compensatory state. Epinephrine is also administered by caregivers in cases of anaphylaxis, severe airway disease, and cardiac arrest.

Release of epinephrine improves CO by increasing the pulse rate and strength. The alpha-1 response to its release includes vasoconstriction, increased peripheral vascular resistance, and increased afterload from the arteriolar constriction. Alpha-2 effects ensure a regulated release of alpha-1. Beta responses from the release of epinephrine primarily affect the heart and lungs. Increases in pulse rate, contractility, conductivity, and automaticity occur in tandem with bronchodilation.

Effects of norepinephrine are primarily alpha-1 and alpha-2 in nature and centre on vasoconstriction and increasing PVR. This vasoconstriction allows the body to shunt blood from areas of lesser need to areas of greater need; that is, it serves to keep the brain and other vital organs perfused in the early phases of shock. In an effort to maintain circulation to the brain, the body

You are the Paramedic Part 3

You decide that the patient does not have spinal involvement. He reports that he was not blown to the ground, but rather felt dizzy and sat down on his own. You and your partner decide to quickly pick the patient up and load him onto the stretcher, rather than spending the time for spinal immobilization to a backboard. You also decide to insert the IV line en route to the regional trauma centre.

The patient is starting to become confused as you place him into Trendelenburg position and head out the door. He states that he is nauseated and thirsty and asks your partner, "Am I going to die?" When closing the back of the ambulance, you note on your watch that 7 minutes have elapsed on the scene. Your plan for the next few minutes is to redo the initial assessment, get IV fluids running, notify the ED, do the rapid trauma assessment and SAMPLE history, and consider PASG/MAST.

Vital Signs	Recording Time: 5 Minutes
Mental status	V (Responsive to verbal stimuli), confused about place and day
Respirations	26 breaths/min, shallow and laboured
Pulse	120 beats/min, thready (core, only not peripheral)
Blood pressure	106 mm Hg by palpation
Skin	Pale, cool, and moist
Spo$_2$	95% on nonrebreathing mask at 15 l/min of supplemental oxygen
ECG	Sinus tachycardia with no ectopy

6. For this patient, is the Spo$_2$ a helpful indicator?

7. Why weren't the baseline vital signs taken on the scene?

will shunt blood away from the following tissues, in this order: placenta, skin, muscles, gut, kidneys, liver, heart, lungs. The skin and muscles can survive with minimal blood flow from vasoconstriction for a much longer period than can major organs such as the kidneys, liver, heart, and lungs. If the blood supply is inadequate to the major organs for more than 60 minutes, they often develop complications that will lead to death, such as renal failure and shock lung. This concept has been traditionally referred to as the "golden hour of trauma," and it explains why it is so important to address the cause of the shock in as timely a manner as possible.

Failure of compensatory mechanisms to preserve perfusion leads to decreases in preload and CO. Myocardial blood supply and oxygenation decrease, reducing myocardial perfusion. As CO further decreases, coronary artery perfusion also decreases, leading to myocardial ischemia.

Types of Shock

The inadequate oxygen and nutrient delivery to the metabolic apparatus of the cell experienced in shock results in impaired cellular metabolism. Once a certain level of tissue hypoperfusion is reached, cell damage proceeds in a similar manner, regardless of the type of initial insult. Impairment of cellular metabolism results in the inability to properly use oxygen and glucose at the cellular level. The cell converts to anaerobic metabolism, which causes increased lactic acid production and metabolic acidosis, decreased oxygen affinity for hemoglobin, decreased adenosine triphosphate (ATP) production, changes in cellular electrolytes, cellular edema, and release of lysosomal enzymes. The blood glucose level may be elevated due to release of catecholamines and cortisol. In addition, fat breakdown (lipolysis) with ketone formation may occur.

The Weil-Shubin classification considers shock from a mechanistic point of view. From this perspective, two types of shock are distinguished: central shock, which consists of cardiogenic shock and obstructive shock, and peripheral shock, which includes hypovolemic shock and distributive shock.

Regardless of type, shock is characterized by reduced CO, circulatory insufficiency, and tachycardia. Most types of shock also include pallor, except for spinal shock and sepsis. The patient's mental status may be altered. Low BP, although classically associated with shock, is a late sign, especially in children.

Cardiogenic Shock

Cardiogenic shock occurs when the heart is unable to circulate sufficient blood to maintain adequate peripheral oxygen delivery. Circulation of blood throughout the vascular system requires the constant pumping action of a normal and vigorous heart muscle. Many diseases can cause destruction or inflammation of this muscle. Within certain limits, the heart can adapt to these problems. If too much muscular damage occurs, however, the heart no longer functions effectively. Filling is impaired because of a lack of pressure to return blood to the heart (preload), or outflow is reduced by a lack of pumping function.

In either case, direct pump failure is the cause of shock. In the case of ischemic heart disease, pump failure is generally due to a loss of 40% or more of the functioning myocardium.

The most common cause of cardiogenic shock is extensive infarction of the left ventricle, diffuse ischemia, or decompensated congestive heart failure resulting in primary pump failure. The heart damage may be due to a single massive event or result from cumulative damage. Other forms of cardiac dysfunction may result in cardiogenic shock as well—for example, large ventricular septal defect, cardiomyopathy, or hemodynamic significant arrhythmias.

Patients have a poor prognosis when more than 40% of the left ventricle is destroyed. Historically, in about 7.5% of patients with acute myocardial infarction, cardiogenic shock develops, and mortality rates range as high as 80%, even with appropriate therapy.

Obstructive Shock

Obstructive shock occurs when blood flow in the heart or great vessels becomes blocked. In pericardial tamponade, diastolic filling of the right ventricle is impaired, leading to a decrease in CO. Obstruction of the superior or inferior vena cava (such as vena cava syndrome as in third-trimester pregnancy) decreases CO by decreasing venous return. A large pulmonary embolus or tension pneumothorax may prevent adequate blood flow to the lungs, resulting in inadequate venous return to the left side of the heart.

Hypovolemic Shock

Hypovolemic shock occurs when the circulating blood volume does not deliver adequate oxygen and nutrients to the body. It is subdivided into two types, exogenous and endogenous, depending on where the fluid loss occurs.

The most common cause of exogenous hypovolemic shock is external bleeding. Hemorrhage is most prevalent in trauma patients due to blunt or penetrating injuries to vessels or organs, long bone or pelvic fractures, major vascular injuries (as in traumatic amputation), and multisystem injury. The organs and organ systems with a high incidence of exsanguination from penetrating injuries include the heart, liver, spleen thoracic vascular system, abdominal vascular system (such as abdominal aorta, superior mesenteric artery), and venous system (such as inferior vena cava or portal vein).

Endogenous hypovolemic shock occurs when the fluid loss is contained within the body, as in dehydration, burn injury, crush injury, and anaphylaxis. With severe thermal burns, for example, intravascular plasma leaks from the circulatory system into the burned tissues that lie adjacent to the injury. By comparison, crushing injuries may result in the loss of blood and plasma from damaged vessels into injured tissues.

Abnormal losses of fluids and electrolytes (that is, dehydration) may occur through a variety of mechanisms:

- GI losses, especially through vomiting and diarrhea
- Increased loss as a consequence of fever, hyperventilation, or high environmental temperatures (through the lungs)

- Increased sweating
- Internal losses ("third-space" losses), as in peritonitis, pancreatitis, and ileus
- Plasma losses from burns

Other causes of body fluid deficits include ascites, diabetes insipidus, acute renal failure, and osmotic diuresis secondary to hyperosmolar states (such as diabetic ketoacidosis).

In each case, the fluid lost has a unique electrolyte composition, and long-term therapy aims to restore the deficient body chemicals. For treatment in the prehospital environment, however, all excessive fluid losses can be considered to lead to dehydration.

Symptoms of dehydration include loss of appetite (anorexia), nausea, vomiting, and sometimes fainting when standing up (postural syncope). Physical examination of a dehydrated patient reveals poor skin turgor (the skin over the forehead or sternum will "tent" when pinched); a shrunken, furrowed tongue; and sunken eyes. The pulse will be weak and rapid, rising more than 15 beats/min when the patient is raised from a recumbent to a sitting position (a maneuver that may cause the patient to feel faint). When fluid and electrolyte depletion are severe, shock and coma may be present.

A dehydrated patient needs replacement of fluid and electrolytes and should be given an IV infusion of normal saline or lactated Ringer's solution at a rate of 100 to 200 ml/h for an adult, depending on the circumstances. Keep the patient flat to optimize circulation to the brain.

Distributive Shock

Distributive shock occurs when there is widespread dilation of the resistance vessels (small arterioles), the capacitance vessels (small venules), or both. As a result, the circulating blood volume pools in the expanded vascular beds and tissue perfusion decreases. The three most common types of distributive shock are septic shock, neurogenic shock, and anaphylactic shock.

Septic Shock

Sepsis comes from the Greek word meaning "to putrefy." Septic shock is defined as the presence of sepsis syndrome plus a systolic BP of less than 90 mm Hg or a decrease from the baseline BP of more than 40 mm Hg.

Sepsis occurs as a result of widespread infection, usually due to gram-negative bacterial organisms; gram-positive bacteria, fungi, viruses, and rickettsia can also be causative agents. Complex interactions occur between the pathogen and the body's defence systems. Initially, the body's defence mechanisms may keep the infection at bay. The infection activates the inflammatory-immune response, which invokes humoural, cellular, and biochemical pathways. This response results in increased microvascular permeability (leaky capillaries), vasodilation, third-space fluid shifts, and microthrombi formation. In some patients, an uncontrolled and unregulated inflammatory-immune response occurs, resulting in hypoperfusion to the cells, tissue destruction, and organ death. Left untreated, the result is multiple-organ dysfunction syndrome and, often, death.

Septic shock is a complex problem. First, there is an insufficient volume of fluid in the container, because much of the blood has leaked out of the vascular system (hypovolemia). Second, the fluid that leaks out often collects in the respiratory system, interfering with ventilation. Third, a larger-than-normal vascular bed is asked to contain the smaller-than-normal volume of intravascular fluid.

Neurogenic Shock

Neurogenic shock usually results from spinal cord injury, resulting in loss of normal sympathetic nervous system tone and vasodilation.

In neurogenic shock, the muscles in the walls of the blood vessels are cut off from the nerve impulses that cause them to contract. As a consequence, all vessels below the level of the spinal injury dilate widely, increasing the size and capacity of the vascular system and causing blood to pool. The available 5 to 6 l of blood in the body can no longer fill this enlarged vascular system. Perfusion of organs and tissues becomes inadequate, even though no blood or fluid has been lost, and shock occurs. The patient experiences relative hypovolemia, which leads to hypotension (systolic BP usually between 80 and 100 mm Hg). In addition, relative bradycardia occurs because the sympathetic nervous system is not stimulated to release catecholamines. The skin is pink, warm, and dry because of cutaneous vasodilation. There is no release of epinephrine and norepinephrine, which would otherwise produce the classic sign of pale, cool, diaphoretic skin. Instead, a characteristic sign of neurogenic shock is the absence of sweating below the level of injury.

Neurogenic shock is not to be confused with *spinal shock*, which refers to the local neurologic condition that occurs immediately after a spinal injury produces motor and sensory losses (which may not be permanent). Spinal shock is characterized by flaccid paralysis, flaccid sphincters, and absent reflexes. There is an absence of all pain, temperature, touch, proprioception, and pressure below the level of the lesion; absent or impaired thermoregulation; absent somatic and visceral sensations below the lesion; bowel distension; and loss of peristalsis.

Anaphylactic Shock

Anaphylaxis occurs when a person reacts severely to a substance to which he or she has been sensitized. Sensitization means developing a heightened reaction (becoming allergic) to a substance. An allergic reaction typically does not occur, or occurs in a milder form, during sensitization. Do not be misled by a patient who reports no history of allergic reaction to a substance following a first or second exposure: Each subsequent exposure after sensitization tends to produce a more severe reaction.

In anaphylactic shock, there is no loss of blood, no vascular damage, and only a slight possibility of direct cardiac muscular injury. Instead, the patient experiences widespread vascular dilation, resulting in relative hypovolemia.

In anaphylaxis, immune system chemicals, such as histamine and other vasodilator proteins, are released on exposure to an allergen. Their release causes the severe bronchoconstriction that accounts for wheezing if the patient is actually moving enough air. Anaphylaxis is also accompanied by urticaria (hives). The results are widespread vasodilation, which causes distributive shock, and blood vessels that continue to leak. Fluid leaks out of the blood vessels and into the interstitial spaces, resulting in hypovolemia and potentially causing significant swelling. In some cases, this swelling may occlude the upper airway, resulting in a life-threatening condition Figure 18-7 ▶ .

Recurrent large areas of subcutaneous edema of sudden onset, usually disappearing within 24 hours and mainly seen in young women (frequently as a result of allergy to food or drugs), is called angioedema.

Shock-Related Events at the Capillary and Microcirculatory Levels

As perfusion decreases, cellular ischemia occurs. Minimal blood flow passes through the capillaries, causing the cells to switch from aerobic metabolism to anaerobic metabolism, which can quickly lead to metabolic acidosis. With less circulation, the blood stagnates in the capillaries. The precapillary sphincter relaxes in response to the buildup of lactic acid, vasomotor centre failure, and increased amounts of carbon dioxide. The postcapillary sphincters remain constricted, causing the capillaries to become engorged with fluid.

The capillary sphincters—circular muscular walls that constrict and dilate—regulate blood flow through the capillary beds. These sphincters are under the control of the autonomic nervous system, which regulates involuntary functions such as sweating and digestion. Capillary sphincters also respond to other stimuli at the local level such as heat, cold, increased demand for oxygen, and the need for waste removal. Thus, regulation of blood flow is determined by cellular need and is accomplished by vessel constriction or dilation, working in tandem with sphincter constriction or dilation.

The body can tolerate anaerobic metabolism for only a limited time. Anaerobic metabolism is much less efficient than aerobic metabolism and leads to systemic acidosis and depletion of the body's normally high energy reserves (ATP).

During anaerobic metabolism, incomplete glucose breakdown leads to an accumulation of pyruvic acid. Pyruvic acid cannot be converted to acetyl coenzyme A without oxygen, however, so it is transformed in greater amounts to lactate and other acid by-products. Acidosis develops because ATP is hydrolyzed to adenosine diphosphate and phosphate with the release of a proton. Hydrogen ion accumulates, decreasing the pool of bicarbonate buffer. Lactate also buffers protons, and lactic acid accumulates in the body.

At the same time, ischemia stimulates increased carbon dioxide production by the tissues. The higher the body's metabolic rate, the higher the carbon dioxide level in hypoperfused states. The excess carbon dioxide combines with intracellular water to produce carbonic acid. Increased tissue acids will, in

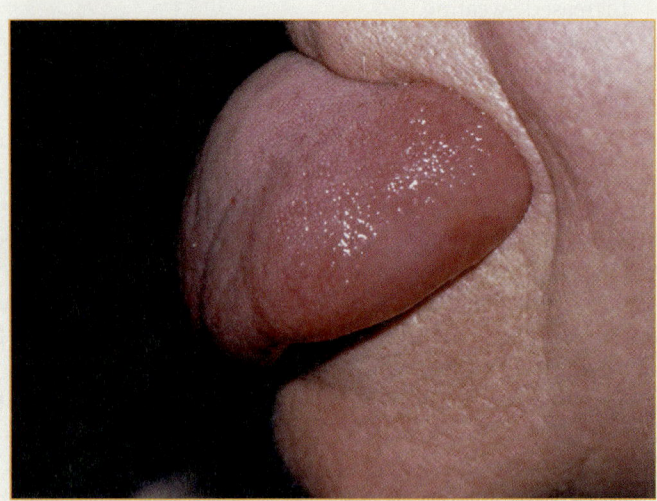

Figure 18-7 In anaphylaxis, interstitial fluid may cause significant swelling. In some cases, this swelling may occlude the upper airway, resulting in a life-threatening condition.

turn, react with other buffers to form more intracellular acidic substances. Thus, acidosis serves as an indirect measure of tissue perfusion. The acidic condition of the blood inhibits hemoglobin in the RBCs from binding with and carrying oxygen. This adds to the cellular oxygen debt, shifting the oxyhemoglobin dissociation curve to the right.

Meanwhile, sodium, which is usually more abundant outside the cells than inside them, is naturally inclined to diffuse into the cells. Normally the sodium-potassium pump acts like a "bouncer" at the cell membrane, sending the sodium back out against the concentration gradient. This mechanism involves active transport and requires an ample supply of ATP. Reduced levels of ATP, however, result in a dysfunctional sodium-potassium pump and alter the cell membrane function. Excessive sodium begins to diffuse into the cells, along with water, which ultimately depletes the interstitial compartment.

The intracellular enzymes that usually help digest and neutralize bacteria introduced into a cell are bound in a relatively impermeable membrane. Cellular flooding damages that membrane and releases these lysosomal enzymes, which then autodigest the cell. If enough cells are destroyed in this way, organ failure will become evident. The release of the lysosomes opens the floodgates for the onset of the last phase of shock, called irreversible shock.

To compound these problems, accumulating acids and waste products act as potent vasodilators, further decreasing venous return and diminishing blood flow to the vital organs and tissues. The arterial pressure falls to the point at which even the "protected organs" such as the brain and heart are no longer being perfused. When aortic pressures fall below a MAP of 60 mm Hg, the coronary arteries no longer fill, the heart is weakened, and the CO falls. Myocardial depressant factor is released from an ischemic pancreas, further decreasing the pumping action of the heart and reducing the CO.

Eventually, the reduced blood supply to the vasomotor centre in the brain results in slowing and then stopping of sympathetic nervous system activity. The metabolic wastes are released into the slower-flowing blood. The blood's sluggish flow coupled with its acidity leads to platelet agglutination and formation of microthrombi. Because the capillary walls are stretched, they lose their ability to retain large molecules, allowing them to leak into the surrounding interstitial spaces. Hydrostatic pressure forces plasma into the interstitial spaces, further increasing the distance from the capillaries to the cells. In turn, oxygen transport decreases, increasing cellular hypoxia.

The continuing buildup of lactic acid and carbon dioxide acts as a potent vasodilator, leading to relaxation of the post-capillary sphincters. The accumulated hydrogen, potassium, carbon dioxide, and thrombosed (clotted) RBCs wash out into the venous circulation, increasing the metabolic acidosis. This has been referred to as the capillary "washout phase." The result is an even greater drop in CO. Ischemia and necrosis ultimately lead to multiple-organ dysfunction syndrome, in which the various organ systems fail.

Systemic Inflammatory Response Syndrome

Systemic inflammatory response syndrome (SIRS) is a systemic inflammatory response to a variety of severe clinical insults. It does not confirm a diagnosis of infection or sepsis because the features of SIRS can be seen in many other conditions, including trauma, burns, and pancreatitis. Simply put, SIRS + infection = sepsis. SIRS is not a diagnosis itself, nor is it a good indicator of outcome.

The definition was proposed in 1991 by the American College of Chest Physicians and the Society of Critical Care to improve the ability of clinicians to make early bedside detection of sepsis, thus allowing early intervention. Also, standardizing the definition allows for improved analysis in research.

The inflammatory response is manifested by two or more of the following conditions: (1) temperature greater than 38°C or less than 36°C; (2) heart rate greater than 90 beats/min; (3) respiratory rate greater than 20 breaths/min or PCO_2 less than 32 mm Hg; and (4) a white blood cell count greater than 12,000/μl or less than 4,000/μl. The SIRS criteria may be considered a crude stratification for patients with systemic inflammation. In a prospective study of SIRS in medical and surgical patients, mortality rates were 3% in patients without SIRS, 6% in those with two criteria, 10% in those with three positive criteria, and 17% in those meeting all four criteria.

The release of cytokines in severe sepsis and injury is central to the development of SIRS. Initially, a central mediator is activated and released, which results in a cascaded secretion of various secondary mediators and the activation of neutrophils, the complement system, and vascular endothelial cells. The outcome of this complex cascade produces the physiologic changes recognized as SIRS.

SIRS affects specific organs and organ systems in the following ways:

- **Cardiovascular.** Manifests as tachycardia and hypotension. Myocardial depression and ischemia lead to pump failure.

Peripheral pulses may be weak or absent, and extremities may be cool and cyanosed.

- **Respiratory.** Manifest as tachypnea and increased minute ventilation. Reduced pulmonary capillary blood flow results in impaired gas exchange. Alveolar cells become ischemic and slow their production of surfactant, resulting in massive atelectasis and a reduction in pulmonary compliance. At the same time, pulmonary capillaries become permeable to water, resulting in edema. The net result is adult respiratory distress syndrome (ARDS) with respiratory failure, severe hypoxemia, and respiratory acidosis.
- **Central nervous system.** Decreased cerebral perfusion results in confusion, progressing to reduced level of consciousness and eventually unresponsiveness.
- **Renal system.** Reduced renal blood flow results in acute tubular necrosis, which in turn leads to oliguria (urine output < 20 ml/h). Toxic waste products cannot be excreted, so they are retained in the blood, worsening metabolic acidosis.
- **Liver and gastrointestinal tract.** Hypoperfusion results in ischemic gut. Impaired liver function and alterations in clotting factors produce coagulopathies, such as disseminated intravascular coagulation, in which clotting and bleeding occur at the same time. Liver cell death is evidenced by an increase in liver enzyme levels.
- **Metabolic.** Respiratory alkalosis is the first acid-base abnormality. Shock progresses with metabolic acidosis.

Uncontrolled SIRS leads to profound hypotension, inadequate perfusion, and death. Both SIRS and sepsis can progress to multiple-organ dysfunction syndrome (MODS), defined as the presence of altered organ function in acutely ill patients such that hemostasis cannot be maintained without intervention. MODS is well established as the final stage in a continuum and carries a high mortality rate of 60% to 90%.

Phases of Shock

Shock occurs in three successive phases (compensated, decompensated, and irreversible). Your goal is to recognize the clinical signs and symptoms of shock in its earliest phase and begin immediate treatment before permanent damage occurs. To do so, you must be aware of the subtle signs exhibited while the body is compensating effectively **Table 18-2 ▶** and treat the patient aggressively. Anticipate the potential for shock from the scene assessment and evaluation of the MOI. Recognize the signs of poor perfusion that precede hypotension, and do not rely on any one sign or symptom to determine the phase of shock the patient is going through. Always err on the side of caution when treating a potential shock patient. Rapid assessment and immediate transportation are essential to preserve any chance of survival.

Compensated Phase of Shock

The earliest stage of shock, in which the body can still compensate for blood loss, is called compensated shock. In this phase, the patient's level of responsiveness is a better indicator of tissue perfusion than most other vital signs. Release of chemical mediators by the autonomic nervous system as it recognizes a potential

Table 18-2	Compensated Versus Decompensated Hypoperfusion	
Compensated Hypoperfusion	**Decompensated Hypoperfusion**	
■ Agitation, anxiety, restlessness	■ Altered mental status (verbal to unresponsive)	
■ Sense of impending doom	■ Hypotension	
■ Weak, rapid (thready) pulse	■ Laboured or irregular breathing	
■ Clammy (cool, moist) skin	■ Thready or absent peripheral pulses	
■ Pallor with cyanotic lips	■ Ashen, mottled, or cyanotic skin	
■ Short of breath		
■ Nausea, vomiting	■ Dilated pupils	
■ Delayed capillary refill in infants and children	■ Diminished urine output (oliguria)	
■ Thirst	■ Impending cardiac arrest	
■ Normal BP		

At the Scene

Regardless of the type of bleeding—whether hidden in the body cavities or visible on the kitchen floor—all patients will proceed through the phases of shock if their bleeding is not controlled. In hemorrhagic shock, the specific phase of shock is a function of the percentage of blood volume lost. Because internal bleeding is more likely to be uncontrolled, stay alert for the subtle signs of shock and be aggressive in your management of its early phase to avoid the slippery downward slope of shock's later phases.

catastrophic event causes the arterial BP to remain normal or slightly elevated. There is an increase in the rate and depth of respirations as the body attempts to bring in more oxygen and remove more carbon dioxide. This effort helps to maintain the acid-base balance by creating respiratory alkalosis to offset the metabolic acidosis.

During the compensated phase of shock, BP is maintained. Blood loss in hemorrhagic shock can be estimated at 15% to 30% at this point. A narrowing of the pulse pressure (the difference between the systolic and diastolic pressures) also occurs. The pulse pressure reflects the tone of the arterial system and is more sensitive to changes in perfusion than the systolic or diastolic BP alone. Patients in the compensated phase will also have a positive orthostatic tilt test result.

Treatment at this stage of shock will typically result in recovery.

Decompensated Phase of Shock

The next stage of shock, when BP is falling, is decompensated shock (also called uncompensated shock or progressive shock). It occurs when blood volume drops by more than 30%. The compensatory mechanisms begin to fail, and signs and symptoms become much more obvious. The CO falls dramatically, leading to further reductions in BP and cardiac function. The signs and symptoms become more obvious as blood is shunted to the

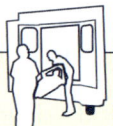

At the Scene

The term orthostatic has to do with positioning. Orthostatic hypotension, for example, is a drop in systolic BP when moving from a sitting to a standing position. An orthostatic tilt test is used to determine dehydration or hypovolemia. Blood pressure and pulse are measured as patients are lying, seated, and standing. A positive tilt test result occurs if the patient becomes dizzy, has a pulse increase of at least 20 beats/min, or has a systolic BP decrease of at least 20 mm Hg.

brain, heart, and kidneys. At this point, vasoconstriction can have a disastrous effect if allowed to continue. Cells in the nonperfused tissues become hypoxic, leading to anaerobic metabolism. Treatment at this stage will sometimes result in recovery.

Blood pressure may be the last measurable factor to change in shock. The body has several automatic mechanisms to compensate for initial blood loss and to help maintain BP. Thus, by the time you detect a drop in BP, shock is well developed. This is particularly true in infants and children, whose BP may be maintained until they have lost more than half of their blood volume.

Irreversible (Terminal) Phase of Shock

The last phase of shock, when this condition has progressed to a terminal stage, is irreversible shock. Arterial BP is abnormally low (typically in hemorrhagic shock there is a 40% or greater blood volume loss). A rapid deterioration of the cardiovascular system occurs that cannot be reversed by compensatory mechanisms or medical interventions. Life-threatening reductions in CO, BP, and tissue perfusion are observed. Blood is shunted away from the liver, kidneys, and lungs to keep the heart and brain perfused. Cells begin to die. Even if the cause of shock is treated and reversed, vital organ damage cannot be repaired, and the patient will eventually die. Even aggressive treatment at this stage does not usually result in recovery.

The Clinical Picture of Hypovolemic Shock

Most of the typical symptoms and signs of shock result from inadequate tissue oxygenation and the body's attempts to compensate for volume loss. Probably the earliest signs of shock are restlessness and anxiety: The patient looks scared! The decline in tissue perfusion is setting off alarms all over the body, to which the patient responds with a feeling of apprehension. If conscious, the patient may complain of thirst, reflecting the deficit of fluids in the body; at the same time, the patient may feel nauseated and even vomit. The diversion of blood flow away from low-priority peripheral tissues causes the skin to become pale, cold, and clammy; sometimes it has a mottled appearance. Meanwhile, the heart speeds up to circulate the remaining RBCs more rapidly, producing a rapid, weak pulse.

While the arteries are constricting and the heart is speeding up, the brain discovers that it is not getting enough oxygen. It assumes that the lungs must be malfunctioning, so the respiratory centre in the brain stem signals the respiratory muscles to speed up their activity. The result is rapid, shallow breathing (tachypnea).

As bleeding continues, the BP finally falls in the shock patient. Do not wait until the BP falls before you suspect shock and begin treatment! Falling BP is a *late* sign in shock, signaling the collapse of all compensatory mechanisms. Furthermore, the BP measured at the arm gives little information about perfusion of vital organs.

The goal in treating shock is to save the brain and kidneys; these organs must remain perfused if the patient is to survive and return to a healthy life. The best indication of brain perfusion is the patient's state of consciousness. If the patient is conscious and alert, the brain is being perfused adequately no matter what the sphygmomanometer says. If the patient is confused, disoriented, or unconscious, perfusion of the brain is likely inadequate. Kidney perfusion can be gauged by urine output in a catheterized patient. Adequately perfused kidneys put out at least 30 to 50 ml of urine per hour; poorly perfused kidneys shut down and stop putting out any urine.

In the prehospital setting—where patients will not ordinarily have urinary catheters—you can estimate the patient's peripheral perfusion by testing for capillary refill, although this is not the most reliable indicator. To do so, press on one of the patient's fingernails until it blanches, then release the pressure. If the skin under the nail doesn't "pink up" within 2 seconds (about as long as it takes to say "good capillary refill"), peripheral perfusion is compromised. To determine how well the *vital* organs are being perfused, you must rely on the patient's state of consciousness.

General Assessment of a Patient With Suspected Shock

The general assessment of a patient who is suspected of having hypoperfusion or shock follows the plan reinforced throughout this book. After sizing up the scene for hazards, taking BSI precautions, and addressing the need for additional help, begin the initial assessment.

Include a quick assessment of the MOI. For a patient with suspected shock, this information can give you clues about the causes and the extent of any bleeding (whether internal or external) or the causes of nonhemorrhagic shock.

Start the assessment by forming an initial diagnosis. Next, assess the patient's mental status (using AVPU) and manage any life threats to airway, breathing, and circulation. In conscious patients, you will usually assess the pulse at the radius; in unconscious patients, you will typically take the carotid pulse in the neck. The radial pulse can give you clues about the phase of shock and the patient's ability to compensate for shock. Ask yourself, "Is the radial pulse strong and regular, or weak and thready, or irregular?" If the radial pulse is barely palpable, yet the patient is sitting up and talking to you with a bullet hole in the abdomen, remember that the purpose of the shock syndrome is to keep the brain perfused—but the reduction in the radial pulse is an indicator that the systolic BP is dropping fast. In such a case, you may even decide that you

simply cannot take the time to measure the patient's BP, because you already know the patient is hypotensive (indicating decompensated shock) and immediate transport to the ED is the best course of action.

Patients with shock will usually be prioritized as "high." If the shock originates from a medical problem, the patient should be fast-tracked through the assessment of the chief complaint (OPQRST). In the more likely case—that the patient has had some sort of trauma—the MOI will guide your rapid trauma assessment of the major body cavities and regions.

Documentation and Communication

> Recording frequent serial vital signs—and observing perfusion indicators such as skin condition and mental status—will give you a window into the progression of shock. Use your documentation to remind you to suspect shock early and treat it aggressively.

The SAMPLE history and the baseline vital signs come next; they can be done en route to the ED along with your ongoing assessment. Time is of the essence in shock cases, so focus on moving toward the ED and keep the on-scene care to the essential items that must be done before moving the patient (that is, ABCs and spinal immobilization). Unless the patient is pinned and there may be a delay in extrication, delay inserting IV lines until en route to the ED.

Shock is considered hypovolemic or hemorrhagic until proven otherwise. **Table 18-3 ▶** summarizes the hemodynamic parameters in the differentiation of shock. The phase of shock in hypovolemic or hemorrhagic shock (compensated, decompensated, or terminal/irreversible) relates to the percentage of blood loss. The percentage blood loss is easily remembered by thinking of the score in a tennis game: 15% to 30% compensated, 30% to 40% decompensated, greater than 40% irreversible.

Management of a Patient With Suspected Shock

As with any patient, airway and ventilatory support take top priority when treating a patient with suspected shock. Maintain an open airway, and suction as needed. Give high-flow supplemental oxygen via nonrebreathing mask or assist ventilation with a bag-valve-mask device. Consider early definitive management in patients who are unable to maintain their own airway. Control any external hemorrhage, and try to estimate the amount of blood lost. Look for signs of internal hemorrhage, and consider the potential for loss in the area of suspected hemorrhage. For example, a patient may lose as much as 1 l of blood in the tissues of the thigh in a closed, uncomplicated femur fracture. Consider the MOI, and maintain a high index of suspicion for occult injuries, especially when the patient has signs of shock with no obvious cause.

Without delaying time at the scene, establish IV access with two large-bore cannulas (14 or 16 gauge) and administer IV fluid to replace blood loss. Isotonic crystalloids, such as normal saline or lactated Ringer's, should be used (synthetic solutions may also be used). Solutions of dextrose in water are not effective for resuscitation of trauma patients. The goal of volume replacement is to maintain perfusion without increasing internal or uncontrollable external hemorrhage. For this reason, most protocols advise administration of IV fluid in boluses of 20 ml/kg until radial pulses return. The presence of radial pulses equates to a systolic BP of 80 to 90 mm Hg, which is generally sufficient to perfuse the brain and other vital organs. In certain cases of shock, especially those caused by penetrating trauma, fluid therapy to maintain the systolic BP at approximately 80 mm Hg may be safer for the patient than to attempt restoration of normotension, which may aggravate ongoing bleeding.

Hypoperfusion with an unstable pelvis is the primary indication for use of the PASG/MAST. Conditions of decreased SVR not corrected by other means, such as increasing fluid volume in cases of neurogenic shock, may also benefit from use of the PASG/MAST. Effects resulting from inflation of the PASG/MAST include an increased arterial BP above the garment, increased SVR, immobilization of the pelvis and possibly the lower extremities, and increased intra-abdominal pressure. Because

use of the device is highly controversial, it is imperative that you follow local protocols.

If the patient exhibits signs of a tension pneumothorax, perform needle chest decompression to improve CO. In cases of suspected cardiac tamponade, you must recognize the need for expeditious transport for pericardiocentesis at the ED. Both of these conditions further impair circulation by compressing the heart and decreasing CO.

Nonpharmacologic interventions for shock include proper positioning of the patient, prevention of hypothermia, and rapid transport. Apply the cardiac monitor, and be alert for possible arrhythmias. When making your transport decision, consider the need for a regional trauma centre. If travel time is lengthy, air medical transportation may be the best option. Provide psychological support en route; speak calmly and reassuringly to the patient throughout assessment, prehospital care, and transport.

Skill Drill 18-2 ▶ provides a review of shock management:

1. Use PPE. Make sure the patient has an open airway, and check breathing and pulse. In general, keep the patient in a supine position. Patients who have experienced a severe heart attack or who have lung disease may find it easier to breathe in the Fowler's or semi-Fowler's position. Always provide supplemental oxygen, assist with ventilation as needed, and continue to monitor the patient's breathing (Step 1).

Table 18-3 Differentiation of Shock

Characteristics

Origin	Etiology	BP	Pulse	Skin	Lungs	EMS Treatment
↓ Pump performance	Cardiogenic	↓	↓ → ↑	Pale, cool, moist	Crackles	Low-dose dopamine
↓ Fluid volume	Hypovolemic, hemorrhagic	↓	↑	Pale, cool, moist	Clear	IV fluids
Vessels or container dilates: maldistribution of blood; low peripheral resistance	Neurogenic	↓	↓	Flushed, dry, warm	Clear	IV fluids, atropine, high-dose dopamine, norepinephrine
	Septic	↓	↑	Flushed or pale, hot or cool, moist	Crackles if pulmonary origin	IV fluids, high-dose dopamine, norepinephrine
	Anaphylactic	↓	↑	Flushed, warm, moist	May have wheezes; may be ↓ with no sounds	Epinephrine, diphenhydramine, salbutamol, ipratropium, corticosteroids

Hemodynamic Parameters

Parameter	Hypovolemic	Cardiac	Neurogenic	Septic
Mean arterial pressure	↓	↓	↓	↓
HR	↑	↑ or ↓	↓	↑
Central venous pressure	↓	variable	↓	↑
CO	↓	↓	↓	↑ then ↓
Peripheral vascular resistance	↑	↑	↓	↑
pH	↓	↓	↓	↓
Pao_2	↓	↓	↓	↓
$Paco_2$	↓	↓	Increase and decrease the rate	↓

2. Control all obvious external bleeding. Place dry, sterile dressings over the bleeding sites, and secure them with pressure bandages (Step 2).

3. Splint bone or joint injuries to minimize pain and bleeding, which can aggravate shock. Splinting also prevents the ends of the broken bone from further damaging adjacent soft tissue and, in general, makes it easier to move the patient. To minimize time spent on the scene, you may use a backboard as a temporary splint until you are headed to the ED. Handle the patient gently and no more than is necessary (Step 3). Use PASG/MAST only with the approval of direct medical control or established local protocols.

4. To prevent the loss of body heat, place blankets under and over the patient. Do not overload the patient with covers or attempt to warm the body too much, however; the goal is to maintain a normal body temperature. Do not use external heat sources, such as hot water bottles or heating pads because they may cause vasodilation and decrease BP even more (Step 4).

5. Once you have positioned the patient on a backboard or a stretcher, place him or her in the Trendelenburg position: Raise the foot of the backboard or stretcher about 30 cm. If the patient is not on a backboard and no lower extremity or back fractures are suspected, place the patient in the shock position: Elevate the patient's legs 30 cm by propping them up on several blankets or other stable objects. These positions help blood return from the extremities to the core of the body, where it is needed most. Patients with respiratory distress do not generally benefit from a Trendelenburg position; it may aggravate breathing because the abdominal organs push against the diaphragm (Step 5).

Skill Drill 18-2: Treating Shock

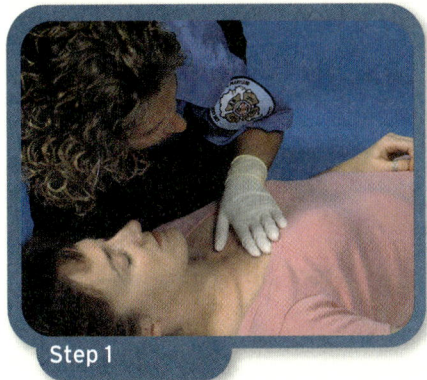

Step 1

Keep the patient supine, open the airway, and check breathing and pulse. Give high-flow supplemental oxygen, and assist ventilations if needed.

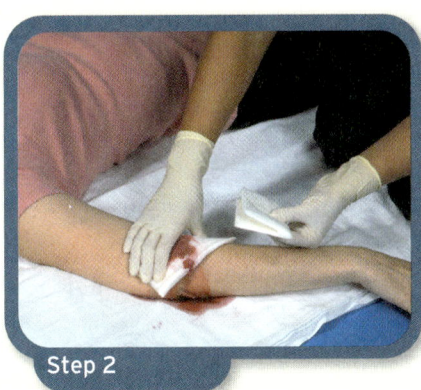

Step 2

Control obvious external bleeding.

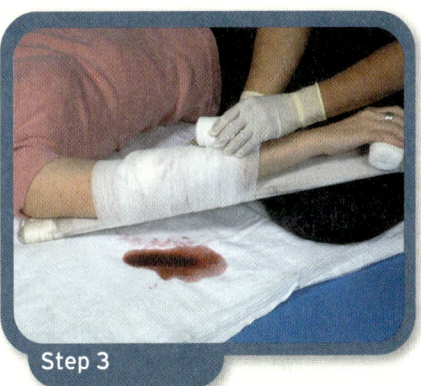

Step 3

Splint broken bones or joint injuries.

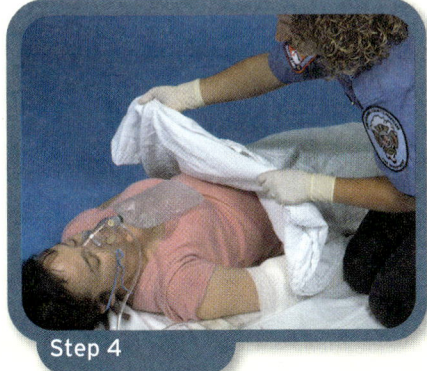

Step 4

Place blankets under and over the patient.

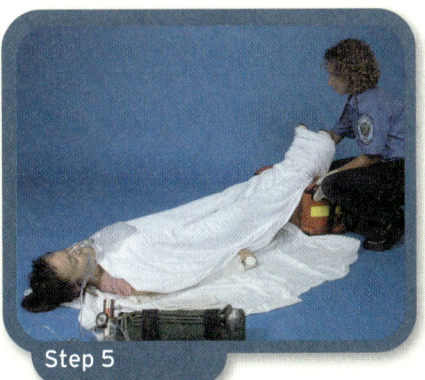

Step 5

If no fractures are suspected, elevate the legs 30 cm. Insert an IV line, and administer warm fluid en route to the ED. Insert an IV line at the scene only if transport of the patient is delayed (such as if the patient is pinned).

IV Therapy

Intravenous lines are inserted for one of two general purposes: to provide a route for immediate replacement of fluid in patients who have already lost significant volumes or to provide a route for potential fluid replacement in patients who are at risk of losing significant volumes of fluid or blood. The IV fluid of choice will be normal saline or lactated Ringer's.

Specifically, all patients in hypovolemic shock need IV fluid replacement. In addition, IV access should be obtained in patients who are likely to develop hypovolemic shock because they have one or more of the following conditions: profuse external bleeding, internal bleeding, vaginal bleeding, blunt trauma to the abdomen, fracture of the pelvis or femur, severe or widespread burns, heat exhaustion, intractable vomiting or diarrhea, and neurogenic shock or septic shock. As always, consult your local or regional protocols regarding access and fluid administration in the setting of shock.

In case of need for emergency administration of drugs, IV lines should also be inserted to keep a vein open. When a patient has poor CO (as in shock), blood is shunted away from the skin and skeletal muscles. Thus, drugs administered subcutaneously or intramuscularly are absorbed at a low and unpredictable rate. Giving a drug directly into the vein ensures that the desired dose of the drug reaches the circulation. Patients who need a vein kept open include those at risk of cardiac arrest (it's easier to start the IV before the arrest) and patients who may need parenteral medication (such as patients with seizures, diabetes, congestive heart failure, or coma).

The IV flow rate is typically determined by local protocol. The decision on flow rates usually reflects the patient's presumptive diagnosis and the condition of his or her lungs (wet or dry), and takes into account whether the IV line was inserted for fluid administration to keep the vein open for future medication administration. **Table 18-4** shows the BP indicators that are often referenced when determining IV flow rates for patients with dry lungs (not pulmonary edema).

Table 18-4	IV Fluid Therapy for Adult Patients in Suspected Shock
Adult Systolic BP (mm Hg)	**Fluid Volume (presumes dry lungs)***
Normotensive (100 to 130; higher end depends on age)	Fluid challenge of 250 ml normal saline, and reevaluate patient
Hypotensive (80 to 90)	Fluid challenge of 500 ml normal saline, and reevaluate patient
Severe hypotension (50 to 80)	Fluid challenge of 1 l normal saline, then titrate additional fluid to achieve low end or normotensive state

*Fluid therapy for burn patients should follow the Parkland formula (see Chapter 20).

Volume Expanders and Plasma Substitutes

Hypovolemic shock should be treated with volume expanders to replace what has been lost or to "fill the container" in relative hypovolemia. For cardiogenic shock, cautious use of volume expanders may increase preload and, subsequently, CO. Positive cardiac inotropic drugs may be administered to increase the strength of contractions, along with rate-altering medications to further enhance perfusion. An example is epinephrine, which serves both purposes with its beta-1 effects.

The vasodilation that accompanies distributive shock creates relative hypovolemia. Treatment involves volume expanders and positive cardiac inotropic drugs. Volume expanders are also indicated for obstructive shock and spinal shock.

A variety of macromolecular solutions have colloidal and osmotic properties similar to those of plasma and are used to maintain circulatory volume in the emergency treatment of shock. Although such solutions cannot replace the RBCs, platelets, or plasma proteins lost in hemorrhage, they are more readily available than whole blood or plasma in an emergency because they do not require typing and can be carried in the ambulance. Furthermore, during multiple-casualty incidents, the supply of blood and blood products may not be adequate, and substitutes must be used. Available plasma substitutes and volume expanders include dextran, plasma protein fractions, and polygeline.

Given that prehospital research has yet to show dextran as superior to crystalloid solution administration, medical directors are not likely to approve its use in the prehospital setting at this time.

Crystalloids

Crystalloids are solutions that do not contain proteins or other large molecules; that is, they are noncolloids. Their effects in restoring volume in shock are usually quite transitory because the fluid rapidly equilibrates across the capillary walls into the tissues. For example, approximately 60% of infused normal saline, when given as a bolus, diffuses out of the intravascular space within 20 minutes of administration. Thus, when noncolloid solutions are used in the treatment of hemorrhagic shock, you need to give two to three times the volume of blood lost.

Crystalloids are clearly the fluids of choice when only salt and water have been lost, such as in dehydration. Where debate continues, however, is about the role of crystalloids versus colloids in the treatment of shock. Despite a great deal of research on the subject, no overwhelming evidence supports one therapeutic approach over the other. Until such evidence is forthcoming, practical considerations will continue to favour the use of crystalloids for initial fluid resuscitation in the prehospital setting.

The crystalloids most commonly used for that purpose are normal saline and lactated Ringer's solution. Normal saline is simply sodium chloride (0.9% NaCl) in water at a concentration isotonic with the extracellular fluid. Lactated Ringer's solution is similarly constituted but includes small amounts of potassium and calcium. Lactated Ringer's solution contains 28 mEq of lactate as well, which is added as a buffer (the liver breaks lactate down into bicarbonate). None of these solutions is superior to the others for acute resuscitation, so the choice remains a matter of the physician's preference.

Recently, there has been considerable interest in the use of hypertonic saline solution (7.5% NaCl solution) for emergency treatment of blood loss. Infusing a hypertonic solution should, in theory, attract interstitial fluid into the vascular space, so such solutions should, at least temporarily, improve intravascular volume. This solution seems to be an effective plasma expander, with infusion of 250 ml producing the same effect as infusion of 2 to 3 l of isotonic crystalloid solution. The effectiveness of this regimen in humans and its ability to improve survival rates over those seen with use of isotonic solution remain to be demonstrated.

Management of Specific Types of Shock

The following sections provide guidance for treatment of specific types of shock. In all cases, be aggressive during the compensated phase of shock to avoid the need to make up for fluid loss if the patient moves into the decompensated phase of shock. If the patient may be in cardiogenic shock, fluids are still indicated, but you must be diligent about monitoring the lung sounds so as to not overload the patient.

Hypovolemic and Hemorrhagic Shock

The priorities in treating a patient in hemorrhagic or hypovolemic shock are the same as in treating any other patient—namely, the ABCs. Establish and maintain an open airway. Keep suction at hand to clear the mouth and pharynx if the patient should vomit. Administer supplemental oxygen, and assist ventilation as needed. Control bleeding, if present, by using direct pressure over the site of external bleeding. Apply the PASG/MAST, if it is part of your local protocol, and begin transport.

Insert at least one, and preferably two, large-bore peripheral IV lines (14 to 16 gauge). Give normal saline or lactated Ringer's solution. For guidance, refer to the IV fluid flow rates in Table 18-4 and to your local protocol. Run in the first 500-ml "fluid challenge" as fast as it will flow, and then reassess the patient to see the impact of the intervention. If warmed fluids are available, consider their use as well. There is growing evidence that aggressive use of crystalloid to resuscitate a patient with hypovolemic shock due to blunt trauma may actually be harmful. While not definitive, recent research suggests that allowing the systolic blood pressure to remain low, in the range of 70 to 80, may actually improve survival compared to resuscitating the patient until their blood pressure is in the normal range. While this evidence is new, local and regional EMS protocols and paramedic practice may change to conservative use of crystalloid resuscitation in patients with hypovolemic shock due to blunt trauma. Paramedics should consult their protocols to determine fluid resuscitation guidelines in their service.

Do not give the patient anything by mouth because he or she is very likely to vomit. Keep the patient at normal temperature, which usually means covering the patient with a blanket—patients in hypovolemic shock are often unable to conserve body heat effectively and are easily chilled. Place the patient in a position with the head elevated 15° to 30° and the legs propped up 30° on pillows (injuries permitting).

Monitor the ECG rhythm because any critically ill or injured patient is apt to have arrhythmias. Also monitor the state of consciousness, pulse, and BP. In a patient with substantial vasoconstriction, the BP sounds may be difficult to hear, especially in the

You are the Paramedic Part 4

Luckily, a paramedic from another unit was able to drive your ambulance, so you and your paramedic partner can focus on the patient for the entire 15-minute trip to the hospital. You insert a large-bore IV cannula and give normal saline, with a pressure infuser attached to the bag. You have just enough time to repeat the initial assessment before you call the ED to report the patient's condition. The physician advises you to hold off on inflation of the PASG/MAST and insert a second IV line. Meanwhile, your partner prepares to begin ventilatory assistance with a bag-valve-mask device. The patient's mental status has diminished, signaling he is truly fighting for his life.

Reassessment	Recording Time: 15 Minutes
Skin	Pale, cool, clammy
Pulse	120 beats/min; thready and getting difficult to palpate
ECG	Sinus tachycardia with occasional premature ventricular contractions
Blood pressure	Unobtainable
Respirations	28 breaths/min, shallow
Sao$_2$	86% with bag-valve-mask ventilation and supplemental oxygen
Pupils	Midsize and sluggish

When you return to the ED after another call, about 4 hours later, you check on the young man. According to the ED physician, the patient is still holding on after a few hours of intensive surgery. Apparently, he had major internal bleeding and damage to his stomach and spleen and major vessel damage from a bullet fragment. The ED physician states that in this case, the patient's best chance is a dose of the "bright lights and cold steel" of the operating suite. Because of your quick judgment about how to save time on the scene and your willingness to call ahead so the ED was ready, the patient made it to the operating suite about 35 minutes after the shooting.

8. Without interventions in the prehospital setting, how long would this patient have lived?

9. What is the benefit of calling ahead and focusing on the time factor?

prehospital setting. If you can feel a pulse over the femoral artery but not over the radial artery, for example, the systolic BP is probably somewhere between 70 and 80 mm Hg.

Cardiogenic Shock

Prolonged efforts to stabilize the condition of a patient in cardiogenic shock in the prehospital setting are not recommended. Because this is a time-sensitive patient, you should expedite transport as quickly as possible. Place the patient in a supine position, secure the airway, monitor the SpO2, and administer supplemental oxygen via a nonrebreathing mask at 12 to 15 l/min. Apply ECG electrodes, and document the initial rhythm. Your IV access should be with a crystalloid solution. Auscultate the lungs; if they are clear and protocols allow, try a fluid challenge of 200 ml to increase the preload and evaluate the effects on the BP and lung sounds.

Some EMS systems advocate the use of dopamine (Intropin) at low doses in the beta range (5 µg/kg/min) if the patient has a MAP of less than 60 mm Hg. Elevating the BP by using high-dose dopamine in the alpha range may be temporarily ordered by direct medical control at the expense of other target organs. In such a case, anticipate very rapid tachycardia that could adversely impact ventricular filling. Combination drug therapy is often needed at the hospital (eg, dopamine plus dobutamine, or norepinephrine) while awaiting cardiac catheterization, hemodynamic monitoring catheters, and insertion of an intra-aortic balloon pump.

Neurogenic Shock

The prehospital care of a patient with suspected neurogenic shock is similar to the general management approach for any patient with shock. In addition, the patient should be immobilized to minimize further movement and injury to the spine. Specific concerns relate to keeping the patient warm because a spinal injury can disrupt the thermoregulatory mechanisms and leave the patient vulnerable to hypothermia.

Another specific concern relates to the issue of fluid therapy. Determine the necessity for IV fluids based on the patient's hemodynamic status. Maintain adequate hydration and volume status to keep the systolic BP at 90 mm Hg or higher. General hemodynamic resuscitation includes volume loading with normal saline IV fluid boluses in 200-ml increments up to 2 l through a large-bore IV cannula. If possible, use warm fluid to prevent hypothermia.

In pure neurogenic shock not associated with hypovolemic shock, vagal blockers—such as atropine, 0.5 mg, by rapid IV push (up to a maximum of 3 mg) if the pulse remains bradycardic—and pressor agents—such as a dopamine drip beginning at 10 µg/kg/min and titrating to 20 µg/kg/min—may be used to better advantage than overhydrating the patient. Monitor the patient's response to vasopressors because it may be less than expected owing to the compromise of the sympathetic nervous system.

Anaphylactic Shock

In a case involving shock due to a severe allergic reaction, you need to act fast. Remove the inciting cause if possible. Resolve any immediate life threats to the ABCs, which may require aggressive airway management and supplemental oxygen administration. Evaluate the patient's ventilatory status and the need for bag-valve-mask device assistance.

Provide cardiovascular support with IV fluid challenges of crystalloid solution. Reverse the target-organ effect by administering epinephrine or a vasopressor such as dopamine (Intropin) in high doses. Consider the need for a bronchodilator such as salbutamol or ipratropium (Atrovent). Impede further mediator release with an antihistamine such as diphenhydramine (Benadryl). If the patient has an epinephrine injector, such as an Epi-Pen, consider using it and taking a spare along to the hospital because its effect will wear off quickly.

▌ Transportation of Patients With Suspected Shock

If a patient is suspected to be in shock, transport is inevitable; the questions to be asked are simply when and where. Consideration for the priority of the patient and the availability of a regional trauma centre should be your concerns, and local transport protocols may specifically deal with these issues. Patients who have suspected shock, whether compensated or decompensated, will benefit from early surgical intervention and should be transported to a facility with those capabilities. Patients with cardiogenic shock may need to go to a hospital with comprehensive cardiac care capabilities (that is, a catheterization lab and heart surgery program). If a facility of this type is not readily available, direct medical control should help you make the transport decision. In some communities, this will involve transport to a local facility and transfer (often aeromedical) to a tertiary care facility with the appropriate facilities and staff to handle the patient's complex needs.

▌ Prevention Strategies

Of course the best prevention of shock would involve not having the incident that led to the shock in the first place! Probably the number one strategy that would prevent many lost lives is simply wearing seatbelts whenever driving or riding in a motor vehicle!

Prevention of shock and its deadly effects begins with your immediate assessment of the MOI, initial assessment findings, and the patient's clinical picture. Be alert, and search for early signs of shock. Don't rationalize irregularities away because they will soon become much more obvious if the patient truly is in shock—but by then it may be too late to stop the patient from sliding down the slippery slope. For example, at the scene of a motor vehicle collision where the patient's brand-new car has a dented driver's door, don't say to yourself, "The patient has tachycardia because he is upset!" Instead, consider the MOI and decide to manage the suspected shock aggressively now.

You are the Paramedic Summary

1. Does the lack of significant visible bleeding and the fact that he is alert indicate that this patient is not bleeding seriously?

No—don't get caught in that trap! The purpose of the compensatory mechanism in the early phase of shock is to ensure the brain is well perfused. If this mechanism is working, as one would expect early in blood loss, the patient would be alert. Don't confuse nervousness or anxiousness with an altered mental state, which implies diminished brain perfusion. As for the lack of visible bleeding, be aware that a patient can lose most of his or her blood volume into large cavities (such as the thigh, chest, or abdomen) without a drop of external blood.

2. What is the significance of time in this type of incident?

Set the timer on your digital watch because this patient does not have a lot of time to spare. In the "golden hour of trauma," a lot of things need to occur, so paramedics in the prehospital setting do not have any more than a "platinum 10 minutes" for the initial assessment and prehospital management of the patient.

3. On the basis of the information you have so far, and remembering that the patient weighs approximately 80 kg, how much blood did he have before the incident? How much could he have lost so far?

Based on 6% to 8% of the total body weight, this patient would have about 4.8 to 6.4 l of blood before the incident. Given that he has no palpable radial (peripheral) pulse but is still alert (and, thus, has a carotid pulse), one could estimate that his systolic BP is between 60 and 90 mm Hg. Rather than take the time at this point to ponder the exact reading, simply note that the patient is hypotensive—that is, he is in decompensated shock. In decompensated shock, this patient may have lost 30% of his blood volume, in this case some 4 units of blood.

4. What phase of shock is this patient in?

Because the patient has no radial pulse, he is hypotensive. He is therefore in the decompensated phase of shock.

5. Which BLS and ALS interventions would be most appropriate for this patient at this time? Should you insert an IV line at the scene?

The BLS treatment for this patient would be to administer high-concentration supplemental oxygen and consider the PASG/MAST if permitted by local protocols. If you suspect a spinal injury, rapidly immobilize the patient on a backboard; if no spinal injury is suspected, place the patient on the stretcher and take him to the ED. Perform the rapid trauma assessment and detailed physical examination en route to the hospital. The ALS interventions would involve two large-bore IV lines with normal saline wide open, ECG monitoring, and calling ahead to the ED so staff are prepared.

A paramedic could certainly provide another set of trained hands to help care for this patient and get him away from the scene quickly. The insertion of an advanced airway can help in the management of the patient should his level of consciousness decrease en route to the hospital. Critical trauma patients often have severe hypoxia and vomiting. A well-managed airway can help control these problems.

Intravenous access for fluid resuscitation is helpful but should not delay transport of a trauma patient in critical condition. Insert the large-bore IV lines en route to the ED; alternatively, you may insert them on the scene, but only while the paramedics are simultaneously packaging the patient for transport. Two arguments are put forth to explain why you should not wait at the scene to insert the IV line in a trauma patient.

First, paramedics usually infuse lactated Ringer's or normal saline, but what the patient in this late phase of hemorrhagic shock really needs is a colloid fluid expander followed by whole blood and likely a trip to the operating room to control bleeding. Although the fluid infused will expand the patient's circulating volume temporarily until it leaks out of the vascular space, it does not contain hemoglobin and, therefore, cannot carry oxygen. Most experts recommend switching to a colloid solution when 2 to 3 l of crystalloid solution is not enough to restore blood volume and whole blood is unavailable.

Second, if the patient was found in decompensated shock, you cannot catch up with the ongoing blood loss by inserting one or two large-bore lines at the scene. The mere time it takes to prep the site and equipment and make a successful venipuncture can add dramatically to the scene time as the patient continues to bleed. For the patient in this case, the paramedic unit should be called, and initiation of one or two IV lines is appropriate en route to the hospital. If the patient becomes unconscious, you should intubate the patient to ensure an adequate airway.

6. For this patient, is the Sp_{O_2} a helpful indicator?

This measurement has limited usefulness in this case. The Sp_{O_2} is only one of many indicators but is sometimes not accurate in low perfusion states. Go with the clinical signs and symptoms, and move fast!

7. Why weren't the baseline vital signs taken on the scene?

In the initial assessment, you discovered that the patient had a pulse and you "guesstimated" that he was hypotensive based on the location of the pulse. You also have a handle on his respirations, so the formal baseline vital signs can be delayed until you get going with this patient.

8. Without interventions in the prehospital environment, how long would this patient have lived?

If it took about 10 minutes for the patient to lose 30% of his blood volume into his belly, he has very little time. At 40% blood loss, his pulse is apt to be lost. He would be dying without your rapid interventions.

9. What is the benefit of calling ahead and focusing on the time factor?

With this patient bleeding so severely, time is precious and any intervention at the scene must be absolutely justified as essential and lifesaving. Otherwise, do it en route to the ED. Let the ED personnel know you are on the way so they can be ready to move the patient through the ED and to the "bright lights and cold steel" of the operating room and expertise of the surgeons.

Prep Kit

Ready for Review

- The cardiovascular system is designed to carry out one crucial job: keep blood flowing between the lungs and the peripheral tissues.
- Hemorrhage simply means bleeding.
  - Bleeding can range from a "nick" to a capillary while shaving, to a severely spurting artery from a deep slash with a knife, to a ruptured spleen from striking the steering column during a car collision.
  - External bleeding can usually be easily controlled by using direct pressure or a pressure bandage.
  - Internal bleeding is usually not controlled until a surgeon locates the source and sutures it closed.
- The assessment of any patient begins with a good scene assessment and proceeds to your general impression and initial assessment.
  - Once the scene is deemed safe to enter, you will need to wear the appropriate level of PPE.
  - Depending on the severity of bleeding and your initial diagnosis, this will entail gloves, mask, eyeshield, and, when the patient is very bloody or blood is spurting, a gown.
- In case of hemorrhage, the issue is not whether the patient will be transported, but rather how fast the transport decision should be made and where the patient should be taken for definitive care.
- Hypoperfusion occurs when the level of tissue perfusion decreases below normal.
  - Early decreased tissue perfusion may result in subtle changes, such as altered mental status, long before a patient's vital signs (that is, BP, pulse, respiratory rate) appear abnormal.
  - Shock refers to a state of collapse and failure of the cardiovascular system that leads to inadequate circulation, creating inadequate tissue perfusion.
- As with any patient, airway and ventilatory support take top priority when treating a patient with suspected shock.
- If a patient is suspected to be in shock, transport is inevitable; the questions to be asked are simply when and where.
  - Consideration for the priority of the patient and the availability of a regional trauma centre should be your concerns, and local transport protocols may specifically deal with these issues.
  - Patients who have suspected shock, whether compensated or decompensated, will benefit from early surgical intervention and should be transported to a facility with those capabilities.

- Prevention of shock and its deadly effects begins with your immediate assessment of the MOI, initial assessment findings, and the patient's clinical picture.
  - Be alert, and search for early signs of shock.

Vital Vocabulary

aerobic metabolism Metabolism that can proceed only in the presence of oxygen.

afterload The pressure in the aorta against which the left ventricle must pump blood.

anaerobic metabolism Metabolism that takes place in the absence of oxygen.

anaphylaxis A severe life-threatening allergic reaction to foreign protein or other substances.

angioedema Recurrent large areas of subcutaneous edema of sudden onset, usually disappearing within 24 hours, which is seen mainly in young women, frequently as a result of allergy to food or drugs.

blood The fluid that is pumped by the heart through the arteries, veins, and capillaries and consists of plasma and formed elements or cells, such as red blood cells, white blood cells, and platelets.

capacitance vessels The smallest venules.

cardiac output (CO) The amount of blood pumped through the circulatory system in 1 minute.

cardiogenic shock A condition caused by loss of 40% or more of the functioning myocardium; the heart is no longer able to circulate sufficient blood to maintain adequate oxygen delivery.

central shock A condition that consists of cardiogenic shock and obstructive shock.

compensated shock The early stage of shock, in which the body can still compensate for blood loss. The systolic blood pressure and brain perfusion are maintained.

decompensated shock The late stage of shock, when blood pressure is falling.

distributive shock A condition that occurs when there is widespread dilation of the resistance vessels, the capacitance vessels, or both.

ejection fraction The portion of the blood ejected from the ventricle during systole.

epistaxis A nosebleed.

erythrocytes Red blood cells.

hematochezia Passage of stools containing bright red blood.

hemoglobin The oxygen-carrying pigment in red blood cells.

hemorrhage Profuse bleeding.

hemostasis Stopping hemorrhage.

hypoperfusion A condition that occurs when the level of tissue perfusion decreases below that needed to maintain normal cellular functions.

hypovolemic shock A condition that occurs when the circulating blood volume is inadequate to deliver adequate oxygen and nutrients to the body.

irreversible shock The final stage of shock, resulting in death.

leukocytes White blood cells.

melena Passage of dark, tarry stools.

multiple-organ dysfunction syndrome (MODS) A progressive condition usually characterized by combined failure of several organs, such as the lungs, liver, and kidney, along with some clotting mechanisms, which occurs after severe illness or injury.

neurogenic shock Circulatory failure caused by paralysis of the nerves that control the size of the blood vessels, leading to widespread dilation; seen in spinal cord injuries.

obstructive shock Shock that occurs when there is a block to blood flow in the heart or great vessels, causing an insufficient blood supply to the body's tissues.

orthostatic hypotension A drop in systolic blood pressure when moving from a sitting to a standing position.

perfusion The delivery of oxygen and nutrients to the cells, organs, and tissues of the body.

peripheral shock A condition that consists of hypovolemic shock and distributive shock.

plasma The fluid portion of the blood from which the cells have been removed.

platelets Small cells in the blood that are essential for clot formation.

pulse pressure The difference between the systolic and diastolic pressures.

resistance vessels The smallest arterioles.

sensitization Developing sensitivity to a substance that initially caused no allergic reaction.

septic shock Shock caused by severe infection, usually a bacterial infection.

shock An abnormal state associated with inadequate oxygen and nutrient delivery to the metabolic apparatus of the cell.

stroke volume The amount of blood that the left ventricle ejects into the aorta per contraction.

systemic inflammatory response syndrome (SIRS) The systemic inflammatory response to a variety of severe clinical insults.

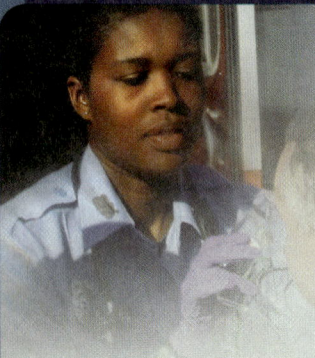

Assessment in Action

You are called to a shopping centre by security on a Friday night for a person who was assaulted. When you arrive, you see a man in his late 20s who is sitting on a bench holding a towel to his face. There is a trail of blood from the men's restroom, and the towel is dripping with blood. According to the security officer, there was a fight in the restroom and they found this man, Joey, stumbling and drenched in blood. Apparently, a couple of gang members beat him up and slashed his face and neck with razors.

You quickly don PPE and ensure that the scene is safe. The police are just arriving behind you. The initial assessment reveals an alert and oriented but anxious patient who has an open and clear airway, has 26 shallow breaths/min and has a very weak and thready radial pulse. He has external bleeding from the face and neck, which your partner is attempting to control with direct pressure. His carotid pulse is 120 beats/min, and his skin is pale, cool, and clammy. You begin to administer supplemental oxygen with a nonrebreathing mask at 15 l/min and lay the patient down with his feet raised so you can do a rapid trauma assessment.

Meanwhile, your supervisor arrives with the stretcher so the patient can be rapidly removed from the scene. The assessment reveals that there may also be potential for internal bleeding because the patient was kicked in the ribs and abdomen when he was down on the floor. You quickly load the patient and decide to insert two IV lines en route to the regional trauma centre. Your supervisor locks his vehicle so you can have plenty of personnel working up your patient en route to the ED because there is much to do to save his life.

1. **This patient has one very obvious injury involving:**
   A. a flail chest.
   B. the facial and neck lacerations.
   C. a ruptured spleen.
   D. an injured left kidney.

2. **With a patient who has so much obvious external bleeding, you should don which PPE?**
   A. Disposable gloves
   B. An eye shield
   C. A disposable mask
   D. All of the above

3. **An example of an injury that is potentially life threatening yet difficult to see in this patient would be:**
   A. internal bleeding.
   B. the facial laceration.
   C. the neck laceration.
   D. head trauma.

4. **What is the significance of the weak radial pulse in this patient?**
   A. It demonstrates he is generally physically fit.
   B. It demonstrates that his bleeding is actually minimal.
   C. It indicates that his systolic blood pressure is already dropping.
   D. It indicates that his body is compensating well for the injuries.

5. **What is the significance of the pale, cool, and clammy skin in this patient?**
   A. It demonstrates that he was on a cold floor.
   B. It shows that the vessels in the skin have been constricting.
   C. It shows that the vessels in the skin have been dilating.
   D. It shows that he has an adequate supply of blood to the brain.

6. **With the patient alert and oriented at this point, how serious is his condition?**
   A. Not very serious at all once a bandage is applied to the face and neck.
   B. The lacerations are serious and will need to be sutured in the ED.
   C. Very serious owing to the combination of external and internal bleeding.
   D. Very serious owing to the symptoms of a head injury.

7. **With deep lacerations to the face and neck, how should the bleeding be controlled?**
   A. Pressure point
   B. Tourniquet
   C. Cold application
   D. Direct pressure

8. **What phase of shock is this patient in at this point?**
   A. Terminal
   B. Decompensated
   C. Compensated
   D. Guarded

9. **What type of shock does this patient potentially have?**
   A. Septic
   B. Neurogenic
   C. Hemorrhagic
   D. Anaphylactic

10. **Aside from controlling the external bleeding, giving supplemental oxygen, and using the Trendelenburg position, what other treatment would be appropriate for this patient en route to the regional trauma centre?**
    A. Two large-bore IV lines for normal saline
    B. The PASG/MAST inflated until the Velcro crackles
    C. Cooling the patient with chilled IV fluid
    D. A dopamine drip in the alpha dose range

Challenging Question

11. **If the patient weighed 90 kg and you obtained a BP of 86 on palpation en route to the ED, what phase of shock is he in, how much blood did he have (roughly) before the assault, and how much blood has he already lost?**

Points to Ponder

You respond to the scene of a single motor vehicle collision in which a 45-year-old woman is walking around the scene. It is obvious from the spiderlike crack in the windshield and her forehead laceration that she struck the glass with her head. She is nervous that she will get in trouble and states she was wearing a seatbelt and did not hit the windshield. You also note the smell of alcohol on her breath, and she denies any medical history. She allowed you to feel her weak rapid radial pulse but now is refusing to let you do any further assessment. Her head lacerations are no longer bleeding, although she has plenty of blood on her white blouse. She is refusing to go to the hospital, stating there is nothing wrong with her. The police officer, who has been dealing with the traffic congestion, states he is going to administer a breathalyzer test.

How should you deal with this patient's refusal to go to the hospital?

Issues: MOI for Internal Injury, Recognition of Shock, Estimating Phases of Shock, Compensation Versus Decompensation During Shock, Treatment Plan for a Patient With Suspected Shock, and Patient Refusal.

19 Soft-Tissue Injuries

Competency Areas

Area 4: Assessment and Diagnostics

4.3.a Conduct primary patient assessment and interpret findings.

4.3.b Conduct secondary patient assessment and interpret findings.

4.3.i Conduct integumentary system assessment and interpret findings.

Area 5: Therapeutics

5.6.d Treat penetration wound.

Area 6: Integration

6.1.a Provide care to patient experiencing illness or injury primarily involving cardiovascular system.

6.1.c Provide care to patient experiencing illness or injury primarily involving respiratory system.

6.1.f Provide care to patient experiencing illness or injury primarily involving integumentary system.

6.1.g Provide care to patient experiencing illness or injury primarily involving musculoskeletal system.

6.1.j Provide care to patient experiencing illness or injury primarily involving eyes, ears, nose, or throat.

6.1.n Provide care to patient experiencing illness or injury due to extremes of temperature or adverse environments.

6.1.o Provide care to patient based on understanding of common physiological, anatomical, incident, and patient-specific field trauma criteria that determine appropriate decisions for triage, transport, and destination.

Appendix 4: Pathophysiology

B. **Neurologic System**
Traumatic Injuries: Hematoma (epidural, subdural, subarachnoid)

G. **Integumentary System**
Traumatic Injuries: Lacerations/avulsions/abrasions

H. **Musculoskeletal System**
Soft Tissue Disorders: Amputation
Soft Tissue Disorders: Compartment syndrome
Soft Tissue Disorders: Contusions
Soft Tissue Disorders: Neocrotizing fasciitis
Inflammatory Disorders: Osteomyelitis

J. **Multisystem Diseases and Injuries**
Trauma: Crush Injuries

L. **Ears, Eyes, Nose, and Throat**
External, Middle, and Inner Ear Disorders: Traumatic ear injuries

Introduction

The skin is the largest organ of the human body and serves as the interface between the body and outside world. For that reason, injuries involving the skin are common. Injuries to the skin are often the most immediately obvious of a person's injuries, although not necessarily the most serious. An inexperienced paramedic is apt to be distracted by dramatic external wounds and neglect to check for higher-priority problems, such as an obstructed airway or significant hypotension. Paramedics can avoid making this critical mistake by ensuring that they have a thorough understanding of the anatomy and physiology of the skin.

This chapter describes each layer of this vital organ along with its function. It also describes soft-tissue injuries along with factors that inhibit normal healing. Finally, it looks at how to assess and manage crush injuries.

Incidence, Mortality, and Morbidity

The soft tissues of the body can be injured through a variety of mechanisms. A blunt injury occurs when the energy exchange between the patient and an object is more than the tissues can tolerate, as can happen in a motor vehicle collision that leads to the person striking the steering wheel. A penetrating injury occurs when an object, such as a bullet or knife, breaks through the skin and enters the body. Barotrauma injuries occur from sudden or extreme changes in air pressure, such as can occur during a scuba diving emergency. Burns may also result in soft-tissue injuries.

Soft-tissue trauma is the leading form of injury. In fact, wound care is one of the most frequently performed procedures in EDs. Most of these injuries require basic interventions

such as wound irrigation, dressing, bandaging, and limited suturing.

Death due to soft-tissue injury is often related to hemorrhage or infection. Uncontrolled hemorrhage can quickly lead to shock and death. When the skin barrier is breached, invading pathogens—bacteria, fungi, and viruses—can cause local or systemic infection. Infection can be life or limb threatening, especially in people with diabetes. Preventing soft-tissue injuries and their associated complications involves simple protective actions. The use of gloves when working with abrasive materials, for example, can prevent skin injuries. Workplace safety measures to reduce injury include use of safety devices to prevent interaction between machine parts and body parts. Teaching children to avoid using sharp objects also helps prevent injury. Plastic scissors, plastic knives, and plastic drinking cups are all designed to reduce the risk of cuts and other skin injuries among children.

Structure and Function of the Skin

The human skin is much more than a wrapping. Rather, skin, or integument, is a complex organ with a crucial role in maintaining the constancy of the internal environment (homeostasis):

- The skin protects the underlying tissue from injury, including that caused by extremes of temperature, ultraviolet radiation, mechanical forces, toxic chemicals, and invading microorganisms.
- The skin aids in temperature regulation, preventing heat loss when the core body temperature starts to fall and facilitating heat loss when core temperature rises.
- As a watertight seal, the skin prevents excessive loss of water from the body and drying of tissues, thereby helping

You are the Paramedic Part 1

While standing by at a high school football game, you and your partner witness a running back injure his right leg after a linebacker fell on him during a tackle. The patient, a 16-year-old male, has an open deformity to his right leg. The injury is actively bleeding and a bone is protruding through the skin. With the appropriate PPE in place, your partner stabilizes the injury site and applies direct pressure to control the bleeding. You perform an initial assessment.

Initial Assessment	Recording Time: 0 Minutes
Appearance	In severe pain
Level of consciousness	A (Alert to person, place, and day)
Airway	Patent; clear of secretions
Breathing	Increased respirations; adequate depth
Circulation	Open injury to leg (bleeding controlled); pulse, rapid and strong; skin, pink and diaphoretic

1. Does this patient require spinal motion restriction precautions? Why or why not?
2. What are your main concerns regarding this patient's injury?

maintain the chemical stability of the internal environment.

- The skin serves as a sense organ, keeping the brain informed about the external environment. Changes in temperature, touch, and body position and sensations of pain are mediated through the sense receptors in the skin.

Significant damage to the skin may make the body vulnerable to bacterial invasion, temperature instability, and major disturbances of fluid balance—precisely what happens when an injury results in an opening in the skin.

Epidermis

The skin is composed of two layers: the epidermis and the dermis Figure 19-1 ▾ . The epidermis, or outermost layer, is the body's first line of defence, the principal barrier against water, dust, microorganisms, and mechanical stress. It consists of five layers: an outermost layer (stratum corneum) of hardened, non-living cells, which are continuously shed through a process called desquamation; and four inner layers of living cells that constantly divide to give rise to the cells of the stratum corneum.

The deeper layers of the epidermis also contain variable numbers of cells bearing melanin granules; these cells are known as melanocytes. The darkness of a person's skin is directly proportional to the amount of melanin present.

Dermis

Underlying the epidermis is a tough, highly elastic layer of connective tissues called the dermis. This complex material is composed chiefly of collagen fibres, elastic fibres, and a mucopolysaccharide gel. Numerous fibroblasts—cells that secrete collagen, elastin, and ground substance—are found within the dermis as well. Collagen, a fibrous protein with a high tensile strength, gives the skin high resistance to breakage under mechanical stress. Elastin, as the name implies, imparts elasticity to the skin, allowing the skin to spring back to its usual contours. Ground substance, which is found in connective tissues in differing amounts, is a transparent mucopolysaccharide gel that gives the skin resistance to compression.

The dermis is subdivided into the papillary dermis and a reticular layer. The vasculature inside the papillary dermis serves two functions: It provides nutrients to the epidermis, and it aids in thermoregulation. Dilation of these vessels increases blood flow to the skin, allowing heat to dissipate. Conversely, blood vessel constriction results in retention of heat. The reticular layer is made of dense, irregular connective tissue, which provides strength and elasticity.

Macrophages and lymphocytes are also found within the dermal layer. Both are part of the inflammatory process and are responsible for combating microorganisms that breach the epidermal layer. Once a pathogen enters the dermis, macrophages and lymphocytes destroy the invading microorganism and signal other cells to migrate into the area. Physical injury will trigger mast cells to degranulate and synthesize special chemical mediators. The result is increased blood flow to the affected area, manifested as redness and warmth.

Several specialized structures can be identified in the dermis:

- **Nerve endings**—mediate the senses of touch, temperature, pressure, and pain.
- **Blood vessels**—carry oxygen and nutrients to the skin and remove carbon dioxide and metabolic waste products. Cutaneous blood vessels also have a crucial role in regulating body temperature by regulating the volume of blood that flows from the body's warm core to its cooler surface.
- **Sweat glands**—produce sweat and discharge it through ducts passing to the surface of the skin. Sweat consists of water and salts, and sweating is regulated through the action of the sympathetic nervous system. The average volume of sweat lost during 24 hours under normal conditions ranges from 500 to 1,000 ml; during strenuous exercise, however, sweat glands may secrete as much as

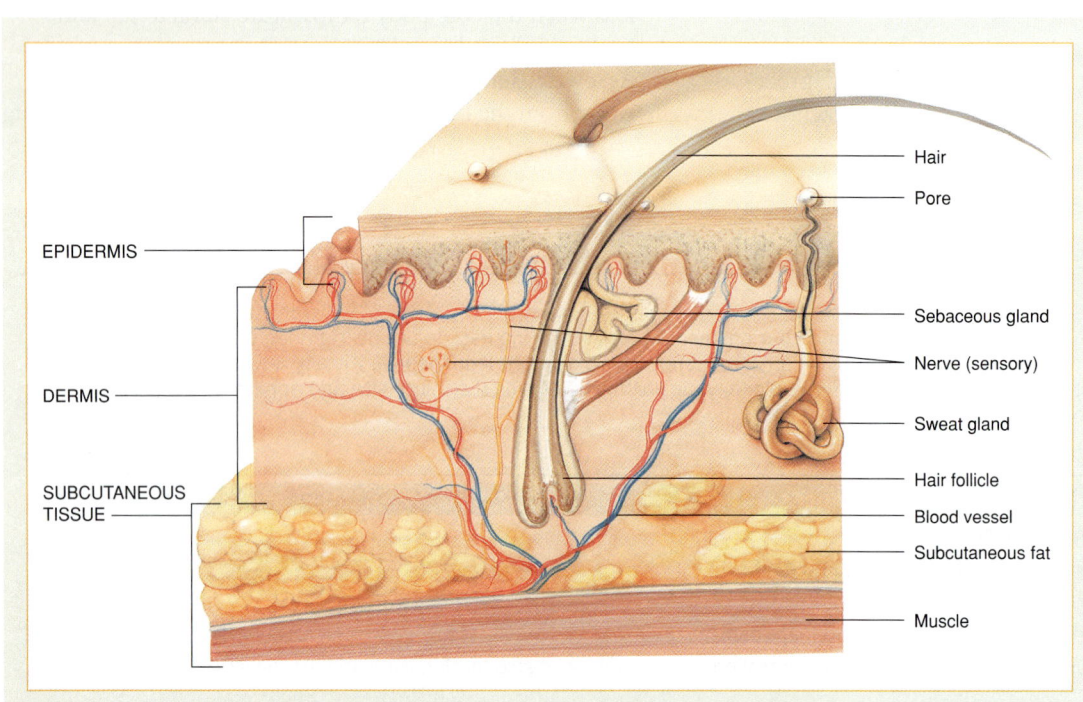

EPIDERMIS

DERMIS

SUBCUTANEOUS TISSUE

Hair
Pore
Sebaceous gland
Nerve (sensory)
Sweat gland
Hair follicle
Blood vessel
Subcutaneous fat
Muscle

Figure 19-1 The skin is composed of a tough external layer called the epidermis and a vascular inner layer called the dermis.

1,000 ml in an hour. This evaporation of water from the skin surface is one of the body's major mechanisms for shedding excess heat.

- **Hair follicles**—produce hair and enclose the hair roots. Each follicle contains a single hair. Attached to the hair follicle is a small muscle that, on contraction, causes the follicle to assume a more vertical position. Hairs in each part of the body have definite periods of growth, after which they are shed and replaced; scalp hair, for example, has a life span of 2 to 5 years and grows 1.5 to 3.9 mm per week.
- **Sebaceous gland**—located at the neck of each hair follicle, is a specialized secretory mechanism that produces an oily substance called sebum. The secretions of the sebaceous glands empty into the hair follicles and from there reach the surface of the skin. The precise function of sebum is not well understood, although it may keep the skin supple so that it doesn't crack.

Notes from Nancy

Sensations such as cold and fright stimulate the autonomic nervous system, which in turn brings about contraction of those muscles; the result is the appearance of the skin called "gooseflesh."

Subcutaneous Tissue

The layer of tissue beneath the dermis—that is, the subcutaneous layer (superficial fascia)—consists mainly of adipose tissue (fat). Blood vessels, lymph vessels, and hair follicle roots are also found in this layer. Subcutaneous fat insulates the underlying tissues from extremes of heat and cold. It also provides a cushion for underlying structures and an energy reserve for the body.

Deep Fascia

Below the subcutaneous tissue is a thick, dense layer of fibrous tissue known as the deep fascia. The deep fascia is composed of tough bands of tissue that ensheath muscles and other internal structures. It supports and protects underlying structures from injury. Muscles and bones are found below this layer.

Skin Tension Lines

The skin is arranged over the body structures in a manner that provides tension. This tautness varies by body region but occurs in patterns known as tension lines. Static tension develops over areas that have limited movement, such as the scalp. Lacerations occurring parallel to the skin tension lines may remain closed with little or no intervention. Larger wounds may be pulled open by the normal tension and require closure with sutures, staples, or a biodegradable "glue." Even small lacerations that lie perpendicular to the tension lines result in a wound that remains open. Healing occurs more slowly in an open wound, and abnormal scar formation is more likely.

Dynamic tension is found in areas that lie over muscle. The tension varies according to the contraction of the underlying muscle and subsequent movement of the skin. Open injuries to dynamic tension lines interfere with healing because they disrupt the clotting process and the tissue repair cycle, resulting in slowed healing and a tendency toward abnormal scar formation.

An abnormal scar may prompt the patient to seek scar revision—surgery to improve its appearance. The surgeon takes skin tension into account when determining the best procedure for revision. This factor must also be considered when wound debridement is necessary or when hospital personnel must remove an impaled object.

Wound Healing

A wound is any injury to the soft tissues—that is, an injury to the skin with or without involvement of the subcutaneous tissues and muscle. Most soft-tissue wounds are relatively low-priority injuries. Although they may be the most obvious and dramatic injuries, they are seldom the most serious of the patient's problems unless they compromise the airway or are associated with massive bleeding. Always search systematically and thoroughly for other injuries or life-threatening conditions before tending to soft-tissue trauma. *Don't let dramatic soft-tissue injuries distract you from thorough initial assessment!*

Pathophysiology of Wound Healing

Healing of wounds is a natural process that involves several overlapping stages, all directed toward the larger goal of maintaining homeostasis. Ultimately, the goal is for the body to return to a functional state, although the injured area may not always be restored to the preinjury condition.

Hemostasis

Among the primary concerns in wound healing is the cessation of bleeding. Loss of blood, internal or external, hinders the provision of vital nutrients and oxygen to the affected area. It also impairs the tissue's ability to eliminate wastes. The end result is abnormal or absent function, which interferes with homeostasis. To stop the flow of blood, the vessels, platelets, and clotting cascade must work in unison.

Injury to soft tissue causes chemicals in the vessel wall to be released. These chemicals constrict the blood vessels, resulting in less space through which blood can flow. The muscular layer in the arteries, arterioles, and some veins constricts to reduce the size of the lumen. Skeletal muscles also have a role in the constriction process. Because capillaries lack smooth muscle, bleeding continues, albeit at a slower rate.

Platelets are also activated by the release of these chemicals. Activated platelets adhere to the affected area and to other platelets. This aggregation of platelets forms a platelet plug.

Although not the permanent repair, the plug temporarily stops the blood loss and is the beginning of blood clot formation.

Inflammation

In inflammation (the next stage of wound healing), additional cells move into the damaged area to begin repair. White blood cells migrate to the area to combat pathogens that have invaded exposed tissue. Chemicals and proteins known as chemotactic factors are released and call repairing cells into the area. Granulocytes and macrophages, among the first restoration cells to arrive, engulf bacteria through phagocytosis, which involves ingestion of damaged cellular parts. Foreign products and bacteria can also be removed from the body by phagocytosis. Similarly, lymphocytes (a type of white blood cell) destroy bacteria and other pathogens.

Mast cells release histamine as part of the body's response in the early stages of inflammation. Histamine causes dilation of blood vessels, increasing blood flow to the injured area and resulting in a reddened, warm area immediately around the site. Histamine makes capillaries more permeable, and swelling may occur as fluid seeps out of these "leaky" capillaries.

Inflammation ultimately leads to the removal of foreign material, damaged cellular parts, and invading microorganisms from the wound site. Reconstruction of the injured region through epithelialization, neovascularization, and collagen synthesis can then begin.

Epithelialization

In the outer layer of skin, epithelial cells are stacked in layers. To replace the area damaged in a soft-tissue injury, a new layer of epithelial cells must be moved into this region—a process known as epithelialization. Cells from the stratum germinativum quickly multiply and redevelop across the edges of the wound. Except in cases of clean incisions, the appearance of the restructured area seldom returns to the preinjury state. For example, large wounds or injuries that result in significant disruption of the skin will often have incomplete epithelialization.

In persons with lightly pigmented skin, a pink line of scar tissue may signal the presence of collagen, a structural protein that has reinforced the damaged tissue. Despite the changed appearance, the function of the area may be restored to near normal.

Neovascularization

In neovascularization, new blood vessels form as the body attempts to bring oxygen and nutrients to the injured tissue. New capillaries bud from intact capillaries that lie adjacent to the damaged skin. These vessels provide a conduit for oxygen and nutrients and serve as a pathway for waste removal. Because they are new and delicate, bleeding might result from a very minor injury. It may take weeks to months for the new capillaries to be as stable as preexisting vessels.

Collagen Synthesis

Collagen is a tough, fibrous protein found in scar tissue, hair, bones, and connective tissue. This vital structural repair unit is synthesized by fibroblasts, repair cells that migrate into damaged tissue. In wound healing, collagen provides stability to the damaged tissue and joins wound borders, thereby closing the open tissue. Unfortunately, collagen cannot restore the damaged tissue to its original strength.

Alterations of Wound Healing

Wound healing does not always follow the pattern described previously. Infection or an abnormal scar may develop, excessive bleeding may occur, or healing may be slow. This section discusses altered wound healing and potential complications.

Anatomical Factors

Areas of the body subjected to repeated motion throughout the day, such as the fingers, tend to heal slowly. One strategy used to speed healing in such cases is to splint the affected part, preventing movement. The arrangement of an open wound in relation to skin tension lines also affects how the wound will heal and determines whether an abnormal scar will form.

You are the Paramedic Part 2

After bandaging and splinting the patient's leg, you assess pulse, motor, and sensory functions; they are grossly intact. The remainder of your focused physical examination is unremarkable. After placing the patient onto the stretcher and loading him into the ambulance, your partner gathers SAMPLE history information from the patient while you obtain a set of baseline vital signs.

Vital Signs	Recording Time: 8 Minutes
Skin	Pink and diaphoretic
Pulse	120 beats/min; strong and regular at the radial artery
Blood pressure	148/88 mm Hg
Respirations	24 breaths/min; adequate depth
Sp_{O_2}	98% on room air
Pain scale	10 on a scale of 0 to 10

3. Is this patient in shock?
4. What additional care should you provide to this patient?

Some medications can delay healing—namely, corticosteroids, nonsteroidal anti-inflammatory drugs, penicillin, colchicine, anticoagulants, and antineoplastic agents. Likewise, a variety of medical conditions may interfere with normal healing—advanced age, severe alcoholism, acute uremia, diabetes, hypoxia, severe anemia, peripheral vascular disease, malnutrition, advanced cancer, hepatic failure, and cardiovascular disease.

High-Risk Wounds

Wounds that carry a high risk for developing infection include human and animal bites. Because the mouth is warm and constantly moist, it offers a hospitable environment for growth of bacteria. Injection of human saliva into tissue can result in significant infection. In particular, rabies is a serious infection that can develop from the bite of an infected animal (such as wild raccoons, dogs, and cats).

Cases in which a foreign body or organic matter is embedded in an open wound are considered high-risk injuries because of the likelihood that the material involved is impregnated with microorganisms. Once the material breaches the skin barrier, the pathogen has easy entry into the rest of the body. A foreign body that remains in place on evaluation should be left in place because a lacerated blood vessel may not be bleeding freely because of the foreign body's position. *Do not remove an impaled object in the prehospital environment unless it interferes with the airway.*

Other high-risk wounds include injection wounds, wounds with significant devitalized tissue, crush wounds, wounds in immunocompromised patients, and injuries to patients with poor peripheral circulation.

Abnormal Scar Formation

Excessive collagen formation can occur if the healing process is not balanced between the building up and breaking down phases of healing. A hypertrophic or keloid scar may develop from the excess protein. Hypertrophic scar formation occurs in areas subject to high tissue stress, such as the elbow and knee. Such a scar does not extend past the borders of the wound margins and tends to form in people with lightly pigmented skin. In contrast, a keloid scar typically develops in people with darkly pigmented skin. It grows over the wound margins and can become larger than the wound area. Keloid scars tend to form on the ears, upper extremities, lower abdomen, and sternum.

Pressure Injuries

Pressure injuries may occur when a patient is bedridden or when pressure is applied for a prolonged period in an unconscious patient or a patient immobilized on a backboard. The involved tissues are deprived of oxygen, which leads to localized hypoxia and cell deterioration. Prevention involves determining the risk and providing a mechanism to reduce or release the pressure on the skin.

Wounds Requiring Closure

Many open wounds heal without intervention from caregivers, but some require closure with sutures, staples, or medical glue (octyl-2-cyanoacrylate). Closure involves bringing the wound edges together to allow for optimal healing. Open injuries that require closure include those that affect cosmetic areas, such as the lips, face, or eyebrows. Such injuries should be considered for closure because scarring often has psychological implications. Gaping wounds and those over tension lines also require closure. Degloving injuries require substantial irrigation and debridement before closing by an emergency practitioner. Closure is also indicated for ring injuries and skin tears.

Open injuries should be closed within 6 to 8 hours in most cases, although there is some variation based on body region. Initial hospital management for open wounds involves assessment for foreign material followed by irrigation. The practitioner can then determine appropriate wound closing options.

Three types of wound closure are performed: primary closure, secondary intention, and tertiary closure. In primary closure, the wound margins are brought together as neatly and evenly as possible. Secondary intention entails dressing high-risk wounds and allowing them to heal through normal body processes over time. Tertiary closure, also known as delayed primary closure, is applied to wounds that would have a poor cosmetic appearance if treated by secondary intention. In this case, wounds are irrigated and dressed initially and closure is performed later.

Patients who receive sutures need appropriate follow-up care to determine whether healing is normal or abnormal. Serious complications, including localized or systemic infection, can arise without adequate follow-up care. In some cases, sutures may need to be removed early to allow a wound to drain infectious material.

Infection

Because the skin serves as an initial barrier against microorganisms, any break can lead to infection. Larger openings, deeper penetrations, and heavily contaminated wounds result in a higher level of risk for developing an infection. Not only will there be a delay in healing from the infection, but additional complications or systemic infection can result.

Once in the body tissues, pathogens begin to grow and multiply, although clinical signs of infection may not appear for several days. Visible clues of infection include erythema, pus, warmth, edema, and local discomfort. Red streaks adjacent to the wound indicate that the patient has developed lymphangitis, an inflammation of the lymph channels. More serious infections can cause systemic signs, such as fever, shaking, chills, joint pain, and hypotension.

Gangrene

Clostridium perfringens is an anaerobic, toxin-producing bacterium that leads to the development of gangrene. Sixty percent of cases result from trauma and 25% end in the patient's death. Once it enters deeply into tissue, it causes the production of a foul-smelling gas. If the gangrene is not treated, the skin will become necrotic and the infection may lead to sepsis. Prompt recognition and early, aggressive hospital therapy offer the best chance for reducing morbidity and mortality.

Tetanus

Tetanus is caused by infection with an anaerobic bacterium, *Clostridium tetani* (a member of the same family that causes gangrene). This bacterium causes the body to produce a potent toxin, which results in painful muscle contractions that are strong enough to fracture bones. Muscle stiffness may be noted first in the jaw ("lockjaw") and neck, with progression down the remainder of the body. Early recognition is important because conventional therapy does not result in rapid recovery.

Tetanus has become rare, thanks to the availability of a vaccine. In Canada, vaccination against tetanus is part of childhood immunization programs. A booster is needed every 10 years, although an inoculation is typically provided to patients who are injured and have not been immunized in the last 5 years. Given the severity of tetanus, you should ask injured patients about the last time they received a tetanus booster.

Necrotizing Fasciitis

Necrotizing fasciitis involves the death of tissue from bacterial infection. This disease is caused by more than one infecting organism—most commonly, *Staphylococcus aureus* and hemolytic streptococci. Although necrotizing fasciitis is rare, the mortality rate ranges from 70% to 80%. Antibiotic therapy and surgical debridement are among the available treatments.

Closed Versus Open Wounds

Closed Wounds

In a closed wound, soft tissues beneath the skin surface are damaged, but there is no break in the epidermis. The characteristic closed wound is a contusion Figure 19-2 ▾. In a contusion (bruise), the skin is intact, but damage has occurred beneath the epidermis. Trauma to the nerve endings produces pain, and leakage of fluid into spaces between the damaged cells produces swelling (edema). If small blood vessels in the dermis are disrupted, a black-and-blue mark (ecchymosis) will cover the injured area; if large blood vessels are torn beneath the contused area, a hematoma—a collection of blood beneath the skin—will be evident as a lump with a bluish discolouration Figure 19-3 ▸.

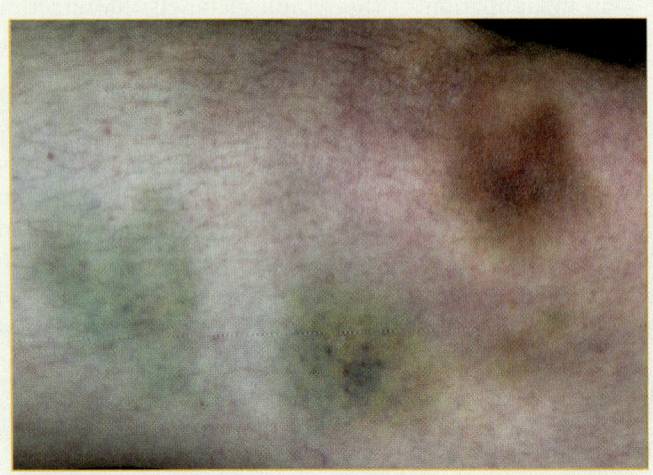

Figure 19-2 A contusion, or bruise, produces characteristic black-and-blue discolouration (ecchymosis).

Open Wounds

An open wound is characterized by a disruption in the skin. Open wounds are potentially much more serious than closed wounds for two reasons. First, they are vulnerable to infection. An open wound is contaminated—that is, microorganisms enter it. Whether the contamination produces infection depends in large measure on how the wound is managed. Second, open wounds have a greater potential for serious blood loss. When the skin is unbroken, bleeding from a disrupted blood vessel is limited. Although a significant volume of blood—up to about 2 units—can be lost into the soft tissues of the leg, eventually the increasing pressure within the leg will prevent further bleeding. In an open wound, the patient's entire blood volume may be lost.

Certain wounds should always be evaluated by a physician. The injuries in Table 19-1 ▾ require transport, even if they appear minor.

Abrasions

An abrasion Figure 19-4 ▸ is a superficial wound that occurs when the skin is rubbed or scraped over a rough surface and part of the epidermis is lost. So-called brush burns or mat burns are good examples. Abrasions typically ooze small amounts of blood and may be quite painful. They may also be contaminated with dirt and debris—for example, from "road rash" caused by sliding on the pavement in a motorcycle collision. Because the skin has been disrupted, infection is a danger.

Don't try to clean an abrasion in the prehospital environment; you don't have the means to do so properly. If you feel compelled to do *something*, cover the wound lightly with a sterile dressing.

Lacerations

A laceration Figure 19-5 ▸ is a cut inflicted by a sharp instrument, such as a knife or razor blade, that produces a clean or jagged incision through the skin surface and underlying structures. Sometimes the word *laceration* is reserved for jagged or irregular cuts, and incision is used to refer to a clean (linear) cut. Incisions tend to heal better than lacerations because of their relatively even

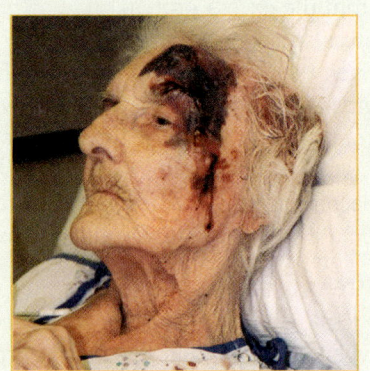

Figure 19-3 A hematoma.

Table 19-1	Conditions That Require Transport

- Compromise of:
  - Nerves
  - Vessels
  - Muscles
  - Tendons or ligaments
- Foreign body or cosmetic complications
- Heavy contamination

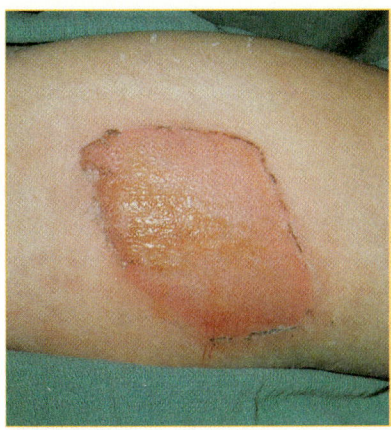
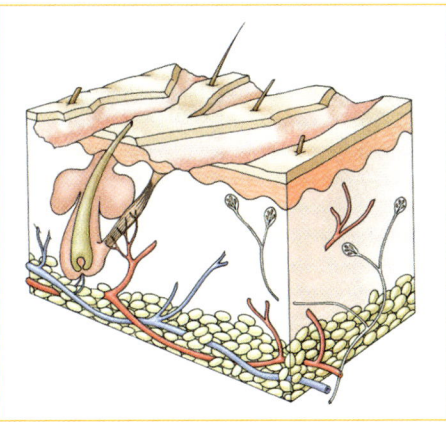

Figure 19-4 Abrasions usually do not penetrate completely through the dermis, but blood may ooze from the capillaries. These wounds are typically superficial and result from rubbing or scraping across a hard, rough surface.

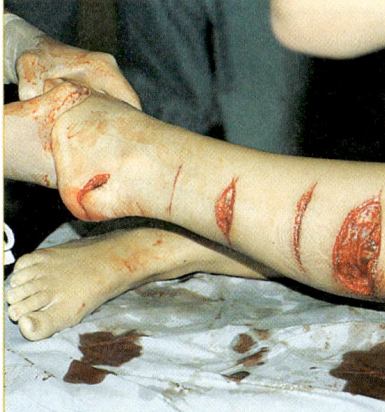
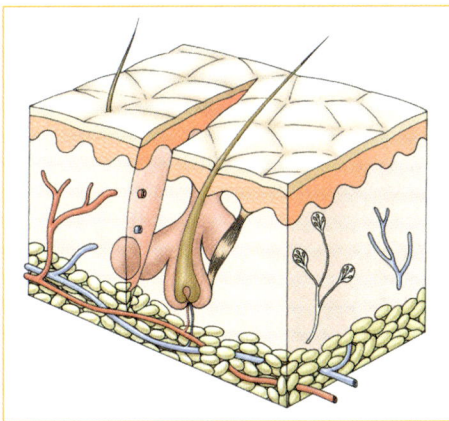

Figure 19-5 Lacerations can vary in depth and can extend through the skin and subcutaneous tissue to the underlying muscles, nerves, and blood vessels. These wounds can be smooth or jagged as a result of a cut by a sharp object or a blunt force that tears the tissue.

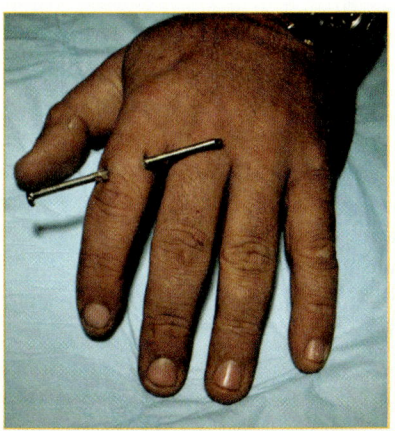
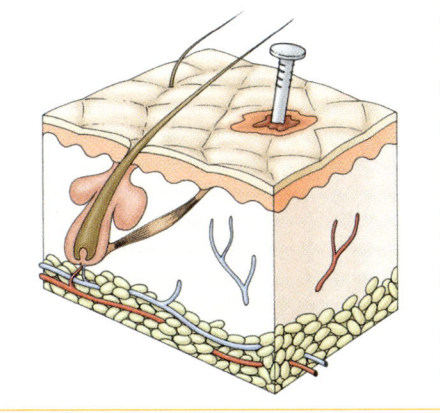

Figure 19-6 Penetrating wounds may cause very little external bleeding but can damage structures deep in the body.

wound margins. The seriousness of a laceration will depend on its depth and the structures that have been damaged. Lacerations may be the source of significant bleeding if they disrupt the wall of a blood vessel, particularly in regions of the body where major arteries lie close to the surface (as in the wrist). The first priority in treating a laceration is to control bleeding, initially by applying direct manual pressure over the wound. Laceration of a major artery can be fatal due to the severe bleeding that can occur.

Puncture Wounds

A puncture wound **Figure 19-6 ◂** is a stab from a pointed object, such as a nail or a knife. Technically speaking, a bullet wound is a puncture wound. Most puncture wounds do not cause significant external bleeding, but they may produce extensive—even fatal—internal bleeding and wreak other havoc that cannot be seen from the outside of the body.

A special case of the puncture wound is the impaled foreign object **Figure 19-7 ▸**. When the instrument that caused the injury remains embedded in the wound, immobilize the object in the position found, and transport the patient.

Avulsions

An avulsion occurs when a flap of skin is torn loose, partially **Figure 19-8 ▸** or completely. Depending on where the avulsion occurs, it may or may not be accompanied by profuse bleeding. The principal danger in this type of injury—besides blood loss and contamination—is loss of the blood supply to the avulsed flap. If the part of the flap that connects it to the body (the pedicle) is folded back or kinked, circulation to the flap will be compromised and that piece of skin will die if the circulation is not restored quickly.

Amputations

An amputation is an avulsion involving the complete loss of a body part, typically one or more of the extremities. If the amputation was produced by a sharp object, blood loss is often much less than expected because the blood vessels retain the ability to constrict. In contrast, a crushing or tearing amputation can result in exsanguination (excessive blood loss due to hemorrhage) if the paramedic does not intervene rapidly.

Wound edges in an amputation are commonly jagged, and sharp bone edges may protrude **Figure 19-9 ▸**. During wound care,

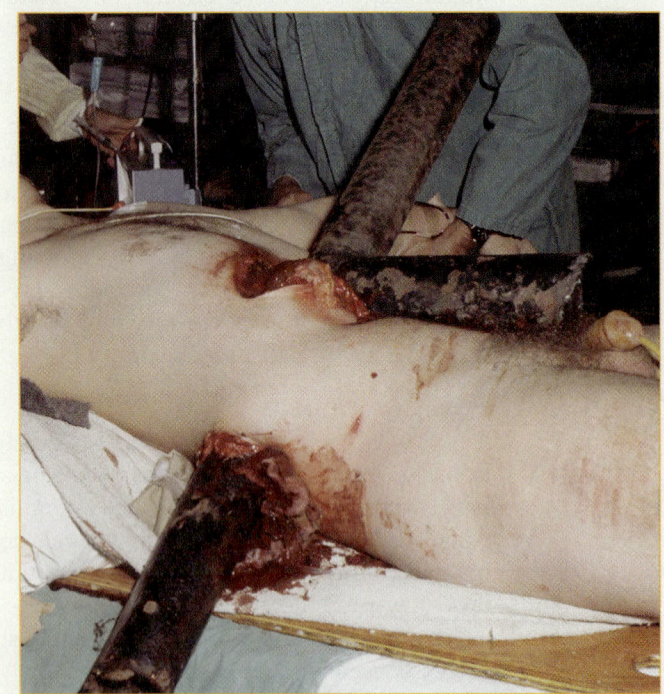

Figure 19-7 An impaled object remains embedded in the wound.

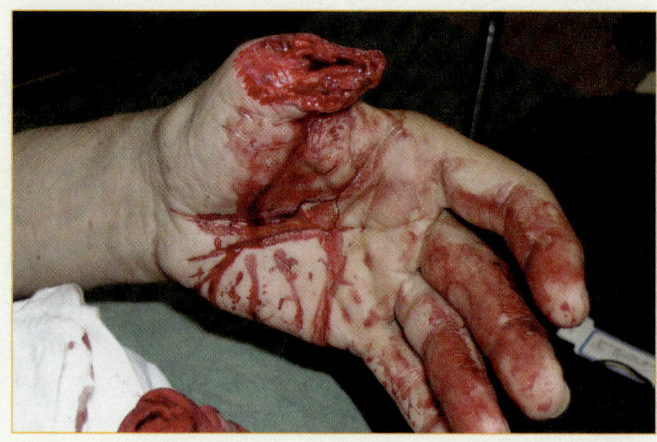

Figure 19-9 An amputation involving the thumb.

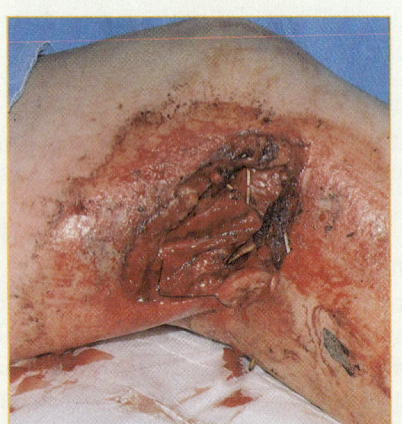
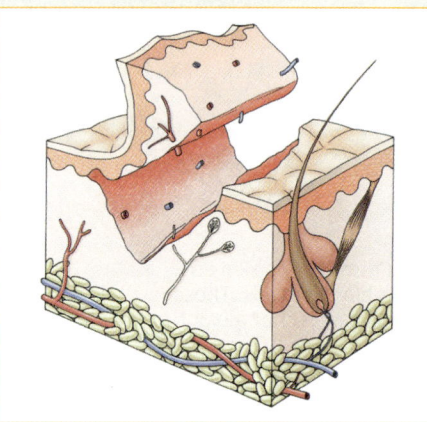

Figure 19-8 Avulsions are characterized by complete separation of tissue or tissue hanging as a flap. Significant bleeding is common.

be aware of any sharp bone protrusions that may lead to an exposure. Large, thick dressings should be used to cover the site. In some cases, the body part will be completely detached. In a partial amputation, soft tissues remain attached. A degloving injury is a specific form of amputation that involves unraveling of skin from the hand, much like partial removal of a glove.

Crush Injuries

When a body part is crushed between two solid objects, a <u>crush injury</u> may occur to the underlying soft tissues and

bones **Figure 19-10 ▸**. Such injuries range from an innocuous finger injury to a life-threatening entrapment of the torso. The latter is likely to be encountered in cases involving structural collapse (such as in collapse of masonry or steel structures, earthquakes, tornadoes, construction accidents, mudslides, motor vehicle collisions, warfare injuries, and industrial accidents). A crush injury can also occur when an unconscious patient has an upper extremity pinned between the body and the floor for a prolonged period. Likewise, a crush injury may develop when a pneumatic antishock garment (PASG) is left in place for an excessive period or a cast is applied too tightly.

The forces involved in a crush injury may be great enough to rupture internal organs. You must rapidly assess the mechanism of injury and determine the likelihood for massive internal trauma. Also, note that the longer an injured area remains compressed, the greater the chance for systemic complications.

In a crush injury, the external appearance may not adequately represent the level of internal damage. An upper extremity that merely appears swollen may, in fact, have enough muscle destruction to cause systemic problems, especially if the extremity has been trapped for longer than 4 hours, which is enough time to develop crush syndrome. In other cases, the injured region may be mangled beyond recognition. Remember that grotesque injuries may not necessarily be the primary problem. Always concentrate on threats to life before addressing injured extremities, no matter how bad the initial appearance.

One of the body's first responses to a vessel injury is localized vasoconstriction that reduces the flow of blood. When vessels are crushed and torn, they often lose the ability to constrict, resulting in a free flow of blood from any unnatural opening. Crush injuries tend to result in hemorrhage that

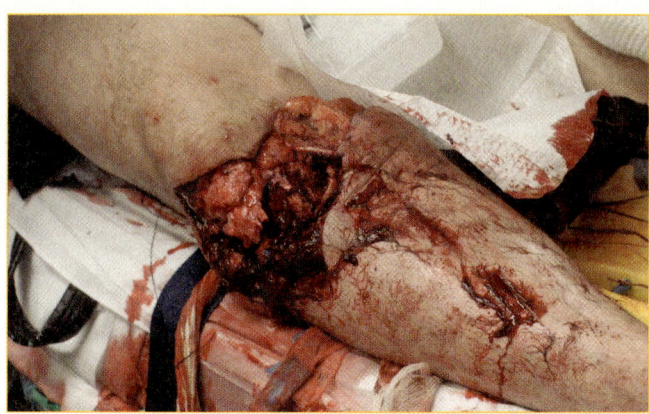

Figure 19-10 A crush injury is characterized by extensive tissue damage and deformity that is often accompanied by swelling and extreme pain.

Table 19-2	The Progression of Crush Syndrome

1. A body part is trapped for more than 4 hours.
2. Rhabdomyolysis occurs.
3. The trapped body part is freed.
4. By-products of metabolism and harmful products from tissue destruction are released, possibly resulting in cardiac arrest, dysrhythmias, kidney damage, hyperkalemia, and hyperphosphatemia.

cannot easily be controlled by standard methods. Inability to precisely locate bleeding or massive extremity trauma may also lead to difficulty in controlling hemorrhage.

Crush Syndrome

When an area of the body is trapped for longer than 4 hours and arterial blood flow is compromised, crush syndrome can develop Table 19-2 ▲ . When muscles are crushed beyond repair, tissue necrosis develops and leads to release of harmful products, a process known as rhabdomyolysis. As muscle cells are destroyed, they experience an influx of water, sodium chloride, and calcium from extracellular fluid. In addition, the body develops an efflux of potassium, purines (from disintegrating nuclei), phosphate, lactic acid, myoglobin, thromboplastin, creatine, and creatine kinase. The compressing force prevents the return of blood from the injured body part, so the release of these products into the systemic circulation does not occur until *after* the limb is freed from entrapment. For this reason, rescuers must intervene *before* lifting the crushing object off the body.

Freeing the limb or other body part from entrapment not only results in release of by-products of metabolism and harmful products of tissue destruction, but also involves the potential for cardiac arrest. In prolonged entrapment, "smiling death" may occur if paramedics do not take proactive measures. In this situation, the trapped person is alert and conversing with rescuers; however, when the entrapped body part is freed, cardiac arrest is almost instantaneous. Life-threatening arrhythmias may develop from increased blood potassium levels (hyperkalemia).

Renal failure is another serious complication that may develop after release of the crushing force. Glomerular filtration can be impaired when the kidneys do not receive enough blood, such as when hypotension develops from bleeding. In addition, the release of large quantities of myoglobin into the central circulation can clog the filtering tubules. The high levels of acids and phosphates can directly damage the kidneys. This problem is compounded by the development of oxygen free radicals. These products travel throughout the affected area, scavenging oxygen molecules and damaging and destroying cells that might otherwise survive the initial injury.

Increased levels of uric acid, lactic acid, and potassium may also cause metabolic acidosis.

Compartment Syndrome

Compartment syndrome develops when edema and swelling result in increased pressure within soft tissues. Within a limb, groups of muscles are surrounded by an inelastic membrane called *fascia*. Thus, the muscles are confined to an enclosed space, or compartment, that can accommodate only a limited amount of swelling. When bleeding or swelling occurs within a compartment, as the result of a fracture or severe soft-tissue injury, pressure increases within the compartment, which in turn leads to compromised circulation. Compartment syndrome commonly develops in the extremities and may occur in conjunction with open or closed injuries (although it is more likely with closed injuries due to the buildup of pressure inside the body). As pressure develops, delivery of nutrients and oxygen is impaired and by-products of normal metabolism accumulate. The longer this situation persists, the greater the chance for tissue necrosis.

Compartment syndrome presents with the six Ps: Pain, Paresthesia, Paresis, Pressure, Passive stretch pain, and Pulselessness. Many of these signs may be delayed or nonspecific. Distal perfusion, sensation, and motor function may be intact.

Compartment syndrome that persists for more than 8 hours carries a serious risk for death of local tissues. In such cases, extensive and disfiguring wound debridement that can leave visible and psychologic scars is required. There is also a risk of sepsis. In-hospital intervention includes a surgical procedure called fasciotomy, or incision of the skin and underlying fascia. This limb-saving procedure also prevents a Volkmann contracture—a deformity of the hand, fingers, and wrist resulting from damage to forearm muscles—and preserves cutaneous sensation. In rare cases, medical direction may authorize prehospital caregivers to perform a fasciotomy.

Blast Injuries

While terrorist attacks clearly illustrated the devastating power of an explosive force, many other circumstances can lead to an explosion—dust buildup in grain silos, sawdust in wood factories, and explosive products transported by rail, sea, or air Figure 19-11 ▸. You must be mentally and physically prepared to respond to an incident involving an explosion.

Blast injuries occur in four phases: primary, secondary, tertiary, and quaternary.

Primary Phase

When an explosion occurs, a pressure wave rapidly develops; this tremendous but concentrated pressure results from air displacement and heat originating from the centre of the blast. The pressure wave damages air-filled cavities (such as the ears and lungs). Burns may occur.

All origins of the pressure wave carry a high risk of injury or death. Explosions from a bomb start at the centre and move outward, so persons closer to the device will be affected to a greater extent. Explosions from fumes or dust involve an entire area, so there is no "safe" region. Underwater blasts have a three times greater range because of the near incompressibility of water. Explosions that occur within a confined space result in more force applied to the body.

Secondary Phase

A blast wind occurs as combustible gases move across the affected area. Although less forceful than the pressure wave, the blast wind is longer lasting. Projectiles also present serious hazards—flying debris may cause blunt and penetrating injuries. With bombs, the casing fragments rip apart with monumental force, spreading in all directions. Structural elements can break apart and travel at high rates of speed. Nails,

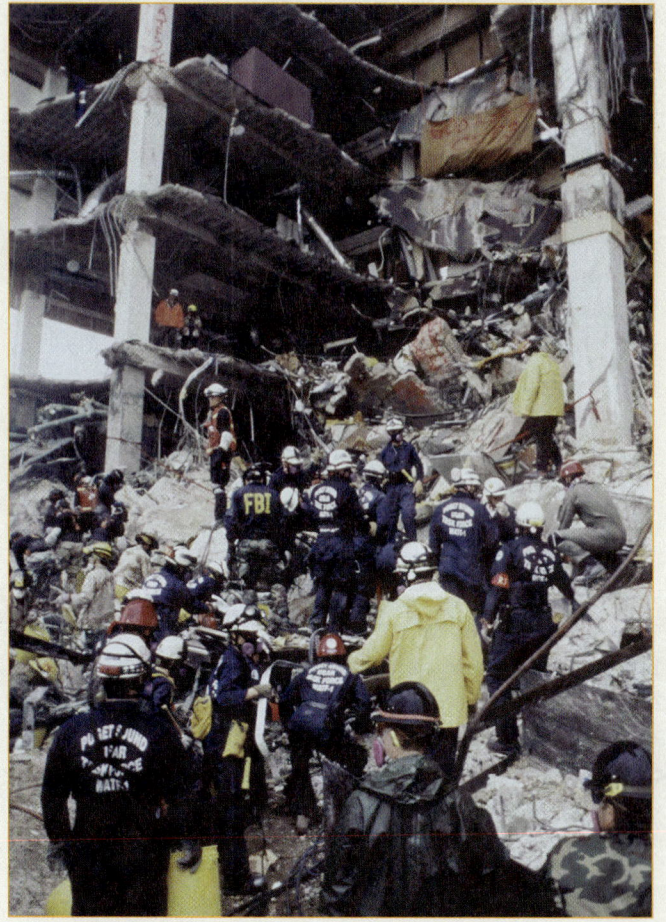

Figure 19-11 The Alfred P. Murrah building's destruction in Oklahoma City killed hundreds.

You are the Paramedic Part 3

After establishing an IV line of normal saline and administering further treatment, you begin transport to a hospital located approximately 24 km away. The patient remains conscious and alert and states that his pain is not as severe as it was initially. With an estimated time of arrival at the hospital of 10 minutes, you reassess the patient.

Reassessment	Recording Time: 15 Minutes
Skin	Pink and diaphoretic
Pulse	94 beats/min; strong and regular at the radial artery
Blood pressure	122/68 mm Hg
Respirations	18 breaths/min; adequate depth
Spo2	99% on room air
Pain scale	5 on a scale of 0 to 10

5. What is compartment syndrome and is this patient at risk for it?

6. What are the signs and symptoms of compartment syndrome?

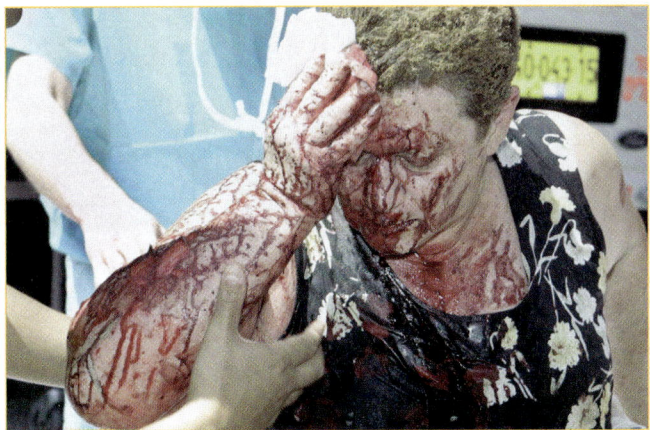

Figure 19-12 Nails, wood splinters, and glass shards can impale victims of a blast explosion.

wood splinters, and glass shards can impact victims located in the area of the blast Figure 19-12.

Tertiary Phase

Victims may be injured from displacement away from the blast site or from collapse of the surrounding structure. Displacement occurs when a person is in proximity to the explosion; survival in this circumstance is highly unlikely. Falling structural beams, walls, and other heavy items may lead to crush injuries that compound the conditions already present. Injuries develop when the person is thrown against rigid surfaces, such as the ground, walls, or other rigid objects. There is also a risk for entrapment that can be prolonged for days. In addition, there may be multiple victims (as in the World Trade Center bombings).

Quaternary Phase

Injuries result from the miscellaneous events that occur during an explosion. For example, the heat generated during an explosion may cause burns, ranging from superficial flash burns to full-thickness burns involving the entire or large areas of the body.

Assessment of Soft-Tissue Injuries

Although skin trauma is often dramatic, it rarely is immediately life threatening. It is important to stay focused on the assessment format used throughout this book to first identify threats to you and your crew using the scene assessment and then identify life threats to the patient using the initial assessment.

The skin is more than just a wrapper; it performs important functions that are altered by trauma. When conducting your initial assessment, you need to determine the nature and mechanism of the injury. The severity of the injury may not be

initially apparent, but it will be revealed as you do your rapid trauma assessment or focused physical examination.

Scene Safety and Assessment

The first aspect to address in any scenario is safety. If you are responding to a vehicle collision, ensure that traffic is controlled and personnel are operating with protective measures in place. When responding to a reported explosion, wait for police personnel to secure the scene and declare it safe before you approach any victims. When a blast seems to be intentional, look for possible secondary devices. Responders have been injured and killed by other explosive devices planted away from the original detonation site.

Once you have determined that the scene is safe, begin evaluating the mechanism of injury. Maintain a high index of suspicion whenever a significant mechanism of injury is present, even if external injuries appear minor. Carefully consider the forces involved as you determine the likelihood of internal damage.

Next, determine how many patients are involved. Diligently search for ejected patients in the case of a significant vehicle collision.

As a part of your scene assessment, be aware that skin injuries typically result in a risk of exposure to blood and other bodily fluids. Significant exposures include contact with body fluids through open wounds or mucous membranes. Less worrisome exposures include body fluid contact with intact skin. Be sure to protect yourself and the patient, and review Chapters 2 and 36 regarding infection control procedures.

Initial Assessment

When the scene has been secured and personal protective equipment measures have been taken, rapidly determine whether threats to life are present. First, note your general impression as you approach the patient. Much information can be obtained from simply looking at the patient and the immediate surroundings. For example, a patient who is lying prone on the ground in a large pool of blood is clearly in worse shape than a patient who meets you at the door with a cut finger.

Many patients have potential injuries to the neck or spine. In such cases, you should assign a crew member to manually immobilize the head and neck. This is an important step because it will determine which maneuvers are used to open the airway.

Evaluation of the patient's initial level of consciousness is also important. Determine whether the patient is alert, responsive to verbal stimuli, responsive to painful stimuli, or completely unresponsive. This assessment may reveal a potential brain injury even when the patient has a seemingly innocuous soft-tissue injury to the head.

Assess the airway as soon as you arrive at the patient's side. When present, immediately suction blood, vomit, or any other product from the airway. If direct airway trauma is present, it may severely compromise the airway. Soft-tissue injuries that result in a flow of blood into the airway can also prove extremely challenging. Immediately correct anything

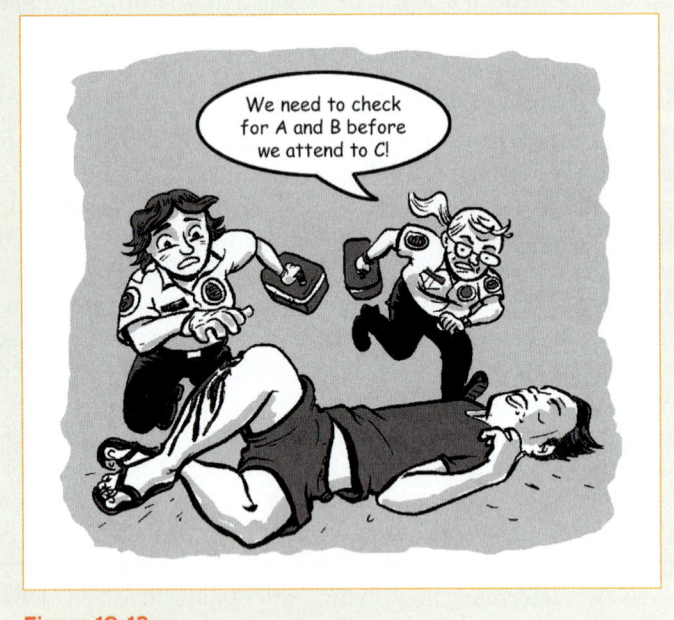

Figure 19-13

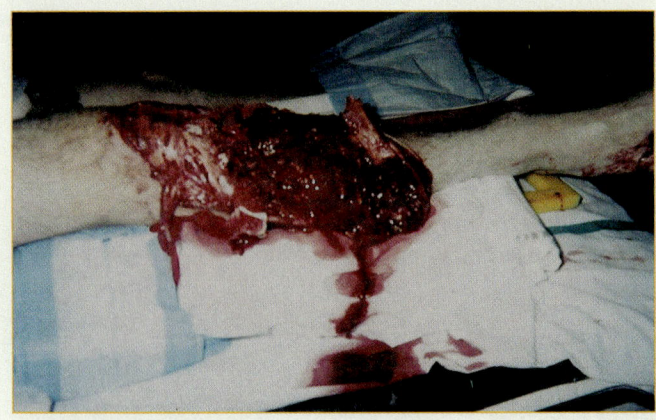

Figure 19-14 A high-velocity gunshot wound to the leg.

that interferes with airway patency; failure to provide a patent airway can quickly lead to the patient's death **Figure 19-13 ▲**.

Assess the patient's breathing. During the initial assessment, it is not important to obtain an exact rate—just determine whether the patient's breathing is abnormally slow or rapid or excessively deep or shallow. Address a significant alteration in breathing by using a nonrebreathing mask with oxygen at 15 l/min or a bag-valve-mask device and supplementary oxygen. An inadequate depth or rate that results in compromised breathing should prompt you to take immediate action.

Assessment of circulatory status involves palpating a pulse and checking the skin signs. In an unresponsive adult, assess the carotid pulse; in a conscious patient, assess the radial pulse. If no pulse is present, take resuscitative measures (see Appendix A). When a pulse is palpated, determine whether it is abnormally fast or slow (an exact rate will be calculated later). The goal at this step is to determine if immediate intervention is necessary.

Palpate and inspect the skin (CTC—Colour, Temperature, and Condition). Pale or ashen skin points to inadequate perfusion. Cool, moist skin is an early indicator of shock. When present, determine if the skin is cool and moist only in the extremities or over the entire body.

Ensure that the patient is adequately exposed during the initial assessment. Sometimes, you need to look at only the chest area. On more serious calls, the patient may need to be completely exposed from head to toe. Gunshot wounds and stab wounds, for example, warrant complete removal of the patient's clothing **Figure 19-14 ▶**.

Once the initial assessment has been completed, you will need to make a priority decision to rapidly package and transport or to stabilize and treat on scene. Patients with significant trauma (significant mechanism of injury [MOI]) should be rapidly transported in accordance with the "golden hour" principle. Patients with isolated injuries (no significant MOI) are often better managed by carefully treating the injuries on scene.

Focused History and Physical Examination
Physical Examination

Patients are stratified into two categories: patients with a significant MOI and patients with no significant MOI. When serious trauma is present, soft-tissue injuries take a lower priority than airway control, breathing inadequacy, and bleeding. *Do not let soft-tissue injuries distract you from life threats that may not be readily apparent.* Patients with less serious injuries will need an examination focused on the specific body part and its function but probably will not need a detailed physical examination.

Significant MOI

Serious trauma is indicated by an altered level of consciousness, lack of airway protection or lack of patency, inadequate breathing, uncontrolled bleeding, and a significant MOI. If any are present or your analysis points to a possibility for serious injury, perform a rapid trauma assessment. Life threats should have been addressed during the initial assessment; if additional life threats are found now, manage them immediately. For example, if examination of the chest reveals absent breath sounds on one side, the chest may need ventilation, sealing with an occlusive dressing, and decompression if there is a tension pneumothorax. Interventions can occur simultaneously during the initial assessment of the patient.

The rapid trauma assessment involves a head-to-toe assessment that focuses on detecting serious injury to major body compartments. Rapidly assess the head, neck, chest, abdomen, pelvis, lower extremities, upper extremities, and posterior. Identify deformities, discolourations, impaled objects, open injuries, and other trauma that demands immediate attention. The mnemonic DCAP-BTLS is a useful reminder of what to look at: Deformities, Contusions, Abrasions, Punctures or penetrations, Burns, Tenderness, Lacerations, and Swelling. Assess areas with alterations in sensation, uneven temperature, or abnormal muscle tone. Note if any blood appears on your gloves. For example, hair can conceal hemorrhage, but if you find blood on your gloves during your examination of the head, you have identified an injury.

Address airway compromises, breathing inadequacies, and uncontrolled hemorrhage that may have been missed in the initial assessment. Trauma patients are often critically injured, and life threats evolve over time, so reassessments may reveal problems not found in the initial examination. Airway takes priority over breathing issues, and both take precedence over active bleeding. In practice, you will work as a part of a team to manage each issue as it is found rather than addressing each life threat sequentially. For example, the paramedic positioned at the head can manage the airway while another paramedic performs bleeding control. Prioritize the injuries that need to be addressed first. Remember that optimal on-scene time is less than 10 minutes, and any intervention that can be done en route should be delayed until in the ambulance.

Once the head and neck have been assessed, you can apply a cervical collar to limit motion and prevent secondary injury. Collars are designed to allow assessment of the front of the neck while in place but do not offer a means to assess the back of the neck without their removal. Completely assess the neck before applying a cervical collar. Once it is in position, a rescuer must continue to stabilize the neck until the patient's torso and head are properly fixed to a backboard. Be diligent about ensuring that the airway stays open and clear. If the collar is in the way, you may need to resort to manual immobilization of the neck while maintaining an open airway with a jaw-thrust maneuver.

At the conclusion of the rapid trauma assessment, you must decide whether to rapidly transport or remain on scene for more detailed care. The detailed physical examination, which is conducted on trauma patients with a significant MOI, is typically performed en route to the ED. Completion of the rapid trauma assessment should prompt you to reconsider or reconfirm the initial transport priority. A complete set of baseline vital signs and the SAMPLE history should also be obtained on concluding this assessment.

No Significant MOI

A complete head-to-toe examination is not always warranted. Patients with isolated extremity trauma do not require a full body evaluation. If you are unsure whether a significant MOI exists, conduct a complete rapid trauma assessment and then perform a detailed physical examination en route to the ED. In all other cases, direct your attention to assessing the chief complaint and area with outward signs of injury.

When local protocols allow, some patients can be treated on scene and released. For example, a patient at a rock concert with a minor laceration; good distal pulses, motor response, and sensation; and recent history of a tetanus shot might be able to be released to a sober adult. Some systems have established a means for referring the patient for further medical care at a local emergency clinic or other suitable medical facility. Release or referral may be preferred for a patient with relatively minor injuries,

such as a simple laceration or abrasion. Paramedics must still provide basic care, such as dressing and bandaging.

History

Gathering information is also an important step in determining how the patient was injured. Ask the patient (if conscious and able to respond) or family members and bystanders about the events leading to injury:

- Was the patient wearing a seatbelt?
- How fast was the vehicle travelling?
- How high is the location from which the patient fell?
- Was there a loss of consciousness?
- What type of weapon was used?

When time and patient condition permit, determine when the last tetanus booster was given. Record the information on the patient care record, and relay it during patient transfer at the hospital. Ask the patient about prescribed and over-the-counter medications, paying particular attention to those that interfere with hemostasis. A higher priority should be given to patients taking warfarin (Coumadin) or other anticoagulants. Other medications that can lead to continued bleeding include aspirin, ticlodipine (Ticlid), and clopidogrel bisulfate (Plavix). To obtain a complete history, use the mnemonic SAMPLE described in previous chapters.

Detailed Physical Examination

After the focused history and physical examination is complete, a more thorough examination should generally be conducted en route when there is a significant MOI and adequate time and the patient is in stable condition. This detailed assessment examines every anatomical region, looking for hidden injuries and clinical signs. A detailed physical examination is an excellent way to gather information but should never delay transport of a patient in critical condition. In most cases, this assessment is completed while travelling to the ED.

Documentation and Communication

Most people charged with shooting another person end up in court at some point, and you may be called to testify. In cases of gunshot wounds, it is even more important than usual that you carefully document the circumstances surrounding the scene, the injury, the patient's condition, and the treatment you give.

Ongoing Assessment

Frequent reassessments of the patient's conditions should be made en route to the hospital and in conjunction with any necessary interventions. A patient in stable condition should be reassessed every 15 minutes; a more serious condition warrants reexamination every 5 minutes. As part of this assessment, vital signs should be obtained and evaluated, any interventions checked, and the patient monitored. Document all findings, and track trends in the patient's condition.

Management of Soft-Tissue Injuries

Management of soft-tissue trauma varies according to the injury present; however, some basic management principles apply to nearly every scenario. Although attending to clinical issues is important, paramedics must also tend to the patient's feelings about the injury. Be empathetic, because the injury may be perceived very differently in the patient's eyes. From a clinical standpoint, bleeding is controlled using direct pressure, elevation, pressure points, and, occasionally, a tourniquet. Irrigate wounds to reduce the risk of infection. Immobilization of an injury site can also be helpful in caring for soft-tissue damage. Once all assessments and interventions are complete and patient care has been transferred, thoroughly document any care provided.

Treatment of Closed Wounds

Small contusions do not require any special treatment. When an extensive closed injury is present, however, bleeding beneath the skin may reach significant proportions, and swelling may compromise vital structures. In such cases, take steps to minimize the bleeding and swelling by following the ICES mnemonic:

- **I** Apply *Ice* or cold packs to the injured area. Cold will stimulate blood vessels to constrict, slowing the bleeding. Do not apply ice or anything very cold directly on the skin.
- **C** Apply firm *Compression* over the injured area to decrease bleeding. Compression may be manual initially, but is most effectively applied with an air splint thereafter.
- **E** *Elevate* the injured part to a level above the heart, to encourage drainage and decrease swelling.
- **S** Apply a *Splint* to an injured extremity. By preventing motion, a splint decreases bleeding. An air splint gives a double benefit—splinting *and* compression.

Treatment of Open Wounds: General Principles

Two general principles govern the treatment of all open wounds:

- Control bleeding by whatever method is most effective.
- Keep the wound as clean as possible. Cut away clothing covering the wound. Wash away loose dirt and debris by pouring sterile water or tap water over the area. Do *not* try to pick out foreign matter embedded in a wound. Simply irrigate the site copiously, and then cover the wound with a dry, sterile dressing.

Determine the magnitude of the injury and relay the findings to the receiving facility. If bleeding is present, determine the colour of the blood, amount lost, and site of origin. Obtaining an accurate history is important when bleeding has stopped before EMS arrival. Ask the patient to describe the bleeding in terms of colour and type of flow.

For wounds already in the healing stage, examine the edges to determine if the wound is closing properly or if the edges are separating. Inspect the area to identify signs of infection, such as redness, swelling, and pain. Discoloured pus may also be present. Signs of systemic infection—fever, general malaise, and altered mental status—warrant transport to a hospital for further examination.

Bandaging and Dressing Wounds

Dressing and bandage materials are used to cover the wound, control bleeding, and limit motion. Simple application of a dressing over an open wound will help prevent infection by providing an artificial barrier against microorganisms. Using bleeding control techniques with dressings will stop all but the most serious active blood loss. Correct application of bandage material will limit motion of the affected area, helping the body to recover from the insult.

A variety of materials are used to dress and bandage wounds. A <u>dressing</u> directly covers a wound and controls bleeding, whereas a <u>bandage</u> keeps the dressing in place. When properly applied, both keep pathogens from entering the open injury.

Sterile and Nonsterile Dressings

Sterile dressings are completely free of microorganisms. These materials are used when a high probability of infection is present, particularly in cases of large open wounds. Each such dressing comes individually wrapped and is marked as being sterile. Because sterility is lost when the package is opened, it is important to quickly dress open wounds when using sterile dressings.

Nonsterile dressings are used when there is a lower risk of infection. Although they are not completely devoid of microorganisms, they are packaged in a clean manner. Nonsterile dressings often come packaged as one large unit without the individual wrapping found in sterile packaging. The prehospital caregiver would first dress the wound with a sterile dressing and then apply multiple nonsterile dressings to increase the ability to absorb blood.

Occlusive and Nonocclusive Dressings

Occlusive dressings are used when it is important to keep air from passing through the material—for example, with open wounds to the neck or thorax where negative pressure would draw air into lacerated blood vessels or the pleural cavity. When an occlusive dressing is applied to an open wound in the thorax, it should be sealed on three sides to allow air to escape. Allowing one corner to remain open helps prevent development of a tension pneumothorax. Because most open wounds do not present a risk for air entering the body, the majority of dressing materials are nonocclusive.

Adherent and Nonadherent Dressings

Adherent dressings allow exudate from the wound to mesh with dressing material. This action facilitates clotting and aids in bleeding control. Because the material becomes bound to exudates, removal of the dressing is painful and may precipitate bleeding.

Nonadherent dressings allow the products of wound repair to pass through the material. This design allows for easy removal of dressing material but does not aid in clot formation. A nonadherent dressing would be applied after a wound closure.

Wet and Dry Dressings

Dry dressings are the most commonly used options in prehospital care. Because wet dressings provide a medium for bacteria and other pathogens to grow, their use is limited in the prehospital environment. Moist dressings can be of benefit for burn care, although commercial burn dressings made with a water-based gel better facilitate pain relief. This sterile form of wet dressing does not stick to open wounds.

Roller and Gauze Bandages

Bandage material is often self-adherent (for example, Kling or Kerlix). As a consequence, when you roll the bandage material over the dressing, the overlapping material will adhere to it and keep the bandage in place. A roller bandage is ideal for wrapping extremity injuries. It is available in a variety of sizes, although the 2.5- and 10-cm versions are the most popular.

A gauze bandage also works well for wrapping dressings into place but is a nonadherent bandage. Although it does not remain in position as readily as roller gauze, it is still an effective means to secure a dressing. This material does not offer much stretch, which can result in excess pressure to areas that begin to swell.

Roller and gauze bandages are considered absorbent bandage materials. Nonabsorbent bandages, which do not absorb fluid but prevent leaking, are also commercially available.

Absorbent Gauze Sponges

When heavy bleeding is present, a thicker, bulkier dressing is needed. An absorbent gauze sponge assists in controlling hemorrhage while providing a dressing. Sponges are available in a variety of sizes and may be sterile or nonsterile.

Elastic Bandages

Elastic bandage material stretches to allow some pressure to be applied. This characteristic is useful to control bleeding. Elastic bandages are also used in musculoskeletal trauma to facilitate healing of damaged tendons and ligaments. Be careful to avoid applying excessive pressure with such bandages because blood flow may be compromised.

Triangular Bandages

Triangular bandages (cravats) are an ideal shape for making slings and swathes. They are typically made of cotton and come packaged with safety pins. Because they do not stretch, there is little conformance to body contours, which is not ideal if pressure must be applied. These bandages can be wrapped into a thin strip to be used as a tourniquet.

Taping

A dressing may be secured with tape alone or in conjunction with bandage material. Several types of medical tape are available, ranging in size from a 2.5- to a 10-cm roll. Be cautious when using tape on patients with skin conditions that might lead to damage upon the tape's removal (such as older patients, who often have very thin skin).

Complications of Improperly Applied Dressings

Improper application of dressing and bandage material can result in significant complications. It is important to learn how to properly dress a wound in the laboratory, clinical, and prehospital settings to avoid causing harm.

Although it is not always possible to use sterile technique, make every effort to avoid further wound contamination. Irrigate open wounds with normal saline to flush out contaminants. If available, apply antibiotic ointment to smaller open wounds to help avoid infection. Large open injuries should not have ointment applied but should be irrigated. Once the wound is irrigated, apply a dressing over the site. Clean blood around the dressing site, and neatly wrap a bandage over the dressing.

Hemodynamic complications include the possibility for continued bleeding. Once a dressing has been placed, it should not be removed because of the risk of disrupting clot formation. If a wound continues to bleed, additional dressings should be applied in conjunction with bleeding control interventions. Frequent reassessments will help prevent unchecked blood loss and hemodynamic complications. Exsanguination is a possibility when a pressure dressing does not stop blood loss; the same is true for an improperly applied tourniquet. If a tourniquet occludes only venous flow, bleeding may actually increase. A properly applied dressing in conjunction with direct pressure is often sufficient to stop blood loss. Conversely, a dressing applied too tightly can occlude distal flow when blood loss is not a concern.

Structural elements—blood vessels, nerves, tendons, muscles, skin, and internal organs—can be damaged, particularly when dressings are excessively tight. Prevention of damage entails assessing and readjusting the dressing and bandage as necessary. Distal pulses, motor, and sensation should be assessed when extremity dressings are in place. Tight dressings may cause pain in a patient who already has an injury.

Control of External Bleeding

External bleeding is bleeding that can be seen coming from a wound when the integrity of the skin has been violated. Theoretically, bleeding can be characterized according to the type of blood vessel that has been damaged **Figure 19-15 ▶** . Arterial bleeding occurs in spurts, and the blood is usually bright red because of the fully saturated hemoglobin. Venous bleeding is more likely to be slow and steady, and the colour of the blood is darker. In reality, most open wounds show a combination of arterial and venous bleeding. Capillary bleeding is characterized by a slow, even flow of bright or dark red blood and is present in minor injuries, such as abrasions or superficial lacerations.

Five methods are used in the prehospital environment to control external bleeding: direct pressure, elevation, pressure point control, immobilization, and a tourniquet.

Notes from Nancy

Steady, direct pressure against the bleeding site is the most effective means to control bleeding.

Direct Pressure

Application of pressure over a bleeding wound stops blood from flowing into the damaged vessels, allowing the platelets to seal the vascular walls.

If possible, use a sterile dressing to exert pressure, and then use your gloved hand to apply pressure over the bleeding site. The steps for controlling bleeding are shown in Skill Drill 19-1 ▶ :

1. Apply a dry, sterile dressing over the entire wound. Apply pressure to the dressing with your gloved hand (Step 1).
2. Maintain the pressure, and secure the dressing with a roller bandage (Step 2).
3. If bleeding continues or recurs, leave the original dressing in place. Apply a second dressing on top of the first, and secure it with another roller bandage (Step3).

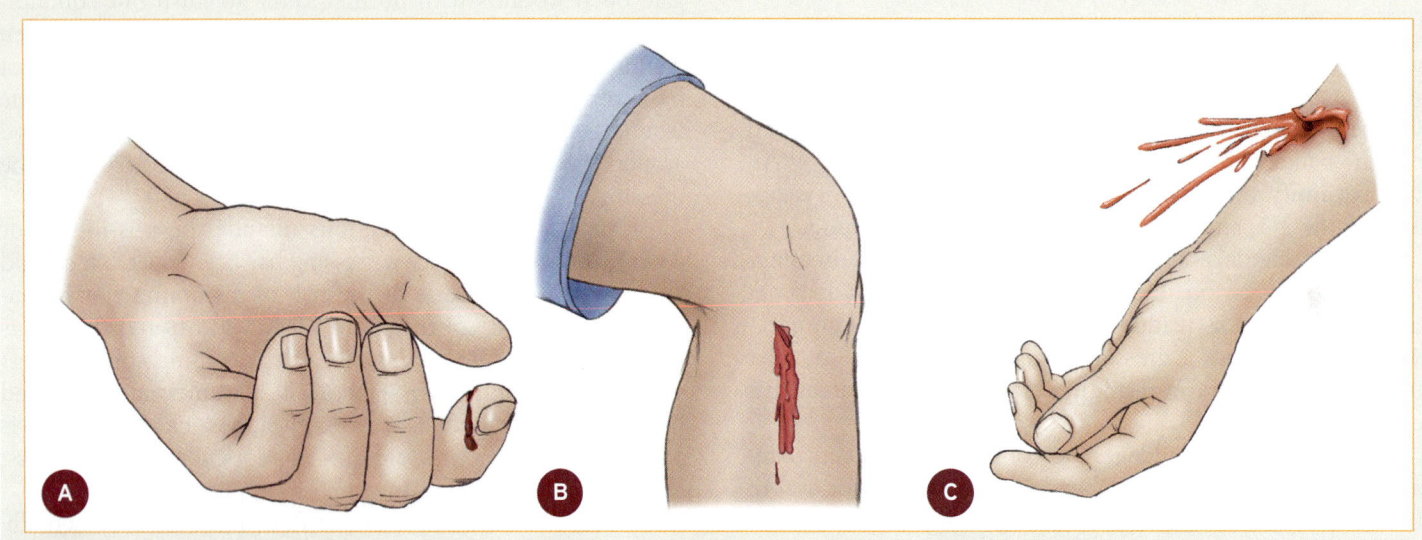

Figure 19-15 A. Capillary bleeding is dark red and oozes from the wound slowly but steadily. **B.** Venous bleeding is darker than arterial bleeding and flows steadily. **C.** Arterial bleeding is characteristically brighter red and spurts in time with the pulse.

You are the Paramedic Part 4

The patient remains hemodynamically stable throughout transport; however, he tells you that his leg is still hurting. You reassess his vital signs and consider the need for additional treatment. Your estimated time of arrival at the hospital is 5 minutes.

Reassessment	Recording Time: 20 Minutes
Skin	Pink and diaphoretic
Pulse	100 beats/min; strong and regular at the radial artery
Blood pressure	124/70 mm Hg
Respirations	18 breaths/min; adequate depth
Spo₂	98% on room air
Pain scale	5 on a scale of 0 to 10

7. Is further treatment indicated for this patient?

8. Are there any special considerations regarding the treatment you have provided to this patient?

Skill Drill 19-1: Controlling Bleeding From a Soft-Tissue Injury

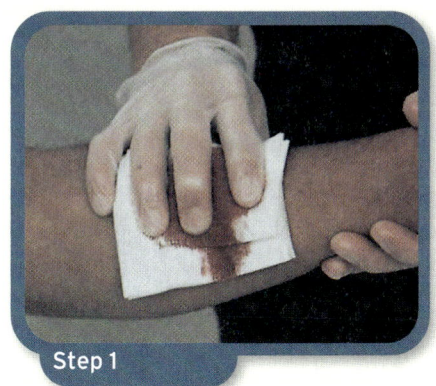

Step 1

Apply direct pressure with a sterile bandage.

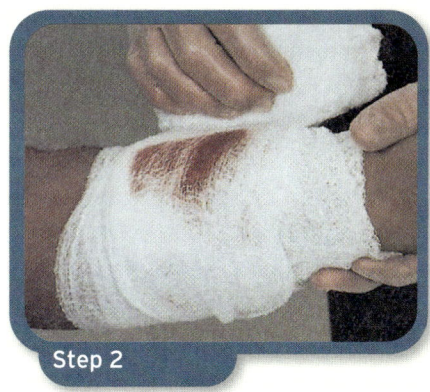

Step 2

Maintain pressure with a roller bandage.

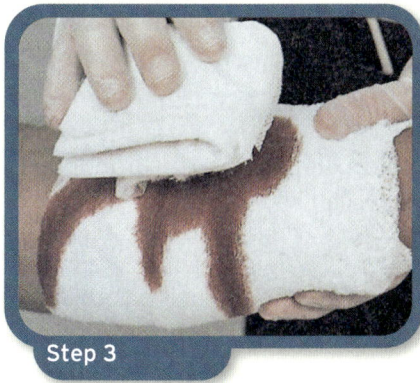

Step 3

If bleeding continues, apply a second dressing and roller bandage over the first.

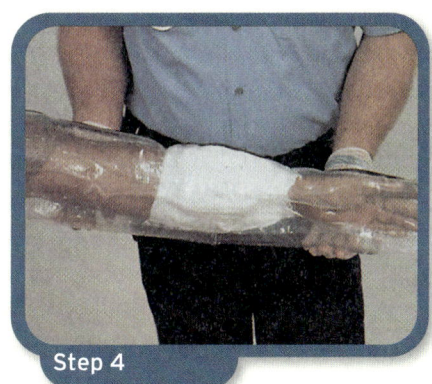

Step 4

Splint the extremity.

allow you to focus on other tasks while pressure is applied. Always assess distal circulation before and after you apply a pressure dressing. Adjust the dressing as needed in case of a complication, such as loss of distal pulse, diminished sensation, or change in skin colour and temperature distal to the dressing.

Elevation

In cases of venous bleeding from an extremity, the rate of bleeding can be substantially slowed by elevating the extremity above the level of the heart. This measure alone will not control bleeding, but it may be helpful in conjunction with other measures, such as direct pressure.

Pressure Point Control

When direct pressure is not sufficient to control bleeding or when the same artery is associated with a number of bleeding points, pressure point control **Figure 19-16 ▾** may help slow the bleeding. The artery chosen must be fairly superficial and overlie a hard structure against which it can be compressed. Three pressure points are typically used: (1) the temporal artery, which overlies the temporal bone of the skull and is used to control bleeding from the scalp; (2) the brachial artery, which overlies the humerus and is used to control bleeding from the forearm; and (3) the femoral artery, which can be compressed against the pelvis and is used to control bleeding from the leg.

Immobilization

Any movement of an extremity, even an uninjured extremity, promotes blood flow within that extremity. When the extremity is

4. Splint the extremity to stabilize the injury, even if there is no suspected fracture, which helps to minimize movement, further control the bleeding, and keep the dressing in place **Step 4**.

To maintain pressure, apply a pressure dressing over the site. On an extremity, one effective way of maintaining uniform pressure on a bleeding site is to apply an air splint over the dressed wound. If one or both of the lower extremities are bleeding, and if allowed by your local protocols, you can use the PASG to apply pressure, as discussed in Chapter 18. Maintain pressure over the bleeding site until the bleeding stops or until the patient reaches the hospital and other personnel take responsibility for care.

Some commercially available pressure dressings allow for simultaneous dressing of the wound and application of pressure. If one of these products is not available, standard dressing material may be used in conjunction with triangular bandages to create localized pressure. This type of dressing will often

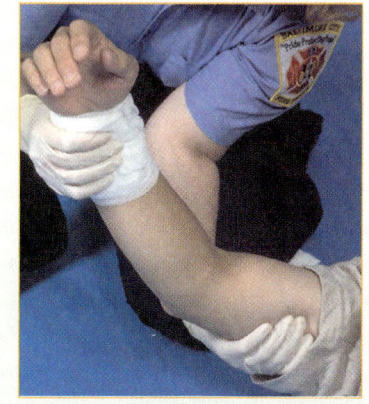

Figure 19-16 Applying pressure at the appropriate pressure point while holding direct pressure may slow difficult-to-control bleeding.

also injured, motion may disrupt the clotting process and lacerate more blood vessels. It follows that preventing motion of an injured extremity will have the opposite effects. Advise the patient to make every effort to minimize movement. If that is not possible and conditions warrant, apply a splint to prevent motion.

An air splint or padded board works well to keep an upper or lower extremity immobilized. Use of an air splint gives a double benefit—splinting *and* direct pressure. Remember to assess distal pulses, motor function, and sensation distal to the splint before and after application.

Tourniquet

In the civilian setting, it is rarely, if ever, necessary to use a tourniquet for control of external hemorrhage. Bleeding control can almost always be achieved by one or more of the methods already described. Furthermore, use of a tourniquet is associated with potential hazards, including damage to nerves and blood vessels and, when the tourniquet is in place for an extended period, loss of the distal extremity. A tourniquet applied too loosely, by contrast, may increase bleeding if it occludes venous return without hampering arterial inflow. *Use a tourniquet only as a last resort, when it is the only way to save the patient's life.*

In military settings, application of a tourniquet would occur more often owing to the nature of injuries experienced during battle. In addition, rapid transport to a medical facility is typically more difficult on the battlefield than in civilian situations. In such a scenario, a tourniquet may be lifesaving, particularly in patients with a traumatic partial amputation of a limb.

Some tourniquets can be applied with one arm (Figure 19-17 ▾), although you may not have access to them. If a tourniquet is required, observe the following application guidelines (Skill Drill 19-2 ▸):

1. Use wide, flat materials, such as a cravat or folded handkerchief. Never use rope, wire, or other narrow materials that might cut into the skin and damage underlying tissues. A blood pressure cuff inflated above the systolic reading works well for upper extremities.

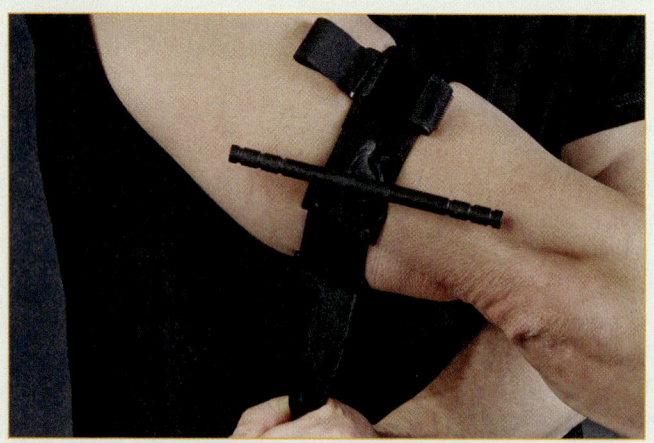

Figure 19-17 A tourniquet that can be applied using only one arm has been developed.

2. Apply a pad over the artery to be compressed.
3. Wrap the tourniquet twice around the extremity, at a point about 10 cm distal to the axilla or groin, and tie a half-knot (Step 1).
4. Place a stick, pencil, or similar object on top of the half knot, and complete the square knot above the stick (Step 2).
5. Twist the stick to tighten the tourniquet just until the bleeding stops (Step 3).
6. Secure the stick in that position so that it will not unwind. Never cover a tourniquet with a bandage or anything else, lest it escape notice when the patient arrives at the hospital. To make doubly sure that the tourniquet is not overlooked, write "TK" and the exact time you applied the tourniquet on a piece of adhesive tape, and fasten the tape to the patient's forehead (Step 4).
7. Do not remove a tourniquet, removal can result in release of an embolus, significant rebleeding, or tourniquet shock.
8. Record on the patient care report the time at which the tourniquet was applied.

Pain Control

Application of a cold compress will help reduce pain and diminish blood flow to an open wound. Once the dressing is in place, apply the cold pack. Avoid placing the compress directly on the site, because excessively cold temperature may do further harm. A pressure dressing may alleviate pain and minimize swelling.

If basic life support measures fail to relieve pain, consider administering morphine sulfate or other agents as allowed by protocol. The common dosage for morphine is .05 mg/kg intravenously every 5 minutes as needed. As with all medications, carefully assess the patient for allergies, and document pertinent information.

Managing an Avulsion

In treating a partially avulsed piece of skin, quickly irrigate any dirt or debris out of the wound and then gently fold the skin flap back onto the wound so that it is more or less normally aligned. Hold the flap in place with a dry, sterile compression dressing.

Preservation of Amputated Parts

When a part of the body is completely avulsed (torn off) or amputated (cut off)—whether a section of skin or an entire limb—it is important to try to preserve the amputated part in optimal condition to maximize the chances of it being successfully reimplanted. Once the patient's injuries have been stabilized, turn your attention to the amputated part, which will also require meticulous care. Follow these guidelines:

- Rinse the amputated part free of debris with cool, sterile saline.
- Wrap the part loosely in saline-moistened sterile gauze.

Skill Drill 19-2: Applying a Tourniquet

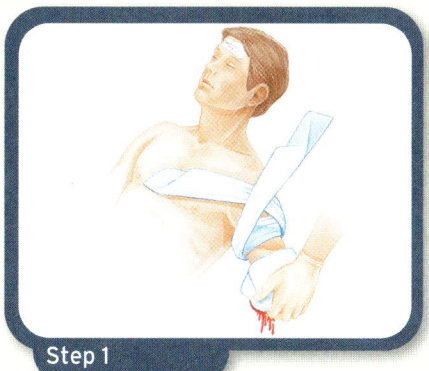

Step 1

Create a 10-cm, multilayered bandage. Wrap the bandage twice around the extremity, just above the bleeding site, and tie a half-knot.

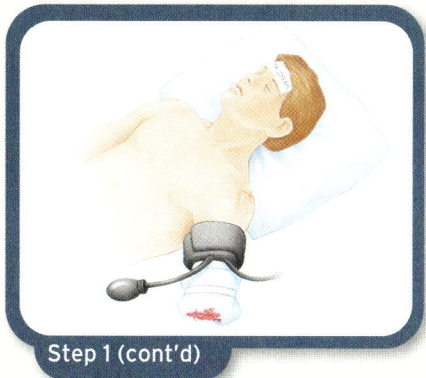

Step 1 (cont'd)

You can also use a blood pressure cuff as an effective tourniquet.

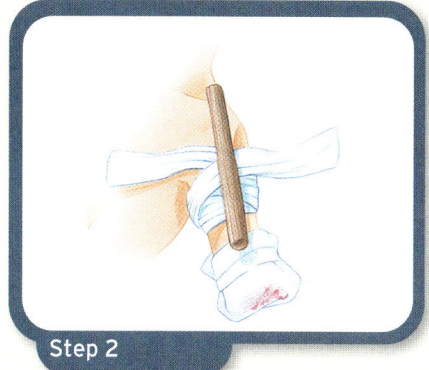

Step 2

Place a stick on top of the half-knot and tie a square knot over the stick.

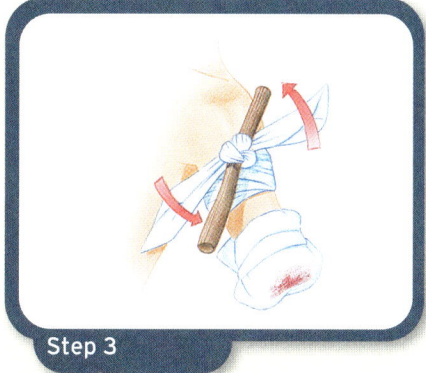

Step 3

Twist the stick until the bleeding stops.

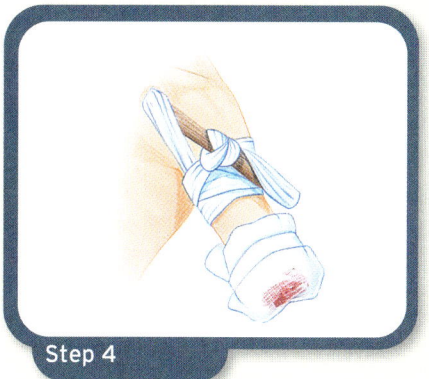

Step 4

Secure the stick so that it will not unwind. Write "TK" and the exact time you applied the tourniquet on a piece of adhesive tape, fasten the tape to the patient's forehead, and notify hospital personnel on arrival.

- Seal the amputated part inside a plastic bag, and place it in a cool container (such as a Styrofoam cooler). Keep it cold, but do not allow it to freeze.
- Never warm an amputated part.
- Never place an amputated part in water.
- Never place an amputated part directly on ice.
- Never use dry ice to cool an amputated part.

Transport the patient and the amputated part as expeditiously as possible. When the amputated part is a limb or part of

a limb, notify emergency department staff in advance of the type of case you are transporting and your estimated time of arrival so that a surgical team can be mobilized while you are en route.

Managing Impaled Objects

The following are basic points regarding management of an impaled object:

- Do not try to remove an impaled object. Efforts to do so may precipitate uncontrolled internal hemorrhage, which may lead to exsanguination or further injury to underlying structures.
- Control hemorrhage by direct compression, but do not apply pressure on the impaled object itself or on immediately adjacent tissues.
- Do not try to shorten an impaled object unless it is extremely cumbersome (such as a fence post impaled in

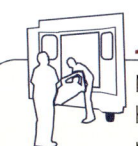

At the Scene

Never place an amputated part directly on ice, because this may cause frostbite and prevent reattachment.

the chest); any motion of the object may damage surrounding tissues.

- Stabilize the object in place with a bulky dressing, and immobilize the extremity (if the object is impaled in an extremity) with a splint to prevent motion.

The goal for prehospital care is to limit motion of the impaled object as soon as possible to minimize additional damage. One technique that is effective for thin objects is to use gauze pads cut midway through the centre. Stack several pads vertically, and arrange the cut portions so that each stack of pads overlaps. Once it is determined that enough pads are in place for stabilizing, tape or bandage them securely. This technique has the dual benefits of providing stabilization and aiding in bleeding control. Larger objects that are impaled in the body can be secured with rolled towels or splinting materials.

Impaled objects in the eye can be managed using gauze pads, a paper or Styrofoam cup, and bandage material. Do not apply pressure to the eye because pressure may cause vital fluids (the vitreous humour) to leak out. First, stabilize the object by hand. Once that is accomplished, use gauze pads cut midway into the centre, as outlined previously. Place the cup on top of the stacked pads after the height is sufficient. Bandage or tape the cup into place. It is important to cover both eyes because consensual movement may cause additional damage **Figure 19-18** . In such cases, it is particularly important to continually provide reassurance to the patient, who may be anxious because of the object and the blocked vision.

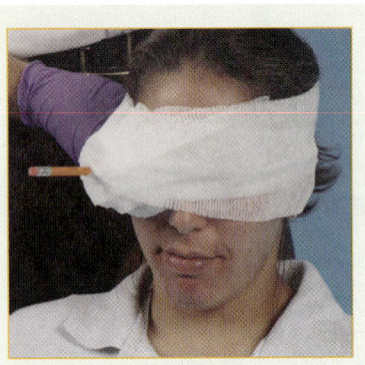

Figure 19-18 Stabilize an object impaled in the eye using gauze pads, a paper or Styrofoam cup, and bandage material.

Whatever presentation you may encounter, it is important to avoid causing additional harm. Secure the object as best as possible, and be creative in using securing materials. Provide reassurance to the patient and family. Constantly assess the risk for developing threats to life, such as airway compromise, breathing inadequacy, and uncontrolled hemorrhage.

On rare occasions, removal of an impaled object may be the best course of action. If the object directly interferes with airway control and the patient's condition is deteriorating rapidly, direct medical direction may authorize removal. It may also be necessary to remove an object that interferes with chest compressions in a patient who is in cardiac arrest and deemed viable. In severe cases, it may be impossible to leave the object in place, such as when the patient is impaled on an immovable object. Establish contact with direct medical control immediately in such cases, and ask for guidance.

Managing Wound Healing and Infection

In the prehospital setting, management of altered wound healing and infection entails basic measures. Wounds that are not healing properly or show signs of infection should be dressed and bandaged appropriately. In severe cases, pain control measures may be indicated.

Dressing Specific Anatomical Sites

Dressing and bandaging wounds is not the same for every part of the body. This section describes the various factors that need to be considered for a given body region.

Scalp Dressings

Scalp injuries tend to bleed profusely owing to their rich blood supply. When bleeding is present, application of direct pressure is often effective owing to the rigid skull that lies under the scalp. Be careful to accurately determine the extent of the injury because significant trauma may lead to skull damage. In that case, control of bleeding must be balanced against the issue of not causing additional damage. When the skull has been compromised and bleeding must be controlled, apply pressure to the areas around the break. Use a bulky dressing that assists in stopping blood loss and helps prevent excessive direct pressure on the already fractured cranium.

The shape of the skull is a consideration when dressing wounds that involve the scalp. Improperly applied dressings can easily slide up or down the scalp, becoming ineffective. In addition, hair may interfere with securing dressings in place.

Facial Dressings

Facial injuries tend to cause significant anxiety for patients and family. While tending to the clinical needs, take the time to reassure the patient. Application of direct pressure is an effective means to control bleeding from soft-tissue disruption along the face. If an avulsed piece of tissue is present, attempt to replace the pedicle to its normal anatomical location as closely as possible. Note that bleeding tends to be quite heavy owing to the rich blood supply in this area.

Assess the patient for the presence of or potential for airway compromise early in your encounter. Blood pouring into an unprotected airway is a recipe for disaster. Be prepared to suction and position the patient to facilitate drainage. Do not allow a gruesome facial injury to distract you from attending to life threats.

Ear or Mastoid Dressings

Trauma to the ear is commonly external, although internal injury is a possibility. Never place a dressing in the ear canal, but loosely apply it along the entire length of the external ear. Gauze sponges work well to aid in stopping blood loss. If blood is flowing from the ear canal, do not attempt to control it directly. Cerebrospinal fluid may be leaking, and halting the blood flow may increase pressure within the skull. Place a bulky dressing to the external ear, and transport the patient rapidly.

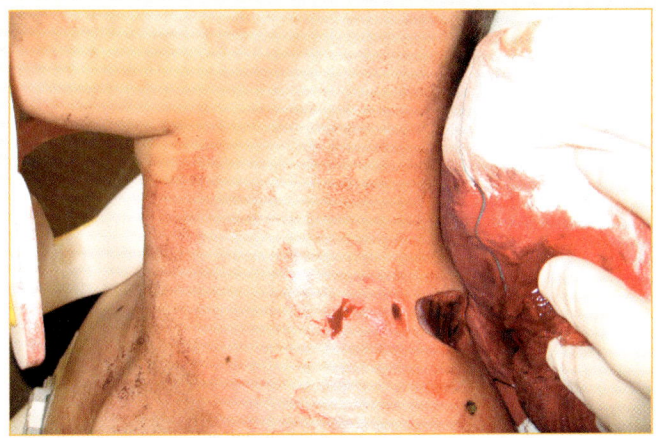

Figure 19-19 Neck wounds can lead to other serious situations such as air embolism and airway problems. Seal with an occlusive dressing right away.

Neck Dressings

Important anatomical structures in the neck include large blood vessels, the airway, and the cervical spine. There is little room for error when trauma is present in this area. A minor neck laceration can lead to an air embolism, a small puncture can penetrate the spinal canal, and an anterior open wound can disrupt the airway **Figure 19-19 ▲**. Pay close attention to the clinical signs that accompany the external trauma.

Open injuries to the neck require use of an occlusive dressing to prevent the drawing of air into the circulatory system. Apply dressings carefully so that they do not interfere with blood flow or movement of air through the trachea.

Shoulder Dressings

The shoulder is relatively easy to dress and bandage. Apply direct pressure to control external hemorrhage in this region. If immobilization is indicated, a sling and swathe will prevent motion of the shoulder girdle.

Truncal Dressings

Injuries to the torso require vigilant assessment for underlying internal trauma. A seemingly innocuous hole may be the only indication that a gunshot wound is present. Cover open wounds with an occlusive dressing that is taped on three sides. Assessment of breath sounds becomes a high priority when you find an open chest wound because a pneumothorax or hemothorax may develop from penetrating trauma to the thorax. Continually reassess a patient with thoracic soft-tissue injuries.

The best choice for securing a truncal dressing in place is medical tape. Wrapping the entire torso may interfere with air movement.

Groin and Hip Dressings

Soft-tissue injuries to the groin and hip do not present a significant challenge to paramedics. Typically, application of a dressing and bandage in combination with direct pressure work well to control blood loss in this region. Injuries to the genitalia are best managed by a paramedic of the same sex, whenever feasible.

In many cases, it is possible to provide the patient with a dressing and allow self-directed care. This makes an uncomfortable scenario easier for patient and paramedic. If proper care cannot be accomplished by working directly with the patient, you must be exceedingly professional and respect the patient's modesty in all but the most serious of cases.

Hand, Wrist, and Finger Dressings

The hands, wrists, and fingers are among the easiest sites to properly dress and bandage. A dressing is applied over any open wound, and bandage material is wrapped completely around the affected area. When possible, the hand should be placed in the position of function. This is accomplished by placing a roll of gauze in the patient's hand **Figure 19-20 ▶**. If limited motion is necessary, the hand and wrist can be easily splinted.

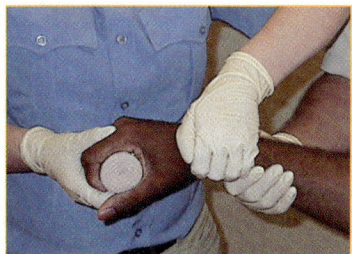

Figure 19-20 The position of function for the hand.

Elbow and Knee Dressings

Joints are not difficult to dress and bandage, but movement may cause the materials to shift from their original position. It is a good practice to provide immobilization of the elbow or the knee when a larger wound is present. Even smaller wounds may be difficult to manage because of skin tension lines and high tissue stress in these areas. When either of these joints is injured, it becomes very important to assess distal neurovascular status. Elbow injuries have a higher risk for neurovascular compromise because of the limited space available for blood vessels and nerves.

Ankle and Foot Dressings

The ankle and foot are simple to dress and bandage. Control of bleeding is accomplished by direct pressure and may be augmented by elevation and pressure points in cases involving significant bleeding. Application of a bandage must not be so tight that it interferes with circulation or sensation. Always assess distal neurovascular function before and after caring for the wound.

Crush Syndrome Management

Crush syndrome has been widely studied in recent years. In January 1995, a massive earthquake shook the southern part of Hyogo Prefecture, Japan, producing 41,000 casualties and 5,500 deaths. When researchers evaluated 372 patients who were diagnosed with crush syndrome, they found that most had lower extremity injuries that led to development of crush syndrome. Upper extremity injuries and trunk entrapment also caused some cases of crush syndrome, albeit to a much lesser extent.

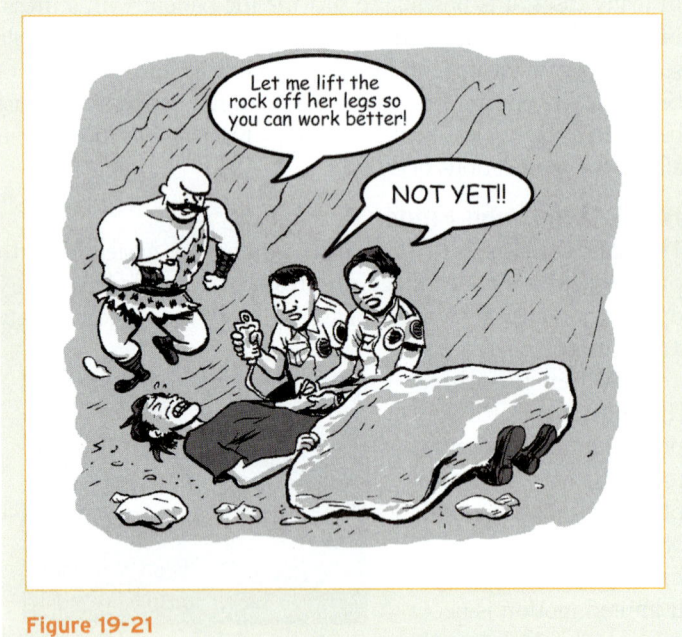

Figure 19-21

Paramount to the issue of managing a case involving crush syndrome is making every effort to treat the patient before removing the crushing object **Figure 19-21 ▲**. Failure to do so can result in significant hypotension and release of harmful products resulting in death. Among the early causes of death are hypovolemia and hyperkalemia. It is possible to treat both problems in the prehospital setting by using a proactive approach.

The first issue to consider in dealing with crush syndrome is scene safety. Given that most instances of crush syndrome involve building collapse, rescuers face a serious risk. Interaction with technical rescue professionals will often be necessary when called to the scene of a collapsed building, irrespective of whether the cause was a natural or human-made disaster. On the scene of an intentional explosion, there is an added danger of a secondary device. Paramedics must work closely with law enforcement officials to determine the relative risk to everyone at the scene.

After scene safety has been ensured, the first step is to conduct as much of the initial assessment as possible given the nature of the entrapment. If debris can be removed by hand, it should be cleared away on gaining access to the patient. Larger items may require removal by technical rescue teams; removal should be conducted after intervention from caregivers, particularly if the patient has been trapped for longer than 4 hours.

Renal failure—a key complication of crush syndrome—can be prevented with aggressive fluid therapy. In some cases, 8 to 24 l has been provided in the first day to prevent kidney failure. In the out-of-hospital setting, intravenous (IV) access should be obtained before removing the object. Although two large-bore IV lines should be established, the entrapment scenario may rule out typical IV sites. If access to the extremities is not possible, caregivers can establish access at the external jugular veins. When available, a sternal intraosseous needle can be inserted in unconscious patients.

Once IV access is established, normal saline should be infused. Lactated Ringer's solution contains potassium, so it is not recommended for use in cases of crush syndrome.

Alkalinizing the blood and urine with sodium bicarbonate helps prevent kidney failure, treats hyperkalemia, and reverses metabolic acidosis. High potassium levels released from damaged muscles can be expected on removal of the crushing item. To prevent this complication, sodium bicarbonate may be administered as part of the IV fluid. Mannitol may be used for its diuretic effect. Furosemide is not indicated because it acidifies the urine. If pretreatment with medicines is not possible, apply a tourniquet above the crush site. The tourniquet will not prevent crush syndrome, but it will reduce some of the reperfusion damage.

Severe hyperkalemia may be treated with 25 ml of $D_{50}W$ followed by 10 units of regular insulin IV. Although caregivers in the prehospital environment typically do not administer insulin, a medical team may potentially be deployed to the site equipped to provide additional medications. Calcium chloride is not indicated to treat hyperkalemia except in cases of significant dysrhythmia.

Once the patient is freed, rapid transport is indicated. En route to the facility, complete a rapid trauma assessment and care for injuries not treated on scene. Open injuries can be handled with dressings and bandaging, and fractures can be splinted, if time permits. Be prepared to administer additional fluids as indicated by patient condition or via direct medical direction. Measure vital signs every 5 minutes at a minimum. Attach an electrocardiographic monitor to detect dysrhythmias due to acidosis, hyperkalemia, hypotension, or other related conditions.

In some cases, a mangled extremity must be amputated on scene to facilitate extrication. When this procedure is performed in the prehospital environment, there is a higher risk for infection. The benefit must clearly outweigh the risk to warrant this step. Except in the most desperate situations, an on-scene emergency practitioner (physician, osteopath, or authorized physician assistant) should perform the amputation.

When you transport the patient, consult with direct medical control regarding the use of a hyperbaric chamber. The physician may opt to have the patient undergo hyperbaric oxygen therapy to aid in tissue recovery and facilitate management of anaerobic bacteria. Hyperbaric therapy, especially when performed early in the course of care, has been shown to decrease muscle necrosis for crush-injured patients and decrease muscle edema.

Blast Injury Assessment and Management

When dealing with an explosion, expect significant trauma and multiple patients. The forces generated have the potential to cover a wide area with devastating effect. If the explosion was intentional, examine the immediate area for a secondary device. When scene safety cannot be ensured, evacuate to a safe distance until qualified personnel advise that it is safe to approach the patient. Also assess the scene for other hazards that may lead to injury, such as exposed electrical wiring, structural instability, and sharp objects.

Wearing appropriate PPE, form a general impression as you approach the patient. Rapidly perform an initial assessment to detect and manage life threats. Immobilize the cervical spine, and assess the airway by performing the jaw-thrust maneuver. Determine if the airway is patent, and correct airway compromises immediately on their discovery. Identify whether breathing is abnormally fast or slow or deep or shallow, and note the gross respiratory pattern. Determine whether circulation is present by assessing the carotid and radial pulses. Reassess the patient's mental status while exposing and examining the patient for injury.

Pulmonary injuries are common when an explosion occurs and can be life threatening. Assess breath sounds frequently throughout care because the pressure wave generated by an explosion can lead to a pneumothorax. Should the air within the chest cavity continue to collapse the affected lung, a tension pneumothorax can develop. Needle decompression is a lifesaving intervention in such a case.

Noncardiogenic pulmonary edema can develop after an explosion. A massive pulmonary contusion can lead to microhemorrhage within the lungs, further compromising ventilation and respiration. Ask the patient about the ease or difficulty of breathing early in your assessment. Have your fellow caregivers examine the patient rapidly for the presence of DCAP-BTLS, and manage life threats rapidly. Establish a baseline pulse oximetry value, and reassess this measure frequently. Although pulse oximeter readings are important, administer high-flow supplemental oxygen even in the presence of a high reading. Patient compromise is likely to develop, even if the initial symptoms are not severe.

Abdominal trauma commonly found in the blast-injured patient includes ruptured organs and internal hemorrhage. The pressure wave can cause air-filled cavities, such as the small and large bowels, to burst. Although these injuries can be catastrophic, they often take time to emerge. An absence of overt signs of abdominal injury should not lead you to conclude that an injury is not present. Recall the kinetic forces involved during an explosion, and maintain a high index of suspicion.

Ask the patient about the presence of abdominal pain. If he or she reports discomfort, use the OPQRST mnemonic to guide your history taking. Examine all quadrants for the presence of DCAP-BTLS, noting tenderness on the patient care report.

During the blast, victims' ears are often adversely affected by the pressure wave. The likelihood of rupture of the tympanic membrane is high. Hearing loss is common when the patient is in proximity to the blast. Because the ears are essential in establishing body position, dizziness can occur when they are affected. Such dizziness can lead to vomiting, which may interfere with airway patency and protection.

Projectiles can lead to penetrating wounds during the secondary blast phase. If you discover an impaled object, leave it in place unless it *directly* interferes with lifesaving care. An object lodged in the airway may have to be removed, but this action should be taken only if it is clearly allowed by protocol or through direct medical direction.

Management of Soft-Tissue Injuries to Specific Anatomical Sites

Soft-tissue injuries that involve the face and neck, thorax, or abdomen deserve special attention. Because the underlying structures in these regions are vital to life, additional concerns arise when they are involved in a traumatic event.

Face and Neck

Injuries to the face and neck may involve the airway or large blood vessels. Airway compromise can arise from substantial bleeding or disruption of soft tissue. In such cases, suctioning and patient positioning may become necessary to maintain airway patency. Open injuries involving the jugular or carotid vessels can result in exsanguination if they are not rapidly addressed. These factors, combined with the psychological impact of facial damage, can create challenging scenarios.

As always, the airway is the first priority. Immediate assessment of patency, protection, and flow of oxygen with removal of carbon dioxide is paramount. Suction secretions or blood as indicated by patient presentation. Ensure delivery of high-flow oxygen with a nonrebreathing mask or, if ventilations are compromised, with a bag-valve-mask device. More invasive management may require use of an advanced airway such as an endotracheal tube, a double-lumen airway, or a laryngeal mask airway. When neither ventilation nor intubation is possible, a surgical airway is indicated.

Control of bleeding can be accomplished while airway control is underway. If only one paramedic is available, bleeding control is addressed only after ensuring an open airway. Manage significant bleeding by applying bulky dressings and direct pressure. Open wounds to the neck require occlusive dressings to prevent air emboli. Realign avulsed skin along the face or neck to its original anatomical position, if possible.

Thorax

Thoracic injuries that appear minor may lead you to believe that minimal trauma is present. This is a serious mistake. In reality, gunshot and stab wounds may present as very small openings yet produce internal damage that can quickly lead to death. It is important to determine the MOI while conducting the initial assessment to detect life threats.

Assessment includes four steps: inspection, palpation, auscultation, and percussion. Examine the entire chest for signs of visible injury. Listen to breath sounds in at least two sites on each side of the chest. If breath sounds are diminished or absent on one side, suspect a pneumothorax. Palpate the entire chest wall, noting any abnormalities. Subcutaneous emphysema is indicative of a disruption in the tracheobronchial tree. Percussion along the chest wall can help you differentiate between a pneumothorax and a hemothorax—either of which can lead to the patient's death.

Open wounds to the thorax require the application of an occlusive dressing to prevent a pneumothorax or at least stop its progression. Tape the dressing on only three sides to allow air to escape. Failure to provide a small opening for relief of pressure can result in a tension pneumothorax, which can be fatal.

Abdomen

Abdominal injuries range from minor abrasions to evisceration. Inspect the abdomen for visible signs of injuries. Palpate the area to identify pain, rigidity, and distension. Cover open wounds that are higher on the abdominal wall with an occlusive dressing to accommodate diaphragmatic movement. As the diaphragm travels downward during inspiration, the relative sizes of the thoracic and abdominal cavities change. This process increases the risk of drawing air into the pleural space when an open wound is present.

Maintain a high index of suspicion when an abdominal injury is readily evident. Blunt or penetrating trauma can lead to laceration of solid organs or rupture of hollow organs. Solid organs tend to bleed profusely, whereas hollow organs spill their contents into the peritoneum. Either can be fatal.

Documentation

Written documentation must be completed for every patient contact. When filling out the patient care report, include all relevant scene findings, such as a severely damaged vehicle or calibre of weapon used. Also record patient findings, including patency of airway, ventilation, and circulation, and any interventions administered. Describe the patient's presentation on your arrival at the scene, and note the body position on arrival (for example, prone or supine).

Note specific injuries. Describe wounds in terms of size, location, depth, and associated complications. Note your assessment findings for distal neurovascular status, range of motion, and presence or absence of infection. Obtain patient demographic information, such as age, date of birth, and home address. Include the patient's medical history, medications, and allergies.

If you performed an intervention, record it on the patient care report. Note how the patient responded to therapy (ie, the same, better, or worse condition). Also document the patient's level of understanding for each intervention. Finally, note which paramedic attended to the patient en route to the receiving facility.

You are the Paramedic Summary

1. Does this patient require spinal motion restriction precautions? Why or why not?

The mechanism of injury—an isolated injury to the leg—does not suggest a high potential for a spinal injury; therefore, spinal motion restriction precautions are likely not necessary. However, it is important to conduct a careful assessment of the patient to determine if any other injuries are present. Football is arguably one of the roughest organized sports; players may experience injuries to multiple parts of their body, especially during a rough tackle.

2. What are your main concerns regarding this patient's injury?

Your patient has an open fracture of his leg, which should raise concern for several potential problems. First, you must control the external bleeding. The fractured bone may have damaged a large blood vessel in the patient's leg and may make bleeding difficult to control—especially if an artery is involved. Second, the bone has broken through the skin, which has placed this patient at risk for infection of the bone and adjacent muscle (osteomyelitis). Although this will not present acutely in the out-of-hospital setting, preventing further contamination (ie, covering the wound with sterile dressings) will certainly reduce the risk of infection.

3. Is this patient in shock?

On the basis of the mechanism of injury, the patient's vital signs—tachycardia, tachypnea, and hypertension—represent pain, not shock. Isolated distal long bone fractures (open or closed) typically do not cause shock in adolescent and adult patients unless they are associated with prolonged uncontrolled bleeding. Nonetheless, careful patient assessment and close monitoring remain essential elements in the overall care of the patient. As noted earlier, football is a rough sport; occult injury cannot be ruled out in the prehospital setting.

4. What additional care should you provide to this patient?

Primary treatment for an open fracture consists of controlling external bleeding, preventing further contamination, and splinting the injury. However, you must not overlook the aspect of pain relief in patients with such injuries. Your patient is in severe pain (10/10); to overlook this would be inappropriate (and inhumane), especially considering the fact that he is hemodynamically stable. Therefore, a narcotic analgesic is clearly indicated. Morphine and fentanyl are the two most commonly administered medications for this purpose. Follow local protocols regarding the appropriate doses of these medications.

5. What is compartment syndrome and is this patient at risk for it?

Compartment syndrome is seen commonly when a part of the body is entrapped for a lengthy period of time—usually greater than 4 hours. However, it can also occur as the result of a fracture. Compartment syndrome can occur following open or closed fractures.

Compartment syndrome develops when hemorrhage and edema cause increased pressure within the osteofascial compartment. Increased compartment pressure results in ischemia and further tissue swelling. As pressure increases, venous return is compromised first, followed by arterial inflow. This causes two significant problems: cellular and tissue damage within the injured compartment and the accumulation of metabolic waste products (ie, lactic acid). Left untreated, compartment syndrome can result in permanent muscle and tissue damage and necrosis of the muscles within the affected compartment.

6. What are the signs and symptoms of compartment syndrome?

Signs and symptoms of compartment syndrome include pain that is disproportionate to the injury, firmness of the area around the injury, a feeling of "pressure" expressed by the patient, and pain when the affected muscles are passively stretched. Later signs include parasthesia, pallor, and loss of the pulse distal to the injury.

7. Is further treatment indicated for this patient?

Your patient remains hemodynamically stable, yet because he is still in pain (5/10), it would not be unreasonable to administer a second dose of a narcotic analgesic (eg, fentanyl, morphine). Again, follow locally established protocols regarding initial and repeat dosing of these medications.

8. Are there any special considerations regarding the treatment you have provided to this patient?

As noted earlier, you should monitor this patient for signs of compartment syndrome and circulatory compromise distal to the injury (just as you would any patient who you have bandaged and splinted). Additionally, because you have administered a narcotic analgesic, it would be prudent to have naloxone (Narcan)—a narcotic antagonist—readily available in the event that the patient experiences central nervous system (CNS) depression (ie, hypotension, bradycardia, hypoventilation). If signs of CNS depression become apparent, administer an appropriate dose of naloxone—usually 0.4 to 2 mg via slow IV push. If IV access is not available, you can administer naloxone intramuscularly.

Prep Kit

Ready for Review

- The skin is a complex organ that fulfills several crucial roles, including maintaining homeostasis, protecting tissue from injury, and regulating temperature.
- The main layers of the skin are the epidermis and the dermis. The epidermis, the outer layer, serves as the principal barrier. The dermis, the inner layer, includes collagen, elastin, and ground substance, which contribute to the skin's strength. It also contains nerve endings, blood vessels, sweat glands, hair follicles, and sebaceous glands.
- The subcutaneous layer lies beneath the dermis and contains adipose tissue. Below the subcutaneous layer is the deep fascia, which offers support and protection to underlying structures such as muscle and bone.
- The skin is arranged in patterns of tautness known as tension lines. Wounds that occur parallel to skin tension lines may remain closed. Wounds that run perpendicular to tension lines may remain open.
- Soft-tissue injuries may be dramatic but are seldom the most serious. Don't let them distract you from thorough initial assessment!
- The first stage of wound healing is cessation of bleeding. The body uses several mechanisms to control bleeding, such as constricting the size of vessels and releasing platelets to form a blood clot.
- The second stage of healing is inflammation, in which additional cells enter the damaged area in an effort to repair it. Epithelialization (creation of a new layer of epithelial cells) occurs, followed by neovascularization (formation of new vessels).
- Wound healing is affected by factors such as the amount of movement the part is subjected to, medications, and medical conditions. A wound is more likely to become infected if it is caused by a human or an animal bite or if a foreign body has been impaled. Pressure injuries can develop when a patient is bedridden or remains on a backboard for too long.
- Signs of infection include redness, pus, warmth, edema, and local discomfort. Gangrene, tetanus, and necrotizing fasciitis are serious infection-related conditions that must be recognized early.
- In a closed wound, the skin is not broken but soft tissues beneath the skin are damaged. An example is a bruise. A hematoma (collection of blood beneath the skin) can also form.
- In an open wound, the skin is broken. Such an injury can become infected and can result in serious blood loss. Open wounds include abrasions, lacerations, puncture wounds, avulsions, and amputations.
- In a crush injury, a body part is crushed between two solid objects, resulting in damage to soft tissues and bone. The patient's external appearance may not adequately represent the level of internal damage.
- Crush syndrome may develop after a body part has been trapped for more than 4 hours. Necrosis occurs in crushed muscles, and harmful products are released in a process called rhabdomyolysis. Freeing the trapped body part can cause these harmful products to be released into the circulation, which can prove fatal. Kidney damage, cardiac arrest, and arrhythmias can also result.
- Compartment syndrome results when pressure increases in the injured area. Tissue necrosis and sepsis may then develop. Patients present with the six Ps: Pain, Paresthesia, Paresis, Pressure, Passive stretch pain, and Pulselessness.
- Blasts (explosions) can result in soft-tissue injuries. A blast wind from the gases released can be very forceful, and projectiles can impale victims; both cause injuries. Falling structures can injure patients, and burns can also occur.
- Observe scene safety before assessing patients with soft-tissue injuries; hazards that caused the injury may still be present. Regardless of the grotesqueness of the injury, assess the ABCs first.

- While taking the history, ask about the event that caused the injury, such as whether a weapon was used or whether the patient lost consciousness. Find out when the patient last had a tetanus booster. Pay attention to whether the patient is taking any medications that may affect hemostasis.
- Depending on whether the mechanism of injury is significant or not, complete your physical examination en route or at the scene, respectively. Direct your attention to the chief complaint and area of injury, and perform frequent reassessments.
- Be empathetic to patients with soft-tissue injuries.
- Managing soft-tissue injuries includes controlling bleeding. With closed injuries, follow the ICES mnemonic: Ice, Compression, Elevation, and Splinting.
- When managing open wounds, control bleeding and keep the wound as clean as possible by irrigating and using sterile dressings. Try to determine the colour and type of bleeding and the amount of blood the patient has lost.
- Dressings and bandages are used to cover the wound, control bleeding, and limit motion. Types of dressings include sterile and nonsterile, occlusive and nonocclusive, adherent and nonadherent, and wet and dry. Types of bandages include roller and gauze, absorbent gauze sponges, elastic, and triangular bandages.
- Medical tape may be used to secure a bandage in place, except for patients with thin skin such as older patients because it can cause damage on removal. Do not apply dressings too tightly.
- Methods of bleeding control include direct pressure, elevation, pressure point control, immobilization, and tourniquets. Cold compresses may help reduce pain. IV medications may be administered if basic measures do not relieve pain.
- Tourniquets are rarely needed in the civilian setting but may be used as a last resort. They can damage nerves and blood vessels and lead to loss of an extremity.
- Management of an avulsion includes irrigation, gently folding the flap back onto the wound, and applying a dry, sterile compression dressing. If the wound is an amputation, preserve the amputated part and transport it.
- Do not remove impaled objects in the prehospital environment. Instead, stabilize the object in place with a bulky dressing. Control bleeding with direct compression, but do not apply pressure on the object or on the immediately adjacent tissues.
- Dressing and bandaging techniques vary for different parts of the body. For example, the shape of the skull and the presence of hair make dressing the scalp challenging.
- Trapped patients must be managed before being freed from the crushing object because this approach improves their chances of survival after experiencing crush syndrome. Aggressive fluid therapy can help prevent kidney failure. Normal saline should be infused. Administration of sodium bicarbonate may help prevent an efflux of potassium. Rapidly transport the patient once freed.
- Blast injuries can include pulmonary damage such as tension pneumothorax and pulmonary contusion, abdominal trauma such as ruptured organs and internal hemorrhage, damage to the ears, and penetrating wounds. Use the DCAP-BTLS guideline to assess the patient rapidly.
- Soft-tissue injuries of the face, neck, thorax, and abdomen deserve special attention because these areas contain vital structures. Do not underestimate the seriousness of these injuries, and maintain a high index of suspicion.
- Document scene findings, including vehicle damage or the calibre of weapon used and patient presentation and position; size, location, depth, and complications of injuries; assessment findings; and interventions.

Vital Vocabulary

abrasion An injury in which a portion of the body is denuded of epidermis by scraping or rubbing.

adipose Referring to fat tissue.

amputation An injury in which part of the body is completely severed.

avulsion An injury that leaves a piece of skin or other tissue partially or completely torn away from the body.

bandage Material used to secure a dressing in place.

chemotactic factors The factors that cause cells to migrate into an area.

closed wound An injury in which damage occurs beneath the skin or mucous membrane but the surface remains intact.

collagen Protein that gives tensile strength to the connective tissues of the body.

compartment syndrome A condition that develops when edema and swelling result in increased pressure within soft tissues, causing circulation to be compromised, possibly resulting in tissue necrosis.

contaminated Containing microorganisms.

contusion A bruise; an injury that causes bleeding beneath the skin but does not break the skin.

crush injury An injury in which the body or part of the body is crushed, preventing tissue function and, possibly, resulting in permanent tissue damage.

crush syndrome Significant metabolic derangement that can lead to renal failure and death. It develops when crushed extremities or other body parts remain trapped for prolonged periods.

deep fascia A dense layer of fibrous tissue below the subcutaneous tissue; composed of tough bands of tissue that ensheath muscles and other internal structures.

degloving A traumatic injury that results in the soft tissue of the hand being drawn downward like a glove being removed.

degranulate To release granules into the surrounding tissue.

dermis The inner layer of skin, containing hair follicle roots, glands, blood vessels, and nerves.

dressing Material used to directly cover a wound.

ecchymosis Extravasation of blood under the skin to produce a "black-and-blue" mark.

elastin A protein that gives the skin its elasticity.

epidermis The outermost layer of the skin.

epithelialization The formation of fresh epithelial tissue to heal a wound.

erythema Reddening of the skin.

fasciotomy A surgical procedure that cuts away fascia to relieve pressure.

gangrene An infection commonly caused by *C perfringens*. The result is tissue destruction and gas production that may lead to death.

glomerular filtration The first step in the formation of urine; calculated to determine renal function.

granulocytes Cells that contain granules.

ground substance Material between cells.

hematoma A localized collection of blood in the soft tissues as a result of injury or a broken blood vessel.

homeostasis The tendency to constancy or stability in the body's internal environment.

hyperkalemia An increased level of potassium in the blood.

hypertrophic scar An abnormal scar with excess collagen that does not extend over the wound margins.

impaled object An object that has caused a puncture wound and remains embedded in the wound.

incision A wound usually made deliberately, as in surgery; a clean cut, as opposed to a laceration.

integument The skin.

keloid scar An abnormal scar commonly found in people with darkly pigmented skin. It extends over the wound margins.

laceration A wound made by tearing or cutting tissues.

lymphangitis Inflammation of a lymph channel.

lymphocytes White blood cells that function to remove invading pathogens.

macrophages Cells that are responsible for protecting the body against infection.

melanin The pigment that gives skin its colour.

mucopolysaccharide gel A key component of ground substance that is a polysaccharide that forms complexes with proteins.

myoglobin A protein found in muscle that is released into the circulation after crush injury or other muscle damage and whose presence in the circulation may produce kidney damage.

neovascularization Development of vessels to aid in healing an injured soft tissue.

open wound An injury in which there is a break in the surface of the skin or the mucous membrane, exposing deeper tissue to potential contamination.

pedicle A narrow strip of tissue by which an avulsed piece of tissue remains connected to the body.

puncture wound A stab injury from a pointed object, such as a nail or a knife.

rhabdomyolysis The destruction of muscle tissue leading to a release of potassium and myoglobin.

scar revision A surgical procedure to improve the appearance of a scar, reestablish function, or correct disfigurement from soft-tissue damage, surgical incision, or lesion.

sebaceous gland The gland located in the dermis that secretes sebum.

sebum An oily substance secreted by the sebaceous glands.

subcutaneous Beneath the skin.

tension lines The pattern of tautness of the skin, which is arranged over body structures and affects how well wounds heal.

Volkmann contracture Deformity of the hand, fingers, and wrist resulting from damage to forearm muscles; develops from muscle ischemia and is associated with compartment syndrome.

www.Paramedic.EMSzone.com/Canada

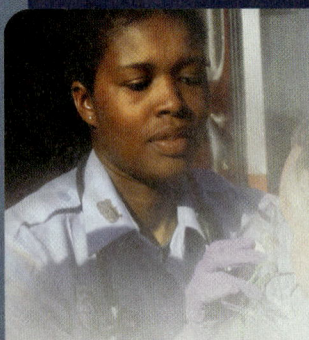

Assessment in Action

You are dispatched to the outside of a private residence for a dog bite. When you arrive, you notice that the patient is sitting upright, speaking in full sentences. She is conscious, alert, oriented, and complaining of pain in both of her arms and head. The family has wrapped towels over both arms and one over her head.

When you unwrap the right arm, you note two large lacerations greater than 10 cm long and multiple puncture wounds. When you examine the upper arm, you notice white material that looks like muscle fascia. You control the bleeding with bandages. The left arm is not as bad, but it is bleeding. When you begin to check out the head, you notice that a piece of the scalp is missing. The family hands you a plastic bag with the missing piece.

1. A "wound" is defined as:
   A. any injury to the soft tissues, with or without involvement of the subcutaneous tissues and muscle beneath.
   B. any injury to the soft tissues that requires special care to stop the bleeding.
   C. any injury to the soft tissues, with involvement of the subcutaneous tissues and muscle beneath.
   D. any injury to the soft tissues that extends into the bone.

2. What are the two types of wound classifications?
   A. Open wounds and lacerations
   B. Lacerations and incisions
   C. Contusions and closed wounds
   D. Closed and open wounds

3. A laceration is defined as:
   A. a superficial wound that occurs when the skin is rubbed or scraped over a rough surface so that part of the epidermis is lost.
   B. a cut inflicted by a sharp instrument, such as a knife or razor blade, that produces a clean or jagged incision through the skin surface and underlying structure.
   C. a clean (linear) cut.
   D. a stab from a pointed object, such as a nail or a knife.

4. A puncture wound is defined as:
   A. a superficial wound that occurs when the skin is rubbed or scraped over a rough surface so that part of the epidermis is lost.
   B. a cut inflicted by a sharp instrument, such as a knife or razor blade, that produces a clean or jagged incision through the skin surface and underlying structure.
   C. a clean (linear) cut.
   D. a stab from a pointed object, such as a nail or a knife.

5. An avulsion is defined as:
   A. a superficial wound that occurs when the skin is rubbed or scraped over a rough surface so that part of the epidermis is lost.
   B. a cut inflicted by a sharp instrument, such as a knife or razor blade, that produces a clean or jagged incision through the skin surface and underlying structure.
   C. a flap of skin that has been torn loose, partially or completely.
   D. a complete loss of a body part, typically involving the extremities.

6. Evaluation of the skin involves:
   A. inspection and auscultation.
   B. auscultation and circulation.
   C. inspection and palpation.
   D. palpation and auscultation.

7. Bleeding may be controlled by using:
   A. direct pressure.
   B. elevation.
   C. pressure point control.
   D. all of the above.

8. It is important to preserve the amputated part because this:
   A. maximizes the chances of it being successfully reimplanted.
   B. allows it to be donated.
   C. minimizes the chances of it being unsuccessfully reimplanted.
   D. all of the above.

9. Scalp injuries tend to bleed more because:
   A. there is no blood supply to this area.
   B. there is a rich blood supply in this area.
   C. there is an excessive number of veins in the scalp.
   D. these are life-threatening injuries.

10. Written documentation must be completed for every patient contact. It should include all of the following, EXCEPT:
   A. ABCs.
   B. relevant scene findings.
   C. interventions and how the patient responded to them.
   D. paraphrasing of the patient's statements.

Challenging Questions

You are dispatched to a scene involving a man caught between a car and a low-end loader. When you arrive, you see that the man is pinned between the two vehicles. He complains of pain in his lower abdomen and pelvic region.

11. What type of injury is this?

12. What treatment do you need to administer?

Points to Ponder

You are dispatched to the site of a motorcycle collision on the off ramp of a major highway. When you arrive on scene, you see a man lying on his right side. You've carried your backboard and cervical collar with you, so you begin to provide full cervical-spine stabilization. You note a tremendous amount of "road rash" and numerous lacerations. While you are placing the board and collar on this patient, your partner begins to attend to the obvious wounds. After you log roll the patient onto the backboard, you note copious amounts of blood in the patient's airway and determine that he has agonal respirations at about 8 breaths/min. You do not feel a radial pulse; however, you are able to obtain a weak and thready carotid pulse at about 110 beats/min. The patient is nonverbal. Your partner is cleaning the patient's arm of debris and glass.

What are your priorities supposed to be in this situation? What do you need to do for this patient?

Issues: Priorities Regarding Life-Threatening Injuries and Wound Closure, The Value of the Written Report.

20 Burns

Competency Areas

Area 1: Professional Responsibilities

1.1.k   Function as patient advocate.
1.3.a   Comply with scope of practice.

Area 2: Communication

2.1.d   Provide information to patient about their situation and how they will be treated.
2.1.g   Use appropriate terminology.

Area 3: Health and Safety

3.3.a   Assess scene for safety.
3.3.b   Address potential occupational hazards.
3.3.e   Conduct procedures and operations consistent with Workplace Hazardous Materials Information System (WHMIS) and hazardous materials management requirements.
3.3.f   Practice infection control techniques.

Area 4: Assessment and Diagnostics

4.2.f   Obtain information regarding incident through accurate and complete scene assessment.
4.3.a   Conduct primary patient assessment and interpret findings.
4.3.b   Conduct secondary patient assessment and interpret findings.
4.3.i   Conduct integumentary system assessment and interpret findings.
4.4.a   Assess pulse.
4.4.b   Assess respiration.
4.4.c   Conduct non-invasive temperature monitoring.
4.4.d   Measure blood pressure by auscultation.
4.4.e   Measure blood pressure by palpation.
4.4.f   Measure blood pressure with non-invasive blood pressure monitor.
4.4.g   Assess skin condition.
4.4.h   Assess pupils.
4.4.i   Assess level of mentation.
4.5.d   Conduct peripheral venipuncture.

Appendix 4: Pathophysiology

C.   **Respiratory System**
Traumatic Injuries: Burns
Traumatic Injuries: Toxic inhalation
G.   **Integumentary System**
Traumatic Injuries: Burns
Infections and Inflammatory Illness: Infections
J.   **Multisystem Diseases and Injuries**
Environmental Disorders: Hyperthermal injuries
Environmental Disorders: Radiation exposure
Shock Syndromes: Hypovolemia
L.   **Ears, Eyes, Nose, and Throat**
Eyes: Burns/chemical exposure

Area 5: Therapeutics

5.1.a   Use manual maneuvers and positioning to maintain airway patency.
5.1.h   Utilize airway devices requiring visualization of vocal cords and introduced endotracheally.
5.4.b   Recognize indications for mechanical ventilation.
5.5.c   Maintain peripheral intravenous (IV) access devices and infusions of crystalloid solutions without additives.
5.5.d   Conduct peripheral intravenous cannulation.
5.6.b   Treat burn.

Appendix 5: Medications

A.   **Medications affecting the central nervous system.**
A.1   Opioid Antagonists

Area 6: Integration

6.1.f   Provide care to patient experiencing illness or injury primarily involving integumentary system.
6.1.n   Provide care to patient experiencing illness or injury due to extremes of temperature or adverse environments.
6.1.o   Provide care to patient based on understanding of common physiological, anatomical, incident, and patient-specific field trauma criteria that determine appropriate decisions for triage, transport, and destination.
6.2.b   Provide care for pediatric patient.
6.2.c   Provide care for geriatric patient.
6.3.a   Conduct ongoing assessments based on patient presentation and interpret findings.
6.3.b   Re-direct priorities based on assessment findings.

Introduction

Approximately 82% of all civilian fire-related deaths occur in residential constructions Figure 20-1 ▾. The incidence of burn injuries and death in North America has decreased somewhat with the advent of stricter building codes and widespread use of smoke detectors. Other effective burn prevention techniques include reducing domestic water heater temperatures to 50°C to prevent severe scalds and making disposable lighters child-safe. Unfortunately, some 400 people still die of fire-related causes in Canada each year. Children younger than 5 years and elderly people are at particularly high risk of dying in fires.

Just as code enforcement and smoke detectors have decreased fire-related deaths, our ability to treat large burns effectively has steadily improved. Before the medical advances of the 20th century, death was "almost inevitable" when more than one third of the body was burned. Now, however, better understanding of "burn shock," advances in the use of fluid therapy and antibiotics, improved ability to excise dead tissue, and the use of biological dressings to aid early wound closure have vastly improved burn care. The formation of specialized teams to resuscitate patients from burn shock, delay infection, and achieve wound closure has resulted in impressive gains in survival rates.

Deaths and serious injuries also occur from electrical and chemical burns. As a consequence, numerous public safety campaigns have focused on the use of smoke detectors and the dangers that surround the use of flammable liquids, petroleum products, solvents, propane, and fireworks.

Although you probably won't see moderate or severe burns on a daily basis, you will encounter some serious burn injuries during your career, and you might encounter serious electrical, chemical, and radiation injuries as well. Accurate recognition of the severity of burn injuries can dramatically enhance the prehospital care of burned patients by allowing you to institute proper care at the scene and notify the receiving facility so personnel can be better prepared to care for the patient and by allowing triage to or consultation with a specialized burn centre.

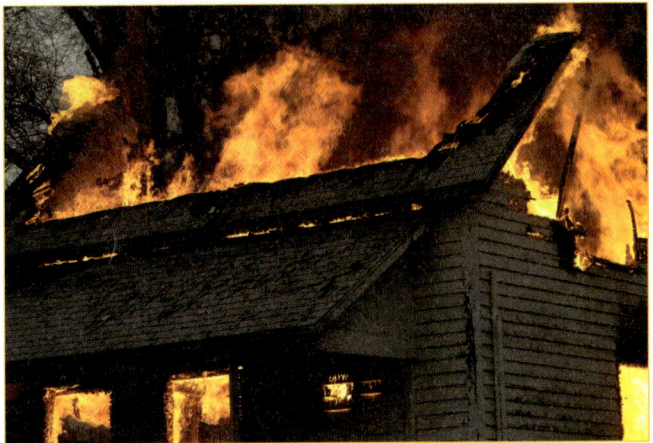

Figure 20-1 Of all civilian fire fatalities, 82% occur in the home.

Anatomy and Function of the Skin

The human skin is much more than a wrapping that keeps the inside of the body from falling out. The skin, also known as the integument, is the largest and one of the most complex organs in the body. It has a crucial role in maintaining homeostasis (balance) within the body. The skin is durable, flexible, and usually able to repair itself. It varies in thickness from almost 1 cm on the heel to 1 mm on the eye's surface. The skin has four functions:

- It acts as an all-purpose fortress to protect the underlying tissue from injury and exposure from extremes of

You are the Paramedic Part 1

You are dispatched to assist the fire department with a structure fire at 9116 East Leesburg Way. Within a few minutes, you hear radio traffic from an interior crew indicating they have found a fire victim. The crew members announce which side of the structure they will exit, and you take your equipment and wait for them there.

Within a few moments, the firefighters emerge with a child who appears to be approximately 8 years old. She is crying, coughing, and holding up her forearm. As you approach, you can see that the young girl has what seems to be a partial-thickness burn to her right arm.

Initial Assessment	Recording Time: 0 Minutes
Appearance	Tearful and upset
Level of consciousness	A (Alert to person, place, and day)
Airway	Patent, loud crying
Breathing	Tachypneic but with good tidal volume
Circulation	Not yet assessed, skin covered with soot

1. What are your patient care priorities?
2. What are patient care concerns when dealing with structure fire victims?

temperature, ultraviolet radiation, mechanical forces, toxic chemicals, and invading microorganisms.

- The skin aids in temperature regulation (thermoregulation), preventing heat loss when the core body temperature starts to fall and facilitating heat loss when core temperature rises.
- As a watertight seal, the skin prevents excessive loss of water from the body and drying of tissues, thereby helping maintain the chemical stability of the internal environment. Without skin, a person would become waterlogged after the first rain and would resemble a prune after the first hot day of summer.
- The skin serves as a sense organ, keeping the brain informed about the external environment. Changes in temperature and sensations of pain are mediated through skin sense receptors.

Significant damage to the skin may make the body vulnerable to bacterial invasion, temperature instability, and major disturbances of fluid balance. People who survive serious burns must live with the ramifications of the damage to large portions of the integument:

- Difficulty with thermoregulation
- Inability to sweat from the scarred portions of the skin
- Impaired vasoconstriction and vasodilation in the areas of severe damage
- Little or no melanin (pigment) in the scar tissue, which makes the skin susceptible to sunburn
- Inability to grow hair on the injured site and little or no sensation in the scarred areas

All of these factors may restrict a person's ability to function even many years after the burn trauma has healed **Figure 20-2 ▶**. Patients who survive serious burns also have a high rate of depression.

Underlying the epidermis is a tough, highly elastic layer of connective tissues called the dermis. The dermis is a complex material composed chiefly of collagen fibres, elastin fibres, and a mucopolysaccharide gel. Collagen is a fibrous protein with a very high tensile strength, so it gives the skin high resistance to breakage under mechanical stress. Elastin imparts elasticity to the skin, allowing it to spring back to its usual contours. The mucopolysaccharide gel gives the skin resistance to compression.

Enclosed within the dermis are several specialized skin structures. Nerve endings mediate the senses of touch, temperature, pressure, and pain, for example. Blood vessels carry oxygen and nutrients to the skin and remove the carbon dioxide and metabolic waste products. Cutaneous blood vessels also

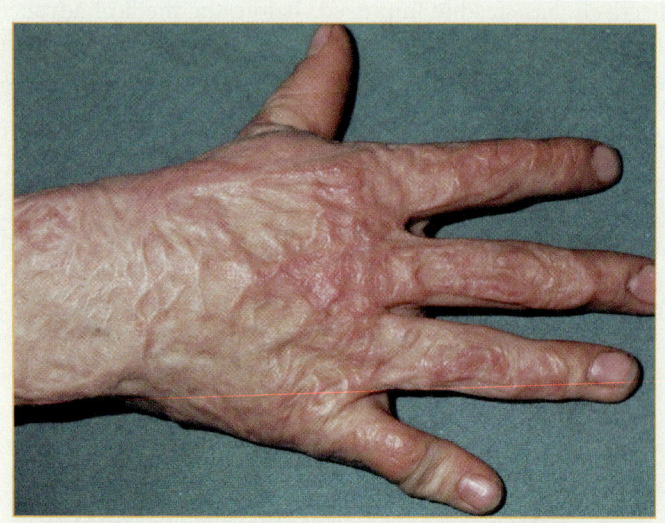

Figure 20-2 People who survive serious burns must live with the ramifications of their injury.

Layers of the Skin

To carry out its functions, the skin needs a specialized structure **Figure 20-3 ▶**. The skin is composed of two principal layers: the epidermis and the dermis.

The epidermis, or outermost layer, is the body's first line of defence, constituting the major barrier against water, dust, microorganisms, and mechanical stress. The epidermis is itself composed of several layers: an outermost layer of hardened, nonliving cells, which are continuously shed through a process called desquamation, and three inner layers of living cells that constantly divide to give rise to new "dead layer" skin cells. The deeper layers of the epidermis also contain variable numbers of cells bearing melanin granules. The darkness of a person's skin is directly proportional to the amount of melanin present.

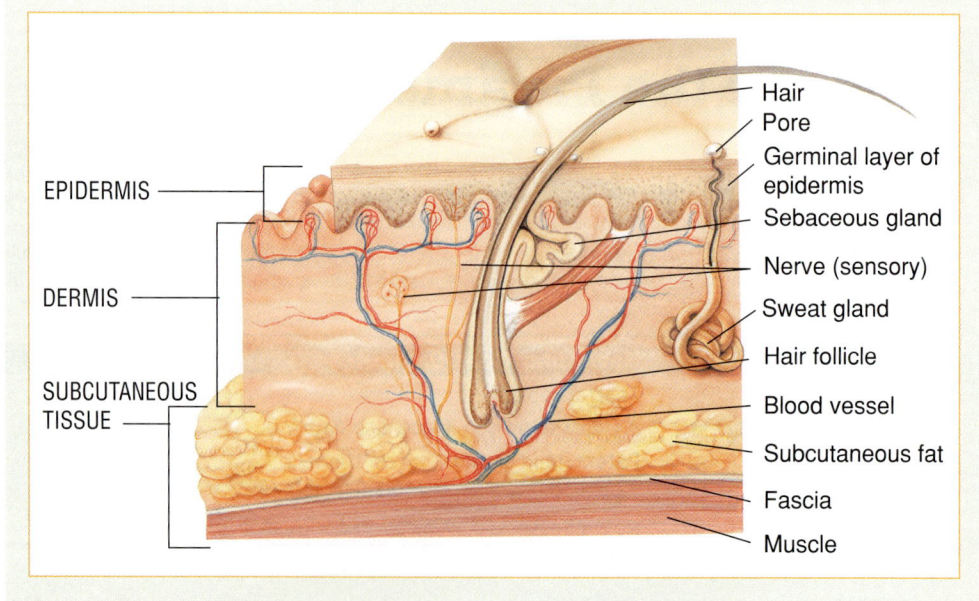

Figure 20-3 The skin has two principal layers: the epidermis and the dermis.

serve a crucial role in regulating body temperature by regulating the volume of blood that flows from the body's warm core to its cooler surface.

Also in the dermis, sweat glands produce sweat and discharge it through ducts passing to the surface of the skin in a process regulated by the sympathetic nervous system. Sweat consists of water and salts. The average volume of sweat lost during 24 hours under normal conditions ranges from 500 to 1,000 ml. During strenuous exercise, sweat glands may secrete as much as 1,000 ml in an hour. Evaporation of water from the skin surface is one of the body's major mechanisms for shedding excess heat.

Hair follicles are structures that produce hair and enclose the hair roots. Each follicle contains a single hair. Attached to the hair follicle is a small muscle that, on contraction, causes the follicle to assume a more vertical position. Sensations such as cold and fright stimulate the autonomic nervous system, which in turn brings about contraction of those muscles and results in "gooseflesh." Hairs in each part of the body have definite periods of growth, after which they are shed and replaced; scalp hair, for example, has a life span of 2 to 5 years and grows at an average rate of 1.5 to 3.9 mm per week. Hair melts when it burns, yet sometimes appears to remain on the patient. When you brush your hand over it, you may find that what you thought was a mustache is now simply a streak of ash. Closely observe nasal hair, eyebrows, and eyelashes in burn patients because damage to them may indicate airway injury. When hair on the arms or legs "falls out" or can be removed without pain, deeper skin structures have been damaged.

At the neck of each hair follicle is a sebaceous gland that produces an oily substance called sebum. The secretions of the sebaceous glands empty into the hair follicles and ultimately reach the surface of the skin. Sebum is believed to keep the skin supple so it doesn't dry out and crack. When sebaceous glands become obstructed, a hard comedo forms, which may serve as the base of an acne pimple.

The tissue beneath the dermis, called the subcutaneous layer, consists mainly of adipose tissue (fat). Subcutaneous fat insulates the underlying tissues from extremes of heat and cold. It also provides a substantial cushion for underlying structures, while serving as an energy reserve for the body.

Finally, beneath the subcutaneous layer are the muscles, tendons, bones, and vital organs. Muscles have thick, fibrous capsules that are prone to hypoxia and anaerobic metabolism in a burn state. Bones are living tissue that can be severely affected by burn injury. Vital organs may also be damaged by thermal, chemical, or electrical energy.

The Eye

The specific anatomy and physiology of the eye are covered in Chapter 21. Clearly, the eyes are sensitive to burn injuries—from a flame, superheated gases, light source (such as a welder's torch), or chemicals. The tear ducts and eyelids combine to constantly lubricate the surface of the eyes **Figure 20-4 ▶** . Unfortunately, intense heat, light, or chemical

reactions on the surface of the eye can quickly burn the thin membrane or skin covering the surface of the eye. Ocular damage is a common result of alkali (base) injury: The higher the pH of the substance, the more severe the damage to the eye. When a patient gets a substance like lime in the eyes, the damage is worsened by repeatedly rubbing the eyes as opposed to initiating copious irrigation and essential treatment in the emergency department (ED).

Pathophysiology

Burns are diffuse soft-tissue injuries created by destructive energy transfer via radiation, thermal, or electrical energy. Thermal burns can occur when skin is exposed to temperatures higher than 44°C. In general, the severity of a thermal injury correlates directly with temperature, concentration, or amount of heat energy possessed by the object or substance and the duration of exposure. For example, solids generally have higher heat content than gases, so exposure to a hot solid (such as the rack inside an oven) typically causes a more significant burn than exposure to hot gases (such as those coming out of an oven). Burns are a progressive process: The greater the heat energy, the deeper the wound.

Exposure time is another important factor. Thermal injury can occur to unresponsive or paralyzed patients from seemingly innocuous heat sources such as heating pads, transcutaneous oxygen sensors, and heat lamps left unattended for long periods.

It may be difficult to evaluate the amount of heat energy or the amount of exposure time in many cases. The temperature of a fire may vary tremendously from the floor to the ceiling.

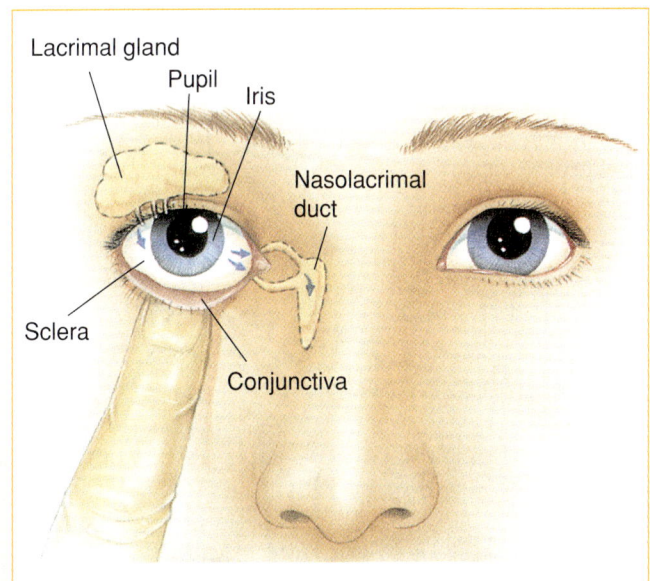

Figure 20-4 Tears act as lubricants and keep the front of the eye protected.

Although most people reflexively limit the amount of time exposed to such heat, if clothing is on fire or the person is trapped or unconscious, exposure time will be longer.

Thermal Burns

A thermal burn is caused fire or other causes of heat injury (electricity, chemical, radiation) **Figure 20-5 ▾**. All of these different situations can cause thermal burns and pose a safety hazard to responding paramedics.

Flame Burns

Most commonly, thermal burns are caused by open flame. A flame burn is very often a deep burn, especially if a person's clothing catches fire **Figure 20-6 ▸**. The fire is fanned by running—hence the adage "stop, drop, and roll" that is taught in schools. Flame burns may also be associated with inhalation injuries.

Scald Burns

Hot liquids produce scald injuries. A scald burn is most commonly seen in children and handicapped adults but can happen to anyone, particularly while cooking. Scald burns often cover large surface areas because liquids can spread quickly. Hot liquids can soak into clothing and continue to burn until the clothing is removed. Some hot liquids, such as oil and grease, adhere to the skin, causing particularly deep scald injuries. Scalds are sometimes associated with child abuse **Figure 20-7 ▸**.

Thousands of scald burns result annually from spilled food and beverages. A child may pull a pot or other container of hot liquid off the stove or counter, a toddler may bump into an adult carrying or holding a hot beverage or food, or a toddler may pull the tablecloth, spilling a hot food or beverage off the table. An important feature of a scald burn is that the severity and the depth of the burn are often not appreciable within the

first 24 to 48 hours. Early appropriate management followed by close observation over time allows one to elucidate the extent of the burn injury.

Contact Burns

Coming in contact with hot objects produces a contact burn. Ordinarily, reflexes protect a person from prolonged exposure to a very hot object, so contact burns are rarely deep unless the patient was prevented from drawing away from the hot object (for example, unconscious, intoxicated, restrained, or impaired). Prolonged contact with something that is just moderately hot can eventually result in a severe burn, however. A patient who has a stroke and falls against a household radiator, for example, may end up with severe burns.

Burns in children, older people, and people with disabilities may be signs of abuse. Burns with formed shapes or unusual patterns and burns in atypical places such as the genitalia, buttocks, and thighs are often consistent with abuse.

Steam Burns

A steam burn can produce a topical (scald) burn. Minor steam burns are common when microwaving food covered with plastic wrap. When the plastic is peeled away, hot steam escapes directly onto the hand of the hungry chef. Steam (that is, gaseous water) is also notorious for

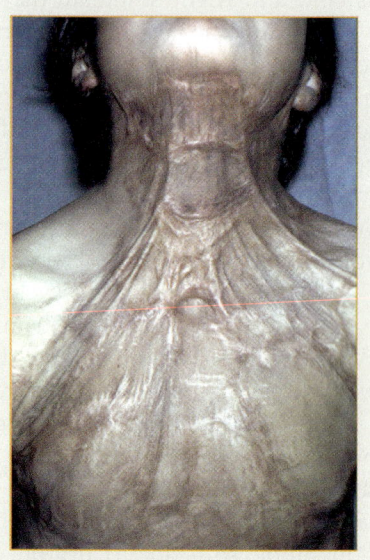

Figure 20-6 Flame burns are often very deep burns.

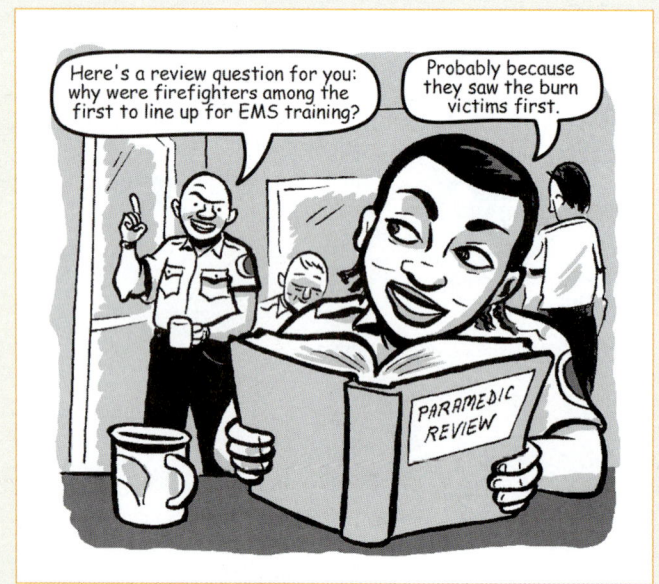

Figure 20-5

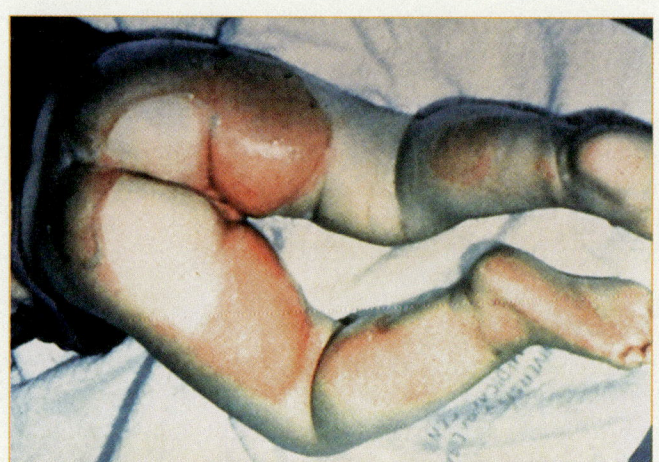

Figure 20-7 Scalds are sometimes associated with child abuse.

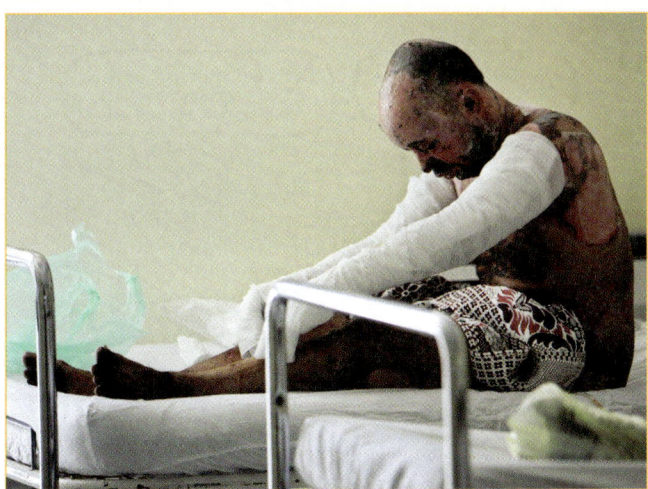

Figure 20-8 Flash burns may be minor compared with the additional trauma inflicted by an explosion.

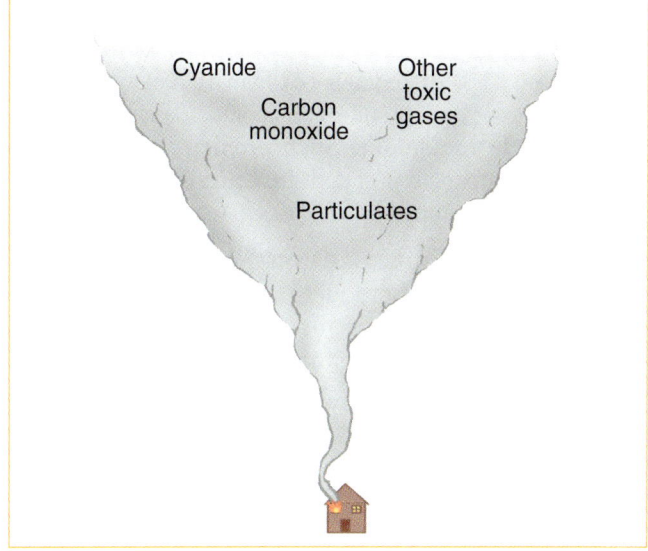

Figure 20-9 Smoke from fires contains many toxins.

causing airway burns. Inhalation of other hot gases may cause supraglottic (upper airway) trauma but rarely leads to burns in the lower airway. Steam is unique because the minute particles of hot water *can* cause significant injury to the lower airway.

Flash Burns
A relatively rare source of thermal burns is the flash produced by an explosion, which may briefly expose a person to very intense heat. Lightning strikes can also cause a flash burn. These injuries are usually minor compared with the potential for trauma from whatever caused the flash **Figure 20-8 ▲**.

Burn Shock
Burn shock occurs because of two types of injury: fluid loss across damaged skin and a series of volume shifts within the rest of the body. Capillaries become leaky, so intravascular volume oozes out of the circulation and into the interstitial spaces. The cells of normal tissues then take in increased amounts of salt and water from the fluid around them.

Burn shock involves the entire body, not just the area burned, and is a result of massive fluid shifts and electrolyte disturbances. Just as in other forms of shock, these changes limit the effective distribution of oxygen and nutrients to the tissues and hamper the circulation's ability to remove waste products from healthy and damaged tissues. Adequate fluid resuscitation is essential to avoid the devastating consequences of burn shock.

Burn shock sets in during a 6- to 8-hour period, so you will not typically witness it in the prehospital environment. Therefore, if an acutely burned patient is in shock in the prehospital phase, look for another injury as the source of shock. People who are caught in fires may fall through floors, jump out of windows, and have things fall on them. There are ample opportunities for traumatic injuries at fire and explosion scenes, so you must be diligent in your assessment.

Airway Burns
Inhalation burns can cause rapid and serious airway compromise. Heat can be an irritant to the lungs and the airway, causing coughing, wheezing, and swelling of the upper airway tissues, often evidenced by stridor. Infraglottic (vocal cords and larynx) and lower airway damage is more often associated with the inhalation of steam or hot particulate matter. Supraglottic (upper airway) damage is more often associated with the inhalation of superheated gases. In rare cases, you may encounter severe upper airway swelling, requiring intervention immediately after a severe burn, although this problem may not manifest itself until transport.

Aggressive airway management may be necessary if supraglottic tissue swelling threatens the patient's airway. In addition, heat inhalation may produce laryngospasm and bronchospasm in the lower airway. Patients sometimes experience pulmonary damage from direct thermal injury. Later pulmonary involvement may be from toxic inhalation injury.

Smoke Inhalation
The vast majority of deaths from fires are not from burns, but rather from inhalation of toxic gases, upper airway compromise, or pulmonary injury. When materials such as plastic, polyvinyl chloride pipes, and synthetic carpets burn, they release toxic chemicals **Figure 20-9 ▲**. Firefighters routinely

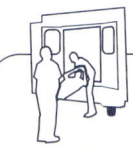

At the Scene

Many fires generate toxic compounds such as cyanides (thiocyanate), which are produced as a result of the combustion of synthetic fabrics and furniture.

protect themselves from these toxins by wearing self-contained breathing apparatus. Anyone who is exposed to smoke from a fire, however, may experience thermal burns to the airway, hypoxia from lack of oxygen (oxygen is consumed by the burning process), and tissue damage and toxic effects caused by chemicals in the smoke. Such problems are particularly common when a person is caught in a burning building, stands up, and breathes in superheated gases.

Carbon Monoxide Intoxication

The combustion process produces a variety of toxic gases. The less efficient the combustion process, the more toxic the gases—such as carbon monoxide (CO) and carbon dioxide (CO_2)—that may be created. When furnaces, kerosene heaters, and other heating devices are in poor repair, they may emit unsafe levels of these toxic gases. Internal combustion engines may emit many of the same gases and, consequently, should always have their exhaust vented to the outdoors. A common cause of CO exposure is running a small engine in an enclosed space like a garage or basement. For this reason, many ambulance services and fire departments have added CO detectors to their garages or ambulance bays. Firefighters who are performing an overhaul after a fire may be exposed to high levels of CO, as may people who are exposed to large amounts of car exhaust (such as toll takers and auto mechanics). Methylene chloride (found in some paint removers) may also produce CO gas.

CO intoxication should be considered whenever a group of people in the same place all complain of headache or nausea (a malfunctioning furnace or car exhaust being sucked into the air-handling system can cause CO intoxication in groups of people). Similarly, you should be suspicious when people complain of feeling sick at home but not when they go to work or school.

CO can displace oxygen from the alveolar air and the blood hemoglobin. Because CO binds to receptor sites on hemoglobin at least 250 times more easily than oxygen (O_2), the patient's hemoglobin may become saturated with the wrong chemical. Being exposed to relatively small concentrations of CO (such as in cigarette smoke) will result in progressively higher blood levels of CO. Most people have approximately 2% CO attached to their hemoglobin, but these levels may be as high as 4% to 8% in heavy smokers. Levels of 50% or higher may be fatal.

Traditional wisdom tells us that patients with CO intoxication will appear "cherry red." Most practitioners agree that this cherry red skin is most commonly seen in people who have died, not living people. So, never rule out CO intoxication because the patient's skin isn't cherry red.

Patients with severe CO intoxication usually present with an O_2 saturation of normal or better. For this reason, you should never trust a pulse oximeter when dealing with a suspected CO poisoning case **Figure 20-10 ▶**. New devices that can measure CO levels will soon be common in prehospital care; they will allow us to find and treat low-level CO intoxication far more readily than we can today.

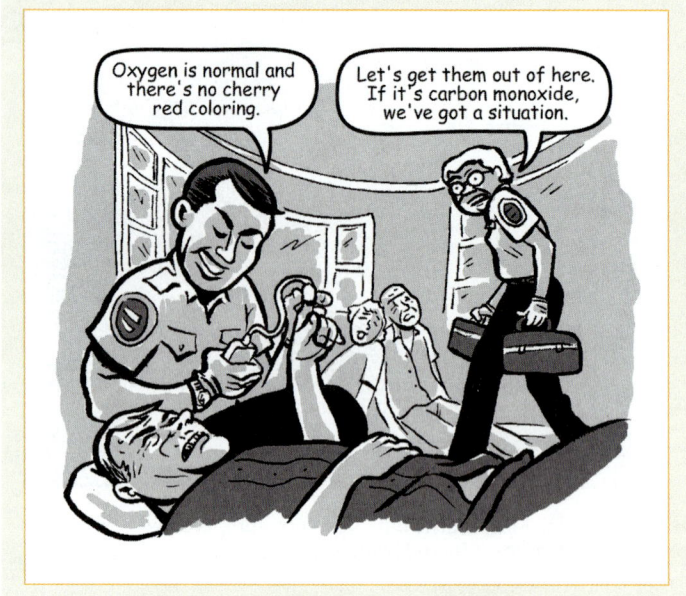

Figure 20-10

At the Scene

Regardless of the cause, hyperbaric oxygen therapy for CO inhalation may be beneficial because it decreases the time it takes for hemoglobin to become saturated with oxygen. The treatment of patients with fairly low levels of CO may also be helpful.

Chemical Burns

Chemical burns occur when the skin comes in contact with strong acids, alkalis or bases, or other corrosive materials 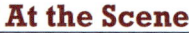 **Table 20-1 ▶**. The burn progresses as long as the corrosive substance remains in contact with the skin. The cornerstone of therapy is, therefore, removal of the chemical from contact with the patient's body.

Skin destruction is determined by the chemical's concentration and duration of contact. Systemic toxicity is determined by the degree of absorption. Immediately removing the patient's clothing will often remove the majority of the chemical from skin contact. Most chemicals are most efficiently removed by washing with copious amounts of low-pressure water (such as in a shower, sink, or eye-wash station). Have the patient bend over when washing the hair and head to avoid having residual chemicals run over the rest of the body. Chemicals can collect in skin folds, where they remain in contact with the tissue and continue to cause more severe damage. Care must be taken to meticulously wash the skin folds at joints and between fingers and toes. Once you think washing is complete, wash the body again. Some chemicals may adhere to the skin, and a mild detergent (dishwashing liquid) will aid in removal. Rinse and wash gently to avoid abrading the skin and exacerbating the injury or absorption of the chemical.

Table 20-1	Chemical Burns	
Chemical Type	**Examples**	**Injury**
Acids	Battery acid (sulfuric acid), hydrochloric acid, hydrofluoric acid	Coagulative necrosis
Bases and alkalis	Potassium hydroxide, sodium hydroxide, lime, drain cleaner, oven cleaner, lye	Liquefactive necrosis
Oxidizing agents	Hydrogen peroxide, sodium chlorate	Exothermic (heat) reaction in addition to tissue destruction; could cause systemic poisoning
Phosphorous	White phosphorous, tracer ammunition, fireworks	Burns when exposed to air; could cause systemic poisoning
Vesicants	Lewisite, sulfur mustard (mustard gas), phosgene oxime	Blister agents; respiratory compromise if inhaled

Some chemicals react violently with water, which obviously precludes irrigation. Such chemicals are usually powders, so it is reasonable to brush off as much dry powder as possible before irrigating any chemical exposure.

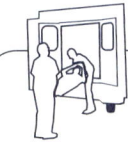

At the Scene

Continue the irrigation until the patient experiences absence of or a significant decrease in pain or burning in the wound.

Injuries From Chemical Burns

Six mechanisms of injury may damage the body's tissues in case of chemical burns:

- **Reduction.** Protein denaturation caused by the reduction of the amide linkages following exposure to a reducing agent (such as alkyl mercuric compounds, diborane, lithium aluminum hydride and other metallic hydrides)
- **Oxidation.** Caused when a chemical inserts oxygen, sulfur, or a halogen (such as chlorine) atoms (such as from sodium hypochlorite, potassium permanganate, peroxides, chromic acid) into the body's proteins
- **Corrosion.** Chemicals that corrode the skin and cause massive protein denaturing (such as phenols, hydroxides, sodium, potassium, ammonium, and calcium)
- **Protoplasmic poisons.** Chemicals that form esters with proteins (such as formic acid and acetic acid) or that bind or inhibit the inorganic ions needed for the body's normal functions (such as oxalic acid and hydrofluoric acid)
- **Desecration.** Desiccants that damage the body by extracting water from tissues (such as concentrated or fuming sulfuric acid); reaction often causes heat (exothermic), which adds insult to the injury
- **Vesication.** Vesicants rapidly produce cutaneous blisters and typically are referred to as chemical warfare agents or weapons of mass destruction (such as mustard gas).

With a chemical burn injury, it is difficult to estimate the extent of the burn—it may have penetrated deep into the

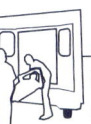

At the Scene

Hydrofluoric acid is a corrosive, inorganic acid used in the manufacture of plastics, pottery glazing, the petroleum industry, and rust removers. Pain and erythema at the site of exposure are the symptoms of exposure to this chemical. After irrigation, paramedics in some services apply topical calcium gluconate gel based on their local or regional protocols.

body's tissues. By using the rule of nines, estimate the body surface area affected, but be aware that the extent of the injury may be much more severe. Do not underestimate the power of a small quantity of chemical. Chemicals such as phenols and highly corrosive acids can cause considerable damage to the skin and its underlying tissues very quickly. Flush, flush, and then flush some more!

When contacting direct medical control for advice on handling specific chemical substances, you will need to identify the chemical and estimate the depth (superficial, partial thickness, or full thickness) of the chemical burn injury.

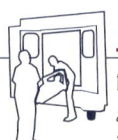

At the Scene

Prolonged contact with petroleum products such as gasoline or diesel fuel may produce a chemical injury to the skin that is actually a full-thickness burn but initially appears to be only a partial-thickness injury. Sufficient absorption of the hydrocarbon may cause organ failure and even death.

Typically, chemical burns react with the skin and tissues quickly. In some cases, however, the injury may take time to develop, as in a person who is exposed to cement (calcium oxide). Cement tends to penetrate through clothing and can react with sweat on the surface of the skin. Hours later, the patient may notice that a burn injury has occurred.

Considerations that influence the management and affect the prognosis of a patient with a chemical burn injury include

At the Scene

The agent, concentration, volume, and duration of contact determine the severity of the chemical injury. The concentration and volume of the chemical influence not only the depth of the injury, but also the extent of body surface involved.

the specific chemical involved, the duration and amount of exposure, and the delay in neutralizing the chemical or decontaminating the patient. This is especially important when considering an injury that may have occurred to the patient's eyes.

Chemical Burns of the Eye

Chemicals known to cause burning injuries to the eyes include acids (such as concentrated liquid chlorine), alkalis (such as cement powder or a strong cleaning agent), dry chemicals (such as lye or lime), and phenols. Always wear eye protection when working with chemicals!

Electricity-Related Injuries

Electricity-Related Burns

Electricity can cause three types of burns 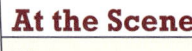 , designated as I, II, and III. The most common is the type I burn, or contact burn. In this true electrical injury, the current is most intense at the entrance and exit sites. At those points, you may see a characteristic bull's-eye lesion, with a central, charred zone of full-thickness burns; a middle zone of cold, grey, dry tissue; and an outer, red zone of coagulation necrosis. The contact burn, while usually not in itself very serious, may signal devastating injury inside the body.

The type II burn, or flash burn, is an electrothermal injury caused by the arcing of electric current. A person who passes close enough to a source of high-voltage current will reach a point where the resistance of the air between the current source and the person is sufficiently low that current arcs through the air, from the current source to the passerby. This arc has a temperature from 3,000°C to 20,000°C—high enough to produce significant charring. Victims standing near an object that was struck by lightning, for example, may get "splashed" and have areas of burns that resemble a fine red rash.

The type III electrical burn, or flame burn, is another thermal injury. It occurs when electricity ignites a person's clothing or surroundings.

At the Scene

When tear gas or pepper spray has been used, the burning sensation may affect you as well as the patient. Take special precautions in such scenarios. Some law enforcement agencies carry an antidote to pepper spray.

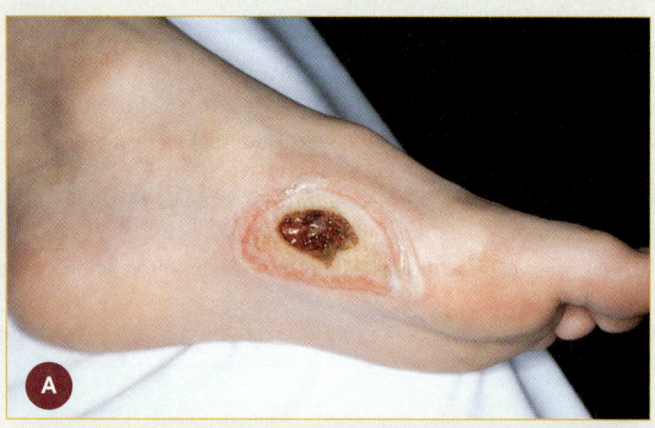

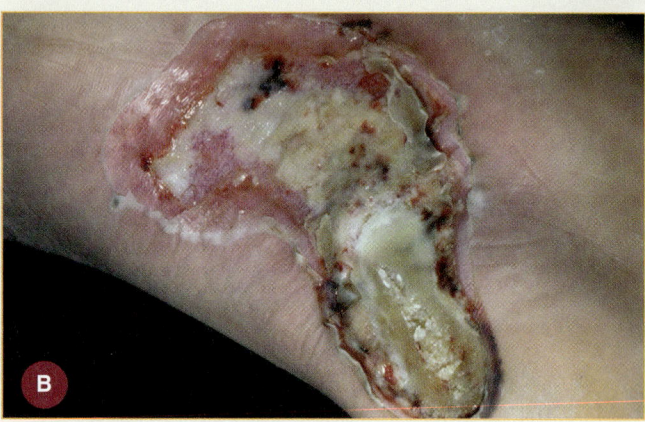

Figure 20-11 Electrical burns have entrance and exit wounds. **A.** The entrance wound is often quite small. **B.** The exit wound can be extensive and deep.

Before beginning your assessment and management of an electrical burn, first and foremost you must assess the scene and ensure that it is safe. If the power could still be on and the patient still energized (such as lying on a live wire), do not approach the patient. Instead, call the power company to turn off all power and make the scene safe.

Electrical burns are most often classified as critical burns because there is a strong possibility of severe internal injury between the point of entry and the point of exit from the body. In some cases, the electricity may have flowed across the chest, potentially injuring the cardiac conduction system.

At the Scene

Many electrical injuries are obvious. Even so, you should always consider the possibility of an "occult" electrical exposure in patients with findings suggesting injury and no obvious mechanism of injury.

Nonburn Injuries From Electricity

Burns may be only one of the problems experienced by a patient who has come in contact with an electrical source—and not necessarily the most serious. The two most common causes of death from electrical injury are asphyxia and cardiac arrest.

Asphyxia may occur when prolonged contact with alternating current induces tetanic contractions of the respiratory muscle. It may also result from current passing through the respiratory centre in the brain and knocking out the impulse to breathe.

Cardiac arrest may occur secondarily, from hypoxia, or as a direct result of the electrical shock. Even currents as small as 0.1 ampere (amp) can trigger ventricular fibrillation if they pass directly through the heart, as when current travels across the body from hand to hand. When cardiac arrest does not occur, cardiac damage may still be manifest in various rhythm disturbances on the electrocardiogram tracing.

A host of neurologic complications have been reported in connection with electrical injury, including seizures, delirium, confusion, coma, and temporary quadriplegia. Damage to the kidneys after electrical injury resembles the syndrome seen after a crush injury, which occurs when the breakdown products of damaged muscle (myoglobin) are liberated into the circulation.

Severe, tetanic muscle spasms may lead to fractures and dislocations, which are often overlooked because of the preoccupation with the electrical injury. Posterior dislocation of the shoulder and fracture of the scapula—otherwise rare injuries—have been reported in several cases of electrocution. And don't forget the cervical spine, especially in a worker who has fallen from a utility pole.

All of these potential injuries conspire to make the victim of an electrical contact a very complex assessment challenge. Never let obvious injuries distract you from a complete assessment, including the neurologic, respiratory, cardiac, and musculoskeletal systems. In dealing with a patient who has an electrical injury, the usual priorities apply.

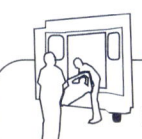

At the Scene

Dysrhythmias commonly seen with electrical injury include atrial fibrillation and atrial flutter.

Injuries From Lightning

One special case of electrical injury deserves specific mention—the injury sustained from lightning. Lightning kills an average of six Canadians each year.

Lightning strikes when a massive discharge of electricity occurs between two bodies that have different charges—for example, between a thundercloud and the ground. The stream of current travels from its origin to its destination and directly to the ground. If any object projects above the surface of the earth that is a better conductor of electricity than the air—such as a building, a light pole, an antenna, a flagpole, or a tree—that object will "attract" the lightning bolt.

A person need not sustain a direct hit from lightning to be injured; in fact, most victims are not struck directly. Much more commonly, the victim is splashed by lightning striking a nearby tree or other projecting object. Ground current produced by lightning striking the ground near the victim can also cause severe injury and accounts for incidents in which there are multiple casualties in an extended area, such as on a golf course.

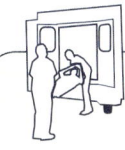

At the Scene

A "stride potential" develops if a person is standing with the legs apart and the current enters the leg closest to the strike, travels up the trunk, and exits through the opposite leg.

The best treatment for lightning injuries is prevention, and all health care professionals have a responsibility to educate the public in preventive measures. Clearly, the most effective precaution is to come in out of the rain, but that is not always possible. Bear in mind that a lightning strike may happen before or after the actual storm has passed, and it can strike up to 15 km away from the storm. Lightning tends to strike the tallest objects that are good conductors. The following rules can help avoid lightning injuries:

Rule 1. *Don't be the tallest object that is a good conductor.* Stay away from the middle of fields, lakes, golf courses, and other large, open areas. If you are stuck in the middle of an open area, try to be as small as you can. Don't hold up an umbrella, golf club, or lightning rod. Don't fly a kite.

Rule 2. *Don't stand under or near the tallest object that is a good conductor.* Although you don't want to be in the middle of the field, you also do not want to be under the tallest tree, radio antenna, or golf umbrella.

Rule 3. *Take shelter in the most substantial structure that you can to remain safe if it is hit by lightning.* A large building with a lightning suppression system is the best choice. An enclosed building is better than an open one (shed, lean-to). Close the shelter as much as possible. If in a car, keep the windows rolled up. Lightning tends to flash over the outside of objects (and people). It can travel substantial distances through conductors, however.

Rule 4. *Avoid touching good conductors during a lightning storm.* Examples of good conductors include plumbing fixtures, fences, and electrical appliances, particularly those connected to wires outside (such as the telephone, TV, and computer).

Lightning carries enormous electrical power—its energy can reach 100 *million* volts, and peak currents can be in the range of 200,000 amps. Unlike other high-voltage electric current, it is *direct*—not alternating—current, and the duration of exposure is measured in milliseconds. Thus, lightning injuries tend to resemble blast injuries more than they do high-voltage injuries, with damage to the tympanic membranes of the ears and air-containing internal organs. Many reports of lightning strikes indicate victims' clothes were "blown off" of their bodies. Muscle damage may occur, and the release of myoglobin from injured muscle may jeopardize the kidneys.

For the cardiovascular system, lightning acts as a cosmic defibrillator, delivering a massive direct-current countershock that depolarizes the entire heart. The heart may resume beating spontaneously shortly after the shock or after approximately 2 minutes of CPR that is started immediately. Because respiratory arrest is apt to persist in patients who have been struck by lightning, continued ventilatory support may be required. The phenomenon of someone regaining a pulse after a lightning strike and having respiratory arrest is known to lead to a secondary cardiac arrest if left untreated. The central nervous system is almost invariably affected by a lightning strike. At least 70% of victims will lose consciousness for some period, and nearly 90% will have some confusion or amnesia (loss of memory). Temporary paralysis of the legs has occurred, and permanent paralysis and quadriplegia have been reported in a few cases.

A lightning burn may have a feathery or zigzag appearance caused by the splash effect. Despite its unique appearance, the immediate threats to life caused by a lightning strike are the same as those caused by a high-voltage power line injury: airway obstruction, respiratory arrest, and cardiac arrest.

Radiation Burns

Acute radiation exposure has become more than a theoretical issue as use of radioactive materials increases in industry and medicine, and you must understand it to function effectively in the prehospital arena. Potential threats include incidents related to the use and transportation of radioactive isotopes and intentionally released radioactivity in terrorist attacks. To be effective, you must first suspect radiation and attempt to determine whether ongoing exposure exists. Increasingly, special response units are equipped with pager-sized radiation detectors, or such detection may be provided by other public safety services.

There are three types of ionizing radiation: alpha, beta, and gamma **Figure 20-12 ▶**. Alpha particles have little penetrating energy and are easily stopped by the skin. Beta particles have greater penetrating power and can travel much farther in air than alpha particles. They can penetrate the skin but can be blocked by simple protective clothing designed for this purpose. The threat from gamma radiation is directly proportional to its wavelength. This type of radiation is very penetrating and easily passes through the body and solid materials.

Radiation is measured in units of radiation absorbed dose (rad) or radiation equivalent in man (rem): 100 rad = 1 gray (Gy). Small amounts of everyday background radiation are measured in rad; the amount of radiation released in a major incident may be measured in gray. The average human exposure from background radiation is 0.36 rem per year. Mild radiation sickness can be expected with exposures of 1 to 2 Gy (100 to 200 rad), moderate sickness at 2 to 5 Gy, and severe sickness at 4 to 6 Gy. Exposure to more than 8 Gy is immediately fatal.

The vast majority of ionizing radiation accidents involve gamma radiation, or x-rays. People who have suffered a radiation exposure generally pose no risk to the people around them. However, in some types of incidents—particularly those

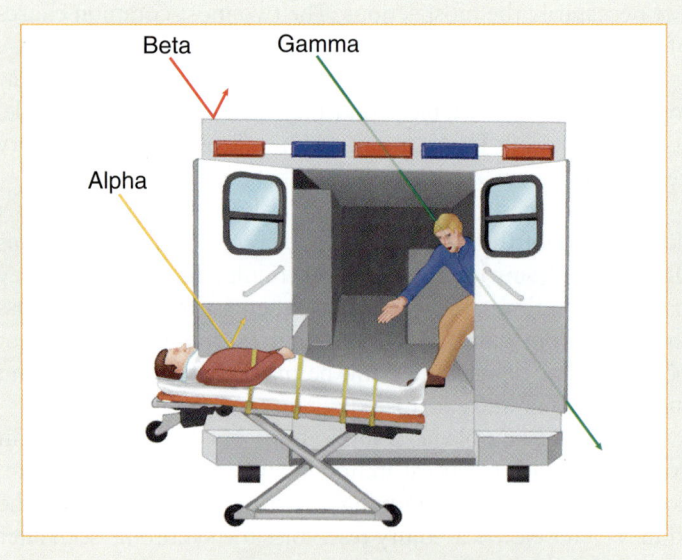

Figure 20-12 Alpha, beta, and gamma radiation shielding.

involving explosions—patients may be contaminated with radioactive particulate matter. It is speculated that after a nuclear explosion, most patients will have sustained some type of trauma in addition to the radiation exposure.

Acute Radiation Syndrome

Acute radiation syndrome causes hematologic, central nervous system, and gastrointestinal changes. Many of these changes occur over time and so will not be apparent during contact with paramedics. Patients who are rendered unconscious by radiation or who manifest vomiting within 10 minutes of exposure will not survive. Those who manifest vomiting in less than an hour have severe exposure and a 30% to 80% survival rate. Many people with moderate exposure will vomit within 1 to 2 hours and have a 95% to 100% survival rate. Clearly, the onset of vomiting soon after exposure is a predictor of poor outcomes. Consider this fact when triaging patients or considering the risks of entering a high-radiation environment to attempt rescue.

Radiation Contact Burns

A person who handles a radioactive source briefly may sustain a local soft-tissue injury without a lot of total body irradiation. This scenario might arise, for example, in a collision involving a vehicle transporting radioactive material or after the detonation of a "dirty bomb." The injury could resemble anything from a superficial sunburn to a chemical burn. Although chemical burns usually become apparent almost immediately after exposure, radiation burns could appear hours or even days after exposure.

▮ General Assessment of Burns

Burns can fool paramedics, because we expect critically injured patients to act sick. Most severely injured and dying cardiac and trauma patients are hypotensive, unresponsive, or in obvious distress. In contrast, patients with an isolated severe burn injury may walk up to you on a scene. The chief complaint may be "I'm terribly cold," and the severity of the injuries may not become apparent until you complete your assessment and realize that the person fits criteria for transfer to a burn centre. Many paramedics have been surprised to find that the moderately burned patient they delivered to the hospital was intubated and transferred to a burn centre within a few hours of arrival.

In other cases, burns may occur in remote locations, and you may not meet the patient until hours after the traumatic burn event. Such patients may present with an entirely different spectrum of problems than you are used to dealing with. Sometimes the patient doesn't realize the ramifications of a burn injury until hours later. Some patients will have additional traumatic injuries from falling debris, explosions, or their attempts to get away from the source of the burn. Seriously burned patients may need to be transferred from tertiary facilities to larger burn centres, and you may need to deal with complex issues such as an escharotomy, a surgical cut through the burned tissue to allow swelling, and advanced fluid management during the transport.

The many types of burns, coupled with the many possible presentations of burn patients, can challenge your assessment skills. As with any trauma patient, it is important to address burned patients in a consistent, efficient, and systematic manner so you don't develop tunnel vision for the major burn trauma and miss other occult injuries that could affect the patient's outcome.

Scene Assessment

Should you run into a burning building to save a patient? Only if you are a trained and properly equipped firefighter. Be wary of entering closed spaces if you see evidence of a recent fire. Toxic gases are often present, even if the fire is out. Never enter a burning building—there is the danger of flashover, when the contents of a room rise in temperature to the point where they all ignite at once. Remember also that plastics contain cyanide, which may be released when they burn.

With modern building construction, be concerned about structural damage to the building. Burning (or recently burned) buildings are notoriously dangerous places; the floors, roofs, beams, and walls may collapse at any time. Electrical wires, gas lines, and plumbing and heating systems can be unstable and dangerous. Look for placards indicating hazardous materials or other signs that hazardous materials may be present. Never enter an area that may contain hazardous materials—only properly trained and protected personnel should enter such areas.

Safety is a primary concern whenever you are operating near a fire scene. Stage yourself and others in a place where it is safe to provide prehospital care—this distancing allows you to stay far enough from the scene to keep a global focus. Remember that your role may include treating victims of the fire and providing rehabilitation for firefighters and other emergency personnel. When paramedics are too close to the hot zone, it is detrimental to their own safety, the prehospital care they provide, and the overall medical response to the situation.

When a recently burned patient comes before you, your initial actions must include extinguishing the flame and cooling the burn. That step may seem obvious, but it is remarkable how many patients arrive by ambulance at hospital emergency departments with clothes still smouldering. A person whose clothing is on fire should not be permitted to run because running fans the flames; nor should the person remain standing because inhaling flame and igniting hair are more likely in the upright position. Rather, have the patient stop, drop to the ground, and roll. If the patient cannot roll, lower the patient to the ground, cover with a blanket, and pat the fire out.

Remove all smouldering clothing and any articles that may retain heat. Watchbands, zippers, and rings not only can retain enough heat to continue burning the patient, but also can melt through your gloves and burn you as well. Make sure that any jewelry on a patient has been cooled appropriately. If the person's hands are burned, they will swell considerably and rings may become tourniquets if not removed quickly enough. If bits of smouldering cloth adhere to the skin, do not pull them off, but rather cut them away. Let burn centre or hospital personnel deal with materials that are melted to the flesh.

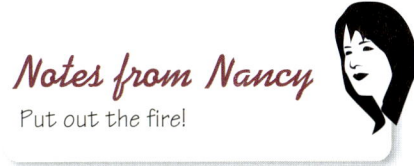

Notes from Nancy
Put out the fire!

If possible, determine the mechanism of injury. As mentioned earlier, patients who have been burned also often have sustained other trauma. Consider and examine other mechanisms associated with the burn: Did the patient jump from a high window to escape flames? Does the patient have musculoskeletal trauma from tetanic spasms after an electrical burn? Was the patient trapped in an enclosed space? Did the patient lose consciousness?

As a part of your scene assessment, do not forget to wear the most appropriate personal protective equipment, perhaps including gloves and a combination mask/eye shield. The burned patient may be "leaking" body fluids and is highly susceptible to infection. Use the most appropriate personal protective equipment to ensure that you are not exposed and the patient is not exposed to you!

Initial Assessment

As you approach a burn trauma patient, simple clues may help identify how serious the injuries are and how quickly you need to assess and treat the patient. If the patient greets you with a hoarse voice and a chief complaint of "trouble breathing," your general impression might be that the patient has a potential airway and/or breathing problem. In the absence of hypoxia or other trauma, a patient with a severe burn may be conscious and is often able to hold a conversation. Although burns are often painful, the more serious burns may present with little or no pain. Indeed, the chief complaint is often "I'm cold." What may first appear to be tattered clothing could turn out to be sheets of the patient's own skin hanging from his burned limbs. Recently burned patients may appear dazed or disconnected from events around them.

Despite what the injuries may look or smell like, you must use compassion when approaching the patient. Burns are obviously traumatic for the patient; if the person survives, he or she may face significant hospitalization and years of rehabilitation. But burns are also traumatic for you, the paramedic. Focusing on the basic principles of emergency care—the ABCs—can help you perform properly in this chaotic situation.

Evaluate Mental Status

Patients with a burn injury may demonstrate varied mental status responses. Combative patients should be considered hypoxic until proven otherwise. Because partial-thickness burns are extremely painful, a patient with this type of injury may be awake and in pain. Even patients with excessive burns will often be awake and attempting to communicate. Isolated burns do not cause unconsciousness (although toxic inhalations can). Unresponsive burn patients must be carefully assessed for the presence of other deadly injuries.

Ensure an Open Airway

As in any other seriously ill or injured patient, airway management is a priority in a patient with a burn. The airway may be in particular jeopardy because the same heat and flames that caused the external burn may have produced potentially life-threatening damage to the airway.

Although rare, laryngeal edema can develop with alarming speed in burn patients, especially in infants and children. Early endotracheal intubation—before the airway has closed off—could be lifesaving in such cases and should be performed by the most experienced paramedic on your team. To intervene early, however, you need to spot the problem early. Airway management is discussed in greater detail later in this chapter.

Assess for Adequate Breathing

Listen to lung sounds, with special attention to stridor, which may be a sign of impending upper airway compromise. Note that patients with preexisting lung disease may have bronchospasm after even relatively minor exposure to smoke; they may respond well to inhaled beta-2 agonists.

Anyone suspected of having a burn to the upper airway may benefit from humidified, cool oxygen. If you do not carry a high-output humidifier (a bubble humidifier is *not* a high-output humidifier), consider using a nebulizer to administer nebulized normal saline. This approach will not provide a high concentration of oxygen, so you will need to balance the need for a high O_2 concentration against the desire for cool humidity. Keep in mind that the patient's oxygen saturation may be suspect if there is the possibility of CO intoxication.

Notes from Nancy

Every person burned in a fire should receive oxygen.

Ensure Adequate Circulation

During the first 24 to 48 hours of a patient's burn care, a great deal of emphasis is placed on fluid resuscitation to prevent burn shock. Burn shock is caused by fluid shifts that typically occur 6 to 8 hours after the burn. Severely burned patients will ultimately require large volumes of fluid, but they don't need it during the first minutes of prehospital care unless their burn injury occurred some time ago. Most patients will ultimately require central venous access, and most intravenous (IV) lines placed in the prehospital setting will be removed owing to tissue swelling and infection risk. If the patient is not grossly hypotensive, do not delay transport by making multiple attempts at vascular access. Of course, if the patient has an obvious peripheral vessel, your early vascular access will be put to good use by hospital or burn centre staff for fluid replacement and pain management.

Patients with other trauma may require immediate vascular access just like any other trauma patient. Although it is preferable to avoid starting IV lines through burned tissue, it isn't frankly contraindicated. Burn patients may challenge your vascular access skills. New options for intraosseous access may provide you with more choices than were available to your predecessors.

Notes from Nancy

If a burned patient is in shock in the prehospital phase, look for another injury as the source of shock.

Burn Severity

The burn wound is categorized by the degree of injury. Historically, such an injury has been described by three pathologic progressions or zones, which radiate from the central zone of greatest damage. Skin nearest the heat source suffers the most profound cellular changes. The central area of the skin, which suffers the most damage, is called the zone of coagulation. There is little or no blood flow to the injured tissue in this area. The peripheral area surrounding the zone of coagulation has decreased blood flow and inflammation; it is known as the zone of stasis. This area may undergo necrosis within 24 to 48 hours after the injury, particularly if perfusion is compromised by burn shock. Last, the zone of hyperemia is the area least affected by the thermal injury. In this area, cells will typically recover in 7 to 10 days.

How Deep Is the Burn?

During your initial assessment, your goal is to identify and manage life threats, as well as to determine the level of care the patient requires (burn centre, trauma centre, local hospital). This means you will need to get an idea of the burn's size and severity to report to the receiving facility. The nature of the patient's burns will evolve during the next 24 hours, and estimations of their size and severity will inevitably change, so little is to be gained by conducting a comprehensive and time-consuming evaluation of every centimetre of the patient's body in the prehospital environment. Nevertheless, a reasonably accurate estimation of the scope of the patient's injuries is helpful for determining the appropriate care.

The traditional labels given to burns were first, second, and third degree. Many centres have expanded that concept, describing burns as fourth, fifth, and sixth degree as tissue destruction goes into the deeper tissues, muscle, and bone. Paramedics should limit their assessment to partial- versus full-thickness burns (described later) to simplify the process and avoid confusion and miscommunication. Multiple paramedics may disagree on the extent of a given burn in the prehospital environment, and reaching a consensus isn't important enough to justify spending time on the discussion. The hospital staff need to know, for example, that they are getting an *x*-year-old male with approximately *x*% full-thickness and *x*% mixed partial-thickness burns with possible airway decompensation.

Quickly assess the burns while considering the presence or absence of pain, swelling, skin colour, capillary refill time, moisture and blisters, the appearance of the wound edges, the presence of foreign bodies, debris, and contaminants, bleeding, and circulatory adequacy. Make sure you assess for concomitant soft-tissue injury.

Determination of burn depth is a subjective assessment that depends on paramedic judgment. Based on this assessment, the burn injury should be classified as superficial, partial thickness, or full thickness **Figure 20-13 ▸** .

A superficial burn (first-degree burn) involves the epidermis only. The skin is red and, when touched, the colour will blanch and return. Usually blisters are not present. Patients will experience pain because nerve endings are exposed to the air. Such a burn will heal spontaneously in 3 to 7 days. The most common example is a sunburn.

A partial-thickness burn (second-degree burn) involves the epidermis and varying degrees of the dermis. This category can be subdivided into superficial partial-thickness and deep partial-thickness burns. With a *superficial partial-thickness burn,* the skin is red; when touched, the colour will blanch and return. Usually there are blisters or moisture present, and the patient may experience extreme pain. Hair follicles remain intact. A superficial partial-thickness burn will heal spontaneously but may scar or have a changed appearance. In contrast, a *deep partial-thickness burn* extends into the dermis, damaging the hair follicle and sweat and sebaceous glands. Hot liquids, steam, or grease are often to blame for these injuries. In the out-of-hospital setting, the delineation between deep partial thickness and full thickness may be difficult to determine.

A full-thickness burn (third-degree burn) involves destruction of both layers of the skin, including the basement membrane of dermis that produces new skin cells. In such an injury, the skin is white and pale, brown and leathery, or charred. Dry and leathery skin is referred to as eschar. No capillary refill occurs with this type of burn because the capillaries have been destroyed. Sensory nerves are destroyed as well, so there may be no pain in the full-thickness section. Because patients usually have mixed depths of burns, they will often experience significant pain in the areas surrounding the full-thickness burns. Treatment of a full-thickness burn will usually require skin grafting because the dermis has been destroyed.

How Much Surface Area Is Burned?

While evaluating the patient's burns, you must approximate the total body surface area (TBSA) burned. Most practitioners advocate counting only the areas of partial- and full-thickness burns (ignoring the areas of superficial burns). The most universal mechanism of calculating the area burned is the rule of nines, which is based on dividing the body into 9% segments. The paramedic adds the portions of the body to obtain a total of the body area affected by the burn injury. Because our proportions change as we grow, different rules of nines apply to infants, children, and adults **Figure 20-14 ▸** .

Another mechanism of assessing the TBSA is the rule of palm. This assessment uses the size of the patient's palm (excluding the fingers) to represent about 1% of the patient's body surface area. This calculation is helpful when the burn covers less than 10% of the body surface area or is irregularly shaped. The Lund and Browder chart is an even more specific method used to estimate the burned area by dividing the body into even smaller and more specific regions **Figure 20-15 ▸** .

You must balance the need for accuracy against the time required to make an estimate of the TBSA. The out-of-hospital estimation is used to guide the patient to the correct place for treatment. The ED estimation of burned area may be used to initiate fluid therapy. The burn centre's estimation of injured area will undoubtedly be more accurate and specific.

Focused History and Physical Examination

With burn patients, proceed through the steps of physical assessment in the usual sequence, starting with the general appearance and moving on to the vital signs. Obtaining vital signs may be challenging if the patient has extensive burns on the arms. Nevertheless, you should try to document vital signs accurately because the management of shock, airway compromise, and pain control depends on them to some degree.

When you have finished your brief inspection of the patient's skin, you have only just begun the head-to-toe examination. The detailed physical examination is intended to make sure that no other injuries have higher priority for treatment. Often such injuries may be obscured by the burn itself, so you need to pay attention to the circumstances of the burn and the possible mechanisms of injury. If the patient jumped from a

At the Scene

Signs and symptoms of vascular compromise in a burned extremity that may necessitate an escharotomy include cyanosis, pallor, deep tissue pain, progressive paresthesia, progressive decrease or absence of the pulse, or sensation of a cold extremity.

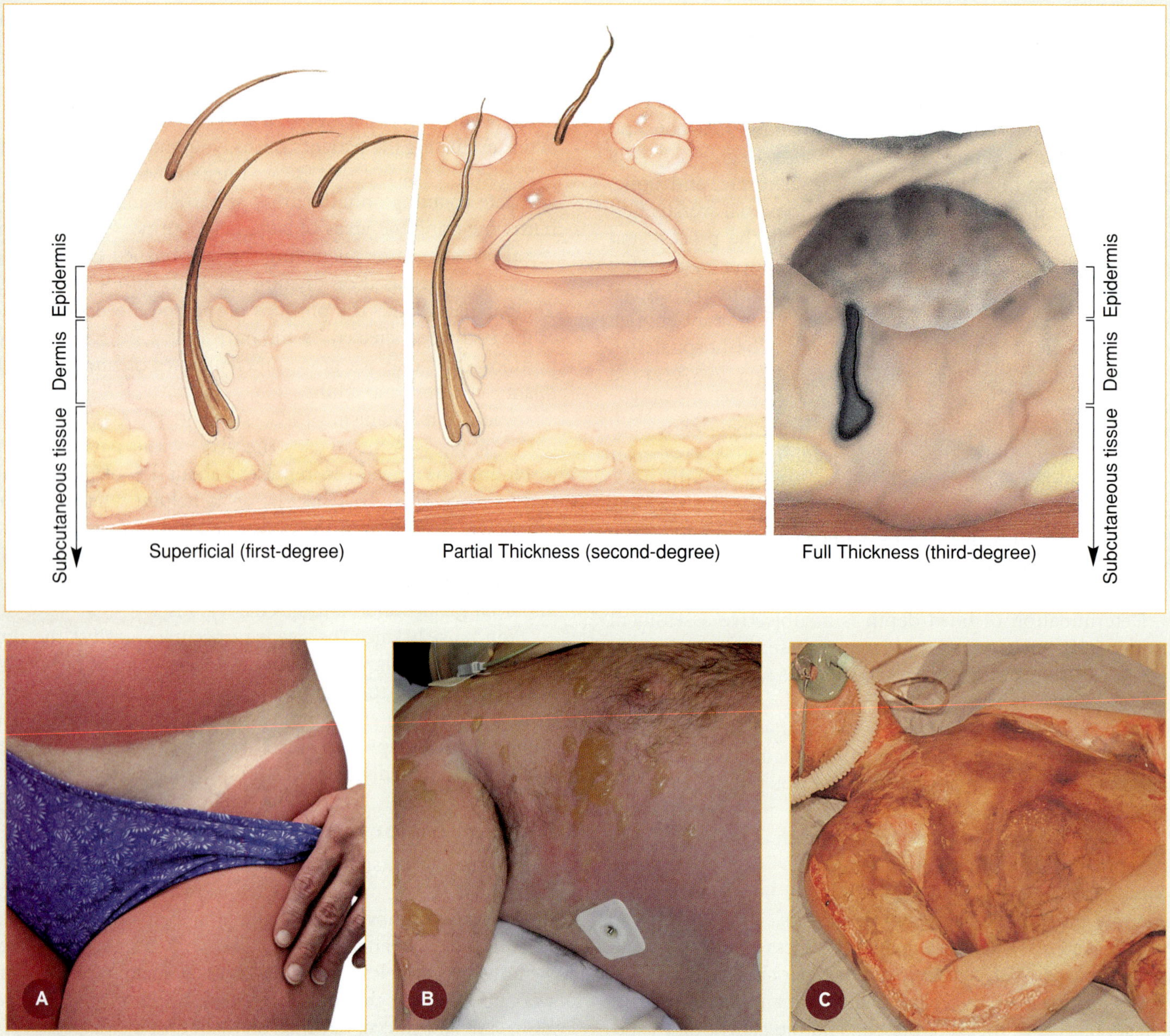

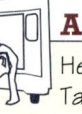

Figure 20-13 Classification of burns. **A.** Superficial (first-degree) burns involve only the epidermis. **B.** Partial-thickness (second-degree) burns involve some of the dermis but do not destroy the entire thickness of the skin. The skin is mottled, white to red, and often blistered. **C.** Full-thickness (third-degree) burns extend through all layers of the skin and may involve subcutaneous tissue and muscle. The skin is dry, leathery, and often white or charred.

second-story window, for example, there may be fractures beneath the obvious burns on the legs.

Look for injuries to the eyes, and cover injured eyes with moist, sterile pads. Check the neck, chest, and extremities for circumferential burns. Progressive edema beneath a circumferential burn—especially when the burned skin has become leathery and unyielding—may act as a tourniquet. In the neck, a circumferential burn may obstruct the airway; in the chest, it may restrict respiratory excursion; and in an extremity, it may cut off the circulation and put the extremity in jeopardy.

At the Scene

Heat loss is a critical problem for burn patients. Take immediate steps to prevent hypothermia, such as heating the ambulance until it's uncomfortable for the crew and using warm blankets and fluids.

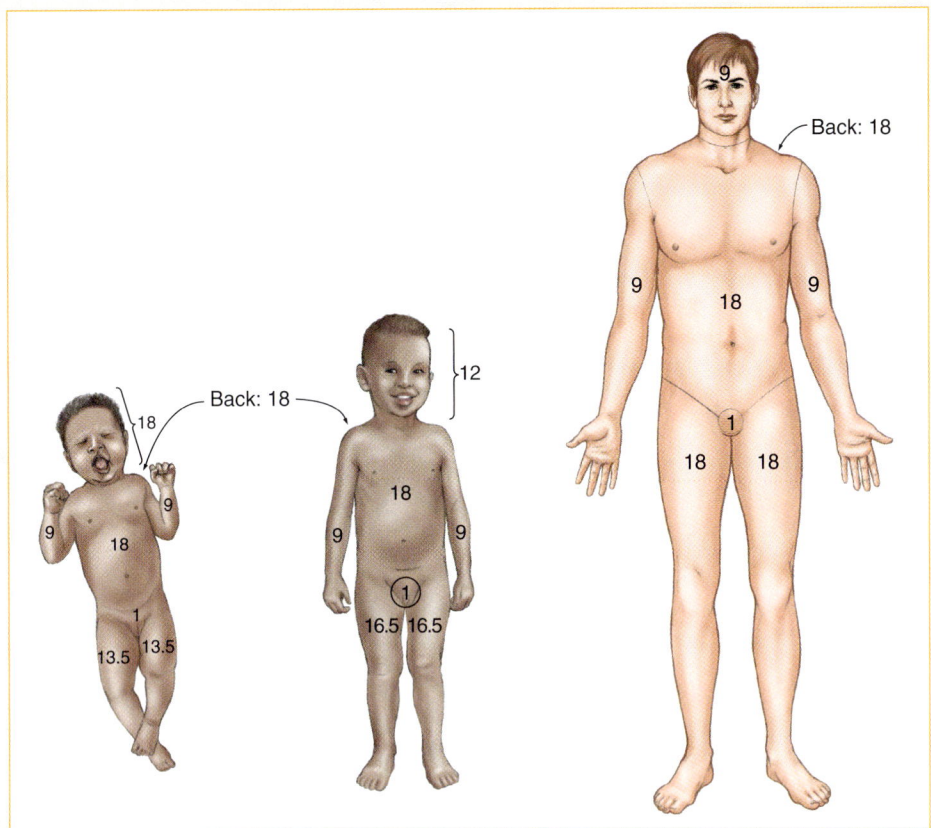

Figure 20-14 The rule of nines is a quick way to estimate the amount of surface area that has been burned. It divides the body into sections, each representing approximately 9% of the total body surface area. The proportions differ for infants, children, and adults.

Patients with circumferential burns must reach a medical facility quickly because it may be necessary to make an incision into the burned area to decompress it. Check and document the distal pulses in burned extremities often.

To the degree possible, get a brief history from the patient. Patients with preexisting diseases, such as chronic obstructive pulmonary disease or acute coronary syndromes, may be triaged as critical burns even if the burn injury is small. As in any other trauma, allergies, medications, and other pertinent medical history may influence the patient's care plan.

Detailed Physical Examination and Ongoing Assessment

If the patient is considered to have a significant mechanism of injury, en route to the ED, you should perform a detailed physical examination and ongoing assessment (see Chapters 13 and 14). Reassessment of vital signs to establish trends is done every 5 minutes for critical patients and every 15 minutes for lower priority patients (in stable condition).

You are the Paramedic Part 2

You immediately begin treating your patient, who tells you her name is Pamela. When you ask what happened, the patient says that she was playing with gasoline and matches with her older brother (who escaped the house unharmed and now is with police officers). As she reached to light a pile of gasoline-soaked rags, the vapours flashed, and she burned her right arm. She is able to talk without difficulty, and there is no indication of burns to her face or airway. She has no other apparent injuries.

By using the rule of palm, you estimate the size of Pamela's burn to be approximately 4% to 5% involving her right arm and hand. You administer supplemental oxygen. Your partner initiates an IV line in the unburned arm while you irrigate the area with cool, sterile saline and assess the right arm. Pulse and motor and sensory functions are present.

Vital Signs	Recording Time: 5 Minutes
Level of consciousness	Alert, with a Glasgow Coma Scale score of 15
Skin	Warm, pink, dry with some soot on skin and clothing
Pulse	Radial pulse, 120 beats/min, strong and regular
Blood pressure	116 by palpation
Respirations	36 to 42 breaths/min, clear and equal breath sounds bilaterally
Spo2	100% while breathing room air

3. Why is pulse oximetry unreliable in these circumstances?
4. Are your transport considerations affected by the location of her burn?
5. What are common complications of burns?

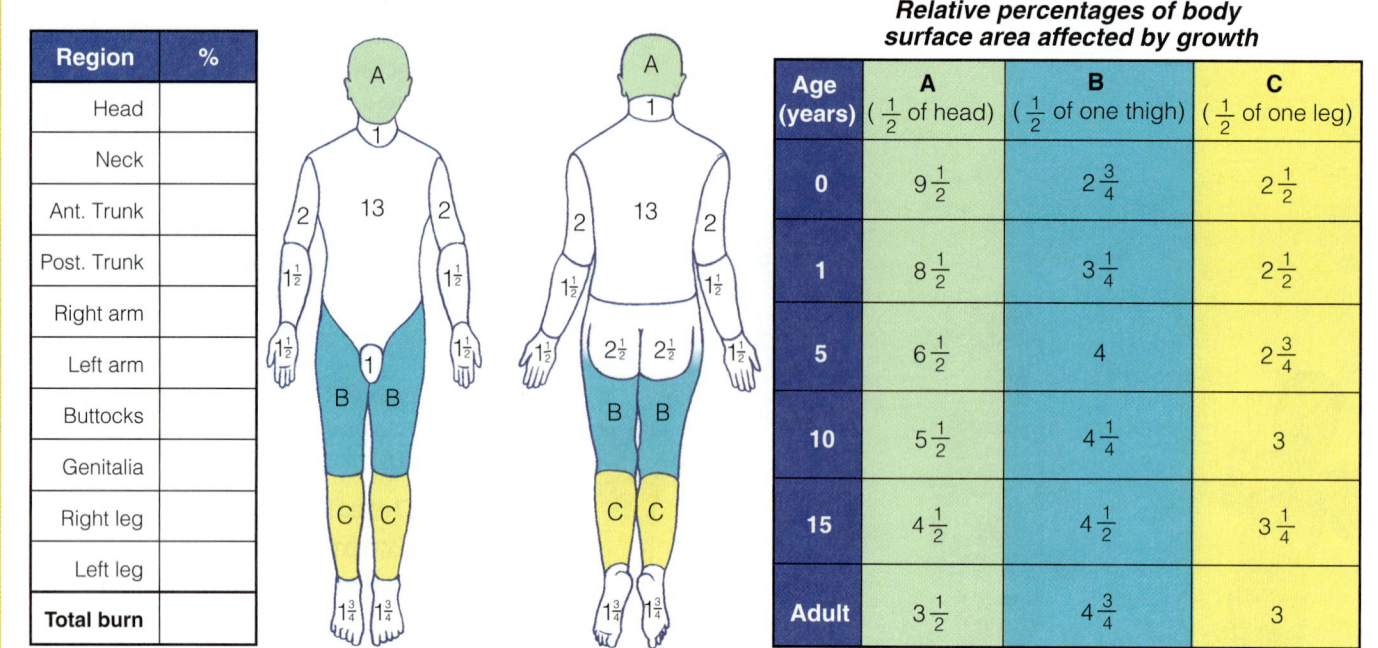

Region	%
Head	
Neck	
Ant. Trunk	
Post. Trunk	
Right arm	
Left arm	
Buttocks	
Genitalia	
Right leg	
Left leg	
Total burn	

Relative percentages of body surface area affected by growth

Age (years)	A ($\frac{1}{2}$ of head)	B ($\frac{1}{2}$ of one thigh)	C ($\frac{1}{2}$ of one leg)
0	$9\frac{1}{2}$	$2\frac{3}{4}$	$2\frac{1}{2}$
1	$8\frac{1}{2}$	$3\frac{1}{4}$	$2\frac{1}{2}$
5	$6\frac{1}{2}$	4	$2\frac{3}{4}$
10	$5\frac{1}{2}$	$4\frac{1}{4}$	3
15	$4\frac{1}{2}$	$4\frac{1}{2}$	$3\frac{1}{4}$
Adult	$3\frac{1}{2}$	$4\frac{3}{4}$	3

Figure 20-15 The Lund and Browder chart.

Source: Adapted from Lund CC, Browder NC. *Surg Gynecol Obstet.* 1944; 79:352-358.

Assessment of Radiation Burns

First and foremost, the assessment of a patient who may have been exposed to radiation involves a scene assessment to determine if the scene is safe for rescuers to enter. In some cases, it may be appropriate to contact the hazardous materials response team so they may determine the appropriate precautions, including exposure-limiting suits, and the most appropriate ED for the patient's treatment. Not all EDs are set up to handle a patient who has been exposed to radiation, so learn the capabilities of your hospitals before an incident occurs! EMS agencies that operate in an area where there is a nuclear power plant or other research facility typically have additional training offered by the facility and regularly practice responding to radiation-related emergencies.

Once the scene is deemed safe, you may proceed with your initial assessment of the patient. Assess the patient's mental status and ABCs, and then prioritize the patient's prehospital care. Unfortunately, patients who have sustained a significant radiation exposure and a major burn are unlikely to survive, even with major resources expended to keep them alive (a burn of > 70% of the TBSA is probably fatal by itself; a burn and radiation of > 30% of the TBSA are probably fatal). When confronted with large numbers of patients who have been exposed to radiation and simultaneously received thermal burns, keep the 30% rule in mind when triaging and making transport decisions. Of course, you should also consult with direct medical control in these complicated cases. In the prehospital environment, it is difficult to determine the extent of the patient's internal injuries due to radiation.

■ Management of Burns

Definitive burn care can be divided into four phases. While paramedics will be most heavily involved in the first phase, it is important to appreciate the magnitude of care that a patient with a severe, or even moderate, burn must receive. Early actions of the paramedic may dramatically affect the patient's long-term outcome. Paramedics may also find themselves transporting patients to specialty or rehabilitation facilities at later stages of their care.

Unlike many emergencies you will encounter, burn patient care is measured in weeks, not hours. Burns are devastating multisystem traumatic injuries that dramatically alter a person's life. You should recognize not only the massive physical trauma caused by burns, but also the emotional, psychological, and financial burdens these horrific injuries impose. Once these costs are appreciated, it is easy to understand the importance of teaching injury prevention strategies to the people we serve.

General Management

Management of a burned patient begins with the steps taken during the scene assessment and initial assessment to extinguish the fire and ensure adequate ABCs. Only when the ABCs are under control should you turn your attention to the burn itself. It is important to have all resuscitative equipment ready for use when treating a burn patient, including advanced airway equipment and heart monitors.

Immediate Management

Stop the burning. When a person burns a hand on a hot oven rack at 230°C, the person will usually stick the hand under cool running water for a few seconds. Is that long enough to cool the tissues and stop the burning? Usually not. It often takes several minutes to completely cool the burned area and achieve some pain relief. All jewelry, metal buttons, zippers, and hooks should be cool to the touch as well. Of course, never use ice on a burn.

After cooling the burns, *keep the patient warm.* This seems like a contradiction, because it is. The trick is to stop the burning process without making the patient hypothermic. Remember, people with large burned areas have lost their primary mechanism for thermoregulation. Keep the patient covered and move him or her into the ambulance as soon as possible to minimize hypothermic stress.

Don't forget other injuries. If the patient is at risk for spinal trauma from a fall or explosion, address this injury the same way you would in any other trauma patient. The same is true for gross bleeding and other traumatic injuries. Burns can also exacerbate a patient's underlying medical conditions, such as chronic obstructive pulmonary disease, asthma, and cardiac conditions. Follow the same priorities for these emergencies as you would for any other patient.

Airway Management

Many burn patients will ultimately require intubation, even though they were talking to you and in no distress in the prehospital environment. Although it is obviously preferable to have such patients intubated in a controlled environment with a full complement of anesthesia agents, a few patients will absolutely require an emergency advanced airway in the prehospital environment. Burn patients fall into four general categories for airway management.

1. **The patient with an acutely decompensating airway who requires intubation in the out-of-hospital environment.** This group includes burn patients who are in cardiac or respiratory arrest and conscious patients whose airways are swelling before your eyes. In these chaotic and difficult situations, you need to plan for the possibility that you cannot intubate. Supraglottic swelling or complete obstruction can occur in some burn scenarios. Surgical airways or rescue devices may be necessary if intubation is not possible and bag-mask ventilation fails.

2. **The patient with a deteriorating airway from burns and toxic inhalations who might require intubation.** It is obviously better for the patient to defer treatment of this airway problem to hospital teams with anesthesia, surgery, specialized equipment, and a fully stocked pharmacy. Patients will often be conscious and may become combative with attempts to place them supine, let alone intubate them. "Awake" techniques, such as nasal intubation, are dramatically more complicated in victims of upper airway burns and should be avoided. Attempt to intubate only if left with no other choice. If the patient's airway continues to swell and intubation will become impossible if you wait for arrival at the hospital, you have little choice but to attempt intubation. Try to consult direct medical control for advice.

Intubation of an awake, scared patient in the prehospital environment is difficult, and considerable damage may be inflicted on the airway if the patient continues to struggle. If intubation becomes necessary under such circumstances, explain carefully to the patient what is to be done, why it is necessary, and how he or she can best cooperate. Have all equipment set up at your side so that intubation, once begun, can proceed rapidly and smoothly. Serious consideration should be made toward performing rapid-sequence intubation if you have been trained in this procedure, carry the appropriate medications, and have direct medical control authorization. The procedure for rapid-sequence intubation is discussed in Chapter 11. It is also advised that the "most experienced" intubator perform this procedure because the swelling can make for a difficult intubation.

An airway compromised by advancing edema represents another classic scenario in which administering a neuromuscular blocker to provide respiratory paralysis may be extremely dangerous. It places the paramedic in the dangerous position of having a patient with no gag reflex or ability to breathe and an airway you may be unable to control.

The choice of endotracheal (ET) tube may present another conundrum. It would obviously be beneficial to use the largest tube possible. Sometimes the ET tube will clog with soot from the patient's airway, causing complete occlusion. At the same time, a smaller than usual ET tube may be necessary owing to airway edema. Select the largest ET tube that will not cause additional trauma during insertion. Never cut the ET tube down to make it shorter. Edema of the face can actually cause ET tube dislodgment on postburn day 2 or 3.

3. **The patient whose airway is currently patent but who has a history consistent with risk factors for eventual airway compromise.** Cool, humidified oxygen from a high-output nebulizer (not a bubble humidifier) is appropriate. Alternatively, you may use an aerosol nebulizer with saline. The patient will probably *not* require acute interventions in the prehospital environment, but make sure you report the patient's history to hospital personnel. Many patients will ultimately undergo elective intubation.

4. **The patient with no signs of or risk factors for airway compromise who is in no distress.** It is reasonable to provide supplemental oxygen to burn patients, even if they are not in distress. It is safe to oxygenate until you are comfortable with the situation surrounding the burn and have completed a full assessment.

Fluid Resuscitation

An IV line may be inserted in the prehospital setting to administer fluids and/or pain medications. A large-bore IV cannula should be inserted as early as possible in any patient who has been severely burned. Do not delay transport to do so, but try to get a large-bore IV cannula into a large vein, and give lactated Ringer's solution or normal saline. You can use the burned extremity for the IV site if you cannot find another site—an IV line in a burned upper extremity is still preferable to an IV line in a lower extremity.

Approximate the amount of fluid the burned patient will need by using the Parkland formula, which states that *during the first 24 hours,* the burned patient will need:

> 4 ml × body weight (in kg) × percentage of body surface burned

Half of that amount needs to be given during the first 8 hours. For example, if a 70-kg man has sustained burns to 30% of his body, his fluid needs during the first 24 hours will be:

> 4 ml × 70 kg × 30 = 8,400 ml

Half of the 8,400 ml—that is, 4,200 ml—should be administered during the first 8 hours.

As aggressive as the Parkland formula may seem, current trends actually lean toward delivering *more* fluid than the Parkland formula indicates (Table 20-2 ▾). Of course, you do not need to attempt to deliver the entire initial amount in the prehospital environment. Most seriously burned patients will need central venous access, and IV lines placed in the prehospital setting will most often be lost as peripheral swelling begins.

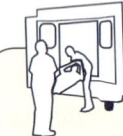

At the Scene

The adequacy of resuscitation is based on monitoring the vital signs, the patient's mentation, and the urine output.

Pain Management

With any patient with burns, you should provide aggressive pain management. Assess the patient's pain before administering any analgesia. Reassessment should be completed using the same scale (for example, 1 to 10) every 5 minutes.

Burn patients may require higher than usual doses of pain medications to achieve relief. Their metabolism rates are accelerated, which creates the need for higher than normal doses of analgesics. Consult your protocols or contact direct medical control for guidance in administering analgesics.

Management of Superficial Burns

Although superficial burns can be very painful, they rarely pose a threat to life unless they involve nearly the entire surface of the body. If you reach a patient with superficial burns within the first hour after the injury occurred, immerse the burned area in cool water or apply cold compresses to the burn. Burned hands or feet may be soaked directly in cool water; and towels soaked in cold water may be applied to burns of the face or trunk.

The objectives of this exercise are twofold: stop the burning process and relieve pain. Commercial products are available that meet both objectives (Figure 20-16 ▸). However you cool the burn, take care not to cool the whole body—don't let the patient become chilled. A dry sheet or blanket applied over the wet dressings will help prevent systemic heat loss.

Do not use salves, ointments, creams, sprays, or any similar materials on any type of burn. They will just have to be scrubbed off in the ED or burn unit, causing the patient further pain. Never apply ice to burns because it can exacerbate the tissue injury.

No further treatment should be necessary in the prehospital setting for an uncomplicated, superficial burn. Simply transport the patient in a comfortable position to the hospital.

Table 20-2	Parkland Formula Chart									
% Burn	**10 kg**	**20 kg**	**30 kg**	**40 kg**	**50 kg**	**60 kg**	**70 kg**	**80 kg**	**90 kg**	**100 kg**
10	25	50	75	100	125	150	175	200	225	250
20	50	100	150	200	250	300	350	400	450	500
30	75	150	225	300	375	450	525	600	675	750
40	100	200	300	400	500	600	700	800	900	1,000
50	125	250	375	500	625	750	875	1,000	1,125	1,250
60	150	300	450	600	750	900	1,050	1,200	1,350	1,500
70	175	350	525	700	875	1,050	1,225	1,400	1,575	1,750
80	200	400	600	800	1,000	1,200	1,400	1,600	1,800	2,000
90	225	450	675	900	1,125	1,350	1,575	1,800	2,025	2,250
20 ml/kg	200	400	600	800	1,000	1,200	1,400	1,600	1,800	2,000

This table represents the fluid recommended in the *first hour* (⅛ of the initial 8-hour dose) by the Parkland formula. The final row represents the amount of a 20-ml/kg bolus.

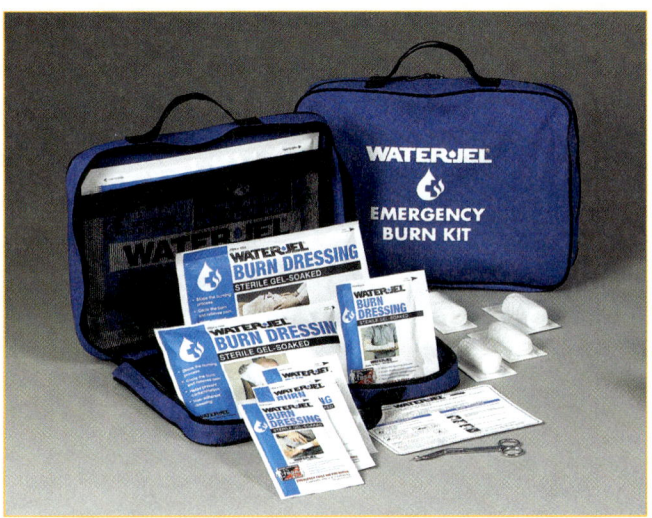

At the Scene

Pain medication is best given via the IV route. Owing to changes in fluid volume and tissue blood flow, absorption of any intramuscular or subcutaneous drug is unpredictable. Accurately measure and assess the patient's pain, and continuously monitor response to pain medication.

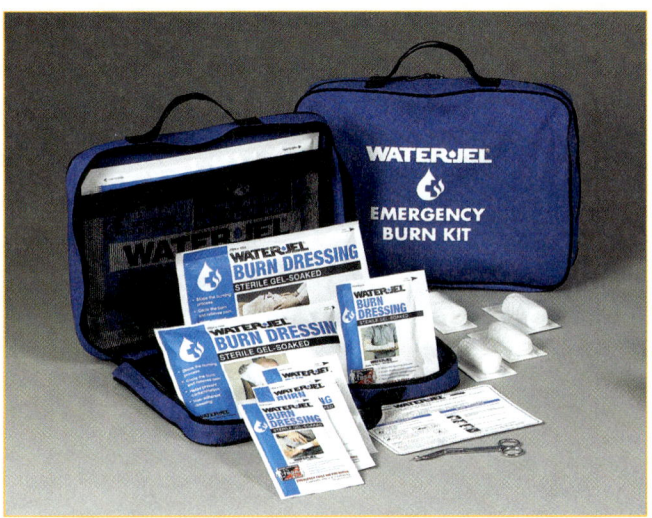

Figure 20-16 Burn dressing (Water-Jel) kits.

Management of Partial-Thickness Burns

Treatment of partial-thickness burns in the prehospital environment is similar to that of superficial burns. Cooling the burned area with water or application of wet dressings within the first hour can diminish edema and provide significant pain relief. Burned extremities should be elevated to minimize edema formation.

Do not attempt to rupture blisters over the burn; they initially act as a physiologic burn dressing. Establish IV fluids with lactated Ringer's solution or normal saline as dictated by local protocol. Pain in partial-thickness burns may be severe, so complete a pain assessment and administer pain medication as allowed by your protocols.

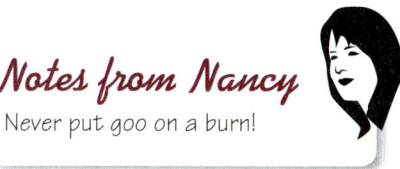

Notes from Nancy
Never put goo on a burn!

Management of Full-Thickness Burns

Although full-thickness burns may not cause pain, most patients will have varying degrees of burns within the affected region of injury. For this reason, a pain assessment should be completed and pain medication should be administered as described earlier. Usually, dry dressings are used after the fire is out. Check with your burn centre or medical centre on their view on wet dressings or analgesia.

Management of Chemical Burns

Speed is essential when treating chemical burns. Begin flushing the exposed area of the patient's body immediately with copious quantities of water **Figure 20-17 ▶**. If the patient is in or

You are the Paramedic **Part 3**

As you are en route to the appropriate facility, your partner works with the local police department in an attempt to contact the patient's parents. One relative is found—the patient's grandmother, who consents to Pamela's treatment and transport and adds that she is a normally healthy child with no medications or allergies. You address the patient's pain by providing an analgesic (morphine sulfate, 2 mg via slow IV push), elevate her arm with pillows, cover her with a blanket, and place her in a comfortable position. You also reassess the affected extremity for the presence of pulse and motor and sensory functions throughout transport.

Reassessment	Recording Time: 10 Minutes
Level of consciousness	Alert, with a Glasgow Coma Scale score of 15
Skin	Warm, pink, and dry
Pulse	Radial pulse, 118 beats/min, strong and regular
Blood pressure	116 by palpation
Respirations	28 to 36 breaths/min
SpO2	100%
Blood glucose	5 mmol/l
ECG	Sinus tachycardia without further ectopy

6. What is appropriate fluid resuscitation for a pediatric patient?
7. Given the nature of burns, what is another important consideration regarding burn care?

near the home, the shower or a garden hose is ideal. In an industrial setting, use the decontamination shower or a hose. While flushing, rapidly remove the patient's clothing, especially shoes and socks that may have become contaminated with the offending agent, taking care not to get any of the hazardous chemicals on your own clothing or skin.

Do not waste time looking for specific antidotes; copious flushing with water is more effective and more immediately available **Figure 20-18 ▶**. Flushing is preferable for 30 minutes before moving the patient; for chemical burns caused by strong alkalis (such as oven and drain cleaners), 1 to 2 *hours* of flushing has been recommended. Paramedics must weigh the realities of flushing on the scene for long periods against the benefits of transport and their ability to continue flushing en route. After flushing, limit hypothermia by keeping the patient covered and warm.

Special Cases of Chemical Burns

If you do not know the identity of the chemical that caused the burn, assume it is *not* a special case, and flush the burn wound with copious water as described.

In alkali burns caused by dry lime, combination with water will produce a highly corrosive substance. For that reason, when a patient has been in contact with dry lime, *first* remove the patient's clothing and *brush* as much lime as you can from the skin (wear gloves!). *Then* start flushing copiously with a garden hose or shower. Your intention is to completely overwhelm any damaging chemical reaction with a deluge of water.

Sodium metals produce considerable heat when mixed with water and may explode. Cover this type of burn with oil, which will stop the reaction by preventing the sodium from coming in contact with the atmosphere.

Hydrofluoric (HF) acid is used in drain cleaners in the home and for etching glass and plastic in industrial settings. HF acid burns that exceed 3% to 5% of the TBSA can be fatal. The patient will complain bitterly of pain, and the pain will not improve even with continuous flushing—a sign that the process of tissue destruction is ongoing. Calcium chloride (CaCl) jelly may be available in an industrial setting that uses HF acid; this jelly is placed on small-area HF acid burns (small burns from splashing or pinholes in gloves) to help reduce continued pain and injury. An ampule of CaCl (10 ml of a 10% CaCl solution) can be mixed with a water-based lubricant to make CaCl jelly in an emergency. Direct medical control may order IV CaCl for HF acid burns.

Hot tar burns are, strictly speaking, thermal burns, not chemical burns, although they tend to be classified with chemical burns. The most important step in the prehospital phase is to immerse the affected area in cold water to dissipate the heat from the tar and speed up the hardening process. Once the tar has cooled, it will not do further damage, and there is no need to try to remove it in the prehospital environment.

Chemical Burns of the Eye

If chemicals have splashed into the patient's eyes, flush the eyes with copious amounts of water. It may be most expeditious to simply support the patient's head under a faucet or at

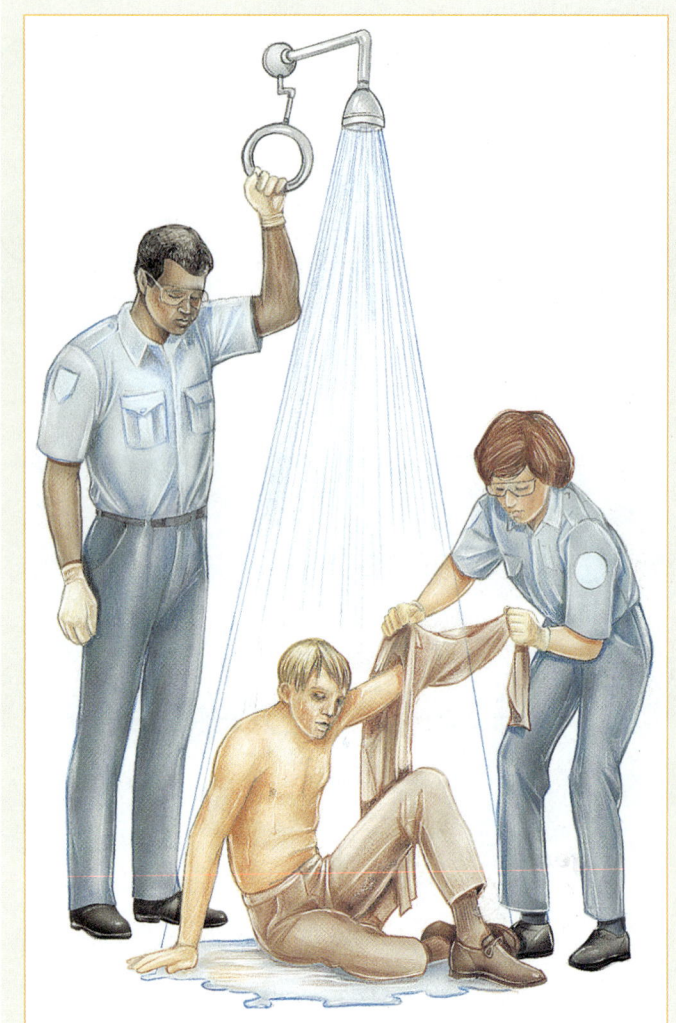

Figure 20-17 Flush the burned area with large amounts of water.

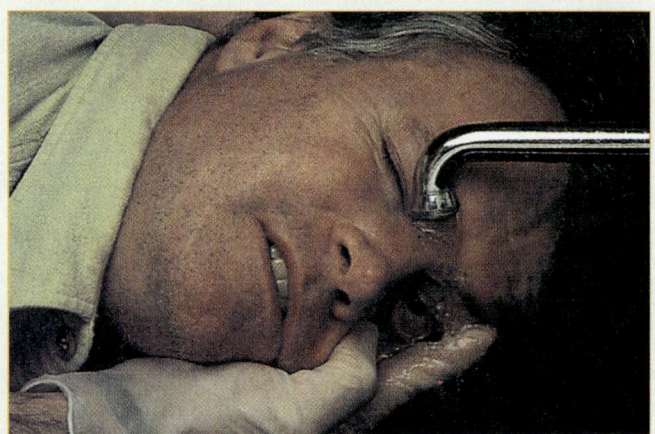

Figure 20-18 Flood the affected eye with a gentle stream of water. Hold the eyelids open—a challenging task because the patient's reflex is to keep the eye shut. Take care to prevent the chemical from getting into the other eye during the flushing.

an eye-wash station, directing a steady stream of lukewarm tap water into the affected eye (Figure 20-18). If the patient wears contact lenses and the stream of water does not flush them out, pause after a minute or two of irrigation to allow the patient to remove the contact lenses—if they remain in place, they will prevent water from reaching the cornea underneath. Be sure to irrigate well underneath the eyelids.

Never use chemical antidotes (such as vinegar or baking soda) in the eyes. Irrigate with water only. After irrigating, patch the patient's eyes with lightly applied dressings and begin transport to the hospital for evaluation.

Eye irrigation is extremely important whenever a chemical has gotten into the eye **Figure 20-19** . It may be uncomfortable and inefficient to attempt to irrigate an eye by prying it open and rinsing with a standard normal saline IV set.

Another option is the Morgan lens, which may make eye irrigation more comfortable, efficient, and effective. It is essentially a plastic contact lens with IV tubing attached to it, which allows IV fluids to flow directly over the surface of the eye. Ocular anesthetic drops are preferable, but care must be taken when the eye is "numb" to keep the patient from scratching or rubbing it. It is important to keep fluid running through the Morgan lens during insertion and removal. Suction can occur between the lens and the eye if the fluid flow is stopped before removal.

Management of Electrical Burns

One of every five construction deaths is caused by electrical contact. Statistics indicate that electrocution is the fifth leading cause of death in the workplace. Children are involved in the majority of electrocutions in the home, which tend to be lower-voltage exposures **Figure 20-20** .

The first priority at the scene of an electrical injury is to protect yourself and bystanders from becoming the next victims. Do *not* use a rope, wooden pole, or any other object to try to dislodge the patient from the current source. Do *not* try to cut the wire. Do *not* go anywhere near a high-tension line.

Many parts of the electrical grid are protected by automatically resetting breakers. When the wind blows a branch into wires or a rambunctious squirrel bridges the gap between two wires, it is desirable to have the breaker reset after a few moments to avoid power outages. As a consequence, a downed wire that "looks dead" can jump back to life, perhaps several times. There is only one safe way to deal with a downed high-tension wire: Call the electric company. Wait until a qualified person has shut off the power before you approach the patient. This can be a traumatic event for paramedics, who will feel helpless waiting for the power to be shut down while a possibly critical patient lies on the ground nearby. But remember—*rescuers die in these situations.* You can help the greatest number of people by being cautious and safe in this circumstance.

Once the electric hazard has been neutralized, proceed to the ABCs. Open the airway using the jaw-thrust maneuver, keeping in mind the possibility of cervical spine injury. Start

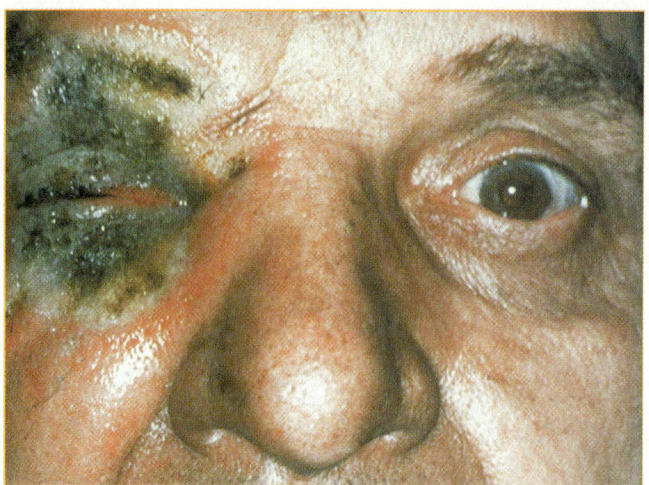

Figure 20-19 The eyes are particularly vulnerable to chemical burns.

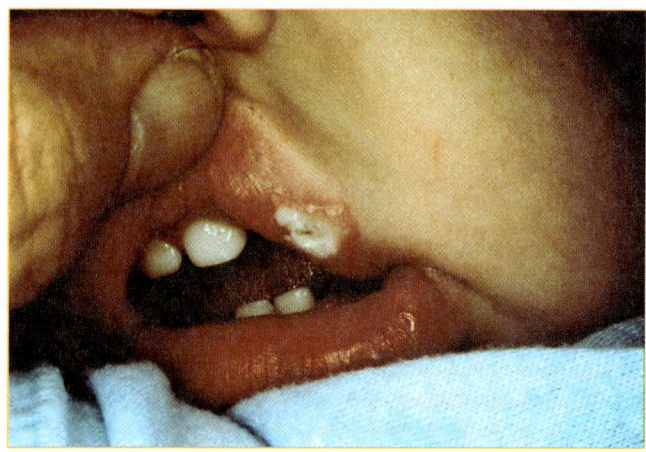

Figure 20-20 Children often sustain electrical burns from chewing on electrical cords.

CPR as indicated, and attach the monitor to identify ventricular fibrillation. If the patient is not in cardiac arrest, dysrhythmias remain a risk, and cardiac monitoring is indicated for 24 hours after the injury.

Make careful note of the patient's state of consciousness, and record his or her vital signs. Try to determine the path the current has taken through the body by looking for entrance and exit wounds and by carefully palpating the skin and soft tissues. When deep tissues have been seriously damaged by heat, the surrounding muscle may swell and become hard. Thus, a rigid abdomen or rigid extremity may indicate a serious internal injury. Be alert for fractures or dislocations, and check the distal pulses in all four extremities.

Electrical burns may produce devastating internal injuries with little external evidence. The degree of tissue injury is related to the resistance of the body tissues, the intensity of current that passes through the victim, and the duration of exposure.

When a person comes in contact with an electrical source, the amount of current delivered to the inside of the body depends to some extent on the resistance of the skin. Wet, thin, clean skin offers less resistance than dry, thick, dirty skin; thus a moist inner surface of the forearm will have much less resistance than a dry, callused palm.

As electric current travels from the contact site into the body, it is converted to heat, which follows the current flow—usually along blood vessels and nerves—causing extensive damage to the tissues in its path. The greater the current flow, the greater the heat generated. When the voltage is low (< 1,000 volts, as in household sources), current follows the path of least resistance, generally along blood vessels, nerves, and muscles. When the voltage is high (as from high-tension lines), current takes the shortest path.

Alternating current is considerably more dangerous than direct current because the alternations cause repetitive muscle contractions, which may "freeze" the victim to the conductor until the current source is turned off. Furthermore, alternating current is more likely than direct current to induce ventricular fibrillation. The direction of current flow is also significant. Current moving from one hand to the other is particularly dangerous because current may then flow across the heart; a current of only 0.1 amp to the heart can provoke ventricular fibrillation.

Management of an electrical burn injury includes initial assessment focusing on the mental status and ABCs and prioritizing care of the patient. If the patient has life-threatening injuries, begin related prehospital care and prepare to transport the patient as soon as practical. Generally, aside from the fluid therapy for the care of a burn injury, no specific pharmacologic interventions are indicated, other than the normal medications used to manage a cardiac dysrhythmia or extreme pain (if authorized by direct medical control). Early oxygen therapy is helpful, as is managing the patient for impending shock. Transport decisions should be made early and take into consideration the regional resources for the care of a patient with a severe (electrical) burn. Contact direct medical control for advice in making a transport decision or regarding the need to use aeromedical evacuation directly to the burn centre. The patient will be very anxious and scared, so be sure to talk calmly. Explain what you are doing and how you plan to obtain the best care.

Management of Lightning-Related Injuries

When you reach the scene of a lightning strike, all the usual priorities apply, but there are two special considerations to keep in mind.

First, if the electrical storm is still going on, your first priority is to get any patients and rescuers to a safe place, preferably indoors, or at least inside the ambulance. Lightning *can* strike twice in the same place. There is, however, no hazard in touching the victim of a lightning strike—contrary to what your grandmother may have told you, electricity does not remain within the body of a person who has been hit by lightning.

Second, be aware that a lightning strike is apt to injure more than one person. Therefore, the first thing you need to do on arrival at the scene—before you leave the safety of the ambulance—is a rapid assessment of the entire scene to determine the number of patients.

Carry out the initial assessment as usual, and start CPR when necessary. When establishing an airway, bear in mind the possibility of cervical spine injury, and do not hyperextend the neck; use the jaw-thrust maneuver.

> **Notes from Nancy**
> In a lightning strike with multiple victims, priority goes to the victims who are not breathing.

Patients with cardiac arrest caused by a lightning strike deserve aggressive, continuing CPR. The chances of a successful resuscitation in such a case are good, even when the patient appears beyond help initially and even when there is a long delay in the return of spontaneous breathing. Minimize the interruption in compressions, and push hard and fast with full chest recoil!

> **Notes from Nancy**
> Don't give up quickly on a patient in cardiac arrest due to a lightning strike.

Treatment of lightning injuries is similar to that of injuries sustained from high-voltage lines:

- Make sure the scene is safe. Move the victim to a safer location if necessary.
- Priority for treatment goes to patients who are not breathing.
- Establish an airway, with cervical spine precautions. Perform CPR as needed.
- Administer supplemental oxygen.
- Monitor cardiac rhythm.
- Insert a large-bore IV cannula and run in normal saline solution wide open to keep the kidneys flushed out.
- Cover any surface burns with dry, sterile dressings.
- Splint fractures.
- If the patient has fallen, immobilize the cervical spine.

Management of Radiation Burns

Patients with radiation burns may be contaminated with radioactive material, so they should be decontaminated before transport. The majority of contaminants can be removed by simply disrobing the patient.

Irrigate open wounds. Washing should be gentle to avoid further damage to the skin, which could result in additional internal radiation absorption. The head and scalp should be irrigated the same way. The ED should be notified as soon as practical if you are transporting a potentially contaminated patient. In contrast with other types of contamination, radioactive particulate matter probably poses a relatively small risk to the rescuer. Consider providing basic care to the patient before decontamination if you are wearing protective clothing.

Radiation injury follows the "inverse square law": Exposure drops exponentially as distance is increased. Increasing your (and your patient's) distance from the source by even a few feet may dramatically decrease your exposure, so it is important to identify the radioactive source and the length of the patient's exposure to it. You must try to limit your duration of exposure, increase your distance from the source, and attempt to place shielding between yourself and sources of gamma radiation.

With contact radiation burns, decontaminate the wound as if it were a chemical burn to remove any radioactive particulate matter. You may then treat it as a burn.

Many radioactive isotopes are used in medicine and industry, some of which can be absorbed or have their toxic effects blunted by another substance. Like their radioactive effects, the toxic effects of these isotopes vary. Antidotes may help bind an isotope, enhance its elimination from the body, or reduce the toxic effects on other organs. Such antidotal therapy should be considered only under the guidance of a knowledgeable physician or public health agency.

Potassium iodide is distributed to people who live near a nuclear power plant and may help protect the thyroid gland if taken within 6 hours of exposure. Contrary to popular belief, however, it is effective only for radionuclides released from fission products from nuclear power plants and would be of little value for exposure to medical radiation.

Management of Burns in Pediatric Patients

Escaping from a fire can be difficult for children. More than half of the fire-related deaths and injuries in children involve preschoolers. Research suggests that young children are not as effectively awakened by smoke detectors, and they are often disoriented immediately after waking. The "reliable waking rate" in children younger than 15 years may be as low as 6%. Young children are also more likely to sustain severe scald injuries. Children's thin skin and delicate respiratory structures are more easily damaged by thermal insults than are those of older children and adults.

In children, fluid resuscitation may be more challenging because of their increased body surface/weight ratio. As a consequence, children may require more fluid per kilogram than adults. You may start with the Parkland formula in children, only to find that direct medical control orders additional fluids for severe burns. Also, because of poor glycogen stores, children may require dextrose-containing solutions earlier than adults. Blood glucose monitoring should be routinely performed in seriously ill children.

Burns may raise the suspicion of child abuse. Pay careful attention to the mechanism of injury, and relay this information to the hospital staff.

Management of Burns in Geriatric Patients

Approximately 1,200 older adults die of fire-related causes each year, making it the sixth leading cause of death in this population. Some 13% of older adults smoke, and smoking is the leading cause of fires that lead to death of elderly people. Burns from fires caused by smoking while wearing supplementary

You are the Paramedic Part 4

As you arrive at the hospital, the patient seems much more comfortable. She is no longer crying as vigorously and occasionally gives you a glimpse of a smile. The grandmother meets you at the hospital and informs you that Pamela's mother is nowhere to be found. You provide a report including the history of events (including the home situation) to the ED staff.

Reassessment	Recording Time: 20 Minutes
Level of consciousness	Alert, with a Glasgow Coma Scale score of 15
Skin	Warm, pink, and dry
Pulse	Radial pulse, 98 beats/min, strong and regular
Blood pressure	108/58 mm Hg
Respirations	24 breaths/min
SpO_2	100%
Temperature	37°C
ECG	Normal sinus rhythm without ectopy

8. What is burn shock, and how does it relate to the prehospital setting?
9. What other considerations must be made when dealing with a pediatric burn patient?

oxygen are the leading sentinel event in home care. Cooking fires represent another distinct hazard to elderly people, who may be less able to smell a gas leak or a fire in the kitchen. Elderly patients are also particularly sensitive to respiratory insults. Relatively small fires can produce toxic fumes before detection or suppression devices are activated.

Geriatric patients may also have poor glycogen stores, so their blood glucose levels should be checked to assess for hypoglycemia. Cardiac monitoring should, of course, be implemented. Although fluid resuscitation is important, pulmonary edema is more likely to develop in geriatric patients. Routinely assess lung sounds.

Transfer to a Burn Specialty Centre

Patients with the following injuries should be transferred to a specialized burn centre:

- Partial-thickness burns of more than 10% of the body surface area
- Burns that involve the face, hands, feet, genitalia, perineum, or major joints
- Full-thickness burns in any age group
- Electrical burns, including lightning
- Chemical burns
- Inhalation burns
- Burn injuries in conjunction with preexisting medical conditions that could complicate management, prolong recovery, or affect mortality
- Burns and concomitant trauma in which the burn injury poses the greatest risk of morbidity or mortality
- Burn injury that requires special social, emotional, or long-term rehabilitation

The following classifications of burn severity are typically used:

- **Minor burns**
  - Superficial—body surface area less than 50% (such as sunburns)
  - Partial thickness—body surface area less than 15%
  - Full thickness—body surface area less than 2%
- **Moderate burns**
  - Superficial—body surface area greater than 50%
  - Partial thickness—body surface area less than 30%
  - Full thickness—body surface area less than 10%
- **Critical burns**
  - Partial thickness—body surface area greater than 30%
  - Full thickness—body surface area greater than 10%
  - Inhalation injury
  - Partial- or full-thickness burns involving hands, feet, joints, face, or genitalia

All critical burns should be transported to a specialty burn centre, if available locally. However, paramedics should consult their local and regional policies to determine if a prehospital bypass for patients with critical burns exists. If a bypass policy does not exist, the paramedic should take the burn patient to the nearest appropriate facility.

Consequences of Burns

The Patient

Serious burn injuries are devastating events that leave patients with long-term physical and psychological challenges. People with major injuries average about 1 day of inpatient treatment for each 1% of the TBSA burned. Extensive rehabilitation may also be necessary to regain function. Survivors of serious burns are left with a host of long-term consequences, including problems with thermoregulation, motor function, and sensory function. Although tremendous improvements in the care of critical burn patients have made long-term survival possible for many who would have died of their injuries a decade ago, large surface area burns remain a critical care challenge on par with other forms of severe multisystem trauma.

The Paramedic

Caring for patients with severe burn emergencies can be one of the most horrifying tasks undertaken by paramedics. Fire scenes are chaotic and dangerous. Patients are often in severe pain. The smell of burned hair and flesh permeates your clothes and equipment. Sheets of tissue may peel off the patient when you perform simple tasks like attempting to take vital signs or moving the patient. Despite the traumatic circumstances, with the proper training and the right mix of confidence and courage, you can make a tremendous impact in the treatment and overall survival of burn patients.

You are the Paramedic Summary

1. What are your patient care priorities?

Your patient care priorities, after ensuring the safety of the scene, are the ABCs. For fire victims, issues of maintaining a patent airway with good ventilation and oxygenation can present a particular challenge for paramedics.

2. What are patient care concerns when dealing with structure fire victims?

Superheated gases and by-products of combustion can cause airway irritation and severe edema. It is essential to act quickly if you believe your patient has inhalation burns—time is of the essence in obtaining and maintaining a patent airway. The presence of soot or burns around the nose or mouth, singed facial hair, wheezing, and stridor are ominous signs. Be prepared to provide advanced airway management.

3. Why is pulse oximetry unreliable in these circumstances?

By-products of incomplete combustion include noxious gases such as CO, formaldehyde, sulfur dioxide, nitrogen dioxide, hydrogen sulfide, cyanide, and particulates. Inhalation of these gases (particularly CO) can be deadly because hemoglobin's affinity for CO is roughly 240 times greater than its affinity for oxygen. The excess CO causes severe tissue hypoxia despite the possibility of acceptable or somewhat normal readings on the pulse oximeter.

4. Are your transport considerations affected by the location of her burn?

Yes. This child should be taken to a burn centre because her right hand is burned. Accepted criteria for transport to a burn centre include partial-thickness burns on greater than 10% of the TBSA; any full-thickness burns; burns involving the hands, feet, face, major joints, or groin; burns involving the airway; circumferential burns (especially involving the chest or neck); electrical burns (including lightning and high-voltage electricity injuries); chemical burns; underlying medical conditions and/or traumatic injuries that could be exacerbated; or the lack of facilities capable of appropriately treating burn patients.

5. What are common complications of burns?

Depending on the area affected (usually when an area greater than 10% of the TBSA is involved) and the thickness of the burn,

patients may experience difficulties with thermoregulation. For this reason, you should take steps to preserve body temperature.

6. What is appropriate fluid resuscitation for a pediatric patient?

The Parkland formula provides guidelines for fluid resuscitation of burn patients. During the first 24 hours, the burn patient will receive 4 ml × body weight (in kilograms) × percentage of body surface burned. Half of that amount needs to be given during the first 8 hours. However, pediatric patients may need more fluids than their adult counterparts, so be prepared to make adjustments accordingly.

7. Given the nature of burns, what is another important consideration regarding burn care?

Beyond estimating the extent of the burn and cooling and covering the area, be aware that burns are extremely painful. As health care professionals, we must be prepared to provide appropriate pain management. Morphine sulfate is highly effective at 0.05 to 0.1 mg/kg, with repeated doses as needed.

8. What is burn shock, and how does it relate to the prehospital setting?

Burn shock occurs because of fluid loss through the damaged skin and a series of volume shifts within the body. Capillaries become leaky, so intravascular fluid oozes out of the circulation and into the interstitial spaces. Meanwhile, cells of normal tissues take in increased amounts of salt and water from the fluid around them. This process occurs during a 6- to 8-hour period. Therefore, if a burned patient is in shock in the prehospital phase, look for another injury as the source of shock. In particular, make sure that you auscultate lung sounds before administration of fluid therapy.

9. What other considerations must be made when dealing with a pediatric burn patient?

Monitor the patient's blood glucose level, and be prepared to administer dextrose as needed. Also, when dealing with minors or older people, be aware of the potential for child or elder abuse. It is your responsibility to report suspected abuse or neglect to the proper authorities.

Prep Kit

Ready for Review

- Although you probably won't see moderate or severe burns on a daily basis, you will encounter some serious burn injuries during your career.
- The skin has four functions:
  - Protect the underlying tissue from injury and exposure
  - Regulate temperature
  - Prevent excessive loss of water from the body
  - Act as a sense organ
- Significant damage to the skin may make the body vulnerable to bacterial invasion, temperature instability, and major disturbances of fluid balance.
- Burns are diffuse soft-tissue injuries created from destructive energy transferred via radiation, thermal, or electrical energy.
- The many types of burns, coupled with the many possible presentations of burn patients, can challenge your assessment skills. Address a burned patient in a consistent, efficient, and systematic manner so you don't develop tunnel vision for the major burn trauma and miss other occult injuries that could affect the patient's outcome.
- Although you will be most heavily involved in the first phase of burn care, it is important to appreciate the magnitude of care that a patient with a severe or even moderate burn must receive. Early actions of paramedics may dramatically affect the patient's long-term outcome.
- Serious burn injuries are devastating events that leave patients with long-term physical and psychological challenges.

Vital Vocabulary

acute radiation syndrome The clinical course that usually begins within hours of exposure to a radiation source. Symptoms include nausea, vomiting, diarrhea, fatigue, fever, and headache. The long-term symptoms are dose-related and are hematopoietic and gastrointestinal.

adipose tissue Fat tissue.

anaerobic metabolism The metabolism that takes place in the absence of oxygen; the principal product is lactic acid.

burn shock The shock or hypoperfusion caused by a burn injury and the tremendous loss of fluids.

circumferential burns Burns on the neck or chest that may compress the airway or on an extremity that might act like a tourniquet.

collagen A protein that gives tensile strength to the connective tissues of the body.

comedo A noninflammatory acne lesion.

contact burn A burn produced by touching a hot object.

cutaneous Pertaining to the skin.

dermis The inner layer of skin containing hair follicle roots, glands, blood vessels, and nerves.

desquamation The continuous shedding of the dead cells on the surface of the skin.

elastin A protein that gives the skin its elasticity.

epidermis The outermost layer of the skin.

escharotomy A surgical cut through the eschar or leathery covering of a burn injury to allow for swelling and minimize the potential for development of compartment syndrome in a circumferentially burned limb or the thorax.

flame burn A thermal burn caused by flames touching the skin.

flash burn An electrothermal injury caused by arcing of electric current.

full-thickness burn A burn that extends through the epidermis and dermis into the subcutaneous tissues beneath; previously called a third-degree burn.

homeostasis A tendency to constancy or stability in the body's internal environment.

integument The skin.

Lund and Browder chart A detailed version of the rule of nines chart that takes into consideration the changes in body surface area brought on by growth.

melanin The pigment that gives skin its colour.

mucopolysaccharide gel One of the complex materials found, along with the collagen fibres and elastin fibres, in the dermis of the skin.

Parkland formula A formula that recommends giving 4 mL of normal saline for each kilogram of body weight, multiplied by the percentage of body surface area burned; sometimes used to calculate fluid needs during lengthy transport times.

partial-thickness burn A burn that involves the epidermis and part of the dermis, characterized by pain and blistering; previously called a second-degree burn.

rule of nines A system that assigns percentages to sections of the body, allowing calculation of the amount of skin surface involved in the burn area.

rule of palm A system that estimates total body surface area burned by comparing the affected area with the size of the patient's palm, which is roughly equal to 1% of the patient's total body surface area.

scald burn A burn produced by hot liquids.

sebaceous gland A gland located in the dermis that secretes sebum.

sebum An oily substance secreted by sebaceous glands.

steam burn A burn that has been caused by direct exposure to hot steam exhaust, as from a broken pipe.

subcutaneous layer Beneath the skin.

superficial burn A burn involving only the epidermis, producing very red, painful skin; previously called a first-degree burn.

supraglottic Located above the glottic opening, as in the upper airway structures.

thermal burn An injury caused by radiation or direct contact with a heat source on the skin.

thermoregulation The ability of the body to maintain temperature through a combination of heat gain by metabolic processes and muscular movement and heat loss through respiration, evaporation, conduction, convection, and perspiration.

total body surface area (TBSA) Used in the calculation of a burn injury to determine the percentage of the surface of the patient's body that has been injured. This is commonly estimated by using the rule of palm or the rule of nines.

zone of coagulation The reddened area surrounding the leathery and sometimes charred tissue that has sustained a full-thickness burn.

zone of hyperemia In a thermal burn, the area that is least affected by the burn injury.

zone of stasis The peripheral area surrounding the zone of coagulation that has decreased blood flow and inflammation. This area can undergo necrosis within 24 to 48 hours after the injury, particularly if perfusion is compromised due to burn shock.

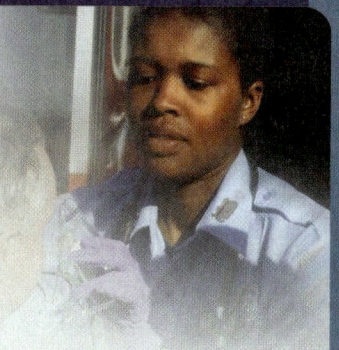

Assessment in Action

You are dispatched to a private residence to for an unconscious victim with possible smoke inhalation. You arrive on scene to find an 81-year-old woman outside being attended to by fire department personnel. The firefighters report that the patient was found on the floor in the kitchen. The patient is conscious but combative and asking repetitive questions. The firefighters transfer the patient to the ambulance, where you begin your assessment.

The patient's blood pressure is 150/90 mm Hg, respirations are 18 breaths/min, heart rate is 110 beats/min, and pulse oximetry is 95% while breathing room air. You notice a significant amount of soot around the patient's face, especially in the nostrils, mouth, and oral airway. The patient remains conscious but does not recognize her family and continues to ask repetitive questions. You insert an IV line, give lactated Ringer's solution, and begin your transport to the local burn centre, which is approximately 25 minutes away.

En route to the hospital, you sedate the patient and successfully intubate her with a 7.0 ET tube. You notice a significant amount of soot around the vocal cords. You transfer the patient to the emergency department. Later, the patient is admitted to the intensive care unit for respiratory failure secondary to an inhalation injury.

1. **What type of burn is described in this scenario?**
   A. Thermal burn
   B. Scald burn
   C. Contact burn
   D. Airway burn

2. **Anyone exposed to smoke from a fire may have _____ burns.**
   A. thermal
   B. scald
   C. contact
   D. radiation

3. **_____ airway damage is more often associated with the inhalation of superheated gases.**
   A. Upper airway
   B. Lower airway
   C. Upper and lower airway
   D. None of these

4. **In the lower airway, _____ and _____ may result from heat inhalation.**
   A. laryngospasm, pulmonary damage
   B. pulmonary damage, bronchospasm
   C. laryngospasm, bronchospasm
   D. mild, severe damage

5. **True or false? If your patient greets you with a hoarse voice and a chief complaint of "trouble breathing," your general impression should be that there is probably nothing wrong with this patient.**
   A. True
   B. False

6. **Combative patients should be considered:**
   A. as having head trauma.
   B. intoxicated.
   C. diabetic.
   D. hypoxic.

7. **_____ can develop with alarming speed in burn patients, especially in infants and children.**
   A. Laryngeal edema
   B. A pulmonary injury
   C. An inhalation burn
   D. Bronchial edema

8. **After listening to lung sounds, you hear _____, a sign of impending upper airway compromise.**
   A. wheezing
   B. stridor
   C. rhonchi
   D. rales

9. **Burn patients fall into several general categories for airway management. They include:**
   A. the patient with the acutely decompensating airway who requires field intubation.
   B. the patient with the deteriorating airway from burns and toxic inhalations.
   C. the patient with no signs of or risk factors for airway compromise who is in no distress.
   D. all of the above.

Challenging Questions

It is 2:00 hrs and you are sent to a "structure fire." The patient was inside the burning house and was standing on the roof when the firefighters arrived. Firefighters had the patient drop and roll. The patient is still smouldering and is in a great deal of pain. You call for a medical helicopter and transfer the patient to the landing zone. You estimate that the burn involves 30% of the TBSA.

10. **What is your treatment while you are driving to the landing zone?**

11. **How do you assess the TBSA burned?**

12. **How much fluid will this patient require?**

▮ Points to Ponder

You and your crew are called to the scene of a fire. When you arrive, you find the patient is a man in his mid 30s. He has dark, discoloured patches of skin on his chest, lower right arm, and lower back. He also has a circumferential burn on his left upper arm. His voice is slightly hoarse, and twice he coughs up dark-coloured sputum. However, he denies having difficulty breathing or having much pain. He is sitting up at the scene, watching all that is going on around him.

Why is this patient of particular concern? What must you make sure to do in treating this patient?

Issues: The Impact of Managing a Burn-Injured Patient, Mortality and Morbidity Based on Pathophysiology and Assessment Findings.

21 Head and Face Injuries

Competency Areas

Area 4: Assessment and Diagnostics

4.3.d Conduct neurological system assessment and interpret findings.

4.3.e Conduct respiratory system assessment and interpret findings.

4.3.n Conduct multisystem assessment and interpret findings.

4.4.h Assess pupils.

4.4.i Assess level of mentation.

Area 5: Therapeutics

5.5.b Control external hemorrhage through the use of direct pressure and patient positioning.

5.6.c Treat eye injury.

Area 6: Integration

6.1.b Provide care to patient experiencing illness or injury primarily involving neurological system.

6.1.j Provide care to patient experiencing illness or injury primarily involving the eyes, ears, nose or throat.

Appendix 4: Pathophysiology

B. **Neurologic System**
Traumatic Injuries: Hematoma (epidural, subdural, subarachnoid)

H. **Musculoskeletal System**
Soft Tissue Disorders: Contusions

L. **Ears, Eyes, Nose, and Throat**
Eyes-Traumatic Injuries: Corneal injuries
Eyes-Traumatic Injuries: Hyphema
Eyes-Traumatic Injuries: Penetrating injury
Eyes-Medical Illness: Cataracts
Eyes-Medical Illness: Glaucoma
Eyes-Medical Illness: Infection
Eyes-Medical Illness: Retinal detachment
External, Middle, and Inner Ear Disorders: Traumatic ear injuries
Face and Jaw Disorders: Dental abscess
Face and Jaw Disorders: Trauma injury
Face and Jaw Disorders: Trismus
Nasal and Sinus Disorders: Epistaxis
Nasal and Sinus Disorders: Trauma injury
Oral and Dental Disorders: Dental fractures
Oral and Dental Disorders: Penetrating injury

Head and Face Injuries

As a paramedic, you will commonly encounter patients with injuries to the head, neck, and face, ranging in severity from a broken nose to traumatic brain injury. The first part of this chapter provides a detailed review of the anatomy and physiology of the head and face. The second part discusses head and face injuries, including their respective signs and symptoms and the appropriate prehospital care for maxillofacial injuries, eye and ear injuries, oral and dental injuries, injuries to the anterior part of the neck, and head and traumatic brain injuries.

The Skull and Facial Bones

The Scalp

The brain—the most important organ in the body—requires maximum protection from injury. The human body ensures that it receives this protection by housing the brain within several layers of soft and hard wrappings.

Starting from the outside and proceeding inward toward the brain, the first protective layer is the scalp, which consists of the following layers, given in descending order:

- Skin, with hair
- Subcutaneous tissue, which contains major scalp veins that bleed profusely when lacerated
- Galea aponeurotica, a tendon expansion that connects the frontal and occipital muscles of the cranium
- Loose connective tissue (alveolar tissue), which is easily stripped from the layer beneath in "scalping" injuries. This loose alveolar layer also provides room for blood to accumulate after blunt trauma between the scalp and skull bone (subgaleal hematoma).
- Periosteum, the dense fibrous membrane covering the surface of bones

The Skull

At the top of the axial skeleton is the skull, which consists of 28 bones in three anatomical groups: the auditory ossicles, the cranium, and the face. The six auditory ossicles function in hearing and are located, three on each side of the head, deep

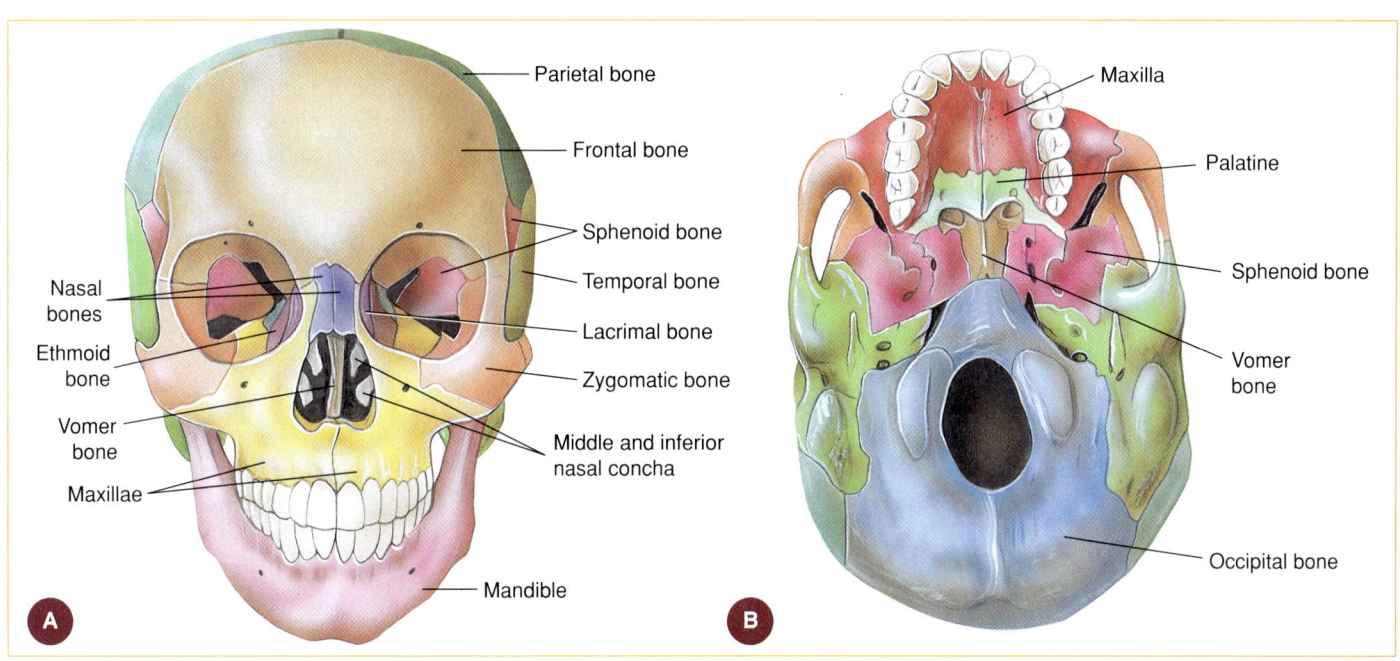

Figure 21-1 The skull and its components. **A.** Front view. **B.** Bottom view.

Front view labels: Parietal bone, Frontal bone, Sphenoid bone, Temporal bone, Lacrimal bone, Zygomatic bone, Middle and inferior nasal concha, Mandible, Nasal bones, Ethmoid bone, Vomer bone, Maxillae

Bottom view labels: Maxilla, Palatine, Sphenoid bone, Vomer bone, Occipital bone

You are the Paramedic Part 1

You respond to the scene of a motorcycle collision. The patient, a young male, was ejected from his motorcycle when it struck a tree; he was not wearing a helmet. The scene is safe, and two police officers are at the scene directing the flow of traffic, as well as the local fire department. As you approach the patient, you note that he is lying in a supine position. His eyes are closed, and he is not moving.

1. What should be your initial concern about this patient?
2. How should you direct your initial care of this patient?

within the cavities of the temporal bone. The remaining 22 bones constitute the cranium and the face Figure 21-1 ◂ .

The cranial vault consists of eight bones that encase and protect the brain: the parietal, temporal, frontal, occipital, sphenoid, and ethmoid bones. The brain connects to the spinal cord through a large opening at the base of the skull called the foramen magnum.

The bones of the skull are connected at special joints known as sutures Figure 21-2 ▾ . The paired parietal bones join together at the sagittal suture. The parietal bones abut the frontal bone at the coronal suture. The occipital bone attaches to the parietal bones at the lambdoid suture. Fibrous tissues called fontanelles, which are soft in infants, link the sutures. The tissues felt through the fontanelles are layers of the scalp and thick membranes overlying the brain. Under normal conditions, the brain may not be felt through the fontanelles. By the time a child is 18 months old, the sutures should have solidified and the fontanelles closed.

At the base of each temporal bone is a cone-shaped section of bone known as the mastoid process. This area is an important site for attachment of various muscles. In addition, a portion of the mastoid process contains hollow mastoid air cells Figure 21-3 ▾ .

The Floor of the Cranial Vault

Viewed from above, the floor of the cranial vault is divided into three compartments: the anterior fossa, middle fossa, and posterior fossa Figure 21-4 ▸ . The crista galli forms a prominent bony ridge in the centre of the anterior fossa and is the point of attachment of the meninges, the three layers of membranes that surround the brain and spinal cord. On the other side of the crista galli is the cribriform plate of the ethmoid bone, a horizontal bone that is perforated with numerous openings (foramina) allowing the passage of the olfactory nerve filaments from the nasal cavity. The olfactory nerves, the cranial nerves for smell, send projections through the foramina in the cribriform plate and into the nasal cavity, the chamber inside the nose that lies between the floor of the cranium and the roof of the mouth.

The Base of the Skull

When the mandible is removed, the base of the skull appears amazingly complex, with numerous foramina visible Figure 21-5 ▸ . The occipital condyles on the occipital bone, which are the points of articulation between the skull and the vertebral column, lie on either side of the foramen magnum. Portions of the maxilla and the palatine bone, the irregularly shaped bone in the posterior nasal cavity, form the hard palate, which is the bony anterior part of the palate, or roof, of the mouth. The zygomatic arch is the bone that extends along the front of the skull below the orbit.

The Facial Bones

The frontal and ethmoid bones are part of the cranial vault and the face. The

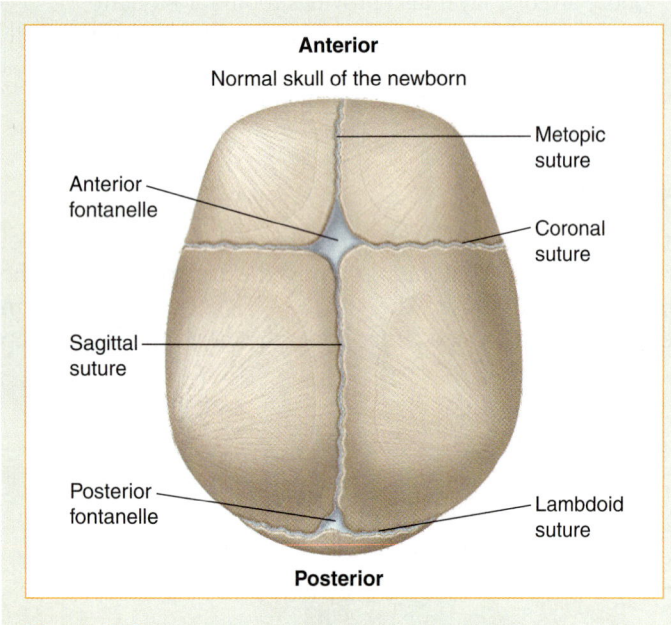

Anterior
Normal skull of the newborn

- Metopic suture
- Anterior fontanelle
- Coronal suture
- Sagittal suture
- Posterior fontanelle
- Lambdoid suture

Posterior

Figure 21-2 The sutures of the skull in a newborn.

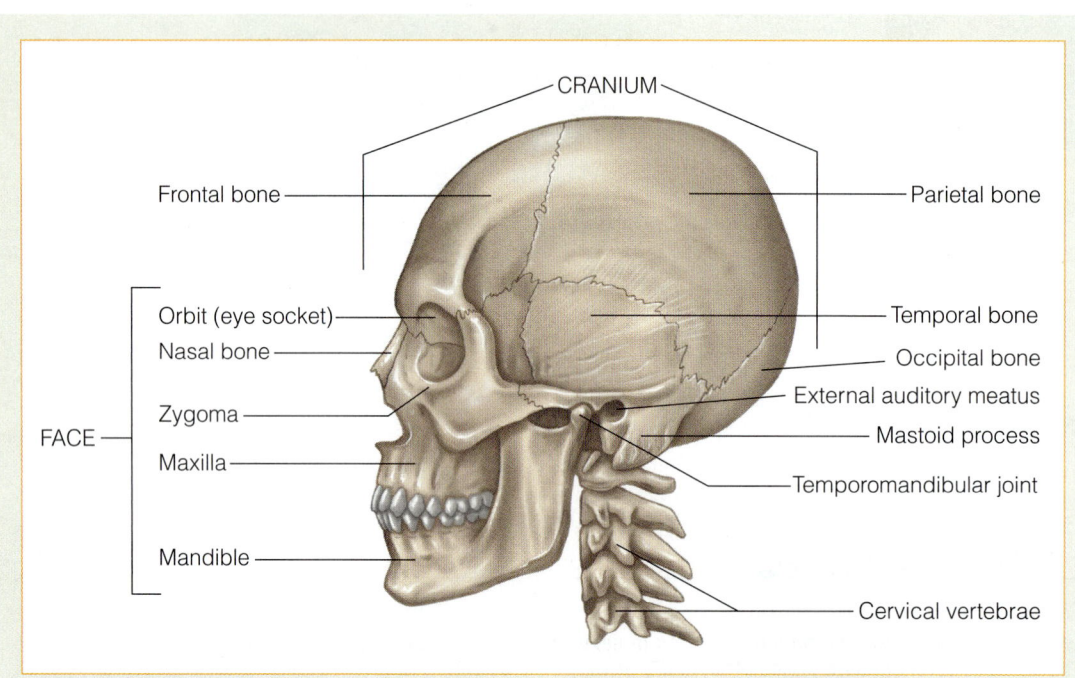

CRANIUM

- Frontal bone
- Parietal bone
- Orbit (eye socket)
- Nasal bone
- Temporal bone
- Occipital bone
- External auditory meatus
- Zygoma
- FACE
- Mastoid process
- Maxilla
- Temporomandibular joint
- Mandible
- Cervical vertebrae

Figure 21-3 The mastoid air cells are located in the mastoid process. Just anterior to the mastoid is the external auditory treatus, which is associated with the ear canal.

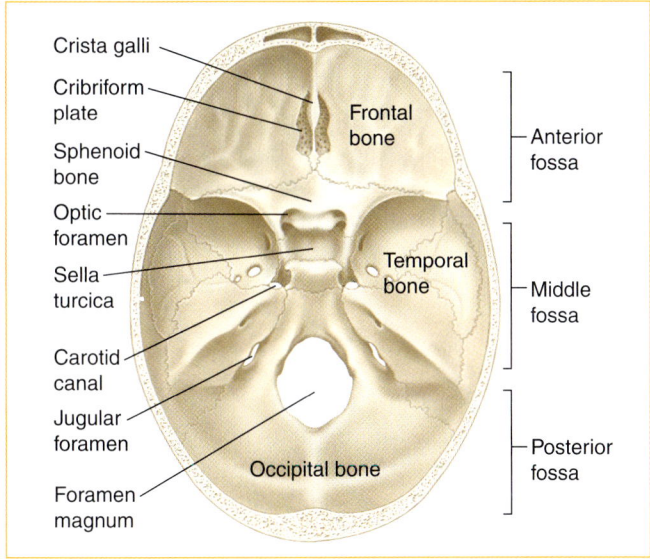

Figure 21-4 The floor of the cranial vault and its anatomy.

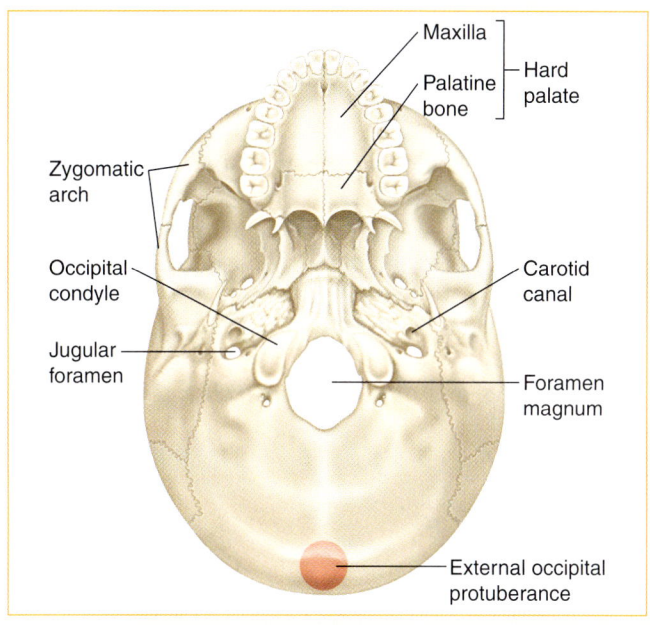

Figure 21-5 The base of the skull from below.

14 facial bones form the structure of the face, without contributing to the cranial vault. They include the maxillae, vomer, inferior nasal concha, and the zygomatic, palatine, nasal, and lacrimal bones (see Figure 21-1A).

The facial bones protect the eyes, nose, and tongue; they also provide attachment points for the muscles that allow chewing. The zygomatic process of the temporal bone and the temporal process of the zygomatic bone form the zygomatic arch **Figure 21-6 ▶**, which lends shape to the cheeks.

Two major nerves provide sensory and motor control to the face: the trigeminal nerve (fifth cranial nerve) and the facial nerve (seventh cranial nerve). The trigeminal nerve branches into the ophthalmic nerve, maxillary nerve, and mandibular nerve. The ophthalmic nerve (a sensory nerve) supplies the skin of the forehead, upper eyelid, and conjunctiva. The maxillary nerve (another sensory nerve) supplies the skin on the posterior part of the side of the nose, lower eyelid,

cheek, and upper lip. The mandibular nerve (a sensory and motor nerve) supplies the muscles of chewing (mastication) and skin of the lower lip, chin, temporal region, and part of the external ear. The facial nerve supplies the muscles of facial expression.

Blood supply to the face is provided primarily through the external carotid artery, which branches into the temporal, mandibular, and maxillary arteries. Because the face is highly vascular, it tends to bleed heavily when injured.

The Orbits

The orbits are cone-shaped fossae that enclose and protect the eyes. In addition to the eyeball and muscles that move it, the orbit contains blood vessels, nerves, and fat.

A blow to the eye may result in fracture of the orbital floor because the bone is most thin here and breaks easily.

You are the Paramedic **Part 2**

As your partner maintains manual stabilization of the patient's head and simultaneously opens his airway with the jaw-thrust maneuver, you perform an initial assessment.

Initial Assessment	Recording Time: 0 Minutes
Appearance	Supine, not moving, massive facial trauma
Level of consciousness	P (Responsive to painful stimuli)
Airway	Blood is draining from the patient's mouth
Breathing	Respirations are gurgling, slow, and irregular
Circulation	Radial pulses are rapid and bounding; bleeding from the mouth; no other gross bleeding

3. How will you manage this patient's airway?

4. Would it be appropriate to intubate this patient? If so, when?

A so-called <u>blowout fracture</u> **Figure 21-7 ▾** results in transmission of forces away from the eyeball itself to the bone. Blood and fat then leak into the maxillary sinus.

The Nose

The nose is one of the two primary entry points for oxygen-rich air to enter the body. The <u>nasal septum</u>—the separation between the nostrils—is located in the midline. Often, it bulges slightly to one side or the other. The external portion of the nose is formed mostly of cartilage.

Several bones associated with the nose contain cavities known as the <u>paranasal sinuses</u> **Figure 21-8 ▸** . These hollowed sections of bone, which are lined with mucous membranes, decrease the weight of the skull and provide resonance for the voice. The contents of the sinuses drain into the nasal cavity.

The Mandible and Temporomandibular Joint

The <u>mandible</u> is the large movable bone forming the lower jaw and containing the lower teeth. Numerous muscles of chewing attach to the mandible and its rami. The posterior condyle of the mandible articulates with the temporal bone at the <u>temporomandibular joint (TMJ)</u>, allowing movement of the mandible (see Figure 21-3).

The Hyoid Bone

The <u>hyoid bone</u> "floats" in the superior aspect of the neck just below the mandible. Although it is not actually part of the skull, it supports the tongue and serves as a point of attachment for many important neck and tongue muscles.

▎The Eyes, Ears, Teeth, and Mouth

The Eye

The <u>globe</u>, or eyeball, is a spherical structure measuring about 3 cm in diameter that is housed within the eye socket, or orbit. The eyes are held in place by loose connective tissue and several muscles. These muscles also control eye movements. The <u>oculomotor nerve</u> (third cranial nerve) innervates the muscles that move the eyeballs and upper eyelids. It also carries parasympathetic nerve fibres that cause constriction of the pupil and accommodation of the lens. The <u>optic nerve</u> (second cranial nerve) provides the sense of vision **Figure 21-9 ▸** .

The structures of the eye **Figure 21-10 ▸** include the following:

- The <u>sclera</u> ("white of the eye") is a tough, fibrous coat that helps maintain the shape of the eye and protects its contents. In some illnesses, such as hepatitis, the sclera become yellow (icteric) from staining by bile pigments.
- The <u>cornea</u> is the transparent anterior portion of the eye that overlies the iris and pupil.
- The <u>conjunctiva</u> is a delicate mucous membrane that covers the sclera and internal surfaces of the eyelids. Cyanosis can be detected in the conjunctiva when it is not easily assessed on the skin of dark-skinned patients.

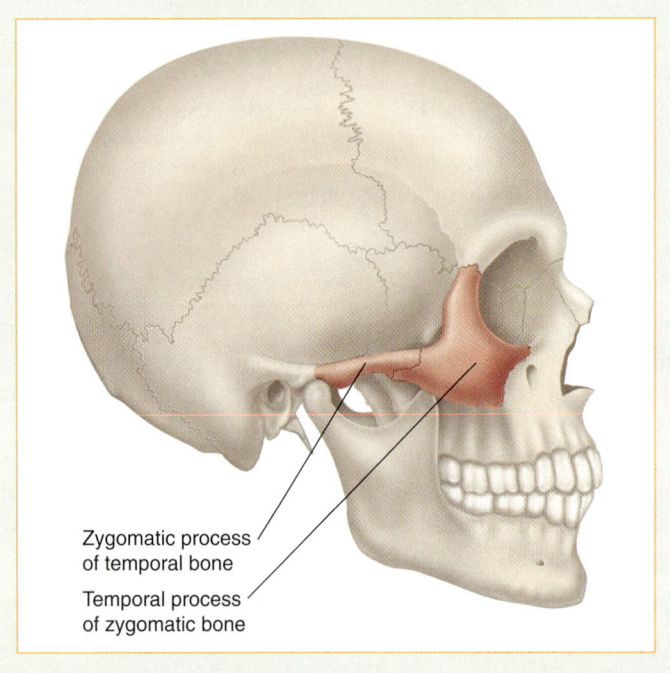

Zygomatic process
of temporal bone

Temporal process
of zygomatic bone

Figure 21-6 The zygomatic arch.

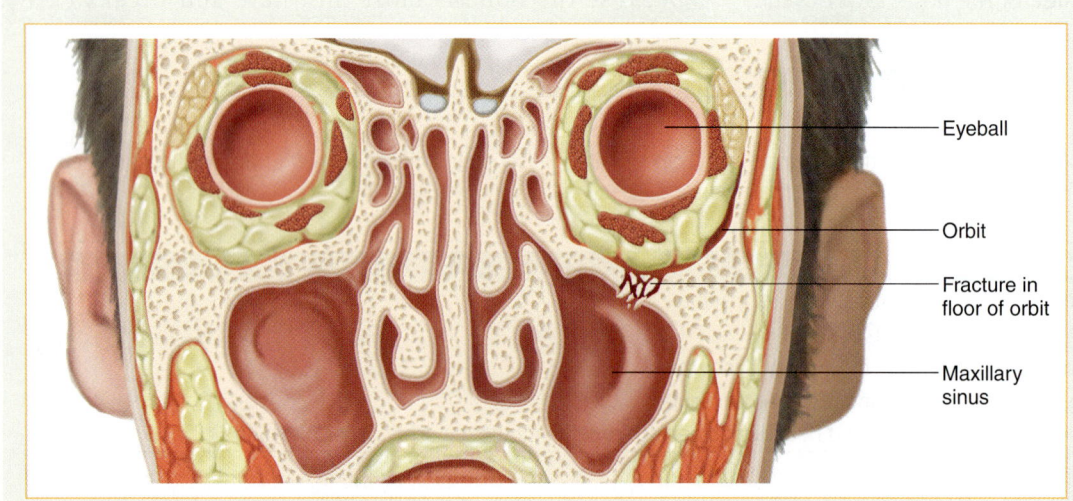

Eyeball

Orbit

Fracture in
floor of orbit

Maxillary
sinus

Figure 21-7 A blowout fracture of the left orbit.

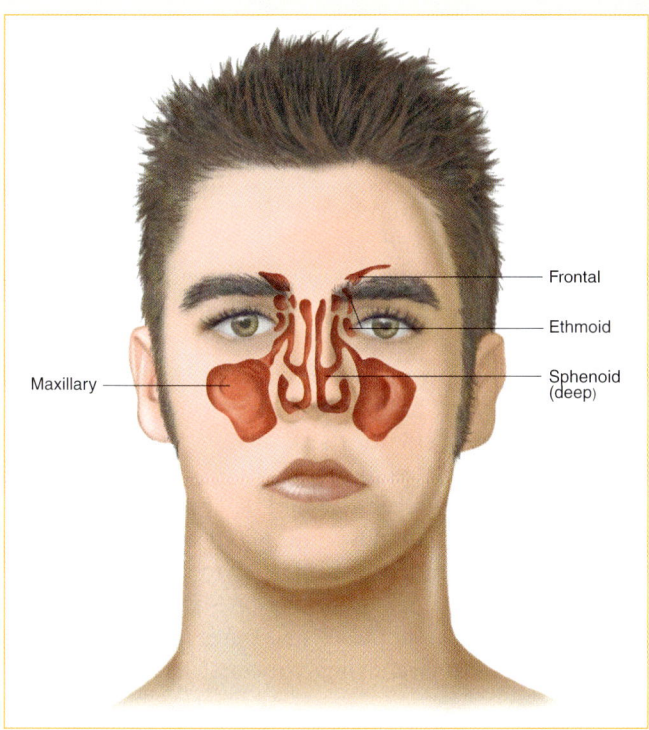

Figure 21-8 The paranasal sinuses.

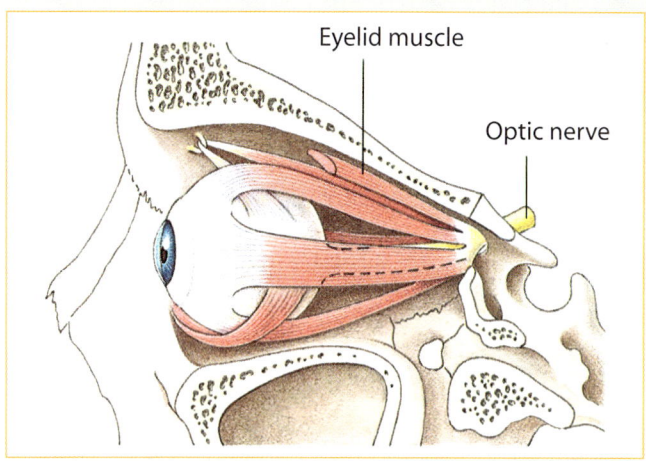

Figure 21-9 The optic nerve.

- The iris is the pigmented part of the eye that surrounds the pupil. It consists of muscles and blood vessels that contract and expand to regulate the size of the pupil.
- The pupil is the circular adjustable opening within the iris through which light passes to the lens. A normal pupil dilates in dim light to permit more light to enter the eye and constricts in bright light to decrease the light entering the eye.
- Behind the pupil and iris is the lens, a transparent structure that can alter its thickness to focus light on the retina at the back of the eye.
- The retina, which lies in the posterior aspect of the interior globe, is a delicate, 10-layered structure of nervous tissue that extends from the optic nerve. It receives light impulses and converts them to nerve signals that are conducted to the brain by the optic nerve and interpreted as vision.

The anterior chamber is the portion of the globe between lens and the cornea. It is filled with aqueous humour, a clear watery fluid. If aqueous humour is lost through a penetrating injury to the eye, it will gradually be replenished.

The posterior chamber is the portion of the globe between the lens and the retina which is filled with vitreous humour, a jellylike substance that maintains the shape of the globe. If vitreous humour is lost, it cannot be replenished, and blindness may result.

Light rays enter the eyes through the pupil and are focused by the lens. The image formed by the lens is cast on the retina, where sensitive nerve fibres form the optic nerve. The optic nerve transmits the image to the brain, where it is converted into conscious images in the visual cortex.

There are two types of vision: central and peripheral. Central vision, facilitates visualization of objects directly in front

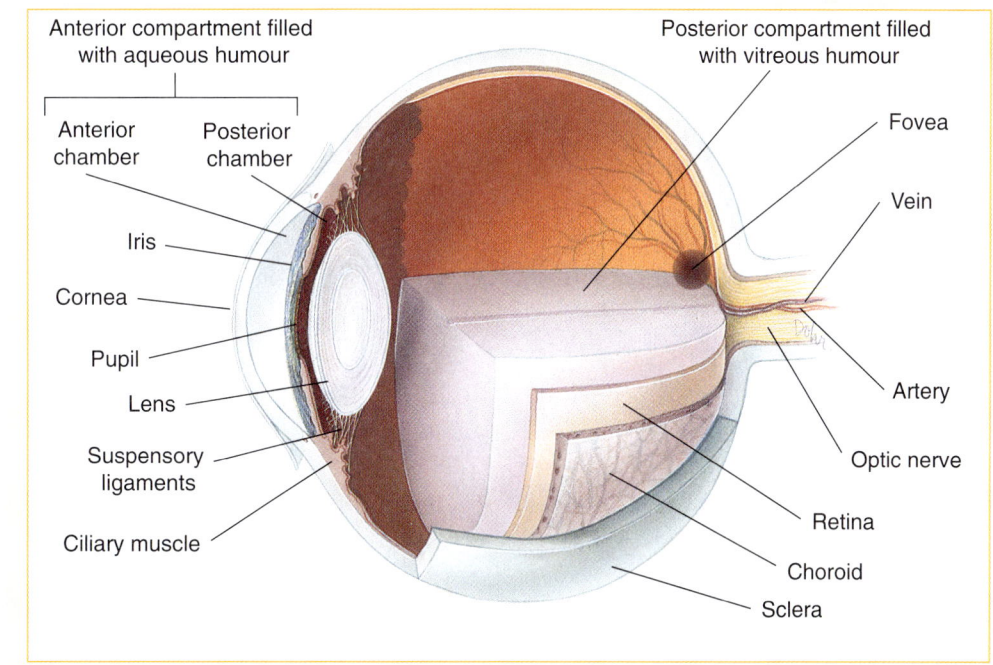

Figure 21-10 The structures of the eye.

of you, and is processed by the macula, the central portion of the retina. The remainder of the retina processes peripheral vision, which gives us visualization of lateral objects while looking forward.

The lacrimal apparatus secretes and drains tears from the eye. Tears produced in the lacrimal gland drain into lacrimal ducts, then into lacrimal sacs that pass into the nasal cavity via the nasolacrimal duct. Tears moisten the conjunctivae **Figure 21-11 ▼** .

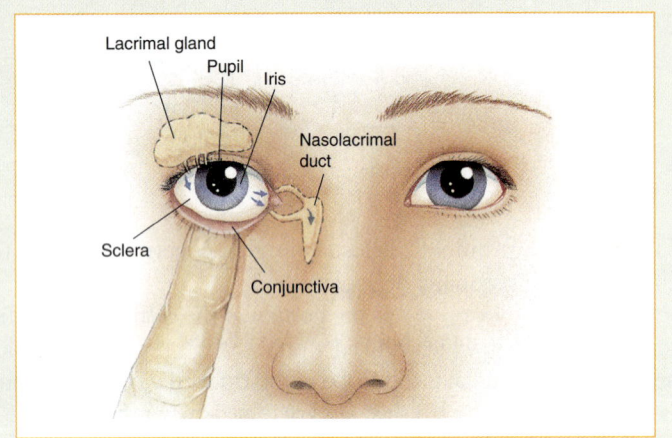

Figure 21-11 The lacrimal system consists of tear glands and ducts. Tears act as lubricants and keep the anterior part of the eye from drying.

The Ear

The ear is divided into three anatomical parts: external, middle, and inner **Figure 21-12 ▼** . The external ear consists of the pinna, external auditory canal, and the exterior portion of the tympanic membrane or what is commonly known as the eardrum. The middle ear consists of the inner portion of the tympanic membrane and the ossicles while the inner ear consists of the cochlea and semicircular canals.

Sound waves enter the ear through the auricle, or pinna, the large cartilaginous external portion of the ear. They then travel through the external auditory canal to the tympanic membrane. Vibration of sound waves against the tympanic membrane sets up vibration in the ossicles, the three small bones on the inner side of the tympanic membrane. These vibrations are transmitted to the cochlear duct at the oval window, the opening between the middle ear and the vestibule. Movement of the oval window causes fluid within the cochlea, a shell-shaped structure in the inner ear, to vibrate. Within the cochlea at the organ of Corti, vibration stimulates hair movements that form nerve impulses that travel to the brain via the auditory nerve. The brain then converts these impulses into sound.

The Teeth

The normal adult mouth contains 32 permanent teeth. The primary or deciduous teeth are lost during childhood. Adult teeth are distributed about the maxillary and mandibular arches. The teeth on each side of the arch are mirror images of each other and form four quadrants: right upper, left upper, right lower, and left lower. Each quadrant contains one central incisor, one lateral incisor, one canine, two premolars, and three molars **Figure 21-13A ▶** . The third molars, called wisdom teeth, do not appear until late adolescence.

The top portion of the tooth, external to the gum, is the crown, containing one or more cusps. Below the crown lie the neck and the root. The pulp cavity fills the centre of the tooth and contains blood vessels, nerves, and specialized connective tissue, called pulp. Dentin and enamel surround the pulp cavity and protect the tooth from damage.

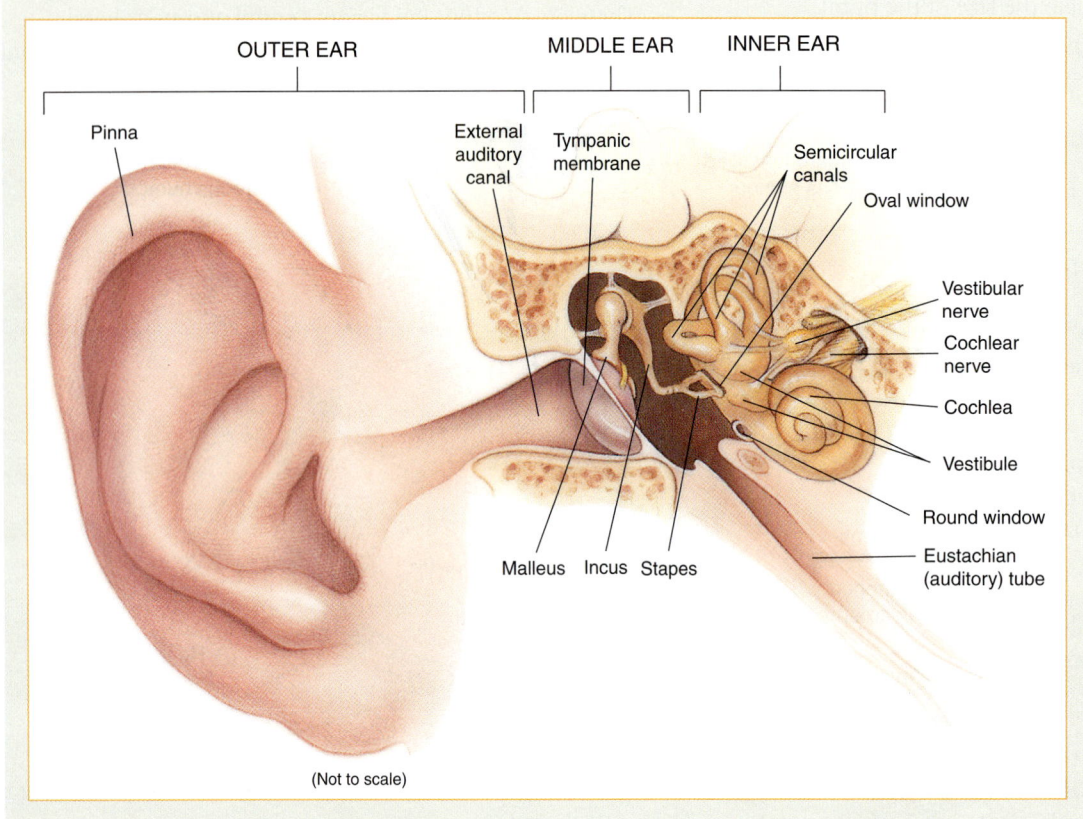

Figure 21-12 The structures of the ear.

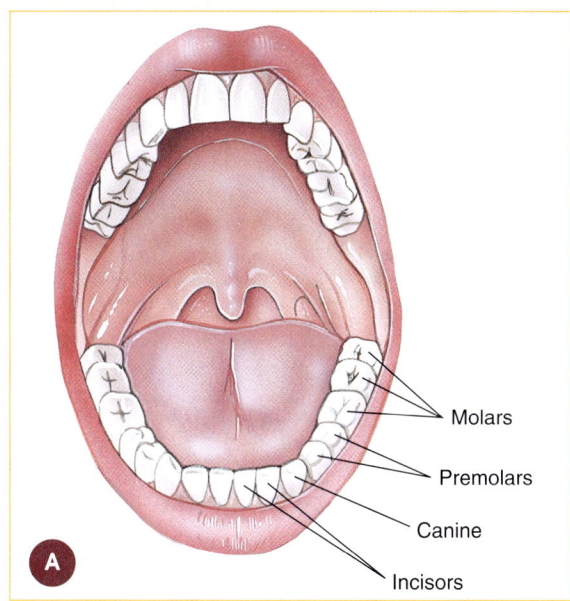

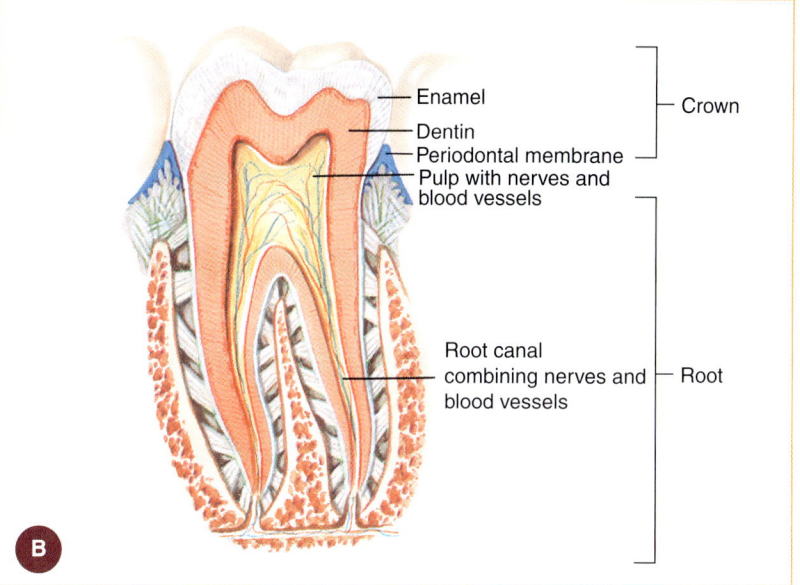

Figure 21-13 The teeth of the adult mouth. **A.** The incisors are used for biting. Canines are used for tearing food. The premolars and molars are used for grinding and crushing. **B.** Each tooth contains nerves and blood vessels.

Dentin, forms the principal mass of the tooth, while the enamel, which is much denser and stronger than bone, covers the tooth. The bony sockets for the teeth that reside in the mandible and maxilla are called alveoli. The ridges between the teeth, the alveolar ridges, are covered by the gingiva, or gums, which are thickened connective tissue and epithelium. Teeth are attached to the alveolar bone by a periodontal membrane Figure 21-13B ▲ .

The Mouth

Digestion begins in the mouth with mastication, or the chewing of food by the teeth. During mastication, food is mixed with secretions from the salivary glands.

The tongue is the primary organ of taste; it is also important in the formation of speech and in chewing and swallowing of food. The tongue is attached at the mandible and hyoid bone, is covered by a mucous membrane, and extends from the back of the mouth upward and forward to the lips Figure 21-14 ▶ .

The hypoglossal, glossopharyngeal, trigeminal, and facial nerves supply the mouth and its structures. The hypoglossal nerve (12th cranial nerve) provides motor function to the muscles of the tongue. The glossopharyngeal nerve (ninth cranial nerve) provides taste sensation to the posterior portions of the tongue and carries parasympathetic fibres to the salivary glands on each side of the face. The mandibular branch of the trigeminal nerve (fifth cranial nerve) provides motor innervation to the muscles of mastication. The facial nerve (seventh cranial nerve), in addition to supplying motor activity to all muscles of facial expression, provides the sense of taste to the anterior two thirds of the tongue and cutaneous sensations to the tongue and palate.

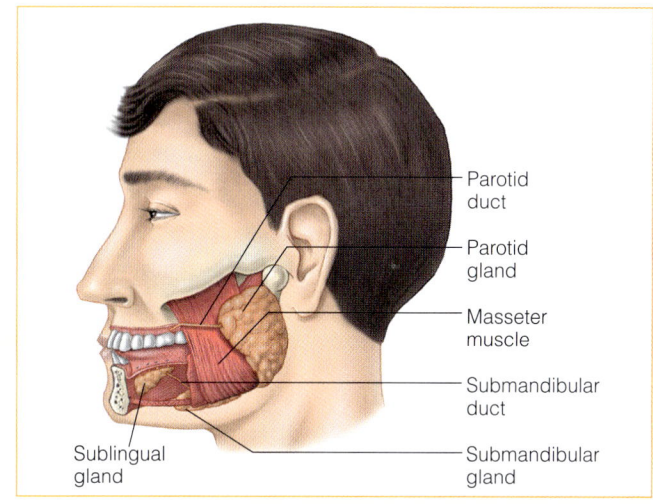

Figure 21-14 The glands and muscles of the mouth.

The Anterior Part of the Neck

The principal structures of the anterior part of the neck include the thyroid and cricoid cartilage, trachea, and numerous muscles and nerves Figure 21-15 ▶ . The major blood vessels in this area are the internal and external carotid arteries Figure 21-16 ▶ and the internal and external jugular veins Figure 21-17 ▶ . The vertebral arteries run laterally to the cervical vertebrae in the posterior part of the neck.

The major arteries of the neck—the carotid and vertebral arteries—supply oxygenated blood directly to the brain. Therefore, in addition to causing massive bleeding and hemorrhagic shock, injury to any of these major vessels can produce

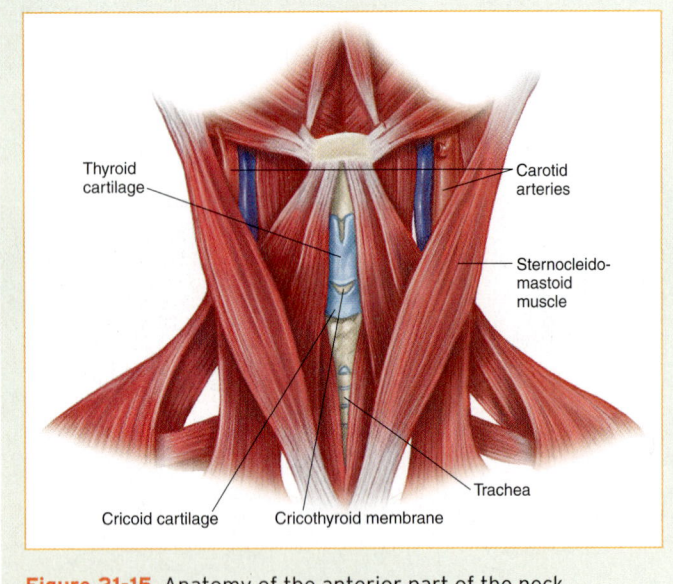

Figure 21-15 Anatomy of the anterior part of the neck.

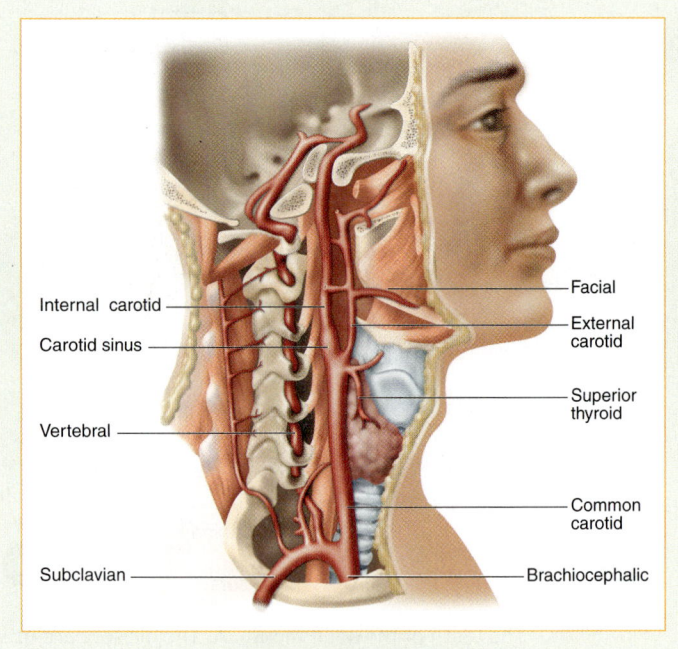

Figure 21-16 The arteries of the neck.

cerebral hypoxia, infarct, air embolism and/or permanent neurologic impairment.

Other key structures of the anterior part of the neck that may sustain injury from blunt or penetrating mechanisms include the vagus nerves, thoracic duct, esophagus, thyroid and parathyroid glands, lower cranial nerves, brachial plexus (which is responsible for function of the lower arm and hand), soft tissue and fascia, and various muscles.

The Brain

The brain, which occupies 80% of the cranial vault, contains billions of neurons (nerve cells) that serve a variety of vital functions   Figure 21-18 ▸ . The major regions of the brain are the cerebrum, diencephalon (thalamus and hypothalamus), brain stem (medulla, pons, midbrain [mesencephalon]), and the cerebellum. The remaining intracranial contents include cerebral blood (12%) and cerebrospinal fluid (8%).

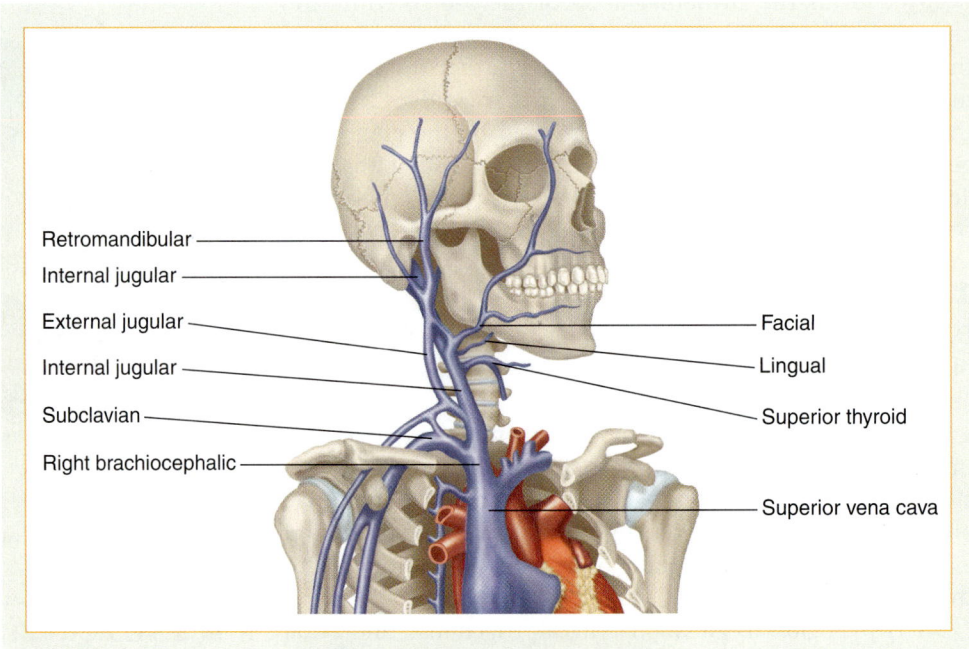

Figure 21-17 The veins of the neck.

The brain accounts for only 2% of the total body weight, yet it is the most metabolically active and perfusion-sensitive organ in the body. The brain metabolizes 25% of the body's glucose, burning approximately 60 mg/min, and consumes 20% of the total body oxygen. Because the brain has no storage mechanism for oxygen or glucose, it is totally dependent on a constant source of both fuels via cerebral blood flow provided by the carotid and vertebral arteries. As such, the brain will continually manipulate the physiology as needed to guarantee that a ready supply of oxygen and glucose are available.

The Cerebrum

The largest portion of the brain is the cerebrum, which is responsible for higher functions, such as reasoning. The cerebrum is divided into right and left hemispheres by a longitudinal fissure. The hemispheres of the cerebrum are not entirely equivalent functionally. In a right-handed person, for example,

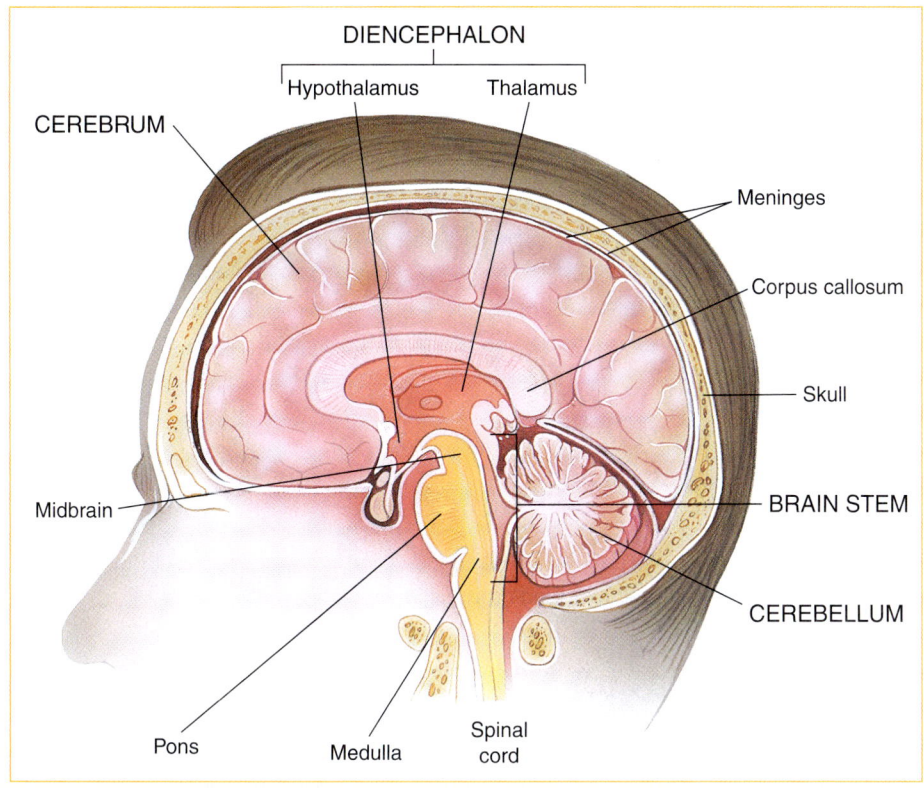

Figure 21-18 The major regions of the brain.

the speech centre is usually located in the left cerebral hemisphere, which is then said to be the dominant hemisphere.

The largest portion of the cerebrum is the cerebral cortex, which regulates voluntary skeletal movement and the level of awareness. Injury to the cerebral cortex may result in paresthesia, weakness, and paralysis of the extremities.

Each cerebral hemisphere is divided functionally into specialized areas called lobes ▶ Figure 21-19 ▶ . The frontal lobe is important for voluntary motor action and personality traits. Injury to the frontal lobe may result in seizures or placid reactions (flat affect). The parietal lobe controls the somatic or voluntary sensory and motor functions for the opposite (contralateral) side of the body, as well as memory and emotions; it is separated from the frontal lobe by the central sulcus. Posteriorly, the occipital lobe, from which the optic nerve originates, is responsible for processing visual information. After a blow to the back of the head, a person may "see stars" which results when the occipital lobe impacts against the back of the skull.

The speech centre is located in the temporal lobe. In approximately 85% of the population, the speech centre is located on the left side of the temporal lobe. The temporal lobe also controls long-term memory, hearing, taste, and smell. It is separated from the rest of the cerebrum by a lateral fissure.

The Diencephalon

The diencephalon, which is located between the brain stem and the cerebrum, includes the thalamus, subthalamus, hypothalamus, and epithalamus ▶ Figure 21-20 ▶ . The thalamus processes most sensory input and influences mood and general body movements, especially those associated with fear and rage. The subthalamus controls motor functions. The functions of the epithalamus are unclear. The most inferior portion of the diencephalon, the hypothalamus, is vital in the control of many body functions, including heart rate, digestion, sexual development, temperature regulation, emotion, hunger, thirst, vomiting, and regulation of the sleep cycle.

The Cerebellum

The cerebellum is located beneath the cerebral hemispheres in the inferoposterior part of the brain. It is sometimes called the "athlete's brain" because it is responsible for the maintenance

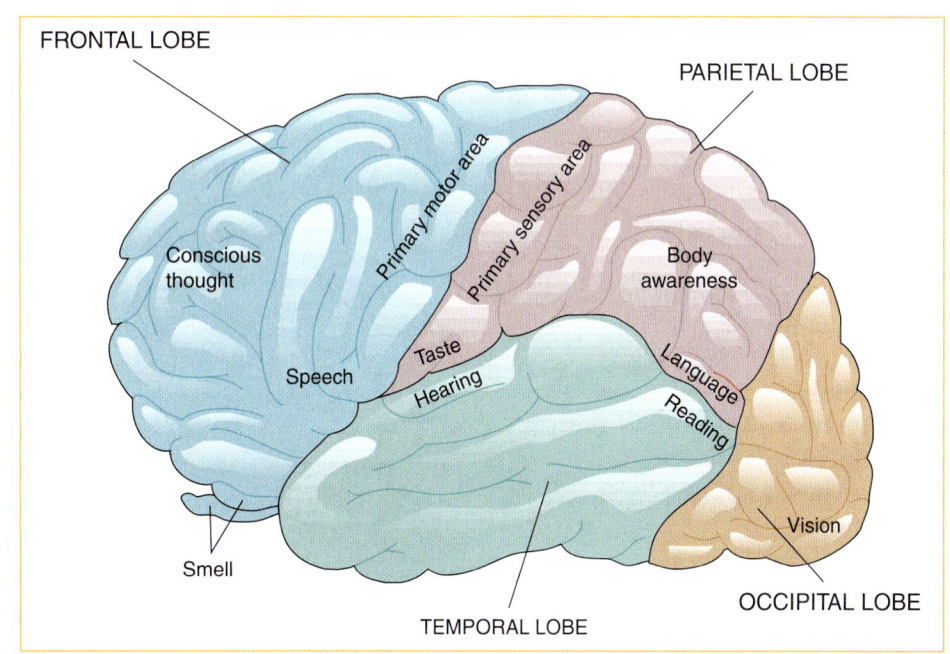

Figure 21-19 Lobes of the cerebrum.

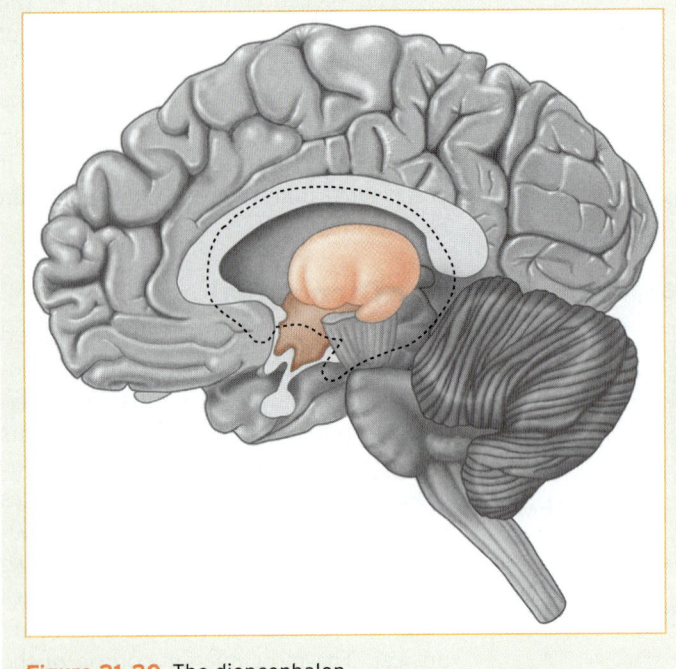

Figure 21-20 The diencephalon.

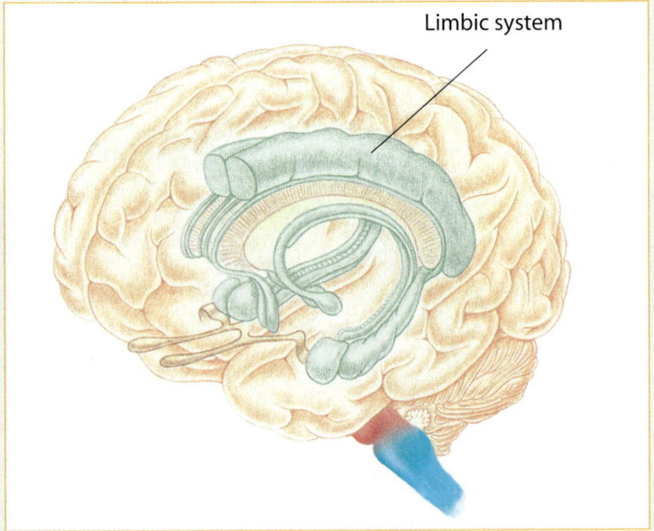

Limbic system

Figure 21-21 The limbic system is the seat of emotions, instincts, and other functions.

of posture and equilibrium and the coordination of skilled movements.

The Brain Stem

The brain stem consists of the midbrain, pons, and the medulla. It is located at the base of the brain and connects the spinal cord to the remainder of the brain. The brain stem houses many structures that are critical to the maintenance of vital functions. High in the brain stem, for example, is the reticular activating system (RAS), which is responsible for maintenance of consciousness, specifically one's level of arousal. The centres that control basic but critical functions—heart rate, blood pressure, and respiration—are located in the lower part of the brain stem. Damage to this area can easily result in cardiovascular derangement, respiratory arrest, or death.

The midbrain lies immediately below the diencephalon and is the smallest region of the brain stem. Deep within the cerebrum, diencephalon, and midbrain are the basal ganglia, which have an important role in coordination of motor movements and posture. Portions of the cerebrum and diencephalon constitute the limbic system, which influences emotions, motivation, mood, and sensations of pain and pleasure **Figure 21-21 ▶**.

The pons, which lies below the midbrain and above the medulla, contains numerous important nerve fibres, including those for sleep and respiration.

The inferior portion of the midbrain, the medulla, is continuous inferiorly with the spinal cord (see Figure 21-18). It serves as a conduction pathway for ascending and descending nerve tracts. It also coordinates heart rate, blood vessel diameter, breathing, swallowing, vomiting, coughing, and sneezing. The vagus nerve (tenth cranial nerve), a bundle of nerves that primarily innervates the parasympathetic nervous system, originates from the medulla.

The Meninges

The meninges are protective layers that surround and enfold the entire central nervous system—specifically the brain and spinal cord **Figure 21-22 ▾**. The outermost layer is a strong, fibrous

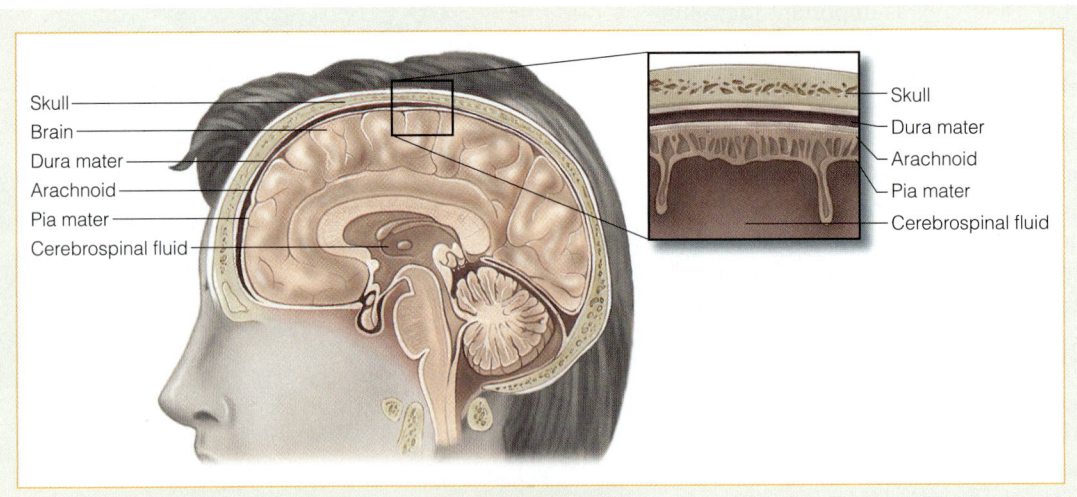

Skull
Brain
Dura mater
Arachnoid
Pia mater
Cerebrospinal fluid

Skull
Dura mater
Arachnoid
Pia mater
Cerebrospinal fluid

Figure 21-22 The meninges.

wrapping called the dura mater (meaning "tough mother"). The dura mater covers the entire brain, folding in to form the tentorium, a structure that separates the cerebral hemispheres from the cerebellum and brain stem. The dura mater is firmly attached to the internal wall of the skull. Just beneath the suture lines of the skull the dura mater splits into two surfaces and forms venous sinuses. When those venous sinuses are disrupted during a head injury, blood can collect beneath the dura mater to form a subdural hematoma.

The second meningeal layer is a delicate, transparent membrane called the arachnoid. It is so named because the blood vessels it contains resemble a spider web. The third meningeal layer, the pia mater ("soft mother"), is a thin, translucent, highly vascular membrane that firmly adheres directly to the surface of the brain.

The meningeal arteries are located between the dura mater and the skull. When one of these arteries (usually the middle meningeal artery) is disrupted, bleeding occurs above the dura mater, resulting in an epidural hematoma.

Cerebrospinal fluid (CSF), which is manufactured in the ventricles of the brain, flows in the subarachnoid space, located between the pia mater and the arachnoid.

CSF is manufactured by cells within the choroid plexus in the ventricles, hollow storage areas in the brain. These areas normally are interconnected, and CSF flows freely between them. CSF is similar in composition to plasma. The meninges and CSF form a fluid-filled sac that cushions and protects the brain and spinal cord.

Face Injuries

Soft-Tissue Injuries

Although open soft-tissue injuries to the face—lacerations, abrasions, and avulsions—by themselves are rarely life threatening, their presence, especially following a significant mechanism of injury, suggests the potential for more severe injuries (eg, closed head injury, cervical spine injury). Furthermore, massive soft-tissue injuries to the face, especially if associated with oropharyngeal trauma and bleeding, can compromise the patient's airway and lead to ventilatory inadequacy.

Maintain a high index of suspicion when a patient presents with closed soft-tissue injuries to the face, such as contusions and hematomas **Figure 21-23 ▾** . These indicators of blunt force trauma suggest the potential for more severe underlying injuries.

Impaled objects in the soft tissues or bones of the face may occur in association with facial trauma. Although these objects can damage facial nerves, the risk of airway compromise is of far greater consequence. This is especially true when an

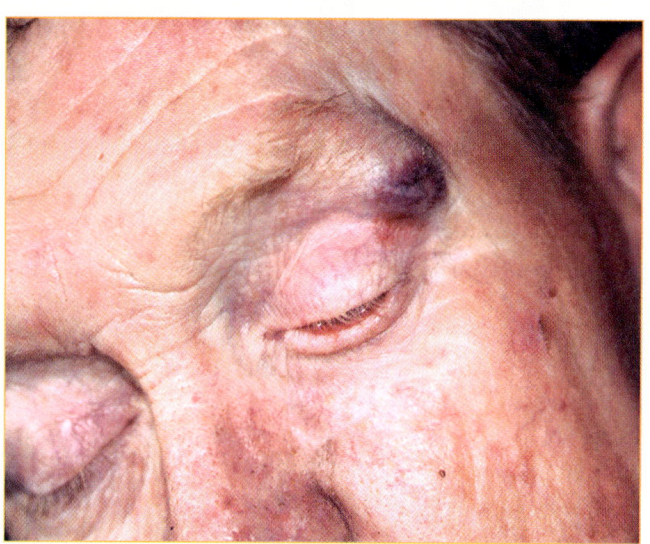

Figure 21-23 Closed soft-tissue injuries to the face may indicate more severe underlying injuries.

You are the Paramedic Part 3

Your partner is appropriately managing the patient's airway. You perform a rapid trauma assessment, which reveals a hematoma to the patient's forehead, massive soft-tissue trauma to the face, unstable facial bones, and bilaterally angulated femurs.

Vital Signs	Recording Time: 5 Minutes
Level of consciousness	Glasgow Coma Scale score of 6
Respirations	6 breaths/min and irregular (baseline); your partner is providing bag-valve-mask ventilation at a rate of 10 breaths/min and 100% oxygen
Pulse	110 beats/min; regular and bounding
Skin	Warm and dry
Blood pressure	140/90 mm Hg
Sao₂	96% (with assisted ventilation and 100% oxygen)

5. How can facial trauma complicate airway management?

6. Is this patient in hypovolemic shock? Why or why not?

impaled object penetrates the cheek, because massive oropharyngeal bleeding can result in airway obstruction, aspiration, and ventilatory inadequacy. In addition, blood is a gastric irritant. For many people, just swallowing a couple of tablespoons of blood can make them vomit, further increasing the likelihood of aspiration.

Maxillofacial Fractures

Maxillofacial fractures commonly occur when the facial bones absorb the energy of a strong impact. The forces involved may be massive. For example, a force up to 150g (g = acceleration of the body due to gravity) is required to fracture the maxilla; a force of that magnitude will likely produce closed head injuries and cervical spine injuries as well. Therefore, when assessing a patient with a suspected maxillofacial fracture, you should protect the cervical spine and monitor the patient's neurologic signs, specifically their level of consciousness.

The first clue to the presence of a maxillofacial fracture is usually ecchymosis, so bruising on the face should alert you to this possibility. A deep facial laceration should likewise increase your index of suspicion that the underlying bone may have been fractured, and pain over a bone tends to support the suspicion of fracture. General signs and symptoms of maxillofacial fractures include ecchymosis, swelling, pain to palpation, crepitus, dental malocclusion, facial deformities or asymmetry, instability of the facial bones, impaired ocular movement, and visual disturbances.

Nasal Fractures

Because the nasal bones are not as structurally sound as the other bones of the face, nasal fractures are the most common facial fracture. These fractures are characterized by swelling, tenderness, and crepitus when the nasal bone is palpated. Deformity of the nose, if present, usually appears as lateral displacement of the nasal bone from its normal midline position.

Nasal fractures, like any maxillofacial fracture, are often complicated by the presence of an anterior or a posterior nosebleed (epistaxis), which can compromise the patient's airway.

Mandibular Fractures and Dislocations

Second only to nasal fractures in frequency, fractures of the mandible typically result from massive blunt force trauma to the lower third of the face; they are particularly common following an assault injury. Because significant force is required to fracture the mandible, this structure may be fractured in more than one place and, therefore, unstable to palpation. The fracture site itself is most commonly located at the angle of the jaw.

Mandibular fractures should be suspected in patients with a history of blunt force trauma to the lower third of the face who present with dental malocclusion (misalignment of the teeth), numbness of the chin, and inability to open the mouth. There will likely be swelling and ecchymosis over the fracture site, and teeth may be partially or completely avulsed.

Although temporomandibular joint (TMJ) dislocations may occur as the result of blunt force trauma to the lower third of the face, this outcome is rare. Mandibular dislocations are most often the result of yawning extravagantly or otherwise opening the mouth very widely. The patient commonly feels a "pop" and then cannot close his or her mouth; it is locked in a wide-open position. The jaw muscles eventually go into spasm, causing severe pain.

Maxillary Fractures

Maxillary fractures to the midface area are most commonly associated with mechanisms that produce massive blunt facial trauma, such as motor vehicle collisions, falls, and assaults. They produce massive facial swelling, instability of the midfacial bones, malocclusion, and an elongated appearance of the patient's face. Midfacial structures include the maxilla, zygoma, orbital floor, and nose.

Le Fort fractures **Figure 21-24 ▾** are classified into three categories:

- **Le Fort I fracture.** A horizontal fracture of the maxilla that involves the hard palate and inferior maxilla
- **Le Fort II fracture.** A pyramidal fracture involving the nasal bone and inferior maxilla
- **Le Fort III fracture** (craniofacial disjunction). A fracture of all midfacial bones, separating the entire midface from the cranium.

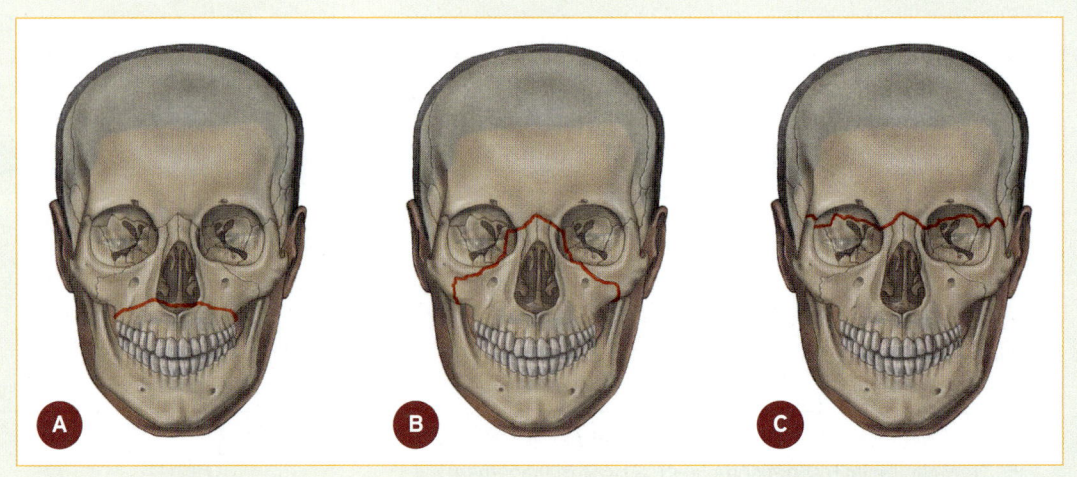

Figure 21-24 Le Fort fractures. **A.** Le Fort I. **B.** Le Fort II. **C.** Le Fort III.

Le Fort fractures can occur as isolated fractures (Le Fort I) or in combination (Le Fort I and II), depending on the location of impact and the amount of trauma.

Orbital Fractures

The patient with an orbital fracture (such as a blowout fracture [see Figure 21-7]) may complain of double vision (diplopia) and lose sensation above the eyebrow or over the cheek secondary to associated nerve damage. Fractures of the inferior orbit are the most common type and can cause loss of upward gaze (the patient's injured eye will not be able to follow your finger *above* the midline).

> *Notes from Nancy*
> Check eye movements in all planes in the patient with possible facial fractures.

Zygomatic Fractures

Fractures of the zygomatic bone (cheek bone) commonly result from blunt trauma secondary to motor vehicle collisions and assaults. When the zygomatic bone is fractured, that side of the patient's face appears flattened, and there may be paresthesia or loss of sensation over the cheek, nose, and upper lip; loss of upward gaze may also be present. Other injuries commonly associated with zygomatic fractures include orbital fractures, ocular injury, and epistaxis.

> *Notes from Nancy*
> Any patient with significant head injury also has cervical spine injury until proven otherwise.

▌Assessment and Management of Face Injuries

Table 21-1 ▶ summarizes the characteristics of various maxillofacial fractures. It is not important to distinguish among the various maxillofacial fractures in the prehospital setting; this determination requires radiographic evaluation in the emergency department. Rapid patient assessment, management of life-threatening conditions, airway management, full spinal precautions, and prompt transport are far more important considerations.

Management of the patient with facial trauma begins by protecting the cervical spine. Because many severe facial injuries are complicated by a spinal injury, you must assume that one exists.

If the patient is semiconscious or unconscious, open the airway with the jaw-thrust maneuver while simultaneously maintaining manual stabilization of the head in the neutral position unless the patient complains of severe pain or discomfort upon movement. Should that occur, the head/neck should be immobilized in the position found. Inspect the mouth for fragments of teeth, dentures, or any other foreign bodies that

Table 21-1	Summary of Maxillofacial Fractures
Injury	**Signs and Symptoms**
Multiple facial bone fractures	• Massive facial swelling • Dental malocclusion • Palpable deformities • Anterior or posterior epistaxis
Zygomatic and orbital fractures	• Loss of sensation below the orbit • Flattening of the patient's cheek • Loss of upward gaze
Nasal fractures	• Crepitus and instability • Swelling, tenderness, lateral displacement • Anterior or posterior epistaxis
Maxillary (Le Fort) fractures	• Mobility of the facial skeleton • Dental malocclusion • Facial swelling
Mandibular fractures	• Dental malocclusion • Mandibular instability

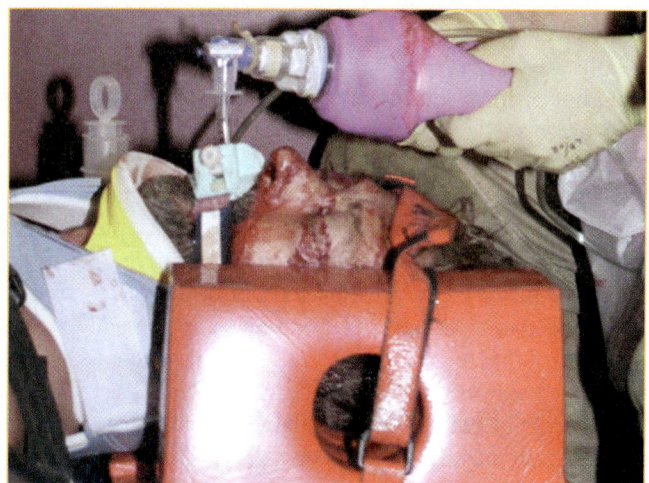

Figure 21-25 Airway management can be especially challenging in patients with massive facial injuries.

could obstruct the airway, and remove them immediately. Suction the oropharynx as needed to keep the airway clear.

Insert an airway adjunct as needed to maintain airway patency. However, *do not insert a nasopharyngeal airway or attempt nasotracheal intubation in any patient with suspected nasal fractures or in patients with CSF or blood leakage from the nose.* After establishing and maintaining a patent airway, assess the patient's breathing and intervene appropriately. Apply 100% oxygen via nonrebreathing mask if the patient is breathing adequately. Patients who are breathing inadequately (ie, fast or slow rate, reduced tidal volume [shallow breathing], irregular pattern of breathing) should receive bag-valve-mask ventilation with 100% oxygen. Maintain the patient's oxygen saturation at greater than 95%.

Airway management can be especially challenging in patients with massive facial injuries **Figure 21-25 ▲**.

At the Scene

Blood or CSF drainage from the nose (cerebrospinal rhinorrhea) suggests a skull fracture. Do not make any attempt to control this bleeding; doing so may increase intracranial pressure (ICP) if the patient has a concomitant brain injury. Furthermore, the insertion of nasal airway adjuncts and nasotracheal intubation should be avoided in patients with suspected nasal fractures, especially if CSF rhinorrhea is present. A nasally inserted airway device could enter the cranial vault through an occult fracture (such as a base of skull fracture) and penetrate the brain further worsening the situation.

Oropharyngeal bleeding poses an immediate threat to the airway, and unstable facial bones can hinder your ability to maintain an effective mask-to-face seal for bag-valve-mask ventilation. Therefore, perform tracheal intubation of patients with facial trauma, especially those who are unconscious, to protect their airway from aspiration and to ensure adequate oxygenation and ventilation. Cricothyrotomy (surgical or needle) may be required for patients with extensive maxillofacial injuries when endotracheal intubation is extremely difficult or impossible to perform (ie, in cases of unstable facial bones, massive swelling, severe oral bleeding).

Treat facial lacerations and avulsions as you would any other soft-tissue injury. Control all bleeding with direct pressure, and apply sterile dressings. If you suspect an underlying facial fracture, apply just enough pressure to control the bleeding. Leave impaled objects in the face in place and appropriately stabilize them, unless they pose a threat to the airway (such as an object impaled through the cheek). When removing an object from the cheek, carefully remove it from the same side that it entered. Next, pack the inside of the cheek with sterile gauze and apply counterpressure with a dressing and bandage firmly secured over the outside of the wound. If profuse bleeding continues, position the patient on his or her side—while maintaining stabilization of the cervical spine—to facilitate drainage of secretions from the mouth and suction the airway as needed.

For severe oropharyngeal bleeding in patients with inadequate ventilation, suction the airway for no more than 15 seconds and provide ventilatory assistance for 2 minutes; continue this alternating pattern of suctioning and ventilating until the airway is cleared of blood or secured with an endotracheal (ET) tube. Monitor the pulse oximeter during this process to keep the patient from becoming hypoxic.

Epistaxis following facial trauma can be severe and is most effectively controlled by applying direct pressure to the nares. If the patient is conscious and spinal injury is not suspected, instruct the patient to sit up and lean forward as you pinch the nares together. Unconscious patients should be positioned on their side, unless contraindicated by a spinal injury. Proper positioning of the patient with epistaxis is important to prevent blood from draining down the throat and compromising the airway either by occlusion or by vomiting and then aspirating

gastric contents. If the conscious patient with severe epistaxis is immobilized on a backboard, you should consider pharmacologically assisted intubation (eg, rapid-sequence intubation [RSI]) to gain definitive control of the airway.

Although facial lacerations and avulsions can contribute to hemorrhagic shock, they are rarely the sole cause of this condition in adults. Severe epistaxis, however, can result in significant blood loss. To counter this problem, you should carefully assess the patient for signs of hemorrhagic shock and administer intravenous (IV) crystalloid fluid boluses as needed to maintain adequate perfusion.

If the facial fracture is associated with swelling and ecchymosis, cold compresses may help minimize further swelling and alleviate pain. Do not apply a compress to the eyeball (globe) if you suspect that it has been injured following an orbital fracture; doing so may increase the intraocular pressure (IOP) and further damage the eye. Other than protecting the airway, little can be done to treat facial instabilities; however, firmly applying a self-adhering roller bandage (such as Kerlix or Kling) can stabilize the mandible. Make sure that you do not compromise the airway when stabilizing the mandible.

After addressing all life-threatening injuries and conditions, you should attempt to ascertain the events that preceded the injury and determine whether the patient has any significant medical problems. The incident that caused the injury may have been preceded by exacerbation of an underlying medical condition (such as acute hypoglycemia, cardiac dysrhythmia, seizure). For unconscious patients, medications that the patient is taking may provide information about his or her medical history. Determine the approximate time that the injury occurred, and ask about any drug allergies and the last oral intake during your SAMPLE history **Figure 21-26** ▶ .

Special Considerations

Relative to younger, healthy adults, elderly patients are at high risk for severe epistaxis following even minor facial injuries, especially in those with a history of hypertension or anticoagulant medication use (such as warfarin [Coumadin]). This bleeding often originates in the posterior nasopharynx and may not be grossly evident during your assessment.

▮ Eye Injuries

By conservative estimates, over 100,000 eye injuries occur annually in Canada. Because trauma to the eyes is so common and the potential consequences are so serious, you must know how to assess and manage ocular injuries.

Eye injuries are frequently caused by blunt trauma, penetrating trauma, or burns. Blunt mechanisms of injury may

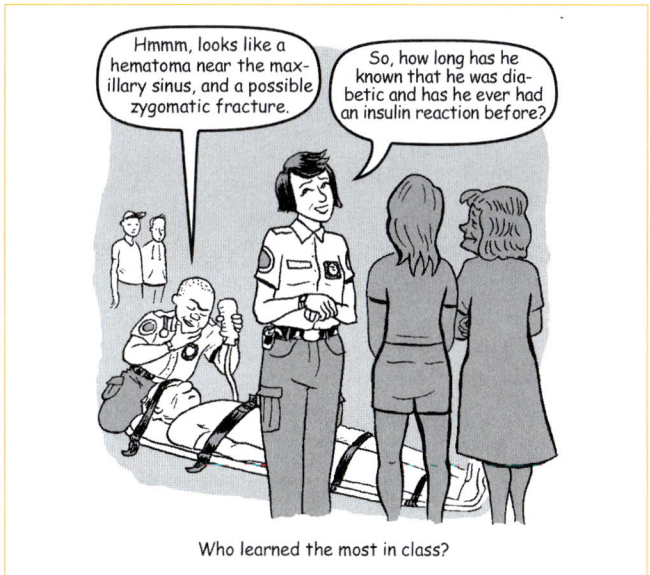

Figure 21-26

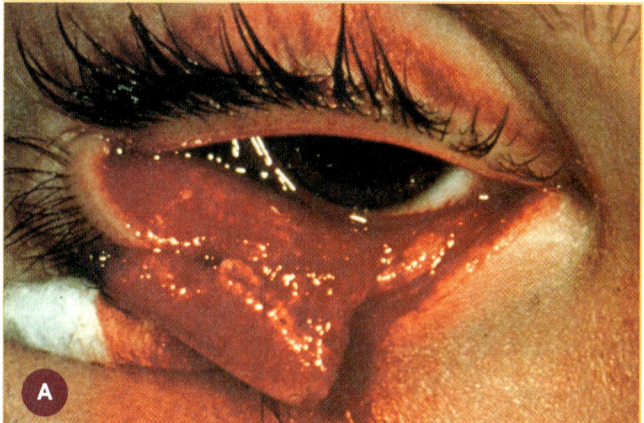

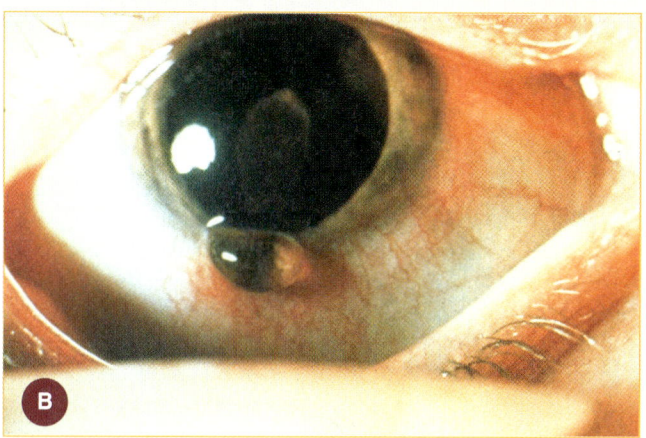

Figure 21-27 Eye lacerations are serious injuries that require prompt transport. **A.** Although bleeding can be heavy, never exert pressure on the eye. **B.** Pressure may squeeze the vitreous humour, iris, lens, or retina out of the eye.

include motor vehicle collisions, motorcycles collisions, falls, and assaults. Penetrating injuries are often secondary to foreign bodies on the surface of the eye (such as sand) or an object impaled in the globe. Burns to the eye can result from a variety of corrosive chemicals or during industrial accidents (such as welding burns).

Lacerations, Foreign Bodies, and Impaled Objects

Lacerations of the eyelids require meticulous repair to restore appearance and function. Bleeding may be heavy, but it usually can be controlled by gentle, manual pressure. *If there is a laceration to the globe itself, apply no pressure to the eye;* compression can interfere with the blood supply to the back of the eye and result in loss of vision from damage to the retina. Furthermore, pressure may squeeze the vitreous humour, iris, lens, or even the retina out of the eye and cause irreparable damage or blindness Figure 21-27 ▸ .

The protective orbit prevents large objects from penetrating the eye. However, moderately sized and smaller foreign objects can still enter the eye and, when lying on the surface of the eye, produce severe irritation Figure 21-28 ▸ . The conjunctiva becomes inflamed and red—a condition known as conjunctivitis—almost immediately, and the eye begins to produce tears in an attempt to flush out the object Figure 21-29 ▸ . Irritation of the cornea or conjunctiva causes intense pain. The patient may have difficulty keeping the eyelids open, because the irritation is further aggravated by bright light.

Foreign bodies ranging in size from a pencil to a sliver of metal may be impaled in the eye Figure 21-30 ▸ . Clearly, these objects must be removed by a physician. Prehospital care involves stabilizing the object and preparing the patient for

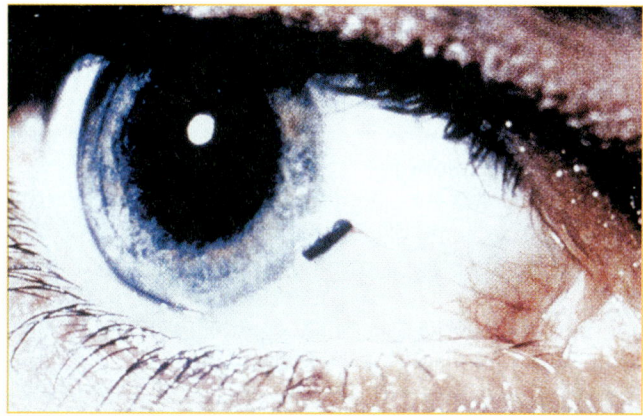

Figure 21-28 A foreign object on the surface of the eye.

transport. The greater the length of the foreign object sticking out of the eye, the more important stabilization becomes in avoiding further damage. Whenever possible, cover both eyes to limit unnecessary movement as the patient tries to use the uninjured eye to compensate for the loss or limited vision of the injured eye.

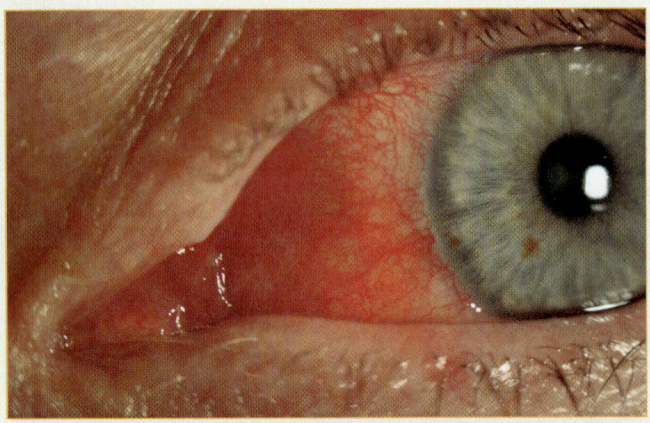

Figure 21-29 Conjunctivitis is often associated with the presence of a foreign object in the eye.

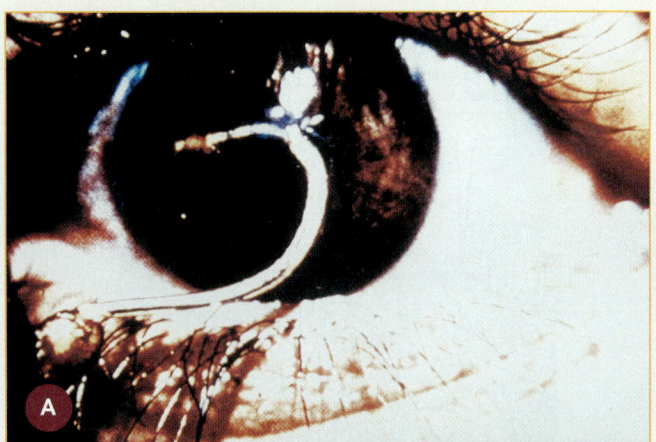
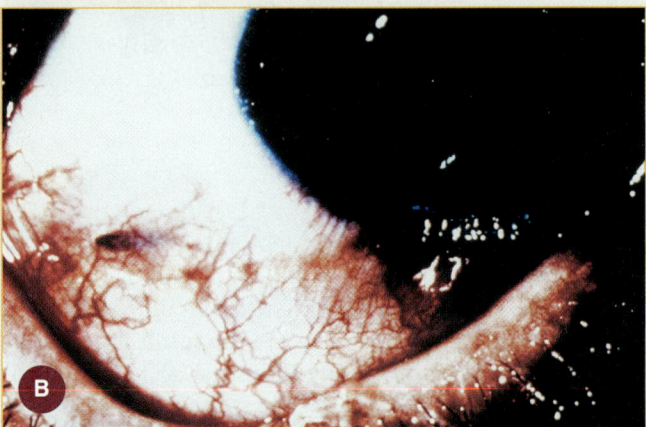
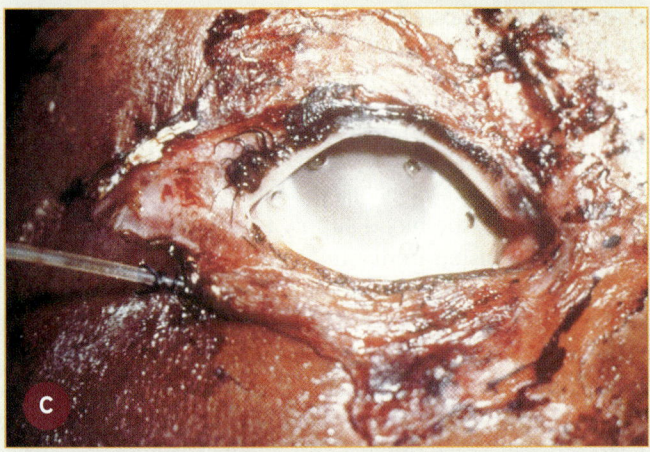

Figure 21-30 Any number of objects can be impaled in the eye. **A.** Fishhook. **B.** Sharp, metal sliver. **C.** Knife blade.

At the Scene

Large and small foreign bodies, particularly small metal fragments, can become completely embedded in the globe. The patient may not even be aware of the cause of the problem. Patients often complain of a foreign body sensation to the eye. Suspect such an injury when the history includes metal work (such as hammering, exposure to splinters, grinding, vigorous filing) and when you observe signs of ocular injury (such as redness, irritation, inflammation).

Blunt Eye Injuries

Blunt trauma can cause serious eye injuries, ranging from swelling and ecchymosis [Figure 21-31 ▶] to rupture of the globe. Hyphema is bleeding into the anterior chamber of the eye that obscures vision, partially or completely [Figure 21-32 ▶]. It often follows blunt trauma and may seriously impair vision. Approximately 25% of hyphemas are associated with globe injuries.

In orbital blowout fractures, the fragments of fractured bone can entrap some of the muscles that control eye movement, causing double vision (diplopia) especially with upward gaze [Figure 21-33 ▶]. Any patient who reports pain, double vision, or decreased vision following a blunt injury about the eye should be assumed to have a blowout fracture and should be promptly transported to an appropriate medical facility.

Another potential result of blunt eye trauma is retinal detachment, or separation of the inner layers of the retina from the underlying choroid (the vascular membrane that nourishes the retina). Retinal detachment is often seen in sports injuries, especially boxing. This painless condition produces flashing lights, specks, or "floaters" in the field of vision and a cloud or shade over the patient's vision. Because it can cause devastating damage to vision, retinal detachment is an ocular emergency and requires *immediate* medical attention.

Burns of the Eye

Chemicals, heat, and light rays can all burn the delicate tissues of the eye, often causing permanent damage. Your role is to stop the burning process and prevent further damage.

Chemical burns, which are usually caused by acid or alkali solutions, require immediate emergency care [Figure 21-34 ▶]. Flush the eye with water or a sterile saline

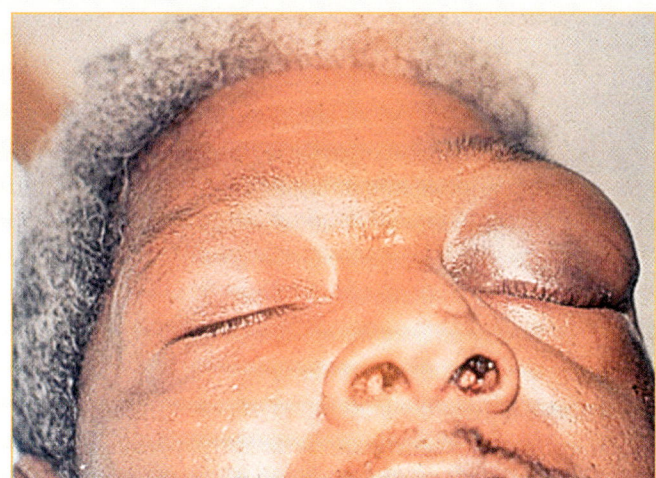

Figure 21-31 Swelling and ecchymosis are hallmark findings associated with blunt trauma to the eye.

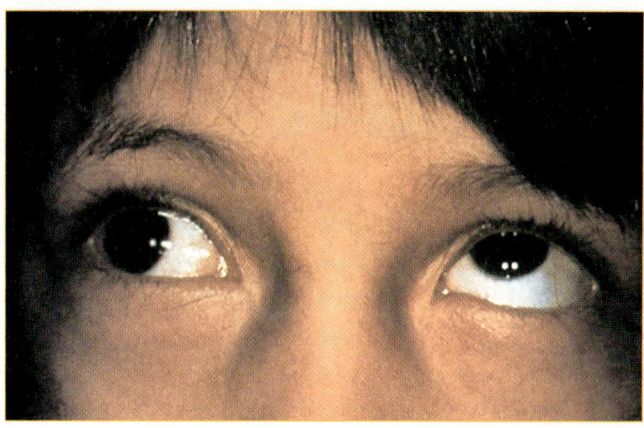

Figure 21-33 In a patient with a blowout fracture, the eyes may not move together because of muscle entrapment, so the patient sees double images of any object.

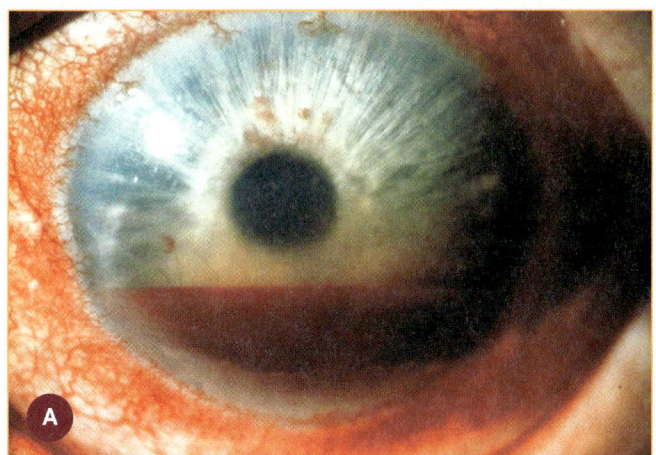

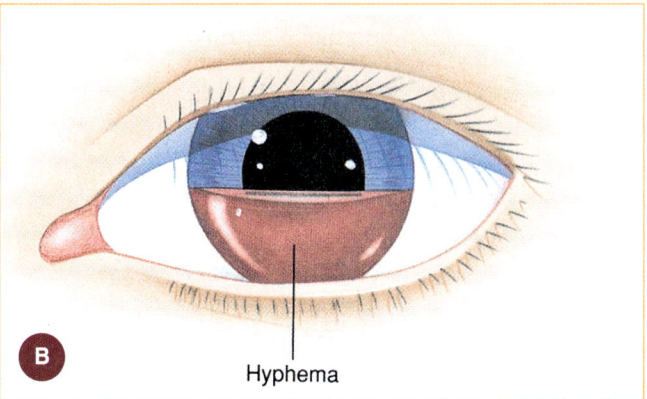

Hyphema

Figure 21-32 A hyphema, characterized by bleeding into the anterior chamber of the eye, can occur following blunt trauma to the eye. This condition should be considered a sight-threatening emergency. **A.** Actual hyphema. **B.** Illustration.

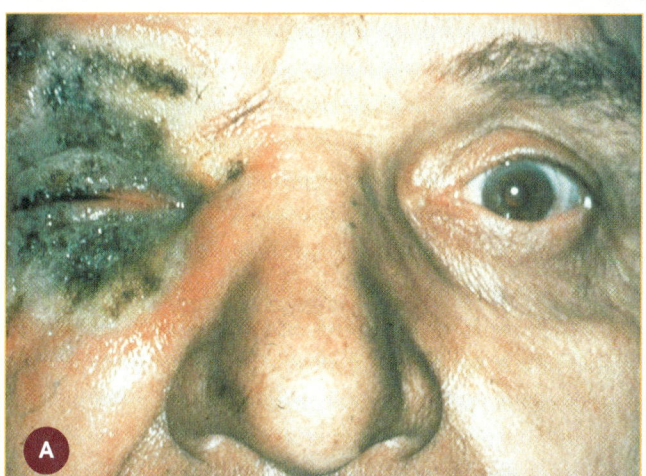

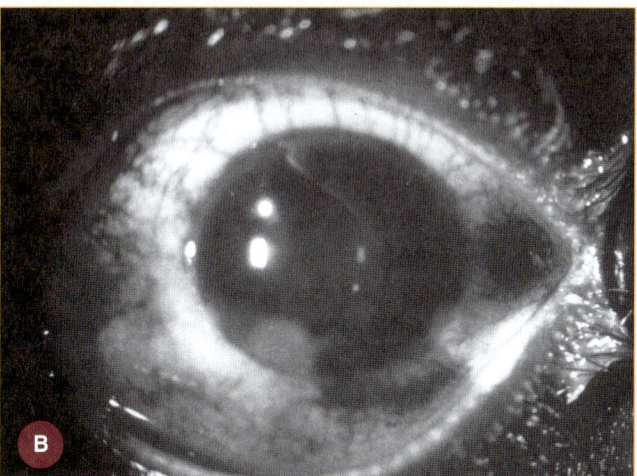

Figure 21-34 **A.** Chemical burns typically occur when an acid or alkali is splashed into the eye. **B.** A chemical burn from lye, an alkaline solution.

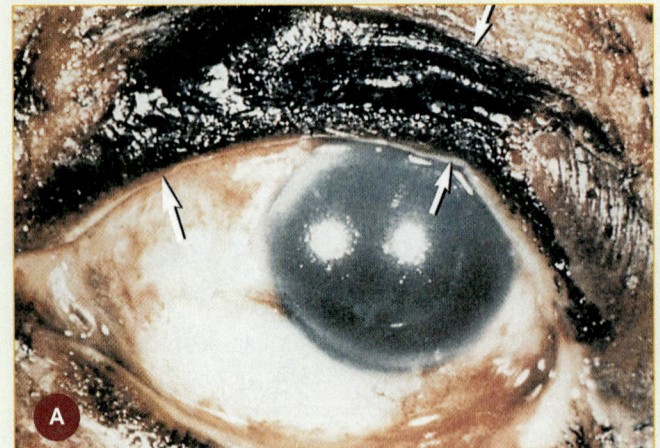

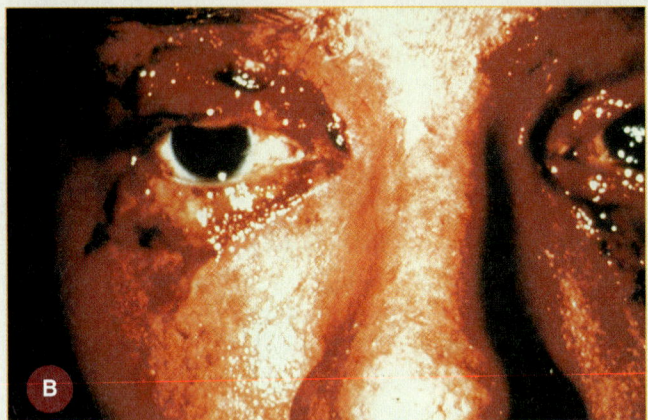

Figure 21-35 Thermal burns occasionally cause significant damage to the eyelids. **A.** Arrows show some full-thickness burns. **B.** Burns of the eyelids require immediate hospital care.

solution. If sterile saline is not available, you can use any clean water. Specific techniques for irrigating the eyes are discussed later in this chapter.

Thermal burns occur when a patient is burned in the face during a fire, although the eyes usually close rapidly because of the heat. This reaction is a natural reflex to protect the eyes from further injury. However, the eyelids remain exposed and are frequently burned   **Figure 21-35 ▲** .

Infrared rays, eclipse light (if the patient has looked directly at the sun), and laser burns can cause significant damage to the sensory cells of the eye when rays of light become focused on the retina. Retinal injuries that are caused by exposure to extremely bright light are generally not painful but may result in permanent damage to vision.

Superficial burns of the eye can result from ultraviolet rays from an arc welding unit, prolonged exposure to a sunlamp, or reflected light from a bright snow-covered area (snow blindness). This kind of burn may not be painful initially but may become so 3 to 5 hours later, as the damaged cornea responds to the injury. Severe conjunctivitis usually develops, along with redness, swelling, and excessive tear production.

Assessment and Management of Eye Injuries

The first step in assessing a patient with an eye injury is to note the mechanism of injury (ie, blunt or penetrating trauma, burn). If it suggests the potential for a spinal injury, use spinal motion restriction precautions. Ensure a patent airway and adequate breathing, and control any external bleeding. If the mechanism of injury is significant, or if the patient's clinical status dictates it, perform a rapid trauma assessment.

When obtaining the history, determine how and when the injury happened, when the symptoms began, and what symptoms the patient is experiencing. Were both eyes affected? Does the patient have any underlying diseases or conditions of the eye (such as glaucoma)? Does the patient take medications for his or her eyes?

A variety of symptoms may indicate serious ocular injury:

- *Visual loss* that does not improve when the patient blinks is the most important symptom of an eye injury. It may indicate damage to the globe or to the optic nerve.
- *Double vision* usually points to trauma involving the extraocular muscles, such as a fracture of the orbit.
- *Severe eye pain* is a symptom of a significant eye injury.
- A *foreign body sensation* usually indicates superficial injury to the cornea or the presence of a foreign object trapped behind the eyelids.

During the physical examination of the eyes, evaluate each of the visible ocular structures and ocular function:

- **Orbital rim:** for ecchymosis, swelling, lacerations, and tenderness
- **Eyelids:** for ecchymosis, swelling, and lacerations
- **Corneas:** for foreign bodies
- **Conjunctivae:** for redness, pus, inflammation, and foreign bodies
- **Globes:** for redness, abnormal pigmentation, and lacerations
- **Pupils:** for size, shape, equality, and reaction to light

At the Scene

Anisocoria, a condition in which the pupils are not of equal size, is a significant finding in patients with ocular injuries or closed head trauma. However, simple or physiologic anisocoria occurs in approximately 20% of the population. Usually, the patient's pupils differ in size by less than 1 mm; however, approximately 4% of people have pupils that vary in size by more than 1 mm. In this case, it is not a clinically significant finding.

Unilateral cataract surgery may also cause inequality of pupil size. The pupil of the eye affected by the cataract will be nonreactive to light.

- **Eye movements in all directions:** for paralysis of gaze or discoordination between the movements of the two eyes (dysconjugate gaze)
- **Visual acuity:** Make a rough assessment by asking the patient to read a newspaper or a hand-held visual acuity chart. Test each eye separately and document the results.

Treatment for specific eye injuries begins with a thorough examination to determine the extent and nature of any damage. Always perform your examination using appropriate personal protective equipment (PPE), taking great care to avoid aggravating the injury.

Although isolated eye injuries are usually not life threatening, they should be evaluated by a physician. More severe eye injuries often require evaluation and treatment by an ophthalmologist.

Injuries to the eyelids—lacerations, abrasions, and contusions—require little in the way of prehospital care other than bleeding control and gentle patching of the affected eye. No eyelid injury is trivial, however, so every patient with eyelid trauma should be transported to the hospital.

Most injuries to the globe—including contusions, lacerations, foreign bodies, and abrasions—are best treated in the emergency department, where specialized equipment is available. Aluminum eye shields (not gauze patches) applied over *both* eyes are generally all that are necessary in the prehospital environment. Follow these three important guidelines in treating penetrating injuries of the eye:

1. *Never exert pressure* on or manipulate the injured globe in any way.
2. If part of the globe is exposed, gently apply a moist, sterile dressing to prevent drying.
3. *Cover the injured eye* with a protective metal eye shield, cup, or sterile dressing. Apply soft dressings to both eyes, and provide prompt transport to the hospital.

If hyphema or rupture of the globe is suspected, take spinal motion restriction precautions. Such injuries indicate that a significant amount of force was applied to the face and, thus, may include a spinal injury. Elevate the head of the backboard approximately 40° to decrease IOP and discourage the patient from performing activities that may increase IOP (eg, coughing). For the same reason, consider giving an antiemetic drug to reduce the incidence of vomiting.

On rare occasions following a serious injury, the globe may be displaced (avulsed) out of its socket **Figure 21-36**. Do not attempt to manipulate or reposition it in any way! Cover the protruding eye with a moist, sterile dressing and stabilize it along

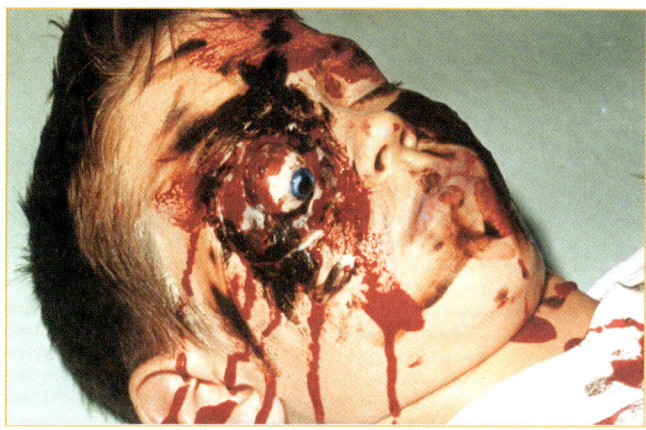

Figure 21-36 Cover an avulsed eye with moist, sterile dressings and protect it from further injury.

with the uninjured eye to prevent further injury due to sympathetic eye movement, the movement of both eyes in unison. Place the patient in a supine position to prevent further loss of fluid from the eye, and provide prompt transport to the hospital.

Burns to the eye that are caused by ultraviolet light are most effectively treated by covering the eye with a sterile, moist pad and an eye shield. The application of cool compresses *lightly* over the eye may afford the patient pain relief if he or she is in extreme distress. Place the patient in a supine position during transport, and protect the patient from further exposure to bright light.

Chemical burns to the eye—acid or alkali—can rapidly lead to total blindness if not immediately treated. The most important prehospital treatment in such cases is to begin immediate irrigation with sterile water or saline solution. *Never use any chemical antidotes (such as vinegar, baking soda) when irrigating the patient's eye; use sterile water or saline only.* Neutralizing the acid or alkali causes a chemical reaction that creates much heat, thereby worsening the burn injury.

The goal when irrigating the eye is to direct the greatest amount of solution or water into the eye as gently as possible. Because opening the eye spontaneously may cause the patient pain, you may have to force the lids open to irrigate the eye adequately. Ideally, you should use a bulb or irrigation syringe, a nasal cannula, or some other device that will allow you to control the flow **Figure 21-37**. In some circumstances, you may have to pour water into the eye by supporting the patient's head under a gently running faucet. You can have the patient immerse his or her face in a large pan or basin of water and rapidly blink the affected eyelid. If only one eye is affected, take care to avoid contaminated water getting into the unaffected eye.

Irrigate the eye for at least 5 minutes. If the burn was caused by an alkali or a strong acid, irrigate the eye continuously for 20 minutes because these substances can penetrate deeply. One common possibility occurs where anhydrous ammonia is used during the process of cooking methamphetamine. If the eyes are not irrigated promptly and efficiently, permanent damage is

At the Scene

As soon as you cover both of the patient's eyes, he or she can no longer see. Therefore, you will have to serve as the patient's eyes, keeping him or her constantly reassured and oriented to your location and what you are doing. Communication is imperative to calm the patient and reduce IOP.

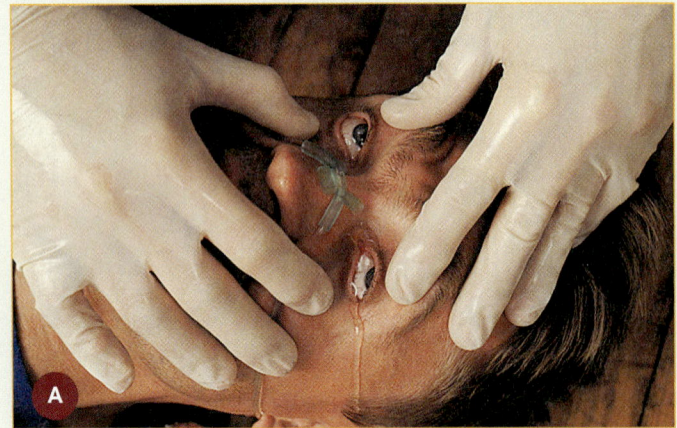
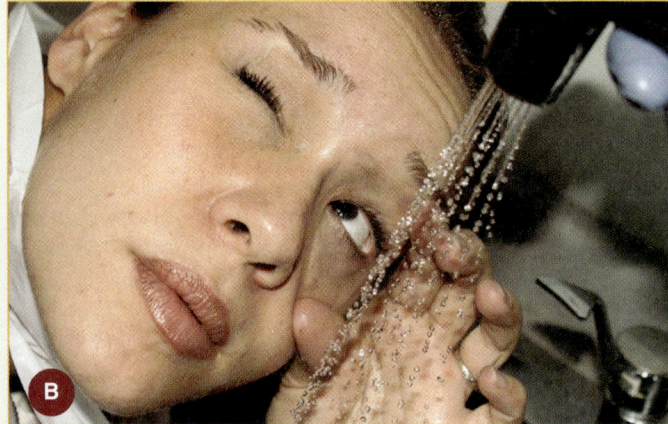
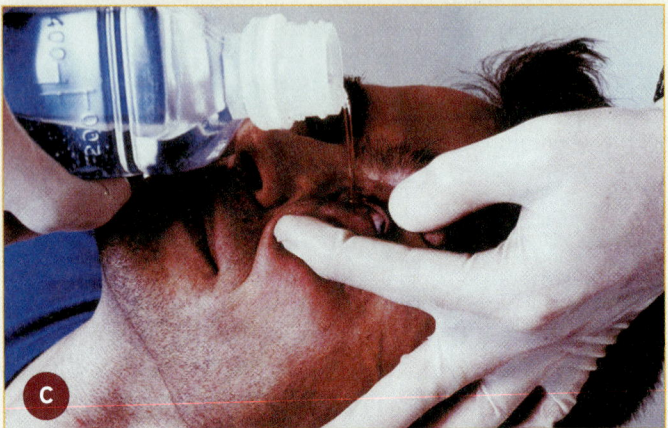
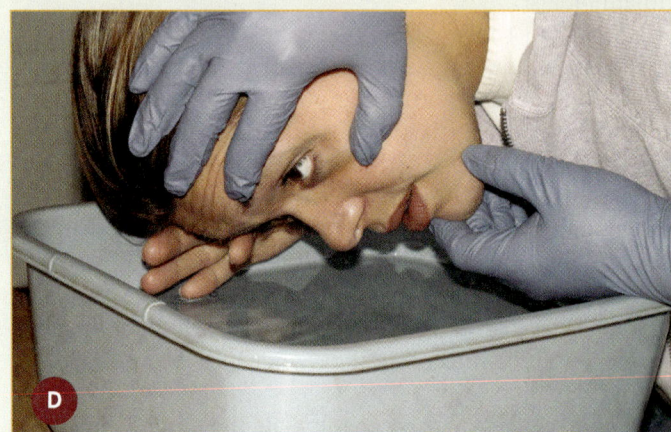

Figure 21-37 Four ways to effectively irrigate the eye: **A.** Nasal cannula. **B.** Shower. **C.** Bottle. **D.** Basin. Always protect the uninjured eye from the irrigating solution to prevent exposure to the substance.

likely. Whenever you have to irrigate the eye(s), continue to irrigate the eye en route to the hospital if possible.

Irrigation with a sterile saline solution will frequently flush away loose, small foreign objects lying on the surface of the eye. Always flush from the nose side of the eye toward the outside to avoid flushing material into the other eye. After its removal, a foreign body will often leave a small abrasion on the surface of the conjunctiva, which leads to continued irritation; for this reason, you should transport the patient to the hospital for further assessment and treatment.

Gentle irrigation usually will not wash out foreign bodies that are stuck to the cornea or lying under the upper eyelid. To examine the undersurface of the upper eyelid, pull the lid upward and forward. If you spot a foreign object on the surface of the eyelid, you may be able to remove it with a moist, sterile, cotton-tipped applicator. *Never attempt to remove a foreign body that is stuck or imbedded in the cornea.*

When a foreign body is impaled in the globe, *do not remove it!* Stabilize it in place. Cover the eye with a moist, sterile dressing; place a cup or other protective barrier over the object, and secure it in place with bulky dressing **Figure 21-38 ▶**. Cover the unaffected eye to prevent further damage caused by sympathetic eye movement, and promptly transport the patient to the hospital.

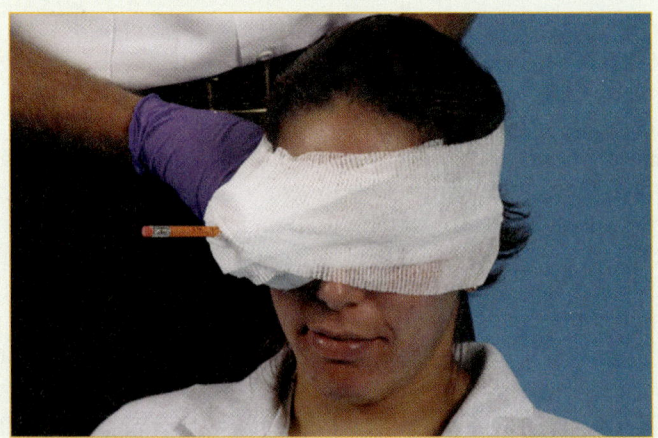

Figure 21-38 Securing an impaled object in the eye with a protective barrier and bulky dressing.

Ear Injuries

Injuries to the ear may be isolated, or they may occur in conjunction with other injuries to the head or face. Although isolated ear injuries are typically not life threatening, they can result in sensory impairment and permanent disfigurement.

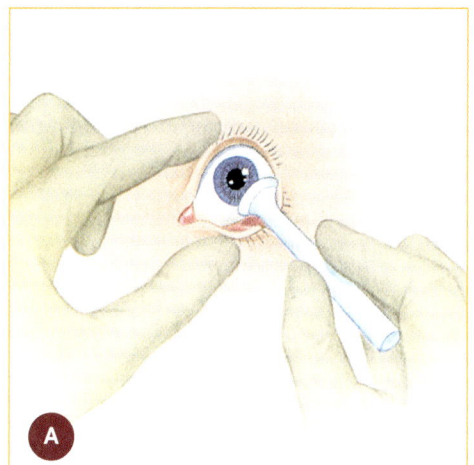
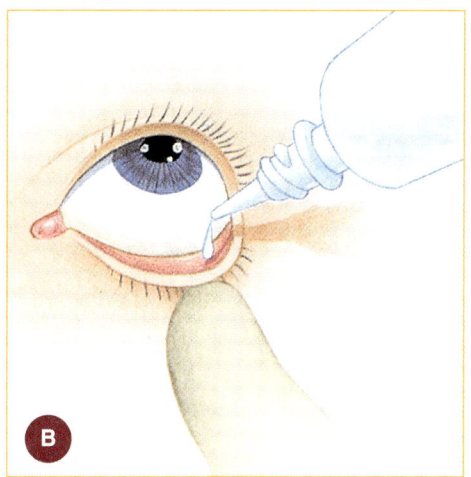
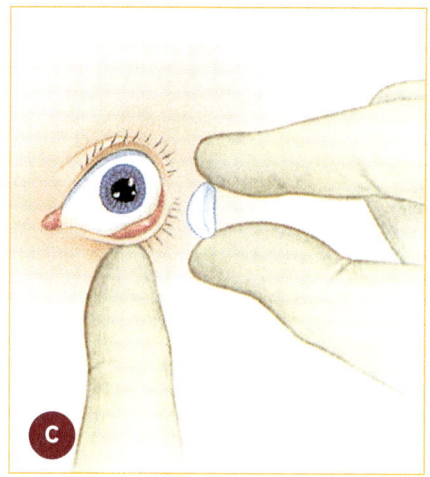

Figure 21-39 Removing contact lenses should be limited to patients with chemical burns to the eye. **A.** To remove hard contact lenses, use a specialized suction cup moistened with sterile saline solution. **B.** To remove soft contact lenses, instill 1 or 2 drops of saline or irrigating solution. **C.** Pinch off the lens with your gloved thumb and index fingers.

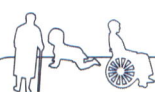

Special Considerations

Contact Lenses and Artificial Eyes

There are three types of contact lenses: hard, rigid gas-permeable, and soft (hydrophilic). Small, hard contact lenses usually are tinted, making them relatively easy to see. Large, soft contact lenses are clear and can be very difficult to see even more so if they "float" up or down under an eyelid.

In general, you should not attempt to remove contact lenses from a patient with an eye injury, lest you aggravate the injury. The only indication for removing contact lenses in the prehospital setting is a chemical burn of the eye. In this situation, the lens can trap the offending chemical and make irrigation difficult thus worsening the injury.

To remove a hard contact lens, use a small suction cup, moistening the end with saline **Figure 21-39A ▲**. To remove soft lenses, place one to two drops of saline in the eye **Figure 21-39B ▲**, gently pinch the lens between your gloved thumb and index finger, and lift it off the surface of the eye **Figure 21-39C ▲**. Place the contact lens in a container with sterile saline solution. Always advise emergency department staff if a patient is wearing contact lenses.

Occasionally, you may provide prehospital care for a patient who is wearing an eye prosthesis (artificial eye). You should suspect an eye of being artificial when it does not respond to light, move in concert with the opposite eye, or appear quite the same as the opposite eye. If you are unsure as to whether the patient has an eye prosthesis, ask him or her. Although no harm will be done if you care for an artificial eye as you would a normal one, you need to be totally clear about the patient's eye function. In addition, it can be quite embarrassing to pass on information during your radio report that the patient has a nonreactive pupil only to find out at the ED that the patient has a prosthetic eye.

Soft-Tissue Injuries

Lacerations, avulsions, and contusions to the external ear can occur following blunt or penetrating trauma. The pinna can be contused, lacerated, or partially or completely avulsed. Trauma to the earlobe can result in similar injuries.

The pinna has an inherently poor blood supply, so it tends to heal poorly. Healing of the cartilaginous pinna is often complicated by infection.

Ruptured Eardrum

Perforation of the tympanic membrane (ruptured eardrum) can result from foreign bodies in the ear or from pressure-related injuries, such as blast injuries resulting from an explosion, or diving-related injuries that result in barotrauma to the ear. Signs and symptoms of a perforated tympanic membrane include loss of hearing and blood drainage from the ear. Although the injury is extremely painful for the patient, the tympanic membrane typically heals spontaneously and without complication. Nevertheless, a careful assessment should be performed to detect and treat other injuries, some of which may be life threatening.

Assessment and Management of Ear Injuries

Assessment and management of the patient with an ear injury begins by ensuring airway patency and breathing adequacy. If the mechanism of injury suggests a potential for spinal injury, apply full spinal motion restriction precautions.

An adequate assessment of the external ear canal and middle ear cannot be performed in the prehospital environment. In general, the ears' poor blood supply limits the amount of external bleeding. If manual direct pressure does not control this bleeding, first place a soft, padded dressing between the ear and the scalp since bandaging the ear against the scalp can be painful. Then apply a roller bandage to secure the dressing in place [Figure 21-40 ▾]. An icepack can also help reduce swelling and pain.

If the pinna is partially avulsed, carefully realign the ear into position and gently bandage it with sufficient padding that has been slightly moistened with normal saline. If the pinna is completely avulsed, attempt to retrieve the avulsed part, if possible, for reimplantation at the hospital. If the detached part of the ear is recovered, treat it as any other amputation; wrap it in saline-moistened gauze, place it in a plastic bag, and place the bag on ice. If a chemical icepack is used, it is recommended to shield the avulsed part with several gauze pads to diffuse the cold, as chemical icepacks are actually colder than ice and inadvertent freezing of the part can occur.

If blood or CSF drainage is noted, apply a loose dressing over the ear—taking care *not* to stop the flow—and assess the patient for other signs of a basal skull fracture.

Do not remove an impaled object from the ear. Instead, stabilize the object and cover the ear to prevent gross movement and to minimize the risk of contamination of the inner ear.

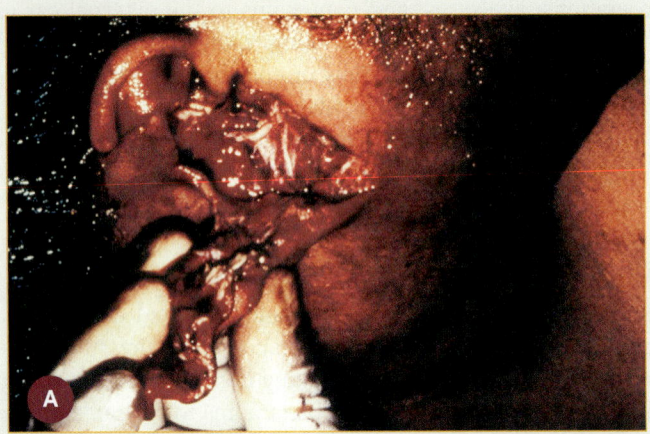

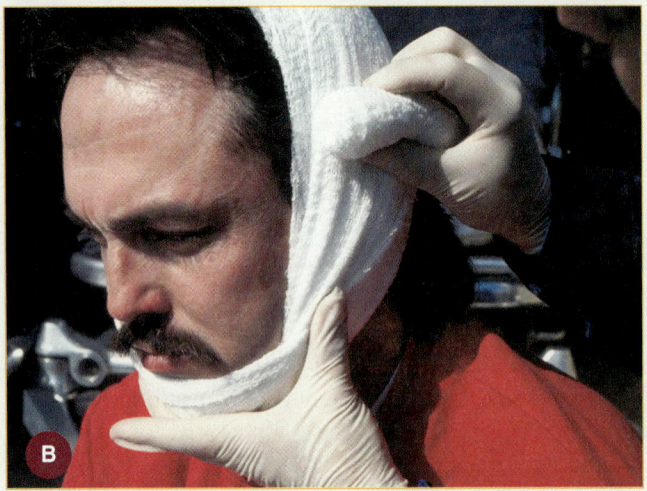

Figure 21-40 A. A major laceration of the ear. **B.** Place a soft, sterile pad behind the ear, between it and the scalp. Then wrap a roller gauze bandage (ie, Kling, Kerlex, etc.) around the head to include the entire ear.

Because isolated ear injuries are typically not life threatening, you must perform a careful assessment to detect or rule out potentially more serious injuries. You may then proceed with specific care of the ear, provide emotional support, and transport the patient to an appropriate medical facility.

Oral and Dental Injuries

Oral and dental injuries are commonly associated with trauma to the face. Blunt mechanisms are commonly the result of motor vehicle collisions or direct blows to the mouth or chin. Penetrating mechanisms are commonly the result of gunshot wounds.

The primary risk associated with oral and dental injuries is airway compromise from oropharyngeal bleeding, occlusion by a displaced dental appliance such as a bridge or partial plate, or possibly by the aspiration of avulsed or fractured teeth. Any patient with significant facial trauma should be carefully assessed for injuries to the mouth and teeth.

Soft-Tissue Injuries

Lacerations and avulsions in and around the mouth are associated with a risk of intraoral hemorrhage and subsequent airway compromise. Therefore, your assessment of any patient with facial trauma should include a careful examination of the mouth, including the teeth. Fractured or avulsed teeth and lacerations of the tongue may cause profuse bleeding into the upper airway [Figure 21-41 ▾]. A conscious patient with severe oral bleeding is often unable to speak unless he or she is leaning forward—this position facilitates drainage of blood from the mouth.

Patients may swallow blood from lacerations inside the mouth, so the bleeding may not be grossly evident. Because blood irritates the gastric lining, the risks of vomiting and aspiration are significant. Objects that are impaled in or through

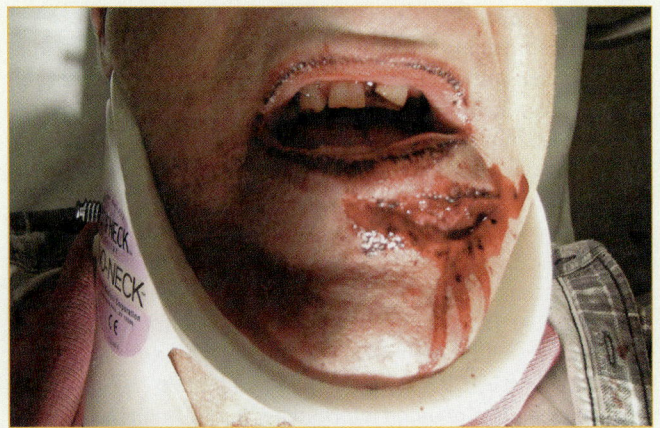

Figure 21-41 Soft-tissue injuries around the mouth can be associated with profuse oral bleeding and airway compromise.

the soft tissues of the mouth (such as the cheek) can also result in profuse bleeding and once again, the threat of vomiting with aspiration.

Dental Injuries

Fractured and avulsed teeth—especially the anterior teeth—are common following facial trauma. Dental injuries may be associated with mechanisms that cause severe maxillofacial trauma (such as motor vehicle collisions), or they may occur in isolation (such as a direct blow to the mouth from an assault).

You should always assess the patient's mouth following a facial injury, especially in cases of fractured or avulsed teeth. Teeth fragments (or even whole teeth) can become an airway obstruction and should be removed from the patient's mouth immediately.

At the Scene

When assessing a patient with fractured or avulsed teeth following an assault, you should also assess the individual who struck the patient, preferably at a distance from the assaulted patient. This should occur only if it is safe to do so. The human mouth is filled with bacteria and other microorganisms, and lacerations to the person's hands or knuckles can easily become infected without proper care. This is called a clenched-fist injury. Occasionally, you may encounter fragments of broken teeth impaled in a person's knuckles! It is important to examine the hand while clenched, not outstretched, otherwise it might be difficult to appreciate the involvement of the metacarpophalangeal (MCP) joint.

Assessment and Management of Oral and Dental Injuries

Ensuring airway patency and adequate breathing are the priorities of prehospital care when managing patients with oral or dental trauma. Suction the oropharynx as needed, and remove fractured tooth fragments to prevent airway compromise. Apply spinal motion restriction precautions as dictated by the mechanism of injury. If profuse oral bleeding is present and the patient cannot spontaneously control his or her own airway (such as with a decreased level of consciousness), pharmacologically assisted intubation may be necessary.

Impaled objects in the soft tissues of the mouth should be stabilized in place unless they interfere with the patient's breathing or your ability to manage the patient's airway. In those cases, remove the impaled object from the direction that it entered, and control bleeding with direct pressure.

An avulsed tooth may be successfully reimplanted even if it has been out of the mouth for up to 1 hour. Direct medical control may sometimes ask you to reimplant the tooth in its

Table 21-2	Care for an Avulsed Tooth

- Handle the tooth by the crown only. Avoid touching the root surface of the tooth.
- Gently rinse the tooth with sterile saline or water. Avoid the use of soap or chemicals, and do not scrub the tooth!
- Do not allow the tooth to dry. Place it in one of the following:
  - Emergency tooth preservation system (commercially available): a break-resistant storage container with soft inner walls and a pH-balanced solution that nourishes and preserves the tooth
  - Cold whole milk
  - Sterile saline solution (for storage periods of less than 1 hour)
- Transport the tooth with the patient, and notify the hospital of the situation.

original socket. Carefully place the tooth in its socket, and hold it in place with your fingers or have the patient gently bite down. If prehospital reimplantation of a tooth is not possible, follow the guidelines outlined in Table 21-2 ▲.

Retrieval and reimplantation or storage of an avulsed tooth is a low priority if the patient is in a clinically unstable condition (such as compromised airway or shock). In such cases, aggressive airway management, spinal precautions, and rapid transport of the patient are obviously more important with the dental problem being addressed at a later time.

Injuries to the Anterior Part of the Neck

The neck is a very vulnerable stretch of anatomy because it houses a critical portion of the airway (ie, larynx, trachea), the major blood vessels to and from the head, and the spinal cord. Other structures contained within the neck that are also vulnerable to injury include muscles, nerves, and glands. Any injury to the anterior part of the neck—blunt or penetrating— must be considered critical until proven otherwise.

Soft-Tissue Injuries

Blunt and penetrating mechanisms can damage the soft tissues of the anterior part of the neck and its associated structures. In both cases, you must be alert for the possibility of cervical spine injury and airway compromise.

Common mechanisms of blunt trauma include motor vehicle collisions, direct trauma to the neck, and hangings. Such injury often results in swelling and edema; injury to the various structures such as the trachea, larynx, or esophagus; or injury to the cervical spine. Less commonly, blunt injuries may damage the vasculature of the anterior part of the neck. Because blunt trauma to the neck is associated with a high incidence of airway compromise and ventilatory inadequacy, you must carefully assess the patient and be prepared to initiate aggressive management.

Common mechanisms of penetrating trauma include gunshot wounds, stabbings, and impaled objects. The lacerations

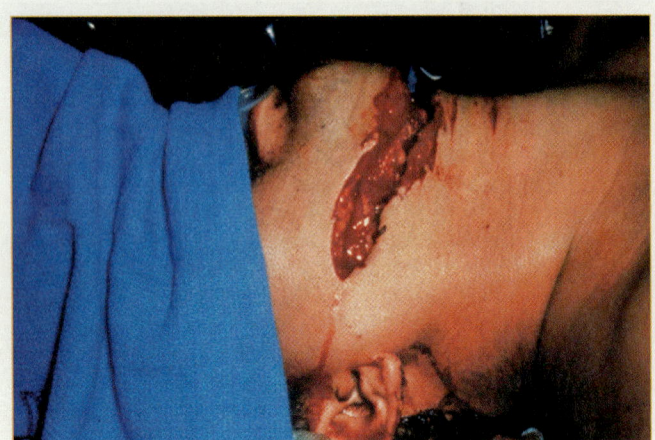

Figure 21-42 Open injuries to the neck can be very dangerous. If veins are exposed to the environment, they can suck in air, resulting in a potentially fatal air embolism.

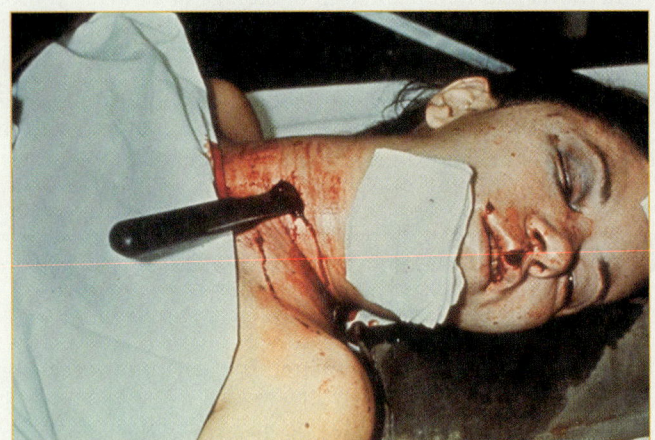

Figure 21-43 Impaled objects in the neck can cause profuse bleeding, if the major blood vessels are damaged, and direct injury to the larynx, trachea, esophagus, or cervical spine.

or puncture wounds produced may be superficial and involve only the fascia or fatty tissues of the neck, or they may be deep and involve injury to the larynx, trachea, esophagus, nerves, or major blood vessels. The primary threats from penetrating neck trauma are massive hemorrhage from major blood vessel disruption and airway compromise secondary to soft-tissue swelling or direct damage to the larynx or trachea.

A special danger associated with open neck injuries is the possibility of a fatal air embolism. If the jugular veins of the neck are exposed to the environment, they may entrain air into the vessel and occlude the flow of blood to the lungs **Figure 21-42 ▲** . As such, open neck wounds should be sealed with an occlusive dressing immediately.

Impaled objects in the neck can present several life-threatening problems for the patient—namely, injury to major blood vessels with massive hemorrhage; damage to the larynx, trachea, or esophagus; or injury to the cervical spine **Figure 21-43 ▲** .

Impaled objects should not be removed but rather stabilized in place and protected from movement. The *only* exception is if the object is obstructing the airway or impeding your ability to effectively manage the airway. In some cases, an emergency cricothyrotomy may be necessary to establish and maintain airway patency.

Injuries to the Larynx, Trachea, and Esophagus

A variety of life-threatening injuries can result if the structures of the anterior part of the neck are crushed against the cervical spine following blunt trauma or if they are penetrated by a knife or similar object. The larynx and its supporting structures (ie, hyoid bone, thyroid cartilage) may be fractured, the trachea may be separated from the larynx (tracheal transection), or the esophagus may be perforated. Many injuries to the larynx, trachea, and esophagus are occult; because they are not as obvious and dramatic as penetrating neck injuries, they can be easily overlooked. Therefore, you must maintain a high index of suspicion and perform a careful assessment of *any* patient with blunt trauma to the anterior part of the neck.

Significant injuries to the larynx or trachea pose an *immediate* risk of airway compromise due to disruption of the normal passage of air, soft-tissue swelling, or aspiration of blood into the lungs. In addition, esophageal perforation can result in mediastinitis, an inflammation of the mediastinum often due to leakage of gastric contents into the thoracic cavity. Mediastinitis is associated with a high mortality rate if not surgically repaired in a timely manner.

At the Scene

Any force that is powerful enough to disrupt the larynx, trachea, or esophagus is powerful enough to injure the cervical spine, so the use of spinal motion restriction precautions is important. Carefully assess the patient for signs of a spinal injury: vertebral deformities (step-offs), paralysis, paresthesia, and signs of neurogenic shock (hypotension, normal or slow heart rate, lack of diaphoresis).

Patients with injuries to the anterior part of the neck may experience concomitant maxillofacial fractures, which can make bag-valve-mask ventilation difficult (usually because of an inadequate mask-to-face seal). Likewise, endotracheal intubation may be extremely challenging, if not impossible, owing to distortion of the normal anatomy of the upper airway. If basic and advanced techniques to secure the patient's airway are unsuccessful or impossible, a surgical or needle cricothyrotomy may be your only means of establishing a patent airway and ensuring adequate oxygenation and ventilation. Prior to deciding to perform a surgical airway, use of a lighted stylette or a gum elastic bougie may get the airway secure in a timely fashion while avoiding more risky procedures.

Assessment and Management of Injuries to the Anterior Part of the Neck

Begin your assessment by noting the mechanism of injury and maintaining a high index of suspicion, especially if the patient has experienced blunt or penetrating trauma between the upper part of the chest and head. Fractures of the first rib are associated with close to 50% mortality, not because of the rib fracture, but because the force it takes to fracture such a short, stout bone takes so much force that significant face, head, and neck trauma are almost always present as well. Remember that obvious and dramatic-appearing soft-tissue injuries may mask occult injuries to the larynx, trachea, or esophagus. Also, the patient may have experienced trauma to multiple body systems, especially following a significant mechanism of injury.

At the Scene

On any call, ensure that the scene is safe before entering it. If the patient's injury is the result of an assault, be aware that the assailant may still be present. Make radio contact with an on-scene law enforcement officer, and do not enter the scene until he or she states that it is safe to do so. Remember this: The life you save may **take** your own!

As you begin your initial assessment, manually stabilize the patient's head in a neutral in-line position and simultaneously open the airway with the jaw-thrust maneuver if the patient is semiconscious or unconscious. Use suction as needed to clear the airway of blood or other liquids. Assess the patient's breathing—rate, regularity, and depth—and intervene immediately. If the patient is breathing adequately, apply a nonrebreathing mask at 15 l/min. If breathing is inadequate (ie, reduced tidal volume, fast or slow respirations), assist with bag-valve-mask ventilation and 100% oxygen.

Your primary focus is always treating the injuries that will be the *most rapidly fatal*. Because death following trauma to the anterior part of the neck is usually the result of airway compromise or massive bleeding, aggressive airway

At the Scene

Never use a flow-restricted, oxygen-powered ventilation device (ie, a manually triggered ventilator) on a patient with trauma to the anterior part of the neck and signs of laryngeal or tracheal injury. The high pressure delivered by such devices can cause barotrauma and potentially exacerbate the patient's injury. If ventilatory support is necessary, use bag-valve-mask ventilation.

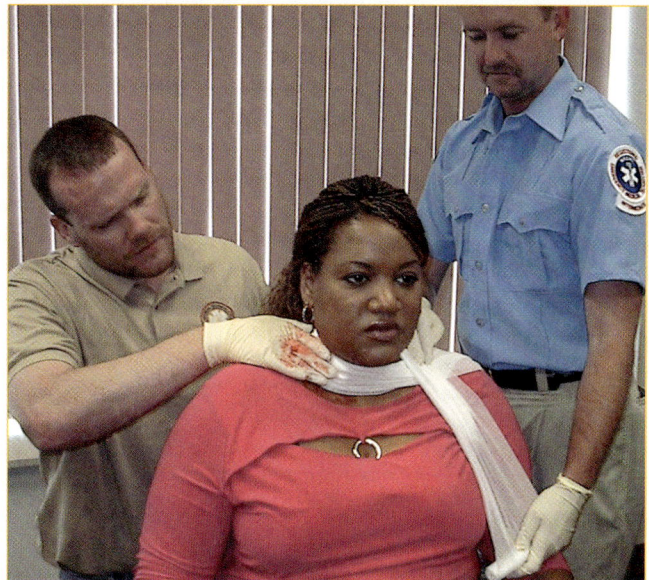

Figure 21-44 Cover open neck wounds with an occlusive dressing, and apply manual pressure to control bleeding. Do not compress both carotid arteries simultaneously because this will impair cerebral perfusion.

management and external bleeding control are the highest priorities of prehospital care. After addressing any life-threatening or other serious problems with the ABCs during the initial assessment, you may perform a rapid trauma assessment to detect and treat other injuries.

To control bleeding from an open neck wound and prevent air embolism, immediately cover the wound with an occlusive dressing. In the case of a small wound, or wounds, ECG electrodes can be fast and effective ways to seal a small hole or holes. Apply manual direct pressure over the occlusive dressing with a bulky dressing. As a last resort, you can secure a pressure dressing over the wound by wrapping roller gauze loosely around the neck and then firmly through the opposite axilla **Figure 21-44 ▲** . *Do not* circumferentially wrap bandages around the neck to secure the dressing in place. This is contraindicated and could even be fatal, because they may impair cerebral perfusion by occluding both carotid arteries or interfere with the patient's breathing. Monitor the patient's pulse for reflex bradycardia, which indicates parasympathetic nervous stimulation due to excessive pressure on the carotid artery.

Bruising or redness to the overlying skin and palpable tenderness are common signs associated with injuries to the anterior part of the neck. **Table 21-3 ▶**   summarizes the signs and symptoms of specific injuries.

If signs of shock are present, keep the patient warm, establish vascular access with at least one large-bore IV en route to the hospital if possible, or on-scene if indicated, and infuse an isotonic crystalloid solution (such as lactated Ringer's or normal saline) as needed to maintain adequate perfusion.

Table 21-3	Signs and Symptoms of Injuries to the Anterior Part of the Neck
Injury	**Signs and Symptoms**
Laryngeal fracture, tracheal transection	• Laboured breathing or reduced air movement • Stridor • Hoarseness, voice changes • Hemoptysis (coughing up blood) • Subcutaneous emphysema • Swelling, edema
Vascular injury	• Gross external bleeding • Signs of shock • Hematoma, swelling, edema • Pulse deficits
Esophageal perforation	• Dysphagia (difficulty swallowing) • Hematemesis • Hemoptysis (suggests aspiration of blood)
Neurologic impairment	• Signs of a stroke (suggests air embolism or cerebral infarct) • Paralysis or paresthesia • Cranial nerve deficit • Signs of neurogenic shock

Many patients with serious laryngeal trauma require a surgical airway. Endotracheal intubation may be hazardous in such cases because you cannot see the tip of the ET tube once it passes between the vocal cords; it may pass straight through a defect in the laryngeal or tracheal wall or could result in the complete transection of the trachea. Signs of this complication include increased swelling of the neck and worsening subcutaneous emphysema during assisted ventilation.

If the patient has experienced an open tracheal wound, you may be able to pass a cuffed ET tube directly through the wound to establish a patent airway. Use caution, however: The trachea may be perforated anteriorly *and* posteriorly, which would increase the risk of false passage of the ET tube outside the

Controversies

Some clinicians advocate aiming for air bubbles, which indicate the *general* location of the glottis, when attempting to intubate a patient with a head, face, or neck injury and severe oropharyngeal bleeding. While this practice is dangerous, it can also be both practical and potentially the best approach! Whenever possible, suction the airway as needed to facilitate an adequate view of the vocal cords. If this is unsuccessful, you should consider performing a cricothyrotomy without delay if the "tube the bubbles" approach doesn't work or doesn't seem practical.

trachea. It is critical to use *multiple* techniques for confirming correct tube placement: frequently monitor breath sounds, use end-tidal capnometry, assess for adequate chest rise, and assess for vapour mist in the ET tube during exhalation.

Head Injuries

A head injury is a traumatic insult to the head that may result in injury to soft tissue, bony structures, or the brain. Approximately 50,000 people experience head injuries of varying severity in Canada each year. Over 20,000 Canadians are hospitalized annually as a result of traumatic brain injury. More than 50% of all traumatic deaths result from a head injury. When head injuries are fatal, the cause is invariably associated injury to the brain.

Motor vehicle collisions are the most common mechanism of injury, with more than two thirds of people involved in motor vehicle collisions experiencing a head injury. Head injuries also occur commonly in victims of assault, when elderly people fall, during sports-related incidents, and in a variety of incidents involving children.

You are the Paramedic Part 4

You apply full spinal motion restriction precautions and quickly load the patient into the ambulance. You and your partner agree that the patient should be intubated. After placing the patient on cardiac monitor and establishing an IV line, you administer the appropriate drugs and place the ET tube. You confirm ET tube placement by seeing the tube pass through the cords, auscultation, and end-tidal CO_2 capnography.

Reassessment	Recording Time: 10 Minutes
Level of consciousness	Sedated with a Glasgow Coma Scale score of 3
Respirations	Intubated and ventilated at a rate of 10 breaths/min
Pulse	70 beats/min; regular and bounding
Skin	Warm and dry
Blood pressure	160/100 mm Hg
Spo_2	98% (intubated and ventilated with 100% oxygen)

7. What do the patient's vital signs indicate?

8. What else should you assess for in this patient?

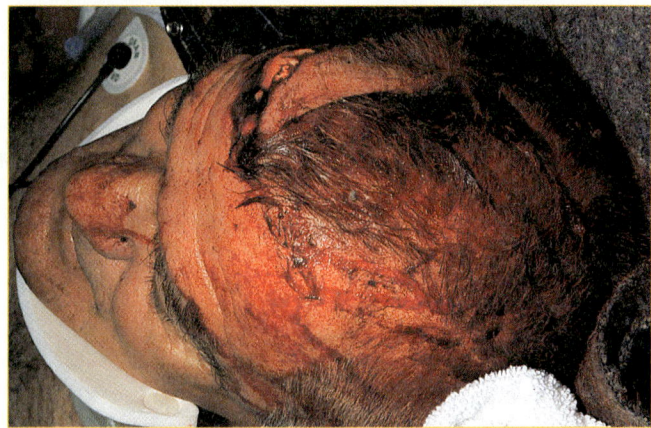

Figure 21-45 The scalp has a rich blood supply, so even small lacerations can lead to significant blood loss.

There are two general types of head injuries: open and closed. A closed head injury (the most common type) is usually associated with blunt trauma. Although the dura mater remains intact and brain tissue is not exposed to the environment, closed head injuries may result in skull fractures, focal brain injuries, or diffuse brain injuries. Furthermore, these injuries are often complicated by increased ICP.

With an open head injury, the dura mater and cranial contents are penetrated, and brain tissue is open to the environment. Gunshot wounds—the most common penetrating mechanism of injury—have a high mortality rate, and for those who survive there is almost always significant neurologic deficit and a decreased quality of life.

Scalp Lacerations

Scalp lacerations can be minor or very serious. Because of the scalp's rich blood supply, even small lacerations can quickly lead to significant blood loss **Figure 21-45 ▲**. Hypovolemic shock in adults is rarely caused by scalp lacerations alone; this is more common in children. However, bleeding from the scalp can contribute to hypovolemia in any patient, especially one with multiple injuries. In addition, because scalp lacerations usually result from direct blows to the head, they often indicate deeper, more severe injuries.

Skull Fractures

Four types of skull fractures are distinguished: linear, depressed, basilar, and open **Figure 21-46 ▶**. The significance of a skull fracture is directly related to the type of fracture, the amount of force applied, and

the area of the head that suffered the blow. Skull fractures are most commonly seen following motor vehicle collisions and significant falls. They may or may not be associated with soft-tissue scalp injuries. Potential complications of any skull fracture include intracranial hemorrhage, cerebral damage, and cranial nerve damage, among others.

Linear Skull Fractures

Linear skull fractures (nondisplaced skull fractures) account for approximately 80% of all fractures to the skull; approximately 50% of linear fractures occur in the temporal-parietal region of the skull (see Figure 21-46A). Radiographic evaluation is required to diagnose a linear skull fracture because there are often no gross physical signs (such as deformity or depression). If the brain is uninjured and the scalp is intact, linear fractures are relatively benign. However, if a scalp laceration occurs in conjunction with a linear fracture—making it an open fracture—there is a risk of infection. In addition, if the fracture occurs over the temporal region of the skull, injury to the middle meningeal artery may result in epidural bleeding, which can rapidly become catastrophic.

Depressed Skull Fractures

Depressed skull fractures result from high-energy direct trauma to a small surface area of the head with a blunt object (such as

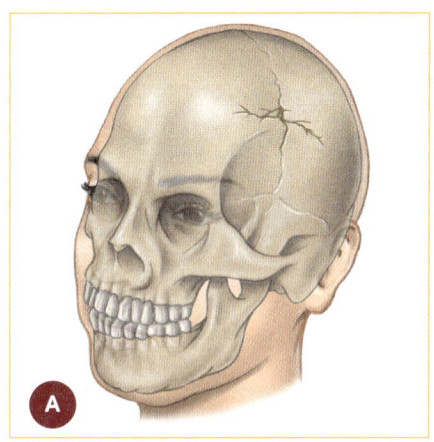
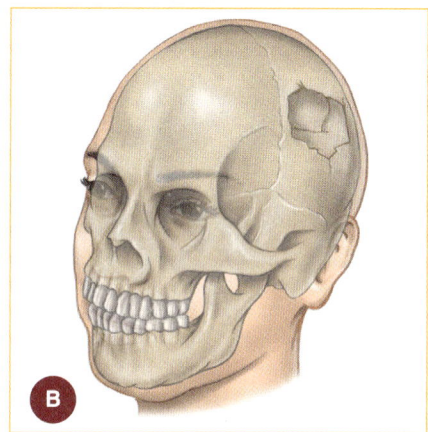
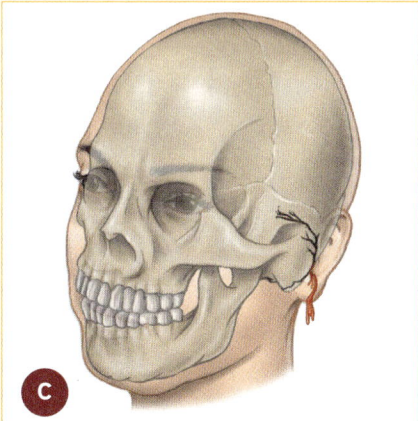
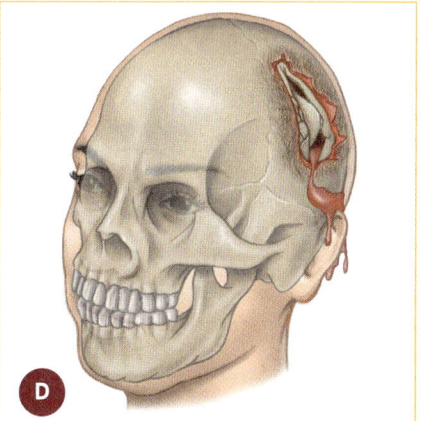

Figure 21-46 Types of skull fracture. **A.** Linear. **B.** Depressed. **C.** Basilar. **D.** Open.

a baseball bat to the head) (see Figure 21-46B). The frontal and parietal regions of the skull are most susceptible to these types of fractures because the bones in these areas, compared with other bones of the skull, are relatively thin. As a consequence, bony fragments may be driven into the brain, resulting in underlying injury. The overlying scalp may or may not be intact. Patients with depressed skull fractures often present with neurologic signs (such as loss of consciousness).

Basilar Skull Fractures

Basilar skull fractures also are associated with high-energy trauma, but they usually occur following diffuse impact to the head (eg, falls, motor vehicle collisions). These injuries generally result from extension of a linear fracture to the base of the skull and can be difficult to diagnose with plain x-rays (see Figure 21-46C).

Signs of a basilar skull fracture include CSF drainage from the ears **Figure 21-47** ▾ , which indicates rupture of the tympanic membrane and freely flowing CSF through the ear. Patients with leaking CSF are at risk for bacterial meningitis.

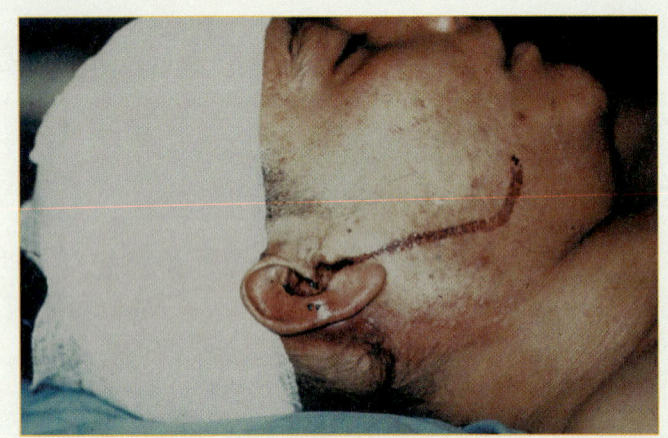

Figure 21-47 Blood draining from the ear after a head injury may contain CSF and suggests a basilar skull fracture.

Other signs of a basilar skull fracture include periorbital ecchymosis that develops under or around the eyes, which is also known as raccoon or panda eyes **Figure 21-48A** ▾ , or ecchymosis behind the ear over the mastoid process known as Battle's sign **Figure 21-48B** ▾ . Depending upon the extent of the damage, raccoon eyes and Battle's sign may appear relatively quickly, but in many cases, they may not appear until up to 24 hours following the injury, so their absence in the prehospital setting does not rule out a basilar skull fracture.

Open Skull Fractures

Open fractures of the cranial vault result when severe forces are applied to the head and are often associated with trauma to multiple body systems (see Figure 21-46D). Brain tissue may be exposed to the environment, which significantly increases the risk of a bacterial infection (such as bacterial meningitis). Open cranial vault fractures have a high mortality rate.

▌Traumatic Brain Injuries

The National Head Injury Foundation defines a traumatic brain injury (TBI) as "a traumatic insult to the brain capable of producing physical, intellectual, emotional, social, and vocational changes." Traumatic brain injuries are classified into two broad categories: primary (direct) injury and secondary (indirect) injury. Primary brain injury is injury to the brain and its associated structures that results instantaneously from impact to the head. Secondary brain injury refers to the "after effects" of the primary injury; it includes abnormal processes such as cerebral edema, intracranial hemorrhage, increased ICP, cerebral ischemia and hypoxia, and infection. Secondary brain injury can occur anywhere from a few minutes to several days following the initial injury.

The brain can be injured directly by a penetrating object, such as a bullet, knife, or other sharp object. More commonly,

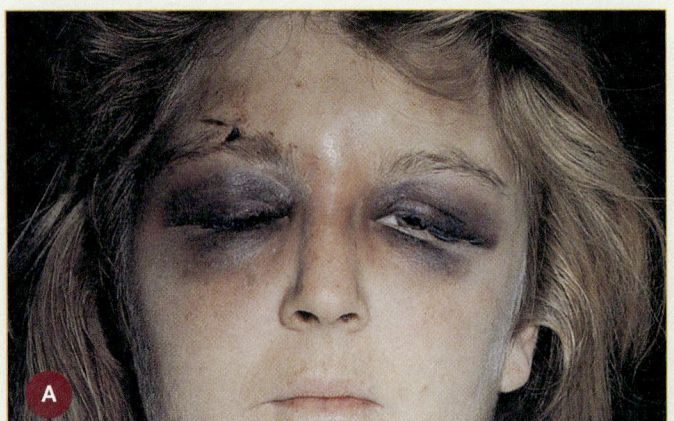

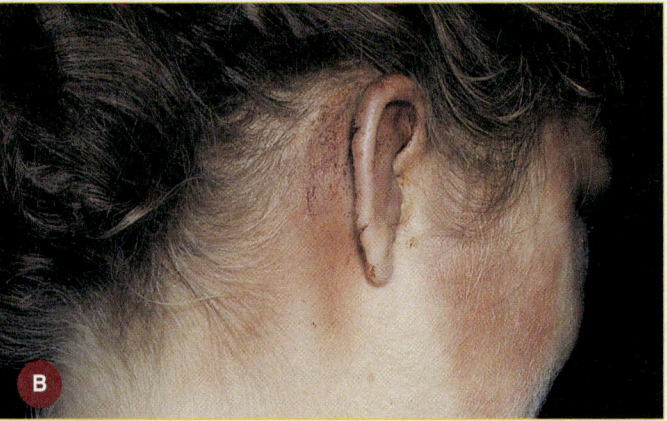

Figure 21-48 Suspect a basilar skull fracture if a head trauma patient has ecchymosis. **A.** Ecchymosis under or around the eyes (raccoon or panda eyes). **B.** Ecchymosis behind the ear over the mastoid process (Battle's sign).

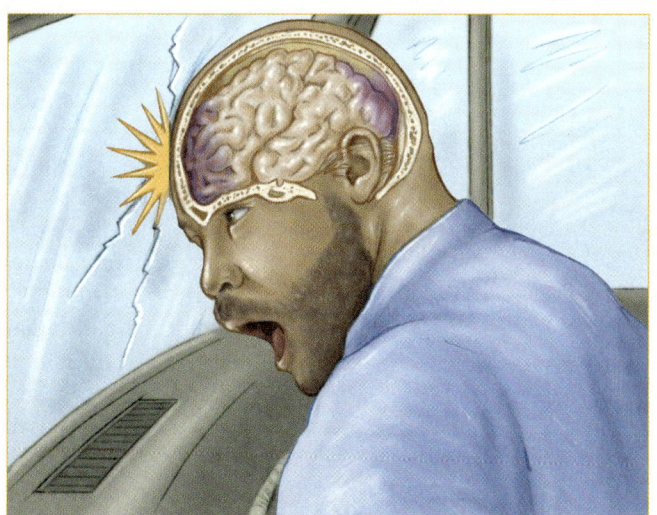

Figure 21-49 For the unrestrained victim in a motor vehicle collision, the brain continues its forward motion and strikes the inside of the skull, resulting in compression injury to the anterior portion of the brain and stretching of the posterior portion.

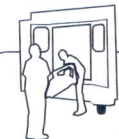

At the Scene

The brain accounts for 80% of the intracranial contents, the cerebral blood volume accounts for 12%, and the CSF volume accounts for the remaining 8%.

such injuries occur indirectly, as a result of external forces exerted on the skull. Consider the most common cause of brain injury, the motor vehicle collision. When the passenger's head hits the windshield on impact with a fixed object, the brain continues to move forward until it comes to an abrupt stop by striking the inside of the skull. This rapid deceleration results in compression injury (or bruising) to the anterior portion of the brain along with stretching or tearing of the posterior portion of the brain (Figure 21-49 ▲). As the brain strikes the front of the skull, the body begins its path of moving backward. The head falls back against the headrest and/or seat, and the brain impacts against the rear of the skull. This type of front-and-rear injury is known as a coup–contrecoup injury. The same type of injury may occur on opposite sides of the brain in a lateral collision.

The injured brain starts to swell, initially because of cerebral vasodilation. An increase in cerebral water (cerebral edema) then contributes to further brain swelling. Cerebral edema may not develop until several hours following the initial injury, however.

Intracranial Pressure

For adults the skull is a rigid, unyielding globe that allows little, if any, expansion of the intracranial contents. It also provides a hard and somewhat irregular surface against which brain tissue and its blood vessels can be injured when the head suffers trauma.

Accumulations of blood within the skull or swelling of the brain can rapidly lead to an increase in intracranial pressure (ICP), the pressure within the cranial vault. Increased ICP squeezes the brain against bony prominences within the cranium.

Normal ICP in adults ranges from 0 to 15 mm Hg. An increase in ICP (such as from cerebral edema or intracranial

hemorrhage) decreases cerebral perfusion pressure and cerebral blood flow. Cerebral perfusion pressure (CPP), the pressure of blood flow through the brain, is the difference between the mean arterial pressure (MAP), the average (or mean) pressure against the arterial wall during a cardiac cycle, and ICP (CPP = MAP – ICP). Obviously, decreasing cerebral blood flow is a potential catastrophe because the brain depends on a constant supply of blood to furnish the oxygen and glucose it needs to survive.

The critical minimum threshold, or minimum CPP required to adequately perfuse the brain, is 60 mm Hg in the adult. A CPP of less than 60 mm Hg will lead to cerebral ischemia, potentially resulting in permanent neurologic impairment or even death. In fact, according to the Brain Trauma Foundation, a *single* drop in CPP below 60 mm Hg *doubles* the brain-injured patient's chance of death!

The body responds to a decrease in CPP by increasing MAP, resulting in cerebral vasodilation and increased cerebral blood flow; this process is called autoregulation. However, an increase in cerebral blood flow causes a further increase in ICP. As ICP continues to increase, CSF is forced from the cranium into the spinal cord.

Clearly, the patient with increased ICP is caught in the midst of a vicious cycle. As ICP increases, cerebral blood flow increases secondary to autoregulation, which in turn leads to a potentially fatal increase in ICP. Conversely, if cerebral blood flow decreases, CPP decreases as well, and the brain becomes ischemic.

CPP cannot be calculated in the prehospital setting. Therefore, prehospital treatment must focus on maintaining MAP, while mitigating ICP rise as much as possible—a very fine balance to maintain.

If increased ICP is not promptly treated in a definitive care setting, cerebral herniation may occur. In herniation, the brain is forced from the cranial vault, either through the foramen magnum or over the tentorium.

You must closely monitor the head-injured patient for signs and symptoms of increased ICP. The exact clinical signs encountered depend on the amount of pressure inside the skull and the extent of brain stem involvement. Early signs and symptoms include vomiting (often without nausea), headache, an altered level of consciousness, and seizures. Later, more ominous signs include hypertension (with a widening pulse pressure), bradycardia, and irregular respirations (Cushing's triad), plus a unilaterally dilated and nonreactive pupil (caused by oculomotor nerve compression), coma, and posturing. Decorticate (flexor) posturing is characterized by flexion of the

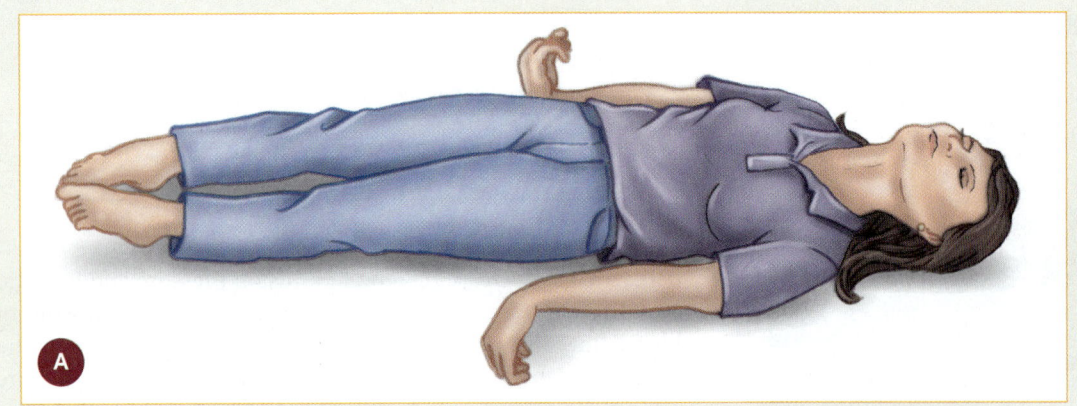

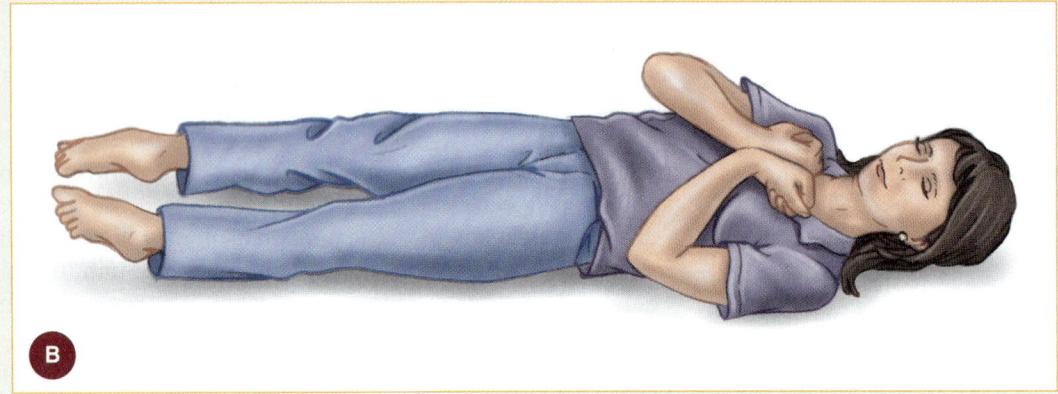

Figure 21-50 Posturing indicates significantly elevated ICP. **A.** Decerebrate (extensor) posturing. **B.** Decorticate (flexor) posturing. You can remember this by thinking of the arms being pulled into the "core" of the body.

Diffuse Axonal Injury

Diffuse axonal injury (DAI) is associated with or similar to a concussion. Unlike a concussion, however, this more severe diffuse brain injury is often associated with a poor prognosis. DAI involves stretching, shearing, or tearing of nerve fibres with subsequent axonal damage. An axon is a long, slender extension of a neuron (nerve cell) that conducts electrical impulses away from the neuronal soma (cell body) in the brain.

DAI most often results from high-speed, rapid acceleration–deceleration forces (such as motor vehicle collisions, significant falls). The severity and, thus, the prognosis of DAI depends on the degree of axonal damage (ie, stretching versus shearing or tearing); DAI is classified as being mild, moderate, or severe **Table 21-4 ▶**.

arms and extension of the legs; decerebrate (extensor) posturing is characterized by extension of the arms and legs **Figure 21-50 ▲**.

Diffuse Brain Injuries

Brain injuries are broadly classified as diffuse or focal. A diffuse brain injury is any injury that affects the entire brain. These injuries include cerebral concussion and diffuse axonal injury.

Cerebral Concussion

A cerebral concussion occurs when the brain is jarred around in the skull. This kind of mild diffuse brain injury is usually caused by rapid acceleration–deceleration forces (coup–contrecoup), such as those seen following motor vehicle collisions or falls.

A concussion injury results in transient dysfunction of the cerebral cortex; its resolution is usually spontaneous and rapid and is not associated with structural damage or permanent neurologic impairment. Signs of a concussion range from transient confusion and disorientation to confusion that may last for several minutes. Loss of consciousness may or may not occur. Retrograde amnesia, a loss of memory relating to events that occurred before the injury, or anterograde (posttraumatic) amnesia, a loss of memory relating to events that occurred after the injury, may follow a concussion.

Focal Brain Injuries

A focal brain injury is a specific, clearly defined brain injury (ie, it can be seen on a CT scan). Such injuries include cerebral contusions and intracranial hemorrhage.

Cerebral Contusion

In a cerebral contusion, brain tissue is bruised and damaged in a local area. Because a cerebral contusion is associated with physical damage to the brain, greater neurologic deficits (such as prolonged confusion, loss of consciousness) are more commonly observed than with a concussion. The same mechanisms of injury that cause concussions—acceleration–deceleration forces and direct blunt head trauma—also cause cerebral contusions.

The area of the brain most commonly affected by a cerebral contusion is the frontal lobe, although multiple areas of contusion can occur, especially following coup–contrecoup injuries. As with any bruise, the reaction of the injured tissue will be to swell. This swelling inevitably leads to increased ICP and the negative consequences that accompany it.

Intracranial Hemorrhage

The closed globe of the skull has no extra room for accumulation of blood, so bleeding inside the skull also increases ICP. Bleeding can occur between the skull and dura mater, beneath

Table 21-4	Diffuse Axonal Injury		
Pathophysiology	**Incidence**	**Signs and Symptoms**	**Prognosis**
Mild DAI			
Temporary neuronal dysfunction; minimal axonal damage	Most common result of blunt head trauma; concussion is an example	Loss of consciousness (brief, if present); confusion, disorientation, amnesia (retrograde and/or anterograde)	Minimal or no permanent neurologic impairment
Moderate DAI			
Axonal damage and minute petechial bruising of brain tissue; often associated with a basilar skull fracture	20% of all severe head injuries; 45% of all diffuse axonal injuries	Immediate loss of consciousness: secondary to involvement of the cerebral cortex or the reticular activating system of the brain stem; Residual effects: persistent confusion and disorientation; cognitive impairment (eg, inability to concentrate); frequent periods of anxiety; uncharacteristic mood swings; sensory/motor deficits (such as altered sense of taste or smell)	Survival likely, but permanent neurologic impairment common
Severe DAI			
Severe mechanical disruption of many axons in both cerebral hemispheres with extension into the brain stem; formerly called "brain stem injury"	16% of all severe head injuries; 36% of all diffuse axonal injuries	Immediate and prolonged loss of consciousness; posturing and other signs of increased ICP	Survival unlikely; most patients who survive never regain consciousness but remain in a persistent vegetative state

At the Scene

It is generally not possible, or necessary, to distinguish between a cerebral contusion and intracranial hemorrhage in the prehospital setting. Instead, you should recognize the signs of increasing ICP and appreciate that those signs represent a critically injured patient who needs immediate treatment and prompt transport to an appropriate facility.

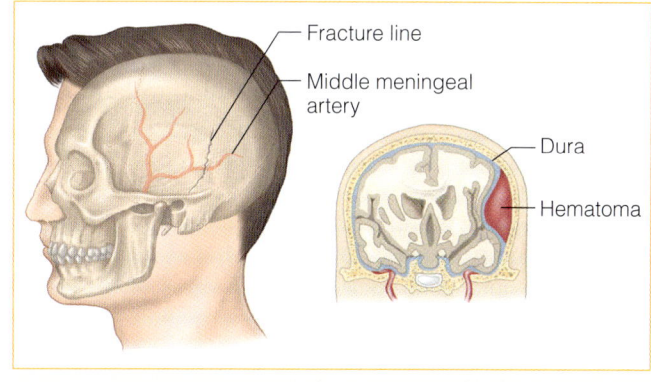

Figure 21-51 An epidural hematoma is usually the result of a blow to the head that produces a linear fracture of the temporal bone and damages the middle meningeal artery. Blood accumulates between the dura mater and the skull.

the dura mater but outside the brain, within the parenchyma (tissue) of the brain itself (intracerebral space), or into the CSF (subarachnoid space).

Epidural Hematoma

An epidural hematoma is an accumulation of blood between the skull and dura mater; it occurs in approximately 0.5% to 1% of all head injuries Figure 21-51 . An epidural hematoma is nearly always the result of a blow to the head that produces a linear fracture of the thin temporal bone. The middle meningeal artery courses along a groove in that bone, so it is prone to disruption when the temporal bone is fractured. In such a case, brisk arterial bleeding into the epidural space will result in rapidly progressing symptoms.

Often, the patient loses consciousness immediately following the injury; this is often followed by a brief period of consciousness ("lucid interval"), after which the patient lapses back into unconsciousness. Meanwhile, as ICP increases, the oculomotor nerve (third cranial nerve) is compressed against the tentorium, and the pupil on the side of the hematoma becomes fixed and dilated. Death will follow very rapidly without surgery to evacuate the hematoma.

Subdural Hematoma

A subdural hematoma is an accumulation of blood beneath the dura mater but outside the brain Figure 21-52 . It usually occurs after falls or injuries involving strong deceleration forces and occurs in approximately 5% of all head injuries. Subdural hematomas are more common than epidural hematomas and may or may not be associated with a skull fracture. Bleeding within the subdural space typically results from rupture of the veins that bridge the cerebral cortex and dura.

A subdural hematoma is associated with venous bleeding, so this type of hematoma—and the signs of increased ICP—typically develops more gradually than with an epidural hematoma. The patient with a subdural hematoma often

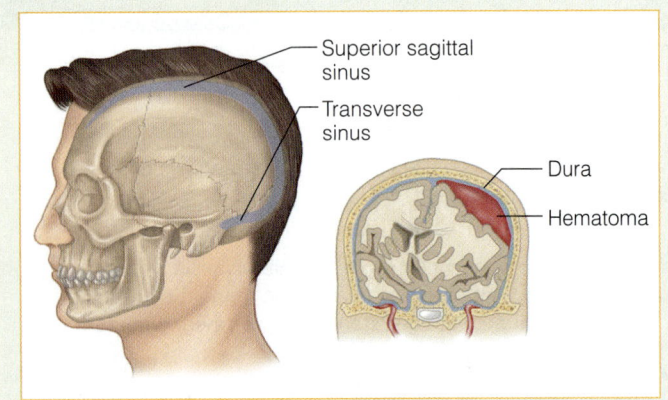

Figure 21-52 In a subdural hematoma, venous bleeding occurs beneath the dura mater but outside the brain.

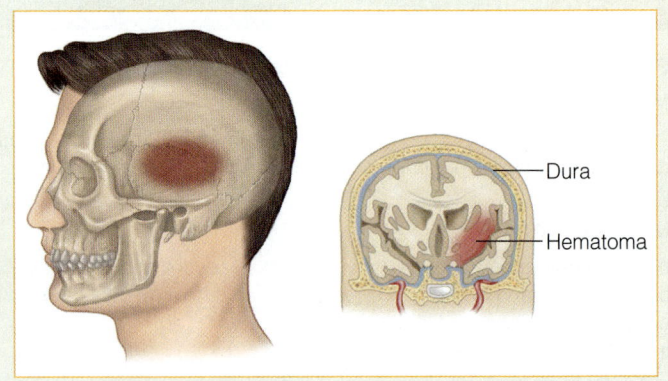

Figure 21-53 An intracerebral hematoma involves bleeding within the brain tissue itself.

experiences a fluctuating level of consciousness, focal neurologic signs (such as unilateral hemiparesis), or slurred speech.

Subdural hematomas are classified as acute (clinical signs developing within 24 hours following injury) or chronic (symptoms may not appear for as long as 2 weeks). Chronic subdural hematomas are more common in elderly patients, patients with alcoholism, patients with bleeding diatheses (such as hemophilia), and patients taking anticoagulants (such as warfarin).

Intracerebral Hematoma

An intracerebral hematoma involves bleeding within the brain tissue itself **Figure 21-53 ▶**. This type of injury can occur following a penetrating injury to the head or because of rapid deceleration forces.

Many small, deep intracerebral hemorrhages are associated with other brain injuries, such as DAI. The progression of increased ICP and neurologic deficit depends on several factors, including the presence of other brain injuries, the region of the brain involved (frontal and temporal lobes are most common), and the size of the hemorrhage. Once symptoms appear, the patient's condition often deteriorates quickly. Intracerebral hematomas have a high mortality rate, even if the hematoma is surgically evacuated.

Subarachnoid Hemorrhage

In a subarachnoid hemorrhage, bleeding occurs into the subarachnoid space, where the CSF circulates. It results in bloody CSF and signs of meningeal irritation (such as nuchal rigidity, headache). Common causes of a subarachnoid hematoma include trauma or rupture of an aneurysm or arteriovenous malformation.

The patient with a subarachnoid hematoma typically presents with a sudden, severe headache. This headache is often localized initially but later becomes diffuse secondary to increased meningeal irritation. As bleeding into the subarachnoid space increases, the patient experiences the signs and symptoms of increased ICP: decreased level of consciousness, pupillary changes, posturing, vomiting, and seizures.

You are the Paramedic Part 5

Your patient's condition is clearly critical, so you ask one of the fire fighters to drive the ambulance to a trauma centre located approximately 24 km away to free up your partner to work in the back with you. En route to the hospital, you establish a second large-bore IV line with normal saline. The patient's pupils are bilaterally dilated and sluggish to react.

Reassessment	Recording Time: 15 Minutes
Level of consciousness	Sedated with a Glasgow Coma Scale score of 3
Respirations	Intubated and ventilated at a rate of 10 breaths/min
Pulse	50 beats/min; regular and bounding
Skin	Warm and dry
Blood pressure	180/90 mm Hg
Spo$_2$	98% (intubated and ventilated with 100% oxygen)

9. Should this patient receive IV fluid boluses? When are IV fluid boluses indicated in a head-injured patient?

10. When is hyperventilation indicated for a head-injured patient? What ventilation rate defines hyperventilation in an adult?

Table 21-5	Signs and Symptoms of Head Injury

- Lacerations, contusions, or hematomas to the scalp
- Soft area or depression noted on palpation of the scalp
- Visible fractures or deformities of the skull
- Battle's sign or raccoon eyes
- CSF rhinorrhea or otorrhea
- Pupillary abnormalities
  - Unequal pupil size
  - Sluggish or nonreactive pupils
- A period of unresponsiveness
- Confusion or disorientation
- Repeatedly asking the same question(s) (perseveration)
- Amnesia (retrograde and/or anterograde)
- Combativeness or other abnormal behaviour
- Numbness or tingling in the extremities
- Loss of sensation and/or motor function
- Focal neurologic deficits
- Seizures
- Cushing's triad: hypertension, bradycardia, and irregular or erratic respirations
- Dizziness
- Visual disturbances, blurred vision, or double vision (diplopia)
- Nausea or vomiting
- Posturing (decorticate and/or decerebrate)

At the Scene

Ensure that any scene is safe before you enter it, regardless of the nature of the call, and don appropriate PPE before making physical contact with the patient. Once patient prehospital care begins, you must remain constantly aware of your surroundings and appreciate the fact that even the most docile scene can quickly turn dangerous.

A sudden, severe subarachnoid hematoma usually results in death. People who survive often have permanent neurologic impairment.

Assessment and Management of Head and Brain Injuries

Prehospital assessment and management of the head-injured patient should be guided by factors such as the severity of the injury and the patient's level of consciousness. As with any patient, your treatment priorities must be based on what will kill the patient *first*.

Assessment of Head and Brain Injuries

Motor vehicle collisions, direct blows, falls from heights, assault, and sports-related injuries are common causes of head and traumatic brain injuries. A patient who has experienced any of these events should immediately elevate your index of suspicion and prompt a search for signs and symptoms of these types of injuries 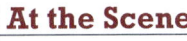 Table 21-5 ▲ . A deformed windshield or

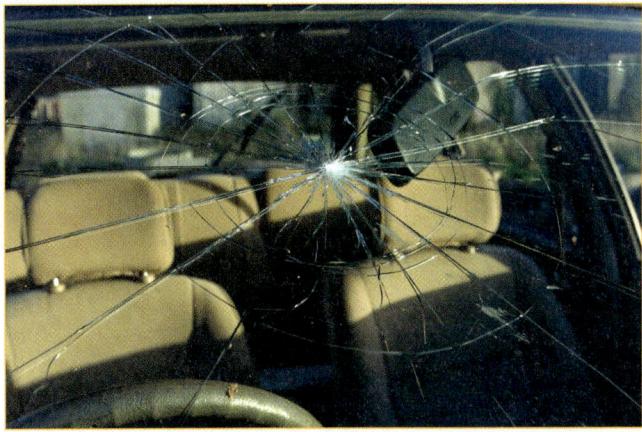

Figure 21-54 The classic "star" on the windshield after a motor-vehicle collision is a significant indicator of injury. Be alert for the signs and symptoms of head and cervical spine injury.

dented or cracked helmet indicates a major blow to the head Figure 21-54 ▲ .

Level of Consciousness

A change in the level of consciousness is the single most important observation that you can make when assessing the severity of brain injury. The level of consciousness usually indicates the extent of brain dysfunction. Whenever you suspect a head injury, you should perform a baseline neurologic assessment using the AVPU scale (Alert; responsive to Verbal stimuli; responsive to Pain; Unresponsive) and record the time.

Notes from Nancy

The most important single sign in the evaluation of a head-injured patient is a changing level of consciousness.

Use the more detailed Glasgow Coma Scale (GCS) when performing serial neurologic assessments of a head-injured patient Figure 21-55 ▶ . The GCS—a widely accepted method of assessing level of consciousness—is based on three independent measurements: eye opening, verbal response, and motor response. The GCS score is used to classify the severity of the patient's brain injury Table 21-6 ▶ and is a reliable predictor of the brain-injured patient's outcome.

Documentation and Communication

A single assessment of the patient's GCS score cannot reliably capture his or her clinical progression. Obtain a baseline GCS score and frequently (at least every 5 minutes if possible) reassess it in a head-injured patient. Document all GCS scores and the times they were obtained on the patient care report. The physician will compare his or her neurologic assessment with those you performed in the prehospital environment.

GLASGOW COMA SCALE

Eye Opening

Spontaneous	4
To Voice	3
To Pain	2
None	1

Verbal Response

Oriented	5
Confused	4
Inappropriate Words	3
Incomprehensible Words	2
None	1

Motor Response

Obeys Command	6
Localizes Pain	5
Withdraws (pain)	4
Flexion (pain)	3
Extension (pain)	2
None	1

Glasgow Coma Score Total	**15**

Figure 21-55 Glasgow Coma Scale scores should be assessed frequently in head-injured patients. The lower the score, the more severe the extent of brain injury.

Table 21-6	Brain Injury Classification Based on the GCS

- **13 to 15.** Mild traumatic brain injury
- **8 to 12.** Moderate traumatic brain injury
- **3 to 8.** Severe traumatic brain injury

Pupillary Assessment

Frequently monitor the size, equality, and reactivity of the patient's pupils. The nerves that control dilation and constriction of the pupils are very sensitive to ICP. When you shine a light into the eye, the pupil should briskly constrict. A pupil that is slow (sluggish) to constrict is a relatively early sign of increased ICP; a sluggish pupil could also indicate cerebral hypoxia.

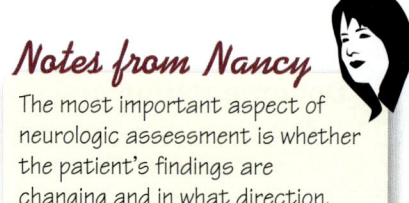

Notes from Nancy

The most important aspect of neurologic assessment is whether the patient's findings are changing and in what direction.

Unequal or bilaterally fixed and dilated ("blown") pupils are later, more ominous signs of increased ICP and indicate pressure on one or both oculomotor nerves **Figure 21-56 ▶**.

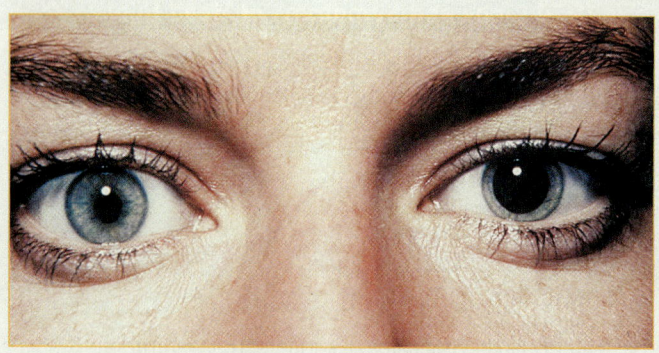

Figure 21-56 Unequal (shown above) or bilaterally fixed and dilated pupils in a head-injured patient are ominous signs and indicate a significantly increased ICP.

Table 21-7	Levels of ICP
Mild elevation	• Increased blood pressure; decreased pulse rate • Pupils still reactive • Cheyne-Stokes respirations (respirations that are fast and then become slow, with intervening periods of apnea) • Patient initially attempts to localize and remove painful stimuli; this is followed by withdrawal and extension • Effects are reversible *with prompt treatment*
Moderate elevation	• Widened pulse pressure and bradycardia • Pupils are sluggish or nonreactive • Central neurogenic hyperventilation (deep, rapid respirations; similar to Kussmaul, but without an acetone breath odour) • Decerebrate posturing • Survival possible but not without permanent neurologic deficit
Marked elevation	• Ipsilaterally fixed and dilated ("blown") pupil • Ataxic respirations (Biot respirations; characterized by irregular rate, pattern, and volume of breathing with intermittent periods of apnea) or absent respirations • Flaccid paralysis • Irregular pulse rate • Changes in the QRS complex, ST segment, or T wave • Fluctuating blood pressure; hypotension common • Most patients do not survive this level of ICP

Assessing ICP

Although ICP cannot be quantified (assigned a numeric value) in the prehospital setting, the severity of increase can be estimated based on the patient's clinical presentation **Table 21-7 ▲**. Critical treatment decisions for brain-injured patients are based on the presence or absence of certain key findings—specifically, posturing, hypotension or hypertension, and abnormal pupil signs. Use serial assessments of the patient's GCS scores and pupillary assessment as indicators of the progression of ICP.

Management of Head and Brain Injuries

Patients with head injuries often have cervical spine injuries as well. Therefore, as you begin your initial assessment of a head-injured patient, manually stabilize the cervical spine in a neutral, in-line position. Avoid moving the neck unnecessarily, and continue manual stabilization until full spinal motion restriction precautions have been applied.

Managing Airway and Breathing

The most important step in the treatment of any type of head injury is to establish and maintain a patent airway. Open the airway with the jaw-thrust maneuver if the patient is semiconscious or unconscious or is otherwise unable to maintain his or her own airway spontaneously.

Patients with a head injury often vomit (especially children). Therefore, after opening the airway, you must be prepared to roll the patient to the side—while maintaining spinal stabilization—to prevent aspiration. If it is safe to do so, manually remove any large debris from the patient's mouth by sweeping the oropharynx with your gloved finger. Use suction to clear secretions, such as blood or thin secretions from the oropharynx. *Mortality increases significantly if aspiration occurs.*

If the patient has a decreased level of consciousness, insert a basic airway adjunct (ie, oral or nasal airway). *Do not insert a nasal airway if CSF or rhinorrhea is present or if you suspect a nasal or basilar skull fracture.*

After you have cleared the airway, assess the patient's ventilatory status. Cerebral edema and ICP are aggravated by hypoxia and hypercarbia; therefore, you must constantly ensure adequate oxygenation and ventilation in any patient with a head injury.

Administer 100% oxygen via nonrebreathing mask if the patient is breathing adequately (ie, adequate rate and depth [tidal volume], regular respiratory pattern). An injured brain is even less tolerant of hypoxia than a healthy one, and research has demonstrated that prompt administration of supplemental oxygen can reduce the amount of brain damage and improve neurologic outcome.

If the respiratory centre of the brain (pons, medulla) has been injured, the rate, depth, or regularity of breathing may be ineffective. Ventilation may also be impaired by concomitant chest injuries or, if the spinal cord is injured, by paralysis of some or all of the respiratory muscles. Patients with inadequate ventilation, especially if associated with a decreased level of consciousness, should receive bag-valve-mask ventilation and 100% oxygen. Ventilate a brain-injured adult at a rate of 10 breaths/min or as dictated by local protocols. *Avoid routine hyperventilation of brain-injured patients.* Although hyperventilation causes cerebral vasoconstriction, which will shunt blood from the cranium and lower ICP, this outcome will merely provide additional room for the injured brain to swell or for more blood to accumulate in the skull. Most important, cerebral vasoconstriction shunts oxygen away from the brain and results in a drop in CPP, causing cerebral ischemia. The BTF recommends hyperventilation (20 breaths/min for adults) *only* if signs of cerebral herniation are present (**Table 21-8 ▾**). In such brain-injured patients, brief periods of hyperventilation may be beneficial. If available, end-tidal carbon dioxide ($EtCO_2$) should be monitored with digital capnometry. Optimally, you should

Table 21-8	**Signs of Cerebral Herniation**

Unresponsive patient with both of the following:

- Asymmetric (unequal) pupils *or* bilaterally fixed and dilated pupils
- Decerebrate (extensor) posturing *or* no motor response to painful stimuli

You are the Paramedic Part 6

Your estimated time of arrival at the trauma centre is 5 minutes. Without time to perform a detailed physical examination, you reassess the patient's vital functions and call in your radio report to the receiving facility.

Reassessment	Recording Time: 20 Minutes
Level of consciousness	Sedated with a Glasgow Coma Scale score of 3
Respirations	Intubated and ventilated at a rate of 10 breaths/min
Pulse	70 beats/min; regular and bounding
Skin	Warm and dry
Blood pressure	170/80 mm Hg
SpO_2	98% (intubated and ventilated with 100% oxygen)

11. Should you be concerned with the exact etiology of this patient's head injury? Why or why not?
12. What are the most important interventions you can perform to maintain cerebral perfusion in this patient?

ventilate the patient to maintain $EtCO_2$ of 35 to 40—an approximation of arterial $PaCO_2$ between 30 and 35 mm Hg. Under no circumstances should the $EtCO_2$ be allowed to ever drop below 30 mm Hg corresponding to $PaCO_2$ below 25 mm Hg as the subsequent vasoconstriction will almost assuredly result in brain death due to anoxia.

Endotracheal intubation of a head-injured patients in the prehospital environment is controversial. The decision to intubate requires special precautions or it may precipitate dangerous increases in ICP. The paramedic may need to factor in such issues as distance from destination centre, his or her skill set, and local medical protocols. This must be balanced against the potential for hypercarbia, hypoxia, or hypotension that can occur during the intubation process. This is especially possible if pharmacology is used to facilitate intubation. If intubation of a head-injured patient is required (eg, unresponsive, unable to effectively perform bag-valve-mask ventilation), observe the following guidelines:

1. Preoxygenate with 100% oxygen for at least 2 to 3 minutes or to a saturation of 100%.

2. Administer 1 to 1.5 mg/kg of lidocaine IV push. Lidocaine has been shown to blunt an acute increase in ICP, which may occur during intubation.

3. Perform intubation with the patient's head in a neutral in-line position. Intubation of a head-injured patient or any patient with significant trauma should be performed by two people: one to maintain manual stabilization of the patient's head and the other to intubate.

If a head-injured patient requires intubation but will otherwise not tolerate laryngoscopy and ET tube placement (for example, because of combativeness or clenched teeth [trismus]), perform pharmacologically assisted intubation (ie, RSI). This procedure involves using a sedative-hypnotic drug (such as midazolam [Versed]) and a neuromuscular blocking drug (such as succinylcholine) to facilitate placement of the ET tube. (Refer to Chapter 11 for more on pharmacologically assisted intubation.)

At the Scene

Effectively managing a brain-injured patient's airway and ensuring adequate oxygenation and ventilation are absolutely critical to the patient's survival. Of course, severe bleeding can also result in death. Therefore, airway management and bleeding control should be performed simultaneously by you and your partner.

Closely monitor the patient's oxygen saturation (SpO$_2$), and maintain it at 95% or higher.

Managing Circulation

After you have secured the patient's airway and ensured adequate oxygenation and ventilation, you must turn your attention to supporting the patient's circulation. Control major bleeding with direct pressure, taking care not to apply excessive pressure to scalp lacerations in which an underlying fracture is present or suspected. Active bleeding will cause or

worsen hypoxia, as well as decrease CPP, by reducing the number of oxygen-carrying red blood cells.

An isolated closed head injury will not cause hypovolemic shock in an adult because the skull does not have enough room to accommodate large volumes of blood. If signs of shock are present (ie, persistent hypotension, tachycardia, diaphoresis), carefully assess the patient for occult injuries, such as intra-abdominal or intrathoracic hemorrhage.

Establish at least one large-bore IV with normal saline or lactated Ringer's solution. Do not administer dextrose-containing solutions (such as 5% dextrose in water [D$_5$W]) because they may worsen cerebral edema. The *only* indication for administering glucose to a head-injured patient is confirmed hypoglycemia (ie, a glucometer reading < 4 mmol/l).

Patients with a severe closed head injury are often hypertensive—a sign of the body's autoregulatory response. Restrict your use of IV fluids for these patients to minimize cerebral edema and ICP, typically at a rate of 25 to 50 ml/hr. However, if hypotension develops, infuse fluids as needed—usually 20 ml/kg boluses or as directed by direct medical control—to maintain a systolic BP of at least 90 mm Hg. Hypotension in a brain-

At the Scene

When assessing and managing an adult with a severe head injury, remember the Brain Trauma Foundation's "90-90-9 rule":

- A *single* drop in the patient's oxygen saturation (SpO$_2$) to less than 90% doubles his or her chance of death.
- A *single* drop in the patient's systolic BP to less than 90 mm Hg doubles his or her chance of death.
- A *single* drop in the patient's GCS score to less than 9 doubles his or her chance of death. A drop in the GCS score of two or more points, at any time, also doubles mortality.

injured patient can be lethal because it may decrease CPP with resultant cerebral ischemia, permanent brain damage, and death.

Severe head injuries, especially if the lower brain stem is involved, can produce a variety of cardiac rhythm disturbances, so use a cardiac monitor for any critically injured patient. Use of a cardiac monitor also allows you to monitor the patient for acute heart rate changes. If cardiac arrest occurs, follow the ACLS pulseless arrest protocol.

Other Management
Thermal Management

Do not allow the patient to become overheated. Patients with head injury, unlike those with shock, can develop a very high body temperature (hyperpyrexia), which in turn may worsen the condition of the brain. Do not cover the patient with blankets if the ambient temperature is 21°C or higher.

Treatment of Associated Injuries

If the patient has an open fracture of the skull with brain tissue exposed, cover it *lightly* with a sterile dressing that has been moistened with sterile saline. Likewise, for leakage of CSF from the ears or nose, apply loose sterile dressings, just to keep the area clean. Objects impaled in the skull should be stabilized in place and protected from being jarred.

Pharmacologic Therapy

Pharmacologic therapy, other than that used to facilitate intubation or treat seizures, is usually not indicated for brain-injured patients in the prehospital setting. However, if transport will be prolonged, direct medical control may order the administration of certain medications, such as mannitol (Osmitrol) and/or furosemide (Lasix) to reduce cerebral edema and decrease ICP.

Seizures in a brain-injured patient must be terminated as soon as possible, lest they provoke further increases in ICP or body temperature. Benzodiazepines, such as diazepam (Valium) or lorazepam (Ativan), should be used to control seizure activity in brain-injured patients. Follow local protocol or contact direct medical control regarding the doses of these drugs.

Transport Considerations

Prompt transport to a definitive care facility (ie, a trauma centre) is crucial to survival of a brain-injured patient. If available, consider air transport if your transport time will be prolonged. If transporting the patient by ground, do so expeditiously, yet cautiously.

Many patients with severe brain injuries and increased ICP require neurosurgical intervention. The extra time it takes to move the patient from one hospital to another could mean the difference between life and death. Therefore, transport the patient directly to a trauma centre that has neurosurgical capabilities, even if it means bypassing the nearest hospital. Every paramedic should know their local and regional hospital bypass policies for brain injured patients to ensure the patient is transported to the most appropriate facility as expeditiously as possible.

You are the Paramedic Summary

1. What should be your initial concern about this patient?

Any motorcycle collision is a significant mechanism of injury, but the fact that the patient was not wearing a helmet dramatically increases his risk of mortality due to a severe head injury. This should be your primary concern, especially considering your general impression of the patient (lying on the ground, not moving).

2. How should you direct your initial care of this patient?

Your first action is to manually stabilize the patient's head while simultaneously opening his airway with the jaw-thrust maneuver. Then, you should perform an initial assessment to identify and treat life-threatening injuries and/or conditions.

3. How will you manage this patient's airway?

This patient's airway is in serious jeopardy! He has two major airway problems that must be addressed promptly: blood in the oropharynx, which places him at *immediate* risk for aspiration, and slow, irregular respirations that are clearly not adequate. You should suction his oropharynx for no more than 15 seconds and then provide bag-valve-mask ventilation with 100% oxygen for 2 minutes. Continue this alternating pattern of suctioning and ventilating until his airway is clear or has been secured with an ET tube.

4. When would it be appropriate to intubate this patient?

Do not immediately intubate! Endotracheal intubation should not be performed before adequate oxygenation and ventilation have been achieved with basic means (ie, bag-valve-mask ventilation and airway adjunct). Furthermore, you must clear this patient's airway with suction first because (1) blood in the airway will make for a difficult intubation and (2) attempting to intubate when you know it will be difficult—especially if the attempt would clearly be facilitated by clearing the airway with suction—will merely increase the risk of hypoxia. Few situations necessitate immediate intubation in any patient; this patient is no exception.

5. How can facial trauma complicate airway management?

Many factors can complicate airway management in a patient with facial trauma, including blood in the airway and unstable facial bones (makes for a difficult mask-to-face seal). You should, therefore, anticipate a difficult intubation and be prepared to secure the airway with other means (such as cricothyrotomy) if intubation is unsuccessful or impossible.

6. Is this patient in hypovolemic shock? Why or why not?

Although the mechanism of injury and bilaterally deformed femurs are clearly a recipe for hypovolemic shock, the patient's present vital signs are not suggestive of this diagnosis. Typical signs of shock include rapid, shallow respirations while this patient's are slow and irregular; a rapid, weak pulse (his pulse quality is bounding); and cool, clammy skin (his skin is warm and dry). Although hypotension is a late sign of shock—and a normal BP does not rule out shock—your patient's BP (140/90 mm Hg) is higher than one would expect, even in a state of compensated shock. Perform a careful assessment to detect any early signs of shock, and implement immediate treatment should they appear, before the patient's condition deteriorates.

7. What do the patient's vital signs indicate?

Hypertension, a slowing pulse rate, and irregular respirations, especially with a mechanism of injury that suggests head injury (motorcycle collision without a helmet), constitute the Cushing's triad, a classic sign of raised intracranial pressure. When the brain is injured, the body's autoregulatory mechanism shunts more blood to the injured brain, which causes a rise in systemic arterial BP and reflex bradycardia. Brain stem involvement results in a variety of abnormal respiratory patterns (such as Cheyne-Stokes respirations, central neurogenic hyperventilation, Biot respirations).

8. What else should you assess for in this patient?

In addition to closely monitoring the patient's BP and pulse rate, you should perform and document serial assessments of his GCS scores. Other signs to assess for in the head-injured patient include cranial deformities or depressions; pupil size, equality, and reactivity; abnormal posturing (decorticate and/or decerebrate); CSF rhinorrhea or otorrhea; Battle's sign; and raccoon eyes. (Battle's sign and raccoon eyes are often not evident in the prehospital setting.)

9. Should this patient receive IV fluid boluses? When are IV fluid boluses indicated in a head-injured patient?

In the absence of hypotension, IV fluids should be restricted in a head-injured patient to avoid increasing ICP; set your IV line(s) to keep vein open at between 25 to 50 ml/hour. Persistent hypotension in a head-injured adult indicates lower brain stem herniation or occult hemorrhage elsewhere in the body. Regardless of the etiology, a single episode of hypotension in a head-injured adult (systolic BP < 90 mm Hg) can be lethal; it results in decreased CPP and cerebral ischemia and doubles mortality. Closely monitor the patient's BP, and be prepared to infuse isotonic crystalloids to maintain a systolic BP of at least 90 mm Hg.

10. When is hyperventilation indicated for a head-injured patient? What ventilation rate defines hyperventilation in an adult?

Brief periods of hyperventilation in a brain-injured adult (20 breaths/min) may be beneficial and are indicated *only* if signs of cerebral herniation are present. Signs of cerebral herniation include an unresponsive patient with *both* of the following: (1) unequal pupils *or* bilaterally fixed and dilated pupils *and* (2) decerebrate (extensor) posturing *or* no motor response to painful stimuli. Do not routinely hyperventilate brain-injured patients because doing so will cause cerebral vasoconstriction. Although hyperventilation may transiently decrease ICP by shunting blood from the brain, it may also decrease CPP and may cause cerebral ischemia.

11. Should you be concerned with the exact etiology of this patient's head injury? Why or why not?

It is not possible to determine the exact etiology of this patient's head injury in the prehospital setting. The underlying injury that is causing his increased ICP can be determined only in a trauma centre with a computed tomographic (CT) scan of the head. Your role is to recognize the signs of increased ICP, provide aggressive prehospital treatment to maintain CPP, and rapidly transport the patient to an appropriate facility.

12. What are the most important interventions you can perform to maintain cerebral perfusion in this patient?

Three factors will cause CPP (and cerebral blood flow) to fall: hypoxia, hypercarbia, and hypotension. Therefore, the most important prehospital interventions for a brain-injured adult with increased ICP include *constantly* maintaining adequate oxygenation and ventilation and maintaining a systolic BP of at least 90 mm Hg. To do so, you must ensure that the patient's airway remains patent and monitor his or her oxygen saturation and blood pressure closely. Ventilation rates should be dictated by the presence or absence of signs of brain herniation. $ETco_2$ monitoring can assist you in approximating the patient's $Paco_2$ level. The $ETco_2$ should be maintained in a range of 35 to 40 mm Hg (slightly decreased from normal). This will approximate a $Paco_2$ level of 30 to 35 mm Hg.

Prep Kit

Ready for Review

- A strong working knowledge of anatomy and physiology of the face, head, and brain is essential to accurately assess and manage patients with injuries to these locations.
- Personal safety is your primary concern when treating any patient with head or face trauma; never enter an unsafe scene.
- Head and face trauma most often result from direct trauma or rapid acceleration–deceleration forces.
- Trauma to the face can range from a broken nose to more severe injuries, including massive soft-tissue trauma, maxillofacial fractures, oral or dental trauma, and eye injuries.
- Your primary concerns with assessing and managing a patient with facial trauma are to ensure a patent airway and maintain adequate oxygenation and ventilation.
- Remove impaled objects in the face or throat *only* if they impair airway patency or breathing or if they interfere with your ability to effectively manage the airway. Otherwise, stabilize them in place and protect them from being jarred.
- Never remove impaled objects from the eye; stabilize them in place and put a protective cone (such as a cup) over the object to prevent accidental movement along with bandaging the unaffected eye to prevent sympathetic movement.
- Flush burns to the eye with copious amounts of sterile saline or sterile water. Never use chemical antidotes when treating burn injuries to the eye.
- The primary threat from oral or dental trauma is oropharyngeal bleeding and aspiration of blood or broken teeth. Keep the airway clear, and ensure adequate oxygenation and ventilation. Endotracheal intubation may be required.
- Any patient with head or face trauma should be suspected of having a spinal injury. Apply spinal motion restriction precautions as indicated.
- The skull is a rigid, unyielding container that does not accommodate a swelling brain or accumulations of blood.
- Normal ICP is 0 to 15 mm Hg in adults. Increased ICP can squeeze the brain against the interior of the skull and/or press it into sharp edges within the cranium. If severely increased ICP is not promptly treated, cerebral herniation will occur.
- CPP is the pressure of blood flowing through the brain; it is the difference between the MAP and ICP.
- If CPP drops below 60 mm Hg in the adult, cerebral ischemia will likely occur, resulting in permanent brain damage or death.
- Begin treatment of a head-injured patient by stabilizing the cervical spine, opening the airway with the jaw-thrust maneuver, and assessing the ABCs.
- All head-injured patients should receive 100% oxygen as soon as possible. If the patient is breathing adequately, apply a nonrebreathing mask set at 15 l/min. If the patient is breathing inadequately, assist ventilation and consider intubation.
- Ventilate a brain-injured adult at a rate of 10 breaths/min. Avoid routine hyperventilation unless signs of cerebral herniation are present. Hyperventilation in a brain-injured adult is defined as a ventilation rate of 20 breaths/min.
- Restrict IV fluids in a head-injured patient unless hypotension (systolic BP < 90 mm Hg) is present. Hypotension in a brain-injured patient should be treated with crystalloid fluid boluses in a quantity sufficient to maintain a systolic BP of at least 90 mm Hg.
- Frequently monitor a head-injured patient's level of consciousness, and document your findings. The GCS is an effective, reliable tool. The GCS must be repeated frequently if it is to be a reliable indicator of the patient's clinical progression.
- Intubation of a brain-injured patient may require pharmacologic adjuncts (such as sedation, neuromuscular-blocking drugs).
- Seizures may occur in a brain-injured patient and can aggravate ICP and cause or worsen cerebral ischemia. Treat seizures with a benzodiazepine (such as diazepam, lorazepam).
- A brain-injured patient's survival depends on recognition of the injury, prompt and aggressive prehospital care, and rapid transport to a trauma centre that has neurosurgical capabilities. Consider air transport if ground transport time will be prolonged.

Vital Vocabulary

alveolar ridges The ridges between the teeth, which are covered with thickened connective tissue and epithelium.

alveoli Small pits or cavities, such as the sockets for the teeth.

anisocoria A condition in which the pupils are not of equal size.

anterior chamber The anterior area of the globe between the lens and the cornea that is filled with aqueous humour.

anterograde (posttraumatic) amnesia Loss of memory relating to events that occurred after the injury.

aqueous humour The clear, watery fluid in the anterior chamber of the globe.

arachnoid The middle membrane of the three meninges that enclose the brain and spinal cord.

auditory ossicles The bones that function in hearing and are located deep within cavities of the temporal bone.

auricle The large outside portion of the ear through which sound waves enter the ear; also called the pinna.

autoregulation An increase in mean arterial pressure to compensate for decreased cerebral perfusion pressure; compensatory response of the body to shunt blood to the brain; manifests clinically as hypertension.

axon Long, slender extension of a neuron (nerve cell) that conducts electrical impulses away from the neuronal soma.

basal ganglia Structures located deep within the cerebrum, diencephalon, and midbrain that have an important role in coordination of motor movements and posture.

basilar skull fractures Usually occur following diffuse impact to the head (such as falls, motor vehicle collisions); generally result from extension of a linear fracture to the base of the skull and can be difficult to diagnose with a radiograph (x-ray).

Battle's sign Bruising over the mastoid bone behind the ear commonly seen following a basilar skull fracture; also called retroauricular ecchymosis.

Biot respirations Characterized by an irregular rate, pattern, and volume of breathing with intermittent periods of apnea; also called ataxic respirations.

blowout fracture A fracture to the floor of the orbit usually caused by a blow to the eye.

brain Part of the central nervous system located within the cranium; contains billions of neurons that serve a variety of vital functions.

brain stem The midbrain, pons, and medulla, collectively.

central neurogenic hyperventilation Deep, rapid respirations; similar to Kussmaul, but without an acetone breath odour; commonly seen following brain stem injury.

central vision The visualization of objects directly in front of you.

cerebellum The region of the brain essential in coordinating muscle movements in the body; also called the athlete's brain.

cerebral concussion Occurs when the brain is jarred around in the skull; a mild diffuse brain injury that does not result in structural damage or permanent neurologic impairment.

cerebral contusion A focal brain injury in which brain tissue is bruised and damaged in a defined area.

cerebral cortex The largest portion of the cerebrum; regulates voluntary skeletal movement and one's level of awareness—a part of consciousness.

cerebral edema Cerebral water; causes or contributes to swelling of the brain.

cerebral perfusion pressure (CPP) The pressure of blood flow through the brain; the difference between the mean arterial pressure (MAP) and intracranial pressure (ICP).

cerebrospinal fluid (CSF) Fluid produced in the ventricles of the brain that flows in the subarachnoid space and bathes the meninges.

cerebrospinal rhinorrhea Cerebrospinal fluid drainage from the nose.

cerebrum The largest portion of the brain; responsible for higher functions, such as reasoning; divided into right and left hemispheres, or halves.

Cheyne-Stokes respirations The respirations that are fast and then become slow, with intervening periods of apnea; commonly seen following brain stem injury.

choroid plexus Specialized cells within the hollow areas in the ventricles of the brain that produce CSF.

cochlea The shell-shaped structure within the inner ear that contains the organ of Corti.

cochlear duct A canal within the cochlea that receives vibrations from the ossicles.

conjunctiva A thin, transparent membrane that covers the sclera and internal surfaces of the eyelids.

conjunctivitis An inflammation of the conjunctivae that usually is caused by bacteria, viruses, allergies, or foreign bodies; should be considered highly contagious; also called pink eye.

cornea The transparent anterior portion of the eye that overlies the iris and pupil.

coronal suture The point where the parietal bones join with the frontal bone.

coup-contrecoup injury Dual impacting of the brain into the skull; coup injury occurs at the point of impact; contrecoup injury occurs on the opposite side of impact, as the brain rebounds.

cranial vault The bones that encase and protect the brain, including the parietal, temporal, frontal, occipital, sphenoid, and ethmoid bones; also called the cranium or skull.

craniofacial disjunction A Le Fort III fracture; involves a fracture of all of the midfacial bones, thus separating the entire midface from the cranium.

cribriform plate A horizontal bone perforated with numerous foramina for the passage of the olfactory nerve filaments from the nasal cavity.

crista galli A prominent bony ridge in the centre of the anterior fossa and the point of attachment of the meninges.

critical minimum threshold Minimum cerebral perfusion pressure required to adequately perfuse the brain; 60 mm Hg in the adult.

crown The part of the tooth that is external to the gum.

Cushing's triad Hypertension (with a widening pulse pressure), bradycardia, and irregular respirations; classic trio of findings associated with increased ICP.

cusps Points at the top of a tooth.

decerebrate (extensor) posturing Abnormal posture characterized by extension of the arms and legs; indicates pressure on the brain stem.

decorticate (flexor) posturing Abnormal posture characterized by flexion of the arms and extension of the legs; indicates pressure on the brain stem.

dentin The principal mass of the tooth, which is made up of a material that is much more dense and stronger than bone.

depressed skull fractures Result from high-energy direct trauma to a small surface area of the head with a blunt object (such as a baseball bat to the head); commonly result in bony fragments being driven into the brain, causing injury.

diencephalon The part of the brain between the brain stem and the cerebrum that includes the thalamus, subthalamus, and hypothalamus.

diffuse axonal injury (DAI) Diffuse brain injury that is caused by stretching, shearing, or tearing of nerve fibres with subsequent axonal damage.

diffuse brain injury Any injury that affects the entire brain.

diplopia Double vision.

dura mater The outermost layer of the three meninges that enclose the brain and spinal cord; it is the toughest meningeal layer.

dysconjugate gaze Paralysis of gaze or lack of coordination between the movements of the two eyes.

dysphagia Difficulty swallowing.

epidural hematoma An accumulation of blood between the skull and dura.

epistaxis Nosebleed.

external auditory canal The area in which sound waves are received from the auricle (pinna) before they travel to the eardrum; also called the ear canal.

external ear One of three anatomical parts of the ear; it contains the pinna, the ear canal, and the external portion of the tympanic membrane.

facial nerve The seventh cranial nerve; supplies motor activity to all muscles of facial expression, the sense of taste to the anterior two thirds of the tongue and cutaneous sensation to the external ear, tongue, and palate.

focal brain injury A specific, well-defined brain injury.

fontanelles The soft spots in the skull of a newborn and infant where the sutures of the skull have not yet grown together.

foramen magnum The large opening at the base of the skull through which the spinal cord exits the brain.

foramina Small natural openings, perforations, or orifices, such as in the bones of the cranial vault; plural of foramen.

frontal lobe The portion of the brain that is important in voluntary motor actions and personality traits.

galea aponeurotica Tough, tendinous layer of the scalp.

Glasgow Coma Scale (GCS) A widely accepted method of assessing level of consciousness that is based on three independent measurements: eye opening, verbal response, and motor response.

globe The eyeball.

glossopharyngeal nerve Ninth cranial nerve; supplies motor fibres to the pharyngeal muscle, providing taste sensation to the posterior portion of the tongue, and carrying parasympathetic fibres to the parotid gland.

hard palate The bony anterior part of the palate, which forms the roof of the mouth.

head injury A traumatic insult to the head that may result in injury to soft tissue, bony structures, or the brain.

hemoptysis Coughing up blood.

herniation Process in which tissue is forced out of its normal position, such as when the brain is forced from the cranial vault, either through the foramen magnum or over the tentorium.

hyoid bone A bone at the base of the tongue that supports the tongue and its muscles.

hyperpyrexia A very high body temperature.

hyphema Bleeding into the anterior chamber of the eye; results from direct ocular trauma.

hypoglossal nerve Twelfth cranial nerve; provides motor function to the muscles of the tongue and throat.

hypothalamus The most inferior portion of the diencephalon; responsible for control of many body functions, including heart rate, digestion, sexual development, temperature regulation, emotion, hunger, thirst, and regulation of the sleep cycle.

inner ear One of three anatomical parts of the ear; it consists of the cochlea and semicircular canals.

intracerebral hematoma Bleeding within the brain tissue (parenchyma) itself; also referred to as an intraparenchymal hematoma.

intracranial pressure (ICP) The pressure within the cranial vault; normally 0 to 15 mm Hg in adults.

iris The pigmented portion of the eye.

lacrimal apparatus The structures in which tears are secreted and drained from the eye.

lambdoid suture The point where the occipital bones attach to the parietal bones.

Le Fort fractures Maxillary fractures that are classified into three categories based on their anatomical location.

lens A transparent body within the globe that focuses light rays.

limbic system Structures within the cerebrum and diencephalon that influence emotions, motivation, mood, and sensations of pain and pleasure.

linear skull fractures Account for 80% of skull fractures; also referred to as nondisplaced skull fractures; commonly occur in the temporal-parietal region of the skull; not associated with deformities to the skull.

malocclusion Misalignment of the teeth.

mandible The movable lower jaw bone.

mandibular nerve A sensory and motor nerve that supplies the muscles of chewing and skin of the lower lip, chin, temporal region, and part of the external ear.

mastication The process of chewing with the teeth.

mastoid process A cone-shaped section of bone at the base of the temporal bone.

maxillary nerve A sensory nerve; supplies the skin on the posterior part of the side of the nose, lower eyelid, cheek, and upper lip.

mean arterial pressure (MAP) The average (or mean) pressure against the arterial wall during a cardiac cycle.

mediastinitis Inflammation of the mediastinum, often a result of the gastric contents leaking into the thoracic cavity after esophageal perforation.

medulla Continuous inferiorly with the spinal cord; serves as a conduction pathway for ascending and descending nerve tracts; coordinates heart rate, blood vessel diameter, breathing, swallowing, vomiting, coughing, and sneezing.

meninges A set of three tough membranes, the dura mater, arachnoid, and pia mater, that encloses the entire brain and spinal cord.

middle ear One of three anatomical parts of the ear; it consists of the inner portion of the tympanic membrane and the ossicles.

nasal cavity The chamber inside the nose that lies between the floor of the cranium and the roof of the mouth.

nasal septum The separation between the right and left nostrils.

nasolacrimal duct The passage through which tears drain from the lacrimal sacs into the nasal cavity.

neuronal soma The body of a neuron (nerve cell).

occipital condyles Articular surfaces on the occipital bone where the skull articulates with the atlas on the vertebral column.

occipital lobe The portion of the brain that is responsible for the processing of visual information.

oculomotor nerve Third cranial nerve; innervates the muscles that cause motion of the eyeballs and upper eyelid.

olfactory nerves Participates in the transmission of scent impulses.

ophthalmic nerve A sensory nerve that supplies the skin of the forehead, the upper eyelid, and conjunctiva.

optic nerve The second cranial nerve that enters the eyeball posteriorly, through the optic foramen.

orbits Bony cavities in the frontal part of the skull that enclose and protect the eyes.

organ of Corti A structure located in the cochlea that contains hairs that are stimulated by vibrations to form nerve impulses that travel to the brain and are perceived as sound.

ossicles The three small bones in the inner ear that transmit vibrations to the cochlear duct at the oval window.

oval window An oval opening between the middle ear and the vestibule.

palatine bone An irregularly shaped bone found in the posterior part of the nasal cavity.

paranasal sinuses The sinuses, or hollowed sections of bone in the front of the head, that are lined with mucous membrane and drain into the nasal cavity.

parietal lobe The portion of the brain that is the site for reception and evaluation of most sensory information, except smell, hearing, and vision.

periorbital ecchymosis Bruising under or around the orbits that is commonly seen following a basilar skull fracture; also called raccoon eyes.

peripheral vision Visualization of lateral objects while looking forward.

pia mater The innermost and thinnest of the three meninges that enclose the brain and spinal cord; rests directly on the brain and spinal cord.

pinna The large outside portion of the ear through which sound waves enter the ear; also called the auricle.

pons Lies below the midbrain and above the medulla and contains numerous important nerve fibres, including those for sleep, respiration, and the medullary respiratory centre.

posterior chamber The posterior area of the globe between the lens and the iris.

primary brain injury An injury to the brain and its associated structures that is a direct result of impact to the head.

pulp Specialized connective tissue within the pulp cavity of a tooth.

pupil The circular opening in the centre of the eye through which light passes to the lens.

raccoon or panda eyes Bruising under or around the orbits that is commonly seen following a basilar skull fracture; also called periorbital ecchymosis.

reticular activating system (RAS) Located in the upper brain stem; responsible for maintenance of consciousness, specifically one's level of arousal.

retina A delicate 10-layered structure of nervous tissue located in the rear of the interior of the globe that receives light and generates nerve signals that are transmitted to the brain through the optic nerve.

retinal detachment Separation of the inner layers of the retina from the underlying choroid, the vascular membrane that nourishes the retina.

retrograde amnesia Loss of memory relating to events that occurred before the injury.

sagittal suture The point of the skull where the parietal bones join.

sclera The white part of the eye.

secondary brain injury The "after effects" of the primary injury; includes abnormal processes such as cerebral edema, increased intracranial pressure, cerebral ischemia and hypoxia, and infection; onset is often delayed following the primary brain injury.

skull The structure at the top of the axial skeleton that houses the brain and consists of 28 bones that comprise the auditory ossicles, the cranium, and the face.

subarachnoid hemorrhage Bleeding into the subarachnoid space, where the cerebrospinal fluid (CSF) circulates.

subarachnoid space The space located between the pia mater and the arachnoid mater.

subdural hematoma An accumulation of blood beneath the dura but outside the brain.

subthalamus The part of the diencephalon that is involved in controlling motor functions.

sympathetic eye movement The movement of both eyes in unison.

temporal lobe The portion of the brain that has an important role in hearing and memory.

temporomandibular joint (TMJ) The joint between the temporal bone and the posterior condyle that allows for movements of the mandible.

tentorium A structure that separates the cerebral hemispheres from the cerebellum and brain stem.

thalamus The part of the diencephalon that processes most sensory input and influences mood and general body movements, especially those associated with fear or rage.

tracheal transection Traumatic separation of the trachea from the larynx.

traumatic brain injury (TBI) A traumatic insult to the brain capable of producing physical, intellectual, emotional, social, and vocational changes.

trigeminal nerve Fifth cranial nerve; supplies sensation to the scalp, forehead, face, and lower jaw and innervates the muscles of mastication, the throat, and the inner ear.

trismus Clenching of the teeth owing to spasm of the jaw muscles.

tympanic membrane A thin membrane that separates the middle ear from the inner ear and sets up vibrations in the ossicles; also called the eardrum.

ventricles Specialized hollow areas in the brain.

visual cortex The area in the brain where signals from the optic nerve are converted into visual images.

vitreous humour A jellylike substance found in the posterior compartment of the eye between the lens and the retina.

zygomatic arch The bone that extends along the front of the skull below the orbit.

Assessment in Action

Your unit is dispatched to a residence for an assault. An on-scene police officer advises you that the scene is safe to enter. Your response time to the scene is approximately 7 minutes. When you arrive, a police officer escorts you to the patient, a man in his late 30s. According to witnesses, the patient was struck in the side of the head with a steel pipe during an altercation with his neighbour. As you approach the patient, you note that he is lying in a supine position and is not moving; there is no gross bleeding. The neighbour is in police custody.

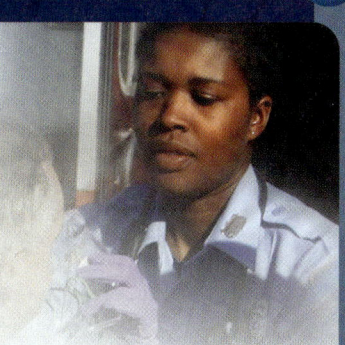

1. **After your partner manually stabilizes the patient's cervical spine, you should:**
   A. vigorously shake the patient to determine his level of consciousness.
   B. open his airway with the head tilt–chin lift maneuver or tongue jaw lift.
   C. suction his oropharynx for 30 seconds to ensure that it is clear of blood.
   D. determine his level of consciousness, and ensure that his airway is clear.

2. **Your initial assessment reveals that the patient is unconscious and unresponsive. You insert an oropharyngeal airway and assess his respirations, which are slow and shallow. His radial pulses are slow and bounding. What must you do next?**
   A. Perform immediate endotracheal intubation.
   B. Provide bag-valve-mask ventilation and 100% oxygen.
   C. Apply a nonrebreathing mask, and reassess him.
   D. Start an IV line and administer atropine sulfate.

3. **The patient's BP is 170/100 mm Hg, his pulse rate is 50 beats/min and bounding, and his baseline respirations are 6 breaths/min and have now become irregular. What is the pathophysiology of this patient's vital signs?**
   A. An increase in mean arterial pressure, cerebral vasodilation, and pressure on the brain stem
   B. Cerebral vasoconstriction, shunting of blood from the brain, and complete brain stem herniation
   C. A decrease in mean arterial pressure, cerebral vasodilation, and a decrease in cerebral perfusion pressure
   D. Cerebral vasodilation, a decrease in cerebral blood flow, and increased parasympathetic tone

4. **All of the following are clinical signs of pressure on the upper brain stem, EXCEPT:**
   A. Cheyne-Stokes respirations.
   B. an increase in the patient's BP.
   C. a marked increase in heart rate.
   D. bilaterally fixed and dilated pupils.

5. **Which of the following are indications for hyperventilation of a brain-injured patient?**
   A. A systolic BP that exceeds 200 mm Hg
   B. Bilaterally dilated and slowly reactive pupils
   C. An absent motor response to painful stimuli
   D. Withdrawal from pain with flexor posturing

6. **Your patient has been intubated and ventilations are continuing. Further assessment reveals that the patient is unresponsive to all stimuli, has unequal pupils, and shows extensor posturing. How many ventilations per minute should this patient receive?**
   A. 10
   B. 20
   C. 25
   D. 30

7. **Which of the following is the most appropriate IV fluid regimen for a head-injured patient with a BP of 70/50 mm Hg?**
   A. An amount sufficient to maintain a systolic BP of at least 90 mm Hg
   B. 1,000 ml to 2,000 ml followed by a reassessment of the patient's BP
   C. A crystalloid solution infusion set to run at approximately 120 ml/h
   D. Set the IV line(s) to keep vein open, because fluids will worsen cerebral edema

8. **Which of the following drugs would you be *least* likely to use when treating a patient with a severe head injury?**
   A. Lorazepam (Ativan)
   B. Lidocaine
   C. 50% dextrose
   D. Normal saline

9. **Which of the following parameters does the Glasgow Coma Scale (GCS) measure?**
   A. Pupil size, eye opening, verbal response
   B. Eye opening, motor response, heart rate
   C. Verbal response, pupil size, motor response
   D. Eye opening, verbal response, motor response

10. You have arrived at the hospital and have transferred patient care to the attending physician. You later learn that the patient had bleeding between the outer meningeal layer and the skull. This is called a(n):
    A. subdural hematoma.
    B. epidural hematoma.
    C. subarachnoid hemorrhage.
    D. intraparenchymal hematoma.

Challenging Questions

A 27-year-old highly intoxicated male was riding in the back of a pickup truck, when he fell out and struck his head on the pavement. Your assessment reveals that the patient is unconscious and unresponsive. His respirations are slow and irregular and his pulse rate is slow and bounding. The only visible injuries are a non-bleeding laceration to his right temporal region and blood draining from his right ear. Your partner manually stabilizes the patient's c-spine and begins ventilation assistance with a bag-valve-mask device and 100% oxygen. Suddenly, the patient begins regurgitating massive amounts of liquid.

11. What is the most effective way to initially manage this patient's airway?

12. What is the pathophysiology of the patient's vital signs? What would you expect his blood pressure to be?

▄▄ Points to Ponder

You are transporting a 30-year-old woman with blunt head trauma. She is conscious but persistently confused. You have applied 100% oxygen via nonrebreathing mask, started an IV line of normal saline and set the flow rate to keep vein open, and applied the cardiac monitor. Because of the mechanism of injury, full spinal motion restriction precautions have been applied. The patient's BP is 138/88 mm Hg, pulse rate is 100 beats/min, and respirations are 20 breaths/min and regular. As you are conversing with the patient, you note that her level of consciousness is progressively decreasing. You reassess her airway, which is still patent, but her respirations are now slow. The patient's pupils have increased in size but are still equal and reactive to light. She responds to pain by pushing your hand away. Noting these changes, you insert an airway adjunct and begin hyperventilating by bag-valve-mask ventilation at a rate of 24 breaths/min and continue to do so until you arrive at the hospital 20 minutes later. After delivering the patient to the hospital and returning to service, you learn that the patient experienced an anoxic brain injury.

Why did this occur? Could you have done something to prevent it?

Issues: Recognizing Clinical Signs of the Different Levels of Intracranial Pressure, Knowing the Appropriate Ventilation Rates for Head-Injured Patients, Understanding the Importance of Maintaining Cerebral Perfusion Pressure.

22 Spine Injuries

Competency Areas

Area 4: Assessment and Diagnostics

4.3.d Conduct neurological system assessment and interpret findings.

Area 5: Therapeutics

5.7.b Immobilize suspected fractures involving axial skeleton.

Area 6: Integration

6.1.b Provide care to patient experiencing illness or injury primarily involving neurological system.

Introduction

Spinal cord injury (SCI) is one of the most devastating injuries encountered by paramedics. Unfortunately, treatment options for SCIs are currently limited, with therapy relying heavily on rehabilitation over acute intervention. Preventive measures directed toward reducing the incidence of primary and secondary SCIs are the health care provider's best option for decreasing the morbidity and mortality associated with SCI.

In the United States, an estimated 40 new cases of SCI per million people, or 11,000, occur each year. In Canada the incidence is 35 new cases of SCI per million people, or 1,050, each year. Approximately 36,000 Canadians live with SCI. The average age at the time of injury is 32 years; 80% of patients are younger than 40 years old and 55% are between the ages of 16 and 30. Several different causes of injury are recognized, which are classified into five major categories: motor vehicle collisions (35%–40%); acts of violence (24.5%); falls, especially in the elderly (21.8%); recreational/athletic activities, especially diving (7.2%); and other causes, including diseases such as polio, spina bifida, and Friedreich's ataxia.

At the Scene

Patients with SCI face dramatic changes in lifestyle. A simple walk in the park, a trip to the shopping centre, or the commute to work becomes much more difficult. Caring for the SCI patient also brings significant financial costs. The annual cost is estimated to be $1.5 billion in Canada.

The overall in-hospital mortality rate is 7% for isolated SCI. In the first few months after injury, the mortality is as high as 20%, a rate that increases with age. The leading causes of death for SCI patients who are discharged from the hospital are pneumonia, pulmonary embolism, and septicemia.

Anatomy and Physiology

An understanding of the form and function of spinal anatomy coupled with a high level of suspicion for SCI is required to decipher the often subtle findings associated with a possible SCI.

The Spine

The spine consists of 33 vertebrae articulating to form the vertebral column, which is the major structural component of the axial skeleton Figure 22-1 ▶ . These skeletal components are stabilized by both ligaments and muscle. Together these components support and protect neural elements while allowing for fluid movement and erect stature.

Vertebrae are identified according to their location as cervical, thoracic, lumbar, sacral, or coccyx. The vertebral body, the anterior weight-bearing structure, is made of bone that provides support and stability. Components of the vertebra include the lamina, pedicles, and spinous processes Figure 22-2 ▶ . Each vertebra is unique in appearance and, with the exception of the atlas and axis (C1 and C2) Figure 22-3 ▶ , shares basic structural characteristics.

The inferior border of each pedicle contains a notch forming the intervertebral foramen. This space in the middle of the vertebra allows the exit of a peripheral nerve root and spinal vein as well as the entrance of a spinal artery on both sides at each vertebral junction.

You are the Paramedic Part 1

On your first day of work as a paramedic, you are dispatched to 9121 Floyd Trail for an "aircraft crash." En route to the scene, dispatch informs you that a witness saw a single-passenger gyrocopter fly into some power lines, then plummet to the ground.

You arrive to find a small rotary wing aircraft that has crashed in the middle of a large field of tall grass. You see power lines lying across the craft and an entrapped occupant who appears pale. A technician from the power company determines that the power lines are not energized so you approach the patient.

Initial Assessment	Recording Time: 0 Minutes
Appearance	Eyes open, anxious, holding lower back
Level of consciousness	A (Alert to person, place, and day)
Airway	Patent; calling for help
Breathing	Rapid and deep
Circulation	Fast, regular radial pulse

1. What is your primary concern?
2. What additional resources (if any) would you request and when?
3. How can you immediately assess and communicate with this patient in a safe manner?

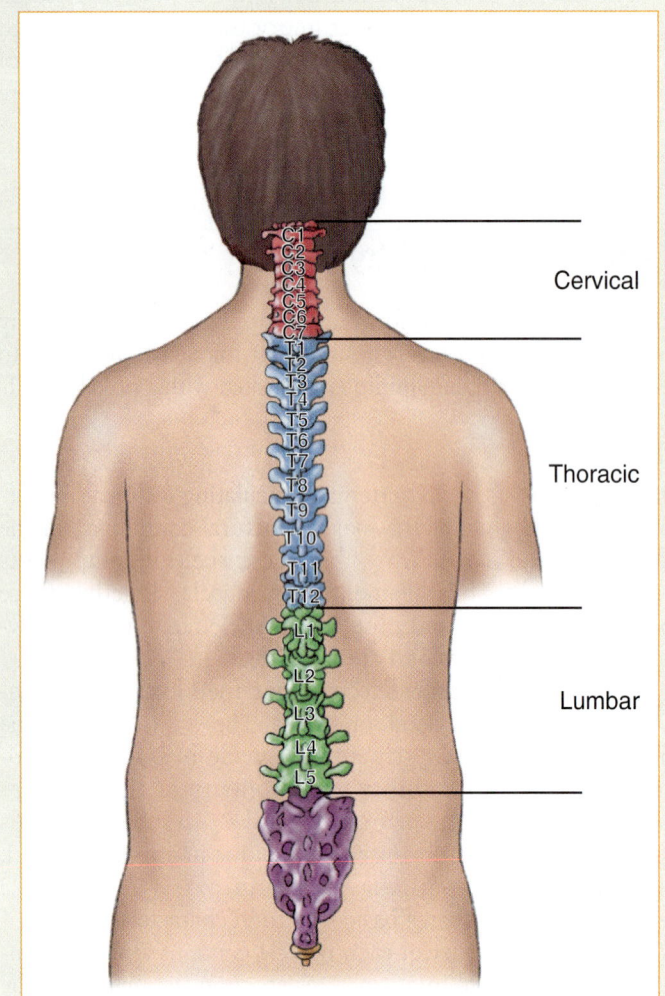

Figure 22-1 The spinal column consists of 33 bones divided into five sections. Each vertebra is numbered and referred to by a letter corresponding to the section of the spine where it is located plus its number. For example, the fifth thoracic vertebra is referred to as T5.

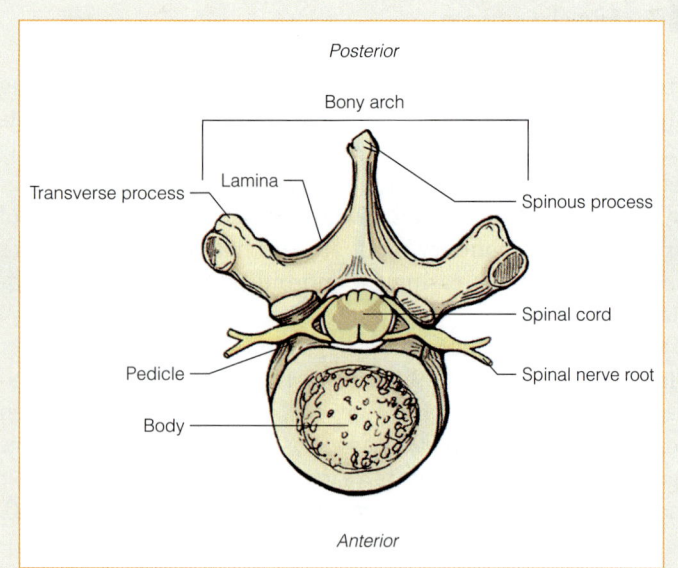

Figure 22-2 The human vertebra. Vertebrae in different sections of the spinal column vary in shape; this is a general representation. The space through which the spinal cord passes is called the canal, and the space through which a nerve root passes is called a foramen.

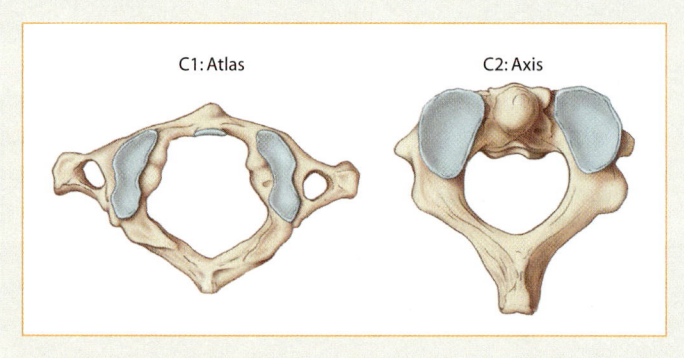

Figure 22-3 Structure of the atlas and axis.

The transverse spinous processes comprise the junction of each pedicle and lamina on each side of a vertebra. They project laterally and posteriorly and form points of attachments for muscles and ligaments. The posterior spinous process is formed by the fusion of the posterior lamina and serves as an attachment site for muscles and ligaments.

The cervical spine includes the first seven bones of the vertebral column and its supporting structures. In addition to protecting the vital cervical spinal cord, the cervical spine supports the weight of the head and permits a high degree of mobility in multiple planes. The atlas (C1) and axis (C2) are uniquely suited to allow for rotational movement of the skull.

The thoracic spine consists of 12 vertebrae in addition to the supporting muscles and ligaments found in the vertebral column; the thoracic spine is further stabilized by the rib attachments. The spinous processes are slightly larger, reflecting their role as attachment points for muscles that hold the upper body erect and assist with the movement of the thoracic cavity during respiration.

The lumbar spine includes the five largest bones in the vertebral column, and is integral in carrying a large portion of the upper body weight. The lumbar spine is especially susceptible to injury because of this weight-bearing capacity.

The sacrum is composed of five fused vertebrae that form the posterior plate of the pelvis. The coccyx is made up of three to five small fused vertebrae. Coccyx injuries, although often extremely painful, are typically clinically insignificant.

Each vertebra is separated and cushioned by intervertebral disks that limit bone wear and act as shock absorbers. As the body ages, these disks lose water content and become thinner, causing the height loss associated with aging. Stress on the vertebral column may cause a disk to herniate into the spinal canal, resulting in a spinal cord or nerve root injury **Figure 22-4 ▶** .

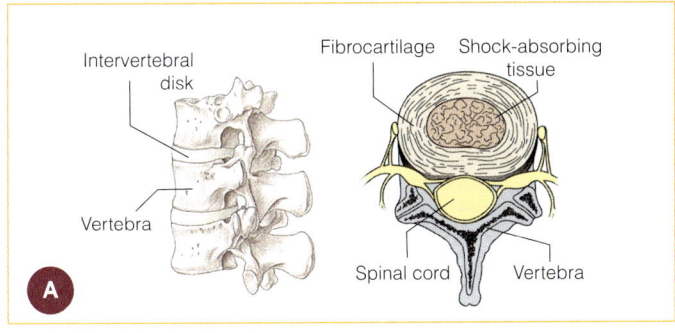

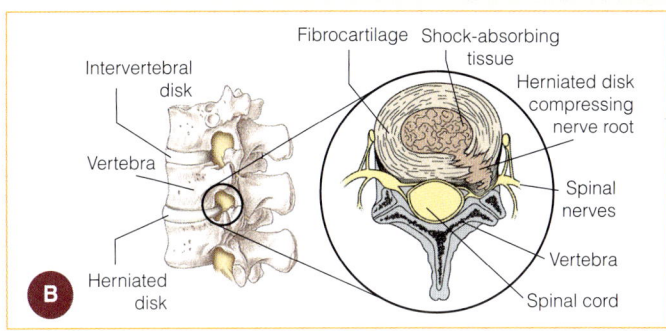

Figure 22-4 **A.** Normal, uninjured vertebral disk. **B.** Herniated disk.

At the Scene

The lumbar spine is a common site of injury. Many of these injuries involve muscle spasm and do not threaten the integrity of the spinal cord and its roots. Nonetheless, low back pain is a common problem, as well as a major cause of impairment and disability.

The muscles, tendons, and ligaments that connect the vertebrae allow the spinal column a degree of flexion and extension, limited to an extent by the stabilization they must provide to the spinal column. The vertebral column can sustain normal flexion and extension without stressing the spinal cord. Flexion or extension beyond normal limits may damage structural ligaments and allow excess vertebral movement that could expose the spinal cord to injury.

The Brain and Meninges

The central nervous system (CNS) consists of the brain and the spinal cord, both of which are encased in and protected by bone. The brain, located within the cranial cavity, is the largest component of the CNS. It contains billions of neurons that serve a variety of vital functions.

The brain stem, which consists of the medulla, pons, and midbrain, connects the spinal cord to the remainder of the brain. The brain stem is vital for numerous basic body functions. Damage to this critical structure can easily result in death. All but two of the 12 cranial nerves exit from the brain stem.

The entire CNS is enclosed by a set of three membranes collectively known as the meninges **Figure 22-5 ▶**. The outer membrane, called the dura mater, is tough and fibrous. The middle layer, called the arachnoid, contains blood vessels that have the appearance of a spider web. The innermost layer, resting directly on the brain or spinal cord, is the pia mater. The meninges float in cerebrospinal fluid (CSF). The meninges and CSF form a fluid-filled cushion that protects the brain and spinal cord.

The Spinal Cord

The spinal cord transmits nerve impulses between the brain and the rest of the body. Beginning at the base of the brain, it

You are the Paramedic Part 2

You request additional resources to aid you in safely treating and transporting the patient. After the known hazards have been addressed, you approach the patient, who says her name is Lynn Chase, to begin your hands-on assessment. As you near her, you notice a strong odour of gasoline and the patient says, "I stink! I have gasoline all over me!"

Reassessment	Recording Time: 10 Minutes
Level of consciousness	A (Alert to person, place, and day)
Skin	Cool, slightly pale, and dry
Pulse	110 beats/min, strong and regular
Blood pressure	140/74 mm Hg
Respirations	36 breaths/min
Spo$_2$	98% on 15 l/min via nonrebreathing mask

4. Given the information your patient has provided, have your priorities changed?

5. Given the mechanism of injury and other factors, what injuries do you suspect?

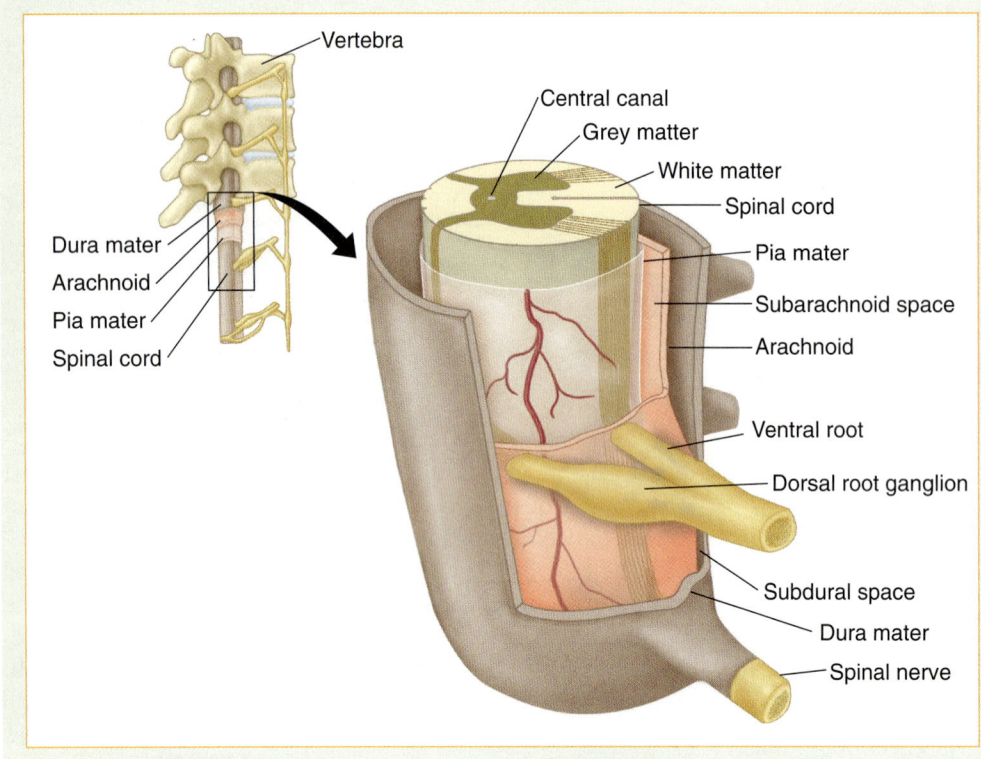

Figure 22-5 The spinal cord and its layers. The meninges enclose the brain and spinal cord.

thoracic nerve roots have varying functions; the upper thoracic nerves supply muscles of the chest that help in breathing and coughing, while the lower thoracic nerves provide abdominal muscle control and contain nerves of the sympathetic nervous system. The five lumbar nerve roots supply hip flexors and leg muscles, as well as provide sensation to the anterior legs. The five sacral nerves provide for bowel and bladder control, sexual function, and sensation in the posterior legs and rectum. The coccyx has a single nerve root.

Nerve roots occasionally converge in a cluster called a plexus that permits peripheral nerve roots to rejoin and function as a group **Figure 22-6 ▶** . For example, the cervical plexus includes C1 through C5; the phrenic nerve (C3–C5) arises from this plexus and innervates the diaphragm. The brachial plexus (C5–T1) joins nerves controlling the upper extremities; the main nerves arising from this plexus are the axillary, median, musculocutaneous, radial, and ulnar. The lumbar plexus (L1–L4) supplies the skin and muscles of the abdominal wall, external genitalia, and part of the lower limbs. The sacral plexus (L4–S4) gives rise to the pudendal and sciatic nerves and supplies the buttocks, perineum, and most of the lower limbs.

represents the continuation of the CNS. This bundle of nerve fibres leaves the skull through a large opening at its base called the foramen magnum. The spinal cord extends from the base of the skull to L2; here it separates into the cauda equina, a collection of individual nerve roots. Thirty-one pairs of spinal nerves arise at different levels along the spinal cord; each pair is named according to its corresponding level.

A cross-section of the spinal cord (see Figure 22-5) reveals a butterfly-shaped central core of grey matter that is composed of neural cell bodies. This grey matter is divided into posterior (dorsal) horns, which carry sensory input, and anterior (ventral) horns, which innervate the motor nerve of that segment. Surrounding the grey matter on each side are three columns of peripheral white matter composed of myelinated ascending and descending fibre pathways. Messages are relayed to and from the brain through these spinal tracts.

Specific groups of nerves are named based on their source of origin and point of termination. Ascending tracts carry information to the brain, and descending tracts carry information to the rest of the body **Table 22-1 ▶** .

Spinal Nerves

The 31 pairs of spinal nerves emerge from each side of the spinal cord and are named for the vertebral region and level from which they arise. The eight cervical roots perform different functions in the scalp, neck, shoulders, and arms. The 12

Table 22-1	Major Spinal Tracts
Anterior Spinal Tracts	
Anterior spinothalamic tracts (ascending)	Carry sensation of crude touch and pressure sensation to the brain
Lateral spinothalamic tracts (ascending)	Carry pain and temperature sensation
Spinocerebellar tracts (ascending)	Coordinate impulses necessary for muscular movements by carrying impulses from muscles in the legs and trunk to the cerebellum
Corticospinal tracts (descending)	Voluntary motor commands
Reticulospinal tracts (descending)	Muscle tone and sweat gland activity
Rubrospinal tracts (descending)	Muscle tone
Posterior Spinal Tracts	
Fasciculus gracilis and cuneatus	Proprioception, vibration, light touch, deep pressure, two-point discrimination, and stereognosis

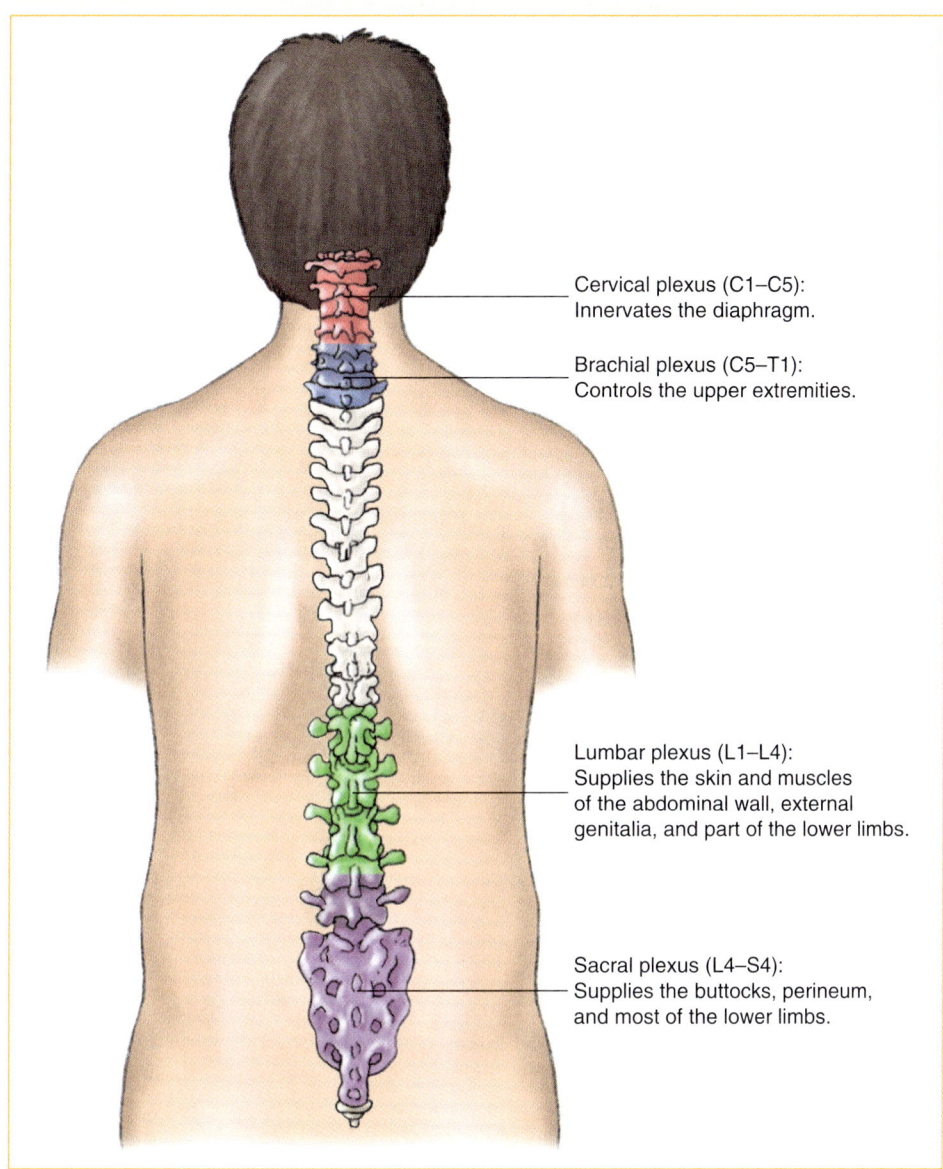

Figure 22-6 Nerve roots converge in plexuses, allowing them to function as a group.

Cervical plexus (C1–C5):
Innervates the diaphragm.

Brachial plexus (C5–T1):
Controls the upper extremities.

Lumbar plexus (L1–L4):
Supplies the skin and muscles
of the abdominal wall, external
genitalia, and part of the lower limbs.

Sacral plexus (L4–S4):
Supplies the buttocks, perineum,
and most of the lower limbs.

nervous system is also responsible for sweating, pupil dilation, and temperature regulation, as well as the shunting of blood from the periphery to the core—the "flight or fight" responses.

A spinal cord injury at or above the level of T6 may disrupt the flow of sympathetic communication. Loss of sympathetic stimulation can disrupt homeostasis and leave the body poorly equipped to deal with changes in its environment. Stimulation of sympathetic nerves without parasympathetic input can cause sympathetic overdrive, resulting in autonomic dysreflexia; this complication of SCI is discussed later in this chapter.

The Parasympathetic Nervous System

The parasympathetic nervous system includes fibres arising from the brain stem and upper spinal cord that carry signals to organs of the abdomen, heart, lungs, and the skin above the waist. The vagus nerve travels from its origins outside of the medulla to the heart via the carotid arteries, thus vagal tone remains intact following a spine injury. When the sympathetic nerves are stimulated and produce autonomic dysreflexia, the parasympathetic nerves attempt to control the rapidly increasing blood pressure by slowing the heart rate. Parasympathetic nerves that supply the reproductive organs, pelvis, and leg begin at the sacral level (S2–S4). Disruption of the lower parasympathetic nerves in the sacrum results in the loss of bowel/bladder tone and sexual function.

The Sympathetic Nervous System

The sensory (afferent) and motor (efferent) nerves are responsible for the somatic functions of the spinal cord and often overshadow the role of the spinal cord in the involuntary autonomic nervous system. The sympathetic nervous system is controlled by the brain's hypothalamus. Information from the brain is transmitted through the brain stem and the cervical spinal cord and then exits at the thoracic and lumbar levels of the spine to reach target structures. The thoracolumbar system provides sympathetic stimulation to the periphery largely through alpha and beta receptors. Alpha receptor stimulation induces smooth muscle contraction in blood vessels and bronchioles. Beta receptors respond with relaxation of smooth muscles in blood vessels and bronchioles, and have chronotropic and inotropic effects on myocardial cells. The sympathetic

Pathophysiology

Mechanism of Injury

Acute injuries of the spine are classified according to the associated mechanism, location, and stability of the injury. Vertebral fractures can occur with or without associated SCI. Because stable fractures do not involve the posterior column, they pose less risk to the spinal cord. Unstable injuries involve the posterior column of the spinal cord and typically include damage to portions of the vertebrae and ligaments that directly protect the spinal cord and nerve roots. Unstable injuries carry a higher risk of complicating SCI and progression of injury without appropriate treatment.

Flexion Injuries

Flexion injuries at the cervical level result from forward movement of the head, typically as the result of rapid deceleration (eg, in a vehicle collision) or from a direct blow to the occiput. At the level of C1–C2, these forces can produce an unstable dislocation with or without an associated fracture. Farther down the spinal column, flexion forces are transmitted anteriorly through the vertebral bodies and can result in an anterior wedge fracture. Depending on their severity, anterior wedge fractures can be stable or unstable. Loss of more than half the original size of the vertebral body or multiple levels of injury suggest involvement of the posterior column, with increasing risk of SCI.

Hyperflexion injuries of greater force can result in teardrop fractures—avulsion fractures of the anterior–inferior border of the vertebral body. The injuries to ligaments associated with teardrop fractures raise concern for possible SCI and qualify as unstable fractures. Severe flexion can also result in a potentially unstable dislocation of vertebral joints. This situation does not involve fracture but can severely injure the ligaments. Strong forces can result in the anterior displacement of facet joints. A bilateral facet dislocation is an extremely unstable injury.

Rotation with Flexion

The only area of the spine that allows for significant rotation is C1–C2. Injuries to this area are considered unstable due to its high cervical location and scant bony and soft-tissue support. Rotation–flexion injuries often result from high acceleration forces. Rotation with abrupt flexion can produce a stable dislocation in the cervical spine. In the thoracolumbar spine, rotation–flexion forces typically cause fracture rather than dislocation.

Vertical Compression

Vertical compression forces are transmitted through vertebral bodies and directed either inferiorly through the skull or superiorly through the pelvis or feet. They typically result from a direct blow to the crown (parietal region) of the skull or rapid deceleration from a fall through the feet, legs, and pelvis. Forces transmitted through the vertebral body cause fractures, producing a "burst" or compression fracture with or without associated SCI **Figure 22-7 ▶**. Compression forces can cause the herniation of disks, subsequent compression on the spinal cord and nerve roots, and fragmentation into the canal.

Although most fractures resulting from these injuries are stable, primary SCI can occur when the vertebral body is shattered and fragments of bone become embedded in the cord. Some compression injuries may be associated with significant retropharyngeal edema, and serious airway compromise is a consideration.

Hyperextension

Hyperextension of the head and neck can result in fractures and ligamentous injury of variable stability. The hangman's fracture (C2) results from hyperextension and distraction due to rapid deceleration of the skull, atlas, and axis as a unit. The resulting bilateral pedicle fracture of C2 is an unstable fracture but is rarely associated with SCI. A teardrop fracture of the anterior–inferior edge of the vertebral body results from hyperextension, resulting in rupture of the anterior longitudinal ligament. The injury is stable with the head and neck in flexion, but unstable in extension due to loss of structural support.

Categories of Spinal Cord Injuries

Primary Spinal Cord Injury

Primary spinal cord injury is injury that occurs at the moment of impact. Penetrating trauma typically results in transection of nonregenerative neural elements and complete injuries. Blunt trauma may displace ligaments and bone fragments, resulting in compression of points of the spinal cord. Hypoperfusion and ischemia may also result from this type of injury to the spinal vasculature. Necrosis from prolonged ischemia leads to permanent loss of function.

Spinal cord concussion, which is characterized by a temporary dysfunction that lasts from 24 to 48 hours, accounts for 3% to 4% of all SCIs. Cord concussion is considered an incomplete injury and may present in patients with simple compression fractures or in those without radiologic evidence of a fracture. The temporary dysfunction may be due to a short-duration shock or pressure wave within the cord.

Spinal cord contusions are caused by fracture, dislocation, or direct trauma. They are associated with edema, tissue damage, and vascular leakage. Hemorrhagic disruption may cause temporary to permanent loss of function despite normal radiographs.

Cord laceration usually occurs when a projectile or bone enters the spinal canal. Such an injury is likely to result in hemorrhage into the cord tissue, swelling, and disruption of some portion of the cord and its associated communication pathways.

Secondary Spinal Cord Injury

Secondary spinal cord injury occurs when multiple factors permit a progression of the primary SCI; the ensuing cascade of inflammatory responses may result in further deterioration. These effects can be exacerbated by exposing neural elements to further hypoxemia, hypoglycemia, and hypothermia. Although some SCI may be unavoidable, the paramedic should minimize further injury through stabilization—that is, through spinal motion restriction and neutral alignment. In addition,

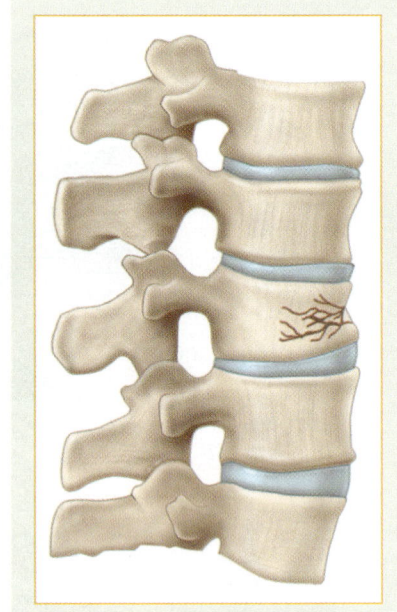

Figure 22-7 A compression fracture.

minimizing heat loss and maintaining oxygenation and perfusion are key elements in the prehospital care of a patient with a possible SCI.

Regardless of the mechanism of injury, all SCIs are classified as complete or incomplete depending on the degree of damage. Complete spinal cord injury involves complete disruption of all tracts of the spinal cord, with permanent loss of all cord-mediated functions below the level of transection. When the injury affects the patient high in the cervical spine, quadriplegia results. A similar injury in the high thoracic area would result in paraplegia. In an incomplete spinal cord injury, the patient retains some degree of cord-mediated function. The degree of SCI is best determined 24 hours after the initial injury; the initial dysfunction may be temporary, and there is some potential for recovery.

Anterior cord syndrome results from the displacement of bony fragments into the anterior portion of the spinal cord, often due to flexion injuries or fractures. The anterior spinal artery provides blood to the anterior two thirds of the spinal cord; disruption of this flow will present as an anterior cord syndrome. Physical findings include paralysis below the level of the insult with loss of sensation to pain, temperature, and touch.

In central cord syndrome, hyperextension injuries to the cervical area present with hemorrhage or edema to the central cervical segments. This type of damage is rarely associated with fractures or bone disruption but more often occurs in conjunction with tears to the anterior longitudinal ligament. Central cord syndrome is frequently seen in older patients, who may already have a significant degree of cervical spondylosis and stenosis due to arthritic changes. A brief episode of hyperextension can exert pressure on the spinal cord within the relatively diminished spinal canal. Within the central cord, motor (efferent) fibres are distributed in a unique fashion, with more cervical and thoracic motor and sensory tracts than in the periphery of the cord. The patient with central cord syndrome will present with greater loss of function in the upper extremities than in the lower extremities, with variable loss of sensation to pain and temperature. The patient may also have some bowel and bladder dysfunction. The prognosis for central cord syndrome is typically good; many patients regain all motor function or have only some residual weakness in the hands.

Posterior cord syndrome is associated with extension injuries. This relatively rare syndrome produces dysfunction of the dorsal columns, presenting as decreased sensation to light touch, proprioception (the ability to perceive the position and movement of one's body), and vibration, while most other motor and sensory functions remain intact. Recovery of function is less prevalent than with central cord syndrome, but the overall prognosis remains good with therapy and rehabilitation.

Brown-Sequard syndrome occurs when penetrating trauma is accompanied by hemisection of the cord and complete damage to all spinal tracts on the involved side. Injury to the corticospinal motor tracts causes motor loss on the same side as the injury, but below the lesion. Damage to the dorsal column causes loss of sensation to light touch, proprioception, and vibration on the same side as the injury (below it). Disruption of the spinothalamic tracts causes loss of sensation to pain and temperature on the opposite side of injury, below the lesion.

Spinal shock refers to the temporary local neurologic condition that occurs immediately after spinal trauma. Swelling and edema of the cord begin within 30 minutes of the initial insult and can lead to a physiologic transection, mechanically disrupting all nerve conduction distal to the injury. The patient may present with variable degrees of acute spinal injury, potentially with flaccid paralysis, flaccid sphincters, and absent reflexes. Sensory function below the level of injury will be impaired, as will thermoregulation and visceral sensation below the lesion, resulting in bowel distension from a loss of peristalsis. Spinal shock usually subsides in hours to weeks, depending on the severity of injury.

Neurogenic shock results from the temporary loss of autonomic function, which controls cardiovascular function, at the level of injury. Marked hemodynamic and systemic effects are seen: hypotension occurs due to absent or impaired peripheral vascular tone with the loss of alpha receptor stimulation; blood pools in the enlarged vascular space, causing a relative hypovolemia and making the patient extremely sensitive to sudden position changes; and cardiac preload decreases, resulting in decreased stroke volume and cardiac output. Bradycardia results as well. The adrenal gland loses its sympathetic stimulation and does not produce epinephrine or norepinephrine. Hypothermia and absence of sweating are also seen because of the loss of sympathetic stimulation. The classic case of neurogenic shock is a hypotensive, bradycardic patient whose skin is warm, flushed, and dry below the level of the spinal lesion.

Patient Assessment

Limiting the progression of secondary SCI is a major goal of prehospital management of SCI. You should be familiar with the circumstances that commonly produce SCI and try to determine, through history-taking and examination of the scene, whether any of these circumstances exist.

Special Considerations

Spinal cord injury without radiographic abnormalities (SCIWORA) can occur in children because their vertebrae lie flatter on top of each other **Figure 22-8 ▶**; in adults, the vertebrae are more curved. A child's vertebrae can easily dislocate and quickly relocate back into their normal positions. The radiograph of a child who has experienced SCIWORA may have no evidence of fracture and will show a perfectly aligned vertebral column, yet the cord itself has been compressed or transected. SCIWORA cannot be diagnosed in the prehospital setting. Even in the emergency department, sophisticated studies such as MRI may be required.

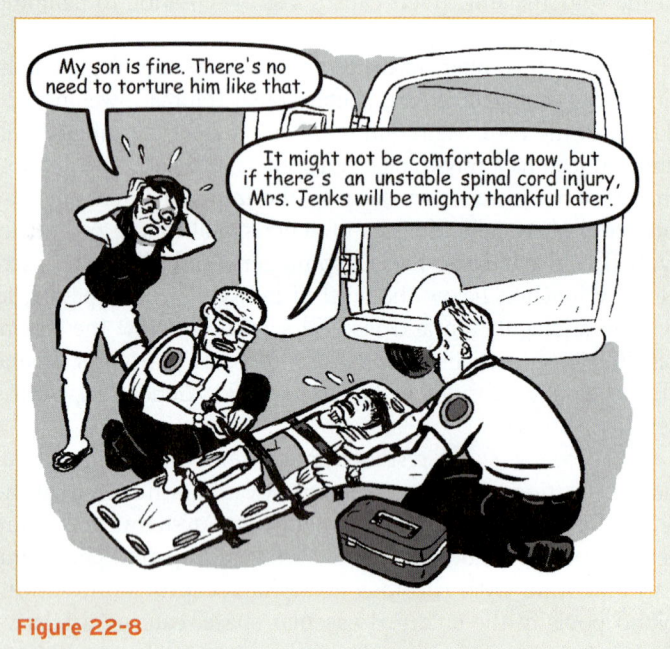

Figure 22-8

When to Suspect a Spinal Cord Injury

The history of present illness typically provides most of the information necessary to reach a diagnosis. Maintain a high index of suspicion in any case for which the mechanism of injury suggests the possibility of SCI. Associated injuries, especially those that reflect involvement of massive forces, may also provide clues of the presence of SCI. Treat all patients who experience multiple trauma or those who are found unconscious after trauma as if a spine injury exists, because the majority of cervical spine injuries are associated with head injury. Patients with evidence of major trauma above the clavicle should be considered at risk for an associated spine injury.

The following high-risk mechanisms of injury strongly suggest spine injury and require full spine immobilization regardless of the physical examination findings:

- High-velocity collision (> 60 km/h) with severe vehicle damage
- Unrestrained occupant of moderate- to high-speed motor vehicle collision
- Vehicular damage with compartmental intrusion (30 cm) into the patient's seating space
- Fall from three times the patient's height
- Penetrating trauma near the spine
- Ejection from a moving vehicle
- Motorcycle collision > 30 km/h with separation of rider from vehicle
- Diving injury
- Vehicle–pedestrian or vehicle–bicycle collision > 10 km/h
- Death of occupant in the same passenger compartment
- Rollover collision (unrestrained)

Mechanisms of uncertain risk for spine injury include the following events:

- Moderate- to low-velocity motor vehicle collision (< 60 km/h)
- Patient involved in a motor vehicle collision has an isolated injury without positive assessment findings for SCI
- Isolated minor head injury without positive mechanism for spine injury
- Syncopal event in which the patient was already seated or supine
- Syncopal event in which the patient was assisted to a supine position by a bystander

Notes from Nancy

Any patient with significant head injury also has cervical spine injury until proven otherwise.

You are the Paramedic Part 3

Firefighters aid you in decontaminating the patient as well as applying spinal precautions. She finds it difficult to lie flat on the board, and tells you that her back hurts a lot. She reports, "It feels better if I hold it." She denies any weakness, numbness, or tingling in her extremities.

Reassessment	Recording Time: 15 Minutes
Level of consciousness	A (Alert to person, place, and day)
Skin	Cool, slightly pale, and dry
Pulse	110 beats/min, strong and regular
Blood pressure	142/76 mm Hg
Respirations	36 breaths/min
Spo₂	100% on 15 l/min via nonrebreathing mask

6. What other factors can impact a patient's ability to handle the stress of trauma?
7. What other information beyond the history of events should you obtain from your patient?
8. If you must decontaminate a patient in the open, how can you preserve patient modesty?

Determine as precisely as possible the circumstances of the incident and types of energy imparted to the patient, including the degree of force and the speed and trajectory of impact. Was there blunt or penetrating trauma? Was it a flexion injury, such as the classic diving accident? Was there torsion on the neck? In the case of a fall, estimate the height of the fall and determine whether anything was struck on the way down, how the patient landed, and what the patient landed on. In vehicular collisions, note the use and positioning of restraints, the patient's position in the vehicle, and the degree of damage to the vehicle. Find out the exact time of the initial injury and record any times and changes in the patient's presentation throughout the prehospital phase.

Special Considerations

The indications for backboard spinal immobilization of infants and toddlers are unknown. Infants and young children cannot verbally communicate symptoms such as weakness, numbness, or pain, so the threshold for immobilization must be lower than for older children and adults. However, restraining a conscious child on a backboard will cause pain and agitation in a short time. Reassure nervous children that the immobilization is necessary but only temporary. Try distraction techniques.

Modify the physical examination of any patient with suspected SCI based on the patient's level of consciousness, reliability as a historian, and mechanism of injury. In cases of high- or intermediate-risk mechanisms, whenever possible complete the physical examination with the patient in a neutral position without any movement of the spine. Apply manual stabilization while asking the patient not to move unless specifically asked to do so. The neck and trunk must not be flexed, extended, or rotated. Frequent reassessments are necessary to determine whether the patient is stabilizing, improving, or deteriorating. Also, be sure to document suspected spinal cord injury, noting the area involved, sensation, dermatomes (discussed in the next section), motor function, and areas of weakness.

Controversies

Several provinces and EMS systems have instituted prehospital spinal clearance protocols with good initial results. In Canada, research on extending the use of the Canadian c-spine rule to the prehospital setting is ongoing. Always follow local protocols and direct medical control regarding protecting the c-spine and clearing it when indicated.

Scene Assessment

After donning PPE, the initial step of any assessment should be a determination of scene safety and the need for any additional resources. Decide whether the trauma system should be activated (eg, air evacuation of the patient to a Level I trauma centre). Note the general age and gender of the patient. Observe the position in which the patient is found and determine if the patient's condition is life-threatening. While maintaining the head and neck in a neutral position through manual stabilization, determine the level of consciousness, using AVPU initially and then the Glasgow Coma Scale (GCS score—a standardized method of relaying information regarding a patient's overall level of consciousness) as time allows. A cervical collar may be applied as soon as the assessment of the airway and neck are complete. Sedation or rapid sequence intubation (RSI) procedures, depending on local protocols, may be required for a combative patient to ensure the patient's protection and spine stabilization.

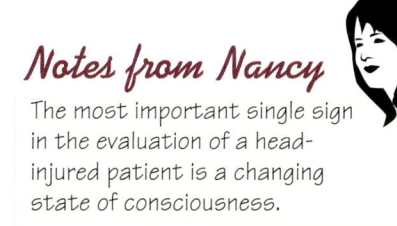

Notes from Nancy

The most important single sign in the evaluation of a head-injured patient is a changing state of consciousness.

Initial Assessment

Airway

After confirming that the scene is safe and determining the patient's mental status, the next priority is to ensure an open airway. Sonorous respirations usually indicate a positional problem, while gurgling respirations often indicate a need for suction. The oropharynx may become occluded by the tongue, secretions, blood, vomitus, foreign bodies, or improperly inserted airways. A retropharyngeal hematoma associated with injury of the upper cervical spine (C2) may also compromise the airway.

While maintaining the head and neck in neutral alignment, clear the mouth and carefully but quickly suction if necessary. Use a jaw-thrust maneuver to open the airway; if this technique is successful, insert an oropharyngeal airway or a nasopharyngeal airway as appropriate. An intact gag reflex is a contraindication for an oropharyngeal airway, because vomiting will increase the likelihood of airway compromise and increase the risk of aspiration. Facial fractures and physical findings or suspicion for a basilar skull fracture are relative contraindications for a nasopharyngeal airway.

A definitive airway with in-line orotracheal intubation should follow the placement of any temporary airway device. If the patient is awake with an impaired airway or has a deteriorating GCS score (8 or less), consider sedative-facilitated orotracheal intubation or rapid sequence intubation (RSI) with in-line stabilization. Local airway protocols may vary from sedative-facilitated intubation to RSI. Log roll the patient to the side in case of vomiting when secured to a backboard or while you maintain manual in-line stabilization of the head and neck. Follow up with suction to remove the secretions.

Breathing

Evaluate the patient's breathing, noting the rate, depth, and symmetry of each respiration. The diaphragm is innervated by the phrenic nerve (C3–C5). Lesions occurring at or above C3–C4, may consequently lead to diaphragmatic paralysis, which is seen clinically as abdominal breathing with use of the accessory muscles of the neck. An injury involving the lower cervical or upper thoracic spinal cord (T2) may result in paralysis of the intercostal muscles, leaving the patient dependent on the diaphragm and accessory muscles of the neck for breathing. Inadequate respirations with or without evidence of decreased oxygenation will require assisted ventilation with a bag-valve-mask device with 12 to 15 l/min of supplementary oxygen flowing, at 10 to 12 breaths/min. If a head injury is suspected, use $EtCO_2$ monitoring to maintain CO_2 levels at 35 to 45 mm Hg.

Circulation

To assess perfusion, compare the radial and carotid pulses for their presence, rate, quality, regularity, and equality, and examine the patient's skin colour, temperature, and moisture. Patients with significant sensory loss from SCI may equilibrate to the surrounding environmental temperature due to the lack of input from the periphery for temperature control. In neurogenic shock, the skin is usually warm, dry, and flushed due to vasodilation and the absence of sweating. These findings should be correlated with the patient's mental status.

In the absence of a pulse, immediately initiate CPR. Control any external bleeding with direct pressure or pressure dressings. Volume resuscitation may be necessary in patients with absent or diminished pulses, especially in the setting of multisystem trauma with hypovolemic shock. Patients with SCI in pure neurogenic shock may not require large amounts of volume resuscitation but may need vagolytic drugs (eg, atropine) and vasopressors (such as dopamine) to reverse the uninhibited vagal stimulation and alpha receptor blockade associated with this type of shock.

Transport Decision

Early on in the initial assessment, you must decide whether to complete the focused history and physical examination on scene or to transport the patient immediately with interventions en route. The unstable or potentially unstable patient should be transported as soon as possible to the most appropriate hospital according to local trauma guidelines or direct medical control instruction.

Focused History and Physical Examination

An accurate history and physical examination are critical for directing management of patients with potential SCIs. A patient's reliability as a historian must always be assessed before performing a focused or detailed assessment. To assess for spinal injury the patient must be nonimpaired and able to perform cognitive functions appropriately. Patients who present with an acute stress reaction, distracting injuries (eg, long-bone fractures, rib fractures, pelvic fractures, or clinically significant abdominal pain), or an alteration in mental status due to brain injury or intoxication from drugs and/or alcohol must be considered unreliable in terms of the neurologic examination. Patients with suspected spinal injury should have continuous spinal protection until the receiving physician clinically and, when indicated, radiographically clears the spinal precaution at the receiving hospital.

The focused physical examination should begin with baseline vital signs and a SAMPLE history. In case of potential spine injuries, the examination includes rapid inspection and palpation of the head, neck, chest, abdomen, pelvis, extremities, and back for injuries. Use the mnemonic DCAP-BTLS—Deformity, Contusion, Abrasion, Puncture/penetration wounds, Bruising, Tenderness, Laceration, and Swelling—to help you remember specific points. An evaluation of neurovascular integrity should include distal PMS (pulse, motor, and sensory function) for all four extremities. Any deficits in the neurologic examination must be noted and monitored.

In addition to evaluating responsiveness with AVPU during your initial assessment, also obtain a GCS score because it

You are the Paramedic Part 4

As soon as your patient is packaged, you begin transport. You establish vascular access, apply the cardiac monitor, and reassess your patient. Her mental status and vital signs remain stable throughout transport, and you transfer patient care to the hospital staff without incident.

Reassessment	Recording Time: 20 Minutes
Level of consciousness	A (Alert to person, place, and day)
Skin	Warm, pink, and dry
Pulse	106 beats/min, strong and regular
Blood pressure	138/70 mm Hg
Respirations	30 breaths/min
Spo2	100% on 15 l/min via nonrebreathing mask
ECG	Sinus tachycardia

The patient experienced compression fractures of her lumbar spine, but no spinal cord damage. She underwent surgery and made a recovery that did not limit her quality of life, including her ability to function as a pilot.

9. What is an appropriate maximum on-scene time for any patient with significant traumatic injury?

10. How does prompt, appropriate prehospital care affect the patient beyond immediate survival of the injuries sustained?

provides more specific clinical information. Assess the pupils for their size, shape, equality, and reactivity to light. If possible, obtain a glucose level in patients who show evidence of alterations in sensation. Perform a brief motor and sensory examination, including PMS in all four extremities, in patients with potential SCI.

During the examination, you should carefully cut away the clothes to minimize motion of the spine. Directly observe the back by log roll to assess for penetrating trauma. Palpate the spine to assess for deformity or displacement (step off) of vertebral bodies. Once the examination is completed, recover the patient with a blanket to maintain normal body temperature. Hypothermia will impair the patient's ability to unbind oxygen from hemoglobin and increase the risk of mortality and morbidity. In colder climates, move the patient to a warmer environment, such as the ambulance, as quickly as possible without compromising the spine further.

Placement on the Backboard

Before you immobilize a patient, be sure you have documented your assessment thus far. It will also be important to document your findings after the patient has been immobilized.

Most patients can be log rolled with visualization for deformity or injury as well as palpation over each posterior spinous process for pain, deformity, or step off. The absence of pain or tenderness along the spine, coupled with a normal neurologic examination and low-risk mechanism of injury, may eliminate the need for manual in-line spinal immobilization. In contrast, patients with clinical suspicion of spinal injury should always be protected with appropriate backboard and stretcher immobilization.

Patients in severe pain may require an alternative method of transfer to a backboard. Use of a scoop stretcher often results in less movement of the patient. Once the scoop is in place, another paramedic can slide the backboard or air mattress underneath the patient. Although the patient can still be palpated with this method, inability to conduct visual inspection of the area is a limitation.

Time on a backboard should be kept to a minimum because skin breakdown can be a major complication of SCI **Figure 22-9 ▶**. This problem occurs as a result of excessive pressure over the bones of the buttocks, the scapular ridges, and the base of the occiput. These five areas are the primary points supporting the patient's weight. The initial stages of pressure lesions may occur in a matter of hours; 32% of patients with SCI develop a skin lesion within 24 hours of injury. Blood distribution shifts to the skin and subcutaneous tissues, and decreased muscle tone and sensation predispose the SCI patient to these injuries.

Several new devices have been developed to enhance patient comfort. The Back Raft takes pressure off specific areas of the back and fills voids that may otherwise allow patient movement. This low-profile air mattress fits under the patient from the shoulders to the waist **Figure 22-10 ▶**. Slightly flexing the knees with towel rolls or a blanket and slightly separating the legs with a pillow or blanket increases patient

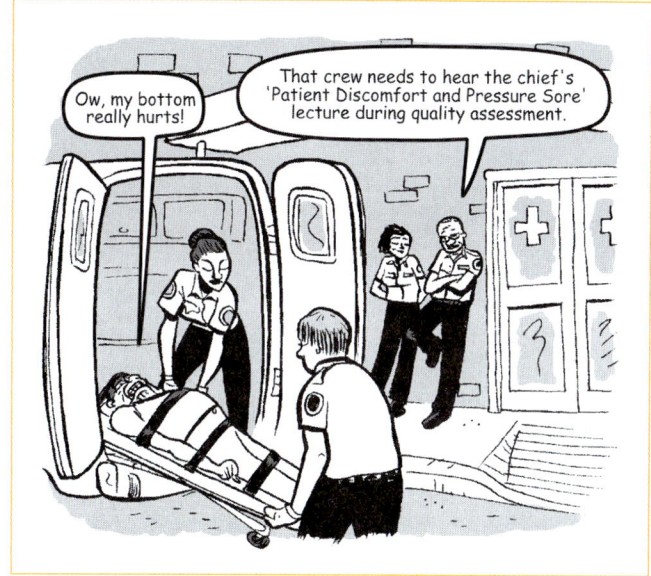

Figure 22-9

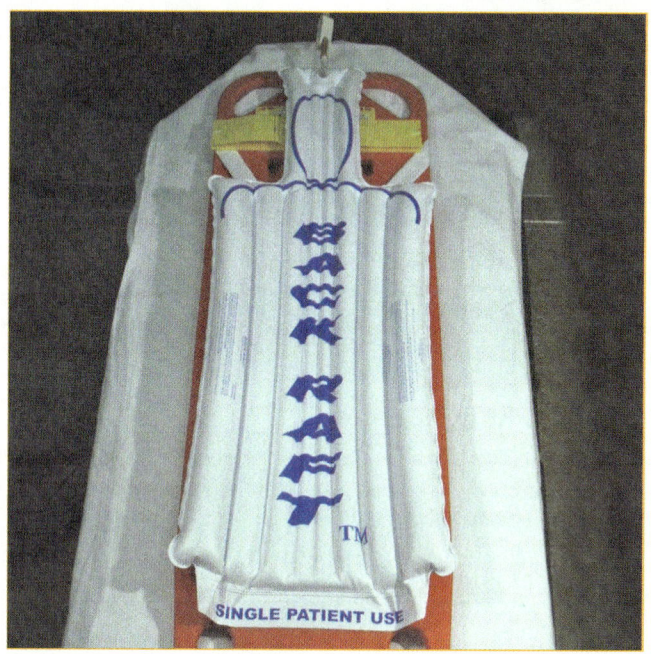

Figure 22-10 The Back Raft.

comfort and decreases the likelihood of postimmobilization problems, yet still provides adequate immobilization of the patient **Figure 22-11 ▶**. Concave backboards also conform more closely to a patient's anatomy than do flat boards. Spider straps should be used to properly immobilize a patient.

Detailed Physical Examination

A detailed physical examination for a trauma patient with a significant MOI should take place while en route to the hospital.

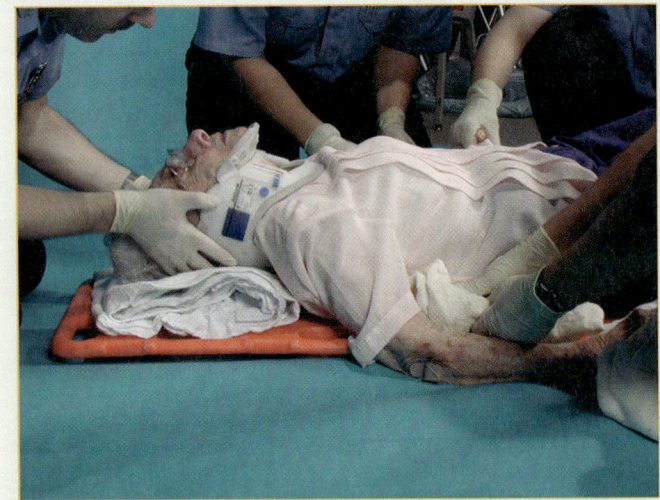

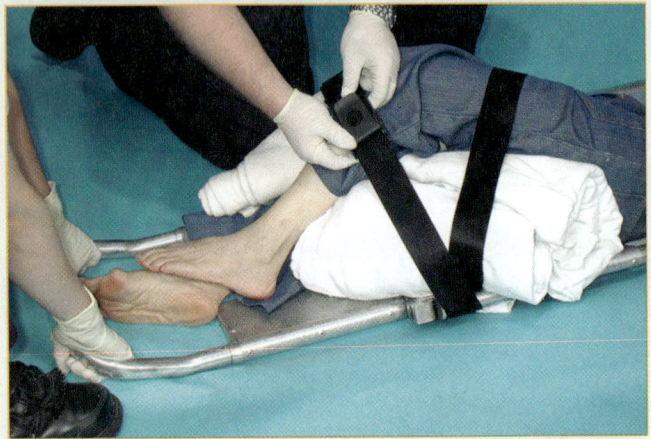

Figure 22-11 Using towel rolls or blankets to pad the backboard will increase patient comfort and can minimize problems resulting from immobilization of the older patient.

At the Scene

Always palpate over the spinous process before concluding that a patient "has no neck pain." Some paramedics simply ask the patient and never perform a physical examination.

Closely examine the head, neck, chest, abdomen, pelvis, extremities, back, and buttocks. A detailed head-to-toe examination can often reveal significant findings, especially in patients with questionable reliability, unclear mechanisms, or multisystem trauma.

Thoroughly assess the head and neck, because many SCI patients will have associated head and facial injuries; a complaint of pain is most predictive of a spine injury. Examination of the neck should include gentle palpation of the cervical spine for pain, deformity, or dislocation (step off).

Evaluate the chest and abdomen for both internal and external injuries. Fractures of the ribs, sternum, clavicle, scapula, or pelvis are often associated with SCI in patients with multisystem trauma. Visualization and palpation are the mainstays of this

evaluation. Bear in mind that the physical examination in the SCI patient may be skewed due to potentially decreased sensation below the level of the spine injury. Assess the chest wall visually for symmetry of chest wall movement, work of breathing, and use of accessory muscles. Auscultation to assess breath sounds may reveal a shortened inspiratory phase. Inadequate ventilation, accessory muscle use, or paradoxical respirations may indicate diaphragmatic impairment due to SCI.

Continually monitor the cardiovascular system for signs of shock. Neurogenic shock may require pharmacologic management, volume replacement, and/or transcutaneous pacing.

Examination of the gastrointestinal system may be unreliable in the presence of a neurologic deficit. First, inspect the abdomen for evidence of trauma, noting its contour. Severe gastric distension may impair respiration and lead to airway compromise due to vomiting. Palpate all four quadrants for tenderness, guarding, or rigidity, but remember that patients may be insensitive to pain and may not develop a rigid abdomen because of absence of muscle tone. Lower abdominal distension with or without suprapubic tenderness may be due to urinary retention. When performing a genital examination on a male, assess for evidence of urethral injury (ie, blood in the meatus, scrotal swelling, and scrotal ecchymosis), which may be present with pelvic fractures. In addition, take note of priapism, which may suggest SCI.

Inspect all extremities for deformity, contusion, abrasions, punctures, lacerations, and edema. Palpate for deformity, tenderness, instability, or crepitus. Look for any abnormal posturing, and assess the patient for potential long bone or other significantly distracting painful injuries that may mask a potential spine or cord injury.

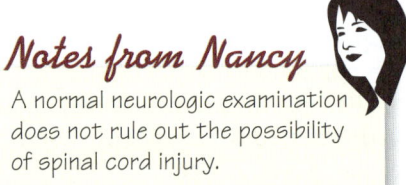

Notes from Nancy

A normal neurologic examination does not rule out the possibility of spinal cord injury.

Neurologic Examination

The focused neurologic evaluation in the prehospital environment is intended to establish a baseline level of the lesion for later comparison. It is also used to determine the completeness of the lesion and to identify cord syndromes if the lesion is incomplete. A normal neurologic examination does not rule out the possibility of SCI. Patients who experienced vehicular trauma have been known to walk away from the collision only to become totally paralyzed hours later, when a casual nod of the head squeezed an unstable vertebral column down against the spinal cord. Accordingly, when the mechanism of injury indicates that the patient could have sustained SCI, treat the individual as having a spine injury regardless of the neurologic findings. The neurologic assessment is intended not only to determine whether the patient should be immobilized, but also to furnish data to the hospital about the precise initial presentation of the patient so that personnel there may evaluate any changes in condition and determine further investigations and treatment.

The initial step of any neurologic assessment is a determination of the level of consciousness. First note the patient's AVPU in the initial assessment, and then address the GCS level

Table 22-2	Landmark Myotomes		
Nerve Root	Muscle Group	Nerve Root	Muscle Group
C3-C5	Diaphragm	L2	Hip flexors: iliopsoas
C5	Elbow flexors: biceps, brachialis, brachioradialis	L3	Knee extensors: quadriceps
C6	Wrist extensors	L4	Ankle dorsiflexors: tibialis anterior
C7	Elbow extensors: triceps	L5	Long toe extensors: extensor hallucis longus
C8	Finger flexors: flexor digitorum profundus to middle finger	S1	Ankle plantar flexors (gastrocnemius, soleus)
T1	Hand intrinsics: interossei, small finger abductors	S4-S5	Anus, bowel, bladder
T2-T7	Intercostal muscles		

Table 22-3	Landmark Dermatomes		
Nerve Root	Anatomical Location	Nerve Root	Anatomical Location
C2	Occipital protuberance	T10	Umbilicus
C3	Supraclavicular fossa	L1	Inguinal line
C5	Lateral side of antecubital fossa	L2	Mid anterior thigh
C6	Thumb and medial index finger (6-shooter)	L3	Medial aspect of the knee
C7	Middle finger	L5	Dorsum of the foot
C8	Little finger	S1-S3	Back of leg
T2	Apex of axilla	S4-S5	Perianal area
T4	Nipple line		

during further assessment. When assigning the GCS, do not score the patient as having no motor response if limbs are paralyzed. Ask the patient to blink or move some facial muscles that would be innervated by a cranial nerve. Remember that an unconscious patient is always at risk for having a spinal injury.

Motor components of spinal nerves innervate discrete tissues and muscles of the body in regions called myotomes Table 22-2 ▲. The examination of these myotomes should take place in the typical head-to-toe fashion, starting with an assessment of the cranial nerves. Cranial nerve assessment is especially important in circumstances suggestive of a high cervical injury. Observe the patient for drooping of the upper eyelid (ptosis), a small pupil (miosis), and ipsilateral anhydrosis (Horner's syndrome) that would indicate an injury to the sympathetic pathway.

Bilaterally assess each major motor group from the top down to identify the lowest spinal segment associated with normal voluntary motor function. Because of the possibility of incomplete spinal cord lesions, it is important to determine the extent of function in segments below this level. Monitor for possible ascending lesions, paying special attention to alterations in respiratory patterns with cervical lesions.

Ask the patient to flex (C5) and extend (C7) both elbows and then both wrists (C6). Have the patient abduct the fingers and keep them open against resistance, and then adduct the fingers and attempt to close them against resistance (T1) Figure 22-12 ▶. As an alternative maneuver, have the patient curl all four fingers while the examiner applies opposing pull with his or her fingers to determine strength against resistance. This will test the finger flexors (C8).

To evaluate the lower extremities, ask the patient to bend and extend the knees. Next ask the patient to plantar flex the feet and ankles as if pressing down on the gas pedal of a car (S1–S2) and to dorsiflex the toes against resistance (L5) Figure 22-13 ▶.

Assessment of motor integrity in an unconscious patient is largely based on the patient's response to a painful stimulus. Spine injury with loss of motor function is likely if an unconscious patient grimaces, vocalises, or opens his or her eyes to a painful response above the level of the neurologic deficit but does not move the limbs. Pain responses should be tested at several locations before assuming an absence of response. If the motor examination cannot be completed due to local injury, the examination is considered unreliable and spine motion restriction is necessary.

Sensory components of spinal nerves innervate specific and discrete areas of the body surface called dermatomes Table 22-3 ▲. In addition to testing a general loss of sensation, ask the patient about abnormal sensations in these areas such as "pins and needles," electric shock, or hyperacute pain to touch (hyperesthesia). As with the motor examination, sensory integrity must be assessed bilaterally but from the feet up. Determine the lowest level of normal sensation and any areas of intact or "spared" sensation below this level. In the conscious patient, a thorough evaluation will include perception of light touch, pin prick, temperature, and position (proprioception).

Reflexes are usually not assessed in the prehospital environment but can provide valuable information regarding sensory input, especially in the unconscious patient. In significant SCIs, reflexes are usually absent but return several hours to several weeks after injury. If reflexes are intact, the preservation of motor and sensory activity in the same spinal cord segment is likely. A positive Babinski reflex occurs when the toes move upward in response to stimulation of the sole of the foot. Under normal circumstances, the toes move downward.

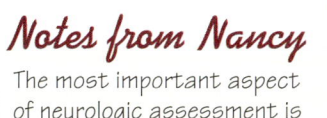

Notes from Nancy

The most important aspect of neurologic assessment is whether the patient's findings are changing and in what direction.

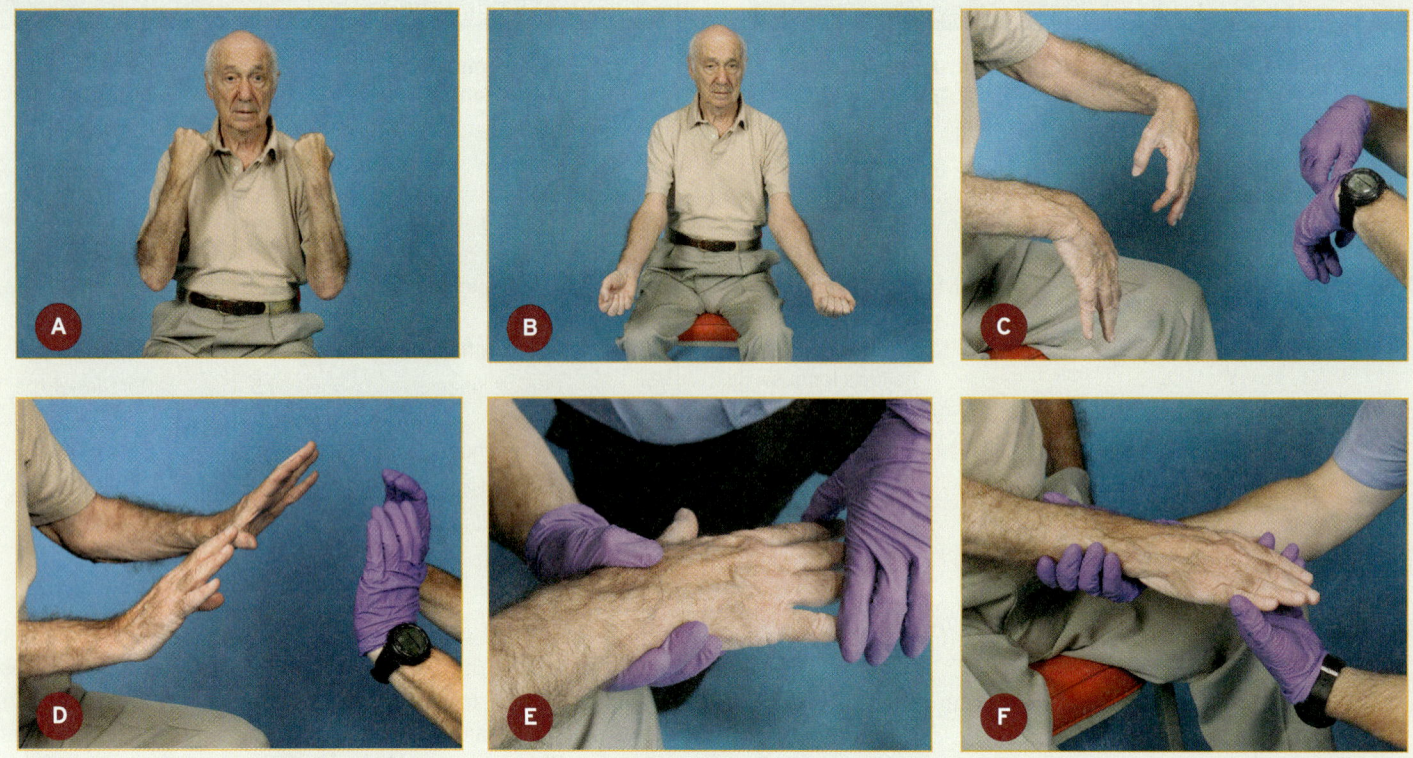

Figure 22-12 Neurologic evaluation of the upper extremities. Ask the patient to flex (**A**) and then extend (**B**) both elbows. Ask the patient to flex (**C**) and then extend (**D**) both wrists. Have the patient abduct the fingers and keep them open against resistance (**E**). Have the patient adduct the fingers and attempt to close them against resistance (**F**).

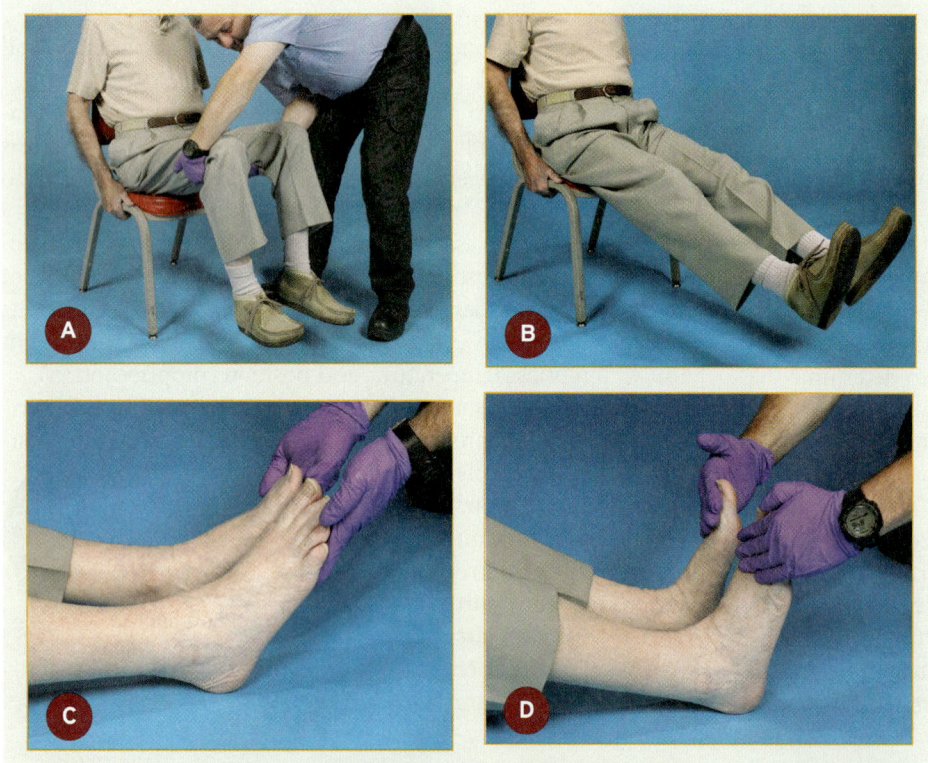

Figure 22-13 Neurologic evaluation of the lower extremities. Ask the patient to bend (**A**) and extend (**B**) the knees. Ask the patient to flex the feet and ankles downward (**C**) and flex the toes upward (**D**).

Ongoing Assessment

Vital signs should be monitored every 5 minutes (unstable patients) to 15 minutes (stable patients), with special attention to the patient's cardiovascular status. Be alert for hypotension without other signs of shock. The combination of hypotension with a normal or slow pulse and warm skin is highly suggestive of neurogenic shock. The SCI responsible for neurogenic shock also generally produces a flaccid paralysis and complete loss of sensation below the level of the injury. In contrast to neurogenic shock, hypovolemic shock is associated with pale, cold, clammy skin and tachycardia.

Check interventions such as oxygen flow and spinal immobilization to ensure that they are still effective. Some EMS systems may administer an antiemetic or corticosteroid per direct medical control. The use of steroids in acute spinal cord injury remains controversial; you should repeat the physical examination and reprioritize the patient as necessary.

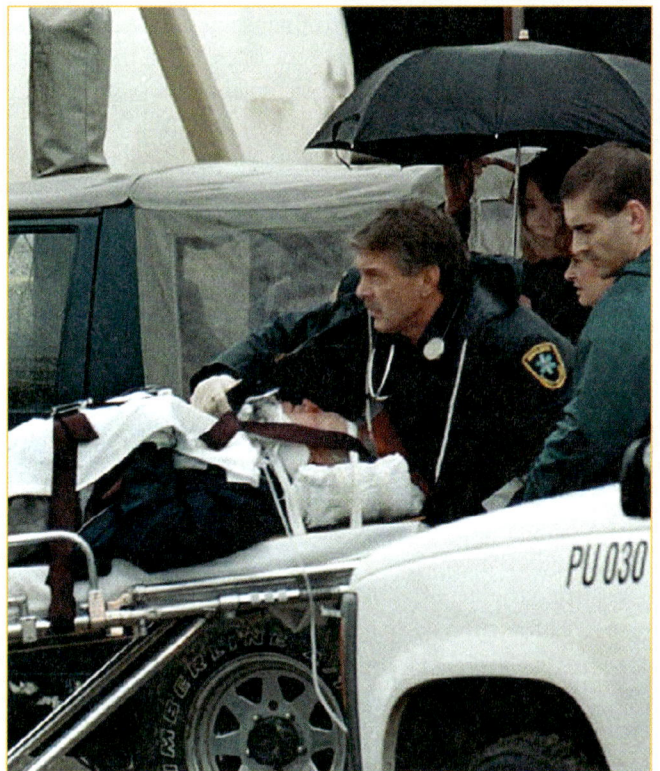

Figure 22-14 Spend no more than 10 minutes on scene unless lengthy extrication is underway or you are awaiting pending arrival of an air ambulance.

Special Considerations

When immobilizing pregnant patients, tilt the backboard 15° to 20° to the left using a pillow or blankets. If this is not possible, manually displace the uterus to the left side.

determine whether complete immobilization is necessary should be reviewed by medical directors for efficacy. If the patient has no neurologic deficit; is not under the influence of alcohol, drugs, or medications; has no distracting injuries; has no motor or sensory deficit; and has no pain or tenderness upon movement or palpation, then he or she may not require immobilization. If there is any doubt, the patient should be immobilized. As always, follow local protocols as determined by the medical director.

Spinal Splinting Procedures

For splinting purposes, the spine should be considered one long bone articulating with the head and the pelvis at either end. Thus the paramedic cannot isolate and splint at only one level of the spinal column; there is simply *no such thing as partial spinal immobilization.*

Special Considerations

In most instances, a toddler can be immobilized in a child seat. If the child and seat need to be placed in a supine position, the child must be extricated from the car seat to avoid placing extra pressure on the abdomen and reducing the lung expansion.

Management

Current principles of spine trauma management include recognition of potential or actual injury, appropriate immobilization (ie, spinal motion restriction), and reduction or prevention of the incidence of secondary injury. The primary goal of spinal immobilization is to prevent further injuries. Unfortunately, studies have shown that complete spinal immobilization can be painful, especially at pressure points of the occiput and lumbrosacral areas, and can produce a restriction on ventilation. Spinal motion restriction also increases the risk for aspiration. Rigid cervical collars have been implicated as contributing to elevated intracranial pressure. Prolonged scene times can also be an issue, as with any trauma patient. The goal of all paramedics, no matter what level, should be to spend no more than 10 minutes on the scene before the patient is transported to the most appropriate facility unless lengthy extrication is taking place or the team is awaiting pending arrival of an air ambulance **Figure 22-14**.

Although a definitive prehospital clinical spine clearance protocol has not yet been established, current practices reflect the principles of hospital-based models. Specific criteria to

Supine Patients

A supine patient can be effectively immobilized by securing him or her to a backboard. The preferred procedure for moving a patient from the ground to a backboard is the four-person log roll; this method is recommended whenever you suspect a spinal injury. In other cases, you may choose to slide the patient onto a backboard or use a scoop stretcher. The patient's condition, the scene, and available resources will dictate which method you choose. Ideally, the patient should be log rolled away from the side of injury. Another technique that limits movement of the spine is the use of a scoop stretcher to lift a patient a few inches off the floor or ground while another paramedic slides a backboard under the patient.

Your job is to ensure that the head, torso, and pelvis move as a unit, with your teammates controlling the movement of the body. If necessary, you may recruit bystanders to the team, but instruct them fully before moving the patient.

To immobilize a patient on a backboard, follow these steps:

1. *Using appropriate PPE, begin manual in-line stabilization* from a kneeling position at the patient's head. Hold the head firmly with both hands. The paramedic at the head directs all patient movement.

2. *Support the lower jaw with your index and long fingers, and support the head with your palms.* If the patient's head is not facing forward, gently move it until the patient's eyes are looking straight ahead and the head and torso are in line (neutral alignment). Never twist, flex, or extend the head or neck excessively. Do not remove your hands from the patient's head until the patient is properly secured to a backboard and the head is immobilized.

3. *Assess distal PMS function in each extremity.*

4. *Apply an appropriately sized cervical collar.* A cervical collar is used in addition to—not instead of—manual in-line cervical spine (also called c-spine) immobilization. Select the collar based on the manufacturer's specifications, and make sure it fits correctly. An improperly sized immobilization device could cause further injury. If you do not have the correct size, use a rolled towel; tape it to the backboard around the patient's head, and provide continuous manual support **Figure 22-15 ▼** . Place the chin support snugly underneath the chin. While maintaining manual in-line stabilization, wrap the collar around the neck and secure the collar to the far side of the chin support. Recheck that the patient is in a neutral in-line position.

5. The other team members should *position the immobilization device* (backboard) and place their hands on the far side of the patient to increase their leverage. Instruct them to use their body weight and their shoulder and back muscles to ensure a smooth, coordinated pull, concentrating their pull on the heavier portions of the patient's body **Figure 22-16A ▸** .

6. On command from the paramedic at the head, the rescuers should *roll the patient* toward themselves. One rescuer should then quickly examine the back while the patient is rolled on the side, then slide the backboard behind and under the patient. The team should then roll the patient back onto the board, avoiding rotation of the head, shoulders, and pelvis **Figure 22-16B ▸** .

7. *Make sure the patient is centred on the board.*

8. *Secure the upper torso to the board* once the patient is centred on the backboard **Figure 22-16C ▸** .

9. *Secure the pelvis and upper legs,* using padding as needed. For the pelvis, use straps over the iliac crests and/or groin loops (leg straps).

10. *Immobilize the head* to the board by positioning a commercial immobilization device or towel rolls. Secure the head to the board only after spider straps or something comparable have secured the torso. If the head is secured first and the body shifts, the spine may be compromised. Securing the majority of the body weight first provides better protection.

11. *Secure the head* by taping the head-immobilization device across the forehead. To prevent airway problems and maintain access to the airway, do not tape over the throat or chin. Instead, tape across the cervical collar just under the chin without covering the opening **Figure 22-16D ▸** .

12. *Check and readjust straps* as needed to ensure that the entire body is snugly secured and will not slide during movement of the board or patient transport.

13. *Reassess distal PMS function* in each extremity, and continue to do so periodically.

Do not force the head into a neutral, in-line position if the patient has muscle spasms in the neck; increased pain with movement (ie, interlocked facets); numbness, tingling, or weakness. In these situations, immobilize the patient in the position in which you found him or her.

The patient should be maintained in the neutral position unless pain or resistance to movement prevent it, in which case you should maintain the patient in the position found. Neutral positioning provides the most space for the spinal cord and may reduce cord hypoxia and excess pressure on the tissue. Do not place pillows under the patient's head. MRI studies, however, have revealed that the adult cervical spinal canal is anatomically aligned if the head is elevated by padding under the occiput with a folded towel or pad. About 80% of adult

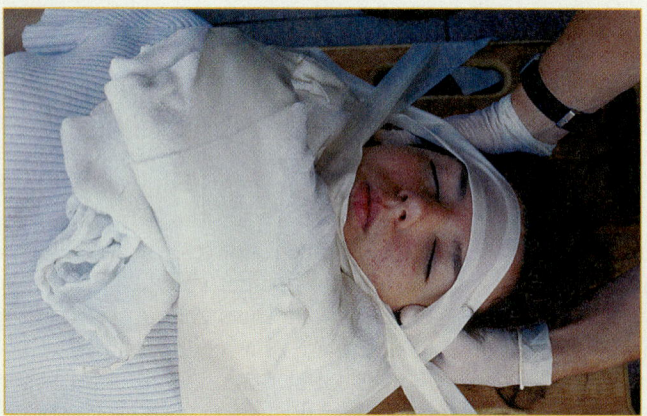

Figure 22-15 If you don't have an appropriately sized cervical collar, use a rolled towel. Tape it to the backboard around the patient's head and provide continuous manual support.

Special Considerations

Do not accept the labeled sizes ("pediatric" or "infant") for cervical collars. Measure each patient individually. Never place tape across the child's neck; it may obstruct the airway. Also, remember to add padding so that the child is as wide as the board.

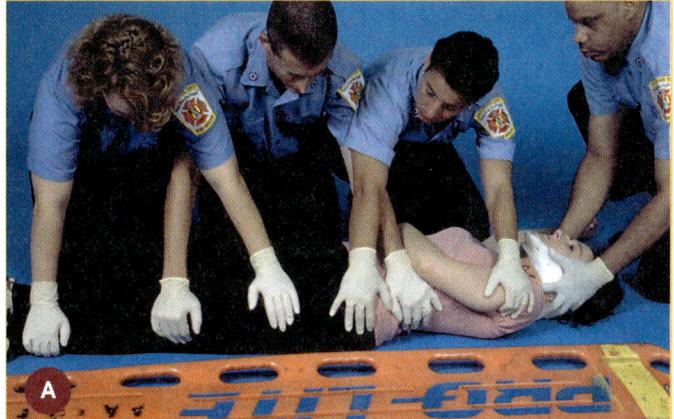
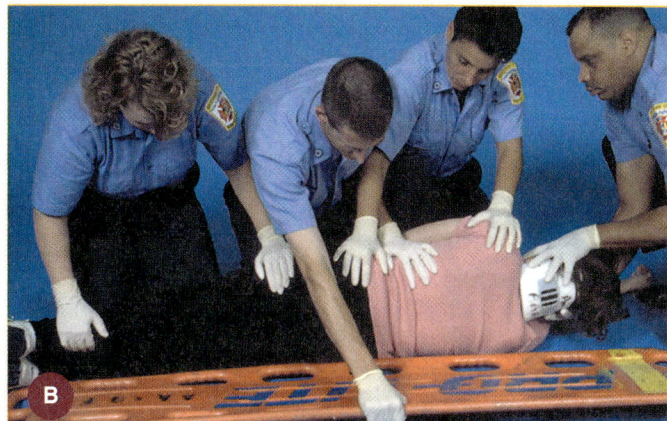
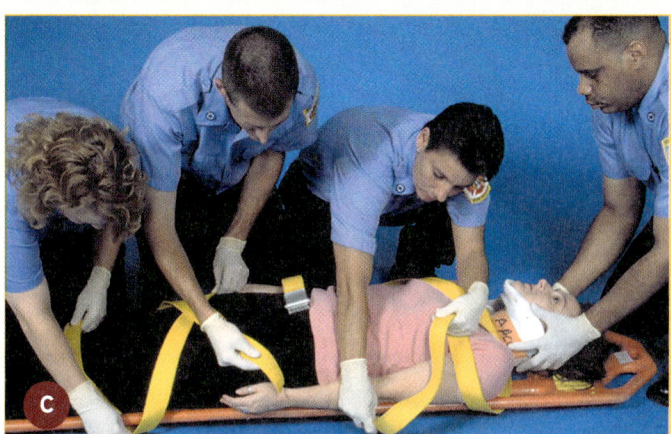
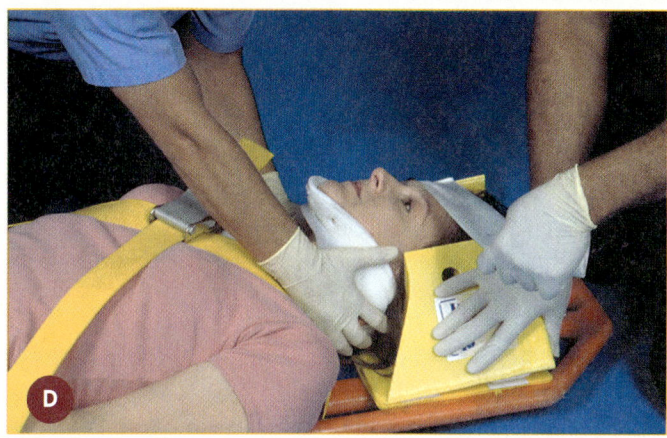

Figure 22-16 Immobilizing a patient to a backboard. **A.** Placing hands on the far side of the patient. **B.** Rolling the patient and examining the back. **C.** Securing the upper and lower torso. **D.** Securing the head.

patients placed flat on a backboard will be in extension and will require 1 cm to 5 cm of padding to achieve neutral positioning. Pediatric patients have relatively larger heads, so they need padding under the torso to maintain alignment and prevent neck flexion if immobilized on an adult backboard. Newer pediatric backboards include a recessed portion that accommodates the head or they have torso padding.

Patients who are found in a prone position or on their side should be log rolled into the supine position with the head and neck manually stabilized in the position in which they were found, and then immobilized as described earlier. One rescuer should take control of the cervical spine using a crossed-hand position to roll the patient. The second rescuer should be positioned at the torso, with any additional help at the pelvis and legs. The rescuer at the head counts, and the patient is rolled as a unit into a supine position. Assessment and immobilization should then continue as usual.

An unconscious patient whose head and neck are passively rotated to one side should be maintained in this position unless respiration is compromised. In case of respiratory distress, attempt to bring the head into axial alignment with gentle traction. A conscious and reliable patient can be asked to turn the head if there are no overt signs of injury or neurologic deficit. If the patient experiences neck pain or nervous system complaints, this movement should be halted and the patient should be transported in the position of comfort.

Seated Patients

Patients found in a sitting position (eg, after a motor vehicle collision) who are without cardiorespiratory compromise but require spine immobilization should also be approached with manual stabilization of the head and neck. A rigid cervical collar should be measured and placed appropriately, and a vest-type extrication device should be used to facilitate the transfer of the patient onto a backboard. Exceptions to this rule include the following situations in which you do not have time to first secure the patient to the short board:

- You or the patient is in danger.
- You need to gain immediate access to other patients.
- The patient's injuries justify urgent removal.

In these situations, your team should lower the patient directly onto a backboard, using the rapid extrication technique discussed later in this chapter. Provide manual stabilization of the cervical spine as you move the patient. Rapid extrication is indicated only in cases of life- or limb-threatening injury. In all other cases, follow these steps to immobilize a sitting patient:

1. *Stabilize the head* and then maintain manual in-line stabilization until the patient is secured to the backboard.
2. *Assess distal PMS function* in each extremity.
3. *Apply the rigid cervical collar.* Because the cervical collar does not provide complete stabilization of the cervical spine, continue manual stabilization of the patient's head and neck until the patient is fully immobilized on a backboard.

4. *Insert a short spine immobilization device* between the patient's upper back and the seat back.
5. *Open the board's side flaps* (if present) and position them around the patient's torso, snug to the armpits **Figure 22-17A** .
6. Once the device is properly positioned, *secure the upper torso straps.*
7. *Position and fasten both groin loops* (leg straps). Pad the groin as needed. Check all torso straps and make sure they are secure. Make any adjustments necessary without excessive movement of the patient.
8. *Pad any space* between the patient's head and the device.
9. *Secure the forehead* strap or tape the head securely, then fasten the lower head strap around the rigid cervical collar **Figure 22-17B** .
10. *Place the backboard* next to the patient's buttocks, perpendicular to the trunk.
11. *Turn the patient* parallel to the long board, and slowly lower him or her onto it.
12. *Lift the patient* and the vest-type device together as a unit (without rotating the patient), and slip the backboard under the patient and device **Figure 22-17C** .

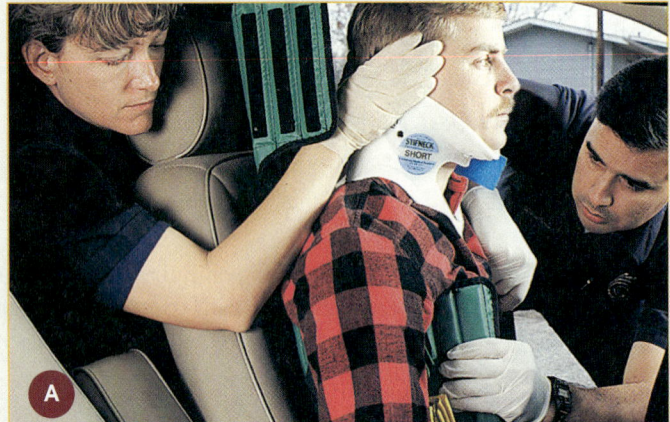

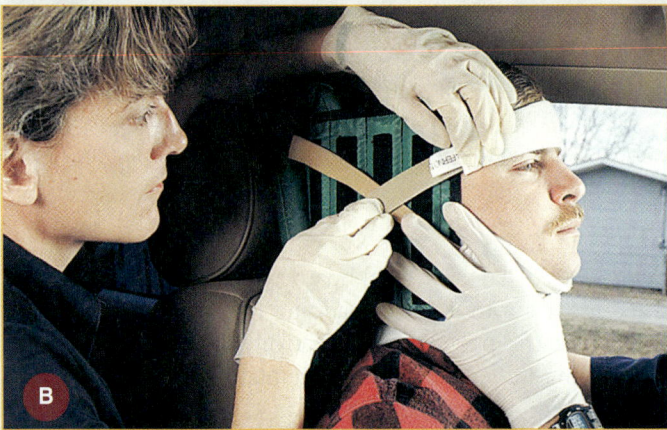

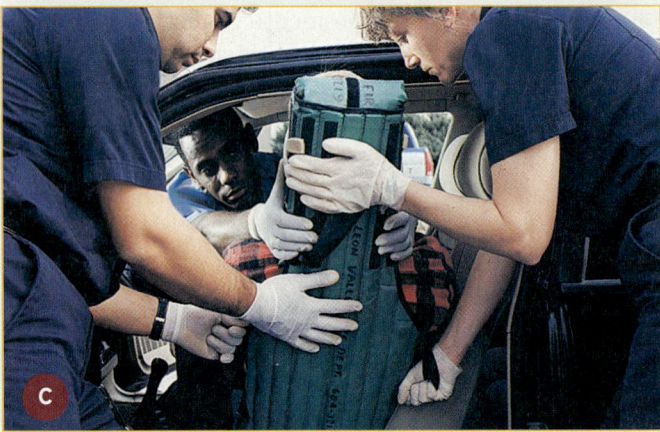

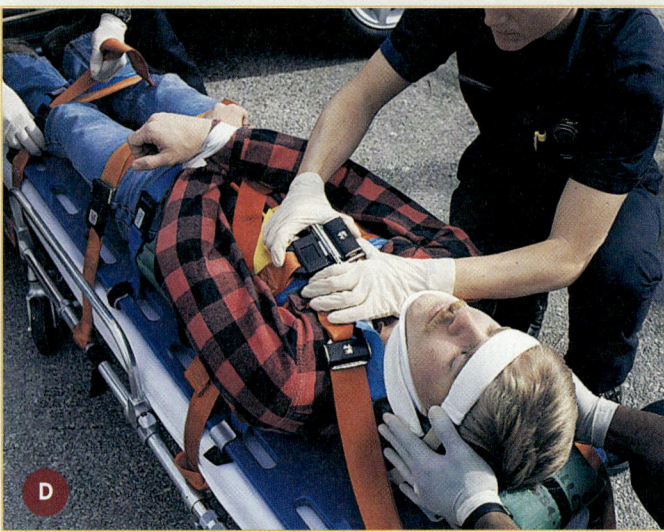

Figure 22-17 Immobilizing a patient found in a sitting position. **A.** Positioning around the patient's torso. **B.** Securing the head straps. **C.** Lowering the patient onto the backboard. **D.** Securing immobilization devices.

Special Considerations

Osteoporosis in the thoracic and lumbar spine contributes to a high rate of injury in older patients. Three types of fractures are commonly encountered in these individuals:

- **Compression fractures**—stable injuries that often result from minimal trauma, eg, simply bending over, rising from a chair, or sitting down forcefully.
- **Burst fractures**—unstable fractures that typically result from a high-energy mechanism of injury such as a motor vehicle collision or a fall from substantial height. They may lead to neurologic injury secondary to shifting of the vertebrae with damage to the spinal cord.
- **Seatbelt-type fractures (Chance fractures)**—involve flexion and cause a fracture through the entire vertebral body and bony arch. These injuries typically occur in individuals who are wearing only a lap belt without a shoulder harness.

13. *Release the leg straps* and loosen the chest strap to allow the legs to straighten and give the chest room to fully expand.
14. *Secure the short device and backboard together.* Do not remove the vest-type device from the patient.
15. *Reassess distal PMS function* in all four extremities. Note your findings on the patient care report, and prepare for transport **Figure 22-17D ◄**.

Rapid Extrication

With the rapid extrication technique, the patient can be moved from sitting in a car to lying supine on a backboard in approximately 2 minutes. You should use the rapid extrication technique in the following situations:

- The vehicle or scene is unsafe.
- The patient cannot be properly assessed before being removed from the car.
- The patient needs immediate intervention that requires a supine position.
- The patient's condition requires immediate transport to the hospital.
- The patient blocks the paramedic's access to another seriously injured patient.

In such cases, the delay that results from applying an extrication-type vest or half-board is contraindicated and unacceptable. Unfortunately, the manual support and immobi-

Special Considerations

To immobilize kyphotic patients, several blankets and pillows or vacuum splints may be required to provide support to the head and upper back. Make sure that the empty spaces under the patient's knees or lumbar spine are padded as well.

lization that you provide when using the rapid extrication technique carry a greater risk of spine movement. You should not use the rapid extrication technique if no urgency exists.

The rapid extrication technique requires a team of three paramedics who are knowledgeable and practiced in the procedure. Follow these steps:

1. The first rescuer provides manual in-line stabilization of the patient's head and cervical spine from behind. Support may be applied from the side, if necessary, by reaching through the driver's door.
2. The second rescuer serves as a team leader and gives the commands to coordinate the team's moves until the patient is supine on the backboard. Because the second rescuer lifts and turns the patient's torso, he or she must be physically capable of moving the patient. The second rescuer works from the driver's doorway. If the first rescuer is also working from that doorway, the second rescuer should stand closer to the door hinges toward the front of the vehicle. The second rescuer applies a rigid cervical collar and performs an initial assessment.
3. The second rescuer provides continuous support of the patient's torso until the patient is supine on the backboard. Once the second rescuer takes control of the torso, usually in the form of a body hug, he or she should not let go of the patient for any reason. Some type of cross-chest shoulder hug usually works well, but you must decide which method will work best for any given patient. You cannot simply reach into the car and grab the patient, because this will twist the patient's torso. You must rotate the patient as a unit.
4. The third rescuer works from the front passenger seat and rotates the patient's legs and feet as the torso is turned, ensuring that they are free of the pedals and any other obstruction. The third rescuer should first carefully move the patient's nearer leg laterally, without rotating the patient's pelvis and lower spine. The pelvis and lower spine rotate only as the third rescuer moves the second leg during the next step. Moving the nearer leg first makes it much easier to move the second leg in concert with the rest of the body. Once the third rescuer moves the legs together, they should be moved as a unit **Figure 22-18A ►**.
5. The patient is rotated 90° so that the back faces out the driver's door and the feet are on the front passenger's seat. This coordinated movement is done in three or four short, quick, one eighth to one quarter turns. The second rescuer coordinates the sequence of moves and the first rescuer directs each quick turn by saying, "Ready, turn" or "Ready, move." Hand position changes should be made between moves.
6. In most cases, the first rescuer will be working from the back seat. At some point, either because the doorpost is in the way or because he or she cannot reach farther from the back seat, the first rescuer will be unable to follow the torso rotation. At that time, the third rescuer should assume temporary manual in-line stabilization of the head and neck until the first rescuer can regain control of the

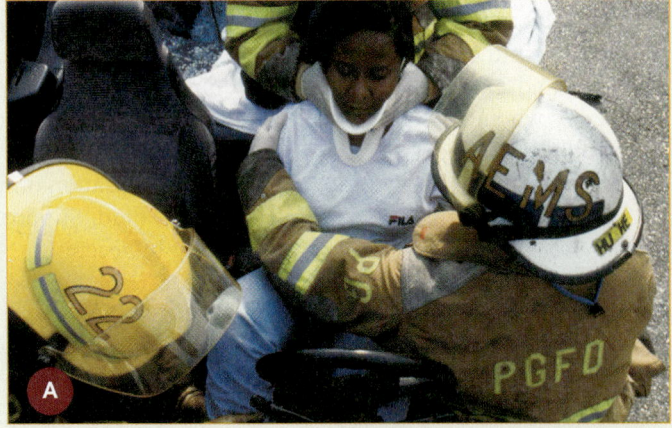
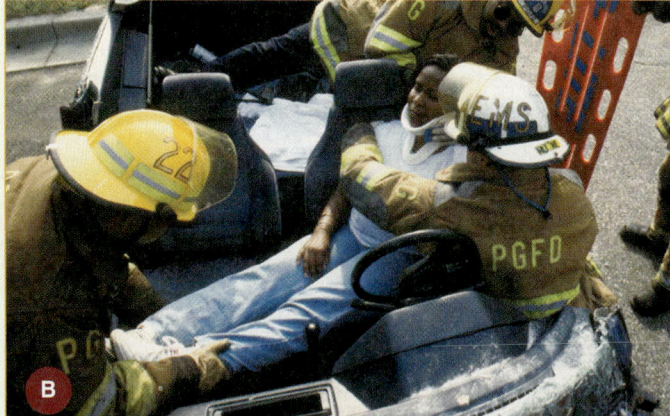
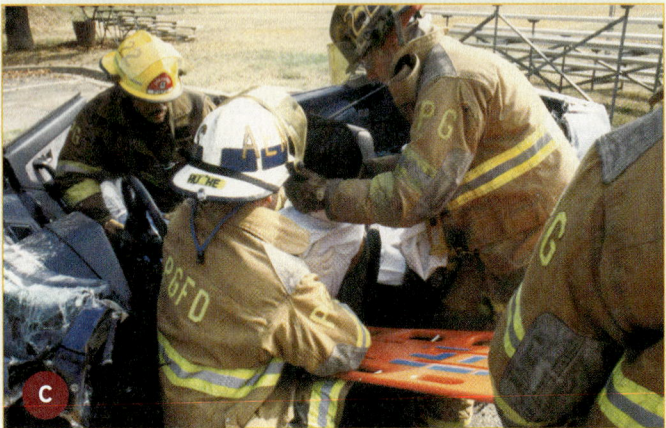
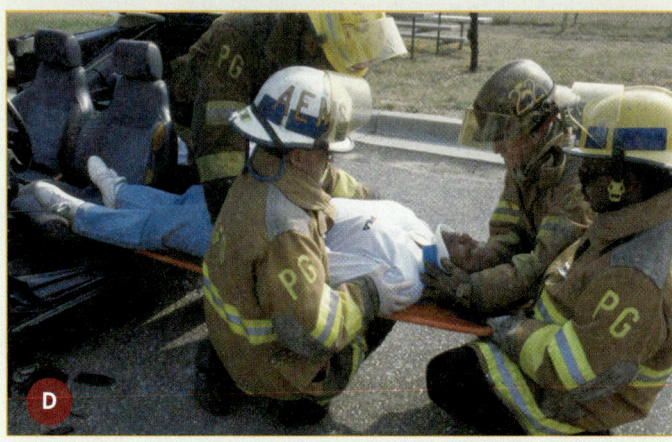

Figure 22-18 Rapid extrication technique. **A.** Moving the patient's legs without moving the pelvis or spine. **B.** Rotating the patient as a unit. **C.** Placing the backboard on the seat. **D.** Sliding the patient onto the board.

head from outside the vehicle. If a fourth rescuer is present, the fourth rescuer stands next to the second rescuer. The fourth rescuer takes control of the head and neck from outside the vehicle without involving the third rescuer. As soon as the change has been made, the rotation can continue **Figure 22-18B ▲**.

7. Once the patient has been fully rotated, the backboard is placed against the patient's buttocks on the seat. Do not try to wedge the backboard under the patient. If only three rescuers are present, place the backboard within arm's reach of the driver's door before the move so that the board can be pulled into place when needed; the far end of the board can be left on the ground. When a fourth rescuer is available, the first rescuer exits the rear seat of the car, places the backboard against the patient's buttocks, and maintains pressure in toward the vehicle from the far end of the board. When the door opening allows, some rescuers prefer to insert the backboard onto the car seat before the patient is rotated.

8. As soon as the patient has been rotated and the backboard is in place, the second and third rescuers lower the patient onto the board while supporting the head and torso so that neutral alignment is maintained. The first rescuer holds the backboard until the patient is secured **Figure 22-18C ▲**.

9. The third rescuer moves across the front seat to be in position at the patient's hips. If the third rescuer stays at the patient's knees or feet, he or she will be ineffective in helping to move the body's weight. The knees and feet follow the hips.

10. The fourth rescuer maintains in-line support of the head and takes over giving the commands. If a fourth rescuer is not present, you can direct a volunteer to assist you. The second rescuer maintains direction of the extrication; this rescuer stands with his or her back to the door, facing the rear of the vehicle. The backboard should be immediately in front of the third rescuer. The second rescuer grasps the patient's shoulders or armpits. On command, the second and third rescuers slide the patient 20 cm to 30 cm along the backboard, repeating this slide until the patient's hips are firmly on the backboard.

11. The third rescuer gets out of the vehicle and moves to the opposite side of the backboard, across from the second rescuer. The third rescuer takes control at the shoulders, and the second rescuer moves back to take control of the hips. On command, these two rescuers move the patient along the board in 20 cm to 30 cm slides until the patient is completely on the board **Figure 22-18D ▲**.

12. The first (or fourth) rescuer continues to maintain manual in-line support of the head. The second and third rescuers

grasp their side of the board, and then carry it and the patient away from the vehicle onto the prepared stretcher nearby.

In some cases, you will be able to rest the head end of the backboard on the stretcher while the patient is moved onto the backboard; in others, you will not. Once the backboard and patient have been placed on the stretcher, you should begin lifesaving treatment immediately. If you used the rapid extrication technique because the scene was dangerous, you and your team should immediately move the stretcher a safe distance away from the vehicle before you assess or treat the patient.

The steps of the rapid extrication technique must be considered a general procedure to be adapted as needed. Every situation will be different—a different car, a different size and priority patient, and a different crew. Your resourcefulness and ability to adapt are necessary elements of a successful rapid extrication.

Standing Patients

Ambulatory patients found on the scene may require immobilization after examination and determination of mechanism and reliability. If you suspect underlying head, neck, or spine injuries, carefully take down the patient using the standing takedown (described below), then immobilize the patient to a backboard. This will require a minimum of three rescuers, undertaking the following steps:

1. Establish manual, in-line stabilization, apply a rigid cervical collar, and instruct the patient to remain still.
2. Position the board upright, directly behind the patient.
3. Two rescuers stand on either side of the patient; the third is directly behind the patient, maintaining immobilization.
4. The two rescuers grasp the handholds at shoulder level or slightly above by reaching under the patient's arms while standing at either side **Figure 22-19A ▶**.
5. Prepare to lower the patient to the ground **Figure 22-19B ▶**.

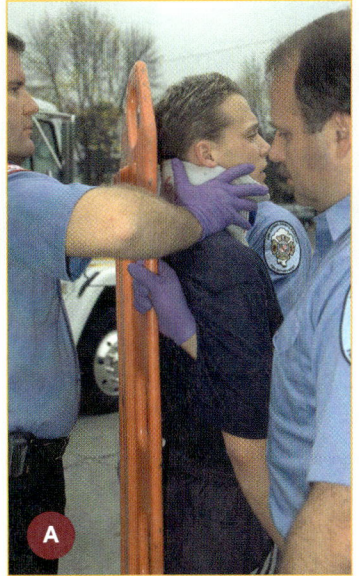

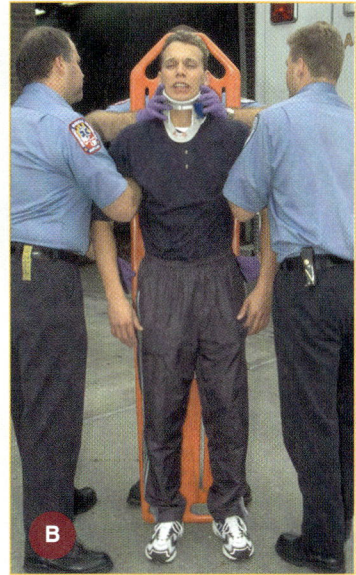

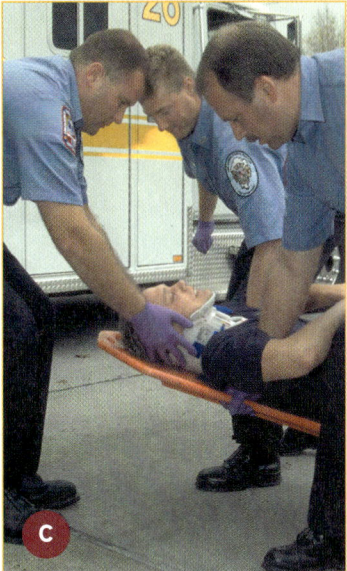

Figure 22-19 Immobilizing a patient found in a standing position. **A.** Positioning rescuers at the sides of the backboard. **B.** Preparing to lower the patient. **C.** Lowering the patient to the ground. Once the patient's head is on the board, do not lift it off the board!

6. Carefully lower the patient as a unit under the direction of the rescuer at the head. The rescuer at the head must make sure the head stays against the board and carefully rotate his or her hands while the patient is being lowered to maintain in-line stabilization **Figure 22-19C ▲**.

Packaging and Removal of Injured Patients From the Water

Whatever the type of accident, the principles of packaging and removal are the same: Keep the head, neck, and trunk in alignment. When the patient may have sustained a spine injury in a confirmed diving accident, spinal immobilization must be initiated even before the patient is removed from the water. If respiratory arrest is suspected, ventilation can be done while still in the water; in case of cardiac arrest, however, the rescuer should quickly evaluate the mechanism of injury. If a spine injury is not obvious, immediately remove the patient from the water and

At the Scene

Most patients who have just sustained a potential spine injury and are standing up at a collision scene still need to be immobilized. Use of the standing takedown technique is strongly recommended. They are not backboarded in the standing position because many of these patients will not stand still for the amount of time it takes to complete the immobilization. Some may be dizzy, weak, or intoxicated. Patients who have sustained head trauma may have a head injury. Also, if the backboard is applied and the patient is then placed in the supine position, the straps and padding may loosen as the patient lies down.

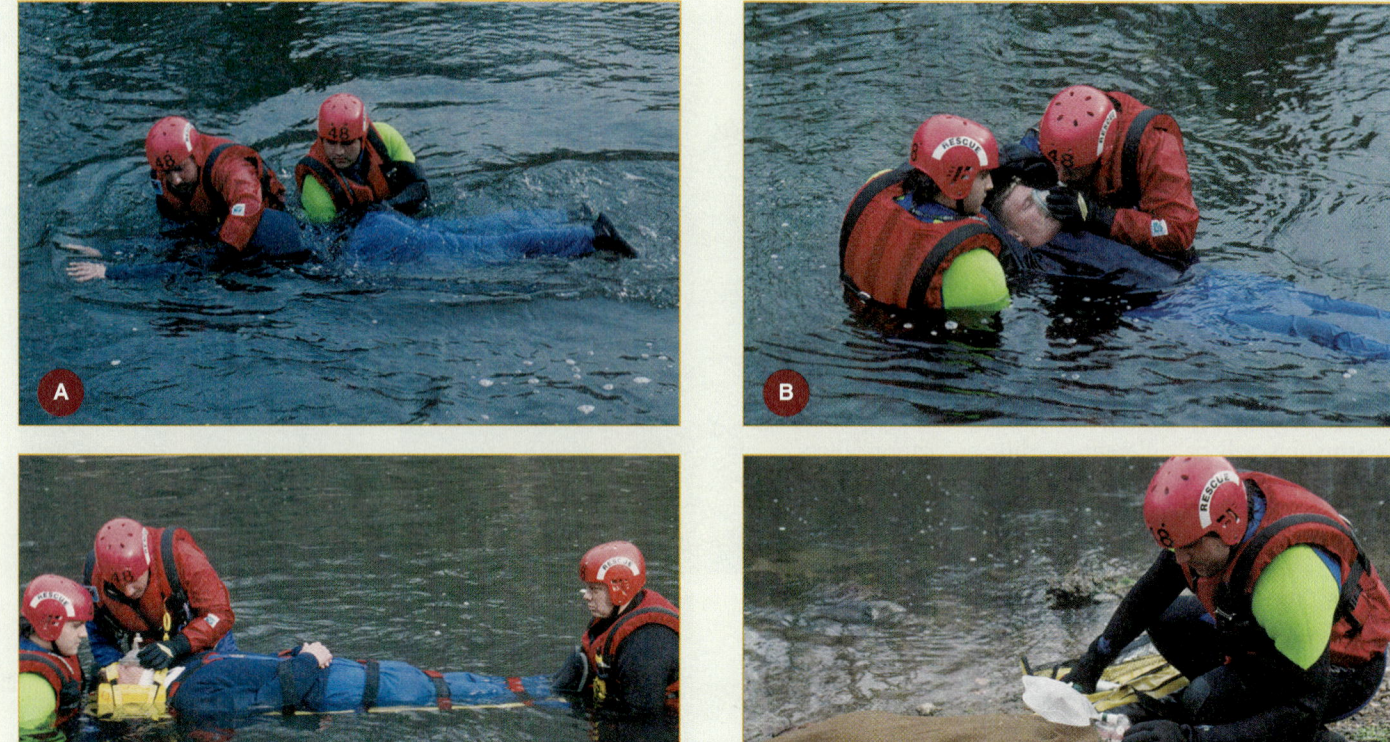

Figure 22-20 Stabilizing a suspected spine injury in the water. **A.** Turning the patient to a supine position in the water. **B.** Providing artificial ventilation. **C.** Securing the patient to a backboard. **D.** Providing prehospital care once out of the water.

begin CPR. However, if there is any indication of a spine injury, follow these steps to stabilize the patient in the water:

1. If the patient is prone in the water, *approach the individual from the top of the head*, and place one arm under the body so that the head is supported on your arm and the chest on your hand. Place your other arm across the head and back to splint the head and neck between your arms. Continuing to support the patient's head and neck in that fashion, take a step backward and smoothly turn the patient to the supine position **Figure 22-20A ▲** .

   Two rescuers are usually required to turn the patient safely, but in some cases one rescuer will suffice. Always rotate the entire upper half of the patient's body as a single unit. Twisting only the head, for example, may aggravate any injury to the cervical spine.

2. *Open the airway and begin ventilation.* Immediate ventilation is the primary treatment of all drowning and submersion patients. As soon as the patient is face up in the water, use a pocket mask if it is available. Have the other rescuer support the head and trunk as a unit while you open the airway and begin artificial ventilation **Figure 22-20B ▲** .

3. *Float a buoyant backboard under the patient* as you continue ventilation.

4. *Secure the head and trunk* to the backboard to eliminate motion of the cervical spine. Do not remove the patient from the water until this step is complete **Figure 22-20C ▲** .

5. *Remove the patient from the water*, on the backboard.

6. *Remove wet clothes*, and cover the patient with a blanket. Give supplementary oxygen if the patient is breathing adequately; give positive-pressure ventilation if the patient is apneic or breathing inadequately. Begin CPR if there is no pulse. Effective chest compressions cannot be performed when the patient is still in the water **Figure 22-20D ▲** .

7. *Consider using an advanced airway device* to maintain the airway if needed. Place the patient on a cardiac monitor and treat dysrhythmias according to the ACLS algorithms (discussed in other chapters).

Patients Wearing Helmets

Helmets are a relatively common finding in motor vehicle and sports-related injuries. The use of helmets has been shown to reduce both the incidence and the severity of brain injuries associated with trauma, and their use is widely encouraged. Most helmets consist of an inner foam layer surrounded by a durable plastic shell. Helmets can inhibit full exposure of the patient and could hinder the paramedic's efforts at airway management and spinal stabilization. Unfortunately, the removal of most types of helmets can result in some spinal motion even under the best circumstances. However, a securely fitting helmet can provide a degree of stabilization and under the proper circumstances can actually assist in maintaining the spine in a neutral position.

The Inter-Association Task Force for the Appropriate Care of the Spine-Injured Athlete (convened in 1999) recommended helmet removal in the following situations:

- The helmet and chin strap fail to hold the head securely, as with a loose-fitting helmet.
- The helmet and chin strap design prevent adequate airway control, even after the removal of a face mask.
- A helmet with a face mask cannot be removed after a reasonable amount of time.
- The helmet prevents proper immobilization for transport.

Only paramedics who are familiar with the procedure should attempt helmet removal. A single rescuer should not attempt helmet removal, because the maneuver requires two paramedics:

1. *Kneel at the patient's head.* Leave enough room between your knees and the helmet so that you can remove the helmet. Your partner should kneel on one side of the patient, at the shoulder area.

2. *Stabilize the helmet* by placing your hands on either side of it, with your fingers on the patient's lower jaw to prevent movement of the head. Once your hands are in position, your partner can loosen the face strap.

3. Your partner should open the face shield, if there is one, and *assess the patient's airway and breathing.* Remove eyeglasses if the patient is wearing them.

4. Once the strap is loosened, your partner should place one hand on the patient's lower jaw at the angle of the jaw and the other behind the head at the back of the helmet. You may then pull the sides of the helmet away from the patient's head **Figure 22-21A ▶** .

5. *Gently slip the helmet partly off the patient's head,* stopping when the helmet reaches the halfway point.

6. Your partner then slides his or her hand from the back of the helmet to the occiput, preventing the head from falling back once the helmet is completely removed **Figure 22-21B ▶** .

7. Once your partner's hand is in place, remove the helmet and provide manual in-line cervical spine stabilization **Figure 22-21C ▶** .

8. *Apply a rigid cervical collar* and secure the patient to the backboard.

👥 Controversies

Considerable controversy exists regarding whether to remove helmets in the prehospital setting. The key considerations boil down to the urgency of airway management, the fit of the helmet, and the best-trained hands to take it off.

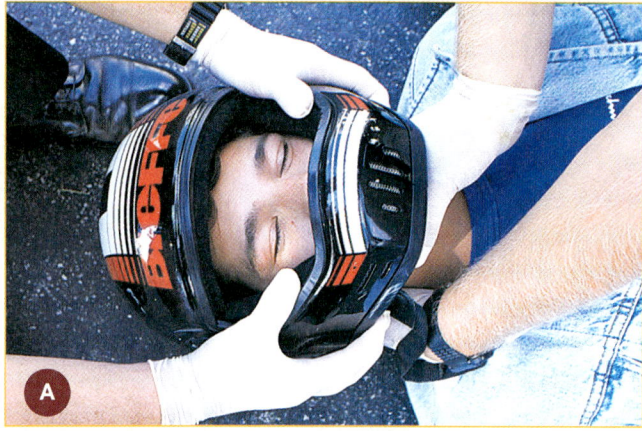

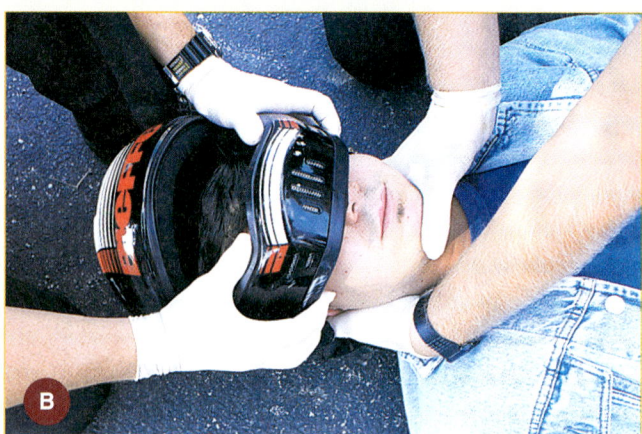

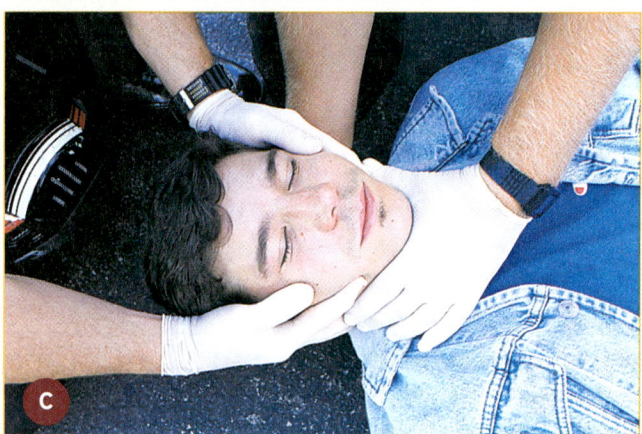

Figure 22-21 Removing a helmet. **A.** Hand positioning for removing a helmet. **B.** Supporting the occiput. **C.** Removing the helmet while stabilizing the head.

9. With large helmets or small patients, you may need to add padding under the shoulders to prevent flexion of the neck. If the patient is wearing shoulder pads or a heavy jacket, you may need to pad behind the head to prevent extension of the neck.

You do not need to remove a helmet if you can access the patient's airway, the head is snug inside the helmet, and the helmet can be secured to an immobilization device.

Pharmacotherapy of Spinal Cord Injury

Short-acting, reversible sedatives are recommended for the acute agitated patient after a correctible cause of agitation (eg, hypoxia) has been excluded. The risk of secondary injury due to movements from acute agitation must be balanced with potential airway and ventilatory compromise as well as a reliable neurologic examination. Pain medication may also be necessary.

The use of steroids in the acute phase of SCI remains controversial. The National Acute Spinal Cord Injury Study II and III (NASCIS) in the United States supports the use of methylprednisolone in acute nonpenetrating SCI. The study regimen includes a 30 mg/kg bolus of methylprednisolone over 15 minutes. After a 45-minute interval, start an infusion of 5.4 mg/kg/h, which continues over the next 23 hours. If treatment with methylprednisolone begins within 3 to 8 hours after injury, the infusion is typically continued for 48 hours.

This practice has been reviewed systematically by the Canadian Spine Society and the Canadian Neurosurgical Society. The committee concluded the following:

- There is insufficient evidence to support the use of high-dose methylprednisolone within 8 hours following an acute closed spinal cord injury as a treatment standard or as a guideline for treatment.
- Methylprednisolone prescribed as a bolus intravenous infusion of 30 mg/kg of body weight over 15 minutes within 8 hours of acute closed spinal cord injury, followed 45 minutes later by an infusion of 5.4 mg/kg of body weight per hour for 23 hours is a treatment option for which there is weak clinical evidence (Level II and III).
- There is insufficient evidence to support extending methylprednisolone infusion beyond 23 hours, if chosen as a treatment option.

The use of steroids in the acute phase of SCI is not routinely practiced in Canada.

Complications of Spinal Cord Injury

The complications of SCI are a consistent cause of the high morbidity and mortality—and high financial cost—associated with this type of injury. Many of the acute-phase complications of SCI have already been addressed in this chapter, such as the potential for aspiration or respiratory arrest, especially with high cervical injuries. Lower cervical lesions may preserve the diaphragm, but the loss of intercostal muscles ultimately impairs coughing and deep breathing, predisposing the patient to atelectasis and pneumonia. Deep-vein thrombosis and pulmonary embolism are late complications that may result from immobility and can become potentially life-threatening.

Autonomic dysreflexia, also called autonomic hyperreflexia, is typically a late complication of SCI but can occur acutely. This potentially life-threatening emergency most commonly occurs with injuries above T4–T6 and results from the loss of

Table 22-4	Signs and Symptoms of Autonomic Dysreflexia
■ Hypertension	■ Rebound hypotension
■ Headache	■ Flushing and sweating above SCI
■ Nasal congestion	■ Erect hairs above SCI
■ Dilation of the pupils	■ Chills without fever
■ Anxiety	■ Bronchospasm
■ Bradycardia	■ Seizures, stroke, and death

parasympathetic stimulation. Patients present clinically with evidence of a massive, uninhibited, uncompensated cardiovascular response due to some stimulation of the sympathetic nervous system below the level of injury Table 22-4. The irritated area sends a signal that is not able to reach the brain, and unabated sympathetic nervous system stimulation results in vasoconstriction as evidenced by cool, pale extremities, systolic blood pressures greater than 200 mm Hg, and diastolic blood pressures of 130 mm Hg or greater. Hypertension leads to parasympathetic stimulation from activation of the vasomotor centre in the medulla. Vagal compensation causes bradycardia and vasodilation of peripheral and visceral vessels above the level of the lesion, although vessels below the SCI remain constricted. Selective vasodilation results in flushed, diaphoretic skin and nasopharyngeal vessel congestion.

Autonomic dysreflexia can be precipitated by any noxious stimuli below the level of a cervical or high thoracic SCI. Common precipitators include skin lesions such as insect bites, constrictive clothing, or sharp objects compressing the skin. Sharp objects should be removed from pockets or seat cushions. Localized wounds such as lacerations, abrasions, decubitus ulcerations, or ingrown toenails are often the source of stimulation. Irritation from skin lesions should be minimized with cold packs. Distension of the bladder due to obstructed urine outflow from spasm or kinked Foley catheters as well as bladder infection, constipation, or bowel impaction must be suspected. Catheters should be irrigated and obstructions removed. In men, tight condom catheters can pinch genitalia and should be checked and removed if necessary. In women, menstrual cramps or pregnancy can be a source of the stimulation.

Management of autonomic dysreflexia is usually not a prehospital intervention. If the source cannot be found or minimized to an effective extent, it may be necessary to reduce blood pressure with vasodilators.

Nontraumatic Spinal Conditions

Back pain is one of the most common physical complaints in emergency departments. An estimated 60% to 90% of the population is afflicted with some form of low back pain. Expenses related to back pain are high due to the extensive costs of therapy and lost wages from missed work days. Upright posture brings a significant amount of weight to bear on the lumbar spine—specifically at L4–L5, where the natural bend in the spine's curvature changes. As a consequence, most people are

Table 22-5	Common Causes of Low Back Pain
■ Muscle or ligament strains ■ Fractures ■ Osteomyelitis—bone infection ■ Degenerative joint/disk disease	■ Spondylolysis ■ Bursitis/synovitis ■ Disk herniation ■ Tumour

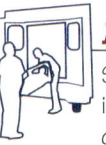

At the Scene

Spondylolysis is a structural defect of the spine involving the lamina or vertebral arch. It usually occurs between the superior and inferior articulating facets. In most people, it is congenital and may be hereditary. A radiograph is necessary to confirm spondylolysis.

susceptible to injury or degenerative disease. Spinal tumours can also be a cause of pain and debilitation. Occupations that require repetitive lifting, exposure to vibrations from vehicles or industrial machinery, and comorbid diseases such as osteoporosis are all risks for developing low back pain.

Most cases of low back pain are idiopathic, and making a precise diagnosis can be difficult. When evaluating nontraumatic back pain, it is important to consider disease processes that can result in significantly debilitating lesions, including SCI **Table 22-5 ▲** . In the absence of trauma, the patient who presents with the complaint of lower back pain must be assessed with the anatomy and neurophysiology of the spine and spinal cord in mind. Pay particular attention to the medications the patient is taking, because patients with chronic back pain and tumours may require very high levels of narcotics to control the intense pain.

Pain may result from strain or sprain of paravertebral muscles and supporting ligamentous structures without significant injury to nerve elements. Older patients (especially women) with a history of osteoporosis are at high risk for spontaneous compression fractures of the spine; these typically stable fractures are not associated with SCI. Furthermore, tumours in the spine from a variety of metastatic carcinomas can cause pathologic spine fractures, with extension of bone fragments or the tumour itself into the spinal canal causing SCI.

Degenerative disk disease is a common entity in patients older than age 50 years. Over time, biomechanical alterations of the intervertebral disk will result in loss of height and reduce the shock-absorbing effect of the disk. Significant narrowing may result in variable segment stability.

Disk herniation is usually caused by some degree of trauma in patients with preexisting disk degeneration. It typically affects men between the ages of 30 and 50 years, and often results from poor lifting technique. Herniation most commonly occurs at L4–L5 and L5–S1 but may also occur in C5–C6 and C6–C7. Patients will present with pain, usually with straining; they may have tenderness of the spine and often have limited range of motion. Alterations in sensation and motor functions may exist as well. Cervical herniations may present with upper extremity pain or paresthesias that worsen with neck motion. Motor weakness may also occur due to spinal cord compression.

Definitive diagnosis of back pain may require multiple modalities of radiographic imaging. Prehospital management of low back pain in the absence of trauma is primarily palliative, directed at decreasing any pain or discomfort with movement. Patients who experience significant pain with movement or have neurologic deficits may benefit from spinal immobilization for greater comfort and to prevent irritation of neural elements.

Controversies

Classic education holds that intervertebral disks have no sensory nerve fibres. In reality, sensory nerves extend into the disk over at least one third the radius of the outer rim, the anulus fibrosis. In the clinical setting, it is impossible to tell whether low back pain is coming solely from the irritation of these nerves. However, this etiology is always a possibility, even if MRI and CT show no damage. Injury to these nerves occurs at a microscopic level that is undetectable on standard tests.

At the Scene

Some patients with acute low back spasm are literally paralyzed with pain. To move them, use a "scoop-type" metal stretcher that fits under the patient. Administration of IV benzodiazepine may be extremely helpful in relieving severe muscle spasm.

You are the Paramedic Summary

1. What is your primary concern?

Scene safety is always your primary concern. Many factors can create an unsafe scene when dealing with downed aircraft. You must address those concerns before undertaking prehospital care. To do otherwise can result in injury or death of yourself, your fellow responders, or the patients in your care.

2. What additional resources (if any) would you request and when?

Unless you are cross-trained as a firefighter and are responding with other fire department apparatus, you must request fire department personnel. This scene may potentially involve fire (including the aircraft, grass, and other structures), extrication, and hazardous materials. You also need to request assistance from the utility companies. Until the power has been shut off, it is unsafe to engage in prehospital care.

3. How can you immediately assess and communicate with this patient in a safe manner?

You can assess your patient using binoculars at a safe distance. You should attempt to gain as much information regarding her overall condition, taking note if she is alert, shows signs of distress through either posture or facial expression, or has a visible skin condition. Communication with your patient is possible with a vehicle-mounted loudspeaker system or bullhorn. If these are not available, hand signals can be used to communicate the need for the patient to stay inside the craft or vehicle.

4. Given the information your patient has provided, have your priorities changed?

Again, you face a safety issue. You must take steps to decontaminate the patient to prevent the possibility of ignition and serious burns.

5. Given the mechanism of injury and other factors, what injuries do you suspect?

You can obtain a wealth of information from the patient's posture, guarding, and facial expression. This patient has a mechanism of injury consistent with a spinal column compression fracture. She is also attempting to stabilize her lumbar spine through her posture and her use of self-splinting. This is the body's natural response to prevent further pain and injury.

6. What other factors can impact a patient's ability to handle the stress of trauma?

Many factors can play a role in the patient's ability to compensate for the stressors of trauma: extremes of age, diseases, certain medications, and environmental conditions. For example, a patient who has a previous history of myocardial infarction and suffers significant blood loss will lack the compensatory mechanisms or "cardiac reserves" that a young, healthy adult will possess. These patients may succumb to the effects of trauma more quickly, and their injuries may be masked.

7. What other information beyond the history of events should you obtain from your patient?

Obtaining a SAMPLE history is important even when caring for trauma patients. Pertinent past medical history will give you an overall sense of your patient and his or her ability to compensate in the presence of blood loss and injury.

8. If you must decontaminate a patient in the open, how can you preserve patient modesty?

If you cannot move a patient to a private location to decontaminate or perform assessments that require visualization of injuries, you can create a visual barrier by using sheets and other responders (facing outward). Consider creating such a visual barrier whenever your examination may compromise patient modesty.

9. What is an appropriate maximum on-scene time for any patient with significant traumatic injury?

Most responders know about the "golden hour" and its impact on caring for the trauma patient. To significantly lessen morbidity and mortality rates, patients with significant trauma require the definitive care of the trauma surgeon and trauma surgical suite available at trauma centres. This equates to the "platinum 10 minutes" for paramedics: Ideally, no more than 10 minutes should be spent on-scene preparing a patient for transport. Every effort should be made to adhere to this time standard. If you must deviate from it, then detailed documentation is required.

10. How does prompt, appropriate prehospital care affect the patient beyond immediate survival of the injuries sustained?

For emergency medical personnel, it is sometimes difficult to think beyond the acute situation at hand. It is important, however, to realize how responders' actions (or lack thereof) can affect the patient and his or her quality of life beyond the short span of the prehospital encounter. If they are treated inappropriately, patients may need weeks or even months in the ICU to recover. Responders should be concerned with their patients' ability to return to the quality of life they are accustomed to. Beyond focusing on prevention measures, responders cannot change what has happened to patients; however, they can review the prehospital care in terms of how it affected the patient over the long term.

Prep Kit

Ready for Review

- SCIs are among the most devastating injuries encountered by paramedics.
- In order to decipher the often subtle findings associated with SCI, you need to understand the form and function of spinal anatomy.
- Acute injuries of the spine are classified according to the associated mechanism, location, and stability of injury.
- Vertebral fractures can occur with or without associated SCI.
- Stable fractures do not involve the posterior column and pose lower risk to the spinal cord.
- Unstable injuries involve the posterior column of the spinal cord and typically include damage to portions of the vertebrae and ligaments that directly protect the spinal cord and nerve roots.
- Primary SCI occurs at the moment of impact.
- Secondary SCI occurs when multiple factors permit a progression of the primary SCI. The ensuing cascade of inflammatory responses may result in further deterioration.
- Limiting the progression of secondary SCI is a major goal of prehospital management of SCI.
- Current principles of spine trauma management include recognition of potential or actual injury, appropriate immobilization, and reduction or prevention of the incidence of secondary injury.
- Short-acting, reversible sedatives are recommended for the acute patient after a correctable cause of agitation has been excluded.
- The use of corticosteroids in the acute phase of SCI remains controversial.
- The complications of SCI are a consistent cause of the high morbidity and mortality associated with this type of injury.
- Back pain is one of the most common physical complaints to present to emergency departments. Most cases of low back pain are idiopathic and difficult to precisely diagnose.

Vital Vocabulary

anterior cord syndrome A condition that occurs with flexion injuries or fractures resulting in the displacement of bony fragments into the anterior portion of the spinal cord; findings include paralysis below the level of the insult and loss of pain, temperature, and touch sensation.

arachnoid The middle membrane of the three meninges that enclose the brain and spinal cord.

autonomic dysreflexia A potentially life-threatening late complication of spinal cord injury in which massive, uninhibited uncompensated cardiovascular response occurs due to stimulation of the sympathetic nervous system below the level of injury. Also known as autonomic hyperreflexia.

Babinski reflex When the toe(s) moves upward in response to stimulation to the sole of the foot. Under normal circumstances, the toe(s) moves downward.

brain Part of the central nervous system, located within the cranium and containing billions of neurons that serve a variety of vital functions.

brain stem The portion of the brain that connects the spinal cord to the rest of the brain, and contains the medulla, pons, and midbrain.

Brown-Sequard syndrome A condition associated with penetrating trauma with hemisection of the spinal cord and complete damage to all spinal tracts on the involved side.

cauda equina The location where the spinal cord separates, composed of nerve roots.

central cord syndrome A condition resulting from hyperextension injuries to the cervical area that cause damage with hemorrhage or edema to the central cervical segments; findings include greater loss of function in the upper extremities with variable sensory loss of pain and temperature.

central nervous system (CNS) The system containing the brain and spinal cord.

cerebrospinal fluid (CSF) Fluid produced in the ventricles of the brain that flows in the subarachnoid space and bathes the meninges.

complete spinal cord injury Total disruption of all tracts of the spinal cord, with all cord mediated functions below the level of transection lost permanently.

dermatomes Areas of the body innervated by sensory components of spinal nerves.

dura mater The outermost of the three meninges that enclose the brain and spinal cord, it is the toughest membrane.

facet joint The joint on which each vertebra articulates with adjacent vertebrae.

flexion injury A type of injury that results from forward movement of the head, typically as the result of rapid deceleration, such as in a vehicle collision, or with a direct blow to the occiput.

foramen magnum A large opening at the base of the skull through which the spinal cord exits the brain.

hyperesthesia Hyperacute pain to touch.

hyperextension Extension of a limb of other body part beyond its usual range of motion.

incomplete spinal cord injury Spinal cord injury in which there is some degree of cord-mediated function; initial dysfunction may be temporary and there may be potential for recovery.

lamina Arise from the posterior pedicles and fuse to form the posterior spinous processes.

myotomes Regions of the body innervated by the motor components of spinal nerves.

neurogenic shock Shock caused by massive vasodilation and pooling of blood in the peripheral vessels to the extent that adequate perfusion cannot be maintained.

parasympathetic nervous system Subdivision of the autonomic nervous system, involved in control of involuntary, vegetative functions, mediated largely by the vagus nerve through the chemical acetylcholine.

pedicles Thick lateral bony struts that connect the vertebral body with spinous and transverse processes and make up the lateral and posterior portions of the spinal foramen.

pia mater The innermost of the three meninges that enclose the brain and spinal cord, it rests directly on the brain and spinal cord.

plexus A cluster of nerve roots that permits peripheral nerve roots to rejoin and function as a group.

posterior cord syndrome A condition associated with extension injuries with isolated injury to the dorsal column; presents as decreased sensation to light touch, proprioception, and vibration while leaving most other motor and sensory functions intact.

posterior spinous process Formed by the fusion of the posterior lamina, this is an attachment site for muscles and ligaments.

primary spinal cord injury Injury to the spinal cord that is a direct result of trauma, for example transection of the spinal cord from penetrating trauma or displacement of ligaments and bone fragments, resulting in compression of the spinal cord.

proprioception The ability to perceive the position and movement of one's body or limbs.

rotation-flexion injury A type of injury typically resulting from high acceleration forces; can result in a stable unilateral facet dislocation in the cervical spine.

secondary spinal cord injury Injury to the spinal cord, thought to be the result of multiple factors that result in a progression of inflammatory responses from primary spinal cord injury.

spinal cord The part of the central nervous system that extends downward from the brain through the foramen magnum and is protected by the spine.

spinal shock The temporary local neurologic condition that occurs immediately after spinal trauma; swelling and edema of the spinal cord begin immediately after injury, with severe pain and potential paralysis.

sympathetic nervous system Subdivision of the autonomic nervous system that governs the body's fight-or-flight reactions by inducing smooth muscle contraction or relaxation of the blood vessels and bronchioles.

transverse spinous process The junction of each pedicle and lamina on each side of a vertebra; these project laterally and posteriorly and form points of attachment for muscles and ligaments.

vertebral body Anterior weight-bearing structure in the spine made of cancellous bone and surrounded by a layer of hard, compact bone that provides support and stability.

vertical compression A type of injury typically resulting from a direct blow to the crown of the skull or rapid deceleration from a fall through the feet, legs, and pelvis, possibly causing a burst fracture or disk herniation.

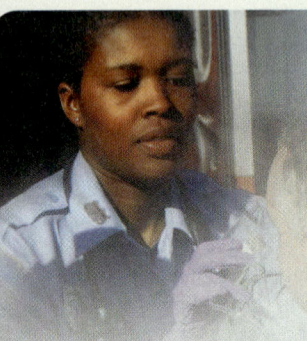

Assessment in Action

You and your partner respond to a patient who has fallen. On arrival, you find a 42-year-old man lying conscious and supine on the ground outside a home. A ladder is lying beside him, with paint spilled on the lawn. Neighbours say the patient fell at least 8 m while painting the second-floor windows. On initial assessment, he complains of pain in his neck area and lower back. His respirations are 22 breaths/min; pulse, 58 beats/min; and blood pressure, 94/58 mm Hg. The skin is warm, red, and dry. He has no sensation below the navel. He cannot move his lower extremities and has no reflexes below the hip.

1. **After the initial assessment reveals adequate ABCs, you should:**
   A. inquire about history.
   B. notify the local hospital.
   C. apply manual in-line cervical spine immobilization.
   D. perform a neurologic examination.

2. **You apply oxygen and apply a long backboard and rigid cervical collar. Now you must decide whether to treat on scene or transport. Which factor should you base your decision on?**
   A. Distance of fall
   B. Patient preference
   C. Vital signs
   D. Mechanism of injury

3. **You are beginning the transport. Where should the patient be transported to?**
   A. The closest hospital
   B. A trauma centre
   C. A local medical centre
   D. None of the above

4. **What is the maximum scene time for this patient?**
   A. 5 minutes
   B. 10 minutes
   C. 15 minutes
   D. However long it takes to immobilize the patient safely

5. **Based on the vital signs and mechanism, what should you suspect is causing the hypotension?**
   A. Blood loss
   B. Head injury
   C. Neurogenic shock
   D. All of the above

6. **What should your treatment actions be?**
   A. Continue assessment and seek out other injuries.
   B. Determine the Glasgow Coma Scale score.
   C. Initiate IV therapy.
   D. All of the above

7. **Based on the level of sensation, what area of the spine may be injured?**
   A. C7
   B. L3
   C. T10
   D. S1

Challenging Questions

You respond to a motor vehicle collision. The vehicle struck a bridge abutment on the highway, resulting in substantial damage to the car. The driver is unconscious and slumped over the steering wheel. He is breathing with difficulty. You suspect partial airway obstruction by his tongue. Smoke is coming from the car's engine compartment.

8. **What should you do?**

Points to Ponder

You respond to a call about a fall. On arrival, you find the patient at the foot of a staircase at the local community college. The patient reports that he slipped while running up the steps, and fell backward from the top to the bottom. The patient is conscious, alert, and oriented, complaining only of pain in his left leg. He has several bruises on the head, legs, and arms. No serious bleeding is noted, and the patient denies loss of consciousness. You immediately secure the cervical spine and begin a neurologic assessment. The patient's pupils are equal and reactive. He has good pulse, motor, and sensation in all extremities, and his reflexes are normal. You find no neurologic abnormalities.

Should you immobilize this patient?

Issues: Thorough Assessment, Proper Management of Spine Injuries.

Competency Areas

Area 4: Assessment and Diagnostics

4.3.j   Conduct musculoskeletal assessment and interpret findings.

Area 5: Therapeutics

5.5.s   Conduct needle thoracostomy.

Area 6: Integration

6.1.a   Provide care to patient experiencing illness or injury primarily involving cardiovascular system.

6.1.c   Provide care to patient experiencing illness or injury primarily involving respiratory system.

Introduction

Thoracic (chest) trauma is not a disease of modern society. For as long as humans have been capable of falling or injuring one another, damage to the thoracic cavity has been a significant concern in the management of the trauma patient **Figure 23-1 ▾** . As more rapid forms of transportation and more lethal weapons continue to evolve, the incidence and severity of thoracic trauma is not likely to diminish, nor is the need for its rapid assessment and treatment.

Today, thoracic trauma accounts for a significant number of serious injuries and fatalities each year. According to the Centers for Disease Control and Prevention (CDC), thoracic trauma causes more than 700,000 emergency department visits and more than 18,000 deaths in the United States annually. Only head trauma and traumatic brain injuries account for

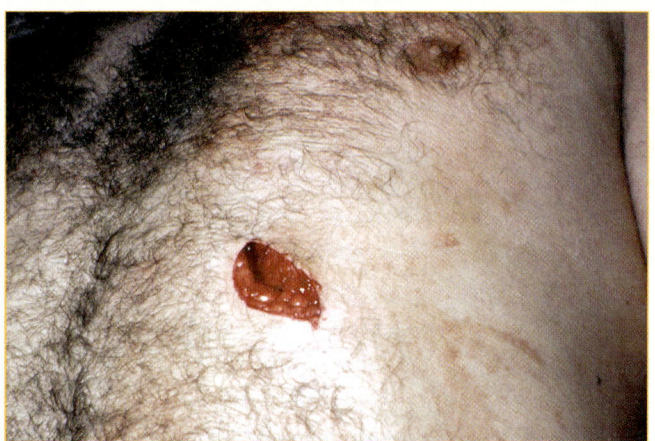

Figure 23-1 Thoracic trauma is a significant concern in the management of the trauma patient.

more deaths among trauma victims. An estimated one in four trauma deaths is directly due to thoracic injuries, and thoracic trauma is a contributing factor in another 25% of trauma patients who die of their injuries.

In a review of the Ontario Trauma Registry's Comprehensive Data Set from 1994 to 1998, 42% of 13,355 trauma patients with an injury severity score greater than 12 had sustained blunt chest injuries and another 3% had penetrating chest injuries. Of those patients with blunt chest injuries, 47% required chest tubes and 19% required chest surgery. Conversely, 75% of patients with penetrating chest injuries required chest tubes and 55% required chest surgery. The overall mortality rate in patients with blunt chest injuries was 15% and 18% in patients with penetrating chest injuries.

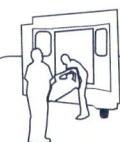

At the Scene

Thoracic injuries, whether severe or seemingly minor, often give rise to elusive findings that are overshadowed by associated injuries.

Given the specific organs that are housed within the thoracic cavity, it is not surprising that these injuries can be so deadly. In addition, the mechanism producing these injuries often involves a great deal of force transmitted to the body, with motor vehicle collisions accounting for seven of every ten patients with blunt thoracic trauma.

Anatomy

The thorax consists of a bony cage overlying some of the most vital organs in the human body. The dimensions of the thorax

You are the Paramedic Part 1

While you are working as a paramedic for a local air medical service, your helicopter is requested by a nearby township to assist with a motor vehicle collision. After lifting off from the helipad, you are informed that you are en route to a head-on collision on a major highway. Two people have already been pronounced dead at the scene.

You arrive to find an 18-year-old male passenger who was partially ejected from the vehicle; he was not wearing a seatbelt. Fire department personnel have extricated the patient from the vehicle, applied full spinal precautions, and are currently assisting his ventilations with a bag-valve-mask device.

Initial Assessment	Recording Time: 0 Minutes
Appearance	Secured to a backboard
Level of consciousness	U (Unresponsive)
Airway	Patent with an oropharyngeal airway inserted
Breathing	Assisted ventilations with 100% supplemental oxygen
Circulation	Pale skin, with a fast, regular radial pulse

1. What will your initial priorities be when assessing and managing this patient?
2. Given the mechanism of injury for an unrestrained passenger in a car and this patient's vital signs, what kinds of injuries should you think about during your assessment?

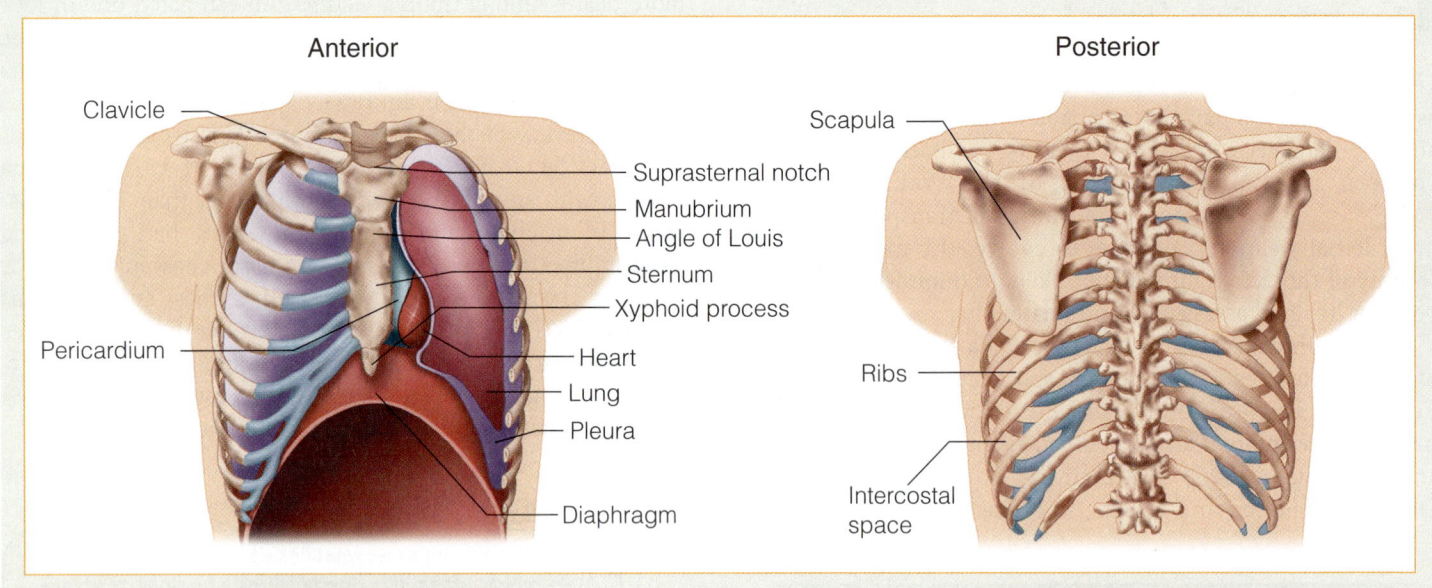

Figure 23-2 The thorax, front and back views.

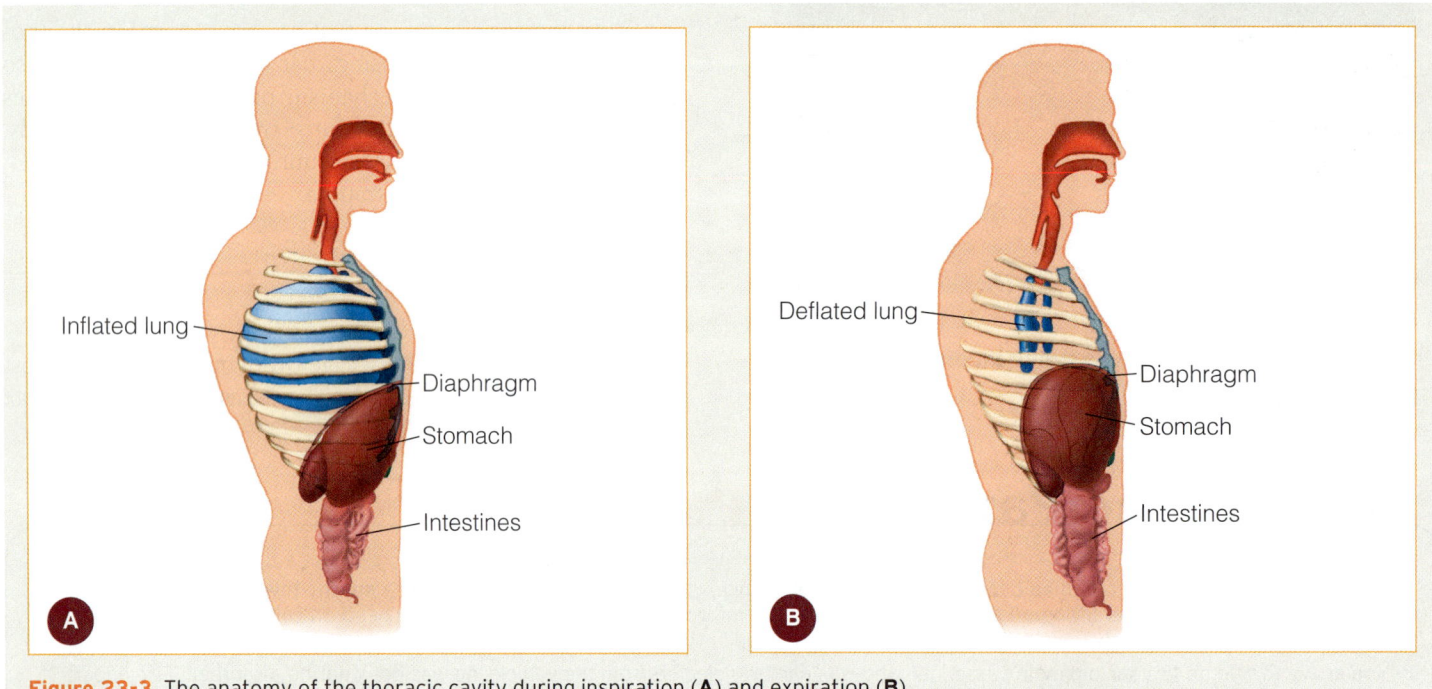

Figure 23-3 The anatomy of the thoracic cavity during inspiration (**A**) and expiration (**B**).

are defined posteriorly by the thoracic vertebrae and ribs, inferiorly by the diaphragm, anteriorly and laterally by the ribs, and superiorly by the thoracic inlet **Figure 23-2 ▲**.

The dimensions of this area of the body are of great importance in the physical assessment of the patient. Although the thoracic cavity extends to the twelfth rib posteriorly, the diaphragm inserts into the anterior thoracic cage just below the fourth or fifth rib. With the movement of the diaphragm during respiration, the size and dimensions of the thoracic cavity will vary **Figure 23-3 ▲**, which could in turn affect the organs or cavities (thoracic versus abdominal) injured in trauma.

The bony structures of the thorax include the sternum, clavicle, scapula, thoracic vertebrae, and 12 pairs of ribs. The sternum consists of three separate portions: the superior manubrium, the central sternal body, and the inferior xyphoid process. The space superior to the manubrium is termed the suprasternal notch; the junction of the manubrium and sternal body is referred to as the angle of Louis.

The clavicle is an elongated, S-shaped bone that connects to the manubrium medially and overlies the first rib as it proceeds laterally toward the shoulder. Beneath the clavicle lies the subclavian artery and vein. Laterally, the clavicle connects to the acromion process of the scapula, the triangular bone that overlies the posterior aspect of the upper thoracic cage.

Each of the 12 matched pairs of ribs attach posteriorly to the 12 thoracic vertebrae. Anteriorly, the first seven pairs of ribs attach directly to the sternum via the costal cartilage. The costal cartilage then continues inferiorly from the seventh ribs and provides an indirect connection between the anterior portions of the eighth, ninth, and tenth ribs and the sternum. The eleventh and twelfth ribs have no anterior connection and, therefore, are known as the "floating ribs."

Between each rib lies an intercostal space. These spaces are numbered according to the rib superior to the space (ie, the space between the second and third ribs is the second intercostal space). These spaces house the intercostal muscles and the neurovascular bundle, which consists of an artery, vein, and nerve.

The central region of the thorax is the mediastinum, which contains the heart, great vessels, esophagus, lymphatic channels, trachea, mainstem bronchi, and paired vagus and phrenic nerves. The heart resides within a tough fibrous sac called the pericardium. Much like the pleura, the pericardium has two surfaces—the inner visceral layer, which adheres to the heart and forms the epicardium, and the outer parietal layer, which comprises the sac itself. The pericardium that covers the inferior aspect of the heart is directly attached to the diaphragm. The heart is positioned so that the most anterior portion is the right ventricle, which has relatively thin chamber walls. The pressure within the right ventricle is approximately one fourth of the pressure within the left ventricle. Most of the heart is protected anteriorly by the sternum. With each beat, the apex

of the heart can be felt in the fifth intercostal space along the midclavicular line, a phenomenon known as cardiac impulse. The average cardiac output for an adult (heart rate times the stroke volume) is $70 \times 70 = 4,900$ ml/min, though it varies depending on the patient's size.

The aorta is the largest artery in the body. As it exits the left ventricle, it ascends toward the right shoulder before turning to the left and proceeding inferiorly toward the abdomen. This artery has three points of attachment—the anulus at its origin from the aortic valve, the ligamentum arteriosum, and the aortic hiatus. These attachments represent sites of potential injury when the vessel is subject to significant shearing forces, such as those seen during sudden deceleration mechanisms.

The lungs occupy most of the space within the thoracic cavity. Like the pericardium, the lungs are lined with a dual layer of connective tissue known as the pleura. The parietal pleura lines the interior of each side of the thoracic cavity. The visceral pleura lines the exterior of each lung.

A small amount of viscous fluid separates the two layers of pleura. This fluid allows the two layers of connective tissue to move against each other without friction or pain. It creates a surface tension that holds the layers together, thereby keeping the lung from collapsing away from the thoracic cage on exhalation. If this space becomes filled with air, blood, or other fluids, the surface tension is lost and the lung collapses.

The diaphragm, the primary muscle of breathing, forms a barrier between the thoracic and abdominal cavities. It works in conjunction with the intercostal muscles to increase the size of the thoracic cavity during inspiration, creating the negative pressure that pulls air in via the trachea. In times of distress, this breathing effort can be aided by other accessory muscles of the thoracic cavity, including the trapezius, latissmus dorsi, rhomboids, pectoralis, and sternocleidomastoid Figure 23-4 ▶ .

You are the Paramedic Part 2

As you assume patient prehospital care, you begin by reassessing the patient's airway. As the bag-valve-mask ventilations continue, you find the patient has a patent airway. His mental status remains unresponsive with a Glasgow Coma Scale score of 5 and some decorticate posturing. You and your partner decide to manage the patient's airway with endotracheal intubation, while still maintaining manual in-line immobilization of the cervical spine.

The patient is intubated without difficulty, the placement of the endotracheal tube is confirmed, and assisted ventilation is continued. As you prepare for transport, your partner starts an IV to administer a fluid bolus of crystalloid. After moving the patient, you reassess his ventilation and note that his breath sounds are absent on the right side. His neck reveals jugular vein distension, and you're not really sure if the trachea is deviated to the left side.

Vital Signs	Recording Time: 10 Minutes
Level of consciousness	Unresponsive, with a Glasgow Coma Scale score of 5
Pulse	Radial pulse, 128 beats/min
Blood pressure	70/38 mm Hg
Respirations	Intubated; ventilating with 100% supplemental oxygen
Skin	Cool, pale, and diaphoretic
SpO_2	88% on room air

3. Why does the patient remain hypoxic despite confirmed airway patency and the effective delivery of high-concentration oxygen?

4. Do his vital signs and physical examination suggest any threats to his breathing that may be correctable?

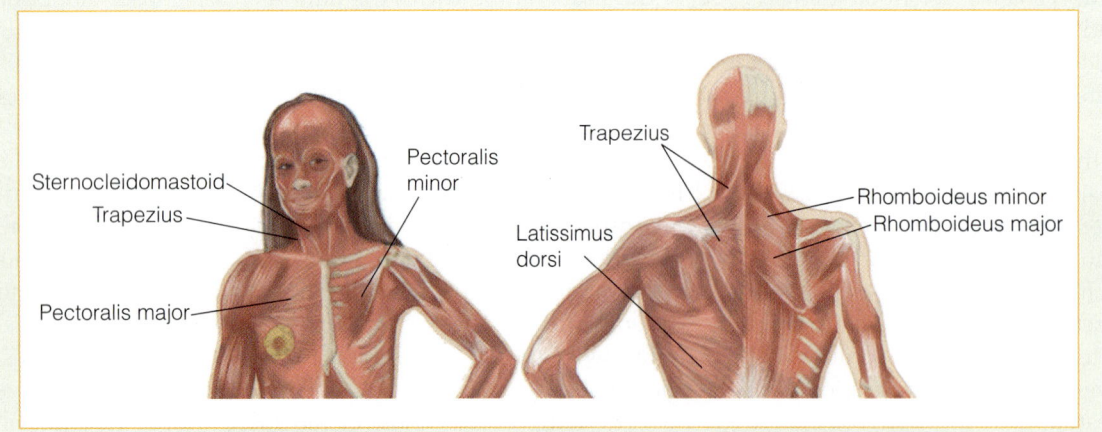

Figure 23-4 The muscles of the thoracic cavity include the trapezius, latissimus dorsi, rhomboid, pectoralis, and sternocleidomastoid muscles.

Physiology

The primary physiologic functions of the thorax and its contents are to maintain oxygenation and ventilation and (via the heart) to maintain circulation.

The process of breathing includes both the delivery of oxygen to the body and the elimination of carbon dioxide from the body. While these processes are often accomplished simultaneously, they are, in fact, different aspects of the breathing process.

First, however, the brain must stimulate the person to breathe. This stimulation occurs via chemoreceptors that are located in the carotid sinus and aortic arch. These receptors are in essence "little chemists" that analyze the arterial blood. When the level of carbon dioxide gets too high, the receptors send a message to the brain, which responds by increasing the respiratory rate in an effort to "blow off the CO_2." Some patients with end-stage chronic obstructive pulmonary disease (COPD) may employ a secondary mechanism called hypoxic drive for this function because they retain excess CO_2 on a chronic basis.

As the diaphragm contracts downward, the intercostal and accessory muscles pull the chest wall out and away from the centre of the body. The resulting negative pressure within the thoracic cavity draws air in through the mouth and nose, down the trachea, passing through smaller and smaller bronchioles until finally it reaches the alveolar spaces. The new air both mixes with and replaces the air contained within the alveoli.

While respiration is occurring, blood is being delivered via the pulmonary circulation to the capillaries that lie adjacent to the alveoli. This blood has returned to the heart after traversing the body, having delivered its oxygen to the cells and removed the cellular waste products such as CO_2. As a result, the blood entering the capillaries adjacent to the alveoli has a low O_2 concentration and a high CO_2 concentration.

The process of oxygenation includes the delivery of oxygen from the air to the blood, where it is carried to cells and tissues throughout the body. Because the air entering the alveoli contains a higher concentration of O_2 (ranging from 21% in room air to as much as 100% in a nonrebreathing mask or bag-valve-mask under ideal circumstances) than the blood in the nearby capillaries, the oxygen will follow its concentration gradient and enter the blood. Most of the oxygen binds to hemoglobin within the red blood cells, and the oxygen returns to the heart with the blood, where it is then pumped throughout the body.

Ventilation is the process by which CO_2 is removed from the body. The air in our environment contains very little CO_2 (0.033%). As a result, when air enters the alveoli, it contains very little CO_2 compared to the blood in the nearby capillaries. The CO_2 diffuses down its concentration gradient, leaving the blood and entering the air within the alveoli.

As the diaphragm and the chest wall relax, positive pressure is created within the thorax. The air from which oxygen has been absorbed and into which carbon dioxide has been diffused is then exhaled. With each subsequent respiration (inhalation and exhalation), the process is repeated.

Proper functioning of the heart is essential to the delivery of blood to the body's tissues. As blood returns from the body via the inferior and superior vena cavae, it is pumped from the right side of the heart to the lungs, where the processes of oxygenation and ventilation take place. As oxygenated blood returns from the lungs, it enters the left side of the heart and is then pumped out to the body.

The ability to pump blood depends on having a functional pump (the heart), an adequate volume of blood to be pumped, and a lack of resistance to the pumping mechanism (afterload)—properties that are collectively known as cardiac output. Cardiac output is the volume of blood delivered to the body in 1 minute. The volume is identified by counting the number of times the heart beats in a minute (heart rate) and determining the amount of blood delivered to the body with each beat (stroke volume). Thus cardiac output equals the heart rate (beats/min) multiplied by the stroke volume (millilitres of blood per beat). Any injury that limits the heart's pumping ability, the delivery of blood to the heart, the blood's ability to leave the heart, or the heart rate will affect cardiac output.

Pathophysiology of Thoracic Injuries

Traumatic injury to the thoracic cavity presents the possibility of compromise of ventilation, oxygenation, or circulation. Accordingly, the assessment of the thoracic cavity becomes an integral part of the overall assessment of the patient's ABCs, the initial assessment, and the continuing assessment. These injuries, if missed or inappropriately treated, could contribute significantly to the patient's morbidity or even cause death.

The patient's ventilation may be affected by both mechanical and functional impairments. Air or blood entering the pleural space may result in the loss of airspace in which ventilation normally occurs. Similarly, injuries to the chest wall or diaphragm may limit the movement of the thorax, thereby constraining the patient's ability to ventilate. Finally, ventilation may be affected simply by a painful injury that limits the patient's ability or willingness to fully ventilate his or her lung tissue with each breath.

Within the lung itself, loss of alveolar space may result in the inability to exchange gases such as oxygen, ultimately leading to clinical hypoxemia. This problem may be caused by alveolar collapse (atelectasis) due to incomplete chest wall and lung expansion, hemorrhage into the lung tissue itself, or airway obstruction.

Within the cardiovascular structures of the thoracic cavity, acute blood loss from vascular injury may result in systemic hypoperfusion. Also, localized blood loss within the pericardium may result in immediate cardiovascular collapse.

Chest Wall Injuries
Flail Chest

Flail chest **Figure 23-5 ▾**, a major injury to the chest wall, may result from a variety of blunt force mechanisms such as falls, motor vehicle collisions, assaults, and even birth trauma. It occurs in as many as 20% of admitted trauma patients. The associated mortality rates range from 50% in some series to even higher rates in patients older than age 60. Mortality rates are directly related to the underlying and associated injuries.

Patients are more likely to suffer a mortal injury if they are elderly, have seven or more rib fractures or three or more associated injuries, present with shock, or have associated head trauma.

A flail segment is defined as two or more adjacent ribs that are fractured in two or more places. The segment between those two fracture sites becomes separated from the surrounding chest wall, leaving it free to succumb to the underlying pressures—hence the name "free-floating segment." Both the location and the size of the segment can affect the degree to which the flail segment impairs chest wall motion and subsequent air movement. In a flail sternum (the most extreme case), the sternum is completely separated from the ribs because of fractures or ruptured costal cartilage. This type of injury results in mechanical dysfunction of both sides of the chest and more severe respiratory impairment.

Once a flail segment has occurred, the underlying physiologic pressures cause paradoxical movement of the segment when compared to the rest of the chest wall. Expansion of the chest wall on inspiration results in negative pressure within the thoracic cavity, which in turn draws the flail segment in toward the centre of the chest. As the chest relaxes or is actively contracted (depending on the degree of dyspnea), the resulting positive pressure forces air from the lungs and also forces the flail segment out away from the thoracic cavity. Because of these movements, the lung tissue beneath the flail segment is not adequately ventilated. Clearly, a flail segment can quickly become life-threatening, which explains why it is managed in the initial assessment of the patient. The concern is not the flail segment itself, but rather the underlying lung injury. The initial treatment is to provide supplemental oxygen. A flail segment does not mandate assisted ventilation or intubation unless supplemental oxygen by itself fails to provide adequate oxygenation.

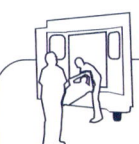

At the Scene

Pulmonary contusion is the main cause of hypoxemia seen with flail chest injuries.

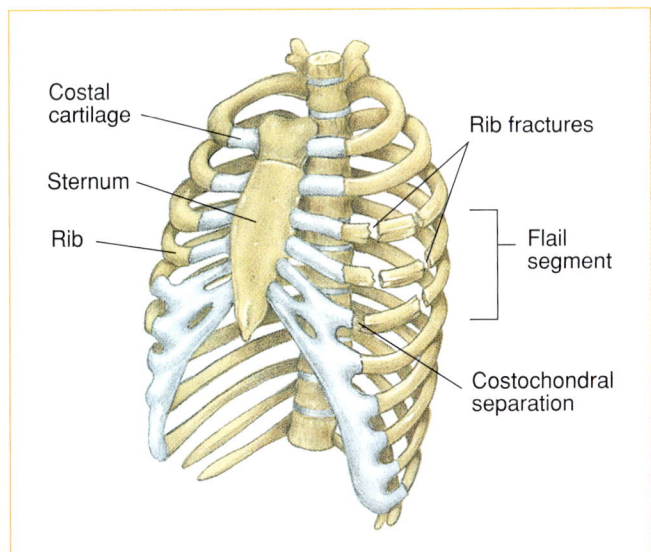

Figure 23-5 In flail chest injuries, two or more adjacent ribs are fractured in two or more places. A flail segment will move paradoxically when the patient breathes.

Costal cartilage
Sternum
Rib
Rib fractures
Flail segment
Costochondral separation

The blunt force trauma that causes the flail segment can also produce a pulmonary contusion **Figure 23-6 ▸**, an injury to the underlying lung tissue that inhibits the normal diffusion of oxygen and carbon dioxide. Three physics principles contribute to the formation of a pulmonary contusion: the Spalding effect, inertial effects, and implosion. With the Spalding effect, the pressure waves generated by either penetrating or blunt trauma disrupt the capillary–alveolar membrane, resulting in hemorrhage. Inertial effects are created by tissue density differences between the alveoli and the larger bronchioles. These tissues accelerate and decelerate at different rates, causing them to tear and hemorrhage. Finally, the positive pressure created by the trauma compresses the gases within the lung, which quickly re-expand.

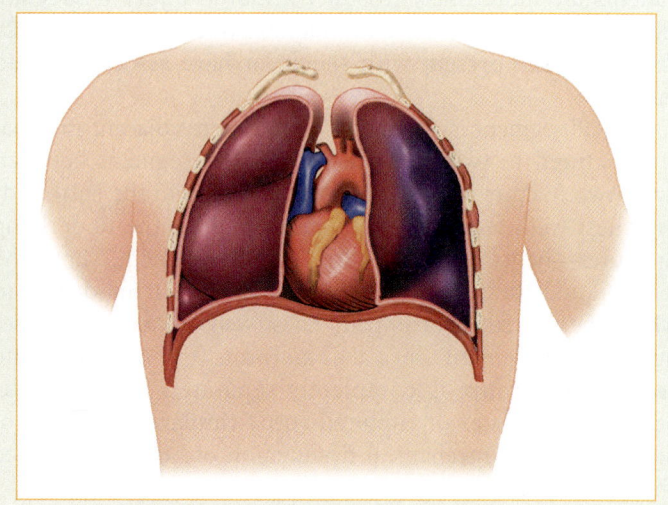

Figure 23-6 Pulmonary contusion.

If this re-expansion is too great, the lung tissue will suffer an implosion injury.

If the blunt force that fractures the ribs drives those bone fragments farther into the body, a pneumothorax or hemothorax may result. In addition, the pain associated with the fractures may prevent the patient from taking in adequate tidal volume because he or she is consciously trying to minimize the movement of that segment of the chest. This "self-splinting" action uses the intercostal muscles and purposefully limited chest wall movement to minimize pain. Unfortunately, it further limits the pulmonary system's ability to compensate for the injury.

Rib Fractures

Rib fractures—the most common thoracic injuries—are seen in more than half of all thoracic trauma patients. Even when the patient experiences no underlying or associated injury, the pain produced by the broken ribs can result in significant morbidity as it contributes to inadequate ventilation, self-splinting, atelectasis, and the possibility of infection (pneumonia) due to inadequate respiration.

When you are examining the chest of a patient who has sustained either blunt or penetrating injury, palpate for subcutaneous emphysema (air under the skin), which can indicate a potential pneumothorax. It has been described as a "snap, crackle, pop" sensation under the skin or a feeling like popping the plastic bubbles in the wrap used to protect fragile items during shipping.

Special Considerations

The incidence of rib fractures varies with age. The ribs of children are pliable, so they may injure underlying structures without being fractured. In older patients, the frail nature of the bones makes the ribs more likely to fracture.

In blunt trauma, the force applied to the thoracic cage results in a fracture of the rib in one of three areas: the point of impact, the edge of the object, or the posterior angle of the rib (weak point). Because they are less well protected by other bony and muscular structures, ribs 4 through 9 are the most commonly fractured.

The ribs are part of a ring that helps to expand and contract the thoracic cavity. Because a fracture of one or more ribs destroys the integrity of this ring, the patient's ability to adequately ventilate is diminished. Just as importantly, the patient will attempt to limit the pain caused by these injuries by using shallow breathing. This tendency results in atelectasis and may lead to hypoxia or pneumonia.

The presence of rib fractures is also suspicious for other associated injuries. When the clinical examination suggests a fracture of ribs 4 through 9, you should be concerned about associated aortic injury, tracheobronchial injury, pneumothorax, vascular injury, or other more serious injuries. Similarly, fractures of the lower ribs (9 through 11) should raise your concern for an associated intra-abdominal injury.

Sternal Fractures

Approximately one in 20 patients with blunt thoracic trauma will suffer a sternal fracture. Although this injury is of little consequence by itself, it is associated with other injuries that cause more than one fourth of patients with this fracture to die. Specifically, findings of myocardial contusions, flail sternum, pulmonary contusions, head injuries, intra-abdominal injuries, and myocardial rupture increase the likelihood of death.

At the Scene

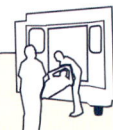

The sternum is a very thick bone. If the thorax receives enough force to fracture the sternum, you must assume that the same force was transmitted to the heart, great vessels, lungs, and diaphragm.

Lung Injuries
Simple Pneumothorax

Small pneumothoraces that are not under tension are a frequent occurrence in the blunt trauma patient, occurring in almost half of patients with thoracic trauma. Patients with penetrating trauma to the chest almost always have a pneumothorax—that is, the accumulation of air or gas in the pleural cavity.

Injuries may result in pneumothoraces either by direct injury to the lung (ie, rib fracture, gunshot, stabbing) or through barotrauma. In the latter case, pressure (eg, from the steering wheel during a motor vehicle collision) is applied to the chest at a time when the patient has inhaled and closed the glottis in anticipation of the trauma and/or pain. This increased pressure is translated to the intrathoracic cavity, where it results in rupture of the lung. In both direct injury and barotrauma, air is allowed to escape into the pleural space, causing a pneumothorax **Figure 23-7 ▶**.

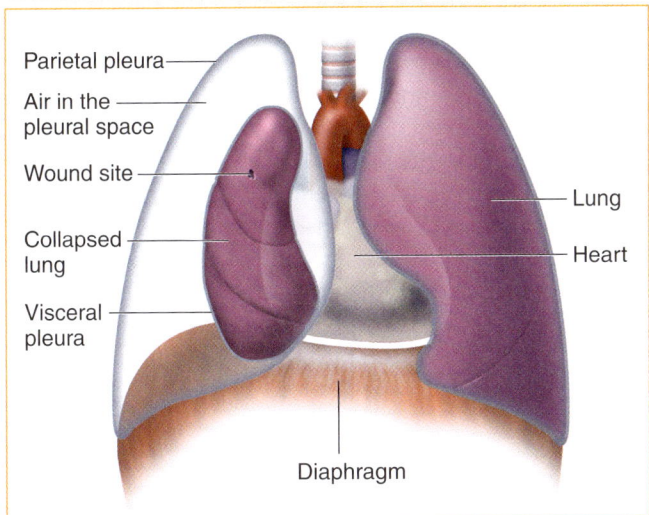

Figure 23-7 Pneumothorax occurs when air leaks into the space between the pleural surfaces from an opening in the chest or the surface of the lung. The lung collapses as air fills the pleural space.

Parietal pleura
Air in the pleural space
Wound site
Collapsed lung
Visceral pleura
Lung
Heart
Diaphragm

Open Pneumothorax

An open pneumothorax occurs when a defect in the chest wall allows air to enter the thoracic space. It results from penetrating chest trauma—for example, gunshot/knife wounds or other impaled objects. The penetrating injury creates a link between the external environment and the pleural space. With each inspiration, the negative pressure created within the thoracic cavity draws more air into the pleural space, resulting in a pneumothorax. As the pneumothorax increases in size, the lung on the involved side loses its ability to expand. Also, if the "hole" is larger than the glottic opening, the air is more likely to enter the chest wall rather than entering via the trachea. As a consequence, the respiratory effort moves air in through the chest wound rather than through the lung, creating the sucking chest wound **Figure 23-8 ▸** .

The collapse of the involved lung creates a mismatch between ventilation and perfusion. If you assume that the pulmonary vasculature on the involved side remains intact, the heart will continue to perfuse the involved lung while the pneumothorax prevents adequate ventilation. The result is an inability to deliver oxygen to the involved lung (hypoxia) and an inability to eliminate carbon dioxide (hypercarbia).

Tension Pneumothorax

A tension pneumothorax **Figure 23-9 ▸** is a life-threatening condition that results from continued air accumulation within the intrapleural space. Air may enter the pleural space from an open thoracic injury, an injury to the lung parenchyma due to blunt trauma (the most common cause of tension pneumothorax), barotrauma due to positive-pressure ventilation, or tracheobronchial injuries due to shearing forces. Although the exact incidence of this injury is unknown, it has been estimated that 10% to 30% of patients transported to

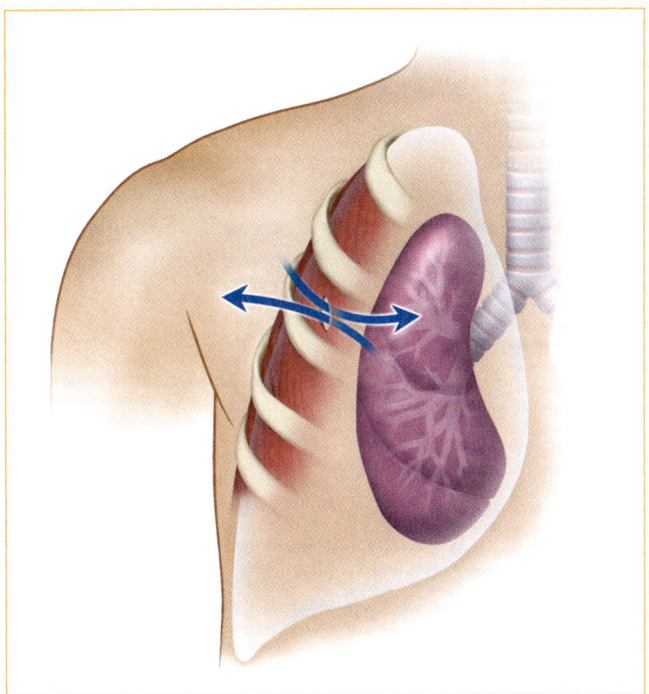

Figure 23-8 With a sucking chest wound, air passes from the outside into the pleural space and back out with each breath, creating a sucking sound. The size of the defect does not need to be large to compromise ventilation.

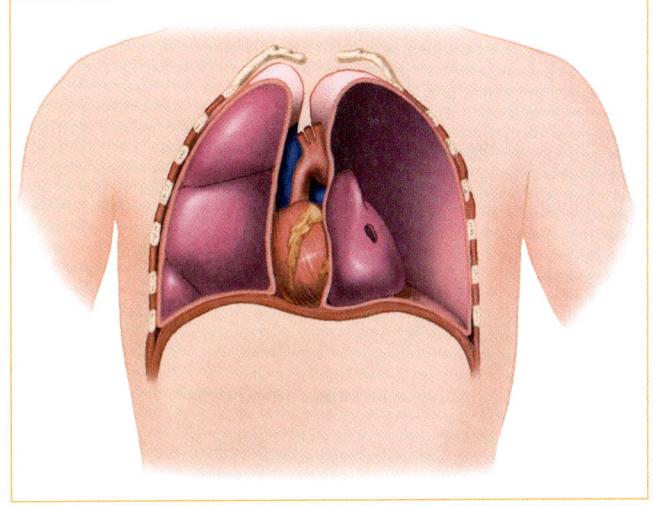

Figure 23-9 In a tension pneumothorax, air accumulates in the pleural space, eventually causing compression of the heart and great vessels.

level 1 regional trauma centres receive emergent treatment for this condition.

An injury to the lung can cause a one-way valve to develop, allowing air to move into the pleural space but not to exit from it. As it continues to accumulate, the air exerts increasing pressure against the surrounding tissues. This growing pressure compresses the involved lung, diminishing its ability to oxygenate blood or eliminate carbon dioxide from the blood. Eventually, the lung will both collapse and push toward the mediastinum, shifting the mediastinum away from the injured side.

This pressure increase may even exceed the pressure within the major venous structures, decreasing venous return to the heart, diminishing preload, and eventually resulting in a shock state. As venous return decreases, the patient's body attempts to compensate by increasing the heart rate in an attempt to maintain cardiac output.

Massive Hemothorax

A hemothorax occurs when the potential space between the parietal and visceral pleura is violated and blood begins to accumulate within this space Figure 23-10 ▾ . Hemothorax occurs in approximately 25% of patients with chest trauma. Although it is most commonly caused by tears of lung parenchyma, it may also result from penetrating wounds that puncture the heart or major vessels within the mediastinum or from blunt trauma with deceleration shearing of major vessels. Rib fractures and injuries to the lung parenchyma are the most common sources of injury in the case of a hemothorax. Other causes include injury to the intercostal arteries (which can lose up to 50 ml of blood per minute) and other intrathoracic vessels.

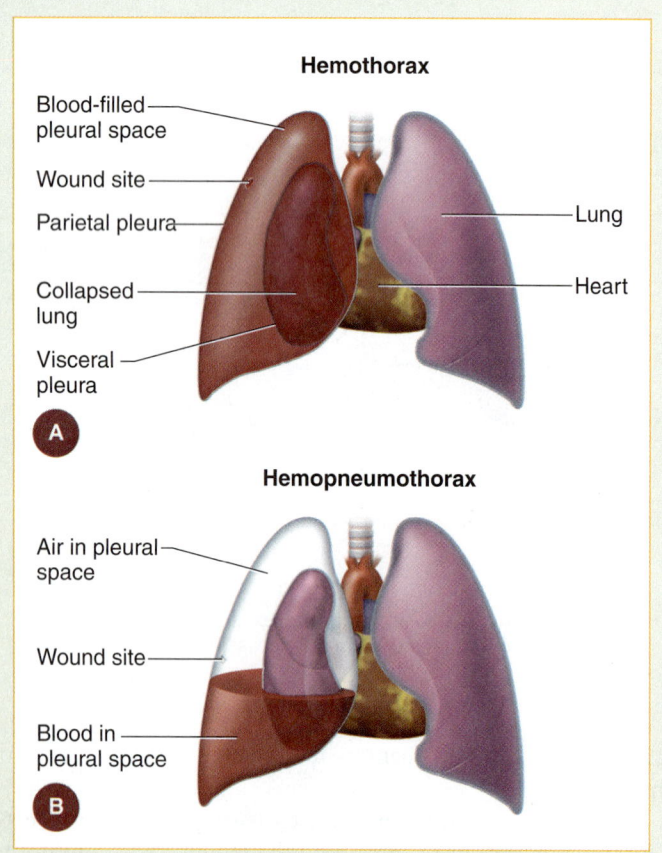

Figure 23-10 A. A hemothorax is a collection of blood in the pleural space produced by bleeding within the chest. **B.** In a hemopneumothorax, both blood and air are present.

The collection of blood within the pleural space compresses and displaces the surrounding lung, limiting the patient's ability to adequately oxygenate and ventilate. Unlike a pneumothorax, this injury has the added potential of causing hypovolemia. A hemopneumothorax occurs when both blood and air are present in the pleural space.

A massive hemothorax is defined as accumulation of more than 1,500 ml of blood within the pleural space. For the average adult, this amount represents a nearly 25% to 30% blood volume loss, meaning that the patient will have progressed to decompensated shock. Because each lung can hold up to 3,000 ml, it is possible for a patient to completely bleed out into the thoracic cavity.

Pulmonary Contusion

The position of the lungs just beneath the thoracic cage places them at increased risk for injury with thoracic trauma. As the lung tissue is compressed against the chest wall by force or by the positive pressure within the chest during a thoracic injury, alveolar and capillary damage results. It leads immediately to a loss of fluid and blood into the involved tissues, followed by white blood cell migration into the area, and local tissue edema.

This local tissue injury and edema dilute the local surfactant in the alveoli, diminishing their compliance and causing alveolar collapse (atelectasis). The edema also reduces the delivery of oxygen across the capillary–alveolar interface, resulting in hypoxia. The hypoxia then worsens the situation by thickening the mucus produced, which may in turn lead to bronchiolar obstruction and further atelectasis.

If the contusion is large, the body compensates by vasoconstricting pulmonary blood flow and increasing cardiac output. This is an attempt to shunt blood from the injured area and increase its delivery to pulmonary tissue that may be able to oxygenate the blood. This pulmonary shunting decreases the functional reserve capacity and leads to mixed venous blood being returned to the heart, further worsening the hypoxemia.

Myocardial Injuries

Pericardial Tamponade

Pericardial tamponade Figure 23-11 ▸ is defined as excessive fluid in the pericardial sac, causing compression of the heart and decreased cardiac output. The hemodynamic effects of cardiac tamponade are determined by the size of the perforation in the pericardium, the rate of hemorrhage from the cardiac wound, and the chamber of the heart involved. The injury may be caused by a blunt or (more commonly) penetrating mechanism. Very few patients with blunt thoracic trauma experience pericardial tamponade, whereas almost all patients with cardiac stab wounds develop this condition.

The mortality associated with tamponade varies, with high-velocity injuries (gunshots) carrying a higher risk of death than low-velocity injuries (stabbings). If pericardial tamponade is the only injury, mortality is greatly reduced.

Pericardial tamponade can occur in both medical and trauma patients. In the medical setting, inflammatory processes (ie, pericarditis, uremia, myocardial infarction) lead to the slow collection of fluid within the pericardial sac and the gradual distension of the parietal pericardium. Through this process, 1,000 to 1,500 ml of fluid may accumulate in the pericardial sac. Conversely, the bleeding in the trauma patient is rapid, with blood loss from the coronary vasculature or the myocardium itself quickly collecting between the visceral and parietal pericardium. Because the parietal pericardium is not able to stretch in such a case, as little as 50 ml of blood may lead to pericardial tamponade.

As the pericardium fills, the continued bleeding increases the pressure within the pericardium. The more pliable structures within the pericardium—namely, the atria and the vena cavae—become compressed, which drastically reduces the preload being delivered to the heart and thereby diminishes stroke volume. The heart initially attempts to compensate for this reduction in preload by increasing the heart rate. This attempt to maintain cardiac output is only temporary, as the continued bleeding will further restrict preload and diastolic filling. The pressure within the pericardial sac will also reduce the perfusion in the myocardium, resulting in global myocardial dysfunction. The combination of these two processes leads to the development of hypotension.

Myocardial Contusion

The heart's anterior and unprotected position just behind the sternum puts it in a potentially precarious position during a blunt force mechanism. At speeds of greater than 30 km/h, the sudden deceleration of the chest wall may cause the heart to move forward until it collides with the posterior aspect of the sternum, leading to the blunt cardiac injury known as myocardial contusion. This type of injury is characterized by local tissue contusion and hemorrhage, edema, and cellular damage within the involved myocardium. Direct damage to the epicardial vessels (coronary arteries and veins) may compromise the blood flow to the heart. Damage to the myocardial tissue at a cellular level may result in ectopic activity, re-entry pathways, and dysrhythmias.

Complications of myocardial contusions are similar to the complications seen in patients who experience a myocardial infarction. Dysrhythmias may occur (although they are uncommon in children) due to cellular membrane injury and changes in the myocardial action potential. Structural changes may include the development of a ventricular septal defect, myocardial rupture or aneurysm formation, and coronary artery occlusion.

Myocardial Rupture

Myocardial rupture is an acute perforation of the ventricles, atria, intraventricular septum, intra-atrial septum, chordae, papillary muscles, or valves. The application of severe blunt force to the chest compresses the heart between the sternum and the vertebrae, which can rupture the myocardium. In penetrating trauma, a foreign object or bony fragment may be propelled into the heart, resulting in a laceration of the myocardial wall. Whether it occurs from a penetrating injury or blunt trauma, a ruptured myocardium is a life-threatening condition that accounts for 15% of fatal chest injuries.

Commotio Cordis

If the thorax receives a direct blow during the critical portion of the heart's repolarization period, the result may be immediate cardiac arrest. This phenomenon, termed commotio cordis, has been documented to have occurred after patients were struck with softballs, baseballs, bats, snowballs, fists, and

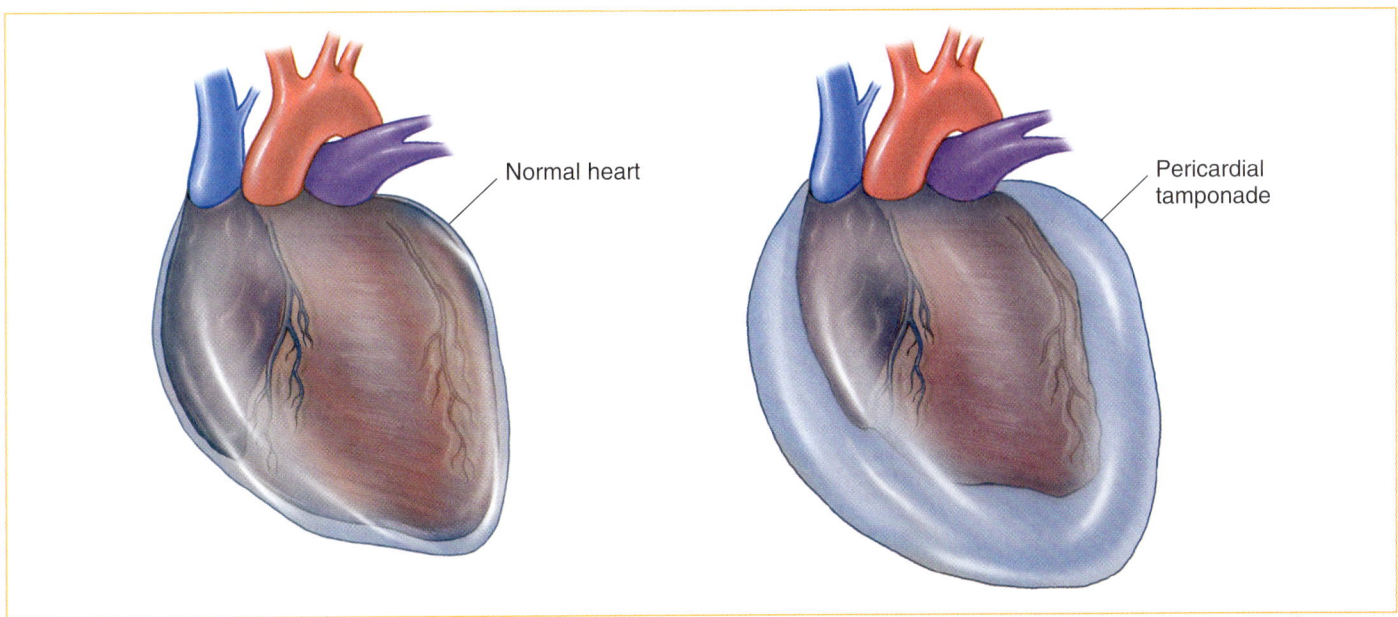

Normal heart

Pericardial tamponade

Figure 23-11 Pericardial tamponade is a potentially fatal condition in which fluid builds up within the pericardial sac, compressing the heart's chambers and dramatically impairing the ability for chambers to fill and pump blood.

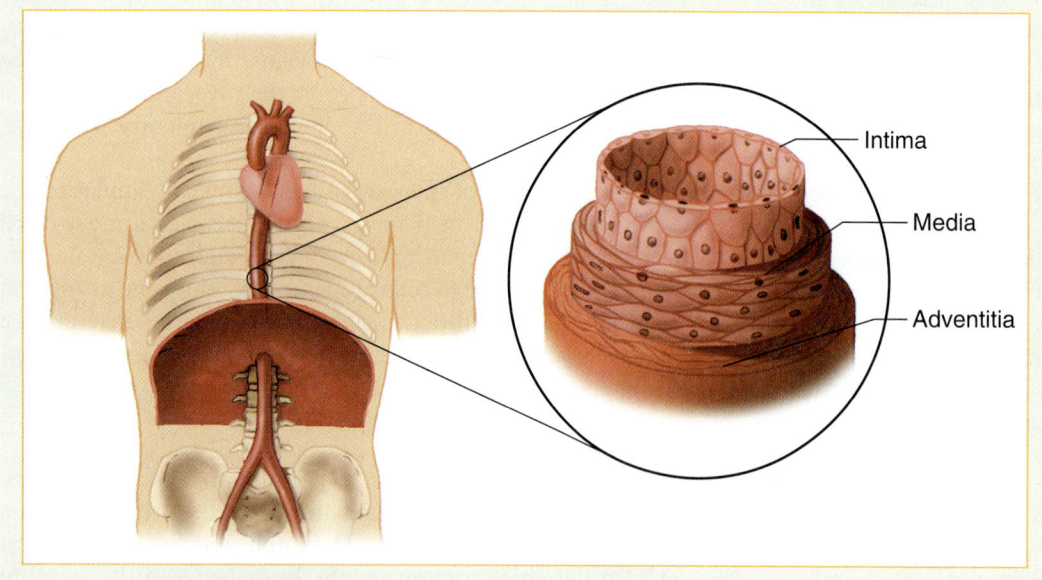

Figure 23-12 The aortic arch, descending aorta, and layers of the aorta.

Intima

Media

Adventitia

even kicks during kickboxing. Such a patient may present with ventricular fibrillation that responds positively to early defibrillation if provided within the first 2 minutes. For this reason, public access to defibrillators in schools and sports venues is essential.

Vascular Injuries
Thoracic Aortic Dissection/Transection
One in every five deaths due to blunt trauma includes a transection of the aorta; the most common causes are high-speed motor vehicle collisions and falls from a height. Given that the body's entire blood volume passes through this vessel, the high mortality associated with such an injury comes as no surprise. Of those patients who experience an aortic injury, only a few will survive until paramedics arrive; most of the individuals reached by paramedics can survive with prompt management including surgical intervention.

The most widely accepted theory of how this injury evolves holds that the aorta is injured at its fixed points due to shearing forces. The high-velocity, high-energy impacts that result in these injuries cause the aortic arch to swing forward. The resulting tension, along with rotation and torque on the area, causes the descending aorta to rupture at its point of attachment to the posterior thoracic wall **Figure 23-12 ▲** .

The aorta includes three layers—the intima, the media, and the adventitia. If the injury tears the intima, the high pressure within the aorta allows the blood to dissect along the media. More severe injuries damage all three layers of the aorta, allowing blood to leak from the aorta into the surrounding tissues. If these tissues can't stop the bleeding, the patient

may survive with prompt intervention. Otherwise, the injury will be fatal.

Great Vessel Injury
With the exception of the aorta, the great vessels are located in areas that offer protection from adjacent bony structures and other tissues. As a consequence, injury to these vessels is much more likely with penetrating trauma. In rare instances, blunt trauma may damage the overlying structures or produce a severe rotational injury (such as that caused by machinery).

Some great vessel injuries may result in occlusion or spasm of the involved artery. These injuries will present with ischemic changes (pain, pallor, paresthesias, pulselessness, paralysis) in the area with a blood supply coming from the involved artery.

Other Thoracic Injuries
Diaphragmatic Injuries
Diaphragmatic injury occurs in a relatively small percentage of all trauma patients, yet the potential for this injury has prompted a change in the management of penetrating trauma in recent years. For example, some surgeons manage penetrating trauma between the midaxillary lines, below the clavicle, and above the iliac crests by undertaking surgical exploration to ensure that the diaphragm is intact. This conservative approach reflects the possibility that a missed diaphragmatic injury may result in significant complications in the years following the injury.

Injury to the diaphragm may result from direct penetrating injury or blunt force trauma leading to diaphragmatic rupture. Because the diaphragm is protected by the liver on the right side, most diaphragmatic injuries (particularly those due to blunt trauma) occur on the left side. Once the diaphragm has been injured, the healing process is inhibited by the natural pressure differences between the abdominal and thoracic cavities.

Injury to the diaphragm and the associated physical findings have been separated into three phases: acute, latent, and

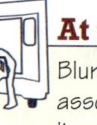

At the Scene

Blunt disruptions of the diaphragm are usually associated with herniation of all or part of the liver into the right side of the chest and the stomach into the left side of the chest. Blunt diaphragmatic injuries occur most commonly on the left side.

obstructive. The acute phase begins at the time of injury and ends with recovery from other injuries (which may overshadow the diaphragmatic injury and serves to explain why less than one fourth of these injuries are identified during the acute phase). In the latent phase, the patient experiences intermittent abdominal pain due to the periodic herniation or entrapment of abdominal contents in the defect. The obstructive phase occurs when any abdominal contents herniate through the defect, cutting off their blood supply (infarct) or causing a bowel obstruction in the process.

A very rare but ultimate complication of a diaphragmatic injury is the herniation of sufficient abdominal contents into the thoracic cavity. The resulting increased intrathoracic pressure both compresses the lung on the affected side and compromises circulatory function; this finding is called a tension gastrothorax.

Esophageal Injuries

Esophageal injuries are one of the most rapidly fatal injuries to the gastrointestinal tract, particularly if the diagnosis is not made early, due to the development of mediastinitis. Fortunately, even with penetrating trauma, such injuries are rare. Because of the location of the esophagus, however, it is often associated with other significant injuries.

Tracheobronchial Injuries

Injuries to the major airways are rare. In most instances, they are caused by penetrating injuries, but they may occasionally be seen in severe deceleration injuries. Tracheobronchial injuries have high mortality due to the associated airway obstruction.

As with aortic injuries, the site of a tracheobronchial injury is often close to a point of attachment—namely, the carina. The injury to the trachea or mainstem bronchi allows for rapid movement of air into the pleural space, resulting in a pneu-

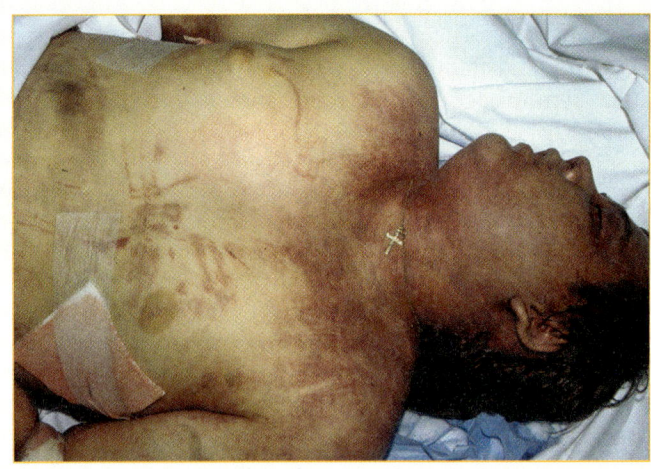

Figure 23-13 Traumatic asphyxia.

mothorax. As this injury progresses to a tension pneumothorax, a needle thoracentesis is often insufficient because the rate of air entry into the pleural space exceeds the rate at which the air can escape from the inserted angiocath.

Traumatic Asphyxia

Traumatic injuries that suddenly and forcefully compress the thoracic cavity may induce traumatic asphyxia **Figure 23-13 ▲** . The sudden compression of the chest causes pressure to be translated into the major veins of the head, neck, and kidneys. This massive increase in pressure then passes into the capillary beds, resulting in their rupture.

You are the Paramedic Part 3

After determining that the patient has a tension pneumothorax, you perform a needle chest decompression. You hear a rapid "rush" of air as the cannula enters the thoracic cavity. You place the patient on a cardiac monitor and reassess the vital signs.

Reassessment	Recording Time: 15 Minutes
Skin	Pale, cool, diaphoretic extremities with a pinker core
Pulse	114 beats/min, somewhat irregular
Blood pressure	98/54 mm Hg
Respirations	Intubated; ventilating with 100% supplemental oxygen
Spo₂	95%
ECG	Sinus tachycardia with occasional premature ventricular contractions and premature atrial contractions

5. What further injuries within the thorax could account for the patient's persistent hypotension and tachycardia?

6. Are there interventions that you can provide in the prehospital environment if such injuries are identified?

Traumatic asphyxia is characterized by a series of dramatic physical findings. There will be cyanosis of the head, the upper extremities, and the torso above the level of the compression. Ocular hemorrhage may be mild, such as bleeding into the anterior surface of the eye (subconjunctival hematoma), or extremely dramatic, causing the eyes to protrude from their normal position (exopthalmos). Other facial structures, including the tongue and lips, may also become dramatically swollen and cyanotic.

General Assessment

Scene Assessment

When you arrive on the scene, your first responsibility is to ensure the safety of both you and your partner. Make sure that the scene is safe to enter and that you are using the appropriate personal protective equipment. After you identify the number of patients, triage those patients, and request any additional resources needed, you should begin assessment of your assigned patient.

Initial Assessment

As with any patient, your initial assessment begins with an assessment of his or her mental status, airway, breathing, and circulation. Pay special attention to the identification and management of any injuries that may jeopardize the patient's vital functions. Such injuries present an immediate threat to the life of the patient and must be managed as soon as they are identified.

Mental Status and the Airway

The initial assessment begins with evaluation of the patient's mental status using AVPU. Assess the patient's level of consciousness and airway status while providing manual in-line immobilization of the cervical spine.

While considering the mechanism of injury and its contribution to the thoracic injuries (ie, the unrestrained passenger who strikes the anterior part of the neck on the dashboard of the vehicle), you should assess for injuries that may result in either obstruction or impairment of the airway. The most common cause of airway obstruction is the tongue's posterior displacement in the setting of altered mental status. Other foreign bodies that may obstruct the airway include the patient's teeth, dentures, blood, mucus, or vomitus. Additionally, the trauma may either directly injure the airway or result in secondary obstruction due to inflammation or edema.

Patients with airway compromise may present in a variety of ways, depending on the severity of the impairment, its duration, and other associated injuries. The airway itself may manifest signs of obstruction—for example, stridor, hoarseness or other changes in the voice, gurgling or snoring respirations, or coughing. Patients may also demonstrate signs of either hypoxia or hypercarbia. Alterations in mental status may range from anxiety to stupor to unresponsiveness. Abnormal respiratory

findings may include tachypnea, coughing, hemoptysis, accessory muscle use, and retractions.

When a patient has airway impairment, you must take immediate action to remedy the situation. Any patient with an airway issue should be assumed to have a simultaneous cervical spine injury and should be manually immobilized. Because of the potential for compromising the cervical spine, the head tilt–chin lift should be avoided in favour of the jaw-thrust maneuver. Suction, basic airway adjuncts (ie, oropharyngeal or nasopharyngeal airways), advanced airway adjuncts (ie, endotracheal intubation, laryngeal mask airway, or a Combitube), or surgical airway management should be used as needed to ensure adequate airway management and protection.

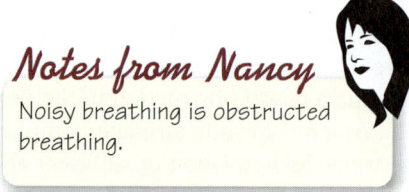

Notes from Nancy

Noisy breathing is obstructed breathing.

Breathing

Once the airway has been assessed and managed appropriately, the assessment should turn to the patient's breathing. The goal here is to identify and manage any impairment of the patient's oxygenation and ventilation **Figure 23-14 ▾**. Such problems may result from deficiencies in diffusion due to pulmonary injuries, preexisting disease, or deficiencies in air movement due to pulmonary, musculoskeletal, or neurologic impairments.

To adequately assess the patient's breathing, the patient's clothing must be removed to expose the thoracic cavity. A systematic approach to assessment will then help to identify both obvious and subtle injuries or impairments.

The breathing assessment begins with an inspection of the patient's thorax. Consider the contour, appearance, and symmetry of the chest wall. Signs of soft-tissue injury (contusions,

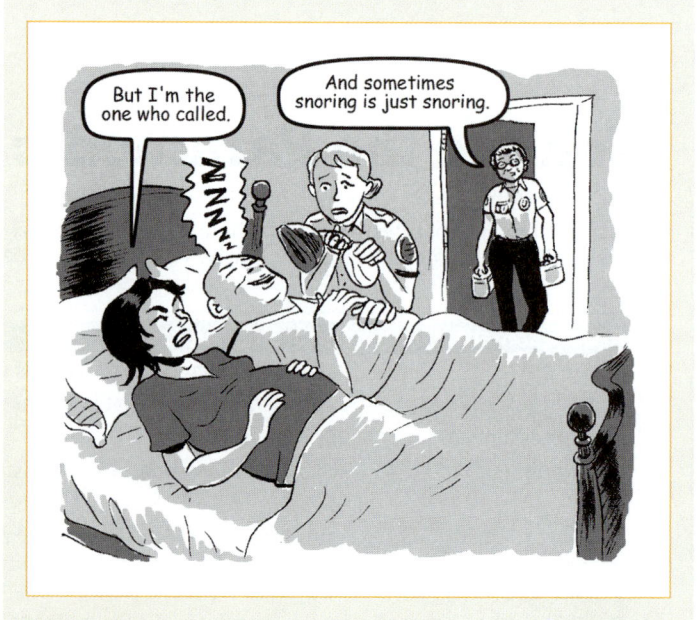

Figure 23-14

abrasions, lacerations, or deformity) suggest the possibility of an underlying injury. Paradoxical motion of a section of the chest wall, retractions, subcutaneous air or edema, impaled objects, or penetrating injuries also suggest an underlying injury with the potential to compromise the patient's breathing.

Consider the adequacy of both ventilation and oxygenation. To assess ventilation, examine the patient's respiratory rate, depth, and effort. Reliance on accessory muscles or findings such as nasal flaring suggest ventilatory compromise. Inadequate oxygenation may be inferred from findings such as cyanosis or altered mental status. The use of monitoring equipment such as capnography and pulse oximetry can aid in the assessment.

The final steps in the assessment of the patient's breathing entail the palpation, percussion, and auscultation of the chest. While palpating the chest, assess for any evidence of point tenderness, bony instability, crepitus, subcutaneous emphysema, edema, and tracheal position. Percussion can help to identify either hyperresonance (suggesting pneumothorax) or dullness (suggesting hemothorax). Auscultation includes the usual assessment for adventitious lung sounds (ie, wheezing, crackles or rales, rhonchi) plus confirmation that lung sounds are present in all lung fields.

Circulation

The next step in the initial assessment involves evaluating your patient's circulatory status. The first insight into the adequacy of the patient's circulation is his or her mental status. Once you have corrected any hypoxia or ventilatory cause leading to altered mental status, circulatory impairment should be suspected when your patient presents in a restless, agitated, confused, irrational, or comatose state. If the patient is well oxygenated and ventilating adequately, these signs may indicate inadequate cerebral perfusion.

A rapid assessment of your patient's pulses can provide a great deal of information about the patient's circulatory status. For example, absent peripheral pulses suggest that the blood pressure is low. The pulses should be assessed for their rate, quality, rhythm, location, and respiratory-induced changes.

While tachycardia is frequently associated with hypovolemia, this is not always the case. Pain, hypoxia, psychological stress related to the incident, and other factors may manifest as tachycardia. A low heart rate does not exclude the possibility of hypovolemia or shock. Neurogenic shock, severe hypoxia, Cushing's reflex, use of beta blockers, and myocardial injury may all result in bradycardia and mask simultaneous hypovolemia. Similarly, while a "thready" or "weak" pulse quality may suggest volume loss, its presence does not guarantee such a state and its absence does not exclude it.

An irregular pulse first raises the possibility of ectopic activity, suggesting hypoxia or hypoperfusion. An irregular pulse noted during the initial assessment should raise your suspicion of serious underlying injuries or shock. Although an ECG monitor may be applied to evaluate the rhythm at this time, this step is recommended only if it does not cause any delay in completing the initial assessment (eg, your partner could perform this task while you continue the initial assessment).

A patient's blood pressure can also serve as a clinical guide to patient assessment and management. Hypotension alone or in combination with tachycardia may suggest hypovolemia. In case of thoracic trauma, however, consideration must be given to both tension pneumothorax and pericardial tamponade as sources of this clinical finding. Regardless of the etiology of the hypotension, this finding suggests a critically injured patient in need of immediate transport, ideally to a certified trauma centre.

Jugular vein distension (JVD) suggests increased intravenous pressure—perhaps resulting from a tension pneumothorax, volume overload, right-sided heart failure, or cardiac tamponade. Because true jugular vein distension is measured with the patient in a 45° semi-Fowler's position, it may be difficult to assess when cervical spine precautions have been implemented. Nevertheless, a lack of jugular vein distension in the supine position in combination with other physical findings (eg, tachycardia, altered mental status, thready pulses, poor skin perfusion) may suggest a hypovolemic state **Figure 23-15 ▾**.

Auscultation of the heart sounds is another important part of the circulatory assessment. For patients with potential intrathoracic injuries, note whether their heart sounds are easily heard or whether they are muffled. Performing such an assessment may prove difficult in the back of a moving or running ambulance or because of other noise on the scene. Even so, the presence of muffled heart tones is an important diagnostic clue to the presence of either a tension pneumothorax (because of its resultant mediastinal shift) or a pericardial tamponade.

Even if the assessment of the patient's circulatory status suggests hypovolemic shock, you should recognize that the cause of that state may not lie within the thorax. Only one in four patients with a combination of thoracic trauma and shock

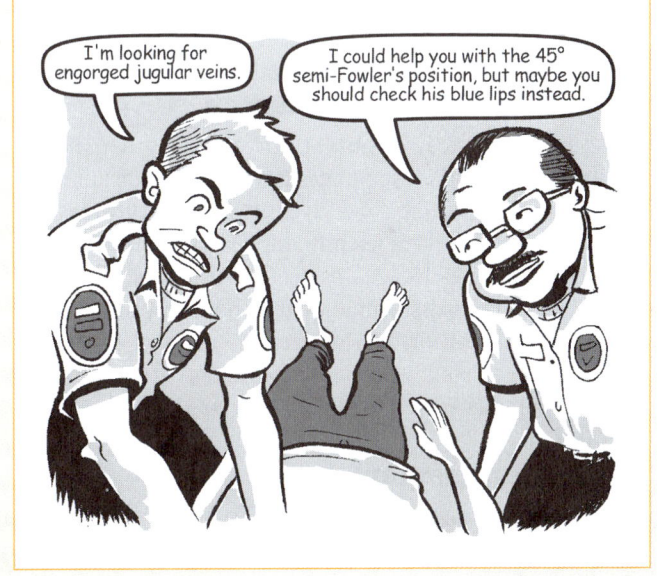

Figure 23-15

Notes from Nancy

It is not necessary to make a specific diagnosis to appreciate that a patient is critically injured.

will have a significant source of hemorrhage within the chest. For this reason, after completing the initial assessment, managing any immediate life-threatening conditions, and prioritizing the patient, you must perform a complete physical examination to identify other significant injuries.

Focused History and Physical Examination

Depending on the severity of the injuries identified up to this point, the focused history and physical examination may need to be done en route to the emergency department. If you have not already done so, obtain a full set of vital signs—including pulse rate, blood pressure, respirations, oxygen saturation, and mental status.

A relevant patient history should be obtained, including a SAMPLE history. Ask the usual questions related to the patient's symptoms, allergies, medications, past medical history, and last oral intake. Questions about the events surrounding the incident should focus on the mechanism of injury: the speed of the vehicle or height of the fall, the use of safety equipment (helmet, airbag, seatbelt, life jacket), the type of weapon used, the number of penetrating wounds, and so on.

During the focused history and physical examination, look for injuries with the potential to compromise the ABCs—namely, aortic transsections, great vessel injuries, bronchial disruptions, myocardial contusions, pulmonary contusions, simple pneumothoraces, rib fractures, and sternal fractures.

Notes from Nancy

Any thoracic injury below the level of the nipples is an abdominal injury as well as a chest injury.

Detailed Physical Examination

The detailed physical examination, which is usually done en route to the hospital for patients with a significant mechanism of injury, should include a complete head-to-toe assessment of the patient. This examination allows you to identify any physical injuries as well as reassess injuries identified in the rapid trauma assessment. For the thoracic trauma patient, pay particular attention to the patient's cervical spine, back, and abdomen, as well as the neurologic and circulatory function in the patient's extremities.

Ongoing Assessment

In your ongoing assessment of the thoracic trauma patient, obtain repeated assessments of the patient's vital signs, oxygenation, circulatory status, and breath sounds. Because the progression from pneumothorax to tension pneumothorax can

Table 23-1	Deadly Dozen Thoracic Injuries
Immediately life-threatening chest injuries that must be detected and managed during the initial assessment:	
1. Airway obstruction	
2. Bronchial disruption	
3. Diaphragmatic tear	
4. Esophageal injury	
5. Open pneumothorax	
6. Tension pneumothorax	
7. Massive hemothorax	
8. Flail chest	
9. Cardiac tamponade	
Potentially lethal chest injuries that may be identified during the focused history and physical examination:	
10. Thoracic aortic dissection	
11. Myocardial contusion	
12. Pulmonary contusion	

occur quite rapidly, all patients with a presumptive diagnosis of a pneumothorax should be considered unstable and reassessed at least every 5 minutes for worsening dyspnea, tachycardia, and the development of JVD. Similarly, other thoracic injuries may suggest the presence of more serious underlying pathologic conditions. Because these injuries may have been overlooked during the initial examinations, you need to maintain a high degree of clinical suspicion during the on-scene treatment and transport of these patients. **Table 23-1 ▲** lists the "deadly dozen" thoracic injuries.

General Management

As with any trauma patient, your management of identifiable thoracic injuries must focus on maintaining the patient's airway, ensuring oxygenation and ventilation, supporting the circulatory status, and expeditiously transporting the patient to an appropriate facility.

With one exception, airway management of the patient with thoracic trauma should proceed the same as with any other trauma patient. The jaw-thrust maneuver should be used rather than the head tilt–chin lift, as the former technique better limits cervical spine motion. Nasal airways should be avoided in patients with signs of facial injury. Instead, endotracheal intubation should be performed while maintaining manual in-line immobilization of the cervical spine. When a patient with thoracic trauma has a possible tracheal injury, however, endotracheal intubation should be reconsidered. With a partial tracheal tear, you run the risk of completing the tracheal tear when passing the endotracheal tube, a complication that can result in an unmanageable airway. Consequently, patients you suspect of having partial tracheal tears should be managed with the least invasive airway management techniques possible.

As part of airway management, you must ensure that the patient maintains adequate oxygenation and ventilation. Oxygenation is accomplished by providing patients with high-flow oxygen via a nonrebreathing mask or, if necessary, with bag-valve-mask ventilation. Ventilation is a more delicate issue in light of the potential complications that can arise from underlying thoracic injuries; you must provide ventilatory assistance in a highly vigilant fashion. Delivery of positive pressure could potentially hasten the expansion of a pneumothorax, convert a pneumothorax into a tension pneumothorax, or increase the dissection of air through a tracheobronchial injury. Positive-pressure ventilation should not be withheld, however; rather, it should be delivered in a fashion that minimizes the degree of pressure used. Watch your patient's chest closely—you're looking for visible chest rise without excessive overinflation!

Assessment of the ability of the circulatory system to provide oxygenation and ventilation to the body tissues is the next step in the management of any trauma patient. The patient whose circulatory status is compromised (as evidenced by tachycardia, hypotension, or end-organ dysfunction) requires supportive measures until definitive care can be delivered. Placing the patient in a supine or Trendelenburg position will deliver blood otherwise held in the venous system of the lower extremities to the central circulation. The provision of judicious intravenous fluids may also help to expand the intravascular volume while maintaining the oxygen-carrying capacity of the blood.

Pharmacologic agents have a very limited role in the management of a trauma patient. With the exception of those medications necessary to ensure appropriate airway management, the only drugs currently used are agents for pain management. Narcotic and nonnarcotic analgesics are essential components of the appropriate and compassionate treatment of any trauma patient. As a responsible paramedic, you will take the proper steps to minimize the pain of your patients, although you may often be limited by local protocols, short transport times in more urban settings, and the clinical status of the patient (including appropriate concern about narcotic suppression of the respiratory drive in thoracic trauma patients). Nonpharmaceutical approaches may include appropriate splinting, application of cold packs, and careful handling.

Finally, the global assessment and management of patients with thoracic trauma include deciding the appropriate facility to which the patient should be transported. Trauma centres designated to provide multisystem evaluation and management of trauma patients would be the first choice for most patients with thoracic trauma, particularly those with potentially life-threatening injuries. Sometimes, however, such facilities may not be readily available or may be physically too distant to allow for timely transport (eg, in a rural environment).

The principle of the golden hour holds that the management of the trauma patient is best accomplished if the patient is delivered to a facility capable of definitive surgical intervention within an hour from the time of injury. Achieving this goal may require the use of alternative means of transportation (ie, air medical care). Ultimately, this decision is best made in advance, whether through written protocols, policies, or discussions with the system medical director and administration.

Assessment and Management of Specific Injuries

There are a select few injuries that you must be able to identify and treat during your assessment of the patient's breathing—namely, open pneumothorax, tension pneumothorax, and flail chest. These injuries, if missed, may claim the patient's life.

Chest Wall Injuries
Flail Chest

Physical assessment is the key to identifying a patient with a flail segment. Beginning with general inspection of the chest, you will note evidence of soft-tissue injury to the chest. On further examination, you may observe paradoxical chest wall movement, although the patient's efforts to splint the injury may prevent its visibility.

On palpation, crepitus and tenderness may be noted at the site, and dissection of air into the tissues should raise your clinical suspicion for this injury and an underlying pneumothorax. Auscultation will reveal decreased or even absent breath sounds on the affected side, depending on the degree of underlying injury, splinting, and pneumothorax.

As the injury begins to affect the patient's physiology, the expected signs and symptoms of hypoxia, hypercarbia, and pain will become apparent. The patient would be expected to have one or more of the following associated findings: complaints of pain, tenderness on palpation, splinting, shallow breathing, agitation/anxiety (hypoxia) or lethargy (hypercarbia), tachycardia, and cyanosis.

Flail segments pose a threat to the patient's ability to breathe and should be treated immediately. When the patient has progressive respiratory failure, intubation and positive-pressure ventilation are indicated. Intubating the patient uses positive-pressure ventilation as a means of expanding the collapsed alveoli. That portion of the lung parenchyma is then able to contribute to the oxygenation and ventilation of the patient.

If intubation is not required, you must provide the patient with supplementary oxygen in the form of high-flow oxygen via a nonrebreathing mask. This step will increase the partial pressure of oxygen delivered to the functional parts of the lung, thereby increasing oxygen delivery to the body as a whole.

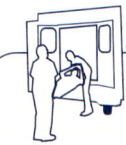

At the Scene

If a patient requires ventilatory support, it is much safer to apply it before actual ventilatory failure develops.

External stabilization of the flail segment is no longer recommended. Such efforts actually decrease aeration of the underlying lung tissue, increase the degree of alveolar collapse (atelectasis), and worsen the patient's pulmonary function.

Rib Fractures

Patients with rib fractures typically complain of pleuritic chest wall pain and mild dyspnea. The physical examination may reveal chest wall tenderness and overlying soft-tissue injury. Crepitus and subcutaneous emphysema may also be noted. When assessing the adequacy of the patient's respiratory effort, watch for shallow ventilations as the patient attempts to limit the movement of the affected area of the thoracic cage. The patient may also lean toward the injury site to reduce muscular tension on the fracture(s).

The management of rib fractures focuses on the ABCs and evaluating the patient for other, more lethal injuries. Administer supplemental oxygen and gently splint the patient's chest wall by having the individual hold a pillow or blanket against the area; this measure may allow the patient to take deeper breaths, something that should be encouraged despite the pain. Intravenous analgesics may also assist in this regard.

Sternal Fractures

On examination, the patient with a sternal fracture will complain of pain over the anterior part of the chest. Palpation of the area may reveal tenderness, deformity, crepitus, overlying soft-tissue injury, and the possibility of a flail segment. Given the risk of an underlying myocardial contusion, ECG rhythm analysis should be performed.

The treatment of sternal fractures is supportive only. Assess the patient's ABCs, and manage associated injuries accordingly. Analgesics in doses sufficient to provide pain relief without suppressing the respiratory drive may aid the patient's ventilatory efforts.

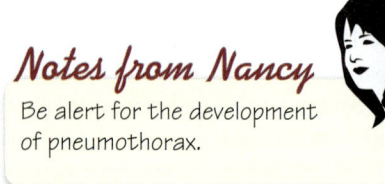

Notes from Nancy

Be alert for the development of pneumothorax.

Lung Injuries

Simple Pneumothorax

The presentation and physical findings in a patient with a simple pneumothorax depend on the size of the pneumothorax and the degree of resulting pulmonary compromise. With a small pneumothorax, the patient may complain only of mild dyspnea and pleuritic chest pain on the affected side. Diminished breath sounds may be heard on auscultation, a finding that is best heard anteriorly if the patient is in the supine position or in the apices if the patient is upright. (Air will accumulate at the highest point and diminish lung sounds in that area.) Hyperresonance to percussion may also be found on the affected side.

As the pneumothorax increases in size, the degree of compromise likewise increases. Patients with larger pneumothoraces will complain of increasing dyspnea and demonstrate

signs of more serious respiratory compromise and hypoxia: agitation, altered mental status, tachypnea, tachycardia, cyanosis, lowered pulse oximetry readings, and even absent breath sounds on the affected side.

The management of the patient with a simple pneumothorax begins with the ABCs and the delivery of high-concentration oxygen. Supplemental oxygen not only aids the patient in overcoming any degree of hypoxia that may exist, but it also helps the body absorb the air from the pleural space, thereby either reducing the size of the pneumothorax or potentially slowing its rate of expansion. The most critical intervention for these patients is repeated assessments to ensure that the injury has not progressed to a tension pneumothorax. Most pneumothoraces result from a small pulmonary injury that seals itself off, preventing further air loss. For those that do progress, however, rapid recognition and management of this condition can be lifesaving.

Open Pneumothorax

On physical assessment, exposure of the chest will reveal a chest wall defect or impaled object. If air is being drawn into the chest by the negative inspiratory pressure, a sucking chest wound may be noted. If air is being forced out of the chest with the positive pressure of expiration, the result may be a bubbling wound. The movement of air in and out of the open wound may also lead to dissection of that air within the subcutaneous tissue, resulting in subcutaneous emphysema.

With any injury that has the potential to violate the integrity of the thoracic cavity, your assessment should focus on evaluating the patient for the presence of a pneumothorax. Due to the decreased ability to oxygenate and ventilate, the patient will experience tachycardia, tachypnea, and restlessness. These symptoms may be simply a manifestation of the pain from the injury, but other findings may confirm an underlying pneumothorax.

As the air within the interpleural space (the pneumothorax) increases, the patient's breath sounds will diminish on the affected side. Because this expanding volume consists of air, percussion of the chest will aid in the assessment by demonstrating a hyperresonant sound. These physical findings should confirm your suspicion of an open pneumothorax.

Sucking chest wounds must be treated immediately **Figure 23-16 ▶**. The injury should first be converted to a closed injury to prevent further expansion of the pneumothorax. To do so, immediately place a gloved hand over the injury and then replace that hand with an occlusive dressing (ideally three to four times the size of the wound). Because of the possibility that an underlying lung injury may continue to contribute to the pneumothorax, this dressing should only be secured on three sides to facilitate the release of increased pressure, should it develop.

All patients with open pneumothoraces, regardless of their oxygenation status as determined by pulse oximetry, should be placed on high-flow supplemental oxygen via a nonrebreathing mask. If oxygenation or ventilation remains inadequate, endotracheal intubation may be required. You

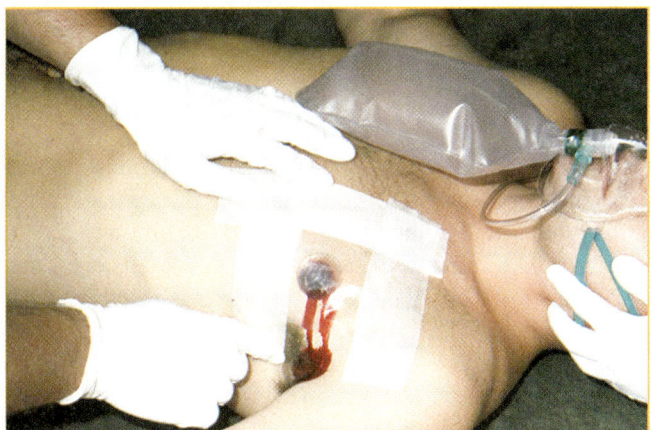

Figure 23-16 A sucking chest wound should be covered with a large occlusive dressing that seals on three sides with the fourth left open as a flutter valve.

may use sedation or neuromuscular blockade to facilitate this process, depending on your local protocols.

An open pneumothorax rarely progresses to a tension pneumothorax. If it does, you should remove the patient's occlusive dressing to allow the pneumothorax to "vent" through the opening in the thoracic cavity. If this measure does not relieve this life-threatening condition, treatment should progress as described in the next section.

Tension Pneumothorax

The classic signs of a tension pneumothorax are an absence of breath sounds on the affected side, tachycardia, jugular vein distension, and tracheal deviation. While tachycardia may not be a unique finding in the trauma patient, tension pneumothorax induces this change—not because of a hypovolemic state, but rather because of the inability of blood to easily return to the heart from the venous system. The increasing pressure within the thoracic cavity leads to the accumulation of blood within the great vessels just outside the thoracic cavity. As the pressure is translated into the most superficial of these veins—the jugular veins—they become distended with blood. Such jugular vein distension is usually a late sign of tension pneumothorax.

The jugular veins, which exit the thoracic cavity from beneath the clavicles and cross over the sternocleidomastoid muscles as they move superiorly, are considered to be distended when they are engorged to a level 1 to 2 cm above the clavicle. This assessment is properly done with the patient in a 45° Fowler's position; however, this is something that can't be accomplished during the initial assessment of the patient in the prehospital environment.

Because of the mediastinal shift caused by the increasing pressure, palpation or visualization of the trachea may manifest

You are the Paramedic **Part 4**

An assessment of the patient's circulation reveals no evidence of muffled heart tones, jugular vein distension, dullness to chest percussion, or evidence of traumatic asphyxia. After loading the patient into the helicopter, you complete a detailed physical examination, establish a second IV line, and continue fluid resuscitation.

Your physical assessment reveals crepitus and palpable deformity over the ninth and tenth ribs on the left, as well as a rigid abdomen. Deformity of the left lower leg is evident, and the patient has multiple soft-tissue injuries on all extremities.

Reassessment	Recording Time: 20 Minutes
Skin	Pale, cool extremities with a pink core
Pulse	108 beats/min
Blood pressure	104/58 mm Hg
Respirations	Intubated; ventilating with 100% supplemental oxygen
Sao$_2$	98%
ECG	Sinus tachycardia without further ectopy

7. What additional injuries might your physical findings suggest?
8. What additional treatments may be needed for this patient?

in a deviation of the trachea away from the affected side. Nevertheless, this late finding in a tension pneumothorax may not be present despite the rapid decompensation of the patient's clinical status. For this reason, you must be vigilant in watching for the cardiopulmonary findings associated with a tension pneumothorax and not rely on the presence of all the classic physical findings in making the diagnosis.

The accumulation of air within the pleural space decreases the lung volume and diminishes the breath sounds on the affected side when you auscultate the chest. The chest will be resonant (like a bell) when percussed, as opposed to the dull sensation expected with fluid or blood.

Due to the injury and the collapsing lung, a patient with a tension pneumothorax often complains of pleuritic chest pain and dyspnea. The resulting hypoxia may cause the patient to become anxious, tachycardic, tachypneic, and even cyanotic.

Hypotension, as a late finding of tension pneumothorax, should not be used to either confirm or exclude the possibility of a tension pneumothorax. Its presence may suggest that the pneumothorax has produced such significant pressure as to severely impede preload, or it may represent a simultaneous shock state due to other injuries. Normal blood pressure suggests that, when other signs of a tension pneumothorax are present, the heart is adequately compensating for the diminished venous return.

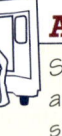

At the Scene

Shock (a late sign), decreased breath sounds, and hyperresonance to percussion on the same side of the chest mean a tension pneumothorax until proven otherwise.

All patients presenting with signs of a tension pneumothorax should immediately be placed on high-flow supplemental oxygen (12 to 15 l/min) via a nonrebreathing mask. Immediate relief of the elevated pressures must then be accomplished through a needle decompression, also referred to as a "needle thoracentesis." The steps for performing a needle decompression are described below Skill Drill 23-1 ▶:

1. Assess the patient to ensure that the presentation matches that of a tension pneumothorax Step 1 :
   - Difficult ventilation despite an open airway
   - Jugular vein distension (may not be present with associated hemorrhage)
   - Absent or decreased breath sounds on the affected side
   - Hyperresonance to percussion on the affected side
   - Tracheal deviation away from the affected side (this late sign is not always present)
2. Prepare and assemble the necessary equipment Step 2 :
   - Large-bore IV cannula, preferably 10- to 14-gauge and at least 5 cm long
   - Alcohol or povidone iodine (Betadine) preps

- Cut off one finger of a glove to use as a substitute if you don't have a commercial device or condom available.
- Adhesive tape
3. Obtain orders from direct medical control, if required.
4. Locate the appropriate site Figure 23-17 ▼ Step 3 . Find the second or third rib, as you'll need to insert the needle just above the third rib into the intercostal space at the midclavicular line on the affected side. If there is significant trauma to the anterior portion of the chest, use the intercostal space between the fourth and fifth ribs at the midaxillary line on the affected side. However, the midclavicular line approach is preferred because it's usually easier to access with less chance of dislodging the needle.
5. Cleanse the appropriate area using aseptic technique Step 4 .
6. Make a one-way valve, or flutter valve, by inserting the cannula through the end of a condom or use a commercially prepared device or the finger of a medical glove, cut off from the glove Step 5 .
7. Insert the needle at a 90° angle, and listen for the release of air Step 6 . Insert the needle just superior to the third rib, midclavicular, or just above the sixth rib, midaxillary. (The nerves, arteries, and veins run along the inferior borders of each rib.)
8. Advance the cannula over the needle, and place the needle in the sharps container Step 7 .

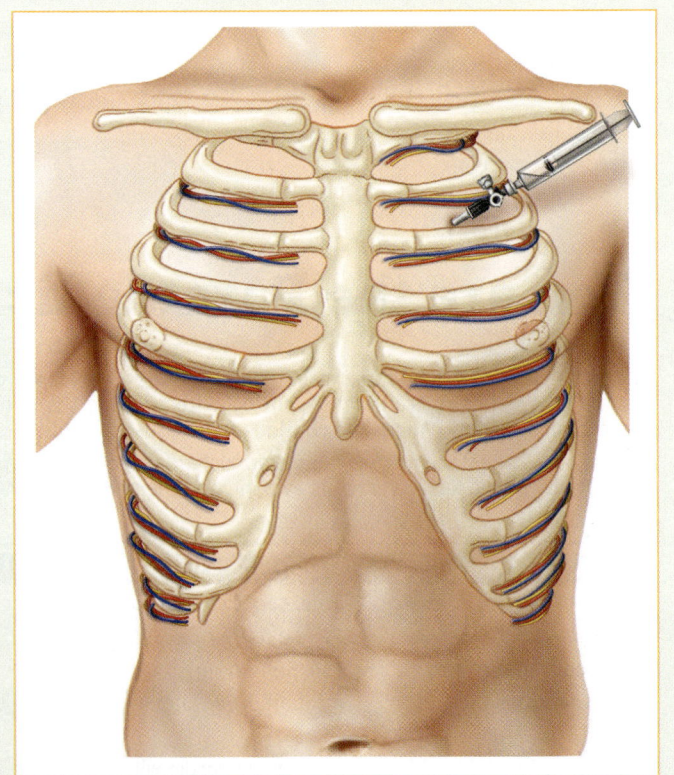

Figure 23-17 Correct placement of needle for decompression. The position of nerves, arteries, and veins are shown in relation to the ribs.

Skill Drill 23-1: Needle Decompression (Thoracentesis) of a Tension Pneumothorax

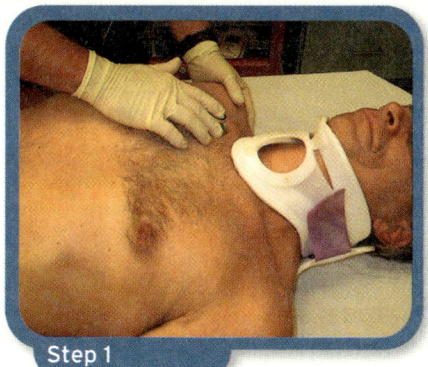

Step 1

Assess the patient.

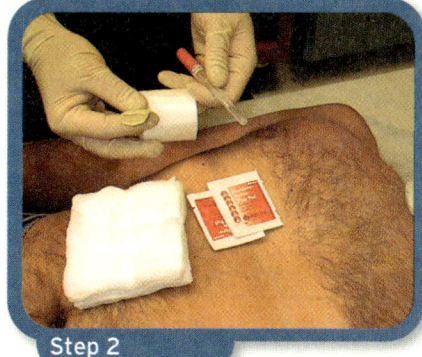

Step 2

Prepare and assemble all necessary equipment. Obtain orders from direct medical control.

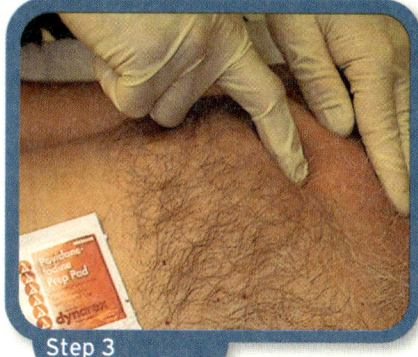

Step 3

Locate the appropriate site between the second and third rib.

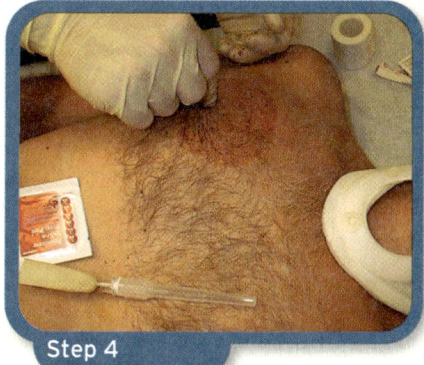

Step 4

Cleanse the appropriate area using aseptic technique.

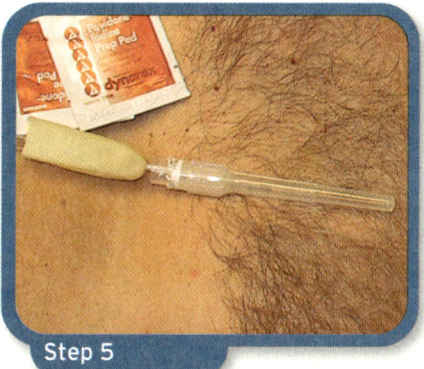

Step 5

Make a one-way valve or flutter valve.

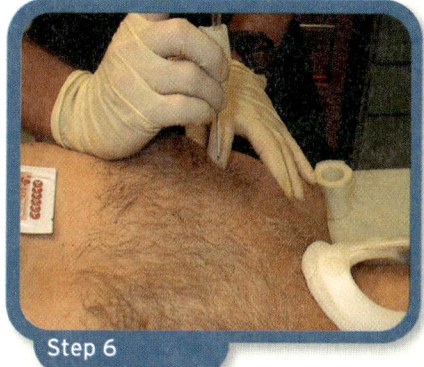

Step 6

Insert the needle at a 90° angle.

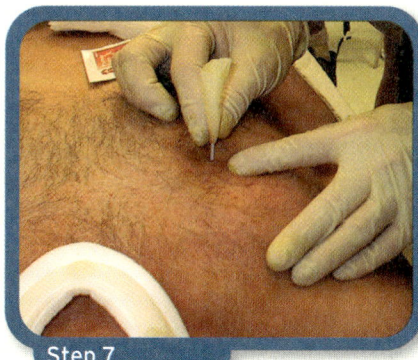

Step 7

Remove the needle and listen for release of air. Properly dispose of the needle in the sharps container.

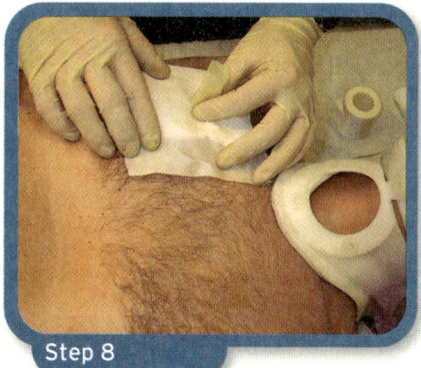

Step 8

Secure the cannula in place. Monitor the patient closely for recurrence of the tension pneumothorax.

9. Secure the cannula in place in the same manner you would use to secure an impaled object (Step 8).

10. Monitor the patient closely for recurrence of the tension pneumothorax. This procedure may need to be repeated several times before arrival at the emergency department.

The performance of a needle decompression is not without risk. If the needle is improperly placed (ie, not inserted over the top of the rib), injury to the intercostal vessels may result in significant hemorrhage. Similarly, passing the needle into the chest may injure the lung parenchyma. However, failure to treat a tension pneumothorax will cause the patient to progress to pulseless electrical activity and cardiopulmonary arrest.

Massive Hemothorax

Physical assessment of the massive hemothorax will reveal signs of both ventilatory insufficiency (hypoxia, agitation, anxiety, tachypnea, dyspnea) and hypovolemic shock (tachycardia, hypotension, pale and clammy skin). The physical findings that help to differentiate this hemothorax from other injuries include the lack of jugular vein distension, the lack of tracheal deviation, possible bloody sputum (hemoptysis), and dullness that may be noted on percussion of the affected side of the chest.

The prehospital management of a suspected hemothorax is supportive. If the airway does not require intervention, place the patient on high-flow supplemental oxygen via a nonrebreathing mask. Initiate two large-bore peripheral IVs, with fluid resuscitation being guided by local protocols and directed at limiting the duration of hypotension. Hypovolemic shock with hypotension that persists for more than 30 minutes raises the mortality from one in ten patients to as high as one in two. For individuals older than age 65, that risk jumps dramatically, to nine out of ten patients.

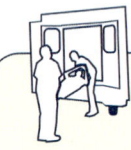

At the Scene

The major problem following a massive hemothorax is the development of hypovolemic shock and respiratory compromise.

Pulmonary Contusion

The assessment of the patient with a pulmonary contusion may not initially reveal the presence or severity of the injury as it may take 24 hours before the severity of the injury becomes clinically evident. Because not every trauma patient presents immediately (eg, cases involving domestic violence, assaults, injuries that occur while intoxicated, patients in remote areas who are not immediately located, or search and rescue operations), it is important to be familiar with the clinical presentation of this injury.

Hypoxia and carbon dioxide retention lead to respiratory distress, dyspnea, tachypnea, agitation, and restlessness. Due to the capillary injury and the hemorrhage into the pulmonary parenchyma, the patient may present with hemoptysis (coughing up blood). Evidence of overlying injury may include

contusions, tenderness, crepitus, or paradoxical motion. Auscultation may reveal wheezes, crackles or rales, or diminished lung sounds in the affected area. In severe cases, cyanosis and low oxygen saturations may be found.

The treatment of pulmonary contusion begins with the assessment and, as needed, management of the patient's airway. Both high-concentration oxygen and positive-pressure ventilation may be used to overcome the pathologic changes described earlier. Because edema may exacerbate the injury, use caution when administering IV fluids. In some cases, the administration of small amounts of analgesics may aid the patient in maximizing ventilatory function without suppressing ventilatory drive.

Myocardial Injuries
Pericardial Tamponade

Beck's triad is the classic combination of physical findings in patients with pericardial tamponade: muffled heart tones, narrowed pulse pressures, and jugular vein distension. Even so, this triad is seen in only 30% of patients diagnosed with cardiac tamponade.

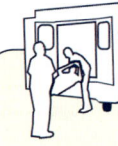

At the Scene

Hypotension and distended neck veins in the presence of normal lung sounds (which rules out pneumothorax), combined with an appropriate history, suggest cardiac tamponade.

Another classic finding in pericardial tamponade (albeit one that is not always present) is the ECG finding of electrical alternans. As fluid accumulates within the pericardial sac, the heart begins to oscillate with each beat. As the heart swings back and forth within the pericardium, its electrical axis changes. Electrical alternans is not commonly seen in acute pericardial tamponade and must be differentiated from bigeminal ectopy, but it is a classic sign of pericardial tamponade.

The reduced cardiac output, hypoperfusion, and hypotension observed in pericardial tamponade produce the findings typical of a patient in shock: weak or absent peripheral pulses, diaphoresis, dyspnea, cyanosis, altered mental status, tachycardia, tachypnea, and agitation. Although these symptoms by themselves do not suggest or exclude the presence of pericardial tamponade, identifying them can flesh out the physical assessment.

Physical findings in a patient with pericardial tamponade are not significantly different than those of a tension pneumothorax—namely, hypotension, jugular vein distension, tachycardia, altered mental status, and signs of tissue hypoperfusion. (Table 23-2 ▶) compares the physical findings of these two emergencies.

The treatment of the patient with pericardial tamponade begins by ensuring adequate oxygen delivery and establishing intravenous access. Giving IV fluids might appear to slow the

Table 23-2	Physical Findings of Pericardial Tamponade Versus Tension Pneumothorax	
Physical Finding	Pericardial Tamponade	Tension Pneumothorax
Presenting sign/ symptom	Shock	Respiratory distress
Neck veins	Distended	Distended
Trachea	Midline	Deviated
Breath sounds	Equal on both sides	Decreased or absent on side of injury
Chest percussion	Normal	Hyperresonant on side of injury
Heart sounds	Muffled	Normal

patient's deterioration by momentarily increasing preload. The patient with a pericardial tamponade should be transported rapidly to a trauma centre for a pericardiocentesis—a procedure in which blood is removed from the pericardial sac via an intracardiac needle inserted through the chest wall. Definitive management occurs in the operating room, in the hands of a cardiothoracic surgeon.

Myocardial Contusion

Sharp, retrosternal chest pain is the most common complaint among patients with myocardial contusion. Inspection of the area may reveal soft-tissue or bony injury in the area. Crackles or rales (due to pulmonary edema from left ventricular dysfunction) may be heard on auscultation.

At the Scene

Many patients with myocardial contusion are relatively asymptomatic, at least initially. Accompanying injuries may present more dramatically. Helpful signs are ECG changes, and persistent sinus tachycardia without obvious hypovolemia.

The ECG in a patient with a myocardial contusion is often abnormal. Sinus tachycardia is the most common ECG abnormality seen in cardiac contusion patients. Additional ECG changes may include atrial fibrillation or flutter, premature atrial contractions (PACs) or premature ventricular contractions (PVCs), a new right bundle branch block, AV blocks, nonspecific ST-segment and T-wave changes, and ventricular tachycardia or fibrillation. In the event of a coronary artery injury (likely the right coronary artery), ischemic changes consistent with those seen in myocardial infarction may also occur.

The treatment of patients with possible myocardial contusion begins with nonspecific, supportive prehospital care, including oxygen administration, frequent assessment of vital signs, cardiac monitoring, and establishing IV access. Fluid resuscitation should be instituted as needed to maintain the patient's blood pressure. Unless allowed by local protocols, consultation with direct medical control should precede the administration of antiarrhythmic agents to trauma patients.

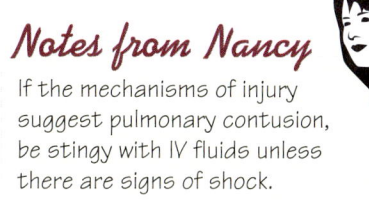

Notes from Nancy

If the mechanisms of injury suggest pulmonary contusion, be stingy with IV fluids unless there are signs of shock.

Myocardial Rupture

Remember that myocardial rupture is life-threatening. Patients may present with acute pulmonary edema or signs of cardiac tamponade. Unless the latter is present and a pericardiocentesis can be done, patients with myocardial rupture should receive supportive prehospital care and be rapidly transported to a facility where a thoracotomy can be performed.

Vascular Injuries
Thoracic Aortic Dissection/Transection

Depending on the exact nature of the injury, the symptoms and physical examination in cases of thoracic aortic dissection or transection will vary from an unstable patient to one with no physical

You are the Paramedic Part 5

The patient's vital signs are monitored en route to the hospital with no further deterioration. You administer IV fluids to maintain perfusion. You and your partner provide prehospital care for the patient's injuries en route to the trauma centre.

When you arrive at the trauma centre, the trauma team takes over the patient's care. You and your partner provide a concise, complete report to the team, including the mechanism of injury, the deaths of two other passengers, your initial physical assessment, the interventions you performed, and the patient's response to those treatments.

During the emergency department evaluation, the patient is found to have a right-sided pneumothorax, a left-sided pulmonary contusion, fractures of left ribs 8 through 11, a lacerated spleen, a fractured left tibia and fibula, and multiple soft-tissue injuries. A tube thoracotomy is performed in the emergency department. The patient is taken to surgery for repair of his abdominal and orthopaedic injuries and, after a 15-day hospitalization, is discharged home with no permanent disability.

complaints. However, most patients will have a complaint of pain behind the sternum or between the scapulae. Other findings may include signs of hypovolemic shock, dyspnea, and altered mental status. If a hematoma forms in the area of the esophagus, trachea, or larynx, the patient may present with dysphagia, stridor, and hoarseness, respectively. A harsh murmur may be noted due to the turbulence created as the blood passes the site of the injury to the intima in the aorta.

Assessment of the patient's pulses in all extremities is an important key to the identification of these injuries. As the dissection or rupture compresses the aorta and progresses along its branch vessels, blood flow to the extremities may be compromised. This phenomenon results in diminished pulses compared to those closer to the injury. On examination, you will note a stronger pulse (and higher blood pressure) in the right arm than in the left arm or the lower extremities.

Because of the high energy involved with aortic injuries, associated injuries are to be expected. They may include multiple rib fractures, flail segment, sternal or scapular fracture, pericardial tamponade, hemothorax or pneumothorax, and clavicle fracture.

Controversies

It has long been taught that first or second rib fractures (which are often a radiographic finding rather than a physical examination finding) are indicative of aortic injuries, but this association has lately come into question.

The prehospital management of potential aortic injuries is symptomatic. After assessment and management of the ABCs, the patient should receive gradual IV hydration for the treatment of hypotension.

Notes from Nancy

Suspect aortic rupture in any accident involving powerful deceleration forces.

ment of hypotension. Aggressive fluid administration may result in sudden changes in the intra-aortic pressure that could worsen the injury. Expedited transport to a trauma centre with an available cardiothoracic surgeon is essential.

Great Vessel Injury

If the vessel is not injured in such a way that bleeding is prevented, the patient will present with signs and symptoms of hypovolemic shock, hemothorax, or cardiac tamponade. If the bleeding results in formation of a hematoma, the compression of adjacent structures (ie, esophagus, trachea) may produce additional signs and symptoms.

The management of potential injuries to the great vessels is no different from the management of any other form of acute blood loss. Establish IV hydration en route to the emergency department. Don't use a pneumatic antishock garment, as it will increase the pressures within the involved vessels and may contribute to greater blood loss.

Other Thoracic Injuries
Diaphragmatic Injuries

Although diaphragmatic injuries are not likely to be identified in the prehospital setting, you should still maintain clinical suspicion for such injuries **Figure 23-18 ▾**. You are most likely to provide prehospital care for the patient during the acute phase, but delayed presentations in the obstructive phase are also possible.

In the acute phase, the patient may present with hypotension, tachypnea, bowel sounds in the chest, chest pain, or absence of breath sounds on the affected side. These signs indicate a large diaphragmatic injury that may be followed by herniation of the abdominal contents into the thoracic cavity.

In the obstructive phase, as the bowel obstructs or as the blood supply to the herniated organs becomes compromised, symptoms will include nausea, vomiting, abdominal pain, constipation, dyspnea, and abdominal distension. In many cases, these symptoms are severe and unrelenting. The most severe findings may be consistent with a tension gastrothorax.

In both the acute and obstructive phases, management of diaphragmatic injury focuses on maintaining adequate

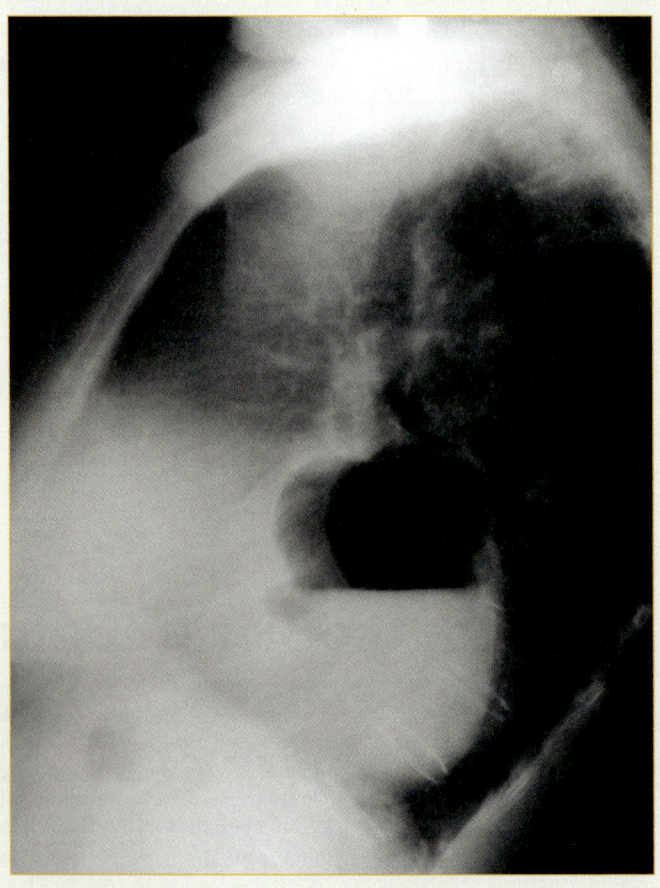

Figure 23-18 Radiograph of a diaphragmatic rupture.

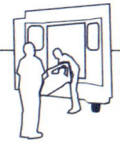

At the Scene

Nitrous oxide should be avoided in patients with a possible diaphragmatic injury because it can greatly increase the volume of gas within entrapped viscera.

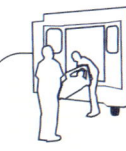

At the Scene

Patients who have been aggressively and improperly restrained by law enforcement, by EMS, or in an altercation situation may experience traumatic asphyxia.

oxygenation and ventilation and rapid transport to the hospital. In prehospital systems that allow for such procedures, nasogastric tube placement may improve the patient's condition by decompressing the involved gastrointestinal organs.

Esophageal Injuries

Esophageal injuries often present with other thoracic and spinal injuries due to the location of the esophagus within the thorax. The patient may experience pleuritic chest pain, and particularly pain that is made worse by swallowing or flexion of the neck. Subcutaneous emphysema may occur, but more than half of esophageal injury patients with this finding have an associated tracheal injury.

No specific therapy for esophageal injuries is possible in the prehospital setting. Definitive care occurs once the patient is evaluated in the hospital and an appropriate surgical consultation is achieved. In the meantime, ensuring that the patient is given nothing orally will help to minimize complications related to this injury.

Tracheobronchial Injuries

The clinical presentation of tracheobronchial injuries may vary from mildly symptomatic to severe respiratory compromise. Expected physical findings include hoarseness, dyspnea and tachypnea, respiratory distress, and hemoptysis. Look for findings of a pneumothorax or tension pneumothorax.

The treatment of a patient with a suspected tracheobronchial injury centres on adequate assessment and management of the patient's ABCs. The patient with a tenuous airway who can be managed with bag-valve-mask ventilation should not be intubated, because introducing an endotracheal tube may complete a partial tracheal injury and result in complete airway obstruction. Similarly, because of the rapid loss of air into the pleural space, high ventilatory pressures should be avoided when providing positive-pressure ventilation (bag the patient gently and slowly).

Traumatic Asphyxia

Although the term "asphyxia" implies a uniformly fatal outcome for patients, this is not always the case. Given the significant force required to produce traumatic asphyxia, however, your suspicion for associated injuries should be high. Don't let the dramatic physical findings in the head and neck, which are not immediately life-threatening, distract you from those injuries that are.

After other life-threatening injuries are managed, the treatment of patients exhibiting traumatic asphyxia is relatively brief. In the absence of intubation, provide high-flow supplemental oxygen via a nonrebreathing mask. Take cervical spine precautions, including spinal immobilization. IV access should be obtained with two large-bore IVs. Transport to the nearest trauma centre or other facility as dictated by local protocols should then be expedited.

You are the Paramedic Summary

1. What will your initial priorities be when assessing and managing this patient?

Assessment of airway, breathing, and circulation with interventions to correct any life-threatening conditions are the assessment and treatment priorities of all paramedics. You can't have good ALS without good BLS.

2. Given the mechanism of injury for an unrestrained passenger in a car and this patient's vital signs, what kinds of injuries should you think about in your assessment?

This case involves a significant mechanism of injury, given the head-on collision and highway speeds, plus the presence of other fatalities. If your patient outwardly appeared to be uninjured, you would still be extremely suspicious of internal bleeding and injuries. Because the patient is unconscious and was unrestrained and partially ejected, you should suspect significant head, chest, abdominal, pelvic, and long bone injuries.

3. Why does the patient remain hypoxic despite confirmed airway patency and the effective delivery of high-concentration oxygen?

The patient remains hypoxic because he has developed a tension pneumothorax. This life-threatening condition must be recognized and corrected immediately. The presence of jugular vein distension and tracheal deviation are late signs of tension pneumothorax.

4. Do his vital signs and physical examination suggest any threats to his breathing that may be correctable?

His hypotension, tachycardia, decreased breath sounds, JVD, and tracheal deviation all point to tension pneumothorax. This requires an emergency needle thoracentesis.

5. What further injuries within the thorax could account for the patient's persistent hypotension and tachycardia?

The patient has hypotension and tachycardia due to increased intrathoracic pressures induced by a tension pneumothorax. This pressure prevents adequate cardiac preload, and therefore decreased cardiac output with resultant hypotension and tachycardia.

6. Are there interventions that you can provide in the prehospital environment if such injuries are identified?

A tension pneumothorax is a correctable condition that requires the release of built-up pressures through the introduction of a large-bore needle into the intercostal space between the second and third ribs, at the midclavicular line of the affected side.

7. What additional injuries might your physical findings suggest?

Given the location of the rib fractures, hypotension, and rigid abdomen, you should be highly suspicious of injury to the spleen. Splenic injuries are among the most common forms of abdominal injury and can result in significant, life-threatening blood loss.

8. What additional treatments may be needed for this patient?

Obviously, once the major life-threatening conditions are addressed, then injuries such as lower extremity fractures can be addressed. Splinting and management of the affected lower extremity as well as managing any soft-tissue injuries would be appropriate at this time.

Prep Kit

Ready for Review

- The thorax contains the ribs, thoracic vertebrae, clavicle, scapula, sternum, heart, lungs, diaphragm, great vessels (including the aorta), esophagus, lymphatic channels, trachea, mainstem bronchi, and nerves.
- Oxygenation and ventilation (delivery of oxygen and removal of carbon dioxide) take place within the thorax, as well as some aspects of circulation.
- Injuries to the thorax can cause air or blood to enter the lungs, or may prevent the organs from being able to move properly, inhibiting oxygenation and ventilation.
- Chest wall injuries include flail chest, rib fractures, and sternal fractures.
- In flail chest, two or more ribs are broken in two or more places. It can result in a free-floating segment of rib that can move paradoxically in comparison to the rest of the chest wall. The lung tissue beneath the flail segment is not adequately ventilated as a result.
- Rib fractures produce significant pain and can prevent adequate ventilation. Sternal fractures are also problematic in that they are usually associated with other serious injuries.
- Lung injuries include simple pneumothorax, open pneumothorax, tension pneumothorax, massive hemothorax, and pulmonary contusion.
- A pneumothorax occurs when air leaks into the space between the pleural surfaces from an opening in the chest or the surface of the lung. The lung collapses as air fills the pleural space. The result is a mismatch between ventilation and perfusion.
- A tension pneumothorax is life-threatening and results from collection of air in the pleural space. The air exerts increasing pressure on surrounding tissues as it accumulates, compromising ventilation, oxygenation, and circulation.
- A hemothorax is the accumulation of blood between the parietal and visceral pleura. It results in compression of structures around the collection of blood and compromises ventilation, oxygenation, and circulation.
- A hemopneumothorax is the collection of both blood and air in the pleural space.
- Pulmonary contusion occurs from compression of the lung. It results in alveolar and capillary damage, edema, and hypoxia.
- Myocardial injuries include pericardial tamponade, myocardial contusion, myocardial rupture, and commotio cordis.
- Pericardial tamponade occurs when excessive fluid builds up in the pericardial sac around the heart. The heart becomes compressed and stroke volume is compromised.
- Myocardial contusion is essentially blunt trauma to the heart. Hemorrhage, edema, and cellular damage result. Dysrhythmias may occur.
- Myocardial rupture is perforation of one or more elements of the anatomy of the heart, such as the ventricles, atria, or valves. It can occur from blunt or penetrating trauma.
- Commotio cordis occurs from a direct blow to the chest during a critical portion of the heart's repolarization period, resulting in possible cardiac arrest.
- Vascular injuries include thoracic aortic dissection/transection and great vessel injury. Thoracic aortic dissection/transection is literally ripping of the aorta. Injuries to other great vessels may cause similar problems of potentially fatal bleeding.
- Other thoracic injuries include diaphragmatic injuries (abdominal contents may herniate through the injury and cut off the blood supply); esophageal injuries, which can be rapidly fatal; tracheobronchial injuries (injury to the airways); and traumatic asphyxia (sudden compression of the chest leading to pressure on the head, neck, and kidneys, causing capillary beds to rupture).
- Begin the assessment of a thoracic trauma patient as you would any other patient—with a scene assessment and assessment of the ABCs.
- In assessing breathing, note any signs of injury to the thorax, which could indicate additional underlying injuries. Look for paradoxical motion, retractions, subcutaneous emphysema, impaled objects, or penetrating injuries.
- Consider adequacy of ventilation and oxygenation. Watch for signs of hypoxia, an irregular pulse, changes in blood pressure, and jugular vein distension.
- Because the mechanism of injury that caused the thoracic problem may have been traumatic, always consider cervical spine stabilization in such cases.
- Several chest injuries may have similar signs and symptoms, such as hypoxia, pain, tachycardia, cyanosis, and shock. Managing the various chest injuries involves several common steps: maintaining the airway, ensuring oxygenation and ventilation, supporting circulatory status, and transporting quickly. Learning the subtle differences between various chest injuries can help you manage them more specifically.
- The one exception to airway management in patients with thoracic trauma is the decision to endotracheally intubate a patient with a possible tracheal injury. Such a decision could further tear the trachea. These patients should be managed with minimal invasion to the airway.
- Management of flail chest includes airway management and possibly positive-pressure ventilation, if the patient experiences respiratory failure. Intubation may also be necessary.
- Management of rib fractures should focus on the ABCs and gentle splinting of the patient's chest by having the patient hold a pillow or blanket against the area.
- Management of a pneumothorax begins with the ABCs and high-concentration oxygen. Cover a sucking chest wound with an occlusive dressing secured on three sides.
- Patients with a tension pneumothorax should be placed on high-flow supplemental oxygen by nonrebreathing mask, and a needle decompression should be performed.
- For patients with pulmonary contusions or pericardial tamponade, follow general management (ABCs) and consider administering IV fluids.
- Management of patients with myocardial contusion should be supportive, but also includes cardiac monitoring and intravenous access.
- Prehospital care for patients with thoracic aortic dissection focuses on symptom control. Management of patients with great vessel injuries is no different from those with acute blood loss.
- Prehospital care for patients with tracheobronchial injuries entails assessment and management of the ABCs.
- Don't be distracted by the dramatic appearance of patients with traumatic asphyxia. Care for the ABCs, obtain IV access, and transport.
- Management of these chest injuries is supportive only: sternal fractures, hemothorax, and myocardial rupture.

Vital Vocabulary

angle of Louis Prominence on the sternum that lies opposite the second intercostal space.

atelectasis Alveolar collapse that prevents use of that portion of the lung for ventilation and oxygenation.

cardiac output The volume of blood delivered to the body in 1 minute.

cardiac tamponade A condition in which the atria and right ventricle are collapsed by a collection of blood or other fluid within the pericardial sac, resulting in a diminished cardiac output.

clavicle An S-shaped bone, also called the collarbone, that articulates medially with the sternum and laterally with the shoulder.

commotio cordis An event in which an often fatal cardiac dysrhythmia is produced by a sudden blow to the thoracic cavity.

crepitus A grating sensation made when two pieces of broken bone are rubbed together or subcutaneous emphysema is palpated.

diaphragm Large skeletal muscle that plays a major role in breathing and separates the chest cavity from the abdominal cavity.

electrical alternans An ECG pattern in which the QRS vector changes with each heart beat. This pattern is pathognomonic for cardiac tamponade.

exopthalmos Protrusion of the eyes from the normal position within the socket.

flail chest An injury that involves two or more adjacent ribs fractured in two or more places, allowing the segment between the fractures to move independently of the rest of the thoracic cage.

hemopneumothorax A collection of blood and air in the pleural cavity.

hemothorax The collection of blood within the normally closed pleural space.

intercostal space The space between two ribs, named according to the number of the rib above it, that contains the intercostal muscles and neurovascular bundle.

jugular vein distension (JVD) A prominence of the jugular veins due to increased volume or increased pressure within the central venous system or the thoracic cavity.

manubrium The superior segment of the sternum; its lower border defines the angle of Louis.

mediastinum Space within the chest that contains the heart, major blood vessels, vagus nerve, trachea, and esophagus; located between the two lungs.

myocardial contusion Blunt force injury to the heart that results in capillary damage, interstitial bleeding, and cellular damage in the area.

myocardial rupture An acute traumatic perforation of the ventricles, atria, intraventricular septum, intra-atrial septum, chordae, papillary muscles, or valves.

needle decompression Also referred to as a needle thoracentesis, this procedure introduces a needle or angiocath into the pleural space in an attempt to relieve a tension pneumothorax.

neurovascular bundle A closely placed grouping of an artery, vein, and nerve that lies beneath the inferior edge of a rib.

open pneumothorax The result of a defect in the chest wall that allows air to enter the thoracic space.

oxygenation The process of delivering oxygen to the blood by diffusion from the alveoli following inhalation into the lungs.

pericardial sac The potential space between the layers of the pericardium.

pericardial tamponade Accumulation of excess fluid or blood in the pericardial sac to the extent that it interferes with cardiac function.

pericardiocentesis A procedure in which a needle or angiocath is introduced into the pericardial sac to relieve cardiac tamponade.

pericardium Double-layered sac containing the heart and the origins of the superior vena cava, inferior vena cava, and the pulmonary artery.

pleura Membrane lining the outer surface of the lungs (visceral pleura), the inner surface of the chest wall, and the thoracic surface of the diaphragm (parietal pleura).

pneumothorax The collection of air within the normally closed pleural space.

pulmonary contusion Injury to the lung parenchyma that results in capillary hemorrhage into the tissue.

scapula A large, flat, triangular bone along the posterior thorax that articulates with the clavicle and humerus.

sternum Also known as the breastbone, this bony structure along the midline of the thorax provides a point of anterior attachment for the thoracic cage.

subconjunctival hematoma The collection of blood within the sclera of the eye, presenting as a bright red patch of blood over the sclera but not involving the cornea.

subcutaneous emphysema A physical finding of air within the subcutaneous tissue.

suprasternal notch The indentation formed by the superior border of the manubrium and the clavicles, often used as a landmark for procedures such as subclavian vein access.

tension pneumothorax A life-threatening collection of air within the pleural space; the volume and pressure have both collapsed the involved lung and caused a shift of the mediastinal structures to the opposite side.

thoracic inlet The superior aspect of the thoracic cavity, this ring-like opening is created by the first vertebral vertebra, the first rib, the clavicles, and the manubrium.

thorax The part of the body between the neck and the diaphragm, encased by the ribs.

traumatic asphyxia A pattern of injuries seen after a severe force is applied to the thorax, forcing blood from the great vessels and back into the head and neck.

ventilation The process of eliminating carbon dioxide from the blood by diffusion into the alveoli and exhalation from the lungs.

xyphoid process An inferior segment of the sternum often used as a landmark for CPR.

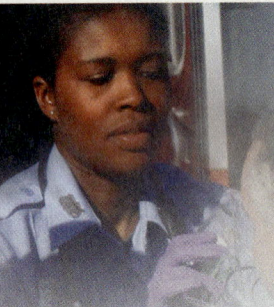

Assessment in Action

You are dispatched to an office building for a patient who has fallen from a ladder. On arrival, you find a 34-year-old man who is in a left lateral recumbent position. He complains of chest pain and shortness of breath. While maintaining in-line stabilization, you notice some bruising to his upper back that extends into his left flank area. Looking at the ladder, you note that he fell at least 6 m.

1. **With a fall victim who is complaining of shortness of breath and chest pain, you should suspect which of the following injuries?**
   - **A.** Tension pneumothorax
   - **B.** Flail segment
   - **C.** Pulmonary contusion
   - **D.** All of the above

2. **_____ is the most common cause of a tension pneumothorax.**
   - **A.** Barotrauma
   - **B.** Blunt force trauma
   - **C.** Tracheobronchial injury
   - **D.** Open thoracic injury

3. **Traumatic injury to the thoracic cavity presents the possibility of compromise of:**
   A. ventilation.
   B. oxygenation.
   C. circulation.
   D. all of the above.

4. **Which injuries must be identified and treated during assessment of the patient's breathing?**
   A. Flail chest, tension pneumothorax, and cardiac tamponade
   B. Open pneumothorax, tension pneumothorax, and flail chest
   C. Aortic injuries, open pneumothorax, and flail chest
   D. Open pneumothorax, tension pneumothorax, and myocardial contusion

5. **All of the following are classic signs of a tension pneumothorax, EXCEPT:**
   A. absence of breath sounds on the affected side.
   B. absence of breath sounds on the unaffected side.
   C. tachycardia.
   D. jugular vein distension.

6. **Traumatic injuries that result in the sudden and forceful compression of the thoracic cavity may cause:**
   A. traumatic asphyxia.
   B. traumatic pneumothorax.
   C. exopthalmos.
   D. hematoma.

7. **The pathology of a tension pneumothorax includes all of the following, EXCEPT:**
   A. the lung collapses on the affected side with mediastinal shift to the contralateral side.
   B. a serious reduction in cardiac output by the deformation of the vena cavae, reducing preload.
   C. the lung collapse leads to right-to-left intrapulmonary shunting and hypoxia.
   D. the lung collapse leads to left-to-right intrapulmonary shunting and hypercarbia.

8. **Muffled heart tones, hypotension, and jugular vein distension—a classic combination of findings in patients with pericardial tamponade—are collectively called:**
   A. Beck's triad.
   B. Circle of Wills.
   C. pulsus paradoxus.
   D. myocardial contusion.

9. **The pathology of a myocardial contusion may include any of the following, EXCEPT:**
   A. development of a hemopericardium when the epicardium or endocardium is lacerated.
   B. clear demarcation of the areas of contusion.
   C. undefined areas of contusion.
   D. conduction defects on the ECG caused by the areas of contusion.

Challenging Question

You are dispatched to the private residence of a 45-year-old woman. The call came in as a stabbing. At the scene, you perform a scene assessment and determine that it is safe to enter the residence. The patient is located upstairs in the bedroom, where she is lying prone on the floor. She is not breathing, and a small quantity of blood is pooling beneath her. She has no pulse.

Maintaining in-line stabilization, you roll the patient over onto a backboard (after examining her back for any obvious injuries). You open her airway and begin ventilating with 100% oxygen. You immediately begin high-quality CPR (pushing hard, fast, and allowing full chest recoil). Your partner successfully intubates the patient, and you hear good breath sounds on the right side. There is no tracheal deviation, but there is jugular vein distension. The monitor shows a narrow-complex pulseless electrical activity at a rate of 100 beats/min.

The police tell you that the patient was in a verbal argument with her husband, who then stabbed her with a 30-cm steak knife. The knife is by her side. You notice a wound just under her left clavicle and feel some subcutaneous emphysema surrounding the wound. When you intubate the patient, you don't hear any breath sounds on the left side. You believe she has a tension pneumothorax.

You properly perform a chest decompression. You hear a rush of air exit the angiocath.

10. **What type of injury is this?**

11. **What other injuries should you expect?**

Points to Ponder

You are dispatched to a local highway for a motor vehicle collision—a car has run into a wall. When you arrive, the fire department is in the process of extricating the patient. During your initial scene assessment, you determined that it was safe to enter the zone. You also noticed a midsize car with severe front-end damage and damage to the top of the roof. The A-post was completely bent down. You have no real access to the patient other than to see that he is unconscious, has agonal respirations, and is grossly diaphoretic. Blood is coming out of his mouth.

You ask witnesses if they saw anything. They tell you that the car was moving at a high rate of speed (in excess of 100 km/h). When it was going around the curve, the car slid on an ice patch and the driver lost control of the vehicle. He drove into the cement abutment head on. The vehicle then flipped up, and its roof struck the wall. The vehicle landed on its wheels. There is significant damage to the driver's compartment, including the steering wheel.

The patient is finally extricated from the vehicle, and the fire department provides spinal precautions.

What will you as the paramedic do for this patient?

Issues: Thorough Assessment to Determine Diagnosis and Treatment Plan, Thorough Scene Assessment to Determine Forces Involved, Proper Treatment of a Patient With Thoracic Trauma.

24 Abdomen Injuries

Competency Areas

Area 4: Assessment and Diagnostics

4.3.g Conduct gastrointestinal system assessment and interpret findings.

4.3.h Conduct genitourinal system assessment and interpret findings.

Area 6: Integration

6.1.d Provide care to patient experiencing illness or injury primarily involving genitourinary/reproductive system.

6.1.e Provide care to patient experiencing illness or injury primarily involving gastrointestinal system.

Appendix 4: Pathophysiology

C. **Respiratory System**
Traumatic Injuries: Diaphragmatic injuries

E. **Gastrointestinal System**
Traumatic Injuries: Abdominal injury–penetrating/blunt
Traumatic Injuries: Esophageal disruption
Traumatic Injuries: Evisceration

Introduction

The abdominal cavity is the largest cavity in the body. It extends from the diaphragm to the pelvis, making the evaluation and management of patients with abdominal trauma challenging for the paramedic. There is great variability in the presentation of conditions, which are rarely resolved in the prehospital setting. Abdominal injuries may be life threatening, and assessment should be rapid so management and transport to an appropriate facility can be started.

The abdominal cavity contains several vital organ systems such as the digestive, urinary, and genitourinary systems. These organ systems are vulnerable to trauma partly because of their location but they also lack some of the protective structures afforded by the skeletal system. Abdominal trauma may be caused by blunt or penetrating forces and ranges from minor single-system injuries to the more complicated and potentially devastating multisystem injuries. Abdominal injuries can be difficult to prevent.

Because of the broad spectrum of abdominal injuries, assessments and interventions should be made quickly and cautiously. Delays in the recognition and management of abdominal injuries can have disastrous consequences. Assessments in the prehospital environment can be difficult because of other system injuries that may lead to changes in a patient's mental status and sensation. For example, an unconscious patient or a patient who does not feel pain after spinal trauma may not be able to communicate, leaving the determination of existing injuries to be based solely on presenting signs and the mechanism of injury.

In recent years, there has been a concerted effort to reduce morbidity and mortality resulting from abdominal trauma. This process has taken shape at several different levels. The education of paramedics in recognizing the need for rapid transport has made a significant reduction in the time from injury to definitive care. The advances in hospital care, such as improved diagnostic equipment (eg, ultrasound), surgical techniques, and postoperative care have also improved patient outcomes. Furthermore, trauma system development has played a large role in providing advanced interventions and detection of traumatic injuries.

The purpose of this chapter is to supply the information necessary to assess and begin managing the trauma patient as quickly and with as much confidence as possible. This chapter provides the concepts and vocabulary for the effective understanding and communication of critical data that will improve the assessment of the trauma mechanism. Your account from the scene is the only source for physicians and surgeons to understand the events and mechanism that led to any given trauma presentation. This information is critical in visualizing and searching for injuries that may not be obviously apparent on physical examination, as is often seen with abdominal trauma.

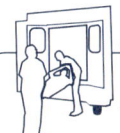

At the Scene

Late recognition of abdominal trauma can be a fatal mistake. Abdominal trauma often goes unrecognized because the mechanism of injury is often not fully appreciated or noticed.

You are the Paramedic Part 1

As you walk into the fire department for the start of your shift, you hear the front doorbell. When you answer the door, you find a neighbourhood child who tells you that, while he was waiting across the street for the school bus, he saw a man lying in the alleyway. You alert your crew, grab a first-in bag, and follow the child, who takes you directly to the man.

As you approach, you see a man lying in the alleyway between two houses, curled in a ball and holding his left ankle. He appears dirty, disheveled, and pale, and you recognize him as a homeless man, Mr. Campbell (Stan), you've seen on previous calls involving drugs, alcohol, and assaultive behaviour. When you ask him what is wrong, he mutters something about tripping and hurting his leg.

Initial Assessment	Recording Time: 0 Minutes
Appearance	Eyes closed; fetal position
Level of consciousness	V (Responsive to verbal stimuli)
Airway	Patent; patient is moaning
Breathing	Rapid and shallow
Circulation	Rapid radial pulse

1. What are your immediate concerns?
2. What about this patient immediately grabs your attention?
3. At this point, what are your treatment priorities?

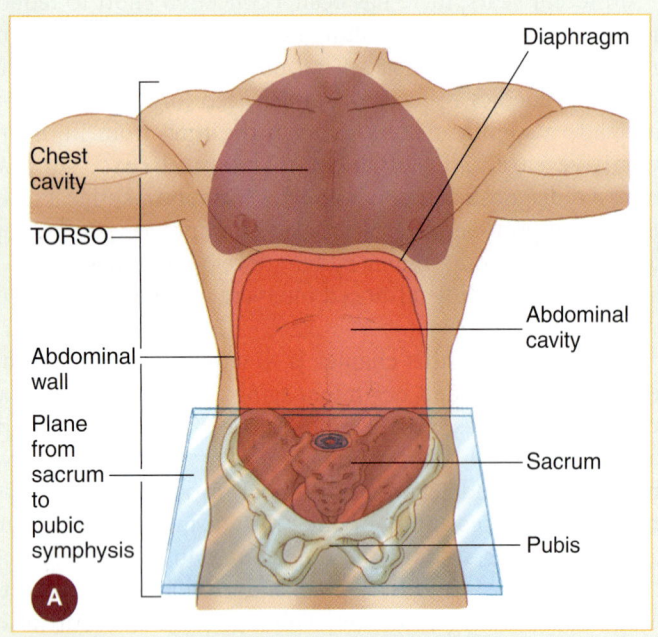

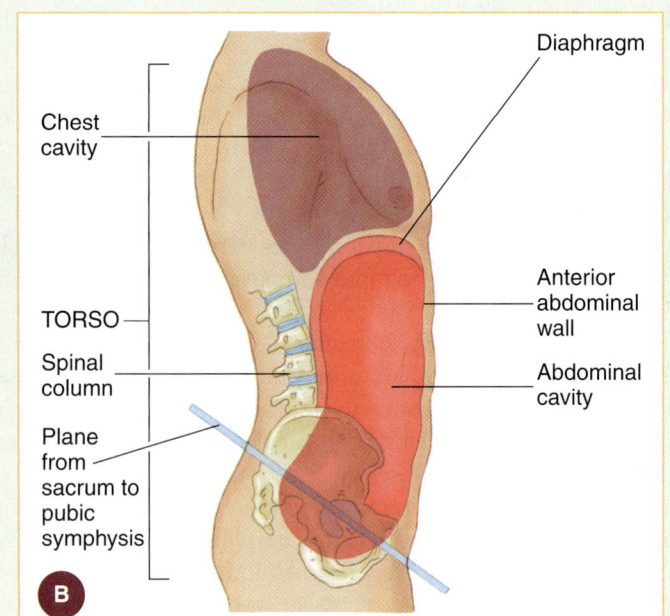

Figure 24-1 The external abdomen consists of the anterior abdomen, the flanks, and the back (retroperitoneal area). The boundaries of the abdomen are the anterior and posterior abdominal cavity walls, the diaphragm, and an imaginary plane from the pubic symphysis to the sacrum. **A.** Anterior view. **B.** Lateral view.

Anatomy Review

Knowledge of the anatomical boundaries of the abdomen is important as we discuss potential injury patterns, such as hollow organ injury, vascular injury, solid organ injury, or injuries to the retroperitoneal area. The oval-shaped abdominal cavity extends from the dome-shaped diaphragm, a large muscle separating the thoracic cavity from the abdomen, to the pelvic brim. The pelvic brim stretches at an angle from the intervertebral disks between L5 and S1 to the pubic symphysis.

The abdomen is divided into three sections, the anterior abdomen, the flanks, and the posterior abdomen or back **Figure 24-1 ▲** . The outer boundary of the abdominal cavity is the abdominal wall on the front of the body and the peritoneal surface on the back of the body. The abdomen extends upward into the lower thorax at about the level of the nipples or the fourth intercostal space. The anterior part of the abdomen extends inferiorly to the inguinal ligaments and symphysis pubis, and laterally to the front of the axillary line. The flanks include the regions between the anterior and posterior axillary lines from the sixth intercostal space to the iliac crest. The back extends posteriorly between the posterior axillary lines, from the scapula to the iliac crests. The flanks and the back are protected by thick abdominal wall muscles that protect that region from low-velocity penetrating trauma.

To describe a location in the abdomen, or a source of pain found when conducting your assessment, the quadrant system

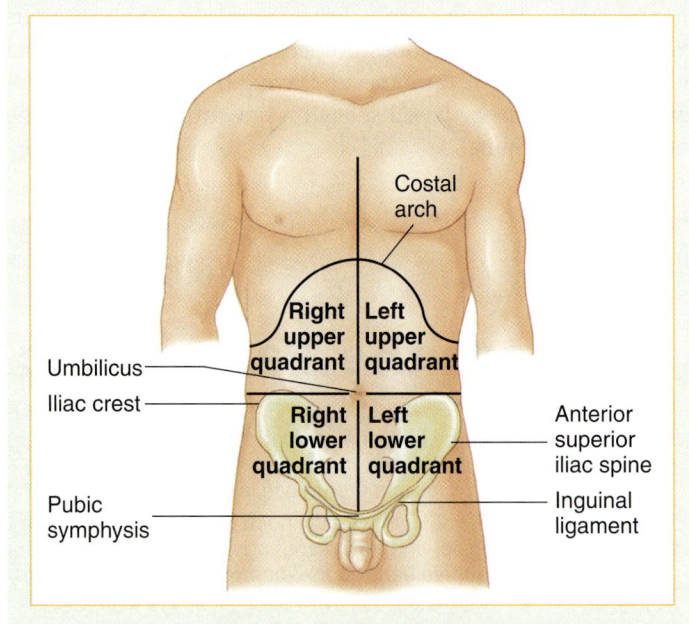

Figure 24-2 The abdomen is often referred to by quadrants.

is generally used **Figure 24-2 ▲** . If you were to place a large imaginary "+" sign with the centre directly on the umbilicus (navel) with the vertical axis extending from the symphysis pubis to the xiphoid process and the horizontal axis extending to both flanks, this would create four quadrants. These four regions are as follows: the right upper quadrant (RUQ), the right lower quadrant (RLQ), the left lower quadrant (LLQ), and the left upper quadrant (LUQ). The area around the umbilicus is referred to as the periumbilical area.

The abdominal cavity is lined with a membrane called the peritoneum, which is similar to the pleura that line the thoracic cavity. The mesentery is a membranous double fold of tissue in the abdomen that attaches various organs to the body wall. The internal abdomen is structurally divided into three regions: the peritoneal space, the retroperitoneal space, and the pelvis (Figure 24-3 ▶). Intraperitoneal structures, encased in the peritoneum, include the liver, spleen, stomach, small bowel, colon, gallbladder, and, in women, the female reproductive organs. The retroperitoneal space contains the aorta, vena cava, pancreas, kidneys, ureters, and portions of the duodenum and large intestine. The rectum, ureters, pelvic vascular plexus, major vascular structures, pelvic skeletal structures, and reproductive organs lie in the pelvis.

Abdominal Organs

The abdomen contains many organs.

The liver is a solid organ and is the largest organ in the abdomen. It lies in the right upper quadrant (extending to the epigastrium), superior and anterior to the gallbladder and the hepatic and cystic ducts. Among its many functions, the liver detoxifies the blood and produces bile (which is necessary to break down ingested fats) that drains into the small intestines.

The gallbladder is a saclike organ located on the lower surface of the liver that acts as a reservoir for bile, one of the digestive enzymes produced by the liver. The liver continually secretes bile, and the gallbladder stores it until it is released through the cystic duct during the digestive process.

Like the liver, the spleen is a solid organ in the abdomen. This highly vascular organ lies in the left upper quadrant and is partially protected by the left lower rib cage. It functions to clear bloodborne bacteria.

The pancreas is an organ located in the retroperitoneal space in the middle of the abdomen. It secretes enzymes into the bowel that aid in digestion. The pancreas also secretes the hormone insulin, which is responsible for helping glucose enter the cells.

The stomach is an intraperitoneal hollow organ that lies in the left upper quadrant and epigastric region. The esophagus passes through the diaphragm and opens into the stomach. The stomach secretes an acid that assists in the digestive process.

The small and large intestines run from the end of the stomach to the anus. The majority of the intestines are in the intraperitoneal area. They digest and absorb water and nutrients. The first part of the small intestine, the duodenum, is retroperitoneal. As contents pass through the stomach, they move through the pylorus, a circumferential muscle at the end of the stomach that acts as a valve between the stomach and the duodenum. Finally, stool passes through the rectum and out of the body through the anus.

The abdomen also contains organs of the urinary system. The kidneys are located in the retroperitoneal space. They filter blood and excrete body wastes in the form of urine. The kidneys

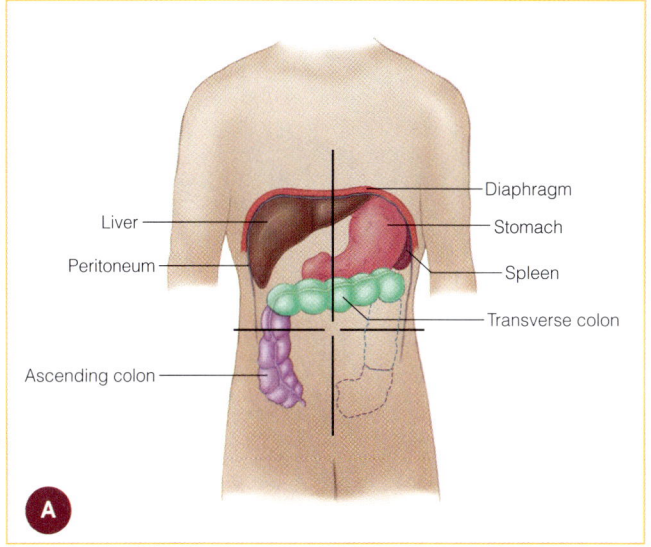

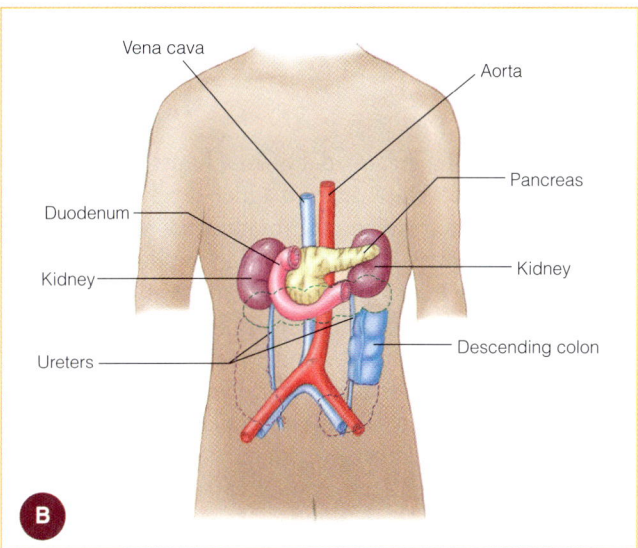

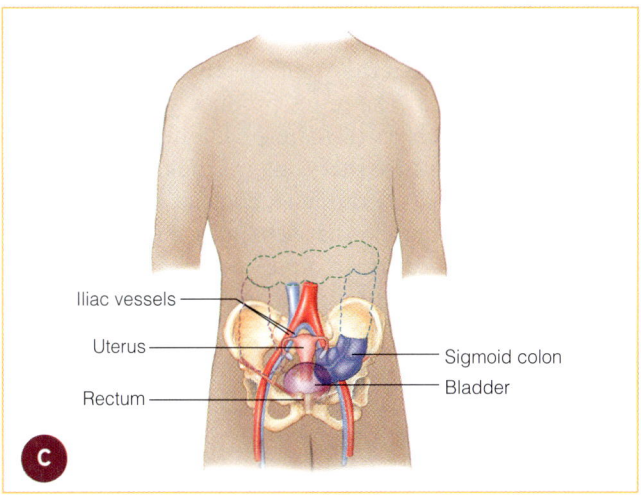

Figure 24-3 Different organs of the abdomen are contained in the peritoneum (**A**), the retroperitoneal space (**B**), and the pelvis (**C**).

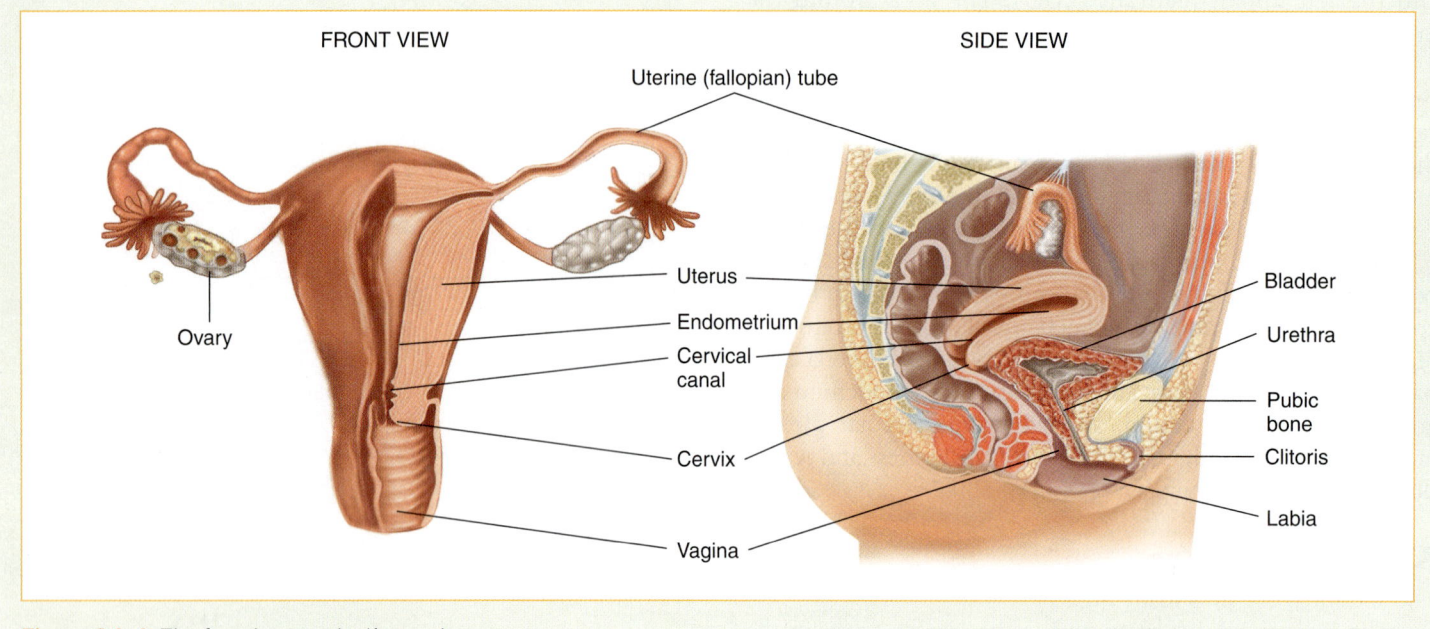

Figure 24-4 The female reproductive system.

will be discussed in greater detail in Chapter 32, *Renal and Urologic Emergencies*. The urinary bladder is a hollow, muscular sac situated in the pelvis along the midline that stores urine until it is excreted. The ureters are a pair of thick-walled, hollow tubes that carry urine from the kidneys to the urinary bladder.

The abdomen also contains organs of the reproductive system. The female reproductive system (Figure 24-4 ▲) contains the uterus, a pear-shaped organ located in the midline of the lower abdomen that allows the implantation, growth, and nourishment of a fetus during pregnancy. The female reproductive system also contains the ovaries, located one on each side of the lower abdominal quadrants. The ovaries produce the precursors to mature eggs, and produce hormones that regulate female reproductive function.

The male reproductive system (Figure 24-5 ▶) includes the penis, the male external reproductive organ, as well as the testes, or testicles. The testes produce sperm and secrete male hormones such as testosterone. The scrotum is the pouch of skin and muscle that contains the testes.

Last but not least, the abdomen contains the diaphragm—the domed-shaped muscle that separates the thoracic cavity from the abdominal cavity. It curves from its point of attachment in the flanks at the twelfth rib and peaks in the centre at the fourth intercostal space.

Physiology Review

When abdominal trauma occurs, the places where enough blood can be lost to cause shock include the abdominal cavity, retroperitoneal space, and the pelvis, (as well as the street, as a result of bleeding from open wounds) (Figure 24-6 ▶).

Because the abdomen and retroperitoneum can accommodate large amounts of blood, the bleeding may produce few signs and symptoms of the trauma. Even the patient's vital signs and physical examination may not indicate the bleeding.

The organs that are most frequently injured after a blunt trauma are the spleen (in approximately 50% of the cases), followed by the liver (in approximately 30%). Because of its size, the liver is the organ that is most frequently injured in penetrating trauma. Solid organs, such as the liver or spleen, can easily be crushed by external blunt trauma. They both have a large blood supply and can bleed profusely. If a trauma patient has unexplained symptoms of shock, you should suspect abdominal trauma.

Hollow organs are more resilient to blunt trauma and less likely to be injured unless they are full. The danger of bursting hollow organs is that they hold toxins (such as urine, bile, stomach acids, or fecal material) that can spill out into the abdominal cavity. This spillage can cause peritonitis, an inflammation of the lining of the abdomen (the peritoneum). Leakage of bacteria from hollow organ rupture can lead to contamination of the normally sterile peritoneal cavity. Peritonitis is a life-threatening infection.

Injury to the abdominal organs is not always evident based on the history and physical examination. You must have a high index of suspicion and a clear understanding of the mechanism of injury (MOI) your trauma patient was exposed to.

Mechanism of Injury

Trauma is a significant cause of death in adults and is the leading cause of death in patients from 1 to 44 years of age. The

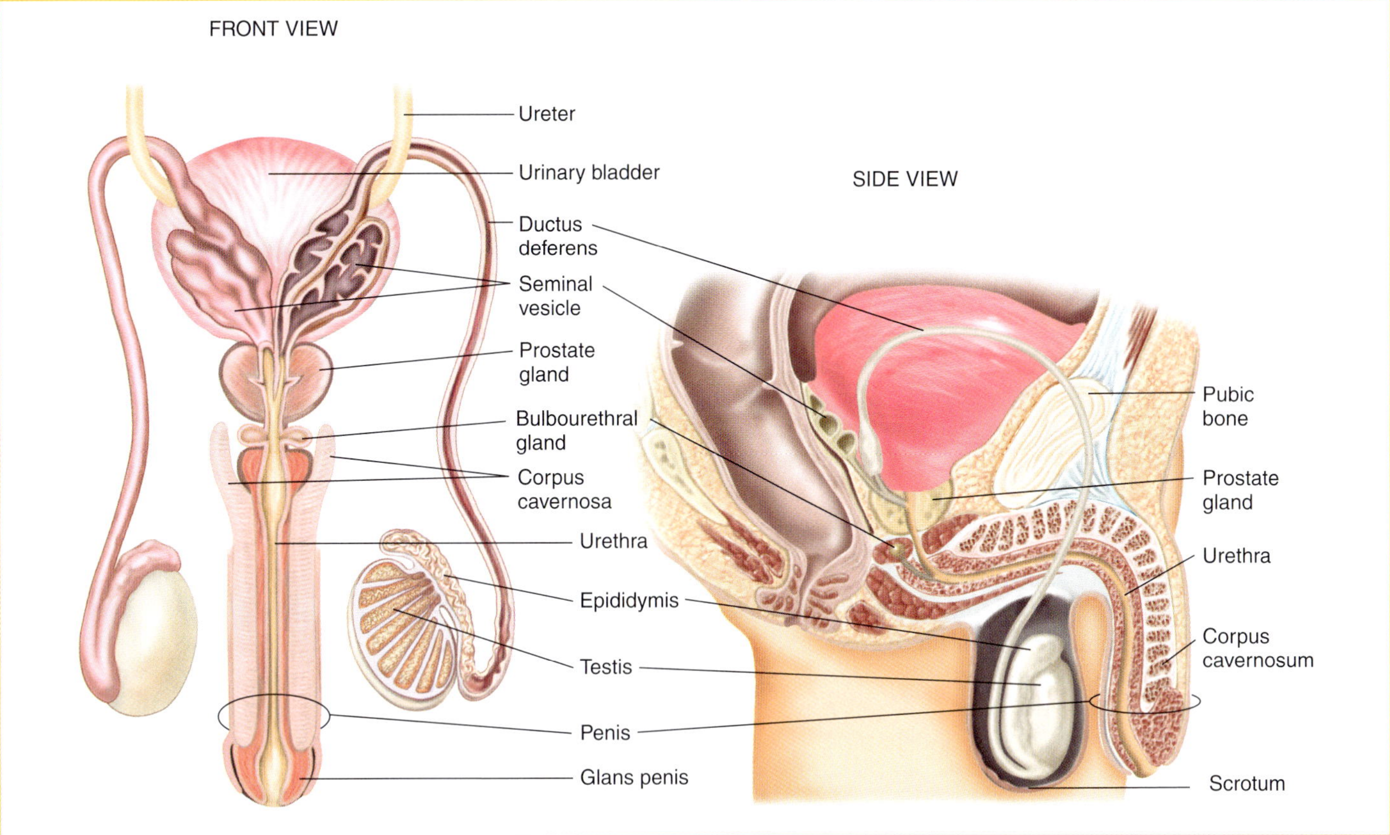

FRONT VIEW

- Ureter
- Urinary bladder
- Ductus deferens
- Seminal vesicle
- Prostate gland
- Bulbourethral gland
- Corpus cavernosa
- Urethra
- Epididymis
- Testis
- Penis
- Glans penis

SIDE VIEW

- Pubic bone
- Prostate gland
- Urethra
- Corpus cavernosum
- Scrotum

Figure 24-5 The male reproductive system.

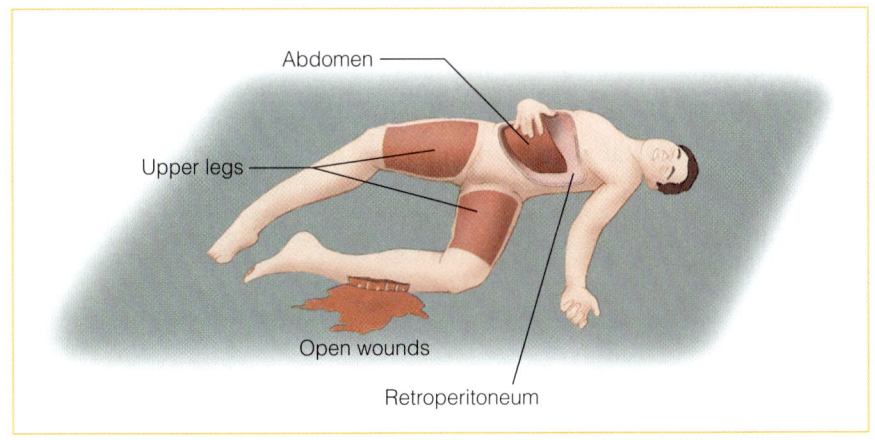

- Abdomen
- Upper legs
- Open wounds
- Retroperitoneum

Figure 24-6 The places where enough blood can be lost to cause shock.

(94%); 4.5% had a penetrating injury; and 2% had a burn injury. Unrecognized abdominal trauma is the leading cause of unexpected deaths because it results in a delay in surgical intervention.

Blunt Trauma

The majority of significant abdominal injuries in Canada involve blunt trauma. Most of these injuries occur during motor vehicle collisions Figure 24-7 ▶, with a resulting mortality of about 11%. Blunt trauma to the abdomen results from compression or deceleration forces and can often lead to a closed abdominal injury—one in which soft-tissue damage occurs inside the body, but the skin remains intact. When assessing the abdominal cavity in a patient who has received blunt trauma, consider three common mechanisms of injury: shearing, crushing, and compression. In the rapid deceleration of a patient during a motor vehicle collision or fall from a height, a shearing force can be created as the internal organs continue their forward motion. This will cause hollow, solid, and visceral organs and vascular structures to tear, especially at their points of attachment to the abdominal wall.

leading cause of injury among all major injury cases was motor vehicle collisions, which were responsible for almost half of the cases (45%), followed by unintentional falls (32%). Homicide and purposely inflicted injury was the third leading cause. Other causes included being unintentionally struck by an object or person and incidents caused by machinery. The most common type of major injury was an internal organ injury (76%). Most cases had a blunt injury

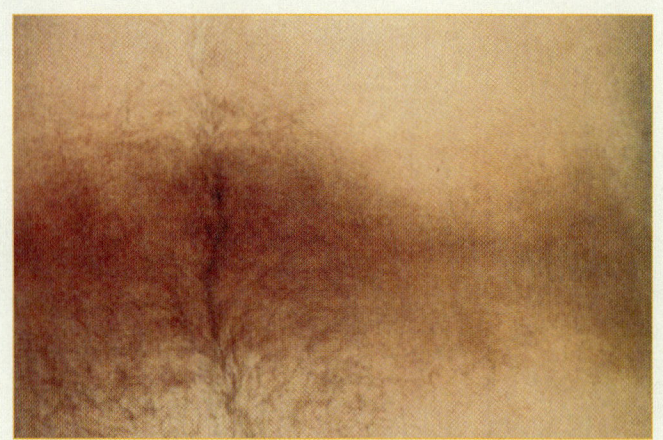

Figure 24-7 Blunt trauma occurs most frequently in vehicle collisions, and typically leads to closed abdominal injury—the internal organs are injured, but the skin remains intact.

Organs that shear or tear would include the liver, kidneys, small and large intestines, and spleen. In motor vehicle collisions, this MOI has been described as the third collision (such as the car into the wall, the patient into the steering column, or the internal organs into the patient's inner rib cage).

Crush injuries are the result of external factors at the time of impact, when abdominal contents are crushed between the anterior abdominal wall and the spinal column (or other structures in the rear). They differ from decelerating injuries that occur before impact. Solid organs like the kidneys, liver, and spleen are at the greatest risk of injury from this mechanism. Direct application of crushing forces to the abdomen would come from things like the dashboard or by the steering wheel striking the abdominal cavity of an unrestrained driver as the person is propelled forward.

The last MOI to consider is compression injury resulting from a direct blow or external compression from a fixed object (such as a lap belt or air bag). These compression forces will deform hollow organs, increasing the pressure within the abdominal cavity. This dramatic change in abdominal pressure can cause a rupture of the small intestine or diaphragm. Rupture of organs can lead to uncontrollable hemorrhage and peritonitis.

Penetrating Trauma

Penetrating trauma results most commonly from low-velocity (< 70 m per second) gunshot or stab wounds. Penetrating trauma causes an open abdominal injury—one in which a break in the surface of the skin or mucous membrane exposes deeper tissue to potential contamination. In general, gunshot wounds cause more injury than stab wounds because bullets travel deep into the body and have more kinetic energy. Gunshot wounds most commonly involve injury to the small bowel, colon, liver, and vascular structures; the extent of injury is less predictable than the injury caused by stab wounds because gunshot wounds depend mostly on the characteristics

of the weapon and the characteristics of the bullet. In penetrating trauma from stab wounds, the liver, small bowel, diaphragm, and colon are the organs most frequently injured.

The extent of damage from a penetrating injury is often a function of the energy that has been imparted to the body. Remember:

$$\text{Kinetic energy} = \frac{\text{Mass}}{2} \times \text{Velocity}^2$$
$$\text{or, KE} = \frac{m}{2} \times v^2$$

Thus, the permanent injury as well as the temporary injury from the tract of the projectile can be considerable with high-velocity penetrations. The velocity delivered during penetrating trauma is typically divided into three levels. Low velocity (< 70 m per second) such as from a knife, ice pick, or handgun; medium velocity (70 to 700 m per second) such as from a 9-mm gun or shotgun; and high velocity (> 700 m per second) such as from a high-powered sporting rifle or military weapon. The trajectory or direction the projectile travelled and the distance it had to travel, as well as the profile of the bullet, can contribute considerably to the extent of the injury.

Motor Vehicle Collisions

In motor vehicle collisions there are five typical patterns of impact (frontal, lateral, rear, rotational, and rollover), which are discussed in depth in Chapter 17. Each of these different mechanisms, with the exception of the rear impact, has the potential to cause significant injury to abdominal organs. In a rear impact collision, the patient is less likely to have an injury to his or her abdomen if he or she has been restrained properly. However, if restraints are improperly worn or not used at all, all bets are off—the potential for injury is great.

Rollover impacts present the greatest potential to inflict lethal injuries. Unrestrained occupants may change direction several times with an increased risk of ejection from the vehicle. The occupants involved in a rollover may collide with each other as well as with the vehicle interior, producing a wide range of probable injuries.

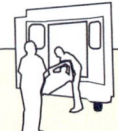 **At the Scene**

Always remember the concept of associated injuries. On the basis of the MOI, some of the following syndromes are common:
- Fractures of the lower rib cage → suspect spleen and/or liver injuries
- Upper abdominal injuries → suspect chest trauma
- Pelvic fractures → suspect intra-abdominal trauma (bladder laceration)
- Penetrating thoracic wounds below the nipple line → suspect intra-abdominal injury

Motorcycle Falls or Collisions

With the popularity of motorcycles and the production of high-performance racing bikes that are most attractive to younger and inexperienced riders, motorcycle collisions continue to increase. In a motorcycle collision, any structural protection from a steel cage, as is the case in an automobile, does not exist. The motorcyclist's only protection are those protective devices worn by the rider, such as the helmet and abrasion-resistant or leather pants, gloves, jacket, and boots. Although helmets are designed to protect against impact to the head, they transmit any impact to the cervical spine so they do not protect against severe cervical injury.

Falls From Heights

When an adult falls from a height, the fall usually occurs in the context of criminal activity, attempted suicide, or intoxication. The position or orientation of the body at the moment of impact will help determine the type of injuries sustained and their survivability. The surface onto which the person has fallen, and the degree to which that surface can deform (plasticity) under the force of the falling body can help in dissipating the forces of sudden deceleration.

Blast Injuries

Although most commonly associated with military conflict, blast injuries are also seen in civilian practice in mines, shipyards, chemical plants, and increasingly in association with terrorist activities. Blast injuries, particularly those from weapons designed specifically for antipersonnel effects (such as mines or grenades) can generate fragments travelling at velocities of 1,500 m per second. This is nearly double the velocity of a projectile from a high-speed rifle. Any energy transmitted from a blast fragment will cause extensive damage to tissue. People who are injured in explosions may be injured by any of four different mechanisms. The primary blast injury is an injury from the pressure wave. The secondary blast injury is caused by debris or fragments from the explosion. The tertiary blast injury is produced when a victim is propelled through the air and strikes another object. There are also injuries called miscellaneous blast injuries that include burns and respiratory injuries from hot gases or chemicals.

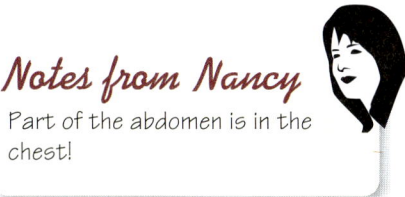

Notes from Nancy

Part of the abdomen is in the chest!

Pathophysiology

Hemorrhage is a major concern in abdominal trauma. It can occur when there is external or internal blood loss. When we deal with abdominal trauma, especially blunt abdominal trauma, the estimation of the volume of blood lost is difficult. Signs and symptoms will vary greatly depending on the volume of blood lost and the rate at which the body is losing blood. Key indicators of hemorrhagic shock will become apparent with the assessment of the neurologic and cardiovascular systems.

You are the Paramedic Part 2

The child's parents are alerted, and he is escorted to his school bus. Police officers quickly arrive and stand ready to assist you if necessary. The patient tells you he's unsure exactly how he ended up in the alleyway, but remembers having an argument with a friend. In fact, he cannot tell you where he is other than the name of the town. He does not know the current day, month, or year. In your past experience with him, this is very unusual.

Before moving your patient, you perform an initial assessment and a rapid trauma examination from head-to-toe and find that he is guarding his abdomen. You see bruising from his right upper quadrant, extending from his anterior axillary line across his left upper quadrant, midclavicular line. He also has noticeable swelling and deformity of his left ankle.

Reassessment	Recording Time: 5 Minutes
Level of consciousness	Verbal, oriented only to person and place
Skin	Cool, pale, and slightly moist
Pulse	130 beats/min; weak and regular
Blood pressure	102/60 mm Hg
Respirations	40 breaths/min
Spo2	96% while receiving 15 l/min oxygen via nonrebreathing mask

4. What do these signs indicate to you?
5. What does abdominal guarding usually indicate?
6. Is this condition an early or late finding?

As hypovolemia increases, the patient will become tachycardic and the respiratory rate will increase. The pulse pressure (difference between systolic and diastolic pressures) will decrease, followed by frank hypotension if the blood loss continues. Patients may become anxious or agitated. Finally, patients with severe hemorrhage will have marked tachycardia and hypotension; cool, clammy skin; and altered mental status.

Injuries to hollow or solid organs can result in the spillage of their contents into the abdominal cavity. When the enzymes, acids, or bacteria leak from hollow organs into the peritoneal or retroperitoneal space, they cause irritation of the nerve endings. As the inflammation affects these nerve endings, localized pain will result. Pain is localized if the extent of the contamination is confined; pain becomes generalized if the entire peritoneal cavity is involved.

Injuries to Solid Abdominal Organs

The solid organs in the abdomen include the liver, spleen, kidneys, and pancreas. When a solid organ in the abdomen is injured during blunt or penetrating trauma, the organ bleeds into the peritoneal cavity. This can cause nonspecific signs such as tachycardia and hypotension. Because these signs may not develop until a patient has lost a significant volume of blood, normal vital signs do not rule out the possibility that there has been a significant intra-abdominal injury. Bleeding into the peritoneal cavity from solid organ injuries can also produce abdominal tenderness or distension even though the distension may not be evident until the patient has lost nearly all the blood into the abdomen. Palpation of the abdomen may reveal localized or generalized tenderness, rigidity, or rebound tenderness, all of which suggest a peritoneal injury. (Kidney injuries are discussed in Chapter 32.)

Liver Injuries

The superior border of the liver can be as high as the patient's nipples, so a liver injury must be suspected in all patients who have right-sided chest trauma as well as abdominal trauma. When injured, the liver releases blood and bile into the peritoneal cavity. The blood loss can be massive, resulting in hypotension, tachycardia, shock, and even death. In addition, the release of bile into the peritoneum can produce abdominal pain and peritonitis.

Spleen Injuries

Falls and motor vehicle collisions can injure the spleen. However, less obvious injury patterns in activities such as sports (for instance, tackling in football or checking in lacrosse) can also cause injury to the spleen. There are case reports of patients who have a ruptured spleen even though the contact was relatively minor. This is especially true if the spleen is enlarged from mononucleosis or other underlying disease. When the spleen ruptures, blood spills into the peritoneum, which can ultimately cause shock and death. As with other intra-abdominal organ injuries, the signs and symptoms of splenic rupture are nonspecific, and as many as 40% of patients have no symptoms. Some patients report only pain in

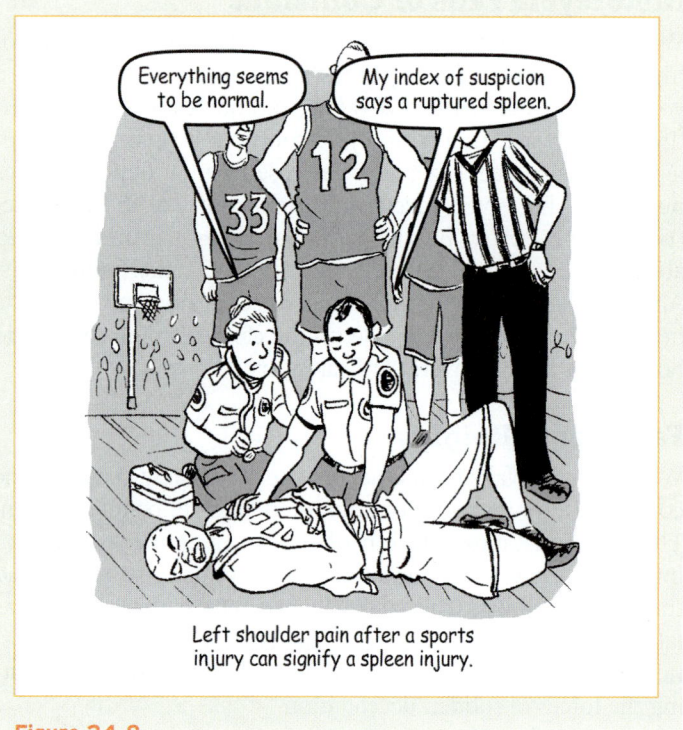

Left shoulder pain after a sports injury can signify a spleen injury.

Figure 24-8

the left shoulder (Kehr's sign) because of referred pain from diaphragmatic irritation **Figure 24-8 ▲**.

Pancreas Injuries

Pancreatic injury occurs in less than 5% of all major abdominal trauma. Because of the anatomical position of the pancreas in the retroperitoneum, it is relatively well protected. It typically takes a high-energy force to damage the pancreas. These high-energy forces are most commonly produced by penetrating trauma (for example, from a bullet) but can also be caused by blunt trauma (such as from a motor vehicle collision). In blunt trauma, an unrestrained driver who hits the steering column or a bicyclist who hits the handlebars is at risk of pancreatic injury.

At the Scene

In the past, the complete removal of the spleen (splenectomy) was routine for any splenic injury. The surgical approach has changed radically in recent years. The spleen provides an important immune function; without it, people are susceptible to life-threatening infections from organisms that would otherwise not be a problem. Surgeons will often opt for conservative management, but have also devised numerous methods of salvaging the spleen, ranging from simply suturing lacerations to grinding up residual splenic tissue and re-implanting it into the omentum (splenosis). Both splenic preservation techniques limit the risk of sepsis (overwhelming infection).

Injuries to the pancreas have subtle or absent signs and symptoms initially but should be suspected in any rapid decelerating injury. Over the course of hours to days, pancreatic injuries result in the spillage of enzymes into the retroperitoneal space, which can damage surrounding structures and lead to infection and retroperitoneal abscess. Injury should be suspected after a localized blow to the midabdomen. These patients usually experience a vague upper and midabdominal pain that radiates to the back. Peritoneal signs may develop several hours after the injury. Patients have been known to develop a form of diabetes after a severe injury to the pancreas.

Diaphragm Injuries

The diaphragm plays the primary role in a patient's ventilatory process. Injury to the diaphragm may cause signs and symptoms of ventilatory compromise. Diaphragmatic injuries or ruptures are not isolated incidents; patients often have associated thoracic, abdominal, head, and extremity injuries.

Injuries to the diaphragm are rare, and result from both blunt trauma (typically high-speed motor vehicle collisions) and from penetrating trauma. A lateral impact during a motor vehicle collision is most likely to cause a diaphragmatic rupture because of the twisting or distortion of the chest wall that may shear or tear the diaphragm. In frontal motor vehicle collisions, the patient may strike the steering wheel or column. This may cause a significant change in abdominal pressure, which may also tear the diaphragm.

Injuries to Hollow Intraperitoneal Organs

The hollow organs of the abdomen include the stomach, small and large intestines, and bladder. Hollow visceral injuries produce most of their symptoms from peritoneal contamination. When a hollow organ such as the stomach or bowel is injured, it releases its contents into the abdomen, which irritate the peritoneum, producing symptoms. When the patient has the seatbelt sign—a contusion or abrasion across the lower abdomen—this usually means that he or she also has intraperitoneal injuries.

Injuries to the Small and Large Intestines

The intestines are commonly injured from penetrating trauma, although they can be injured from severe blunt trauma as well. When ruptured, the intestines spill their contents (which contain fecal matter and a large amount of bacteria) into the peritoneal or retroperitoneal cavities, resulting in peritonitis.

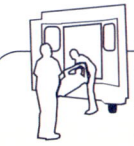

At the Scene

The best way to prevent hollow organs (such as the intestines or bladder) from bursting during a motor vehicle collision is to empty them before you get in the car!

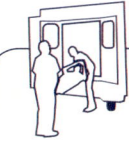

At the Scene

During a collision, improperly placed lap belts cause compression, potentially resulting in the rupture of the small intestine, large intestine, or bladder.

Stomach Injuries

Most injuries to the stomach result from penetrating trauma; the stomach is rarely injured from blunt trauma. When rupture of the stomach does occur after blunt trauma, it is usually associated with a recent meal or inappropriate use of a seatbelt. Trauma to the stomach frequently results in the spillage of acidic material into the peritoneal space, creating a chemical irritation that produces abdominal pain and peritoneal signs relatively quickly.

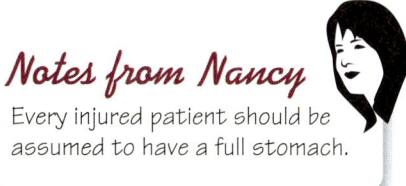

Notes from Nancy

Every injured patient should be assumed to have a full stomach.

Bladder Injuries

Bladder injuries occur as a result of penetrating and blunt abdominal trauma. The likelihood of a bladder injury varies by the severity of the mechanism, but also by the degree of the bladder distension. The fuller the bladder, the greater the opportunity for injury. Bladder injuries are usually associated with pelvic injuries from motor vehicle collisions, falls from heights, and physical assaults to the lower abdomen. These MOI may perforate the bladder.

The signs and symptoms of bladder injuries are generally nonspecific but may present as gross hematuria, suprapubic pain and tenderness, difficulty voiding, and abdominal distension, guarding, or rebound tenderness. The presence of signs of peritoneal irritation may also indicate the possibility of an intraperitoneal bladder rupture.

Retroperitoneal Injuries

Structures contained within the retroperitoneal cavity are the pancreas, kidneys, vascular structures, and duodenum. Injuries confined to the retroperitoneum can be very difficult to diagnose because, in general, they produce few visible signs or symptoms. Because the blood or other contaminants are held in the retroperitoneal space, they do not frequently cause abdominal pain, peritoneal signs, or abdominal distension. Occasionally, retroperitoneal bleeding can lead to ecchymosis of the flanks (Grey Turner's sign) or around the umbilicus (Cullen's sign). This ecchymosis is usually delayed hours to days, however, and is unreliable in the prehospital setting.

Vascular Injuries

Besides the kidneys, the vascular structures found in the retroperitoneal space include the descending aorta (and its branches), the superior phrenic artery, the inferior phrenic artery, the inferior vena cava, and the mesenteric vessels.

Injuries to these structures occur with both blunt and penetrating trauma, but penetrating trauma is the major cause. Penetrating trauma that causes injury to the great vessels of the abdomen will also be associated with injuries to multiple intra-abdominal organs. Blunt trauma can cause injuries to vascular structures as they are sheared from their points of attachment.

Notes from Nancy

Blunt abdominal injury may be much more serious than it looks. Don't dawdle at the scene!

The patient could have an abdominal aortic aneurysm that has become worse as a result of abdominal trauma. The specifics on abdominal aortic aneurysm are discussed in Chapter 27.

Assessment findings in a patient with vascular injuries depend on whether the bleeding is contained (a hematoma) or there is active hemorrhage. In active hemorrhage, the patient will present with significant hypotension, tachycardia, and shock.

Duodenal Injuries

In abdominal trauma, the duodenum can rupture, spilling its contents into the retroperitoneum, usually because of high-speed deceleration injuries **Figure 24-9 ▶**. Contamination of the retroperitoneum with duodenal contents may ultimately produce abdominal pain or fever, although symptoms will not likely develop for hours to days. Abdominal pain, nausea, and vomiting may develop, although belatedly. Because of the delayed presentation and variable symptoms, a high degree of suspicion for duodenal injury must be maintained in any abdominal trauma, but especially in high-speed deceleration collisions.

Assessment

During the evaluation of the abdominal cavity, you must look for evidence of hemorrhage (shock) or spillage of bowel contents (pain or tenderness) into the abdominal space. Have a high index of suspicion and understand that intra-abdominal injuries are likely with trauma to the chest or abdomen. Priorities in resuscitation begin with providing adequate tissue perfusion and oxygen delivery. In 10% of mortalities after trauma, the abdominal injury proves to be the primary cause of death; however, in a substantial number of cases, the exact cause of death is not clear.

The evaluation of a patient who has abdominal trauma must be systematic, keeping the entire patient in mind and prioritizing injuries accordingly. Approximately 20% of all patients with significant hemoperitoneum—collection of blood in the abdominal cavity—have a benign abdominal examination upon initial assessment. The abdomen should be examined closely for bruising, localized swelling, lacerations, distension, or pain. Clues to intra-abdominal trauma will include symptoms of shock not proportional to obvious external evidence or estimated blood loss. Retroperitoneal hemorrhage may be present because of lacerated or avulsed kidneys and injuries to the blood vessels. All abdominal organs have a generous blood supply, making them susceptible to significant

You are the Paramedic Part 3

Given the unclear events surrounding this situation, you take spinal precautions with the patient, apply high-flow supplemental oxygen, and establish a large-bore IV en route to the emergency department.

You are very concerned about internal bleeding and organ damage associated with this apparent blunt trauma and initiate immediate transport to the local trauma centre. En route to the hospital, you start a second large-bore IV and splint his left ankle. You administer normal saline wide open with frequent reassessment. You place him on a cardiac monitor. His chief complaint remains pain in his left leg.

Reassessment	Recording Time: 10 Minutes
Level of consciousness	Verbal, still oriented only to person and place
Skin	Cool, pale, and slightly moist
Pulse	130 beats/min, weak and regular
Blood pressure	102/60 mm Hg
Respirations	42 breaths/min
Spo$_2$	96% while receiving 15 l/min via nonrebreathing mask
ECG	Sinus tachycardia

7. Why is it important to provide rapid transport and interventions such as IVs en route to the hospital?

8. Are patients' chief complaints and primary problems always identical?

9. Which organs are at risk of injury given the apparent location of this patient's injury?

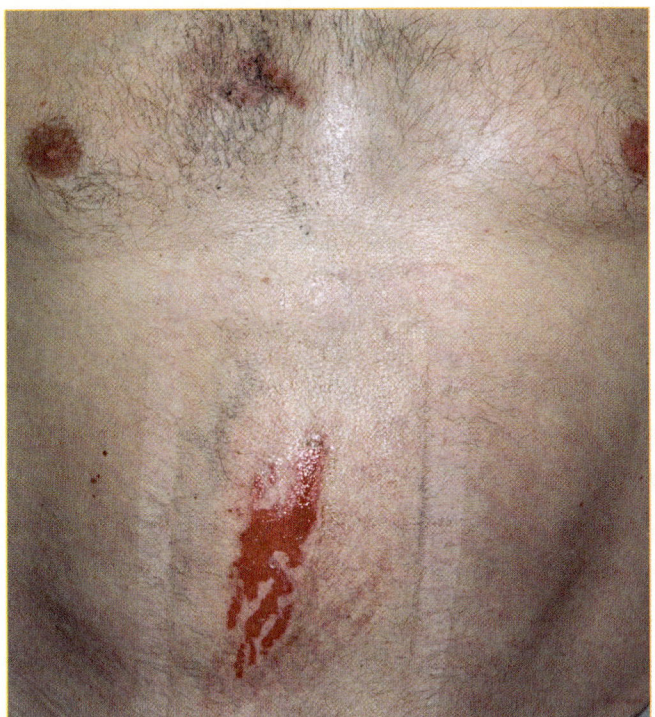

Figure 24-9 Remember that abdominal injury can be severe even in the absence of symptoms. Contamination of the intra-abdominal space may not produce pain or fever for hours or even days.

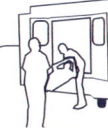

At the Scene

All trauma patients should be assumed to have a full stomach, even if they deny recent ingestion of food or liquids.

DCAP-BTLS). Often the injury to the abdomen involves ecchymosis, abrasions, or lacerations.

Blood, gastrointestinal contents, and urine that have spilled into the peritoneum may produce peritonitis that could result in decreased or absent abdominal sounds, but auscultation of bowel sounds is not a useful assessment tool in the prehospital setting. The next steps in the abdominal examination are percussion and palpation. With these maneuvers, look for tenderness and signs of peritonitis (such as the patient guarding his or her abdomen or experiencing pain while being gently moved to the stretcher). Carefully palpate all four quadrants of the abdomen while assessing the patient's response and noting abdominal masses and deformities.

Controversies

Listening to bowel sounds in the prehospital setting may not be helpful. To properly auscultate bowel sounds, it is necessary to listen for several minutes. This is not practical in the prehospital environment, and the ambient noise may be too great to determine the presence or absence of bowel sounds.

A common misconception is that patients without abdominal pain or abnormal vital signs are unlikely to have serious intra-abdominal injuries. Keep in mind that peritonitis can take hours to days to develop. Similarly, nonspecific symptoms such as hypotension, tachycardia, and confusion may not develop until the patient has lost more than 40% of his or her circulating blood volume. Always maintain a high index of suspicion in any patient who has a mechanism of injury consistent with abdominal trauma, regardless of the examination findings. Abdominal distension is a late indication of abdominal trauma. Patients must have a significant volume of blood enter the abdominal cavity to fill it and produce distension.

Try to obtain as many details about an injury as possible, keeping in mind that trauma patients should be transported to the

bleeding as a result of blunt forces causing a shearing-type injury. An injury to the abdomen can be fatal primarily because of hemorrhage. The injury can be slow to develop, and may be subtle and difficult to locate and assess.

Scene Assessment

As with all other aspects of prehospital care, scene safety remains the priority before providing any patient care. It is always important to remember that if a patient has penetrating or blunt trauma, some external force caused this injury. These cases could also potentially be dangerous to the paramedic.

Initial Assessment

Once you have sized up the scene and determined that it is safe, the first patient priorities are those of the initial assessment: mental status, airway with c-spine precautions, breathing, circulation, and prioritizing the patient. Once the initial assessment is complete and overtly life-threatening conditions have been addressed, a focused history and physical examination may uncover more subtle signs and symptoms of abdominal injury.

Focused History and Physical Examination

The first step in the focused history and physical examination is inspection of the abdomen. This means you will need to expose the abdomen and inspect for signs of trauma (such as

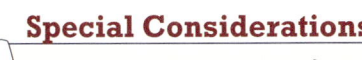

Special Considerations

Patients at the extremes of age have more flaccid abdominal walls (containing less muscle and more fat) and may be at increased risk for intra-abdominal injury. In obese patients or those with increased abdominal wall size, it may be necessary to apply greater pressure during examination to assess for injury. In these patients, a higher-than-usual index of suspicion for internal organ injury is warranted if they complain of abdominal pain.

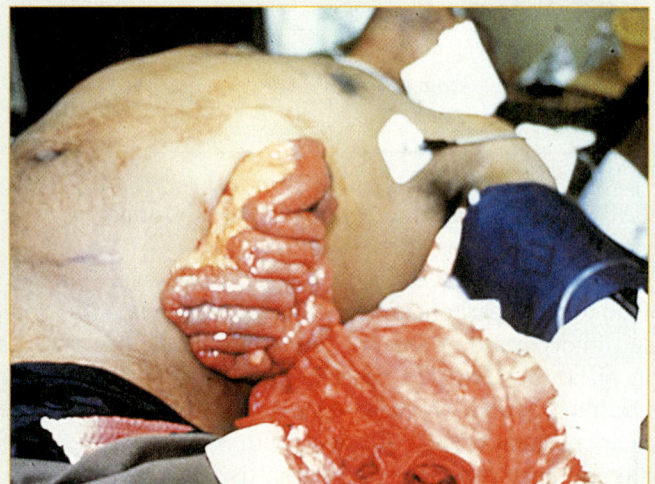

Figure 24-10 An abdominal evisceration is an open abdominal wound from which internal organs or fat protrude.

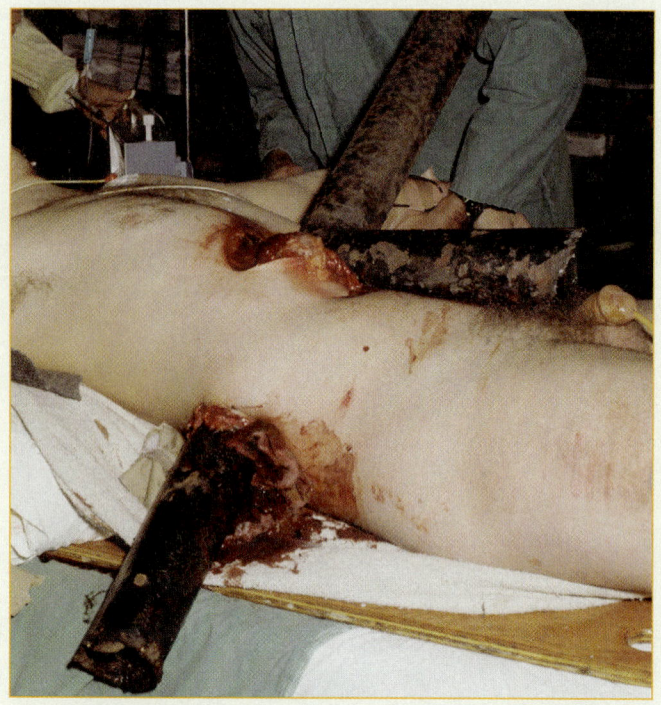

Figure 24-11 An object impaled in the abdomen.

hospital quickly. In other words, in addition to getting information about the patient (such as the SAMPLE history), it is important to obtain details on how the injury occurred, whether from the patient, witnesses, police, or other paramedics.

In blunt trauma caused by a motor vehicle collision, determine the types of vehicles involved, the speed at which they were travelling, and how the cars collided. You should also try to find out other information about the event, such as the use of seatbelts, the deployment of air bags, and the patient's position in the vehicle.

In penetrating trauma, it's helpful to identify the type of weapon used. However, this is often impossible because assailants usually leave with their weapon. In a gunshot case, determine the type of gun and the number of shots, if possible. Paramedics should try to ascertain an estimated distance between the victim and the assailant whenever possible. In stab wounds, determine the type of knife, possible angle of the entrance wound, and number of stab wounds.

As part of the focused history and physical examination of a trauma patient, you may be faced with a number of challenges associated with abdominal trauma. You may discover the presence of an abdominal <u>evisceration</u>—displacement of an organ outside the body 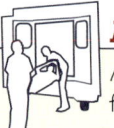 **Figure 24-10 ▲** . This is where the abdominal organs are found protruding through a wound in the abdominal wall. Generally, little pain is associated with this type of injury; do not apply any material that will adhere to the abdominal structures. Paramedics may also be confronted with impaled objects 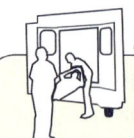 **Figure 24-11 ▶** . Impaled objects are stabilized and transported in the position they were found. Stabilization of impaled objects can be impractical under some prehospital conditions, but effective stabilization and safe transportation can help reduce serious tissue damage.

If you suspect injury to the diaphragm, focus on the airway, breathing, and circulatory status of the patient. Remember

At the Scene

Always examine the back of the patient as carefully as you examine the front. Gunshot wounds or stab wounds can easily be missed in creases of the body, especially if the patient is obese or has large quantities of body hair.

that the diaphragm plays a large role in the mechanical process of breathing. Examine the patient's neck and chest, paying particular attention to the trachea (tracheal deviation due to mediastinal shift), symmetry of the chest during expansion, and absence of breath sounds.

Detailed Physical Examination

Perform a detailed physical examination on a patient who has abdominal trauma and was found to have a significant MOI.

At the Scene

Cullen's sign is a black-and-blue discolouration (ecchymosis) in the umbilical region caused by peritoneal bleeding. Grey Turner's sign includes ecchymosis present in the lower abdominal and flank regions. They are both caused by intra-abdominal bleeding and are found 12 to 24 hours after the initial injury. The presence of these signs is helpful, but their absence does not rule out life-threatening abdominal hemorrhage.

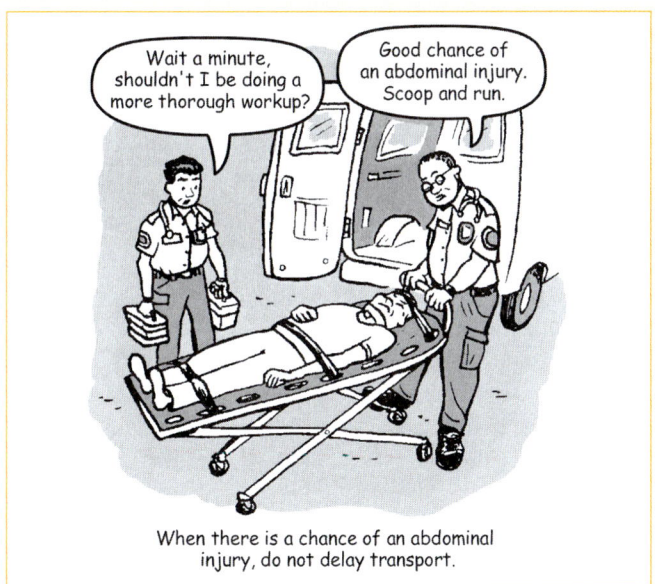

When there is a chance of an abdominal injury, do not delay transport.

Figure 24-12

Because, at this point, you will have completed the initial assessment as well as the rapid trauma examination, the detailed physical examination should be conducted en route to the emergency department to avoid any unnecessary delays **Figure 24-12 ▲** . Basically, the detailed physical examination assesses the same structures as the rapid trauma examination, except more methodically. Close examination may uncover additional findings that were either not picked up during the rapid trauma examination or are only now starting to develop (such as hematoma, bruises, or tender areas). As long as you can ensure that the problems

Notes from Nancy

An injury to the chest anywhere below the nipples is also an injury to the abdomen.

Documentation and Communication

Pertinent documentation of the abdominal trauma assessment should include the following: whether or not seatbelts were worn, which type, and their position on the patient; the location, intensity, and quality of pain; whether or not nausea or vomiting is present; the contour of the abdomen; any ecchymosis or open areas present on the soft-tissue inspection; the presence or absence of rebound tenderness, guarding, rigidity, or localized pain; any changes in the level of consciousness and serial vital signs; other injuries found; the presence or absence of alcohol, narcotics, or any type of analgesic; and the results of your ongoing assessment.

found in the initial assessment have been attended to, and there is time en route, perform a very thorough detailed physical examination on your patient.

Ongoing Assessment

The ongoing assessment includes reassessment of the initial assessment as well as retaking vital signs and checking interventions on the patient.

Management Overview

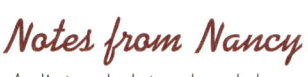

In general, the prehospital management of patients who have abdominal trauma is straightforward. As always, ensuring an open airway while taking spinal precautions is the first step. Administer high-concentration oxygen to the patient via a nonrebreathing mask. Establish IV access with two large-bore lines, and start replacing fluid with lactated Ringer's solution or normal saline. Do not delay transport to initiate IV therapy; establish IV lines whenever possible during transport. Minimize external hemorrhage by applying pressure dressings. Apply a cardiac monitor. Transport the patient to the appropriate hospital or regional trauma centre, depending on your local transport protocols. Note that the assessment should also not delay patient prehospital care and transport. Repeated abdominal examinations are the key to discovering a patient's worsening condition before vital signs change. Perform your examinations en route during the ongoing assessment.

In some cases of penetrating injury, part of an abdominal organ may protrude outside of the body (evisceration). If this occurs, do not attempt to place the organ back into the body. Rather, cover it with a sterile dressing moistened with saline, and protect the organ from damage during transport. Administer pain medication, remembering it may be contraindicated because of the patient's hypotension. Follow your local protocols or consult with direct medical control en route to the hospital to discuss analgesia.

Notes from Nancy

A distended, tender abdomen after injury means internal bleeding. Treat for shock and transport immediately.

Pelvic Fractures

The pelvis is best thought of as a ring, with its sacral, iliac, ischial, and pubic bones held together by ligaments. Large forces are required to damage this ring. The majority of pelvic

At the Scene

There is an old medical school scenario of a patient who was shot in the head who is hypotensive. The puzzle is, "What's wrong with the patient?" The answer, as we have learned in this chapter, is that the patient was probably shot in the belly with a second bullet! Always remember that hemorrhaging will continue until controlled in the operating room under "bright lights and cold steel." Survival may be determined by the length of time from the injury to definitive surgical control of the hemorrhage. Delays in the prehospital environment may negatively impact the patient's long-term survival. So, if you are not the solution to this patient's problem, don't add to the problem. Get the patient to the trauma centre!

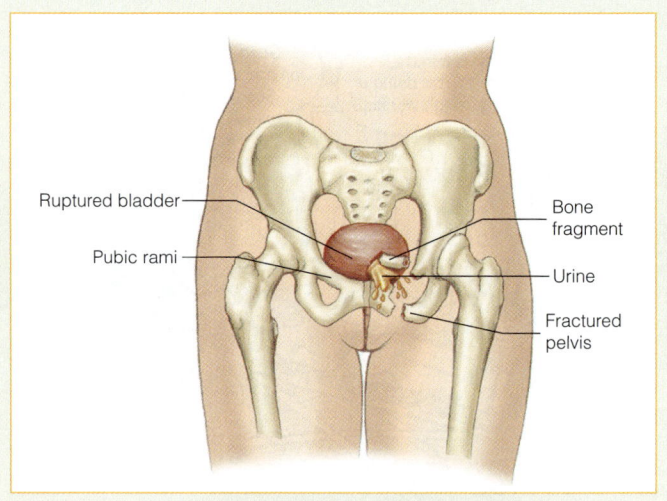

Figure 24-13 Pelvic fractures occasionally cause laceration of the bladder as a result of penetration by bony fragments. Externally, pelvic fractures can cause severe bruising and swelling.

fractures are a result of blunt trauma from motor vehicle collision or from vehicles striking pedestrians.

Because of the forces required to break the pelvis, suspect multisystem trauma if your patient has a pelvic injury (until proven otherwise). Commonly associated injuries are urethral disruptions, bladder rupture, and abdominal, thoracic, and head trauma **Figure 24-13 ▶**. Signs and symptoms of blunt trauma to the pelvis include pain in the pelvis, groin, or hips; hematomas or contusions to the pelvic region; obvious external bleeding; or hypotension without obvious external bleeding.

Special Considerations

Pediatric trauma patients are less likely to have pelvic fractures than adults.

Anteroposterior compression, which can result from a head-on collision, may lead to an "open-book" pelvic fracture in which the pubic symphysis spreads apart. The subsequent increase in volume of the pelvis means a patient with internal pelvic bleeding may lose a much larger amount of blood than someone without an open-book fracture. Such patients will require IV fluids with lactated Ringer's solution or normal saline but may still remain hypotensive in the prehospital environment.

Lateral compression of the pelvis results from a side impact. It generally does not result in an unstable pelvis. Because the volume in the pelvis is reduced, not increased, life-threatening hemorrhage is less of a concern in such cases.

Vertical shear is seen in falls from heights. It results in one side of the pelvis moving superiorly or inferiorly compared to the other, disrupting the bony or ligamentous structures. This unstable fracture results in an increased pelvic volume.

Saddle injuries result from falling on an object. They may result in fractures of the bones that are directly under the female and male genitalia (pubic rami fractures).

Although penetrating trauma to the pelvis may result in bony fractures, the more worrisome injury is to the major vascular structures, which can cause life-threatening hemorrhage. Open fractures (not to be confused with open-book fractures) may result from either penetrating or blunt trauma and frequently result in chronic pain and disability that persist for years after the initial injury.

Assessment and Management

Properly evaluating and treating the patient is more important than identifying the specific type of pelvic fracture. A search for entry and exit wounds for a penetrating trauma is helpful but

You are the Paramedic **Part 4**

Upon your arrival at the hospital, the patient's condition is immediately evaluated and he is taken to surgery. You later learn that he had significant blood loss from liver lacerations and a ruptured spleen. He also had multiple fractures of his left distal tibia and fibula as a result of several blows from a baseball bat.

10. How can age and medical problems make traumatic injuries worse?

Controversies

Anecdotal cases of the successful use of the pneumatic antishock garment (PASG) in the treatment of ruptured aortic aneurysms and ectopic pregnancy abound, especially in areas with prolonged transport times. Always follow your local protocols.

an extended search should never delay quick transport and treatment of hypotension. In both blunt and penetrating trauma, the presence of thoracic trauma may result in a life-threatening tension pneumothorax. In addition, if you suspect an open-book pelvic fracture in a patient with hypotension, tie a sheet around the patient's hips at the level of the superior anterior iliac crests, thereby decreasing the pelvic volume. There are several devices specific to the management of this type of injury that provide superior immobilization and are faster to apply.

The pneumatic antishock garment (PASG) is a controversial treatment that can be used to stabilize the pelvis during rapid transports. It can potentially decrease pain by causing less movement of the fractured bones and decrease bleeding by reducing pelvic volume, although some emergency medicine specialists believe that the PASG may increase bleeding by putting pressure on pelvic vessels. Follow your local protocols for use of PASG. For a review of this skill, see Chapter 18.

You are the Paramedic Summary

1. What are your immediate concerns?

Your first priority is always scene safety. Given your previous exposure to the patient and your knowledge of his history of drugs, alcohol, and assaultive behaviour, you should discretely request police response as well as ask one of your department members to locate the child's parents. If the child's parents are not available, he should be moved to a safe location (possibly to school) until his parents or his legal guardian can be contacted.

2. What about this patient immediately grabs your attention?

The patient's location, his level of consciousness, and his body position are immediate causes for concern. Given the time of day, question how long he has been lying in this location. You should also wonder about the possibilities of alcohol and/or drug use and their effects in limiting your patient's ability to accurately perceive pain and injury.

3. At this point, what are your treatment priorities?

Assessing and managing life-threatening conditions is always your top priority. A patient who exhibits a decreased level of consciousness, tachycardia, and tachypnea should be treated swiftly and appropriately.

4. What do these signs indicate to you?

Given the patient's decreased level of consciousness, skin signs, tachycardia, and hypotension in the presence of abdominal guarding, he has likely lost a significant amount of blood.

5. What does abdominal guarding usually indicate?

Abdominal guarding usually indicates peritonitis, an inflammation of the lining of the abdomen that results from either blood or hollow organ contents spilling into the abdominal cavity.

6. Is this condition an early or late finding?

Peritonitis is a late finding. It can take hours or even days to develop. Blood loss significant enough to produce signs and symptoms of shock may not develop until 40% or more of the patient's blood volume is lost. For this reason, you should be highly suspicious of injuries resulting from significant blunt or penetrating trauma. Patients with these injuries can appear to have normal vital signs in the presence of significant injuries in the early stages.

7. Why is it important to provide rapid transport and interventions such as IVs en route to the hospital?

Definitive care for the trauma patient is available at the nearest appropriate trauma centre. To delay transport so as to initiate IVs, splint fractures, and the like would delay the prehospital care the patient ultimately needs. Be aware of scene times, striving to keep these to 10 minutes or less. Obviously, if extra time has to be spent on the scene for issues such as extrication, provide interventions as required and document the reasons for the delayed transport.

8. Are patients' chief complaints and primary problems always identical?

Your patients may or may not complain of pain or discomfort associated with the source of their primary problem. In this scenario, the patient is more concerned about his leg and ankle pain; you should be more concerned about the internal bleeding in his abdomen. This is an important lesson for any paramedic—don't allow yourself to become consumed with the outward, most obvious injuries, as they may or may not be life threatening.

9. Which organs are at risk of injury given the apparent location of this patient's injury?

You should be worried that the liver and spleen could have significant damage given the patient's skin condition and vital signs. Injury to one or both of these organs can produce significant bleeding. The liver can suffer lacerations as well as contusions in blunt trauma, and the spleen is at great risk of rupture.

10. How can age and medical problems make traumatic injuries worse?

Geriatric and pediatric patients do not have the same compensatory mechanisms that healthy young and middle-aged adults possess. Extremes of age (and disease processes such as diabetes, heart conditions, and high blood pressure, along with their accompanying medicines) can mask signs and symptoms in otherwise healthy patients. Also, mechanisms of injury and their associated damage can change with age. Children who are struck by cars have different injury patterns than those of adults. Older patients on beta-blockers are not able to compensate for blood loss with increased heart rates in the same way that younger patients can. For this reason, whenever possible, you should obtain a trauma patient's medical history, including medications and allergies.

Prep Kit

Ready for Review

- Unrecognized abdominal trauma is the leading cause of unexpected death in trauma patients. Recognizing abdominal injuries and providing rapid transport is one of the best contributions you can make to a patient who has these injuries.
- The abdomen contains many vital organs and structures, including the kidneys, liver, spleen, pancreas, diaphragm, small and large intestines, stomach, bladder, and several great vessels.
- The quadrant system is generally used to describe a location in the abdomen. These are the right upper quadrant (RUQ), the right lower quadrant (RLQ), the left lower quadrant (LLQ), and the left upper quadrant (LUQ).
- The peritoneum is a membrane that lines the abdominal cavity. Abdominal trauma can lead to peritonitis, an inflammation of the peritoneum that results from either blood or hollow organ contents spilling into the abdominal cavity. This may lead to a life-threatening infection.
- The retroperitoneal space is the area behind the peritoneum and contains the aorta, vena cava, pancreas, kidneys, ureters, and portions of the duodenum and large intestine.
- When a patient has experienced trauma to the chest or abdomen, suspect that he or she also has additional internal abdominal injuries. Also suspect abdominal trauma in patients who have unexplained symptoms of shock.
- Injury to the abdomen can be slow to develop, and can be fatal. An injury may be subtle and difficult to locate and assess.
- Solid organs such as the liver and spleen have a large blood supply and can easily be crushed by blunt trauma. The abdomen and retroperitoneum can accommodate large amounts of blood but produce few signs and symptoms.
- Injury to hollow organs can cause the release of toxins such as urine, bile, or stomach acid into the abdominal cavity, causing peritonitis.
- The majority of all abdominal injuries involve blunt trauma, occurring mostly during motor vehicle collisions. Blunt trauma can often lead to a closed abdominal injury.
- Penetrating trauma most commonly results from stab wounds or low-velocity gunshot wounds. Penetrating trauma causes open abdominal injury.
- During the assessment, try to obtain as many details about an injury as possible. Also note the use of seatbelts, deployment of air bags, and the patient's position in the vehicle. If a weapon was involved, note the type of weapon if this information is available.
- Peritonitis can take hours to days to develop. Shock, tachycardia, and confusion may not develop until the patient has lost a significant amount of blood. Maintain a high index of suspicion for a patient who has a mechanism of injury consistent with abdominal trauma, regardless of vital signs and other findings.
- Generally, management of patients with abdominal trauma is straightforward:
  - Ensure a secure airway with c-spine precautions.
  - Establish intravenous access and fluid replacement without delaying transport.
  - Minimize hemorrhaging with pressure dressings.
  - Apply a cardiac monitor and oxygen therapy, and then transport.
- Assessment should never delay patient prehospital care and transport!
- Pelvic fractures can result in damage to the major vascular structures, which can cause life-threatening hemorrhage.
- Because of the forces required to break the pelvis, if the patient has a pelvic fracture, suspect multisystem trauma.

Vital Vocabulary

blunt trauma Injury resulting from compression or deceleration forces, potentially crushing an organ or causing it to rupture.

closed abdominal injury An injury in which there is soft-tissue damage inside the body, but the skin remains intact.

duodenum The first part of the small intestine.

evisceration Displacement of an organ outside the body.

hemoperitoneum The presence of extravasated blood in the peritoneal cavity.

Kehr's sign Left shoulder pain that may indicate a ruptured spleen.

mesentery A membranous double fold of tissue in the abdomen that attaches various organs to the body wall.

open abdominal injury An injury in which there is a break in the surface of the skin or mucous membrane, exposing deeper tissue to potential contamination.

penetrating trauma An injury in which the skin is broken; direct contact results in laceration of the structure.

peritoneum A membrane in the abdomen encasing the liver, spleen, diaphragm, stomach, and transverse colon.

peritonitis Inflammation of the peritoneum (the lining around the abdominal cavity) that results from either blood or hollow organ contents spilling into the abdominal cavity.

periumbilical Pertaining to the area around the umbilicus.

pylorus A circumferential muscle at the end of the stomach that acts as a valve between the stomach and duodenum.

retroperitoneal space The area in the abdomen containing the aorta, vena cava, pancreas, kidneys, ureters, and portions of the duodenum and large intestine.

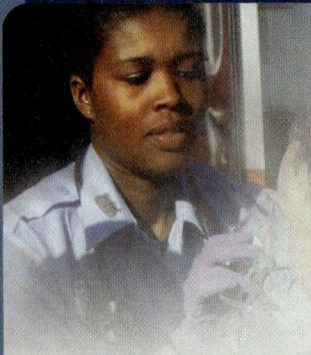

Assessment in Action

You are dispatched to a motor vehicle collision at an intersection. When you arrive, you find two vehicles, one which is broadsided on the driver's side. The driver is still in the vehicle and the fire department is in the process of extricating her. You notice that the damage to the driver's side door is significant with extensive damage to the B post. There is approximately 45-cm intrusion.

The driver is conscious, alert, and oriented. She is complaining only of pain in the left upper quadrant of her chest, just below her rib cage. Her vital signs are: respirations, 20 breaths/min; pulse, 130 beats/min; blood pressure, 100/60 mm Hg; and pulse oximetry, 98% on room air. The patient's c-spine is immobilized and she is removed from the vehicle. In the ambulance, you perform a complete assessment. Everything is unremarkable except she has pain on palpation to her left upper quadrant and pain in her left shoulder. Her abdomen is soft, and she is not guarding it. You initiate two large-bore IVs, apply oxygen, and transport the patient to the nearest trauma-designated hospital.

1. **What type of injury should you suspect?**
   A. Lacerated liver
   B. Ruptured spleen
   C. Contusion of the heart
   D. Ruptured appendix

2. **What type of impact did this patient receive?**
   A. Frontal impact
   B. Rear impact
   C. Lateral or side impact
   D. Rotational impact

3. **Which are solid organs of the abdomen?**
   A. Liver, spleen, kidneys, and pancreas
   B. Liver, spleen, and pancreas
   C. Large intestine, small intestine, and kidneys
   D. Liver, spleen, kidneys, and intestines

4. **On-scene care of a patient who has signs of shock from abdominal injury should include which of the following?**
   A. Comprehensive physical examination
   B. Initiation of IV fluid therapy
   C. Ongoing assessment
   D. Oxygen administration

5. **When the spleen ruptures, blood spills into the:**
   A. duodenum.
   B. peritoneum.
   C. stomach.
   D. pylorus.

6. **Some patients who have a splenic injury may report only left shoulder pain. This is called:**
   A. Cullen's sign.
   B. Grey Turner's sign.
   C. Peritoneal's sign.
   D. Kehr's sign.

7. **The abdominal cavity is lined with a membrane called the:**
   A. retroperitoneal space.
   B. pylorus.
   C. peritoneum.
   D. periumbilical.

8. **The spleen is a highly vascular organ that lies in the _____ quadrant.**
   A. right upper
   B. left lower
   C. left upper
   D. right lower

9. **Rupture of an organ can lead to hemorrhage and:**
   A. peritoneum.
   B. peritonitis.
   C. hemoperitoneum.
   D. internal bleeding.

10. **True or false? Patients without abdominal pain or abnormal vital signs are unlikely to have serious intra-abdominal injuries.**
    A. True
    B. False

Challenging Questions

You are dispatched to the local bar for an assault victim. On arrival you find a 38-year-old man on the ground, conscious, and alert and orientated to person, place, and time. He is in the right lateral recumbent position. You notice a large pool of blood under him. He has a weak radial pulse and his skin is cool, pale, and diaphoretic. His vital signs are: respirations, 40 breaths/min; pulse, 120 beats/min with sinus tachycardia on the monitor; systolic blood pressure, 80 mm Hg; and pulse oximetry, 92% on room air. He is complaining of pain to his stomach and is becoming very agitated. There is a 30-cm knife lying next to him. You check his back for wounds and then quickly log roll him onto a backboard and provide c-spine precautions. On examination of the abdomen, you see a stab wound to the upper right quadrant. You immediately move the patient to your ambulance.

11. **What type of injury should you suspect?**

12. **What are the major complications of a lacerated liver?**

13. **What is your further treatment for this patient?**

Points to Ponder

You are called to the scene of a minor vehicle collision in which a car has hit a telephone pole. When you arrive, you immediately notice that the driver is not inside the car. The air bag has deployed, but the windshield appears intact. The steering wheel appears slightly deformed. Bystanders say the car was not travelling very fast when it hit the pole. They do not think the driver was wearing a seatbelt.

You approach the driver to ask him about the collision. He is sitting on the grass, with no apparent external injuries. Even though it is early afternoon, you smell what you think is alcohol as you speak with him. He tells you he doesn't know how the collision happened, but he insists he is fine and doesn't want to be examined or questioned.

Though you can see no injuries, he is guarding his abdomen, and grimaces as though he's in pain as you're speaking. The more you try to encourage him to be examined by either you or a doctor, the more defensive and angry he gets. You tell him the risks of not being examined, and tell him he can sign a consent form to not be treated. He agrees to let you take his vital signs and then signs the consent form to refuse treatment. His blood pressure is 80/60 mm Hg; pulse, 130 beats/min; and respirations, 27 breaths/min.

When you find this, what do you do?

Issues: Thorough Scene Assessment, Thorough Assessment, Patient Refusal of Treatment.

Competency Areas

Area 4: Assessment and Diagnostics

4.3.j Conduct musculoskeletal system assessment and interpret findings.

Area 5: Therapeutics

5.5.b Control external hemorrhage through the use of direct pressure and patient positioning.

5.6.a Treat soft tissue injuries.

5.7.a Immobilize suspected fractures involving appendicular skeleton.

Area 6: Integration

6.1.f Provide care to patient experiencing illness or injury primarily involving integumentary system.

6.1.g Provide care to patient experiencing illness or injury primarily involving musculoskeletal system.

Appendix 4: Pathophysiology

H. **Musculoskeletal System**
Soft Tissue Disorders: Amputation
Soft Tissue Disorders: Compartment syndrome
Soft Tissue Disorders: Dislocations
Soft Tissue Disorders: Sprains
Soft Tissue Disorders: Strains
Soft Tissue Disorders: Subluxations
Skeletal Fractures: Open, closed

J. **Multisystem Diseases and Injuries**
Environmental Disorders: Systemic hypothermia

Introduction

Musculoskeletal injuries are one of the most common reasons that patients seek medical attention. Complaints related to the musculoskeletal system lead to almost 6 million visits to physicians annually in Canada, more than for any other reason. Approximately 1 in 7 Canadians will experience some type of musculoskeletal impairment, leading to millions of missed days of work or school and costing billions of dollars yearly. In Canada, unintentional falls account for the majority of these injuries, followed by motor vehicle collisions. An estimated 70% to 80% of all patients with multiple system trauma have one or more musculoskeletal injuries. Some areas of public policy, legislative changes, and public education have been effective in reducing the injury problem. For example, efforts related to cell phone use by drivers, child safety seat use and availability, and falls in older people have had positive impacts.

Injuries related to the musculoskeletal system are usually easily identifiable because of the associated pain, swelling, and deformity. Although these injuries are rarely fatal, they often result in short- or long-term disability. By providing prompt temporary measures, such as splinting and analgesia, paramedics may help reduce the period during which patients are disabled. However, despite the sometimes dramatic appearance of these injuries, you should not focus on the musculoskeletal injury without first determining that no life-threatening injury exists. *Never forget the ABCs!*

Anatomy and Physiology of the Musculoskeletal System

The musculoskeletal system gives the body its shape and allows for its movement. It is essential that you understand its basic anatomy and physiology.

Functions of the Musculoskeletal System

The musculoskeletal system performs many important functions within the body. Bones help *support* the soft tissues of the body and form a framework that gives the human body its shape and allows it to maintain an erect posture. *Movement* is generated because muscles are attached to bones by tendons. (Reminder: Muscles-To-Bones [MTB] means Muscles–Tendons–Bones.) When a muscle contracts, the force generated by the muscle is transferred to a bone on the opposite side of the joint from the muscle, leading to motion. Bones also offer *protection* to the more fragile organs and structures beneath them—for example, the skull's protection of the brain, the rib cage's protection of the heart and lungs, and the spinal column's protection of the spinal cord.

Another important function of the musculoskeletal system is hematopoiesis—the process of generating blood cells. In adults, it most commonly occurs in the red bone marrow of the sternum, ribs, vertebral bodies, pelvis, and the proximal portions of the femur and humerus. Each day, the body produces new red blood cells, white blood cells, and platelets from the stem cells that are present in the bone marrow, thereby replacing those that have been lost or that are no longer functional.

The Body's Scaffolding: The Skeleton

The integrated structure formed by the 206 bones of the body is called the skeleton. It may be divided into two distinct portions: the axial skeleton and the appendicular skeleton. The axial skeleton is composed of the bones of the central part, or axis, of the body; its divisions include the vertebral column, skull, ribs, and sternum. The skull is composed of the cranium, basilar skull, face, and inner ear Figure 25-1 ▶ .

The spine is composed of 33 spinal vertebrae: 7 cervical, 12 thoracic, 5 lumbar, 5 sacral, and 4 coccygeal. Moving anteriorly, the thorax is formed by the sternum and 12 pairs of

You are the Paramedic Part 1

You are dispatched to a private residence for a man who has fallen off a ladder. En route to the scene, dispatch advises you that a neighbour witnessed the incident and estimated the fall to be 5 to 7 m. The witness also reports the man appears to be awake and breathing and looks to be in great pain.

On arrival, you find a 63-year-old man on the ground next to a ladder that is leaning against the house. He complains of pain in his left leg and left wrist, is slow to respond to your questions, but remembers what happened.

Initial Assessment	Recording Time: 0 Minutes
Appearance	Wincing and holding his left arm
Level of consciousness	A (Alert to person, place, and day)
Airway	Patent
Breathing	Rapid with adequate tidal volume
Circulation	Blood-soaked left sleeve, rapid radial pulse

1. What are your initial assessment and treatment priorities?
2. What other information should be obtained about the patient and the incident?

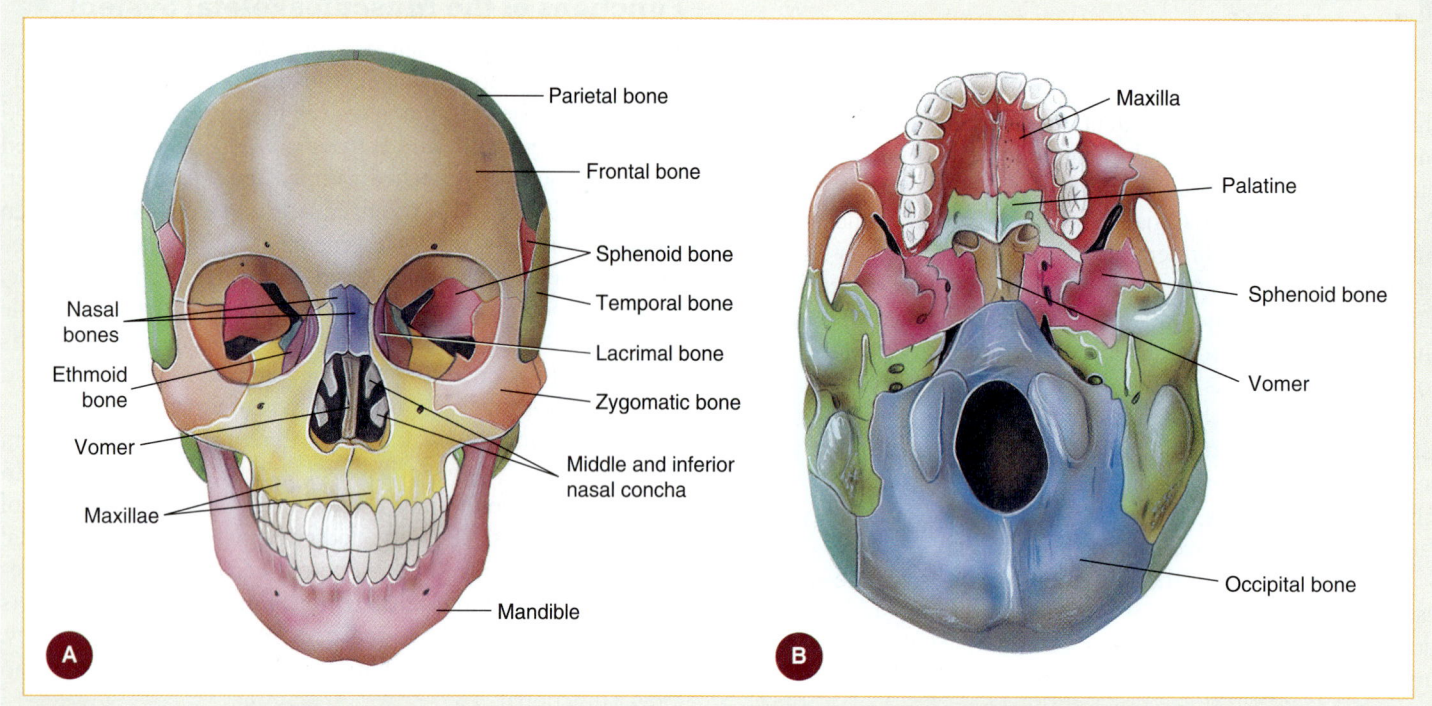

Figure 25-1 The skull and its components. **A.** Front view. **B.** Bottom view.

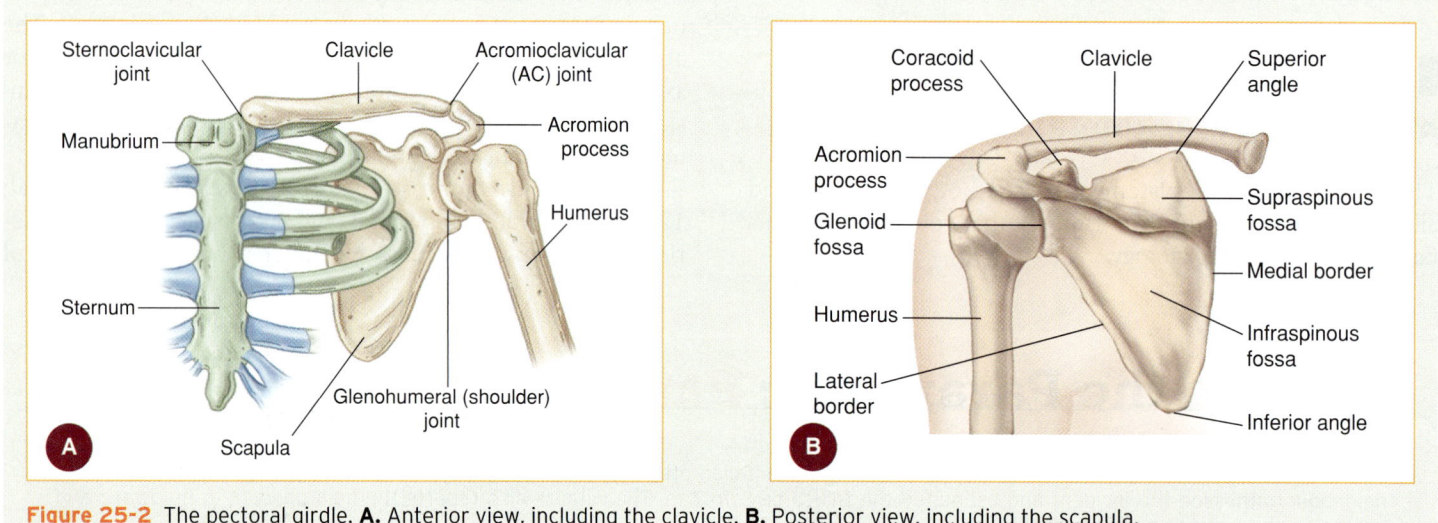

Figure 25-2 The pectoral girdle. **A.** Anterior view, including the clavicle. **B.** Posterior view, including the scapula.

ribs. The appendicular skeleton is divided into the pectoral girdle, the pelvic girdle, and the bones of the upper and lower extremities.

Shoulder and Upper Extremities

The pectoral girdle **Figure 25-2 ▲** , also referred to as the shoulder girdle, consists of two scapulae and two clavicles. The scapula (shoulder blade) is a flat, triangular bone held to the rib cage posteriorly by powerful muscles that buffer it against injury. The clavicle (collarbone) is a slender, S-shaped bone

attached by ligaments at the medial end to the sternum and at the lateral end to the raised tip of the scapula, called the acromion. The clavicle acts as a strut to keep the shoulder propped up; however, because it is slender and very exposed, this bone is vulnerable to injury.

The upper extremity **Figure 25-3 ▶** joins the shoulder girdle at the glenohumeral joint. The proximal portion contains the humerus, a bone that articulates proximally with the scapula and distally with bones of the forearm—the radius and ulna—to form the hinged elbow joint.

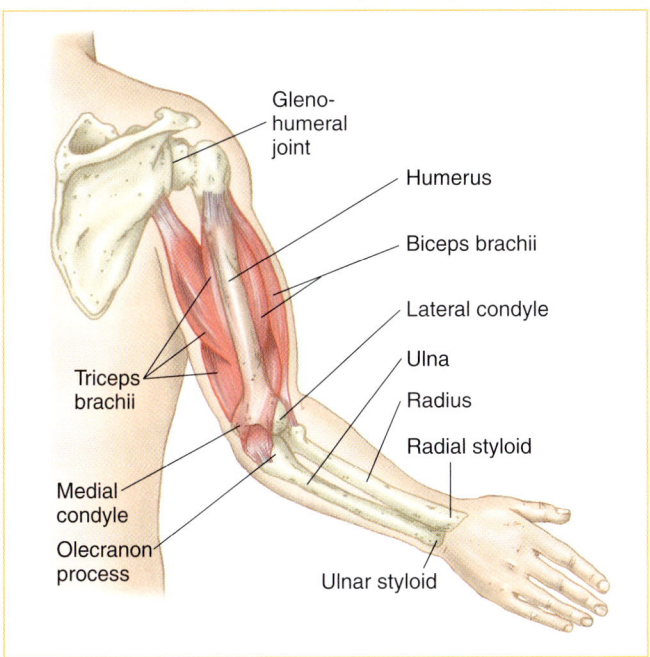

Figure 25-3 The anatomy of the arm.

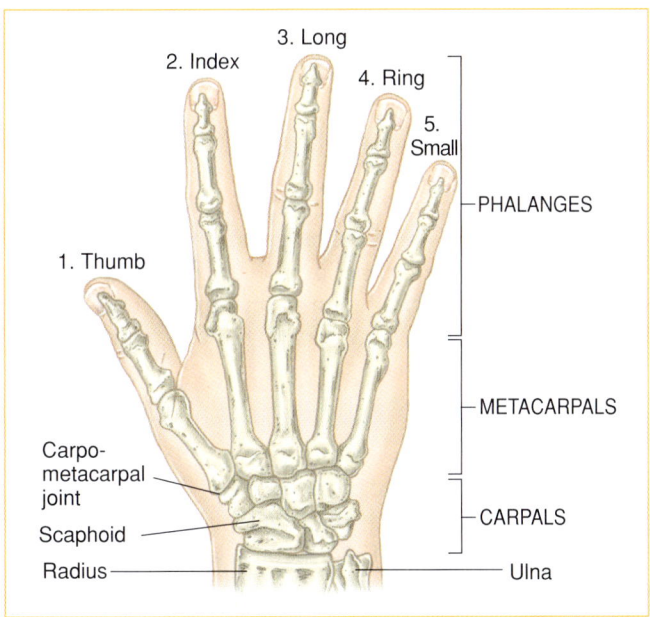

Figure 25-4 The anatomy of the wrist and hand.

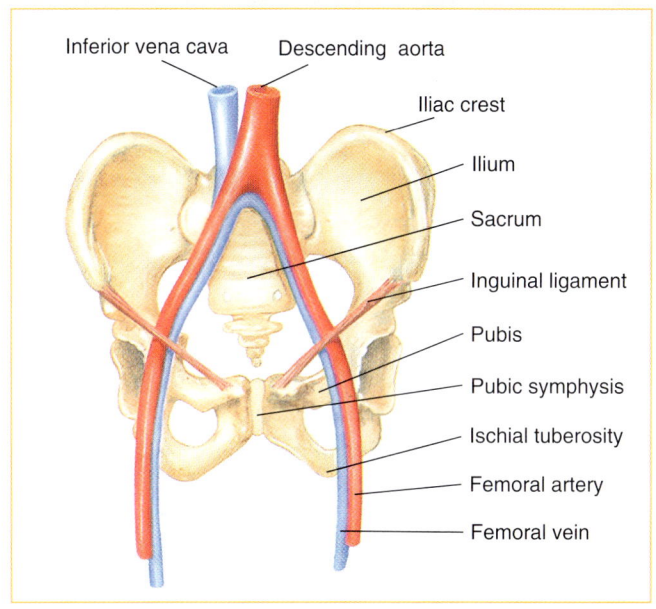

Figure 25-5 The pelvic girdle.

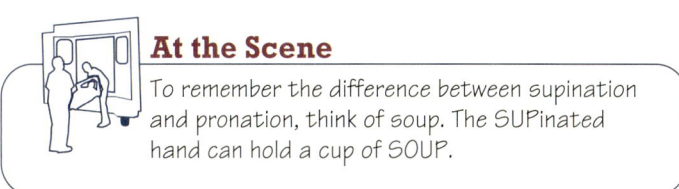

At the Scene

To remember the difference between supination and pronation, think of soup. The SUPinated hand can hold a cup of SOUP.

The radius and ulna make up the forearm. The radius, the larger of the two forearm bones, lies on the *thumb* side of the forearm. Distally, the ulna is narrow and is on the small-finger side of the forearm. It serves as the pivot around which the radius turns at the wrist to rotate the palm upward (supination) or downward (pronation). Because the radius and the ulna are arranged in parallel, when one is broken, the other is often broken as well.

The hand (**Figure 25-4** ▲) contains three sets of bones: wrist bones (carpals), hand bones (metacarpals), and finger bones (phalanges). The carpals, especially the scaphoid, are vulnerable to fracture when a person falls on an outstretched hand. Phalanges are more apt to be injured by a crushing injury, such as being slammed in a car door.

Pelvis and Lower Extremities

The pelvic girdle (**Figure 25-5** ▲) is actually three separate bones—the ischium, ilium, and pubis—fused together to form the innominate bone. The two iliac bones are joined posteriorly by tough ligaments to the sacrum at the sacroiliac joints; the two pubic bones are connected anteriorly by equally tough ligaments to one another at the pubic symphysis. These joints allow very little motion, so the pelvic ring is strong and stable.

The lower extremity consists of the bones of the thigh, leg, and foot (**Figure 25-6** ▸). The femur (thigh bone) is a long, powerful bone that articulates proximally in the ball-and-socket joint of the pelvis and distally in the hinge joint of the knee. The *head* of the femur is the ball-shaped part that fits into the acetabulum. It is connected to the *shaft*, or long tubular portion of the femur, by the femoral *neck*. The femoral neck is a common site for fractures, generally referred to as hip fractures, especially in the older population.

The lower leg consists of two bones, the tibia and the fibula. The tibia (shin bone) forms the inferior component of the knee joint. Anterior to this joint is the patella (kneecap), a bone that is important for knee extension. The tibia runs down the front of

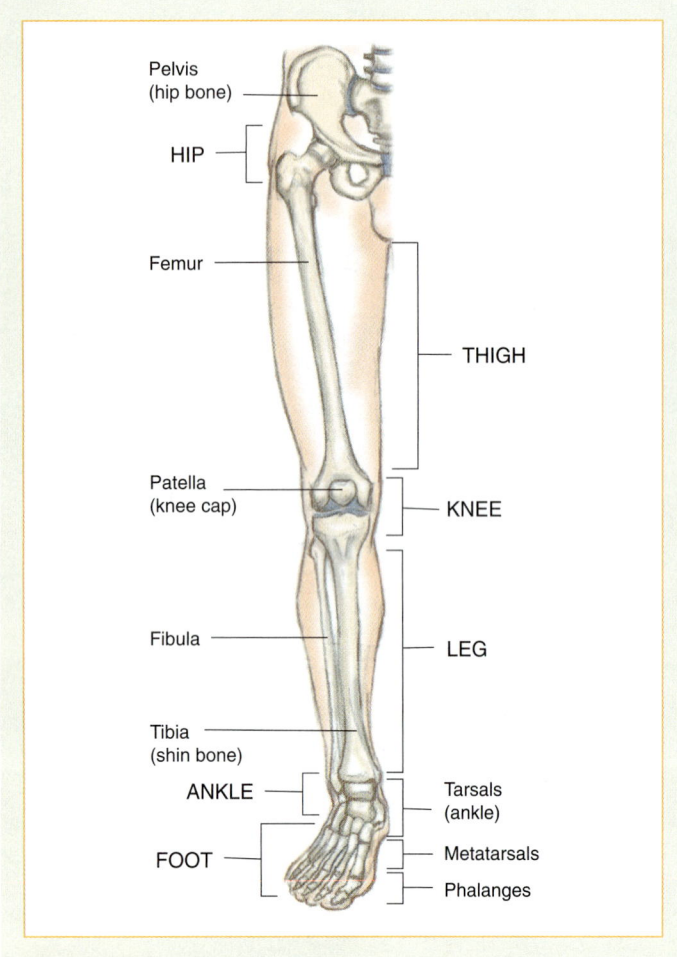

Figure 25-6 The bones of the leg.

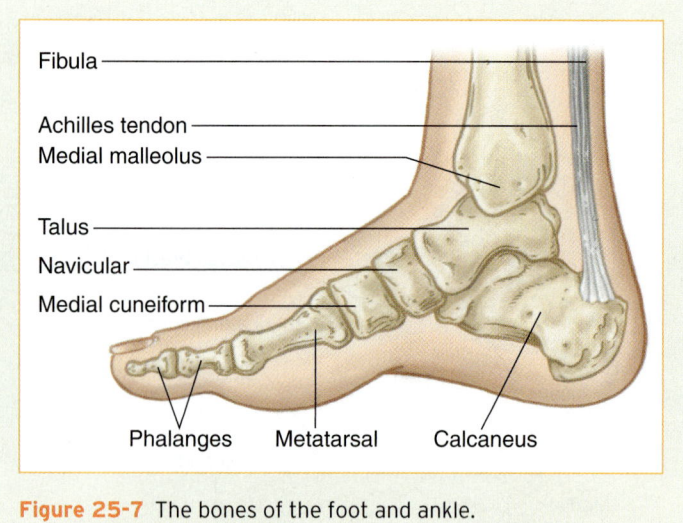

Figure 25-7 The bones of the foot and ankle.

At the Scene

Here's a tip to help remember which bones are carpal (hand bones) and which bones are tarsal (foot bones): "I steer my CAR (pal) with hands and walk through TAR (sal) with my feet."

At the Scene

Fractures that occur through the growth plate in a bone of a child may affect the future growth of that bone.

the lower leg, where it is vulnerable to direct blows, and can be felt just beneath the skin. The much smaller fibula runs posteriorly and laterally to the tibia. The fibula is not a component of the knee joint, but it does make up the lateral knob of the ankle joint (lateral malleolus) at its distal articulation.

The foot consists of three classes of bones: *ankle bones* (tarsals), *foot bones* (metatarsals), and *toe bones* (phalanges) **Figure 25-7 ▶**. The largest of the tarsal bones is the heel bone, or calcaneus, which is subject to injury when a person jumps from a height and lands on the feet.

Characteristics and Composition of Bone
Bone Shapes
Bones may be classified based on their shape. Long bones are longer than they are wide; examples include the femur,

humerus, tibia, fibula, radius, and ulna. Short bones are nearly as wide as they are long; they include the phalanges, metacarpals, and metatarsals. Flat bones are thin, broad bones; they include the sternum, ribs, scapulae, and skull. Irregular bones do not fit into one of the other categories but rather have a shape that is designed to perform a specific function, such as the bones of the vertebral column and the mandible. Round bones are generally found in proximity to a joint and help with movement. They are often referred to as sesamoid bones because of their location within a tendon. The patella is the largest of these bones.

Typical Long Bone Architecture
Long bones have several distinct regions and anatomical features **Figure 25-8 ▶**. These bones can grow to such long lengths because of the presence of the growth plate, or physis, in children. Once a person reaches adulthood, the growth plate closes and the mature adult bone is complete. The long bone is divided into three regions: the diaphysis, the epiphysis, and the metaphysis.

The articular surfaces of a long bone come in contact with other bones to form articulations (joints). These regions of the bone are covered by articular cartilage, a substance that acts as a cushion to protect the bone from damage and wear.

The portion of bone that is not covered by articular cartilage is, instead, covered by the periosteum. This dense, fibrous membrane contains capillaries and cells that are important for bone repair and maintenance. In the inner portion of the long bone, blood comes from the nutrient artery of the bone. Once

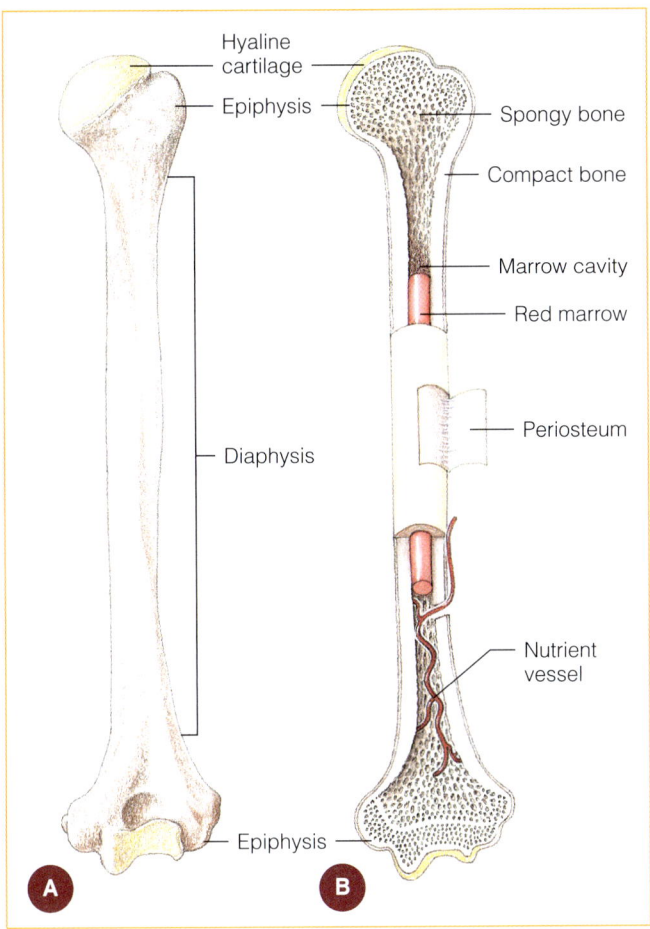

Figure 25-8 Anatomy of the long bone. **A.** The humerus. Notice the long shaft and dilated ends. **B.** Longitudinal section of the humerus showing compact bone, spongy bone, and marrow.

Labels on figure: Hyaline cartilage, Epiphysis, Spongy bone, Compact bone, Marrow cavity, Red marrow, Diaphysis, Periosteum, Nutrient vessel, Epiphysis

it penetrates the bone's outer cortex, the artery enters the medullary canal, the hollow inner portion of the shaft that is lined by the endosteum (similar to the periosteum, but on the inside) and contains yellow (fatty) marrow in adults.

Age-Associated Changes in Bone

Bone ages just like any other tissue of the body, decreasing in density after the age of 35 years, leading to a loss of height, and producing changes in facial structure. In women, this decrease in density is further accelerated once menopause is reached because of the loss of estrogen, a hormone that helps promote bone formation. A significant decrease in bone density, called osteoporosis **Figure 25-9 ▶** , is associated with a higher risk of fracture. People with osteoporosis are at risk for incurring a fracture, especially in the hip, spine, and wrist.

Other changes associated with aging of bone include aging of muscles, cartilage, and other connective tissues that may also lead to degradation of joints and disk herniation. For example, the water content of the intervertebral disks

decreases, increasing the risk of disk herniation. In some joints, the cartilage may become degraded, leading to arthritis and pain; in others, the cartilage becomes calcified, leading to restricted motion.

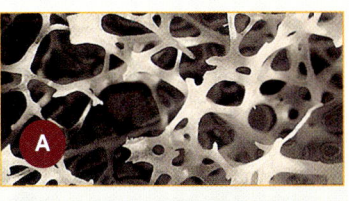
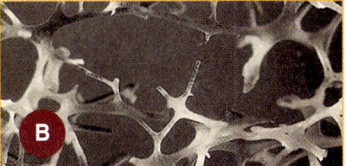

Figure 25-9 The structural difference between normal and osteoporotic bone. **A.** Normal bone in a 29-year-old woman. **B.** Osteoporotic bone in a 92-year-old-woman.

Joints

When two bones come together, they articulate with one another to form a joint. Some joints are fused and allow for no motion, such as the joints of the skull. Other joints allow for motion by permitting movement between the two bones, typically within a certain plane of motion that is defined by the structure of the bones that form it. The various motions that a joint may allow include flexion, extension, abduction, adduction, rotation, circumduction, pronation, and supination **Figure 25-10 ▶** .

Types of Joints

The three general types of joints are fibrous, cartilaginous, and synovial **Figure 25-11 ▶** . Fibrous joints, also referred to as synarthroses or fused joints, contain dense fibrous tissue that does not allow for movement. Examples include the bones of the skull and the distal tibiofibular joint.

Cartilaginous joints, also called amphiarthroses, allow for very minimal movement between the bones. The pubic symphysis and the joints connecting the ribs to the sternum are examples of this type of joint.

Synovial joints, or diarthroses, are the most mobile joints of the body. They are surrounded by an extension of the periosteum called the joint capsule, with the bones that form them being held in place by very strong ligaments. Within the joint are the articular cartilage and the synovial membrane, which secretes synovial fluid into the joint cavity to lubricate it.

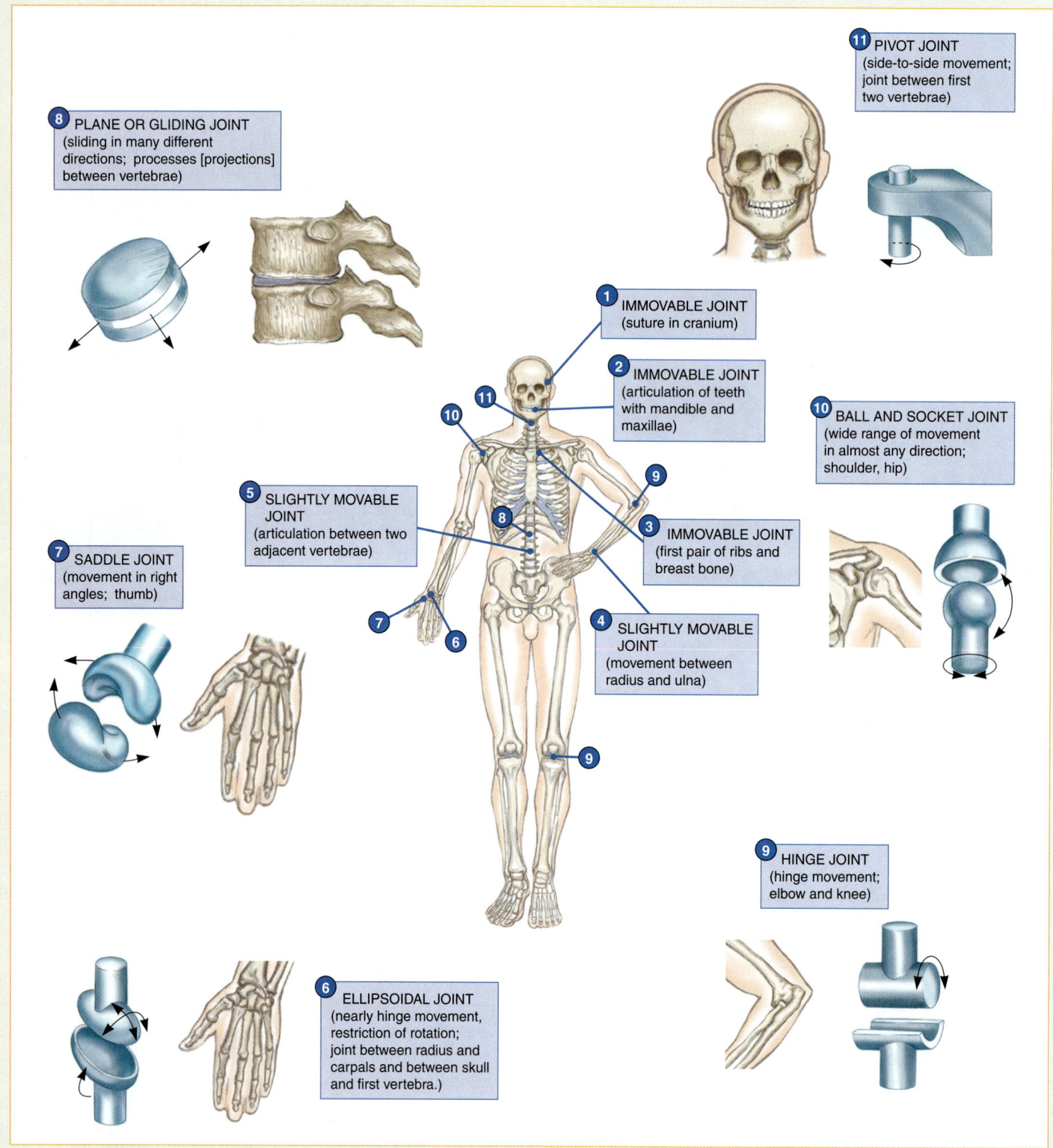

Figure 25-10 Joints in the body.

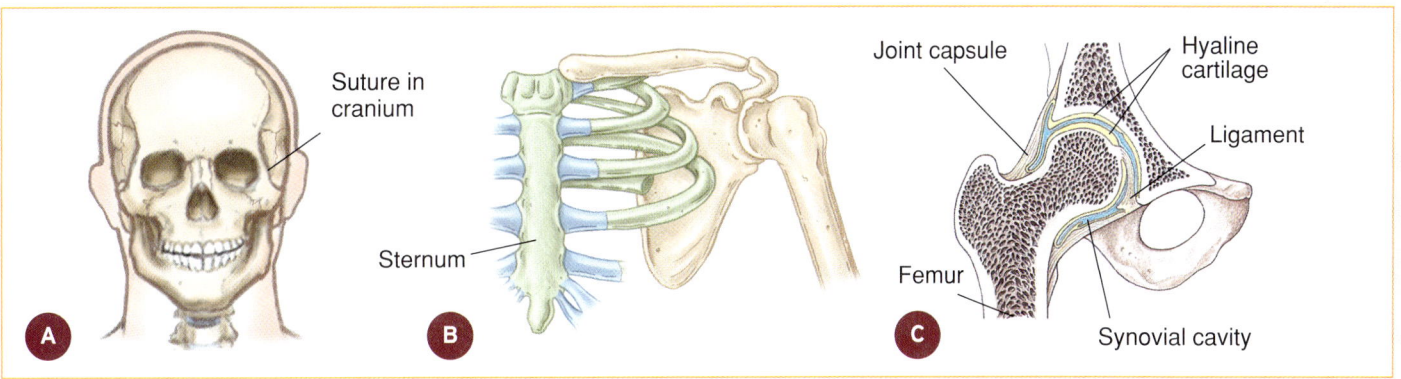

Figure 25-11 Types of joints. **A.** Fibrous. **B.** Cartilaginous. **C.** Synovial.

Bursa

A bursa is a padlike sac or cavity located within the connective tissue, usually in proximity to a joint. It may be lined with a synovial membrane and typically contains fluid that helps reduce the amount of friction between a tendon and a bone or between a tendon and a ligament. Examples include the olecranon bursa of the elbow and the prepatellar bursa of the knee. Bursitis is inflammation of a bursa.

Skeletal Connecting and Supporting Structures

Tendons connect muscle to bone. These flat or cordlike bands of connective tissue are white and have a glistening appearance.

 Ligaments connect bone to bone and help maintain the stability of joints and determine the degree of joint motion. These inelastic bands of connective tissue have a structure similar to that of tendons.

 Cartilage consists of fibres of collagen embedded in a gelatinous substance. This flexible connective tissue forms the smooth surface over bone ends where they articulate, provides cushioning between vertebrae, gives structure to the nose and external ear, forms the framework of the larynx and trachea, and serves as the model for the formation of the skeleton in children. Cartilage has a very limited neurovascular supply—it receives nutrients through diffusion from the outer covering of the cartilage or from the synovial fluid—so it does not heal well if it is injured.

The Moving Forces: Muscles

Muscles are composed of specialized cells that contract (shorten) when stimulated to exert a force on a part of the body. Three types of muscle are found in the body: smooth muscle, cardiac muscle, and skeletal muscle **Figure 25-12 ▸**.

Skeletal Muscle

Skeletal muscle **Figure 25-13 ▸** is also called voluntary muscle, because its contractions are largely under voluntary control, or striated muscle, because striations can be seen in it during microscopic examination. Skeletal muscle includes all

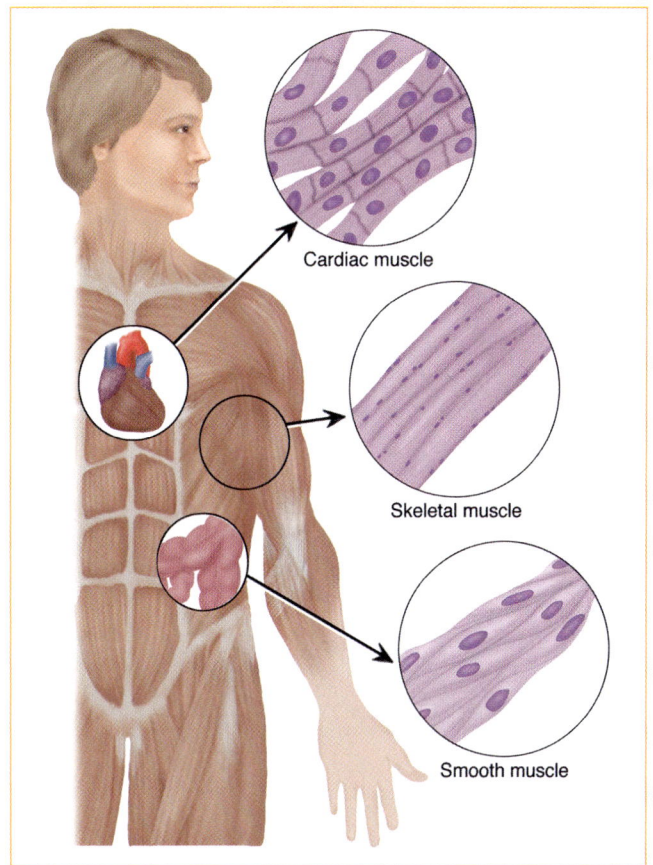

Figure 25-12 The three types of muscle are skeletal, smooth, and cardiac.

of the muscles attached to the skeleton and forms the bulk of the tissue of the arms and legs. It is also found along the spine and buttocks. By maintaining a state of partial contraction, this type of muscle allows the body to maintain its posture and to sit or stand. It varies greatly in size and shape, from thin strands to the large muscles of the thigh and back. It also constitutes the muscles of the tongue, soft palate, scalp, pharynx, upper esophagus, and eye. About 40% to 50% of normal body

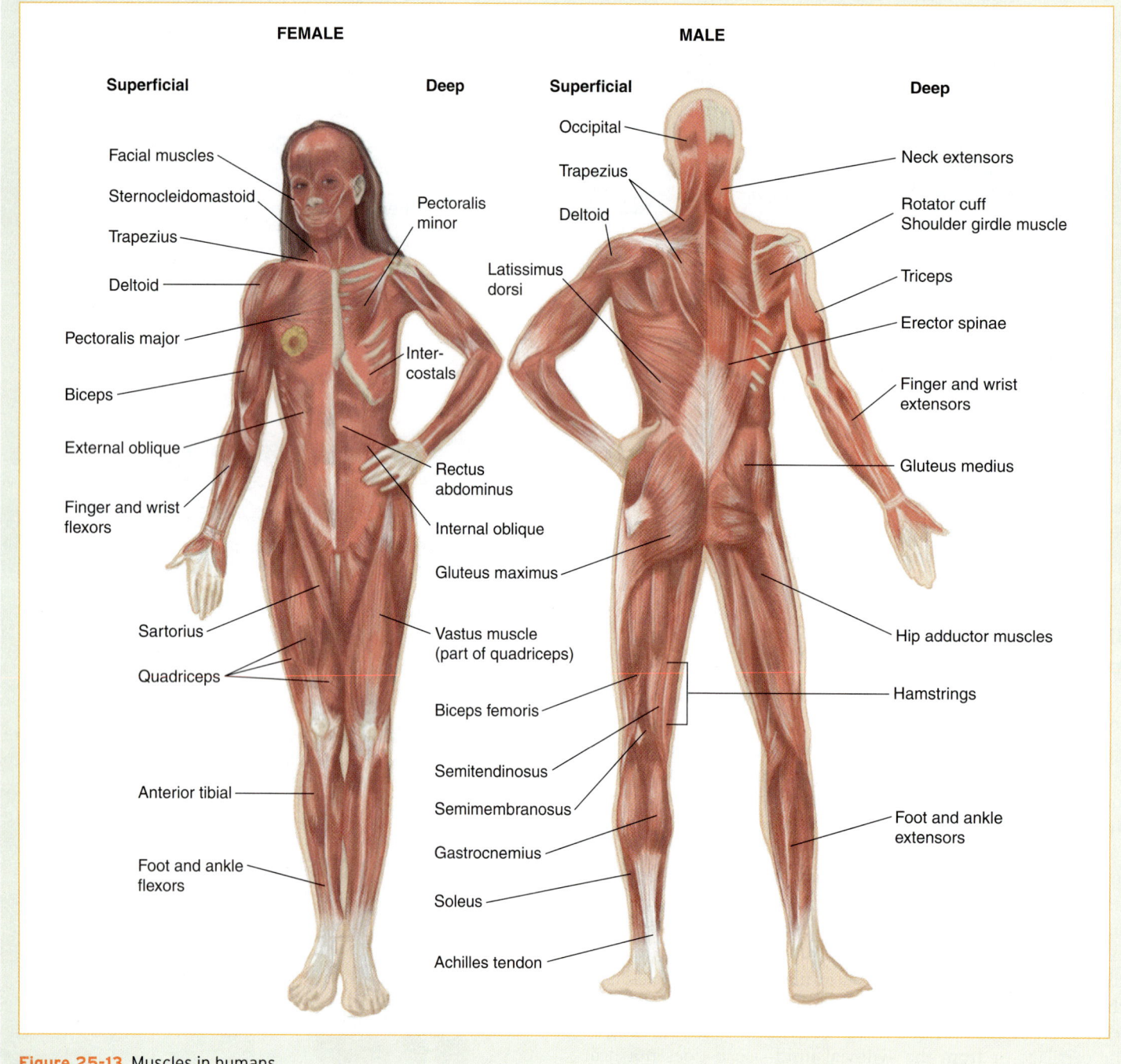

Figure 25-13 Muscles in humans.

weight is skeletal muscle, as it has a high water content. In addition, because of its high metabolic rate and demand for energy and oxygen, skeletal muscle has a very rich blood supply, which causes it to bleed significantly when injured.

Skeletal muscles are profoundly affected by the amount of training and work to which they are subjected. Unused muscles tend to atrophy (shrink or waste away), whereas physical training promotes hypertrophy (increase in size).

Skeletal muscles are attached to bones by tendons. Tendons cross joints to create a pulling force between two bones

when a muscle contracts. The biceps muscle, for example, has its origin on the scapula; the biceps tendon passes over the head of the humerus, where it fuses with the body of the biceps muscle; at the distal end of the biceps, a tendon passes over the anterior surface of the elbow and inserts on the radius. Thus, when the biceps muscle contracts, the force causes the elbow to bend (flex).

Muscle contraction requires energy. This energy is derived from the metabolism of glucose and results in the production of lactic acid (lactate). Lactic acid, in turn, must be converted

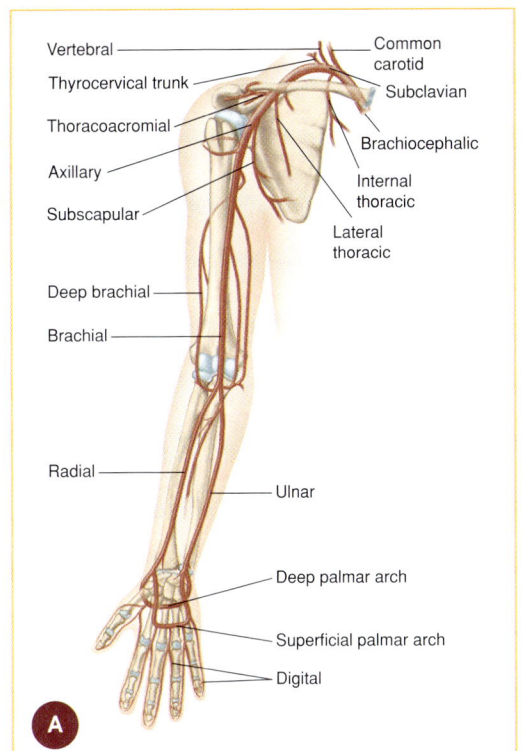

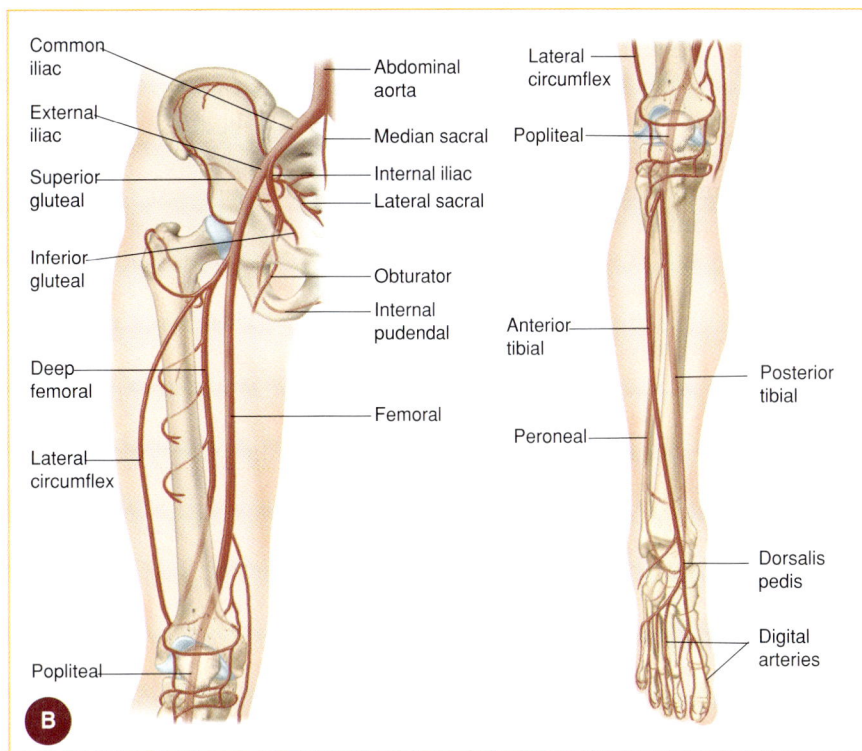

Figure 25-14 The arterial supply of the extremities. **A.** Upper extremities. **B.** Lower extremities.

into carbon dioxide and water, a process that requires oxygen. For that reason, vigorous muscular activity is often followed by an increased respiratory rate, which increases oxygen delivery to and carbon dioxide removal from the tissues.

The sensation of muscle fatigue occurs when the energy supply to the muscle is inadequate to meet the energy demands. If muscle fatigue occurs as a result of excessive muscular activity, rest produces quick recovery. However, if it occurs from a lack of oxygen or essential nutrients or electrolytes (such as sodium or calcium), rest will not lead to such a quick recovery.

Muscle Innervation

Skeletal muscle is innervated by somatic motor neurons. These neurons transmit electrical stimuli to a muscle that cause it to contract. The combination of the muscle and the neuron that innervates it constitutes a motor unit. A motor unit that receives a signal to contract responds as forcefully as possible or does not contract at all: It is an all-or-nothing response. To generate a more forceful contraction, more neurons need to signal more muscle cells to contract, a process called recruitment.

Innervation of the upper extremities arises from the brachial plexus. The brachial plexus is formed by a network of nerves that originate from the spinal cord at the C5–T1 levels.

After the fibres of these nerves network with one another, five distinct nerves are formed: the axillary, radial, musculocutaneous, ulnar, and median. Innervation of the lower extremities is provided by the lumbar and lumbosacral plexuses, which are formed by the spinal nerves that originate from L1–S4. The networking of nerves within these two plexuses leads to the formation of multiple distinct nerves, including the femoral nerve and the sciatic nerve, which branches in the popliteal fossa to form the peroneal and tibial nerves.

Musculoskeletal Blood Supply

When a person has a musculoskeletal injury, the arteries that supply the injured region may also be damaged. Therefore, it is important to realize which arteries are present in each part of the extremity **Figure 25-14 ▲** .

The upper extremity's blood supply originates from the subclavian artery. When the subclavian artery reaches the axilla, it is referred to as the axillary artery. After giving off several branches that supply the shoulder region with blood, the artery leaves the axilla and becomes the brachial artery. After the brachial artery passes through the elbow, it divides into the radial artery and ulnar artery. In the hand, the radial and ulnar arteries form superficial and deep arcades of blood vessels that branch to form the arteries of each finger, the digital arteries.

In the lower extremity, the blood supply originates from the external iliac artery. When the external iliac artery reaches the leg, it becomes the femoral artery. When it reaches the knee, the femoral artery turns posteriorly and laterally and is referred to as the popliteal artery. The popliteal artery divides into the anterior tibial artery and posterior tibial artery. The anterior tibial artery travels along the anterior and lateral surface of the tibia until it reaches the ankle, where it proceeds along the dorsal surface of the foot toward the great toe and becomes the dorsalis pedis artery. The posterior tibial artery travels along the posterior aspect of the tibia until it reaches the ankle, where it follows a path just behind the medial malleolus until it reaches the plantar aspect of the foot. Within the foot, arcades of arteries supply the various structures with blood and give off branches that form the digital arteries of the toes.

Patterns and Mechanisms of Musculoskeletal Injury

Skeletal injuries result from blunt and penetrating trauma. In some cases, a force that might not generally cause harm to normal healthy bone produces a fracture. Such a pathologic fracture occurs when a medical condition causes the bone to become abnormally weak. In adults and children, motor vehicle collisions, falls, and athletic activities are common causes of injury. Among infants and children, intentional trauma or maltreatment is a common cause of fractures and musculoskeletal injuries.

Sports account for a significant number of musculoskeletal injuries Figure 25-15 ▸ .

Injury Forces and Motions
Direct Force
An object that strikes a person will transfer its energy to its point of impact. This energy is first absorbed by the soft tissues in the region of the impact. When the amount of force is so great that the soft tissues cannot fully dissipate it, a fracture occurs.

Penetrating injuries may also lead to a fracture or other musculoskeletal injury. A high-velocity injury, such as that caused by a high-power rifle, typically shatters bone and causes extensive soft-tissue damage.

An impalement injury commonly causes a soft-tissue injury similar to that seen in a low-velocity penetrating injury. If the impaled object happens to strike a bone, it may cause a fracture. In any case of impalement, it is essential to stabilize the object to protect the soft tissues from further injury.

Indirect Force
An indirect injury occurs when a force is applied to one region of the body but causes an injury in another region of the body. In this type of injury, the force is transmitted through the skeleton until, at some point, it reaches an area that is structurally

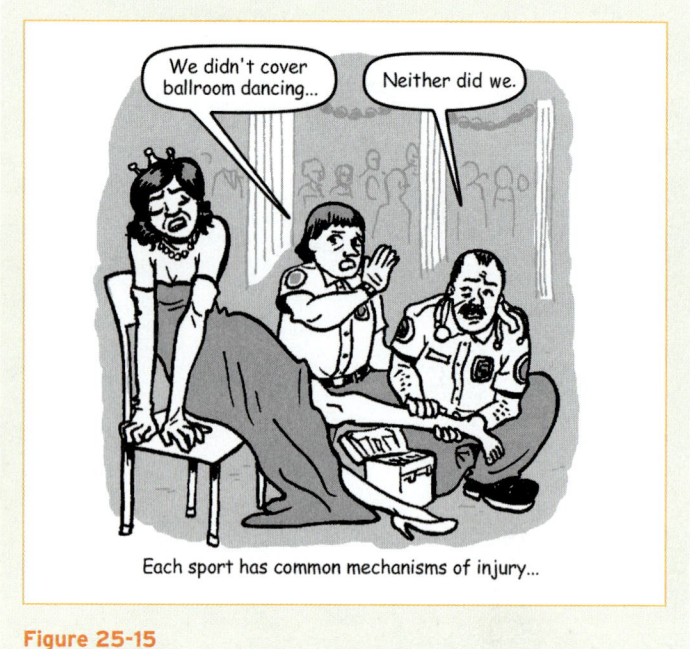

Figure 25-15

weak in comparison with the other parts of the musculoskeletal system through which the force has travelled.

For example, a hip fracture may occur when a person's knee strikes the dashboard during a motor vehicle collisions. In this case, the force is applied to the knee and travels proximally along the femur. When this force reaches the femoral neck, it causes the femoral neck to fracture.

Forces may be transmitted along the entire length of a bone or through several bones in series and may cause an injury anywhere along the way. Thus, a person falling on an outstretched hand may have one or more injuries as the result of forces transmitted proximally from the point of impact: (1) fracture of the scaphoid bone of the hand (direct blow); (2) fracture of the distal radius (Colles fracture Figure 25-16 ▸); (3) fracture-dislocation of the elbow; (4) fracture-dislocation of the shoulder; or (5) fracture of the clavicle.

Twisting injuries, like those that commonly occur in football or skiing, result in fractures, sprains, and dislocations. Typically, the distal part of the limb remains fixed, as when cleats or a ski holds the foot to the ground, while torsion develops in the proximal section of the limb; the resulting force causes tearing of tendons and ligaments and spiral fractures of bone. Fatigue fractures, also called march fractures, are caused by repetitive stress and most commonly occur in the feet after prolonged walking.

Pathologic fractures are seen in patients with diseases that weaken areas of bone, such as metastatic cancer, and may occur with minimal force. Older people, particularly those with osteoporosis, also have weaker, more brittle bones and are more susceptible to fractures than younger people.

Some injuries are commonly encountered together because of the way the causative forces are transmitted; thus, if you find one, look for the others (Table 25-1 ▶). Pain and swelling over the scaphoid bone of the wrist, for example, means that the patient fell hard against an outstretched hand, so he or she may have other injuries anywhere along the axis from the hand to the shoulder.

Fractures

A fracture is a break in the continuity of a bone. Fractures occur when the magnitude of the force applied to a bone (a single application or an accumulation of repetitive applications)

Documentation and Communication

Some services take digital pictures at collision scenes to include in reports to the receiving hospital. These images allow emergency department staff to better understand the forces involved.

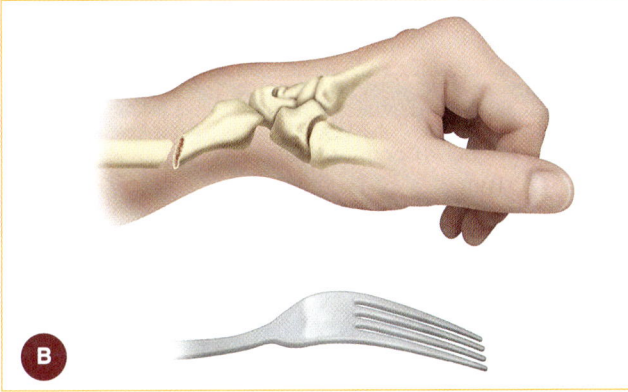

Figure 25-16 A. Fractures of the distal radius produce a characteristic Colles fracture (dinner fork deformity). **B.** An artist's illustration of the injury.

Table 25-1	Musculoskeletal Injuries That Commonly Occur Together	
If You Find	**Look For**	
Scapular fracture	Rib fracture, pulmonary contusions, pneumothorax	
Scaphoid fracture	Wrist, elbow, or shoulder fracture	
Pelvic fracture	Lumbosacral spine and other long bone fractures, intra-abdominal or genitourinary injury	
Hip dislocation	Fracture of the acetabulum or femoral head	
Femoral fracture	Dislocation of ipsilateral hip	
Patellar fracture	Fracture-dislocation of ipsilateral hip	
Knee dislocation	Tibial fracture; distal pulse may be absent	
Calcaneal fracture	Fracture of the ankle, leg, hip, pelvis, spine, and the other calcaneus	

You are the Paramedic Part 2

As you continue your initial assessment, an engine company arrives and assists with application of spinal precautions and high-flow supplemental oxygen. Soon afterward, the neighbour approaches and identifies himself. He says that the patient seemed to have lost his balance while painting and may have struck the air conditioner during his fall. On further assessment, you note that the patient appears to have an open fracture of his left arm, which is bleeding significantly.

Vital Signs	Recording Time: 2 Minutes
Level of consciousness	A (Alert to person, place, and day)
Skin	Pink, warm, and slightly moist
Pulse	110 beats/min, full and regular
Blood pressure	144/90 mm Hg
Respirations	42 breaths/min
Spo₂	96% with 15 l/min via nonrebreathing mask

3. What are the potential complications of an open fracture?
4. Why are open fractures prone to bleeding more than closed fractures?
5. Would your treatment priorities change if the patient complained of abdominal pain in the presence of hypotension?

overcomes the strength of the bone. The strength of a bone is affected by age, osteoporosis, nutritional status, and disease processes.

Fracture Classification
Fracture Type

A fracture may be classified based on the direction that the fracture line travels through a bone, number of fractures on the bone, or number of cortices involved Table 25-2 ▾ .

> **Special Considerations**
>
> Children with fractures may not want you to see, touch, or splint the injured extremity. You should always be honest with children about what you are doing and whether it will hurt. In particular, splinting is a necessary and sometimes painful intervention for a child with a fracture. Once the splint is in place, cold is applied, and analgesia is considered, the child will likely have less pain because the fracture is stabilized.

Fracture Classification Based on Displacement

Fractures may be classified based on the type of displacement Table 25-3 ▸ .

Angulation of a fracture means that each end of the fracture is not aligned in a straight line and that an angle has formed between them. Angulation may occur in the frontal plane, sagittal plane, or both.

Open Versus Closed Fractures

In an open fracture Figure 25-18 ▸ , sometimes called a compound fracture, a break in the overlying skin allows the fracture to communicate with the outside environment. In a closed fracture, the skin over the fracture site remains intact.

In addition to having a higher risk of infection, open fractures have the potential for more blood loss than a closed fracture for two reasons. First, open fractures usually result from high-energy injuries, so they typically involve more soft-tissue damage. Second, in most fractures, the periosteal vessels and the vessels supplying the surrounding soft tissues are disrupted, leading to the formation of a hematoma. In a closed

Table 25-2	Fracture Classification Based on Fracture Type		
Type of Fracture	**Description**	**Common Causes**
Direction the Fracture Line Travels Through a Bone Figure 25-17 ▸		
Linear fracture	Parallel to the long axis of the bone	Low-energy stress injuries
Transverse fracture	Straight across a bone at right angles to each cortex	Direct, low-energy blow
Oblique fracture	At an angle across the bone	Direct or twisting force
Spiral fracture	Encircles the bone	Twisting injury
Impacted fracture	End of one bone becomes wedged into another bone	Fall from a significant height
Number of Fractures on One Bone		
Comminuted fracture	> 2 fracture fragments located in one area of the bone	High-energy injury (such as crush injury)
Segmental fracture	> 2 fracture fragments, but breaks occur in different parts of the bone	High-energy injury
Number of Cortices Injured		
Complete fracture	Break through both cortices	High-energy injury
Incomplete fracture	Break through one cortex	Low-energy injury
■ Greenstick fracture	Typically occurs in the proximal metaphysis or diaphysis of the tibia, radius, or, when this fracture occurs in the shaft, the cortex on the convex side of the deformity is broken, but the cortex on the concave side remains intact	Usually occurs in children
■ Buckle fracture (torus fracture)	Occurs in the metaphysis of long bones in response to excessive compression loading on one side of the bone; the compressed cortex buckles, and the opposite cortex is pulled away from the physis	Unique to children; most commonly seen in the distal radius, usually resulting from a fall on an outstretched hand
■ Bowing fracture	When a compression force is applied to a bone, numerous small fractures on the compressed side of the bone cause it to bend	Often occurs in children and young adults; most commonly affects the radius, ulna, tibia, fibula, or clavicle
■ Fatigue fracture (stress fracture)	Occurs when the muscle develops faster than the bone and places exaggerated stress on the less developed bone; may also be due to repetitive small injuries that eventually lead to bone failure	Usually occurs in the legs or feet of people who engage in strenuous, repetitive activities (such as dancers, joggers, military recruits)

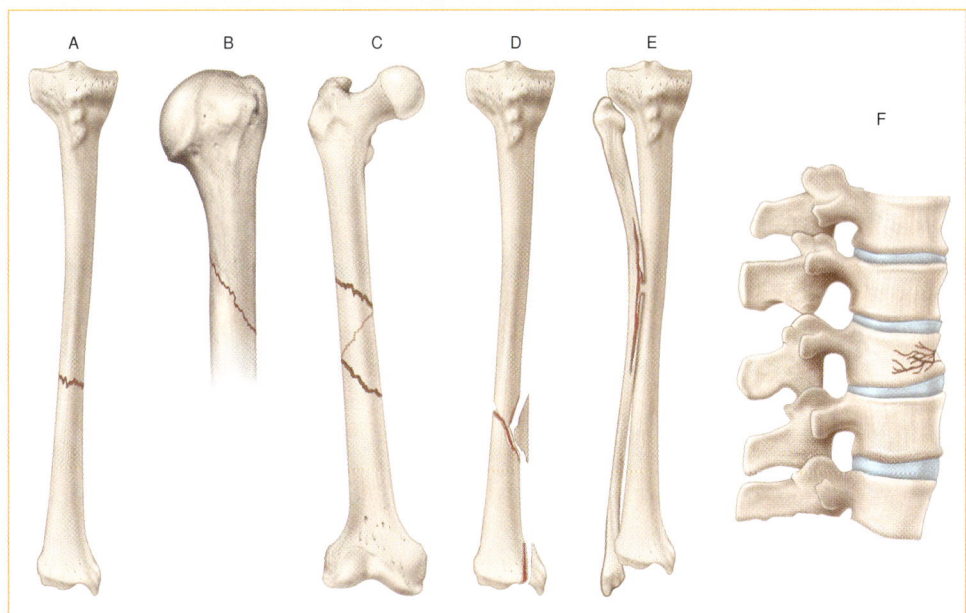

Figure 25-17 Types of fractures. **A.** Transverse fracture of the tibia. **B.** Oblique fracture of the humerus. **C.** Spiral fracture of the femur. **D.** Comminuted fracture of the tibia. **E.** Greenstick fracture of the fibula. **F.** Compression fracture of a vertebral body.

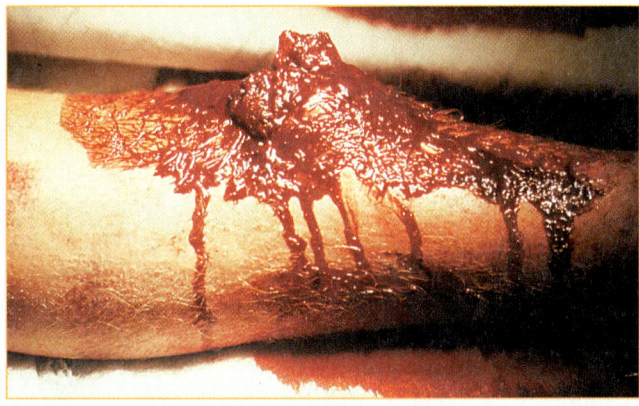

Figure 25-18 An open fracture.

fracture, the increased interstitial pressure within the hematoma compresses the blood vessels, limiting the size of the hematoma. In a closed femur fracture, the blood loss may exceed 1 litre before enough pressure develops to tamponade the bleeding. In contrast, open fractures allow much of the blood to escape, so tamponade does not occur as readily or at all.

Signs and Symptoms of a Fracture

The primary symptom of a fracture is *pain* that is usually well localized to the fracture site. In addition, the patient may report hearing a snap or feeling a break. Signs of fracture detected on physical examination include the following:

- *Deformity* is one of the most reliable signs of a fracture. The limb may be found in an unnatural position or show motion at a place where there is no joint. Compare the deformed limb with the extremity on the other side **Figure 25-19 ▶**.
- *Shortening* occurs in fractures when the broken ends of a bone override one another. It is characteristic of femur fractures, for example, because the broken femur can no longer serve as a strut to oppose spasm in the powerful thigh muscles.

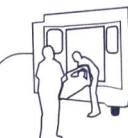

At the Scene

The ends of a fractured bone are sharp. Use caution whenever bone ends are exposed to prevent a puncture injury to yourself, your crew, or the splint.

Table 25-3	Fracture Classification Based on Displacement	
Type of Fracture	**Description**	**Common Causes**
Nondisplaced fracture	Bone remains aligned in its normal position, despite the fracture.	Low-energy injury
Displaced fracture	Ends of the fracture move from their normal positions.	High-energy injury
■ Overriding	Muscles pull the distal fracture fragment alongside the proximal one, leading them to overlap; the limb becomes shortened.	Only occurs when a fracture is fully displaced and there is no bone contact
■ Distraction injury	A powerful tensile force is rapidly applied to a bone, causing it to fracture—the bone ends are pulled apart.	Industrial equipment, machinery
■ Impacted fracture (impaction injury)	A massive compressive force is applied to a bone, causing it to become wedged into another bone.	More likely to happen in cancellous bone
■ Avulsion fracture	A powerful muscle contraction causes the insertion site of the muscle to be fractured off of the bone.	Sudden "jerking" of a body part
■ Depression fracture	Blunt trauma to a flat bone (such as the skull) causes the bone to be pushed inward.	Blunt injury

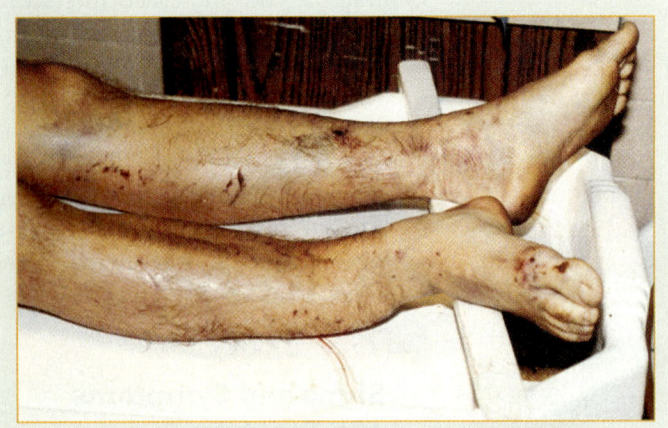
Figure 25-19 Obvious deformity is a sign of bone fracture.

- Visual inspection will usually reveal *swelling* at the fracture site due to bleeding from the broken bone and the accumulation of fluid. As blood infiltrates the tissues around the broken bone ends, *ecchymosis* will become apparent.
- *Guarding* and *loss of use* characterize most fractures. The patient will try to keep a fractured bone still and will avoid putting any stress on it. Sometimes the measures a patient takes to protect a fractured bone from movement are so characteristic that one can almost diagnose the fracture without examining the extremity. A patient who walks to the ambulance holding the dorsum of one wrist in the other hand, for example, almost certainly has a Colles fracture. A patient standing with the head cocked toward a "knocked-down shoulder" probably has a fracture of the clavicle on the side to which the head is leaning.
- A fractured bone is almost invariably *tender to palpation* over the fracture site.
- Palpation may reveal crepitus, a grating sensation, over the broken bone ends. Crepitus may be noted as an incidental finding during splinting attempts. Do *not* try to elicit this sign, because your efforts may result in further injury to the bone and surrounding soft tissues, not to mention severe pain.

Notes from Nancy

The best way to detect deformity or any other abnormality in an extremity is to compare it to the extremity on the other side.

- In an open fracture, *exposed bone ends* may be visible in the wound.

Ligament Injuries and Dislocations

The shapes of the bones that form a joint and the tightness of the ligaments that hold them in place are key factors in determining a joint's range of motion. When forced beyond their normal limit, the bones that form a joint may break or become displaced and the supporting ligaments and joint capsule may tear.

Dislocations, Subluxations, and Diastases

In a dislocation, a bone is totally displaced from the joint. Typically, at least part of the supporting joint capsule and some of the joint's ligaments are disrupted. Dislocations occur when a body part moves beyond its normal range of motion and the articular surfaces are no longer in contact. The dislocated bones are then locked in this abnormal position by muscle spasms. Evaluation of the patient usually reveals an obvious and significant deformity, a significant decrease in the joint's range of motion (ROM), and severe pain. In all cases of a dislocation, a fracture should be suspected until ruled out by radiographs.

The partial dislocation of a joint is a subluxation. In this type of injury, the articular surfaces of the bones that form the joint remain partially, but not completely, in contact. In some cases, part of the joint capsule and supporting ligaments may be damaged. Despite the subluxation, the patient may be able to move the joint to some degree. Failure to recognize and treat a subluxation may lead to persistent joint instability and pain.

When the ligaments that hold two bones in a fixed position with respect to one another are disrupted and the space between them increases, a situation known as a diastasis occurs. An example of this would be an injury to the ligaments that hold the pubic symphysis together, causing the width of the joint to increase (diastasis of the pubic symphysis).

The principal symptom of a dislocation is pain or a feeling of pressure over the involved joint, plus loss of motion of the joint. A patient with a posterior dislocation of the shoulder, for example, is unable to raise the arm but holds it against the side instead. Sometimes the joint will seem "frozen." The principal sign of dislocation is deformity.

A dislocation is considered an urgent injury because of its potential to cause neurovascular compromise distal to the site of injury. If the dislocated bone presses on a nerve, there may be numbness or weakness distally; if an artery is compressed, there may be absent distal pulses (such as in a knee dislocation). For these reasons, you should always assess the patient's neurovascular status distal to the site of dislocation (check pulse and motor and sensory functions [PMS]).

Sprains

Sprains are injuries in which ligaments are stretched or torn. They usually result from a sudden twisting of a joint beyond its normal range of motion that also causes a temporary subluxation. The majority of sprains involve the ankle or the knee because most occur after a person misjudges a step or landing. Evasive moves, like those done during a sporting event, commonly cause sprains in athletes. Sprains are typically characterized by pain, swelling, and discolouration over the injured joint and unwillingness to use the limb. In contrast with fractures and dislocations, sprains usually do not involve deformity and joint mobility is usually limited by pain, not by joint incongruity.

Because it may be difficult to differentiate among the various types of injuries in the prehospital environment, it is best to

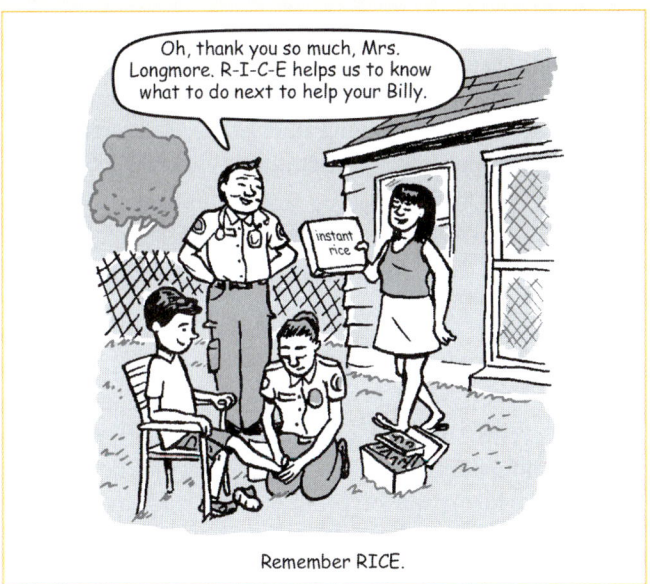

Remember RICE.

Figure 25-20

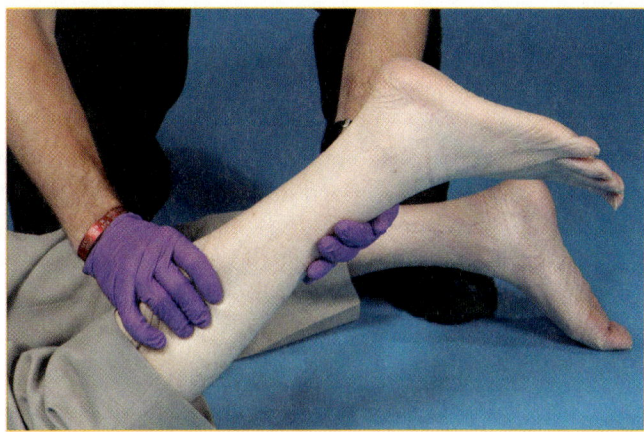

Figure 25-21 The Thompson test.

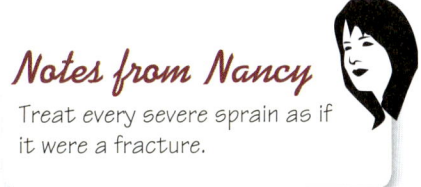

Notes from Nancy

Treat every severe sprain as if it were a fracture.

err on the side of caution and treat every severe sprain as if it were a fracture. General treatment of sprains is similar to that of fractures and includes the following (numbers 1 through 4 form the mnemonic RICE) **Figure 25-20 ▲** :

1. **Rest.** Immobilize or splint injured area
2. **Ice** or cold pack over the injury
3. **Compression** with an elastic bandage (usually applied at the hospital once radiography rules out a fracture)
4. **Elevation**
5. Reduced or protected weight bearing
6. Pain management as soon as practical

Muscle and Tendon Injuries

Strains

A strain (pulled muscle) is an injury to a muscle and/or tendon that results from a violent muscle contraction or from excessive stretching. Often no deformity is present and only minor swelling is noted at the site of injury. Some patients may complain of increased pain with passive movement of the injured extremity.

Achilles Tendon Rupture

A rupture of the Achilles tendon usually occurs in athletes older than 30 years who are involved in start-and-stop sports such as basketball or football. The most immediate indications are pain from the heel to the calf and a sudden inability for plantar flexion of the foot. As time passes, the calf muscles begin to contract

proximally and a gap may be felt in the Achilles tendon. The Thompson test can be performed in the prehospital setting to identify an Achilles tendon rupture. To perform this test, have the patient assume a prone position and then squeeze the calf muscles of the injured leg **Figure 25-21 ▲** . If the foot plantar flexes while squeezing, the tendon is most likely intact. If there is no movement of the foot, the Achilles tendon has likely been torn. Management of an Achilles tendon injury includes RICE and pain control. These injuries are treated with surgery or multiple casts and can require up to 6 months for recovery.

Inflammatory Processes

When a muscle is subjected to frequent and repetitive use, its tendon or nearby bursa are at risk for becoming inflamed. When inflammation of the tendon causes pain, the patient is said to have tendinitis. There will typically be point tenderness on the inflamed tendon with pain often increasing if the person performs the movement that led to the inflammation. When a bursa becomes painful and inflamed, it is called bursitis. Patients with bursitis often complain of pain in the region of the inflamed bursa, especially with motions that cause the space where the bursa sits to become smaller. Examination of the site may reveal tenderness, swelling, erythema, and warmth. Tendinitis and bursitis are treated with RICE, pain relievers, and, in many cases, steroid injections.

Arthritis

Arthritis means inflammation of a joint. The three most common types of arthritis are osteoarthritis, rheumatoid arthritis, and gouty arthritis.

Osteoarthritis (OA) is a disease of the joints that occurs as they age and begin to wear. It is characterized by pain and stiffness, which typically get worse with use, and "cracking" or "crunching" of the affected joints. The spine, hands, knees, and hips are the most commonly affected sites. In general, the risk of developing OA increases with age, but other factors also increase the risk, such as obesity and prior joint injury. Treatment of OA involves low-impact physical therapy, pain control, anti-inflammatory medications, joint injections, and, in severe cases, joint replacement surgery.

Rheumatoid arthritis (RA) is a systemic inflammatory disease that affects joints and other body systems. In RA, significant bone erosion at the affected joints makes them more susceptible to fractures and dislocations. Of particular concern is the cervical spine, which is at high risk of subluxating following trauma or during intubation. Give extra attention to the cervical spine of a patient with RA to prevent further injury.

Gout is a condition in which the body has difficulty eliminating uric acid. When the concentration of uric acid in the blood becomes too great, the uric acid may crystallize within a joint. The patient will then have a hot, red, swollen joint with decreased range of motion. Prehospital treatment involves immobilization, pain relief, and transportation to an emergency department (ED) where the fluid in the joint can be aspirated to search for the characteristic crystals of gouty arthritis.

Injuries That May Signify Fractures

Amputations

An amputation is the separation of a limb or other body part from the remainder of the body **Figure 25-22 ▾**. The amputation may be incomplete, leaving only a small segment of tissue connecting the part, or it may be complete, causing the part to be fully separated. Hemorrhage from complete or incomplete amputations can be severe and life threatening. Fractures may also be present with amputations. Amputations are discussed in more detail in Chapter 19.

Lacerations

A laceration is a smooth or jagged cut caused by a sharp object or a blunt force that tears the tissue. The depth of the injury

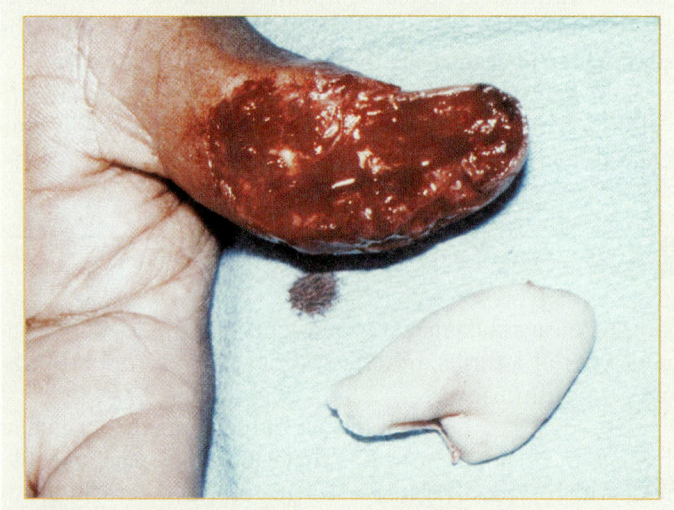

Figure 25-22 A partial avulsion involving the thumb.

can vary, extending through skin and subcutaneous tissue and even into the underlying muscles and adjacent nerves and blood vessels. Lacerations involving damaged arteries or veins may result in severe bleeding. The presence of lacerations may also be a sign of an underlying fracture. Deep lacerations may injure the muscle nerves, or vasculture, so distal PMS functions should always be evaluated.

Vascular Injuries

When blood vessels are damaged following a musculoskeletal injury, devascularization of the body part that is supplied by the vessel may occur. The types of injuries that a vessel may sustain include a contusion of the vessel wall, laceration, kinking or bending, and formation of pseudoaneurysms. In addition, a blood vessel may thrombose (become occluded by a clot) when the injury causes blood flow to become very slow. Regardless of the type of vascular injury involved, it is important to assess and reassess pulses, control bleeding, and maintain adequate intravascular volume by using intravenous (IV) fluid.

General Principles of Assessment and Management

When assessing an injured patient, *do not be distracted by visually impressive injuries!* It is essential to complete the initial assessment of the patient before focusing on the extremities. In cases of musculoskeletal injuries, patients may be classified based on the presence or absence of associated injuries:

- Life- or limb-threatening injury or condition, including life- or limb-threatening musculoskeletal trauma
- Life-threatening injuries and only simple musculoskeletal trauma
- Life- or limb-threatening musculoskeletal trauma and no other life-threatening injuries
- Isolated, non–life- or non–limb-threatening injuries

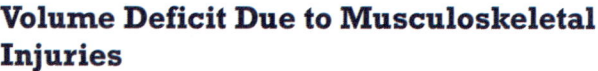

Notes from Nancy

Musculoskeletal injuries are rarely, if ever, an immediate threat to life. A fracture can wait. The airway cannot.

Volume Deficit Due to Musculoskeletal Injuries

Fractures may lead to significant blood loss from damage to vessels within the bone and musculature around the bone and, in some cases, from damage to large blood vessels in the region of the fracture. When caring for patients with fractures, undertake interventions such as applying direct pressure, splinting,

Table 25-4	Potential Blood Loss from Fracture Sites
Fracture Site	**Potential Blood Loss (ml)**
Pelvis	1,500–3,000
Femur	1,000–1,500
Humerus	250–500
Tibia or fibula	250–500
Ankle	250–500
Elbow	250–500
Radius or ulna	150–250

and administering IV fluids to prevent hypotension and unstable condition of the patient. **Table 25-4 ▲** lists the potential blood loss from various fracture sites and may serve as a guideline for estimating the amount of resuscitation required. The goal of prehospital management should be to keep the patient's volume, vital signs, and mental status normal.

Principles of Assessment

As with all patients, you should conduct a scene assessment, focusing on safety and body substance isolation precautions and then proceed to an initial assessment focusing on the patient's mental status, ABCs, and priority. If the initial assessment indicates that the patient has no immediately life-threatening condition and only localized musculoskeletal trauma, continue with a focused history and physical examination. If the patient has a significant mechanism of injury, complete a rapid trauma assessment and perform a detailed physical examination en route to the ED. The priorities throughout the assessment and management of musculoskeletal injuries should include identifying the injuries, preventing further harm or damage to the injured structures and surrounding tissues, supporting the injured area, and administering pain medication if necessary.

History of Present Injury

Obtain information about the incident that led to the injury from the patient and any bystanders who witnessed it. In particular, determine the condition of the patient immediately before the incident, the details of the incident, and the patient's position after the incident. Also, ask the patient for a subjective description of the injury: How did this happen? Did you hear a pop? Do you have pain? What functional limitations do you now have?

Medical History

Obtain the patient's medical history using the standard SAMPLE format. This history should also identify any preexisting musculoskeletal disorders and attempt to learn more about the injury. Some information obtained will be very relevant to the injury (such as the patient is taking anticoagulant medications).

Examination

When examining the patient, obtain a baseline set of vital signs. The focus can then shift to evaluating the injured extremity. One of the simplest ways to assess an extremity is to compare one side with the other, noting any discrepancy in length, position, or skin colour. Next, complete an examination noting DCAP-BTLS (Deformity, Contusions, Abrasions, Penetrating injury–Burns, Tenderness, Lacerations, Swelling) as you observe and palpate the soft tissue from head to toe and assess the patient for limitations, such as inability to move a joint. While performing the examination, be sure to cover the 6 Ps of musculoskeletal assessment: Pain, Paralysis, Paresthesias (numbness or tingling), Pulselessness, Pallor (pale or delayed capillary refill in children), and Pressure.

Pain

A person experiences acute pain when peripheral pain receptors (nocioceptors) convert painful stimuli into electrical impulses that are transmitted via the peripheral nerve fibres to the spinal cord. The signal ascends along the spinal cord to the pain-sensing region of the brain. When a tissue is injured, various chemical mediators are released that facilitate the conduction of the painful stimulus to the brain.

When assessing a patient's pain, remember the OPQRST mnemonic: Onset of the pain; Provoking or Palliating factors; Quality of the pain (such as sharp, pressure, crampy); Region of the pain, including its primary location and areas where pain radiates or refers; Severity of the pain; and the Time (duration) that the patient has been experiencing pain. It is also useful to have the patient quantify the severity of the pain by using a scale of 1 to 10 or with visual images such as faces that appear to be happy or in pain.

Inspection

When inspecting an injured extremity, always evaluate the joint above and the joint below the site of injury because the injuring force may have affected these sites as well. In particular, compare the injured side with the uninjured side. While inspecting a patient's injuries, look for the following signs:

- Deformity, including asymmetry, angulation, shortening, and rotation
- Skin changes, including contusions, abrasions, avulsions, punctures, burns, lacerations, and bone ends
- Swelling
- Muscle spasms
- Abnormal limb positioning
- Increased or decreased range of motion
- Colour changes, including pallor and cyanosis
- Bleeding, including estimating the amount of blood loss

Palpation

Palpation of an injured extremity should include the injury site and the regions above and below it. Regions of point tenderness should be identified. Reassess any tender areas frequently to determine whether there are changes in the location or severity of the pain or tenderness. Note that while point tenderness is one of the best indicators of an injury, it may be absent in patients who are intoxicated or who have an injury to the spinal cord.

When palpating an injured site, attempt to identify instability, deformity, abnormal joint or bone continuity, and displaced bones. Feel for crepitus, which is commonly found at the site of a fracture. Palpate distal pulses on all extremities, with special attention to comparing the strength of the pulses in the injured extremity with those in a normal one.

On occasion, an arterial injury may be identified while palpating an extremity. Signs of an arterial injury include a pulsatile expanding hematoma, diminished distal pulses, a palpable thrill (vibration) over the site of injury that correlates with the patient's heartbeat, and difficult-to-control bleeding.

The purpose of palpating the pelvis is to identify instability and point tenderness. Gently apply pressure over the pubic symphysis to evaluate for tenderness and crepitus. Next, gently press the iliac wings toward the midline and then posteriorly. Any gross instability found during this examination should be reported to hospital personnel because it may indicate a severe pelvic injury. Do not repeatedly examine the pelvis if instability is found because the manipulation may disrupt blood clots and cause further bleeding.

The upper and lower extremity examination should include palpation of the entire length of each arm and leg to identify any sites of injury. The most efficient way to accomplish this is to place your hands around the extremity and squeeze. Repeat this procedure every few centimetres until you reach the end of the extremity. When evaluating the upper extremities, always examine the cervical spine and shoulder because complaints within the arm may be caused by a more proximal disorder. Likewise, with the lower extremities, always conduct an examination of the lower back, pelvis, and hip if the patient complains of pain in the leg.

Motor Function and Sensory Examination

It is essential to assess a patient's distal pulse, as well as motor and sensory function, in the case of a musculoskeletal injury. A motor function examination should be performed whenever a patient has an injury to an extremity, provided the patient does not also have a life-threatening injury. When assessing motor function, consider the preinjury level of function. In some cases, weakness or motor deficits may be due to prior injuries or medical problems. For this reason, you should perform a careful review of the patient's history whenever a patient complains of being weak or unable to move an extremity.

While performing a motor examination, carry out each test with and without resistance because some patients may be too weak to overcome any outside resistance. Also, perform the test on both sides of the body simultaneously so that each extremity can be compared.

A sensory examination should be performed on all patients who have an injury or complaint related to an extremity, assuming that it does not take attention away from a potentially fatal condition. The sensory examination and history should attempt to identify any preexisting deficits in function or other disorders, including diabetes and nerve disorders that may cause changes in sensation. It is important to assess not only for the presence or absence of sensation, but also for the quality and symmetry of sensation.

To perform a sensory examination, first ask the patient if he or she feels any abnormal sensations, such as numbness, tingling, or burning. Next, conduct a gross sensory examination by lightly touching the injured extremity and the unaffected side simultaneously; have the patient report whether the two sides feel the same or different. In some cases, a patient may complain of an abnormally severe sensation of pain when just lightly touched. Such hyperesthesia may be a sign of an injury to the spinal cord.

To perform a motor function and sensory examination, follow the steps shown in **Skill Drill 25-1 ▶** :

1. Have the patient abduct his or her arms at the elbow to test axillary nerve motor function (**Step 1**).
2. Evaluate the patient's ability to extend the arms at the elbow to test musculocutaneous nerve motor function (**Step 2**).
3. Have the patient extend the thumbs (thumbs up) to test radial nerve motor function (**Step 3**).
4. Assess the patient's ability to make an "okay" sign to test median nerve motor function (**Step 4**).
5. Check the patient's ability to spread his or her fingers apart to test ulnar nerve motor function (**Step 5**).
6. Instruct the patient to extend his or her legs at the knee to test femoral nerve motor function (**Step 6**).
7. Have the patient plantarflex his or her feet to test tibial nerve motor function (**Step 7**).
8. Assess the patient's ability to dorsiflex the feet to test peroneal nerve motor function (**Step 8**).
9. Check light touch over the lateral surface of the shoulder (over the deltoid) to test axillary nerve sensory function (**Step 9**).
10. Evaluate light touch on the anterolateral surface of the forearm to test musculocutaneous nerve sensory function (**Step 10**).
11. Assess light touch on the dorsal surface of the web space of the thumb to test radial nerve sensory function (**Step 11**).
12. Lightly touch the volar surface of the distal thumb, index, and middle fingers to test median nerve sensory function (**Step 12**).
13. Lightly touch the distal volar surface of the small finger to test ulnar nerve sensory function (**Step 13**).
14. Examine the patient's sense of light touch over the anteromedial surface of the thigh to test femoral nerve sensory function (**Step 14**).
15. Evaluate light touch on the plantar surface of the toes to test tibial nerve sensory function (**Step 15**).
16. Assess light touch in the web space between the great toe and the second toe to test peroneal nerve sensory function (**Step 16**).

Documentation and Communication

Always document the findings of a neurovascular examination, even if they are normal. When an abnormality is identified, document the specific deficit—for example, the patient was unable to extend the thumb or the wrist.

Skill Drill 25-1: Performing a Motor Function and Sensory Examination

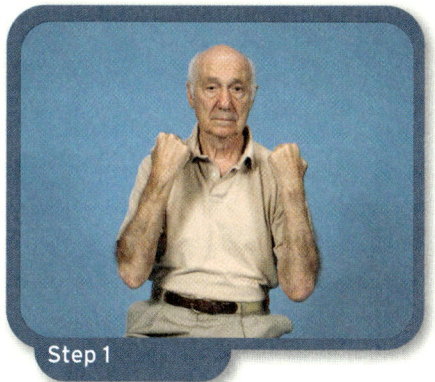

Step 1

Have the patient flex his or her arms at the elbow.

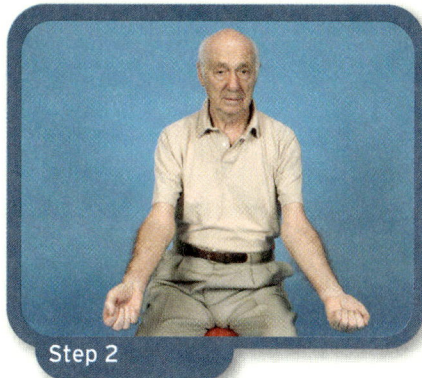

Step 2

Have the patient extend the arms at the elbow.

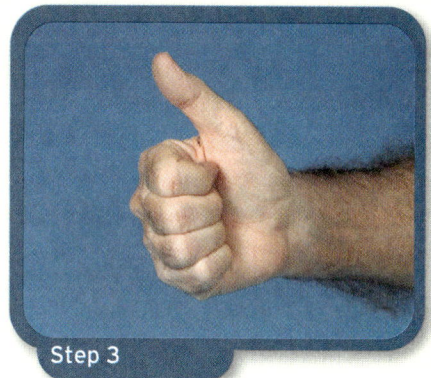

Step 3

Have the patient extend the thumbs (thumbs up).

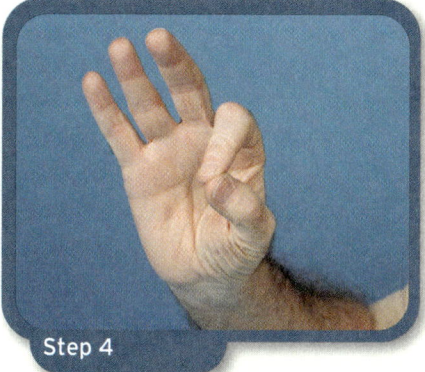

Step 4

Have the patient make an "okay" sign.

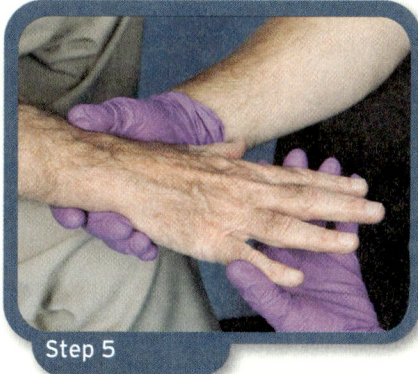

Step 5

Have the patient spread his or her fingers apart.

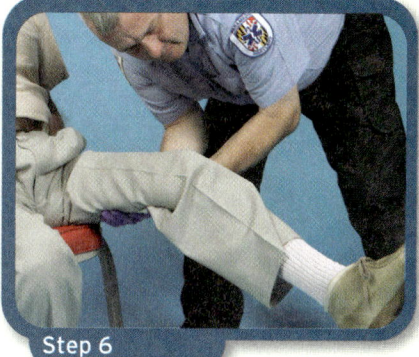

Step 6

Instruct the patient to extend his or her leg at the knee.

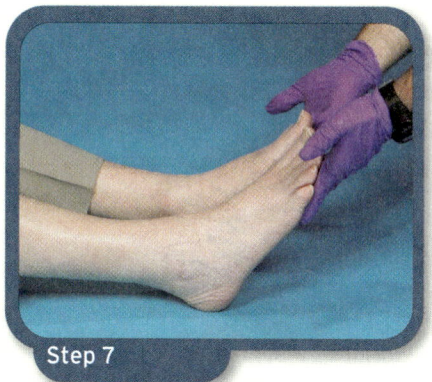

Step 7

Have the patient flex his or her feet and ankles downward.

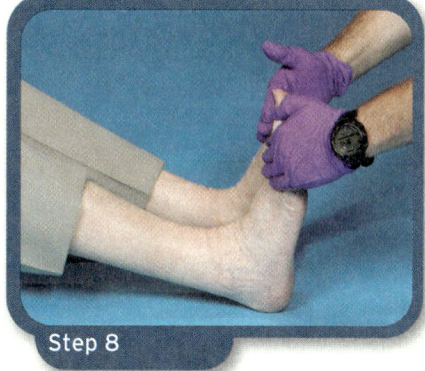

Step 8

Instruct the patient to flex the ankles upward.

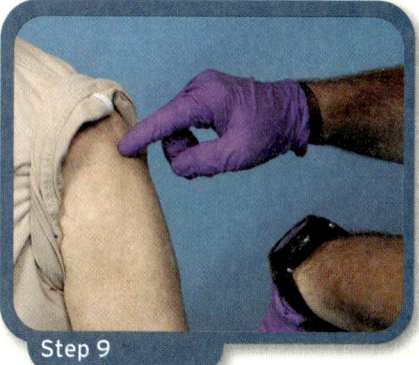

Step 9

Check light touch over the lateral surface of the shoulder (over the deltoid).

Skill Drill 25-1: Performing a Motor Function and Sensory Examination (*continued*)

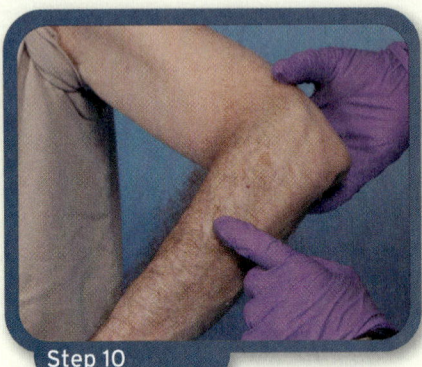

Step 10

Evaluate light touch on the anterolateral surface of the forearm.

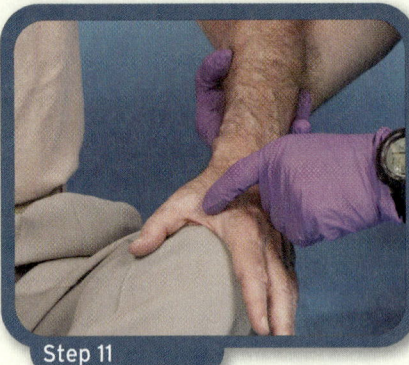

Step 11

Assess light touch on the dorsal surface of the web space of the thumb.

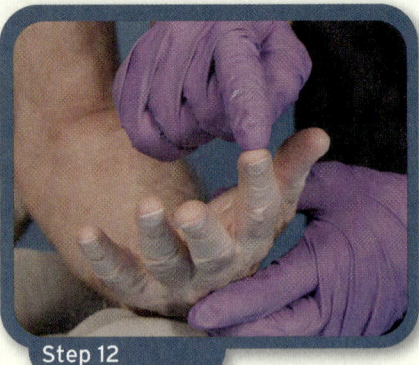

Step 12

Lightly touch the volar surface of the distal thumb, index, and middle fingers.

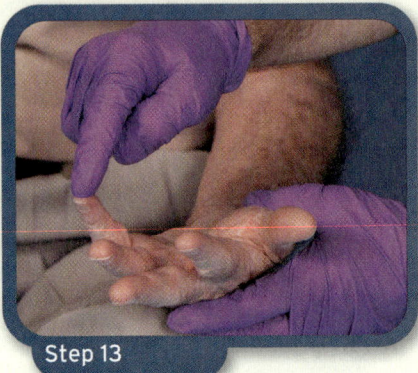

Step 13

Lightly touch the distal volar surface of the small finger.

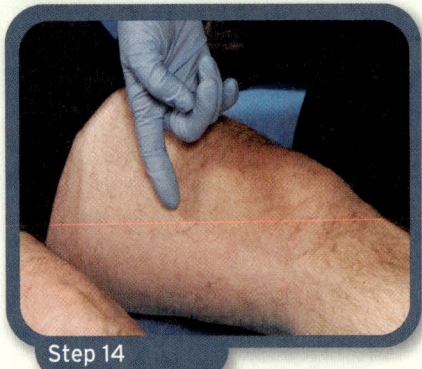

Step 14

Examine the patient's sense of light touch over the anteromedial surface of the thigh.

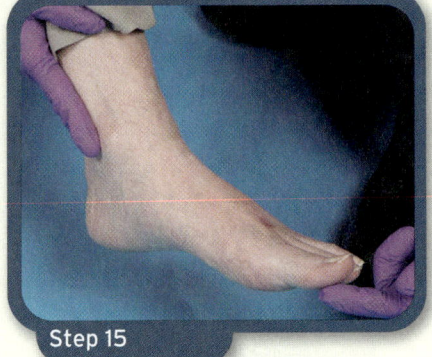

Step 15

Evaluate light touch on the plantar surface of the toes.

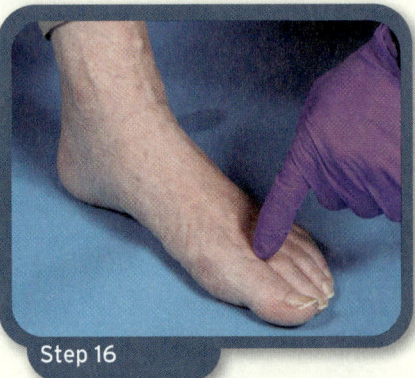

Step 16

Assess light touch in the web space between the great toe and the second toe.

General Interventions

The overall goal in the treatment of a musculoskeletal injury is to identify the type and extent of the injury and to create a biological environment that maximizes the normal healing process of the injured structure. This process begins in the prehospital environment with a thorough assessment of the patient and proper immobilization of injuries to prevent further harm.

Pain Control

A patient who has sustained a musculoskeletal injury may experience pain for a number of reasons. Pain may be caused by a fracture or continued movement of an unstable fracture, muscle spasm, soft-tissue injury, nerve injury, or muscle ischemia. Orthopedic injuries are often extremely painful, so the goal of prehospital pain control should be to diminish the patient's pain to a tolerable level.

A number of interventions may be performed in the prehospital setting to control pain from a musculoskeletal injury. The first step is to assess the level of pain. Establishing a baseline level of pain and reassessing it after each intervention allows you to determine the effectiveness of the treatment being provided. Simple methods for controlling pain include splinting, resting and elevating the injured part, and applying ice or heat packs.

When simple procedures do not effectively control a patient's pain, consider the administration of an analgesic or antispasmodic agent. Analgesics used in the prehospital environment include narcotics, such as fentanyl and morphine, and nitrous oxide; antispasmodic agents include diazepam and lorazepam. These agents should be reserved for patients in hemodynamically stable condition who have an isolated musculoskeletal injury. It is important to obtain vital signs before and after administering any medication for pain and spasm and to monitor the patient's respiratory status for signs of respiratory depression. After pain medication is administered, reassess the patient's pain to ensure that pain relief is adequate.

Administering pain medication before splinting may allow the extremity to be immobilized more effectively. Remember, *it hurts* to have an injured extremity held in the proper position for splinting. Pain medication may make it possible for the patient to tolerate that position longer and allow the splint to be applied properly.

Cold and Heat Application

Cold packs are useful for treating patients during the initial 48 hours following an injury and are very effective at decreasing pain and swelling. Cooling the injured area causes vasoconstriction of the blood vessels in the region and decreases the release of inflammatory mediators. As a result, swelling and inflammation are reduced when ice packs are used during the acute stage of an injury.

Conversely, heat therapy should not be used during the initial 48 to 72 hours following an injury because it may actually increase pain and swelling during this period. Once the acute

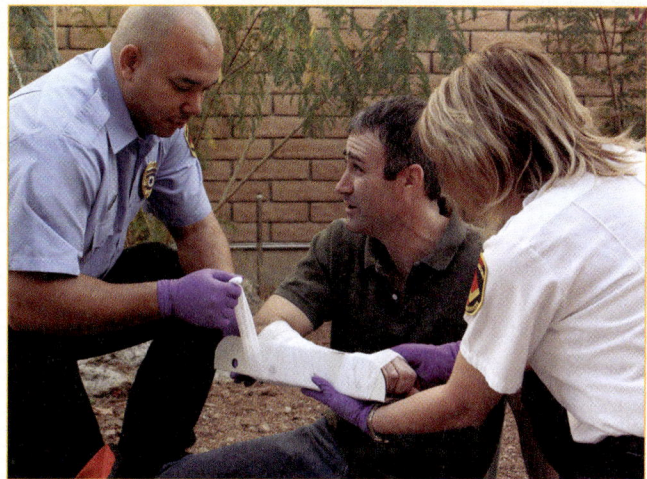

Figure 25-23 Splinting reduces pain and helps prevent additional damage to the extremity.

phase of the injury ends and the damaged blood vessels become clotted, heat is useful for increasing blood flow to the region to decrease stiffness and to promote healing. As a consequence, heat packs may be beneficial for patients who report an injury that occurred several days before contacting paramedics.

Splinting

Splinting is intended to provide support to and prevent motion of the broken bone ends **Figure 25-23 ▲** . Correctly splinting an injured extremity not only decreases the pain a patient experiences, but also reduces the risk of further damage to muscles, nerves, blood vessels, and skin. In addition, splinting helps to control bleeding by allowing clots to form where vessels were damaged.

When a patient with multiple orthopedic injuries must be transported immediately, you will not have time to splint each fracture one by one. The best way to stabilize multiple fractures when the patient's overall condition is critical is to splint the axial skeleton by using a backboard and straps or an alternative device, such as a vacuum mattress. This will serve two purposes: (1) It will protect against a spinal injury. (2) It will reduce the movement of injured extremities by securing them to the board.

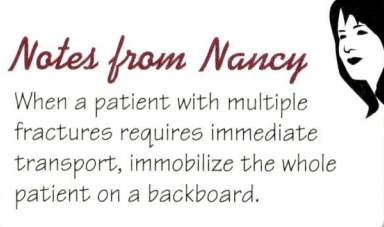

Notes from Nancy

When a patient with multiple fractures requires immediate transport, immobilize the whole patient on a backboard.

Principles of Splinting

Splinting is one of the most crucial skills to learn when caring for patients with musculoskeletal injuries. Failure to properly splint an injured extremity leads to unnecessary discomfort and the possibility of further injury or harm. Allowing a closed fracture in the distal tibia to become an open fracture owing to mishandling or improper splinting will result in the need for surgery and a hospital stay and may increase the patient's complication rate and rehabilitation time. Keep the following points in mind when applying a splint:

1. The injured area must be adequately visualized before splinting. Remove clothing as necessary so that you can inspect the area thoroughly.

2. Assess and *record* distal PMS functions before and after splinting.

3. Cover all wounds with a dry, sterile dressing before applying the splint. Do not attempt to push exposed bone ends back under the skin.

4. Do not move the patient before splinting unless an immediate hazard exists.

5. *For fractures,* the splint must immobilize the bone ends and the two adjacent joints. *For dislocations,* the splint must extend along the entire length of the bone above and the entire length of the bone below the dislocated joint.

6. Pad the splint well to prevent local pressure and to provide optimal motion restriction.

7. Support the injured site manually with one hand above and one hand below the injury, and minimize movement until the splint is applied and secured.

8. If a long bone fracture is severely angulated, gently apply longitudinal traction (tension) to attempt to realign the bone and improve circulation. Use a smooth, firm grip to apply manual traction, and take care to avoid any sudden, jerky movements of the limb. *Do not attempt to straighten fractures involving joints without first obtaining medical direction.* In fact, there is no need to straighten or manipulate the joint unless it has no distal pulse.

9. Splint the knee straight if not directly injured and angulated; splint the elbow at a right angle. (The patient may not be able to tolerate this procedure, and rapid transport should be initiated.)

10. If the patient complains of severe pain or offers resistance to movement, discontinue applying traction, splint in the position of deformity, and carefully monitor the distal neurovascular status (PMS).

11. Splint firmly, but not so tightly as to occlude the distal circulation.

12. If possible, do not cover fingers and toes with the splint to allow for monitoring of skin CTC (colour, temperature, and condition).

Notes from Nancy

Always check the pulses, strength, and sensation distal to a musculoskeletal injury.

13. If possible, apply cold packs and elevate the splinted limb to minimize swelling.

14. When the patient has a life-threatening injury, individual splint application for possible fractures must not delay transportation and might not be accomplished.

Documentation and Communication

Document the neurovascular examination and distal PMS functions before and after splinting.

Types of Splints

Any device used to immobilize a fracture or dislocation is considered a splint. Commercially available splints include board splints, inflatable or vacuum splints, and traction splints. Lack of a commercially made splint should never prevent proper immobilization of an injured patient; multiple casualties may tax the resources of even the best-equipped ambulance, requiring improvisation.

Rigid Splints

A rigid splint is any inflexible device that may be attached to a limb to maintain stability—a padded board, a piece of heavy cardboard, or an aluminum "ladder" or SAM splint moulded to fit the extremity. More elaborate rigid splints are designed to quickly fit around two or three sides of an extremity and be secured with Velcro straps or cravats. Some rigid splints are made of a radiolucent material that allows radiographs to be obtained without removal of the splint. Whatever its construction, the splint must be generously padded to ensure even pressure along the extremity and long enough to be secured well above and below the fracture site (beyond the proximal and distal joints).

When applying a rigid splint, grasp the extremity above and below the fracture site, and apply gentle traction. Another paramedic should then place the splint alongside the limb. While one paramedic maintains traction, the other wraps the limb and splint in self-adhering bandages that are tight enough to hold the splint firmly to the extremity but not so tight as to occlude circulation **Figure 25-24 ▾** . (If the splint has its

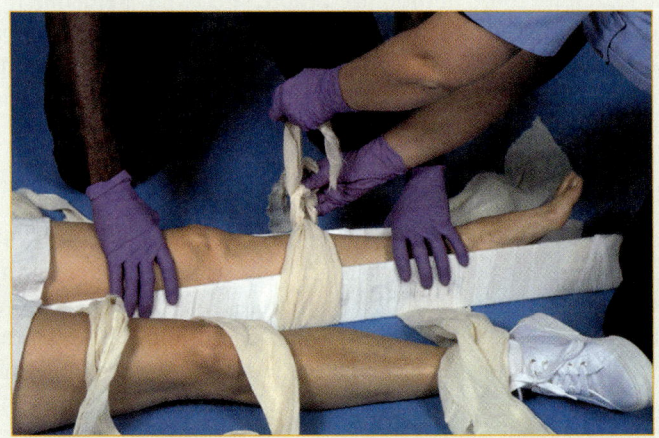

Figure 25-24 In applying a rigid splint, wrap the limb and splint so that the splint is firmly in place but does not cut off circulation.

own straps that are used to secure it to the extremity, this step is not required.) Leave the fingers or toes out of the bandage so that distal circulation can be monitored.

Sling and Swath

An arm sling may be fashioned from a triangular bandage and is useful to immobilize injuries that involve the shoulder or as an adjunct to a rigid splint of the upper extremity. The sling holds the injured part against the chest wall and takes some of the weight off the injured area.

To apply a sling, place the splinted extremity in a comfortable position across the chest and lay the long edge of a triangular bandage along the patient's side opposite the injury. Bring the bottom edge of the bandage up and over the forearm, and tie it *at the side* of the neck to the other end. Tie or pin the pointed end of the sling, at the elbow, to form a cradle. Secure the sling so that the hand is carried higher than the elbow and the fingers are visible for checking peripheral circulation (**Figure 25-25 ▾**).

An arm that is splinted with a sling can be further immobilized by adding a swath. Create a swath by using one or more triangular bandages to secure the arm firmly to the chest wall. This technique is particularly useful for injuries to the clavicle

and for anterior dislocations of the shoulder. Do not use a sling if the patient has a neck injury.

Pneumatic Splints

Pneumatic splints (also known as air splints or inflatable splints) are useful for immobilizing fractures involving the lower leg or forearm. They are not effective for angulated fractures or for fractures that involve a joint because they will forcefully attempt to straighten the fracture or joint. Likewise, air splints should not be used on open fractures in which the bone ends are exposed.

Air splints offer two distinct advantages: They can help slow bleeding and minimize swelling by applying pressure over fracture sites to decrease small-vessel bleeding. For injuries involving the pelvis or femur, the pneumatic antishock garment (PASG) may be used as an air splint and can potentially tamponade bleeding from larger vessels (see Chapter 18). If a PASG is used for this purpose, it is necessary to use high pressure in the device (106 mm Hg or until the pop-off valves for the compartments blow off).

The method of application for an air splint depends on whether it is equipped with a zipper. If it is not, gather the splint on your own arm so that its proximal edge is just above your wrist. Grasp the patient's hand or foot while an assistant maintains proximal countertraction, then slide the air splint over your hand and onto the patient's extremity. Position the air splint so that it is free of wrinkles. Then, while you continue to maintain traction, instruct your assistant to inflate the splint with a commercially available device that is compatible with the splint system—do *not* use a compressed air tank to inflate an air splint. If the air splint has a zipper, apply it to the injured area while an assistant maintains traction proximally and distally; then zip it up and inflate (**Figure 25-26 ▾**). In either case, inflate the splint just to the point at which finger pressure will make a slight dent in the splint's surface.

You must watch air splints carefully to ensure that they do not lose pressure or become overinflated. Overinflation is particularly

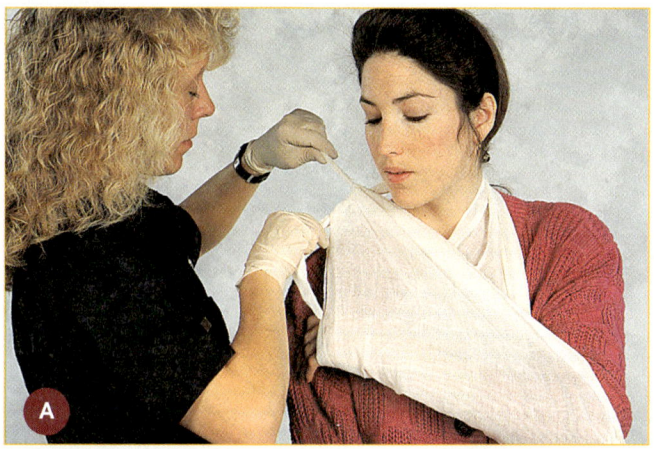
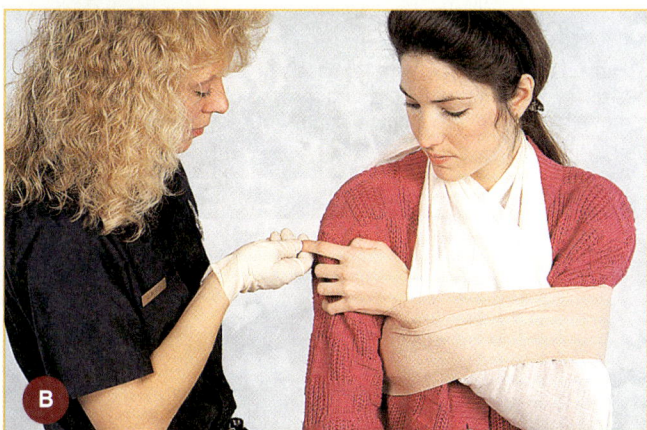

Figure 25-25 **A.** Apply the sling so that the knot is tied at one side of the neck. **B.** Secure the sling. Leave the fingers exposed to allow for circulation checks.

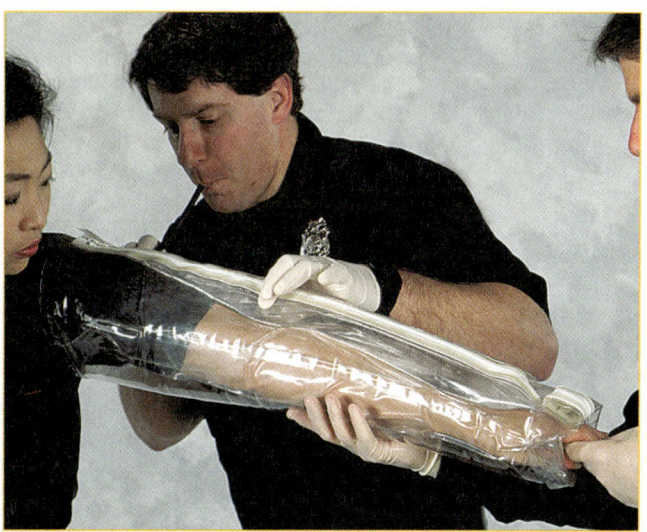

Figure 25-26 Positioning an air splint that features a zipper.

likely when the splint is applied in a cold area and the patient is subsequently moved to a warmer area because the air inside the splint will expand as it gets warmer. Air splints will also expand when going to a higher altitude if the patient compartment is unpressurized, a factor that must be considered when patients are transported by air ambulance.

Vacuum Splints

A vacuum splint consists of a sealed mattress that is filled with air and thousands of small plastic beads. The mattress is laid out on the stretcher, and the patient is placed on top of it and allowed to settle into a comfortable position. A suction pump attached to the mattress is then used to evacuate the air from inside the mattress. The resulting vacuum inside the mattress compresses the beads in such a way that the whole splint becomes rigid, much like a plaster cast that has been moulded to conform to the contours of the patient's entire posterior surface.

The vacuum mattress is an excellent splint, but there are a few factors that may limit its broad appeal. The splint is quite bulky, so it not only takes up a lot of storage room in the vehicle, but also can be difficult to work with in cramped quarters. Furthermore, like all vacuum splints, it requires a mechanical suction pump, yet another piece of equipment to grab.

A smaller vacuum splint is available to splint individual limbs. This type of splint is applied by positioning the injured limb on the splint and then evacuating the air from inside of it. The result is a splint that is moulded to the extremity (Figure 25-27 ▶). This type of vacuum splint requires less space than a mattress-style vacuum splint but is still relatively expensive compared with standard rigid splints.

Pillow Splints

A pillow is an effective means to immobilize an injured foot or ankle. Simply mould an ordinary pillow around the affected foot and ankle in a position of comfort, then secure the pillow in place with several cravats. Pillows can also be moulded around an injured knee or elbow and are invaluable for padding backboards when they are used to immobilize patients with dislocated hips.

Special Considerations

Because vacuum mattresses conform to the body, they may be the best choice to immobilize older patients who have abnormal curvatures of the spine and are suspected of having spinal column injuries.

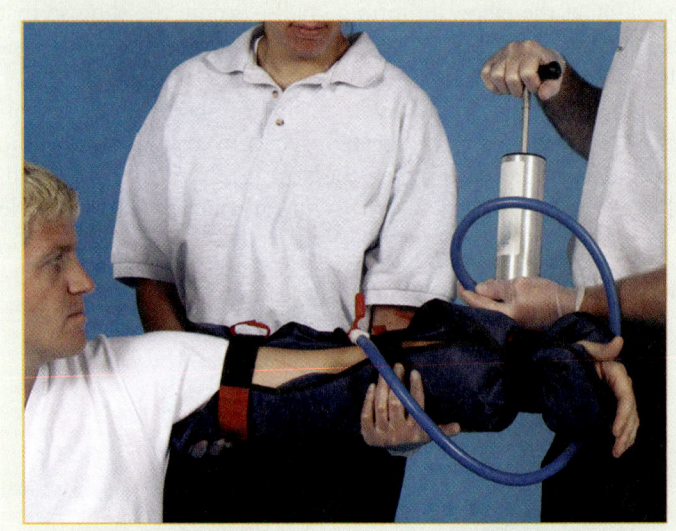

Figure 25-27 Applying a vacuum splint to a limb.

You are the Paramedic Part 3

You have assessed the patient's airway, breathing, and circulation and have controlled significant bleeding found on the left arm. During this time, your partner has inserted a large-bore IV cannula in the right arm.

As you continue your rapid trauma examination, you find that the left pedal pulse is absent. When you expose the leg, you see significant deformity of the knee consistent with a posterior dislocation. The patient has difficulty feeling his foot and moving his toes. This is a true emergency. With your patient immobilized on the backboard, you decide to move him to the ambulance as per your local protocols.

Reassessment	Recording Time: 7 Minutes
Skin	Pink, warm, and slightly moist; pale and cool left foot
Pulse	110 beats/min, full and regular
Blood pressure	144/92 mm Hg
Respirations	40 breaths/min
Spo₂	100% on 15 l/min via nonrebreathing mask
ECG	Sinus tachycardia with no ectopy

6. Why would this dislocation be considered a true emergency?

7. What is an important consideration before manipulating a dislocation?

Traction Splints

Following a femur fracture, the strong muscles of the thigh go into spasm and this often leads to significant pain and deformity. Traction splints provide constant pull on a fractured femur, thereby preventing the broken bone ends from overriding as a result of unopposed muscle contraction. In addition, these splints help maintain alignment of the fracture pieces and provide effective immobilization of the fracture site. As a result, patients are likely to experience less pain.

Traction splints also reduce blood loss. Normally, the thigh is shaped like a cylinder. In a femur fracture, the thigh is shortened and becomes spherical. The volume of a sphere can be substantially greater than that of a cylinder, so a person with an untreated femur fracture can accumulate more blood in the thigh than a person whose thigh is pulled out to length by a traction splint.

Traction splints are indicated for the treatment of most femur fractures. They should not be used when the patient has an additional fracture below the knee on the same extremity. The most commonly used traction splints are the Sager and the Hare traction splints. The basic principles of application are the same for both. After assessing the injured extremity for distal PMS functions, place the splint next to the uninjured leg to determine the proper length. The traction splint should extend 15 cm to 20 cm beyond the foot.

Support and stabilize the leg to minimize movement while another rescuer applies the ankle hitch. When the hitch is secure, the second rescuer will apply gentle longitudinal traction using enough force to realign the extremity. The initial rescuer can then place the splint into position and connect the upper attachment point of the splint and then the ankle hitch **Figure 25-28 ▾**. After applying the splint, reassess PMS functions before securing the patient and splint for transport.

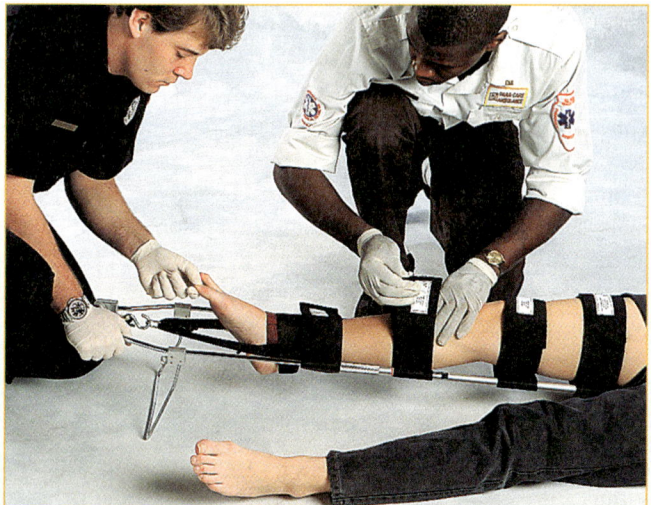

Figure 25-28 A Hare traction splint is shown here. One rescuer connects the straps and another checks distal pulse, motor function, and sensation.

Buddy Splinting

Buddy splinting is used to splint injuries that involve the fingers or toes. With this technique, an adjacent uninjured finger or toe serves as a splint to the injured one. To buddy splint, tape the injured digit to an uninjured one. Place a gauze pad between the digits that are taped together, and ensure that the tape does not pass over joints.

Complications of Musculoskeletal Injuries

Musculoskeletal injuries can lead to numerous complications—not just those involving the musculoskeletal system, but also systemic changes or illness. It is essential to not focus all of your attention on the musculoskeletal injury: Keep in mind that there is a patient attached to the injured extremity!

The likelihood of having a complication is often related to the strength of the force that caused the injury, the injury's location, and the patient's overall health. Any injury to a bone, muscle, or other musculoskeletal structure is likely to be accompanied by bleeding. In general, the greater the force that caused the injury, the greater the hemorrhage that will be associated with it.

Following a fracture, the sharp ends of the bone may damage muscles, blood vessels, arteries, and nerves, or the ends may penetrate the skin and produce an open fracture. A significant loss of tissue may occur at the fracture site if the muscle is severely damaged or if the bone's penetration of the skin causes a large defect. To prevent infection following an open fracture, you should brush away any obvious debris on the skin surrounding an open fracture before applying a dressing. Do not enter or probe the open fracture site in an attempt to retrieve debris because this may lead to further contamination.

Long-term disability is one of the most devastating consequences of a musculoskeletal injury. In many cases, a severely injured limb can be repaired and made to look almost normal. Unfortunately, many patients cannot return to work for long periods because of the extensive rehabilitation required and because of chronic pain. Paramedics have a critical role in mitigating the risk of long-term disability. By preventing further injury, reducing the risk of wound infection, minimizing pain by the use of cold and analgesia, and transporting patients with musculoskeletal injuries to an appropriate medical facility, they help reduce the risk or duration of long-term disability.

Neurovascular Injuries

The skeletal system normally protects the neurovascular structures within the limbs from injury. These critical structures typically lie deep within the limb and close to the skeleton. For example, the brachial plexus is situated within the axilla and the inner aspect of the arm, shielded from injury by the shoulder girdle. When the shoulder girdle or proximal humerus is fractured, displaced fracture fragments may lacerate or impale the nerves of the plexus, leading to a neurologic deficit. Neurovascular injuries are also likely to occur following a joint dislocation because the nerves and vessels in the region of a joint tend to be more securely tethered to the soft tissues and are less likely to escape injury.

Compartment Syndrome

Within a limb, groups of muscles are surrounded by an inelastic membrane called fascia. Thus, the muscles are confined to an enclosed space, or compartment, that can accommodate only a limited amount of swelling. When bleeding or swelling occurs within a compartment as the result of a fracture or severe soft-tissue injury, the pressure within it rises. Too-high pressure may impair circulation and lead to pain, sensory changes, and progressive muscle death. This condition, known as compartment syndrome, is one of the most devastating consequences of a musculoskeletal injury.

External and internal factors can lead to the development of compartment syndrome. External factors include bandages, splints or casts that are applied too tightly and restrict circulation. A number of internal factors can also increase the amount of material within a compartment. For example, bleeding within a compartment may occur because of a fracture, dislocation, crush injury, vascular injury, soft-tissue injury, or bleeding disorder. Alternatively, fluid leakage or edema may occur secondary to ischemia, excessive exercise, trauma, burns, or any condition associated with the leakage of proteins and fluid from vessels into the interstitial space. A common misconception is that open fractures are safe from compartment syndrome—a notion that is not true.

Signs and symptoms of compartment syndrome include early and late findings. Typically, the first complaint will be of a searing or burning *pain* that is localized to the involved compartment and out of proportion to the injury. This pain is often severe and typically not relieved with pain medication, including narcotics. When examining the patient, passive stretching of an ischemic muscle will result in severe pain. In the lower extremities, test for this condition by flexing and extending the great toe and by dorsiflexion and plantar flexion of the foot. In the upper extremity, use finger and hand flexion and extension.

During examination of the patient, the affected area may feel very firm and there may be skin pallor. Typical neurologic changes include paresthesias, such as a burning sensation, numbness, or tingling, and paralysis of the involved muscles, which occurs late in the condition. Another late sign of compartment syndrome is pulselessness. By the time the pressure within the compartment reaches the point where it totally occludes the artery passing through it, significant muscle necrosis has probably occurred.

The goal of prehospital care is to deliver the patient to an emergency facility before the extremity is pulseless. Thus, management should include elevating the extremity to heart level (*not above!*), placing ice packs over the extremity, and opening or loosening constrictive clothing and splint material.

Crush Syndrome

Crush syndrome occurs because of a prolonged or severe compressive force that impairs muscle metabolism and circulation—actually, following the extrication or release of an entrapped limb. This condition happens not only in trauma patients, but also in patients who have been lying on an extremity for an extended period (4–6 hours of compression)—for example, when a drug overdose or stroke victim is not found for an extended period.

After severe or prolonged compression, the muscle cells begin to die and release their contents into the localized vasculature. When the force compressing the region is released, blood flow is reestablished and the material from the cells that was released into the local vasculature quickly enters the systemic vasculature. The primary substances that are of concern are lactic acid, potassium, and myoglobin. In particular, the return of myoglobin is likely to result in decreased blood pH, hyperkalemia, and renal dysfunction.

Treatment of crush syndrome, which aims to prevent complications due to toxin release, should always be performed with medical direction. A number of steps must be taken *before* releasing the compressing force. As with all patients, assess the ABCs in case of suspected crush syndrome. Ensure that the patient is being given high-flow supplemental oxygen, and then administer a bolus of crystalloid solution to increase the intravascular volume and to protect the kidneys from the forthcoming myoglobin load. Establish cardiac monitoring to evaluate for electrocardiographic (ECG) changes related to hyperkalemia (such as peaked T waves, widening QRS complex, prolonged P-R interval, dysrhythmia). To protect against the surge of potassium, a nebulizer treatment with salbutamol may be given during extrication (beta-2 agonists promote the movement of potassium into cells). Once the patient is freed, if the ECG shows changes consistent with hyperkalemia, administer calcium to stabilize the myocardium; also give sodium bicarbonate to promote the intracellular shift of potassium. Insulin may also be given intravenously with dextrose, in the hospital, to facilitate the intracellular movement of potassium. Compressive devices should not be applied.

Thromboembolic Disease

Thromboembolic disease, including deep vein thrombosis (DVT) and pulmonary embolism, is a significant cause of death following musculoskeletal injuries, especially injuries to the pelvis and lower extremities that lead to prolonged immobilization.

Signs and symptoms of DVT include disproportionate swelling of an extremity, discomfort in an extremity that worsens with use, and warmth and erythema of the extremity. When

At the Scene

A patient who shows evidence of compartment syndrome must be transported on an emergency basis to the hospital. There is no treatment for this syndrome other than surgery—do not delay transport.

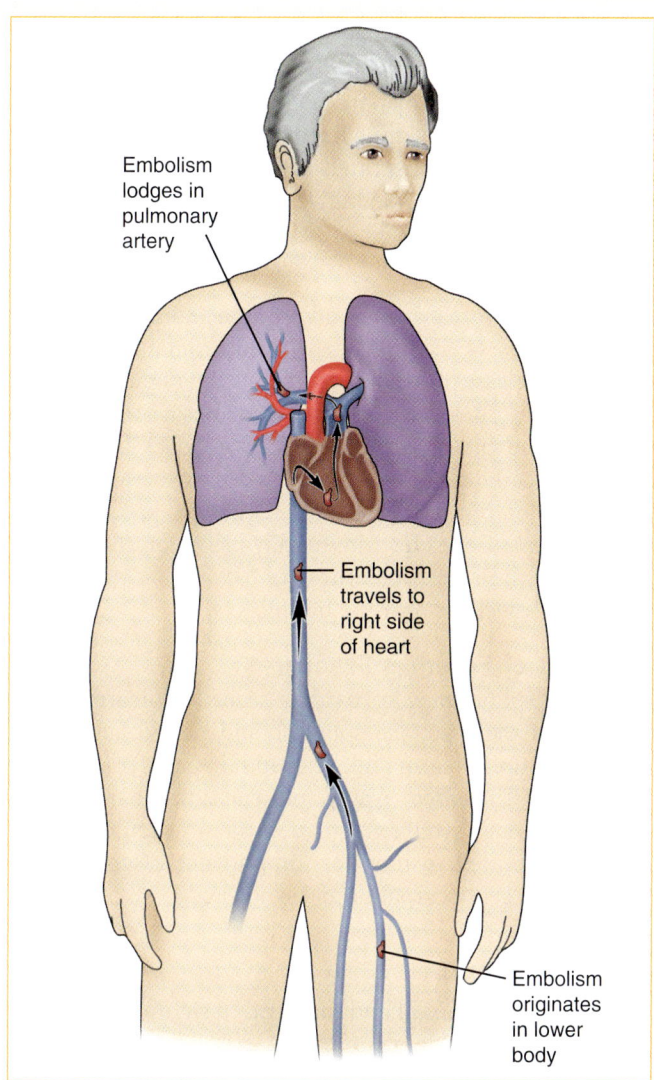

Figure 25-29 When a portion of a DVT dislodges, it may travel to the pulmonary arteries and inhibit blood flow from the heart to the lungs.

a portion of a DVT dislodges, it may cause a pulmonary embolism—a blood clot that travels to and occludes a portion or all of the pulmonary arteries **Figure 25-29** . Signs and symptoms of a pulmonary embolism include a sudden onset of dyspnea, pleuritic chest pain, dyspnea, tachypnea, tachycardia, right-sided heart failure, shock, and, in some cases, cardiac arrest.

In addition to the risk of DVT, patients with long bone or pelvic fractures are at risk for developing a fat embolism. In this condition, fat droplets enter the circulation and become lodged in the vasculature of the lungs. Affected patients have inflammation of the vasculature of the lungs and other blood vessels where fat is deposited. Generally, symptoms begin within 12 to 72 hours of injury; they include tachycardia, dyspnea, tachypnea, pulmonary congestion, fever, petechiae, change in mental status, and organ dysfunction.

Treatment for thromboembolic disease in the prehospital setting is limited to maintaining an airway, adequate oxygenation, and intravascular volume and rapid transportation to an ED.

Specific Fractures

Shoulder Girdle

The shoulder girdle consists of the clavicle, shoulder, and scapula.

Clavicle

Clavicle fractures are very common and often occur in children. In most cases, the clavicle fractures in the middle third of the bone, typically from a fall onto an outstretched hand or from direct lateral trauma to the shoulder (as in contact sports, snowboarding, and cycling). Patients have pain in the region of the shoulder, swelling, unwillingness to raise the arm, and tilting of the head toward the injured side.

Shoulder

Fractures of the shoulder include those that involve the glenoid fossa of the scapula, the humeral head, and the humeral neck. Most shoulder fractures are caused by a fall onto an outstretched hand and usually occur in elderly patients (younger patients tend to dislocate the shoulder because they have stronger bones). Patients with a shoulder fracture rarely have evidence of a significant deformity, but instead have considerable swelling, ecchymosis, and pain with movement of the arm. In some cases, an associated injury to the brachial plexus may be identified during the neurologic examination.

Scapula

Injuries to the scapula usually result from violent, direct trauma. Therefore, when a scapular injury is suspected, it is essential to look for associated injuries—particularly intrathoracic injuries, such as pneumothorax, hemothorax, and fractured ribs. Signs and symptoms of a scapular fracture include pain that increases with arm abduction and swelling in the region of the scapula. Potential complications include axillary artery or nerve injury, brachial plexus injury, pulmonary contusion, and clavicle fractures.

Treatment of Shoulder Girdle Fractures

Fractures in the shoulder region may usually be treated by using a sling and swath. These bindings should be applied to maintain the extremity in the position of comfort, keeping the arm against the chest wall to allow the body to act as a splint. In cases of suspected scapula fractures, full spinal immobilization is usually warranted given the amount of force required to cause a fracture.

Midshaft Humerus

Fractures of the shaft of the humerus usually occur in younger patients secondary to high-energy injuries, such as motor vehicle collisions. Unlike fractures that occur more proximally, these injuries typically have substantial deformity. Examination of the extremity usually reveals a significant amount of swelling, ecchymosis, gross instability of the region, and crepitus. If the force that caused the injury is severe enough, the nerves and blood vessels in the upper arm may also be damaged. Of particular concern is the radial nerve, which may be injured by the force itself or could become entrapped within the fracture site. The classic sign of a radial nerve injury is wrist drop.

Treatment of Midshaft Humerus Fractures

If the fracture is angulated, longitudinal traction may be applied to correct the deformity, but efforts should be halted if the patient's pain is too severe or if neurovascular status worsens. Once the extremity is in the desired position, apply a rigid splint that extends from the axilla to the elbow. Next, apply a sling and swath to immobilize the arm to the chest wall, and place cold packs over the fracture site to decrease the patient's pain and swelling.

Elbow

Distal Humerus

Supracondylar fractures of the humerus occur most often in children. The typical mechanism is a fall onto an outstretched hand with the elbow in extension, thereby breaking the distal humerus; as a result, the distal fragment of the humerus is pushed posteriorly and the humeral shaft is pulled anteriorly, where it compresses the brachial artery and the radial and median nerves. If the brachial artery is compromised, the patient could develop compartment syndrome in the forearm. When this complication occurs, the patient is at risk for a Volkmann ischemic contracture, a condition in which muscles of the forearm degenerate from prolonged ischemia. The patient's muscles that allow for movement of the fingers become contracted and nonfunctional, and the patient loses the ability to use the hand. Patients with a distal humerus fracture will complain of pain in the area of the elbow and typically have a significant degree of swelling and ecchymosis.

Proximal Radius and Ulna

Radial head fractures may result from a fall onto an outstretched hand or from a direct blow to the bone. This injury causes the patient to have significant pain when he or she attempts supination or pronation. In either case, the patient is likely to have pain and ecchymosis in the region of the injury. Similar to distal humerus fractures, these injuries may lead to an injury of the nerves or blood vessels in proximity to the fracture site. Therefore, a careful neurovascular examination should be performed.

Treatment of Elbow Fractures

Treatment of injuries in the region of the elbow is the same regardless of the exact location of the injury. The injured extremity must be repeatedly assessed for evidence of compartment syndrome. Before splinting the extremity, it is mandatory to document a neurovascular examination. The injured extremity should be splinted in the position that it is found if

the patient has a strong distal pulse, and ice packs should be used only if there is no evidence of compartment syndrome. If the patient has an absent distal pulse or neurologic deficits, consult with the appropriate medical facility to determine whether you should attempt fracture reduction. In any event, the patient must be transported urgently to the closest appropriate medical facility for definitive treatment.

Forearm

Fractures of the forearm may involve the radius, the ulna, or, more commonly, both. Injury may result from a direct blow to the bone, the classic example of which is the nightstick fracture of the ulna. In other cases, injury occurs because of a fall onto an outstretched hand, as in the case of a Colles fracture. This fracture typically occurs in older patients with osteoporosis who have fallen but may be found in younger patients as well. A patient with a Colles fracture usually has a dorsally angulated deformity of the distal forearm (the "dinner fork deformity") and pain and swelling near the injured site.

Treatment of Forearm Fractures

A variety of splints may be used to secure a forearm fracture. Regardless of the type, the splint should provide immobilization of the entire forearm and wrist and, in cases of more proximal fractures, the elbow. Apply cold packs to the injury site to decrease pain and swelling. Frequent neurovascular examinations are warranted to monitor for evidence of compartment syndrome and acute carpal tunnel syndrome.

Wrist and Hand

Injuries to the wrist and hand may lead to significant long-term disability, especially in people who rely on the use of their hands to earn a living. Sometimes these injuries occur while working; in other cases they result from a fall or during a sporting event. Careful splinting of the injured site is essential to help reduce the risk of long-term disability.

Scaphoid

The scaphoid, also called the carpal navicular, is located just distal to the radius. It may be injured from a fall onto an outstretched hand, for which the classic finding is pain and tenderness in the anatomical snuffbox. To identify the anatomical snuffbox on yourself, extend your thumb. Two tendons will be visible at the base of the thumb on the radial aspect of the wrist. The region between these two tendons is the snuffbox **Figure 25-30 ▶** . The major complication of a scaphoid fracture is avascular necrosis of the bone, or poor fracture healing because of the limited blood supply to this bone.

Boxer's Fracture

A boxer's fracture is a fracture of the neck of the fifth metacarpal (small finger). It commonly occurs after punching a hard object, such as a wall or a door. The patient typically has pain over the ulnar aspect of the hand and may have noticeable swelling.

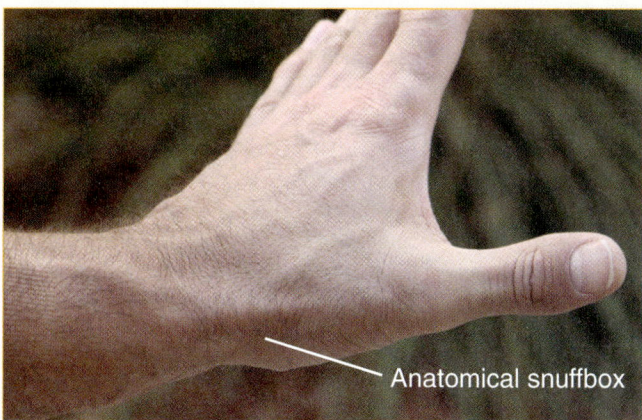

Figure 25-30 The region between the two tendons shown is the anatomical snuffbox.

Metacarpal Shaft

Fractures of the metacarpals may result from a crush injury or from direct trauma. Assessment of the injured hand may reveal abnormal rotation or alignment of the fingers, swelling of the palm, and pain and tenderness in the region of injury. You should assess the neurovascular function of the hand and fingers following a crush injury, because development of compartment syndrome is possible within the hand.

Mallet Finger (Baseball Fracture)

A mallet finger occurs when a finger is jammed into an object, such as a baseball or basketball, resulting in an avulsion fracture of the extensor tendon from the distal phalanx. The patient will not be able to extend the distal phalanx of the finger and will maintain it in a flexed position.

Treatment of Wrist and Hand Fractures

Splint the injured hand in the position of function by placing the wrist in about 30° of dorsiflexion with fingers slightly flexed (a roll of gauze approximately 5 to 10 cm in diameter accomplishes this nicely). Next, secure the extremity to an armboard or other rigid splint that extends proximally to the elbow and is slightly elevated to help reduce swelling **Figure 25-31 ▶**. For injuries that are isolated to the digits, use a foam-padded flexible aluminum splint to splint the injured digit, if available. In the case of penetrating injuries, regardless of whether a fracture is present, apply bulky dressings to the site of injury and splint the injured hand in the position of function.

Pelvis

Pelvic fractures are relatively uncommon injuries, accounting for fewer than 3% of all fractures. Despite their low incidence, these injuries are responsible for a significant number of deaths in blunt trauma patients. The risk of death following a pelvic fracture ranges from 8% to 50%, depending on the severity of the injury; when the fracture is open, the mortality rate rises to 25% to 50%. Death after a pelvic fracture commonly results

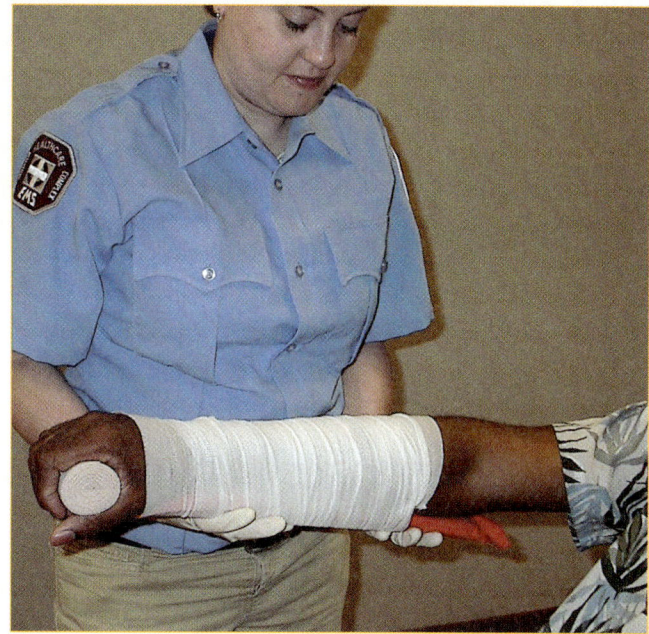

Figure 25-31 Splinting the hand and wrist.

from massive hemorrhage caused by damage to the arteries and veins of the pelvis.

Disruptions of the pelvic ring occur secondary to high-energy trauma such as crush injuries, motorcycle collisions, and falls from a significant height. A number of structures within the pelvis are at risk for injury when it is fractured—the bladder, urethra, rectum, vagina, and sacral nerve plexus. The blood vessels that are most prone to damage are the veins within the pelvis, but there may be damage to the internal or external iliac and arteries in the lumbar region. The nerves at greatest risk of injury are those in the lumbar and sacral regions and the sciatic and femoral nerves.

Patients with pelvic ring disruptions who have a stable injury, such as a minimal lateral compression injury, may complain of pain in the pelvis and difficulty bearing weight. Patients with a more severe injury may show evidence of profound shock, gross pelvic instability, and diffuse pelvic and lower abdominal pain. There may also be bruising or lacerations in the perineum, scrotum, groin, suprapubic region, and flank and hematuria (blood in the urine) or blood coming from the meatus of the penis, vagina, or rectum.

Lateral Compression Pelvic Ring Disruptions

Lateral compression injuries result from an impact on the side of the body (such as being struck by a car from the side or falling from a significant height and landing on one side of the body). The side of the pelvis that sustains the impact becomes internally rotated around the sacrum, and the actual volume within the pelvis decreases **Figure 25-32 ▶**. Although this injury is not commonly associated with massive hemorrhage into the pelvis, it is often associated with injuries in other regions of the body.

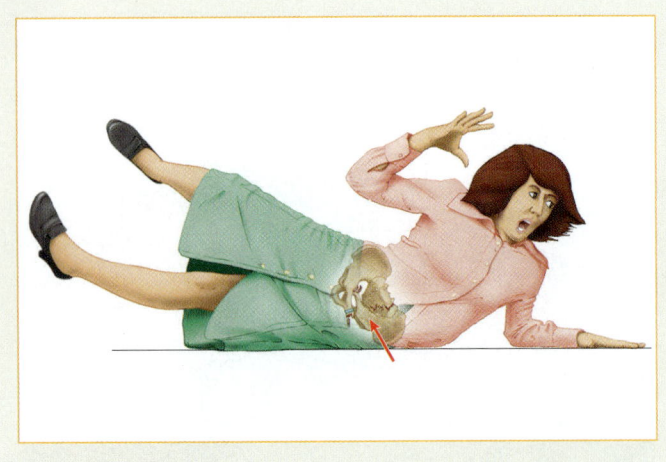

Figure 25-32 A lateral compression injury to the pelvis.

Anterior-Posterior Compression Pelvic Ring Disruptions

These injuries may occur following a head-on motor vehicle collision, motorcycle collision, or in a pedestrian who is struck head-on by a vehicle. The force of the impact compresses the pelvis in the anterior-to-posterior direction, causing the pubic symphysis and posterior supporting ligaments to be disrupted and tear apart. The pelvis then spreads apart and opens like a book—hence the name open book pelvic fracture. Such an injury has the potential for massive blood loss because the volume of the pelvis is greatly increased.

Vertical Shear

Vertical shear injuries occur when a major force is applied to the pelvis from above or below, such as when a person falls from a significant height and lands on the feet. On landing, the force is transmitted through the legs to the pelvis, leading to the complete displacement of one or both sides of the pelvis toward the head. Thus, this kind of injury has anterior and posterior components. The anterior component involves a fracture of the rami or disruption of the symphysis pubis. The posterior component involves a fracture of the ilium or sacrum or a disruption of the sacroiliac joint. The patient is likely to have significant shortening of the limb on the affected side and is at risk for massive hemorrhage into the pelvis.

Straddle Fracture

A straddle fracture occurs after a fall when a person lands in the region of the perineum and sustains bilateral fractures of the inferior and superior rami. This injury does not interfere with weight bearing, but it does carry a risk owing to its associated complications, particularly those of the lower genitourinary system.

Open Pelvic Fractures

Open pelvic fractures are life-threatening injuries. Such an injury is defined by the presence of a laceration of the skin in the pelvic region, vagina, or rectum. This uncommon fracture is caused by a high-velocity injury with subsequent massive hemorrhage and has a mortality rate of 25% to 50%. Even small amounts of blood found during a vaginal or rectal examination should raise your suspicion for an open fracture.

Treatment of Pelvic Fractures

Assessment of the patient with a possible pelvic fracture should begin as in any other trauma patient—with an initial assessment of the mental status, ABCs, and taking spinal precautions. During the rapid trauma examination of the patient, you should search for injuries typically associated with pelvic fractures. Assess the pelvis for bleeding, lacerations, bruising, and instability. To assess for instability, apply pressure over the iliac wings in a medial direction and in a posterior direction. Once instability of the pelvis is identified, the pelvis should not be reassessed for instability to avoid causing increased bleeding.

Treatment should include careful monitoring of the ABCs, spinal immobilization, and IV access with at least one (if not two) large-bore cannulas. Management of the pelvic injury is aimed at reducing the amount of bleeding and decreasing the degree of instability. It is often appropriate to seek medical direction for the management of these patients, especially for determining how to best stabilize the pelvis. Methods used to accomplish this may include application of a PASG or pelvic binder or simply tying a sheet around the pelvis, depending on local protocols. Applying pressure to the iliac wings and forcing them to shift toward the midline reduces the potential space within the pelvis, which may allow for tamponade of the bleeding vessels. Once packaged, the patient should be rapidly transported to a trauma centre, and IV fluid should be administered to maintain adequate tissue perfusion but avoiding hypertension.

Hip

A hip fracture involves a fracture of the femoral head, femoral neck, intertrochanteric region, or proximal femoral shaft. Fractures of the femoral head are uncommon injuries that are usually associated with a hip dislocation. Femoral neck and intertrochanteric fractures typically occur in older patients with osteoporosis who have fallen and sustained direct trauma to the hip. They may occur in younger patients with healthy

At the Scene

Controlling bleeding from a severely injured pelvis is a major challenge, even to the most experienced trauma surgeon. Nevertheless, reducing the volume of an unstable pelvis can decrease bleeding and be a lifesaving intervention. This may be accomplished by using a PASG, depending on local protocols, applying a commercially made pelvic binder, or applying a sheet. When a sheet or pelvic binder is used, place it around the iliac wings and secure it while a paramedic on each side of the patient applies medially directed pressure. Paramedics often make the mistake of placing this device too low on the pelvis, which decreases its effectiveness in reducing the pelvic volume.

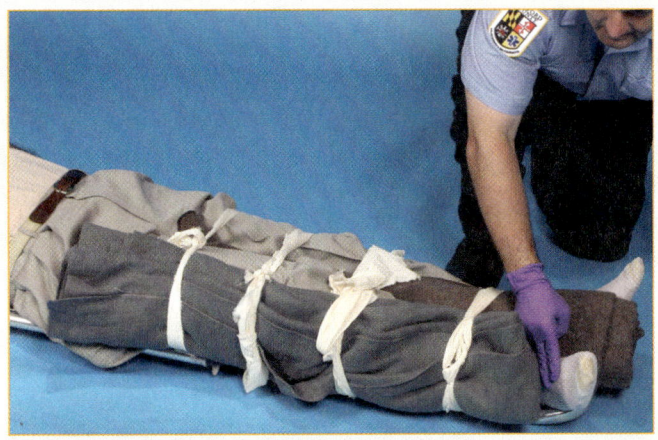

Figure 25-33 An acceptable method for splinting a hip fracture.

bone, typically as the result of a high-energy mechanism. Proximal femoral shaft fractures can occur in patients of any age and result from a high-energy mechanism.

Patients with a hip fracture will complain of pain in the affected hip, especially with attempts at movement, and report an inability to bear weight. They may also report hearing or feeling something snap. If the fracture is displaced, the patient almost always has an externally rotated and shortened leg. If there is no displacement, the leg may appear normal. Examination of the injury site usually finds tenderness to palpation, and there may be noticeable swelling, deformity, or ecchymosis.

Treatment of Hip Fractures

The treatment of hip fractures depends on the mechanism of injury. Hip fractures in older patients who sustained a low-energy injury, such as a fall from a standing position, do not require traction splints. Treat these injuries by supporting the injured extremity in the position in which it is found. This may be accomplished by placing pillows or blankets under the affected extremity and securing them in place **Figure 25-33 ▲** .

In younger patients and in those with high-energy injuries, place the injured extremity in a traction splint to reduce the amount of bleeding. Treat the patient as you would any other trauma patient: Fully immobilize the patient, establish vascular access, monitor for shock, and transport to a trauma centre.

Special Considerations

A hip fracture in an elderly patient can be a debilitating and life-altering injury. In many cases, these injuries occur in the home after slipping on a throw rug, tripping over an object that extends into the walkway, or stumbling because of poor lighting. To help prevent this injury and other fall-related problems, you should point out any safety hazards in the home to the patient or a family member. It takes only a minute, and most patients and families appreciate the advice.

Definitive treatment of a hip fracture almost always requires surgery. If possible, the bone is repaired with plates, rods, or screws. Sometimes, however, the hip must be replaced.

Femoral Shaft

Femoral shaft fractures occur following high-energy impacts. Thus, the presence of a fracture of the femoral shaft should alert you to the risk of other injuries. Patients with femoral shaft fractures will complain of severe pain. The fracture may be severely angulated or lead to significant limb shortening, or it may be open. Examination may identify significant thigh edema, bruising, crepitus, and muscle spasm.

There is often significant blood loss (perhaps 500–1,500 ml) at the fracture site. In addition, damage to the neurovascular structures of the thigh is possible. Femoral shaft fractures also place the patient at risk for fat emboli.

Treatment of Femoral Shaft Fractures

Management of femoral shaft fractures includes monitoring for evidence of shock, full spinal immobilization, and establishing vascular access. Place the injured extremity in a traction splint. Use a PASG, if allowed by local protocols, if further stability and hemorrhage control are needed. Because these injuries may be extremely painful, consider the administration of pain medication.

Knee

Fractures of the knee may involve the distal femur, proximal tibia, or patella. An injury to this region may result from a direct blow to the knee, an axial load of the leg, or powerful contractions of the quadriceps. Assessment of the patient generally reveals significant pain in the knee, decreased range of motion, pain with movement and weight bearing, ecchymosis, swelling, and, in the case of displaced fractures, deformity.

Treatment of Knee Fractures

Management of knee fractures depends on the position of the leg and the status of distal pulses. If the patient has a good distal pulse, splint the extremity in the position that it is found. If there is no distal pulse, seek medical consultation to determine whether you should attempt manipulation before transportation. In all cases, elevate the leg to the heart level and apply cold packs. Frequent neurovascular checks are mandatory, given the high incidence of compartment syndrome and neurovascular injury in cases of knee fracture.

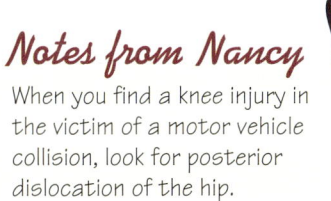

Notes from Nancy

When you find a knee injury in the victim of a motor vehicle collision, look for posterior dislocation of the hip.

Tibia and Fibula

Fractures of the tibia and/or fibula may result from direct trauma to the lower leg or from application of rotational or compressive forces. These injuries often present with significant deformity and soft-tissue injury. Complications may include compartment syndrome, neurovascular injury, infection, poor healing, and chronic pain.

Treatment of Tibia and Fibula Fractures

Apply a rigid, long leg splint, and administer pain medication as necessary. If there is gross angulation, attempt to align the leg after giving pain medication, documenting the premanipulation and postmanipulation neurovascular status. Monitor the patient closely for evidence of compartment syndrome, elevate the extremity to heart level, and apply cold packs.

Ankle

Fractures of the ankle `Figure 25-34` ▸ usually result from sudden and forceful movements of the foot that damage the malleoli and sometimes produce dislocation (called a fracture-dislocation). In other cases, an axial load is transmitted through the foot and causes the talus (the bone of the foot that articulates with the tibia) to impact the distal tibia, leading to a fracture. Signs and symptoms of an ankle fracture include pain, deformity, and swelling. Ankle fractures may lead to damage of the nerves and blood vessels that supply the foot, the development of compartment syndrome, and chronic ankle pain and arthritis.

Treatment of Ankle Fractures

All ankle fractures should be immobilized using a commercially available splint or a pillow splint. The toes should be exposed to allow for frequent checks of distal neurovascular function. Elevate the extremity to the heart level, and apply cold packs to reduce swelling.

If an ankle fracture-dislocation is associated with a pulseless foot, medical direction may recommend that you

attempt reduction. To reduce a fracture-dislocation of the ankle, first relax the calf muscles to allow the foot to move more freely by flexing the patient's leg at the knee. With the leg flexed, grasp the heel and the foot just proximal to the toes and apply gentle traction. Next, rotate the foot back into its normal position without forcing it. If this procedure is successful, reassess the distal neurovascular status and splint the extremity in the reduced position, using care not to allow the ankle to dislocate again. If the fracture-dislocation cannot be reduced, notify direct medical control and expedite

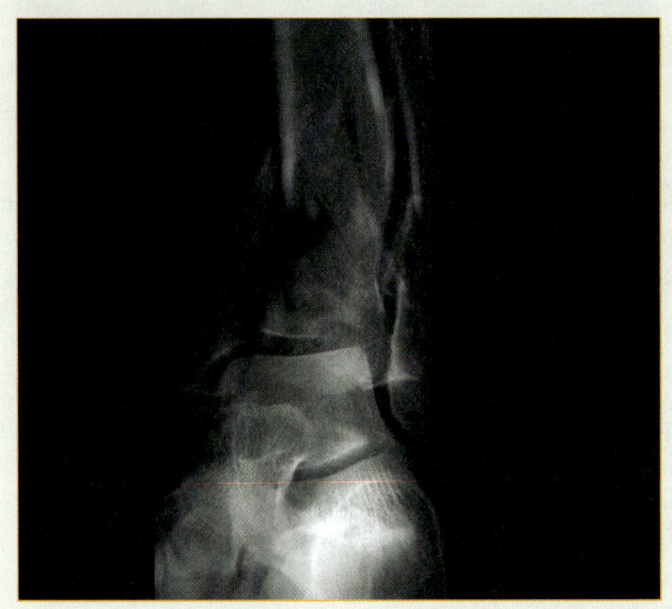

Figure 25-34 A severe fracture of the ankle.

You are the Paramedic Part 4

You have set the IV of normal saline to keep vein open. After consulting with direct medical control, you receive an order to administer 1 mg of midazolam (Versed) and 50 µg of fentanyl to take the edge off the pain and permission to carefully attempt manipulation of the knee to restore its circulation. After movement of the tibia, PMS functions are restored distal to the knee. You carefully splint the leg and notice improvement of local skin signs. You reassess the splint on the left arm and note no changes. The patient tells you his pain is much less, and he thanks you for taking care of him. You place blankets on the patient and continue to monitor him throughout transport.

Reassessment	Recording Time: 15 Minutes
Skin	Pink, warm, and dry
Pulse	90 beats/min, full and regular
Blood pressure	134/76 mm Hg
Respirations	28 breaths/min
Spo$_2$	100% while breathing 10 l/min via nonrebreathing mask
ECG	Sinus rhythm with no ectopy

8. Why should a joint that has just been manipulated be splinted immediately?

9. What facts should be relayed to the emergency department staff in your radio report?

transportation after splinting the ankle in the position in which it was found.

Calcaneus

The calcaneus may be fractured when a patient jumps from a height and lands on the feet or when a powerful force is applied directly to the heel. These injuries present with foot pain, swelling, and ecchymosis and should alert paramedics to the possibility of injuries in the knee, pelvis, and spine.

Treatment of Calcaneus Fractures

When a calcaneus fracture is suspected, splint the injured extremity with a pillow and apply ice packs to help decrease swelling. Any patient with a suspected calcaneus fracture requires spinal immobilization given the high risk of an associated spine injury.

Joint Injuries and Dislocations

Shoulder Girdle Injuries and Dislocations

Acromioclavicular Joint Separation

Separation of the acromioclavicular (AC) joint **Figure 25-35 ▶** usually occurs from a direct blow to the superior aspect or point of the shoulder, as may happen during contact sports and falls. Patients generally complain of pain and tenderness in the region of the AC joint, and the prominence of the distal clavicle may lead to a noticeable protrusion.

Posterior Sternoclavicular Joint Dislocation

Posterior dislocation of the clavicle at its junction with the sternum most often occurs as a result of a direct blow to the clavicle but is sometimes seen after strong pressure is applied to the posterior shoulder (as when a football player ends up at the bottom of a pile-up). This injury is rarely difficult to identify because there is pain and swelling at the sternoclavicular joint. What makes this a potentially dangerous and even potentially fatal injury is not the dislocation itself, but the possible damage to underlying structures—specifically, the trachea, esophagus, jugular vein, subclavian vein and artery, carotid artery, and other vascular structures. Any symptoms that suggest such underlying injury—such as *dyspnea, pain on swallowing, a sensation of choking, loss of pulses,* or a *sensory deficit* in the upper extremity on the same side—are *danger signals* and should prompt rapid transport of the patient to the hospital.

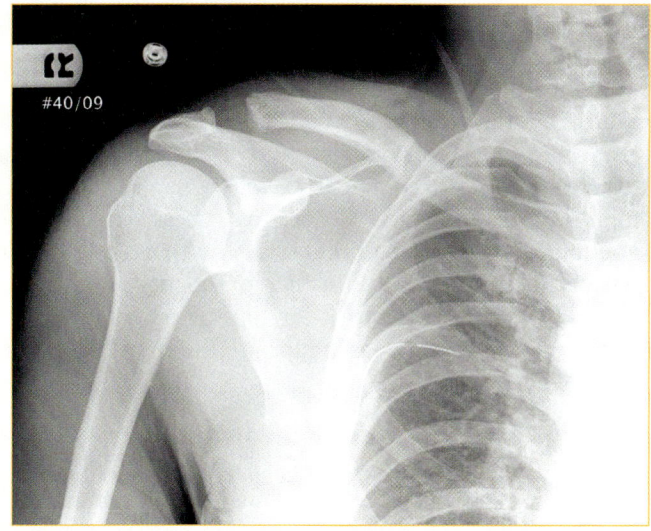

Figure 25-35 Separation of the AC joint. This space is wider than it should normally be.

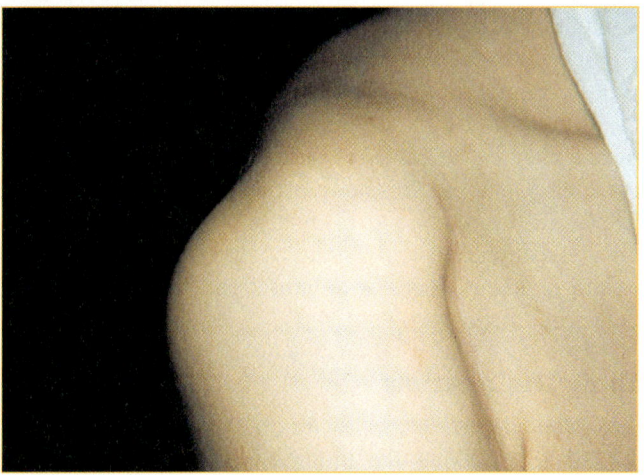

Figure 25-36 The typical appearance of an anterior shoulder dislocation.

Shoulder Dislocation

Roughly 90% of shoulder dislocations are anterior dislocations. Usually, anterior shoulder dislocations are caused by a fall onto an outstretched arm that is abducted and externally rotated. Patients complain of severe pain and have significantly decreased range of motion at the shoulder. The arm is usually held by the side, supported by the patient's other arm, and any efforts at moving it result in extreme pain **Figure 25-36 ▲**. A prominent bulge from the acromion is often noted on the anterior surface of the shoulder, the humeral head may be palpable in the axilla, and the patient may experience frequent and painful muscle spasms.

Posterior shoulder dislocations are much less common and are often caused by massive muscle contractions such as those seen with electrical shocks and seizures. These injuries present with the same complaints of pain and limited motion, but the arm is maintained in internal rotation and adduction.

In some patients, a shoulder dislocation will produce a tear of the rotator cuff or a fracture of the glenoid. Some patients may have a concomitant injury to the brachial plexus, axillary artery, or axillary vein. The axillary nerve is also prone to injury during a shoulder dislocation; assess sensation over the deltoid muscle to determine whether there is a sensory deficit in the distribution of this nerve. Patients with a shoulder dislocation are also at risk for future dislocations, especially during the first 2 years following the injury and if the patient is young.

Treatment of Joint Injuries Involving the Shoulder Girdle

In cases of an AC joint separation, a sling and swath will often provide significant pain relief. In case of a posterior sternoclavicular joint dislocation, position the patient supine with the arm on the affected side abducted and place a rolled towel under the shoulder blade, a position that may take some of the pressure off the structures beneath the sternoclavicular joint. Pay close attention to the patient's airway, and keep airway equipment readily available.

For a dislocated shoulder, splint the injured extremity in the position in which it was found by using blankets, pillows, and, when possible, a sling and swath. When applying the swath, it may be necessary to connect two cravats together so as to encircle the patient's body, extremity, and pillows or blankets. Given the likelihood of muscle spasm and pain, use of pain medication and antispasmodic agents may be necessary. Perform neurovascular assessments frequently to monitor for changes in function.

Elbow Dislocation

Elbow dislocations are medical emergencies because of the high risk of neurovascular injury. The vast majority of elbow dislocations are posterior injuries that result from a fall onto an outstretched hand or from hyperextension of the elbow joint. Patients usually complain of significant pain in the region of the elbow and may have a large degree of swelling and ecchymosis. A palpable deformity may be present at the elbow from the prominence of the olecranon process `Figure 25-37 ▶`, and there is typically locking or resistance to movement of the joint. Major complications of an elbow dislocation include an associated fracture in the region of the joint, brachial artery injury, median nerve injury, and injury to the ulnar nerve.

> *Notes from Nancy*
> When there is injury to a joint, splint the extremity in the position in which it is found.

Radial Head Subluxation

Subluxation of the radial head is also referred to as nursemaid's elbow. It commonly occurs in children younger than 6 years

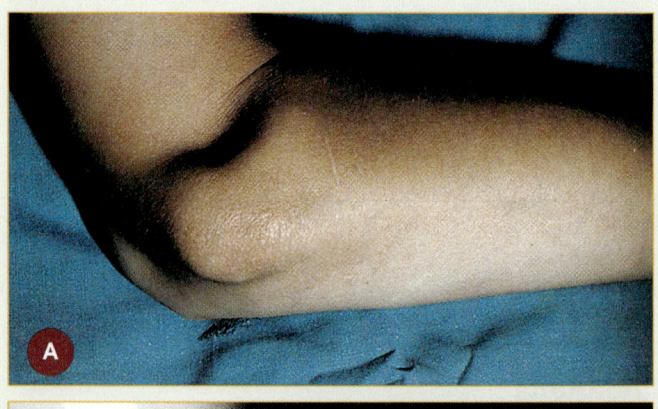
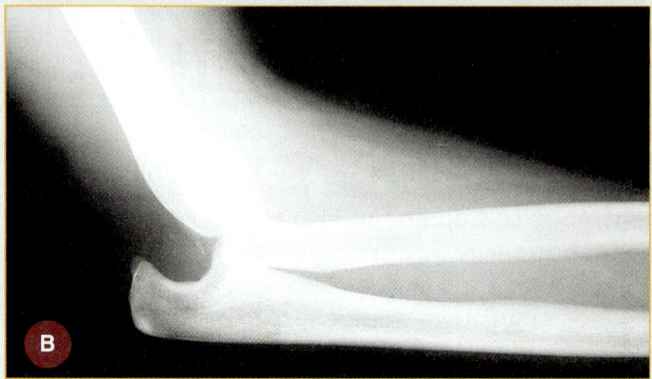

Figure 25-37 A posteriorly dislocated elbow. **A.** The clinical appearance of an elbow dislocation. **B.** Radiographic appearance of the same elbow.

and is caused by a sudden pull on the child's arm. Clinically, the injured arm is held in flexion and the child will often refuse to move the hand or elbow on the injured side. In general, there is only mild swelling in the region of the elbow.

Treatment of Elbow Dislocation

When you suspect a dislocation or subluxation in the elbow, splint the injured extremity in the position in which it was found. A sling and swath may be applied to provide additional stabilization to the injured elbow.

Finger Dislocation

Finger dislocations are caused by a sudden "jamming" force or from extension of the fingers beyond the normal range of motion. There is generally pain and deformity at the affected joint, and there may be compromise of the neurovascular structures of the digit, leading to paresthesias.

Treatment of Finger Dislocation

Manage the dislocated finger by splinting the entire hand in the position of function and using soft dressings as needed to support the digit. Do not attempt to relocate the injured digit in the prehospital setting unless you are directed to do so by direct medical control. To reduce a dislocated digit, if the digit is dislocated to the dorsal side, extend the digit; if it is dislocated to the volar side, flex the digit. Next, use gentle longitudinal traction to bring the digit back into its normal position. It may be helpful to apply pressure at the dislocated joint to push the distal part into position. Following reduction, the neurovascular status of the digit should be reassessed and the digit should be fully immobilized to prevent it from dislocating again.

Hip Dislocation

More than 90% of all hip dislocations involve posterior dislocation. The majority of these occur due to deceleration injuries, in which a flexed knee strikes an immobile object with a great degree of force   **Figure 25-38 ▾** . When a patient has a posterior hip dislocation, the leg of the affected side is typically found in flexion, adduction, and internal rotation, and it is noticeably shorter. Patients complain of severe pain and inability to move the leg, and significant soft-tissue swelling may be evident. Complications arising from such injuries include sciatic nerve injury, avascular necrosis of the hip, and associated fractures of the acetabulum.

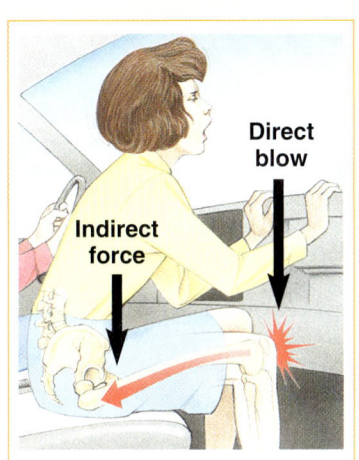

Figure 25-38 When a flexed knee strikes a dashboard, the force may be transmitted to the femur causing it to be driven posteriorly. The hip may dislocate, and the acetabulum may fracture.

Anterior hip dislocations usually follow a forceful spreading injury that occurs while the hip is flexed. The affected leg is usually flexed, abducted, and externally rotated, and the patient complains of severe pain. Major complications of this type of injury include injury to the femoral artery or nerve and avascular necrosis of the hip.

Treatment of Hip Dislocation

Because the majority of hip dislocations are associated with a high-energy mechanism, a full trauma assessment should be conducted and the patient fully immobilized. Splint the injured extremity in the position in which it is found by using blankets and pillows. Perform and document frequent neurovascular checks on your PCR. Once at the hospital, the patient generally requires sedation and muscle relaxants to allow the hip to be reduced.

Knee Dislocation

Dislocations of the knee are true emergencies that may threaten the limb. When the knee is dislocated, the ligaments that provide support to it may be damaged or torn. The knee may be dislocated by high-energy trauma (as in motor vehicle collisions), or it may dislocate secondary to powerful twisting

forces (as when athletes attempt to avoid another player). In most cases, the knee will spontaneously reduce following the injury and there may be no obvious evidence of injury.

The direction of dislocation refers to the position of the tibia with respect to the femur. Anterior knee dislocations, which result from extreme hyperextension of the knee, are the most common, occurring in almost half of all cases. Commonly, the anterior and posterior cruciate ligaments are damaged, but there is also a high risk of injury to the popliteal artery.

In posterior dislocations, a direct blow to the knee forces the tibia to shift posteriorly. There is also the possibility of damage to the cruciate ligaments and injury to the popliteal artery.

Medial dislocations result from a direct blow to the lateral part of the leg. Because the deforming force causes the medial aspect of the knee to stretch apart, there is a high likelihood of injury to the medial collateral and cruciate ligaments. When the force is applied from the medial direction, a lateral dislocation occurs and the lateral part of the knee is stretched apart, injuring the lateral collateral ligament. Lateral and medial dislocations happen less commonly and have a lesser risk of injuring the popliteal artery.

Patients with a knee dislocation will typically complain of pain in the knee and report that the knee "gave out." If the knee did not spontaneously reduce, there may be evidence of significant deformity and decreased range of motion. Complications may include limb-threatening popliteal artery disruption; injuries to the popliteal, peroneal, and tibial nerves; and joint instability. Do not confuse this injury with a relatively minor patella dislocation.

Treatment of Knee Dislocation

In all cases of knee dislocation, distal neurovascular function must be assessed frequently and will often guide the management. If a pulse is palpable in the foot, splint the knee in the position in which it is found. If there is no palpable pulse, you may need to reduce the knee to restore circulation. A number of factors, including time to the hospital and duration of dislocation, will affect this decision, so you should always seek medical direction before reducing a dislocated knee.

To reduce a dislocated knee, apply longitudinal traction to the tibia in the direction of the foot. While the first rescuer is applying traction, a second paramedic should apply pressure to the distal femur and proximal tibia. If the knee is dislocated anteriorly, apply pressure to the femur in the anterior direction and to the tibia in the opposite direction. In the case of a posterior dislocation, apply pressure in the opposite manner, with the tibia pressed anteriorly and the femur pressed posteriorly. Once the reduction has been accomplished, check the patient's neurovascular status and splint the leg securely. If the attempt at reduction fails, splint the knee in the position in which it is found and undertake rapid transportation to an appropriate facility.

You are the Paramedic Summary

1. What are your initial assessment and treatment priorities?

As with any trauma patient, after ensuring that the scene is safe, the initial assessment priorities for this patient are the mental status, the ABCs, and prioritizing the patient. Then proceed with a rapid trauma examination to identify the patient's injuries. Because this patient fell from a significant height, it is also important to protect his spine. During the initial assessment, you note that he has a site of bleeding from his arm; this bleeding should be controlled. Once this is accomplished, IV access should be obtained and the assessment should continue in a systematic and orderly manner.

2. What other information should be obtained about the patient and the incident?

Obtain information about the events that led the patient to fall, such as how he felt before falling and why he thought he fell. It is also important to learn details about the fall, such as how his extremities were positioned when he landed or whether he struck any other objects while falling. Obtain any other information related to the patient's status after the fall, such as loss of consciousness, mental status, and movement of extremities, from the patient or anyone who witnessed the fall. Also obtain information about any allergies the patient may know he has, any medication he takes, and the last time he had anything to eat or drink.

3. What are the potential complications of an open fracture?

One of the most significant complications following an open fracture is infection of the bone or soft tissues. To reduce the risk of infection, do not probe open fractures, brush away any debris on the surface of the skin, and cover the wound with a sterile dressing. Other complications of open fractures include poor healing of the fracture, soft-tissue loss, neurovascular injury, and long-term disability.

4. Why are open fractures prone to bleeding more than closed fractures?

In general, open fractures are higher-energy injuries than closed fractures, so they are likely to have more soft-tissue damage and, hence, more bleeding. Also, because the fracture is open, the blood that would normally accumulate within the closed fracture site is allowed to escape, so there is no tamponade of the bleeding vessels.

5. Would your treatment priorities change if the patient complained of abdominal pain in the presence of hypotension?

If the patient were found to be in unstable condition with evidence of an intra-abdominal injury, immediate and rapid transportation to a trauma centre would be warranted. For a trauma patient in unstable condition who has a fracture, place the patient on a backboard and fully immobilize the patient. While immobilizing the spine, the injured extremities may be immobilized as well by securing them to the board. The result is a compromise: The injured extremity is secured in place and protected from further movement without dedicating precious time to applying a formal splint.

6. Why would this dislocation be considered a true emergency?

When a patient with a dislocated knee has a pulseless foot, medical direction should be obtained and consideration should be given to reducing the dislocation. Some paramedics may have a standing order to deal with this type of situation. Factors that will influence this decision include the duration of the dislocation, time to the hospital, the patient's vital signs, and the patient's overall condition.

7. What is an important consideration before manipulating a dislocation?

If the patient has no contraindications (such as hypotension), sedation should be considered before attempting manipulation of the extremity. This can be a very painful procedure, and without determining the appropriate use of analgesics such as morphine, you will not be addressing an important patient care issue—comfort.

8. Why should a joint that has just been manipulated be splinted immediately?

A dislocation is often associated with damage to the ligaments and capsule that support the affected joint, making it susceptible to recurrent dislocations. Once a dislocated joint has been reduced, it should be splinted to prevent movements that may allow for it to once again dislocate.

9. What facts should be relayed to the emergency department staff in your radio report?

The presence of a dislocation and/or fracture with compromised neurovascular status should be relayed immediately to the receiving facility. Any attempts to correct the impairment should be explained, along with any changes or responses to treatment. Paint a clear picture of the mechanism of injury and the patient's condition. Remember, the only information the emergency department staff have to plan for your arrival is based on your brief radio report.

Prep Kit

◼ Ready for Review

- Injuries and complaints related to the musculoskeletal system are one of the most common reasons that patients seek medical attention.
- Musculoskeletal injuries are sometimes very dramatic, but attention should not be focused on them until life-threatening conditions have been excluded.
- You have a vital role in reducing the complications associated with musculoskeletal injuries by promptly and effectively splinting injured extremities.
- Assume the existence of a fracture whenever a patient who complains of a musculoskeletal injury has deformity, bruising, decreased range of motion, or swelling.
- Always perform and record an accurate neurovascular examination before and after splinting an injured extremity.
- When a dislocation is associated with absent distal pulses, obtain medical direction to determine whether the injury should be reduced.
- Look for injuries to the chest and abdomen, and fully immobilize the spine when patients have evidence of a high-energy injury, such as a femoral shaft or scapular fracture.
- Because fractures may be associated with significant blood loss, resuscitation with IV fluid may be necessary.
- Pelvic fractures are potentially lethal injuries owing to the massive potential for blood loss.
- *Never forget the ABCs!* Do not become distracted; the fracture can wait, if airway, breathing, or circulation problems are noted.

◼ Vital Vocabulary

6 Ps of musculoskeletal assessment Pain, Paralysis, Parasthesias, Pulselessness, Pallor, and Pressure.

abduction Movement *away* from the midline of the body.

acetabulum The cup-shaped cavity in which the rounded head of the femur rotates.

acromion Lateral extension of the scapula that forms the highest point of the shoulder.

adduction Movement *toward* the midline of the body.

amputation Severing of a part of the body.

angulation The presence of an abnormal angle or bend in an extremity.

anterior tibial artery The artery that travels through the anterior muscles of the leg and continues to the foot as the dorsalis pedis.

appendicular skeleton The part of the skeleton comprising the upper and lower extremities.

arthritis Inflammation of the joints.

articulations The locations where two or more bones meet; *joints*.

atrophy Wasting away of a tissue.

avascular necrosis Tissue death resulting from the loss of blood supply.

avulsion fracture A fracture that occurs when a piece of bone is torn free at the site of attachment of a tendon or ligament.

axial skeleton The part of the skeleton comprising the skull, spinal column, and rib cage.

axilla The armpit.

axillary artery The artery that runs through the axilla, connecting the subclavian artery to the brachial artery.

bowing fracture An incomplete fracture typically occurring in children in which the bone becomes bent as the result of a compressive force.

boxer's fracture A fracture of the head of the fifth metacarpal that usually results from striking an object with a clenched fist.

brachial artery The artery that runs through the arm and branches into the radial and ulnar arteries.

buckle fracture A common incomplete fracture in children in which the cortex of the bone fractures from an excessive compression force.

buddy splinting Securing an injured digit to an adjacent uninjured one to allow the intact digit to act as a splint.

bursa A fluid-filled sac located adjacent to joints that reduces the amount of friction between moving structures.

bursitis Inflammation of a bursa.

calcaneus The heel bone; the largest of the tarsal bones.

cancellous bone Trabecular or spongy bone.

carpals The eight small bones of the wrist.

cartilage Tough, elastic substance that covers opposable surfaces of moveable joints and forms part of the skeleton.

cartilaginous joints Joints that are spanned completely by cartilage and allow for minimal motion.

clavicle The collar bone.

closed fracture A fracture in which the skin is not broken.

comminuted fracture A fracture in which the bone is broken into three or more pieces.

compartment syndrome An increase in tissue pressure in a closed fascial space or compartment that compromises the circulation to the nerves and muscles within the involved compartment.

complete fracture A fracture in which the bone is broken into two or more completely separate pieces.

compound fracture An open fracture; a fracture beneath an open wound.

crepitus A grating sensation felt when moving the ends of a broken bone.

crush syndrome A condition that arises after a body part that has been compressed for a significant period is released, leading to the entry of potassium and other metabolic toxins into the systemic circulation.

deep vein thrombosis (DVT) The formation of a blood clot within the larger veins of an extremity, typically following a period of prolonged immobilization.

depression fracture A fracture in which the broken region of the bone is pushed deeper into the body than the remaining intact bone.

devascularization The loss of blood to a part of the body.

diaphysis The shaft of a long bone.

diastasis An increase in the distance between the two sides of a joint.

digital arteries The arteries that supply blood to the fingers and toes.

dinner fork deformity The dorsal deformity of the forearm that results from a Colles fracture.

dislocation The displacement of a bone from its normal position within a joint.

distraction injury An injury that results from a force that tries to increase the length of a body part or separate one body part from another.

dorsal Referring to the back or posterior side of the body or an organ.

dorsiflex To bend the foot or hand backward.

endosteum The inner lining of a hollow bone.

fascia A strong, fibrous membrane that covers, supports, and separates muscles.

fatigue fractures Fractures that result from multiple compressive loads.

femoral artery The main artery supplying the thigh and leg.

femoral shaft fractures A break in the diaphysis of the femur.

femur The proximal bone of the leg that extends from the pelvis to the knee.

fibrous joints The joints that contain dense fibrous tissue and allow for no motion.

fibula The smaller of the two bones of the lower leg.

flat bones Bones that are thin and broad, such as the scapula.

fracture A break or rupture in the bone.

glenoid fossa Socket in the scapula in which the head of the humerus rotates.

gout A painful disorder characterized by the crystallization of uric acid within a joint.

greenstick fracture A type of fracture occurring most frequently in children in which there is incomplete breakage of the bone.

hematopoiesis The generation of blood cells.

humerus The bone of the upper arm.

hypertrophy An increase in size.

ilium The broad, uppermost bone of the pelvis.

impacted fracture A broken bone in which the end of one bone becomes wedged into another bone, as could be the case in a fall from a significant height.

incomplete fracture A fracture in which the bone does not fully break.

indirect injury An injury that results from a force that is applied to one region of the body but leads to an injury in another area.

intertrochanteric fractures Fractures that occur in the region between the lesser and greater trochanters.

irregular bones Bones with unique shapes that allow them to perform a specific function and that do not fit into the other categories based on shape.

ischium The lowermost dorsal bone of the pelvis.

joint The point at which two or more bones articulate, or come together.

joint capsule A saclike envelope that encloses the cavity of a synovial joint.

lactic acid A metabolic end product of the breakdown of glucose that accumulates when metabolism proceeds in the absence of oxygen.

lateral compression A force that is directed from the side toward the midline of the body.

ligaments Tough bands of tissue that connect bone to bone around a joint or support internal organs within the body.

linear fracture A fracture that runs parallel to the long axis of a bone.

long bones Bones that are longer than they are wide.

malleolus The large, rounded bony protuberance on either side of the ankle joint.

mallet finger An avulsion fracture of the extensor tendon of the distal phalynx caused by jamming a finger into an object.

march fractures *See* fatigue fractures.

medullary canal The hollow centre portion of a long bone.

metacarpals The five bones that form the palm and back of the hand.

metaphysis The region of the long bone between the epiphysis and diaphysis.

metatarsals The five long bones extending from the tarsus to the phalanges of the foot.

muscle fatigue The condition that arises when a muscle depletes its supply of energy.

neurovascular compromise The loss of the nerve supply, blood supply, or both to a region of the body, typically distal to a site of injury; characterized by alterations in sensation, including numbness and tingling, or by a loss or decrease of motor function; vascular compromise is indicated by weak or absent pulses, poor skin colour, and cool skin.

nondisplaced fracture A break in which the bone remains aligned in its normal position.

nursemaid's elbow The subluxation of the radial head that often results from pulling on an outstretched arm in children.

oblique fracture A fracture that travels diagonally from one side of the bone to the other.

olecranon The proximal bony projection of the *ulna* at the elbow; the part of the ulna that constitutes the "funny bone."

open book pelvic fracture A life-threatening fracture of the pelvis caused by a force that displaces one or both sides of the pelvis laterally and posteriorly.

open fracture Any break in a bone in which the overlying skin has been damaged.

osteoarthritis (OA) The degeneration of a joint surface caused by wear and tear that leads to pain and stiffness.

osteoporosis A condition characterized by decreased bone density and increased susceptibility to fractures.

overriding The overlap of a bone that occurs from the muscle spasm that follows a fracture, leading to a decrease in the length of the bone.

paresthesias Abnormal sensations such as burning, numbness, or tingling.

patella The kneecap.

pathologic fracture A fracture that occurs in an area of abnormally weakened bone.

pectoral girdle The shoulder girdle.

pelvic girdle The large bone that arises in the area of the last nine vertebrae and sweeps around to form a complete ring.

periosteum The fibrous tissue that covers bone.

phalanges The bones of the fingers or toes.

physis The growth plate in long bones.

plantar Referring to the sole of the foot.

plantar flexion Bending of the foot toward the ground.

point tenderness The tenderness that is sharply localized at the site of the injury, found by gently palpating along the bone with the tip of one finger.

popliteal artery The artery in the area or space behind the knee joint.

posterior tibial artery The artery that travels through the calf muscles to the plantar aspect of the foot.

pronation The act of turning the palm of the hand backward or downward, performed by internal rotation of the forearm.

pubic symphysis The midline articulation of the pubic bones.

pubis One of two bones that form the anterior portion of the pelvic ring.

pulmonary embolism Obstruction of a pulmonary artery or arteries by solid, liquid, or gaseous material swept through the right side of the heart into the lungs.

radial artery The artery pertaining to the wrist.

radius The bone on the thumb side of the forearm.

range of motion (ROM) The arc of movement of an extremity at a joint in a particular direction.

recruitment The process of signaling additional muscle fibres to contract to create a more forceful contraction.

rheumatoid arthritis (RA) An inflammatory disorder that affects the entire body and leads to degeneration and deformation of joints.

round bones The small bones that are found adjacent to joints that assist with motion.

sacroiliac joints The points of attachment of the *ilium* to the sacrum.

scaphoid The wrist bone that is found just beyond that most distal portion of the radius.

scapula The shoulder blade.

segmental fracture A bone that is broken in more than one place.

short bones The bones that are nearly as wide as they are long.

skeletal muscle Muscle that is attached to bones and usually crosses at least one joint; striated or voluntary muscle.

snuffbox The region at the base of the thumb where the scaphoid may be palpated.

somatic motor neurons The nerve fibres that transmit impulses to a muscle.

spiral fracture A break in a bone that appears like a spring on a radiograph.

sprains Injuries, including a stretch or a tear, to the ligaments of a joint that commonly lead to pain and swelling.

straddle fracture A fracture of the pelvis that results from landing on the perineal region.

strain Stretching or tearing of a muscle by excessive stretching or overuse.

stress fracture A fracture that results from exaggerated stress on the bone caused by unusually rapid muscle development.

striated muscle Skeletal muscle that is under voluntary control.

subclavian artery The artery that travels from the aorta to each upper extremity.

subluxation A partial or incomplete dislocation.

supination To turn the forearm laterally so that the palm faces forward (if standing) or upward (if lying supine).

supracondylar fractures Fractures of the distal humerus that occur just proximal to the elbow.

synovial joints Joints that permit movement of the component bones.

synovial membrane The lining of a joint that secretes synovial fluid into the joint space.

talus The bone of the foot that articulates with the tibia.

tarsals The ankle bones.

tendinitis Inflammation of a tendon that most commonly results from overuse.

tendons The fibrous portions of muscle that attach to bone.

Thompson test Squeezing of the calf muscle to evaluate for plantar flexion of the foot to determine whether the Achilles tendon is intact.

thromboembolic disease The condition in which a patient has a DVT or pulmonary embolism.

tibia The shin bone.

torus fracture *See* buckle fracture.

transverse fracture A fracture that runs in a straight line from one edge of the bone to the other and that is perpendicular to each edge.

twisting injuries Injuries that commonly occur during athletic activities in which an extremity rotates around a planted foot or hand.

ulna The larger bone of the forearm, on the side opposite the thumb.

ulnar artery The artery of the forearm that travels along its medial aspect.

vertical shear The type of pelvic fracture that occurs when a massive force displaces the pelvis superiorly.

volar Pertaining to the palm or sole; referring to the flexor surfaces of the forearm, wrist, or hand.

Volkmann ischemic contracture Contraction of the fingers and, sometimes, the wrist, with loss of muscular power, that sets in rapidly after severe injury around the elbow joint.

voluntary muscle Muscle that can be controlled by a person.

www.Paramedic.EMSzone.com/Canada

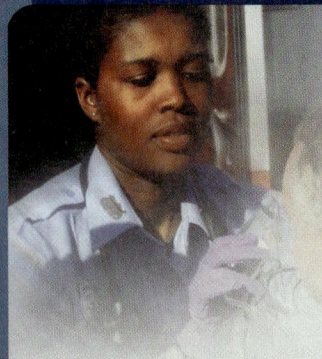

Assessment in Action

You are dispatched to the home of a 13-year-old boy with pain in his foot. When you arrive, the boy is sitting in his mother's car complaining of severe pain in his left foot, ankle, and leg. On assessment, he has a distal pulse; his foot is cold and has limited range of motion. There is swelling noted in ankle region. There is no discolouration or obvious deformity. The remainder of his vital signs are within normal limits.

He tells you that he was in the mountains and was snowboarding. He went down a hill when suddenly, a tree was in the way. He struck the tree with the bottom of his left foot (travelling approximately 30 km/h). He felt immediate pain in his foot and then began to feel a burning sensation up his left leg. His mother drove him back to their house, approximately 45 minutes away. He had no pain while travelling, but when he attempted to step out of the vehicle, the pain soared through him. You provide comfort care for the young man and transport him to the hospital. He tells you that his pain is about 7 on a 1 to 10 scale. You follow-up at the hospital and are told that he has a comminuted fracture in his heel and a fractured ankle.

1. **What type of injury force did this young man sustain?**
   A. Tapping injury force
   B. Crush injury force
   C. Penetrating injury force
   D. Indirect injury force

2. **With the complaint of pain in his left leg, what other type of injury should have been suspected?**
   A. Indirect injury
   B. Direct injury
   C. Twisting injury
   D. March fracture

3. **The foot consists of three classes of bones. Which are they?**
   A. Tarsals, metatarsals, and calcaneus
   B. Tarsals, metatarsals, and phalanges
   C. Tarsals, calcaneus, and tibia
   D. Tibia, fibula, and malleolus

4. **Signs and symptoms of extremity trauma that have a high urgency include which of the following?**
   A. Absent distal pulses
   B. Crepitus
   C. Decreased range of motion
   D. Swelling and deformity

5. **Flexion, extension, abduction, and circumduction are all movements allowed by what type of joint?**
   A. Hinge
   B. Synovial
   C. Saddle
   D. Ball and socket

6. **Muscles are composed of specialized cells that contract when stimulated to exert a force on a part of the body. Three types of muscles found in the body are:**
   A. smooth, cardiac, and skeletal.
   B. smooth, cardiac, and striated.
   C. ligaments, cartilage, and smooth.
   D. cardiac, skeletal, and cartilage.

7. **When a person sustains a musculoskeletal injury, the arteries that supply the injured region may be damaged as well. What arteries supply the ankle and the foot?**
   A. Tibial artery; anterior tibial artery
   B. Popliteal artery; anterior tibial artery
   C. Anterior tibial artery; posterior tibial artery
   D. Popliteal artery; posterior tibial artery

8. **What is the *primary* symptom of a fracture?**
   A. Pain
   B. Deformity
   C. Shortening
   D. Loss of use

9. **When assessing the patient's pain, you should use the mnemonic:**
   A. PQRST.
   B. OPRST.
   C. OPQRST.
   D. OPRST.

Challenging Questions

You are dispatched to the home of a 60-year-old man found by neighbours. On your arrival, you find the man in a right lateral recumbent position and he is moaning. You're not sure how long he has been on the ground, but there is 4 days worth of mail in the mailbox. You apply a backboard and cervical collar because you are not sure of the reason the patient is on the ground. His blood pressure is 100/60 mm Hg and the heart rate is 120 beats/min with sinus tachycardia, he has strong radial pulses, and his respirations are 12 breaths/min. He is verbally responsive by moaning. He is unable to tell you what happened or if anything hurts.

You provide supportive and comfort care en route to the hospital. His body is very stiff and you have difficulty manipulating his extremities. When you perform an assessment, you note that there is a nickel embedded in his head. There are large areas of ecchymosis along his right pelvic area and his right leg. His right shoulder has open wounds. He is incontinent of urine and feces. This man was admitted to the intensive care unit with a diagnosis of acute sepsis and crush syndrome.

10. **What signs and symptoms would you recognize for the crush syndrome?**

11. **How would you treat this type of injury?**

12. **What will be the concerns of the hospital staff for this patient?**

Points to Ponder

You are responding to a call at an assisted care facility for an older woman who has fallen out of bed while attempting to get up. When you arrive, the woman is still on the floor next to her bed. She tells you that her left leg and back hurt, but she is mentally alert and denies any other symptoms. She is sitting up, and it does not seem that she has bumped her head or injured herself in any other way besides the fall. Your physical examination reveals tenderness and pain in her left leg and crepitus and instability in her left hip. The staff tells you that the woman has osteoporosis but no other major medical problems.

How would you best treat this patient?

Issues: Thorough Assessment of Musculoskeletal Injuries, Pain Management.

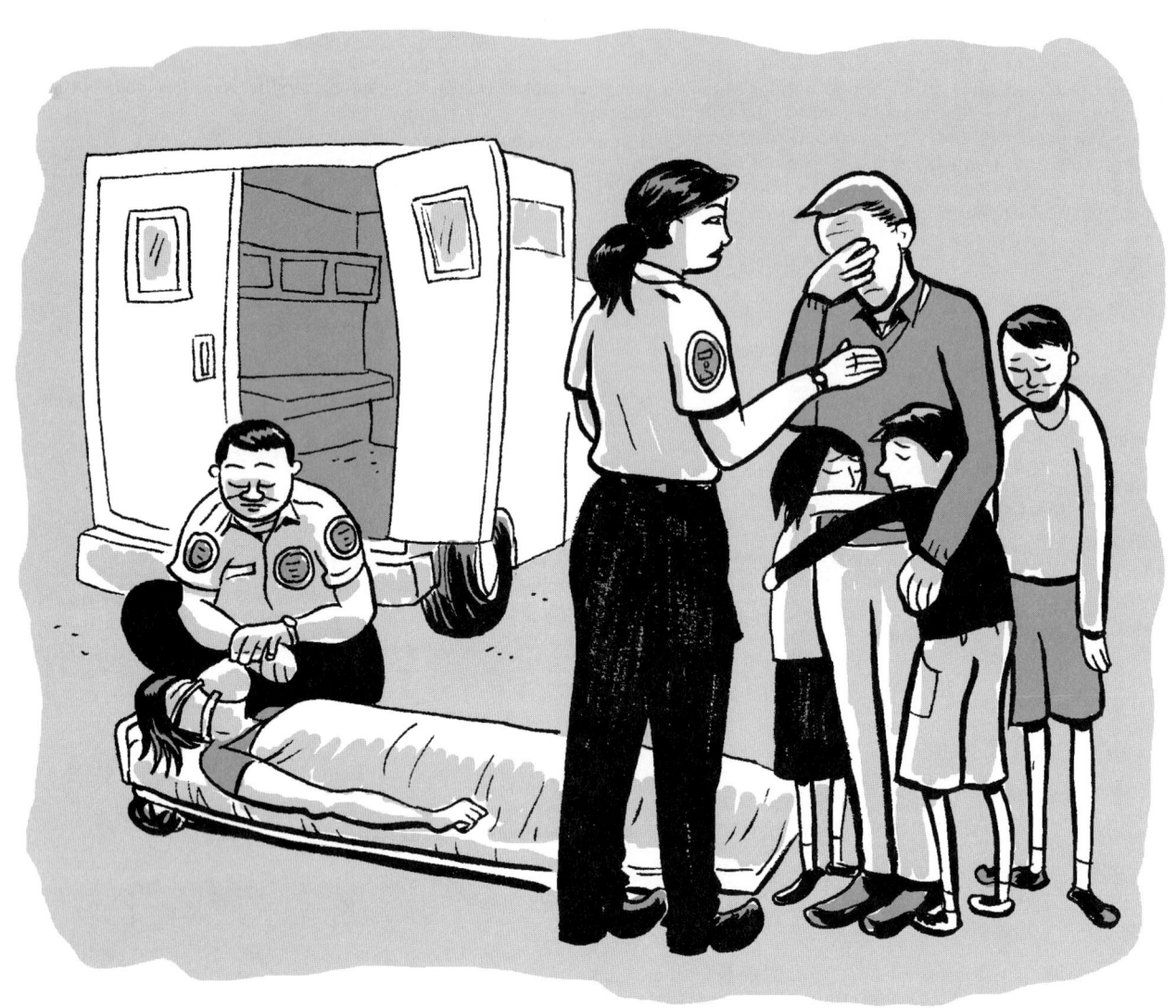

"
Remember, behind every medical emergency is a person."

—Mickey Eisenberg, MD, PhD

Medical

Section Editors: Jeffrey M. Singh, MD, MSc, FRCPC
Randy S. Wax, MD, MEd, FRCPC

26 Respiratory Emergencies

Competency Areas

Area 2: Communication

2.2.a   Record organized, accurate, and relevant patient information.

Area 4: Assessment and Diagnostics

4.2.a   Obtain list of patient's allergies.
4.2.b   Obtain list of patient's medications.
4.2.c   Obtain chief complaint and/or incident history from patient, family members, and/or bystanders.
4.2.d   Obtain information regarding patient's past medical history.
4.2.f   Obtain information regarding incident through accurate and complete scene assessment.
4.3.a   Conduct primary patient assessment and interpret findings.
4.3.b   Conduct secondary patient assessment and interpret findings.
4.3.e   Conduct respiratory system assessment and interpret findings.
4.4.a   Assess pulse.
4.4.b   Assess respiration.
4.4.d   Measure blood pressure by auscultation.
4.4.g   Assess skin condition.
4.4.h   Assess pupils.
4.4.i   Assess level of mentation.

Area 5: Therapeutics

5.1.a   Use manual maneuvers and positioning to maintain airway patency.
5.2.a   Recognize indications for oxygen administration.
5.3.b   Administer oxygen using low concentration mask.
5.3.d   Administer oxygen using high concentration mask.
5.4.a   Provide oxygenation and ventilation using bag-valve-mask.
5.4.b   Recognize indications for mechanical ventilation.
5.4.c   Prepare mechanical ventilation equipment.
5.4.d   Provide mechanical ventilation.
5.8.a   Recognize principles of pharmacology as applied to the medications listed in Appendix 5.
5.8.c   Administer medication via subcutaneous route.
5.8.d   Administer medication via intramuscular route.
5.8.e   Administer medication via intravenous route.
5.8.g   Administer medication via endotracheal route.

Area 6: Integration

6.1.c   Provide care to patient experiencing illness or injury primarily involving respiratory system.

Appendix 4: Pathophysiology

A.   **Cardiovascular System**
Cardiac Conduction Disorder: Life-threatening arrhythmias
B.   **Neurologic System**
Infectious Disorders: Guillian Barre syndrome
Traumatic Injuries: Head injury
C.   **Respiratory System**
Medical Illness: Acute respiratory failure
Medical Illness: Adult respiratory disease syndrome
Medical Illness: Aspiration
Medical Illness: Chronic obstructive pulmonary disorder
Medical Illness: Hyperventilation syndrome
Medical Illness: Pleural effusion
Medical Illness: Pneumonia/bronchitis
Medical Illness: Pulmonary edema
Medical Illness: Pulmonary embolism
Medical Illness: Reactive airways disease/asthma
Traumatic Injuries: Aspirated foreign body
Traumatic Injuries: Pneumothorax (simple, tension)
Pediatric Illness: Croup
J.   **Multisystem Diseases and Injuries**
Cancer: Malignancy
L.   **Ears, Eyes, Nose, and Throat**
Neck and Upper Airway Disorders: Obstruction
Neck and Upper Airway Disorders: Peritonsillar abscess
Neck and Upper Airway Disorders: Retropharyngeal abscess
Neck and Upper Airway Disorders: Tonsillitis

Appendix 5: Medications

A.   **Medications affecting the central nervous system**
A.8   Opioid Analgesics
B.   **Medications affecting the autonomic nervous system**
B.4   Cholinergic Antagonists
C.   **Medications affecting the respiratory system**
C.1   Bronchodilators
D.   **Medications affecting the cardiovascular system**
D.3   Diuretics
I.   **Medications used to treat/prevent inflammatory responses and infections**
I.1   Corticosteroids

Introduction

There are few incentives to dial 9-1-1 more powerful than having difficulty breathing (dyspnea). In the majority of cases, that distressing feeling is caused by a problem in the respiratory system itself. In this chapter, we examine some of the respiratory problems that produce dyspnea. We begin by reviewing the anatomy and physiology of the respiratory system. We next consider the assessment of a patient whose chief complaint is dyspnea—namely, which aspects to emphasize in taking the history and carrying out the physical examination. Then we look at various problems that may affect the normal functioning of the respiratory system—from the respiratory control centres in the brain to the alveolus, the smallest functional unit of respiration in the lung.

Review of Respiratory Anatomy and Function

The primary components of the respiratory system are often compared to an inverted tree, with the trachea representing the tree's trunk and the alveoli resembling the tree's leaves. This image is simple to understand, but in reality a respiratory tree would have to branch 24 times and have nearly a billion leaves **Figure 26-1 ▾** .

The Upper Airway

Air enters the upper airway primarily through the nares (nostrils) of the nose. Nares are lined with nasal hairs. The hairs serve as filters that catch particulate matter in the air we breathe. The external nares are separated by the nasal septum.

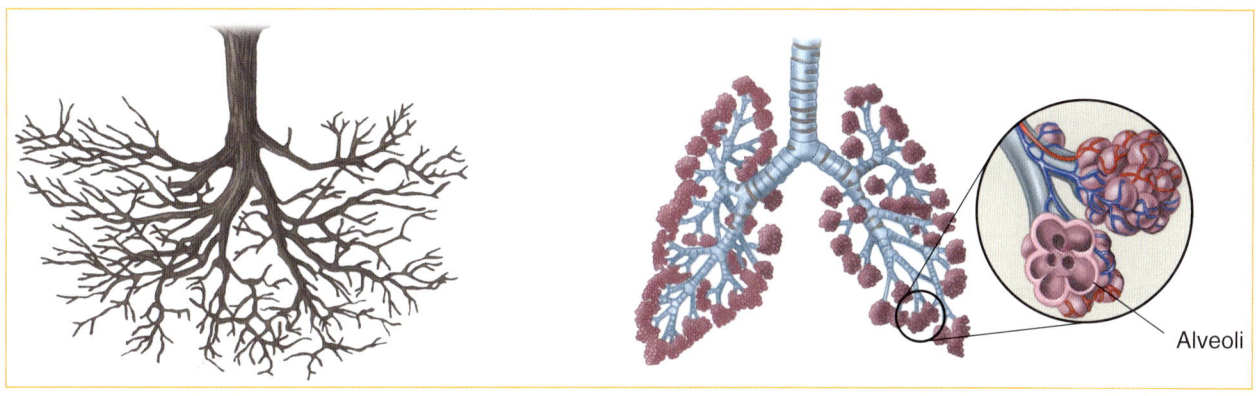

Alveoli

Figure 26-1 The tracheobronchial tree branches in much the same way as a tree, except that even the most branched tree has only half as many branchings as those inside the lung.

You are the Paramedic Part 1

You are dispatched to 275 Thomas Lane to help an older man who is having difficulty breathing. You arrive to find a 65-year-old man sitting in the tripod position at his kitchen table. As you speak with him, you notice that he is struggling to breathe and can give you only one- or two-word responses. His extremities are pale and his face is flushed. As you attempt to obtain more information regarding his medical history, the patient grabs your arm and says, "I'm so tired!"

Initial Assessment	Recording Time: 0 Minutes
Appearance	Anxious, tired
Level of consciousness	V (Responsive to verbal stimuli)
Airway	Open; accessory muscle use
Breathing	Rapid and laboured
Circulation	Weak radial pulse

1. What about this patient's presentation gives you cause for concern?
2. What are your assessment and treatment priorities?
3. If you are unable to gather much information from your patient about his medical history, what other ways can you obtain this information?

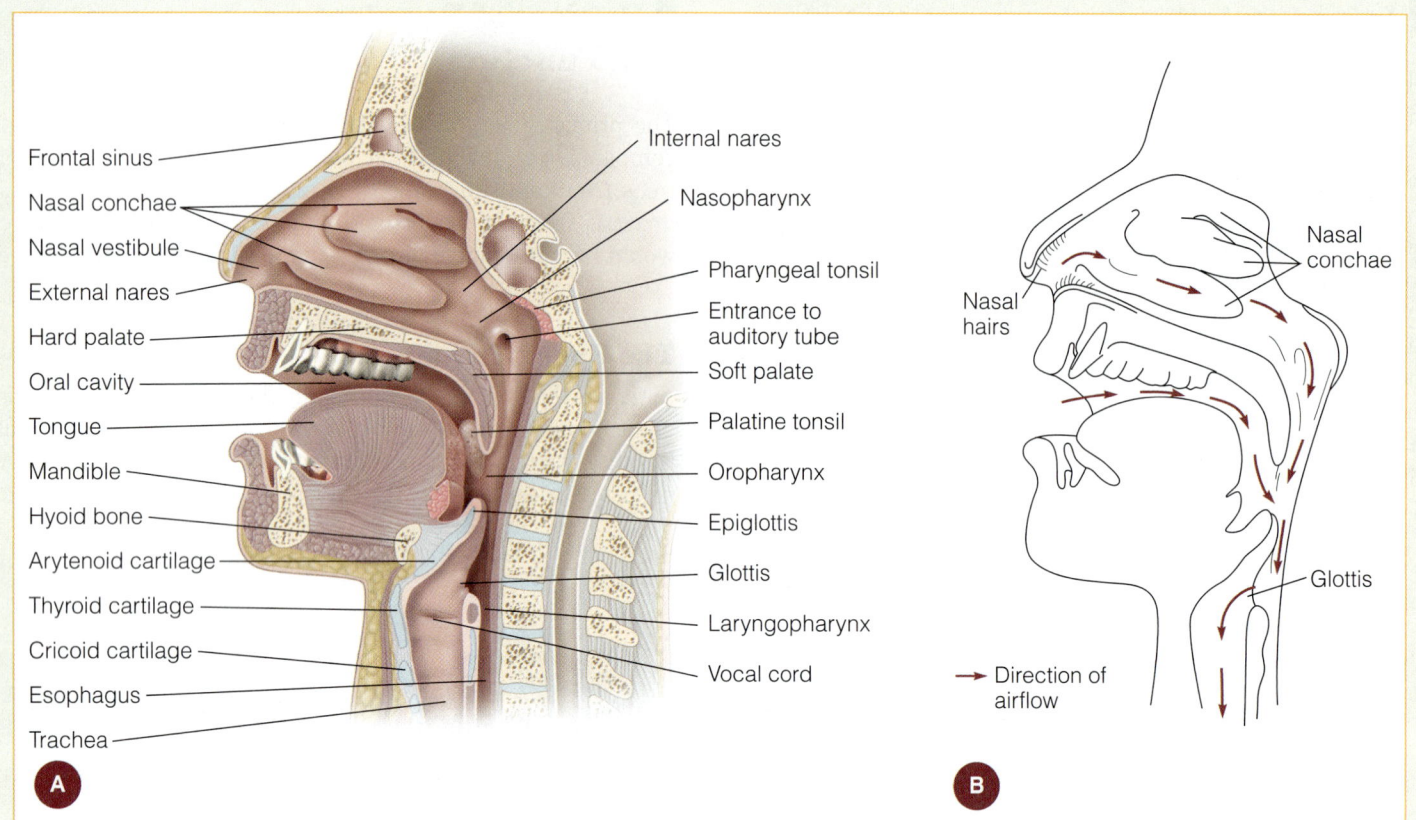

Figure 26-2 **A.** The upper airway contains many blood vessels and serves to heat and humidify the air we breathe. **B.** Note that an important filter is lost when we bypass the upper airway via intubation.

After passing through the nares, air is pulled over the turbinates. These ridges of tissue are covered with a mucous membrane and contain many blood vessels. The mucous membrane traps more particulate matter, and the large surface area of the turbinates warms and humidifies the air we breathe as the air passes over it. Processes such as intubation or a tracheostomy allow inhaled air to skip this trip through the nose, bypassing the humidification and filtering. Because the turbinates contain many blood vessels, they easily swell (causing a stuffy nose) or bleed. It is very important to understand the orientation of the turbinates when passing a nasogastric (NG) tube. The passage of an NG tube should follow an axis parallel to the base of the nose, and not be directed upward toward the fragile cribiform plate.

Anyone with hay fever can attest to the severe swelling that can occur in the nasal cavity. In children, foreign bodies such as pencil erasers, candy, and beans frequently obstruct a nostril. These items often sit in the nose for a day or two before the child presents with pain and a foul-smelling nasal discharge. Don't try to remove the obstruction yourself, because this process can occasionally be painful. It is better to attempt foreign-body removal in the controlled setting of an emergency department.

Quiet breathing typically allows air to flow through the nose (**Figure 26-2 ▲**). Even people who breathe through their mouth usually have some nasal airflow.

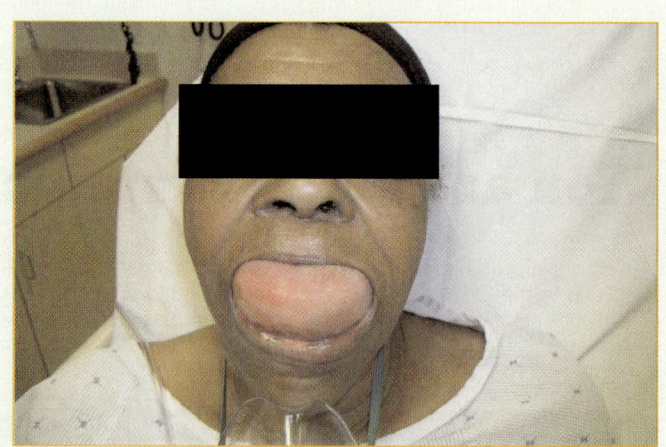

Figure 26-3 Angioedema presents as acute swelling, usually of the lips, mouth, or tongue, often secondary to an allergic reaction. Some medications, such as ACE inhibitors, are known to cause angioedema.

The mouth and oropharynx also contain many blood vessels and are covered by a mucous membrane. Swelling can be extreme, and potentially dangerous. Bee stings to the lips or tongue can cause profound swelling. Angioedema (**Figure 26-3 ▲**) is a type of allergic reaction that may cause severe swelling of the mouth, tongue, or lips. Always ask patients who may be experiencing an allergic reaction if their tongue "feels thick." Monitor their speech for symptoms (such as low volume or a raspy voice) of oral or laryngeal swelling, and examine the upper airway for early signs of edema, such as swelling of the uvula.

The oropharynx and nasopharynx meet in the back of the throat at the hypopharynx (sometimes called the posterior pharynx). The gag reflex is most profound in this area. Triggering the gag reflex, on purpose or by accident, can cause vagal bradycardia (a slow heartbeat caused by stimulation of the vagus nerve), vomiting, and increased intracranial pressure. A strong gag reflex may make the use of many airway devices difficult or inappropriate **Figure 26-4 ▸**. Conversely, patients with a diminished or absent gag reflex may require endotracheal intubation to help isolate and protect the airway from foreign materials.

The larynx (voicebox) **Figure 26-5 ▾** and glottis (opening at the top of the trachea) are typically considered the dividing line between the upper airway and the lower airway. The thyroid cartilage is the most obvious external landmark of the larynx. The glottis and vocal cords are found in the middle of the thyroid's cartilaginous structure.

Several cartilages that support the vocal cords may be visible when intubating the patient. The arytenoid cartilages appear as two pearly white lumps at the inferior end of each vocal cord. On either side of the glottis, tissue forms a pocket called the piriform fossa **Figure 26-6 ▸**. Sometimes NG tubes or endotracheal (ET) tubes will get stuck here during placement, causing "tenting" that is visible externally on the neck. Any device stuck in a piriform fossa must be withdrawn a few centimetres and reinserted.

The glottic opening is covered by the epiglottis. Most of us were taught that the epiglottis covers the glottis like a trap door when we swallow, keeping food and liquid from entering the trachea. In reality, many people aspirate around their epiglottis, but others seem to swallow just fine even after their epiglottis has been surgically removed. Because the epiglottis can make it difficult to see the vocal cords, one of your primary tasks during endotracheal intubation is to identify the epiglottis and use

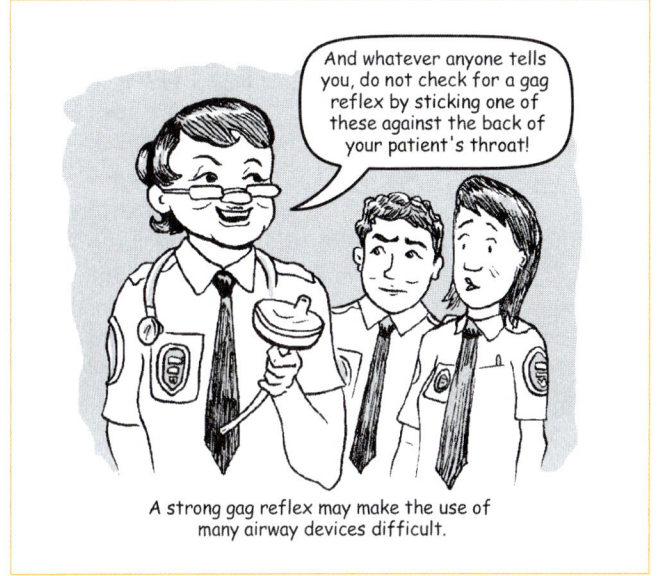

A strong gag reflex may make the use of many airway devices difficult.

Figure 26-4

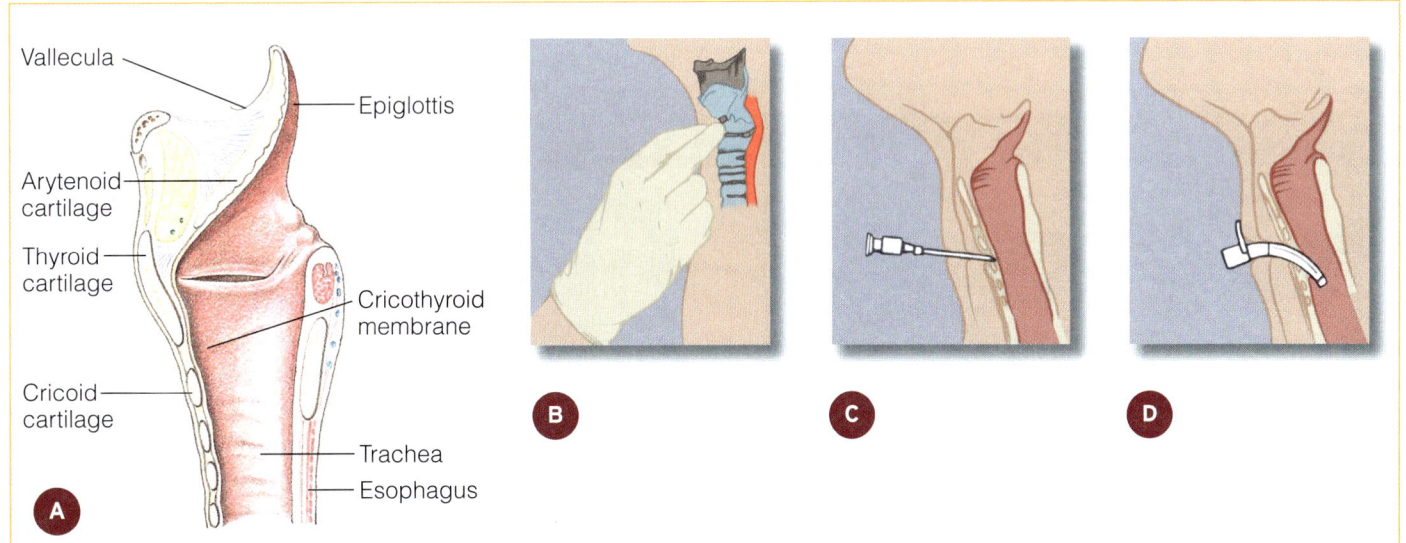

Figure 26-5 It is imperative that you completely understand the anatomy of the larynx in order to perform a number of airway management skills. **A.** Anatomy of the larynx. **B.** Applying pressure to the cricoid cartilage (Sellick maneuver) compresses the esophagus and may help prevent aspiration, while allowing the trachea to remain open. **C.** An IV cannula is inserted into the cricothyroid membrane. **D.** A tracheostomy tube is inserted below the cricoid cartilage.

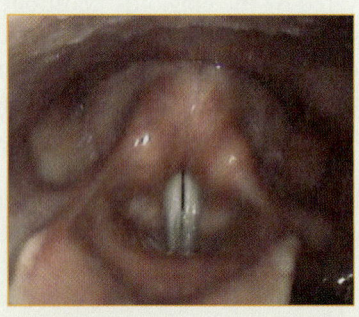

Figure 26-6 The arytenoid cartilages and piriform fossae are sometimes the only landmarks visible during a difficult intubation. The arytenoid cartilages are a pair of small pyramid-shaped cartilages to which the vocal cords are attached.

the laryngoscope to move it out of the way.

The cricoid cartilage can be palpated just below the thyroid cartilage in the neck. It forms a complete ring and maintains the trachea in an open position. Pressing on the anterior portion of this ring compresses the esophagus against the anterior aspect of the body of the sixth cervical vertebra while keeping the trachea open.

The palpable gap between the thyroid and cricoid cartilages is the location of the cricothyroid membrane. The membrane doesn't contain many blood vessels and is covered only by skin and minimal subcutaneous tissue. It is the site for performing a cricothyrotomy (an incision through the skin and cricothyroid membrane to relieve difficulty breathing caused by an obstruction in the airway) if you are unable to secure the airway with an advanced airway device. The rest of the neck contains large blood vessels, important nerves, and other critical anatomical structures that you must avoid cutting when performing a cricothyrotomy. Cricothyrotomies look easy when performed by skilled clinicians, but this procedure can turn into a bloody disaster if you aren't absolutely certain of anatomical landmarks, or have poor technique.

Trauma or swelling of any of the laryngeal structures can create a life-threatening airway obstruction **Figure 26-7** ▾. In the worst-case scenario, this entire anatomical region may

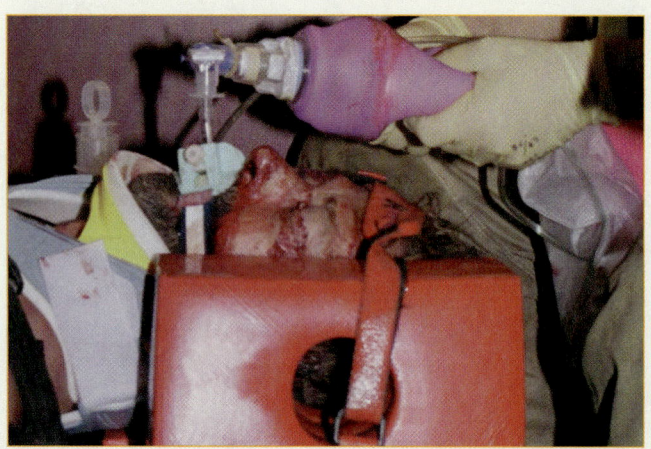

Figure 26-7 Trauma to the head and neck can completely obscure your view of the anatomy of the airway. You must be comfortable enough with airway anatomy to manage the airway, even when it has been significantly altered.

be bypassed by a tracheostomy (a surgical opening into the trachea). By their very nature, traumatic injuries may alter the typical anatomy of the upper airway. Procedures such as a cricothyrotomy can prove highly challenging when the airway is filled with blood or vomit, or when the anatomical landmarks are obscured by swelling or subcutaneous air.

The Lower Airway

Inspired gas is distributed to the millions of alveoli by a network of conducting airways. Gas in these tubes does not come into close contact with capillaries, so it does not participate in ventilation. This wasted ventilation is called anatomical dead space. Typically, anatomical dead space is about 2 ml per pound of ideal body weight (a 75-kg person has about 150 ml of anatomical dead space). This dead space remains relatively constant. If a 75-kg patient took an average breath (tidal volume [V_T]) of 700 ml, about 550 ml would participate in ventilation at the alveolar level; the other 150 ml would fill the tubes and would never be exposed to blood flow. If the same patient were to drop his or her V_T to 500 ml, only 350 ml would participate in ventilation, because 150 ml is still filling the anatomical dead space.

The trachea is about 10 to 13 cm long and extends from the level of the sixth cervical vertebra to its point of bifurcation (carina) at roughly the fifth thoracic vertebra (approximately nipple level) **Figure 26-8** ▸. At this point, it forks into the right and left mainstem bronchi. In adults, the right mainstem bronchus typically branches at a less acute angle than the left. Thus, if you advance an ET tube too far into an adult, it almost always goes down the right mainstem bronchus. Similarly, aspirated foreign bodies often end up in the right mainstem bronchus.

The mainstem bronchi branch into lobar bronchi, segmental bronchi, subsegmental bronchi, and bronchioles. These structures account for approximately 15 branchings of the airway and are lined with ciliated epithelium. Cilia are little hair-like structures that rhythmically wave in a pattern that helps move particulate matter up and out of the airway **Figure 26-9** ▸.

Goblet cells are also found in the lining of these airways. These cells produce a blanket of mucus that covers the entire lining of the conducting airways. The mucus covers the cilia and forms a two-layered blanket that is thick at the surface (gel layer) and thin and watery next to the cilia (sol layer). The gel layer of the mucous blanket is thick and floats over the sol layer. Cilia constantly push the gel layer up and out of the airway in the healthy individual. As the cilia beat, they reach out into the gel layer, pushing it up and toward the glottis. On the return stroke, the cilia collapse into the sol layer, so that they don't pull the gel layer back down. In this manner, the cilia slowly move the entire gel layer up and out of the tracheobronchial tree, where it is either swallowed or expectorated.

Smooth muscle surrounds the conducting airways down to the subsegmental level. Bronchoconstriction occurs when the smooth muscle constricts around these larger airways.

Below this level, bronchodilator medications have little effect upon the airways. Wheezing that is resolved with bronchodilator medication was probably caused by constriction of the smooth muscles. Wheezing that is not resolved with these medications may be caused by a variety of pathologic conditions, including inflammation.

The terminal airways and alveoli include branches 16 through 24 of the tracheobronchial tree, the so-called terminal bronchioles. The tracheobronchial tree ends with the alveoli, but the transfer of oxygen and carbon dioxide can nevertheless take place across both the alveoli and the terminal bronchioles. It is often helpful to think of alveoli as little balloons at the end of a straw. Alveoli cluster around the terminal bronchioles, and capillaries cover the alveoli and bronchial tubes from level 16 to level 24. The alveoli and terminal bronchioles actually make up the majority of the lung mass.

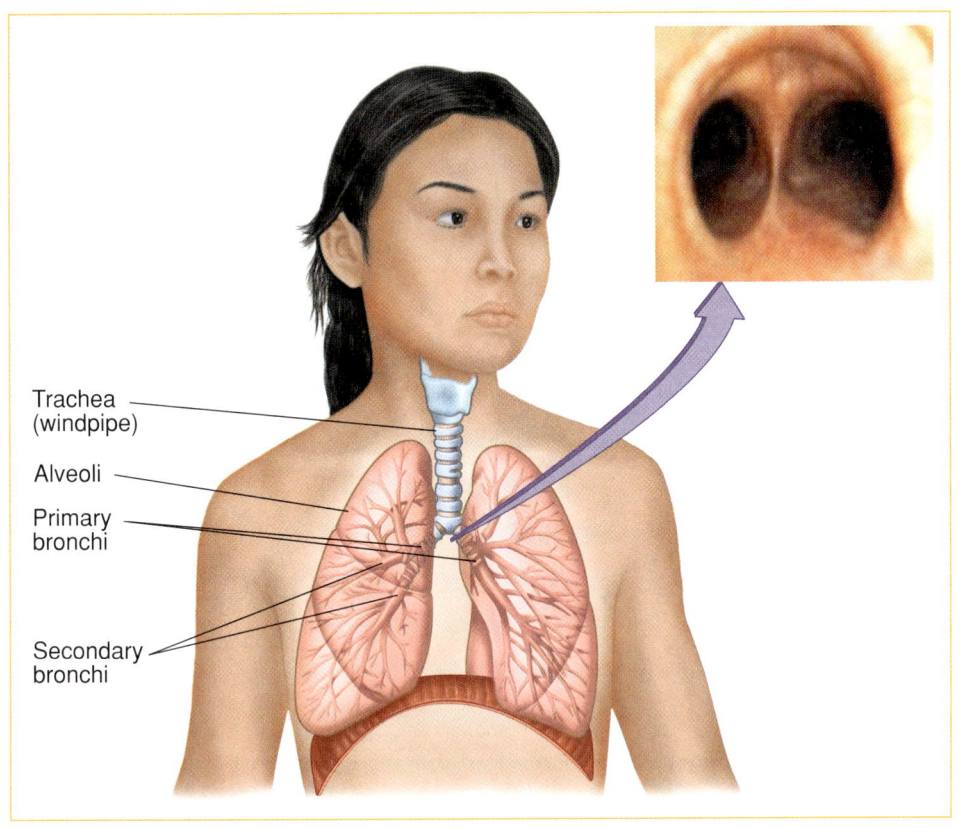

Figure 26-8 The carina is the point of bifurcation of the right and left mainstem bronchi. In an adult, it is located at roughly the fifth intercostal space.

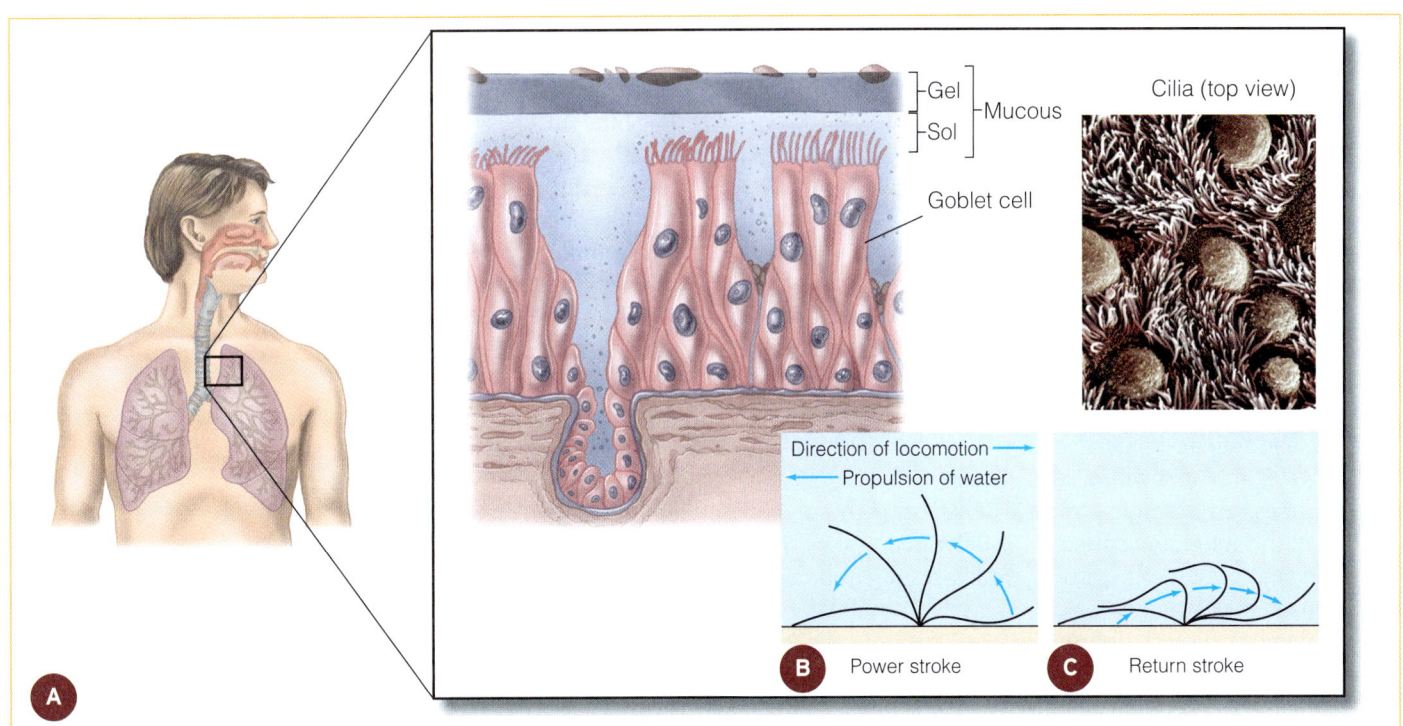

Figure 26-9 Cilia line the larger airways of the respiratory tract (**A**). Their regular pattern of movement between the gel and sol layers of mucus helps move foreign material out of the tracheobronchial tree (**B** and **C**).

Inset photo: © Dr. Kessel & Dr. Kardon/Tissue & Organs/Visuals Unlimited

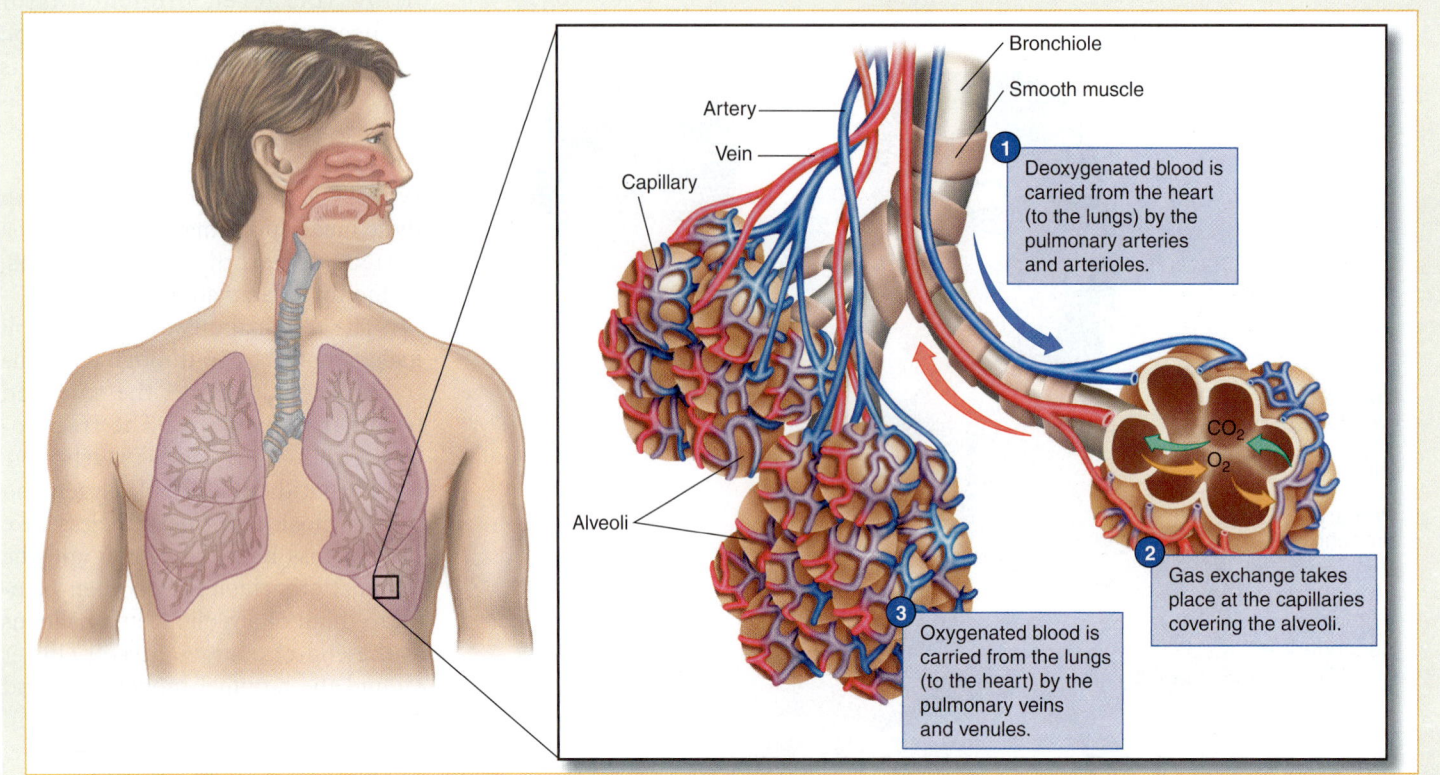

- Bronchiole
- Smooth muscle
- Artery
- Vein
- Capillary
- Alveoli

1 Deoxygenated blood is carried from the heart (to the lungs) by the pulmonary arteries and arterioles.

CO_2
O_2

2 Gas exchange takes place at the capillaries covering the alveoli.

3 Oxygenated blood is carried from the lungs (to the heart) by the pulmonary veins and venules.

Figure 26-10 The respiratory bronchioles, sometimes called terminal bronchioles, include the alveoli and the last several branches of the tracheobronchial tree. Gas exchange occurs over this entire area, not just the alveoli.

Gas transfer is most efficient in the alveoli, but a significant amount of gas is also exchanged across the respiratory bronchioles (**Figure 26-10 ▲**). These terminal bronchioles are very thin and have little structure. This is helpful for gas exchange, but it also means that these bronchioles lack cilia, a mucous blanket, smooth muscle, or rigid structures. Once foreign material gets into the terminal bronchioles and alveoli (parts of the lung collectively known as the lung parenchyma), it may cause significant damage. Emphysema may affect this area of the lung, destroying the few structural components that are present. When that happens, the terminal branches of the tracheobronchial tree become so weak that they collapse during exhalation, and trap air in the alveoli.

The alveoli are lined with a substance known as surfactant, which reduces surface tension and helps keep the alveoli expanded. If the amount of surfactant is decreased or the alveoli are not inflated, the alveoli collapse, which results in a condition known as atelectasis.

If smoking or disease destroys certain types of cells in an alveolus, it cannot repair itself. Conversely, alveoli can repair significant damage if certain cells survive an illness.

The pulmonary circulation begins at the right ventricle where the pulmonary artery (the only artery that usually carries deoxygenated blood) branches into increasingly smaller vessels until the pulmonary capillary bed surrounds the alveoli and terminal bronchioles (**Figure 26-11 ▶**). There is significantly more circulation to the lung bases than there is to the lung apices.

Like all the capillaries in the body, the pulmonary capillaries are very narrow, and typically allow only red blood cells to pass through in single-file fashion. People whose lung tissue has been destroyed by smoking (emphysema) have fewer and smaller capillaries, which increases the resistance to blood flow across the lungs and strains the right side of the heart. In addition, people with chronic lung disease and chronic hypoxia often make a surplus of red blood cells over time (polycythemia), which makes their blood thick. Pushing this thicker-than-normal blood through the tiny pulmonary capillaries can also put a significant strain on the right side of the heart. Right heart failure secondary to chronic lung disease is known as cor pulmonale.

Airway Problems Versus Breathing Problems

From your first cardiopulmonary resuscitation (CPR) class, the differences between maintaining the airway and breathing for the patient are highlighted. Unfortunately, a paramedic can still easily become confused between pathologic conditions that affect one versus the other. Many patients present with an airway that can use a little assistance. No one should be snoring, gurgling, squeaking, or using accessory muscles to inhale. You must remain vigilant that secretions, soft tissue, blood, or vomit do not compromise an airway that you initially thought was open.

At the same time, an open airway does not ensure that an adequate volume of gas is moving in and out of the lungs. Proper ventilation is necessary to provide adequate oxygen to the bloodstream and to remove carbon dioxide. Increasing the amount of available oxygen ensures that even a patient who is not moving adequate volumes of gas (eg, hypoventilating) can still maintain adequate oxygen saturation. Unfortunately, if ventilation remains inadequate, carbon dioxide levels will increase. Hypoventilating patients become hypercapneic (have too much carbon dioxide in their blood) and acidemic (the pH of their arterial

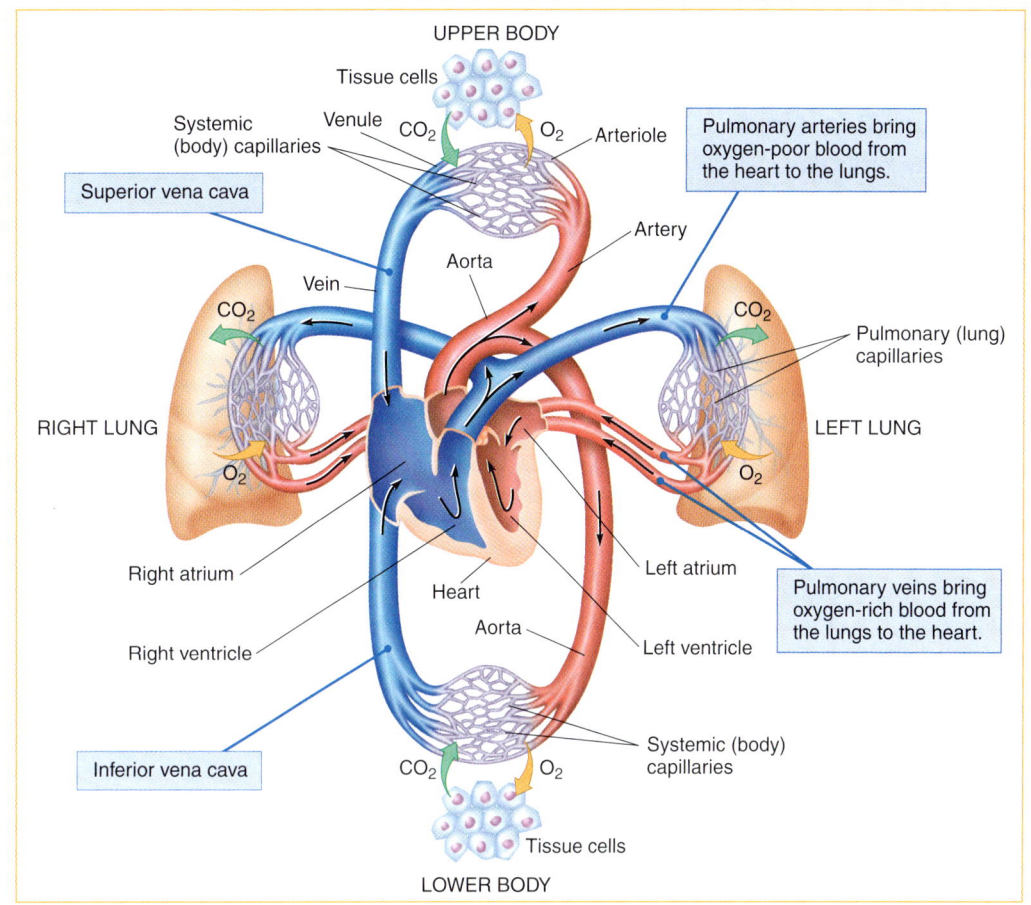

Figure 26-11 Pulmonary circulation begins as blood leaves the right ventricle via the pulmonary artery. The pulmonary capillary bed brings red blood cells very close to the terminal bronchioles. There is more perfusion to the bases of the lungs than to the apices. After picking up oxygen, the blood returns to the left atrium via the pulmonary veins.

You are the Paramedic Part 2

As you apply oxygen and obtain vital signs, you notice that the nail beds and oral mucosa of your patient are bluish (cyanosis). You adjust the sensor location of the pulse oximeter and obtain a reading. The patient's wife tells you that her husband has been running a fever, has experienced progressive weakness, and has had a productive cough (with thick, yellowish green sputum) for the past 4 to 5 days. She also tells you that her husband has been up all night struggling to breathe. He also has COPD and has smoked two packs of cigarettes a day since he was 15 years old. On auscultation of the chest, you note rhonchi in all lung fields on both inspiration and expiration.

Vital Signs	Recording Time: 5 Minutes
Level of consciousness	A (Alert to person, place, and day)
Skin	Pale, cool extremities, diaphoretic
Pulse	110 beats/min, weak; occasionally irregular
Blood pressure	108/54 mm Hg
SpO_2	75% (receiving 100% oxygen via nonrebreathing mask)
Temperature	38.2°C (reported by wife)
ECG	Sinus tachycardia with occasional premature ventricular contractions

4. Given the patient's presentation, which assessment tools should you use to obtain a greater understanding of the patient's medical condition?

5. What was likely the initial problem with obtaining a pulse oximetry reading?

blood falls too low). Both conditions can interrupt important body systems and, if uncorrected over a period of time, can result in death.

Ventilation Revisited

Many airway problems can be bypassed by inserting an ET tube. By contrast, alterations in breathing can be much more complex. They can involve problems with the conducting airways (branches), such as asthma or bronchitis; difficulties at the alveolar level, such as pneumonia or emphysema; problems with the muscles and nerves that make breathing work, as in Guillain-Barré syndrome or spinal cord injury; or problems with the rigid structure of the thorax that allows the pressure changes that make breathing work, such as flail chest.

We are usually negative-pressure breathers (air suckers). The expansion of the chest and downward movement of the diaphragm create negative pressure in the thorax. Air is pulled in through the mouth and the nose, over the turbinates, and around the complex terrain of the epiglottis and glottis. Air typically does not enter the esophagus and stomach because it is preferentially sucked into the trachea (Figure 26-12 ▾).

This negative-pressure vacuum effect occurs because the thorax is essentially an airtight box with a flexible diaphragm (the major muscle of breathing) at the bottom and an open tube (the trachea) at the top. During quiet breathing, when the diaphragm flattens, the overall size of the container increases, and air is sucked in through the tube at the top to fill the increasing space inside the thorax. You can increase the amount of air you move each minute (minute ventilation) by taking bigger breaths (hyperpnea) or by breathing more rapidly (tachypnea). To breathe even more deeply, you can

use additional muscles to pull the ribs up and out, further increasing both the size of the thoracic cavity as well as increasing the negative-pressure environment and moving larger volumes of air. Clearly, disruptions of the thoracic cage will hinder your ability to move air by this mechanism.

Holes in the thorax provide another place for air to be sucked in, resulting in a sucking chest wound (Figure 26-13 ▾). When multiple ribs are broken in more than one place (flail chest), free-floating sections of the thorax get pulled in when you breathe, limiting the amount of air that can be sucked in through the trachea. Infants and small children may exhibit retraction, or indrawing, of the intercostals and ribs when airflow is restricted by disease processes. The normal expansion of the chest without the ability of air to move easily results in greater negative pressure in the thorax. This draws the intercostals inward with each chest expansion.

When you ventilate someone with positive-pressure (ie, with a pocket mask or bag-valve-mask ventilation), air is forced into the upper airway and flows into both the trachea and esophagus unless steps are taken to help direct it into the trachea (Figure 26-14 ▸). Indeed, positive-pressure ventilation with bag-valve-mask ventilation or a pocket mask is physiologically the opposite of normal (negative-pressure) ventilation.

Exhalation is usually a passive process. After the size of the thorax has increased during inhalation, the components of the respiratory system return to their original places, and air is pushed out of the trachea under positive pressure. When a patient has trouble exhaling, for example, in asthma, reactive airway disease, or COPD, he or she may need to use the

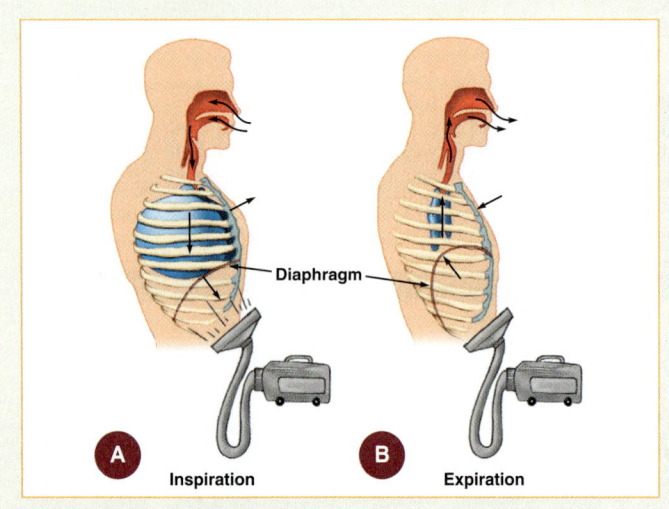

Figure 26-12 Normal ventilation is negative-pressure ventilation, meaning that we suck air into our lungs, much as a vacuum cleaner sucks in air. The negative pressure pulls down the diaphragm, causing the lungs to fill (**A**). When the pressure is released, the diaphragm relaxes and the lungs empty (**B**). Compare with positive-pressure ventilation, shown in Figure 26-14.

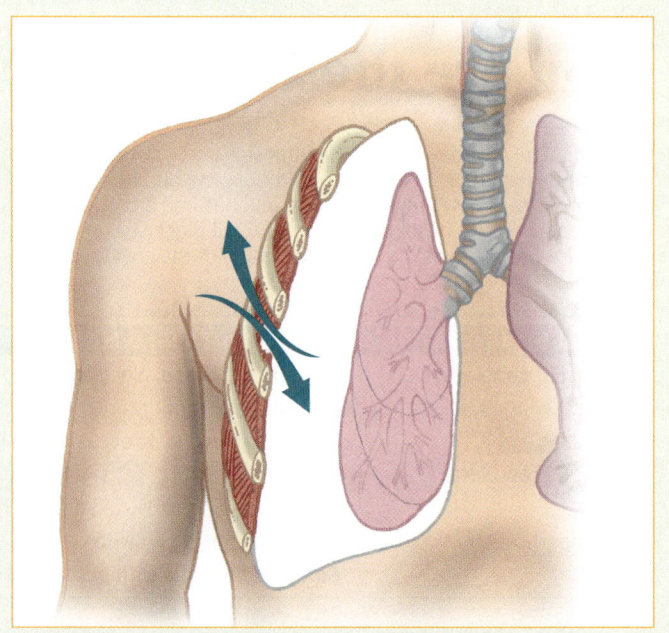

Figure 26-13 A sucking chest wound reduces ventilation by allowing air to enter the thorax during the inspiratory or negative-pressure phase of ventilation.

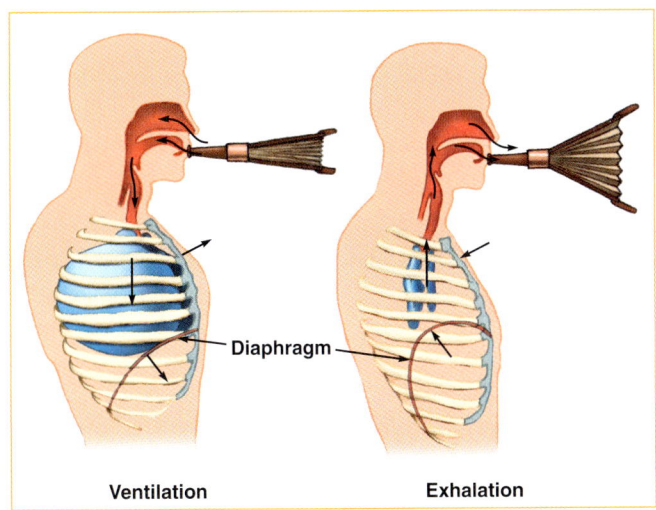

Figure 26-14 Positive-pressure ventilation is physiologically the opposite of normal ventilation. Air is pushed into the respiratory tract with bag-valve-mask ventilation and can go into the esophagus and stomach unless careful technique is applied. Compare with negative-pressure ventilation, shown in Figure 26-12.

Ventilation

Exhalation

Diaphragm

abdominal muscles to push air out. When this occurs, exhalation is no longer a passive process. Watch your patient work as he or she breathes. Is the patient having trouble pulling air in or pushing air out? Difficulty in exhalation usually indicates obstructive disease; difficulty in inhalation may indicate upper airway obstruction.

The neurologic control of respiration is complex. At least four parts of the brain are responsible for the smooth, rhythmic respirations that we take for granted—one area helps control rate, another depth, another inspiratory pause, and yet another rhythmicity. Patients with traumatic brain injuries may exhibit bizarre respiratory patterns when one or more of these respiratory centres are damaged or deprived of adequate blood flow. Table 26-1 ▸ summarizes the various breathing patterns.

Most of these respiratory centres are in and around the brain stem Figure 26-15 ▾ . Patients who suffer serious trauma to the upper cerebral hemispheres (such as from a gunshot wound) are often still breathing despite mortal wounds. Apneustic breathing results from damage to the apneustic centre in the brain, which regulates inspiratory pause. A patient exhibiting apneustic respirations will have a short, brisk inhalation with a long pause before exhalation. This pattern is indicative of severe pressure within the cranium or direct trauma to the brain. Similarly, Biot respirations are seen when the centre that controls breathing rhythm is damaged. This respiratory pattern is grossly irregular, sometimes with lengthy apneic periods.

Cheyne-Stokes respirations are more of a high-brain function. Many deep sleepers or intoxicated people will exhibit this type of respiratory pattern. The depth of breathing (or volume of snoring) gradually increases, then decreases (crescendo-decrescendo), followed by an apneic period. The apneic period is usually brief in the relatively healthy patient. Exaggerated Cheyne-Stokes respirations may be seen in patients who have a severe brain injury, where the crescendo-decrescendo is much more prominent. The apneic period may last 30 to 60 seconds.

Stretch receptors in the lungs are responsible for the Hering-Breuer reflex, which limits inspiration and may cause coughing if you take too deep a breath. Paramedics become accustomed to ventilating unresponsive patients. When called

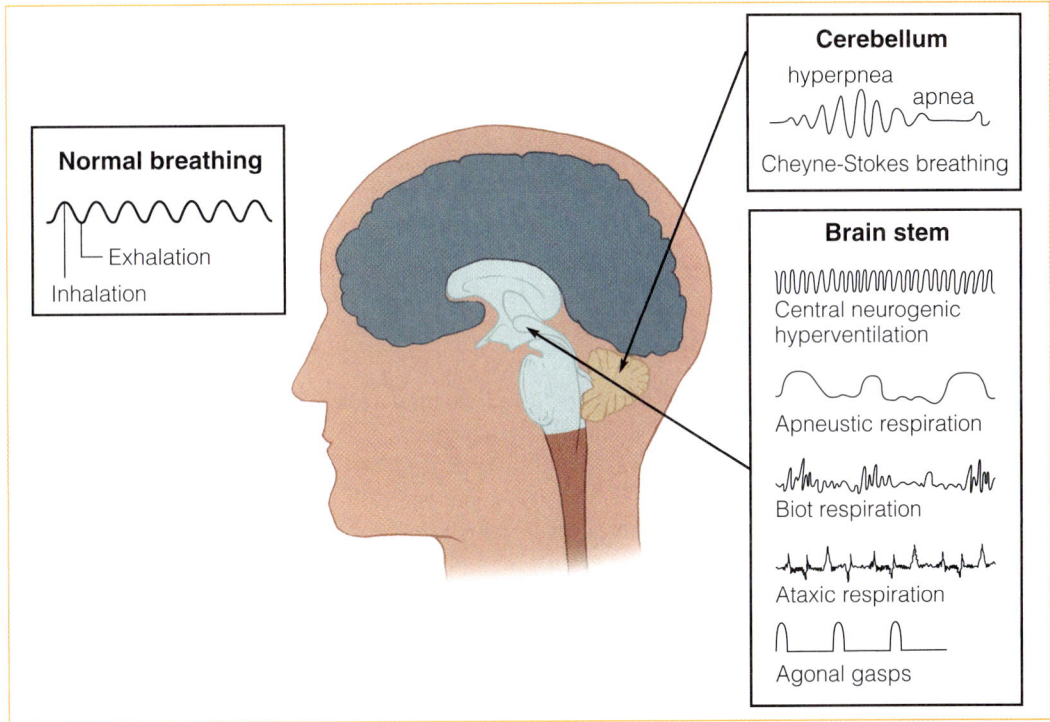

Figure 26-15 The neurologic control of respiration is complex, and many variations in the respiratory pattern may be noted in the scenario of brain injury. The respiratory patterns shown—each recorded for 1 minute—have been documented using an end-tidal carbon dioxide detector. Note that most irregular breathing patterns are controlled by the brain stem.

Table 26-1	Breathing Patterns
Pattern	**Comments**
Agonal	Irregular gasps that are few and far between. Usually represent stray neurologic impulses in the dying patient. It is not unusual for patients who are pulseless to have an occasional agonal gasp.
Apneustic	When the pneumotaxic centre in the brain is damaged, the apneustic centre causes a prolonged inspiratory hold (fish breathing). This ominous sign indicates severe brain injury.
Ataxic	Completely irregular respirations that indicate severe brain injury or brain-stem herniation.
Biot respirations	Respirations with an irregular pattern, rate, and depth with intermittent patterns of apnea. Indicative of severe brain injury or brain-stem herniation.
Bradypnea	Unusually slow respirations.
Central neurogenic hyperventilation	Tachypneic hyperpnea. Rapid and deep respirations caused by increased intracranial pressure or direct brain injury. Drives carbon dioxide levels down and pH levels up, resulting in respiratory alkalosis.
Cheyne-Stokes respirations	Crescendo-decrescendo breathing with a period of apnea between each cycle. It is not considered ominous unless grossly exaggerated or in the context of a patient who has brain trauma.
Cough	Forced exhalation against a closed glottis; an airway-clearing maneuver. Also seen when foreign substances irritate the airways. Controlled by the cough centre in the brain. Antitussive medications work on the cough centre to reduce this sometimes-annoying physiologic response.
Eupnea	Normal breathing.
Hiccup	Spasmodic contraction of the diaphragm causing short exhalations with a characteristic sound. Sometimes seen in cases of diaphragmatic (or phrenic nerve) irritation from acute myocardial infarction, ulcer disease, or endotracheal intubation.
Hyperpnea	Unusually deep breathing. Seen in various neurologic or chemical disorders. Certain drugs may stimulate this type of breathing in patients who have overdosed. It does not reflect respiratory rate—only respiratory depth.
Hypopnea	Unusually shallow respirations.
Kussmaul respirations	The same pattern as central neurogenic hyperventilation, but caused by the body's response to metabolic acidosis; the body is trying to rid itself of blood acetone via the lungs. Kussmaul respirations are seen in patients who have diabetic ketoacidosis, and are accompanied by a fruity (acetone) breath odour. The mouth and lips are usually cracked and dry.
Sighing	Periodically taking a very deep breath (about twice the normal volume). Sighing forces open alveoli that close in the course of day-to-day events.
Tachypnea	Unusually rapid breathing. This term does not reflect depth of respiration, nor does it mean that the patient is hyperventilating (lowering the carbon dioxide level by breathing too fast and too deep). In fact, patients who breathe very rapidly frequently move only small volumes of air and are *hypo*ventilating (much like a panting dog).
Yawning	Yawning seems to be beneficial in the same manner that sighing is.

upon to assist a conscious patient's respirations, as may happen when a patient is breathing shallowly, many paramedics give breaths that are too large, causing repeated coughing and discomfort to the patient. Assisting the spontaneously breathing patient with bag-valve-mask ventilation can be a complex skill, requiring practice.

Respiration Revisited

Respiration is the process by which oxygen is taken into the body, distributed to the cells, and used by the cells to make energy. Respiration takes place in each cell. It involves using oxygen and glucose to make energy that allows the cell to do its work. The oxygen must be supplied by the lungs and circulatory systems. The primary byproduct of this process is carbon dioxide.

The respiratory system is involved in the delivery of the oxygen to the bloodstream and the removal of the waste carbon dioxide from the body. If the lungs are not functioning appropriately, both of these vital functions may be impaired. Failure to deliver oxygen efficiently results in cellular hypoxia. Hypoxia kills cells by making it impossible for them to make enough energy to do their work; it also causes acidosis. We can often help the patient with hypoxia by providing additional oxygen.

Under normal circumstances, the carbon dioxide evolved during cellular respiration is returned to the lungs by the circulatory system, where it is exhaled during ventilation. When the lungs are not working adequately, carbon dioxide is not efficiently disposed of and accumulates in the blood. This carbon dioxide combines with water to form bicarbonate ions and hydrogen (H^+) ions, also known as acid (pH is an expression of how many free H^+ ions are in a solution). The result is acidosis. By contrast, in hyperventilation, the person breathes faster or deeper than normal and blows off more carbon dioxide than usual, resulting in alkalosis.

A Systems Approach to Respiratory Emergencies

Evaluation of the respiratory organs is clearly an important component of assessing respiratory emergencies. However, the job performed by the respiratory system so dramatically impacts other body systems that a thorough respiratory assessment includes much more than listening to the patient's lungs.

Neurologic Status

The brain is very sensitive to reduced levels of oxygen. For this reason, any alteration in level of consciousness could represent a degree of respiratory compromise. Anxiety can be an early sign of hypoxia, while confusion, lethargy, and coma are typically later signs. A brief seizure often accompanies a hypoxic event or cardiac arrest. Dizziness and tingling extremities could signify hyperventilation. Major neurologic insults may also manifest themselves with some altered respiratory pattern.

Brain trauma or anything else that disturbs the function of the brain may depress the respiratory control centres in the medulla. For example, the increasing intracranial pressure in closed head trauma may literally put the squeeze on the medulla to produce a variety of respiratory abnormalities, including apnea. A stroke may have a similar effect by depriving portions of the brain of circulation (see Chapter 28). Overdose with drugs that depress the central nervous system (such as narcotics or barbiturates) may also severely depress the activity of the respiratory centre.

Injury high in the spinal cord may paralyze the intercostal muscles and even the diaphragm. Polio attacks the nerves that supply the respiratory muscles, but certain chronic illnesses, such as myasthenia gravis, weaken the respiratory muscles themselves. The net effect of these conditions is the inability of the respiratory muscles to function normally in response to the respiratory drive. As a consequence, the tidal volume is shallow, and the minute volume is correspondingly decreased. Patients with such conditions often need assisted ventilation to increase the tidal volume and, thus, minute volume.

Cardiovascular Status

Think of the lungs as lying between the right and left sides of the heart (in terms of function). Although an anatomical drawing may not depict the lungs in this way, the description is a very accurate concept when reviewing blood flow through the body. The right side of the heart pumps blood to the lungs, while the left side of the heart receives blood from the lungs and then pumps it around the body. Any major change in the function of the lungs, right side of the heart, or left side of the heart almost always affects the other components. The

body's immediate response to mild hypoxemia is to increase the heart rate (tachycardia), in order to deliver a higher volume of blood to tissues to compensate for lower blood oxygen levels. Severe hypoxia often causes bradycardia. Any uncorrected hypoxic insult may result in lethal cardiac arrhythmias, such as ventricular fibrillation or ventricular tachycardia. Changes in fluid balance, right-heart pumping pressures, or left-heart pumping pressures can cause various forms of congestive heart failure. A thorough evaluation of the cardiovascular system is requisite in the evaluation of the respiratory patient.

Muscles and Mechanics

Muscles have to work to allow you to breathe under normal circumstances, and they have to work a lot harder when oxygen needs are higher or when there is a problem with the normal mechanics of breathing. This extra work comes at a cost. People who have asthma, for instance, can often compensate for their respiratory distress by devoting lots of energy to their breathing. They can maintain their oxygen and carbon dioxide levels in an acceptable range as long as they continue to apply their muscles to this effort. The tremendous workload causes them to use tremendous amounts of energy, which requires even more oxygen and ventilation. Such patients are typically not in a position to eat and drink normally, so they continue to get more dehydrated, more malnourished, and more tired. At some point they will tire out and be unable to continue doing the necessary work of breathing; they will then look sleepy, the rate and depth of their respirations will slowly drop, and they will decompensate (respiratory failure).

Other things may interfere with the mechanics of breathing. Placing a patient in the Trendelenburg position, or even laying the patient flat, especially if the patient is overweight, causes the abdominal organs to push up against the diaphragm. With each breath, the patient must move the abdominal contents out of the way to expand the thorax and breathe. This explains why most people seek a sitting position when they are short of breath (orthopnea). If the abdomen is distended with air or blood, the situation is compounded. Things that bind the chest or abdomen (such as tight clothing or undergarments, a pneumatic antishock garment, or backboard straps) can also make it very difficult to breathe. Diseases that cause muscle weakness (such as botulism, amyotrophic lateral sclerosis, or Guillain-Barré syndrome) can be fatal when they render the patient unable to breathe.

Renal Status

Fluid balance, acid-base balance, and blood pressure are controlled, in part, by the kidneys. Each of these factors also affects the pulmonary mechanics and hence the delivery of oxygen to the tissues. Patients with severe renal disease often present with respiratory signs and symptoms, so the paramedic should always note signs of severe renal disease when evaluating the conditions of such patients. The conditions of patients who have congestive heart failure secondary to renal disease can be difficult to manage because diuresis may be difficult or impossible for them. Patients who have renal disease may also have acid-base disturbances that cause them to hyperventilate and that are sometimes mistaken for respiratory disorders. Often, a patient's need for emergency dialysis may influence your transport decisions and options.

Assessment of the Patient With Dyspnea

As always, remember that recognizing and treating life threats is the priority in the initial assessment, and throughout prehospital care.

Initial Assessment

Your first glance at a patient may identify a body type associated with a particular pathologic condition. The classic presentation of a patient with emphysema includes a barrel chest (a chest that is rounded and bulging, like the shape of a barrel, from years of having air trapped in the thorax), muscle wasting (the patient has cannibalized his or her own body mass for energy), and pursed-lip breathing (a technique often used to improve breathing in patients with obstructive lung disease). Such patients are often tachypneic and do not typically present with profound hypoxia and cyanosis—hence the term pink puffer.

Patients who have chronic bronchitis tend to be more sedentary and thus may be obese. These patients are often encountered in a chair or recliner, where they sleep in an upright position. They may be surrounded by a wastebasket overflowing with tissues, a cup into which they spit their copious secretions, a urinal to avoid frequent trips to the bathroom, and an overflowing ashtray. The table next to their chair may have several medications, inhalers, or an aerosol nebulizer. Such a scene can disclose volumes of information about the patient and his or her history long before the paramedic ever places a stethoscope on the chest.

Severely ill patients with end-stage diseases, cancer, or immune system disorders are often easy to spot, as are the sickly appearance, rigors, and chills of a patient with pneumonia. A spontaneous pneumothorax tends to occur in tall, thin young adults, and women who smoke and take birth-control pills are predisposed to pulmonary embolus. Clues to a variety of pathologic conditions may be evident from your very first impression of a patient, but keep in mind that they are only clues. Avoid making a hasty initial diagnosis based on minimal information. The patient's presentation may make you suspicious about a particular condition, but make sure you confirm your suspicions with a thorough assessment.

Position and Degree of Distress

Patients in respiratory distress tend to seek the sitting position. The tripod position involves leaning forward and rotating the scapulae outward by placing the arms on a table or by placing the hands on the knees **Figure 26-16**. This stabilizes the

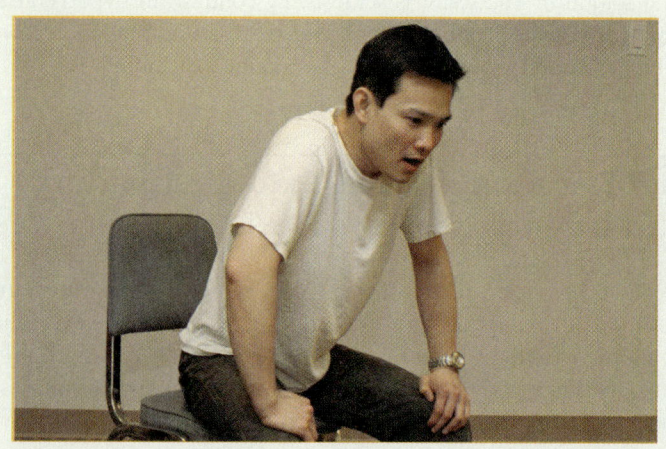

Figure 26-16 The tripod position (elbows out) allows better diaphragmatic movement by getting the abdomen out of the way, as well as a little more airflow to the apices, by rotating the scapulae laterally. This takes work, which requires more oxygen.

shoulder girdle, improves efficiency of the accessory breathing muscles, and decreases the total work of breathing. Beware of the patient in respiratory distress who is willing to lie flat; this could be a sign of sudden deterioration.

Purposeful hyperextension occurs when a patient maximizes airflow through the upper airway. Such patients essentially hold their heads in the head tilt–chin lift or "sniffing" position. This position may indicate upper airway swelling, but it is also commonly seen in patients who are trying to maximize airflow. Maintaining this position uses up valuable energy. As a patient who is severely ill with respiratory disease begins to feel fatigue, he or she may hold the head up in this position only during inhalation, letting it fall into flexion during exhalation. This head bobbing is a very ominous sign, signaling the potential for imminent decompensation. Head bobbing is frequently preterminal behaviour!

Work of Breathing

Patients who are using lots of muscles to breathe are in danger of tiring out, so it is important to note the use of accessory muscles. Is the patient using the muscles of the abdomen to push air out (as in asthma or COPD), or is the patient using muscles in the chest and neck to pull air in? Patients who are using a lot of extra muscles to breathe may cause dramatic pressure changes within the thorax and exhibit the following signs and symptoms:

- **Chest-wall retractions.** These are most common in infants and small children, where the rigid structure of the thorax is still flexible. On inhalation, the child may pull (or retract) the sternum or ribs into the chest, causing a visible deformity with each breath **Figure 26-17**.
- **Soft-tissue retractions.** In most patients, the bones are rigid and don't move, but the soft tissue is pulled in around the bones. Dramatic retractions can be seen during inhalation in the supraclavicular, intercostal, and subxiphoid areas.

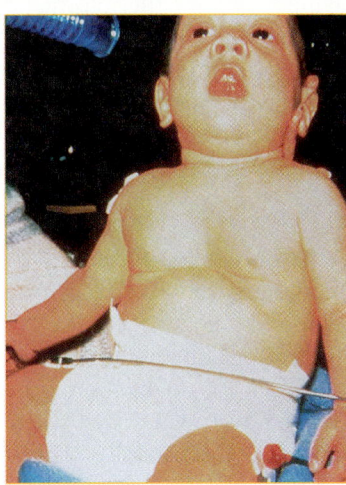

Figure 26-17 Chest-wall retractions are not only a sign of severe distress and increased work of breathing, they also contribute to respiratory failure. With inhalation, the lower sternum is pulled into the lungs. Every cubic centimetre of space displaced by the retraction is a cubic centimetre of air that cannot get into the chest.

- **Nasal flaring.** The nostrils are pulled wide open on inhalation.
- **Tracheal tugging.** The thyroid cartilage is pulled upward and the area just above the sternal notch is sucked inward with inhalation.
- **Paradoxical respiratory movement.** The epigastrium is pulled in with inhalation while the abdomen pushes out, creating a see-saw appearance as the two move in opposing directions.
- **Pulsus paradoxus.** Profound intrathoracic pressure changes cause the peripheral pulses to weaken (or disappear!) on inspiration; these pulses are easier to palpate during exhalation. This is rare.

Assessing breathing for rate and depth is an obvious component of a respiratory assessment, but one that is often not accurately determined. Respiratory rate may be a commonly "guessed" vital sign, but respiratory depth is even more commonly misjudged. A patient with an adequate rate but a low volume will still have a pitifully low minute volume (respiratory rate × tidal volume = minute volume). While assessing the respirations, note their pattern (see Table 26-1) and the inspiratory-to-expiratory (I:E) ratio. Is the patient working hard to inhale, to exhale, or both? Does the breath have a peculiar odour (such as the acetone breath odour associated with diabetic ketoacidosis)? Are there any audible abnormal respiratory noises? As a general rule, *any* respiratory noises that you can hear without a stethoscope are abnormal noises.

Notes from Nancy

Noisy breathing is obstructed breathing.

Snoring indicates partial obstruction of the upper airway by the *tongue*—a form of obstruction that is easily corrected by head tilt maneuvers. Gurgling signals the presence of fluid in the upper airway. Stridor, a harsh, high-pitched sound heard on inhalation, indicates narrowing, usually as a result of swelling (laryngeal edema).

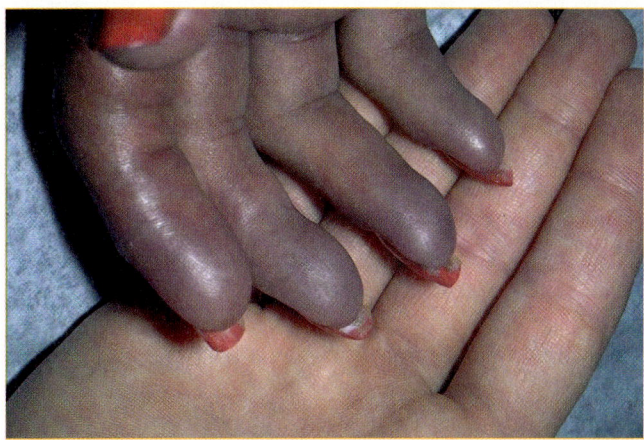

Figure 26-18 Skin colour can provide an early, fast indication of several disease processes. Cyanosis (shown here) presents as bluish skin and indicates at least 50 g/l of unoxygenated hemoglobin. Carbon monoxide intoxication can present as cherry-red skin, though this is a very late sign. When making any preliminary diagnosis, allow for the wide variation in patients' skin colour and tone.

Quiet breathing should also be of interest. The patient with tachypnea who has crystal-clear breath sounds may have hyperventilation syndrome but may also be breathing fast because of acidosis. Quiet tachypnea should prompt you to consider shock. Paramedics occasionally mistake tachypnea caused by pain, anxiety, or metabolic disorders as the patient's primary problem, and administer aerosol treatments for diabetic crisis or sepsis. Obviously, aerosol bronchodilators don't help those conditions.

Neurologic Assessment

Assessing the level of consciousness is enormously important in patients with dyspnea. Although you cannot measure the patient's arterial blood gases in the prehospital environment, the patient's brain is constantly doing precisely that. Any decline in Pa_{O_2} (hypoxemia) will manifest initially as restlessness, confusion, and in worst case scenarios, as combative behaviour. An increase in Pa_{CO_2}, by contrast, usually has sedative effects, making the patient sleepy and hard to rouse.

Skin Colour

Assessing skin colour is a fast way to begin forming an early impression of the patient's condition **Figure 26-18 ▲**. While it is obviously important to note the generalized cyanosis of oxygen desaturation or the profound pallor of shock, more subtle information can be gained by assessing the patient's mucous membranes. The tissue inside the mouth, under the eyelids, and even under the nail beds is usually the same pink colour in all healthy patients. A few notable variations are described below:

- **Cyanosis.** Healthy adults have a hemoglobin level of 120 to 140 g/l. Under those conditions, a person will begin to exhibit the blue discolouration of cyanosis when about 50 g/l is desaturated (does not have oxygen attached).

That means their oxygen saturation would be roughly 65%! If a person's hemoglobin level were only 100 g/l, 50% of it (50 of the 100 g/l) would have to be desaturated before the patient would look cyanotic. Some patients in cardiac arrest are a deep blue, while others are simply pale. Similarly, patients with high hemoglobin levels (those who have chronic respiratory disease) may develop cyanosis earlier than patients who have normal hemoglobin levels. Of course, there are slight variations in what is considered normal. Also, some patients who have chronic respiratory conditions who have an artificially low oxygen saturation may also have a low level of chronic cyanosis (which explains the use of the term blue bloater to describe patients who have chronic bronchitis).

■ **Chocolate brown skin.** High levels of methemoglobin derived from nitrates and some toxic exposures may turn the mucous membranes brown. This transformation is typically more evident in the patient's venous blood than in the skin and mucous membranes.

■ **Pale skin.** Pale skin and mucous membranes are caused by a reduction of blood flow to the small vessels near the surface of the skin. The source of this condition could be hypoxia, shock, catecholamine release, such as from epinephrine or norepinephrine, or a cold environment.

While you are noting the colour of the mucous membranes, also note their moistness. Dehydration can be seen in the mucous membranes of the mouth and eyes. Dry, cracked lips; a dry, furrowed tongue; and dry, sunken eyes point to obvious dehydration. The skin of an older patient may always look dry with poor turgor, so skin assessment may be of less value in some older people.

The Focused History: Elaboration on the Chief Complaint

One challenge in assessing respiratory patients is that they may not be able to talk to you because of having difficulty breathing. While it is usually best to ask open-ended questions and allow patients to tell their own stories, dyspneic patients may be able to speak only in short sentences, or may be reduced to nodding in response to a series of yes-or-no questions. In some cases, the bulk of your history-taking may have to be hastily obtained from a family member, or gleaned from the few clues (such as medications) immediately available. You often have to institute basic therapy (such as oxygen or nebulizer therapy) before getting the complete story from patients. Sometimes, you must immediately intubate patients, which will eliminate your ability to get a history from them from that point on.

When it is possible to discuss the history of the present illness with patients, several lines of questioning can provide important data. Utilizing the OPQRST mnemonic can help you elaborate on the chief complaint.

Reason for Calling for Help

Have patients explain in their own words what they are feeling. Many patients will identify their problem and tell you the best way to treat it without you having to dig for the information. Patients who have chronic respiratory conditions are often knowledgeable about their disease or disorder and may have tried several potential treatment options already. If they have been intubated and placed on a ventilator in past episodes, that is important information for you to have.

Onset and Duration

The speed with which the patient's distress has worsened is an important consideration in determining the underlying cause. Rapid-onset dyspnea may be caused by acute bronchospasm, anaphylaxis, pulmonary embolism, or pneumothorax. Left heart failure typically progresses much faster than right heart failure. Right heart failure may slowly worsen over many days, whereas left heart failure resulting from a massive AMI can kill a patient in a matter of minutes! Infectious diseases sometimes present very rapidly, but at other times may occur at the end of a lengthy battle with a low-grade infection. Did this problem arise suddenly, or did it get worse over time? How long has it been this bad?

Paroxysmal nocturnal dyspnea—dyspnea that comes on suddenly in the middle of the night is an ominous sign. It may signal left heart failure, worsening of COPD, or both. It occurs because of accumulation of fluid in the alveoli or pooling of secretions in the bronchi during sleep.

The position of comfort and difficulty speaking may also help you gauge the degree of distress. A patient who is comfortable while lying flat and speaking in full sentences can be deemed to be in little distress. A patient who is sitting in a Fowler's position (90°) speaking only in two- or three-word statements is probably in considerable distress, possibly even life-threatening distress.

History of the Problem

Asthma attack, congestive heart failure, pneumonia in immunocompromised patients, and even spontaneous pneumothorax are often repeating pathologic conditions. If the patient has some experience with these types of events, they can serve as a baseline to assess the current condition. Ask these questions: Do you feel better or worse than last time? How often does this happen to you? What did the doctor tell you it was? What helped you or what happened last time?

Attempts at Treatment

When respiratory disorders are chronic or recurring, patients may already have strategies to manage their crises. Determine what the patient may have already tried, and whether it had any effect (positive or negative). By following this simple line of questioning, you can determine which medications the patient is supposed to be taking (which often gives valuable clues to other problems) and whether the patient is taking those medications correctly. Patients also often know exactly what caused their problems.

Associated Symptoms

Respiratory difficulty must always be evaluated in light of the patient's cardiovascular and renal status. Many acute myocardial infarctions present as congestive heart failure, as do renal crises. Tachypnea can signal anxiety, diabetes, or shock. In addition, the vast majority of chronically ill patients have a respiratory component to their disease. A whole host of pathologic conditions can masquerade as respiratory distress, especially in patients who have underlying respiratory disease. Don't be too quick to conclude that your patient's *only* problem is a relatively straightforward respiratory issue. Always dig deeper to determine what else may be triggering or worsening the patient's respiratory distress.

The Focused Physical Examination

By the time you have elicited the history of a patient who has respiratory complaints, you should already have some important information about the patient's physical signs. In particular, you should have observed the patient's level of consciousness, position, degree of distress, and so forth. This section presents the components of the physical examination in sequence, noting at each step the points of particular relevance to the dyspneic patient.

Neck Examination

In the neck, look for jugular venous distension when a patient is in a semi-sitting position. Jugular venous distension is a condition in which the jugular veins are engorged with blood. Cardiac tamponade, pneumothorax, heart failure, and COPD can all cause jugular venous distension. It is common all of the time in patients who have an obstructive lung disease such as asthma or COPD. Healthy young adults often demonstrate jugular venous distension when they are supine (lying on their back), and it is common to see gross jugular venous distension when people are laughing or singing **Figure 26-19 ◂** . When jugular venous distension is present in patients who are sitting upright, it can provide a rough measure of the pressure in the right atrium of the heart. Distended neck veins may implicate cardiac failure as the source of the patient's dyspnea. Jugular venous distension may also indicate high pressure in the thorax, which keeps the blood from draining out of the head and neck. Hepato-

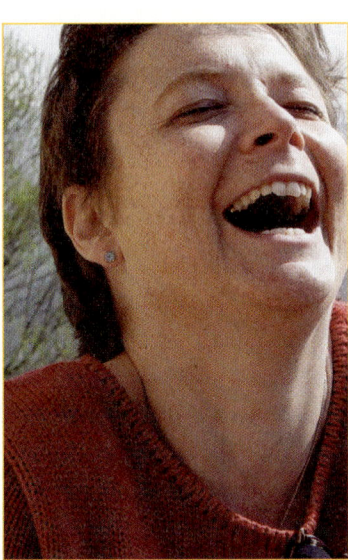

Figure 26-19 Jugular venous distension may be a normal finding in a healthy young adult who is supine or laughing. But in an adult who is sitting upright, it may indicate blood backing up as it tries to enter the thorax or the right atrium.

jugular reflux occurs when mild pressure on the patient's liver causes the jugular veins to engorge further. This is a specific sign of right heart failure.

Obviously, jugular venous distension must be interpreted in light of the patient's position and other vital signs. The trauma patient who demonstrates grossly distended jugular veins despite a blood pressure of 80/40 mm Hg should cause considerable concern and could be a sign of tamponade or tension pneumothorax. A healthy 20 year old who has jugular venous distension when lying flat (but not while sitting) is of little concern.

While looking at the neck, note the trachea. Tracheal deviation is a classic—albeit late and uncommon—sign of a tension pneumothorax **Figure 26-20 ▾** . Tension pneumothorax is very difficult to see except in extreme cases. On a radiograph, the trachea can be seen deviating because of a tension

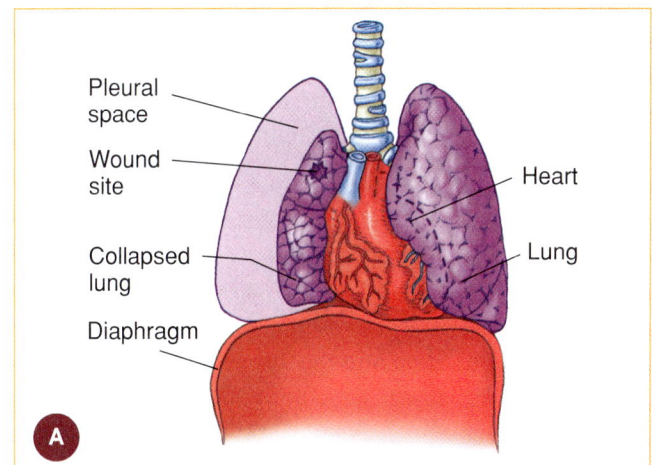

Pleural space

Wound site

Collapsed lung

Diaphragm

Heart

Lung

A

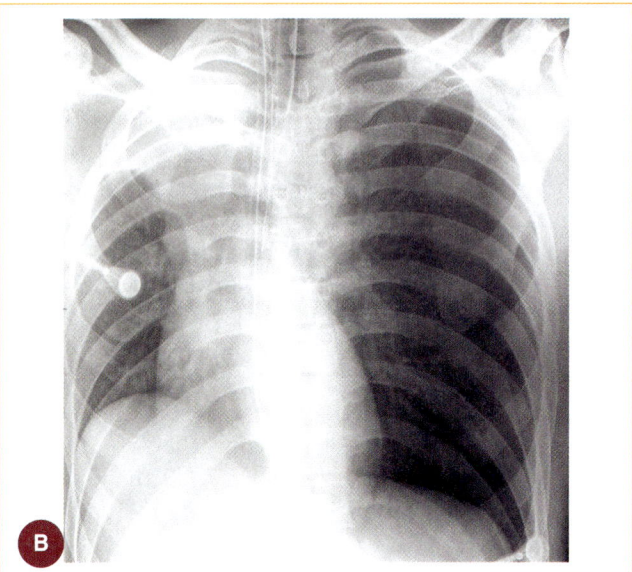

B

Figure 26-20 A pneumothorax occurs when air leaks into the pleural space between the lung and the chest wall (**A**). The radiograph (**B**) shows a collapsed lung on the right, which appears darker.

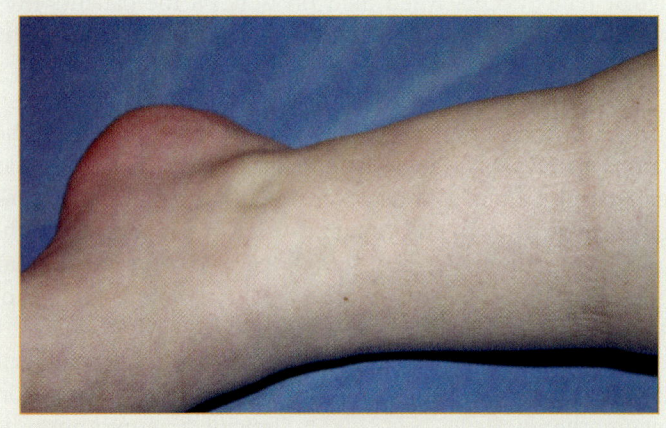

Figure 26-21 Pitting edema is present when you palpate the area, and your fingers leave temporary depressions in the tissue.

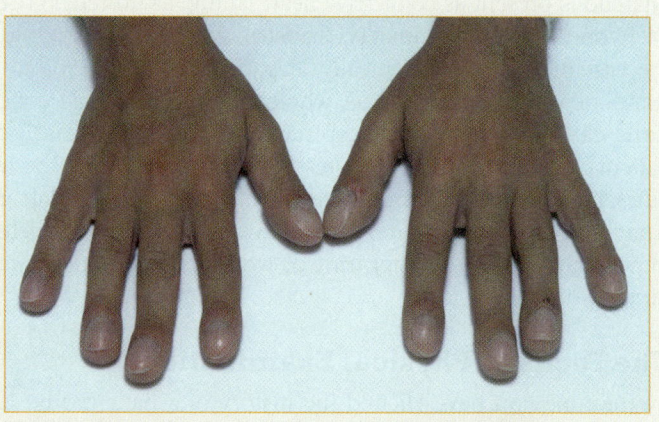

Figure 26-22 Digital clubbing is a sign of chronic hypoxia. It is seen in young people who have congenital heart disease and in older people who have severe chronic lung disease.

pneumothorax. The deviation occurs behind the sternum, so it may not be seen or even felt. Consider palpating the trachea at the suprasternal notch. When the trachea does deviate, it often does so at a point behind the sternum, so it may not be palpable or visible.

Chest and Abdominal Examination

Hepatojugular reflux is specific to right heart failure. When the right ventricle is not pumping effectively, blood backs up, making it difficult for the jugular veins and the large reservoir of blood in the liver to drain into the thorax. As a result, the combination of jugular venous distension and hepatomegaly (distended liver) may present in right heart failure. If you gently press on the liver, the blood you squeeze out will back up behind the failing ventricle and the jugular veins will engorge further. When a patient in respiratory distress is sitting up in a semi-Fowler's (45°) position, it is easy to check for hepatojugular reflux.

Feel the chest for vibrations as the patient breathes (tactile fremitus); secretions in the large airways are usually easy to feel and to hear. Some people recommend percussing the chest. With experience, you can tell the difference between a normal chest and a bad pneumothorax, but this remains a difficult procedure to perform in the prehospital setting because of ambient noise around you and the patient.

Examination of the Extremities

Does the patient have edema of the ankles or lower back? If so, does it pit, and leave a depression, when you push your finger into the edema **Figure 26-21 ▲** ? Is there peripheral cyanosis? Check the pulse. Is the patient profoundly tachycardic (from exertion or hypoxia)? Is there pulsus paradoxus? Also note the patient's skin temperature. Does the patient have an obvious fever, or is he or she cool and clammy from shock? Is there distal clubbing (from chronic hypoxia) **Figure 26-22 ▶** ?

Data Collection

As appropriate to your patient care plan, attach any monitors that are immediately available to you. Repeated vital signs, ECG, and pulse oximetry readings are the data most commonly collected. In some situations, depending on available equipment, you might also record peak expiratory flow, end-tidal carbon dioxide, or even transcutaneous carbon monoxide levels. (Monitoring devices are discussed later in the chapter.)

The Stethoscope

As far as stethoscopes go, the following guideline applies: the longer the tubing, the more extraneous the noise you will probably hear. Avoid overly long stethoscopes. Higher-quality stethoscopes have a tubing-within-the-tubing design that limits its external noise interference. Although the Sprague-Rappaport design is popular **Figure 26-23 ▶** , its two parallel tubes often bang against each other while moving, which can create extra noise.

Practically speaking, your stethoscope is the single most important investment you will make as a paramedic. Buy the best you can afford and take good care of it. Periodically check to make sure the

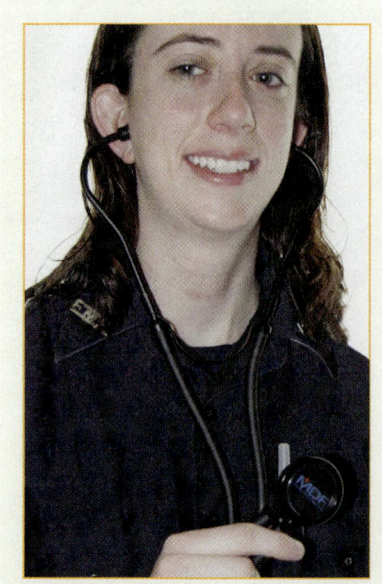

Figure 26-23 Earpieces should follow the normal (forward) slant of your ear canals. Note the Sprague-Rappaport–style stethoscope.

earpieces are clean and clear of earwax. On a regular basis, wipe down the length of the main tubing with an all-purpose cleaner. This helps slow the breakdown of the tube from the oils it picks up when you place it around your neck.

The diaphragm of the stethoscope is for high-pitched sounds (breath sounds); the bell (if present) is for low-pitched sounds (some heart tones). If you press the bell firmly against the skin, it stretches the skin beneath it and makes it act like a diaphragm. Hence, the bell should be placed lightly against the skin if you hope to hear the lower-pitched sounds. Some newer stethoscopes take advantage of this principle, allowing a single head to help transmit high- and low-pitched sounds based upon the pressure exerted by the operator. In older style stethoscopes, the bell rotates, allowing you to better hear the sounds you are trying to assess.

Your ear canals tend to point anteriorly in your skull (toward your eyes). You may wish to tilt the earpieces on your scope more forward for a better fit. But be careful: you may hear little or nothing if you accidentally place your scope in your ears backward, causing the earpieces to hit the sides of your ear canal.

Auscultation

Whenever possible, auscultate the lungs systematically. While we tend to compare the left and right sides, the lungs are not symmetrical. The right lung has three lobes: right upper lobe (RUL), right middle lobe (RML), and right lower lobe (RLL). The left lung has only two lobes: left upper lobe (LUL) and left lower lobe (LLL). Understand where you must listen to hear the various lobes **Figure 26-24 ▸** . Some of the pathologic conditions you will listen for are gravity-dependent, meaning most pneumonias and congestive heart failure will tend to be found in the lung bases. In the case of wheezing, it may be diffuse and spread throughout the lung fields. The bases are almost exclusively heard by listening to the patient's back. The upper lobes, which rarely have abnormalities, are heard by listening to the anterior part of the chest. The right middle lobe can best be heard by listening just beneath, or lateral to, the right breast. The best left-right differentiation can be appreciated in the midaxillary line; this is the best place to listen for ET tube placement. If you listen to the anterior part of the chest, you are very close to the noise-maker (the endotracheal tube), whether it is in the trachea or the esophagus.

Specific Breath Sounds

The breath sounds you hear are made by turbulent flow in the large airways as they are transmitted through the chest to your stethoscope. Tracheal breath sounds are not commonly auscultated, but note how harsh and tubular they sound. Bronchial breath sounds are also quite loud, but note that exhalation predominates. Moving farther toward the periphery, bronchovesicular sounds are softer, and have equal inspiratory and expiratory sides. Finally, the most commonly heard breath sounds are the soft, breezy vesicular sounds heard in the periphery. They have a much more obvious inspiratory compo-

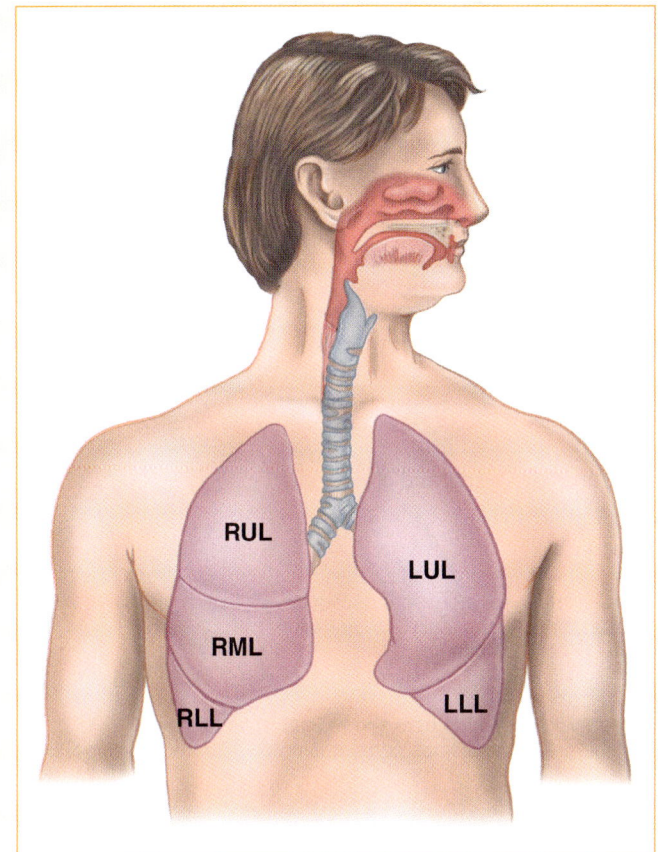

Figure 26-24 The lungs are not symmetrical. Most acute pathologic conditions are best heard in the lung bases, requiring you to listen to the patient's back. The right middle lobe is best heard beneath the right breast, or just lateral to it. LUL, left upper lobe; LLL, left lower lobe; RUL, right upper lobe; RML, right middle lobe; RLL, right lower lobe.

nent. You will want to listen to a large number of healthy lungs to become familiar with the four different sounds **Figure 26-25 ▸** . Pathologic conditions may cause you to hear some normal breath sounds in abnormal places!

Sound moves better through fluid than it does through air. Thus, the more air that is present in a patient's chest (as in COPD or asthma), the more distant, diminished, or absent the breath sounds will be in the periphery. Conversely, the more "wet" the patient's lungs are (as in pneumonia; consolidation, when fluid causes the lungs to become firm; or congestive heart failure), the louder the sounds will be in the periphery. If a patient has pneumonia in the right middle lobe, you may hear bronchovesicular (equal inspiration and expiration) or even bronchial (greater expiration than inspiration) in the periphery, instead of the expected vesicular sounds (greater inspiration than expiration).

The quality of the breath sounds also depends on the amount of extra tissue you must listen through and the patient's respiratory effort. For this reason, it is often helpful to

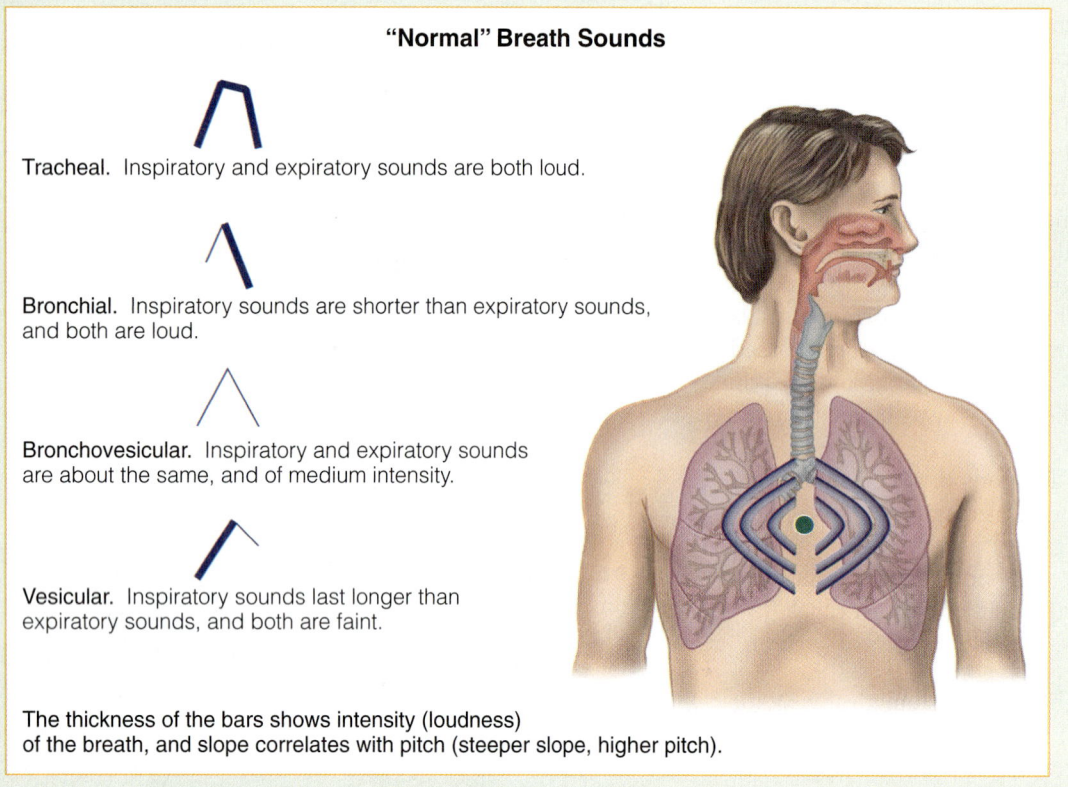

"Normal" Breath Sounds

Tracheal. Inspiratory and expiratory sounds are both loud.

Bronchial. Inspiratory sounds are shorter than expiratory sounds, and both are loud.

Bronchovesicular. Inspiratory and expiratory sounds are about the same, and of medium intensity.

Vesicular. Inspiratory sounds last longer than expiratory sounds, and both are faint.

The thickness of the bars shows intensity (loudness) of the breath, and slope correlates with pitch (steeper slope, higher pitch).

Figure 26-25 Normal breath sounds are heard over different parts of the chest. As you move away from the largest airways, breath sounds will become softer. The character of inspiration versus exhalation also changes.

ing. Have the patient cough and listen again if you hear a sound on only one side; it could be caused by the movement of secretions. A wheeze may begin at the start of exhalation and continue until the end of exhalation.

Crackles are any discontinuous noises heard on auscultation of the lungs and are caused by the popping open of air spaces. They are usually associated with increased fluid in the lungs. These sounds are often referred to as crackles (rales) or rhonchi. A rhonchus is classically defined as a low-pitched continuous sound (such as a low wheeze or death rattle), but the term is sometimes used to mean a low-pitched crackle (thick secretions in the large airways).

The most ominous breath sounds are no breath sounds at all. They mean the patient is not moving enough air to ventilate the lungs. *Silence means danger!*

Sputum

It is probably not productive to discuss specific pathologic conditions suggested by various sputum colours, but it is appropriate to note whether the patient is coughing up colourful sputum **Table 26-3 ▶**. Many smokers or patients who have chronic respiratory diseases cough up sputum every day (especially first thing in the morning), so determine if the colour or amount of this sputum has changed. Many patients don't spit their sputum out, whereas others will keep a cup or emesis

compare breath sounds on the right versus the left. The breath sounds of a patient who has a one-sided pathologic condition (such as pneumonia) will sound *louder* over the side with the abnormality than they will over the healthy side.

Both breath sounds and vocalisations travel more efficiently through a firm, fluid-filled lung than through a healthy lung, but travel poorly through a hyperinflated lung. If a patient speaks while you are auscultating the chest, you cannot usually understand what he or she is saying through your stethoscope. If you can, it may mean consolidation from pneumonia or atelectasis. You will likely hear these sounds directly only over the consolidated lobe. **Table 26-2 ▶** lists tests that indicate consolidation.

Adventitious (abnormal) breath sounds are the extra noises that you may hear on top of the breath sounds described previously. Continuous sounds (for example, a wheeze) can be heard across some portion of each breath. Discontinuous sounds are the instantaneous pops, snaps, and clicks that we often identify as crackles **Figure 26-26 ▶**.

Wheezes are high-pitched, whistling sounds made by air being forced through narrowed airways, which makes them vibrate, much like the reed in a musical instrument. Wheezing may be diffuse, as in asthma and congestive heart failure, or localized, as when a foreign body obstructs a bronchus. Pathologic conditions such as asthma rarely cause one-sided wheez-

Table 26-2	Signs of Consolidation
Sign	**Test**
Bronchophony	When the patient says "99" repeatedly, it sounds like a hum through the normal lung. Through the consolidated lung, you can understand the words "99."
Egophony	The patient says "eeeeee" while you are auscultating, and you hear "aaaaaa." The sound may be heard particularly well over a pleural effusion.
Whispered pectoriloquy	The patient whispers while you are auscultating, and you can understand what is said.

Table 26-3	Classic Sputum Types
Type of Sputum	**Causes**
Frothy, sometimes with a pink tinge	Congestive heart failure
Thick	Dehydration or antihistamine use
Purulent	Infectious process (because the pus contains dead white blood cells)
Yellow, green, brown	Older secretions in various stages of decomposition
Clear or white	Bronchitis
Blood streaked	Tumour, tuberculosis, pulmonary edema, or trauma from coughing

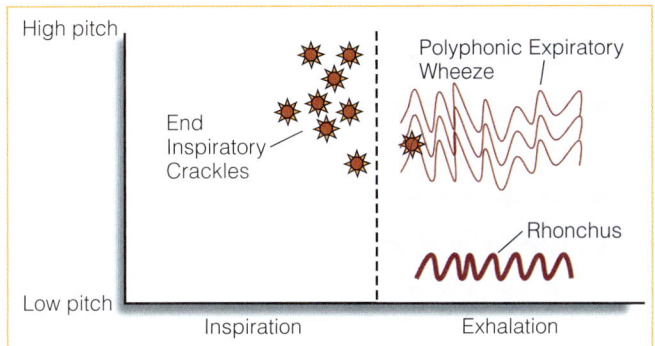

Figure 26-26 Adventitious sounds can be described as either continuous (wheezes and rhonchi) or discontinuous (crackles). They can also be characterized by their pitch (such as high or low), by where they are in the respiratory cycle (end inspiration or forced exhalation), and by their complexity (monophonic versus polyphonic).

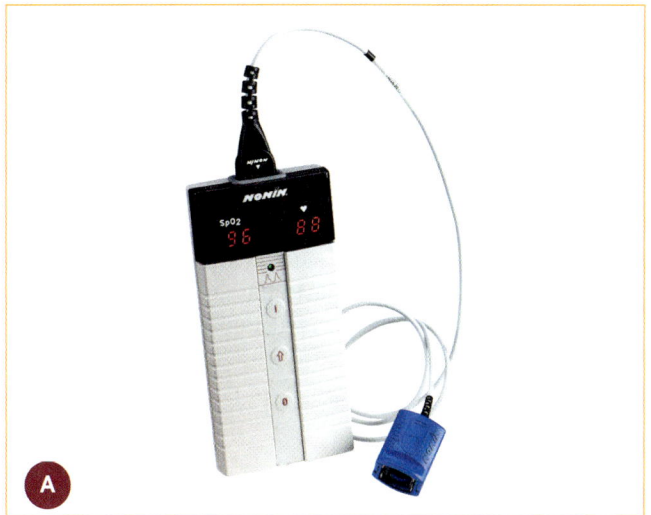

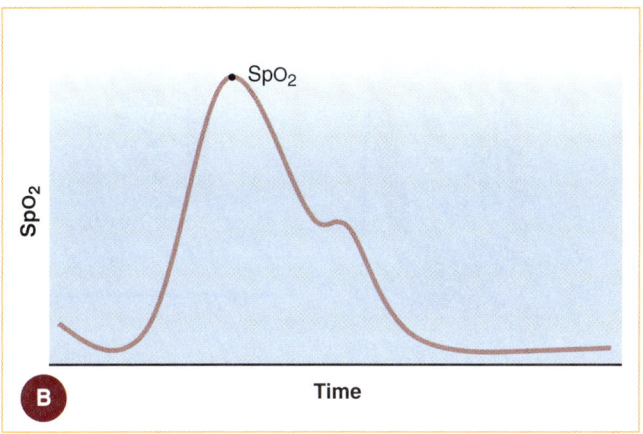

Figure 26-27 Pulse oximeters come in many sizes and, increasingly, are built into cardiac monitors (**A**). Some oximeters provide a waveform (**B**), which should demonstrate this characteristic shape when the oximeter is properly sensing.

basin next to their chair to spit in. Blood-tinged sputum may be a warning sign of tuberculosis or pulmonary edema, or it may mean the patient has been coughing forcefully and broken small blood vessels in the airway. Also note if mucus is purulent (puslike). Ask the patient these questions: Have you been coughing up anything colourful? Is that different for you?

Monitoring Devices
Pulse Oximetry
Under normal circumstances, a pulse oximeter is a noninvasive device that tells us what percentage of the patient's hemoglobin has oxygen attached to it **Figure 26-27 ▸**. For example, an oxygen saturation of 97% indicates that 97% of the patient's hemoglobin has oxygen attached to it. An oxygen saturation greater than 95% is considered normal. Most healthy people would feel short of breath at a saturation rate of less than 90%.

A pulse oximeter must "see" a pulsatile capillary bed to read properly. If the patient is wearing nail polish, you may need to remove it with an acetone nail polish remover before obtaining a reading (although some research indicates that if you are getting a consistent reading through nail polish, the reading is probably accurate). Poor peripheral perfusion, cold extremities, or patient movement (tremors or shivering) can make the reading inaccurate. Most pulse oximeters also display the patient's heart rate; this reading should match the patient's palpated heart rate.

Pulse oximetry does not recognize the difference between an oxygen molecule attached to hemoglobin and a carbon monoxide molecule attached to hemoglobin. From living in an industrialized society, most of us have a 1% to 2% carbon monoxide level all of the time. Smokers may have a 3% to 4% level. Thus a 97% pulse oximetry reading may actually consist of 95% oxygen and 2% carbon monoxide. Patients who have toxic or even fatal levels of carbon monoxide may show normal or high pulse oximetry values. Portable devices, called *pulse CO-oximeters*, that specifically measure carbon monoxide levels are poised to become important tools, enabling paramedics to readily assess for carbon monoxide poisoning in the prehospital setting **Figure 26-28 ▸**.

The oxyhemoglobin dissociation curve **Figure 26-29 ▾** describes the relationship between oxygen saturation and the amount of oxygen dissolved in the plasma (PaO_2). It demonstrates that when present at very low levels, oxygen molecules bind easily to the hemoglobin, so that small changes in PaO_2 result in relatively large changes in oxygen saturation. As the hemoglobin begins to fill with oxygen molecules, larger changes in PaO_2 (shown on the horizontal axis) are required to produce changes in oxygen saturation. Placing a healthy patient on a nonrebreathing mask may increase the saturation level from 96% to 99%, whereas placing a hypoxic patient on a nasal cannula at 2 l/min may increase the oxygen saturation from 80% to 92% (a much bigger change). Conversely, the more hypoxic patients become, the faster they will desaturate as they fall off the steep part of the oxyhemoglobin dissociation curve. Other factors, such as acid-base balance, body temperature, and amount of hemoglobin, can also affect the entire system and shift the entire curve to the left or the right.

End-Tidal Carbon Dioxide Detector

Carbon dioxide is returned to the lungs in the venous blood, where it is exhaled during ventilation. We can measure this exhaled carbon dioxide by various methods.

Colorimetric end-tidal carbon dioxide ($EtCO_2$) detecting does not measure the exact amount of carbon dioxide exhaled, but it does indicate whether carbon dioxide is present in *reasonable* amounts in the exhaled breath of the patient **Figure 26-30 ▾** . This type of monitoring helps in identifying placement of an ET tube. Air exhaled through an ET tube that has been properly placed in the trachea of a normally perfused patient should contain 4% to 5% carbon dioxide (a yellow reading on the colorimetric device). If the tube has been mistakenly placed in the esophagus, less than 0.5% carbon dioxide will be present in the exhaled gas (a purple reading). Note that the monitor might be fooled if the patient has carbon dioxide trapped in the stomach from the ingestion of carbonated beverages, so confirm the reading over at least six breaths to be certain it isn't a false positive.

The exact percentage of carbon dioxide contained in the last few millilitres of the patient's exhaled air can be measured by a special sensor. For example, some electronic end-tidal carbon dioxide detectors use a photoelectric sensor that relies on absorption of infrared light by carbon dioxide to provide this measurement. The sensor can evaluate $EtCO_2$ in the spontaneously breathing patient via a specialized nasal cannula–type device, or it can be attached to the end of an ET tube. These devices typically display a waveform **Figure 26-31 ▸** that can give additional data about the patient's respiratory status.

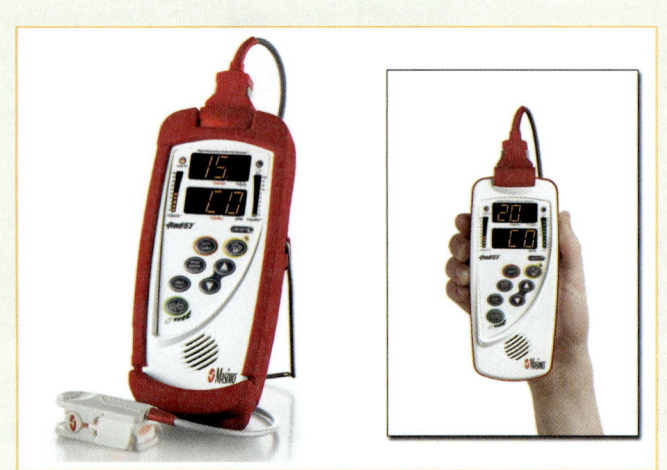

Figure 26-28 Pulse CO-oximeter devices can measure oxygen saturation as well as carbon monoxide levels.

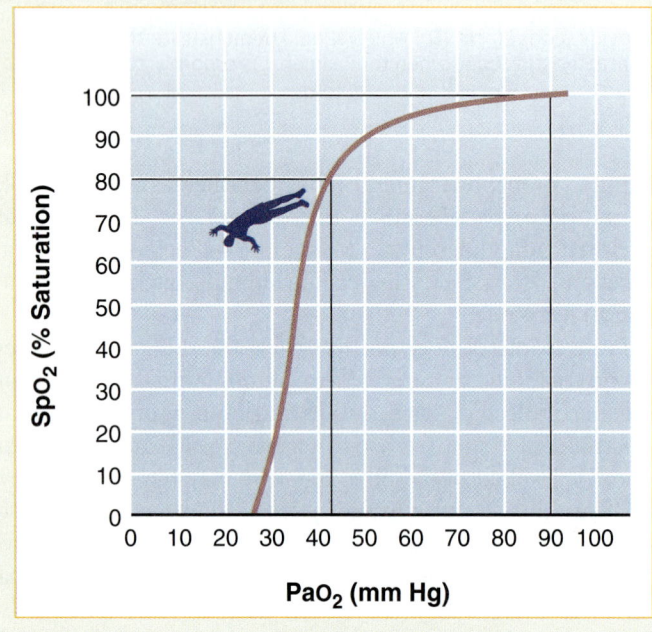

Figure 26-29 The oxyhemoglobin dissociation curve. As patients become increasingly hypoxic (lower percentage of SpO_2), they may "fall off" the curve and drop their saturation rapidly.

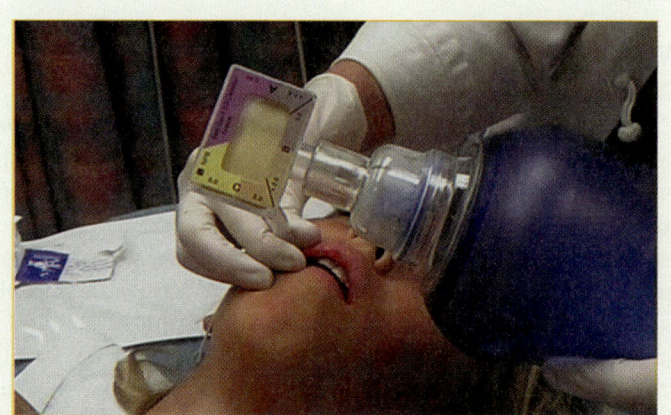

Figure 26-30 Carbon dioxide detectors are common devices used to help confirm endotracheal placement.

In addition, such monitors serve as alarms that can alert paramedics to changes in respiratory rate or depth.

Peak Expiratory Flow

The peak flow is the maximum flow rate at which the patient can expel air from the lungs. (Skill Drill 11-1 in Chapter 11 describes the use of a peak expiratory flowmeter.) A lower value indicates that the patient's larger airways are narrowed by bronchial constriction or bronchial edema. Many patients who have pulmonary disease check their peak flow themselves and chart the results. They may present this chart to you upon your arrival. Normal peak flow values vary by age, sex, and height, but generally run from about 350 to 700 l/min. The current Canadian guidelines for the assessment and treatment of adult asthma (from the Lung Association, the Canadian Thoracic Society, and the Canadian Association of Emergency Physicians) define a moderate exacerbation of asthma as less than 300 l/min; a peak flow below 200 l/min is considered severe and signals significant distress. Some people with chronic asthma have a peak flow that never exceeds 100!

Upper Airway Obstruction

Anatomical Obstruction

The most common cause of upper airway obstruction in the semiconscious or unconscious patient is the tongue. Indeed, this problem results in the death of some trauma patients, diabetics, patients who have had a seizure, or intoxicated patients every year. There seems to be an inherent urge on the part of bystanders to place a pillow behind the head of an unresponsive individual, which merely exacerbates this problem. If the patient is snoring, take away the pillow and reposition the patient's airway!

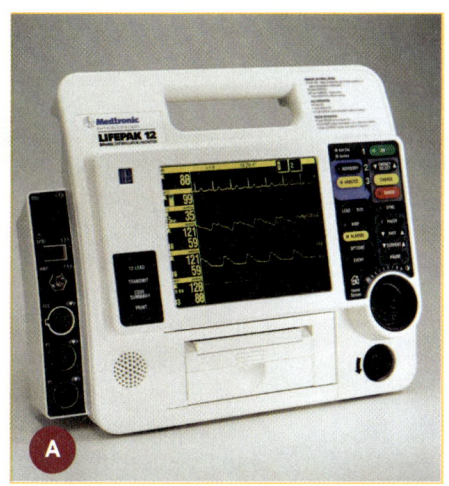

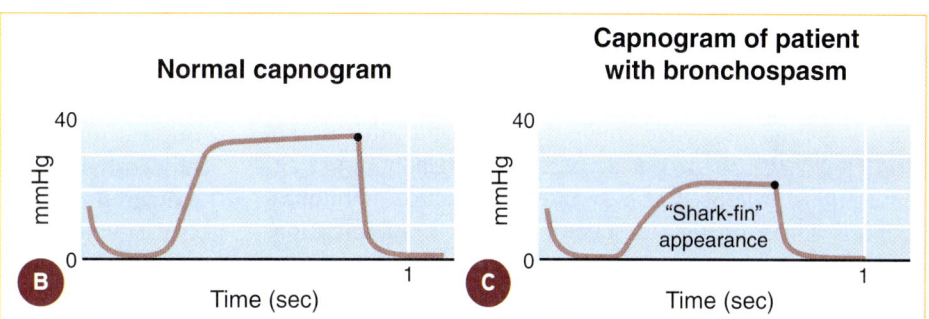

Figure 26-31 The waveform supplied by end-tidal carbon dioxide detectors (**A**) provides important data in addition to the actual Etco$_2$ value. Variations in waveform shape—normal is shown in graph (**B**) may help identify air-trapping disorders such as asthma (**C**) and COPD. It may also document altered respiratory patterns and serve as an alarm for apnea, bradypnea, or tachypnea.

You are the Paramedic Part 3

Your patient is not interacting with you, but rather stares blankly around the room and only responds by withdrawing from painful stimuli. His pulse oximetry reading continues to fall, and he is unable to sit upright without assistance. The patient accepts a nasal airway, but still has a gag reflex. You begin to provide ventilations with a bag-valve-mask ventilation device and 100% supplemental oxygen, but the patient's condition continues to worsen rapidly. You establish an 18-gauge IV of normal saline in the right antecubital vein.

Reassessment	Recording Time: 10 Minutes
Level of consciousness	Responsive to pain, with a Glasgow Coma Scale score of 9
Skin	Pale, cool, perspiring
Pulse	106 beats/min; weak; occasionally irregular
Blood pressure	102 mm Hg by palpation
Respirations	30 breaths/min; shallow
Spo$_2$	72% via bag-valve-mask ventilation and 100% supplemental oxygen
Capnography	65 mm Hg
ECG	Sinus tachycardia with occasional premature ventricular contractions

6. Do you believe that your patient is able to maintain his airway?

7. What options do you have available to maintain this patient's airway?

Excess soft tissue in the airway is one cause of obstructive sleep apnea, and some people go so far as to have tissue surgically removed from their pharynx to limit this anatomical obstruction. Fortunately, you can manually displace the soft tissue of the upper airway with a variety of simple maneuvers; these maneuvers were discussed in Chapter 11. Also, whenever you do not have a concern for spinal motion restriction, unconscious patients may be positioned on their side (the recovery position) to avoid blocking the airway. Many post-seizure, intoxicated, or hypoglycemic patients can be transported most safely on their side, which also reduces the risk of aspiration if they vomit.

The Hot (Infected) Airway

A variety of infections can cause swelling in the upper airway. The most common is probably <u>croup</u>, a distressing viral infection of the upper airway that most commonly occurs in small children. Poiseuille's law tells us that, as the diameter of a tube decreases, resistance to flow increases exponentially. This phenomenon explains why children—who have inherently narrow airways—get croup when a viral infection causes a little swelling in their upper airway, while adults with the same virus do not Figure 26-32 ▾ . In recent decades, many deadly upper airway infections have become very rare as a result of immunization efforts. Unfortunately, the rate of childhood immunizations has begun to decline as the general public becomes complacent about these diseases, so paramedics must remain vigilant for these pathologic conditions. Table 26-4 ▸ lists infections that can impair the upper airway.

Croup and tonsillitis are common, especially in children, but the other conditions are rare. When these pathologic conditions do occur, they are critical emergencies, because the airway could swell shut with little warning, making orotracheal intubation extremely difficult or impossible. *Avoid manipulating the airway* in these patients unless absolutely necessary. It is usually possible to ventilate such patients with bag-valve-mask ventilation by paying careful attention to technique. If intubation is essential because of an inability to effectively ventilate the patient with bag-valve-mask ventilation, you may find that the airway is entirely obscured by the swelling, and your attempts at laryngoscopy may merely make the swelling worse. Try to have a partner press on the patient's chest while you look for a stream of bubbles coming from the airway (use an ET tube at least two full sizes smaller than what you would typically choose for that patient). If this effort fails after a single attempt, a needle or surgical cricothyrotomy will be necessary.

Aspiration

Aspirating stomach contents into the lungs carries a significantly high mortality rate. It is a common but profoundly dangerous complication in patients who have had a cardiac arrest or in unresponsive patients who have had trauma or who overdosed. Follow these guidelines when treating such patients:

1. Aggressively reduce the risk of aspiration by avoiding gastric distension when ventilating and by decompressing the stomach with an NG tube whenever appropriate.

2. Aggressively monitor the patient's ability to protect his or her own airway, and seek to protect the patient's airway with an advanced airway if this is impossible.

3. Aggressively treat aspiration with suction and airway control if steps 1 and 2 fail!

If basic life-support maneuvers fail to clear an obstructed airway, use laryngoscopy and Magill forceps and, if necessary, perform a needle or surgical cricothyrotomy.

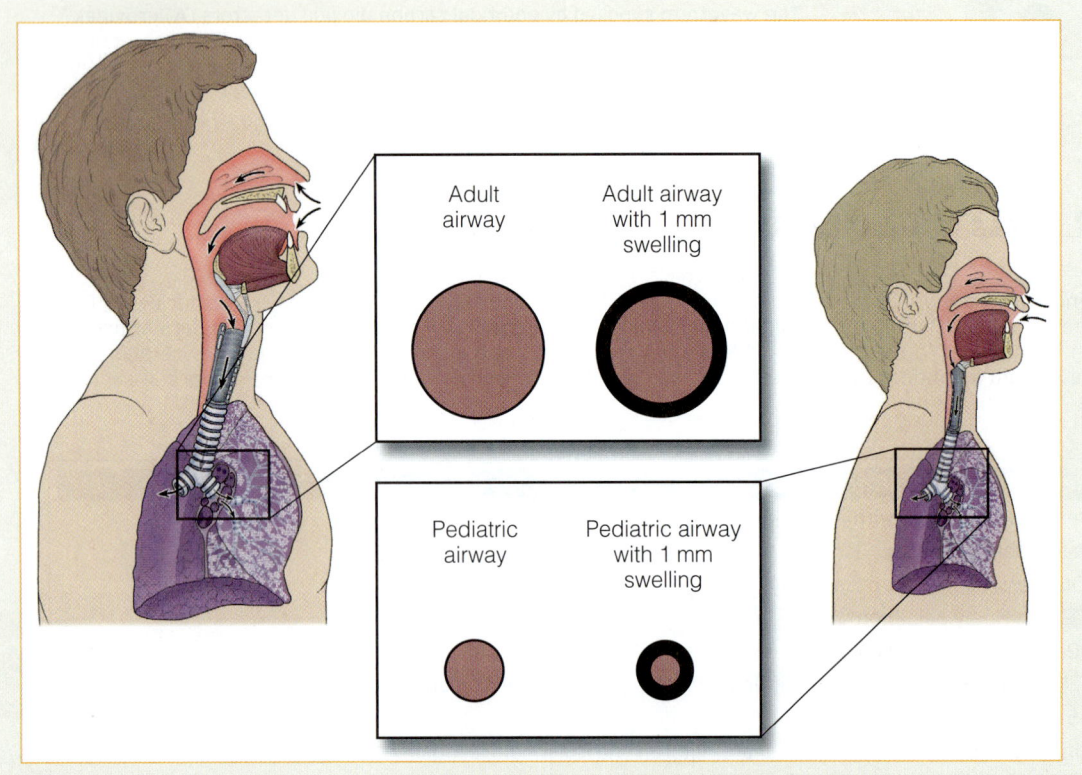

Figure 26-32 Any constriction of an airway (caused by a condition such as asthma) can cause a severe reduction in the volume of airflow, especially in children. Pouiselle's law explains conditions such as croup and presents implications for the choice of the size of an endotracheal tube.

Adult airway

Adult airway with 1 mm swelling

Pediatric airway

Pediatric airway with 1 mm swelling

Table 26-4	Infections That Can Impair the Upper Airway
Infection	**Comments**
Croup	Viral infection of area around glottis. Most common in children between 6 months and 3 years of age. Child has classic seal-bark cough. May be distressing but is not typically fatal. Also called laryngotracheobronchitis. Typically occurs in winter and early spring. May improve with exposure to cool air and humidity. Do not manipulate the airway.
Epiglottitis	Severe, rapidly progressive infection of epiglottis and surrounding tissues that may be fatal because of sudden respiratory obstruction. Most common infectious organism is *Haemophilus influenzea* type b. Vaccination has helped make acute epiglottitis rare. Unlike croup, patients may present at any age and at any time of year. Patients typically drool and have a fever, hoarse voice, and purposeful hyperextension. Epiglottitis is a true emergency. Do not manipulate the airway.
Peritonsillar abscess	Uncommon in children (more common in young adults). Abscess forms behind pharyngeal tonsil on one side. Patient has fever and sore throat. May be mistaken for epiglottitis until you look in throat and see lateral abscess (instead of enlarged epiglottis). Do not manipulate the airway.
Retropharyngeal abscess	Most common in children, in whom infections from retropharyngeal lymph nodes can flourish. May also be caused by direct trauma to pharynx. Patient may have fever and sudden stridor. May be mistaken for epiglottitis until laryngoscope examination reveals huge retropharyngeal pus sack (instead of cherry-red epiglottis). Do not manipulate the airway.
Diphtheria	Causative bacterium attacks and kills layer of epithelial tissue, creating pseudomembrane that is often seen in tonsillar area. Membrane (and swelling of upper airway caused by disease) can obstruct upper airway. Most children receive diphtheria, tetanus, and pertussis (DTP) immunization and receive boosters. Do not manipulate the airway.
Enormous tonsils	Palatine tonsils can swell excessively, resulting in fever, difficulty swallowing, and throat pain. Tonsils can grow to golf-ball size in some individuals. Severely swollen tonsils rarely compromise the airway but can cause snoring or stridor. Do not manipulate the airway.

Aspiration could also refer to foreign body airway obstruction. Remember that most adults choke when they are intoxicated or traumatized or have a reduced gag reflex from stroke or aging. Chronic aspiration of food is also a common cause of pneumonitis in older patients. Make sure you don't make the situation worse by allowing these patients to eat when they are having difficulty breathing.

Obstructive Airway Diseases

Obstructive airway diseases are characterized by diffuse obstruction to airflow within the lungs. The most common obstructive airway diseases are emphysema and chronic bronchitis (chronic diseases), and asthma (an acutely episodic syndrome); these three conditions collectively affect as many as 10% to 20% of adults. Emphysema and chronic bronchitis are collectively classified as COPD because the changes in pulmonary structure and function are chronic, progressive, and irreversible. Asthma is considered a separate entity because—at least in its early stages—it is a condition of *reversible* airway narrowing.

Obstructive disease occurs when the positive pressure of exhalation causes the small airways to pinch shut, trapping gas in the alveoli. The harder the patient tries to push air out, the more it gets trapped in the alveoli **Figure 26-33 ▸**. Hence, patients with obstructive disease end up with large amounts of gas trapped in their lungs that they can't effectively expel. Patients with obstructive disease learn that if they push the gas out slowly at a low pressure, they can exhale more than if they try to push it out hard and fast.

Patients with obstructive airway disease may demonstrate a variety of physical findings that can alert you to the nature of their disease:

- **Pursed-lip breathing.** Breathing in this way allows patients to push a breath out slowly under controlled pressure.
- **Increased inspiratory-to-expiratory (I:E) ratio.** The I:E ratio is typically 1:2 in healthy people breathing quietly (it takes about twice as long to exhale as it does to inhale). Patients who are very sick with obstructive disease may have an I:E ratio of 1:6 or 1:8.
- **Abdominal muscle use.** We use abdominal muscles to push air out (exhalation). Patients with obstructive disease must work to push air out with every breath. Patients who have asthma often complain of abdominal pain after an attack. They do the equivalent of hundreds of sit-ups as they force each exhalation.
- **Jugular venous distension.** The trapped air creates a higher pressure in the thorax. Blood draining into the superior vena cava from the head and neck can back up in the jugular veins, causing jugular venous distension.

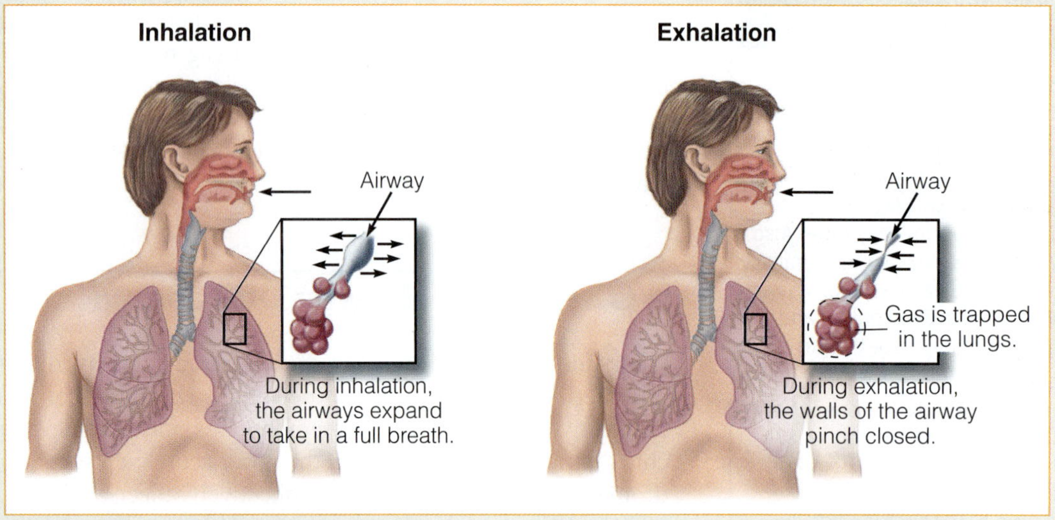

Inhalation

Airway

During inhalation, the airways expand to take in a full breath.

Exhalation

Airway

Gas is trapped in the lungs.

During exhalation, the walls of the airway pinch closed.

Figure 26-33 Obstructive disease involves changes to the smaller airways that cause them to pinch closed during exhalation, trapping air inside the patient's lungs. Healthy airways narrow during exhalation but not to the extent that causes obstruction or air trapping.

Asthma

The name asthma (from Greek, meaning "panting") was first given to this disease by the second-century Greek physician Aretaeus "because in the paroxysms, the patients also pant for breath." Asthma is characterized by an inflammation in the bronchiole airways due to a variety of stimuli. This inflammation results in widespread, reversible narrowing of the airways, or bronchospasm Figure 26-34 ▶ . Sometimes we refer to this condition as reactive airway disease to indicate that the patient experiences bronchospasm when exposed to certain triggers, such as dust, cold, or smoke.

Asthma characteristically occurs in acute attacks of variable duration. Between attacks, the patient may be relatively asymptomatic.

According to the Asthma Society of Canada, more than 3 million Canadians reported having asthma in 2005, and 60% of them do not have adequate control. Asthma is the most common diagnosis in emergency departments in Canada, and the frequency is increasing. Approximately 500 adults and 20 children (1 in 100 admissions) will die each year because of asthma in Canada.

The death rates from asthma are increasing across Canada, although not equally across all populations. The fastest-growing asthma rates are observed in children younger than

At the Scene

Asthma is a term describing paroxysmal narrowing of the airways due to inflammation of the bronchi and bronchospasm from contraction of bronchial smooth muscle. It may present differently in different people, but it is a very common pathologic condition.

5 years. Overall death rates from asthma are also higher in those under 35 years. Asthma is more common in males but tends to be more severe in females. First Nations and visible minorities have higher rates and severity of asthma as well.

Bronchospasm

Bronchospasm is caused by the constriction of smooth muscle that surrounds the larger bronchi in the lungs Figure 26-35 ▶ . This may occur because of stimulation by an allergen or irritants such as dust, perfume, cat dander, or cold temperatures or by other stimuli such as exercise or stress. When air is forced through the constricted tubes, it causes them to vibrate, which creates wheezing. Bronchospasm can also reduce the peak expiratory flow caused by a turbulent airflow. The primary treatment of bronchospasm is the administration of bronchodilator medication (beta-2 agonist such as salbutamol). Anticholinergic medications (ipratropium/tiotropium) are less commonly used. For life-threatening asthma, epinephrine is sometimes used to help reverse bronchoconstriction. Other treatments, such as magnesium for severe asthma, are generally reserved for the emergency department setting.

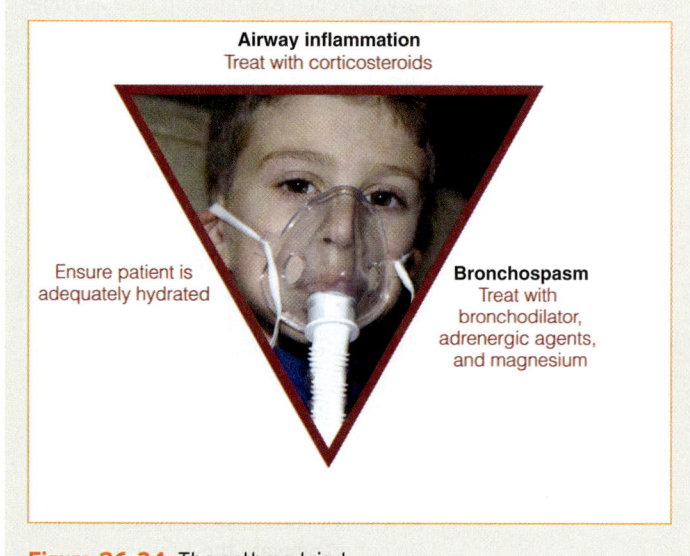

Airway inflammation
Treat with corticosteroids

Ensure patient is adequately hydrated

Bronchospasm
Treat with bronchodilator, adrenergic agents, and magnesium

Figure 26-34 The asthma triad.

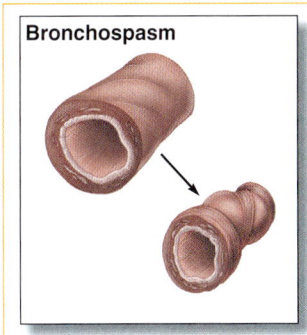

Bronchospasm	Inflammation
With bronchospasm, the muscle contracts, causing the entire tube to narrow.	With inflammation, the wall of the tube swells, causing only the lumen to narrow.

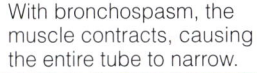

Figure 26-35 Bronchospasm is a constriction (narrowing) of the entire airway, whereas bronchial inflammation is a swelling of the airway wall. Both cause the functional diameter of airways to be reduced.

Bronchial Inflammation

Inflammation of the bronchi is the underlying cause of asthma. Therefore, the vast majority of asthma patients will need steroids, which are sometimes administered in the prehospital environment. Unlike bronchodilators, steroids may take longer before their action is seen.

Potentially Fatal Asthma

Patients who have potentially fatal asthma often have severely compromised ventilation all of the time. Such patients are at serious risk if something triggers acute bronchospasm or if they get an infection. A patient who has asthma is at high risk of respiratory arrest if he or she has a history consistent with any of the factors in **Table 26-5 ▶**. Medication noncompliance also predisposes a patient to asthma.

Table 26-5 | Potentially Fatal Asthma

- Previous intubation for respiratory failure or respiratory arrest
- Previous ICU admissions
- Recent emergency department visits, and patient on maximal therapy
- Altered mental status, hypoxia, silent chest

COPD

COPD comprises at least two distinct clinical entities: emphysema and chronic bronchitis.

Emphysema

Emphysema is the destruction of the airway distal to the terminal bronchioles and alveoli. Some people have emphysema caused by a congenital enzyme deficiency (alpha$_1$-antitrypsin deficiency), but the most common cause of emphysema is cigarette smoking.

In pure emphysema, the breakdown of the connective tissue structure of the terminal airways results in groups of alveoli merging into large blebs or bullae, which are far less efficient at exchanging oxygen and collapse far more easily (causing obstruction) than does normal lung tissue. Although little can be done in the prehospital environment to help this condition, many patients have associated bronchospasm, inflammation, or infections that can be relieved, helping improve the patient's overall situation. Many patients who have emphysema have a barrel chest caused by chronic lung hyperinflation. These patients are often tachypneic, as they attempt to maintain a normal carbon dioxide level despite their dysfunctional lungs. They often use extreme amounts of energy attempting to breathe, cannibalizing their own muscle mass in the process.

Notes from Nancy

Status asthmaticus is a severe, prolonged asthmatic attack that cannot be broken with conventional treatment. It is a dire medical emergency. Just as the patient with COPD ordinarily does not call for an ambulance unless there has been a marked change in his condition, so, too, the average asthmatic does not dial 9-1-1 unless the attack is much worse than those he usually has to deal with. So it is a reasonably safe assumption that any asthmatic who feels sick enough to call an ambulance is in status asthmaticus until proved otherwise.

On examining the patient in status asthmaticus, you will find him fighting desperately to move air through his obstructed airways, with prominent use of accessory muscles of respiration. The chest is maximally hyperinflated. Breath sounds and wheezes may be entirely inaudible because air movement is negligible, and the patient is usually exhausted, severely acidotic, and dehydrated.

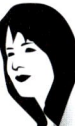

Notes from Nancy

All that wheezes is not asthma.

Among the other causes of diffuse wheezing are acute left heart failure ("cardiac asthma"), smoke inhalation, chronic bronchitis, and acute pulmonary embolism. Localized wheezing reflects an obstruction, by foreign body or tumour, in a specific area. Only a careful history and physical examination will enable you to reach the correct diagnosis. It is particularly important to distinguish the wheezing of asthma from that caused by left heart failure, because the treatment of the two conditions is markedly different.

In the acute asthmatic attack, silence is not golden—it's deadly!

Chronic Bronchitis

Chronic bronchitis is officially defined as sputum production most days of the month for 3 or more months out of the year for more than 2 years. The hallmark of this disease is excessive mucous production in the bronchial tree, which is nearly always accompanied by a chronic or recurrent productive cough (a cough that produces phlegm). The typical patient who has chronic bronchitis is almost invariably a heavy cigarette smoker.

Notes from Nancy

Patients with COPD ordinarily come to some sort of modus vivendi with their disease. Over the years, they learn how much exertion they can tolerate, in what position sleep is possible, and so forth. So when a patient with COPD calls for an ambulance, it nearly always means that something has changed—and changed for the worse.

He or she is usually somewhat obese, congested, and sometimes has a bluish complexion. His or her blood gases tend to be abnormal, with elevated Pa_{CO_2} (hypercapnia) and decreased Pa_{O_2} (hypoxemia) levels. Often he or she has associated heart disease and right heart failure (cor pulmonale).

The pink puffer (emphysema) and blue bloater (chronic bronchitis) represent two extremes of the COPD spectrum. In reality, as the disease progresses, most patients with COPD fall somewhere between these two clinical extremes, showing signs and symptoms of both disease processes.

Typical Presentations of COPD

Patients who have COPD are often very sick people, with little or no respiratory reserves to help them deal with any additional respiratory insults. You must actively search for what has pushed them over the edge from a relatively stable state to the insufficiency that caused them to call 9-1-1. The following are some common issues that conspire to cause the patient who has COPD to decompensate.

COPD With Pneumonia

Because they are chronically ill, have poor secretion clearance, and sometimes have excessive mucous production (which acts like a culture medium for nasty bugs), these patients often get infections in their bronchi and lungs. Do they have a fever? Has the colour or amount of their sputum production changed? Do they have other signs of infection (such as body aches, general malaise, or pain when breathing)? Are auscultated breath sounds (such as localized rhonchi) consistent with pneumonia? COPD exacerbations with signs of infection are typically treated with antibiotics.

COPD With Right Heart Failure

It is very difficult for the right side of the heart to push the patient's thick blood through lungs destroyed by emphysema and through capillaries squashed by hyperinflated alveoli. This commonly causes right heart failure secondary to the patient's lung disease (cor pulmonale). If patients take in too much salt or fluid, or if they do not get rid of fluid (because of renal failure or insufficient diuretic use), they may have an episode of congestive heart failure. Do they have peripheral edema? Jugular venous distension with hepatojugular reflux? End inspiratory crackles? (It may be difficult to tell the difference between the crackles of congestive heart failure and the crackles that these patients always have secondary to their COPD.) Do they say they have had a progressive increase in dyspnea over several days? Have they taken in more fluid than usual, or run out of their diuretics?

COPD With Left Heart Failure

Patients with COPD are at high risk of having a sudden cardiac event. Any sudden left ventricular dysfunction such as an AMI or cardiac rhythm disturbance (dysrhythmia) can cause them to have sudden-onset left heart failure. Don't allow your initial impression of COPD to prevent you from identifying the patient who is also having an acute myocardial infarction!

Acute Exacerbation of COPD

In the acute exacerbation, no co-pathologic condition such as congestive heart failure or pneumonia clearly accounts for the patient's sudden decompensation. Instead, the patient's condition suddenly becomes worse, often because of some environmental change such as weather, humidity, or sudden activation of the heating or cooling system. An acute exacerbation can also be prompted by the inhalation of trigger substances. Did your patient decide to go through some old boxes today? Did a neighbour just visit with a cat? Is someone painting in the next room?

End-Stage COPD

Patients with severe COPD will eventually reach a point when their lungs simply cannot support oxygenation and ventilation any longer. You may come to know these patients well as their calls to 9-1-1 become more frequent. Some will be in hospice care. In the end stages of the disease, it can be difficult to determine whether a patient has an exacerbation that can be resolved or if he or she has reached the end of the disease process. Unfortunately, endotracheal intubation may result in a situation where the patient cannot make his or her wishes known. In addition, the more frequently the patient has to be intubated and placed on a ventilator, the more difficult it becomes to wean the patient off the ventilator. Having this knowledge increases the anxiety level of the patient, thus increasing his or her cardiac workload and cardiac oxygen consumption—a potentially lethal combination for the end-stage COPD patient.

All EMS systems have their own ways of dealing with do-not-resuscitate orders. It is important to secure documentation of the patient's wishes as the terminal phase of the disease begins. Follow local protocol or contact direct medical control as needed regarding such issues.

Hypoxic Drive

Hypoxic drive is a rare phenomenon that affects only a very small percentage of patients who have the most chronic forms of pulmonary disease in the end stage of their disease. As a paramedic, you will routinely provide prehospital care for the sickest of the sick, so you should understand this concept. You will likely encounter patients whose respiratory drive can be decreased by high levels of oxygen. However, 100% supplemental oxygen is foundational therapy for most patients, so it makes no sense to withhold oxygen from anyone who needs it for fear of decreasing the respiratory drive of those few individuals who might have this complication.

When a patient has chronic hypoventilation, bicarbonate (HCO_3) ions are retained to compensate for respiratory acidosis. The patient might then switch to a hypoxic drive, meaning that the primary stimulus to breathe comes from decreased levels of oxygen, *not* increased levels of carbon dioxide. This places the paramedic in the position of having to decide whether the administration of oxygen is appropriate. In making this decision, consider the following points:

Notes from Nancy

The best protection against TB is personal protection.

At the Scene

Bagged to Death

Not everyone should be ventilated the same way.

If you are ventilating a patient who has severe obstructive disease, such as those with either decompensated asthma or COPD, remember that *these patients have difficulty exhaling*. If each breath is not allowed to come back out before the delivery of the next, then pressures in the thorax will continually go up. This phenomenon, which is called auto-PEEP (positive end-expiratory pressure), can eventually cause a pneumothorax or cardiac arrest. Increased pressure in the chest reduces the amount of blood returning to the heart, thus limiting venous return and worsening the overall ability to pump oxygenated blood.

Such patients should be ventilated as little as four to six breaths per minute to avoid "bagging them to death." This is very difficult to do when your partner, bystanders, the BLS crew, and your own epinephrine release are all telling you to hyperventilate the patient, but it is an absolute necessity if you hope to avoid the dire consequences of raising the thoracic pressure more with each breath. Seek guidance from your medical director and local protocols when you encounter patients who have severe COPD or asthma who are in cardiac arrest or near-arrest. However, also remember that the standard ventilation rate for adults is only 10 to 12 breaths/min.

1. Only a small subset of patients with COPD breathe because of hypoxic drive, but you cannot tell who they are just by looking at them.
2. Such patients do not suddenly become apneic after a whiff of oxygen. High levels of oxygen slowly depress their respiratory drive, and their respiratory rate slowly declines. They become sleepy and, eventually, their respiratory rate falls into the single digits before they become apneic. Although the paramedic is likely to be close enough to the patient to recognize this phenomenon, the real concern is the in-hospital patient who receives 100% supplemental oxygen but then is left by himself or herself for a prolonged period.
3. If the patient becomes apneic, provide artificial ventilation and consider intubation.
4. While oxygen saturation (SpO_2) may be a valuable adjunct to your decision, SpO_2 numbers are a little different for patients with COPD and tell you nothing about their carbon dioxide levels.

At the Scene

Tuberculosis Presentation

The classic presentation of tuberculosis (TB) includes weight loss, night sweats, fever, and cough with blood-tinged sputum. This clinical presentation should raise a red flag. The best protection against TB is good airflow through your environment. Don't let the patient cough in your face, and keep the rear windows of the ambulance open, if possible. Consider using an oxygen mask on the patient instead of a nasal cannula. You can deliver the same FIO_2 while limiting the spread of droplets when the patient coughs. Also, you should wear a high-efficiency particulate air (HEPA) filter mask that meets NIOSH N95 or Occupational Safety and Health Administration (OSHA) criteria (ie, a TB or duckbill mask).

Common Respiratory Presentations

Asthma With Fever

When patients with reactive airways begin wheezing, their inhalers usually will help for only a little while before their symptoms return. The typical asthma attack that responds to treatment but occurs again in a few hours is sometimes caused by an underlying infection (such as pneumonia or bronchitis) that continually triggers the asthmalike symptoms. The asthma attack won't go away until the patient receives treatment of the trigger. Does your patient have a fever or chills? Is he or she coughing up colourful sputum?

Failure of a Metered-Dose Inhaler

Metered-dose inhalers indicate how many actuations (puffs) they are designed to deliver, but most patients don't keep track of their usage very well. Often the medication may be exhausted even though some propellant remains in the canister. The patient may have been sucking nothing but propellant for days, which explains why their wheezing isn't getting better. Similar problems can occur when patients use grossly outdated medications or medications that have been overheated (left in a hot car or similar environment). In this case, your bronchodilator may work well, even though theirs has failed. Another problem that can occur is that patients who do not fully understand how to use the device do not inhale at an appropriate point and then end up spraying the medicine on the inside of their mouths. This is one reason why physicians often prescribe a spacer device to be added to the metered-dose inhaler for children and for adults who have difficulty using the device.

Dyspnea Triggers

Just because someone knows that their reactive airways are triggered by cats, perfume, cigarette smoke, cold, or pollen doesn't mean that they can always avoid these triggers. Sometimes a social or family situation is important enough that patients are willing to risk experiencing an episode of dyspnea. Sometimes people who are allergic to cats will hold a cat, and people who are on strict fluid restriction will drink excessively.

Seasonal Issues

Many ugly things grow in heating ducts and air conditioners during their off-seasons. When the weather suddenly changes, and heating systems or air conditioners begin turning on in houses all over your district, you can expect an increase in calls from chronically ill respiratory patients. Excessive heat, humidity, cold, pollen, dust, and smog can all conspire to push someone over the edge and experience a flare-up of respiratory disease.

Noncompliance With Therapy

Many patients who have chronic respiratory disease will rebel against their therapy as a means of seeming to regain some control over their lives. Sometimes, the long-term nature of their therapy isn't fully understood, and they attempt to wean themselves off of their medications, oxygen, or respiratory support devices. Unfortunately, this may cause them to have a crisis.

Many patients have been prescribed home oxygen, nebulizer therapy, continuous positive airway pressure (CPAP), bilevel positive airway pressure (BiPAP), and a variety of medications that they refuse to use or use only sporadically. Some

medications, such as oral corticosteroids, can cause dangerous complications if their use is terminated abruptly.

Failure of Technology/Running Out of Medicine

Advances in technology have allowed patients who have chronic respiratory disease much more freedom to get out of the house and to travel. This creates the risk that you will be called to assist someone whose oxygen tank has run dry, whose portable ventilator has suddenly malfunctioned, or whose medications were left behind.

Exertion-Related Problems

Oxygen demand increases with any kind of exertion. If patients' conditions are stable at rest, compare their condition during typical exertion. Do they get dyspneic when they move from their chair to your stretcher, go to the bathroom, or eat? Note oxygen saturation while at rest and during any simple exertion. Check babies while they are eating or after they cry.

■ Other Causes of Respiratory Problems

Pulmonary Infections

Bacteria, viruses, fungi, mycoplasmas, and a host of other agents cause infections. The respiratory tract is particularly vulnerable to a variety of airborne agents, as well as those that set up shop in the nose or throat and subsequently migrate into the bronchi and lungs. Infections of the upper airway may require aggressive approaches to airway management. Infections in the lower airway are usually treated with supportive prehospital care and by transport to the hospital.

In general, infectious diseases cause swelling of the respiratory tissues, an increase in mucous production, and the production of pus. Swelling in the well-perfused respiratory tissues can be dramatic, particularly in the upper airway. This is problematic because the resistance to airflow goes up exponentially when tube diameter is narrowed (Pouiselle's law). Alveoli can also become nonfunctional if they fill up with pus, as occurs in pneumonia. Like collapsed or fluid-filled alveoli, pus-filled alveoli do not participate in gas exchange. Instead, these alveoli contribute to shunt, in which oxygen does not reach the bloodstream, perhaps resulting in hypoxemia. Problems with ventilation, perfusion, or both can prevent oxygen from reaching the bloodstream **Table 26-6 ▶**.

Pneumonia may be caused by any of a variety of bacterial, viral, and fungal agents. Bacterial pneumonia is most frequently caused by *Streptococcus pneumoniae* bacillus, for which an effective vaccine is now available. This type of pneumonia is responsible for about 10% of hospital admissions in Canada

Table 26-6	Potential Problems With Alveoli and Capillary Supply
Normal Function	• Good ventilation • Good perfusion
Dead Space	• Good ventilation • Poor perfusion (as in pulmonary embolus or shock)
Shunt	• Poor ventilation • Good perfusion (as in pneumonia or atelectasis)
Silent	• Poor ventilation • Poor perfusion (as in cardiac arrest)

and approximately 50% of patients who become septic with their pneumonia. Even in this era of antibiotics, in Canada patients with pneumonia have an 11% in-hospital and a 26% one-year mortality rate.

Older people, patients with chronic illnesses, and smokers are at greater risk of contracting this illness. In fact, anyone who is not moving air well, who has excessive secretions (such as patients with COPD or asthma or who are postoperative, bedridden, or sedentary), or who is immunocompromised (from human immunodeficiency virus or other illnesses) is at risk of developing pneumonia. Patients with acquired immunodeficiency syndrome are particularly susceptible to Pneumocystis pneumonia caused by *Pneumocystis carinii* (also called PCP); it is a primary cause of morbidity and mortality in such patients. All high-risk patients are strongly encouraged to get the pneumonia vaccine annually.

The patient with pneumonia usually reports several hours to days of weakness, productive cough, fever, and sometimes chest pain made worse by a cough. The illness may have started abruptly with a shaking chill (rigor) or came on more gradually with progressive weakness. As you obtain your history of recent illness, be particularly tuned in for comments regarding something akin to, ". . . and I just got over the flu about a week ago." Frequently, pneumonia is a secondary infection that follows a bout of the flu, and is one of the leading causes of death under those circumstances.

On physical examination, the patient with pneumonia often appears very ill (has a toxic appearance). He or she may or may not be coughing. Crackles may be heard on auscultation of the chest, and there may also be increased tactile fremitus and sputum production. In advanced cases, areas of diminished or absent breath sounds are noted, due to consolidation. Sputum may be either thick (because of dehydration) or purulent (puslike).

Pneumonia often occurs in the lung bases, typically on only one side. Sometimes patients' oxygen saturation will be significantly lower when they lie on one side versus the other. In pneumonia, this is typically when the good lung is down, although this is not always the case.

Patients with pneumonia are often dehydrated, which contributes to V/Q mismatch, and intravenous hydration is often required. Supportive prehospital care includes oxygenation, secretion management (suctioning), and transport to an appropriate facility. Bronchodilators will not help the pneumonia, but they may slightly improve the patient's ability to ventilate, especially if they have underlying asthma or COPD.

Alveolar Dysfunction

The alveoli are vulnerable to a number of disorders. They may collapse (atelectasis) from obstruction somewhere in the proximal airways or from external pressures produced, for example, by pneumothorax or hemothorax. They may fill with pus in pneumonia, with blood in pulmonary contusion, or with fluid in near drowning or congestive heart failure.

Atelectasis

In healthy lungs, most alveoli do not collapse on exhalation. Instead, the healthy individual employs a variety of methods to keep them open, such as sighing and coughing. However, after operations, when people are sick, or when there is injury or damage to the chest wall, lungs, or surrounding tissues, the alveoli and lung segments may collapse, which is called *atelectasis*. Deep breathing, sighing, yawning, and coughing are all mechanisms through which our bodies keep alveoli open and avoid atelectasis. Like balloons, alveoli are more difficult to blow reopen once they have completely collapsed.

In the hospital, patients are encouraged to take deep breaths. A device called an incentive spirometer helps patients quantify how deep their breaths are **Figure 26-36 ▾**. These devices are often sent home with patients for continued use after they have been discharged from the hospital (ie, rib fracture, chest surgery).

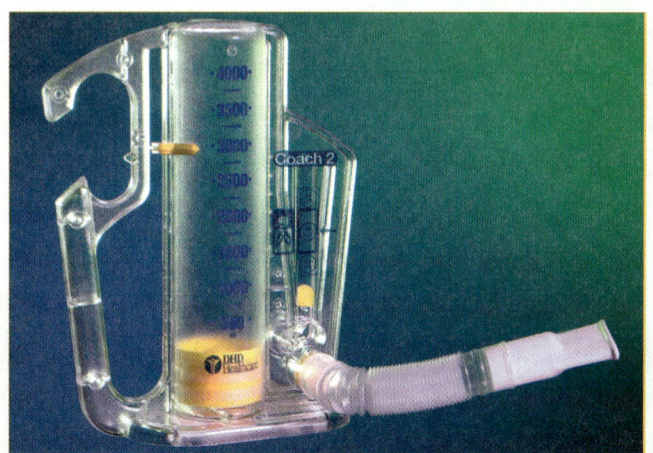

Figure 26-36 An incentive spirometer helps patients quantify how deep their breathing is. It helps them take deep breaths to avoid atelectasis.

Cancer

Lung cancer is one of the most common forms of cancer, especially in cigarette smokers or in people exposed to occupational lung hazards, such as asbestos, coal dust, or second-hand smoke. Lung cancer is the leading cause of death due to cancer in Canada, representing an estimated 30% of the cancer deaths in males and 25% of the cancer deaths in females. The vast majority of cases are caused by smoking.

Lung cancer may present with a variety of symptoms, including hemoptysis (blood in the sputum) and uncontrollable coughing, shortness of breath due to cancerous fluid accumulating around the lung, or pneumonias because tumours compress and block a major airway. Because many patients with lung cancer are smokers, these symptoms may be accompanied by COPD and impaired lung function. The lungs are also common sites for the metastasis of cancers from other parts of the body.

Other cancers may invade the lymph nodes in the neck, producing tumours that threaten to occlude the upper airway. Patients with various types of cancers may experience pulmonary complications from their chemotherapy or radiation therapy. Lung irradiation, for example, may be associated with some degree of pulmonary edema. Tumours or treatment may also cause pleural effusions, which can present with rapidly progressing dyspnea.

Paramedics are sometimes called to assist with end-of-life issues for cancer patients. Patients in hospice care, for example, may present with depressed respirations caused by the large amounts of narcotics administered to them or that they have administered to themselves. In this type of narcotics overdose, remember to titrate naloxone *only* to improve respirations—do not completely reverse the patient's primary pain control as you can abruptly leave them in complete misery. In the past, the respiratory depressant effects of narcotics and antianxiety agents may have been overemphasized, but now these agents are gaining increased popularity in the management of chronic pain, chronic cough, and anxiety in end-of-life scenarios. For instance, fentanyl, a strong narcotic, is sometimes dispersed through an aerosol to suppress a chronic cough in patients who have end-stage lung cancer.

Toxic Inhalations

Many potentially toxic substances can be inhaled into the lungs. The type of damage done depends in large part on the water solubility of the toxic gas. Highly water-soluble gases like ammonia will react with the moist mucous membranes of the upper airway and cause swelling and irritation. If the substance gets in the patient's eyes, they will also burn and feel inflamed and irritated.

Less water-soluble gases may get deep into the lower airway, where they may do damage over time. Such toxins have been used in war to disable the enemy, because they do not cause immediate distress but rather cause pulmonary edema up to 24 hours later. Gases such as phosgene and nitrogen dioxide will present in this manner.

Table 26-7	Toxic Gases	
Type of Toxic Gas	**Example**	**Effect**
Highly water soluble	Ammonia	Acute upper airway irritation
Moderately water soluble	Chlorine	Depends on concentration and amount of exposure. Coughing, wheezing, rales, pulmonary edema, and chemical burns.
Minimally water soluble	Phosgene	Delayed pulmonary edema

Some common gases, like chlorine, are moderately water soluble and present somewhere between the two extremes. Severe exposure may present with upper airway swelling, whereas lower-level exposure may present with the classic delayed-onset, lower airway damage. **Table 26-7** ▲ details the different categories of toxic gases.

A patient who has been exposed to such a substance must be removed from contact with the toxic gas immediately and provided with 100% supplemental oxygen or assisted ventilation if breathing is impaired (there is reduced tidal volume). If the upper airway is compromised, aggressive airway management (such as intubation or a cricothyrotomy) may be required.

Pulmonary Edema

Swelling of the lungs occurs when fluid from the blood plasma migrates into the lung parenchyma (the tissues that make up the walls of the capillaries and alveoli). This pulmonary edema compromises gas exchange long before this fluid spills into the alveoli and becomes noticeable (usually presenting with pink, frothy sputum).

One of the most common causes of pulmonary edema is heart failure resulting from a left side AMI. Inhaled toxins can damage alveolar tissue and cause fluid to seep into the lungs. Other infection-mediated substances may also damage the pulmonary capillaries and cause the same effect. Sometimes trauma or even altitude changes can lead to acute respiratory distress syndrome or high-altitude pulmonary edema.

Early in pulmonary edema, you will hear crackles in the bases of the lungs at the end of inspiration. This sound is caused by fields of alveoli popping open as the lungs reach maximal inflation. Always listen to the lower lobes of the lungs through the patient's back.

As pulmonary edema worsens, you may begin to hear crackles higher in the patient's lung fields—often described as "crackles up to the subscapular level" or "crackles up to the apices." As fluid migrates into the larger airways and mixes with mucus, you will begin to hear coarse crackles on inspiration and exhalation. You may also feel tactile fremitus. Ultimately, the patient will begin to cough up watery sputum that often has a pink tinge (from red blood cells). As air is forced in and out of the fluid-filled lungs, the fluid may bubble and foam. Coughing up pink and foamy or blood-tinged sputum is a classic danger sign of severe pulmonary edema.

Acute Respiratory Distress Syndrome

You won't see acute respiratory distress syndrome very often in the prehospital setting unless you are involved in doing interfacility transfers. However, you can play a vital role in preventing this devastating pathologic condition in many patients. This syndrome is caused by diffuse damage to the alveoli, as a result of trauma, shock, aspiration of gastric contents, pulmonary edema, toxicity, or hypoxic events. It seems to be worse when there is some direct damage to the lungs, as in trauma patients who have severe pulmonary contusions.

Alveoli become stiff (noncompliant) and difficult to ventilate. Patients may ultimately require mechanical ventilation under very high pressure, which causes even more damage. Studies have shown that the way people are ventilated in the prehospital and early hospital setting may impact their likelihood of developing acute respiratory distress syndrome later. You can play an important role in reducing the risk of developing ARDS by avoiding high airway pressures and supraphysiologic volumes in patients who have pneumonia, trauma, or hypoxemic respiratory failure.

Problems Outside the Lung Parenchyma

Pneumothorax

When a patient has a pneumothorax, air collects between the visceral and the parietal pleura that line the inside of the chest cavity. Some people have blebs in their lung parenchyma that are congenital or that result from COPD, and which leave them prone to developing this condition. Blebs are weak spots that can rupture when under stress, causing a spontaneous pneumothorax. The stress that ruptures the bleb may be as simple as coughing, or as severe as aggressive bag-valve-mask ventilation. People who have severe asthma are prone to blebs, as are tall, thin people, especially those who smoke.

Some patients have had multiple simple pneumothoraces in their life and may actually present with the chief complaint: "I'm having another pneumothorax." They may describe feeling a sharp pain after they cough, followed by increasing dyspnea over the subsequent minutes or hours. Most of these patients will not require acute intervention such as needle chest decompression, but you should at the very least administer high concentrations of oxygen and monitor their respiratory status closely while en route to the hospital.

Pleural Effusion

When fluid collects between the visceral and parietal pleura, it is called a pleural effusion **Figure 26-37** ▶. Effusions can be caused by infections, tumours, CHF, or trauma. Pleural effusions can impair breathing by limiting lung expansion and causing partial or complete lung collapse.

Some pleural effusions can contain several litres of fluid. A large effusion will obviously decrease lung capacity and make the patient dyspneic.

It may be difficult to hear any breath sounds through the effusion. Because the effusion is filled with fluid, the patient's position will affect his or her ability to breathe. Shifting positions may make patients significantly more dyspneic, and they usually will fight being placed into anything other than Fowler's position. Supportive prehospital care, including proper positioning and aggressive supplemental oxygen administration, should be used until you can get the patient to an appropriate facility where the effusion can be definitively treated.

Disruption of the Pulmonary Circulation

The pulmonary circulation may be compromised by a blood clot (thromboembolism), a fat embolism from a broken bone, an amniotic fluid embolism from leakage of amniotic fluid from the amniotic sac of a pregnant woman, or even an air embolism resulting from air entering the circulation from a laceration in the neck or an IV administration set that was

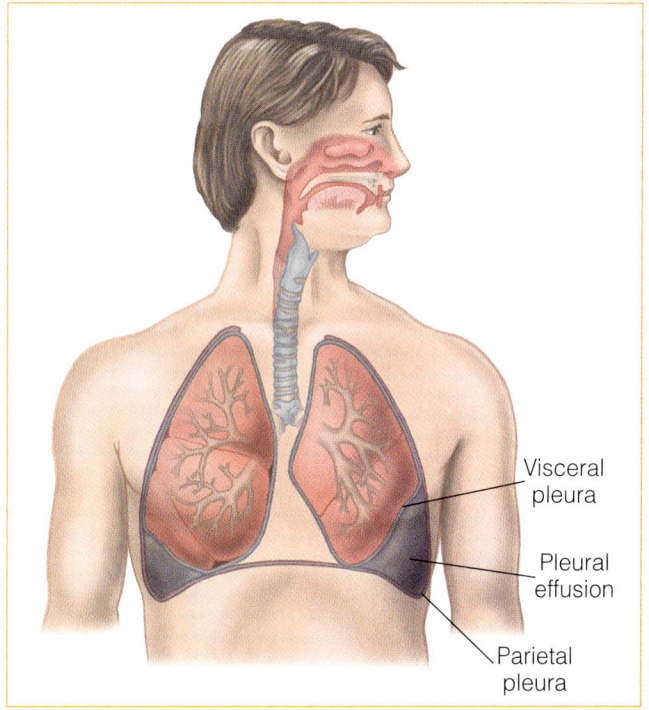

Figure 26-37 A pleural effusion is a buildup of fluid between the visceral and parietal pleura. It is like a blister growing between the pleura.

improperly or not flushed. A large embolism, of whatever type, may lodge in a major branch of the pulmonary artery and act as a plug and prevent any blood flow through that branch. Adequate gas exchange in the lungs requires functional alveoli to provide oxygen and take up carbon dioxide, as well as intact pulmonary vessels to convey oxygen-poor blood to the alveoli. Normal alveoli will be of little use if the venous blood cannot reach them, as is the situation in pulmonary embolism.

Pulmonary embolism is considered one of the most frequently misdiagnosed conditions in emergency medicine. As such, it is often a very confusing presentation, because it is not immediately evident that anything is wrong with the patient's lung. The story of sudden dyspnea, perhaps with a sharp pain in the chest, should make you think about pulmonary embolism.

Most pulmonary emboli come from the large veins in the legs, particularly the greater saphenous veins, where clots can form a deep vein thrombosis (DVT) and subsequently break off and migrate through the venous circulation, through the right side of the heart, and into the pulmonary circulation **Figure 26-38 ▾** . Patients with thrombophlebitis (inflammation of the veins in the legs) are at high risk of pulmonary embolism. They may exhibit leg swelling or calf tenderness.

Many patients with DVT or PE have an identifiable risk factor (recent surgery, immobilization, air travel, or blood-clotting disorder), although a large proportion of those with DVT or PE do not have an identifiable risk factor and are deemed idiopathic. Certain cancers predispose patients to clots, as does pregnancy and oral contraceptive use. Clots may also form when patients are immobile for long periods of time.

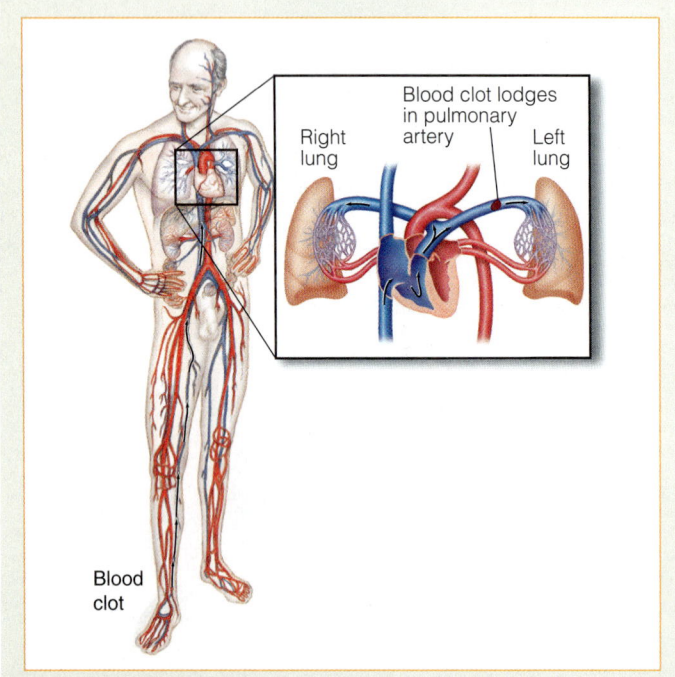

Figure 26-38 Pulmonary emboli are most common in immobilized patients, where DVTs may form in the legs and pelvis. The resultant blood clot goes through the right side of the heart and lodges in the pulmonary artery, blocking blood flow to a portion of the lungs.

Sudden pulmonary embolisms sometimes occur in people after long car trips or lengthy airplane flights. Bedridden patients are often prescribed anticoagulants or wear special stockings or other devices to reduce the formation of blood clots in the legs. Treatment for deep venous thrombosis is usually anticoagulants with blood thinners (heparin or warfarin), although if this is not possible then a Greenfield filter may be inserted. This device, which opens like a mesh umbrella in the main vein that returns blood to the heart, is intended to catch any clots that break loose and travel from the legs.

Very large pulmonary emboli can lodge at the bifurcation of the right and left pulmonary arteries. These are called a saddle embolus and may be immediately fatal. If there is a very large saddle embolus and the patient is unstable, fibrinolytic therapy may break-up the clot and prevent cardiac arrest. If the patient suffers a cardiac arrest due to the clot, resuscitation is not likely to be successful with few patients surviving the cardiac arrest. Cardiac arrest caused by a large pulmonary embolus is a very difficult situation that few patients survive. You may note ongoing cyanosis—deep cyanasis of the face, neck, chest, and back—despite good-quality CPR and ventilation with 100% supplemental oxygen in this scenario.

Disorders of Ventilation

Ventilation is the movement of gas in and out of the lungs. With the use of supplemental oxygen, reasonable and even high oxygen levels are easy to maintain in patients who have healthy lungs, even if ventilation is severely compromised. The best measurement of ventilation, however, is the carbon dioxide level. Under normal circumstances, the volume of ventilation (minute volume) is regulated by the need to maintain the $Paco_2$ in the range of 35 to 45 mm Hg. In a person at rest, that goal is usually accomplished by breathing a tidal volume of around 500 ml at a rate of 12 to 16 breaths/min—that is, with a minute volume in the range of 6 to 8 l. During deep sleep, a smaller minute volume may suffice, while the muscular exertion associated with exercise may require a larger minute volume. As long as the $Paco_2$ remains in the normal range, ventilation is considered normal.

The carbon dioxide level is also directly related to pH (acid-base balance). Patients who are hypoventilating usually have respiratory acidosis. As their carbon dioxide level goes up, their pH level goes down. Patients who are hyperventilating are usually in respiratory alkalosis. As their carbon dioxide level goes down, their pH level goes up.

Respiratory Failure Resulting From Hypoventilation

Many different problems can cause patients to hypoventilate:

- Conditions that impair lung function
- Conditions that impair the mechanics of breathing
- Conditions that impair the neuromuscular apparatus
- Conditions that reduce respiratory drive

In these circumstances, you must often provide aggressive treatment to help the patient's respiratory efforts.

Conditions That Impair Lung Function

When the patient is breathing but gas exchange is impaired, carbon dioxide levels rise. This can happen in severe cases of atelectasis, pneumonia, pulmonary edema, asthma, or COPD.

Conditions That Impair the Mechanics of Breathing

A high cervical fracture, flail chest, diaphragmatic rupture, severe retractions, an abdomen full of air or blood, abdominal or chest binding (using a pneumatic antishock garment or immobilization straps), or anything else that impairs the pressure changes that allow breathing can result in reduced gas flow.

Pickwickian syndrome is the name given to respiratory compromise secondary to extreme obesity. One of the earliest descriptions of the combination of obesity, respiratory compromise, and sleep apnea can be found in the character of "Joe the fat boy" in Charles Dickens's *Pickwick Papers*. Poor Joe would fall asleep in midsentence, snore loudly, and generally exhibit signs of hypercapnia. This syndrome is on the rise in today's society given the increased prevalence of obesity.

Conditions That Impair the Neuromuscular Apparatus

Patients who have had head trauma, intracranial infections, or brain tumours may have damage to the respiratory centres of the brain, which in turn may compromise ventilation. Serious injury to the spinal cord (above C5) may block the nerve impulses that cause breathing to occur. Guillain-Barré syndrome causes progressive muscle weakness and paralysis. If the paralysis reaches the nerves supplying the diaphragm, the patient will be unable to breathe effectively. Amyotrophic lateral sclerosis also causes progressive muscle weakness. This disease is fatal, with death usually coming from respiratory failure as the muscles of respiration become unable to maintain adequate ventilation. Botulism is caused by the bacterium *Clostridium botulinum*. Though somewhat uncommon, it is usually the result of food poisoning or from an unknowing mother giving her infant or young child raw honey. In northern Canada, it may be seen in Inuit patients who ingest raw or improperly processed seal or walrus meat. Botulism can cause muscle paralysis and is typically fatal when it reaches the muscles of respiration.

Conditions That Reduce Respiratory Drive

Perhaps the most common hypoventilation crisis seen by EMS systems is the acute opiate (heroin, OxyContin) overdose. Intoxication with alcohol, narcotics, and a host of other drugs or toxins can reduce the respiratory drive. Head injury, hypoxic drive, or asphyxia can all present with grossly low respiratory rates and volumes. Of course, the ultimate expression of hypoventilation is respiratory and then cardiac arrest.

Hyperventilation

Hyperventilation occurs when people breathe in excess of metabolic need. This typically occurs when they increase the rate or depth of breathing enough to cause a decrease in their CO_2 level. Interestingly, a falling carbon dioxide level may make the patient feel short of breath, so they tend to become anxious and breathe even more rapidly and deeply. In acute hyperventilation syndrome, patients usually feel as if they cannot breathe at all. The continued fall in their carbon dioxide level leads to a rise in their pH level (respiratory alkalosis) that in turn causes numbness or tingling in the hands and feet and around the mouth. The patient may eventually lose consciousness if the patient is unable to control his or her breathing.

The traditional therapy for hyperventilation called for patients to rebreathe their own carbon dioxide by breathing into a paper bag, or by applying a partial rebreather mask at 21% oxygen. This a very dangerous practice for important reasons:

- Patients quickly exhaust the oxygen in the gas they are breathing (and rebreathing). Remember, hyperventilation does not mean that the patient has too much oxygen, but rather that he or she is blowing off too much carbon dioxide. Do not cause the patient to become hypoxic while trying to stop a relatively benign hyperventilation episode.
- Any patient who is acidotic might be hyperventilating in an attempt to drive their pH level down to normal levels. In diabetic ketoacidosis, for example, the patient's body is making too much acid because of inadequate glucose metabolism, so the body attempts to compensate for the acidosis by hyperventilating (Kussmaul respirations). It would be a grave error to force such a patient to breathe into a paper bag. A variety of overdoses, toxic exposures, and metabolic abnormalities can also result in acidosis and compensatory hyperventilation, and none of them have the kind of hyperventilation that should be treated by rebreathing carbon dioxide. You should never come to the conclusion that your patient is just hyperventilating until you have ruled out all other potential causes for their presentation, which would be very difficult if not impossible to do in the prehospital environment.

Frequently, hyperventilation will follow some emotional stressor. Speak calmly with the patient and explain the cause of the physical symptoms. Other techniques include breathing *with* the patient, having the patient count to two between each breath (increasing to higher numbers as he or she is successful), and various distraction techniques (such as asking the patient to recite his or her life stories). Hyperventilation that is not caused by some metabolic crisis is usually self-limiting. Explain to the patient that the physical symptoms will pass with normal breathing patterns.

Notes from Nancy

Not every patient who is breathing deeply or rapidly is hyperventilating.

Managing the Patient Who Has Dyspnea

The paramedic has a relatively short list of tools to treat respiratory compromise. At the most basic level, we provide supportive prehospital care, ensure airway adequacy, administer high-concentration supplemental oxygen therapy, and provide monitoring and transport for many patients. In actuality, there is little we can do in the prehospital setting to alter their pathologic conditions (such as COPD, pneumonia, or pulmonary contusion).

The primary exception is the treatment of bronchoconstriction. A whole host of bronchodilators are available to help relax bronchial smooth muscle. This therapy can be extremely helpful if the patient's primary problem is bronchial muscle spasm resulting from anaphylaxis or asthma. Bronchodilator therapy may be somewhat helpful to many other patients as well.

At the other end of the spectrum of prehospital care are the patients who are in overt respiratory failure. The primary approach to this population is to take over the work of breathing completely by intubating them and manually ventilating them.

Ensure an Adequate Airway

The first part of assessing and managing any respiratory problem is to ensure an open and maintainable airway. Get rid of any food, gum, chewing tobacco, or like items out of the patient's mouth. Suction if necessary, and keep the airway in the optimal position, which typically is the position that makes the patient most comfortable.

Decrease the Work of Breathing

Remove constricting clothing (such as belts or tight collars). Reduce the patient's breathing workload. Help the patient sit up if they feel that position is more comfortable. *Don't make the person walk.* Don't let a big abdomen get in the way of the diaphragm. Relieve gastric distension (perhaps with a nasogastric tube). Don't bind the chest or make the patient lie on the good lung.

Provide Supplemental Oxygen

It is essential to deliver supplemental oxygen to any patient who needs it. If the patient is breathing adequately, administer 100% oxygen via a nonrebreathing mask. Patients who are not breathing adequately should receive bag-valve-mask ventilation and 100% oxygen. Closely reassess the patient's breathing status and adjust your treatment accordingly.

Bronchodilate

Many patients who have respiratory distress can benefit a little from bronchodilation, and some patients can benefit a lot. Today's aerosol bronchodilators rarely hurt patients, so we tend to use them aggressively in the prehospital setting. Patients who do not have bronchospasm will probably benefit only a little from aerosol bronchodilators, and you may have to drop their delivered oxygen concentration during a typical aerosol treatment. In these circumstances, the nonrebreathing mask trumps the aerosol treatment. Follow local protocol.

Consider Fluid Balance

Rehydration is supplemental therapy for patients with respiratory problems who are dehydrated (for example, some patients who have pneumonia or asthma). It is common practice to give a fluid bolus to younger patients in these scenarios. Any elderly patient or patient who has a cardiac dysfunction could be pushed into pulmonary edema by too much fluid. Always

You are the Paramedic Part 4

Your protocols allow for rapid sequence induction, and you choose to perform this procedure on your patient. You successfully place the airway after administering 20 mg of etomidate, 50 µg of fentanyl, and 120 mg of succinylcholine (Anectine). Next, you administer a bolus of 500 ml of normal saline. You notice marked improvement in his pulse oximetry and skin signs throughout your transport to the hospital.

Reassessment	Recording Time: 20 Minutes
Level of consciousness	Sedated, pharmacologically paralyzed
Skin	Improving in colour; pinker, no cyanosis noted in mucosa or nail beds
Pulse	98 beats/min, regular
Blood pressure	110/60 mm Hg
Respirations	Intubated; ventilated at 15 breaths/min
SpO2	92% with bag-valve-mask ventilation and 100% supplemental oxygen
Capnography	45 mm Hg
ECG	Sinus rhythm

8. Beyond inadequate ventilation and oxygenation, what must you take into consideration before attempting intubation?
9. If capnography, pulse oximetry, and other similar pieces of assessment equipment are unavailable, how can you determine whether your interventions are improving the patient's condition?
10. What other techniques can you use to improve ventilation and oxygenation?

assess breath sounds *before* and *after* giving a fluid bolus to make certain you have not volume overloaded the patient. Of course, patients who have respiratory problems can become very sick in a hurry, and you will almost always want to have an IV lifeline in place, in case of further deterioration.

Provide Diuresis

Many elderly patients who have respiratory disease have a component of congestive heart failure and might benefit from a loop diuretic such as furosemide (Lasix). Of course, not every patient who has crackles has pulmonary edema. Giving diuretics to patients who have pneumonia or asthma may actually worsen their overall condition. As always, careful assessment and interpretation must lead you to a correct diagnosis. If transport time is short and the patient's condition is not dire, perhaps the emergency department can make a better decision after seeing a radiograph and some labwork.

Support/Assist Ventilation

If the patient becomes fatigued, you may need to support breathing in a more aggressive fashion. Therapy with CPAP and BiPAP is becoming increasingly common and can allow you to avoid intubation in many patients. Some patients may simply require bag-valve-mask ventilation for a short period to reoxygenate, improve their hemoglobin saturation, and reduce Pa_{CO_2} levels.

You must be confident in your bag-valve-mask ventilation technique so that you don't make a patient's condition worse. Trying to supplement breathing in a patient who is *already breathing on his or her own* is one of the most difficult interventions to pull off. Gastric distension and vomiting from overaggressive ventilation can be disastrous in a patient who is already compromised. As always, *do no harm*. The same is true when providing sedation to anxious or combative patients. The need to control them must be balanced against the possibility of depressing their respirations further. Agitation from dyspnea needs to be corrected with proper oxygenation and ventilation, not sedation.

Take Over Ventilation

Ultimately, you may need to intubate and ventilate patients who are in respiratory failure. Intubation can be lifesaving, and many patients can be extubated within a day or two and go on to have excellent outcomes. However, there are some issues to consider when intubating a patient. The paramedic must weigh these issues along with the protocols, medical direction, and any expression of the patient's wishes. Keep these issues in mind:

- Intubation should be the last option for patients who have severe asthma. These patients are extremely difficult to ventilate and are prone to pneumothoraces.
- Be proactive; ventilate patients *before* cardiac arrest occurs. When in doubt, attempt to ventilate. If they fight you, they may not be ready for intubation. If they allow you to bag them, they probably are ready for intubation. Patients who

are conscious, however, yet still in respiratory distress, will often require sedation and neuromuscular blocking medications (through rapid sequence intubation) to facilitate intubation.

- Some patients who have diabetes or have overdosed present with an obvious need for intubation. However, if an ampule of 50% dextrose or naloxone (Narcan) is likely to completely change that picture, it might be better to use bag-valve-mask ventilation for a few minutes to monitor the effect of the initial therapy, assuming you can do so without causing gastric distension and vomiting. Remember to ventilate slowly (more than 1 second), and use only enough ventilation to produce visible chest rise.

Respiratory Pharmacology

Medication Delivery

Pharmaceutical therapy for respiratory problems is delivered via a variety of methods, some of which are discussed here.

Metered-Dose Inhalers

When properly used, the metered-dose inhaler should be at least as effective as an aerosol treatment. This device is small, easy for the patient to carry and use, and convenient. Because it does not require additional equipment (such as a nebulizer or air compressor), it is usually the delivery method of choice for both bronchodilators and corticosteroids in the home setting **Figure 26-39 ▶**.

Metered-dose inhalers do have some drawbacks. First, using such a device requires a cooperative patient who is able (and willing) to perform the maneuver correctly. Because the entire dose is delivered in one or two breaths, improper technique may result in little or no medication actually getting into the lungs. Also, patients may not realize when they are using an empty inhaler, ie, some propellant remains but there is no medication.

The metered-dose inhalers that you carry on the ambulance should ideally be equipped with spacers. A spacer is a device that collects the medication as it is released from the canister, allowing more to be delivered to the lungs and less to be lost to the environment. Remember, the mist you see coming out of the inhaler isn't what reaches the patient's alveoli; rather, the 5-μm particles, which stay suspended in the spacer for several minutes, are pulled deep into the lungs by smooth laminar flow. When a spacer is used, the patient does not have to worry about timing the inhalation to coincide with the discharge of the inhaler. Spacers also reduce deposition of the drug into the mouth and oropharynx, which is a problem with the inexperienced user.

Achieving the proper technique when using a metered-dose inhaler isn't difficult, but it requires constant reinforcement. The steps for administering medication with a metered-dose inhaler are demonstrated in Chapter 8.

Following are some tips on common errors when using or administering a metered-dose inhaler, and how to avoid them:

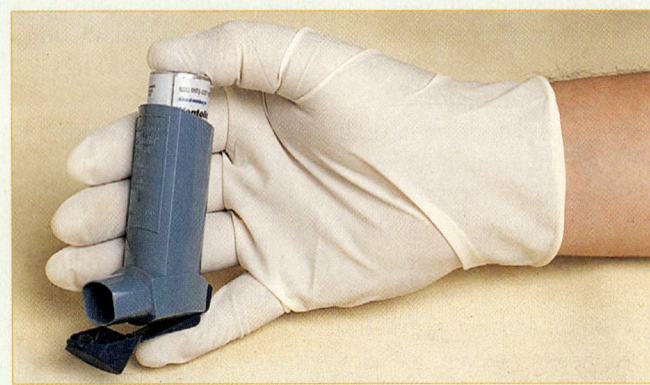

Figure 26-39 Metered-dose inhalers are a common delivery platform for respiratory medications. Their effectiveness is greatly increased by the use of a spacer, which regulates the release of medication into the inhaler.

- Patients need to deeply inhale as they discharge the inhaler to suck the medication deep into their lungs. Placing the inhaler directly into the patient's mouth (without a spacer) often causes much of the medication to fall on the posterior pharynx, from where it is swallowed and digested, thus negating its intended effect.
- Some patients mistakenly blow into the spacer. Tell them to think of the spacer as a big straw, and they should try to suck the medication out of the bottom.
- Many spacers will make a harmonica-like sound if the patient sucks too hard. The best particle deposition comes from smooth, low-pressure, laminar flow. Sucking too hard causes turbulent flow, which makes a lot of the particles stick to the trachea and large bronchi, where they aren't as effective.
- Patients should try to inhale the medication deeply, and then hold their breath for a few seconds. This is a lot to ask of someone who is dyspneic, and it isn't always possible. Sometimes the inhaler causes the patient to cough immediately after inhaling the medication, which also doesn't result in the best delivery, but may be unavoidable.
- Let the first puff open up the airways a little, so the second puff gets in deeper a minute or two later.
- Give the bronchodilator first. Many patients have multiple inhalers. A common package might include a rapid-acting beta-2 agonist (rescue inhaler), a corticosteroid, and a slow-acting bronchodilator. Always use the rescue inhaler first. It will dilate the bronchi so that subsequent medications are more effective. In an emergency situation, the slow-acting branchodilators will not have any immediate effect, so they would not be given.
- After using a corticosteroid inhaler, patients are encouraged to rinse out their mouth with water or mouthwash. Residual corticosteroid in the pharynx can predispose the patient to thrush, an annoying fungal infection in the pharynx or mouth.

- Make sure the inhaler contains medication. Most inhalers list the number of puffs of medication in the canister on the label. Patients should be encouraged to keep track of how many times they have used the inhaler, and to discard it when they reach the recommended number of uses. Just because you can hear fluid in the canister when you shake it does not mean that there is medication left.
- Keep the spacer and canister holder clean and dry.

Nebulizer Therapy

Aerosol nebulizers deliver liquid medications in the form of a fine mist **Figure 26-40 ▾**. Recall that 5-μm or smaller particles ride laminar airflow into the lower respiratory tract. Larger particles rain out in the mouth and pharynx and get swallowed, so they have little ultimate effect. To generate the optimal particle size, most nebulizers need to have gas flow of at least 6 l/min.

In the home, most people run their aerosol treatments off of a small air compressor; in the ambulance, we typically run this therapy off of either our tanked oxygen or off a wall unit attached to the main oxygen supply. As a result, you might be giving only 35% to 40% oxygen via an aerosol treatment, but this is still more than the 21% oxygen contained in room air.

A nebulizer can be attached to a mouthpiece (pipe), a face mask, a tracheostomy collar, or simply held in front of the patient's face (blow-by technique). The less the patient breathes in the mist, the less medication he or she actually receives. Blow-by and mouthpiece treatments are not very effective if patients keep turning their head or removing the mouthpiece to answer your questions. As such, once the decision is made to deliver a breathing treatment, try to stop the conversation and let the patient focus on breathing in the medication.

Although bronchodilators are the drugs most commonly delivered by aerosolization, corticosteroids, anesthetic agents, antitussives, and mucolytics can all be dispersed through an

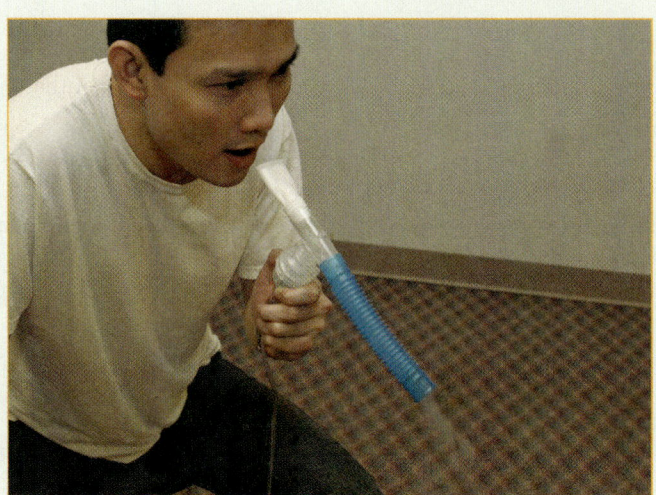

Figure 26-40 Aerosol nebulizers are often used to deliver medications directly to the respiratory tract. Unfortunately, they may give only 35% oxygen during a treatment. Flow rate is an important factor in how much medication makes it into the lungs.

aerosol. Aerosol lidocaine is an extremely effective method of numbing the upper airway before procedures, and aerosol fentanyl is used to reduce chronic coughing in patients who are terminally ill with lung cancer.

The newer aerosol bronchodilators cause far less tachycardia than the older, less beta-2 specific ones. As a result, it has become possible to give repeated treatments to patients with bronchospasm. Continuous nebulizers are available that hold up to 10 times the usual medication dosages, and run for an hour or more. The steps for administering medications via small-volume nebulizer were demonstrated in Chapter 8.

Dry Powder Inhalers

Some respiratory medications are most stable in the form of a very fine powder. Such medications are often placed inside a plastic device that the patient places in his or her mouth and from which he or she inhales deeply. These devices are reasonably convenient and easy to use, but they are rarely used during emergency care.

Several common corticosteroids and slow-acting bronchodilators are routinely packaged in a disc-like device, which holds about 1 month's medication. Each time the device is opened, the small plastic blister that holds a dose is rotated into position. The patient then pushes a small lever to puncture the blister and sucks the powder out of the device. The device is then closed. The device is used to deliver reasonably expensive medications, so be careful not to open and close it repeatedly; you would be wasting several days' worth of medication as the blisters rotate into, and then past, their turn to be punctured.

Other devices require the patient to insert a capsule of powdered medication, which is then pierced when the patient compresses a button or lever on the device. The patient sucks the powder out in a similar fashion to that described above.

Intramuscular Injections

Drug administration methods that require the patient to inhale the medication may become unreliable or ineffective when the patient's breathing effort is inadequate (reduced tidal volume). In some circumstances, it may be beneficial to give intramuscular epinephrine. These medications are not as beta-2 specific as their aerosol cousins and have many more systemic effects but, when the patient's airways are severely closed, they are sometimes needed.

Direct Instillation

Under certain circumstances, such as cardiac arrest when prompt vascular access is delayed, the administration of select drugs via the endotracheal tube is an option. The dose usually is 2 to 2½ times the usual dose, because much of the drug sticks to the inside of the ET tube or drains onto the carina. Newer devices "mist" the drug into the tube, allowing this process to occur without interrupting CPR. While research has shown that this is clearly an inferior delivery model for medications, it is still an option to consider if all else fails.

Fast-Acting Bronchodilators

The most commonly used and fastest-acting bronchodilators work by stimulating the beta-2 receptors in the lungs—part of the sympathetic nervous system. These so-called rescue inhalers provide almost instant relief, a property that sometimes leads to their misuse. Present-day bronchodilators are very beta-2 specific, meaning that they stimulate only beta-2 receptors without acting on other parts of the body, but many patients still use older, less specific medications. Salbutamol (Proventil, Ventolin), which is currently the most common beta-2 agonist, is routinely given every 4 hours, but more frequent treatments, and even continuous therapy for hours at a time are commonly used.

Anticholinergics

In general, the sympathetic and parasympathetic nervous systems act as opposites. In terms of heart rate and bronchodilation, it is reasonable to think of them as the gas (sympathetic stimulation speeds up heart rate [beta-1] and produces bronchodilation [beta-2]) and the brake (parasympathetic stimulation slows heart rate and causes bronchoconstriction). Anticholinergic medications block the parasympathetic response, so they are like taking the foot off the brake. Just as it is hard to drive your car if someone has constant pressure on the brake pedal, so we can see how bronchodilation can be enhanced by specifically blocking the bronchoconstriction mechanism **Figure 26-41 ▶**.

In the past, the strategy was to disperse atropine (the most common parasympathetic blocker) through an aerosol. Today, we have a medication specifically designed for aerosol use, ipratropium; also available in a metered-dose inhaler). The combination of salbutamol (beta-2 agonist) and ipratropium (anticholinergic) is also available as a pre-mixed cocktail, marketed as an aerosol or a metered-dose inhaler.

Anticholinergics have emerged as a very important component in the management of COPD. Tiotropium, a once-a-day anticholinergic for this indication, is taken via a type of dry powder inhaler. Patients taking tiotropium would not typically also use aerosol ipratropium.

Long-Acting Bronchodilators

A variety of bronchodilators exist that work by mechanisms other than beta-2 stimulation. Although most of these medications do not provide immediate relief of symptoms, if taken daily they can reduce the frequency and severity of asthma attacks. Patients who are used to the immediate change in their symptoms after using beta-2 agonists often complain that these agents don't work and have to be encouraged to take them as prescribed until they note the long-term benefits.

Popular long-acting bronchodilators include salmeterol (Serevent) and cromolyn (Intal, NasalCrom). Such agents have dramatically improved the quality of life for many patients who have respiratory illness and who use the drugs correctly.

Leukotriene Modifiers

Some patients with asthma release bronchoconstricting chemicals called leukotrienes. Such patients often benefit from a

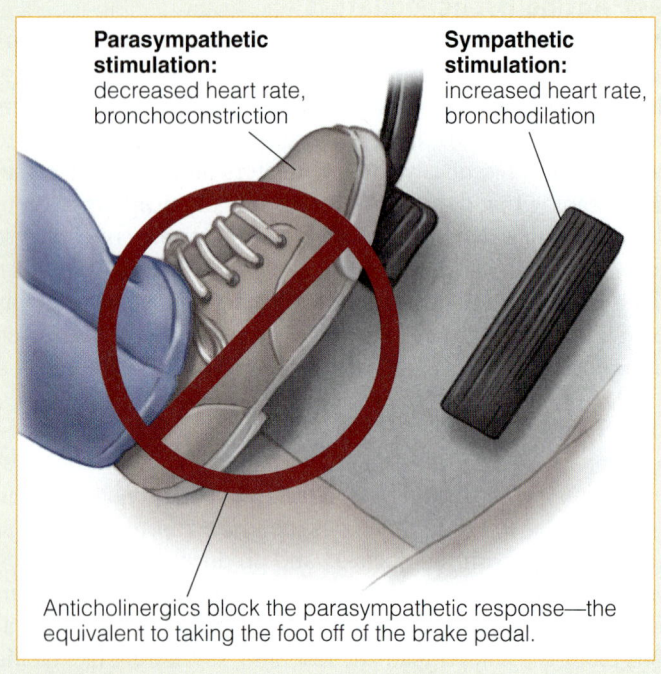

Parasympathetic stimulation: decreased heart rate, bronchoconstriction

Sympathetic stimulation: increased heart rate, bronchodilation

Anticholinergics block the parasympathetic response—the equivalent to taking the foot off of the brake pedal.

Figure 26-41 Blocking the parasympathetic nervous system (the anticholinergic effect) is like pulling your foot off the brake pedal, whereas giving sympathetic nervous system stimulators is like stepping on the gas.

leukotriene blocker such as montelukast (Singulair), which is usually taken via a dry powder inhaler.

Methylxanthines

Methylxanthines, which include aminophylline and theophylline, were once the mainstay of asthma and COPD therapy. Their popularity has declined in recent years because their adverse effects (particularly cardiac effects) are significant and their monitoring is more onerous compared to the many new drugs available. Some patients who have long-term COPD, however, still take aminophylline or theophylline. These drugs can be administered orally (in tablet form or in sprinkles that are placed in food); they can also be given intravenously. Overdose with these agents may cause cardiac dysrhythmias and hypotension, and the level of the drugs in the bloodstream must be closely monitored.

Magnesium

Studies indicate that magnesium plays a role in bronchodilation. In moderate and severe asthma attacks, some physicians give 1 to 2 g of magnesium sulfate over 20 minutes. Consult with direct medical control or follow local protocols regarding this therapy.

Corticosteroids

Corticosteroids are used to reduce bronchial swelling (edema). Although these are not the anabolic corticosteroids that may be abused by athletes, the corticosteroids used in respiratory medicine do have a variety of adverse effects. Long-term corticosteroid use can cause Cushing's syndrome, which is characterized by the classic moon face and generalized edema. Corticosteroids also make blood glucose go out of control and can blunt the immune system, allowing any infections to flourish. Patients taking long-term corticosteroids such as prednisone must taper their use gradually. Because of these adverse effects with prolonged use, most patients are prescribed a short course of corticosteroid therapy that lasts 5 to 7 days with no taper.

Inhaled Corticosteroids

Fortunately, inhaled corticosteroids do not appear to have the same adverse effects as their oral counterparts. For that reason, inhaled corticosteroids are a mainstay of asthma treatment and are common adjuncts to the treatment of COPD. Reviewing the asthma triad, you can see how a slow-acting bronchodilator can reduce bronchial constriction, while an inhaled corticosteroid can reduce bronchial swelling.

IV Corticosteroids

In an emergency, it is reasonably common to give corticosteroids intravenously. A single bolus of IV corticosteroids does not appear to cause any negative long-term consequences and is reasonably safe. Methylprednisolone and hydrocortisone are both IV corticosteroid preparations given as an IV bolus, usually for acute asthma exacerbations. Steroid administration in the setting of a COPD exacerbation is reserved for patients who do not have an underlying respiratory infection, such as pneumonia. Their onset of action takes hours, so you will not see any results in the prehospital environment. As always, consult your local protocols and medical direction before administering these agents.

Antitussives

Antitussives are designed to stop a cough. Coughs can be very annoying, particularly if they interrupt the patient's sleep. However, the need for comfort must be weighed against the need to get rid of excess secretions. Overuse of antitussives can sedate the patient, reduce respiratory drive, and cause excessive plugging of secretions. Many over-the-counter cough syrups also contain antihistamines that can cause problems if not used appropriately.

Aerosol fentanyl is sometimes used to stop the severe coughing associated with tracheobronchial cancers.

Diuretics

Diuretics are used to help reduce blood pressure and to maintain fluid balance in patients who have heart failure. Patients who present with pulmonary edema may benefit from diuretics to remove excess fluid from the circulation, which ultimately keeps it out of the lungs. Loop diuretics, such as furosemide (Lasix) are the most commonly used agents in emergent situations. Thiazide diuretics are also commonly taken orally to treat high blood pressure or heart failure. Many diuretics cause the patient to lose not only fluid but also potassium. Patients who do not take their potassium supplements may have low potassium levels, and a subsequent predisposition to cardiac dysrhythmias and chronic muscle cramping.

Don't give diuretics to patients who have pneumonia or to patients who are already dry—try to reserve them for those who clearly have pulmonary edema. In fact, some EMS systems reserve furosemide (Lasix, a diuretic) on standing orders for patients with wet lungs and peripheral edema. Patients who have some degree of renal failure may require very large doses of diuretics, or they may be completely unresponsive to diuretics. If your patient requires dialysis for renal failure, trying to induce diuresis is unlikely to be an effective strategy.

Vasodilators

Another common treatment of pulmonary edema is nitroglycerine. It is a strong vasodilator that reduces the cardiac preload, and may rapidly improve pulmonary edema. Morphine, a strong narcotic, also reduces pain and anxiety, and may also help with vasodilation. It can be very helpful in the scenario of respiratory distress. Too much morphine, however, can decrease respiratory drive and cause a drop in blood pressure. Use morphine carefully, titrating it based on blood pressure and respiratory status.

▮ Assisted Ventilation

Continuous Positive Airway Pressure

Continuous positive airway pressure (CPAP) is used in two distinctly different ways.

Many people who have been diagnosed with obstructive sleep apnea wear a CPAP unit at night to maintain their airways while they sleep. This type of CPAP may be applied via nasal pillows, a nasal mask, a face mask that resembles a typical mask used for bag-valve-mask ventilation, or a mask that covers the entire face. Note that this is *not* the type of CPAP that you will apply to the critically ill patient. The positive pressure delivered maintains the stability of the posterior pharynx, thereby preventing obstruction of the upper airway when the person sleeps. This limits both hypoxic episodes and snoring.

The CPAP used as therapy for respiratory failure is almost always delivered via a face mask that is held to the head with some type of strapping system. You should ensure that there is a good seal with minimal leakage **Figure 26-42 ▸**. In the prehospital setting, 100% supplemental oxygen is the most common driving gas for the positive pressure. Be vigilant about monitoring your gas supply—depending on the flow and the patient's respiratory rate, some CPAP units may empty a D cylinder in as little as 5 to 10 minutes. The mask is fitted with a pressure-relief valve that determines the amount of pressure delivered (such as 5 cm H_2O). The end effect is similar to having a gale-force wind blowing in your face (high inspiratory flow) and having to push a pressure valve open with exhalation. This would appear to require a great deal of effort, and to tire out the already-decompensating patient who is in respiratory failure. Miraculously, many patients who appear to be preparing to take their last breath will make a dramatic turnaround when CPAP is applied.

Some patients find the CPAP mask claustrophobic, and will fight its application. You will be able to talk some of these patients through the process with good results, but other patients simply cannot tolerate the mask. If your CPAP equipment permits, apply the mask with free-flowing supplemental oxygen but no positive pressure. If the patient tolerates the mask, then apply the positive pressure based on your local or regional protocols. Do not fight with your patient if he or she is unwilling to apply the mask, as you will only increase the patient's anxiety, cardiac workload, and cardiac oxygen consumption. That is a bad trade off. When CPAP works as planned, it can provide dramatic relief and the patient avoids intubation. When CPAP fails, you need to recognize if the patient's condition is deteriorating and be prepared to move to the next step (usually intubation). Within several minutes of application, the patient's oxygen saturation should increase, and the respiratory rate should decrease. The success of CPAP is grossly related to the patient's respiratory rate soon after its application. If this rate *increases,* the therapy is likely to fail; if this rate *decreases,* then the therapy is likely to succeed.

Administering CPAP increases pressure in the chest. If the patient's blood pressure is already low, too much CPAP can decrease venous return to the heart and make the patient's blood pressure suddenly drop. This isn't common with lower levels of CPAP, but blood pressure should be carefully monitored whenever CPAP is applied (especially at levels above 10 cm H_2O). Keep in mind that CPAP can also turn a simple pneumothorax into a tension pneumothorax in a few breaths.

Experts have not determined whether CPAP is useful in the prehospital setting. Initial small EMS studies suggest that CPAP may provide symptom relief for patients with acute respiratory failure. Large emergency department and hospital-based studies have demonstrated that noninvasive ventilation methods, such as CPAP, improve respiratory distress symptoms and can avert the need for tracheal intubation, but there is no effect on mortality. Services that carry out interfacility patient transport are equipped to manage patients receiving noninvasive ventilation, such as CPAP. These patients are typically more stable than emergency response patients, and noninvasive ventilation is a useful method to support oxygen and ventilation needs in this patient population. Although CPAP is useful in this situation or as a bridge to more definitive airway management, the overall role and benefit of CPAP in this prehospital setting has yet to be determined.

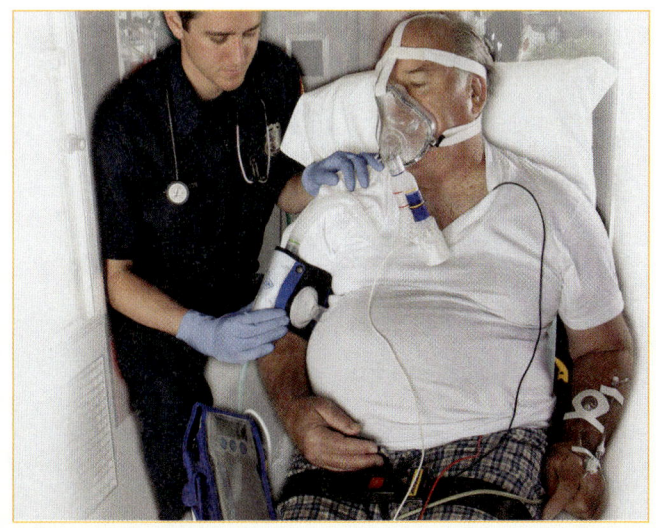

Figure 26-42 The CPAP used in the acute setting is usually administered via face mask, which must make a tight seal to function properly.

Bilevel Positive Airway Pressure

Bilevel positive airway pressure (BiPAP) is just CPAP with IPAP and EPAP: it can deliver one pressure during inspiration (inspiratory positive airway pressure [IPAP]) and a different pressure during exhalation (expiratory positive airway pressure [EPAP]). Instead of applying 8 cm H_2O of CPAP, you might set the BiPAP at 16/8 (16 cm H_2O on inspiration and 8 cm H_2O during exhalation). This may reduce the patient's work of breathing and increase his or her tidal volumes, improving ventilation and CO_2 elimination. It is also a more complex and expensive device, and one that is not commonly used in the prehospital setting.

Automated Transport Ventilators

Automated transport ventilators are essentially flow-restricted oxygen-powered ventilation devices (FROPVDs) with timers on them. They can be set to deliver a particular volume at a particular rate, which can be very helpful when you need an extra pair of hands **Figure 26-43 ▸**. They are particularly good for replacing the role of bag-valve-mask ventilation when the patient is in cardiac or respiratory arrest. Basic automated transport ventilators may lack any alarms, the ability to control flow rate, or the ability to provide various modes of ventilatory support. They are *not* little ventilators and are *not* intended to ventilate patients without direct observation and attention by a skilled paramedic.

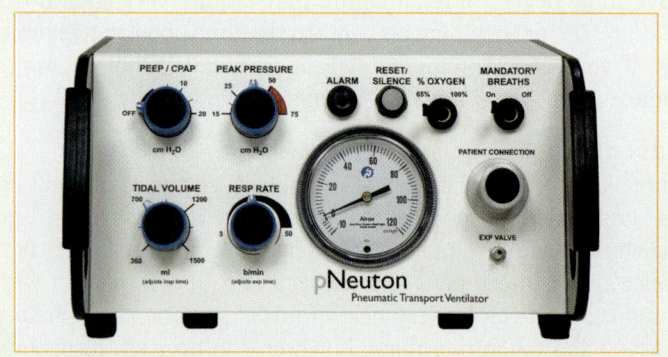

Figure 26-43 Automated transport ventilators are flow-restricted oxygen-powered ventilation devices. They can be very helpful during a cardiac arrest, but the preset flow of 40 l/min is not appropriate for conscious patients.

Conscious patients require up to 150 l/min of flow to comfortably breathe. Most automated transport ventilators are permanently set to deliver 40 l/min, which would be extremely uncomfortable for the spontaneously breathing patient. Both FROPVDs and automated transport ventilators are preset to 40 l/min, which is the optimal flow for ventilating a patient who has had a cardiac arrest—via face mask, and without causing gastric distension.

You are the Paramedic Summary

1. What about this patient's presentation gives you cause for concern?

The patient's body position, facial expression, increased work of breathing, accessory muscle use, and cries for help are very worrisome. All of these signs point to a patient who is in severe respiratory distress. This patient will need appropriate, aggressive prehospital care to prevent his condition from significantly and rapidly worsening.

2. What are your assessment and treatment priorities?

As always, assessment and treatment priorities involve airway, breathing, and circulation. These priorities are learned as a primary care paramedic. No matter how advanced you become in your certifications and knowledge as a medical professional, you must always remember that the fundamentals of emergency medicine are built upon the principles of basic life support—that is, assessment and treatment of life-threatening illness and injury inherently related to a problem with airway, breathing, and circulation.

3. If you are unable to gather much information from your patient about his medical history, in what other ways can you obtain this information?

Utilize the scene or—better yet—the patient's family members or friends. Significant others are usually highly aware of acute changes in the patient's condition. They may be the first to offer information that can clarify the patient's condition or provide new insight that the patient had not noticed. If no family member is available, you should look for medical identification tags or bracelets and prescription bottles, and assess the scene to gain a better understanding of your patient's medical history. Use resources wisely to avoid delaying lifesaving patient prehospital care by searching throughout the home.

4. Given the patient's presentation, which assessment tools should you use to obtain a greater understanding of the patient's medical condition?

Listening to lung sounds is a given and, as a well-trained medical professional, you will likely have many other assessment tools at your disposal. It is critical that you understand when and how to use tools such as tactile fremitus, egophony, bronchophony, whispered pectoriloquy, and percussion. It is not always wise to spend precious minutes using these assessment tools on a patient whose condition is deteriorating rapidly. As a paramedic, you must determine how to best use your time and your resources in accordance with your patient's condition. For example, to delay transport to check the function of all 12 cranial nerves in the presence of an obvious cerebrovascular accident is inappropriate and could cost the patient his or her life.

5. What was likely the initial problem with obtaining a pulse oximetry reading?

In cases of shock, the body shunts blood away from the extremities and directs it to the vital organs. Therefore, when the body is poorly perfused or when the extremities are cold, this will affect the oximeter's ability to obtain a reading. Choose alternative sites in which to place the sensor, such as the ear or the bridge of the nose.

6. Do you believe that your patient is able to maintain his airway?

Given the information regarding his level of consciousness; his respiratory rate, depth, and quality; his skin signs; and the oximetry reading, it is obvious that this patient is not ventilating or oxygenating adequately.

7. What options do you have available to maintain this patient's airway?

The most important skills for successfully maintaining a patient's airway are basic life support measures—specifically, bag-valve-mask ventilation and use of airway adjuncts. The importance of these skills becomes painfully obvious in the event of failed intubations or failure of alternative airways.

Controversy exists in the medical community regarding the appropriateness of prehospital rapid sequence induction. The medical director must determine whether his or her paramedics should use this advanced airway management tool. If the medical director has decided that rapid sequence induction is an appropriate skill for his or her personnel, you must commit to maintaining the knowledge and skills required to safely and successfully perform this procedure.

For those agencies that do not have the capabilities to perform rapid sequence induction or intubation, nasal airways can be an appropriate choice, assuming your patient has no contraindications such as head trauma. If you are unable to manage the airway with either of these procedures, and the patient continues to have an intact gag reflex, then alternate advanced airways such as the laryngeal mask airway, King Airway, or Combitubes will not be an option. In these cases, use nasogastric or orogastric tubes to remove the stomach contents, ventilate the patient using bag-valve-mask ventilation and 100% oxygen, and continually monitor the airway for the need to suction secretions.

8. Beyond inadequate ventilation and oxygenation, what must you take into consideration before attempting intubation?

You must always consider the patient's anatomy and your ability to place the ET tube correctly. Patients with small mouths or short necks or who are obese can be quite difficult to intubate.

9. If capnography, pulse oximetry, and other similar pieces of assessment equipment are unavailable, how can you determine whether your interventions are improving the patient's condition?

Almost anyone who has worked with a seasoned partner has likely heard that new medics are too dependent on gadgets. Some of this disdain could be rooted in fear of change, but it still makes a valid point. Paramedics can become overly dependent on equipment to provide information that can and should be validated in the patient's signs and symptoms. Reassess the patient for signs of improvement.

10. What other techniques can you use to improve ventilation and oxygenation?

Another advantage of obtaining a definitive airway is your ability to provide tracheal suctioning. This patient definitively would benefit from the removal of secretions.

Prep Kit

■ Ready for Review

- The primary components of the respiratory system are like an inverted tree, with the trachea representing the tree's trunk and the alveoli resembling the tree's leaves.
- Swelling in the mouth and oropharynx can be profound and potentially dangerous.
- The larynx and glottis are typically considered the dividing line between the upper airway and the lower airway. The thyroid cartilage is the most obvious external landmark of the larynx. The glottis and vocal cords are found in the middle of the thyroid cartilage.
- The cricoid cartilage can be palpated just below the thyroid cartilage in the neck. It forms a complete ring and maintains the trachea in an open position. Applying cricoid pressure or Sellick maneuver may be helpful in preventing aspiration.
- The small space between the thyroid and cricoid cartilages is the cricothyroid membrane. It is a good choice for providing oxygen via an IV cannula or a small breathing tube.
- Pulmonary circulation begins after blood leaves the right ventricle, where the pulmonary artery branches into increasingly smaller vessels until it reaches the pulmonary capillary bed, which surrounds the alveoli and terminal bronchioles.
- Patients who have traumatic brain injuries may exhibit bizarre respiratory patterns, including agonal gasps; apneustic and ataxic patterns; Cheyne-Stokes, and Kussmaul respirations; as well as central neurogenic hyperventilation, bradypnea, hyperpnea, hypopnea, and tachypnea.
- The respiratory system delivers oxygen to the body and removes the primary waste product of metabolism, carbon dioxide. If the lungs are not functioning appropriately, both of these vital functions may be impaired. Hypoxia, cell death, and acidosis can then occur.
- The brain is very sensitive to reduced levels of oxygen. It requires a regular supply of both oxygen and glucose to function, but can store neither. Alteration in level of consciousness could represent respiratory compromise.
- A patient who has respiratory disease may not be able to talk because he or she is having difficulty breathing. You may have to obtain the history from a family member or from only a few clues.
- It is critical to evaluate how hard your patient is working to breathe. Patients in respiratory distress may be able to compensate at first, but will eventually become sleepy, have a decreased respiratory rate and depth, and then, decompensate.
- Patients who have chronic respiratory disease are often knowledgeable about their disease and may have tried several potential treatment options already. Ask them about these efforts and what results, if any, they produced.
- Onset and duration of distress are important considerations in determining the underlying cause. Find out if the problem happened suddenly or gradually worsened over time.
- Assessing the patient's position of comfort and difficulty speaking may help you gauge the patient's degree of distress. A patient sitting in a Fowler's position and speaking only in two- or three-word statements is probably in considerable distress.
- Patients in respiratory distress tend to seek the tripod position. The condition of a patient in respiratory distress who is willing to lay flat may be quickly deteriorating. Head bobbing is also an ominous sign.
- Find out if the patient's condition is a recurrence of a past condition. If so, compare the current situation with other episodes.
- Note any audible abnormal respiratory noises. Noisy breathing is obstructed breathing.
- Snoring indicates partial obstruction of the upper airway by the tongue. Stridor indicates narrowing of the upper airway, usually as a result of swelling (laryngeal edema).
- Assessing the level of consciousness is enormously important in dyspneic patients.
- Assess the patient's mucous membranes for cyanosis, pallor, and moisture.
- Look for jugular venous distension in the neck, with the patient in a semi-sitting position. Distended neck veins may be caused by cardiac failure, tension pneumothorax, or tampony.
- Feel the chest for vibrations as the patient breathes. Check for edema of the ankles or lower back. Check for peripheral cyanosis. Check the pulse and note the patient's skin temperature. Attach any available monitors.
- Auscultate the lungs whenever possible. Adventitious breath sounds are the extra noises that you may hear; they include wheezing or crackles.
- Crackles are any discontinuous noises heard on auscultation of the lungs. They are caused by the popping open of air spaces and are usually associated with increased fluid in the lungs.
- Wheezes are high-pitched, whistling sounds made by air being forced through narrowed airways, which makes them vibrate. Wheezing may be diffuse in conditions such as asthma and congestive heart failure or localized when caused by a foreign body obstructing a bronchus.
- *Silence means danger!* If you don't hear anything with your stethoscope, the patient is not moving enough air to ventilate the lungs.
- Note whether the patient is coughing up colourful sputum, if the colour or amount of sputum has changed, and if it contains blood or pus.
- A pulse oximeter indicates what percentage of the patient's hemoglobin has oxygen attached to it. An oxygen saturation level greater than 95% is considered normal.
- The peak flow is the maximum flow rate at which the patient can expel air from the lungs. Normal peak flows run from about 350 to 700 l/min. A peak flow of less than 200 l/min is very low and signals significant distress.
- A variety of infections can cause swelling in the upper airway. Croup is one of the most common, though it usually occurs in small children.
- Pulmonary aspiration of stomach contents is very dangerous. Avoid causing gastric distension when bagging the patient, and monitor the patient's ability to protect his or her airway. If you determine that the patient can't protect his or her airway, one of your primary jobs is to protect it for them, by intubation.
- Common obstructive airway diseases include emphysema, chronic bronchitis, and asthma. Emphysema and chronic bronchitis are collectively classified as COPD.
- Asthma is caused by allergens or irritants and is characterized by widespread, reversible narrowing of the airways (bronchospasm) and inflammation. It can cause significant airway obstruction.
- Primary treatment of bronchospasm is bronchodilator medication. Primary treatment of bronchial edema is corticosteroids, which may or may not be administered in the prehospital setting.
- Status asthmaticus is a severe, prolonged asthmatic attack that cannot be broken with conventional treatment. It is a dire medical emergency. Any person with asthma who feels sick enough to call an ambulance is in status asthmaticus until proved otherwise.
- When a patient has recurring asthma attacks, his or her inhaler could be empty or the medication could no longer be effective. Try administering a new bronchodilator.
- Emphysema is a chronic weakening and destruction of the walls of the terminal bronchioles and alveoli. A patient with emphysema classically has a barrel chest, muscle wasting, and pursed-lip breathing. Such patients are often tachypneic.
- Chronic bronchitis is characterized by excessive mucous production in the bronchial tree, nearly always accompanied by a chronic

or recurrent productive cough. A patient with chronic bronchitis tends to be sedentary and obese, sleep in an upright position, use many tissues, have copious secretions, and be cyanotic.

- In assessing patients who have COPD, search for what pushed them over the edge. Look for signs of infection, peripheral edema, jugular venous distension with hepatojugular reflux, and crackles. Find out if the onset of dyspnea was sudden or gradual.

- Not everyone should be ventilated the same way. Allow each breath to come back out before the delivery of the next breath. If you don't, pressures in the thorax will rise, eventually causing pneumothorax or cardiac arrest. Patients with severe obstructive diseases should be ventilated as little as 4 to 6 breaths/min.

- Noncompliance could trigger an asthma attack. Ask what the patient was doing when the asthma attack began. Ask if the patient took his or her medications today. Ask if movement worsens the dyspnea.

- Pneumonia may be caused by a variety of bacterial, viral, and fungal agents. The patient with pneumonia usually reports weakness, productive cough, fever, and sometimes chest pain that worsens with coughing. Supportive prehospital care includes oxygenation, suctioning, and transport to an appropriate facility.

- Pulmonary edema occurs when fluid enters the alveoli in the lungs. The patient expectorating pink and foamy secretions probably has severe pulmonary edema.

- When a patient has a pneumothorax, air collects between the visceral pleura and the parietal pleura. Administer supplemental oxygen and monitor the patient's respiratory status closely.

- Pleural effusion will make the patient dyspneic. Supportive prehospital care, including proper positioning and aggressive oxygen administration, should be given.

- A pulmonary embolism occurs when a blood clot breaks off in the deep venous circulation and travels to the lungs, blocking blood flow and nutrient exchange. Bedridden patients, those with cancer, and patients with clotting disorders are at risk of pulmonary embolism.

- Respiratory failure, or insufficient ventilation, can occur from a multitude of pathologic conditions, from injuries to the lungs, heart, and neurologic system to overdoses. Prehospital care includes providing supplemental oxygen.

- In hyperventilation syndrome, ventilation is excessive. If it continues, the patient may experience chest pain and syncope. Psychological support techniques such as counting breaths, and distraction work best and help calm the patient.

- In managing the condition of a patient who is in respiratory distress, begin by ensuring that there is an open and maintainable airway. Suction if necessary and keep the airway optimally positioned. Remove constricting clothing. Reduce the patient's effort to breathe.

- Patients in respiratory failure may ultimately need to be intubated. There are major drawbacks and risks to intubating in the prehospital setting, but it can also be lifesaving. Weigh these issues along with protocols, medical direction, and the patient's wishes.

- Metered-dose inhalers deliver medication as an aerosol treatment. They are usually the delivery method of choice for both bronchodilators and corticosteroids in the home setting. Improper technique may result in little or no medication actually getting into the lungs.

- Aerosol nebulizers deliver liquid medications in the form of a fine mist to the respiratory tract. Weigh the potential benefits of nebulizer therapy against the lower FIO_2 delivered during the treatment.

- Drug administration methods that require the patient to inhale the medication may become unreliable or ineffective when the patient's airways are severely compromised. Some cases may warrant delivering medications such as epinephrine.

- Medications can be instilled directly into the tracheobronchial tree when patients are intubated or have a tracheotomy.

- Continuous positive airway pressure (CPAP) can often be used as therapy for respiratory failure. Within several minutes of application, the patient's oxygen saturation should increase, and the respiratory rate should decrease. Intubation can often be avoided if CPAP is attempted early.

- Bilevel positive airway pressure (BiPAP) is CPAP that delivers one pressure during inspiration and a different pressure during exhalation. It is more like normal breathing and may decrease the patient's work of breathing.

- Automated transport ventilators are essentially flow-restricted oxygen-powered breathing devices with timers on them. They are particularly good choices for filling the role of the bag-valve-mask ventilator when the patient is in cardiac or respiratory arrest, but are not intended to ventilate patients without direct observation and attention from a skilled practitioner.

Vital Vocabulary

abscess A collection of pus in a sac, formed by necrotic tissues and an accumulation of white blood cells.

adventitious A type of breath sound that occurs in addition to the normal breath sounds; examples are crackles and wheezes.

alveoli Sac-like units at the end of the bronchioles where gas exchange takes place (singular: alveolus).

angioedema An allergic reaction that may cause profound swelling of the tongue and lips.

arytenoid cartilages One of the paired, pitcher-shaped cartilages at the back of the larynx, at the upper border of the cricoid cartilage.

atelectasis Collapse of the alveolar air spaces of the lungs.

beta-2 agonists Pharmacologic agents that stimulate the beta-2 receptor sites found in smooth muscle; include common bronchodilators like salbutamol.

botulism Poisoning from eating food containing botulinum toxin.

bronchospasm Severe constriction of the bronchial tree.

carina Point at which the trachea bifurcates into the right and left mainstem bronchi.

chronic bronchitis Chronic inflammatory condition affecting the bronchi that is associated with excess mucous production that results from overgrowth of the mucous glands in the airways.

cilia Hairlike microtubule projections on the surface of a cell that can move materials over the cell surface.

cor pulmonale Heart disease that develops secondary to a chronic lung disease, usually affecting primarily the right side of the heart.

crackles Abnormal breath sounds that have a fine, crackling quality; previously called rales.

cricoid cartilage Ringlike cartilage forming the lower and back part of the larynx.

cricothyroid membrane Membrane between the cricoid and thyroid cartilages of the larynx.

croup Common disease of childhood characterized by a barking cough and wheezing due to inflammation of the larynx and upper airway.

dead space The portion of the tidal volume that does not reach the alveoli and thus does not participate in gas exchange.

diuresis Increased urine production by the kidney.

emphysema Infiltration of any tissue by air or gas; a chronic obstructive pulmonary disease characterized by distension of the alveoli and destructive changes in the lung parenchyma.

end-tidal carbon dioxide The numeric percentage of carbon dioxide contained in the last few millilitres of the patient's exhaled air.

Fowler's position A sitting position with the head elevated to 90° (sitting straight upright).

glottis Opening between the vocal cords.

goblet cells Cells that produce a protective mucous lining.

Greenfield filter A mesh filter placed in the inferior vena cava to catch blood clots in patients who are at high risk of pulmonary embolus.

Guillain-Barré syndrome A disease of unknown etiology that causes paralysis that progresses from the feet to the head (ascending paralysis). If the paralysis reaches the diaphragm, the patient may require respiratory support.

hemoglobin Oxygen-carrying pigment of the red blood cells. When hemoglobin has absorbed oxygen in the lungs, it is bright red and is called oxyhemoglobin. After hemoglobin has given up its oxygen in the tissues, it is purple and is called reduced hemoglobin.

hemoptysis Coughing up blood.

Hering-Breuer reflex The nervous system mechanism that terminates inhalation and prevents lung overexpansion.

hypoventilate To not move adequate volumes of gas; underventilate.

hypoxic drive A situation in which a person's stimulus to breathe comes from a fall in Pa_{O_2} rather than the normal stimulus, a rise in Pa_{CO_2}.

jugular venous distension The visible bulging of the jugular veins when the patient is in semi-Fowler's or full Fowler's position. This is indicative of inadequate blood movement through the heart and/or lungs.

Kussmaul respirations A respiratory pattern characteristic of the person with diabetes who is in ketoacidosis, with marked hyperpnea and tachypnea.

larynx The organ of voice production.

ongoing cyanosis Deep cyanosis of the face and neck and across the chest and back; associated with little or no blood flow; it is particularly ominous.

oropharynx The area behind the base of the tongue between the soft palate and the upper portion of the epiglottis.

orthopnea Severe dyspnea experienced when recumbent and relieved by sitting or standing up.

palatine tonsils One of three sets of lymphatic organs that comprise the tonsils; located in the back of the throat, on each side of the posterior opening of the oral cavity; help protect the body from bacteria introduced into the mouth and nose.

parenchyma The substance of a gland or solid organ.

paroxysmal nocturnal dyspnea Severe shortness of breath occurring at night after several hours of recumbency, during which fluid pools in the lungs.

piriform fossa Hollow pockets on the lateral sides of the glottic opening.

pleural effusion Excessive accumulation of fluid in the pleural space.

pneumonitis Inflammation of the lung. Implies lung inflammation from an irritant such as a chemical, dust, or radiation, or from aspiration. When lung inflammation is caused by an infectious agent, it would typically be called pneumonia.

polycythemia The production of more red blood cells over time, making the blood thick; a characteristic of people who have chronic lung disease and chronic hypoxia.

pseudomembrane A false membrane formed by a dead tissue layer. Seen in the posterior pharynx of patients with diphtheria.

pulsus paradoxus Weakening or loss of a palpable pulse during inhalation, characteristic of cardiac tamponade and severe asthma.

purulent Full of pus; having the character of pus.

rales Old terminology for abnormal breath sounds that have a fine, crackling quality; now called crackles.

reactive airway disease A term used to describe any condition that causes hyperreactive bronchioles and bronchospasm.

retraction Drawing in the intercostal muscles and the muscles above the clavicles in respiratory distress.

rhonchus A coarse, low-pitched breath sound heard in patients who have chronic mucus in the airways (plural: rhonchi).

Sellick maneuver Pressure applied over the cricoid to prevent reflux of gastric contents.

shunt Situation in which a portion of the output of the right side of the heart reaches the left side of the heart without being oxygenated in the lungs; may be caused by atelectasis, pulmonary edema, or a variety of other conditions. In hemodialysis, an anastomosis between a peripheral artery and vein.

smooth muscle Nonstriated involuntary muscle found in vessel walls, glands, and the gastrointestinal tract.

snoring Noise made on inhalation when the upper airway is partially obstructed by the tongue.

spacer A device that collects medication as it is released from the canister of a metered-dose inhaler, allowing more to be delivered to the lungs and less to be lost to the environment.

status asthmaticus A severe, prolonged asthma attack.

stridor Harsh, high-pitched sound associated with severe upper airway obstruction, such as that caused by laryngeal edema.

surfactant A liquid protein substance that coats the alveoli in the lungs.

tactile fremitus Vibrations in the chest as the patient breathes.

tidal volume The amount of air inhaled or exhaled during one breath.

tracheostomy Surgically opening the trachea to create an airway.

tuberculosis A chronic bacterial disease caused by *Mycobacterium tuberculosis* that usually affects the lungs but can also affect other organs such as the brain or kidneys.

turbinates A set of bony convolutions formed by the conchae in the nasopharynx.

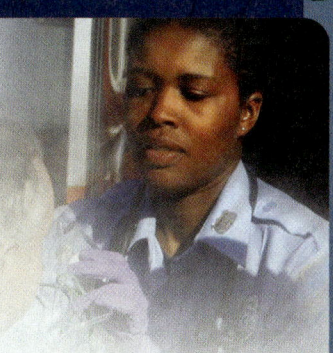

Assessment in Action

You arrive on the scene and find a 63-year-old woman in moderate respiratory distress. She is in the tripod position, using some accessory muscles, and is speaking in three- to four-word sentences. The patient is conscious, alert, and orientated to person, place, and time. Her blood pressure is 134/70 mm Hg; heart rate is 118 beats/min and regular; and her respiratory rate is 28 breaths/min. The pulse oximeter reads 90%. The patient's skin is warm and her nail beds are slightly cyanotic. She has been taking her salbutamol inhaler all day and it hasn't worked. She states this all began 2 days ago and has not gotten any better. She is wheezing in all lung fields.

1. **Which of the following is essential for normal ventilations to occur?**
   A. Functional diaphragm and intercostal muscles
   B. Interstitial space that is not filled with fluid
   C. Adequate blood volume
   D. Pulmonary capillaries that are not occluded

2. **What is chronic obstructive pulmonary disease?**
   A. A recurring condition of partially reversible airflow obstruction
   B. An acute inflammation of the lungs
   C. An absence of breath sounds on one side
   D. A progressive and irreversible disease of the airway

3. **What might bring about an exacerbation in an underlying respiratory condition?**
   A. Stress and infections
   B. Cigarette smoking
   C. Exercising
   D. All of the above

4. **What are important questions to ask this patient?**
   A. Has this happened before?
   B. Have you ever been intubated in the past?
   C. Is breathing uncomfortable when you lie down (more comfortable when you are sitting up or standing)?
   D. All of the above.

5. **What is usually the most reliable indicator of the patient's severity of respiratory distress?**
   A. One-word sentences
   B. Gross diaphoresis and pale colour
   C. Patient's description of respiratory distress
   D. Tachycardia

6. **What are wheezes?**
   A. High-pitched, whistling sounds
   B. Noises heard on auscultation of lungs, caused by popping open of air spaces
   C. Absent breath sounds
   D. Bubbling sounds heard at bases of the lungs

7. **What is emphysema?**
   A. Reversible narrowing of the airways
   B. Chronic weakening and destruction of the walls of the terminal bronchioles and alveoli
   C. An acute inflammatory condition of the lungs
   D. The leading cause of respiratory illnesses in children

8. **What is the hypoxic drive?**
   A. To not move adequate volumes of gas
   B. A respiratory pattern characterized by ketoacidosis
   C. A situation in which a person's stimulus to breathe comes from a fall in Pao_2 rather than the normal stimulus, a rise in $Paco_2$
   D. The portion of tidal volume that does not reach the alveoli

9. **True or false? You should withhold oxygen from a patient who has been diagnosed with COPD.**
   A. True
   B. False

10. **What is peak expiratory flow?**
    A. Maximum flow rate at which patients can expel air from their lungs
    B. Partial obstruction of the upper airway by the tongue
    C. Adventitious breath sounds when auscultating the lungs
    D. Silent lung fields

Challenging Questions

You are dispatched to the train station. Arriving on the scene, you find a 54-year-old man in respiratory distress. Upon auscultation of his lungs, you note wheezing in all lung fields. The patient is unable to talk to you.

11. **Is this patient having an asthma attack?**

▬ Points to Ponder

Your shift is just beginning and you are dispatched to the home of a 90-year-old man who has respiratory problems. It's a cold winter evening and the BLS crew is about ready to bring him to the ambulance. You enter the house and immediately hear audible crackles coming from the next room. The crew has the patient on 100% oxygen via nonrebreathing mask. The patient is conscious, alert, and oriented to person, place, and time. Blood pressure is 220/110 mm Hg, respiratory rate is 40 breaths/min, heart rate is 85 beats/min, pulse oximetry is 91%. The patient has jugular venous distension and peripheral edema.

The patient appears to be in severe respiratory distress, using accessory muscles, speaking in one-word sentences, and grossly diaphoretic. Family states that this all began while he was watching TV approximately 45 minutes ago, and has gotten progressively worse. The patient's medications include metoprolol, pravastatin, furosemide, potassium, and digoxin. The family cannot tell you much about his medical history.

What do you know about this patient, based on his presentation and medications?

Issues: Recognizing a Respiratory Emergency, Timely and Correct Treatment, Determining Medical History Based on Medications.

27 Cardiovascular Emergencies

Competency Areas

Area 4: Assessment and Diagnostics

4.2.a Obtain list of patient's allergies.

4.2.b Obtain list of patient's medications.

4.2.c Obtain chief complaint and/or incident history from patient, family members, and/or bystanders.

4.2.d Obtain information regarding patient's past medical history.

4.2.f Obtain information regarding incident through accurate and complete scene assessment.

4.3.a Conduct primary patient assessment and interpret findings.

4.3.b Conduct secondary patient assessment and interpret findings.

4.3.c Conduct cardiovascular system assessment and interpret findings.

4.3.n Conduct multisystem assessment and interpret findings.

4.4.a Assess pulse.

4.4.b Assess respiration.

4.4.d Measure blood pressure by auscultation.

4.4.e Measure blood pressure by palpation.

4.4.g Assess skin condition.

4.4.h Assess pupils.

4.4.i Assess level of mentation.

4.5.d Conduct peripheral venipuncture.

4.5.l Conduct 3-lead electrocardiogram (ECG) and interpret findings.

4.5.m Obtain 12-lead electrocardiogram and interpret findings.

Area 5: Therapeutics

5.1.g Utilize airway devices not requiring visualization of vocal cords and introduced endotracheally.

5.1.h Utilize airway devices requiring visualization of vocal cords and introduced endotracheally.

5.2.a Recognize indications for oxygen administration.

5.3.a Administer oxygen using nasal cannula.

5.3.d Administer oxygen using high concentration mask.

5.3.e Administer oxygen using pocket mask.

5.4.a Provide oxygenation and ventilation using bag-valve-mask.

5.5.a Conduct cardiopulmonary resuscitation (CPR).

5.5.c Maintain peripheral intravenous (IV) access devices and infusions of crystalloid solutions without additives.

5.5.d Conduct peripheral intravenous cannulation.

5.5.i Conduct automated external defibrillation.

5.5.j Conduct manual defibrillation.

5.5.k Conduct cardioversion.

5.5.l Conduct transcutaneous pacing.

5.8.a Recognize principles of pharmacology as applied to the medications listed in Appendix 5.

5.8.b Follow safe process for responsible medication administration.

5.8.e Administer medication via intravenous route.

5.8.h Administer medication via sublingual route.

Area 6: Integration

6.1.a Provide care to patient experiencing illness or injury primarily involving cardiovascular system.

6.3.a Conduct ongoing assessments based on patient presentation and interpret findings.

6.3.b Re-direct priorities based on assessment findings.

Appendix 4: Pathophysiology

A. **Cardiovascular System**
Vascular Disease: Aneurysm
Vascular Disease: Arteriosclerosis
Vascular Disease: Deep vein thrombosis
Vascular Disease: Hypertension
Vascular Disease: Peripheral vascular disease
Acute Coronary Syndromes: Infarction
Acute Coronary Syndromes: Ischemia/angina
Heart Failure: Left-sided
Heart Failure: Pericardial tamponade
Heart Failure: Right-sided
Cardiac Conduction Disorder: Benign arrhythmias
Cardiac Conduction Disorder: Lethal arrhythmias
Cardiac Conduction Disorder: Life-threatening arrhythmias

C. **Respiratory System**
Medical Illness: Acute respiratory failure
Medical Illness: Pulmonary edema
Medical Illness: Reactive airways disease/asthma

J. **Multisystem Diseases and Injuries**
Shock Syndromes: Cardiogenic
Shock Syndromes: Hypovolemic

Appendix 5: Medications

A. **Medications affecting the central nervous system.**

A.8 Opioid Analgesics

B. **Medications affecting the autonomic nervous system.**

B.1 Adrenergic Agonists

B.2 Adrenergic Antagonists

B.3 Cholinergic Agonists

B.4 Cholinergic Antagonists

B.5 Antihistamines

D. **Medications affecting the cardiovascular system.**

D.1 Antihypertensive Agents

D.2 Cardiac Glycosides

D.3 **Diuretics**

D.4 Class 1 Antidysrhythmics

D.5 Class 2 Antidysrhythmics

D.6 Class 3 Antidysrhythmics

D.7 Class 4 Antidysrhythmics

D.8 Antianginal Agents

E. **Medications affecting blood clotting mechanisms.**

E.1 Anticoagulants

E.2 Thrombolytics

E.3 Platelet Inhibitors

Introduction

Cardiovascular disease (CVD) has been the number one killer in Canada almost every year since 1900. It was for the purpose of providing early, definitive treatment for patients with acute myocardial infarction (AMI) that the job of paramedic first came into being more than 30 years ago. Even with paramedic availability, more than 72,000 Canadians die every year of coronary heart disease; approximately half die in an emergency department (ED) or before reaching a hospital, during the first minutes and hours after the onset of symptoms. It is easy to see why the recognition and management of cardiovascular emergencies continue to receive strong emphasis in paramedic education.

This chapter is intended to prepare you to integrate pathophysiologic principles and assessment findings to formulate an initial impression and implement the treatment plan for patients with CVD. We begin by looking at the epidemiology of CVD in terms of its prevalence, mortality and morbidity, risk factors, and prevention strategies. After reviewing the anatomy and function of the cardiovascular system, we examine some of the clinical manifestations of CVD. Considerable emphasis is given to the interpretation of cardiac arrhythmias and their management within the context of the patient's overall clinical condition. Finally, we examine the pharmacologic and other treatment modalities that make up advanced cardiac life support (ACLS).

Epidemiology

According to the Heart and Stroke Foundation of Canada, CVD was the cause of about 32% of all deaths in Canada. Every 7 minutes someone in Canada dies from heart disease or stroke. Canadian acute care hospitals handled almost 3 million hospitalizations in 2004. However, there is good news: between 1994–1995 and 2003–2004, the rate of hospitalizations for ischemic heart disease has declined 25% and for acute heart attack the rate has declined 9%. However, the leading cause of hospitalization in Canada continues to be circulatory diseases (heart disease and stroke), accounting for 15.4% of all hospitalizations. Heart disease and stroke cost the Canadian economy more than $18 billion every year in physician services, hospital costs, lost wages, and decreased productivity. The many risk factors for coronary artery disease (CAD) include age, family history, hypertension, elevated cholesterol level, smoking, and carbohydrate intolerance. It was previously thought that CAD was a man's disease, but we now realize that more women die of a cardiac event than men. Other factors contributing to CAD include diet, obesity, oral contraceptive use, sedentary lifestyle, stress, and personality type.

A healthy lifestyle may be all a person with a low risk needs to ward off CAD. High-risk people may be treated by using a combination of drug and nondrug therapies. This aggressive approach can reduce the risk of heart attack by 50%. Patients classified as being at intermediate risk may benefit from further testing for signs of atherosclerosis, which is an indicator of heart disease.

Education and early recognition are also important prevention strategies. Making people aware of the risk factors and signs and symptoms of CVD may decrease its prevalence. This is an area of interest for paramedics who are involved in community heath promotion. **Table 27-1 ▾** lists goals for decreasing CVD risks.

Table 27-1	Goals for Decreasing CVD Risks

- Quit smoking
- Lower and control blood pressure
- Lower total cholesterol level
- Lower LDL cholesterol level
- Increase HDL cholesterol level
- Lower weight, if overweight
- Increase aerobic exercise

LDL indicates low-density lipoprotein; and HDL, high-density lipoprotein.

You are the Paramedic Part 1

You and your partner are enjoying the rare treat of a quiet Sunday shift. You are watching television, and your partner is studying for final examinations. You are about to drift off when the pager disrupts the tranquility. You are dispatched to the medical school library for an unknown medical emergency. On arrival, you and your partner are led to the third floor stacks where you find a 22-year-old man complaining of palpitations.

Initial Assessment	Recording Time: 0 Minutes
Appearance	Young, well-nourished man; appears anxious and nervous
Level of consciousness	A (Alert to person, place, and day)
Airway	Open
Breathing	Normal rate, adequate volume
Circulation	Strong and rapid radial pulses with pink, warm, diaphoretic skin

1. What are some potential causes of palpitations?
2. What questions would you like to ask your patient at this time?

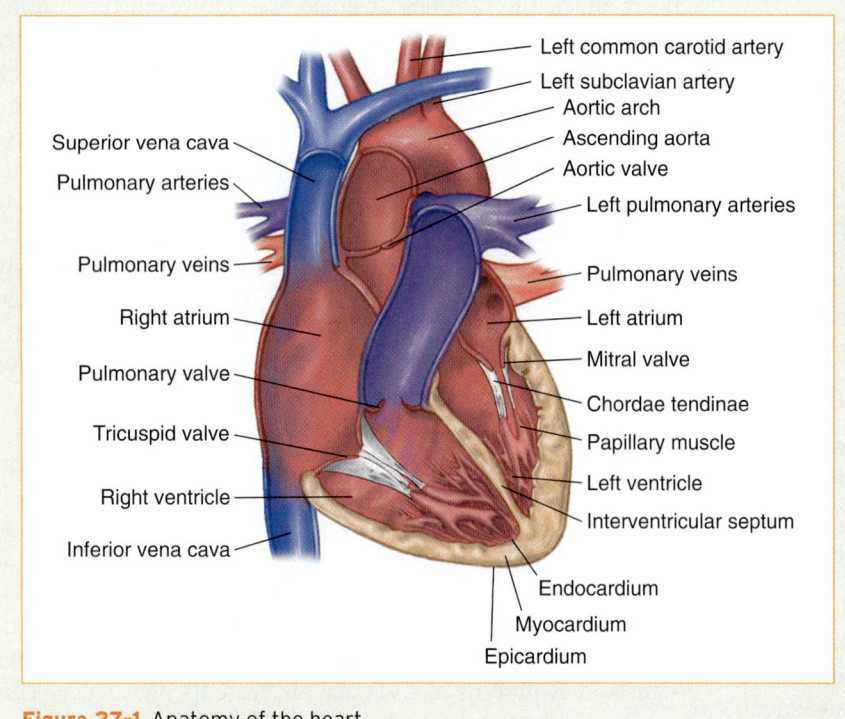

Left common carotid artery
Left subclavian artery
Aortic arch
Ascending aorta
Aortic valve
Left pulmonary arteries

Superior vena cava
Pulmonary arteries

Pulmonary veins
Right atrium
Pulmonary valve
Tricuspid valve
Right ventricle
Inferior vena cava

Pulmonary veins
Left atrium
Mitral valve
Chordae tendinae
Papillary muscle
Left ventricle
Interventricular septum
Endocardium
Myocardium
Epicardium

Figure 27-1 Anatomy of the heart.

Cardiovascular Anatomy and Physiology

Structure and Function

The cardiovascular system is composed of the heart and blood vessels. Its primary function is to deliver oxygenated blood and nutrients to every cell in the body. It is also responsible for delivering chemical messages (hormones) within the body and for transporting the waste products of metabolism from the cells to sites of recycling or waste disposal.

The Heart

The driving force behind this extensive pickup and delivery service is the heart **Figure 27-1 ▲**, a remarkable little pump that sits in the chest, above the diaphragm, behind and slightly to the left of the lower sternum (retrosternal). The heart is not much larger than a man's fist and weighs only 250 to 300 g. Despite its relatively small size, it is big and strong enough to move 7,000 to 9,000 l of blood around the body every day of our lives!

On visualisation of the chest, one may be able to see the apical thrust or point of maximal impulse (PMI). The PMI is normally located on the left anterior part of chest, in the midclavicular line, at the fifth intercostal space. This thrust occurs when the heart's

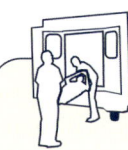

At the Scene

Three components are required to have adequate tissue perfusion: pump (heart), container (vessels) and fluid (blood).

apex rotates forward with systole, gently beating against the chest wall and producing a pulsation.

Surrounding the heart is a tough, fibrous sac called the pericardium. The pericardium normally contains about 30 ml of serous fluid, which serves as a lubricant—that is, it enables the heart muscle, as it contracts and relaxes, to slide easily within the pericardial sac. The pericardium does not stretch readily, so it cannot accommodate sudden accumulations of fluid.

The wall of the heart consists of three layers:

- The epicardium, the outermost surface layer, is a thin serous membrane.
- The endocardium is the innermost smooth layer of connective tissue.
- The myocardium is the muscular layer of the cardiac wall found between the epicardium and endocardium.

Endocarditis is a rare but potentially serious infection of the internal linings and valves of the heart. People who have predisposing cardiac diseases may acquire this disorder. Myocarditis is a less severe infection of the myocardial tissues that may present with or without symptoms. Most people recover completely.

Like all cells in the body, myocardial cells require an uninterrupted supply of oxygen and nutrients. Indeed, the cardiac demand for oxygen is particularly unremitting because the heart never stops to rest (not without catastrophic consequences), so it is essential that the heart have an absolutely reliable blood supply. Oxygenated blood reaches the heart through the coronary arteries **Figure 27-2 ▶**, which branch off the aorta at the coronary ostia, just above the leaflets of the aortic valve. There are two main coronary arteries—left and right. The left main coronary artery subdivides into the left anterior descending and circumflex coronary arteries, both of which branch widely to supply the more muscular left ventricle of the heart along with the interventricular septum and part of the right ventricle. The right coronary artery (RCA) supplies the right atrium and ventricle and part of the left ventricle. The numerous connections (anastomoses) between the arterioles of the various coronary arteries allow for the development of alternative routes of blood flow (collateral circulation) in case of blockage. Unfortunately, the coronary arteries are also vulnerable to narrowing in atherosclerotic heart disease. When the lumen (channel) of one of those arteries becomes so narrowed that blood flow through it is impeded, the symptoms of angina occur.

The arteries and the main coronary vein cross the heart in a groove, called the coronary sulcus, that separates the atria from the ventricles. Venous blood empties into the coronary sinus, a large vessel in the posterior part of the coronary sulcus, which in turn ends in the right atrium of the heart.

Structurally, the heart consists of four chambers (see Figure 27-2). The upper chambers of the heart, or atria, are separated from their respective lower chambers, or ventricles, by atrioventricular (AV) valves, which prevent backflow during ventricular contraction. The tricuspid valve separates the right atrium

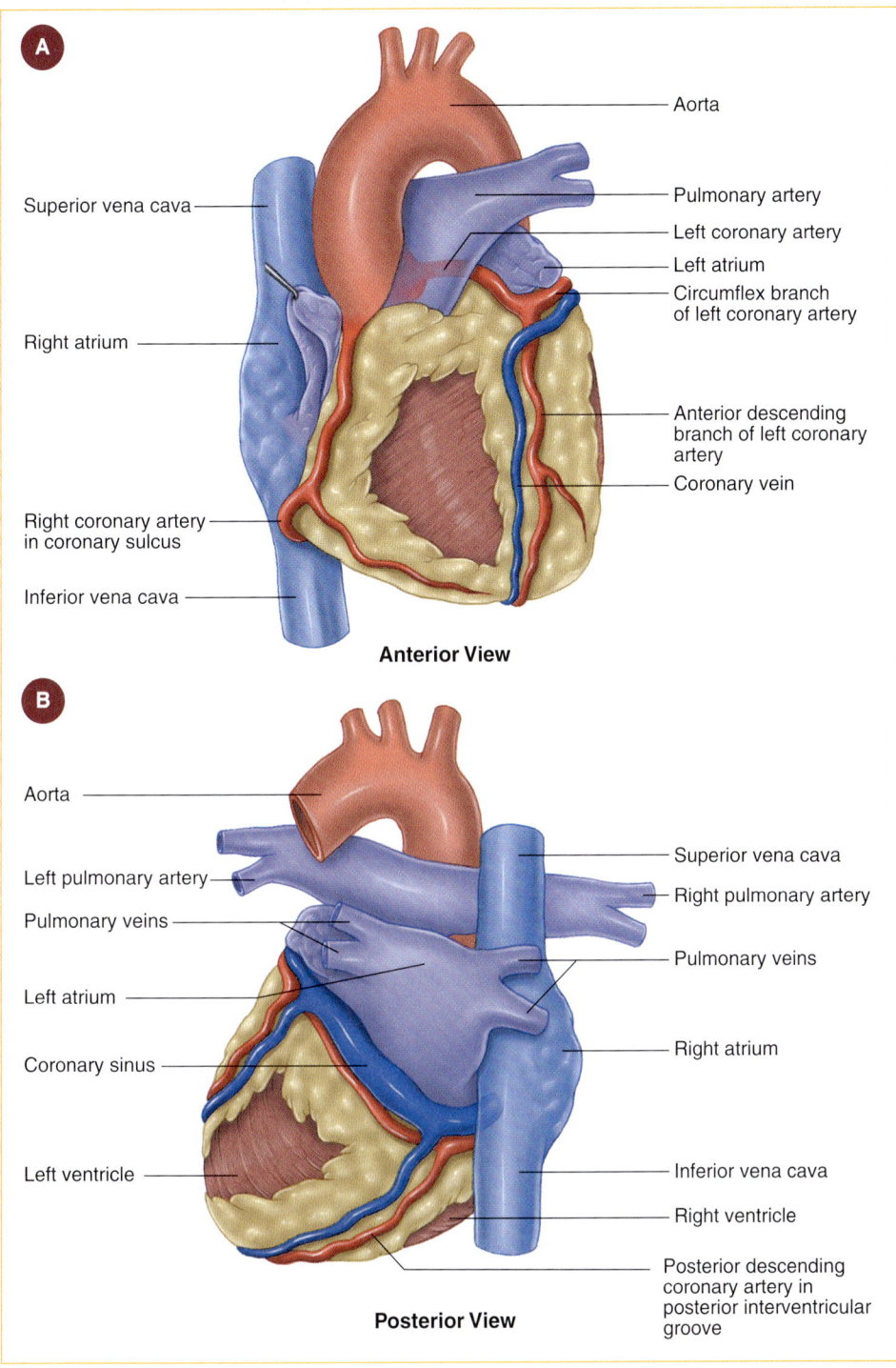

Figure 27-2 Coronary arteries. **A.** Anterior view, showing takeoff point of left and right main coronary arteries from the aorta. **B.** View from below and behind, showing the coronary sinus.

from the right ventricle; the mitral valve separates the left atrium from the left ventricle. Anatomical guide wires, called chordae tendineae, attached to papillary muscles within the heart anchor those two valves and keep them from inverting (prolapsing) during ventricular contraction. Injury or disease, however, may disrupt the chordae tendineae and permit a valve leaflet to prolapse, allowing blood to regurgitate from the ventricle into the atrium.

Two other valves in the heart **Figure 27-3 ▸**, which are collectively known as semilunar valves because of their half-moon shape, are found at the junction of the ventricles and the pulmonary and systemic circulation. The pulmonic valve separates the right ventricle from the pulmonary artery, preventing backflow from the artery into the right ventricle. The aortic valve serves the same function for the left ventricle, preventing blood that has already entered the aorta from flowing back into the left ventricle.

Heart Sounds

The purpose of listening to heart sounds is to identify the "lub-dub" that indicates the cardiac valves are operating properly. The major heart sounds are the two normal sounds, S_1 and S_2 **Figure 27-4 ▸**, and the two abnormal sounds, S_3 and S_4 **Figure 27-5 ▸**.

S_1 occurs near the beginning of ventricular contraction (systole), when the tricuspid and mitral valves close. The closing of these two valves should occur simultaneously as the pressure within the ventricles increases. Any delay in the closing of these two valves, heard as a split sound, is considered abnormal.

S_2 occurs near the end of ventricular contraction (systole), when the pulmonary and aortic valves close. As the ventricles relax, these valves close because of backward flow in the pulmonary artery and aorta. The two valves can close simultaneously or with a slight delay between them under normal physiologic circumstances.

S_3 is the result of the end of the rapid filling period of the ventricle during the beginning of diastole. An S_3 sound should occur 120 to 170 milliseconds (ms) after S_2, if it is heard at all.

At the Scene

The mitral valve is on the left side of the heart. The left side has higher pressure than the right. Because the mitral valve is involved in the higher pressure side, remember it as the "mighty" valve.

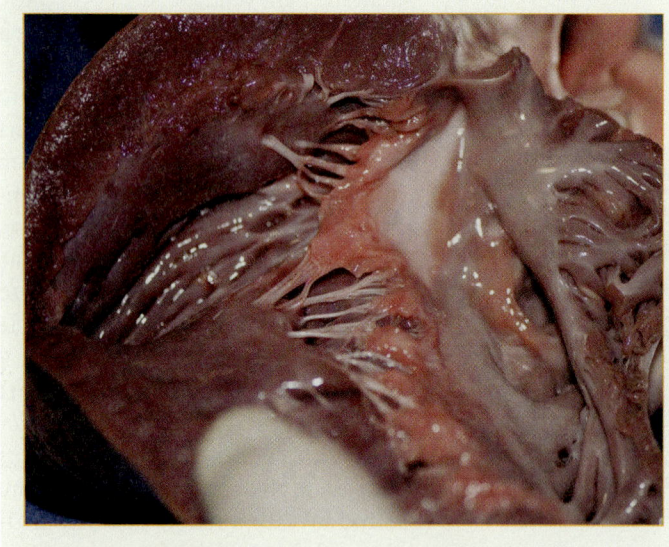

Figure 27-3 Heart valves.

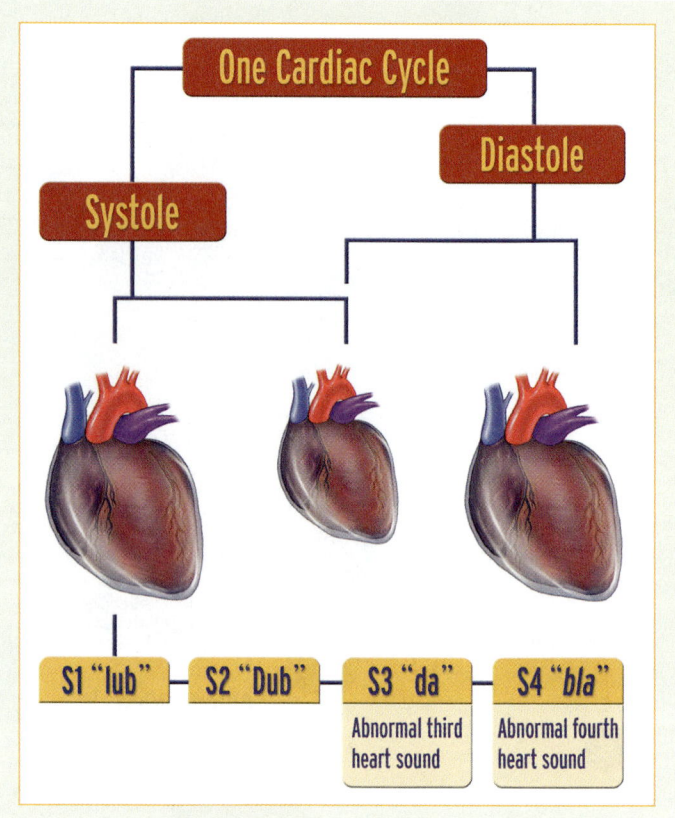

S1 "lub" — S2 "Dub" — S3 "da" — S4 "bla"

S3 "da" Abnormal third heart sound

S4 "bla" Abnormal fourth heart sound

Figure 27-5 The abnormal S₃ and S₄ heart sounds.

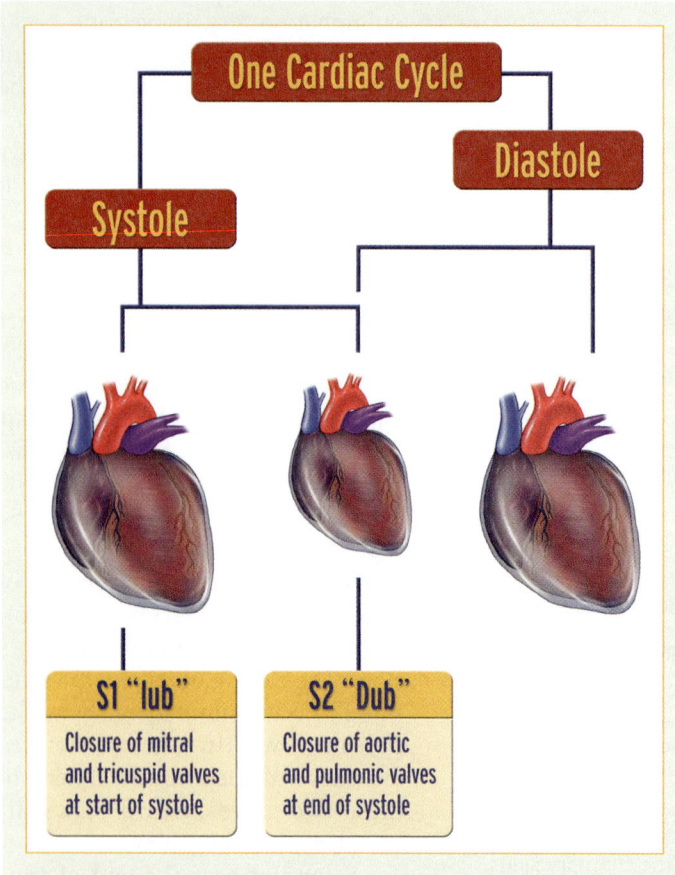

S1 "lub"

Closure of mitral and tricuspid valves at start of systole

S2 "Dub"

Closure of aortic and pulmonic valves at end of systole

Figure 27-4 The normal S₁ and S₂ heart sounds.

S_3 is generally heard in children and young adults. When it is heard in older adults, it often signifies heart failure.

S_4, if heard, coincides with atrial contraction at the end of ventricular diastole. If heard at any other time, it usually occurs in patients who have resistance to ventricular filling, as seen in patients with a thickened left ventricular muscle wall due to hypertension or those with active, ongoing cardiac ischemia.

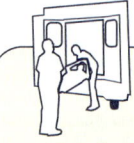 **At the Scene**

Atrial kick describes approximately 20% of blood flow that comes from the atria to the ventricles by contraction. The other 80% gets from the atria to the ventricles passively via gravity.

The Cardiac Cycle

The cardiac cycle comprises one complete phase of atrial and ventricular relaxation (diastole), followed by one atrial and ventricular contraction (systole).

During the relatively longer relaxation phase (normally 0.52 second [s]), the left atrium fills passively with blood, under the influence of venous pressure. Approximately 80% of ventricular filling also occurs during this time as blood flows through the open tricuspid and mitral valves.

With atrial contraction (normally both atria contract at the same time), the contents of each atrium are squeezed into the respective ventricle to complete ventricular filling. The contribution to ventricular filling made by contraction of the atrium is referred to as atrial kick—it is the amount of blood "kicked in" by the atrium. At the beginning of ventricular contraction, the AV valves snap shut, the two ventricles contract (ventricular systole), and the semilunar valves are forced open. Blood squeezed out of the right ventricle moves forward, through the pulmonic valve, and into the pulmonary arteries. Blood from the left ventricle is pushed through the aortic valve and out

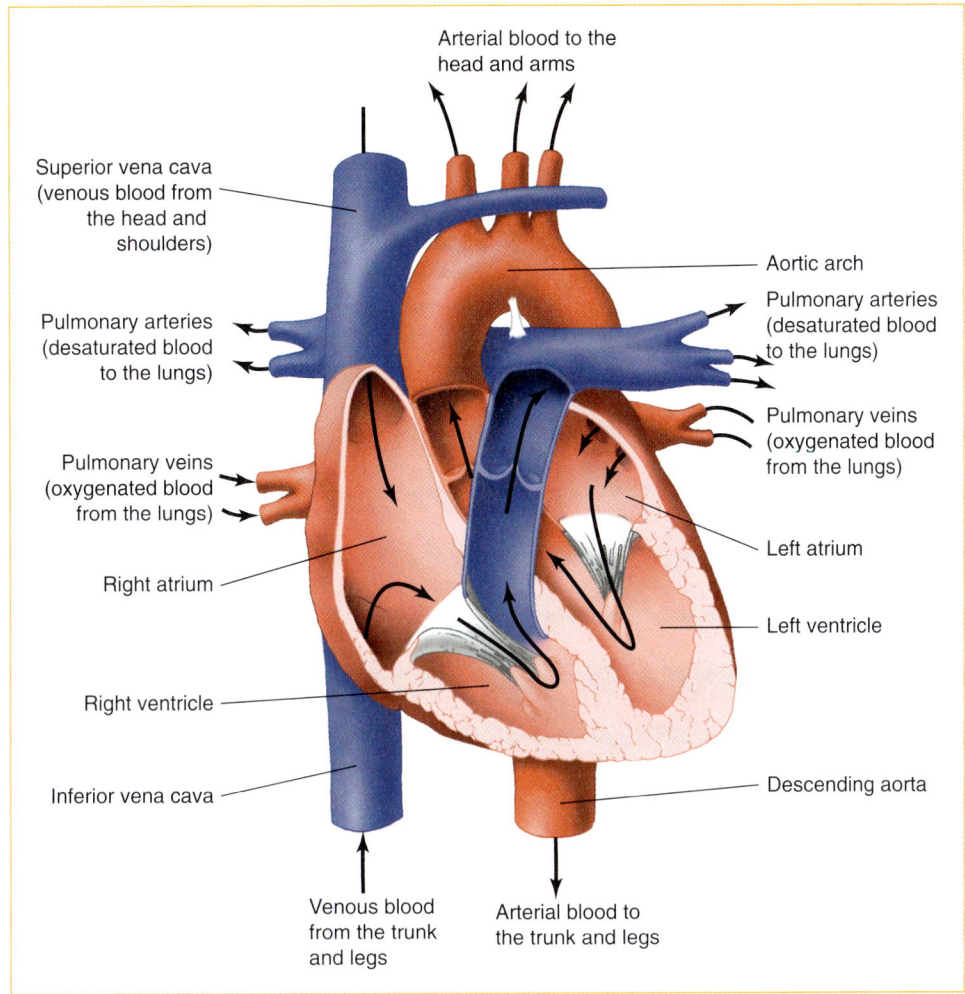

Arterial blood to the head and arms

Superior vena cava (venous blood from the head and shoulders)

Aortic arch

Pulmonary arteries (desaturated blood to the lungs)

Pulmonary arteries (desaturated blood to the lungs)

Pulmonary veins (oxygenated blood from the lungs)

Pulmonary veins (oxygenated blood from the lungs)

Right atrium

Left atrium

Left ventricle

Right ventricle

Inferior vena cava

Descending aorta

Venous blood from the trunk and legs

Arterial blood to the trunk and legs

Figure 27-6 Blood flow through the heart. Desaturated blood enters the right atrium from the venae cavae, proceeds to the right ventricle, and from there moves via the pulmonary arteries to the lungs. Oxygenated blood enters the left atrium from the pulmonary veins, proceeds to the left ventricle, and then goes out to the body via the aorta.

into the aorta. Systole is usually accomplished in a little more than half the time it takes to fill the ventricles, about 0.28 s.

Two Pumps in One

Although we called the heart a pump, that description is not entirely accurate. Functionally, the heart is actually *two* pumps—a right pump and a left pump, separated by a thin wall (the interventricular septum)—that just happen, for purposes of efficiency, to be housed in one organ and to work in parallel **Figure 27-6 ▲**.

The right side of the heart, which is composed of the right atrium and right ventricle, is a *low-pressure* pump: It pumps against the relatively low resistance of the pulmonary circulation. The right atrium collects oxygen-poor venous blood from the venae cavae and the coronary sinus and pumps it into the right ventricle, which pumps the blood into the pulmonary artery for distribution to the alveoli and oxygenation in preparation for delivery to the left side of the heart.

The pulmonary veins collect the now oxygen-rich blood and return it to the left side of the heart—specifically, to the left

atrium, which pumps it into the powerful left ventricle. The left side of the heart is a *high-pressure* pump: It drives blood out of the heart against the relatively high resistance of the systemic arteries.

Because there are two pumps, there must be two sets of tubing into which the pumps empty. Thus, the human body, in effect, has two circulations. The systemic circulation **Figure 27-7A ▶** consists of all blood vessels beyond the left ventricle up to the right atrium, which receive the output of the left side of the heart. The pulmonary circulation **Figure 27-7B ▶** comprises the blood vessels between the right ventricle and left atrium, which receive the output of the right side of the heart.

At any given time, a major proportion of the body's blood flow may be shunted into one of these two circulations. If, for example, the right side of the pump fails and cannot squeeze out its contents efficiently, blood will back up behind the right atrium into the systemic veins, which then become engorged and distended. The most readily visible of the systemic veins are the external jugular veins, which reflect the condition of all the other systemic veins. Distension of the external jugular veins signals that there is considerable back pressure from the right side of the heart throughout the systemic circulation. As pressure increases within the systemic veins, fluid starts to leak into the surrounding tissues, causing the tissues to swell. When enough fluid has leaked into the interstitial spaces, that swelling becomes visible as edema in the subcutaneous tissues; it is less readily visible, but equally present, in the liver, walls of the intestine, and other internal tissues.

By contrast, if the left side of the pump fails, blood backs up behind the left atrium into the pulmonary circulation. As pressure builds up in the pulmonary veins, fluid is squeezed into the alveoli, producing the characteristic signs and symptoms of pulmonary edema: dyspnea, bubbling crackles, and frothy sputum. Although the heart has two distinct pumping circuits, left and right, the heart functions as a single organ with a single conduction system. In other words, what affects one side of the heart will affect the other side.

The Blood Vessels

Besides the "cardio" component (the heart), the cardiovascular system includes a second, "vascular" component—that is, the blood vessels. There are two principal types of blood vessels in

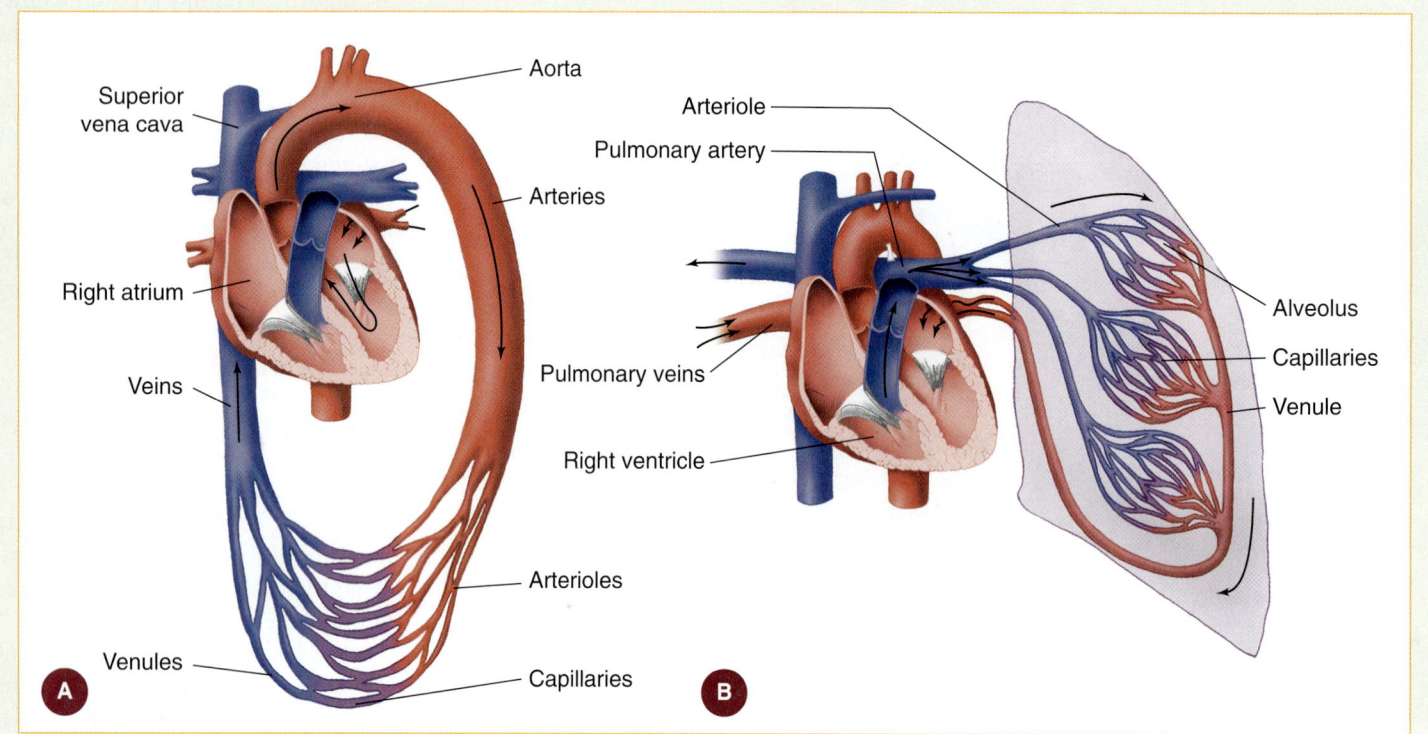

Figure 27-7 Dual human circulation. **A.** The systemic circulation consists of all blood vessels distal to the left ventricle. **B.** The pulmonary circulation consists of all blood vessels between the right ventricle and the left atrium.

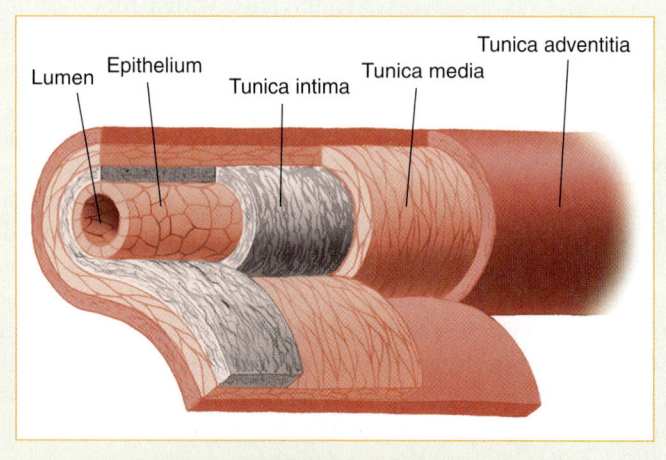

Figure 27-8 Structure of a blood vessel.

the human body—arteries and veins—both of which share a common structure (**Figure 27-8 ▲**). A protective outer layer of fibrous tissue, the tunica adventitia, provides blood vessels with the strength needed to withstand high pressure against their walls. A middle layer of elastic fibres and muscle, the tunica media, gives strength and contractility to blood vessels. This medial layer is much thicker and more powerful in arteries than in veins. The innermost layer of the blood vessel, the tunica intima, is a smooth inner lining that is only one cell thick. The opening within the blood vessel is referred to as the lumen.

Arteries are thick-walled, muscular vessels—befitting pipes operating in a high-pressure system—that carry blood away

from the heart. Usually, arteries carry *oxygenated* blood; the only exceptions are the pulmonary arteries, which carry oxygen-depleted blood from the right ventricle to the lungs (they carry blood away from the heart). Arteries range in size from the largest artery in the body, the aorta, to the tiniest arterial branch, or arteriole. (**Figure 27-9 ▸**) depicts the major arteries in the body.

Arterial walls are highly sensitive to stimulation from the autonomic nervous system. Indeed, in response to that stimulation, their diameter may change significantly as the arteries contract and relax. In that manner, the arteries help to regulate blood pressure—that is, the pressure exerted by the blood against the arterial walls. Blood pressure is generated by repeated forceful contractions of the left ventricle, which keep blood flowing through the body. The magnitude of the blood pressure is influenced not only by the output of the heart and the volume of blood present in the system, but also by the relative constriction or dilation of arteries.

Veins, which operate on the low-pressure side of the system, have thinner walls than arteries and, consequently, less capacity to decrease their diameter. The thinner walls also make the veins much more likely to distend when exposed to small increases in "backpressure." Veins carry blood to the heart—as a rule, oxygen-poor blood. The only exceptions are the pulmonary veins, which carry oxygenated blood to the left side of the heart. The smallest veins, or venules, gradually empty into larger and larger veins, terminating in the two largest veins of the body, the inferior and superior venae cavae. Veins also

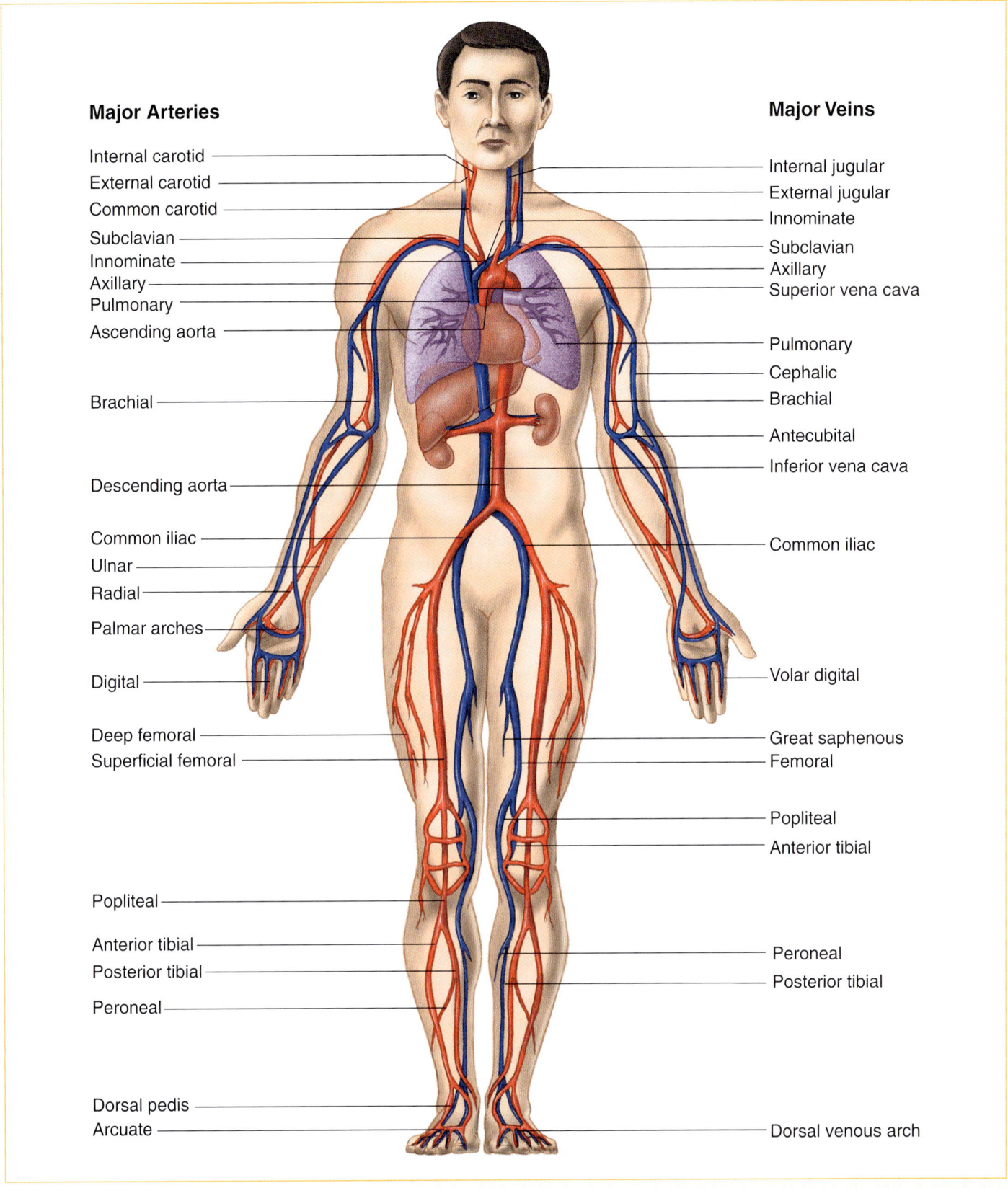

Major Arteries

Internal carotid
External carotid
Common carotid
Subclavian
Innominate
Axillary
Pulmonary
Ascending aorta

Brachial

Descending aorta

Common iliac
Ulnar
Radial

Palmar arches

Digital

Deep femoral
Superficial femoral

Popliteal

Anterior tibial
Posterior tibial

Peroneal

Dorsal pedis
Arcuate

Major Veins

Internal jugular
External jugular
Innominate
Subclavian
Axillary
Superior vena cava

Pulmonary
Cephalic
Brachial

Antecubital
Inferior vena cava

Common iliac

Volar digital

Great saphenous
Femoral

Popliteal
Anterior tibial

Peroneal
Posterior tibial

Dorsal venous arch

Figure 27-9 The major arteries and veins.

contain valves (which are unnecessary in arteries); these valves keep the blood flowing in the forward direction only.

Between the tiny arterioles and venules at the tissue level is a network of microscopic blood vessels called capillaries. The walls of capillaries are extremely thin—only one cell thick—enabling the exchange of gases and nutrients across them; the capillary diameter is so small that red blood cells must pass through them single file.

The Pump at Work

To understand how the heart functions as a pump, it is necessary to learn some technical terms:

- **Cardiac output (CO).** The amount of blood that is pumped out by either ventricle. The left and right ventricles are approximately equal in interior size, so the two ventricles have relatively equivalent outputs. Normal CO for an average adult is 5 to 6 l/min.
- **Stroke volume (SV).** The amount of blood pumped out by either ventricle in a single contraction (heartbeat). Normally, the SV is 60 to 100 ml, but the healthy heart has considerable spare capacity and can easily increase SV by at least 50%.
- **Heart rate (HR).** The number of cardiac contractions (heartbeats) per minute—in other words, the pulse rate. The normal HR for adults is 60 to 100 beats/min.

$$CO = SV \times HR$$

The volume of blood that either ventricle pumps out per minute equals the volume of blood it pumps out in a single contraction times the number of contractions per minute:

To meet changing demands, the heart must be able to increase its output several times over in response to the body's increased demand for oxygen—for example, during exercise. The CO equation tells us that the heart can increase its output by increasing its SV, increasing its rate, or both.

In a mechanical piston pump, the SV is a fixed quantity related to the distance travelled by the piston and the size of the cylinder. The heart, by contrast, has several ways of increasing SV. One characteristic of cardiac muscle is that, when it is stretched, it contracts with greater force to a limit—a property called the Frank-Starling mechanism. If an increased volume of blood is returned from the systemic veins to the right side of the heart or from the pulmonary veins to the left side of the heart, the muscle surrounding the cardiac chambers must stretch to accommodate the larger volume. The more the cardiac muscle stretches, the greater the force of its contraction, the more completely it empties, and, therefore, the greater the SV. From the CO equation, it is clear that any increase in SV, with the HR held constant, will cause an increase in the overall CO. However, this relationship between volume, stretch, and CO continues only until the heart becomes overfilled and the muscle fibres become overstretched. At this point, further volume does not result in increased CO.

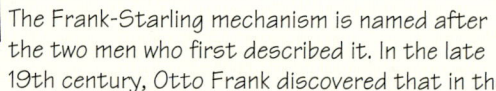

At the Scene

The Frank-Starling mechanism is named after the two men who first described it. In the late 19th century, Otto Frank discovered that in the frog heart, the strength of ventricular contraction was increased when the ventricle was stretched before contraction. In the 20th century, Ernest Starling expounded on this information with studies finding that increasing venous return, and, therefore, the filling pressure of the ventricle, led to increased stroke volume in dogs.

The pressure under which a ventricle fills is called the preload and is influenced by the volume of blood returned by the veins to the heart. In situations of increased oxygen demand, the body returns more blood to the heart (preload increases), and CO consequently increases through the Frank-Starling mechanism. In a diseased heart, the same mechanism is used to achieve a normal resting CO (which explains why some diseased hearts become enlarged).

The heart can also vary the degree of contraction of its muscle *without* changing the stretch on the muscle—a property called contractility. Changes in contractility may be induced by medications that have a positive or negative inotropic effect. The ventricles are never completely emptied of blood with any single beat. However, if the heart squeezes into a tighter ball when it contracts, a larger percentage of the ventricular blood will be ejected, thereby increasing SV and overall CO. Nervous controls regulate the contractility of the heart from beat to beat. When the body requires increased CO, nervous signals increase myocardial contractility, thereby augmenting SV.

The heart can also increase its CO, given a constant SV, by increasing the number of contractions per minute—that is, by increasing the HR (positive chronotropic effect). As an example, consider a heart that has a resting SV of 70 ml/beat and a resting rate of 70 beats/min:

$$CO = 70 \text{ ml} \times 70 \text{ beats/min} = 4{,}900 \text{ ml}$$

Suppose that the owner of that heart begins to exercise. Oxygen demand increases, and nervous mechanisms stimulate the heart to increase its rate. If, for example, the HR increases to 110 beats/min without any change in the SV, the CO would increase as follows:

$$CO = 70 \text{ ml/beat} \times 110 \text{ beats/min} = 7{,}700 \text{ ml/min}$$

The Frank-Starling mechanism is an intrinsic property of heart muscle—that is, it is not under nervous system control. By contrast, contractility and changes in HR are regulated by the nervous system.

The Electrical Conduction System of the Heart

Heart muscle is unique among body tissues because it can generate its own electric impulses without stimulation from nerves, a property known as automaticity. In addition, the heart is endowed with specialized conduction tissue that can rapidly propagate electrical impulses to the muscular tissue of the heart. The area of conduction tissue in which the electrical activity arises at any given time is called the pacemaker, because it sets the pace (that is, rate) for cardiac contraction. This system as a whole is termed the electrical conduction system.

The Dominant Pacemaker: The Sinoatrial Node

Theoretically, any cell within the heart's electrical conduction system can act as a pacemaker. In the normal heart, however, the dominant pacemaker is the sinoatrial (SA) node, which is located in the right atrium, near the inlet of the superior vena cava **Figure 27-10 ◄**. The SA node normally receives blood from the RCA. If the RCA is occluded, as in a myocardial infarction (MI), the SA node will become ischemic. The subsequent death of the conduction cells will prevent the SA node from firing.

The SA node is the fastest pacemaker in the heart. Electric impulses generated in this node spread across the two atria through internodal pathways (including the Bachman bundle) in the atrial wall in about 0.08 s, causing the atrial tissue to depolarize as they pass. The blood supply to the SA node comes from a branch of the right coronary artery. From there, they move to the atrioventricular (AV) node in the region of the AV junction (which includes the AV node and its surrounding tissue along with the bundle of His). The AV node serves as a "gatekeeper" to the ventricles. In 85% to 90% of humans, its blood supply comes from a branch of the RCA; in 10% to 15%, it comes from a branch of the left circumflex artery. The conduction of the impulse is delayed in the AV node for about 0.12 s so that the atria can empty into the ventricles. Approximately 70% to 90% of the blood in the atria fills the ventricles by gravity; the remaining 10% to 30% comes from atrial contraction (atrial kick).

When the atrial rate becomes very rapid, not all atrial impulses can get through the AV junction. Normally, however, impulses pass through it into the bundle of His and then move rapidly into the right and left bundle branches located on either side of the interventricular septum. Next, they spread into the Purkinje fibres, thousands of fibrils distributed through the ventricular muscle. It takes about 0.08 s for an electric impulse to spread across the ventricles, during which time the ventricles contract simultaneously. The effect on the velocity of conduction is referred to as the dromotropic effect.

Depolarization and Repolarization

Depolarization—the process by which muscle fibres are stimulated to contract—comes about through changes in the concentration of electrolytes across cell membranes **Figure 27-11A ►**. Myocardial cells, like all cells in the body,

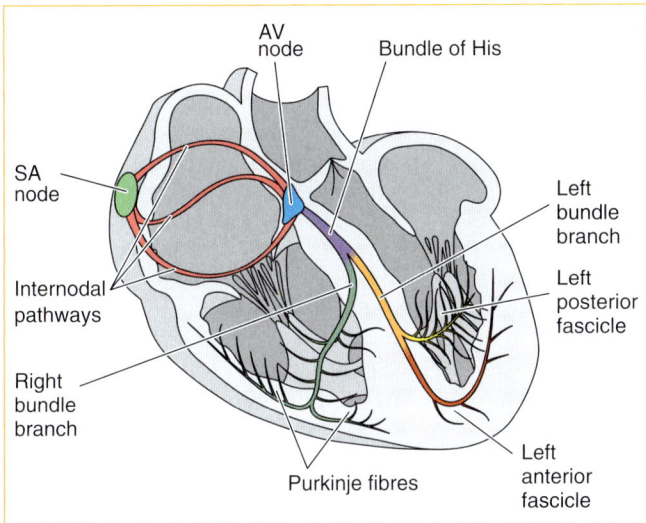

Figure 27-10 Electrical conduction system of the heart. Impulses that originate in the SA node spread through the atria and along the internodal pathways to the AV node. From the AV node, they travel down the bundle of His and right and left bundle branches and into the Purkinje network of the ventricles.

You are the Paramedic Part 2

You ask your partner to obtain an initial set of vital signs while you begin your patient assessment. When asked about the palpitations, the patient tells you that they began about 45 minutes ago while he was studying for finals. He is a first-year medical student and needs to do well on finals to avoid being placed on academic probation. He admits to being awake for the past 36 hours with the help of "Monster" energy drinks and caffeine pills. His last oral intake was pizza last night around 23:00 hours. He denies any medical history or allergies and emphatically denies the use of any drugs other than the caffeine pills.

Vital Signs	Recording Time: 5 Minutes
Skin	Pink, warm, and diaphoretic
Pulse	210 beats/min, regular; strong radial pulses
Blood pressure	104/62 mm Hg
Respirations	20 breaths/min, nonlaboured
Spo_2	95% on room air

3. What are some of your concerns based on this information?
4. Which interventions should you consider at this point?

are bathed in an electrolyte solution. Chemical pumps inside the cell maintain the concentrations of ions within the cell, in the process creating an electric gradient across the cell wall. As a consequence, a resting (polarized) cell normally has a net charge of −90 millivolts (mV) with respect to the outside of the cell (Figure 27-11, part A1). When the myocardial cell receives a stimulus from the conduction system (Figure 27-11, part A2), the permeability of the cell wall changes through opening of specialized channels in such a way that sodium ions (Na^+) rush into the cell, causing the inside of the cell to become more positive. Calcium ions (Ca^{++}) also enter the cell—albeit more slowly and through a different set of specialized channels—helping maintain the depolarized state of the cell membrane and supplying calcium ions for use in contraction of the cardiac muscle tissue. This reversal of electric charge—depolarization—starts at one spot in the cell and spreads in a wave along the cell until the cell is completely depolarized (Figure 27-11, part A3). As the cell depolarizes and calcium ions enter, mechanical contraction occurs.

If the cell were to remain depolarized, it could never contract again! Fortunately, the cell is able to recover from depolarization through a process called repolarization **Figure 27-11B ▾**. Repolarization starts with the closing of the sodium and calcium channels, which stops the rapid inflow of these ions. Next, special potassium channels open, allowing a rapid escape of potassium ions (K^+) from the cell. This helps restore the inside of the cell to its negative charge; the proper electrolyte distribution is then reestablished by pumping sodium ions out of the cell and potassium ions back in. After the potassium channels close, this sodium-potassium pump helps move sodium and potassium ions back to their respective locations. For every three sodium ions this pump moves out of the cell, it moves two potassium ions into the cell, thereby maintaining the polarity of the cell membrane. To accomplish this task, the sodium-potassium pump moves ions against the natural gradient by a process called active transport, which requires the expenditure of energy.

Table 27-2 ▾ summarizes the roles of the various electrolytes in cardiac function.

A myocardial cell cannot respond to an electric stimulus from the conduction system normally unless it is fully polarized.

Table 27-2	**Role of Electrolytes in Cardiac Function**
Electrolyte	**Role in Cardiac Function**
Sodium (Na^+)	Flows into the cell to initiate depolarization
Potassium (K^+)	Flows out of the cell to initiate repolarization *Hypokalemia* → increased myocardial irritability *Hyperkalemia* → decreased automaticity/conduction
Calcium (Ca^{++})	Has a major role in the depolarization of pacemaker cells (maintains depolarization) and in myocardial contractility (involved in contraction of heart muscle tissue) *Hypocalcemia* → decreased contractility and increased myocardial irritability *Hypercalcemia* → increased contractility
Magnesium (Mg^{++})	Stabilizes the cell membrane; acts in concert with potassium, and opposes the actions of calcium *Hypomagnesemia* → myocardial irritability, ventricular arrhythmias *Hypermagnesemia* → myocardial irritability, heart block, and possible asystole

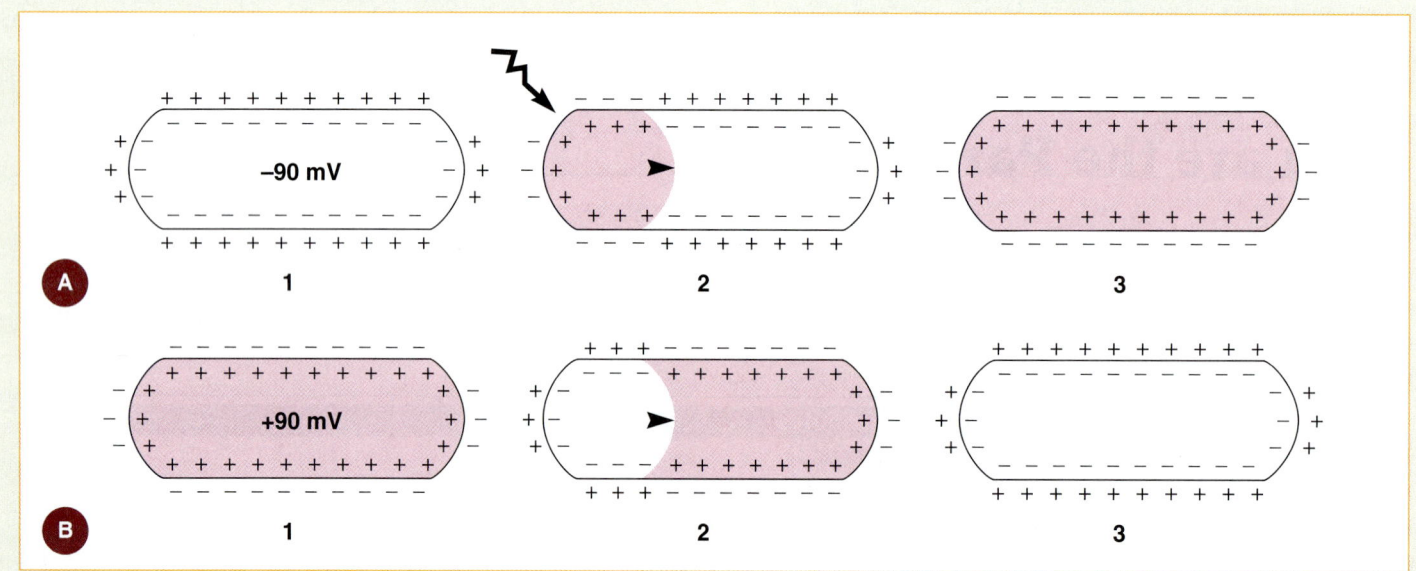

Figure 27-11 Movement of ions to produce a net current flow. **A.** Depolarization. (1) At rest, the cellular interior has a net charge of −90 mV. (2) The wave of depolarization begins as sodium ions pour into the cell. (3) Depolarized cell. **B.** Repolarization. (1) Depolarized cell. (2) The wave of repolarization begins as potassium ions leave the cell. (3) Repolarized cell.

The period when the cell is depolarized or in the process of repolarizing—the so-called refractory period—consists of two phases. In the absolute refractory period, the heart muscle has been drained of energy and needs to recharge; it will not contract during this period. In the relative refractory period, the heart is partially charged, albeit not strongly enough to create a full contraction.

Secondary Pacemakers

The SA node normally has the most rapid intrinsic rate of firing (60 to 100 times/min), so it will literally outpace any slower conduction tissue. If it becomes damaged or is suppressed, any component of the conduction system may act as a secondary pacemaker. The farther removed the conduction tissue is from the SA node, the slower its intrinsic rate of firing. Thus, the AV junction will spontaneously fire 40 to 60 times/min, whereas the ventricular Purkinje system, which is farther removed from the SA node, will spontaneously fire only 20 to 40 times/min.

Suppose that the SA node is damaged by ischemia (tissue injury caused by hypoxemia) and does not fire. When it fails to receive impulses from the SA node, the AV junction might then begin firing at its own rate; thus, an electrocardiogram (ECG) would show a "junctional rhythm" at a rate of 40 to 60 beats/min. If both nodes fail to initiate an impulse, the Purkinje fibres will initiate an impulse, resulting in a "ventricular rhythm" at a rate of 20 to 40 beats/min Table 27-3 ▾ .

Measuring the Heart's Electrical Conduction Activity

The electrical conduction events in the heart can be recorded on an ECG as a series of waves and complexes Figure 27-12 ▸ . The depolarization of the atria produces the P wave. It is followed by a brief pause as conduction is momentarily slowed through the AV junction. Next, the QRS complex occurs, representing depolarization of the ventricles. Repolarization of the atria and ventricles produces T waves; however, the atrial repolarization wave is small and is buried within the QRS complex, so it isn't seen Table 27-4 ▸ . The larger, ventricular T wave follows the QRS complex.

The intervals between waves and complexes also have names. The P-R interval is the distance from the beginning of the P wave to the beginning of the QRS complex. It represents the time required for an impulse to traverse the atria and AV junction and is normally 0.12 to 0.20 s (three to five little squares on standard ECG paper). The ST segment is the line from the end of the QRS complex to the beginning of the T wave (the beginning of which is referred to as the J-point). The ST segment should

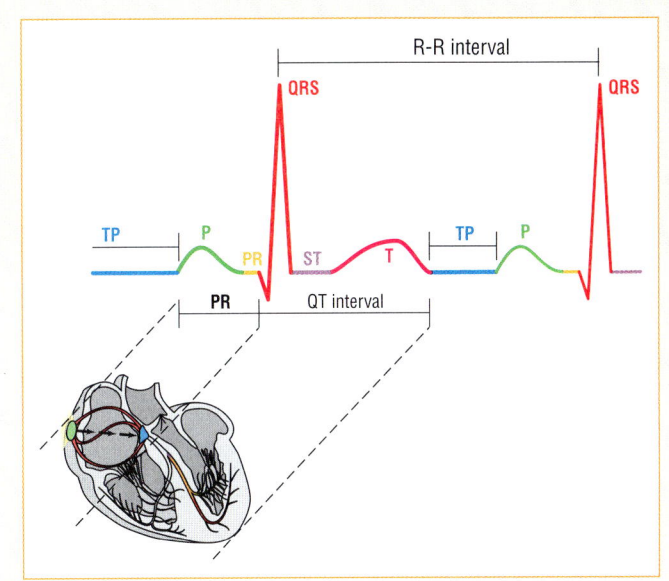

Figure 27-12 The ECG and cardiac events.

Table 27-4	Components of the ECG
ECG Representation	**Cardiac Event**
P wave	Depolarization of the atria
P-R interval	Depolarization of the atria and delay at the AV junction
QRS complex	Depolarization of the ventricles
ST segment	Period between ventricular depolarization and beginning of repolarization
T wave	Repolarization of the ventricles
R-R interval	Time between two ventricular depolarizations

normally be at the same level as the baseline (isoelectric line). An elevated or depressed ST segment may indicate myocardial ischemia or injury. The R-R interval is the time between two successive QRS complexes. It represents the interval between two ventricular depolarizations and gives an indication of the HR.

The Autonomic Nervous System and the Heart

The autonomic nervous system is the part of the human nervous system that controls automatic (that is, involuntary) actions. Its importance can be gauged by considering the alternative: Suppose all body functions were solely under voluntary control. Sixty times a minute, 24 hours a day, you would have to remind your heart to beat. Twelve times a minute, 24 hours a day, you would be required to order your lungs to inflate and relax. You would have to warn your stomach that food was on the way, tell your pancreas and gallbladder to step up their activities, and urge your gut to speed up or slow down as necessary. Whenever you changed your level of activity—for example, during exercise—you would be forced to issue a

Table 27-3	Pacemaker Rates
Pacemaker	**Rate (beats/min)**
SA node	60 to 100
AV junction	40 to 60
Purkinje fibres	20 to 40

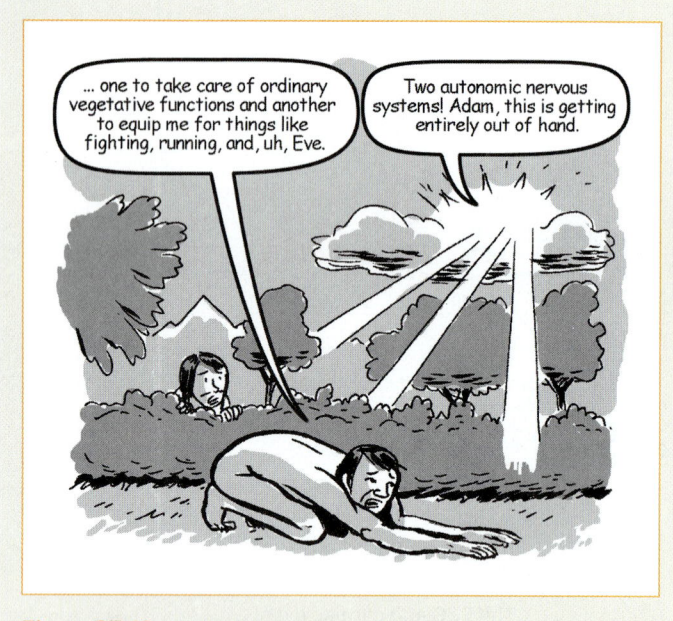

Figure 27-13

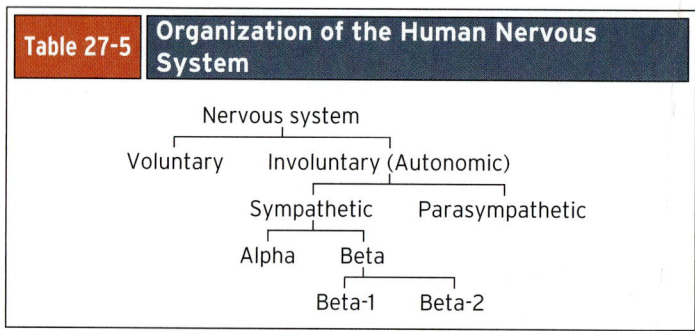

| Table 27-5 | Organization of the Human Nervous System |

Nervous system

Voluntary   Involuntary (Autonomic)

Sympathetic   Parasympathetic

Alpha   Beta

Beta-1   Beta-2

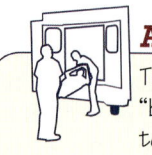

At the Scene

The parasympathetic nervous system is your "brake pedal," and the sympathetic nervous system is your "gas pedal."

complex series of orders to your cardiovascular system to ensure that CO increased sufficiently to meet increased metabolic demands.

Fortunately, this administrative work is accomplished for us, without conscious effort on our part. It happened more or less like this:

In the beginning, when God was working out the circuitry for humans, Adam persuaded Him to include an autonomic nervous system **Figure 27-13 ▲** . "Look," said Adam, "I don't want to spend all my time thinking about my CO and ventilation and digestion. I want to think great philosophic thoughts and maybe have a little fun on the side."

"I'll see what I can do," said God.

After some debate, they worked out a compromise. "I tell you what I'll do for you, Adam. I'll give you *two* nervous systems. One will be fully automatic—an autonomic nervous system—so that your body functions can proceed without your having to bother yourself about them. The other will be voluntary, so that you can consciously control the movement of your muscles."

That seemed reasonable, and Adam agreed. So it came to pass that humans have two nervous systems.

One day God noticed that Adam was looking sad.

"What's the matter, Adam?" asked God.

"It's my autonomic nervous system," said Adam. "It's not quite right yet."

"What do you mean, it's not quite right? I designed it according to our agreement, didn't I?"

"I know. But I've noticed that my life is divided into two kinds of activity. I do a lot of rather vegetative things, like sleeping and digesting my food, during which my heart needs to slow down. But I also do really exciting things—especially since Eve arrived—during which my heart needs to speed up. What I really need are two autonomic nervous systems—one

to take care of ordinary vegetative functions and another to equip me for things like fighting, running, and, uh, Eve."

"*Two* autonomic nervous systems! Adam, this is getting entirely out of hand."

"This is supposed to be Eden, isn't it? And everything's supposed to be perfect, isn't it? If You were really concerned about my welfare, You'd give me two autonomic nervous systems like it says in the medical textbooks."

"All right, all right," said God. "I'll see what I can do."

The next day, God said to Adam, "I've got everything fixed up. From now on, you'll have a voluntary nervous system and *two* autonomic nervous systems. One of them will be called the parasympathetic nervous system, and it will regulate your vegetative functions: It will slow your HR, help you digest your food, and all that stuff. The other will be called the sympathetic nervous system: It will speed up your heart, constrict your blood vessels, dilate your bronchi and pupils, and so forth."

"Why do they have to have such funny names?" asked Adam.

"Because I said so," said God, "and I'm still Boss around here, in case you've forgotten."

Thus, the human nervous system consists of a voluntary and an involuntary system. The latter, also called the autonomic nervous system, is further divided into the sympathetic and parasympathetic systems, as shown in **Table 27-5 ▲** . **Table 27-6 ▶** provides a review of the properties of the autonomic nervous system.

The Parasympathetic Nervous System

The parasympathetic nervous system is concerned primarily with vegetative functions and sends its messages mainly through the vagus nerve. Think of it as the "rest and digest" nervous system. The vagus can be stimulated in a number of ways, including pressure on the carotid sinus, straining against a closed glottis (Valsalva maneuver), and distension of a hollow organ (such as the bladder or stomach).

Suppose that the brain decided the heart should slow a little; perhaps someone applied pressure over the carotid or

Table 27-6	Autonomic Nervous System	
Features	**Parasympathetic**	**Sympathetic**
Other name	Cholinergic; "rest and digest"	Adrenergic; "fight or flight"
Natural chemical mediator	Acetylcholine	Norepinephrine, epinephrine
Primary nerve(s)	Vagus	Nerves from the thoracic and lumbar ganglia of the spinal cord
Effect of stimulation	Decreases contractility (negative inotropic effect) Slows conduction velocity (negative dromotropic effect) Slows the heart* (negative chronotropic effect) Constricts pupils Increases salivation Increases gut motility	Increases contractility (positive inotropic effect) Speeds conduction velocity (positive dromotropic effect) Speeds the heart (positive chronotropic effect) Dilates pupils Constricts blood vessels Slows the gut Dilates the bronchi
Stimulating drugs	Neostigmine, reserpine	Alpha: phenylephrine Beta: isoproterenol Beta-2: salbutamol Alpha + beta: norepinephrine, epinephrine, dopamine, dobutamine
Blocking drugs	Atropine	Alpha: chlorpromazine, phentolamine Beta: propranolol, metoprolol, labetalol, atenolol, esmolol

* Slowing occurs mostly in the atria.

strained during a bowel movement. A message in the form of an electric impulse would go barreling down the vagus nerve to the place where this nerve abuts on the SA node of the heart. There, the electric impulse would cause the release of a naturally occurring chemical, acetylcholine (ACh). (The parasympathetic nervous system derives its other name, the *cholinergic* nervous system, from this chemical.) The ACh would cross over to the SA node of the heart and say, "Listen, SA node, the brain says you ought to slow down; I just heard it from the vagus." Just to be on the safe side, another ACh molecule would wander down to talk to the AV node of the heart: "We've just instructed the SA node to slow down; just in case, it didn't get the message, we want you to make sure that no extra impulses get through to the ventricles, understand?"

"Sure thing," says the AV node, which is more sensitive to criticism from the vagus nerve. "They shall not pass."

"Okay," says the ACh, as it is escorted away by cholinesterase. (Cholinesterase is an enzyme that cleaves, or breaks apart, ACh, rendering it unable to continue its action on the receptors.)

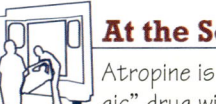

At the Scene

Atropine is also referred to as an "anticholinergic" drug with "vagolytic" properties.

"No kidding?"

"No kidding."

So the SA node speeds up. Meanwhile, the atropine reaches the AV node. "How are you doing, AV?" asks the atropine.

"Oh, it's kind of slow lately. The vagus ordered me to close down two lanes southbound."

"The vagus again. Listen, AV node, if you keep paying attention to the vagus, before you know it, that nerve will close down the entire highway to the ventricles, and they'll go off merrily on their own."

"Gee whiz," says the AV node. "What should I do?"

"Take my advice, bud, and open the gates wide. Let all the impulses through."

"Are you sure that's a good idea? The vagus said . . ."

"Forget about the vagus. He's just an old obstructionist."

"Okay," says the AV node, always eager to please when atropine is around. And he opens all southbound lanes.

The Sympathetic Nervous System

The sympathetic nervous system prepares the body to respond to various stresses; it is the fight-or-flight system mentioned earlier. The parasympathetic nervous system works well for routine activities such as keeping the heart beating during rest or coordinating digestion, but it provides no mechanism for the body to adapt to changing demands. By contrast, the sympathetic nervous system increases the HR, strengthens the force of cardiac muscle contractions, and provides other adaptive responses to ensure that the tissues' increased oxygen demands are satisfied with increased CO.

The only drug with which we shall be concerned that interacts directly with the parasympathetic nervous system is atropine. Atropine is a parasympathetic blocker; that is, it opposes the action of ACh on the heart and elsewhere, thereby allowing the body's natural sympathetic system to increase the HR.

Suppose the heart is plodding along at a rate of 50 beats/min, and you administer 0.5 mg of atropine intravenously. The atropine will travel through the bloodstream until it reaches the SA node.

"You're firing a little slowly today, aren't you?" says atropine.

"Just following orders," says the SA node. "The vagus told me to take it easy."

"The vagus, the vagus—that's all I ever hear. Why do you want to listen to that old stick-in-the-mud? Listen, stick with me, and I'll add a little excitement to your life."

Suppose you start running to catch a bus. After a few seconds, your muscles will have used up all the oxygen and nutrients immediately on hand. "It's getting awfully stuffy down here," says one muscle to another.

"You said it!"

"I wish the heart would increase the delivery of oxygen."

So the muscles send a message to the brain: "HELP! We can't breathe!"

In response to their pleas, the brain sends a message through sympathetic nerves, passing through the thoracic and lumbar ganglia, ultimately arriving at the heart. Whereas the vagus nerve releases ACh, sympathetic nerves convey their commands through release of norepinephrine. Norepinephrine travels to the SA node, AV node, and ventricles, spreading the command from the sympathetic nerves: "Let's speed this operation up," says norepinephrine. "The muscles are suffocating and threatening to bomb the circulation with lactic acid if they don't get more oxygen." So the heart speeds up, increasing CO and, therefore, delivering more oxygen and nutrients throughout the body.

When intense stimulation of the sympathetic nervous system occurs, a special hormone—epinephrine—may be mobilized to spread the alarm and command the heart to speed up. Epinephrine is produced in the adrenal gland and is also called adrenaline, leading to the other name of the sympathetic system—the *adrenergic* system.

Drugs That Act on the Sympathetic Nervous System

Drugs that influence the sympathetic nervous system are classified according to the receptors with which they interact. A drug receptor can be visualised as analogous to the ignition switch in a car. When the proper key is inserted into the car's ignition and turned, a predictable sequence of events follows: The battery sends a current to the starter and the spark plugs, which fire; combustion of gasoline and air occurs; and the engine starts. Although many keys may fit into a specific car's ignition, not every key that fits will turn and start the car—but all that do turn cause the same reaction. Likewise, the organs of the body have a number of "ignition switches." In the sympathetic nervous system, those switches, or receptors, are labeled alpha and beta. Whenever one of those switches is activated by a "key" (a drug or hormone), a predictable sequence of responses will occur **Table 27-7 ▸**.

The heart has one primary ignition switch for a beta agent. Any beta agent will have the same effect on the heart—that is, it will increase the heart's rate, force, and automaticity. The arteries, by contrast, have receptors for alpha and beta agents. An alpha drug will turn on the switch that

causes vasoconstriction; a beta agent will activate the switch that causes vasodilation. Similarly, the lungs have alpha and beta receptors. Alpha agents don't have much effect on the lungs; at most, they cause minor bronchoconstriction. By contrast, beta agents (such as drugs used to treat asthma) trigger significant bronchodilation. **Figure 27-14 ▾** represents these concepts schematically.

Drugs that have alpha or beta sympathetic properties are called sympathomimetic drugs because they imitate (mimic) the actions of naturally occurring sympathetic chemicals. If we know whether a sympathomimetic drug is an alpha or beta agent, we can predict the response by the heart, lungs, and arteries.

Consider isoproterenol (Isuprel). It is a pure beta agent. Armed with this knowledge, we can immediately recognize that isoproterenol acts in the manner shown in **Figure 27-15 ▸**—it stimulates the heart, dilates the bronchi, and dilates the arteries.

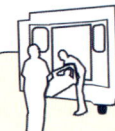

At the Scene

To remember the difference between beta-1 and beta-2, ask yourself, "How many hearts do I have?" One heart—beta-1. "How many lungs do I have?" Two lungs—beta-2.

Table 27-7	Responses to Sympathetic Stimulation
Organ	**Sympathetic Stimulation**
Heart	Increased HR (positive chronotropic effect) (beta-1) Increased force of contraction (positive inotropic effect) (beta-1) Increased conduction velocity (positive dromotropic effect) (beta-1)
Arteries	Constriction (alpha); dilation (beta-2)
Lungs	Bronchial muscle relaxation (beta-2)

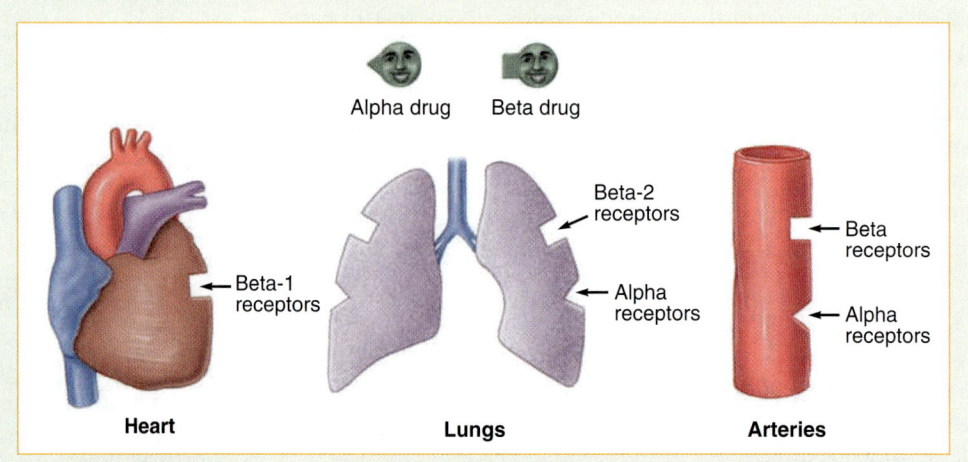

Figure 27-14 Receptor sites of the sympathetic nervous system in the heart, lungs, and arteries.

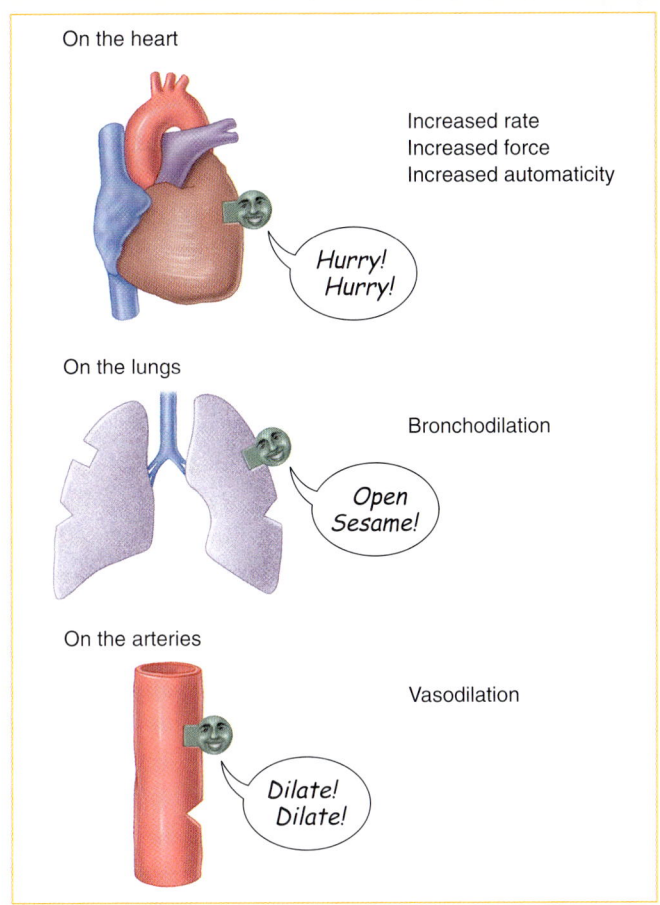

Figure 27-15 Beta sympathetic agents increase the rate, force, and automaticity of the heart; dilate the bronchi; and dilate peripheral arteries.

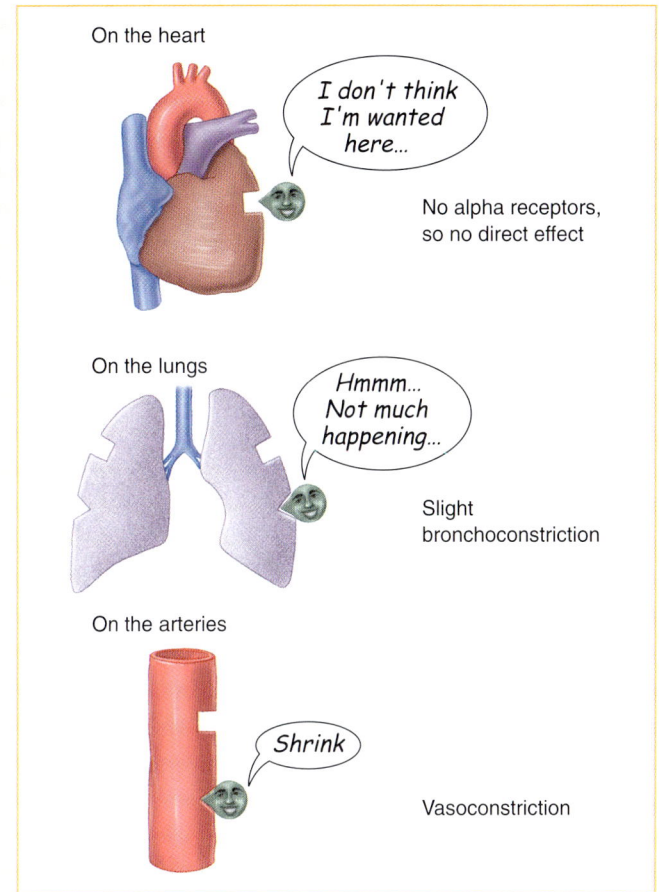

Figure 27-16 Alpha agents have no direct effect on the heart; they cause slight bronchoconstriction and marked vasoconstriction.

Phenylephrine (Neo-Synephrine), by contrast, is a pure alpha agent. It has no direct effect on the heart but causes slight bronchoconstriction and marked vasoconstriction **Figure 27-16 ▶**.

In reality, things are not always so simple. Although isoproterenol and phenylephrine are pure beta and alpha agents, respectively, most other sympathomimetic drugs have varying degrees of alpha and beta activity **Figure 27-17 ▶**. Norepinephrine (Levophed) is chiefly an alpha agent, and its alpha effects predominate; because it also has some beta activity, however, it will have effects on the heart. Conversely, epinephrine (Adrenalin) is chiefly a beta agent, and its beta effects predominate; nevertheless, when administered in high doses, epinephrine will produce some alpha effects, especially on the arteries.

Table 27-8 ▶ lists several sympathomimetic agents that are commonly encountered in the prehospital environment. Two of the drugs, norepinephrine and epinephrine, are also naturally occurring chemicals of the sympathetic nervous system. Their actions are the same whether they are produced in the body and released from the nervous system or manufactured in a factory and injected.

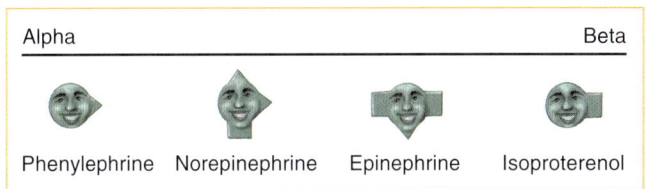

Figure 27-17 Many sympathomimetic agents have alpha and beta properties.

Beta sympathetic agents can be classified into two groups based on the subtle differences between the beta receptors in the heart and the lungs. Drugs that act primarily on cardiac beta receptors are called beta-1; those that act chiefly on pulmonary beta receptors are called beta-2. Some newer bronchodilators—such as salbutamol, isoetharine, and terbutaline—are selective beta-2 agents, so they provide effective bronchodilation with far fewer cardiac side effects.

Another class of drugs that acts on the sympathetic nervous system comprises the sympatholytic or sympathetic blockers. As their name implies, they block the action of sympathetic

Table 27-8	Common Sympathomimetic Agents
Alpha	**Phenylephrine (Neo-Synephrine)**
Alpha ↓ Beta	Norepinephrine bitartrate (Levophed) Dopamine Epinephrine, dobutamine
Beta	Salbutamol (Proventil; beta-2-specific) Isoproterenol (Isuprel; pure beta-specific)

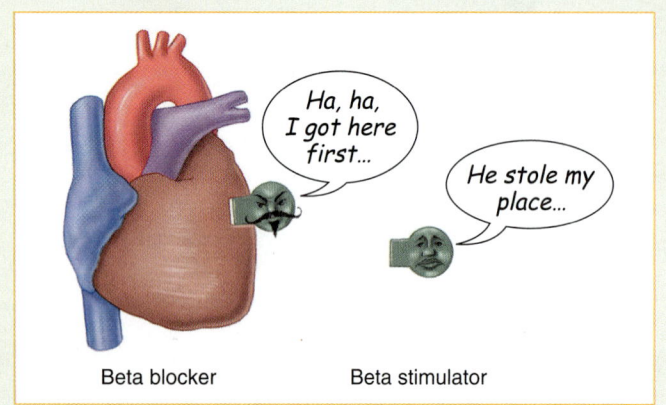

Ha, ha, I got here first...

He stole my place...

Beta blocker   Beta stimulator

Figure 27-18 A sympathetic blocker occupies the receptor site for the stimulating drug, thereby preventing the stimulating drug from exerting its usual effect.

agents by beating them to the receptor sites and preventing these agents from turning on the ignition. The receptor sites, which aren't very smart, cannot distinguish a blocker from a stimulator until it is too late. With the blocker occupying the receptor site, the stimulating agent cannot get in to turn on the switch Figure 27-18 ▲ .

Beta blockers occupy beta receptors in the heart, lungs, and arteries, as well as elsewhere in the body Figure 27-19 ▶ . Thus beta agents, whether released from sympathetic nerve endings or given intravenously, cannot exert their full effects when a beta blocker such as metoprolol has been administered previously Figure 27-20 ▶ .

Beta blocker

Figure 27-19 A beta blocker is a sympathetic blocking agent.

The indications for the major autonomic stimulating and blocking agents can be deduced once we know the properties of the drugs and the manner in which they interact with the autonomic nervous system:

- **Atropine.** Parasympathetic blocker, opposing the vagus nerve. It is used to speed the heart when excessive vagal firing has caused bradycardia.
- **Norepinephrine.** Sympathetic agent (primarily alpha), causing vasoconstriction. It is used to increase the blood pressure when hypotension is caused by vasodilation (as in neurogenic shock).
- **Isoproterenol.** Sympathetic agent (almost pure beta), causing a strong increase in HR and dilation of bronchi. It is used in extreme cases to increase CO and to dilate bronchi in asthma.
- **Epinephrine.** Sympathetic agent (predominantly beta), with actions similar to those of isoproterenol, but having an additional, primarily peripheral vasoconstrictor effect. Indications for epinephrine are similar to those for isoproterenol, but also include asystole, pulseless electrical activity (PEA), and ventricular fibrillation (to increase the

You are the Paramedic Part 3

Your partner has applied the cardiac monitor and is giving oxygen at 4 l/min via nasal cannula. The cardiac monitor displays a narrow complex tachycardia at a rate of 212 beats/min. While looking for a site to insert an intravenous (IV) line, you ask the patient to bear down hard as if he were having a bowel movement. There is no change in his rate and rhythm. You insert an 18-gauge IV cannula in his right forearm and prepare to administer 6 mg of adenosine (Adenocard). You rapidly administer the 6 mg of adenosine, followed by a 20-ml fluid bolus. The monitor showed a transient decrease in the HR to 165 beats/min, which quickly picked back up to a rate of 206 beats/min. Anthony tells you that he experienced "the strangest sensation" in his chest when you gave him the medication and asks what you gave him.

Reassessment	Recording Time: 11 Minutes
Skin	Pink, warm, and diaphoretic
Pulse	206 beats/min, regular; strong distal pulses
ECG	Supraventricular tachycardia
Blood pressure	102/64 mm Hg
Respirations	20 breaths/min, nonlaboured
Spo2	99% on nasal cannula at 4 l/min of oxygen
Pupils	Equal and reactive to light

5. How does adenosine work?

6. What should you tell your patient before you administer adenosine?

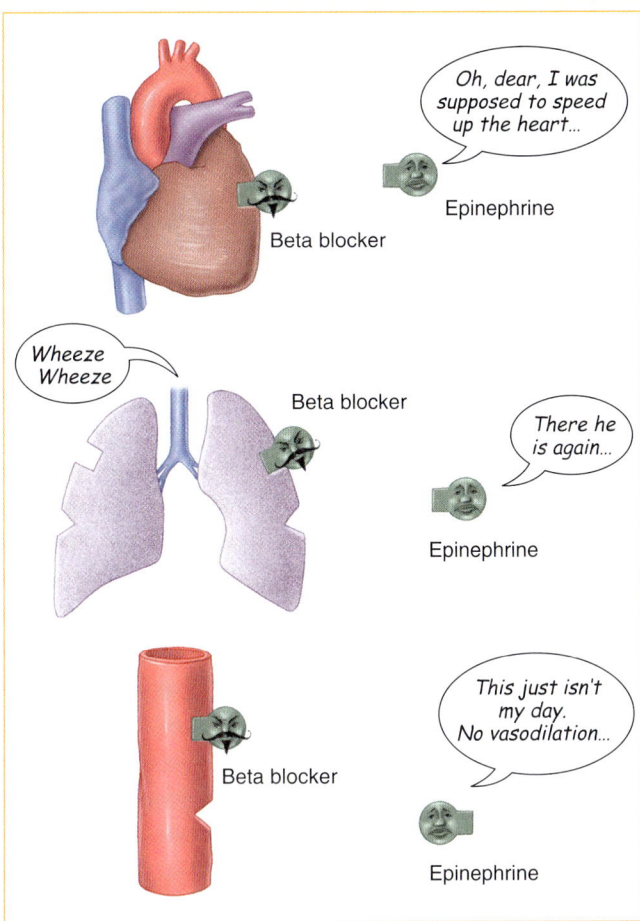

Figure 27-20 By occupying beta receptor sites, the beta blocker prevents epinephrine from exerting its usual effects on the heart, lungs, and blood vessels.

automaticity of the heart and vasoconstriction); and anaphylactic shock (for all of its effects—bronchodilation, vasoconstriction, increased CO).

- **Dopamine.** Sympathetic agent, used at low (beta) doses to increase the force of cardiac contractions in cardiogenic shock. Its dilation (beta) effects on renal and mesenteric arteries mean that dopamine may help maintain urine flow and good perfusion to abdominal organs.
- **Salbutamol.** Sympathetic beta-2 agents that act on the lungs. These agents are used to induce bronchodilation in asthma, chronic obstructive pulmonary disease, and other bronchospastic conditions.

- **Metoprolol.** Sympathetic beta blocker, opposing the actions of beta-stimulating agents. It is used clinically to slow the HR in certain tachyarrhythmias, to decrease the pain of chronic angina (by decreasing the work of the heart), and to depress irritability in the heart (by decreasing the tendency of the heart to fire automatically). Its use is contraindicated in asthma.

The Sympathetic Nervous System and Blood Pressure Regulation

The body attempts to maintain a fairly constant blood pressure to ensure perfusion of vital organs. At any given moment, the blood pressure is influenced by the CO and the resistance (degree of constriction) of the arterioles:

$$Blood\ Pressure = CO \times Peripheral\ Resistance$$

Thus, the blood pressure can be increased by increasing the CO, the peripheral resistance, or both.

Under normal circumstances, the body balances flow and resistance to maintain a stable blood pressure. That is, alterations in one variable bring about compensatory changes in the other variable to restore blood pressure toward normal. Consider, for example, a situation in which CO decreases suddenly, as in hemorrhage. The fall in CO will inevitably lead to a fall in blood pressure unless the peripheral resistance is altered. The falling CO activates the sympathetic nervous system, however, which in turn causes the arterioles to constrict. Vasoconstriction increases the peripheral resistance, thereby tending to restore the blood pressure back toward normal.

The resistance against which the ventricle contracts is termed the afterload. The greater the afterload, the harder the ventricle must work to pump the blood. In conditions of chronically high afterload, such as arteriosclerosis-induced high blood pressure, the left ventricle may eventually grow exhausted from the extra work and cease pumping efficiently or even fail.

Patient Assessment

Patients experience a variety of symptoms when they have a cardiovascular problem. The most common complaints are chest pain, dyspnea, fainting, palpitations, and fatigue. If the patient is pulseless or breathless, basic life support (BLS) measures may be used. In some cases, ALS procedures may be necessary. This section reviews the organized approach to assessing patients by focusing on their cardiac and pulmonary systems. For this assessment, we will assume the patient is conscious and breathing and has a pulse.

Scene Assessment

The initial assessment begins with scene assessment and ensuring scene safety. In addition, you should try to anticipate the need for other resources such as extra personnel.

Initial Assessment

Observe the patient's general appearance as you approach him or her, and assess for apparent life threats. The initial assessment is fairly consistent for all patients, but this discussion has a cardiac focus. Sometimes assessing the ABCs can be accomplished easily by merely greeting the patient and introducing yourself, assuming that the patient can answer you, is conscious, has an open airway, is breathing, and has a pulse. Determine the patient's level of consciousness (LOC) based on his or her response to your greeting, and use the AVPU scale.

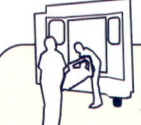

At the Scene

Just by shaking someone's hand and introducing yourself, you can learn a lot about the patient.

Determine the patency of the patient's airway. If the patient is talking to you, the airway is patent. The patient may be able to maintain an open airway or, depending on the LOC, may need help with clearing obstructions (debris, blood, or teeth) by properly positioning the head and/or placing an airway adjunct. Note the rate, quality, and effort of the breathing, and consider initiating oxygen therapy at this time.

Assessment of circulation is done primarily by checking the patient's pulse. For a conscious patient, you will typically check the radial pulse; if the patient is unconscious, check the carotid pulse. While checking the pulse, note the rate, regularity, and overall quality. Is it weak, bounding, or irregular?

While holding the patient's hand in yours, assess the skin colour and condition. The skin is the largest organ of the body, so a good indication that the rest of the body is getting adequate circulation is that the skin and mucous membranes are pink and the skin is warm and dry. Is there edema, poor turgor, or skin "tenting"?

The initial assessment ends with making a transport decision for your patient. Based on your findings to this point, you should be able to determine whether the patient requires immediate transport. If you are unsure, continue with the focused assessment, and the correct decision may become more apparent.

Focused History and Physical Examination

During the focused history and physical examination, you will perform a focused assessment. This inquiry into the patient's medical history and a physical examination are based on the patient's chief complaint; the inquiry is also referred to as the history of present illness. The SAMPLE history is included in this assessment. In patients with acute coronary syndromes (ACS), the most common chief complaints are chest pain, dyspnea, fainting, palpitations, and fatigue.

Symptoms

Chest pain is often the presenting symptom of an AMI. The patient's description of the pain is important for assessing its significance. The OPQRST format can be used to elaborate on the patient's chief complaint:

O What is the *Onset* or origin of the pain—that is, how did it begin (suddenly or gradually)? Has anything like this ever happened before?

P What *Provoked* the pain—that is, what, if anything, brought it on? Is it exertional or nonexertional? What was the patient doing at the time? Sitting in a chair? Changing a tire? Having an argument with the boss? Does anything make it worse? What palliates the pain—that is, does anything make it better? Patients with chronic CAD may take nitroglycerin for episodes of chest pain. Ask whether the patient did so and, if so, whether it helped.

Q What is the *Quality* of the pain—that is, what does it feel like? Get the patient's narrative description. Dull? Sharp? Crushing? Heavy? Squeezing? Note the exact words the patient uses to describe the pain, and observe the patient's body language as he or she does so. Try not to lead the patient's description unless he or she is unable to describe the pain. In such cases, try to give alternatives, such as "Is it sharp or dull?"

R Does the pain *Radiate*? From where to where? To the jaw? Down the left arm? Into the back?

S What is the *Severity* of the pain—that is, how bad is it? Use the pain scale of 1 to 10, with 10 being the worst. If the patient has chronic angina, ask him or her to compare the pain with the usual angina pain.

T What was the *Timing* of the attack—that is, when did it start? How long did it last? What time did it get worse or better? Was it continuous or intermittent?

Another chief complaint among patients with an ACS is dyspnea. In the context of ACS, dyspnea may be the first clue to failure of the left side of the heart. To explore this possibility, ask the following questions:

- When did the dyspnea start? Did it awaken the patient from sleep? Paroxysmal nocturnal dyspnea (PND) is an acute episode of shortness of breath in which the patient suddenly awakens from sleep with a feeling of suffocation. Often the patient will report going to a window to get "more air" or will move from the bed to a recliner. PND is one of the classic signs of left-sided heart failure, although it may also occur in chronic lung diseases.
- Did the dyspnea come on gradually or suddenly?
- Is it continuous or intermittent?
- Does it happen during activity or while at rest?

- Does any position make the dyspnea better or worse? The dyspnea of pulmonary edema usually worsens when the patient is lying down (orthopnea), because blood pools in the lungs when the body is horizontal. Patients with significant orthopnea will often sleep with several pillows, or even sitting in a recliner, to maintain a semi-upright position.
- Has the patient ever had dyspnea like this before? If so, under what circumstances?
- Does the patient have a cough? Is it dry or productive?
- Any fever or travel history to suggest an infectious, noncardiac cause of symptoms?
- Were there any associated symptoms?

Fainting (syncope) occurs when CO suddenly declines, leading to a reduction in cerebral perfusion. Cardiac causes of syncope include arrhythmias, increased vagal tone, and heart lesions. There are also numerous noncardiac causes of syncope (discussed in Chapter 28). As part of taking a history from someone who has fainted, try to sort out whether the patient fainted from cardiac or noncardiac causes:

- Under what circumstances did the syncopal episode occur? What was the patient doing at the time? A 20-year-old who faints at the sight of blood is unlikely to have significant underlying cardiac disease; a 60-year-old who faints after feeling some "fluttering" in the chest may have a dangerous cardiac arrhythmia.
- Were there any warning feelings before the episode, or did the fainting spell occur suddenly and unexpectedly?
- What position was the patient in when he or she fainted? Standing? Sitting? Lying down? Losing consciousness while sitting or lying down has more ominous implications than fainting while standing up.
- Has the patient fainted before? If so, under what circumstances?
- Were there any associated symptoms, such as nausea, vomiting, urinary incontinence, or seizures?

Finally, patients with cardiac problems may present with a chief complaint of palpitations. Palpitations refer to the sensation of an abnormally fast or irregular heartbeat—except after extreme exertion, a person normally remains blissfully unaware of his or her heartbeat. The cause of palpitations is often a cardiac arrhythmia, such as premature ventricular contractions (PVCs) or paroxysmal supraventricular tachycardia (PSVT). The patient may not use the word "palpitations" but may report feeling the heart "skip a beat" or use words to that effect. In such a case, inquire about the onset, frequency, and duration of this symptom and previous episodes of palpitations. Also ask about the presence of associated symptoms (such as chest pain, dizziness, and dyspnea).

Patients may report a variety of other related symptoms as you explore their history of present illness. They may have a "feeling of impending doom" or a sense that they will soon experience a life-changing event. Some patients relate feeling nauseous or having vomited. Listen carefully for indications that trauma may be involved or that their activity has been limited as a result of their condition. Observe their faces as you listen to them tell their stories. Do you see a look of fear or anguish? Are they holding their chest? Most of the other associated complaints your patients may have are related to hypoxia or poor perfusion resulting from inadequate CO—for example, decreased LOC, diaphoresis, restlessness and anxiety, fatigue, headache, behavioural changes, and syncope.

After exploring the patient's chief complaint, inquire briefly about pertinent aspects of the patient's other medical history:

- Is the patient under treatment for any serious illnesses or conditions? Ask specifically whether he or she has ever been diagnosed with any of the following:
  - Coronary artery disease
  - Atherosclerotic heart disease: angina, previous MI, hypertension, congestive heart failure (CHF)
  - Valvular disease
  - Aneurysm
  - Pulmonary disease
  - Diabetes
  - Renal disease
  - Vascular disease
  - Inflammatory cardiac disease
  - Previous cardiac surgery (such as coronary artery bypass graft or valve replacement)
  - Congenital anomalies
- Is the patient taking any medications regularly? The focused history is a great opportunity to ask about which drugs have been prescribed and whether the patient is taking them as instructed. Be sure to ask when the patient took the medications last. Is he or she taking medications that were prescribed for someone else (borrowed)? Also ask about any over-the-counter medications or any herbal supplements the patient uses. It may be appropriate to ask about recreational drug use. Take particular note of the groups of medications prescribed for the treatment of cardiac problems listed in **Table 27-9 ▶**. If you are unfamiliar with any medication, ask the patient what it was prescribed for. It is also a good idea to ask if the patient takes any medication for each medical condition he or she reports as part of the history and to verify these medical conditions match the medications the patient is actually taking.
- Does the patient have known allergies to foods or medications? If so, ask what kind of reaction the patient has with each one.
- Ask the patient when he or she last had anything to eat or drink, and note the time that occurred. This information will prove helpful later in many situations.
- If you haven't asked already, find out the history of the current event. Get any extra information about what was happening when the problem started and what was done before your arrival.

Vital Signs

Pulse

When you take the vital signs, make a careful assessment of the patient's pulse. Is it regular or irregular? Abnormally fast or slow? Strong or weak? An irregular pulse signals a disturbance

Table 27-9	Medicines Prescribed to Treat or Prevent Heart Disease
Category	**Drug**
Angiotensin-converting enzyme inhibitors	Captopril (Capoten); enalapril (Vasotec); lisinopril (Prinivil, Zestril); fosinopril (Monopril); ramipril (Altace); quinapril (Accupril); perindopril (Aceon)
Calcium channel blockers	Amlodipine (Norvasc); felodipine (Plendil); diltiazem (Cardizem, Cardizem CD, Cardizem SR, Dilacor XR, Diltiazem XT, Tiazac); verapamil (Calan, Calan SR, Covera-HS, Isoptin, Isoptin SR, Verelan, VerelanPM); nifedipine (Adalat, Adalat CC, Procardia, Procardia XL); nicardipine (Cardene, Cardene SR); nisoldipine (Sular); bepridil (Vascor)
Angiotensin II receptor blockers	Losartan (Cozaar); valsartan (Diovan); irbesartan (Avapro); candesartan (Atacand)
Cholesterol-lowering drugs	Statins: lovastatin (Altacor, Mevacor); fluvastatin (Lescol); pravastatin (Pravachol); atorvastatin (Lipitor); simvastatin (Zocor) Niacins: nicotinic acid (Niacor); extended-release niacin (Niaspan) Bile acid resins: colestipol (Colestid); cholestyramine (Questran) Fibrates: clofibrate (Atromid); gemfibrozil (Lopid); fenofibrate (Tricor)
Antiarrhythmics	Amiodarone (Cordarone); sotalol (Betapace)
Cardiac glycoside	Digoxin (Lanoxin, Lanoxi-caps)
Antiplatelet agents	Clopidogrel (Plavix); ticlopidine (Ticlid); aspirin
Diuretics	Furosemide (Lasix); bumetamide (Bumex); torsemide (Demadex); hydrochlorothiazide (Esidrix); metolazone (Zaroxolyn); spironolactone (Aldactone)
Beta blockers	Acebutolol (Sectral); bisoprolol (Zebeta); esmolol (Brevibloc); propranolol (Inderal); atenolol (Tenormin); labetalol (Normodyne, Trandate); carvedilol (Coreg); metoprolol (Lopressor, Toprol-XL)
Vasodilators	Isosorbide dinitrate (Dilatrate-SR, Iso-Bid, Isonate, Isorbid, Isordil, Isotrate, Sorbitrate); isosorbide mononitrate (Imdur); hydralazine (Apresoline)
Coumarin anticoagulant	Warfarin (Coumadin)

in cardiac rhythm. A very rapid pulse (tachycardia) may simply indicate anxiety, but it can also occur secondary to severe pain, CHF, or a cardiac arrhythmia. A weak, thready pulse suggests a reduction in CO.

You should be familiar with the potentially abnormal pulse findings. For example, the patient may have a pulse deficit. A deficit occurs when the palpated radial pulse rate is less than the apical pulse rate; it is reported numerically as the difference between the two. To assess for a deficit, check the peripheral radial pulse while listening to an apical pulse.

Another abnormal pulse finding is pulsus paradoxus. Pulsus paradoxus is an excessive drop (> 10 mm Hg) in the systolic blood pressure with each inspired breath. Pulsus paradoxus can sometimes be palpated as a decrease in the amplitude of the pulse waveform, which makes the affected pulse beats feel weaker than the others. This observation can best be made when the rhythm is regular. If the variation is slight, it can be detected only by use of a blood pressure cuff and stethoscope.

Finally, you might recognize pulsus alternans. This pulse alternates in strength from one beat to the next.

Blood Pressure

In patients older than 50 years, a systolic blood pressure of more than 140 mm Hg is a much more important risk factor for CVD than the diastolic pressure. Patients with a systolic blood pressure of 120 to 139 mm Hg or a diastolic blood pressure of 80 to 89 mm Hg are considered "prehypertensive" and need to adopt a healthier lifestyle to prevent CVD.

In emergency situations, an elevated blood pressure may reflect the patient's anxiety or pain. A systolic blood pressure of less than 90 mm Hg might suggest serious hypotension and shock, depending on the patient's overall condition and chief complaint. The pulse pressure (the difference between the systolic and diastolic pressures) gives a rough indication of the elasticity of the arterial walls and the SV. In patients with arteriosclerosis, the arterial walls are stiffened, and the pulse pressure is increased. In cardiogenic shock or cardiac tamponade, the SV is reduced because the heart cannot pump effectively, so the pulse pressure is narrowed accordingly. A very low diastolic pressure may indicate a drop in systemic vascular resistance due to causes such as septic shock, anaphylaxis, or sedative drugs.

It may be beneficial to take the blood pressure in both arms and compare the readings. Some conditions such as stroke or aortic aneurysm may cause blood pressures to vary from the right to the left side.

Respirations

Note the rate and quality of the patient's respirations. Is the respiratory rate abnormally rapid (tachypnea)? Is the patient labouring to breathe? Respiratory distress in a cardiac patient suggests the possibility of CHF, with fluid in the lungs. Remember the old saying, "Look, listen, and feel"? In this physical examination, it is called inspection, auscultation, and palpation.

Cardiac Monitoring and Pulse Oximetry

As part of taking the vital signs, attach the cardiac monitor and pulse oximeter if you have not done so already. Use the ECG interpretation and oxygen saturation measurement just as you do other vital signs—that is, as tools to help you in your assessment and not as the only guide to treatment (treat the patient, not the monitor). Supplemental oxygen is needed for the patient in respiratory distress. However, it is not needed for patients without evidence of respiratory distress if the oxygen saturation is at least 94%. Note that very low cardiac output may lead to a failure to obtain a pulse oximeter reading; this is a good clue to check for low cardiac output. When caring for a patient in relatively stable condition who does not require rapid assessment, the physical examination may be done at this point.

Focused Physical Examination

The focused physical examination is similar for many medical patients. Nevertheless, certain aspects warrant greater emphasis in the patient whose chief complaint suggests a cardiac problem.

When observing the patient's general appearance, pay particular attention to the LOC, which is an excellent indicator of the adequacy of cerebral perfusion. If a patient is alert and oriented, the brain is getting enough oxygen, which in turn means the heart is doing its job as a pump. Conversely, stupor or confusion may indicate poor CO, which may be the result of myocardial damage or dysfunction. Skin colour and temperature are also valuable indicators of the state of the patient's circulation: The cold, sweaty skin of many patients with MI reflects massive peripheral vasoconstriction.

Physical Examination

In continuing the physical examination, begin by inspecting the neck and tracheal position. Is the trachea midline and mobile to gentle manipulation? Press down with your finger in the patient's suprasternal notch to verify that the trachea is midline.

What about the adjacent structures such as the neck veins? The external jugular veins reflect the pressure within the patient's

systemic circulation. Normally, they are collapsed when a person is sitting or standing. If the function of the right side of the heart is compromised, however, blood will back up into the systemic veins behind the right side of the heart and distend those veins. To estimate the patient's venous pressure, place the patient in a semisitting position (45° angle) with the head slightly rotated away from the jugular vein you are examining; observe the height of the distended fluid column within the vein, and note how far up the distension extends above the sternal angle.

Continue the assessment by inspecting and palpating the chest. Look for surgical scars that might indicate previous cardiac surgery. Is there a nitroglycerin patch on the patient's skin? Is there a bulge under the patient's skin indicating a pacemaker or an automated implanted cardioverter defibrillator (AICD)? These devices are implanted just below the right or left clavicle and are about the size of a one-dollar coin **Figure 27-21 ▾**.

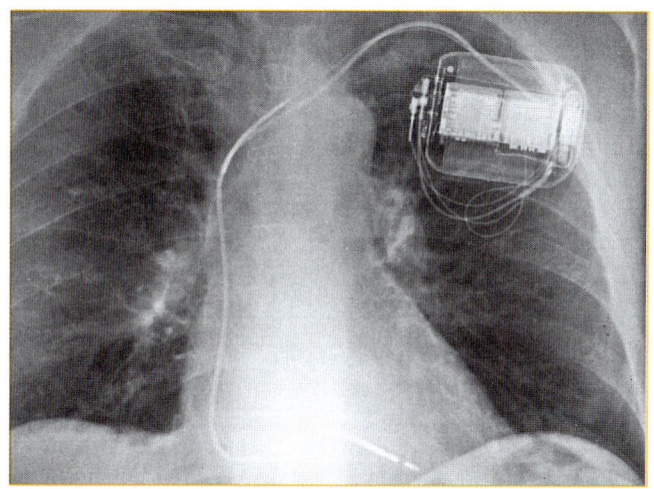

Figure 27-21 An AICD is attached directly to the heart and continuously monitors heart rhythm, delivering shocks as needed. The electricity from the AICD is so low that it has no effect on rescuers.

You are the Paramedic Part 4

Since the initial dose of adenosine caused a transient drop in the HR, you decide to administer 12 mg of adenosine after 2 minutes has passed. This time, you let Anthony know that you will be administering the medication and give it followed by a 20-ml flush. The monitor showed a 3-second period of asystole followed by a sudden increase in the HR back to approximately 210 beats/min. After waiting 2 minutes, you administer another 12 mg of adenosine, the third and final dose, with similar results.

Reassessment	Recording Time: 17 Minutes
Skin	Pink, warm, and diaphoretic
Pulse	210 beats/min; regular, with strong distal pulses
ECG	Supraventricular tachycardia
Blood pressure	104/66 mm Hg
Respirations	18 breaths/min, nonlaboured
Spo2	99% on nasal cannula at 4 l/min of oxygen
Pupils	Equal and reactive to light

7. How should your treatment proceed?

Is the anterior-posterior diameter of the chest enlarged, as in a barrel-chested patient with COPD? On palpation, do you observe any sign of crepitus?

Listen carefully to the chest with your stethoscope. Crackles or wheezes may be suggestive of left-sided heart failure with pulmonary edema. Listen for a third heart sound ("lub da-da" instead of "lub-dub"), known as an S₃ gallop, which again gives evidence of CHF. Examine the extremities and back for edema, a sign of failure of the right side of the heart.

Ongoing Assessment

Once the history and vital signs have been taken and the physical examination has been completed, treatment of the patient should be continued and transportation initiated. The ongoing assessment is accomplished en route to the hospital. It begins with a repeated initial assessment (LOC and ABCs). The vital signs should be taken every 5 to 15 minutes during this time as well. A repeated physical examination should be accomplished to see if any changes have occurred or if any conditions were missed in the initial physical examination. Finally, all the effectiveness of interventions implemented should be assessed. For example, is the IV fluid still flowing or has the pain diminished after nitroglycerin administration?

Pathophysiology and Management of Cardiovascular Problems

CAD and Angina

Coronary artery disease (CAD) is the most common form of heart disease and the leading cause of death in adults in Canada. The coronary arteries supply oxygen and nutrients to the myocardium. If one of these blood vessels becomes blocked, the muscle it supplies will be deprived of oxygen (ischemia). If this oxygen supply is not quickly restored, the ischemic area of heart muscle will eventually die (undergo infarction).

Atherosclerosis is of particular concern because it affects the inner lining of the aorta and cerebral and coronary blood vessels, leading to the narrowing of those vessels and reduction of blood flow through them. The atherosclerotic process begins, probably in childhood, when small amounts of fatty material are deposited along the inner wall (intima) of arteries, usually at points of turbulent blood flow (such as where the arteries bifurcate or where the arterial wall has been damaged). As the streak of fat enlarges, it becomes a mass of fatty tissue, an atheroma, which gradually calcifies and hardens into a plaque. The atheromatous plaque infiltrates the arterial wall and decreases its elasticity. At the same time, it narrows the arterial lumen and interferes with blood flow through the lumen. The narrowed, roughened area of the arterial intima provides a locus for the formation of a fixed blood clot, or thrombus, which may then obstruct the artery altogether (when in a coronary artery is known as a coronary thrombosis). In addition, calcium may precipitate from the bloodstream into the arterial walls, causing arteriosclerosis, which greatly reduces the elasticity of the arteries.

Risk Factors for Atherosclerosis

Although atherosclerosis is widespread in industrialized countries, certain factors increase the risk of developing atherosclerosis and CAD: hypertension (high blood pressure), cigarette smoking, diabetes, high serum cholesterol levels (which may be related to a high dietary intake of saturated fats and calories), lack of exercise, obesity, family history of heart disease or stroke, and male sex. Clearly, these risk factors include some things we can't do anything about (other than thank our parents). We cannot, for example, select our parents and grandparents or choose to be born female. Nevertheless, we can do something about nearly half the risk factors for CAD, which are, therefore, called modifiable risk factors:

- Cigarette smoking is the most significant cause of preventable death in Canada, and a smoker's chances of sudden death are several times greater than those of a nonsmoker. The good news is that smokers who quit return very rapidly to the same risk level as nonsmokers.
- Hypertension cannot be prevented or cured, but it can be controlled with changes in diet and with medications. A person with uncontrolled hypertension has two to three times the risk of CAD as a person with normal blood pressure.
- The levels of serum cholesterol are at least in part a consequence of dietary intake of saturated fats. In populations with low fat intake, the incidence of CAD is also low. Furthermore, lowering the serum cholesterol levels has been shown to reduce the incidence of heart attacks and other dangerous cardiac events. Cholesterol may also be controlled with medications, if necessary.
- One behaviour that may have a role in elevating serum cholesterol is lack of exercise, which also has a variety of other untoward effects on the body. Exercise improves overall fitness, cardiac reserve, and collateral coronary circulation.
- Obesity may go hand in hand with several other risk factors (such as diabetes and hypertension). But obesity by itself also may contribute to an increased risk of CAD. Weight reduction, through consumption of a sensible diet and increased physical exercise, can reap several lifelong and life-extending benefits. Normalizing body weight will lower elevated blood pressure, elevated serum cholesterol levels, elevated blood glucose levels, and the risk of CAD.

Data suggest that risk factor modification can make a difference in the impact of CAD. Accordingly to the Heart and Stroke Foundation of Canada, between 1994–1995 and 2003–2004, hospitalizations for ischemic heart disease declined by 25%. Acute heart attack deaths declined by 9%. However, there are still an estimated 72,000 heart attacks each year in Canada.

Approximately 19,000 Canadians die each year as the result of a heart attack. Most of these deaths occur out of the hospital. The number of heart attack-related hospitalizations has increased steadily over the past decade (1994–1995 to 2003–2004).

The number of Canadians living with some form of heart disease or stroke (based on self-report) remains high and increases with age (see **Table 27-10 ▶**). Finally, 8 in 10 Canadians (80%) have at least one risk factor for heart disease or stroke (smoking, alcohol, physical inactivity, obesity, high blood pressure, high blood cholesterol, or diabetes).

Peripheral Vascular Disorders

Although atherosclerosis is rarely the primary cause of medical emergencies, it is a major contributor to other conditions that may become medical emergencies. For example, arterial bruits or "swishing" sounds (heard with a stethoscope placed over the carotid arteries) signal the presence of atherosclerosis and contraindicate the use of carotid sinus massage. Atherosclerosis can also contribute to claudication, a severe pain in the calf muscle caused by narrowing of the arteries in this muscle and leading to a painful limp. Finally, atherosclerosis may be associated with phlebitis—swelling and pain along the veins that can lead to the formation of blood clots (thrombophlebitis). If dislodged, these thrombi become emboli that could travel to the heart and through its right side, lodging in the pulmonary arterial tree and causing a pulmonary embolism.

An estimated 2 million Canadians are affected by significant peripheral vascular disorders annually. Risk factors for peripheral vascular disorders include age, oral contraceptive use, smoking, recent surgery, recreational IV drug use, trauma, and extended immobilization. The most dangerous complication of these disorders is pulmonary embolism. In an average year, approximately 50,000 serious pulmonary embolisms occur in Canada, leading to about 5,000 deaths. An embolus, usually formed in the leg, lodges in one of the arteries of the lungs. Identification of these risk factors has a significant role in diagnosing peripheral vascular occlusions. Signs of peripheral vascular occlusion may include pain, redness, swelling, warmth, and tenderness in the extremity; these signs are present in only about half of all cases, however. The presence of claudication indicates a significant narrowing of the peripheral arteries associated with peripheral vascular disorders. Arterial bruits are another sign of vascular narrowing that can contribute to ischemia or stroke.

Because peripheral vascular disorders can have serious consequences, such as pulmonary embolism or loss of limb through arterial occlusions, you must be familiar with the signs, symptoms, and risk factors for these conditions. Unfortunately, prehospital treatment of peripheral vascular conditions is limited. Beyond supplementary oxygen, IV access, and, possibly, aspirin administration, little can be done in the prehospital setting if you suspect a peripheral vascular disorder. If a pulmonary embolism is suspected, however, the treatment involves an anticoagulant or thrombolytic medications. Anticoagulants prevent further clotting, and thrombolytics help the body to dissolve the original clot.

Acute Coronary Syndrome

Acute coronary syndrome (ACS) is the term used to describe any group of clinical symptoms consistent with acute myocardial

Table 27-10	Self-Reported Heart Attacks in Canada
Age Group	**Percent (%) Reporting Heart Attack**
20-49	0.3
50-64	3.4
65-79	8.2
80+	11.8
Total (20+)	**2.5**

ischemia, from stable angina to myocardial infarction. It typically presents as chest pain due to insufficient blood supply to the heart muscle, which itself is a result of CAD.

ACS includes a continuous spectrum of disease. Patients experiencing symptomatic, acute myocardial ischemia should receive a 12-lead ECG to determine whether they have an ST-segment elevation. Most patients whose ECG displays ST-segment elevation will ultimately develop what was formerly known as a Q-wave AMT (heart attack), now referred to as a STEMI (ST-elevation myocardial infarction). Patients who have ischemic discomfort (chest pain) without an ST-segment elevation are having unstable angina or a non–ST-segment elevation MI (formally referred to as a non–Q-wave MI); these conditions are now collectively known as UA/NSTEMI (unstable angina/non–ST-elevation myocardial infarction).

Angina Pectoris

The principal symptom of CAD is angina pectoris (literally "choking in the chest"). Angina occurs when the supply of oxygen to the myocardium is insufficient to meet the demand. As a result, the cardiac muscle becomes ischemic, and a switch to anaerobic metabolism leads to the accumulation of lactic acid and carbon dioxide. The concept of "supply and demand" is critical here. When at rest, a person with heart disease may have an adequate supply of oxygen to the heart to meet these sedentary needs, despite some narrowing of the coronary arteries. When the same person exercises or experiences some other stress, however, the blood flow to the myocardium may not be able to satisfy the heart's increased demand for oxygen; in that case, angina will result. Clearly, the patient who experiences angina at rest, when oxygen needs are minimal, has more severe CAD than a person who experiences angina only with vigorous exercise.

When taking the history from a patient with chest pain, it is important to distinguish between stable angina and unstable angina. Stable angina follows a recurrent pattern: A person with stable angina experiences pain after a certain, predictable amount of exertion, such as climbing one flight of stairs or walking for three blocks. The pain also has a predictable location, intensity, and duration. The patient may report, for example, "Every time I walk up the hill to the bus stop, I get a squeezing pain under my breast bone, and I have to sit down for 2 or 3 minutes until it goes away."

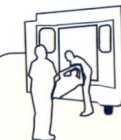

At the Scene

ACS includes a continuum of disease, ranging from stable angina at one end of the spectrum to acute myocardial infarction at the other.

Patients with chronic, stable angina often take nitroglycerin or some other form of "nitrate" for relief of anginal pain. In its usual formulation, nitroglycerin is supplied as a white tablet, which is placed under the tongue (sublingual) and allowed to dissolve there, or in a spray form that is sprayed under the tongue. It may also be given as sustained-release capsules taken two or three times a day, as a cream rubbed into the skin (topical), or as a patch worn on the skin. Regardless of which form is used, nitroglycerin will have a predictable effect in stable angina, producing relief of symptoms within a few minutes.

Unstable angina is much more serious than stable angina and indicates a greater degree of obstruction of the coronary arteries. It is characterized by noticeable changes in the frequency, severity, and duration of pain and often occurs without predictable stress. The patient may report that the anginal attacks have grown more frequent and severe during the past several days or weeks or that they awaken him or her from sleep or occur when otherwise at rest. Such attacks are often warning signs of an impending MI.

Management Considerations

Of course, not all chest pain is caused by cardiac ischemia or injury. Many other conditions—such as pulmonary embolism, pneumothorax, pneumonia, pericarditis, aortic dissection, indigestion, and peptic ulcer—may cause chest pain that can be mistaken for angina or an MI. It is important to perform a thorough physical examination, including a focused history, to determine whether the cause of the complaint is likely cardiac in origin.

Notes from Nancy

When a patient with chest pain calls for an ambulance, it means that the patient never had chest pain before or that his or her chronic chest pain has changed. Either way, it's serious.

As a general rule, it is safe to assume that any patient who has called for an ambulance because of chest pain has, at the least, unstable angina and perhaps an evolving AMI. Patients with chronic, stable angina rarely call for help unless something has changed—often dramatically—for the worse. Because it is difficult and sometimes impossible to differentiate between angina and an MI in the prehospital environment, the treatment of angina should be the same as for an MI. It is far better to overtreat angina as an MI than to undertreat an MI by assuming it is angina.

Acute Myocardial Infarction

An acute myocardial infarction (AMI), or heart attack, occurs when a portion of the cardiac muscle is deprived of coronary blood flow long enough that portions of the muscle die (undergoes necrosis, or infarcts). Several things can diminish flow through coronary vessels, especially if the vessels are already narrowed by atherosclerotic disease: occlusion of a coronary artery by a blood clot (thrombus), spasm of a coronary artery, or reduction of overall blood flow from any cause (such as shock, arrhythmias, or pulmonary embolism).

The location and size of a myocardial infarct depend on which coronary artery is blocked and where along its course the blockage occurred. The majority of infarcts involve the left ventricle. When the anterior, lateral, or septal walls of the left ventricle are infarcted, the source is usually occlusion of the left coronary artery or one of its branches. Inferior wall infarcts are usually the result of RCA occlusion. When the ischemic process affects only the inner layer of muscle, the infarct is referred to as subendocardial. When the infarct extends through the entire wall of the ventricle, it is a transmural MI. The infarcted tissue is invariably surrounded by a ring of ischemic tissue—an area that is relatively deprived of oxygen but still viable. That ischemic tissue tends to be electrically unstable and is often the source of cardiac arrhythmias.

Notes from Nancy

For purposes of treatment outside the hospital, the patient with chest pain must be assumed to be suffering an acute myocardial infarction until proven otherwise and should therefore be treated as any other patient with a suspected AMI.

Cardiovascular disease leading to acute myocardial infarction is the leading cause of death in Canada, accounting for more than 72,000 deaths each year. Of all deaths from AMI, 90% are due to arrhythmias, usually ventricular fibrillation, which typically occur during the early hours of the infarct. Arrhythmias can be prevented or treated, so *most deaths from AMI are preventable.*

Symptoms of AMI

Although there is no "typical AMI patient," when most Canadians think about the symptoms of an AMI, they envision the classic pain presentation usually associated with men. In fact, AMIs can occur in younger and older people and in men and women. The patient may be slightly overweight and may have recently overindulged at the dinner table or perhaps on the tennis court. Nevertheless, many heart attacks occur at rest or just after arising in the morning.

The most common symptom of AMI is chest pain. This pain is similar to that of angina but can be much more severe and last more than 15 minutes. A patient with chronic angina will be aware that something very different from previous anginal attacks is happening. The pain of AMI is typically felt just beneath the sternum and is variously described as heavy, squeezing, crushing, or tight. Often the patient unconsciously clenches a fist when describing the pain (Levine sign) to convey in body language the squeezing nature of the pain. In 25% of cases, the pain radiates to the arms (most often the left arm) and into the fingers; it may also radiate to the neck, jaw, upper back, or epigastrium. Occasionally, a patient will mistake the pain of AMI for indigestion and may take antacids in an attempt to relieve the discomfort. The pain of AMI is not influenced by coughing, deep breathing, or other body movements.

Not every AMI patient has chest pain, however. In fact, 10% to 20% of patients with AMI *do not experience any chest pain.* Diabetics, older people, and heart transplant patients, for example, generally do not present with chest pain, a condition referred to as "silent MI." Instead, these patients may present with symptoms related to a drop in CO. It is not unusual for them to develop sudden dyspnea, progressing rapidly to pulmonary edema, a sudden loss of consciousness, an unexplained drop in blood pressure, an apparent stroke, or simply confusion.

Women with an AMI may present differently from men with the same condition. Women may experience nausea, lightheadedness, epigastric burning, or sudden onset of weakness or unexplained tiredness. Because they are not experiencing the typical chest pain expected with an AMI, many women ignore their symptoms. Unfortunately, CVD accounts for one third of all female deaths in Canada. It is the number one cause of death for women in Canada.

At the Scene

More men have heart disease, but more women die of heart disease, in part because their symptoms are less clear-cut.

When obtaining the history from a patient whose chief complaint is chest pain, ask the usual OPQRST questions to elabourate on the chief complaint, but also ask whether the patient has taken anything for the pain and, if so, whether it helped. If the patient reports having taken nitroglycerin without relief, it is important to establish *why* the patient did not obtain relief.

Two reasons might explain this failure. One possibility is that the patient is, indeed, having an AMI, for which nitroglycerin would not provide complete pain relief. The other possibility is that the nitroglycerin has simply gone stale. To retain its potency, nitroglycerin must be stored in a dark, airtight container; if it is left out in the open for any period (for example, if the patient stores the medicine on the window sill above the kitchen sink), it loses its therapeutic effectiveness. To distinguish between the two explanations, ask the patient whether he or she noticed the usual effects of the nitroglycerin. Nitroglycerin tablets that are therapeutically active cause a slight burning under the tongue, may make the patient feel flushed,

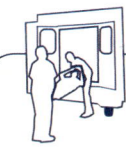

Notes from Nancy

Start treatment immediately for any patient with chest pain.

or may give the patient a transient throbbing headache. If the patient confirms that he or she felt one of those effects but the chest pain still wouldn't go away, then you know there was nothing wrong with the nitroglycerin but there may be something very wrong with the patient.

As soon as you have elicited a chief complaint of a cardiac nature, you will need to start treatment of the patient; obtaining a focused history and physical examination can wait. For purposes of discussion, though, we shall continue here to proceed through the history and physical examination. Besides pain (or, sometimes, instead of pain), a number of other symptoms are associated with AMI:

- Diaphoresis (sweating), often profuse, is principally the result of massive discharge by the autonomic nervous system. The patient may soak through his or her clothing and complain of a cold sweat.
- Dyspnea may be a warning of impending left-sided heart failure.
- Anorexia (loss of appetite), nausea, vomiting, or belching frequently accompanies MI. Hiccups may occasionally occur as well, due to irritation of the diaphragm by an inferior wall MI.
- Weakness may be profound, and the patient may describe this feeling with phrases such as "a limp rag."
- If CO is significantly diminished, dizziness may reflect the reduced circulation to the brain.
- Palpitations are sometimes experienced by patients with cardiac arrhythmias as a sensation that the heart has skipped a beat.
- A feeling of impending doom is common among patients having an MI. The patient is frightened, looks frightened, and expresses his or her fear to other people—all of which adds to a general atmosphere of panic and dread.

Signs of AMI

Although patients with AMI often have abnormalities in the physical examination, many have relatively normal physical examination findings, and the diagnosis in the prehospital environment (and, indeed, in the ED) depends chiefly on the history. Nevertheless, it is important to take note of a few specific things during the physical examination to detect the development of complications to AMI, such as heart failure or cardiogenic shock.

- Pay attention to the patient's general appearance. Does the patient appear anxious? Frightened? In obvious pain?
- What is the patient's state of consciousness? Is he or she fully alert? Confused? Remember: Poor perfusion creates confusion. If the patient does not seem "all there," it may be because the heart is giving out and not enough oxygenated blood is reaching the brain.
- Is the skin pale, cold, and clammy?
- Assess the patient's vital signs. Is the pulse strong or weak? Regular or irregular? Is the respiratory rate abnormally rapid? Is the blood pressure abnormally high or low?
- Are there signs of left-sided heart failure (wheezes or crackles)? Signs of right-sided heart failure (distended neck veins, pedal or presacral edema)?

A typical patient with an AMI is very apprehensive, with an ashen-grey pallor and cold, wet skin. He or she *looks* scared. The pulse may be rapid unless heart block has occurred. The blood pressure may be decreased, reflecting decreased CO from the damaged heart, or it may be elevated from pain and anxiety.

Prehospital Management of ACS

On your arrival at the scene, start treatment at once for any middle-aged or older patient with chest pain, even before you complete the history and physical examination. The longest delay in treatment seems to be the phase from onset of symptoms to patient recognition, so your prehospital care must begin immediately. The goals of treatment are to limit the size of the infarct, to decrease the patient's fear and pain, and to prevent the development of serious cardiac arrhythmias.

Place the Patient at Physical and Emotional Rest

The stress response causes the adrenal glands to squeeze out a surge of catecholamines (epinephrine and norepinephrine), which in turn can send the damaged heart racing. At the same time, the massive discharge throughout the fight-or-flight system puts the peripheral circulation in a state of severe vasoconstriction; thus, not only is the heart being flogged to go faster and faster, but it also has to work harder and harder against the increased afterload. The heart's need for oxygen, therefore, soars precisely when it is already in a state of marked oxygen deprivation. This cycle can lead quickly to arrhythmias and death. Prehospital deaths are related to arrhythmias (often ventricular fibrillation), and most occur during the first 4 hours after onset of symptoms. Nevertheless, this deadly cycle can be interrupted by community education programs designed to assist citizens in early recognition of symptoms, early activation of EMS, and, if needed, CPR and early access to an automated external defibrillator (AED).

To begin your treatment, put the patient physically at ease. Recall that one goal of treatment is to try to limit the size of the infarct; one way to do so is to decrease the amount of work that the heart must do, which will begin to decrease the patient's myocardial oxygen requirements immediately. The position in which cardiac work is minimal is the semi-Fowler's position—that is, reclining on the stretcher with the back of the stretcher raised about 30°. Of course, the patient has to get to the stretcher and must not be permitted to do so alone. From the time you arrive, the patient must not do anything, including walking to the ambulance.

Administer Oxygen and Aspirin

The mnemonic MONA is used to help remember the supportive treatments of Morphine, Oxygen, Nitroglycerin, and Aspirin for a patient with an ACS—but these treatments are not to be given in that order. MONA is administered in the following order, provided these measures are not contraindicated by hypotension: (1) oxygen, (2) aspirin, (3) nitroglycerin, and (4) morphine.

Oxygen may limit ischemic myocardial injury and reduce the amount of ST-segment elevation. Its effects on morbidity

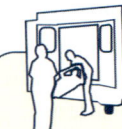

At the Scene

Oxygen is the first drug in the treatment of ACS.

and mortality in acute infarction are unknown. The recommendation is to initiate oxygen at a rate of 4 to 6 l/min via nasal cannula, although a nonrebreathing mask that provides oxygen at a rate of 12 to 15 l/min is also acceptable. Monitor the SpO_2 and titrate until the patient is in stable condition or the hypoxemia is corrected (that is, $SpO_2 > 90\%$).

In most EMS systems, as long as the patient has no aspirin allergy or gastrointestinal bleeding, dispatchers may advise patients to chew baby aspirin (160 to 325 mg). If this has not been done before your arrival or the patient has not already taken aspirin on his or her own, then give the patient 160 to 325 mg of non–enteric-coated aspirin to chew.

Provide Pain Relief

Some form of pain relief must be provided because the pain of AMI is very severe and places enormous stress on the patient's autonomic nervous system—stress that may contribute to complications. Nitroglycerin is a good place to start, but make sure the patient's blood pressure is adequate before its administration. In particular, before giving this medication, it is imperative that you ascertain whether the patient is taking phosphodiesterase-5 (PDE-5) inhibitors for erectile dysfunction **Table 27-11 ▾**. These drugs may worsen certain medical conditions and interact with a number of drugs, especially nitrate medications (such as nitroglycerin) prescribed to prevent or treat acute angina. Both types of medication dilate blood vessels, and their combined effects can cause dizziness, low blood pressure, and loss of consciousness.

Place a 0.4-mg tablet (or spray) of nitroglycerin under the patient's tongue. If the patient is experiencing an AMI and not simply angina, this medication is unlikely to relieve his or her pain, but it may help to reduce the size of the infarction. Do *not* give nitroglycerin if there is hypotension or bradycardia, and do *not* give it to patients having epigastric symptoms ("indigestion") or hiccups. Nitroglycerin may be repeated every 3 to 5 minutes, up to a total of three doses as long as the patient's condition remains stable.

If nitroglycerin provides no relief of pain and if authorized by your protocols or direct medical control, morphine sulfate may be titrated in IV doses according to local protocols. Give this medication in 2- to 4-mg IV doses as needed for pain,

Table 27-11 **PDE-5 Inhibitors**		
Brand Name	**Generic Name**	**Duration of Effect**
Viagra	Sildenafil citrate	Up to 4 h
Levitra	Vardenafil	Up to 4 h
Cialis	Tadalfil	24 to 36 h

being sure to reassess the patient's blood pressure, pulse, and respiratory rate after each dose, until the patient experiences relief of pain or experiences a drop in pulse or blood pressure. If bradycardia occurs, notify the physician immediately. Remember that morphine should *not* be given to patients with low blood pressure (less than about 100 mm Hg systolic or according to local protocol), dehydrated patients, or patients suspected of having an AMI involving the inferior wall of the heart. At least half of all patients with MI of the inferior wall will also experience a right ventricular infarction; as a consequence, they may already be hypotensive or the administration of nitroglycerin and morphine may cause hypotension.

In some EMS medical protocols, fentanyl is favoured over morphine for pain not relieved with nitroglycerin because of its rapid onset and relatively short duration. Fentanyl also has fewer side effects than morphine.

Perform Cardiac Monitoring

Apply the ECG monitor, and run a strip to document the initial rhythm. As long as you are applying electrodes to the chest, also place your anterior chest leads in anticipation of doing a 12-lead ECG. Ideally, your monitor should have an audible tone that beeps with each QRS complex (also called systole beep), so that you can keep track of the patient's cardiac rhythm even when you have to take your gaze from the monitor to do other things. The ear, in any case, is far more sensitive than the eye to slight irregularities in rhythm, so the chances are that you will *hear* the beginning of a cardiac arrhythmia much sooner than you will see it on the monitor. Keep the other cardiac drugs that you carry close at hand so you can reach them quickly if a cardiac arrhythmia develops.

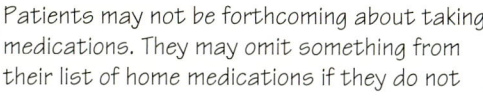

At the Scene

Patients may not be forthcoming about taking medications. They may omit something from their list of home medications if they do not take the medicine daily. Be sure to ask.

Record the Vital Signs

Obtain vital signs, including pulse, respirations, blood pressure, and oxygen saturation. Measure the blood pressure, and repeat that measurement at least every 5 minutes. Measure the pulse. The ECG monitor provides information only about the electrical activity of the heart; it gives no information about the strength of the heartbeat (muscular activity) or even about whether the heart is beating at all! It is, therefore, necessary to monitor the patient's pulse to assess peripheral blood flow, especially during transport, when blood pressure measurements are difficult and unreliable.

Perform a Detailed History and Physical Examination

After you have completed the preceding steps (as appropriate), you should obtain a more detailed history and perform a physical examination. Find out if the patient has a history of cardiac disease; takes any heart medications, such as beta-blockers, angiotensin-converting enzyme inhibitors, diuretics, or nitroglycerin (nitrates); or has had a previous heart attack or any heart surgery (such as coronary artery bypass graft). Also obtain a more complete description of the present symptoms, especially regarding their onset. Gathering that information should not, however, delay transport to the hospital. Once you have taken

You are the Paramedic **Part 5**

The adenosine did not work, and your patient continues to be in hemodynamically stable condition, which gives you the opportunity to continue treating Anthony pharmacologically. In accordance with department protocols you reach into the drug box, grab a pre-filled syringe of diltiazem, and wipe the sweat off of your brow. Before administering the diltiazem, you recheck the protocol book and confirm the dose as 25 mg by IV push. You administer the diltiazem, knowing that at any time Anthony's condition can become unstable. After about a minute passes, you note that the HR on the cardiac monitor begins to steadily decrease, finally stabilizing at 94 beats/min. Both you and Anthony can breathe a sigh of relief. You contact the receiving ED, give your report, and receive no further orders.

On arrival at the ED, a diltiazem drip is started. He is admitted overnight for observation on the telemetry floor. After an uneventful night, Anthony is discharged home with strong suggestions not to overindulge in energy drinks and caffeine pills and to find healthier study habits!

Reassessment	Recording Time: 25 Minutes
Skin	Pink, warm, and dry
Pulse	94 beats/min, regular; strong distal pulses
ECG	Normal sinus rhythm
Blood pressure	124/76 mm Hg
Respirations	18 breaths/min, nonlaboured
Spo₂	99% on nasal cannula at 4 l/min of oxygen
Pupils	Equal and reactive to light

8. What type of medication is diltiazem?

9. How does diltiazem work?

the necessary precautions to stabilize the patient's condition (aspirin, oxygen, IV saline lock, monitor/12-lead ECG, analgesia), there is no reason to remain any longer at the scene unless a cardiac arrest or arrhythmia requires immediate treatment. Take the rest of the history en route to the hospital. Remember that "time is muscle": Heart cells are being destroyed during the infarction before reperfusion is started in the hospital.

Prehospital 12-lead ECG

An important component of ACS care is performance of out-of-hospital 12-lead ECG with transmission or interpretation by paramedic personnel and advance notification to the receiving facility. The goal is to reduce time to reperfusion, with either fibrinolytic therapy or primary PCI. Out-of-hospital 12-lead ECG has been shown to reduce the time to primary PCI and can help triage patients with acute STEMI to a hospital with interventional cardiac care facilities. When paramedics activate the cardiac care team, reductions in reperfusion times are observed.

Transport the Patient

Once the patient is in stable condition, transport him or her to an appropriate hospital in a semi-Fowler position (unless the patient is in shock, in which case he or she should be supine). Do all you can to ensure that the patient is as relaxed and as comfortable as possible. En route, some additional treatment measures may be worthwhile, especially when transport will take a long time.

Safe and appropriate transport is the name of the game. *Do not rush* and *do not use sirens* when transporting the patient to the hospital, unless absolutely necessary. High speed and sirens send two clear messages to the patient: (1) Something is terribly wrong. (2) The personnel on the ambulance don't feel capable of dealing with the situation. Those are *not* the messages you want to convey to a frightened patient with a damaged heart! The patient needs to feel confident that those caring for him or her are in control of the situation.

If a serious arrhythmia occurs during transport, institute treatment immediately, and notify direct medical control. Except under unusual circumstances, treatment of life-threatening situations should not be attempted in a moving ambulance. Whenever possible, the driver should pull over to the side of the road and go to the back of the vehicle to help the other paramedic.

Reperfusion Techniques for ACS

The majority of AMIs occur as a result of thrombus (fixed blood clot) formation at the site of a preexisting atherosclerotic plaque. The thrombus occludes the coronary artery, preventing further blood flow through it. Thus, it seems reasonable to try to restore circulation through the occluded coronary artery, thereby restoring perfusion to the ischemic myocardium. Simply put, that is reperfusion.

The most immediate forms of reperfusion are fibrinolytic therapy and percutaneous intervention (PCI). All paramedics should be alert for patients who are good candidates for reperfusion, should know which hospitals in their area carry out fibrinolytic therapy and/or PCI, and should provide early notification (along with 12-lead ECG results) to the ED that a candidate for such therapy is en route.

Fibrinolysis

One way in which to reperfuse the blocked coronary artery is to try to dissolve the occluding blood clot, thereby restoring circulation to the ischemic heart. That idea is the essence of fibrinolytic therapy.

In fact, this concept is not altogether new. Attempts to use fibrinolytic agents in the treatment of AMI were reported at least 40 years ago, albeit without success. In retrospect, we realize that one reason the early attempts failed was that fibrinolytic therapy was started too late, after irreversible damage to the myocardium had already occurred. With that realization came the concept that "time is myocardium": The longer a segment of myocardium remains unperfused, the smaller the chances of salvaging that tissue and restoring its normal function. The obvious corollary is that the sooner fibrinolytic therapy can begin with respect to the onset of the blockage, the better the chances for saving the affected distal myocardium. Indeed, fibrinolytic treatment given within 30 to 60 minutes of the onset of symptoms can sometimes abort the MI altogether.

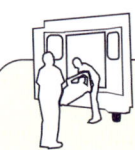

At the Scene

Time is muscle (myocardium)!

In the 1980s, fibrinolytic therapy was given to AMI patients as soon as they reached the ED, rather than waiting until the patient was admitted to the coronary care unit. Inevitably, applying the doctrine that time is myocardium led to the idea of starting fibrinolytic treatment even earlier, in the prehospital phase of care.

Recent clinical trials have shown the benefit of starting fibrinolysis as soon as possible after the onset of ischemic-type chest pain in patients with STEMI or new or presumably new left bundle branch block. Several prospective studies have also documented reduced time to administration of fibrinolytics and decreased mortality rates when out-of-hospital fibrinolytics were given to patients with STEMI and no contraindications to fibrinolytics. Some EMS systems may opt to start fibrinolytic treatment in the prehospital environment, and in rural areas with very long transport times, prehospital initiation of fibrinolytic therapy may make a lot of sense. Even in EMS systems in which paramedics do not give fibrinolytic therapy, their ability to identify candidates for such therapy has a decisive role in helping ED personnel administer fibrinolytic therapy early enough to make a difference. For these reasons, all paramedics should thoroughly understand the principles of fibrinolytic therapy for AMI.

Fibrinolytic therapy seeks to administer, during the early hours of AMI, an agent that will activate the body's own internal system for dissolving clots, the fibrinolytic system. Once activated, that system can begin to dissolve the clot that has formed within the coronary artery, thereby reopening the artery (recanalization) and allowing the resumption of blood flow through it (reperfusion). Unfortunately, if an agent capable of promoting clot dissolution is given intravenously, its effects cannot be limited to the clot in the coronary artery; it can also act

Table 27-12	ST-Segment Elevation or New or Presumably New LBBB: Evaluation for Reperfusion

Step 1: Assess time and risk

- Time since onset of symptoms
- Risk of STEMI
- Risk of fibrinolysis
- Time required to transport to skilled PCI catheterization suite

Step 2: Select reperfusion (fibrinolysis or invasive) strategy

Note: If presentation < 3 hours and no delay for PCI, then no preference for either strategy.

Fibrinolysis is generally preferred if:

- Early presentation (≤ 3 hours from symptom onset)
- Invasive strategy is not an option (eg, lack of access to skilled PCI facility or difficult vascular access) or would be delayed
  —Medical contact-to-balloon or door-balloon > 90 min
  —(Door-to-balloon) minus (door-to-needle) is > 1 hour
- No contraindications to fibrinolysis

An invasive strategy is generally preferred if:

- Late presentation (symptom onset > 3 hours ago)
- Skilled PCI facility available with surgical backup
- Medical contact-to-balloon or door-balloon < 90 min
- (Door-to-balloon) minus (door-to-needle) is < 1 hour
- Contraindications to fibrinolysis, including increased risk of bleeding and ICH
- High risk from STEMI (CHF, Killip class is ≥ 3)
- Diagnosis of STEMI is in doubt

anywhere else in the body where clots are being formed and, therefore, may lead to bleeding. Thus, the benefit of fibrinolytic therapy—the possible salvage of myocardium—must always be weighed against its risks—principally, the risk of bleeding.

To determine the appropriate candidates for fibrinolytic agents, we need to be as certain as possible that we are really dealing with a patient who is having an AMI. A patient having chest pain from another source would receive no potential benefit from fibrinolytic therapy—so he or she would be subjected to this therapy's risks for no reason. Although it is difficult in the early hours of an AMI to be certain of the diagnosis, inclusion criteria have been established to help select patients most likely to be having an AMI. At the same time, exclusion criteria are used to identify patients for whom the risk of fibrinolytic therapy is unacceptably high—for example, patients most likely to experience hemorrhagic complications. **Table 27-12 ▲** summarizes typical inclusion and exclusion criteria for fibrinolytic therapy.

Most treatment regimens for fibrinolysis include one of three agents: tenecteplase, alteplase (Activase; a tissue plasminogen activator), or reteplase (Retavase; recombinant tissue). All of them work by converting, in one way or another, the body's own clot-dissolving enzyme from its inactive form, plasminogen, to its active form, plasmin.

The key to realizing the benefits of fibrinolysis is to start early. A prehospital fibrinolytic program is recommended only in systems with well-established protocols, checklists, experience in ACLS, ability to communicate with the receiving institution, and a medical director with training and experience in the management of STEMI.

Percutaneous Intervention

Many institutions now perform emergent primary PCI as an alternative to fibrinolysis. Primary PCI involves emergent opening of the blocked coronary artery by mechanical means with a balloon-tipped catheter, instead of delivering a fibrinolytic agent. Studies have shown that patients undergoing rapid primary PCI have better outcomes than those receiving fibrinolytic therapy. This is true for patients with STEMI and cardiogenic shock. The key to better outcomes is rapid response—the artery is opened by a balloon within 90 minutes of first contacting the health care system. This is only possible in well-organized hospital systems with interventional cardiac care facilities available and standing by for such a patient.

Canadian studies have also demonstrated that paramedics can reliably identify patients with STEMI with 12-lead ECG, utilize a hospital bypass protocol, and transport patients with STEMI directly to a hospital with interventional cardiac care facilities. Programs that integrate EMS, emergency department, and cardiology services are improving patient outcomes. Paramedics should be aware of their local or regional protocols for ACS and STEMI patients, including 12-lead ECG interpretation and hospital bypass.

Congestive Heart Failure

Congestive heart failure (also known as chronic heart failure) occurs when the heart is unable, for any reason, to pump powerfully enough or fast enough to empty its chambers; as a result, blood backs up into the systemic circuit, the pulmonary circuit, or both. Although CHF may develop in situations other than AMI—for example, in a patient with chronic high blood pressure—the basic principles of diagnosis and treatment are similar, whatever the precipitating factors. It is estimated that 400,000 Canadians are living with congestive heart failure. Depending on the symptom severity, heart dysfunction, age, and other factors, congestive heart failure can be associated with an annual mortality of between 5% and 50%. The average annual mortality rate for congestive heart failure is 10% per year, with a 50% 5-year survival rate. Up to 40% to 50%

Table 27-13	Differentiation and Treatment of Asthma and Left-Sided Heart Failure	
	Asthma	**Left-Sided Heart Failure**
History	Often a younger patient May have allergic history or family history of allergy Previous attacks of acute, episodic dyspnea May have had recent respiratory infection Unproductive cough	Often an older patient May have history of heart problems, hypertension Dyspnea worse when lying down (orthopnea) Recent rapid weight gain Cough with watery or foamy sputum
Possible physical findings	Wheezing Chest hyperinflated and hyperresonant Use of accessory muscles to breathe If bronchospasm severe, chest may be silent	Wheezing Crackles S_3 gallop Distended neck veins Pedal or presacral edema
Treatment	Oxygen (humidified) Intermittent positive-pressure breathing Monitor IV: normal saline Selective beta-2 adrenergic medications	Oxygen Intermittent positive-pressure breathing Monitor IV: normal saline to keep open or saline lock (adrenergics and bicarbonate usually contraindicated) Morphine Nitroglycerin

of people with congestive heart failure die within 5 years of diagnosis.

Left-Sided Heart Failure

The left ventricle is most commonly damaged during an AMI. Likewise, in chronic hypertension, the left ventricle tends to suffer the long-term effects of having to pump against an increased afterload (constricted peripheral arteries). In both cases, the right side of the heart continues to pump relatively normally and to deliver normal volumes of blood to the pulmonary circulation. By comparison, the left side of the heart may no longer be able to pump the blood being delivered from the pulmonary vessels. As a result, blood backs up behind the left ventricle, and the pressure in the left atrium and pulmonary veins increases. As the pulmonary veins become engorged with blood, serum is forced out of the pulmonary capillaries and into the alveoli. The serum mixes with air in the alveoli to produce foam (pulmonary edema).

When fluid occupies the alveoli, oxygenation is impaired. The patient experiences that impairment as shortness of breath (dyspnea), particularly in the recumbent position (orthopnea). If left ventricular failure is the result of chronic overload (as opposed to AMI), the patient is likely to give a history of a week or two of PND. To compensate for the impairment in oxygenation, the patient's respiratory rate increases (tachypnea); even so, if the patient's condition is advanced enough, cyanosis may become evident. In some patients with pulmonary edema, especially elderly patients, Cheyne-Stokes respirations may be present.

Fluid from the pulmonary vessels also leaks into the interstitial spaces in the lungs, and increasing interstitial pressure causes narrowing of the bronchioles. Air passing through the narrowed bronchioles creates wheezing noises, whereas air bubbling through the fluid-filled alveoli produces crackles.

Furthermore, the patient may cough up the edema fluid in the form of foamy, blood-tinged sputum. As the airways narrow and the lungs grow heavier from the accumulation of fluid, the work of breathing increases, which puts an even greater strain on the already floundering heart. Dyspnea and hypoxemia produce a state of panic, which induces the release of epinephrine from the adrenals. The heart is pushed even harder, and its oxygen demand is increased precisely when fluid in the alveoli is reducing the amount of oxygen available.

To make matters worse, the sympathetic nervous system response produces peripheral vasoconstriction: Peripheral resistance (afterload) increases, and the weakened, hypoxic heart finds itself trying to push blood out into smaller and smaller pipes. Clinically, peripheral vasoconstriction is apparent as pallor and elevated blood pressure. The massive sympathetic discharge also produces sweating of the pale, cold skin.

It is not unusual for a patient with left-sided heart failure to become frantic from air hunger. He or she may pace or thrash about or may even be combative and struggle with the rescue team. Furthermore, hypoxemia results in inadequate oxygen supply to the brain, often manifested as confusion or disorientation. If hypoxemia is severe, cardiac arrest may follow quickly.

Signs and Symptoms of Left-Sided Heart Failure

The signs and symptoms of left-sided heart failure include extreme restlessness and agitation, confusion, severe dyspnea and tachypnea, tachycardia, abnormally high or low blood pressure, crackles and possibly wheezes, and frothy, pink sputum. Sometimes, it may be difficult to distinguish the wheezing of asthma from that of left-sided heart failure. **Table 27-13 ▲** presents some of the features that can help you differentiate the two conditions.

Management of Left-Sided Heart Failure

Prehospital treatment of left-sided heart failure is aimed at improving oxygenation, decreasing the workload of the heart, and reducing the volume of venous blood returned to the heart (the preload) so that the left ventricle is less overburdened.

Administer 100% supplementary oxygen and monitor oxygenation with pulse oximetry. For a patient with severe respiratory distress, this is preferably done via a bag-valve-mask device with positive end-expiratory pressure (with an attached PEEP valve), because positive pressure is helpful in driving fluid out of the alveoli. Positive airway pressure also reduces work for the heart, leading to improved stroke volume and improvement of heart failure symptoms. Many EMS programs are now introducing simplified continuous positive airway pressure (CPAP) devices with tightly fitting masks to improve oxygenation in patients with severe pulmonary edema and hypoxemia that does not respond to a nonrebreathing mask. If the patient will not tolerate either of those modalities or has only mild to moderate distress, then use a nonrebreathing mask.

Position the patient sitting up with the feet dangling, if possible. This position encourages venous pooling in the legs, thereby reducing venous return to the heart. The sitting position also makes breathing easier for a patient in respiratory distress.

Start a saline lock or an IV with normal saline at a TKVO rate. Also, attach cardiac monitoring electrodes, because patients in CHF are prone to arrhythmias.

Decisions regarding prehospital pharmacologic therapy of left-sided heart failure may vary slightly between regions, but the traditional drug therapy includes the drugs mentioned below. Some of these therapies will be guided by vital signs, specifically blood pressure, and thus this should be monitored closely. Refer to your local protocols/directives for specific therapies and dosing in your area.

Nitroglycerin is the mainstay of treatment for acute CHF exacerbation and the single medication that may reduce mortality, intubation rate, ICU admission rate, and myocardial infarction rate. This medication is usually given sublingually (supplied as 0.4-mg spray or 0.3-, 0.4-, or 0.6-mg tablets) as a single or double dose depending on the patient's blood pressure. It can also be delivered via an intravenous infusion (primarily in the hospital).

Nitroglycerin's direct effects are to first cause venodilation; at higher doses it causes arterial dilation. Indirectly, this may lead to a reduction in cardiac work and an improvement in cardiac output. The venodilation may result in venous pooling, thereby reducing the volume of blood returned from the periphery to the heart. This may reduce the amount of pulmonary edema being produced. The arterial dilation reduces the afterload, or the force the heart pumps against. This will reduce the strain on the heart and secondarily improve cardiac output. The initial dose of 0.4 mg or 0.8 mg may be repeated at 3- to 5-minute intervals with frequent blood pressure checks.

Furosemide (Lasix) is a diuretic that is used for symptomatic benefit in chronic heart failure, but it should be used cautiously in acute heart failure. As a diuretic, it removes excess fluid from the body by promoting its excretion by the kidneys. This may be useful if the patient is fluid overloaded, but it may take 30 minutes to have an effect. Large doses in acute CHF may lead to a reflexive increase in afterload, making the patient worse, in addition to worsening hypokalemia and causing hypovolemia. Rapid IV bolus of furosemide may also cause hypotension. Prehospital studies have shown that large doses can be deleterious; therefore, this medication should be used with caution in the prehospital setting. If ordered, furosemide is given in a dose of 20 to 40 mg or 0.5 to 1 mg/kg by IV bolus.

Morphine sulfate has long been part of the standard treatment of cardiogenic pulmonary edema, but it appears to have little benefit and may cause some harm. Morphine works as a vasodilator, increasing the pooling of blood in the periphery, and it also has a calming effect on a frantic patient. Prehospital studies have shown that the sedation may be detrimental and lead to a greater likelihood of intubation. Because vasodilation can be easily accomplished by nitroglycerin, this medication is rarely indicated. If morphine is ordered, first check the patient's blood pressure (do not give morphine if the patient is hypotensive). Then give approximately 2 mg slowly by IV bolus, and recheck the blood pressure. If the blood pressure remains stable, another 2 mg may be given. Proceed in that manner until the total dose ordered by the physician has been administered.

The presence of wheezing is common and may indicate that bronchoconstriction has developed from the excessive fluid. However, if the patient does not show substantial evidence of bronchoconstriction, bronchodilators should be avoided, because they all cause tachycardia, which can worsen the patient in CHF. If bronchoconstriction is significant, bronchodilator drugs such as salbutamol (Ventolin) or ipratropium bromide (Atrovent) may be ordered.

Under special circumstances, when transport will be prolonged and the patient's blood pressure is low, direct medical control may order an inotrope (drug that increases cardiac contractility) such as dopamine, which will increase blood pressure and/or CO. The dose is 5 to 20 mcg/kg/min by IV drip titrated to the desired blood pressure.

Transport the patient to the hospital in a sitting position, with legs dangling down.

Right-Sided Heart Failure

Right-sided heart failure most commonly occurs as a result of left-sided heart failure. As blood backs up from the left side of the heart into the lungs, the right side has to work increasingly harder to pump blood into the engorged pulmonary vessels. Eventually, the right side of the heart is unable to keep up with the increased workload, and it, too, fails. Right-sided heart failure may also occur as a result of pulmonary embolism or long-standing COPD, especially chronic bronchitis. The presence or absence of pulmonary edema on physical examination can often provide a helpful clue as to whether right-sided heart failure is secondary to left-sided heart failure (pulmonary edema present) or due to primary lung or right-sided heart problems (no pulmonary edema).

When right-sided heart failure occurs, blood backs up behind the right ventricle and increases the pressure in the systemic veins, causing them to become engorged. Distension can be seen in the veins visible on the surface of the body, such as the external jugular veins. Over time, as the pressure within the systemic veins increases, serum is forced out of the veins and into the surrounding tissues, producing edema. Edema is most likely to be visible in dependent parts of the body, such as the feet in a person who is sitting or standing or the lower back in a bedridden patient. Edema is also present in parts of the body that are *not* visible; a painful liver easily palpable in the right upper quadrant, for example, signals engorgement and swelling within that organ (hepatomegaly).

Right-sided heart failure, by itself, is seldom a life-threatening emergency. Usually it develops gradually over days to weeks; likewise, it requires days to weeks to reverse the process by slowly ridding the body of excess salt and water. Treatment in the prehospital environment of a patient with right-sided heart failure, therefore, is simply to make the patient comfortable, preferably in the semi-Fowler's position. Monitoring is always indicated in any patient with significant cardiac disease. If signs of associated left-sided heart failure are present, treat them as outlined in the previous section.

Cardiac Tamponade

The pericardium is a tough, fibrous membrane with the ability to stretch only up to a point. Normally, a small amount of pericardial fluid separates the pericardium and the outer surface of the heart. Cardiac tamponade occurs when excessive fluid accumulates within the pericardium, limiting the heart's ability to expand fully after each contraction and resulting in reduced CO. If unrecognized and untreated, this condition will reduce cardiac filling to the point that the heart is unable to circulate the blood.

Cardiac tamponade occurs when an effusion (fluid buildup) either occurs quickly or to such an extent that it causes hemodynamic compromise. It can occur as a result of tumours, pericarditis, or trauma to the chest. Pericarditis, for example, is an inflammatory or infectious process that can gradually result in excessive amounts of fluid accumulating in the pericardial space. Blunt or penetrating trauma can result in bleeding into the pericardial space, causing abrupt accumulation of blood.

Signs and Symptoms of Cardiac Tamponade

Signs and symptoms of cardiac tamponade vary depending on its cause. If the onset is gradual (as with pericarditis), the initial complaints might be dyspnea and weakness. If the cause is traumatic, the chief complaint might be chest pain. As the volume of fluid increases in the pericardium, the SV decreases, causing an initial drop in the systolic blood pressure. Eventually, the diastolic pressure will slowly rise, resulting in the classic symptom of narrowing pulse pressure. The initial drop in blood pressure is usually followed by an increase in HR, which leads to tachycardia. The heart sounds may be muffled or quieter than usual owing to the buildup of fluid, although this sign may be difficult to identify in the prehospital environment. The patient may experience jugular venous distension as well, owing to the backup of blood from the right side of the heart. The combination of narrowing pulse pressure (hypotension) along with jugular venous distension and muffled heart sounds is commonly known as the Beck's triad.

When cardiac tamponade is suspected, the most helpful clue on examination is to look for pulsus paradoxus. Pulsus paradoxus is an exaggeration of the usual drop in systolic blood pressure during inspiration. This can be noted by a drop in systolic blood pressure of more than 10 mm Hg or a weakening pulse with the patient's inspiration. Pulsus paradoxus can occur in conditions other than cardiac tamponade, but you should consider the diagnosis if it is present.

The ECG is of limited value in identifying cardiac tamponade. Aside from tachycardia, you might rarely see electrical alternans (alternating small- and large-amplitude QRS complexes). In addition, you might identify pulsus alternans (alternating strong and weak pulses). Muffled heart sounds, pulsus alternans, electrical alternans, and pulsus paradoxus are not common signs and so may be easily overlooked.

In trauma patients, you may have difficulty distinguishing between cardiac tamponade and tension pneumothorax as the cause of hypotension. One way to differentiate between the two is to remember that in cardiac tamponade the breath sounds will be equal and the trachea will be midline because the lungs are not affected.

Management of Cardiac Tamponade

The ultimate treatment for cardiac tamponade is pericardiocentesis, which involves inserting a needle or drain into the pericardium and then withdrawing fluid. Often, withdrawal of as little as 50 ml of fluid will result in significant improvement in the patient's condition. This technique is risky, and usually performed under ultrasound guidance in the ED or operating room. In the prehospital setting, treatment that will significantly enhance the patient's survival is rapid transport to a facility that can perform this procedure.

Supporting the patient's airway, breathing, and oxygenation during transport are essential. An IV fluid bolus of 500–1000 ml of saline might be ordered by direct medical control. When reporting to direct medical control, make sure that you identify all signs and symptoms that led you to believe the patient has cardiac tamponade so that the receiving hospital will be prepared to manage the patient.

Cardiogenic Shock

Cardiogenic shock occurs when the heart is so severely damaged that it can no longer pump a volume of blood sufficient to maintain tissue perfusion. An AMI nearly always produces some impairment of left ventricular function. When 25% of the left ventricular myocardium is involved in the AMI, left-sided heart failure usually develops. When 40% or more of the left ventricle has been infarcted, cardiogenic shock may occur. Thus, cardiogenic shock indicates extensive injury to the myocardium; accordingly, there is a high mortality rate. Transient cardiogenic shock can occur after resuscitation, for example, following return of spontaneous circulation (ROSC) after defibrillation

Table 27-14	Vasopressor Agents			
Drug	**Preparation**	**Concentration (mcg/ml)**	**Rate**	
Dopamine (Intropin)	400 mg in 250 ml normal saline	1,600	5 to 20 mcg/kg/min For 70 kg at 5 mcg/kg/min: 350 mcg/min (13 microdrops/min)	
Norepinephrine (Levophed)	4 mg in 250 ml D_5W	16	0.5 to 1.0 mcg/min (2–4 microdrops/min)	
Epinephrine (Adrenalin)	1 ml (1 mg) in 250 ml normal saline	4	2 to 10 mcg/min (30–150 microdrops/min)	

for VF. Other causes of cardiogenic shock can cause nonischemic problems, such as overdose of cardiac drugs (eg, beta blocker or calcium channel blocker), viral myocarditis, and peripartum cardiomyopathy of pregnancy.

Signs and Symptoms of Cardiogenic Shock

The signs and symptoms of cardiogenic shock are similar to those of most other kinds of shock. Because of the reduced cerebral perfusion, the patient is often confused or even comatose; if awake, he or she is likely to be restless and anxious. Massive peripheral vasoconstriction results in pale, cold skin, and poor renal perfusion is reflected in minimal or absent urine output. Pulse oximeter readings are frequently difficult to obtain in patients with cardiogenic shock, because the fingers and toes are barely perfused due to the intense vasoconstriction. Respirations are rapid and shallow, so auscultation usually reveals crackles throughout the chest, and the pulse is racing and thready.

As these compensatory mechanisms begin to fail, the blood pressure will fall, sometimes to less than 90 mm Hg systolic. However, this vital sign may be deceptive. In patients with preexisting hypertension, systolic pressures higher than 90 mm Hg may still be associated with cardiogenic shock. The goal in treatment of cardiogenic shock is to identify and support the patient before the blood pressure drops to the point where the shock becomes irreversible.

Management of Cardiogenic Shock

Treatment of cardiogenic shock focuses on improving oxygenation and peripheral perfusion without adding to the work of the heart. Administer 100% supplemental oxygen by mask or bag-valve-mask device. An advanced airway may be necessary if the patient is comatose. The addition of continuous positive airway pressure (CPAP) using a PEEP valve attached to a bag-valve-mask device or a CPAP/mask delivery system may be helpful to improve oxygenation in cases of cardiogenic shock associated with pulmonary edema, although the blood pressure may worsen when applied. Place the patient in a supine position unless pulmonary edema is present; in that case, the patient should be placed in the semi-Fowler's position.

Start an IV with normal saline at a TKVO rate. Direct medical control may order a trial of fluids to determine whether the shock includes a hypovolemic component if pulmonary edema is absent or mild. If so, rapidly infuse 100 to 200 ml of saline,

and closely monitor the patient's pulse, blood pressure, and LOC. Report those observations to the physician.

Apply monitoring electrodes and obtain a 12-lead ECG if available. Arrhythmias may bring about hypotension by causing severe disturbances in CO; thus, until major arrhythmias are corrected, you cannot be certain that the patient's hypotension is due to cardiogenic shock.

Depending on the distance to the hospital and local protocols, you may be asked to administer a vasopressor drug, such as one of those listed in **Table 27-14** ◂ . Dopamine is the most commonly used vasopressor by paramedics. In addition to increasing the blood pressure, most vasopressors will also act as an inotrope, which increases cardiac contractility. The infusion rate will depend on the patient's weight and response, but it is usually initiated at 5 mcg/kg/min, with a range of 5–20. The administration of dopamine or any other vasopressor drug requires careful titration and frequent monitoring of the blood pressure. Measure the blood pressure at least every 5 minutes. Slow the infusion if the systolic pressure rises to more than 90 or 100 mm Hg; speed up the infusion if the systolic pressure falls below 80 mm Hg.

Transport the patient expeditiously to the hospital. Except for the correction of life-threatening arrhythmias, there are no measures that can stabilize the condition of a patient in cardiogenic shock in the prehospital environment. Thus, a short scene time is essential.

Aortic Emergencies

The two most concerning aortic emergencies are aneurysm and dissection. The word aneurysm comes from a Greek word for *widening*; it refers to the dilation or outpouching of a blood vessel. The most common concern for paramedics is an expanding or ruptured aneurysm of the abdominal aorta and is not all that uncommon, especially in patients older than 50 years of age.

Dissection is a tear in the innermost wall of the artery, which leads to blood flow between the layers of the artery. It can block or restrict flow to branches of the artery and may eventually rupture. It is usually not associated with an aneurysm and is commonly found in the thoracic aorta. It is very rare, with fewer than 200 patients diagnosed in Canada annually.

Acute Dissection of the Aorta

The proximal aorta is subject to enormous hemodynamic forces. Anywhere from 60 to 100 times a minute, 60 minutes an hour, 24 hours a day—that is, around 40 million times a year—pulsatile waves of blood come pounding out of the left ventricle against the aortic walls. Over the years, that pounding takes its toll, producing degenerative changes in the media (the middle layer) of the aorta, especially the ascending aorta

Table 27-15	AMI Versus Aortic Dissection	
	AMI	**Aortic Dissection**
Onset of pain	Gradual, with prodromal symptoms	Sudden, without prodromal symptoms
Severity of pain	Increases with time	Maximal from the outset
Timing of pain	May wax and wane	Does not abate once it has started
Location of pain	Substernal; back is rarely involved	Back is often involved, between the shoulder blades
Clinical signs	Peripheral pulses equal	Blood pressure or pulse strength discrepancy between arms or decrease in a femoral or carotid pulse
	No neurologic signs	May have stroke symptoms

(the part of the aorta that rises from the heart toward the aortic arch). The degenerative changes are more pronounced with advancing age, in people with chronic high blood pressure, and in younger patients with connective tissue disorders (such as patients aged 20 to 40 years with Marfan syndrome). The resulting effect is to "unglue" the layers of the aortic wall from one another.

Eventually, the degenerative changes in the aortic media may lead to a disruption of the underlying intima (innermost layer of the artery). Tearing of the intima is most likely to occur in the portions of the thoracic aorta that are under the greatest stress—specifically, the ascending aorta just distal to the aortic valve (approximately 65% of cases) and the descending aorta just beyond the takeoff point of the left subclavian artery.

Once the intima is torn, the process of dissection, or separation of the arterial wall, often begins. With each ventricular systole, a jet of blood is forced into the torn arterial wall, creating a false channel between the intimal and medial layers of the wall. This channel is propagated distally and sometimes proximally along the length of the wall. If the dissection progresses back into the aortic valve, it may prevent the valve from closing, so that blood regurgitates back from the aorta into the left ventricle during systole. Recall that the coronary arteries branch off from the aorta just above the leaflets of the aortic valve; thus, if the valve is affected, coronary blood flow will likely be affected as well and may result in an AMI. If the dissection involves the takeoff point of the innominate, left common carotid, or left subclavian artery, blood flow through the affected artery or arteries will be compromised and may cause a stroke or arm ischemia.

Signs and Symptoms of Acute Dissection of the Aorta

The typical patient with a dissection is a middle-aged or older man with chronic hypertension, although dissection may occur during pregnancy and in younger patients with Marfan syndrome. By far, the most common chief complaint is chest pain, which is usually described as "the worst pain I have ever experienced," or as "ripping," "tearing," "sharp," or "like a knife." This pain comes on very suddenly and may be located in the anterior part of the chest or in the back between the shoulder

blades, and/or radiate into the posterior chest, back, or abdomen.

On the basis of the patient's description, it may be difficult to differentiate the chest pain of a dissection from that of an AMI, but a number of distinctive features may help. The pain of an AMI is often accompanied or preceded by other symptoms—nausea, "indigestion," weakness, and sweating—and tends to come on gradually, getting more severe with time and often being described as "pressure" rather than "stabbing." By contrast, the pain of aortic dissection usually becomes maximal within 1 minute, without prodromal symptoms, and often includes radiation into the back. **Table 27-15** summarizes the differences in the clinical presentations of AMI and aortic dissection.

Other signs and symptoms of dissection will depend on the site of the intimal tear and the extent of the dissection. In dissections of the ascending aorta, which tend to occur in younger patients previously in good health, one or more of the vessels of the aortic arch are usually compromised. Disruption of flow through the innominate artery, for example, is likely to produce a difference in blood pressure between the two arms. (If you don't routinely check the blood pressure in both arms, you'll never pick up that sign!) You may also find that one femoral or carotid pulse is missing or weak. Disruption of blood flow into the left common carotid artery may produce signs and symptoms of a stroke. When the dissection extends proximally to the ostia of the coronary arteries, coronary blood flow is apt to be compromised, and ECG changes of myocardial ischemia are likely. Death from dissection of the ascending aorta is nearly always a result of aortic rupture into the pericardium and resultant cardiac tamponade. In such a case, you will see the characteristic signs of cardiac tamponade: distended neck veins, hypotension, narrow pulse pressure, and muffled heart sounds.

Dissection of the descending aorta occurs more commonly in older patients, especially those with a history of hypertension. The pain is apt to be somewhat less severe when the descending aorta is involved; indeed, the patient may wait a few days before seeking help. The dissection usually proceeds distally, so the aortic arch is spared, which means that blood pressure discrepancies between the two arms are not part of the picture. The pulses in the lower extremities, however, may be affected.

Management of Acute Dissection of the Aorta

The goal of prehospital management in a suspected aortic dissection is primarily to provide adequate pain relief. In the hospital setting, medications will be given to lower the patient's blood pressure and reduce myocardial contractility to take some of the hemodynamic load off the aorta. Only in very unusual circumstances would such therapy be started in the prehospital environment, however, because it requires careful monitoring of intra-arterial pressure.

The steps of prehospital management in suspected aortic dissection are as follows:

- Calm and reassure the patient.
- Administer 100% supplemental oxygen by nonrebreathing mask.
- Insert an IV with a crystalloid solution.
- Apply monitoring electrodes and obtain an ECG rhythm strip.
- If the patient is not hypotensive, administer IV morphine sulfate, 2 mg at a time, up to a total dose of 10 mg during 10 to 15 minutes.
- Transport without delay. Nothing can be done to stabilize the patient's condition in the prehospital setting. He or she will need aggressive therapy in the intensive care unit and possibly surgery, so don't dawdle!

Expanding and Ruptured Abdominal Aortic Aneurysms

Abdominal aortic aneurysms (AAAs) affect approximately 2% of the population older than 50 years and account for 300 deaths each year in Canada. Most commonly, the aneurysm is located just distal to the renal arteries. An expanding aneurysm is, as the name implies, an aneurysm that is getting larger and producing symptoms by compressing on adjacent structures, although the aortic wall remains intact. When an aneurysm starts expanding and producing symptoms, one can assume that rupture is imminent.

Signs and Symptoms of Expanding and Ruptured AAAs

The typical patient with an AAA is a man in his late 50s or 60s. So long as the aneurysm is stable, the patient will usually be asymptomatic. When the aneurysm starts to expand, however, the patient becomes symptomatic, with the sudden onset of abdominal or back pain. When the pain is principally in the abdomen, it tends to centre on the umbilicus. Often, the pain may be located solely in the lower back, leading the patient to think he or she has "pulled a muscle" or otherwise injured the back. The pain is constant and moderate to severe; it cannot be relieved by changes in position. It tends to radiate into the thigh and groin. If the aneurysm is leaking blood into the retroperitoneal space, the patient may complain of an urge to defecate. In some patients, an episode of syncope heralds the onset of symptoms.

The most characteristic physical finding in an AAA is a pulsatile mass palpable in the abdomen. The patient is likely to be normotensive when first seen, but signs of shock, with or without hypotension, may develop rapidly if the aneurysm has ruptured.

Management of Expanding and Ruptured AAAs

Prehospital management of an expanding or ruptured aortic aneurysm is aimed at getting the patient to the hospital as expeditiously as possible because the definitive treatment requires urgent surgery. The key is to maintain a high index of suspicion whenever a middle-aged or older person presents with sudden back pain and a pulsatile abdominal mass. The

more likely problem in the prehospital environment in a conscious patient is a leaking aneurysm that has yet to rupture.

The steps of prehospital management in expanding or ruptured aortic aneurysm are as follows:

- Administer supplemental oxygen.
- Transport without delay.
- Insert an IV line en route (large-gauge cannula), and give normal saline or lactated Ringer's. Use a large-gauge cannula, but maintain the flow to keep the vein open unless signs of shock appear. If there are signs of shock, treat as for any other case of shock, with IV fluids only to bring the blood pressure up to 90 mm Hg (higher may cause more blood loss).

Hypertensive Emergencies

Hypertension (high blood pressure) afflicts nearly 1 in 5 Canadians, about 6 million people, yet almost half of those with hypertension do not know it because they have no symptoms. In addition, it is a major contributing cause in many cases of MI, CHF, and stroke. Most hypertension is the result of and in return causes advanced atherosclerosis or arteriosclerosis, which decreases the lumen of the arteries and reduces their elasticity. The resulting high afterload on the heart leads to an increase in filling volume and stimulates the Frank-Starling reflex, which raises the pressure behind the blood leaving the heart.

Hypertension is present when the blood pressure at rest is consistently greater than 140/90 mm Hg. Normal blood pressure is below 120/80 mm Hg. Many conditions, such as anxiety or pain, can transiently elevate a person's blood pressure (especially the systolic blood pressure), so a single blood pressure measurement taken during an emergency scarcely constitutes adequate grounds for telling a patient that he or she is hypertensive. Instead, one may say something like this: "Sir, your blood pressure is a little high right now. That may be because of the stress you are under and may not have any real significance. To be safe, you should have your blood pressure rechecked a couple of times in the next few months under less stressful circumstances."

Persistent elevation of the diastolic pressure, by contrast, is indicative of hypertensive disease. If left untreated, hypertension significantly shortens the life span and predisposes the patient to a variety of other medical problems. The most common complications of hypertension include renal damage, stroke, and heart failure—the last a result of the left ventricle having to pump for years against a markedly increased afterload.

Signs and Symptoms of Hypertensive Disease

In the majority of cases, hypertension is entirely asymptomatic and is detected during routine examination. By the time symptoms start to occur, hypertension is already in a more advanced stage and has probably produced at least some damage to organs such as the heart, kidneys, and brain.

The symptoms that occur in advanced hypertensive disease may be related to the elevated blood pressure or to secondary complications. Headache is the most common symptom directly related to blood pressure elevation; hypertensive headache is usually localized to the occipital region of the head and occurs when the patient first awakens in the morning, then subsides gradually over the next few hours. Other symptoms of moderately severe hypertension include dizziness, weakness, epistaxis, and blurring of vision. Often a patient with these hypertension-related signs and symptoms has already been prescribed medication for hypertension but it still may not be adequately controlled.

Management of Hypertensive Diseases

Hypertensive emergencies occur in about 1% of all hypertensive patients. A hypertensive emergency is defined as an acute elevation of blood pressure with evidence of end-organ damage. That last phrase is important, because it is the evidence of end-organ dysfunction that determines the urgency of the situation, not the reading on the sphygmomanometer. Two end-organ emergencies that may result from uncontrolled hypertension were discussed earlier in this chapter: left-sided heart failure and aortic dissection. A rare but just as devastating complication of hypertension is hypertensive encephalopathy.

Hypertensive encephalopathy (also known as acute hypertensive crisis) may complicate any form of hypertension. Hypertensive crisis is usually signaled by a sudden, marked rise in blood pressure to levels greater than 200/130 mm Hg. The determining factor for hypertensive encephalopathy is usually the mean arterial pressure (MAP). The MAP is calculated by adding one third of the difference between the systolic blood pressure (SBP) and diastolic blood pressure (DBP) to the diastolic blood pressure.

$$MAP = DBP + \tfrac{1}{3}(SBP - DBP)$$

When the MAP exceeds 150 mm Hg, the pressure may breach the blood-brain barrier with resultant fluid leaking out, increasing intracranial pressure. Usually the first symptoms noticed are severe headache, nausea, and vomiting. They are followed by seizures and alternations in mental status (that is, confusion to unresponsiveness). Sometimes patients may show focal neurologic signs, such as sudden blindness, aphasia (disturbances in speech production or comprehension), or hemiparesis. Widespread neuromuscular irritability may be signaled by muscle twitching. It is often difficult in the prehospital environment to differentiate hypertensive encephalopathy from intracerebral hemorrhage or other causes of coma.

The goal of treatment in hypertensive encephalopathy is to lower the blood pressure no more than one third in a controlled manner during a 30- to 60-minute period so that cerebral blood flow is restored to normal. Excessive lowering of the blood pressure can cause complications and must be avoided. That is best accomplished under controlled conditions in a hospital.

Thus, if you are within 20 to 30 minutes of the nearest hospital, provide supportive treatment only:

- Administer supplemental oxygen by nasal cannula or nonrebreathing mask and secure the airway if required.
- Establish an IV with normal saline at a TKVO rate.
- Apply monitoring electrodes, and run an ECG rhythm strip (consider running a 12-lead ECG en route to the ED).
- Transport without delay. Be prepared to deal with seizures en route, and have a benzodiazepine, such as diazepam (Valium) ready.

In some settings where the diagnosis is known, such as an interfacility transfer, paramedics may continue antihypertensive therapy initiative by the sending hospital. A commonly used drug for this purpose is labetalol, which has alpha- and beta-blocking properties. It can only be given if it is within your paramedic scope of practice, part of your medical directive, and with direct medical control. This drug should not be used by a paramedic for whom it is not within scope of practice, and only on orders from direct medical control. As an alpha blocker, labetalol prevents vasoconstriction, thereby decreasing the overall peripheral vascular resistance. Meanwhile, its beta-blocking actions prevent the reflex tachycardia that would otherwise occur in response to a drop in blood pressure. As a beta blocker, however, labetalol is relatively contraindicated in patients with asthma and COPD.

Labetalol can be given initially by slow IV push at 10–20 mg, repeated in 10 minutes as necessary, or an IV drip can be started. If delivered by infusion, watch the infusion like a hawk! A runaway IV could prove disastrous. Monitor the patient's blood pressure every 2 to 3 minutes. When the blood pressure has fallen to the target level specified by medical control physician, modify subsequent doses or the infusion rate.

The other drug that may be ordered to lower a dangerously high blood pressure is nitroglycerin, 0.4 mg sublingual. This drug is not the first choice for this indication, but its use is acceptable if labetalol is not available. Once again, use of nitroglycerin for this purpose depends on your medical directives and direct medical control.

Whenever you give a drug to lower a patient's blood pressure, keep the patient supine, and measure his or her blood pressure at least every 3 to 5 minutes. Record each measurement on a flowchart.

■ Cardiac Arrhythmias

Cardiac rhythm disturbances or arrhythmias **Table 27-16 ▶** may arise from a variety of causes; they are not solely caused by AMI. A cardiac arrhythmia is simply a disturbance in the normal cardiac rhythm, which may or may not be clinically significant. Sometimes arrhythmias are caused by ischemia, electrolyte imbalances, disturbances or damage in the electrical conduction system resulting in escape beats, circus reentry, or enhanced automaticity. Thus, it is always necessary to evaluate the arrhythmia in the context of the patient's overall clinical condition. Indeed, it is the patient's clinical condition—not the

Table 27-16	Causes of Cardiac Arrhythmias

- Myocardial ischemia or infarction
- Other forms of heart disease
- Rheumatic heart disease
- Cor pulmonale
- Generalized hypoxemia from any cause
- Autonomic nervous system imbalance
- Increased vagal tone
- Increased sympathetic output
- Distension of cardiac chambers (as in heart failure)
- Electrolyte disturbances, especially those involving
- potassium, calcium, or magnesium
- Drug toxicity
- Certain poisons (such as organophosphate insecticides)
- Central nervous system damage
- Hypothermia
- Metabolic imbalance
- Normal variations
- Trauma (such as cardiac contusions)

lines and squiggles on a piece of paper—that should ultimately determine whether treatment is necessary. Treat the patient, not the monitor!

One of the most important tasks in the prehospital care of a patient with an AMI is to anticipate, recognize, and treat life-threatening arrhythmias. Arrhythmias develop after an AMI for two principal reasons. First, irritability of the ischemic heart muscle surrounding the infarct may cause the damaged muscle to generate abnormal currents of electricity that cause abnormal cardiac contractions. When the arrhythmia arises from irritable spots in the myocardium (ectopic foci), it is usually a rapid arrhythmia (tachyarrhythmia), such as (VT), premature atrial contractions, or premature ventricular contractions (PVCs). Second, arrhythmias may occur after an AMI because the infarct damages the conduction tissues. In such a case, the abnormal rhythm is usually a block or a bradyarrhythmia.

Very slow HRs (< 40 to 50 beats/min) frequently lead to inadequate CO and often precede electrical instability of the heart. Furthermore, when the sinus rate becomes very slow, ectopic pacemakers in the AV node or ventricles may fire and produce escape beats to assist in maintaining CO.

Conversely, very rapid HRs (> 120 to 140 beats/min) increase the work of the heart, causing further myocardial ischemia and damage. Tachycardias may also be associated with decreased CO secondary to decreased SV because the ventricles have less time to fill between beats. Hypoxia, metabolic alkalosis, hypokalemia, and hypocalcemia can lead to electrical instability; cells that usually do not have automaticity may then begin to fire impulses. This kind of enhanced automaticity may occur with the use of drugs such as digoxin or atropine and is manifested by ectopic beats anywhere in the heart. The result is the potential for tachycardias, flutters, and fibrillations in the atria or ventricles, heralding grave rhythms such as VT and VF. Circus reentry can also be a serious problem **Figure 27-22 ▶** . The AV node may be bombarded by more than one impulse—potentially blocking the pathway for one impulse

and allowing the other to stimulate cardiac cells that have already depolarized. The danger here comes when these impulses get "stuck" in a pattern of repetition, causing multiple ectopic beats or VF.

ECG analysis is indicated in any patient who might have a cardiac-related condition or rapid or slow heart rate. Any patient with a chest pain should certainly undergo ECG analysis, but this monitoring should also be instituted for any patient with a history of heart problems. Given that age is a contributing factor to heart disease, ECG analysis is appropriate for elderly patients in many situations. Indeed, the ECG should be thought of as another vital sign, similar to the blood pressure or pulse oximetry.

ECG Monitoring: Placement of Leads and Electrodes

How reliable would ECG tracings or 12 leads be if the electrodes were placed anywhere on the patient? To maintain consistency in monitoring and obtaining a useful ECG, there are predetermined locations to place electrodes and leads.

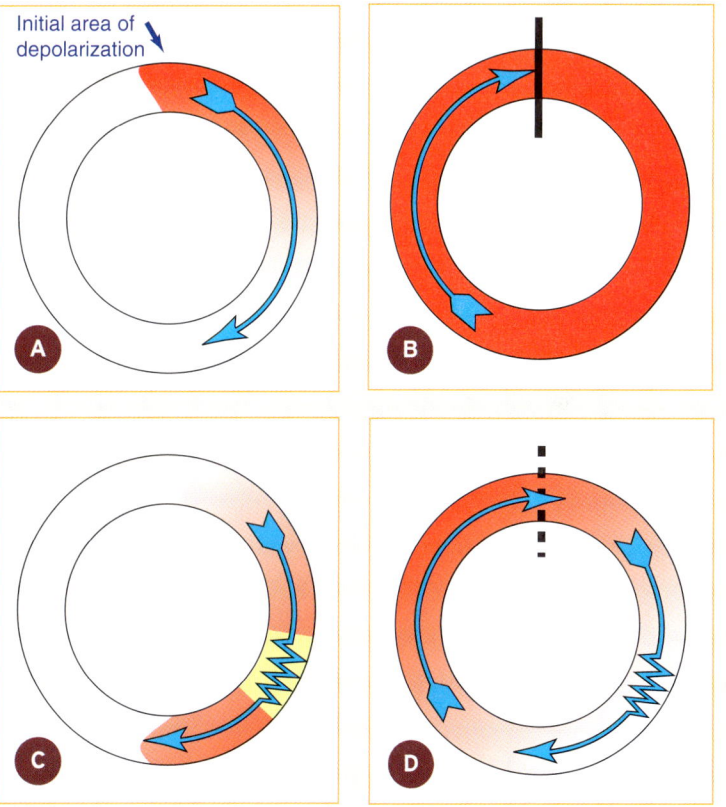

Figure 27-22 A. The original impulse site fires and triggers a depolarization wave that spreads throughout the rest of the cells in the direction shown. **B.** By the time the depolarization wave reaches the original site (represented by the black line) the original site is still refractory and cannot accept the new impulse. The depolarization wave essentially dies at this point. **C.** The area in yellow represents an area of slow conduction. The depolarization wave slows down as it traverses this area. **D.** By the time the depolarization wave reaches the original site (represented by the dotted black line) the original site is now ready to receive a new impulse. The result is a circus movement that is self-perpetuating.

Electrodes used in the prehospital setting are generally adhesive and have a gel centre to aid in skin contact. Some manufacturers offer a "diaphoretic" electrode that sticks to a sweating patient more effectively. Whichever type is used, certain basic principles should be followed to achieve the best skin contact and minimize artifact in the signal:

- To maintain the correct lead placement, it may be necessary to shave body hair from the electrode site. Don't be fooled by a hairy chest. It may appear that you have great skin contact initially, but the electrode will rise off the skin and stick to the hair. Shaving should also be done when using hands-free adhesive defibrillation pads.
- To remove oils and dead tissues from the surface of the skin, rub the electrode site briskly with an alcohol swab before application. Wait for the alcohol to dry before electrode application or dry it with a quick wipe of a gauze pad.
- Another trick of the trade to provide excellent skin contact is to gently scrape the electrode site with the disposable plastic backing of the electrode to "rough up" the skin cells before application.
- Attach the electrodes to the ECG cables before placement. Confirm that the appropriate electrode is attached to the appropriate cable (each cable is marked and colour coded as to the correct location for placement).
- Once all electrodes are in place, switch on the monitor, and print a sample rhythm strip. If the strip shows any "interference" (artifact), verify that the electrodes are firmly applied to the skin and the monitor cable is plugged in correctly.

Artifact on the monitor can be tricky. A straight-line ECG in an alert, communicative patient indicates a loose or disconnected lead, not asystole (flat line). Similarly, a wavy baseline resembling VF may be caused by patient movement or muscle tremor. Before you lunge for the defibrillator paddles, look at the patient! If he or she is alert and in no obvious distress, recheck the leads and equipment.

Although acquisition of a 12-lead ECG in the prehospital setting is becoming a standard of care, you will still need to monitor the patient's heart rhythm using one of three leads. A lead offers an electrical snapshot of certain parts of the heart. The standard is to use one of the "bipolar" leads for monitoring purposes—that is, lead I, II, or III. Generally, lead II will give the best overall view of the PQRST complexes. Bipolar leads (that is, "limb leads") consist of two electrodes, one positive and one negative, that are placed on two different limbs. When using bipolar leads, any impulse in the body moving to a positive electrode will cause a positive deflection on the ECG.

At the Scene

Here are two easy ways to remember cable placement: "White is on the right, smoke (black) is over fire (red)" (on the left) or (starting on the right) "salt (white), pepper (black), ketchup (red)."

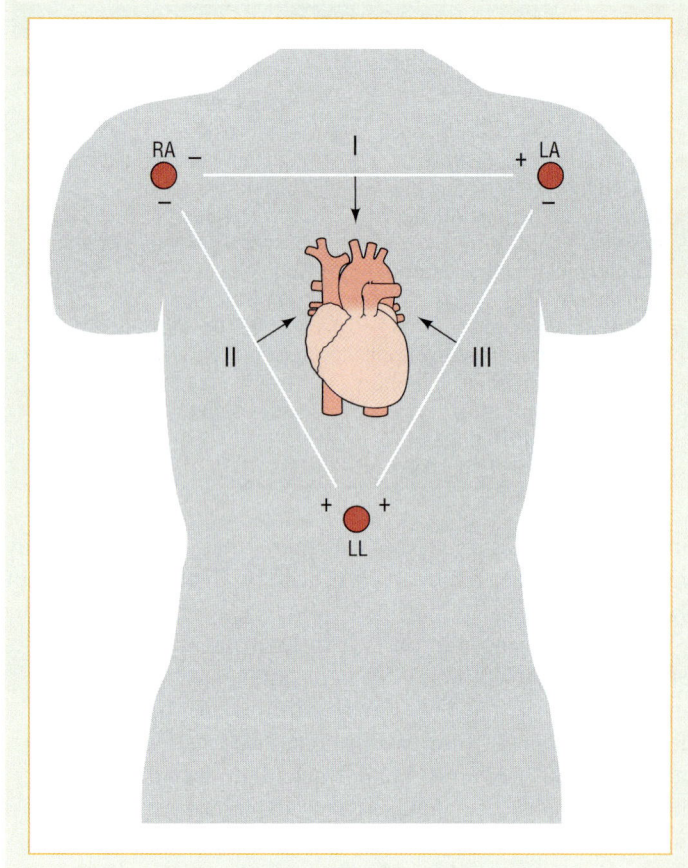

Figure 27-23 The Einthoven triangle.

Conversely, if an impulse is moving toward a negative electrode, it will result in a negative deflection on the ECG tracing. If the electrical impulse changes direction, you may see a "biphasic" waveform, which is above and below the isoelectric baseline. A lack of electrical impulse or an impulse that is perpendicular to the lead will produce an isolectric or flat line.

When correctly positioned on the chest, these leads form a triangle around the heart, called the Einthoven triangle **Figure 27-23 ▲**. Today, it is not necessary to change the electrical poles of the electrodes to get a different lead. ECG monitors have the ability to change the polarity of the leads so that we can view leads I, II, and III by turning a knob or pressing a button.

Reading an ECG Rhythm Strip

The most reliable method of analyzing a rhythm strip is to use a systematic approach and examine every strip the same way. By using such an approach, you will find in most cases that even the most complex-appearing arrhythmias can be reduced to simple terms and can be identified correctly.

ECGs are recorded on standardized graph paper, which is moved past a stylus at a standardized speed (25 mm/s). Thus, a given distance on the graph paper represents a given time. Specifically, one small (1 mm) square is equivalent to 0.04 second

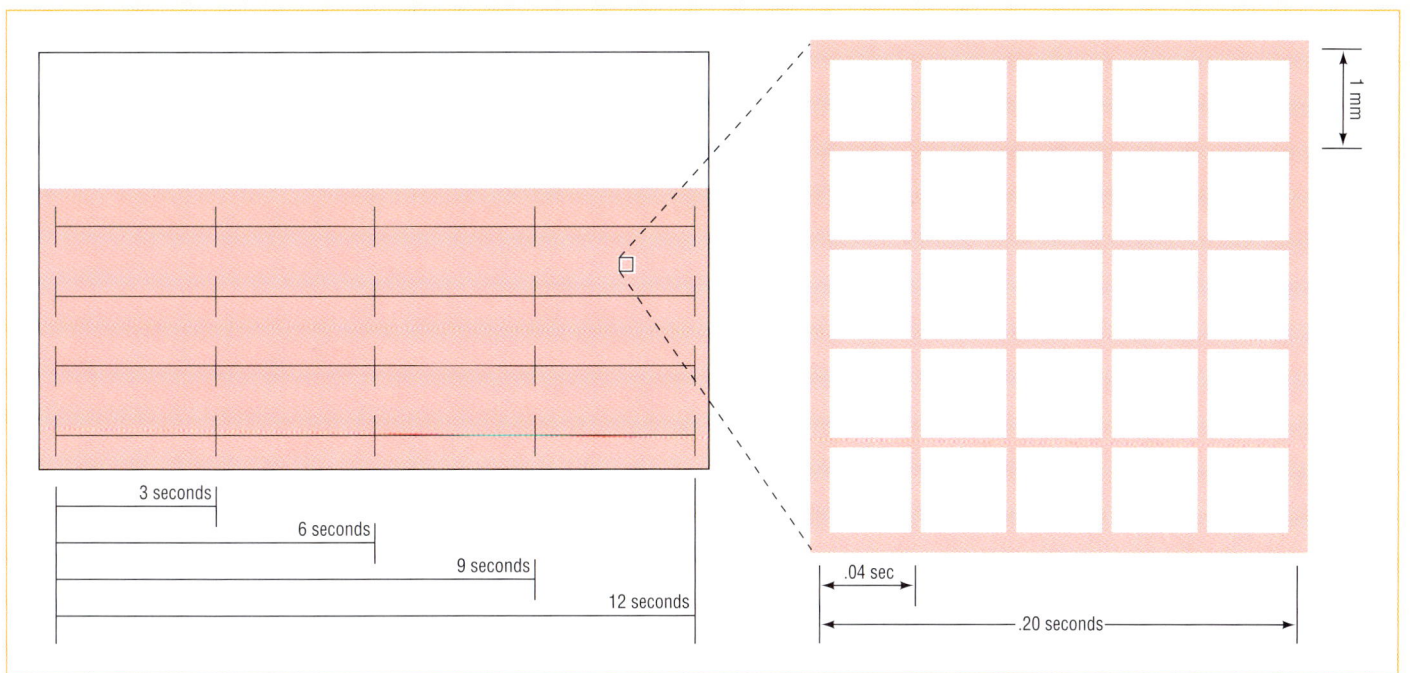

Figure 27-24 ECG paper. Height (amplitude) is measured in millimeters (mm) and width in seconds (s).

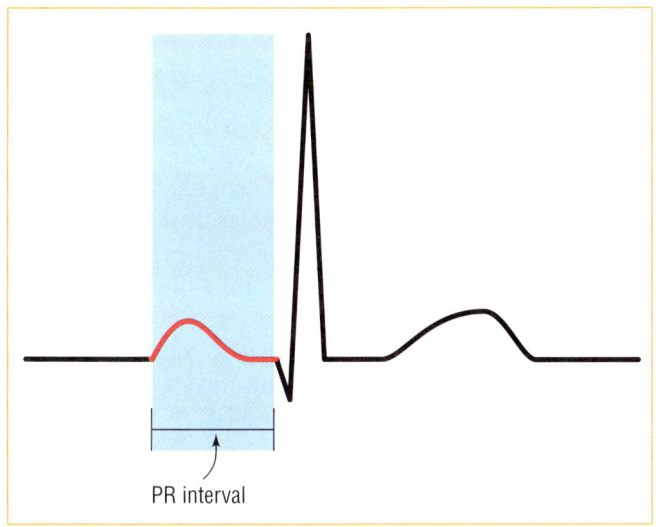

Figure 27-25 The normal P-R interval is 0.12 to 0.20 s.

(1/25th of a second), and one large square (which consists of five small squares) is equivalent to 0.20 second (0.04 × 5 = 0.20) **Figure 27-24** .

Components of an ECG Complex

Let's break down the ECG waveforms into their individual components.

P Wave

The P wave is normally a small, upright waveform (in leads I and II). It immediately precedes the QRS. The P wave is formed as the impulse is generated by the SA node in the right atrium and spreads over the atria, causing depolarization. Typically lasting only 0.06 to 0.11 s, P waves can give clues to the pacemaker site if they are missing or do not have a uniform appearance.

If there are no P waves, the pacemaker for the heart is not in the SA node, and one must consider the possibility of atrial fibrillation or a junctional or ventricular rhythm. If a P wave is present but not followed by a QRS complex, a block is present somewhere in the AV junction or below and is preventing conduction from the atria to the ventricles. P waves that vary in size and configuration mean that there are several pacemaker sites at different locations throughout the atria.

P-R Interval

The PRI includes atrial depolarization and the conduction of the impulse through the AV junction. It includes the slight delay that normally occurs when the impulse is held in the AV node, allowing time for ventricular filling **Figure 27-25** .

The PRI is measured from the start of the P wave to the point at which the QRS complex begins. Although it normally lasts 0.12 to 0.20 s (three to five small squares on the ECG strip), the PRI may be prolonged and give clues that the AV node is diseased or damaged, as in an MI **Figure 27-26** . A PRI that exceeds 0.20 s (five small squares), for example, is called first-degree AV block and may indicate injury to the AV junction. A PRI may also be shorter than 0.12 s in cases of Wolff-Parkinson-White syndrome, when the AV node is bypassed altogether.

QRS Complex

The QRS complex, which consists of one to three waveforms, represents depolarization of two simultaneously contracting ventricles. It is measured from the beginning of the Q wave to

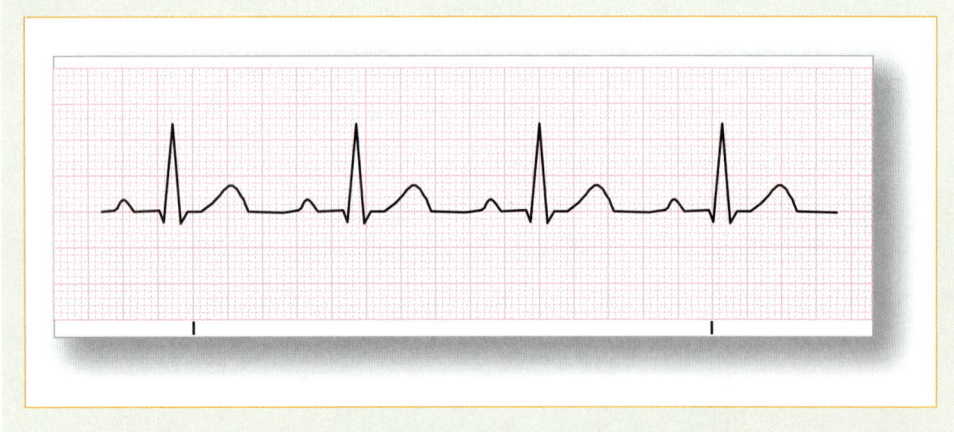

Figure 27-26 A P-R interval greater than 0.20 s is considered prolonged.

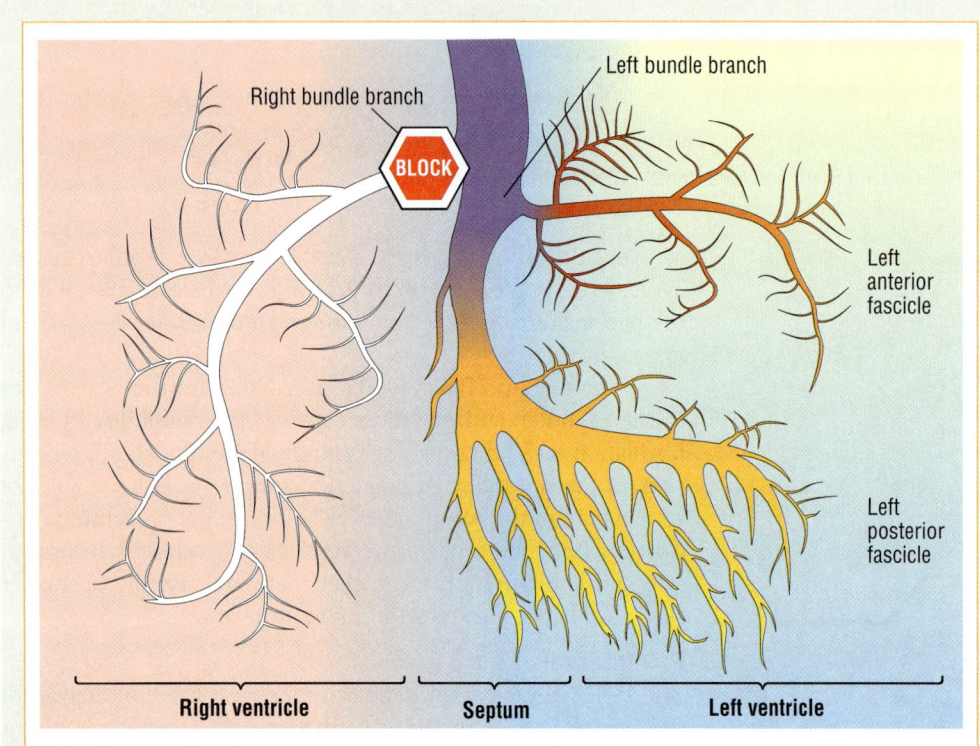

Figure 27-27 Bundle branch block.

septum. The electricity spreads from right to left through the septum. The first upward deflection of the QRS is referred to as the R wave. Most of both ventricles are depolarized during the R wave. The R wave may be wide if the ventricle is enlarged and may be abnormally high if ventricular hypertrophy is present. The S wave is any downward deflection after the R wave. If the S wave is abnormally large, it may indicate hypertrophy of the ventricles. If there is a second upward deflection, it is called an R-prime (R′) wave. R-prime waves are never normal, and they indicate trouble in the conduction system of the ventricle.

Q waves are abnormal or pathologic if they are one small square (0.04 s) wide on the ECG strip. Likewise, if they are deeper than one third of the total height (amplitude) of the QRS complex (in lead II), they are abnormal. This finding is significant when looking at 12-lead ECGs because it may indicate a current or previous AMI.

J Point

The J point is the point in the ECG where the QRS complex ends and the ST segment begins. Thus, it represents the end of depolarization and the apparent beginning of repolarization. In some cases, locating the J point may make it easier to identify the ST segment when you are looking for elevation (another clue to an AMI).

ST Segment

The ST segment, which is the line between the QRS complex and the beginning of the T wave, is normally isolectric. An ST segment that is significantly (> 1 mm or one small square) above or below the isoelectric line is highly suggestive of myocardial ischemia or injury, although a full 12-lead ECG is required to determine the precise significance of ST segment elevation or depression.

T Wave

A T wave represents ventricular repolarization, but may also show abnormalities such as those found with electrolyte disturbances. In hyperkalemia, for example, the T wave may be tall and sharply peaked.

The T wave represents a time when the conduction system is in a state of relative refractoriness, which means that the cells are partially repolarized. Early in the T wave, the cells will not

the end of the S wave and should follow each P wave in a consistent manner.

In healthy people, the QRS complex is narrow, with sharply pointed waves, and has a duration of less than 0.12 s (three small squares on the ECG strip). Such a complex indicates that conduction of the impulse has proceeded normally from the AV junction, through the bundle of His, left and right bundles, and the Purkinje system. If abnormal, the complex has a bizarre appearance and a duration longer than 0.12 s. It signifies some abnormality in conduction through the ventricle as in a bundle branch block **Figure 27-27**.

The first downward deflection in the QRS is called a Q wave; this wave represents conduction through the ventricular

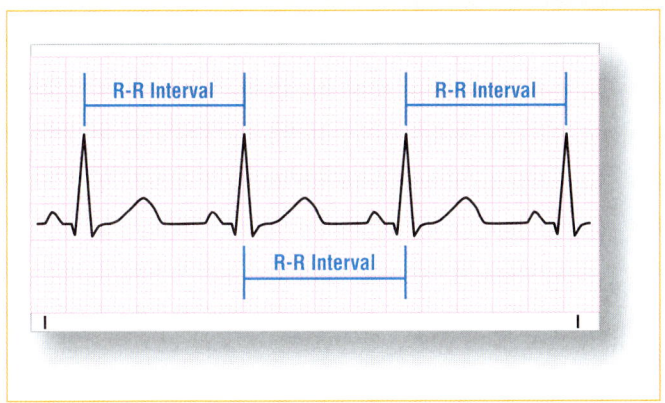

Figure 27-28 When the rhythm is regular, the R-R intervals are the same.

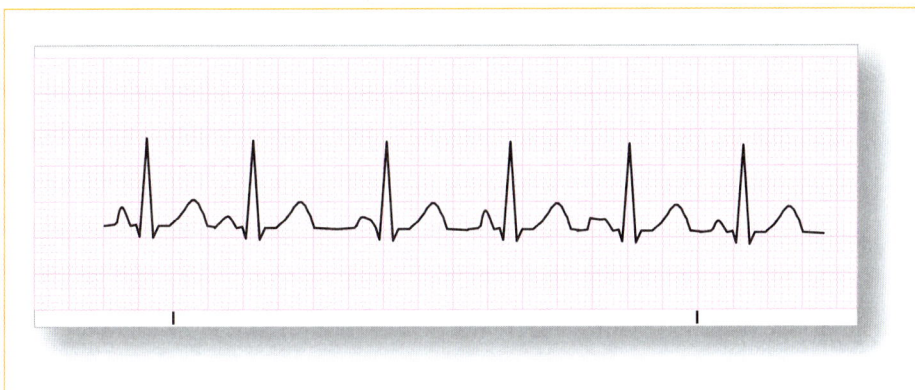

Figure 27-29 In an irregular rhythm, not all R-R intervals are the same.

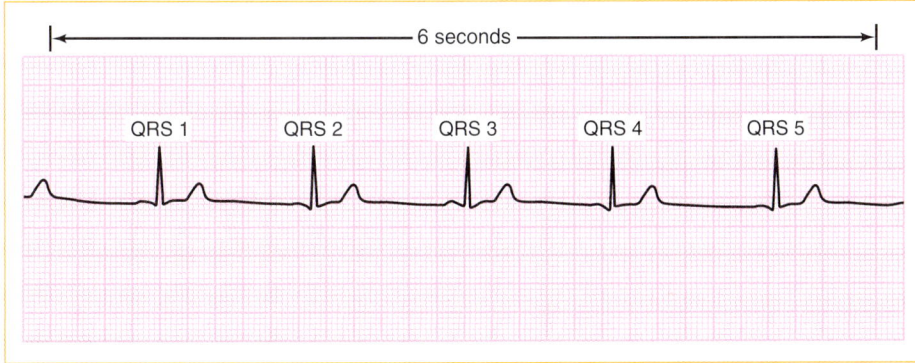

Figure 27-30 Calculation of rate. To calculate the rate, multiply the number of QRS complexes in a 6-second strip by 10.

accept another impulse. However, on the down slope (the vulnerable period), a strong impulse could cause depolarization, overpowering the primary pacemaker to take over the pacemaker control. The supernormal phase is the time near the end of the T wave (the last one third), just before the cells become completely repolarized. During this period, a stimulus weaker

than normally required can cause depolarization, resulting in a dangerous heart rhythm.

This behaviour of the T wave is the main reason there are "synch" (synchronize) buttons on monitors and defibrillators. When using the cardioversion technique on a rhythm that has regular T waves, you must press the synch button so that the shock will be delivered during the safest period of the ECG, away from the T wave.

Q-T Interval

The Q-T interval includes all activity that occurs during the QRS complex and T wave (that is, ventricular depolarization and repolarization). It begins with the onset of the Q wave and ends with the T wave as it comes back to the isoelectric line. If there is no Q wave, measurements begin with the R wave.

The Q-T interval normally lasts 0.36 to 0.44 s. A prolonged Q-T interval (long Q-T syndrome) indicates that the heart is experiencing an extended refractory period, making the ventricle more vulnerable to arrhythmias. Such prolongation may occur with administration of some drugs, hypocalcemia, an AMI, pericarditis or congenital conditions. Conversely, the Q-T interval may be shortened in hypercalcemia and in patients taking digoxin.

Regular or Irregular: That Is the Question!

What makes a rhythm irregular? When the rhythm is regular, the R-R intervals are the same. How much variability is allowed within R-R intervals? The distinction between regular and irregular rhythms is not always clear-cut. It is acceptable to have less than 0.12 s (three small squares) variance between the shortest and longest R-R interval to be able to call a rhythm regular **Figure 27-28**. If there is a gap of 0.12 s or more between the shortest and longest R-R intervals, however, the rhythm is considered irregular **Figure 27-29**.

Determining Heart Rate

This section describes some of the more common methods of determining the rate of a cardiac rhythm strip.

The 6-Second Method

The 6-second method is the simplest and most accurate method when the rhythm is irregular or very slow (< 60 beats/min):

■ Count the number of QRS complexes in a 6-second strip, and multiply that number by 10 to obtain the rate per minute **Figure 27-30**.

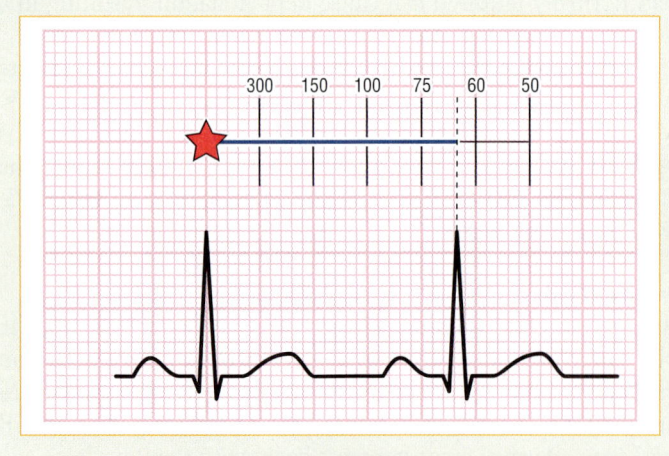

Figure 27-31 The sequence method.

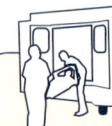
The Sequence Method

The sequence method **Figure 27-31 ▲** is commonly used for regular rhythms and strips less than 6 s long:

- Calculate the rate by first memorizing the following sequence: 300, 150, 100, 75, 60, 50.
- Find an R wave on a heavy line (large square), and count off "300, 150, 100, 75, 60, 50" for each large square you land on until you reach the next R wave. (Estimate the rate if the second R wave doesn't fall exactly on a heavy black line.)
- If the R-R interval spans fewer than three large squares, the rate is greater than 100 (tachycardia). If it covers more than five large squares, the rate is less than 60 (bradycardia).

The Grid Method

The grid method is completely accurate only when the rhythm is absolutely regular:

- Calculate the rate by counting the number of large squares between any two QRS complexes (the R-R interval), and then divide that number into 300.
- In Figure 27-32, for example, there are approximately 5.6 large squares between two successive QRS complexes; 300/5.6 = 54, so the rate would be about 54 beats/min.

Systematic Analysis of the ECG Rhythm Strip

So, now we are to the point of using a systematic approach to the ECG and examining every strip the same way. When examining the rhythm strip, proceed in the following, stepwise manner:

1. Are QRS complexes present? Are they normal or abnormal in shape and duration (or width)? Are they all the same?
2. Are there P waves? Is there a P wave before every QRS complex and a QRS complex after every P wave? Do all of the P waves look

the same? Based on the information on P and QRS waves, what is the pacemaker site?
3. What is the PRI? Is it prolonged? Shortened? Does it vary?
4. Is the rhythm regular or irregular? Are the R-R intervals equal? Often one can determine whether the rhythm is irregular at a casual glance, but sometimes it will be necessary to measure the R-R intervals and compare them (special ECG calipers are available for that purpose).
5. What is the rate? The normal HR is considered to be between 60 and 100 beats/min. Rates less than 60 per minute are generally called bradycardia **Figure 27-32 ▾** ; rates greater than 100 per minute are called tachycardia **Figure 27-33 ▶** .

Specific Cardiac Arrhythmias

Cardiac arrhythmias can be induced by a variety of events. Many can be traced to ischemia in the heart, especially in areas related to the cardiac conduction system. Often ischemia will cause a particular area of the heart to spontaneously depolarize, resulting in a premature complex. These premature complexes interfere with the normal conduction of impulses and produce arrhythmias. In other situations, the ischemia occurs within the conduction system itself, causing it to malfunction directly.

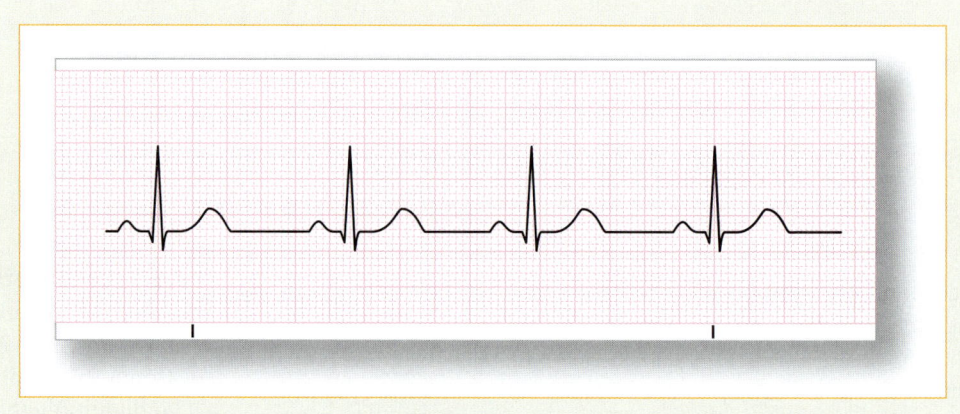

Figure 27-32 A HR less than 60 beats/min is considered bradycardia.

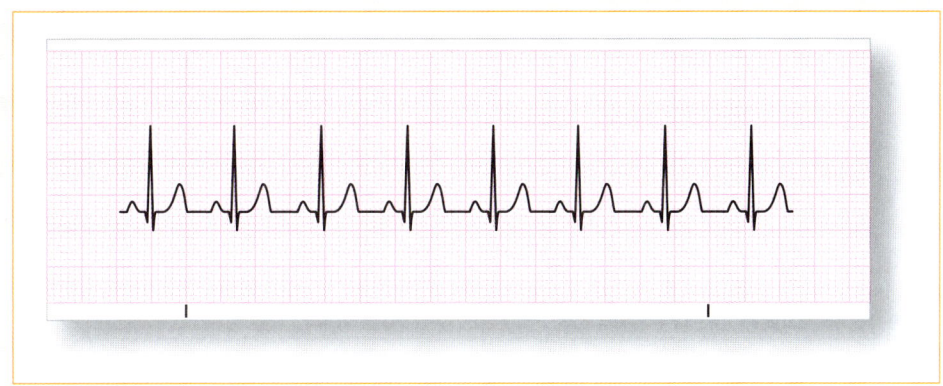

Figure 27-33 A HR greater than 100 beats/min is considered tachycardia.

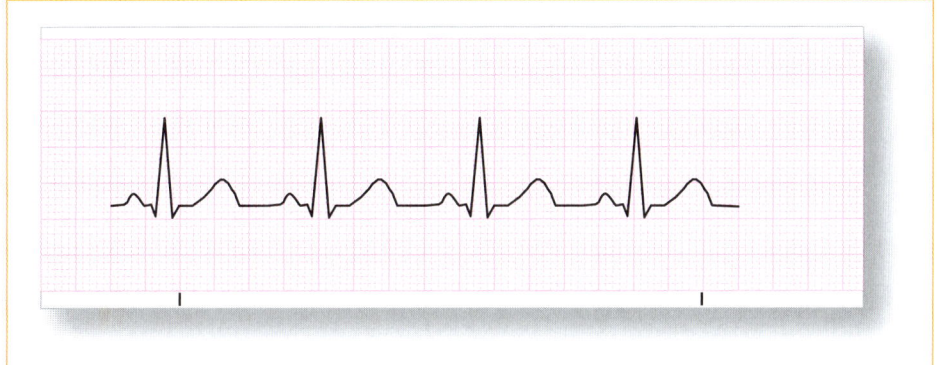

Figure 27-34 Normal sinus rhythm.

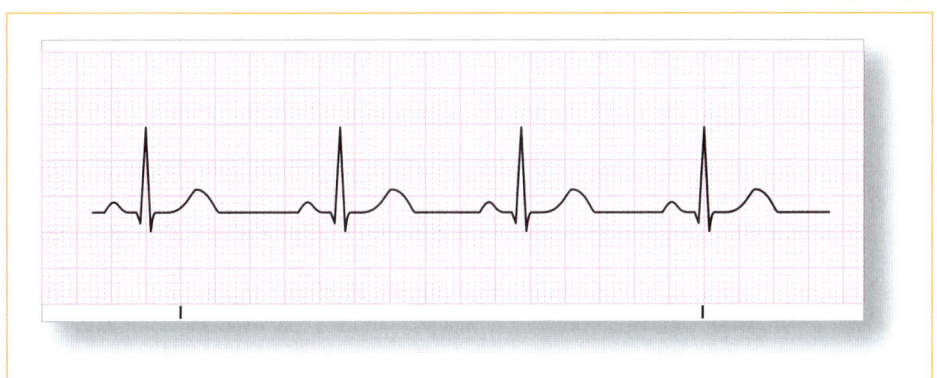

Figure 27-35 Sinus bradycardia.

according to whether they are disturbances of automaticity or disturbances of conduction, whether they are tachyarrhythmias or bradyarrhythmias, or whether they are life threatening or non–life threatening. In this text, we will study the cardiac arrhythmias based on the site from which they arise (and as they appear in lead II). After looking at a normal sinus rhythm for comparison, we will consider the arrhythmias that arise in the SA node, those that arise in the atrial tissue, those that arise in the AV junction, and so on, down the conduction pathway.

Rhythms of the SA Node

Normal Sinus Rhythm

The SA node is the primary pacemaker for the heart. A normal sinus rhythm Figure 27-34 ◀ has an intrinsic rate of 60 to 100 beats/min. The rhythm is regular, with minimal variation between R-R intervals. The P wave is present, is upright, and precedes each QRS complex. The PRI will measure 0.12 to 0.20 s. The QRS complex will measure 0.04 to 0.12 s.

Sinus Bradycardia

In sinus bradycardia, the pacemaker is still the SA node, but with a rate of less than 60 beats/min Figure 27-35 ◀. The rhythm is regular, and P waves are present and upright, preceding every QRS complex. The PRI is 0.12 to 0.20 s. The QRS complex is 0.04 to 0.12 s.

Sinus bradycardia can be an asymptomatic phenomenon in healthy adults and conditioned athletes and may be exhibited during sleep. More serious causes include hypothermia; SA node disease; AMI, which may stimulate vagal tone (parasympathetic stimulation); increased intracranial pressure; and use of beta blockers, calcium channel blockers, morphine, quinidine (including interactions between quinidine and some calcium channel blockers), or digoxin.

In general, treatment focuses on the patient's tolerance to the bradycardia and looking for causative factors. Atropine may be necessary. Patients who are symptomatic and do not respond to atropine may require a transcutaneous pacemaker to assist the heart in increasing its ventricular rate.

It is difficult to estimate the number of people affected by cardiac arrhythmias because many arrhythmias are well tolerated and cause no serious effects. It is well documented, however, that cardiac arrhythmias are the most common cause of cardiac arrest.

There are nearly as many systems for classifying cardiac arrhythmias as there are cardiologists who have written books on the subject. Arrhythmias may, for example, be categorized

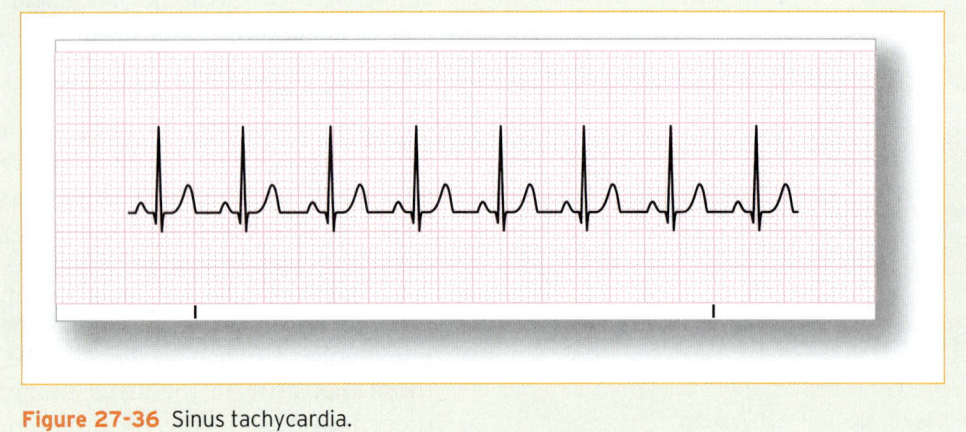

Figure 27-36 Sinus tachycardia.

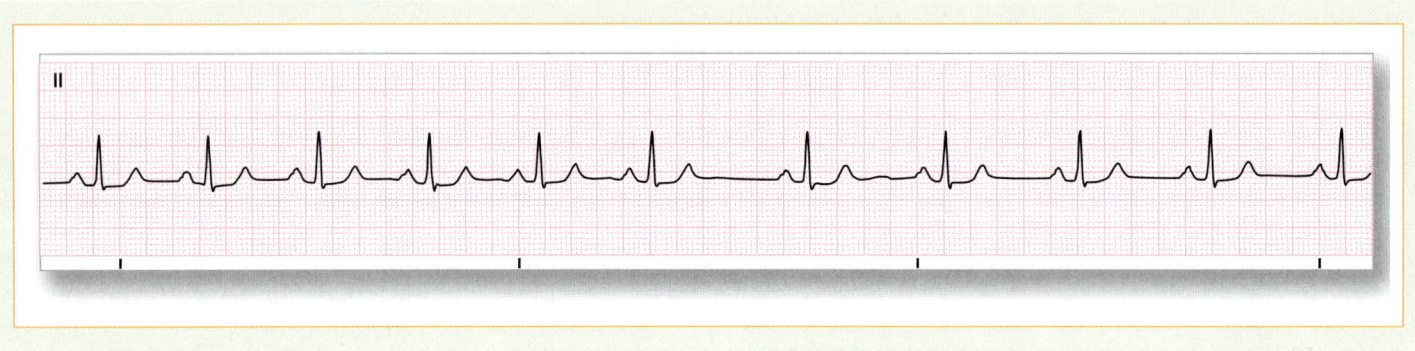

Figure 27-37 Sinus arrhythmia.

Sinus Arrhythmia

Sinus arrhythmia is defined as a slight variation in cycling of a sinus rhythm, usually one that exceeds 0.12 s between the longest and shortest cycles **Figure 27-37 ▾**. The SA node is still the pacemaker; P waves are present and upright, preceding every QRS complex; and a PRI of 0.12 to 0.20 s still exists. The QRS complex is 0.04 to 0.12 s.

Sinus arrhythmia is often somewhat more prominent with fluctuation in the respiratory cycle because the HR accelerates with inspiration and slows with expiration. Increased filling pressures of

Sinus Tachycardia

The SA node is still the pacemaker in sinus tachycardia but demonstrates a rate of more than 100 beats/min **Figure 27-36 ▴**. The rhythm is regular, and P waves are present and upright, preceding every QRS complex (although they may occasionally be difficult to see if they are partially buried in the T wave of the beat before them). The PRI is 0.12 to 0.20 s. The QRS complex is 0.04 to 0.12 s.

Sinus tachycardia may result from a variety of causes, including pain, fever, hypoxia, hypovolemia, exercise, stimulation of the sympathetic nervous system (such as by stress, fright, or anxiety), an AMI, pump failure, or anemia. In addition, certain drugs (such as atropine, epinephrine, amphetamines, and cocaine), caffeine, nicotine, and alcohol can cause tachycardia.

Prolonged tachycardia will increase the work of the heart, leading to further ischemia and infarction during an AMI. In addition, CO may be significantly reduced when the HR exceeds 120 to 140 beats/min because the ventricles do not have enough time between contractions to fill completely with blood. The treatment of sinus tachycardia is related to the underlying cause. The use of medications to reduce the heart rate in sinus tachycardia without treating the underlying cause can be dangerous, so take care to think about why the patient has sinus tachycardia.

the heart during inspiration stimulate the Bainbridge reflex, which increases the HR and is partially responsible for respiratory sinus arrhythmia. The increased filling pressure on the heart increases SV (remember the Frank-Starling mechanism) and blood pressure. The increase in blood pressure stimulates the baroreceptor reflex (baroreflex), which attempts to block the rate increase caused by the Bainbridge reflex. In this way, the baroreflex inhibits the respiratory sinus arrhythmia.

Sinus arrhythmia is often a normal finding in children and young adults and tends to diminish or disappear with age.

Sinus Arrest

Sinus arrest occurs when the SA node fails to initiate an impulse, eliminating the P wave, QRS complex, or/and T wave for one cardiac cycle **Figure 27-38 ▸**. After this missed set of complexes, the SA node resumes normal functioning just as if nothing ever happened. In sinus arrest, the atrial and ventricular rates are usually within normal limits and the rhythm is regular except for the absent complexes. P waves are present and upright, preceding every QRS complex, and the PRI, when present, is 0.12 to 0.20 s. The QRS complex, when present, is 0.04 to 0.12 s.

Common causes of sinus arrest include ischemia of the SA node, increased vagal tone, carotid sinus massage, and use of drugs such as digoxin and quinidine. Occasional episodes of sinus arrest are not significant; however, if the HR drops below

30 to 50 beats/min, the CO may fall and an ectopic focus from the ventricles may take over. In such a case, treatment is based on the overall HR and tolerance by the patient and may include a temporary pacemaker (a transcutaneous pacer in the prehospital environment and/or a transvenous pacer in the ED) or a permanent pacemaker once the patient is admitted to the hospital.

Sick Sinus Syndrome

Sick sinus syndrome (SSS) encompasses a variety of rhythms that involve a poorly functioning SA node and is common in elderly patients. On an ECG, SSS announces itself in many ways, including sinus bradycardia, sinus arrest, SA block, and alternating patterns of extreme bradycardia and tachycardia (bradycardia-tachycardia syndrome). As a result of SSS, some patients may experience a syncopal or near-syncopal episode, dizziness, and palpitations. Other patients remain asymptomatic. This is often managed with a permanent implanted pacemaker.

Rhythms of the Atria

Although the SA node is normally the pacemaker for the heart, any area in the atria may originate an impulse, thereby usurping the pacemaking authority of the SA node within the body's electrical conduction system. Rhythms originating from the atria will have upright P waves that precede each QRS complex but that are not as well rounded as those coming from the SA node. Atrial rhythms generally result in HRs of 60 to 100 beats/min.

Wandering Atrial Pacemaker

In wandering atrial pacemaker, as the name suggests, the pacemaker of the heart **Figure 27-39 ▸** moves from the SA node to various areas within the atria. Wandering atrial pacemaker usually has a rate of 60 to 100 beats/min. The rhythm is slightly irregular, with variations between R-R intervals based on the site of the pacemaker for that particular complex. The P wave is present and upright and precedes each QRS complex; however, the shapes of the P waves vary as an indication of their different sites of origin. The definition of wandering atrial pacemaker depends on having at least three different shapes of P waves within one ECG strip. The PRI will measure 0.12 to 0.20 s, but will also vary slightly based on the origin of the particular complex. The QRS complex will measure 0.04 to 0.12 s.

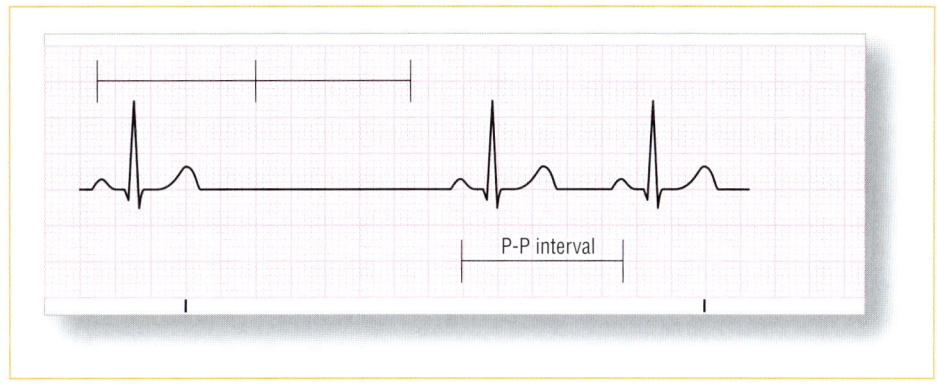

Figure 27-38 Sinus arrest.

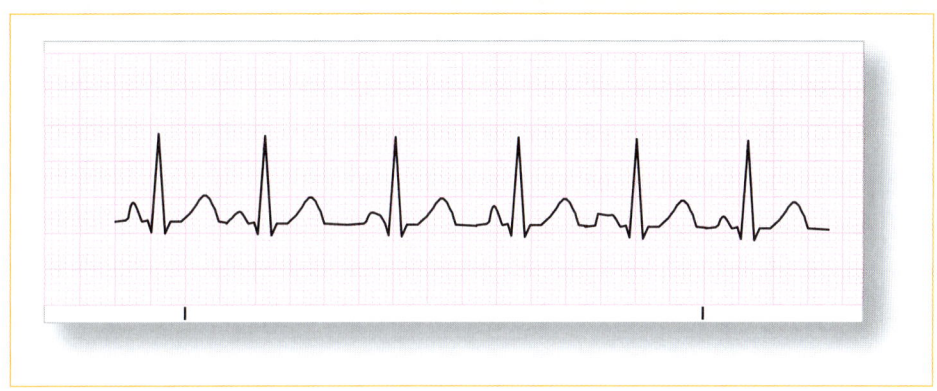

Figure 27-39 Wandering atrial pacemaker.

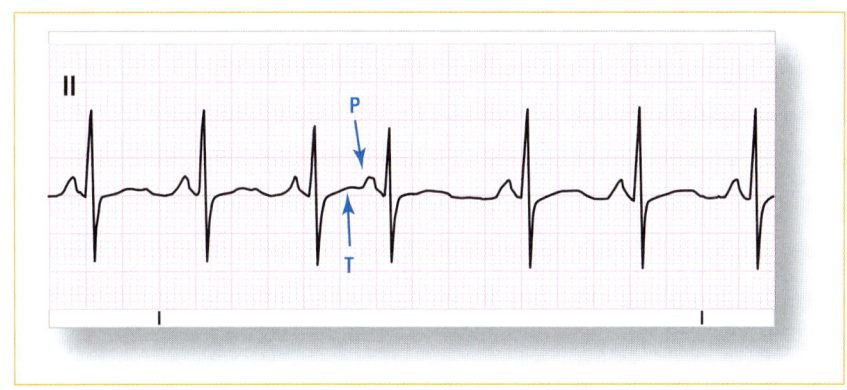

Figure 27-40 Premature atrial complex.

Wandering atrial pacemaker is most commonly seen in patients with significant lung disease. Treatment is usually not indicated in the prehospital setting, although the rhythm is an indication of likely future cardiac complications.

Premature Atrial Complex

A premature atrial complex (PAC) is not, strictly speaking, an arrhythmia, but rather the existence of a particular complex within another rhythm **Figure 27-40 ▲**. Premature atrial complexes are also known as ectopic complexes, meaning that they occur out of the normal location. A PAC occurs earlier in time than the next expected sinus complex, leading to an abnormally short R-R interval between it and the previous complex. Because the HR depends on the underlying rhythm, the presence of a PAC will make the rhythm irregular. The P wave is present and upright and precedes each QRS complex; however, its shape differs from the shapes of the P waves originating from the SA node, as an indication of its different site of origin. The PRI will measure 0.12 to 0.20 s but may vary slightly based on the origin of the premature complex. The QRS complex will measure 0.04 to 0.12 s.

A PAC can be caused by use of a variety of drugs (including caffeine), or it may result from organic heart disease. It is not usually treated in the prehospital setting but may be a predictor of future cardiac arrhythmias.

Supraventricular Tachycardia

Supraventricular tachycardia (SVT) is defined as a tachycardic rhythm originating from a pacemaker above the ventricles **Figure 27-41 ▾**. Once called atrial tachycardia, it occurs when the true origin of a tachycardia is unknown (which is why the name was changed).

When tachycardias reach 150 to 180 beats/min, the P waves (if present) may be completely obscured by the T wave of the preceding beat. To be considered SVT, a rhythm should have a rate exceeding 150 beats/min. The rhythm is regular, with essentially no variation between R-R intervals. SVT is known to originate from a point above the ventricles because the QRS complexes are of normal width. The PRI may be not measurable because the P wave may be obscured. The QRS complex will measure 0.04 to 0.12 s.

PSVT is a specific rhythm reflecting its tendency to begin and end abruptly (*paroxysmal* means "occurring in spasms"), which does not normally have visible P waves. It should be differentiated from sinus tachycardia. Technically, to call this arrhythmia a PSVT, you would need to witness the rhythm speed up on the ECG. The most up-to-date terminology is AV-nodal reentry SVT.

When the ventricular rate exceeds 150 beats/min, the ventricular filling time is greatly diminished, which will in turn greatly reduce the CO. For this reason, nonsinus SVT should be treated promptly. The treatment, which is discussed later in this chapter, includes using medication or electrical therapy to slow the HR.

Multifocal Atrial Tachycardia

In multifocal atrial tachycardia (MAT), the pacemaker of the heart moves within various areas of the atria **Figure 27-42 ◂**. Multifocal atrial tachycardia is characterized by a rate of more than 100 beats/min and is, in effect, a tachycardic wandering atrial pacemaker. The rhythm is irregular, with variation between R-R intervals based on the site of the pacemaker for that particular complex. The P wave is present and upright and precedes each QRS complex; however, the shapes of the P waves vary as an indication of their different sites of origin. The PRI will measure 0.12 to 0.20 s, but also varies slightly based on the origin of the particular complex. If the MAT increases to a rate exceeding 150 beats/min, the P waves may no longer be visible; thus, the only indication of the rhythm may be the irregularity associated with the varying sites of origin within the atria. The QRS complex will measure 0.04 to 0.12 s.

Like a wandering atrial pacemaker, MAT is most commonly seen in patients with significant lung disease. Treatment is usually not attempted in the prehospital setting, and therapies aimed at correcting SVT are usually ineffective with MAT.

Atrial Flutter

Atrial flutter is a rhythm in which the atria contract at a rate much too rapid for the ventricles to match **Figure 27-43 ▸**. The atrial complexes in atrial flutter are known as flutter or F waves rather than P waves.

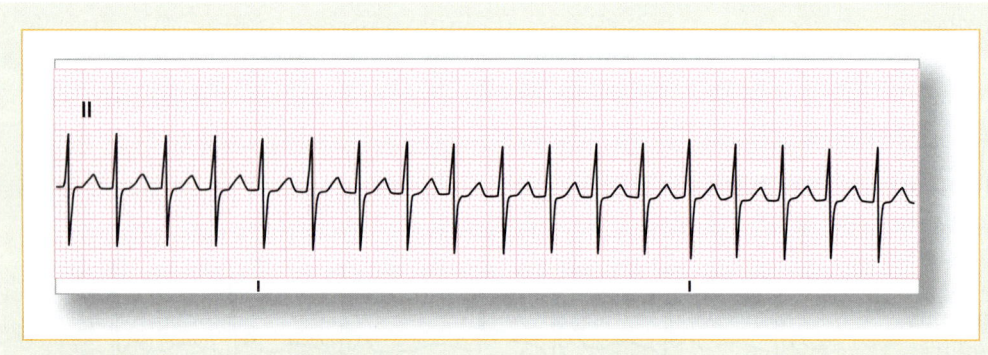

Figure 27-41 Supraventricular tachycardia.

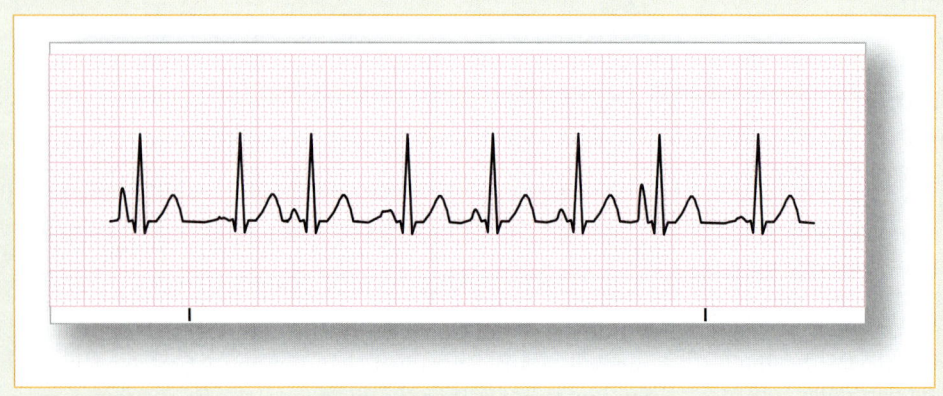

Figure 27-42 Multifocal atrial tachycardia.

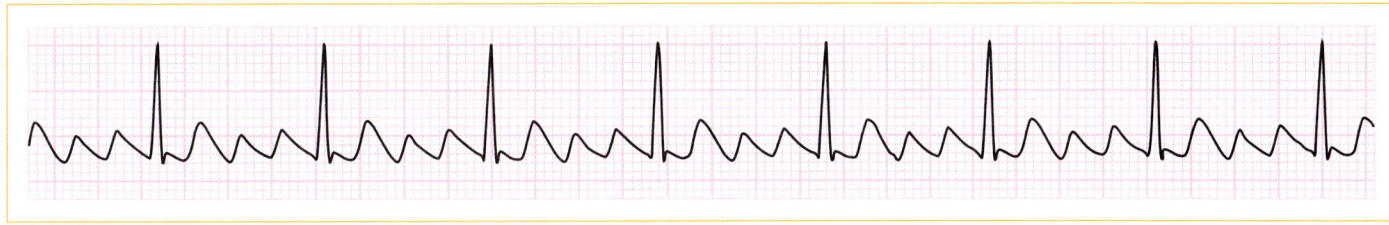

Figure 27-43 Atrial flutter.

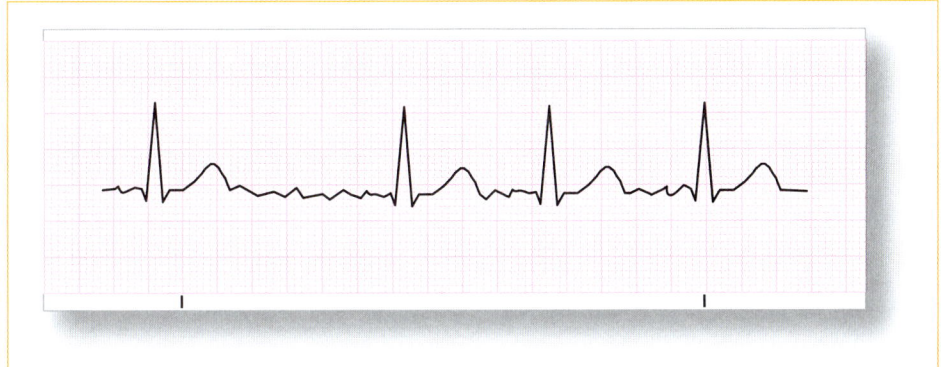

Figure 27-44 Atrial fibrillation.

F waves have a distinctive shape, resembling a sawtooth or picket fence.

In atrial flutter, one or more of the F waves is blocked by the AV node, resulting in several flutter waves before each QRS complex. The rhythm may be regular (most common), with a constant (usually 2:1) conduction (typically at a rate of exactly 150), or irregular if the conduction of impulses to the ventricles varies. The PRI will measure 0.12 to 0.20 s for conducted complexes. The QRS complex will measure 0.04 to 0.12 s.

Atrial flutter is usually a sign of a serious heart problem. In many cases, it is a transient rhythm that degenerates into atrial fibrillation. Treatment generally consists of medication or electrical cardioversion, although neither of these measures is usually attempted in the prehospital environment unless the patient's condition is very critical and transport time is long.

Atrial Fibrillation

Atrial fibrillation is a rhythm in which the atria no longer contract but rather fibrillate or quiver without any organized contraction **Figure 27-44 ▲**. It occurs when many different cells in the atria depolarize independently rather than in response to an impulse from the SA node. The result of this random depolarization, which occurs throughout the atria, is a fibrillating or chaotic baseline.

In atrial fibrillation, there are usually no visible P waves on the ECG strip and, hence, no PRI to measure. Instead, one of the keys to identifying this condition is its "irregularly irregular" appearance. Because the AV node is bombarded with impulses from the fibrillating atria, it allows impulses to pass on to the ventricles in a random manner, which results in the highly irregular ventricular rhythm. The QRS complex will measure 0.04 to 0.12 s.

Atrial fibrillation is usually a sign of a serious heart problem and is a fairly common rhythm among elderly patients. One of the main hazards associated with this arrhythmia is that the blood moving through the fibrillating atria has a tendency to form small clots, which may then become emboli and block circulation elsewhere in the body. Because of this risk, many elderly patients whose normal rhythm is atrial fibrillation take an anticoagulant medication such as warfarin (Coumadin), as well as other medications, such as digoxin, to regulate the rate of ventricular response. Prehospital treatment of atrial fibrillation is usually limited to control of a rapid ventricular rate in a patient with severe symptoms and a prolonged transport time, which may include medications or electrical cardioversion.

Rhythms of the AV Node or AV Junction

If the SA node—the body's dominant pacemaker—fails to initiate an impulse, the AV node may take over as pacemaker of the heart. Rhythms originating from the AV node are commonly referred to as "junctional" rhythms owing to the proximity of the AV node to the junction of the atria and ventricles. Junctional rhythms feature inverted or missing P waves but normal, narrow QRS complexes.

When an impulse is generated in the AV node, it travels down through the conduction system into the ventricles as if it had come from the SA node, resulting in normal QRS complexes. At the same time, the impulse travels upward through the atria and the internodal pathways toward the SA node. There are then three possible cases, none of which includes an upright P wave, but in which the QRS complex appears normal:

- If the impulse begins moving upward through the atria before the other part of it enters the ventricles, an upside-down P wave will be visible (upside down because the impulse is travelling in the opposite direction from that which causes normal upright P waves). This P wave is usually followed immediately by the QRS complex, without any pause between the two.

- If the impulse moving through the atria occurs at the exact same time as the impulse is travelling through the ventricles, the smaller inverted P wave will be buried within the larger QRS complex. This will give the appearance of a missing P wave—that is, the baseline remains flat until the beginning of a normal QRS complex.
- The impulse may start late through the atria and result in an inverted P wave appearing after the QRS complex.

Because the intrinsic rate of the AV node is 40 to 60, junctional rhythms normally present with rates of 40 to 60 beats/min.

Junctional (Escape) Rhythm

A junctional rhythm occurs when the SA node ceases functioning and the AV node takes over as the pacemaker of the heart Figure 27-45 ▾ . Because this allows the heart to "escape" from stopping completely, junctional rhythms are sometimes referred to as junctional escape rhythms. A normal junctional escape rhythm has a rate of 40 to 60 beats/min owing to the intrinsic rate of the AV node as a pacemaker. A junctional escape rhythm is usually regular, with little variation between R-R intervals. The P wave, if present, is inverted or upside down but may appear to be absent. The PRI, if an inverted

P wave is present, will measure less than 0.12 s. The QRS complex will measure 0.04 to 0.12 s.

Junctional rhythms are most commonly seen in patients with significant problems with the SA node. Treatment usually consists of a surgically implanted pacemaker. Thus, little can be done in the prehospital environment other than to institute transcutaneous pacing (TCP) if the patient's condition is severely compromised.

Accelerated Junctional Rhythm

Occasionally, a junctional rhythm will present with a rate that exceeds its normal upper rate of 60 beats/min but remains less than 100 beats/min. Because the rhythm is greater than 60 beats/min, it cannot be considered a "normal" junctional rhythm; because it is less than 100 beats/min, it cannot be called tachycardia either. In this case, the name given the rhythm is accelerated junctional rhythm.

An accelerated junctional rhythm is also regular, with little variation between R-R intervals Figure 27-46 ▾ . The P wave, if present, is inverted or upside down but may appear to be absent. The PRI, if an inverted P wave is present, will measure less than 0.12 s. The QRS complex will measure 0.04 to 0.12 s.

Accelerated junctional rhythms are serious, but they seldom require treatment in the prehospital setting because the rate is usually fast enough to maintain a reasonable CO.

Junctional Tachycardia

Occasionally, a junctional rhythm will present with a rate that exceeds 100 beats/min. Any rhythm that results in a ventricular rate greater than 100 beats/min is referred to as tachycardia. In this case, the rhythm is termed junctional tachycardia.

Junctional tachycardia is also regular, with little variation between R-R intervals Figure 27-47 ▸ . The P wave, if present, is inverted or upside down but may appear to be absent. The PRI, if an inverted P wave is present, will measure less than 0.12 s. The QRS complex will measure 0.04 to 0.12 s.

Junctional tachycardia is serious, but it seldom requires treatment in the prehospital setting because the rate is usually fast enough to maintain a reasonable CO. If the rate exceeds 150 beats/min, however, the CO could suffer. In such a case, the rhythm is rarely junctional and is referred to as SVT.

Premature Junctional Complex

Premature junctional complex (PJC) is not, strictly speaking, an arrhythmia (just as PAC is not), but rather the

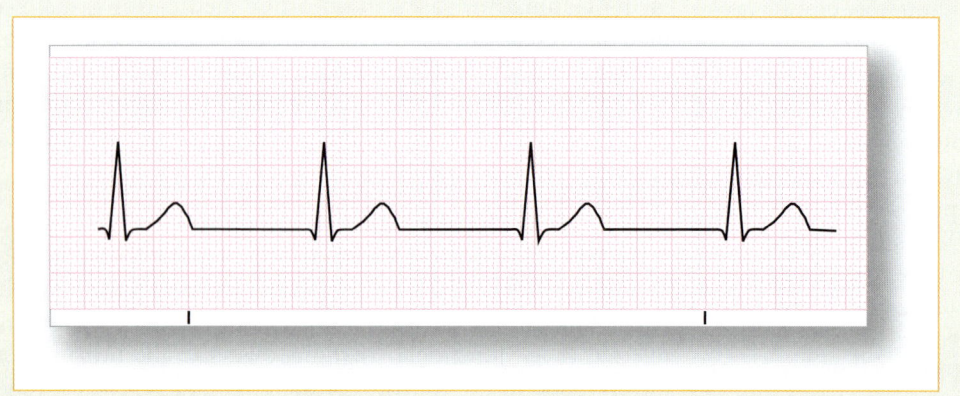

Figure 27-45 Junctional rhythm.

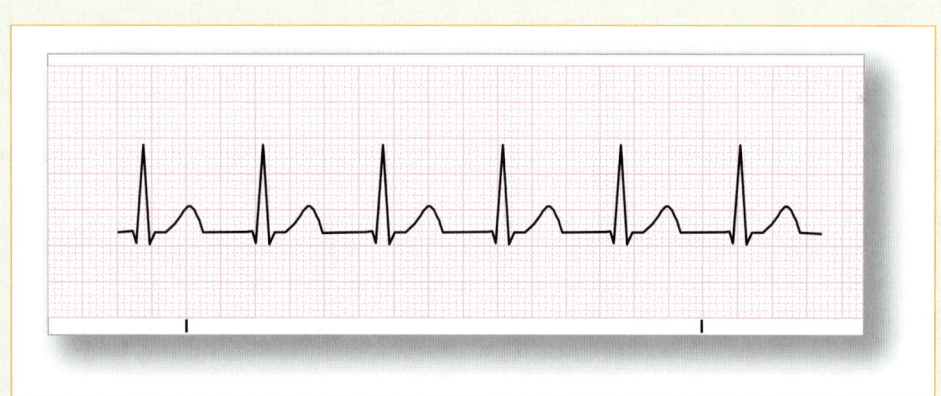

Figure 27-46 Accelerated junctional rhythm.

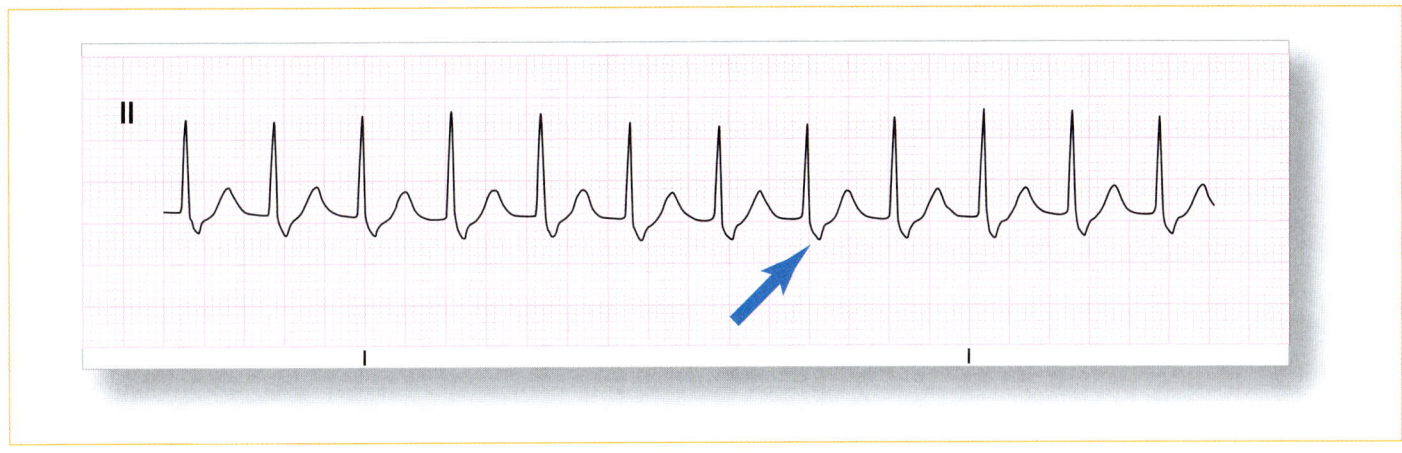

Figure 27-47 Junctional tachycardia. The blue arrow points to an inverted P wave after the QRS wave.

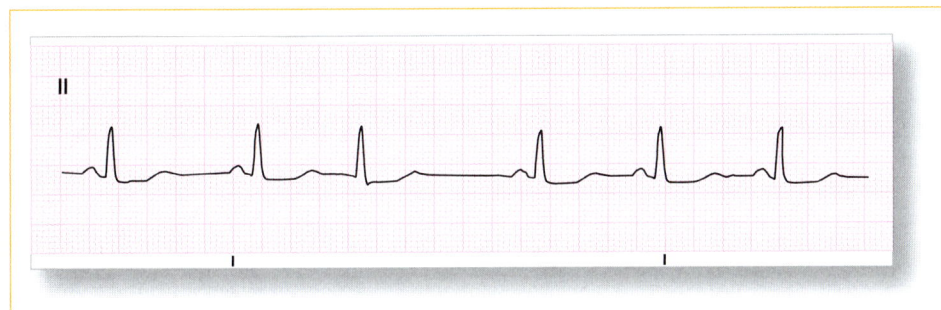

Figure 27-48 Premature junctional complexes.

existence of a particular complex within another rhythm **Figure 27-48 ▲**. Premature junctional complexes are also known as ectopic complexes, meaning that they occur out of the normal location. A PJC also occurs earlier in time than the next expected sinus complex, causing the R-R interval to be less between it and the previous complex.

The rate depends on the underlying rhythm, and the PJC will make the rhythm irregular. The P wave, if present, will be inverted or upside down, and it may precede or follow the QRS complex. The PRI, if present, will measure less than 0.12 s. The QRS complex will measure 0.04 to 0.12 s.

Premature junctional complexes can be caused by many of the same problems that cause premature atrial contractions. They are rarely treated in the prehospital setting but may be a predictor of future cardiac arrhythmias.

Heart Blocks

After the SA node initiates impulses, the impulses proceed through the atria and ventricles and result in contraction of the heart. When they reach the AV node, the impulses are delayed to allow the atria to contract and fill the ventricle. This delay is a normal function of the AV node and usually causes no problems. Occasionally, however, the impulses travelling through the AV node are delayed more than usual, resulting in heart blocks.

Heart blocks are classified into different degrees based on the seriousness of the block and the amount of myocardial damage. The least serious heart block is a first-degree heart block; the most serious is a third-degree block. In between are two types of second-degree block.

First-Degree Heart Block

A first-degree heart block occurs when each impulse reaching the AV node is delayed slightly longer than is expected and results in a PRI greater than 0.20 s. Because each impulse eventually passes through the AV node and causes a QRS complex, this block is considered the least serious. Nevertheless, it is often the first indication of damage that has occurred to the AV node.

Because it originates from the normal pacemaker of the heart, first-degree heart block usually has an intrinsic rate of 60 to 100 beats/min, although it typically occurs at the low end of this range **Figure 27-49 ▶**. The rhythm is regular, with minimal variation between R-R intervals. The P wave is present and upright, and it precedes each QRS complex. The PRI will measure greater than 0.20 s. The QRS complex will measure 0.04 to 0.12 s. The only difference between first-degree heart block and normal sinus rhythm is the prolonged PRI.

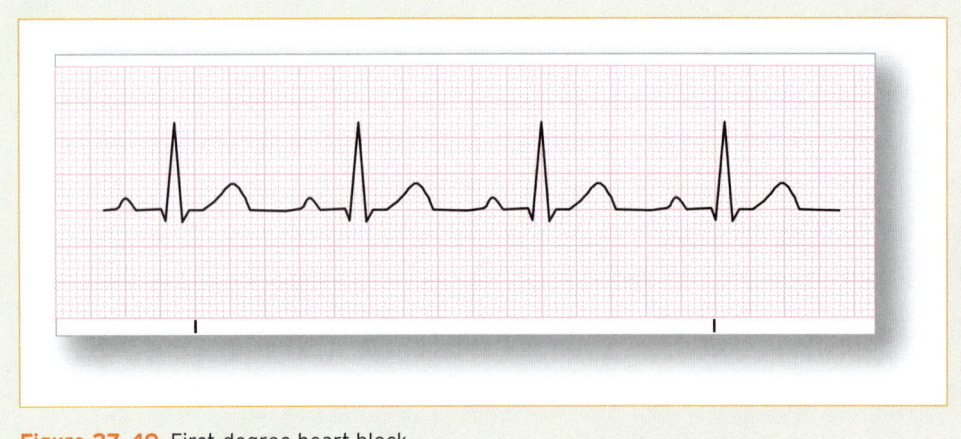

Figure 27-49 First-degree heart block.

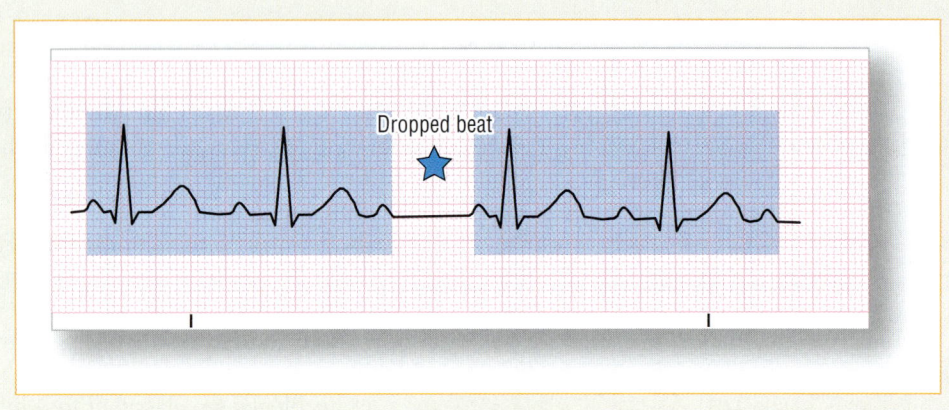

Figure 27-50 Second-degree heart block, Mobitz type I.

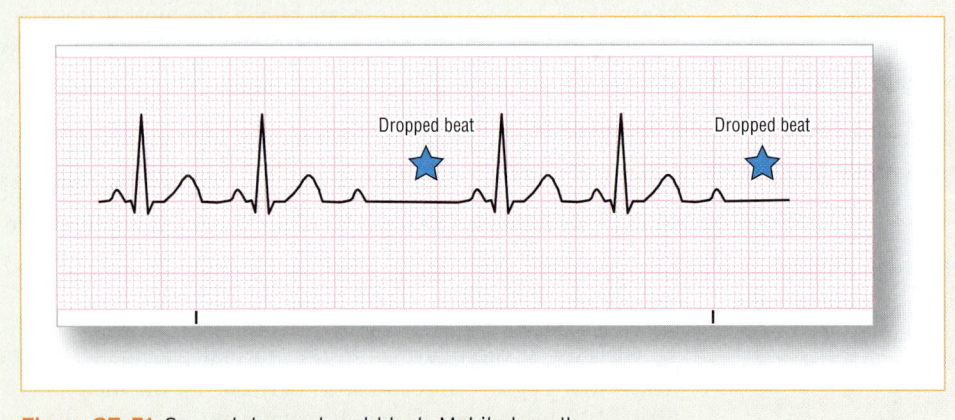

Figure 27-51 Second-degree heart block, Mobitz type II.

ventricles and causing a QRS complex. Second-degree heart block, Mobitz type I (Wenckebach), occurs when each successive impulse is delayed a little longer, until finally one impulse is not allowed to continue.

Because it begins from the normal pacemaker of the heart, second-degree heart block, type I, usually has an intrinsic rate of 60 to 100 beats/min, although it typically occurs at the low end of this range Figure 27-50 ◂ . The rhythm is irregular, with a prolonged R-R interval occurring between the last QRS complex before the blocked P wave and the QRS complex after the first unblocked P wave. The P wave is present and upright, and it precedes most QRS complexes. The PRI starts out within the normal limits of 0.12 to 0.20 s but, with each successive P wave, grows longer. It finally results in a P wave that is followed not by a QRS complex, but by another P wave; this P wave is then followed by a QRS complex with a normal PRI. This pattern repeats over and over in the rhythm. The QRS complex will measure 0.04 to 0.12 s.

The key to identification of second-degree type I heart block is the recognition of the increasing PRI followed by the P wave without a QRS complex. This rhythm is always irregular, and you can often easily see the wide R-R interval with the "extra" P wave located there.

Second-degree type I heart blocks are treated in the prehospital setting only if they are associated with bradycardia that results in significantly reduced CO.

Second-Degree Heart Block: Mobitz Type II (Classical)

Second-degree heart block, Mobitz type II, occurs when several impulses are not allowed to continue. It is sometimes called classical because it was well known before the Wenckebach heart block was discovered.

Because it originates from the normal pacemaker of the heart, second-degree heart block, type II, usually has an intrinsic rate of 60 to 100 beats/min, although it typically occurs at the low end of this range Figure 27-51 ◂ . The rhythm may be regular, with every other P wave blocked, or irregular, with a prolonged R-R interval between the last

First-degree heart block is rarely treated in the prehospital setting unless it is associated with bradycardia that results in significantly reduced CO.

Second-Degree Heart Block: Mobitz Type I (Wenckebach)

A second-degree heart block occurs when an impulse reaching the AV node is occasionally prevented from proceeding to the

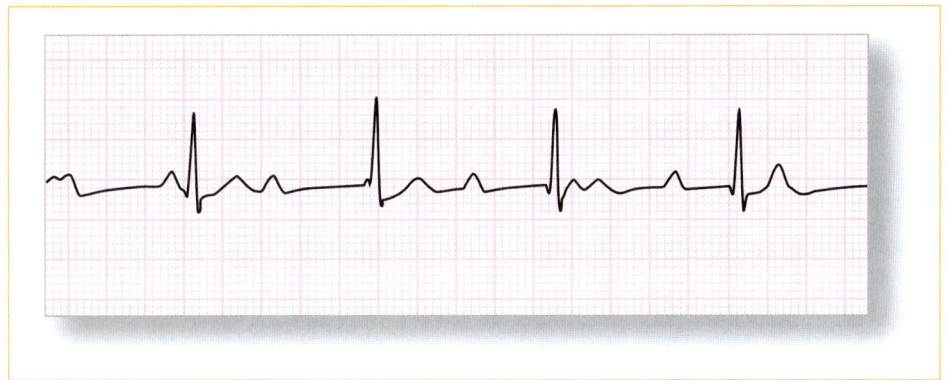

Figure 27-52 Third-degree heart block.

QRS complex before the blocked P wave and the QRS complex after the first unblocked P wave. The P wave is present and upright, and it precedes some QRS complexes. The PRI is always constant. In fact, this is the easiest way to identify a second-degree type II heart block. If you see a rhythm with some nonconducted P waves, but the PRI is constant among all conducted P waves and their corresponding QRS complexes, you have identified a second-degree type II heart block.

It is important to remember that this block can be regular or irregular. Sometimes several normal beats will occur without a nonconducted P wave; sometimes two or more nonconducted P waves may appear before one P wave is conducted. In other situations, a pattern develops that consists of one conducted P wave followed by one nonconducted P wave.

Second-degree type II heart blocks are treated in the prehospital setting only if they are associated with bradycardia that results in significantly reduced CO. Although second-degree type II heart block with symptoms may respond to medications, transcutaneous pacing is occasionally required.

Third-Degree Heart Block (Complete Heart Block)

A third-degree heart block occurs when all impulses reaching the AV node are prevented from proceeding to the ventricles and causing a QRS complex. Unlike in first- and second-degree heart blocks, in a third-degree heart block *all* impulses from the atria are prevented from travelling to the ventricles. As a consequence, this block is also known as a complete heart block. Because all impulses from the atria are blocked, the ventricles will develop their own pacemaker to continue circulation of blood, albeit at a greatly reduced rate.

Because it originates from the normal pacemaker of the heart, third-degree heart block usually has an intrinsic atrial rate of 60 to 100 beats/min, but the ventricular rate—which depends on the activity of a ventricular pacemaker—is less than 60 beats/min **Figure 27-52 ▲**. The rhythm is usually regular, with the P-P and R-R intervals being consistent. The P wave is present and upright. The PRI in this type of heart block is nonexistent.

The classic way of identifying a third-degree heart block is to identify the presence of nonconducted P waves and then to be unable to identify a relationship between the P waves and the QRS complexes. Because the ventricular rate depends on the presence of a ventricular pacemaker, it is common to see the QRS complexes in a third-degree heart block that are wider than 0.12 s. When you see a rhythm with wide QRS complexes (and no narrow QRS complexes) along with P waves, you should suspect a third-degree heart block. If the rhythm is regular and the PRI is not constant, it is almost certainly a third-degree heart block. One challenge in diagnosing third-degree heart blocks to be regular is the fact that if a premature ventricular complex (described later) occurs within the block, it will make the block appear irregular.

Third-degree heart blocks are treated in the prehospital setting only if they are associated with bradycardia that results in significantly reduced CO. In such a case, the patient will usually require transcutaneous pacing.

Rhythms of the Ventricles

If the SA node fails to initiate an impulse, the AV node will usually take over as pacemaker. If the AV node cannot perform this duty, however, the ventricles may begin to originate their own impulses and become the pacemaker of the heart. Such ventricular rhythms will have missing P waves and wide QRS complexes.

If an impulse is generated in the ventricles, it must travel through the ventricles in a cell-to-cell manner because the cell originating the impulse is unlikely to be located on the conduction system. Because impulses travel more slowly via cell-to-cell transmission than when they travel on the conduction system, ventricular-initiated impulses result in very wide QRS complexes—more than 0.12 s in duration. Because the intrinsic rate of the ventricles is 20 to 40, ventricular rhythms normally demonstrate rates of 20 to 40 beats/min.

Idioventricular Rhythm

An idioventricular (meaning only the ventricles or produced by the ventricles) rhythm occurs when the SA and AV nodes fail and the ventricles must takes over pacing the heart **Figure 27-53 ▶**. It has a rate of 20 to 40 beats/min owing to the intrinsic rate of the ventricles as pacemakers. An idioventricular rhythm is usually regular, with little variation between R-R intervals. P waves are absent owing to the failure of the SA and AV nodes. Because there is no P wave, there is no PRI. The QRS complex will measure greater than 0.12 s because it originates in the ventricles.

Idioventricular rhythms are serious and may or may not result in a palpable pulse. Treatment is geared toward improving

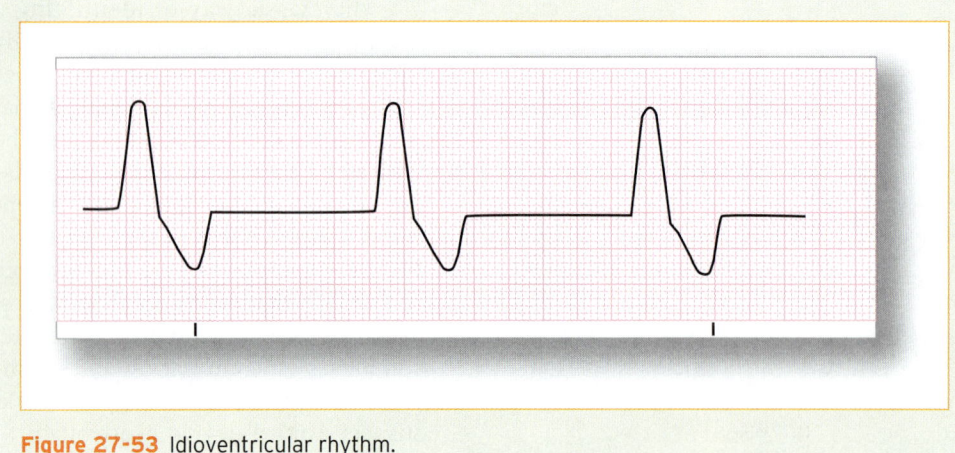

Figure 27-53 Idioventricular rhythm.

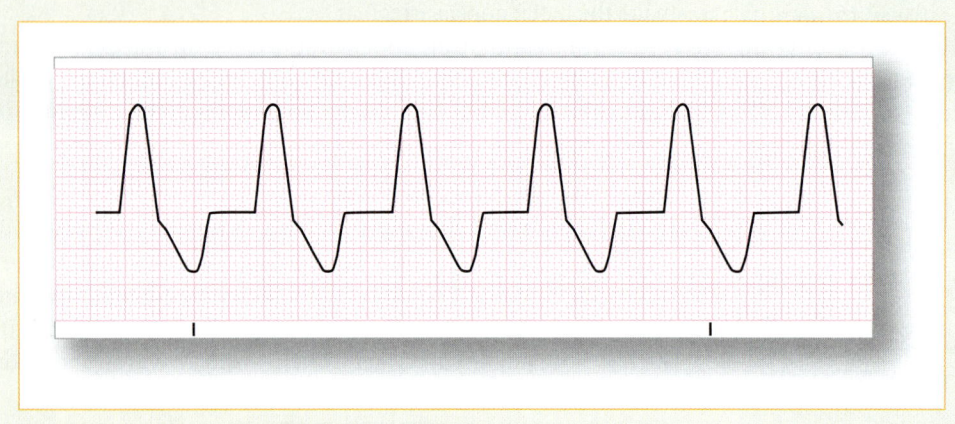

Figure 27-54 Accelerated idioventricular rhythm.

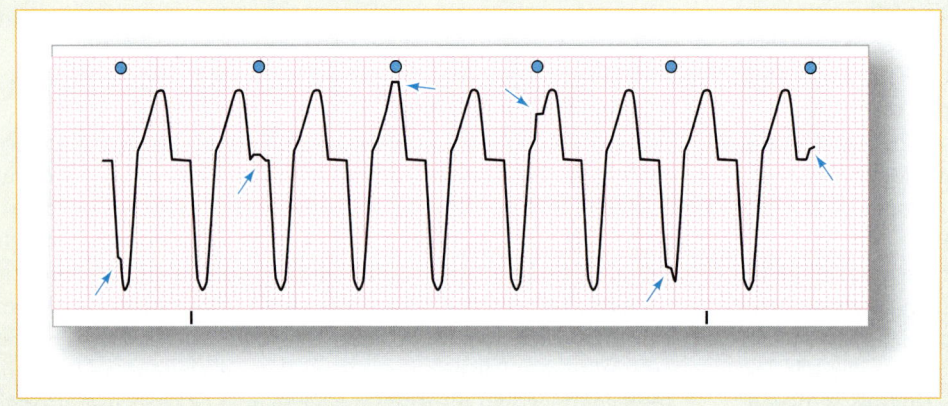

Figure 27-55 Monomorphic ventricular tachycardia.

the CO by increasing the rate and, if possible, treating the underlying cause. In such a case, the patient's condition is usually severely compromised.

Accelerated Idioventricular Rhythm (AIVR)

Occasionally, an idioventricular rhythm exceeds its normal upper rate of 40 beats/min but remains less than 100 beats/min. Because the rhythm is greater than 40 beats/min, it cannot be considered a "normal" ventricular rhythm; because it is less than 100 beats/min, it cannot be called tachycardia either. In this case, the rhythm is called accelerated idioventricular rhythm.

An accelerated idioventricular rhythm is also regular, with little variation between R-R intervals. The P waves are absent, so the PRI does not exist   Figure 27-54 ◀ . The QRS complex will measure greater than 0.12 s.

Accelerated idioventricular rhythms may represent serious cardiac disease, although they are most frequently seen following fibrinolysis for acute myocardial infarction and suggest reopening of the occluded coronary artery. Antiarrhythmic medications are usually not indicated for AIVR, particularly in the prehospital setting.

Ventricular Tachycardia

Ventricular rhythms occur when the SA and AV nodes fail as the pacemakers of the heart. Occasionally, a ventricular rhythm has a rate that exceeds 100 beats/min. Any rhythm that results in a ventricular rate greater than 100 beats/min is considered tachycardia. In this case, the rhythm is termed ventricular tachycardia.

Ventricular tachycardia is regular, with no variation between R-R intervals. The P waves are absent, so the PRI also does not exist. The QRS complex will measure greater than 0.12 s.

Ventricular tachycardia usually presents with QRS complexes that have uniform tops and bottoms; this type of VT is referred to as monomorphic (having one common shape of QRS complex)   Figure 27-55 ◀ . Occasionally,

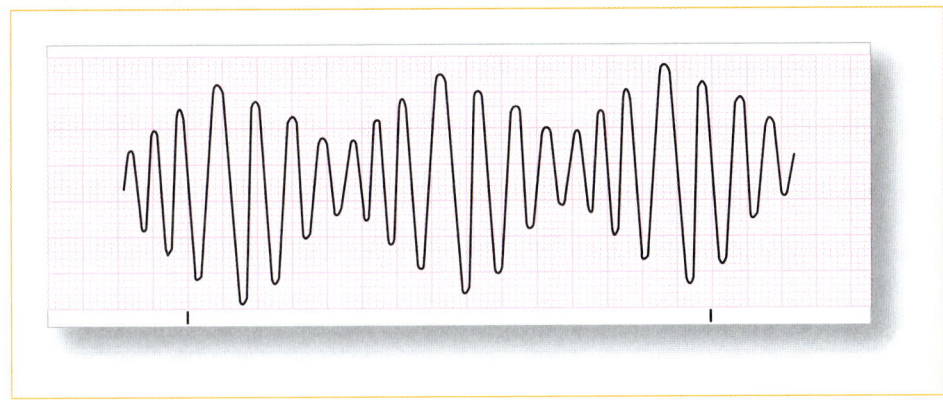

Figure 27-56 Polymorphic ventricular tachycardia.

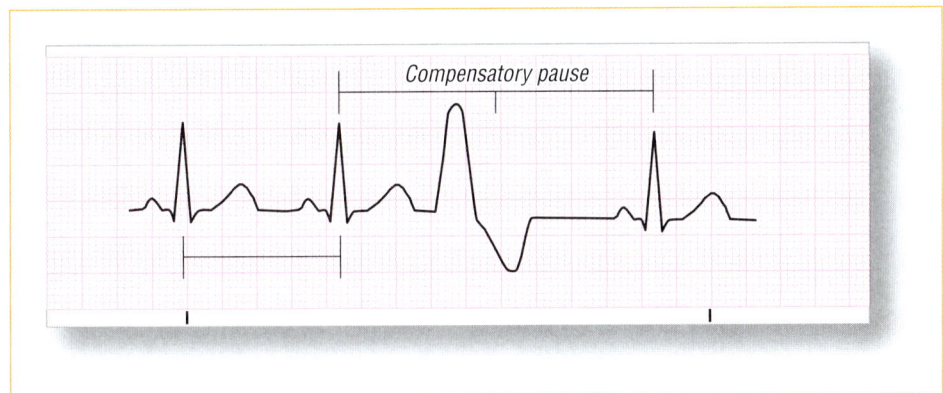

Compensatory pause

Figure 27-57 Premature ventricular complex.

usually too fast to maintain adequate CO. This reduced CO, in conjunction with the increased workload of the heart due to the tachycardia, usually leads to ventricular failure or fibrillation if not treated promptly. Pulseless VT requires an immediate unsynchronized shock with supportive CPR. Unstable VT (with associated hypotension, pulmonary edema, or chest pain) typically requires synchronized cardioversion, either in the prehospital environment or upon arrival to the ED, depending on the extent of instability. Stable VT may be treated with medication, although treatment may be deferred until arrival to the ED when transport times are short.

Premature Ventricular Complex

Premature ventricular complex is not, strictly speaking, an arrhythmia (just as premature atrial and junctional complexes are not), but rather the existence of a particular complex within another rhythm **Figure 27-57 ◄**. Premature ventricular complexes are also known as ectopic complexes, meaning that they occur out of the normal location. A premature ventricular complex also occurs earlier than the next expected sinus complex, causing the R-R interval to be less between it and the previous complex.

Because the rate depends on the underlying rhythm, the premature ventricular complex will make the rhythm irregular. There is no P wave associated with the premature ventricular complex, so there is no PRI. The QRS complex will measure greater than 0.12 s.

Premature ventricular complexes may also be further distinguished as unifocal or multifocal. Unifocal premature ventricular complexes originate from the same spot or "focus" within the ventricle and will appear the same on the ECG **Figure 27-58 ►**. Two premature ventricular complexes with different appearances are multifocal, meaning there is more than one focus initiating ventricular impulses **Figure 27-59 ►**.

Sometimes two premature ventricular complexes may occur together without any pause between them. This pair of complexes is referred to as a couplet **Figure 27-60 ►**. If three or more premature ventricular complexes occur in a row, they constitute a "run" of ventricular tachycardia. Occasionally, these complexes will become so frequent that they

VT will present with QRS complexes that vary in height in an alternating pattern; this type of VT is called polymorphic VT **Figure 27-56 ▲**. The most common polymorphic VT is torsade de pointes, which is usually seen in patients who have a condition of a prolonged Q-T interval. Torsade de pointes may be related to a congenital prolonged Q-T interval or it may be precipitated by medications or drugs such as antibiotics, antipsychotics, or quinidine. Torsade de pointes with a normal Q-T interval prior to the arrhythmia is frequently associated with cardiac ischemia.

Polymorphic VT is usually considered more challenging to treat than monomorphic VT and converts spontaneously back to a normal rhythm or degenerates into VF.

Ventricular tachycardia is extremely serious, and it may require treatment in the prehospital setting because the rate is

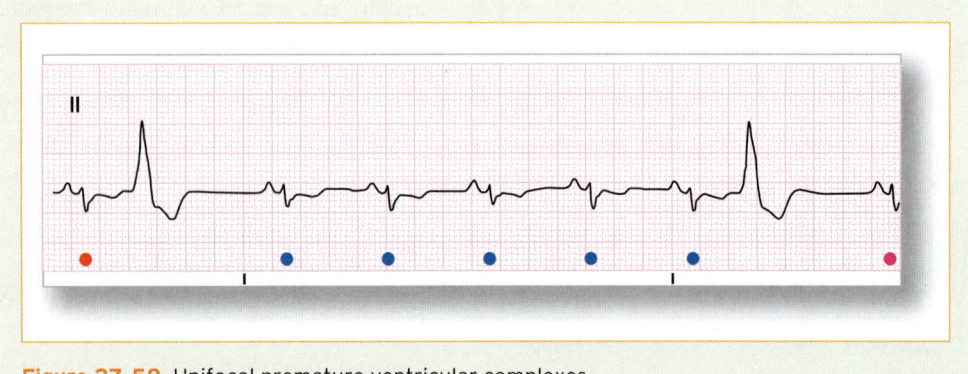

Figure 27-58 Unifocal premature ventricular complexes.

alternate with normal complexes, causing a normal–premature ventricular complex–normal–premature ventricular complex pattern. This pattern is called bigeminy of premature ventricular complexes **Figure 27-61 ▸** . If every third beat is a premature ventricular complex (normal–normal–premature ventricular complex), the pattern is called trigeminy.

Premature ventricular complexes can be caused by many of the same problems that cause premature atrial and junctional contractions, but they most commonly originate from ischemia

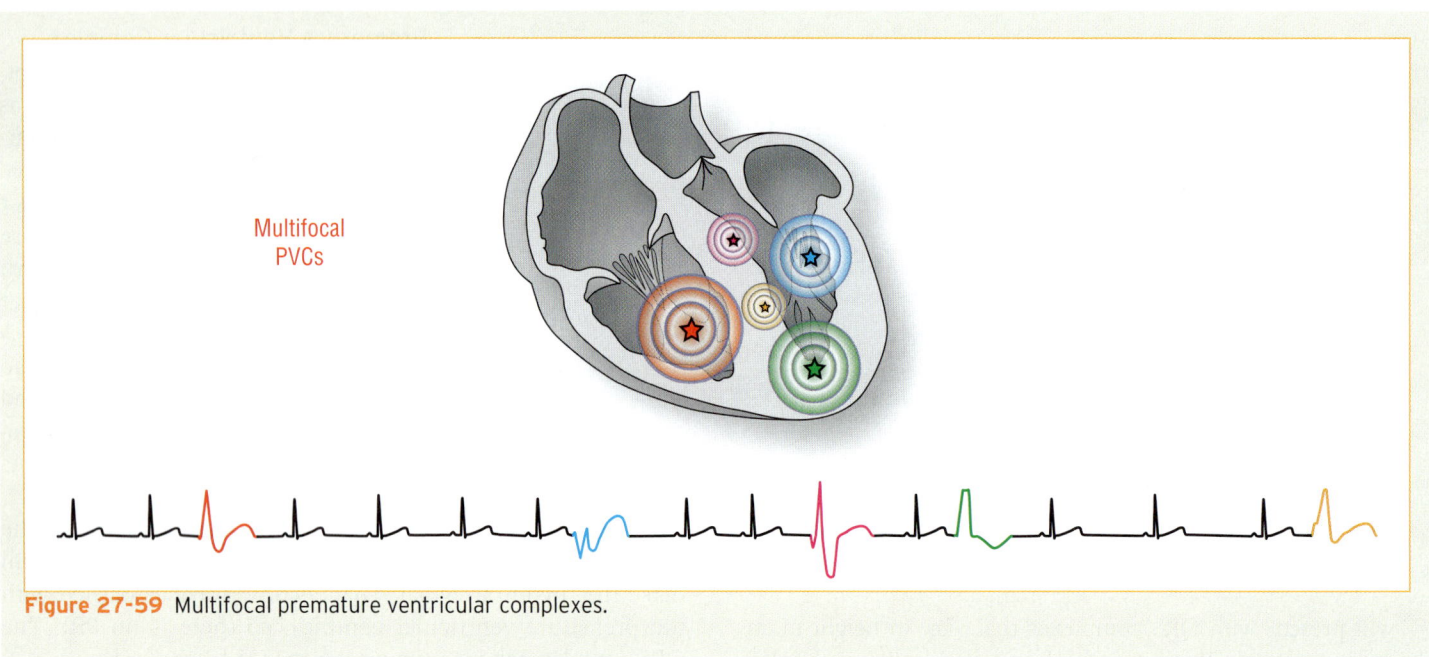

Multifocal
PVCs

Figure 27-59 Multifocal premature ventricular complexes.

in the ventricular tissue. They are generally considered more serious than premature atrial or junctional complexes. Multifocal, couplet, and bigeminy premature ventricular complexes are considered more serious than unifocal premature ventricular complexes. One of the principal hazards of premature ventricular complexes is that they might occur at a time when the ventricles are not fully repolarized (as indicated by the T wave). This so-called R-on-T phenomenon often results in VF. For this and other reasons, premature ventricular complexes are considered serious and

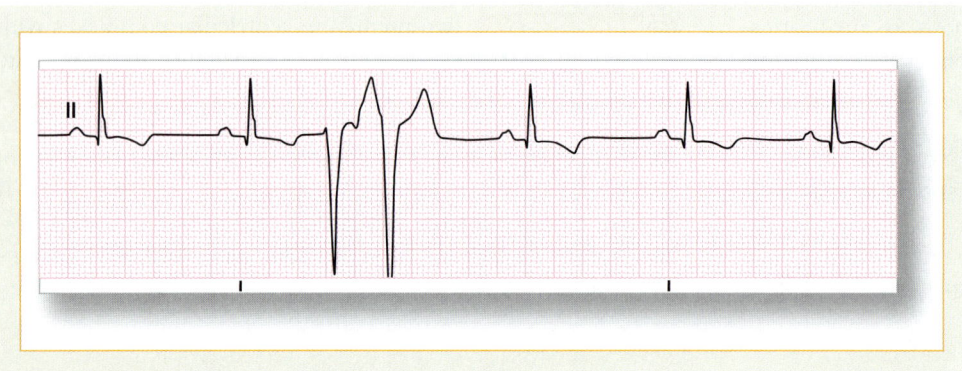

Figure 27-60 Couplet premature ventricular complexes.

an indication of serious underlying heart conditions. Nevertheless, this condition is not usually treated in the prehospital setting, unless it is significantly affecting CO, and even then it must be treated with caution. Treatment of the underlying causes of the premature ventricular complexes, such as relief of ischemic chest pain, may be appropriate and should be considered prior to any use of antiarrhythmic drugs.

Ventricular Fibrillation

Ventricular fibrillation is a rhythm in which the entire heart is no longer contracting but rather fibrillating or quivering without any organized contraction. It occurs when many different cells in the heart become depolarized independently rather than in response to an impulse from the SA node **Figure 27-62 ◂**. The result of this random depolarization is a fibrillating or chaotic baseline without indication of organized activity. As opposed to atrial fibrillation, there are no P waves, no PRI, and no QRS complexes.

Early in VF, the cardiac cells have energy reserves that allow a consider-

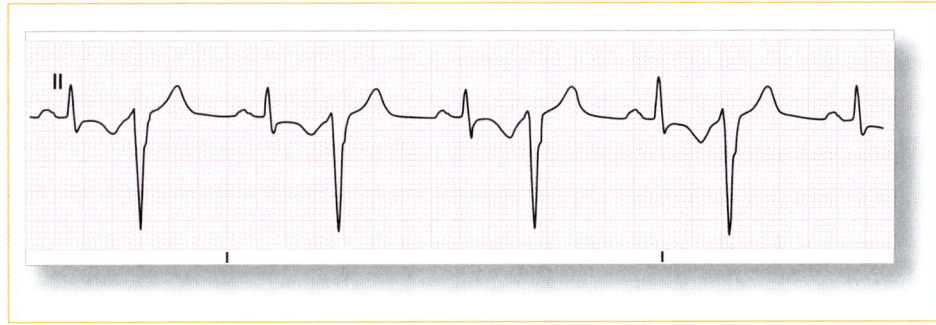

Figure 27-61 Bigeminy premature ventricular complexes.

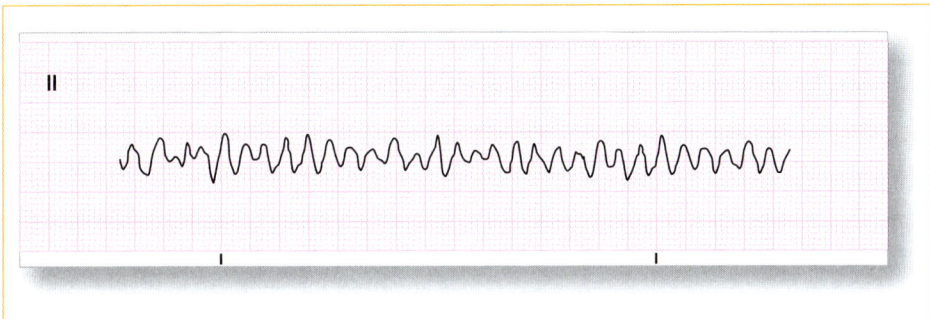

Figure 27-62 Ventricular fibrillation.

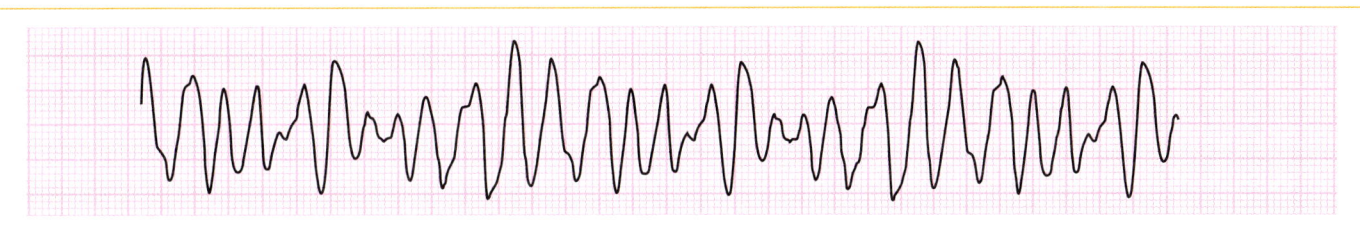

Figure 27-63 Coarse ventricular fibrillation.

able amount of electrical energy to be expended and cause the height of the chaotic waves to be large. These large waves are sometimes referred to as "coarse" VF **Figure 27-63 ▴**. As the ventricles continue to go without circulation, the energy reserves of the cardiac cells are gradually used up, leading to a great reduction of the height of the chaotic waves. This phenomenon is sometimes called "fine" VF **Figure 27-64 ◂**. Effective chest compressions during CPR can delay the deterioration to "fine" VF.

Ventricular fibrillation is the rhythm most commonly seen in adults who go into cardiac arrest. Fortunately, it responds

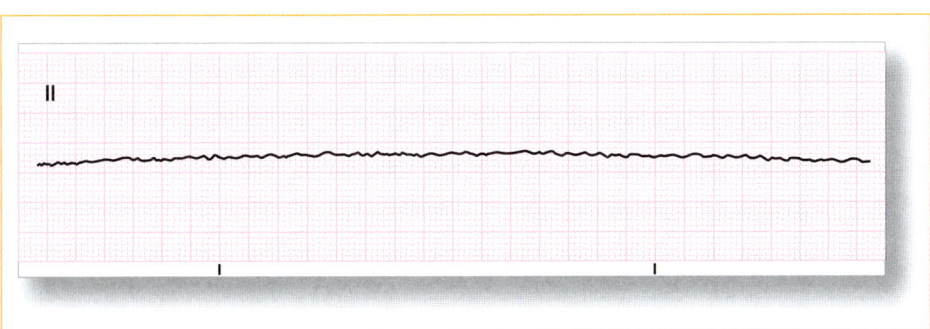

Figure 27-64 Very fine ventricular fibrillation.

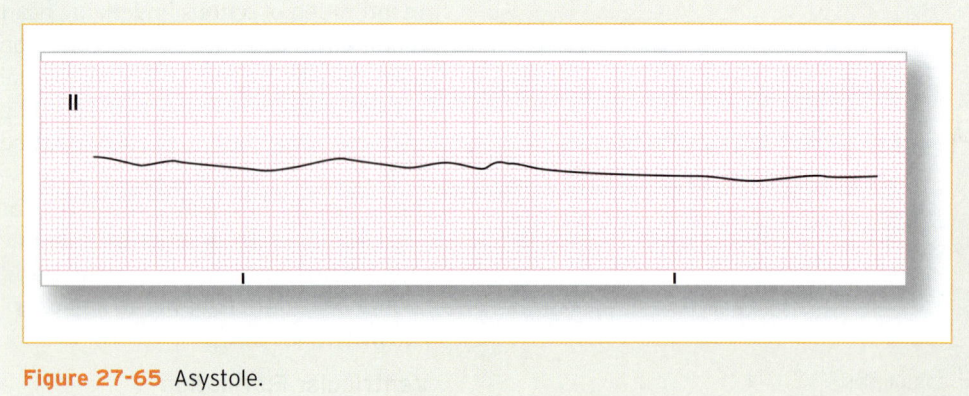

Figure 27-65 Asystole.

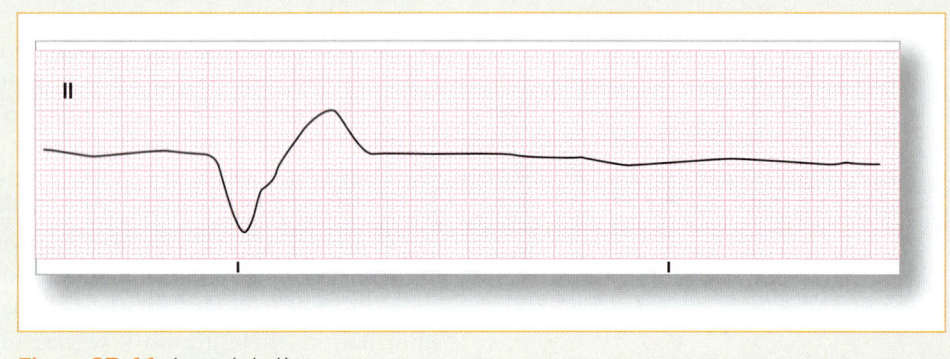

Figure 27-66 Agonal rhythm.

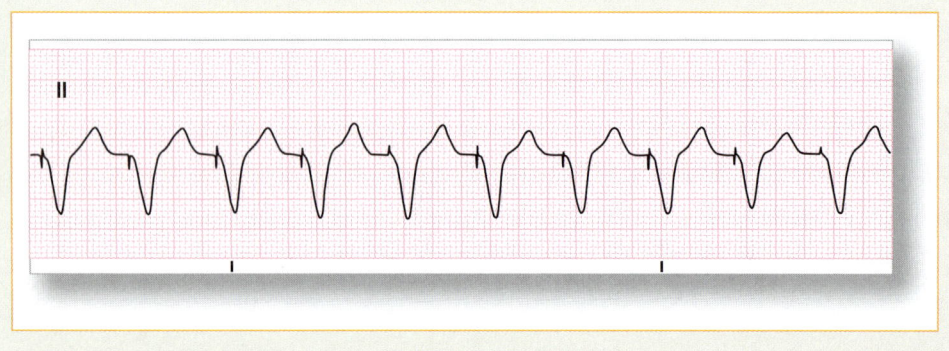

Figure 27-67 Artificial pacemaker rhythm.

In one variation of asystole, the flat baseline associated with asystole is interrupted by a small sinusoidal complex at a rate of less than 20 beats/minute. This condition, which is termed agonal rhythm, is probably a result of residual electrical discharge from a dead heart. Agonal rhythm should not be confused with an idioventricular rhythm Figure 27-66 ◂ . An idioventricular rhythm may result in a palpable pulse, but an agonal rhythm will not.

Asystole is generally considered a confirmation of death, although in certain circumstances, it may be treated (as discussed later in this chapter).

Artificial Pacemaker Rhythms

Many of your patients will have experienced problems with their cardiac conduction systems and had artificial pacemakers implanted in their chest. When these patients are connected to the heart monitor, the presence of the artificial pacemaker is obvious. The firing of an artificial pacemaker causes a unique vertical spike on the ECG tracing Figure 27-67 ◂ . When you attach the cardiac monitor to a patient and see these sharp vertical spikes on the ECG, you can assume the patient has an artificial pacemaker Figure 27-68 ▸ .

Many types of artificial pacemakers exist, and more are being developed. Some are termed ventricular pacemakers, which are attached to the ventricles only; they cause a sharp pacemaker spike followed by a wide QRS complex resulting from the impulse travelling through the ventricles. Another type of pacemaker is attached to the atria and the ventricle (dual chamber); it produces a pacemaker spike that is followed by a P wave and another pacemaker spike followed by a wide QRS complex. Pacemakers are equipped with sensors that can identify the rate of spontaneous depolarization of the heart. These "demand" pacemakers begin to generate pacing impulses only when they sense that the natural pace of cardiac impulses has slowed below a specific number (usually 60 per minute) Figure 27-69 ▸ .

Occasionally, a patient may experience a problem with his or her pacemaker. If the patient's pacemaker is failing (eg, due to battery failure), the pacemaker spikes may still be visible, but they will not be followed by a QRS complex. This loss of capture indicates the pacemaker is not operating properly. A loss of capture may also occur if the wire connecting the pacemaker to the patient's heart becomes dislodged. In either of these cases,

well to defibrillation performed with an automated or manual defibrillator within the first 4 minutes of an arrest. After 4 minutes or so, it is necessary to provide CPR compressions to help make the heart more susceptible to defibrillation and to increase the oxygen to the myocardial cells. Prehospital treatment of VF is common and will be discussed in detail later in this chapter.

Asystole

Asystole ("flat line") is a rhythm in which the entire heart is no longer contracting but rather is sitting still within the thorax without any organized activity Figure 27-65 ▴ . It occurs when many cells of the heart have been hypoxic for so long that they no longer have any energy for any kind of contraction. Asystole presents with a complete absence of electrical activity: no P waves, no PRIs, no QRS complexes, and no T waves.

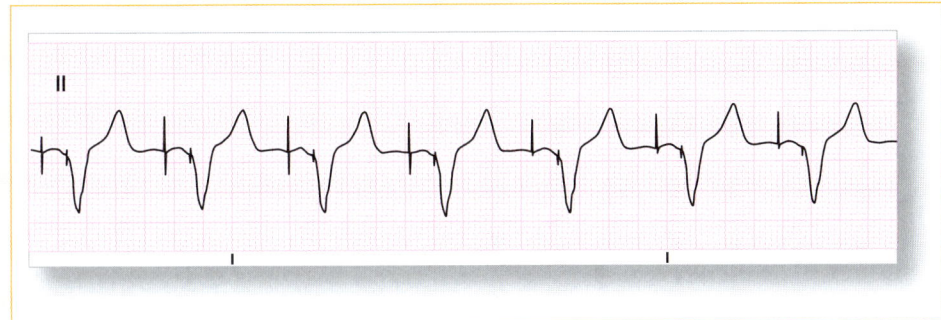

Figure 27-68 Artificial pacemaker rhythm (AV sequential).

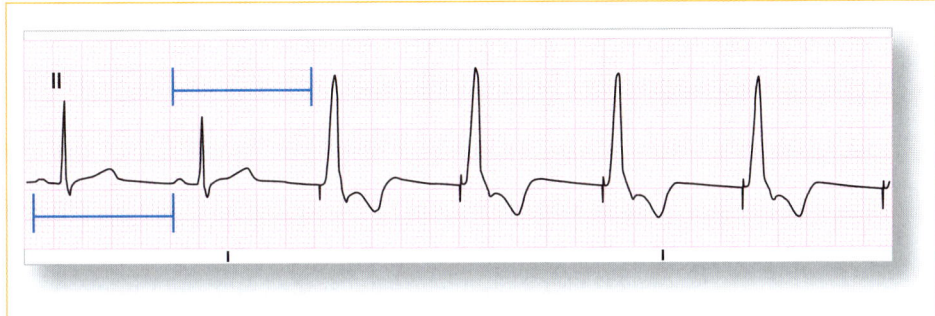

Figure 27-69 Artificial pacemaker rhythm (demand pacemaker).

Other ECG Abnormalities

A few other ECG abnormalities are not identified as arrhythmias but are indicative of significant cardiac conditions. For example, a delta wave is an indication of Wolff-Parkinson-White (WPW) syndrome. Patients with WPW syndrome have an accessory pathway between the atria and the ventricles called the bundle of Kent. This bundle of conductive tissue bypasses the AV node and begins ventricular depolarization early, resulting in a rapid up slope to the R wave immediately after the end of the P wave **Figure 27-70 ◂**. This early up slope can be interpreted as a widened QRS complex (more than 0.12 s), and a short PRI. This situation, which is referred to as aberrant conduction, can lead to the misinterpretation of SVTs as ventricular in origin. Patients with WPW syndrome are highly susceptible to SVTs.

Another important abnormality is an Osborne, or J, wave. It occurs in cases of hypothermia and presents as what appears to be a P wave at the end of the QRS complex **Figure 27-71 ▾**. The J wave may also be accompanied by ST-segment depression and T-wave inversion. Generally, the more serious the hypothermia, the larger the J wave. Evidence of a J wave should be considered only an indication of hypothermia; it is not enough to make a definitive diagnosis. Electrolyte imbalances can also cause changes in the ECG that are not arrhythmias but can be indicators of serious conditions. The two most common of these electrolyte imbalances are hyperkalemia and hypokalemia. Hyperkalemia often presents with very tall, pointed T waves; these T waves may be as tall or taller than the QRS complex **Figure 27-72 ▸**. The rhythm strip for someone with profound, severe hyperkalemia has the appearance of a sine wave **Figure 27-73 ▸**. By contrast, hypokalemia

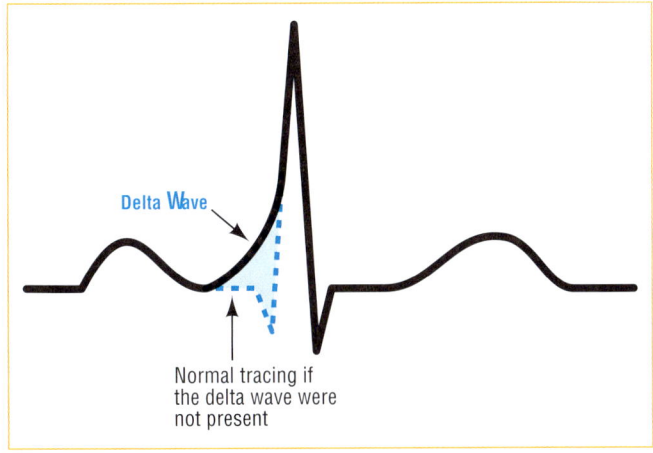

Figure 27-70 Delta wave: WPW syndrome.

the patient's heartbeat now depends on the natural pacemaker (usually the ventricles), resulting in greatly reduced CO. In such cases, patients need TCP instituted as quickly as possible.

Another type of pacemaker failure involves a "runaway" pacemaker. A runaway pacemaker presents as a very tachycardic pacemaker rhythm that must be slowed to preserve the patient's cardiac function. Usually a strong magnet placed over the pacemaker will "reset" a runaway pacemaker to a preset regular rate at 60 to 80 beats/min.

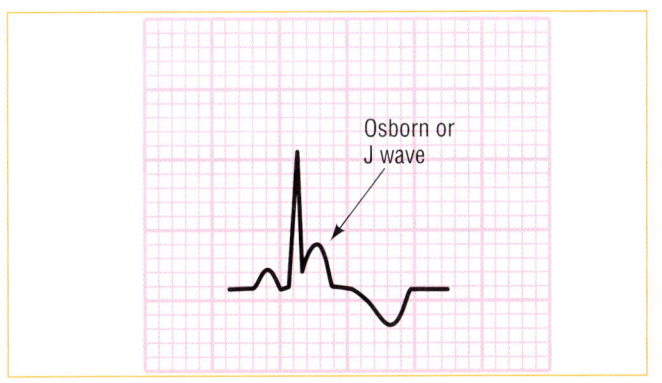

Figure 27-71 Osborne (J) wave.

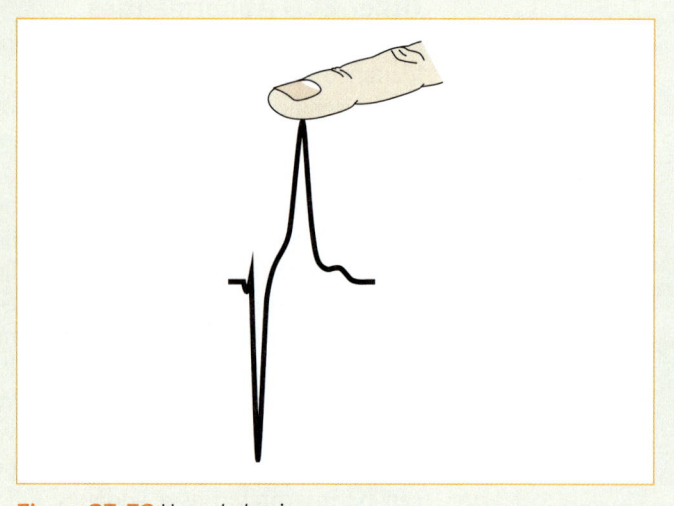

Figure 27-72 Hyperkalemia.

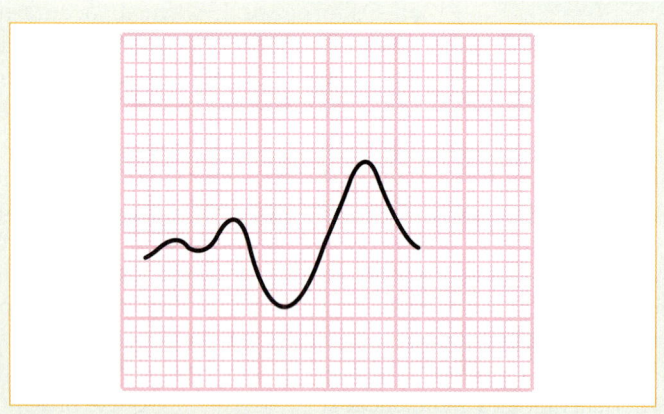

Figure 27-73 The rhythm strip for someone with profound, severe hyperkalemia has the appearance of a sine wave.

usually presents with flat or apparently absent T waves along with the development of a U wave. The U wave is a small wave (smaller even than a P wave) that occurs after a T wave but before the next P wave. U waves are very uncommon and may often be mistaken for extra P waves or another unknown abnormality.

Other electrolyte imbalances do not cause such obvious changes in the ECG. Hypercalcemia may cause a shortened Q-T interval, for example, whereas hypocalcemia may slightly lengthen the Q-T interval. These changes would likely not be obvious in the prehospital environment.

12-Lead ECGs

Up to now, we have considered ECG rhythm strips obtained from monitoring a single lead. For purposes of rhythm interpretation, a single lead (usually lead II) is usually sufficient. To localize the site of injury to heart muscle, however, we must be able to look at the heart from several angles. That is precisely the purpose of a 12-lead ECG.

What Is a 12-Lead ECG?

Suppose you wanted to check out the condition of a used car you were thinking of buying. If you needed to know only whether the motor was running, you could stand anywhere near the car and listen (just as you can use any one lead to monitor the cardiac rhythm). But if you wanted to know what kind of shape the car body is in, you would have to walk around the car and look at it from all sides. The driver's side might be in mint condition, but if you stroll around to the passenger's side, you might see that the entire door frame is caved in from a road accident.

Similarly, each ECG lead looks at the heart from a different angle. Although one lead may see a normal myocardium, another may be looking at major damage.

What Do ECG Leads Record?

What does a lead "see" when it looks at the heart? The word *lead*, as it is used in electrocardiography, can be somewhat confusing. Sometimes the word is used to refer to one of the cables and monitoring electrodes that connect the ECG machine to the patient (such as the "right arm lead"). A lead provides an electrical picture of the heart taken from a specified vantage point. Lead I, for example, "looks" at the heart from the left, so it "sees" the left side of the heart. Lead aVF looks up at the heart from the feet (F stands for "foot"), so it "sees" the bottom of the heart. In the standard ECG, we record 12 leads—that is, 12 different pictures of the electrical activity of the heart.

Six of the leads—I, II, III, aVR, aVL, and aVF—are called limb leads because the pictures taken by those leads are derived from attaching cables to the patient's limbs. The limb leads look at the heart from the sides and from the feet, in the vertical plane. **Figure 27-74 ▶** shows the viewpoint of each of the limb leads. For example, lead II has a direct view of the bottom of the heart (the inferior or diaphragmatic wall of the heart), whereas aVL (L stands for "left") looks at the heart from the vantage point of the left shoulder.

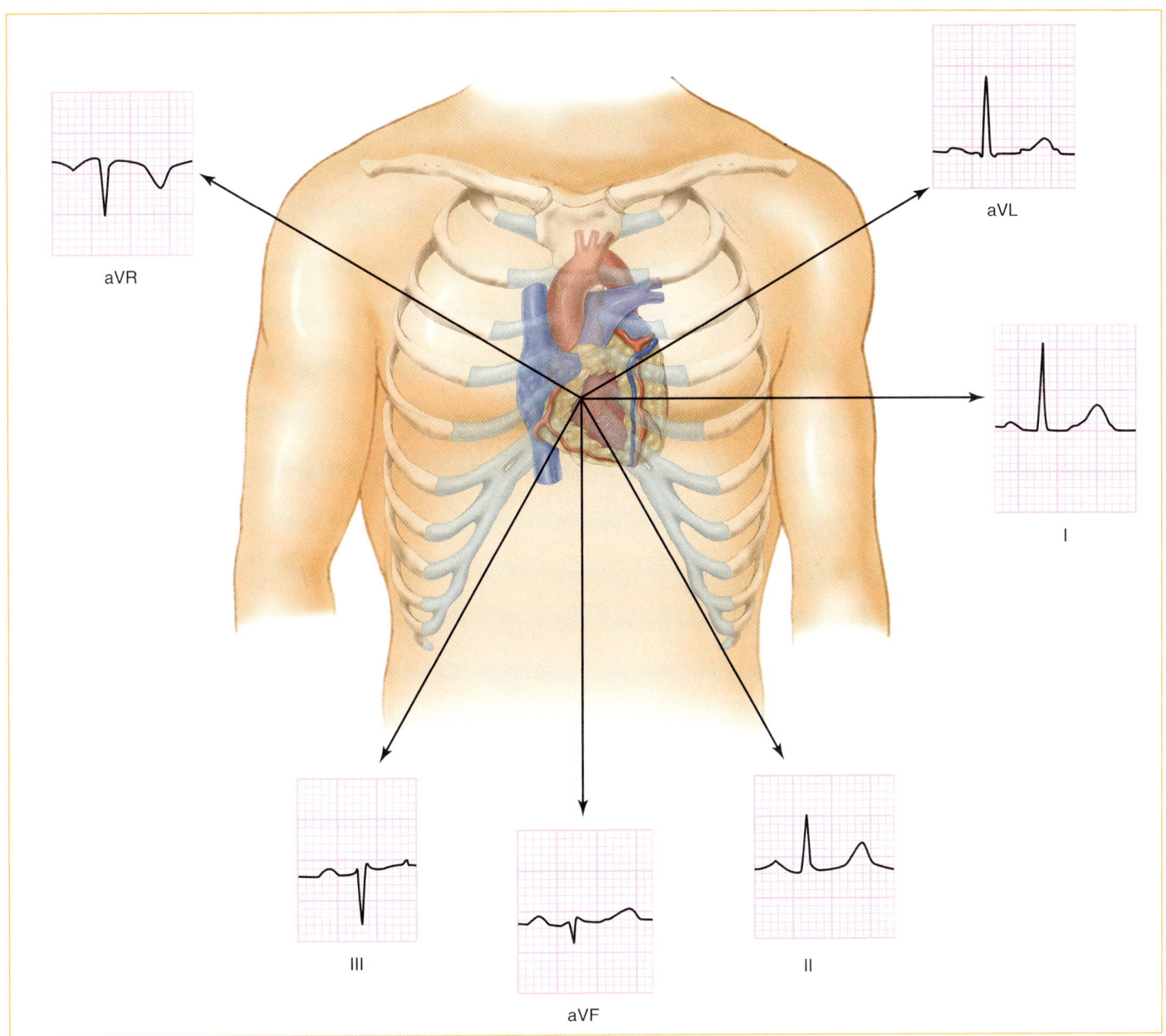

Figure 27-74 Limb leads look at the heart in the vertical plane. Leads II, III, and aVF give us a picture of the wall of the heart that rests on the diaphragm, the inferior wall.

In addition to the limb leads, there are six precordial leads (V_1 to V_6), also called chest leads, anterior leads, or V leads. The six precordial leads are placed on the anterior and lateral chest walls, usually with adhesive electrodes, in the positions shown in **Figure 27-75 ▶**. These leads look at the heart in the horizontal plane (as shown in the inset to Figure 27–80), so they provide a picture of the heart taken from the front (anterior wall of the heart) and from the left side (anterolateral). More specifically, leads V_1 and V_2 look at the septum; V_3 and V_4 look at the anterior wall of the left ventricle; and V_5 and V_6 look at the lateral wall of the left ventricle.

12-Lead ECG Lead Placement

How reliable would 12-lead ECGs be if you could place the electrodes anywhere on the chest? When a 12-lead ECG is read, it is assumed that the person who performed the recording placed the electrodes correctly on the chest. Correct placement is important because the 12-lead ECGs are compared with previous ECGs. For the comparison to be reliable for identifying existing problems or highlighting the appearance of new problems (such as ST-segment elevation), the electrodes must be placed consistently. **Table 27-17 ▶** outlines where the different leads look.

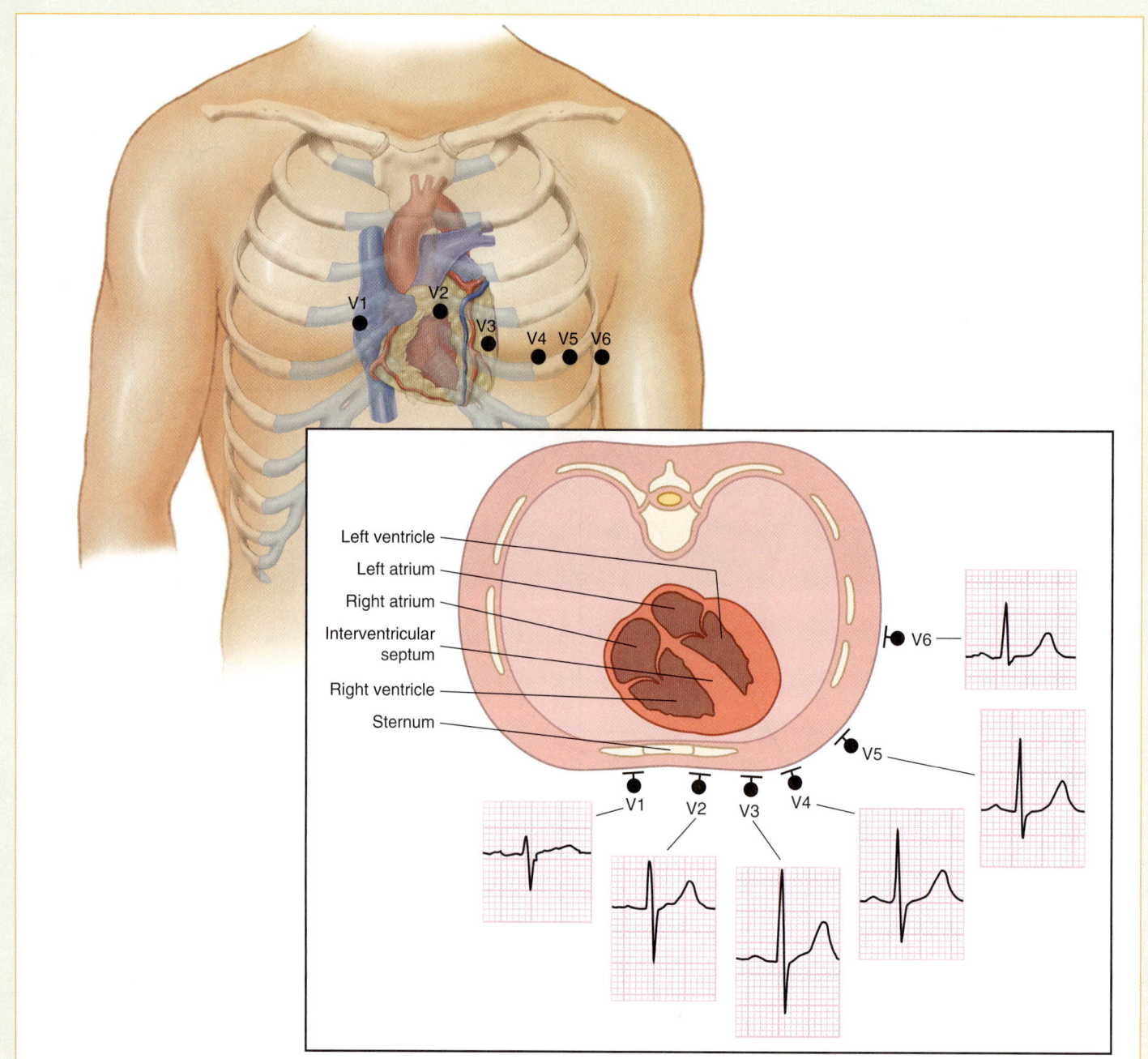

Figure 27-75 Precordial leads (chest leads) look at the heart in the horizontal plane. Inset: V₁ and V₂ look at the interventricular septum. V₃ and V₄ "see" the anterior left ventricle. V₅ and V₆ see the anterior and lateral left ventricle.

Table 27-17	Focus of ECG Leads		
Leads	**Area of Damage**	**Coronary Artery Involved**	**Possible Complications**
II, III, and aVF	Inferior wall LV	RCA: posterior descending	Hypotension, LV dysfunction
V₁ and V₂	Septum	LCA: LAD, septal	Infranodal blocks and BBBs
V₃ and V₄	Anterior wall LV	LCA: LAD, diagonal	LV dysfunction, CHF, BBBs, complete heart block, PVCs
V₅, V₆, I, and aVL	Lateral wall LV	LCA: circumflex	LV dysfunction, AV nodal block in some
V₄R (II, III, aVF)	RV	RCA: proximal	Hypotension, supranodal and AV nodal blocks, atrial fibrillation, PACs

LV indicates left ventricle; LAD, left anterior descending; BBB, bundle branch block; RV, right ventricle; RCA, right coronary artery; LCA, left coronary artery; PAC, premature atrial contraction; PVC, premature ventricular contraction; CHF, congestive heart failure.

When a current is moving toward a lead, it creates a positive (upright) deflection on the ECG tracing of that lead. Thus, in **Figure 27-76 ▾**, the current depolarizing the ventricles is moving toward lead II, so what we see in lead II is an upright QRS complex (recall that the QRS complex is produced by depolarization of the ventricles). If the depolarizing current is moving toward lead II, then it must be moving away from lead aVR, so we would expect to see a negative deflection in aVR. And, indeed, the QRS complex in aVR is a downward deflection. That makes intuitive sense. If you and a friend are standing facing each other at opposite ends of a football field, a ball thrown toward your friend will look bigger and bigger to the friend as it approaches; the same ball will meanwhile look smaller and smaller to you as it travels the same course. Similarly, leads II and aVR, being nearly opposite each other, will present nearly opposite pictures of the same wave of electrical depolarization. If a depolarizing wave is coming toward lead II, it will be going away from aVR.

The 12-Lead ECG in a Normal Heart

The gold standard for multilead ECGs is the 12-lead ECG. In special situations, a 15- or 18-lead ECG may also be performed. Any ECG that is recorded electronically always has the same layout on the paper, meaning that the leads will be plotted out in the same manner every time **Figure 27-77 ▸**.

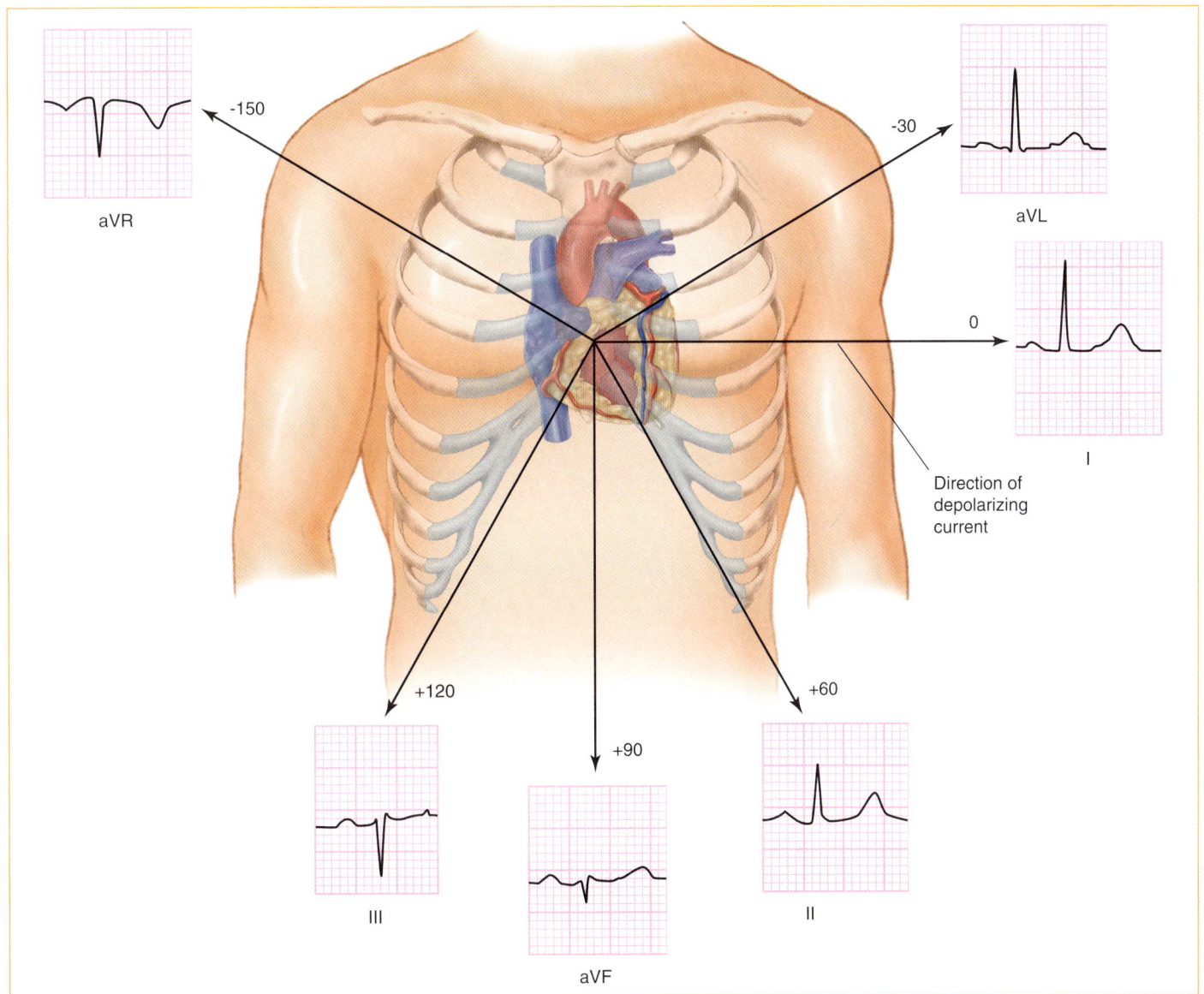

Figure 27-76 The morphology of QRS complexes varies based on the lead position and the direction of the electrical impulse movement within the heart. If the electrical impulses are moving primarily toward lead II, it will be upright as shown, while lead aVR will be inverted since the impulse is moving away from it.

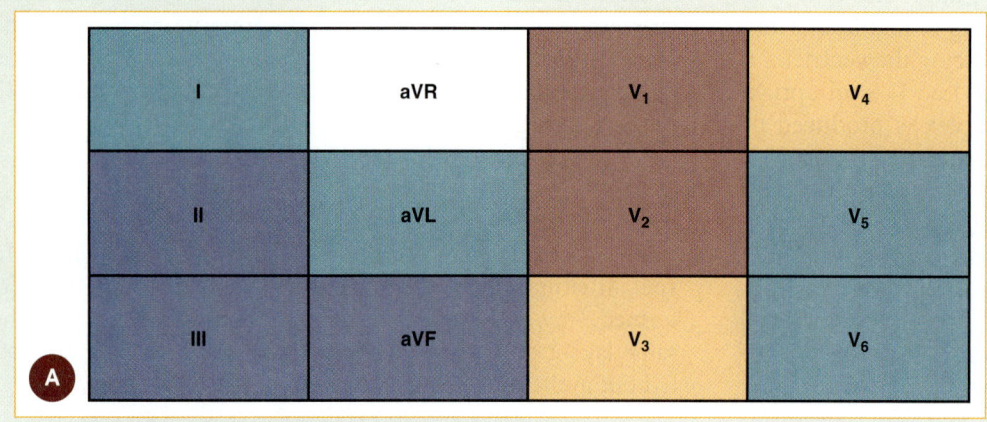

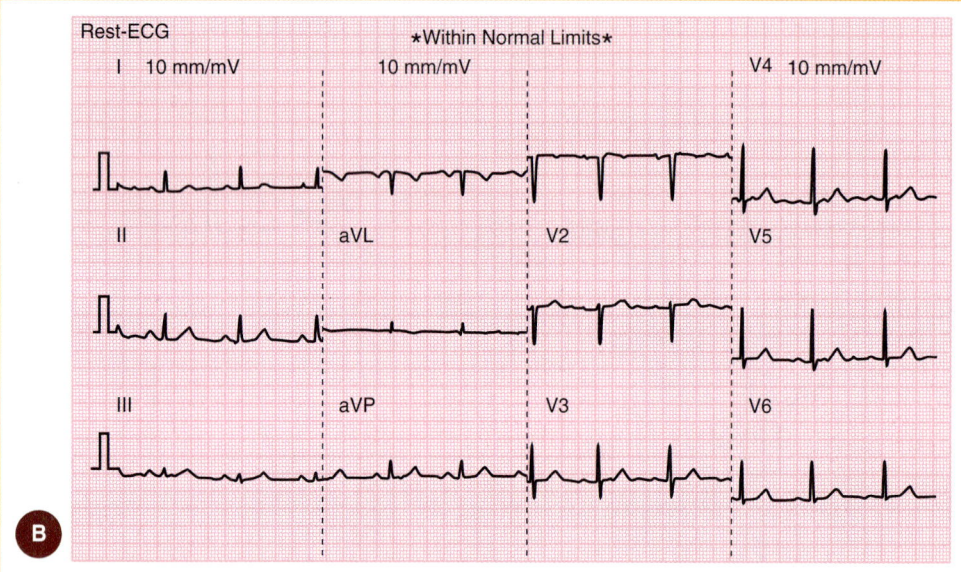

Figure 27-77 A. The areas on a 12-lead ECG correlate to different leads. **B.** A normal ECG with standard 12-lead format.

completely. Those leads are anatomically contiguous—that is, the leads look at the same general area of the heart. When we are looking for evidence of injury to the heart and we must see it in two or more contiguous leads, then the following information will be important:

Contiguous Inferior Leads

- Lead II is contiguous with lead III.
- Lead III is contiguous with leads II and aVF.
- Lead aVF is contiguous with lead III.

Contiguous Septal-Anterior-Lateral Leads

- V_1 is contiguous with V_2.
- V_2 is contiguous with V_1 and V_3.
- V_3 is contiguous with V_2 and V_4.
- V_4 is contiguous with V_3 and V_5.
- V_5 is contiguous with V_4 and V_6.
- V_6 is contiguous with V_5 and lead I.
- Lead I is contiguous with V_6 and aVL.
- aVL is contiguous with lead I.

The 12-Lead ECG in a Damaged Heart

The ECG tells the practitioner many things about a patient's heart. For our purposes in the prehospital environment, we will keep it simple and look for any evidence that the patient is having an AMI. To do so, we must focus on three parts of the ECG: the ST segment, the Q wave, and the T wave.

Recall the sequence of events in an AMI. As the blood supply to the affected area of heart muscle slows to a trickle, the muscle no longer receives sufficient oxygen. In other words, the muscle becomes ischemic (deprived of blood). If ischemia persists more than a few minutes, it leads to actual injury to the heart muscle, which in turn will be followed by infarction (death of muscle) if the circulation to the area is not rapidly restored.

The ECG can provide a graphic record of that sequence of events (Table 27-18 ▶). Ischemia commonly causes ST-segment depression and may also lead to T-wave inversion. Injury may initially cause a transient peaking of T waves quickly, followed by ST-segment elevation. Infarction (indicative of dead cardiac tissue) often results in the development of a pathologic Q wave. A Q wave that is wider than 0.04 s (one small square on the ECG strip) or deeper than one third of the height of the R wave that follows it and that is seen in two or more contiguous leads generally indicates an infarction has happened at some time in the past (Figure 27-79 ▶).

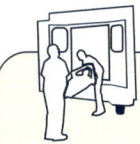

At the Scene

If the PQRST configuration is upright in lead aVR, the limb leads are on wrong! Specifically, the arm leads have been switched.

Each of the colours in (Figure 27-78A ▶) has a purpose; that is, each colour represents the leads that look at a particular wall of the heart. Lead aVR is not used for this purpose, so no colour is assigned to it.

(Figure 27-78B ▶) depicts an ECG. (Some information has been added to help you out.) Notice that the specific wall of the left ventricle is listed along with the coronary artery that supplies that wall for each lead. The left ventricle is the stronger and more muscular of the two ventricles; it will be the first to let its owner know that it is not getting enough oxygen. If the left ventricle becomes damaged, in addition to pain, the patient may develop deadly arrhythmias such as ventricular fibrillation. Each wall requires two to four leads or views to see its image

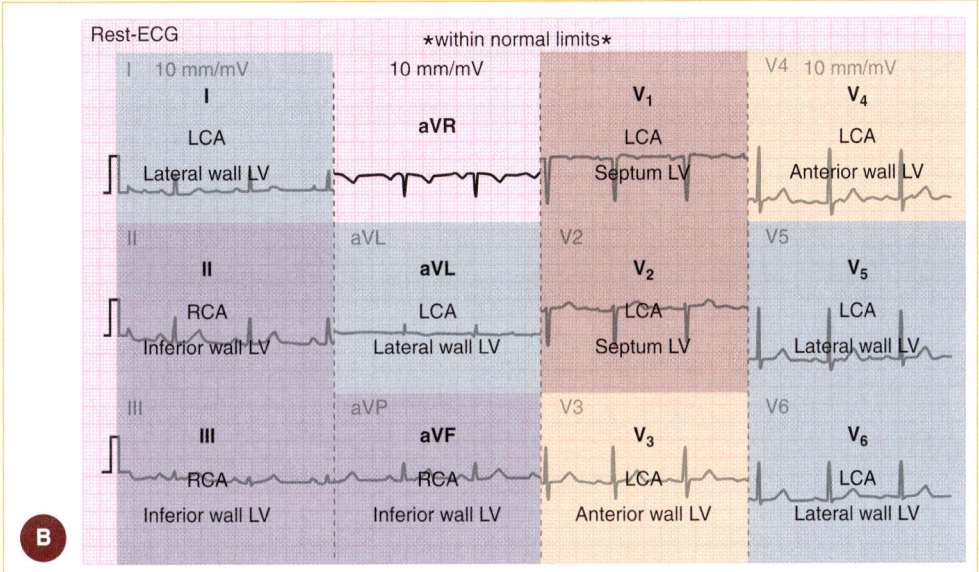

I	aVR	V$_1$	V$_4$
LCA		LCA	LCA
Lateral wall LV		Septum LV	Anterior wall LV
II	**aVL**	**V$_2$**	**V$_5$**
RCA	LCA	LCA	LCA
Inferior wall LV	Lateral wall LV	Septum LV	Lateral wall LV
III	**aVF**	**V$_3$**	**V$_6$**
RCA	RCA	LCA	LCA
Inferior wall LV	Inferior wall LV	Anterior wall LV	Lateral wall LV

A

B (Rest-ECG, *within normal limits*)

Figure 27-78 A. A schematic representation of a 12-lead ECG. **B.** A normal ECG with standard 12-lead format.

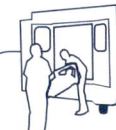

At the Scene

When a doctor reads an ECG and sees pathologic Q waves, he or she will usually ask when the patient had his MI. These changes represent an evolved MI of unknown age.

elevation of greater than 1 mm in the V$_4$R lead on this second ECG, there is a high likelihood that you have identified a right ventricular MI. Of course, the ECG monitor does not know that this V$_4$ is a right-sided one, so on printing this ECG tracing, you should add an "R" next to the "V$_4$," and circle the V$_4$R to make it stand out.

Patients who are experiencing an MI of the right ventricle may already be hypotensive or may become extremely hypotensive if nitroglycerin is given. For this reason, you are well advised to perform a second 15-lead ECG or 12-lead ECG every time you find a patient with an inferior wall MI. You may be ordered by the physician to give 1 to 2 l of saline IV before administering any nitroglycerin.

Patients with inferior AMIs may also have posterior wall involvement (or a posterior AMI may occur in isolation). This may be noted by reciprocal changes in V$_1$ and V$_2$ (tall R waves and ST depression). This can be confirmed by performing a 15-lead ECG using leads V$_8$ and V$_9$.

A 15-lead ECG can be performed after the first 12-lead ECG for the following indications: ST elevation in the inferior leads (II, III, aVF) and/or ST depression in the septal leads (V$_1$, V$_2$). Repeat the 12-lead ECG by moving the V$_4$–V$_6$ to the positions of V$_4$R, V$_8$, and V$_9$ **Table 27-19 ▸** . After acquiring this new 15-lead ECG, ensure that you label it appropriately with V$_4$R, V$_8$, and V$_9$ instead of V$_4$–V$_6$.

Figure 27-80 ▸ depicts an injury (ST-segment elevation) in the leads that look at the anterior wall of the heart, leads V$_3$ through V$_5$. **Figure 27-81 ▸** shows the signs of ischemia (T-wave inversion) in the leads that look at the anterolateral wall of the heart, leads V$_4$ through V$_6$.

Sometimes, the ischemia or injury extends from one wall to the next. Such ischemia is evidenced by inverted (or flipped) T waves in leads V$_3$ through V$_6$. Table 27-19 summarizes the leads corresponding to different locations of myocardial injury.

Table 27-18	Evolution of an AMI on the ECG	
Stage	**ECG Changes in Overlying Leads***	**Timing**
Ischemia	T-wave inversion	With the onset of ischemia
	ST-segment depression	
Injury	Peaked T waves	Minutes to hours
	ST-segment elevation	
Infarction	Q waves appear	Within several hours to several days

*Reciprocal changes will be seen in opposite leads.

In 40% of patients who experience an inferior wall MI, a right ventricular MI will eventually develop as well. To verify this, a 15-lead ECG can be done or an electrode can be placed in the fifth intercostal space at the midclavicular line on the right side of the chest (V$_4$R). Unsnap the original V$_4$ on the left side of the chest and snap it onto the new lead on the right side, leaving all the other electrodes in place. Now press "acquire" on the 12-lead ECG monitor. If you see ST-segment

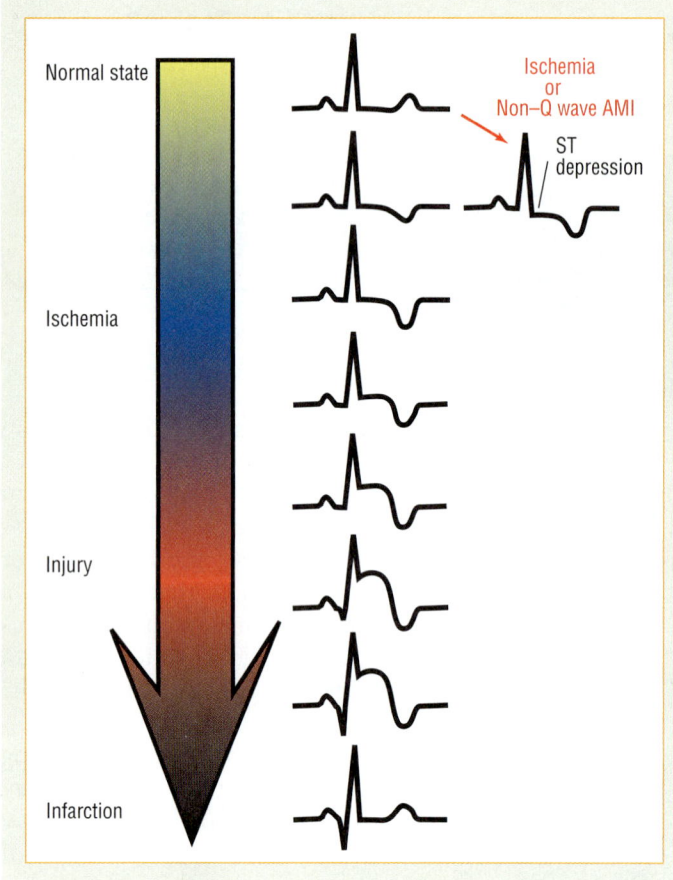

Figure 27-79 Evolutionary pattern or indicative changes of MI.

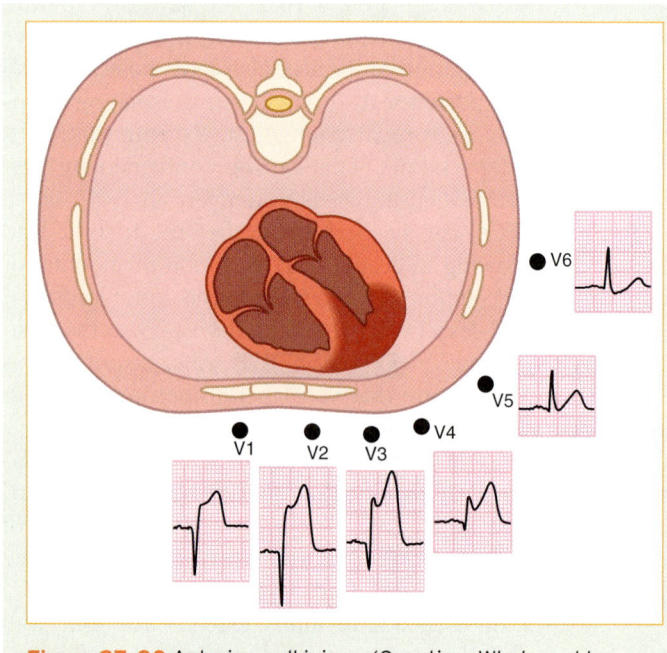

Figure 27-80 Anterior wall injury. (Question: What would *ischemia* in the anterior wall look like?)

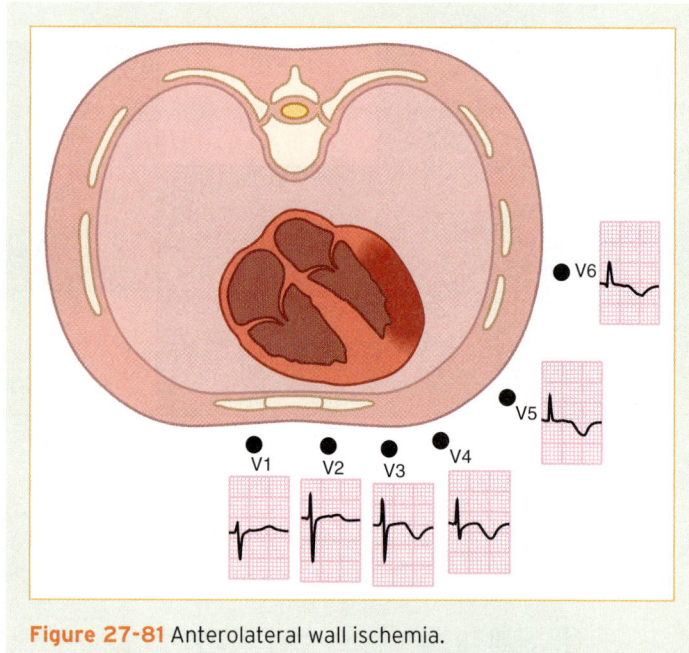

Figure 27-81 Anterolateral wall ischemia.

Table 27-19	Localization of AMI
Site of Infarction	**Primary ECG Changes Seen in Leads**
Inferior (diaphragmatic) wall	II, III, and aVF
Anteroseptal	V_1 to V_3
Anterolateral	V_4 to V_6
Extensive anterior wall	V_1 to V_6, I, and aVL
Posterior wall	V_1 to V_2 (tall R waves with ST depression; or V_8 to V_9; reciprocal changes) (15-lead ECG)

Benefits of Using 12-Lead ECGs

The most important 12-lead finding in the prehospital phase of care is simply the answer to the following question: Does this patient have ECG evidence of ischemia, injury, or infarction? This information will help the receiving hospital decide whether to mobilize the necessary resources for reperfusion. Meanwhile, the 12-lead ECG provides you with information that can help you choose the most appropriate emergency management in the prehospital environment. For example, patients who have an inferior wall MI and possibly a right ventricular infarction will not respond well to nitroglycerin or morphine. If we know which leads to check for signs of injury to the inferior wall of the heart (and do a V_4R), we should be able to identify patients who might need a fluid bolus and avoid nitroglycerin administration to prevent extreme hypotension.

Prehospital 12-lead ECGs and advanced notification to the receiving hospital can lead to faster diagnosis, decrease the time until fibrinolysis is administered or primary angioplasty is performed, and, perhaps, decrease mortality rates. In some EMS systems, field diagnosis of ST-elevation MI may allow bypass of the emergency department and allow paramedics to take the patient directly to the catheterization lab. The time savings in door-to-reperfusion therapy in most studies ranges from 10 to 60 minutes. As we have learned, "Time is myocardium." Paramedics can efficiently acquire and transmit (or communicate their findings) to the ED with only a minimal increase (0.2 to 5.6 minutes) in their scene time. The decision of where to transport patients with ACS should be based on current guidelines and recommendations from national groups. The 2005 guidelines suggest that a checklist be used to assist in the triage of patients with ACS **Figure 27-82 ▼** .

Remember—the absence of an MI on the ECG doesn't mean that the patient isn't having one. It may take hours for changes to appear in the ECG.

You should be equipped with portable ECG machines, monitors, and defibrillators that provide computerized ECG interpretation. Even if you're a whiz at reading 12-lead ECGs, computer ECG interpretations provide consistency and a high degree of accuracy. (They also provide on-the-job refresher training in ECG interpretation!) As soon as you have the ECG printout, contact the receiving hospital and read the computer ECG interpretation to the emergency physician there. If you have something to add to what the computer says, by all means do so (briefly!). And, of course, provide details of the patient's history and the physical examination findings.

Notes from Nancy

Every patient with a story of heavy, crushing, squeezing, or choking chest pain must be treated for AMI even if the ECG is perfectly normal.

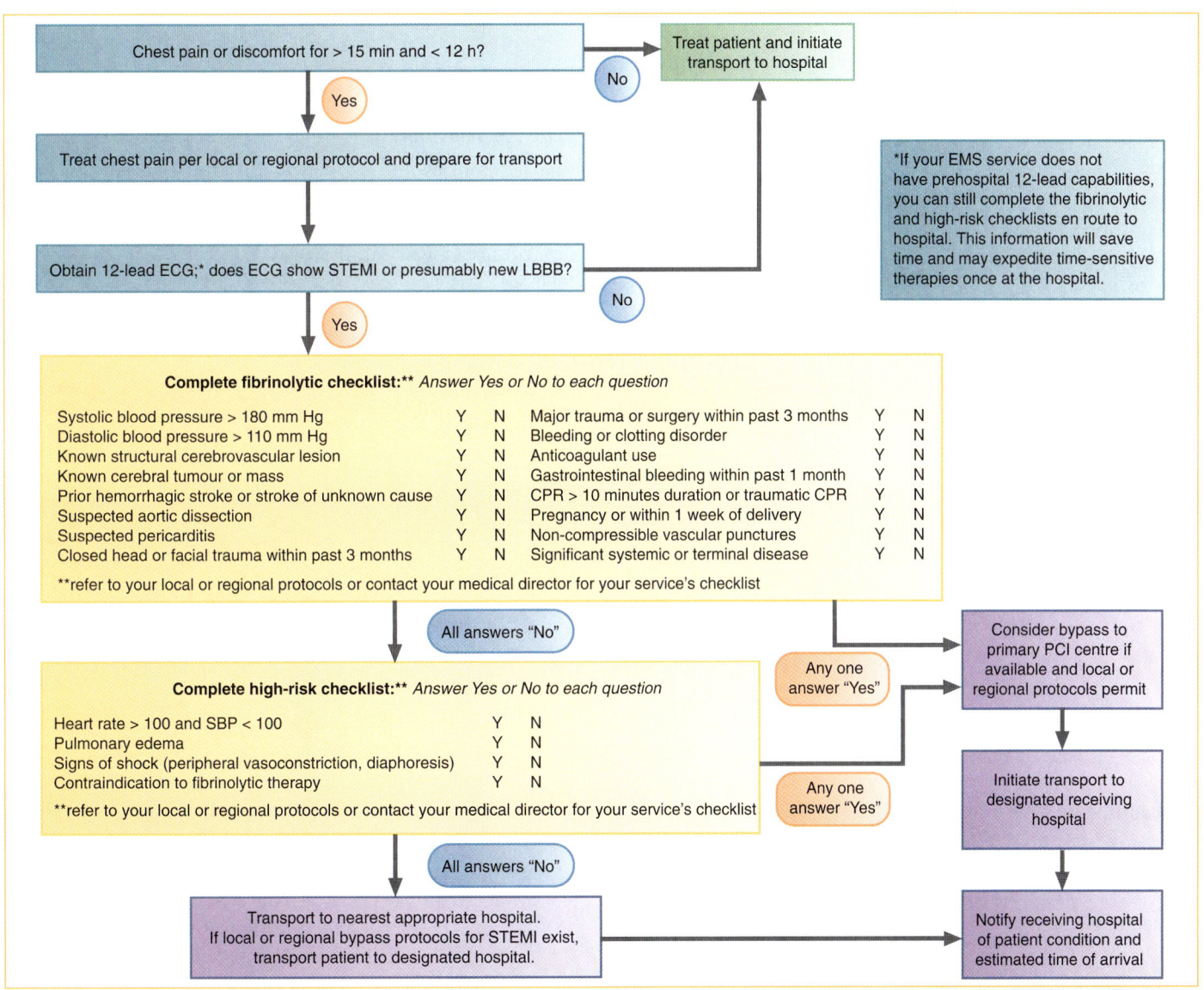

Figure 27-82 Chest pain checklist.

Guidelines for Performing a 12-Lead ECG

The only way to learn how to obtain a 12-lead ECG is to practice with the equipment itself. Here are some guidelines to help ensure that the ECGs you obtain are of the highest quality possible.

- The patient should be supine. If the patient feels short of breath in that position, you may elevate the back of the stretcher about 30°.
- Make sure the patient does not become chilled, because shivering will produce artifact in the ECG tracing. Note that 12-lead ECGs are more sensitive to artifact than 3-lead monitoring ECGs.
- Prepare the patient's skin as you would for placing monitoring electrodes.
- Connect the four limb electrodes. Double-check that the correct electrode is on each limb (the "LA" electrode on the left arm, the "RA" electrode on the right arm, and so on). Confirm that the limb electrodes are on the arms and legs and *not* on the trunk of the body, as sometimes is the case in a 3-lead ECG.
- Connect and apply the precordial leads as indicated in **Table 27-20 ▾**.
- Ensure the patient remains very still and the arms and legs are resting. The 12-lead ECG is more susceptible to movement artifact.
- Record the ECG.
- Acquiring a 12-lead tracing should not normally prolong scene time or transport more than 2 minutes.

Table 27-20	Applying the Precordial Leads
Lead	**Placement**
Standard 12-lead	
V_1	Fourth intercostal space at right sternal border
V_2	Fourth intercostal space at left sternal border
V_3	Equidistant between V_2 and V_4
V_4	Fifth intercostal space in left midclavicular line
V_5	Anterior axillary line (same horizontal plane as V_4)
V_6	Midaxillary line (same horizontal plane as V_4)
Modified 15-lead ECG	
V_4 becomes V_4R	Fifth intercostal space at right midclavicular line (same as V_4 but on right side of chest)
V_5 becomes V_8	Level with V_{4-6} at left midscapular line
V_6 becomes V_9	Level with V_{4-6} at left paravertebral

■ Management of Adult Cardiac Arrest

Nothing gets the adrenaline pumping more furiously—in paramedics, even if not in the patient—than a "code," or cardiopulmonary arrest. Most adult cardiac arrest victims have evidence of atherosclerosis or other underlying cardiac disease. However, cardiac arrest can also occur after electrocution, drowning, and other types of trauma. Indeed, many cardiac arrest victims have no warning before the event occurs. No matter what the cause, cardiac arrest is a stressful event for paramedics.

Management of cardiac arrest requires you to deploy a great many of the advanced life support (ALS) skills that you have learned and to do so under very urgent circumstances in which minutes may mean the difference between life and death. It is very difficult to think clearly in such stressful circumstances, especially when there are likely to be other stressed and panicky people at the scene (the patient's family, for example). For these reasons, it is absolutely essential for you to follow an orderly, systematic approach to cardiac arrest emergencies. That approach needs to be rehearsed repeatedly in a team setting, until it is nearly automatic, and must include the steps of BLS and ALS.

BLS: A Review

The techniques and sequences of adult BLS should be very familiar to all paramedic students. Here, we will simply review the guidelines for ensuring maximally effective (and minimally damaging) CPR to adults in cardiac arrest. For a complete review of this skill, see Appendix A.

- Concentrate on high-quality compressions (deep enough, fast enough, and with full chest recoil) with a minimum of interruptions.
- Avoid excessive inflation pressures in artificial ventilation. Inflate just enough to observe visible chest rise.
- Keep your compressions smooth, regular, and uninterrupted.
  1. The compression depth must be at least 5 cm in adults, maintaining each compression for at least half the compression-release cycle.
  2. Avoid bouncing or jerky compressions,
  3. Keep your shoulders directly over the patient's sternum, and keep your elbows straight.
  4. Maintain proper hand position: fingers off the chest, and hands coming up off the sternum slightly between compressions to allow for complete chest recoil.
  5. Change the person doing the compressions every 2 minutes to ensure that fatigue does not affect the quality of compressions.
- As a single rescuer, give 30 compressions to two ventilations at a rate of at least 100 compressions per minute. Once an advanced airway is placed, compressions continue at a rate of at least 100 beats/min uninterrupted with 8 to 10 ventilations given with 100% supplemental oxygen.
- Do not interrupt CPR compressions except for advanced airway placement, defibrillation, or moving the patient. In all cases, minimize the duration of the interruption to as close

to 10 to 15 seconds as possible. Any stop in compressions also stops perfusion—and perfusion is what it is all about!

We shall now consider how to integrate these well-rehearsed steps of BLS into the sequences of ACLS.

Advanced Cardiac Life Support

We defined BLS as maintenance of the airway, breathing, and circulation—the ABCs—without adjunctive equipment. Basic life support is a holding action only and is unlikely to restore the heart to effective activity. You will be called on to deliver more definitive therapy as well, so the skills of ACLS must also become second nature, to be deployed swiftly and systematically in the event of cardiac arrest.

What Is ACLS?

The Heart and Stroke Foundation has defined ACLS for a patient in cardiac arrest (or a patient at immediate risk of cardiac arrest) as consisting of the following elements:

- Effective and minimally interrupted chest compression (for cardiac arrest)
- Use of adjunctive equipment for ventilation and circulation
- Cardiac monitoring for arrhythmia recognition and control
- Establishment and maintenance of an IV or IO (intraosseous) infusion line
- Use of definitive therapy, including defibrillation and drug administration, to:
  1. Prevent cardiac arrest
  2. Aid in establishing an effective cardiac rhythm and circulation when cardiac arrest occurs
  3. Stabilize the patient's condition
- Transportation with continuous monitoring

We have already discussed the use of airway adjuncts and equipment for artificial ventilation. In this section, we focus on the sequence of actions in ACLS. The last section of the chapter will describe some of the specific techniques—such as defibrillation—for restoring an effective cardiac rhythm.

The Universal Algorithm

The approach to every patient in cardiac arrest will start with the same steps. These basic steps are always deployed as soon as a person is found unresponsive and possibly in cardiac arrest. The BLS health care provider algorithm includes measures that bystanders should take before your arrival (such as "phone 9-1-1 or emergency number"), so we need to modify the universal algorithm a bit to make it applicable to emergency medical services personnel.

Whenever you are called for a case that might be a cardiac arrest (such as "man down," "unconscious woman," "choking," "stopped breathing"), carry the defibrillator with you on your first trip from the ambulance to the patient. You should also carry a portable oxygen cylinder and a "jump kit" that contains equipment for managing the airway. If you have enough help—for example, a three-person crew—by all means take the intubation kit, the IV equipment, and the drug box as well. But if you're shorthanded, don't spend the time carting every piece of equipment from the ambulance to the patient. You can send someone to the ambulance for other equipment later.

As soon as you reach the patient, one paramedic should ready the monitor-defibrillator while the other carries out the following steps:

1. **Assess responsiveness.** If the patient is *not responsive and there is no pulse, start CPR.* CPR should continue for 2 minutes or 5 cycles of 30 compressions and two ventilations. As CPR continues, the second paramedic should attach the monitor-defibrillator. At the end of 2 minutes, pause CPR and:

2. **Check the rhythm on the monitor.** At this point, all you want to know is the answer to one question: Is *VF or VT* present?
   - *If VF or VT is present* on the monitor-defibrillator, follow the VF/VT arm of the algorithm.
   - *If VF or VT is not present* on the monitor-defibrillator, *resume CPR immediately.*

What you see on the monitor at this point will determine which side of the algorithm you will now follow. If the patient is still in cardiac arrest, he or she may be in any of the following situations:

- VF or pulseless VT
- PEA (that is, you can see an organized rhythm on the monitor, but there is no detectable pulse)
- Asystole

Each of these situations requires a different, specific approach (a different pathway down the pulseless arrest algorithm).

Experienced paramedics will note that rescue breathing and ventilation are deemphasized. The traditional "ABC" approach to basic and advanced cardiac life support maneuvers has changed to "CAB." Chest compressions can be started immediately, whereas positioning the head and achieving a seal for bag-valve-mask rescue breathing takes time. Animal studies have shown that delaying chest compressions reduces survival, so such delays should be avoided. If there is only one rescuer, starting compressions is the priority. If there is more than one rescuer, the first rescuer starts compressions and subsequent rescuers can open the airway and begin rescue breathing. Rescue breathing no longer needs to be synchronized to chest compressions.

Treatment for VF or Pulseless VT

Managing VF or pulseless VT is probably the most important pathway down the algorithm for you to know because patients found in VF or VT are the most likely to be successfully resuscitated—*if* they receive timely and appropriate treatment. The steps in managing VF and pulseless VT are as follows:

- *Initiate resuscitation* based on the BLS algorithm (see Appendix A).
- *Perform CPR for 2 minutes while the defibrillator is being attached.*
- *Confirm VF or VT on the monitor-defibrillator.*
- *Resume CPR while charging the defibrillator.*
- *Clear the patient and then defibrillate* the VF or VT:
  1. If using a biphasic defibrillator, set it to 120 to 200 joules (J). This energy level depends on the

manufacturer's recommendation. If the recommendation is unknown and the defibrillator is biphasic, use 200 J for all shocks.

2. If using a monophasic defibrillator, set it to 360 J for all shocks.

As soon as the defibrillator discharges, immediately resume CPR. It is important not to delay resuming CPR at this time to determine the rhythm or check for a pulse. Continue CPR for 2 minutes or 5 cycles. Recent research indicates that even if an organized rhythm appears in the postresuscitation period, the presence of an immediate pulse is unlikely. It has also been shown that 2 minutes of postresuscitation CPR is unlikely to cause a return of VF. Only stop CPR during this 2 minutes if you have obvious signs of life. After 2 minutes or five cycles, stop CPR, and assess the patient's circulation and check the rhythm on the monitor.

- If a rhythm other than VF or VT appears on the monitor screen:
  1. *Identify the new rhythm.*
  2. If there is no pulse, move to the asystole-PEA pathway down the algorithm and resume CPR immediately.
  3. If there is a pulse, move to the appropriate algorithm for the new rhythm.
- If the rhythm is persistent VF or VT, *resume CPR while charging the defibrillator.*
- *Clear the patient and then defibrillate* the VF or VT:
  1. Use the same energy setting as previously discussed.
  2. *Resume CPR immediately,* and continue for 2 minutes after the shock. The CPR compressor and ventilator should change positions at the end of each 2-minute session of CPR (while the rhythm and pulse are being checked) to avoid fatigue, which can reduce the effectiveness of chest compressions.
  3. During this 2 minutes of CPR, you should *insert an advanced airway if the BLS airway is not adequate.* Advanced airways include the endotracheal tube, laryngeal mask airway, laryngeal tube, and Combitube. After intubation, verify placement using multiple methods and secure the tube. Once the patient has been intubated, it is no longer necessary to pause CPR compressions for ventilation to be administered. Ventilations should be administered at a rate of 8 to 10 breaths per minute (one breath every 6 to 8 seconds). The rate of compressions is at least 100/min.
  4. *Start an IV* with normal saline.
  5. *If unable to establish IV access, consider establishment of intraosseous (IO) access* via an adult IO access system. If IV access is not obtained but IO access is, all drugs and fluids that would normally be administered via IV should be administered via IO until IV assess is established.
  6. As soon as IV or IO has been established, *administer a vasopressor drug.* The two recommended vasopressor drugs are epinephrine and vasopressin. *Epinephrine (1:10,000) is given as 1 mg IV push;* this dose should be repeated every 3 to 5 minutes as long as a pulse is absent. *Vasopressin is an alternative given as 40 units IV*

push, one time only. Vasopressin can be given in place of the first or second dose of epinephrine (but not both). Whenever you give a medication through a peripheral IV line during CPR, follow it immediately with a 20- to 30-ml bolus of IV fluid and then elevate the extremity to facilitate delivery of the medication to the central circulation (which may take 1 to 2 minutes).

- *At the end of 2 minutes of CPR, pause compressions to check for circulation and check the rhythm on the monitor.*
- If VF or VT is still present, *resume CPR while charging the defibrillator.*
- *Clear the patient and then defibrillate* the VF or VT:
  1. Use the same energy setting as before.
  2. Resume CPR immediately, and continue for 2 minutes after the shock. Remember to change CPR compressors after each rhythm check.
  3. During this 2 minutes of CPR, you should *consider the administration of an antiarrhythmic medication.* The preferred antiarrhythmic medication is *amiodarone,* which is given as a 300-mg bolus during CPR. Amiodarone may be repeated once at 150 mg in 3 to 5 minutes after the initial dose. If amiodarone is unavailable, you may administer *lidocaine,* 1 to 1.5 mg/kg IV push. Lidocaine can be repeated at 0.5 to 0.75 mg/kg every 5 to 10 minutes until the maximum dose of 3 mg/kg has been reached. It is important not to combine these two antiarrhythmic medications because this practice can actually cause arrhythmias.
- *At the end of 2 minutes of CPR, pause compressions to check for circulation and check the rhythm on the monitor.*
- If VF or VT is still present, *resume CPR while charging the defibrillator.*
- *Clear the patient and then defibrillate* the VF or VT:
  1. Use the same energy setting as the third shock.
  2. Resume CPR immediately, and continue for 2 minutes after the shock. Remember to change CPR compressors after each rhythm check.
  3. If VF or VT is still present, consider making a transport decision with the advice of direct medical control. Continue the cycle of defibrillation followed by immediate CPR for 2 minutes while administering repeated doses of medications.
- If at any point during this sequence there is a return of spontaneous circulation:
  1. Assess the patient's vital signs.
  2. Support the airway and breathing, as required.
  3. Provide medications as indicated for regulating the HR, controlling cardiac arrhythmias, and maintaining the blood pressure.

The steps of the VF/VT pathway down the pulseless arrest algorithm are presented schematically in **Figure 27-83 ▶**.

Treatment for Pulseless Electrical Activity

The term pulseless electrical activity (PEA) refers to an organized cardiac rhythm (other than VT) on the monitor that is not accompanied by any detectable pulse. This category includes what was once called electromechanical dissociation and

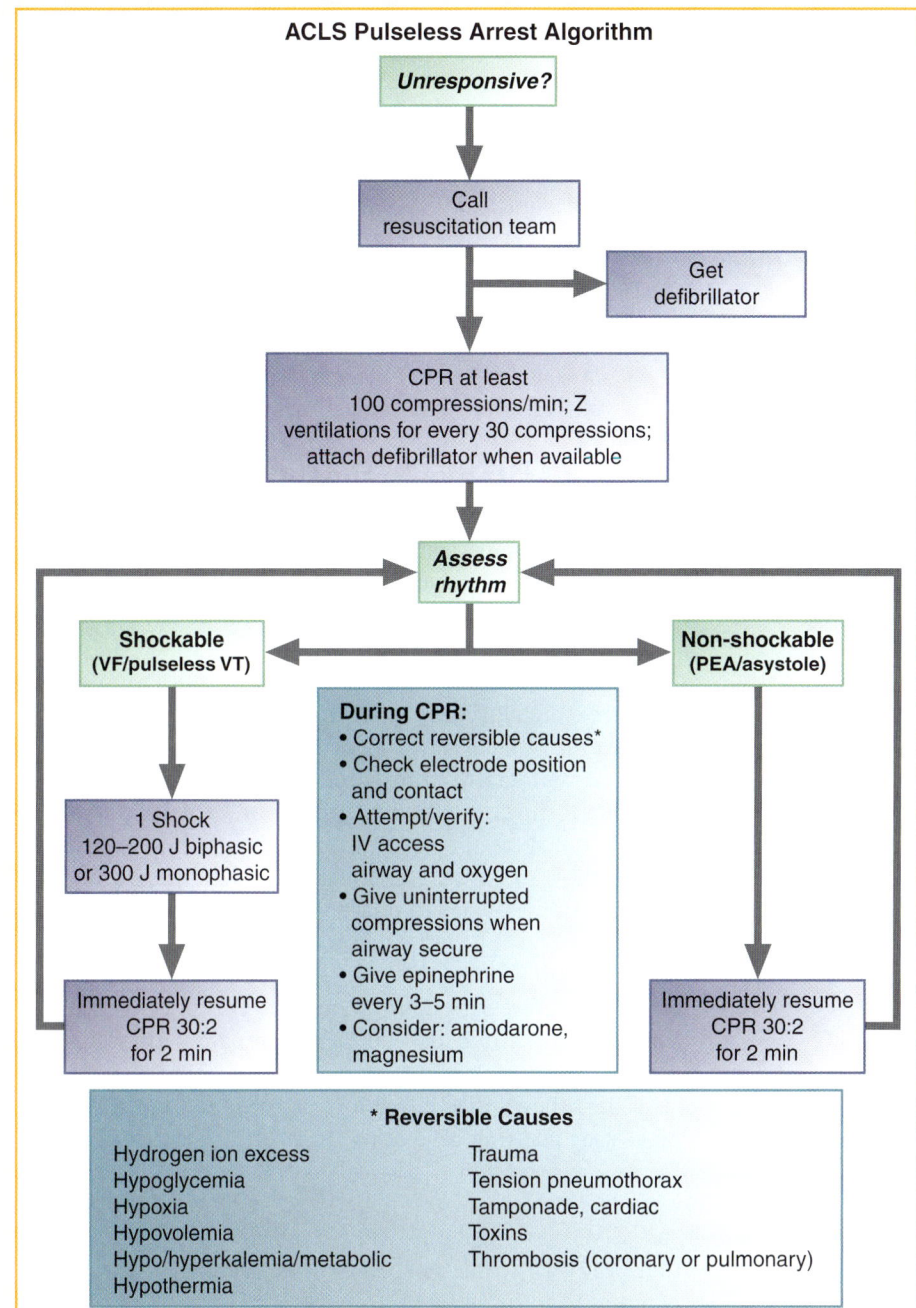

Figure 27-83 ACLS Algorithm for Pulseless Arrest.

Modified from *Adult Advanced Life Support Algorithm*. Copyright European Resuscitation Council. www.erc.edu
Approval #2009/011.

1. *Immediately resume CPR.*
2. *Insert an advanced airway if the BLS airway is not adequate.*
3. *Start an IV* with normal saline.
4. *If you are unable to establish IV access, consider establishing IO access.*
5. As soon as IV or IO access has been established, *administer a vasopressor drug.* The two recommended vasopressor drugs are epinephrine and vasopressin. *Epinephrine (1:10,000) is given as 1 mg IV push;* this dose should be repeated every 3 to 5 minutes for as long as a pulse is absent. *Vasopressin is an alternative and is given as 40 units IV push, one time only.* Vasopressin can be given in place of the first or second dose of epinephrine (but not both). Whenever you give a medication through a peripheral IV line during CPR, follow it immediately with a 20- to 30-ml bolus of IV fluid and then elevate the extremity to facilitate delivery of the medication to the central circulation (which may take 1 to 2 minutes).
6. Search for and treat the possible causes **Table 27-21 ▶**. If you are unable to identify and treat the possible underlying causes, the patient is unlikely to survive.
7. *At the end of 2 minutes of CPR, pause the compressions to check for circulation and check the rhythm on the monitor.*
8. If PEA is still present:
   ▪ *Continue CPR immediately.*
   ▪ Repeat epinephrine every 3 to 5 minutes, as indicated.
   ▪ If no reversible cause is found, consider termination of resuscitation with consultation from direct medical control.

conditions in which the heart beats so weakly that it cannot produce a palpable pulse, which may occur, for example, in cardiogenic or hypovolemic shock, cardiac tamponade, massive pulmonary embolism, disturbances of electrolyte imbalance, or drug overdose. Providing the appropriate treatment depends on identifying the cause of PEA in a specific case.

When the monitor is applied to a pulseless patient and a rhythm (other than VF or VT or asystole) is seen:

Asystole Treatment

A flat line on an ECG monitor may or may not be asystole. Thus, one of the first things to do when you see a flat-line ECG is to rule out causes other than asystole. Possible causes of a flat-line ECG include leads that are not connected to the patient, loose leads, leads that are not connected to the monitor-defibrillator, an incorrect monitor setting, very-low-voltage VF, and true asystole.

Table 27-21	Possible Causes and Treatment of PEA	
Possible Cause of PEA	**Clues to Cause**	**Treatment**
Hypovolemia	Patient history	Volume infusion
Hypoxemia	Cyanosis, airway problem	Intubation and ventilation with 100% oxygen
Hypoglycemia	Blood glucose level, < 4 mmol/l	Dextrose 50% in water, 25 g (50 ml of $D_{50}W$)
Hypothermia	History of exposure to cold	See hypothermia algorithm
Hyperkalemia, hypokalemia, hydrogen ions (acidosis)	History, ECG changes	Immediate transport Consider sodium bicarbonate if certain of acidosis. Consider calcium chloride if hyperkalemia is strongly suspected.
Tension pneumothorax	History, no pulse with CPR, unequal breath sounds with hyperresonance to percussion on affected side	Needle decompression of the affected side of the chest
Cardiac tamponade	History, no pulse with CPR, jugular venous distension	Pericardiocentesis (immediate transport)
Others: Drug overdose, trauma, massive MI, pulmonary embolism	History	Immediate transport

When the monitor is applied to a pulseless patient and asystole is seen:

1. *Immediately resume CPR,* assuming you are not presented with a valid advance directive indicating *not* to perform CPR ("do not resuscitate" orders).
2. *Confirm asystole by checking for other causes of the flat line.* Make sure that all monitoring electrodes are firmly fastened to the patient and that the cables are hooked into the monitor. Switch to another lead to detect low-voltage VF. If the rhythm is asystole, you need to be aware that the prognosis is grim and the chances for successful resuscitation are poor.
3. *Insert an advanced airway if the BLS airway is not adequate.*
4. *Start an IV* with normal saline.
5. *If unable to establish IV access, consider establishing IO access.*
6. As soon as IV or IO access has been established, *administer a vasopressor drug.* The two recommended vasopressor drugs are epinephrine and vasopressin. *Epinephrine (1:10,000) is given as 1 mg IV push;* this dose should be repeated every 3 to 5 minutes for as long as a pulse is absent. *Vasopressin is an alternative and is given as 40 units IV push, one time only.* Vasopressin can be given in place of the first or second dose of epinephrine (but not both).

Whenever you give a medication through a peripheral IV line during CPR, follow it immediately with a 20- to 30-ml bolus of IV fluid and then elevate the extremity to facilitate delivery of the medication to the central circulation (which may take 1 to 2 minutes).

7. *At the end of every 2 minutes of CPR, pause the compressions to check for circulation and to check the rhythm on the monitor.*
8. If asystole is still present:
   - *Immediately resume CPR.*
   - Search for and treat possible causes. Possible causes are the same as for PEA and are listed in Table 27-21.
   - *Seriously consider termination of the resuscitation with advisement from direct medical control.*

Postresuscitative Prehospital Care

If an effective cardiac rhythm is restored in the prehospital environment, your next task is to make sure that the rhythm *stays* restored and that optimal conditions are provided to promote recovery of the patient's brain from the hypoxic insult of cardiac arrest.

First, the HR should be stabilized. If the rhythm is bradycardic or tachycardic in the postresuscitation period, the bradycardia or tachycardia algorithms should be followed.

Next, cardiac rhythm should be stabilized to the degree possible. If the arrest rhythm was VF or VT, consider administering a bolus of an antiarrhythmic drug, followed by an infusion of the same drug. Historically, lidocaine has been given in this situation, but if amiodarone was given to the patient in arrest, then an infusion of amiodarone should be started and lidocaine should not be used. If severe bradycardia is present in the postarrest period, atropine or TCP may be required, and the hospital should be alerted to prepare a transcutaneous pacemaker.

Once the cardiac rhythm is stable, attention turns to the brain itself and to ameliorating the effects of cardiac arrest on it. Marked hypotension needs to be corrected rapidly because the brain will not be adequately perfused so long as the blood pressure is very low. If the patient has marked hypotension and the transport time to the hospital will be prolonged, the physician may order an infusion of dopamine or norepinephrine. In an intubated patient, avoid tracheal suctioning unless absolutely necessary; suctioning tends to increase intracranial pressure. Finally, consider elevating the patient's head to about 30° to increase cerebral venous drainage. Therapeutic hypothermia of comatose patients with return of spontaneous circulation may be very beneficial, with initiation typically taking place upon arrival to the ED. Some EMS systems may consider initiation of cooling with cold IV fluids and ice packs during transport.

Postresuscitative care is complex and best carried out in a critical care setting where careful monitoring and titrated therapy can most effectively be given. Thus, transport to the hospital should not be delayed for patients who are resuscitated from cardiac arrest. If an effective cardiac rhythm is restored in the prehospital environment, transport immediately. Only when transport will be significantly prolonged (such as a cardiac arrest occurring far from the hospital) should additional postresuscitative measures be started in the prehospital environment as directed by medical control.

The following is a summary of usual postresuscitative prehospital care to be used en route:

1. Stabilize the cardiac rhythm (give an antiarrhythmic drug for post–VF or post–VT; give atropine or use a transcutaneous pacemaker for symptomatic bradycardia).

2. Normalize the blood pressure (give a dopamine or norepinephrine infusion to raise the systolic pressure to at least 100 mm Hg).

3. Elevate the patient's head to 30° if the blood pressure allows.

4. Monitor oxygen saturation and titrate inspired oxygen concentrations to maintain a saturation of at least 94%.

When to Stop CPR

Since the dawn of paramedic-staffed ambulances in the early 1970s, many communities have *not* permitted the termination of CPR in the prehospital environment. That policy was established because, in most jurisdictions, only a physician is authorized to declare a person dead (stopping CPR is considered equivalent to declaring a person dead). Cardiac arrest patients who were not successfully resuscitated at the scene were invariably transported urgently to the hospital, with some semblance of CPR occurring en route.

With the accumulation of vast experience from EMS systems throughout the United States and Canada, it soon became clear that transport to the ED of adults who did not respond to an adequate trial of prehospital ACLS was an exercise in futility. Fewer than 1% who did not respond to prehospital ACLS ultimately survived. This policy was also given as the example of an unethical practice in the guidelines because it instills false hope in the family. Furthermore, rapid transport of patients in cardiac arrest, with CPR en route, involves considerable hazards to paramedics. The risks of vehicular crashes or of injuries while working in a moving ambulance are greatly increased during urgent transport.

Many EMS systems in Canada allow paramedics to contact direct medical control after failed initial ACLS resuscitation (eg, 10 to 20 minutes or 2 to 3 rounds of medications) for consideration to cease resuscitation in the prehospital environment. Where this is in place, the physician and paramedic discuss the specific case to determine if the resuscitation is truly futile (< 1% chance of survival) prior to ceasing resuscitation.

There may also be a role for ceasing resuscitation in certain situations with a provider equipped with an AED but no other ACLS care. A Canadian-derived Termination of Resuscitaton prediction rule outlines a subgroup of out-of-hospital cardiac arrests managed by AED-trained paramedics where futility may exist and it may be appropriate to stop resuscitative efforts in the prehospital setting. This rule found that only 0.5% of cardiac arrest patients survived if the arrest was not witnessed by paramedics, no shocks were administered, and there was no return of spontaneous circulation in the prehospital environment (three analyses). This rule would reduce the number of transports by 50%. Contact with direct medical control in these situations allows the paramedic and physician to discuss the specific patient and situation prior to ceasing resuscitation.

Provincial legislation and/or medical authority approval is required to permit cease of resuscitation at the scene by a paramedic. Each EMS system will have to formulate its own criteria and protocols for the termination of resuscitation in the prehospital setting.

Gaining permission to stop CPR in the prehospital environment will not necessarily make your life easier. Delicate issues are involved, such as the expectations of the patient's family, breaking bad news, and the disposition of the body. You may face pressure from bystanders to continue resuscitative efforts long after there is any medical justification for doing so. Stopping CPR may also be difficult for you; you will find yourself in the unaccustomed role of having to tell a family, "Your husband [or father, and so forth] is dead; there is nothing more that can be done." It is much easier to go careening off to the hospital with red lights flashing and sirens blaring and leave the ED staff with the "expectation of providing a miracle" and the unpleasant business of breaking bad news.

If your EMS system is allowed to terminate CPR in the prehospital environment, it will be a good idea to meet with your medical director and "walk through" some of the scenes you may have to face. Role-play exercises can be particularly useful in helping you to pinpoint situations in which you feel uncomfortable and develop strategies in advance for dealing with those situations.

Management of Symptomatic Bradycardia

A patient who presents with or develops symptomatic bradycardia needs to be treated in a manner that will increase the HR and improve CO. Symptoms such as altered mental status and hypotension are common indications for treatment of bradycardic patients. If the patient is asymptomatic, then the bradycardia does not require immediate therapy and should be monitored en route. Assuming that airway and breathing have been supported:

1. Establish an IV line of normal saline.

2. Administer atropine, 0.5-mg IV bolus (unless the patient is in a second-degree type II or third-degree heart block, then you should proceed directly to step 3). You may repeat this dose every 3 to 5 minutes until the heart reaches the desired rate (usually 60 beats/min or faster) or until the maximum total dose of 0.04 mg/kg has been reached.

3. If the patient is in a severely compromised condition or doesn't respond to the administration of atropine, establish TCP as quickly as possible. If the patient is in a second-degree type II or third-degree heart block, TCP is the first-line treatment.

4. If atropine and TCP are unsuccessful (or if TCP is unavailable), consider the administration of a sympathomimetic drug—most commonly, dopamine or epinephrine, albeit only as a drip in this situation. Dopamine is administered at its usual dose of 5 to

20 mcg/kg/min. Dopamine is available in premixed bags, which simplifies initiation of the infusion. The epinephrine drip rate is 2 to 10 mcg/min. To mix an epinephrine drip, put 1 mg of epinephrine into a 250-ml bag of normal saline, start the drip at approximately 30 drops/min with a microdrip administration set, and titrate to the desired HR.

5. Transport the patient to hospital, and prealert the facility so they can prepare for pacing of the patient.

Patients who are symptomatic and require TCP in the prehospital environment often require a transvenous and ultimately the surgical implantation of a pacemaker in the hospital Figure 27-84. Early identification and hospital notification can often speed this process.

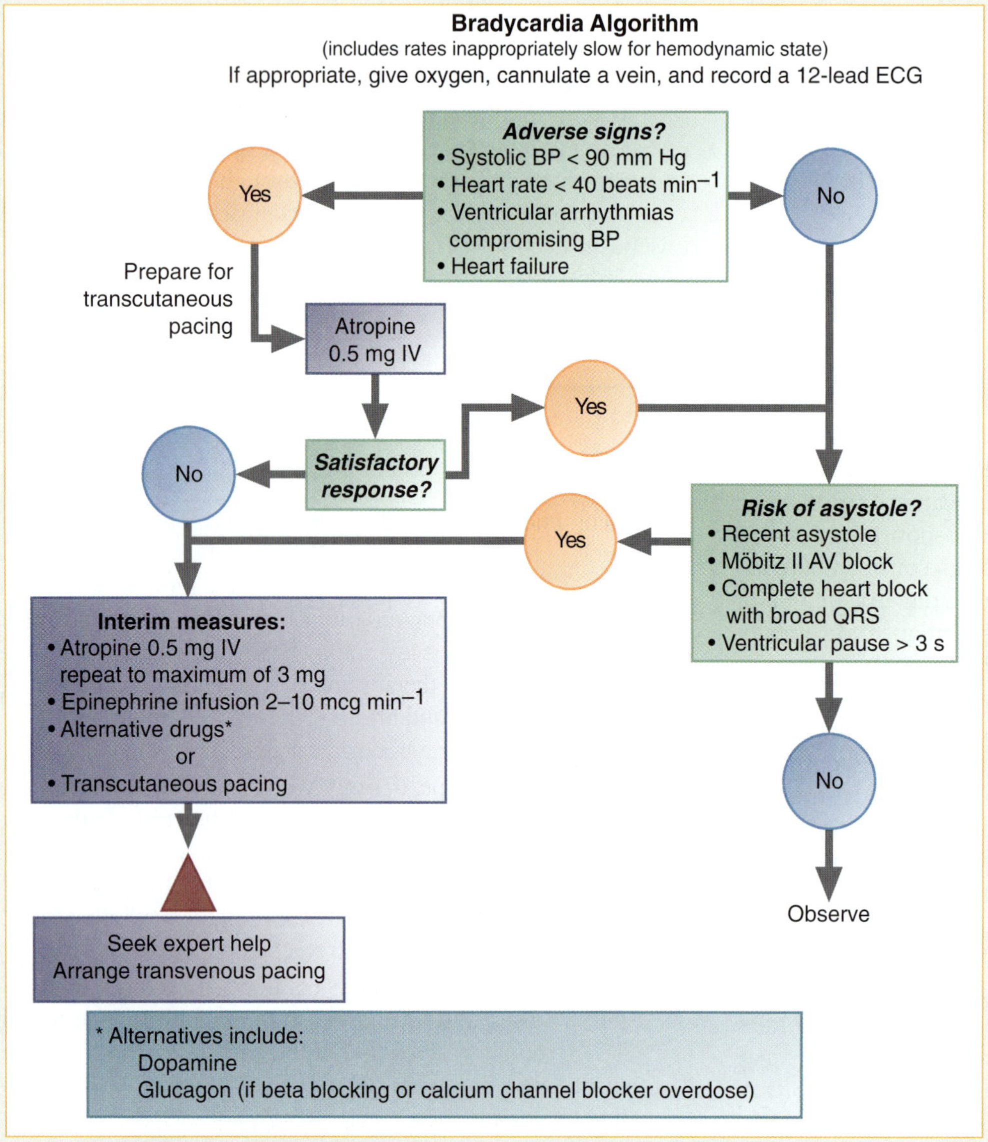
Bradycardia Algorithm
(includes rates inappropriately slow for hemodynamic state)
If appropriate, give oxygen, cannulate a vein, and record a 12-lead ECG
Adverse signs?
• Systolic BP < 90 mm Hg
• Heart rate < 40 beats min−1
• Ventricular arrhythmias compromising BP
• Heart failure
Yes
No
Prepare for transcutaneous pacing
Atropine 0.5 mg IV
Yes
Satisfactory response?
No
Risk of asystole?
• Recent asystole
• Möbitz II AV block
• Complete heart block with broad QRS
• Ventricular pause > 3 s
Yes
Interim measures:
• Atropine 0.5 mg IV repeat to maximum of 3 mg
• Epinephrine infusion 2–10 mcg min−1
• Alternative drugs*
or
• Transcutaneous pacing
No
Observe
Seek expert help
Arrange transvenous pacing
* Alternatives include:
Dopamine
Glucagon (if beta blocking or calcium channel blocker overdose)

Figure 27-84 Algorithm for bradycardia.

Modified from *Bradycardia Algorithm*. Copyright European Resuscitation Council. www.erc.edu Approval #2009/011.

Management of Tachycardia

A patient who presents with or develops tachycardia presents a more complicated situation than one in bradycardia. Tachycardia can have a supraventricular pacemaker site or may be ventricular in origin. In addition, the patient may be mildly or severely symptomatic owing to the tachycardia or another condition. Because of the many possible variations in tachycardic patients, several judgments and determinations must be made before treatment is begun.

The first decision relates to the seriousness of the signs or symptoms the patient is exhibiting. Patient who present with serious signs and symptoms such as chest pain, dyspnea, hypotension, or altered mental status should be considered in unstable condition and may need immediate treatment. First, however, you must determine whether these signs and symptoms are the result of the tachycardia or whether the tachycardia and signs and symptoms are the response to another condition.

Tachycardias with rates of less than 150 beats/min are rarely fast enough to cause serious signs and symptoms. For example, a patient who is experiencing an MI is likely to be mildly tachycardic, but obviously the MI—not the tachycardia—is causing the signs and symptoms. Conversely, a patient who was previously asymptomatic but becomes symptomatic only after the onset of the tachycardia is more likely presenting with symptoms resulting from the tachycardia. This brings to mind the adage: "Treat the patient, not the monitor." It is critical to make this distinction before beginning treatment, because slowing the HR of a patient whose heart is compensating for a medical condition may be a fatal mistake.

A patient in unstable condition whose signs and symptoms are determined to be the result of tachycardia needs synchronized cardioversion. Electrical cardioversion (described in detail later in the chapter) is similar to defibrillation and, as such, is a serious intervention. For this reason, it is limited to patients whose condition is so serious as to make them likely to arrest if the treatment is not administered quickly. Most of these patients will be unconscious. In the unlikely case in which a conscious patient needs cardioversion, sedation (usually with diazepam or midazolam) is a necessity. Wait an appropriate amount of time for the drugs to take effect before cardioversion. Should the patient become unconscious, sedation is no longer a concern. Be prepared for side effects of sedation medications used during cardioversion, mainly a drop in blood pressure or suppression of respiratory rate.

When a patient in tachycardia has limited or mild signs and symptoms, a slower but safer treatment regimen is recommended. In these cases, it becomes necessary to determine the origin of the tachycardia or the pacemaker site of the rhythm. Generally speaking, wide QRS complexes are presumed to be ventricular in origin, whereas narrow QRS complexes (< 0.12 s) are presumed to be supraventricular in origin. SVTs may originate in the SA node, elsewhere else in the atria, or in the AV node (junctional rhythms). The differentiation among these three pacemaker sites requires examining the P wave and rhythm. In tachycardias with rates exceeding 150 beats/min, however, the P waves may be difficult to visualise and are occasionally "buried" within the T wave of the preceding beat. The inability to see P waves limits us to labeling these tachycardias as supraventricular rather than giving a specific site of origin. In is important to identify sinus tachycardia, because this rhythm should not be treated specifically in the prehospital environment, but rather the underlying cause should be determined (eg, pain, fear, illness) and treated, if possible.

Occasionally, aberrant conduction of a supraventricularly originated beat will make it difficult to identify a tachycardia as truly ventricular or supraventricular. In most cases of uncertainty, a wide rhythm should be treated as VT. In either case, you should administer oxygen and establish an IV line for normal saline.

In SVTs, you can attempt to stimulate the patient's vagus nerve. Many vagal stimulation techniques exist, but the most common is having the patient bear down against a closed glottis. The patient is instructed to perform this technique as if attempting to have a bowel movement. The stimulation of the vagal nerve in turn stimulates the parasympathetic nervous system to slow the heart. If this technique is successful, the patient should still be transported for hospital evaluation because the condition is likely to recur. If it reappears, instruct the patient to repeat the vagal maneuver. If at any time the vagal stimulation proves unsuccessful, pharmacologic treatment should be attempted. Another vagal stimulation technique, carotid sinus massage, should not be performed without direct medical control authorization, because it has a risk of causing a stroke in a patient with atherosclerotic disease.

If the vagal maneuvers were unsuccessful, the next step is to administer adenosine, 6 mg, by rapid IV push. Adenosine is recommended in the initial diagnosis and treatment of stable, undifferentiated, regular, monomorphic, wide-complex tachycardia. Before you begin this treatment, you should always recheck the history for allergies and contraindications and advise the patient of the possible adverse effects of adenosine administration. Adenosine is contraindicated in patients with asthma, because it can cause bronchoconstriction. Adenosine is also contraindicated

in patients with irregular, wide-complex tachycardia because it may cause degeneration of the rhythm to VF. Additionally, it typically causes the patients to experience a flush, slight chest pressure, and a feeling of "doom." To administer the medication, choose the closest IV site to the patient and insert the syringe of adenosine. In the same site, insert another syringe containing at least 20 ml of normal saline solution. After clamping off the IV line above the site, push the adenosine as rapidly as possible and then push the saline as soon as the adenosine plunger hits bottom. Be prepared to see a short run of asystole with the administration of adenosine (although this response does not always occur). If the first dose of adenosine is unsuccessful, you may administer it again in 1 to 2 minutes up to two times at 12 mg each. If the adenosine is unsuccessful in converting the patient's rhythm, transport expeditiously to the hospital without further treatment as long as the patient remains in stable condition. Adenosine frequently causes a transient slowing of the rhythm that allows easier identification rather than rhythm conversion, so ensure that the rhythm strip is being printed during drug administration to allow for careful review.

If at any time the condition of a patient with SVT becomes unstable, you should move to the "unstable" or cardioversion algorithm. Remember that when cardioversion of SVT is required, you should start at a lower energy setting than with a ventricular rhythm.

If the patient is in stable condition but the rhythm is ventricular in origin, the patient should be transported to the hospital while you watch carefully for the development of serious signs and symptoms. If they appear, the patient should undergo cardioversion according to the unstable tachycardia algorithm. If your transport time to the hospital is long, direct medical control may order the administration of a ventricular antiarrhythmic medication such as amiodarone or lidocaine. In cases involving a short transport time, administration of these medications may be delayed until hospital admission.

Any patient with a tachycardic rhythm should be monitored carefully **Figure 27-85 ▸**. A heart that is stressed by the requirements of excessive tachycardia is very likely to become ischemic and is at high risk for arrest.

▌ Techniques of Management in Cardiac Emergencies

This section profiles some of the devices and methods used in the treatment of patients with cardiac emergencies. Not all of the techniques or devices described are used in every EMS system, and not all are required for certification as a paramedic. Direct your attention to the material that is relevant to your local practice.

Defibrillation

Defibrillation is the process by which a surge of electric energy is delivered to the heart. Recall that when the heart fibrillates, its individual muscle fibres get "out of synch" with one another and begin contracting individually. As a result, the heart as a whole ceases any useful movement. Indeed, if you were to look

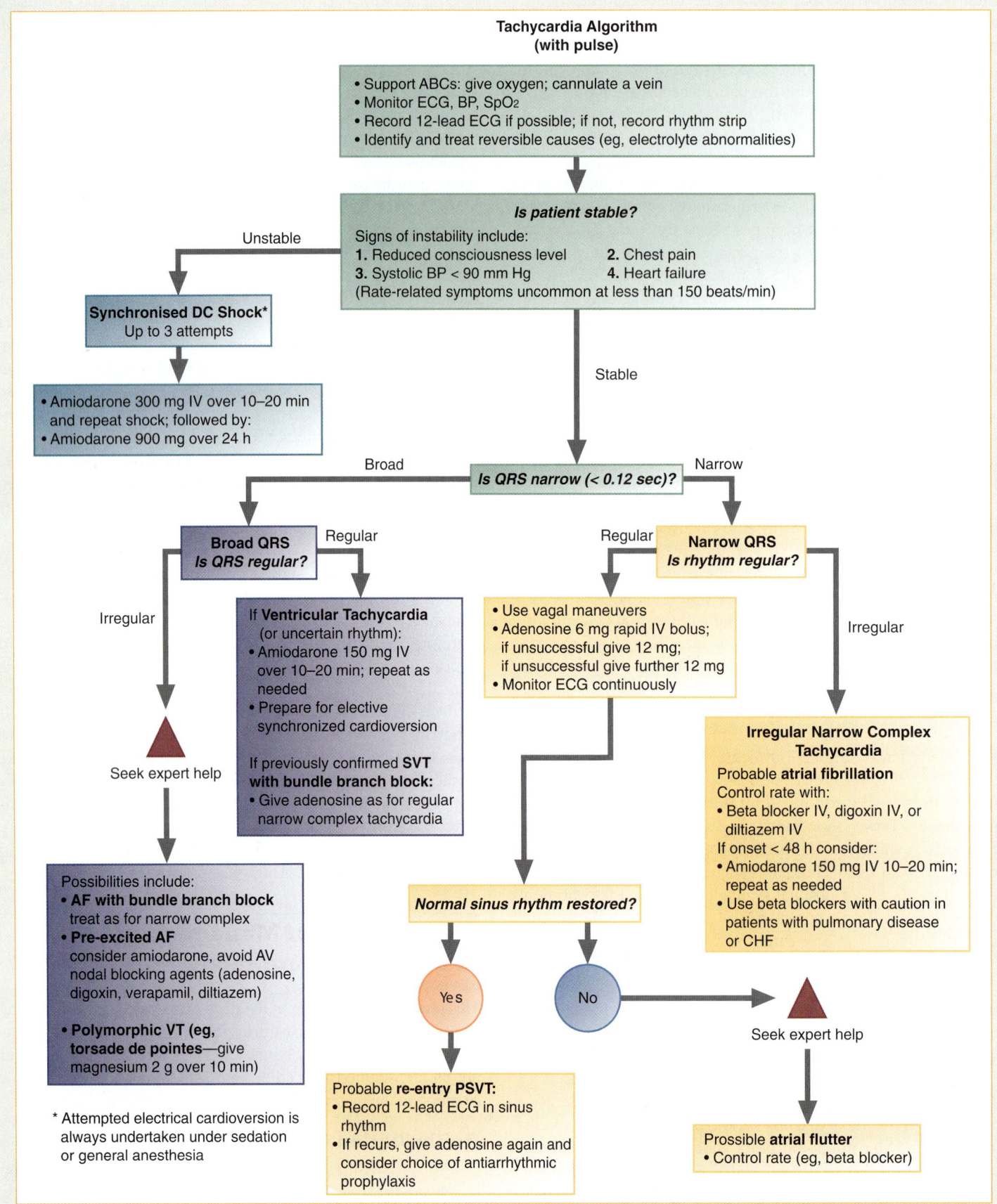

Figure 27-85 Algorithm for tachycardia.

at a fibrillating heart, you would see movement resembling that of a bag of energetic worms. The idea behind defibrillation is to deliver a current to the heart that is powerful enough to depolarize all of its component muscle cells; ideally, when those cells repolarize after the shock, they will respond to an impulse from the SA node and begin organized depolarization, leading to cardiac contraction.

Defibrillation needs to be carried out as soon as possible in VF or pulseless VT because the likelihood of its success declines rapidly with time. If the arrest is not witnessed and CPR is not in progress, immediately start CPR and continue for at least 2 minutes before delivering the first shock. If the patient's rhythm converts to VF or pulseless VT and the defibrillator is already attached, perform CPR only long enough to charge the defibrillator and then defibrillate. Defibrillation is *not* useful in asystole because there is no evidence that the myocardial cells are spontaneously depolarizing. Defibrillation of asystole is unlikely to be beneficial and may be harmful. Thus, if you are unsure about asystole after checking more than one lead, resume CPR and follow the asystole pathway in the pulseless arrest algorithm until the next pulse and rhythm check.

Defibrillation Algorithm

To perform defibrillation, attach the adhesive defibrillation pads to the chest as instructed on the package. One option is to position one pad anteriorly left of the lower sternum and the other pad posteriorly just below the left scapula. The second option is to position one pad anteriorly left of the lower sternum, with the second pad in the same position on the patient's back. As with ECG electrode placement, you may have to dry the skin before placing the defibrillation pads. Once they are in place, turn the main power switch on. Set the energy level to 200 J (for biphasic defibrillation of unknown type), or follow the defibrillator manufacturer's recommendations regarding the appropriate energy level. Monophasic monitors should be charged to 360 J for the first and all successive shocks. Charge the defibrillator.

If using paddles instead of adhesive hands-free pads, it will be necessary to reduce the resistance of the patient's skin to passage of electric current by applying a conductive medium to the paddles; otherwise, the energy will be delivered largely to the skin itself, resulting in burns to the skin and ineffective energy delivery to the heart. Use electrode paste or saline gel pads to make good electric contact between the paddles and the skin. Apply about 11 kg of pressure to hold the paddles in contact with the chest. Many paddles have a visual guide to indicate whether contact is adequate. This should be checked, and subsequent paddle adjustments made as needed.

Whichever method you choose—saline pads or electrode paste—take care to prevent contact (bridging) between the two conductive areas on the chest wall. If the saline or paste from one paddle comes in contact with that from the other paddle, the electric current will simply pass along the skin from one paddle to the other. Effective current will thus bypass the heart, causing superficial burns of the skin instead.

If there is a nitroglycerin patch on the patient's chest, remove it and wipe the skin dry before you apply the defibrillator paddles. Although nitroglycerin does not—contrary to popular legend—explode, the backing used on some nitroglycerin patches can support electrical arcing during defibrillation, producing smoke, noise, and burns to the patient.

Position the paddles so that the negative (sternum) paddle is just to the right of the upper part of the sternum below the right clavicle and the positive (apex) paddle is just below and to the left of the left nipple **Figure 27-86 ▾** . Exert firm pressure (8 to 10 kg) on each paddle to make good skin contact. Inadequate contact is another cause of burns and ineffective countershock.

When the defibrillator is charged, clear the area so that no one—including the operator—is in contact with the patient or stretcher. The operator should then announce, "All clear!" At this point, discharge the defibrillator by pressing the button on each handle simultaneously or pressing the button on the machine if using a hands-free system. If current has reached the patient, contraction of the chest and other muscles will be evident. If you do not see contraction, check the defibrillator to be certain the synchronizing switch is off and the battery is charged.

Immediately after delivering the defibrillating current, resume CPR. Continue CPR for 2 minutes or 5 cycles, and then pause to check for a pulse and reevaluate the rhythm. If at any point you see signs of life, check for a pulse.

An implanted artificial pacemaker—which you may detect from the pacemaker-produced spikes on the ECG or the bulge where its battery pack has been implanted under the patient's skin—is *not* a contraindication to defibrillation. Just avoid

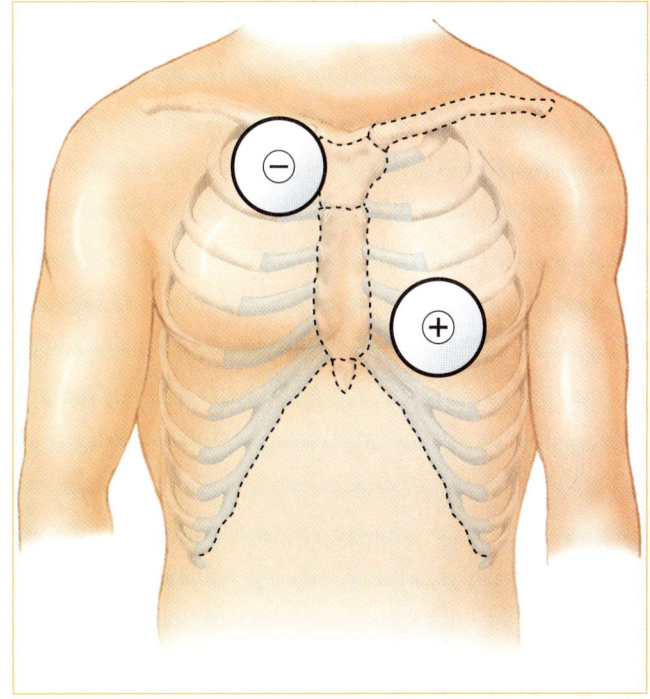

Figure 27-86 Position the paddles for defibrillation.

placing the electrode paddles or pads directly over the pacemaker battery.

The defibrillator should be inspected at the beginning of each shift, using a checklist to cover all aspects of the apparatus and its gear. Inspection should include the paddles, cables and connectors, power supply, monitor, ECG recorder, and any ancillary supplies (such as electrode gel, pads, spare battery). Your service should have a standard checklist procedure that you follow at the beginning of every shift. This will ensure your equipment, including your defibrillator, is in proper working order.

The following list summarizes the procedures for defibrillation:

1. Turn the main power on, and make sure the synchronize switch is off.
2. Set the energy level at 200 J (or the appropriate setting for your defibrillator).
3. Place the hands-free pads on the chest or apply paddles to patient with conduction gel pads between paddle and patient.
4. Charge the defibrillator.
5. Clear the area with a verbal warning to rescuers and a visual confirmation that no one is touching the patient.
6. Discharge the defibrillator.
7. Resume CPR, and recheck the rhythm in 2 minutes.

Automated External Defibrillator

The AED is a "smart" defibrillator that can—thanks to sophisticated computer chips—analyze the patient's ECG rhythm and determine whether a defibrillating shock is needed. The semiautomatic AED identifies the rhythm and then instructs the rescuer what to do about it. If, for example, the AED detects VF, a voice prompt may say, "Shock advised. Press to shock." The rescuer must then depress the shock button to defibrillate the patient. Thus the "A" in AED is *automated* and not *automatic*.

These are the basic sequence of steps for using an AED in a patient without a pulse:

1. Turn on the AED. (This should always be the first step as the device will start providing audio prompts to help you remember the next steps required.)
2. Expose the patient's chest.
3. Attach the two self-adhesive electrode pads firmly to the patient's chest—the sternal pad at the junction of the right clavicle and upper border of the sternum; the apex pad along the left lower rib margin at the anterior axillary line.
4. Stop CPR, and instruct everyone to get clear of the patient.
5. The AED assesses the rhythm (for 6 to 20 s) and determines whether it is "shockable" (that is, whether the rhythm is one that will respond to defibrillation).
6. If the AED detects a shockable rhythm, it automatically starts charging, which takes 5 to 10 seconds.
7. The defibrillator indicates if a shock is advised, and the rescuer pushes the button to deliver the shock.

8. The defibrillator may indicate, "No shock advised," which means that the patient has asystole or pulseless electrical activity. A "No shock advised" indication after repeated shocks may mean that the patient has gone back into sinus rhythm, and therefore a pulse check will also be required to determine whether CPR should be resumed.

New AEDs appear on the market all the time, and each model comes with its own operating manual. If you will be using an AED, train with the specific apparatus carried by your service, using the manufacturer's instructions for that machine.

Cardioversion

Cardioversion is the use of the defibrillator to terminate arrhythmias other than VF. In cardioversion, unlike defibrillation, the current is synchronized with the ECG so that it will not be delivered during the vulnerable period (that is, on top of the T wave). Electrical cardioversion is performed just as defibrillation except that the synchronize setting on the defibrillator is selected first. When the defibrillator is "fired" in the synchronize mode, the machine monitors the R waves of the QRS complexes and delivers the shock at a time when the R-on-T phenomenon is least likely to occur. The R-on-T phenomenon occurs when the defibrillator fires at the top of the T wave and usually results in the rhythm changing to VF. Although this can happen with the synchronizer on, it is much less likely to occur when the shock is "synchronized."

Emergency cardioversion is indicated for rapid ventricular and supraventricular rhythms that are associated with severely compromised CO—causing symptoms such as hypotension, decreased level of awareness, chest pain, or pulmonary edema. Emergency cardioversion should not be used outside the hospital to convert rapid rhythms that result from digoxin toxicity (for practical purposes, that means any tachyarrhythmia in any patient taking digoxin).

In the prehospital environment, cardioversion is carried out *only* for patients whose CO is severely impaired. These patients are usually unconscious, so premedication is not necessary. When cardioversion is performed electively on a conscious patient, the patient *must* be sedated first; cardioversion is a painful and terrifying experience for an awake patient. Medications commonly used for sedation in these circumstances include benzodiazepines such as diazepam or midazolam (follow your medical director's instructions). Be prepared for side effects of sedation given during cardioversion, such as hypotension or decreased respiratory rate.

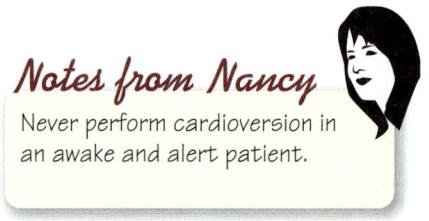

Notes from Nancy

Never perform cardioversion in an awake and alert patient.

The following is the procedure for cardioversion:

1. Turn the main power on, and ensure synchronization is on (unlike for defibrillation). Watch for markings on the ECG rhythm display indicating successful synchronization.

2. Prepare and apply the pads or paddles as described for defibrillation.

3. Set the energy level as ordered by the physician. Energy levels required for cardioversion vary depending on the type of arrhythmia and the type of defibrillator. Supraventricular tachycardia, for example, can often be converted with energy levels as low as 50 J; by contrast, VT will usually require at least 100 J. In emergencies, if an initial attempt to convert a rapid rhythm with a low energy level fails, immediately turn the setting up (stepwise to 100, 200, 300, and then 360 J) and repeat the shock as needed. The energy recommended for cardioversion using a biphasic defibrillator may differ depending on the manufacturer of the device.

4. Charge the defibrillator.

5. Clear the area by announcing, "All clear!"

6. Depress the shock buttons, and keep them depressed until the defibrillator discharges. That may take a few seconds because the charge is synchronized to fire about 10 ms after the peak of the R wave.

7. Reassess the patient's condition (ECG rhythm and pulse). Repeat the cardioversion if necessary (ensure that synchronization is turned on each time).

8. If a cardioversion shock produces VF, immediately:
   - Recharge the defibrillator to the setting for defibrillation.
   - Ensure synchronization is off if it has not defaulted to that position.
   - Deliver the defibrillation.

Transcutaneous Cardiac Pacing

Artificial pacemakers deliver repetitive electric currents to the heart. Like the tiny electric currents generated by natural pacemakers, the current from an artificial pacemaker can cause the myocardial tissue to depolarize. In this way, the artificial pacemaker can substitute for a natural pacemaker that has become blocked or nonfunctional.

The artificial pacemakers first developed for emergency use consisted of a small battery pack and a wire that had to be threaded through a vein into the right ventricle of the heart. Insertion of those transvenous pacemakers is a tricky and often time-consuming job, usually best undertaken in a coronary care unit. Recently, however, effective transcutaneous pacemakers—that is, pacemakers that deliver their current through the skin of the chest—have been developed and have come into widespread use. Indeed, most prehospital monitor-defibrillators now come equipped with TCP capability.

In TCP, a small electrical charge is passed through the patient's skin across the heart between one externally placed pacing pad and another. The pacer is set for a specific rate, and the energy is increased until the heart just begins to respond to the stimulus. This phenomenon, which is termed "capture," is usually associated with depolarization of the ventricles, which appears as a wide QRS complex on the ECG and results in a corresponding pulse.

TCP may have several useful applications in prehospital care:
- Interhospital transfer of patients needing pacemaker implantation (for example, a patient with complete heart block admitted to a small community hospital that does not have the facilities to implant a permanent pacemaker)
- Symptomatic patients with artificial pacemaker failure
- Patients with bradyarrhythmias or blocks associated with severely reduced CO and that are unresponsive to atropine, before cardiac arrest

In any of those circumstances, TCP may buy time for the patient and enable him or her to reach the hospital in a state of optimal perfusion rather than in or near cardiac arrest.

Many brands of transcutaneous external cardiac pacemakers are available, and you must become familiar with the particular pacemaker used in your local EMS system. In general, the steps in initiating TCP are as follows:

1. Apply the pacing electrodes. Often the same pads can be used for defibrillation and pacing. The best position is to place one pad anteriorly left of the lower sternum and the other pad posteriorly just below the left scapula. If pads have already been placed in the sternum/apex position, it is usually not necessary to switch to an anterior/posterior configuration if need for pacing develops in an unstable patient. Note that the 3-lead cable must be attached to the patient in addition to pacing pads for the defibrillator to allow pacing to take place.

2. Switch the pacer power on.

3. Set the pacing rate (60 to 80 beats/min is commonly chosen).

4. Start increasing the current. Raise the current by 10 to 20 milliamps every few seconds.

5. Check for electrical capture; that is, look for every pacemaker spike being followed by a (usually wide) QRS complex **Figure 27-87 ▶** . If the QRS is not present, the pacemaker current is not depolarizing the ventricles. Increase the current gradually until there is consistent electrical capture.

6. Check for mechanical capture—a palpable pulse with each electrical beat.

7. Once capture is achieved, briefly lower the current until capture is lost, and then increase it by the smallest amount possible to restore capture. The purpose of this action is to find the lowest energy setting that achieves consistent capture.

8. Immediately transport the patient.

Transcutaneous pacemakers depolarize not only cardiac muscle, but also muscles in the chest wall beneath the pacing electrode. As a result, patients who are conscious when TCP is initiated (or who regain consciousness during pacing) usually experience chest discomfort and sometimes severe pain from the procedure. Some form of analgesia and sedation (such as midazolam or morphine) should be given to conscious patients when transcutaneous pacemakers are used.

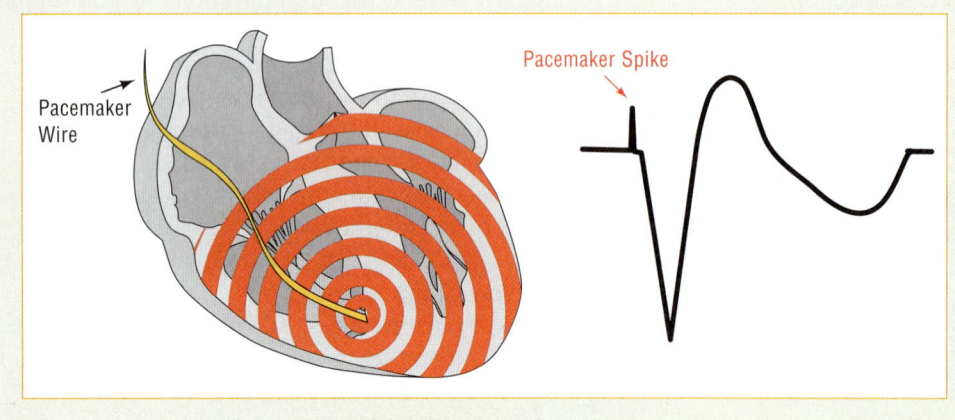

Figure 27-87 Pacemaker spike followed by QRS complex.

Medications Commonly Prescribed to Patients With Cardiovascular Diseases

Patients with diseases affecting the cardiovascular system may be taking a wide variety of medications for a variety of reasons, and it is not always possible to identify the patient's specific problem on the basis of a medication that he or she is taking. Beta blockers, for example, are prescribed for relief of angina, to lower blood pressure in hypertension, and to prevent recurrence of AMI. Similarly, diuretic medications may be given simply to help rid the body of excess fluid in CHF or because of their effects in lowering blood pressure. Thus, one needs to look at any given medication the patient is taking in the context of the patient's clinical history and the other medications he or she is taking **Figure 27-88 ▶**.

Digoxin Preparations

Digoxin preparations are prescribed for the treatment of chronic CHF or for certain rapid atrial arrhythmias (such as rapid atrial flutter, atrial fibrillation, supraventricular arrhythmias). Digoxin acts by increasing the strength of cardiac contractions, thereby improving CO, and slowing conduction through the AV junction (such as in atrial fibrillation or flutter, allowing fewer impulses to be conducted through to the ventricles so the overall HR slows). In at least 30% of patients taking digoxin, some symptoms of toxic effects of the drug develop—for example, loss of appetite, nausea, vomiting, headache, blurred vision, yellow vision, or various cardiac arrhythmias. *Virtually any cardiac arrhythmia may be caused by the toxic effects of digoxin,* so it is important to ask all patients with disturbances in cardiac rhythm to determine whether they are taking digoxin.

Patients taking digoxin are very sensitive to calcium preparations. They are also highly sensitive to a decline in the serum potassium level, so caution must be exercised in giving agents that might reduce the body's potassium stores (such as diuretics or large quantities of sodium bicarbonate).

Antianginal Agents

Three major classes of drugs are used to relieve the pain of angina: nitrates, beta blockers, and calcium channel blockers. All of them work exclusively or primarily on the demand side of the oxygen supply-demand equation; that is, all of them diminish, in one way or another, myocardial oxygen demand.

Nitrates

Nitrates were the first drugs to be used for the relief of angina. The prototype of this group is nitroglycerin, which comes as sublingual spray, rapid-acting sublingual tablets, sustained-release oral tablets, topically applied ointment, and skin patches **Table 27-22 ▾**. If a patient reports that he or she takes a medicine that is put under the tongue, that medicine is mostly likely nitroglycerin.

Nitroglycerin is thought to exert its therapeutic effect by decreasing the work of the heart. The heart's need for oxygen is, therefore, decreased, as is the anginal pain that results from

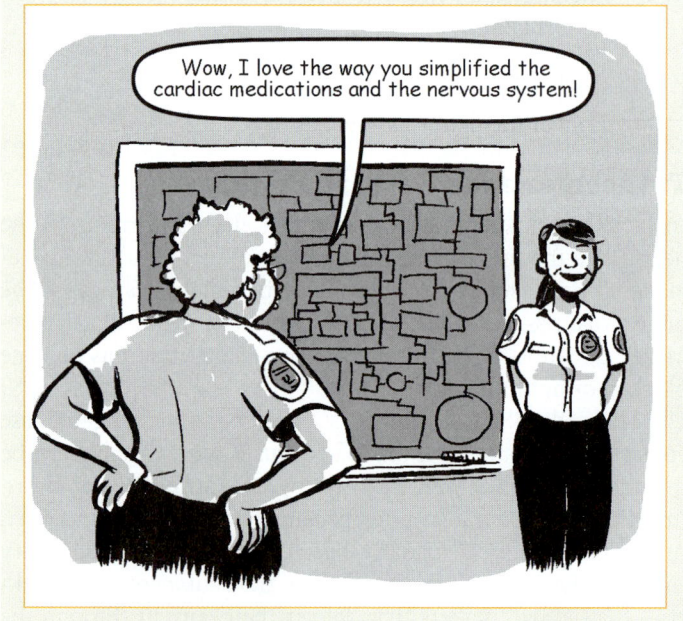

Figure 27-88

Table 27-22	Commonly Prescribed Nitrates
Generic Name	**Trade Name**
Nitroglycerin	Minitran, Nitrostat, Nitrolingual, Nitrogard, Nitroglycerin, Nitrong, Nitro-Bid, Nitro-Dur, Nitrol, Nitroglyn, Nitroject, Transderm-Nitro, Trinipatch
Isosorbide dinitrate	Isordil, Sorbitrate, Imdur, nitrates, apo-ISDN

insufficient oxygenation. Nitroglycerin usually takes effect within 3 to 5 minutes of administration.

Nitroglycerin also causes significant vasodilation. For that reason, it is sometimes used in the prehospital environment as an adjunctive therapy in the treatment of pulmonary edema secondary to left-sided heart failure. Used in that circumstance, nitroglycerin produces an "internal phlebotomy"—that is, a pooling of blood within the venous vessels that reduces the blood volume in the pulmonary vasculature just as if blood had been physically withdrawn from the body (phlebotomy).

When a patient reports taking nitroglycerin for chest pain, you need to find out the answers to two questions: (1) How much nitroglycerin did the patient take? (2) Did the nitroglycerin relieve the pain? Failure of nitroglycerin to relieve anginal pain can occur for one of two reasons—the pain is of extraordinary severity, is from infarction rather than angina, or the nitroglycerin has been open too long and is no longer effective. Fresh, potent nitroglycerin has certain distinct side effects, including a transient, throbbing headache; a burning sensation under the tongue; and a bitter taste. If the patient did not experience the bitter taste or did not experience a headache when he or she took the nitroglycerin, chances are the drug was outdated or ineffective. If the patient experienced a throbbing headache but still got no relief from the chest pain, suspect that the patient is having an AMI.

Beta Blockers

Drugs that block beta sympathetic receptors are also prescribed for the relief of angina Table 27-23 ▼. They work by decreasing the rate and strength of cardiac contractions, thereby decreasing the heart's demand for oxygen. Taking beta-blocking drugs on a regular basis usually leads to resistance to the action of beta-stimulating agents, such as epinephrine. Therefore, when such patients have a cardiac arrest, the administration of epinephrine during resuscitation attempts may not have the desired beta-agonist effect, because the beta effects of epinephrine may be blocked. The alpha-agonistic effects of epinephrine, namely vasoconstriction, are not blocked, thus making it a useful drug in resuscitation of cardiac arrest patients, even if they are taking beta blockers.

Calcium Channel Blockers

Calcium channel blockers, as their name implies, block the influx of calcium ions into cardiac muscle. These agents relieve angina in two ways: (1) by preventing spasm of the coronary arteries and (2) by decreasing the force of the cardiac contraction, thereby decreasing myocardial oxygen demand. Hypotension may be a significant side effect. Table 27-24 ▼ lists calcium channel blockers.

Antiarrhythmic Drugs

Antiarrhythmic drugs are used to control chronic disturbances in cardiac rhythm. Thus, when you encounter a patient taking one of these agents, you know the patient has had significant arrhythmias in the past, which justifies particular surveillance for recurrent rhythm disturbances. Patients taking antiarrhythmic drugs should be monitored while under your care.

Some of the drugs mentioned under other categories are also used for their antiarrhythmic activity. Digoxin preparations, for example, are used to suppress atrial arrhythmias. Beta blockers are sometimes prescribed for their suppressive effect on myocardial excitability, as are some of the calcium channel blockers. Table 27-25 ▼ lists commonly used antiarrhythmic drugs.

Table 27-24	Calcium Channel Blockers
Generic Name	**Trade Name**
Diltiazem	Cardizem
Verapamil	Calan, Isoptin
Amlodipine	Norvasc
Felodipine	Plendil, Renedil
Nifedipine	Adalat, Procardia

Table 27-23	Beta blockers
Generic Name	**Trade Name**
Acebutolol	Rhotral, Sectral
Atenolol	Tenormin
Bisoprolol	Monocor
Carvedilol	Coreg
Esmolol	Brevibloc
Labetalol	Normodyne, Trandate
Metoprolol	Lopressor, Betaloc
Nadolol	Corgard, Nadol
Pindolol	Pindol, Visken
Propranolol	Inderal, Pranol
Sotalol	Sotacor, Sotamol
Timolol	Timol

Table 27-25	Commonly Used Antiarrhythmic Drugs	
Generic Name	**Trade Name**	**Indications**
Amiodarone	Cordarone	Ventricular tachycardia and other life-threatening ventricular arrhythmias
Digoxin	Lanoxin	Atrial flutter or fibrillation
Disopyramide	Rhythmodan	Ventricular arrhythmias
Flecainide	Tambocor	Life-threatening ventricular arrhythmias
Mexiletine	Mexitil	Ventricular arrhythmias
Procainamide	Procan, Pronestyl	Ventricular arrhythmias
Quinidine	Cardioquin, Duraquin, Biquin Durules	Ventricular arrhythmias, some atrial arrhythmias
Tocainide	Tonocard	Ventricular arrhythmias
Verapamil	Calan, Isoptin	Ventricular tachycardias

Diuretics

Diuretics ("water pills") are prescribed to patients with chronic fluid overload, principally patients with chronic CHF, but are also used as primary or adjunctive therapy in the treatment of hypertension. Diuretics trick the kidneys into excreting more sodium and water than usual (the desired effect). Depending on the diuretic, the kidneys may also tend to dump out potassium along with the sodium (an undesired effect). Thus, patients taking diuretics often become depleted of potassium if they are not given potassium supplements. Patients in whom potassium deficits (hypokalemia) develop are prone to cardiac arrhythmias—especially if they are also taking digoxin. **Table 27-26 ▸** lists commonly prescribed diuretics.

Antihypertensive Drugs

As the name implies, antihypertensive agents are used to treat hypertension (high blood pressure). Many of the diuretic agents already mentioned are also used as antihypertensives or in combination with antihypertensives for a synergistic effect. Similarly, beta blockers are used in the treatment of hypertension.

It is often difficult to regulate the dosage of antihypertensives so that the patient's blood pressure is lowered enough but not too much. As a consequence, some patients taking these agents may have symptoms of hypotension, including weakness and dizziness. Many will experience a feeling of lightheadedness with a change in position (such as when moving from a recumbent to a sitting or standing position); this phenomenon is termed orthostatic hypotension. Every patient taking antihypertensive drugs, therefore, should have his or her blood pressure checked in the recumbent and sitting positions to detect orthostatic hypotension. **Table 27-27 ▸** lists commonly prescribed antihypertensive agents.

Anticoagulant Drugs

Anticoagulant drugs ("blood thinners") diminish the ability of the blood to clot. They are prescribed to patients who have had recurrent problems with blood clots (such as patients who have had pulmonary emboli) and to patients who might be prone to develop clots (such as some patients who have had a MI in the past; patients with artificial heart valves or valvular heart disease; patients whose normal heart rhythm is atrial fibrillation). Patients who take anticoagulants are apt to bleed excessively from minor trauma or even venipuncture, so you should be alert to that possibility. The principal oral anticoagulant drug is warfarin (Coumadin). Patients undergoing home dialysis may be taking the IV anticoagulant, heparin, during their dialysis cycle.

Table 27-26 | Commonly Prescribed Diuretics

Generic Name	Trade Name
Bumetanide	Burinex
Chlorthalidone	Chlorthalidone
Ethacrynic acid	Edecrin
Furosemide	Lasix
Hydralazine	Hydralazine
Indapamide	Lozide
Metolazone	Zaroxolyn
Spironolactone	Aldactone, Spiroton
Thiazides Hydrochlorothiazide	HCTZ
Combination drugs	
Hydrochlorothiazide and spironolactone	Aldatazide, Spirozine
Triamterene and hydrochlorothiazide	Dyazide, Triazide, Triamzide

Table 27-27 | Commonly Prescribed Antihypertensive Agents

Generic Name	Trade Name
Captopril	Capoten
Clonidine	Catapres, Dixarit
Enalapril	Vasotec
Guanethedine	Ismelin
Labetalol*	Normodyne, Trandate
Lisinopril	Prinivil, Zestril
Methyldopa	Methyldopa
Prazosin	Apo-Prazo, Novo-Prazin
Propranolol*	Inderal

*Beta blocker.

Antiplatelet Drugs

Antiplatelet drugs ("blood thinners") interfere with platelet aggregation and clot formation, impeding the ability of the blood to clot. They are prescribed to patients with coronary artery and cerebrovascular disease, as well as to those with a coronary artery stent. They are also very useful in the setting of an acute myocardial infarction, because they prevent more platelets from being recruited to form a new clot. Patients who take antiplatelet drugs are apt to bruise easily or bleed excessively from minor trauma. Clopidrogrel (Plavix) is a common antiplatelet agent.

You are the Paramedic Summary

1. What are some potential causes of palpitations?

Palpitations can be caused by a wide variety of things. Using our patient as an example, his palpitations can be caused by fatigue, stress, excessive caffeine intake, dehydration, or hypoglycemia. Other things to consider would be exercise, fever, smoking, use of other stimulant medications, ischemia, or an underlying cardiac problem.

2. What questions would you like to ask your patient at this time?

SAMPLE! SAMPLE! SAMPLE! Did we mention SAMPLE? To effectively treat Anthony, you need to try to identify the cause of his palpitations. In addition to the SAMPLE questions you may consider asking about the use of any other drugs legal or illegal, prior occurrences, and, if this is not the first time he has experienced palpitations, what was done to correct the problem.

3. What are some of your concerns based on this information?

Your first thought might be, "How long can Anthony hemodynamically compensate for an HR of 210 beats/min?" The HR definitely needs to be brought back down. The question is how. Because Anthony is currently in stable condition, you may treat the problem pharmacologically. Drug selection can be made once you have identified the rhythm on the cardiac monitor. Your goal should be to reduce the HR while the patient is in stable condition.

4. Which interventions should you consider at this point?

The monitor shows a narrow complex tachycardia. With no P waves and a regular rhythm, it is most likely PSVT, also known as AV-nodal reentry tachycardia. Multitasking works well here. While you are trying to establish IV access, ask the patient to perform a vagal maneuver such as bearing down as if having a bowel movement. The worst that can happen is that it doesn't work. In that case, it is time to bring out the arsenal. For narrow complex tachycardia, your first medication would be adenosine. If adenosine is unsuccessful in converting the rhythm and the patient remains in stable condition, you can move on to other drugs such as diltiazem.

5. How does adenosine work?

Adenosine works both the SA and AV nodes. It causes a decrease in impulse formation from the SA node and then slows conduction through the AV node. It is this combined effect that produces the slowing of the HR. Because adenosine slows impulse formation and conduction, don't be surprised to see a brief period of asystole on the cardiac monitor after it is administered. So beware!

6. What should you tell your patient before you administer adenosine?

Before administering adenosine, tell the patient that he or she may experience some side effects. Patients may experience chest pain, nausea, flushing, lightheadedness, or an "empty-feeling" sensation in their chest. This empty feeling usually coincides with the brief period of asystole on the monitor. The good news is the side effects will come and go in a matter of seconds owing to the brief half-life (< 10 s) of the drug.

7. How should your treatment proceed?

When treating a stable narrow complex tachycardia, the use of diltiazem is recommended if the rhythm was not converted using adenosine.

8. What type of medication is diltiazem?

Diltiazem is a calcium channel blocker. Other examples of calcium channel blockers include verapamil, felodipine (Plendil), and amlodipine (Norvasc).

9. How does diltiazem work?

Calcium channel blockers work by inhibiting the flow of calcium across the cell membrane of cardiac and vascular tissue. This inhibition of calcium results in a decrease of electrical impulse formation from the SA node, decreased conduction of electrical impulses across the AV node, and relaxation of the arterial smooth muscle. Clinically, the patient will present with a lower HR and blood pressure.

Prep Kit

■ Ready for Review

- Cardiovascular disease has been the number one killer in Canada almost every year since 1900.
- The cardiovascular system is composed of the heart and blood vessels. Its primary function is to deliver oxygenated blood and nutrients to every cell.
- Patients experience a variety of symptoms when they have a cardiovascular problem.
- Coronary artery disease is the most common form of heart disease and the leading cause of death in adults in Canada.
- Cardiac rhythm disturbances or arrhythmias may arise from a variety of causes—they are not solely caused by AMI.
- Most cardiac arrest victims have evidence of atherosclerosis or other underlying cardiac disease. However, cardiac arrest can also occur secondary to electrocution, submersion, and other types of trauma. Indeed, many cardiac arrest victims have no warning before the event occurs.
- A patient who presents with or develops symptomatic bradycardia needs to be treated in a manner that will increase the HR and improve CO.
- A patient who presents with or develops tachycardia presents a more complicated situation than one in bradycardia. Tachycardia can have a supraventricular pacemaker site or may be ventricular in origin. In addition, the patient may be mildly or severely symptomatic owing to the tachycardia or another condition. Because of the many possible variations in tachycardic patients, several judgments must be made before treatment is begun.
- Patients with diseases affecting the cardiovascular system may be taking a wide variety of medications for a variety of reasons, and it is not always possible to identify the patient's specific problem on the basis of a medication that he or she is taking.

■ Vital Vocabulary

aberrant conduction The abnormal conduction of the electrical impulse through the heart.

absolute refractory period The early phase of cardiac repolarization, wherein the heart muscle cannot be stimulated to depolarize.

acetylcholine A chemical mediator of the parasympathetic nervous system.

acute coronary syndrome Term used to describe any group of clinical symptoms consistent with acute myocardial ischemia.

acute myocardial infarction (AMI) A condition present when a period of cardiac ischemia caused by sudden narrowing or complete occlusion of a coronary artery leads to death (necrosis) of myocardial tissue.

adrenaline The hormone produced by the adrenal gland with alpha and beta sympathomimetic properties.

afterload The resistance against which the ventricle contracts.

agonal Pertaining to the period of dying.

agonal rhythm A cardiac dysrhythmia seen just before the heart stops altogether; essentially asystole with occasional QRS complexes that are not associated with cardiac output.

aneurysm A sac or bulge resulting from the weakening of the wall of a blood vessel or ventricle.

angina pectoris The sudden pain from myocardial ischemia, caused by diminished circulation to the cardiac muscle. The pain is usually substernal and often radiates to the arms, jaw, or abdomen and usually lasts 3 to 5 minutes and disappears with rest.

aorta The largest artery in the body, originating from the left ventricle.

aortic valve The valve between the left ventricle and the aorta.

arrhythmias Disturbances in cardiac rhythm.

arteries The muscular, thick-walled blood vessels that carry blood away from the heart.

arteriole A small blood vessel that carries oxygenated blood, branching into yet smaller vessels called capillaries.

arteriosclerosis A pathologic condition in which the arterial walls become thickened and inelastic.

artifact An artificial product; in cardiology, is used to refer to noise or interference in an ECG tracing.

asystole The absence of ventricular contractions; a "straight-line ECG."

atherosclerosis A common type of arteriosclerosis affecting the coronary and cerebral arteries.

atrial kick The addition to ventricular volume contributed by contraction of the atria.

atrioventricular (AV) node A specialized structure located in the AV junction that slows conduction through the AV junction.

atrioventricular (AV) valves The mitral and tricuspid valves.

atropine A parasympathetic blocker; opposes the action of acetylcholine on the heart and elsewhere, thereby allowing the body's natural sympathetic system to speed up the heart rate.

automaticity Spontaneous initiation of depolarizing electric impulses by pacemaker sites within the electric conduction system of the heart.

autonomic nervous system A subdivision of the nervous system that controls primarily involuntary body functions. It comprises the sympathetic and parasympathetic nervous systems.

AV junction The atrioventricular junction; the portion of the electric conduction system of the heart located in the upper part of the interventricular septum that conducts the excitation impulse from the atria to the bundle of His.

bigeminy An arrhythmia in which every other heartbeat is a premature contraction.

blood pressure The pressure exerted by the pulsatile flow of blood against the arterial walls.

bradycardia A slow heart rate, less than 60 beats/min.

bronchoconstriction Narrowing of the bronchial tubes.

bronchodilation Widening of the bronchial tubes.

bruits Abnormal whooshing sounds indicating turbulent blood flow within a blood vessel.

bundle branch block A disturbance in electric conduction through the right or left bundle branch from the bundle of His.

bundle of His The portion of the electric conduction system in the interventricular septum that conducts the depolarizing impulse from the atrioventricular junction to the right and left bundle branches.

capillaries Extremely narrow blood vessels composed of a single layer of cells through which oxygen and nutrients pass to the tissues. Capillaries form a network between arterioles and venules.

cardiac cycle The period from one cardiac contraction to the next. Each cardiac cycle consists of ventricular contraction (systole) and relaxation (diastole).

cardiac output (CO) Amount of blood pumped by the heart per minute, calculated by multiplying the stroke volume by the heart rate per minute.

cardiac tamponade Restriction of cardiac contraction, failing cardiac output, and shock, caused by the accumulation of fluid or blood in the pericardium.

cardiopulmonary arrest The sudden and often unexpected cessation of adequate cardiac output.

cardioversion The use of a synchronized direct current (DC) electric shock to convert tachyarrhythmias (such as atrial flutter) to normal sinus rhythm.

chordae tendineae Fibrous strands shaped like umbrella stays that attach the free edges of the leaflets, or cusps, of the atrioventricular valves to the papillary muscles.

chronotropic effect The effect on the rate of contraction of the heart.

circumflex coronary artery One of the two branches of the left main coronary artery.

collateral circulation The mesh of arteries and capillaries that furnishes blood to a segment of tissue whose original arterial supply has been obstructed.

contractility The strength of heart muscle contractions.

coronary arteries The blood vessels of the heart that supply blood to its walls.

coronary artery disease (CAD) A pathologic process caused by atherosclerosis that leads to progressive narrowing and eventual obstruction of the coronary arteries.

coronary sinus A large vessel in the posterior part of the coronary sulcus into which the coronary veins empty.

coronary sulcus The groove along the exterior surface of the heart that separates the atria from the ventricles.

couplet Two premature ventricular contractions occurring sequentially.

defibrillation The use of an unsynchronized direct current (DC) electric shock to terminate ventricular fibrillation.

delta wave The slurring of the upstroke of the first part of the QRS complex that occurs in Wolff-Parkinson-White syndrome.

depolarization The process of discharging resting cardiac muscle fibres by an electric impulse that causes them to contract.

diastole The period of ventricular relaxation during which the ventricles passively fill with blood.

digoxin preparation Medication prescribed for the treatment of chronic CHF or for certain rapid atrial arrhythmias.

dissection In references to blood vessels, an aneurysm, or bulge, formed by the separation of the layers of an arterial wall.

dromotropic effect The effect on the velocity of conduction.

electrical conduction system In the heart, the specialized cardiac tissue that initiates and conducts electric impulses. The system includes the SA node, internodal atrial conduction pathways, atrioventricular junction, atrioventricular node, bundle of His, and the Purkinje network.

endocardium The thin membrane lining the inside of the heart.

epicardium The thin membrane lining the outside of the heart.

fibrinolytic therapy The therapy that uses medications that act to dissolve blood clots.

first-degree heart block A partial disruption of the conduction of the depolarizing impulse from the atria to the ventricles, causing prolongation of the P-R interval.

heart rate (HR) The number of heart contractions per minute.

hyperkalemia An excessive amount of potassium in the blood.

hypertension High blood pressure, usually a diastolic pressure greater than 90 mm Hg.

hypocalcemia A low level of calcium in the blood.

hypokalemia An abnormally low concentration of potassium in the blood.

infarction Death (necrosis) of a localized area of tissue caused by the cutting off of its blood supply.

internodal pathways The three pathways of the electrical conduction system found in the atria that transmit the impulse from the SA node to the AV node.

interventricular septum A thick wall that separates the right and left ventricles.

ischemia Tissue anoxia from diminished blood flow to tissue, usually caused by narrowing or occlusion of the artery.

isoelectric When referring to a wave, the wave is neither positive nor negative.

isoelectric line The baseline of the ECG.

junctional rhythm An arrhythmia arising from ectopic foci in the area of the atrioventricular junction; often shows an absence of the P wave, a short P-R interval, or a P wave appearing after the QRS complex.

lead Any one of the conductors, composed of two or more electrodes, in the ECG that shows the electrical conduction in the heart.

left atrium The upper left chamber of the heart; receives blood from the pulmonary veins.

left ventricle The thick-walled, muscular, lower left chamber of the heart; receives blood from the left atrium and pumps it out through the aorta into the systemic arteries.

limb leads The ECG leads attached to the limbs and that form the hexaxial system, dividing the heart along a coronal plane into the anterior and posterior segments.

lumen The inside diameter of an artery or other hollow structure.

mitral valve The valve located between the left atrium and the left ventricle of the heart.

monomorphic Having one common shape of QRS complex.

multifocal Arising from or pertaining to many foci or locations.

myocardium The cardiac muscle.

necrosis The death of tissue, usually caused by a cessation of its blood supply.

norepinephrine A neurotransmitter and drug sometimes used in the treatment of shock; produces vasoconstriction through its alpha stimulator properties.

normal sinus rhythm The normal rhythm of the heart, wherein the excitation impulse arises in the SA node, travels through the internodal pathways to the atrioventricular junction, down the bundle of His, through the bundle branches, and into the Purkinje network without interference.

orthopnea Severe dyspnea experienced when lying down and relieved by sitting up.

orthostatic hypotension A fall in blood pressure when changing to an erect position.

P wave The first wave of the ECG complex, representing depolarization of the atria.

pacemaker The specialized tissue within the heart that initiates excitation impulses; an electronic device used to stimulate cardiac contraction when the electric conduction system of the heart is malfunctioning, especially in complete heart block. An electronic pacemaker consists of a battery-powered pulse generator and a wire that transmits the electric impulse to the ventricles.

palpitations A sensation felt under the left breast of the heart "skipping a beat," usually caused by a premature ventricular contraction.

papillary muscles Protrusions of the myocardium into the ventricular cavities to which the chordae tendineae are attached.

parasympathetic nervous system A subdivision of the autonomic nervous system that is involved in control of involuntary, vegetative functions, mediated largely by the vagus nerve through the chemical acetylcholine.

paroxysmal nocturnal dyspnea (PND) Severe shortness of breath occurring at night after several hours of recumbency, during which fluid pools in the lungs; the person is forced to sit up to breathe. PND is caused by left heart failure or decompensation of chronic obstructive pulmonary disease.

pericardium The double-layered sac containing the heart and the origins of the superior vena cava, inferior vena cava, and pulmonary artery.

phlebitis Inflammation of the wall of a vein, sometimes caused by an IV line, manifested by tenderness, redness, and slight edema along part of the length of the vein.

phlebotomy The withdrawal of blood from a vein.

plaque In cardiology, the white to yellow lesion found in atherosclerosis that is made up of lipids, cell debris, and smooth muscles cells; in older people, may also include calcium.

plasmin A naturally occurring clot-dissolving enzyme, usually present in the body in its inactive form, plasminogen.

point of maximal impulse (PMI) The palpable beat of the apex of the heart against the chest wall during ventricular contraction; normally palpated in the fifth left intercostal space in the midclavicular line.

P-R interval The period between the beginning of the P wave (atrial depolarization) and the onset of the QRS complex (ventricular depolarization), signifying the time required for atrial depolarization and passage of the excitation impulse through the atrioventricular junction.

precordial leads Another term used to describe the chest leads in an ECG.

preload The pressure under which the ventricle fills.

pulmonary artery One of two arteries that carry deoxygenated blood from the right ventricle to the lungs.

pulmonary circulation The flow of blood from the right ventricle through the pulmonary arteries and all of their branches and capillaries in the lungs and back to the left atrium through the venules and pulmonary veins; also called the lesser circulation.

pulmonary edema Congestion of the pulmonary air spaces with exudate and foam, often secondary to left heart failure.

pulmonary veins The vessels that carry oxygenated blood from the lungs to the left atrium.

pulmonic valve The valve between the right ventricle and the pulmonary artery.

pulsus paradoxus A weakening or loss of a palpable pulse during inhalation, characteristic of cardiac tamponade and severe asthma.

Purkinje fibres A system of fibres in the ventricles that conducts the excitation impulse from the bundle branches to the myocardium.

QRS complex Deflections of the ECG produced by ventricular depolarization.

recanalization The opening up of new channels through a blocked artery.

receptors Specialized areas in tissues that initiate certain actions after specific stimulation.

refractory period A short period immediately after depolarization in which the myocytes are not yet repolarized and are unable to fire or conduct an impulse.

relative refractory period That period in the cell-firing cycle at which it is possible but difficult to restimulate the cell to fire another impulse.

reperfusion The resumption of blood flow through an artery.

retrosternal Situated or occurring behind the sternum.

right atrium The upper right chamber of the heart; receives blood from the venae cavae and supplies blood to the right ventricle.

right ventricle The lower right chamber of the heart; receives blood from the right atrium and pumps blood out through the pulmonic valve into the pulmonary artery.

R-R interval The period between the onset of one QRS complex and the onset of the next QRS complex.

semilunar valves The two valves, the aortic and pulmonic, that divide the heart from the aorta and pulmonary arteries.

sinoatrial (SA) node The dominant pacemaker of the heart, located at the junction of the superior vena cava and the right atrium.

sinus arrhythmia A slight irregularity of the heart rate caused by changes in parasympathetic tone during breathing.

sinus bradycardia A sinus rhythm with a heart rate less than 60 beats/min.

sinus tachycardia A sinus rhythm with a heart rate greater than 100 beats/min.

stable angina Angina pectoris characterized by periodic pain with a predictable pattern.

ST segment The interval between the end of the QRS complex and the beginning of the T wave; often elevated or depressed with respect to the isoelectric line when there is significant myocardial ischemia.

stroke volume (SV) The volume of blood pumped forward with each ventricular contraction.

sympathetic nervous system A subdivision of the autonomic nervous system that governs the body's fight-or-flight reactions, stimulating cardiac activity.

syncope Fainting; brief loss of consciousness caused by transiently inadequate blood flow to the brain.

systemic circulation The flow of blood from the left ventricle through the aorta, to all of its branches and capillaries in the tissues, and back to the right atrium through the venules, veins, and venae cavae; also called the greater circulation.

systole The period during which the ventricles contract.

T waves The upright, flat, or inverted wave following the QRS complex of the ECG, representing ventricular repolarization.

tachycardia A rapid heart rate, more than 100 beats/min.

tricuspid valve The valve between the right atrium and right ventricle of the heart.

trigeminy A premature complex in every third heartbeat.

tunica adventitia The outer layer of tissue of a blood vessel wall, composed of elastic and fibrous connective tissue.

tunica intima The smooth, thin, inner lining of a blood vessel.

tunica media The middle and thickest layer of tissue of a blood vessel wall, composed of elastic tissue and smooth muscle cells that allow the vessel to expand or contract in response to changes in blood pressure and tissue demand.

U wave A small flat wave sometimes seen after the T wave and before the next P wave.

unifocal Arising from a single site.

unstable angina Angina pectoris characterized by a changing, unpredictable pattern of pain, which may signal an impending acute myocardial infarction.

vagus nerve The 10th cranial nerve, the chief mediator of the parasympathetic nervous system.

Valsalva maneuver Forced exhalation against a closed glottis, the effect of which is to stimulate the vagus nerve and, thereby, slow the heart rate.

vasoconstriction Narrowing of the diameter of a blood vessel.

vasodilation Widening of the diameter of a blood vessel.

veins The blood vessels that carry blood to the heart.

venae cavae The largest veins of the body; they return blood to the right atrium.

venules Very small veins.

Wolff-Parkinson-White (WPW) syndrome A syndrome characterized by short P-R intervals, delta waves, nonspecific ST-T wave changes, and paroxysmal episodes of tachycardia caused by the presence of an accessory pathway.

Assessment in Action

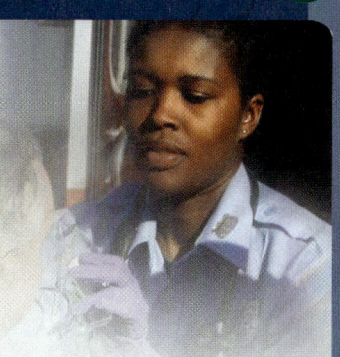

You are dispatched to the private residence of an 88-year-old man who is complaining of shortness of breath. When you arrive on scene, you find the patient in severe respiratory distress, speaking in two- to three-word sentences. He is grossly diaphoretic and complains of chest tightness. The patient tells you that he has no medical problems and does not take any medications. His vital signs are as follows: respiratory rate, 42 breaths/min with a room air pulse oximetry of 88%; blood pressure, 220/110 mm Hg; heart rate, 130 beats/min. The ECG monitor shows rapid atrial fibrillation.

1. **What differential diagnosis can you make?**
   A. Pneumonia
   B. Angina
   C. Congestive heart failure
   D. Acute myocardial infarction

2. **Cardiac output is:**
   A. the amount of blood that is pumped out by either ventricle, measured in litres per minute.
   B. the pressure exerted by the blood against the arterial walls.
   C. the contribution to ventricular filling made by contraction of the atrium.
   D. one complete phase of atrial and ventricular relaxation.

3. **What is the most common form of heart disease and is the number one killer of men and women?**
   A. Angina
   B. Pulmonary edema
   C. Myocardial infarction
   D. Coronary artery disease

4. **What is the principal symptom of CAD?**
   A. Pulmonary edema
   B. Myocardial infarction
   C. Angina pectoris
   D. Unstable myocardium

5. **The term that describes when a portion of the cardiac muscle is deprived of coronary blood flow long enough that the muscle dies is:**
   A. unstable angina.
   B. stable angina.
   C. CAD.
   D. acute myocardial infarction.

6. **What term describes the situation when the heart is so severely damaged that it can no longer pump a volume of blood sufficient to maintain tissue perfusion?**
   A. Acute myocardial infarction
   B. Cardiogenic shock
   C. Unstable angina
   D. Pulmonary edema or congestive heart failure

Challenging Question

7. **Given the patient's age, are there any special considerations that you should keep in mind?**

Points to Ponder

You are dispatched to an assisted-living facility for a 78-year-old woman who is feeling weak, dizzy, and nauseous. When you arrive, you find the patient resting comfortably. She tells you that while she was trying to have a bowel movement, she suddenly became very dizzy. There was no diaphoresis or shortness of breath. Her vital signs are as follows: respiratory rate, 18 breaths/min with a room air pulse oximetry reading of 97%; blood pressure, 90/58 mm Hg; pulse rate, 40 beats/min. When you apply the ECG to monitor her pulse rate, you notice a third-degree block. The patient's medical history includes hypertension, congestive heart failure, and renal failure secondary to type 1 diabetes. Her medications consist of metoprolol, furosemide, potassium, digoxin, and insulin. She tells you that she has taken all of her medicines this morning as prescribed.

What steps should you take to manage this patient's condition?

Issues: Understanding the Importance of a Complete Physical Examination, Understanding the Importance of ECG Rhythm Analysis, Understanding When to Apply the Transcutaneous Pacer.

www.Paramedic.EMSzone.com/Canada

Neurologic Emergencies

Competency Areas

Area 4: Assessment and Diagnostics

4.3.a   Conduct primary patient assessment and interpret findings.
4.3.b   Conduct secondary patient assessment and interpret findings.
4.3.d   Conduct neurological system assessment and interpret findings.
4.4.a   Assess pulse.
4.4.b   Assess respiration.
4.4.d   Measure blood pressure by auscultation.
4.4.e   Measure blood pressure by palpation.
4.4.g   Assess skin condition.
4.4.h   Assess pupils.
4.4.i   Assess level of mentation.
4.5.c   Conduct glucometric testing and interpret findings.
4.5.d   Conduct peripheral venipuncture.

Area 5: Therapeutics

5.2.a   Recognize indications for oxygen administration.
5.3.d   Administer oxygen using high concentration mask.
5.4.a   Provide oxygenation and ventilation using bag-valve-mask.
5.5.c   Maintain peripheral intravenous (IV) access devices and infusions of crystalloid solutions without additives.
5.5.d   Conduct peripheral intravenous cannulation.

Area 6: Integration

6.1.b   Provide care to patient experiencing illness or injury primarily involving neurological system.

Appendix 4: Pathophysiology

B.   **Neurologic System**
Convulsive Disorders: Febrile Seizures
Convulsive Disorders: Generalized seizures
Convulsive Disorders: Partial seizures (focal)
Headache and Facial Pain: Infection

Headache and Facial Pain: Intracranial hemorrhage
Headache and Facial Pain: Migraine
Headache and Facial Pain: Tension
Cerebrovascular Disorders: Ischemic/hemorrhagic stroke
Cerebrovascular Disorders: Transient ischemic attack
Altered Mental Status: Metabolic
Altered Mental Status: Structural
Chronic Neurologic Disorders: Alzheimers
Chronic Neurologic Disorders: Amyotrophic lateral sclerosis (ALS)
Chronic Neurologic Disorders: Bell's palsy
Chronic Neurologic Disorders: Cerebral palsy
Chronic Neurologic Disorders: Multiple sclerosis
Chronic Neurologic Disorders: Muscular dystrophy
Chronic Neurologic Disorders: Parkinson's disease
Chronic Neurologic Disorders: Poliomyelitis
Infectious Disorders: Guillian Barre syndrome
Infectious Disorders: Meningitis
Tumors: Structural
Tumors: Vascular
Pediatric: Spina bifida
J.   **Multisystem Diseases and Injuries**
Cancer: Malignancy
Shock Syndromes: Neurogenic

Appendix 5: Medications

A.   **Medications affecting the central nervous system.**
A.3   Anticonvulsants
A.5   Anxiolytics, Hypnotics, and Antagonists
J.   **Medications used to treat poisoning and overdose.**
J.1   Antidotes or Neutralizing Agents

Introduction

Many paramedics love the challenge of trauma and the excitement of dealing with its sudden nature. Trauma injuries can be graphic and attract your attention easily. By contrast, the medical patient is an entirely different animal. These patients require a keen eye, sharp assessment skills, and—above all—critical thinking to determine the nature of the problem. Medical patients can be very challenging as they often have complaints that are not apparent.

According to the Health and Stroke Foundation of Canada, cardiovascular disease, which includes heart disease and stroke, is the leading cause of death among Canadians (32% of deaths). Clearly, the paramedic will encounter many neurologic emergencies.

Neurologic patients can be extremely vulnerable or even helpless. Many of the reflexes that protect an awake person may not function when the nervous system is depressed. The eyelids don't blink away dust and irritants. The larynx doesn't gag and cough in reaction to secretions oozing down the airway. The body doesn't seek a more comfortable position in response to compression of a limb in an awkward position. The tongue goes slack. The airway is at risk.

In this chapter, the anatomy and physiology of the nervous system are reviewed first. Then the general pathology of neurologic conditions is explored, laying the proper foundation for discussion of their assessment and treatment.

Anatomy and Physiology

The nervous system is the most complex organ system within the human body. It consists of two major structures, the brain and spinal cord, plus thousands of nerves allowing every part of the body to communicate. This system is responsible for fundamental functions such as controlling breathing, heart rate, and blood pressure. But the real beauty of the nervous system is found in its higher level activity. Reading a good book (like this one), enjoying music, having a discussion with a friend, and even watching television require the brain to engage memory, understanding, and thought. Here is where the true complexity of this system can be seen.

Figure 28-1 ▶ shows the basic structure of the nervous system. The major structures are divided into two main categories: the central nervous system (CNS), which is responsible for thought, perception, feeling, and autonomic body functions; and the peripheral nervous system (PNS), which transmits commands from the brain to the body and receives feedback from the body.

Consider the case of Justin—a child riding a bicycle. This common and seemingly simple activity is rich with both conscious and unconscious functions. It's a beautiful summer morning, so Justin goes to the garage to get his bike. Already the brain is hard at work. As Justin enters the garage, the brain must determine which object is a bike. Justin scans the garage. The images produced by his eyes are transmitted via the optic nerve to the occipital lobe of the brain **Figure 28-2 ▶** . There the image, which is transmitted upside down, is reoriented. The occipital lobe then pores through tens of thousands of stored images. Has this image been seen before?

Once the image is recognized, an existing pathway is accessed to the temporal lobe, where language and speech are stored. Now, as Justin walks through the garage, he is able to put names to what he sees—a car, a workbench, a bike. When Justin was learning to speak, he often became confused about the names of objects. As he practiced, he received reinforcement for the correct names and redirection for the incorrect

You are the Paramedic Part 1

You are dispatched to 16600 Courage Court for an older man who has fallen. You arrive to find Mr. Hishari, an 81-year-old man, lying on the floor. His two sons explain that they visited their father last night and left around 1900 hrs. When they returned this morning, they found their father lying on the floor next to the chair in which he was sitting when they last saw him. He has been unable to explain what happened and, because he lives alone, no one is sure how long he's been on the floor.

The patient is awake and responding to his sons, but they say he is "not acting right." They describe him as "very sharp," but today he keeps getting their names confused. They say this only happens when his blood glucose level is low. The patient has type 2 diabetes.

Initial Assessment	Recording Time: 0 Minutes
Appearance	Lying on the floor, appears clean
Level of consciousness	V (Responsive to verbal stimuli), oriented to person and place, but not day
Airway	Patent
Breathing	Nonlaboured
Circulation	Strong radial pulse

1. What do you suspect as the reason(s) why Mr. Hishari is on the floor?
2. How would you prioritize those reasons?

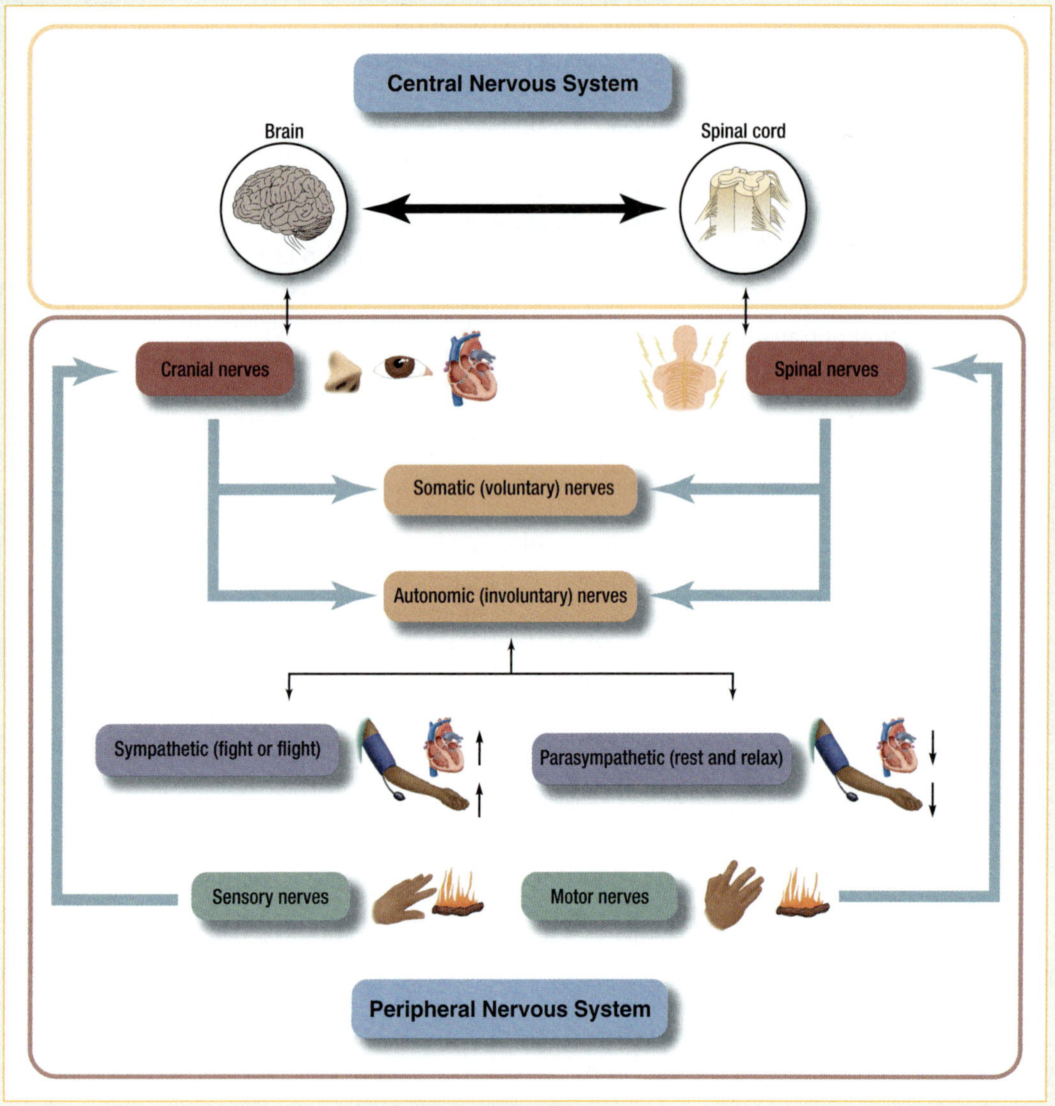

Central Nervous System

Brain

Spinal cord

Cranial nerves

Spinal nerves

Somatic (voluntary) nerves

Autonomic (involuntary) nerves

Sympathetic (fight or flight)

Parasympathetic (rest and relax)

Sensory nerves

Motor nerves

Peripheral Nervous System

Figure 28-1 Organization of the nervous system.

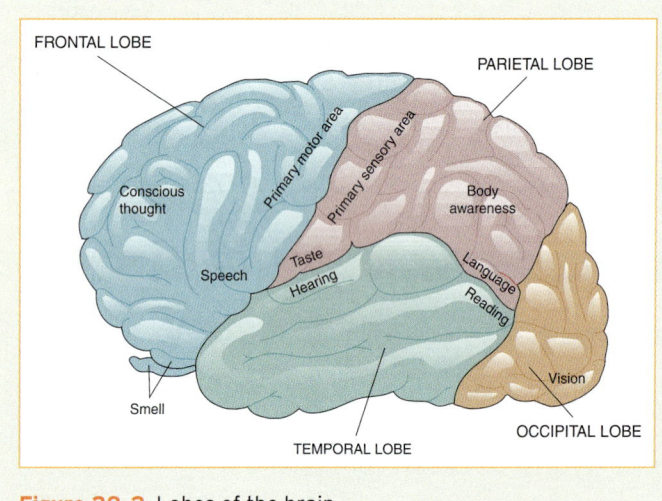

FRONTAL LOBE

PARIETAL LOBE

Primary motor area

Primary sensory area

Conscious thought

Body awareness

Speech

Taste

Hearing

Language

Reading

Smell

Vision

OCCIPITAL LOBE

TEMPORAL LOBE

Figure 28-2 Lobes of the brain.

names. In his brain, more pathways were established between the image of an object with two wheels, a seat, and pedals, which was stored in the occipital lobe, and the word for that object (bike), which was stored in the temporal lobe.

As Justin retrieves his helmet, the frontal lobe of his brain springs into action. The frontal lobe, which controls voluntary motion, sends signals out of the CNS along efferent nerves to the arms, shoulders, chest, and hands to perform the task of picking up the helmet. The efferent nerves leave the brain through the PNS and convey commands to other parts of the body.

Which way should the helmet be applied? This motor memory is stored in the frontal lobe; the brain stores memories in the areas that are initially stimulated. As he places the helmet on his head, Justin needs to make fine adjustments to its position. His brain is receiving impulses from nerves within the skull and muscles of his head, indicating that the helmet is uncomfortable. Justin senses pressure and possibly pain from the improperly positioned helmet. The afferent nerves (that send information to the brain) transmit signals of discomfort to the parietal lobe, where the body's sense of touch and pain perception are found. Signals sent from the parietal lobe to the frontal lobe make the body adjust the helmet until the pressure signals have stopped.

As you have been reading this tale, huge amounts of information have been pouring from your PNS into your CNS. Signals are sent from organs, muscles, and areas of the skin to the spinal cord until they reach the lower portions of the CNS. The position of your legs, the distribution of your body weight, the sensation of the pages in your fingers, the state of your renal arteries—all of these data are being sent to the CNS. How does the brain manage this massive amount of information without confusion and misdirection? By using the diencephalon and brain stem **Figure 28-3 ▶**.

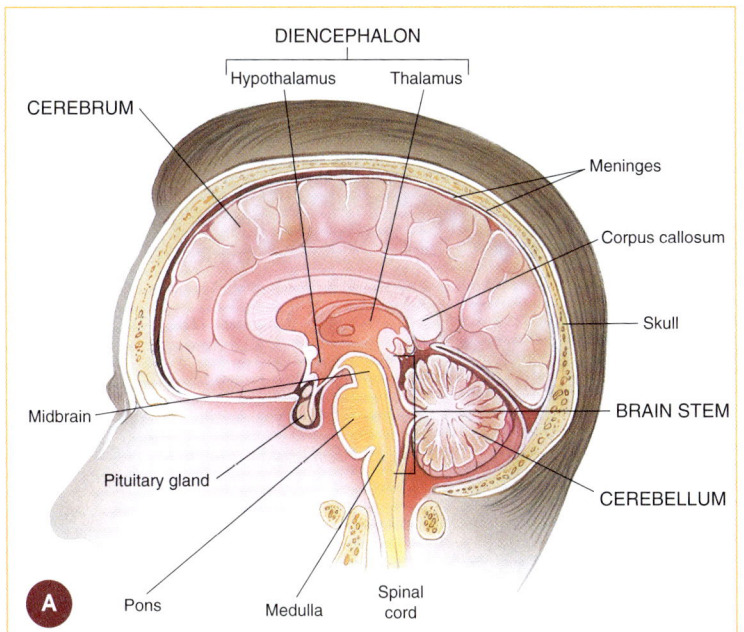
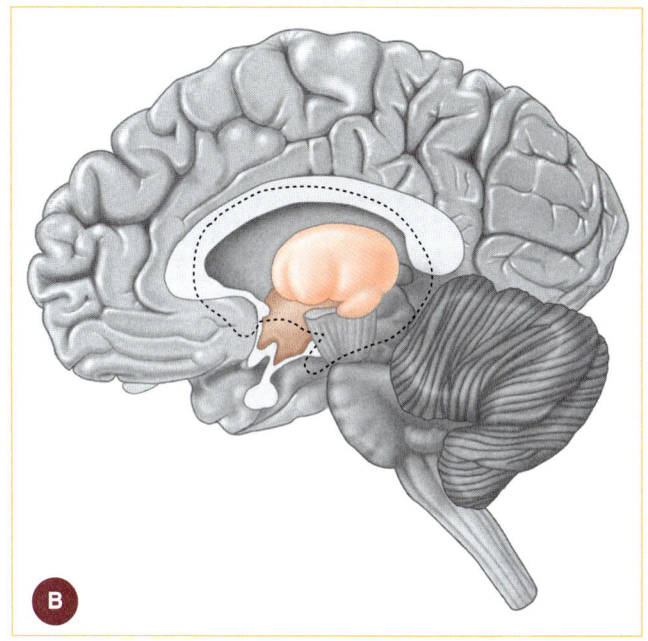

Figure 28-3 **A.** Areas of the brain, including the brain stem. **B.** The diencephalon.

One major role of the diencephalon is to filter out unneeded information from the cerebral cortex. Imagine if you had to "think" about shifting your weight on a chair when it became uncomfortable. The signals of pressure or pain being sent via the peripheral nerves initially stop in the diencephalon. The body's administrative assistant then decides whether the big boss (the cerebral cortex) needs to be bothered with this information. In the case of an uncomfortable bottom, the diencephalon simply sends commands so that you move slightly. Unless you were concentrating on how you were sitting, you would never even know that you moved.

How did Justin know it was time to get up this morning? His internal alarm clock went off, of course. The midbrain (part of the brain stem) is responsible for regulating the level of consciousness (LOC). You often get tired at the same time each day due to the functions of the reticular activating system (RAS). Justin is wide awake and thinking clearly thanks to his RAS.

How are blood pressure, heart rate, respiratory rate, and breathing pattern controlled? Again, the brain stem is responsible. The pons 〔**Figure 28-4** ▶〕, which is located just inferior to the midbrain, regulates your respiratory pace and the depth at which you breathe. The medulla oblongata controls the blood pressure and heart rate. Of course, these functions need to occur constantly, but Justin couldn't ride his bike if he needed to spend time and energy consciously controlling his pulse. The brain stem frees the cerebral cortex up to engage in higher level activities.

Justin now mounts his bike and begins to ride. The smile on his face reveals that he is having fun. Emotions come from two main areas within the brain: the limbic system

〔**Figure 28-5** ▶〕, where rage and anger are generated; and the hypothalamus (a part of the diencephalon), where pleasure, thirst, and hunger are found. All emotions are then mediated by the prefrontal cortex so people can choose how they are going to act in relation to how they feel.

Justin begins to pick up speed. As he approaches a corner, he must turn or risk crashing into a tree. The excitement increases his heart rate and blood pressure. The hypothalamus communicates to the pituitary gland, a member of the endocrine system. The pituitary gland, in turn, sends chemical commands to the adrenal glands to release epinephrine and norepinephrine. The release of these chemicals by the sympathetic nervous system gives Justin the increased strength and cardiovascular reserves that he needs to handle the bike in a tight turn. Just as quickly as these chemicals act, they are shut off to prevent the body from depleting its reserves. Too much epinephrine and norepinephrine can also be damaging over the long term.

Justin shifts his weight and makes the turn successfully, due in large part to his cerebellum. This lobe of the brain (located in the posterior, inferior area of the skull) manages complex motor activity. When Justin first learned to ride a bike, he had to think about what to do, where to shift his weight, and how to hold his upper body. Eventually, the frontal lobe of the brain got tired of sending the same commands again and again, so this task was transferred to the cerebellum. This lobe keeps track of Justin's body position at all times and helps to manage activities such as walking, swimming, and riding a bike.

All of this wonderfully complex activity is made possible by the synapses. Nerve cells don't actually come in direct contact with one another. Instead, a slight gap separates the cells,

Cerebral cortex
- Receives sensory information from skin, muscles, glands, and organs
- Sends messages to move skeletal muscles
- Integrates incoming and outgoing nerve impulses
- Performs associative activities such as thinking, learning, and remembering

Basal nuclei
- Plays a role in the coordination of slow, sustained movements
- Suppresses useless patterns of movement

Thalamus
- Relays most sensory information from the spinal cord and certain parts of the brain to the cerebral cortex
- Interprets certain sensory messages such as those of pain, temperature, and pressure

Hypothalamus
- Controls various homeostatic functions such as body temperature, respiration, and heartbeat
- Directs hormone secretions of the pituitary

Cerebellum
- Coordinates subconscious movements of skeletal muscles
- Contributes to muscle tone, posture, balance, and equilibrium

Brain stem
- Origin of many cranial nerves
- Reflex centre for movements of eyeballs, head, and trunk
- Regulates heartbeat and breathing
- Plays a role in consciousness
- Transmits impulses between brain and spinal cord

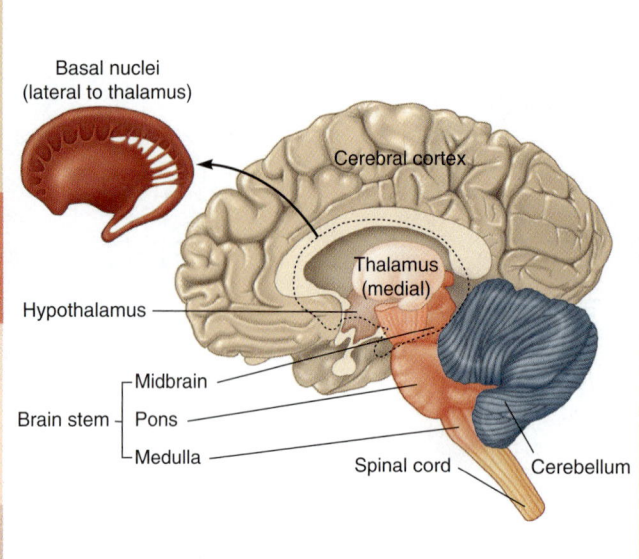
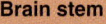

Figure 28-4 The pons.

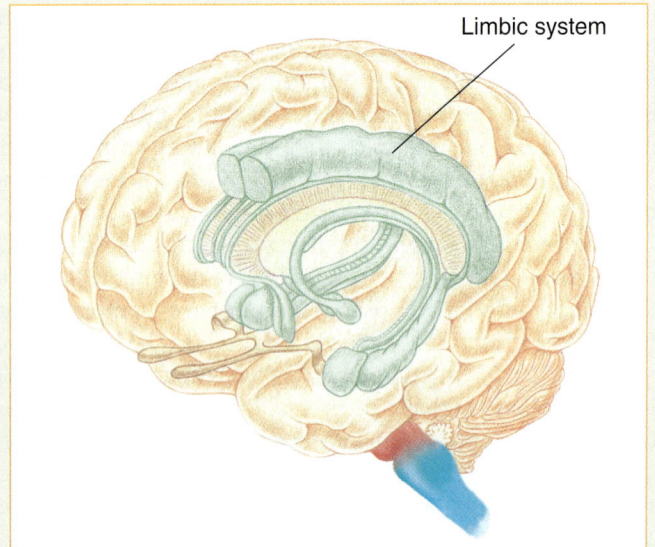

Figure 28-5 The limbic system is the seat of emotions, instincts, and other functions.

which allows for a far greater level of fine control. The synapse, which is present wherever a nerve cell terminates, "connects" to the next cell via chemicals called <u>neurotransmitters</u>. A host of neurotransmitters are present in the brain and throughout the body. Dopamine, acetylcholine, epinephrine, and serotonin are all examples of neurotransmitters. These chemicals take the electrically conducted signal from one nerve cell (a neuron) and relay it to the next cell. Nerve cells respond to these signals in an "all or nothing" fashion: They either fire or they don't. A neuron can't fire weakly.

How do the neurotransmitters achieve a greater degree of control than that permitted by simply wiring the cells together? The answer lies in the connections made as the signal travels from the cell to the synapse **Figure 28-6 ▸**.

1. The first neuron fires and sends a signal along its <u>axon</u> to the axon terminal.

2. The impulse reaches the axon terminal, where neurotransmitters are released and trickle across the synapse.

3. Dendrites detect these chemicals and are triggered to send the signal to the cell's nucleus, which then transmits it down that axon, and so on.

4. Dendrites release neurotransmitter deactivators so that one impulse from cell 1 generates one response from cell 2.

The complexity in the system derives from how the cells are connected. In Figure 28-6, each cell is connected in a straight-line fashion. Although this is a reliable method of getting a signal from point A to point B, gaining more control requires more complexity. In **Figure 28-7 ▸**, three cells are brought together to connect with the same cell. Cell 4 will not respond unless it receives simultaneous stimulation from cells 1, 2, and 3. The same concept can be extended to the situation in which one cell sends signals to many different cells. In Figure 28-7, for example, cell 4 stimulates cells 5 and 6. As a consequence of this joint action, Justin is able to see his bike, recognize the object, know its name, instantly know how to use it, know how to make the muscles of his mouth say the word "bike," and appreciate how it will feel to ride the bike.

Neurons may or may not have <u>myelin</u> around their axons. Myelin, a protein wrapped around the nerve cells, acts as an insulator. It helps prevent the electrical signal from leaving the nerve cells and entering the surrounding tissues, but its major function is to increase the speed of conduction. Myelinated nerve fibres are predominantly found in vertebrates and higher organisms, all of which rely on rapid nerve conductions to allow higher thought and brain function.

Table 28-1 ▶ summarizes the structures of the nervous system and their functions.

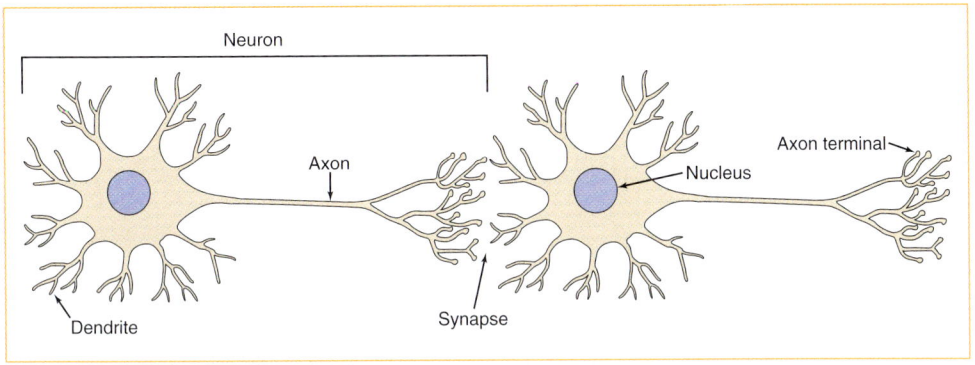

Figure 28-6 Neuron and synapse.

Pathophysiology

The pathophysiology of the nervous system can be examined from several angles. Discussion of cancerous, degenerative, developmental, infectious, vascular, and multifactorial causes of neurologic conditions will be followed by a review of increased intracranial pressure and its effects on the nervous system.

Neoplastic (Cancerous) Causes

<u>Neoplasms</u> (the medical term for cancer) are caused by the abnormal and unregulated growth of cells in the body. Many neoplasms are related to errors that occur during cellular reproduction, especially during the unwinding and reproduction of the DNA during cell duplication. These errors are not critical enough to cause cell death, but allow the unchecked multiplication of the cell, and thus the development of a neoplasm.

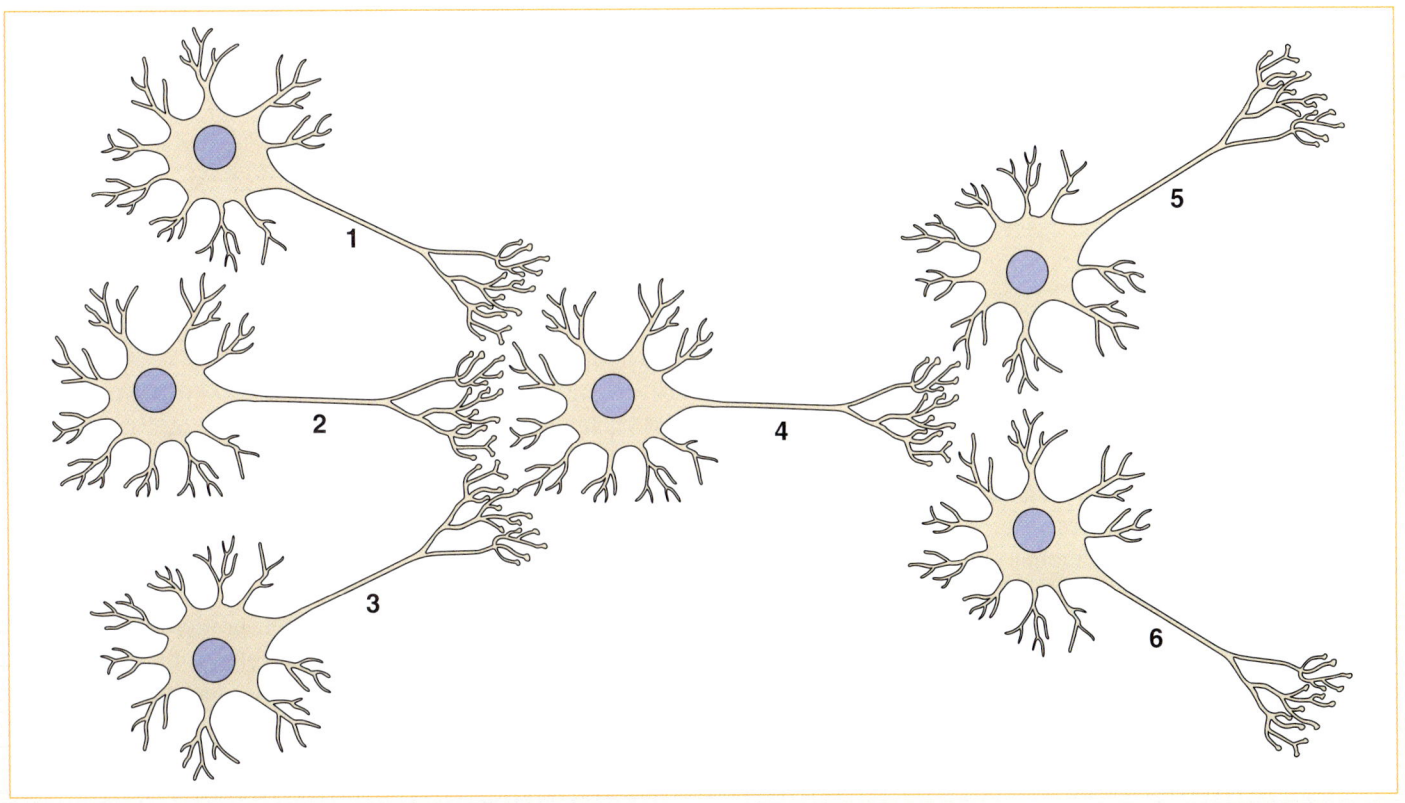

Figure 28-7 Complex synapse. Many cells (1, 2, 3) are brought together to connect with one cell (4). Cell 4 then connects with cells 5 and 6.

Table 28-1 | **Structures of the Nervous System and General Functions**

Major Structure	Subdivision	General Function
Central nervous system		
Brain	Occipital	Vision and storage of visual memories
	Parietal	Sense of touch and texture; storage of those memories
	Temporal	Hearing and smell; language; storage of sound and odour memories
	Frontal	Voluntary muscle control; storage of those memories
	Prefrontal	Judgment and predicting consequences of actions; abstract intellectual functions
	Limbic system	Basic emotions; basic reflexes (eg, chewing, swallowing)
	Diencephalon (thalamus)	Relay centre; filters important signals from routine signals
	Diencephalon (hypothalamus)	Emotions; temperature control; interaction with endocrine system
Brain stem	Midbrain	LOC; RAS; muscle tone and posture
	Pons	Respiratory patterning and depth
	Medulla oblongata	Heart rate; blood pressure; respiratory rate
Spinal cord		Reflexes; relays information to and from body
Peripheral nervous system		
Cranial nerves		Brain to body part communication; special peripheral nerves that connect directly to body parts
Peripheral nerves		Brain to spinal cord to body part communication; receive stimuli from body; send commands to body

Neoplasms can be categorized as either benign (noncancerous) or malignant (cancerous). Essentially, benign neoplasms are not very aggressive. They tend to remain within a capsule, so their growth is limited. In addition, these tumours are usually relatively easy to remove. By contrast, malignant neoplasms may forcefully take over blood supplies, grow unchecked, and move to other sites within the body (metastasis). They create finger-like projections into surrounding tissue, spreading and invading new areas. This growth without regard to other cells explains why many malignancies are fatal.

Degenerative Causes

Degenerative conditions result when a normal structure is altered over time. Such damage can occur in several ways—for example, due to wear and tear. Consider the effects of osteoarthritis on the knee joint. Every time a person falls on the knee, a small amount of damage is done to this joint. If the damage is not completely repaired, it may continue to accumulate until the patient experiences pain. With enough damage, the patient experiences limited mobility and pain to the joints.

Degenerative conditions may also occur through autoimmune effects. The body has the ability to determine which proteins are "self" and which are "nonself." This recognition enables the immune system to attack the bacteria in a cut yet leave the surrounding skin cells alone. In autoimmune disorders, the body begins to attack its own cells. The immune system is no longer able to distinguish friend from foe. Under normal conditions, myelin coats the axons of most nerve cells and allows for smooth transmission of signals to

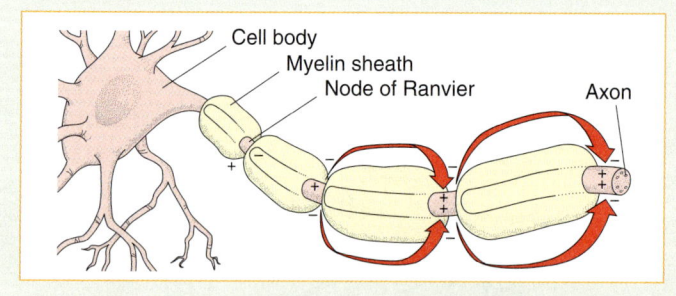

Figure 28-8 The myelin sheath normally allows impulses to jump from node to node, greatly accelerating the rate of transmission.

their target cell **Figure 28-8 ▲**. In multiple sclerosis (MS), however, the body believes that the proteins making up this insulation are foreign. It therefore attacks the myelin, creating gaps in the insulation that produce the signs and symptoms of MS.

Developmental Causes

Developmental conditions arise when portions of the nervous system are not formed correctly. Such an error can occur at any point in the development from embryo to fetus. The earlier the error occurs, the more severe the damage. In the case of spina bifida, embryonic growth does not proceed correctly.

Soon after conception, the fetus is a ball of cells—each cell identical to all the others. Within just 8 days, however, the once uniform ball of cells is ready to give rise to an embryo.

One of the critical changes that must occur is the formation of the neural tube. Around days 15 to 20, a layer of cells will fold in and form a hollow tube that will eventually become the entire nervous system. In spina bifida, some cells do not fold correctly and remain outside the neural tube. This creates an outcropping of nervous system cells that expands as the embryo grows. The ultimate result is a child born with part of its nervous system outside the body.

Even if the fetus is formed correctly, other problems may occur. If an infection or chemical agent is able to gain access to the growing fetus, it may damage areas of the brain. Likewise, a temporary decrease in oxygen may lead to brain damage. These mechanisms are postulated as the causes of cerebral palsy.

Genetics appear to play a role in many diseases, which has implications for developmental causes of neurologic disorders. DNA provides the recipe for building every part of the body and outlining every process that should occur. If the recipe is perfect, then the body part will function normally. If the recipe is only slightly off, the final product may function normally but may not be able to handle stress or wear and tear as easily. However, if the recipe is very wrong, a person has an obvious disease.

This concept helps to explain why some people seem to get diseases very easily while others do not. Consider a man who has been smoking for many years. Although smoking often leads to cardiovascular disease, this man lives to be 90 years old. Another man who eats correctly, exercises every day, and never smokes dies of a heart attack at age 45. Why?

Some of the answer lies in how their coronary arteries were created. Perhaps the smoker had larger, more resilient arteries than those of the 45-year-old heart attack victim. Even though the first man makes many unhealthy lifestyle choices, he benefits from the greater capacity of his coronary arteries, which prevents them from narrowing dramatically. The second man, even though he follows a much healthier lifestyle, has narrower arteries at the beginning, so even a small amount of narrowing has a more profound impact on coronary perfusion. This basic concept is becoming more important in understanding disease incidence and severity.

Infectious Causes

Infectious diseases result when bacteria, viruses, fungi, or prions (a certain type of protein) gain access to the body, where they reproduce and cause damage. These organisms have the same basic goal as humans do—to continue to live. When they begin to attack the body, they are simply looking for fuel so that they can create the next generation of bacteria, viruses, or other organisms. The damage that these invaders inflict occurs due to one of two mechanisms—the body's reaction to the infection or the activities of the attacking organisms.

The most common sign of infectious disease is the presence of a fever. Many organisms prefer to grow in a very narrow temperature range, so even a 1° or 2°C increase in body temperature can slow down the reproduction of some viruses or bacteria. This allows the immune system to get the upper hand. It also provides valuable time for neutrophils (the body's soldiers) to find and kill the invading organisms. Finally, it signals the rest of the body that an attack is under way. In response, more white blood cells are produced and chemical mediators are released to improve the body's effectiveness at finding and eliminating the organisms.

If the temperature of the body becomes too high, however, the brain can be affected. The increased temperature may make a person's thinking dull, make it difficult to concentrate, and lead to a headache. Neurons are highly sensitive to temperature changes. As the temperature rises, the effects on the neurons can become more profound. Eventually, a person may hallucinate, become delusional, or lose consciousness. The random firing of neurons might also produce a febrile seizure.

Infectious agents may also damage the body by destroying cells. These organisms may produce endotoxins or exotoxins that alter living cells. Endotoxins are proteins that are released by gram-negative bacteria when they die. Exotoxins are proteins that are secreted by some bacteria or fungi to aid in the death and digestion of other cells. In poliomyelitis, for example, the virus responsible for the disease attacks the axons directly and destroys them. This virus shows a preference for motor axons—the neurons responsible for making muscles contract. Without these axons, the patient can experience weakness, paralysis, and respiratory arrest.

Vascular Causes

Blood vessels are needed to supply nutrients and oxygen to cells and to remove waste products **Figure 28-9 ▶**. If a blood vessel suddenly becomes blocked, as in an embolism, the cells beyond the blockage may become ischemic. As oxygen and glucose levels drop, brain cells resort to anaerobic metabolism to stay alive. Unfortunately, this mechanism is only a stop-gap measure. Anaerobic metabolism creates minuscule amounts of energy for the cell and produces acidic by-products. If circulation is not restored quickly, the cell will not have enough fuel to survive.

Vascular emergencies may occur either suddenly or gradually over time. Sudden occurrences typically result from emboli or aneurysms. Emboli are insoluble objects that float in the bloodstream until they reach a point in the artery that is too narrow for them to pass through. Common types of emboli include pieces of a thrombus that have broken off or small clots that are produced by turbulent blood flow within the heart. Patients with atrial fibrillation, for example, need to have their heart rhythm controlled and take anticoagulants to

Notes from Nancy

Once brain cells are destroyed, from whatever cause, they cannot be regenerated. Clearly, then, it is of enormous importance to provide the brain with maximum protection from harm.

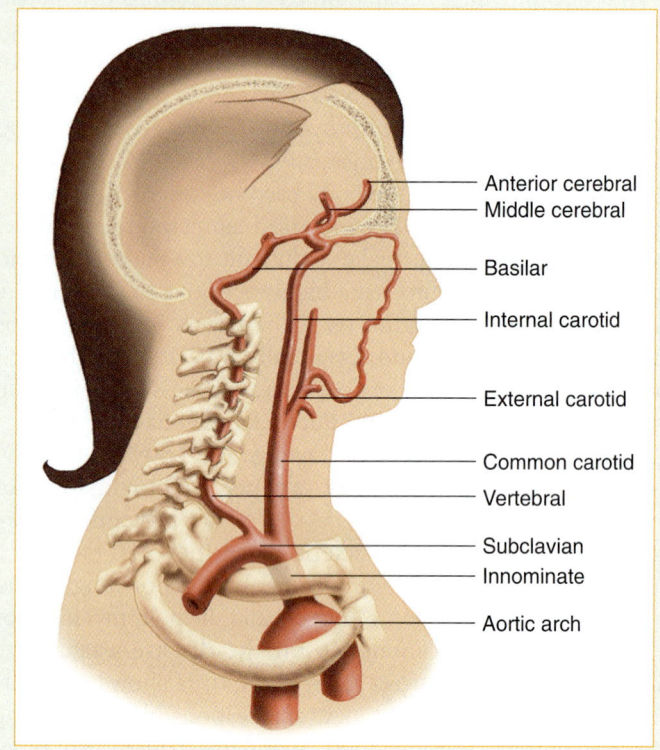

Anterior cerebral
Middle cerebral
Basilar
Internal carotid
External carotid
Common carotid
Vertebral
Subclavian
Innominate
Aortic arch

Figure 28-9 Blood supply to the brain.

prevent clots from forming in the heart and travelling to the brain, which could cause a stroke. Other types of emboli include globules of fat from long bone fractures, air bubbles infused from an IV, or a portion of an IV cannula that has been sheared off during insertion. These objects stop blood flow distal to the blockage, causing ischemia and necrosis of tissue **Figure 28-10 ▶** .

Artery walls consist of three layers of tissue. Aneurysms, which are weaknesses in those walls, occur in the following circumstances:

1. A small tear or defect occurs within the wall of an artery.
2. Blood penetrates between the layers of the artery.
3. Pressure builds up and the initial small tear increases in size.
4. If the buildup continues, the wall will become so damaged that it can no longer withstand the normal pressure of blood within it. A bulge may then develop. If the weakness is severe, the bulge may leak or fail catastrophically, causing an intracranial hemorrhage.

Gradual processes occur as plaque accumulates in blood vessels over the years. This buildup creates turbulence within the artery, allowing small clots (called thrombi) to form on its walls. The amount of plaque buildup reflects a combination of lifestyle choices (how we eat, exercise, and relieve stress) and family history (how we process food, manage fats, and the elasticity of our blood vessels). Over time, the buildup narrows the diameter of the arterial lumen. Eventually, the narrowing becomes so severe that blood flow is either diminished or cut off.

Even the blood vessel itself may cause difficulties for some patients. In trigeminal neuralgia, the normal functioning of facial blood vessels produces severe pain. As the blood vessels change in diameter to meet the needs of the surrounding tissue, their pulsations can irritate the trigeminal nerve. This nerve is responsible for receiving signals related to pain, temperature, and pressure on the face.

Multifactorial Causes

Most diseases or conditions are multifactorial, meaning that they have multiple causes. Just because a person gets an infection, that doesn't mean that the individual will experience tissue damage. Just because someone eats unhealthy foods, it doesn't mean that his or her arteries will definitely become blocked. The following factors explain why many people get diseases:

- How well the body system was created during development as an embryo/fetus
- How effective the body's defence and repair mechanisms are
- How severe or prolonged the factors trying to damage the body are

Thus a health-conscious person may have a body that is less effective at repair and maintenance. In contrast, a person who smokes, drinks alcohol, and does not pursue a healthy lifestyle may have a body that is very effective at repair, which can help minimize the impact of those unhealthy activities.

Intracranial Pressure

Hemorrhagic strokes that cause bleeding into the brain place patients at risk for increased intracranial pressure (ICP). Treatment of these patients is directed at providing some degree of control over this potentially deadly effect.

The skull (cranial vault) is filled with three substances: brain, blood, and cerebrospinal fluid (CSF). These substances exert a pressure (ICP) against the skull, and the skull in turn exerts a reflected pressure. This balanced exchange allows the brain to fit snugly within the skull without permitting any voids. If the skull contained empty spaces, with head movement the brain would slam into the skull and cause damage.

When the pressure within the cranial vault begins to climb and remains high, it creates two major problems. The brain may either become ischemic due to lack of blood supply or herniate (push through the ligaments that compartmentalize the brain, such as the tentorium).

As ICP rises, the amount of blood available to the brain decreases. Cerebral perfusion pressure (CPP), the pressure of blood within the cranial vault, then begins to fall. CPP can be calculated by the following equation:

$$CPP = MAP - ICP$$

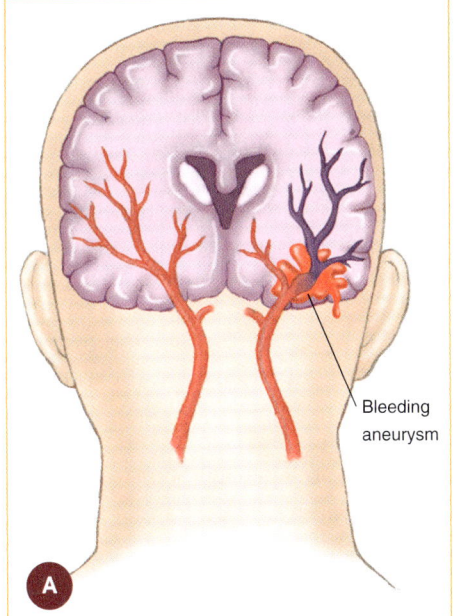
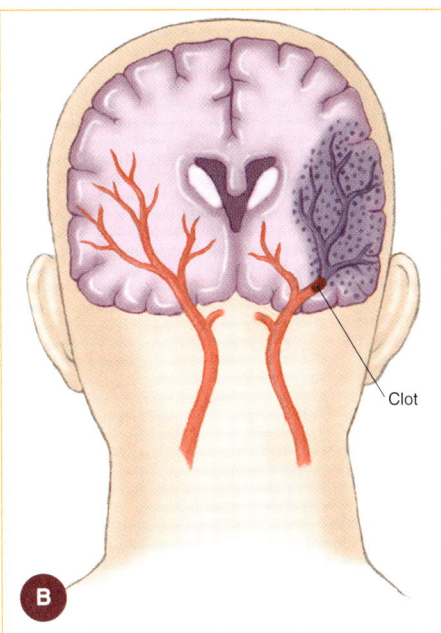
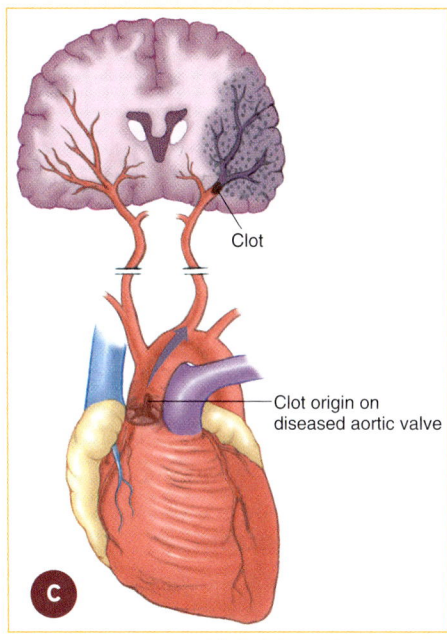

Figure 28-10 Vascular causes of neurologic conditions. **A.** Aneurysms are areas of weakness in the walls of arteries that can dilate (bulge out) and eventually rupture or leak. **B.** Atherosclerosis can damage the wall of a cerebral artery, producing narrowing and/or a clot. When the vessel is completely blocked, blood flow may be blocked and cells begin to die. **C.** An embolus, a blood clot usually formed on a diseased heart valve, can travel through the body's vascular system, lodge in a cerebral artery, and cause a stroke.

The mean arterial pressure (MAP) is the average (mean) pressure within the blood vessels. The average pressure is typically 80 to 90 mm Hg. Normal ICP usually ranges from 1 to 10 mm Hg. Normal CPP is, therefore, in the range of 70 to 80 mm Hg. The lower end of normal CPP is around 50 to 60 mm Hg. With CPP below 50 mm Hg, the brain begins to become ischemic.

ICP changes constantly. Coughing, vomiting, and bearing down, for example, will increase ICP. These momentary spikes in ICP are not harmful. By contrast, if there is blood, swelling, pus, or a tumour within the cranial vault, ICP will increase and remain high. Because the volume of the cranial vault is limited and inflexible, pressure increases as more substances squeeze into this space. As long as there is no significant drop in blood pressure or significant rise in ICP, the heart will still be able to get blood into the brain. However, if ICP rises sharply or blood pressure falls critically, patients may experience serious problems.

Consider a patient with meningitis (an infection of the membranes that cover the brain and spinal cord). The battle between the infecting organism and the immune system causes fluid to accumulate around the brain, which in turn causes ICP to climb. As long as the increase remains moderate, the brain will continue to receive adequate oxygen and nutrients. If the infection goes unchecked and travels to the general circulatory system, however, sepsis and septic shock may occur. Then, as the organism continues to grow and feed, capillaries may begin to leak. Eventually, the blood pressure will decline and the MAP will fall. At a certain point, CPP may drop so low that the brain starts to become ischemic.

This concept dictates the priorities for treatment. Given how critical normal perfusion of the brain is, blood pressure must be closely monitored in any patient with a potential ICP problem. Frequent assessment becomes even more essential when a decrease in blood pressure is also present. For any patient at risk for ICP, the paramedic needs to ensure a blood pressure of at least 110 to 120 mm Hg systolic.

Another potential outcome of ICP is herniation, or displacement of the brain out of the cranial vault. Herniation results when pressure increases within the skull and the brain is pressed down through the foramen magnum (the "large hole" at the inferior portion of the skull where the spinal cord exits). Pressure on the medulla oblongata (located directly superior to the spinal cord) can result in rather bizarre vital signs and other findings, including slowed heart and respiratory rates.

Oxygen and carbon dioxide levels are important factors to consider in preventing deterioration of the brain during neurologic emergencies. Optimizing oxygenation through adequate airway management will reduce ongoing ischemia. In the past, it was believed that lowering the CO_2 through hyperventilation would also reduce ICP and improve patient outcomes. However, we

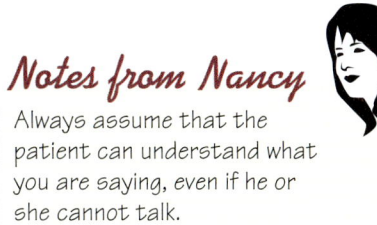

Notes from Nancy

Always assume that the patient can understand what you are saying, even if he or she cannot talk.

now realize that hyperventilation may cause more harm than good by causing constriction and decreasing cerebral perfusion.

General Assessment

The brain is the organ that is most sensitive to fluctuating levels of oxygen, glucose, and temperature; it responds to alterations in these levels with changes in its function. The difficulty for the paramedic is that the brain is relatively resilient to internal environmental changes: It doesn't simply shut down when oxygen levels fall. The key to identifying a neurologic problem is to look for both the gross or obvious changes and the subtle, sometimes hidden changes that can indicate disease.

This section reviews the assessment process for the neurologic patient. As with all patients, begin with the scene assessment.

Scene Assessment

PPE and routine precautions are taken for granted in many EMS systems. Its purpose is to protect the paramedic from exposure to potentially harmful organisms or environments. Patients having tonic-clonic seizures, for example, may be incontinent.

Some unconscious patients may be suffering from overdoses. With the use of illegal drugs, the presence of weapons, money, and crime increases. This potentially places the paramedic close to armed criminals.

Patients with altered levels of consciousness may not be able to walk, may be combative, or may be completely unresponsive. You may need additional assistance with lifting and moving these patients. Special circumstances can be overcome easier if additional resources—such as helicopter transportation, rescue equipment, or fire suppression—are requested early in the call.

Examine the scene to ascertain the number of patients. Clues can be obtained from the dispatch information. Also consider the mechanism of injury or history of present illness. Motor vehicle collisions typically involve more than one vehicle and, therefore, more than one patient. If many patients exhibit similar signs and symptoms, you should be very cautious. One patient with a headache does not stand out. If an entire family in the same house complains of a headache, then you should consider the possibility of carbon monoxide exposure. In such a case, the house may be an unsafe scene, so ensure that you have the correct PPE.

Weapons of mass destruction can follow similar patterns. If you encounter several patients who all exhibit the same signs and symptoms, all within the same general time frame and geographic location, you should consider immediate evacuation, donning appropriate PPE and contacting the dispatcher to begin a more in-depth investigation.

Initial Assessment

Begin assessing the neurologic patient as you would any other patient. Assess and secure the ABCs. Use the AVPU system to determine LOC. If the patient does not respond to verbal stimuli, consider whether he or she may be displaying some abnormal posturing; these unconscious movements may indicate severe brain dysfunction. There are two main abnormal postures that the patient may demonstrate with painful stimulation— decorticate and decerebrate. If you see either posture, you should immediately consider the patient to be critical.

In decorticate posturing, the patient flexes the arms and curls them toward the chest. At the same time, he or she points her toes. Finally, the wrists are flexed. This posture, which is

You are the Paramedic Part 2

You obtain the patient's vital signs. As your partner obtains his blood glucose level, you continue your assessment and determine that he is quite confused. He is alert and oriented to person and place, but is unsure as to what day it is and cannot describe the events leading up to your arrival.

The patient shows no signs of trauma. During your assessment of his pupils, however, he takes your penlight and tries to shave his face with it. He also seems to use inappropriate words for common, household objects and appears frustrated that you can't understand him.

Vital Signs	Recording Time: 5 Minutes
Level of consciousness	Verbal, oriented to person and place, but not day, with a Glasgow Coma Scale score of 14
Skin	Pale, warm, and dry
Pulse	90 beats/min and irregular
Blood pressure	142/86 mm Hg
Respirations	26 breaths/min
Spo2	98% on 15 l/min via nonrebreathing mask
Blood glucose	6.5 mmol/l

3. Given the information you have now, what do you think could be this patient's underlying illness, injury, or condition?

4. Do your assessment and treatment priorities ever change?

5. What are appropriate interventions?

also called abnormal flexion, may indicate damage to the area directly below the cerebral hemispheres **Figure 28-11 ▸** .

In decerebrate posturing, the patient again points the toes, but now extends the arms outward and rotates the lower arms in a palms-down manner (called pronation). The wrists are again flexed. This posture is a more severe finding than decorticate posturing, as the level of damage is within or near the brain stem (diencephalon/pons/midbrain) **Figure 28-12 ▸** .

Airway

The trigeminal, glossopharyngeal, vagus, and hypoglossal nerves are responsible for airway control. These nerves allow for swallowing, controlling the tongue, and ensuring that the muscles in the hypopharnyx are slightly contracted. Alteration in the signals from these nerves can produce too much relaxation or too much constriction of the airway **Figure 28-13 ▸** .

Trismus, in which the teeth are clenched closed, can make managing the airway very difficult. Trismus can occur in conscious or unconscious patients. In an unconscious patient, it can indicate a seizure in progress, severe head injury, or cerebral hypoxia. The patient may need to be sedated or paralyzed to relax the clenched teeth and allow you to better control the airway.

Breathing

As part of your assessment of the neurologic patient, you need to check the rate and rhythm of breathing. Rhythms can have subtle changes or be dramatically different from normal. Generally, the greater the deviation from normal, the more severely the nervous system is affected.

Circulation

Evaluate the peripheral and central pulse pressures. Are they the same? The absence of a peripheral pulse with a central pulse present should cause the paramedic to suspect shock. What is the characteristic of the skin? Do you see evidence of gross bleeding? Is the pulse bounding? Remember, shock is rarely caused solely by a neurologic problem.

If a patient suffers from increased pressure within the cranium, the vital signs may provide evidence of this problem. **Table 28-2 ▸** shows the vital signs associated with increased ICP. Notice how the blood pressure rises, the heart/respiratory rates fall, and the pulse pressure widens (systolic hypertension) in increased ICP. This set of conditions—known as Cushing's reflex—are the opposite of what is expected in shock.

As ICP rises, blood flow to the brain diminishes. To compensate, the medulla oblongata sends signals to the heart to increase the force of contraction. This causes systolic pressure to rise. If the ICP continues to increase, downward forces on the brain stem begin to damage the medulla's ability to send signals to the body. The diastolic blood pressure falls as the blood vessels relax or dilate, which in turn results in a widened pulse pressure. Finally, this pressure damages the ability to control respiratory and heart rate; consequently, both decrease.

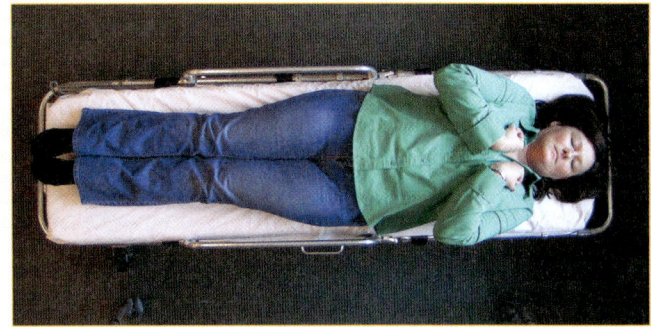

Figure 28-11 Decorticate posturing.

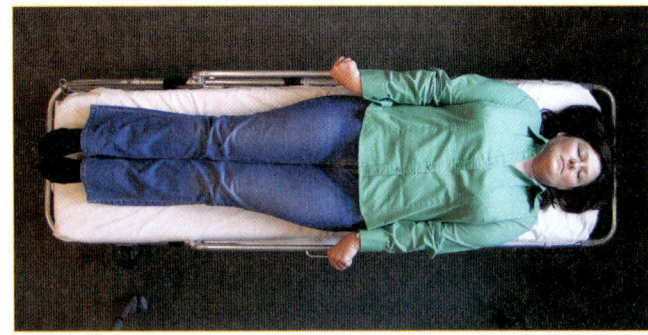

Figure 28-12 Decerebrate posturing.

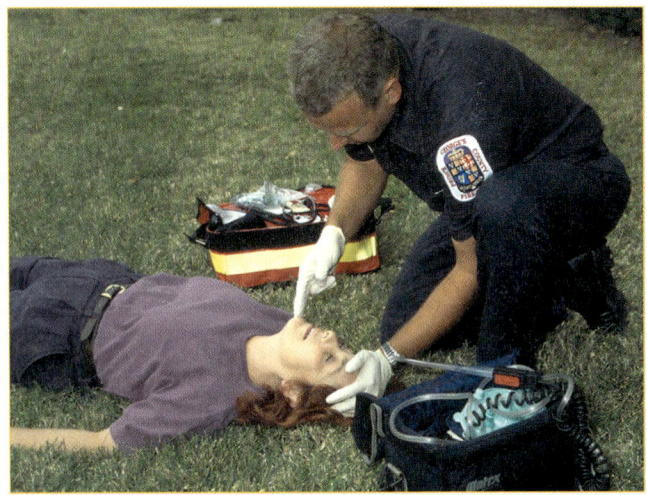

Figure 28-13 Securing and maintaining the airway in a patient who is unconscious is critical. Be sure to have suction readily available in the event that the patient vomits.

Table 28-2	Vital Signs for Shock Versus Increased ICP			
	Heart Rate	Respiratory Rate	Blood Pressure	Pulse Pressure
Shock	↑	↑	↓	Narrowed
Increased ICP	↓	↓	↑	Widened

Transport Decision

At this point in the examination, the paramedic may make a broad decision about whether to "load and go" or "stay and play." Critical patients—those with alterations in their initial assessment or significant mechanism of injury (MOI) and history of present illness—should be transported urgently to an emergency department. Defer gathering very detailed information about these patients; instead, focus on stabilizing and maintaining ABCs. With stable patients—those with normal initial assessments and minor MOI/history of present illness—you have more time to gather detailed information at the scene. You can question family and bystanders to gain valuable insight into your patient's complaint.

Special Considerations

When you are working with geriatric patients, take their past medical history into account. Patients with a history of dementia will be very complicated to manage. The primary question is: How much change has occurred in the patient's LOC? Don't assume that the patient's baseline LOC is what you would consider "normal"; speak to family, friends, or other caregivers to determine the patient's baseline LOC. Document that level clearly, using active language.

Focused History and Physical Examination

Rapid Trauma Assessment

Once the initial assessment is complete, you need to decide how to proceed. Is the patient stable or unstable? Do you suspect a major problem just below the surface? How should you transport this patient? At this point, you have two choices:

- Complete a rapid assessment using a full head-to-toe approach
- Perform a focused history and physical examination (ie, evaluate only the area of patient complaint)

You should perform a rapid assessment for any patient who has an abnormal initial assessment, has a significant MOI/history of present illness, or whom you suspect may have a major problem. Examples would include individuals who are

Documentation and Communication

Avoid using terms that can have multiple meanings, such as "lethargic," "sleepy," "obtunded," or "out of it." Instead, describe the patient using active language.

Potentially confusing: "Arrive to find male patient who is out of it."

Better: "Arrive to find a male patient disoriented to place and day."

Potentially confusing: "Caring for a 43-year-old obtunded male."

Better: "Caring for a 43-year-old male who is very slow to respond to painful stimulation."

Special Considerations

In the pediatric population, consider the developmental stage of the child. A 1-year-old should cry when assessed; that's a normal reaction to strangers. A 5-year-old who normally talks freely may be rather tight-lipped with a stranger.

unconscious, are seizing, or experience a sudden loss of movement of the body. The focused history and physical examination is done on patients who are stable and have narrow complaints. These individuals have a completely normal initial assessment and a minor MOI/history of present illness, and you suspect a very local problem. Examples would include patients with headaches or nontraumatic back pain.

Be cautious. If a patient has a headache, stress may not be the cause. Stroke patients can also experience headaches. If you suspect a more complicated problem, perform a rapid assessment to ensure that you give the patient the best possible prehospital care.

History

History taking in the patient with a potential neurologic complaint should follow the same process followed for any other medical or trauma patient. For example, if weakness is a symptom found in a medical patient with no trauma, use the OPQRST mnemonic to elaborate on the complaint of general body weakness. The physical examination for this complaint should investigate potential cardiac, neurologic, respiratory, metabolic, or infectious causes. Appropriate tests and serial vital signs such as blood glucose levels, ECG, vital signs, lung sounds, and temperature will also help you rule out potential causes of the weakness.

Detailed Physical Examination

The detailed physical examination examines all of the areas covered within the rapid assessment, but looks at them more closely.

Head

The head is the area where you will spend the most time, gathering critical information on the functioning of the nervous system. Of course, you want to assess the head for trauma. Deformities, Contusion, Abrasions, Penetrations, Burns, Tenderness, Lacerations, and Swelling (DCAP-BTLS) are the trauma assessment components you should assess on every body area.

There are many shades of LOC and many ways to evaluate LOC. A patient may be interacting appropriately with the environment or not at all. **Figure 28-14 ▸** shows a continuum that ranges from what most would consider to be normal behaviour to no response whatsoever. The point on the extreme right side of the continuum is coma, a state in which the patient does not respond to verbal or painful stimuli. The points in between (guide markings) are not intended to imply that every patient will stop at every point as his or her LOC increases or decreases, but rather

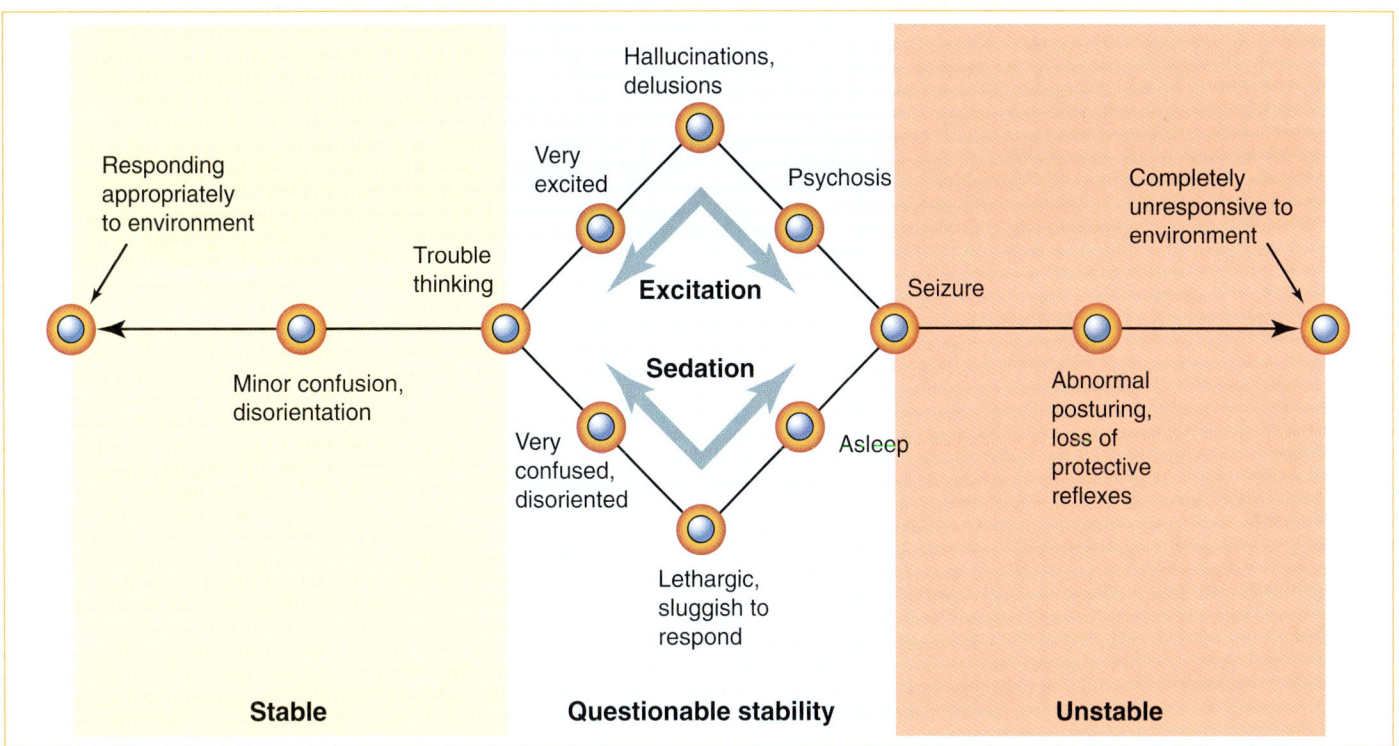

Figure 28-14 Level of consciousness continuum.

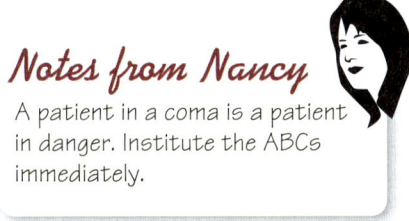

Notes from Nancy

A patient in a coma is a patient in danger. Institute the ABCs immediately.

illustrate the relationships between various levels of consciousness. While the extremes are easy to understand, the points in the middle (the shades of grey) can be more confusing.

One tool to assist with the consistent evaluation of LOC is the Glasgow Coma Scale (GCS) **Table 28-3 ▶** . This assessment tool provides a basis to determine a patient's degree of illness or injury. It is used to determine the patient's LOC and evaluate responses to eye opening as well as verbal and motor skills **Figure 28-15 ▶** . To determine the GCS score, add the three numbers together from each of the subsections of the GCS.

The GCS score can provide information as to what prehospital care should be given and where the patient should be transported. **Table 28-4 ▶** provides general guidelines for using these scores. Patients with mild conditions need standard prehospital care; usually the paramedic can honour their request to be transported to a particular hospital. Patients with moderate conditions are very difficult to manage. They are not stable enough for you to relax, and not critical enough to completely get your attention. With this group, close assessment and transport to the nearest appropriate facility are prudent. Critical patients need airway management and rapid transport to the closest appropriate hospital.

Table 28-3	Glasgow Coma Scale	
	Adult	**Pediatric Patient (< 5 y)**
Eye opening	4. Spontaneous	4. Spontaneous
	3. Voice	3. To shout/voice
	2. Pain stimulation	2. Pain stimulation
	1. None	1. None
Verbal	5. Oriented	5. Cry, smile, coo, words correct for age
	4. Disoriented	4. Cries, inappropriate words for age
	3. Inappropriate words	3. Inappropriate scream or cry
	2. Incomprehensible	2. Grunts
	1. None	1. None
Motor	6. Obeys	6. Spontaneous
	5. Localizes pain	5. Localizes pain
	4. Withdraws from pain	4. Withdraws from pain
	3. Decorticate	3. Decorticate
	2. Decerebrate	2. Decerebrate
	1. None	1. None

Changes in the patient's mood or tempo of the nervous system should alert you to changes in neurologic status. Oxygen levels or blood pressure could be falling. Body temperature

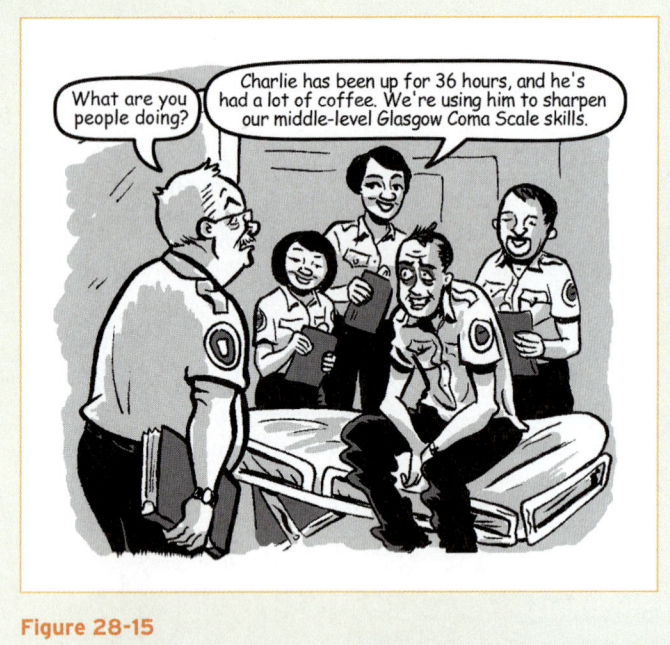

Figure 28-15

Table 28-4	Interpretations of Glasgow Coma Scale Scores		
GCS Score	Interpretation	Treatment	Facility
13–15	Mild	Standard pre-hospital care	Patient/family choice
9–12	Moderate	Close airway assessment, watch for decreasing consciousness	Closest appropriate facility
8 or less	Critical	Intubation, decrease scene time (less than 8, intubate)	Closest appropriate facility

could be climbing. A psychiatric condition could be escalating. Blood glucose levels could be too high or too low. Regardless of the underlying cause, your observation of a change should prompt further evaluation to ensure the appropriate level of prehospital care. Mood or affect is another attribute that provides insight into the patient's condition. Ask the patient how he or she feels. Frustration, anger, or aggression can be caused by low glucose or oxygen levels.

Ask the patient how easy it is for him or her to think. Patients who have decreased blood glucose levels or who are taking narcotics can experience difficulty concentrating. Lower blood glucose levels and narcotics tend to produce sedation of the nervous system. In contrast, patients who are taking cocaine may experience difficulty concentrating due to excitement or mania. Cocaine, a sympathomimetic, increases nervous system activity, causing thoughts to come very

quickly. If the speed of nervous system activity continues to increase, the patient may hallucinate or become delusional or psychotic.

Visual Findings

Perform the DCAP-BTLS assessment. Look at the symmetry of the face. Is there an obvious facial droop? Look at the eyes. Are the eyelids even bilaterally? Ptosis (drooping eyelids) can indicate Bell's palsy or a stroke. **Figure 28-16 ▶** demonstrates what happens when such a patient is asked to smile; weakness to one side of the face causes facial droop and slight ptosis.

Assess the cranial nerves, the peripheral nerves that control various portions of the body (see Chapter 13). Look for the ability to respond, strength of response, and symmetry. Patients with stroke, trigeminal neuralgia, myasthenia gravis, or other neurologic conditions may demonstrate abnormal cranial nerve functioning.

Speech

Listen to the quality of the speech. Is it slurred? Slurring is a classic finding with stroke. Is the speech appropriate? Focus on not only the quality of the words that are spoken, but also the appropriateness of those words. Sometimes speech may be clear but word choice is incorrect. Assess the patient's object recognition abilities.

Patients may be able to speak clearly, yet have subtle knowledge deficits. In agnosia (*a* = without, *gnosis* = knowledge), patients will be unable to name common objects because connections between visual interpretation of objects and the words that name them have become damaged. Apraxia (*a* = without, *praxia* = movement) refers to the inability to know how to use a common object.

To test for these signs, simply show the patient your pen, scissors, or a set of keys. Ask the patient to name the object. If the individual responds correctly, hand the object to the patient and ask him or her to demonstrate the object's use. The patient should write with the pen, cut with the scissors, and turn a lock with the keys. Patients may have one of these signs without the other. One is not a more severe finding than the other. They simply indicate that some degree of misfiring of neurons is occurring between the occipital lobe and the temporal lobe (agnosia) or between the temporal lobe and the frontal lobe (apraxia).

Language can be affected by injury or disease. In aphasia, speech is affected. There are three main forms of aphasia:

- **Receptive aphasia.** The patient cannot understand (receive) speech, but is able to speak clearly. This form of aphasia indicates damage to the temporal lobe. Ask patients questions to which both you and they know the answer: "Who is the president?" "What month is it?" Do not ask yes/no questions. If the patient speaks clearly but gives incorrect answers, he or she may have receptive aphasia.
- **Expressive aphasia.** The patient can't speak (express themselves) clearly, but is able to understand speech. This form of aphasia indicates damage to the frontal lobe, which controls the motor portion of speech. Ask patients

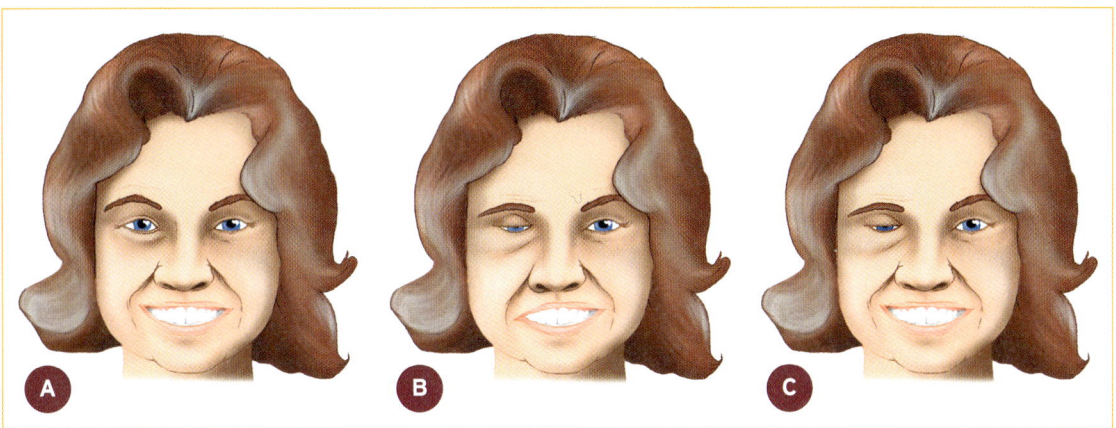

Figure 28-16 A. A normal smile. **B.** Facial droop, including a drooping eyelid (ptosis), which may or may not be present. **C.** A normal smile with ptosis present.

to raise an arm. If they respond correctly, they can understand you. Ask patients their name. If they can't respond or their responses are slurred, they have expressive aphasia.

- **Global aphasia.** This form of aphasia is a combination of expressive and receptive aphasia. In this setting, the patient will not follow commands and can't answer your questions. Nevertheless, patients with global aphasia can often think clearly. They have needs, anxieties, and discomforts, but no

way to express them. This can be incredibly frightening for patients who can't understand anything that you're saying and can't speak to you. Be sensitive to this state. Move slowly and purposely. Use therapeutic touch and good eye contact to reassure the patient.

Pupils

Pupillary shape can be changed by trauma, glaucoma, or increased ICP. Cocaine, metham- phetamines, and hallu- cinogens tend to cause dilation of the pupils. Depressants usually lead to constriction of the pupils.

Equality of pupils is an important observation. Unequal pupils, called anisocoria, can be a sign of increased ICP Figure 28-17 ⌄ . Many people have a slight inequality in pupillary size. Anything greater than a 1-mm difference is worth noting, however. As pressure increases within the skull, the brain stem can be squeezed. This squeezing can interrupt sig- nals to one pupil, resulting in dramatically different-size pupils.

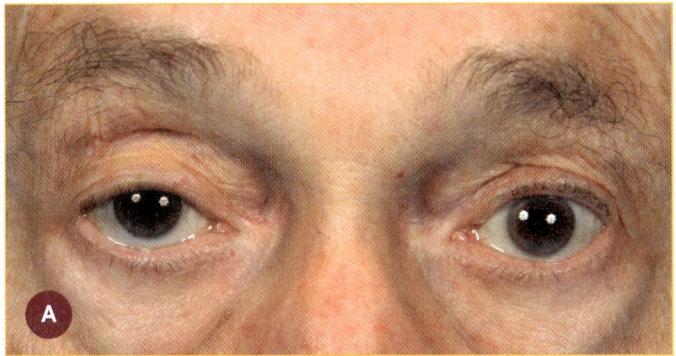
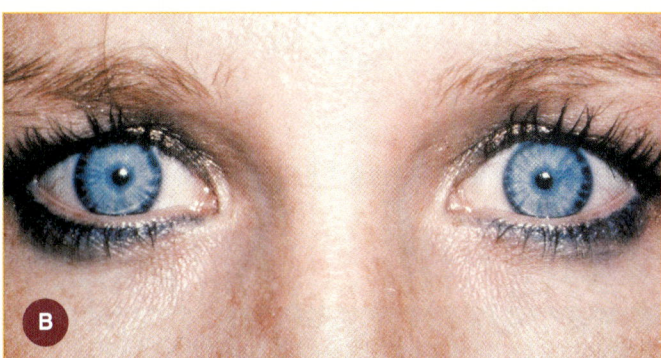
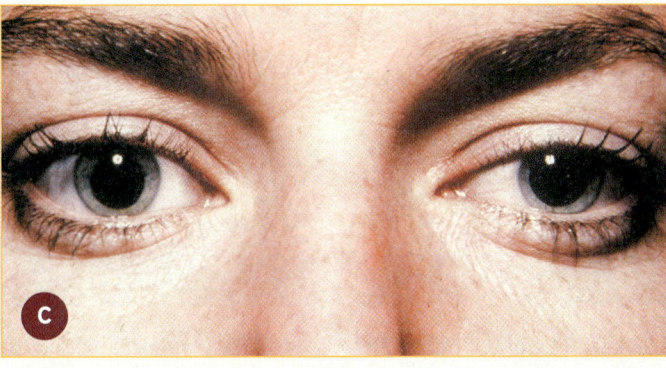
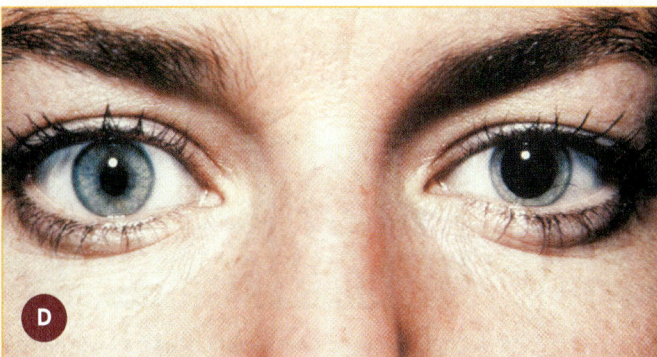

Figure 28-17 Pupil responses. **A.** Normal. **B.** Constricted (pinpoint). **C.** Dilated. **D.** Unequal.

Finally, determine whether the eyes are twitching. <u>Nystagmus</u> (the involuntary, rhythmic movement of the eyes) can be caused by seizures, vertigo, and MS.

Movement of the Body

Observe how the patient moves. Does the body move equally on both sides? Patients with strokes may suffer from weakness (<u>hemiparesis</u>) or paralysis (<u>hemiplegia</u>) of one side of the body. Sometimes you may discover patients with weakness on one side of their body but facial droop on the other side. This condition may be caused by <u>decussation</u>, in which nerves cross as they leave the cerebral cortex, move through the brain stem, and arrive at the spinal cord. Nerves that decussate start on one side of the brain and then cross to control the opposite side of the body. Some nerves do not decussate—facial nerves, for example. The left side of the brain controls the right side of the body, but the left side of the face. A left cerebral stroke would therefore result in right-sided arm and leg weakness, but left-sided facial droop.

Examining the function of the cerebellum can also allow you to gather information about potential damage to the brain. Have the patient close his or her eyes and hold out the arms in front of the body at the same level. With the eyes closed, the patient's only way to tell where the arms are located is from the sensations being processed by the cerebellum. If the individual has suffered a stroke, one of the arms may drift away from the other **Figure 28-18 ▾**.

Have the patient walk for several steps (unless some medical reason rules the activity out). Assessing <u>gait</u> (walking patterns) is another way to test the activity of the cerebellum. Walking is really a controlled fall. As your centre of gravity moves forward, you must move a leg forward to catch yourself. Once you learn how to walk, your cerebellum controls these mechanics, so you can focus on where you want to walk, not how to walk. Damage to the cerebellum may be manifested as erratic walking, stumbling, or even losing the ability to walk.

Several medical conditions cause alterations in the patient's gait. <u>Ataxia</u> is the term used to describe changes in a person's ability to perform coordinated motions like walking. Patients with Parkinson's disease exhibit a classic gait in which they place their feet very close together and shuffle. Their stride is short, and they have great difficulty changing direction. Such a patient will shuffle-walk in a straight line and, when asked to turn, will take very small steps until the turn is complete. With this kind of <u>bradykinesia</u>, routine motions may slow dramatically. In contrast, patients with cerebral palsy may walk with a scissors gait. In the spastic form of this disease, the person will point the toes inwardly, have a stiff gait, and nearly touch the knees together while walking.

In addition to the patient's gait, you should assess the posture. Have the individual stand straight. Place one hand on the patient's chest and the other hand behind the back (to catch the patient in the event that he or she can't do so), and then push on the chest. Normally, as you push backward, the patient will compensate quickly and take a step forward to prevent a fall. In Parkinson's disease, the patient's posture is so rigid that they can't compensate quickly enough and will fall over.

Bizarre movements may indicate a disruption within the nervous system. <u>Myoclonus</u> is a type of involuntary contraction of the muscles that is rapid and jerky in nature. Most people have suffered myoclonic jerks at some point. Have you ever seen a seated person who is very tired? As the person gets closer to falling sleep, the head will begin to sag. Often the person will involuntarily jerk the head upward (myoclonic jerk) and wake up.

Another form of bizarre movement is <u>dystonia</u>, in which a part of the body contracts and remains contracted. A foot cramp where the great toe extends while the other toes curl under is an example of a common dystonia. Alternatively, the face may become extremely distorted as one side contracts. The head can twist to one side. An arm or leg can become frozen in a contracted position. Dystonia can be caused by brain injuries or medication reactions.

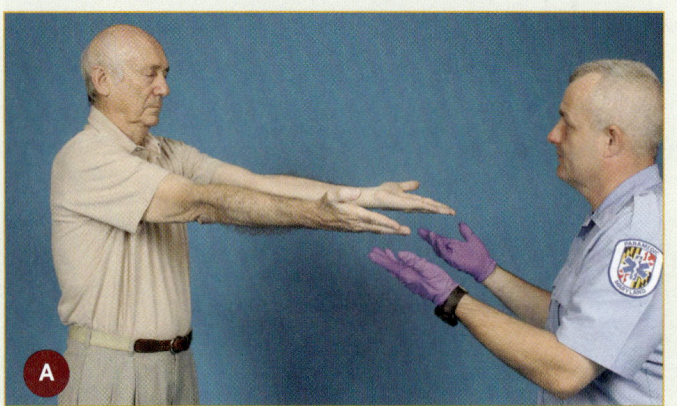 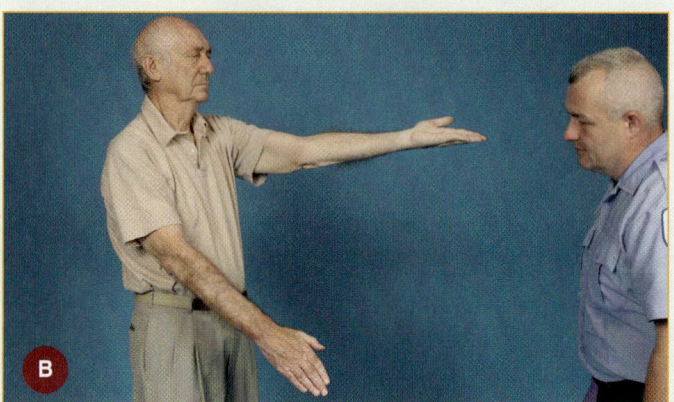

Figure 28-18 A. A person who has not experienced a stroke will be able to hold both hands in front of the body and maintain them there. **B.** If a person has had a suspected stroke, he or she may not be able to maintain this position. Instead, one arm will drift down and turn toward the body.

When you are watching the patient, does he or she move smoothly? This kind of motion requires proper functioning of the frontal lobe, cerebellum, brain stem, spinal cord, and peripheral nerves. When they are functioning correctly, muscle groups will alternately contract and relax, allowing the body to move smoothly. Patients with Parkinson's disease suffer from rigidity in which this fine balance is upset, so they move in fits and spurts.

Tremors are another potential alteration in smooth motion. These fine oscillating (back-and-forth) movements are usually found in the hands and head.

- **Rest tremors**—occur with the patient at rest and not in motion. They are common in Parkinson's disease.
- **Intension tremors**—occur when the patient tries to reach out and grab an object. These tremors may increase as the patient gets closer to the object to be grabbed. Intension tremors are common in MS.
- **Postural tremors**—occur when a body part is required to maintain the same position for a long period of time. Most people have experienced this type of tremor when they were working hard for a long time. As they tire, their worked body parts begin to shake. A postural tremor can also occur when a person is standing and the head oscillates back and forth. Patients with Parkinson's disease also experience these tremors.

Seizures may appear very similar to tremors. Generally, tremors are fine movements while seizures are larger, less focused types of movement. There are two basic types of movements that patients can perform while seizing:

- **Tonic activity** is a very rigid, contracted body posture. The arms, legs, neck, and back can contract so tightly that the body part will shake slightly from the intensity of the contraction.
- **Clonic activity** is a rhythmic contraction and relaxation of muscle groups. It may appear as bizarre, nonpurposeful movements of any body part. Arms and legs may flail, teeth may clench, the head may bob, and the torso may move wildly.

Sensation

Many neurologic conditions can alter the ability to feel pain, temperature, pressure, or light touch. A sensation of numbness or tingling is called paresthesia. If the patient can feel nothing within a body part, the condition is called anesthesia.

Blood Glucose Level

Glucose is the fuel that runs the brain. The brain uses glucose faster than any other part of the body, but it has no means to store glucose. For this reason, all patients with a change in LOC should have their blood glucose level checked. A normal blood glucose reading is 4 to 7 mmol/l. As glucose levels fall below 4 mmol/l, LOC begins to decrease. LOC can also be affected by a high blood glucose level, although a significant increase is required before LOC is altered. Glucose levels below 0.6 mmol/l are incompatible with brain functioning and typically lethal. Generally, if levels are below 2 mmol/l, confusion or uncon-

sciousness will occur. Blood glucose monitoring is standard pre-hospital care for the patient with an altered LOC.

Chest

Evaluate the chest for DCAP-BTLS. Look for symmetry in its shape. Does the chest rise and fall equally? Apply the cardiac monitor and evaluate the ECG. Many cardiac dysrhythmias can cause neurologic disorders by decreasing the blood supply to the brain. Perform a 12-lead ECG in all patients with sudden loss of consciousness. How much effort must the patient make to breathe? Do you observe any degree of respiratory distress? Listen to lung sounds. Evaluate for the presence of adventitious sounds and equality of sounds. Determine the pulse oximeter reading, remembering that normal readings are 95% to 100% and that this number is affected by the amount of hemoglobin within the body and the presence of carbon monoxide.

Abdomen

Examine the abdomen for DCAP-BTLS. Do you note any masses? Are there any pulsations within the abdomen? Does the patient have any complaints related to the abdomen? Signs of nausea and vomiting are common with some neurologic conditions, such as headaches or increased ICP.

Pelvis

Examine the pelvis for DCAP-BTLS. Is it stable to stress? If the patient is able to walk without assistance, the pelvis should be stable. Does the patient have any incontinence? Urinary or fecal incontinence are common findings with seizures or syncope. Incontinence also serves as a relatively objective marker for the severity of the unconsciousness. When we sleep, we are not incontinent. Thus if incontinence is present, the LOC has decreased below that of sleep.

Extremities

Examine the limbs for DCAP-BTLS. Do you see any signs of edema? Look for venipuncture marks and note whether these marks are at various stages of healing. Such marks may indicate recent illegal drug use.

Ongoing Assessment

The ongoing assessment is intended to monitor patients for changes. Talk with them. Ask them how they're feeling. Ask about their children. Ask if they caught the game last night. Casual conversation will allow you to closely monitor brain functions. It also communicates a caring environment. If the patient is nonverbal, keep a close eye on respiratory patterns and eye and body movements, and monitor for seizure activity.

Routine monitoring should include heart rate, ECG, blood pressure, respiratory rate and pattern, pulse oximetry, and repeat glucose (if the level was low and sugar was given to the patient). Continue

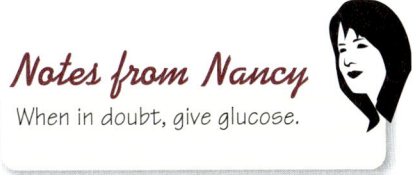

Notes from Nancy
When in doubt, give glucose.

oxygenation and ventilation support. Monitor IVs closely to ensure that accidental fluid overload does not occur. If the patient's condition undergoes a sudden dramatic change, repeat the rapid assessment and detailed physical examination as if this were a new patient. This will give you a chance to modify your prehospital care so as to manage the new development.

General Management

This management guideline should be followed with all patients who experience a change in LOC. The focus of prehospital care for neurologic patients is directed at ensuring that the body has an adequate internal environment to allow for optimal brain function. The three major elements that the brain needs to function are *oxygen, glucose,* and *normal temperature.* The general management techniques discussed in this section—the standard prehospital care—serve as the foundation on which additional prehospital care for specific neurologic problems is built.

As always, provide for routine precautions and scene safety. Ensure that you and your partner are safe and you have routine precautions in place.

Evaluate the patient's airway and effectiveness of breathing. If necessary, secure the airway, and provide ventilatory support to make sure oxygen saturation remains higher than 90%. Routine hyperventilation of neurologic patients can be harmful, so provide hyperventilation only to those patients with documented unconsciousness *and* signs of increased ICP.

Establish IV access, and then administer normal saline or lactated Ringer's solutions. Consider drawing blood samples for later analysis at the hospital. Don't use solutions containing dextrose. Check the patient's blood pressure and heart rate. Support hypotension to ensure adequate CPP; the target is a systolic blood pressure of 110 to 120 mm Hg.

Table 28-5	Hallmarks of Increased ICP	
Cushing's Reflex	**Other Signs**	
■ Bradycardia	■ Decorticate posturing	■ Biot respirations
■ Bradypnea	■ Decerebrate posturing	■ Apneustic respirations
■ Widened pulse pressure (systolic hypertension)	■ Anisocoria	■ Cheyne-Stokes respirations

Continuously monitor the patient on an ECG. Perform 12-lead ECG monitoring if permitted to do so.

Check the blood glucose level. If it's low, administer dextrose 50%, 25 g IVP. Be very cautious when you can't check the patient's blood glucose level. If the patient is unresponsive or has a decreased LOC and no blood glucose monitor is available, administer 12.5 g (½ syringe) and then reassess the response. Proceed with additional dextrose cautiously, based on responses to previous doses. Hyperglycemia can increase the morbidity rate among stroke patients.

Look for the hallmarks of increased ICP **Table 28-5 ▲**. In patients who are unconscious *and* demonstrate other signs of increased ICP, ensure a systolic blood pressure of 110 to 120 mm Hg. Administer fluids as needed. Unless you are concerned about possible cervical spine fracture, elevate the head 30°.

Special Considerations

When assessing for ICP in infants, consider the quality of the cry. As ICP increases, the pitch of the cry will increase until a shriek similar to that of a cat can be heard. At the same time, the shape of the pupils can change from round to more oval. These two findings lead to the saying related to infants and ICP: "cats' eyes and cats' cries."

You are the Paramedic Part 3

In the interest of time, you place your patient on the stretcher, obtain IV access and administer normal saline TKVO, draw blood, and perform an ECG. You also complete a fibrinolytic screen while en route to the hospital. You ask one of the patient's sons to accompany you and provide more information regarding his medical history. The patient's son tells you that his medical history includes atrial fibrillation (which you confirm on the monitor) and that the patient takes aspirin, diltiazem, Coumadin, and glucophage. The patient has no known drug allergies, has no recent history of illness, and has been compliant with his medications and diet.

Reassessment	Recording Time: 10 Minutes
Level of consciousness	Alert, with a Glasgow Coma Scale score of 14
Skin	Pale, warm, and dry
Pulse	92 beats/min, strong and irregular
Blood pressure	140/84 mm Hg
Respirations	24 breaths/min
Spo2	100% on 15 l/min via nonrebreathing mask

6. Would you choose to place this patient in manual in-line spinal precautions?

7. What places this patient at greater risk for cerebrovascular accident?

Provide ventilatory support at 16 to 20 breaths/min. Don't increase the rate any higher than 30 breaths/min, as hyperventilation will cause vasoconstriction and decrease perfusion to the brain. Ensure that the airway is clear, but don't suction vigorously. Stimulating the cough and gag reflexes will increase ICP.

A patient with increased ICP may be bradycardic. Atropine and pacing are not indicated, however, due to the systolic hypertension that accompanies the bradycardia. The ICP is causing the bradycardia, not the reverse. Instead, notify the hospital and provide rapid transport.

Check for drug use. If the patient may have taken a narcotic, consider administering naloxone, 0.4 to 2 mg IVP. Watch for seizures. If the seizure is prolonged, administer diazepam or lorazepam.

Evaluate the patient's temperature. If it is low, cover the patient, turn on the heat, and prevent heat loss. If it is high, remove clothing, cover the naked patient in a sheet, and turn the heat off in the patient compartment.

Provide emotional support for the patient and family. Neurologic emergencies can produce confusion, fear, anger, and helplessness. Consider giving a therapeutic gentle touch on the shoulder. Touch can communicate compassion. Use a calm, reassuring voice to show that you're there to help. Try to reorient the patient, as confusion is often present in these cases.

Administration of Dextrose/Glucose

Consult your local protocol to determine whether the blood glucose reading is considered low. One guideline states that if the blood glucose level is below 4 mmol/l, then glucose is needed. Two medications are available for prehospital treatment of hypoglycemia: dextrose 50% ($D_{50}W$) and glucagon. When administering $D_{50}W$, you must establish an IV line. This access site should be within a large vessel (18-gauge or larger is preferred), because $D_{50}W$ is quite thick. Ensure that the IV is patent *before* you attempt to give the $D_{50}W$. Extravasation of $D_{50}W$ into the interstitial space can cause severe damage to muscles, nerves, and skin or even death. The usual dose is 25 g of $D_{50}W$ or one full syringe. The effects from $D_{50}W$ typically begin in 30 seconds to 2 minutes. If no effect is apparent or the patient's blood glucose level remains low, ensure adequate IV access and administer a second dose of $D_{50}W$.

You may need to give thiamine before administration of $D_{50}w$ begins. Patients who are severely malnourished, such as chronic alcoholics, may have insufficient supplies of vitamin B1 (thiamine) to adequately metabolize dextrose. Thiamine allows the body to convert its store of glycogen into glucose as part of the Krebs cycle. The typical dose in an emergent situation is 50 mg via slow IV bolus and 50 mg IM. Thiamine can cause hypotension if administered too quickly. If you cannot obtain vascular access, administer 0.5 to 1 mg of glucagon subcutaneously or IM. The LOC and blood glucose levels should increase within 20 minutes after administration. If the blood glucose levels remain low, repeat the glucagon in a maximum of three doses.

There is currently no safe way to lower high blood glucose levels in the prehospital setting. Administration of insulin can be very problematic and can easily overshoot the mark, sending the patient into a hypoglycemic state. For these patients, provide standard prehospital care and ensure adequate blood pressure. Hyperglycemic patients are often dehydrated and usually need volume support.

Oral glucose administration is another option for the patients with a decreased LOC who can swallow safely. Assess these patients carefully, confirming that they are awake enough to follow commands. First give them a small amount of water to drink—say, 10 ml. If they can swallow that amount, then consider administering oral glucose 25 g (one tube). Alternatives to oral glucose include cake icing, a plain chocolate bar (without nuts), or orange juice with sugar added. Administration of sugar by mouth will take longer to raise blood glucose levels. Constantly supervise patients as they consume the sugar. Make sure they don't aspirate.

Airway Management

Sometimes patients may not be able to adequately protect the airway or ventilate themselves. The use of a bag-valve-mask, laryngeal mask airway, Combitube, or endotracheal intubation should be initiated to provide sufficient oxygen, ventilation, and airway protection in such cases. Endotracheal intubation is the most effective means by which you can isolate and protect the trachea from aspiration. Ensure that the pulse oximeter reading is higher than 90%. Provide oxygen via nasal cannula or mask as necessary. Provide ventilatory assistance as needed.

If the patient has trismus, determine how effectively the patient can be ventilated with a bag-valve-mask. If ventilation is poor or unsuccessful, you may attempt to place a nasotracheal airway. If this is unsuccessful, consider using a paralytic agent to relax the mouth and allow for airway management. If paralytics are not available or contraindicated and the patient can't be ventilated, transtracheal airway management is the only option to prevent hypoxia and death.

Administration of Naloxone

Naloxone is used for the treatment of unconscious/unknown patients or those with suspected narcotic overdose. The initial dose is 0.4 to 2.0 mg IVP. You may repeat this dose until you reach 10 mg. This narcotic antagonist will compete with any circulating narcotic, displacing it from its receptors and allowing the LOC to increase. Naloxone can have quite a dramatic effect: Patients with a GCS score of 3 can move to a score of 15 within 30 seconds. This rapid change in LOC may cause patients to become fearful and potentially angry or aggressive. Make sure that you have adequate resources to restrain the patient or that you have the ability to leave the scene quickly *before* you administer naloxone. It may be advisable to push the drug in small increments until an improvement in LOC or respiration is noted. If the medication does not produce a response, then intubation may be needed. Some EMS systems are modifying or restricting use of naloxone use to decrease the risks of precipitating narcotic withdrawal seizures in narcotic-dependent patients and paramedic safety due to patients emerging from narcotic-induced states in a violent manner. Paramedics are advised to consult their local and regional protocols, and exercise caution in naloxone use.

Airway management in relation to the narcotic overdose can also be tricky. Airway and ventilation are the focus of much of the prehospital care provided to unconscious patients. When you encounter a severely bradypneic, cyanotic patient, you reflexively want to establish an airway and intubate the patient quickly. When considering administering naloxone, however, a slightly different approach is recommended.

Ensure airway control and adequate ventilation but don't immediately intubate the patient. As you are oxygenating the patient, establish an IV and administer the naloxone carefully. Given the drug's quick onset of action and the potential for a dramatic response, an intubated patient may quickly wake up after the naloxone, grab the endotracheal tube, and yank it out. The result of this violent extubation may be vocal cord or tracheal trauma. If the medication doesn't produce a response, then intubation may be needed.

Temperature Assessment

The patient's temperature can be difficult to determine in the prehospital environment. If you suspect hypothermia or hyperthermia, the standard of prehospital care is to use a thermometer to establish the patient's temperature. Oral, otic, transdermal, or rectal temperature can be measured. Avoid using the axillary method of measurement due to its inaccuracy.

Not all EMS systems have the ability to check a patient's temperature. In such a situation, you can still gather information about the history of present illness that can lead to a conclusion of temperature alteration. Was the patient in water for a long period of time? Has the patient been out in the snow? Did the patient fall and lie on the floor of a cold home, unable to get up for several days? In these cases, hypothermia should be considered. It would be reasonable to cover the patient in blankets and turn the heat up in the patient compartment.

Has the patient been out in the hot sun for several hours? Is the skin hot and dry? Is there a history of fever? In these cases, it would be prudent to remove the patient's clothing, place a sheet over the individual, and at least turn the heat off in the patient compartment.

Assessment and Management of Specific Injuries and Illnesses

Table 28-6 ▶ will help you better classify specific neurologic conditions based first on the part of the nervous system they affect and then on the type of condition.

Table 28-6	Neurologic Disease by Type of Condition	
Major System	**Disease**	**Type of Condition**
Central nervous system	Neoplasm	Cancer (malignant or benign)
	Alzheimer's disease	Degenerative
	Amyotrophic lateral sclerosis	Degenerative
	Parkinson's disease	Degenerative
	Cerebral palsy	Developmental
	Spina bifida	Developmental
	Abscess	Infectious
	Poliomyelitis	Infectious
	Dystonia	Various causes
	Headaches	Various causes
	Seizures	Various causes
	Cerebral vascular accidents	Vascular
	Transient ischemic attacks	Vascular
Peripheral nervous system	Bell's palsy	Infectious
	Guillain-Barré syndrome	Degenerative
	MS	Degenerative
	Myasthenia gravis	Degenerative
	Trigeminal neuralgia	Various
Muscles	Muscular dystrophy	Degenerative

One way to manage these conditions is to try to create a patient profile that describes the circumstances that typically characterize a particular disease. How old is the typical patient? What sex and race is the patient? What are the common signs and symptoms of the condition? Are any unusual signs present that are uncommon in other conditions? How does the condition develop over time? If the patient profile indicates that men are most commonly affected by the condition, remember that females may also suffer from it.

The patient profile is intended to distill the condition down to its core elements. You can use this valuable system to create flash cards that you can study. This summary of typical age, sex, race, history of present illness, signs and symptoms, and treatment will be provided for each condition discussed in the remainder of this chapter.

Stroke

Cerebrovascular accidents (CVAs) or strokes represent a serious medical condition in which the blood supply to areas of the brain becomes interrupted, resulting in ischemia. Today nearly half of all patients who suffer from brain attacks or strokes deny their symptoms. Many will not activate EMS and subsequently delay seeking prehospital care. The goal of treatment is early recognition and rapid, appropriate intervention. The longer the CVA continues without intervention, the less likely the patient will have a promising outcome. "Time is brain."

Two basic types of strokes are distinguished: <u>ischemic</u> and <u>hemorrhagic</u>. **Figure 28-19** ▾ provides some insight into the evolution of strokes.

The majority of the time (75%), strokes are ischemic rather than hemorrhagic. In ischemic stroke, a blood vessel is blocked, so the tissue distal to the blockage becomes ischemic. Eventually that tissue will die if blood flow is not restored. This pathology is self-limiting; only the tissue beyond the blockage is affected, so the areas of the brain involved are limited. The signs and symptoms eventually stop increasing and then plateau, indicating that the area of the brain involved is no longer working. The extent and severity of the stroke will be dictated by which artery is involved and which portion of the brain is denied oxygen. An ischemic CVA to the brain stem is life-threatening.

In contrast, hemorrhagic CVAs tend to worsen over time due to bleeding within the cranium. This bleeding may increase ICP and leads to herniation of the brain stem. One hallmark of a hemorrhagic CVA is the "worst headache of my life" complaint. If the patient complains of a very severe headache, later cannot speak, becomes difficult to arouse, and

Documentation and Communication

Patients with strokes can present a wide range of communication difficulties.

- Patients who are multilingual may lose understanding of only one language.
- Patients may be able to visually understand the written word but not the spoken word.
- Patients may not be able to understand any form of communication.
- Be open to trying various ways to communicate. Remember, communication problems do not indicate that the patient is not thinking, just that the patient can't get you to understand those thoughts.

Controversies

The mission of hospitals is to provide high-quality patient care. But how can they provide quality care without seeing patients? The CVA patient provides an excellent example of this potential dilemma.

Suppose a 62-year-old woman is having a stroke. Your assessment reveals left-sided weakness, slurred speech, and an arm drift. These changes began around 08:15 hrs. It's now 08:45 hrs, and you are caring for the patient, who says that she has the worst headache of her life. She's getting very sleepy and becoming more difficult to arouse. You place the patient in the ambulance and begin transport to the local hospital, but the patient begins to have decorticate posturing. What should you do?

Appropriate prehospital care for this patient should include excellent airway management and rapid transport. But transport to where? Given the patient history, physical findings, and rapid deterioration of LOC, this patient appears to be suffering from a CVA. If your initial diagnosis is correct, she will ultimately need a facility capable of managing a patient with a stroke. Her family wants her to go to the closest hospital, which is 15 minutes away but does not have stroke centre capability. The closest facility with this capability is 30 minutes away. Which is better for the patient: immediate transfer to a facility that may not be able to completely manage the patient or a lengthened transport time?

Your main objective is to provide quality prehospital care, which includes acting as a patient advocate. One way to advocate for quality patient prehospital care is to engage in discussions with your EMS medical director about the idea of triaging patients to appropriate hospitals. Before your discussion, you need to do your homework:

- Gather information about how different types of strokes present.
- Research acute stroke and its prehospital care.
- Identify the capabilities of the hospitals in your area.
- Create a template guideline to be discussed with the medical director.

During the conversation with the medical director, control your emotions and be prepared to compromise. Speak from facts. Speak from good patient prehospital care. Whatever guideline or template you create, ensure that it leaves room for later modification. If you present yourself well, you'll pave the way for more responsibility as a paramedic and increased respect for the profession. You will also improve patient prehospital care.

If, however, your EMS service and medical director have already identified care of the acute stroke patient as one of the possible patient categories that require bypassing the local facility and redirection to a designated stroke centre, this controversy would be a nonissue. Many jurisdictions in Canada have redirection policies and procedures to ensure that a patient with a suspected acute stroke is transported directly to a designated stroke centre. As a paramedic, it is your responsibility to know your local and regional destination policies to ensure you are an advocate for your patient.

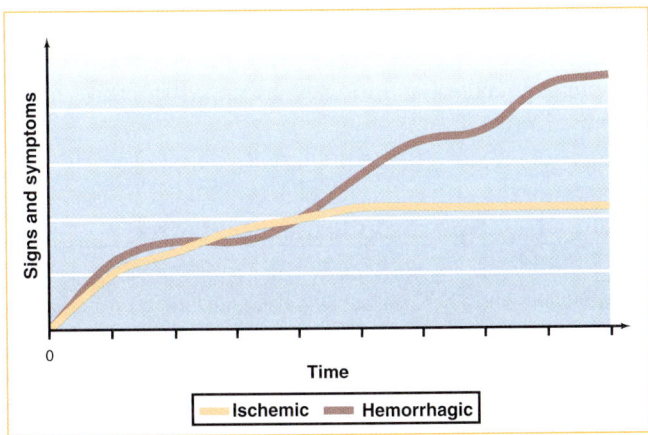

Figure 28-19 Symptom patterns for hemorrhagic versus ischemic CVA.

finally shows signs of increased ICP, you should strongly consider a diagnosis of hemorrhagic CVA.

Patients with a suspected stroke or transient ischemic attack (TIA; discussed in the next section) are usually older than age 65. Although men have more strokes, women die from them more often. First Nation and Inuit experience a greater rate of stroke than other groups within the population.

Presentation

Patients with stroke can exhibit a variety of signs and symptoms. Language effects may include slurred speech, aphasia, agnosia, and apraxia. Movement effects—hemiparesis, hemiplegia, arm drifting, facial droop, ptosis, and ataxia—may be observed as well. Sensation effects may include headache (in hemorrhagic CVA), sudden blindness, and sudden unilateral paresthesia. Consciousness problems, such as decreasing LOC, difficulty thinking, seizures, and coma, may be noted. The patient may also develop hypertension.

The hospital will take different paths of care for each type of stroke. In any event, speedy treatment is essential. For ischemic strokes, fibrinolytics must be administered within 3 hours of onset of symptoms. In hemorrhagic stroke, the more the patient bleeds into the cranium, the greater the potential for increased ICP and brain stem damage.

Prehospital Management

Paramedics need to be involved in educating the community about stroke signs and symptoms, the effects of strokes, and EMS. Too many patients deny their complaints or drive themselves to emergency departments. Reinforce with the public the common signs and symptoms of a stroke and how to activate the EMS system in their community.

Prehospital care of the stroke patient should begin with the standard prehospital care outlined previously. Ensure adequate ABCs and blood pressure. Establish the patient's oxygen and glucose level. Establish IV access in case fluids or medications are needed.

During the assessment phase, use a stroke assessment tool—such as the Cincinnati Prehospital Stroke Scale **Table 28-7 ▶**, the Los Angeles Prehospital Stroke Screen **Table 28-8 ▶** or Ontario Paramedic Prompt Card for Acute Stroke Protocol **Table 28-9 ▶**—to increase the accuracy of your working diagnosis. Rapid identification is imperative.

In some cases, pinning down the exact time the stroke began can be very difficult, such as with patients who live alone. In those cases, ask family or care providers when the patient last seemed "normal." Do not administer aspirin in the field; it will help the ischemic CVA, but hurt the hemorrhagic CVA. Aspirin should be administered only after a computed tomography (CT) scan or magnetic resonance imaging (MRI) has been completed in the hospital. Protect any impaired limbs from injury. Patients may not be able to move their arms or legs if they begin to get injured. If local or regional protocols permit it, transport the patient to an appropriate facility with a stroke team that is trained in the administration of fibrinolytics.

Transient Ischemic Attack

Transient ischemic attacks (TIAs) are episodes of cerebral ischemia that do not inflict any permanent damage. Any of the typical presentations associated with a CVA can occur with TIAs, but the TIA signs and symptoms resolve within 24 hours without any residual damage to brain tissue. These ministrokes are often signs of a serious vascular problem that requires medical evaluation. More than one third of patients with TIAs will suffer a CVA soon afterward.

As with strokes, management of TIAs begins with standard prehospital care. Follow the same management guidelines as for CVA. Close neurologic assessment is needed. Patients may experience multiple TIAs in a short time frame—coming and going.

Strongly encourage the patient to be transported. If the individual refuses transportation, appeal to the patient's family for assistance. Encourage the patient to seek medical care very soon. It is important to reinforce the message that the TIA is a warning sign of a very serious and potentially deadly problem with the blood vessels within the brain. In fact, hypertension is the number one preventable cause of strokes and TIAs. Encourage the patient to talk with his or her doctor about blood pressure control and to take any antihypertensive medications prescribed.

Notes from Nancy

Just because the patient is a known alcoholic or because his breath smells of alcohol, it does not mean that he cannot be in a coma from other causes.

Documentation and Communication

Stroke documentation points:
- When did the patient last seem "normal"?
- When did the signs and symptoms begin?
- Was there any change in the patient during transport?
- Document the reason for the choice of hospital.

Special Considerations

Many medications can alter LOC. Explore all medications that the patient is taking, including prescription, nonprescription, herbal, supplements, homeopathic substances, and illegal drugs. Geriatric patients may have many physicians, many conditions, and many medications. Combinations of medications can result in unexpected neurologic effects.

Table 28-7	Cincinnati Prehospital Stroke Scale		

Assessment	Normal	Abnormal
Facial Droop. Ask the patient to smile and show the teeth.	Both sides of the face move equally well.	One side of the face does not move as well as the other.
Arm Drift. Ask the patient to close the eyes and hold the arms out with palms up for 10 seconds.	Both arms move the same, or both arms do not move.	One arm does not move, or one arm drifts down compared with the other.
Abnormal Speech. Ask the patient to say, "The sky is blue in Cincinnati" or "You can't teach an old dog new tricks."	The patient uses the correct words with no slurring.	The patient slurs words, uses inappropriate words, or is unable to speak.

Interpretation: If any assessment criterion is abnormal, the probability of a stroke is 72%.

Table 28-8	Los Angeles Prehospital Stroke Screen		

Criteria	Yes	Unknown	No
1. Age > 45	❏	❏	❏
2. History of seizures or epilepsy absent	❏	❏	❏
3. Symptoms < 24 hours	❏	❏	❏
4. At baseline, patient is not wheelchair-bound or bedridden	❏	❏	❏
5. Blood glucose between 3 and 22 mmol/l	❏	❏	❏
6. Obvious asymmetry (right versus left) in any of the following three examination categories (must be unilateral):	❏	❏	❏
	Equal	**Right Weak**	**Left Weak**
Facial smile/grimace	❏	❏ Droop	❏ Droop
Grip	❏	❏ Weak grip	❏ Weak grip
		❏ No grip	❏ No grip
Arm strength	❏	❏ Drifts down	❏ Drifts down
		❏ Falls rapidly	❏ Falls rapidly

Interpretation: If criteria 1–6 are marked yes, the probability of a stroke is 97%.

Table 28-9	Indications for Patient Transport to a Designated Stroke Centre		

Transport to a Stroke Centre must be considered for patients who:

present with a new onset of at least one of the following symptoms suggestive of the onset of an acute stroke;

- unilateral arm/leg weakness or drift
- slurred or inappropriate words or mute
- facial droop

  AND

can be transported to arrive within two (2) hours of a clearly determined time of symptom onset or the time the patient was "last seen in a usual state of health."

Contraindications for Patient Transport Under Stroke Protocol:

Any of the following conditions exclude a patient from being transported under Stroke Protocol:

- CTAS Level 1 and/or uncorrected airway, breathing, or significant circulatory problem
- symptoms of the stroke have resolved
- blood glucose ≤ 4 mmol/l
- seizure at onset of symptoms or observed by paramedic
- Glasgow Coma Scale score < 10
- terminally ill or palliative care patient

Dispatch centre will authorize the transport once notified of the patient's need for transport under the Stroke Protocol.

Altered Level of Consciousness/Coma

Altered mental status has many possible causes, so these calls are relatively common. One way to remember the most common causes is to use the mnemonic AEIOU-TIPS (Alcohol/acidosis, Epilepsy, Insulin, Overdose, Uremia, Trauma, Infection, Psychosis, and Stroke). As with most medical complaints, the history of present illness is vital to identifying the underlying cause of the patient's complaints. An easy approach is to determine when the patient was last seen functioning normally.

Presentation

Evaluate the speed of onset for the altered LOC; this may help distinguish its cause. It is very rare that a person would be absolutely healthy one minute and be unresponsive from infection the next, for example. By contrast, seizures can cause unresponsiveness almost instantly. The common signs and symptoms for altered LOC/coma are thought effects (decreasing LOC, confusion, hallucinations, delusions, psychosis, difficulty thinking, overly sleepy), speech effects (slurred speech, agnosia, apraxia, aphasia), movement effects (ataxia, seizures, posturing), and total unresponsiveness or coma.

Prehospital Management

In the case of altered LOC, prehospital care proceeds in two stages. First, the paramedic needs to support vital functions, including securing and maintaining ABCs. Second, the paramedic needs to gather information about the possible cause of the altered LOC. Determine past medical history, evaluate medications, look for signs of trauma, and determine the history of present illness. Does the patient have a medic alert tag? Was drug paraphernalia found near the patient? How was the patient acting before you were called?

In-hospital care will focus on supporting ABCs and attempting to discover the underlying problem. Patients will routinely need blood and urine specimens, radiographs, and CT/MRI scans.

Seizure

Seizures involve sudden, erratic firing of neurons. Patients who have epilepsy commonly have seizures, for example. Patients may experience a wide array of signs and symptoms when having seizures, ranging from one hand shaking or having a taste of pennies in the mouth to movement of every limb or the complete loss of consciousness. They may be aware of the seizure, or they may wake up afterward not knowing what happened.

The paramedic should try to determine the cause of the seizure. In particular, ask about medication compliance. Phenytoin, lorazepam, carbamezapine, and valproic acid are common anticonvulsant medications, but patients may be taking them in insufficient levels to prevent seizures. Patients may feel that they are cured because they haven't suffered a seizure in many months, and stop taking their medications. Children may outgrow their anticonvulsant dosage. Older patients may be unable to afford the medication.

Infants who have a fever may suffer a febrile seizure. Diabetics may have low blood glucose levels and consequently seize. Knowing the cause will help direct management. **Table 28-10 ▶** lists many of the causes of seizures.

Classification of Seizures

Seizures can be classified as generalized (affecting large portions of the brain) or partial (affecting a limited area of the brain). The classifications of seizures are outlined in **Table 28-11 ▶**.

You are the Paramedic Part 4

During transport, the patient's condition did not change. You continue to monitor his mentation, vital signs, and deficits while en route to the hospital. You provide a prompt radio report to the receiving facility, and deliver your patient to the emergency department without incident.

Reassessment	Recording Time: 15 Minutes
Level of consciousness	Alert, with a Glasgow Coma Scale score of 14
Skin	Pale, warm, and dry
Pulse	88 beats/min, strong and irregular
Blood pressure	140 by palpation
Respirations	24 breaths/min
SpO_2	100% on 15 l/min via nonrebreathing mask

8. What other important considerations relate to total patient prehospital care?

Table 28-10 Causes of Seizures

- Abscess
- AIDS
- Alcohol
- Birth defect
- Brain infections (meningitis, encephalitis)
- Brain trauma
- Diabetes mellitus
- Fever
- Idiopathic (no known cause)
- Inappropriate medication dosage
- Organic brain syndromes
- Recreational drugs
- Stroke or TIA
- Systemic infection
- Tumour
- Uremia (kidney failure)

Within the category of generalized seizures are the tonic-clonic and absence types. Tonic-clonic seizures also called tonic-clonic seizures present the paramedic with the most challenges. Most tonic-clonic seizures follow a pattern, travelling through each of the following steps in order, although sometimes skipping a step:

1. **Aura.** A sensation the patient experiences before the seizure occurs (eg, muscle twitch, funny taste, seeing lights, hearing a high-pitched noise).

2. **Loss of consciousness.**

3. **Tonic phase.** Body-wide rigidity.

4. **Hypertonic phase.** Arched back and rigidity.

5. **Clonic phase.** Rhythmic contraction of major muscle groups. Arm, leg, head movement; lip smacking; biting; teeth clenching.

6. **Postseizure.** Major muscles relax, nystagmus may still be occurring. Eyes may be "rolled back."

7. **Postictal.** Reset period of the brain. This can take several minutes to hours before the patient gradually returns to the preseizure LOC **Figure 28-20**. During this time patients are often initially aphasic (unable to speak), confused or unable to follow commands, very emotional, and tired or sleeping. They may present with a headache. Gradually the brain will begin to function normally.

During the seizing process, respirations may become very erratic, loud, and obviously abnormal. Alternately, the patient may stop breathing and become cyanotic. These periods of apnea are usually very short-lived and do not require assistance. If the patient is apneic for more than 30 seconds, immediately begin ventilatory assistance. Another disconcerting aspect of seizures, particularly for the patient, is incontinence.

In contrast to tonic-clonic seizures, absence seizures present with little or any movement. The typical patient with absence seizures is a child. Classically the child will simply stop moving; he or she may be walking and just stop, may be speaking and stop midsentence, or may be playing and freeze with a toy in the hand. The child will rarely fall. These seizures usually last no more than several seconds. There is no postictal period and no confusion. These may be brought on by flashing lights or hyperventilation.

Partial seizures may be classified as either simple partial or complex partial. Such seizures involve only a limited portion of the brain. They may be localized to just one spot within the brain or they may begin in one spot and move in wave-like fashion to other locations. Such a Jacksonian March wave is akin to the ripples that occur from dropping a pebble in a still pond.

Table 28-11 Seizure Classifications

Generalized Seizures	Characteristics
Absence seizure	- Staring episodes or "absence spells," during which the patient's activity ceases; loss of motor control is uncommon, although eye blinking or lip smacking may occur. - Most common in children between 4 and 12 years of age; rarely occurs after age 20. - Typically lasts less than 15 seconds, after which the child's LOC immediately returns to normal.
Tonic-clonic seizure	- Characterized by a loss of consciousness, followed by generalized (entire-body) muscle contraction (tonic phase) alternating with rhythmic "jerking" movements (clonic phase). - Often preceded by an aura—a strange taste, smell, or other abnormal sensation—that warns the patient of the impending seizure. - Can occur at any age. - Often lasts several minutes; may progress to status epilepticus—a prolonged seizure or two consecutive seizures without an intervening lucid interval. - Typically followed by a postictal phase, during which the patient is confused, appears sleepy, and may be agitated or combative.

Partial (Focal) Seizures	Characteristics
Simple partial seizure	- Also referred to as focal motor or "Jacksonian March" seizures. - Characterized by tonic-clonic activity localized to one part of the body; may spread and progress to a generalized tonic-clonic seizure. - No aura or associated loss of consciousness.
Complex partial seizure	- Also referred to as temporal lobe or psychomotor seizures. - Manifests as changes in behaviour (mood changes, abrupt bouts of rage). - Often preceded by an aura. - Usually lasts less than 1 to 2 minutes, after which patient quickly regains normal mental status (no postictal phase).

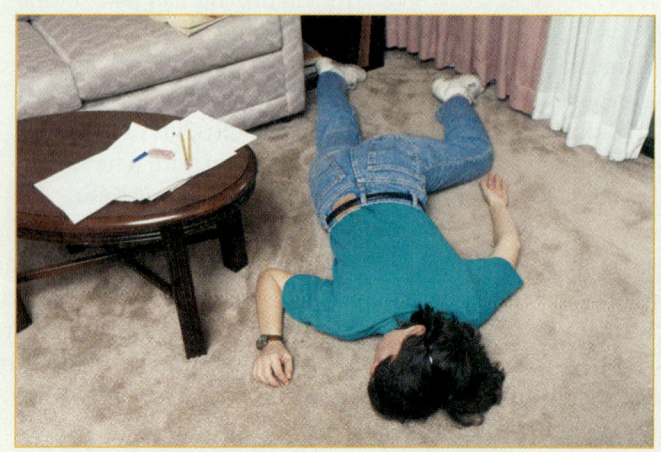

Figure 28-20 A patient who has had a seizure may be found in the postictal state when you arrive. In such a case, ask family members or bystanders to verify that a seizure has occurred and describe how the seizure developed.

Simple partial seizures involve either movement of one part of the body (frontal lobe) or altered sensations in one part of the body (parietal lobe). An example of a Jacksonian March in a simple partial seizure would be shaking of the left hand, which moves to the left arm, then to the shoulder, then to the head, then to the right arm, then to the right hand, and finally stops. Complex partial seizures involve subtle LOC changes. The patient may become confused, lose alertness, suffer hallucinations, or be unable to speak. The head or eyes may make small movements. Patients typically do not become unresponsive.

Documentation and Communication

Seizure documentation points:
- Was any aura noted by the patient?
- Which body parts were in motion?
- Was the patient awake during the seizure?
- How long did it last?
- How was the patient after the seizure?
- What was the response to your therapy?

Prehospital Management

Most seizures are self-limiting, so you simply need to monitor and protect patients from injuring themselves. Prehospital management of patients with seizure begins with standard prehospital care. Quickly determine whether trauma is a concern.

- Where was the patient before the seizure?
- What was the patient doing before the seizure?
- How did the patient get to the current position?
- If the situation is unclear or there is confirmed trauma, perform manual in-line immobilization.

Prehospital care during the seizure includes calmness on your part. Don't restrain the patient or try to stop the seizing

movement. Prevent the patient from striking objects and becoming injured. Place nothing within the patient's mouth while the seizure is ongoing. If bystanders have placed objects (eg, spoons, butter knives) in the mouth, remove them.

Provide ventilatory assistance only if the seizure or apnea is prolonged. Ventilation of the actively seizing patient will be very difficult. Oral or nasotracheal intubation will be next to impossible during a seizure.

In the postseizure phase, emotional support is very important. Provide privacy. Speak calmly and slowly. Be prepared to repeat yourself. Reorient the patient to place and time. If a child is febrile, encourage parents to administer a drug for fever reduction (acetaminophen or ibuprofen).

Unless a clear and easily reversible cause for the seizure is found, all patients should be transported because seizures can be a warning sign of more serious nervous system problems. If the patient has a known history of seizures, he or she may not wish to go to the hospital. Advise the patient to follow up with the family doctor within 24 hours. The diabetic who is awakened after glucose administration may not wish to be transported. Advise this patient to eat a good meal and follow up with the family doctor.

Any patient who you suspect could seize should have the following prehospital care.

- Establish IV access. Diazepam and lorazepam are the drugs of choice to stop seizures. In patients who are seizing and in whom IV access cannot be established, diazepam can be administered rectally at 0.2 mg/kg.
- Place blankets over the rails of the ambulance stretcher.
- Place blankets over hard surfaces near the patient.
- Ensure that the patient's stretcher straps are not too tight.

In-hospital management will seek to identify the cause of the seizure. Blood studies, including drug and blood glucose determinations, will be done. CT or MRI scans may be performed.

Status Epilepticus

Status epilepticus is a seizure that lasts for longer than 4 to 5 minutes or consecutive seizures that occur without consciousness returning between seizure episodes. This time frame is arbitrary, however, and some authors suggest that status epilepticus does not occur until 20 minutes of uninterrupted seizing. Refer to your local protocols for guidelines on how long a seizure can continue before you should intervene.

During a seizure, neurons are in a hypermetabolic state (using huge amounts of glucose and producing lactic acid). For a short period, this state does not produce long-term damage. If the seizure continues, however, the body can't remove the waste products effectively or ensure adequate glucose supplies. Such a hypermetabolic state can result in neurons being damaged or killed. The goal of prehospital care is to stop the seizure and ensure adequate ABCs.

Management of status epilepticus begins with standard prehospital care. Administer benzodiazepines (diazepam, 5.0 mg IV, or lorazepam, 0.05 mg/kg [maximum 4 mg]). You may repeat diazepam every 10 to 15 minutes to a total dose of 30 mg. If you are unable to obtain IV access, you may give diazepam rectally. You may repeat the lorazepam dose in 10 to 15 minutes, with a maximum dose of 8 mg in 12 hours.

Be prepared to completely control airway and ventilation, as benzodiazepines can cause respiratory depression and arrest. Continue to use airway positioning and bag-valve-mask ventilations until the seizure stops. If benzodiazepines do not quickly control the seizure and the patient can't be ventilated, paralytics may be needed to allow for adequate airway management.

Syncope

Syncope (fainting) is the sudden and temporary loss of consciousness with accompanying loss of postural tone. It affects mainly adults and accounts for nearly 3% of all emergency department visits. The brain uses glucose at a high rate and has no ability to store glucose, so even a 3- to 5-second interruption in blood flow can cause loss of consciousness. The question then becomes, What caused the sudden decrease in cerebral perfusion? ◖ Table 28-12 ▾ ◗ lists the common causes of syncope.

Presentation

Classically, the patient with syncope is in a standing position when the event occurs. With young adults, the pattern is usually one of vasovagal syncope. The person will experience fear, emotional stress, or pain. Suddenly the room will seem to spin, and the individual will pass out. (This is why you should always seat a patient before drawing blood or starting an IV.) In older adults, cardiac dysrhythmia is a more typical cause of syncope. The patient experiences a sudden run of ventricular tachycardia, the blood pressure drops, and the person falls to the floor. The rhythm terminates, the blood pressure rises, and the individual regains consciousness. In either case, the whole process takes less than 60 seconds.

Patients with syncope usually experience prodrome, signs or symptoms that precede a disease or condition. For syncope, prodromal complaints include feelings of dizziness, weakness,

Table 28-12	Causes of Syncope	
Category	**Causes**
Cardiac rhythm	Bradycardia of any type
	Sick sinus syndrome
	Supraventricular tachycardia
	Torsade de pointes
	Transient asystole
	Transient ventricular fibrillation
	Ventricular tachycardia
Cardiac muscle	Cardiomyopathy
	Myocardial infarction
Others	Dehydration
	Hypoglycemia
	Vasovagal

Table 28-13	Differentiating Syncope from Seizure	
Characteristic	**Syncope**	**Seizure**
Position of patient before event	Standing	Any position
Prodromal signs and symptoms	Dizziness, visual changes, shortness of breath, weakness	Aura: funny taste, seeing lights, hearing sound, twitching
Activity during event	Relaxed	Generalized body movement
Response after event	Quick return of orientation	Slow return of orientation

shortness of breath, chest pain, headache, or visual disturbances. Incontinence is possible with syncope, though uncommon. Seizures and syncope can be difficult to differentiate; ◖ Table 28-13 ▴ ◗ provides some guidelines for making this distinction.

Prehospital Management

Begin with standard prehospital care. Determine if the patient may have experienced trauma during the fall, and take cervical spine precautions as needed. Focus on blood glucose level and likely cardiac causes. Obtain orthostatic vital signs if possible.

Provide emotional support, as syncope can be very embarrassing. Transport the patient to the hospital. Syncope can be a sign of life-threatening cardiac dysrhythmias, stroke, or another serious medical condition.

Headache

Almost everyone has suffered a headache at one time or another. What exactly is hurting? The brain and skull don't have pain receptors. Headache pain originates from the nerves within the scalp, face, blood vessels, and muscles of the neck and head.

Several types of headaches may be identified. Muscle tension headaches—the most common type—are caused by life stress (tension) that results in residual muscle contractions within the face and head. The pain tends to occur on both sides of head and travels from back to front; it is a dull ache or squeezing in nature. The jaw, neck, or shoulders may be stiff or sore.

Migraine headaches are thought to be caused by changes in blood vessel size within the base of the brain. The patient may experience an aura (eg, seeing bright lights) and unilateral, focused pain that then spreads over time. The pain is throbbing, pounding, or pulsating in nature. Nausea or vomiting may be present. These patients prefer dark, quiet environments. Migraines can last several days.

Cluster headaches are rare vascular headaches that start in the face. They occur in groups or clusters. They last only 30 to 45 minutes, but a patient may have several each day. The headaches may recur for days and then stop entirely. They may return the next month. The pattern consists of minor pain around one eye, pain that quickly intensifies and spreads to one side of the face, and a feeling of anxiety.

Sinus headaches are caused by inflammation or infection within the sinus cavities of the face. The pain, which is located in the superior portions of the face, increases with bending the head forward. It's worse when first waking. The patient may have postnasal drip, a sore throat, and nasal discharge.

Other, rare types of headaches include those caused by tumours, inflammation of the temporal artery, strokes, CNS infections, or hypertension. Their presentations vary depending on the underlying cause.

Headaches can be frustrating calls for paramedics. Many may feel that such calls are a waste of EMS resources—at least, until they experience a migraine of their own **Figure 28-21 ▼** . One problem faced by paramedics is that the complaint is entirely subjective; there is no way to "prove" the person is or is not having a severe headache. Try to determine the patient's level of stress, possible infections, and history of headaches. The patient can have various locations and intensity of pain, and may have nausea, vomiting, or light and sound phobia.

The majority of patients have real pain and need assistance from EMS. Others, however, may be drug-seeking, addicted, or abusing medications. Here are some clues to drug-seeking behaviour:

- Does the patient have a history of calling 9-1-1 for headaches?
- Do the patient's allergies limit him or her to a small number of narcotic medications?
- Is the patient very reluctant to try other pain management options besides narcotics?

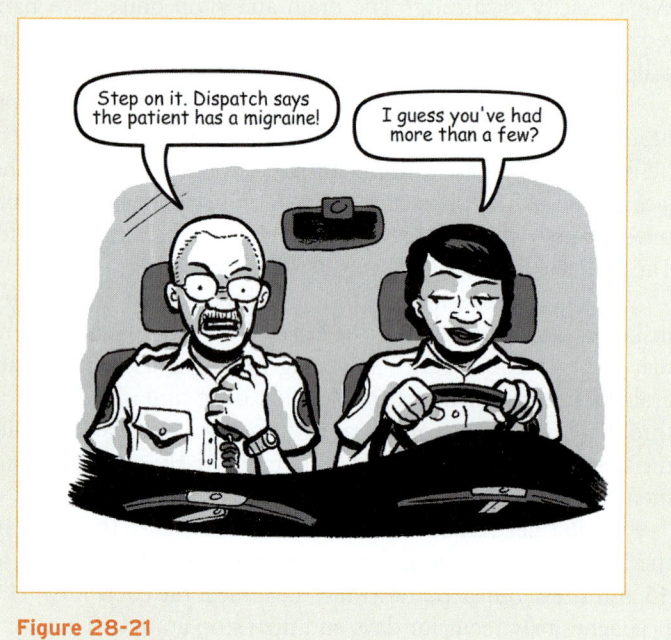

Figure 28-21

- Does the patient suddenly relax after being told that narcotics are on the way?

No single presentation characteristic should lead you to classify the patient as drug-seeking. Instead, consider the entire environment. What has the patient done to manage this headache? When did it start? How bad is it? Even if you suspect drug-seeking behaviour, it would be inappropriate to withhold medication from the patient without first communicating with medical direction. Upon arrival at the hospital, relay your concerns to emergency department personnel in a fact-based conversation. Point out specifics of behaviour, comments, history, and other factors that have led you to suspect possible drug-seeking.

Be cautious, as headaches can indicate a more serious problem. Give standard prehospital care. Consider stroke, abscess, tumour, hypertension, and CNS infections. Ask which medications the patient has taken. Many patients will appreciate a darkened, quiet environment, so don't use lights and sirens if transporting. Medications for pain management could include meperidine, morphine, and ketorolac. Also consider promethazine for nausea or vomiting. In-hospital management would include analgesics and ruling out serious medical problems.

Abscess

Abscesses result when an infectious agent invades the brain or spinal cord. The bacteria or fungi then attack brain cells and destroy tissue. In response, the immune system attempts to kill the infectious agent but fails to do so. To prevent the bacteria or fungi from spreading, the body erects a barrier around the area. The area within the barrier contains the infectious agent, dead or dying brain cells, dead white blood cells, and white blood cells that continue fighting the infection. Over time, with the continued destruction of tissue and the immune system's ongoing attempts to kill the agent, swelling can occur.

The underlying cause of an infection within the brain may be an infection of the sinuses, throat, gums, or ears that has spread. The organism can also be injected during trauma to the head. Such an infection has two major consequences: damage to the brain tissue and the presence of an abscess within the cranial vault that leads to increased ICP. These two factors may result in low- or high-grade fever, persistent headache (often localized), drowsiness, confusion, general or focal seizures, nausea and vomiting, focal motor or sensory impairments, and hemiparesis. Abscess usually occurs in people younger than 50 years of age and has a gradual onset.

Prehospital management starts with standard prehospital care. Although no specific prehospital care is available for the abscess patient in the prehospital setting, the paramedic needs to pay close attention for evidence of increased ICP. Look for changes in LOC, respiratory patterns, and posturing. If needed, begin hyperventilation. Notify the hospital of the critical nature of your patient. Take seizure precautions and be ready to administer diazepam if needed.

In-hospital management will likely involve antibiotics, seizure precautions, and potentially surgical removal of the abscess.

Multiple Sclerosis

Multiple sclerosis (MS) is an autoimmune condition in which the body attacks the myelin sheath of the neurons in the brain and spinal cord, leading to areas of scarring. This disease is more prevalent in temperate regions than in tropical regions. Some evidence suggests that an environmental trigger—perhaps a virus, although none have been identified—begins to focus the attention of the immune system on the myelin. MS typically affects people between the ages of 20 and 40.

The presentation of MS usually follows a pattern of attacks and remissions. The attacks can vary in intensity and the remissions can vary in length. Patients may recover or have long-term complaints. In the initial attack, double vision and blurred vision are common complaints. Other symptoms include muscle weakness; impairment of pain, temperature, and touch senses; pain (moderate to severe); ataxia; intension tremors; speech disturbances; vision disturbances; vertigo; bladder or bowel dysfunction; sexual dysfunction; depression; euphoria; cognitive abnormalities; and fatigue during attacks.

Prehospital management is supportive. Give standard prehospital care. In-hospital treatment will be directed at controlling the symptoms. Anti-inflammatory medications may be administered to decrease the length of the attack. There is currently no cure for MS.

Neoplasm

For the purposes of this chapter, a neoplasm is defined as cancer within the brain or spinal cord. Two basic types of cancer are identified: primary and metastatic. Primary neoplasms begin within the nervous system. Metastatic neoplasms begin in some other part of the body, gain access to the bloodstream or lymphatic system, and then take up residence within the nervous system. Lung and breast cancers are the cancers that most commonly metastasize to the CNS. Once mature, neurons no longer divide, so only rarely do they become cancerous. Primary CNS cancers are usually caused by mitosis errors in the support structures of the CNS.

Headache, nausea and vomiting, seizures, changes in mental status, and stroke-like signs and symptoms are common in cases of neoplasm. The rate and intensity of these signs and symptoms depend on the cancer's growth rate and location. Patients may have months of headaches, or suddenly experience a seizure without any prior complaints.

Prehospital management is supportive. Watch for status epilepticus and increased ICP. All patients with new-onset seizures or chronic headaches that cannot be managed need medical evaluation. In-hospital management is complex and depends on the type of cancer and location.

Dystonia

Dystonia are marked by severe, abnormal muscle spasms that cause bizarre contortions, repetitive motions, or postures. These movements are involuntary and often painful. The initial episode usually occurs before the patient is in his or her 40s.

Sudden onset may be precipitated by stress or continuous use of a muscle group. Patients tend to have normal intelligence and no psychiatric medical history.

Dystonia is both a sign and a condition. Some patients who take antipsychotic medications may suffer a sudden onset of bizarre contortions of the face or body; this is considered a secondary dystonia. Primary dystonias occur for unknown reasons, although a defect in the body's ability to process neurotransmitters is thought to lie at the heart of this problem. Spasmodic torticollis is a primary dystonia in which the neck muscles contract, twisting the head to one side and pulling it forward or backward. The head then remains painfully frozen in that position.

Prehospital management should focus on ruling out other problems such as seizures, strokes, or psychiatric medication reaction. If you suspect a dystonic reaction to antipsychotics, diphenhydramine is the drug of choice to stop the contraction. Unfortunately, this medication is ineffective in primary dystonias. Give standard prehospital care. Regardless of the underlying cause, dystonias are socially upsetting as patients suddenly twist and writhe uncontrollably. Providing compassionate prehospital care is critical. In-hospital management involves a variety of medication options to control the condition. There currently is no cure for dystonia.

Parkinson's Disease

In Parkinson's disease, the substantia nigra (the portion of the brain that produces dopamine) becomes damaged. Dopamine is the neurotransmitter that, among other things, ensures smooth muscular contractions. Parkinson's disease symptoms have a gradual onset that spans months to years. The initial signs are often unilateral tremors. Over time, as dopamine levels fall, more areas of the body become involved. Genetics play an important role in this disease. Parkinson-like activity can be observed in head injuries and some overdose patients, in which progression of the symptoms occurs more rapidly. The average age of onset is 60 years, and more men are affected than women.

The classic presentation of Parkinson's disease includes four characteristics: tremor, postural instability, rigidity, and bradykinesia. Rest tremors and postural tremors are also common. Other symptoms include depression, difficulty swallowing, speech impairments, and fatigue. Prognosis is poor as the condition advances. Patients in later stages are at a much greater risk of death from aspiration, pneumonia, falls, or complications due to immobility.

Prehospital management involves standard prehospital care and emotional support. In-hospital management will include levodopa, which may temporarily restore dopamine levels. Other medications, surgery, and modification of diet and exercise are also options.

Trigeminal Neuralgia

Trigeminal neuralgia, also called tic douloureux, is an inflammation of the trigeminal nerve (fifth cranial nerve). The trigeminal nerve receives sensory information from the face. The usual cause of trigeminal neuralgia is irradiation by an artery lying too close to the nerve. Over time, as the artery changes diameter to meet blood supply needs, this motion grates the myelin sheath off the nerve. With its insulation gone, the nerve may "short out," causing pain without trauma to the area. Patients are usually older than age 50, and more women are affected than men.

Patients experience severe shock-like or stabbing pain, usually on one side of the face. These attacks can last for several minutes to several months. They may be triggered by touching the face, speaking, brushing the teeth, eating, putting on clothing, the wind—essentially any activity that stimulates the face. There is typically no loss of taste, hearing, or facial sensation with this condition. Likewise, there is no loss of motor control over the face, so facial droop, ptosis, and difficulty controlling the airway are very uncommon.

Although not life-threatening, this condition can be quite debilitating. Patients experience severe pain. Some will stay indoors, eat softer foods, or stop washing their faces in an effort to prevent an attack. These patients need compassion and understanding.

Prehospital care consists of standard care. Meperidine, morphine, or ketorolac may be indicated to help with pain management. Try to limit conversations to decrease facial movement. Administer oxygen if the patient is in respiratory distress or has a low pulse oximeter reading. Use of a nasal cannula or a nonrebreathing mask can instigate an attack. Even trying to administer blow-by oxygen could be painful to the patient. Long-term treatment for this condition is medication (carbamazepine or phenytoin) to calm the trigeminal nerve and sometimes surgery to place a barrier between the nerve and the artery.

Bell's Palsy

Bell's palsy is a temporary paralysis of the facial nerve (seventh cranial nerve). The facial nerve controls the muscles on each side of the face, including those used in eye blinking and facial expressions such as smiling and frowning. It also controls the tear glands and the saliva glands. Finally, the facial nerve transmits taste sensations from the tongue.

Patients typically experience a minor infection before Bell's palsy appears. The attack is very sudden and can easily be confused with a stroke. Signs and symptoms include ptosis, facial droop or weakness, drooling, and loss of the ability to taste. This condition strikes all races and both sexes equally. It is more common in middle-aged people (between 15 and 60 years old).

Bell's palsy will often resolve within 2 weeks. Prehospital management involves standard care. Make sure that these patients are not suffering from a stroke. Complete a full assessment. When in doubt, treat the case as if it were a stroke. In-hospital treatment for Bell's palsy includes corticosteroids (eg, prednisone) and acyclovir, which helps manage viral infections.

Amyotrophic Lateral Sclerosis

Amyotrophic lateral sclerosis (ALS), also known as Lou Gehrig's disease, is a disease that involves the death of voluntary motor neurons, for unclear reasons. One theory suggests that the body's immune system selectively attacks and kills these motor neurons. Some evidence indicates that genetics may play a role. ALS is more common in middle-aged males of any race.

Initially, this condition is rather subtle and progresses without drawing notice. Fatigue, general weakness of muscle groups, and difficulty performing routine activities such as eating, writing, and dressing are early signs. Patients may also experience difficulty speaking. As ALS progresses, the patient loses his or her ability to walk, move the arms, eat, and speak. The speed of progression differs for every patient. Because this condition affects only the motor neurons, patients remain completely aware of their surroundings.

The average person who is diagnosed with ALS will die within 3 to 5 years. As the destruction of motor neurons continues, eventually patients are unable to breathe effectively without ventilatory assistance. Patients die of respiratory infections or other complications related to immobility.

Prehospital treatment for these patients is standard care. Assess the ability to swallow, and monitor the airway closely. Patients may be surrounded by a variety of home medical technology, including feeding pumps, IV pumps, long-term IV access ports, and ventilators. Transportation becomes complicated by the management of this technology. General guidelines include asking for guidance from the family or home health care provider related to the operation of the technology. If necessary, disconnect the patient from the technology, after consulting medical direction, and transport.

In-hospital care for ALS is geared toward supporting vital functions. Patients will undergo physical therapy to help strengthen their remaining neurons and muscles. Medications can be given to assist with some of the symptoms; however, there is no cure for ALS.

You are the Paramedic Part 5

A CT scan showed a mild stroke in the parietal lobe. The patient was not a candidate for fibrinolytics because the onset of his stroke couldn't be determined. He soon returned home with the support of his family and full-time nursing care. Because you rapidly recognized his stroke and transported him with the appropriate sense of urgency, the emergency department nurses and doctors were able to promptly confirm the type of stroke and begin appropriate care.

Guillain-Barré Syndrome

Guillain-Barré syndrome is a rare condition that is rather scary for most patients. It begins as weakness and tingling sensations in the legs. This weakness moves up the legs and begins to affect the thorax and arms. It can quickly become severe and lead to paralysis. In fact, the transition from being able to walk and speak to needing a ventilator to breathe may take as little as several hours. Most patients will experience maximum muscle weakness and paralysis within 2 weeks.

The cause of this condition is unclear, although some degree of immune response appears to be present. Patients usually report having a minor respiratory or gastrointestinal infection prior to the onset of weakness. One theory is that the infectious agent creates a situation in which the body attacks its own neurons. This attack damages the myelin, thereby causing "shorting" of the signals travelling along the axon.

The reversal of this disease can be almost as dramatic as its onset. Some patients will have a complete recovery without residual weakness in as little as several weeks. About one third retain some degree of weakness after 3 years. Some patients will require ventilatory assistance for the remainder of their lives.

Prehospital management includes standard care and close assessment of the patient's ability to effectively protect the airway and ventilate. Because of the sheer terror that patients can experience, a comforting voice and use of therapeutic touch are important.

In-hospital management includes plasmapheresis (exchanging the plasma within the blood) and immunoglobulin injections. These therapies decrease the time until recovery.

Poliomyelitis

Poliomyelitis is a viral infection that is transmitted by the fecal-oral route. Its incidence in Canada peaked in the post–World War II era of the late 1940s and 1950s. With the introduction of the Salk vaccine in 1955, the number of new polio victims in Canada declined dramatically. Polio vaccination has been available free to all Canadians since 1955. The Americas were certified polio-free by the Pan American Health Organization in 1994. In May 1988, the World Health Organization set a goal to eradicate polio from the planet by 2000. Unfortunately, delivering and administering the vaccine to countries in conflict have hampered this goal, but with fewer than 2,000 new cases each year, the goal is within sight. The vast majority of patients who contract the virus do not become ill. Polio can occur at any age, but very young and older patients are at greatest risk. Signs and symptoms may begin as soon as one week after infection. In the most severe cases, they include sore throat, nausea, vomiting, diarrhea, stiff neck, and weakness or paralysis of muscles.

Prehospital management consists of standard care. In severe cases, patients will need ventilatory assistance. In-hospital care for patients with the acute illness is directed at hydration, ventilation, and calorie support until the immune system gains control over the infection.

The way the virus damages the nervous system places patients at risk for problems decades after the initial infection. In the initial infection, the virus attacks motor neurons within the brain and brain stem, which causes the classic signs of weakness and paralysis. The remaining neurons then begin to send out new axons to try to compensate for this loss, which allows the patient to regain function. Over time, these neurons maintain their unusually high workload. When they begin to break down and die, the patient may develop postpolio syndrome. As a consequence, some patients who suffered polio in the early part of the 20th century (most are older than 60 years) are now having difficulty swallowing, weakness, fatigue, or breathing problems. Typically, wherever patients had symptoms when they were originally infected, they experience symptoms again, albeit in a milder form. Prehospital treatment is standard care, with emphasis on possible airway obstruction due to swallowing difficulties. In-hospital treatment includes physical therapy and experimental medications.

Cerebral Palsy

Cerebral palsy (CP) is a developmental condition in which damage is done to the brain (often the frontal lobe). Although it was believed that perinatal (around the time of birth) hypoxia was the primary cause, research has shown that this actually accounts for less than 10% of cases. Infections, jaundice, or Rh incompatibility also appear to be possible causes. The condition is self-limiting and does not worsen over time. Babies who are low birth weight, premature, delivered breech, or from multiple births (eg, twins or triplets) are at higher risk for CP.

The presentation of CP begins in infancy. Developmental milestones such as walking or crawling may be delayed. The type and extent of damage soon become apparent. In spastic CP (70% to 80% of cases), the muscles are in a near-constant state of contraction. If both lower legs are affected, patients will have a classic scissors walk in which the lower legs turn inward, with the legs remaining stiff and the knees almost touching. Other types of CP involve slow, uncontrolled writhing movements; tremors; or difficulties with coordination.

Prehospital management is supportive. Provide standard prehospital care. Patients may have ambulatory assistive devices (eg, wheelchairs, walkers, crutches, canes, leg braces) that will need to be transported along with them. In-hospital management is based on the particular set of symptoms. There is no cure or correction for the damage. Instead, care is directed at maximizing the child's abilities through surgery on affected limbs and physical/occupational therapy.

Spina Bifida

Spina bifida is a developmental condition resulting from a neural tube defect. Because the neural tube does not close (for unknown reasons), a portion of the spinal cord remains outside its normal location. The severity of the condition depends on where the defect lies on the cord and how much it is displaced from normal. In spina bifida occulta, one small section of vertebrae is malformed and slightly displaced. The mildest form of spina bifida, it rarely has any significant clinical features and patients may not even know the malformation is present. In the most severe form, known as myelomeningocele, a portion of the spinal cord remains completely outside the vertebral column and outside of the skin. There are also two intermediary forms of spina bifida.

Consequences of spina bifida can range from no complications to complete loss of motor and sensory functions below the defect. Patients may have muscle problems ranging from mild defects to paralysis, experience seizures, or have severe neurologic impairments. In the most severe forms, the defect interferes with normal movement of CSF. CSF is made within the brain, circulates, and is then reabsorbed. Hydrocephalus (water on the brain) is common in severe spina bifida because the CSF continues to be produced but cannot circulate effectively. Pressure builds within the brain, causing increased ICP problems and seizures.

EMS may be called for problems with spina bifida patients related to medical technology, seizures, trauma, or infections. Prehospital management is standard care. Be aware that many of these patients have latex allergies. In the most severe cases of spina bifida, children are in need of multiple types of medical technology, including feeding tubes, long-term IV access, ventilatory support, ambulatory assistive devices, and intraventricular shunts (designed to drain excess CSF from within the brain's ventricles). To avoid complications, consult with family and other home health care personnel when attempting to transport the patient. In-hospital management will be supportive. It is possible to reimplant the spinal cord, even while the fetus remains within the uterus, but the damage to the nerve tissue is permanent.

Myasthenia Gravis

Acetylcholine is an important neurotransmitter needed to allow for muscular contraction. In myasthenia gravis, the body creates antibodies against the acetylcholine receptors. The thymus gland (where T-cells mature) is believed to play a role in the production of these antibodies. As acetylcholine levels fall, muscle weakness begins. This weakness most commonly affects the eyes, eyelids, and facial muscles. Some patients will have difficulty swallowing or speaking, or leg or arm weakness. Patients suffer no sensory impairment. Myasthenia gravis usually affects women younger than 40 and men older than 60.

Myasthenia crisis is a sudden increase in the destruction of acetylcholine, resulting in weakness in the respiratory muscles. As a result, patients can become hypoxic. Infections, emotional stress, or reactions to medications can trigger this crisis.

Standard prehospital care will effectively manage these patients in the prehospital environment. Be prepared to assist with ventilations in patients with crisis. In-hospital management includes removal of the thymus gland, medications to boost neurotransmitter levels, and immunosuppressants.

Alzheimer's Disease

Alzheimer's disease (discussed in more detail in Chapter 42) is the most common form of dementia. Dementia is a chronic deterioration of a person's personality, memory, and ability to think. Alzheimer's disease is a progressive organic condition in which neurons die; there is no definitive treatment for the destroyed neurons. Prehospital management is standard care.

Peripheral Neuropathy

Peripheral neuropathy comprises a group of conditions in which the nerves leaving the spinal cord become damaged. As a consequence, the signals moving to or from the brain become distorted. Causes of peripheral neuropathy include trauma, toxins, tumours, autoimmune attacks, and metabolic disorders. Trigeminal neuralgia and Guillain-Barré syndrome are examples. The remainder of this discussion focuses on the most common form, diabetic neuropathy. Diabetic neuropathy is frequently seen in diabetic patients older than age 50; more males than females are affected. Its onset is gradual, occurring over months and years.

As blood glucose levels rise, the peripheral nerves may become damaged, resulting in misfiring and shorting of signals. Affected individuals may then experience sensory or motor impairment. Loss of sensation, numbness, burning sensations, pain, paresthesia, and muscle weakness are common. Patients may eventually lose the ability to feel their feet or other areas.

Management in the prehospital setting is supportive. Provide standard prehospital care. In-hospital management will include pain medication. The use of antidepressants and anticonvulsants seems to have a positive effect on calming the peripheral nerves.

Muscular Dystrophy

Muscular dystrophy (MD) is a nonneurologic condition of genetic origin marked by the degeneration of muscular tissue. The defective DNA causes an error in muscle tissue, such that the malformed muscle cells rupture more easily. MD is diagnosed at age 2 to 5 years and occurs only in males. Its onset is gradual, with progression over months to years.

Several forms of MD exist, each distinguished by the involvement of a particular gene and a unique set of characteristics. Generally, MD presents with progressive muscle weakness, delayed development of muscle motor skills, ptosis, drooling, and poor muscle tone. The most common type of MD, Duchenne's, manifests itself in childhood and can include damage to the respiratory and cardiac muscles. These patients have a much shortened life expectancy, rarely living beyond their middle 20s. They often die from pneumonia or cardiogenic shock.

Standard prehospital care is effective in these patients. In severe cases, ventilatory support may be necessary. Blood pressure support may be required; fluids and dopamine may be needed to manage damaged heart muscle. These severely ill patients will have extensive use of home medical technology. In-hospital management is supportive, as there is no cure for MD.

Conclusion

Neurologic patients can present a major challenge to the para-medic. To avoid becoming overwhelmed, follow a methodical and systematic approach to the assessment and prehospital care of these patients. Use the same format for all of your physical examinations. Focus your prehospital care on providing an environment that will facilitate optimal nervous system functioning. Reassess the patient after your interventions to note any changes. You are part of a health care team, so be aware of how your prehospital care will affect later activities within the emergency department. Know the material within this book. When you have mastered this information, you should be able to provide your patients with the highest level of prehospital care and your profession with an example of excellence.

You are the Paramedic Summary

1. What do you suspect as the reason(s) why Mr. Hishari is on the floor?

This patient could be on the floor for any number of reasons, including, but not limited to, a syncopal episode, loss of balance with a fall, sudden onset of weakness, or exacerbation of an underlying medical condition. At this point, there are many possibilities, which will require further investigation in both history-taking and physical assessment.

2. How would you prioritize those reasons?

As a paramedic, it's your job to recognize and treat life-threatening conditions. In some instances, definitive care can be provided; in other cases, treatment options are limited. With some underlying traumatic and medical emergencies, your job is to simply recognize the signs and symptoms, provide prompt transport to the nearest appropriate facility, and initiate supportive prehospital care without delay to definitive care.

3. Given the information you have now, what do you think could be this patient's underlying illness, injury, or condition?

Given the new information obtained, you believe the patient is experiencing a CVA. This life-threatening condition requires immediate recognition and prompt transport. There is no sure way of knowing what sort of stroke this patient is experiencing, so the goal of the paramedic is to ensure the fastest possible time to the hospital.

4. Do your assessment and treatment priorities ever change?

Although concern with ABCs is first, assessment and treatment priorities must be flexible to avoid tunnel vision and misappropriate initial diagnosis. At first, the patient appeared to have confusion most likely as a result of a low blood glucose level. After you assessed his blood glucose level and found it to be within appropriate levels, your overall impression changed, causing you to consider other reasons for his decreased LOC.

5. What are appropriate interventions?

Appropriate prehospital care would include placing the patient on high-flow oxygen, obtaining an ECG, initiating at least one IV for the purposes of collecting blood samples and providing a port for administration of fibrinolytics if deemed necessary by emergency department staff, and completing a fibrinolytic checklist prior to arrival at the hospital.

6. Would you choose to place this patient in manual in-line spinal precautions?

Keeping in mind that "time is brain," you'll have to make the determination as to whether to place the patient in spinal precautions. If the mechanism of injury indicates risk for spinal fracture, if you are unsure, or if your local protocols dictate it, you should immobilize this patient. As with any intervention, you should consider whether this step is appropriate.

7. What places this patient at greater risk for cerebrovascular accident?

His history of atrial fibrillation places your patient at greater risk for ischemic stroke. Clots could develop in his atria and travel to the brain, resulting in stroke.

8. What other important considerations relate to total patient prehospital care?

For patients who are unable to communicate, this experience can be quite frustrating and frightening. If possible, use other forms of communication. If you are unable to obtain information or understand the patient, do everything you can to ease his or her anxiety and fear.

Prep Kit

Ready for Review

- The nervous system is responsible for thought, judgment, personality, memory, emotions, voluntary motor activity, interpretation of sensory stimulation, and various autonomic activities within the body.
- Blood flow to the brain is described by the equation CPP = MAP − ICP.
- The nervous system is critical in maintaining airway control.
- Two abnormal postures that indicate brain damage in an unconscious patient are decorticate posturing (moving arms toward the core) and decerebrate posturing (moving arms away from body).
- Use the Glasgow Coma Scale to help determine a patient's level of consciousness, evaluate his or her responses to eye opening and verbal and motor skills, and guide prehospital care.
- Facial droop on one side of the face or a drooping eyelid can indicate a neurologic condition.
- Problems such as slurring or difficulty recognizing objects can signify a neurologic problem. Three forms of language problems are receptive aphasia, expressive aphasia, and global aphasia.
- Pupil shape, size, motion, and reactivity are indicators of nervous system functioning.
- Have the patient hold the arms out in front of the body and close the eyes. If one arm drifts away, the patient may have experienced a stroke.
- Abnormal, involuntary muscle contractions, such as tremors and seizures, can indicate a neurologic problem.
- Sensation can also be affected by nervous system conditions.
- The three major elements that the brain needs to function are oxygen, glucose, and normal temperature.
- Managing the neurologic patient includes administering IV solutions, monitoring the ECG, checking blood glucose levels, managing intracranial pressure, evaluating the patient's temperature, and providing emotional support.
- You may be able to administer dextrose or glucagon to treat low blood glucose levels, depending on your local protocol.
- Naloxone may be given to treat unconscious patients or those with suspected narcotic overdose.
- If you can't take the patient's temperature, use patient history to determine it. Don't actively warm or cool patients.
- Stroke is a serious medical condition in which blood supply to areas of the brain is interrupted. Ischemic stroke results from a blocked blood vessel. Hemorrhagic stroke results from bleeding within the brain.
- Patients with stroke can be affected in their language, movement, sensation, level of consciousness, and blood pressure.
- Time is essential in managing strokes. Fibrinolytics can be administered for ischemic strokes, but must be administered within 3 hours of stroke onset.
- Use the Cincinnati Prehospital Stroke Scale or Los Angeles Prehospital Stroke Screen during assessment of a potential stroke patient. You may also use a fibrinolytic checklist.
- Stroke patients should be transported to facilities trained in the administration of fibrinolytics, and to facilities with CT or MRI equipment.
- A TIA looks like a stroke but will resolve without damage; however, one third of patients with a TIA will eventually experience a stroke.
- Management of TIAs is the same as for stroke. Encourage the patient to be transported.
- Use the AEIOU-TIPS mnemonic to assess a patient with an altered level of consciousness. Evaluate the speed and onset. Common effects of altered LOC are changes in thought, speech, and movement. Total unresponsiveness can also result.

- Prehospital care for a patient with an altered LOC includes the ABCs and gathering information about the possible cause.
- Seizures are the sudden erratic firing of neurons, generally characterized by involuntary shaking. They are classified as generalized (affecting large areas of the brain) or partial (affecting limited areas of the brain).
- Generalized seizures include tonic-clonic and absence seizures. Tonic-clonic seizures generally consist of an aura, loss of consciousness, tonic-clonic movement, and the postictal phase. Absence seizures involve little or no movement. Instead, the person—usually a child—simply "freezes."
- Partial seizures are categorized as simple or complex. Simple partial seizures involve movement or altered sensation in one part of the body. Complex partial seizures involve subtle changes in level of consciousness.
- When caring for a patient with a seizure, don't try to stop the seizing movement. Prevent the patient from injuring himself or herself. Once the seizure has ceased, provide prehospital care and emotional support.
- Status epilepticus is a seizure lasting more than 4 or 5 minutes or consecutive seizures without return of consciousness between events.
- Prehospital care for a patient with status epilepticus includes administration of benzodiazepines and management of airway and ventilation.
- Syncope (fainting) is the sudden loss of consciousness and postural tone. It can be caused by cardiac problems, dehydration, hypoglycemia, or a vasovagal reaction.
- Prehospital care for patient who experienced syncope includes standard prehospital care and emotional support.
- Types of headaches include muscle tension headaches, migraines, cluster headaches, sinus headaches, and headaches caused by a tumour, stroke, infections, hypertension, or inflammation of the temporal artery.
- Prehospital care for patients with headaches includes standard prehospital care, a thorough history, potentially medication administration, and providing a dark, quiet environment.
- An abscess is a walled-off infectious area within the cranial vault. Symptoms include a fever, persistent headache, drowsiness, confusion, general or focal seizures, nausea and vomiting, focal motor or sensory impairments, and hemiparesis. Provide standard prehospital care.
- Multiple sclerosis is an autoimmune disorder that damages myelin of the brain and spinal cord. Patients can experience attacks and remissions, muscle weakness, changes in sensation, pain, ataxia, intension tremors, and speech and vision changes. Prehospital management is supportive.
- Neoplasm, for the purposes of this chapter, is cancer in the brain or spinal cord. It can have a gradual or sudden onset. Symptoms include headaches, seizures, change in mental status, and stroke-like signs and symptoms. Prehospital care is supportive.
- Dystonia is the sudden onset of severe, sometimes painful, abnormal muscle contractions. Prehospital care involves ruling out other causes and administering diphenhydramine if you suspect the dystonia is a result of a reaction to antipsychotics.
- In Parkinson's disease, the brain cannot produce dopamine. These patients have tremors, bradykinesia, postural instability, and rigidity. Prehospital management is standard care.
- Trigeminal neuralgia is irritation of the trigeminal nerve. Patients experience severe electric shock-like pain in the face, which can be triggered by any activity that stimulates the face. Prehospital management is standard care.

- Bell's palsy is a temporary, sudden paralysis of the facial nerve triggered by an infection. The patient may have ptosis, facial droop, facial weakness, drooling, and loss of the ability to taste. Prehospital management is standard care.
- Amyotrophic lateral sclerosis is a disease in which the motor neurons die. It has a gradual onset with fatigue, weakness, ataxia, severe body-wide weakness, and eventual immobility. Prehospital management is standard care.
- Guillain-Barré syndrome is a rare condition characterized by a sudden onset of weakness and paresthesia ascending from the toes to the head. Patients usually have an infection prior to the attack. Prehospital management is standard care with airway management.
- Poliomyelitis is a viral infection that attacks the myelin of motor neurons in the brain and brain stem. Symptoms include a sore throat, nausea, vomiting, diarrhea, a stiff neck, and weakness or paralysis of muscles. Prehospital management is standard care with careful attention to the airway.
- Patients who had poliomyelitis in the past may develop postpolio syndrome later in life in which they experience the same symptoms as in the original infection, only milder.
- Cerebral palsy is a developmental condition in which the frontal lobe of the brain suffers damage. Infants may have developmental delays in walking and standing, muscles in constant contraction, a scissors walking gait, and tremors. Prehospital management is supportive.
- Spina bifida is a developmental condition in which the neural tube fails to close completely and part of the spinal cord or vertebrae are damaged and misplaced outside the normal position. Prehospital management is standard care.
- Myasthenia gravis is a condition in which the body creates antibodies against acetylcholine receptors, causing acetylcholine levels to fall. Symptoms include weakness of the face and eyes, difficulty swallowing, and leg weakness. Prehospital management is standard care.
- Peripheral neuropathy is a group of conditions characterized by damage to the peripheral nerves. Diabetic neuropathy occurs from high blood glucose levels. Patients may have paresthesia, burning sensation, and muscle weakness. Prehospital care is supportive.
- Muscular dystrophy is a group of nonneurologic conditions in which muscle tissue degenerates. It generally presents with progressive muscle weakness, delayed development of muscle motor skills, ptosis, drooling, and poor muscle tone. Prehospital management is standard care, possible with ventilatory support.

■ **Vital Vocabulary**

abscesses Areas created as a result of infection within the brain or spinal cord, in which brain cells have been attacked and tissue destroyed. The immune system erects a wall to prevent spread of the infection, which results in a pus-filled area buried in tissue.

adrenal glands Endocrine glands located on top of the kidneys that release adrenaline when stimulated by the sympathetic nervous system.

agnosia Inability to connect an object with its correct name.

Alzheimer's disease A progressive organic condition in which neurons die, causing dementia.

amyotrophic lateral sclerosis (ALS) Also known as Lou Gehrig's disease, this disease strikes the voluntary motor neurons, causing their death. It is characterized by fatigue and general weakness of muscle groups; eventually, the patient will not be able to walk, eat, or speak.

anesthesia Lack of feeling within a body part.

anisocoria Unequal pupils (difference greater than 1 mm).

apraxia Inability to connect an object with its proper use.

ataxia Alteration in the ability to perform coordinated motions like walking.

aura Sensations experienced before an attack occurs. Common in seizures and migraine headaches.

axon A projection from a neuron that makes connections with adjacent cells.

Bell's palsy A temporary paralysis of the facial nerve (7th cranial nerve), which controls the muscles on each side of the face.

bradykinesia The slowing down of voluntary body movements. Found in Parkinson's disease.

brain stem The area of the brain between the spinal cord and cerebrum, surrounded by the cerebellum; controls functions that are necessary for life, such as respirations.

central nervous system (CNS) The brain and spinal cord.

cerebellum The region of the brain essential in coordinating muscle movements of the body.

cerebral palsy (CP) A developmental condition in which damage is done to the brain. It presents during infancy as delays in walking or crawling, and can take on a spastic form in which muscles are in a near constant state of contraction.

cerebrovascular accident (CVA) An interruption of blood flow to the brain that results in the loss of brain function.

clonic activity Type of seizure movement involving the contraction and relaxation of muscle groups.

coma A state in which one does not respond to verbal or painful stimuli.

decerebrate posturing Abnormal extension of the arms with rotation of the wrists along with toe pointing. This indicates brain stem damage.

decorticate posturing Abnormal flexion of the arms toward the chest with the toes pointed. This indicates lower cerebral damage.

decussation Movement of nerves from one side of the brain to the opposite side of the body.

dementia The slow onset of progressive disorientation, shortened attention span, and loss of cognitive function.

diencephalon The part of the brain between the brain stem and the cerebrum that includes the thalamus, the subthalamus, hypothalamus, and epithalamus.

dystonia Contractions of the body into a bizarre position.

endotoxin A toxin released by some bacteria when they die.

exotoxin A toxin that is secreted by living cells to aid in the death and digestion of other cells.

expressive aphasia Damage to or loss of the ability to speak.

gait Walking pattern.

Glasgow Coma Scale (GCS) Evaluation tool used to determine level of consciousness. Effective in determining patient outcomes.

global aphasia Damage to or loss of both the ability to speak and the ability to understand speech.

Guillain-Barré syndrome A rare condition that begins as weakness and tingling sensations in the legs and moves to the arms and thorax; it can lead to paralysis within 2 weeks.

hemiparesis Weakness of one side of the body.

hemiplegia Paralysis of one side of the body.

hemorrhagic One of the two main types of stroke; occurs as a result of bleeding inside the brain.

hypothalamus The most inferior portion of the diencephalon, it is responsible for control of many bodily functions, including heart rate, digestion, sexual development, temperature regulation, emotion, hunger, thirst, and regulation of the sleep cycle.

idiopathic Of no known cause.

intension tremors Tremors that occur when trying to accomplish a task.

ischemic One of the two main types of stroke; occurs when blood flow to a particular part of the brain is cut off by a blockage (eg, a clot) inside a blood vessel.

Jacksonian March The wave-like movement of a seizure from a point of focus to other areas of the brain.

limbic system Structures within the cerebrum and diencephalon that influence emotions, motivation, mood, and sensations of pain and pleasure.

medulla oblongata The inferior portion of the midbrain, which serves as a conduction pathway for both ascending and descending nerve tracts.

midbrain The part of the brain that is responsible for helping to regulate level of consciousness.

multiple sclerosis (MS) An autoimmune condition in which the body attacks the myelin of the brain and spinal cord, leading to gaps in the insulation normally provided by the myelin, causing scarring.

muscular dystrophy (MD) A nonneurologic condition of genetic origin in which defective DNA causes an error in the creation of muscle tissue, resulting in the degeneration of muscular tissue. This presents with progressive muscle weakness, delayed development of muscle motor skills, ptosis, drooling, and poor muscle tone.

myasthenia gravis A condition in which the body creates antibodies against the acetylcholine receptors, causing muscle weakness, often in the face.

myelin An insulating-type substance present in some neurons that allows the cell to consistently send its signal along the axon without "shorting out" or losing electricity to surrounding fluids and tissues.

myoclonus Jerking motions of the body.

neoplasms Tumours.

neurotransmitters Chemicals produced by the body that stimulate electrical reactions in adjacent neurons.

nystagmus The rhythmic shaking of the eyes.

paresthesia Sensation of tingling, numbness, or "pins and needles" in a body part.

Parkinson's disease A neurologic condition in which the portion of the brain responsible for production of dopamine is damaged or overused, resulting in tremors.

peripheral nervous system (PNS) The part of the nervous system that consists of 31 pairs of spinal nerves and 12 pairs of cranial nerves. These nerves may be sensory nerves, motor nerves, or connecting nerves.

peripheral neuropathy A group of conditions in which the nerves leaving the spinal cord are damaged, resulting in distortion of signals to or from the brain. One type is diabetic, in which the peripheral nerves are damaged as blood glucose levels rise, causing loss of sensation, numbness, burning, pain, paresthesia, and muscle weakness.

pituitary gland The gland that secretes hormones that regulate the function of many other glands in the body; also called the hypophysis.

poliomyelitis A viral infection that attacks the axons, especially motor axons, and destroys them, causing weakness, paralysis, and respiratory arrest. An effective vaccine has been developed and this disease is now rare.

pons The portion of the brain stem that lies below the midbrain and contains nerve fibres that affect sleep and respiration.

postictal The period of time after a seizure during which the brain is reorganizing activity.

postpolio syndrome A result of polio in which neurons break down and die, resulting in difficulty swallowing, weakness, fatigue, or breathing problems even after the patient has healed.

postural tremors Tremors that occur as the person holds a body part still.

prodrome The early signs and symptoms that occur before a disease or condition fully appear, eg, dizziness before fainting.

pronation Turning of the lower arms in a palm-downward manner.

psychosis Breaking with common reality and existing mainly within an internal world.

ptosis Drooping of an eyelid.

receptive aphasia Damage to or loss of the ability to understand speech.

rest tremors Tremors that occur when the body part is not in motion.

spina bifida A development defect in which a portion of the spinal cord or meninges may protrude outside of the vertebrae and possibly even outside of the body, usually at the lower third of the spine in the lumbar area.

status epilepticus A condition in which seizures recur every few minutes, or last more than 30 minutes.

synapses Gaps between nerve cells across which nervous stimuli are transmitted.

syncope Fainting spell or transient loss of consciousness.

tonic activity Type of seizure movement involving the constant contraction and trembling of muscle groups.

transient ischemic attack (TIA) A disorder of the brain in which brain cells temporarily stop working because of insufficient oxygen, causing stroke-like symptoms that resolve completely within 24 hours of onset.

trismus The involuntary contraction of the mouth resulting in clenched teeth. Occurs during seizures and head injuries.

uremia Severe kidney failure resulting in the buildup of waste products within the blood. Eventually brain functions will be impaired.

www.Paramedic.EMSzone.com/Canada

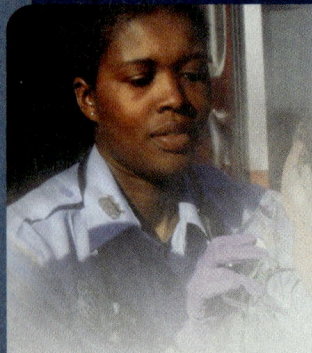

Assessment in Action

You're just walking in the door to start your shift when you are sent to a diabetic emergency. En route to the call, the fire department delivers an update: The patient is a 78-year-old man who is unconscious and unresponsive. On arrival, you find the patient supine on his bed. The fire department is preparing to move him to the ambulance. You notice that he has sonorous respirations; his skin is warm, dry, and normal in colour; blood pressure is 240/140 mm Hg; respirations are 24 breaths/min and shallow; pulse oximetry is 95% on room air; and heart rate is 78 beats/min. The patient has a left-side eye gaze and doesn't respond to painful or verbal stimuli.

When you interview the family, they report that the patient woke up today with no complaints and took a shower. After the shower, he collapsed onto the bed. They called 9-1-1 at approximately 08:00 hrs. The patient has type 2 diabetes. You immediately perform a blood glucose check, which comes back as 191 mg/dl. The patient is unable to control his airway; however, his mouth is clenched shut and you are unable to insert an oral airway. While the patient is being transferred to the ambulance, his respiratory rate decreases, allowing you to insert an oral airway. You prepare to intubate the patient and ventilate him with 100% oxygen via a bag-valve-mask device. En route to the hospital, you successfully intubate and secure the endotracheal tube.

Arriving at the hospital, you give your report to the emergency department. When you do your end-of-shift report, you are told the patient had a "huge cerebellum bleed." His prognosis is poor and the emergency department staff is speaking with the family about removing him from the ventilator.

1. _____ is a serious medical condition in which blood supply to areas of the brain is interrupted, resulting in ischemia.
   A. Myocardial infarction
   B. Pulmonary embolism
   C. Cerebrovascular accident
   D. Bell's palsy

2. The two basic types of strokes are ischemic and:
   A. neurologic.
   B. hemorrhagic.
   C. pathologic.
   D. neoplasm.

3. A hallmark of a hemorrhagic CVA is the:
   A. "worst headache of my life."
   B. "worst chest pain of my life."
   C. "worst blurred vision of my life."
   D. "worst weakness of my life."

4. The nervous system is the most complex organ in the human body. It consists of two major structures the_____ and_____ and thousands of nerves allowing every part of the body to communicate.
   A. brain, myocardium
   B. pulmonary, embolism
   C. brain, spinal cord
   D. spinal cord, myocardium

5. The major structures are divided into two main categories: the central nervous system and the:
   A. parasympathetic nervous system.
   B. sympathetic nervous system.
   C. peripheral nervous system.
   D. autonomic nervous system.

6. Weakness on one side of the body is called:
   A. hemiplegia.
   B. decussation.
   C. nystagmus.
   D. hemiparesis.

7. The _____ is located in the posterior, inferior area of the skull.
   A. medulla oblongata
   B. cerebellum
   C. midbrain
   D. cerebrum

8. The synapse, which is present wherever a nerve cell terminates, connects to the next cell through chemicals called:
   A. synapse.
   B. dendrites.
   C. neurotransmitters.
   D. axon terminals.

9. A hallmark of increased ICP is Cushing's reflex, which means:
   A. bradycardia, bradypnea, and widened pulse pressure.
   B. tachycardia, tachypnea, and narrowing pulse pressure.
   C. bradycardia, tachypnea, and widened pulse pressure.
   D. tachycardia, bradypnea, and widened pulse pressure.

10. Time is essential in treating either kind of stroke. The American Heart Association states:
    A. Time is muscle.
    B. Time is brain.
    C. Time is essential.
    D. Time doesn't matter.

Challenging Questions

You're dispatched to an assisted living home for an 83-year-old woman with an altered mental status. When you arrive and the patient is speaking to you, she appears confused and repeats her statements. Her vital signs are all within normal limits: blood pressure, 130/70 mm Hg; heart rate, 84 beats/min; respiratory rate, 18 breaths/min; and pulse oximetry, 99% on room air. The staff taking care of her reports that she "hasn't been right all day." The paperwork provided to you by the staff is incomplete; however, the medication list is there and you see Aricept.

11. What type of medical history do you suspect based on this medication?

12. How should you provide prehospital care for this patient?

Points to Ponder

You and your partner are dispatched to a private residence for a seizure. When you arrive on scene, you find a 24-year-old man who is responsive to verbal stimuli but is nonverbal. The family reports that the patient had a seizure, which lasted approximately 3 minutes. It was a full-body, normal seizure for the patient. He is in his normal postictal state as well. There is positive incontinence to urine and no tongue laceration. His blood pressure is 130/90 mm Hg; heart rate is 93 beats/min; respiratory rate is 16 breaths/min; and pulse oximetry is 98% on room air.

During transport to the hospital, the patient slowly becomes more responsive. He appears scared and keeps asking, "What happened?" You explain that he apparently had a seizure. You keep reassuring him throughout the transport to the hospital. On arrival, he is less apprehensive and you give your report to the emergency department. During your follow-up, you find out he was treated and released from the hospital. The patient apparently did not take his Dilantin for several days.

How can you narrow down the cause of a seizure in the prehospital environment? What benefits does this provide for patient prehospital care?

Issues: Understanding and Implementing Treatment of a Patient Who Experienced a Seizure, Empathy for the Patient Who Regains Consciousness Among Strangers.

29 Endocrine Emergencies

Competency Areas

Area 4: Assessment and Diagnostics

4.2.a   Obtain list of patient's allergies.

4.2.b   Obtain list of patient's medications.

4.2.c   Obtain chief complaint and/or incident history from patient, family members, and/or bystanders.

4.2.d   Obtain information regarding patient's past medical history.

4.2.f   Obtain information regarding incident through accurate and complete scene assessment.

4.3.a   Conduct primary patient assessment and interpret findings.

4.3.l   Conduct assessment of the endocrine system and interpret findings.

4.5.c   Conduct glucometric testing and interpret findings.

Area 5: Therapeutics

5.5.c   Maintain peripheral intravenous (IV) access devices and infusions of crystalloid solutions without additives.

Area 6: Integration

6.1.i   Provide care to patient experiencing illness primarily involving endocrine system.

Appendix 4: Pathophysiology

I.   **Endocrine System**
Addison's disease
Cushing's disease
Diabetes mellitus
Thyroid disease

Appendix 5: Medications

H.   **Medications used to treat electrolyte and substrate imbalances.**

H.2   Antihypoglycemic Agents

H.3   Insulin

Introduction

Few other systems in the body share the level of responsibility assigned to the endocrine system. This system directly or indirectly influences almost every cell, organ, and function of the body. Consequently, patients with an endocrine disorder often present with a multitude of signs and symptoms that require a thorough assessment and immediate treatment to interrupt life-threatening emergencies.

Anatomy and Physiology

The endocrine system comprises a network of glands that produce and secrete chemical messengers called hormones. The main function of the endocrine system and its hormone messengers is to maintain homeostasis and promote permanent structural changes. Maintaining homeostasis requires a response to any change in the body, such as low glucose or calcium levels in the blood.

Exocrine glands (*exo* means "outside") excrete chemicals for elimination. These glands have ducts that carry their secretions to the surface of the skin or into a body cavity. Sweat glands, salivary glands, and the liver are examples of exocrine glands.

Endocrine glands (*endo* means "inside") secrete or release chemicals that are used inside the body. These glands lack ducts, so they release hormones directly into the surrounding tissue and blood. Hormones act on the body's cells by increasing or decreasing the rate of cellular metabolism. They transfer information from one set of cells to another to coordinate bodily functions, such as the regulation of mood, growth and development, metabolism, tissue function, and sexual development and function.

Whereas the nervous system—the body's major controlling system—uses nerve impulses to activate and monitor the faster processes of the body, hormones of the endocrine system—considered the body's second great controlling system—are released directly into the bloodstream and act more slowly to achieve their effects. The hormones travel in the bloodstream to target tissues Figure 29-1 ▶ . Each target cell has specific receptor sites on the cell membrane, or inside the cell, to which the specific hormone can attach or bind. These receptors have two main functions: to recognize and bind to their particular hormones and to initiate an appropriate signal. Once the hormone has attached to the receptor site of the cell, the "message" to alter the cellular function is delivered.

Many cells contain multiple receptors and act as targets for several hormones—or for molecules introduced into the body as therapy. Agonists are molecules that bind to a cell's receptor and trigger a response by that cell; they produce some kind of action or biological effect. Antagonists are molecules that bind to a cell's receptor and block the action of agonists. Hormone antagonists are widely used as drugs.

Hormonal Regulation Mechanism

Hormones operate within feedback systems (either positive or negative) to maintain an optimal internal operating environment in the body. Release of hormones is regulated by chemical

You are the Paramedic Part 1

You and your partner are among the millions of national television viewers watching the high-profile murder trial that is taking place in your city in which a physician is accused of murdering his wife. Currently on the stand is the medical examiner, explaining the autopsy protocol and describing photos from the crime scene and autopsy. In the middle of her testimony, the judge unexpectedly calls for a 15-minute recess and your pager goes off. You are dispatched to the county courthouse for an unknown medical emergency. As you and your partner approach the courthouse, a police escort meets you and guides you and your partner through a sea of news vehicles and reporters. You safely enter the building from a restricted back entrance. You are then met by a deputy, who escorts you to a judge's chambers where you find your patient.

Lying on the couch is a middle-aged, well-nourished female patient. She appears to be extremely lethargic, pale, and diaphoretic. A fellow member of the jury explains that as the photos of the autopsy were being shown, the woman, Ms. Engle, suddenly went pale and passed out. She was immediately brought to the judge's chambers and placed on the couch. It is estimated that she was unconscious for approximately 1 to 2 minutes.

Initial Assessment	Recording Time: 0 Minutes
Appearance	Looks ill
Level of consciousness	V (Responsive to verbal stimuli)
Airway	Open
Breathing	Adequate chest rise and volume
Circulation	Weak, rapid radial pulse

1. What are some potential differential diagnoses?
2. When do symptoms of hypoglycemia occur?

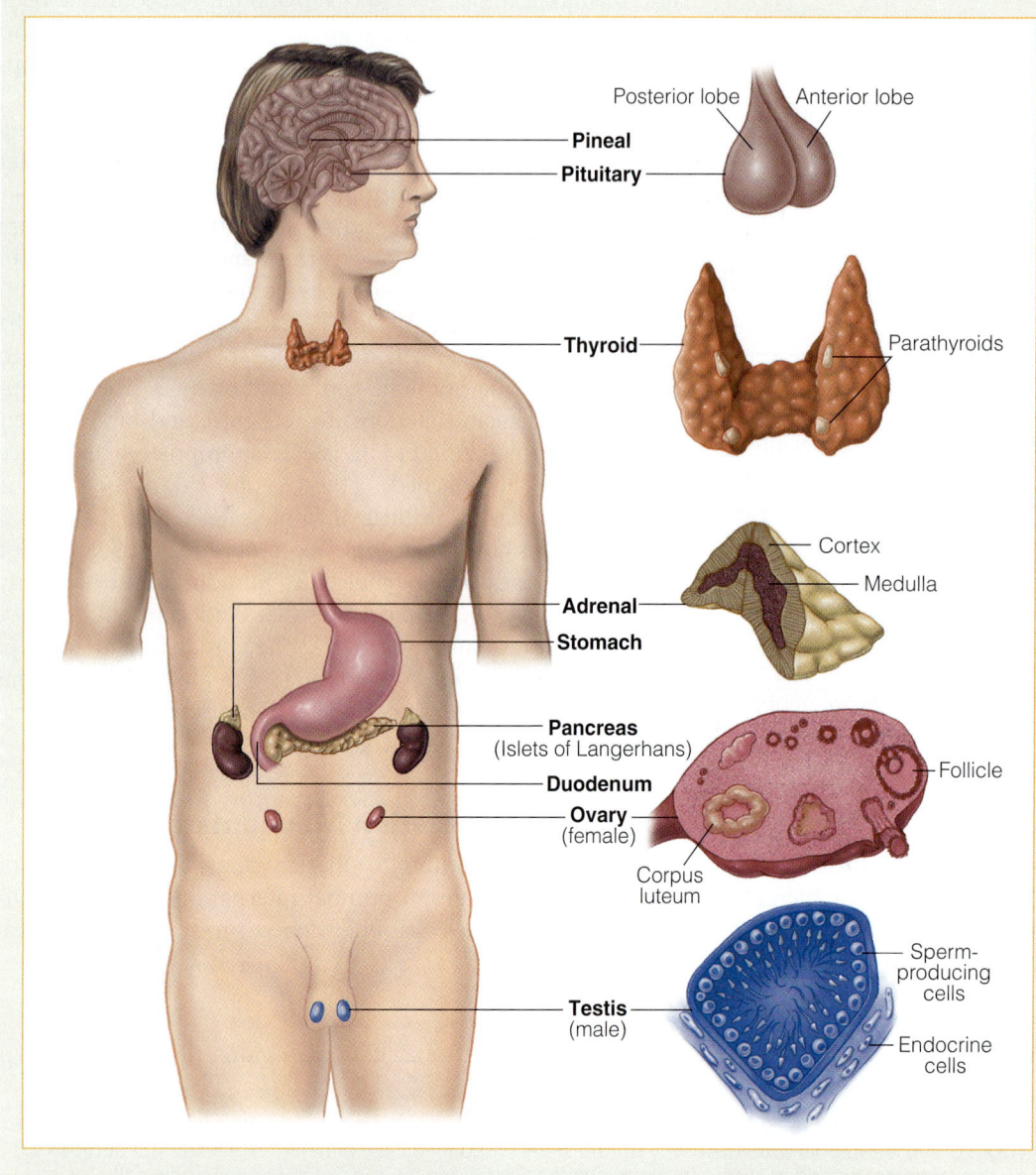

Posterior lobe   Anterior lobe

Pineal
Pituitary

Thyroid — Parathyroids

— Cortex
— Medulla
Adrenal
Stomach

Pancreas
(Islets of Langerhans)
Duodenum
Ovary
(female)
— Follicle

Corpus
luteum

Sperm-
producing
cells
Testis
(male)
Endocrine
cells

Figure 29-1 The endocrine system uses the various glands within the system to deliver chemical messages to organ systems throughout the body.

inappropriate cell function, which can cause harm to the organ or to the entire body. Cell signaling is covered in more detail in Chapter 6.

The hypothalamic–pituitary system controls the function of multiple peripheral endocrine organs (eg, thyroid, adrenal cortex, gonads, breasts). It is often considered a part of the endocrine system, because it sends signals to the adrenal gland to release the hormones epinephrine and norepinephrine. It also produces its own hormones: antidiuretic hormone (ADH), oxytocin, and regulatory hormones. The regulatory hormones control the release of hormones by the pituitary gland.

Some of these hormones have pharmacologic effects that depend on their concentration. For example, if there is a low or physiologic level of ADH in the bloodstream, the renal tubules are stimulated to reabsorb sodium and water. At the same time, ADH acts as a vasopressor, causing constriction of smooth muscle in arteries leading to increased blood pressure.

factors, other hormonal factors, and neural control. Endocrine regulation, through negative feedback, is the most important method by which hormonal secretion is maintained within a physiologic range.

One example of this negative feedback mechanism is the release of epinephrine from the adrenal medulla in response to stress. When stress stimulates the body's neural regulation (via the sympathetic nervous system), it releases epinephrine into the bloodstream from the adrenal medulla to assist the body's response to the stress stimuli. When the stress is removed, the nervous system stimulation decreases and less epinephrine is released   **Figure 29-2** ▶ .

Disease occurs when normal cell signaling is interrupted and the usual feedback mechanisms are disrupted, leading to

Components of the Endocrine System

The major components of the endocrine system are the hypothalamus, pituitary, thyroid, parathyroid, adrenals, and reproductive organs (gonads). The pancreas is also part of this system; it has a role in hormone production as well as in digestion.

Hypothalamus

The hypothalamus is a small region of the brain (not a gland) that contains several control centres for the body functions and emotions. It is the primary link between the endocrine system and the nervous system.

Pituitary Gland

The pituitary gland is often referred to as the "master gland" because its secretions control, or regulate, the secretions of other endocrine glands. It is located at the base of the brain and is about the size of a grape. The pituitary is attached to the

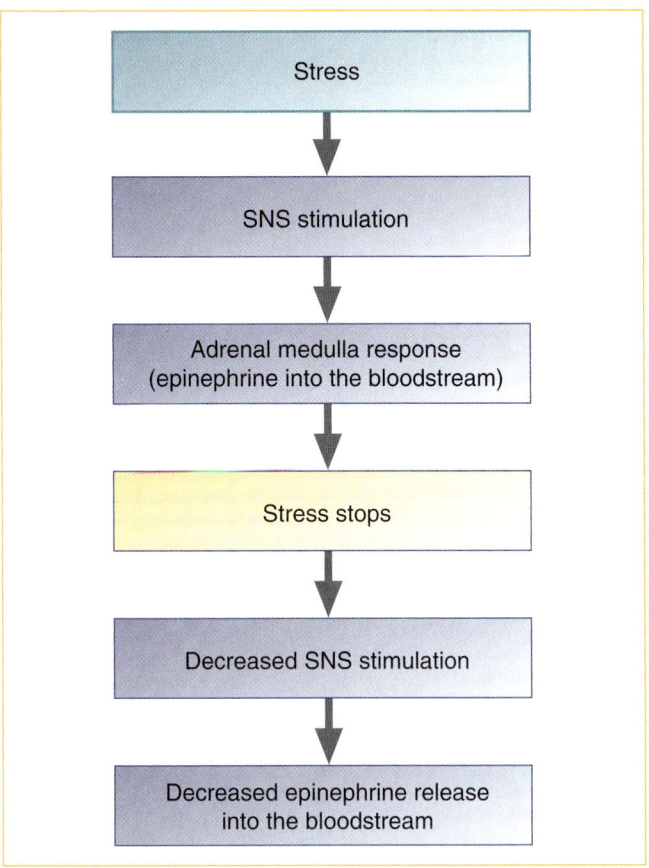

Figure 29-2 Stress stimulates the sympathetic nervous system (neural regulation) to signal the adrenal medulla to release epinephrine into the bloodstream to assist the body's "flight or fight" response. When the stimulus is eliminated, the neural regulating mechanism decreases its signals to the adrenal medulla and less epinephrine is released (negative feedback loop).

hypothalamus by a very thin piece of tissue. This gland is divided into two regions, or lobes: (1) the anterior pituitary, which produces and secretes six hormones (growth hormone, thyroid-stimulating hormone, adrenocorticotropin hormone, and three gonadotropic hormones); and (2) the posterior pituitary, which secretes two hormones (ADH and oxytocin) but does not produce them **Figure 29-3 ▸**. ADH and oxytocin are synthesized in hypothalamic neurons but are stored in the posterior pituitary gland until the hypothalamus sends nerve signals to the pituitary to release them.

Table 29-1 ▸ lists the eight hormones secreted by the pituitary gland. Six of these hormones stimulate other endocrine glands and are referred to as "tropic" (from the Greek *tropos*, meaning "to turn" or "change") hormones. The other two hormones control other bodily functions. The production and secretion of pituitary hormones can be influenced by factors such as emotions and seasonal changes.

Thyroid

The thyroid secretes thyroxine when the body's metabolic rate decreases. Thyroxine, the body's major metabolic hormone, stimulates energy production in cells, which increases the rate at which cells consume oxygen and use carbohydrates, fats, and proteins. When the body gets cold, for example, the increased cellular metabolism creates heat. Iodine is an important component of thyroxine. Without the proper level of dietary iodine intake, thyroxine can't be produced, and the individual's physical and mental growth are diminished. Thyroxine production is regulated by a negative feedback mechanism that prevents the hypothalamus from stimulating the thyroid.

The thyroid gland also secretes calcitonin, which helps maintain normal calcium levels in the blood. This hormone is secreted directly into the bloodstream when the thyroid detects high levels of calcium. Calcitonin travels to the bones, where it stimulates the bone-building cells to absorb the

You are the Paramedic Part 2

You ask your partner to obtain a set of vital signs and perform a blood glucose check while you begin your assessment of the patient. Your initial assessment reveals that she is responsive to verbal stimuli; however, she is unable to answer questions appropriately. The only other significant finding is a weak, rapid regular pulse. Your partner whispers to you that the blood glucose level came back at 1.8 mmol/l.

Vital Signs	Recording Time: 5 Minutes
Level of consciousness	Verbal
Pulse	130 beats/min, weak and regular
Blood pressure	122/68 mm Hg
Respirations	22 breaths/min, regular
Skin	Pale, cool, and diaphoretic
Sao_2	97% on room air

3. What are some of the causes of hypoglycemia?

4. How may a person with hypoglycemia present?

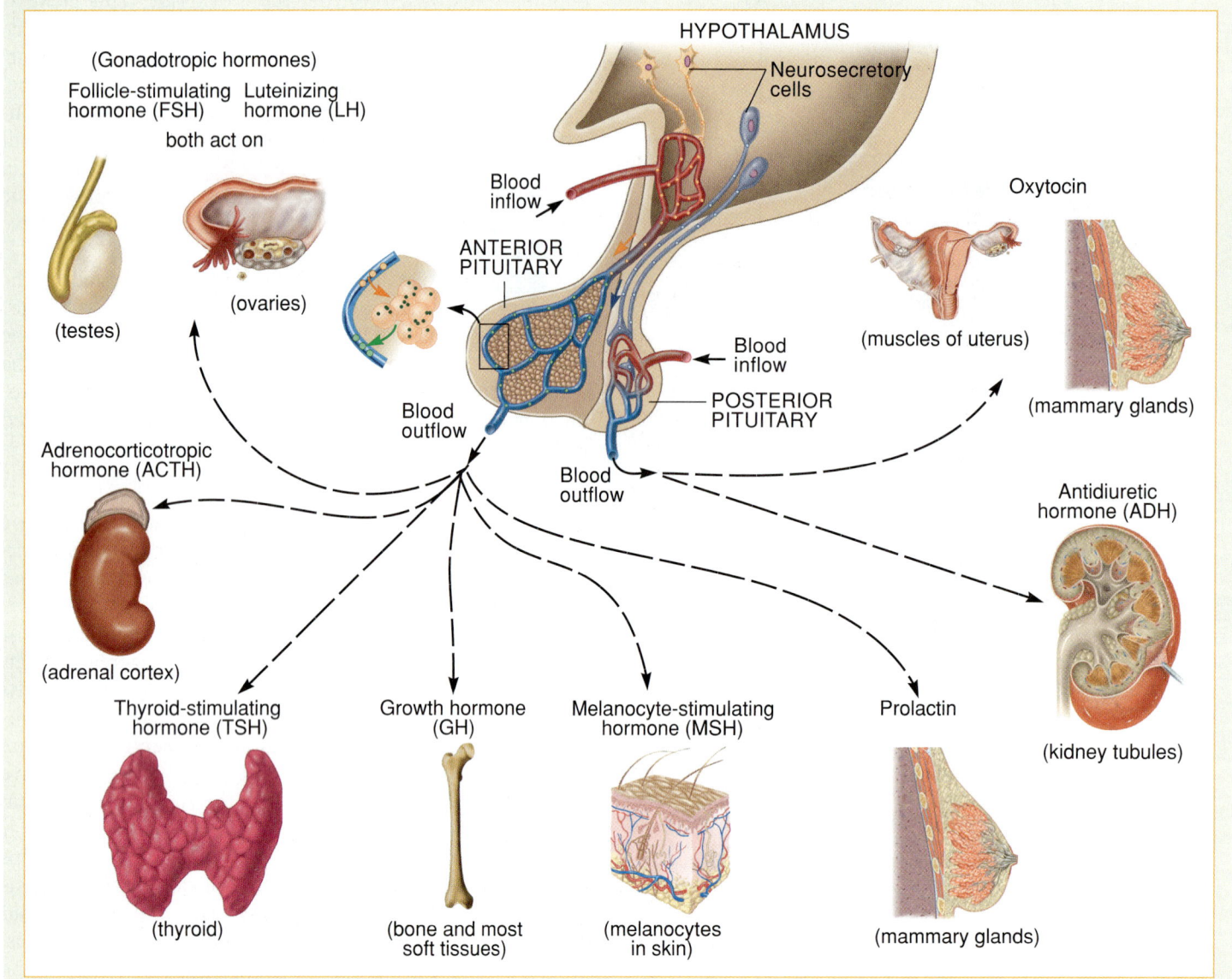

Figure 29-3 The pituitary gland secretes hormones from its two regions, the anterior pituitary lobe and the posterior pituitary lobe.

excess calcium. It also stimulates the kidneys to absorb and excrete excess calcium.

Parathyroid

The parathyroid gland also assists in the regulation of calcium. However, the parathyroid hormone (PTH), when secreted by the parathyroid, acts as an antagonist to calcitonin. PTH is secreted when calcium blood levels are low. It stimulates the bone-dissolving cells to break down bone and release calcium into the bloodstream. In the kidneys, PTH decreases the amount of calcium released in the urine. The secretion of PTH is regulated by the calcium level in the blood.

Adrenal Glands

The adrenal glands consist of two parts: an outer part, called the adrenal cortex, and an inner part, called the adrenal medulla Figure 29-4 ▸ . Both parts produce hormones Table 29-2 ▸ . The adrenal cortex produces two families of hormones called corticosteroids, and mineralocorticoids, which regulate the body's metabolism, its balance of salt and water, the immune system, and sexual function. The adrenal medulla produces hormones called catecholamines (epinephrine and norepinephrine), which assist the body in coping with physical and emotional stress by increasing the heart and respiratory rates and the blood pressure.

Table 29-1	Hormones Secreted by the Pituitary Gland
Growth hormone (GH)	Regulates metabolic processes related to growth and adaptation to physical and emotional stressors
Thyroid-stimulating hormone (TSH)	Increases production and secretion of thyroid hormone
Adrenocorticotropic hormone (ACTH)	Stimulates the adrenal gland to secrete cortisol and adrenal proteins that contribute to the maintenance of the adrenal gland
Luteinizing hormone (LH)	In women: ovulation, progesterone production In men: regulates spermatogenesis, testosterone production
Follicle-stimulating hormone (FSH)	In women: follicle maturation, estrogen production In men: spermatogenesis
Prolactin	Milk production
Antidiuretic hormone (ADH)	Controls plasma osmolality; increases the permeability of the distal renal tubules and collecting ducts, which leads to an increase in water reabsorption
Oxytocin	Contracts the uterus during childbirth and stimulates milk production

Table 29-2	Hormones of the Adrenal Glands
Cortisol	Increases metabolic rate, using fat and protein for energy
Aldosterone	Reabsorbs sodium and water from the urine, and excretes excess potassium
Epinephrine/norepinephrine	Stimulates sympathetic nervous system receptors

production. Cortisol is also necessary to maintain vascular smooth muscle tone.

If the body experiences a drop in blood pressure or volume, a decrease in sodium level, or an increase in the potassium level, the adrenal cortex is stimulated to secrete aldosterone (a mineralocorticoid). Aldosterone stimulates the kidneys to reabsorb sodium from the urine and excrete potassium by altering the osmotic gradient in the blood. When sodium is reabsorbed into the blood, water follows; this action increases both blood volume and blood pressure. Aldosterone also reduces the amount of salt and water lost through the sweat and salivary glands.

The body's reaction to physical or emotional stress is referred to as the "fight or flight" response. Following stimulation from the hypothalamus, the adrenal medulla secretes small amounts of norepinephrine and large amounts of epinephrine. Norepinephrine raises blood pressure by causing blood vessels and skeletal muscles to constrict. Epinephrine stimulates sympathetic nervous system receptors throughout the body. In addition, it stimulates the liver to convert glycogen to glucose for use as energy in the cells. The action of both hormones results in increased levels of oxygen and glucose in the blood and faster circulation of blood to the brain, heart, and muscles, which in turn enables the body to respond to the short-term emergency situation.

Pancreas

The pancreas is a digestive gland that is considered both an endocrine gland and an exocrine gland. It secretes digestive enzymes into the duodenum through the pancreatic duct. The exocrine component is responsible for the secretion of the digestive enzymes. The endocrine component comprises the islets of Langerhans. These cell groups within the pancreas act like "an organ within an organ." The main hormones they secrete—glucagon (produced by alpha cells) and insulin (produced by beta cells)—are responsible for the regulation of blood glucose levels Figure 29-5 ▶.

When the body's blood glucose level falls, such as between meals, glucagon is secreted to raise the glucose level and bring the body's energy back to normal. When it enters the bloodstream, glucagon stimulates the liver to change glycogen (a starch form of the sugar glucose made up of thousands of glucose units) into glucose, which is secreted into the bloodstream for distribution as an energy source for cells throughout the body.

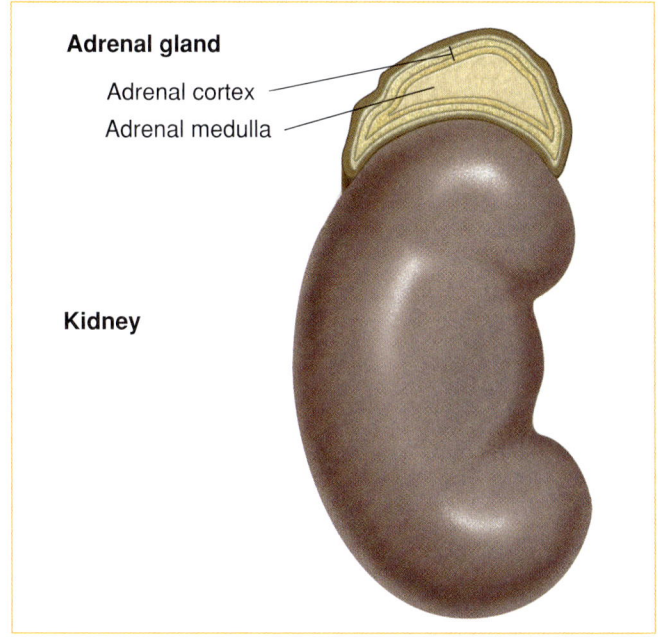

Adrenal gland
Adrenal cortex
Adrenal medulla

Kidney

Figure 29-4 The adrenal glands, which sit on top of the kidney, consist of two parts—the adrenal cortex and the adrenal medulla.

During times of stress, the hypothalamus secretes a hormone that stimulates the anterior pituitary to release adrenocorticotropic hormone (ACTH). ACTH targets the adrenal cortex and causes it to secrete cortisol (a glucocorticoid). Cortisol stimulates most body cells to increase their energy

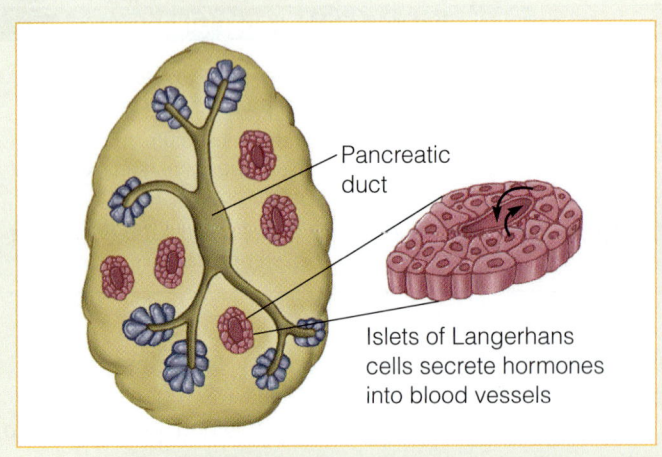

Pancreatic duct

Islets of Langerhans cells secrete hormones into blood vessels

Figure 29-5 The islets of Langerhans secrete hormones into blood vessels.

Table 29-3	Hormones of the Gonads
Male	
Testosterone	Main sex hormone in males Responsible for secondary sex characteristics: voice deepening, growth of facial hair, muscle development, pubic hair, growth spurts
Female	
Estrogen	Responsible for secondary sex characteristics: breast growth, fat accumulation at hips and thighs, pubic hair, growth spurts Involved in pregnancy Regulation of menstrual cycle
Progesterone	Involved in pregnancy Regulation of menstrual cycle Prevents maturation of additional egg during ovulation

Insulin enables cells to uptake glucose and allows for the storage of glycogen, fats, and protein. When blood glucose levels are elevated, beta cells of the islets of Langerhans secrete insulin, which is carried by the bloodstream to the cells. The cells then take in more glucose and use it to produce energy. Insulin also stimulates the liver to take in more glucose and store it as glycogen for later use by the body. Insulin is essential for transporting glucose into cells. Insulin is the *only* hormone that decreases blood glucose levels. Once the blood glucose levels have returned to normal, the islets of Langerhans stop secreting insulin.

Gonads

The gonads are the main source of sex hormones Table 29-3 ▲ . In men, the gonads, or testes, are located in the scrotum and produce hormones called androgens. The most important androgen in men is testosterone. Androgens regulate body changes associated with sexual development (puberty), including growth spurts, deepening of the voice, growth of facial and pubic hair, and muscle growth and strength.

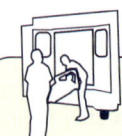

At the Scene

Although specific pathophysiology varies for each disease, endocrine emergencies are usually due to:
- Failure of normal hormone production
- Excessive hormone production
- Cellular resistance to hormones
- Failure of feedback inhibition systems involving the hypothalamus, pituitary gland, endocrine gland, and the target organ

In women, the gonads are the ovaries, which release the eggs and secrete the hormones estrogen and progesterone. Estrogen signals the anterior pituitary gland to secrete luteinizing hormone (LH) when an egg is developing in an ovarian follicle. Estrogen and progesterone also assist in the regulation of the menstrual cycle. At puberty, estrogen also supports development of the secondary sex characteristics: enlargement of the breasts, uterine enlargement, fat deposits in the hips and thighs, and development of hair under the arms and in the pubic area.

▌Pathophysiology

Endocrine disorders can be caused by hormone hypersecretion, leading to excessive target-gland activity. Target-organ underactivity can be caused by insufficient secretion of a hormone by a gland or resistance to a hormone at the target organ.

The effects of a disturbance of endocrine gland function are determined by the degree of dysfunction of the gland, as well as by the age and sex of the patient. All degrees of glandular dysfunction are possible, ranging from barely detectable variations to extreme dysfunction.

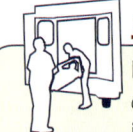

At the Scene

Despite their intricate pathophysiology, most clinically significant endocrine emergencies result in alterations of the ABCs, fluid balance, mental status, vital signs, and blood glucose level.

Diabetes Mellitus

The word *diabetes* is derived from the Greek word *diabainein,* meaning "to pass through," referring to excessive urination. *Mellitus* means "honey-sweet" and refers to the excessive glucose content of urine from patients with an impaired ability to regulate glucose levels. Glucose (also known as *dextrose,* referring to the biologically active form of glucose) is one of the basic sugars in the body and, along with oxygen, is the primary fuel for cellular metabolism.

Medically, the term diabetes mellitus refers to a metabolic disorder in which the body's ability to metabolize simple carbohydrates (glucose) is impaired. It is characterized by the passage of large quantities of urine containing glucose, significant thirst, and deterioration of body function.

This disease is characterized by an inability to sufficiently metabolize glucose. It occurs either because the pancreas does not produce enough insulin or because the cells do not respond to the effects of the insulin that is produced. Both cases result in elevated glucose levels in the blood and glucose in the urine. Glucose builds up in the blood, overflows into the urine, and flows out of the body. Thus cells can starve even though the blood contains large amounts of glucose Figure 29-6 ▶ . Note that another disease state, *diabetes insipidus*, also describes excessive urination, but this condition is related to problems with antidiuretic hormone (ADH) function that lead to excessive water loss in the urine. It should not be confused with diabetes mellitus.

In 2005, the Public Health Agency of Canada estimated that the total prevalence of diabetes in the Canada was 1.8 million people (5.5% of the population), equivalent to 1 out of every 18 Canadians. The rates increased with age—from about 2% of individuals in the third decade of life to about 21% of those aged 75 years or older. The distribution of diabetes differs across Canada, with a higher prevalence in Newfoundland and Labrador, Nova Scotia, New Brunswick, Manitoba, and Ontario. Quebec, British Columbia, Yukon, Alberta, and Nunavut have a lower prevalence compared with other provinces and territories.

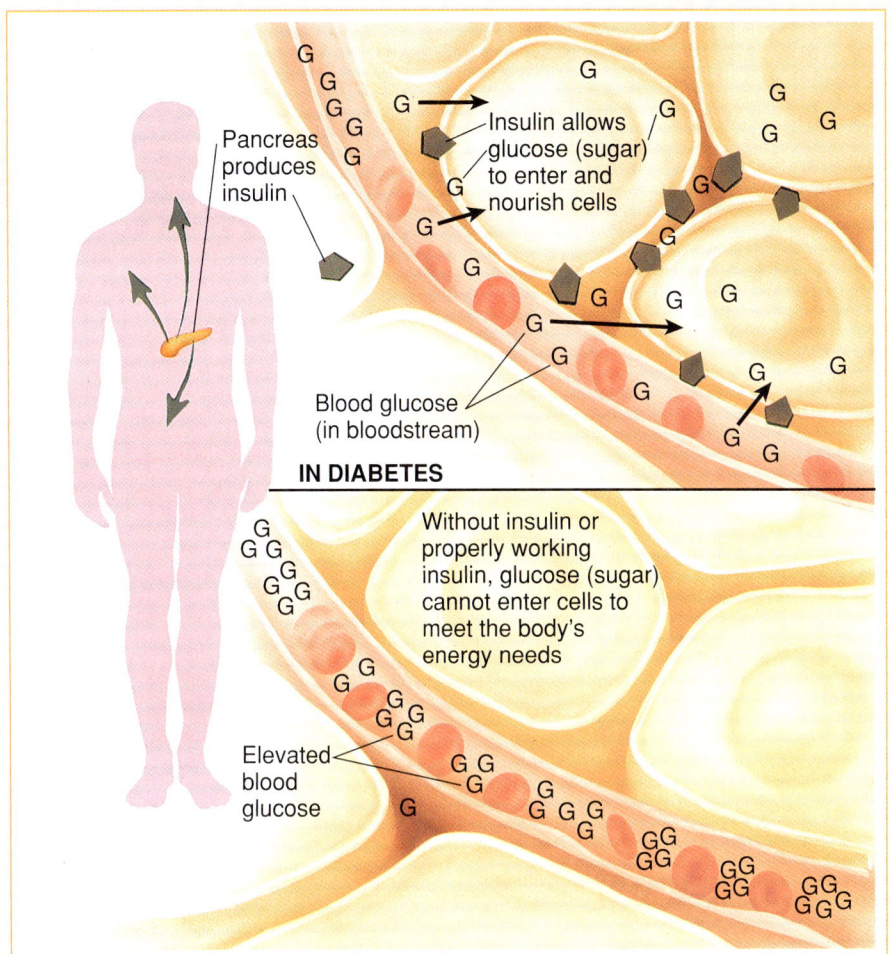

Figure 29-6 Diabetes is defined as a lack of or ineffective action of insulin. Without insulin, cells begin to "starve" because insulin is needed to allow glucose to enter and nourish the cells.

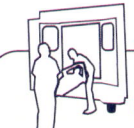

At the Scene

Macrovascular complications of diabetes include:
- Coronary artery disease/myocardial infarction (MI)
- Hypertension
- Dyslipidemia
- Peripheral vascular (foot ulcers/amputations)
- Cerebrovascular (stroke)

Microvascular complications of diabetes include:
- Retinopathy
- Nephropathy (end-stage renal disease)
- Neuropathy (paresthesias, sexual impotence, neurogenic bladder, constipation, diarrhea)

Left untreated, diabetes leads to wasting of body tissues and death. Even with medical care, some patients with particularly aggressive forms of diabetes will die relatively young from one or more complications of the disease. The severity of diabetic complications is related to how high the average blood glucose level is and how early in life the disease begins. Although most patients live a normal life span, they must be willing to adjust their lives to the demands of the disease, especially their eating habits and activities. There is no cure for the disease, so treatment focuses on maintaining blood glucose levels within the normal range.

Two forms of diabetes exist: type 1 and type 2. Both types are serious conditions that affect many tissues and functions other than the glucose-regulating mechanism, and both require life-long medical management.

Type 1 Diabetes Mellitus

Type 1 diabetes generally strikes children as opposed to adults, so it has been referred to as "juvenile diabetes." Although type 1 diabetes has a hereditary predisposition, it is now believed that environmental factors may be part of the cause—for example, an infection that triggers an autoimmune disorder (ie, antibodies destroy the islets of Langerhans).

In type 1 diabetes, most patients do not produce insulin at all. They require daily injections of supplementary, synthetic insulin throughout their lives to control blood glucose. Patients with type 1 diabetes also require insulin to inhibit production of ketoacids in the body. Failure to take insulin can lead to dangerous, and occasionally fatal, levels of ketoacids in the blood (known as *diabetic ketoacidosis,* or DKA), which is discussed later in detail. In addition to daily insulin injections, strict diet control must be observed; this can be difficult with young children. Increased activity and alcohol consumption can lead to low blood glucose levels. It is important to consider

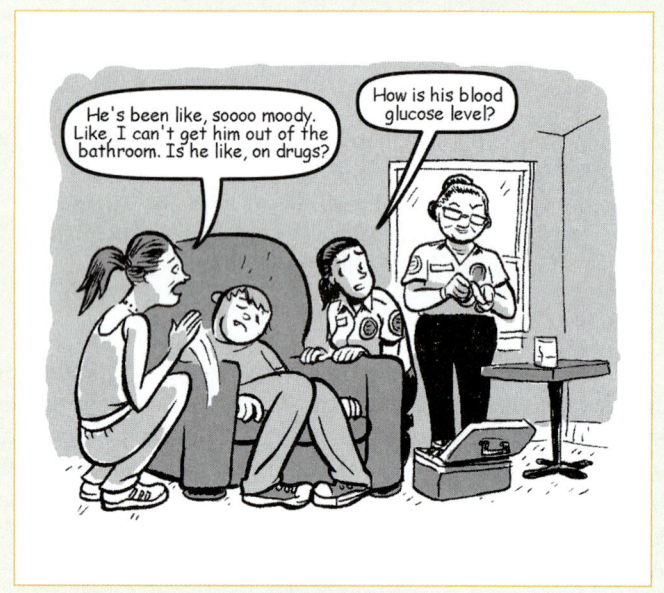

Figure 29-7

low blood glucose as a cause of altered mental status **Figure 29-7 ◄** . Complications of diabetes include kidney problems, nerve damage, blindness (diabetes is the number one cause of blindness), heart disease, and stroke.

Type 2 Diabetes Mellitus

The most common form of diabetes is type 2 diabetes (sometimes called adult-onset diabetes), in which blood glucose levels are elevated. The vast majority of diabetics in Canada suffer from type 2 diabetes, which typically develops later in life, usually when the patient is middle-aged, although the disease is becoming more common in younger people. Type 2 diabetes may be related to *metabolic syndrome,* a cluster of characteristics including excessive fat in the abdominal area, elevated blood pressure, and high levels of blood lipids. Risk factors for developing metabolic syndrome include excess weight, lack of physical activity, and genetic factors.

In many people with type 2 diabetes, the pancreas actually produces enough insulin; however, for reasons not fully understood, the body cannot effectively utilize it. This condition is known as insulin resistance. One possible explanation is that the insulin receptor cells located on the target cells have changed in some way and are no longer able to receive the insulin when it arrives at the target cell. Type 2 diabetes can also be caused by a deficiency in insulin production.

Symptoms of type 2 diabetes may include fatigue; nausea; frequent urination; thirst; unexplained weight loss; blurred vision; frequent infections and slow healing of wounds; being cranky, confused, or shaky; unresponsiveness; and seizure. These symptoms tend to develop gradually and usually become noticeable in middle age. In fact, the onset of type 2 diabetes may be so insidious that patients may not realize they suffer from the disorder. In some instances, the symptoms can develop over several years in overweight adults older than 40 years or even younger in patients with severe obesity. A small percentage of people do not display any symptoms.

Weight loss is an important factor in helping to control type 2 diabetes. Exercise and a well-balanced, nutritious diet are key components in combating the complications of diabetes. To maintain glucose levels within the normal range, food intake must be spread throughout an entire day, with a limit on simple carbohydrates. When diet and weight loss alone cannot control blood glucose levels, patients with type 2 diabetes may be started on oral medications to increase their sensitivity to insulin. In some cases, insulin injections are also used at high doses to overcome receptor resistance. These patients usually do not develop diabetic ketoacidosis when insulin is withheld, in contrast to type 1 diabetes patients.

Hypoglycemia

Hypoglycemia in the diabetic patient is often the result of having taken too much insulin or oral diabetes medication, too little food, or both. Unlike other organs, which can usually metabolize fat or protein in addition to glucose, the cells of the central nervous system (including the brain) depend entirely on glucose as their source of energy. If the level of glucose in the blood drops dramatically, the brain is starved. The patient will experience trembling, a rapid heart rate, sweating, and a feeling of hunger—a result of the actions of epinephrine. These symptoms reflect both the disordered function of hungry brain cells and the alarm reaction (sympathetic nervous system discharge) set off by the brain's distress. If hypoglycemia persists, cerebral dysfunction progresses very quickly to permanent brain damage. Additional signs and symptoms associated with hypoglycemia include headache, mental confusion, memory loss, incoordination, slurred speech, irritability, dilated pupils, and seizures and coma in severe cases.

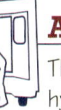

At the Scene

The longer a patient remains unconscious from hypoglycemia, the more likely there will be permanent brain damage! Severe hypoglycemia of longer than 30 minutes duration may lead to production of toxic compounds in the brain that can cause permanent neuronal damage.

Normal blood glucose is approximately 4 to 8 mmol/l, hypoglycemia occurs when blood glucose drops below 4 mmol/l. Hypoglycemia can develop *very rapidly*, from minutes to a few hours. It should be suspected in any patient with diabetes who presents with bizarre behaviour, neurologic signs, or coma. Often the hypoglycemic patient appears intoxicated, because of slurred speech and lack of coordination, and may be paranoid, hostile, and aggressive.

Of course, diabetics are not the only individuals who are prone to episodes of hypoglycemia. Alcoholics, patients who have ingested certain poisons or overdosed with certain drugs (notably aspirin), and patients with certain cancers, liver disease, kidney disease, and some other conditions may also suffer hypoglycemic episodes. Don't discount the possibility of hypoglycemia in a comatose patient just because the individual is not known to have diabetes. Conversely, don't let a known diagnosis of diabetes prevent you from considering other causes of coma. Diabetics are not immune to head injury, stroke, seizures, meningitis, and other traumatic injuries or conditions. Keep an open mind and assess the patient thoroughly. Hypoglycemia is one of the simplest causes of changes in level of awareness to fix.

Whenever you suspect hypoglycemia, treat it *immediately*: A hungry brain is a very unhappy brain, and permanent cerebral damage may ensue if blood glucose levels are not restored rapidly. Measure the patient's blood glucose, especially if his or her age or clinical history suggests that the problem may be stroke. Patients with severe hypoglycemia may present with strokelike symptoms. Hyperglycemia is associated with worse neurologic outcome after a stroke; therefore, it is important to detect hyperglycemia for subsequent treatment after arrival at the hospital 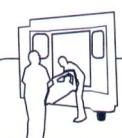 **Figure 29-8** ▶. When the comatose patient is older than 55 years or the family gives a history of recent transient ischemic attacks, perform a glucose test at the scene (Dextrostix, Chemstrip BG) to rule out hypoglycemia.

At the Scene

If uncertain of a patient's blood glucose level, always err on the "low side" and assume that hypoglycemia is present. A period of hypoglycemia is more dangerous to the patient than an equivalent period of hyperglycemia.

If the patient is alert, is able to swallow, and has an intact gag reflex, administer glucose by mouth. Provide a candy bar, a glass of warm water to which a few teaspoons of glucose have been added, a nondiet cola drink—any of those should do the trick. Do *not* give anything by mouth to a patient whose level of consciousness is depressed!

If the patient is in a coma, treat him or her as any other comatose patient, with attention to the airway and supplemental oxygen. Hold off on use of an advanced airway (ie, endotracheal tube, Combitube, laryngeal mask airway) if hypoglycemia is suspected, until you have given the patient $D_{50}W$ (50% dextrose); if the $D_{50}W$ works, the patient will pull out the endotracheal tube as soon as he or she wakes up!

Start an IV with a *large-bore cannula* (no smaller than 18-gauge) in a *big vein,* and hook up a 0.9% normal saline (NS) infusion. Check the IV carefully to confirm that it's patent and flowing freely. Inject a test bolus of 10 to 20 ml of NS infusion fluid, making sure the IV is not prone to infiltration. Recheck its status by lowering the IV bag and looking for backflow of blood into the infusion set. $D_{50}W$ is both hypertonic and acidic, and it can do a lot of damage if it infiltrates out of the vein and enters the surrounding tissue.

If you are certain the IV is reliable, open the IV wide (don't pinch it shut) and administer 25 g of $D_{50}W$ *slowly,* over at least 3 minutes. To ensure the patency of the line, draw back on the $D_{50}W$ syringe to observe a blood return. If the cause of coma is hypoglycemia, the patient will often waken with dramatic rapidity—although in cases of very severe hypoglycemia, another 25 g of $D_{50}W$ may be required to restore a normal level of consciousness.

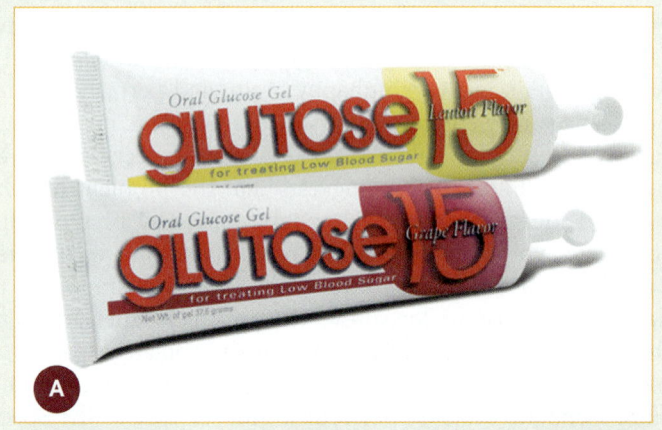

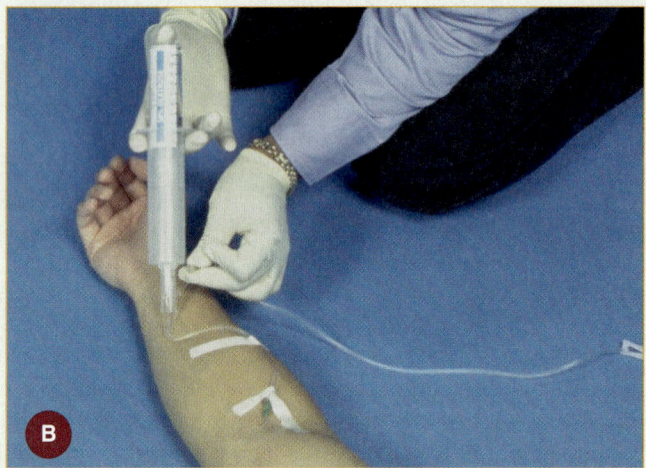

Figure 29-8 Administering glucose is appropriate in diabetic emergencies unless you have a reliable blood glucose measurement indicating normal or high blood glucose levels. Available forms include (**A**) oral glucose paste and (**B**) 50% glucose solution for IV administration.

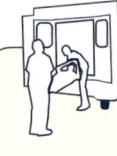 **At the Scene**

The exact value for the blood glucose is not extremely helpful. It is far more important to know the general range (very high, very low, or normal) plus the patient's clinical presentation.

If vascular access is not available, glucagon, 1 mg by intramuscular injection, should be given.

Hyperglycemia and Diabetic Ketoacidosis

Hyperglycemia (high blood glucose level) is one of the most common presenting features of diabetes mellitus. Common early symptoms also include frequent and excessive thirst, accompanied by frequent and excessive urination. A hyperglycemic condition without other classic symptoms does not confirm a diagnosis of diabetes mellitus, because hyperglycemia is also an independent medical condition with other causes. The signs and symptoms of hypoglycemia and hyperglycemia overlap, and therefore the paramedic should check blood glucose levels if *any* of the symptoms or signs of hyperglycemia or hypoglycemia are present   Table 29-4 ▶ .

Hyperglycemia occurs when levels of glucose in the blood exceed normal range. Doctors tend to try to keep the glucose levels of their diabetic patients at less than 8 mmol/l. Hyperglycemia can be caused by excessive food intake, insufficient insulin dosages, infection or illness, injury, surgery, and emotional stress. Onset may be rapid (within minutes) or gradual (hours to days), depending on the cause. For example, excessive food intake may cause blood glucose to rise quickly, whereas an infection or illness will result in hyperglycemia over the course of several days.

If left untreated, hyperglycemia will progress to diabetic ketoacidosis (DKA). A life-threatening condition, DKA occurs when certain acids accumulate in the body because insulin is not available   Figure 29-9 ▶ . Patients who suffer from this condition tend to be young—teenagers and young adults. In DKA, the deficiency of insulin prevents cells from taking up the extra glucose. From the viewpoint of the cells, famine is at hand, and a distress signal goes out over the sympathetic nervous system, causing the release of various stress hormones. Because the body can't utilize glucose, it turns instead to other sources of energy—principally, fat. The metabolism of fat generates *acids* and *ketones* as waste products. (The ketones give the characteristic fruity odour to the breath of a patent in DKA.) Because glucose must be excreted in the urine in solution, the body loses excessive amounts of water and electrolytes (sodium and potassium). This may lead to disturbances in water balance and acid–base balance. Disturbances in acid–base balance and the compensatory role of the kidneys are covered in more detail, in Chapter 6.

Meanwhile, glucose continues to accumulate in the blood. As the blood glucose rises, the patient undergoes massive osmotic diuresis (passing large amounts of urine because of the high solute concentration of the blood); this, together with vomiting, causes dehydration and even shock.

At the Scene

There is no predictable correlation between the increase in a patient's blood glucose level and the degree of ketoacidosis in the blood. Rely on the patient's clinical presentation rather than the "number."

These processes usually progress slowly, over a period of 12 to 48 hours, with the patient's level of consciousness deteriorating only gradually. Patients in DKA are seldom deeply comatose, so if the patient is totally unresponsive, look for another source of the coma, such as head injury, stroke, or drug overdose.

The signs and symptoms of DKA are generally predictable from the underlying pathophysiology:

- Polyuria (excessive urine output), because of osmotic diuresis
- Polydipsia (excessive thirst), because of dehydration
- Polyphagia (excessive eating), probably related to inefficient utilization of nutrients
- Nausea and vomiting, the latter worsening dehydration

Table 29-4	Characteristics of Hyperglycemia and Hypoglycemia	
	Hyperglycemia	**Hypoglycemia**
History		
Food intake	Excessive	Insufficient
Insulin dosage	Insufficient	Excessive
Onset	Gradual (hours to days)	Rapid, within minutes
Skin	Warm and dry	Pale and moist
Infection	Common	Uncommon
Gastrointestinal tract		
Thirst	Intense	Absent
Hunger	Absent	Intense
Vomiting	Common	Uncommon
Respiratory system		
Breathing	Rapid, deep (Kussmaul respirations)	Normal or rapid
Odour of breath	Sweet, fruity	Normal
Cardiovascular system		
Blood pressure	Normal to low	Low
Pulse	Normal or rapid and full	Rapid, weak
Nervous system		
Consciousness	Restless merging to coma	Irritability, confusion, seizure, or coma
Urine		
Glucose	Present	Absent
Acetone	Present	Absent
Treatment		
Response	Gradual, within 6 to 12 hours following medical treatment	Immediately after administration of glucose

At the Scene

Common causes of DKA include infection, injury, alcohol use, emotional discord, and illness, such as stroke or MI. Many of these conditions will lead patients to decide not to use their insulin as prescribed, which, in combination with physiologic stress, is a frequent setup for DKA.

- Tachycardia as a consequence of dehydration
- Deep, rapid respirations (Kussmaul respirations)—the body's attempt to compensate for metabolic acidosis by blowing off carbon dioxide
- Warm, dry skin and dry mucous membranes, also reflecting dehydration
- Fruity odour of ketones on the breath
- Sometimes fever, abdominal pain, and hypotension

The treatment of DKA in the prehospital setting depends on making the correct diagnosis. If the patient's history and physical examination are consistent with DKA and your measurement of the patient's glucose level reveals that it is markedly elevated (more than 16 mmol/l), the physician will probably order treatment for DKA. The goals of prehospital treatment are to begin rehydration and to correct the patient's electrolyte and acid–base abnormalities. In most instances, specific treatment with insulin should await the patient's arrival at the hospital, where therapy can be closely monitored with laboratory determinations of blood glucose, ketones, etc.

Follow the procedure for any comatose patient with regard to airway maintenance and oxygen. Be particularly alert for *vomiting*, and have suction ready.

Start an IV and infuse up to 1 l of NS over the first half hour or at the rate suggested by protocol or direct medical control. Remember, a patient in DKA is severely dehydrated, often to the point of shock, and needs volume, usually at a rate of about 1 l/h for at least the first few hours.

Monitor cardiac rhythm. Changes in serum potassium caused by DKA can lead to marked myocardial instability. Note the contour of the T waves on the rhythm strip; if they are sharply peaked, the patient's potassium level may be dangerously high, and you may need to administer sodium bicarbonate. If ordered to do so, proceed with extreme caution—even a little too much can cause serious problems, including death. Insulin will also cause potassium to shift into cells and drop blood potassium levels, so be aware that you may face very low or very high levels of potassium, which can change rapidly with treatment.

Hyperosmolar Nonketotic Coma

Hyperosmolar nonketotic coma (HONK), also called hyperosmolar hyperglycemic nonketotic coma (HHNC), is a metabolic derangement that occurs principally in patients with type 2 diabetes. This condition is characterized by hyperglycemia, hyperosmolarity, and an absence of significant ketosis.

Oddly enough, coma is present in fewer than 10% of cases. Instead, most patients present with severe dehydration and focal or global neurologic deficits. In addition, acute MI is frequently associated with HONK/HHNC. The clinical features of HONK/HHNC and DKA tend to overlap and are often observed simultaneously.

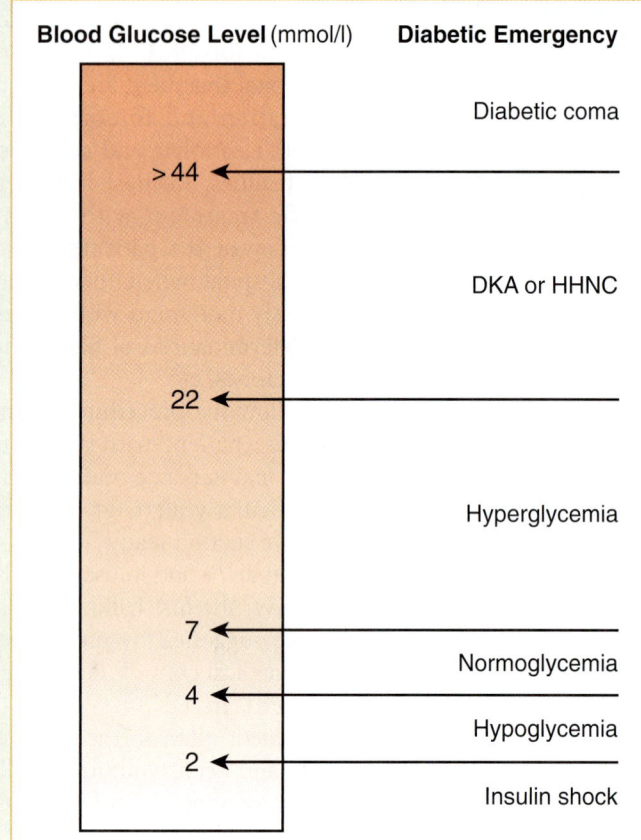

Figure 29-9 The two most common diabetic emergencies, diabetic ketoacidosis and insulin shock, develop when the patient has too much or too little glucose in the blood, respectively.

HONK/HHNC often develops in patients with diabetes who have some secondary illness that leads to reduced fluid intake. Although infection (in particular, pneumonia and urinary tract infection) is the most common cause, many other conditions can cause altered mentation or dehydration. In most cases, the secondary illness is not identified.

Hyperglycemia and hyperosmolarity lead to osmotic diuresis and an osmotic shift of fluid to the intravascular space, resulting in further intracellular dehydration. Unlike patients with DKA, patients with HONK/HHNC do not develop ketoacidosis. Although most patients diagnosed with HONK/HHNC have a known history of diabetes (usually type 2), approximately 30% do not have a prior diagnosis of diabetes. The stress

At the Scene

Certain medications may contribute to the development of HONK/HHNC by raising serum glucose, inhibiting insulin, or causing dehydration: diuretics, beta blockers, histamine-2 (H₂) blockers, dialysis, total parenteral nutrition, and dextrose-containing fluids.

At the Scene

Not all patients with increased blood glucose levels have DKA or HONK/HHNC. Many people have glucose intolerance and hyperglycemia with absolutely no symptoms. Look at the patient, not at the number.

response to any acute illness tends to increase hormones that favour elevated glucose levels; cortisol, catecholamines (epinephrine and norepinephrine), glucagon, and many other hormones have effects that tend to counter those of insulin. Various neurologic changes may be found, including drowsiness and lethargy, delirium and coma, focal or generalized seizures, visual disturbances, hemiparesis, and sensory deficits.

The treatment of HONK/HHNC in the prehospital setting follows the pathway for dehydration and altered mental status. Airway management is the top priority. The comatose patient is often unable to maintain and protect his or her airway. For this reason, endotracheal intubation may be indicated and should be completed as early as possible. Cervical spine immobilization should be used for all unresponsive patients found down, unless witnesses can validate that no fall occurred. Large-bore IV access should be gained as soon as possible, but do not delay transfer while initiating the IV. If necessary, obtain IV access during the transport to the emergency department. Also obtain a blood glucose level as soon as possible.

At the Scene

Although oral steroid therapy is the most common cause of exogenous adrenal suppression, inhaled steroids (used for asthma or chronic obstructive pulmonary disease) may also have a similar effect.

Once you have initiated the IV, a bolus of 500 ml 0.9% NS is appropriate for nearly all adults who are clinically dehydrated. In patients with a history of congestive heart failure and/or renal insufficiency, a 250-ml bolus may be a more appropriate starting point. Fluid deficits in HONK/HHNC patients may amount to 10 l or more. These patients may receive 1 to 2 l within the first hour. If the glucose level is less than 4 mmol/l (which is highly unusual in HONK/HHNC) and is the patient is symptomatic, then (depending on your local protocols), administer 25 g of D₅₀W as soon as possible.

Adrenal Insufficiency

Adrenal insufficiency is characterized by decreased function of the adrenal cortex and consequent underproduction of cortisol and aldosterone. A decrease in either of these adrenal hormones will result in weakness, dehydration, and the body's inability to maintain adequate blood pressue or to properly respond to stress.

Cortisol affects almost every organ and tissue in the body. Although its primary role is to assist with the body's response to stress, this adrenal hormone also helps maintain blood pressure and cardiovascular function; regulates the metabolism of carbohydrates, proteins, and fats; affects glucose levels in the blood by balancing the effects of insulin; and functions as an anti-inflammatory agent by slowing the inflammatory response.

Aldosterone regulates and maintains the salt and potassium balance in the blood. Secretion of this adrenal hormone is primarily regulated by the renin–angiotensin system, but is also stimulated by increased serum potassium concentrations.

Abnormal adrenal cortical function produces abnormalities in the metabolism of carbohydrates and protein as well as disturbances of salt and water metabolism. This condition is usually well tolerated unless there are coexisting factors (eg, infection, stress).

Primary Versus Secondary Adrenal Insufficiency

Adrenal insufficiency is classified as either primary or secondary. Primary adrenal insufficiency (also known as Addison's disease) is caused by atrophy or destruction of both adrenal glands, leading to deficiency of all the steroid hormones produced by these glands. A rare disease, it is most frequently the result of idiopathic atrophy, an autoimmune process in which the immune system creates antibodies that attack the adrenal cortex, which leads to its gradual destruction. This phenomenon accounts for most cases of Addison's disease cases in Canada. Adrenal insufficiency occurs when at least 90% of the adrenal cortex has been destroyed. Less commonly (approximately 30% of cases), the adrenal destruction is caused by tuberculosis; bacterial, viral (including HIV), or fungal infections; adrenal hemorrhage; or cancer of the adrenal glands.

Patients with Addison's disease who receive treatment have a normal life expectancy.

In patients with Addison's disease, the body fails to properly regulate the content of sodium, potassium, and water in body fluids. Blood volume and pressure fall, as does the concentration of sodium in the blood; blood potassium rises. The blood volume may become so reduced that the circulation can no longer be maintained efficiently. The smooth muscle tone in blood vessels can also be reduced, leading to vasodilatory shock in extreme cases. Patients with Addison's disease also frequently exhibit increased pigmentation of the skin, which is caused by the increased secretion of hormones **Figure 29-10 ▶** .

At the Scene

Signs of chronic adrenal insufficiency include unexplained weight loss, fatigue, vomiting, diarrhea, anorexia, salt craving, muscle and joint pain, abdominal pain, postural dizziness, and increased pigmentation in the extensor surfaces, palm creases, and oral mucosa.

Secondary adrenal insufficiency (a relatively common condition) is defined as a lack of ACTH secretion from the pituitary gland. ACTH, a pituitary messenger, stimulates the adrenal cortex to manufacture and secrete cortisol. If ACTH secretion is insufficient, cortisol production is not stimulated. Patients who abruptly stop taking corticosteroids (eg, oral prednisone, inhaled steroids for COPD/asthma, excessive doses of nasal steroids for sinusitis) may also experience secondary

You are the Paramedic Part 3

You quickly begin to look for an IV site as your partner prepares the equipment and a prefilled syringe of $D_{50}W$. An 18-gauge cannula is successfully inserted into the right antecubital fossa and you administer 25 grams of $D_{50}W$. Within a minute, your patient becomes more alert and is confused and scared about her surroundings.

You explain to the patient what happened while she was in the courtroom. She blushes and becomes embarrassed. She admits to being diabetic and tells you that the trial has been making her stressed and as a result she has not been eating properly and trying to self-regulate her insulin. She denies any other medical history, medications, or allergies.

Reassessment	Recording Time: 11 Minutes
Skin	Pink, warm, and dry
Pulse	85 beats/min, strong and regular
Blood pressure	116/74 mm Hg
Respirations	18 breaths/min, regular
Spo2	98% on room air
ECG	Sinus rhythm with no ectopy
Pupils	PERLA
Blood glucose	8 mmol/l

5. Which medications besides insulin can be used to control diabetes?

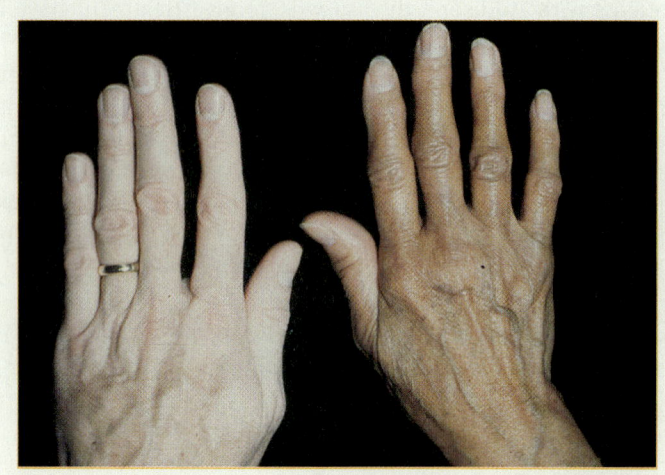

Figure 29-10 The hand of a patient with Addison's disease (right) compared with the hand of a normal subject (left).

adrenal insufficiency. Corticosteroid treatments suppress natural cortical production; however, aldosterone production is usually not affected with this form of adrenal insufficiency.

Addisonian Crisis

Signs and symptoms of acute adrenal insufficiency may appear suddenly and are referred to as an Addisonian crisis. They may result from an acute exacerbation of chronic insufficiency, usually brought on by a period of stress, trauma, surgery, or severe infection. Overly rapid reduction of prescribed steroids, or abrupt withdrawal, is the most common cause of acute adrenal crisis.

Although most patients with adrenal insufficiency experience symptoms that are severe enough to seek medical treatment prior to a crisis, approximately 25% of patients will develop their first symptoms during an Addisonian crisis. The primary clinical manifestation of adrenal crisis is shock. Patients may also manifest nonspecific symptoms, including

weakness; lethargy; confusion or loss of consciousness; low blood pressure (vascular collapse); elevated temperature; severe pain in the lower back, legs, or abdomen; and severe vomiting and diarrhea that leads to dehydration.

Treatment of Adrenal Insufficiency

Adrenal insufficiency is a potentially fatal disease if unrecognized and untreated. Death usually results from hypotension or cardiac dysrhythmias due to hyperkalemia. The treatment for adrenal insufficiency is based on the clinical presentation and findings, and is geared toward maintaining the airway, breathing, and circulation until arrival at the emergency department. Other goals of prehospital treatment are to begin rehydration of the patient and to correct the electrolyte and acid–base abnormalities. Ultimately, the patient's adrenal insufficiency and electrolyte abnormalities will require steroid hormone and possibly electrolyte replacement. This is done in the emergency department and not typically addressed in the prehospital setting.

Follow the procedure for a patient with altered mental status or comatose patient with regard to airway maintenance and supplemental oxygen. Be alert for *vomiting,* and have suction ready.

Start an IV and infuse up to 1 l of 0.9% NS. If the patient is hypotensive, administer an NS bolus at 20 ml/kg. Remember, a patient in adrenal insufficiency may be severely dehydrated, often to the point of shock, and needs volume.

Check the patient's glucose level. Administer 25 to 50 g of $D_{50}W$ to correct the hypoglycemia. D_5NS is the preferred IV fluid, but a second IV, administering D_5W, can be used to maintain the patient's blood glucose level. Monitor cardiac rhythm, as changes in serum electrolytes can lead to marked myocardial instability.

Cushing's Syndrome

Cushing's syndrome is caused by an excess of cortisol production by the adrenal glands or by excessive use of cortisol or other similar steroid (glucocorticoid) hormones. Tumours of

You are the Paramedic Part 4

Concerned about the attention she has brought to herself, your patient requests not to be transported to the hospital. She does not want to cause any further delays in the court proceedings or be removed from the jury. You explain to her that although her blood glucose level has returned to normal, it's still very important for her to be transported to the hospital to ensure that it will remain stable. Still hesitant about going to the hospital, the patient asks if she could contact her physician to get his opinion. You agree and help her place the call. After much convincing from her physician, she agrees to be transported to the hospital for observation.

Reassessment	Recording Time: 20 Minutes
Skin	Pink, warm, and dry
Pulse	84 beats/min, strong and irregular
Blood pressure	118/74 mm Hg
Respirations	18 breaths/min, regular
SpO_2	98% on room air
ECG	Sinus rhythm with no ectopy

6. Does diabetes affect other organ systems?

Table 29-5	Comparison of Major Effects of Hypothyroidism and Hyperthyroidism	
	Hypothyroidism	**Hyperthyroidism**
Cardiovascular effects	Slow pulse, reduced cardiac output	Rapid pulse, increased cardiac output
Metabolic effects	Decreased metabolism, cold skin, weight gain	Increased metabolism, skin hot and flushed, weight loss
Neuromuscular effects	Weakness, sluggish or absent reflexes	Tremor, hyperactive reflexes
Mental, emotional effects	Mental processes sluggish, personality placid	Restlessness, irritability, emotional lability
Gastrointestinal effects	Constipated	Diarrhea
General somatic effects	Cold, dry skin	Warm, moist skin

At the Scene

Patients with severe hyperthyroidism and severe hypothyroidism may require supplemental oxygen. Hyperthyroid metabolic activity increases oxygen demand and may have high-output cardiac failure. Hypothyroid conditions may lead to diminished respiratory effort that may require positive-pressure ventilation.

the pituitary gland or adrenal cortex can stimulate the production of excess hormone, for example, and lead to Cushing's syndrome. Administration of large amounts of cortisol or other glucocorticoid hormones (eg, hydrocortisone, prednisone, methylprednisolone, or dexamethasone) for the treatment of life-threatening illnesses, such as asthma, rheumatoid arthritis, systemic lupus, inflammatory bowel disease, and some allergies, can also cause this syndrome.

Regardless of the cause, excess cortisol causes characteristic changes in many body systems. Metabolism of carbohydrate, protein, and fat is disturbed, such that the blood glucose level rises. Protein synthesis is impaired so that body proteins are broken down, which leads to loss of muscle fibres and muscle weakness. Bones become weaker and more susceptible to fracture. Other common signs and symptoms related to excess cortisol include the following:

- Weakness and fatigue
- Depression and mood swings
- Increased thirst and urination
- High blood glucose level
- Hypertension
- Weight gain, especially on the abdomen, face ("moon face"), neck, and upper back ("buffalo hump")
- Thinning of the skin, with easy bruising and pink or purple stretch marks (striae) on the abdomen, thighs, breasts, and shoulders
- Increased acne, facial hair growth, and scalp hair loss in women, and cessation of menstrual periods
- Darkening of skin (acanthosis) on the neck
- Obesity and poor growth in height in children

The incidence of Cushing's syndrome is about 5 to 25 cases per 1 million people per year. It generally affects people between the ages of 25 and 45.

Prehospital treatment is generally supportive. Obtain a glucose level, monitor the patient's blood pressure, and treat abnormalities as they present.

Hypothyroidism and Hyperthyroidism

The hypothalamus secretes thyrotropin-releasing hormone (TRH), which acts on the anterior pituitary gland, causing it to release thyroid-stimulating hormone (TSH). The TSH then stimulates the thyroid gland to release thyroid hormone. Inadequate or excessive thyroid hormone results in hypothyroidism or hyperthyroidism, respectively. **Table 29-5** summarizes the major effects of hypothyroidism and hyperthyroidism.

Myxedema Coma

Thyroid hormones are critical for cell metabolism and organ function. If their supply becomes inadequate, organ tissues don't grow or mature (due to the decreased metabolic rate), energy production declines (a cause of the decreased metabolic rate), and the actions of other hormones are affected.

Many patients have silent hypothyroidism, which causes nonspecific symptoms, such as weight gain and fatigue. Severe adult hypothyroidism is sometimes called *myxedema*. The condition is manifested by a general slowing of the body's metabolic processes due to the reduction or absence of thyroid hormone. All organ systems may exhibit symptoms in such a case, with the severity of the symptoms reflecting the degree of hormone deficiency. Frequently, there are localized accumulations of mucinous material in the skin, which gives the disease its name (*myx* = mucin; *edema* = swelling) **Figure 29-11**.

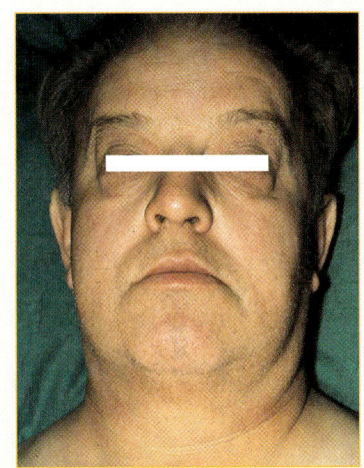

Figure 29-11 Localized accumulations of mucinous material in the neck of a hypothyroid patient.

Symptoms of hypothyroidism include fatigue, feeling cold, weight gain, dry skin, and sleepiness. Because these symptoms are often subtle and can be mistaken for other conditions, the disease may go undiagnosed. Continued decrease of the hormone levels may lead to myxedema coma, an extreme manifestation of untreated hypothyroidism that is accompanied by physiologic decompensation. When hypothyroidism is long standing, physiologic adaptations occur, such as reduced metabolic rate and decreased oxygen consumption, which in turn lead to peripheral vasoconstriction. Triggers such as infection (especially lung and urine infections), exposure to cold, trauma, surgery, and certain medications are often precipitating factors in the progression to myxedema coma.

The hallmark of myxedema coma is deterioration of the patient's mental status. Although family members may not be overly concerned about more subtle changes, such as apathy or decreased intellectual function, more obvious changes, such as confusion, psychosis, and coma, will most certainly elicit a call for emergency assistance.

Most cases of myxedema coma occur during the winter in women older than age 60. The condition is 4 to 8 times more common in women than in men. Just as the incidence of hypothyroidism increases with age, myxedema coma occurs primarily in elderly patients. One consistent finding is hypothermia, and you may need to use a thermometer that records temperatures of less than 32° C in cases of myxedema coma. Thus absence of fever in the presence of infection is a common finding.

Hypothyroidism decreases intestinal motility, and the decreased metabolic rate associated with this condition can lead to drug toxicity, especially in the elderly. A slower metabolic rate causes the levels of medications, especially those that affect the central nervous system, to rise to toxic levels in the blood. This accidental overdose in the hypothyroid patient can actually precipitate myxedema coma.

Myxedema coma is a metabolic and cardiovascular emergency. If not diagnosed and treated immediately, the mortality rates are approximately 50%. Thus the patient's condition must be stabilized as soon as possible.

Administer supplemental oxygen therapy to correct hypoxia. Intubation and ventilation are indicated for patients with diminished respiratory drive or those who are unable to protect their airway; these measures will help prevent respiratory failure.

Monitor the patient's cardiac status. Hypotension may respond to crystalloid therapy, and vasopressor agents may be necessary (eg, dopamine). Administer 25 to 50 g of $D_{50}W$ if glucose levels are less than 4 mmol/l and the patient is symptomatic.

Treat hypothermia with passive rewarming methods, as aggressive rewarming may lead to vasodilation and hypotension.

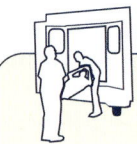

At the Scene

Protrusion of the eyeballs (exophthalmos) is common in chronic hyperthyroidism.

Hemodynamically unstable patients with profound hypothermia, however, will require active rewarming. Avoid sedatives, narcotics, and anesthetics because of the delayed metabolism.

Thyrotoxicosis

Thyrotoxicosis is a toxic condition caused by excessive levels of circulating thyroid hormone. Although hyperthyroidism can cause thyrotoxicosis in some patients, the two conditions are not identical. Thyrotoxicosis may also be caused by goiters, autoimmune disease (Grave's disease—the most common cause of hyperthyroidism), and thyroid cancer. Grave's disease, which has an incidence of 1.4 cases per 1,000 persons, has a chronic course with remissions and relapses. If left untreated, it may be fatal.

At the Scene

Both hyperthyroidism and hypothyroidism can adversely affect the electrical status of the myocardium. Application of the cardiac monitor may reveal tachyarrhythmias in hyperthyroidism or bradyarrhythmias in hypothyroidism. Treat all arrhythmias according to your local protocols, while keeping in mind that these arrhythmias may be difficult to correct without first fixing the underlying disorder.

A thyroid storm is a rare, life-threatening condition that may occur in patients with thyrotoxicosis. The condition is usually triggered by a stressful event or increased volume of thyroid hormones in the circulation. In addition to the normal signs and symptoms of hyperthyroidism, patients may present with fever, severe tachycardia, nausea, vomiting, altered mental status, and possibly heart failure. The management of thyroid storm is complex because it affects multiple organ systems. Paramedics should focus on and manage immediate threats to life, provide supportive care, and transport the patient promptly to the nearest emergency department.

General Assessment

The difficult part of assessing patients with endocrine emergencies is that their problems tend to affect many organ systems and the seriousness of their presentations varies greatly. Many of the patients will have had their conditions for some time and may already be receiving treatment. These patients or their family members will likely share with you that there is a history of an endocrine problem; this information, in addition to the common signs and symptoms associated with each endocrine emergency, should help you determine the cause of the current problem. In any event, don't take these calls lightly, as poor outcomes can result very quickly.

Scene Assessment

Your initial scene assessment will vary depending on the rate of the progression of deterioration and the patient's symptoms

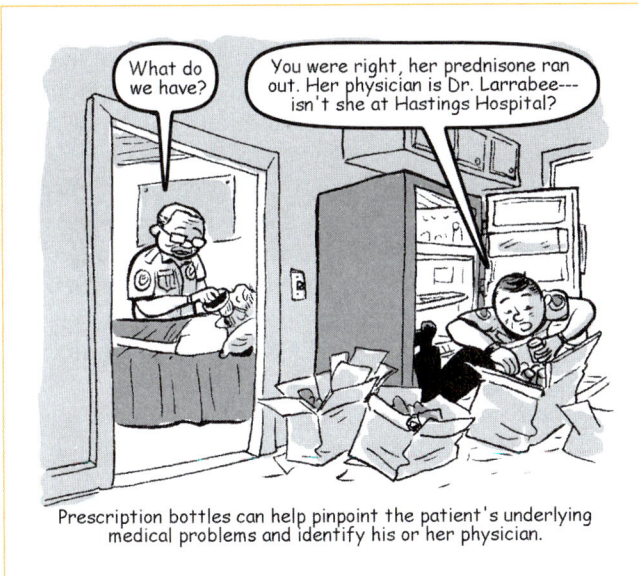

Prescription bottles can help pinpoint the patient's underlying medical problems and identify his or her physician.

Figure 29-12

when you arrive. Regardless of the patient's condition or the cause, airway, breathing, and circulation must always be assessed first.

Your observations of the scene in which the patient is found can also furnish valuable information regarding what might have happened. Check bureau tops, bedside tables, and medicine cabinets for medications that might give a clue as to the patient's underlying illness. Check the refrigerator for insulin **Figure 29-12 ▲**. Bring any medication bottles along with the patient to the hospital. They can help pinpoint the patient's underlying medical problems and identify his or her physician, who should be able to provide more information.

Initial Assessment

The initial assessment begins with the basics: airway, breathing, and circulation. Patients in the middle of any endocrine emergency may be in serious distress, so be prepared to assist them if your initial assessment reveals any of these basics to be abnormal.

When patients present with an altered level of consciousness, they may be unable to protect the airway. Many will be very ill and have chronic episodes of vomiting. Maintain the airway as needed through patient positioning, suctioning, or basic airways.

Patients with endocrine emergencies may present with varied respiratory status. Supplemental oxygen is recommended in all cases of suspected respiratory involvement. Do not hesitate to provide supplemental oxygen even in the presence of a normal oxygen saturation reading if you have any concerns about the patient's respiratory status.

Assess the patient's skin colour, moisture, and temperature, and take his or her blood pressure. Because endocrine emergencies may affect the body's ability to compensate for illness, IVs or blood component replenishment may be necessary. Follow your local protocols.

Many patients with endocrine disorders are being treated by specialists, and they should be transported to a facility that specializes in these conditions. If the patient is unstable or shows signs of becoming unstable, take him or her to the closest facility for stabilization first.

Focused History and Physical Examination

In diabetic emergencies in particular, the family history can provide very important information. Because genetics can influence the development of diabetes (passed down through family members), learning that a parent or grandparent has a diabetic history is a major clue, and may prove to be invaluable in your treatment decision. This is especially true if the patient is a child and has a new onset of altered mental status.

The goals of the physical examination in the comatose patient are twofold. First, you want to determine the patient's level of consciousness with precision, so that other examiners who assess him or her later can readily determine whether the patient's condition is improving or deteriorating. Second, you should look for signs that might provide clues to the source of coma.

Begin the physical assessment by observing the patient's general appearance and the position in which he or she is found. Patients found in awkward positions often have brain stem damage; conversely, a natural posture tends to be a good sign. Decorticate or decerebrate posturing should also be noted, if present; both are *bad* signs.

Your physical examination should be geared toward identifying as many atypical findings as possible. Using this information, you can make a more educated decision about treatment. Unless the patient had an endocrine emergency that caused some form of trauma, a rapid trauma assessment is usually not necessary.

Detailed Physical Examination

The detailed physical examination will reveal the finer abnormalities that will provide you with the final determining factors for your treatment.

The condition of the skin may be very informative. Cold, clammy skin is classically a sign of shock but may also signal severe hypoglycemia, as from an insulin reaction. Cold, dry skin may indicate overdose of sedative drugs or alcohol. Hot, dry skin suggests fever or, if the circumstances are appropriate, heat stroke.

In checking the vital signs, look for the combination of hypertension and bradycardia, which suggest increased intracranial pressure. Be alert for abnormal respiratory patterns. Cheyne-Stokes breathing usually points to a nonneurologic source of the coma. More worrisome are other abnormal breathing patterns, such as central neurogenic ventilation or huffing and puffing that doesn't seem to move much air. Look for "pararespiratory" motions, such as sneezing and yawning. An intact brain stem is required to produce a sneeze or a yawn, so both of those actions have positive prognostic significance. Hiccupping and coughing, by contrast, may indicate brain stem damage.

Ongoing Assessment

Once you've initiated your treatment plan, continually reassess the patient to check for obvious, and subtle, changes. For every action you take, there should be a response. No response *is* a response. Document your findings along the way.

■ General Management

Management of the ABCs should have been carried out during the initial assessment. Remember that a patient whose gag reflex is absent can't protect his or her own airway from aspiration and should be intubated at the earliest opportunity. If breathing is abnormally slow or shallow, assist breathing with bag-valve-mask ventilation. Give supplemental oxygen whether the patient is breathing spontaneously or being ventilated.

If the patient has altered mental status, establish an IV with 0.9% NS or a saline lock. Make an immediate determination of the blood glucose level and initiate treatment if the reading is less than 4 mmol/l. Give 25 g of $D_{50}W$; this dose will reverse most cases of hypoglycemia. If the patient doesn't come around after a dose of $D_{50}W$ or if you have any other reason to suspect narcotics overdosage (pinpoint pupils, needle tracks on the arms, depressed respirations), then consider administration of naloxone (Narcan).

Monitor the cardiac rhythm of every comatose patient. For the neurologic assessment, the most important consideration is not a single measurement at a single point in time but rather the *trend* shown by several measurements. Recheck vital signs, pupils, and level of consciousness (every 5 minutes in unstable patients and every 10 minutes in stable patients) and *record your findings* immediately.

Transport the comatose patient *supine* if he or she is intubated; otherwise, you may transport the patient in the stable side position (unless injuries preclude that position). If the patient must be supine (eg, because of suspected spine injury) and can't be intubated, keep the mouth and pharynx suctioned free of secretions, vomitus, and blood.

At the Scene

Obtaining blood specimens early is particularly important in the diabetic patient because any administration of prehospital dextrose or other medications will significantly change the chemical makeup of subsequent blood samples.

You are the Paramedic Summary

1. What are some potential differential diagnoses?

On the basis of the signs and symptoms, your patient's potential differential diagnoses can include hypotension, drug overdose, arrhythmias, and hypoglycemia.

2. When do symptoms of hypoglycemia occur?

Signs and symptoms of hypoglycemia usually occur once the blood glucose level falls below 4 mmol/l. However, if the drop in glucose levels is rapid, they can be seen at higher levels.

3. What are some of the causes of hypoglycemia?

The causes of hypoglycemia are very diverse. The more common causes of hypoglycemia in patients with diabetes are taking too much insulin or oral hypoglycemic medications, not eating enough, and unusual or extreme exercise without adequate food intake. Hypoglycemia may also be found in patients who are chronic alcoholics, suffer from malnutrition, or have pancreatic disorders, liver disease, hypothermia, cancer, or sepsis. Be on the lookout for intentional overdoses on insulin and oral hypoglycemic medications. People with a history of eating disorders may take insulin to burn off the "extra calories" of desserts or other foods that may be considered high calorie.

4. How may a patient with hypoglycemia present?

Why, you may actually be exhibiting signs and symptoms of hypoglycemia as you are studying this section! Are you hungry, irritable, shaky, or have a headache? Are you having glucose cravings? These are all signs and symptoms of hypoglycemia. Others include changes in mental status, appearance of intoxication, seizures, and coma. Vital sign changes will include a weak, rapid pulse and pale, cool, diaphoretic skin.

5. Which medications besides insulin can be used to control diabetes?

Patients with type 2 diabetes may be prescribed oral hypoglycemic agents to help regulate their glucose levels. Type 2 diabetics are able to use these medications because they work with the body's own insulin (they have working beta cells). Examples of commonly prescribed oral hypoglycemic agents include chlorpropamide, tolazide, tolbutamide, glipizide, and glyburide. Two newer medications include pioglitizone and metformin.

6. Does diabetes affect other organ systems?

Unfortunately, the answer to this question is yes. Diabetic patients are at risk for developing blindness, kidney disease, peripheral neuropathy, hypertension, atherosclerosis, heart disease, and peripheral vascular disease.

Prep Kit

Ready for Review

- The endocrine system directly or indirectly influences almost every cell, organ, and function of the body.
- Patients with an endocrine disorder often present with a multitude of signs and symptoms that require a thorough assessment and immediate treatment to interrupt life-threatening emergencies.
- The endocrine system comprises a network of glands that produce and secrete hormones. The main function of the endocrine system and its hormone messengers is to maintain homeostasis and promote permanent structural changes.
- Hormones travel in the bloodstream to target tissues.
- The major components of the endocrine system are the hypothalamus, pituitary, thyroid, parathyroid, adrenals, and reproductive organs (gonads). The pancreas is also part of this system; it has a role in hormone production as well as in digestion.
- The pituitary gland is often referred to as the "master gland" because its secretions control, or regulate, the secretions of other endocrine glands.
- The thyroid secretes thyroxine when the body's metabolic rate decreases. Thyroxine, the body's major metabolic hormone, stimulates energy production in cells, which increases the rate at which cells consume oxygen and use carbohydrates, fats, and proteins. The thyroid gland also secretes calcitonin, which helps maintain normal calcium levels in the blood.
- The adrenal glands produce hormones that regulate the body's metabolism, its balance of salt and water, the immune system, and sexual function. Adrenal hormones also help the body cope with physical and emotional stress by increasing the pulse and respiratory rates and the blood pressure.
- The pancreas secretes digestive enzymes as well as the hormones glucagon and insulin, which are responsible for the regulation of blood glucose levels.
- The gonads are the main source of sex hormones (Table 29-3). In men, the gonads, or testes, are located in the scrotum and produce hormones called androgens. The most important androgen in men is testosterone. Androgens regulate body changes associated with sexual development (puberty), including growth spurts, deepening of the voice, growth of facial and pubic hair, and muscle growth and strength.
- In women, the gonads are the ovaries, which release the eggs and secrete the hormones estrogen and progesterone.
- Diabetes is a metabolic disorder in which the body's ability to metabolize glucose is impaired. It is characterized by the passage of large quantities of urine containing glucose, significant thirst, and deterioration of body function.
- In type 1 diabetes, most patients do not produce insulin at all. They require daily injections of supplemental synthetic insulin throughout their lives to control blood glucose levels.
- The most common form of diabetes is type 2 diabetes (sometimes called adult-onset diabetes), in which blood glucose levels are elevated.
- Hypoglycemia in the insulin-dependent diabetic is often the result of having taken too much insulin, too little food, or both. The patient will experience trembling, a rapid pulse rate, sweating, and a feeling of hunger—a result of the actions of epinephrine.
- Hyperglycemia (high blood glucose level) is one of the classic symptoms of diabetes mellitus. Common early signs include frequent and excessive thirst, accompanied by frequent and excessive urination.
- If left untreated, hyperglycemia progresses to the life-threatening condition known as diabetic ketoacidosis (DKA). DKA occurs when certain acids accumulate in the body because insulin is not available. DKA usually occurs in patients with type 1 diabetes.

- Hyperosmolar nonketotic coma (HONK), also called hyperosmolar hyperglycemic nonketotic coma (HHNC), is a metabolic derangement that occurs principally in patients with type 2 diabetes. This condition is characterized by hyperglycemia, hyperosmolarity, and an absence of significant ketosis.
- Adrenal insufficiency is characterized by underproduction of cortisol and aldosterone, which leads to weakness, dehydration, and the body's inability to maintain adequate blood pressure or to properly respond to stress. Primary adrenal insufficiency (also known as Addison's disease) is caused by atrophy or destruction of both adrenal glands, leading to deficiency of all the steroid hormones produced by these glands. Secondary adrenal insufficiency is defined as a lack of ACTH secretion from the pituitary gland.
- Acute adrenal insufficiency is referred to as an Addisonian crisis, which may result from an acute exacerbation of chronic insufficiency, usually brought on by a period of stress, trauma, surgery, or severe infection.
- Cushing's syndrome is caused by an excess of cortisol production by the adrenal glands or by excessive use of cortisol or other similar steroid (glucocorticoid) hormones.
- Thyroid hormones are critical for cell metabolism and organ function. If their supply becomes inadequate, organ tissues don't grow or mature (due to the decreased metabolic rate), energy production declines (a cause of the decreased metabolic rate), and the actions of other hormones are affected.
- Symptoms of hypothyroidism include fatigue, feeling cold, weight gain, dry skin, and sleepiness. Continued decrease of the hormone levels may lead to myxedema coma.
- Thyrotoxicosis is a toxic condition caused by excessive levels of circulating thyroid hormone. A thyroid storm is a rare, life-threatening condition that may occur in patients with thyrotoxicosis.
- Assessing patients with endocrine emergencies can be difficult because their conditions tend to affect many organ systems and the seriousness of their presentations varies greatly. Don't take these calls lightly, as poor outcomes can result very quickly.

Vital Vocabulary

adrenal cortex The outer part of the adrenal glands that produces corticosteroids.

adrenal glands The two glands, each one located in the region of the upper poles of each kidney and made up of an adrenal cortex and adrenal medulla.

adrenal medulla The inner part of the adrenal glands that produces catecholamines (epinephrine and norepinephrine).

adrenocorticotropic hormone (ACTH) Hormone that targets the adrenal cortex to secrete cortisol (a glucocorticoid).

agonists Molecules that bind to a cell's receptor and trigger a response by that cell. Agonists produce some kind of action or biological effect.

aldosterone Hormone that stimulates the kidneys to reabsorb sodium from the urine and excrete potassium by altering the osmotic gradient in the blood.

androgens Male sex hormones that regulate body changes associated with sexual development (puberty), including growth spurts, deepening of the voice, growth of facial and pubic hair, and muscle growth and strength.

antagonist Molecules that bind to a cell's receptor and block the action of agonists. Hormone antagonists are widely used as drugs.

antidiuretic hormone (ADH) A hormone secreted by the posterior pituitary lobe of the pituitary gland, ADH constricts blood vessels and raises the blood pressure; also called vasopressin.

calcitonin A hormone released by the thyroid gland that inhibits the release of calcium from bone and lowers calcium levels in blood.

catecholamines Catechol hormones, epinephrine and norepinephrine, produced by the adrenal gland.

corticosteroids Hormones that regulate the body's metabolism, the balance of salt and water in the body, the immune system, and sexual function.

cortisol Hormone that stimulates most body cells to increase their energy production.

Cushing's syndrome A condition resulting from excessive production and release of cortisol.

diabetes mellitus Disease characterized by the body's inability to sufficiently metabolize glucose. The condition occurs either because the pancreas doesn't produce enough insulin or the cells don't respond to the effects of the insulin that's produced.

diabetic ketoacidosis (DKA) A form of acidosis in uncontrolled diabetes in which certain acids accumulate when insulin is not available.

endocrine glands Glands that secrete or release chemicals that are used inside the body. Endocrine glands lack ducts and release hormones directly into the surrounding tissue and blood.

epinephrine A catecholamine secreted by the adrenal medulla in response to stress; stimulates autonomic nerve action.

estrogen One of the three major female hormones. At puberty, estrogen brings about the secondary sex characteristics.

exocrine glands Glands that excrete chemicals for elimination.

glands Cells or organs that selectively remove, concentrate, or alter materials in the blood and then secrete them back into the body.

glucagon Hormone produced by the pancreas that is vital to the control of the body's metabolism and blood glucose level. Glucagon stimulates the breakdown of glycogen to glucose.

gonads The reproductive glands; the main source of sex hormones.

hormones Chemicals secreted by the body that regulate many body functions, such as growth, reproduction, temperature, metabolism, and blood pressure.

hyperglycemia Abnormally high blood glucose level.

hyperosmolar hyperglycemic nonketotic coma (HHNC), also known as hyperosmolar nonketotic coma (HONK), is a metabolic derangement that occurs principally in patients with type 2 diabetes. The condition is characterized by hyperglycemia, hyperosmolarity, and an absence of significant ketosis.

hyperosmolar nonketotic coma (HONK), also known as hyperosmolar hyperglycemic nonketotic coma (HHNC), is a metabolic derangement that occurs principally in patients with type 2 diabetes. The condition is characterized by hyperglycemia, hyperosmolarity, and an absence of significant ketosis.

hypoglycemia Abnormally low blood glucose level.

hypothalamus A small region of the brain that contains several control centres for the body functions and emotions. It is the primary link between the endocrine system and the nervous system.

insulin Hormone produced by the pancreas that's vital to the control of the body's metabolism and blood glucose level. Insulin causes glucose, fatty acids, and amino acids to be taken up and metabolized by cells.

insulin resistance Condition in which the pancreas produces enough insulin but the body can't effectively utilize it.

iodine An essential element in the diet and an important component of thyroxine. Without the proper level of iodine intake, thyroxine can't be produced, and physical and mental growth are diminished.

islets of Langerhans A specialized group of cells in the pancreas where insulin and glucagon are produced.

luteinizing hormone (LH) Hormone that regulates the production of both eggs and sperm, as well as production of reproductive hormones.

mineralocorticoids Any of a group of steroid hormones, such as aldosterone, that are secreted by the adrenal cortex and regulate the balance of water and electrolytes in the body.

myxedema coma A rare condition that can occur in patients who have severe, untreated hypothyroidism.

norepinephrine A catecholamine secreted by adrenal medulla in response to stress.

ovaries Female gonads; ovaries release eggs and secrete the female hormones.

pancreas The digestive gland that secretes digestive enzymes into the duodenum through the pancreatic duct. The pancreas is considered both an endocrine gland and an exocrine gland.

parathyroid hormone (PTH) A hormone secreted by the parathyroids that acts as an antagonist to calcitonin. PTH is secreted when calcium blood levels are low.

pituitary gland Gland whose secretions control, or regulate, the secretions of other endocrine glands. Often called the "master gland."

primary adrenal insufficiency Also known as Addison's disease. A rare condition in which the adrenal glands produce an insufficient amount of adrenal hormones.

progesterone One of the three major female hormones.

target tissues Tissues to which hormones are directed to act on.

testes Male gonads located in the scrotum that produce hormones called androgens.

testosterone The most important androgen in men.

thyroid Large gland located at the base of the neck that produces and excretes hormones that influence growth, development, and metabolism.

thyroid-stimulating hormone (TSH) Hormone that controls the release of thyroid hormone from the thyroid gland.

thyroid storm A rare, life-threatening condition that may occur in patients with thyrotoxicosis. The condition is usually triggered by a stressful event or increased volume of thyroid hormones in the circulation.

thyrotoxicosis A toxic condition caused by excessive levels of circulating thyroid hormone.

thyrotropin-releasing hormone (TRH) A hormone secreted by the hypothalamus that stimulates the release of thyrotropin.

thyroxine The body's major metabolic hormone. Thyroxine stimulates energy production in cells, which increases the rate at which the cells consume oxygen and use carbohydrates, fats, and proteins.

type 1 diabetes The type of diabetic disease that usually starts in childhood and requires daily injections of supplemental synthetic insulin to control blood glucose. Sometimes called juvenile or juvenile-onset diabetes.

type 2 diabetes The type of diabetic disease that usually starts in later life and often can be controlled through diet and oral medications. Sometimes called adult-onset diabetes.

Assessment in Action

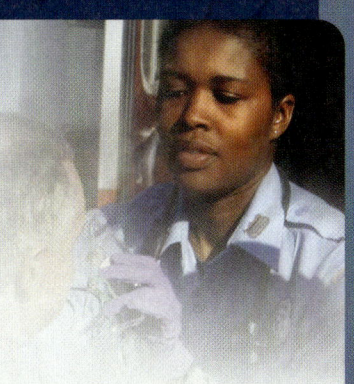

You are dispatched to a warehouse for an unconscious man. You arrive on scene and are greeted by the plant manager. He walks you through the plant and advises you that the patient is an insulin-dependent diabetic who got caught up working and was unable to eat lunch on time. When you arrive to the patient's side, you find the patient unresponsive to verbal stimuli; however, he does withdraw purposefully when you attempt to perform your physical assessment. You obtain a baseline set of vitals, which are within normal limits. You initiate an IV of normal saline and you perform a glucose test, which gives a reading of 1.8 mmol/l. Under the standing orders for your department, you give the patient 25 g of 50% dextrose. The patient slowly responds to the glucose and initially appears lethargic. As the glucose metabolizes through his body, the patient becomes conscious, alert, and oriented and refuses transport to the hospital. After you advise the patient that he should go to the hospital and he still refuses, you advise him that he needs to eat a meal with carbohydrates and explain to him that the dextrose you gave him is short acting.

1. **Glucagon is a hormone that:**
   A. is produced in the pancreatic alpha cells and facilitates the process of glycogenolysis.
   B. is released by the beta cells of the pancreas and facilitates the cellular uptake of glucose.
   C. causes a decrease in circulating blood glucose levels by blocking the conversion of glycogen to glucose.
   D. is typically administered by the paramedic in a dose of 25 g via rapid IV push.

2. **The term *diabetes mellitus* refers to:**
   A. a metabolic disorder in which the body's ability to metabolize simple glucose is normal.
   B. a metabolic disorder in which the body lacks the ability to produce hormones that stimulate the sympathetic nervous system.
   C. glands that secrete or release chemicals that are utilized inside the body.
   D. a disease that is characterized by an inability to sufficiently metabolize glucose.

3. **The _____ is a digestive gland that is considered both an endocrine gland and an exocrine gland.**
   A. gonad
   B. liver
   C. kidney
   D. pancreas

4. **What is insulin responsible for?**
   A. The removal of glucose from the blood for storage as glycogen, fats, and protein
   B. The maintenance of glucose levels in the blood for storage as glycogen, fats, and protein
   C. The main source of sex hormones
   D. The hormones that regulate the body's metabolism

5. **What causes diabetes mellitus?**
   A. The liver does not produce enough insulin.
   B. There is not enough glucose in the bloodstream.
   C. The pancreas does not produce enough insulin or the cells do not respond to the effects of the insulin produced.
   D. The pancreas produces too much insulin and the cells respond appropriately to the effects of the insulin produced.

6. **What is type 1 diabetes mellitus?**
   A. The type of diabetic disease that usually starts in childhood and requires daily injections of supplemental, synthetic insulin to control blood glucose
   B. The type of diabetic disease that usually starts in later life and often requires daily injections of supplemental, synthetic insulin to control blood glucose
   C. The type of diabetic disease that usually starts later in life and often can be controlled through diet and oral medications
   D. The type of diabetic disease that usually starts in childhood and can often be controlled through diet and oral medications

7. **What is type 2 diabetes mellitus?**
   A. The type of diabetic disease that usually starts in childhood and requires daily injections of supplemental, synthetic insulin to control blood glucose
   B. The type of diabetic disease that usually starts in later life and often requires daily injections of supplemental, synthetic insulin to control blood glucose
   C. The type of diabetic disease that usually starts in later life and often can be controlled through diet and oral medications
   D. The type of diabetic disease that usually starts in childhood and can often be controlled through diet and oral medications

8. _____ in the insulin-dependent diabetic is often the result of having taken too much insulin, too little food, or both and often presents with an altered mental status.
   A. Hyperglycemia
   B. Increase in blood glucose
   C. Hypoglycemia
   D. Hypotension

9. A normal blood glucose level is approximately:
   A. 2 to 7 mmol/l.
   B. 4 to 7 mmol/l.
   C. 4 to 11 mmol/l.
   D. 9 to 30 mmol/l.

Challenging Question

You are dispatched to a private home for a person with weakness. When you arrive, the patient tells you that she has been feeling weak and fatigued for approximately 1 week. She called today because she "can't take it anymore." She states that she has been depressed lately and does not understand why. Her vital signs are within normal limits. Her medical history includes hypertension, cardiac problems (unable to specify), and lupus. Her medications include metoprolol and hydrocortisone. You question her as to whether she has had any increased thirst or urination, and she states yes.

10. What initial diagnosis can you make?

▬ Points to Ponder

You are dispatched to a private residence for a patient with an altered level of consciousness. When you arrive, you are greeted by the patient's husband, who tells you that his wife is "not acting right." When you begin to assess her, she does not answer questions appropriately, and she has erratic respirations. She is hot to the touch, dry, and appears pink. Her pulse rate is 132 beats/min, with sinus tachycardia on the monitor; her blood pressure is 140/70 mm Hg. After you initiate an IV of normal saline, you perform a glucose test that reads "high" on your monitor. In your head you understand that this means her glucose is greater than 28 mmol/l. Her husband states that she has not been feeling well for the last 2 days, and they believed she was coming down with the flu. He called today because she appeared confused to him.

What are your priorities in this situation? What do you need to do for this patient?

Issues: Understanding the Importance of the Endocrine System, Understanding the General Assessment Findings Associated With an Endocrine Emergency.

30 Allergic Reactions

Competency Areas

Area 4: Assessment and Diagnostics

4.2.a	Obtain list of patient's allergies.
4.2.b	Obtain list of patient's medications.
4.2.c	Obtain chief complaint and/or incident history from patient, family members, and/or bystanders.
4.2.d	Obtain information regarding patient's past medical history.
4.2.e	Obtain information about patient's last oral intake.
4.3.a	Conduct primary patient assessment and interpret findings.
4.3.b	Conduct secondary patient assessment and interpret findings.
4.3.c	Conduct cardiovascular system assessment and interpret findings.
4.3.e	Conduct respiratory system assessment and interpret findings.
4.3.i	Conduct integumentary system assessment and interpret findings.
4.3.k	Conduct assessment of the immune system and interpret findings.
4.4.a	Assess pulse.
4.4.b	Assess respiration.
4.4.d	Measure blood pressure by auscultation.
4.4.g	Assess skin condition.
4.4.h	Assess pupils.
4.4.i	Assess level of mentation.

Area 5: Therapeutics

5.1.a	Use manual maneuvers and positioning to maintain airway patency.
5.2.a	Recognize indications for oxygen administration.
5.5.c	Maintain peripheral intravenous (IV) access devices and infusions of crystalloid solutions without additives.
5.5.d	Conduct peripheral intravenous cannulation.
5.8.d	Administer medication via intramuscular route.
5.8e	Administer medication via intravenous route.

Area 6: Integration

6.1.h	Provide care to patient experiencing illness primarily involving immune system.

Appendix 4: Pathophysiology

G.	**Integumentary System**
	Infectious and Inflammatory Illness: Allergy/urticaria
J.	**Multisystem Diseases and Injuries**
	Environmental Disorders: Anaphylaxis/Anaphylactoid reactions
	Environmental Disorders: Stings and Bites
	Shock Syndromes: Anaphylactic

Appendix 5: Medications

Medications Affecting the Autonomic Nervous System: Andrenergic Agonists

Medications Affecting the Autonomic Nervous System: Antihistamines

Medications Used to Treat/Prevent Inflammatory Responses and Infections: Corticosteroids

Introduction

Allergic reactions and anaphylaxis have been documented for many years. One of the earliest accounts may have been noted by the late 17th century clergyman Increase Mather:

> Some men also have strange antipathies in their natures against that sort of food which others love and live upon. I have read of one that could not endure to eat either bread or flesh; of another that fell into a swooning fit at the smell of a rose . . . There are some who, if a cat accidentally comes into the room, though they neither see it, nor are told of it, will presently be in a sweat, and ready to die away.

Although these cases cannot be proven to be anaphylaxis, the descriptions suggest some type of reaction was present—possibly an allergic or anaphylactic reaction given the severity and fatality of the descriptions. This chapter explores these types of reactions, including their typical signs and symptoms, and the steps you should take to manage such patients. In addition, it discusses the common causes of "swooning fit" so we can be better prepared to provide prehospital care for affected patients.

The first task is to clarify the many terms associated with allergic and anaphylactic reactions. An allergen is a substance that produces allergic symptoms in a patient. Most allergens are usually harmless substances that do not pose a threat to other people—for example, milk, eggs, chocolate, and strawberries. An antibody is a protein the body produces in response to an antigen. This protein (globulin) is found in the plasma—hence, its other name *immunoglobulin* (Ig). **Table 30-1 ▼** lists the common antibodies, their actions, and locations.

An allergic reaction is an abnormal immune response the body develops when the person is reexposed to a substance or allergen. In most people, exposure to this substance would not be a problem; in a person with an allergic reaction, however, a local or systemic reaction may occur. In a local reaction, the body limits its response to a specific area after being exposed to a foreign substance; the swelling around an insect bite would be an example. A systemic reaction occurs throughout the body, possibly affecting multiple body systems. It is seen when a person who is allergic to shellfish, for example, has swelling and hives all over his body after eating shrimp paste used to make the sauce of a

Table 30-1	Antibodies or Immunoglobulins	
Antibody	**Action**	**Location**
IgA	Provides localized protection to mucous membranes.	Tears, saliva, mucus, breast milk, gastrointestinal secretions, blood, and lymph
IgD	Thought to stimulate antibody-producing cells to make antibodies	Blood, lymph, and the surfaces of B cells
IgE*	Responds in allergic reactions	Located on mast and basophil cells
IgG	Provides protection against bacteria and viruses; enhances phagocytosis, neutralizes toxins, triggers the complement system	Blood, lymph, intestines
IgM	One of the first to appear; causes agglutination and lysis of microbes. ABO agglutinins are IgM antibodies.	Blood, lymph, and surface of B cells

*The primary antibody you need to be concerned with during allergic and anaphylactic reactions is the IgE antibody.

You are the Paramedic Part 1

You are dispatched to a private residence for a 26-year-old man with "trouble breathing." On arrival, you find a young man, Matthew Weil, in the living room of his home, holding his throat and working hard to breathe. You hear wheezes without the use of a stethoscope and notice that he is leaning far forward on the edge of the couch.

His wife tells you that the patient has been sick with "pneumonia." She just picked up a new prescription for him, azithromycin, which he took just a few minutes ago. She said her husband is normally very healthy, has no other medical history, and is not taking any other medications.

Initial Assessment	Recording Time: 0 Minutes
Appearance	Sitting on the edge of the couch, appears very anxious
Level of consciousness	A (Alert to person, place, and day)
Airway	Coughing, hoarse voice, and audible wheezing
Breathing	Rapid and laboured
Circulation	Weak, fast radial pulse

1. How would you categorize this patient and why?
2. What must you do to correct life-threatening conditions?

toxin. After the second dose of the toxin, one of the dogs died. Because this response was the opposite of protection, it was referred to as anaphylaxis (meaning "without protection").

In Canada, it is estimated that up to 3 million people are at risk of anaphylaxis, and approximately 1 person per 3 million population die each year due to anaphylaxis. Unfortunately, no exact cause for anaphylaxis can be determined in up to two thirds of patients. To anticipate anaphylaxis, of course, it would be useful to be able to identify people at greatest risk. Neither race nor sex seems to affect the incidence of anaphylaxis. The incidence of insect sting anaphylaxis tends to be higher in men. Women have a greater incidence of anaphylactic reactions to latex, aspirin, and intravenous (IV) muscle relaxants. Anaphylactic reactions have been documented in children as young as 6 months and adults as old as 89 years. Children are more likely to have severe food allergies, whereas adults tend to have anaphylactic reactions to insect stings, anesthetics, and radiocontrast media. **Table 30-2 ▼** lists the common substances associated with anaphylaxis.

curry. Hypersensitivity occurs when a patient reacts with exaggerated or inappropriate allergic symptoms after coming into contact with a substance perceived by the body to be harmful. Anaphylaxis is an extreme systemic form of an allergic reaction involving two or more body systems. This term was first used in 1902, when Portier and Richet were vaccinating dogs with sea anemone

Table 30-2	**Common Causes of Anaphylactic Reactions**	
General Type of Antigen	**Specific Antigen**	**Examples/Comments**
Drugs	Penicillin (antibiotic)	Causes most IgE-mediated drug interactions
	Beta-lactam antibiotics (cephalosporins)	Possibly a cross-reaction in patients allergic to penicillin
	Other antibiotics	Ampicillin
	Sulfa drugs (antibiotic)	Sulfanomide, sulfisoxazole
	Muscle relaxants, hypnotics, opioids	Acetaminophen with codeine, morphine, meperidine
	Salicylates and NSAIDs	Aspirin
	Colloids	Pentaspan, gelofusine
	Local anesthetics	Procaine
	Enzymes	Chymotrypsin, penicillinase
	Mismatched blood transfusion	
	Intravenous radiocontrast dyes used in taking radiographs	Intravenous pyelogram, contrast computer tomography
	Biological extracts and hormones	Insulin, heparin
	Vaccines	
Insect stings	Bees, yellow jackets, hornets, wasps, ants	0.5%–3% of the population will have a systemic reaction after being stung.
Foods (problem worldwide—most common cause of anaphylaxis)	Peanuts	As little as 100 μg of peanut protein can cause a reaction.
	Tree nuts, fish, and shellfish	Most common to all age groups
	Some fruits	Mango, strawberries
	Egg, soy, and milk	Most common in children
Latex (may be seen in myelodysplasia, genitourinary anomalies, patients with frequent exposure to latex, and sensitized health care workers)	Gloves and other materials made from latex	The incidence rate is decreasing owing to awareness and better manufacturing practices. People with allergies to bananas, kiwi, and strawberries may have a cross-reaction to latex.
Immunotherapy	Allergen immunotherapy, skin testing (Note: Patients with atopic diseases are at greater risk for anaphylaxis.)	Rare, associated with asthma, errors in administration, overdose, and beta-blocker use during immunotherapy
Animals	Dander	Long-haired animals
	Animal serum products	Horse serum, gamma globulins

Adapted from Dreskin et al, Anaphylaxis, eMedicine, *www.emedicine.com/med/topic128.htm*. Accessed 5/26/06.

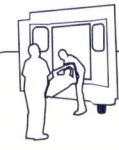

At the Scene

It is important to be prepared for latex allergies in the prehospital environment and to consider a latex-free or latex-safe environment.

Diseases related to allergies, such as allergic rhinitis, asthma, and atopic dermatitis increase the potential for anaphylactic reactions. One third to one half of patients with anaphylaxis have a history of atopic diseases.

The other major factors associated with anaphylaxis are the route of exposure to the allergen and time between exposures. When a substance is ingested (taken by mouth), it is less likely to cause an anaphylactic reaction, and, if a reaction occurs, it usually is not fatal. By contrast, if a substance is injected, the reaction is more likely to be severe. Also, the longer the time between exposures to a substance, the less likely a severe anaphylactic reaction will occur. This is thought to be due to the decreased production of the specific Ig (antibody) cells in the body over time.

Anatomy and Physiology

The Normal Immune Response

The immune system protects the human body from substances and organisms that are considered foreign to the body. Without our immune system for protection, life as we know it would not exist. We would be under constant attack from any bacterium, virus, or other type of invader that wanted to make our bodies their home. Luckily, for the majority of the population, the body is equipped with an amazing immune system that is on patrol 24 hours a day, 7 days a week, to detect unauthorized visits or invading attacks by foreign substances.

The body protects itself via two types of systems: cellular immunity and humoural (that is, related to the body's fluids) immunity. In cellular immunity, the body produces special white blood cells called T cells that attack and destroy invaders. In humoural immunity, the body uses the antibodies dissolved in the plasma and lymph to wage war on invading organisms. The cells producing immunity are located throughout the body in the lymph nodes, spleen, and gastrointestinal tract. Their goal is to intercept foreign forces as they enter the body, thereby limiting the invaders' spread and damage.

Routes of Entry for Allergens

Substances can invade the body through the skin, the respiratory tract, or the gastrointestinal tract. Invasion through the skin may come in the form of injection or absorption. In injection, the invading substance pierces the skin and deposits foreign material into the skin. Bees and hornets prefer this method of invasion. Absorption occurs when foreign material is deposited on the skin and slowly absorbed through the skin. Invasion by absorption may occur when lotions or therapeutic medicinal creams are applied to the skin. Invaders do not stop at the skin, but may also enter the respiratory tract as the patient quietly breathes; this type of raid is referred to as an inhalation exposure. The foreigners advance through the respiratory system and launch their attack from the lungs. Cats, peanuts, and many plants attack in this way. The final way invading armies attack the body is through the gastrointestinal tract via ingestion. That is, invaders may camouflage themselves as some tempting delicacy such as strawberry shortcake, a mushroom-and-cheese omelet, or a peanut butter pie **Figure 30-1 ▶** .

You are the Paramedic Part 2

You take Mr. Weil's vital signs, and your partner immediately applies high-flow oxygen via nonrebreathing mask and obtains a blood pressure while you gain IV access. As you begin your series of interventions, you explain to the patient what is happening to him and what you need to do to correct it. You then administer epinephrine and diphenhydramine via IV per local protocols. You are mentally prepared to aggressively manage this patient's airway but hope that your treatments will result in quick, significant patient improvement. You administer IV normal saline at a wide-open rate using a 16-gauge cannula and 0.3 mg of epinephrine 1:10,000 and 25 mg of diphenhydramine.

Vital Signs	Recording Time: 5 Minutes
Level of consciousness	Alert, with a Glasgow Coma Scale score of 14
Skin	Flushed, hives
Pulse	130 beats/min, weak and slightly irregular
Blood pressure	88/40 mm Hg
Respirations	50 breaths/min
Spo_2	90% with oxygen at 15 l/min via nonrebreathing mask

3. Why does the order of the medications matter?
4. Why is knowing all of the medication administration routes important?
5. Would your prehospital care change if this patient were geriatric?

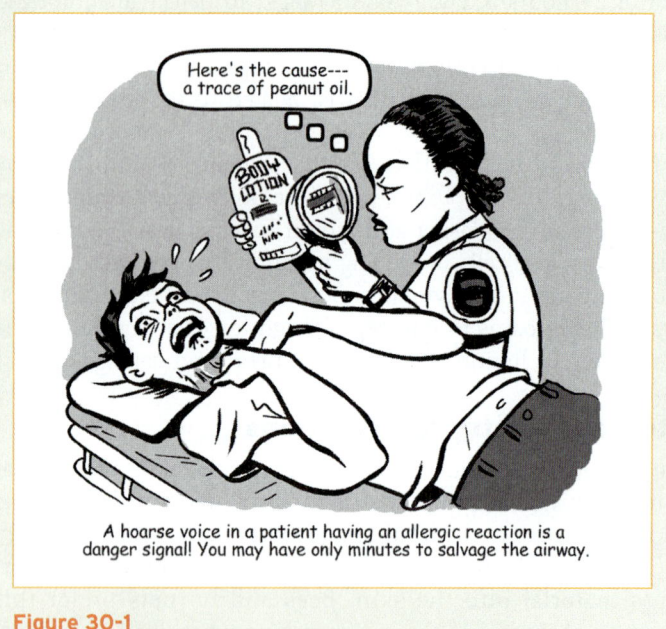

A hoarse voice in a patient having an allergic reaction is a danger signal! You may have only minutes to salvage the airway.

Figure 30-1

The basophils and mast cells produce the body's "chemical weapons"—that is, chemical mediators Table 30-3 ▸ . These cells contain granules filled with a host of powerful substances that are ready to be released to fight invading forces of antigens. As long as the body is not invaded by one of the previously identified foreign substances, the granules are kept encapsulated in their protective walls and remain inactive. If an antigen invades the body and combines with one of the antibodies, however, the granules are ejected from the mast cells and detonated. The chemical mediators are then released into the surrounding tissue and the bloodstream Figure 30-2 ▾ .

The chemical mediators launch and maintain the immune response. They summon more white blood cells to the area to battle the invading force. They also increase blood flow to the area under attack by dilating the blood vessels and increasing the capillary permeability. These actions are useful when a small invasion occurs to a limited area but can be extremely dangerous when they spread throughout the body. When they have systemic effects, the chemical mediators cause the signs and symptoms of the allergic and anaphylactic reactions seen in the body.

Physiology

Once a foreign substance invades the body, the body goes on alert and initiates a series of responses. The first encounter with the foreign substance begins the primary response. Cells (macrophages) immediately greet, confront, and engulf the invaders to check their papers or passports to see if they can legally be present in the body. If the body is unable to identify the substance or determines the papers are not in order, it starts a file on the outsider. It fingerprints the invader or takes a "mug shot" of the suspect for later identification by using immune cells to record the salient features of the outside substance. These cells record one or two of the proteins on the surface of the invading substance and then design specific proteins to match each substance. These proteins—called antibodies—are intended to match up with the invader—the antigen—and inactivate it.

Through the primary response, the body develops sensitivity—that is, the ability to recognize the foreigner the next time it is encountered. To determine whether the substance is "one of us," the body records enough details to assist in future identification of the substance and production of antibodies to perfectly fit the invading antigen. The body then sends out these details to the rest of the body, much like sending out "Wanted" posters to "post offices" throughout the body. The Wanted posters are distributed by placing the specific antibodies on two types of cells: basophils and mast cells. Basophils are stationed like guards in specific sites within the tissues. Mast cells are on patrol like police cruisers or bounty hunters through the connective tissues, bronchi, gastrointestinal mucosa, and other vulnerable border areas that act as barriers to foreign invaders.

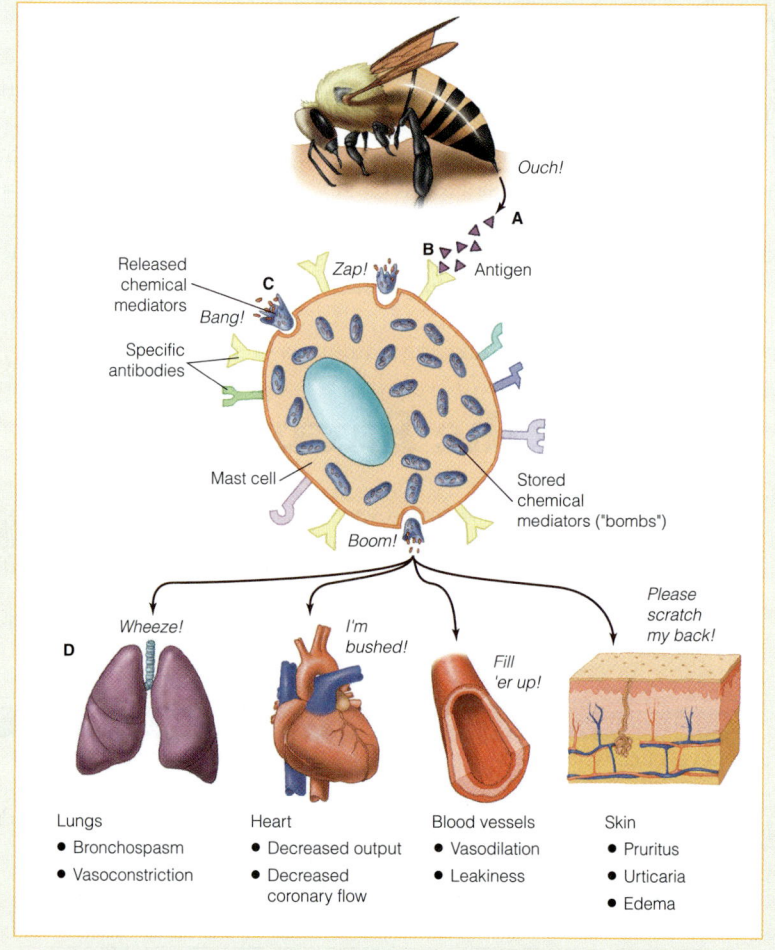

Figure 30-2 The sequence of events in anaphylaxis. **A.** The antigen is introduced into the body. **B.** The antigen-antibody reaction at the surface of a mast cell. **C.** Release of mast cell chemical mediators. **D.** Chemical mediators exert their effects on end organs.

Table 30-3	Chemical Mediators
Mediator	**Physiological Effects**
Histamine	• Systemic vasodilation • Increased permeability of blood vessels • Decreased cardiac contractility • Decreased coronary blood flow • Dysrhythmias • Bronchoconstriction • Pulmonary vasoconstriction
Eosinophil chemotactic factor	• Attracts eosinophils and neutrophils
Arachidonic acid (precursor of the following):	These factors act to produce other inflammatory mediators:
Prostaglandin	• Smooth muscle contraction

Leukotrienes (slow reaction substance of anaphylaxis [SRS-A])	• Vascular permeability
	• Bronchoconstriction
	• Decreased force of cardiac contraction
	• Decreased coronary blood flow
	• Dysrhythmias
	   – More potent than histamine (thousands of times)
	   – React more slowly than histamine

Platelet-activating factor	• Platelet aggregation • Causes histamine release
Serotonin	• Pulmonary vasoconstriction • Bronchoconstriction

Proteoglycans:
  Heparin
  Chondroitin sulfate
  Chemokines
  Cytokines
	• Control the release of histamine. These mediators as a whole work to activate the kinin system and are thought to contribute to prolonged and biphasic reactions.
	• These mediators trigger inflammatory pathways and increase the recruitment of inflammatory cells.

Kinins	• Bradykinin is one of the stronger kinins and is responsible for increased vascular permeability.

As paramedics, we exploit the body's ability to protect itself. For example, we administer vaccines to produce immunity against a disease. The body develops antibodies in response to the vaccine so it can produce an immune response to neutralize the invading disease before it can establish itself and damage the body. Thus, the body develops antibodies in a controlled way. When the hepatitis B vaccine is administered, for example, a small amount of the hepatitis B virus (HBV) enters the body. The body identifies this virus and produces antibodies to it; these antibodies are then distributed throughout the body. Should an immunized person later be exposed to HBV, the virus will invade the body. Once in the body, the virus begins to set up residency and reproduce. At this point, the officer on patrol (the wandering immune cell) identifies the HBV as something that does not belong in the area. It remembers seeing the HBV Wanted poster and radios for backup (activates the immune system). The alarm is sounded, and the body begins aggressive production of the "antihepatitis" antibodies, sending in platoons of immune system soldiers to kill the HBV and clean up residual traces of the invasion. This intense response to the invading virus is called the secondary response. Meanwhile, the "contaminated," immunized person remains blissfully unaware of the battle raging inside his or her body.

This battle is termed acquired immunity. In this type of immunity, the administration of a vaccine allows the body to produce antibodies without having to experience the disease. Vaccinations against measles, mumps, and polio are examples of acquired immunity. In natural immunity, by contrast, the body encounters the antigen and experiences a full immune response with all the pathology of the disease. Having the measles, for example, causes the body to produce antibodies to this pathogen, but the drawback is that the person has the itching, rash, and high fever associated with the disease.

Use of the polio vaccine has resulted in herd immunity, which occurs when a group of individuals are immunized against a substance. This immunization protects vulnerable people in the group and the entire group by decreasing the number of people able to contract the disease, thus protecting the group.

Pathophysiology

Abnormal Immune Reactions

An ever-watchful and responsive immune system is essential to life and health. Unfortunately, sometimes the immune system becomes overzealous in defending the body. The resulting

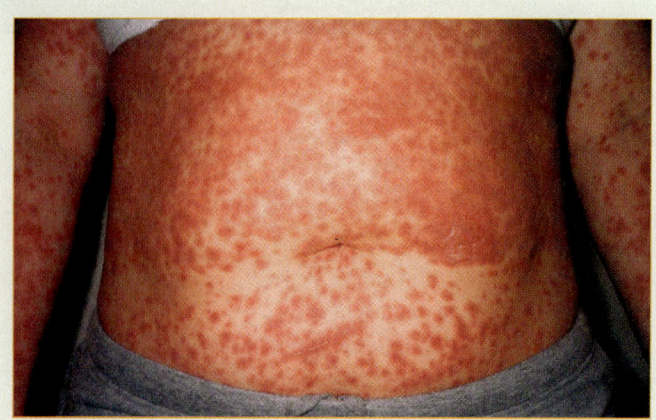

Figure 30-3 A severe allergic reaction to medication. This patient was allergic to penicillin and most other antibiotics.

begin releasing chemical mediators. Histamine, one of the primary chemical weapons, causes the blood vessels in the local area to dilate and the capillaries to leak. Leukotrienes, which are even more powerful, are released and cause additional dilation and leaking. White blood cells are called to the area to help engulf and destroy the enemy, and platelets begin to collect and clump together. In most cases, this overreaction to harmless invaders is usually restricted to the local area being invaded. The runny, itchy nose and swollen eyes associated with hay fever are examples of a local allergic reaction.

In the case of anaphylaxis, the person is not so lucky. The body not only has out-of-control border guards, but also has out-of-control special forces units that do not restrict their activities to the local area. They take their chemical weapons to the remainder of the body and detonate them, causing widespread havoc. Although the same chemical mediators are released, the effect involves more than one system throughout the body. An initial effect may be seen from the histamine release, with secondary effects following a few hours later when the remainder of the chemicals are released.

Histamine release causes immediate vasodilation, which often presents as flushed skin and hypotension. It also increases vascular permeability, which results in tissue swelling and fluid secretion. The tissue swelling can present as hives **Figure 30-4 ▶**, narrowing of the airway, and increased fluids in the airway. Histamine likewise causes smooth muscle contraction, especially in the respiratory system and gastrointestinal system. This results in laryngospasm or bronchospasm and abdominal cramping. Finally, histamine decreases the contractility of the heart. When this effect is coupled with vasodilation, the person may experience profound hypotension. Dysrhythmias due to hypoperfusion and hypoxia are also common.

Later responses from the much more powerful leukotrienes compound the effects of histamine. The person's respiratory status will become even more dire as these highly potent

problems may range in severity from hay fever to anaphylaxis and exist along the spectrum from a simple annoyance to a life-threatening crisis. During these abnormal reactions, the immune system becomes hypersensitive to one or more substances. The body often has these reactions to substances that should not be identified as harmful by the immune system—substances such as ragweed, strawberries, and penicillin **Figure 30-3 ▲**. The immune cells of the allergic person are more sensitive and jumpier than the immune cells of a person without allergies. Although these cells are able to recognize and react to dangerous invaders such as bacteria and viruses, they also identify harmless substances as posing a threat. They behave like border guards gone berserk, shooting the smugglers and the tourists!

Not only do the border guards go berserk, but they also call in the special forces. When the invading substance enters the body, the mast cells recognize it as potentially harmful and

You are the Paramedic Part 3

Mr. Weil's condition is improving rapidly. He is able to communicate with you and seems fully alert. He still has some shortness of breath, which you treat with a beta-2 agonist. You begin transport, apply the cardiac monitor, and administer epinephrine subcutaneously.

Your quick action and proficient skills saved this patient's life. He is later released, with no permanent deficits. He now wears a medical ID bracelet that identifies his severe allergy to azithromycin.

Reassessment	Recording Time: 15 Minutes
Level of consciousness	Alert, with a Glasgow Coma Scale score of 15
Skin	Warm, pink, and slightly diaphoretic
Pulse	110 beats/min, weak and slightly irregular
Blood pressure	106/70 mm Hg
Respirations	36 breaths/min
Spo_2	95% with oxygen at 15 l/min via nonrebreathing mask

6. If the initial dose of epinephrine was successful, why administer another dose subcutaneously?

7. What other options are available should your patient begin to have the same signs and symptoms you noted initially?

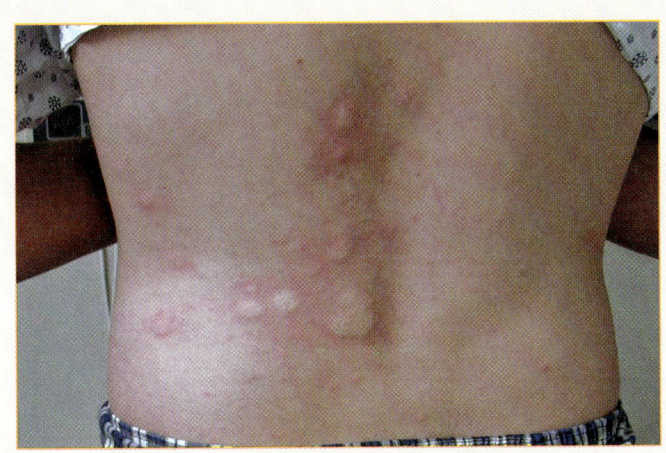

Figure 30-4 Urticaria, or hives, may appear following a sting and are characterized by multiple, small, raised areas on the skin.

bronchoconstrictors are released. In addition, leukotriene release causes coronary vasoconstriction, which contributes to a worsening cardiac condition and myocardial irritability. Leukotrienes are also associated with increased vascular permeability, contributing to a further state of hypoperfusion.

The remaining chemical mediators continue to worsen the situation as they undertake what they see as steps to protect the body from this foreign invader. As a result of these activities, when the body undergoes an anaphylactic reaction, it may not survive without immediate intervention.

Clinical Symptoms of Anaphylaxis

The skin is the body's first line of defence against would-be invaders, so skin symptoms are often the first indications of anaphylaxis. Initially, the person may be aware of feeling warm and flushed. Pruritus (itching) is another early sign, which is due to vasodilation and capillary leaking. The area around the eyes is often susceptible to this effect, which causes swollen, red eyes. Swelling of the face and tongue may contribute to airway compromise. You may also note swelling of the hands and feet. Histamine is responsible for the urticaria (hives) experienced by the anaphylactic patient.

The most common complaints are usually respiratory symptoms, which often present as shortness of breath or dyspnea and tightness in the throat and chest. You may also note stridor and/or hoarseness. These signs and symptoms are often due to upper airway swelling in the laryngeal and epiglottic areas. Affected patients may complain of a lump in the throat. The lower airway is often involved as well. Bronchoconstriction and increased secretions may result in wheezes and crackles. It is not uncommon for the patient to cough or sneeze as the body tries to clear the airway. These symptoms may progress slowly or alarmingly fast. You may have only 1 or 3 minutes to halt this rapid, life-threatening process.

Cardiovascular symptoms are serious complications of anaphylaxis. As noted earlier, histamine and leukotrienes work directly on the heart to decrease its contractility. The resulting

decrease in cardiac output is complicated by vasodilation and increased capillary permeability, which further decrease the amount of fluid returned to the heart. As cardiac output declines, perfusion decreases, leading to ischemia and bringing the potential for cardiac dysrhythmias. As the fluid leaks out of the capillaries, the intravascular system is left short on fluid. (As much as 50% of the vascular volume can be shifted to the extravascular space within 10 minutes of exposure to an antigen.) Instead of responding normally to the fluid loss and constricting, the blood vessels do just the opposite: They dilate. The already low vascular volume becomes totally inadequate, and hypotension reigns. In response to the low blood pressure, the heart rate increases, putting stress on an already compromised heart. In this situation, tachycardia, flushed skin, and hypotension are synonymous with anaphylactic shock.

> ### Notes from Nancy
>
> Flushing (from vasodilation) and tachycardia are so characteristic of anaphylactic shock that it is very questionable to make the diagnosis without these two signs being present.

Gastrointestinal symptoms may also be part of an anaphylactic response, particularly if the offending antigen has been ingested. Abdominal cramping is a common presentation, but nausea, bloating, vomiting, abdominal distension, and profuse, watery diarrhea may also be present.

Patients may present with central nervous system symptoms in response to decreased cerebral perfusion and hypoxia. These symptoms include headache, dizziness, confusion, and anxiety. A sense of "impending doom" aptly represents the patient's sense of being near death. This observation may be more fact than fiction.

Table 30-4 ▶ summarizes the signs and symptoms of anaphylaxis. Anaphylaxis may present as affecting any two or more of these body systems, so the picture can be confusing at times. Think of a patient with anaphylaxis as experiencing three types of shock: (1) cardiogenic shock due to decreased cardiac output, (2) hypovolemic shock due to fluids leaking into the tissues, and (3) neurogenic shock due to inability of the blood vessels to constrict. You will need to use your assessment skills to identify the potential for anaphylaxis and take aggressive action to manage the patient and stop the anaphylactic process as rapidly as possible.

■ Assessment of a Patient With Anaphylaxis

Assessment of a patient with an anaphylactic reaction can be highly challenging. You may have to simultaneously assess the patient, identify the problem, and intervene within seconds of arriving on the scene to save the patient's life. Index of suspicion for anaphylaxis must be high on your list if any of the symptoms discussed previously are present. You may not have

Table 30-4	Signs and Symptoms of Anaphylaxis*
System	**Signs and Symptoms**
Skin	• Warm • Flushed • Itching (pruritus) • Swollen, red eyes • Swelling of the face and tongue • Swelling of the hands and feet • Hives (urticaria)
Respiratory	• **Dyspnea** • Tightness in the throat and chest • Stridor • Hoarseness • Lump in throat • Wheezes • Crackles • Coughing • Sneezing
Cardiovascular	• Dysrhythmias • **Hypotension** • **Tachycardia**
Gastrointestinal	• Abdominal cramping • Nausea • Bloating • Vomiting • Abdominal distension • Profuse, watery diarrhea
Central nervous	• Headache • Dizziness • Confusion • Anxiety and restlessness • Sense of impending doom • Altered mental status

*Key indicators are represented by bold type.

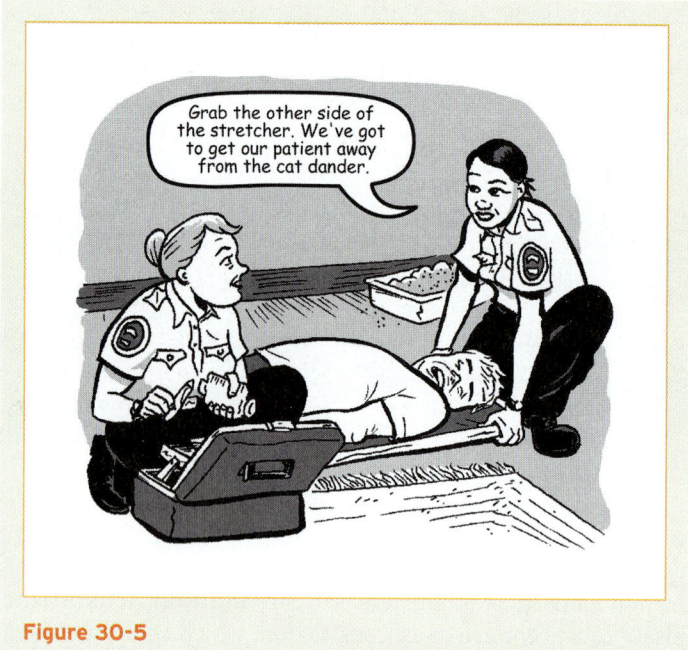

Figure 30-5

a second opportunity because the patient's condition may deteriorate before your eyes.

Scene Assessment

When you arrive on scene, you should observe it for any potential exposure problems. For example, if the patient was out gardening, a bee sting might be a cause of the problem. Dinner at a seafood restaurant might make you suspicious of the shellfish menu items. Because anaphylaxis is a life-threatening event, taking the time to survey the scene for potential anaphylactic hazards is important   Figure 30-5 ▶ .

Initial Assessment
Level of Consciousness

The status of the brain is a direct reflection of the patient's oxygenation status. A restless, confused, anxious, or combative patient is most likely hypoxic. As the patient's condition deteriorates and the oxygen level decreases or the carbon dioxide level increases, you are likely to find a patient with a decreased level of consciousness or completely unresponsive. If the

patient is unable to speak, assess the airway for patency before assuming a neurologic problem. Any change in mental status in an anaphylactic patient should direct you to immediate airway evaluation and management.

Upper Airway

A noisy upper airway is a concern in any patient, but even more so in an anaphylactic patient because it may be an early sign of impending airway occlusion due to swelling. You should listen for stridor and hoarseness. In addition, the patient may complain of a tight feeling or a "lump in the throat."

Lower Airway

Observe the patient for tachypnea, laboured breathing, accessory muscle use, abnormal retractions, and prolonged expiration. The severity of these findings predicts the stability of the patient's condition. Lung sounds are also a predictor of severity. Initially, you will hear wheezing. As the patient's condition deteriorates and the lungs become tighter and less ventilated (hypoventilation), the diminished lung sounds will be present and the chest may become silent. A silent chest is an ominous finding.

Circulation

Evaluate the skin for redness, rashes, edema, moisture, itching, and urticaria—these symptoms are more commonly associated with an anaphylactic reaction due to histamine release. Pallor and cyanosis may be present as well.

Focused History and Physical Examination
History

Does the patient have any allergies? Has the patient ever had an allergic or anaphylactic reaction? If so, how severe was the incident and how rapidly did it progress? You may want to interview the patient to determine whether he or she had a previous exposure to the antigen. A severe reaction may occur at the second exposure to an antigen, so the patient might not know about the allergy. In some cases, you may not be able to identify the offending antigen. When in doubt, in the presence of a severe reaction, intervention takes precedence over identifying the antigen. To identify where you are in the process, ask when the symptoms began. Because the airway is a major concern, ask about feelings of dyspnea.

You should also determine whether the patient or first responders have administered any treatment before your arrival. This may include using an EpiPen, taking diphenhydramine (Benadryl), or using an inhaler with a beta agonist (such as salbutamol) **Figure 30-6 ▶**.

Vital Signs

A patient with an allergic reaction will often present with tachypnea, tachycardia, and hypotension. When these signs are noted in conjunction with flushed skin and hives, anaphylaxis should be one of the major considerations. Obviously, the more abnormal the vital signs, the more aggressively you should treat the patient.

Physical Examination

The classic presentation of anaphylaxis includes respiratory symptoms and hypotension. Gastrointestinal symptoms such as abnormal cramping, nausea, vomiting, and diarrhea may be present.

You should use tools such as a cardiac monitor in your assessment because dysrhythmias may be associated with anaphylaxis. A 12-lead electrocardiogram should be considered during the assessment to monitor for cardiac ischemia.

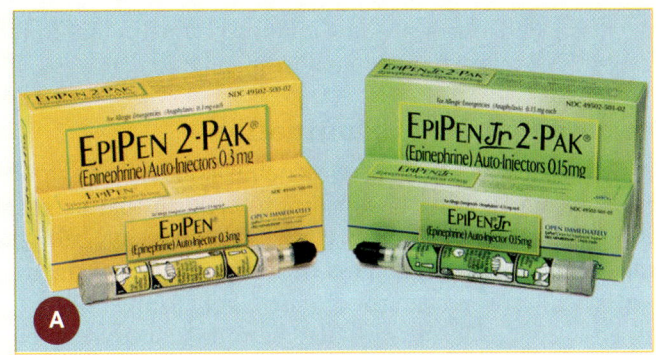

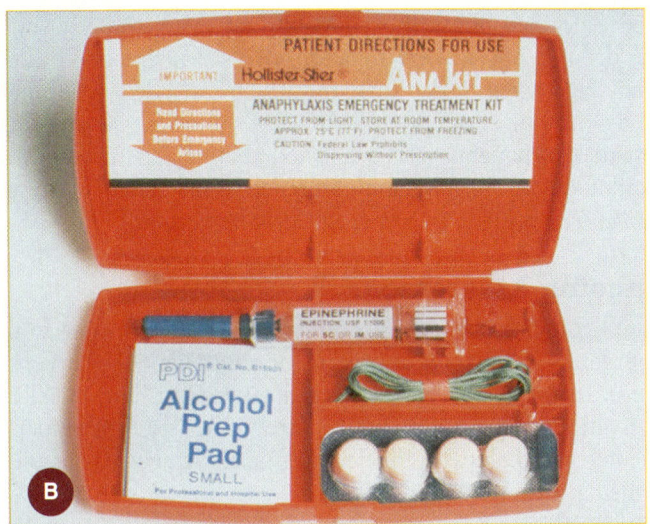

Figure 30-6 Patients who experience severe allergic reactions often carry their own epinephrine, which comes predosed in an auto-injector or a standard syringe. **A.** EpiPen auto-injectors (adult and pediatric sizes). **B.** AnaKit with epinephrine syringe.

You are the Paramedic Part 4

Mr. Weil's condition remains stable throughout transport. You note ectopy on the electrocardiogram, but this subsides and your patient tells you that he can breathe much more easily. You decide to place a second IV line in case his condition deteriorates, and you administer 2.5 mg of salbutamol. You release the patient to emergency department staff who keep close watch on his condition.

Reassessment	Recording Time: 20 Minutes
Level of consciousness	Alert, with a Glasgow Coma Scale score of 15
Skin	Warm, pink, and dry with some hives still noted
Pulse	110 beats/min, weak and regular
Blood pressure	106/70 mm Hg
Respirations	36 breaths/min
SpO_2	95% with oxygen at 15 l/min via nonrebreathing mask

8. If your patient had not responded to initial treatment, what would you have anticipated in terms of interventions related to airway management?

9. If you had been unable to obtain IV access, how would this have affected the call?

Monitoring pulse oximetry may alert you to low oxygen saturation. End-tidal carbon dioxide should be monitored because the level may be elevated in anaphylaxis.

Detailed Physical Examination

A patient with a minor allergic reaction will most likely require further examination by paramedics to confirm that no other problems are contributing to his or her condition. Typically, the detailed physical examination is done on trauma patients who have a significant mechanism of injury. For example, a patient with an allergic reaction who may have developed symptoms of anaphylaxis and who has sustained significant trauma will need a detailed physical examination en route to the hospital. The detailed physical examination involves examination of the head, face, eyes, nose, ears, mouth, neck, chest, abdomen, pelvis, all four extremities, back, and buttocks. Do not delay transport of patients with suspected anaphylaxis to perform a detailed physical examination on scene. If the patient has a second EpiPen bring it with you as it may be needed.

Ongoing Assessment

The ongoing assessment is conducted typically en route to the emergency department. In case of anaphylaxis, it involves reassessment of the patient, serial vital signs, and checking interventions (such as the need for another dose of epinephrine, oxygen therapy, Trendelenburg position, and reassessment of the patient's lung sounds).

Management of Anaphylactic Reactions

An anaphylactic reaction is a life-threatening emergency and must be treated as such. It takes rapid recognition and rapid intervention to reverse the anaphylactic process and save the patient's life. Although the actions to reverse anaphylaxis will be reviewed here in an orderly manner, in reality, these interventions may be performed simultaneously, especially if multiple paramedics are available.

Remove the offending agent. When possible, remove the patient from the situation involving the antigen or the antigen from the patient. For example, if the patient is allergic to peanuts and is being exposed to peanuts through inspiration, you may need to remove the patient from the room because you may not be able to eliminate the peanut allergen from the air. If the patient has a stinger from a bee sting still in place, you may need to remove the stinger. Remember to scrape the stinger off because you can inject more venom into the patient if you pinch or squeeze the stinger **Figure 30-7 ▸** .

Maintain the airway—the airway is always a priority regardless of the situation. You will need to be prepared to intubate. If the airway is already swollen shut, you may need to perform a cricothyrotomy to ventilate the patient. Assessing for the presence of stridor and hoarseness should indicate the severity of the

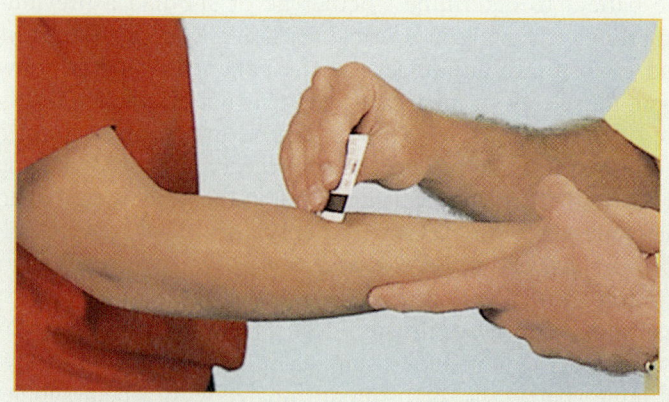

Figure 30-7 To remove the stinger of a honeybee, gently scrape the skin with the edge of a sharp, stiff object such as a credit card.

At the Scene

In the absence of an IV site, intramuscular (IM) administration of epinephrine is preferred because it provides more rapid absorption. Subcutaneous (SQ) administration of epinephrine is unpredictable and may have delayed effects in the presence of shock.

airway compromise. If the patient is still awake, allow him or her to assume a position that does not compromise breathing. Use an appropriate oxygen device for supplemental oxygen administration, and consider early transport. Be prepared to assist breathing as needed. *Early administration of epinephrine should be a priority.*

Because epinephrine has immediate action, it can rapidly reverse the effects of anaphylaxis. Administer epinephrine by the IM, SQ, or IV route as soon as possible if airway or respiratory compromise and/or hypotension are present. Epinephrine is the drug of choice for anaphylactic reactions because it stops the process of mast cell degranulation. In addition, epinephrine reverses the effects of the chemical mediators released via this degranulation. The alpha-adrenergic properties cause the blood vessels to constrict, which reverses vasodilation and hypotension. This, in turn, elevates the diastolic pressure and improves coronary blood flow. The beta-1 adrenergic effects increase cardiac contractility, reversing the depressing effects on the heart and improving the strength of cardiac contractions. The beta-2 adrenergic effects cause bronchodilation, relieving bronchospasm in the lungs. Many patients and paramedic crews carry epinephrine in the form of an EpiPen and may have administered it before your arrival. The patient may have taken other medications as well, so it is important to obtain a medication history.

Maintain circulation by inserting at least one large-bore IV cannula to give an isotonic solution (lactated Ringer's or normal saline) at a wide-open rate. Ideally, you should place two IV lines en route to the ED. This step is crucial, especially if the patient is hypotensive and does not respond to the epinephrine.

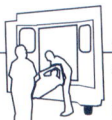
Initially, 1 to 2 l should be administered. If there is no response, you may need to administer up to 4 l. If the patient does not respond after 4 l of fluid, consider a vasopressor in conjunction with fluid administration.

Initiate pharmacologic therapy: oxygen, epinephrine, antihistamines, anti-inflammatory and immunosuppressant agents, and a vasopressor. Administer high-flow oxygen, and be prepared to assist ventilation. Patients who receive epinephrine must be monitored closely for adverse effects. You can do so by using a cardiac monitor to watch for dysrhythmias and reassessing vital signs frequently.

Allergic reactions that are *not* accompanied by signs of cardiovascular collapse (that is, hypotension) or airway compromise can be adequately treated with epinephrine 1:1,000 via the SQ route. For adults, give 0.3 to 0.5 mg of epinephrine; for children, give 0.01 mg/kg.

The adult EpiPen **Figure 30-8 ▾** delivers the medication intramuscularly in a dose of 0.3 mg of a 1:1,000 solution. The EpiPen Jr, which is used for children who weigh less than 15 kg, is also administered intramuscularly, but the concentration is 1:2,000 and the dose is 0.15 mg.

Epinephrine should be administered intravenously as soon as possible if hypotension or a reaction involving the airway or respiratory system is suspected or occurring. With IV epinephrine, give adults 0.1 to 0.5 mg of a 1:10,000 solution (during 5 minutes); give children 0.01 mg/kg of the same (1:10,000)

solution. An IV infusion of epinephrine should be administered at 1 to 4 μg/min (that is, 1 mg in 250 ml of saline = 4 μg/ml concentration). The advantage of an IV infusion is that the dose can be more easily controlled if the patient reacts negatively to the epinephrine (such as a geriatric patient or a patient with coronary artery disease). This approach may eliminate the need for repeated doses.

Antihistamine administration should be considered only after epinephrine has been administered. Antihistamines block the histamine 1 (H_1) and 2 (H_2) receptor sites. The antihistamine diphenhydramine (Benadryl) is commonly used in the prehospital setting following the administration of epinephrine. This medication does not prevent histamine release, but rather blocks histamine effects at the H_1 receptor sites. The typical dose of Benadryl is 25 to 50 mg administered slowly via the IM or IV route. H_2 blockers such as cimetidine (Tagamet) and ranitidine (Zantac) are also indicated but are more commonly used in the in-hospital setting. It is recommended that H_1 and H_2 blockers be administered until the anaphylactic symptoms resolve.

Corticosteroids do not have an immediate effect but are useful in preventing late-phase anaphylactic reactions and should be administered early in the treatment process. Common corticosteroids include methylprednisolone (Solu-Medrol), hydrocortisone (Solu-Cortef), and dexamethasone (Decadron).

Glucagon may also be indicated for an anaphylactic patient, especially if the patient does not respond to epinephrine or is taking a beta blocker. The usual dose is 1 to 2 mg IM or IV every 5 minutes. Glucagon increases cardiac contractility.

Vasopressors such as dopamine or levophed should be considered if the patient does not respond to fluid administration to treat the hypotension.

Inhaled beta-adrenergic agents such as salbutamol may also be included as part of the prehospital care regimen if bronchospasm is present.

Psychological support is a crucial component of management. Anaphylaxis can progress rapidly and has the potential to be a life-threatening event. Patients and their families will

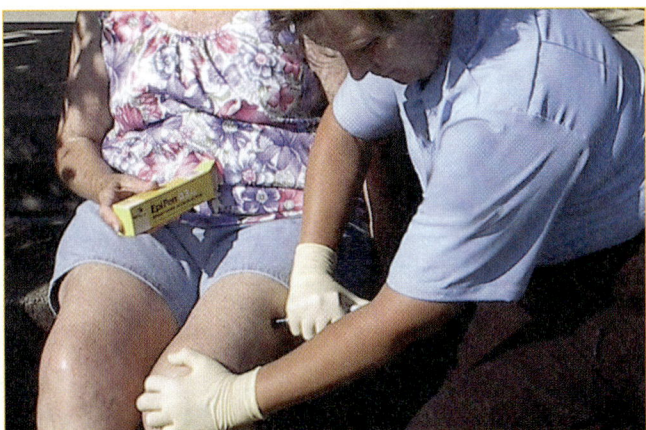

Figure 30-8 Administration of epinephrine with an auto-injector involves stabilizing the leg, pushing the auto-injector firmly against the thigh, and holding it in place until all of the medication is injected.

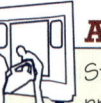

need reassurance as you perform the necessary interventions. Many of the patients have experienced similar events and may recognize how serious their condition has become. For others, this may be a first-time event. You need to be professional and reassuring and focus on early intervention and transport.

Consider early transport if the patient needs resources beyond your capabilities. Even if you are able to stop the reaction and the patient begins to recover, it is recommended that patients be observed in a medical facility. As many as 20% of patients will have a recurrence of the symptoms within the next 8 hours, even if they have been symptom-free for a time. Once the patient has been symptom-free for 4 hours, he or she can be released from the facility but should be instructed to return or call an ambulance if the symptoms recur.

Management of Allergic Reactions

People having allergic reactions are separated into two groups for management purposes. The first group includes patients who have signs of an allergic reaction—for example, hives—but no respiratory distress or dyspnea. The drug of choice is diphenhydramine. Continue to monitor for changes in condition, but most in this group will recover with no further problems.

The second group includes patients with signs of an allergic reaction and dyspnea. Patients require oxygen, epinephrine, and antihistamines (usually diphenhydramine). Whenever dyspnea is present with signs of an allergic reaction, you should administer epinephrine and monitor the patient for the development of anaphylaxis.

Patient Education

The best management of anaphylaxis and allergic reactions is to educate patients about prevention and self-preservation. At a minimum, discuss the following topics:

- **How to avoid the antigen.** Review information on the offending item. For example, if the patient is allergic to penicillin, he or she should be provided with a list of drugs that include penicillin and the alternative names for penicillin. Drugs that may produce a cross-reaction should also be discussed.
- **Notify all health personnel of the allergy.** Review the need to alert health personnel to the allergy. This is important because people often think only the doctor would need this information, not the paramedic.
- **Wear identification tags or bracelets.** These items notify paramedics of allergies in case the patient is unable to do so.
- **Carry an anaphylaxis kit.** A reaction may happen rapidly or worsen before help can arrive. Make sure the patient and his or her family know how to use the kit.
- **Report symptoms early.** Ideally, intervention should begin before the situation becomes life threatening. The patient should recognize that reactions can occur more rapidly and with greater severity with repeated exposures.

You are the Paramedic Summary

1. How would you categorize this patient and why?

Without always realizing it, you formulate your initial impression in a matter of moments. Factors such as facial expression, body position, and skin signs are noted immediately and provide valuable information about your patient's condition. Owing to this patient's anxious expression, tripod position, flushed skin, and audible wheezing, you know in 10 seconds or less that he is experiencing a life-threatening emergency.

2. What must you do to correct life-threatening conditions?

Given his tachypnea, tachycardia, hypotension, and recent history, you recognize this case as anaphylactic shock. You must apply high-flow oxygen and definitive prehospital care by administering epinephrine and diphenhydramine. These drugs will stop the production and absorption of histamine.

3. Why does the order of the medications matter?

Epinephrine should be administered first, because it will stop the production of histamine and correct the hypotension and continued edema, which could affect the airway. Diphenhydramine (Benadryl) should follow immediately. It binds the histamine receptor sites, minimizing the effects from histamine already present in the bloodstream.

4. Why is knowing all of the medication administration routes important?

If you cannot use your first choice of access for drug administration, you must be aware of alternatives. If you are unaware of these choices, you will cause unnecessary delays in prehospital care.

5. Would your prehospital care change if this patient were geriatric?

Because epinephrine has positive beta-1 and alpha-1 properties, its administration increases myocardial oxygen demand. With the current patient, his heart will be able to compensate for this increase without much difficulty. For a patient with a diseased heart, you must provide these interventions judiciously and be prepared for adverse reactions.

6. If the initial dose of epinephrine was successful, why administer another dose subcutaneously?

Like all drugs, epinephrine has a half-life. Providing another dose of epinephrine subcutaneously will maintain the therapeutic level in your patient.

7. What other options are available should your patient begin to have the same signs and symptoms you noted initially?

Initiating an epinephrine drip via IV piggyback is a choice you should anticipate. This will also provide a continual supply of epinephrine that may be required to counteract the histamine response, particularly because this patient took an oral medication that will likely continue to be released in the body for minutes to hours.

8. If your patient had not responded to initial treatment, what would you have anticipated in terms of interventions related to airway management?

Patients experiencing airway edema can be a particular challenge for paramedics. Endotracheal intubation can become impossible if laryngeal edema is too severe. Anticipate a narrowed glottis, which may require the choice of a smaller tube than would be normally used. If you cannot use bag-valve-mask ventilation and intubation is unsuccessful, you must consider implementing a surgical airway in accordance with your local protocols.

9. If you had been unable to obtain IV access, how would this have affected the call?

All of the medications used in this case could have been administered intramuscularly or subcutaneously. Doing so would have been less effective, however. Certain calls demand skill proficiency; they are literally a matter of life and death. As a paramedic, you must keep your skills sharp. If your call volume is high, you will not struggle as much with this issue. If you work in a location that does not respond to many calls, you must make up for this infrequency with constant practice and training. Regardless, do not delay initiating transport if you are unable to establish IV access. The patient with an anaphylactic reaction is a true medical emergency, and should be transported to the emergency department without delay.

Prep Kit

▬ Ready for Review

- An antigen is a substance the body recognizes as foreign. This recognition causes the body to produce antibodies to destroy the foreign substance.
- The immune system is responsible for the antigen–antibody response.
- An allergic response occurs when the body produces the antigen–antibody response when exposed to a substance that is usually harmless. An allergic response is usually limited to one body system or a local area.
- Anaphylaxis is an extreme form of systemic allergic response involving two or more body systems.
- A person must be sensitized to an antigen before an allergic or anaphylactic reaction can occur.
- The routes of exposure to an antigen include injection, absorption, inhalation, and ingestion.
- Mast cells release chemical mediators to stimulate the allergic reaction.
- Chemical mediators produce signs and symptoms through their effects on the skin, cardiovascular, respiratory, neurologic, and gastrointestinal systems.
- Skin effects include flushing, hives, and itching. Cyanosis and pallor may also be present.
- Cardiovascular effects include vasodilation, hypotension, decreased cardiac output, cardiac ischemia, and dysrhythmias.
- Respiratory effects include upper airway edema and stridor, hoarseness, bronchoconstriction, increased bronchial secretions, wheezes, hypoxia, and hypercapnea.
- Neurologic symptoms include altered level of consciousness, anxiety, restlessness, combativeness, and unconsciousness.
- Gastrointestinal symptoms include nausea, vomiting, diarrhea, and cramping.
- As part of your assessment, you should evaluate the scene, patient history, level of consciousness, upper airway, lower airway, skin, and vital signs. Assessment tools such as a pulse oximeter, cardiac monitor, and capnography are useful.
- Treatment of anaphylaxis includes removing the offending agent; maintaining the airway; administering medications such as epinephrine, antihistamines (diphenhydramine, cimetidine, ranitidine), corticosteroids, inhaled beta-adrenergic agents, and vasopressors; resuscitating with IV fluids; and initiating rapid transport.
- Epinephrine is first-line drug therapy for anaphylaxis.
- Patient education to prevent reexposure, to understand symptoms, and to understand the need to use an anaphylaxis kit is essential.

▬ Vital Vocabulary

absorption In allergic reactions, when foreign material is deposited on and moves into the skin.

acquired immunity The immunity the body develops as part of exposure to an antigen.

allergen A substance that produces allergic symptoms in a patient.

allergic reaction An abnormal immune response the body develops when reexposed to a substance or allergen.

anaphylaxis An extreme systemic form of an allergic reaction involving two or more body systems.

antibody A protein the body produces in response to an antigen; an immunoglobulin.

antigen An agent that, when taken into the body, stimulates the formation of specific protective proteins called antibodies.

basophils White blood cells that work to produce chemical mediators during an immune response.

cellular immunity The immunity provided by special white blood cells called T cells that attack and destroy invaders.

chemical mediators Chemicals that work to cause the immune or allergic response, for example, histamine.

histamine A chemical found in mast cells that, when released, causes vasodilation, capillary leaking, and bronchiole constriction.

humoural immunity The use of antibodies dissolved in the plasma and lymph to destroy foreign substances.

hypersensitivity Occurs when a patient reacts with exaggerated or inappropriate allergic symptoms after coming into contact with a substance the body perceives as harmful.

immune system The system that protects the body from foreign substances.

immunity The body's ability to protect itself from acquiring a disease.

ingestion Eating or drinking materials for absorption through the gastrointestinal tract.

inhalation In allergic reactions, foreign substances are breathed in through the respiratory system.

injection In allergic reactions, when the skin is pierced, and foreign material is deposited into the skin.

local reaction When the body limits a response to a specific area after being exposed to a foreign substance.

mast cells Basophils that are located in the tissues.

natural immunity The immunity the body develops as part of being exposed to an antigen and developing antibodies, for example, exposure to measles, having the measles, and developing immunity to the measles.

primary response The first encounter with the foreign substance to begin the immune response.

pruritus Itching.

secondary response The body's reaction when it is exposed to an antigen for which it already has antibodies, in which it responds by killing the invading substance.

sensitivity The ability to recognize a foreign substance the next time it is encountered.

systemic reaction A reaction that occurs throughout the body, possibly affecting multiple body systems.

urticaria Hives or reddened elevated patches on the skin.

Assessment in Action

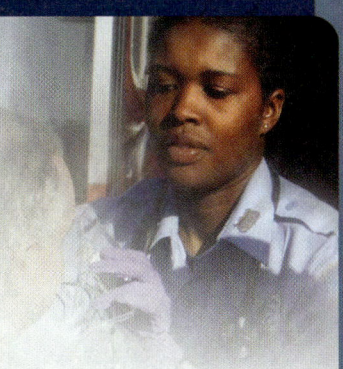

You are dispatched to the home of a 30-year-old woman who called because of an allergic reaction. When you enter the home, you see that the patient has bright red hives on her arms and upper part of the chest. She is in obvious respiratory distress. Her friend says that she is being treated for a recent strep infection. Her doctor gave her an antibiotic, and the patient has been taking it for approximately 4 days. When you ask her about allergies, she says that she was allergic to penicillin when she a teenager. She noticed her face and arms were turning red approximately 2 days ago; last night, her eyes began to swell. She called today because she felt as if her throat were closing up and she began having trouble breathing. She also complains of chest tightness. Her vital signs are a heart rate of 104 beats/min, sinus tachycardia on the monitor, pulse oximetry of 93% while breathing room air, blood pressure of 80/64 mm Hg, and a respiratory rate of 28 breaths/min.

1. An _____ is an overreaction by the body's immune response to normally harmless foreign substances, which cause damage to body tissues.
   A. antigen
   B. antibody
   C. allergic reaction
   D. allergy

2. In the preceding scenario, what type of reaction is the patient experiencing?
   A. Local reaction
   B. Systemic reaction
   C. Hypersensitivity reaction
   D. Allergen reaction

3. The most common causes of anaphylaxis include all of the following, EXCEPT:
   A. drugs.
   B. insect stings.
   C. blood products.
   D. IV fluids.

4. What are the routes of entry by which substances can invade?
   A. Skin, respiratory tract, and gastrointestinal tract
   B. Skin, respiratory tract, and cardiovascular system
   C. Skin, cardiovascular system, and gastrointestinal tract
   D. Skin, respiratory tract, and urinary tract

5. White blood cells that work to produce chemical mediators during an immune response are:
   A. mast cells.
   B. antibodies.
   C. basophils.
   D. histamines.

6. When an antigen enters the body, it binds to the IgE antibodies on the mast cells. This stimulates the mast cells to release:
   A. chemical mediators.
   B. granules.
   C. antihistamines.
   D. cellular immunity.

7. Itching or pruritus is an early sign of an allergic reaction. What is it caused by?
   A. Vasoconstriction
   B. Vasodilation
   C. Antigens
   D. Bronchodilation

8. What is the preferred route for administering epinephrine to a patient in anaphylactic shock?
   A. IV
   B. IM
   C. SQ
   D. SL

9. What is the IM adult dose of epinephrine?
   A. 1:1,000, 0.3–0.5 mg
   B. 1:10,000, 0.3–0.5 mg
   C. 1:1,000, 1 mg
   D. 1:10,000, 1 mg

Challenging Question

You are dispatched to the local high school to treat an allergic reaction. When you arrive on scene, you find a 17-year-old girl complaining of itchiness and hives. There is no respiratory distress. Her vital signs are all within normal ranges.

10. Is this patient having an allergic reaction or an anaphylactic reaction?

▬ Points to Ponder

You are treating a 46-year-old man for chest pain. You administer nitroglycerin and 325 mg of "baby" aspirin. En route to the hospital, you notice that the patient's skin is beginning to turn red and urticaria is developing. His lips are beginning to swell. You ask the patient about these signs, and he says that he forgot to tell you he is allergic to aspirin. His blood pressure has dropped significantly, his respiratory rate has increased, and his heart rate is increasing.

How urgent is this patient's emergency, and how will you provide prehospital care for it?

Issues: Understanding the Pathophysiology of an Allergic or Anaphylactic Reaction, Knowing Your Treatment Protocols for an Allergic Reaction and Anaphylactic Shock.

31 Gastrointestinal Emergencies

Competency Areas

Area 3: Health and Safety

3.3.a Assess scene for safety.
3.3.f Practice infection control techniques.
3.3.g Clean and disinfect equipment.
3.3.h Clean and disinfect an emergency vehicle.

Area 4: Assessment and Diagnostics

4.2.a Obtain list of patient's allergies.
4.2.b Obtain list of patient's medications.
4.2.c Obtain chief complaint and/or incident history from patient, family members, and/or bystanders.
4.2.d Obtain information regarding patient's past medical history.
4.2.e Obtain information about patient's last oral intake.
4.2.f Obtain information regarding incident through accurate and complete scene assessment.
4.3.a Conduct primary patient assessment and interpret findings.
4.3.b Conduct secondary patient assessment and interpret findings.
4.3.g Conduct gastrointestinal system assessment and interpret findings.
4.4.a Assess pulse.
4.4.b Assess respiration.
4.4.d Measure blood pressure by auscultation.
4.4.e Measure blood pressure by palpation.
4.4.i Assess level of mentation.
4.5.a Conduct oximetry testing and interpret findings.

Area 5: Therapeutics

5.2.a Recognize indications for oxygen administration.
5.5.b Control external hemorrhage through the use of direct pressure and patient positioning.
5.5.c Maintain peripheral intravenous (IV) access devices and infusions of crystalloid solutions without additives.

5.5.d Conduct peripheral intravenous cannulation.
5.8.a Recognize principles of pharmacology as applied to the medications listed in Appendix 5
5.8.b Follow safe process for responsible medication administration.

Appendix 4: Pathophysiology

E. **Gastrointestinal System**
Esophagus/Stomach: Esophageal varices
Esophagus/Stomach: Esophagitis
Esophagus/Stomach: Gastritis
Esophagus/Stomach: Gastrointestinal reflux
Esophagus/Stomach: Upper gastrointestinal bleed
Liver/Gall Bladder: Cholecystitis/biliary colic
Liver/Gall Bladder: Cirrhosis
Liver/Gall Bladder: Hepatitis
Pancreas: Pancreatitis
Small/Large Bowel: Appendicitis
Small/Large Bowel: Diverticulitis
Small/Large Bowel: Gastroenteritis
Small/Large Bowel: Inflammatory bowel disease
Small/Large Bowel: Lower gastrointestinal bleed
Small/Large Bowel: Obstruction
Traumatic Injuries: Esophageal disruption

I. **Endocrine System**
Thyroid disease

J. **Multisystem Diseases and Injuries**
Toxicologic Illness: Food poisoning
Immunologic Disorders: Autoimmune disorders
Shock Syndromes: Hypovolemic

Appendix 5: Medications

A. **Medications affecting the central nervous system.**
A.7 Non-narcotic analgesics
A.8 Opioid analgesics

Introduction

Gastrointestinal (GI) problems are rarely life threatening. This fact does not minimize the systemic problems that can erupt from untreated or undertreated diseases of the GI system. The appendix—a small, inconsequential portion of the intestine—has no known function, and its removal places the patient at no great health risk. Yet, if this little dangling outcropping becomes infected, the consequences can be deadly.

Almost everyone has suffered from abdominal pain at some point. Pain, diarrhea, nausea, and vomiting are common symptoms, but they should be regarded as signs and symptoms of an underlying condition. These symptoms can cause a wide range of conditions. Gastrointestinal disorders are common, as indicated by the data in Table 31-1 ▸. For example, it is estimated that 10% to 20% of people in Canada suffer from symptoms of gastroesophageal reflux disease (GERD).

Patients may have risk factors that can predispose them to GI disorders. Elements of a patient's history, such as age, previous illnesses or surgery, family history, medications, and use of cigarettes, alcohol, and illicit drugs may provide important clues to the etiology of a patient's symptoms. For example, alcohol consumption and smoking increase a person's risk for developing stomach disorders. Smoking can increase gastric acid secretion, and alcohol can help break down the gastric mucosal barrier to acid, putting the individual at risk for peptic

ulcers within the upper GI tract. Table 31-2 ▸ lists other activities that place patients at increased risk. Many people incorrectly believe that spicy foods can cause problems of the esophagus and stomach, but this is not known to be a risk factor for GI disease.

Table 31-1	Prevalence of Gastrointestinal Disorders in Canada
Disorder	**Prevalence**
All GI disorders	60 to 70 million (234,000 deaths per year, US data)
Constipation	63 million in North America
Crohn's disease	112,000
Diverticulitis	53 in every 100,000
Acute cholecystitis	88 in every 100,000
GERD	10% to 20% of Canadians
Hepatitis A	15 in every 100,000
Hepatitis B	2.3 in every 100,000
Hepatitis C	0.8% of Canadians
Infectious diarrhea	11 million cases in Canada each year
Irritable bowel syndrome	6% of Canadians
Pancreatitis	17 new cases in every 100,000
Peptic ulcer disease	14.5 million (US data)
Ulcerative colitis	88,500

You are the Paramedic Part 1

It is 01:00 hours on a busy Friday, and you and your partner are finally returning to the station for the first time since lunch. You barely get your boots off and rub your feet when the tones play that familiar song. Dispatch is sending you to a popular bar for a patient with uncontrolled bleeding. No other information is available at this time.

You walk into a dimly lit bar. The bartender waves you over and shouts that the patient is in the men's bathroom. You push your way through the crowd and slowly open the door. Your partner points to an open stall in the corner where a man is slumped over the toilet bowl with bright red blood trickling from the corner of his mouth. He responds appropriately but slowly when you speak to him.

Initial Assessment	Recording Time: 0 Minutes
Appearance	Ill-appearing middle-aged man
Level of consciousness	V (Responsive to verbal stimuli)
Airway	Patent
Breathing	Adequate chest rise and volume: good air entry bilaterally
Circulation	Weak, rapid radial pulse

1. What is your first priority in this situation?
2. What are some of the potential differential diagnoses?

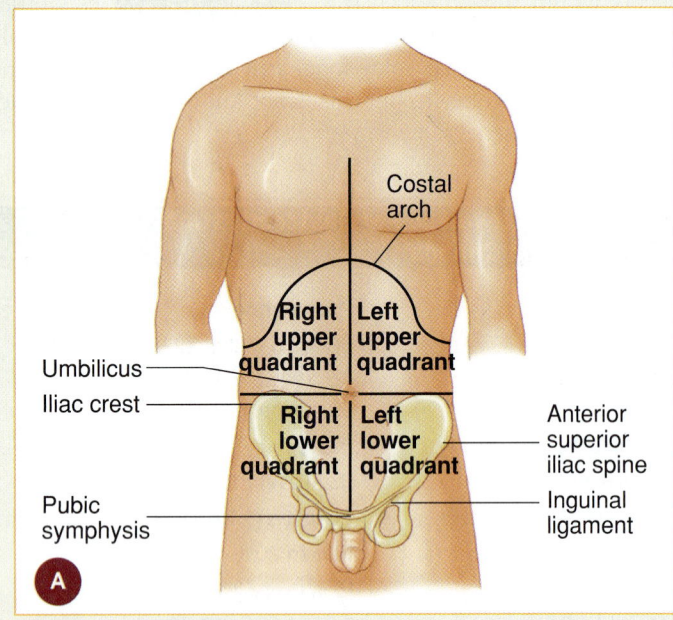

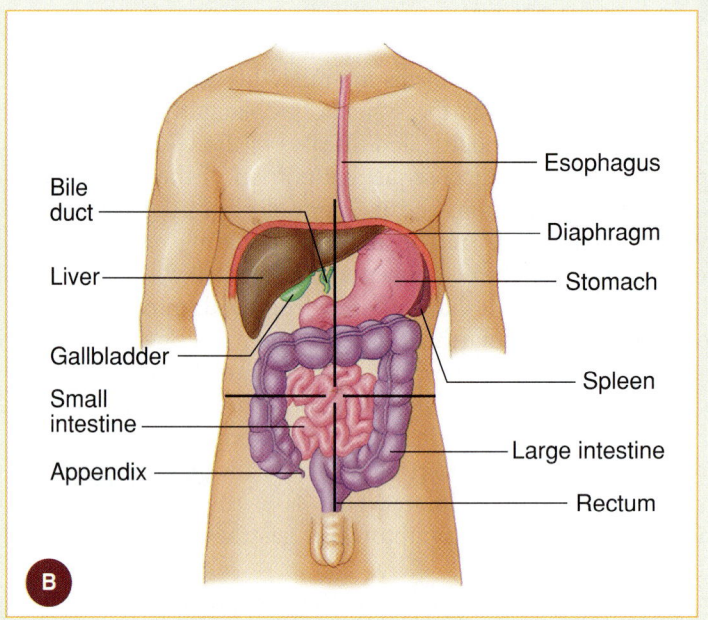

Figure 31-1 The anatomy of the abdomen. **A.** The four quadrants of the abdomen. **B.** Abdominal organs can lie in more than one quadrant.

Table 31-2	Risk Factors for GI Diseases
Behaviour	**Risk of GI Disease**
Smoking	Gastroesophageal reflux, stomach cancer
Ingestion of caustic agents	GI tract ulceration/perforation
Helicobacter pylori infection	Peptic ulcer, stomach cancer
Low-fibre diet	Constipation, diverticular disease
Alcohol	Esophageal varices, peptic ulcers, pancreatitis
Ingestion of nonsteroidal anti-inflammatory drugs (NSAIDs), anticoagulants	GI bleeding
High consumption of pickled foods	Stomach cancer

Anatomy and Physiology

It's dinner time, and Miranda is enjoying one of her favourite meals—a garden salad with lettuce, tomatoes, cucumbers, raisins, peanuts, croutons, carrots, and shrimp with ranch dressing. Examining the journey from food intake to elimination will illuminate the normal anatomy and physiology related to the GI system   Figure 31-1 ▲ .

In anticipation of eating, the salivary glands produce saliva, which contains water and mucous. Saliva helps to lubricate the food during chewing and swallowing. Miranda takes a bite of her salad. The lettuce, carrots, and cucumbers feel cool and crisp in her mouth, and this pleasant sensation encourages her to chew, a process called *mastication*   Figure 31-2 ▲ .

Miranda's front teeth are mainly used to tear or cut the food. At the back of her mouth, her molars pound and grind

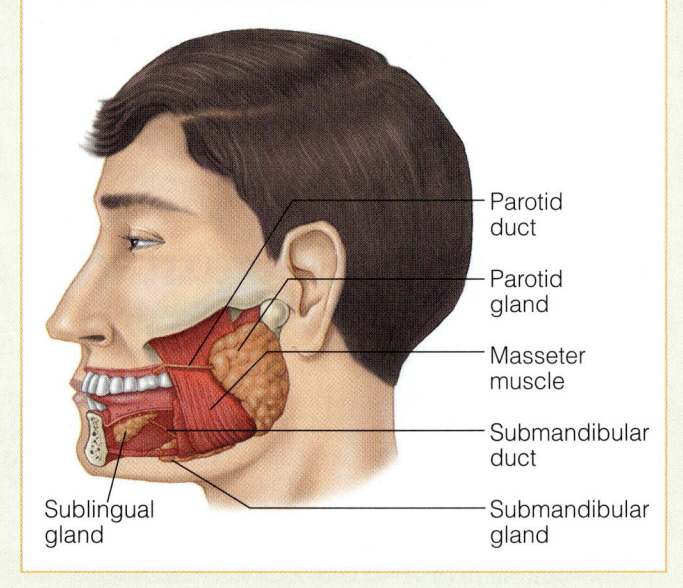

Figure 31-2 Mastication—the first step in the journey of the garden salad.

the food into a more easily swallowed consistency. This mechanical activity prepares food to travel down the esophagus more easily and prevents aspiration. As food is propelled to the back of the mouth by the tongue, it triggers a swallowing reflex.

Saliva also contains enzymes that begin the chemical breakdown of foods, in particular, starches. These complex carbohydrates can be disassembled into simple sugars that are more easily absorbed. As Miranda eats the raisins, the simple sugars are released and rapidly absorbed by capillaries within her tongue and mouth. In addition, some initial breakdown of triglycerides occurs.

Now Miranda prepares to swallow. The swallowing process is actually a complex, coordinated reflex that is mediated by a group of neurons in the brainstem. The proximal esophagus is located at the posterior portion of the hypopharynx. This muscular tube is typically collapsed (ie, closed in on itself), which allows for air to easily flow into the lungs but not into the stomach. The proximal esophagus rises and opens to receive the food bolus, while the glottis closes to prevent aspiration.

This collapsed tube idea also explains how gastric dilation and impairment of lung expansion can occur during ventilation. If a person needs positive-pressure ventilation, bag-valve-mask ventilation can push air into the lungs. If the pressure of the breath is too high, then the esophagus dilates; air then follows the path of least resistance. Given the choice between moving through a large tube into a large open space (the stomach) or moving down a series of progressively smaller tubes (the trachea into the right or left mainstem bronchus), air will flow into the stomach.

As Miranda swallows, a sequential series of muscle contractions propels the food toward the stomach. Although the esophagus is normally collapsed at rest, swallowing, reflux, and forceful ventilation with a bag-valve-mask device can all open this muscular organ. As the food moves more distally, the esophagus contains its own neurons that mediate sequential contractions, known as peristalsis, that propel the food bolus toward the stomach without involvement of the brainstem. As the food bolus nears the lower esophageal sphincter, this muscular segment relaxes to admit the food to the stomach. Some acid may be refluxed at this point. Saliva also contains a small amount of bicarbonate ions, which can neutralize small amounts of refluxed acid.

Intertwined around the esophagus are veins that drain into an even more complex series of veins, which ultimately join together to form the portal vein. The portal vein transports venous blood from the GI tract directly to the liver for processing of the nutrients that have been absorbed. If blood flow through the liver slows for any reason, the blood may back up throughout the entire GI system, because this series of veins lacks any valves. The veins surrounding the stomach and esophagus then become dilated. Even a low amount of pressure can cause leaking or rupture of these vessels.

The esophagus does not absorb nutrients, but rather pushes the food along using rhythmic contractions called *peristalsis*. The food travels in the esophagus past the diaphragm and comes to a doorway, the sphincter located at the junction of the esophagus and the stomach. The cardiac sphincter (which earns its name because people who have regurgitation of acid out of their stomach into their esophagus often feel they are having a heart attack) controls the amount of food that moves back up the esophagus.

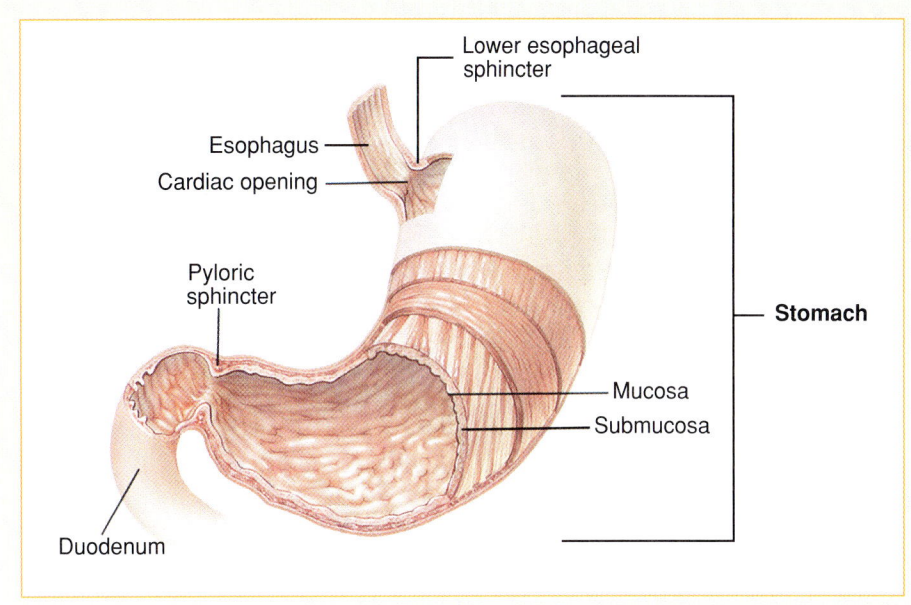

Figure 31-3 The stomach.

When empty, the stomach is rather small, but it is capable of stretching many times beyond its normal size to accommodate meals **Figure 31-3 ▲**. As the food enters this muscular organ, the stomach begins to secrete hydrochloric acid and pepsin, which help to break down the food. To mix the acid with the food more evenly, the stomach also contracts, churning the acid and food mixture together until a relatively smooth consistency is achieved. The material that exits the pyloric sphincter, the doorway at the inferior portion of the stomach, is called chyme.

Miranda eats a fairly large helping of salad. This is far too much food for the duodenum, the portion of the small intestine that will begin the very active stage of absorption. The stomach is designed to release only small amounts of the food into the duodenum, thereby enabling the small intestine to better manage digestion.

The stomach absorbs some materials, such as water and fat-soluble substances (eg, alcohol). If Miranda decided to have a glass of wine with her meal, the absorption of the alcohol would begin, slowly, within the stomach. Alcohol is absorbed rapidly within the duodenum. The longer the alcohol remains within the stomach, the slower the rate of its absorption into the bloodstream. Drinking alcohol with a fatty meal will delay gastric emptying, as the stomach works to digest the difficult fats. Miranda's meal is relatively low in fats, however, so she will feel the effects of the alcohol relatively quickly.

The real purpose of the digestive system is revealed in the next portion of the GI system. Why is Miranda eating in the first place? As the levels of nutrients available to her cells begin to drop, she feels hungry. She eats to replenish her resources, keeping her cells supplied with proteins, sugars, fats, electrolytes, and vitamins. The main function of the GI system is to absorb these resources for use by other cells in the body.

The duodenum is the first part of the small intestine. It is where the pancreas, liver, and gallbladder connect to the digestive system. The exocrine portion of the pancreas secretes several enzymes into the duodenum that assist with digestion of fats, proteins, and carbohydrates. In addition, pancreatic juice contains bicarbonate, which helps to neutralize gastric acids.

The liver creates bile, which is then stored in the gallbladder. Bile is an enzyme used by the body to help break down fats. Miranda's salad included shrimp and ranch dressing, both of which contain fat that must be broken down before it can be absorbed into the bloodstream. Bile is released into the duodenum, where it helps to emulsify (ie, dissolve into solution) the fats.

The liver receives blood with all the absorbed nutrients through the portal vein, and is responsible for a large part of the body's carbohydrate metabolism. The liver also affects the GI system indirectly, through carbohydrate metabolism. The brain cells can burn only one fuel source—glucose. If blood sugar falls, the liver can convert its glycogen stores into glucose.

Dramatic drops in sugar stores will cause the liver to convert fats and proteins into sugar. As blood flows through the liver, fat and protein metabolism continues. Without a functioning liver, Miranda would soon die, because she would not be able to use any of the proteins that were absorbed from the GI system. In addition, the liver detoxifies drugs, completes the breakdown of dead white blood cells and the heme component of dead red blood cells, and stores vitamins and minerals.

The real absorptive workhorse of the digestive system is the small intestine: 90% of all nutrient absorption occurs there. This 7-metre long structure is divided into three sections: the duodenum, the jejunum, and the ileum. The small intestine produces additional enzymes that work with the pancreatic enzymes and bile to turn chyme into smaller molecules that can be absorbed by the capillaries of the small intestine and move into the bloodstream Figure 31-4 ◄.

Blood loaded with nutrients exits the intestinal circulation and heads to the liver, where additional metabolism of fats and proteins takes place. The blood then leaves the liver and enters the systemic circulation. The water-soluble vitamins from the tomatoes and cucumbers in Miranda's salad are absorbed into the bloodstream for use by cells.

The large intestine, or colon, is the next destination for the remnants of the salad Figure 31-5 ▾. The substance that arrives in this 2-metre long structure is no longer called chyme, but feces. The valve between the ileum and the first portion of the large intestine is called the ileocecal valve. The first portion of the large intestine in the right lower quadrant is called the cecum. The appendix, a blind, wormlike pouch leading off the cecum can contain small amounts of fecal material. Occasionally, the appendix becomes impacted with material or infected and can become inflamed, resulting in appendicitis.

Rising up from the cecum is the ascending colon. It is continuous with the transverse colon, which runs from right to left. After another 90° turn, it becomes the descending colon. In the left lower quadrant, the colon then takes an "S" turn, where it is referred to as the sigmoid colon, which aligns its most inferior portion in the centre of the abdomen. The sigmoid colon continues as the rectum, the last portion of the colon. The colon

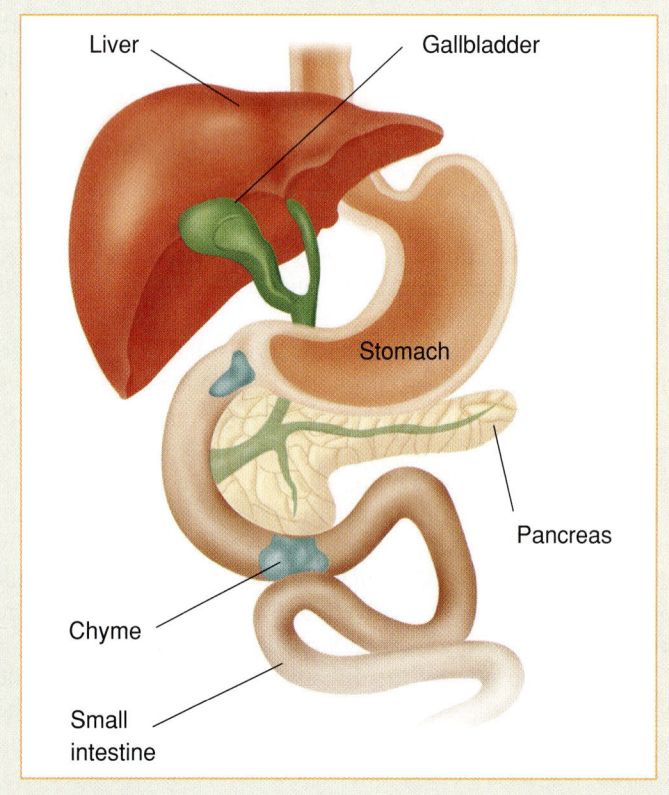

Figure 31-4 The garden salad is broken down into nutrients that the body can use.

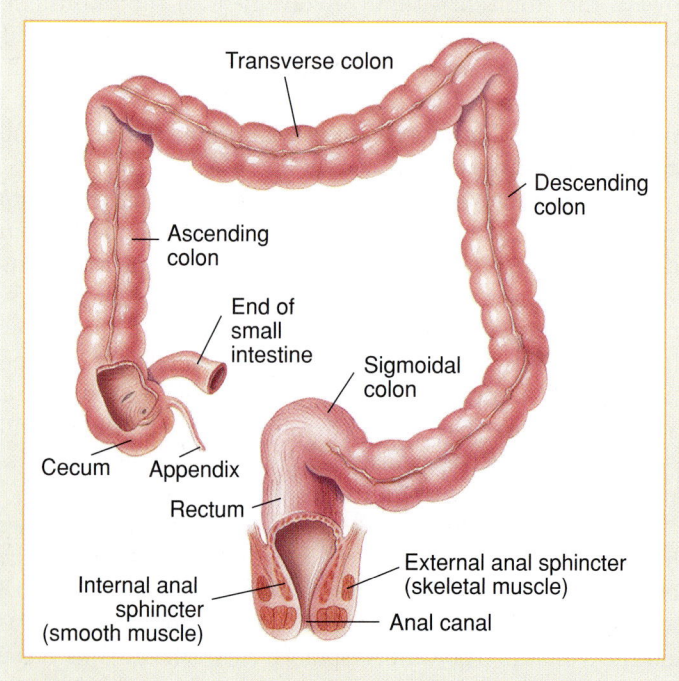

Figure 31-5 The colon is the next destination for the garden salad.

terminates at a sphincter called the anus, where feces are expelled from the body.

The primary role of the large intestine is to complete the reabsorption of water. Although the majority of water is reabsorbed in the small intestine, the osmotic function within the colon helps to solidify the digested material into a formed stool. Excess fluid secretion in the intestine or failure of this portion of the bowel can lead to a soft stool, or diarrhea.

The colon is also the site of bacterial digestion. Bacteria normally found within the colon help to finish the breakdown of chyme. This breakdown produces gas as a by-product. Flatulence may be considered impolite, but it is certainly normal. Loss of normal bacterial flora can lead to diarrhea or overgrowth of pathogenic bacteria such as *Clostridium difficile*.

Table 31-3 ▾ summarizes the organs involved in digestion. The entire digestion process takes 8 to 72 hours. At this pace, bowel movements range from three movements per day to one movement every three days. Of course, this number varies based on the types of food eaten, the amount of water consumed, exercise, and stress.

General Approach to GI Diseases

Diseases of the GI tract present with certain common symptoms. The most common symptoms are pain, fluid losses (vomiting and/or diarrhea), bleeding, and alterations in bowel habits. Less common symptoms relate to alterations of liver or pancreatic function, such as jaundice or malabsorption. Taking a brief, but appropriate, history; conducting a focused physical examination; and deciding on appropriate prehospital interventions are key in dealing with a patient presenting with GI disease.

Table 31-3 | Abdominal Organs, Location, and Functions

Organ/Structure	Location	Function
Mouth	Head	Mechanical breakdown of food. Begins chemical breakdown with saliva.
Esophagus	Substernal, epigastric	Tube that moves food from the mouth to the stomach. Muscular and vascular structure.
Stomach	Left upper quadrant, epigastric	Performs mechanical and chemical breakdown of food. Food in, chyme out.
Small intestine: duodenum	Central, upper umbilical	Major site for chemical breakdown of food and major absorption of water, fats, proteins, carbohydrates, and vitamins.
Small intestine: jejunum	Central, umbilical	
Small intestine: ileum	Central, hypogastric to lower right abdomen	
Large intestine: ascending colon	Right lower quadrant, hypogastric into epigastric	Water reabsorption, formation of feces, bacterial digestion of food.
Large intestine: transverse colon	Right to left upper quadrant, epigastric	
Large intestine: descending colon	Left upper and lower quadrant, epigastric to umbilical	
Large intestine: sigmoid colon	Left lower quadrant, hypogastric	
Large intestine: rectum	Superpubic, hypogastric	
Anus	Most inferior portion of the large intestine	Sphincter to control release of feces.
Liver	Upper abdomen. Mainly right with central upper abdomen.	Production of bile; assists with carbohydrate, protein, and fat metabolism of nutrients within the bloodstream; vitamin storage and manufacture; detoxification of blood; elimination of waste.
Pancreas	Posterior to the stomach	Exocrine: enzymes for protein, carbohydrate, and fat breakdown within duodenum. Endocrine: insulin, somatostatin, glucagons.
Gallbladder	Inferior surface of the liver	Storage of bile.
Spleen	Left upper abdomen	Filtering of blood, recycling of dead red blood cells.
Aorta	Central upper abdomen	Main artery to lower body.
Bladder	Suprapubic area	Storage of urine.
Uterus	Suprapubic area	Reproduction.
Iliac arteries	Central abdomen and lower right/left quadrants	Blood supply to legs and pelvis.

Abdominal Pain

Abdominal pain can be a nonspecific indicator of gastrointestinal disease, although certain characteristics of the pain can provide important clues to the underlying etiology. In addition, organs that are not part of the GI tract can also cause abdominal pain. The paramedic should consider whether the patient's pain could relate to non-GI organs, such as the urinary system, aorta, or reproductive system.

As with all types of pain, obtaining a good patient history includes defining the nature and time course of the pain, the pain's location, aggravating and relieving factors, and associated symptoms. The internal organs of the GI tract are poorly innervated for conscious sensation, thus the patient may initially have poorly localized abdominal pain. This is typical of visceral sensations, which are carried through neurons of the autonomic nervous system. Associated symptoms such as fever, nausea, vomiting, or alterations of bowel function—either constipation or diarrhea—may provide additional clues as to the source of the pain. Sometimes visceral pain arising from a muscular organ such as the bowel or gallbladder will wax and wane with contractions of the organ.

Referred pain is pain that is distant to the site of the problem, usually because of the way in which the body's autonomic nervous system has pain nerves arising from a large area. For example, pain radiating to a shoulder may herald a problem with an organ close to the diaphragm, such as the gallbladder, which shares innervation with the shoulder. Pain in the back sometimes arises from retroperitoneal organs, such as the kidneys, aorta, and pancreas.

As the disease progresses, it may cause irritation of the peritoneal lining close to the organ. The peritoneal is richly innervated, thus the development of well-localized, somatic pain may point to the source of the problem. This typical progression sometimes occurs in appendicitis, which can start as pain in the umbilical region and then become localized to the right lower quadrant.

Perforation of an organ of the GI tract can occur as the result of obstruction or an inflammatory process, such as an ulcer. With a perforation, the bowel contents spill into the peritoneal cavity and irritate the nerves of the peritoneal lining. The generalized abdominal pain that ensues, along with reflux contraction of the abdominal wall muscles, is referred to as *peritonitis*. Peritonitis can also result from the irritating effect of bleeding into the peritoneal cavity. The presence of bacterial-laden fecal contents into the peritoneal cavity is also associated with the development of fever, and sometimes septic shock. This can be seen in patients who develop a perforation as a complication of appendicitis.

Fluid Losses

Dehydration may result from vomiting, diarrhea, poor oral intake, or malabsorption of water in the large intestine. As the patient loses fluid, the body continues to shift water from the interstitial fluid to the vascular space and from the intracellular space to the interstitial space in an attempt to maintain vascular volume for perfusion of organs. A patient may initially present with normal vital signs and thirst. Progressive dehydration can lead to tachycardia. The development of hypotension heralds severe dehydration, because the patient is no longer capable of mobilizing fluid into the vascular space.

Electrolyte balance is also affected by GI fluid losses. Both vomiting and diarrhea are known to deplete potassium. Depending on how much sodium is lost, dehydration can also result in low or high sodium levels. **Table 31-4** ▾ summarizes the effects of electrolyte imbalances. Depending on the speed at which these losses occur, symptoms may range from mild to severe and life threatening.

GI Bleeding

Hypovolemia may also be a consequence of hemorrhage. The GI tract's generous blood supply helps to ensure that nutrients can be absorbed rapidly, but it also makes it more vulnerable to severe hemorrhage. The location of the hemorrhage can sometimes be ascertained from the nature of the bleeding. Upper GI bleeding in the esophagus or stomach will sometimes present with vomiting of blood or a material that resembles coffee grounds. This latter material represents hemoglobin that has been exposed to gastric acid. Rectal blood loss may take the form of obvious bleeding or a black, tarry material called melena. This latter material represents blood after it is transformed by passage through the GI tract. Finally, some blood loss is termed *occult*, because it is only determined by fecal testing and is not obvious to the patient or caregiver. Obvious blood loss through the rectum can result from either a lower GI bleed or a particularly brisk upper GI bleed.

Most bleeding from the rectum results from erosion of blood vessels near the surface of the mucosa. This sometimes occurs in peptic ulcers, diverticular disease, or cancer. Other causes of bleeding arise from severe inflammation of the GI tract. For example, patients with inflammatory diseases of the bowel such as Crohn's disease or ulcerative colitis may develop bleeding ulcers of the intestines. These patients will usually report additional symptoms, such as pain and fever, in addition to bloody diarrhea. Trauma is an obvious but rarely seen mechanism for bleeding from within the GI system. Common causes of GI

Table 31-4	Electrolyte Imbalances Caused by Diarrhea	
Condition	**Effects**	**Signs and Symptoms**
Hyponatremia (low sodium)	Swelling of cells	Muscle weakness, cramping, coma, convulsions
Hypernatremia (high sodium)	Shrinking of cells due to excessive water loss	Coma, convulsions
Hypokalemia (low potassium)	More stimulation needed to fire nerve/muscle cells	Muscle cramps, weakness, paralysis, heart failure, dysrhythmia
Hyperkalemia (high potassium)	Less stimulation needed to fire nerve/muscle cells	Muscle weakness and cramps, bradycardia, asystole

Table 31-5	Gastrointestinal Bleeding by Organ and Cause			
Organ	**Causes**		**Location**	**Substances**
Esophagus	Inflammation (esophagitis) Varices (varicose veins) Tear (Mallory-Weiss syndrome) Cancer Dilated veins (cirrhosis, liver disease)		Upper GI	Melena, hematemesis, vomit with gross blood
Stomach	Ulcers Cancer Inflammation (gastritis)		Upper GI	Melena, hematemesis, vomit with gross blood
Small intestine	Ulcer (duodenal)		Upper GI	Melena, hematemesis, vomit with gross blood
	Cancer Inflammation (inflammatory bowel disease, Crohn's disease)		Upper or lower GI	Melena, hematemesis, vomit with gross blood
Large intestine	Infections Inflammation (ulcerative colitis) Colourectal polyps Colourectal cancer Diverticular disease		Lower GI	Hematochezia
Rectum	Hemorrhoids		Lower GI	Hematochezia, gross bleeding

bleeding are listed in **Table 31-5 ▲**. Because the blood loss from the GI tract cannot be controlled by the application of pressure, GI bleeding can sometimes be fatal.

With either severe diarrhea or hemorrhage, the patient may suffer from shock. As discussed in Chapter 18, the body compensates for shock by releasing catecholamines. In an effort to maintain blood pressure, these neurotransmitters increase the heart rate, force contractions of the heart, and increase vasoconstriction. During compensated shock, organ perfusion and blood pressure remain near normal. Signs of compensated shock may include tachycardia and pale, cool, clammy skin as the body shunts blood away from the skin and muscles. The pulse pressure narrows, because epinephrine causes vasoconstriction, and respirations increase. As shock progresses, compensatory mechanisms begin to fail. The blood pressure may drop, and there may be ominous signs of loss of end organ perfusion, such as changes in mental status and decreased urine output.

Altered Bowel Habit

Although food contains a variety of bacteria, viruses, and fungi, most of these are destroyed through cooking or pasteurization of food. The organisms that remain are usually killed by stomach acid and digestive juices. However, small amounts of organisms sometimes get past the immune system's defences, which can lead to gastrointestinal infection. In the majority of affected patients, GI infections often present with diarrhea and/or vomiting. In the United States, an estimated 76 million people get a foodborne illness each year, but only 5,000 die of this cause—a mere 0.007% of those who become ill. In Canada, estimates suggest that up to one sixth of the population suffers from a foodborne illness each year, but deaths due to this illness are rare. People who are immunocompromised (eg, patients who have acquired

immunodeficiency syndrome [AIDS] or certain types of cancers, patients who are undergoing chemotherapy, and transplant recipients), the very old, and the very young generally have a harder time fighting off an infection of any type and are more likely to have a poor outcome from foodborne illness. Travelling to other countries can also place a person at greater risk for food intolerances or food-borne infections. "Traveller's diarrhea" affects as many as 33% of all people who travel to countries where food cleanliness is less than adequate, such as in parts of South America, Asia, and Africa.

The opposite change in bowel habit, decreased stool frequency, can result from constipation or bowel obstruction. Constipation is a common complaint and sometimes results in calls to EMS when it is associated with severe pain or discomfort. Constipation may result from changes to medications, use of opioids, immobility or lack of physical activity (sometimes seen in the bedridden elderly), and may be acute or chronic. The longer the stool remains in the colon, the harder it becomes as the colon works to reabsorb water. Despite the discomfort, these patients rarely suffer from vomiting and are still able to pass flatus.

Bowel obstruction occurs when there is failure of peristalsis due to diseases of the bowel, systemic illness, medications, or mechanical blockage of passage of material through the intestine. The most common reason is when the intestines, which are normally free to move or slide internally in the peritoneal cavity, become twisted or entrapped. This can occur in patients who have scar tissue from previous surgery or hernias. Volvulus is a complete twisting of the bowel on itself. Finally, cancers may cause narrowing or complete blockage of the lumen of the intestine. Bowel obstructions present with crampy, poorly localized abdominal pain, absence of stool and flatus, and sometimes vomiting.

Altered Organ Function

Symptoms attributable to the liver can sometimes result in right upper quadrant pain. More often, it is difficult to distinguish organ involvement without specific testing or imaging unless there are specific signs of failure of the involved organ. Patients with liver failure, once it reaches an advanced stage, may develop yellow skin and sclerae from jaundice. Other signs and symptoms of advanced liver failure include altered mental status from the buildup of bilirubin, ammonia, and other toxins and itchy skin. A distended abdomen

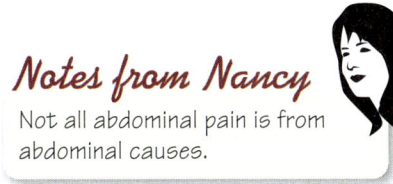

Notes from Nancy

Not all abdominal pain is from abdominal causes.

may be the result of cirrhosis, which causes blood to back up in the GI organs and fluid to accumulate in the abdomen. The pancreas may become acutely inflamed and painful in pancreatitis, but poor pancreatic function can be more subtle, with diarrhea and fat droplets in the stool due to fat malabsorption.

Special Considerations

The geriatric population presents paramedics with a number of complicating factors. For example, older adults tend to have more than one disease, they may take several medications, and the function of their organ systems is declining. In addition, the perception of pain by an older patient may be affected by dementia or diabetic neuropathy, preventing the patient from feeling or responding to pain in a typical manner. For example, an elderly patient with altered mental status, vomiting, and vague abdominal pain may actually be suffering from acute appendicitis.

Patients who have decreased immune function may have altered illness presentation. These patients may include very young infants, the elderly, patients taking immune-suppressant medications such as chemotherapy agents or steroids, and patients with AIDS. The reaction of the body to illness is to mount an inflammatory response with fever and pain from peritoneal irritation, as white blood cells migrate to the site of the problem. Patients with decreased immune function may lack many of the classic symptoms and yet have severe or overwhelming disease.

The prudent paramedic will perform a detailed assessment of the conscious geriatric patient to detect even subtle changes related to bowel habits, eating habits, new foods, travel, new medications, low-grade fevers, or other factors. Gathering information may be more challenging, but your efforts will convey your sense of compassion and caring to a population that is sometimes marginalized or dismissed.

Specific Conditions

Table 31-6 ▶ summarizes the major diseases of the GI system.

Esophageal Varices

Esophageal varices occur when the pressure within the blood vessels of the distal esophagus increases due to liver damage or cirrhosis. In industrialized countries, alcohol is the main cause of portal hypertension. Chronic alcohol consumption damages and scars the interior of the liver (cirrhosis), leading to slower blood flow and higher venous pressures. These higher pressures are the cause of increased risk of bleeding. In developing countries, viral hepatitis is the main cause of liver damage. Esophageal varices can present with massive, life-threatening upper GI bleeding.

Mallory-Weiss Syndrome

Mallory-Weiss syndrome may lead to severe hemorrhage. With this condition, the esophageal lining tears during severe vomiting. In addition to bleeding, a frank rupture of the esophagus can rarely occur (known as Boerhaave's syndrome). Spillage of gastric contents into the mediastinum can result in pneumothorax and overwhelming sepsis. Mallory-Weiss syndrome affects both men and women equally, but it is more prevalent in older adults and older children.

Hemorrhoids

Hemorrhoids are caused by swelling and inflammation of the blood vessels surrounding the rectum. They are a common problem, with almost half the population having at least one hemorrhoid by age 50. Hemorrhoids may result from conditions that increase pressure on the rectum or irritation of the

You are the Paramedic Part 2

You begin your assessment while your partner takes a set of vital signs. You are able to find out that the patient's name is Rob and that he is 47 years old. When asked what happened this evening, all he is able to tell you is that he was drinking at the bar minding his own business when he felt a horrible pain in his stomach. He felt like he needed to throw up, so he went to the bathroom. That is the last thing he remembers. You observe a significant amount of bright red blood (approximately 1 litre) on the floor around the toilet.

The patient says that he is still very nauseous and is in extreme pain. He rates his pain as 10 out of 10 on the pain scale. His pain is located in the epigastric area and does not radiate. He describes the pain as knifelike. He denies having any past medical condition or allergies. When questioned about his alcohol intake for the night, he says that he lost count at five whiskey on the rocks and about 10 beers since 20:00 hours.

Vital Signs	Recording Time: 5 Minutes
Level of consciousness	Verbal
Pulse	118 beats/min, weak and regular
Blood pressure	88/64 mm Hg
Respirations	26 breaths/min, regular
Skin	Warm, jaundiced, slightly diaphoretic
Spo$_2$	97% on room air

3. What are the signs and symptoms of ruptured esophageal varices?

4. What is the most common cause of esophageal varices?

Table 31-6	Gastrointestinal Diseases by Condition Type and Presenting Problem	
Disease	**Condition Type**	**Common Presenting Problems**
Acute gastroenteritis	Infectious	Pain, diarrhea, dehydration
Acute hepatitis	Infectious	Pain, liver failure
Appendicitis	Acute inflammation	Pain, sepsis
Bowel obstruction	Decreased motility	Pain, vomiting, sepsis
Cholecystitis	Acute inflammation	Pain
Colitis	Chronic inflammation	Pain, diarrhea, bleeding, dehydration
Crohn's disease	Chronic inflammation	Pain, diarrhea, dehydration
Diverticulitis	Acute inflammation	Pain, sepsis
Esophageal varices	Hemorrhagic	Pain, hemorrhage
Gastroenteritis	Erosive	Pain, diarrhea, dehydration
Hemorrhoids	Hemorrhagic	Pain, hemorrhage
Pancreatitis	Acute inflammation	Pain, hemorrhage
Peptic ulcer disease	Erosive/infectious	Pain, hemorrhage

rectum. Pregnancy, straining at stool, and chronic constipation cause increased pressure. Anal intercourse and diarrhea cause irritation.

Peptic Ulcer Disease

The stomach and duodenum are subjected to high levels of acidity. To prevent damage to these organs, protective layers of mucus line both organs. In peptic ulcer disease (PUD), the protective layer is eroded, allowing the acid to eat into the mucosal lining of the stomach.

In the past, PUD was thought to be related to the types of foods eaten. Today, it is known to have a variety of etiolotigies. The major risk factors are *Helicobacter pylori* infection and use of nonsteroidal anti-inflammatory drugs (NSAIDs). Alcohol and smoking can also exacerbate PUD.

PUD affects both men and women equally, but tends to occur more often in older adults. In addition to having an increased prevalence of *H pylori* infection, the geriatric population also uses NSAIDs more frequently for arthritis and other musculoskeletal complaints.

Cholecystitis

Cholecystitis is caused by obstruction of the cystic duct leading from the gallbladder to the duodenum, usually by gallstones. Gallstones are believed to form either due to increased production of bile or decreased emptying of the gallbladder.

The gallbladder stores bile, an enzyme used to break down fat; when it contracts, it releases this bile. When fatty foods are present within the duodenum, the contraction will occur, but if a blockage is present the patient may experience severe extreme right upper quadrant pain, radiating to the right shoulder. In addition to the pain, the patient may demonstrate a positive Murphy's sign. This can be elicited by asking the patient to breathe in deeply while pressing deeply

on the right upper quadrant near the costal margin. As the diaphragm descends, the inflamed gallbladder is pushed distally toward the examiner's fingers. If the patient stops the inspiration suddenly due to pain, this is considered a positive Murphy's sign. Pain alone is characteristic of biliary colic. Progression with development of fever, jaundice, and tachycardia suggests inflammation of the gallbladder, called cholecystitis.

Females suffer from cholecystitis two to three times more often than do males. Older adults are more prone to this condition than their younger counterparts. Caucasians have a higher prevalence than African Canadians. People who are overweight or have had a recent extreme weight loss are also at greater risk. The profile of the "classic" cholecystitis patient is fair, fat, female, and 50.

Appendicitis

Appendicitis begins with the accumulation of material, usually feces, within the appendix. Once this organ is obstructed, pressure may build within the appendix. This pressure decreases the flow of blood and lymph fluid, which in turn hinders the body's ability to fight infection in the local area. If left unchecked, the appendix may eventually rupture, causing peritonitis, sepsis, and death.

Adolescents have the highest incidence of appendicitis, with the number of cases dropping as age increases. Although older adults suffer from appendicitis less often, they have a higher mortality with this condition compared to their younger counterparts. Males are slightly more prone to developing appendicitis than females.

Diverticulitis

Diverticulitis was first recognized around 1900, when it was noted that people in Western societies tended to eat more foods containing processed grains and less dietary fibre. Diets low in fibre tend to result in more solid stools and increased intraluminal pressures in the colon. Small defects within the colonic wall are normally present at points where the arteries enter. The increased intraluminal pressures result in bulges in the colon wall at the points of entry of the arteries. These small outcroppings eventually turn into pouches, called diverticula.

As feces travel through the colon, some may become trapped within these pouches. When bacteria grow there, they cause localized inflammation and infection. As the body attempts to manage this infection, scarring can occur, along with adhesions and fistulas. A fistula is an abnormal connection between two cavities. In the case of diverticulitis, fistulas are typically between the colon and the bladder, increasing their vulnerability to infection.

The typical patient with diverticulitis is older than age 40. More important than sex or race is the amount of fibre in the patient's diet. Decreased fibre increases the risk for this disease. Interestingly, people in Western societies are more likely to develop diverticulitis than those from Africa and Asia.

Pancreatitis

The pancreas produces several enzymes that help break down food into substances that can be absorbed by the intestines. If the duct carrying these enzymes becomes blocked, the enzymes become activated and begin to break down the protein and fat of the pancreas itself, a process referred to as autodigestion of the pancreas. Factors contributing to the development of pancreatitis include increased alcohol consumption and gallstones. Other causes include medication reactions, trauma, cancer, and very high triglyceride levels.

Pancreatitis can occur suddenly, or it may persist over many months. Patients can have singular attacks or recurrent episodes. The condition is more common in men than women. It also occurs more often in African Canadians aged 35 to 64 years.

Ulcerative Colitis

Ulcerative colitis is caused by generalized inflammation of the colon. It is unclear what causes this chronic inflammation, but genetics, stress, and autoimmunity have been speculated to contribute to its etiology. In ulcerative colitis, the inflammation causes a thinning of the wall of the intestine, resulting in a weakened, dilated colon. The damaged lining of the colon is then prone to bacterial infections and bleeding.

Ulcerative colitis is a disease of the young; most patients are between 15 and 30 years of age. It occurs with equal incidence in men and women. The disease has a strong hereditary component; 20% of patients have a family member with this disease. Ulcerative colitis is also more prevalent in Caucasians and people of Jewish descent.

Crohn's Disease

Crohn's disease is similar to ulcerative colitis, but it may affect the entire GI tract. In this condition, the immune system attacks the GI tract, and the activity of the white blood cells damages all layers of the portion of the GI tract involved. The most likely site of inflammation is the ileum, the final portion of the small intestine before it joins the large intestine. The result is a scarred, narrowed, stiff, and weakened portion of the small intestine; this damaged patch is found among areas of intestine that are perfectly normal.

To date, no definitive cause for Crohn's disease has been identified. However, the presence of signs and symptoms outside the GI system supports the hypothesis that there is an autoimmune component. Perhaps the presence of antigens within the GI tract triggers an immune response, or perhaps the immune system itself is not working correctly. Another hypothesis is that the immune system creates antibodies for an antigen that does not exist, initiating a cascade of reactions to a ghost invader.

Most patients with Crohn's disease are between the ages of 20 and 30 years. Men are diagnosed as often as women. People of African descent tend not to suffer from this condition, whereas people of Jewish descent have an increased incidence. Many of the people with this condition have a blood relative with some type of inflammatory bowel disease, suggesting that these conditions have a genetic component.

Acute Gastroenteritis

Acute gastroenteritis comprises a family of infectious conditions presenting with diarrhea, nausea, and vomiting. Bacterial, viral, and parasitic organisms that can cause this condition include *Escherichia coli, Salmonella, Shigella, Giardia*, the Norwalk virus, *Clostridium difficile*, and rotavirus. These agents typically enter the body through contaminated food or water or through fecal–oral contact with ill patients. Patients may begin to experience cramps, vomiting, diarrhea, and sometimes fever and chills several hours to several days after contact with the organism. The disease then either runs its course in 2 to 3 days or continues for several weeks.

Certain organisms secrete toxins that cause destruction of the intestinal mucosa, leading to bloody diarrhea. Immune-compromised patients are at risk of more severe infections, including systemic infections and even death.

Cholera, a type of acute gastroenteritis that is relatively unknown in Canada, is encountered frequently in the developing world. The Norwalk virus is responsible for the majority of acute viral gastroenteritis in adults, whereas rotavirus causes the same condition in children. These latter two infections are usually self-limited and resolve with supportive care and oral or intravenous hydration.

Noninfectious causes of nausea, vomiting, and diarrhea include medications or chemotherapy, toxins found in some shellfish or contaminated foods, or certain poisons.

Acute Hepatitis

Acute hepatitis is the result of damage to the liver caused by one of several viruses. In Canada, the hepatitis A, B, and C viruses are the predominant causes of acute hepatitis. Hepatitis D is a co-infection with hepatitis B, but is rare in developed countries. Similarly, hepatitis E is primarily found in Southeast Asia, Africa, and Central America. Two other strains, F and G, are also being investigated for their role in causing liver damage. Other causes of acute hepatitis include the Epstein-Barr virus, cytomegalovirus, certain bacterial infections, and liver cancer.

Hepatitis viruses are transmitted in a variety of ways. Types A and E move from patient to patient by the fecal–oral route (ie, feces from an infected person is released into the environment and then contaminates either the food or water consumed by another individual). Types B, C, and D are transmitted by person-to-person contact, typically either by sexual intercourse or parenterally (ie, blood-to-blood contact, usually by blood transfusion, accidental needlesticks, or sharing of dirty needles). IV drug users and prostitutes are at higher risk for acquiring hepatitis B, C, and D, whereas people travelling to countries where food and water safety are not adequate are at risk for developing hepatitis A and E.

The time from the initial infection to the emergence of clinical signs and symptoms can range from 14 to 180 days with acute hepatitis. Acute hepatitis can cause abdominal pain, vomiting, fever, and jaundice. Chronic infection or complications of an acute infection can lead to cirrhosis, with all its attendant complications.

■ Assessment and Evaluation

Scene Assessment

Scene safety is the paramount concern for all types of calls. Although there are no specific concerns related to patients with GI emergencies, you need to exercise caution to ensure that all personnel remain safe. In terms of additional resources, these patients often need some type of assistance with hygiene, because GI complaints routinely involve body substances. Because many GI diseases have the potential to cause transmission of communicable diseases, additional resources for the GI patient may include extra gloves, mask, gowns, change of uniform, suction equipment, extra linens, blankets, wash rags, towels, and adult and child diapers.

The mechanism of injury or nature of illness, as with most medical complaints, will contribute to your initial impression. Early in the call, the only information available may have come from the dispatch centre. Use this information determine the amount of equipment you will take into the scene. Note that most calls for GI problems will not involve multiple patients. However, a call for assistance at an office building where several people are complaining of GI symptoms should lead you to suspect release of an agent. Biological or chemical agents, for example, can cause people to have abdominal pain, nausea, vomiting, diarrhea, and other GI signs and symptoms.

The last component of the scene assessment is the use of personal protective equipment (PPE) and routine precautions. This consideration is particularly important for GI patients. Gloves are needed, as with most calls. Given that you may need to manage vomit, diarrhea, and soiled patient clothing in these calls, additional PPE resources may be called upon. Gowns can be helpful when dealing with patients who have become incontinent. Masks can help with noxious odours.

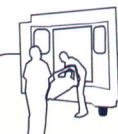
Notes from Nancy
Severe abdominal pain that comes on suddenly and lasts longer than 6 hours must be considered serious and will often require surgery.

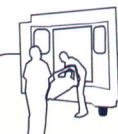
At the Scene
All paramedics should have a clear understanding of the medical terms used to describe findings from a GI patient to avoid confusion.

Initial Assessment

In forming your general impression, closely examine the location where the patient is found, because it can provide hints about what happened. Was the patient walking to the bathroom when he or she passed out? Has the patient been sick for several days and camped out on the couch? Was the patient at work when a sudden bout of pain doubled him or her over
Figure 31-6 ▾ ?

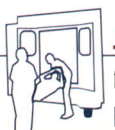
At the Scene
Patients tend to assume the most comfortable position. Flexion of the hips reduces movement of the psoas muscle and decreases pain. Ask the patient whether movement, walking, or deep breathing relieves or intensifies the pain. Peritoneal pain intensifies with movement. Patients with colicky pain (ie, renal, biliary, bowel) often present with restlessness, pacing, or writhing in pain.

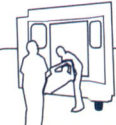
At the Scene
Remain alert to the four causes of acute abdominal pain that are immediate life threats: acute myocardial infarction (AMI), ruptured abdominal aortic aneurysm, ruptured ectopic pregnancy, and a ruptured viscus (any hollow organ).

One aspect of the general impression that is different for the GI patient is odour. What is the smell of the room or location of the patient? The foul-smelling melena stool that accompanies an upper GI bleed can be an important clue to the disease, and these smells should be noted and reported even though they can make even experienced paramedics nauseous. When dealing with these strong odours, the key is to hold your ground. The sense of smell

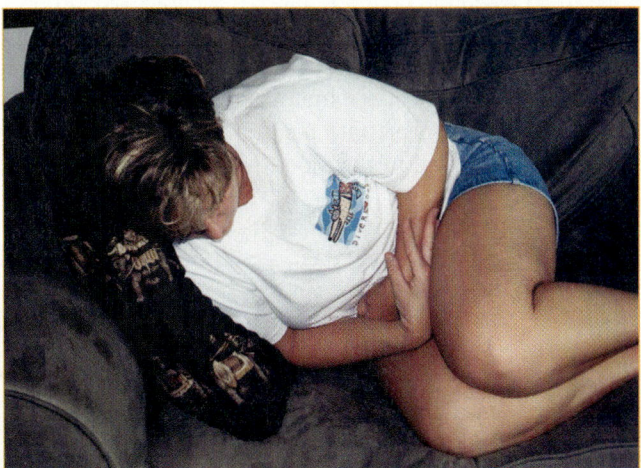
Figure 31-6 A patient experiencing abdominal pain will often curl up into a fetal position to relieve the pressure on the abdomen.

is the most acute for about a minute, but then more than 50% of the intensity of an odour is lost due to the olfactory nerve becoming tired of sending the same signal. If you are faced with a strong odour on a call, stay in the environment. After 2 to 5 minutes, the smell may be less noticeable.

Airway patency becomes a more pertinent concern with the GI patient. A patient who is vomiting has a greater chance to aspirate. Open the airway using the appropriate maneuvers, and closely inspect it for foreign bodies. Remove or suction any obstructions that are found. While evaluating the airway, notice any unusual odours emanating from the mouth. Patients who have extremely advanced bowel obstructions can have feculent breath, smelling of stool.

GI problems rarely affect breathing directly. If a breathing problem or altered breathing is encountered, it typically stems from a systemic complication. Ensure that the airway is clear. Suspect aspiration if a vomiting patient has difficulty maintaining oxygenation and ventilation.

The assessment of the circulatory system is essential in understanding how the GI disease is affecting the body. As with all patients, assess skin colour, temperature, and condition (ie, moisture content). Note findings consistent with shock. Determine the heart rate. Evaluate the peripheral pulses and compare them to the central pulses.

Many GI diseases involve pain and/or hemorrhage. As blood volume begins to drop, the body tries to compensate for this change by releasing catecholamines in the form of epinephrine and norepinephrine. These agents attempt to stabilize blood pressure through vasoconstriction, increased heart rate, and increased force of left ventricular contraction. Pain stimulates similar body responses. Either problem can leave the patient with tachycardia, pallor, and diaphoresis.

Check the patient's blood pressure. To ensure this measurement's accuracy, obtain a manual pressure before you use an automated blood pressure machine.

Orthostatic vital signs will help you determine the extent of bleeding that has occurred. First, have the patient lie down or recline in a position of comfort. Take an accurate blood pressure and heart rate. Next, have the patient sit or stand. Use caution, because the patient may potentially lose consciousness with a positional change. Wait a minute or two, and then repeat the blood pressure and heart rate measurements. Normally, there should be little change in the blood pressure or heart rate with

At the Scene

Ask your patient about their recent food intake. Fatty foods cause the gallbladder to contract, releasing bile. In the patient with gallbladder disease, this leads to distension and pain. Spicy foods can act as an irritant on the GI tract; when eaten in large amounts, they may cause pain even though they do not cause any damage. Milk products contain the sugar lactose, which is digested by an enzyme in the small intestine. Lactose intolerance is very common, and patients affected by it will experience bloating, pain, and often violent diarrhea within minutes of ingestion of dairy products.

At the Scene

Orthostatic changes usually occur when there has been a 15% to 20% loss in circulating volume. Shock is almost always present when the patient loses more than 30% of the blood volume.

such a positional change. When a patient has a significant loss of fluid within the vascular space, however, there may be a 10-beat increase in the heart rate and/or a 10-mm Hg drop in blood pressure.

When you examine the GI patient for gross bleeding, it is not unusual to find large amounts of blood. Take note of the amount of blood lost, focusing on being accurate. Many people grossly exaggerate the volume lost due to the emotional effects of seeing large amounts of blood. The amount of blood in a toilet is particularly difficult to estimate due to dilution. To practice volume estimation, measure the amount of water in a glass and then spill it on a carpet; note the size of the puddle. Spill another volume of water on a hard surface such as a tile floor; again note the size of the puddle.

When making your transport decision, integrate the information gathered from the initial assessment. If the patient has an orthostatic change in vital signs, then thoughtfully consider how the patient will be moved. Can the patient tolerate sitting in a stair chair, or will he or she pass out? Is the patient critical, so that he or she needs to be moved urgently?

In females of childbearing age, consider possible non-GI sources of disease, such as ectopic pregnancy, spontaneous or threatened abortion, ovarian cyst, or pelvic inflammatory disease. Your history should include addressing the gynecological system and the risk factors for these patients. In pediatrics, consider common causes such as gastroenteritis, appendicitis, and intussusception of the small bowel. Always maintain an index of suspicion for child maltreatment. The elderly can be poor historians, have muted symptoms, atypical pain, and low or absent fever.

Focused History and Physical Examination

For the unstable patient, a rapid head-to-toe examination will provide you with ample opportunities to discover clues as to the underlying problem. Beginning at the head, perform the standard DCAP-BTLS examination. With a GI problem, examination of the head, neck, and chest will often not reveal any major changes. Instead, the major effects from GI disease typically relate to the nervous, cardiovascular, and respiratory systems and result from pain, hypovolemia, and infection.

Examination of the abdomen can be uncomfortable for the patient with abdominal pain. In addition, respect for the patient's privacy should permit deferral of the examination until the patient is protected from curious onlookers. As you prepare for the abdominal examination, if the patient is stable, place a pillow under his or her knees. Have the patient relax the arms at his or her side. Maintaining straight legs and arms over the head can result in flexed abdominal muscles, which can distort your examination **Figure 31-7 ▸**. Make sure your hands are warm before you touch the abdomen. If the patient is uncomfortable

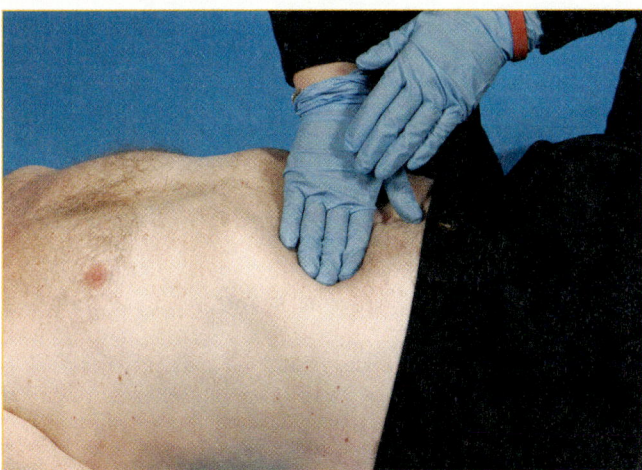

Figure 31-7 Examining a patient's abdomen.

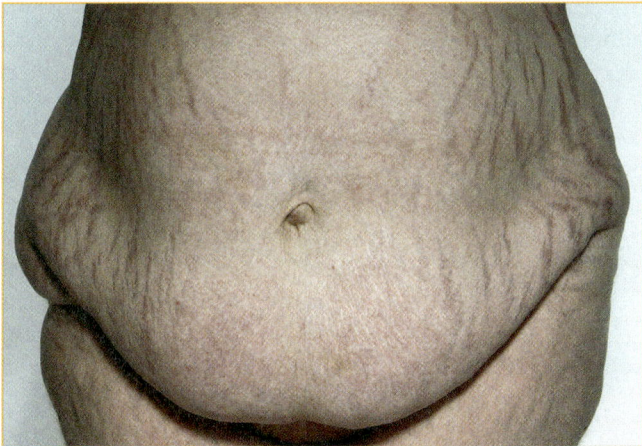

Figure 31-8 Striae.

with this examination, try to distract him or her by having a casual conversation. If the patient is unstable, then proceed with the examination in a quick and compassionate manner.

Examine the skin for irregularities. Do you see scars indicating trauma or past surgery? If so, ask the patient about the scarring. Do you notice stretch marks (striae)? These indicate a change in the size of the abdomen over a short period of time. Recent increases or decreases in weight, pregnancy, and severe abdominal edema can all cause striae **Figure 31-8 ▲**.

Is the abdomen symmetric? Looking down at a supine patient, the abdomen should lie flat and gently slope off of the ribs with a gentle upward slope as you approach the pelvis. Tumors, hernia, enlarged or distended organs, pregnancy, and other masses can cause asymmetry.

What is the shape of the abdomen? Is it flat, round, protuberant, or scaphoid? As people gain weight, the weight can be localized to the abdomen, producing a round abdomen. If weight becomes extreme, the abdomen may protrude. Other causes of protuberance include fluid buildup in the abdomen (such ascites in liver failure), pregnancy, and organ enlargement.

A scaphoid (concave) abdomen may result from decreased abdominal volume, such as would happen with malnutrition from malabsorption or chronic disease.

Listen to the abdomen before you touch it, because palpation of the abdomen can alter the bowel sound patterns. Bowel sounds are transmitted easily through the abdominal cavity. Place your stethoscope lightly on the abdominal wall and listen. Listening to one location, such as the right lower quadrant, is usually all that is needed.

Normal bowel sounds sound like gurgles and clicks and occur 5 to 30 times per minute **Table 31-7 ▶**. In your examination, you are merely listening for the presence or absence of these sounds. Sometimes you may hear loud prolonged sounds. This "stomach growling" (borborygmi) indicates strong contractions of the intestines; it can be normal or it may present with diarrhea. Interestingly, hyperperistalsis (enhanced bowel sounds) can also be heard in patients with early bowel obstruction, as the bowel contracts forcefully in an effort to overcome the obstruction.

Decreased bowel sounds—that is, listening over the right lower quadrant and not hearing anything for 15 to 20 seconds—can indicate decreased peristalsis of the intestines. This lack of movement can lead to bowel obstruction. True absent bowel sounds, which are characterized by no sounds heard for 2 minutes, are typically not practical to discover in the out-of-hospital setting. The absence of bowel sounds means that the intestines are not contracting, so any material within them is not in motion.

To palpate the abdomen, place your hand flat on the wall of the abdomen with your fingers together. Choose the quadrant farthest away from where the patient is having the complaint to start your assessment, and systematically palpate each quadrant, finally making your way to the quadrant where the complaint is located. Such a cautious approach to an abdominal assessment will decrease the patient's anxiety, help to reveal more accurate information, and allow the patient to focus his or her attention on other portions of the abdomen that he or she may not have considered because of the current discomfort.

With your hand sitting on the wall of the abdomen, raise your wrist so that you indent the abdominal wall with your fingers about 5 to 10 cm. As you are palpating, assess the abdomen for the presence of rigidity, discomfort, or masses. Sometimes patients may feel ticklish or otherwise guard the abdomen with flexed muscles, which can make it difficult to determine if the abdomen is rigid or just muscularly guarded. A rigid abdomen may indicate peritonitis due to hemorrhage or infection.

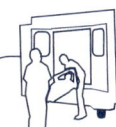

At the Scene

The noisy prehospital environment makes it difficult to assess for bowel sounds. Although some recommend listening for bowel sounds for anywhere from 1 to 5 minutes in each quadrant, this is rarely done in practice. Follow your local protocols. Most important, note whether bowel sounds are present or absent—their absence is more clinically significant than the variations in sounds that are present.

Have the patient breathe with an open mouth. It is more difficult to hold the stomach contracted during mouth breathing, so this technique can help to relax the abdomen and allow for a more accurate assessment. You can also hold your fingers slightly depressed into the abdomen during the respiratory cycle.

When the patient exhales, the abdomen typically relaxes. You can also try to coach the patient to relax the abdomen. It isn't always possible to get the patient to relax the abdomen, however. Nevertheless, if you are going to report a rigid abdomen, you should take reasonable steps to ensure that your assessment finding is accurate.

Pain is often a finding of importance with GI patients, because it can indicate trauma, hemorrhage, infection, or obstruction. As with the initial assessment, determine the OPQRST of the complaint. **Table 31-8 ▾** describes the types of pain that may be experienced with an abdominal problem.

As with all pain evaluations, you also need to determine *when* the patient has pain. Does he or she have pain when the abdomen is not being touched? Does the palpation of the abdomen increase the pain? What is the character of the pain? Does the pain change in character or location during your palpation?

Rebound tenderness (parietal pain) may sometimes accompany abdominal pain and is suggestive of a serious and potentially life-threatening pathology. It occurs when the peritoneum is irritated due to either hemorrhage or infection. The peritoneum is a thin layer of tissue lining the abdominal cavity and normally contains only a tiny amount of fluid.

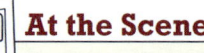

At the Scene

Be aware of common pain referral patterns:
- Biliary pain commonly radiates around to the right side of the back and angle of the scapula.
- Pancreatic pain goes straight through from the epigastrium to the back in the midline.
- Blood/pus under the diaphragm may present as pain in the top of the shoulder.
- A leaking or ruptured aneurysm causes abdominal pain and back pain in the lumbosacral area, which may radiate to the upper thighs.
- Renal colic (kidney stones) pain originates in either flank and radiates to the groin and external genitalia.
- Uterine and rectal pain will be present in the suprapubic region, the lower back, or both.

To demonstrate the rebound tenderness of peritoneal irritation, your examination goal is to have the peritoneum vibrate or move rapidly. Once you discover an area of maximal tenderness, depress the skin with your fingertips about 5 to 10 cm and then quickly pull your fingers off the abdominal wall. Speed is essential—if you pull the fingers off too slowly, you won't be able to get the desired movement of the peritoneum.

The abdomen should be rather smooth when subjected to light palpation **Figure 31-9 ▸**. Although assessment of internal organs by palpation can be conducted, this is rarely employed within the prehospital setting. However, if as you palpate the abdomen you note the presence of any bumps or masses, these may signal the presence of an engorged liver, bowel distension, aortic aneurysm, a pregnant uterus, or cancerous tumors.

The SAMPLE history will help the paramedic elicit the relevant current and past medical history **Figure 31-10 ▸**. When asking patients about their complaints, you may need to reframe your questions in everyday language. It is important

Table 31-7	Bowel Sounds	
Sound	**Description**	**Possible Causes**
Normal	Soft gurgles or clicks occurring 5 to 30 times a minute.	Normal movement of material through the intestines.
Borborygmi	Loud gurgles, often heard without a stethoscope and occurring at greater than 30 times a minute.	Hyperperistalsis. Can be normal. If prolonged, can indicate increased intestinal contractions as with diarrhea of any cause.
Decreased	Quiet sounds occurring at less than 1 sound every 15 to 20 seconds.	Hypoperistalsis. Can indicate impending obstruction of the intestines.
Absent	No sounds after 2 minutes of continuous listening.	Bowel obstruction/intestinal paralysis.

Table 31-8	Types of Abdominal Pain		
Type of Pain	**Origin**	**Description**	**Cause**
Visceral pain	Hollow organs	Difficult to localize; described as burning, cramping, gnawing or aching; usually felt superficially.	Organ contracts too forcefully or is distended (stretched).
Parietal pain/ rebound pain	Peritoneum	Steady, achy pain; more easy to localize than visceral. Pain increases with movement.	Inflammation of the peritoneum (blood and/or infection).
Somatic pain	Peripheral nerve tracts	Well localized pain, usually felt deeply.	Irritation or injury to tissue, causing activation of peripheral nerve tracts.
Referred pain	Peripheral nerve tracts	Pain originating in the abdomen and causing "pain" in distant locations. Due to similar paths for the peripheral nerves of the abdomen and the distant location.	Usually occurs after an initial visceral, parietal, or somatic pain.

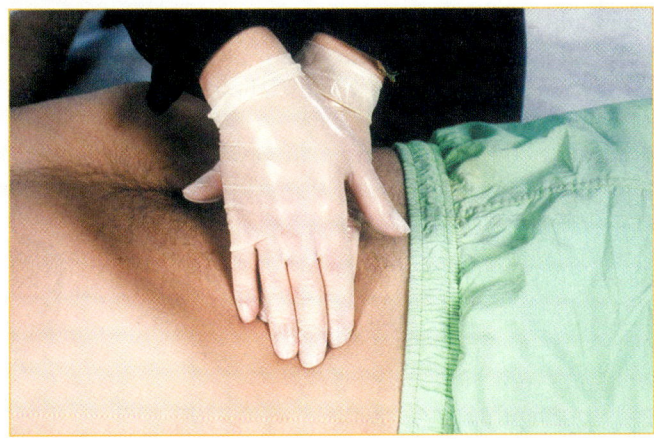

Figure 31-9 Check tenderness by gently palpating each of the four quadrants.

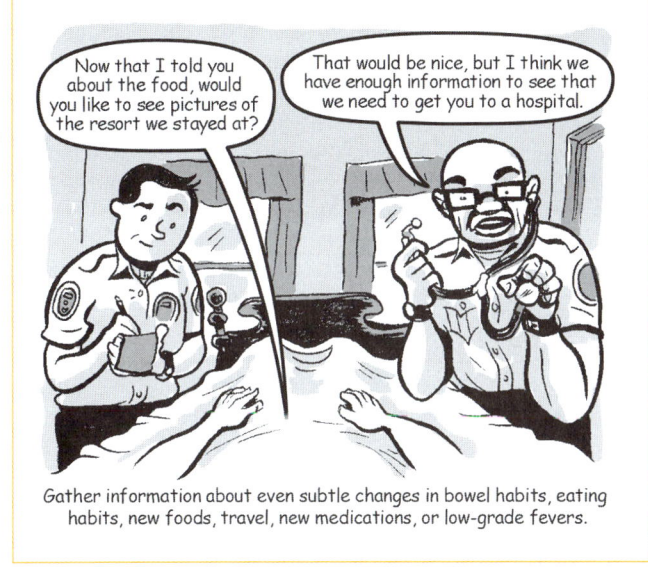

Gather information about even subtle changes in bowel habits, eating habits, new foods, travel, new medications, or low-grade fevers.

Figure 31-10

that you and your patient have a common frame of reference. For example, one person's "diarrhea" may be another person's "soft stool." You may also need to use colloquial words to ask about bodily functions. "Poop" is sometimes better understood by nonmedical individuals than "bowel movements." **Table 31-9 ▾** suggests ways to standardize language regarding excreted substances so that

Notes from Nancy
Don't spend a lot of time poking at the belly of a patient with abdominal pain.

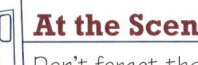 **At the Scene**
Don't forget that atypical cardiac pain may radiate or even originate in the abdomen. Patients may describe the pain as aching, sharp, "gassy," or indigestion-like.

Substance	Description	Possible Cause
Table 31-9	**Bodily Substances from the GI Tract**	
Vomit	Food and partially digested food. Strong acid odour mixed with odour of food eaten.	Gastroenteritis, ingested toxins, bowel obstruction.
Hematemesis or coffee-ground emesis	Dark, granular material that is the black or very dark red. This slurry of material may have food within it. The food and blood are indistinguishable.	Blood from the mouth, esophagus, or stomach that has been digested by stomach acids and then vomited.
Vomit with gross blood	Vomit with obvious red blood. In this setting, there is distinct food and blood that are not incorporated into each other.	Bleeding from the mouth or esophagus that has not been exposed to stomach acids.
Diarrhea	Liquid stool that is the consistency of water. It can range in colour from clear to dark brown.	Intestinal infections, partial bowel obstructions, colitis.
Acholic stools	Light, tan-coloured, formed stools. May be softer than typical.	Liver or biliary tract disease. Bile gives stool its usual brown colour.
Steatorrhea	Foamy, foul-smelling, mushy, yellow to grey stools. These oily stools will usually float within water.	Malabsorption of fat, usually from liver or pancreatic disease, causing excessive excretion of fat within the stool.
Soft stools	Formed stools that the patient describes as less firm than their usual consistency; may resemble the consistency of soft-serve ice cream.	Normal variant for some people. Can be caused by new foods or rapid change in diet.
Hematochezia	Frank red blood in stool.	Bleeding from the lower GI tract. May also occur from very rapid upper GI bleeding.
Melena	Stool that contains blood that has been altered by digestion in the intestine. These are black, tarry, sticky, and have a distinctive odour.	Bleeding from the upper GI tract.

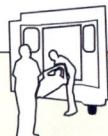

At the Scene

When recording information about the character and quantity of a patient's bodily substances, be as accurate as possible. Describe the substances in detail. Saying the patient had feces covering the legs is adequate if melena is not present. If you see the diarrhea, describe how liquid it is. This information can help to determine the nature of the patient's illness, degree of blood loss, or hydration status.

At the Scene

The following factors may complicate the abdominal assessment:

- **Young age:** Poor historians; fear
- **Old age:** poor historians, muted symptoms, atypical presentations
- **Obesity/pregnancy:** large abdomen can displace or hide abdominal organs
- **Compromised immune systems:** don't mount a typical immune response to infection or inflammatory disease.

the health care providers taking over care from you will have the same understanding of the patient's condition as you do.

Ongoing Assessment

The goal of the ongoing assessment is to monitor your patient for changes en route to the hospital. Routine monitoring should include heart rate, ECG, blood pressure, respiratory rate, and pulse oximetry. If the patient is suffering from a GI

bleed, continue to assess for signs of shock. Equally important, you should determine what effect your treatment is having. Before giving additional fluid boluses, listen to the patient's lung sounds to determine whether he or she is developing acute pulmonary edema.

Also monitor the patient's pain level. Many patients with abdominal pain may be receiving pain medication. How effective was your treatment? Does the patient need more medication? What are the patient's blood pressure and respiratory rate?

If the patient's condition undergoes a sudden dramatic change, repeat the rapid and detailed assessments as if this case were a new patient. This will give you the best chance of adjusting your prehospital care to adequately manage this new development.

Notes from Nancy

It is not necessary to diagnose the specific cause of a patient's abdominal pain in order to appreciate that the patient is in a serious condition.

Assessment of Specific Conditions

Gastrointestinal Bleeding

Presentation of GI bleeding is variable, because it can reflect the presence of a number of diseases. Each of these conditions has its own pattern of disease progression. For example, diverticular disease has a rather gradual onset and tends to strike

You are the Paramedic Part 3

Your physical examination is significant for jaundiced skin and eyes, jugular venous distension while sitting, and a swollen abdomen with a palpable liver. You are able to smell an alcohol-like odour on the patient's breath. While completing your examination, the patient leans forward and vomits an additional 250 ml of bright red blood on the floor.

You and your partner decide to load Rob onto the stretcher and initiate treatment in the back of the ambulance. While you insert two 18-gauge needles in the left and right antecubital region and hang 1,000-ml bags of normal saline running wide open, your partner applies 100% oxygen via a nonrebreathing mask and attaches the cardiac monitor. A nasogastric tube is inserted in his right nare and returns an additional 100 ml of blood into the suction canister.

Reassessment	Recording Time: 13 Minutes
Skin	Cool, jaundiced, and diaphoretic
Pulse	130 beats/min; weak and regular
Blood pressure	80/56 mm Hg
Respirations	26 breaths/min, regular
SpO$_2$	98% on nonrebreathing mask at 12 to 15 l/min of oxygen
ECG	Sinus tachycardia with no ectopy
Pupils	Pupils equal and reactive to light and accommodation

5. What does this patient need to be monitored for?

6. Is it possible that your patient has aspirated blood? Why or why not?

people in their 50s, 60s, or later decades. Mallory-Weiss syndrome has a very sudden onset and affects people of all ages. Gathering the information about how the patient progressed from initial symptoms to calling an ambulance is critical in forming your initial impression.

The patient's medical history and other possible events of abdominal pain or bleeding from the GI tract may also provide important information. Find out which medications the patient is taking; many drugs can irritate the GI tract, precipitating bleeding. Determine how long the patient has had the problem.

The most important component of the physical examination is to determine how much bleeding has occurred. Do you see evidence of bleeding in the environment? If so, try to estimate the amount of liquid present. Focus your assessment on evaluation for shock. Determine whether the patient is compensating for the fluid loss. Orthostatic vital signs are the key to gauging the degree of fluid loss in the prehospital setting.

Esophageal Varices

Initially, the esophageal varices are asymptomatic but the patient may show other subtle signs of liver disease, such as fatigue, weight loss, jaundice, anorexia, edema in the abdomen, and pruritis. Once there is a variceal bleed, the presentation is quite dramatic. The patient may complain of sudden-onset discomfort in the throat. There is often copious vomiting of bright red blood, hypotension, and signs of shock. If the bleeding is less severe, then hematemesis and melena predominate. Bleeding esophageal varices can be life threatening.

Mallory-Weiss Syndrome

Mallory-Weiss syndrome develops due to repeated, severe vomiting. In women, this syndrome may occur with hyperemesis gravidarum (ie, severe vomiting related to pregnancy). The extent of the bleeding can range from very minor, resulting in very little blood loss, to severe bleeding and extreme hypovolemia. In extreme cases, patients may suffer from signs and symptoms of shock, epigastric abdominal pain, hematemesis, and melena.

Hemorrhoids

Hemorrhoids present as bright red rectal bleeding. This hematochezia tends to be minimal and is easily controlled. However, the blood loss appears dramatic to the patient, because the water in the toilet turns red with only a few drops of blood. Additionally, patients may experience pain or itching and a

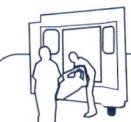

At the Scene

Many patients who bleed from a peptic ulcer have had no prior symptoms or history of ulcer disease. When obtaining a history, ask about recent ingestion of alcohol, ibuprofen, aspirin, or other NSAIDs.

At the Scene

Missed appendicitis is more common in the young, the elderly, and in pregnant patients because the symptoms are often atypical.

small mass on the rectum. Typically, this mass is a clot formed in response to the mild bleeding.

Peptic Ulcer Disease

Patients with peptic ulcers experience a classic sequence of burning or gnawing pain in the abdomen that subsides or diminishes immediately after eating and then reemerges 2 to 3 hours later. Nausea, vomiting, belching, and heartburn are common as well. If the erosion is severe, gastric bleeding can occur, resulting in hematemesis and melena. Perforation of the stomach or intestine will result in signs of peritonitis.

Cholecystitis

Patients with biliary colic typically develop severe right upper quadrant pain after large or fatty meals. The development of fever and tachycardia is suggestive of inflammation of the gallbladder wall, which occurs in cholecystitis.

Appendicitis

Patients with appendicitis classically present with periumbilical visceral pain that eventually migrates to the right lower quadrant. Rebound tenderness suggests possible perforation of the appendix with resultant peritonitis. Additionally, these patients often develop anorexia, nausea, and fever.

Diverticulitis

Diverticulitis presents with abdominal pain, which tends to be localized to the left side of the lower abdomen. Classic signs of infection include fever, malaise, body aches, chills, nausea, and vomiting. Diverticular disease may also be a source of lower GI bleeding, often without pain. Due to the local infections of these pouches, adhesions may develop, narrowing the diameter of the colon, resulting in constipation and bowel obstruction.

Pancreatitis

The pain of pancreatitis tends to be localized to the epigastric area or right upper abdomen. It can be sharp and may be quite severe. Radiation of the pain to the back is common. Patients may also experience nausea, vomiting, fever, tachycardia, hypotension, and muscle spasms in the extremities as a result of hypocalcemia (low blood calcium). Both the inflammatory condition caused by pancreatitis as well as erosion of nearby blood vessels causing internal bleeding can cause shock or hemodynamic instability. If there is severe internal hemorrhage, Grey Turner's sign (bruising in the flanks) and Cullen sign (bruising around the umbilicus) indicate that retroperitoneal bleeding may be present.

Ulcerative Colitis

Ulcerative colitis presents with bloody diarrhea (hematochezia) and abdominal pain, which can range from mild to severe. Other signs and symptoms may include joint pain and skin lesions, possibly due to the systemic nature of the autoimmune response thought to be responsible for this disease. Patients may also experience fever, fatigue, and loss of appetite as a consequence of the infections occurring within the colon.

Crohn's Disease

Crohn's disease presents with recurrent flares of abdominal pain. Rectal bleeding, weight loss, diarrhea, arthritis, skin problems, and fever may also be present. There may be blood loss, but this bleeding tends to be small amounts over a long period of time. Acute severe hemorrhage is rare, but chronic bleeding resulting in anemia can occur. Patients may experience repeated episodes of mild to severe signs and symptoms.

Gastroenteritis

The presentation of acute gastroenteritis involves vomiting and diarrhea. Certain organisms cause inflammation of the intestines resulting in blood, mucous, or pus in the stool. Abdominal cramping is frequent as hyperperistalsis continues. Fever, nausea, and anorexia are often also present.

If the vomiting and diarrhea continues, dehydration and hemodynamic instability will result. As the volume of fluid loss increases, the likelihood of potassium and sodium imbalance increases. Watch for orthostatic changes in heart rate and blood pressure and changes in level of consciousness and other signs of shock, because they indicate a critical volume loss.

Acute Hepatitis

Acute hepatitis, regardless of etiology, is often associated with a number of signs and symptoms. Clinically, the disease occurs in two phases. In the first phase, patients experience symptoms suggestive of a mild viral illness, such as joint aches, weakness, fatigue, fever, nausea, abdominal pain that is often mild, vomiting and anorexia. At this point in the course of the disease, the patient may sometimes be misdiagnosed as having gastroenteritis.

In the later phase of hepatitis, symptoms of liver failure predominate. This can occur days to years after the initial infection. This is characterized by acholic stools, darkening of the urine, and the yellow skin and sclerae of jaundice. Abdominal pain in the right upper quadrant and an enlarged liver also become apparent at this time. Depending on the disease progression, total liver failure may be only days away.

Bowel Obstruction

The presentation of bowel obstruction varies according to the underlying cause. If this condition is caused by a twisting of the bowels around a fixed point, then obstruction can manifest within hours. If it is caused by cancer, then the narrowing may take months to become apparent.

Signs of this problem include abdominal pain and fullness. Initially, diarrhea will occur as small amounts of stool bypass the obstructed area. Peristalsis increases as the body tries to overcome the obstruction, which may be perceived by the patient as crampy abdominal pain. If this effort is unsuccessful, constipation results, with decreased bowel sounds. Nausea and vomiting are common in the later stages, with both the emesis and the patient's breath having a feculent odour. Eventually, perforation of the bowel may occur, leading to peritonitis and sepsis.

Management

General Management Guidelines

Often there is little the paramedic can do about the GI disease itself, but you can provide prehospital care for the effects of the disease. Patients may be in extreme pain; they may be suffering from severe dehydration, hypotension, or extreme nausea. Your main goals are to maintain routine precautions and PPE, manage the ABCs, and attend to the patient's pain and nausea.

With GI patients, PPE is essential due to the high likelihood of coming into contact with infectious agents. Be prepared to deal with large amounts of vomit, feces, and blood. The following equipment will be essential to ensure your safety:

- Gloves, gowns, eye protection, surgical mask
- Towels and wash rags
- Extra linen
- Absorbent pads
- Emesis basin
- Disposable basin
- Biohazard bags
- Sterile water for irrigation

Helping to clean the patient helps to return some degree of dignity to a person who is often humiliated by the circumstances of his or her disease.

The main airway concern for the GI patient is the potential for aspiration or obstruction of the airway due to vomit or blood. Although these complications are rare, they pose real concerns for the paramedic. Effective positioning of the patient will ensure adequate drainage of material out of the mouth. If the patient has suffered trauma, be prepared to tilt the backboard. In such a case, the patient needs to be packaged and padded well so that spinal movement is minimized during the board movement. Portable suction should be part of every department's first-in equipment.

At the Scene

Patients with abdominal emergencies should be maintained NPO (nothing by mouth) until evaluated by a physician. First, the risk of aspiration is decreased if the stomach remains empty. Second, food causes the release of digestive enzymes that can worsen some abdominal conditions. Also, it is helpful to minimize stomach contents in the event that surgery is required.

If breathing problems are present in association with GI problems, they are often associated with decreased hemoglobin due to bleeding. Be liberal in delivering oxygen to patients with GI bleeds. Don't rely on oxygen saturation readings as evidence that oxygen is not needed. A patient who has been bleeding internally may have a severely decreased hemoglobin level. Although the oxygen saturation may read 96%, if the hemoglobin is low, the patient still needs oxygen.

Oxygen masks can cause some patients to experience a sense of confinement, especially if they're experiencing nausea. Monitor patients with whom you use a mask to ensure they can get the mask off quickly if they need to vomit.

Listen to lung sounds. This baseline and continuing information is paramount to the safe administration of fluids. Blood or fluid losses should prompt the placement of one or two large bore intravenous cannulas, if protocol permits. In patients who are suffering from dehydration, the degree of hemodynamic instability combined with evidence of pulmonary edema will dictate the aggressiveness of fluid resuscitation. The goal of management is to provide enough volume to keep vital organs from becoming hypoxic, but not so much volume as to precipitate pulmonary edema or increase the bleeding. If the patient is hypotensive, a rapid bolus of 10 to 20 ml/kg of an isotonic crystalloid such as normal saline or lactated Ringer's should be initiated.

Maintaining peripheral perfusion as evidenced by normal mentation, skin condition, and presence of a radial pulse should be adequate to allow for adequate perfusion of the brain, kidneys, and other vital organs. Once the patient arrives within the hospital, blood administration will be critical to stabilization.

Pain management of the GI patient is a controversial subject. Although some have suggested that analgesia may mask symptoms of disease or disease progression, it is now generally agreed that analgesia is humane and does not delay accurate hospital diagnosis of GI problems. Your system protocols should provide guidance as to which medications, if any, are to be used in this setting. In any event, controlling pain should be a priority with GI patients. The only true contraindication to pain management in the prehospital setting for the GI patient is hypotension. Analgesia to decrease pain should be used judiciously, because it may result in hemodynamic compromise.

The following five medications provide the paramedic with tools to manage abdominal pain:

- Morphine, 2 to 5 mg IV/IO/IM. As with all opioids, this narcotic can cause hypotension and respiratory depression.
- Ketorolac (Toradol), 15 to 60 mg IV/IO/IM (IV dose not in excess of 30 mg). This medication is non-narcotic, so it does not cause hypotension or respiratory depression. Because it is an NSAID, it should be avoided if peptic ulcer disease is suspected.
- Fentanyl (Sublimaze), 0.5 to 1 mcg/kg is a popular opioid agonist because it is rapid acting, very potent, and has a relatively short duration of action. In rare instances, rapid infusion of fentanyl has been reported to cause chest wall rigidity, potentially leading to respiratory compromise.

At the Scene

Certain medications vary in their effectiveness on specific conditions. Pain arising from inflammation of abdominal organs responds well to ketorolac (Toradol). Most pain responds well to opioids, although caution needs to be maintained because of side effects, particularly in patients with hemodynamic compromise.

At the Scene

Saving samples of vomitus may provide significant diagnostic clues, especially in cases of unknown ingestions, GI bleeding, or an abdominal disease of unknown origins. Follow your local protocols.

- Dimenhydrinate (Gravol), 25 to 50 mg IV/IO/IM, may be administered for management of nausea. This medication has anticholinergic side effects and can cause drowsiness and a decline in blood pressure.

Proper cleaning and maintenance of equipment and uniforms soiled by bodily fluids from patients with GI diseases is essential. Hepatitis B, for example, can remain infectious even in dried blood for longer than a week.

Gastrointestinal Bleeding

Care for the patient with hemorrhage is directed at maintaining perfusion of vital organs. Internal hemorrhage cannot be controlled in the prehospital setting. Although volume replacement is critical to ensure adequate circulation to the vital organs, very aggressive volume replacement can result in dramatic hemodilution (ie, dilution of the blood), and potentially death. Establish secure IV lines with 1,000 ml of normal saline solution or lactated Ringer's solution with large-bore cannulas and macrodrip chambers to allow rapid fluid resuscitation, if merited by the patient's condition.

Esophageal Varices

Treatment for patients with esophageal varices in the prehospital setting should follow the general management guidelines.

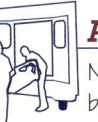

At the Scene

Nasogastric (NG) tube placement, if permitted by local protocols, may be beneficial in patients with GI bleeding. It can relieve the nausea associated with a large volume of blood in the stomach and may confirm that the blood loss is from an upper GI source. Iced saline lavage to control ongoing bleeding via vasoconstriction has been described, but this has significant risks with little proven benefit.

As with any GI bleeding disorder, accurate assessment of the extent of blood loss is critical. Be prepared for a very hemodynamically unstable patient who needs volume resuscitation and aggressive suctioning. If the patient's level of consciousness begins to deteriorate, consider inserting an advanced airway to minimize the potential for aspiration.

In-hospital treatment involves aggressive fluid resuscitation and control of bleeding. The latter may be achieved endoscopically or by placement of a large esophageal balloon to tamponade the bleeding varices.

Mallory-Weiss Syndrome

Management of Mallory-Weiss syndrome is the same as for esophageal varices and is directed at determining the extent of blood loss. The patient may be dehydrated from both repeated vomiting and blood loss. In-hospital management includes volume resuscitation, as needed; endoscopy to visualize the extent of the damage; and possibly an attempt to repair the damage. In most cases, Mallory-Weiss syndrome resolves spontaneously.

Hemorrhoids

Prehospital management of hemorrhoids is largely supportive. In isolation, hemorrhoids are more of an inconvenience than a life-threatening condition. Rarely, some patients suffer severe lower GI bleeds, and a hemorrhoidal source for the bleeding may not be apparent. Ensure that the patient is hemodynamically stable using orthostatic vital signs, and fluid resuscitate, if necessary.

The majority of hemorrhoids resolve in 2 to 3 days with only conservative management, such as creams, to shrink the inflamed tissues and stool softeners. Rarely, surgical removal may be necessary to stop bleeding and prevent recurrence. The best prevention for hemorrhoids is to maintain soft stools by eating a high-fibre diet.

Peptic Ulcer Disease

The major focus for the prehospital management of patients with peptic ulcers is to accurately assess the extent of blood loss and to prepare to manage any hypotension that is present. Orthostatic vital signs are critical in determining fluid needs and transportation/packaging issues.

In-hospital management includes administration of medication to neutralize stomach acids and reduce acid secretion. Antibiotic therapy directed at *H pylori* can prevent many new cases from occurring. Patients will often need an endoscopic examination to assess the stomach wall for damage. Long-term acid suppressive therapy is often effective in treating peptic ulcer disease.

Cholecystitis

Prehospital treatment for cholecystitis is directed at making the patient comfortable and treating hypovolemia if there is a fever and indications of septic shock. Medications given to control pain include morphine and meperidine. Morphine has been reported to cause a contraction of the sphincter of Oddi, the valve controlling bile movement out of the gallbladder; in most cases, morphine is used with no adverse effects. To control nausea, use one of the medications mentioned in the standard management guidelines. IV fluids are also indicated, because these patients are often vomiting. In-hospital treatment may include antibiotics, pain medication, ultrasound, and surgical removal of the gallbladder.

Appendicitis

Prehospital management for appendicitis includes remaining vigilant for signs of perforation or septic shock. Volume resuscitation may not be adequate to restore blood pressure. Be prepared to use dopamine if crystalloids are not effective. Administration of pain and antinausea medications is clearly indicated with these patients. At the hospital, these patients will receive antibiotics and typically undergo surgical removal of the appendix.

Diverticulitis

Management of diverticulitis is directed at making the patient comfortable. Examine the patient closely to ensure that severe infection is not present, because sepsis can occur, as well as complications such as fistulas to the urinary bladder. Patients with diverticulitis may also need large amounts of fluids and/or dopamine to maintain blood pressure. In-hospital treatment includes antibiotics, allowing the GI tract to rest by giving the patient a liquid diet, and possibly surgery if there is perforation or fistula formation.

Pancreatitis

Management for the prehospital patient with pancreatitis should follow the general management guidelines. Pay special attention to assessing the patient for signs of severe hemorrhage or shock. If they are present, begin fluid resuscitation.

In-hospital management includes GI rest, analgesia, and fluid resuscitation. In some cases, antibiotics and surgery can be helpful. Although the pancreas cannot be removed, surgery may be performed to control bleeding or manage the gallstones and subsequent blockage of bile from the liver.

Ulcerative Colitis

Management of ulcerative colitis consists of determining the degree of hemodynamic instability. Look for signs of shock. If the diarrhea and bleeding have caused sufficient volume loss to make the patient unstable, administer fluids to return the patient to a near-normal volume balance. Otherwise, provide supportive care and follow the general management guidelines.

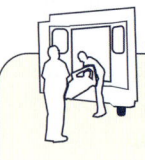

At the Scene

Remember to follow routine precautions and PPE procedures with these patients. Some of the causative organisms for gastroenteritis are highly contagious.

In-hospital care for these patients will include anti-inflammatory or immunosuppressive medications, antibiotics, antidiarrheals, and, potentially, surgical resection of the diseased sections of the colon. Many patients with ulcerative disease suffer for years with periods of diarrhea and abdominal pain, and nearly one third will eventually have part of their colon removed.

Crohn's Disease

Management of Crohn's disease in the prehospital setting should follow the general management guidelines. Volume resuscitation may be needed because of diarrhea and chronic hemorrhage. Measures to control nausea and pain are commonly needed.

In-hospital care focuses on stopping the inflammation, correcting any fluid imbalances, managing infections, and creating an environment where the GI tract can heal itself. The damage to the intestines can be so severe that surgical resection of portions is sometimes needed.

Acute Gastroenteritis

Prehospital management of gastroenteritis follows the general management guidelines. Pay special attention to the problem of determining the degree of fluid deficit. Indeed, patients often feel markedly better after rehydration. Take the orthostatic vital signs to determine the need for fluid resuscitation. Analgesic and antiemetic medications are sometimes also indicated for these patients.

In the emergency department, care is directed to rehydration, control of vomiting and diarrhea, identification of the organism involved, antibiotic therapy if a bacteria or parasite is implicated, and stabilization of electrolyte imbalances. The patient will have blood evaluation of electrolytes before electrolyte replacement or stabilization therapies are initiated. Once hemodynamically stable, the patient may receive an oral rehydration solution containing water, sodium, potassium, and sugar.

One of the most critical issues when managing acute gastroenteritis is education. It is a food- and waterborne illness, so patients need to be instructed on safe food and water use to prevent future infections.

Acute Hepatitis

Prehospital management for acute hepatitis is supportive and follows the general management guidelines for GI patients. Two important areas on which to focus during patient prehospital care are infection control and medication administration.

Patients with acute hepatitis are infectious, so you should take adequate precautions to limit contact with bodily fluids. Use good hand washing and equipment cleaning techniques, remembering that hepatitis B can remain infectious in dried blood for at least a week. A vaccine for hepatitis A and B is also available.

One of the liver's functions is to detoxify medications. When patients have hepatitis, any drug that is given may remain active within the body for longer than anticipated. When administering medications to patients with signs of liver failure, consider using lower dosages and at longer intervals. Watch for signs of cumulative effects.

Without a functioning liver, the patient will die within a few days. Although many cases of hepatitis resolve spontaneously, antiviral medications may be needed to slow the effects of the virus. In extreme cases, a liver transplant is the only effective treatment.

Bowel Obstruction

Management of bowel obstruction follows the general management guidelines. This disease is rarely life threatening in the prehospital setting. In-hospital management focuses on decompressing the intestines, determining the cause of the obstruction, and treating any side effects, such as infection or intestinal perforation. Surgery is sometimes required to relieve the obstruction.

You are the Paramedic Part 4

Just as your partner pulls into traffic upon leaving the parking lot, your patient loses consciousness. A quick reassessment reveals shallow breathing at a rate of 10 breaths per minute and an absent radial pulse. You are relieved to discover that a strong carotid pulse is present. Work of breathing is taken over using bag-valve-mask ventilation with 100% oxygen. Both IV lines are patent. The emergency department is contacted and notified of your impending arrival in approximately 8 minutes.

The emergency room staff is awaiting your arrival in the resuscitation room. The patient is intubated, has a central line inserted for fluid resuscitation, receives 2 units of packed red blood cells, and is taken to the endoscopy suite for diagnosis and treatment. He is diagnosed with bleeding esophageal varices, which were managed medically with vasopressin injected at the site of the bleed. He is admitted to the medical intensive care for 3 days and is discharged from the hospital after the 7th day on propranolol (Inderal).

Reassessment	Recording Time: 20 Minutes
Skin	Cool, jaundiced, and diaphoretic
Pulse	134 beats/min (carotid)
Blood pressure	76/50 mm Hg
Respirations	12 manual ventilations/min via bag-valve-mask ventilation
Spo2	99% on 100% oxygen
ECG	Sinus rhythm without ectopy

7. Why was the patient discharged on propranolol?

You are the Paramedic Summary

1. What is your first priority in this situation?

This is an easy one! Scene safety should always be your priority. In this situation, you are entering a dimly lit bar late at night; many of the customers are more than likely happy to "assist" you in a variety of ways. You are also working in a confined space inside of this establishment, which increases the possibility of something going wrong. It wouldn't be a bad idea to have additional personnel, or even law enforcement, on scene with you.

2. What are some of the possible differential diagnoses?

The differential diagnoses for upper GI bleeding include peptic ulcer disease, esophageal varices, Mallory-Weiss syndrome, and tumors.

3. What are the signs and symptoms of ruptured esophageal varices?

Patients with esophageal varices may present with bright red hematemesis, melena, and signs of shock.

4. What is the most common cause of esophageal varices?

In the adult patient, the most common cause of esophageal varices is cirrhosis of the liver, which is most often caused by alcohol abuse.

5. What does this patient need to be monitored for?

Rob is exhibiting classic signs and symptoms of decompensated shock: altered mental status, increased heart rate, and decreased blood pressure. We know that he no longer has a radial pulse. He does, however, have a strong carotid pulse. It is vital to frequently reassess the presence of the carotid pulse to ensure that Rob has not developed pulseless electrical activity. His airway is currently being managed by manual ventilations with bag-valve-mask ventilation. Protection of the airway is paramount! Perhaps you thought of other ways that the airway should have been managed, but at the end of the day you need to make sure that the airway remains secure, no matter how it's done.

6. Is it possible that the patient has aspirated blood? Why or why not?

Absolutely! When you arrived on scene, Rob was already experiencing an altered mental status. There is no guarantee that he didn't aspirate blood prior to your arrival. Always assume the worst and be pleasantly surprised with the best!

7. Why was the patient discharged on propranolol?

You might still be scratching your head on this one! Propranolol is a beta blocker. A review of the properties of beta blockers should remind you that they reduce blood pressure, including in the portal veins. Therefore, a lower pressure should help prevent a recurrence of bleeding by lowering the pressure within the esophageal veins.

Prep Kit

Ready for Review

- Gastrointestinal (GI) problems can present with apparently mild symptoms even though they may herald the presence of life-threatening disease.
- Three major pathologies are responsible for diseases of the GI tract: hypovolemia, infection, and inflammation.
- Bleeding within the GI tract is a symptom of another disease, not a disease itself.
- Presentation of GI bleeding is variable, because it can reflect the presence of a number of diseases. Each of these conditions has its own pattern of disease progression.
- Often there is little the paramedic can do about the GI disease itself, but you can provide prehospital care for the effects of the disease.
- Patients may be in extreme amount of pain; they may be suffering from severe dehydration, hypotension, or extreme nausea.
- Your main goals are to maintain routine precautions and PPE, manage the ABCs, and attend to the patient's pain and nausea.

Vital Vocabulary

acholic stools Light, clay-coloured stools caused by liver failure.

ascites Abdominal edema typically caused by liver failure.

borborygmi A bowel sound characterized by increased activity within the bowel.

chyme The partially digested food that exits the stomach, entering the duodenum.

diarrhea Liquid stool.

endoscopy The insertion of a flexible tube into the esophagus with the intent of visualizing and repairing damage or disease.

epigastric The right upper region of the abdomen directly inferior to the xyphoid process and superior to the umbilicus.

feculent Smelling of feces.

hematemesis Vomit with blood; either like coffee grounds in appearance, indicating partially digested blood, or bright red, indicating current active bleeding.

hematochezia Blood with the stool that is separate; caused by lower GI bleeds.

hyperperistalsis Increased movement within the bowel.

hypoperistalsis Decreased bowel movement.

melena Dark, tarry, very odourous stools caused by upper GI bleeds.

Murphy's sign Pain when pressure is applied to the right upper quadrant of the abdomen in a specific manner; helps detect gallbladder problems.

orthostatic vital signs Assessing vital signs in two different patient positions to determine the degree of hypovolemia.

peptic ulcer disease (PUD) Abrasion of the stomach or small intestine.

peristalsis The rhythmic contractions of the intestines and esophagus that allow material to move.

periumbilical Located around the navel.

portal vein A large vessel created by the intersection of blood vessels from the GI system. The portal vein empties into the liver.

protuberant A convex, or distended, shape of the abdomen. This can be caused by edema.

scaphoid A concave shape of the abdomen. This can be caused by evisceration.

steatorrhea Foamy, fatty stools caused by liver failure or gallbladder problems.

striae Stretch marks on the abdomen caused by size changes.

suprapubic The region of the abdomen superior to the pubic bone and inferior to the umbilicus.

umbilical The region of the abdomen surrounding the umbilicus.

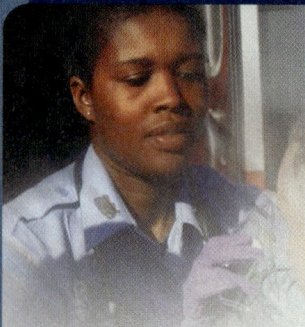

Assessment in Action

You are dispatched to the assisted-living facility for someone who is "bleeding." When you arrive on scene you find the patient supine on the floor. The smell to you indicates lower GI bleeding and you immediately walk into the bathroom to check out the toilet bowl, where you see approximately 200 ml of a substance that resembles coffee grounds. The patient's vital signs are as follows: pulse rate, 120 beats/min; sinus tachycardia on the cardiac monitor; blood pressure, 70 mm Hg by palpation; respiratory rate, 26 breaths/min; and pulse oximetry, 97% on room air.

1. **What are the three main conditions responsible for diseases of the GI tract?**
   A. Hypovolemia, infection, inflammation
   B. Hypertension, hypovolemia, tachycardia
   C. Hypovolemia, infection, hypertension
   D. Hypovolemia, inflammation, gallstones

2. **From what organs does an upper GI bleed originate?**
   A. Small intestine, large intestine, rectum, stomach
   B. Esophagus, stomach, rectum
   C. Rectum, stomach, large intestine
   D. Esophagus, stomach, small intestine

3. **An aspect of the general impression that is often different for the patient with GI bleeding is:**
   A. patient colour.
   B. patient vital signs.
   C. odour.
   D. restlessness.

4. **_____ becomes more pertinent with the GI patient.**
   A. Airway patency
   B. Breathing
   C. Circulation
   D. Bleeding

5. **As blood volume begins to drop, the body begins to compensate by releasing:**
   A. antihistamines.
   B. ketoacidosis.
   C. catecholamines.
   D. insulin.

6. **What is the dark red or black granular material called?**
   A. Hematemesis, or coffee ground emesis
   B. Vomit
   C. Diarrhea
   D. Steatorrhea

7. **What is the most important component of the physical exam?**
   A. The length of time the patient has been having complaints
   B. How much bleeding has occurred
   C. Where the abdominal pain, if any, is located
   D. Noting when the last bowel movement occurred

8. **_____ are the key to gauging the degree of fluid loss in the prehospital setting.**
   A. Normal vital signs
   B. Orthostatic vital signs
   C. Abnormal vital signs
   D. No vital signs

Challenging Question

You are dispatched to a private residence for a person with abdominal pain. When you arrive on scene, the patient is doubled over in pain and complains of point tenderness to the upper right quadrant. The patient's vital signs are as follows: pulse rate, 108 beats/min with sinus tachycardia; blood pressure, 110/70 mm Hg; respiratory rate, 24 breaths/min; and pulse oximetry, 100% on room air.

9. **What management is required for this patient with an acute abdomen?**

Points to Ponder

You are dispatched to the home of a 37-year-old woman. When you arrive, you find her doubled over in pain, complaining of left upper quadrant pain that radiates to the right upper quadrant. You take the following set of vital signs: pulse rate, 118 beats/min; sinus tachycardia on the cardiac monitor; blood pressure, 140/82 mm Hg; respiratory rate, 24 breaths/min; and pulse oximetry, 99% on room air. Your patient tells you that her last menstrual cycle ended 4 days ago. She also tells you that the pain has been intermittent for approximately 2 weeks. The pain is sharp, like a knife cutting away her abdomen. You initiate IV therapy and administer 15 l/min of oxygen by nonrebreathing mask. You transport her to the hospital in a position of comfort and give your patient care report to the emergency department staff. Towards the end of your shift, you call the hospital and find out she was admitted with acute pancreatitis.

What are some common causes of abdominal pain? How can pancreatitis affect other body systems?

Issues: Understanding the Importance of a Complete Abdominal Assessment, Appropriate Medical Response to Gastrointestinal Emergencies.

32 Renal and Urologic Emergencies

Competency Areas

Area 2: Communication

2.4.b   Exhibit empathy and compassion while providing care.

Area 4: Assessment and Diagnostics

4.3.a   Conduct primary patient assessment and interpret findings.
4.3.b   Conduct secondary patient assessment and interpret findings.
4.3.h   Conduct genitourinary system assessment and interpret findings.

Area 5: Therapeutics

5.3.a   Administer oxygen using nasal cannula.
5.3.d   Administer oxygen using high concentration mask.
5.5.c   Maintain peripheral intravenous (IV) access devices and infusions of crystalloid solutions without additives.
5.5.d   Conduct peripheral intravenous cannulation.
5.5.o   Provide routine care for patient with urinary catheter.
5.5.q   Provide routine care for patient with non-catheter urinary drainage system.
5.8.a   Recognize principles of pharmacology as applied to the medications listed in

Appendix 5

5.8.b   Follow safe process for responsible medication administration.

Area 6: Integration

6.1.d   Provide care to patient experiencing illness or injury primarily involving genitourinary/reproductive systems.
6.1.l   Provide care to patient experiencing non-urgent medical problem.
6.3.a   Conduct ongoing assessments based on patient presentation and interpret findings.
6.3.b   Re-direct priorities based on assessment findings.

Appendix 4: Pathophysiology

A.   **Cardiovascular System**
Cardiac Conduction Disorder: Lethal arrhythmias
B.   **Neurologic System**
Altered Mental Status: Metabolic
C.   **Respiratory System**
Medical Illness: Pulmonary embolism
F.   **Genitourinary System**
Reproductive Disorders: Testicular torsion
Renal/Bladder: Colic/calculi
Renal/Bladder: Infection
Renal/Bladder: Obstruction
Renal/Bladder: Renal failure
Traumatic Injuries: Traumatic injuries
I.   **Endocrine System**
Thyroid disease
J.   **Multisystem Diseases and Injuries**
Shock Syndromes: Hypovolemic

Appendix 5: Medications

A.   **Medications affecting the central nervous system.**
A.7   Non-narcotic analgesics
A.8   Opioid Analgesics

Introduction

The urinary system performs two main functions for the body. It acts as the body's accounting firm, keeping track of the electrolytes, water content, and acids of the blood; and it acts as the blood's sewage treatment plant, removing metabolic wastes, drug metabolites, and excess fluids. The kidneys perform these functions continuously, filtering 200 l of blood each day.

The most common renal disorder is kidney disease. Kidney disease has a tremendous impact on the health of Canadians. Every day, an average of 14 Canadians are told their kidneys have failed, and each year there is a 7% increase in the number of people diagnosed with kidney disease. The number of Canadians living with kidney disease is expected to double within the next 10 years. Today, almost 30,000 Canadians are being treated for kidney failure. The cost of caring for Canadians with kidney disease is substantial. Dialysis treatment and care of patients who have received a kidney transplant cost the Canadian health care system approximately $2 billion annually. Kidney disease also contributes to the risk of cardiovascular disease, including hypertension and other chronic diseases that shorten lifespan.

Anatomy and Physiology

The urinary system consists of the kidneys, which filter the blood and produce urine; the urinary bladder, which stores the urine until it is released from the body; the ureters, which transport the urine from the kidneys to the bladder; and the urethra, which transports the urine from the bladder out of the body. The bean-shaped kidneys are found in the retroperitoneal space (behind the peritoneum), which extends from the twelfth thoracic vertebra to the third lumbar vertebra. The right kidney is slightly lower than the left due to the position of the liver. The medial side of the kidney is concave, forming a cleft called the hilum, where the ureters, renal blood vessels, lymphatic vessels, and nerves enter and leave the kidney Figure 32-1 ◂ .

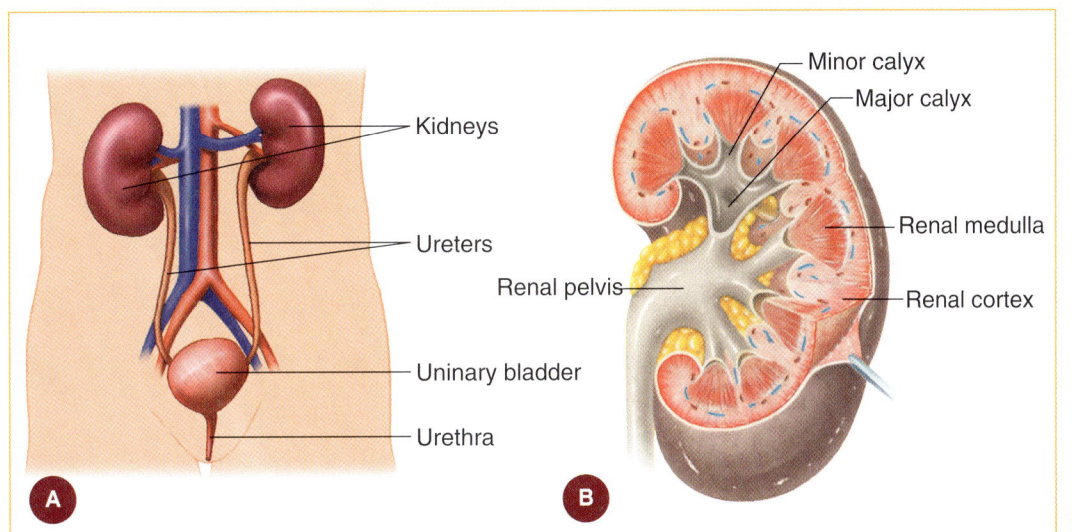

Figure 32-1 The urinary system. **A.** Anterior view showing the relationship of the kidneys, ureters, urinary bladder, and urethra. **B.** Cross-section of the human kidney showing the renal cortex, renal medulla, and renal pelvis.

You are the Paramedic Part 1

You arrive at a residence of a 71-year-old woman with severe weakness. As you enter the residence, you find the patient seated in a chair in her living room. She is conscious, but somewhat confused, and she clearly appears ill. She tells you that she has missed her last few dialysis treatments because her friend—who usually takes her to and from her treatments—is out of town. Your initial assessment findings are as follows:

Initial Assessment	Recording Time: 0 Minutes
Appearance	Looks ill; hands and feet are edematous
Level of consciousness	V (Responsive to verbal stimuli), somewhat confused
Airway	Patent
Breathing	Tachypneic; adequate tidal volume
Circulation	Radial pulses are rapid and irregular

1. What is the purpose of dialysis?
2. What are the two types of dialysis?

A fibrous capsule covers the kidney and protects it against infection. Surrounding this capsule is a fatty mass of adipose tissue, which cushions the kidney and holds it in place in the abdomen. A layer of dense fibrous connective tissue called the renal fascia anchors the kidney to the abdominal wall.

The internal anatomy of the kidney can be divided into three distinct regions: the cortex, the medulla, and the pelvis. The cortex is the lighter-coloured outer region closest to the capsule. The medulla (middle layer) includes the cone-shaped renal pyramids (parallel bundles of urine-collecting tubules), and inward extensions of cortical tissue that surround the pyramids, called the renal columns. The renal pelvis is a flat, funnel-shaped tube that fills the sinus at the level of the hilum. The major and minor calyces branch off the pelvis and connect with the renal pyramids to receive the urine draining from the collecting tubules. This arrangement has been described as several strands of uncooked spaghetti (the collecting tubules) sitting in a thimble (the papilla, or tip, of the pelvis). The collected urine flows through the pelvis and into the ureter on its way to the bladder.

Approximately one fourth of the body's systemic cardiac output of blood flows through the kidney each minute. The blood flows from the abdominal aorta into the kidney by way of the renal artery. Once it enters the kidney at the hilum, the artery branches several times to become the afferent arteriole. The afferent arteriole quickly branches into a tuft of capillaries called a glomerulus, which is the main filter for the blood in the kidney. From the glomerulus, the blood enters the efferent arteriole, which branches into the peritubular capillaries, where tubular resorption occurs. This secondary set of capillaries is unique to the kidney; no other organ in the body has two distinct capillary beds. The capillaries then merge, forming venules and veins, until the renal vein leaves the hilum, carrying the cleansed blood to the inferior vena cava.

Nephrons, found in the cortex, are the structural and functional units of the kidney that form urine. Each nephron is composed of the glomerulus; the glomerular (Bowman's) capsule, which surrounds the glomerulus; the proximal convoluted tubule (PCT); the loop of Henle; and the distal convoluted tubule (DCT), which connects with the kidney's collecting tubules). Each kidney contains approximately 1.25 million nephrons **Figure 32-2 ▾** .

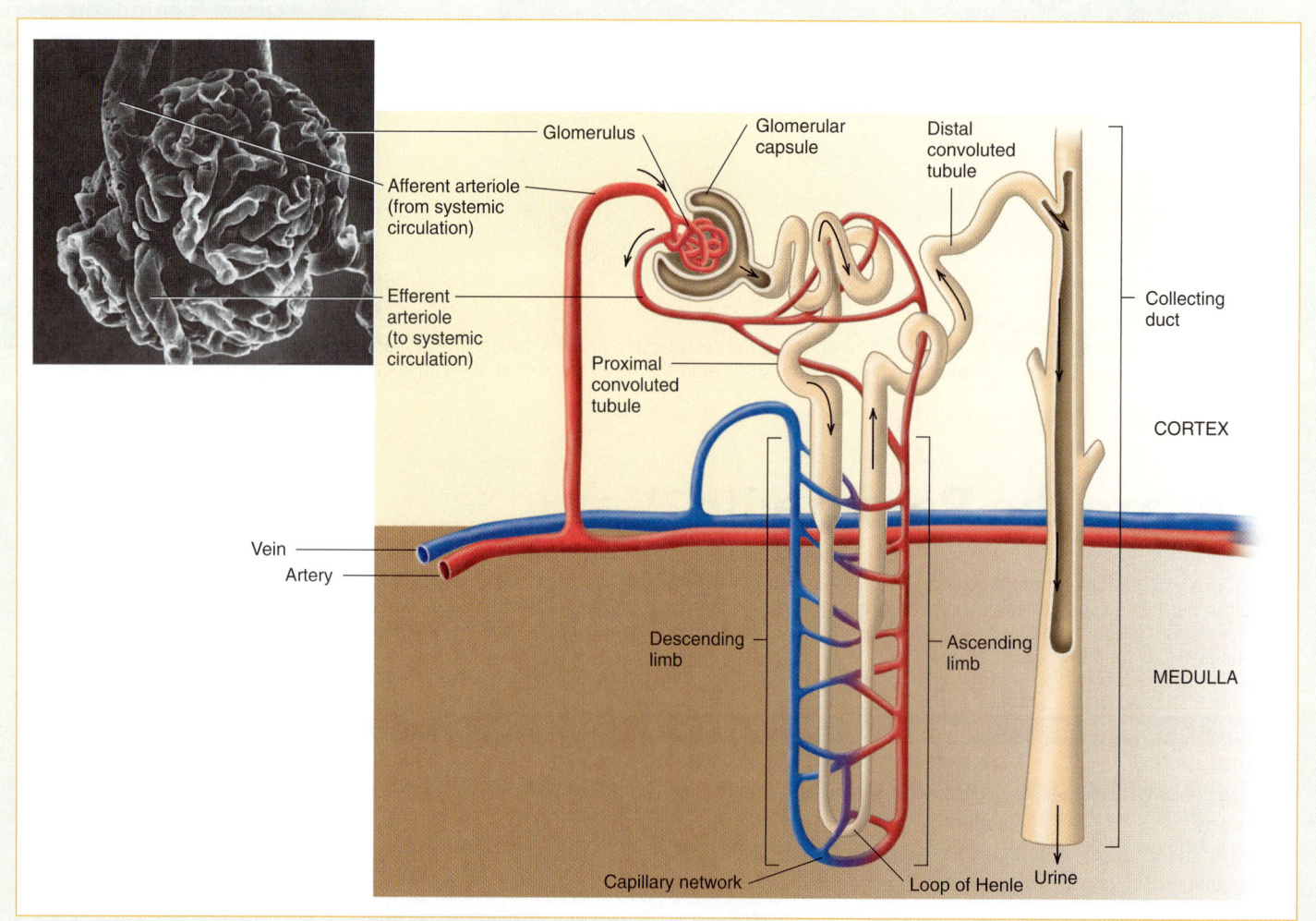

Figure 32-2 The nephrons of the kidney. Part of the nephron is located in the cortex, and part is located in the medulla. Inset at left, Electron micrograph of a glomerulus from a human nephron.

The glomerular capsule is a double-layered cup in which the inner layer infiltrates and surrounds the capillaries of the glomerulus. Special cells in the inner membrane called podocytes wrap around the capillaries in the glomerulus, forming filtration slits. The filtrate passes through these slits, across the filtration membrane, and into the capsule. In this manner, the filtration membrane prevents large molecules, such as proteins, from entering the capsule (**Figure 32-3** ▾).

The amount of filtrate produced, called the glomerular filtration rate (GFR), is maintained at a relatively constant rate of 125 ml/min in healthy adults. Changes in the GFR cause many of the renal emergencies encountered in the prehospital setting.

Initially, the filtrate contains everything that can pass through the filtration membrane: salts, minerals, glucose, water, and metabolic wastes. As the filtrate passes through the rest of the nephron, tubular resorption and tubular secretion convert the filtrate into urine. As the fluid passes through the PCT, the cells lining the PCT remove all organic nutrients and plasma proteins, as well as some ions from the filtrate. These compounds are deposited in the interstitial fluid surrounding the PCT. As these solutes accumulate, the concentration of the surrounding fluid becomes higher than that of the filtrate. Water will then move from the filtrate by osmosis. The fluid and nutrients in the interstitial fluid, in turn, move into the peritubular capillaries around the PCT. This process reestablishes the homeostatic balance in the blood and reduces the volume of the tubular filtrate.

Additional resorption of water and electrolytes occurs in the loop of Henle. The loop of Henle has two sections—the descending limb, extending toward the medulla, and the ascending limb, moving toward the cortex. The cells in the descending limb are permeable to water, but impermeable to sodium and chloride ions; the cells in the ascending limb are permeable to sodium and chloride ions, but impermeable to water. As a consequence, when the sodium and chloride ions move out of the ascending limb, they increase the solute concentration of the fluid surrounding the descending limb. Water moves by osmosis from the descending limb into the surrounding tissue and eventually into the vasa recta, a series of peritubular capillaries that surround the loop of Henle. This countercurrent multiplier process allows the body to produce either concentrated or diluted urine, depending on the body's needs.

After leaving the loop of Henle, the fluid enters the DCT. At this point, approximately 80% of the water and 85% of the solutes originally forced out of the glomerulus have been reabsorbed. As the urine passes through the DCT and the collecting ducts to which it is attached (both of which are impermeable to solutes), its composition undergoes its final adjustments. Ions are actively secreted or reabsorbed, and the body alters the permeability of the DCT and collecting ducts to water as necessary, depending on the body's homeostatic needs. These adjustments to the final composition of the urine facilitate the removal of metabolic wastes while maintaining the body's fluid-electrolyte balance.

At the site where the efferent arteriole comes in contact with the DCT, a structure called the juxtaglomerular apparatus is formed. The cells in the efferent arteriole (called juxtaglomerular cells) are pressure-sensitive, and monitor the blood pressure. The cells in the DCT (called macula densa cells) are sensitive to chemical changes and monitor the concentration of the filtrate in the DCT. When triggered by changes in the blood pressure of filtrate content, the juxtaglomerular cells release renin. This enzyme initiates a cascade of reactions in the body by converting the plasma protein angiotensinogen into angiotensin I. Other enzymes present in the blood then convert angiotensin I into angiotensin II. A potent vasoconstrictor, angiotensin II promotes smooth muscle contraction in the arterioles throughout the body. This constriction raises the blood pressure by increasing peripheral resistance. Angiotensin II also increases the resorption of sodium from the PCT. Given that water tends to follow sodium, by increasing sodium resorption, the kidney increases water resorption and, in turn, blood pressure.

The final adjustments to the composition of the urine at the DCT and collecting duct are controlled primarily by two hormones: antidiuretic hormone (ADH) and aldosterone. ADH is produced by the hypothalamus and stored in the posterior lobe of the pituitary; aldosterone is produced in the adrenal glands.

Neurons in the hypothalamus monitor the solute concentration of the blood. When the solute concentration of the blood increases (eg, due to sweating or decreased fluid

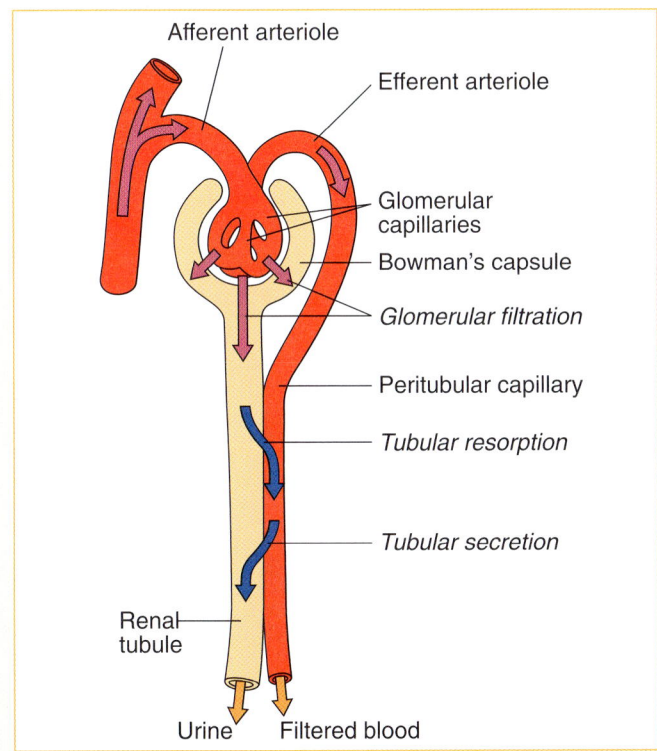

Figure 32-3 The glomerulus of the kidneys. The nephron carries out three blood-filtering processes: glomerular filtration, tubular resorption, and tubular secretion.

intake), ADH is released into the bloodstream. This hormone travels to the DCT and collecting ducts, increasing these structures' permeability to water. Water therefore leaves the DCT and collecting ducts, and reenters the bloodstream. As the solute concentration returns to normal, secretion of ADH will stop.

Aldosterone increases the rate of active resorption of sodium and chloride ions into the blood; a corresponding increase occurs in water resorption. This hormone also decreases the resorption of potassium ions, resulting in excess potassium being secreted in the urine.

Diuretics, chemicals that increase urinary output, work in a variety of ways. A substance that is not reabsorbed from the filtrate, for example, will increase the amount of water retained in the urine. An example of such an osmotic diuretic is glucose in a patient with diabetes mellitus. Alcohol encourages diuresis by inhibiting the production of ADH. Other diuretics, including caffeine and the diuretics commonly prescribed for hypertension and congestive heart failure (Lasix, Diuril), inhibit the sodium importers in the DCT and collecting ducts.

Once the urine enters the collecting ducts (the renal pyramids of the medulla), it passes through the minor calyx, into the major calyx, and then into the renal pelvis. From there, the urine moves through the ureter (one ureter from each kidney) and is stored in the urinary bladder. Most of the bladder sits in the anterior abdominal cavity, but the dome of the bladder sits in the posterior abdominal cavity, or retroperitoneum, where the ureters and kidneys reside. When empty, the bladder collapses, and the muscular walls fold over onto themselves. In contrast, as urine accumulates, the bladder expands and becomes pear-shaped. The stretching of the bladder walls

ultimately stimulates nerve impulses to produce the micturition reflex. This spinal reflex causes contraction of the bladder's smooth muscles, which in turn produces the urge to void as pressure is exerted on the internal urinary sphincter. Normally, the brain exerts control over this urge, keeping the external urinary sphincter contracted until conditions are favourable for urination. At this point, the inhibition of the external urinary sphincter is reduced and the urine passes from the urinary bladder into the urethra.

The beginning of the urethra, through which urine is expelled, sits at the inferior aspect of the bladder. In females, the urethra exits at the site of the external genitalia. The female urethra is shorter than the male urethra (4 cm versus 20 cm) **Figure 32-4 ▸**. The male urethra can be divided into three regions:

- The *prostatic urethra* begins at the bladder and extends through the prostate gland.
- The *membranous urethra* extends from the prostate gland through the abdominal wall and into the penis.
- The *spongy, or penile, urethra* passes through the penis to the external urethral opening.

Pathophysiology

Diseases and problems of the renal and urologic system range from mild (urinary tract infections) to true emergencies (acute renal failure). Although the prehospital care for many urologic diseases is supportive, your ability to recognize the signs and symptoms of the true emergencies is critical to provide your patients with the best chance of a positive outcome.

You are the Paramedic Part 2

You have placed the patient on oxygen via a nonrebreathing mask set at 12 l/min. During your focused history, the patient tells you that she has been taking dialysis treatments for over a year for "kidney failure." Additionally, she takes numerous medications and has a history of high blood pressure. Your physical examination reveals scattered crackles in her lungs and edema to her hands and feet. As you apply a cardiac monitor, your partner obtains baseline vital signs.

Vital Signs	Recording Time: 5 Minutes
Level of consciousness	V (Responsive to verbal stimuli), somewhat confused
Skin	Cool and dry
Pulse	110 beats/min and irregular
Blood pressure	104/58 mm Hg
Respirations	24 breaths/min; adequate tidal volume
Spo$_2$	97% (on supplemental oxygen)
Blood glucose	7 mmol/l

The 3-lead ECG reveals sinus tachycardia at 110 beats/min with premature ventricular complexes (PVCs) and tall peaked T-waves. The patient denies having any heart problems or diabetes.

3. What condition do you suspect this patient is experiencing?
4. What special concerns should you have regarding the patient's condition?

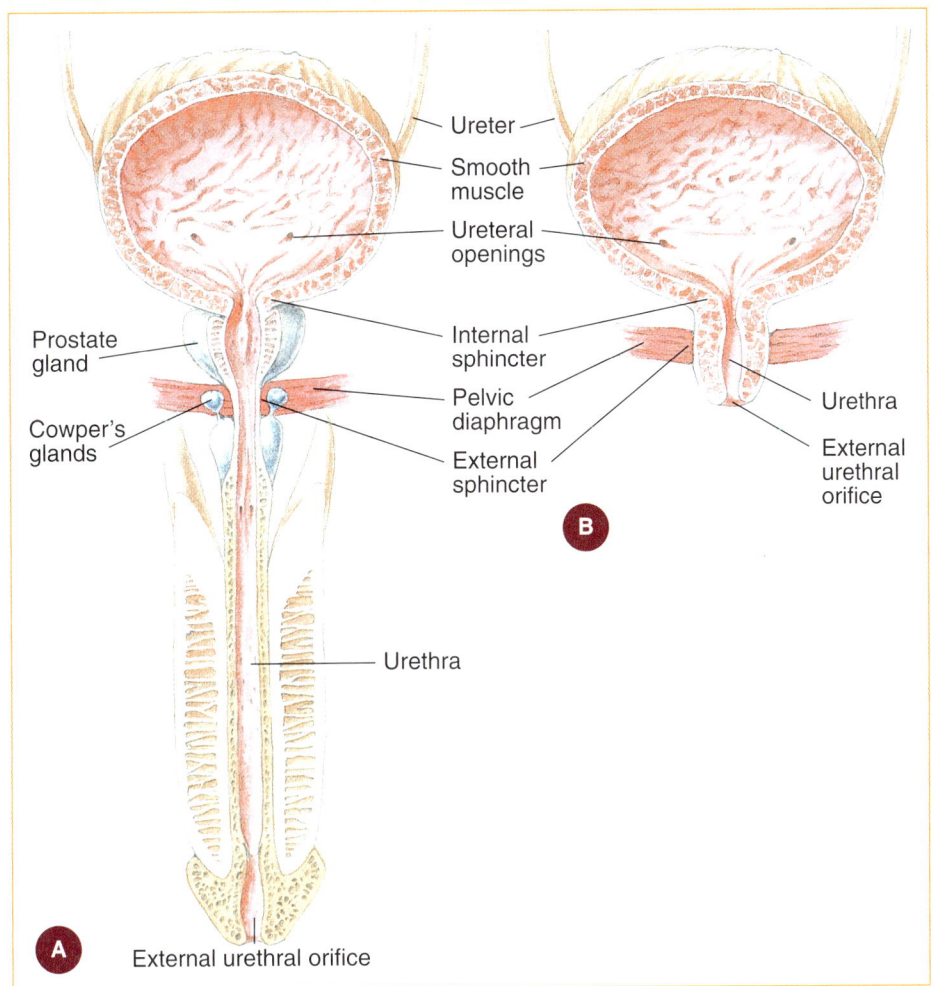

Figure 32-4 The differences in the urethras of (**A**) men and (**B**) women.

Urinary Tract Infections

Urinary tract infections (UTIs) usually develop in the lower urinary tract (urethra and bladder) when normal flora bacteria, which exist naturally on the skin, enter the urethra and grow. These infections are more common in women due to the relatively short urethra and the close proximity of the urethra to the vagina and rectum. UTIs in the upper urinary tract (ureters and kidneys) occur most often when lower UTIs go untreated. Upper UTIs can lead to pyelonephritis (inflammation of the kidney linings) and abscesses, which eventually reduce kidney function. In severe cases, untreated UTIs can lead to sepsis.

Common symptoms in patients with a lower UTI include painful urination, frequent urges to urinate, and difficulty in urination. The pain usually begins as a visceral discomfort, but then converts to an extreme burning pain, especially during urination. The pain, which remains localized in the pelvis, is often perceived as bladder pain in women and as prostate pain in men. Sometimes the pain may be referred to the shoulder or neck. In addition, the urine will have a foul odour and may appear cloudy.

Renal Calculi (Kidney Stones)

Kidney stones originate in the renal pelvis and result when an excess of insoluble salts or uric acid crystallizes in the urine Figure 32-5 ▾ . This excess of salts is typically due to water intake that is insufficient to dissolve the salts. The stones consist of different types of chemicals, depending on the precise imbalance in the urine.

The most common stones—calcium stones—occur more frequently in men than in women and may have a hereditary component. These stones also occur in patients with metabolic disorders such as gout or with hormonal disorders. Struvite stones are more common in women, and may be associated with chronic UTI or frequent catheterization. Uric acid and cystine stones are the least common. Uric acid stones tend to run in families, especially those with a history of gout. Cystine stones are associated with a condition that causes large amounts of amino acids and proteins to accumulate in the urine.

Patients who have kidney stones will almost always be in pain (many rate kidney stone pain as 11 on a scale of 1 to 10). The pain usually starts as a vague discomfort in the flank, but becomes very intense within 30 to 60 minutes. It may migrate forward and toward the groin as the stone passes through the system.

Some patients will be agitated and restless as they walk and move in an attempt to relieve the pain. Others will attempt to remain motionless and guard the abdomen. Either behaviour makes palpation of the abdomen difficult. Vital signs will vary, depending on the severity of pain. The greater the pain, the higher will be the blood pressure and pulse.

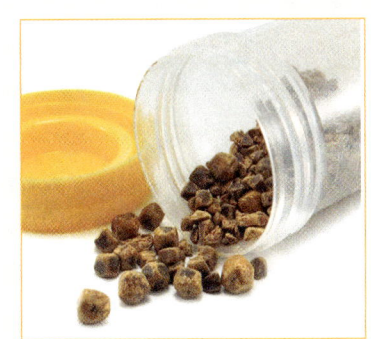

Figure 32-5 Kidney stones.

If a stone has become lodged in the lower ureter, signs and symptoms of a UTI (frequency and urgency of urination, painful urination, and/or hematuria) may be present, but the patient will not have a fever. If a kidney stone is suspected, be sure to obtain both a patient history and a family history; both can supply important information.

Acute Renal Failure

Acute renal failure (ARF) is a sudden (possibly over a period of days) decrease in filtration through the glomeruli. It is accompanied by an increase of toxins in the blood. Approximately 5% to 6% of all patients admitted to an ICU suffer from ARF. Sepsis is the most common contributing factor to ARF. Patients who are admitted to an ICU with ARF have an overall mortality rate of 50% to 60%. However, the disease is reversible if diagnosed and treated early and survival is more likely. For those who survive, approximately one in eight will require long-term dialysis.

If the urine output drops to less than 500 ml/day, the condition is called oliguria. If urine production stops completely, the condition is called anuria. Whenever ARF occurs, the patient may experience generalized edema, acid buildup, and high levels of nitrogenous and metabolic wastes in the blood. If left untreated, ARF can lead to heart failure, hypertension, and metabolic acidosis.

ARF is classified into three types, based on the area where the failure occurs: prerenal, intrarenal, and postrenal. The signs and symptoms of each type are summarized in Table 32-1 ▼.

Prerenal ARF is caused by hypoperfusion of the kidneys. In other words, not enough blood passes into the glomeruli for them to produce filtrate. The most common causes of prerenal ARF are hypovolemia (hemorrhage, dehydration), trauma, shock, sepsis, and heart failure (congestive heart failure, myocardial infarction). Prerenal ARF is often reversible if the underlying condition can be treated and perfusion restored to the kidney.

Intrarenal acute renal failure (IARF) involves damage to one of three areas in the kidney: the glomeruli capillaries and small blood vessels, the cells of the kidney tubules, or the renal parenchyma (the interstitial cells around the nephrons). Damage to the small vessels and glomeruli hinders blood flow through these vital parts of the nephrons. This damage is often caused by immune-mediated diseases (eg, type 1 diabetes mellitus). Tubule damage can be caused by prerenal ARF or toxins (eg, heavy metals). Chronic inflammation of the interstitial cells surrounding the nephrons (interstitial nephritis) can also produce IARF. This type of renal failure may be caused by medications such as antibiotics, anticancer drugs, alcohol, and drugs of abuse (eg, cocaine).

Postrenal ARF is caused by obstruction of urine flow from the kidneys. The source of this obstruction is often a blockage of the urethra by prostate enlargement, renal calculi, or strictures. This blockage causes pressure on the nephrons to increase, which eventually causes the nephrons to shut down. At this point, the kidneys can no longer carry out their cleansing functions, resulting in the development of hyperkalemia (an increase in the blood potassium levels) and/or metabolic acidosis (an increase in the hydrogen ion content of the blood). Both conditions are life-threatening emergencies that can lead to fatal dysrhythmias of the heart.

Chronic Renal Failure

Chronic renal failure (CRF) is progressive and irreversible inadequate kidney function due to permanent loss of nephrons. This disease develops over months or years. More than half of all cases are caused by systemic diseases, such as diabetes or hypertension. CRF can also be caused by congenital disorders or prolonged pyelonephritis.

As the nephrons become damaged and cease to function, scarring occurs in the kidneys. The tissue begins to shrink and waste away as the scarring progresses, leading to a loss of nephrons and renal mass. As kidney function diminishes, waste products and fluid build up in the blood. Uremia (increased urea and other waste products in the blood) and azotemia (increased nitrogenous wastes in the blood) develop, leading to systemic complications such as hypertension, congestive heart failure, anemia, and electrolyte imbalances.

Patients with CRF exhibit several signs and symptoms, beginning with an altered level of consciousness due to the electrolyte imbalance and the resulting effects on nerve transmission in the brain. In the late stages, seizures and coma are possible. The patients may also present with lethargy, nausea, headaches, cramps, and signs of anemia.

Table 32-1	Signs and Symptoms of Acute Renal Failure
Acute renal failure	Hypertension Shortness of breath and edema (volume overload) Hyperventilation (acidosis) Confusion Lethargy (uremia) Chest pain (pericarditis)
Prerenal acute renal failure	Hypotension Tachycardia Dizziness Thirst, oliguria
Intrarenal acute renal failure	Rash Purpura Inflammatory arthritis
Postrenal acute renal failure	Suprapubic or flank pain Distended bladder Hematuria

In a case of CRF, the patient's skin will be pale, cool, and moist, and the individual may appear jaundiced due to the buildup of nitrogenous wastes. A powdery accumulation of uric acid called uremic frost may also be present, especially around the face. The skin may appear bruised, and muscle twitching may be present.

Patients with CRF exhibit edema in the extremities and face due to fluid imbalances; they will also be hypotensive and have tachycardia. As hyperkalemia develops, the heart's electrical conduction will decrease. The ECG monitor will show increasing PR and QT intervals. As the hyperkalemia progresses, these dysrhythmias may evolve into an idioventricular rhythm. Pericarditis and pulmonary edema are also common and should be evaluated during auscultation of the chest.

Notes from Nancy

Patients with renal failure have impaired ability to metabolize or excrete medications, and the medication's effects may be more prolonged or pronounced. Do not give medications to patients with chronic renal failure unless it is specifically permitted in your protocols or you are instructed to do so by medical control.

Renal Dialysis

Although not truly a urologic disorder, renal dialysis and problems associated with it may require prehospital interventions. Renal dialysis is a technique for "filtering" toxic wastes from the blood, removing excess fluid, and restoring the normal balance of electrolytes **Figure 32-6 ▾**.

There are two types of dialysis—peritoneal dialysis and hemodialysis. In peritoneal dialysis, large amounts of specially formulated dialysis fluid are infused into (and back out of) the abdominal cavity. This fluid stays in the cavity for 1 to 2 hours, allowing equilibrium to occur. Peritoneal dialysis is very effective but carries a risk of peritonitis; consequently, aseptic technique is essential. With proper training, however, peritoneal dialysis can be performed in the home.

In hemodialysis, the patient's blood circulates through a dialysis machine that functions in much the same way (albeit not as elegantly) as the normal kidneys. Most patients undergoing chronic hemodialysis have some sort of shunt, ie, a surgically created connection between a vein and an artery. The patient is connected to the dialysis machine through this shunt, which allows blood to flow from the body into the dialysis machine and back to the body. A Scribner shunt, for example, consists of two plastic tubes: one fastened in the radial artery, the other in the cephalic vein. These two tubes are joined together near the wrist with a Teflon connector. A Thomas shunt is similar, but this device is usually placed in the groin. Other patients will have a small, button-shaped device, a Hemasite, with a rubber septum that can be punctured with dialysis needles during treatment. Hemasites are usually placed in the upper arm or proximal anterior thigh. Finally, some patients have an internal shunt (an arteriovenous [AV] fistula), which is an artificial connection between a vein and an artery that is usually located in the forearm or upper arm **Figure 32-7 ▾**.

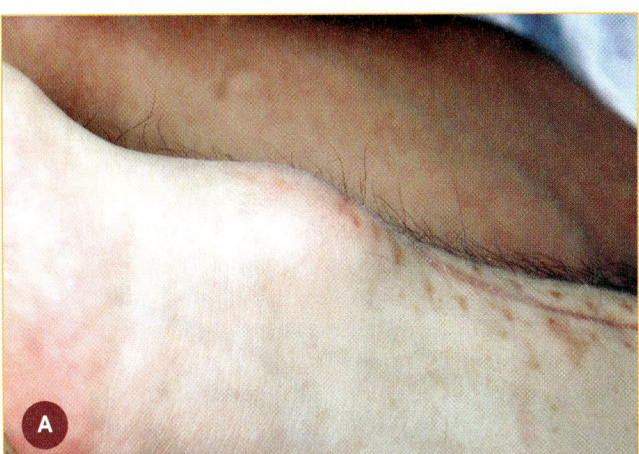

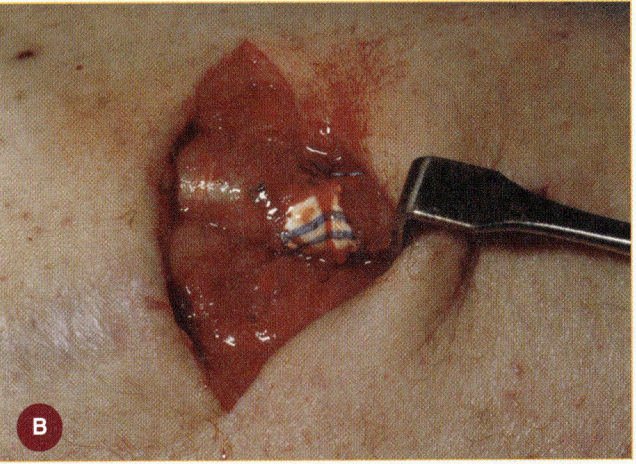

Figure 32-7 A. With an AV fistula, a bulge is created by arterial pressure. **B.** An AV graft creates a raised area that looks like a large vessel.

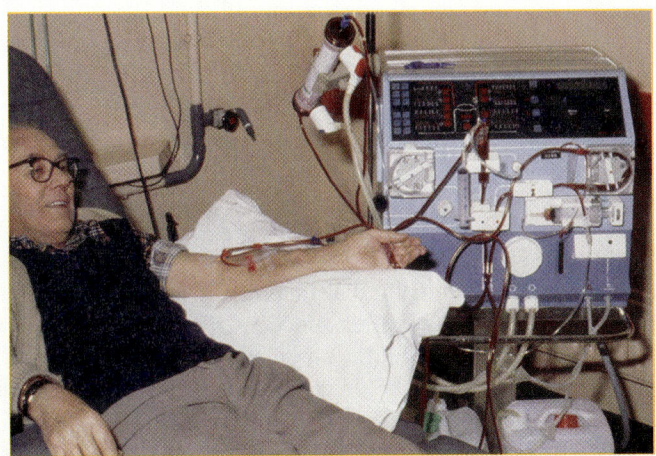

Figure 32-6 A patient undergoing dialysis.

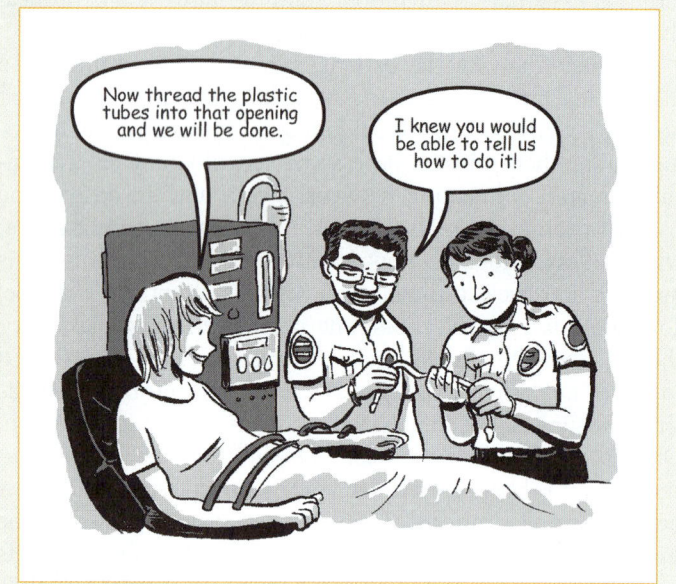

Figure 32-8

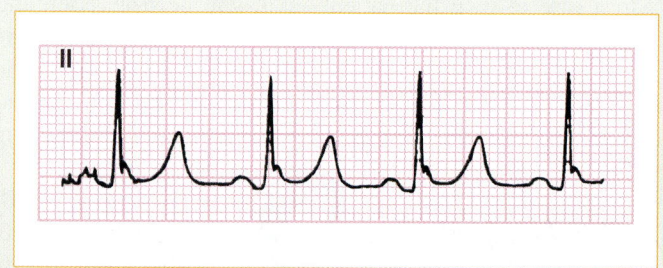

Figure 32-9 Peaked T waves, as shown in this rhythm strip, are a classic sign of hyperkalemia.

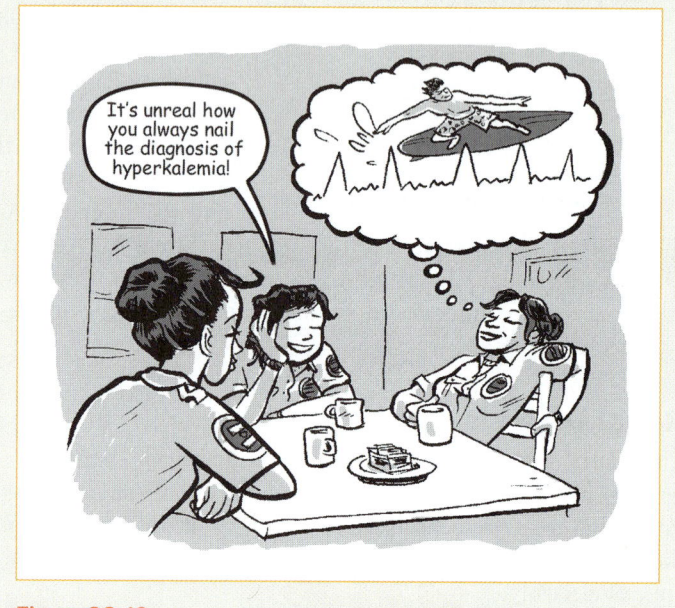

Figure 32-10

Patients requiring chronic dialysis usually go "on the machine" every 2 or 3 days for a period of 3 to 5 hours. Many receive dialysis in the hospital or in community dialysis facilities, but a significant number have home dialysis units. Patients undergoing dialysis at home usually have extensive training in the procedures, and often someone else in the home has also been trained. If a problem with the machine occurs, the patient may know a lot more about it than you do, so always ask what the patient has done prior to your arrival **Figure 32-8**!

Patients undergoing chronic dialysis can suffer the same spectrum of illnesses and injuries as any other patients. Dialysis patients, however, are particularly vulnerable to certain problems, either because of the dialysis itself or because of the underlying renal failure. Problems associated with dialysis may result from accidental disconnection from the machine, malfunction of the machine, or rapid shifts in fluids and electrolytes that produce hypotension, potassium imbalances, and disequilibrium syndrome.

Notes from Nancy

When you measure the blood pressure in a dialysis patient, use the arm that doesn't have the shunt!

Hypotension and Shock

A sudden drop in blood pressure is not uncommon during or immediately after dialysis, but it can lead to cardiac arrest if not promptly detected and treated. The patient may feel light-headed or become confused, and often he or she yawns more than usual. Because dialysis alters the blood's chemistry, the patient may develop an electrolyte imbalance. For this reason, you should always monitor dialysis patients for cardiac

dysrhythmias. Shock secondary to bleeding is also possible from any number of causes. Patients with CRF, for example, are very prone to duodenal ulcers; bleeding from those ulcers is not unusual. Bleeding may also occur from the dialysis cannula.

When you find a shunt leaking during the dialysis cycle, see if you can tighten up the connection. If it has become disconnected at the vein, clamp the cannula and disconnect the patient from the machine. In a suicide attempt, the patient may open up the cannula and allow himself or herself to exsanguinate. Keep in mind that these patients have often endured numerous medical interventions to simply survive. If you encounter this situation, immediately *clamp off the cannula* and apply direct pressure.

Potassium Imbalance

One consequence of renal impairment is the inability to excrete ingested potassium. As a consequence, CRF patients are prone to developing hyperkalemia, especially in circumstances of increased potassium intake or catabolic stress. Such a patient may present with profound muscular weakness. On the ECG, the classic signs of hyperkalemia are peaked T waves (**Figure 32-9** and **Figure 32-10**), a prolonged QRS complex, and sometimes disappearance of the P waves. Complete heart block and asystole may occur. If you see these signs, treatment is urgently required and must be undertaken in the prehospital environment if your transport time to the emergency department is long.

Hypokalemia may also occur as a consequence of overaggressive dialysis. It is most likely to be seen during or immediately after a dialysis cycle. The patient may be hypotensive, and cardiac dysrhythmias are almost always present (usually bradycardias). Treat the dysrhythmia if it is hemodynamically significant (see Chapter 27).

Disequilibrium Syndrome

During dialysis, the concentration of urea in the blood is lowered rapidly, while the solute concentration of the cerebrospinal fluid (CSF) remains high. Water, of course, moves by osmosis from a solution of lower concentration into a solution of higher concentration. Thus, as a consequence of dialysis, water initially shifts from the bloodstream into the CSF, thereby increasing intracranial pressure. In such a circumstance, the patient may experience typical symptoms of mildly increased intracranial pressure, including nausea, vomiting, headache, and confusion. After a few hours, the fluid will re-equilibriate between the blood and CSF, and the patient's symptoms will improve on their own. In the prehospital environment, however, it may be impossible to distinguish between disequilibrium syndrome and subdural hematoma, to which dialysis patients are particularly prone. In such a case, transport the patient to the hospital immediately for a full neurologic evaluation.

Air Embolism

If any of the fittings and connections in the dialysis system are loose, air may enter the system and produce an air embolism. Symptoms of air embolism include sudden dyspnea, hypotension, and cyanosis. If you have reason to suspect air embolism, disconnect the patient from the dialysis machine, place him or her in the left lateral recumbent position with about 10° of head-down tilt, and transport immediately.

Tumour of the Adrenal Gland

Pheochromocytoma is a tumour of the adrenal gland, usually in the medulla, that causes excess release of the hormones epinephrine and norepinephrine. Less than 10% of the tumours are malignant (cancerous).

The tumours may occur at any age, but they are most common in young to mid-adult life. A common clinical presentation is a combination of symptoms (ie, hypertension, anxiety, chest pain, abdominal pain, fatigue, weight loss, vision problems, and potentially seizures) that may be frequent but sporadic, and may increase in frequency, duration, and severity.

Genitourinary Trauma

Trauma to the genitourinary (GU) system—ie, the kidneys, ureters, bladder, and male and female reproductive organs—may result from either blunt or penetrating trauma. Such injuries are found in 10% to 20% of major trauma patients and 2% to 5% of all trauma patients. Eighty percent of all injuries to the GU system involve the kidneys. Paramedics should consider trauma to the GU system whenever a patient has sustained injuries to the lower rib cage, abdomen, pelvis, or upper legs.

Kidney

Renal (kidney) trauma is seen in less than 5% of all trauma patients, with about 75% of such cases involving patients younger than age 45. Injuries to the kidneys generally involve large forces, eg, falls from height, high-speed motor vehicle collisions, or sports-related injuries.

Blunt renal trauma results when the kidney becomes compressed against the lower ribs or lumbar spine (as is seen in sports injuries, also known as kidney punch) or when the

You are the Paramedic Part 3

You and your partner package the patient and load her into the ambulance. As you prepare to start an IV of normal saline, you notice that the patient has an AV shunt on her left forearm. The patient tells you that you *must* start the IV in her right arm. After securing the IV in place, you begin transport to the hospital. En route, you reassess the patient.

Reassessment	Recording Time: 12 Minutes
Level of consciousness	V (Responsive to verbal stimuli), somewhat confused
Skin	Cool and dry
Pulse	112 beats/min and irregular
Blood pressure	106/60 mm Hg
Respirations	24 breaths/min; adequate tidal volume
SpO_2	98% (on supplemental oxygen)
ECG	Sinus tachycardia with PVCs and tall, peaked T waves

5. What types of shunts are used for patients who require dialysis?

6. Why should you *not* take a blood pressure in the arm that has a shunt?

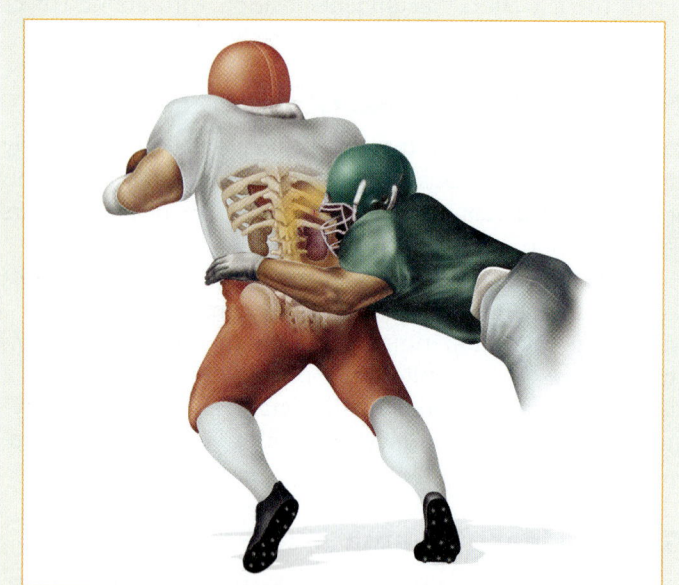

Figure 32-11 A football tackle that results in blunt trauma to the lower rib cage or flank can cause renal injury.

upper abdomen becomes compressed just below the rib cage (such as when a child is run over by a car). Contact sports such as football, soccer, hockey, boxing, and rugby are some of the more common culprits in renal injury **Figure 32-11**.

The most frequent presentation of blunt renal trauma is flank pain and hematuria (blood in the urine), which usually goes undetected until evaluation in the emergency department. Suspicion for renal injuries should be high whenever a patient has obvious hematomas or ecchymoses over the upper abdomen, lateral aspects of the middle back, or lower rib cage. Fractures of the lower rib cage should also raise the suspicion for renal trauma.

Penetrating renal trauma can occur with gunshot or stab wounds in the abdomen or lower chest. A high suspicion for significant injury must be maintained regardless of the site of the entry wound. Penetrating renal trauma is more likely to be associated with injury to the liver, lung, and spleen. For instance, the upward motion of stabbing may cause a renal laceration as well as a pneumothorax. A gunshot wound may result in direct injury to the kidney, but produce greater surrounding tissue destruction due to the expanding cavity created by the travelling bullet.

Prehospital care of renal injuries relies on the basics of abdominal trauma. Any obvious external abdominal hemorrhage must be addressed. If hemorrhage is not readily apparent but the patient has a large abdominal bruise in the region of the kidneys or is hypotensive, the astute paramedic may surmise that the patient has significant internal hemorrhage and begin intravenous hydration in the prehospital environment as per protocol.

Ureter

Ureteral injuries are difficult, if not impossible, to identify in the prehospital setting. However, they rarely lead to an immediate life-threatening condition.

Bladder and Urethra

Trauma to the bladder or urethra is often associated with other significant injuries. For instance, 27% of urethral injuries occur in conjunction with other intra-abdominal injuries.

A blunt or penetrating injury to the bladder may result in bladder rupture or laceration, usually as a result of blunt trauma. Bladder injury should be suspected in any patient with trauma to the lower abdomen or pelvis. In particular, obvious pelvic fractures are frequently associated with bladder injury. A seatbelt that causes contusions to the lower abdomen may also cause blunt trauma to the bladder. This type of injury is seen more frequently in drunk drivers, who are more likely to have a full bladder.

Bladder rupture is associated with a high mortality rate because the trauma required to pierce the bladder frequently damages other organs or vascular structures. If a bladder rupture results from sudden deceleration forces, such as those occurring in motor vehicle collisions, urine may be spilled into either part of the abdominal cavity, leading to either intraperitoneal, extraperitoneal, or retroperitoneal rupture.

Bladder injury may be suspected in the prehospital setting if a patient complains about an inability to urinate, blood is noted at the penile opening during the focused history and physical examination, or the patient has tenderness upon palpation of the suprapubic region. Prehospital care of such injuries follows basic trauma principles; secure the airway, address breathing issues, support the circulatory system, and immobilize the spine if necessary.

Injuries to the Male Genitalia
Testicle and Scrotal Sac

The testicles have two layers of covering—the tunica albuginea and the tunica vaginalis—and are held outside the body in the scrotal sac **Figure 32-12**. The testicles can be retracted into a more protected position by the cremaster muscles. Due to their mobility and natural position, severe injuries to the testicles are rare. Although loss of fertility is the major concern when a patient sustains a testicular injury, the exact outcome depends on whether the testicle can be preserved via definitive treatment in the hospital setting.

Blunt trauma to the testicles or scrotal sac can result from motor vehicle collisions, physical assaults, or sports injuries. Blunt testicular trauma can result in simple contusions, rupture of the testicle, and, in rare cases, torsion (twisting) of the testicle. More than half of all testicular ruptures occur in sports participants. Testicular injuries frequently present following trauma to the thighs, buttocks, penis, lower abdomen, and pelvis. Contusions result in painful hematomas that may respond to application of ice packs. Rupture of the testicle is difficult to identify in the prehospital setting, although tender scrotal swelling should be a presenting complaint. Similarly, paramedics will not know if a particular blunt trauma has resulted in a testicular torsion. Although serious injury to the testicles is rare, it does not require much force to cause intrascrotal bleeding. If enough bleeding or concomitant

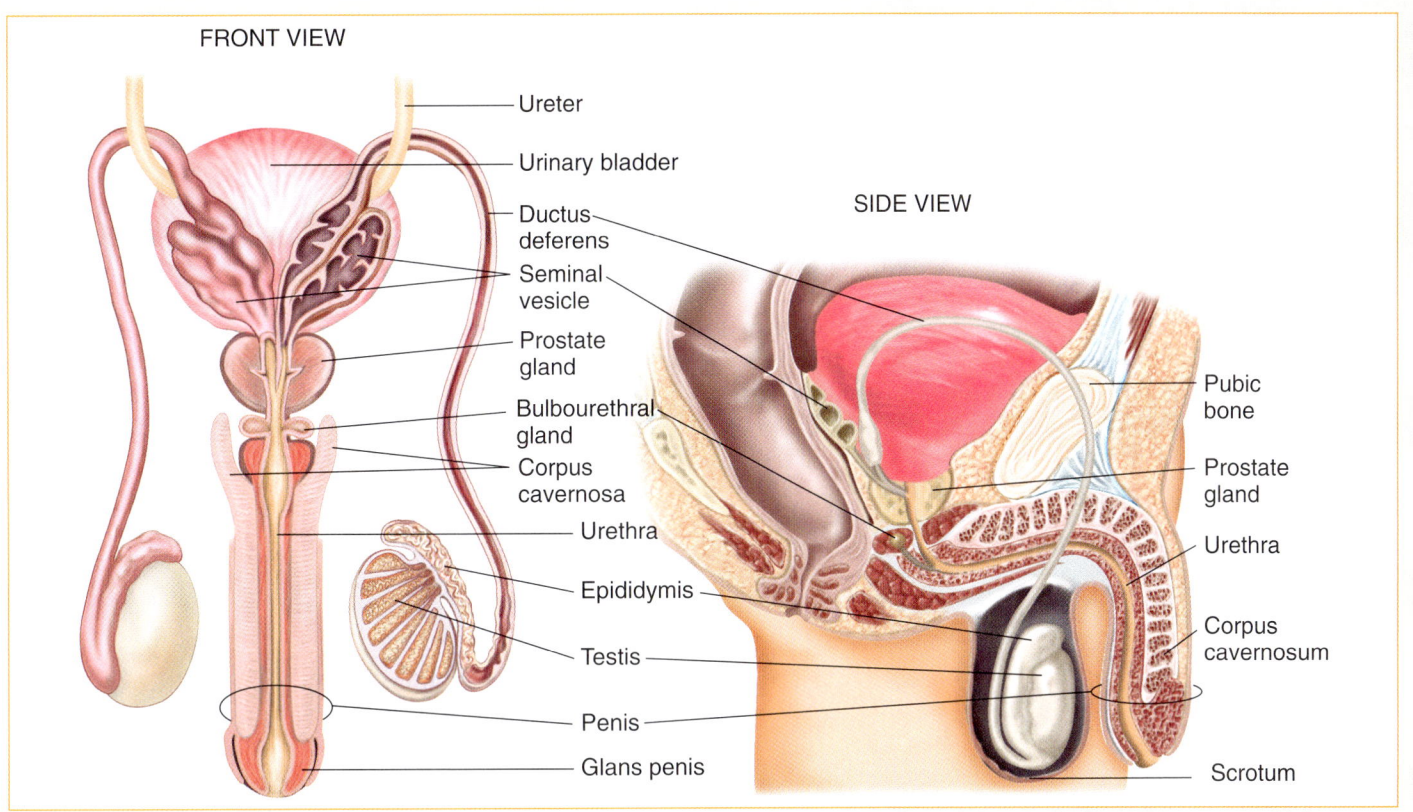

FRONT VIEW

Ureter
Urinary bladder
Ductus deferens
Seminal vesicle
Prostate gland
Bulbourethral gland
Corpus cavernosa
Urethra
Epididymis
Testis
Penis
Glans penis

SIDE VIEW

Pubic bone
Prostate gland
Urethra
Corpus cavernosum
Scrotum

Figure 32-12 The male genitalia includes the testicles, vasa deferentia, seminal vesicles, urethra, and penis.

swelling occurs, pressure necrosis (tissue death) may result. For this reason, you should not ignore testicular complaints even in the face of other trauma, and should communicate this concern to the emergency department staff.

Penetrating trauma to the testicles or scrotal sac may result from stab wounds, gunshot wounds, blast wounds, or animal bites. A high suspicion for other associated injuries is well advised in cases of obvious penetrating trauma.

Scrotal lacerations or avulsions should be treated with proper attention to any hemorrhage or eviscerated testicle. Gentle compression and the application of ice packs may help decrease bleeding, swelling, and pain.

Penis

The penis is vital for both proper urination and sexual function. Injuries to the penis may result from blunt or penetrating trauma but also may arise from sexual behaviour or self-mutilation. Physiologically, a penis becomes erect when blood fills the corpus cavernosa. Priapism—a sustained, painful penile erection—can be caused by conditions such as spinal injury and the use of erectile dysfunction drugs (eg, Viagra, Levitra, Cialis).

A fractured penis may occur when an erect penis is accidentally impacted against the partner's pubic symphysis or bent too far via self-manipulation. The wall of the corpora cavernosa is torn in these blunt trauma cases; pain and a large hematoma are the presenting signs and symptoms.

In the pediatric population, penile contusions have been reported to occur when a toilet seat falls unexpectedly and compresses the child's penis. Ice packs can help decrease swelling. Note that penile trauma in a child may be a sign of abuse, and an evaluation for other injuries may be warranted.

Penetrating trauma to the penis most often results from gunshot wounds. Attention should be paid to controlling hemorrhage and assessment for other injuries resulting from the trauma.

Reports in the medical literature describe self-mutilation or amputation of the penis. Typically this type of injury occurs in patients with significant psychiatric disorders. Attempts should be made to recover the amputated penis because surgical repair is often possible.

In addition, a number of reports have described people who have placed objects around the penis, testicles, or both. Inability to remove the object can result in incarceration of the organ, with tissue death being the most feared consequence. No attempt to remove the object should be made in the prehospital environment. Instead, the patient should be transported to the hospital for proper evaluation and treatment, which may necessitate the use of cutting devices or aspiration of the distal edema.

Injuries to the Female Genitalia

In females, the uterus lies behind the bladder and is well protected within the pelvis **Figure 32-13** . On either side of the uterus are the ovaries; in nonmenopausal women, these release an egg every month that travels to the uterus through the fallopian tubes. In the nonpregnant female, the uterus then sheds its lining each month, as evidenced by bleeding through the vaginal canal.

Vaginal trauma may be the result of blunt or penetrating trauma or may be self-inflicted. Blunt trauma may result from motor vehicle collisions in which high-energy impacts cause significant abdominal and pelvic trauma or from saddle-type injuries, eg, falling on the handlebars of a bicycle. Lacerations to the vaginal wall can occur, as well as uterine rupture or ovarian contusion. Trauma to the external genitalia may produce contusions to the vulva or labia. Signs of trauma may include hematomas and ecchymoses in the lower pelvic area and on the external female genitalia, bleeding from the vagina, and tenderness upon palpation of the lower pelvis.

Penetrating trauma to the reproductive organs may result from stabbings to the lower pelvis or gunshot wounds. Because the path of a bullet cannot be predicted from the entry wound alone, any injuries to the abdomen or upper legs may have also damaged the reproductive organs. Use packing and compression to stem any external hemorrhage, and administer replacement fluids to treat the hypotensive patient. Use any pain medication with extreme caution in the hypotensive patient.

Self-inflicted trauma has been reported in female children and in psychiatric patients who insert foreign bodies into their genitalia. Occasionally, women of reproductive age can cause vaginal lacerations by using devices or tools to remove

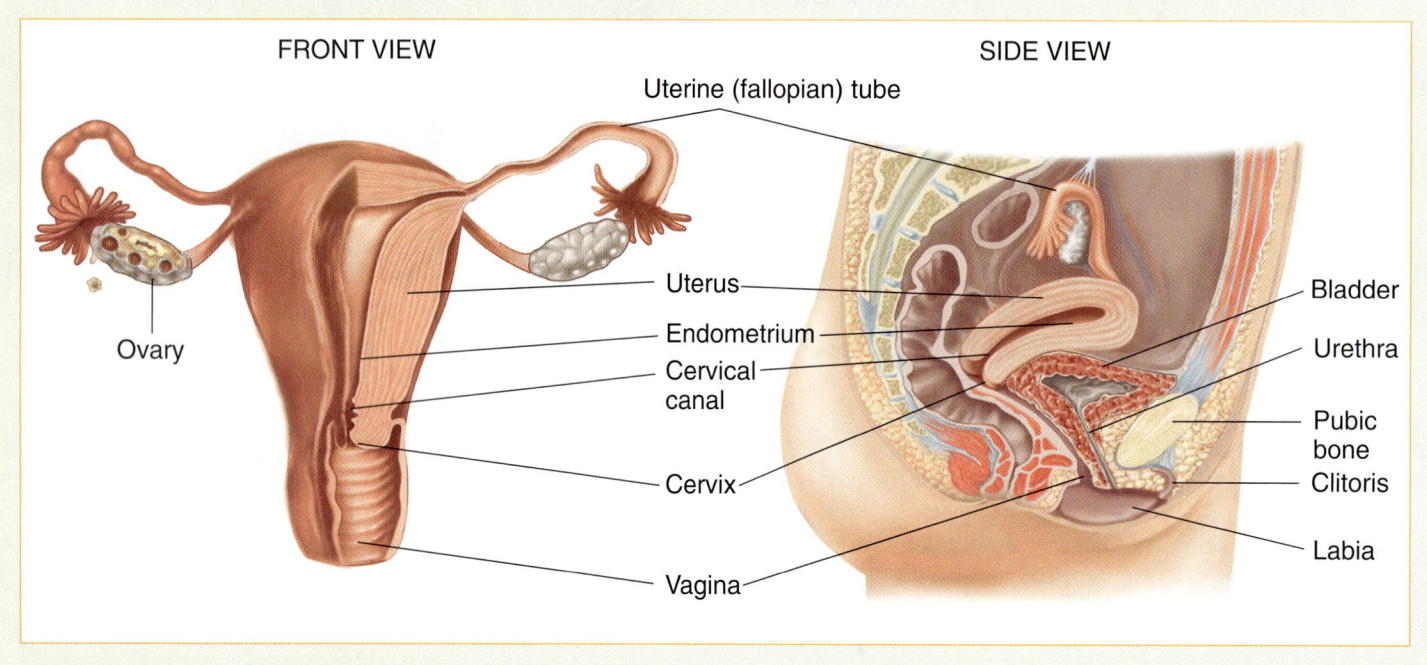

Figure 32-13 The female genitalia include the ovaries, fallopian tubes, uterus, cervix, and vagina.

You are the Paramedic Part 4

The patient's condition remains unchanged during transport. She remains conscious although confused, and still complains of severe weakness. With an estimated time of arrival at the hospital of 5 minutes, you reassess the patient and then call in your radio report.

Reassessment	Recording Time: 20 Minutes
Level of consciousness	V (Responsive to verbal stimuli), somewhat confused
Skin	Cool and dry
Pulse	108 beats/min and irregular
Blood pressure	104/64 mm Hg
Respirations	22 breaths/min; adequate tidal volume
Spo$_2$	97% (on supplemental oxygen)
ECG	Sinus tachycardia with PVCs and tall, peaked T waves

7. What medications, if any, may be indicated for this patient in the prehospital setting?

tampons, pads, and other products that they could not digitally remove from the vaginal canal. Do not attempt to remove any objects; immediately transport the patient for treatment at the hospital.

Assessment

Assessment of a patient with renal and urologic emergencies is the same as with any other medical patient. Begin with the scene assessment, perform an initial assessment, obtain a focused history and physical examination, form an initial impression and make a treatment decision, and perform ongoing assessments en route to the hospital. Patients who are experiencing renal problems may exhibit many of the same symptoms as a patient with other abdominal problems—nausea and vomiting, constipation or diarrhea, weight loss, loss of appetite, chest pain, and abdominal pain.

Because pain is a common symptom in both abdominal and urologic ailments, it is often difficult to determine the source of the pain. Urologic pain can have many origins, eg, bacterial infection, extension of the ureter by a kidney stone, or distension of the bladder due to prostate enlargement. However, assessment of urologic emergencies, as with all abdominal emergencies, is designed to detect and prevent life threats and provide supportive prehospital care for the patient. Don't waste valuable time trying to determine the exact cause of the pain in the prehospital setting.

When receptors at the affected organs are stimulated, they send impulses along the nerves to the brain, where the impulses are evaluated and interpreted as pain. Visceral pain—the type of pain most commonly associated with urologic problems—usually occurs when receptors in the hollow structures such as the ureters, urinary bladder, and urethra become stimulated. It is described as crampy, aching pain, deep within the body. Pinpointing the source of such pain is challenging because only a few nerve fibres may be involved in the pain transmission.

Because many different nerve fibres travel to the brain through the spinal cord, pain that originates in one area of the body (eg, the urinary bladder) may be interpreted by the brain as coming from a different area of the body (eg, the neck or shoulder). This referred pain can be used as a diagnostic tool in some urologic and renal diseases.

Scene Assessment

In the scene assessment, you should not only ensure that the scene is safe for you and your fellow paramedics, but also take routine precautions, consider the mechanism of injury, assess for hazards and the need for additional help, and determine the number of patients. Is the patient in obvious pain? Does he or she appear pale or jaundiced? What is the patient's level of consciousness? This general impression will be continually reevaluated, but it's important to establish your "baseline impression" early in the assessment process.

Initial Assessment

In the initial assessment, you form your general impression of the patient and check for life-threatening conditions with the assessment of the patient's mental status and ABCs. A patient with urologic or renal problems may exhibit extremes of activity. Is the patient constantly changing positions in an attempt to find a comfortable position ("the kidney stone dance")? Or is the patient sitting very still with the knees drawn to the chest? Now check for life threats. Do you see signs of respiratory distress or failure? Are there signs of profuse bleeding or circulatory compromise? Is the abdomen distended or rigid? If you discover any life-threatening conditions, take immediate steps to correct them.

Focused History and Physical Examination/Detailed Physical Examination

In urologic patients, the patient history and physical examination will provide the information needed to successfully manage the patient. Because 80% of all medical diagnoses are based on the patient's history, it is imperative that you ask the right questions during this examination. Determining that the pain actually started in the flank and not in its present location of the lower right quadrant could mean the difference between a correct initial diagnosis of a kidney stone and an incorrect initial diagnosis of appendicitis. Similarly, determining that the patient has a history of diabetes and hypertension along with signs of uremia can help confirm your impression of chronic kidney failure.

The SAMPLE mnemonic can guide you in obtaining pertinent historical information from the patient. For example, a patient who complains of flank pain and is agitated (S); who has had two previous kidney stone attacks (P); who had bacon, eggs, and coffee for breakfast 7 hours ago (L); and who has been working in the sun all day (E) has presented a history that would lead you to suspect kidney stones. You would obviously want to assess allergies (A) and any medications (M) the patient has taken before proceeding with treatment.

The OPQRST mnemonic is used to evaluate the type and severity of pain, such as the flank pain mentioned earlier. *Onset* involves questions about when the pain started and what the patient was doing at the time. Visceral pain, such as from a kidney stone, often begins as a vague discomfort and then gradually increases. Next, determine what, if anything, *Provokes* the pain (eg, the kidney stone dance or statue stillness). To help rule out other abdominal causes of pain, take note of any relationship between food consumption and the pain.

After determining the onset and provocation, assess the *Quality* of the pain. As stated earlier, pain from a kidney stone usually begins as a vague discomfort but, within 30 to 60 minutes, becomes extremely sharp. The *R* stands for Region (location), Radiation, or Referral; the pain in our example has moved from the flank anteriorly toward the groin. The fact that the pain has moved also suggests that a kidney stone is passing through the system.

To evaluate the *Severity* of the pain, ask the patient, "On a scale of 1 to 10, with 10 being the worst pain you have ever

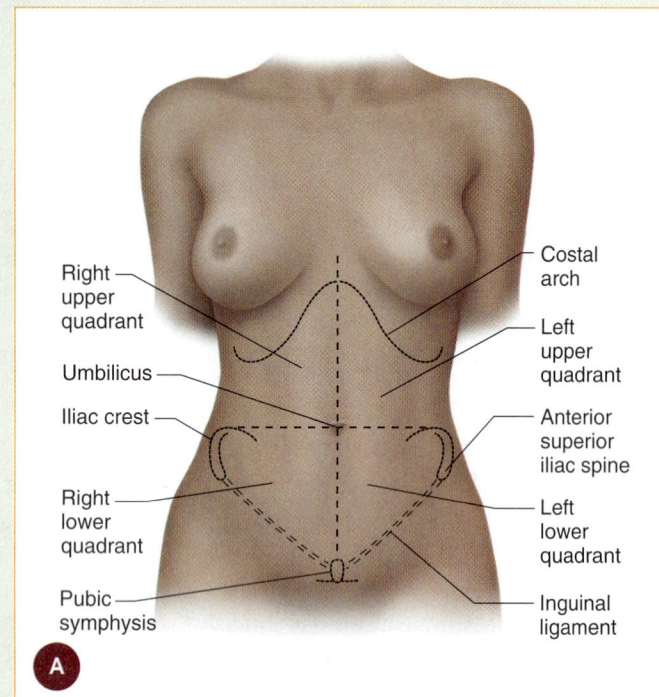

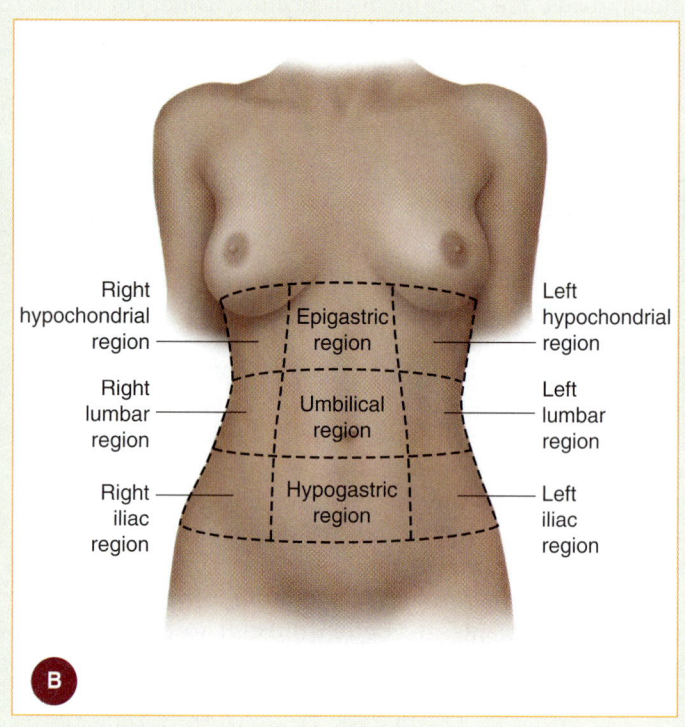

Figure 32-14 **A.** The four-quadrant system. **B.** Abdominal region mapping in nine sections.

experienced, how would you rate the pain?" Although this number is helpful, by itself it tells you very little. The severity of the pain may not correspond with the severity of the problem. Especially in older patients who have a higher pain threshold, a pain considered very severe (10+) by younger individuals may be reported as 3 or 4. It is important to repeat this severity assessment to look for trends or to verify efficacy of the treatments.

The final pain evaluation is the *Timing* of the pain. Did the pain come on suddenly, or more gradually? Has it been constant, or does it come and go? In the case of a kidney stone, you would expect fairly constant pain that varies in severity and moves as the stone moves through the system.

The physical examination includes monitoring and vital signs. ECG monitoring is extremely important in any patient with a suspected urologic emergency due to the possible electrolyte imbalances and their effect on the heart. The examination itself may be focused, or go from head to toe, depending on the presentation of signs and symptoms. Figure 32-14 ▲ shows the four-quadrant system overlying the internal organs and the nine sections of abdominal region mapping. A more detailed physical examination may be performed en route if not done at the scene.

Initial Impression and Treatment Plan

Once you have completed the focused history and physical examination, you must use the information obtained to form an initial impression and create a treatment plan. This could be as simple as monitoring the ABCs and giving circulatory support for a patient with a UTI, or as complex as adjusting medications and support in patients with renal failure due to

changes in the ECG (with medical consultation and direction). The treatment plan includes the transport decision, which may be made at any time during the assessment process. If the disease process requires immediate medical procedures that go beyond the scope of the prehospital setting, the treatment plan can be carried out en route to the hospital.

Ongoing Assessment

Patients with urologic emergencies, especially those with signs and symptoms of renal failure, need ongoing assessment. The electrolyte imbalances caused by the buildup of toxins can cause major, rapid changes in the functioning of the body's organs. The heart is particularly susceptible to electrolyte changes, so cardiac monitoring should be established for every renal patient. Serial vital signs should be obtained and documented on the prehospital care report, at least every 5 minutes in cases of possible renal failure. Note any trends in the vital signs and level of consciousness, as they can be indicators of disease progression. Patients with possible urologic disease

At the Scene

Patients with renal failure who miss their dialysis treatments are prone to, among other conditions, hyperkalemia. Suspect hyperkalemia if the patient presents with severe muscle weakness and tall, peaked T waves on the ECG.

should not be given anything by mouth because this may induce vomiting or complicate surgical procedures. Document all vital signs and report noted trends to the receiving facility in your transfer report.

Management

The management of patients with a UTI or renal calculi centres on comfort and support. Once you have checked and established adequate airway, breathing, and circulation (ABCs), allow the patient to assume a position of comfort. Patients in severe pain may have nausea and vomiting, so be prepared to suction and be ready for the possibility of aspiration. Analgesia may be provided if necessary, but remember that the masking of abdominal pain is not a desired result of prehospital care. Consult with direct medical control before administering pain medication. Establish an IV line. If kidney function is present, administer a bolus of fluid to the patient with a UTI as well as to the patient with a kidney stone. The fluid will rehydrate the UTI patient, and increased urine will help flush the infection from the system. For the patient suffering from renal calculi, the increased urine formation will help move the stone though the system.

ARF and CRF can lead to life-threatening emergencies. Support of the ABCs is imperative. Because of the possible toxic buildup and electrolyte problems, medications to regulate acidosis and electrolyte imbalance as well as fluids for volume regulation may be required. With either of these treatments, you must monitor the patient's reaction because drastic shifts in electrolytes, although rare, may occur. Emergent transport and supportive prehospital care are often preferred over aggressive management in these patients.

The management of medical emergencies resulting from dialysis is summarized in **Table 32-2 ▶**.

Assessment and Management of Specific Emergencies

This section considers how the specifics of the more common renal and urologic emergencies lead to the appropriate management plan.

Urinary Tract Infections

Patients with UTIs display a classic triad of symptoms: painful urination, frequency of urination, and difficulty of urination. They will appear restless and uncomfortable. The skin will range from pale, cool, and moist in a patient with a lower UTI to warm and dry in a patient with an upper UTI, such as pyelonephritis. Vital signs will vary with the degree of illness, but palpation of the abdomen will usually reveal tenderness over the pubis or pain in the flank, depending on the area of the infection.

Table 32-2	**Medical Emergencies in Dialysis Patients**
Problem	**Prehospital Management**
Problems related to dialysis itself:	
Hypotension	Give 50 ml of normal saline IV
Hemorrhage from the shunt	If the shunt cannot be reconnected, clamp it off; check for signs of shock
Potassium imbalance	For hypokalemia: treat bradycardia with atropine For hyperkalemia: calcium and bicarbonate may be considered
Disequilibrium syndrome	Supportive treatment only
Air embolism	Left lateral recumbent position in about 10° of head-down tilt
Machine dysfunction	Turn off machine; clamp ends of shunt; disconnect patient from machine; transport
Problems to which dialysis patients are more vulnerable:	
Congestive heart failure	Oxygen; sitting position; rapid transport to dialysis facility
Myocardial infarction and cardiac dysrhythmias	Treat as any other patient, but use caution in administering any medications
Hypertension	Transport only; the treatment is dialysis
Pericardial tamponade	Emergency transport as soon as detected
Uremic pericarditis	Oxygen; position of comfort; transport
Subdural hematoma	Oxygen; urgent transport

Management of patients with UTIs consists mainly of supportive prehospital care of the ABCs. Allow the patient to ride in a position of comfort, but be prepared for nausea and vomiting. Analgesics will probably be needed only in severe cases of pyelonephritis. For most patients, nonpharmacologic pain management with breathing and relaxation techniques is usually sufficient. Establish an IV and administer a fluid bolus, which will promote blood flow through the kidney and dilute the urine. Transport the patient to the nearest appropriate facility for evaluation.

Kidney Stones

The prehospital management of kidney stones centres on pain relief. After ensuring the ABCs, allow the patient to assume a position of comfort. Consider analgesia, but remember that narcotics should not be given if there is a possibility of a gastrointestinal condition. Pain management may also be accomplished by using breathing techniques like those used for women during labour. Establish an IV line and administer fluids to promote movement of the stone through the system. Transport the patient to an appropriate facility with a lithotripsy unit if possible, providing supportive prehospital care, as necessary **Figure 32-15 ▶**.

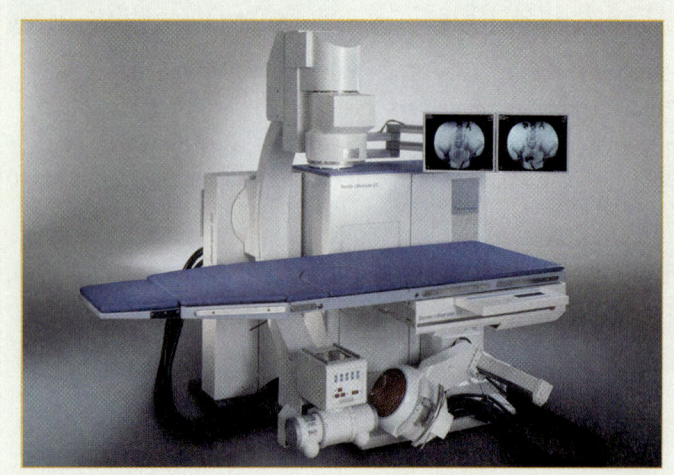

Figure 32-15 A lithotripsy unit, where kidney stones are disintegrated.

Acute Renal Failure

The toxic buildup of nitrogenous wastes and salts in the blood associated with ARF causes impaired mentation, hypotension, fluid retention, tachycardia, and increased PR and QT intervals associated with hyperkalemia. The patient's skin will be pale, cool, and moist, and edema will appear on the extremities and face. When inspecting the abdomen, look for any scars, ecchymosis, or distension. If the abdomen is distended, note whether the swelling is symmetric. Palpate the abdomen for any pulsing masses, which could indicate an aortic aneurysm. A hematocrit and urinalysis (if available) may be helpful to identify such causes as acute anemia, chronic hemorrhage, or pyelonephritis.

Because the metabolic changes caused by ARF can be life-threatening, it is imperative that the treatment plan supports the ABCs. Provide the patient with high-flow supplemental oxygen and, if necessary, provide ventilatory support with bag-valve-mask ventilation. Place the patient in the shock position with the feet elevated to increase blood flow to the brain and vital organs. Consider an IV bolus if the patient exhibits signs of shock, but use caution to prevent pulmonary edema. If possible, and with medical direction, you may perform a fluid lavage for patients who undergo peritoneal lavage.

The reduction of materials in cases of ARF may be toxic to the kidneys. Many medications can be nephrotoxic, including many analgesics and antibiotics. Consult with direct medical control if you suspect ARF and are transporting a patient with antibiotic or analgesic drips. If direct medical control is unavailable, discontinue the medication and transport the patient to the nearest appropriate facility.

As with any medical patient, patients with ARF need psychological support. Talk with your patient and inform him or her of what you are doing and what is occurring. Be confident and calm in your responses to questions, and reassure the patient that he or she is receiving the best prehospital care possible.

Chronic Renal Failure

Patients with CRF will exhibit an altered level of consciousness. In the late stages, seizures and coma are possible. Patients may also present with lethargy, nausea, headaches, cramps, and signs of anemia. The skin will be pale, cool, and moist, and may appear jaundiced with uremic frost present around the face. Bruising of the skin and muscle twitching may also be present. Edema in the extremities and face will be apparent, and patients will be hypotensive and tachycardic. The ECG monitor will show increasing PR and QT intervals. As hyperkalemia increases, these dysrhythmias may become an idioventricular rhythm. Pericarditis and pulmonary edema are also common and should be evaluated during auscultation of the chest.

Management of a CRF patient is initially similar to managing an ARF patient. Support the ABCs. Provide the patient with high-flow supplemental oxygen and, if necessary, ventilatory support with bag-valve-mask ventilation. Place the patient in the shock position with the feet elevated to increase blood flow to the brain and vital organs. If there are no signs of pulmonary edema, consider an IV bolus if the patient shows signs of shock. Because CRF patients are prone to third-space shock (due to fluid shifts) and major electrolyte changes, treatment strategies should centre on the regulation of fluid imbalances and cardiovascular function. For example, if hypotension occurs, a vasopressor may be administered, or direct medical control may order the administration of sodium bicarbonate to correct acidosis. Ultimately, patients with CRF will require renal dialysis. After life threats are addressed, transport the patient to the appropriate facility for treatment.

Because patients in CRF are already suffering from electrolyte imbalances in their blood, be conservative with your treatment plans for these individuals. Transport should be undertaken in a calm manner; talk quietly and confidently with the patient. If the patient has an altered mental status, be sure to assess his or her orientation frequently and record any changes.

You are the Paramedic Summary

1. What is the purpose of dialysis?

Renal dialysis is a technique for "filtering" toxic wastes from the blood, removing excess fluid, and restoring the normal balance of electrolytes. Although dialysis is most commonly used to replace the function of the kidneys in patients with acute or chronic renal failure, it is also used to remove other toxins from the blood, such as those caused by a drug overdose. Without dialysis, patients with renal failure (acute or chronic) would experience uremia and azotemia—conditions in which nitrogenous wastes accumulate in the blood. These conditions lead to systemic complications, such as hypertension, anemia, electrolyte imbalances, and circulatory overload.

2. What are the two types of dialysis?

There are two types of dialysis: peritoneal and hemodialysis. With peritoneal dialysis, large amounts of specially formulated dialysis fluid are infused into (and back out of) the abdominal cavity. This fluid remains in the abdominal cavity for one to two hours, allowing equilibrium to occur. With hemodialysis, the patient's blood circulates through a dialysis machine—much in the same way that it circulates through the kidneys. Unlike peritoneal dialysis, hemodialysis utilizes a shunt—a surgical connection between a vein and an artery. Patients requiring chronic dialysis usually receive treatments every 2 or 3 days for a period of 3 to 5 hours.

3. What condition do you suspect this patient is experiencing?

Given the patient's history of dialysis treatments for over a year, it is clear that her baseline problem is chronic renal failure (CRF). CRF is the progressive and irreversible failure of the kidneys due to permanent loss of nephrons—the cells that comprise the kidneys. CRF develops over months or years; hypertension—which your patient has a history of—is a common cause of CRF. Because the patient has missed her last few dialysis treatments, you should suspect that she is uremic; this would explain her jaundiced skin colour (indicates nitrogenous waste accumulation in the blood). As evidenced by her edematous hands and feet and crackles in her lungs, you should also suspect fluid retention. Furthermore, her severe weakness and ECG changes (ie, tall, peaked T waves) should lead you to suspect hyperkalemia—an increased serum potassium level.

4. What special concerns should you have regarding the patient's condition?

Definitively, this patient requires dialysis to restore her body to a state of equilibrium; she will no doubt receive this in the hospital. During transport, however, you should be most concerned with the fact that she is at increased risk for cardiac arrest secondary to hyperkalemia. T waves that are tall and peaked are a classic sign of hyperkalemia—especially in a patient with CRF who has missed dialysis treatments—and the PVCs she is experiencing indicate ventricular irritability. Close monitoring of the patient's cardiac rhythm is essential. As potassium levels continue to rise, other ECG changes may occur, such as PR interval prolongation, disappearance of P waves, and widened QRS complexes. You must be prepared to treat this patient for ventricular fibrillation, pulseless ventricular tachycardia, asystole, or pulseless electrical activity (PEA).

5. What types of shunts are used for patients who require dialysis?

As noted earlier, a shunt is a surgical connection between a vein and an artery and is used in patients undergoing hemodialysis. There are several types of shunts used. A Scribner shunt consists of two plastic tubes—one fastened in the radial artery and the other in the cephalic vein. These two tubes are joined together near the wrist with a Teflon catheter. A Thomas shunt—similar to a Scribner shunt—is usually placed in the groin. A Hemasite is a small, button-shaped device with a rubber septum that is punctured with dialysis needles during treatment. Hemasites are usually placed in the upper arm or proximal anterior thigh. An arteriovenous (AV) fistula, an internal shunt, is an artificial connection between a vein and artery. AV fistulas are usually located in the forearm or upper arm.

6. Why should you *not* take a blood pressure in the arm that has a shunt?

A shunt can become occluded by a thrombosis (blood clot). Decreased blood flow is a common cause of thrombosis. Anything that impairs circulation to the extremity with the shunt—even for a few minutes—can result in thrombosis. For this reason, you should avoid taking a blood pressure in the arm that has a shunt.

7. What medications, if any, may be indicated for this patient in the prehospital setting?

If the patient experiences cardiac arrest, epinephrine (or vasopressin) administration is indicated. Other medications, such as amiodarone or lidocaine and atropine, may be indicated, depending on the patient's cardiac arrest rhythm. In this patient, you should suspect that severe hyperkalemia is the underlying cause of cardiac arrest if it occurs. Hyperkalemic cardiac arrest is treated with calcium chloride and sodium bicarbonate. Calcium chloride is used for hyperkalemia to stabilize the cell membrane. Sodium bicarbonate is used to force potassium from the serum (blood) back into the cell, thus decreasing serum potassium levels. Depending on your transport time to the hospital, direct medical control may order you to administer calcium chloride and sodium bicarbonate if severe hyperkalemia is suspected (ie, frequent PVCs, widened QRS interval, PR interval prolongation). Follow locally established protocols regarding pre-arrest pharmacologic treatment for hyperkalemia.

Prep Kit

Ready for Review

- Kidney disease is the most common renal disorder. Kidney stones and urinary tract infections also impact many people.
- The genitourinary system includes the kidneys, urinary bladder, ureters, urethra, male and female reproductive organs, and specific structures within the kidneys.
- Blood flows through the kidney into the afferent arteriole and then the glomerulus, the main filter. It then enters the efferent arteriole, followed by the peritubular capillaries, where it is reabsorbed.
- Urine forms in the nephrons. The nephrons are composed of the glomerulus, the glomerular capsule, the proximal convoluted tubule, loop of Henle, and the distal convoluted tubule.
- In the glomerular capsule, filtrate from the blood—which contains salts, minerals, glucose, water, and metabolic wastes—passes through a membrane. Next, it passes through the rest of the nephron; after which it is converted into urine. This urine passes through the proximal convoluted tubule and loop of Henle to be further concentrated.
- In the distal convoluted tubule, the composition of urine is further refined based on the body's needs. Two hormones, antidiuretic hormone and aldosterone, are involved in adjusting the urine composition.
- The juxtaglomerular apparatus in the kidneys can release renin, an enzyme that can cause reactions in the body such as an increase in blood pressure.
- Diuretics are chemicals that increase urinary output.
- As urine collects in the bladder, the micturition reflex causes it to contract, producing the urge to void.
- Urinary tract infections can move into the upper urinary tract when a bacterial infection in the lower urinary tract is not treated.
- The anatomy of the urethra is different in males and females. The female urethra is shorter and therefore more prone to urinary tract infection.
- Symptoms of urinary tract infection include painful urination, frequent urges to urinate, difficulty urinating, and possibly referred pain to the shoulder or neck. The urine may have a foul odour and be cloudy.
- Kidney stones result when an excess of insoluble salts or uric acid crystallizes in the urine. Symptoms include severe pain in the flank that may migrate forward to the groin. The pain may cause an increased blood pressure and pulse.
- Acute renal failure is a sudden decrease in filtration through the glomeruli, resulting in a release of toxins into the blood. The three types of acute renal failure are prerenal, intrarenal, and postrenal. Signs and symptoms range from hypotension, tachycardia, dizziness, and thirst, to pain, oliguria, distended bladder, hematuria, and peripheral edema.
- Chronic renal failure is progressive and irreversible inadequate kidney function. Nephrons become damaged, losing their functionality and causing a buildup of wastes and fluid in the blood. Symptoms include an altered level of consciousness, lethargy, nausea, headaches, cramps, anemia, bruised skin, edema in the extremities and face, hypotension, tachycardia, or possibly seizures or coma. A powdery buildup of uremic acid (uremic frost) may appear on the skin. Hyperkalemia may be noted on the ECG.
- Renal dialysis is a procedure for removing toxic wastes and excess fluids from the blood. Dialysis patients usually have a shunt through which they are connected to the dialysis machine. They are vulnerable to problems such as hypotension, a potassium imbalance, disequilibrium syndrome, or air embolism.
- Kidney trauma can cause flank pain and hematuria. Management is the same as for other types of abdominal trauma.
- Suspect a bladder injury in any patient who has trauma to the lower abdomen or pelvis. Symptoms include inability to urinate, blood at the urethral opening, and tenderness of the suprapubic region. Management follows basic trauma principles.
- Blunt trauma to the testicles can cause painful hematomas, testicular rupture, or testicular torsion. The scrotum may be tender and swollen. Lacerations or avulsions should be treated with gentle compression and ice packs.
- Blunt trauma to the penis can cause a large hematoma and pain. Management follows basic trauma principles.
- Vaginal trauma can cause hematomas and ecchymoses in the lower pelvic area and on the external female genitalia, bleeding from the vagina, and tenderness on palpation of the lower pelvis.
- Assessment of renal and urologic emergencies is the same as with other medical patients. It may be difficult to determine the source of pain, as it may be visceral (cramp, aching) or referred (in another area of the body). Focus on addressing life threats and providing supportive prehospital care.
- Note whether the patient seeks a particular position that reduces the pain. Determine where the pain began. Obtain a thorough history using the SAMPLE and OPQRST mnemonics. In the physical examination, use the four-quadrant system and abdominal region mapping. Perform cardiac monitoring, and do not give urologic patients anything by mouth.
- Consult with direct medical control to administer pain medication. Patients with a urinary tract infection or kidney stone should receive a bolus of IV fluid. Allow kidney stone patients to assume a position of comfort.
- For patients with acute or chronic renal failure, support the ABCs. It may be necessary to administer medications to regulate acidosis, electrolyte imbalances, and fluid volume. Provide psychological support and transport in a calm fashion.

Vital Vocabulary

acute renal failure (ARF) A sudden decrease in filtration through the glomeruli.

afferent arteriole The structure in the kidney that supplies blood to the glomerulus.

aldosterone One of the two main hormones responsible for adjustments to the final composition of urine, aldosterone increases the rate of active resorption of sodium and chloride ions into the blood and decreases resorption of potassium.

antidiuretic hormone (ADH) One of the two main hormones responsible for adjustments to the final composition of urine, ADH causes ducts in the kidney to become more permeable to water.

anuria A complete stop in the production of urine.

azotemia Increased nitrogenous wastes in the blood.

calyces (singular: calyx) Large urinary tubes that branch off the renal pelvis and connect with the renal pyramids to collect the urine draining from the collecting tubules.

chronic renal failure (CRF) Progressive and irreversible inadequate kidney function due to permanent loss of nephrons.

cortex Part of the internal anatomy of the kidney; the lighter-coloured outer region closest to the capsule.

countercurrent multiplier The process in which the body produces either concentrated or diluted urine, depending on the body's needs.

distal convoluted tubule (DCT) Connects with the kidney's collecting tubules.

diuretics Chemicals that increase urinary output.

efferent arteriole The structure in the kidney where blood drains from the glomerulus.

glomerular (Bowman's) capsule A double-layered cup with the inner layer infiltrating and surrounding the capillaries of the glomerulus.

glomerular filtration rate (GFR) The rate at which blood is filtered through the glomerula.

glomerulus A tuft of capillaries located in the kidney that serve as the main filter for the blood in the kidney.

hematuria The presence of blood in the urine.

hilum A cleft where the ureters, renal blood vessels, lymphatic vessels, and nerves enter and leave the kidney.

internal shunt Also called an arteriovenous (AV) fistula, this device is an artificial connection between a vein and an artery, usually in the forearm or upper arm.

interstitial nephritis A chronic inflammation of the interstitial cells surrounding the nephrons.

intrarenal acute renal failure (IARF) A type of acute renal failure due to damage in the kidney itself, often caused by immune-mediated diseases, prerenal ARF, toxins, heavy metals, some medications, or some organic compounds.

juxtaglomerular apparatus A structure formed at the site where the efferent arteriole and distal convoluted tubule meet.

kidneys Solid, bean-shaped organs located in the retroperitoneal space that filter blood and excrete body wastes in the form of urine.

kidney stones Solid crystalline masses formed in the kidney, resulting from an excess of insoluble salts or uric acid crystallizing in the urine; may become trapped anywhere along the urinary tract.

loop of Henle The U-shaped portion of the renal tubule that extends from the proximal to the distal convoluted tubule; concentrates the filtrate and converts it to urine.

medulla Part of the internal anatomy of the kidney; the middle layer.

micturition reflex A spinal reflex that causes contraction of the bladder's smooth muscles, producing the urge to void as pressure is exerted on the internal urinary sphincter.

nephrons The structural and functional units of the kidney that form urine; composed of the glomerulus, the glomerular (Bowman's) capsule, the proximal convoluted tubule (PCT), loop of Henle, and the distal convoluted tubule (DCT).

oliguria A decrease in urine output to the extent that total urine output drops below 500 ml/day.

peritubular capillaries A set of capillaries unique to the kidney that branch off from the efferent arteriole; the site of tubular resorption.

podocytes Special cells in the inner membrane of the glomerulus that wrap around the capillaries in the glomerulus, forming filtration slits.

postrenal ARF A type of acute renal failure caused by obstruction of urine flow from the kidneys, commonly caused by a blockage of the urethra by prostate enlargement, renal calculi, or strictures.

prerenal ARF A type of acute renal failure that is caused by hypoperfusion of the kidneys, resulting from hypovolemia (hemorrhage, dehydration), trauma, shock, sepsis, and heart failure (congestive heart failure, myocardial infarction); often reversible if the underlying condition can be found and perfusion restored to the kidney.

priapism A sustained, painful erection of the penis.

proximal convoluted tubule (PCT) One of two complex sections of the nephron, the PCT includes an enlargement at the end called the glomerular capsule.

pyelonephritis Inflammation of the kidney linings.

referred pain Pain that originates in one area of the body but is interpreted as coming from a different area of the body.

renal columns Inward extensions of cortical tissue that surround the renal pyramids.

renal dialysis A technique for "filtering" the blood of its toxic wastes, removing excess fluids, and restoring the normal balance of electrolytes.

renal fascia Dense, fibrous connective tissue that anchors the kidney to the abdominal wall.

renal pelvis Part of the internal anatomy of the kidney; a flat, funnel-shaped tube filling the sinus at the level of the hilum.

renal pyramids Parallel cone-shaped bundles of urine-collecting tubules that are located in the medulla of the kidneys.

renin A hormone produced by cells in the juxtaglomerular apparatus when the blood pressure is low.

uremia The presence of excessive amounts of urea and other waste products in the blood.

uremic frost A powdery buildup of uric acid, especially around the face.

ureters A pair of thick-walled, hollow tubes that transport urine from the kidneys to the bladder.

urethra A hollow, tubular structure that drains urine from the bladder, passing it outside of the body.

urinary bladder A hollow, muscular sac in the midline of the lower abdominal area that stores urine until it is released from the body.

urinary tract infections (UTIs) Infections, usually of the lower urinary tract (urethra and bladder), which occur when normal flora bacteria enter the urethra and grow.

urine Liquid waste products filtered out of the body by the urinary system.

vasa recta A series of peritubular capillaries that surround the loop of Henle, into which water moves after passing through the descending and ascending limbs of the loop of Henle.

visceral pain Crampy, aching pain deep within the body, the source of which is usually hard to pinpoint; common with urologic problems.

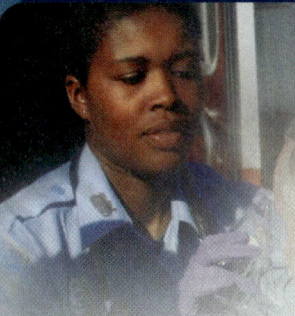

Assessment in Action

You are dispatched to the home of a 54-year-old man complaining of abdominal pain. When you arrive, you find the patient doubled over in pain and he states that this began approximately 2 hours ago. It is the worst pain he has ever had and he tells you that it "burns" when he urinates. His blood pressure is 140/90 mm Hg; pulse rate, 110 beats/min; and respiratory rate, 24 breaths/min. His rhythm on the monitor indicates sinus tachycardia. His pulse oximetry reading on room air is 100%. He has no medical problems and has no allergies.

1. **Which of the following conditions originates in the renal pelvis and is the result of an excess of insoluble salts or uric acid crystallizing in the urine?**
   A. Gallstones
   B. Urinary tract infections
   C. Kidney stones
   D. Pyleonephritis

2. **What is the most common type of stone?**
   A. Struvite
   B. Calcium
   C. Uric
   D. Cystine

3. **If a stone becomes lodged in the lower ureter, signs and symptoms of a _____ may be present.**
   A. UTI
   B. uric event
   C. URI
   D. MRSA

4. **Patients who are experiencing renal problems may exhibit many of the same symptoms as a patient with other abdominal problems. These symptoms include nausea and vomiting, constipation or diarrhea, weight loss, abdominal pain, and:**
   A. chest pain.
   B. headache.
   C. dizziness.
   D. back pain.

5. **What is the most common type of pain associated with urologic problems?**
   A. Referred pain
   B. Pain in the urethra
   C. Visceral pain
   D. Pain that can be pinpointed to a specific location

6. **Pain that may be interpreted by the brain as coming from another area of the body is called:**
   A. visceral pain.
   B. urethra pain.
   C. pleurisy.
   D. referred pain.

Challenging Questions

You are dispatched to the high school for a football player who was injured. When you arrive on scene, you find the patient complaining of right flank pain. You find out that the patient was running with the football and was tackled from the side. He was jolted and immediately felt a sharp pain in his side. He thought the pain would subside, but it hasn't. You observe his abdominal area and see a contusion in the right flank region and some bruising near his spine. You provide spinal precautions and begin transport to the hospital. His vital signs appear to be within normal limits; however, he is in a great deal of pain.

7. **What do you suspect is wrong with the patient?**

8. **How would you begin treatment of this patient?**

Points to Ponder

You and your partner are dispatched to the dialysis centre in your town for an unconscious patient. When you arrive on scene, you find a patient sitting in the chair in the dialysis centre and the staff tells you that after the patient received dialysis, he had an episode of syncope. The patient's blood pressure is 80/40 mm Hg; pulse rate, 64 beats/min; respiratory rate, 18 breaths/min; and pulse oximetry reading on room air, 97%.

Why might a patient who had received dialysis experience syncope?

Issues: Understanding the Role of the Kidneys, Treating Patients Who Received Dialysis, Understanding Renal Dialysis.

33 Toxicology: Substance Abuse and Poisoning

Competency Areas

Area 4: Assessment and Diagnostics

4.2.a   Obtain list of patient's allergies.
4.2.b   Obtain list of patient's medications.
4.2.c   Obtain chief complaint and/or incident history from patient, family members, and/or bystanders.
4.2.d   Obtain information regarding patient's past medical history.
4.2.e   Obtain information about patient's last oral intake.
4.2.f   Obtain information regarding incident through accurate and complete scene assessment.
4.3.a   Conduct primary patient assessment and interpret findings.
4.3.b   Conduct secondary patient assessment and interpret findings.
4.3.p   Conduct psychiatric assessment and interpret findings.
4.5.a   Conduct oximetry testing and interpret findings.
4.5.c   Conduct glucometric testing and interpret findings.

Area 5: Therapeutics

5.1.a   Use manual maneuvers and positioning to maintain airway patency.
5.1.b   Suction oropharynx.
5.1.c   Suction beyond oropharynx.
5.1.h   Utilize airway devices requiring visualization of vocal cords and introduced endotracheally.
5.2.a   Recognize indications for oxygen administration.
5.3.d   Administer oxygen using high concentration mask.
5.4.a   Provide oxygenation and ventilation using bag-valve-mask.
5.5.c   Maintain peripheral intravenous (IV) access devices and infusions of crystalloid solutions without additives.
5.5.d   Conduct peripheral intravenous cannulation.
5.8.a   Recognize principles of pharmacology as applied to the medications listed in Appendix 5.
5.8.b   Follow safe process for responsible medication administration.

Area 6: Integration

6.1.k   Provide care to patient experiencing illness or injury due to poisoning or overdose.
6.3.a   Conduct ongoing assessments based on patient presentation and interpret findings.

Appendix 4: Pathophysiology

B.   **Neurologic System**
      Convulsive Disorders: Generalized seizures
E.   **Gastrointestinal System**
      Liver/Gail Bladder: Cirrhosis
J.   **Multisystem Diseases and Injuries**
      Toxicologic Illness: Prescription medication
      Toxicologic Illness: Non-prescription medication
      Toxicologic Illness: Recreational
      Toxicologic Illness: Poisons (absorption, inhalation, ingestion)
      Toxicologic Illness: Acids and alkalis
      Toxicologic Illness: Hydrocarbons
      Toxicologic Illness: Asphyxiants
      Toxicologic Illness: Cyanide
      Toxicologic Illness: Organophosphates
      Toxicologic Illness: Alcohols
      Toxicologic Illness: Food poisoning
      Alcohol Related: Chronic alcoholism
      Alcohol Related: Delirium tremens
      Alcohol Related: Korsakov's psychosis
      Alcohol Related: Wernicke's encephalopathy
      Environmental Disorders: Stings and bites
K.   **Psychiatric Disorders**
      Cognitive Disorders: Delirium

Appendix 5: Medications

A.   **Medications affecting the central nervous system.**
A.1   Opioid Antagonists
A.3   Anticonvulsants
A.5   Anxiolytics, Hypnotics, and Antagonists
A.8   Opioid Analgesics
B.   **Medications affecting the autonomic nervous system.**
B.5   Antihistamines
H.   **Medications used to treat electrolyte and substrate imbalances.**
H.1   Vitamin and Electrolyte Supplements
J.   **Medications used to treat poisoning and overdose.**
J.1   Antidotes or Neutralizing Agents.

Introduction

Paramedics provide prehospital care to patients who are on medications, who take over-the-counter substances, who take supplements, or who take preparations for pleasurable purposes, whether these are licit (as in alcohol) or illicit (as in cocaine) Figure 33-1 ▾ . Other exposures can occur in the workplace and the home through ingestion, inhalation, or by contact. All of these scenarios can lead to morbidity, whether through interactions with underlying diseases or with other substances; because of the inherent toxicity of the involved substance; or because of excessive dosing, whether intentional or inadvertent. The objective of this chapter is to give the paramedic an informed approach to the patient with toxic exposure.

Types of Toxicologic Emergencies

Toxicologic emergencies usually fall under one of two general headings: intentional and unintentional. Poisoning in adults is commonly intentional. In particular, suicide is often accomplished with the use of drugs.

An unintentional toxicologic emergency can occur in many ways. For example, medication dosing errors are common problems in clinical practice.

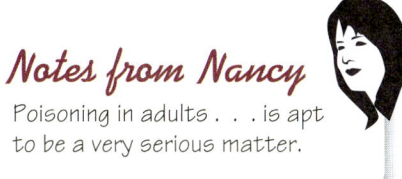

Notes from Nancy

Poisoning in adults . . . is apt to be a very serious matter.

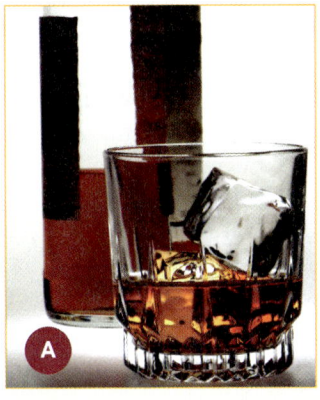 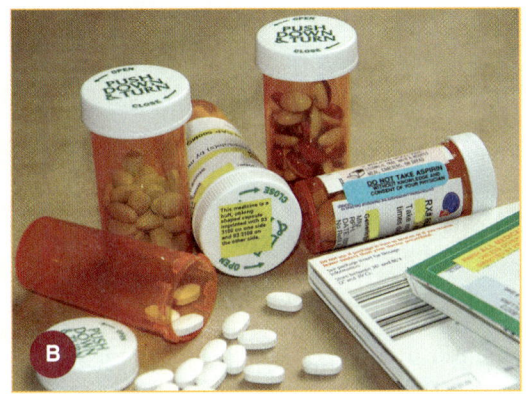 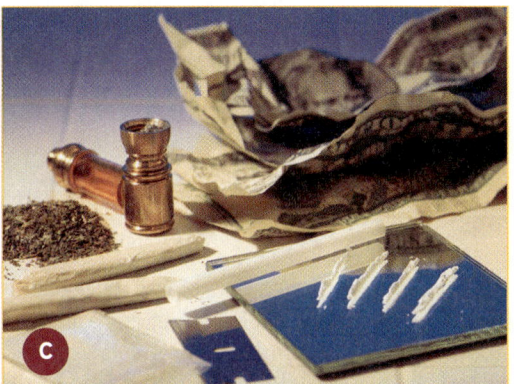

Figure 33-1 **A.** Alcohol is a legal substance that is a drug. **B.** Medications are legal substances that can be abused. **C.** Illegal drugs can also be abused.

You are the Paramedic Part 1

You and your partner respond to the local high school for an unknown medical emergency. You are met at the school entrance by the girls' physical education coach, who escorts you to the gymnasium. There, your attention is drawn to a group of young girls surrounding one of their peers, who is lying motionless on the floor.

Your partner makes room for the two of you to reach the patient. You find a 14-year-old girl lying supine on the floor and unresponsive to verbal stimuli. When you apply a sternal rub, she mumbles incoherently. A student steps forward and introduces herself as the patient's best friend. She says that Julie has been sleepy all morning, becoming drowsy during lunch and passing out while getting ready to play volleyball.

Initial Assessment	Recording Time: 0 Minutes
Appearance	Unconscious, no apparent distress
Level of consciousness	P (Responsive to painful stimuli), mumbles incoherently
Airway	Open
Breathing	Adequate rate and volume
Circulation	Radial pulse present

1. What are your priorities at this point?
2. What information do you need to obtain?

In some cases the event may be idiosyncratic: 2 mg of midazolam may simply relax one patient but cause respiratory arrest in another.

Childhood poisonings are quite common, especially in younger children who may put anything into their mouths **Figure 33-2 ▾** , such as colourful berries on a house or garden plant that draw a child's attention. A parent's prescription medication may be mistaken for candy. Indeed, many pediatric medications are formulated as candy look-alikes to improve compliance.

Even nature is fraught with toxicologic perils, as any hiker who has inadvertently wandered through a patch of poison ivy would attest. Wild mushrooms, once in the body, can produce a wide spectrum of results—from being a tasty treat, to being nauseating, to being deadly. Most therapeutic medications were originally derived from natural sources. Chemical substitution gives these substances more specific effects. For example, digoxin is derived from the foxglove plant.

The workplace also harbors its share of toxic hazards. Carbon monoxide, hydrogen sulfide, acids, and alkalis are some of the exposures to be expected in the occupational setting, all of which the paramedic must protect him- or herself against. Unfortunately, some of these hazards are not identified until after the exposure has occurred. For example, thousands of people developed asbestosis after continued exposure to asbestos in the workplace.

Unintentional toxicologic emergencies can also occur from simple neglect or oversight. Consider a geriatric person with diabetes, possibly combined with early-onset dementia or Alzheimer's disease, who takes his or her insulin in the morning and later cannot remember whether the dose was taken, so takes another dose. The result: a call to 9-1-1 for an "unconscious, unresponsive" person in need of assistance.

Biological warfare has drawn increasing attention in recent years owing to the heightened awareness of bioterrorism, but intentional poisoning or overdose may also commonly occur during more intimate crimes. In recent years, "date rape" drugs such as flunitrazepam have been used to facilitate sexual assault. Chloral hydrate ("knockout drops") has been used to commit assault for decades, and pharmacologic agents are used in homicide as well.

■ Poison Centres in Canada

Given the variety of illicit drugs coupled with the continued growth of licit drugs, even the most well-read veteran paramedic may find it difficult to keep current with the myriad drugs sold in the streets today. For this reason, Poison Centres may be an indispensable aid.

Suppose you are called to a home where a frantic mother is hovering over a toddler who sits beside the remains of a potted philodendron, most of which he apparently just ate. Is the plant poisonous? How poisonous? Should you make the child vomit? Is an antidote available? In such a scenario, you can call the Poison Centre to get information on the ingestion, its toxic potential, and steps to negate its effects, thereby providing proper prehospital care. (In fact, philodendrons are not poisonous per se, but contain tiny spicules of insoluble calcium oxalate crystals. Biting a leaf will cause immediate oral burning but no systemic toxicity. It is highly unlikely that a child will take more than a bite.)

Poison Centres are a virtual gold mine of information that you should add to your toolbox. Never hesitate to tap these resources when confronted with *any toxin* for which you have limited or no familiarity. At the same time, your call helps the centre collect data on poisonings in your region. These data may be analyzed to help detect trends, spot developing public health problems, and evaluate current treatment protocols for different poisonings. There is no universal number to contact Poison Centres in Canada. In fact, some provinces and territories do not even have such a centre. In some provinces and territories, calls from the public are hosted by 9-1-1, others by a regional hospital, in New Brunswick by Telehealth. In Manitoba, the number is only accessible to callers local to Winnipeg. In these provinces, the advice is not offered to members of the health care profession. The following is a list of numbers to provincial centres, accessible within the designated province only:

- Alberta Poison and Drug Information Services: 1-800-322-1414
- British Columbia Drug and Poison Centre: 1-800-567-8911
- Centre Anti-Poison du Quebec: 1-800-463-5060
- Manitoba: 204-787-2591 (Winnipeg only)
- Newfoundland: 709-722-1110
- Nova Scotia and Prince Edward Island: 1-800-565-8161
- Ontario Poison Centre: 1-800-268-9017
- Saskatchewan: 1-800-454-1212

Notes from Nancy

Record all your findings about a poisoned patient, even if you don't know their significance. Someone at the Poison Centre will know.

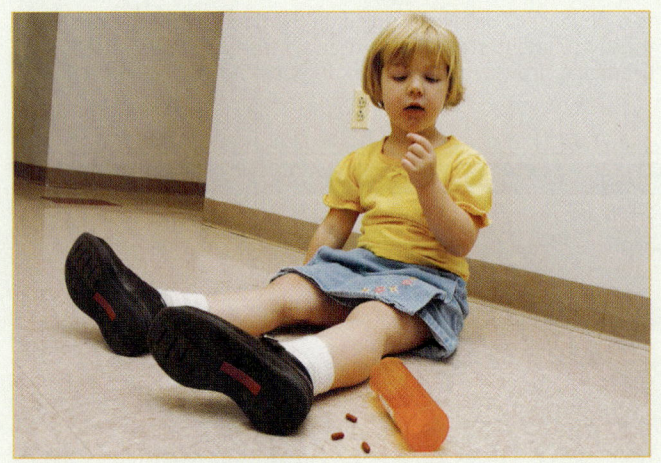

Figure 33-2 Toddlers will put anything into their mouths, including dangerous medications.

Where a provincial Poison Centre is available, specially trained registered nurses and/or pharmacists answer the phone lines 24 hours a day, 7 days a week. In Canada, the respective Colleges of Nurses and Pharmacists have standards for the practice of telephone medicine. A registered nurse or pharmacist may give telephone information to a registered health professional only. In the case of a paramedic, the nurse or pharmacist may provide advice upon which you may act directly, but he or she cannot give you information to relay to the hospital. For example, you may be told that the substance can cause loss of consciousness and seizures so that you may be prepared. The poison specialist will not tell you that the substance is also one that may be able to be dialyzed, because you will not be able to carry out that intervention yourself.

Routes of Absorption

As nasty as they are, toxins cannot exert their effects until they enter the human body. The four primary methods of entry are ingestion, inhalation, injection, and dermal absorption. Just as each of these methods of entry is unique, so is the rate at which a given toxin is absorbed into the body. Once a toxin is in the body, the combination of the amount of toxin and the relative speed at which it is metabolized affect the bioavailability of the toxin and the excretion rate.

Poisoning by Dermal Absorption

Some poisons gain access to the body by being absorbed through the skin. Of the poisonings that occur by dermal absorption, those caused by pesticides such as organophosphates and similar substances are often the most serious.

Poisoning by Ingestion

Ingested poisons may produce immediate damage to tissues, or their toxic effects may be delayed for several hours. Ingestions of a caustic substance (that is, a strong acid or alkali) can cause immediate damage. By contrast, some poisons must be absorbed into the bloodstream before they can produce their toxic effects. Medications around the home and household chemicals (such as cleaning agents) are the most common sources of poisoning by ingestion.

Poisoning by ingestion is marked by a wide range of possibilities regarding *what* is ingested and *why* it was ingested. Consider the curious child who eats a few bright red berries from the holly

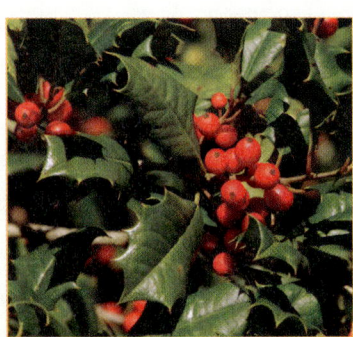

Figure 33-3 Certain berries and flowers are poisonous, such as those of the holly plant.

plant [**Figure 33-3** ◂] or the patient with pain who inadvertently increases the amount of analgesia taken from every 4 hours to every 2 hours to get relief. Both of these scenarios are considered accidental. Minor gastrointestinal discomfort may result from the former, whereas if the analgesia was acetaminophen, fulminant hepatic failure could result. Intentional poisonings occur as well. The suicidal patient may take a full prescription of a benzodiazepine with little consequence. A teen may attempt to get high one night, take a single tablet of ecstasy, and die.

Assessment clues pointing toward ingestion can be as obvious as a plant with partially chewed leaves or a section of plant with berries missing. Stained fingers, lips, or tongue are also worth noting. Any patient complaining of a sudden onset of stomach cramps with or without nausea, vomiting, or diarrhea may have an ingestion-related problem. Empty pill bottles are another obvious clue, as is the date on which the prescription was filled. The bottle for a prescription filled 6 months ago likely wasn't full today; an empty bottle for a prescription filled yesterday is far more ominous. A thorough search for substances, including medications, should be made and all should be brought with the patient to the emergency department if patient stability allows.

A toxin that enters the body by the oral route generally provides a more forgiving time frame for treatment. Little absorption occurs in the stomach; indeed, the ingested substance may stay there for a variable period, with the vast majority of absorption actually taking place in the small intestine. As a consequence, much of the management of poisoning by ingestion aims to remove or neutralize the poison before it gains access to the intestines.

Poisoning by Inhalation

A person can be poisoned by inhalation only if the poison is present in the surrounding atmosphere. That fact, obvious as it seems, has important implications. First, so long as the patient remains in the toxic environment, he or she will keep inhaling the poison—and so will you, if you enter that environment without the appropriate protective breathing apparatus. Second, when poisoning occurs because of a toxic environment, you are likely to encounter more than one patient at the emergency scene. Household chemical products (such as bleach and cleaning agents) are responsible for the most common types of inhalation emergencies.

Poisoning by inhalation may be accidental or intentional. Consider carbon monoxide (CO) poisoning. Leaving the garage door shut while seated in an automobile with the engine running provides a quick, painless method of suicide. Similarly, an automatic damper on a furnace that fails to open or a bird nest that blocks a chimney may fill a house with colourless, odourless CO, quietly and efficiently poisoning those inside.

From the anatomical and physiologic perspective, inhaled toxins quickly reach the alveoli, providing almost instant access to the circulation. CO, for example, binds to hemoglobin in the red blood cells (RBCs) about 250 times more avidly than do oxygen molecules. As a result, rapid systemic distribution can occur with an equally rapid onset of signs and symptoms. For this reason, the window of opportunity for treatment is limited.

When dealing with an inhalation emergency, the first general management consideration is that of scene safety. After donning the appropriate breathing apparatus, remove the patient(s) to a safe environment before beginning any treatment.

At the Scene

Scene safety is your primary concern when you are called to an inhalation incident. Whenever you encounter more than one patient but find no evidence of the mechanism of injury (MOI), be suspicious. Toxic fumes may be odourless and colourless, and they do not discriminate between rescuers and victims. Be suspicious of toxic fumes when encountering patients with changes in level of consciousness (LOC), especially at an industrial site or enclosed space.

Inhaled toxins produce a wide range of signs and symptoms, many of which are unique to the toxin involved. A patient with CO poisoning does not exhibit the same signs and symptoms as a person who has sniffed glue, who in turn looks nothing like a patient poisoned by a furniture stripper containing methylene chloride. Frequently, the emergency scene itself contains the clues to the identification of the toxin that is making the patient ill. That information, coupled with the assistance of the Poison Centre and direction from the direct medical control physician, will drive your treatment plan. Correction of hypoxia is a must, so administer a high concentration of supplemental oxygen. Establish vascular access, apply an electrocardiographic (ECG) monitor, and perform pulse oximetry and capnography.

Poisoning by Injection

Injected poisons usually gain access to the body as the result of stings or bites from a variety of unpleasant creatures. Abuse of intravenously administered drugs such as heroin, cocaine, amphetamines, and "speedballs" (heroin and cocaine together) is also common in the prehospital setting.

In Canada, the risk of poisoning by injection from natural products is limited. Three venomous species of snakes exist. In British Columbia, one might encounter the Northern Pacific rattlesnake; in Alberta, the prairie rattlesnake; and in selected areas of Ontario, the Massasauga rattlesnake. Paramedics should remember that an underground zoo of venomous snakes and lizards also exist where pet owners have exotic animals not native to Canada. Wasps, yellow jackets, hornets, and bees have a ubiquitous distribution throughout Canada. Stings from these insects can occur anywhere.

In Canada, the manifestations of a bite from most of these injected natural venoms can be local, allergic, or occult systemic. When a bite or sting hits a vein or artery and results in a toxin immediately entering the bloodstream, the outcome is much more dangerous than when the same toxin enters a muscle mass, such as the calf, from which absorption and distribution is much slower.

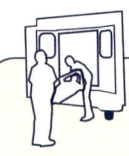

At the Scene

Treat all tools used to inject substances as biohazards. These needles or devices may have been shared with other drug users and may carry the human immunodeficiency virus or other pathogens.

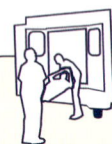

At the Scene

Always treat the patient and not the diagnostic tool. Pulse oximeters may give false readings when patients have been exposed to CO.

You are the Paramedic Part 2

You conduct your initial assessment of the patient. A rapid trauma assessment reveals no life-threatening conditions. As you prepare to perform a detailed physical examination, you ask the coach to find out if the patient has any relevant medical history and to get a contact number for her mother. You also ask the patient's friend if she knows of any information that might be helpful. She says that Julie has been depressed lately over problems with her boyfriend and thinks that she might be taking some medication to help her cope. The friend seems to remember something and suddenly runs off.

Vital Signs	Recording Time: 5 Minutes
Skin	Flushed, warm, and dry
Pulse	140 beats/min, regular, and weak
Blood pressure	88/58 mm Hg
Respirations	10 breaths/min
Spo$_2$	93% on nonrebreathing mask at 12 l/min of supplemental oxygen

3. What are some potential differential diagnoses?

4. Which interventions should you consider at this point, if any?

When assessing bites and stings, physical findings will usually provide the most clues, especially local reactions such as pain at the wound site. Depending on the specific toxin, signs and symptoms can vary greatly. Frequently, the patient may be able to identify the source, greatly simplifying the assessment process.

At the Scene

Absorption of toxic substances through the skin is a common problem in agriculture and manufacturing. Most solvents and "cides"—insecticides, herbicides, and pesticides—are toxic and can be readily absorbed through the skin.

Understanding and Using Toxidromes

Although the sheer number of substances of abuse may seem daunting, the good news is that many drugs, on entering the body, result in similar signs and symptoms. Consider narcotics. Irrespective of whether it is a natural product derived from opium (that is, an opiate) or a synthetic, non–opium-derived narcotic (that is, an opioid), all drugs in this group work in a similar manner, so they produce similar signs and symptoms. The syndrome-like symptoms of a poisonous agent are termed a toxic syndrome or toxidrome. Toxidromes are useful for remembering the assessment and management of different substances that fall under the same clinical umbrella. The major toxidromes are produced by narcotics, cholinergics, anticholinergics, sympathomimetics (stimulants), and sedative and hypnotics Table 33-1 ▾ .

Table 33-2 ▶ lists common signs and symptoms of poisoning. If you look at your history and physical examination findings in conjunction with the vital signs, more often than not you can develop an initial diagnosis that will allow you to provide appropriate prehospital care until you can deliver the patient to the receiving facility.

Overview of Substance Abuse

Human beings have a long history of abusing drugs and alcohol. With the passing of time, the physiologic and societal effects of alcohol abuse have become well known and thoroughly documented. Unfortunately, the area of medicine dealing with drugs of abuse is highly challenging because of uncertainty about the prevalence of the problem and the continual evolution of the substances themselves. In the 1980s, creative chemists took existing pharmacologic agents and structurally manipulated them to create new or different drugs ("designer drugs") that were often far more potent than the original drugs.

Substance abuse can be broadly defined as the self-administration of licit or illicit substances in a manner not in accord with approved medical or social practice. Part of that definition is cultural—and there is great variation in what is considered substance abuse. In our society, for example, it is acceptable to administer narcotics under medical supervision for the relief of pain; conversely, self-administration of the same drugs for the purpose of inducing euphoria is regarded as drug abuse.

Any given society's definition of abuse may have little relation to the potential harm from the abused substance. For example, our culture places no restrictions on the long-term and compulsive use of tobacco, even though it is a major contributor to cardiovascular and respiratory disease Figure 33-4 ▶ .

Table 33-1	Major Toxidromes	
Toxidrome	**Drug Examples**	**Signs and Symptoms**
Stimulant	Amphetamine, methamphetamine, cocaine, diet aids, nasal decongestants	Restlessness, agitation, incessant talking; insomnia, anorexia; dilated pupils, tachycardia; tachypnea, hypertension or hypotension; paranoia, seizures, cardiac arrest
Narcotic (opiate and opioid)	Heroin, opium, morphine, hydromorphone (Dilaudid), fentanyl, oxycodone-aspirin combination (Percodan)	Constricted (pinpoint) pupils, marked respiratory depression; needle tracks (IV abusers); drowsiness, stupor, coma
Sympathomimetic	Pseudoephedrine, phenylephrine, phenylpropanolamine, amphetamine, and methamphetamine	Hypertension, tachycardia, dilated pupils (mydriasis), agitation and seizures, hyperthermia
Sedative and hypnotic	Phenobarbital, diazepam (Valium), thiopental	Drowsiness, disinhibition, ataxia, slurred speech, mental confusion, respiratory depression, progressive central nervous system depression, hypotension
Cholinergic	Diazinon, orthene, parathion, sarin, tabun, VX	Increased salivation, lacrimation, gastrointestinal distress, diarrhea, respiratory depression, apnea, seizures, coma
Anticholinergic	Atropine, scopolamine, antihistamines, antipsychotics	Dry, flushed skin, hyperthermia, dilated pupils, blurred vision, tachycardia; mild hallucinations, dramatic delirium

Table 33-2	Common Signs and Symptoms of Poisoning	

Sign or Symptom	Type	Possible Causative Agents
Odour	Bitter almonds	Cyanide
	Garlic	Arsenic, organophosphates, phosphorous
	Acetone	Methyl alcohol, isopropyl alcohol, aspirin, acetone
	Wintergreen	Methyl salicylate
	Pears	Chloral hydrate
	Violets	Turpentine
	Camphor	Camphor
	Alcohol	Alcohol
Pupils	Constricted	Narcotics, organophosphates, Jimson weed, nutmeg, propoxyphene (Darvon)
	Dilated	Barbiturates, atropine, amphetamine, glutethimide (Doriden), lysergic acid diethylamide (LSD), cyanide, CO
Mouth	Salivation	Organophosphates, arsenic, strychnine, mercury, salicylates
	Dry mouth	Atropine (belladonna), amphetamines, diphenhydramine (Benadryl), narcotics
	Burns in mouth	Formaldehyde, iodine, lye, toxic plants, phenols, phosphorous, pine oil, silver nitrate, acids
Skin	Pruritis	Jimson weed, belladonna, boric acid
	Dry, hot skin	Atropine (in belladonna), botulism, nutmeg
	Sweating	Organophosphates, arsenic, aspirin, amphetamines, barbiturates, mushrooms, naphthalene
Respiratory	Depressed respirations	Narcotics, alcohol, propoxyphene, CO, barbiturates
	Increased respirations	Aspirin, amphetamines, boric acid, cyanide, kerosene, methyl alcohol, nicotine
	Pulmonary edema	Organophosphates, petroleum products, narcotics, CO
Cardiovascular	Tachycardia	Alcohol, amphetamines, arsenic, atropine, aspirin, cocaine, some antiasthma drugs
	Bradycardia	Digitalis, gasoline, nicotine, mushrooms, narcotics, cyanide, mistletoe, rhododendron
	Hypertension	Amphetamines, lead, nicotine, antiasthma drugs
	Hypotension	Barbiturates, narcotics, tranquilizers, house plants, mistletoe, nitroglycerin, antifreeze
Central nervous system	Seizures	Amphetamines, camphor, cocaine, strychnine, arsenic, CO, petroleum products, scorpion sting
	Coma	All depressant drugs (such as narcotics, barbiturates, tranquilizers, alcohol), CO, cyanide
	Hallucinations	Atropine, LSD, mushrooms, organic solvents, phencyclidine (PCP), nutmeg
	Headache	CO, alcohol, disulfiram (Antabuse)
	Tremors	Organophosphates, CO, amphetamine, tranquilizers, poisonous marine animals
	Weakness or paralysis	Organophosphates, botulism, eel, hemlock, puffer fish, pine oil, rhododendron
Gastrointestinal	Cramps, nausea, vomiting, and/or diarrhea	Many, if not most, ingested poisons

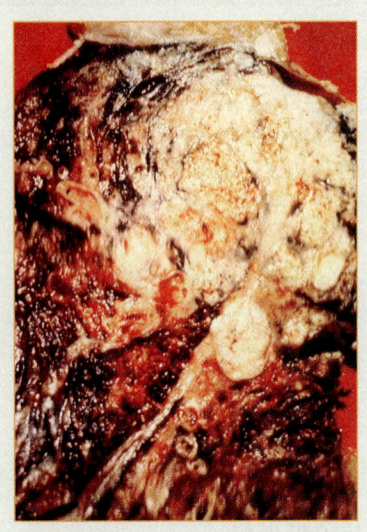

Figure 33-4 A diseased lung as a result of tobacco use.

Let's formally define some basic terms and concepts related to substance abuse:

- **Drug abuse.** Any use of drugs that causes physical, psychological, economic, legal, or social harm to the user or to others affected by the drug user's behaviour.
- **Habituation.** Psychological dependence on a drug or drugs.
- **Physical dependence.** A physiologic state of adaptation to a drug, usually characterized by tolerance to the drug's effects and by a withdrawal syndrome if the drug is stopped, especially if it is stopped abruptly.
- **Psychological dependence.** The emotional state of craving a drug to maintain a feeling of well-being.
- **Tolerance.** Physiologic adaptation to the effects of a drug such that increasingly larger doses of the drug are required to achieve the same effect.
- **Withdrawal syndrome.** A predictable set of signs and symptoms, usually involving altered central nervous system (CNS) activity, which occurs after the abrupt cessation of a drug or after rapidly decreasing the usual dosage of a drug.
- **Drug addiction.** A chronic disorder characterized by the compulsive use of a substance resulting in physical, psychological, or social harm to the user, who continues to use the substance despite the harm.
- **Antagonist.** Something that counteracts the action of a substance.

- **Potentiation.** Enhancement of the effect of one drug by another drug.
- **Synergism.** The action of two substances, such as drugs, in which the total effects are greater than the sum of the independent effects of the two substances (that is, 2 + 2 = 5).

Drug abuse is not limited to members of the younger generation or to any particular stratum of society. It occurs in all age groups and at all social levels.

Alcoholism

Alcohol is the most widely abused drug in Canada. In one survey, 79.3% of the Canadian population indicated that they used alcohol in the past year. In the same survey, 8.8% of Canadians, on average, indicated that they were alcoholic, using the definition that they had come to harm because of their alcohol drinking pattern in the last year. Furthermore, because of its harmful effects on organs, including the liver, stomach, heart, pancreas, brain, and CNS, alcoholism decreases a person's life span by 10 to 20 years. In addition, people with alcoholism tend to have chronic malnutrition and fall frequently, increasing the likelihood of head injury or other trauma.

Alcoholism usually consists of two distinct phases. The first phase is problem drinking, during which alcohol is used increasingly more often to relieve tensions or other emotional difficulties. Because of the disinhibition, relaxation, and sense of well-being mediated by alcohol, some degree of psychological dependence often develops with its use. Unfortunately, many people become so dependent on the psychological influences of alcohol that they become compulsive consumers. As a person becomes more dependent on drinking, his or her performance at work and relationships with friends, family, and colleagues may deteriorate. Increased absence from work, emotional disturbances, and automobile crashes become more frequent.

Physical dependence also results from the regular consumption of large quantities of alcohol. This becomes apparent when a person abruptly stops consuming alcohol and withdrawal symptoms result. The severity of the withdrawal can vary according to the length and intensity of the alcoholic habit.

Notes from Nancy

The patient found stuporous with alcohol on his or her breath must not be assumed to be intoxicated.

Minor withdrawal is characterized by restlessness, anxiousness, sleeping problems, agitation, and tremors.

In the second phase of alcoholism, true addiction, abstinence causes major withdrawal symptoms—for example, increased blood pressure, vomiting, and hallucinations. Delirium tremens, or alcohol withdrawal delirium, results in fever, disorientation, confusion, seizures, and possibly death.

Alcoholism occurs in all social strata. Red flags pointing to alcohol abuse include the following:

- Drinking early in the day
- Drinking alone or in "secret"
- Periodic binges
- Loss of memory or "blackouts"
- Tremulousness and anxiety
- Chronically flushed face and palms

Medical Consequences of Alcohol Abuse

Because of the toxic effects of alcohol, a person with alcoholism is considerably more prone to a number of serious illnesses and injuries Table 33-3 ▾ . Chronic damage to the CNS, for

Table 33-3	Medical Problems to Which People With Alcoholism Are Particularly Susceptible
Condition	**Contributing Factors**
Subdural hematoma	Frequent falls; impaired clotting mechanisms
GI bleeding	Irritant effect of alcohol on the stomach lining (leading to gastritis); impaired clotting mechanisms; cirrhosis of the liver, leading to engorgement of esophageal veins (esophageal varices)
Pancreatitis	Indirect effect on alcohol of the pancreas
Hypoglycemia	Damage to the liver, which normally mobilizes sugar into the blood
Pneumonia	Aspiration of vomitus occurring during intoxication and coma; suppression of immune system by alcohol
Burns	Relative insensitivity to pain occurring during intoxication; falling asleep with a lit cigarette while intoxicated
Hypothermia	Insensitivity to extremes of temperatures while intoxicated; falling asleep outside in the cold
Seizures	Effect of withdrawal from alcohol
Arrhythmias	Toxic effects of alcohol on the heart
Cancer	Mechanism not known (perhaps related to suppression of the immune system), but people with alcoholism are 10 times more likely than the general population to have cancer
Esophageal varices (abnormally enlarged veins in the lower part of the esophagus)	Develop when normal blood flow to the liver is blocked and blood backs up into smaller, more fragile blood vessels in the esophagus; do not produce symptoms unless they rupture and bleed (a life-threatening condition that requires immediate medical care; can be fatal when not controlled)

example, leads to deterioration in higher mental functions, such as memory and logical thinking. Damage to the cerebellum affects balance, which in turn contributes to frequent falls. Damage to the peripheral nerves leads to decreased sensation in the extremities, making one prone to burns and similar injuries that an intact pain sense would ordinarily prevent.

As alcohol travels through the digestive system, it irritates tissue and can damage the lining of the stomach by causing acid imbalances, inflammation, and acute gastric distress. Often, the result is gastritis (an inflamed stomach) and heartburn. The more frequently consumption takes place, the greater the irritation. One in three heavy drinkers has chronic gastritis. Heavy drinkers also have double the risk of cancer of the mouth and esophagus. Prolonged heavy use of alcohol may cause ulcers, hiatal hernias, and cancers throughout the digestive tract.

The toxic effects of alcohol on the liver produce a variety of complications, such as coagulopathies (easy bleeding and poor clotting ability), hypoglycemia, and cirrhosis. In addition, people with alcoholism are at high risk of acute pancreatitis, pneumonia, and cardiomyopathy.

Alcohol-Related Emergencies

Any of the conditions previously mentioned may contribute to an emergency. In addition, acute consumption of and acute abstinence from alcohol may produce serious problems, including withdrawal seizures.

Acute Alcohol Intoxication

Severe alcohol intoxication is a form of poisoning and carries the same lethal potential as poisoning with any other CNS depressant. Death from alcohol intoxication has been reported with blood alcohol levels of 87 mmol/l, which can be attained by the relatively rapid consumption of as little as a half-pint of whiskey. The most immediate danger to an acutely intoxicated person is death because of respiratory depression and/or aspiration of vomitus or stomach contents secondary to a suppressed gag reflex. Remember that the legal blood alcohol level is 17.2 mmol/l in most provinces and territories in Canada.

If an intoxicated patient is unconscious, treat him or her as you would any unconscious patient. As always, first establish and maintain the airway. With an intact gag reflex, place the patient in left lateral recumbent position with suction ready. If there is no gag reflex, intubate the patient. In addition, give high-concentration supplemental oxygen, and assist ventilation as needed. Establish vascular access. Monitor the ECG rhythm. Assess the patient's blood glucose level, treating hypoglycemia if it is found. Thiamine 100 mg via slow intravenous (IV) push may be administered upon arrival to the ED. Finally, transport the patient to an appropriate facility.

Notes from Nancy

The patient with alcohol on his or her breath may be ill or injured from other causes. Don't let the smell of alcohol impair your judgment as well as the patient's.

Alcohol Withdrawal Seizures

A person who has been drinking heavily for an extended period and suddenly stops drinking may have a variety of withdrawal phenomena. Seizures usually occur within about 12 to 48 hours of the last drink. Use the same prehospital care plan described for alcohol intoxication, and consult with direct medical control about giving benzodiazepines for seizure control. Simple withdrawal seizures usually are short-lived and self-resolving. With delirium tremens, however, the seizures may mimic that of status epilepticus and require massive amounts of benzodiazepines for improvement.

Delirium Tremens

One of the most serious and lethal complications of alcohol withdrawal is delirium tremens (DTs). Symptoms usually start 48 to 72 hours after the last alcohol intake, although a week to 10 days may pass before the onset of symptoms in some cases. Delirium tremens is a serious and potentially fatal syndrome with mortality reported as high as 15%. Signs and symptoms are typically related to excess catecholamine release and can include confusion, tremors and restlessness, tachycardia, fever and diaphoresis, hallucinations (extremely frightening—such as snakes, spiders, and rats), and hypotension, often secondary to dehydration. Hypertension is often seen initially, but hypotension may later ensue because patients are typically dehydrated.

The treatment for a patient in DTs is aimed at protecting him or her from injury and providing supportive prehospital care. The often-terrifying hallucinations associated with DTs typically make for an agitated, often combative patient. Try to keep the patient calm. In addition, you should administer supplemental oxygen by nasal cannula and establish vascular access. Benzodiazipines are the treatment of choice for signs and symptoms associated with the excess catecholamines. If the patient is hypotensive due to dehydration or benzodiazepine use, or if dehydration is noted clinically, then the treatment of choice is infusion of normal saline. The paramedic should ensure that the patient is assessed frequently and maintain an ongoing dialogue with the patient throughout transport to help orient and reassure the patient.

General Principles of Assessment and Management for Toxicologic Emergencies

Generally, patients with toxicologic emergencies are considered medical patients, although toxicologic emergencies may also lead to trauma. The general assessment approach is the same for all patients: scene assessment, initial assessment, and then focused history and physical examination. If the mental status is altered, monitor the patient's airway and breathing diligently to ensure that he or she does not aspirate and is adequately filling the chest with air. If the patient is responsive, use the OPQRST mnemonic to elaborate on the chief complaint, take the patient's vital signs, take a SAMPLE history, and perform a focused physical examination. If the patient is not responsive, obtain vital signs and complete a rapid medical assessment; obtain the OPQRST and SAMPLE history from bystanders and family members, if possible.

To choose the appropriate course of action in a toxicologic emergency, obtain at least the following specific information:

- *What is the agent?* If the patient has overdosed on a prescription drug, bring the pill bottle and the remaining pills with the patient **Figure 33-5 ▾** . If the substance was a commercial product, take the closed container and its remaining contents to the emergency department (ED). (Remember that the container should be capped or kept in another closed container). If the patient ingested a plant, find out what part (roots, leaves, stem, flower, or fruit) and take a sample of the plant to the ED for identification. If the patient vomits, save a sample of the vomitus in a clean, closed container, and take it with you to the emergency department **Figure 33-6 ▸** . Vomitus can rarely be analyzed except in the incidence of mushroom ingestions. Do not delay transport of an ill patient to obtain this sample.
- *When was the poison ingested, injected, dermally absorbed, or inhaled?* The decision to decontaminate the gastrointestinal

📻 Documentation and Communication

While at the scene, make thorough (and legible) notes about the nature of the poisoning. You can then quickly state the type and amount of substance and the time and route of exposure in your radio, verbal, and written reports. Clear notes that can be handed over on arrival will be appreciated by busy hospital staff.

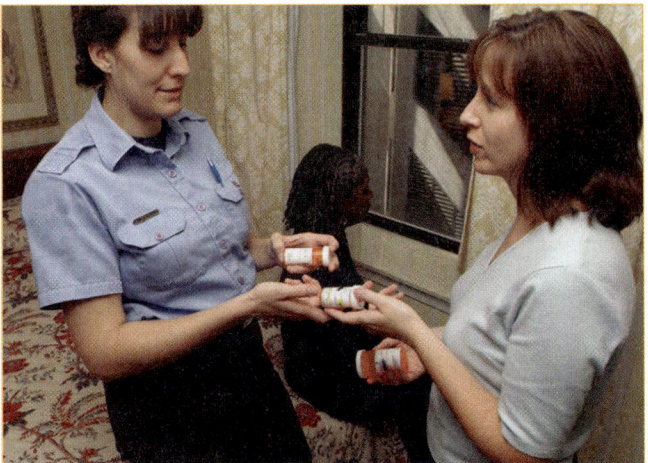

Figure 33-5 Take any bottles, containers, and their remaining contents to the ED.

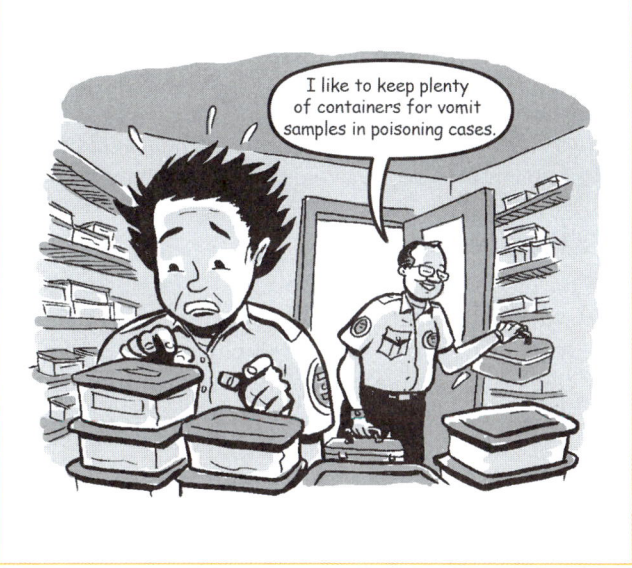

Figure 33-6

tract is strongly influenced by the amount of time that has elapsed since the exposure. The likelihood of binding significant quantities of the poison in the stomach decreases rapidly after the first 30 to 60 minutes in most circumstances.

- *How much was taken, injected, dermally absorbed, or inhaled?* Street drugs are commonly sold in single-dose "hits" or "tabs" (tablets). If the patient says he has taken "three hits of acid," you know he has taken three times the "normal dose" of LSD. If the patient says that she took 4 tabs of ecstasy, that's four times a single dose. There is almost always a distinct correlation between dose and toxic effects.
- *What else was taken?* A majority of intentional self-poisonings (suicide attempts) or illicit drug overdoses involve polydrug ingestions, often with alcohol as one of the drugs. The patient may also have tried to take something as an antidote (that is, something to counteract the effect of the poison). This information can be invaluable to ED staff when deciding which tests to order.
- *Has the patient vomited or aspirated?* If so, how soon after the ingestion or exposure did the vomiting occur? How much? Was there evidence of toxin, tablets, or pills in the vomitus?
- *Why was the substance taken?* Although you may not get a reliable answer from someone abusing illicit drugs, this is still a question worth asking. Don't assume that every patient is trying to get high. Drug use could be a coping mechanism for a person who is being abused, or it could be a suicide attempt. Put the reason in "quotation marks" on your patient care report.

Scene Assessment

Patients who have taken an overdose may be extremely dangerous, so make sure you do a scene assessment in every case. If necessary, call for law enforcement backup or a crisis unit to minimize potential for injury to paramedics. Pay particular attention to the safety of the prehospital environment if you suspect an accidental inhaled or a dermal route of absorption. In some cases, PPE will be required or the patient will require decontamination prior to contact (eg, gross contamination of the patient with organophosphate-based insecticide). Cooperation with HazMat teams may be required to safety extricate and decontaminate patients prior to detailed assessment.

Initial Assessment

The initial assessment of a drug-overdosed or poisoned patient begins with your general impression. It can be as simple as "a young adult man snoring in a public bathroom stall." The initial assessment seeks to rapidly identify concerns with mental status, airway, breathing, and circulation. Threats to life need to be quickly managed by measures such as a head tilt–chin lift, suctioning, or ventilation assistance with a bag-valve-mask device. The initial assessment may identify the MOI or nature of illness and the need for additional units and set the priority and "tone" of the call.

Focused History and Physical Examination

After completing the initial assessment, begin the focused history and physical examination. With a trauma case, you will need to classify the patient as having a significant or nonsignificant MOI. With a significant MOI, you must quickly perform a rapid trauma assessment of the major body regions—head, neck, chest, abdomen, pelvis, back, buttocks, and four extremities. Obtain a set of baseline vital signs and a SAMPLE history. This patient should also receive a detailed physical examination en route to the hospital. If the patient does not have a significant MOI, perform a focused exam of the injured body part—that is, evaluate distal pulse, motor, and sensory functions, and range of motion.

Special Considerations

In an accidental overdose or poisoning, a geriatric patient may have become confused about his or her drug regimen. The person may have forgotten that the medication had been taken and repeat the dose one or more times. The patient could also have forgotten the doctor's instructions to discard leftover medication and might have taken the current and the older drug, resulting in increased effects or unwanted drug interactions. A geriatric patient may also intentionally overdose in a suicide attempt.

Most poisoning and overdose cases involve patients with medical conditions, so you will need to elaborate on their chief complaint using the OPQRST questions. If the patient is not responsive, perform a rapid medical assessment (basically the same as the rapid trauma assessment), obtain baseline vital signs, and ask the SAMPLE history questions of the family or bystanders, if possible. If the patient is responsive, complete the SAMPLE history, obtain the baseline vital signs, and conduct a focused examination targeting the body system most relevant to the complaint (for example, cardiovascular, pulmonary, neurologic, trauma).

Controversies

If a pediatric patient is in stable condition and has a history of a single small ingestion of a low-risk agent, some EMS systems allow the transport to be cancelled after agreement from direct medical control. Although this approach may be medically sound, it eliminates an opportunity for assessment of psychosocial and risk factors in the ED.

Detailed Physical Examination

The detailed physical examination should be conducted en route to the ED, unless you are delayed on the scene and have the time to complete it there. Such an examination is usually conducted on a patient who has trauma with a significant MOI—as may occur in an overdosed or a poisoned patient who fell, was assaulted, or decided he or she could "fly." The detailed physical examination is similar to the rapid trauma assessment except that it is slower, is more involved, and looks more closely at the head. After completing the detailed physical examination, prioritize the injuries, manage them appropriately, and document your findings on the patient care report.

Ongoing Assessment

The ongoing assessment includes reassessment, reprioritizing, and checking the effectiveness of interventions provided. It is done en route to the ED. Continually monitor all patients who have ingested, injected, absorbed, or inhaled a poisonous substance, and be aware that they may vomit at any point. A stable patient may become unstable en route as more toxin is absorbed over time.

Documentation and Communication

Have someone count the medications left in the prescription bottle to figure out the maximum number the patient might have taken.

Assessment and Management of Overdose With Specific Substances

From a management perspective, ALS care builds on the basics:

- Ensure the scene is safe for access and egress.
- Maintain the airway.
- Ensure that breathing is adequate.
- Ensure that circulation isn't compromised (that is, by hypoperfusion or arrhythmia).
- Administer high-concentration supplemental oxygen.
- Establish vascular access.
- Be prepared to manage shock, coma, seizures, and arrhythmias.

- Transport the patient as soon as possible. Place the patient in the left lateral recumbent position if there is any risk of vomiting to reduce the risk of aspiration.

Drugs of Abuse

Stimulants

Few drugs compare with stimulants in potential for abuse—particularly cocaine and amphetamines. A first-time user may become an addict to one of these substances within just a few days. Very few of those who are addicted to stimulants successfully complete treatment and stay sober for the remainder of their life.

Depending on the formulation, stimulant drugs may be taken orally, smoked, or injected intravenously. The clinical presentation of the stimulant abuser includes excitement, delirium, tachycardia, hypertension or hypotension, and dilated pupils. As toxic levels are reached, the patient may develop outright psychosis, hyperpyrexia, tremors, seizures, and cardiac arrest.

The chronic user may appear wild-eyed and cachectic with nervous or jittery movements. Week-long stretches without sleeping are not unusual, with little attention paid to normal nutrition or self-care. As the days pass, increasing paranoia makes encounters risky. Patients can be very agitated; it often takes very little to provoke someone.

Cocaine

Cocaine is a naturally occurring alkaloid that is extracted from the *Erythroxylon coca* plant leaves found in South America. In the sixth century, the chewing of coca leaves was a daily event for people living in the coca-growing region of South America. With a relative purity of only about 2%, the leaves served as a mild stimulant, with no real potential for overdose. Chewing coca leaves also produced anorexia, euphoria, and improved energy. Once processed into cocaine hydrochloride, however, the active ingredient in the leaves goes from 2% to 100% pure, drastically increasing its toxic potential.

During the 1800s, cocaine and opium were commonly found in the elixirs, potions, and syrups sold by travelling medicine shows. Although neither substance cures anything, the people who used these products did not complain, given the drugs' euphoria-producing capabilities.

In more recent times, use of cocaine has had devastating effects on the Canadian population. The Canadian Addiction Survey (2004) found that the lifetime rate use of cocaine and/or crack has increased from 3.8% of the population in 1994 to 10.6% in 2004. Lifetime rate use is defined as having ever used or tried cocaine. In 2005, a total of 2,556 kg of cocaine were seized at border crossings in Canada, the bulk entering via passenger and commercial aircraft. This represents only a minute portion of drug that is delivered undetected. Over 15,500 convictions related to possession, trafficking, and smuggling of cocaine/crack were made in 2005 in Canada. No data are available that quantifies direct costs due to cocaine use and abuse alone. However, approximately 950 deaths occurred

in Canada in 2002 from overdose of illegal drugs of abuse and 300 from drug-facilitated suicides.

Cocaine is a local anesthetic and a CNS stimulant. It also has the ability to create a euphoria that features enhanced alertness and a tremendous sense of well-being. Collectively, this constellation of effects makes cocaine a very psychologically addictive drug.

Today, cocaine has limited use in clinical medicine, mostly in ear, nose, throat, and eye surgery. This water-soluble hydrochloride salt is quickly absorbed across all mucosal membranes, allowing it to be applied topically, swallowed, or injected intravenously. Cocaine powder (hydrochloride) is usually insufflated (snorted) or injected. Crack cocaine is simply cocaine mixed with two inexpensive ingredients: baking soda and water. After being mixed together into a paste-like slurry and cooked or baked, the end result is smokeable cocaine (crack).

When cocaine is snorted nasally, effects are felt within 1 to 2 minutes, and peak effects occur in 20 to 30 minutes. After the intense, initial high, only 15 to 30 minutes passes before the user wants to redose. When cocaine is smoked and the alveoli are literally bathed in cocaine-laden smoke, the onset of effects is much more rapid (in the 8- to 10-second range) and the high is even more intense than when cocaine is snorted.

When the effects of cocaine wear off, a predictable cycle of events occurs. The user experiences a "crash," which is characterized by depression, irritability, sleeplessness, and exhaustion. To avoid this crash, the user will often seek more cocaine.

Adding to the problem, a cocaine addict who is trying to escape the unpleasant effects of a crash often takes a sedative (such as diazepam, alcohol, or heroin). Thus, a chronic cocaine user might practice polypharmacy and may be dependent on more than cocaine, increasing the likelihood that he or she will need EMS prehospital care, possibly overdosed on uppers, downers, or both.

A person who has overdosed on cocaine may exhibit any of the signs and symptoms for stimulants in general (discussed earlier). Furthermore, cocaine has been reported to cause a variety of serious—sometimes fatal—complications: lethal ECG arrhythmias, acute myocardial infarction, seizures, stroke, apnea, and hyperthermia. In addition, a crack smoker risks pneumothorax and pneumomediastinum.

Give particular attention to the ECG rhythm in the case of a suspected cocaine overdose. Cocaine has membrane-stabilizing effects on cardiac conduction, causing widening of the QRS. With increased dosing levels, cocaine exerts potentially deadly effects on the myocardium, which may present as wide-complex arrhythmias, negative inotropic effects with decreased cardiac output, hypotension, or tachycardia initially, followed by bradycardia. For these reasons, use of beta or calcium channel blockers is contraindicated in managing tachyarrhythmias due to cocaine intoxication.

A speedball is a combination of heroin and cocaine. Heroin addicts may use cocaine to withdraw or detoxify themselves from heroin by gradually decreasing the amounts of heroin taken while increasing the amounts of cocaine used. Addicts claim that cocaine provides relief from the unpleasant withdrawal effects that accompany heroin abstinence in a dependent user.

Amphetamine, Methamphetamine, and Amphetamine-like Drugs

Amphetamines are structurally similar to the derivatives of phenylethylamine and include methamphetamine (crank or ice), methylenedioxyamphetamine (MDA, Adam), and methylenedioxymethamphetamine (MDMA, ecstasy). Amphetamine and amphetamine-like drugs have a number of legitimate clinical applications. Most nasal decongestants and diet pills are members of this family, as are the drugs used to treat narcolepsy, attention-deficit disorder, and attention-deficit/hyperactivity disorder **Figure 33-7 ▾**.

Methamphetamine is problematic because it is a low-cost, long-acting (up to 12 hours) stimulant that is extremely addictive. Although methamphetamine use is increasing across the country, with use the greatest in the west and the least in the east, the methamphetamine epidemic has not influenced Canada to the same degree as in the United States. It is true that "cooking" methamphetamine is easily done from common ingredients. For this reason, many decongestant cold medications have been placed "behind the counter" in attempts to limit its manufacture. "Meth labs" are dangerous and should be treated as hazardous materials incidents (see Chapter 50).

The clinical presentation of the patient abusing amphetamine or methamphetamine is almost identical to that of a person abusing cocaine, with the primary exception that the effects of the former drugs last many hours longer than those of cocaine. Patient management remains the same as well. In the majority of cases, prehospital management is primarily supportive. Never forget about the potential emotional and psychological instability, particularly in patients who have been on a "binge." With each passing day of no sleep and little or no food, the users become increasingly paranoid and even psychotic. Be prepared to contact law enforcement for support. (Chapter 37 deals with the issue of restraint in detail.)

Management of Stimulant Abuse

The treatment for patients abusing cocaine, amphetamine, or methamphetamine is fundamentally the same: maintain maximum oxygen saturation levels, prevent seizures with adequate sedation, and monitor serial vital signs.

- Establish and maintain the airway. Consider an advanced airway as needed.
- Give high-concentration supplemental oxygen.
- Establish vascular access.
- Apply the ECG monitor, pulse oximeter, and capnometer.
- Manage hypotension with a fluid infusion of normal saline.
- Benzodiazepines are first-line treatments for hypertension, tachycardia, anxiety, and seizures.
- Transport to the appropriate facility.
- The administration of beta-adrenergic antagonist agents is *absolutely contraindicated* for patients abusing stimulants.

In severe cases of stimulant overdose, the patient may present with hyperthermia, which can be lethal. Application of ice packs or misting the patient's skin may reduce his or her temperature.

Marijuana and Cannabinoids

When the leaves and flower buds of the *Cannabis sativa* plant are harvested and dried, the end product is referred to as marijuana (also known as weed, pot, dope, and smoke **Figure 33-8 ▾**). The resin produced by the maturing flower tops can also be harvested and used to produce hashish (also known as hash). Clinical uses of marijuana are limited but include the treatment of glaucoma and relief of nausea and appetite loss for patients undergoing chemotherapy.

The primary psychoactive ingredient in marijuana and hashish is delta 9-tetrahydrocannabinol. Marijuana is usually smoked but can be ingested (such as when baked in cookies or brownies). The onset of effects from smoking marijuana is a matter of minutes; oral ingestion slows the onset time to several hours. When smoked, the effects generally last 2 to 4 hours. When ingested, the effects can last twice as long.

Although classified as a hallucinogen, marijuana does not produce true hallucinations (unlike PCP, LSD, and mescaline), but users may have a distorted sense of time and space and, occasionally, a feeling of unreality. Smoking marijuana results in bronchodilation and slight tachycardia. Other signs and symptoms of marijuana use include euphoria, drowsiness, decreased short-term memory, diminished motor coordination, increased appetite, and injected conjunctiva.

Management focuses on supportive prehospital care because the likelihood of a serious medical complication is small. A novice user may exhibit some behavioural symptoms such as paranoia and (rarely) psychosis. Psychological first aid and reassurance generally suffice to address

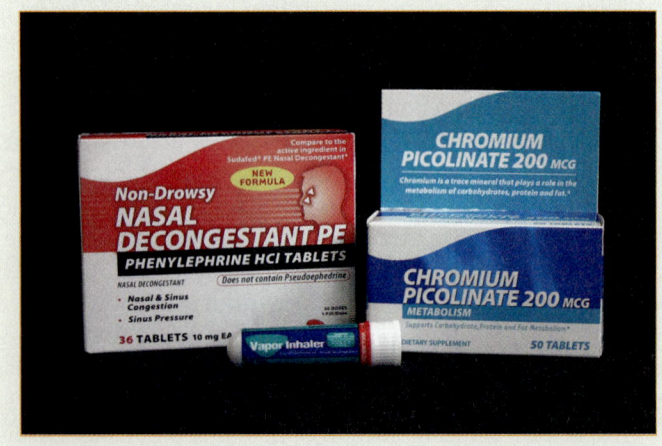

Figure 33-7 Drugs such as nasal decongestants and diet pills generally fall into the category of amphetamines.

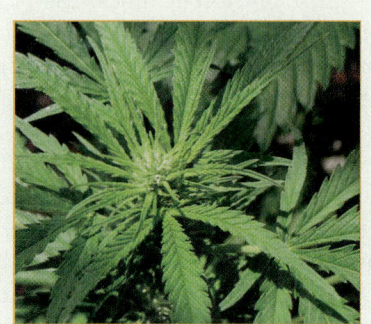

Figure 33-8 A marijuana plant.

either issue. If the patient remains anxious, low-dose benzodiazepines may be administered. Transport for continued evaluation is rarely warranted, but providing information for support and counseling services can be helpful.

Hallucinogens

A hallucinogen is a substance that causes some distortion of sense perception—seeing, hearing, or feeling things that are not actually present. These outcomes are termed psychedelic effects. Experiences involving hallucinogens can vary markedly, with people taking the same dose of the same drug from the same batch experiencing totally different effects. The overall drug experience is affected by the user's previous drug experience, the dose taken, the user's expectations, and the social setting.

A wide variety of substances have been used over the centuries for their hallucinogenic properties, and these substances can be classified into two categories: synthetic and naturally occurring. The synthetic class includes LSD, PCP, and ketamine. The naturally occurring hallucinogens include marijuana, mescaline, psilocybin containing mushroom, and the seeds of the Jimson weed plant.

LSD

In 1947, Dr. Albert Hoffman discovered what would be the prototype for synthetic hallucinogens, LSD. Use of this drug peaked in the 1960s and then faded, and resurfaced in the 1990s. LSD is considered a non–habit-forming drug, although tolerance can occur if it is taken for several days in a row.

LSD primarily affects the senses. Synthesthesias (crossing of the senses) often prompt a user to respond to the question "What were you doing?" with a reply such as "I was watching the music play" or "I was listening to that painting." Users often experiment with LSD for self-exploration, for religious reasons, or to experience its often stunning visual and auditory effects.

Because of LSD's high potency, as little as 25 μg can produce CNS effects. A single dose or "hit" is 25 to 100 μg, although many users take three or more hits. As dosing increases to about 1,000 μg, there is a proportional increase in the drug's effects, which may last as long as 12 hours, although 3 to 4 hours is more typical.

From a physiologic perspective, the effects of LSD are mostly sympathomimetic, often consisting of tachycardia, mild hypertension, and dilated pupils. In a "bad trip," the user has a frightening experience, resulting in an acute anxiety attack and the physical effects secondary to increased anxiety.

The treatment for a patient using LSD is primarily supportive, focusing on the psychological aspects of the drug experience. For a person having a bad trip, think of it as being in a living nightmare or a dream that is as real as reality; this dream doesn't end until the drug wears off, however. Try to limit sensory stimulation as much as possible—for example, by avoiding the use of emergency lights and sirens. Routine transport to the appropriate facility plus psychological support are usually all that is required in the prehospital setting.

Phencyclidine (PCP)

PCP, also called angel dust or dust, was developed in the late 1950s as a potential anesthetic. In clinical trial, problems with the drug—namely, delirium and psychotic-like symptoms—led to PCP to be relegated to use as an animal tranquilizer (Syrnalan). PCP abuse was first noted in the 1970s. Very little PCP is available on the streets of Canada today, because most people are now aware of its significant untoward effects. What is available is manufactured in clandestine laboratories, so variations in potency and purity are common. PCP can be a contaminant of other street drugs.

Although PCP is grouped with the hallucinogens here, it is actually classified as a dissociative anesthetic, as is ketamine. It is typically smoked or snorted, although it can be injected. Small doses (25–50 mg) can produce signs and symptoms of intoxication in an adult, with the high from a single dose typically lasting 4 to 6 hours. Slurred speech, staggering gait, tachycardia, hypertension, staring blankly for extended periods, and horizontal nystagmus (involuntary, rhythmic movement of the eyes) are common with PCP use. This is the prototypical substance of abuse that can cause opisthotonus, a severe form of muscle rigidity where the occiput and heels of the patient touch the bed when supine, but the neck, back, and pelvis are severely arched above the horizontal.

More problematic are the mind-body separation, related hallucinations, and violent outbreaks that are hallmarks of PCP use. Users may make bizarre comments such as "I can fly" and then jump off a balcony to prove it. Users have an almost unfathomable ability to take pain with no reaction and exhibit almost superhuman strength.

PCP can cause some of the most violent and difficult behaviour you will encounter in the prehospital environment, so prehospital care focuses on protecting the patient and the EMS team from attacks involving poor judgment and impaired behaviour. Supportive prehospital care includes oxygen, cardiac monitoring, and intravenous access, if possible, without provoking the patient and benzodiazepines for sedation. If an intravenous access cannot be established, then lorazepam may be given intramuscularly.

Ketamine

Ketamine (special K, vitamin K; also discussed in Chapter 38) is an analogue of PCP and another dissociative anaesthetic. Most ketamine available on the streets is diverted from veterinary clinics, although this drug is used in clinical medicine, primarily for pediatrics. Liquid ketamine is colourless and odourless. Ketamine can also be found in a powdered form. It is often mixed in a drink, although it can be snorted. It is physically and psychologically addicting.

Typical oral dosing is 75 to 300 mg. When snorted, the dose is reduced slightly, to 15 to 200 mg. At low doses, a user presents with mild inebriation, dreamy or erotic thoughts, and increased sociability. At higher doses, a patient may have pronounced nausea, difficulty moving, and a complaint of "entering another reality." In extreme cases, users will enter the "K hole," which involves out-of-body experiences, a feeling of being detached from one's surroundings.

Although violent outbreaks are much less likely with ketamine than with PCP, the principles of management are the same for the two drugs. Secure the patient well, assess and manage the ABCs, provide oxygen therapy, and establish vascular access if time and the situation allow as you provide safe transport to the appropriate facility. Keep a close eye on the patient because both agitation and profound sedation with respiratory compromise can occur with this drug.

Psilocybin Mushrooms

Hallucinogenic, or psilocybin-containing, mushrooms are native to both the east and west coasts of Canada, but not central Canada Figure 33-9 ▾ . They can, however, be purchased on the streets as dried caps anywhere in the country. The typical dose is estimated to be 4 to 10 mg (approximately 2–4 mushrooms). Consumption of 100 mushrooms or more as a single dose has been reported.

The onset of symptoms and hallucinogenic effects (similar to LSD but less intense) is within 30 minutes of ingestion, and effects usually last 4 to 6 hours. Signs and symptoms include nausea and vomiting, mydriasis, mild tachycardia, and mild hypertension. As doses increase, frank psychosis, wild agitation, and other sympathomimetic symptoms can occur. The likelihood of any serious medical side effects is low, although the literature describes seizures and hyperthermia in some cases. Because there are many "look-alikes," foraging for magic mushrooms raises the risk of eating hepatotoxic mushrooms. Delayed-onset vomiting, diarrhea, and the absence of hallucinations should alert the caregiver to the possibility of a hepatotoxic mushroom ingestion.

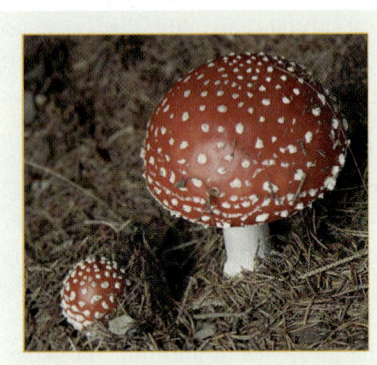

Figure 33-9 Certain mushrooms are hallucinogenic if ingested.

Treat the patient with supportive prehospital care. Attention to the ABCs and monitoring vital signs are usually all that is required, along with safe transport to the appropriate facility. If time and circumstances allow, establish vascular access to facilitate seizure control with benzodiazepines, if necessary.

Sedatives and Hypnotics

The drugs in the sedative-hypnotic category have a wide range of applications. Drugs with sedative qualities are used to reduce anxiety and to calm agitated patients. Drugs with hypnotic qualities are used as sleep aids, helping produce drowsiness and sleep. In either case, sedative-hypnotic drugs function primarily as CNS depressants.

Barbiturates

The barbiturates have a long history of use as sleep aids, antianxiety drugs, and seizure-control medications. Barbiturate use and abuse reached its peak in the late 1970s, when these drugs were tagged with street names that coincided with the colour of the pill or capsule: reds (secobarbital), yellows or yellow jackets (pentobarbital), blues or blue heavens (amobarbital), and rainbows (amobarbital plus secobarbital). The frequent combination of alcohol and barbiturates as a suicide

mechanism, coupled with the high incidence of accidental overdoses, pushed researchers to develop sedative-hypnotic drugs that had fewer depressive effects on the respiratory system and that were less lethal. Today, there is little prescribing or abuse of barbiturates except for phenobarbital, which continues to be used for seizure control.

Barbiturate abusers quickly develop tolerance and require increasing doses to produce the desired effects. Long-term use results in physical addiction. Abrupt cessation in a long-term barbiturate abuser will produce typical signs and symptoms of the withdrawal syndrome in approximately 24 hours, with potentially life-threatening signs and symptoms arising up to a week after abrupt cessation. In the case of minor withdrawal, the patient may present with symptoms similar to those observed in a patient with alcohol withdrawal: restlessness and anxiety, depression, insomnia, diaphoresis, abdominal cramping, nausea, and vomiting. With severe cases of withdrawal, patients commonly experience delirium, hallucinations, psychosis, seizures, hyperthermia, and cardiovascular collapse.

Your assessment of the barbiturate intoxicated patient will include findings similar to those seen with alcohol intoxication. The patient will be drowsy and exhibit decreased inhibitions, ataxia, mental confusion, and staggering gait. As the dose increases, the patient will have more CNS depression until he or she is comatose. Prehospital care for a patient who has overdosed on barbiturates follows a logical and predictable path. Airway protection and ventilatory support are the first management priorities because of the CNS depressant effects of these drugs. The patient may require intubation or other advanced airway maneuver to secure the airway and prevent aspiration should the patient vomit. Supplemental oxygen is needed because patients with altered levels of consciousness typically hypoventilate and are hypoxic before treatment begins. Once the airway and breathing are managed, attention to circulation should include monitoring cardiac rhythm and obtaining intravenous access. The paramedic can follow local or regional protocols or medical directives to manage hypotension or evidence of volume depletion.

Once absorbed, a variety of interventions can be used to cause the phenobarbital to be eliminated more quickly from the body. Although these are best initiated in the emergency department setting, if patient transport times are very long the paramedics may wish to contact direct medical control to discuss further therapy such as activated charcoal or alkalinization of urine. Multiple–dose-activated charcoal has been proven to decrease the half-life of phenobarbital. Although not typically administered in the prehospital setting, it may be useful if administered soon after drug ingestion. The paramedic should take great care in administering charcoal to a patient who has

Notes from Nancy

Consider the possibility of a drug-related problem in any patient presenting with unexplained behavioural changes, stupor, coma, or seizures.

taken a drug that can depress the CNS. If the patient who has received charcoal then requires airway protection or ventilatory support, aspiration of the charcoal will cause significant injury to the lungs. Alkalinization of the patient's urine with intravenous sodium bicarbonate can alter phenobarbital's charge in the blood, thereby trapping it in the urine and promoting its excretion via this route. Although these two therapies, charcoal and alkalinization, may decrease phenobarbital's toxicity, they must not be delivered without permission from direct medical control. There is no evidence that forced diuresis using a diuretic (such as furosemide) decreases the half-life or toxicity of phenobarbital. Finally, the patient with severe phenobarbital poisoning might require dialysis for drug removal.

If you encounter barbiturate withdrawal in the prehospital setting, focus your treatment on immediate threats to life, including seizures, and providing supportive prehospital care. The paramedic should promptly initiate transport to the emergency department, because the patient will require investigations and care that can only be delivered in the hospital.

Benzodiazepines and Other Sedative-Hypnotics

Benzodiazepines are also members of the sedative-hypnotic family. They are most commonly used to treat anxiety, seizures, and withdrawal symptoms. In recent years, other medications have been developed, such as zolpidem, zopiclone, and eszopiclone, for the treatment of insomnia. These drugs are not benzodiazepines, but have effects on the inhibitory neurotransmitter, gamma-aminobutyric acid (GABA), as do benzodiazepines. Although apparently less addictive, they do have the potential to cause a similar clinical

picture of sedation in overdose; dependence can develop in chronic use; and when stopped suddenly after a period of prolonged use, a withdrawal syndrome can occur.

In a single-entity overdose, benzodiazepines have a relatively low rate of morbidity and mortality. The most common clinical effects of benzodiazepine overdose include altered mentation, drowsiness, confusion, slurred speech, ataxia, and general incoordination. For a suspected overdose in which the patient presents with severe respiratory depression, hypotension, or coma, think beyond a simple benzodiazepine event to other CNS depressants and alcohol. Treatment of benzodiazepine overdose is relatively straightforward:

- Assess and manage the airway, inserting an advanced airway as needed.
- Give high-concentration supplemental oxygen.
- Establish vascular access.
- Apply the ECG monitor, pulse oximeter, and capnometer.
- Transport to the appropriate facility.

The specific benzodiazepine antagonist, flumazenil, is not advised in benzodiazepine overdose, because its administration can precipitate acute benzodiazepine withdrawal. In the prehospital environment, this could translate into intractable seizures and no available treatment because benzodiazepine receptors are then blocked.

Gamma-Hydroxybutyrate (GHB)

Gamma-hydroxybutyrate (GHB) is an endogenous metabolite of gamma-aminobutyrate acid, a neuromodulator involved with sleep cycles, memory retention, and emotional control. GHB was initially used as an anesthetic in Europe before it

You are the Paramedic Part 3

Upon completing your detailed physical examination, you determine that the cause of Julie's altered mental status is a possible overdose. As you insert an 18-gauge IV cannula in her right arm, your partner begins to prepare the equipment for intubation. You secure the IV line, begin to run a fluid challenge with normal saline, and turn your attention to securing an airway. Under direct visualization of the vocal cords, you insert a 6.5 endotracheal tube. Correct placement of the endotracheal tube is confirmed with auscultation of bilateral breath sounds, bilateral chest rise, and a positive colour change on the end-tidal carbon dioxide detector. You secure the tube at the 23-cm mark at the teeth and ask your partner to ventilate via a bag-valve-mask device at a rate of 12 breaths/min. You administer 0.4 mg of naloxone (Narcan) in case Julie ingested narcotics, but you do not get a response.

As you begin to package Julie for transport, her friend returns with an empty pill bottle that she found next to Julie's backpack in the locker room. The label reveals a prescription for amitriptyline (Elavil) filled the day before; the prescription was for 60 pills.

Reassessment	Recording Time: 10 Minutes
Skin	Flushed, warm, and dry
Pulse	160 beats/min; regular and weak
ECG	Possible wide complex tachycardia
Blood pressure	80/50 mm Hg
Respirations	12 breaths/min via bag-valve-mask device
Spo$_2$	97% on 100% supplemental oxygen via bag-valve-mask device
Pupils	Dilated
Blood glucose	4 mmol/l

5. Given the current situation, should you consider treating the patient in the prehospital setting or continuing treatment on the way to the hospital?

6. How should your patient management progress?

appeared in North America as a bodybuilding aid. By the late 1980s, GHB had gained popularity with young people as a club drug, earning the name "liquid ecstasy" from its euphoric effects at raves (all-night dance parties). In the mid-1990s, GHB became increasingly associated with sexual assaults.

Although GHB is available as an odourless and colourless liquid, it has a slightly salty taste. Once ingested, GHB quickly crosses the blood–brain barrier, exerting its effects within 30 to 60 minutes. As little as 0.5 mg of GHB can produce a pronounced hypnotic effect along with disinhibition and antegrade amnesia. When taken with alcohol, GHB increases the risk of CNS depression.

GHB intoxication can result in significant, but fluctuating, CNS depression and airway compromise. First, establish and maintain the airway, inserting an advanced airway as needed. Carefully monitor the patient's LOC. Assist breathing as necessary, and give high-flow supplemental oxygen. Establish vascular access. Apply the ECG monitor, pulse oximeter, and capnometer. Finally, provide transport to the hospital.

Narcotics, Opiates, and Opioids

A narcotic is a drug that produces sleep or altered mental status. Historically, narcotics have been classified into two major divisions: opiates and opioids. The term opiate is used to describe natural drugs derived from opium or the poppy; the term opioid refers to non–opium-derived synthetics. We use the term *opioids* to describe licit therapeutic agents and illicit substances in this group.

Opioids have a long history of use and abuse, with writings as far back as the third century BC mentioning the use of poppy juice. Today, abuse of narcotics remains one of the most common causes of overdose deaths reported to Poison Centres.

Opioids include morphine, codeine, heroin, fentanyl, oxycodone, meperidine, propoxyphene, and dextromethorphan. Although these drugs share certain properties, they exhibit highly diverse effects and vary widely in their potency. Opioids are used primarily in clinical medicine for analgesia, whereas the illicit drug heroin is abused for the unique euphoria it produces. In terms of potency, 80 to 100 mg of meperidine (Demerol) produces analgesia for 2 to 4 hours; 10 mg of morphine produces a similar effect for 4 to 5 hours; and just 2 mg of hydromorphone (Dilaudid) has an analgesic effect, which also lasts for 4 to 5 hours.

Opioids produce their major effects on the CNS by binding with receptor sites in the brain and other tissues. The highest concentrations of receptor sites are found in the limbic system, frontal and temporal cortices, thalamus, hypothalamus, midbrain, and spinal cord.

Opioids are readily absorbed from the GI tract but can also be absorbed from the nasal mucosa (when snorted) or from the lungs (opium smoking). When taken orally, the effects of these drugs are lessened owing to their significant first-pass metabolism through the liver compared with their effects when given parenterally. When heroin passes through the liver, it is metabolized into acetyl-morphine, which continues to exert narcotic effects that may outlast the effects of naloxone. Remember that a dose of naloxone has a short half-life as compared to many opioids;

redosing of naloxone is the rule rather than the exception. A patient should not be allowed to refuse transport after a dose of naloxone, because they may lapse back into unconsciousness.

Morphine is a commonly used analgesic in the prehospital setting and is a potent vasodilator. When given to young adults, its half-life is roughly 2 to 3 hours, but it typically takes longer to metabolize in older adults.

Assessment

The classic presentation of opioid use features euphoria, hypotension, respiratory depression, and pinpoint pupils. Depending on the particular agent, nausea, vomiting, and constipation may occur as well. Allergic phenomena may also occur with opioid use, albeit rarely. With increased doses, coma, seizures (usually secondary to hypoxia), and cardiac arrest (usually secondary to respiratory arrest) are common.

Morphine (named after Morpheus, the god of dreams) and heroin produce an impressive dreamlike state. Shortly after injecting heroin, a user will appear to pass out (in street terms, "going on the nod"). However, the user is typically quite lucid and remains aware of what is being done or said.

Management

Because of the CNS depressant effects, patient management initially focuses on establishing and maintaining a patent airway and providing adequate ventilation. A patient who has overdosed on opioids is almost always hypoventilating, sometimes breathing as few as 4 or 5 breaths/min, and is consequently hypoxic and hypercarbic. Rather than moving immediately to intubation, place an oropharyngeal airway and provide bag-mask ventilation with 15 l/min of supplemental oxygen.

Be aware that opioid-induced hypoventilation can cause significant hypercapnea, which can further suppress the patient's level of awareness due to CO_2 narcosis. This may be worsened by partial airway obstruction due to reduced pharyngeal muscle tone and tongue malpositioning. Neurological status may improve with basic airway management and reduction of arterial dioxide levels, independent of other interventions.

Next, establish vascular access and administer small doses of naloxone (0.4 mg). The desired response is improved ventilation so that intubation and ventilation might be avoided. Large doses of naloxone will precipitate acute narcotic withdrawal in a chronic user. These withdrawal symptoms are not life threatening, as is alcohol or benzodiazepine withdrawal. The chronic abuser—abruptly wakened—may become agitated and uncooperative (because he or she is in pain) and refuse to be transported to the hospital. Again, the likelihood is that the effects of the naloxone will wear off imminently and the patient will lapse back into unconsciousness several minutes later.

The patient who does not respond to usual doses of naloxone may have a taken a highly potent drug such as fentanyl, taken a sedative-hypnotic with clinical features similar to an opioid, taken a combination of medications, or have a concomitant head injury as a consequence of inebriation. When naloxone has not been effective, insert an advanced airway, provide other prehospital care as needed, and transport to the hospital.

Carbon Monoxide

CO causes more accidental poisoning deaths than any other toxic substance. It is produced by incomplete combustion of organic fuels, such as a home-heating device. Hence, its presentation is often seasonal, occurring when furnaces are running and flues or ventilation systems become blocked. It is also a major hazard when a running engine in an enclosed space generates the gas. A running engine in a closed garage can generate lethal concentrations of CO within 30 minutes. This is often a mechanism of successful suicide. CO is a major component of smoke in enclosed-space fires and can be responsible for fire-related deaths. The use of carbon monoxide detectors in homes and other locations is a critical preventive health measure that can save lives and should be highly encouraged by all EMS agencies.

CO is a colourless, odourless, tasteless gas. Hence, those exposed to it have no warning of its presence. The toxicity arises primarily from CO's affinity for hemoglobin in RBCs; CO displaces oxygen, thereby preventing the RBCs from carrying oxygen to the tissues and leading to suffocation at the cellular level. Hemoglobin's affinity for CO is more than 250 times its affinity for oxygen, so the atmospheric level of CO does not need to be very high for poisoning to occur. Even relatively small concentrations of CO in the atmosphere can convert a significant proportion of hemoglobin into carboxyhemoglobin (hemoglobin combined with carbon dioxide), making it ineffective as an oxygen carrier.

Because the overall ability of the blood to transport oxygen is so drastically reduced when CO reaches toxic levels, anything that increases the body's oxygen requirements, such as physical exertion or a fever, will increase the severity of the poisoning. Children, whose metabolic rate is intrinsically higher than that of adults, tend to have more severe symptoms at any given level of exposure.

CO poisoning can be difficult to diagnose in the prehospital setting unless it is the direct result of an easily identifiable cause such as a fire or intentional exposure to exhaust fumes from an automobile. Its signs and symptoms are highly variable and quite vague, often resembling early onset of the flu—for example, headache, nausea, and vomiting. With acute CO poisoning, the patient may be confused and unable to think clearly. Physical examination often reveals bounding pulses, dilated pupils, and pallor or cyanosis. Consider the possibility of CO poisoning whenever you are confronted with several (possibly many) people who have shared the same accommodations for any period, especially if they have been quartered together in a closed area, such as one house in the winter.

The cherry red colour of the skin that is mentioned in many textbooks is a very late sign of CO poisoning. Put bluntly, cherry red usually means really dead.

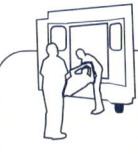

At the Scene

CO is a hazard for rescuers as well as for patients. Multiple patients with medical complaints—at the same time and inside the same building—equals poisoning until proven otherwise!

Note that pulse oximetry at the scene *will not* provide a true assessment of arterial oxygenation because the device cannot determine whether CO or oxygen is bound to the hemoglobin. A reading of 99% on the pulse oximeter would be excellent in a normal environmental setting but would be a grave error in the presence of carboxyhemoglobin because the hemoglobin is saturated with the wrong chemical! Application of the ECG monitor to assess for cardiac ischemia can further support diagnostic and treatment efforts when CO is the suspected culprit. Portable noninvasive oximeters can also measure carbon monoxide levels in the prehospital environment and have the potential to more rapidly identify patients with CO poisoning.

Treatment of CO poisoning in the prehospital setting is aimed at providing the highest concentration of oxygen possible to attempt to displace CO molecules from the hemoglobin. For patients breathing room air, the elimination half-life of carboxyhemoglobin is roughly 4 hours. By comparison, if the patient is breathing 100% oxygen, the half-life can be reduced to about 1.5 hours. Hyperbaric oxygen (HBO) therapy at 2.5 atmospheres of pressure can further reduce the elimination time to 15 to 20 minutes, although its use is controversial. Hyperbaric oxygen may improve neurologic outcome in some situations through mechanisms unrelated to CO elimination.

If you suspect CO poisoning:

- Remove the patient from the exposure environment.
- Establish and maintain the airway, inserting an advanced airway as needed.
- Give high-flow supplemental oxygen by tight-fitting nonrebreathing mask.
- Maintain maximal inspired oxygen concentration regardless of measured arterial oxygen saturation.
- Establish vascular access.
- Keep the patient quiet and at rest to minimize oxygen demand.
- Monitor the ECG rhythm and LOC.
- Transport to your nearest medical facility.
- For patients with injuries or illness from a structural or vehicular fire, consider the possibility of combined CO/cyanide poisoning, especially if the patient has signs of shock.

CO poisoning can be reversed if it is diagnosed and treated in time. Even if the patient recovers, however, acute CO poisoning may result in permanent damage to vital organs and lead to mild to severe neurologic deficits.

Chlorine Gas

Incidents involving chlorine gas are relatively common because of the widespread use of chlorine compounds in the home and occupational settings. Household exposures usually occur upon mixing a cleaning agent containing sodium hypochlorite (such as bleach) with a strong acid in an overzealous attempt to remove a stain **Figure 33-10 ▶**. The resulting chemical reaction releases chlorine gas, often in high concentrations. Most cases of chlorine gas exposure occur outside the home, however. The chlorination of large swimming pools, which tends to

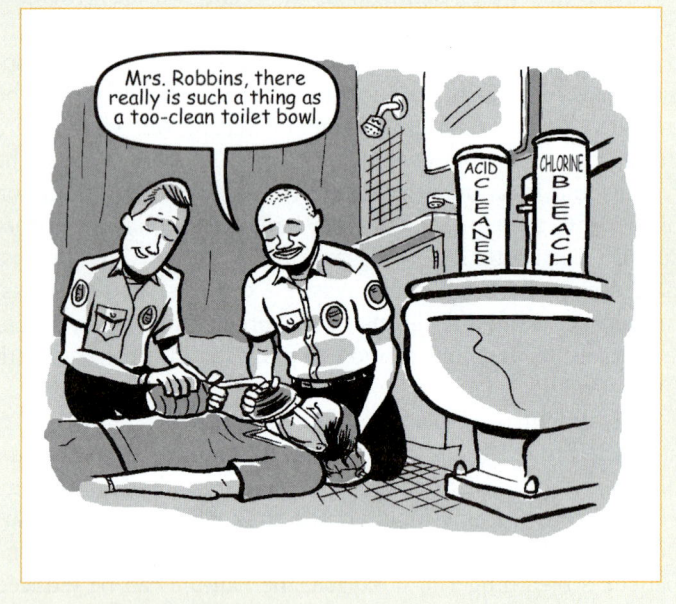

Figure 33-10

rely on gaseous rather than liquid or solid forms of chlorine, has led to mass exposures at hotels and community recreation centres. Leakage of chlorine gas from an industrial storage tank, truck, or rail car can also result in a mass-casualty incident.

The signs and symptoms of chlorine gas exposure depend on the concentration of the inhaled gas and the duration of exposure. Chlorine gas is extremely irritating to all mucous membranes. When it comes in contact with the moisture on those surfaces, it can form hydrochloric and other acids that are damaging to human tissue. With a minor exposure, the patient will experience burning sensations in the eyes, nose, and throat along with a slight cough. More intense exposure to chlorine gas causes chest tightness, choking, paroxysmal cough, headache, nausea and vomiting, and diffuse wheezing. Patients with more severe exposures may also develop cyanosis, crackles in the chest, shock, seizures, and loss of consciousness.

When treating patients who have been exposed to chlorine gas, your first priority is to remove them from the area of exposure. If the incident involves a serious gas spill, an upwind location for parking the ambulance is a must. Also make sure that all rescuers wear protective breathing apparatus.

Once in a safe environment, quickly triage the patients. People with dyspnea, wheezing, severe cough, or other signs of respiratory distress are priority patients and should ideally receive high-concentration, humidified oxygen by mask. Intubation may be necessary due to laryngeal edema and upper airway obstruction or due to refractory hypoxemia secondary to lung inflammation. Irrigate burning or itching eyes with water, as well as any areas of the skin that have come in contact with the chlorine.

Cyanide

Cyanide is used in industry for electroplating, ore extraction, and fumigation of structures. In addition to industrial exposures, poisoning can occur after ingestion of cyanide contained in commercial products such as silver polish or from the seeds of cherries, apples, pears, and apricots. More commonly, cyanide poisoning occurs when a household fire results in the combustion of nitrogen-containing materials (such as plastic items or furnishings, wool carpeting, polyurethane silk).

Cyanide is a rapid-acting and deadly poison. This toxin does its damage by combining with a crucial cellular enzyme, cytochrome oxidase, which in turn blocks the utilization of oxygen at the cellular level. The results are cellular suffocation and death of the patient within seconds if the cyanide was inhaled or within minutes to possibly an hour or two if it was ingested.

Physical examination of a patient who has been poisoned with cyanide may reveal an altered mental state. If awake enough to answer questions, the patient may complain of headache, palpitations, or dyspnea. The classic odour of bitter almonds on the patient's breath is highly suggestive of cyanide poisoning but is not diagnostic. Respirations are rapid and laboured early on; as the poisoning progresses, they become slow and gasping. The pulse is usually rapid and thready. Vomiting, seizures, and coma can occur. The patient's venous blood and sometimes the patient's body may be bright red—even though oxygen is available in the bloodstream, it is not being taken up by the tissues. Thus, a patient who is cyanotic has either not been poisoned with cyanide or is very close to death.

If the cyanide poisoning occurred as the result of a toxic inhalation, remove the patient from the source of the cyanide (the toxic environment). Establish an airway and administer 100% supplemental oxygen, assisting ventilation as necessary. Establish intravenous access. Because the majority of paramedics in Canada do not carry a cyanide antidote, the mainstay of treatment is transportation to the closest hospital emergency department. It is advisable to notify the receiving hospital en route and contact your provincial Poison Centre. Many EDs have a small number of cyanide treatment kits immediately available, but will likely have to locate additional kits from elsewhere in the hospital in the event of a multiple casualty incident.

Different antidotes are available for the treatment of cyanide. A commercially available kit, "the cyanide kit," contains pearls of amyl nitrite to be given only if intravenous access has not been established, as well as sodium nitrite for injection and sodium thiosulfate for injection. Hydroxycobalamin for injection is another antidote, acting as a safer chemical to attract the cyanide from its target enzyme. This antidote, the precursor to vitamin B12, does not have the same toxicity as the nitrites that exist in the commercially available kit and may become the more usual antidote in the future.

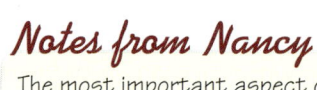

Notes from Nancy

The most important aspect of treatment in toxic inhalations is to remove the patient from the toxic environment, but do not enter a known toxic environment without protective breathing apparatus.

Pesticides

Organophosphates and Carbamates

Organophosphates and carbamates are the active ingredients in many household (low concentration) and farm pesticides. In developing countries, these agents are commonly used in suicide attempts because they are readily available, as compared to pharmaceuticals. Nerve gases, which are used in chemical warfare, are also rapid acting and highly potent organophosphates.

Organophosphates and carbamates exert their toxic effects at junctions (synapses) of the nerve cells of the autonomic nervous system, preventing the breakdown of acetylcholine. The conduction of an impulse from one nerve to another occurs through the release of acetylcholine at the synapse. Acetylcholine works as a chemical messenger, crossing the synapse to depolarize the nerve on the other side of the junction. Once it has delivered its message, the acetylcholine molecule must be inactivated or it would continue to stimulate the target nerve cell indefinitely, leaving the nerve cell unable to receive another message from the brain. The symptoms of organophosphate or carbamate poisoning include CNS and peripheral nervous system manifestations and are the same whether the exposure was by ingestion, inhalation, or dermal absorption.

CNS symptoms can include confusion, restlessness, tremors, seizures, and loss of consciousness. Peripheral manifestations are of cholinergic excess and can be remembered by the mnemonic DUMBELS: Diaphoresis and diarrhea, Urination, Miosis (or mydriasis), Bronchospasm, bronchorrhea, and bradycardia, Emesis, Lacrimation, Salivation. In addition, because acetylcholine is active at motor end plates, with excessive stimulation patients develop marked motor weakness. Remember that commercially available organophosphates and carbamates are usually dissolved in hydrocarbon vehicles. Respiratory toxicity can also occur from aspiration of the hydrocarbon.

Assessment and management of a patient with exposure to a nerve gas or pesticide starts with decontamination and removal of all contaminated clothing *before* initiating care or loading the patient into the ambulance. Wear PPE if the patient has ingested the suspect toxic product, because vomiting after topical decontamination may lead to exposure. Contaminated clothing should be placed in plastic bags and disposed of as hazardous materials. Ideally, the patient should be scrubbed with soap and water. After that, patient care includes the following measures:

- Establish and maintain the airway. Consider an advanced airway, as needed.
- Suction as needed.
- Give high-flow supplemental oxygen.
- Establish vascular access. Place the patient on an ECG monitor, pulse oximeter, and capnometer.
- For an adult patient, administer 2.0 mg atropine IV push. Double the dose every 5 minutes until bronchial secretions dry and bronchospasm (wheezing) resolves. Do not use heart rate as your endpoint.
- Transport to a medical facility.

Poisonous Plants and Mushrooms

Poisonous Plants

Of the thousands of plant species known, few are truly poisonous (ie, causing systemic toxicity). Indeed, many medicinals were originally derived from plants. Certainly many varieties of plants can cause contact dermatitis. Similarly, ingestion of many other varieties of plants can cause gastroenteritis.
Figure 33-11 ▶ shows some common Canadian plants that can cause toxicity. It is not expected that paramedics should be able to identify the plant involved. Remember to attend to symptoms and bring any remaining parts of the plant to the hospital with the patient.

A number of plants in the Araceae family, including household varieties of dieffenbachia, caladium, and philodendron, contain insoluble calcium oxalate crystals, or raphides. If chewed, these raphides cause a painful burning sensation in the mouth. This usually limits the exposure because of pain. However, chewing large amounts can cause edema of the upper airway.

The leaves of rhubarb plants contain soluble calcium oxalate. Eating the leaves can lead to renal failure. This is *not* the case with the insoluble oxalates as in the household plants.

Chewing the pits of a number of fruits, including apricots, choke cherries, and peaches, can result in the release of cyanide, because the amygdalin within them is activated by saliva. Swallowing the pits intact carries no risk. Similarly, one must chew the seeds of the black locust plant, which grows in certain parts of Canada, to release the toxalbumin within. This toxin is the same as that in the castor bean, from which the chemical warfare agent ricin is derived. Exposure to the toxalbumin causes a systemic illness that starts with gastroenteritis but leads in days to multi-organ failure.

A number of plants contain cardiac glycosides. The most familiar is foxglove, from which the cardiac inotrope digoxin is derived. Other plants, including monkshood and yew berries, contain other pro-arrhythmic toxins. Cardiac monitoring is essential in the event of exposure to large quantities of these plants.

Some plants, such as the roots of water hemlock, contain CNS toxins that can cause seizures. Other plants are abused for their hallucinogenic properties. The seeds of the morning glory contain an LSD-like substance. All parts, but especially the seeds, of jimsonweed and deadly nightshade contain atropine-like toxins that lead to the anticholinergic toxidrome of dry mouth, dilated pupils, tachycardia, urinary retention, and hallucinations.

Finally, all parts of the autumn crocus contain the medicinal, or toxin, if taken in large quantities, known as colchicine. This is an antimetabolite used for the treatment of gout. Initial symptoms of overingestion include gastroenteritis. As white cell lines are depleted over time, infection and sepsis occurs.

When you encounter a case of plant poisoning, get all the information you can from the patient or parent and then consult your provincial Poison Centre. What plant and plant parts were eaten? If seeds were ingested, were they chewed? When was the ingestion? What symptoms have developed?

The vast majority of plant exposures are not toxic and do not require treatment more than observation. The decision to allow a

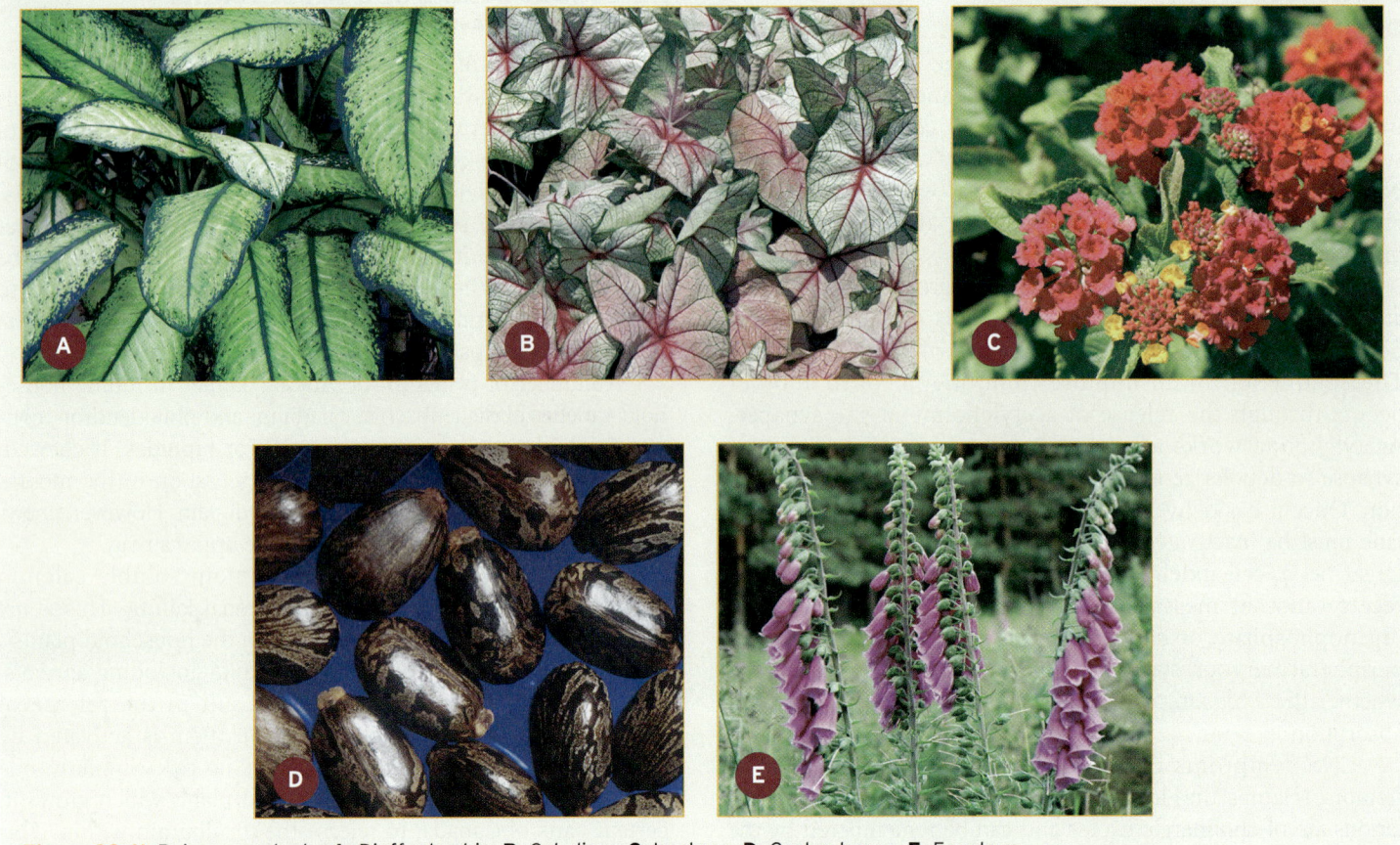

Figure 33-11 Poisonous plants. **A.** Dieffenbachia. **B.** Caladium. **C.** Lantana. **D.** Castor beans. **E.** Foxglove.

patient to remain at home should be made in consultation with direct medical control and the provincial Poison Centre.

Poisonous Mushrooms

Three groups of people are most likely to be the victims of poisoning related to mushroom ingestion: those that forage for their own mushrooms, those looking for hallucinogenic mushrooms, and young children who eat them by accident. Even among educated people who like to gather their own mushrooms in the wild, mistakes can happen.

A variety of factors determine whether a mushroom ingestion will produce toxic results: the age of the mushroom, the season in which it was gathered, the amount ingested, and the preparation method. Toxic effects vary from mild GI signs and symptoms to severe cytotoxic—even lethal—effects. In Canada, almost all deaths due to mushroom ingestion involve hepatotoxic mushrooms of the *Amanita* or *Lepiota* species **Figure 33-12**.

If the patient has ingested a single variety of mushroom, symptom onset can be a predictor of prognosis. Early onset of gastrointestinal complaints, within 2 hours of ingestion, is predictive of a benign exposure. Gastrointestinal complaints that occur greater than 6 hours following ingestion are more ominous. Many other manifestations of mushroom toxicity can occur, although, as with plants, the majority of mushrooms are nontoxic. Some mushrooms cause seizures, others anticholinergic symptoms. Some are abused for their hallucinogenic properties. Rare varieties can cause renal failure.

Management for the symptomatic patient following a mushroom ingestion includes the usual measures. Establish and maintain the airway. Obtain vascular access. For hypotension, administer fluid boluses. Contact your local Poison Centre and direct medical control for local protocols. Transport the patient to the hospital.

Over-the-Counter Products

Analgesics

Acetaminophen

Acetaminophen is a well-tolerated drug with few side effects and few drug interactions. It is available in many preparations on an over-the counter basis. These characteristics have made this drug a popular analgesic. It is, however, a common medication on which to overdose and has been responsible for a number of deaths. Its lethality may be secondary to the perception that acetaminophen is so safe and to the lack of awareness that acetaminophen may be one ingredient of many in many cough, cold, and analgesic preparations so that inadvertent cumulative dosing occurs. A total dose, taken acutely, of greater than 150 to 200 mg/kg can be toxic.

Once ingested, regular-release acetaminophen is rapidly absorbed from the GI tract, producing peak serum levels in 30 to 120 minutes. Absorption slows when taken in combination with medications that slow gastric emptying, such as anticholinergics or narcotics, or when a slow-release preparation is

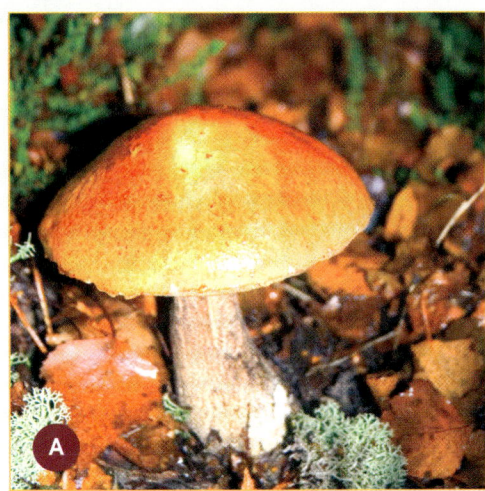
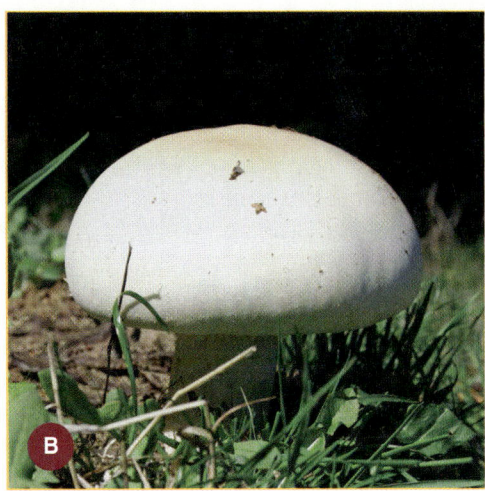

Figure 33-12 **A.** The deadly *Amanita* mushroom. **B.** A nonpoisonous, edible mushroom.

For symptomatic patients, prehospital care is usually supportive. For vomiting, give intravenous fluid boluses as necessary if hypotensive. For rare seizures, treat with benzodiazepines, as for any other seizure protocol. Transport the patient to a health care facility.

A unique side effect of NSAID use is aseptic meningitis, in which a patient presents with complaints of a stiff neck, headache, and fever within several hours after taking an NSAID. Discontinuing the NSAID therapy generally resolves the problem, but patients must be evaluated at the hospital to rule out other causes.

taken. One unique aspect of acetaminophen overdose is that signs and symptoms can occur in four distinct phases. It is also possible that a potentially lethal amount may be taken and the patient may have no symptoms.

It is important to try to accurately estimate the time of ingestion, because this information drives the decision-making process for patient care in the prehospital environment and in the hospital. Although an antidote for acetaminophen exists, *n*-acetylcysteine, its efficacy is greatest when given within 8 to 10 hours of the overdose. Typically, it is administered in the hospital based on laboratory results. As such, it is not a prehospital intervention.

Management of the patient in the prehospital setting focuses on the airway. Give high-flow supplemental oxygen, and establish vascular access. Transport the patient to the hospital if it is established that the ingestion is of a toxic amount and/or the intention was of self-harm.

Nonsteroidal Anti-inflammatory drugs (NSAIDs)

Medications used for pain management comprise a huge part of the over-the-counter drug market. In the OTC and prescription drug markets, NSAIDs are some of the most popular options for pain relief, fever control, and anti-inflammatory action. Their convenient dosing schemes and large therapeutic windows, coupled with their safe track records relative to acute ingestion and overdose, enhance their popularity.

NSAIDs are rapidly absorbed from the GI tract before being eliminated from the body in urine and feces. The half-lives of these agents vary widely, ranging from 2 to 4 hours for ibuprofen to approximately 15 hours for selective cyclooxygenase-2 inhibitors to 50 hours for some long-acting agents. Patients who take lithium and NSAIDs have slowed renal clearance of lithium, increasing the likelihood that they will inadvertently reach a toxic lithium level.

Most of the problems associated with NSAIDs involve long-term use; patients may experience GI bleeding and kidney dysfunction. Acute ingestions and symptomatic overdoses are rare.

Salicylates

Aspirin (acetylsalicylic acid, or ASA) products are almost ubiquitous in over-the-counter medications used for analgesia, fever control, liniments, cough and cold preparations, and prevention of coronary heart disease, to name a few indications. For example, a single 30-ml dose of bismuth subsalicylate (Pepto Bismol) contains 261 mg of salicylate (two thirds the total dose of one aspirin). Similarly, many liniments contain high levels of methyl salicylate; 15 ml of 100% methyl salicylate contains 7,000 mg of salicylate equivalent. With continued use of these products alone or in combination for a period of days, one can be exposed to excessive amounts of salicylate.

The clinical presentation of salicylate overdose can change based on three primary variables: the patient's age, the dose ingested, and the duration of the exposure. Ingestion of 150 mg/kg or less will usually make a person "mildly toxic." At this level, chief complaints are usually nausea, vomiting, and abdominal pain. With a dosing range of 150 to 300 mg/kg, moderate toxicity results with signs and symptoms including vomiting, diaphoresis, hyperpnea, ringing in the ears or tinnitus, and acid-base disturbances. At levels of 300 mg/kg, severe toxicity may produce a combination of respiratory alkalosis and metabolic acidosis and pulmonary and cerebral edema.

Chronic salicylate poisonings are probably the most often missed diagnosis in the confused elderly patient, and acute salicylate poisonings can be so severe as to result in death. No salicylate antidote is available, so prehospital management is primarily supportive. Establish and maintain the airway, inserting an advanced airway as needed. Give high-flow supplemental oxygen, and establish vascular access. If hypotension develops (from volume depletion), administer serial boluses of normal saline. Monitor carbon dioxide levels with capnometry. Transport the patient to a medical facility. Urine alkalinization and dialysis might be instituted at the receiving hospital depending on the severity of the intoxication in your patient.

Household Products

From a toxicologic perspective, the average home is a nightmare. Many houseplants have poisonous leaves or berries. All pesticides and herbicides used in lawn and garden care are potentially poisonous. All hydrocarbon products (such as paint thinners, solvents, gas) can cause permanent neurologic damage or death if inhaled in the right amount; the same is true of glue fumes (often called "huffing"). Many household cleaning agents are also toxic if ingested.

It is not possible within the scope of this chapter to discuss all of the possibilities when it comes to household poisonings. Some of the more likely culprits are included below. As always, keep in mind that your provincial Poison Centre is an invaluable resource.

Caustics

Caustics include strong acids (pH < 2.0) and strong alkalis (pH > 12.0). Both types of chemicals are commonly used in industry, agriculture (anhydrous ammonia), and the home **Table 33-4 ▸** and **Figure 33-13 ▸**. Most cases involve accidental dermal or ocular exposure, although occasionally you may encounter oral ingestions.

The widespread practice of storing such substances in beverage containers (such as soft drink or sports drink bottles), increases the likelihood that a child will regard the substance as a tasty drink. As the liquid enters the mouth and begins to burn, the child may simultaneously remove the bottle and turn the head, resulting in burns to the mouth, tongue, and face. Caustic substances cause direct chemical injury to the tissues that they contact. Signs and symptoms of a caustic exposure can include severe pain, burns, difficulty talking, difficulty swallowing (with oral ingestions), and hypoperfusion or shock (rarely, usually secondary to internal bleeding).

Most patients who have swallowed caustic substances present with severe pain in the mouth, throat, or chest. Respiratory distress can result, due to soft-tissue swelling in the larynx, epiglottis, or vocal cords, which means that the patient is in immediate danger of complete airway obstruction. For a caustic ingestion in an alert patient, give a single glass of water to the patient to drink to dilute the caustic. Never give a substance to neutralize because this will also result in the generation of heat, and thermal burns will complicate the situation. Establish vascular access, usually en route, because immediate transport to the ED is indicated.

With dermal exposure to a strong acid, the result is immediate and excruciating pain. For a strong alkali, the onset of

Notes from Nancy

If a patient who swallowed a caustic agent is in respiratory distress, get moving without further delay to the hospital. Have your cricothyrotomy kit ready.

Table 33-4	Common Caustic Substances	
Substance	**Example**	**Source**
Acids	Hydrochloric acid	Toilet bowl cleaners, swimming pool cleaners
	Sulfuric acid	Battery acid, toilet bowl cleaners (as bisulfate)
	Others	Bleach disinfectants, slate cleaners
Alkalis	Lye (sodium or potassium hydroxide)	Paint removers, washing powders, drain cleaners (such as Drano, Liquid Plumr, Plunge), button-shaped batteries, Clinitest tablets
	Sodium hypochlorite	Bleach (Clorox)
	Sodium carbonate	Bleach (Purex), nonphosphate detergents
	Ammonia	Hair dyes, jewelry cleaners, metal cleaners or polishes, antirust agents
	Potassium permanganate	Electric dishwasher detergents

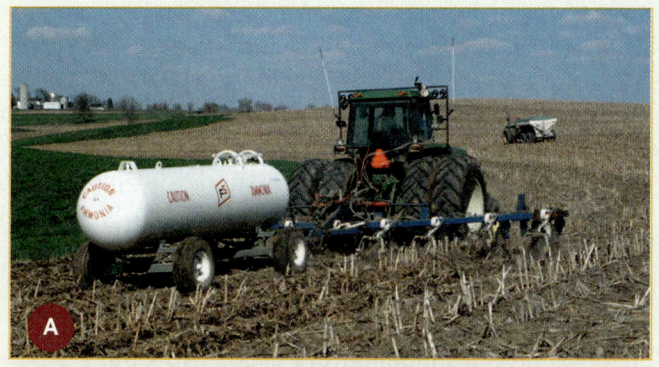

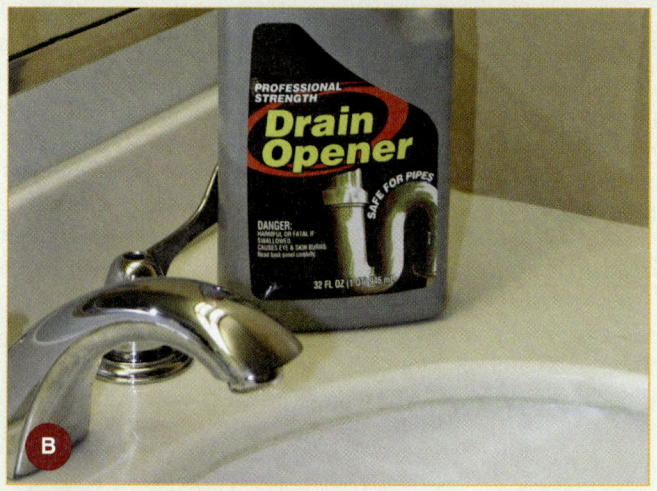

Figure 33-13 Caustic chemicals are commonly used in industry. **A.** Anhydrous ammonia tank used in agriculture. **B.** Plumbing agents used in the home.

At the Scene

Some chemicals react with water. Although small amounts can usually be flushed safely with large quantities of water, larger amounts of such chemicals can give off toxic fumes or explode when wet. Be sure to check the relevant warnings or placards.

pain is somewhat delayed, allowing more time before the patient reacts and increasing the severity of the burn. In such an injury, diluting and flushing away the caustic substance is the main goal of prehospital treatment. Acids tend to be more water-soluble than alkalis, so they are often diluted relatively quickly. With alkalis, it is more important to keep water continually flowing because it usually takes much longer to rinse an alkali away (compared with an acid).

For an eye exposure, cut the prong section off a nasal cannula, place it on the bridge of the patient's nose, and plug in a macro IV administration set and run it wide open to provide continuous irrigation. This also frees you up to perform other tasks. A Morgan lens may also be used after the initial gross flushing has been accomplished.

One of the most common caustic exposures in the agricultural setting involves anhydrous ammonia. The exposure usually occurs during the hook-up or disconnection of a nurse tank. Farmers often keep a small water bottle in the shirt pocket, allowing them to immediately rinse their eyes should an exposure occur. Without treatment, eye exposure to anhydrous ammonia can cause devastating damage in less than a minute, resulting in cataracts or blindness.

Metals

Acute poisonings by metals and metalloids are relatively rare except for that of iron. Many forms of metals exist. The inorganic forms of many are predominantly caustic; symptoms include nausea, vomiting, hematemesis, diarrhea, and melena. Multi-organ manifestations occur later. Prehospital treatment is supportive, as always. Establish and maintain the airway. Give high-flow oxygen and establish vascular access. Treat hypotension with fluid boluses and transport the patient to the hospital.

Iron

Pediatric iron ingestions have, in the past, been a major source of morbidity and mortality. Limiting the concentration of iron in preparations meant for children and the numbers of doses in these containers as well as child-resistant containers have been important public health measures that have led to significantly decreased exposures in Canada. Although only a small amount of iron is required as part of a healthy diet, many adult and pediatric multivitamins contain iron.

A small amount of iron is considered necessary for the normal functioning of the human body; as such, it is an essential mineral. In the average 70-kg adult, the entire iron supply is only 4 g. This iron is bound to proteins in the form of hemoglobin, cytochromes, and myoglobin and is transported in the blood bound to transferrin. No iron is "free," or unbound. Most iron is available in a balanced diet. However, supplemental iron is available in many pediatric and adult multivitamin preparations. When a toxic amount of iron is ingested, free iron is then available to damage target organs. For practical purposes, mild to moderate toxicity can occur with the ingestion of 20 to 60 mg/kg of elemental iron. Severe, potentially fatal, iron overdose symptoms occur with ingestions of greater than 60 mg/kg of elemental iron.

Stages of iron poisoning have been described. Early symptoms are of gastrointestinal irritation with nausea, vomiting, hematemesis, and melena. Significant fluid losses can occur. Later systemic poisoning manifestations include cardiovascular collapse and hepatotoxicity. The mainstays of therapy are as for any other life-threatening illness. Assess and establish a definitive airway and ventilations as necessary, establish intravenous access, and give judicious boluses (10 to 20 ml/kg) of normal saline for hypotension, do a glucose check, and transport the patient to medical care.

Hydrocarbons

Hydrocarbons are compounds made up principally of hydrogen and carbon atoms, with most, but not all, obtained from the distillation of petroleum. Hydrocarbons are found in a variety of products around the home, including cleaning and polishing agents, glues, spot removers, lighter fluids, paints, paint thinners and paint removers, other fuels, and as the diluent in pesticides.

Hydrocarbon Inhalation

The vast majority of intentional hydrocarbon inhalations are "recreational." The rich alveolar capillary network makes the lungs a highly efficient mechanism for providing a quick and inexpensive drug high. Unfortunately, long-term inhalant abuse can lead to permanent loss of mental function as evidenced by a variety of neuropathies, such as loss of hearing, loss of fine motor function, balance and equilibrium disorders, and occasionally death.

The modern epidemic of inhalation began in the early 1960s, when the first reports of glue sniffing and its consequences appeared. Within a short time, the number of agents being inhaled to get high had increased exponentially, as had the techniques for inhalation. Simple sniffing over the opening of a glue bottle did not provide an intense enough exposure for serious abusers. Pouring the volatile material onto a rag, placing it in a plastic bag, and holding the bag over one's face to breathe in the fumes proved far more efficient, producing a more intense high more quickly. Breathing fumes directly off a soaked rag or towel is termed huffing, whereas the use of a plastic bag is termed bagging. **Table 33-5 ▶** lists commonly abused inhaled compounds.

The primary goals when dealing with a patient who has inhaled hydrocarbons focus on removal from the noxious environment, giving high-concentration supplemental oxygen, and prompt transport to the appropriate facility.

Table 33-5	Compounds Commonly Abused by Sniffing and Bagging	
Example	**Sources**	**Signs and Symptoms of Toxicity**
Halogenated hydrocarbons		
1,1,1-Trichloroethane (methylchloroform)	Cleaning solvents, typewriter correction fluid, aerosol propellant	Eye irritation, light-headedness, incoordination, CNS depression, respiratory failure, cardiac arrhythmias, sudden death
Trichloroethylene	Degreasing solvent, aerosol propellant, rubber cement, plastic cement	Euphoria, anesthesia, weakness, vomiting, abdominal cramps, loss of coordination, neuropathy, blindness, cardiac arrhythmias, "degreaser's flush" (flushed face, neck, and shoulders when taken along with alcohol)
Tetrachloroethylene (perchloroethylene)	Solvent, dry cleaning agent	Drunken behaviour, dizziness, lightheadedness, difficulty walking, numbness, sleepiness, visual disturbances, memory impairment, eye irritation, cutaneous flushing, sudden death
Methylene chloride (dichloromethane)	Refrigerant, paint remover, aerosol propellant	Fatigue, weakness, chills, sleepiness, nausea, dizziness, incoordination, pulmonary edema
Carbon tetrachloride	Cleaning fluid	Narcosis, sudden death
Petroleum hydrocarbons		
Benzene	Cable cleaner, industrial solvents, rubber cement	Delirium, agitation, seizures, sudden death
Toluene	Spray paint, model and plastic cements, lacquer thinner	Narcosis, hallucinations, mania; impulsive, destructive, accident-prone behaviour; sudden death
Gasoline	Gas tank	Sudden death

Hydrocarbon Ingestion

Given the ready accessibility of hydrocarbons and the high likelihood that they might be mistaken for potable beverages, it is not surprising that hydrocarbon poisonings are common among children younger than 5 years. The potential hazards of swallowing a given hydrocarbon are directly related to the viscosity of the agent: the lower the viscosity, the higher the risk of pulmonary aspiration and other complications. The vast majority of hydrocarbon ingestions do *not* produce lasting damage. Patients who develop symptoms within a few minutes of ingestion are likely to have aspirated and need immediate attention.

Low-viscosity hydrocarbons (such as kerosene, naphtha, and toluene) can easily enter the lungs during swallowing. If the patient reports coughing, choking, or vomiting immediately after swallowing the substance, assume that aspiration has occurred. Similarly, any signs of respiratory distress—air hunger, intercostal retractions, tachypnea, cyanosis—must be considered danger signals.

Low viscosity also facilitates the uptake of a hydrocarbon by tissues of the CNS and, therefore, its anesthetic effects. At first, the patient may experience excitement and euphoria, followed by weakness, incoordination, drowsiness, confusion, and coma. Some petroleum products—notably gasoline—can produce hypoglycemia and cardiac arrhythmias, so you should always monitor the patient's ECG rhythm.

All symptomatic patients suspected of ingesting a hydrocarbon product—especially patients with respiratory symptoms—should be transported to an emergency department for further evaluation and care. Management should include the following measures:

- Remove contaminated clothing and decontaminate the patient, ideally before placing the patient in the ambulance.
- Establish and maintain the airway, and ensure adequate ventilation.
- Give high-flow supplemental oxygen.
- Establish vascular access.
- Continuously monitor the ECG rhythm; consider running a 12-lead.
- Administer sequential bolus infusions of normal saline to treat hypotension.
- Transport the patient to the most appropriate facility.

Toxic Alcohols

The form of alcohol consumed by humans in alcoholic beverages is ethyl alcohol (or ethanol). It is not conventionally recognized as a poison, even though it has many properties of a poison when ingested in sufficient quantities. Instead, "toxic alcohols," such as methyl alcohol and ethylene glycol Figure 33-14 ▶ , are generally considered alcohols manufactured for purposes other than ingestion and are metabolized by the body to acids via the enzyme alcohol dehydrogenase.

Ethylene Glycol

Ethylene glycol is a colourless, odourless liquid found in a variety of commercial products, including antifreeze, coolant, deicers, polishes, and paints. Because it has a slightly sweet taste, it may be ingested by children accidently. The lethal dose of ethylene glycol is estimated at 2 ml/kg, or as little as 150 ml in the average-size adult.

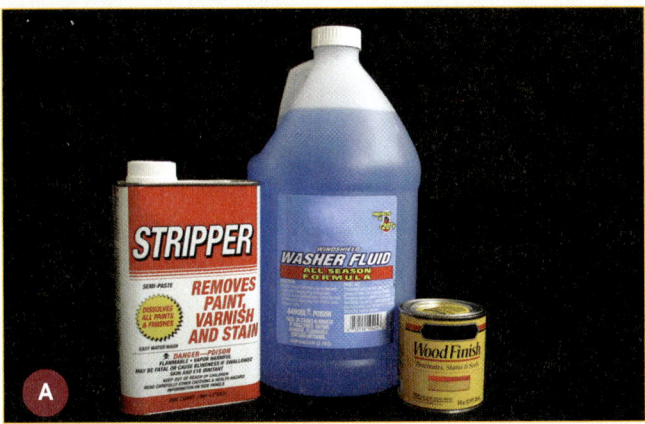

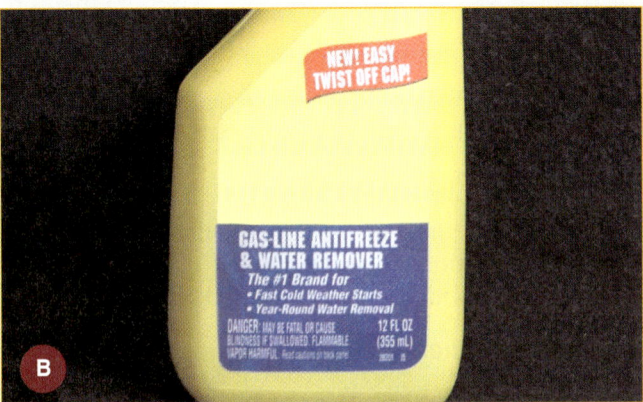

Figure 33-14 Methyl alcohol is present in paints, paint remover, windshield washer fluids, and varnishes (**A**) and in antifreeze and canned fuels (**B**).

Ethylene glycol is very water soluble. With oral intake, it is absorbed rapidly, with peak blood levels attained within 1 to 4 hours after ingestion. The liver and kidneys metabolize ethylene glycol into a number of toxic metabolites, including aldehydes, lactate, and oxalate. In turn, these metabolites produce metabolic acidosis. Metabolism of these toxins takes several hours. Toxic manifestations may not be evident for many hours after ingestion.

Early signs and symptoms of ethylene glycol intoxication are that of inebriation, because it is an alcohol. Later, as the acidic metabolites are formed, the patient can present with a decreased level of awareness, nausea and vomiting, cardiac dysrhythmias from hypocalcemia and acidosis, and tachypnea.

Methyl Alcohol

Methyl alcohol (also known as wood alcohol or methanol) is present in paints, paint remover, windshield washer fluids, varnishes, antifreeze, and canned fuels such as Sterno®. Methanol poisoning can occur after inadvertently drinking contaminated whiskey or moonshine. Methanol is commonly decanted into smaller containers and accidentally ingested because of look-alike properties to sports drinks. Methanol is a popular substitute for ethanol when ethanol is not available.

Methanol itself is not harmful. Rather, its metabolic breakdown products, formaldehyde and formic acid, are responsible for the characteristic signs and symptoms of methanol poisoning. A dose of as little as 30 ml (2 tablespoons) can produce toxicity and even death. Once ingested, methanol is quickly absorbed from the GI tract, with peak blood levels attained within 30 to 90 minutes. In mild toxicity, the half-life of methanol is 14 to 20 hours. As toxicity increases, the half-life increases to 24 to 30 hours. The liver eliminates 90% to 95% of the methanol.

You are the Paramedic Part 4

Now that you have identified the substance that Julie might have taken, you contact the hospital for medical guidance once you are situated in the back of the unit. Once you establish contact with the ED physician, you explain what you found on arrival, your physical assessment findings (including your suspicion of amitriptyline overdose), the interventions undertaken, and the current reassessment findings. The physician agrees with your assessment and orders the IV administration of 50 mEq of sodium bicarbonate.

Reassessment	Recording Time: 18 Minutes
Skin	Flushed, warm, and dry
Pulse	165 beats/min; regular and weak
ECG	Possible wide complex tachycardia
Blood pressure	88/56 mm Hg
Respirations	12 breaths/min via bag-valve-mask device
Spo₂	99% via bag-valve-mask device on 100% supplemental oxygen
Pupils	Dilated

7. Can the information you provide to hospital staff during your radio report contribute to a negative patient outcome?

8. Are there any potential complications that can arise during transport relative to the patient's condition?

As with ethylene glycol, the symptoms of methanol poisoning do not usually appear immediately but begin from 12 to 18 hours, occasionally up to 72 hours, after ingestion. As a consequence, the patient may not connect the symptoms to what he or she drank yesterday or several days ago. Patient complaints include nausea and vomiting (in almost 50% of cases), headache or vertigo, abdominal pain (often from pancreatitis), and blurred vision ("looks like a snowstorm") or, possibly, blindness. Physical examination findings may include altered mental status, ranging from drunken behaviour to seizures or coma; dilated pupils with sluggish or no reaction; hyperpnea and tachypnea from metabolic acidosis; and bradycardia and hypotension (very late signs).

Prehospital Care

Prehospital care for toxic alcohol exposure is primarily supportive. Establish and manage the airway, considering advanced airway placement, as needed. Establish vascular access. Place the patient on a cardiac monitor. Assess the blood glucose level, and administer glucose if the patient has hypoglycemia. Provide immediate transport to an appropriate facility.

Some EMS systems, particularly those carrying out interfacility patient transports, may have treatment protocols for management of patients with toxic alcohol ingestions. The goal of treatment is to overwhelm or inhibit the alcohol dehydrogenase enzyme responsible for converting the alcohols to toxic metabolites. Ethanol infusions, mixed in a dextrose solution, can overwhelm the enzyme and prevent production of the toxic metabolites. The enzyme can also be inhibited by fomepizole, a drug that specifically inhibits alcohol dehydrogenase from breaking down the toxic alcohols. Paramedics should determine whether their local or regional protocols include specific treatment of toxic alcohol ingestions.

Prescription Medications

An exhaustive discussion of all prescription medications is beyond the scope of this chapter. Cardiac, oral hypoglycemic, and psychiatric medications will be highlighted. Ingestion of the former two medications can be potentially lethal in small amounts, because many such drugs have narrow therapeutic indices. The latter is discussed because of the frequency that overdoses occur with these medications.

Cardiac Medications

The medications used to treat patients with cardiac and cardiac-related problems continue to increase in number and sophistication. The major classes of drugs used as part of these treatment regimens include antiarrhythmics, beta blockers, calcium channel blockers, and cardiac glycosides. Many patients take a combination of drugs, sometimes three or more, in attempts to control hypertension, ECG rhythm disturbances, or other problems.

Overdose with these medications leads to the "slow and low" toxidrome; most commonly these patients are bradycardic and hypotensive. Other signs and symptoms of overdose may include weakness or confusion, nausea and vomiting, headache, and dyspnea. As with all emergencies, ensure a patent airway, provide adequate ventilation, and administer high-flow supplemental oxygen.

Establish vascular access in case of overdose with these agents, because several therapeutic interventions and antidotes are available if the specific agent is identified. For hypotension, a fluid bolus is recommended first, as always. Atropine may be beneficial for a digoxin overdose that presents with bradycardia. Calcium gluconate may be of benefit for hypotension due to a calcium channel blocker. For both beta blocker and calcium channel toxicity, high-dose insulin euglycemia is now recommended. Glucagon is now controversial, because it can make hypotension worse. Among the most problematic cardiac medications in propensity to reach toxic levels are the cardiac glycosides (such as digoxin), which typically have very small therapeutic windows. For an overdose with these agents, digoxin immune Fab fragments are the antidote of choice. Antiarrhythmics of the sodium channel blocking family may respond to sodium bicarbonate boluses of 1–2 amps for the adult patient. Because of the complexity of cardiac drugs and the likelihood that the patient may be taking multiple cardiac and other medications, making contact with direct medical control to consult with a physician is prudent.

Psychiatric Medications
Lithium

Despite the major advances made in many areas of psychiatric medicine, lithium remains the cornerstone drug for the treatment of bipolar disorder. In 1949, lithium salts made their debut for the treatment of mania. Eventually, they were found to be much more efficacious for the treatment of bipolar disorder, and they retain their position as first-line treatment for this condition.

Lithium is almost completely absorbed in the GI tract roughly 8 hours after ingestion. Bioelimination occurs relatively slowly, with approximately 95% of the lithium eliminated in the urine; although two thirds of the lithium dose is excreted within 12 hours after ingestion, the remainder is excreted during the next 2 weeks.

Early signs and symptoms of lithium overdose include nausea, vomiting, hand tremors, excessive thirst, and slurred speech. Increased toxicity results in neurologic symptoms: ataxia, muscle weakness and incoordination, blurred vision, and hyperreflexia (twitching). Eventually, the patient may have seizures and become comatose.

Prehospital management of a patient suspected of a lithium overdose is mostly supportive. Establish and maintain the airway, inserting an advanced airway as needed. Give high-flow supplemental oxygen, and ensure vascular access. If the patient experiences hypotension, administer serial boluses of normal saline. Adequate hydration will improve lithium excretion. Maintain continuous ECG monitoring, being alert for AV blocks and ventricular arrhythmias. Finally, transport the patient to a health care facility. In some cases, dialysis may be indicated to enhance the elimination of lithium.

Selective Serotonin Reuptake Inhibitors

Selective serotonin reuptake inhibitors (SSRIs) have a far greater margin of safety than do many other antidepressants. In addition, SSRIs have far fewer anticholinergic and cardiac effects than the tricyclic antidepressants. Some SSRIs or other atypical antidepressants may cause seizures even in therapeutic doses. The most common manifestations of a pure SSRI overdose include gastrointestinal irritant effects and short-lived tonic–clonic seizures. Prehospital treatment is supportive:

- Establish and maintain the airway.
- Administer high-flow supplemental oxygen.
- Establish vascular access.
- Provide continuous ECG monitoring.
- Treat seizure activity with benzodiazepines per local protocol.
- Transport to the appropriate facility.

Serotonin syndrome is an idiosyncratic complication that occasionally occurs with antidepressant therapy. This condition is not limited to patients taking SSRIs, but also can occur when patients take any combination of drugs that increase central serotonin neurotransmission. Because a diagnostic laboratory test for serotonin syndrome is not available and the symptomatology is vague, at best, the ultimate diagnosis is based on clinical suspicion after other psychiatric or medical causes have been ruled out. The syndrome is characterized by vasomotor instability (ie, fever, diaphoresis, hypotension or hypertension, tachycardia), mental status changes, and musculoskeletal abnormalities, especially tremulousness. Rigidity has been described as well.

Tricyclic Antidepressants

In the past, tricyclic antidepressants (TCAs) were the drugs of choice to treat depression. Since the introduction of the safer SSRIs, fewer patients are on the TCAs for depression, although they may be making a therapeutic comeback. As well, there are other therapeutic uses for these medications, including neuropathic pain and enuresis.

Tricyclic antidepressants affect many different neurotransmitters. In low doses, TCAs are anticholinergics, causing dilated pupils and blurred vision, dry mouth, dry skin, fever, urinary retention, confusion and hallucinations, and sinus tachycardia. At higher doses, they have some sympathomimetic effects but eventually lead to depletion of noradrenaline. This contributes first to sinus tachycardia and then to bradycardia and hypotension. Tricyclics can stimulate GABA receptors and cause a decreased LOC. Finally, and most dangerous, in high doses tricyclic antidepressants cause membrane or sodium-blocking channel effects, leading to a widened QRS and ventricular arrhythmias and seizures. These manifestations may be precipitous. At one moment, the patient is somewhat drowsy but otherwise vital signs stable; the next moment the patient is seizing or arresting.

Prehospital management of patients with a TCA overdose includes the following measures:

- Maintain the airway. If the patient's mental status suddenly deteriorates, as is often the case, insert an advanced airway.
- Give high-flow supplemental oxygen.
- Establish vascular access.
- Provide continuous ECG monitoring (watch for widening of the QRS).
- Consult with direct medical control to consider sodium bicarbonate administration (if the QRS is widened).
- Treat hypotension with sequential boluses of normal saline.
- Assess blood glucose levels. Give $D_{50}W$ if the patient is hypoglycemic.
- Rule out head trauma as a possible cause of decreased mental status.
- Seizures require rapid control with benzodiazepines and/or intubation and paralysis. Cardiac arrhythmias often follow.
- Transport to the nearest appropriate facility.

Oral Hypoglycemics

Adult-onset, or type 2, diabetes is treated with a variety of oral medications that act in different ways to achieve glucose control. Those that act to increase insulin release from the pancreas will cause symptomatic hypoglycemia and generally have a prolonged duration of action. These include the sulfonylureas and meglitinides. If a toddler ingested a single tablet of either of these two classifications of oral hypoglycemics, death from hypoglycemia could result. The standard treatment of symptomatic hypoglycemia includes intravenous access, administration of exogenous dextrose, and monitoring until delivery of the patient at the medical facility. In the hospital, an antidote, octreotide, exists to limit the recurrence of hypoglycemia.

■ Occupational and Environmental Toxins

Bites and Stings

Injected poisons usually gain access to the body as the result of stings or bites from a variety of creatures. This section considers the ill effects that may result from unfriendly encounters with creatures from the land, air, and sea.

Arthropod Bites and Stings

If sheer numbers were the sole criterion determining such things, arthropods would rule the world. The phylum Arthropoda includes at least 1.5 million species of "joint-footed" animals, ranging from the lobster to the mite. The classes of arthropods of most medical importance, because of their ability to inject venom, are the arachnids (including spiders, scorpions, and ticks), Chilopoda (centipedes), and insects (including the Hymenoptera).

Scorpion Stings

Scorpions are not native to Canada, although, as with other exotic creatures, it is possible for envenomations to occur when these animals are imported into Canada as unexpected passengers in personal luggage from the Caribbean or Mexico or as hitchhikers on produce from endemic countries. Usually pain relief is the issue. Contact your provincial Poison Centre for specific management guidelines.

Spider Bites

There are an estimated 34,000 species of spiders worldwide. All of these carnivores can bite; most are venomous, using their venom to subdue their prey. The amount of venom injected into a human, proportional to the body size of a human, is usually inconsequential. No spiders native to Canada have venom potent enough to cause medical illness. This is not to say that occasionally an allergic manifestation or local wound infection might not develop. As well, there are incidences where medically significant spiders from other countries arrive in Canada in shipments of imported produce or furniture. A discussion of all venomous spiders in the world is beyond the scope of this text.

Prehospital care of a spider bite victim includes attention to the airway and breathing, giving high-flow oxygen as needed, and establishing intravenous access. If there is no evidence of allergic or anaphylactic manifestations, analgesia may be necessary, because some bites from exotic spiders are extremely painful. Deaths, even from bites of extremely potent exotic spiders, is not instantaneous, and often results as a complication of initial manifestations. Transport the patient to the hospital for a medical assessment.

Hymenoptera Stings

The Hymenoptera family of insects includes bees, wasps, hornets, yellow jackets, and ants **Figure 33-15 ▼**. Collectively, they kill more people each year than any other venomous animals, including snakes. Death from a Hymenoptera sting usually occurs from anaphylaxis, which is covered in detail in Chapter 30.

The diagnosis of a bee sting is usually not difficult—indeed, in most cases, the patient will have already made the diagnosis. There is almost always an immediate local reaction consisting of pain (sometimes extreme), redness and swelling,

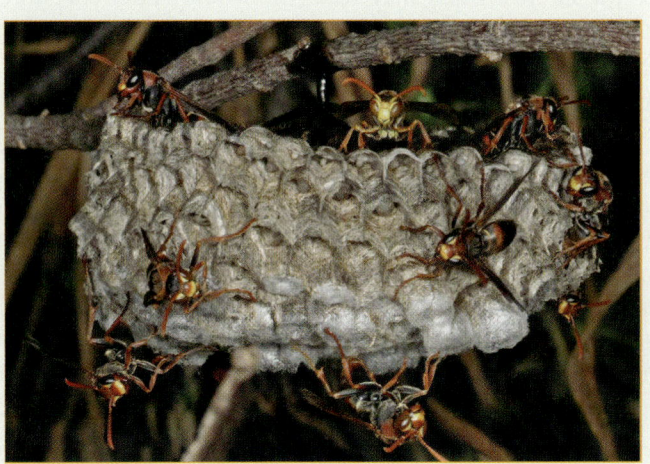

Figure 33-15 Hymenoptera stings include those from bees, wasps, hornets, yellow jackets, and ants.

and sometimes itching at the site of the sting. Honeybees sting once, usually leaving the barbed stinger and the venom sac attached to the patient's skin. By comparison, wasps, hornets, yellow jackets, and fire ants can sting repeatedly until they are chased away or the patient is removed.

If the patient has no history of allergy to bee stings and does not have a systemic reaction, transport to the hospital is usually unnecessary. When this decision is made, advise the patient of the warning signs of anaphylaxis and the urgency of calling 9-1-1 in such an event. Instruct the patient to have the wound checked by a doctor if it does not improve markedly within 24 hours. Bee stings, especially those to the extremities, often become infected and require antibiotic treatment.

Treatment of a Hymenoptera sting focuses primarily on pain relief and minimization of the risk of infection. First, determine whether the stinger and venom sac are still attached to the skin. If so, use a scalpel blade to gently scrape the stinger and venom sac from the wound. Do not try to pluck the stinger out with tweezers or forceps. If you squeeze the stinger or the venom sac, you will pump more venom into the wound!

After removing the stinger, clean the wound thoroughly with soap and water or an antiseptic solution such as povidone-iodine. Apply cold packs to the site for pain relief.

Snakebites

Although venomous snakes cause an estimated 3 million bites and 150,000 deaths worldwide each year, as there are only three species of such snakes in Canada, a snakebite from a native species is a rare poisoning. As mentioned earlier, an underground zoo exists in every part of Canada, where enthusiasts may have venomous snakes in their personal collections. As envenomations are singularly uncommon, a call to the provincial Poison Centre should be made whenever encountering such a patient.

Pit Vipers

The three species of venomous snakes native to Canada are all of the Crotalid family, or pit vipers. The heads of all Canadian pit vipers are triangular, resembling an arrowhead. Just beneath the eyes on either side is an indentation or pit, which is a heat-sensing organ that helps the snake locate its prey **Figure 33-16 ▶**. North American pit vipers also have vertical pupils (most other snakes have round pupils). These physical characteristics cannot be assumed to be similar to exotic snakes. Their long, erectile fangs are used to puncture the skin, leaving a distinctive mark.

Pit vipers are not naturally aggressive, but will attack in self-defence or when surprised, such as when a hiker accidentally steps on a snake. A variable amount of venom, ranging from no venom to a potentially lethal dose, might be injected. This venom is composed of a mixture of metalloenzymes that cause local tissue damage, hemolysis, increased permeability of the vasculature, coagulopathy, and neuromuscular dysfunction.

One of every four pit viper bites is "dry"; that is, no venom is injected. This determination cannot be made in the prehospital setting. Even without envenomation, the most

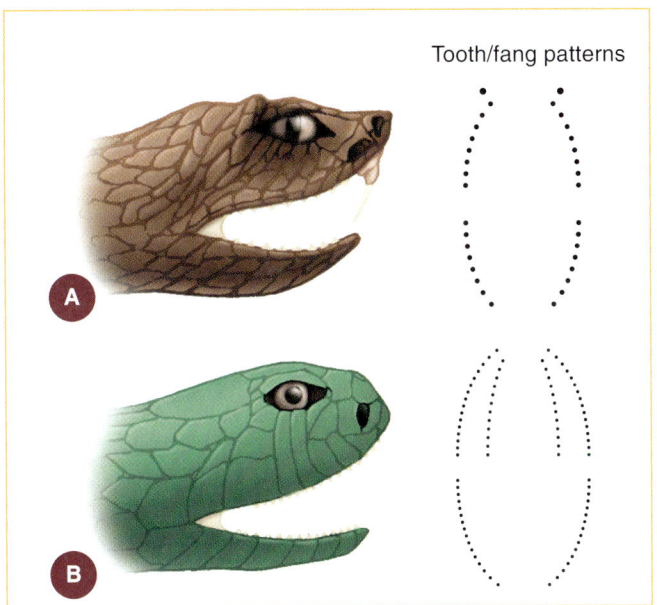

Tooth/fang patterns

Figure 33-16 Characteristics of pit vipers and nonpoisonous snakes. **A.** Pit vipers have vertical pupils, a pit between the eye and the nostril, a single row of teeth, and two erectile fangs. **B.** Nonpoisonous snakes have round pupils and often a double row of upper teeth; they do not leave fang marks.

common initial symptoms are fang marks and localized pain. Signs and symptoms of envenomation include a metallic taste in the mouth, nausea and vomiting, tachycardia, hypotension, tachypnea, and edema developing around the area of the bite.

Prehospital care of the bitten patient includes attention to the airway, breathing, and circulation, as with any patient. Give high-flow supplemental oxygen, establish vascular access, and give a fluid bolus of normal saline if the patient is hypotensive. Keep the patient calm, supine, and motionless to decrease venom spread and absorption. Immobilize the extremity with the bite in a neutral position. Do *not* apply constricting bands. Do not apply ice. Finally, begin immediate transport to a medical facility. Antivenin does exist for the treatment of Crotalid bites when envenomation has occurred.

Tick Bites

Ticks are blood-sucking arthropods found around the world, often in rural, wooded areas **Figure 33-17** ▾. Ordinarily, tick bites are not a medical emergency, but they are of concern because ticks serve as disease vectors. Bacteria, viruses, and protozoa can be transmitted via a tick bite, and they are linked to a variety of serious illnesses. With the exception of Lyme disease, these are rarely seen in Canada.

In the unlikely event that you are called to a patient with a tick bite, the principal treatment is careful removal of the tick. Ticks attach themselves tenaciously to their victims using their mouth parts and a cement-like adhesive. If you try to pull the tick away from the skin, the mouth parts may remain embedded. To remove the tick, after putting on gloves, use a curved forceps to grasp the tick by the head as close to the skin as possible and pull straight upward using steady gentle traction. Use even pressure as you pull, and avoid twisting or jerking the tick. Do not squeeze or crush the tick's body. Dispose of the tick in a container of alcohol.

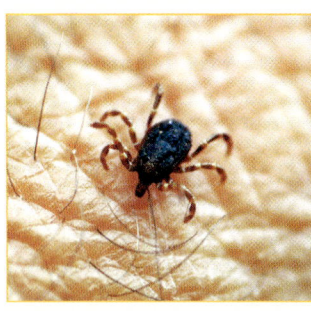

Figure 33-17 Ticks typically attach themselves directly to the skin.

Once you have removed the tick, wash the area around the bite with soap and water. There is no reason to transport the patient if he or she remains asymptomatic. In case of tick paralysis, transport the patient with spinal motion restriction to an appropriate facility.

You are the Paramedic Summary

1. What are your priorities at this point?

Safety is the main priority at all times. In this scenario, crowd control might be a factor. Once you are confident of scene safety, turn your attention to addressing the patient's ABCs. Additional priorities include obtaining as much pertinent information as possible and appointing someone to contact the patient's parents or caregivers.

2. What information do you need to obtain?

This scenario emphasizes the need to obtain as much information related to SAMPLE as possible. Because the patient cannot provide information, your sources will be her friends and the coach. Patients with altered mental status can have a wide variety of problems, and SAMPLE will be one of the keys to providing successful treatment.

3. What are some potential differential diagnoses?

Although your rapid trauma survey did not reveal life-threatening injuries, you cannot rule out a head injury as the cause of Julie's altered mental status. Based on the information you have at this point, other differential diagnoses include overdose, hypoglycemia, and infection.

4. Which interventions should you consider at this point, if any?

By now, you should have delegated the role of cervical spine immobilization. The patient is already receiving supplemental oxygen. While you perform a detailed physical assessment, you can ask your partner to obtain a glucose level and apply the cardiac monitor. Until you obtain more information, no further interventions are needed.

5. Given the current situation, should you consider treating the patient treating on the scene, or continuing treatment on the way to the hospital?

In this case, it is best to package the patient and continue treatment on the way to the hospital. If the patient's condition continues to deteriorate, the optimal place for treatment to be given would be the ED.

6. How should your patient management progress?

Maintenance of the ABCs should take priority. Now that you have ruled out trauma as a potential MOI, the patient no longer requires cervical spine immobilization. Prehospital management for a tricyclic antidepressant overdose such as amitryptalline is administration of sodium bicarbonate. Depending on your department's protocol, you might have to contact the receiving hospital for orders. Remember to bring the medication bottle to the hospital. Also, keep a watchful eye on the cardiac monitor for the development of ventricular rhythms associated with the drug's toxicity.

7. Can the information you provide to the hospital staff during your radio report contribute to a negative patient outcome?

Absolutely! Not providing the proper information to the hospital staff can lead to mistreatment of your patient. In this case, not making the ED staff aware of the ingestion of amitriptyline, including the dose and number of pills taken, might delay life-saving treatment or lead to the administration of incorrect treatment that produces unwanted complications, including death. You are the eyes and ears of the ED physician—it is your responsibility to paint an accurate picture that enables the physician to make proper treatment decisions.

8. Are there any potential complications that can arise during transport relative to the patient's condition?

Tricyclic antidepressants are extremely toxic medications. Life-threatening events potentially include the development of ventricular arrhythmias, seizures, and pulmonary edema. Sound knowledge of the effects of tricyclic antidepressants and good assessment skills are paramount to the delivery of effective prehospital care.

Prep Kit

Ready for Review

- Toxicologic emergencies usually fall under one of two general headings: intentional and unintentional.
- Given the variety of illicit drugs coupled with the continued growth of licit drugs, even the most well-read veteran paramedic may find it difficult to stay current with the myriad drugs sold in the streets today. For this reason, Poison Centres may be an indispensable aid.
- The four primary methods whereby a toxin commonly enters the body are ingestion, inhalation, injection, and absorption.
- Although the sheer number of substances of abuse may seem daunting, the good news is that many drugs, on entering the body, produce similar signs and symptoms.
- Human beings have a long history of abusing drugs and alcohol. With the passing of time, the physiologic and societal effects of alcohol abuse have become well known and thoroughly documented. Unfortunately, the area of medicine dealing with drugs of abuse is challenging because of uncertainty about the prevalence of the problem and the continual evolution of the substances themselves.
- Alcohol is the most widely abused drug in Canada.
- Generally, patients with toxicologic emergencies are considered medical patients, although toxicologic emergencies may lead to trauma, too.
- From a management perspective, ALS care builds on the basics:
  - Ensure the scene is safe for access and egress, paying careful attention to the possibility of exposure to residual toxin depending on the agent suspected.
  - Maintain the airway.
  - Ensure that breathing is adequate.
  - Ensure that circulation isn't compromised (by hypoperfusion or arrhythmia).
  - Administer high-concentration supplemental oxygen.
  - Establish vascular access.
  - Be prepared to manage shock, coma, seizures, and arrhythmias.
  - Transport the patient as soon as possible. Place the patient in the left lateral recumbent position if there is any risk of vomiting to reduce the risk of aspiration.

Vital Vocabulary

alcoholism A state of physical and psychological addiction to ethanol.

amphetamines A class of drugs that increase alertness and excitation (that is, stimulants); includes methamphetamine (crank or ice), methylenedioxyamphetamine (MDA, Adam), and methylenedioxymethamphetamine (MDMA, Eve, ecstasy).

antagonist Something that counteracts the action of something else; in relation to drugs, a drug that is an antagonist has an affinity for a cell receptor and, by binding to it, the cell is prevented from responding.

barbiturates Potent sedative-hypnotics historically used as sleep aids, antianxiety drugs, and as part of the regimen for seizure control.

benzodiazepines The family of sedative-hypnotics most commonly used to treat anxiety, seizures, and alcohol withdrawal.

caustics Chemicals that are acids or alkalis; cause direct chemical injury to the tissues they contact.

delirium tremens (DTs) A severe withdrawal syndrome seen in people with alcoholism who are deprived of ethyl alcohol; characterized by restlessness, fever, sweating, disorientation, agitation, and seizures; can be fatal if untreated.

drug abuse Any use of drugs that causes physical, psychological, economic, legal, or social harm to the user or others affected by the user's behaviour.

drug addiction A chronic disorder characterized by the compulsive use of a substance that results in physical, psychological, or social harm to the user who continues to use the substance despite the harm.

habituation The situation in which there is a physical tolerance and psychological dependence on a drug or drugs.

hallucinogen An agent that produces false perceptions in any one of the five senses.

hydrocarbons Compounds made up principally of hydrogen and carbon atoms, mostly obtained from the distillation of petroleum.

illicit In relation to drugs, illegal drugs such as marijuana, cocaine, and LSD.

licit In relation to drugs, legalized drugs such as coffee, alcohol, and tobacco.

lithium The cornerstone drug for the treatment of bipolar disorder.

marijuana The dried leaves and flower buds of the *Cannabis sativa* plant that are smoked to achieve a high.

methamphetamine A drug in the amphetamine family.

narcotic The generic term for opiates and opioids, drugs that act as a CNS depressant and produce insensibility or stupor.

opiate Various alkaloids derived from the opium or poppy plant.

opioid A synthetic narcotic not derived from opium.

organophosphates A class of chemical found in many insecticides used in agriculture and in the home. Capable of irreversibly binding to acetylcholinesterase and producing the cholinergic toxidrome.

physical dependence A physiologic state of adaptation to a drug, usually characterized by tolerance to the drug's effects and a withdrawal syndrome if use of the drug is stopped, especially abruptly.

potentiation Enhancement of the effect of one drug by another drug.

psychological dependence The emotional state of craving a drug to maintain a feeling of well-being.

sedative-hypnotic A drug used to reduce anxiety, calm agitated patients, and help produce drowsiness and sleep (CNS depressants).

selective serotonin reuptake inhibitors (SSRIs) A class of antidepressants that inhibit the reuptake of serotonin.

serotonin syndrome An idiosyncratic complication that occurs with antidepressant therapy in which patients have lower extremity muscle rigidity, confusion or disorientation, and/or agitation.

synergism The action of two substances such as drugs, in which the *total effects are greater than the sum of the independent effects* of the two substances.

tolerance Physiologic adaptation to the effects of a drug such that increasingly larger doses of the drug are required to achieve the same effect.

toxidrome The constellation of signs and symptoms attributable to the effects of a class of substances.

tricyclic antidepressants (TCAs) A group of drugs used to treat severe depression and manage pain; minimal dosing errors can cause toxic results.

withdrawal syndrome A predictable set of signs and symptoms, usually involving altered central nervous system activity, that occurs after the abrupt cessation of a drug or after rapidly decreasing the usual dosage of a drug.

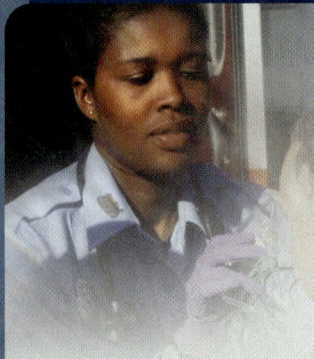

Assessment in Action

You and your partner have arrived on the scene of a reported diabetic emergency. When you arrive at the patient's side, you see a 50-year-old man who seems to be unconscious on the floor. The patient's wife states that her husband had been at work all day. When he arrived at home, he stated he had a very bad headache and then collapsed to the floor. The wife confirms that the patient has type 1 diabetes.

As you and your partner begin your assessment, you notice that he is drooling severely, is diaphoretic, and has been incontinent. You direct your partner to obtain a blood glucose level, which comes back as 10 mmol/l. You were assuming that this call was for a diabetic emergency, but now that does not seem to be the case. As you return to your assessment, the patient vomits a large amount, which has a distinct chemical smell. You suction the patient aggressively and complete airway management measures. When you ask the wife what the patient may have been around at work, she says that her husband works at a landscaping business.

1. **What are the two types of toxicologic emergencies?**
   A. Licit and illicit
   B. Prescribed and OTC
   C. Intentional and unintentional
   D. Drug or poison

2. **The patient in this scenario may be experiencing signs and symptoms of which toxidrome?**
   A. Stimulant
   B. Narcotic
   C. Sedative-hypnotic
   D. Cholinergic

3. **You determine through further questioning that the patient was using some kind of chemical at work, but the wife does not know what it was. What is your primary concern at this point in your assessment?**
   A. Determine what your crew and bystanders have potentially been exposed to.
   B. Move the patient quickly to your ambulance and transport immediately.
   C. Obtain IV access and administer naloxone per protocol.
   D. Determine the potential for the patient to become violent.

4. **A patient with salivation and lacrimation may have been exposed to:**
   A. carbon monoxide.
   B. organophosphates.
   C. barbiturates.
   D. chlorine.

5. **Organophosphates exert their toxic effects on which body system?**
   A. Integumentary
   B. Cardiac
   C. Nervous
   D. Endocrine

6. **The approach to a patient with organophosphate poisoning should start with:**
   A. decontamination and removal of contaminated items.
   B. administering atropine 2.0 mg IV push immediately.
   C. contacting law enforcement personnel to prevent violence.
   D. obtaining an oxygen saturation level on your patient.

Challenging Question

7. **Given that your crew and the patient's wife have potentially been contaminated through contact with the patient's clothing and emesis, which component becomes the most important part of decontamination—the patient or everyone else in the room?**

Points to Ponder

You and your partner are called to a single-family residence near a college campus. When you arrive in front of the residence, you notice a large number of college-age people gathered around someone lying supine on the front lawn. A law enforcement officer arrives on the scene at the same time you do. You approach the patient and find a female who looks to be in her late teens or early 20s. You hear snoring respirations and notice that the patient is covered in emesis. As your partner is rolling the patient to her side and clearing her airway, you ask some of the bystanders what happened. They back away, saying, "We were just having a party, and she wasn't feeling good so we brought her outside." Your partner reports that the patient is breathing and responds to deep painful stimuli but does not have a gag reflex.

What is your first treatment priority? Can you immediately assume that the signs and symptoms you are seeing are caused by alcohol ingestion? What other assessment points should you consider?

Issues: Assessing a Potential Alcohol Overdose, Obtaining Information From Bystanders.

34 Hematologic Emergencies

Competency Areas

Area 4: Assessment and Diagnostics

4.3.n   Conduct multisystem assessment and interpret findings.

Appendix 4: Pathophysiology

J.   **Multisystem Diseases and Injuries**
Hematologic Disorders: Anemia
Hematologic Disorders: Bleeding disorders
Hematologic Disorders: Leukemia
Hematologic Disorders: Lymphomas (Hodgkins, non-Hodgkins)
Hematologic Disorders: Multiple myeloma
Hematologic Disorders: Sickle cell disease

Introduction

Hematologic emergencies are not common in most EMS systems. Hematologic disorders can be complex, difficult to assess, and challenging to treat in the out-of-hospital setting. Although you may be able to provide only limited interventions, your actions may not only offer support, but actually save the patient's life. As a paramedic, you should have a basic understanding of the hematopoietic system (the blood components and the organs involved in their development and production) and hematologic disorders, and you should know how to respond to these kinds of emergencies appropriately.

Anatomy and Physiology

Blood and Plasma

Blood is "the fluid of life": Without it, we would not be able to live. Blood performs the following functions:

- **Respiratory function.** Transports oxygen from the lungs to the tissues and carbon dioxide from the tissues to the lungs
- **Nutritional function.** Carries nutrients (glucose, proteins, and fats) from the digestive tract to cells throughout the body
- **Excretory function.** Ferries the waste products of metabolism from the cells where they are produced to the excretory organs
- **Regulatory function.** Transports hormones to their target organs and transmits excess internal heat to the surface of the body to be dissipated
- **Defensive function.** Carries defensive cells and antibodies, which protect the body against foreign organisms

Blood is made up of two main components: plasma and formed elements (cells). Plasma is essentially 92% water and 6% to 7% proteins; the remainder consists of a variety of other elements (including electrolytes, clotting factors, glucose). Plasma accounts for 55% of the total blood volume. It has a specific gravity of around 1.03. Specific gravity is a substance's weight relative to that of water. Anything with a specific gravity greater than 1.0 is "heavier" than water, and anything with a specific gravity less than 1.0 is "lighter."

The formed elements account for 45% of the total blood volume. These elements include red blood cells (RBCs) or erythrocytes, white blood cells (WBCs) or leukocytes, and platelets or thrombocytes   **Figure 34-1 ▾** . Most of these elements (99%) are RBCs.

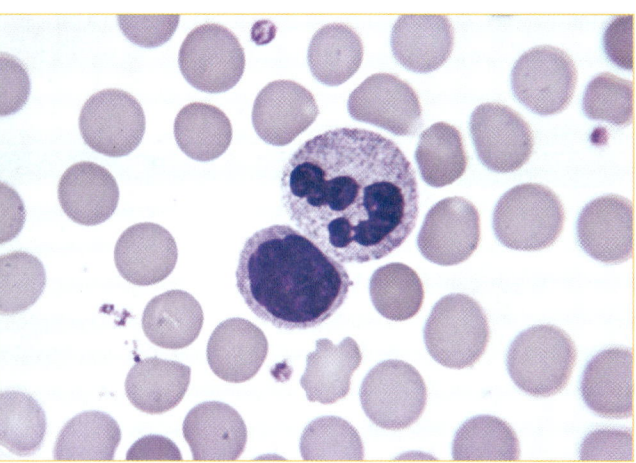

Figure 34-1 The components of blood include RBCs, WBCs, platelets, and plasma.

You are the Paramedic Part 1

It is early evening, and you have just been dispatched to 1355 Northwest Lane for a 30-year-old man complaining of shortness of breath and severe abdominal pain. The fire department's first responders have also responded and can provide additional assistance.

When you arrive, you are greeted at the front door by a concerned family member. The woman points to the bedroom and says, "He's in there! He's having another attack!" When you enter the bedroom, you see an African-American man sitting on the edge of the bed holding his stomach.

Initial Assessment	Recording Time: 0 Minutes
Appearance	Eyes open with pained expression
Level of consciousness	A (Alert to person, place, and day)
Airway	Patent
Breathing	Fast, laboured, and shallow
Circulation	Weak, fast radial pulse; diaphoretic skin

1. What, if anything, about his appearance gives you cause for concern?
2. What information do you already have at your disposal?

RBCs are derived from stem cells within the bone marrow. RBC production is stimulated by erythropoietin, a protein produced by the kidneys in response to circulatory need. RBC production will not be able to keep up with demand if the kidneys fail to produce sufficient erythropoietin, such as in patients with chronic renal failure. RBCs may take as long as 5 days to mature and have an average life of about 4 months. Their specific gravity is approximately 1.09. Within the RBCs, iron-rich hemoglobin is responsible for carrying oxygen to the tissues. Oxygen attached to hemoglobin gives blood its characteristic red colour, although many other factors can change the colour of blood (such as carbon monoxide poisoning).

Three laboratory tests are commonly performed on blood: RBC count, hemoglobin level, and hematocrit. The RBC count measures the number of RBCs in a sample of blood. The hemoglobin level identifies the concentration of hemoglobin found within the RBCs. The hematocrit is the proportion of blood volume that is composed of red blood cells. The hematocrit can be estimated as three times the hemoglobin level (measured in g/l),

and the RBC count can be estimated as one third the hemoglobin level. **Table 34-1 ▼** describes these tests in more detail.

WBCs, which are larger than RBCs, provide the body with immunity against "foreign invaders." They are derived from the stem cells, or cells that develop into other types of cells in the body. Several types of WBCs exist, each of which performs a specific task in relation to maintaining the immune system.

At the Scene

Platelets help form the initial plug following vascular injury. The clotting proteins that interact with platelets then toughen and complete the blood clot.

Platelets are the smallest of the formed elements and are responsible for the clotting of the blood. (The coagulation process or hemostasis is described in more detail in Chapter 6.)

Table 34-1	RBC and WBC Tests		
Name	**Normal Values**	**Conditions Associated With Low Readings**	**Conditions Associated With High Readings**
Complete Blood Count Test			
RBC count	4.5–5.8×10^{12}/l adult 3.3–5.5×10^{12}/l child	Anemia, hemorrhage, certain leukemias, overhydration, chronic infections	Polycythemia, cardiovascular disease, hemoconcentration, dehydration
Hemoglobin (Hgb)	12.0–16.0 g/l female 14.0–18.0 g/l male 10.7–17.1 g/l child	Anemia, hyperthyroidism, liver disease, hemorrhage, hemolytic reactions	COPD, CHF, polycythemia, high altitude sickness
Hematocrit (HCT)	0.36–0.46 female 0.41–0.53 male 0.32–0.55 child	As above, including leukemia, lupus, endocarditis, rheumatic fever, nutritional disorders	Polycythemia and usually anything that produces severe dehydration
WBC Count and Differential			
WBC count	4.5–11.0×10^9/l adult 4.5–15.0×10^9/l child 9.4–34.0×10^9/l infant	Viral infections, bone marrow diseases or disorders, leukemia, radiation, late-stage AIDS, severe sepsis	Viral and bacterial infections, hemorrhage, traumatic tissue injuries, leukemia, cigarette smoking
Neutrophils (segmented and unsegmented)	0.40–0.70*	Leukemia, infections, rheumatoid arthritis, vitamin B12 deficiency, enlarged spleen	Bacterial infections, tissue breakdown, hemolytic reactions, tumours, MI, surgical stress, and cancer
Basophils (also known as mast cells)	0–0.3*	Allergic reactions, hyperthyroidism, MI, bleeding ulcers, stress	Certain leukemias, inflammations, allergy, polycythemia, hemolytic anemia
Eosinophils	0–0.8*	Mononucleosis, CHF, Cushing's disease	Addison's disease, tumours, skin infections, allergies
Lymphocytes	0.22–0.44*	Hodgkin's disease, burns, trauma, lupus, Cushing's disease, immunodeficiency states	Numerous bacterial and viral infections, hepatitis, leukemia, toxoplasmosis, Graves' disease
Monocytes	0.04–0.11*	Steroid use, infections, rheumatoid arthritis, HIV	Numerous bacterial and parasitic infections, recovery of acute infections, TB, hematologic disorders
Thrombocytes (platelets)	150–350×10^9/µl	Thrombocytopenia, certain cancers, certain leukemias, sickle cell disease, systemic lupus erythematosus	Pulmonary embolism, polycythemia, acute hemorrhage, metastatic cancer, surgical stress

COPD indicates chronic obstructive pulmonary disease; CHF, congestive heart failure; MI, myocardial infarction; and TB, tuberculosis.
*Proportion of the total WBC count.

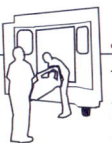

At the Scene

To check whether your patient might have a low RBC count, look for conjunctival pailor. If present, the hematocrit (or RBC count) may be low! This test works only on normal-temperature skin.

Approximately two thirds of the platelets circulate throughout the blood; the rest are stored in the spleen. Platelets are also derived from stem cells. They have an average life span of up to 11 days.

Blood-Forming Organs and RBC Production

Although many parts and organs of the human body can alter or affect the hematologic system, the major players are the bone marrow, liver, and spleen **Figure 34-2 ▾**.

The bone marrow is the primary site for cell production within the human body. Bone marrow may be found in most of the long bones plus the pelvis, skull, and vertebrae.

The liver produces the clotting factors found in the blood. The liver filters the blood, removing toxins, and is essential to normal metabolism and homeostasis. As old RBCs enter the liver, they are broken down into bile. The liver is a highly vascular organ that also stores some blood within itself.

At the Scene

Fibrinolytic therapy, also known as "clot busters," is given when an artery supplying blood to a vital organ (ie, heart, brain, or lung) is blocked by a clot. Acute myocardial infarction, acute ischemic stroke, and large pulmonary embolism are examples of when fibrinolytic therapy is given. These agents activate the body's fibrinolytic system, resulting in clot breakdown, also known as lysis. Patients given a fibrinolytic therapy must be monitored closely, because fibrinolysis may cause excess bleeding.

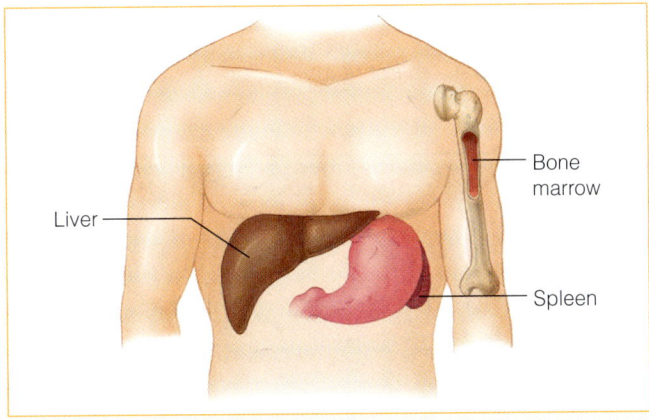

Figure 34-2 The bone marrow, liver, and spleen are the main components of the body related to the blood system.

The spleen is also quite vascular. It is involved with the filtering and breakdown of erythrocytes, assists with the production of lymphocytes, and has an important role in providing homeostasis and infection control. The spleen stores about one third of the platelets. If the spleen is removed, the platelets return to the blood.

Inflammatory Response

Many of the body's proteins are antigens, substances capable of eliciting an immune response. Typically, the body is tolerant to its own antigens and does not initiate a reaction against these proteins (see Chapter 6). However, when the body is exposed to something it cannot identify as its own (ie, from invading bacteria or viruses), it produces antibodies to counteract the foreign or unidentified antigen. For unknown reasons, patients with an autoimmune disorder may develop a reaction and produce antibodies to their own proteins.

The Immune System

The primary component of the immune system is the WBCs. Like other blood cells, WBCs are produced in the bone marrow. A small number of WBCs are always circulating in the bloodstream, but a larger reserve is ready to spring into action whenever infectious-type material is detected in the blood. Specific laboratory values relating to WBCs and measurement of essential subcomponents—namely, neutrophils, lymphocytes, basophils, and eosinophils—can provide valuable information about the status of the immune system (see Table 34-1).

The baseline WBC count is measured when the body is in a normal state (during times of no known infection or inflammation). The normal range is 4.5 to $11.0 \times 10^9/l$ cells.

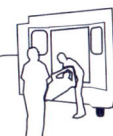

At the Scene

The life cycle of a WBC begins when the bone marrow releases a type of cell called granulocytes, which remain in the circulation for 6 to 12 hours. If the cells travel to tissues, they live for a few more days. Otherwise, WBCs are recycled by the reticuloendothelial system, as are RBCs.

Blood Classifications

To ensure compatibility and prevent medical problems during blood component replacement, blood type classifications have been developed. In the ABO system, the RBC classification types are "O," "A," "B," and "AB"; they indicate which antigens are found in the plasma membrane **Table 34-2 ▸**.

Blood contains a secondary antigen, known as the Rh antigen (the name signifies that the antigen was first found in the Rhesus monkey). Approximately 85% to 90% of the population have this antigen. Thus, if an individual has the blood type A-positive (A+), the blood contains the Rh antigen.

Some patients may be receiving or have previously received a blood transfusion. It is important to determine a

Table 34-2	Blood Types		
Blood Type	**ABO Antigens**	**ABO Antibodies**	**Acceptable Blood Donor Types**
A	A	Anti-B	A, O
B	B	Anti-A	B, O
AB	A, B	None	A, B, AB, O
O	None	Anti-A Anti-B	O

patient's blood type and the type of blood received. When a patient receives blood or plasma that matches his or her classification (A+ into A+) or the universal donor blood type (O), problems rarely arise. However, if a patient receives a blood type that is different than his or her own—for example, a patient with type A receives type B—a transfusion reaction will occur due to ABO incompatibility. Also, if a patient with A–blood receives an A+ transfusion, a transfusion reaction could occur, but a reaction due to Rh incompatibility is not as common. One exception to this is in pregnant women. Rh-negative women who develop antibodies because they were exposed to Rh-positive blood may have problems with pregnancy if they conceive a baby who is Rh positive. In such instances, the mother's antibodies attack the baby's blood cells in the womb, causing severe life-threatening fetal anemia. This is why young women are typically given O-negative blood (universal donor) in emergent situations when full blood matching is not possible. Blood reactions are similar to an anaphylactic reaction—they occur rapidly and can cause severe circulatory collapse and even death. When a patient receives a blood transfusion, it is important to monitor the patient very closely for the first 30 to 60 minutes because transfusion reactions typically begin within this time frame.

Epidemiology

Anemia

Anemia is defined as a hemoglobin or erythrocyte level that is lower than normal **Figure 34-3 ▸**. Usually it is associated with some type of underlying disease process. Anemia may also result from blood loss or a decrease in production or increase in destruction of erythrocytes. Finally, anemia may be an outcome of a preexisting hemolytic disorder—a disorder related to the breakdown of RBCs.

Iron Deficiency Anemia

Iron deficiency anemia, the most common type of anemia, affects 50 of 1,000 men and 140 of 1,000 women. Typical causes include gastrointestinal blood loss, blood loss from menstrual bleeding (a common cause of anemia in women), and blood loss due to frequent donations or diagnostic tests for patients hospitalized for long periods.

Hematologic Disorders

Hemolytic disorders can be caused by genetic (hereditary) problems within the RBC. Some diseases affect the production of hemoglobin, such as thalassemia, and some affect the

You are the Paramedic Part 2

When you introduce yourself, the patient tells you his name and that he has sickle cell anemia. He reports that he has had similar episodes in the past and is afraid he is having another "flare-up." The patient looks frightened and tells you his grandfather died of sickle cell anemia at a relatively young age. You apply supplemental oxygen at 15 l/min via nonrebreathing mask. Your assessment reveals the following:

Vital Signs	Recording Time: 5 Minutes
Level of consciousness	Alert, with a Glasgow Coma Scale score of 15
Skin	Diaphoretic and feverish with pale mucous membranes
Pulse	Radial pulse, 112 beats/min, weak and regular
Blood pressure	108/46 mm Hg
Respirations	28 breaths/min and shallow
Spo_2	92% while breathing room air

3. What complications are common with sickle cell anemia?

4. What are your treatment priorities given your understanding of patients with sickle cell anemia?

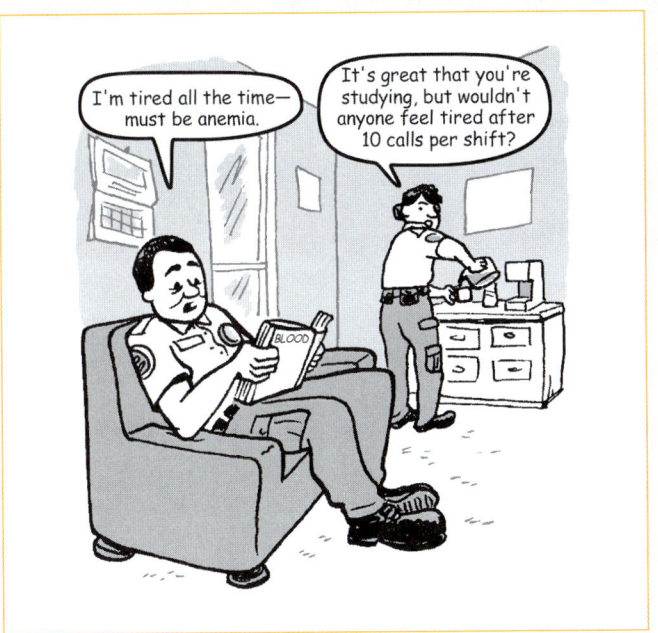

Figure 34-3

hemoglobin itself, such as sickle cell disease. In these disorders, the abnormal hemoglobin causes RBC deformation or shortens the RBC lifespan. The deformed RBCs may then become lodged in small blood vessels, leading to thrombosis (a blood clot). In many hematologic disorders, the defective RBCs migrate to the spleen, where they are destroyed. Anemia may also result from a deficiency of an enzyme known as glucose-6-phosphate dehydrogenase; this enzyme helps protect cells during infections. When levels of this enzyme are low, cells can become damaged. Although glucose-6-phosphate dehydrogenase deficiency is commonly seen in Africans and Southern Europeans, it can arise in individuals of any race.

Anemia can have serious consequences for people who travel to high-altitude areas. The combination of the lower number of RBCs and reduced oxygen levels in the atmosphere can lead to serious conditions that a healthy individual would not experience, such as hypoxia, difficulty breathing, and chest pain.

Leukemia

Leukemia is a disease that develops in the lymphoid system. In this type of cancer, blood cells—particularly WBCs—develop abnormally and/or excessively. Leukemia can cause anemia and thrombocytopenia (decrease in platelets). Leukemia can also cause an overproduction of some specific types of white blood cells, resulting in overall white cell counts that are extremely high (severe leukocytosis). Patients with leukemia experience frequent bleeding, bruising, infections, and fever **Figure 34-4 ▶**.

Leukemia can be classified as acute or chronic. Chronic leukemias tend to develop more frequently in older populations (65 years or older), whereas acute leukemias can develop in children or the elderly. In acute leukemia, bone marrow is replaced with

abnormal lymphoblasts, which spill over into the peripheral blood. In chronic leukemia, abnormal mature lymphoid cells accumulate in the bone marrow, lymph nodes, spleen, and peripheral blood. This form of leukemia is typically found by chance during routine blood tests; suspicions are raised when the tests reveal a high lymphocyte count.

Survival of leukemia depends on factors such as the stage at which the disease is detected, the patient's underlying medical condition, and

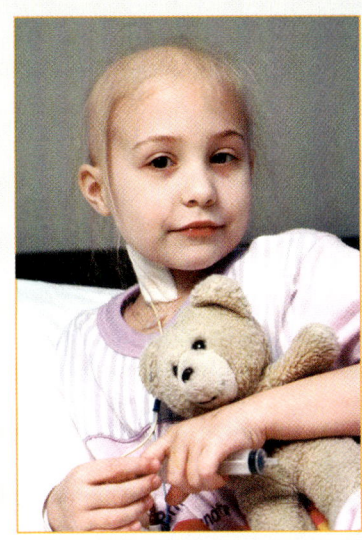

Figure 34-4 People with leukemia may have frequent bleeding, bruising, infections, and fever.

the response to treatment. Acute and chronic leukemia are treated with chemotherapy and radiotherapy. After receiving treatment, most patients will go into remission, especially when their conditions are identified early. Indeed, approximately 80% of children will be cured when their leukemia is diagnosed and treated early. Owing to the higher occurrence of genetic abnormalities and leukemic lymphoblasts as a result of the aging process, the adult cure rate is, at best, 30% to 40%.

At the Scene

When abnormalities of the blood cells are suspected, note the following:
1. Anemia commonly results in complaints of fatigue, lethargy, and dyspnea.
2. Low WBC counts (leukopenia) often lead to infection and fever.
3. Low platelet counts (thrombocytopenia) often cause cutaneous bleeding (including petechiae) and bleeding from mucous membranes (nosebleeds, rectal bleeding).

Lymphomas

Lymphomas are a group of malignant diseases that arise within the lymphoid system. They are classified in two categories: non-Hodgkin lymphoma (accounting for the majority of cases) and Hodgkin lymphoma.

Non-Hodgkin lymphoma can occur at any age in any person and can be hereditary. Furthermore, these types of cancer may be characterized based on the progression of the disease: indolent, aggressive, or highly aggressive. With very slow (indolent) progression, the disease may never leave the lymphoid system. In the highly aggressive form, the disease may affect multiple organs in a relatively short period, usually within several months. How well a patient responds to treatment depends on how early the disease is recognized and classified.

Hodgkin lymphoma is a painless progressive enlargement of the lymphoid glands, most commonly affecting the spleen and the lymph nodes. It is a highly rare form of lymphoma and is suspected to have some hereditary components. The incidence of Hodgkin lymphoma has two peaks: one between 15 and 35 years of age and a second peak after age 55 to 60 years. The disease is twice as common in men as in women. Patients may not show any symptoms for many years, with the disease being discovered only after patients complain of night sweats, chills, persistent coughs, and swelling of various lymph nodes (usually in the neck first). They may also note loss of appetite for an unknown reason, significant weight loss, generalized itching, fatigue, and/or bone pain. With aggressive treatment, symptoms may disappear for long periods; 60% to 90% of patients may actually be cured. Hodgkin lymphoma was one of the first cancers to be cured by radiation and combination chemotherapy.

Polycythemia

Polycythemia is characterized by an overabundance or overproduction of RBCs. The increased RBC production can be caused by a rare disorder originating in a single stem cell or an existing disease such as congestive heart failure or emphysema. It can also arise in individuals who live in high-altitude areas for long periods. The disease can cause the blood to become too thick (hyperviscosity).

The overabundance of the blood products associated with polycythemia may lead to many other signs and symptoms, such as strokes, transient ischemic attacks, headaches, and abdominal pain (usually associated with an enlarged spleen). Many times this disease is found accidentally when blood cell counts are performed after a patient complains of frequent episodes of the previously mentioned signs and symptoms. Cases of polycythemia are more frequently found in middle-aged adults (50 years and older).

Clinical treatment usually includes phlebotomy to try to maintain hematocrit levels at less than 45% in men and less than 42% in women. Other treatments have included cancer-type therapy intended to slow the production of new RBCs within the bone marrow. Survival is less than 18 months when the disease goes untreated but can be as long as 15 years for treated patients.

Disseminated Intravascular Coagulopathy

Disseminated intravascular coagulopathy (DIC) may result from any number of life-threatening conditions such as massive injury and hypotension due to trauma, sepsis, and obstetric complications Figure 34-5 .

The condition progresses in two stages. First, free thrombin and fibrin deposits in the blood increase, and platelets begin to aggregate. In this stage of the condition, owing to excessive bleeding, massive blood loss, or tissue injury, the coagulation system and fibrinolytic system become over-

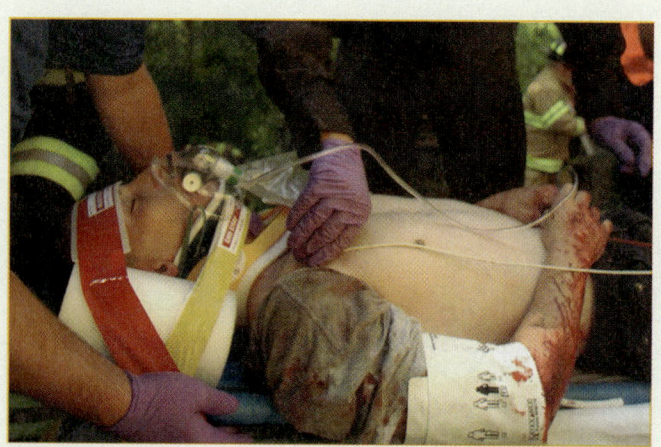

Figure 34-5 Severe trauma and extended hypotension can result in DIC.

whelmed. The fibrinolytic system is activated, which causes a breakdown of the fibrin clots, a process known as defibrination. In the second stage of the condition, uncontrolled hemorrhage results from the severe reduction in clotting factors.

The mortality of DIC is quite high, especially in acute cases; some studies have shown it to be 75%. The primary causes of death relate to uncontrolled bleeding, hypotension, and shock.

Hemophilia

Hemophilia is a bleeding disorder in which there is a defect in a clotting factor. It is usually associated with an X-linked recessive inheritance pattern, albeit one that is poorly understood. The disease is classified into two primary types: type A, which is due to low levels of factor VIII (antihemophilic globulin and antihemophilic factor), and type B, which is associated with a deficiency of factor IX (plasma thromboplastin component, also known as the Christmas factor). This disease is primarily found in the male population. The levels of factors VIII and IX determine the severity of the disease.

Both type A and type B have the same signs and symptoms. Acute and chronic bleeding can occur at any time and may or may not be life-threatening. Any injury or illness that can cause bleeding must not be taken lightly in a person with hemophilia. Spontaneous intracranial bleeding is common in hemophilia and is a major cause of death. Patients with significant acute bleeding episodes require hospitalization for transfusion and often require infusion of factors VIII and IX. If a patient has just had or needs surgery, these factors should be at 100% at the beginning of the procedure and should be maintained to a level up to 50% for several weeks thereafter.

Sickle Cell Disease

Sickle cell disease is a common inherited blood disorder in certain populations. Although it primarily affects those of African, Caribbean, and Southern European descent, it can occur in anyone. The Sickle Cell Association of Ontario estimates that the black population of Canada is approximately 700,000 and growing. The carrier frequency of the sickle cell gene is cited at 1 in 10 in the United States. The carrier rate is at least 1 in 10 in Canada, because most blacks in Canada come from areas of the world where the carrier rate is higher than 10%. The Caribbean carrier rate is 10% to 14% and the West African carrier rate is 20% to 25%. There are an estimated 67 black infants affected with sickle cell disease born annually in Canada. Mortality in patients with sickle cell disease peaks between 1 and 3 years of age, usually due to sepsis caused by *Streptococcus pneumoniae*. After infancy, patients with sickle cell disease are usually anemic and may experience painful crises.

Sickle cell disease starts with a gene defect of the adult-type hemoglobin (HgbA) gene. This mutation can be inherited from both parents (HbSS or sickle cell disease) or one parent (HgbS or sickle cell trait). In sickle cell disease, the abnormal hemoglobin stick together and alter the shape of the RBC, changing it from a round disk to a pointed sickle or spindle shape **Figure 34-6 ▶**. These abnormal RBCs are destroyed or broken down faster than normal; thus patients with sickle cell disease have anemia (low hemoglobin levels). The odd shape may also cause RBCs to lodge in the small blood vessels, decreasing oxygen delivery to tissues. In addition, hypoxia makes the RBC deformation worse. These events can lead to crises due to blockage of blood vessels: painful crises (thrombosis or strokes), sequestration crises (acute enlargement of the spleen), and chest crises (lung injury with severe hypoxia). Sickle cell disease may also be complicated by aplastic crises, in which RBC production is temporarily stopped by viral infections, or to hemolytic crises, in which RBCs break down quickly due to exposure to drugs, toxins, or other stressors.

Thalassemias

The thalassemias are hereditary conditions due to mutations causing decreased or absent production of the alpha-globin or beta-globin chains of hemoglobin. Beta-thalassemia major occurs in offspring of parents who are both carriers for thalassemia; each parent passes a defective copy of the gene producing beta-globin to the offspring. Infants with beta-thalassemia are usually born healthy and may remain healthy for up to 3 years. They then develop severe anemia, requiring regular transfusions. Later, they can develop iron overload from the many blood transfusions they receive and subsequently require iron chelation therapy. Affected individuals usually die in the third decade of life.

Alpha-thalassemia results from deletions in one or more of the four genes responsible for alpha-globin synthesis. It is common in persons of Southeast Asian descent, but also occurs in persons of African and Mediterranean origin. Fetuses with a four-gene deletion develop hydrops fetalis secondary to severe anemia and die before or soon after birth. Mothers of these infants are at risk for toxemia during pregnancy, for operative

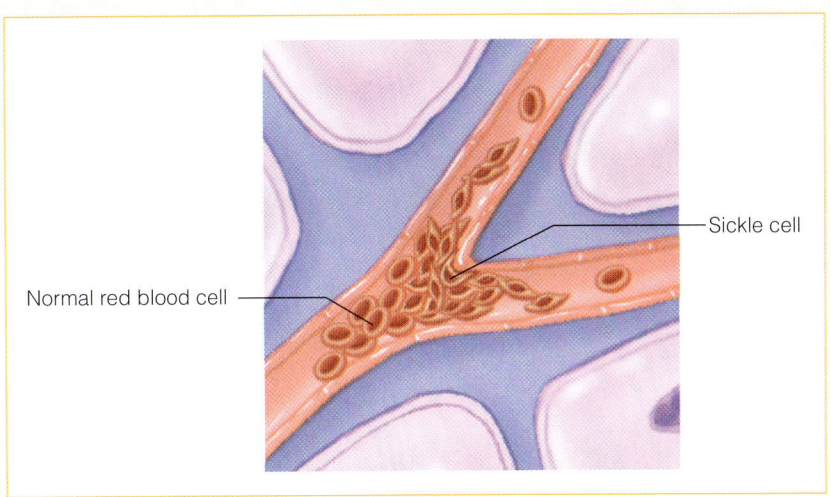

Figure 34-6 Normal RBCs and sickle cells.

delivery, and for postpartum hemorrhage. The exact prevalence of alpha-thalassemia is uncertain, but it is estimated to be 5% to 30% among African-Americans and 15% to 30% among Southeast Asians.

Multiple Myeloma

Multiple myeloma is a cancer of the plasma cells, the cells that produce antibodies that fight bacterial infections. The affected plasma cells multiply excessively and infiltrate the bone marrow. They may also overproduce antibody proteins, which can be found in the blood and lead to organ failure (primarily the kidneys) and eventually death. This disease rarely occurs early in life—most patients are older than 40 years. Men tend to have this disease more frequently than do women.

The sole presence of myeloma proteins in the blood (monoclonal gammopathy of unknown significance) does not mean a patient has multiple myeloma, but these patients may be at risk for the development of myeloma later in life (at a rate of approximately 1% per year). As the disease progresses, tumours grow or become numerous, and patients may develop weakness in the bones, resulting in spontaneous fractures. In advanced cases of myeloma, chemotherapy and other anti-cancer treatments may be given, which may slow or temporarily stop the disease, but myeloma is not curable. Morbidity and mortality primarily depend on the extent of the disease and on any underlying medical conditions.

General Assessment and Management

Assessment of a patient suspected of having a hematologic disorder should be no different from assessment of any other patient, albeit with a few additional items to consider and questions to ask. During your initial assessment, note any signs

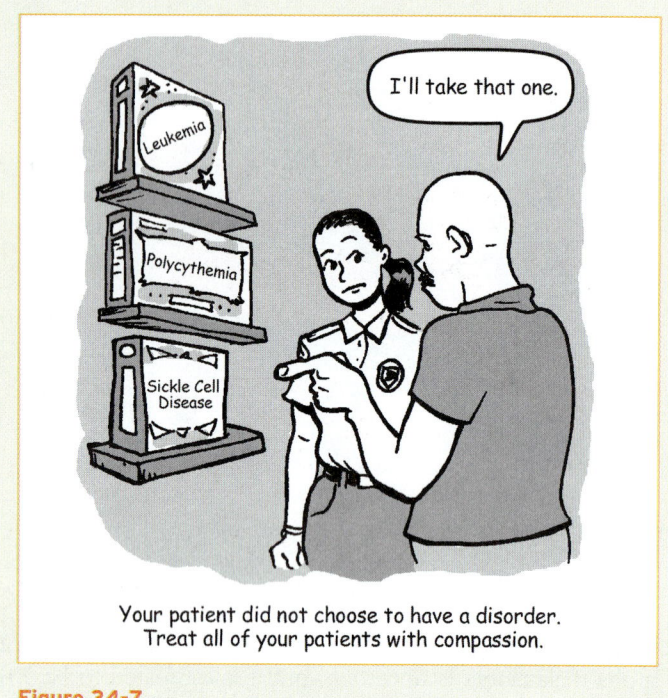

Your patient did not choose to have a disorder.
Treat all of your patients with compassion.

Figure 34-7

Table 34-3	Common Findings With Blood Disorders
System	**Common Findings**
Skin	Uncontrolled bleeding, unexplained or chronic bruising, itching, pallor or jaundice (yellow appearance usually indicates liver problems)
Gastrointestinal	Epistaxis (bloody nose), bleeding or infected gums, ulcers, melena (blood in the stool), and liver failure (causes jaundice)
Skeletal	Chronic joint or bone pain or rigidity
Cardiovascular	Dyspnea, tachycardia, chest pain, hemoptysis (coughing up blood)
Genitourinary	Hematuria, menorrhagia, chronic or recurring infections

- **Electrocardiogram (ECG).** Monitor and treat symptomatic cardiac rhythm disturbances as needed.
- **Transport.** Transport to the closest, most appropriate facility.
- **Pharmacology.** Pain management is sometimes necessary, especially in the case of a sickle-cell crisis.
- **Psychological support.** Be supportive and communicate with the patient.

Assessment and Management of Anemia

Your basic assessment should be the same for all patients, although you may want to ask some specific questions when anemia is suspected. Most commonly, patients with anemia will complain of feeling worn down, having no energy, or feeling as if they have overexerted themselves. Patients may also complain that they "can't catch their breath." Owing to the reduction of hemoglobin, some may develop anginal-type chest pain related to the reduction in oxygen availability to the heart muscle. Also common in anemic patients are leukopenia (reduction in WBCs) and thrombocytopenia (reduction in platelets); both conditions can induce more frequent infections, fevers, cutaneous bleeding, and frequent nosebleeds.

In cases of anemia, check and monitor the airway and the patient's breathing closely, administering high-flow oxygen when necessary. Check vital signs frequently. In cases of chest pain, apply a cardiac monitor and closely watch the rhythm. A 12-lead ECG may also be warranted to make sure the chest pain is not related to a new-onset myocardial infarction. Blood pressure management may also be needed, along with fluid replacement therapy. Monitor patients closely during fluid replacement. Do not be surprised if you have to control significant nosebleeds or other external hemorrhages in any patient with low platelets.

Allow the patient to rest in a comfortable position and transport him or her to the closest, most appropriate facility. In most cases, a gentle, easy transport is appropriate. However, if the patient experiences an abrupt change in the level of consciousness, hypotension develops, or other significant perfusion inadequacies arise, consider rapid transport.

and symptoms that may be immediately life-threatening. When performing the focused history and physical examination, it is extremely important to understand the chief complaint; to do so, you may need to be very inquisitive about the patient's history and SAMPLE history. Also, be very supportive of the patients and their families—some patients with a blood disorder may not be willing to disclose the condition because they may feel that they will be treated differently (**Figure 34-7 ▲**).

During the focused history and physical examination, look for changes in level of consciousness and symptoms such as vertigo, feelings of fatigue, or syncopal episodes. Does the patient have any complaints of dyspnea, chest pain, changes in heart rate and rhythm, or coughing up of blood? Has the patient experienced visual disturbances, muscle pain, or stiffness? Skin changes such as colour changes, burning, or itching? Bleeding problems from the nose, gums, and ulcers? Any history of liver problems or pain for unknown reasons? Problems with the genitourinary system?

When treating a patient with a known or suspected blood disorder, you will need to perform a physical examination. In such cases, it will be extremely important to have a basic understanding of some of the common findings in blood disorders (**Table 34-3 ▶**).

General management for any patient with problems related to a blood disorder should include the following elements:

- **Oxygen.** The amount needed and how it is given (that is, bag-valve-mask ventilation, nonrebreathing mask) depends on the severity of the patient's condition and respiratory status.
- **Fluids.** Initiate intravenous (IV) fluid replacement as indicated for the specific disorder or chief complaint.

Assessment and Management of Leukemia

How patients with leukemia present depends on the stage of the leukemia and the patient's current treatment. Patients typically complain of fatigue, headaches, or dyspnea or have signs of neurologic defects. During the detailed physical examination, fever, bone pain, and diaphoresis may be evident. Patients may complain of feeling full, soreness in the mid part of the chest, and unexplained bleeding. You should monitor vital signs (blood pressure, pulse, respirations, and temperature) and the cardiac rhythm. Do not be surprised if the vital signs indicate shock because the common signs of hypotension and tachycardia are often present. Be aware that fever in a patient with leukemia or following chemotherapy can be very serious, because the immune system is severely suppressed. These patients can deteriorate very rapidly with infections and may not exhibit the typical signs and symptoms of an infection until it is well advanced.

Management includes providing airway support and oxygen therapy as appropriate. IV fluid therapy and analgesics for comfort may be needed as well. Patients typically need constant positive support because many have a negative outlook toward their condition. The patient's loved ones may be quite concerned, especially when the patient is in the advanced stages of the disease; be supportive to them as well. In some cases, you may be called because the patient's condition has deteriorated and the family is uncertain about what to do. In such a scenario, your assessment may indicate normal findings for the patient. The patient or family may change their minds about transport or may have never truly wanted transport but rather professional insight and support. Discuss this situation with direct medical control, document all findings before leaving, and have a refusal and/or release form signed.

Few calls for patients with leukemia require extreme measures or rapid transport, but be alert to rapid changes in the patient's condition. If you transport, be aware that the patient could have a cardiorespiratory arrest. Make sure you find out the patient's and family's wishes about what to do in this situation.

Assessment and Management of Lymphomas

Generally speaking, lymphomas require specialized levels of treatment involving some form of chemotherapy or radiation therapy. How well a patient responds to these treatments depends on the stage of disease and its classification. As a rule, lymphomas respond well to chemotherapy; in fact, aggressive lymphomas respond better than indolent ones. Even if an indolent lymphoma is not cured with chemotherapy, many patients may survive as long as 10 years.

When assessing patients with lymphoma, ask specific questions such as "What type of lymphoma (cancer) do you have?" and "What type of treatment are you receiving?" As you perform your assessment, you will usually note pallor. The airway will usually be patent and breathing adequate, although sometimes you may note some congestion in the lower lung fields. The patient may complain of being first hot and then

You are the Paramedic Part 3

As your partner obtains IV access, applies 12 l of oxygen by nonrebreathing mask, and readies the patient for transport, you perform a quick examination. When you ask the patient to point to the area of pain, he puts his hand over his left upper quadrant and says that he has vomited a few times this evening. He also mentions that he has had chills and feels like he cannot catch his breath. You note the presence of dullness when percussing the lowest intercostal space in the anterior axillary line on the left side. On gentle palpation and observation of the patient's face, you note that he has some tenderness in his left upper quadrant, and you can feel a portion of the spleen.

Your partner inserts an 18-gauge IV cannula in the left antecubital vein and begins to administer a 250-ml bolus of normal saline, after confirming that the patient has clear breath sounds.

Reassessment	Recording Time: 10 Minutes
Level of consciousness	Alert, with a Glasgow Coma Scale score of 15
Skin	Diaphoretic and feverish with pale mucous membranes
Pulse	Radial pulse, 116 beats/min, weak and regular
Blood pressure	108/44 mm Hg
Respirations	20 breaths/min and shallow
Spo2	95%
Blood glucose level	7 mmol/l
ECG	Sinus tachycardia without ectopy

5. What, if anything, is abnormal about your physical assessment findings?
6. Given your assessment, what do you think are potential sources of the patient's complaints?

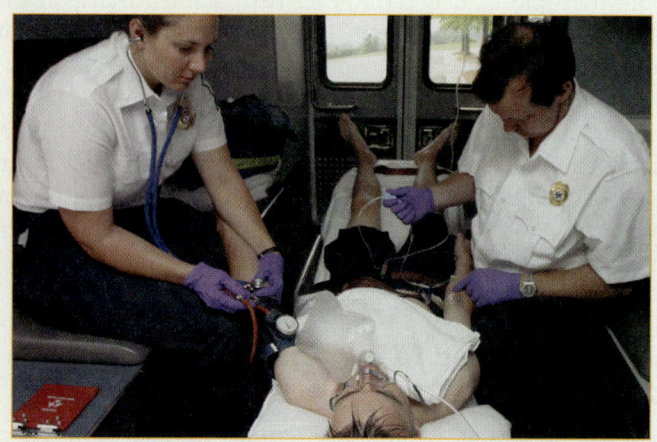

Figure 34-8 Patients with lymphoma who are in extreme pain should receive fluid therapy, oxygen, and analgesics.

cold or even both in different areas of the body. Signs of inadequate perfusion are common, including low blood pressure accompanied by an elevated heart rate. Abnormal ECG rhythms may also be evident.

Patients with lymphoma may be in constant extreme pain; therefore, if pain management is needed and available, it should be provided. Treat inadequate perfusion with fluid therapy, and provide supplemental oxygen 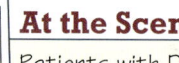. If necessary, treat abnormal heart rhythms. If the patient's condition does not improve or even deteriorates following these measures, initiate rapid transport to the closest facility. As with leukemia, you may be called to offer support but no transport. Be supportive, discuss your findings with direct medical control, explain the options to the patient and family, and allow them to make a decision.

Assessment and Management of Polycythemia

Owing to the nature of polycythemia and its plethora of symptoms, your assessment findings may vary widely. Altered levels of consciousness may be evident due to stroke or transient ischemic attack-like events or hypoxia secondary to poor circulation from lesions within the circulatory system. Respiratory distress is common, as are changes in peripheral pulses, heart rate, and skin colour. Tachycardia is the most common change in heart rhythm. Patients also tend to have purplish skin with red hands and feet.

As you assess the patient, note the extent and duration of dyspnea. Has the patient experienced uncontrolled itching (pruritus) or noted changes in skin temperature? Make sure to obtain a thorough medical history in cases of known or suspected polycythemia.

Prehospital care largely consists of supportive care and transporting the patient to an appropriate facility. Administer oxygen as needed. Establish IV access for possible pharmacologic

interventions for pain or heart rate control as appropriate. Be supportive to the patient and family.

Assessment and Management of DIC

As you assess and provide prehospital care for critically injured or ill patients, keep in mind the issues that may lead to DIC. Your goal is to identify signs and symptoms commonly associated with DIC or progression toward it. In cases involving severe trauma, patients may have episodes of respiratory difficulty, signs of shock, and skin changes, ranging from cold and clammy to pallor to small black-and-blue marks (purpura) on the chest and abdomen.

It is important to identify the cause underlying the patient's presenting condition and establish treatment early, while not delaying transport to an appropriate facility. Maintain an airway, administer supplemental oxygen, and treat the patient for shock (keep the patient warm, control bleeding, administer IV fluids for hypotension) per local protocol. Pharmacologic interventions may include pain management and treatment for abnormal heart rhythms, although treatment for altered heart rhythms should come last. Patients who have DIC due to severe trauma have a poor survival rate; they and family members need strong support. Be optimistic but honest with patients and family, and don't give false impressions regarding survival.

At the Scene

Patients with DIC have a failure of multiple organs (kidneys, lungs, heart) at once, accompanied by bleeding from IV sites, bleeding into joints, and, possibly, intracranial hemorrhage.

Assessment and Management of Hemophilia

When taking the patient's history, you may discover previous or current hemophilia conditions. In addition to taking care of the ABCs, be alert for signs of acute blood loss (pallor, weak pulse, and hypotension). Note any bleeding of unknown origin, such as nosebleeds, bloody sputum, and blood in the urine or stool (melena). Owing to blood loss, patients may exhibit signs of hypoxia due to the reduction in oxygen-carrying capacity. Any patient who complains of respiratory problems should receive high-flow oxygen.

Note ECG findings, and treat symptomatic dysrhythmias as appropriate. IV therapy may be necessary in cases of unstable hypotension, but understand that the patient actually needs a transfusion or plasma. Some patients will have significant pain, so analgesics may be appropriate. Although you may be called to treat someone with bleeding of unknown cause only to find that the bleeding stopped before you arrived on scene or the patient has treated themselves with replacement clotting factors, you should suggest that the patient get immediate hospital or physician follow-up.

Assessment and Management of Sickle Cell Disease

Do not take a call for a person having a sickle cell crisis lightly. Patients are often in life-threatening situations, characterized by shortness of breath and signs of pneumonia. Their skin will show signs of inadequate perfusion, accompanied by hypotension. They may show signs of jaundice and yellowing in the eye (icteric sclera). High levels of oxygen are recommended to prevent further deformation of the RBCs due to hypoxia. Patients may complain of multiple system involvement, including chest, abdominal, and arthritic-type pain, although some may report only fatigue or achiness along with fever.

Besides providing oxygen therapy and rapid transport to an appropriate facility, you may need to give IV fluid therapy to counter the patient's dehydration. Remember that patients may have lived with the disease for a long time and, thus, may have a very high pain threshold. As a consequence, they often require a higher level of analgesia.

Assessment and Management of Multiple Myeloma

Findings during your assessment and management of multiple myeloma depend on the patient's stage of disease. Early-stage complaints may be as simple as fatigue or mild pain. Later-

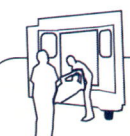

At the Scene

Sickle cell disease may mimic appendicitis or opiate withdrawal.

stage disease may be evidenced by unexplained hemorrhage and significant weight loss, frequent bone fractures, and elevated pain in any number of locations.

Management is similar to that for other blood disorders: IV fluid therapy, pain management, and supportive prehospital care. Do not assume that the patient is ready to or is going to die; he or she may just be having a complication of the myeloma. On receiving definitive care at an appropriate facility, the patient's condition may improve.

You are the Paramedic Part 4

You gently transport the patient to the nearest appropriate facility and continue to monitor his condition en route. Although he reports that his feeling of shortness of breath has decreased, he continues to have abnormal skin signs. When you give your report to the emergency department nurse, she indicates that she is familiar with this patient because he has had periodic exacerbations of sickle cell anemia. One such incident required multiple blood transfusions secondary to an aplastic crisis.

Reassessment	Recording Time: 20 Minutes
Level of consciousness	Alert, with a Glasgow Coma Scale score of 15
Skin	Diaphoretic and warm with improved colour of mucous membranes
Pulse	Radial pulse, 98 beats/min, weak and regular
Blood pressure	116/60 mm Hg
Respirations	20 breaths/min
Spo₂	98%
Temperature	38°C
ECG	Normal sinus rhythm without ectopy

7. Should this patient receive analgesics? Why or why not?
8. Would this call change if the patient had the same or similar signs and symptoms in the presence of trauma?

You are the Paramedic Summary

1. What, if anything, about his appearance gives you cause for concern?

The patient is showing signs of hypoperfusion. He is sweaty, his breathing is laboured, and his facial expression and body position suggest that he is experiencing moderate to severe abdominal pain.

2. What information do you already have at your disposal?

The patient has a medical history that has significantly affected him in the past and could be related to his chief complaint. It is important to absorb all possible information provided by the patient. Information from family, friends, and bystanders may also be helpful.

3. What complications are common with sickle cell anemia?

Patients struggle with oxygenation and tissue perfusion. They are at high risk for hypoxia because the deformed RBCs cannot deliver oxygen and do not return to their normal shape, causing vascular injury. They may experience cessation of RBC production and/or RBC breakdown.

4. What are your treatment priorities given your understanding of patients with sickle cell anemia?

Recognize the potential seriousness of the patient's condition by conducting an appropriate physical examination and history taking, administer high-flow supplemental oxygen and IV fluids (as needed), and provide prompt transport to the nearest appropriate facility.

5. What, if anything, is abnormal about your physical assessment findings?

Physical findings point to splenic enlargement or splenomegaly. The spleen can become enlarged for many reasons, including viral, bacterial, and parasitic infections; cancer; and hemolytic anemias. Patients with sickle cell anemia are at greater risk for splenic sequestration (enlargement of the spleen as a result of the trapping of RBCs). Patients with left upper quadrant pain should be examined for enlargement of the spleen. These patients must be transported quickly and the receiving facility notified immediately.

6. Given your assessment, what do you think are potential sources of the patient's complaints?

His abdominal pain could be the result of splenic crisis or his enlarged spleen could be the result of an infection (especially in the presence of fever). No matter what its underlying cause, the patient's condition should be treated as very serious with prompt transport and frequent reassessments for changes in the patient's condition.

7. Should this patient receive analgesics? Why or why not?

Pain management is an essential part of patient prehospital care. When dealing with abdominal pain in the prehospital setting, some physicians may not want you to administer medications such as morphine because it can mask the source of pain. In these situations, make every attempt to consult with direct medical control before administration of analgesics. If it has been determined that analgesics are inappropriate, make every attempt to address the patient's pain through body position and gentle handling and transport.

8. Would this call change if the patient had the same or similar signs and symptoms in the presence of trauma?

An enlarged spleen with the added history of trauma can equate to a fatal patient outcome. What makes this case even more serious is that this patient may have underlying anemia due to sickle cell disease, which would put him or her at risk for hypoxia. Worsening hypoxia could, in turn, precipitate a sickle cell chest or painful crises. Bleeding, especially at the volume seen in splenic rupture, is an especially life-threatening situation for a patient with sickle cell anemia.

Prep Kit

Ready for Review

- Most EMS systems rarely respond to hematologic emergencies.
- Blood performs respiratory, nutritional, excretory, regulatory, and defensive functions.
- Blood disorders include anemia, iron deficiency anemia, hematologic disorders, leukemias, lymphomas, polycythemia, DIC, hemophilia, sickle cell disease, and multiple myeloma.
- During the initial assessment of a patient with a hematologic disorder, note any signs and symptoms that may be immediately life threatening.
- During the focused history and physical examination, look for changes in level of consciousness such as vertigo, feelings of fatigue, or syncopal episodes.
- General management for any patient with problems related to a blood disorder should include the following elements: oxygen, fluids, ECG, transport, pharmacology, and psychological support.

Vital Vocabulary

ABO system The antigen classification given to blood.

anemia A lower than normal hemoglobin or erythrocyte level.

antibodies Molecules in the body that react against foreign antigens in the body.

antigens Substances (usually protein) identified as foreign to the body.

autoimmune disorder Disorder in which the body identifies its own proteins as a foreign body and activates the inflammatory system.

clotting factors Substances in the blood that are necessary for clotting; also called coagulation factors.

coagulation Clotting.

disseminated intravascular coagulopathy (DIC) A life-threatening condition commonly found in severe trauma.

erythrocytes Red blood cells.

fibrin A white, insoluble protein formed in the clotting process.

fibrinolytic system The mechanism by which fibrin undergoes dissolution owing to the action of enzymes; clots are destroyed.

hematocrit The percentage of RBCs in total blood volume.

hematopoietic system The system that includes all blood components and the organs involved in their development and production.

hemoglobin The iron-rich protein in the blood that carries oxygen.

hemolytic disorder A disorder relating to the breakdown of RBCs.

hemophilia A bleeding disorder that is primarily hereditary, in which clotting does not occur or occurs insufficiently.

iron deficiency anemia The most common type of anemia in which iron stores are low or lacking and the serum iron concentration is low.

leukemia Cancer or malignancy of the blood-forming organs, particularly affecting the WBCs that develop abnormally and/or excessively at the expense of normal blood cells.

leukocytes White blood cells.

leukopenia Reduction in the number of WBCs.

lymphoblasts Lymphocytes transformed because of stimulation by an antigen.

lymphoid system The system primarily made up of the bone marrow, lymph nodes, and spleen that participates in formation of lymphocytes and immune responses.

lymphomas Malignant diseases that arise within the lymphoid system; includes non-Hodgkin and Hodgkin lymphomas.

melena Blood in the stool.

multiple myeloma A disease in which an abnormal plasma cell infiltrates the bone marrow with a cancerous (neoplastic) cell, causing tumours to form inside the bones.

petechiae Tiny purple or red spots that appear on the skin due to bleeding within the skin or under mucous membranes.

phlebotomy Making an incision into a vein to remove blood.

plasma A component of blood, made of 92% water, 6% to 7% proteins, and electrolytes, clotting factors, and glucose; this makes up 55% of the total blood volume.

polycythemia An overabundance or production of RBCs, WBCs, and platelets.

pruritus Unspecified itching.

reticuloendothelial system The system in the body that is primarily used to defend against infection.

sickle cell disease A disease that causes the RBCs to be misshapen, resulting in poor oxygen-carrying capability and potentially resulting in lodging of the RBCs in blood vessels or the spleen.

specific gravity The weight of a substance compared with water.

stem cells Cells that can develop into other types of cells in the body.

thalassemia A type of anemia in which not enough hemoglobin is produced, or the hemoglobin is defective.

thrombin An enzyme that causes the conversion of fibrinogen to fibrin, which binds to the platelet plugs, forming the final mature blood clot.

thrombocytes Platelets.

thrombocytopenia Reduction in the number of platelets.

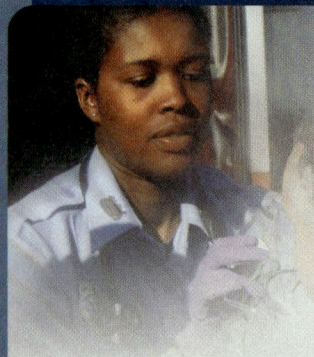

Assessment in Action

You are dispatched for a "sick person." When you arrive on scene, you find a 32-year-old woman lying supine on her couch. She called 9-1-1 because she has not been feeling "right" for about 1 week and just can't move today. During your assessment, you note that she is very pale; her skin is warm and dry. Her vital signs seem to be within normal limits. The patient says that she is tired all the time and has lost approximately 9 kg during the past 3 to 4 weeks. She denies any chance of pregnancy but reports that her menstrual cycles have been heavier. She denies any medical history of disease and tells you that she takes a daily vitamin and an iron supplement.

You apply oxygen via a nasal cannula at 4 l/min, begin an IV line at a to keep vein open rate, and transport the patient to the hospital. While you are obtaining your patient's disposition, an emergency department staff member tells you that the patient was admitted to a regular floor with anemia.

1. **What is anemia?**
   - A. Reduction below the normal levels of RBCs, as shown by a decreased hemoglobin or hematocrit level
   - B. A malignant tumour of blood-forming tissue
   - C. Overproduction of RBCs and platelets
   - D. A malignant tumour of lymphatic tissues

2. **What is the name of the body system that produces blood cells?**
   - A. Circulatory system
   - B. Respiratory system
   - C. Hematopoietic system
   - D. Hepatic system

3. **What are the blood-forming organs in an adult?**
   - A. Liver
   - B. Bone marrow
   - C. Spleen
   - D. Lungs

4. **What is the normal life cycle of an RBC?**
   - A. 1 month
   - B. 3 months
   - C. 4 months
   - D. 1 year

5. **Hematocrit (Hct) is:**
   - A. an iron-rich compound responsible for carrying oxygen to the tissues.
   - B. a measure of RBCs per unit of blood volume.
   - C. the pulse oximetry reading.
   - D. the number of leukocytes per unit of blood volume.

6. **Hemoglobin (Hgb) is:**
   - A. an iron-rich compound responsible for carrying oxygen to the tissues.
   - B. the proportion of RBC volume in a given volume of blood.
   - C. the pulse oximetry reading.
   - D. the number of leukocytes per unit of blood volume.

7. **Cells that can develop into or produce other types of cells in the body are:**
   - A. stem cells.
   - B. erythrocytes.
   - C. fibrin.
   - D. plasma.

8. **_____ are the smallest of the formed elements and are responsible for the clotting of the blood.**
   - A. Leukocytes
   - B. Erythrocytes
   - C. Platelets
   - D. Stem cells

9. **Blood transports oxygen from the lungs to the tissues and carbon dioxide from the tissues to the lungs. This is the_____ function.**
   - A. respiratory
   - B. nutritional
   - C. excretory
   - D. regulatory

10. **Blood carries glucose, proteins, and fats from the digestive tract to cells through the body. This is the_____ function.**
    - A. respiratory
    - B. nutritional
    - C. excretory
    - D. regulatory

11. **Blood ferries the waste products of metabolism from the cells where they are produced to excretory organs. This is the _____ function.**
    - A. respiratory
    - B. nutritional
    - C. excretory
    - D. regulatory

12. **Blood brings hormones to their target organs and transmits excess internal heat to the surface of the body to be dissipated. This is the _____ function.**
    - A. respiratory
    - B. defensive
    - C. excretory
    - D. regulatory

13. **Blood carries defensive cells and antibodies that protect the body against foreign organisms. This is the _____ function.**
    - A. respiratory
    - B. defensive
    - C. excretory
    - D. regulatory

Challenging Questions

You are dispatched to the local mall for a fall victim. On arrival, you find a 42-year-old man sitting at the base of the steps. According to witnesses, he tripped up the steps, lost his balance, and then fell down four steps. He is alert to his name but is confused about what happened. The patient complains of pain to his left axillary area and his left knee. During your assessment, you find him to be tachycardic, tachypneic, and grossly diaphoretic. His blood pressure is 70/30 mm Hg, pulse rate is 118 beats/min, and respiratory rate is 30 breaths/min. While you and your partner are providing the patient with full cervical-spine precautions, you note a bruise on his left flank area. You provide the patient with 100% supplemental oxygen via a nonrebreathing mask and take him to the ambulance for transport to the emergency department.

During your focused examination, you note a medical ID tag that reads "Hemophilia A." You initiate IV therapy and provide a fluid bolus. The patient is transported to the hospital without any further incident. You give report to the emergency department nurse and physician. You overhear the physician order "factor VIII" from the pharmacy.

14.   **What is your care in the prehospital setting for a patient with hemophilia?**

15.   **What would your prehospital care be for any patient with a hematopoietic problem?**

Points to Ponder

You respond to a private residence, where you find a 28-year-old West African woman lying in bed. She complains of pain in her chest with associated shortness of breath. You note swelling of her hands and feet. The patient says that she has had the flu for the past 2 days and has vomited at least four times. She has also had a low-grade fever and generalized body aches. Your physical examination reveals nothing truly remarkable. The patient has a history of high blood pressure and sickle cell disease.

What is happening with this patient physiologically? What, if any, treatment should you administer?

Issues: Understand the Urgency for Assessment and Intervention in Patients With Hematologic Crises.

35 Environmental Emergencies

Competency Areas

Area 1: Professional Responsibilities

1.1.c   Dress appropriately and maintain personal hygiene.
1.1.g   Utilize community support agencies as appropriate.
1.5.c   Work collaboratively with other emergency response agencies.

Area 3: Health and Safety

3.3.a   Assess scene for safety.
3.3.b   Address potential occupational hazards.

Area 4: Assessment and Diagnostics

4.2.c   Obtain chief complaint and/or incident history from patient, family members, and/or bystanders.
4.2.f   Obtain information regarding incident through accurate and complete scene assessment.
4.4.c   Conduct non-invasive temperature monitoring.

Area 5: Therapeutics

5.6.e   Treat local cold injury.

Area 6: Integration

6.1.n   Provide care to patient experiencing illness or injury due to extremes of temperature or adverse environments.

Appendix 4: Pathophysiology

J.   **Multisystem Diseases and Injuries**
Environmental Disorders: Barotrauma
Environmental Disorders: Air embolism
Environmental Disorders: Decompression sickness
Environmental Disorders: Descent, ascent barotraumas
Environmental Disorders: Heat cramps
Environmental Disorders: Heat exhaustion
Environmental Disorders: Heat stroke
Environmental Disorders: High altitude cerebral edema
Environmental Disorders: High altitude pulmonary edema
Environmental Disorders: Local cold injuries
Environmental Disorders: Near drowning and drowning

Introduction

According to Statistics Canada, 491 people died of hypothermia-related causes from 2000 to 2004. During 2000 to 2004, 67 deaths were classified as heat-related. Environmental emergencies are medical conditions caused or worsened by the weather, terrain, or unique atmospheric conditions such as high altitude or underwater. Most paramedics would recognize the obvious problem of a child who has fallen into an icy lake. The challenge lies in recognizing patients with environmental emergencies in the unusual settings of endurance sports events or at mass gatherings, and even acutely confused older patients Figure 35-1 ▾.

Unique to environmental emergencies are the conditions that directly cause harm or complicate treatment and transport considerations. Wind, rain, snow, temperature extremes, and humidity may all affect the body's ability to adapt to its environment. Unprepared hikers can experience cold illnesses during summer rainstorms as easily as overdressed snow sports enthusiasts can die of heat illnesses during strenuous outings. The locations of these outings can also have a huge impact on the ability to know about, respond to, and rescue people in remote settings Figure 35-2 ▾.

Certain generic risk factors predispose people to environmental emergencies. In addition, very young and old people have unique disadvantages when it comes to thermoregulation. Conditions such as diabetes, cardiac disease (for example, coronary artery disease, congestive heart failure), restrictive lung disease, thyroid disease, and psychiatric illnesses can alter the body's ability to compensate for environmental extremes.

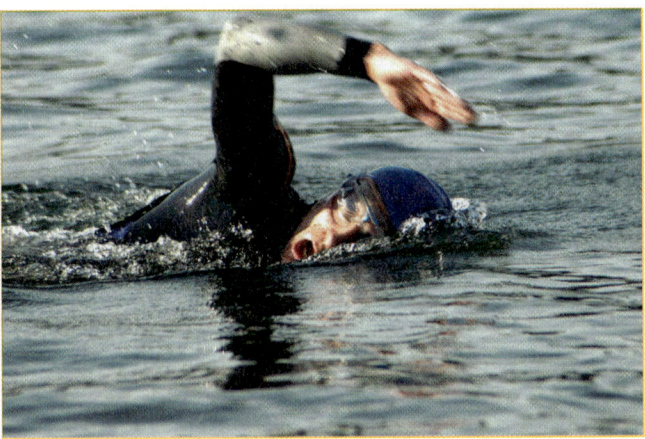

Figure 35-1 Environmental emergencies can occur in a variety of settings, including endurance sports events.

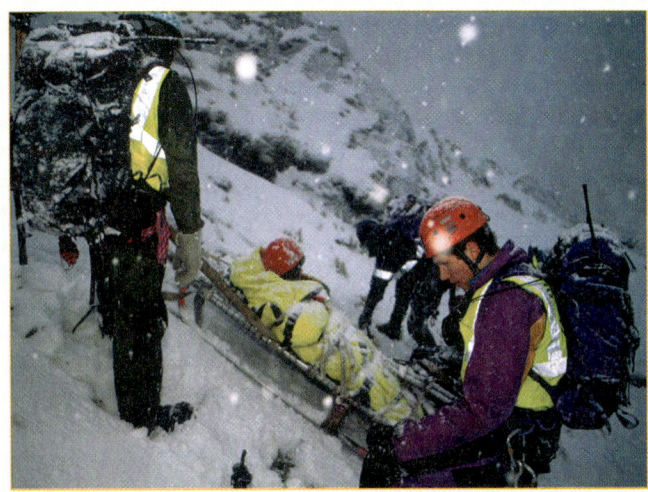

Figure 35-2 Medical attention may be needed in some extreme environments.

You are the Paramedic Part 1

You and your partner are called to the public library because of a man "acting strangely." You notice that the spring day has turned cooler as you respond and begin to consider why someone would be acting strangely at the library.

When you arrive, you run through the downpour and wind to the entrance. You recognize one of the police officers. She tells you, "I think he's just drunk," and notes that she arrested the man a month ago after a bar disturbance. After you confirm that the police officer has checked the man for weapons, you ask the bystander who has given up his coat to the patient what is going on. He reports that the patient was standing outside trying to remove his shirt and pants. The patient told him that he was "too hot."

Initial Assessment	Recording Time: 0 Minutes
Appearance	Eyes open, no obvious distress
Level of consciousness	V (Responsive to verbal stimuli); slurs words
Airway	Open; odour of alcohol on breath
Breathing	Adequate rate and tidal volume
Circulation	Radial pulse present; cold hands

1. What are three things that could medically harm this man in the next hour?
2. Do you believe the scene to be adequately secured?
3. Where do you believe is the best place to properly assess the patient?

Finally, the patient's overall health and fitness status and ability to acclimatize (that is, adjust to the new environment) can mean the difference between life and death.

This chapter first describes the techniques that the healthy body uses to respond to changes in temperature. It then assesses factors that can interfere with the body's ability to shed or gain heat, thereby increasing a person's risk of experiencing an environmental emergency. Next, it examines the pathophysiology, recognition, and treatment of environmental illnesses. Finally, the chapter considers preventive measures for environmental illnesses.

Homeostasis and Body Temperature

Homeostasis refers to body processes that balance the supply and demand of the body's needs. Ensuring the balance between heat production and heat loss (thermoregulation) is the job of thermosensitive neurons in the anterior hypothalamus. Like a car thermostat, the hypothalamus—the "master thermostat" in the brain—operates according to the principle of negative feedback control: A rise in core body temperature elicits responses that increase heat loss and shut off normal heat production pathways (thermogenesis); a fall in core body temperature prompts heat production and conservation and turns off normal heat-liberating pathways (thermolysis) **Figure 35-3 ▼** .

The human body stubbornly defends a constant core temperature of approximately 37°C that represents a balance

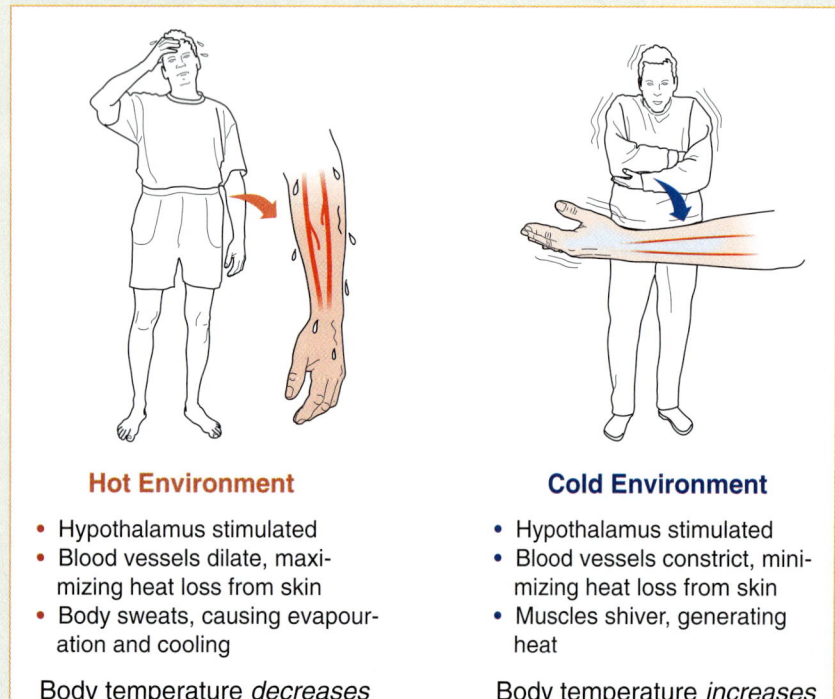

Hot Environment

- Hypothalamus stimulated
- Blood vessels dilate, maximizing heat loss from skin
- Body sweats, causing evapouration and cooling

Body temperature *decreases*

Cold Environment

- Hypothalamus stimulated
- Blood vessels constrict, minimizing heat loss from skin
- Muscles shiver, generating heat

Body temperature *increases*

Figure 35-3 Like a car thermostat, the hypothalamus notes a rise or fall in core body temperature mend elicits responses to regulate it.

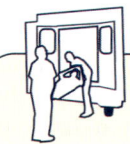

At the Scene

Do not become a victim yourself. Dress for the weather.

between the heat produced or absorbed by the body and the heat eliminated to the outside. At this temperature, the metabolic reactions of the body proceed at their optimal level. Temperatures in the core (the brain and thoracoabdominal organs) remain relatively constant. The temperature of the periphery (the skin) can fluctuate a great deal, so this part of the body has a major role in thermoregulation. The lowest body temperature at which human survival of accidental hypothermia has been reported is 13.7°C. More generally, hypothermia is defined as a body temperature lower than 35°C and heat stroke at temperatures above 40°C.

In the prehospital environment, the oral temperature is commonly used and is a suitable measurement for general medical conditions such as suspected pneumonia. It can vary dramatically from the core temperature if the patient has been mouth breathing or drinking hot or cold liquids. The axillary temperature, taken in the armpit, is typically 0.5°C cooler than the oral temperature. Tactile temperatures taken by parents are remarkably accurate but only in terms of knowing whether a child has a fever, not in determining the actual temperature. In environmental situations, the most accurate means of determining core temperatures is to use a rectal thermometer capable of measuring extremes of temperatures **Figure 35-4 ▶** . Tympanic temperatures, which are taken with a device that measures the heat reflected off the eardrum, also provide accurate core measurements.

Thermoregulatory Mechanisms

The body's main thermoregulatory centre is located in specialized tissue found in the hypothalamus. The thermogenic (heat-generating) tissues in the hypothalamus are mediated by the sympathetic nervous system; the thermolytic (heat-liberating) tissues are mediated by the parasympathetic nervous system. The hypothalamus receives signals from peripheral receptors (located primarily in the skin and muscles) and central receptors (triggered by changes in blood temperature; located in the core).

At rest, the body produces heat chiefly by the metabolism of nutrients (carbohydrates, fats, and rarely proteins), with the subsequent liberation of primarily water and carbon dioxide. Liver and skeletal muscles are the major contributors to the basal metabolic rate (BMR), the heat energy produced at rest from normal body metabolic reactions. The BMR can be thought of as the minimal caloric energy requirement to sit on

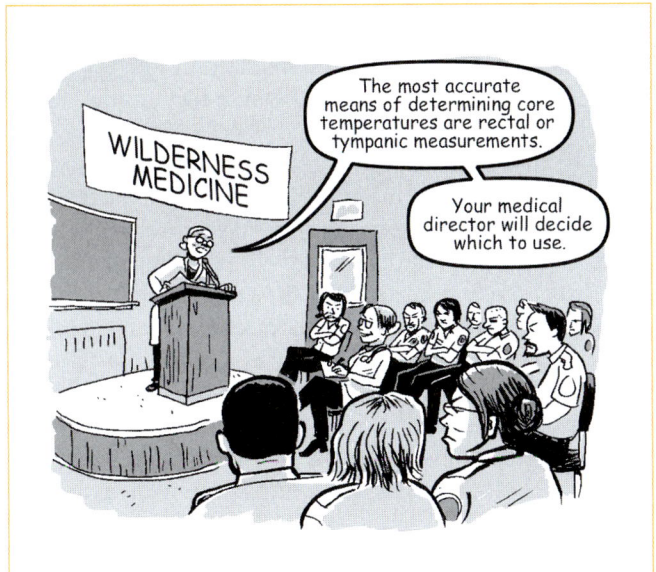

Figure 35-4

the couch all day! The BMR of the average 70-kg adult is in the range of 60 to 70 kcal per hour. Many factors affect this rate, including age, sex, stress, and hormones. The most important factor, however, is body surface area. As the ratio of body surface area to body volume increases, heat loss to the environment increases. Thus, when two people have the same weight, the shorter person will have a higher BMR.

Exertion also affects the metabolic rate. A brisk walk can produce heat totaling 300 kcal/h, for example. The recommended daily caloric intake is 2,000 to 2,500 kcal (a food "calorie" is actually a kilocalorie).

Some of the heat generated by metabolism and glycogen breakdown for muscular work is used to warm the body; the excess is excreted, ordinarily by taking advantage of the temperature gradient between the body and the outside environment. If the environmental temperature is higher than the body temperature, there is a third potential source of body heat: absorption of heat from the outside. Standing in bright sunshine on a hot, breezeless day, for example, can add up to 150 kcal/h to the internal heat load.

Physiologic Responses to Heat and Cold
Thermolysis

The body reacts to its daily production of heat energy and to hot environmental conditions in much the same way— thermolysis, the release of stored heat and energy from the body. An increase in core temperature causes the hypothalamus to send signals via efferent pathways in the parasympathetic nervous system, causing vasodilatation and sweating.

Because of cutaneous vasodilation, the effective volume of the vascular system is increased (when the diameter of a tube, such as an artery, is increased, its volume increases); the heart must increase its output to compensate for this effect. Heart

rate and stroke volume increase, but the work of the heart is markedly increased. If vasodilation increases dramatically, the person may have a complete loss of vasomotor control (that is, the ability of the arteries to constrict in response to sympathetic stimulation). In that case, blood pools in the periphery, and the patient could experience neurogenic shock.

When warmed blood from the core and overheated muscles heads for the peripherally dilated cutaneous vessels, it may be cooled in four major ways (in addition to behavioural changes, such as slowing down or seeking shade):

- **Radiation**, the transfer of heat via electromagnetic waves, accounts for more than 65% of heat loss in a cooler setting. Heat loss through the head is especially notable. If the ambient temperature is high (20°C or greater), body heat will be gained.
- **Conduction** is the transfer of heat from a hotter object to a cooler object by direct physical contact. Air is a poor conductor of heat (only 2% of body heat is lost to it), whereas the ground is a good conductor. Water is the best conductor. A person who falls into a cold lake will lose heat 25 times faster than a dry person exposed to air of the same temperature. Clothing soaked with rain, snow, or perspiration can be just as dangerous.
- **Convection** refers to the loss of heat that takes place when moving air picks up heat and carries it away. A person instinctively uses this principle when blowing on hot food to cool it. Likewise, air moving across the body surface can pick up heat and carry it away. The faster the air is moving, the faster it can remove heat from the body. The windchill factor measures the chilling effect of a given temperature at a given wind speed. For example, the chilling effect of a 1°C temperature with a 58 kph wind is −20°C.
- **Evapouration**, the conversion of a liquid to a gas, liberates 1 kcal per 1.7 ml of sweat. Sweating and heat dissipation by evapouration normally account for about 30% of cooling. Evapouration is the main mode of cooling in higher temperatures until a high humidity level slows the rate of evapouration. It has a minor role via respiration. This phenomenon is also behind the evapourative method of cooling for heat stroke patients. In cold conditions, wet clothes can cause heat loss by conduction and, as they dry, further heat loss by evapouration.

These four mechanisms require a thermal gradient between the body and its surroundings; that is, the mechanisms work only as long as the temperature of the skin surface is higher than that of the outside environment (and metabolism does not produce an overwhelming heat load). When the outside temperature approaches or exceeds skin surface temperature, however, heat loss by radiation and convection diminishes and finally ceases. When the environmental temperature exceeds the skin temperature, the body absorbs heat. In those circumstances, the increase in blood flow to the skin becomes counterproductive because it promotes increased heat absorption.

The only way the body can dissipate heat when the ambient temperature approaches body temperature is by the evapouration of sweat, up to a point. A healthy adult can sweat a maximum of about 1 l/h but cannot maintain that rate for more than a few hours at a time. Furthermore, for effective evapouration of sweat, the ambient air must be relatively unsaturated with water. As the relative humidity increases, the rate of evapouration decreases; effective sweat evapouration ceases when the relative humidity reaches about 75%.

Thermogenesis

In a cold environment, the skin serves as the body's thermostat. If your skin is cold, your body will shiver even if your core body temperature is not lowered. Thermogenesis, the production of heat and energy for the body, is the main method of dealing with cold stressors. In addition to normal heat production from the BMR and physical exertion, the sympathetic nervous system can increase muscle tone and initiate shivering in the short-term and increase thyroid hormone levels in the long-term. The hypothalamus also stimulates peripheral vasoconstriction, thereby shunting blood to the core. Sweating decreases. The thicker the outer shell, the better the insulation. All other factors being equal, heavier people are more effectively insulated from the cold. This conservation of heat for the sake of the core continues until the body's ability to generate heat becomes overwhelmed, resulting in hypothermia.

■ Heat Illness

Heat illness is an increase in core body temperature (CBT) due to inadequate thermolysis. The fundamental problem is the inability to get rid of the heat buildup in the body, often because of hot and humid conditions. A person's general state of health, clothing, mobility, age, preexisting illnesses, and certain medications (Table 35-1 ▶) can add to the problem. When the thermoregulatory system is taxed beyond its limits or fails for any reason, the core body temperature soars, sometimes rising from normal to about 41°C in less than 15 minutes. That is the situation in heat stroke, for example.

Risk Factors for Heat Illness

Certain factors increase a person's risk for ill effects from any given heat stress; the factors are summarized in (Table 35-2 ▾). Older people are at particular risk because they do not adjust as well to the heat: They perspire less; they acclimatize more slowly; they feel thirst less readily in response to dehydration; and decreased mobility may make getting a glass of water difficult. Older people are also more likely to have chronic conditions, such as diabetes and cardiovascular disease, that interfere with normal heat excretion. In addition, they are more apt to be taking medications that disrupt the body's mechanisms for dissipating heat. For example, diuretics taken for hypertension may result in an older person being dangerously close to dehydration and electrolyte disturbances and interfere with the peripheral vasodilation necessary for heat transfer. Beta blockers can lessen a tachycardic response to heat stress, as can normal age-related decreased

Table 35-1	Medications Contributing to Heat Illness
■ Alcohol	■ Laxatives
■ Alpha agonists	■ Lithium
■ Amphetamines	■ Lysergic acid diethylamide (LSD)
■ Anticholinergic medications (atropine sulfate, scopolamine, benztropine mesylate, belladonna, and synthetic alkaloids)	■ Monoamine oxidase inhibitors
	■ Phencyclidine hydrochloride
	■ Phenothiazines (prochlorperazine, chlorpromazine, promethazine)
■ Antihistamines	
■ Antiparkinsonian agents	
■ Antipsychotics (such as haloperidol)	■ Sympathomimetic medicines (amphetamines, epinephrine, ephedrine, cocaine, norepinephrine)
■ Beta blockers	
■ Calcium channel blockers	
■ Cocaine	■ Thyroid agonists (levothyroxine)
■ Diuretics (furosemide, hydrochlorothiazide, bumetanide)	■ Tricyclic antidepressants (amitriptyline, imipramine, nortriptyline, protriptyline)
■ Heroin	

Table 35-2	Factors That Predispose to Heat Illness		
Factors That Increase Internal Heat Production		**Factors That Interfere With Heat Dissipation**	
■ Physical exertion		■ High ambient temperature	
■ Response to infection (fever)		■ High humidity	
■ Hyperthyroidism		■ Obesity (insulation effect, less efficient dissipation)	
■ Agitated and tremulous states (Parkinson, psychosis, mania, drug withdrawal—opiate and alcohol)		■ Impaired vasodilation	
		■ Diabetes	
■ Drug overdoses (such as sympathomimetics, cocaine, caffeine, lysergic acid diethylamide, phencyclidine hydrochloride, methamphetamine, ecstasy)		■ Alcoholism	
		■ Drugs: diuretics, tranquilizers, beta blockers, antihistamines, phenothiazines	
		■ Impaired ability to sweat (cystic fibrosis, skin diseases, healed burns)	
		■ Heavy or tight clothing	
Factors That Increase Heat Absorption		**Factors That Impair the Body's Response to Heat Stress**	
■ Confined, unventilated, hot living quarters		■ Dehydration	
■ Working in hot conditions (bakeries, steel mills, construction sites)		■ Prior heat stroke	
		■ Hypokalemia	
■ Being in parked cars in summer		■ Cardiovascular disease	
		■ Previous stroke or other central nervous system lesion	

Table 35-3	Comparing Conditions Resulting From Heat Stress		
Variable	**Heat Cramps**	**Heat Exhaustion**	**Heat Stroke**
Pathophysiology	Sodium and water loss	Sodium and water loss, hypovolemia	Failure of heat-regulating mechanisms
Mental status	Normal	Normal or mild confusion	Altered, delirium, seizures
Temperature	May be mildly elevated	Usually mildly elevated	> 40.5°C
Skin	Cool, moist	Pale, cool, moist	Dry, hot, but sweating may persist, especially with exertional heat stroke
Muscle cramping	Severe	May or may not be present	Absent

maximum heart rates. Acclimatazation can decrease the likelihood of heat illness, but it takes days of progressive exertion in a hot environment to be effective.

Among the young and healthy, people most vulnerable to heat stress include infants and young children exposed to a hot environment. Children, compared with adults, have proportionately higher metabolic heat production, have a CBT that rises faster during dehydration, and do not dissipate heat as well owing to their smaller organ and vascular systems. Athletes and military recruits engaging in heavy exertion in hot conditions are also at increased risk.

The following subsections discuss the major types of heat illness   Table 35-3 ▲ .

Heat Cramps

Heat cramps are acute and involuntary muscle pains, usually in the lower extremities, the abdomen, or both, that occur because of profuse sweating and subsequent sodium losses in sweat. Three factors contribute to heat cramps: salt depletion, dehydration, and muscle fatigue. Heat cramps most often afflict people in good physical condition—for example, athletes, military personnel, and physical labourers. In fact, British coal miners would add salt to their beer to prevent cramps. A recent study of US college football players showed a twofold increase in sweat sodium losses in athletes prone to heat cramps. Usually a person exerting himself or herself in a hot environment will become thirsty and increase the intake of fluids. But if the person is sweating heavily, he or she is losing fluids and salt through the skin. If the person drinks plain water, he or she will not replace sweat sodium losses   Figure 35-5 ▶ . Hence, the rehabilitation sector at a fire should have watered-down sports drinks available instead of just water.

Heat cramps usually start suddenly during strenuous and/or prolonged physical activity. They may be mild, characterized by only slight abdominal cramping and tingling in the extremities. More often, however, they present with severe, incapacitating pain in the extremities and abdomen. The patient may become hypotensive and nauseated but remains alert. The pulse is generally rapid, the skin pale and moist, and the temperature normal.

Treatment of heat cramps aims to eliminate the exposure and restore lost salt and water to the body:

- Move the patient to a cool environment. Have the patient lie down if he or she feels faint.

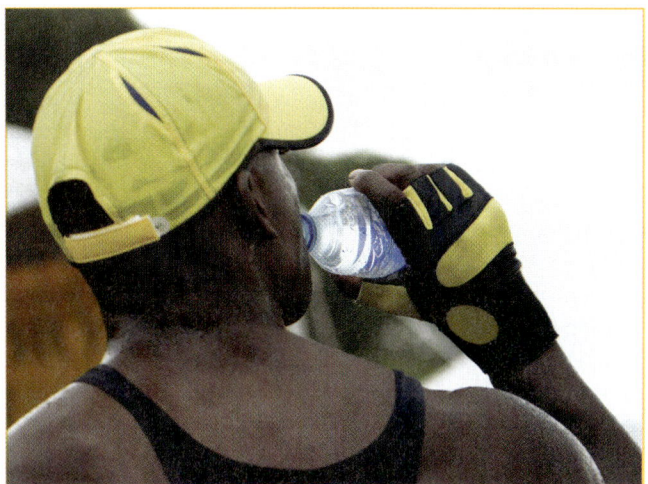

Figure 35-5 If you drink plain water, you will not replace the sweat sodium losses.

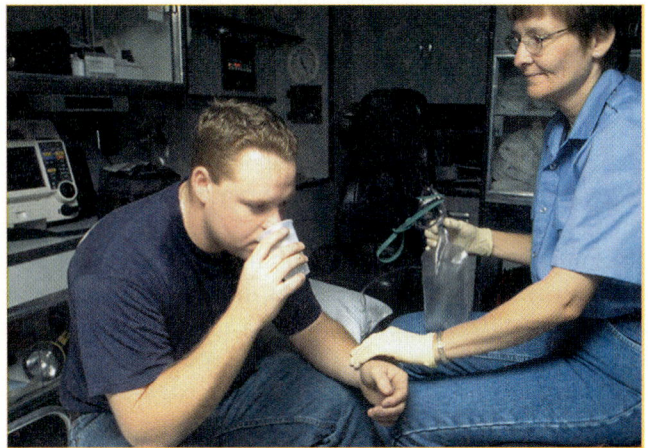

Figure 35-6 Give the patient with heat cramps one or two glasses of a salt-containing solution if he or she is not nauseated.

- If the patient is not nauseated, give one or two glasses of a salt-containing solution (such as lemonade with ½ teaspoon of salt added or a commercial sports drink)   Figure 35-6 ▲ . Instruct the patient to drink the solution slowly. Have the patient munch on salty chips or pretzels. Salt tablets can irritate the stomach lining and may precipitate or worsen nausea.

- If the patient is too nauseated to take liquids by mouth, insert an intravenous (IV) cannula and infuse normal saline rapidly. (Consult your local protocols or direct medical control for the IV rate.)
- Do not massage the cramping muscles. That tactic may actually aggravate the pain.
- As the patient's salt balance is restored, the symptoms will abate and the patient may want to resume activity. In the prehospital setting, this decision is best made with direct medical control.

Heat Syncope

Heat syncope is an orthostatic syncopal, or near-syncopal, episode that typically occurs in nonacclimated people who may be under heat stress. It can occur with prolonged standing, as in mass outdoor gatherings, or when standing suddenly from a sitting or lying position. Peripheral vasodilatation, possibly exacerbated by some degree of dehydration, is thought to be the cause. Treatment involves placing the patient in a supine position and replacing fluid deficits. If the patient does not recover quickly in the supine position, suspect heat exhaustion or heat stroke.

Heat Exhaustion

Heat exhaustion is a clinical syndrome thought to represent a milder form of heat illness on a continuum leading to heat stroke. Its hallmarks are volume depletion and heat stress. Classically, two forms are described: water-depleted and sodium-depleted. Water-depleted heat exhaustion occurs primarily in geriatric patients owing to immobility, medications that contribute to dehydration, and decreased thirst sensitivity and in active younger workers or athletes who do not adequately replace fluids in a hot environment. Sodium-depleted heat exhaustion may take hours or days to develop and results from huge sodium losses from sweating but replacing only free water, not sodium.

A concept closely related to sodium-depleted heat exhaustion is exertional hyponatremia. Studies from the Boston Marathon, the Grand Canyon National Park, and the U.S. military point to a common thread: prolonged exertion in a hot environment coupled with excessive hypotonic fluid intake. This phenomenon leads to nausea, vomiting, weight gain, and, in severe cases, mental status changes, cerebral edema, and seizures. The practical concern in the prehospital environment is older, debilitated patients and patients who participate in extreme endurance sports events such as marathons and Ironman competitions.

Symptoms of heat exhaustion may include headache, fatigue, dizziness, nausea, vomiting, and, sometimes, abdominal cramping. The patient is usually sweating profusely, and the skin is pale and clammy. He or she may be slightly disoriented. The temperature may be normal or slightly elevated ($< 40°C$). Tachycardia is present, although this response may be blunted if the patient is taking a beta blocker. Respirations are fast and shallow. Tachypnea may produce symptoms of hyperventilation: carpopedal spasm, perioral numbness, and a low end-tidal carbon dioxide

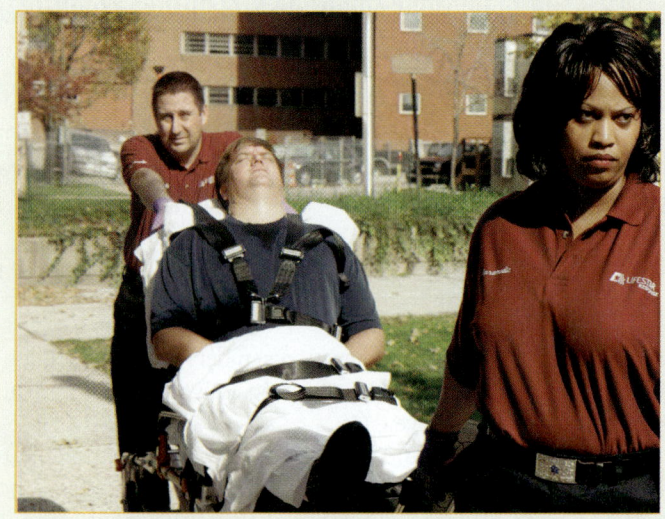

Figure 35-7 Remove the patient from the heat.

level. Blood pressure may be decreased due to peripheral pooling of blood or volume depletion; if not decreased at rest, blood pressure will almost certainly drop when the patient tries to sit or stand from a recumbent position (orthostatic hypotension). If the patient reports brown urine, suspect rhabdomyolysis (the destruction of muscle tissue leading to a release of potassium and myoglobin).

Heat exhaustion is sometimes mistaken for "summer flu," and the condition may be misdiagnosed. If untreated, heat exhaustion may progress to heat stroke. The treatment of heat exhaustion is aimed at removing the patient from exposure to heat and repairing the derangement in fluid and electrolyte balance:

- Move the patient to a cool environment **Figure 35-7 ▲** ; remove excess clothing, and place supine with legs elevated.
- If the patient's temperature is elevated, sponge, spray, or drip the patient with tepid water and fan gently to make him or her more comfortable—but don't overdo it. Heroic measures to lower body temperature rapidly are unnecessary, and chilling the patient can cause shivering and thermogenesis.
- Consider specially designed cooling chairs for hand and forearm immersion in cold water for rehabilitation at fire scenes, mass gatherings, and endurance sports.
- Oral hydration with sports drinks may be appropriate. If nausea and vomiting are present, start a normal saline IV and draw blood for electrolyte determinations. Use the heart rate and blood pressure to guide the fluid amounts administered.
- If exertional hyponatremia is suspected, do not give fluids by mouth. Instead, draw blood for checking the blood sodium level and administer IV normal saline.
- Monitor cardiac rhythm, vital signs, temperature, and end-tidal carbon dioxide.
- If you cannot determine whether the patient has heat exhaustion or heat stroke, treat for heat stroke.

Controversies

Prehospital care of endurance sports athletes is controversial. We no longer automatically give them fluids via large-bore IV and lots of oral fluid without first ruling out hypoglycemia and letting them lie down for a few minutes because they may actually be hyponatremic. In that case, the IV fluid would cause iatrogenic hyponatremia, irritable heart, and dysrhythmias.

Heat Stroke

Of all heat illnesses, heat stroke is the least common but the most deadly. It is caused by a severe disturbance in the body's thermoregulation and is a profound emergency, with mortality rates as high as 10% in treated patients and 30% to 80% in untreated patients. Experts typically rely on two findings to make this diagnosis: core temperature more than 40°C and altered mental status.

Two heat stroke syndromes are distinguished: classic and exertional Table 35-4 ▼ . Classic heat stroke (passive heat stroke), which usually occurs during heat waves, is most likely to strike very old, very young, or bedridden people. Patients with chronic illnesses, such as diabetes or heart disease, are particularly susceptible, as are people with alcoholism and patients taking certain medications (diuretics, sedatives, anticholinergics). In this syndrome, high environmental temperatures initially elicit thermolysis, but the CBT eventually soars, and the typical signs and symptoms of heat stroke appear.

Exertional heat stroke is typically an illness of young and fit people exercising in hot and humid conditions. When the ambient temperature approaches body temperature, radiation and convection are no longer effective means of shedding excess heat. If the relative humidity rises above 75%, evapourative cooling becomes ineffective. A person who continues exercising in such conditions will continue generating heat without any means of excreting that heat. Heat will then build up within the body, causing the CBT to skyrocket.

Table 35-4	Classic Versus Exertional Heat Stroke	
Characteristic	Classic Heat Stroke	Exertional Heat Stroke
Age	Older	Younger
General health	Chronic diseases, schizophrenia	Healthy person
Medications	Beta blockers, diuretics, anticholinergics	Often none, consider stimulant abuse
Activity	Very little to bedridden	Strenuous
Sweating	Absent	Present
Skin	Hot, red, dry	Moist, pale
Blood glucose level	Normal	Hypoglycemic
Rhabdomyolysis	Rare	Common
Acute renal failure	Rare	Common

The Clinical Picture of Heat Stroke

Both types of heat stroke present with similar signs and symptoms, which may or may not be recognized as the consequence of heat exposure. Patients almost certainly won't be able to give a coherent history because they will be confused, delirious, or comatose. Often the very earliest signs of heat stroke are changes in behaviour—irritability, combativeness, signs the patient is hallucinating—which may mislead bystanders and paramedics into thinking the patient is having a behavioural or substance-related emergency. Older patients with heat stroke may present with signs resembling those of a suspected stroke. Other central nervous system disturbances—including tremors, seizures, constricted pupils, and decerebrate or decorticate posturing—may also be prominent features of heat stroke.

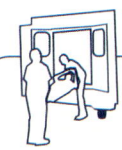

At the Scene

Suspect heat stroke and check a core temperature in any person behaving strangely in a hot environment.

The diagnostic vital sign is, of course, a markedly elevated temperature, usually greater than 40°C. Signs of a hyperdynamic state are usually present: tachycardia, hyperventilation with an end-tidal carbon dioxide of less than 20 mm Hg, and lowered peripheral vascular resistance from efforts of the body to cool itself with vasodilation. Heat stroke is characterized by some degree of dehydration, which worsens the problem by decreasing the body's ability to get the hotter core blood to the periphery for thermolysis. Blood pressure can be normal or decreased depending on the level of dehydration. The skin can be dry, red, and hot in classic heat stroke or pale and sweaty in exertional heat stroke.

The diagnosis of heat stroke is easy to miss. It may develop rapidly in a patient whose heat exhaustion was mistaken for the flu, or it may present as coma of unknown origin. Unless you keep the possibility of heat stroke constantly in mind during the hot months of the year and routinely take the temperature as part of the vital signs, you may waste precious time searching for some other cause of the patient's symptoms.

Fever and Conditions That Mimic Heat Stroke

New paramedics may face a perplexing challenge: Why is this nursing home patient's temperature elevated? Is it heat stroke, a febrile illness, or sepsis? Neurologic changes can be present in either case. The history, however, may suggest infectious causes. For example, a change in the urine colour in a catheter bag, a recent complaint of cough and dyspnea, an obvious skin infection, or complaints of a fever, rash, photophobia, and stiff neck may point to meningitis. An intermittent shaking chill also favours infectious causes of increased temperature.

A fever can signal that the body is fighting an infection by inhibiting reproduction of harmful toxins. Pyrogens (proteins secreted by infective organisms and the body's immune system) act on the hypothalamus by increasing the thermal set point, which results in a fever. The body then uses its thermoregulatory tools to maintain the new temperature setting. The patient with a reset temperature may adapt to this change by wearing more clothes, and sometimes the body creates more heat via shivering. Although aspirin and nonsteroidal anti-inflammatory drugs can lower a fever (by blocking prostaglandins), they are not usually effective in treating heat-related illness and may cause harmful side effects when organ failure is present.

Anticholinergic poisoning presents with an elevated temperature; dry, red skin; mental status changes; and tachycardia. Anticholinergic poisonings usually cause dilated pupils, whereas patients with heat stroke usually have constricted pupils.

Two rare syndromes must also be considered. Neuroleptic malignant syndrome (NMS) is caused by antipsychotic and some antiemetic medications and presents with hyperthermia, muscular rigidity, altered mental status, and a hyperdynamic state. A similar state, neuroleptic malignant-like syndrome (NMLS), can occur when medications to control Parkinson's are abruptly withdrawn. Malignant hyperthermia can occur as a result of common anesthesia medications (notably succinylcholine) and presents similarly to NMS. Researchers are exploring a common genetic contributor to malignant hyperthermia and heat stroke.

Treatment of Heat Stroke

If you are unsure about what exactly is causing the elevated temperature, the prudent step is to treat for heat stroke given the deadly consequences of missing it. Direct medical control may also help with treatment plans.

Treatment of heat stroke aims at removing the patient from the environment and promoting rapid cooling. Two main methods are used for rapid cooling: ice water body immersion and evapourative cooling by spraying tepid water over the patient accompanied by the use of fans to promote convection. Placing ice packs on the neck, groin, and axillae can augment the evapourative method. Research has shown that ice water immersion is probably the more effective means of rapid cooling but has obvious limitations in the back of an ambulance, including the need for ice. Conscious patients do not tolerate this measure well, and patients with altered mental status can be challenging to manage in an ice bath. You must also monitor CBT to avoid overshoot, resulting in shivering and even hypothermia.

- Evaluate the ABCs, administer supplemental oxygen, and be prepared to intubate.
- Move the patient to a cool environment, and strip the patient to underclothing. Monitor the rectal temperature every 10 minutes. Cooling efforts should continue until the rectal temperature has fallen below about 39°C.
- Cool as rapidly as possible by the most expeditious means available.
  - Spray the patient with tepid water while fanning constantly to promote rapid evapouration. The ambulance should carry a portable fan during the summer months for this purpose. Apply ice packs to the patient's neck, groin, and axillae to aid in cooling from evapourative techniques.

- Consider ice water immersion in cases of prolonged transport or delayed evacuation. Cooling with ice water–soaked blankets and fanning is nearly as effective as immersion. Pay close attention to airway status; watch for seizures and CBT to avoid overcooling.
- Start an IV line, give normal saline, and check the blood glucose level. Be careful with fluids—pulmonary edema is a known complication of heat stroke. Remember that cooling promotes peripheral vasoconstriction that can raise the blood pressure.
- Monitor cardiac rhythm, and remember that rhabdomyolysis can occur with resultant hyperkalemia.
- Be prepared to treat seizures with common antiseizure medicines (lorazepam, midazolam, or diazepam).

A few measures are *not* helpful: Covering the patient with wet sheets may impede heat loss by evapouration. Dantrolene, a medication once thought to aid in lowering the temperature, has not been shown to be effective. Last, massaging muscles to combat cutaneous vasoconstriction from overcooling is not beneficial.

Prevention of Heat Illness

The following measures can help protect you, your colleagues, and the communities you serve from heat illness:

- Paramedics working in hot climates should have appropriate summer uniforms.
- If you are standing by at a post or street location, park the ambulance in the shade and make sure the air conditioning works.
- Increase your daily intake of fluid. Do not rely on thirst to gauge your need. Try to drink something every hour during very hot weather, aiming for urination every 2 hours. Dark urine is concentrated, indicating that the body is dehydrated. Avoid beverages with a high sugar content and those that promote diuresis (such as caffeinated or alcoholic drinks).
- Install or carry a portable fan in the ambulance to improve convection, supplement the air conditioning, and treat patients with heat illness.
- Carry a portable cooler or—if you are lucky enough—an onboard refrigerator for hot weather. Fill the cooler about half full with crushed ice, and stock it with sports drinks or other salt-containing drinks for patients and the ambulance crew.
- Review **Figure 35-8 ▶** outlining the relationship of heat and humidity to heat stress.
- Conduct community-based programs aimed at high-risk populations—for example, nursing home risk assessments.

Be alert for early symptoms of heat illness, such as headache, nausea, cramps, and dizziness. If you experience any of those symptoms, get out of the hot environment immediately and get medical attention.

Environment Canada uses the humidex to report how hot and humid the weather feels to a person. The humidex was invented in Canada and is widely used. It combines the temperature and humidity level into one number, which is the perceived temperature **Table 35-5 ▶**. It is rare for the humidex to reach extreme levels in Canada. The highest humidex on record was in Windsor, Ontario, on June 20, 1953, when it reached 52.1.

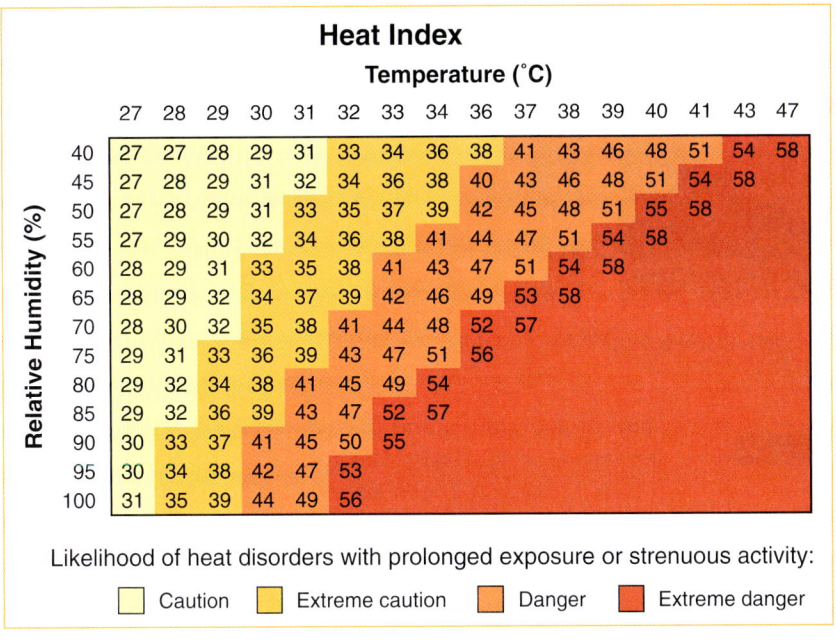

Heat Index

Temperature (°C)

	27	28	29	30	31	32	33	34	36	37	38	39	40	41	43	47
40	27	27	28	29	31	33	34	36	38	41	43	46	48	51	54	58
45	27	28	29	31	32	34	36	38	40	43	46	48	51	54	58	
50	27	28	29	31	33	35	37	39	42	45	48	51	55	58		
55	27	29	30	32	34	36	38	41	44	47	51	54	58			
60	28	29	31	33	35	38	41	43	47	51	54	58				
65	28	29	32	34	37	39	42	46	49	53	58					
70	28	30	32	35	38	41	44	48	52	57						
75	29	31	33	36	39	43	47	51	56							
80	29	32	34	38	41	45	49	54								
85	29	32	36	39	43	47	52	57								
90	30	33	37	41	45	50	55									
95	30	34	38	42	47	53										
100	31	35	39	44	49	56										

Relative Humidity (%)

Likelihood of heat disorders with prolonged exposure or strenuous activity:

☐ Caution ☐ Extreme caution ☐ Danger ☐ Extreme danger

Figure 35-8 Likelihood of heat disorders.
Reprinted from: US National Weather Service. Available at: http://www.nws.noaa.gov/om/heat/index.shtml. Accessed April 2009.

Local Cold Injury

Environment Canada uses a wind chill index that is expressed in temperature-like units. The index likens the way your skin feels to the temperature on a calm day. For example, if the outside temperature is −10°C and the wind

chill is −20, it means that your face will feel as cold as it would on a calm day when the temperature is −20°C.

Most injuries from the cold are localized to the extremities or exposed parts of the body, such as the tips of the ears, nose, upper cheek, and tips of the fingers or toes Figure 35-9 ▶. Local freezing injuries fall under the general heading of frostbite. Frostbite is an ischemic injury that is classified as superficial or deep depending on whether tissue loss occurs. With a wind chill index of −25°C, there is a risk of frostbite. When the wind chill index drops to −45°C, the skin can freeze in minutes.

A very mild form of frostbite, sometimes called frostnip, comes on slowly and generally is not painful, so the victim tends to be unaware of its occurrence. This problem is easily treated by placing a warm hand firmly over the chilled nose or ear or, when the fingers are frost-nipped, by placing the fingers into the armpit. The return of warmth to a frost-nipped area is usually signaled by some redness and tingling. Windmilling involves rapidly making a large circle with your hand, starting with your hand next to your side, raising it backward and up until you are reaching straight up, and moving it rapidly down frontward. This technique forces blood into the cold hand.

Deeper degrees of frostbite involve freezing of tissues and can occur only in ambient temperatures well below the freezing point. Cells are composed chiefly of water, so when they are subjected to low enough temperatures, the water within them turns into ice

You are the Paramedic Part 2

You ask the patient what is going on as you assist him to the ambulance. His gait is unsteady. Your partner obtains an initial set of vital signs. The patient takes a moment and tells you that he had been drinking earlier and got caught in the rain. You notice that the coat he is wearing is dry. When you ask him if it is his coat, the patient says "no." Your partner informs you that the coat belongs to the bystander who initially helped him and that his identification says he is 44 years old.

As you begin to undress the patient, you notice that his clothes are wet and his appearance is unkempt. The patient states that his head hurts. He says "no" when asked about dizziness, visual disturbances, chest pain, and trouble breathing. He says that his stomach "always hurts," and that he has trouble with his pancreas but can offer no more clarification on his pain or history. There is no nausea, vomiting, diarrhea, or unusually coloured stools. The patient states he has been drinking most of the afternoon but does not know where he is or what day it is. He denies any psychiatric history.

Vital Signs	Recording Time: 5 Minutes
Skin	Pink, cool, and dry
Pulse	112 beats/min; irregular and weak
Blood pressure	108/60 mm Hg
Respirations	24 breaths/min
Sp_{O_2}	Not reading

4. Does the additional information narrow the diagnostic possibilities?
5. What prehospital interventions might benefit the patient?
6. Why is the pulse oximetry not working?

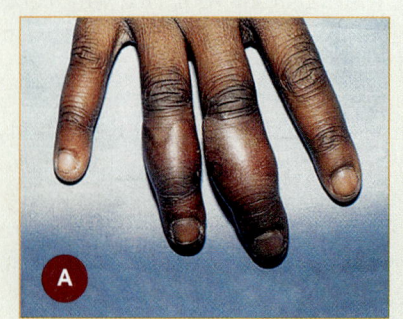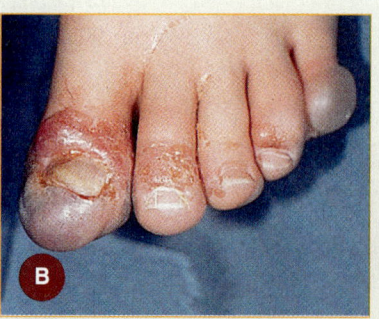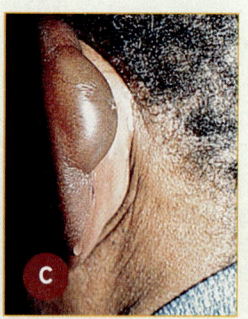

Figure 35-9 The extremities (**A** and **B**) and the ears (**C**) are particularly susceptible to frostbite.

Superficial Frostbite

The most common symptom of frostbite is an altered sensation: numbness, tingling, or burning. The skin typically appears white and waxy and has been compared with frozen halibut Figure 35-10 ▾ . Because it is frozen, the skin is firm to palpation, but the underlying tissues remain soft. Once thawing occurs, the injured area turns cyanotic, and the patient experiences a hot, stinging sensation. Capillary leakage produces edema in the frostbitten area, and blebs develop within a few hours after thawing. Dull or throbbing pain may persist for days or weeks after the injury.

The prehospital treatment of superficial frostbite differs significantly from that of deep frostbite, so it is very important to distinguish between the two. Usually it is difficult to determine the depth of the injury when you first see it—even a shallow frostbite injury can appear to be frozen solid. If the tissues beneath the skin are soft when you press down on the skin surface, the frostbite is probably superficial. If not, or if there is any doubt, treat the injury as deep frostbite.

Mild cold injuries are generally managed by a combination of dressing, rest, food, and limiting exposure to the cold. Once you have determined that the patient has superficial frostbite only, proceed as follows:

- *Get the patient out of the cold.* Take the patient indoors or into a heated ambulance so the body can stop hoarding its warm blood in the core and instead send some warm blood to the periphery, where it is urgently needed.
- *Rewarm the injured part with body heat.* If an ear, nose, or foot is frostbitten, apply firm, steady pressure against the

Table 35-5	Humidex
Humidex	**Degree of Comfort**
< 29	No discomfort
30 to 39	Some discomfort
40 to 45	Great discomfort, avoid exertion
> 45	Dangerous
> 54	Heat stroke imminent

crystals, which can damage or destroy the cells. This problem is further complicated by increased viscosity accompanied by "sludging," poor flow, capillary leakage, and resultant thrombus and ischemic injury.

Risk Factors for Frostbite

Several factors predispose a person to frostbite:

- Going out on a cold, windy day without earmuffs, mittens, a scarf, or a hat.
- Impeding the circulation to the extremities:
  - Wearing tight gloves and shoes and too many socks.
  - Lacing boots very tightly and remaining in a cramped position for a while.
  - Wearing plastic boots that won't expand. Preferably, boots should be lined with felt, which will expand when wet.
  - Smoking, which constricts arteries.
  - Drinking, which helps peripherally dilate blood vessels, helping the person to get colder.
- Going out in the cold when tired, dehydrated, or hungry.
- Coming in direct contact with cold objects.
- Not staying hydrated, which would otherwise promote increased blood flow.
- Allowing oneself to become thoroughly chilled. Generalized hypothermia is the most effective way to sustain local cold injury.

To avoid getting frostbite, avoid all of the preceding behaviours! Note the windchill, and always cover your face when you are outside for a long time (such as when skiing). Keep your feet dry and warm, and come in often to warm up. This precaution is especially important for children.

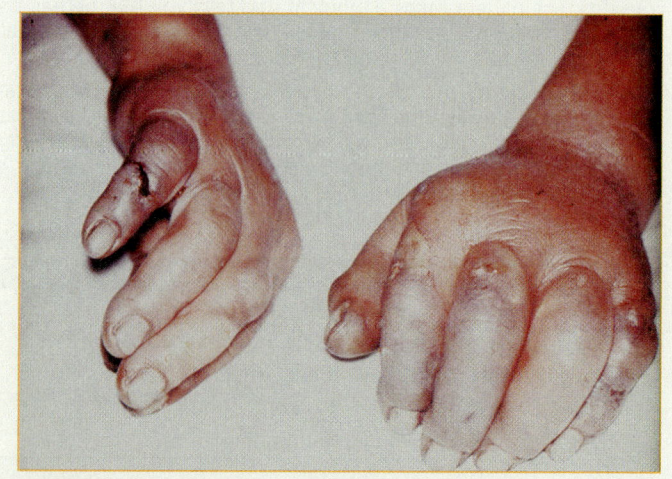

Figure 35-10 Frostbitten parts are hard and usually waxy to the touch.

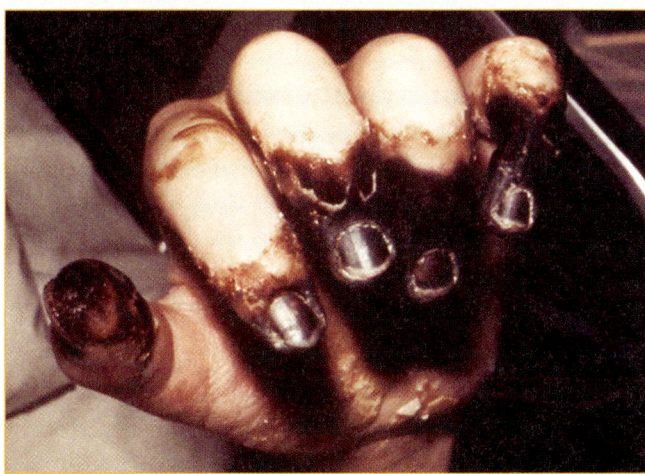

Figure 35-11 Gangrene can occur when tissue is frozen and chemical changes occur in the cells.

area with a warm hand. If a hand is frostbitten, have the patient insert the hand into the armpit and hold it there without moving. Do not try to rewarm a frostbitten part with radiant or dry heat.

- *Do not rub or massage the frostbitten area;* massage will cause further damage to injured tissues.
- *Cover blisters with a dry, sterile dressing,* and protect the area from further injury.
- *Transport the patient to the hospital* with the injured area elevated and protected from the cold.

Deep Frostbite

Deep frostbite usually involves the hands or the feet. A frozen extremity looks white, yellow-white, or mottled blue-white, and it is hard, cold, and without sensation. The major tissue damage occurs not from the freezing of the tissues, but rather when the tissues thaw out, particularly if thawing occurs gradually. When tissues thaw slowly, partial refreezing of melted water may occur. Because these new ice crystals tend to be much larger than those formed during the original freeze, they cause even greater tissue damage. As thawing occurs, the injured area turns purple and becomes excruciatingly painful. Gangrene (permanent cell death) may set in within a few days, requiring amputation of all or part of the injured limb **Figure 35-11 ▲** .

The prehospital treatment of deep frostbite depends on two factors: (1) whether the injured extremity has been partially or completely thawed before you arrive and (2) how far the patient is from the hospital.

- If the extremity is still frozen when you find the patient, leave it frozen until the patient reaches the hospital; rapid rewarming is extremely difficult to carry out properly in the prehospital environment. If you are within about an hour's drive of a medical facility:
  1. Leave the frozen extremity frozen. As long as the limb is not thawed, the patient may even walk on it if necessary.

  2. Once you get the patient into the ambulance, pad the injured extremity to protect the tissues from further trauma, and keep the extremity away from the heater or any other sources of dry heat.
  3. Do not massage the extremity. The cells are full of ice crystals, and massaging the extremity will cause the ice crystals to lacerate delicate tissues.
  4. Transport without delay.
- If the extremity is already partially thawed or if the evacuation or transport will be delayed, contact direct medical control to discuss rewarming in the out-of-hospital setting.
  1. Rewarm the injured extremity before transport. To do so, you will need a water bath—a large, clean container in which the extremity can be immersed without touching the container's side or bottom. Water should be heated in a second container and then stirred into the water bath until the temperature of the bath is between 35°C and 40°C. While you are heating the water, administer intravenous analgesia such as fentanyl or morphine. The patient will experience very severe pain as the limb thaws out, and you want to mitigate that pain as much as possible.
  2. When the water bath has reached the appropriate temperature, gently immerse the injured extremity. Keep a thermometer in the water. When the water temperature falls below 38°C, temporarily remove the injured extremity from the bath while you add more hot water to the container. Stir the water around and keep adding more hot water until the bath is again in the appropriate temperature range; then reimmerse the injured extremity.

     The rewarming procedure typically takes 10 to 30 minutes. It is complete when the frozen area is warm to the touch and is deep red or bluish (and remains red when you remove the limb from the water bath). While rewarming is in progress, the patient should be kept warm, preferably indoors, with insulated clothing and blankets. Do not permit the patient to smoke, because nicotine causes vasoconstriction and, therefore, interferes with blood flow to the injured area.
  3. Once rewarming is complete, dry the extremity and apply sterile dressings very gently. Use sterile gauze to separate frostbitten fingers and toes.

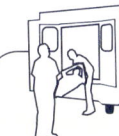

At the Scene

Do not attempt rewarming in the prehospital environment if there is any possibility of refreezing or if the patient must walk on the frostbitten foot.

Trench Foot

Trench foot involves a process similar to frostbite but can occur at temperatures as high as 15.5°C. It is caused by prolonged exposure to cool, wet conditions. The mechanism of injury can be explained by conduction: Wet feet lose heat 25 times faster than dry feet. Vasoconstriction and an ischemic cascade similar to that seen with frostbite then set in. Prevention—keeping the feet dry and warm—is the best treatment.

■ Hypothermia

Hypothermia is defined as a decrease in CBT generally starting at 35°C owing to inadequate thermogenesis and/or excess environmental cold stress. Any temperature below the body's temperature can result in hypothermia. For example, a geriatric patient with alcoholism who has had a stroke and is now living alone can become hypothermic in a 15.5°C home. An unprepared hiker caught in a summer wind and rainstorm is another classic example, as is a person who becomes submerged in icy water Figure 35-12 ▼ .

The body regulates cold stress by increasing thermogenesis, decreasing thermolysis, and pursuing adaptive behavioural changes. Table 35-6 ▼ summarizes the factors contributing to thermoregulation and hypothermia.

Risk Factors for Hypothermia

People at risk for hypothermia have increased thermolysis, decreased thermogenesis, impaired thermoregulation, or other contributing factors. Many issues can lead to the development of a hypothermic condition, including cold temperatures, fatigue, improper gear for adverse conditions, wetness, dehydration, malnutrition, and the length of exposure and intensity of weather conditions Table 35-7 ▼ .

Studies in the 1980s in New York City and other major urban areas showed that alcohol is by far the most common cause of heat loss in urban settings. It predisposes the patient to hypothermia by impairing shivering thermogenesis (decreased thermogenesis) and by promoting cutaneous vasodilatation (increased thermolysis), which hinders the body's attempts to create an insulating shell around its warm core. Liver disease, which leads to inadequate glycogen stores, and the subnormal nutritional status of most people with alcoholism further impair metabolic heat generation. Finally, alcohol impairs judgment,

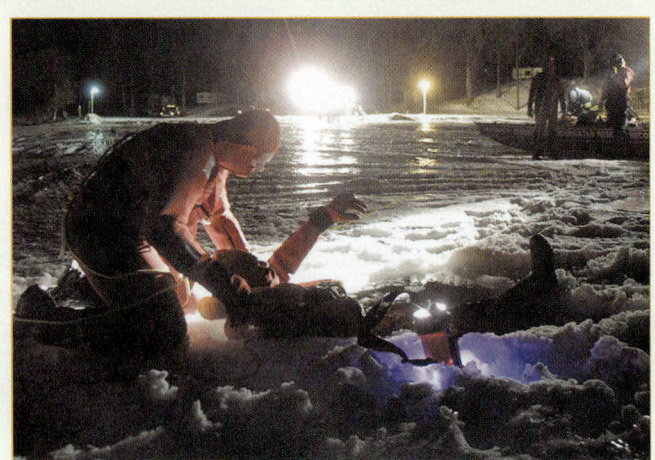

Figure 35-12 Patients who have been submerged in cold water are at high risk for hypothermia.

Table 35-6	Factors Contributing to Thermoregulation and Hypothermia		

If thermogenic factors plus heat retention factors are less than cold factors, then hypothermia results.

Thermogenic Factors	Heat Retention Factors	Cold Factors
Muscular exertion	Vasoconstriction	Radiation • Temperature • Surface areas
Shivering (↑ BMR 2–5 times)	Body surface area	Convection • Windchill
Energy stores	Adipose tissue	Conduction • Wetness

Table 35-7	Factors That Predispose to Cold Illness			

Factors That Increase Heat Loss	Factors That Impair Thermoregulatory Mechanisms	Factors That Decrease Heat Production	Miscellaneous Causes

■ Cold water drowning
■ Wet clothes
■ Windchill
■ Impaired judgment from drugs or alcohol
■ Vasodilation from:
   – Alcohol
   – Acute spinal cord injury
■ Diabetic peripheral neuropathies
	■ Dehydration
	■ Parkinson's disease or dementias
	■ Multiple sclerosis
	■ Anorexia nervosa
	■ Central nervous system bleeding or ischemic cerebrovascular accident
	■ Multisystem trauma
	■ Drugs interfering with vasoconstriction:
	   – Alcohol
	   – Benzodiazepines
	   – Phenothiazines
	   – Tricyclic antidepressants
		■ Hypothyroidism
		■ Age extremes
		■ Hypoglycemia
		■ Malnutrition
		■ Inability to shiver and immobility
			■ Sepsis
			■ Meningitis
			■ Overzealous heat stroke treatment

which often leads to inappropriate behaviour in cold conditions. Impaired thermoregulation can also occur with therapeutic or overdoses of sedative medications, tricyclic antidepressants, and phenothiazines, primarily by interfering with central nervous system (CNS)-mediated vasoconstriction.

Older people often cannot generate heat effectively because of reduced muscle mass and a diminished shivering response. Atrophy of subcutaneous fat also reduces elderly patients' insulation against heat loss. Medications commonly prescribed to older people may interfere with vasoconstriction as well. Hypothyroidism and malnutrition may further contribute to an older person's vulnerability (decreased thermogenesis).

Special Considerations

Older people on fixed budgets should be checked on during cold spells. Infants and toddlers, who have a large head-to-body surface area, should always have their heads covered during the winter.

At the Scene

Simply covering a patient hit by a car and lying in the street is not good enough; body heat continues to be conducted away into the cold pavement. Remove the patient from the street onto a blanket or backboard quickly.

The most important of the other factors contributing to hypothermia is trauma. Hypotension and hypovolemia can interfere with normal thermoregulation. Patients with CNS trauma or shock will not be able to mount a shivering response owing to the nature of their injuries. Last, hypothermia in trauma patients can lead to serious coagulation problems. If you are wearing protective gear in the cold, make sure your ambulance is toasty, ask the patient if he or she is cold, and do what you can to conserve the patient's body heat **Figure 35-13 ▶**.

The Clinical Picture of Hypothermia

The National Institutes of Health in the United States has initiated a public awareness campaign informing the public to watch for "umbles"—stumbles, mumbles, fumbles, and grumbles. These behaviours are good indicators of how the cold affects the cerebral and cognitive functioning of patients in the early stages of hypothermia.

The clinical definition of mild hypothermia is a CBT not lower than 32.2°C. Below this CBT, the condition is considered severe hypothermia. In the early stage of hypothermia, the CBT is not lower than 35°C, but the patient shows obvious signs and symptoms of hypothermia. Luckily, the body may compensate for this condition through thermogenesis until the patient finds a way to increase heat production or the glycogen energy stored in muscles and liver is exhausted.

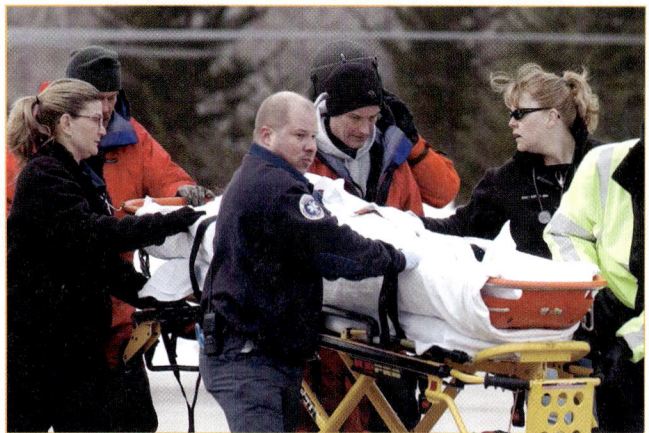

Figure 35-13 Trauma patients need to be moved to the backboard or stretcher with a blanket on it as soon as is safe and medically appropriate.

Hypothermia may also be classified according to the time to onset. Acute occurs rapidly (as in cold water drownings), subacute during a short time (as in exposure to cold conditions during a short time), and chronic that may occur over days (for example, an urban homeless person or a poorly heated home with an elderly resident). In yet another classification, primary hypothermia is caused by cold exposures, whereas secondary hypothermia is due to problems such as severe sepsis.

In mild hypothermia, the shivering is in full force and the umbles are noticeable. Often, however, the initial symptoms are vague. Older people may simply have a more flat affect, be slightly more confused, or develop symptoms suggestive of a possible stroke, including dysarthria and ataxia. No strong correlation has been observed between signs or symptoms and a specific CBT.

The net effect of hypothermia is to slow things down, but different body systems react in different ways. The overall slowdown of function is most dramatically apparent in the CNS, where just about everything slows—thinking, feeling, speaking. A hypothermic patient is typically apathetic and often shows impaired reasoning ability. Speech is slow and may be slurred; coordination is impaired; the gait is ataxic. This picture may closely resemble that associated with stroke, head injury, or alcohol intoxication, which probably explains why so many cases of hypothermia are initially misdiagnosed.

In the cardiovascular system, hypothermia induces several changes. Initially, as peripheral vasoconstriction shunts blood to the body core, the body's volume receptors interpret the increased flow as an increase in volume. They therefore stimulate the kidneys to start producing more urine (cold diuresis). At the same time, cooling of the tissues induces a flow of water from the intravascular to the extravascular spaces. The net effects are to increase the viscosity of the blood, thereby impairing circulation, and to produce a state of hypovolemia. Meanwhile, the heart is suffering from the drop in body temperature.

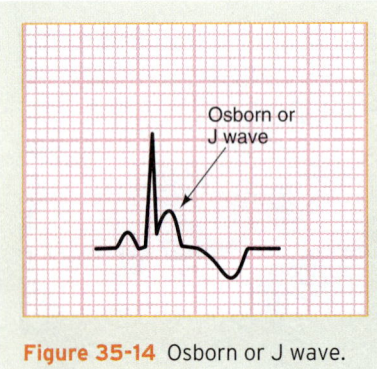

Figure 35-14 Osborn or J wave.

Cold initially speeds up the heart, then slows the rate and disrupts the electric conduction system. At a CBT of approximately 32.2°C, the body experiences cardiac dysrhythmias, including atrial fibrillation. A unique Osborn wave may be observed if shivering does not obscure the tracing **Figure 35-14 ▲** . Of special concern is ventricular fibrillation (VF), to which a hypothermic heart becomes susceptible at a CBT around 28°C. Once the heart fibrillates, repeated defibrillation is not recommended until the CBT is greater than 30°C.

Initially, the respiratory rate speeds up, but later it slows, leading to a decrease in minute volume. Tracheobronchial secretions increase, and bronchospasm may occur. At 32.2°C, hypoventilation is profound, protective airway reflexes decline, and oxygen consumption decreases by about half.

The muscular system also slows down in response to cold. Although the initial muscular reaction to cold is shivering, that reaction is a mixed blessing. It generates heat, but it also makes skilled movements more difficult. Shivering, in any case, ceases when the CBT falls below 32.7°C. Thereafter, cold muscles become progressively weaker and stiffer, impairing the exposed person's ability to save himself or herself.

Finally, cold affects the body's metabolism. Shivering can deplete the body of glucose, leading to hypoglycemia. Meanwhile, insulin levels fall, making further glucose metabolism impossible, so the body switches to the metabolism of fat. The liver's metabolism of drugs is also affected by the cold. Because medications are metabolized more slowly than normal, the effects of those drugs last much longer.

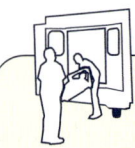

At the Scene

If a patient in a car collision is shivering, this is not a good sign. If you need heavy clothing, remember that the patient will also be cold.

Treatment of Hypothermia

This section first discusses general prehospital care and then explains how to manage cardiac arrest in a hypothermic patient. General prehospital care is aimed at preserving further heat loss and rewarming. The victim should be stripped of wet clothes and insulated from further heat loss. The 2005 Advanced Cardiac Life Support (ACLS) guidelines divide hypothermia into three classes and base treatment on the CBT and the presence (or absence) of a perfusing rhythm.

Breathing Patients With a Pulse
Mild Hypothermia Cases: 34°C

The treatment is passive rewarming, which involves removing wet clothing, drying the patient's skin, moving the patient into a warmed ambulance, and using warm blankets or reflective (space) blankets to prevent further conductive heat loss. Depending on the patient's location and the relative ease of transport, you may have to promote heat generation by feeding the patient, giving warm fluids (not caffeine or alcohol), and getting the person to move about.

Moderate Hypothermia Cases: 30°C to 34°C

The treatment is passive rewarming and active external rewarming of the truncal areas. This approach involves the use of several means to directly warm the patient's skin, including heating blankets or radiant heat from hot packs in the groin, neck, and axillae; forced hot air; and warmed IV fluids. Fluids at temperatures from 39°C to 40.5°C may be infused. It is prudent to administer a 500-ml bolus (unless otherwise contraindicated) to counter the hypovolemia commonly encountered in hypothermia. Commercial warming devices that use special blankets and a heated fan unit can warm patients at a rate of up to 2.4°C per hour, which is twice as fast as warm blankets at a rate of 1.2°C per hour. Carefully monitor the patient for hemodynamic changes and direct thermal tissue injury because active external rewarming measures can cause "afterdrop." Afterdrop, the continued lowering of CBT even after the patient is removed from the cold due to a shift of cold blood from extremities during rewarming, is more common in chronic hypothermia and hypothermia complicated by frostbitten extremities. Nevertheless, forced air rewarming can be effective for some patients, even patients with severe hypothermia.

Paramedics working in regions where winter wilderness rescue operations are routine should carry specialized gear for prehospital management of hypothermia. The hydraulic sarong, for example, is a thin, double-layered blanket with a network of plastic tubing running between the two layers **Figure 35-15 ▶** . This blanket is wrapped around the hypothermia victim, and water heated over a camp stove is pumped through the tubing. Other devices have been developed to help deliver heated, humidified supplemental oxygen to aid in core rewarming. Note that the oxygen must be heated *and* humidified to be effective, which generally requires the use of commercial devices.

Severe Hypothermia Cases: Less Than 30°C

The active internal rewarming sequence used to treat severe hypothermia is accomplished in-hospital using the following modalities: warm IV fluids; warm, humid oxygen; peritoneal lavage (potassium chloride–free fluid); extracorporeal rewarming; and esophageal rewarming tubes. Rewarming should continue until the CBT is greater than 35°C, spontaneous circulation returns, or resuscitative efforts cease.

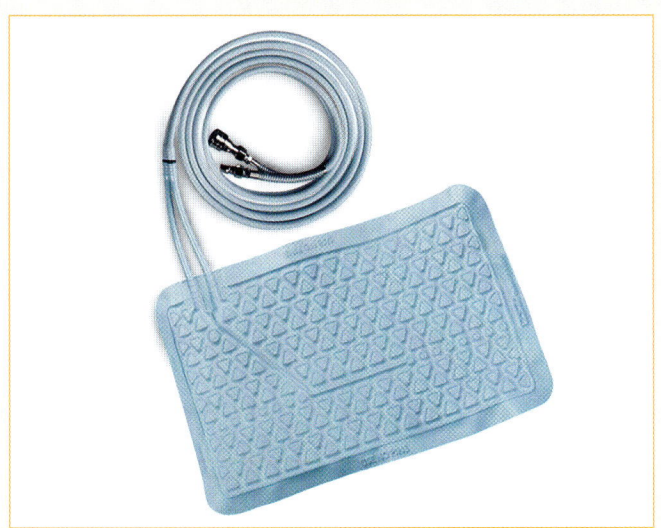

Figure 35-15 The hydraulic sarong can be wrapped around a patient with hypothermia and warms the patient via warm water fed through tubes.

Patients With No Pulse or Not Breathing

You may need to "look, listen, and feel" for a good 60 seconds to determine whether breathing and a pulse are present and, perhaps, use a portable Doppler device. Patients in cardiac arrest require high-quality CPR (push hard and fast, and allow full chest recoil) and a single shock if in VF/VT. Resume CPR immediately. Establish IV access. Infuse warm normal saline. Attempt to insert an advanced airway, and ventilate with warm, humid oxygen.

Cases of Hypothermia Less Than 30°C

Continue CPR, attempt a single defibrillation for VF/VT, establish IV access, withhold IV medications, and transport to the hospital.

Cases of Hypothermia Greater Than 30°C

Continue CPR, and administer IV medications as indicated by the electrocardiographic rhythm, but space them at longer than standard intervals. Repeat defibrillation for VF/VT as the core temperature rises. Transport the patient to the hospital to provide active internal rewarming.

Withholding and Cessation of Resuscitative Efforts

In the prehospital environment, patients with obvious lethal traumatic injuries or those so frozen as to block the airway or chest compression efforts generally are dead. If submersion preceded the arrest, successful resuscitation is unlikely, with the possible exception of immersion in icy waters. Trauma and alcohol and drug overdoses could have led to hypothermia in the first place and can hamper resuscitation efforts. Try to

Controversies

There is a widespread belief that rough handling of a hypothermic heart may cause VF. Although people in severe hypothermia are prone to a VF arrest, it has not been clearly demonstrated that intubation or roughly handling the patient causes VF. Do not let your concern for possible VF prevent you from inserting an advanced airway or moving the patient, unless dictated otherwise by your local or regional treatment protocols.

You are the Paramedic Part 3

After getting the patient out of his wet clothes, you begin your examination. He is barely shivering. He has trouble following your commands but does not seem to have any focal weakness. His pupils are equal, round, and reactive to light. His voice is slurred, but his facial muscles are symmetric and intact. The spine is nontender; the lungs are clear; and there is moderate epigastric tenderness to palpation. You find no evidence of trauma.

You insert an 18-gauge IV cannula, draw a blood sample, and check the patient's glucose level. It is 9 mmol/l. Your partner has hung a bag of warm normal saline. The rectal temperature is 33°C. You begin to remove the patient's clothes and place hot packs in the groin, axillae, and neck. You wrap the IV fluid warmer around the bag of the nonrebreathing mask and wrap the oxygen tubing in a hot pack.

Reassessment	Recording Time: 15 Minutes
Skin	Getting pinker, cold, dry
Pulse	108 beats/min; regular and strong
Blood pressure	110/64 mm Hg
Respirations	24 breaths/min
Spo$_2$	100% on nonrebreathing mask at 10 l/min supplemental oxygen; good waveform

7. What information is important to convey to the emergency department staff when you call?
8. What effect does alcohol have on hypothermia?
9. Why did the patient remove his clothing if he was hypothermic?

factor these conditions into your treatment decisions. For example, a heroin user who was found outdoors and quickly recovers after naloxone administration should have a temperature check and should not be left at the scene.

Some believe that patients who appear dead after prolonged exposure to cold temperatures are not dead until "warm and dead." The effects of hypothermia may essentially protect the brain and organs if hypothermia develops quickly, a fact that is being used to successfully treat some cardiac arrest patients. Sometimes it may be impossible to know which came first—a cardiac arrest and then hypothermia or vice versa. In those situations, it is prudent to attempt resuscitation.

Drowning or Submersion

According to the Lifesaving Society, 551 unintentional drownings occurred in Canada in 1998. Populations that are at high risk of death from drowning are toddlers, youth aged 15 to 19 years, people with seizure disorders, recreational fishermen, and aboriginal men aged 25 to 34 years. Alcohol consumption and not wearing personal flotation devices (PFDs) have been found to be factors in many boating-related drownings. Statistics Canada reported that drowning was the fourth most common cause of death by unintentional injury in Canada from 1991 to 2000, following highway deaths, falls, and poisoning. It is the leading cause of death for recreational and sporting activities. The good news is that these numbers are declining as more groups tout the virtues of prevention.

The first task in understanding drowning is to define this condition. At one point, 33 different definitions existed. In 2002, the first World Congress on Drowning developed the definition now in use: Drowning is the process of experiencing respiratory impairment from submersion/immersion in liquid. The "Utstein style" guidelines were then modified for drowning, and the term "near-drowning" was abandoned.

People may live or die based on what happens when a liquid-air interface occurs at the airway's entrance. Consequently, the drowning continuum progresses from breath holding, to laryngospasm, to the accumulation of carbon dioxide and the inability to oxygenate the lungs, to subsequent respiratory and cardiac arrest from multiple-organ failure due to tissue hypoxia. The victim can be resuscitated at any point along this continuum.

Table 35-8 ▾ lists the risk factors for drowning. Note that toddlers typically drown in bathtubs, school-age children in pools, and teens in lakes or rivers.

Table 35-8	Risk Factors for Drowning and Submersion

- Male gender
- Younger than 20 years (even higher for < 5 years)
- Preexisting conditions, such as seizure disorder
- Alcohol use
- Ineffective safety barriers (gates, locks, or use of a solar cover on a pool)
- Hyperventilation (may lead to shallow water blackout syndrome)

Pathophysiology of Drowning and Submersion

Drowning generally follows a predictable sequence starting when the victim cannot keep his or her face out of the liquid medium:

- The length of breath holding depends on the victim's state of health and fitness, his or her level of panic, and the water temperature.
- As the victim goes under and water enters the mouth and nose, coughing and gasping ensue, and the victim swallows considerable amounts of water. Note that while some theoretical differences distinguish saltwater and freshwater drownings, this information is neither clinically significant nor useful in resuscitating a patient. In fact, 11 ml of water per kilogram of body weight is required to produce significant blood problems, and 22 ml/kg is needed to create electrolyte problems. Both types of water can lead to pulmonary injuries.
- A very small amount of water is aspirated into the posterior pharynx and perhaps the trachea, setting off spasms of the laryngeal muscles (laryngospasm) that effectively seal off and protect the airway—at least temporarily—from further aspiration.
- Laryngospasm leads to asphyxia—that is, a combination of hypoxemia and hypercarbia—and the patient may lose consciousness. Hypoxemia stimulates the body to shift from aerobic to anaerobic metabolism, with the ensuing production of lactate and development of metabolic acidosis. If the patient dies during this phase of laryngospasm, as occurs in 10% to 15% of drowning cases, it is essentially a death from suffocation, because the lungs are still dry ("dry drowning").
- At a certain point, which varies from person to person, water begins to enter the lungs. That event may occur because the hypercarbic and hypoxic drives stimulate inhalation or, if the patient has lost consciousness, because progressive asphyxia causes the laryngeal muscles to relax. In either case, the net effect is to permit water to gain access to the lungs ("wet drowning"). Its entry triggers an increase in peripheral airway resistance along with constriction of pulmonary vessels, all of which decrease the compliance of the lungs. In other words, the lungs become stiff.
- The decompensation stage of drowning occurs next. The victim gasps for air, inhaling yet more water, which mixes with air and chemicals in the lungs to form froth. Apnea recurs, and the patient loses consciousness (if he or she has not already done so). The process of hypoxic brain damage begins, and cardiac arrest occurs.

Response to Drowning and Submersion Incidents

In general terms, the resuscitation of a victim of a submersion is the same as that for any other patient in respiratory or cardiac arrest, albeit with a few new logistic problems.

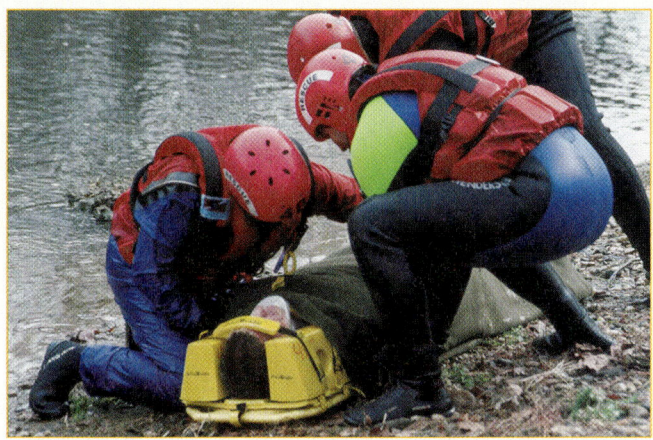

Figure 35-16 Rescuers must wear proper personal protective equipment, including a personal flotation device, when performing a water rescue.

Table 35-9 Management of Drowning and Submersion

- Rescuers trained and practiced in doing so should perform the water rescue.
- Ensure basic life support measures are being carried out with an emphasis on airway and oxygenation.
- Anticipate vomiting.
- Administer supplemental oxygen and intubate if needed.
- Establish IV access.
- Measure core temperature, and prevent or treat hypothermia.
- Give a beta-2 adrenergic by metered-dose inhaler or nebulizer for wheezing.
- Monitor end-tidal carbon dioxide and pulse oximetry.
- Insert a nasogastric tube in intubated patients.
- Transport every submersion patient to the hospital, including patients who seem to recover at the scene.

First, of course, you must reach the victim. People who have specialized training and experience in water rescue are best able to accomplish this task Figure 35-16 . Many fire departments and law enforcement agencies have water rescue teams, as does the Canadian Coast Guard, Canadian Forces, and Search and Rescue.

When you reach the victim, the steps of treatment follow the usual sequence of ABCs. The first priority is establishing the airway. Cervical spine precautions should then be taken if necessary. Routine cervical spine stabilization is not needed in cases involving drowning or submersion. The exceptions are patients who have a history of diving or using a water slide before the drowning or who have obvious traumatic injury signs and when witnesses claim alcohol was involved.

Assist ventilation as soon as possible, even before the patient is removed from the water. Do not perform manual thrusts (Heimlich maneuver) to remove water from the lungs because they may displace water from the stomach into the lungs.

Start supplementary oxygen at the same time that you quickly determine whether a pulse is present. If there is no pulse, begin high-quality CPR. You may need to suction. One Australian study of drowning victims noted that 66% of patients receiving rescue breathing and 86% getting compressions vomited; one of your primary goals will be to prevent vomiting. In any event, protect the airway from aspiration during vomiting. Advanced airway placement may be appropriate if BLS airway interventions fail.

During normal, spontaneous breathing, the pressure in the airways at the end of exhalation is effectively zero. As a result, some alveoli normally collapse during the expiratory phase of the respiratory cycle. When there is widespread atelectasis and shunt—as in drowning—it is desirable to maintain some positive pressure at the end of exhalation to keep alveoli open and to drive any fluid that may have accumulated in the alveoli back into the interstitium or capillaries. The technique called positive end-expiratory pressure (PEEP) focuses on maintaining some degree of positive pressure at the end of the expiratory phase of respiration. In the prehospital environment, PEEP is indicated for intubated patients who must be transported over long distances to the hospital after submersion or who have other conditions that produce significant shunt. Several commercial devices are designed to allow PEEP delivery. PEEP can be delivered to improve oxygenation to either intubated patients or to nonintubated patients who are being bag-valve-mask ventilated. Other simple CPAP delivery devices may also be used via mask, although these are usually not used in patients with an impaired level of consciousness. In addition, portable ventilators usually have a PEEP setting.

If an endotracheal tube has been inserted (not before insertion!), insert a nasogastric tube to decompress the stomach (discussed in Chapter 11). If a pulse is absent, implement advanced life support measures similar to those used in any other case of cardiopulmonary arrest: establish IV access, administer epinephrine and other appropriate ACLS drugs, perform cardiac monitoring, and ensure electric conversion of VF.

Patients rescued from submersion are prone to bronchospasm from the irritation to their airways. If you hear wheezes, administer a beta-2 adrenergic drug, such as salbutamol by nebulizer, as you would for a patient having an acute asthmatic attack.

Do not give up on the victim of submersion, especially if the patient is a child and the incident occurred in icy water Figure 35-17 . Successful resuscitations with complete neurologic recovery have been reported even in cases in which the victim had been submerged for more than an hour in icy water. Remember to consider the effects of hypothermia on a drowning patient, including measuring a core temperature and using the hypothermia algorithm. Studies indicate that the length of submersion and the response to resuscitation in the prehospital environment are major predictors of outcome. In other words, if patients are awake on hospital arrival, they will do better.

Table 35-9 summarizes the management of drowning and submersion.

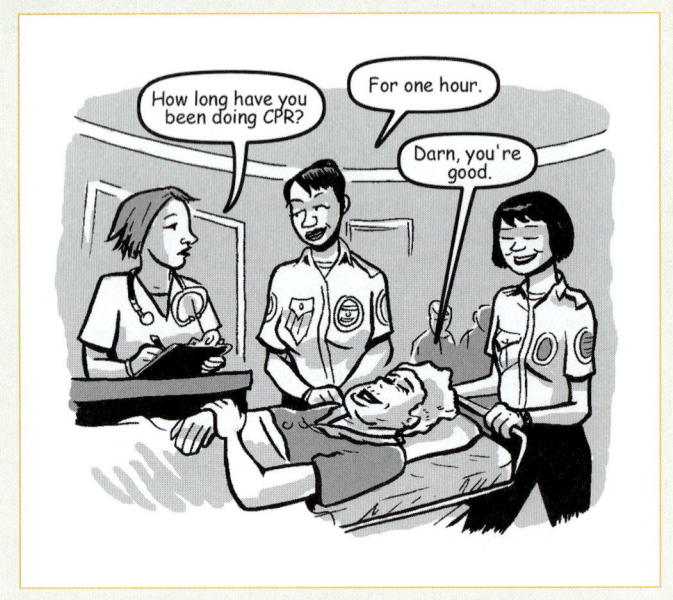

Figure 35-17

Documentation and Communication

In case of a diving emergency, pass along the following information to the emergency department: how long the diver was at the bottom, how many dives were performed, whether the patient was carrying a computer that recorded dive-related data, whether there was a decompression stop before fully ascending, and how deep the diver was.

Postresuscitation Complications

Adult respiratory distress syndrome, chemical or bacterial pneumonitis, and renal failure are common complications that can occur hours to days after a submersion. These factors highlight the importance of an emergency department evaluation of submersion victims. Their symptoms may be subtle (slight cough, mild tachypnea), or they may be asymptomatic.

Diving Injuries

There are millions of recreational scuba divers around the world, not to mention people engaged in diving for commercial and military purposes. Paramedics who work in coastal or lakefront areas are likely to encounter a diving casualty. Paramedics who operate in areas where diving is popular should become at least as conversant with diving medicine as enthusiasts of the sport.

Four modes of diving are distinguished:

- **Scuba diving.** The most popular form of diving, scuba diving is named for the self-contained underwater breathing apparatus that the diver carries on his or her back.
- **Breath-hold diving.** Also called free diving, it does not require any equipment, except sometimes a snorkel.

- **Surface-tended diving.** Air is piped to the diver through a tube from the surface.
- **Saturation diving.** The diver remains at depth for prolonged periods.

All divers, irrespective of the type of diving they do, are subject to the increased ambient pressures that occur under water.

Pressure Effects: Physical Principles

Pressure, which is defined as force per unit area, may be expressed in a number of ways. The weight of air at sea level, for example, can be expressed as 14.7 pounds per square inch (psi), as 760 mm Hg, or as 1 atmosphere absolute (ATA). The latter system—measurement in atmospheres absolute—is used most commonly in diving medicine. Because water is much denser than air, relatively small changes in depth produce large changes in pressure. For every 33 feet of seawater (fsw), the pressure increases 1 ATA. The depth of the dive can be used to estimate the pressure to which the diver was exposed: At a depth of 33 fsw, the pressure is 2 ATA; at 66 fsw, it is 3 ATA; and so forth. The majority of scuba diving is done at depths between 60 and 120 fsw.

The body and its tissues, because they are composed primarily of water, are not compressible and, therefore, are not significantly affected by the pressure changes experienced in descent or ascent through water. Gas-filled organs are another matter, however, because they *are* compressible:

- Nitrogen, an inert gas, is fat-soluble (it prefers to dissolve in fatty or lipid-rich tissues), exists safely as gas nuclei in body tissues, and is found in 79% of the air we breathe. It produces nitrogen narcosis in humans at a depth of 100 fsw. Nitrogen can cause decompression sickness (decompression illness) on ascent because of the bubbles that form on reduction of pressure. For this reason, commercial divers use a decompression schedule. Recreational divers usually adhere to a "no-decompression" limit (a table outlining safe times at various depths) so they do not have to decompress on surfacing.
- Boyle's law states that at a constant temperature, the volume of a gas is inversely proportional to its pressure (if you double the pressure on a gas, you halve its volume): $PV = K$, where P = pressure, V = volume, and K = a constant. This equation tells us that as a diver descends (and the pressure goes up), gas volume is reduced; as the diver ascends (pressure goes down), gas volume increases **Figure 35-18** ▸ . This law explains the problems that can occur in gas-filled spaces in the body (eg, lungs, gastrointestinal tract, sinuses, and parts of the ear).
- Dalton's law deals with the pressures exerted by mixtures of different gases. Dalton's law states that each gas in mixture exerts the same partial pressure that it would exert if it were alone in the same volume and that the total pressure of a mixture of gases is the sum of the partial pressures of all gases in the mixture. Thus, for fresh air:

$$P_{total} = P_{O_2} + P_{CO_2} + P_{N_2}$$

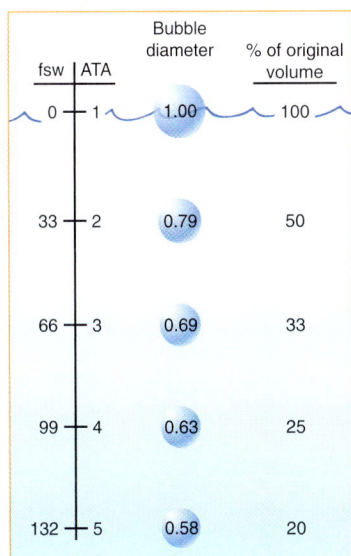

Figure 35-18 Boyle's law: As a bubble descends through water, its volume changes in inverse proportion to the ambient temperature.

This law helps explain nitrogen narcosis, oxygen toxicity, and the dangers of contamination in pressurized breathing systems. It also explains why pulse oximetry readings in divers with nitrogen narcosis remain unaffected.

- Henry's law states that the amount of gas dissolved in a liquid is directly proportional to the partial pressure of the gas above the liquid. A classic example of this law is when a sealed bottle that has dissolved carbon dioxide is opened: The lowering of the pressure of the gas in solution (in this case, a mixture of a liquid and a gas) allows its volume to increase and the gas to escape as bubbles.

Diving History

It is very important to obtain as many details as you can about the dive and the onset of the patient's symptoms. It is helpful to use a special form for taking the diving history that records the following information:

- Onset of symptoms (during ascent or descent). Decompression sickness will usually manifest within the first hour of surfacing and certainly within 6 hours. Symptoms occurring within 10 minutes suggest air embolism, especially when they are accompanied by a loss of consciousness.
- Type of diving and the type of equipment used
- Type of tank used (compressed air or a Nitrox system with distinctive yellow and green stripes on the tank)
- Site of diving and water temperature
- Number of dives made during the past 72 hours, along with the depth, bottom time, and surface interval for each. Was a dive computer used?
- Were safety stops used?
- Were there any attempts at in-water decompression (a no-no!)?
- Dive complications, if any
- Predive and postdive activities

Injuries During Descent

The major problem encountered during descent is barotrauma ("squeeze"). This injury results from a pressure imbalance between gas-filled spaces inside the body and the external atmosphere. Barotrauma can result from two different mechanisms: compression of gases within body spaces during descent or expansion of gases within those spaces during ascent (discussed later). Barotrauma can affect any gas-filled space in the body, including the sinuses, the inner and middle ears, and even teeth. **Table 35-10 ▶** summarizes the types of barotrauma.

A person who is scuba diving is theoretically protected from barotrauma by breathing compressed air, which will match the pressure of the surrounding environment. Thus, as long as the air-filled cavities of the body can equilibrate freely, they will not implode, unless there is an obstruction.

If there is blockage in the eustachian tube, which connects the middle ear with the nasopharynx, or if the diver cannot equalize ear pressures with a Valsalva maneuver, the pressure in the middle ear cannot be equalized with that of the outside water. A characteristic "middle ear squeeze" syndrome then develops with severe ear pain. If the tympanic membrane ruptures, nausea, vomiting, and vertigo may occur. This effect is especially likely in colder waters. At depths, this reaction may cause panic, rapid ascent, and the problems associated with such an ascent. Treatment involves a loose dressing for ear bleeding; some patients may require IV antiemetics or sedatives.

Injuries at Depth

Nitrogen narcosis ("rapture of the deep," "narc'ed") is a state of altered mental status caused by breathing compressed air (including nitrogen) at depth. The human body does not use nitrogen for metabolism; thus, in a breathing gas mixture, nitrogen dilutes the concentration of oxygen. A problem may occur when a diver descends to a depth of 99 ft (30 m), for example, where the ambient pressure is 4 ATA. For the person to be able to breathe, the inspired air pressure must be the same as the ambient pressure. Thus, the inspired partial pressure of nitrogen is 80% times 4 ATA, or 3.2 ATA (per Dalton's law).

Nitrogen narcosis typically occurs around 100 ft, becomes more pronounced at 150 fsw, and is why sport divers should not use compressed air only for dives greater than 120 ft. Signs and symptoms include a euphoric feeling; inappropriate behaviour at depth, including lack of concern for safety, apparent stupidity or inappropriate laughter; and tingling of lips, gums, and legs. Divers report tolerance over their diving lifetime. A diver may suddenly become panicked and spit out the regulator or surface too quickly. The only effective way to counteract the narcotic effect of nitrogen is to lower the nitrogen partial pressure through controlled ascent or by using a Nitrox system.

Injuries During Ascent
Barotrauma

As the diver ascends and the ambient pressure around him or her decreases, the gases within the body's air-filled spaces will expand. For example, the lung volume of a scuba diver who

Table 35-10 Diving Injuries

Mechanisms and Pathophysiology	Body Region	Condition	Clinical Features	Treatment
Barotrauma				
During *descent:* compression of gas in closed spaces	Ear	External ear squeeze (*barotitis externa*)	Otalgia, bloody otorrhea	Keep ear canal dry; no swimming or diving until healed
		Middle ear squeeze (*barotitis media*)	Severe ear pain, tympanic membrane can rupture; emesis, vertigo, nystagmus	Decongestants; no diving until healed, may need IV antinausea medications
		Inner ear squeeze	Tinnitus, vertigo, hearing loss; emesis, pallor, diaphoresis	May need IV antinausea medications, surgical repair
	Paranasal sinuses	Sinus squeeze	Severe pain over affected sinuses and upper teeth, epistaxis	Topical and oral decongestants; antibiotics
	Face	Face mask squeeze	Ecchymoses and petechiae of skin beneath face mask; scleral/conjunctival hemorrhage	Cold compresses, prevent by forced exhalation through nose
During *ascent:* expansion of gas in closed spaces	Gastrointestinal tract	"Gas in gut" (*aerogastralgia*)	Colicky belly pain, belching, flatulence	Rare reports of rupture; usually, no care needed
	Lungs	Pulmonary barotrauma "burst lung," pulmonary overpressurization syndrome (POPS)	Dyspnea, dysphagia, hoarseness, substernal pain; subcutaneous emphysema around neck; pneumothorax, syncope	100% oxygen; decompress pneumothorax
		Arterial gas embolism (AGE)— complication of POPS	Altered mental status, vertigo, dizziness, seizures, dyspnea, pleuritic chest pain, sudden loss of consciousness on surfacing; sudden death	100% oxygen; transport supine; hyperbaric therapy; steroids
Decompression sickness	Skin		Pruritus, subcutaneous emphysema, swelling, rashes	Symptomatic; observe for complications
	Joints and muscles	Bends ("pain-only bends")	Arthralgias, especially in elbows and shoulders, relieved by pressure	Analgesia; observe
	Cerebrum		Multiple sensory and motor disturbances	Hyperbaric therapy; IV fluids
	Cerebellum	The "staggers"	Unsteadiness, incoordination, vertigo	Corticosteroids for all patients with anything more than skin and musculoskeletal involvement
	Spinal cord		Paraplegia, paraparesis, bladder dysfunction (inability to void), back pain	See above
	Lungs	Venous air embolism (the "chokes")	Chest pain, cough, dyspnea, signs of pulmonary embolism	See above
Dissolved nitrogen	Central nervous system	Nitrogen narcosis ("rapture of the deep")	Symptoms like those of alcohol intoxication	Ascent to shallower water
Hyperventilation before dive	Central nervous system	Shallow water blackout (in breath-hold dives)	Loss of consciousness just before reaching surface	100% oxygen; assisted breathing

has inhaled to his total lung capacity at a depth of 33 fsw would double by the time the diver reached the surface if he were to hold his breath during ascent. For that reason, all diving students are trained to exhale constantly as they are ascending so as to vent air from their lungs. A common scenario in which barotrauma occurs involves a diver who has used decongestants before a dive. If the medication begins to wear off before ascent, air may become trapped in the sinuses and ears, creating a "reverse squeeze" in which the increasing pressure cannot equalize during ascent. Symptoms are identical to those observed during descent.

A more dangerous situation can occur in an emergency ascent—for example, when the diver experiences difficulty with his or her equipment and panics—and gives in to the instinctive impulse to hold his or her breath under water. The result is one of the worst forms of barotrauma of ascent—pulmonary overpressurization syndrome (POPS), also known as "burst lung." It can cause pneumothorax, mediastinal and subcutaneous emphysema, alveolar hemorrhage, and a lethal arterial gas embolism (AGE). Because the relative pressure and volume changes are greatest near the surface of the water, which is also the area of greatest danger for burst lung, a very small overpressurization—that produced by breath holding for the last 2 m of ascent, for example—can suffice to rupture alveoli. People with chronic obstructive pulmonary disease and asthma are at increased risk owing to their already-altered air movement dynamics.

When alveoli rupture, the signs and symptoms depend in part on where the air escaping from the lungs ends up. Most commonly, it leaks into the mediastinum and beneath the skin, causing mediastinal and subcutaneous emphysema. The patient may complain of a sensation of fullness in the throat, pain on swallowing (odynophagia), dyspnea, or substernal chest pain. When the patient speaks, he or she may be hoarse or have a brassy quality to the voice. Physical examination may reveal palpable subcutaneous air above the clavicles. Sometimes a crunching noise that is synchronous with the heartbeat may be audible by auscultation. Theoretically, pneumothorax is also a possibility after alveolar rupture, so always look for unequal breath sounds, low pulse oximetry values, and hyperresonance on the affected side of the chest.

By far, the most dangerous possible consequence of POPS is AGE, which is second only to drowning as a cause of death among divers. Air bubbles from ruptured alveoli enter the pulmonary capillaries and coalesce into increasingly larger bubbles as they travel through the pulmonary veins back to the left side of the heart. From the left ventricle, these bubbles may enter the coronary arteries, producing all of the effects of acute myocardial infarction, including cardiac arrest. The vast majority of air emboli, however, proceed to the cerebral circulation simply because the diver's head is usually the highest part of the body during ascent and bubbles rise.

The clinical picture of AGE tends to be dramatic. Symptoms usually appear within seconds or minutes (most commonly within 10 minutes) after surfacing and may involve just about

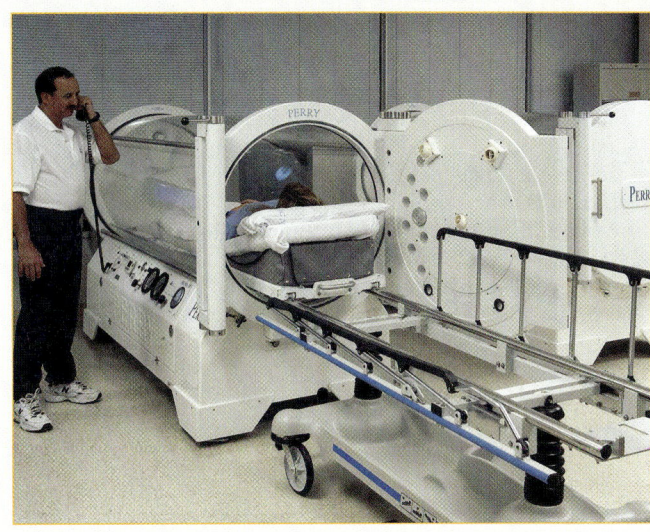

Figure 35-19 A hyperbaric chamber, usually a small room, is pressurized to more than atmospheric pressure and used in the treatment of decompression sickness and air embolism.

any cerebral function. The patient may experience weakness or paralysis of one or more of the extremities, seizure activity, or unresponsiveness. A variety of other neurologic symptoms—including paresthesias, visual disturbances, deafness, and changes in mental status—are also reported.

Notes from Nancy

Any diver who loses consciousness right after a dive has suffered an air embolism until proved otherwise.

The prehospital treatment of a patient with pulmonary barotrauma depends—at least in terms of urgency—on whether the patient has an AGE. A diver with only pneumomediastinum and subcutaneous emphysema will probably be managed symptomatically in the hospital. A pneumothorax may require needle decompression or a chest tube. In the prehospital environment, give 100% oxygen (by nonrebreathing mask; if you must bag the patient be careful—that is, don't give PEEP to POPS!) as it increases oxygen's partial pressure and may decrease bubble size and speed up "off-gassing." If you suspect an AGE, transport the patient to a hyperbaric chamber facility as soon as possible for recompression **Figure 35-19 ▲** . **Table 35-11 ▶** summarizes the treatment of suspected AGE.

Decompression Sickness

Decompression sickness (DCS) refers to a broad range of signs and symptoms caused by nitrogen bubbles in blood and tissues coming out of solution during ascent. Bubbles do their damage in two ways: by interfering mechanically with tissue perfusion and by triggering chemical changes within the body. The ensuing multisystem disorder can potentially affect almost every

Table 35-11	Treatment of Suspected AGE

- Ensure an adequate airway. Intubate an unresponsive patient with an advanced airway, but remember to fill air balloons with saline—not air—to allow for hyperbaric therapy.
- Administer 100% supplemental oxygen by nonrebreathing mask.
- Transport in supine position. Monitor for hypothermia if appropriate.
- Ground transport is preferred to air owing to cabin pressures.
- Establish IV access, and administer normal saline solution.
- Monitor cardiac rhythm, and be prepared to treat dysrhythmias.
- Have drugs ready for immediate use if needed:
  - Seizures may require sedatives (lorazepam, midazolam, or diazepam).
  - Dopamine infusion (10 μg/kg/min) may be needed for hypotension.
- Follow local protocols for direct referral to a hyperbaric chamber facility.

Table 35-12	Treatment of Decompression Sickness

- Ensure an adequate airway.
- Give 100% supplemental oxygen by nonrebreathing mask.
- Insert an IV line for normal saline, and give fluids at the rate ordered. (For long-range transport of a catheterized patient, adjust fluids to produce a urine output of 1 to 2 ml/kg/h.)
- Contact direct medical control regarding the use of steroids or lidocaine.
- Do not use nitrous oxide/oxygen (Nitronox) for analgesia!
- Arrange for transport per protocol to a hyperbaric facility. If you don't know where that is, telephone the Divers Alert Network for assistance: (919) 684-8111.

Source: Adapted from Hacket PH, Roach RC. High-altitude illness. *N Engl J Med* 2001; 345:107-114.

organ in the body. Because nitrogen is highly lipid-soluble, the CNS and the spinal cord are more susceptible to DCS.

As a diver descends, increasing quantities of nitrogen and oxygen become dissolved in the blood (per Henry's law) and are then carried to the tissues. As the diver ascends and ambient pressure decreases, the reverse process occurs: Nitrogen begins to diffuse out of the tissues. If the ascent is slow enough, the amount of nitrogen in the tissues will equilibrate with that in the alveoli. If the ascent takes place more rapidly than nitrogen can be removed, however, the diver's tissues will literally begin to bubble. This effect can be worsened if the diver undertakes multiple dives in a short time without allowing for nitrogen "off-loading."

Another risk factor for DCS is the presence of a patent foramen ovale (PFO), which affects as much as one third of the general population. This congenital defect arises when the foramen ovale between the atria fails to close at birth. Bubbles formed in the venous system may pass through the PFO, bypass the lungs, and travel to body tissues, causing symptoms. Other risk factors for DCS include obesity (more fatty tissues), dehydration, fatigue, and flying (going to higher altitude) within 12 to 14 hours of diving.

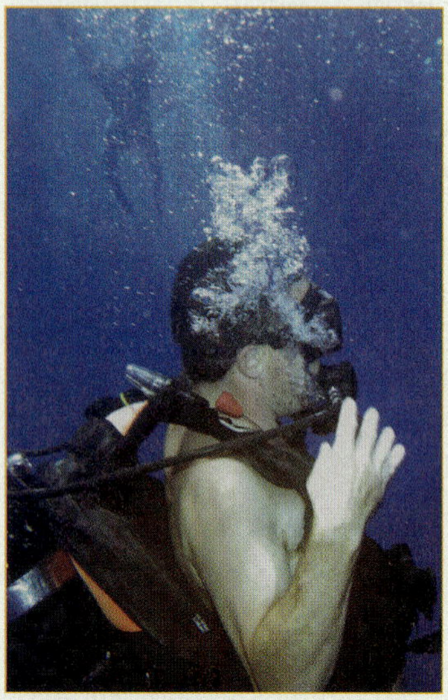

Decompression sickness is classified as type I or type II. Type I refers to mild forms of DCS that involve only the skin, lymphatic

Figure 35-20 Decompression sickness (the "bends") affects divers who ascend to the surface too quickly.

system, and musculoskeletal system. Joint pain, the most common symptom, causes the patient to "bend" over in pain. The skin may become mottled and pruritic. Type II includes all the other organs and is regarded as more serious. A much more informative way to describe DCS is to specify the systems affected and the precise symptoms (see Table 35-10).

It may not always be possible to distinguish between DCS and AGE in the prehospital setting, especially when the patient has neurologic symptoms **Figure 35-20** . As a general rule, symptoms produced by air embolism usually reflect cerebral dysfunction, whereas the spinal cord is more likely to be involved in decompression sickness. A loss of consciousness points to AGE. In terms of prehospital treatment, the distinction between the two is somewhat academic, because management in either case is basically supportive: Get the patient to a hyperbaric facility in optimal condition **Table 35-12** . Hyperbaric oxygen therapy involves intermittent inhalation of pure oxygen under a pressure greater than 1 atm. This treatment mechanically reduces bubble size, reduces nitrogen content, and increases oxygen delivery to ischemic tissues.

Other Gas-Related Problems

Most recreational divers breathe compressed air. Tanks that hold various mixtures of nitrogen and oxygen allow divers to remain underwater for longer periods. Such divers are less likely to develop DCS because they are breathing less nitrogen. Conversely, these divers are more prone to oxygen toxicity, which constitutes a CNS emergency. An affected diver may experience dizziness, lack of coordination, confusion, twitching or paresthesia symptoms, and underwater seizures.

On rare occasions, a scuba tank may be filled with contaminated air, especially if the compressor that fills the tanks malfunctions. Carbon monoxide and carbon dioxide will affect the diver quickly—a characteristic that helps distinguish this condition from DCS.

Shallow Water Blackout

Shallow water blackout is a condition that may be seen by paramedics in any part of the country. It can occur as readily in the backyard swimming pool as in the ocean. The blackout is most frequently seen among adolescent boys competing to see who can remain the longest underwater. One way of extending one's underwater endurance—at least among swimmers who don't know any better—is to hyperventilate just before diving beneath the surface. Hyperventilation decreases Pa_{CO_2} and causes cerebral vasoconstriction. Meanwhile, as the swimmer descends, his or her Pa_{O_2} increases. Because the Pa_{CO_2} is relatively low, the diver's respiratory drive is suppressed, so the person tends to remain underwater longer than normal—and all the while oxygen is being removed from the alveoli. The individual remains conscious because cerebral function is maintained by the increased Pa_{O_2} at depth. On surfacing, however, ambient pressure rapidly decreases, the Pa_{O_2} plummets, and hypoxemia combined with cerebral vasoconstriction causes blackout just before reaching the surface.

Treatment is the same as for any other case of drowning. When the patient regains consciousness, however, a lecture is in order: Explain to the victim and his or her friends that hyperventilation before a breath-hold dive can indeed help a swimmer remain underwater for a long time—sometimes forever.

Getting Help for Diving Injuries

A valuable resource for emergency medical personnel dealing with underwater diving accidents is the Divers Alert Network (DAN), which provides a 24-hour emergency consultation service at (919) 684-8111. Calls are received at DAN headquarters at Duke University Medical Center in Durham, North Carolina. DAN is an international organization that provides medical assistance and information to divers around the world via telephone and Internet. It also funds medical research and diving safety courses. Physicians, nurses, paramedics, and other health care professionals answer these calls and can assist with diagnosis, provide advice for early management of the accident, and supervise referral to an appropriate recompression chamber when necessary. The DAN also produces many excellent training and continuing medical education resources, which are available on its website.

Altitude Illness

Altitude illnesses are illnesses caused by the effects of hypobaric (low atmospheric pressure) hypoxia on the CNS and pulmonary system as a result of unacclimatized people ascending to altitude. It runs the gamut from the common acute mountain sickness (AMS) to the rare deaths from high-altitude cerebral edema (HACE) and high-altitude pulmonary edema (HAPE). It typically occurs in people who rapidly ascend to heights above 2,500 m (8,000′) but can occur at altitudes as low as 2,000 m (6,500′). Symptoms usually occur within 6 to 10 hours. The risk of altitude illness is related to the rate of ascent and altitude. Altitude can be classified into high (1,500 to 3,500 m [4,500′ to 10,500′]), very high (> 3,500 to 5,500 m [10,500′ to 16,500′]), and extreme height (> 5,500 m [16,500′]). Rapid ascent to an altitude of 5,500 m (10,500′), even for only a brief period of time, can lead to severe illness or death.

Altitude illness is a problem of hypoxia caused by low atmospheric pressures. The partial pressure of oxygen in the atmosphere decreases with increasing altitude but remains a constant 21% of the earth's barometric pressure. The barometric pressure at 5,500 m (10,500′) is half of what it is at sea level. For example, the partial pressure of arterial oxygen (Pa_{O_2}) is 103 mm Hg at sea level but only 81 mm Hg in Cypress Hills, Saskatchewan (1,468 m). Barometric pressure varies according to how far north you are located and is typically lower in the winter. Interestingly, local changes in barometric pressures can alter the "relative altitude" by 500 to 2,500′. In addition, the temperature drops approximately 6.5°C for every 1,000 m of elevation, and the penetration of ultraviolet light increases by approximately 4% for every 300 m of elevation, which adds to the risk for illness.

Risk Factors for Altitude Illness

Several factors predispose a person to altitude illnesses. The most important risk factor is a history of AMS, in which case slow ascents and use of prophylactic medicines are recommended. Normal residence below 914 m (3,000′), physical exertion, presence of chronic obstructive pulmonary disease, and sleeping above 2,438 m (8,000′) also increase the risk of developing altitude illness Figure 35-21 ▶ . Physical fitness is not a factor. Indeed, older people may be less likely to develop such an illness. Another individual factor is the hypoxic ventilatory drive. The brain stem normally responds to rising carbon dioxide levels. If you suddenly find yourself at altitude, the brain stem senses the lowered oxygen levels and responds by increasing ventilations.

The Clinical Picture of Altitude Illness

The following definitions have been established for altitude illness:

- **Acute mountain sickness (AMS).** At Lake Louise in 1993, a consensus committee determined a definition for AMS. For a diagnosis of AMS, all three of the following criteria

You are the Paramedic Part 4

As you transfer the patient into the emergency department, a member of the nursing staff comments that she saw him during her last shift. You politely convince her that despite his history, the patient is in moderate hypothermia and may have acute pancreatitis. She is appreciative of the blood draw and the prehospital care you've given. You assist the staff as they place the patient on a commercial hot-air warming blanket. When you follow up later, you learn that the patient was eventually rewarmed but was admitted for pancreatitis and observation.

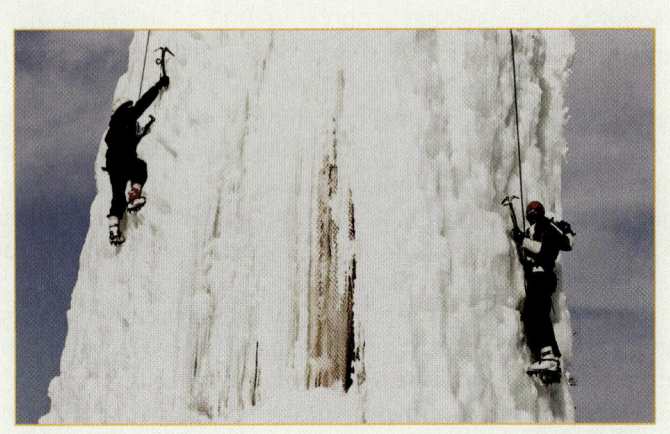

Figure 35-21 Physical exertion is a risk factor for altitude illness.

must be present: a recent gain in altitude; at least several hours at the new altitude; and the presence of headache combined with any one of these symptoms: fatigue or weakness, gastrointestinal symptoms (nausea, vomiting, or loss of appetite), dizziness or lightheadedness, or difficulty sleeping. The headache is often described as throbbing that is worse over the temporal or occipital areas and is exacerbated by the Valsalva maneuver.

- **High-altitude pulmonary edema (HAPE).** At least two of the following symptoms: dyspnea at rest, cough, weakness or decreased exercise performance, or chest tightness or congestion. Also, at least two of the following signs: central cyanosis, audible rales or wheezing in at least one lung field, tachypnea, or tachycardia.
- **High-altitude cerebral edema (HACE).** HACE requires the presence of a change in mental status and/or ataxia in a

Table 35-13	Management and Prevention of Altitude Illnesses		
Clinical Condition	**Signs and Symptoms**	**Management**	**Prevention**
Mild AMS	Headache with nausea, dizziness, and fatigue during first 12 h after rapid ascent to high altitude (> 2,438 m or 8,000´); "hung over"	Descend ≥ 500 m or 1,600´; or rest, and acclimatize; or speed acclimatization with acetazolamide (125–250 mg twice daily); or treat symptoms with analgesics and antiemetics; or use a combination of above.	Slower ascents; spend a night at an intermediate altitude; avoid overexertion; avoid direct transport to ≥ 2,758 m or 9,000´; consider taking acetazolamide (125–250 mg twice daily) beginning 1 day before ascent and continuing for 2 days at high altitude
Moderate AMS	Worsening headache with marked nausea, dizziness, poor sleep, fluid retention at high altitude > 12 h	Descend ≥ 500 m or 1,600´; if unable, use a portable hyperbaric chamber or low-flow supplemental oxygen (1–2 l/min); if descent is not possible and oxygen is not available, give acetazolamide (250 mg twice daily), dexamethasone (4 mg orally or intramuscularly every 6 h), or both until symptoms resolve; treat symptoms; or use a combination of above.	Same as above but treat and monitor AMS early.
High-altitude cerebral edema	AMS for ≥ 24 h, ataxia, severe lassitude, mental confusion	Initiate immediate descent or evacuation; if not possible, use a portable hyperbaric chamber; give supplemental oxygen (2–4 l/min); give dexamethasone (8 mg orally, intramuscularly, or intravenously initially, and then 4 mg every 6 h); administer acetazolamide if descent is delayed.	Avoid direct transport ≥ 2,758 m or 9,000´; slower ascents; avoid overexertion; consider taking acetazolamide (125–250 mg twice daily) beginning 1 day before ascent and continuing for 2 days at high altitude; treat and monitor AMS early.
High-altitude pulmonary edema	Dyspnea at rest and cough, severe weakness, drowsiness; later may see cyanosis, tachycardia, tachypnea, rales	Give supplemental oxygen (4–6 l/min until condition improves, and then ↓ to conserve supplies); descend as soon as possible, with minimal exertion, or use a portable hyperbaric chamber; if descent is not possible or no oxygen, give nifedipine (10 mg orally then 30 mg of extended release orally every 12–24 h); add dexamethasone if neurologic deterioration occurs. No evidence for furosemide or morphine.	Slower ascents; avoid overexertion; consider using nifedipine (20–30 mg of extended release every 12 h) in persons with repeated episodes; long-acting beta-2 agonists.

Source: Adapted from Hackett PH, Roach RC: High-altitude illness. *N Engl J Med* 2001; 345:107–114.

person with AMS or the presence of mental status changes and ataxia in a person without AMS.

Other conditions can mimic AMS, and the emergence of symptoms 3 or more days after being at higher elevations, a lack of a headache, or the failure of descent to improve signs or symptoms points to other causes.

Pathophysiology of Altitude Illness

Hypoxia is the main culprit behind the pathophysiologic responses observed in altitude illness, but the exact mechanism remains poorly understood. The hypoxia is believed to initiate a complex series of reactions (often sympathetically mediated)

that result in overperfusion to the brain and lungs, with resultant increases in capillary pressures, leakage, and then cerebral and pulmonary edema.

Management and Prevention of Altitude Illness

The mainstay of management includes oxygen, descent, and evacuation. Prevention is best accomplished via acclimitazation, slower ascents, and, occasionally, the use of acetazolamide. **Table 35-13 ◄** summarizes the management and prevention of common altitude illnesses.

You are the Paramedic Summary

1. **What are three things that could medically harm this man in the next hour?**

Alcohol abuse has many potential deadly consequences. You should always consider intracranial problems (intracranial bleeding from alcohol-related falls or ischemic stroke), hypoglycemia, and hypothermia.

2. **Do you believe the scene to be adequately secured?**

The presence of the police, the alcohol consumption, the patient's male sex, and the history of mental illness all predict violence toward paramedics. Verify with law enforcement that the patient has been properly searched. If you are uncertain, use your physical examination as a weapons sweep. You must conduct a risk assessment on all potentially violent patients you will be with in the back of the ambulance.

3. **Where do you believe is the best place to properly assess this patient?**

At this point, you do not have enough information to properly formulate a plan. Preserving the patient's dignity and getting the patient into the back of a warm ambulance are key concerns. Standing outside with the public looking on is not conducive to conducting a hands-on examination.

4. **Does the additional information narrow the diagnostic possibilities?**

This patient complains of a headache and abdominal pain. A patient with alcoholism and a headache may have something as dangerous as chronic subdural bleeding or as simple as an alcohol-related headache. The abdominal pain suggests acute or chronic pancreatitis, but also esophageal problems. The fact the patient is wet, is confused, and has been out in the rain and wind suggests hypothermia.

5. **What interventions would benefit the patient?**

A check of the blood glucose level, core temperature, and a rhythm strip are all indicated at this point. The initiation of IV access must be weighed against relative ease, length of transport, and your protocols.

6. **Why is the pulse oximetry not working?**

Hypothermia. Numerous hypothermia-related factors can affect the functioning of the pulse oximetry unit. You must analyze the waveform to know if it is truly malfunctioning or if the patient's condition is causing the inability to obtain a reading.

7. **What information is important to convey to the emergency department staff when you call?**

Your suspicions of hypothermia and pancreatitis, the basics of how the patient was found, and his core temperature should be enough information to alert the staff to a sick patient.

8. **What effect does alcohol have on hypothermia?**

Alcohol promotes vasodilatation, sending more blood to the skin and promoting further heat loss. It also impairs shivering mechanisms, judgment, and decision making.

9. **Why did the patient remove his clothing if he was hypothermic?**

Normally constricted blood vessels beneath the skin can dilate on reaching a certain core temperature, causing the patient to suddenly feel warm. It can be a sign of mental impairment from hypothermia.

Prep Kit

◼ Ready for Review

- Environmental emergencies are medical conditions caused or worsened by the weather, terrain, or unique atmospheric conditions such as high altitude or being underwater.
- Risk factors that predispose people to environmental emergencies include being very young, being elderly, being in a poor state of health, and taking certain medications.
- Thermoregulation is the body's ability to ensure a balance between heat production and elimination. The hypothalamus is the organ involved in regulating this balance. The skin also has a major role.
- The body produces heat through metabolism. The basal metabolic rate (BMR) is the heat energy produced at rest from normal metabolic reactions. Metabolism can be increased through exertion, which also creates body heat. Absorption of heat from the environment can also occur.
- Thermolysis is the release of heat and energy from the body. Thermogenesis is the production of heat and energy for the body.
- The body has four main means of cooling itself: radiation—transfer of heat to the environment; conduction—transfer of heat to a cooler object through direct contact; convection—loss of heat to air moving across the skin; and evapouration—conversion of liquid to a gas (sweating).
- Heat illness is the increase in core body temperature due to inadequate thermolysis; the body cannot get rid of a heat buildup.
- Heat cramps are acute, involuntary muscle pains in the abdomen or lower extremities resulting from profuse sweating and sodium loss. The patient's pulse is usually rapid, the skin pale and moist, and the temperature normal. Treatment includes moving the patient to a cool environment, providing a salt-containing solution if the patient is not nauseated, or administering IV normal saline.
- Heat syncope can occur when an overheated patient suddenly changes position. Treatment includes placing the patient supine and replacing fluids.
- Heat exhaustion can result from dehydration and heat stress. Symptoms include headache, fatigue, dizziness, nausea, vomiting, and abdominal cramping. Skin is usually pale and clammy, and heart rate and respirations are rapid. Treatment consists of removing the patient from heat and providing fluids through sports drinks or an IV line.
- Heat stroke is defined as a core temperature above 40°C and altered mental status. Signs include changes in behaviour, nervous system disturbances (such as tremors), elevated temperature, tachycardia, hyperventilation, and skin that is dry and red or pale and sweaty. Treatment is to remove the patient from the heat, perform cooling measures, administer normal saline, and monitor the cardiac rhythm.
- Fever can mimic heat stroke. Take a thorough history, and treat for heat stroke if in doubt.
- To prevent heat illness, dress appropriately, stay hydrated, and stay in the shade or air conditioning. Community-based programs aimed at high-risk populations can provide valuable education.
- Frostbite is local freezing of a body part; it is classified as superficial or deep. Frostnip is a very mild form of frostbite.
- Superficial frostbite is characterized by numbness, tingling, or burning. The skin is white, waxy, and firm to palpation. When thawed, the skin turns cyanotic and the patient feels a hot, stinging sensation. Treatment is getting the patient out of the cold; rewarming the injured part with body heat; covering with a warm, sterile dressing; and transporting the patient.
- In deep frostbite, the injured body part looks white, yellow-white, or mottled blue-white and is hard, cold, and without sensation. Major tissue damage can occur when the part thaws. Gangrene (permanent cell death) can result in the need for amputation. Treatment includes leaving the part frozen if it is found frozen, or rewarming the part if it is partially thawed.
- Trench foot is similar to frostbite but results from prolonged exposure to cool, wet conditions. Prevention is the best treatment.
- Hypothermia is a decrease in core body temperature. It can be mild, moderate, or severe.
- Mild hypothermia is a core body temperature of greater than 34°C. The patient shivers and may be confused, have slurred speech, or have impaired coordination. Treatment is passive rewarming such as removing wet clothing or drying the patient's skin and possibly providing warm fluids.
- Moderate hypothermia is a core body temperature in the range of 30°C to 34°C. Treatment is passive rewarming, active external rewarming of truncal areas, administering warmed IV fluids, and potentially using special rewarming devices.
- Severe hypothermia is a core body temperature less than 30°C. Treatment is active internal rewarming, such as administering warm IV fluids, and in-hospital measures.
- Hypothermic patients who are not breathing or who do not have a pulse need resuscitation. Patients in cardiac arrest require high-quality CPR and possibly a single shock depending on the heart rhythm. Attempt to insert an advanced airway; deliver ventilation with warm, humidified oxygen; and provide IV fluids.
- Hypothermic patients with obvious lethal traumatic injuries or patients who are so frozen as to block the airway or chest compression efforts generally are dead. If the patient appears dead after prolonged exposure, hypothermia may protect the brain and organs. Resuscitation can be attempted in cases of cardiac arrest and hypothermia.
- Drowning or submersion is the process of experiencing respiratory impairment from submersion or immersion in liquid. Drowning progresses from breath holding, to laryngospasm, to respiratory and cardiac arrest.
- Caring for a submersion patient starts with reaching the patient, a task that should be undertaken by specially trained rescuers. Treatment includes caring for the ABCs and taking cervical spine precautions. Positive end-expiratory pressure may be used to keep the alveoli open and drive fluid out. A nasogastric tube may be inserted to decompress the stomach if the patient is intubated. Submersion patients may develop bronchospasm and may require administration of a beta-2 adrenergic drug.
- In diving injuries, obtain as many details as possible about the patient, including the type of diving, type of tank, number of dives in the past 72 hours, and predive and postdive activities.
- Barotrauma can result during dive descent, owing to a pressure imbalance between the inside of the body and the outside atmosphere. It may result in ear pain. Treatment is a loose dressing for ear bleeding, plus possibly IV antiemetics or sedatives.
- Nitrogen narcosis is a state of altered mental status caused by breathing compressed air at depth. Signs and symptoms include feeling euphoric; exhibiting inappropriate, foolish behaviour; and tingling of the lips, gums, and legs.
- When a diver ascends too quickly, pulmonary overpressurization syndrome (POPS, also known as burst lung) can occur. Signs and symptoms include mediastinal and subcutaneous emphysema, a sense of fullness in the throat, pain on swallowing, dyspnea, and substernal chest pain.
- Arterial gas embolism is a dangerous consequence of POPS. Air bubbles may travel to the coronary arteries, causing cardiac arrest, or to the brain, causing stroke. Symptoms include weakness or paralysis of the extremities, seizure activity, unresponsiveness, and other neurologic symptoms.

- Treatment of barotrauma depends on whether an air embolism is present. A pneumothorax may require needle decompression. With an air embolism, the patient must receive treatment in a hyperbaric chamber.
- Decompression sickness encompasses a broad range of signs and symptoms caused by nitrogen bubbles in blood and tissues coming out of solution on dive ascent. Symptoms include itchy skin, subcutaneous emphysema, swelling, rashes, joint and muscle pain, sensory and motor disturbances, incoordination, paralysis, chest pain, and dyspnea. Treatment is 100% oxygen, IV normal saline, and transport to a hyperbaric facility.
- Shallow water blackout occurs when a person hyperventilates just before diving underwater and passes out before resurfacing. Treatment is the same as for any other submersion.
- The Divers Alert Network is a valuable resource for diving-related injuries. Callers are immediately connected to a physician experienced in diving medicine who can provide advice regarding specific management.
- Altitude illness occurs when unacclimatized people ascend to altitude. Types of altitude illness include acute mountain sickness (AMS), high-altitude cerebral edema (HACE), and high-altitude pulmonary edema (HAPE).
- Symptoms of AMS include headache plus fatigue, weakness, gastrointestinal symptoms, dizziness, lightheadedness, and difficulty sleeping.
- Symptoms of HACE include a change in mental status and/or ataxia in a person with AMS or the presence of both in a person without AMS.
- Symptoms of HAPE include at least two of the following: dyspnea at rest, cough, weakness, or chest tightness or congestion and at least two of the following: central cyanosis, audible rales, wheezing, tachypnea, or tachycardia.
- Treatment of altitude illnesses includes descending or using a portable hyperbaric chamber, providing oxygen, and giving certain IV medications.

▇ Vital Vocabulary

acute mountain sickness (AMS) An altitude illness characterized by headache plus at least one of the following: fatigue or weakness, gastrointestinal symptoms (nausea, vomiting or anorexia), dizziness or lightheadedness, or difficulty sleeping.

afterdrop Continued fall in core temperature after a victim of hypothermia has been removed from a cold environment, due at least in part to the return of cold blood from the body surface to the body core.

altitude illnesses Conditions caused by the effects from hypobaric (low atmospheric pressure) hypoxia on the CNS and pulmonary systems as result of unacclimatized people ascending to altitude; range from acute mountain sickness to high altitude cerebral edema (HACE) and high altitude pulmonary edema (HAPE).

arterial gas embolism (AGE) The resultant gaseous emboli from the forcing of gas into the pulmonary vasculature from barotrauma.

ataxia Inability to coordinate the muscles properly; often used to describe a staggering gait.

atmosphere absolute (ATA) A measurement of ambient pressure; the weight of air at sea level.

barotrauma Injury resulting from pressure disequilibrium across body surfaces.

basal metabolic rate (BMR) The heat energy produced at rest from normal body metabolic reactions, determined mostly by the liver and skeletal muscles.

Boyle's law At a constant temperature, the volume of a gas is inversely proportional to its pressure (if you double the pressure on a gas, you halve its volume); written as PV = K, where P = pressure, V = volume, and K = a constant.

breath-hold diving Also called free diving, this type of diving does not require any equipment, except sometimes a snorkel.

classic heat stroke Also called passive heat stroke, this is a serious heat illness that usually occurs during heat waves and is most likely to strike very old, very young, or bedridden people.

cold diuresis Secretion of large amounts of urine in response to cold exposure and the consequent shunting of blood volume to the body core.

conduction Transfer of heat to a solid object or a liquid by direct contact.

convection Mechanism by which body heat is picked up and carried away by moving air currents.

core body temperature (CBT) The temperature in the part of the body comprising the heart, lungs, brain, and abdominal viscera.

Dalton's law Each gas in mixture exerts the same partial pressure that it would exert if it were alone in the same volume, and the total pressure of a mixture of gases is the sum of the partial pressures of all the gases in the mixture.

decompression sickness (DCS) A broad range of signs and symptoms caused by nitrogen bubbles in blood and tissues coming out of solution on ascent.

deep frostbite A type of frostbite in which the affected part looks white, yellow-white, or mottled blue-white and is hard, cold, and without sensation.

drowning The process of experiencing respiratory impairment from submersion or immersion in liquid.

dysphagia Difficulty in swallowing.

environmental emergencies Medical conditions caused or exacerbated by the weather, terrain, or unique atmospheric conditions such as high altitude or underwater.

evapouration The conversion of a liquid to a gas.

exertional heat stroke A serious type of heat stroke usually affecting young and fit people exercising in hot and humid conditions.

exertional hyponatremia A condition due to prolonged exertion in hot environments coupled with excessive hypotonic fluid intake that leads to nausea, vomiting, and, in severe cases, mental status changes and seizures.

frostbite Localized damage to tissues resulting from prolonged exposure to extreme cold.

frostnip Early frostbite, characterized by numbness and pallor without significant tissue damage.

fsw Abbreviation for feet of seawater, an indirect measure of pressure under water.

gangrene Permanent cell death.

heat cramps Acute and involuntary muscle pains, usually in the lower extremities, the abdomen, or both, that occur because of profuse sweating and subsequent sodium losses in sweat.

heat exhaustion A clinical syndrome characterized by volume depletion and heat stress that is thought to be a milder form of heat illness and on a continuum leading to heat stroke.

heat illness The increase in core body temperature due to inadequate thermolysis.

heat stroke The least common and most deadly heat illness, caused by a severe disturbance in thermoregulation, usually characterized by a core temperature of more than 40ºC and altered mental status.

heat syncope An orthostatic or near-syncopal episode that typically occurs in nonacclimated individuals who may be under heat stress.

Henry's law The amount of gas dissolved in a liquid is directly proportional to the partial pressure of the gas above the liquid.

high-altitude cerebral edema (HACE) An altitude illness in which there is a change in mental status and/or ataxia in a person with AMS or the presence of mental status changes and ataxia in a person without AMS.

high-altitude pulmonary edema (HAPE) An altitude illness characterized by dyspnea at rest, cough, severe weakness, and drowsiness that may eventually lead to central cyanosis, audible rales or wheezing, tachypnea, and tachycardia.

homeostasis Body processes that balance the supply and demand of the body's needs.

hyperthermia Unusually elevated body temperature.

hypothalamus Portion of the brain that regulates a multitude of body functions, including core temperature.

hypothermia Condition in which the core body temperature is significantly below normal.

laryngospasm Severe constriction of the larynx in response to allergy, noxious stimuli, or illness.

lassitude Condition of listlessness and fatigue.

malignant hyperthermia A condition that can result from common anesthesia medications (notably succinylcholine) and present with hyperthermia, muscular rigidity, altered mental status, and a hyperdynamic state.

neuroleptic malignant syndrome (NMS) A condition caused by antipsychotic and even common antiemetic medications that presents with hyperthermia, muscular rigidity, altered mental status, and a hyperdynamic state.

nitrogen narcosis A state resembling alcohol intoxication produced by nitrogen gas dissolved in the blood at high ambient pressure; also called rapture of the deep.

orthostatic hypotension A fall in blood pressure that occurs when moving from a recumbent to a sitting or standing position.

partial pressure The amount of the total pressure contributed by various gases in solution.

pulmonary overpressurization syndrome Also called "POPS" or "burst lung," this diving emergency can occur during ascent and can cause pneumothorax, mediastinal and subcutaneous emphysema, alveolar hemorrhage, and the lethal arterial gas embolism (AGE).

radiation Emission of heat from an object into surrounding, colder air.

saturation diving A type of diving in which the diver remains at depth for prolonged periods.

self-contained underwater breathing apparatus The expansion of the acronym (SCUBA) for specialized underwater breathing equipment.

shallow water blackout A diving emergency that occurs when a person hyperventilates just before submerging underwater and loses consciousness before resurfacing due to hypoxemia and cerebral vasoconstriction.

superficial frostbite A type of frostbite characterized by altered sensation (numbness, tingling, or burning) and white, waxy skin that is firm to palpation, but the underlying tissues remain soft.

surface-tended diving A type of diving in which air is piped to the diver through a tube from the surface.

thermogenesis The production of heat in the body.

thermolysis The liberation of heat from the body.

thermoregulation The process by which the body compensates for environmental extremes, for example, balancing between heat production and heat excretion.

trench foot A process similar to frostbite but caused by prolonged exposure to cool, wet conditions.

windchill factor The factor that takes into account the temperature and wind velocity in calculating the effect of a given ambient temperature on living organisms.

Assessment in Action

You are dispatched to the senior citizen complex for an unconscious person. When you arrive on scene and enter the apartment, you find the patient lying on floor. This is the fourth day of a heat wave and the patient did not have her air conditioning unit on. The patient's heart rate is 120 beats/min; the respiratory rate is 36 breaths/min.

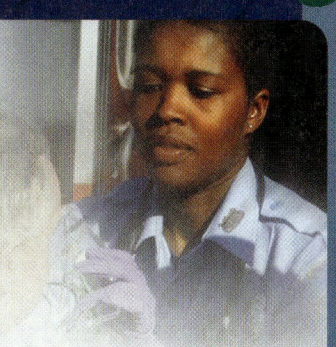

1. **What do you suspect is wrong with this patient?**
   A. Heat exhaustion
   B. Heat cramps
   C. Heat stroke
   D. Frostbite

2. **What are the two types of heat stroke?**
   A. Classic heat stroke and exertional heat stroke
   B. Thermolysis and thermoregulation
   C. Orthostatic hypotension and classic hypotension
   D. Classic heat stroke and orthostatic hypotension

3. **A clinical syndrome thought to represent a milder form of heat illness and on a continuum leading to heat stroke is:**
   A. heat cramps.
   B. classic heat stroke.
   C. hyponatremia.
   D. heat exhaustion.

4. **A condition closely related to sodium-depleted heat exhaustion is:**
   A. classic heat stroke.
   B. exertional heat stroke.
   C. exertional hyponatremia.
   D. heat exhaustion.

5. **Medical conditions caused or worsened by the weather, terrain, or unique atmospheric conditions such as high altitude or underwater are called:**
   A. hypothermia.
   B. hyperthermia.
   C. weather-related emergencies.
   D. environmental emergencies.

6. **Which of the following terms refers to the body processes that balance the supply and demand of the body's needs?**
   A. Homeostasis
   B. Thermoregulation
   C. Hypothalamus

7. **The body's reaction to its daily production of heat energy and to hot environmental conditions is:**
   A. thermogenesis.
   B. thermolysis.
   C. hypothermia.
   D. hyperthermia.

8. **When warmed blood from the core and overheated muscles heads for the peripherally dilated cutaneous vessels, the four major means of cooling it are:**
   A. thermogenesis, thermolysis, hypothermia, and hyperthermia.
   B. radiation, conduction, convection, and evapouration.
   C. hypothermia, radiation, conduction, and hyperthermia.
   D. conduction, convection, evapouration, and thermogenesis.

Challenging Questions

You are treating a severely hypothermic middle-aged male who is in cardiac arrest. The man was found in a wilderness area after being lost for 12 hours. The ambient temperature is −2.2°C. CPR is in progress and the patient has been successfully intubated. Direct medical control orders you to attempt defibrillation one time if indicated, withhold all cardiac medications, and rapidly transport the patient to the closest appropriate facility.

9. **What affect would repeated defibrillation attempts have on this patient?**

10. **Why should medication therapy be withheld in cardiac arrest patients with severe hypothermia?**

▬ Points to Ponder

You are dispatched for a man down outdoors. When you arrive, you find a man lying on the ground responsive to painful stimuli only. It is the middle of winter and is very cold. The patient is wearing only a light jacket and regular clothes. You immediately put the patient in the ambulance and begin assessing the patient. You turn the heat up in the back of the ambulance. The patient is extremely cold to the touch. His heart rate is 50 beats/min; blood pressure is 100/60 mm Hg; and the respiratory rate is 12 breaths/min. You are unable to obtain a pulse oximetry reading.

What are your main concerns for this patient?

Issues: Understanding the Pathophysiology of Environmental Emergencies. Understanding the Treatment Modalities for Hypothermia. Understanding How Young and Old People Are at Risk for Hypothermia.

36

Infectious and Communicable Diseases

Competency Areas

Area 1: Professional Responsibilities

1.1.c   Dress appropriately and maintain personal hygiene.

Area 3: Health and Safety

3.3.b   Address potential occupational hazards.
3.3.f   Practice infection control techniques.
3.3.g   Clean and disinfect equipment.
3.3.h   Clean and disinfect an emergency vehicle.

Area 4: Assessment and Diagnostics

4.3.n   Conduct multisystem assessment and interpret findings.

Appendix 4: Pathophysiology

A.   **Cardiovascular System**
Inflammatory Disorders: Endocarditis
B.   **Neurologic System**
Infectious Disorders: Encephalitis
Infectious Disorders: Meningitis
C.   **Respiratory System**
Medical Illness: Pneumonia/bronchitis
Pediatric Illness: Bronchiolitis
Pediatric Illness: Croup
Pediatric Illness: Epiglottitis
E.   **Gastrointestinal System**
Small/Large Bowel: Gastroenteritis
G.   **Integumentary System**
Infectious and Inflammatory Illness: Infestations
H.   **Musculoskeletal System**
Inflammatory Disorders: Osteomyelitis
J.   **Multisystem Diseases and Injuries**
Infectious Diseases: Acquired immune deficiency syndrome
Infectious Diseases: Antibiotic resistant infection
Infectious Diseases: Influenza virus
Infectious Diseases: Malaria
Infectious Diseases: Tetanus
Toxicologic Illness: Food poisoning

Introduction

In 1913, Randolph Borne said "We can become as much slaves to precaution as we can to fear." This statement is particularly relevant to EMS care in the streets today, because many paramedics are fearful when caring for patients who have or are suspected to have a communicable disease. A paramedic who does not understand how communicable diseases are transmitted and how to take sensible precautions will be hesitant in caring for some patients, no matter what the cause of their illness. This chapter examines the ways in which communicable diseases are transmitted from one person to another. The communicable diseases that paramedics are most likely to encounter in the course of their work are examined, as well as those illnesses that create the greatest anxiety among paramedics and the public at large. Finally, the chapter reviews the measures that a paramedic can take to protect against communicable disease.

Agencies Responsible for Protecting the Public Health

A number of government agencies are responsible for protecting the health of the general public. Agencies at the national level include Health Canada and its public health agency, the Public Health Agency of Canada. In Canada, the federal, provincial, and territorial governments jointly fund health care; however, health care and delivery of health care services is a provincial mandate.

Provincial and territorial governments have different approaches to the delivery of public health services. In some cases, public health is managed at the provincial/territorial level, whereas in others it is managed at the local or regional level with provincial/territorial oversight. Paramedics should be familiar with the public health roles and responsibilities for each level of government in their province or territory.

Regardless of which level of government bears the responsibility, the roles of public health departments and units include protection from disease, prevention of epidemics, and management of outbreaks. Although paramedics may not feel that supervision of water quality, cleanliness of restaurants, and routine inoculation programs relate directly to emergency care, clearly it is beneficial for EMS agencies to know their local public health officials and work with them. When potential threats to a community's health exist—the severe acute respiratory syndrome (SARS) outbreak in Toronto, the West Nile virus outbreak in Winnipeg, or the *E. coli* outbreak in Calgary—a close working relationship between paramedics and public health agencies is essential. If you don't know your local public health professionals and officials, reach out to them and learn who they are.

Host Defence Mechanisms

The human body provides "built-in protection" from pathogenic organisms with several defences that protect you against infection. Bloodborne pathogens are pathogenic microorganisms that are present in human blood and can cause disease in humans. These pathogens include, but are not limited to, hepatitis B virus (HBV) and human immunodeficiency virus (HIV).

Skin, which covers the entire exterior of the body, offers a primary protective barrier blocking pathogens' ability to enter through the intact surface. The normal secretions of the skin also provide an antibacterial property that protects against pathogen entry.

Mucous membranes offer another protective barrier. For example, the eyes produce tears that dilute and remove foreign substances. The mucous membranes that line the urinary,

You are the Paramedic Part 1

You are dispatched to a private residence for an older woman who is "not feeling well." You are greeted by a family member who identifies herself as the 9-1-1 caller. She tells you that she found her 70-year-old grandmother lying on the bathroom floor complaining of "feeling warm, sick, and hurting all over." She thinks that her grandmother has been on the floor since this morning.

You are unable to bring all of your bags and equipment into the bathroom because of the cramped space, and your patient is wedged behind the bathroom door. Before entering, you peek around the door to perform a quick initial assessment. After you squeeze through the doorway, you must close the door to gain complete access to the patient's face and head.

Initial Assessment	Recording Time: 0 Minutes
Appearance	Fetal position, appears tired
Level of consciousness	A (Alert to person, place and day)
Airway	Patent, occasional cough
Breathing	Rapid and shallow
Circulation	Flushed face, sweaty skin, rapid pulse

1. Given your initial findings, what do you know about the patient's overall condition?
2. What are your immediate concerns?

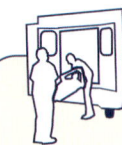

At the Scene

Your body (intact skin) offers the first line of defence against infection.

respiratory, and gastrointestinal (GI) tract also trap and remove organisms. Cells that line the respiratory tract secrete lysozymes that destroy bacteria, and macrophages trap and destroy bacteria; thus these mucous membranes serve as the first line of defence against airborne and droplet-transmitted diseases. Goblet cells lining the GI tract produce highly acidic and alkaline secretions, which form barriers and prevent penetration by bacteria and some viruses.

The immune system contains proteins that kill viruses. Immune response ignites the production of antibodies that are directed against a specific invading organism. Both B cells and T cells work together to fight infection.

The Cycle of Infection

Infection involves a chain of events through which the communicable disease spreads. In some cases, solving the puzzle of why a particular individual or group of individuals developed a specific disease may be as simple as retracing steps to find the source of exposure. In other cases, the puzzle is more difficult to solve, with infectious disease experts taking years to find a pattern in the spread of a disease and then plan a strategy to break the chain of the infection. The study of infectious diseases takes into consideration population demographics that can affect the spread of a disease, such as age distributions; genetic factors; income levels; ethnic groups; workplaces and schools; geographic boundaries; and the expansion, decline, or movement of the disease.

Here is a classic tale that illustrates how easily disease may spread. In a local hospital pediatric unit, a visitor brought a box of candy for a child. Because of the "no food" rule, his attentive nurse placed the candy at the nurses' station. Another nurse had emptied a bedpan of stool from a child admitted for hepatitis A infection, but was in such a rush that she forgot to wash her hands. She then noticed the box of candy, poked a few selections, and finally found one she wanted to eat. The candy, being out in a public place, was consumed throughout the morning. Subsequently, another nurse came down with hepatitis A, a disease that is typically spread by the oral–fecal route. Obviously, the chain of infection in this scenario could have been broken by handwashing and following a few simple rules **Figure 36-1 ▶**.

Transmission of Communicable Diseases

By the very nature of their work, paramedics come in contact with sick people; a certain proportion of those sick people have

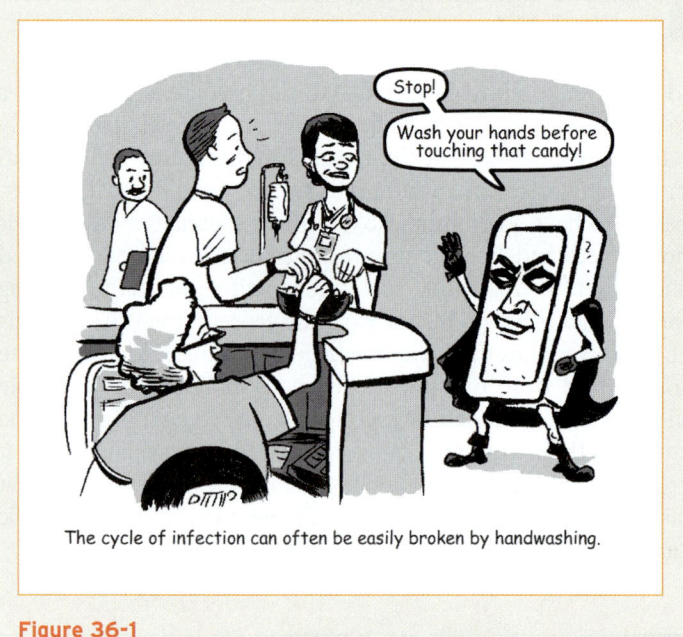

The cycle of infection can often be easily broken by handwashing.

Figure 36-1

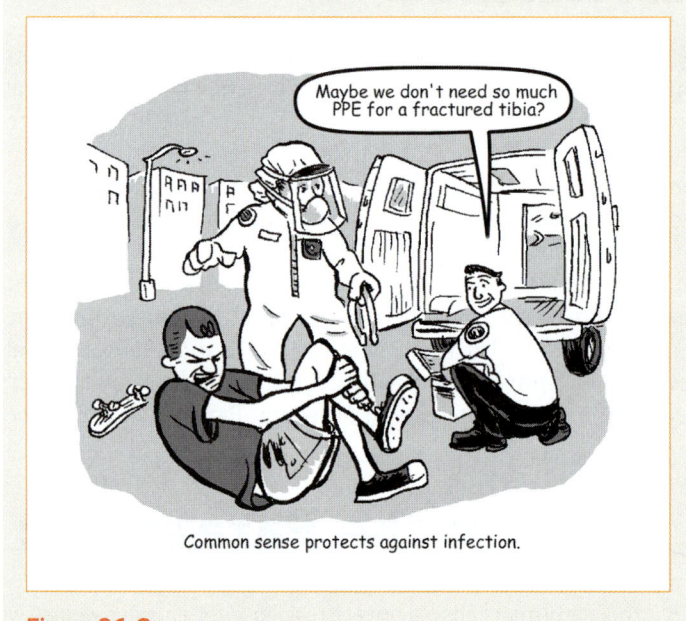

Common sense protects against infection.

Figure 36-2

contagious diseases. Communicable diseases can be transmitted from one person to another under certain conditions **Figure 36-2 ▲**.

To understand the principles of prevention, you must first understand how diseases are spread. Communicable diseases are caused by microorganisms—usually bacteria or viruses, but sometimes fungi and parasites. They spread from person to person by several specific mechanisms:

- **Direct contact** with the infected person—that is, by touching. Direct contact may be as brief as touching one patient after caring for another patient or as intimate as sexual intercourse. Most cases of the common cold are thought to be transmitted through casual direct contact.

Venereal diseases, such as syphilis and gonorrhea, are transmitted principally by sexual contact, and are therefore referred to as sexually transmitted diseases (STDs).

- **Indirect contact**—for example, touching a bloody stretcher railing with an open cut or sore on your hand. Objects that harbor microorganisms and can transmit them to others are called fomites. Towels used by a patient are a good illustration of fomites that could transmit the infection. Fomites, including countertops, bed rails, stethoscopes, and other equipment, can support organisms for as long as 7 days.
- **Inhalation** of infected droplets, such as those released into the surroundings when a person with pulmonary tuberculosis (TB) coughs or sneezes.
- **Puncture by a contaminated needle** or other sharp instrument. Punctures may occur if a paramedic is not using needlesafe or needleless devices.
- **Transfusion** of contaminated blood products. Screening tests for bloodborne disease have vastly reduced the risks of contracting illnesses from contaminated blood. However, donated blood is not 100% safe from bloodborne pathogens.
- **Vectorborne** A vector is a vehicle that transmits infection from a reservoir to a host. For example, a mosquito infected with West Nile virus that bites a susceptible person may transmit the disease.
- **Airborne transmission** occurs when organisms travel on dust particles or on small respiratory droplets that may become aerosolized when people sneeze, cough, laugh, or exhale. They hang in the air and can travel on air currents over considerable distances. These droplets are loaded with infectious particles. With airborne transmission, direct contact with someone who is infected is not necessary to become ill.
- **Droplet transmission** occurs when organisms travel on relatively large respiratory droplets that people sneeze, cough, drip, or exhale. They travel only short distances before settling, usually less than 1 m. These droplets are loaded with infectious particles. They can be spread directly if people are close enough to each other. More often, though, fomites are involved. The droplets land on surfaces where they sometimes remain infectious for hours or days. Hands that come in contact with these surfaces then become contagious. When the infectious hand touches the nose or eyes, the infection is able to enter the body.

Several factors determine a person's actual risk of contracting an infection following an exposure. An organism's mere presence presents a risk. However, other factors influence the level of risk, including the dosage of the organism, the virulence of the organism, its mode of entry, and the host resistance of the paramedic.

Type of Organism

Pathogenic organisms may be bacteria, viruses, fungi, or parasites. Bacteria grow and reproduce outside the human cell in an environment characterized by the appropriate temperature and nutrients. They cause disease when they invade and multiply in the host. Salmonella bacteria, for example, can multiply in potato salad that has been unrefrigerated, leading to human illness when the food is eaten.

Viruses are much smaller than bacteria and can multiply only inside a host. Viruses die when exposed to the environment. For example, the human immunodeficiency virus (HIV) does not multiply or maintain its infectiousness outside a living host.

Fungi are similar to bacteria in that they can grow rapidly in the presence of nutrients and organic material. Most fungal infections are acquired from contact with decaying organic matter or from airborne spores in the environment (eg, moulds).

Parasites live in or on another living creature. They take advantage of their host by feeding off its cells and tissues. Scabies and lice are examples. Parasites include both protozoans—single-celled, usually microscopic, eukaryotic organisms (eg, amoebas, ciliates, flagellates, and sporozoans)—and helminths (commonly called worms), which are invertebrates with long, flexible, rounded or flattened bodies.

Dosage of the Organism

A certain number of organisms must be present for infection to occur. For example, a large number of salmonella organisms (1 to 100 million) are necessary to produce foodborne illness, but as few as 500 *Campylobacter* bacteria can also cause illness.

Virulence of the Organism

Virulence is the ability of an organism to invade and create disease in a host. It also encompasses the organism's ability to survive outside the living host. For example, HIV does not pose a risk outside the human body because it dies upon exposure to light and air.

Mode of Entry

If the organism does not enter the body by the correct route, infection cannot occur. Thus if you suspect a patient has a respiratory communicable disease and you mask the patient, you can't inhale the droplets.

Host Resistance

The healthier you are, the less susceptible you are to infection. Your ability to fight off infection is called host resistance. Your immune system will protect you from acquiring disease even though all of the other risk factors may be present. Wellness programs and vaccine/immunization programs serve to boost host resistance.

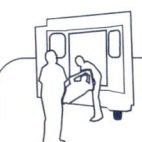

At the Scene

Exposure does not mean infection.

Once a susceptible person has been exposed to an organism, it takes time for the organism to multiply within the body and produce symptoms. That time period—between exposure to the organism and the first symptoms of illness—is called the incubation period. For example, it usually takes 12 to 26 days from a susceptible person's exposure to the mumps virus until the patient begins to feel feverish and unwell. The incubation period for the influenza virus is much shorter—usually 24 to 72 hours.

Most communicable diseases are contagious only during a portion of the illness. A person may be sick with chickenpox for 2 to 3 weeks, but is capable of transmitting the virus to another individual for only about 1 week—from 1 day before the vesicles appear on the skin to about 6 days after. The period during which a person can transmit the illness to someone else is called the communicable period. It is important to note that some diseases may be communicable prior to the onset of signs and symptoms; hence the importance of routine infection control practices whenever potential exposure to body fluids may occur.

Just as exposure and infection are different concepts, we also need to distinguish between contamination and infection. An object that has organisms on or in it is contaminated. This term applies to water, food, dressing materials, linens, sharps, equipment, and even the ambulance. A person is not infected, however, unless the organisms actually produce an illness. With some diseases, such as hepatitis B or C viral infection, a person may have the disease and not be aware of it; there are no signs or symptoms, and the person is not ill. However, such carriers can pass the disease on to others through their blood or through sexual contact.

In the context of communicable disease, a reservoir is a place where organisms may live and multiply. In institutional settings, for example, air-conditioning systems and showerheads have been identified as reservoirs for the bacterium that causes Legionnaires' disease. In ambulances, the oxygen humidifier is commonly implicated as a reservoir for infection. Obviously, paramedics have a responsibility not only to protect themselves from contracting communicable diseases, but also to ensure that they and their equipment do not transmit illness to others.

Precautions for the Paramedic

Although the risk of contracting a communicable disease is real, it should not be exaggerated and certainly should not be a source of fear and stress. Fear comes from lack of proper education and training, and there is no reason a paramedic should not be properly educated about disease issues.

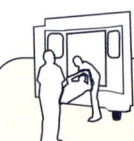

At the Scene

Infection control works for the patient and the paramedic.

Public Health Department

Provincial and local health departments are responsible for many activities related to infectious diseases, including collecting data on the incidence of diseases, performing contact follow-up, and running TB and immunization clinics. Each province also has a list of communicable diseases Table 36-1 ▸ that, if identified, require reporting to public health officials. The goal of immediate reporting of these diseases is to ensure the rapid identification, control, and treatment of specific communicable diseases that may pose a threat to the health of the population as a whole should they occur in

You are the Paramedic Part 2

Because of the problem with access, you decide to carry the patient to the stretcher in the next room using the front cradle method (patient's arms around your neck, your arms under her torso and legs). During your carry, you notice that your patient is quite warm and coughs occasionally. When you ask about her flulike symptoms, she says that she has had fever, chills, and a dry cough since arriving home.

Vital Signs	Recording Time: 7 Minutes
Level of consciousness	A (Alert to person, place, and day)
Skin	Flushed, warm, and sweaty
Pulse	110 beats/min, weak radial pulse
Blood pressure	118/72 mm Hg
Respirations	36 breaths/min, shallow
Spo_2	90% on room air

3. Think of a few potential illnesses that could cause these signs and symptoms.

4. Of those, which are the most serious and why?

the community. Paramedics play a role in reporting diseases to public health officials if they identify any disease on the mandatory reporting list, and each EMS service should have a system to facilitate this reporting. Public health departments (PHDs) also play a major role in outbreak investigations. The PHD acts as a backup for exposure notification and determination of the need for medical follow-up treatment. The PHD Medical Officer of Health, or their designate, serves as a liaison for problems that may arise regarding exposure notification by the medical facility and the sharing of source-patient testing results. The PHD collects all disease statistics for each locality and shares the information with the provincial and federal government.

Routine Practices

Health Canada introduced routine practices in 1999. Routine practices merge aspects of universal precautions and body substance isolation (BSI) into a new, more comprehensive standard of practice that relies on knowledge of signs and symptoms and communicable disease modes of transmission rather than diagnosis. The goal is for paramedics to use appropriate infection control measures when they recognize any potential sign or symptom of a communicable disease. Early recognition and appropriate protection may reduce the risk of acquiring and transmitting a communicable disease. Paramedics should use routine practices for every patient contact because all patients are potentially infectious.

Table 36-1	Mandatory Reportable Diseases in the Province of Ontario	
Acquired Immunodeficiency Syndrome (AIDS)	*3. Other viral causes	*Rubella
Amebiasis	Hepatitis, viral	Rubella, congenital syndrome
*Anthrax	1. *Hepatitis A	Salmonellosis
*Botulism	2. Hepatitis B	*Severe Acute Respiratory Syndrome (SARS)
*Brucellosis	3. Hepatitis C	*Shigellosis
Campylobacter enteritis	4. Hepatitis D (Delta hepatitis)	*Smallpox
Chancroid	Herpes, neonatal	*Streptococcal infections, Group A invasive
Chickenpox (Varicella)	Influenza	Streptococcal infections, Group B neonatal
Chlamydia trachomatis infections	*Lassa Fever	Streptococcal pneumoniae, invasive
Cholera	*Legionellosis	Syphillis
*Cryptosporidiosis	Leprosy	Tetanus
*Cyclosporiasis	*Listeriosis	Transmittable Spongiform Encephalophathy, including:
Cytomegalovirus infection, congenital	Lyme Disease	I. Creutzfeldt-Jakob Disease, all types
*Diphtheria	Malaria	II. Gerstmann-Strassler-Scheinker Syndrome
*Encephalitis, including:	*Measles	III. Fatal Familial Insomnia
*1. Primary, viral	*Meningitis, acute	IV. Kuru
2. Post-infectious	*1. Bacterial	Trichinosis
3. Vaccine-related	2. Viral	Tuberculosis
4. Subacute sclerosing panencephalitis	3. Other	*Tularemia
5. Unspecified	*Meningococcal disease, invasive	*Typhoid Fever
*Food poisoning, all causes	Mumps	*Verotoxin-producing E. coli infections and indicator conditions including Hemolytic Uremic Syndrome (HUS)
*Gastroenteritis, institutional outbreaks	Ophthalmia neonatorum	*West Nile Virus, including:
*Giardiasis, except asymptomatic cases	*Paratyphoid Fever	i. West Nile fever
Gonorrhea	Pertussis (Whooping Cough)	ii. West Nile neurological manifestations
*Haemophilus influenzae b disease, invasive	*Plague	*Yellow Fever
*Hantavirus Pulmonary Syndrome	*Poliomyelitis, acute	Yersiniosis
*Hemorrhagic fevers, including:	Psittacosis/Ornithosis	
*1. Ebola virus disease	*Q Fever	
*2. Marburg virus disease	*Rabies	
	*Respiratory infection outbreaks in institutions	

Note: Diseases marked * (and influenza in institutions) should be reported *immediately* to the PHD Medical Officer of Health by telephone. Other diseases can be reported by the next working day by fax, phone, or mail.

Source: Ministry of Health and Long-Term Care, Government of Ontario, Ontario Regulations 559/91 and amendments under the Health Protection and Promotion Act (and revisions).

The components of routine practices include:

- Hand hygiene
- Personal protective equipment (PPE)
- Sharps safety
- Patient accommodation and transport considerations
- Routine equipment cleaning
- Routine vehicle cleaning and disinfection

Routine practices require that equipment used to care for a patient and the environment in which the patient is cared for are cleaned and disinfected after each and every patient. This reduces the risk of spread of infection to patient and also to paramedics themselves.

Additional precautions may also be needed, depending on the mode of transmission of a known or suspected infectious disease. A good history may identify a known infectious disease, and additional precautions may be necessary. For example, a patient with a cough, weight loss, and night sweats may be suspected of having tuberculosis. To take precautions against tuberculosis, additional precautions to prevent spread of airborne disease are needed. Asking whether a patient has recently travelled outside of the country may identify a patient with a higher risk of unusual infectious diseases. Knowing whether other contacts of the patient have been sick, such as close family members or other residents in a chronic care facility, will also give clues to the presence of a communicable disease requiring additional consideration for infection control precautions.

Each paramedic should have an infection control manual outlining routine practices and additional precautions necessary for specific suspected or known communicable diseases. Paramedics are urged to refer to this manual for specific, detailed procedures to protect themselves and their patients.

Recommended Immunizations and Vaccinations

Keeping current with recommended vaccines and immunizations boosts host resistance and the immune response. It is up to each province and territory to determine a routine schedule of immunization and what parts of the program receive public funding. The federal government's National Advisory Committee on Immunizations and the Canadian Immunization Guide provide detailed information regarding immunizations. The effectiveness of provincial/territorial childhood immunization programs in Canada has eliminated wild-type poliovirus and decreased the incidence of *Haemophilus influenzae* type b and measles infections by 95%.

As a health care provider, you have a responsibility to protect your patients and prevent the spread of communicable disease. One very effective way to do so is to ensure that you are immune to common infectious diseases Table 36-2 . If you are not, vaccination is the best way to get and maintain your immunization status against certain communicable diseases. The regulations regarding immunity and vaccination vary by employer and jurisdiction. It is your responsibility to ensure that you are appropriately immunized. You may have the right to decline immunization, but if you decline

Table 36-2	Recommended Immunizations/ Vaccinations for Health Care Providers (If not already immune)

- Hepatitis B vaccine
- Measles, mumps, rubella (MMR)
- Chickenpox vaccine
- Tuberculosis (TB) testing
- Tetanus (every 10 years)
- Influenza vaccine (annually)

Consult your EMS agency or public health department for specific requirements in your location.

immunization, you may be prevented from working in certain circumstances (such as a communicable disease outbreak) when your nonimmunized status poses a risk to your patients and colleagues.

Personal Protective Equipment

Personal protective equipment (PPE) serves as a secondary protective barrier beyond what your body provides. The selection and use of PPE depends on the task and procedure at hand. Your EMS service's infection control manual should contain a listing of its risk procedures and the recommended use of PPE. All PPE and patient care equipment should be latex-free Table 36-3 .

Health Canada states that, "Handwashing is the single most important procedure for preventing infection." Contaminated hands are a frequent cause of infection in the health care setting. Handwashing includes both washing the hands and proper skin care. Paramedics should pay attention to the condition of their skin and use moisturizers, as required. Moisturizers help prevent dry, cracked skin. Healthy, intact skin is an effective barrier to infection.

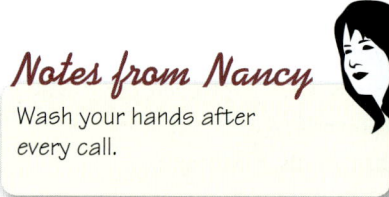

Notes from Nancy

Wash your hands after every call.

One standard for handwashing is the use of antimicrobial soap, alcohol-based foams, or gels Figure 36-3 . However, paramedics should note that most alcohol-based products are not a substitute for handwashing when hands are dirty or grossly contaminated. In addition, alcohol-based products do not remove organisms that form spores, such as *Clostridium difficile*. If *C. difficile* infection is known or suspected, paramedics must wash their hands with soap and water to properly remove the spores and prevent cross-contamination.

The best practices for performing proper hand hygiene include:

- At the beginning and end of the shift
- Before and after patient contact
- During and after PPE removal
- Before any invasive procedures
- After cleaning/disinfecting equipment and the vehicle
- Before leaving the hospital

Table 36-3	**Typical Recommended Personal Protective Equipment for Prevention of Transmission of Communicable and Infectious Diseases in the Out-of-Hospital Setting**			
Task or Activity	**Disposable Gloves**	**Gown**	**Mask**	**Protective Eyewear**
Bleeding control with spurting blood	Yes	Yes	Yes	Yes
Bleeding control with minimal bleeding	Yes	No	No	No
Emergency childbirth	Yes	Yes	Yes, if splashing is likely*	Yes, if splashing is likely*
Blood drawing	Yes	No	No	No
Starting an intravenous line	Yes	No	No	No
Tracheal intubation, laryngeal mask airway, use of Combitube or similar device, bag-valve-mask ventilation, any form of noninvasive ventilation (CPAP/BiPAP)	Yes	No	Yes	Yes
Oral/nasal suctioning, manually cleaning airway	Yes	No	Yes	Yes
Handling and cleaning instruments with microbial contamination	Yes	No, unless soiling is likely	No	No
Measuring blood pressure	No	No	No	No
Measuring temperature	No	No	No	No
Giving an injection	Yes	No	No	No

*Splashing is often likely, so use PPE accordingly.

Consult your EMS agency or public health department for specific requirements in your location.

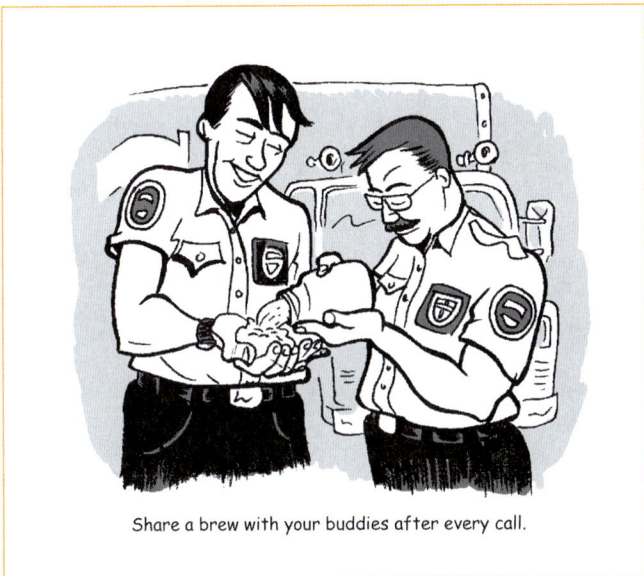

Figure 36-3

Share a brew with your buddies after every call.

- Before and after handling food
- Before and after smoking
- After personal body functions (sneezing, coughing, using the bathroom)
- Any time hands are visibly soiled
- Any time you cannot remember when your hands were last washed

Paramedics should consider the following points when washing their hands:

- Remove all hand and wrist jewelry. Jewelry should be cleaned and disinfected prior to being put back on.
- Do not wear artificial nails.
- Use warm water.
- Use adequate amounts of soap or hand sanitizer.
- Rub the hands vigorously to create friction.
- Wash for at least 15 seconds, ensuring that all parts of the hands and wrists are covered.
- Rinse well with water.
- Refrain from habits such as nail biting.
- Avoid hand contact with the mucous membranes and conjunctiva.

Paramedics who have open cuts or sores on their hands should cover the area with a dressing. If the area is too large to cover, the paramedic should not perform high-risk tasks and procedures.

PPE should consist of, but not be limited to, disposable gloves, protective eyewear, cover gowns, surgical masks, N95 respirators (or similar submicron respirator), waterless hand-washing alcohol-based foam or gel, needlesafe or needleless devices, biohazard bags, and resuscitative equipment.

PPE should never be worn in the driver's compartment of a vehicle because it may contaminate surfaces and equipment. The exception to this is when transporting a patient with signs and symptoms of a respiratory illness such as SARS or a viral hemorrhagic fever. However, paramedics can wear a

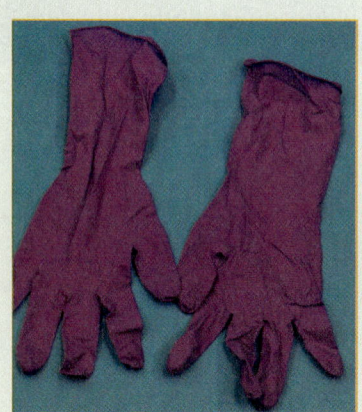

Figure 36-4 Gloves should be nonlatex, vinyl, nitrile, or rubber to reduce the risk for developing latex allergy/sensitivity.

submicron particulate respirator and protective eyewear in the driver's compartment of the ambulance under any circumstance.

Although controversy may exist regarding the necessity of a submicron particulate respirator over a standard surgical mask, many EMS agencies in Canada use this level of respiratory protection. Paramedics should use a submicron particulate respiratory mask (or the mask dictated by local or regional regulations) under the following circumstances:

- Febrile patient without a known source
- Coughing patient
- Patient with a communicable disease transmitted by respiratory droplet or airborne routes
- When blood or body fluid splash is likely
- When performing procedures such as intubation or suctioning that could result in aerosolisation
- When cleaning the vehicle and equipment following the transport of a patient with a known or suspected communicable disease transmitted by the airborne or the respiratory droplet route
- When cleaning gross amounts of blood/body fluids

Gloves should be nonlatex, vinyl, nitrile, or rubber, to help reduce the risk for developing latex allergy/sensitivity 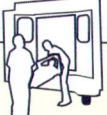 **Figure 36-4 ▲**. Paramedics should use gloves in the following situations:

- When a patient is febrile without a known source
- When there is the possibility of blood/body fluid contact
- When in contact with mucous membranes or nonintact skin
- When there is nonintact skin on the hands
- When performing procedures such as IV insertion, intubation, or any other invasive procedure
- When treating/transporting a patient with a known/suspected communicable disease transmitted by contact, respiratory droplet, or airborne routes
- When cleaning the vehicle and equipment following patient transport

Paramedics should always remember that gloves are an additional measure and *not* a substitute for proper hand hygiene. In addition, hand hygiene should never be performed with gloves on because soap and hand sanitizers break down the integrity of gloves. You should not handle personal items or items in the driver's compartment of the ambulance, because you may contaminate these items.

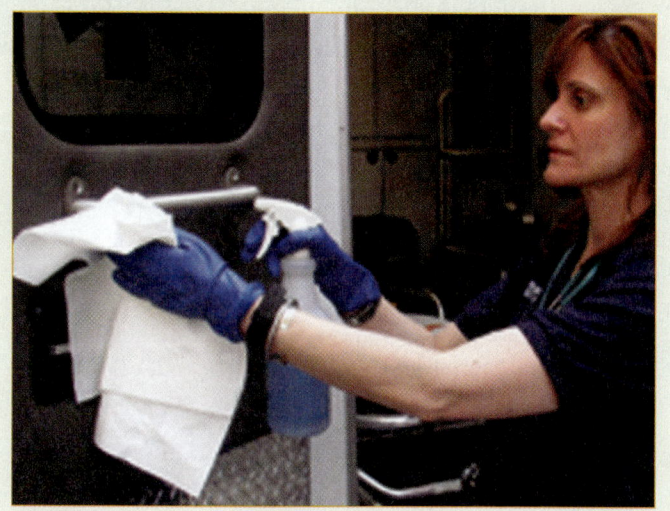

Figure 36-5 Utility-style gloves are washable and reusable as long as they are free of tears or holes.

At the Scene

Other potentially infectious materials (OPIM) include cerebrospinal fluid (CSF), pericardial fluid, amniotic fluid, synovial fluid, peritoneal fluid, and any fluid containing visible blood.

Utility-style gloves (dishwashing gloves or similar) should be used for cleaning activities. These are washable and reusable as long as they are free of tears or holes **Figure 36-5 ▲**. Hands should be washed after glove removal, because gloves are not a primary protection. Many gloves contain holes and absorb viruses and bacteria.

Surgical masks protect against splatter into the mouth or up the nose. They are also placed on patients deemed to have a respiratory or droplet-transmitted disease, because they filter what goes out through the mask.

N95 or P100 respirators are required for severe acute respiratory syndrome (SARS), smallpox, and some TB patients. A full respiratory protection program must be in place if these devices are on EMS vehicles. A respirator filters what comes in through the mask. Note that an ill-fitting respirator provides false assurance and inadequate protection from diseases spread via the airborne route. Paramedics should ensure that they know which mask fits them through appropriate fit-testing. In the event of changes in facial structure, such as due to significant weight loss or gain, fit-testing should be repeated to ensure that the mask selection remains appropriate.

Protective eyewear blocks splatter of blood and body fluids into the eye. Prescription glasses may be worn with disposable or reusable side shields. To prevent contamination, paramedics should not touch their eyes or faces during care for a patient. Remove eye protection carefully to prevent self-contamination.

Finally, perform appropriate hand hygiene after removing eye protection. Goggles should not be worn over prescription glasses because vision may be distorted **Figure 36-6 ▾** . Paramedics who wear contact lenses should be aware that their lenses may become contaminated if goggles or other protective eyewear are not worn.

Some EMS services also provide protective face shields. The face shield provides additional protection for your eyes and face. Face shields are particularly useful when performing advanced airway skills, such as airway insertion and intubation, or when there is a danger of blood or body fluid splash. As with other eye protection, face shields must be removed carefully to prevent self-contamination, and proper hand hygiene is necessary after removal.

Cover garments are recommended for large-splash situations such as childbirth or managing an uncontrolled hemorrhage. Gowns can be washable or disposable. If they are washable, the gowns should be washed in a designated decontamination area at the base or sent out for laundering to a service equipped to handle contaminated clothing. The paramedic should never take contaminated garments home. If using gowns or other cover garments, paramedics must ensure that the gown covers them completely in the front and in the back. Paramedics also must remove the gown once patient care responsibilities are complete and wash or discard it according to local procedures. Gowns and disposable garments must not be worn in the driver's compartment of the ambulance.

Booties and hair covers are not needed in the prehospital setting. Pocket masks and/or respiratory assistive devices (eg, bag-valve-masks) must be readily available. The final part of PPE is knowing how to put it on and remove it properly. Knowing the proper sequence ensures that you are adequately protected and prevents you from self-contamination. When putting on PPE, follow this order: gown or coveralls, submicron particulate respirator mask, eye protection, and then gloves. When removing PPE, remove the gloves first, then the gown or coveralls, eye protection, and finally the submicron particulate respiratory mask. Gloves are removed first because they are likely the most contaminated. When removing PPE, always remember to practice proper hand hygiene. If you suspect that you might have contaminated your hands during the process of removing PPE, do not hesitate to clean your hands with an alcohol hand rinse as often as needed during the process. Pay particular attention to avoiding touching clean clothing or skin with contaminated gloves.

The most frequent cause of bloodborne infection in health care settings is a needlestick injury. There are an estimated 50,000 needlestick injuries to health care workers each year in Canadian hospitals. Paramedics handling sharp devices are at risk of occupational exposure to bloodborne infectious agents. The risk is very low, but it is necessary to have a sharps safety system for handling all sharps to prevent injuries. In order to handle sharps safely and prevent injuries, paramedics should:

- Communicate with other personnel (eg, "sharps out", "sharps clear").
- Count number of sharps used and ensure that all have been disposed of at the end of the procedure.
- Dispose of sharps in an appropriate sharps container immediately after use **Figure 36-7 ▾** .
- Never leave sharps to be disposed by other personnel.
- Never carry uncapped sharps in pockets.
- Never pass exposed sharps from person-to-person.
- Remain clear of the person using the sharp.
- Do not recap needles.
- Never bend or break a needle.
- Use a needleless system and use safety cannulas and needles.
- Dispose of sharps containers in an appropriate biohazard container when the full line is reached.

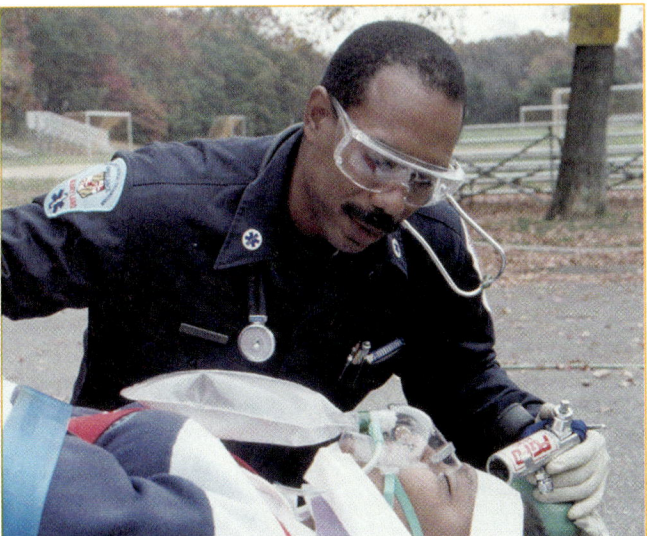

Figure 36-6 Wear eye protection to prevent blood and oral secretions from splattering into your eyes.

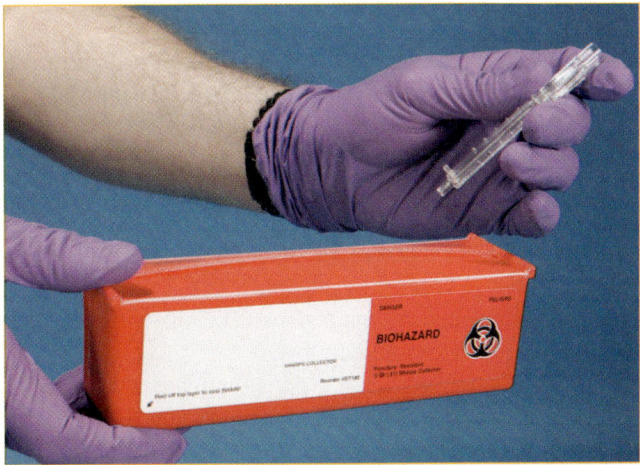

Figure 36-7 All sharps must be placed into containers that are puncture-resistant, closable, leakproof, and contain the biohazard symbol.

All needlestick injuries should be reported to an immediate supervisor. The paramedic should be assessed promptly by a physician at the local emergency department to determine the risk of infection and the need for postexposure prophylaxis.

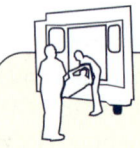

At the Scene

PPE is your second line of protection!

Postexposure Medical Follow-up

Postexposure medical follow-up is your third line of defence against communicable diseases. If all else fails and an exposure occurs, the paramedic should immediately seek medical care in the local emergency department. This will ensure that the paramedic receives proper medical treatment, including counseling and postexposure prophylaxis (if necessary) to protect against the disease to which the paramedic was exposed. Postexposure medical prophylaxis (prevention) is available for many diseases such as HIV and hepatitis B.

Exposure to bloodborne pathogens can happen in a number of different ways:

- A contaminated needlestick injury
- Blood/OPIM splattered into the eye, up the nose, or in the mouth
- Blood/OPIM in contact with an open area of the skin (fresh cut/abrasion/dermatitis)
- Cuts with a sharp object covered with blood/OPIM
- Human bites involving blood exposure (The source is the person who is bleeding, not the biter.)

If one of these events occurs, you should contact your supervisor and seek medical attention immediately.

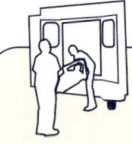

At the Scene

Contaminated laundry has been soiled with blood or OPIM or may contain sharps. A contaminated sharp is any contaminated object that can penetrate the skin.

Postexposure medical management begins with the source individual, not the exposed employee.

Blood work for the source patient includes HIV testing, hepatitis B virus (HBV) antigen, rapid hepatitis C virus (HCV) antibody, and, if the HIV or HCV test is positive, syphilis testing. HIV testing requires patient consent but your jurisdiction may have an exception for occupational exposure of health care providers.

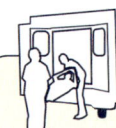

At the Scene

Postexposure medical follow-up is your third protective level.

Postexposure medical counseling and treatment should begin within 24 to 48 hours, unless testing of the source patient yields information that necessitates more rapid follow-up.

Department Responsibilities

Every EMS service should protect its staff from exposure to bloodborne pathogens with a comprehensive infection control manual and plan. This document lays out the specifics of how the service plans to reduce the risk of exposure to infectious agents and provide postexposure medical follow-up if needed. Key elements of the manual and plan include proper education and training related to bloodborne pathogens and TB and establishment of postexposure medical follow-up procedures **Table 36-4 ▾** .

Another key component of the plan is compliance monitoring. Management must make spot checks to ensure that staff members are following the infection control plan and that the plan is working effectively. Although management is responsible for developing and implementing the plan, employees are required to follow the plan.

A part of the infection control plan that will benefit both department personnel and patients is the work restriction guidelines. These guidelines indicate when employees with various illnesses may or may not be at work and when they may not care for high-risk patients. Work restriction guidelines require employees to use sick time unless the illness is the result of an occupational exposure; in which case it is covered under workers' compensation. Paramedics who are experiencing symptoms of a possible infectious illness should not risk exposing patients and colleagues by coming to work ill. Ensure that you understand who to contact in your service to seek advice on whether or not you should come to work.

Table 36-4	Typical Infection Control Plan Components

- Exposure determination
- Education and training
- Hepatitis B vaccine program
- TB testing program
- Personal protective equipment (PPE)
- Engineering controls/work practices
- Postexposure management
- Medical waste management
- Compliance monitoring
- Recordkeeping

Consult your EMS agency or public health department for specific contents of your jurisdiction's plan.

General Assessment Principles

The assessment of a patient suspected to have an infectious disease should be approached much like any other medical patient. First the scene must be evaluated for safety and routine practices taken. Once you can be ensured that the scene is safe, proceed with the initial assessment—assess the patient's mental status, airway, breathing, and circulation and prioritize treatment of the patient. With most patients who have a potentially infectious disease and are being seen in the prehospital setting, the next step will be a focused history and physical examination, using the OPQRST to elaborate on their chief complaint. Typical chief complaints include fever, nausea, rash, pleuritic chest pain, and difficulty breathing. Be sure to take a SAMPLE history and obtain a set of baseline vital signs, paying particular attention to medications the patient is currently taking, and the events leading up to today's problem and also whether the patient has recently travelled. Always show respect for the feelings of patients, family, and others at the scene.

General Management Principles

The general management of the patient with a suspected infectious disease first focuses on any life-threatening conditions that were identified in the initial assessment (airway maintenance, oxygen and ventilatory assistance, bleeding control, and circulatory support). Remember to be empathetic. Because most of these patients will have a fever of an unexplained origin or mild breathing problems, place the patient in the position of comfort on the stretcher and keep him or her warm. If the patient has early signs of dehydration, a preliminary IV and a fluid infusion of normal saline or lactated Ringer's solution may be appropriate. Remember to use standard precautions for your own safety and to properly dispose of sharp, even needlesafe devices. Always follow your agency's infection control plan in cleaning the suction unit and any reusable equipment and properly discard any disposable supplies as well as linens.

Airborne Transmitted Diseases

Common Communicable Diseases of Childhood

The most striking aspect of "common" communicable diseases of childhood is that they are no longer so common, at least not in developed countries. Thirty years ago, few children reached their teens without having had measles, chickenpox, and usually mumps. In Canada, all children are offered a wide range of immunizations against many vaccine-preventable diseases. The majority of these immunizations are provided free of charge by provincial and territorial governments, but which vaccines are free varies by province and territory. Canada has a very high rate of immunization against preventable diseases and has virtually eliminated many of them. Nonetheless, there are still sporadic cases and even occasional epidemic outbreaks of those diseases, including some related to religious waivers from vaccination.

You are the Paramedic Part 3

To gather more information about the patient, you request that her granddaughter ride with you in the ambulance on the way to the hospital. She reveals that her grandmother and grandfather have recently returned home from a month-long trip to visit relatives in China. After a fall, the patient had required several weeks of full-time nursing care that her family was unable to provide. She has been in her own home for about 3 days, and the first flulike symptoms occurred the day she arrived home. Her grandfather is also ill. The patient now complains of headache, weakness, and some difficulty breathing. As you consider her signs, symptoms, and history, you begin to hone your differential diagnosis, and immediately don additional PPE. You administer oxygen at 12 l/min using a special HiOx mask and establish a 20-gauge IV of normal saline in her right hand, giving a 150-ml bolus. You contact the hospital and advise them of your patient's status and estimated time of arrival.

Reassessment	Recording Time: 17 Minutes
Skin	Flushed, warm, and sweaty
Pulse	110 beats/min, weak radial pulse
Blood pressure	118/68 mm Hg
Respirations	36 breaths/min, shallow
SpO_2	94%
Temperature	38°C
Lung sounds	Inspiratory crackles (bilateral lower lobes)
Blood glucose	5 mmol/l
ECG	Sinus tachycardia (no ectopy)

5. Why is it important to periodically reconsider your differential diagnosis throughout the call?
6. Given your updated differential, what would be considered "high-risk" procedures for this patient?

Special Considerations

Because of their relatively immature immune systems, infants and small children are especially susceptible to infectious diseases. Pediatric immunizations prevent disease in children who receive them and protect those who come into contact with unvaccinated individuals. At a minimum, all children should be immunized against the following diseases:

- Measles, mumps, and rubella
- Diphtheria, pertussis, and tetanus
- Hepatitis B virus
- Polio
- *Haemophilus influenzae* type b

Other vaccinations are recommended for children in addition to those listed. Refer to your local public health department for the pediatric immunization schedule in your jurisdiction.

At the Scene

Use a surgical mask on any patient who presents with fever and a rash. Most droplet and airborne disease exposure can be prevented by following this simple rule.

Measles

Measles—also known as rubeola, hard measles, or red measles—is a highly communicable viral disease characterized by fever, conjunctivitis, coughing, a blotchy red rash, and whitish grey spots on the buccal (mouth) mucosa 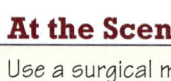 **Figure 36-8** . Transmission occurs by airborne aerosolized droplets or direct contact with the nasal or pharyngeal secretions of an infected person. Less commonly, measles can be spread by contact with articles recently soiled by the patient's nasal or throat sections (tissues). The incubation period is about 10 days. The onset of fever is generally between days 7 to 18 (after exposure) and the rash appears about day 14 after exposure. The communicable period begins when the first symptoms appear (about 4 days before the rash) and then diminishes rapidly to end about 2 days after the rash appears.

Although placing a mask on the patient may prevent droplet transmission, the only certain protection against measles is immunity. Anyone who has had measles or received live virus measles vaccine can be assumed to be immune to measles. If you did not receive live virus vaccine, you should be revaccinated. Postexposure treatment includes a vaccine if you are not immune.

No special disinfection measures are required for the ambulance after carrying a patient known to have measles. Simply washing patient contact areas and laundering any soiled linens is sufficient.

Rubella

Rubella, also known as German measles or three-day measles, is characterized by a low-grade fever, headache, runny nose, swollen

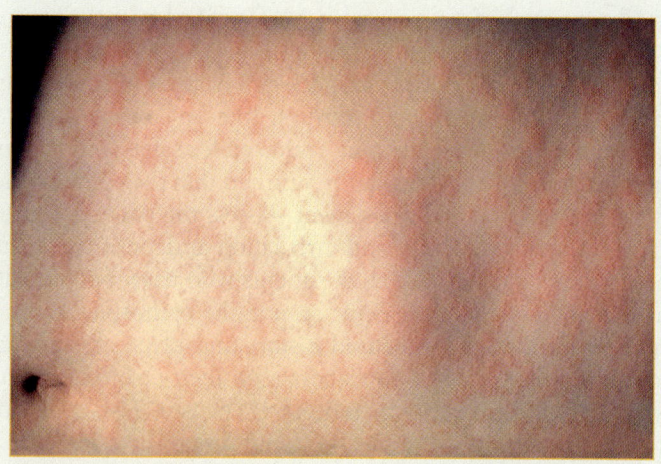

Figure 36-8 A blotchy red rash is characteristic of measles.

lymph glands, and usually a diffuse rash that may look a bit like the rash of measles. When it occurs in children, rubella is ordinarily a mild, uncomplicated illness. When it occurs in women during the first 3 to 4 months of pregnancy, however, rubella may cause severe abnormalities in the developing fetus, including deafness, cataracts, mental retardation, and heart defects.

Rubella occurs most commonly during the winter and spring and is highly communicable to susceptible individuals. Transmission occurs by direct contact with the nasopharyngeal secretions of an infected person—either by droplet spread or by touching the patient or articles freshly contaminated with the patient's secretions. The incubation period is 14 to 23 days. The communicable period starts about a week before the rash appears and continues until 4 days after the rash becomes evident.

As with measles, the only certain protection against rubella is immunity. All paramedics should be immunized against rubella before starting their employment. No special measures are needed to disinfect the ambulance after carrying a patient known to have rubella. Prevention measures include masking the patient with a surgical mask. Postexposure treatment includes a vaccine if you are not immune. Practice standard precautions and routine cleaning after transport of a rubella patient.

Mumps

Mumps is a viral disease that occurs most commonly in winter and spring. Signs and symptoms in children include fever plus swelling and tenderness of one of the salivary glands, usually the parotid. Mumps in males past the age of puberty may have a very painful complication; inflammation of the testicles occurs in up to 25% of cases, but this does not result in sterility. Thus while rubella is a matter of particular concern for female paramedics, mumps should worry any male paramedic who did not have the illness or receive immunization against it as a child. All paramedics should be immunized against mumps before starting employment if they are not already immune.

Transmission of mumps occurs by droplet spread or direct contact with the saliva of an infected person. The incubation period is 12 to 26 days. The communicable period lasts 9 days after the salivary glands swell up. As a precaution, place a surgical mask on the mumps patient. Wear gloves when in contact with drainage, and carry out routine cleaning following patient transport. Postexposure treatment with a vaccine is not recommended. Work restriction will apply.

Chickenpox

Chickenpox, also known as varicella, is a highly contagious viral disease that produces a slight fever, photosensitivity, and a vesicular rash that gradually crusts over, leaving a series of scabs **Figure 36-9 ▾** . The rash comes in crops, moving from the covered areas of the body to uncovered areas. The same virus can lead to herpes zoster ("shingles") in adults. Herpes zoster arises when the chickenpox virus takes up residence in the ganglion of a nerve. When the individual later becomes stressed (physically or emotionally), lesions may appear along the affected nerve pathway. Herpes zoster can be extremely painful.

Transmission of varicella virus occurs by direct contact or droplet spread of respiratory secretions from patients with chickenpox. Contact with the vesicular fluid of patients with either chickenpox or herpes zoster, and probably contact with articles recently contaminated by that fluid, can also transmit the virus. The incubation period for chickenpox is 10 to 21 days. The communicable period starts 1 to 2 days before the appearance of the rash and lasts about 5 days after the first vesicles become apparent.

Having chickenpox as a child usually provides lifelong immunity against infection. All paramedics should have their titres checked to ensure that they are immune. If they are not, then they should be vaccinated. When transporting a patient suspected to have chickenpox, place a surgical mask on the patient. Wear gloves when in contact with discharges or drainage from lesions. Postexposure treatment includes a vaccine if not immune. If the exposed person is pregnant or immunocompromised, varicella zoster immune globulin should be offered.

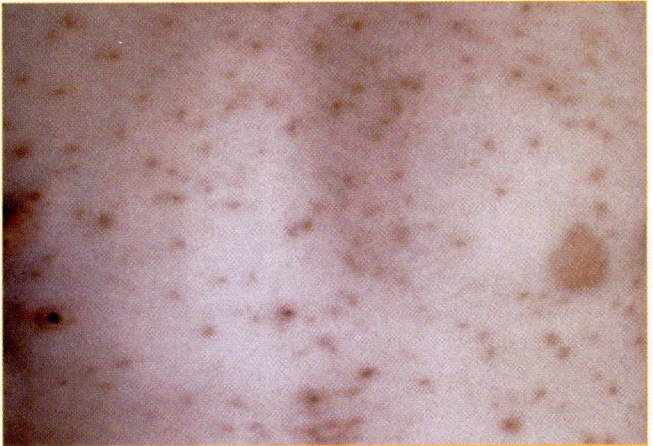

Figure 36-9 The distinctive rash produced by chickenpox.

Pertussis

Pertussis (whooping cough) is a bacterial infection. It has an insidious onset and is characterized by an irritating cough that becomes paroxysmal in about 1 to 2 weeks; this cough may last for 1 to 2 months. In recent years, the incidence of this disease has been increasing in adolescents and young adults. Some cases have occurred in previously vaccinated persons who have diminished immunity.

Transmission takes place through direct contact with discharges from mucous membranes and/or airborne droplets. The incubation period is 7 to 14 days. This disease is highly communicable in its early stages before the cough becomes paroxysmal, and then becomes negligible in about 3 weeks. Prevention includes placing a surgical mask on the patient. If coughing makes this placement difficult, try a nonrebreathing mask. Postexposure care may include antibiotic treatment. Good handwashing and routine cleaning of the vehicle are the only special measures required after transporting a patient with pertussis. All paramedics should be assessed for vaccination with DPT (diphtheria, pertussis, tetanus).

Other Common or Serious Communicable Diseases

Meningitis

Meningitis is an inflammation of the membranes that cover the brain and spinal cord, called the meninges. Two types of meningitis are distinguished: bacterial and viral. The bacterial form is communicable, and the viral form is not. Meningitis is not transmitted through the air, but rather is a droplet-transmitted disease. The most common bacterial organisms implicated in meningitis are *Neisseria meningitidis, Streptococcus pneumoniae,* group B *Streptococcus, Listeria monocytogenes,* and *Haemophilus influenzae.* Although *H. influenzae* used to be a common organism, it is rarely seen in Canada due to widespread vaccination.

The type of meningitis most often involved in epidemic outbreaks is meningococcal meningitis, which is caused by *N meningitidis.* Sporadic cases of meningococcal meningitis occur most frequently during winter and spring, but epidemic outbreaks can occur at any time, especially where young people live together under crowded conditions, such as in college dorms or military barracks. The classic signs and symptoms of meningitis are the same for both the viral and bacterial forms: sudden-onset fever, severe headache, stiff neck, photosensitivity, and a pink rash that becomes purple in colour. The patient almost always experiences changes in mental status, ranging from apathy to delirium. Projectile vomiting is common. Diagnosis is made by Gram's stain.

Transmission occurs following direct contact with the nasopharyngeal secretions of an infected person (mouth-to-mouth, suctioning/intubation with spraying of secretions). The incubation period for meningococcal meningitis lasts between 2 and 10 days. The communicable period is variable, as it lasts as long as meningococcal bacteria are present in the patient's nasal and oral secretions. The microorganisms generally

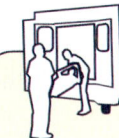

At the Scene

Meningitis is *not* transmitted via airborne means. Viral meningitis is not communicable.

At the Scene

Notify your supervisor if you believe you may have been exposed to TB. The medical facility is required to notify public health officials of any TB-positive patient. Public health should notify the EMS agency if a patient that they transported is later found to have TB.

disappear from the patient's upper respiratory tract within 24 hours after antibiotic treatment begins.

When treating a patient with meningitis, place a surgical mask or nonrebreathing mask on the patient. In addition, if meningitis is suspected, you should don a surgical mask or N95 respirator, if available. Transmission from patient to paramedic is rare. Postexposure treatment typically includes ciprofloxacin (one dose given orally) or rifampin. This treatment is not appropriate if the person is taking birth control pills, and it should not be offered to pregnant personnel. A polyvalent meningitis vaccine is available. It is recommended for college students entering dormitory living for the first time, military recruits, and middle school and high school students. Meningitis vaccine is not routinely recommended for any health care worker group.

Tuberculosis

Tuberculosis (TB) was once widespread in Canada. There are about five new cases of TB for every 100,000 people each year. It remains quite common in high-risk populations such as HIV patients, IV drug abusers, prisoners, and those who frequent homeless shelters. Despite progress in its control in Canada, TB remains an important cause of disability and death in much of the developing world.

TB is *not* a highly communicable disease. Three types of TB exist: typical, which is communicable, and atypical and extrapulmonary (TB of the bone, kidney, lymph glands, and so on), which are not communicable.

TB infection means that the individual has tested positive for exposure to TB but does not have, and may never develop, active disease. People with TB infection do not pose a risk to others. *TB disease* means that the individual has active TB disease verified by laboratory testing and a positive chest radiograph.

TB is becoming increasingly difficult to control with drugs. Multidrug-resistant TB is being identified more frequently, usually in immunocompromised people who have not complied with their full course of treatment. Although it was initially an untreatable disease, multidrug therapies are now available.

Signs and symptoms of TB include a persistent cough for more than 3 weeks plus one of more of the following: night sweats, headache, weight loss, hemoptysis, or chest pain. Transmission occurs by airborne droplets from a person with active untreated disease. In general, that type of spread occurs among people who have continued, prolonged, and intimate exposure to the infected individual (primarily those living in the same household). For the paramedic, such intense exposure is likely to occur only when advanced airway procedures are carried out in a patient with active

untreated TB. Thanks to new medications, 10% of people are no longer communicable after 2 days of treatment.

The incubation period for TB is 4 to 12 weeks. The disease is communicable only when an active lesion develops in the lungs and droplets are expelled into the air by coughing. As a result of medications, 10% of patients are no longer communicable after 2 days of treatment. After 14 days of treatment virtually all patients are no longer communicable.

Early infection with TB can be detected either by a tuberculin skin test or by the QFT-TB Gold blood test. All health care providers, including paramedics, should have a tuberculin test at the beginning of employment, at least yearly, and periodically based on the TB risk assessment. Paramedics should consult their EMS agency for TB screening and testing procedures.

As a preventive measure, place a surgical mask on the suspected TB patient. You should also don an N95 respirator while giving care. If prevention was not taken, report the incident to your supervisor. Given that the incubation period for TB is 4 to 12 weeks, the paramedic who suspects he or she has been exposed to TB should assess the need for baseline testing and then be retested in 8 to 10 weeks. If the test has become positive at that time, the individual will have a

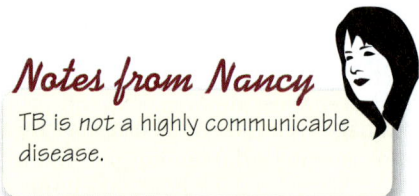

Notes from Nancy

TB is *not* a highly communicable disease.

chest radiograph to rule out infection and usually will be offered a course of antibiotic therapy. Because these drugs can be toxic to the liver, the individual should not consume alcohol while on the drugs and liver function tests should be done monthly.

No special decontamination measures are required after transporting a patient suspected of having active TB. The vehicle should be cleaned as usual.

Pneumonia

Each year, thousands of people in Canada die from pneumonia. Pneumonia is an inflammation of the lungs triggered by bacteria, viruses, fungi, or other organisms. More than 50 types of pneumonia have been identified, ranging from mild to life-threatening. Individuals who are most susceptible to pneumonia are older adults, heavy smokers or alcoholics, individuals with chronic illnesses, and immunocompromised individuals. Worldwide, pneumonia is a leading cause of death in pediatric patients, particularly infants. Although antibiotics have been very successful in treating the most common forms of bacterial pneumonia, some antibiotic-resistant strains pose a very serious therapeutic challenge.

Other Respiratory Conditions

A number of other respiratory conditions may (or may not) be associated with a fever and may (or may not) be infectious. These conditions range from basic annoyance to potentially life-threatening conditions.

Bronchiolitis is an infection of the lungs and airways that usually occurs in children 3 to 6 months of age. The child starts with a runny nose and slight fever. After 2 to 3 days, the child is wheezing and coughing with tachypnea and tachycardia. The cause is usually viral (eg, respiratory syncytial virus, parainfluenza, influenza). Transmission of bronchiolitis generally occurs by inhaling droplets of infected mucus or respiratory secretions.

Bronchitis arises when the inner walls of the bronchioles become infected and inflamed. Symptoms include soreness in the chest and throat, congestion, wheezing, dyspnea, and a slight fever. This condition is caused by the same virus that produces the common cold, as well as by common pollutants and smoking or secondhand smoke. "Chronic" bronchitis patients cough for periods spanning 3 months or more a year, for two or more consecutive years.

Laryngitis is an inflammation of the voice box due to overuse, irritation, or infection. Its cause is usually viral but can be bacterial. Symptoms include hoarseness, weak voice, sore throat, dry throat, and cough.

Croup is the inflammation of the larynx and airway just below it. It primarily affects children 5 years old or younger. Croup comes on strongest in the nighttime and may last 3 to 7 days. Symptoms include a loud, harsh, barking cough; fever; noisy inhalations; hoarse voice; and mild to moderate dyspnea. This infection is caused by a virus, similar to the common cold, as well as by other viruses (eg, parainfluenza, respiratory syncytial virus, measles, adenovirus). It is spread by respiratory secretions or droplets from coughing, sneezing, and breathing.

Epiglottitis is a life-threatening condition that causes the epiglottis and supraglottic tissue to swell. The pus-filled flap of tissue then partially or completely occludes the glottic opening. Although this disease can affect any age group, it is most prevalent in 2- to 7-year-olds. Its incidence has fallen sharply in the past 20 years thanks to routine administration of the Hib vaccine to 2-month-old infants. Symptoms include difficulty breathing and swallowing with stridor and drooling. Patients are very anxious, are cyanotic, and have a muffled voice and fever. Epiglottitis is caused by the *Haemophilus influenzae* type b (Hib) bacteria and is contagious by the droplet route via coughing and sneezing.

The common cold is an infection of the upper respiratory system characterized by a runny nose, sore throat, cough, congestion, and watery eyes. Any one of 200 viruses can cause the cold, so symptoms may vary. Patients do not have a fever. Colds are very common in preschoolers but can occur in patients of all ages. Colds usually last about a week and are spread by droplets, coughing, hand-to-hand contact, and shared utensils.

Respiratory Syncytial Virus

Respiratory syncytial virus (RSV) is the leading cause of lower respiratory tract infections in infants, older people, and immunocompromised individuals. This virus spreads in the hospital environment as well as in the community. In the community setting, outbreaks generally occur in late fall, winter, and early spring.

Signs and symptoms include those of upper respiratory infection—sneezing, runny nose, nasal congestion, cough, and fever. The disease progression moves to the lower respiratory tract, leading to pneumonia, bronchiolitis, and tracheobronchitis. Hypoxemia and apnea are often seen in infants and are usually the leading cause for the child's hospitalization.

Transmission may occur in two ways: (1) by direct contact with large droplets that do not extend more than 3′, or (2) by indirect contact with contaminated hands or contaminated items. Research has shown that RSV can survive on hands for less than 1 hour; however, the virus has been shown to survive on other surfaces for as long as 30 hours. The infection's incubation period ranges from 2 to 8 days.

Prevention of RSV transmission relies on proper use of PPE. Gloves should be worn when caring for the RSV-infected patient, and their removal must be followed by good handwashing. The use of alcohol-based foams or gels is acceptable. Post-transport cleaning of the vehicle is important, but special cleaning solutions are not required.

Postexposure treatment consists of supportive care. Paramedics who develop RSV infection should be placed on work restrictions—in particular, they should not care for immunocompromised patients.

Mononucleosis

Mononucleosis is caused by the Epstein-Barr virus, a herpesvirus. This virus is also suspected of causing a related disease, chronic fatigue syndrome. The virus grows in the epithelium of the oropharynx and sheds into saliva—hence the name "kissing disease" for mononucleosis.

Transmission occurs via direct contact with the saliva of an infected person. Some cases have also been linked to contaminated blood transfusions. The incubation period is 4 to 6 weeks following exposure, with a prolonged communicable period. Pharyngeal excretions may persist for a year or more after infection. Signs and symptoms include sore throat, fever, secretions from the pharynx, and swollen lymph glands, with or without malaise, anorexia, headache, muscle pain, and an enlarged liver and spleen.

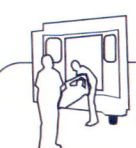

At the Scene

A paramedic with a cold or flu can be extremely hazardous to a patient who is immunocompromised.

Prevention involves the use of gloves and good handwashing techniques when in direct contact with patient oral secretions. No special cleaning solutions are required following patient transport.

Influenza

Influenza (flu) viruses cause acute respiratory illnesses generally presenting as winter epidemics. In Canada, the flu accounts for approximately 60,000 hospital admissions and 8,000 deaths each year. Infection rates are high in children, but the most deaths occur in the over-65 age group, especially in patients with medical conditions such as chronic pulmonary or heart disease.

For this droplet-transmitted disease, transmission occurs from person to person by coughing and sneezing. The incubation period is about 1 to 4 days following exposure. The communicable period in adults lasts from the day before symptoms begin until about 5 days after the onset of the illness. Signs and symptoms include systemic fever, shaking chills, headache, muscle pain, malaise, and loss of appetite. Respiratory symptoms include dry cough, hoarseness, and nasal discharge. The duration of illness is about 3 to 4 days, and complications may include viral or bacterial pneumonia.

New strains of influenza, including the highly pathogenic avian influenza (H5N1), may present an increased risk to patients due to viral factors or changes in the nature of transmission. Any history of travel outside the country to areas of the world with an increased incidence of H5N1 or a history of contact with sick poultry or other animals, should be passed on to receiving facilities so that they can consider further investigation of the nature of the virus strain.

Prevention involves placing a surgical mask or nonrebreathing mask on the patient. Paramedics should also don respiratory PPE (surgical mask or N95 respirator) when caring for suspected influenza patients. The key preventive measure, however, is an annual flu shot. Each year, a new vaccine is developed based on the anticipated strains for that year. The injectable form of the vaccine does not contain live virus, so you cannot get the disease from the flu shot. If you do not receive a vaccine and have an exposure, you may be offered antiviral drugs within 48 hours to reduce the severity of the flu should you contract it. You may have the right to decline immunization, but if you decline immunization, then you may be prevented from working when your nonimmunized status poses a risk to your patients and colleagues.

Sexually Transmitted Diseases

As the name implies, sexually transmitted diseases (STDs) are usually acquired by sexual contact. While the term STD ordinarily conjures up diagnoses such as gonorrhea or syphilis, in fact the range of diseases that are transmitted sexually is very wide and includes such conditions as herpes, hepatitis, and HIV infection. Hepatitis and HIV/AIDS are considered separately in this chapter. This section reviews the features of gonorrhea, syphilis, scabies, and genital herpes infections.

Gonorrhea

Gonorrhea is an infection caused by the gonococcal bacteria, *Neisseria gonorrhoeae*. Transmission occurs sexually, by contact with the pus-containing fluid from mucous membranes of infected persons. The incubation period is usually 2 to 7 days but may be longer. This infection is communicable for months if not treated. If treated, the individual is noncommunicable within hours.

Signs and symptoms of gonorrhea differ between males and females. Males usually see a pus-containing discharge from the urethra and often experience pain on urination (dysuria) starting a few days after the exposure. In females, the initial inflammation of the urethra or cervix may be so mild that it passes unnoticed, and the illness may progress until it presents as pelvic inflammatory disease, with signs and symptoms of an acute abdomen. Depending on the patient's sexual practices, gonorrheal infection may also involve the anus and throat.

The risk of acquiring any STD through a route other than sexual contact is remote. Prevention includes glove use if touching drainage from the genital area and thorough handwashing.

Syphilis

Syphilis is an acute and chronic disease caused by the spiral-shaped bacteria *Treponema pallidum*. Its incidence has been increasing for the past 5 years. The groups with the highest incidence rates are young people aged 20 to 35 years. High numbers of cases are also reported in urban areas.

Transmission occurs by direct contact with the infectious fluids of the primary lesion(s). The bacteria can be transmitted across the placenta from an infected mother to her fetus and by sexual contact. In some cases, transmission has occurred via blood transfusion. The incubation period is 10 days to 3 months; the communicable period has a variable length. If treated with penicillin, the individual is considered noncommunicable within 24 to 48 hours.

The initial infection with syphilis produces an ulcerative lesion, called a chancre, of the skin or mucous membrane at the site of infection **Figure 36-10 ▸**. Chancres are most commonly located in the genital region. "Secondary infection" is the term used to describe the presence of skin rash, patchy hair loss, and swollen lymph glands. Complications of syphilis can include cardiac, ophthalmic, auditory, and central nervous system complications, as well as lesions of the tissues and bone.

Prevention measures include use of gloves and good handwashing techniques. No special cleaning precautions are required.

Genital Herpes

Genital herpes is a chronic, recurrent illness produced by infection with the herpes simplex virus. The herpes simplex virus is

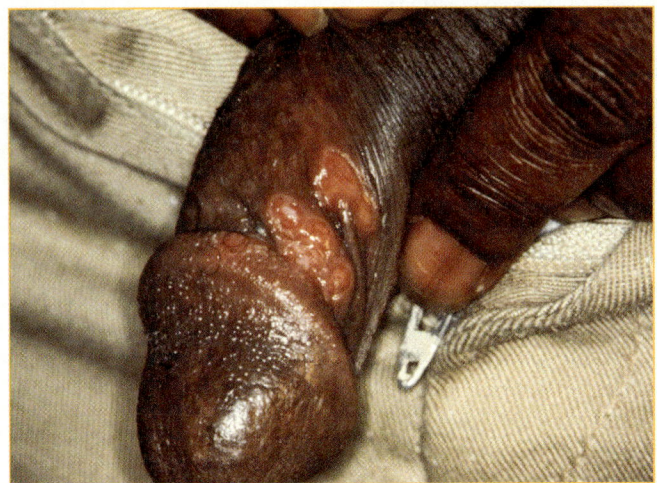

Figure 36-10 A chancre is a sign of syphilis.

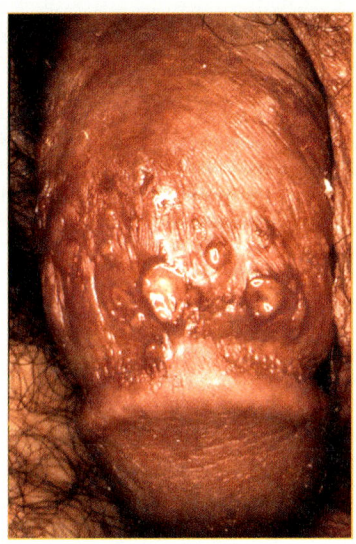

Figure 36-11 Genital herpes.

This disease is elusive; it can suddenly become reactivated, often repeatedly, over many years. Outbreaks are often stress-related. This disease can be treated with acyclovir, valacyclovir, or famciclovir for 7 to 10 days to reduce outbreaks. There is no cure, however. Preventive measures include the use of gloves when touching drainage from lesions and good hand-washing techniques. No special cleaning precautions are necessary.

further classified into two types: type 1 is generally transmitted via contact with oral secretions, and type 2 is spread through sexual contact. Genital herpes is characterized by vesicular lesions **Figure 36-11** . In women, the vesicles occur initially on the cervix; during recurrent infections, vesicles may also appear around the vulva, legs, and buttocks. In men, lesions commonly occur on the penis, as well as around the anus, depending on sexual practices. Lesions may also be present on the mouth as the result of oral sex.

Transmission usually occurs through sexual contact, but infants may become infected if delivered through the birth canal of a woman with active disease. The incubation period is 2 to 12 days. Secretion of the virus in saliva has been noted to persist for up to 7 weeks following the appearance of a lesion. Genital lesions are infectious for 4 to 7 days.

Chlamydia

Chlamydia infections have the highest incidence of all STDs. The incidence is increasing, possibly due to the availability of more sensitive screening tests and the trend toward routine screening. In most women, this infection initially remains asymptomatic. However, many women who are infected with *Chlamydia trachomatis* go on to develop pelvic inflammatory disease. In men, infection may lead to epididymitis, prostatitis, proctitis, and proctocolitis.

Transmission occurs through sexual contact. Perinatal infections may result in premature rupture of membranes, premature birth, or stillbirth. The incubation period is believed to be 7 to 14 days or longer. The communicable period is unknown. Signs and symptoms include inflammation of the urethra, epididymis, cervix, and fallopian tubes when the

You are the Paramedic Part 4

When you arrive at the emergency department, you are met by the staff as you open your ambulance doors. They are wearing full PPE, including gloves, gowns, goggles, and N95 masks. With the information you provided in your radio report, the hospital staff suspect that your patient may have acquired a communicable disease while travelling in China. Your patient will be placed in isolation.

Reassessment	Recording Time: 25 Minutes
Skin	Flushed, warm, and sweaty
Pulse	108 beats/min, weak radial pulse
Blood pressure	116/56 mm Hg
Respirations	36 breaths/min, shallow
Spo₂	94%
ECG	Sinus tachycardia (no ectopy)

7. After the transfer of care, what steps must be taken with regard to exposure?

8. Will this alter your immediate lifestyle or work habits? If so, how?

9. What are some other considerations with respect to this patient's family?

infection is acquired through sexual transmission. Urethral discharge may appear grey or white in colour. The amount of discharge is variable.

Chlamydia infection is treated with antibiotics. Preventive measures include wearing gloves when in contact with discharge from the genital area and using good handwashing techniques. There are no special cleaning requirements for the EMS vehicle or linens.

Scabies

Scabies is caused by infection with *Sarcoptes scabiei,* a parasite. Incidence of this disease has been increasing over the past few years in both North America and Europe. This infection commonly affects families, children, sexual partners, chronically ill patients, and persons in communal living.

Transmission occurs via direct skin-to-skin contact, such as through wrestling, sexual contact, undergarments, towels, and linens. The incubation period is 2 to 6 weeks for persons with no prior exposure to the pathogen. The communicable period lasts until the mites and eggs are destroyed by treatment. Signs and symptoms include nocturnal itching and the presence of a rash involving the hands, flexor aspects of the wrists, axillary folds, ankles, toes, genital area, buttocks, and abdomen Figure 36-12 ▾ .

Prevention consists of wearing gloves and practicing good handwashing techniques. Vehicle linens require only routine washing in hot water, with routine cleaning of the vehicle after patient transport. Lindane is a topical treatment for scabies, but no treatment cream or lotion should be applied on a routine basis because of reports of lindane toxicity. In case of documented exposure, treatment will be undertaken and work restrictions from patient care may be ordered.

Lice

Lice are small insects that live in hair and feed on blood through the skin. There are three types of lice: head lice, body lice, and pubic lice. All types of lice are acquired through direct contact with an infested person. Head and body lice can also be acquired from objects such as hats, combs, or clothes infested with lice. Lice eggs look like small white or tan dots on the skin. The eggs hatch after about one week, and then the new lice mature in 1 to 2 weeks. Head lice can be found in the hair, as well as in other hairy areas of the head such as eyebrows, eyelashes, mustaches, and beards. Body lice is usually found in the seams of clothing, and can transfer certain diseases. Signs and symptoms of lice include itching and irritation, and possibly sores.

When discussing lice as an STD, the focus is on pubic or crab lice. *Phthirus pubis* is a parasite that is usually greyish in colour. Lice are common in individuals with poor hygiene, communal lifestyles, and multiple sexual partners.

Transmission of pubic lice occurs through intimate physical or sexual contact. The incubation period lasts approximately 8 to 10 days after the eggs hatch. The communicable period ends when all lice and eggs are destroyed by treatment. Signs and symptoms include slight to severe itching and visual nits clinging to the pubic, perianal, or perineal hair. Pubic lice can also infest eyelashes, eyebrows, axilla, scalp, and other body hairs.

Preventive measures include wearing gloves and practicing good handwashing techniques. Routine cleaning of the vehicle after transport is sufficient. In case of documented exposure, permethrin cream treatment may be prescribed and restrictions from prehospital care may be indicated until the paramedic is free of lice.

Bloodborne Diseases

Viral Hepatitis

Viral hepatitis is an inflammation of the liver produced by a virus. Five distinct forms of viral hepatitis exist (A, B, C, D, and E) that are produced by different viruses and vary somewhat in their means of transmission. All five types present with the same signs and symptoms, so the type causing illness is ultimately determined by blood testing. Hepatitis A and hepatitis E will be discussed as enteric (intestinal) diseases in this chapter, because they are not bloodborne infections.

Hepatitis B Virus Infection

Hepatitis type B virus (HBV) cases have greatly diminished in Canada due to vaccination programs geared toward health care providers, all children, and young adults. Transmission is through sexual contact, blood transfusion, or puncture of the skin with contaminated needles. Occasionally other objects, such as shared razors, tattoo needles, or acupuncture needles, have been implicated in transmission. HBV is particularly common in intravenous drug users who share needles. Health care providers, especially those involved in surgery, dentistry, and emergency medicine, were deemed to carry a particularly high risk of contracting hepatitis through accidental needlestick injuries until vaccination programs began. Since then, the

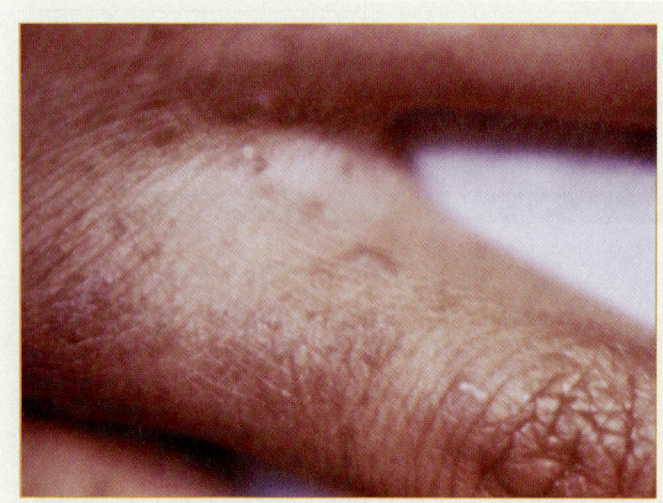

Figure 36-12 Rash produced by scabies.

incidence rate for occupationally acquired HBV infection has fallen by 95%.

Limited data suggest that this virus can survive outside the body in the presence of dried blood for as long as 7 days. The incubation period for HBV varies widely—from 45 to 200 days. The communicable period starts weeks before the first symptoms appear and may persist for years in chronic carriers. It is estimated that 2% to 10% of all HBV-infected individuals will become chronic carriers. Approximately 3% to 5% of infected persons will eventually develop cirrhosis of the liver or liver cancer.

Signs and symptoms of HBV infection include loss of appetite, nausea, vomiting, general fatigue and malaise, low-grade fever, vague abdominal discomfort, and sometimes aching in the joints. The very smell of food may provoke nausea, and smokers often notice a sudden distaste for cigarettes. Signs and symptoms may subside at this point for 50% to 60% of infected persons, which explains why many infected individuals never know that they have acquired the disease. For those who progress into the second phase of the disease, the urine begins to turn dark, and then a day or two later, the patient develops jaundice, a yellowing of the skin, and scleral icterus, a yellowing of the eyes Figure 36-13 ▾ . Type B hepatitis usually lasts several weeks, although complete recovery may take 3 to 4 months.

Table 36-5	Typical Vaccine Series for Hepatitis B

- Initial dose
- Second dose: 4 weeks from first dose
- Third dose: 6 months from first dose
- Titre: 1 to 2 months after completion of the three-dose series to ensure protective antibodies

Prevention of HBV transmission focuses on using gloves when handling blood, OPIM, or materials containing "gross visible" blood. Good handwashing technique is essential. Paramedics should be immunized against HBV when hired. Vaccination, which is both safe and effective, protects only against HBV but offers that protection for life; it indirectly protects against hepatitis D infection because one must be infected with type B to acquire type D. Vaccine is administered in a multi-dose series Table 36-5 ▲ . After the series is completed, you should have a blood test (titre) performed 1 to 2 months later to ensure that you responded to the vaccine.

Practice routine precautions. If you are exposed, notify your supervisor and seek medical attention immediately. Public health or the hospital will verify the source patient's test results. If you have a positive titre on file, no follow-up treatment is needed. If you do not have a titre report on file and the patient is positive for HBV infection, a titre will be ordered on you. Treatment will depend on the results of that titre report. If you have not been vaccinated and the patient is positive for HBV, you will be offered hepatitis B immune globulin and the vaccine series. The risk of infection is 6% to 30% only if you were not vaccinated and did not report the exposure event.

Hepatitis C Virus Infection

The hepatitis C virus (HCV) is the most common chronic bloodborne infection and the leading cause of liver transplantation. Prior to mandatory testing of all blood and blood products in Canada in 1992, hepatitis C was also transferred through transfusion of blood and blood-derived products. An estimated 1% to 4% of health care providers are antibody-positive for HCV. However, this disease is not efficiently transmitted through occupational exposure, and no health care provider group is at increased risk for occupationally acquired HCV infection. Instead, occupational risk is related to a contaminated deep needlestick with visible blood on the sharp, a sharp that has been in the patient's vein or artery, a hollow-bore needle, and a source patient with a high viral load.

Transmission may occur by blood-to-blood contact with an open area of the skin, sexual contact, blood transfusion, organ donation, unsafe medical practices, and from an infected mother to her infant. Transmission through mucous membrane or nonintact skin exposure is rare. The virus cannot survive in the environment long enough to pose a risk for any means of transmission except via bloodborne contact.

Approximately 75% to 80% of HCV-infected individuals progress to long-term chronic infection. The incubation period ranges from 2 to 24 weeks (average is 6 to 7 weeks). Signs and symptoms are the same as those for hepatitis B, and diagnosis

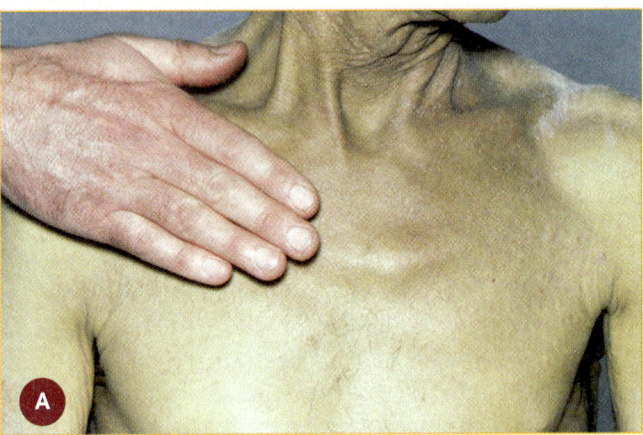

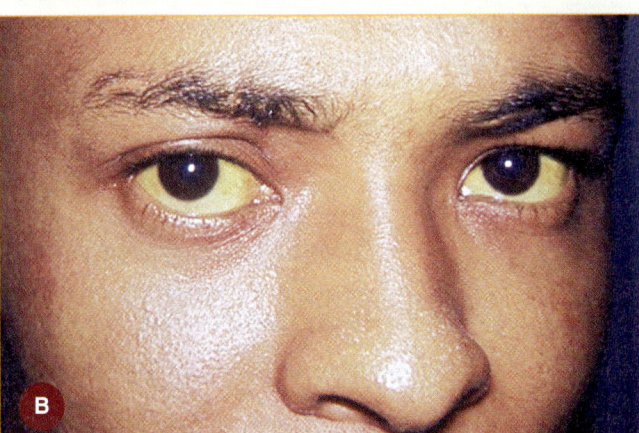

Figure 36-13 Signs of HBV infection. **A.** Jaundice. **B.** Scleral icterus.

is established by testing for HCV antibody. Some 75% of infected persons remain unaware that they acquired the infection because they do not develop phase 2 signs and symptoms.

To prevent HCV transmission, use gloves when in direct contact with blood or OPIM, and use needlesafe or needleless devices. No special cleaning requirements apply—just perform routine cleaning of the vehicle and equipment.

If you have sustained an exposure, testing will begin with the source patient in accordance with your province's testing law. If the source is HCV-positive, you will have a baseline HCV antibody test and liver function test. You should have a repeat test 4 to 6 weeks following the exposure event. If negative, you did not acquire HCV from the exposure. If it is positive, you will begin treatment. There is no vaccine to protect against HCV infection, nor can any medication offer postexposure prevention against infection, however, treatment is available, which is highly successful in preventing chronic infection.

Hepatitis D Virus Infection

Hepatitis type D, also called delta hepatitis, requires that the host be infected with hepatitis B for hepatitis D virus (HDV) infection to occur. For this reason, HDV is considered a parasite for HBV. The highest incidence is noted in IV drug users and those with multiple sexual partners. Transmission is generally by percutaneous exposure, as HDV is not effectively transmitted through sexual contact. Perinatal transmission is rare.

The incubation period for HDV infection ranges from 30 to 180 days. Blood is considered to be infectious during all phases of the illness. Signs and symptoms are the same as those associated with hepatitis B.

To protect against HDV transmission, use gloves when in contact with blood or OPIM, use needlesafe or needleless devices, and perform routine cleaning of the vehicle following patient transport. Remember that you should not go through the pockets of known IV drug users who are found unconscious, as you may get cut with a contaminated sharp. If a documented exposure occurs, testing begins with the source patient in accordance with provincial testing laws. If the source is positive for HDV and you are protected against HBV, no further treatment is indicated.

Notes from Nancy

Assume that every patient you treat is HIV-positive, even your grandmother.

Human Immunodeficiency Virus Infection

Human immunodeficiency virus (HIV) type 1 was first identified in the late 1970s. Today, an estimated 60 million people worldwide are infected with this virus.

Although HIV is primarily a sexually transmitted disease, it is also bloodborne and can be transmitted from mother to infant in the birthing process. The rate of infection from mother to child is only 1% to 3% if infected mothers are treated with antiretroviral drugs beginning in the second trimester. HIV is also transmitted through blood transfusions, albeit at a very low rate since the initiation of testing for the presence of P24 (a protein present from the beginning of the HIV life cycle) in donated blood. With P24 testing, the virus can now be detected 1 to 6 days after infection.

HIV is not transmitted through casual or even household contact. Even among individuals who routinely share eating utensils, toothbrushes, and razors with HIV-infected patients, there is no evidence of an increased rate of HIV infection. This disease is not airborne or droplet transmitted.

The HIV pathogen envelops infected cells and attacks the immune system and other body organs. The immune system is then unable to assist in protecting the infected individual from other diseases. It takes about 7 days for the virus to envelop a cell, and this process may occur 4 to 6 weeks after the exposure event. The communicable period is unknown, but is believed to span from the onset of infection possibly throughout life.

Signs and symptoms may include acute febrile illness, malaise, swollen lymph glands, headache, and possibly rash. Following initial infection, most individuals present with enlargement of the lymph nodes and appear healthy. However, the number of T-helper lymphocytes (CD4 cells) gradually declines. T-helper cells are essential components of the immune system that mediate both cellular and humoural immunity. Seroconversion occurs, meaning that antibodies can be detected in the blood; this usually occurs within the first 3 months. Persons who are seropositive for HIV are placed on antiretroviral drug treatment.

Prevention focuses on the use of gloves when in direct contact with patient blood or OPIM, the use of needlesafe or needleless devices, good handwashing technique, and routine cleaning of the vehicle after transport. Postexposure medical follow-up is covered in the AIDS section that follows.

The risk for acquiring HIV infection is sharps-related. A high-risk exposure to HIV includes *all* of the following: a deep stick with a large-gauge hollow-bore needle, the device has visible blood on it, the patient is HIV-positive with a high viral load, and the device had been in the patient's vein or artery. Following this type of exposure, the risk of transmission is 0.3% for mucous membrane exposure to the eye and 0.09% for nonintact skin.

Acquired Immunodeficiency Syndrome

Acquired immunodeficiency syndrome (AIDS) is the end-stage disease process caused by HIV. The patient with AIDS is extremely vulnerable to numerous bacterial, viral, and fungal infections that would not affect a person with an intact immune system. These *opportunistic infections* include pneumonia in infants or people with compromised immune systems, loss of vision due to cytomegalovirus,

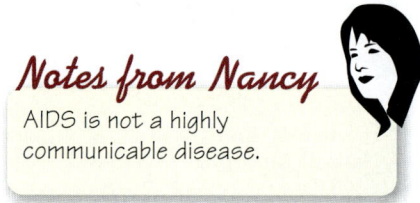

Notes from Nancy

AIDS is not a highly communicable disease.

reddish/purple skin lesions, atypical TB, and cryptococcal meningitis.

The incubation period of AIDS spans the time between documented infection (ie, becoming HIV-positive) and development of the end-stage disease; it is determined by the CD4 cell count and the presence of opportunistic infections. The communicable period is presumed to last as long as the patient is seropositive, *even before clinically apparent AIDS develops.* Surveys of patients presenting to emergency departments have shown that around 6% of seriously ill or injured patients are HIV-positive.

Prevention involves following standard precautions. Use gloves when in contact with blood or OPIM, use needlesafe or needleless devices, and perform routine cleaning of the vehicle and equipment. There is no need to restrict pregnant paramedics from contact with known HIV/AIDS patients.

If an actual exposure occurs, the source patient will be tested in accordance with provincial or territorial law. If the test is negative, then no further testing is indicated for the paramedic. If the source is positive, then blood is sent for assessment of viral load and the paramedic may be offered a combination of antiretroviral drugs for a period of 4 weeks. The criteria for use of these drugs are published by provincial and territorial public health departments.

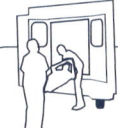

At the Scene

Body fluids that do not transmit bloodborne disease: tears, sweat, urine, stool, vomitus, nasal secretions, and sputum.

Antiretroviral drugs are toxic, so careful and complete counseling should be provided to the exposed health care provider. A physician knowledgeable in the use of these drugs should be consulted to offer counseling and ensure appropriate follow-up is in place. Before initiating antiretroviral therapy, baseline laboratory testing should be done—CBC, liver function, and kidney function. For a female of childbearing age, pregnancy testing is appropriate. These tests should be repeated every 2 weeks while on the drugs.

Enteric (Intestinal) Diseases

Gastroenteritis

Gastroenteritis, also known as the stomach flu, comprises many types of infections and irritations of the gastrointestinal tract. Patients experience symptoms such as nausea and vomiting, fever, abdominal cramps, and diarrhea. In healthy individuals, gastroenteritis is usually not serious. In children, elderly persons, and patients with chronic illness, severe complications such as dehydration may develop.

Hepatitis A Virus Infection

Hepatitis type A is the most common type of hepatitis in Canada. In the past, outbreaks of this disease have been reported in several states. Transmission is by the fecal–oral route—that is, by ingestion of food or water that has been contaminated by infected feces. Epidemic outbreaks are most often traced to contaminated drinking water, milk, sliced meats, and undercooked shellfish. Hepatitis A is often described as a "benign" disease because once you acquire the disease you have lifelong immunity to it. A vaccine is available to protect against hepatitis A, and some provinces and territories now include this vaccination.

The incubation period is usually about 2 to 4 weeks, although it can range from 15 to 50 days after ingestion of the virus. The communicable period probably starts toward the end of the incubation period and continues for a few days after the patient becomes jaundiced. Signs and symptoms in phase 1 include fatigue, loss of appetite, fever, nausea, and abdominal pain; smokers will lose their interest in smoking. In phase 2, patients have jaundice, dark-coloured urine, and whitish stools.

Prevention includes use of gloves and good handwashing technique if in contact with patient stool. No special cleaning of the vehicle is needed. Hepatitis A vaccine is recommended for people who travel overseas to prevent the risk of acquiring it from infected food and water sources.

Hepatitis E Virus Infection

Hepatitis E virus (HEV) infection is enterically transmitted and accounts for an estimated 50% of hepatitis cases in developing countries. Transmission occurs via the fecal–oral route by ingestion of contaminated water. In developing countries, there is a strong association between HEV and floods, poor sanitation, and primitive hygiene. Rare cases of transmission via transfusion have been documented, and sexual transmission is on record.

This disease is not chronic. Its incubation period is about 15 to 64 days. The communicable period is believed to be the same as for hepatitis A. Signs and symptoms are the same as for other forms of hepatitis. Prevention includes the use of gloves when in contact with stool, good handwashing technique, and cleaning contaminated equipment.

Vectorborne Diseases

West Nile Virus

West Nile virus (WNV) is a relatively new disease in Canada. The virus was first discovered in Uganda in the 1930s; its first identified appearance in the Western Hemisphere was in New York City in 1999. WNV has been identified in birds and other animals across Canada. Each year, there are reports of human cases, particularly in Ontario and Manitoba.

Transmission is via bite from a mosquito carrying the virus (only about 1% of mosquitoes carry WNV). This infection is not transmitted from person to person, so there is no period of communicability. WNV has been transmitted via donated blood and organs, as well as during hemodialysis; two cases have involved needlestick injuries in laboratory workers working with this virus. The incubation period is from 3 to 14 days following the bite.

In the majority of cases, this disease is mild and uneventful. Indeed, 80% of persons who acquire WNV infection remain unaware that they have it. The 20% of persons who are symptomatic exhibit fever, headache, body rash, and swollen lymph glands. Mild symptoms appear in older people and immunocompromised persons. In healthy individuals, the immune system fights off the disease. About 1 in 150 symptomatic individuals will go on to develop severe signs and symptoms, which include encephalitis, meningitis that can lead to neurologic complications, and death.

Use needlesafe devices systems to avoid a contaminated sharps injury when WNV infection is suspected. If you sustain a contaminated sharps injury involving a patient with WNV, notify your supervisor. There is no recommended medical follow-up treatment. No special cleaning of the vehicle is needed or recommended.

Lyme Disease

Lyme disease is a common tick-borne disease in certain parts of Canada. Lyme disease is found in southern and eastern Ontario, on British Columbia's west coast, southeastern Manitoba, and Nova Scotia, but its true extent in Canada is not well known. Peak season is between June and August; incidence rates decrease in the early fall.

Lyme disease primarily affects the skin, heart, joints, and nervous system. Some patients remain asymptomatic. This disease occurs more often in children younger than age 10 years and in middle-aged adults. Lyme disease is not transmitted from person to person. Its incubation period ranges from 3 to 32 days.

Lyme disease is usually divided into three stages: early localized, early disseminated, and late manifestations. The early stage is characterized by a round, red skin lesion. This bull's-eye rash (so called because it extends outward with a ring in the centre) is most common in the area of the groin, thigh, or axilla **Figure 36-14 ▶**. If present, it is warm to the touch, and may blister or scab. In the early disseminated stage, secondary lesions may develop within days and the patient may complain of flu-like symptoms—fever, chills, headache, malaise, and muscle pain. Nonproductive cough, testicular swelling, sore throat, enlarged spleen, and enlarged lymph nodes may be present. Neurologic involvement may occur in 15% to 20% of untreated patients within 2 to 8 weeks; cardiac involvement may occur in 10% of untreated patients. In the third phase of the illness, arthritis occurs in about 60% of untreated patients, beginning days to years after the initial infection. Intermittent joint pain affects about 50% of patients, and lasts from days to months. Chronic neurologic symptoms

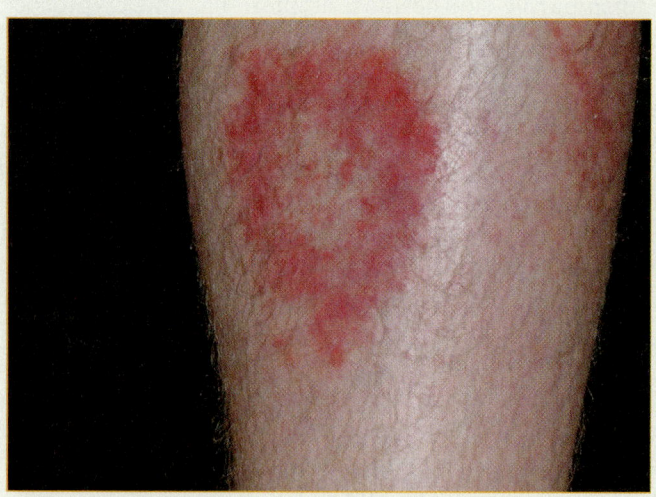

Figure 36-14 The bull's-eye rash of Lyme disease is most common in the area of the groin, thigh, or axilla.

are uncommon. Memory impairment, depressed mood, and severe fatigue are the most common symptoms of Lyme disease.

Prevention includes wearing long sleeves and pants when in tick-infested areas, plus use of insecticides as necessary. Daily inspection of exposed skin, including the scalp, and removal of any ticks is recommended. If you sustain a tick bite, use the proper technique for removing ticks. Routine postexposure prophylactic treatment of a tick bite with antibiotics is not warranted or recommended if the tick is found and removed within 72 hours after attachment. If a tick is not found and not removed within 72 hours after attachment, then prophylaxis is warranted in endemic areas. Because this is a vectorborne illness, there are no additional PPE or equipment cleaning requirements when caring for these patients.

Zoonotic (Animal-borne) Diseases

Hantavirus

Hantavirus, also known as hemorrhagic fever with renal syndrome, is associated with the deer mouse, white-footed mouse, and cotton rat. It has also been found in rats in urban areas. This disease was first identified in Korea in the early 1950s and in Canada's prairie provinces over a decade ago.

Hantavirus is found in the urine, feces, and saliva of chronically infected rodents. Transmission occurs via direct contact with rodent waste matter, often through aerosol inhalation. The incubation period usually lasts 12 to 16 days following exposure but has been noted to range from 5 to 42 days. This disease is not transmitted from person to person, so there is no period of communicability. Signs and symptoms begin with the sudden onset of fever, which lasts 3 to 8 days. It is accompanied by headache, abdominal pain, loss of appetite, and vomiting.

Prevention focuses on standard precautions. Routine cleaning of the vehicle is all that is indicated.

Rabies

Rabies (hydrophobia) is found worldwide but is quite rare in Canada. Since reporting began in 1925, 22 people have died of rabies in Canada. After 1985, there were no reported deaths until 2000. In September 2000, a young boy died of rabies in Quebec. The most likely source of the rabies infection in this case was an unrecognized bat exposure several weeks before the onset of symptoms.

Over the past few years, the incidence of rabies in bats has increased, and of the last five human rabies cases in Canada, four followed exposure to bats. Most of the animal rabies cases reported in Canada are found in Ontario and Manitoba. The most commonly infected animals across the country are bats, skunks, and foxes.

The vaccination of domestic animals and the development of a vaccine and rabies immunoglobulin have greatly reduced the number of deaths in humans who contract rabies. However, as many as 39,000 people worldwide receive postexposure prophylaxis, and an estimated 30,000 to 50,000 die due to rabies worldwide each year. Although deaths due to rabies are rare in Canada, between 1,000 and 1,500 people in Canada receive postexposure prophylaxis each year.

Transmission is primarily related to the direct bite of an infected animal. The virus is shed in the saliva of the infected animal from the time it becomes infected. Other routes of transmission include contamination of mucous membranes (eyes, mouth) and one case suspected to be related to a cornea organ transplant. In general, however, nonbite exposures to rabies—scratches, abrasions, open wounds, or mucous membranes contaminated with saliva or other potentially infectious material from a rabid animal—are rare. There are no documented cases of human-to-human transmission of rabies.

The incubation period is usually 2 to 8 weeks, but varies depending on the severity of the bite and the location of the wound. Signs and symptoms in human infection are generally nonspecific: fever, chills, sore throat, malaise, headache, and weakness. Paresthesia (skin sensation with no apparent cause) may develop at or near the site of exposure. Following these initial signs, the neurologic phase of the disease begins—hyperactivity, seizures, bizarre behaviour, and hydrophobia. Patients also have fear of the sight of water or while drinking it as a result of severe spasms of the throat and masseter (chewing) muscles. As the disease progresses, patients may develop paralysis and deterioration of mental status leading to coma. Although rabies is generally viewed as a fatal disease, several cases of survival have been reported recently.

For prevention, follow standard precautions for prehospital care and cleaning of the vehicle. If you are bitten by or have come in close contact with a suspect animal, you will be offered human rabies vaccine with or without rabies immune globulin if deemed appropriate.

Tetanus

Thanks to immunization programs in Canada, the incidence of tetanus has decreased significantly. During the 1920s and 1930s, 40 to 50 deaths from tetanus were reported annually. With the introduction of tetanus toxoid in Canada in 1940, mortality rapidly declined; only five deaths from tetanus have been reported since 1980. However, tetanus is still seen in Canada, with three cases reported in 1997 and two in 1998. Tetanus is more common in agricultural areas and in underdeveloped areas, where contact with animal waste is common and immunization is inadequate. The tetanus bacillus is found in the intestines of horses and other animals, but some cases have been linked to use of IV drugs.

Transmission occurs when tetanus spores enter the body by either of two means: (1) a puncture wound contaminated with animal feces, street dust, or soil, or (2) contaminated street drugs. Tetanus is not transmitted from person to person. Occasionally, cases have occurred postoperatively or following seemingly minor injuries.

The incubation period is usually about 14 days from the exposure but has been documented to be as short as 3 days. The cases that have short incubation periods tend to feature a higher level of contamination. Signs and symptoms begin at the site of the wound, followed by painful muscle contractions in the neck and trunk muscles. The key sign that suggests tetanus is abdominal rigidity, although this rigidity may be confined to the location of the injury.

Prevention involves the use of gloves when handling any patient wounds and drainage. Paramedics should receive a tetanus booster dose every 10 years. No special cleaning routines are necessary after transport of a patient with tetanus.

◼ Antibiotic-Resistant Organisms

The overuse and misuse of antibiotics has led some pathogens to develop resistance to the antibiotic drugs commonly prescribed to eradicate them. As a consequence, many medical facility pharmacies and provincial governments now restrict the use of certain antibiotics. There has also been an attempt to educate the population regarding the risks associated with the overuse of antibiotics.

Methicillin-Resistant *Staphylococcus aureus*

Staphylococcus aureus became resistant to penicillin in the late 1950s. Today almost 90% of community (CA-MRSA) and hospital isolates are resistant to penicillin. The drug methicillin was made available in the early 1960s to treat infections with this pathogen. By the mid-1970s, methicillin-resistant *S aureus* (MRSA) was present in hospitals; it has since moved into the larger community. MRSA strains are also resistant to some other antibiotics, including cephalosporins, erythromycins, clindamycin, tetracyclines, and aminoglycosides. Although vancomycin has been shown to effectively treat MRSA, some mild strains are showing resistance to this drug as well. Newer drugs are used to treat vancomycin-resistant MRSA, but the options to treat these strains of MRSA are very limited.

In health care settings, MRSA is believed to be transmitted from patient to patient via unwashed hands of health care providers. Studies have shown that 50% to 90% of health care providers carry MRSA in their nares; the pathogen can subsequently be transferred to skin and other areas of the body through a break in the skin. Surfaces contaminated with MRSA do not seem to be important in transmission. Factors that increase the risk for developing MRSA include antibiotic therapy, prolonged hospital stays, a stay in intensive care or a burn unit, and exposure to an infected patient. Many patients who contract MRSA live in long-term care facilities. The incidence of community-based MRSA is also increasing; therefore, antibiotic coverage for MRSA in critically ill patients is often considered when *S. aureus* is isolated while awaiting antibiotic sensitivities.

Patients with MSRA may be either colonized with this organism or infected. The incubation period appears to be between 5 to 45 days. The communicable period varies, as patients who have active infection may carry MRSA for months. MRSA results in soft-tissue infections. Its signs and symptoms may involve localized skin abscesses and cellulites, empyemas, and endocarditis. Sepsis is found in older patients with *S aureus* infections. After bloodstream infection with this organism, secondary infections such as osteomyelitis and septic arthritis may develop at other body sites.

To prevent MRSA transmission, use standard precautions (gloves and good handwashing technique) when in contact with patient wounds and nonintact skin. If you are in direct contact with wound drainage but your skin is intact, no exposure will occur. If you have a true exposure, no postexposure treatment is recommended. The incident must still be documented, however.

Vancomycin-Resistant Enterococci

Enterococcus is a common, normal organism of the GI tract, urinary tract, and genitourinary tract. More than 450 species of enterococci exist, many of which are resistant to antimicrobial agents. These organisms grow under both reduced and oxygenated conditions. When they become resistant to the main drug used for treating enterococcal infection, vancomycin, the patient is said to have vancomycin-resistant enterococci (VRE). VRE is primarily a hospital-acquired (nosocomial) infection. Although a few sporadic cases were previously known, the first outbreak was documented in a renal unit of a Toronto hospital in 1995. Since that time, VRE has been identified in over 100 health care facilities in 10 provinces, and there have been several reported outbreaks of VRE in Canadian hospitals. VRE is not commonly encountered in the community. Patients identified with VRE outside the hospital setting typically reside in nursing homes or visit hemodialysis centres.

VRE may be found in urinary tract infections and bloodstream infections; it has also been identified in livestock stool,

uncooked chicken, and persons who work at farms or processing plants. The infectious organisms can live on surfaces for long periods of time, so transmission may occur by direct contact with contaminated surfaces or equipment. A person can be either colonized or infected with VRE, but only infected patients can transmit this organism. Thus transmission may occur when you have direct contact with wound drainage and an open cut or sore allows entry of the organism.

Prevention relies on the use of standard precautions, gloves, and good handwashing technique when in contact with wound drainage. A cover gown is necessary only if your uniform may come in contact with wound drainage. Post-transport cleaning of all areas that came in contact with the patient is important, but no special cleaning solution is required. If you sustain direct contact with an open wound and VRE body fluids, notify your supervisor and complete an exposure report. No postexposure medical treatment is indicated.

New and Emerging Diseases

In the past, a disease would jump from animals to humans every 20 to 30 years. Today, this transmission is occurring much more frequently. Recent examples include HIV infection, monkeypox, SARS, and avian flu. The latter two are discussed here.

Severe Acute Respiratory Syndrome

Severe acute respiratory syndrome (SARS) is a newly emerged infectious disease that was first reported in November 2002 in Foshan City, Guangdong Province, China. This viral infection presented as an atypical pneumonia, and patients rapidly deteriorated and often died. In February 2003, the Chinese Ministry of Health informed the World Health Organization (WHO) of the outbreak, prompting the WHO to issue a global alert about this new disease. The WHO referred to the disease as severe acute respiratory syndrome (SARS). By early 2003, SARS had spread internationally, via Hong Kong, causing outbreaks in several countries.

The first Canadian death due to SARS occurred in Toronto, Ontario, on March 5, 2003. The index case and her husband were in Hong Kong in late February, staying in the same hotel as a physician from Guangdong Province. A case cluster in Toronto was linked to the index case and a single Toronto hospital in mid-March. This first cluster included relatives of the index case, paramedics, and hospital-based health care workers who cared for the index case and her relatives.

By late March, a large-scale SARS outbreak was underway in the Greater Toronto Area (GTA). The outbreak prompted the Government of Ontario to declare a health care emergency, activate the Provincial Operations Centre, and require all GTA hospitals to initiate their emergency response plans for an external disaster. Public health officials investigating the GTA outbreak determined SARS had spread from the index hospital to several other hospitals and health care institutions, in part,

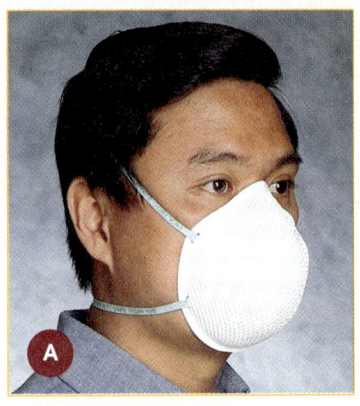

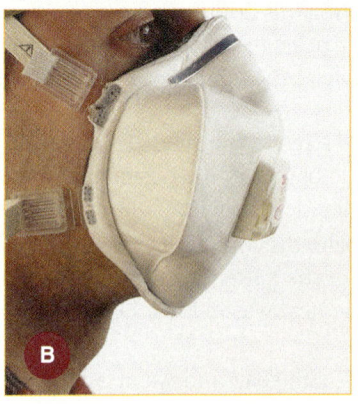

Figure 36-15 Wear an N95 respirator (**A**) or P100 respirator (**B**) that has been properly fit-tested to protect yourself from SARS.

due to interfacility patient transfers. To prevent further spread, an EMS-based command, control, and tracking system was set up to prevent the spread of SARS among health care facilities, health care workers, and patients in Ontario due to interfacility patient transfers.

There were a total of 375 probable and suspect cases of SARS in Toronto, with 44 deaths, including three health care workers. In addition, over 28,000 residents were placed in voluntary 10-day quarantine to prevent the spread of SARS. The WHO reported a total of 8,098 cases worldwide and 774 deaths as a result of the 2003 outbreak. The latest cases of SARS were reported in April 2004 in China and resulted from a laboratory accident.

EMS services and paramedics were affected by the SARS outbreak. EMS services strengthened their infection control practices and set up monitoring systems to protect paramedics and to detect the earliest signs of illness. During the SARS outbreaks, there were five cases of probable SARS and three cases of suspect SARS among paramedics in Toronto. More important, 526 of Toronto's 920 paramedics were quarantined during the SARS outbreaks. Most paramedics required quarantine due to an unprotected exposure to a hospital with a SARS outbreak or exposure to a colleague who had developed SARS-like symptoms following treatment of patients with SARS.

Transmission of SARS is by close personal contact—that is, living with and caring for a person with the disease or having direct contact with respiratory secretions or body fluids of an infected person (eg, kissing or hugging, talking within 1 m, sharing eating utensils). The incubation period is about 10 days from the date of exposure; the communicable period is approximately 10 days. Signs and symptoms include a fever of greater than 38°C, headache, overall feeling of discomfort, and body aches. SARS resembles any general flu-like illness; however, after 2 to 7 days a dry cough appears, and patients with severe illness progress to pneumonia and may need respiratory support.

Prehospital care for a person suspected of having SARS begins with an assessment and taking of a travel history and inquiry as to whether any family members are ill after recent travel. In the setting of a community outbreak, additional history regarding exposure to health care facilities with known SARS is also necessary. Place a surgical mask on a patients who presents with signs and symptoms of SARS in order to contain secretions. The paramedic should wear an N95 or P100 respirator that has been properly fit-tested **Figure 36-15** . Under the current reporting system, medical facilities are required to notify public health officials if a patient transported is later diagnosed with SARS. If an unprotected exposure occurs, notify the EMS supervisor and complete an exposure report form. If a true exposure occurred, a 10-day quarantine may be recommended. This time off will be covered by workers' compensation. The exposed paramedic will be asked to take a temperature check at least daily as well as follow-up with the EMS service and public health officials.

Avian Flu

Avian (bird) flu is caused by a virus that occurs naturally in the bird population. This virus is carried in the intestinal tract of wild birds and does not usually cause illness. However, in domestic bird populations (eg, chickens, ducks, and turkeys), it is very contagious. Birds acquire the illness from contact with contaminated excretions or surfaces that are contaminated with excretions. If an infected bird is used for food and is cooked, it does not pose a risk to those who eat it.

The first cases of avian flu in humans were reported in Hong Kong in 1997; 18 people became infected and 6 died in this outbreak. In the cases that have occurred since then, the death rate is approximately 25%. Human cases of avian flu have occurred, typically when humans have been in prolonged close contact with infected birds. The transmission risk for humans is quite low. There are a few reports of human-to-human transmission of this disease, but this form of transmission is not typical.

Signs and symptoms of avian flu include fever, sore throat, cough, and muscle aches; some eye infections have also been noted. Illness may eventually progress to pneumonia and severe respiratory distress.

Preventive measures include placing a surgical mask on the patient to contain secretions. If the patient's condition does not permit this action, the paramedic can wear a surgical mask for protection. Medical facilities must notify public health officials if a patient is diagnosed with avian flu. If an exposure is

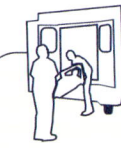

At the Scene

Travel history should be a routine part of your assessment for any patient suspected to have an infectious or communicable disease.

documented, then an antiviral drug may be offered within 48 hours of exposure. Antiviral drugs do not prevent the flu, but rather reduce the severity of the illness. The Canadian federal and provincial governments developed a stockpile of antiviral drugs, and provincial and territorial governments have reserved use of these antiviral drugs to confirmed or suspected outbreaks of avian influenza. In the setting of an outbreak, the antiviral drugs will be released by public health officials. Finally, paramedics should get an annual flu shot to ensure protection from type A viruses. Although this may not prevent avian influenza, it will protect paramedics against common influenza viruses and may provide some reduction in the severity of illness if avian influenza is acquired.

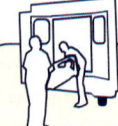

Notes from Nancy

Don't drive a four-wheeled fomite. Clean and air the ambulance after every call.

At the Scene

The lead agencies for responding to potential pandemic diseases are the Public Health Agency of Canada and the Provincial/Territorial Ministries of Health.

Ambulance Cleaning and Disinfection

The paramedic has an obligation to protect patients from nosocomial infections (infections acquired from a health care setting—in this instance, an ambulance). One way to protect patients is by complying with work restriction guidelines: Reporting for work when you have a sore throat or the flu is *not* in the best interests of your patients or your colleagues.

Another way to protect patients from nosocomial infections is to keep the ambulance interior and its equipment clean and disinfected. When cleaning equipment, select cleaning solutions to fit the equipment category:

- **Critical equipment:** items that come in contact with mucous membranes; laryngoscope blades, endotracheal tubes, Combitubes (or similar). Use of single-patient use equipment or high-level disinfection if approved as reusable equipment—that is, use of chemical "sterilants"—is the minimum level for this equipment.
- **Semicritical equipment:** items that come in direct contact with intact skin; stethoscopes, blood pressure cuffs, splints, pneumatic antishock garments. Clean with solutions that have a label claiming to kill HBV. Bleach and water at 1:100 dilution fits this requirement.
- **Noncritical equipment:** cleaning surfaces, floors, ambulance seats, work surfaces. Hospital-grade cleaner or bleach and water mixture is effective for this equipment.

General cleaning routines need to be listed in the service's infection control plan. A simple approach is to do the following after *every* call:

1. Strip used linens from the stretcher immediately after use, and place them in a plastic bag or in the designated receptacle in the emergency department.
2. In an appropriate receptacle, discard all disposable equipment used for care of the patient that meets your province's definition of medical waste. Most items will be considered general trash.
3. Wash contaminated areas with soap and water or a hydrogen peroxide wipe specifically designed for decontamination purposes. For disinfection to be effective, cleaning must be done first.
4. Disinfect all nondisposable equipment used in the care of the patient. For example, disassemble the bag-valve-mask device and place the components in a liquid sterilization solution as recommended by the manufacturer.
5. Clean the stretcher with an approved germicidal/virucidal solution or bleach and water at 1:100 dilution or a specifically designed hydrogen peroxide wipe.
6. If any spillage or other contamination occurred in the ambulance, clean it up with the same germicidal/virucidal or bleach/water solution.
7. Create a schedule for routine full cleaning for the vehicle, as required by the infection control plan. Name the brands of solution to be used.
8. Have a written policy/procedure for cleaning each piece of equipment. Refer to the manufacturer's recommendations as a guide.

You are the Paramedic Summary

1. Given your initial findings, what do you know about the patient's overall condition?

Her flushed, sweaty skin points to the possibility of fever and infection. Depending on her health history, she may or may not be able to compensate for the vasodilation and the resultant increased myocardial workload and oxygen consumption.

2. What are your immediate concerns?

Before moving this patient, you must determine that no trauma has occurred. Also note the length of time that this patient has been on the floor and whether any loss of consciousness occurred.

3. Think of a few potential illnesses that could cause these signs and symptoms.

Viral, bacterial, fungi, and other parasitic infections can result in pneumonia, bronchitis, and influenza, to name just a few.

4. Of those, which are the most serious and why?

Communicable, contagious, or infectious diseases not only place your patient at risk but all those individuals around the patient, including friends, family, health care providers, and the general public.

5. Why is it important to periodically reconsider your differential diagnosis throughout the call?

You must remain mentally flexible and periodically rethink your list of possible causes related to the patient's signs and symptoms. Failure to do so can result in a pigeon-holing of your differentials and can cause you to make errors in prehospital care. Critical thinking skills are the key to delivering good medicine.

6. Given your updated differential, what would be considered "high-risk" procedures for this patient?

Any airway maneuvers, procedures, or treatment that could potentially spread the disease and/or place the paramedic at elevated risk for exposure would be considered "high risk." Examples include endotracheal intubation, laryngeal mask airway, Combitube, CPAP, BiPAP, bag-valve-mask ventilations (without appropriate filtration), delivery of high-flow oxygen, and use of nebulizer treatments.

7. After the transfer of care, what steps must be taken with regard to exposure?

During this call, which included close patient contact in an enclosed space as well as carrying the patient to the stretcher, you may have received a true exposure. Your supervisor and medical director may remove you from duty until the nature of the patient's disease is determined. Because your partner did not receive the same level of exposure, he or she may or may not be removed from active duty.

8. Will this alter your immediate lifestyle or work habits? If so, how?

Yes—being removed from duty means that you will not be going to work on an EMS unit and potentially coming in contact with sick patients (for your sake and theirs).

9. What are some other considerations with respect to this patient's family?

The granddaughter and any other family members will need to be notified and watched by public health officials for signs and symptoms of any similar illness.

Prep Kit

■ Ready for Review

- Government agencies bear the responsibility for protection of the public health, prevention of epidemics, and management of outbreaks.
- The human body offers several defences to protect against infection, such as skin, the mucous membranes, and the immune system.
- Infection involves a typical chain of events through which the communicable disease spreads.
- Communicable diseases can be transmitted from one person to another under certain conditions.
- Precautions against communicable diseases include the designated infection control officer, the public health department, routine practices, immunizations and vaccinations, personal protective equipment, postexposure medical follow-up, and an infection control plan.
- The overuse and misuse of antibiotics has led some pathogens to develop resistance to the antibiotic drugs commonly prescribed to eradicate them.
- New and emerging diseases of concern include SARS and the avian flu.
- Clean and disinfect the ambulance and your equipment to protect patients from infection.

■ Vital Vocabulary

acquired immunodeficiency syndrome (AIDS) The end-stage disease process caused by the human immunodeficiency virus (HIV). A person with this is extremely vulnerable to numerous bacterial, viral, and fungal infections that would not affect a person with an intact immune system.

avian (bird) flu A disease caused by a virus that occurs naturally in the bird population. Signs and symptoms include fever, sore throat, cough, and muscle aches.

bacteria Small organisms that can grow and reproduce outside the human cell in the presence of the temperature and nutrients, and cause disease by invading and multiplying in the tissues of the host.

bloodborne pathogens Pathogenic microorganisms that are present in human blood and can cause disease in humans. These pathogens include, but are not limited to, hepatitis B virus (HBV) and human immunodeficiency virus (HIV).

carrier An individual who harbors an infectious agent and, although not personally ill, can transmit the infection to another person.

chancre The primary hard lesion or ulcer of syphilis that occurs at the entry site of the infection.

chickenpox A very contagious disease caused by varicella zoster virus, which is part of the herpes virus family, occurring most often in the winter and early spring.

Chlamydia A sexually transmitted disease that has the highest incidence. Signs and symptoms include inflammation of the urethra, epididymis, cervix, fallopian tubes, and discharge from the urethra.

communicable disease A disease that can be transmitted from one person to another under certain conditions.

communicable period The period during which an infected person is capable of transmitting illness to someone else.

contaminated The presence or the reasonably anticipated presence of blood or other potentially infectious materials on an item or surface.

enterococcus A common, normal organism of the GI tract, urinary tract, and genitourinary tract, and which may become resistant to vancomycin.

fomite An inanimate object contaminated with microorganisms that serves as a means of transmitting an illness.

fungus (plural: fungi) A small organism that can grow rapidly in the presence of nutrients and organic material, and can cause infection related to contact with decaying organic matter or from airborne spores in the environment such as moulds.

gastroenteritis A term that comprises many types of infections and irritations of the gastrointestinal tract; symptoms include nausea and vomiting, fever, abdominal cramps, and diarrhea.

gonorrhea An sexually transmitted disease which results in infection caused by the gonococcal bacteria, *Neisseria gonorrhea*. Signs and symptoms include pus-containing discharge from the urethra and painful urination in males, and signs and symptoms of an acute abdomen in females.

hantavirus Also known as hemorrhagic fever with renal syndrome, this is a type of virus found in wild rodents, which can also cause disease in humans, characterized by fever, headache, abdominal pain, loss of appetite, and vomiting.

helminths Invertebrates with long, flexible, rounded, or flattened bodies, commonly called worms; a type of parasite.

host resistance One's ability to fight off infection.

human immunodeficiency virus (HIV) AIDS (acquired immunodeficiency syndrome) is caused by HIV, which kills or damages the cells in the body's immune system so that the body is unable to fight infections and certain cancers.

icterus Jaundice; the yellow appearance of the skin and other tissues caused by an accumulation of bile pigments.

incubation period The time period between exposure to an organism and the first symptoms of illness, during which the organism multiplies within the body and starts to produce symptoms.

infection The abnormal invasion of a host or host tissue by organisms such as bacteria, viruses, or parasites, with or without signs or symptoms of disease.

influenza The flu, a respiratory infection caused by a variety of viruses. It differs from the common cold in that the flu involves a fever, headache, and extreme exhaustion.

jaundice The presence of excessive bile pigments in the bloodstream that give the skin, mucous membranes, and eyes a distinct yellow colour; jaundice is often associated with liver disease.

lice Tiny, wingless, parasitic insects that feed on the patient's blood. This infestation is easily spread through close personal contact. Several types exist: head, body, and pubic lice.

Lyme disease A tick-borne disease which primarily affects the skin, heart, joints, and nervous system, and characterized by a round, red lesion or bull's-eye rash.

measles An infectious viral disease that occurs most often in late winter and spring. It begins with a fever followed by a cough, running nose, and pink eye. Then a rash spreads from the face and neck down the back and trunk.

meningitis An inflammation of the meningeal coverings of the brain and spinal cord; it is usually caused by a virus or bacterium.

meningococcal meningitis An infection of the fluid of a person's spinal cord and the fluid that surrounds the brain. Sometimes referred to as spinal meningitis, it is caused by bacteria or virus. The viral type is less severe than the bacterial; the bacterial type can result in brain damage, hearing loss, learning disability, or death.

mononucleosis Infectious mononucleosis or mono (glandular fever), caused by the Epstein-Barr virus, is often called the kissing disease. It is also spread by coughing or sneezing.

mumps A viral infection that primarily affects the parotid glands, which are one of the three pairs of salivary glands, causing swelling in front of the ears.

needleless systems A device that does not use needles for: (1) collection of body fluids or withdrawal of body fluids after initial venous or arterial access is established; (2) administration of medication or fluids; or (3) any other procedure involving the potential for occupational exposure to bloodborne pathogens due to percutaneous injuries from contaminated sharps.

nosocomial infection An infection acquired from a health care setting.

OPIM An acronym that stands for other potentially infectious materials. These include CSF, pericardial fluid, synovial fluid, pleural fluid, amniotic fluid, peritoneal fluid, and any fluid containing gross visible blood.

parasite Any living organism in or on any other living creature; takes advantage of the host by feeding off cells and tissues.

pertussis An acute infectious disease characterized by a catarrhal stage, followed by a paroxysmal cough that ends in a whooping inspiration. Also called whooping cough.

pneumonia An inflammation of the lungs caused by bacteria, viruses, fungi, or other organisms.

protozoans Single-celled, usually microscopic, eukaryotic organisms such as amoebas, ciliates, flagellates, and sporozoans; a type of parasite.

rabies A fatal infection of the central nervous system caused by a bite from an animal that has been infected with the rabies virus.

reservoir In the context of communicable disease, a place where organisms may live and multiply.

respiratory syncytial virus (RSV) A labile paramyxovirus that produces its characteristic fusion of human cells in a tissue culture known as the syncytial effect. Two subtypes, A and B, have been identified. RSV can affect both the upper and lower respiratory tracts but is more prevalent with the lower, causing pneumonias and bronchiolitis.

routine practices Term used to describe infection control practices that merge aspects of universal precautions and body substance isolation and that relies on knowledge of signs and symptoms and communicable disease modes of transmission rather than diagnosis.

rubella A viral disease similar to measles, best known by the distinctive red rash on the skin. It is not nearly as infectious or severe as measles.

scabies An infestation of the skin with the mite *Sarcoptes scabei*. It spreads rapidly when there is skin-to-skin contact.

seropositive Having a positive blood test for an infectious agent, such as HIV or hepatitis B or C virus.

severe acute respiratory syndrome (SARS) Potentially life-threatening viral infection that usually starts with flu-like symptoms.

sexually transmitted diseases (STDs) A group of diseases usually acquired by sexual contact, and which include gonorrhea, syphilis, chlamydia, scabies, pubic lice, herpes, hepatitis, and HIV infection.

source individual Any individual, living or dead, whose blood or other potentially infectious materials may be a source of occupational exposure to the member/volunteer. Examples include, but are not limited to, hospital and clinic patients; clients in institutions for the developmentally disabled; trauma victims; clients of drug and alcohol treatment facilities; residents of hospices and nursing homes; human remains; and individuals who donate or sell blood or blood components.

Staphylococcus aureus A strain of bacteria that became resistant to the drug methicillin, creating a new strain called methicillin-resistant *staphylococcus aureus;* symptoms include infection and possibly localized skin abscesses and cellulites, empyemas, and endocarditis.

syphilis A sexually transmitted disease caused by the spiral-shaped bacteria *Treponema pallidum* and whose signs and symptoms include an ulcerative lesion or chancre of the skin or mucous membrane at the site of infection, commonly in the genital region.

tetanus A disease caused by spores that enter the body through a puncture wound contaminated with animal feces, street dust, or soil, or which can enter through contaminated street drugs, and whose signs and symptoms include pain at the wound site and painful muscle contractions in the neck and trunk muscles.

transmission–airborne The spread of infection by droplet nuclei or dust through the air. Without the intervention of winds or drafts the distance over which airborne infection takes place is short (< 5 m).

transmission–droplet The direct dissemination of a pathogen from a reservoir to a susceptible host's conjunctiva, nose, or mouth by spray with relatively large, short-ranged (± 1 m) aerosols produced by sneezing, coughing, or talking.

tuberculin skin test A test to determine if a person has ever been infected with tuberculosis.

tuberculosis (TB) An infection which can progress to a disease characterized by a persistent cough for 2 to 3 weeks plus night sweats, headache, weight loss, hemoptysis, or chest pain.

vesicle A tiny fluid-filled sac; a small blister.

viral hepatitis An inflammation of the liver produced by one of five distinct forms of the virus—A, B, C, D, and E. The five types differ in transmission but present with the same signs and symptoms.

virulence The ability of an organism to invade and create disease in a host. Also refers to the ability of an organism to survive outside the living host.

virus A small organism that can only multiply inside a host, such as a human, and cause disease.

West Nile virus (WNV) A type of virus that is transmitted by mosquitos, and which usually only causes mild disease in humans, but can cause encephalitis, meningitis, or death. Symptoms, if exhibited, include fever, headache, body rash, and swollen lymph glands.

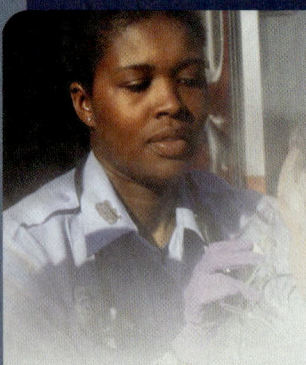

Assessment in Action

A call goes out for a patient complaining of fever, rash, and weakness. The location given is the local university. When the paramedics arrive, they are taken to a dorm room where a student is lying on the sofa. Patient assessment reveals a pinkish-coloured rash, rapid onset of a headache, and stiff neck; also, the patient does not want to be in bright light.

During transport to the local hospital, the patient vomits. The next day, a rumor circulates that the student was diagnosed with bacterial meningitis. The medical facility contacts the supervisor, who then contacts public health. Public health initiates contact tracing and calls the EMS service, which then contacts the crew members who were on the call.

1. **What is meningitis?**
   A. Inflammation of the lining of the myocardium
   B. Inflammation of the meninges, the membranes that cover the brain and spinal cord
   C. Inflammation of the pleura
   D. Inflammation of the endocrine system

2. **What is the transmission mode for influenza?**
   A. Vectorborne
   B. Direct contact with the nasopharyngeal secretions of an infected person
   C. Indirect contact
   D. Inhalation of infected droplets

3. **How is the diagnosis of meningitis made?**
   A. Lumbar puncture
   B. Standard blood work
   C. Chest radiographs
   D. Arterial blood gas analysis

4. **What is the incubation period of meningitis?**
   A. 12 to 24 hours
   B. 8 to 36 hours
   C. 2 to 10 days
   D. 10 to 21 days

5. **Which type of meningitis is communicable?**
   A. Viral
   B. Bacterial

6. **Communicable diseases are caused by microorganisms. How many means of transmission are there?**
   A. 3
   B. 6
   C. 8
   D. 4

7. **What are bacteria?**
   A. Small organisms that can grow and reproduce outside the human cell in the presence of the right temperature and nutrients
   B. Small organisms that multiply inside a host; they die when exposed to the environment
   C. Organisms that grow rapidly in the presence of nutrients and organic material
   D. Small living organisms in or on any living creature

8. **Who does the postexposure medical management begin with?**
   A. Employee
   B. Source individual
   C. Family members
   D. Supervisor

9. **The liaison who handles notification between the hospital and an exposed responder is the:**
   A. medical director.
   B. supervisor.
   C. chief supervisor.
   D. dispatcher.

10. **In an approach to infection control, which of the following is based on the assumption that all blood and body fluids are potentially infectious?**
    A. PPE
    B. Handwashing
    C. Biohazard labeling
    D. Routine practices

Challenging Question

It's 02:00 hr and you are dispatched to a private residence for a man who doesn't feel well. When you arrive on the scene, the patient tells you he has been coughing for approximately 2 weeks. During that time he has had a headache, unexplained weight loss, and night sweats. On the way to the hospital, the patient begins to cough uncontrollably, including in your face.

11. **What are some communicable diseases this patient may possibly have, and how can you prevent becoming exposed to them?**

Points to Ponder

You are dispatched to a private residence for a 42-year-old man complaining of right-sided chest pain. During your assessment you find the patient to be in supraventricular tachycardia at a rate of 220 beats/min, with a blood pressure of 100/70 mm Hg and a respiratory rate of 22 breaths/min. He is pale in colour and slightly diaphoretic. Before starting an IV, your partner practices the appropriate routine precautions. You are helping your partner clean up when you suddenly feel a sharp prick in the palm of your hand. You have just received a needlestick from the used cannula. Your palm has small specks of blood coming from it. When you arrive at the hospital, the patient informs you that he has hepatitis C virus and is currently under treatment for this disease.

What should you do now? Could you have prevented this exposure?

Issues: Safe Management of a Patient With an Infectious and Communicable Disease, Compliance With Routine Precautions and PPE, Managing an Exposure.

37 Behavioural Emergencies

Competency Areas

Area 2: Communication

2.1.e Interact effectively with the patient, relatives, and bystanders who are in stressful situations.
2.3.b Practice active listening techniques.
2.4.b Exhibit empathy and compassion while providing care.
2.4.f Manage and provide support to patients, bystanders, and relatives manifesting emotional reactions.
2.4.h Exhibit conflict resolution skills.

Area 4: Assessment and Diagnostics

4.2.b Obtain list of patient's medications.
4.2.c Obtain chief complaint and/or incident history from patient, family members, and/or bystanders.
4.2.d Obtain information regarding patient's past medical history.
4.2.f Obtain information regarding incident through accurate and complete scene assessment.
4.3.p Conduct psychiatric assessment and interpret findings.

Area 6: Integration

6.1.k Provide care to patient experiencing illness or injury due to poisoning or overdose.
6.1.p Provide care for patient experiencing psychiatric crisis.

Appendix 4: Pathophysiology

K. **Psychiatric Disorders**
Anxiety Disorders: Generalized anxiety disorder
Anxiety Disorders: Panic disorder
Anxiety Disorders: Post-traumatic stress disorder
Childhood Psychiatric Disorders: Attention-deficit disorder
Cognitive Disorders: Delirium
Eating Disorders: Anorexia nervosa
Eating Disorders: Bulimia nervosa
Affective Disorders: Bipolar disorder
Affective Disorders: Depressive disorders
Affective Disorders: Suicidal ideation
Psychotic Disorders: Delusional disorder
Psychotic Disorders: Homicidal ideation
Psychotic Disorders: Schizophrenia

Introduction

Problems related to abnormal behaviour are commonly the result of "mental problems," implying that they originate in some ephemeral place called the mind, as opposed to "real" medical problems, which originate in the solid, tangible structures of the body. In reality, the mind and the body are not separate entities; they are inseparable parts of a whole human being. When a person becomes ill with any disease, that illness will inevitably affect the individual's behaviour—often making him or her anxious or depressed. Similarly, changes in mental state influence the body's physical health. A depressed person, for example, may lose appetite or become more susceptible to bodily disease. Thus, whenever we examine a patient, it is important to view the patient as a whole person and try to understand both the physical and the mental factors that contribute to the patient's distress

Notes from Nancy

Abnormal behaviour may be due to many conditions other than mental illness.

Figure 37-1 ▶ .

What Is a Behavioural Emergency?

The concept of behaviour has been widely debated over the years. Most experts define it as the way people act or perform—for example, how they react to a situation. Behaviour includes all the things people do and the reasons why they do those things. Who defines when the behaviour becomes abnormal is also a source of debate, as is who defines what is normal—society in general, a particular community or social group, a parent, a boss, a friend, or even a stranger. Abnormal behaviour in and of itself may not be a medical problem and is hardly cause for alarm. The real questions are "When does abnormal behaviour require medical intervention?" and "When does it require EMS?" Almost all disordered behaviour represents the individual's effort to adapt to some stress, whether internal or external. In most cases the disruptive behaviour is a temporary action, abating when the individual has managed to mobilize his or her psychological defence mechanisms.

A behavioural disorder is a disorder of mood, thought, or behaviour that interferes with an individual's ability to perform activities of daily living (ADLs), and is caused by organic and/or psychiatric illness. ADLs are normal, everyday activities such as getting dressed and taking out the garbage. When a person becomes so depressed that he or she cannot get up in the morning, shower, and make breakfast, or when someone has

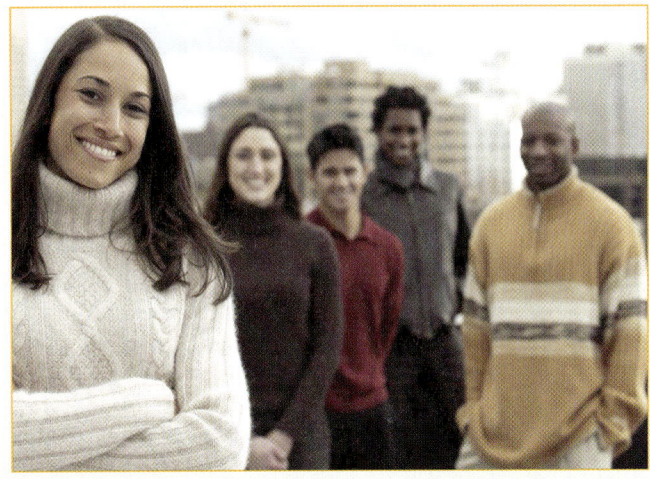

Figure 37-1 Which of these people is battling mental illness?

You are the Paramedic Part 1

You are dispatched to 1022 Pierce Lane for a 39-year-old man who is "acting crazy." Per dispatch protocols, law enforcement officers have been sent as well. You stage two blocks from the scene and wait for an update from law enforcement. A few minutes later, a police officer notifies you that the scene is safe and one man is in custody.

You arrive to find a man in his 30s lying on the ground with his hands cuffed behind his back. He is yelling about seeing flashing green and yellow lights from the sky. After you introduce yourself, he tells you that his name is Eugene.

Initial Assessment	Recording Time: 0 Minutes
Appearance	Sweaty, anxious
Level of consciousness	A (Alert to person, place, and day)
Airway	Patent
Breathing	Fast and deep
Circulation	Fast, slightly irregular pulse

1. What are some medical conditions that can give the appearance of "acting crazy?"
2. What are some considerations to discuss with your partner while you stage the scene?

delusions or hallucinations that prohibit holding a job, a behavioural disorder exists.

A behavioural emergency exists when the abnormal behaviour threatens an individual's health and safety or the health and safety of another. The most extreme examples are psychiatric emergencies in which a person becomes suicidal, homicidal, or has a psychotic episode. In a psychotic episode, a person often experiences delusions (false beliefs) or hallucinations (false perceptions) that result in loss of contact with reality. For example, a patient who has taken illicit drugs may experience an alteration of reality—a "bad trip." Psychotic episodes may be dangerous because the individual's behaviour may become so disorganized due to exaggerated fear or paranoia that they fail to care for him- or herself, undertake risky behaviours, or become violent.

No matter what definition of a behavioural emergency a textbook may furnish, the *operative* definition is provided by the person who dials 9-1-1. Often what makes a behavioural emergency an "emergency" is panic on the part of the patient, the family, bystanders, or all of these parties. That panic, in turn, may translate into a demand for action, and the paramedic may therefore face intense pressure to do something (such as transport the patient to an emergency department with a crisis unit).

Paradoxically, it is precisely in this situation—when the patient is behaving strangely and bystanders are clamoring for action—that the paramedic usually feels least *able* to do something. Most paramedics would much prefer to deal with a train wreck than with the tangle of confused and frayed feelings presented by a behavioural emergency. Most people prefer to operate in areas in which they feel competent. For paramedics, that means dealing with problems like broken legs, cardiac dysrhythmias, or narcotic overdoses. Paramedics feel much less confident of their ability to deal with emotional disturbances—especially because most paramedic training programs don't delve into such matters. Furthermore, paramedics tend to be action-oriented people. They like to see tangible results of what they do—a hypoglycemic patient coming around after a bolus of glucose, a clinically dead patient restored to life by CPR and defibrillation. What tangible rewards can there be in escorting a confused, hallucinating patient to the hospital, let alone in dealing with a belligerent and violent patient who's screaming obscenities?

In fact, prehospital intervention *is* possible and often critical in behavioural emergencies. Paramedics can make a huge difference in the life of a disturbed patient, and the skills for doing so can be learned just like any other skill. Indeed, the skills for dealing with abnormal behaviour may ultimately be much more important to the paramedic's work than skills such as endotracheal intubation. After all, how many calls require placing an advanced airway? Many more calls require the paramedic to deal with people who are angry, depressed, agitated, panicky, or out of control. Clearly, it's worthwhile learning an organized and systematic approach to emergencies that involve abnormal behaviour.

Causes of Abnormal Behaviour

Anyone who has seen a paranoid, belligerent diabetic transformed into a paragon of courtesy and charm by the mere addition of 25 g of glucose to the bloodstream knows that not all behavioural problems are caused by psychiatric illness. Similarly, no one would diagnose mental illness in a person who was stunned and mute after the unanticipated death of a husband or wife. Abnormal behaviour typically results from a complex interaction of biological or organic causes, developmental factors, psychological stressors, emotional stimuli, and sociocultural influences. Those causes can be classified into three broad categories: (1) biological or organic causes, (2) psychosocial causes, and (3) sociocultural causes.

Biological or Organic Causes of Abnormal Behaviour

Many patients presenting with psychiatric symptoms are actually suffering from a physical illness or are under the influence of a substance that interferes with normal cerebral function. Such patients are generally classified as having organic brain syndrome. Diabetes, seizure disorders, severe infections, metabolic disorders, head injury, stroke, alcohol, tumours in the brain, and drugs may all cause derangements in behaviour. When faced with abnormal behaviour, always look for situational and organic causes, as they're the ones you'll be best able to treat in an acute emergency.

The conditions and substances that can produce psychiatric symptoms are summarized in **Table 37-1 ▶**. Probably the most common offenders are alcohol and drugs. Besides intoxication with alcohol or drugs, other common forms of organic brain syndrome include delirium and dementia. Delirium is characterized by a global impairment of consciousness and cognitive function that comes on quite rapidly and may fluctuate in severity over the course of a day. Delirium is almost always a consequence of a general medical condition. Dementia is a more chronic process that produces severe deficits in memory, abstract thinking, and judgment.

Psychosocial Causes of Abnormal Behaviour

Normal individuals may develop abnormal reactions to stressful psychosocial events (eg, childhood trauma) or developmental influences (eg, parents who deprived them of love, caring, support, and encouragement). When a person's basic needs are threatened, that individual faces a crisis. A person in crisis has two alternatives for dealing with this threat: (1) cope with it, finding ways to alter the situation or his or her perception of it so that it is no longer so stressful, or (2) attempt to alleviate the discomfort by escaping from the stress. Escape may take many forms, including alcohol, drugs, psychiatric symptoms, and even suicide.

Table 37-1	Selected Medications and Conditions That May Produce Psychotic Symptoms
Medications	• Digitalis • Steroids • Sedative hypnotics • Analgesic agents/opiates • Antinausea medications • Seizure medications • Antihistamines • Antipsychotic medications • Anticholinergic medications • Polypharmacy in the elderly
Infections	• Sepsis • Syphilis • Parasites • Urinary tract infection • Pneumonia
Neurologic disease	• Seizure disorders (especially temporal lobe seizures) • Primary and metastatic tumours of the brain • Dementia • Cerebrovascular accident • Closed head injury • CNS infections (encephalitis, meningitis, brain abscess)
Cardiovascular disorders	• Low cardiac output (in heart failure) • Hypoxia • Hypercarbia
Endocrine disorders	• Thyroid hyperfunction/hypofunction • Adrenal hyperfunction (Cushing's disease)
Metabolic disorders	• Electrolyte imbalances (after severe diarrhea) • Hypoglycemia • Diabetic ketoacidosis
Illicit drugs	• Amphetamines/stimulants • LSD, PCP, and other psychedelics/hallucinogens • Cannabis • Cocaine
Poisonings and overdose Vitamin deficiencies Liver failure Kidney failure	

Sociocultural Causes of Abnormal Behaviour

Chapter 2 considered the responses of patients, their families, bystanders, and rescue personnel to the stresses of emergencies and the various ways that people react to death and dying. Humans are social animals; we prefer to live in groups. Not surprisingly, then, social and cultural factors directly affect biology, behaviour, and responses to the stress of emergencies. For example, the effects of assault, rape, and racial attacks or the death of a loved one may produce significant changes in an individual's behaviour.

Psychopathology

Many factors contribute to disturbances of behaviour. Some of these influences are easily identified and treated, whereas others may never be clearly understood. The causes, signs, symptoms, and management of abnormal behaviour can be grouped into several common areas of psychopathology:

- Anxiety disorders
- Mood disorders and suicide
- Personality disorders
- Somatoform (a disorder involving excessive concern with one's physical health and appearance) and dissociative disorders
- Eating, impulse control, and substance-related disorders
- Schizophrenia and other psychotic disorders
- Hostile and violent patients

The remainder of this chapter focuses on these areas of psychopathology. Before considering those categories in detail, however, you need to learn about assessing a patient with a behavioural emergency.

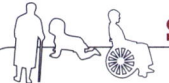

Special Considerations

The American Psychiatric Association (APA) is a scientific and professional organization composed of psychiatrists. Its goals are to promote the highest quality care for individuals with mental disorders, promote psychiatric education and research, and advance and support the profession of psychiatry.

The APA publishes the *Diagnostic and Statistical Manual of Mental Disorders, Fourth Edition, Text Revision (DSM IV TR)*, a comprehensive reference manual focusing on mental health disorders, including symptomatic and diagnostic information.

■ Psychiatric Signs and Symptoms

When an organ begins functioning abnormally, the human body mobilizes various defences to correct the abnormality. The patient experiences those corrective measures as symptoms, and the paramedic observes their effects as signs. Physical symptoms and signs reflect the body's attempts to maintain its balance in the face of physical stress.

Psychiatric signs and symptoms serve the same function for the mind: They reveal the personality trying to maintain the optimal internal balance in the face of a stressor. Like the symptoms and signs of physical illness, psychiatric symptoms and signs can be grouped according to the "systems" they affect. Here, however, the focus is on systems of psychological (rather than physiologic) functioning. The psychological functions involved are consciousness, motor activity, speech, thought, affect, memory, orientation, and perception. Psychiatric signs and symptoms are categorized by disorder in **Table 37-2 ▶**.

Table 37-2	Classification of Psychiatric Signs and Symptoms
Disorder	**Psychiatric Signs and Symptoms**
Disorders of consciousness	Confusion Delirium Stupor and coma
Disorders of motor activity	Restlessness Stereotyped movements Compulsions Retarded movements
Disorders of speech	Retarded speech Acceleration or pressure of speech Neologisms (words the patient invents) Echolalia (the patient echoes words he or she hears) Mutism
Disorders of thinking	Disordered thought progression: • Flight of ideas • Retardation of thought • Perseveration • Circumstantial thinking Disordered thought content: • Delusions • Obsessions • Phobias
Disorders of mood and affect	Anxiety Euphoria Depression Inappropriate affect Flat affect
Disorders of memory	Amnesia Confabulation
Disorders of orientation	Disoriented to person, place, and time
Disorders of perception	Illusions Hallucinations
Disorders of intelligence	Mental retardation

Disorders of Consciousness

Consciousness refers to the degree to which a person is aware of and attentive to the external world. Disorders of consciousness such as delirium, stupor, and coma usually indicate an organic basis for the patient's disorder. Other disorders of consciousness, however, are seen in psychiatric patients. Confusion refers to impaired understanding of one's surroundings.

Disorders of Motor Activity

Motor activity in a disturbed patient may be increased, decreased, or bizarre in some way. Restlessness refers to the situation in which a patient cannot sit still; when restlessness occurs in association with extreme excitement, it's called agitation. At the other end of the spectrum, a very depressed or psychotic patient may exhibit exceptionally slow or retarded movements. In some cases, the patient appears to have little or no control over motor activity. Stereotyped activity involves a repetition of movements that don't seem to serve any useful purpose—for instance, a patient's repetitive touching of the elbow, nose, and forehead in succession. Compulsions are repetitive actions that are carried out to relieve the anxiety of obsessive thoughts.

Disorders of Speech

Like motor activity, speech may be abnormally fast or abnormally slow. Retardation of speech is seen in severely depressed patients, whereas manic patients often show accelerated speech and pressure of speech (ie, words pour out like water escaping under pressure). The words the patient uses may themselves be strange or unusual. Neologisms are words that the patient invents. In echolalia, the patient echoes the words of the examiner. When the patient doesn't speak at all, the condition is called mutism.

Disorders of Thinking

Thinking is the highest of the mental functions, requiring integration of knowledge, perception, and memory. Thinking may be disordered in its progression or in its content.

The *progression* of thought, like motor activity and speech, may be speeded up or slowed down. Flight of ideas, which occurs in some manic conditions, refers to accelerated thinking in which the mind skips so rapidly from one idea to another that the listener finds it difficult to grasp the connection between them. At the other end of the spectrum, depressed patients may experience retardation of thought, in which it seems to take a very long time to get from one thought to the next. In circumstantial thinking, the patient includes many irrelevant details in his or her account of things. Perseveration refers to repetition of the same idea over and over again.

The *content* of thought may also be abnormal in a patient with psychiatric problems. The patient may, for example, express delusions—fixed beliefs that are not shared by others of the same culture or background and that the patient is not willing to change by reasonable explanation. With delusions of persecution, the individual believes that others are plotting against him or her. With delusions of grandeur, the patient believes he or she is someone of great importance. Other delusions that suggest psychoses include thought broadcasting (the belief that others can hear one's thoughts), thought control (the belief that outside forces are controlling one's thoughts), and ideas of reference (the belief that external forms of communication such as television, radio, and newspapers are directed specifically at the individual).

Obsessions are thoughts that will not go away, despite attempts to forget them. Usually the person with an obsession knows that the idea is unreasonable, but can't stop thinking about it. Patients may, for example, have an obsessional belief that the gas stove hasn't been turned off, so they'll return again and again to the kitchen to make sure. Each time they do so,

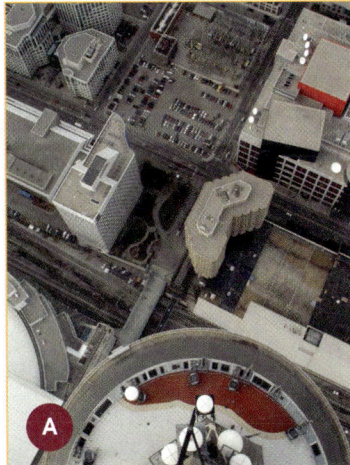

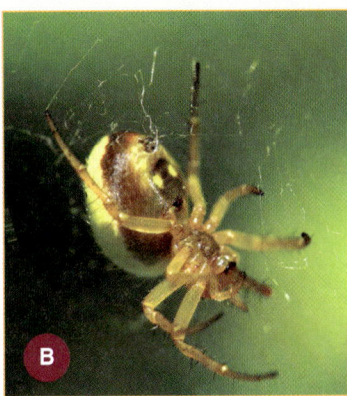

Figure 37-2 Phobias are irrational fears of specific things, such as fear of heights (**A**) or fear of certain animals (**B**).

their anxiety will be relieved for a short time, but then they must go back and check yet again. Phobias are obsessive, irrational fears of specific things or situations, such as fear of heights, fear of open places, fear of confined places, or fear of certain animals Figure 37-2 ◀ .

Disorders of Mood and Affect

Mood refers to a person's sustained and pervasive emotional state; affect is the outward expression of a person's mood. A person's mood may be described as *depressed, euphoric,* or *anxious.* Affect is described as *appropriate* or *inappropriate.* A patient who puts on a waxy smile as he tells you of a parent's death would be considered to be showing inappropriate affect—that is, the emotion expressed is out of synch with the situation. Affect is characterized as labile when it shifts rapidly, as in the patient who is laughing one moment and crying the next. With a flat affect, the patient does not seem to feel much of anything at all.

Disorders of Memory

The most profound disorder of memory is amnesia, the loss of memory. Memory is a complex process consisting of four separate functions: registration, the ability to add new items to the cerebral data bank; retention, the ability to store those items in an accessible place in the mind; recall, the ability to retrieve a specific piece of stored information on demand; and recognition, the ability to identify information that one has encountered before. Amnesia may reflect the disruption of one or several of those functions. In delirium, for example, a person may be unable to register events properly and thus can't recall what happened while he or she was delirious. When painful memories are repressed, recall is impaired.

Sometimes patients with severe memory deficits from organic brain disease will invent experiences to "paper over" the gaps in memory; this behaviour is called confabulation.

Disorders of Orientation

Orientation refers to a person's sense of who one is (person), where one is (place), at what day of the week one finds him- or herself (day), and an understanding of events leading up to where one finds him- or herself (events). A person who is confused about those particulars is said to be disoriented. Disorientation is most common in organic brain syndromes.

Disorders of Perception

Perception refers to the way a person processes the data supplied by the five senses. Two disorders of perception are illusions and hallucinations. An illusion is a misinterpretation of sensory stimuli—for example, mistaking a piece of rope for

You are the Paramedic **Part 2**

After a few minutes, you are able to calm the patient. When you ask why he's upset, he tells you that he came home from work to find the neighbour's dog barking. He tells you that the barking changed into understandable words. The dog said that it would tell his boss that he was stealing at work. Your patient also tells you that things have been stressful at work with many cutbacks and layoffs, and he's afraid he might lose his job if his boss thought he was stealing. After you display concern for his well-being, the patient agrees to let you "check him out."

Vital Signs	Recording Time: 5 Minutes
Skin	Sweaty, flushed, and warm
Pulse	100 to 120 beats/min (dependent on emotional state)
Blood pressure	146/90 mm Hg
Respirations	24 to 42 breaths/min (dependent on emotional state)
Spo₂	99% ambient air

3. What are the medical implications when police control the scene of a violent patient?

4. Is it wise to agree with or validate a patient's hallucinations?

a snake or a cat's meowing for a human voice. A hallucination is a perception that has no basis in reality and occurs without any external stimuli. Hallucinations may involve any of the five senses—a person may hear, see, feel, taste, or smell something that isn't there. Auditory hallucinations (eg, hearing voices) are the most common. Hallucinations involving other senses (eg, the frightening visual hallucinations in delirium tremens) suggest an organic cause.

Disorders of Intelligence

Intelligence refers to a person's intellectual ability. A person's intelligence is not necessarily a function of his or her education. For example, a person with a disorder of intelligence may have been born with mental retardation or may have suffered from a disease that makes it more difficult to process, remember, and communicate information.

At the Scene

Many people have mental disorders, and many individuals who don't currently have such a disorder may develop one at some point in their lives. It's no cause for shame. With so many stressors in today's society, it's quite understandable.

Assessment of the Patient With a Behavioural Emergency

The first step in assessing a patient with a behavioural emergency is directed at ruling out an organic illness. Further evaluation of the patient with a behavioural emergency differs in at least two ways from the methods of patient assessment studied so far. In assessing the patient with trauma or acute illness, you use a variety of diagnostic instruments to measure vital functions and detect abnormalities—a stethoscope to evaluate breath sounds, a sphygmomanometer to measure the blood pressure, and so forth. In assessing the disturbed patient, *you* are the diagnostic instrument. You must use your thinking processes to evaluate someone else's thinking processes, your perceptions to test the validity of someone else's perceptions, and your feelings to measure someone else's feelings.

A second way in which the assessment of a patient with a behavioural emergency differs from that of a patient with a nonmental medical problem is that the assessment is part of the treatment. As soon as you speak to the patient, your voice and manner will influence his or her condition, for better or worse. The very process of listening to the patient describe the issue at hand can also mitigate the problem.

Scene Assessment

The patient's overall condition and the nature of his or her psychiatric problem will determine how much of the assessment you are able to perform. A disturbed patient may prefer not to be touched,

and you must respect that wish unless there's a compelling medical reason for doing otherwise (eg, profuse bleeding from slashed wrists or a decreased level of consciousness from an overdose). At the very least, you should be able to assess the patient's general appearance—for example, the patient's dress, cleanliness, and grooming, all of which provide clues to the way the patient perceives himself or herself. Pay attention to the patient's posture. Does the patient appear frustrated, angry, sobbing, or catatonic (lacking expression or movement, or appearing rigid)? Observe the scene carefully for weapons, remembering that almost anything—a chair, a lamp, or a book—can be used as a weapon. Prior to entering a scene, ensure that you have a clear exit route available for personal safety. If you have any questions about your ability to manage the situation safely, call for assistance.

Initial Assessment

Identify yourself clearly. Tell the patient who you are and what you are trying to do. If the patient is confused or delusional, you may have to explain who you are at frequent intervals. Do so without arguing, in an emotionally neutral tone of voice. ("No, Mr. Jones, I'm not from CSIS. I'm a paramedic with the city ambulance service, and I'm here to help you.")

Attend first to priority problems—airway, breathing, or circulatory concerns. Your assessment must look for signs and symptoms of abnormal functioning as well as abnormal behaviour.

Be prepared to spend time with the disturbed patient. Don't be in a hurry; rather, convey the message that you have the time and concern to learn what's bothering the patient. Assess the patient wherever the emergency occurs. Don't rush off immediately to the hospital, because the hospital is likely to be a strange, intimidating place for the patient; your haste to get there may reinforce the patient's belief that something is terribly wrong. Let the patient recover his or her bearings in familiar surroundings when medically possible.

Patients who are seriously disturbed should be seen by a physician and evaluated for possible hospitalization. Many of these patients will agree to their transport to the hospital. Others may not want your help and try to prevent you from taking them to a hospital. Because this kind of transport deprives the patient of his or her civil liberties, it must never be undertaken lightly. Even an experienced psychiatrist may find it difficult to define what kind of behaviour justifies removing a person from society or what constitutes "dangerous behaviour." Furthermore, laws vary from one region to another, so it's important to be familiar with the legal requirements in your community.

As a general rule, consent is required to take a competent, conscious adult to the hospital. If consent is withheld, a patient may be taken against his or her will if he or she is deemed incompetent and is felt to require hospital care. Additionally, patients expressing thoughts of self-harm or harm to others should be taken against their will to the hospital. In all cases where patients are transported against their will, police must be involved. The same policy applies to the use of forcible restraint. Where such measures are deemed necessary, law enforcement officers should be summoned. In addition, every ambulance service should have clearly defined protocols, drawn up with legal advice, for dealing with patients who require involuntary commitment. Follow those protocols to the letter and consult direct medical control, if present in your system.

Focused History and Physical Examination

Begin your focused history and physical examination for individuals who are behaving abnormally by obtaining both their past medical history and their history of present illness. To gather the needed information, talk with the patient and use your interviewing skills. Set some ground rules for your interview. Let the patient know what you expect, and what he or she may expect of you. ("It's okay to cry or even scream, but we aren't going to let you hurt yourself or anyone else.") Allow the patient tell the story in his or her own way. Don't attempt to direct the conversation, but allow the patient to vent his or her feelings.

Interviewing Techniques

When evaluating a trauma patient, you can generally obtain enough information to provide appropriate initial treatment just from the physical examination, even if the patient is unconscious and can't give a history. When evaluating a patient with a behavioural emergency, by contrast, virtually all of the diagnostic information (and much of the therapeutic benefit) must come from talking with the patient. Skill in interviewing a disturbed person, therefore, is central to dealing with psychiatric emergencies. Here are some guidelines:

- *Begin the interview with an open-ended question.* An open-ended question doesn't provide possible answers for the patient, but rather allows the patient to select the answer. For example, say "It's clear you've been feeling bad. Tell me something about the kind of troubles you've been having." (The only circumstance in which you should begin with more direct questioning is when it is essential to obtain specific information in a hurry, such as "What kind of pills did you take? How many?")
- *Let the patient talk* and tell the story in his or her own way, even if it takes a little more time. Letting patients talk allows them to gain some control over themselves and their situation. At the same time, it enables *you* to assess the patient's speech, affect, and thought processes.
- *Listen, and show that you're listening.* Your facial expression, posture, eye contact, and an occasional nod—all of these things can convey to the patient that you're paying close attention to what he or she is saying **Figure 37-3 ▶** .
- *Don't be afraid of silences*, even though they may seem intolerably long. Maintain an attentive and relaxed attitude until the patient takes up the story again. It's especially important to be silent when the patient stops speaking because of overwhelming emotion. Avoid the temptation to jump into the silence with a hasty "There, there," to forestall the patient's expressions of emotion, such as

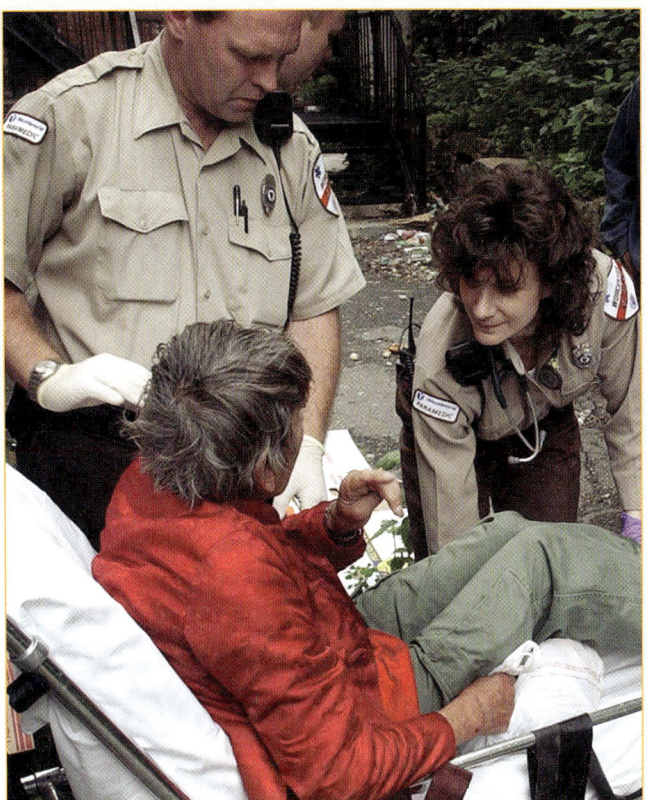

Figure 37-3 Making eye contact with a patient can provide useful clues about his or her emotional state—but don't stare at the patient.

crying. The expression of feelings is often therapeutic in itself—that's why people speak of having "a good cry"—and the patient will likely be better able to express himself after intense emotion has been released. Furthermore, your silence gives patients a chance to get control of themselves in their own way.

- *Acknowledge and label the patient's feelings.* The disturbed patient may feel overwhelmed by intense and chaotic feelings. Identifying those feelings and giving them a name (eg, "You seem very angry") can help the patient gain control over them.
- *Don't argue.* If the patient misperceives reality, make note of the misperceptions, but don't try to talk the patient out of them. When a misperception is very frightening or distressing to the patient, you might try just once to provide a simple and factual statement, in a neutral tone of voice ("Yes, that does look a lot like a snake, but actually it's just a shadow."). But don't get into a dispute on the nature of reality.
- Facilitation is a technique of encouraging the patient to communicate by using gestures or noncommittal words, such as a nod of the head or a phrase like "Go on," "I see," or "What happened after that?" You can also use facilitation to return the patient to a topic on which you'd like some elaboration. For example, a patient may have

made a passing reference to suicidal thoughts and then moved on to another subject. When the patient finishes, you might comment, "You say you've had thoughts of suicide?" This remark tells the patient that you've been paying attention to the story and would like to learn more.

- Confrontation refers to pointing out something of interest in the patient's conversation or behaviour, thereby directing the patient's attention to something he or she may have been unaware of. Confrontations describe how the patient appears to the interviewer based on observations, *not* judgments. For example, the interviewer might remark, "You seem worried" or "You look very sad." Such comments often elicit a freer expression of feelings from the patient. Confrontations must be carefully phrased, so they won't sound nagging or condescending.

- When the patient finishes giving the initial account of the problem, you will have to *ask questions*. Keep the questions as nondirective as possible. Avoid asking questions that can be answered with a yes or no ("Are you very angry?") or asking leading questions ("Do you think that your husband is a part of the problem?"). *How* and *what* questions are preferred ("How did you feel when that happened?").

Some patients find it difficult to deal with the unstructured situation of nondirective questioning and may become very anxious during silences. That response is particularly likely among adolescents, severely depressed patients, and confused or disorganized patients. When your open-ended questions meet with uncomprehending silence, try another approach and perform a more structured interview.

The Mental Status Examination

The mental status examination (MSE) is a key part of your focused physical examination of a patient who is experiencing an acute psychiatric problem. To conduct the MSE, you must check each of the "systems" of mental function in an orderly way. A useful mnemonic for the elements of the MSE is COASTMAP, also discussed in Chapter 14 (Figure 37-4 ▶):

- **Consciousness.** Determine the patient's level of consciousness (alert, confused, responds to pain, unresponsive). Note the patient's ability to *pay attention* to a discussion and *concentrate*. Is the patient easily distracted, or can he or she focus on the events at hand?

- **Orientation.** Ask what the year or month is. Ask the patient to state where he or she is at the moment—the country, province, town, or specific location. If the patient is not sure, have the patient make a best guess. Ask the patient to describe the events leading up to the current circumstance.

- **Activity.** Examine the patient's behaviour. Is the patient restless and agitated, pacing up and down? Experiencing tremors? Sitting very still, scarcely moving at all? Making any strange or repetitive movements (scanning of the environment, odd or repetitive gestures)?

- **Speech.** Identify the form, rather than the content of the patient's speech. Note the rate, volume, flow, articulation, and intonation of speech. Is it too fast or too slow? Too

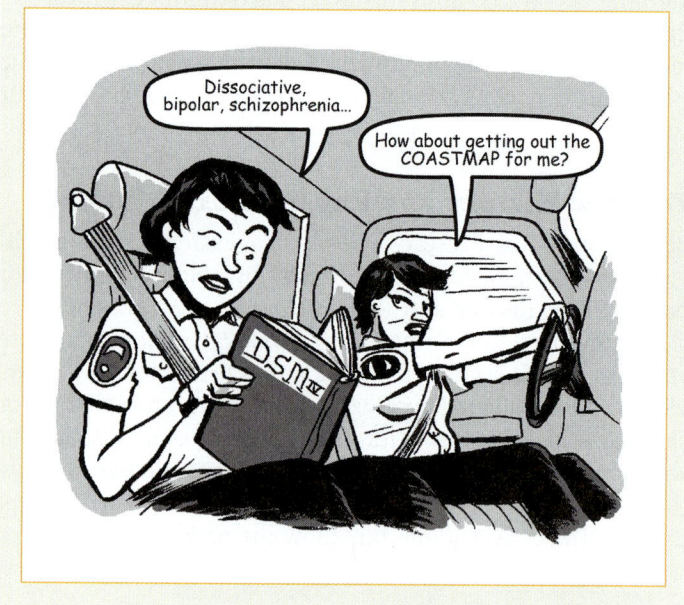

Figure 37-4

loud or too soft? Is the speech garbled or slurred (dysarthria)? Is the patient stuttering or mumbling? Using any strange words?

- **Thought.** Listen to the patient's story. What's on his or her mind? Is the patient making sense? Is there anything unusual about his or her reasoning? Is the patient expressing apparently false ideas (delusions), such as a belief that CSIS is after him/her? Is the patient experiencing any false sensory impressions (hallucinations), such as hearing voices? Is he/she experiencing a flight of ideas?

- **Memory.** Form an impression of the patient's memory—recent, remote, and immediate. If memory loss is present, determine whether it is constant or variable. Some patients may create memories to take the place of things they can't recall (confabulation).

- **Affect and mood.** The patient's mood may be objectively noted via body language. Is the mood euphoric or sad? Is it labile? Does the affect—the expression of inner feelings—seem appropriate to the situation or is it animated, angry, flat, or withdrawn?

- **Perception.** Detecting disorders of perception may be difficult, because patients often hesitate to answer direct questions about hallucinations or illusions. Sometimes it is helpful to ask the patient, "Do you ever hear things that other people can't hear?"

You can conduct nearly all of the MSE just by watching and listening (and knowing what to watch and listen *for!*). Only the assessment of memory, orientation, and perhaps perception requires you to ask some direct questions. Practice being an observer. As you sit in a diner drinking your coffee, eavesdrop on the waitress talking to other customers and systematically go through the COASTMAP sequence to

Documentation and Communication

The mental status examination (MSE) contains many new terms that most health care and mental health professionals use to describe behaviour. Using the same terms will help you avoid ambiguous meanings and communicate a clear description of the behaviour.

At the Scene

The physical assessment of a patient with an acute injury or illness relies on the evaluation of specific criteria. The psychological assessment (MSE) of a patient with an acute behavioural emergency also has specific criteria. Most of the information in the MSE is gathered in the initial assessment and the focused history and physical examination.

evaluate *her* mental status. Get into the habit of *noticing* how other people talk, move, and express their feelings, and practice describing those things to your partner.

Patients with psychiatric problems may be taking any of several types of psychotropic drugs—that is, drugs that affect mood, thought, or behaviour. During your assessment, you should determine which medications have been prescribed for your patient, and whether he or she is actually taking them. Psychotropic drugs are among the most widely prescribed medications in Canada. Most of these medications target the autonomic nervous system by either inhibiting or enhancing the sympathetic or parasympathetic nervous systems. The wise paramedic will have a thorough understanding of these two systems as well as knowledge of how the drugs in the paramedic's kit may potentially interact with these types of medications.

Many acute problems arise when patients fail to take their medications. Acute symptoms can be relieved by transporting the patient to a hospital safely and quickly. In the hospital, crisis workers can assist patients in getting their medications to prevent recurring episodes.

The Rest of the Focused History and Physical Examination

While much of your focused history and physical examination involves interviewing the patient about psychiatric history and performing the MSE, you must also look for signs of an organic cause of the patient's behaviour:

- Measure the **vital signs** for indications of organic illness; perform a bedside glucose measurement, if indicated, to rule out hypoglycemia.
- Examine the **skin** temperature and moisture. Scars may indicate self-mutilation in borderline personality disorders.

- Inspect the **head** for evidence of trauma.
- Check the **pupils** for size, equality, and reaction to light. Pupillary abnormalities may indicate a toxic ingestion or an intracranial process as the source of the patient's behaviour.
- Note any unusual **odours on the patient's breath** such as poisons, alcohol, or ketones from diabetic ketoacidosis.
- In examining the **extremities**, check for needle tracks, tremors, and unilateral weakness or loss of sensation.

Detailed Physical Examination and Ongoing Assessment

Based on your transport time and the patient's mental status, a full head-to-toe assessment may not be practical. However, it is essential to perform a sufficiently detailed physical examination to rule out any medical or trauma problems. Additionally, transport time affords a good opportunity to assess more details of your patient's mental status and provide ongoing reassessment.

Many times patients with abnormal behaviour may have settled down physically, but their minds may still be in a state of flux; this could lead to very impulsive behaviour. Monitor patients vigilantly for sudden changes in thought or behaviour, particularly as you near the hospital. If patients don't want help, they may try to jump from the ambulance or hurt themselves.

General Principles

The following guidelines apply to the care of *any* patient with a psychiatric problem:

- *Be as calm and direct as possible.* Disturbed patients are often frightened of losing self-control. Your behaviour should indicate that you have confidence in the patient's ability to maintain control. Indeed, one of the main purposes of the interview is to help the patient reestablish some self-mastery. If you show anxiety or panic, you merely affirm the patient's conviction that the situation is overwhelming.
- *Exclude disruptive people from the interview.* In most cases, you should interview the patient alone (if scene safety permits), while relatives and bystanders wait in another room (your partner can interview them). Some patients, however, will become anxious if separated from an important person—a parent, or perhaps a friend. If another person has a calming effect on the patient, ask that person to remain present.
- *Sit down* to interview the patient, preferably at a 45° angle from the individual so you don't encroach on the patient's "personal space" **Figure 37-5 ▶**. Paramedics should maintain a clear exit route at all times to allow for a rapid escape should the patient become aggressive.
- *Maintain a nonjudgmental attitude.* Accept the patient's right to have his or her own feelings about things, and don't blame, judge, or criticize him or her for those feelings.
- *Provide honest reassurance.* Give supportive, truthful information—for example, "Many people experience periods of hopelessness like you're having, but today there

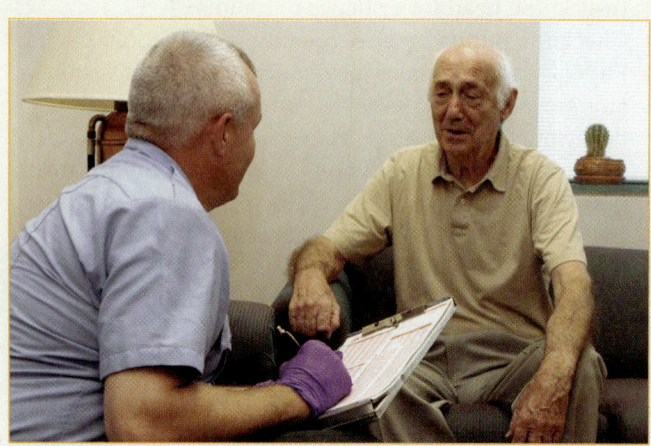

Figure 37-5 When interviewing the patient, sit at a 45° angle to avoid encroaching on personal space.

are effective treatments for those feelings." Avoid excessive reassurance, however, such as "Everything's going to be all right." Such statements will merely convince the patient that you don't understand how bad things are.

- After the patient has finished telling his or her story and you have concluded your assessment, *develop a definite plan of action*. This step gives the patient the feeling that something is being done to help, which in turn relieves anxiety. Furthermore, people in crisis need direction. Don't confront the patient with an array of decisions (eg, "Do you want to go to the hospital, or would you rather stay at home and call your doctor tomorrow?"); rather, state what you think is the best course of action ("I think it's important for you to go to the hospital. There are doctors there who

can help you."). Once the plan is determined and you have begun to carry it out, allow the patient to make choices and thereby exercise some control over the situation. You might ask the patient, for example, whether he or she prefers to be carried on a stretcher or to walk to the ambulance on his or her own. These small decisions may seem minor, but they allow the patient to attain a measure of self-respect.

- *Encourage some motor activity.* Moving about often helps ease anxiety. If you are taking the patient to the hospital, have the patient gather up the things he or she wants to bring along. Let the patients do as much for themselves as possible, to reinforce the feeling that you expect them to improve.

- *Stay with the patient at all times.* Once you have responded to the emergency, the patient's safety becomes your responsibility. If the patient politely excuses himself or herself, locks the bathroom door, and swallows the contents of a bottle of sleeping pills, you'll have a lot of explaining to do—at least to your own conscience.

- *Bring all of the patient's medications to the hospital.* If the patient is receiving treatment for psychiatric problems, knowing which medications have been prescribed can help the doctors at the hospital identify the condition for which the patient has been treated.

- *Never assume that it's impossible to talk with any patient until you've tried.* Even if the patient sits silently and appears unaware of your presence, assume that he or she can hear and understand everything you say.

General Management

General management of the patient with a psychiatric problem follows the approach stressed throughout this text. After ensuring

You are the Paramedic Part 3

Eugene explains that he's been struggling with his finances and may lose his house. His wife divorced him last year after she said he was lazy and a lousy husband. He says, "I still love her and wish I knew how to win her back, but it's been difficult to think clearly for the last couple of years." He starts to cry and whispers to you, "I wish I was dead." Given his behaviour and statements, you suggest that Eugene come with you to the hospital to be evaluated. He hesitantly agrees.

Reassessment	Recording Time: 10 Minutes
Skin	Warm, pink and sweaty
Pulse	100 beats/min, regular
Blood pressure	144/70 mm Hg
Respirations	24 breaths/min
SpO_2	100% ambient air
Blood glucose	4.9 mmol/l

5. How important is police involvement if the patient apparently becomes agreeable?

6. What are the risk factors for suicide, and do they apply in this situation?

7. Would you talk with Eugene about his comment or wait and let the hospital explore these issues?

that the scene is safe, which may require assistance from law enforcement personnel, focus on any life-threatening conditions discovered in the initial assessment. If immediate life threats are not present, perform a focused history and physical examination to uncover any medical abnormalities that should be considered. If the erratic behaviour might possibly be caused by a medical disorder (eg, hypoglycemia, overdose, or hypoxia), treat the individual for the medical disorder before presuming that the patient's behaviour is due to an emotional or psychiatric cause. These measures may include oxygen therapy, testing of the blood glucose level, and administration of $D_{50}W$, as well as general interventions for hypothermia or shock management.

Disorganization and disorientation are *not* diagnoses, but rather ways in which various conditions such as organic brain syndromes (eg, head injury, drug ingestion, and metabolic disorders) or schizophrenia may present themselves. These presentations account for a large number of ambulance calls, particularly those involving older people. While the paramedic doesn't need to make a specific diagnosis in such cases, he or she does need to know how these patients should be managed in the prehospital setting.

Disorganized patients are characterized by uncontrolled and disconnected thought. They are usually incoherent or rambling in their speech, although they may be oriented to person and place. Often such patients are found wandering aimlessly down the centre of the street, dressed peculiarly, uttering meaningless words and sentences. A thorough examination of such a patient is rarely possible. However, if safety permits, it is important to attempt to perform a sufficient medical examination to rule out serious medical conditions. En route to the hospital, the principal objective is to transport the patient in an atraumatic fashion.

The disorganized patient needs structure. The paramedic should explain in very plain language what's being done and what the patient's role will be. Directions should be simple, consistent, and firm. It may be useless to try to take a detailed history; a name and address may be all that can be obtained. Explain to such patients that they need to be seen by a doctor, and that you'll take them to the hospital to get help.

In managing the disoriented patient, the key is to *keep orienting the patient* to time, place, and the people in the environment. Tell the patient who you are, and explain what you're doing. You may have to identify yourself several times en route. Reassure the patient, and point out landmarks that will help the patient orient himself/herself.

Specific Conditions

Anxiety Disorders

Anxiety disorders are mental disorders in which the dominant moods are fear and apprehension. Everyone experiences anxiety occasionally, and a certain amount of anxiety helps people adapt constructively to stress. Patients with anxiety disorders, by contrast, experience persistent, incapacitating anxiety in the absence of external threat. Almost one fifth of adults will experience some form of anxiety disorder in any given year. Several types of anxiety disorders are likely to elicit a call for an ambulance or affect the delivery of prehospital care, including generalized anxiety disorder, phobias, and panic disorder.

Generalized Anxiety Disorder

Although some anxiety in everyday activity is normal, when a person worries about everything for no particular reason, or if that worrying is unproductive and the individual can't decide what to do about an upcoming situation, the person may be suffering from generalized anxiety disorder (GAD). To make a diagnosis of GAD, symptoms (anxiety and worry) must be present more days than not for a period of at least 6 months and the worry must be difficult to turn off or control. GAD is one of the most common anxiety disorders. Patients suffering from GAD are often treated with both pharmacologic agents and counseling. The acute symptoms of anxiety and worry can become overwhelming in GAD, however, prompting the patient, a family member, or colleague to call for an ambulance.

When dealing with a patient with GAD, identify yourself in a calm, confident manner. Listen attentively to the patient and talk with the individual generally about his or her feelings.

Phobias

Phobic disorders involve an unreasonable fear, apprehension, or dread of a specific situation or thing. The patient with a simple phobia focuses all his or her anxieties onto one class of objects (eg, mice, spiders, dogs) or situations (eg, high places, darkness, flying). Almost one tenth of adults have social phobias, or fear of everyday social situations such as fear of going to parties, meeting new people, speaking, eating in public, etc. When confronted with the feared object or situation, the phobic person experiences intolerable anxiety and all of the autonomic symptoms that anxiety brings. The patient usually recognizes that the fear is unreasonable but is unable to do anything about it.

In managing a phobic patient, explain each step of treatment in detail before you carry it out **Figure 37-6 ▾** : "First we'll

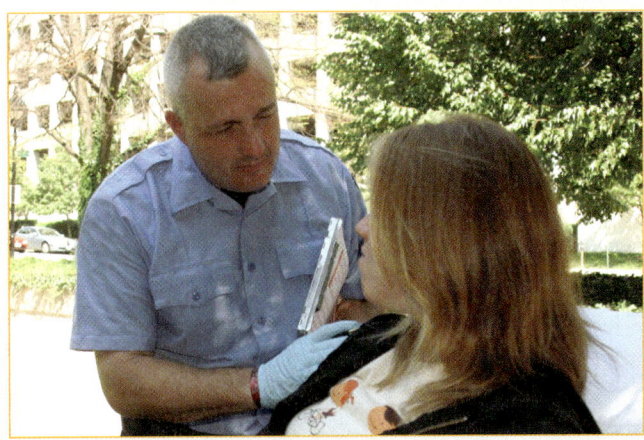

Figure 37-6 With a phobic patient, explain each step of treatment in detail before carrying it out.

Table 37-3	Signs and Symptoms of a Panic Attack
■ Shortness of breath or a sensation of being smothered	■ Dizziness or feeling faint
■ Palpitations or tachycardia	■ Trembling
■ Sweating	■ Feeling of choking
■ Nausea or abdominal distress	■ Paresthesias
■ Flushes or chills	■ Chest pain or discomfort
■ Fear of dying	■ Fear of going crazy
■ Feelings of unreality or of being detached from oneself	

Source: Adapted from American Psychiatric Association, *Diagnostic and Statistical Manual of Mental Disorders, Fourth Edition, Text Revision.* Washington, DC: APA, 2000.

give you oxygen to help you breathe. Then we're going to move you onto the stretcher, so that we can carry you downstairs."

Panic Disorder

Panic disorder is characterized by sudden, usually unexpected, and overwhelming feelings of fear and dread, accompanied by a variety of other symptoms produced by a massive activation of the autonomic nervous system. Women are two thirds more likely to be affected by this condition than are men, and the disorder tends to run in families. The attacks usually begin when the patient is in their 20s. Most affected individuals can identify a stressful event that preceded their first attack, such as an illness or loss of a loved one. Thereafter, the attacks may come "out of the blue," without any apparent precipitating stress. If allowed to continue, panic attacks may cause severe restrictions in the patient's lifestyle. When severe, the individual becomes afraid to go to work, to go shopping, or to leave the house at all, out of fear that an attack will occur away from home. The fear of going into public places is called agoraphobia (literally, "fear of the marketplace").

The classic signs and symptoms of panic disorder are summarized in **Table 37-3 ▲**. A large percentage of the signs and symptoms—such as palpitations and sweating—are a consequence of autonomic nervous system discharge, while others (chest discomfort, paresthesias) may reflect hyperventilation. The symptoms usually peak in intensity within about 10 minutes and last around an hour altogether.

By the time the paramedics arrive at the scene, the patient having a panic attack may be surrounded by a horde of anxious and excited people, who will themselves contribute to the problem. Accordingly, you'll need to take control of the situation quickly:

- *Separate the patient from panicky bystanders.* If you can find a calm friend or member of the patient's family, however, having this person present may be helpful.
- *Provide as calm an environment* as possible as you transport the patient to the hospital.
- *Be tolerant of the patient's disability.* The patient having an anxiety attack may not be able to cooperate or answer questions at first, because of intense fear and distress. Your manner must convey that everything is under control.

- *Reassure the patient that he or she is safe.* The word "safe" can be a magic pill that will often de-escalate symptoms to a more manageable level: "We're going to take you down these stairs on the stretcher. It's going to be okay; we'll go slowly and be very careful to keep you safe while we move you."
- *Give the patient's symptoms a name.* Once you have checked the vital signs and the electrocardiogram (ECG) monitor, you should be in a position to reassure the patient that he or she is not in immediate danger of dying: "I know that your symptoms are very distressing, but they're not a life-threatening condition."
- *Encourage the patient to do things for him- or herself* to the extent that he or she is able, thus allowing the patient to regain a sense of being in control.

Panic attacks may mimic a range of physical disorders in their presentation. Conversely, symptoms of anxiety may be the presenting complaint in medical conditions such as cardiac dysrhythmias, withdrawal states, anaphylaxis, hyperthyroidism, and certain tumours. For that reason, any patient experiencing a panic attack—especially a first panic attack—should be fully evaluated in the hospital. Hyperventilating patients should not be treated with "paper-bag therapy." Patients whose anxiety results from an unsuspected pulmonary embolism or cardiac problem may suffer serious complications and even die from the hypoxemia induced by this treatment. Hyperventilation is best managed by coaching patients to slow their breathing until they regain control.

Posttraumatic Stress Disorder

The number of traumatic events occurring in the general population has increased in both frequency and intensity in recent years. Posttraumatic stress disorder (PTSD) is a severe form of anxiety that stems from a traumatic experience; it is characterized by the patient reliving the stress and nightmares of the original situation. Causes can be as general as combat military service and terrorist attacks or as personal as a motor vehicle collision or sexual assault **Figure 37-7 ▼**.

One symptom commonly associated with PTSD is flashbacks—sudden memories in which the victim relives the

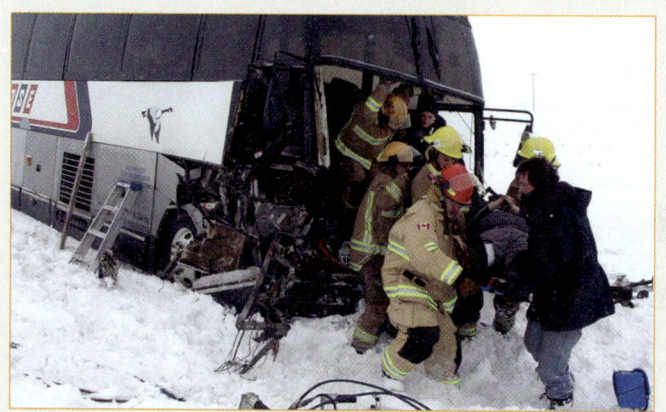

Figure 37-7 Posttraumatic stress disorder can be caused by a traumatic event such as a motor vehicle collision with a fatality.

Table 37-4	Medications for Anxiety	
Class	**Generic Name**	**Trade Name**
Antidepressants		
Selective serotonin reuptake inhibitors	Citalopram	Celexa
	Fluoxatine	Prozac
	Fluvoxamine	Luvox
	Paroxetine	Paxil
	Sertraline	Zoloft
Monoamine oxidase inhibitors	Phenelzine	Nardil
Serotonin-norepinephrine reuptake inhibitors	Venlafaxine	Effexor
Anxiolytics		
Benzodiazepines	Alprazolam	Xanax
	Clonazepam	Rivotril
	Diazepam	Valium
	Lorazepam	Ativan
Nonbenzodiazepines	Buspirone	BuSpar
Other Classes		
Antihistamines	Hydroxyzine	Atarax
Beta blockers	Propanolol	Inderol
Anticonvulsants	Carbamazepine	Tegretol
	Gabapentin	Neurontin
	Valproic acid	Depakene

event. Sleep disturbances, including nightmares, and depression or survivor guilt are other signs and symptoms of PTSD. Treatment in the prehospital setting is intended to protect the patient, support the individual in a positive way, and transfer the individual to a medical facility for a more thorough evaluation.

Medications for Anxiety

Several classes of medications are effective in the treatment of anxiety disorders, including many antidepressants Table 37-4 ▲ . In the past, drugs that exert a tranquilizing or sedative effect, thereby reducing anxiety, were the most commonly prescribed (and overprescribed) psychotropic agents. Today, much safer drugs such as the selective serotonin reuptake inhibitors are more frequently prescribed.

Benzodiazepines serve such functions—as antianxiety agents, muscle relaxants, anticonvulsants, and sedatives. Unfortunately, they are often the source of overdoses. In addition to use of these drugs for chemical restraint, paramedics can administer benzodiazepines to treat status epilepticus, for pain for external pacing or synchronized cardioversion. Beware of the signs and symptoms of potential overdose: severe hypoventilation, severe hypotension, bradycardia, slurred speech, altered mental status, and impaired coordination. Management of a benzodiazepine overdose includes airway management, IV fluids for hypotension, and the potential medical control option of flumazenil to reverse the effects of the benzodiazepine. Flumazenil should not be used in patients with

chronic benzodiazepine use or mixed overdose due to the risk of inducing an acute withdrawal state/seizure.

Mood Disorders

Mood disorders, formally known as affective disorders, are among the most prevalent psychiatric disorders. As much as 10% of the population will experience a mood disorder, such as a major depression at some point in their lives. Although feelings such as depression and joy are universal, mood disorders differ from normal bouts of sadness or happiness. In mood disorders, the changes in affect are accompanied by other symptoms, and the net effect is to cause a major disturbance in the person's ability to function. Patients who experience either depression or mania suffer from a unipolar mood disorder; that is, their mood remains at only one pole of the depression–mania continuum. Patients who alternate between mania and depression (both poles of the continuum) have bipolar mood disorder. The majority of patients with a unipolar mood disorder are depressed. Unipolar mania is relatively rare.

Depression and Suicidal Behaviour

Depression is the leading cause of disability in people between 15 and 44 years of age. It affects women more frequently than men and may occur at any age (the mean age of onset is 32 years). The depressed patient is often readily identified by a sad expression, bouts of crying, and listless or apathetic behaviour. He or she expresses feelings of worthlessness, guilt, and pessimism. These patients may want to be left alone, asserting that no one understands or cares and that their problems are hopeless.

Depression may occur in episodes with a sudden onset and limited duration; this is common in major depressive disorder, in which the patient feels substantial suffering and pain that interfere with social or occupational functioning. In other cases, the onset of depression may be insidious and chronic in nature. When a person experiences signs and symptoms of depression for more days than not for a period of at least two years, he or she may be suffering from a chronic form of depression known as dysthymic disorder. The signs and symptoms of dysthymic disorder cause social and occupational distress but rarely require hospitalization unless the individual becomes suicidal.

The diagnostic features of depression are most easily remembered by the mnemonic GAS PIPES:

- **Guilt** and self-reproach are characteristic features of depression. One way to try to get at the patient's guilt feelings is to ask a question such as "Are you down on yourself?" or "Do you ever feel as if you're worthless?"
- **Appetite** is abnormal in depression. Usually it is *decreased,* but a minority of depressed patients may report increased appetite.
- **Sleep disturbance** usually takes the form of insomnia. The typical depressed patient will report that he or she awakens at 03:00 hr and can't get back to sleep again.
- **Paying attention.** The depressed patient has difficulty paying attention; that is, the ability to concentrate is

impaired, sometimes severely. Ask the patient, "When you're reading a book or a newspaper, can you get all the way through what you're reading, or does your mind start to wander after a couple of minutes?"

- **Interest.** The depressed patient loses interest in things that were once important. He or she can no longer summon enthusiasm for work or hobbies. You might ask the patient, "Are you a [local team name] fan?" If the answer is yes, ask, "How are they doing this season?" The depressed patient will tell you, "Well, I haven't really been following them lately."
- **Psychomotor abnormalities** in the depressed patient can take the form of either retardation or agitation. Although many depressed patients seem to do everything in slow motion, a significant percentage show agitated behaviour, such as pacing, wringing their hands, or picking at themselves.
- **Energy.** Depressed people have no energy. They are tired all the time and don't feel like doing anything.
- **Suicide.** Most worrisome, depressed people tend to have pervasive and recurrent thoughts of suicide.

Medications for Depression

Antidepressants are prescribed to combat the symptoms of depressive illness (Table 37-5 ▸). They are classified into three categories:

- *Selective serotonin reuptake inhibitors (SSRIs)* are the most commonly prescribed medications for depression. Side effects include headaches, sexual dysfunction, and insomnia. Abrupt cessation of SSRIs can cause a discontinuation syndrome that results in flu-like symptoms.
- *Tricyclic antidepressants (TCAs) and related drugs,* like the neuroleptics, produce atropine-like side effects and may cause orthostatic hypotension.
- *Monoamine oxidase (MAO) inhibitors* are usually prescribed when TCAs are not effective. Their most notable side effect is *hypertensive crisis*, which may occur in patients taking MAO inhibitors if they receive certain other drugs (eg, sympathomimetics, narcotics) or if they eat certain foods (eg, cheese, yogurt, sour cream, beer, wine, chopped liver).
- *Other agents* include the very widely prescribed venlafaxine (Effexor).

Suicidal Ideation

Suicide is any willful act designed to end one's own life. It is the third leading cause of death among 15- to 25-year-olds and the fourth leading cause of death in the 25- to 44-year age group. For people aged 45 to 64 years, suicide rates are the eighth leading cause of death. Suicide is more common among men, especially those who are Caucasian and single, widowed, or divorced. The risk of

Notes from Nancy

Evaluate the suicide risk in every depressed patient.

suicide is also high among depressed patients, one sixth of whom will succeed in taking their own lives. Alcoholism is another important risk factor. Notably, more than half of all successful suicides have made a previous attempt, and three fourths have given a clear warning of their intent to kill themselves. The risk factors for suicide are summarized in (Table 37-6 ▾).

Suicide attempts typically occur when a person feels that close emotional attachments are endangered or when the person has lost someone or something important in his or her life. The suicidal person may also have feelings characteristic of depression—feelings of worthlessness, lack of self-esteem, and a sense of being unable to manage his or her life. Like suicide, people may consider homicidal fantasies. Fortunately, most do not act on these thoughts; however, there is a risk when this is associated with other severe forms of psychosis or delusion.

Evaluation of Suicide Risk

The assessment of *every* depressed patient must include an evaluation of the suicide risk. Many paramedics are reluctant to ask a patient directly about suicidal thoughts, because they fear that they might "put ideas into the patient's head" (Figure 37-8 ▸). The paramedic should realize, however, that suicide is not such

Table 37-5	Medications for Depression	
Class	**Generic Name**	**Trade Name**
Selective serotonin reuptake inhibitors	Citalopram	Celexa
	Fluoxatine	Prozac
	Fluvoxamine	Luvox
	Paroxetine	Paxil
	Sertraline	Zoloft
Serotonin norepinephrine reuptake inhibitors	Venlafaxine	Effexor
Tricyclic antidepressants and related drugs	Amitriptyline	Amitril, Elavil
	Desipramine	Norpramin
	Doxepin	Sinequan
	Imipramine	Imavate
	Nortriptyline	
	Trimipramine	Surmontil
MAO inhibitors	Phenelzine	Nardil
	Tranylcypromine	Parnate
Others	Trazodone	Desyrel

Table 37-6	Risk Factors for Suicide
■ Depression, or sudden improvement in depression	■ Expresses suicidal thoughts and concrete plans for carrying them out
■ Male sex, age > 55	■ Caucasian
■ Single, widowed, or divorced	■ Social isolation
■ Alcohol or other drug abuse	■ Previous suicide attempt(s)
■ Recent loss of spouse or significant relationship	■ Financial setback or job loss
■ Chronic, debilitating illness	■ Family history of suicide
■ Schizophrenia	

At the Scene

Patients with suicidal thoughts, especially those who have made a threat or unsuccessful attempt, may not be thinking clearly and may behave in very unpredictable ways. Some recognize that if they get into the ambulance or enter the hospital, they won't have the opportunity to complete their threat or gesture. They may therefore make a last effort to kill themselves. Suicidal and/or homicidal patients won't hesitate to hurt you or your partner. Be very careful how you assess the situation, making certain that you, your team, and the patient are safe.

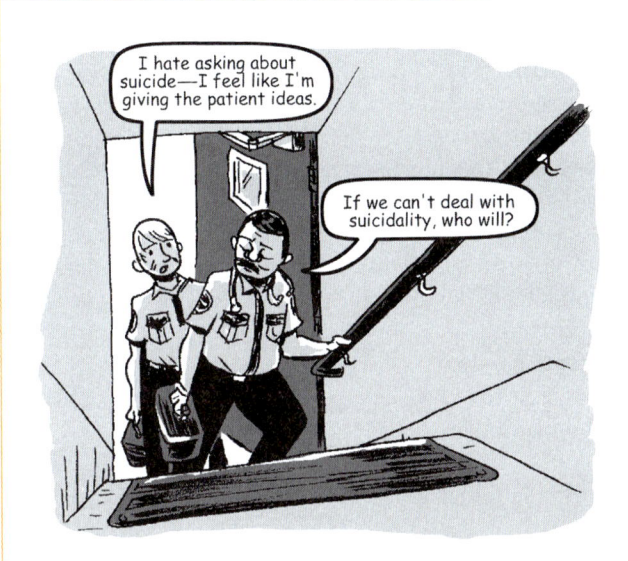

Figure 37-8

an original idea that a depressed patient will not have thought of it. Most depressed patients, in fact, are relieved when the topic is brought up, as this discussion gives them "permission" to talk about their suicidal ideas. Often it is easier for both the paramedic and the patient to broach the subject in a stepwise fashion. You might start by asking, "Have you ever thought that life wasn't worth living?" From there, you may proceed by degrees: "Did you ever feel that you would be better off dead? Have you ever thought of harming yourself? Do you feel that way now? Do you have a plan of how you would go about it? Do you have the things you need to carry out the plan? Has anyone in your family ever committed suicide? Have you ever tried to kill yourself before?" Patients who have made previous attempts; who have fashioned detailed, concrete plans for suicide; or who have a history of suicide among close relatives are at higher risk and must be evaluated at the hospital.

Many patients make last-minute efforts to communicate their suicidal intentions. When an individual phones to threaten suicide, someone should stay on the line until the rescue squad has reached the scene. On arrival, quickly survey the area for any implements that the patient might use to injure himself or herself and discreetly remove those items. Make certain that you account for your own safety. Talk with the patient, and encourage him or her to discuss feelings. Ask the same questions mentioned earlier regarding the patient's suicidal ideas and plans.

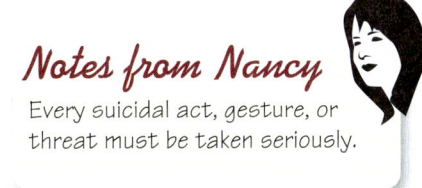

Notes from Nancy
Every suicidal act, gesture, or threat must be taken seriously.

Management of the Patient at Risk of Suicide

Whenever you find a patient to be severely depressed or you have another reason to suspect that a patient is at risk of suicide, follow these guidelines:

- Don't leave the patient alone. The patient's well-being is your responsibility until transferred to the care of another medical professional.
- Bring any pill bottles or substance containers you may have found at the scene to the hospital.
- Acknowledge the patient's feelings. Don't argue with the wish to die, but provide honest reassurance. ("It's not unusual for a person to feel like you do after losing someone close to them. Sometimes it helps to talk about it.")
- If the patient refuses transport, try to involve persons close to him or her in eliciting cooperation. If resistance persists, obtain police assistance in order to facilitate transport to the hospital.

When a person has *attempted* suicide, medical treatment has priority. The patient who has taken an overdose of sedative or depressant drugs must be managed for possible respiratory depression or circulatory collapse; the patient who has slashed his or her wrists must be treated to control bleeding and restore circulating volume. Nonetheless, if the patient is stable and conscious, try to establish communication and ask the patient to talk about the situation.

A person who attempts suicide is in enormous distress. Among the most important skills that any health care provider can acquire is the ability to see beyond another person's behaviour to the underlying distress. When called to treat a person who has attempted suicide, it's worthwhile to say to the person, and to remind yourself, "You must have been very unhappy to do something like this. It's time to get some help."

Manic Behaviour

Mania is one of the most striking psychiatric conditions. Typically a bystander or family member calls for an ambulance, because the patient is unlikely to believe there's anything wrong. To the contrary, the manic patient is more apt to report being "on top of the world—never felt better in my life." Individuals experiencing mania typically have abnormally exaggerated happiness, joy, or euphoria with hyperactivity and insomnia.

Table 37-7	Medications for Mania
Generic Name	**Trade Name**
Lithium carbonate	Lithium, Lithane, Carbolith, Duralith
Lithium citrate	Lithium
Carbamazepine	Tegretol
Valproic acid	Depakene

Medications for Mania

Drug therapy for bipolar (manic-depressive) disorder usually requires multiple medications **Table 37-7 ▲** . Antianxiety drugs may help reduce agitation or anxiety, while antipsychotic drugs may help reduce psychomotor activity and delusions or hallucinations. Antidepressants may help reduce depression. While these agents may be used for a limited period of time, mood stabilizers are considered lifetime therapy for bipolar patients. Lithium carbonate and valproic acid (Depakene) are most often used as first-line therapy. Unfortunately, some patients taking lithium preparations develop symptoms of toxicity, including nausea and vomiting, dysarthria, tremors, and lethargy. Lithium toxicity may lead to brain damage if not treated, so patients showing signs of toxicity require medical attention. Antiepileptic medications such as valproic acid (Depakene) or carbamazepine (Tegretol) are frequently used for lithium nonresponders, who account for 20% to 40% of bipolar patients.

The Mental Status Examination in the Manic Patient

In manic patients, the MSE is likely to reveal the following findings:

- **Consciousness**—awake and alert, but easily distracted. The patient may complain of an inability to concentrate.
- **Orientation to time and place**—commonly disturbed in manic patients.
- **Activity**—markedly hyperactive. Almost all manic patients report a significantly decreased need for sleep, and they may go for days without sleeping.
- **Speech**—pressured and rapid. The patient is also very talkative.
- **Thought**—flight of ideas and delusions of grandeur. Patients may report that their thoughts are racing; their monologues may skip rapidly from one topic to another (tangential thinking). Their ideas are often grandiose, such as unrealistic plans to embark on a large business venture or to run for high public office. Patients may also believe that they have special powers or they are famous and wealthy.
- **Memory**—usually intact in manics, but may be distorted by underlying delusions.
- **Affect**—an apparently elated affect (the hallmark of mania). The patient seems to be on a "high," and is unusually and infectiously cheerful. The good cheer may be quite brittle, however, and the person may quickly become irritable, sarcastic, and hostile with very little provocation.
- **Perception**—may be disturbed. A person having an acute manic episode may show psychotic symptoms such as hallucinations.

You are the Paramedic Part 4

You establish a 20-gauge IV of normal saline in the patient's right hand to keep vein open. You contact the hospital and notify them of your patient's status. Hospital personnel in turn contact the crisis response team and other mental health professionals who will evaluate the patient in the emergency department.

Upon arrival at the emergency department, you are met by a nurse and a security guard. They are very calm and compassionate, and the patient readily trusts both of them. He remains calm throughout your stay there, even falling asleep just before you leave for another call.

Reassessment	Recording Time: 20 Minutes
Skin	Warm, pink and slightly moist
Pulse	90 beats/min, regular
Blood pressure	138/68 mm Hg
Respirations	20 breaths/min
Spo$_2$	100% ambient air
Temperature	37°C
Pupils	4 mm/PEARRL
Blood glucose	4.9 mmol/l
ECG	Sinus rhythm

8. How can your professionalism and general demeanor affect patient care in scenarios such as these?

9. What would you tell the hospital in your radio report to help personnel there prepare for the patient?

Management of the Manic Patient

Individuals experiencing acute manic episodes have a high probability of getting themselves into trouble of one sort or another—for example, going on wild spending sprees, driving recklessly, committing sexual indiscretions, or picking fights. Generally it is when the person has gotten into some sort of trouble, or when his or her behaviour has become intolerably disruptive, that an ambulance is summoned.

Because manic patients are unlikely to consider themselves ill, they may not agree that they need treatment. In dealing with the manic patient, be calm, firm, and patient; don't argue or get into a power struggle. Minimize external stimulation. If scene safety will permit, talk to the patient in a quiet place, away from other people. (Meanwhile, have your partner obtain the history separately from relatives or bystanders.) When it's time to transport, don't use sirens.

If the patient refuses transport, consult direct medical control if available in your service. Obtain police assistance for transport if the patient continues to refuse and hospital evaluation is necessary.

Personality Disorders

According to the American Psychiatric Association, personality disorders are "enduring patterns of perceiving, relating to and thinking about the environment and one's self that are exhibited in a wide range of social and personal contexts" and are "inflexible and maladaptive, and cause significant functional impairment or subjective distress." Common definitions of "personality" include the ways a person behaves or thinks. How people think or behave in the world and with others may be suspicious, outgoing, fearful, or overly dramatic. When these ways of relating to others become dysfunctional or cause distress to other people, that person is considered to have a personality disorder. Many times the person with the personality disorder doesn't feel any subjective distress but such distress may be acutely felt by others. The *Diagnostic and Statistical Manual of Mental Disorders, Fourth Edition, Text Revision (DSM IV TR)*, classifies personality disorders into three categories: odd or eccentric disorders; dramatic, emotional or erratic disorders; and anxious or fearful disorders.

True personality disorders are rare in the general population. When a person does have a personality disorder, another psychiatric illness is likely to be present at the same time. Such patients tend to do poorly during treatment. For example, individuals who are depressed in addition to having a personality disorder usually have more difficulty managing the depression.

Paramedics will have difficulty influencing personality disorders over the long term because of their limited interaction with patients. Nevertheless, they need to understand these abnormal behaviours to be aware of how they should react in the current situation. A patient with an antisocial personality will not think twice about hurting you if agitated. One with a histrionic personality may be demanding and dictate the level of care. Be calm and professional in your interactions with patients exhibiting these traits.

Somatoform Disorders

People who are overly concerned with their physical health and appearance may have a somatoform disorder if their preoccupation dominates their life. A hypochondriac provides the classic example of a somatoform disorder. In hypochondriasis, patients have a great deal of anxiety or fear that they may have a serious disease. They are so convinced that they're ill that even a physician can't convince them otherwise. With somatization disorder, individuals also have multiple complaints, but are more concerned with the symptoms than with their meaning. In conversion disorders, a physical problem (eg, paralysis, blindness, or seizures) has no identifiable pathophysiology, and is often triggered by conflict or other stressors. In conversion disorder, the symptoms are not produced or faked intentionally.

As opposed to conversion disorder, in factitious disorders the symptoms the patient is experiencing are under voluntary control but there is no obvious reason for them except to assume the "sick role" and receive extra attention. This type of behaviour has also been referred to as Munchausen syndrome. When a parent (typically a mother) intentionally makes a child sick to garner attention and pity, it is referred to as factitious disorder by proxy or Munchausen syndrome by proxy. This is an atypical form of child abuse.

Dissociative Disorders

People who have mild feelings of being detached from themselves, as if they were dreaming, are said to be having a dissociative experience. When this dissociation becomes so intense that they lose their identity and assume new ones or are unable to function because they have lost their memory or sense of reality, a dissociative disorder may be present. Somatoform and dissociative disorders have been linked historically and share many common traits. Management of these patients centres on careful observation to prevent injury and management of symptomatic signs and symptoms based on local protocols. Because treatment to correct the disorder is difficult and often unsuccessful, it should be carried out in the safety and security of a hospital. Talk with the patient about what is happening so you have detailed information to report to the hospital staff.

A stressful event, exhaustion, or physical or mental pressures—usually extreme in nature—may cause a feeling of dreaming or slow motion. These alterations in perceptions of reality are often referred to as dissociative experiences; they can be either mild and readily explained or extraordinarily frightening. Two types of experiences are distinguished—depersonalization and derealization. As a paramedic, you may have responded to a horrible motor vehicle collision where a patient described the event as "dreamlike" or "as if time had stopped." In such a case of depersonalization, the patient loses his or her own sense of reality. In derealization, objects seem to change size or shape; people may seem dead or behave like robots. In their most severe forms, dissociative disorders result in abnormal functioning, amnesia, a trance, or even a new identity (formerly known as multiple personality disorder).

Eating, Impulse Control, and Substance-Related Disorders

Disorders of personal control, motivation, and substance use generally evolve over a relatively long period of time. Because of the chronic nature of these problems, EMS will typically be called when an acute exacerbation of the underlying problem occurs—for example, when a bulimic patient experiences electrolyte imbalances that produce a sudden onset of weakness, dizziness, cardiac or respiratory complaints, or seizures, or when an alcoholic suffers respiratory depression from binge drinking. Emergency management of these patients typically focuses on treating symptomatic complaints and the presenting signs and symptoms.

Eating Disorders

Eating disorders have been around for many decades, although their incidence began to increase rapidly in the 1950s and 1960s. Today, eating disorders are widespread in the developed world and are emerging as a problem in developing countries: Some countries are experiencing a fourfold increase in eating disorders. Individuals most likely to be affected by these disorders are young females of upper-middle-class or upper-class socioeconomic status who live in socially competitive surroundings.

There are two major types of eating disorders: bulimia nervosa and anorexia nervosa. In both forms, individuals may experience severe electrolyte imbalances leading to cardiac problems, seizures, and renal failure as well as less severe erosion of dental enamel and salivary gland enlargement. Anxiety, depression, and substance abuse disorders are noted in as many as two thirds of those diagnosed with eating disorders.

Bulimia nervosa is characterized by consumption of large amounts of food, typically more junk food than fruits and vegetables; many individuals with this disorder describe their eating as "out of control." Patients compensate for the binge eating by using purging techniques such as vomiting, laxatives, diuretics, or excessive exercise. Individuals with bulimia are humiliated by both their problem and their lack of control.

People with anorexia differ from those with bulimia in one important characteristic—they are successful at losing weight. Unfortunately, they are so effective at losing weight that they jeopardize their health and even their lives. They may even binge, albeit on smaller quantities of food. These individuals diet by exerting extraordinary control over their eating. The typical anorexic has decreased body weight based on age and height, demonstrates an intense fear of obesity even though the person is underweight, and females may experience amenorrhea (the absence of menstruation).

Impulse Control Disorders

Individuals who have impulse control disorders lack the ability to resist a temptation or can't avoid acting on a drive. Examples of impulse control disorders include intermittent explosive disorder (acting on aggressive impulses involving the destruction of property), kleptomania (acting on the urge to steal things), pyromania (acting on the urge to set fires), and pathological gambling.

Of course, not every arsonist is a pyromaniac, nor is everyone who steals a kleptomaniac. Impulse control disorders are typically associated with other disorders, such as depression, antisocial or borderline personality disorders, and Alzheimer's disease. Treatment relies on cognitive and behavioural interventions to identify underlying triggers and influences. This group of disorders is rare; only 4% of arsonists are diagnosed with pyromania, for example.

Substance-Related Disorders

Substance-related disorders include psychological disorders associated with the use of alcohol, cigarettes, illicit drugs, and other substances that change the way a person feels, behaves, or thinks. These disorders have been known for thousands of years and now cost thousands of lives and billions of dollars annually. It was not until 1980 that substance-related disorders were recognized as a complex biological and psychological problem rather than a sign of moral weakness, however.

Substance-related disorders are regarded on four levels. In substance use, a person may use moderate amounts of a substance without seriously affecting ADLs (eg, a social drinker). Substance intoxication describes use that results in impaired thinking and motor function (eg, a drunk driver). Substance abuse occurs when the use of a substance disrupts ADLs (eg, a person has difficulty with work, school, or relationships). Substance dependence describes a physical or psychological requirement for a substance so strong that it becomes necessary to have the substance to function normally. The person who is physiologically dependent often requires increasingly larger amounts to produce the same effect. An addict may display "drug-seeking behaviours" such as the repeated use of the substance or taking desperate measures to ingest more of the substance (stealing money, standing out in the cold for a smoke).

Determining the most effective treatment for substance-related disorders requires an integrative approach of examining the social, biological, cultural, cognitive, and psychological dimensions of the problem. As a paramedic, it will be difficult to explore these areas during a short transport to the hospital, particularly given that much of your time will be devoted to ensuring the safety of your crew and the patient's ABCs. Understanding the complex nature of substance-related disorders is the first step in providing professional, competent, and compassionate care to the homeless drug addict as well as the substance-dependent businessperson.

Psychosis

Psychosis is a state of delusion in which the individual is out of touch with reality. Affected people are tuned into their own internal reality of ideas and feelings, which they mistake for the reality of the external world. To the person experiencing a psychotic episode, the line differentiating reality from fantasy is blurred—not distinct, as it is in those without psychoses. That internal reality may make patients belligerent and angry toward others. Alternatively, they may become mute and withdrawn as they give all their attention to the voices and feelings within.

Psychoses or psychotic episodes occur for many reasons; the use of mind-altering substances is one of the most common causes, and that experience may be limited to the duration of the substance within the body. Other causes include intense stress, delusional disorders, and, more commonly, schizophrenia. Some psychotic episodes last for brief periods; others last a lifetime.

Schizophrenia

Schizophrenia is a complex disorder that is neither easily defined nor readily treated, yet has a dramatic effect on society. One in 100 people will be affected by schizophrenia in their lifetimes. An estimated 0.2% to 1.5% of the world's population has schizophrenia. The typical onset occurs during early adulthood, with dysfunctional symptoms becoming more prominent over time. Some individuals diagnosed with schizophrenia display signs during early childhood; their disease may be associated with brain damage suffered early in life. Other influences thought to contribute to this disorder include genetics, neurobiological influences, and psychological and social influences.

Persons with schizophrenia may experience positive, negative, or disorganized symptoms. Positive symptoms include delusions and hallucinations. Negative symptoms (a lack of normal behaviour) include apathy, mutism, a flat affect, and a lack of interest in pleasure. Disorganized symptoms include erratic speech, emotional responses, and motor behaviour.

Schizophrenia can be divided into several subclasses. The paranoid type is characterized by delusions or hallucinations usually centred on a specific theme, while cognitive functions remain intact. Individuals with the disorganized type of schizophrenia usually display the wrong emotion for a particular situation and have disorganized speech behaviour. Patients with the catatonic type display odd motor activity, such as strange expressions in their face or remaining rigid, while the undifferentiated type features behaviours that don't fit neatly into another category.

Medications for Psychosis

Antipsychotic drugs are separated into two groups: atypical antipsychotic (AAP) agents and typical (traditional) antipsychotic agents (also known as neuroleptics). Both classes are prescribed to control psychotic symptoms, no matter what their cause. Antipsychotic medications are listed in (Table 37-8 ▸).

Patients taking typical antipsychotic agents may occasionally experience an acute dystonic reaction, in which the individual develops muscle spasms of the neck, face, and back within a few days of starting treatment with the drug. An acute dystonic reaction can be rapidly corrected by giving diphenhydramine (Benadryl), 25 to 50 mg IV, but the muscle spasms are apt to recur after the diphenhydramine wears off. Neuroleptics also have atropine-like effects (anticholinergic effects), so patients taking antipsychotic medications may suffer the side effects associated with atropine use, such as dry mouth, blurred vision, urinary retention, and cardiac dysrhythmias.

The AAP agents are often used as first-line therapy because they not only relieve symptoms such as delusions and

Table 37-8	Antipsychotic Medications	
Type	**Generic Name**	**Trade Name**
Atypical antipsychotic (AAP) agents	Clozapine	Clozaril
	Olanzapine	Zyprexa
	Quetiapine	Seroquel
	Risperidone	Risperidal
Traditional antipsychotics	Chlorpromazine Hydrochloride	Chlorpromazine
	Fluphenazine	Modecate
	Haloperidol	Haldol
	Loxapine	Loxitane, Daxolin
	Perphenazine	Trilafon
	Thioridazine	Thioridazine
	Thiothixene	Navane

hallucinations but also enhance the quality of life for schizophrenics by improving the affective symptoms of anxiety and depression and decreasing suicidal tendencies. However, the AAP medications may cause metabolic side effects such as glucose deregulation, hypercholesterolemia, and hypertension.

The Mental Status Examination of the Psychotic Patient

The most characteristic feature of psychosis is a profound thought disorder, often accompanied by disturbances in mood and perception. The following list outlines disturbances of mood and perception.

- **Consciousness.** The psychotic is awake and alert, but may be easily distracted, especially if paying attention to hallucinations. If the level of consciousness is fluctuating, suspect an organic brain syndrome.
- **Orientation.** Disturbances in orientation are more common in organic disorders than in psychoses, but the severely psychotic patient may be disoriented as to time and place.
- **Activity.** Activity is most commonly accelerated, with agitation and hyperactivity, but can be retarded. Bizarre, stereotyped movements are common.
- **Speech.** Speech may be pressured or sound strange because of unusual words that the patient has invented (neologisms).
- **Thought.** Thought is disturbed in progression and content and may show any of the following disorders:
  - Flight of ideas, the headlong plunge from one thought to another.
  - Loosening of associations, in which the logical connection between one idea and the next becomes obscure, at least to the listener. In extreme cases, the patient's speech may be entirely incomprehensible.
  - Delusions, especially of persecution.
  - Thought broadcasting (the belief that thoughts are broadcast aloud and can be heard by others.)
  - Ideas of reference (the belief that external forms of communication such as television, radio, and newspapers are directed specifically at the individual).

- Thought insertion (the belief that thoughts are being thrust into his or her mind by another person) and thought withdrawal (the belief that thoughts are being removed).

- **Memory.** Memory can be relatively or entirely intact in psychosis. It may be difficult to obtain the cooperation of the patient for formal memory testing.

- **Affect and mood.** Mood is likely to be disturbed in psychosis. The disturbance may take the form of euphoria, sadness, or wide swings in mood; affect may reflect those inner states or be flat. Patients may have an inappropriate affect where they are happy when others would be sad (ie, laughing at a loved one's death) or sad when others would be happy (ie, feeling depressed at winning the lottery).

- **Perception.** Auditory hallucinations are common in psychosis. Patients hear voices commenting on their behaviour or telling them what to do. Suspect that patients are hearing such voices when they seem to be attending a conversation other than yours or talking to themselves.

Management of the Patient With Psychotic Symptoms

Dealing with a psychotic patient is difficult. The usual methods of reasoning with a patient are unlikely to be effective, because the psychotic person has his or her own rules of logic that may be quite different from those that govern nonpsychotic thinking. Furthermore, the paramedic is likely to feel uncomfortable in the presence of a psychotic person. Those uncomfortable feelings are one of your built-in diagnostic instruments. They are elicited by the fear, suspicion, and hostility that the patient is broadcasting through body language. Use your uncomfortable feelings to help make a tentative diagnosis of a psychotic problem. Then proceed as follows:

Notes from Nancy

Warning! The patient who hears voices commanding him to hurt himself or others must be considered dangerous.

- *Assess the situation for danger* to yourself or others.
- *Identify yourself clearly*, and explain your mission. ("I'm Gloria Goodheart. I'm a paramedic with the ambulance service, and this is my partner, Stan Steadfast. We've come to see if we can help. Can you tell us about your problem?")
- *Be calm, direct, and straightforward.* Your calmness and confidence can do a great deal toward calming the patient.
- *Maintain an emotional distance.* Don't touch the patient, and don't be overly friendly or effusively reassuring. Convey an attitude of emotional neutrality.
- *Don't argue.* Don't challenge patients regarding the reality of their beliefs or the validity of their perceptions. Don't go along with their delusions simply to humour them, but don't make an issue of the delusions either. Talk about real things.

- *Explain your expectations of the patient.* ("We're not going to let you hurt anyone with that baseball bat. . . .")
- *Explain each step of management.* ("Let's walk downstairs to the ambulance.")
- *Involve people the patient trusts*, such as family or friends, in managing the patient and gaining cooperation.

Special Considerations

Pediatric Behavioural Problems

Behavioural disorders are estimated to affect as many as one in five children and adolescents, with two thirds of those having a mental health problem not receiving proper treatment. When not treated properly, such a problem will most likely persist into adulthood. Given that suicide is the third leading cause of death in adolescents and the seventh leading cause of death in school-aged children, more attention has been given to mood disorders, anxiety, and other behavioural problems in this population. Children are also more likely to have coexisting problems (eg, attention deficit hyperactivity disorder, conduct disorder, and oppositional defiant disorder) along with the more traditional mental health disorders.

Mental health problems in children are difficult to diagnose because the lines between normal and abnormal behaviour are less clear in this population. Diagnosis and treatment may be difficult when trying to distinguish between organic, genetic, and environmental causes. Cultural and ethnic factors also blur the line between normal and abnormal coping mechanisms. The mental status assessment of the child is similar to that of an adult, but takes the child's developmental level into consideration. Abnormal findings in the developmental and MSE are often related to adjustment disorders and stress rather than the more serious disorders. Your assessment must include an assessment of suicide risk in any child **Figure 37-9 ▶** .

Geriatric Behavioural Problems

As people age, they are exposed to new experiences and alterations to routines that may have become well established over the course of many years. Some of these experiences may result in physical and psychological changes in the older adult. For example, dementia, a gradual loss of mental capabilities, may result from Alzheimer's disease, chronic alcohol abuse, aftereffects of multiple strokes, or nutritional deficiencies. The loss of loved ones or family moving away may cause loneliness. Financial worries, dissatisfaction with living arrangements, or doubts about the significance of one's life accomplishments may become a significant concern as well. These issues often produce psychological distress and physical pain, which may manifest as abnormal behaviour. Anxiety disorders, substance abuse disorders (particularly alcohol abuse), and mood disorders such as depression and even suicide are common among older people.

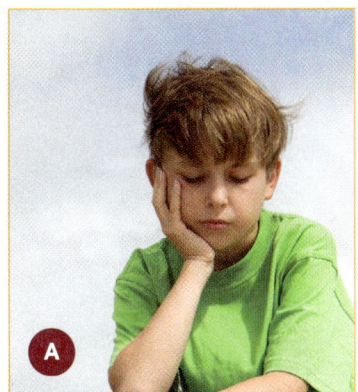

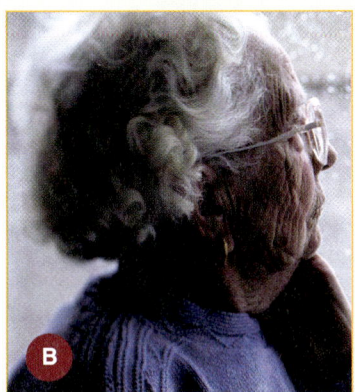

Figure 37-9 Children as well as older adults are affected by behavioural problems.

An elderly person is less likely to be accurately diagnosed with a mental illness than a similarly affected younger person. All too often, anxiety and depression are incorrectly considered a normal part of aging. Agism is discrimination against older people because of their age. To avoid engaging in agism and to provide proper care for the geriatric population, particularly those with mental health issues, you must first take stock of your own attitudes toward older people and the mentally ill. With this awareness, you will be able to perform a complete physical and psychosocial assessment without bias, and will understand the complex issues surrounding the care of older people.

Hostile and Violent Patients

Few situations are as difficult for the paramedic as dealing with a hostile, angry patient. It takes a great deal of maturity and a lot of experience to understand that anger may be a response to illness and aggressive behaviour may be the patient's way of dealing with feelings of helplessness. Sometimes the patient seems to be implying, "There's something very wrong with me, and you're not doing everything possible to help." The temptation is to respond with anger, but doing so rarely serves any useful purpose. Most angry patients can be calmed by a trained person who conveys an impression of confidence that the patient will behave well. It may be helpful to ask the patient directly about his or her anger: "Can you explain why you're so angry with me?" Giving the patient a chance to talk about these feelings often enables the patient to gain mastery over those feelings.

A patient who is violent or threatening violence poses one of the most difficult management problems for paramedics. Most paramedics see themselves as caregivers, not as "heavies," and often find themselves unprepared—both psychologically and tactically—to deal with hostile or violent behaviour. Furthermore, the encounter with a violent patient carries the constant risk that someone may get hurt—the patient, a

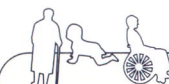

Special Considerations

Many law enforcement agencies use TASER® devices **Figure 37-10 ▶** to immobilize people who are behaving in a violent or aggressive manner. TASER® devices were designed as an alternative to more violent immobilization methods. There is some controversy in the use of these weapons in the in-custody death phenomenon. There is data supporting the assertion that these weapons are temporally, but not causally related to these deaths in custody. EMS personnel need to be aware that many of the patients subjected to a TASER® exposure are at high risk for medical problems due to the underlying condition which is affecting their behaviour. It is important for EMS personnel to identify these underlying conditions and to ensure appropriate medical care. Police officers are not routinely trained to recognize these conditions, and will rely on EMS personnel to make appropriate medical decisions at the scene.

bystander, the paramedics, or all of them. The best way to ensure that no one is harmed is to take preventive action—that is, to assess the potential for violence in *every* call and to take steps to prevent violence from happening.

Assessing the potential for violence is not merely an academic exercise. Canadian data is lacking, however, a 1993 survey of EMS agencies in 25 US cities reported high rates of violence against on-duty paramedics. In Chicago, for example, 92% of the fire department paramedics reported that they had been assaulted at least once while on duty (68% sustained blunt trauma, 33% were cut or stabbed, and 64% were shot at). The paramedic who does *not* look out for a possible violent encounter may become a statistic like those just cited.

Identifying Situations With the Potential for Violence

Preventive action starts with being psychologically prepared for a possible violent encounter and keeping that possibility somewhere in the back of your mind in your response to *every* call. Don't rely too heavily on the information you get from your dispatcher—the "old woman with a possible stroke" may have a disgruntled son with an M-16 rifle! Being psychologically prepared for violence does *not* mean becoming paranoid or treating every patient with distrust. It *does* mean developing a "nose for danger," also known as "survival awareness."

Risk Factors for Violence

Scenarios in which violence is more likely to occur include any situation where alcohol or illicit drugs are being consumed (eg, tavern, party), crowd incidents, and incidents in which violence has already occurred (eg, shooting, stabbing, domestic

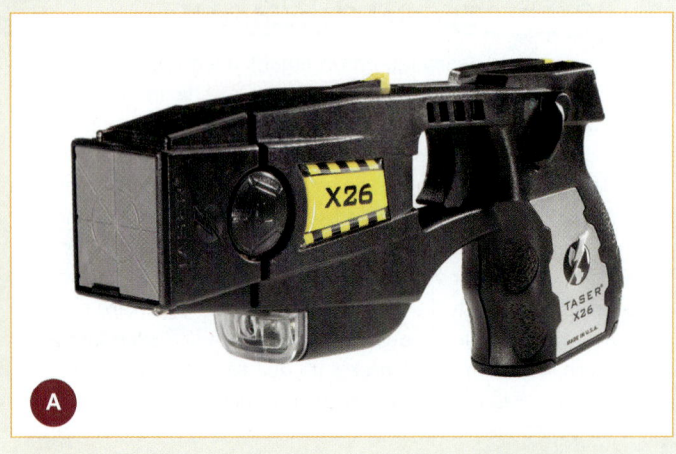 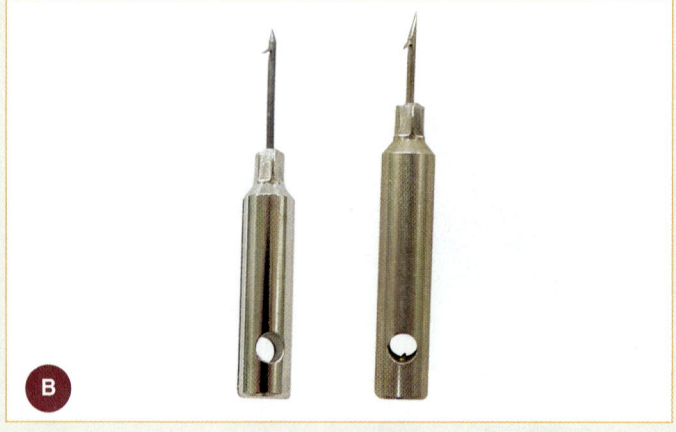

Figure 37-10 **A.** TASER® Electronic Control Device. **B.** TASER® probes.

disturbances). People who are more likely to be violent include those who are intoxicated with alcohol or drugs (especially PCP, LSD, amphetamines, and cocaine), experiencing withdrawal from alcohol or drugs, psychotic (especially manic and paranoid types), or delirious from any cause (eg, hypoglycemia, sepsis).

The most important clues to the patient's potential for violence are found in the individual's behaviour and body language. Look for these warning signals:

- **Posture**—the patient who sits tensely at the edge of the chair or grips at the armrest.
- **Speech**—loud, critical, threatening, full of profanity.
- **Motor activity**—unable to sit still; pacing back and forth or in circles; easily startled.
- **Other body language**—clenched fists, avoidance of eye contact, turning away when spoken to.
- **Your own feelings**—your own "gut" response to the patient. If your instinct tells you that you're in danger, pay attention!

Management of the Violent Patient

Once you have concluded, for *any* reason, that there is a potential for violence in a situation, take the following steps.

Call for back-up. This includes police attendance, if indicated, as well as other personnel who may be needed if a show of force or physical restraint is required.

Assess the situation. Are factors in the surroundings contributing to the escalation of violence (eg, friends who are egging the patient on)? Can those factors be removed? Does evidence suggest drug use, alcohol use, head injury, or diabetes? Can anyone present give you some background information? (Did the patient's behaviour come on gradually or suddenly? Does he or she have a history of violent behaviour? Are there any known medical problems, such as diabetes?)

Observe your surroundings. Make sure you have an escape route. Place yourself between the patient and the door, but

don't move behind an agitated patient. Don't turn your back on the patient—not even for a moment. Note any furniture or other potential barriers. Scan the area for anything that could be used as a weapon (eg, heavy or sharp objects) if the level of violence escalates. If a violent patient is armed with a weapon, don't try to deal with the situation yourself; back off and notify law enforcement authorities. Make sure that others at the scene are not endangered while you await the arrival of the police.

Maintain a safe distance. Moving too close to a potentially violent patient is likely to increase his or her anxiety level. Maintain a safety zone of two arm lengths; if the patient is backing away from you, it's a sign that you're too close. Let the patient find a comfortable distance. Don't position yourself directly face-to-face with the patient but rather slightly to the side at a 45° angle, with your escape route unobstructed.

Try verbal restraints first. Anger and aggressive behaviour are often responses to illness or to feelings of helplessness. Just talking to the angry person in a calm, sympathetic way may defuse some of the anger.

- Take a moment to concentrate your own thoughts so that you can convey an impression of calmness and self-control to the patient.
- Identify yourselves as medical personnel who are there to try to help. Keep your voice low—that forces the patient to stop what he or she is doing to focus on what you are saying.
- Acknowledge the patient's behaviour, and restate your willingness to help. ("You look very upset. How can we help you?").
- Encourage the patient to talk about what is bothering him or her. *Listen* to what is said, and *show* that you are listening by paraphrasing the words back to the patient. ("I think I understand. Are you saying that . . .?")
- Ask the patient specifically if he or she might lose control or is carrying any sort of weapon.
- Define your expectations of the patient's behaviour. Acknowledge his or her potential to do harm ("You could

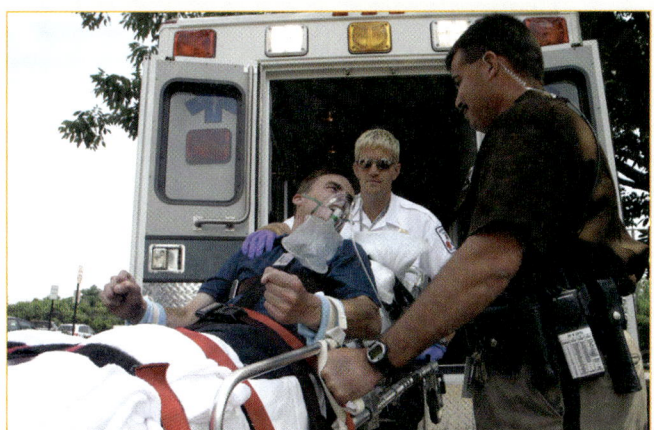

Figure 37-11 You may use physical restraints only to protect yourself or others or to prevent a patient from causing injury to himself or herself.

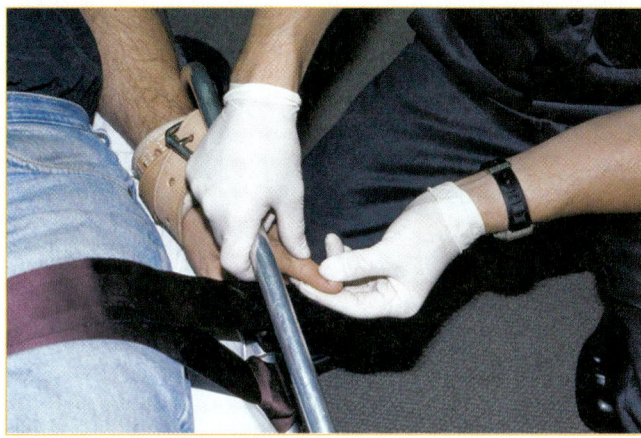

Figure 37-12 Assess circulation frequently while a patient is restrained.

really hurt someone with that crowbar . . ."), but assure the patient that losing control won't be permitted.

- If "verbal de-escalation" isn't working, back off and get help. ("Look, I've been trying to talk to you for the past 15 minutes and we're just going in circles. I'm going to leave you alone for a few minutes and see if you can get hold of yourself. When I come back, we'll try talking again, but if that still doesn't work, I'm going to have some people with me to keep you from hurting anyone.")

When verbal restraint fails, use physical restraint **Figure 37-11 ▲** . Some restraint devices may be improvised from materials on the ambulance; others are commercially made from leather or nylon that is padded for comfort and safety. Most commercial restraints are applied to the wrists and ankles to prevent movement of the arms and legs. Some are placed around the waist to restrict movement of the torso. Vest-type restraints are applied from the front of the patient and may include sleeves to restrain the arms from moving. Make sure you are familiar with the restraints used by your agency before you enter a situation requiring their application.

Make sure you have sufficient personnel before you attempt to overpower the patient. You will need police assistance. You must have overwhelming force to apply a physical restraint, which means a *minimum* of five trained, able-bodied people— one for each limb (assign a specific limb in advance to each responder) and one for the head. Appoint one leader, who will direct the team and maintain verbal contact with the patient.

Sometimes the show of force may be enough to calm the patient. The mere sight of five police officers, for example, has been known to have a remarkably tranquilizing effect on even the most belligerent patient. Don't move toward the patient immediately; give him or her a chance to make a graceful retreat to a nonviolent alternative behaviour.

If the show of force doesn't calm the patient down (eg, someone under the influence of drugs such as PCP), you must move quickly to restrain the patient. First, remove any equipment or jewelry from your own person that could be used as a weapon (eg, name badge, scissors worn on the belt, key chain, earrings). Make sure you have adequate restraining devices— preferably padded leather or nylon restraints—immediately available. Then, at a signal from the leader, move in *fast* from the patient's sides. Grasp the patient at the elbows, knees, and head, and apply restraints to all four extremities. The best position in which to secure the patient to the stretcher is supine, with legs spread-eagled and both arms secured to one side of the stretcher. This position will turn the patient's head to the side, so that he or she won't aspirate in case of vomiting. Never "hog tie" a patient (tying the ankles and wrists together as one); this type of restraint has been known to result in death. Never "hobble tie" a patient (tying just the feet together). Placing a patient face down on a stretcher can also be dangerous and lead to positional asphyxia or aspiration.

Throughout the entire restraint procedure and transport, the leader should maintain verbal contact with the patient, even if the patient does not appear to be paying attention to what you're saying. When only the leader speaks, the patient can focus on what the leader is saying. This will decrease the amount of stimuli experienced by the patient. Avoid being bitten by the patient during the restraining procedure. Once the restraints are in place, don't remove them. Don't negotiate or make deals. If the patient is spitting, you can place an oxygen mask over the face with a normal flow rate.

The patient's clinical condition and vital signs should be reassessed frequently. Additionally, check the patient's peripheral circulation every few minutes to make sure the restraints aren't too tight **Figure 37-12 ▲** . Check the radial pulses in the arms and the dorsalis pedis pulses in the feet.

Document everything in the patient's chart—the reasons for using restraints (be specific, giving examples of the patient's behaviour and the indications of the violence potential); the number of people used to subdue the patient; the restraining devices used; any injuries to the patient or staff that occur during the restraining process; and the patient's clinical status including of the peripheral circulation after restraints were applied.

Proper restraint is summarized in the following steps, shown in **Skill Drill 37-1 ▸**:

1. Assemble five rescuers and have the stretcher or carrying device and soft restraints (wide cloth or commercial leather restraints) nearby **Step 1**.

2. Designate a leader who will communicate with both the team and the patient.

3. Assign positions to each team member: four extremities and the head **Step 2**.

4. If possible, corner the patient in a safe area with the least obstruction and no glass **Step 3**.

5. On the direction of the team leader, who will be talking to the patient calmly, move together toward the patient **Step 4**.

6. Each team member should grasp the assigned body part and carefully, with the least amount of force, bring the patient to the ground **Step 5**.

Controversies

Physical restraint is not without complications and hazards. One alternative is to use chemical restraints, this option should be used only with direct medical control approval or by following local protocols. Until recently, benzodiazepines, droperidol, and haloperidol were the only medications available for chemical restraint in the prehospital arena. The Food and Drug Administration (in the United States) has issued a black box warning for droperidol due to its association with prolonged QT syndromes. Benzodiazepines and haloperidol carry their own risks. Newer atypical antipsychotic (AAP) agents hold promise for preventing injuries to patients and paramedics.

7. Carefully place the patient on the stretcher or carrying device in a face-up position **Step 6**.

8. Tie the patient with soft restraints at each wrist and ankle as well as over the chest and pelvis with sheets **Step 7**. If the patient is spitting, place an oxygen mask on his or her face.

Skill Drill 37-1: Restraining a Patient

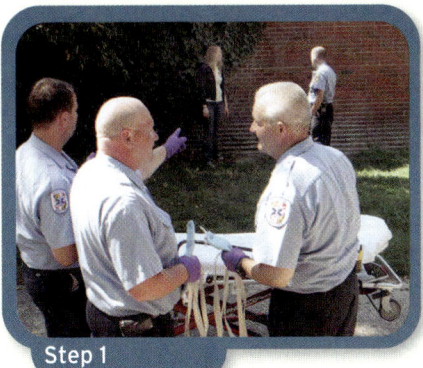

Step 1

Assemble five rescuers and have the stretcher or carrying device and soft restraints nearby. Designate a leader.

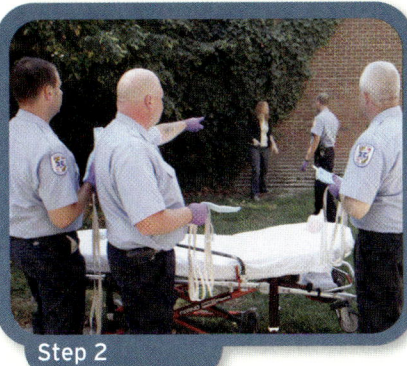

Step 2

Assign positions to each team member: four extremities and the head.

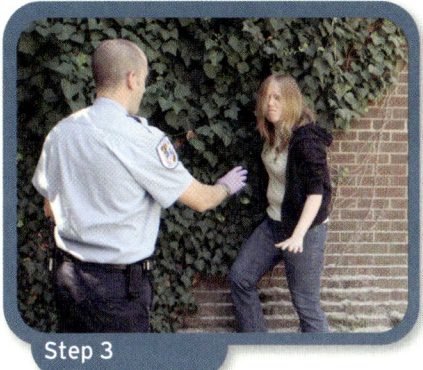

Step 3

If possible, corner the patient in a safe area.

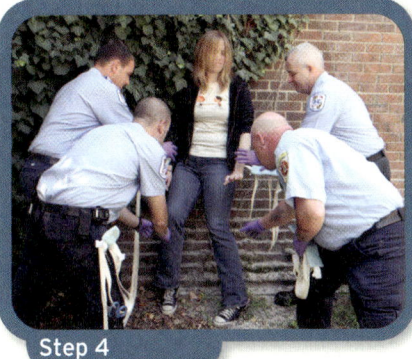

Step 4

On the direction of the team leader, move together toward the patient.

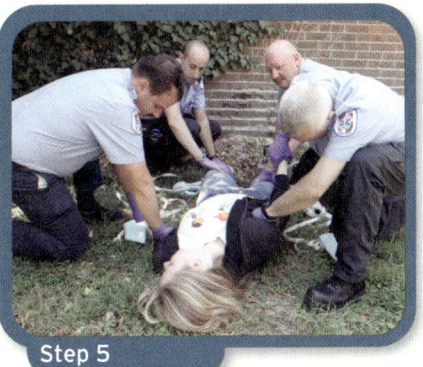

Step 5

Each team member should grasp the assigned body part and carefully, with the least amount of force, bring the patient to the ground.

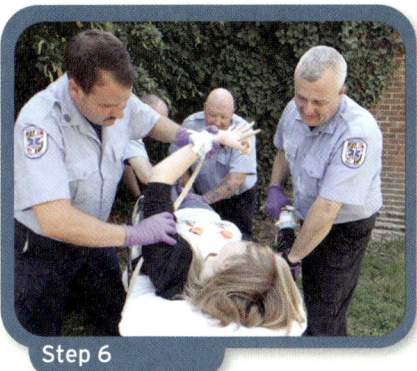

Step 6

Carefully place the patient on the stretcher or carrying device in a face-up position.

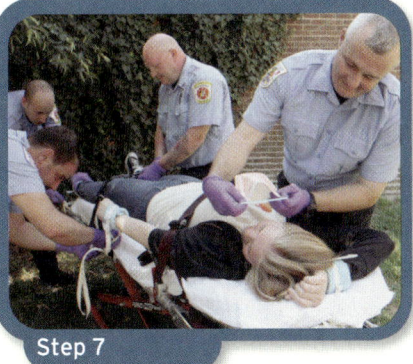

Step 7

Tie the patient with soft restraints at each wrist and ankle as well as the chest and pelvis with sheets. If the patient is spitting, place an oxygen mask on his or her face.

You are the Paramedic Summary

1. What are some medical conditions that can give the appearance of "acting crazy"?

Abnormal behaviour may have many medical causes. It is very important to look at all of the possible reasons that could result in combative and aggressive behaviour. Hypoxia and hypoglycemia are two of the most common underlying medical conditions that can manifest themselves in ways similar to this patient's behaviour.

2. What are some considerations to discuss with your partner while you stage the scene?

Every situation has a potential for danger. Situations you have been asked to stage in which the police are on scene are even more likely to have problems. Good mental preparation and careful observation of the scene are your best defences against harm. Follow the lead of the police, but realize that even they are caught off guard at times.

3. What are the medical implications when police control the scene of a violent patient?

When the police are present, they control the scene. Medical responders should follow their direction on when and how to approach. Police officers are not responsible for medical care unless protocol dictates that they are and they are appropriately trained. The most important rule is for everyone to work together to ensure the safety of the responders and safeguard the best interest of the patient.

4. Is it wise to agree with or validate a patient's hallucinations?

If the patient asks you what a dog is saying, truthfully and neutrally answer that you don't hear it. This response does not deny the patient's own experience, but does inform the patient that others are not having the same experience.

5. How important is police involvement if the patient apparently becomes agreeable?

A patient's attitude and general demeanor can change in a flash. You must always consider this potential for change, especially if you will be providing patient care while alone in the back of the ambulance. Ask for escorts, including an officer in the back if you feel it's appropriate. When the patient is restrained, perform frequent reassessments of vital signs and clinical condition. Additionally, check the extremities every 5 minutes to ensure that circulation and neurologic function are not compromised.

6. What are the risk factors for suicide, and do they apply in this situation?

This man is in danger of losing his job, he has an altered perception of reality, he is recently divorced, and he may be under the influence of drugs. He has several risk factors for suicide even if he doesn't express the intent.

7. Would you talk with Eugene about his comment or wait and let the hospital explore these issues?

Every statement regarding suicide must be taken seriously, even if it's made impulsively or casually. You must determine the patient's seriousness by asking whether he or she has plans or has made preparations. The patient's responses may affect your immediate safety.

8. How can your professionalism and general demeanor affect patient care in scenarios such as these?

Talking with the patient is therapeutic. Take the time to build trust and rapport. Let the patient tell the story in his or her own way. Listen. Don't argue or dispute the nature of reality.

9. What would you tell the hospital in your radio report to help personnel there prepare for the patient?

Hospital personnel need to know the basics of the patient's thinking and state of mind. They also need to know if and why the patient is restrained. If a patient is out of control, the hospital may want additional security or chemical restraints immediately available. Don't bring behavioural emergency patients into the emergency department unannounced.

Prep Kit

Ready for Review

- Behaviour includes the things we do—how we act or react to situations.
- Behaviour may be abnormal as defined by society, your boss, a parent, or friend. Abnormal behaviour by itself may not be an emergency.
- In a behavioural disorder, the individual's presenting problem is a disorder of thought, mood, or behaviour that interferes with the activities of daily living.
- The behavioural disorder becomes a psychiatric emergency when the patient becomes suicidal, homicidal, or acutely psychotic.
- Abnormal behaviour can stem from a situational crisis, organic problems, or psychiatric causes.
- When assessing psychiatric problems, you collect information about the person's state of mind and thinking. Your actions and attitude often provide some of the therapy sought by the patient. Be prepared to spend some time with the patient as you assess his or her thinking.
- Dissociative disorders are characterized by depersonalization (stepping out of one's current experience) and derealization (an altered perception of objects or people in an experience). In the most severe form of dissociative disorders, multiple personalities may emerge.
- The mind generates specific signs and symptoms when it is not functioning well. Paramedics must sharpen their assessment skills to properly identify how the patient is functioning mentally. The COASTMAP mnemonic can be used to remember various disorders of behaviour.
- In anxiety disorders, the dominant mood is fear and apprehension. Fear can turn into a phobia when it becomes unreasonable. Anxiety, when sudden and overwhelming, may become a panic disorder. Anxiety, phobias, and panic disorder may complicate your efforts to treat a person.
- Mood disorders are the most common psychiatric disorders. In mania, the patient often feels great to the point of exaggeration, with hyperactivity, insomnia, and grandiose ideas. Feelings of depression can be accompanied by guilt, apathy, and sleep disturbances. Depression may become so severe that the person may attempt suicide.
- Suicide and attempted suicide are problems affecting all age groups and people of all socioeconomic status. Men are often more successful at suicide because they use more lethal means, although women make more attempts. Every suicidal gesture must be assessed and taken very seriously. Don't be afraid to talk with patients about their suicidal thoughts.
- Personality disorders are exaggerations in how people think about or perceive their environment and surroundings. They are classified into three categories: odd or eccentric behaviours; dramatic, emotional, or erratic behaviours; and anxious or fearful behaviours.
- In somatoform disorders, such as conversion disorders and hypochondriasis, patients are overly concerned with their physical health or appearance to the point that this concern dominates their lives.
- Eating disorders, such as anorexia nervosa and bulimia nervosa, are disorders of personal control related to eating. They can result in acute and chronic problems.
- Impulse control disorders include impulsive gambling, kleptomania, and pyromania. They reflect the inability to resist temptation.
- Substance-related disorders are associated with the use of alcohol and drugs. A variety of social, biological, cultural, and physiologic dimensions define substance-related disorders.
- Psychosis is a state of delusion in which individuals are out of touch with reality. Causes include psychiatric problems (eg, schizophrenia) and drug-induced psychotic states.
- Individuals with schizophrenia may display positive symptoms (hallucinations and delusions), negative symptoms (apathy and a flat affect), or disorganized symptoms (erratic speech or motor function). Dealing with psychotic patients is difficult because their behaviour may be dangerous.
- Disorganization and disorientation describe how conditions may present themselves. Disorganized patients have uncontrolled and disconnected thoughts. They need structure, explanations, and directions. Disoriented patients may not know where they are, what day it is, or even who they are. These patients need continuous orienting.
- Dealing with hostile, combative, and violent patients can be emotionally and physically demanding for paramedics. Be cautious when approaching these individuals and evaluating situations where violent or potentially violent patients may be. Know the specific risk factors and signs of hostile situations and call for police assistance when indicated.
- Combative patients may need to be restrained. In such cases, make sure you have enough experienced people and work quickly. Follow the legal guidelines for restraining patients.

Vital Vocabulary

activities of daily living (ADLs) Normal everyday activities such as getting dressed, brushing teeth, taking out the garbage, etc.

acute dystonic reaction A syndrome that may occur in patients taking typical antipsychotic agents. The patient develops muscle spasms of the neck, face, and back within a few days of starting treatment with the drug.

affect The outward expression of a person's mood.

agitation Extreme restlessness and anxiety.

agoraphobia Literally, "fear of the marketplace"; fear of entering a public place from which escape may be impeded.

amnesia Loss of memory.

anger A strong, negative emotion that may be a response to illness, and which could result in aggressive behaviour on the part of the patient.

anorexia nervosa An eating disorder in which a person diets by exerting extraordinary control over his or her eating, and loses weight to the point of jeopardizing his or her health and life.

antipsychotic drugs Medications used to control psychosis.

anxiety disorder A mental disorder in which the dominant mood is fear and apprehension.

atropine-like effects Results of some antipsychotic medications that include side effects similar to atropine, resulting in dry mouth, blurred vision, urinary retention, and cardiac dysrhythmias.

behaviour The way people act or perform, for example how they react/respond to a situation.

behavioural disorder A situation in which the patient's presenting problem is some disorder of mood, thought, or behaviour that interferes with their ability to perform activities of daily living (ADLs).

behavioural emergency A situation in which abnormal behaviour threatens an individual's health and safety or the health and safety of another.

bipolar mood disorder A disorder in which a person alternates between mania and depression. The alterations in mood are usually episodic and recurrent.

borderline personality disorder A disorder characterized by disordered images of self, impulsive and unpredictable behaviour, marked shifts in mood, and instability in relationships with others.

bulimia nervosa An eating disorder characterized by consumption of large amounts of food, and for which the patient then sometimes compensates by using purging techniques.

catatonic Lacking expression or movement, or appearing rigid.

catatonic type A type of schizophrenia in which the person displays odd motor activity, such as strange facial expression or rigidity.

circumstantial thinking Situation in which a patient includes many irrelevant details in his or her account of things.

compulsion A repetitive action carried out to relieve the anxiety of obsessive thoughts.

confabulation The invention of experiences to cover gaps in memory, seen in patients with certain organic brain syndromes.

confrontation Interviewing technique in which the interviewer points out to the patient something of interest in his/her conversation or behaviour.

confusion An impaired understanding of one's surroundings.

delirium An acute confessional state characterized by global impairment of thinking, perception, judgment, and memory.

delusion A fixed belief that is not shared by others of a person's culture or background and that can't be changed by reasonable argument; a false belief.

delusions of grandeur A state in which a person believes oneself to be someone of great importance.

delusions of persecution A state in which a person believes that others are plotting against him or her.

dementia Chronic deterioration of mental function.

depersonalization A type of dissociative disorder in which a person loses his or her sense of reality, and may experience events as being "dream-like."

depression A persistent mood of sadness, despair, and discouragement; may be a symptom of many different mental and physical disorders, or it may be a disorder on its own.

derealization A symptom of a dissociative disorder in which objects seem to change size or shape; people may seem dead or behave like robots when viewed during a moment of acute stress.

disorganization A condition in which a person is characterized by uncontrolled and disconnected thought, is usually incoherent or rambling in speech, and may or may not be oriented to person and place.

disorganized symptoms Refers to erratic speech, emotional responses, and motor behaviour.

disorganized type A type of schizophrenia in which the person usually displays the wrong emotion for a particular situation, often self-absorbed.

disorientation Confusion regarding a person's sense of who one is (person), where one is (place), and at what point in time one finds oneself (time), and about the events leading up to where one finds oneself (events).

dissociation Feelings of being detached from yourself, as if you were dreaming.

echolalia Meaningless echoing of the interviewer's words by the patient.

facilitation An interviewing technique in which the interviewer uses noncommittal words and gestures to encourage the patient to proceed.

fear Also sometimes referred to as a phobia, this is an anxious feeling, usually about specific things or situations.

flat Used to describe behaviour in which the patient doesn't seem to feel much of anything at all.

flight of ideas Accelerated thinking in which the mind skips very rapidly from one thought to the next.

generalized anxiety disorder (GAD) A disorder in which a person worries about everything for no particular reason, or their worrying is unproductive and they can't decide what to do about an upcoming situation.

hallucination A sense perception not founded on objective reality; a false perception.

ideas of reference The belief that external forms of communication (television, radio, and newspaper) are directed specifically at the individual.

illusion A misinterpretation of sensory stimuli.

impulse control disorders A condition in which an individual lacks the ability to resist a temptation or can't stop acting on a drive.

labile Used to describe a rapid shift in mood.

loosening of associations A situation in which the logical connection between one idea and the next becomes obscure, at least to the listener.

mania A mental disorder characterized by abnormally exaggerated happiness, joy, or euphoria with hyperactivity, insomnia, and grandiose ideas.

mental status examination (MSE) A way of measuring the "mental vital signs" in a disturbed patient. The mnemonic COASTMAP can be used to conduct this examination, assessing consciousness, orientation, activity, speech, thought, memory, affect and mood, and perception.

mood A person's sustained and pervasive emotional state.

mood disorder A group of disorders in which the disturbance of mood is accompanied by full or partial manic or depressive syndrome.

mutism The absence of speech.

negative symptoms Evidence of a disease or condition, noted by lack of normal circumstances, rather than the presence of new physical evidence or a physical change; with regard to schizophrenia, refers to a lack of normal behaviour, and apathy, mutism, a flat affect, and a lack of interest in pleasure.

neologism An invented word that has meaning only to its inventor.

obsession A persistent idea that a person cannot dismiss from his or her thoughts.

organic brain syndrome Temporary or permanent dysfunction of the brain, caused by a disturbance in the physical or physiologic functioning of brain tissue.

orientation A person's sense of who one is (person), where one is (place), and at what day of the week one finds oneself (day), and an understanding of events leading up to where one finds oneself (events).

paranoid type A type of schizophrenia in which the person experiences delusions or hallucinations usually centred around a specific theme, where their cognitive functions remain intact.

perception The way a person processes the data supplied by the five senses.

perseveration Repeating the same idea over and over again.

personality disorder The term used to describe a condition a person has when he or she behaves or thinks in a way that is dysfunctional or causes distress to other people.

phobia An abnormal and persistent dread of a specific object or situation.

positive symptoms Evidence of or physical change due to a disease or condition, which can be physically noted by the patient or health care provider; with regard to schizophrenia, refers to delusions and hallucinations.

posttraumatic stress disorder (PTSD) A severe form of anxiety that stems from a traumatic experience. PTSD is characterized by the reliving of the stress and nightmares of the original situation.

posture The position of one's body.

pressure of speech Speech in which words seem to tumble out under immense emotional pressure.

psychiatric emergency An emergency in which abnormal behaviour threatens an individual's health and safety or the health and safety of another person, specifically for example when a person becomes suicidal, homicidal, or has a psychotic episode.

psychosis A mental disorder characterized by loss of contact with reality.

psychotropic drugs Drugs that affect mood, thought, or behaviour.

recall The ability to retrieve a specific piece of stored information on demand.

recognition The ability to identify information that one has encountered before.

registration The ability to add new items to the cerebral data bank.

restlessness A situation in which the patient can't sit still.

retardation of thought The patient seems to take a very long time to get from one thought to the next.

retention The ability to store items in an accessible place in the mind.

simple phobia A fear that is focused on one class of objects (eg, mice, spiders, dogs) or situations (eg, high places, darkness, flying).

somatoform disorder A condition in which a person is overly concerned with physical health and appearance to the point that it dominates his or her life; an example is hypochondria.

stereotyped activity Repetitive movements that don't appear to serve any purpose.

substance abuse Use of a substance that disrupts activities of daily living.

substance dependence Use of a substance that results in addiction and physiologic dependence on the substance.

substance intoxication Use of a substance that results in impaired thinking and motor function.

substance use Use of moderate amounts of a substance without seriously affecting activities of daily living.

suicide Any willful act designed to bring an end to one's own life.

tangential thinking Leaving the current topic midconversation to talk about something else, inhibiting interpersonal communication.

thought broadcasting The belief that others can hear one's thoughts.

thought control The belief that outside forces are controlling one's thoughts.

thought insertion The belief that thoughts are being thrust into one's mind by another person.

thought withdrawal The belief that thoughts are being removed from one's mind.

undifferentiated type Schizophrenia that does not fit neatly into another category.

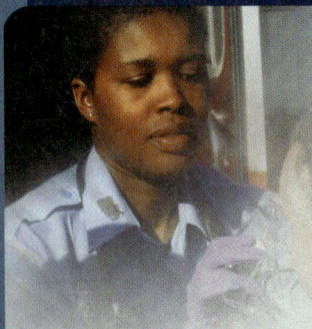

Assessment in Action

Dispatch requests that you respond with the police department to "check the welfare" of an older woman. Dispatch received a call from the woman's niece, who lives in another province. She said her aunt called and told her that her house was being robbed by an "invisible man." This behaviour is not normal for her.

On your arrival, the police department has to use force to gain access to the apartment. You find the patient squatting in the corner. She is belligerent and screaming obscenities to the "invisible robber." You spend some time trying to speak with her, but she isn't cooperative. It is time to transport the patient to hospital, but she refuses to go.

1. **This patient is more than likely having a(n) _____ type of behavioural emergency.**
   A. organic
   B. situational
   C. psychiatric
   D. depressive

2. **What type of psychiatric disorder could this be considered?**
   A. Mood disorder
   B. Eating disorder
   C. Somatoform disorder
   D. Schizophrenic/psychotic disorder

3. **Which of the following statements regarding open-ended questions is not true?**
   A. They can lead patients to give a specific answer.
   B. They give patients an opportunity to express themselves.
   C. They encourage better patient responses.
   D. They are less likely to provoke unwanted answers.

4. **Classifications of psychiatric signs and symptoms include:**
   A. disorders of consciousness.
   B. disorders of motor activity.
   C. disorders of speech.
   D. all of the above.

5. **Delusions of persecution fall under which classification?**
   A. Disorders of thinking
   B. Disorders of orientation
   C. Disorders of perception
   D. Disorders of memory

6. **Disorder of perception refers to a:**
   A. person's sense of who one is, where one is, and what time it is.
   B. person's ability to process the data supplied by the five senses.
   C. person's intellectual ability.
   D. person's sustained and pervasive emotional state.

7. **The patient in the above scenario is having which of the following?**
   A. A hallucination
   B. An illusion
   C. Acute depression
   D. Organic symptoms

8. **When examining a patient's mental status, use the mnemonic:**
   A. SAMPLE.
   B. AMPLE.
   C. MSE.
   D. COASTMAP.

9. **Psychosis is defined as a(n):**
   A. state of delusion and describes individuals who are out of touch with reality.
   B. complex disorder that is neither easily defined nor easily treated, and that dramatically affects today's society.
   C. inability to resist a temptation.
   D. eating disorder.

10. **The best way to deal with a patient having hallucinations is to:**
    A. use physical restraints.
    B. use the talk-down method.
    C. administer antipsychotic medications.
    D. scream at the patient.

Challenging Question

You are dispatched to a private residence for a 96-year-old woman. The patient's daughter found her sitting in a chair, not responding as she would normally. Her daughter initially thought she might have awakened her mother, and her mother was just "a little slow." After approximately 30 minutes, she called 9-1-1. Upon your arrival, you find the patient to be resting comfortably in her chair. She is alert and responsive to her name and address only. She doesn't remember her daughter's name, nor does she know what month or year it is. Her daughter states that she has had a stroke in the past and has a history of high blood pressure. The patient denies any complaints, has no chest pain, and no shortness of breath. During your assessment you find no neurologic deficits, and the patient has equal hand grips, negative facial droop, and negative slurred speech. Her blood glucose level is 6.2 mmol/l. She doesn't remember getting out of bed this morning and doesn't remember going to her chair. She continuously asks you who you are and why you're there.

11. **As the paramedic, what initial differential diagnosis could you make?**

Points to Ponder

Toward the end of your shift, you are dispatched to a private residence for a 24-year-old man having chest pain. When you arrive on scene, you find the young man lying on the ground, complaining of reproducible chest pain and trembling. He appears to be hyperventilating. He does not answer questions, but does follow commands. His vital signs are all within normal limits, except he's breathing approximately 30 times per minute. As you attempt to speak to the patient, his father keeps interrupting, wanting to know whether his son is having a heart attack. The father is upset that you're not transporting right away. While you're attempting to take control of the scene, his sister tells you that the patient was on the phone with his girlfriend and she was breaking up with him. He became very agitated, and then began to breathe "very fast." She called 9-1-1. The patient has a history of anxiety/panic attacks, but this episode was different than in the past.

What are some possibilities for what could be happening with this patient? How can you calm this patient down?

Issues: Empathy for Patients With Behavioural Emergencies, Respectful Approach to Patients and Family Members.

Competency Areas

Area 2: Communication

2.1.d   Provide information to patient about their situation and how they will be treated.

2.1.f   Speak in language appropriate to the listener.

2.1.g   Use appropriate terminology.

2.3.a   Exhibit effective non-verbal behaviour.

2.3.b   Practice active listening techniques.

2.3.c   Establish trust and rapport with patients and colleagues.

2.3.d   Recognize and react appropriately to non-verbal behaviours.

2.4.a   Treat others with respect.

2.4.b   Exhibit empathy and compassion while providing care.

2.4.c   Recognize and react appropriately to individuals and groups manifesting coping mechanisms.

2.4.d   Act in a confident manner.

2.4.e   Act assertively as required.

2.4.f   Manage and provide support to patients, bystanders, and relatives manifesting emotional reactions.

2.4.g   Exhibit diplomacy, tact, and discretion.

2.4.h   Exhibit conflict resolution skills.

Area 4: Assessment and Diagnostics

4.2.a   Obtain list of patient's allergies.

4.2.b   Obtain list of patient's medications.

4.2.c   Obtain chief complaint and/or incident history from patient, family members, and/or bystanders.

4.2.d   Obtain information regarding patient's past medical history.

4.3.a   Conduct primary patient assessment and interpret findings.

4.3.b   Conduct secondary patient assessment and interpret findings.

4.3.h   Conduct genitourinary system assessment and interpret findings.

4.4.a   Assess pulse.

4.4.b   Assess respiration.

4.4.d   Measure blood pressure by auscultation.

4.4.g   Assess skin condition.

4.4.i   Assess level of mentation.

Area 5: Therapeutics

5.5.c   Maintain peripheral intravenous (IV) access devices and infusions of crystalloid solutions without additives.

5.5.d   Conduct peripheral intravenous cannulation.

Area 6: Integration

6.1.d   Provide care to patient experiencing illness or injury primarily involving genitourinary/reproductive systems.

6.1.k   Provide care to patient experiencing illness or injury due to poisoning or overdose.

6.3.a   Conduct ongoing assessments based on patient presentation and interpret findings.

Appendix 4: Pathophysiology

D.   **Female Reproductive System and Neonates**
Pregnancy Complications: Ectopic pregnancy

F.   **Genitourinary System**
Reproductive Disorders: Bleeding/discharge
Reproductive Disorders: Infection
Reproductive Disorders: Ovarian cyst
Renal/Bladder: Obstruction

J.   **Multisystem Diseases and Injuries**
Infectious Diseases: Toxic shock syndrome
Toxicologic Illness: Non-prescription medication
Toxicologic Illness: Recreational
Shock Syndromes: Hypovolemic
Shock S-yndromes: Septic

Appendix 5: Medications

A.   **Medications affecting the central nervous system**

A.8   Opioid Analgesics

Introduction

The *Merriam-Webster Dictionary* defines gynecology as "a branch of medicine that deals with the diseases and routine physical care of the reproductive system of women" and obstetrics as "a branch of medical science that deals with birth and with its antecedents and sequels." Although the medical specialties of obstetrics and gynecology are separate fields of study, the two are so inextricably entwined—as these definitions make clear—that it is virtually impossible to write about one without referencing the other.

Before the 20th century, both fields of study were relegated to the realm of "subjects not discussed in polite society." Despite the work of pioneering doctors dating back as far as 98 AD, most of the knowledge of these two sciences was held by midwives, who jealously guarded the "secrets" of womankind with religious fervour.

One of the earliest medical texts covering obstetrics and gynecology was written by Soranus (98 AD), a Greco-Roman physician. His obstetric textbook, which was used until the 1600s, described podalic version (delivery of the infant feet first), the obstetric chair, and instructions for the newborn: "boiled water and honey for the child for the first two days, then on to the mother's breast." Unfortunately for women, the enlightened science of the Romans did not survive their empire. In 1522, a German physician named Wert masqueraded as a woman to sneak a peek at the mysteries of the birthing room. He was unmasked and burned at the stake for his intellectual curiosity.

Three other physicians of the 1500s fared better than the hapless Dr Wert. Ambrose Pare was a surgeon-barber who apprenticed at the famous Paris Hotel Dieu, the first midwife school in Paris, and was one of the first physicians to record dilating the cervix to induce labour. Thomas Raynalde penned *The Birth of Mankynde* in 1544, which described cesarean section. In 1554, Jacob Rueff published *De Conceptu Generationis Hominis,* which described the whole process of pregnancy.

Despite the advances of these forward-thinking minds, childbirth and female medical conditions remained in the realm of superstition and folk medicine until well into the 1900s. The women's suffrage movement (1848–1920) and the women's liberation movement of the 1960s not only catalyzed progress in equal rights, but also made strides in the scientific study of women's unique medical problems.

It has often been said that human males and females are actually two separate species, which just happen to be able to reproduce. The physiologic, emotional, and mental processes experienced by the two sexes are widely disparate, despite sharing many similarities. The physiologic, chemical, hormonal, and even mental differences between men and women are beyond the scope of this book. The most obvious difference between the two sexes, however, is that women are uniquely designed to conceive and give birth. This difference makes women susceptible to a variety of problems that do not occur in men.

This chapter examines a few of those problems. It first discusses the female anatomy, then outlines issues that are unique to female patients, including problems that may be encountered in the emergency setting. We next consider the gynecologic causes of abdominal pain in women and look in detail at life-threatening conditions. We also briefly examine vaginal bleeding, both traumatic and organic, and discuss how it should be managed in the prehospital environment. Finally, we consider the principles of managing a woman who has been the victim of sexual assault.

Female Anatomy

The female external genitalia, collectively called the pudendum or the vulvar area, are the structures seen from the outside of the body, including the labia, clitoris, urethral, and vaginal openings

You are the Paramedic Part 1

You are dispatched to a private residence for a 40-year-old woman with abdominal pain and vaginal bleeding. You arrive to find an apparently healthy middle-aged woman, Maria Medina, lying on her side on the couch with her knees drawn up.

The patient tells you that she has been experiencing spotting for 10 to 15 minutes and is now having abdominal pain and cramping. She is 6 weeks' pregnant, and this is her first pregnancy. She immediately phoned her doctor when the spotting started and was headed out the door to his office when the pain began.

Initial Assessment	Recording Time: 0 Minutes
Appearance	Anxious and tearful
Level of consciousness	A (Alert to person, place, and day)
Airway	Patent; patient is talking
Breathing	Rapid with adequate tidal volume
Circulation	Strong, slightly fast radial pulse

1. Based on your general impression and initial assessment, how would you categorize this patient?
2. What interventions would you choose to initiate at this point?

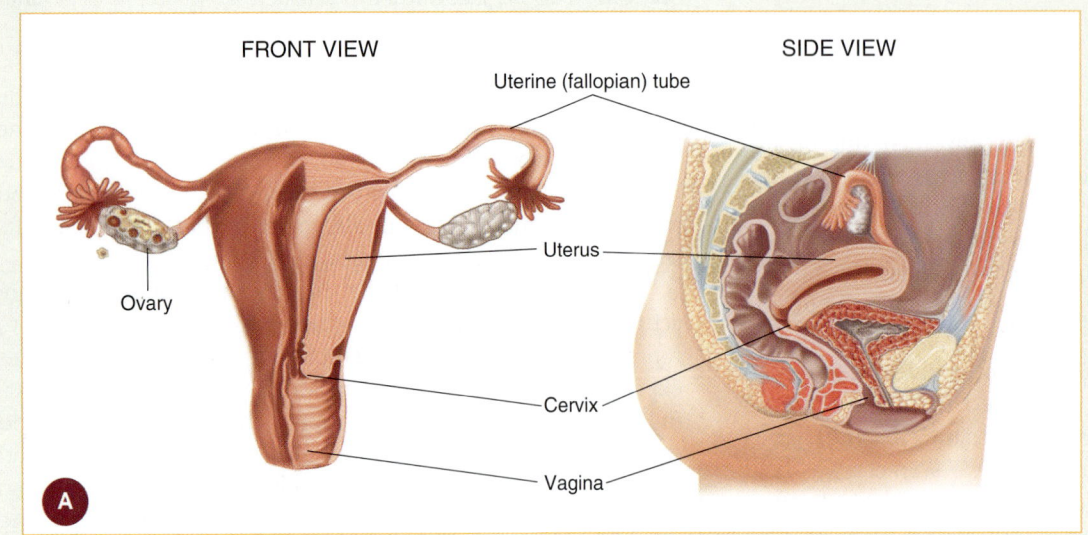

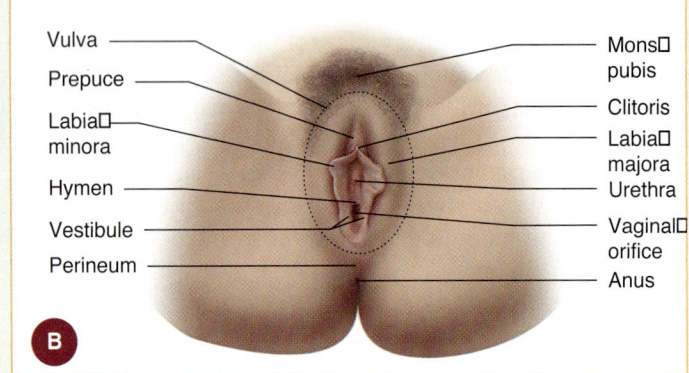

Figure 38-1 The anatomy of the female reproductive system. **A.** Front and side views. **B.** External genitalia.

The vagina, or lower portion of the birth canal, serves as a passage for menstrual flow and as the receptacle of the penis during sexual intercourse. Just inside the lower vagina are two tiny openings that lead to the Bartholin glands. These glands secrete mucus that acts as a lubricant during intercourse. The glands may become blocked by skin or tissue debris, causing cysts to form. This is a common occurrence. Occasionally, the cysts become infected by normal vaginal skin organisms or by sexually transmitted disease organisms, such as gonorrhea, causing abscesses to form.

Before first intercourse, the vaginal orifice is protected by the hymen. This membrane forms a border around the vaginal orifice, partially enclosing it. The hymen may be ruptured before first intercourse by trauma or by such mundane events as horseback riding, gymnastics, or other sports. Pain and vaginal bleeding will generally be present in such an event; because this usually occurs in young women, it may be of concern to the patient and her parents. In some cases, the hymen may completely cover the vaginal orifice, a condition called imperforate hymen. If it remains undetected until puberty, this condition will block the flow of first menses, resulting in relatively acute pain, with severe constipation and low back pain among the presenting symptoms. Such a condition may lead to endometriosis or cause other secondary painful effects as well. Imperforate hymen can also be caused by childhood sexual abuse, in which the imperforation results from scarring from digital or penile penetration.

About an inch below the vaginal opening is the anal opening, which allows for the passage of feces and bowel gases. The area of skin between the vagina and the anus is called the clinical perineum.

Figure 38-1 ▲. The mons veneris (mons pubis) is a rounded pad of fatty (adipose) tissue that overlies the symphysis pubis, located anterior to the urethral and vaginal openings. The mons veneris is not an organ, but rather a "landmark." Coarse, dark hair normally appears over the mons in early puberty, becoming sparser later in life with the advent of menopause. The labia majora and labia minora surround and protect the vaginal opening together with the more anterior opening of the urethra. The labia majora are covered with pubic hair, but the labia minora are devoid of it. The area between the vaginal opening and the anus is called the perineum. The clitoris is located at the anterior junction of the labia minora, just below a layer of skin called the prepuce. The clitoris is a small, cylindrical mass of erectile tissue and nerves that is homologous to the glans penis of the male.

Between the labia minora is a cleft referred to as the vestibule. Located within the vestibule is the urethral opening (orifice), the vaginal opening (orifice), and the hymen. The urethra, which leads to the bladder, allows for passage of urine. The length of the urethra in females averages approximately 3.8 cm. This short length is one reason why women are more prone than men to urinary tract infections and bladder infections.

Menstruation

Of the many emergencies that paramedics are called on to treat, one of the most common calls is bleeding. For gynecologic emergencies, that would translate into "vaginal bleeds." However,

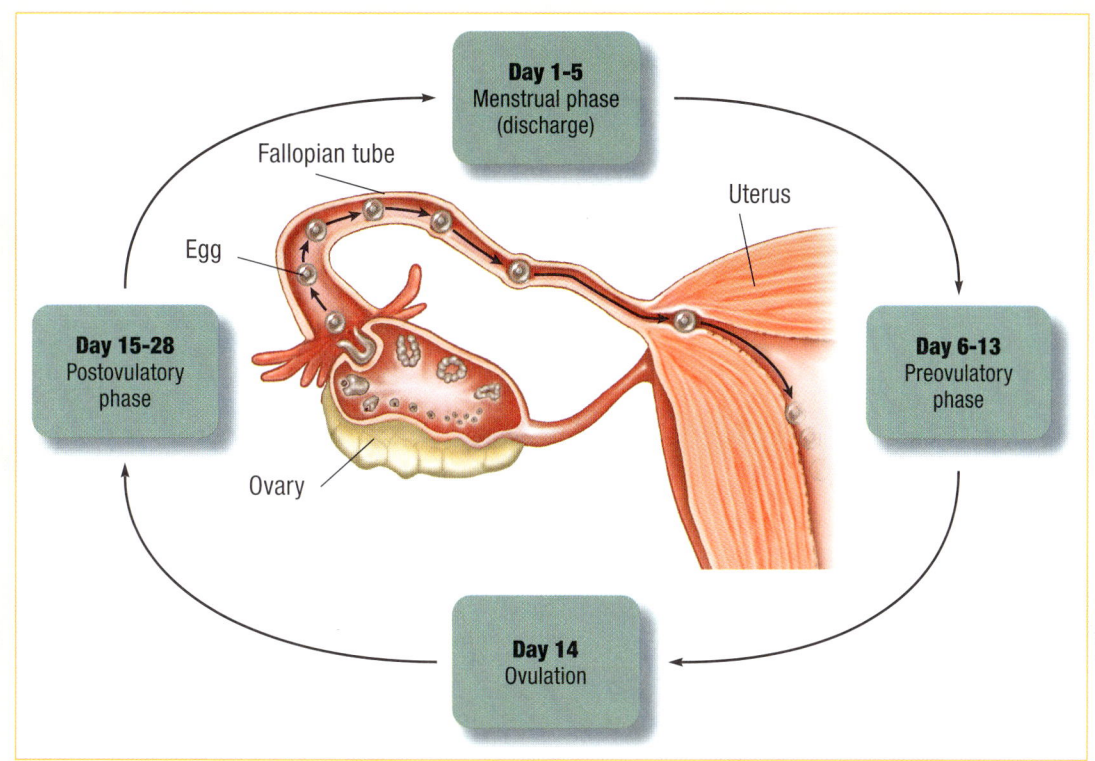

Figure 38-2 The menstrual cycle, based on an average 28-day cycle. The length of the cycle and number of days in each phase vary from woman to woman, but generally fall within a range of 24 to 35 days.

before we embark on the emergency treatment of vaginal bleeding, we must first broach what is "normal" vaginal bleeding.

One way in which women are uniquely different from men is the physiologic phenomenon of menstruation. Also called the menses, period, or menstrual cycle, menstruation is the cyclic and periodic vaginal discharge of 25 to 65 ml of blood, epithelial cells, mucus, and tissue. The duration of the cycle differs from woman to woman, ranging from an average of 24 days to 35 days. Unless told otherwise by the patient, assume the average cycle to be 28 days. Three phases make up the entire menstrual cycle: the menstrual phase (the first phase), the preovulatory phase, and the postovulatory phase. Based on a 28-day cycle, the menstrual (discharge) phase lasts about 5 days. The preovulatory phase lasts from about day 6 to 13, and the postovulatory phase lasts from day 15 to 28 Figure 38-2 ▲.

The onset of first menses, when a female reaches childbearing age, is called menarche. Depending on genetics, socioeconomic factors, and individual health, this event may take place anywhere between the ages of 11 and 14 years. The last menses, when a woman has reached the end of childbearing age, is called menopause. The advent of menopause typically begins between the ages of 40 and 50, with menstrual cycles becoming less frequent. The transitional phase preceding menopause, including the period of life that follows it, is called the climacteric.

Owing to gradually decreasing production of estrogen and other hormones during the climacteric, a woman may experience a range of symptoms due to hormonal imbalance. These symptoms may be as benign as copious diaphoresis, hair loss, and hot flashes (sometimes accompanied by tachycardia) or as ominous as the symptoms seen often in the emergency setting such as severe muscle aches and pains, headache, dyspnea, vertigo, digestive problems, and emotional instability. Postmenopausal women no longer have to deal with the discomfort and irritation of monthly menses, but the decreased hormone production makes them more susceptible to atherosclerosis, osteoporosis, and coronary heart disease. Diminished estrogen may also result in atrophy of genitourinary organs, resulting in vaginal dryness and discomfort. Atrophy of the bladder and urethral mucosa can result in urinary frequency, nocturia, and incontinence.

Menstruation is predominantly related to the discussion of obstetrics, but is also a necessary component of the gynecologic examination. Disorders of the menstrual cycle may be seen in the prehospital setting, actually putting the call for emergency service in motion. Some of these disorders are classified in the following paragraphs.

During the menstrual cycle, a woman experiences several systemic changes as her hormone levels ebb and flow. She may experience a weight gain of several pounds due to extracellular edema (fluid retention), which tends to localize in the abdomen, fingers, and ankles; muscle sensitivity due to the extracellular edema (hypertonicity); vascular alterations that increase susceptibility to bruising; breast pain and tenderness resulting from swelling; mild to severe headache, including "menstrual migraine" (a vascular headache resulting from hormonal changes); severe cramping; and emotional changes, such as agitation, irritability, depression, anger, and moodiness. Premenstrual syndrome (PMS) is a cluster of all or some of these symptoms; in some cases it can be debilitating. It normally occurs 7 to 14 days before the onset of the menstrual flow, then generally subsides once the flow begins. Premenstrual syndrome affects about one third of all reproductive age women, particularly in the 30- to 40-year-old group. Stress, diet, alcohol consumption, and prescription or nonprescription drug use may exacerbate symptoms. Prehospital treatment is predominantly supportive; the root cause of the symptomology must be defined by differential medical diagnosis. Supportive prehospital treatment may include administration of a small dose of analgesics to reduce patient anxiety.

Some women may experience abdominal pain and cramping in the 2 weeks before the beginning of menses. This pain and its accompanying symptoms result from the ovulatory process and are collectively called mittelschmerz (pronounced "MITT-ul-shmurz"; German for "middle pain"). Mittelschmerz, which may start at any time during ovulation (midcycle), affects approximately 20% of women. In most cases, the pain is not severe; it may last only a few minutes or as long as 48 hours (average, 6 to 8 hours). Signs and symptoms include sharp, cramping pain in the lower abdomen, localized to one side, beginning midcycle, with a history of similar pain episodes during previous periods. The pain may also be reported as "switching sides" from month to month. Some women also report feeling nauseated or experiencing minor blood spotting. The condition itself is not serious, and the pain can often be relieved by over-the-counter analgesics. Any persistent pain or any abnormal symptoms are cause for concern and should be evaluated by a physician.

Dysmenorrhea is painful menses. It is classified into two categories: primary and secondary. Primary dysmenorrhea occurs with the advent of the menstrual flow and normally lasts for the first 1 to 2 days with gradual relief. Mild cramping is normal, but some women experience severe cramping, with pain originating in the area of the symphysis pubis and radiating downward to the vulva and outward to the thighs. Nausea, vomiting, and diarrhea may accompany the pain. Primary dysmenorrhea accounts for about 80% of patients presenting with painful menses and accompanies a "regular" period. Secondary dysmenorrhea is pain that is present before, during, and after the menstrual flow. It is generally organic in nature (not hormonal) and may signal an underlying illness or structural abnormality. As with premenstrual syndrome, prehospital treatment is largely supportive.

At this point, you may be asking why this information is important and whether anyone would actually call EMS for "menstrual" problems. If the situation is an emergency to the patient, professionally, it should be an emergency to you as well. Generally, for menstrual-related conditions, EMS is called because (1) the symptoms are new for the patient, (2) the symptoms are worse than in the past, or (3) the patient innately "feels" that something is wrong **Figure 38-3 ▶**. Your history taking and inferences can provide important information for the treating physician and contribute to the overall well-being and recovery of the patient. Of course, for you to ascertain what is "abnormal," you must know what is "normal."

Amenorrhea is divided into two categories: primary and secondary. Primary amenorrhea is the complete absence of menses—the patient has never had a menstrual cycle. Secondary amenorrhea occurs when the patient has menstrual cycles that cease for at least three consecutive months. This condition may be caused by a number of factors, but *the most common cause of secondary amenorrhea is pregnancy.*

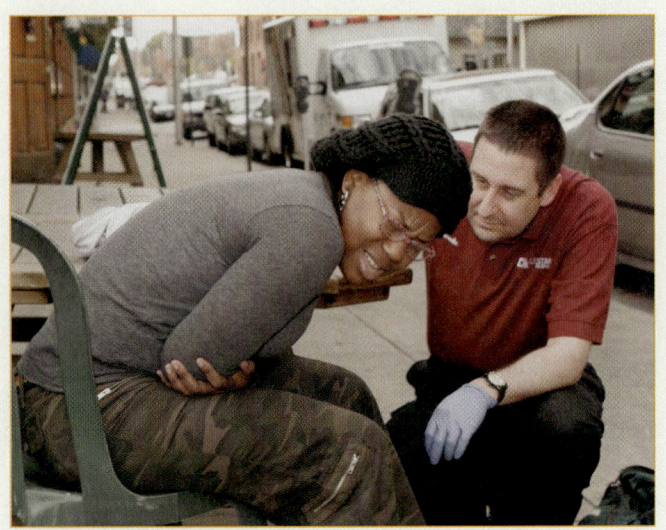
Figure 38-3 A patient may call EMS because she perceives her condition to be an emergency. Make sure you take each call seriously.

Exercise-induced amenorrhea is common in female athletes, particularly those who participate in physically intense sports. Amenorrhea can also be caused by emotional problems or extreme stress. In an adolescent or young adult, the condition may have its origination in anorexia nervosa; in this case, it is a symptom of the patient's malnutrition and emotional state.

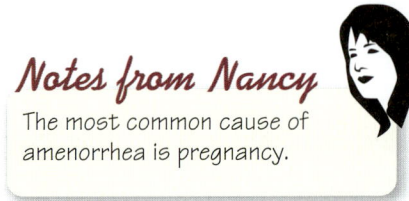
Notes from Nancy
The most common cause of amenorrhea is pregnancy.

Vaginal bleeding is one of the most frequent reasons that women consult a gynecologist. The assessment and management of a patient with this chief complaint depend largely on whether there is a mechanism of injury. Vaginal bleeding, when not in the course of regular menstruation, is always an abnormal finding. The cause may be as benign as emotional stress or as serious as pelvic, cervical, or uterine cancer. Likewise, a disturbance in the normal menstrual cycle is cause for concern. If the flow of blood lasts several days longer than normal or is excessive, the condition is called menorrhagia. If the blood flow occurs more often than a 24-day interval, it is termed polymenorrhea. Menorrhagia and polymenorrhea have four main causes: organic causes (infection, bleeding disorders); endocrine disorders (hypo- or hyperthyroidism, pituitary gland dysfunction); anatomical causes (fibroids, polyps, pregnancy); or iatrogenic causes (intrauterine device [IUD], medications). Blood flow or intermittent spotting of blood occurring irregularly but frequently is termed metrorrhagia. Metrorrhagia is of greatest concern to paramedics because its causes range from hormonal imbalance to malignancies to spontaneous abortion (miscarriage).

Documentation and Communication

Your attempts to obtain accurate, truthful information from the patient may be hindered by the presence of family members, loved ones, or bystanders. Removing nonessential personnel from the area will increase the likelihood that you obtain accurate information.

Pathophysiology

Causes of gynecologic emergencies range from infection to ectopic pregnancy to trauma.

Endometritis

Endometritis is an inflammation of the endometrium (uterine lining), most commonly caused by infection. Sexually transmitted diseases are a frequent cause (gonorrhea and chlamydia, predominantly), but endometritis may also occur after gynecologic surgery, abortion (elective, miscarriage, or therapeutic), or use of an IUD. Postpartum endometritis can occur within the first 24 to 48 hours or up to 6 weeks after delivery. Approximately 1% to 3% of women who have had a vaginal birth develop endometritis as a postpartum complication. The risk is considerably higher in women who have had a caesarean section birth and is estimated to be 10% to 20%. Symptoms may include malaise, fever (high- or low-grade), constipation or uncomfortable bowel movements, vaginal bleeding or discharge (or both), abdominal distension, and lower abdominal or pelvic pain. Abdominal auscultation may reveal decreased bowel sounds, and pain may be elicited by palpation of the abdomen. Left untreated, endometritis may lead to septic shock or cause spontaneous abortion in a pregnant patient.

Endometriosis

Endometriosis affects an estimated 10% to 15% of women of reproductive age in Canada. This condition can be extremely painful, or there may be no symptoms. It results when endometrial tissue grows outside the uterus, generally on the surface of abdominal and pelvic organs. Organs of the pelvic cavity are the most common locations for the ectopic growths, but endometrial tissue can occasionally be found in the lungs or other parts of the body. This condition is one of the leading causes of infertility in women, with 30% to 40% of affected women unable to conceive. Many women do not even realize they have endometriosis until they encounter difficulties trying to get pregnant.

In women who experience symptoms, the most common complaint is pain, generally localized in the lower back, pelvic, and abdominal regions, that may be chronic. Other symptoms include painful coitus (during and after), gastrointestinal pain, dysuria and painful bowel movements during the menstrual cycle, fatigue, extremely painful and escalating menstrual cramping, and very heavy menstrual periods. Patients may also experience bleeding between periods or report premenstrual spotting.

Pelvic Inflammatory Disease

It is estimated that approximately one of every seven women will contract pelvic inflammatory disease (PID) at some point. In Canada, the actual incidence rate is unknown, because most women with PID are treated as outpatients, and PID is not a mandatory reportable disease. Over the past decade, the rate of hospital admissions for PID has declined to roughly 2.5%. These statistics do not account for the many cases of "silent" or asymptomatic PID that can occur. One fourth of the women will require hospitalization. PID is one of the most common causes of women presenting to an emergency service

---

You are the Paramedic Part 2

You administer oxygen to the patient, obtain vital signs, insert an IV line, and apply the cardiac monitor and note sinus rhythm. As you continue your assessment, she says, "Please just take me to the hospital. Please." You can tell that she is very frightened. You assist her to the stretcher, where she finds her original position of comfort.

Vital Signs	Recording Time: 5 Minutes
Level of consciousness	Alert, with a Glasgow Coma Scale score of 15
Skin	Warm, pink, and dry
Pulse	90 beats/min and regular
Blood pressure	110/68 mm Hg
Respirations	30 breaths/min
Spo$_2$	100% with oxygen at 4 l/min via nasal cannula

3. What other information would you like to know?

4. What issues do you foresee that will likely impact patient prehospital care?

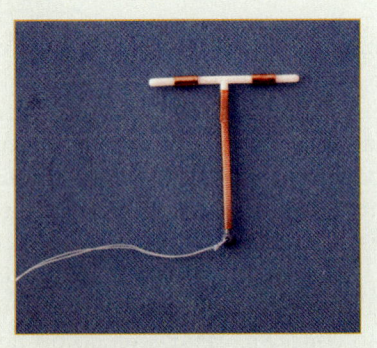

Figure 38-4 The IUD contraceptive device can increase a woman's risk of developing PID and ectopic pregnancy and may cause pain and bleeding.

with a chief complaint of abdominal pain. One of every four women who contract PID will have severe abdominal pain or experience sterility or childbirth complications.

PID is an infection of the female upper organs of reproduction—specifically, the endometrium, ovaries, fallopian tubes, pelvic peritoneum, and contiguous structures—that occurs almost exclusively in sexually active women. Disease-causing organisms enter the vagina, generally by the process of sexual activity, and migrate through the opening of the cervix and into the uterine cavity, where they invade the mucosa. Symptoms vary depending on the pathogenicity of the causative organism and can range from asymptomatic to severe pain, fever, and shock. Chlamydial infection is more likely to present as "silent," or asymptomatic, PID, particularly in the adolescent age group. The infection may expand to the fallopian tubes (producing scarring that can lead to life-threatening ectopic pregnancy or sterility), eventually involving the ovaries (leading to the development of a tubo-ovarian abscess) and the peritoneal cavity. Although PID itself is seldom a threat to life, its ultimate consequences can be lethal, due to the high risk of subsequent ectopic pregnancy.

Risk factors for PID include the use of an IUD as a contraceptive device **Figure 38-4 ▲**, frequent sexual activity with multiple partners, and a history of previous PID. The disease is most prevalent in the collegiate age group (20 to 24 years) and statistically decreases after age 30 years (the typical monogamy and marriage years).

Interstitial Cystitis

In Canada, roughly 3% of all outpatient visits to a urologist are for interstitial cystitis/painful bladder syndrome (IC/PBS). Although this condition affects men and women, 94% of diagnosed cases have been women. IC/PBS is a chronic bladder condition with an unknown cause; it results in an inflamed or irritated bladder wall. In severe cases, the irritation can lead to the formation of ulcers in the bladder and bleeding into the bladder lining. The bladder may become internally scarred and stiff, resulting in markedly reduced bladder capacity. Symptoms vary but may mimic the symptoms associated with urinary tract infections and sexually transmitted diseases: pressure or tenderness in the bladder and surrounding pelvic region, pain that ranges from mild discomfort to severe, and urinary frequency or urgency. Some patients report urinating as many as 60 times per day. Painful coitus is not uncommon, and

many women report that their symptoms become worse during their menstrual cycle.

There is currently no cure for IC/PBS and antibiotics are ineffective. Patients are generally treated to provide symptomatic relief. Some physicians may prescribe antihistamines or antidepressants, whereas others give ibuprofen, aspirin, or even narcotics for severe cases.

Ectopic Pregnancy

The word *ectopic* means "located away from a normal position." In ectopic pregnancy, a fertilized egg is implanted somewhere besides the uterus **Figure 38-5 ▶**. In 97% of cases, the egg is fertilized inside one of the fallopian tubes and has been blocked from passing into the uterus, generally by an obstruction, such as PID-related tubal scarring or as a result of tubal surgery (ligation or reverse ligation). The other 3% of ectopic pregnancies occur in the abdomen, within the cervix, or on an ovary. Ectopic pregnancy is the leading cause of maternal death in the first trimester and accounts for 4% of all pregnancy-related deaths in Canada. Nearly 1 in 66 women who get pregnant will experience an ectopic pregnancy. Fifty percent of all women have known risk factors for ectopic pregnancy. Although PID is the most common cause of ectopic pregnancy, other causes include pelvic surgery, smoking, IUD use (IUDs do not cause ectopic pregnancy but, by blocking uterine pregnancy, may cause fertilization to occur higher up), fibroids, tumours or cysts in the tubes, fallopian endometriosis, hormonal imbalance, and fertility treatments.

With a tubal pregnancy, the fertilized egg implants in the fallopian tube, then begins to grow and produce hormones in the same way a normally implanted egg does, taking nourishment from the maternal blood supply. Owing to the production of hormones, the woman begins to experience the early physiologic changes of pregnancy. Her period stops, her breasts become enlarged and tender, and the uterine environment changes just as it would with a normal pregnancy. The fallopian tube, lacking the expansive muscle capacity of the uterus, has little stretching ability, so the developing embryo will soon run out of growing room. When this occurs, the tube is likely to rupture, causing massive intra-abdominal hemorrhage and shock. Ectopic pregnancies are commonly diagnosed between 6 to 10 weeks of gestation. If a woman has irregular cycles, she may not even realize she is pregnant.

Ruptured Ovarian Cyst and Tubo-ovarian Abscess

Ruptured ovarian cysts and tubo-ovarian abscesses are rarely life threatening, but present with similar findings as an ectopic pregnancy. These clinical entities cannot be differentiated in the prehospital setting and, therefore, should be managed as an ectopic pregnancy.

An ovarian cyst is essentially a fluid-filled sac that forms on or within an ovary. Of the many types of cysts, the most common is the *functional cyst,* which generally develops during

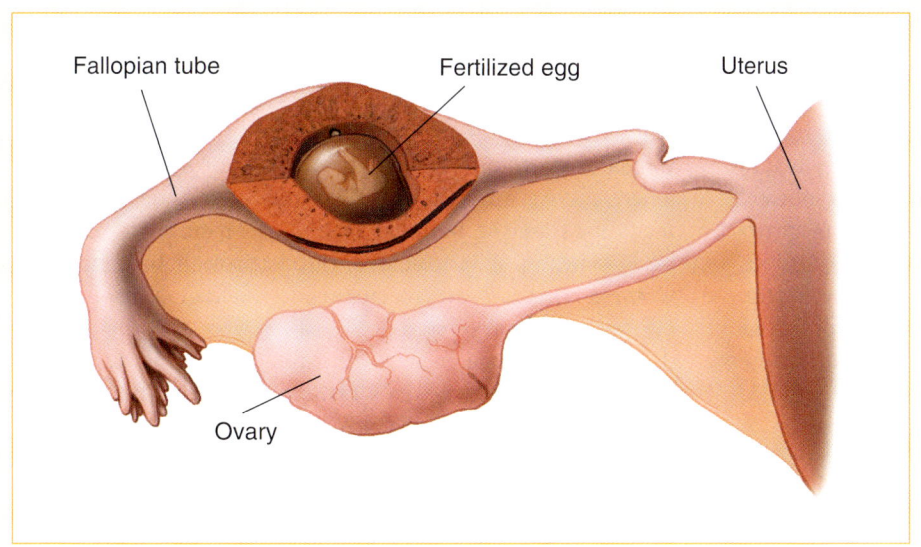

Figure 38-5 In an ectopic pregnancy, a fertilized egg implants somewhere other than the uterus. Here it is implanted in one of the fallopian tubes.

Labels: Fallopian tube, Fertilized egg, Uterus, Ovary

the menstrual cycle. During the cycle, the ovaries form tiny sacs (cysts) to hold the eggs. Once an egg matures, the sac breaks open and releases the egg, which then begins its journey through the fallopian tube for fertilization; the sac itself dissolves. If the sac fails to break open, however, the egg may continue to mature and form a *follicular cyst.* Under normal circumstances, this type of cyst spontaneously disappears within a 1- to 3-month period. A *corpus luteum cyst* develops if the sac seals itself after release of the egg. Fluid then accumulates inside the cyst, and the cyst continues to grow. These cysts usually resolve spontaneously but may grow up to 10 cm. At this size, they can cause ovarian torsion, which can manifest as pain and bleeding as the ovary becomes necrotic from being cut-off from its blood supply. Fertility drugs can increase the chances of corpus luteum cysts developing.

If the cycle of forming sacs is repeated excessively and the eggs do not release, *polycystic ovaries* may develop. This hormonal reproductive disorder is characterized by lack of progesterone and high levels of androgens (male hormone). It can have a negative impact on normal insulin production, leading to diabetes (especially gestational). It can also initiate heart and blood vessel problems, such as hypertension, and produce pelvic pain and irregular menstrual cycles.

Dermoid cysts lead to growths of formational tissue, such as teeth and hair, and may become very large and painful. Large dermoid cysts can also cause ovarian torsion. Endometriomas form in women who have endometriosis, when uterine tissue attaches to the ovaries and begins to grow. Pain from this type of cyst usually manifests during menstruation or sexual intercourse. Cystadenomas are formed from cells on the outer surface of the ovary. These cysts are usually filled with a thick mucus. They can become large and cause pain. A hemorrhagic cyst forms when a blood vessel bursts in the cyst wall and the

blood fills the sac. Occasionally, these cysts will rupture and spill blood into the abdominal cavity, resulting in great pain.

Tubo-ovarian abscess is encountered secondary to a primary infectious agent—typically, the ones that cause PID. The most common underlying cause is gonorrhea. Diverticulitis and appendicitis have also been found to be causative agents. In this condition, the fallopian tubes or ovaries become blocked by an infectious mass, which grows and forms an abscess.

Toxic Shock Syndrome

Toxic shock syndrome (TSS) is a form of septic shock. The disease made headlines in the 1980s, when it was identified as a syndrome affecting women who used tampons. A connection was made between the use of super-absorbancy tampons and a risk of contracting the disease, but the panic that ensued was out of proportion to the actual threat. The disease has been identified as having *Streptococcus pyogenes* (group A strep) or *Staphylococcus aureus* as the causative agent. TSS affects men and women, and it can involve several of the body's systems, including the hepatic, cardiovascular, central nervous, and renal systems. It can result when minor infections of the lungs, sinuses, skin lesions, or the vagina progress to actual TSS, which can be lethal. Menstruating women appear particularly prone to developing TSS—hence, the original association between the syndrome and tampon use. Initial symptoms include syncope, myalgia, diarrhea, vomiting, headache, fever, and sore throat. Other symptoms may include diverse petechiae, light rash, and scleral injection (bloodshot eyes). As the disease progresses, signs of systemic shock will begin to appear. Disseminated intravascular coagulation, severe hypotension, adult respiratory distress syndrome, and dysrhythmias may develop, and the patient may show signs of kidney and liver failure.

Rapid transport is indicated in cases of TSS. Provide high-flow supplemental oxygen, IV therapy, and cardiac monitoring. Little more can be done for a patient with TSS in the prehospital setting because aggressive antibiotic therapy and possible surgical intervention are required.

Common Gynecologic Infections

Two of the most common infections that affect women are bacterial vaginosis and vaginal yeast infections. Although the incidence of these infections is higher in sexually active women, they are not considered to be sexually transmitted.

Bacterial vaginosis is one of the most common conditions to afflict women. In this infection, normal bacteria in the vagina are replaced by an overgrowth of other bacterial forms. Symptoms may include itching, burning, or pain and may be accompanied by a "fishy," foul-smelling discharge. Left untreated, bacterial vaginosis can lead to premature birth or low birth weight in case of pregnancy, make the patient more susceptible to more serious infections, and result in PID. It is treated with metronidazole, an antibiotic.

Vaginal yeast infections are typically caused by the fungus *Candida albicans*. Yeasts are tiny organisms that normally live in small numbers inside the vagina and on the skin. The normal acidic environment of the vagina helps keep yeast from growing. If the vagina becomes less acidic, however, the yeast population may increase dramatically, causing infection. Conditions that may alter the acidic balance of the vagina include oral contraceptives, menstruation, pregnancy, diabetes, and some antibiotics. Moisture and irritation of the vagina also seem to encourage yeast growth. Stress from lack of sleep, illness, or poor diet are other contributing factors. Women with immunosuppressive diseases such as HIV infection or diabetes are also at increased risk. Approximately 75% of all women will likely experience at least one infection during their lifetime. Symptoms include itching, burning, soreness in the vagina and around the vulva and vulvar swelling. Some women may report a thick, white vaginal discharge ("cottage cheese" appearance), pain during sexual intercourse, and burning on urination.

Sexually Transmitted Diseases

As mentioned earlier, PID results from infective organisms crossing the cervix. It is typically a secondary infection, with the primary infection being a sexually transmitted disease (STD)—often chlamydia or gonorrhea. STDs are reviewed briefly here, with the exception of the human immunodeficiency virus (HIV), which is discussed in Chapter 36.

Chancroid is caused by infection with the bacterium *Haemophilus ducreyi*. This highly contagious yet curable disease causes painful soft margin ulcers, usually of the genitals. Swollen, painful lymph glands or inguinal buboes in the groin area may be present as well. Women may be asymptomatic and, thus, unaware they have the disease. Chancroid is known to facilitate the transmission of HIV.

Chlamydia is caused by the bacterium *Chlamydia trachomatis* and is the most common STD in Canada, primarily in the 15- to 24-year-old age group. Although symptoms of chlamydia are usually mild or absent, some women may have symptoms including lower abdominal pain, low back pain, nausea, fever, pain during intercourse, to bleeding between menstrual periods. Chlamydial infection of the cervix can spread to the rectum, leading to rectal pain, discharge, or bleeding. Left untreated, the disease can progress to PID and infertility. In rare cases, chlamydia causes arthritis that may be accompanied by skin lesions and inflammation of the eye and urethra (Reiter syndrome).

Genital herpes is an infection of the genitals, buttocks, or anal area caused by herpes simplex virus, type I or type II. Type I, which is the most common form, infects the mouth and lips, causing cold sores or blisters; it may also produce sores on the genitals. Type II, the more serious infection, can affect the mouth as well, but is more commonly known as the primary cause of genital herpes. Genital herpes infection is more prevalent in women than in men.

In an active herpes infection, symptoms generally appear within 2 weeks of primary infection and can last for several weeks. Symptoms may include tingling or sores near the area where the virus has entered the body, such as on the genital or rectal area, on the buttocks or thighs, or on other parts of the body where the virus has entered through broken skin. In women, the sores may occur inside the vagina, on the cervix, or in the urinary passage. Small red bumps appear first, develop into small blisters, and finally become itchy, painful sores that might develop a crust and heal without leaving a scar. Other symptoms that may accompany the first outbreak, and possibly subsequent outbreaks, include fever, muscle aches and pains, headache, dysuria, vaginal discharge, and swollen glands in the groin area.

Gonorrhea is caused by *Neisseria gonorrhoeae*, a bacterium that can grow and multiply rapidly in the warm, moist areas of the reproductive tract, including the cervix, uterus, and fallopian tubes in women and in the urethra in women and men. The bacterium can also grow in the mouth, throat, eyes, and anus. Symptoms, which are generally more severe in men than in women, appear approximately 2 to 10 days after exposure. Women may be infected with gonorrhea for months but experience virtually no symptoms until the infection has spread to other parts of the reproductive system. When symptoms do appear in women, they generally manifest as dysuria (painful urination), with associated burning or itching, a yellowish or bloody vaginal discharge, usually with a foul odour, and occult blood associated with vaginal intercourse. More severe infections may present with cramping and abdominal pain, nausea and vomiting, and bleeding between periods; these symptoms indicate that the infection has progressed to PID. Rectal infections generally present with anal discharge and itching, plus occasional painful bowel movements with fecal blood spotting. Infection of the throat (for which oral sex is the introducing factor) is called gonococcal pharyngitis. Its symptoms are usually mild, consisting of painful or difficult swallowing, sore throat, swollen lymph glands, and fever. Headache and nasal congestion may also be present. If the infection is not treated, the bacterium may enter the bloodstream and spread to other parts of the body, including the brain—a condition known as disseminated gonococcemia.

Genital warts (also called condylomata acuminata and venereal warts) are caused by the human papillomavirus (HPV). Of the more than 100 types of HPV that have been identified, about 30 types are spread through sexual contact. HPV is the most common viral STD, with almost 6 million new cases being reported every year and more than 20 million open cases being treated. Some infected people have no symptoms. In others, multiple growths develop in the genital areas—that is, the vagina, vulva, cervix, or rectum, or the penis and scrotum in men. HPV has been identified as a causative agent in cervical, vulvar, and anal cancers. In pregnant women, warts may develop that become large enough to impede urination or obstruct the birth canal.

Syphilis is caused by the bacterium *Treponema pallidum*. Because many of its signs and symptoms mimic other diseases, syphilis is sometimes called the "great imitator" by clinicians. The disease manifests in three stages: primary, secondary, and late. Approximately 20,000 to 30,000 cases of syphilis are reported each year in the United States, mostly in the 20- to 40-year-old group; the highest incidence is found in women aged 20 to 24 years. The rates in Canada are not as high, but are on the rise. Transmission occurs through direct contact with open sores, which may arise anywhere on the body, but tend to appear on the genitals, anus, rectum, lips, or mouth. A person with syphilis may remain asymptomatic for years, not realizing that his or her sores are manifestations of a disease.

The primary stage of syphilis is usually marked by the appearance of a single sore (a chancre), although in some people, multiple sores develop. The chancre is usually painless and is small, firm, and round. It usually goes away after 3 to 6 weeks, at which point the disease has progressed to the second stage.

The secondary stage of syphilis is characterized by the development of mucous membrane lesions and a skin rash. The characteristic rash may manifest on the palms of the hands and the bottoms of the feet as rough, red or reddish brown spots. Alternatively, it may be barely discernible or resemble rashes from other diseases. The rash generally does not itch. Symptoms of secondary syphilis may include fever, swollen lymph glands, sore throat, patchy hair loss, headaches, weight loss, muscle aches, and fatigue. Like the chancre of the primary stage, these symptoms will resolve without treatment. Left untreated, the secondary stage invariably leads to tertiary syphilis.

In tertiary, there are no signs or symptoms, but internal damage is accumulating. Symptoms become evident once permanent damage has occurred. Syphilis attacks the brain, nerves, eyes, heart, blood vessels, liver, bones, and joints, although the damage may not become evident for years. Paralysis, numbness, dementia, gradual blindness, and difficulty coordinating muscle movements are possible physical manifestations and may be serious enough to cause death. Pregnant women with syphilis may have stillborn babies, babies who are born blind, developmentally delayed babies, or babies who die shortly after birth.

Trichomoniasis is caused by a single-celled protozoan parasite, *Trichomonas vaginalis*. This parasite is transmitted through sexual contact, with the vagina being the most common site of infection. The infected person may be asymptomatic or may experience signs and symptoms including a frothy, yellow-green vaginal discharge with a strong odour. The infection may also cause irritation and itching of the female genital area, discomfort during intercourse, dysuria, and lower abdominal pain. When present, symptoms usually appear in women within 5 to 28 days of exposure to *T vaginalis*. Left untreated, the infection can lead to low birthweight or premature birth in pregnant women and to increased susceptibility to HIV infection.

Patient Assessment

Obtaining an accurate and detailed patient assessment is of utmost importance when dealing with gynecologic issues. You may not be able to make a specific diagnosis in the prehospital environment, but a thorough detailed examination and patient history will help determine just how sick the patient is and whether lifesaving measures should be initiated. This is especially true when dealing with abdominal pain.

Women have many of the same conditions that cause abdominal pain in men—for example, renal colic, ulcers, gastroenteritis, cholecystitis, diverticulitis, pancreatitis, appendicitis, mesenteric ischemia, and dissecting aneurysm. In addition, there are numerous gynecologic causes of abdominal pain. An old medical axiom states, "Anyone who neglects to consider a gynecologic cause in a woman of childbearing age who complains of abdominal pain will miss the diagnosis at least 50% of the time." Missing the diagnosis may be fatal for the patient.

Scene Assessment

Every emergency call—including calls involving gynecologic emergencies—begins with a thorough scene assessment. Is the scene safe? Will you need assistance? Is it a medical call, a trauma call, or both? How many patients do you have? What is the mechanism of injury or nature of illness? Have you taken proper body substance isolation precautions? Gynecologic emergencies can be very messy, sometimes involving large amounts of blood and body fluids contaminated with communicable diseases.

Where is the patient found? If she is at home, what is the condition of the residence? Is it clean, filthy, or wrecked? Do you see evidence of a fight? Are alcohol, tobacco products, or drug paraphernalia present? Are there pictures of loved ones or, conversely, a noticeable absence of pictures? Does the patient live alone or with other people? All information you obtain will contribute to your assessment of the patient's overall health and the safety of the scene. In case of a crime scene, you may also be required to testify in court regarding the conditions on your arrival.

Initial Assessment

What is the overall presentation of the patient? Are there any obvious life threats? Is she conscious? Does she have obvious breathing difficulty or evidence of injury? Does she appear pale, cyanotic, red, or grey? Is she alert and oriented or confused? Is she calm or not? What is her emotional state? What is her physical appearance—well kept or dirty? Do you find the patient sitting up, lying down, prone, supine, in the fetal position, in the tripod position, in the bathtub, or on all fours?

Once you have answered these basic questions and treated any immediate threats to airway, breathing, or circulation, you can proceed with the focused physical examination, rapid medical assessment, or rapid trauma assessment as the situation dictates. Conduct rapid medical or trauma assessment if the patient is not responsive or has a significant mechanism of injury but life threats are not immediately obvious. In the focused history and physical examination, pay special attention to gynecologic and reproductive history in addition to the usual criteria.

Try to protect the patient's modesty at all times during your history and physical examination. Gynecologic emergencies can be highly embarrassing for the patient, and many women may be extremely uncomfortable about discussing their sexual history in front of strangers or even close family members **Figure 38-6 ▶**. A teenage or adolescent girl may want to keep her sexual history from her parents. Limit the number of personnel required to perform the necessary tasks, and show the patient you respect her by being the advocate for her modesty. If a female paramedic is available, offer the patient the option of having her perform the examination. You also serve as a role model for other paramedics when you act this way.

Notes from Nancy

In the woman with abdominal pain, the most important things to look for are signs of shock.

Documentation and Communication

By properly documenting your general impression, level of consciousness, chief complaint, life threats, and ABCs (the initial assessment), you provide vital information that is necessary for good, ongoing patient care.

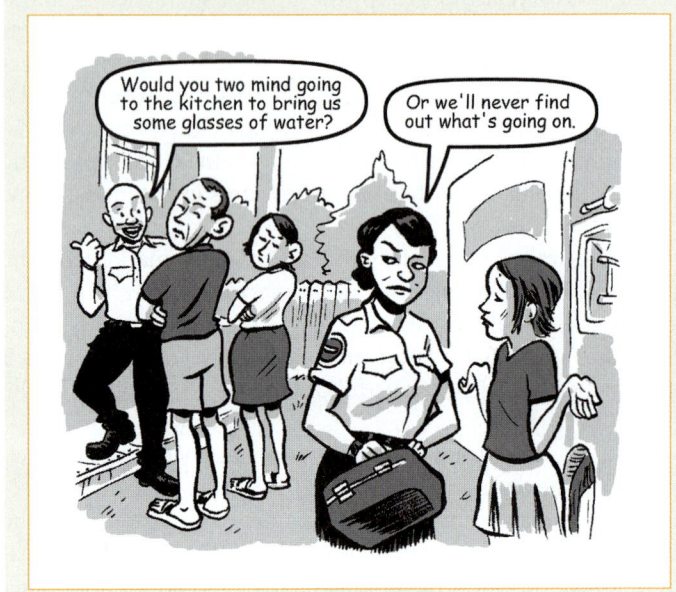

Figure 38-6

You are the Paramedic Part 3

You continue to ask questions about Mrs. Medina's pain and pregnancy using the LORDS TRACHEA mnemonics (see the "Focused Physical Examination" section of this chapter). You obtain her orthostatic vital signs and perform a focused physical examination. No changes in positional vital signs are noted, and you find no signs of shock or trauma. You believe that Mrs. Medina is in stable condition but requires immediate physician evaluation. En route to the receiving facility, you advise emergency department personnel of the patient's signs, symptoms, and other pertinent information regarding your assessment and interventions.

Vital Signs	Recording Time: 15 Minutes
Level of consciousness	Alert, with a Glasgow Coma Scale score of 15
Skin	Warm, pink, and dry
Pulse	86 beats/min and regular
Blood pressure	110/66 mm Hg
Respirations	24 breaths/min
SpO$_2$	100% with supplemental oxygen at 4 l/min via nasal cannula

5. Given the information you have so far, will this patient require aggressive prehospital care?

6. What are the three true life-threatening gynecologic emergencies?

7. Does your differential diagnosis include any of these conditions?

Focused History and Physical Examination

Obtaining the History

What is the patient's chief complaint? If it is excessive bleeding, you can move on to getting the gynecologic history. If the chief complaint is abdominal pain, you need to find out more about the pain itself. Although the OPQRST (Onset; Provoking factors; Quality of pain; Region of pain and whether it radiates or refers; Severity; and Time [duration]) method discussed in previous chapters works well, a more specific approach is the LORDS TRACHEA mnemonic.

L What is the *Location* of the pain? Can the patient point to where the pain originates? Are multiple areas producing pain? Pain located in the midline may indicate spontaneous abortion (miscarriage). An achy pain that is diffused throughout the lower abdomen may be PID. Pain localized to one side of the abdomen may be an ectopic pregnancy.

O What was the *Onset* of the pain? When did the pain start? What activity was the patient performing when the pain started? A patient who reports the pain began during exercise may have a ruptured ovarian cyst.

R Does the pain *Radiate?* That is, does the pain stay centralized or does it travel? Pain that radiates to the shoulder may indicate large amounts of blood in the abdomen.

D What is the *Duration* of the pain? Is it constant or intermittent? If intermittent, how long does the pain last?

S What is the *Severity* of the pain, on a scale of 1 to 10? Is the pain excruciating or tolerable? Excruciating pain usually points to a nongynecologic cause, such as renal colic or aortic dissection.

T What is the *Timing* of the pain? Did it start after the patient took an oral contraceptive? Is there a temporal relationship between the onset of the pain and the last menstrual period? Pain that originates with PID generally starts after the last menstrual flow. Which symptoms presented first? In cases of spontaneous abortion, pain generally *follows* bleeding. With ectopic pregnancy, the pain usually develops *before* bleeding.

R Does anything *Relieve* the pain? Does holding still, posturing a particular way, or lying down diminish the pain? Has the patient taken any medication for the pain? If so, what? Did the medication help?

A What *Aggravates* the pain? Does physical activity such as walking, sitting, or turning make the pain worse? Is the pain aggravated by physiologic activities, such as urinating, defecating, breathing, or swallowing? A patient with PID may (or may not) volunteer that the pain is made worse by sexual intercourse.

C What is the *Character* of the pain? Is it crampy? Aching? Sharp? Dull? Squeezing? Shooting? Stabbing? A patient experiencing a spontaneous abortion generally presents with "cramping" pain. The pain of PID will most likely be dull and steady.

H Is there a *Historic* precedent? Has the patient ever had this pain before? If yes, what was the cause? Is the pain now the same as or different from the earlier pain? What is the difference?

E Has the patient *Eaten* anything? If so, what? How much? How long ago? Did the symptoms appear after eating? If not, did eating alleviate any of the symptoms? Fluctuating hormonal levels frequently give rise to digestive problems, so it is just as important to rule out the obvious (indigestion) as it is to pinpoint the obscure.

A Are there *Associated* symptoms? Ask specifically about bleeding and symptoms of significant blood loss. Has the patient experienced any nausea, vomiting, or vertigo?

Once you have ascertained all that you can about the chief complaint and have developed a feeling for the patient's pain, you can proceed to obtain the gynecologic history. Probably the single most important question to ask is, "When did you have your last menstrual period (LMP)?" If the patient knows for certain, record the beginning and ending dates of the LMP. If she is unsure, record the approximate dates. Ask the patient whether she noticed anything unusual about the LMP. Was it longer or shorter than usual? Was the flow heavier or lighter than usual? Was there more or less cramping involved? Was the period late or on time? Did she have any spotting or bleeding between periods? Was any unusual pain involved?

Does the patient suspect that she might be pregnant, or is there any possibility of pregnancy? Many patients may find this question highly personal and may be uncomfortable answering it. They do not want you making a character judgment of their sexual history. Be patient, reassuring, professional, and non-judgmental in your questioning. If the answer is a strong "No way," find out why. Younger, sexually active women may incorrectly presume that birth control methods are 100% effective against pregnancy; in truth, most current methods are only 98% effective at best, and only if used correctly. If not using any contraceptive, 25% of women will become pregnant within 1 month and 85% within 1 year. If the patient insists she cannot be pregnant, ask about other symptoms such as breast enlargement and tenderness, morning sickness (nausea and vomiting on waking), weight gain, and urinary frequency.

Does the patient use contraception and, if so, what kind? Does the patient use birth control pills and, if so, what kind? (**Table 38-1 ▶** shows several currently used birth control methods.) Are they uniquely prescribed for her or does she borrow them from a friend? Did the patient just start using birth control pills? (Vaginal spotting is sometimes a side effect of a new prescription.) Does she use spermicides, condoms,

At the Scene

Use the mnemonic ACHES-S to help isolate the "symptom cluster" associated with oral contraceptives: Abdominal pain, Chest pain, Headache (severe), Eyes (blurred vision), Spotting, and Sharp leg pain.

or a diaphragm? Does she use an implanted device (such as, Norplant) or an IUD? Woman who use an IUD (also called the "loop" or "coil") are more prone to PID and ectopic pregnancy. The IUD may also perforate the uterus, causing pain and bleeding.

Continuing on with the assessment, determine whether the patient has experienced vaginal bleeding. If yes, try to quantify the amount of blood. Try to obtain an accurate description of the bleeding. Is the blood bright red, dark, or a combination? Are there clots? When did the bleeding start? Is it intermittent or continuous? Is the bleeding excessive? Are signs of shock present? If so, initiate standard fluid therapy with a large-bore IV cannula according to your local medical directives. A fluid bolus may be required for the hypotensive patient. You may wish to contact direct medical control for further assistance in managing the unstable patient.

Has the patient experienced any vaginal discharge? If so, what was its nature? Did the discharge have an odour? What colour was it? Was it clear fluid or mucus? Was it frothy, lumpy, or stringy? Was any blood observed with the fluid? Has the patient or her partner ever had an STD? If yes, which one? Has she ever been treated for an STD?

Notes from Nancy

Abnormal vaginal bleeding is a complication of pregnancy until proved otherwise.

At the Scene

Vaginal bleeding is a sign of internal bleeding and should not be taken lightly. Apply a pad over the vaginal area, and transport all used pads with the patient to the hospital for analysis.

| Table 38-1 | Birth Control Methods |

Type of Contraceptive	Description
Male condom latex/polyurethane	A sheath placed over the erect penis blocking the passage of sperm; the only method that provides good protection against STDs
Female condom	A lubricated polyurethane sheath shaped similarly to the male condom; closed end has a flexible ring that is inserted into the vagina; may give some STD protection
Diaphragm	A dome-shaped rubber disk with a flexible rim that covers the cervix so that sperm cannot reach the uterus; spermicide is applied to the diaphragm before insertion
Lea's shield	A dome-shaped rubber disk with valve and a loop that is held in place by the vaginal wall; covers the upper vagina and cervix so that sperm cannot reach the uterus; spermicide is applied before insertion
Cervical cap	A soft rubber cup with a round rim, which fits snugly around the cervix
Sponge	A disk-shaped polyurethane device containing the spermicide nonoxynol-9
Spermicide	A foam, cream, jelly, film, suppository, or tablet that contains nonoxynol-9, a sperm-killing chemical
Oral contraceptives	Pills that suppress ovulation by the combined actions of the hormones estrogen and progestin; chewable form approved in November 2003 • The progestin-only version reduces and thickens cervical mucus to prevent sperm from reaching the egg. • The 91-day regimen, which contains estrogen and progestin, is taken in 3-month cycles of 12 weeks of active pills followed by 1 week of inactive pills.
Patch	A skin patch worn on the lower abdomen, buttocks, or upper body that releases progestin and estrogen into the bloodstream
Vaginal contraceptive ring	A flexible ring about 5 cm in diameter that is inserted into the vagina and releases progestin and estrogen
Postcoital contraceptives	Pills containing progestin alone or progestin plus estrogen
Injection	An injectable progestin or a combination of progestin and estrogen that inhibits ovulation, prevents sperm from reaching the egg, and/or prevents the fertilized egg from implanting in the uterus
Implant	Six matchstick-size rubber rods that are surgically implanted under the skin of the upper arm, where they steadily release the contraceptive steroid levonorgestrel
IUD	A T-shaped device inserted into the uterus by a health care professional
Periodic abstinence	Deliberately refraining from having sexual intercourse during times when pregnancy is more likely
Transabdominal surgical sterilization—female	Blocking of the woman's fallopian tubes so the egg and sperm cannot meet in the fallopian tube, preventing conception
Sterilization implant—female	Small metallic implant placed into the fallopian tubes; causes scar tissue formation, blocking the fallopian tubes and preventing conception
Surgical sterilization—male	Sealing, tying, or cutting a man's vas deferens so that the sperm cannot travel from the testicles to the penis

Source: Adapted from the U.S. Food and Drug Administration. Available at: www.fda.gov/fdac/features/1997/babytabl.html. Accessed May 11, 2006.

What is the woman's obstetric history? Has she ever been pregnant? How many times? Has she ever had a live birth? How many? (The medical term for pregnancy is gravid or gravidity; the term for live delivery is parity. Thus a woman who has been pregnant three times, with one live birth, one miscarriage, and one abortion would be documented as gravida 3, parity [or para] 1.) Have any of the deliveries been complicated? How? Were any of the pregnancies complicated? How? What kind of deliveries did she experience—vaginal or cesarean? How much time passed between pregnancies? Has she had any miscarriages and, if so, how many? Has she had any abortions? Were they spontaneous or elective? If elective, what form of abortion was used—medical or surgical? Elective abortion statistically increases the risks of future miscarriage, ectopic pregnancy, and development of certain cancers. A recent elective abortion may also be the underlying cause of the current emergency.

Does the patient have a history of gynecologic problems? Any known issues such as bleeding or infections? Any ectopic pregnancies?

Does the patient have any known medical conditions? Any personal or familial history of diabetes, cancer, hypertension, cardiovascular disease, or bleeding disorders? Is the familial history maternal or paternal? Is the patient being treated for a known medical condition? Does she take antihypertensives, anticoagulants, or diuretics? Make sure all of the components of the SAMPLE history are completed at this point.

The Physical Examination

When you are conducting an examination of a woman with abdominal pain, essentially one fundamental question needs to be answered in the prehospital setting: Is the pain a symptom of a life-threatening condition?

Your chief concern is to identify any signs of shock Figure 38-7 ▶ . Thus, the points of emphasis in the focused history and physical examination are as follows:

- What is the patient's general presentation? Does she appear anxious? Is she restless or apprehensive? Is she fatigued? Is she thirsty?
- What is the condition of the skin and mucous membranes? Is the skin warm and dry? Feverish? Diaphoretic? Cold and clammy? Is there pallor or cyanosis? Does the patient appear dehydrated? Are the mucous membranes pale?
- What are the patient's vital signs? Are there any variations in the pulse? Is it fast, slow, or irregular? Strong or weak and thready? Is the blood pressure normal, low, or elevated? What is normal for the patient? Check the pressure in sitting and standing positions. Are there significant orthostatic changes? If yes, the patient must be presumed to be in shock.

Next, examine the patient's abdomen. Examination of the abdomen is a process of inspection, auscultation, percussion, and palpation.

Inspect the abdomen for signs of abuse, such as bruising. The abdomen is a favourite target of abusers, especially if a

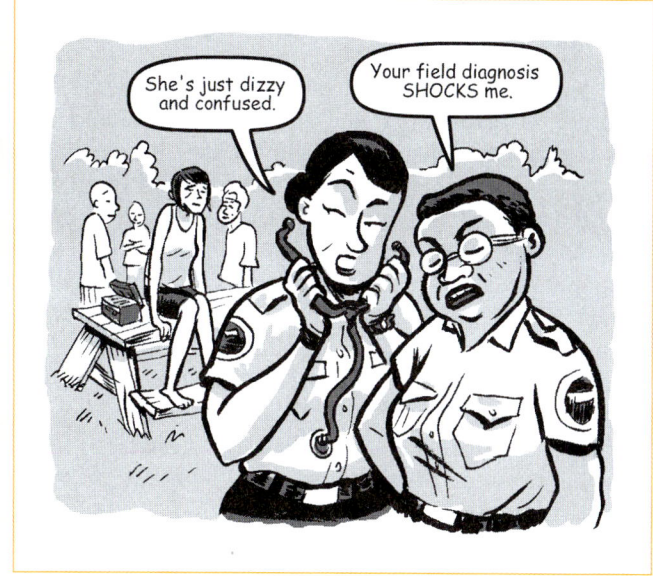

Figure 38-7

woman is pregnant. Note whether there are several bruises in various stages of healing. Do you see any surgical scarring from abdominal surgery or previous cesarean section or stretch marks from previous pregnancies? Is evidence of needle tracks from illicit drug use apparent? The abdomen is a favourite injection spot for chronic drug abusers because clothing hides the evidence. Is the abdomen swollen and distended (possibly indicative of pregnancy, internal bleeding, bowel obstruction, or liver problems)? Is it flat and flaccid? Is there any guarding of the abdomen? Are any rashes or lesions present? Is the abdomen symmetrical? Is the liver or spleen enlarged and protruding from under the rib cage?

Auscultate the abdomen before you undertake palpation or percussion because the latter activities tend to alter the frequency of bowel sounds. The most significant finding in the prehospital setting is *lack of bowel sounds,* which may indicate internal bleeding.

Percussion is a skill not widely practiced by paramedics, but it may yield useful information and guide palpation. Percuss all four quadrants of the abdomen (lightly) to elicit areas of dullness or tympany. Large, dull areas may indicate an underlying mass or enlarged organ. Tympanic areas indicate areas of gas. If the abdomen is distended and tympanic throughout, it generally indicates an intestinal obstruction.

Palpate the abdomen. Examine all quadrants, starting at the quadrant farthest from the pain and working toward the quadrant where the pain is located. Examine this quadrant last. Is the abdomen rigid (possibly indicative of internal bleeding)? Is there point tenderness? Does the palpation elicit more pain? Is rebound tenderness present (indicative of infection, such as may be associated with appendicitis)? Are there masses present? If yes, are they pulsating (abdominal aortic aneurysm)?

Pain Presentations

There are essentially three categories of abdominal pain: visceral pain, parietal pain, and referred pain.

Visceral pain is caused by some dysfunction of the hollow abdominal organs. It is generally poorly localized and diffuse but is typically felt near the midline. Right upper quadrant pain that mediates to the midline may have its origin in the liver or biliary tree. Epigastric pain that mediates to the midline is generally pain from the stomach, pancreas, or duodenum. Midline periumbilical pain typically has its origin in the proximal colon, small intestine, or appendix. Most hypogastric pain is from the colon, bladder, or uterus. Suprapubic pain generally indicates disorders in the rectum or bladder.

Parietal pain is caused by inflammation of the parietal peritoneum. It is generally described as a steady, aching pain that is aggravated by movement (such as coughing). The patient will usually try to lie as still as possible to avoid triggering the pain.

Referred pain develops as pain levels become more intense, and the pain seems to radiate or travel. Gallbladder pain tends to radiate and localize to the right shoulder or posterior part of the chest. Pancreatic or duodenal pain may be referred to the patient's back. Pleuritic pain from lungs or ischemic pain from acute coronary syndrome may be referred to the upper abdominal area; the same is true for pain from the pelvis, chest, and spine.

General management of abdominal pain is mostly psychologically supportive. Local protocols may allow for administration of narcotic analgesics for pain management, but you should always check with the receiving facility first. If you have obtained a complete history, and thorough assessment, the attending physician may feel comfortable enough to allow administration of narcotics in the field. Pain-free or reduced pain transport will greatly reduce your patient's anxiety.

Detailed Physical Examination

The overall detailed physical examination is intended to get a complete picture of your patient's health and needs. When you are conducting this examination, pay special attention to the details that are specific to women.

Starting at the head, examine the condition of the patient's hair. Is it clean, dirty, oily, or dry and brittle? Most women take great care in their physical appearance; failure to do so may indicate depression. Dry and brittle hair may indicate vitamin deficiencies or chronic methamphetamine use. Examine the way the hair is styled. Does it cover one side of the face more than the other, as if the patient is trying to hide signs of physical abuse. Examine the teeth. Rotting teeth may also be a sign of methamphetamine use. Are there any sores on the patient's face? If yes, they may indicate an underlying condition or may signify illicit drug use.

How is the patient dressed? Long sleeves in hot weather may be an attempt to hide signs of abuse. Is the patient dressed too warmly for the season? This may indicate an illness affecting the body's thermoregulation ability. Do you see signs of bruising on the patient's upper torso or linear or odd-shaped bruises in various stages of healing? Again, these are potential signs of abuse. Do not palpate or examine the breasts unless there is a specific and documentable necessity to do so.

Is small scarring present on the abdomen? It may indicate diabetes and daily insulin shots, or it may signal illicit drug use. Examine the abdomen for the presence of bruising as well, then perform the same examination for the hips and legs. If drug use is suspected, inspect the webs between the toes and fingers because these spots may be used as injection sites in an attempt to hide the signs of use.

Last, check distal pulses and motor and sensory function, and note any deficits or remarkable findings.

You are the Paramedic Part 4

The patient's husband greets her as she is brought into the emergency department. She is taken immediately to the obstetric wing, where her physician awaits her. As you transfer care, the husband thanks you for getting her to the hospital so quickly. He said he felt much better knowing she was not alone.

Vital Signs	Recording Time: 20 Minutes
Level of consciousness	Alert, with a Glasgow Coma Scale score of 15
Skin	Pink, warm, and dry
Pulse	82 beats/min and regular
Blood pressure	110/60 mm Hg
Respirations	24 breaths/min
Sao_2	100% with oxygen at 4 l/min via nasal cannula

8. What do you believe is the source of her bleeding, cramping, and pain?

Ongoing Assessment

En route to the hospital, recheck your interventions and note any improvement (or decline) in the patient's condition. Remember to obtain serial vital signs. Pay specific attention to the needs of your patient, and accommodate her desire for conversation or silence. Do not focus on your paperwork. You are caring for a human being—the paperwork can wait until the patient has been delivered to the receiving facility.

General Management

The general management of a gynecologic patient is actually simple because there are few interventions you can initiate in the prehospital setting. Primary management will be directed at mitigating life threats, being supportive and compassionate, and protecting the patient's modesty. In most gynecologic emergencies, your role will be primarily investigatory. The more accurate and detailed the history and examination are, the better you will be at differentiating gynecologic and nongynecologic pathology. For all patients, assess and supply the appropriate oxygen needs. Obtain baseline vital signs, and continue to monitor vital signs throughout patient care for trends. Obtain a baseline electrocardiogram (ECG). Initiate fluid therapy, providing for pharmacologic interventions (pain management) or volume replacement as necessary. Provide transport. Protect the patient's modesty, and provide psychological care with a supportive attitude.

Management of Gynecologic Trauma

The female genital area is highly vascularized and very susceptible to trauma. Trauma sustained from motor vehicle collisions, sporting events, assault, and even consensual sex are common mechanisms of injury. Bleeding from genital trauma may be profuse (and very painful), and, if the patient is currently having her period, trying to differentiate between menstrual blood and trauma-related blood can be difficult.

Applying simple external pressure over the area of the laceration is usually sufficient to control bleeding. Bleeding from the *internal* genitalia, by contrast, can be massive and very difficult to control. Blindly packing the vagina is dangerous and is *not* recommended or even useful. A woman with exsanguinating vaginal hemorrhage must be treated as any other injured patient with exsanguinating hemorrhage—that is, she must be treated for shock and rapidly transported to the hospital.

Assessment of a patient with gynecologic trauma will focus on the following questions: What are her symptoms? Is there a mechanism of injury? Is the patient pale, cool, and diaphoretic? Does she appear fatigued? Anxious? Irritable? Is the patient using sanitary pads or tampons? Can she tell you how many pads have been soaked? An average pad holds about 30 ml of blood and a tampon about 20 ml. Is the blood a normal colour? Is it brighter or darker than normal? Do any clots appear in the

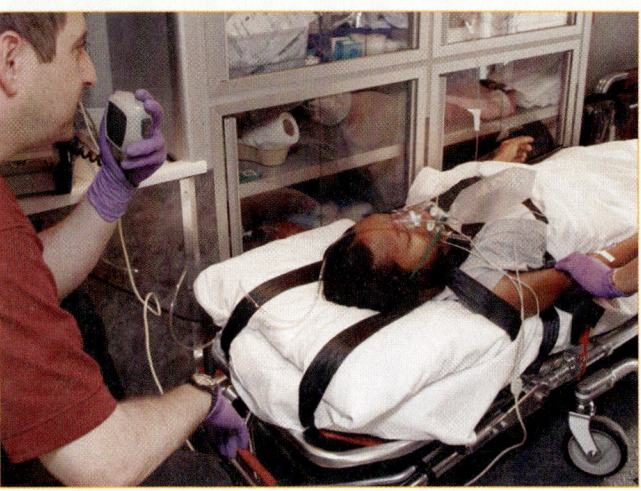

Figure 38-8 A patient with gynecologic trauma should be kept lying down. Manage the airway, administer supplemental oxygen and IV fluids, and monitor the ECG.

flow? Is the abdomen tender or distended? Affirmative answers may indicate that the patient is in the early stages of shock. Keep the patient recumbent. Ensure an adequate airway, administer oxygen, insert a large-bore IV cannula and give normal saline or lactated Ringer's solution, and monitor the ECG **Figure 38-8 ▲** . Assess vital signs frequently. Consider transport in the Trendelenburg position. Do *not* perform an interior vaginal examination. Examination of the external genitalia is warranted in the presence of genital trauma only.

Estimating Blood Loss

Estimating blood volume loss in the prehospital environment is a tricky business and cannot be done accurately, especially in female patients, in whom trauma and the menses may be found together. Nevertheless, some physicians may want you to make an estimate before arrival at the hospital. Visual estimation methods provide a very rough guess of total blood loss and fail to take into consideration blood that may be leaking into an internal cavity. The most reliable out-of-hospital method is based on symptomology and the patient's vital signs. **Table 38-2 ▶** shows estimated blood loss based on the patient's symptoms.

One rule of thumb is that for the average patient, 7% to 8% of body weight is the available circulating blood volume (70 ml/kg body weight). For example, a 70-kg patient has approximately 4,900 ml of available circulating blood. Thus, if the patient has the symptoms listed in Table 38-2 for 30% to 40% blood loss, you would estimate 1,470 to 1,960 ml of blood lost. Even the pulse changes listed in Table 38-2 are not highly reliable indicators—recent military studies have shown that that the heart rate can remain fairly stable even in severe cases of shock. Instead, consider the overall presentation of the patient. What are her symptoms? Is she pale, cool, or diaphoretic? Is she

Table 38-2   Estimating Blood Volume Loss

Grade of Hemorrhage/ Blood Loss	Heart Rate	Respiratory Rate	Blood Pressure	Central Nervous System
First/< 15%	Minor tachycardia	No change	No change	No change
Second/15%–30%	Tachycardia	Tachypnea	Decreased pulse pressure	Anxiety or combativeness
Third/30%–40%	Marked tachycardia	Marked tachypnea	Systolic hypotension	Altered mental status
Fourth/> 40%	Marked tachycardia	Marked tachypnea	Severe systolic hypotension	Comatose/unresponsive

Source: Adapted from United States Department of Defense. *Emergency War Surgery Nato Handbook.* 2004:Table 7-1. Available at: http://www.bordeninstitute .army.mil/emrgncywarsurg/Chp7Shock&Resuscitation.pdf. Accessed May 18, 2006.

thirsty? Do the symptoms include restlessness or nausea? This information paints a fuller picture regarding how much blood the patient has lost.

Assessment and Management of Specific Conditions

Of the several diverse gynecologic conditions that you may be called on to treat, an ectopic pregnancy is the one immediate life-threatening gynecologic emergency. Ruptured ovarian cysts and tubo-ovarian abscesses are rarely life threatening, but present with similar symptoms to an ectopic pregnancy. You may also be called on to treat conditions related to PID.

Pelvic Inflammatory Disease

A patient with PID will present with abdominal pain in virtually every scenario encountered by paramedics. The pain generally starts during or after normal menstruation, so eliciting the LMP is an important component of the history. The pain is typically diffuse and is spread over both quadrants of the lower abdomen. It may be described as "achy," and the patient may volunteer that the pain is made worse by walking or by sexual intercourse. The latter revelation usually indicates cervical involvement in the infective process. Pain localized to the right upper quadrant is indicative of infection that has spread to the abdominal cavity. Associated symptoms may include vaginal discharge, fever and chills, and pain or burning on urination (dysuria).

Notes from Nancy

In ectopic pregnancy, bleeding usually occurs *after* the onset of pain.

Any woman with PID who feels sick enough to call for an ambulance probably has a severe infection and is likely to present as febrile and look ill. Physical examination findings may be sparse or may include the entire textbook profile. Be alert for signs of peritoneal irritation (that is, the patient winces on palpation of the abdomen or every time the ambulance hits a

At the Scene

The ambulance does not carry the appropriate supplies and equipment for a definitive diagnosis in the prehospital setting. Look for life threats, treat for shock, and transport in a position of comfort.

bump). Be very gentle should you decide to palpate this patient's abdomen as part of the examination.

PID cannot be treated in the prehospital environment because it generally requires administration of an appropriate antibiotic for 10 to 14 days. The best you can do is obtain a thorough history, make the patient as comfortable as possible, and transport with as gentle a ride as can be managed.

Ectopic Pregnancy

Nearly all women with ectopic pregnancy will present with a chief complaint of abdominal pain. This pain will generally be localized to one side of the abdomen and, in the early stages, will be described as crampy and intermittent. As the pregnancy progresses, the embryo will abort or the tube will rupture. Either event will produce severe abdominal pain, localized to one side. By the time EMS is involved, the patient is likely to be in constant pain, which will be diffused throughout the abdomen.

In the history, you need to establish the intervals between the manifestations of the various symptoms. Part of the blood volume in ectopic pregnancy originates in the shedding of the uterine lining as the embryo is displaced from its site of implantation and the production of hormones ceases. Vaginal bleeding may itself be light, so it is not a good indicator of internal blood loss. The classic triad for diagnosing ectopic pregnancy is amenorrhea (75% of patients), vaginal bleeding, and abdominal pain. A history of ectopic pregnancy, IUD use, and a history of PID also significantly raise the index of suspicion. Only 50% of women will have a typical presentation. Approximately 20% of women will be hemodynamically unstable on initial presentation. Signs of shock will generally be a pulse greater than 100 beats/min; systolic blood pressure less than 90 mm Hg, cold, moist skin; fatigue; and restlessness and anxiety.

Always treat for shock in any woman presenting with abdominal pain and vaginal bleeding, regardless of whether shock symptoms are actually present **Figure 38-9 ▸** . Follow these steps in the management of a patient with a suspected ectopic pregnancy:

- Ensure an adequate airway, and administer high-concentration supplemental oxygen.
- Insert at least one large-bore IV cannula and administer lactated Ringer's solution or normal saline; be prepared to run it wide open if signs of shock develop.
- Give nothing by mouth, including water.
- Anticipate vomiting. Have an emesis bag and suction close at hand.
- Keep the patient warm.
- Monitor the patient's ECG.
- Transport.
- Notify the receiving hospital of the patient's suspected diagnosis, her condition, and your estimated time of arrival.
- The patient may require IV analgesics. Follow your local medical directives or contact direct medical control for further direction in the unstable patient.
- Recheck vital signs frequently during transport.

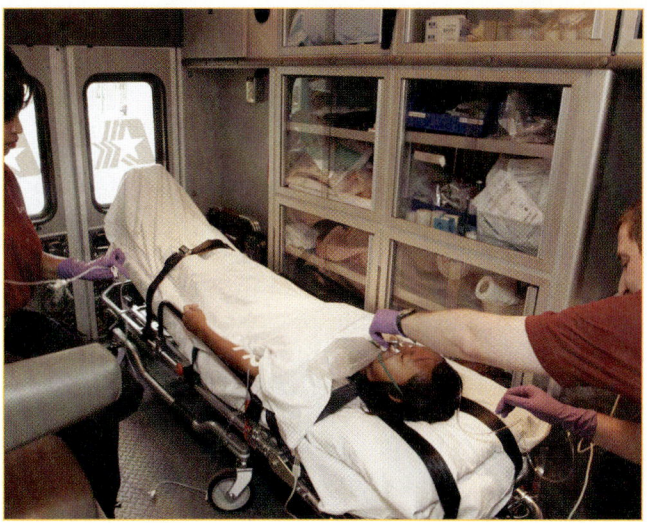

Figure 38-9 Always treat for shock in any woman with abdominal pain and vaginal bleeding.

Ruptured Ovarian Cyst and Tubo-ovarian Abscess

A patient with an ovarian cyst may complain of dull, achy pain in the lower back and thighs, abdominal pain or pressure, nausea and vomiting, breast tenderness, abnormal bleeding and painful menstruation, and painful intercourse. A patient with a tubo-ovarian abscess may present with severe abdominal pain, guarding and rebound tenderness, nausea and vomiting, abdominal distension, and fever. If the abscess ruptures, infectious matter can spread throughout the entire body. Ruptured ovarian cysts and tubo-ovarian abscesses are rarely life threatening, but cannot be differentiated from an ectopic pregnancy in the field. The prehospital management of ruptured ovarian cyst and tubo-ovarian abscess are the same as for ectopic pregnancy.

▍ Sexual Assault

Sexual assault is defined as any unwanted sexual act committed by one person upon another, ranging from unwanted sexual touching to rape. In Canada, approximately 50% of all women have experienced at least one incident of sexual or physical violence. Sixty percent report being under the age of 18 at the time of the assault. Less than 10% of sexual assault victims report the assault to the police.

Paramedics called on to treat a victim of sexual assault, molestation, or actual or alleged rape face many complex issues, ranging from obvious medical ones to serious psychological and legal issues. In particular, you may be the first person the victim has contact with after the encounter, and how the situation is managed from first contact throughout

treatment and transport may have lasting effects for the patient and you. Professionalism, tact, kindness, and sensitivity are of paramount importance.

Because sexual assault is a *crime,* you can generally expect police involvement early in the situation. In many cases, EMS may be called by the police. Police officers generally have rudimentary medical training. Nevertheless, primary training for police officers focuses on *investigation,* not patient care.

A sexual assault victim incurs a significant and overwhelming psychological and physical trauma to their personhood. The act was most likely perpetrated by someone she knew and trusted. The last thing she wants to do is give a concise, detailed report of what she has just experienced, and attempting to elicit information in this manner most likely will cause the victim to "shut down." Whenever possible, a female sexual assault victim should be given the option of being treated by a female paramedic because the patient may be experiencing ambivalent feelings toward men in general; these feelings will hinder assessment and the patient's well-being.

The job of paramedics is to deal with the medical aspects of the case and to act as the patient advocate. In this capacity, it is important for you to focus on several key issues.

The first issue is the medical treatment of the patient. Is she physically injured? Are any life-threatening injuries present? Does the patient complain of any pain?

The second issue is your psychological care of the patient. Do not cross-examine her or attempt to elicit information for the benefit of the police. These issues will be handled later in the ED setting. Do not pass judgment on the patient, and protect her from the judgment of others on the scene.

Last, remember that you are at a crime scene. Although your job is to treat the *medical* aspects of the incident and not collect evidence, you still have a responsibility to *preserve* evidence. Do not cut through any clothing or throw away anything from the scene. Place bloodstained articles in separate paper (not plastic) bags. Obtain evidentiary bags from the police if necessary. Paper bags allow wet items to dry naturally, whereas plastic allows mould to grow and may destroy biological evidence.

It may also be necessary to gently persuade the patient to *not* clean herself up. This will be a natural desire on the part of the patient, stemming from the desire to "wash away" the humiliation and embarrassment of the assault. Valuable evidence can be destroyed in this process. The patient also needs to be discouraged from urinating, changing clothes, moving her bowels, or rinsing out her mouth. She will need to be photographed by law enforcement personnel as well, and the photographic record needs to be as accurate as possible. If the patient cannot be dissuaded from taking these actions, respect her feelings. Some patients may refuse transport altogether, and they have the right to do so. Do not simply accept this refusal and leave. Instead, try to persuade the patient to allow you to call a friend or relative who can stay with her or, better yet, with whom the victim can stay. Getting the patient away from the scene keeps her from having to constantly relive the experience by being subjected to the environment where the assault occurred. Many churches offer pastoral care to rape victims, and the patient may benefit from this resource if she has religious inclinations. Many communities also have rape crisis centres, with victim advocates on-call. Getting a professional advocate to the scene may help the patient deal with the trauma, and the advocate can better explain the necessities of evidence preservation in more compassionate detail. Be aware of the resources available to sexual assault victims in your community and offer to assist the patient in accessing these services if she desires.

Notes from Nancy

Find out if the woman has been injured. Do *not* ask questions about the incident itself.

Documentation and Communication

Just as you might be uncomfortable talking about your last sexual encounter to a total stranger, so your patient might feel a mix of emotions, including shame and frustration after being assaulted. A calm, nonjudgmental approach from a same-sex paramedic will be helpful.

Limit any physical examination to a brief survey for life-threatening injuries. Expose and examine the vaginal area only if there is evidence of bleeding that needs to be treated. Do everything possible to protect the patient's privacy. Examine and interview the patient with a minimum of people present, moving her to the ambulance if necessary.

The patient report is a legal document and, should the case result in an arrest and subsequent trial, may be subpoenaed. Keep the report concise, and record only what the patient stated in her own words. Use quotation marks to indicate that you are reporting the patient's version of events. Do not insert your own "opinion" as to whether the patient was raped or offer any conclusions that would validate or invalidate the patient's account of the event. Focus on the facts. Record all of your observations during the physical examination—the patient's emotional state, the condition of her clothing, obvious injuries, and so forth. Bear in mind that sexual assault is a *legal* diagnosis, not a medical diagnosis. Although sexual assault is a crime, it is up to the victim to decide whether to pursue formal charges and proceed with the investigation, unless the victim is a minor. Sexual assault of a minor requires mandatory reporting to the police.

Sexual Practices and Medical Emergencies

The human race is fascinated by sex. Indeed, the various ways humankind can engage in sexual acts has been a source of intense study and curiosity since the beginnings of recorded history. The Bible records the first sexual act between human beings in the book of Genesis. Other works that record the sexual interactions of men and women range from the *Kama Sutra* of ancient India to the modern lab reports of Masters and Johnson.

The most common sexual gynecologic emergency you may encounter is simply a foreign object that has become stuck in the vagina or anus. For example, a bottle may develop a vacuum inside of the body and stick to an interior structure. Attempts at removal by the patient may result in intense pain or even vaginal bleeding as internal structures tear. Bleeding and pain cause the patient to panic. With this type of call, keep the patient calm, protect her dignity as much as possible, and transport. Overpenetration of any item may lead to internal injury or peritonitis, and should be managed as such.

Some cases of bottle insertion may be associated with sexual assault. Use extreme care and do not move the patient more than necessary to prevent even more internal damage.

Among some of the more bizarre practices you may encounter include a technique known as "fisting" and the insertion of live animals into the vagina or rectum. The patient becomes alarmed when the animal goes in but does not come out. Treat such a case as you would with any other foreign object, remain nonjudgmental, and transport. Do not attempt to retrieve the foreign body from inside the vagina. Transport the patient in a knees-flexed, legs-together position.

Documentation and Communication

"Fisting" involves placing the closed fist and wrist into a body orifice (vagina or rectum) for sexual stimulation. Whether the patient is male or female, organ rupture (rectum, vagina) is likely. Life-threatening peritonitis may result. As with other sexually related injuries, patients are often reluctant to divulge correct historical information.

Drugs Used to Facilitate Sexual Assault

Alcohol was probably the first drug used to facilitate sexual assault and, even in this modern age, remains the most common element to sexual assault scenes. The perpetrator and the victim may be intoxicated; as the central nervous system becomes depressed, the perpetrator becomes more aggressive and the victim more vulnerable. Some of the earliest reports in the United States of a drug other than alcohol used in crimes date back to the late 1800s, when legend has it that a Chicago bar owner named Mickey Finn would slip patrons drops of chloral hydrate in their drinks, for the purpose of knocking them out for robbery. Today, the drugs of choice for commission of the crime of sexual assault are "club drugs" such as gamma-hydroxybutyrate (GHB), ketamine, ecstasy, and Rohypnol.

Gamma-Hydroxybutyrate

Gamma-hydroxybutyrate (GHB) is the best known of the date-rape drugs. During the 1980s, it was available over-the-counter in nutrition stores as a body-building aid, sexual aid, and sleep aid. Illegally produced GHB is very common in the "rave" and "club" crowds. This colourless liquid generally has a salty taste that is disguised when mixed in with a drink. Street names for GHB include Georgia home boy, grievous bodily harm, easy lay, G, scoop, liquid X, soap, and salty water.

GHB is a depressant and has amnestic properties. Symptoms of GHB intoxication range from sleepiness, loss of muscle tone, and forgetfulness to seizurelike activity. Respirations and heartbeat are depressed, progressing to a comalike state that generally last about 2 hours. Prehospital care is supportive, making sure that adequate ventilatory support is initiated for patients in respiratory depression. There is no current antidote for GHB ingestion, and naloxone (Narcan) and flumazenil (a benzodiazepine agonist) are of no benefit.

Ketamine Hydrochloride

Ketamine hydrochloride (Ketalar, Ketaset) is predominantly marketed as a veterinary anesthetic. It works well in this capacity owing to its ability to block pain pathways without affecting respiratory or circulatory function. Ketamine also has some use in human medicine owing to its dissociative effects, and it can be effective in cases of major trauma, such as burn injuries. It creates an "out of body" sensation that removes the patient from the pain stimulus. In some people, it may produce frightening hallucinations. The hallucinatory effects make this drug popular with the club crowd, and the anesthetic and dissociative effects make it a popular date-rape drug. Street names for this agent include special K, vitamin K, cat Valium, and Fort Dodge.

A phencyclidine hydrochloride (PCP) derivative, ketamine has physical effects similar to those of PCP, plus psychedelic effects resembling those associated with LSD (lysergic acid diethylamide). It is available in liquid and powder form and can be inhaled, injected, or mixed into a drink. Symptoms of ketamine use include loss of coordination, muscle rigidity, slurred speech, and a catatonic or "blank" stare. The anesthetic properties may also produce a general sense of "numbness." Like PCP, ketamine can lead to aggressive and violent behaviour and an exaggerated sense of strength. Physiologic symptoms of overdose include nausea and vomiting, hypertension, and respiratory impairment leading to oxygen deprivation of the brain. There is no out-of-hospital antidote for ketamine.

Ecstasy

Methylenedioxymethamphetamine (MDMA), also known as ecstasy, is a methamphetamine derivative with hallucinogenic properties. It is generally sold in capsule or tablet form but can also be found as a powder. It can be injected, snorted, ingested, or smoked. The tablets come in many colours and may be imprinted with the Superman, Batman, Nike, Mercedes, Rolls Royce, or any of many other logos. Street names for ecstasy include XTC, Adam, X, lover's speed, and clarity. Although law enforcement reports cite it as a date-rape drug, ecstasy is actually a stimulant. Mental confusion is a side effect of its ingestion, and overdose can result in unconsciousness and death. Ecstasy affects serotonin levels in the brain, which probably explains the reports of heightened sexual experiences and feelings of tranquility the drug allegedly produces. These effects also explain why it is included in the date-rape category—the powder can be mixed in an alcoholic drink to get the victim "in the mood."

The signs and symptoms of ecstasy use are similar to those of cocaine and speed. The most serious are a rapid heart rate and rapid increase of body temperature, often to deadly levels. Other symptoms include anxiety, hypertension, blurred vision, mental confusion, nausea, and excessive sweating, leading to dangerous levels of dehydration. Rapid eye movement and tremors have also been reported. Bruxism (teeth clenching) is another common side effect, and regular users may use paraphernalia such as rubber or candy pacifiers to ease the effects. A surgical mask smeared with Vicks VapoRub is also a clue of ecstasy use because the vapours reportedly increase the effect of the "rush."

Rohypnol

Rohypnol is one of the latest drugs to hit the club scene and be used as a date-rape drug. Rohypnol is illegal in Canada but is legally marketed in 64 countries around the world by Roche Pharmaceutical as a sedative and preoperative anesthetic. This benzodiazepine has sedative-hypnotic, amnestic, and anesthetic properties. Street names for Rohypnol include roofies, roof, roachies, rocha, and Mexican Valium.

Rohypnol is sold as a white, scored tablet, with the word "Roche" appearing on one side. The tablet can be dissolved in a drink, where it is undetectable. Roche Pharmaceuticals has recently added a colour base of royal blue to the tablet; if the drug is mixed with a drink, the colour will appear.

When ingested, Rohypnol impairs judgment and motor skills, creating a condition in which the victim is unable to resist a sexual attack. Its sedative-hypnotic effects also make victims highly prone to suggestion. Losing social inhibitions (disinhibition) is a reported side effect of Rohypnol when taken alone or in combination with alcohol. The potentiated effect of alcohol on Rohypnol creates a significant danger.

Effects generally begin within 30 minutes after Rohypnol is consumed and last for about 8 hours, with peak effects occurring about 2 hours after ingestion. Symptoms include decreased blood pressure, drowsiness, dizziness, confusion, and memory loss. This last effect makes Rohypnol a particularly popular date-rape drug because the victim has no memory of the last 15 to 20 minutes or longer before blacking out. Overdose can lead to death due to central nervous system depression. Treatment in the prehospital setting is ALS supportive, with possible administration of flumazenil. Naloxone (Narcan) has no effect on Rohypnol, but its administration may be considered because Rohypnol is sometimes used in conjunction with other drugs.

You are the Paramedic Summary

1. Based on your general impression and initial assessment, how would you categorize this patient?

Based on her mentation, skin signs, and vital signs, Mrs. Medina appears to be in no immediate danger. At this point, she is in stable condition, which allows for more thorough history taking and assessment. Be aware that her condition could change, though.

2. What interventions would you choose to initiate at this point?

Although she appears to be well ventilated and oxygenated and shows no signs of shock, your patient will benefit from supplemental oxygen and IV access. Keeping her on her side and covering her to preserve body temperature are other important aspects of prehospital care.

3. What other information would you like to know?

Obtaining a SAMPLE history is very important, as is conducting a thorough physical examination, including inspection, auscultation, and palpation of the abdomen. You also need to estimate blood loss, which can be done by asking your patient about the number and type of pads she has used since the spotting began.

4. What issues do you foresee that will likely impact patient prehospital care?

The patient is understandably very frightened. Your management of her will require gentle care, compassion, and utmost respect for preserving her modesty. When you perform your assessment, explain everything that you are doing and why you are doing it. Establishing and maintaining trust with your patient will go a long way for both of you.

5. Given the information you have so far, will this patient require aggressive prehospital care?

Sometimes your job is to "hover." Because most paramedics have an inherent drive to "take action," sometimes watching and anticipating problems can be quite a challenge.

6. What are the three truly life-threatening gynecologic emergencies?

The three truly life-threatening emergencies discussed in this chapter are ectopic pregnancy, ruptured ovarian cysts, and tubo-ovarian abscesses. None of your findings correspond to those found in any of these conditions. In particular, this patient does not present with signs of shock.

7. Does your differential diagnosis include any of these conditions?

Based on this information, your differential diagnosis would not include ectopic pregnancy, ruptured ovarian cyst, and tubo-ovarian abscess. The patient could be experiencing the onset of a spontaneous abortion, hormonal imbalances, or stress.

8. What do you believe is the source of her bleeding, cramping, and pain?

Sometimes we find ourselves scratching our heads as to the underlying condition that causes a specific patient presentation. Sometimes we are never certain. Focus on recognizing and treating life-threatening emergencies and keep a suspicious eye out for the worst-case scenarios.

Prep Kit

Ready for Review

- Gynecology is the study of and care for diseases of the female reproductive system.
- The external anatomy of the female genitalia, sometimes referred to as the vulvar area, includes the mons veneris, labia majora, labia minora, clitoris, prepuce, and vestibule.
- The internal anatomy of the female genitalia includes the vagina, Bartholin glands, and the hymen (before rupture).
- Menstruation (menses or period) is the vaginal discharge of primarily blood that generally occurs every 25 to 34 days in premenopausal women.
- A woman can experience physical changes during the menstrual cycle that result in fluid retention, breast pain and tenderness, headache, cramping, and more intense emotional states. This premenstrual syndrome can be debilitating.
- The last menses is called menopause; it generally occurs between the ages of 40 and 50 years. Women may experience physical symptoms of menopause, including diaphoresis, hair loss, hot flashes, muscle aches and pains, headache, dyspnea, vertigo, digestive problems, and emotional instability.
- Mittelschmerz is abdominal pain and cramping that occur about 2 weeks before menstruation. Dysmenorrhea is painful menstruation. Prehospital treatment is supportive.
- Amenorrhea is the absence or cessation of menses. The most common cause is pregnancy. Amenorrhea can also occur in athletes and in people with anorexia nervosa or emotional problems.
- Endometritis is inflammation or irritation of the endometrium. Symptoms include malaise, fever, bowel problems, vaginal bleeding, abdominal distension, and lower abdominal or pelvic pain.
- Endometriosis is the growth of endometrial tissue outside of the uterus. It can cause infertility. Symptoms include low back, pelvic, or abdominal pain; painful coitus; elimination problems during menstruation; menstrual cramping; and heavy menstruation.
- Pelvic inflammatory disease (PID) is an infection of the female upper reproductive organs. One of the most common causes of abdominal pain in women, it can cause infertility.
- Interstitial cystitis is a chronically inflamed or irritated bladder wall. Symptoms may mimic those of gynecologic origin.
- In ectopic pregnancy, a fertilized egg implants somewhere other than the uterus, usually in a fallopian tube, which can lead to rupture of the fallopian tube.
- Ruptured ovarian cyst and tubo-ovarian abscess are other gynecologic conditions that can become an emergency.
- Toxic shock syndrome is a form of septic shock that can result from an infection in the body. Symptoms include syncope, myalgia, diarrhea, vomiting, headache, fever, sore throat, petechiae, rash, and bloodshot eyes. Transport patients rapidly.
- Sexually transmitted diseases (STDs) can cause PID. STDs include chancroid, chlamydia, genital herpes, gonorrhea, syphilis, and trichomoniasis.
- Symptoms of STDs can include itching, burning, pain, fishy smelling discharge, sores around the genitals, swollen or painful lymph glands, lower abdominal or back pain, nausea, fever, painful intercourse, bleeding between menstrual periods, fatigue, headache, and painful urination.
- When assessing a patient with a gynecologic emergency, begin by focusing on the ABCs.
- Protect the patient's modesty at all times. Gynecologic emergencies can be very embarrassing for the patient.
- If the chief complaint is abdominal pain, investigate the pain by following the mnemonic LORDS TRACHEA: Location, Onset, Radiation, Duration, Severity, Timing, Relief, Aggravation, Character, History, Eating, and Associated symptoms.

- Determine when the patient had her last menstrual period, if it is unusual in any way, whether she could be pregnant, and whether she uses contraception.
- Vaginal bleeding that does not occur during the course of regular menstruation is cause for concern. Consider whether there is a mechanism of injury. Try to obtain an accurate description of the bleeding.
- During the patient history, obtain the patient's obstetric history, including any previous pregnancies, miscarriages, or abortions. If the patient has a vaginal discharge, obtain a description of it.
- During the physical examination, determine whether there is a life-threatening condition. Inspect the abdomen for signs of abuse. Palpate the painful quadrant last.
- Abdominal pain can be visceral, parietal, or referred. Management should be psychologically supportive.
- General management for gynecologic emergencies is simple, including addressing life threats, being supportive, and protecting the patient's modesty.
- Gynecologic trauma may cause profuse bleeding. Control external bleeding using pressure over the area, but never pack the vagina. Attempt to estimate the patient's blood loss.
- Patients with PID will present with abdominal pain starting during or after menstruation. Take a thorough history and transport gently.
- The three life-threatening gynecologic emergencies are ectopic pregnancy, ruptured ovarian cyst, and tubo-ovarian abscess. Patients will present with abdominal pain and possibly vaginal bleeding, nausea, vomiting, or fever. Identify when each symptom began. Management includes airway maintenance, supplemental oxygen, positioning the patient on the left side, IV fluids, keeping the patient warm, monitoring the ECG, and transporting.
- Sexual assault is a category of crime that includes molestation and rape. Your compassion and professionalism in these situations are of the utmost importance.
- It may be difficult to obtain a history from a victim of sexual assault. Have a female paramedic treat the patient when possible.
- Remember that your job is to medically treat the patient. Ask only medical questions, and do not judge the patient. Limit the physical examination to addressing life-threatening injuries.
- Preserve evidence when possible. Try to persuade the sexual assault victim not to clean herself.
- If a sexual assault victim refuses transport, try to call a friend or relative with whom she can stay.
- Document cases of sexual assault properly and professionally. Report the patient's words in quotation marks. Record facts obtained from the physical examination.
- Sexual emergencies may involve foreign objects stuck in the vagina or anus, which may potentially lead to internal injury. Do not remove the object. Remain professional, and transport the patient.
- Drugs used to facilitate rape include gamma-hydroxybutyrate, acid, ketamine hydrochloride, ecstasy, and Rohypnol. These drugs can cause sleepiness, forgetfulness, numbness, loss of inhibitions, or rapid heart rate and increase in body temperature, depending on the drug.

Vital Vocabulary

amenorrhea Absence of menstruation.

bacterial vaginosis An overgrowth of bacteria in the vagina, characterized by itching, burning, or pain, and possibly a "fishy" smelling discharge.

Bartholin glands The glands that secrete mucus for sexual lubrication.

chancroid A highly contagious sexually transmitted disease caused by the bacteria *Haemophilus ducreyi*, which causes painful sores (ulcers), usually of the genitals.

chlamydia A sexually transmitted disease caused by the bacterium *Chlamydia trachomatis.*

climacteric End phase of a woman's life menstrual cycle.

clitoris A small, cylindrical mass of erectile tissue and nerves located at the anterior junction of the labia minora, homologous to the glans penis of the male.

contraceptive device A device used to prevent pregnancy.

cystadenomas Fluid-filled cysts that form on the outer ovarian surface.

dermoid cysts Ovarian cysts containing formational tissue, such as hair and teeth.

dysmenorrhea Painful menstruation.

ecstasy A drug officially named methylenedioxymethamphetamine (MDMA) that is sometimes used to facilitate date rape; a methamphetamine derivative with hallucinogenic properties; street names include XTC, Adam, X, lover's speed, and clarity.

ectopic pregnancy A pregnancy in which the ovum implants somewhere other than the uterine endometrium.

endometriomas Ovarian cysts formed from endometrial tissue.

endometriosis A condition in which endometrial tissue grows outside the uterus.

gamma-hydroxybutyrate (GHB) A drug used to facilitate date rape; is colourless with a salty taste disguised when mixed with a drink; street names include Georgia home boy, grievous bodily harm, easy lay, G, scoop, liquid X, soap, and salty water.

genital herpes An infection of the genitals, buttocks, or anal area caused by herpes simplex virus (HSV), which may cause sores of the genitals, mouth, or lips.

genital warts Warts caused by the human papillomavirus (HPV), a sexually transmitted disease; also called condylomata acuminata or venereal warts.

gonorrhea A sexually transmitted disease caused by *Neisseria gonorrhoeae.*

gravid Pregnant; the number of times a woman has been pregnant is indicated by gravida, for example, gravida 3 indicates three pregnancies.

hemorrhagic cyst A blood-filled sac that forms when a blood vessel bursts in a cyst wall and the blood fills the sac.

hymen A membrane that protects the vaginal orifice before first intercourse.

imperforate hymen A situation in which the hymen completely covers the vaginal orifice.

ketamine hydrochloride A drug used to facilitate date rape but that is predominantly marketed in Canada as a veterinary anesthetic and is a phencyclidine hydrochloride derivative; street names include special K, vitamin K, cat Valium, and Fort Dodge.

labia majora Outer fleshy skin folds covered with pubic hair that protect the vagina.

labia minora Inner fleshy skin folds devoid of pubic hair that protect the vagina.

menarche The beginning phase of a woman's life cycle of menstruation.

menopause The ending phase of a woman's life cycle of menstruation.

menorrhagia Menstrual blood flow that lasts several days longer than it should or flow that is abnormally excessive.

menstrual cycle The entire monthly cycle of menstruation from start to finish.

menstruation Monthly flow of blood.

metrorrhagia Irregular but frequent vaginal bleeding.

mons veneris Also called the mons pubis, this is a rounded pad of fatty tissue that overlies the symphysis pubis and is anterior to the urethral and vaginal openings.

parietal pain Pain caused by inflammation of the parietal peritoneum that is generally described as steady, aching, and aggravated by movement.

parity Number of live births a woman has had.

perineum The area between the vaginal opening and the anus.

pelvic inflammatory disease (PID) An infection of the female upper organs of reproduction, specifically the uterus, ovaries, and fallopian tubes.

polymenorrhea Menstrual blood flow that occurs more often than a 24-day interval.

premenstrual syndrome (PMS) A cluster of all or some of the troubling symptoms that occur during a woman's menstrual phase that can include fluid retention, breast pain and tenderness, headache, severe cramping, and emotional changes, including agitation, irritability, depression, and anger.

prepuce In the anatomy of the female genitalia, a layer of skin directly above the clitoris.

pudendum The female external genitalia.

rape Sexual intercourse inflicted forcibly on another person, against that person's will.

referred pain Pain that seems to radiate or travel as it becomes more intense.

Rohypnol A benzodiazepine used to facilitate date rape and that can create memory loss; street names include roofies, roof, roachies, rocha, and Mexican Valium.

ruptured ovarian cyst A fluid-filled sac within the ovary that bursts from internal pressure.

sexual assault An attack against a person that is sexual in nature, the most of common of which is rape.

syphilis A sexually transmitted disease caused by the bacterium *Treponema pallidum*, which manifests in three stages—primary, secondary, and late—and is transmitted through direct contact with open sores.

toxic shock syndrome (TSS) A form of septic shock caused by *Streptococcus pyogenes* (group A strep) or *Staphylococcus aureus;* initial symptoms include syncope, myalgia, diarrhea, vomiting, headache, fever, and sore throat.

trichomoniasis A parasitic infection.

tubo-ovarian abscess An infectious mass growing within the ovaries and fallopian tubes.

vagina The lower portion of the birth canal, which also serves as a passage for menstrual flow and as the receptacle of the penis during sexual intercourse.

vaginal bleeding Bleeding from the vagina.

vaginal yeast infection An infection caused by the fungus, *Candida albicans*, in which fungi overpopulate the vagina.

vestibule A cleft between the labia minora, where the urethral opening (orifice), the vaginal opening (orifice), and the hymen are located.

visceral pain Pain caused by some dysfunction of the hollow abdominal organs and is generally poorly localized and diffuse.

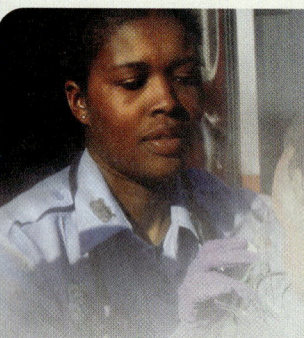

Assessment in Action

You are dispatched to a call for abdominal pain in an office building. When you arrive on scene, you are led to the cubicle of a 21-year-old woman who is bent over at the waist complaining of severe pain in her pelvic region. She states her pain began last night while she was watching TV and states that it's becoming unbearable. Her vital signs are a respiratory rate of 24 breaths/min, blood pressure of 130/74 mm Hg, a heart rate of 120 beats/min, sinus tachycardia on the ECG monitor, and a pulse oximetry reading of 100% while breathing room air. She tells you that she is currently menstruating so there is no chance she is pregnant. Her bleeding is normal. She takes birth control pills.

1. **How long does the normal menstrual cycle last?**
   A. Generally 14 days and occurs at regular intervals from puberty to menopause
   B. Generally 21 days and occurs at regular intervals from puberty to menopause
   C. Generally 28 days and occurs at regular intervals from puberty to menopause
   D. Generally 35 days and occurs at regular intervals from puberty to menopause

2. **When should you ask about sexual activity?**
   A. Whenever you have a patient who might be pregnant
   B. In all patients with abdominal pain
   C. In all adult women but not children
   D. In all women except older women

3. **Some potential causes of this patient's pain include all the following, EXCEPT:**
   A. ectopic pregnancy.
   B. pelvic inflammatory disease.
   C. ruptured ovarian cyst.
   D. none of the above.

4. **An infection in the female reproductive system and surrounding organs that can lead to sepsis and infertility is called:**
   A. ruptured ovarian cyst.
   B. endometriosis.
   C. pelvic inflammatory disease.
   D. spontaneous abortion.

5. **The inflammation of PID frequently follows the onset of menstrual bleeding by:**
   A. 1 to 3 days.
   B. 4 to 6 days.
   C. 7 to 10 days.
   D. 14 to 21 days.

6. **A ruptured ovarian cyst may mimic all of the following, EXCEPT:**
   A. appendicitis.
   B. cholecystitis.
   C. ectopic pregnancy.
   D. salpingitis.

7. **Ectopic pregnancy usually presents with:**
   A. missed periods, watery periods, nausea, vomiting, or frequent urination.
   B. the Kehr sign, breast tenderness, nausea, vomiting, and shortness of breath.
   C. chest pain, low blood glucose level, and frequent urination.
   D. elevated white blood cell count, low SpO_2, and hyperglycemia.

8. **Gynecologic emergencies are classified into which of the following three groups?**
   A. Nontraumatic, traumatic, and sexual assault
   B. Normal, traumatic, and sexual assault
   C. Self-inflicted, nontraumatic, and sexual assault
   D. Sexual assault, nontraumatic, and hereditary

9. **What is mittelschmerz?**
   A. Lower abdominal pain experienced by some women at the time of ovulation
   B. Upper abdominal pain experienced by some women at the time of ovulation
   C. The absence of pain during menstruation
   D. Painful menses but also may be associated with headache, syncope, backache, and leg pain

10. **Endometritis is inflammation of the:**
    A. uterine lining.
    B. ovaries.
    C. fallopian tubes.
    D. endometrial wall.

11. **What are the complications of vaginal bleeding?**
    A. Uncontrolled vaginal bleeding can lead to hypovolemia, shock, and death.
    B. Uncontrolled vaginal bleeding can lead to hypertension.
    C. Uncontrolled vaginal bleeding can lead to endometriosis.
    D. Uncontrolled vaginal bleeding can lead to cystitis.

Challenging Questions

12. **What is the prehospital treatment for a ruptured ectopic pregnancy?**

Points to Ponder

You are dispatched to the local college campus for an assault. When you arrive on scene, you are met by campus security personnel and informed of an alleged assault on a 19-year-old female student. When you begin your assessment, you note that the patient is in a fetal position and appears to be in a catatonic state. She is nonverbal and stares at the wall. The patient does not make any eye contact with you when you call her name. You note that she has bruises on her face and her wrists and is wrapped in a blanket.

How can you interview this patient in a way that will yield the information you need without further upsetting her?

Issues: Protecting a Patient's Modesty and Privacy, Obtaining Necessary Information in a Sensitive Way, Providing Appropriate Care for a Victim of a Sexual Assault.

39 Obstetric Emergencies

Competency Areas

Area 1: Professional Responsibilities

1.1.a	Maintain patient dignity.
1.1.e	Maintain patient confidentiality.
1.1.k	Function as patient advocate.
1.3.b	Recognize "patient rights" and the implications on the role of the provider.

Area 2: Communication

2.1.e	Interact effectively with the patient, relatives, and bystanders who are in stressful situations.
2.1.f	Speak in language appropriate to the listener.
2.1.g	Use appropriate terminology.
2.3.c	Establish trust and rapport with patients and colleagues.
2.4.a	Treat others with respect.
2.4.c	Recognize and react appropriately to individuals and groups manifesting coping mechanisms.
2.4.g	Exhibit diplomacy, tact, and discretion.

Area 4: Assessment and Diagnostics

4.2.c	Obtain chief complaint and/or incident history from patient, family members, and/or bystanders.
4.2.d	Obtain information regarding patient's past medical history.
4.2.e	Obtain information about patient's last oral intake.
4.3.a	Conduct primary patient assessment and interpret findings.
4.3.b	Conduct secondary patient assessment and interpret findings.
4.3.f	Conduct obstetrical assessment and interpret findings.
4.3.o	Conduct neonatal assessment and interpret findings.
4.4.a	Assess pulse.
4.4.b	Assess respiration.

Area 5: Therapeutics

5.1.h	Utilize airway devices requiring visualization of vocal cords and introduced endotracheally.
5.2.a	Recognize indications for oxygen administration.
5.3.c	Administer oxygen using controlled concentration mask.
5.5.c	Maintain peripheral intravenous (IV) access devices and infusions of crystalloid solutions without additives.

Area 6: Integration

6.1.d	Provide care to patient experiencing illness or injury primarily involving genitourinary/reproductive systems.
6.1.q	Provide care for patient in labour.
6.2.a	Provide care for neonatal patient.
6.3.a	Conduct ongoing assessments based on patient presentation and interpret findings.

Appendix 4: Pathophysiology

A.	**Cardiovascular System**
	Vascular Disease: Hypertension
B.	**Neurologic System**
	Convulsive Disorders: Generalized seizures
C.	**Respiratory System**
	Medical Illness: Pulmonary embolism
	Medical Illness: Reactive airways disease/asthma
D.	**Female Reproductive System and Neonates**
	Pregnancy Complications: Abruptio placenta
	Pregnancy Complications: Eclampsia
	Pregnancy Complications: Ectopic pregnancy
	Pregnancy Complications: First trimester bleeding
	Pregnancy Complications: Placenta previa
	Pregnancy Complications: Pre-eclampsia
	Pregnancy Complications: Third trimester bleeding
	Pregnancy Complications: Uterine rupture
	Childbirth Complications: Abnormal presentations
	Childbirth Complications: Post partum complications
	Childbirth Complications: Post partum hemorrhage
	Childbirth Complications: Prolapsed cord
	Childbirth Complications: Uterine inversion
F.	**Genitourinary System**
	Renal/Bladder: Obstruction
I.	**Endocrine System**
	Diabetes mellitus
	Thyroid disease
J.	**Multisystem Diseases and Injuries**
	Hematologic Disorders: Sickle cell disease

Appendix 5: Medications

A.	**Medications affecting the central nervous system.**
A.3	Anticonvulsants
G.	**Medications affecting labour, delivery, and post partum hemorrhage.**
G.1	Uterotonics
G.2	Tocolytics
H.	**Medications used to treat electrolyte and substrate imbalances.**
H.1	Vitamin and Electrolyte Supplements
H.2	Antihypoglycemic Agents
H.3	Insulin

Introduction

In Chapter 38, we discussed gynecology and medical emergencies unique to the female. This chapter goes a step further by discussing obstetric emergencies.

When you are responding to an obstetric crisis, keep several key issues in mind. First, pregnancy itself is not a disease that needs treatment; it is the natural continuation of the human species. Women have been having children without the benefit of emergency departments, painkillers, and enhanced 9-1-1 since time began. For the most part, childbirth is a happy event for all involved. Emotions may run rampant, however, ranging from delirious exuberance to panicked distress. You need to be the eye in the centre of the emotional hurricane, bringing professional calm and control to the scene. Second, the number of patients increases to a minimum of two—the expectant mother and the baby—or perhaps even more if more than one baby is expected.

Although childbirth and pregnancy are both naturally occurring states, they are not without potential complications, including maternal death and fetal death. With the advent of modern medicine, maternal and infant mortality rates have been significantly reduced, and close medical monitoring usually discovers problems long before childbirth. In developing nations, however, mortality remains high. Contributing factors include malnutrition, disease, lack of education, and lack of adequate medical care.

Anatomy of the Female Reproductive System

The female reproductive organs include the external organs that constitute the pudendum: mammary glands (breasts), vagina, uterus (womb), and ovaries and fallopian tubes. The ovaries are the beginning point for reproduction. These paired glands are found next to the uterus, one ovary on either side. They are about the size and shape of an unshelled almond and are homologous to the testes in the male (ie, they are essentially the female gonads). The ovaries are positioned in the upper pelvic cavity but typically descend to the brim of the pelvis during the third month of fetal development.

Each ovary contains about 200,000 follicles, and each follicle contains an oocyte (egg). The human female is born with all the eggs she will ever release (approximately 400,000). Each month, during the menstrual cycle, about 20 of these follicles begin the process of maturation, but only a single follicle ultimately matures and releases an ovum; the other follicles die in a process called atresia. (Chapter 38 covers the menstrual cycle.)

The maturation of an oocyte occurs when the follicular cells respond to follicle-stimulating hormone (FSH) released by the anterior pituitary gland, which is first stimulated by the release of gonadotropin-releasing factor (GnRF) from the hypothalamus. As the preovulatory phase of the menstrual cycle progresses, the anterior pituitary gland releases luteinizing hormone (LH), which stimulates the process of ovulation—that is, the release of the egg (or at this point, the ovum). LH continues to be excreted throughout the ovarian cycle and subsequent pregnancy, should it occur, stimulating the ovarian cells to produce the hormones relaxin, progesterone, and various estrogens.

What is left of the follicle after the egg has been released becomes the corpus luteum, which in turn secretes another female hormone, progesterone. Under the influence of progesterone, the secretory phase (the second phase of the menstrual cycle) takes place. The glands of the endometrium increase in size and secrete the materials on which the fertilized egg will implant and grow. There it will develop into an embryo and then a fetus   Figure 39-1 ▶ . If the ovum is *not* fertilized, however, it dies and degenerates 36 to 48 hours after being released. The corpus luteum also degenerates about 10 days later, and the endometrium then breaks down and is shed as menstrual flow on about the 28th day of the cycle (ie, about 14 days after ovulation).

You are the Paramedic Part 1

You are dispatched to a residence for a woman in labour. Upon arriving at the scene, you are escorted to the patient by her husband, who is clearly excited. He tells you that his wife's water broke about 3 hours ago, and that she is now having contractions. You find the patient lying on her left side on her bed. She is having regular contractions every 3 minutes—each lasting approximately 45 seconds. You perform an initial assessment.

Initial Assessment	Recording Time: 0 Minutes
Appearance	Conscious; holding her lower back; panting
Level of consciousness	A (Alert to person, place, and day)
Airway	Patent
Breathing	Increased respirations; adequate depth
Circulation	Radial pulses, rapid and strong; skin, pink and moist

1. What specific questions should you ask this patient?

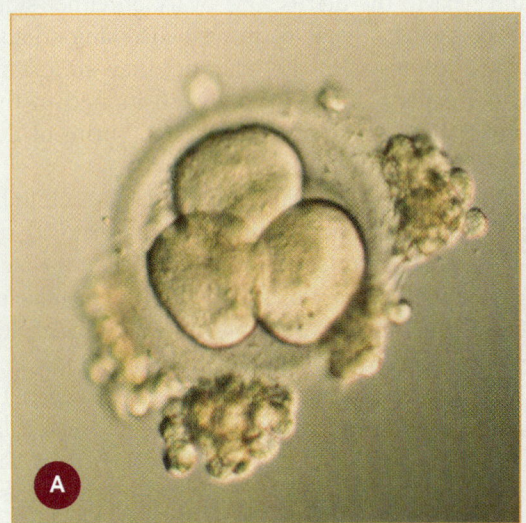 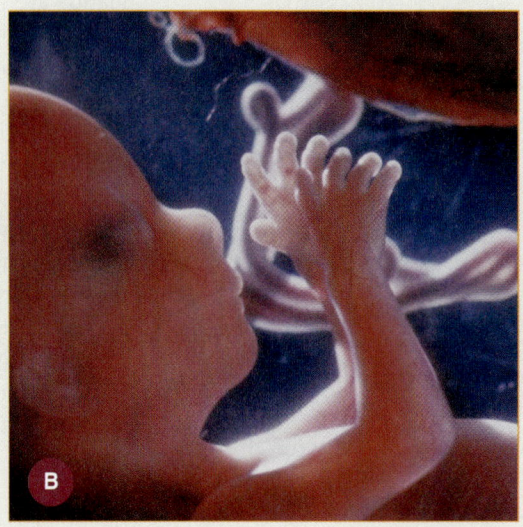

Figure 39-1 A. Embryo. **B.** Fetus.

The ova passes from the ovaries to the uterus through the fallopian tubes, or oviducts. These paired structures measure about 10 cm long. Each tube extends out laterally from the uterus, terminating just short of an ovary. The proximal end of each fallopian tube is very thick and narrow and connects to the uterus itself. Each fallopian tube comprises three layers of tissue: the internal mucosa, the muscularis, and the serosa. The serosa—the outer layer—consists of a serous membrane that protects the tubes. The muscularis—the middle layer—is made of smooth muscle; contractions of this layer help move the ovum through the tube and into the uterus. The internal mucosa—innermost layer—contains secretory cells and ciliated columnar cells, which also move the ovum along and may play a part in providing nutrition to the ovum. In summary, when an ovary releases an egg, the ciliary action of the fimbriae sweeps the egg into the infundibulum, and the actions of the internal mucosa and the muscularis provide the ovum with a short tube ride to the uterus. If the egg collides with a sperm cell somewhere along the length of the ampulla, it may become fertilized. Fertilization can occur at any time within about a 24-hour window following ovulation.

The uterus is a muscular, inverted pear-shaped organ that lies between the urinary bladder and the rectum. The dome-shaped top of the uterus is called the fundus. Below the dome, the uterus begins to taper and narrow, forming the body. The narrowest portion of the uterus, called the cervix, opens into the vagina; the junction of the two is called the external os. The interior of the body of the uterus is the uterine cavity, and the interior of the cervix is the cervical canal.

The uterus is where the fertilized ovum will implant, where the fetus will develop, and where the act of labour takes place. It consists of three layers of tissue: the perimetrium (outer protective layer), the myometrium (middle layer), and the endometrium (inner lining). The myometrium is composed of three layers of muscle fibres; the contractions of these muscles help expel the fetus during childbirth. The endometrium is a mucous membrane

composed of two layers, the stratum basalis and the stratum functionalis. The stratum functionalis, the layer innermost to the uterine cavity, is shed during menstruation. The stratum basalis is permanent and produces a new stratum functionalis following the period. As the follicle starts developing and pumping out estrogen, the endometrium is stimulated to increase its thickness in preparation for the reception and future growth of a fertilized egg (proliferative phase).

The vagina is a highly muscular, tubular organ lined with mucous membranes. It serves as a receptacle for the male penis during sexual intercourse, and allows for the exit of the menstrual flow. The interior of the vagina is acidic owing to the breakdown of glycogen (found in large amounts in the vaginal mucosa), which creates a low-pH environment that inhibits bacterial growth. This acidity, while beneficial, is injurious to sperm cells. Semen is alkaline in nature and likewise has antibacterial properties. The alkalinity of seminal fluid neutralizes the acidity of the vagina, allowing the sperm cells to survive and fertilize the ovum.

The vagina is the lower portion of the birth canal and can stretch widely to accommodate the delivery of a fetus. If the vagina is unable to stretch far enough, then the tissues in and around the perineum may tear, causing much pain and bleeding. In such cases, the attending physician may make an incision in the perineal skin called an episiotomy. In the prehospital setting, you are limited to providing gentle pressure against the infant's head to prevent an explosive birth and give the tissues time to expand.

The mammary glands (breasts) are modified sweat glands that are mainly composed of adipose tissue. Their primary purpose is lactation, or milk secretion, to provide nourishment to the newborn. Milk is carried to the surface of each breast through lactiferous ducts that terminate in a nipple. The nipple of the breast is surrounded by a darker pigmented area called the areola. Breast enlargement, tenderness, and milk excretion are all signs that a woman is most likely pregnant. Unilateral enlargement, discoloured or foul fluid excretion, or pain and tenderness in the breasts may indicate a more serious underlying condition.

Conception and Gestation

Once the egg has been fertilized and implanted in the endometrium of the uterus, both the egg and the pregnant woman begin to undergo major physiologic, hormonal, and chemical changes. The egg, upon entering the uterus, begins absorbing uterine fluid through the cell membrane. As the fluid fills the interior of the egg, cell division increases rapidly, and the cells multiply on the outside of the egg surface, forming layers that will eventually generate the fetal membrane, placenta, and embryo. The egg, now called a blastocyst, will migrate to the endometrial wall and become implanted there approximately 1 week after conception. Upon implantation, the egg will adhere to the endometrium, and enzymatic activity from the egg will dissolve endometrial tissue and provide nourishment for its development. Occasionally, the mechanism of implantation may result in vaginal bleeding that is spotty and painless, but of concern to the patient who does not yet realize her condition.

The implantation and subsequent actions of the blastocyst trigger the development of placental tissues, whose formation stimulates the release of human chorionic gonadotropin hormone, which in turn sends signals to the corpus luteum that pregnancy has begun. The corpus luteum then begins to produce hormones designed to support the pregnancy until the placenta has developed. By the second week after conception, the blastocyst has evolved into an embryonic disc, and the amniotic sac and placenta are starting to differentiate into their specialized duties. The developing placenta produces projections that tap into the external tissue layer (extra-embryonic ectodermal) tissue of the blastocyst, where spaces called lacunae have been formed. These spaces are filled with maternal blood, and the connection allows both the embryo to draw on the maternal circulation for oxygenation and nutrition and embryonic waste products to be shunted safely away. This connection serves as the beginning of the umbilical cord.

In the third week after conception, the egg, now officially the *embryo,* is ready to begin the process of forming specialized body systems. The rudiments of the central nervous system, cardiovascular system, spine, and portions of the skeletal anatomy begin to appear. At the end of this week, an S-shaped tubular heart begins to beat, and blood cells produced in the yolk sac begin to circulate. The pregnant woman, by this point, may notice that she has missed her period and begin to suspect that she is pregnant.

At around the 14th day after ovulation, the placenta begins to develop. Essentially an enlarged endocrine gland, the placenta carries out a number of crucial functions during pregnancy. The placenta serves as an early liver, taking care of the synthesis of glycogen and cholesterol, metabolizes fatty acid, and produces antibodies that protect the fetus. It also provides the following:

- **Respiratory gas exchange.** The placenta functions as the fetal lungs, enabling the fetus to exchange its carbon dioxide-laden blood for oxygen-rich blood.
- **Transport of nutrients** from maternal to fetal circulation.
- **Excretion of wastes,** some of which pass into the maternal circulation and others of which are excreted into the amniotic fluid.

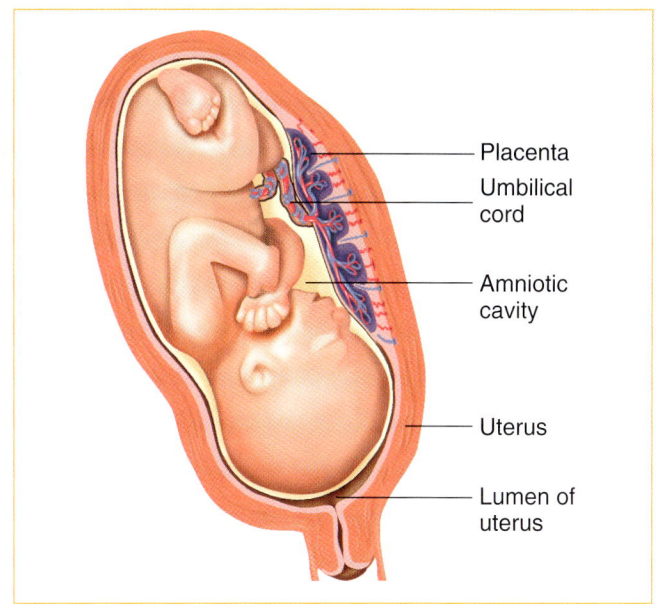

Figure 39-2 The umbilical cord and other structures of the pregnant uterus.

Labels: Placenta · Umbilical cord · Amniotic cavity · Uterus · Lumen of uterus

- **Transfer of heat** from mother to fetus.
- **Hormone production.** The placenta produces chorionic gonadotropin, a hormone that maintains the pregnancy and stimulates changes in the mother's breasts, vagina, and cervix that prepare her for delivery and motherhood.
- **Formation of a barrier** against harmful substances in the mother's circulation, such as chemicals or microorganisms. When the placenta blocks a drug from reaching the fetal bloodstream, we say that the drug "does not cross the placenta." The placenta is not able to exclude every harmful substance, so you need to be very careful about which drugs are administered to women during pregnancy.

The umbilical cord connects the placenta to the fetus via the fetal umbilicus (navel) Figure 39-2 ▲ . The cord is grey, easily compressed, and soft and pliant though structurally tough. The interior of the cord contains a mucoid material (Wharton's jelly—it keeps the umbilical cord from becoming knotted) and a supportive framework of loose connective tissue. The umbilical cord also contains two arteries and one vein. Occasionally, a child will be born with only a single umbilical artery (SUA). SUA may be normal genetically in some children, but may also indicate a congenital abnormality, such as heart or kidney malformations.

Fetal circulation differs from that of the mother. The umbilical *vein* carries oxygenated blood from the placenta to the fetus, while the umbilical *arteries* carry deoxygenated blood to the placenta. Since the fetus obtains its oxygen via the placenta, the fetal circulation bypasses the lungs until birth. A duct connects the umbilical vein and the inferior vena cava, another duct connects the pulmonary artery and the aorta, and an opening connects the right and left atria of the fetal heart.

At birth, the neonate's lungs begin to function, and the arteriovenous shunts close.

The amniotic sac is a membranous bag that encloses the fetus in a watery fluid called amniotic fluid. The amniotic fluid, whose volume reaches about 1 l by the end of pregnancy, provides the fetus with a weightless environment in which to develop. In the latter stages of pregnancy, the fetus swallows amniotic fluid and passes wastes out into the fluid. In this way amniotic fluid assists in fetal excretory function.

The 4th through the 8th weeks of embryonic development are critical for normal development. During this period, the major organs and other body systems are forming and are most susceptible to damage. Some prescription drugs and even over-the-counter medications may have side effects that harm the fetus. Women who use illicit drugs, smoke tobacco, drink alcohol, or are exposed to other toxic substances during their pregnancy also run the risk of creating birth defects in the fetus.

The gestational period is the time that it takes for the infant to develop in utero. The gestational age of the pregnancy, however, can only be estimated from the last menstrual period, because the exact time of conception is often unknown. In a typical pregnancy where the woman has regular menstrual cycles, ovulation occurs about 2 weeks after the first day of the last menstrual period, and conception would occur around then, too. Due to the uncertainty of exactly when conception occurs, pregnancies are dated from the first day of the last menstrual period. It normally takes approximately 40 weeks (dated from the last menstrual period) to reach full-term, with significant developmental progress occurring each week. A full-term pregnancy where the fetus has reached full maturation of all organ systems is defined as between 37 to 42 weeks of gestation.

Physiologic Maternal Changes During Pregnancy

When a woman conceives, carries a baby to term, and then gives birth, several physiologic changes occur within her body. Many of these changes can alter the normal response to trauma or exacerbate or create medical conditions that can threaten the health of both the woman and baby. In particular, hormonal changes precipitate physiologic changes, and the rapidly changing internal environment puts stress on the woman. Metabolic demands increase during pregnancy, and the enlarging uterus with its significant vascularity creates mechanical changes as well.

The most significant physiologic changes occur in the uterus. Before a woman's first pregnancy, the uterus measures about 8 cm long by 5 cm wide and is approximately 2 cm thick. After pregnancy has stretched the uterus, it will rarely return to its previous dimensions. In the nonpregnant patient, the uterus weighs only about 2 g and has a fluid capacity of about 10 ml. By the end of pregnancy, the uterus may weigh as much as 1 kg and have a capacity of about 5,000 ml.

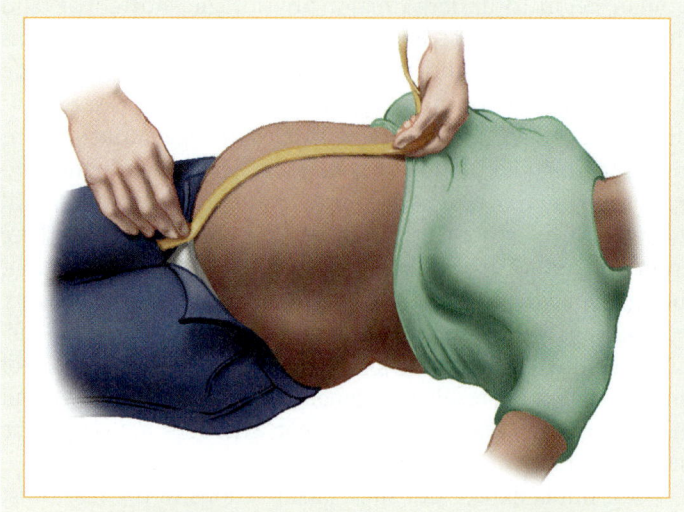

Figure 39-3 Measuring the fundus.

The measurement of the fundus of the uterus (the top portion, opposite the cervix) can indicate possible developmental problems. The fundus is measured in centimetres by running a measuring tape vertically from the top of the pubic bone to the top of the fundus **Figure 39-3 ▲**. The length in centimetres roughly corresponds to length of gestation. For example, if the patient is 32 weeks' pregnant, the measurement would be 32 cm. If the length is longer or shorter than expected, it could indicate uterine growth problems or breech position (if shorter) or the possibility of twins (if longer).

The circulatory system of a woman is impacted by pregnancy in several ways. The average woman has about 4 to 5 litres of blood available as total circulating volume. Blood volume in the pregnant female increases gradually throughout gestation, such that there may be as much as a 40% to 50% overall increase at term. The level of increase depends on such factors as patient size, number of times gravid (total pregnancies, but not necessarily carried to term) and para (pregnancies carried to more than 28 weeks' gestation, regardless of whether delivered dead or alive), and number of fetuses she is carrying. This increase in blood volume is necessary to meet the metabolic needs of the developing fetus, to adequately perfuse maternal organs—especially the uterus and kidneys—and to help compensate for blood loss during delivery. At term, the uterus normally contains 15% to 16% of the mother's total circulating blood volume. During vaginal delivery, a woman may lose as much as 500 ml of blood (1,000 ml in case of cesarean section). The uterus, as it contracts, tends to shunt blood back into maternal circulation (autotransfusion), thereby preserving maternal circulatory hemostasis.

As blood volume increases, so does the number of red blood cells (RBCs), which increase by as much as 33% over the normal count. The increase in RBCs heightens the pregnant woman's need for iron, which is why most women have to take prenatal vitamins. If the woman does not take iron supplements, the fetus will rob maternal stores for its needs, resulting in anemia for the woman—and often leading to preterm labour and spontaneous abortion. Women who live in socioeconomically deprived areas and lack access to prenatal health care are the most likely to experience pregnancy-related anemia.

A woman's white blood cell (WBC) count also increases during pregnancy, with an average of 4,300 to 4,500 cells/μl before pregnancy to as high as 12,000 cells/μl or more in the third trimester of pregnancy. Clotting factors are similarly increased, while fibrinolytic factors are depressed. These issues are important considerations if the paramedic has to deal with obstetric hemorrhage or thromboembolic disease.

As blood volume increases, so does the size of the pregnant woman's heart, by an average of 10% to 15% from prepregnancy levels, with a collateral capacity increase of 70 to 80 ml. Cardiac output increases to about 40% more than before pregnancy, reaching its maximum capacity at about 22 weeks' gestation and then maintaining this level until term. As the uterus enlarges and the diaphragm becomes elevated, internal maternal organs begin to shift to make room. The myocardium is displaced upward and to the left with a slight rotation in its long axis, which causes the apex of the heart to shift laterally (remember this point when auscultating the S_3 and S_4 heart sounds). In addition, the intensity of the "lub-dub" S_1 heart sound increases, while the S_2 heart sound generally remains normal. Increased cardiac output can also cause a benign systolic flow murmur, which results from hypertrophy of the heart and dilation across the tricuspid valve.

A pregnant woman's heart rate gradually increases during pregnancy, by an average of 15 to 20 beats/min by term. ECG changes that can occur during pregnancy include ectopic beats and supraventricular tachycardia, which is often considered normal. Other changes include a slight left axis deviation and lead III changes such as low-voltage QRS, T-wave inversion or flattening, or even occasional Q waves.

As gestation increases, a woman's sensitivity to body positioning increases as well. Resting or lying supine can cause the uterus to impinge upon the inferior vena cava, thereby decreasing venous return to the heart. Pressure by the fetus on the common iliac vein creates this problem as well. Over time, if pressure is not relieved, cardiac output is decreased, blood pressure drops, and lower extremity edema will result. In about the 12th week of gestation, systolic pressure may drop slightly, but diastolic pressure usually declines by 5 to 10 mm Hg. Diastolic pressure usually returns to normal prepregnancy levels at about 36 weeks' gestation.

The pressures exerted upon the circulatory system and the increased blood volume combine to produce venous distension of about 150% of prepregnancy levels. Blood return to the heart is reduced as the venous ends of the capillaries become dilated. Gravid women who are bedridden or who spend a great deal of time lying down are in particular danger of experiencing deep venous thrombosis, which can lead to pulmonary embolism.

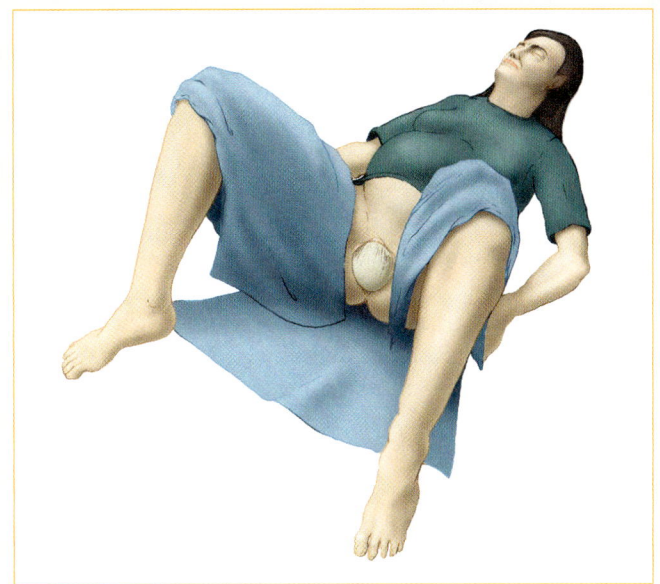

Figure 39-4 Lithotomy position.

The slow return also causes delayed absorption of subcutaneously or intramuscularly injected medications.

When a gravid patient goes into labour, the position she is in stresses the cardiovascular system as well. The standard position is the lithotomy position, in which the woman is supine (on her back) with her knees spread apart, or her feet in stirrups **Figure 39-4 ▲**. Most ambulance stretchers don't have stirrup attachments, so let's assume that birth will occur in the supine or semi-Fowler's position. In the supine position, maternal cardiac output can increase as much as 25% from uterine contractions, with pulse pressure increasing by about the same percentage. Impingement of the uterus on the inferior vena cava may cause the heart rate to decrease about 15%, in turn causing stroke volume to increase as much as 30%. Intra-abdominal pressure combined with the intensity of uterine contractions then causes central venous pressures to rise. Blood volume also increases during contractions to about 300 to 500 ml.

The workload of the heart increases significantly during both gestation and labour. For a healthy woman, this presents no undue complications. For a woman with heart disease or other forms of cardiac compromise, however, the increased work can result in ventricular failure or pulmonary edema, culminating in congestive heart failure. The pain and pressures of labour can further stress the heart, resulting in cardiac arrest.

During pregnancy, the respiratory system undergoes stresses as well. The uterus pushes the diaphragm up toward the abdominal cavity, resulting in about a 4 cm displacement of the diaphragm. To compensate for this change, the rib margins flare outward, increasing the lower thoracic diameter by about 2 cm and the total thoracic circumference by as much as 6 cm. This flaring allows the respiratory system to maintain intrathoracic volume. The abdominal muscles tend to lose their tone during pregnancy, which allows respiration to be more diaphragmatic.

As maternal oxygen demand increases, the respiratory physiology changes to accommodate this need. The hormone progesterone, which is produced early in pregnancy by the corpus luteum and later by the placenta, decreases the threshold of the medullary respiratory centre to carbon dioxide. It also acts on the bronchi, causing them to dilate, and regulates mucus production, causing an overall decrease in airway resistance. Oxygen consumption increases by about 20%, and tidal volume increases gradually to about 40% owing to the effects of progesterone. The increase in tidal volume causes minute ventilation to increase by as much as 50% over prepregnancy values and Paco$_2$ to drop by about 5 mm Hg. The latter change is accompanied by a decrease in blood bicarbonate and a slight increase in plasma pH levels, which in turn affects acid-base balance. Thus, in the pregnant state, respiratory alkalosis is balanced by a metabolic acidosis. The acid-base changes become quite marked during actual labour, but return to normal about 3 weeks postpartum (after birth). Minute ventilation is also affected by a slight increase in maternal respiratory rate, which typically rises to about 10 l/min.

At term, the displacement of the diaphragm by the fully enlarged uterus causes a decrease in expiratory reserve volume, functional residual capacity, and residual volume. Tidal volume and inspiratory reserve volume increase, causing the inspiratory capacity to increase. Structural changes within the respiratory mucous membrane result in increased vascularity and edema. For these reasons, you should avoid nasal intubation in pregnant patients and (if necessary) choose the next smaller size ET tube for oral intubation, to avoid creating additional complications from trauma to the respiratory tract. Estrogen also affects the nasal tract, leading the respiratory membrane to become friable, and making epistaxis a potential emergency condition with the pregnant patient.

As the pregnancy progresses, the maternal metabolism undergoes phenomenal changes—most obviously, weight gain and alterations in physical structure. Weight gain is partly due to increased blood volume and increases in intracellular and extracellular fluid (2.7 to 3 kg), uterine growth (1.4 kg), placental growth (1 kg), fetal growth (3 kg), and increased breast tissue (1 to 1.4 kg). Some weight gain is also attributable to increased proteins and fat deposits, with the average weight gain in pregnancy being 12.3 kg.

The hormone relaxin, which is released during pregnancy, causes collagenous tissues to soften and produces a generalized relaxing of the ligamentous system, especially along the spine; this effect contributes to the characteristic lordosis of latter pregnancy and the increased flexion of the neck, both of which help the pregnant patient compensate for balance. Animal studies have shown that relaxin also appears to enhance mammary gland enlargement, soften the cervix, and increase pelvic joint motility.

Pregnancy increases the demand for carbohydrates, which seems to be based on fetal demand for glucose. Because the insulin molecule is too large to pass through the placental barrier, several fetoplacental and maternal hormones are utilized to compensate for the increased carbohydrate requirement. Women who are predisposed to a diabetic state may become diabetic during pregnancy, but return to a normal carbohydrate metabolism postpartum. During pregnancy, the pancreas secretes insulin in greater amounts and at a faster pace, while cellular sensitivity to insulin declines. The increased production of insulin is the result of increased levels of free cortisol and progesterone. Estrogen has the effect of blunting the action of insulin, whereas progesterone decreases the utilization of insulin by the cells. Human chorionic somatomammotropin (hCS) is released to help stimulate lypolysis; it also acts on glucose to increase peripheral utilization. The net effect is to make glucose available to the fetus from increased energy production from fat. In a healthy woman, these systems work a very fine

You are the Paramedic Part 2

The patient tells you that this is her second pregnancy. She has a healthy 5-year-old boy, and did not have any complications with his pregnancy. She further tells you that she feels as though she needs to move her bowels. The closest appropriate medical facility is approximately 25 minutes away. As you perform a physical examination on the patient, your partner obtains her vital signs.

Vital Signs	Recording Time: 5 Minutes
Level of consciousness	A (Alert to person, place, and day)
Respirations	26 breaths/min; adequate depth
Pulse	110 beats/min; strong and regular at the radial artery
Skin	Pink, warm, and moist
Blood pressure	104/64 mm Hg
Spo$_2$	98% on room air

2. On the basis of what the patient has told you, what do you expect to find during your physical examination?

3. Is there adequate time to transport this patient to the hospital, or should you prepare for imminent delivery?

balancing act to maintain homeostasis. In obese women or women who have been diagnosed with or are predisposed to diabetes, this balance is much harder to achieve. In such cases, gestational diabetes is a possibility.

Gestational diabetes mellitus (GDM) is the inability to process carbohydrates during the pregnancy. Increased maternal insulin production results in increased placental production of human placental lactogen, which leads to an imbalance between the supply of the mother's insulin and glucose production. The patient may be asymptomatic or may exhibit the same signs observed in patients with diabetes mellitus, polyuria, polydipsia, and polyphagia. Treatment consists of diet control and insulin therapy if required. As GDM may occur early in the pregnancy, it is recommended that patients undergo a fasting glucose test as part of routine prenatal testing.

Medical Conditions That Can Be Detrimentally Affected by Pregnancy

Several medical conditions may adversely affect the health of both the woman and the developing fetus. Pregnancy has the tendency to aggravate preexisting medical conditions and give rise to new ones. Pregnancy is also associated with some unique conditions, such as placentitis, a viral or bacterial infection of the placental surface. Only the most common pregnancy-related complications are discussed here.

Heart Disease

Heart disease is of major concern when dealing with a gravid patient. When you are obtaining the patient's medical history, find out the nature and treatment of any heart conditions. Which cardiac medications has the patient been taking? Has she previously been diagnosed with dysrrhythmias or heart murmurs? Has she had a history of rheumatic fever, or was she born with a congenital heart defect? Such heart defects may be benign under normal conditions, but the added stresses of pregnancy could create major problems. Has the patient experienced any episodes of dizziness, lightheadedness, or syncopal episodes with the pregnancy? Such episodes can be indicative of dysrrhythmias that can become critical during the stresses of labour.

Hypertension

A major cause of mortality and morbidity in the pregnant woman is hypertension. Blood pressure is generally lower during the gestational period than at prepregnancy levels, but women who are hypertensive or borderline hypertensive may have their hypertension exacerbated by pregnancy.

Chronic hypertension is a blood pressure that is equal to or greater than 140/90 mm Hg, which exists prior to pregnancy, occurs before the 20th week of pregnancy, or continues to persist postpartum. Diastolic pressures higher than 110 mm Hg place the patient in an increased risk category for stroke and other cardiovascular dangers.

Gestational hypertension develops after the 20th week of pregnancy in women with previously normal blood pressures and resolves spontaneously in the postpartum period. It is more commonly experienced by women who are obese or glucose intolerant. Gestation hypertension has been defined to be inclusive of all hypertensive states in pregnancy and includes chronic hypertension, preeclampsia, and transient hypertension of pregnancy, which was previously described as pregnancy-induced hypertension that did not progress to preeclampsia.

Preeclampsia (also called toxemia of pregnancy) is the most serious of the hypertensive disorders. Women younger than 20 years who are experiencing their first pregnancy are at highest risk, followed by women with advanced maternal age, histories of multiple pregnancies, and risk factors of chronic hypertension, renal disease, and diabetes. Race also tends to play a factor, with black women being most susceptible. The disorder manifests after the 20th week of pregnancy, with the onset of a triad of symptoms: edema, usually of the face, ankles, and hands; gradual onset of hypertension; and protein in the urine. Other symptoms include severe headache, nausea and vomiting, agitation, rapid weight gain, and visual disturbances. Preeclampsia can lead to chronic hypertension, which can retard growth and development of the fetus, impair liver and renal function, cause pulmonary edema, or progress to life-threatening tonic–clonic seizures, a state called eclampsia. Complications that signify severe preeclampsia include liver or renal failure, cerebral hemorrhage, placental abruption, and HELLP syndrome (Hemolysis, Elevated Liver enzymes, Low Platelets), the presence of which necessitates immediate delivery of the fetus to save the woman's life. A systolic pressure exceeding 160 to 180 mm Hg and a diastolic pressure exceeding 105 mm Hg, in the presence of these other risk factors, may require administration of emergency hypertensive medications, such as labetalol or hydralazine. Preeclampsia normally resolves with delivery, but can manifest postpartum. Severe preeclampsia may require treatment with intravenous magnesium sulfate, which can help prevent the development or recurrence of seizures (eclampsia).

Diabetes

Diabetes may be markedly affected by pregnancy. As the hormones of pregnancy alter the insulin-regulating mechanisms, diabetics may experience wildly fluctuating blood glucose levels, manifested as hyperglycemic or hypoglycemic episodes. Unfortunately, oral hypoglycemic agents can cross the placental barrier and affect the fetus, so insulin-dependent diabetics may have to adjust their daily dosing during pregnancy.

Respiratory Disorders

One of the most common complaints of pregnant patients is breathlessness or general dyspnea, which is often precipitated by hormone-related anatomical changes to the respiratory system and is generally only of minor concern and discomfort to the patient. In the pregnant patient, it is important to distinguish between this kind of *physiologic* dyspnea and *pathologic* dyspnea. In the latter case, careful evaluation of the patient, identification of signs and symptoms, or a medical history may reveal an underlying condition that is being aggravated by the pregnancy.

Asthma is one of the most common conditions that can complicate pregnancy. It can either be aggravated as a preexisting illness or occur for the first time during pregnancy, triggered by the effects of stress or respiratory irritants on an already-sensitized respiratory system. Acute asthma attacks render the fetus and woman vulnerable to progressive hypoxia. Maternal complications of an asthma attack may include premature labour, preeclampsia, respiratory failure, vaginal hemorrhage, or eclampsia. Fetal complications may include premature birth, low birth weight, growth retardation, and quite possibly fetal death.

Tuberculosis is not directly aggravated by pregnancy, but the effects of the disease on the respiratory tree can overtax the respiratory system burdened by pregnancy. Women with tuberculosis are more prone to experience premature delivery as well as spontaneous abortion. Endometritis and placentitis with tuberculosis as the causative agent are also potential complications.

Cystic fibrosis (CF) is a hereditary disease that affects the whole body. It results from an autosomal-recessive mutation that impairs the genes responsible for creating sweat, mucus, and digestive juices. CF is basically an exocrine system disorder, whose mechanism causes intense scarring of targeted organs. The lungs are particularly susceptible, such that patients experience frequent lung infections. There is no cure for the disease, and it often proves fatal before a person reaches 40 years of age. CF does not appear to affect pregnancy directly, or vice versa, although women with CF have a greater chance of diabetes developing. The primary effects of CF on pregnancy appear to be collateral, with pregnancy exacerbating other disease processes that CF has affected. Reduced pulmonary function in a patient with CF may also lead to complications in pregnancy.

Pneumonia is an illness of the respiratory system and lungs. It results in alveolar inflammation and edema. Pneumonia can be caused by fungal, viral, or bacterial infection; parasitical infestation; or traumatic or chemical insult to the lungs (eg, aspiration of vomitus). Alcohol abuse is another factor. Pneumonia can be especially virulent during pregnancy, due to the mother's already depressed immune system. In conjunction with disorders such as CF, it can have a significant impact on maternal mortality and morbidity. Low birth weight and premature labour are common complications, with preterm delivery occurring in as many as 43% of cases and before 36 weeks' gestation.

Renal Disorders

As pregnancy progresses, a woman's kidneys increase in length by up to 2 cm, and her ureters get longer, wider, and more curved. Although these changes increase the capacity of the ureters, they can also lead to urinary stasis, resulting in urinary tract infections. These infections can be mild, but they may also progress to states that result in low fetal birth weight and retarded fetal development, premature labour, or even intrauterine fetal death.

Pressure on the bladder as the uterus enlarges can also result in increased urinary frequency. The renal plasma flow rate increases by as much as 25% to 50%, and the glomerular filtration rate increases by about 50%. Patients with preexisting renal disease are likely to experience compounding of associated problems, and those without a diagnosis of renal disease may experience renal malfunctions or failure due to hypertensive disorders or conditions such as hyperemesis gravidarum.

Hemoglobinopathies

According to the 2001 Canadian census, over 3.7 million Canadians (approximately 12.5% of the population) identify their ethnic origin as one known to be at increased risk of thalassemia or hemoglobinopathy. The ethnic origins at increased risk include those from Mediterranean, Middle Eastern, Southeast Asian, Western Pacific, South American, and Caribbean countries. Of note, Japanese, Koreans, Caucasians of Northern European ancestry, First Nations, and Inuit are *not* at increased risk of hemoglobinopathies. The two most clinically significant hemoglobinopathies are sickle cell anemia (SSA) and thalassemia.

In sickle cell disease, under certain physiological conditions the mutation causes the RBCs to become malformed, assuming a sickle shape. This cell alteration inhibits the RBCs from passing smoothly through the small capillaries, which in turn can block blood flow. Complications arising from this blockage include severe acute pain, strokes, and target organ damage, especially the spleen and liver. Because these individuals are anemic, they are prone to infectious states, particularly pneumonia, which is a common cause of death of those with SSA.

Pregnant patients with SSA are prone to pain crises, seizure disorders, and thrombosis. Anemia can also significantly affect fetal growth and mortality. Episodes of SSA can mimic several other conditions (eg, chest pain, abdominal pain) and can cause conditions such as kidney failure and congestive heart failure. Treatment for pregnant patients follows the same modality as for nonpregnant patients. Pain management in the prehospital environment is controversial, and should be determined by local protocol and direct medical control.

Genetic mutations in the thalassemias result in a decrease in the amount of normal hemoglobin. Thalassemias are more common in peoples of Mediterranean descent as well as in African and Middle Eastern populations. The severity of the condition depends on the severity of mutation. In pregnant women with severe cases, the anemia causes such a high level of oxygen deprivation that the fetus cannot survive, and a massive fluid accumulation can manifest in the fetus (hydrops fetalis) resulting in neonatal death. The most severe form of thalassemia, called Cooley's anemia, greatly increases an infant's susceptibility to infection and causes growth retardation and skeletal malformations.

Isoimmunization (Rh Disease)

Rh factor is a protein found on the RBCs of most people. When this factor is absent, the person is said to be Rh negative. When a woman who is Rh negative becomes pregnant by a man who has the Rh factor (Rh positive) and the fetus inherits this factor, the fetal blood can pass into the mother's circulation and produce maternal antibody (isoimmunization) to the factor. Rh disease is normally not a problem in first pregnancies, but in subsequent pregnancies the immune response to an Rh-positive fetus becomes much greater and maternal antibodies will cross the placental barrier to attack the fetal RBCs, which the mother's body identifies as foreign proteins **Figure 39-5 ▲** . This attack can result in death for the fetus or cause hemolytic disease (erythroblastosis fetalis) in a newborn. Newborns with hemolytic disease may present with jaundice, anemia, and hepatomegaly.

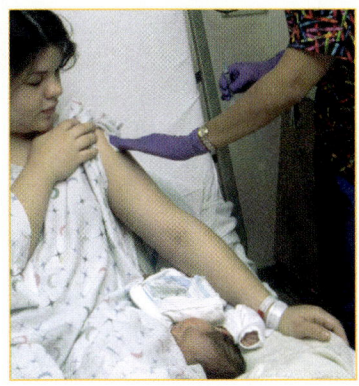

Figure 39-5 An Rh-negative woman who becomes pregnant by an Rh-positive man should receive the Rhogam shot, which prevents the woman's body from attacking subsequent Rh-positive pregnancies.

Rh-negative pregnant women are routinely immunized with Rhogam when there is a risk that a significant amount of fetal RBCs may have crossed into the maternal circulation. Typically, this occurs during spontaneous or therapeutic abortions, during major trauma, or when an invasive procedure such as amniocentesis is performed. Rhogam contains immuglobulins to Rh antigens and will attach to the circulating fetal RBCs and prevent them from triggering the maternal immune system. Rhogam prophylaxis for Rh-negative pregnant women is also routinely performed antepartum at 28 weeks and within 72 hours of delivery of a Rh-positive baby.

Group B Streptococci Perinatal Infections

Group B streptococcus (GBS) is the leading cause of life-threatening infections in newborns, yet remains one of conditions for which pregnant women are not routinely screened. Routine screening has been controversial, because antepartum treatment has not been definitively shown to reduce the incidence of serious neonatal infections by group B streptococci. The only consensus approach remains to have a high index of suspicion for group B streptococci infections in the neonate, particularly those at high risk from prolonged rupture of membranes, preterm labour, and previous known history of group B streptococci infection of the mother or a prior sibling. This infection is caused by *Streptococcus agalactiae,* bacteria that live in the genitourinary and gastrointestinal tracts of healthy individuals, generally without causing any ill effects. In pregnancy, the bacteria can proliferate, resulting in urinary tract infection, infection of the uterus, and stillbirth. If the infection is passed on to the newborn, it can cause respiratory problems, pneumonia, septic shock, and meningitis. Infant illness generally manifests within the first 7 days after birth, but can occur several months later.

Perinatal Viral and Parasitic Infections

Viral and parasitic infections in pregnancy can cause significant problems for the pregnant woman and child. Infections early in pregnancy can affect the formation of the organ systems of the fetus; infections later in pregnancy can result in neurologic impairments, growth disturbances, and heart and respiratory effusions. The most commonly encountered infections include varicella zoster virus, human parvovirus B19 (fifth disease), toxoplasmosis, and cytomegalovirus.

Epilepsy

Most women with epilepsy have normal pregnancies. In women who take medication to control seizures, however, the altered hemodynamics of pregnancy can affect medication levels, possibly resulting in seizures. Nearly one third of epileptic women will experience an increase in seizures, regardless of medication alterations. Generalized tonic–clonic seizures have been known to cause miscarriages, and the onset of labour can trigger seizures in some women, which will ultimately result in fetal distress. Women with epilepsy also tend to have an increased risk of vaginal bleeding, both during and after pregnancy.

Seizures

When a seizure occurs in pregnancy, two patients are involved—the pregnant woman and the fetus. Seizures can be caused by hypertension, toxemia, preeclampsia, or a preexisting seizure disorder. Treatment for a pregnant patient is especially difficult because diazepam (Valium) and phenobarbital—the drugs commonly used to treat seizures—can cross the placental barrier, causing fetal distress. In pregnant patients, magnesium sulfate is the recommended treatment, especially in the patient with eclampsia. In addition, high-flow supplemental oxygen is needed for both patients to counteract the hypoxia that occurs in seizures. Potential complications in such cases may include abruptio placenta, hemorrhage, disseminated intravascular coagulation, and death.

Thyroid Disorders

The thyroid is a butterfly shaped endocrine gland that is located in the neck, directly in front of the trachea. It is responsible for production of several hormones, including thyroxine (T_4) and triiodothyronine (T_3). These hormones regulate the metabolic rate and affect the functions and growth of other organ systems. Calcitonin, which controls calcium blood levels, is also produced in the thyroid. Thyroid disorders affect about

2% of pregnant women and, if left untreated, can lead to complications for both patients. Some pregnant women have pre-existing thyroid conditions, while others experience thyroid problems during or after pregnancy, secondary to metabolic alterations.

When the thyroid produces too much thyroid hormone, hyperthyroidism results. Symptoms of hyperthyroidism in pregnancy include nervousness and irritability, tachycardia, and feeling warm. One of the serious complications of hyperthyroidism is preeclampsia.

When the thyroid produces too little thyroid hormone, the condition is called hypothyroidism. Symptoms of hypothyroidism include fatigue, forgetfulness, constipation, bradycardia, feeling cold, and muscle and joint aches. Hypothyroidism can cause long-term neurologic or developmental deficits in the fetus, and may result in mental retardation.

Cholestasis

Cholestasis is a disease of the liver that occurs during pregnancy. Hormones affect the gallbladder by slowing down or blocking the normal bile flow from the liver. Bile, which aids the process of digestion by breaking down fats, is produced in the liver and stored in the gallbladder. When its normal flow is altered, bile acids build up in the liver, then spill out into the bloodstream. The most common symptom of this condition is profuse, painful itching, particularly of the hands and feet. Patients may also complain of fatigue or depression, nausea, and right upper quadrant pain. They may also notice colour changes in waste elimination—dark urine and light grey or yellow bowel movements. Women who are carrying multiple fetuses are at a higher risk for the development of cholestasis, as are women who have a familial history of cholestasis or who have had previous liver damage.

Cholestasis is relatively benign and transitory for the pregnant woman, but can have serious effects on the fetus. Because the fetus relies on the woman's liver to remove bile acids from the blood, any impediment to this process puts stress on the developing fetal liver. Preterm birth and stillbirth are potential complications of untreated cholestasis.

■ Complications of Pregnancy

Most pregnancies proceed uneventfully, but paramedics are likely to be summoned when they do not.

Abortion

Abortion is defined as expulsion of the fetus, from any cause, before the 20th week of gestation (some sources consider any loss of the pregnancy up to the 28th week of gestation to be an abortion). Most abortions occur during the first trimester, before the placenta is fully mature.

Spontaneous Versus Induced Abortion

Abortions can be broadly classified as spontaneous or induced. A spontaneous abortion (miscarriage) occurs naturally, affecting about 1 of every 5 pregnancies. Causes may include acute or chronic illness in the pregnant woman, maternal exposure to toxic substances (illicit drugs), abnormalities in the fetus, or abnormal attachment of the placenta. In many cases, the cause of a spontaneous abortion cannot be found.

An induced abortion is brought about intentionally. When you are taking a medical history that includes an abortive history, you must be dispassionate and professional regardless of your personal convictions. You may encounter a patient who is experiencing

You are the Paramedic Part 3

Your visual examination of the patient's vaginal area reveals crowning of the baby's head. After ensuring that you and your partner are wearing the appropriate PPE, you open the sterile OB kit, properly position the patient, and prepare for imminent delivery. You ask the patient's husband to sit next to his wife's head.

Reassessment	Recording Time: 10 Minutes
Level of consciousness	A (Alert to person, place, and day)
Respirations	28 breaths/min; adequate depth
Pulse	118 beats/min; strong and regular
Skin	Pink, warm, and moist
Blood pressure	Not obtained; you and your partner are preparing to deliver the baby
Spo2	98% on room air

As the baby's head delivers, you note the presence of a nuchal cord. You instruct the patient to stop pushing so you can correct the situation. Your partner applies oxygen to the patient via nonrebreathing mask.

4. What is a nuchal cord? How should you manage this situation?

complications following an induced abortion, such as vaginal bleeding or sepsis from having parts of the fetus in utero. You may also encounter a patient who has "self-medicated" in an attempt to induce an abortion and is experiencing toxic effects of the herbal remedy as well as a threatened or progressing abortion. Herbal preparations work by making the uterus and bloodstream too toxic for the fetus to survive, which in turn may be too toxic for the woman to survive.

Stages of Abortion

You will most likely find yourself attempting to manage an abortion that is occurring spontaneously. The specific management of such a case depends to some extent on the stage of the abortion when the patient presents for treatment. All pregnant patients presenting with vaginal bleeding or abdominal pain should be transported and evaluated at a definitive care facility.

A threatened abortion is an abortion that is attempting to take place. It is generally characterized by vaginal bleeding during the first half of pregnancy—usually in the first trimester. The patient may present with abdominal discomfort or complain of menstrual cramps. Severe pain is rarely a presenting complaint, as uterine contractions are not rhythmic. The cervix remains closed. An obstetrical ultrasound is required to rule out an ectopic pregnancy. If an intrauterine pregnancy is found, then the ultrasound can help to determine fetal size, development, and heart activity. A threatened abortion can progress to an incomplete abortion, or it may subside, allowing the pregnancy to go to term. There is usually nothing that can be done to prevent a spontaneous abortion. Although patients are usually put off work and advised to avoid strenuous activity, it is unlikely that this will affect the natural course. Patients should continue with their normal activities and have follow-up ultrasounds and serum pregnancy tests to observe the course of the pregnancy, with instructions to return to the hospital should severe pain or bleeding occur. Your role in this case is usually transport and emotional support.

An inevitable abortion is a spontaneous abortion that cannot be prevented. The patient will generally present with severe abdominal pain caused by strong uterine contractions. Vaginal bleeding, often massive, will be present, as well as cervical dilation, as the uterus is preparing to expel the products of conception. When you are treating a patient who is experiencing a spontaneous abortion, your goals are to maintain blood pressure and prevent hypovolemia. Treatment consists of establishing an IV line of normal saline to maintain blood pressure, 100% supplemental oxygen via nonrebreathing mask at 15 l/min, acquiring an ECG, and providing emotional support with rapid transport. Be alert for signs of shock.

An incomplete abortion occurs when part of the products of conception are expelled but some remain in the uterus. (For example, the fetus is expelled but the placenta remains, or only part of the fetus is expelled.) As the cervix has dilated to expel the fetus, vaginal bleeding will be present, which may be slight or profuse, but will be continuous. Be alert for signs and symptoms of shock, and start an IV line of normal saline. If products of conception are protruding from the vagina, consult direct medical

control for instructions; gentle removal of protruding tissues may prevent or relieve signs of shock. You will most often encounter this situation when you find the patient on the toilet, having attempted a bowel movement, with the fetus in the toilet still attached to the umbilical cord hanging from the vagina. The fetus should be gently collected, and emotional support provided to the patient. Fundal massage may be beneficial in stimulating the placenta to deliver. All products of conception need to be collected and presented to the receiving facility. Do not deter the patient from viewing the fetus if she wishes, but be prepared for a strong emotional reaction. A complete abortion has occurred when all the products of conception have been expelled.

In a missed abortion, the fetus dies during the first 20 weeks of gestation but remains in utero. There is no prehospital management of a missed abortion other than transport and emotional support. Management at the hospital will consist of a dilation and curettage (D&C), in which the cervix will be manually dilated and the endometrial lining scraped and suctioned. You should suspect a missed abortion when the patient presents with a history of threatened abortion. The typical history will be a cessation of vaginal bleeding followed by a gradual diminishing of the signs of pregnancy, such as uterine and breast enlargement. The mother may also report having had a brownish vaginal discharge, possibly accompanied by a rank smell. On examination, the uterus may feel like a hard mass in the abdomen, and fetal heart sounds cannot be heard. Missed abortion is generally caused by anembryonic gestation (blighted ovum), maternal disease, uterine anomalies, embryonic anomalies, placental abnormalities, or fetal chromosomal abnormalities. It almost always occurs because of a problem with the fetus, but occasionally a healthy fetus can be expelled by a diseased or damaged uterus. A missed abortion generally precedes a spontaneous abortion.

Septic abortion was once the leading cause of maternal death worldwide. In medical literature, a common complication of childbirth was puerperal fever, which was caused by a streptococcal infection of the genital tract. The incidence of puerperal fever declined significantly in the early 20th century when physicians began routinely washing their hands between patients Figure 39-6 ▸ . Septic abortion occurs when the uterus becomes infected—often by common vaginal bacterial flora—following any type of abortion. The patient will generally give a history of fever and bad-smelling vaginal discharge, usually starting within a few hours after abortion. Physical examination will generally reveal fever and abdominal tenderness. In severe cases, the infection will have progressed to septicemia, resulting ing in septic shock. For this life-threatening emergency, prehospital management consists of starting an IV line of normal saline, administering 100% supplemental oxygen via

Notes from Nancy

Any vaginal bleeding during the third trimester of pregnancy must be regarded as a dire medical emergency until proved otherwise.

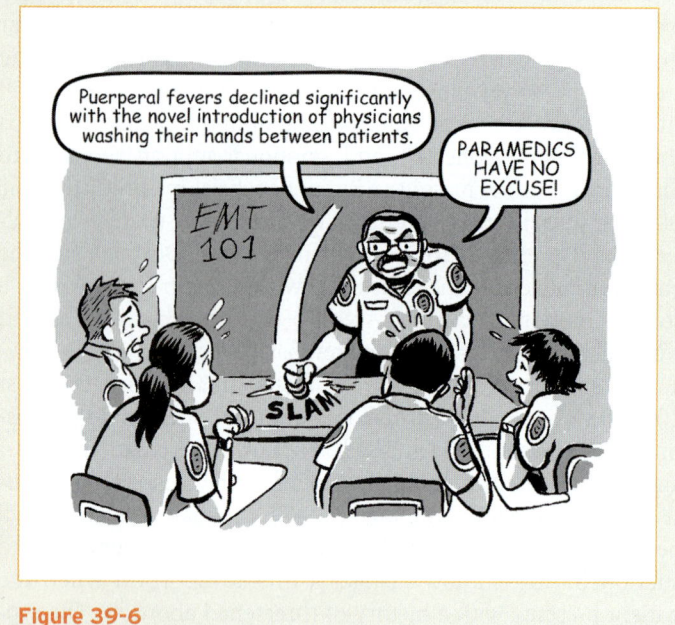

Figure 39-6

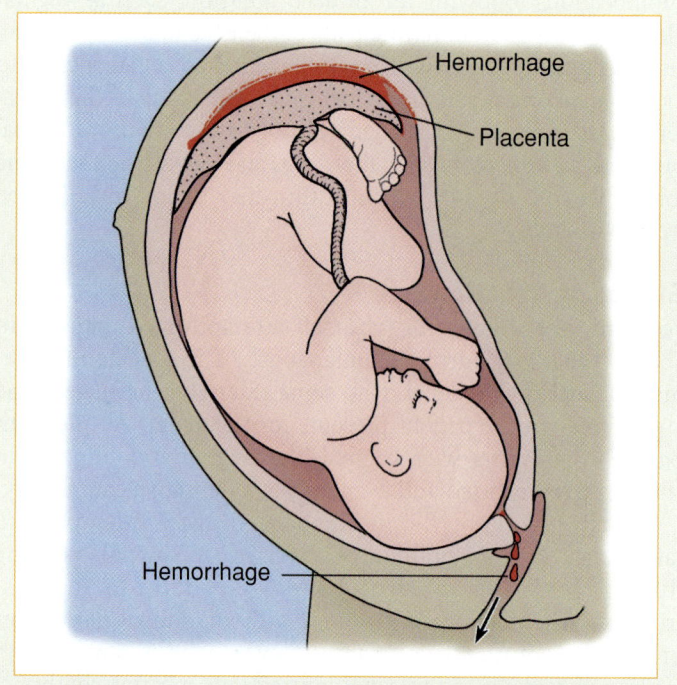

Figure 39-7 In abruptio placenta, the placenta separates prematurely from the wall of the uterus.

nonrebreathing mask, ECG monitoring, and rapid transport. The fluid administration rate should maintain the patient's blood pressure at an acceptable level.

Third-Trimester Bleeding

Abortion accounts for the majority of vaginal bleeding that results in an emergency call. Any detachment of the ovum or embryo from the uterine wall will result in bleeding. The patient may complain of light or heavy bleeding, normally accompanied by cramping abdominal pain. She may also report the passage of tissue or clots. Vaginal bleeding is a serious sign at any stage of pregnancy, but the complications of bleeding increase as the gestation time lengthens.

Third-trimester bleeding presents the greatest danger of hemorrhage, which becomes more acute as the woman approaches term. A complicating factor of third-trimester bleeding is the large volume of blood present within the pregnant woman's body and the compensatory mechanisms that are functioning as a result of pregnancy. A pregnant woman can lose a full 40% of her circulating volume before significant signs and symptoms of hypovolemia become apparent.

Causes of Third-Trimester Bleeding

The three major causes of significant antepartum hemorrhage (hemorrhage before delivery) are abruptio placenta, placenta previa, and uterine rupture.

Abruptio placenta refers to a premature separation of a normally implanted placenta from the wall of the uterus Figure 39-7 ▶ . It most commonly occurs during the last trimester of pregnancy, but can take place in the second trimester as well. Abruptio placenta affects about 1 of every 100 pregnancies that go to term. Maternal hypertension is the most common cause of abruption (44%), followed by trauma

(eg, motor vehicle accidents), assault, falls, and infection. Drug abuse, alcohol use, and smoking are also contributing factors. Incidence is greater among multiparous women and those who have previously experienced abruptio placenta.

The patient with abruptio placenta will usually report vaginal bleeding, with bright red blood, although in some cases the blood does not emerge through the cervix and the bleeding may remain concealed within the endometrium. In any case, the woman will experience the sudden onset of severe abdominal pain, and she may report that she no longer feels the baby moving inside her. Physical examination may reveal signs of shock, often out of proportion to the apparent volume of blood loss. The abdomen will be tender and the uterus rigid to palpation. Fetal heart sounds are often absent because the fetus, being partly or completely cut off from its blood supply, is likely to die. Other complications include severe hemorrhaging. If the hemorrhaging cannot be controlled after delivery, a hysterectomy may be necessary.

In placenta previa, the placenta is implanted low in the uterus and, as it grows, it partially or fully obscures the cervical canal Figure 39-8 ▶ . This condition is the leading cause of vaginal bleeding in the second and third trimesters of pregnancy, with the majority of problems occurring near term, as the cervix begins to dilate in preparation for delivery. Maternal age and multiparity are risk factors, with women older than 30 years being three times as likely to experience the condition as will women in their 20s. Placenta previa occurs in about 5 of every 1,000 births, with a maternal mortality rate of 0.03%. Complications include disseminated intravascular coagulation, hemorrhage, and low fetal birth weight.

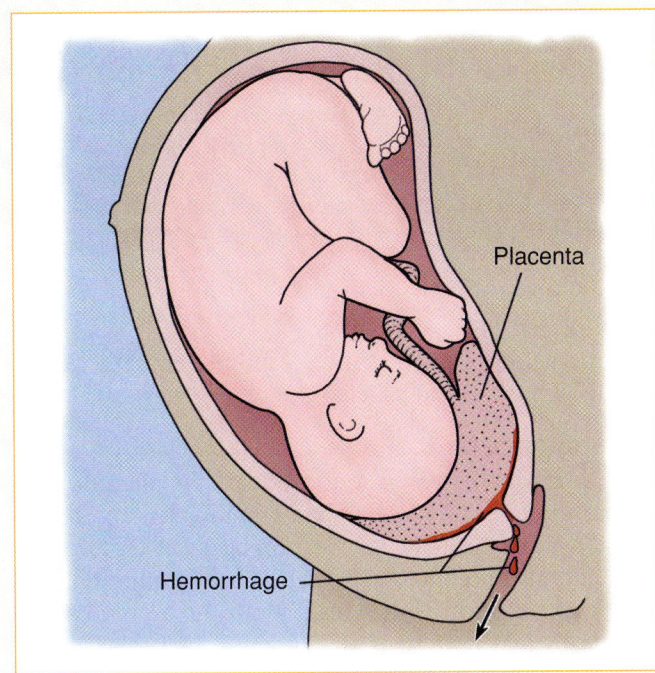

Figure 39-8 In placenta previa, the placenta develops over and covers the cervix.

The chief complaint of a woman with placenta previa is usually painless vaginal bleeding, with the loss of bright red blood. Because the blood supply to the fetus is not immediately jeopardized, fetal movements continue and fetal heart sounds remain audible. On gentle palpation, the uterus is soft and nontender. (Do *not* try to palpate the abdomen deeply in any woman with third-trimester bleeding; if she does have placenta previa, deep palpation may induce heavy bleeding.)

If the uterus ruptures, it will happen during labour. Patients at greatest risk are women who have had many children and those with a scar on the uterus (eg, from a previous cesarean section). Typically, you will be called for a "possible OB," and find a woman in active labour complaining of weakness, dizziness, and thirst. She may tell you that she initially had very strong and painful contractions, but then the contractions slackened off. Physical examination will reveal signs of shock—sweating, tachycardia, and falling blood pressure. Significant vaginal bleeding may or may not be obvious.

Assessment and Management of Third-Trimester Bleeding

Assessment of third-trimester bleeding is much the same as assessment of vaginal bleeding. When the patient presents with the chief complaint of vaginal bleeding, try to determine as much as possible about the nature of the bleeding. When did it start? What activity was the woman engaged in at the onset? Was she active or at rest? How much blood has been lost? (Use the blood loss chart in Chapter 38 to quantify this amount.) Is the patient experiencing abdominal pain? What is the nature of the pain? Sharp? Cramping? Dull? Achy? Use

OPQRST to elaborate on the chief complaint of labour pain. Rate its severity on a scale of 1 to 10. During the physical examination, identify any changes in orthostatic vital signs. Orthostatic changes indicate a significant blood loss, which may be contrary to the physical evidence of bleeding, which may be slight. Look for a positive Grey Turner's sign or Cullen's sign, which can help correlate the presence of internal bleeding.

You do not need to identify the underlying cause of the third-trimester bleeding to treat it. Regardless of the source of hemorrhaging, prehospital management is the same as follows:

1. Keep the woman recumbent, lying on her left side.
2. Administer 100% supplemental oxygen via nonrebreathing mask at 15 l/min.
3. Provide rapid transport to a definitive care facility, notifying the facility of the patient's condition en route.
4. Start an IV line of normal saline with a large-bore IV cannula. Infuse at a rate necessary to maintain blood pressure. An additional IV line may be indicated.
5. Establish an ECG and obtain baseline vital signs. Do not attempt to examine the woman internally or pack the vagina with trauma pads.
6. Use loosely placed trauma pads over the vagina in an effort to stop the flow of blood.
7. If bleeding is severe and signs and symptoms of shock are present, pharmacologic management may be indicated at the discretion of direct medical control. Tocolytics are drugs that are used to delay labour. They may be used to decrease uterine contractions in order to allow time to transport to the receiving hospital prior to delivery. In the case of third-trimester bleeding, they may be helpful in decreasing hemorrhage, particularly in placenta previa. Magnesium sulfate has been used in the past, but it does not appear to be a very effective tocolytic. Ritodrine IV, a beta-agonist, has been effective in the past, but has cardiovascular side effects. Ongoing research suggests that indomethacin and nitroglycerin may be effective. In cases of uterine rupture, oxytocin may be administered at a dose of 20 to 40 units (1,000 ml at 100 ml/h) to encourage uterine contractions.

Disorders of Pregnancy States
Hyperemesis Gravidarum

Hyperemesis gravidarum is a condition of persistent nausea and vomiting during pregnancy. Nearly all women experience the infamous—but normal—"morning sickness," especially during the first several weeks of pregnancy. Hyperemesis gravidarum is a much more serious condition. Prolonged vomiting leads to dehydration and malnutrition, which have negative effects on the woman and fetus. The exact cause of the condition is unknown, but suspects include increased hormone levels—especially estrogen and human chorionic gonadotropin (hCG)—stress, and changes to the gastrointestinal system. Hyperemesis gravidarum is most common in first-time pregnancies, with multiple gestations, and in women who are obese. This condition may also present in conjunction with molar pregnancy (discussed below) and HELLP syndrome. Symptoms include severe and persistent vomiting, in excess of three or four times daily. Vomiting is usually projectile and generally consists of bile and possibly blood. Severe nausea, pallor, and possibly jaundice may also be seen.

Prehospital treatment of hyperemesis gravidarum includes the following steps:

1. Provide 100% supplemental oxygen via nonrebreathing mask.
2. Start an IV line of normal saline and administer the first 250 ml of fluid.
3. If protocols allow, administer dimenhydrinate, 10 to 50 mg IV or deep IM. This drug has both sedative and antiemetic effects, but is contraindicated if the patient is taking MAO inhibitors.
4. Check blood glucose level.
5. Check orthostatic vital signs, and obtain an ECG.
6. Transport. Severe cases will ultimately require hospitalization.

Molar Pregnancy

Molar pregnancy (hydatidiform mole) arises when a malfunction of the egg or sperm creates a problem at the fertilization stage, resulting in an abnormal placenta. A complete mole occurs when an empty egg is fertilized, which triggers the normal progression of pregnancy, but there is no fetus present. A partial mole occurs when two sperm fertilize the same egg; instead of twins, a malfunction occurs resulting in an abnormal placenta and a fetus with an abnormal chromosome count.

In cases involving molar pregnancies, you will most likely be responding to a call for vaginal spotting or bleeding (usually dark brown) or excessive nausea and vomiting. Preeclampsia is also a potential complication. Molar pregnancies are particularly frightening and heartbreaking as well, as the woman truly believes she is having a normal pregnancy. Prenatal screenings tend to find most instances of molar pregnancy, and a D&C is scheduled early on.

Pseudopregnancy

Pseudocyesis ("psychogenic" pregnancy) is a false pregnancy that develops all the typical signs and symptoms of true pregnancy, including weight gain, menstrual cessation, tender breasts, enlarged uterus, and even labour pains. Its exact cause is unknown, but it is presumed to be caused by the emotional desire to be pregnant. There is little for you to do for these cases except provide emotional support.

Ectopic Pregnancy

Ectopic pregnancy is a severe disorder of pregnancy with potentially life-threatening consequences. In an ectopic pregnancy, a fertilized ovum becomes implanted somewhere other than in the uterus, usually in one of the fallopian tubes. All the normal signs and symptoms of pregnancy are usually present. The patient is in severe pain, possibly in hypovolemic shock. Any young female of reproductive age presenting with nontraumatic shock and abdominal pain needs to have a pregnancy test as soon as

possible, because the most concerning diagnosis would be a ruptured ectopic pregnancy, which is a surgical emergency. If a pregnancy test is not available, then ectopic pregnancy remains the top differential diagnosis. It is important for you to be understanding, empathetic, and, above all, supportive and patient.

> **Notes from Nancy**
>
> A pregnant woman may lose a lot of blood before she shows signs of shock. Don't wait for signs and symptoms. Suspect shock from the mechanisms of injury.

Pregnancy and Drugs

When a pregnant woman is a drug addict, the illicit drugs she uses pass through the placenta barrier and enter into the fetal circulation. The fetus may then develop birth defects (see Chapter 44) and also becomes an addict. When you are delivering the baby of a woman with a history of drug abuse, be aware that the baby may have signs of withdrawal after it is born—for example, respiratory depression, bradycardia, tachycardia, seizures, and cardiac arrest. Treatment should revolve around cardiorespiratory support.

General Assessment of the Pregnant Patient

Some Definitions

When you are talking about the characteristics of labour and delivery in women with different obstetric histories, special terminology is used. Gravidity refers to a uterus that contains a fetus, whatever the outcome (ie, abortion, stillbirth, or live birth). Parity refers to delivery of a infant after the 28th week of gestation, irrespective of whether the infant was born alive or dead. We classify a woman, then, according to the number of times her uterus has been occupied (gravidity) and the number of times she has carried a fetus more than 28 weeks (parity).

- **Primigravida**—a woman who is pregnant for the first time.
- **Primipara** ("primip")—a woman who has had only one delivery.
- **Multigravida**—a woman who has had two or more pregnancies, irrespective of the outcome.
- **Multipara** ("multip")—a woman who has had two or more deliveries. A woman who has had more than five deliveries is referred to as a "grand multipara."
- **Nullipara**—a woman who has never delivered.

For example, a woman who has had four pregnancies but carried only one of them to term—the three others ended in miscarriage—would be classified as gravida 4, para 1. The medical shorthand annotation would be G4P1. You could also write the preceding case history as G4P1A3, showing abortive history.

Scene Assessment and Initial Assessment

Proper physical assessment and medical history are an important part in treating the obstetric patient. Perform a scene assessment as with any other call. Likewise, the initial assessment should be the same as with any patient.

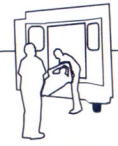

At the Scene

Blood pressure is an unreliable indicator of perfusion in any patient, but it is even less reliable in the pregnant patient because a greater volume of blood can be lost before hypotension develops.

Focused History and Physical Examination

Determine the patient's chief complaint, elaborate on this chief complaint using the OPQRST, and obtain the SAMPLE history. Specifically, you want to know if the patient is pregnant, how many times she has been pregnant (gravida), and how many times she has had a live birth (para). The first question can generally be bypassed if the patiently is obviously pregnant. Asking a woman who is near term if she is pregnant (the unspoken implication is that she is just fat) is not a good way to develop trust or gain a friend—but, if in doubt, ask. The number of times pregnant may also need to be clarified, as many women do not count abortions or miscarriages as pregnancies, and tend to think only of actual deliveries. Also ask about the length of gestation and her estimated due date or date of confinement.

Ask the patient whether she has experienced complications with any of her pregnancies, or whether she has had any obstetric or gynecologic complications. Has she ever had a cesarean section? If so, is the current baby planned for cesarean delivery or does the patient intend to have a vaginal birth after cesarean (VBAC)? Complications of VBAC can include uterine rupture. Is the patient currently under a physician's care? Has she been taking prenatal vitamins? When was her last visit to her physician? Has her physician indicated any concerns about this pregnancy?

Has the patient had a recent ultrasound? What were the findings? Did the ultrasound reveal more than one fetus or any abnormal presentations? Is the patient taking any current medications? Any over-the-counter drugs, recreational drugs, or herbals? Does the patient have any allergies? (This subject should have been covered in the SAMPLE history, but ask again now.)

What is your general impression of the patient's overall health? Has she been smoking, consuming alcohol, or used any illicit drugs during the pregnancy? If yes, how recently? Is the patient currently experiencing pain? If yes, what is the quality and duration? Where is it located and does it radiate? Was the onset gradual or sudden? When did the pain start, and does anything relieve it? Has the patient experienced this type of pain before? When? Is the pain occurring regularly? Is it sporadic or constant?

Has the patient noticed any vaginal bleeding or spotting? If so, what was the amount of bleeding? How long did the bleeding last? What colour was the blood? What was the patient doing prior to the bleeding? Did she use sanitary pads to stop the bleeding? How many pads? Did the bleeding stop? Has the patient passed any clots or tissue? If so, try to obtain samples to give to the emergency department. Has the patient experienced any other type of vaginal discharge? What was the amount, colour, and duration of that discharge? Was any identifiable or disagreeable odour associated with the discharge?

If the patient is in active labour, has her water broken? Does she need to move her bowels or push? If she answers yes to these last questions, delivery may be imminent.

Focused Physical Examination

Your physical examination should be based on the patient's chief complaint. Just because a woman is pregnant, you should not rule out the possibility of asthma, heart attack, or allergic reactions, for example. No matter what the chief complaint, the detailed physical examination should also include fetal heart tones and heart rate. By feeling the abdomen, you can roughly palpate the fetal position. Pay close attention to the vital signs of both patients—the woman and the fetus.

You are the Paramedic Part 4

After successfully managing the nuchal cord, you immediately suction the infant's mouth and nose and deliver the rest of the body. The infant is blue, but begins breathing spontaneously within a few seconds. The mother remains hemodynamically stable. After you pat the infant dry, correctly position the infant, and resuction the infant's mouth and nose, you assess the infant.

Newborn Assessment	Recording Time: 14 Minutes
Respirations	Rapid and irregular; adequate tidal volume
Pulse rate	130 beats/min; strong and regular
Skin	Central and peripheral cyanosis, warm and moist

5. Should the Apgar score be used to determine the need for newborn resuscitation? Why or why not?
6. Is additional treatment required for this infant other than maintaining airway patency and providing thermal management?

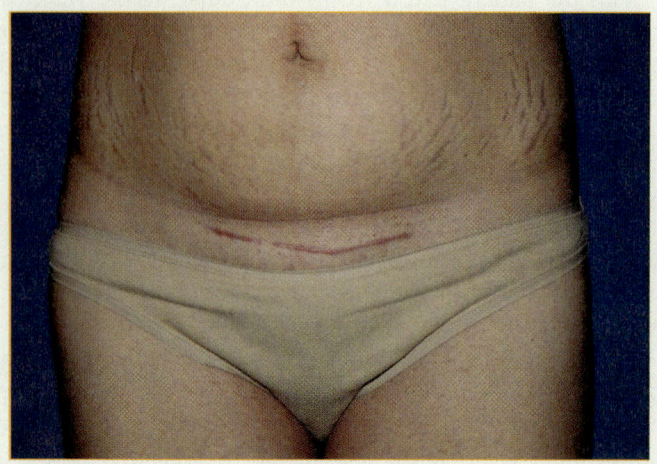

Figure 39-9 A scar from a lower segment transverse cesarean section.

At the Scene

If you note a scar above a woman's pubic hair line **Figure 39-9 ▲**, it may mean she has delivered once before by cesarean. Ask whether she knows of any reason why she would not be able to delivery vaginally, and report her response to direct medical control. Women who have previously delivered by cesarean are not precluded from having a normal, vaginal delivery.

If the patient tells you she has abdominal pain, ask her to describe the pain; this information will help determine whether she is having contractions.

Inspect the vaginal area for crowning or vaginal bleeding or discharge. Crowning indicates that you will need to deliver the baby on scene. If there is no crowning, ask the mother how far apart the contractions are, and then time them. Ask the patient if her water has broken, and, if so, how long ago. First-time mothers (gravida 1) typically take more time to deliver, whereas multigravida and multipara mothers can deliver very quickly.

If you see bleeding or discharge, ascertain when it started and check the abdomen for tenderness and rigidity. Normal abdomens are not rigid during pregnancy. Assessment of the serial vital signs will tell you if the woman or fetus is in distress.

Some women may experience Braxton-Hicks contractions, or intermittent uterine contractions that may occur every 10 to 20 minutes. Usually seen in the third month of the pregnancy, this condition is also known as false labour. Because you have no way of telling in the prehospital environment if a patient's contractions are from a miscarriage or another complication of pregnancy, the patient needs to be transported to the emergency department.

Ongoing Assessment

Ongoing examination should include an assessment of the woman's serial vital signs and the fetal heart rate and heart tones. Also, time the contractions and perform a head-to-toe examination of the woman (if you have not already done so) to avoid missing other possible injuries and complications. Check any interventions and transport to an appropriate facility.

■ Trauma During Pregnancy

Trauma is a serious complicating factor in pregnancy, partly because of the many physiologic changes that occur during pregnancy, but mostly because of the involvement of two patients—the woman and her fetus. Both patients are particularly vulnerable to trauma because of the unique features of pregnancy.

Trauma is the leading cause of maternal death, with 6% to 8% of pregnant women experiencing some type of trauma during the pregnancy, usually in the last trimester. The major causes of injury to pregnant women are motor vehicle collisions, falls, domestic abuse, and penetrating injuries such as gunshot wounds.

At the Scene

Throughout pregnancy, seatbelts should be used with *both* the lap belt and the shoulder harness in place. The lap belt portion should be placed under the abdomen and over the iliac crests and the pubic symphysis. The shoulder harness should be positioned between the breasts.

Vulnerability of the Pregnant Woman to Trauma

In general, abdominal trauma occurs from the same mechanisms in pregnant women as in nonpregnant women. However, because the likelihood of domestic abuse increases greatly during a woman's pregnancy, prehospital personnel should be suspicious for evidence of this crime.

The anatomical changes during pregnancy have important implications for trauma. As the woman approaches term, her abdominal contents are compressed into the upper abdomen. The diaphragm is elevated by about 4 cm, so there is a higher incidence of abdominal injuries in association with chest trauma. Meanwhile, because the peritoneum is maximally stretched, significant abdominal trauma may occur without peritoneal signs.

In the first trimester of pregnancy, the uterus is well protected in the woman's bony pelvis and is rarely damaged from abdominal trauma. In the second and third trimesters of pregnancy, the uterus grows out from the pelvis and extends into the abdomen, making it more vulnerable to blunt and penetrating trauma. In motor vehicle collisions, for example, the use of a lap belt increases the likelihood of uterine damage because the lap belt compresses the uterus. Shoulder restraints, by contrast, decrease the chance of uterine injury. In penetrating injuries, the large uterus protects the other organs from injury. Because the uterus shields the other organs, pregnant women with penetrating wounds have excellent outcomes, although the fetus is often injured by the trauma. In addition to abdominal tenderness, the examination of an injured pregnant woman may reveal an abnormal fetal position, an easily palpated fetus, inability to palpate the top of the uterus, or vaginal bleeding.

As early as the second trimester of pregnancy, the bladder is displaced upward (superior) and forward (anterior) so that it lies outside the pelvic cavity. It is therefore at increased risk of injury, particularly from a deceleration injury caused by a lap seatbelt. Should you encounter a restrained pregnant patient in a motor vehicle collision, make a note of belt placement. If the patient is found with the belt placed over the abdomen or on top of the uterine dome, this positioning should dramatically increase your index of suspicion for internal injuries to the woman and fetus. The uterus also becomes more vulnerable to injury as it increases in size, and deceleration forces, such as those produced by vehicular trauma, may bring about abruptio placenta or uterine rupture.

As noted earlier, pregnancy is accompanied by a significant increase in vascular volume. Normal vascular volume increases by nearly 50% during the first 6 months of pregnancy as a result of the pregnant woman having to perfuse her own circulation and that of the fetus. To meet this demand, normal cardiac output increases by about 40% as a result of the increasing pulse rate and stroke volume. The resting pulse rate increases by 15 to 20 beats/min over the rate in a nonpregnant patient, so the resting pulse may be as high as 100 beats/min by the end of the second trimester of pregnancy. This physiologic change makes it much more difficult to interpret tachycardia. Furthermore, because of the pregnant woman's vastly expanded blood volume, other signs of hypovolemia, such as a falling blood pressure, may not be evident until she has lost as much as 40% of her blood volume. Therefore you need to be aggressive in managing a pregnant woman with a mechanism of injury (MOI) that indicates shock.

A relative redistribution of blood volume also occurs during pregnancy, with blood flow to the pelvic region increasing tenfold. If a pregnant woman sustains a pelvic fracture, her chances of bleeding to death are therefore significantly higher than those of a nonpregnant woman. A good deal of blood volume can be lost before signs and symptoms of shock develop because other mechanisms are compensating for the loss.

Regarding respiration, the pregnant woman has a higher basal metabolism and therefore an increased need for oxygen. At the same time, she has more carbon dioxide to eliminate—hers and that produced by fetal metabolism. She responds by increasing her tidal volume and, therefore, her minute volume. If she should need artificial ventilation, you will have to administer supplemental oxygen at a higher minute volume than usual.

During pregnancy, digestion slows and bowel motility decreases, resulting in the stomach staying full longer. With the gravid uterus placing pressure on the stomach, the chances of aspiration are dramatically increased.

Vulnerability of the Fetus to Trauma

The muscular wall of the uterus acts as a cushion for the fetus against the direct effects of blunt trauma, but fetal injury can occur as a result of rapid deceleration of circulation or may be secondary to impaired fetal circulation. The most common cause of fetal death from trauma is maternal death, but a woman will often survive an incident that proves fatal for the fetus. Blunt trauma resulting in abruptio placenta, for instance, provides a good statistical outcome for the mother but often results in the death of the fetus.

If the pregnant woman has sustained trauma and is bleeding massively, the maternal circulation will shunt blood away from fetal circulation to maintain maternal homeostasis—maternal circulation takes precedence over the requirements of the fetus. Therefore, any injury that involves significant maternal bleeding will threaten the life of the fetus. By the time the woman shows clinical signs of shock, fetal circulation will be so compromised that you can expect a fetal mortality of 70% to 80%.

Notes from Nancy
A fetal heart rate lower than 120 or higher than 160 beats per minute suggests fetal distress.

The best indication of the status of the fetus after trauma is the fetal heart rate. A normal fetal heart rate is between 120 and 160 beats/min. A rate slower than 120 beats/min means fetal distress and signals a dire emergency. To measure the fetal heart rate, listen with the bell of the stethoscope over the pregnant woman's abdomen. You may have to move the stethoscope around the abdomen until you can hear the fetal heart tones. Palpate the woman's pulse at the same time as you count the fetal heart rate. If the fetal heart rate is identical to the maternal pulse, you are probably listening to an echo of the maternal heartbeat and not the fetal heart, so change the position of your stethoscope and try again. It takes a lot of practice to hear fetal heart tones and requires quiet surroundings. Some modern ambulances may be equipped with Doppler stethoscopes, which make assessment of fetal heart sounds much easier.

Notes from Nancy
Every pregnant woman who has been in an accident must be evaluated at the hospital, even if her own injuries appear trivial.

Treatment of the Pregnant Trauma Patient

Although trauma in a pregnant woman involves at least *two* patients, we can treat only one of them directly: the woman. In general, what is good for the woman will be good for the fetus. For example, any effort to improve maternal perfusion will have a collateral effect of improving fetal circulation. Potential damage to the fetus cannot be adequately assessed in the prehospital environment, however, only presumed or suspected. While a decreased fetal heart rate signals an emergency situation, a normal fetal heart rate does not guarantee that all is well. Even minor deceleration forces can cause significant injury to the fetus.

In general, the prehospital management of pregnant women with abdominal trauma is the same as for nonpregnant patients. Airway, breathing, and circulation remain the highest priorities. However, because the large uterus can compress the vena cava (decreasing right atrial preload), a pregnant woman should be transported to the hospital on her left side unless a spinal injury is suspected **Figure 39-10 ▶**. If you must transport a patient in the supine position, elevate her right hip about 15 cm to minimize the pressure of the vena cava. Be aware that because of the physiologic changes that occur in a woman's body during pregnancy, the fetus may lack appropriate circulation even if the woman's vital signs appear normal. In other words, the fetus may be in shock before signs appear in the mother, so initiate early, aggressive fluid resuscitation.

Prehospital treatment of a pregnant trauma patient is as follows:

1. *Ensure an adequate airway.* Regurgitation and aspiration are much more likely in a pregnant woman than in a patient who is not pregnant, so if the patient is unconscious, provide early endotracheal intubation to isolate the airway. Provide cricoid pressure until the airway is secured.

2. *Administer oxygen.* A pregnant woman's oxygen needs are 10% to 20% higher than normal, so provide 100%

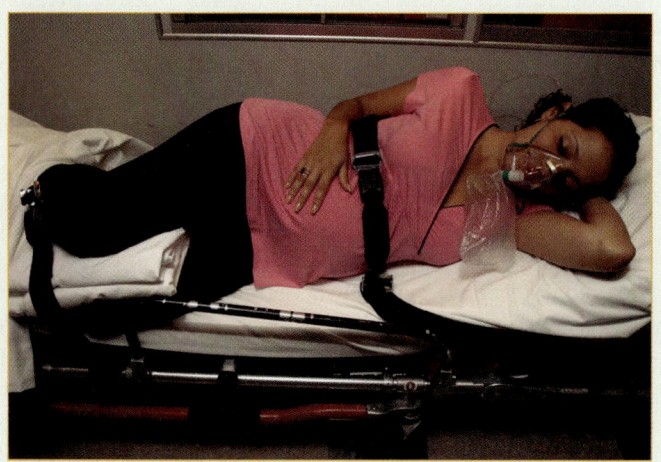

Figure 39-10 Whenever possible, transport a pregnant patient lying on her left side to allow for sufficient circulation through the vena cava.

supplemental oxygen via nonrebreathing mask if the patient is conscious.

3. *Assist ventilations as needed, and provide a higher minute volume than usual.* Because the uterus of a pregnant woman presses up against the diaphragm, she will be more difficult to ventilate. Once the patient is intubated, therefore, you may want to use a positive-pressure ventilator periodically to ensure visible chest rise (representing an adequate tidal volume).

You are the Paramedic Part 5

The infant's trunk is pink following the administration of blow-by oxygen; however, the infant's hands and feet remain somewhat cyanotic. The infant is breathing adequately and has a heart rate of 130 beats/min. After clamping and cutting the umbilical cord, you wrap the infant, a little girl, with a warm blanket and hand her to the mother. As your partner retrieves the stretcher from the ambulance, you quickly reassess the mother.

Reassessment	Recording Time: 21 Minutes
Level of consciousness	A (Alert to person, place, and day)
Respirations	24 breaths/min; adequate depth
Pulse	104 beats/min; strong and regular
Skin	Pink, warm, and moist
Blood pressure	100/60 mm Hg
Spo₂	99% on nonrebreathing mask of 15 l/min oxygen

During transport, you initiate an IV of normal saline and set the flow rate to keep vein open. You reexamine the mother and note a moderate amount of vaginal bleeding. Your estimated time of arrival at the hospital is 20 minutes.

7. How will you treat this patient's postpartum bleeding?
8. Is a crystalloid fluid bolus indicated at this point?

Following your interventions, the patient's bleeding has subsided. The placenta delivers shortly before you arrive at the hospital. The mother and baby remain stable.

4. *Control external bleeding promptly.* Splint any fractures.

5. *Start one or two IV lines of normal saline.* Use large-bore cannulas and macro drip sets. Administer a bolus if signs and symptoms of hemodynamic compromise are present, with the goal of maintaining blood pressure. Remember that a larger volume of fluid is necessary for the pregnant patient.

6. *Notify the receiving hospital* of the patient's status and your estimated time of arrival.

7. *Transport* the woman in the lateral recumbent position. If she is on a backboard, tilt the backboard 30° to the left by wedging pillows beneath it. This will cause the uterus to shift, taking the weight off the inferior vena cava and improving venous return to the heart.

If cardiac arrest occurs, provide CPR and ALS as you would for a nonpregnant patient.

If resuscitation efforts are not effective within 5 minutes, an emergency cesarean section must be performed to save the woman and possibly the baby. Immediate evacuation of the uterine contents provides the most favourable resuscitation scenario for the woman. If a cesarean is done within 5 minutes of maternal death, the fetus at term has a 70% chance of survival. Paramedic cesarean section protocols are not commonplace and remain highly controversial; therefore, your patient requires rapid transport and prior notification to the closest medical facility. Even if the woman is *obviously* dead (eg, in case of decapitation), good CPR and ventilatory support may keep the fetus viable until a cesarean section can be performed.

Normal Childbirth

When you get a chance to assist in childbirth, the event is often a happy one. Of course, pregnant women rarely call 9-1-1

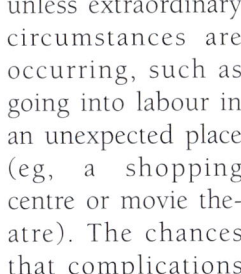

Notes from Nancy

The paramedic's most important job at a delivery is to appear calm.

unless extraordinary circumstances are occurring, such as going into labour in an unexpected place (eg, a shopping centre or movie theatre). The chances that complications will occur increase significantly when delivery occurs unplanned outside of the hospital. You will usually be working in an uncontrolled, nonsterile environment, so having a good working knowledge of potential complications and strategies to resolve them is mandatory.

Labour

Let's start by reviewing the stages of normal labour. Labour refers to the mechanism by which the products of conception—

that is, the baby and the placenta—are expelled from the pregnant woman's uterus. It is called labour because it is *hard work*.

Labour progresses through several well-defined stages, whose durations depend in part on whether the mother is going through her first pregnancy or is a veteran at delivering. Labour starts with the prodromal stage, which often goes unnoticed. In the prodromal stage, the woman begins to feel a relief of pressure in her upper abdomen and a simultaneous increase of pressure in her pelvis as the baby starts its descent toward the birth canal. A plug of mucus, sometimes mixed with blood (called the bloody show), is expelled from the dilating cervix and discharged from the vagina.

The first stage of labour begins with the onset of labour pains—crampy abdominal pains that may radiate into the small of the back and reflect the contractions of the uterus. Those early contractions come at 5- to 15-minute intervals, and they serve to maneuver the baby into position and prepare the cervical opening for the baby's egress. As the uterus contracts, its less muscular lower segment is pulled upward over the presenting part, resulting in effacement (thinning and shortening) of the cervix. Effacement is accompanied by progressive cervical dilation—that is, stretching of the cervical opening until it is wide enough to accommodate passage of a baby. The first stage of labour lasts until the cervix is fully dilated, an average of about 12 hours in a nullipara and anywhere up to 8 hours in a multipara. Toward the end of this first stage of labour, the amniotic sac often ruptures, with a dramatic gush of fluid pouring out of the vagina.

The second stage of labour begins as the baby's head enters the birth canal. The woman's contractions become more intense and more frequent, now occurring 2 to 3 minutes apart. Her pulse rate increases, and sweat appears on her face. She tends to bear down with each contraction and, because of the pressure of the baby's head against her rectum, she may feel as if she has to move her bowels. The cervix meanwhile becomes fully dilated and effaced, and the presenting part of the baby (the part that emerges from the mother first—normally the head) begins bulging out of the vaginal opening, a process called crowning. When crowning occurs, delivery is imminent. The second stage of labour concludes when the baby is fully delivered. Altogether, the second stage of labour takes about an hour in a nullipara and 20 to 30 minutes in a multipara.

The third stage of labour (placental stage) is the period from the delivery of the baby until the placenta has been fully expelled and the uterus has con-

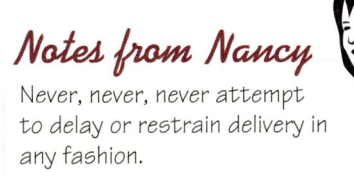

Notes from Nancy

Never, never, never attempt to delay or restrain delivery in any fashion.

tracted. Uterine contraction is necessary to squeeze shut all of the tiny blood vessels left exposed when the placenta separates from the uterine wall. **Table 39-1 ▸** summarizes the stages of labour.

Table 39-1	The Stages of Labour: Nullipara Versus Multipara	
Stage of Labour	**Nullipara**	**Multipara**
First stage	8 to 12 hours	6 to 8 hours
Second stage	1 to 2 hours	30 minutes
Third stage	5 to 60 minutes	5 to 60 minutes

Table 39-2	False Labour Versus True Labour	
Parameter	**True Labour**	**False Labour**
Contractions	Regularly spaced	Irregularly spaced
Interval between contractions	Gradually shortens	Remains long
Intensity of contractions	Gradually increases	Stays the same
Effects of analgesics	Do not abolish the pain	Often abolish the pain
Cervical changes	Progressive effacement and dilation	No changes

Assessment of the Obstetric Patient

In assessing the pregnant woman who has called for an ambulance because of labour pains, you really need to answer only the following two questions:

- Am I going to have to deliver this baby?
- If so, which potential complications, if any, should I anticipate in this particular case?

Always keep in mind that you are a role model when you are discussing or performing steps to assist in childbirth.

Is There Time to Reach the Hospital?

To answer the first question, find out the following:

- Has the woman had a baby before? Labour in a nullipara is usually slower than in subsequent pregnancies, allowing more time for transport.
- What are the contractions like? Some women experience Braxton-Hicks contractions throughout the pregnancy, so it is important to distinguish false labour from the real thing. The pains of true labour are regularly spaced and increase in intensity over time. **Table 39-2 ▶** distinguishes false labour from true labour.
- How frequent are the contractions? If they are more than 5 minutes apart, you generally have enough time to get the woman to a nearby hospital. Contractions that are less than 2 minutes apart signal impending delivery, especially in a multipara.
- Does the woman feel an urge to move her bowels? That sensation occurring during labour is caused by the baby's head in the mother's vagina pressing against the rectum; it indicates that delivery is imminent. If the woman reports an urge to move her bowels, *do not allow the mother to go to the toilet.*

The answers to those questions should give you a good idea of whether there will be time to transport the woman to the hospital. To double-check, *inspect* the mother for crowning—crowning indicates that the baby will be born within the next few minutes.

Is This Likely to Be a Complicated Delivery?

To answer the second question, you need to ask a few more questions and examine the woman further, even as you are setting up for delivery, as follows:

- Has the patient been receiving prenatal care? Obstetric complications are more frequent among women who have not been receiving care.
- What is the actual due date of the baby? Complications are more likely if the baby is coming prematurely. As the baby

has not had time to grow to term, it will be smaller, and the chances for breech delivery or prolapsed umbilical cord are greater.

- Has the patient's water broken? If yes, how long ago did it break? If rupture occurred many hours before, the chances of fetal infection and fetal distress are higher.
- Does the patient have a history of cesarean section? The likelihood of uterine rupture is increased if positive for a previous surgical birth, as scar tissue weakens the uterus.
- Has the patient experienced any previous complications of pregnancy? If so, what were they?
- What number child is this? If the patient is a multipara, your preparation time will be significantly reduced.

If delivery is imminent, you will not have time to conduct an extensive physical examination, but try to do the following:

- *Assess the woman's vital signs.* If the woman's blood pressure is elevated or her hands and face look puffy, test the deep tendon reflexes at the knees ("knee jerks") for hyperactivity. Any of those signs—elevated blood pressure, facial edema, or hyperactive reflexes—strongly suggest that the woman has preeclampsia, and you must be prepared to deal with seizures before, during, or after delivery.
- *Try to estimate the gestational age.* Palpate the abdomen to estimate the height of the uterus. If the top of the uterus (the fundus) is palpable just above the symphysis pubis, the gestational age is 12 to 16 weeks; if the fundus is palpable at the level of the mother's umbilicus, the gestational age is 22 weeks; if the fundus reaches all the way to the xiphoid, the fetus is at or near term.
- *Listen for fetal heart tones.* Anything lower than 120 beats/min suggests fetal distress.

If the history and physical assessment indicate that there is ample time to reach the hospital, place the woman in the lateral recumbent position, remove any of her underclothing that might obstruct delivery in the event that the baby surprises you en route to the hospital, and begin transport.

If you reach the conclusion that there is *not* enough time to get to the hospital, prepare to assist in delivery of the baby at the scene. In a crowded or public place, try to find an area of maximum privacy and cleanliness in which to work. In the patient's

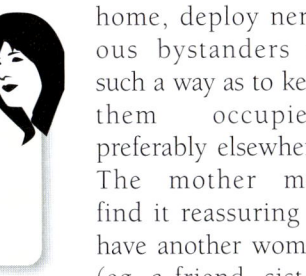

Notes from Nancy

If the baby is coming fast, it is more important to control the delivery than to put on sterile drapes.

home, deploy nervous bystanders in such a way as to keep them occupied, preferably elsewhere. The mother may find it reassuring to have another woman (eg, a friend, sister, mother, or neighbour) or her husband present. But your own behaviour, if calm and reassuring, will be the most effective sedative for patient and bystanders alike.

Setting Up for Delivery Outside the Hospital

When you have to assist in childbirth outside the hospital, it means you didn't have enough time to reach the hospital. Consequently, you generally don't have time to make a lot of preparations. You may have only a minute or two to get the mother into position, open the OB kit, and catch the baby. Thus the sequence of actions in emergency childbirth needs to be well planned and well rehearsed before you use it in the prehospital setting.

Position the pregnant woman. If childbirth is to take place in the patient's home, the baby is usually delivered with the woman lying supine in her bed, preferably with a Reeves stretcher and sheet beneath her to facilitate moving her after delivery. While placing the woman in the supine position makes things much easier for you assisting delivery, it makes things harder for the mother, for she has to push against gravity. Some women therefore prefer to sit at the edge of a chair or to squat for delivery—positions that enable the woman to take advantage of gravity.

Controversies

Some medical personnel feel strongly that in-home delivery should be on the stretcher if at all possible to facilitate quick removal should the situation take a turn for the worse.

Delivery modalities have changed dramatically in recent years. More women are opting for home deliveries versus inhospital care, and the phenomenon of natural childbirth is becoming more popular. The use of nurse midwives, lay midwives, professional birth assistants, chiropractors, and doulas (an assistant who "mothers" the mother) are gradually gaining acceptance within the medical community. As a paramedic, you should be aware that other practitioners may be assisting with home deliveries in your region. You should know how you and your EMS service are meant to interact with these practitioners. The worst possible time to learn how to interact with these other practitioners is when an emergency is taking place during a home birth.

Standing Birth

Birthing from a standing position is an ancient practice, and one that is used in several areas of the world

Figure 39-11 ▶. This position is sometimes used in the active birth model, in which the mother is allowed total freedom to move around and be active up to the point of delivery. Standing birth allows the mother to take advantage of gravity and allows the pelvis to open to a maximal position. The fetal head is moved away from the sacral area as the mother arches her back, a movement that is not easily accomplished while supine. Standing birth purportedly allows breech births to proceed without complications, although no verifiable statistical data are available to quantify this claim.

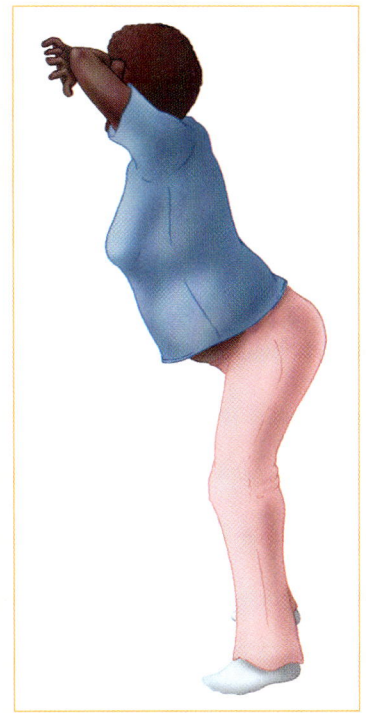

Figure 39-11 The standing position.

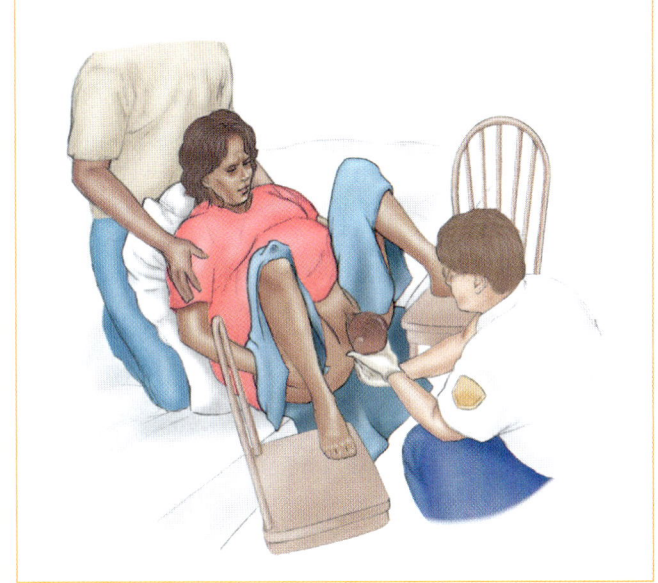

Figure 39-12 Semi-Fowler's position.

Semi-Fowler's Position

The semi-Fowler's position is basically the supine lithotomy position, with the woman's torso propped up to a high Fowler's or Fowler's position **Figure 39-12 ▲**. Sitting up seems to help some women with pushing, as they can lie back to rest in-between contractions.

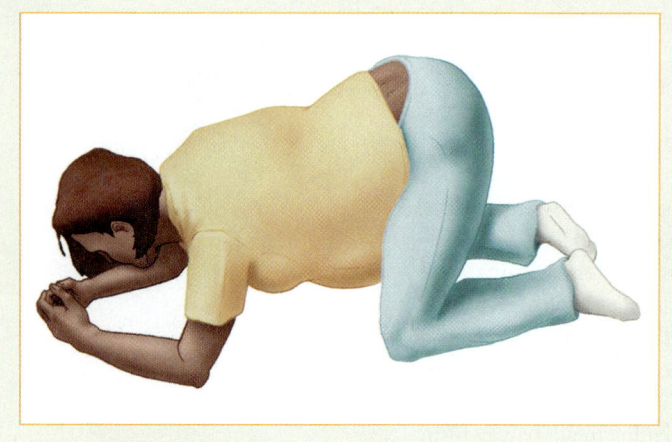

Figure 39-13 Kneeling birth position.

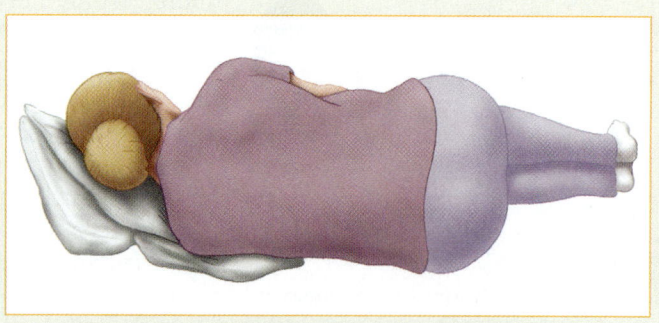

Figure 39-14 Left-Sims position.

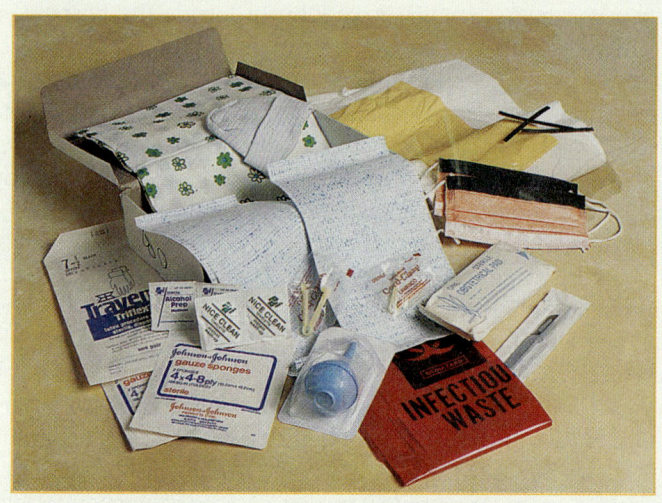

Figure 39-15 Your unit should contain a sterile OB kit. Items usually found in this kit are listed in Table 39-3.

Kneeling Birth

In the kneeling birth position, the woman kneels with her buttocks in the air and usually rests on her elbows **Figure 39-13 ▲** . This position provides some of the same advantages as squatting: It enables the mother to arch her back to assist delivery, which allows the fetal head to move away from the sacrum, thereby facilitating the birth. Some women may use this method in a bathtub full of water (water birth), which is reputed to ease delivery. Unintentional submersion (of the woman and baby) is a possible downside to this method, but is technically a low risk. The baby continues to be oxygenated through the umbilical cord until the face breaks water, or the baby is stimulated.

Side-Lying Position

The side-lying position is essentially a left-Sims position, with the upper torso possibly supported with pillows **Figure 39-14 ▶** . This position ensures that the uterus and the fetus are moved away from the inferior aorta. Some midwives report a significantly reduced incidence of perineal tears using this method. While some women may prefer to have their legs widely spread during birth, the side-lying position allows the knees to be held together, which also purportedly reduces tearing, especially during the crowning stage.

If the woman prefers to be in one of these positions, don't argue with her. She may use whatever position she is most comfortable with, and you need to adapt to the circumstances, as long as the alternative method does not endanger the woman.

Standard Delivery Set-up

In the ambulance, there generally isn't enough working space to permit the woman to sit or squat for delivery. Instead, you will need to position the woman on her back on the stretcher, with a folded sheet under her buttocks. She should then bend her knees and spread her thighs apart.

- Open the sterile obstetric kit, making sure to maintain sterility by touching only the outside **Figure 39-15 ▶** (see **Table 39-3 ▶** for kit contents).

- Wash your hands thoroughly with a povidone-iodine scrub solution.
- Put on sterile gloves, using sterile donning technique.
- Maintain routine precautions. Deliveries are often messy, and the chance of contamination from body fluid exposure is high. Put on a sterile gown and surgical mask, and wear eye protection.
- Prepare the woman for delivery by draping her with towels using the sterile towels in the OB kit. Have the woman lift her buttocks, and place the first towel beneath them. Take care not to touch her or the sheet she has been sitting on so that you do not break your sterile field. Lay a second sterile towel flat on the bed or stretcher between the woman's legs, just below the vaginal opening. Lay a third sterile towel or drape across the woman's abdomen, and drape each thigh as well. When you finish, everything should be covered with sterile drapes except the vaginal opening.

If the baby is coming without giving you the courtesy of time to prepare, forget the drapes and control the delivery. A safe and controlled delivery takes precedence over a nice textbook draping procedure.

Table 39-3	Sterile Obstetrics Kit for Ambulances		
Quantity	**Item**	**Quantity**	**Item**
1	Pair surgical scissors	1 to 2	Surgical masks
4	Cord clamps	12	10 cm × 10 cm gauze sponges
4 to 6	30-cm lengths of umbilical tape	1	Bulb syringe
4 to 6	Towels	1	Baby blanket
2 to 3	Pairs surgical gloves	2	Large plastic bags
1	Surgical gown	3	Povidone-iodine scrub brush

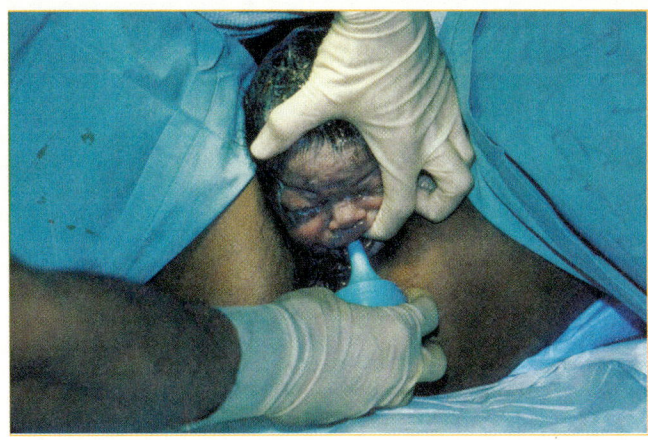

Figure 39-16 Clear the baby's airway.

Do not forget to attend to the emotional needs of the patient and family members who are bystanders. This job should be managed by your partner while you are getting prepared. Emotions tend to run high during deliveries, and additional stress may be experienced if the delivery is occurring in a crowded area. Your partner should take a position at the woman's head to help keep her calm. Your partner should also ensure that an emesis basin and portable suction are at hand. If there is a spare moment, your partner should start an IV line with normal saline to keep a vein open, especially if your provincial or regional protocol calls for giving oxytocin after delivery.

Encourage the woman to rest between contractions and to resist bearing down until you are ready to assist with the delivery. This may be a tall order, because once she is ready to push, she is *going* to push. If she finds it difficult not to bear down, instruct her to "pant like a dog" during each contraction. Panting makes it nearly impossible to push because bearing down requires a closed glottis.

Assisting Delivery

With the woman prepared as described, take up a position just distal to her buttocks (on her right side if you are right-handed and on her left side if you are left-handed) and follow these steps.

1. Control the delivery. When crowning occurs, place *gentle* pressure on the baby's head with the palm of your gloved hand to prevent the head from delivering too quickly and tearing the woman's vagina.

2. As the baby's head begins to emerge from the vagina, it will start to turn. Support the head as it turns. Do *not* attempt to pull the baby from the vagina! If the membranes cover the head after it emerges, tear the amniotic sac with your fingers or forceps to permit escape of amniotic fluid and enable the baby to breathe.

3. Slip your middle finger alongside the baby's head to check for a nuchal cord. In such a case, the umbilical cord becomes wrapped around part of the infant's body, generally the neck and as a single loop. In most cases, a nuchal cord is

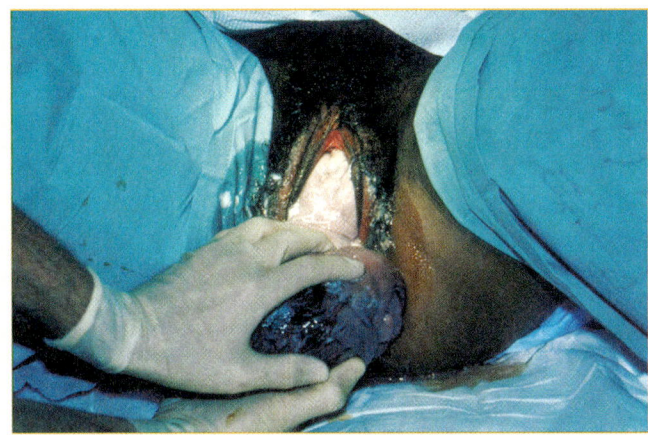

Figure 39-17 Gently guide the baby's head downward to allow delivery of the upper shoulder.

not a significant problem, but as the fetus descends during labour, cord compression may occur, causing the fetal heart rate to slow and resulting in fetal distress.

4. If you find a nuchal cord, try to slip it gently over the baby's shoulder and head. Should this maneuver fail, and if the cord is wrapped tightly around the neck, place umbilical clamps 5 cm apart and cut the cord between the clamps.

5. With the baby's head cradled and supported in your hand, clear the baby's airway by suctioning with the bulb syringe Figure 39-16 ▲ . Suction the mouth first, and then the nose.

6. Gently guide the baby's head downward to allow delivery of the upper shoulder Figure 39-17 ▲ . Do not pull on the baby to facilitate the delivery.

7. Gently guide the head upward to allow delivery of the lower shoulder Figure 39-18 ▶ .

8. Once the shoulders are delivered, the baby's trunk and legs will follow rapidly Figure 39-19 ▶ . Be prepared to grasp

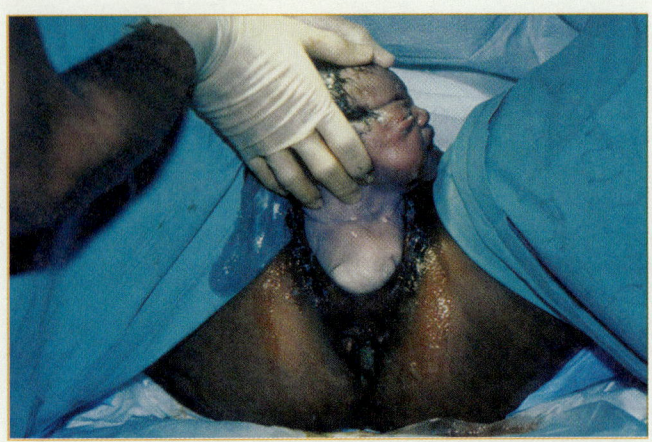

Figure 39-18 Gently guide the head upward to allow delivery of the lower shoulder.

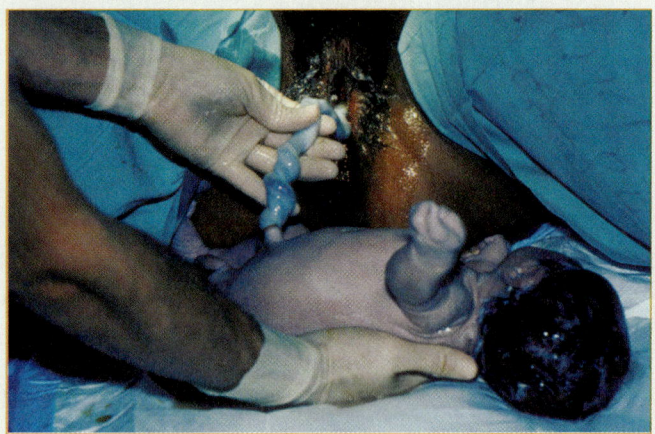

Figure 39-19 Once the shoulders are delivered, the baby's trunk and legs will follow rapidly.

and support the infant as it emerges, keeping in mind an important fact: *Newborn babies are wet and slippery.*

9. Once the baby is delivered, lay the baby along your arm and grasp it like a football, with one arm and shoulder between your fingers and the head held dependent to aid drainage.

10. Wipe any blood or mucus from the baby's nose and mouth with a sterile gauze. Use the rubber bulb aspirator to suction the baby's mouth and nostrils. Be sure to squeeze the bulb *before* inserting the tip, and only *then* place the tip in the baby's mouth or nostril and release the bulb slowly. Withdraw the bulb, expel its contents into a waste container, and repeat suctioning as needed.

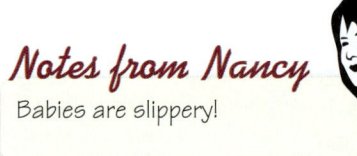

Notes from Nancy

Babies are slippery!

11. Dry the baby with sterile towels (wet babies lose heat faster than dry ones), place the infant in the foil bunting, and wrap with a dry blanket.

12. Record the time of birth for your PCR.

In a normal delivery, the baby will usually be breathing on his or her own, if not shrieking, by the time you finish suctioning the airway. Babies are usually born blue, but with a few good howls they should turn a nice pink, although their extremities may remain dusky.

Apgar Scoring

The Apgar scoring system (devised by Virginia Apgar, MD) is a useful means of evaluating the adequacy of a newborn's vital functions immediately after birth; such information will prove useful to those who take over the care of the baby after your delivery. In this system, five parameters—heart rate, respiratory effort, muscle tone, reflex irritability, and colour—are each given a score from 0 to 2 both 60 seconds and then 5 minutes after birth. The majority of infants are vigorous and have a total score of 7 to 10; they cough or cry within seconds of delivery and require no further resuscitation. Infants with a score in the 4 to 6 range are moderately depressed; they may be pale or

blue 1 minute after delivery, with poorly sustained respirations and flaccid muscle tone. Such infants will require some form of resuscitation (discussed in Chapter 40).

Cutting the Umbilical Cord

Once the infant has been delivered and is breathing well, the umbilical cord can be clamped and cut, as it is no longer necessary for the infant's survival.

1. Handle the umbilical cord with care. It tears easily.

2. Tie or clamp the cord about 20 cm from the infant's navel, with two ties (or clamps) placed 5 cm apart. Cut the cord between the two ties or clamps. There is evidence for delaying cord clamping for at least 1 minute in term and preterm newborns not requiring resuscitation. However, do not delay cord clamping if the newborn requires resuscitation.

3. Examine the cut ends of the cord to be certain there is no bleeding. If the cut end attached to the infant is bleeding, tie or clamp the cord *proximal* to the previous clamp, and examine it again (do *not* remove the first clamp). There should not be any oozing from the infant's end of the cord.

4. Once the cord is clamped and cut, wrap the baby in a dry blanket and place him or her at the mother's breast. This gives the mother a chance to attempt breastfeeding and allows for bonding between the mother and child. The suckling reflex also triggers the uterus to contract, which will speed the delivery of the placenta and reduce bleeding.

Delivery and Management of the Placenta

With the delivery of the baby, the second stage of labour is complete, and the third stage—delivery of the placenta—begins. The placenta is usually delivered within 20 minutes of the baby's arrival. Your job is to make stimulating conversation with the mother and bystanders as you wait patiently for the placenta to begin to separate spontaneously. Do not attempt to speed delivery of the placenta by pulling on the umbilical cord.

The first sign that the placenta is separating from the uterine wall is usually the patient's complaint that her contractions are starting again. The uterus rises in the abdomen and feels hard to palpation. The end of the umbilical cord protruding from the vagina lengthens, and there is usually a gush of blood from the vagina. When these signs occur:

1. Instruct the patient to bear down to expel the placenta.
2. As she does so, hold the placenta with both hands and gently twist it so that the membranes will peel completely off the uterine wall.
3. Gently massage the abdomen over the uterus to aid in its contraction.
4. If your provincial or regional protocol says to do so, add 10 units of oxytocin (Pitocin) to the mother's IV bag and drip it in *slowly,* no faster than about 30 ml/min. Before you start oxytocin, make absolutely sure the woman isn't delivering a second baby!

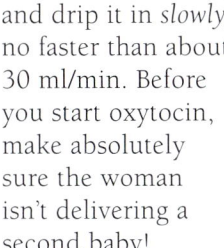

Notes from Nancy
Never pull on the umbilical cord to try to hasten delivery of the placenta.

Once you have the placenta in your hand, examine it for completeness. One side (fetal side) should be grey, shiny, and smooth; the other side (maternal side) should be dark maroon with a rough texture **Figure 39-20**. There may also be a white fringe around the placenta, which is the remnant of the amniotic sac. Pallor of the maternal surface of the placenta may indicate hemorrhage or fetal anemia. Blood clots adhering to the surface suggest abruption. Try to determine whether the placenta is malformed in any way or if pieces are obviously missing; retained pieces of placenta will cause persistent bleeding. Place the placenta in one of the plastic bags from the OB kit, and transport it with you to the hospital for examination by the pathology lab.

Examine the perineum for lacerations and apply pressure to any bleeding tears. Clean up and place a sanitary pad over the mother's vaginal opening, lower her legs, and prepare for transport. If the placenta has not delivered after 15 minutes,

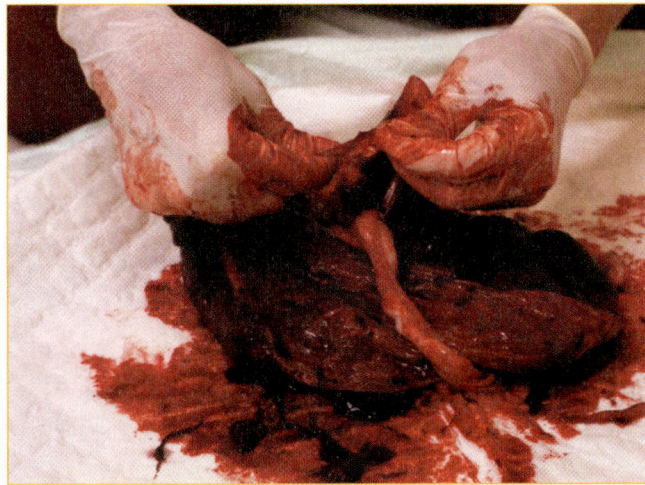

Figure 39-20 A whole placenta.

transport the patient anyway. Transport the patient in the supine recumbent position, with pads and draping in place, maintaining BSI precautions.

Some women may request to keep the placenta. This is standard practice in some parts of the world, where consumption of the placenta is considered a means for the mother to quickly regain her strength. Women from some cultures may want to keep the placenta to bury it and plant a tree over the spot, so that the tree and the child grow together. You need to respect such requests. If the patient refuses transport to the hospital, try to follow local protocol and law as to who should receive the placenta.

Abnormal Deliveries

Most deliveries are normal. The baby arrives headfirst, followed shortly by the placenta; the mother and paramedics come through the event like champs. Occasionally, however, complications arise. To deal with obstetric complications successfully, the paramedic must know when to anticipate them, how to recognize them when they do occur, and what action to take to ensure that everyone makes it through the event successfully.

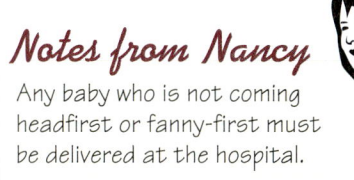

Notes from Nancy
Any baby who is not coming headfirst or fanny-first must be delivered at the hospital.

Breech Presentations

Most term babies enter the world headfirst (vertex presentation). The baby's head serves to open a path through the cervix for the narrower shoulders and hips. In a breech presentation, however, another part of the body leads the way, usually the buttocks (the word *breech* means "buttocks") **Figure 39-21**, but sometimes one of the feet comes first. Breech presentations occur in 4% of all deliveries and are more common with premature births.

The best place for a breech presentation to be delivered is in the hospital. Of course, sometimes you won't realize that you are dealing with a breech until the mother is crowning and you

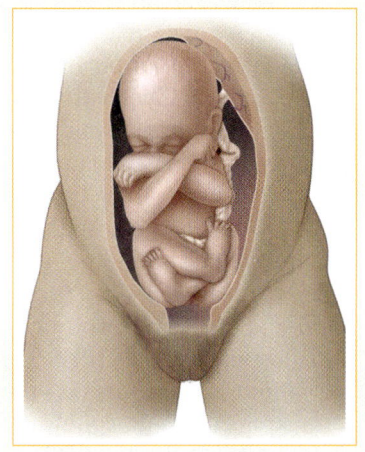

Figure 39-21 In a breech presentation, the buttocks are delivered first. These deliveries are usually slow, so you will often have time to transport the mother to the hospital.

notice that the presenting part does not have any hair but rather has a suspicious indentation down the middle. By the time you have made that astute observation, it's usually too late to get the woman to the hospital.

If you have determined that the buttocks are the presenting part and delivery is imminent, consider initiating immediate transport to the nearest hospital. Delivery of a breech presentation is difficult and may require operative intervention. Initiating transport will get you closer to the hospital in case difficulties are encountered, and proceed as follows:

- Position the woman with her buttocks at the edge of the bed or stretcher and her legs flexed.
- Allow the buttocks and trunk of the baby to deliver spontaneously. *Do not pull on the baby.*
- Once the baby's legs are clear, support the baby's body on the palm of your hand and volar surface of your arm.
- Lower the baby slightly so that it very nearly hangs by its own weight downward; that will help the head pass through the pelvic outlet. You can tell when the head is in the vaginal canal because you'll be able to see the baby's hairline at the nape of his or her neck just below the woman's symphysis pubis.
- Delivery of the head (which is the largest part of the baby) is the most difficult part. Maintaining neck flexion is key to minimizing the diameter of the head that presents to the birth canal. Grasp the baby by the ankles and lift him or her upwards in the direction of the mother's abdomen.
- If the baby's head does not deliver within 3 minutes, the child is in danger of suffocation, and immediate action is indicated. Suffocation may occur when the baby's umbilical cord is compressed by his or her head against the birth canal, which cuts off the baby's supply of oxygenated blood from the placenta, and the face is pressed against the vaginal wall, which prevents the baby from breathing on his or her own. Place your gloved hand in the vagina, with your palm toward the baby's face. Using two fingers form a "V" on the baby's face and try to help flex the neck. Your other hand should be on the baby's posterior shoulders with the middle finger on the posterior occiput flexing it forward. The ALSO manual describes this as the modified Mauriceau-Smellie-Veit maneuver. During delivery of the head, do not apply traction on the body or pull the neck and head out, because this will injure the newborn.
- Remember: *This is a delivery, not an extrication.* Do not attempt to forcibly pull the baby out or allow an explosive delivery. If the head does not deliver within 3 minutes of establishing the airway, provide rapid transport to the hospital, with the mother's buttocks elevated on pillows. Try to maintain the baby's airway throughout transport. En route, alert the hospital so that it can have the appropriate personnel on hand when the mother arrives.

Other Abnormal Presentations

There are a variety of other abnormal ways in which the baby may present for delivery, most of them fortunately quite rare. In a footling breech, one or both feet will dangle down through the vaginal opening **Figure 39-22 ▸** . In a transverse presentation (transverse lie), the fetus lies crosswise in the uterus and may wave at the paramedic with one hand protruding through the vagina. Even the baby who is coming headfirst may deflex the

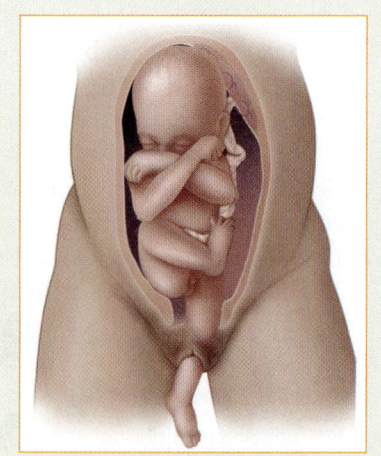

Figure 39-22 In very rare instances, an infant's limb—usually a single arm or leg—presents first. This is a serious situation, and you must provide prompt transport for hospital delivery.

head and present with the face or brow instead of the top of the head (vertex). With all of those abnormal presentations, the most important point is *not to attempt delivery in the prehospital environment.* Nearly all of these abnormal presentations will require delivery by cesarean section, so prehospital management is to provide rapid transport.

Prolapsed Umbilical Cord

With a prolapsed umbilical cord, the cord emerges from the uterus ahead of the baby **Figure 39-23 ▾** . With each uterine contraction, the cord is then compressed between the presenting part and the bony pelvis, shutting off the baby's supply of oxygenated blood from the placenta. Fetal asphyxia may ensue if circulation through the cord is not rapidly reestablished and maintained until delivery. Cord prolapse occurs in 3% of deliveries and is more likely when the presenting part does not completely fill the pelvic brim, such as in abnormal presentations or with small babies (premature births, multiple births).

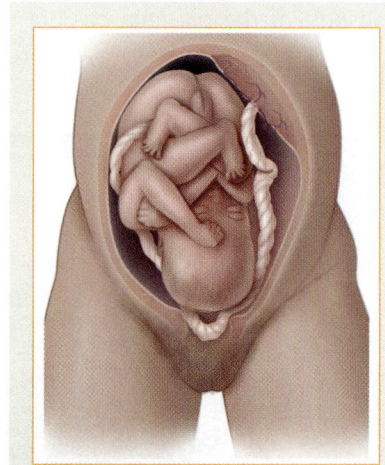

Figure 39-23 A prolapsed umbilical cord, another rare situation, is very dangerous and must be cared for at the hospital.

Treatment of cord prolapse is clearly urgent. Take the following steps:

1. Position the woman supine with her hips elevated as much as possible on pillows.
2. Administer 100% supplemental oxygen via nonrebreathing mask.
3. Instruct the woman to pant with each contraction, which will prevent her from bearing down.
4. With two fingers of a gloved hand, gently push the baby (not the cord) back up into the vagina until the presenting part no longer presses on the cord
5. While you maintain pressure on the presenting part, have your partner cover the exposed portion of the cord with dressings moistened in normal saline.
6. Somehow, you must try to maintain that position, with a gloved hand pushing the presenting part away from the cord, throughout *urgent transport* to the hospital.

Premature and Small Infants

Preterm labour occurs late in the second trimester or early in the third trimester of pregnancy. The pregnant woman will start to experience contractions; she also may have spotting and leakage of amniotic fluid. These babies have less of a chance of survival and more birth defects if they are born before 37 weeks of gestation. The treatment for this condition is to prevent labour from occurring, thereby allowing the fetus to more fully develop and have a better chance of survival. Medications given to halt preterm labour may include indomethacin and nitroglycerine.

Any baby born before 37 weeks' gestation *or* weighing less than 2.5 kg needs special prehospital care. Chapter 40 discusses the prehospital care of neonates in more detail. For our purposes here, follow these guidelines when dealing with small, red, wrinkled babies:

1. Keep the baby warm. Babies lose heat by the same mechanisms that adults do—radiation, convection, conduction, and evapouration. But babies—and especially "premies"—have less natural insulation and a larger surface area in relation to mass, so they are much more vulnerable to rapid heat loss.
   - Dry the baby thoroughly as soon as possible after birth.
   - Wrap the baby in foil bunting, from head to toe.
   - Cover the baby with a dry blanket.
   - Place the baby on the mother's chest, and cover both with another blanket.
2. Keep the ambulance interior nice and warm. If it's comfortable for you, it's too cold for the premie.
3. Maintain the baby's airway. Use a bulb syringe to keep the baby's mouth and nose clear of fluid.
4. Prevent bleeding from the umbilical cord; a very small baby cannot afford to lose even a little bit of blood. If the cord is oozing, apply another clamp.
5. Administer supplemental oxygen through a tent above the infant's head; do *not* blast oxygen directly into the baby's eyes. Use low flow—less than 4 l/min.

6. Prevent contamination. Premature babies are highly susceptible to infection. Wear a surgical gown and mask, and keep bystanders—especially relatives who want to "give the new baby a big kiss"—at a distance.

Shoulder Dystocia

Shoulder dystocia occurs when the infant becomes trapped in between the symphysis pubis and sacrum because its shoulders are larger than its head; it is most often observed in infants with increased birth weight. In shoulder dystocia, the head delivers normally, but then abruptly retracts against the perineum.

If shoulder dystocia occurs, position the mother with her buttocks off the edge of the bed and her thighs flexed upward as much as possible. Apply firm open-hand pressure just above the symphysis pubis bone to facilitate delivery. If delivery does not occur, administer 100% oxygen to the mother, maintain the infant's airway, and transport immediately.

Multiple Births

Multiple gestations occur in about 3% of all pregnancies. Generally, the older a woman is at the time of conception, and the more pregnancies she has had, the higher her chances of a multiple birth. The use of fertility drugs also significantly increases a woman's odds of being pregnant with more than one child, including quadruplets and quintuplets.

The incidence of multiple births in Canada has risen significantly in recent years, so the odds of a paramedic having to assist in the delivery of multiple births is not necessarily a remote one. This is one of the reasons the OB kit has more than you can use with a single birth, and why there should always be a spare OB kit on the unit. As a rule, the delivery of multiple births does not pose any special problems, except that you have to do a few things twice (or three times!). There is a greater chance of encountering breech presentations in such births. Because the babies are usually smaller, however, delivery is easier than in a single breech birth.

The mother is generally aware that she is carrying more than one baby, especially if she has had appropriate prenatal care, and ideally will let you know. In the absence of prenatal care, particularly in socioeconomically depressed areas, the woman may be unaware of her condition. If the mother is still suspiciously large after delivery of the first baby, or another clue presents itself, such as a tiny hand waving at you from the vaginal opening, get ready for another delivery.

If you have reason to suspect there is more than one baby, proceed as follows:
- Repeat the earlier preparations for delivery. If time permits, put on new gloves and a gown from the spare OB kit.
- Twins are usually delivered single file, one after the other. When the first baby is born, clamp and cut the cord in the usual fashion. Inspect *both* ends of the cord for oozing, and apply a second clamp if necessary, to prevent hemorrhage from the twin if there is a shared placenta (you won't know until the placenta delivers). Some twins share a placenta; others may have their own, separate placentas or share two placentas that have fused into one.

- Contractions will usually start again within about 5 to 10 minutes after the birth of the first baby, and the second baby can be expected to arrive within 30 to 45 minutes of its twin. That gap usually gives you time to transport before the birth of the second baby, if you decide to.
- Usually both babies are born before the first placenta is delivered.
- Given that twin babies tend to be smaller than single term babies, treat them as you would premature babies, paying meticulous attention to keeping them warm, well oxygenated, and in as sterile an environment as possible.

Stillborn Babies

On rare occasions, the happiness of childbirth is overshadowed by despair when the baby is born dead. Stillbirth occurs in about 1 of every 200 pregnancies. Good prenatal care most often identifies a stillborn child well before delivery, but in the absence of such care, it may be totally unsuspected. Complications of labour and delivery can also precipitate such an unhappy occurrence, with the baby dying in utero shortly before birth.

Resuscitation should always be attempted, unless the baby is obviously dead (signs of putrification are evident). In such cases, you need to remember that although one patient has been lost, you may have several other patients to deal with as the emotional trauma sets in. Reactions can range from complete silence and pretending the dead baby does not exist, to wailing and screaming. If the family is religious, the grieving parents may want to have the baby baptized and a short eulogy of blessing spoken. Knowing the cultural and ethnic heritage of where you work will help prepare you for this situation. Keep the phone numbers of local religious leaders available to contact.

■ Complications of Labour and Delivery

Postpartum Hemorrhage

The average blood loss during the third stage of labour is normally about 150 ml. When blood loss exceeds 500 ml during the first 24 hours after giving birth, it is considered postpartum hemorrhage (bleeding after birth). Anything that interferes with the contractions of the interlacing uterine muscle fibres after delivery of the placenta will promote postpartum hemorrhage as follows:

- **Prolonged labour or delivery of multiple babies.** They may lead to a "tired" uterus.
- **Retained products of conception.** The uterus cannot contract fully until it is empty.
- **Grand multiparity.** After many pregnancies, the muscle tissue in the uterus is gradually replaced with fibrous tissue, which does not contract.
- **Multiple pregnancy.** The placental site is larger, and the overstretched uterine muscles don't contract as well.
- **Placenta previa.** Muscles in the lower segment of the uterus, where the placenta is implanted, do not contract efficiently.

- **A full bladder.** It may prevent proper placental separation and uterine contraction.

The only measures feasible in the prehospital setting to manage postpartum hemorrhage are those that encourage uterine contraction and help restore circulating volume as follows:

1. Continue uterine massage.
2. Put the baby (or babies) to the mother's breast(s).
3. Add 20 units of oxytocin to the IV bag (1,000 ml), and infuse at a rate of 250 ml/hr. (This treatment should comply with the protocol in your service or region, and may require direct medical control to initiate).
4. Notify the receiving hospital of the mother's status and your estimated time of arrival.
5. Transport without delay.
6. Start another large-bore IV line en route, and infuse normal saline wide open.
7. Do not attempt internal examination of the vagina.
8. Do not attempt to pack the vagina with any form of dressing.
9. Manage *external* bleeding from perineal tears with firm pressure. It may be necessary to open the labia and place packs at the bleeding site.

Meconium Staining

While in utero, the fetus passively ingests several elements—for example, lanugo, mucus, and amniotic fluid. This material is stored in the intestines and constitutes the first stool the infant passes. This first stool, which is called meconium, is odourless, greenish-black, and has a tar-like consistency. Unlike later feces, it is also sterile. In cases of fetal distress, or with the stresses of labour and delivery, the fetus may void the meconium into the amniotic fluid. If this occurs in utero, it may result in chemical pneumonia in the child. Umbilical cord prolapse is one condition that can cause such fetal distress, if compression of the cord has occurred.

There is no way for you to ascertain whether meconium is in the amniotic fluid until the bag of waters breaks. Normally, the waters should be clear. A yellow tint to the amniotic fluid suggests the meconium has been in the amniotic fluid for a while. A greenish-black colour, especially with the presence of particulate matter, indicates recent passage of meconium and is a sign of danger.

You need to be vigilant regarding the need for suctioning if meconium staining is present. Meconium aspiration syndrome can develop if the infant is allowed to take a breath before meconium is suctioned away. The viscosity of meconium can cause the infant's airway to become partially or completely blocked, and meconium trapped in the infant's airways will irritate the respiratory tract, further hampering the infant's efforts to breathe. If meconium is noticed prior to delivery, you should prepare as follows:

- If available, use a suction trap or meconium aspirator to clean out the hypopharynx. Aggressive suctioning is necessary the moment the head appears. Repeat if necessary.

- Tracheal suctioning may be indicated for thick particulate matter, if the neonate is not vigorous. Neonatal resuscitation guidelines now recommend tracheal suctioning of meconium only if the neonate is not vigorous. For meconium-stained amniotic fluid and a nonvigorous infant, prior to stimulation and drying, use endotracheal tube suctioning until clear of meconium. Routine oropharyngeal and nasopharyngeal suctioning on the perenium in infants with meconium-stained fluid is no longer recommended.

Supine Hypotensive Syndrome

When the gravid uterus compresses the inferior vena cava, venous blood return to the heart is diminished or, in some cases, occluded. This problem occurs mainly when a gravid woman assumes a supine position (hence the term supine hypotensive syndrome) but can also occur when the woman is sitting. This condition is usually associated with late-stage pregnancy, when the uterus is at its largest, and patient mobility is significantly impaired. It also occurs more commonly in women who have venous varicosities. The woman is most prone to this syndrome during labour, but may also experience difficulties in sleep states, particularly if she falls asleep on her back. Left uncorrected, supine hypotensive syndrome can result in significant maternal hypotension and potentially lead to fetal distress as the maternal hypotension translates into placental hypoperfusion. It generally takes 3 to 7 minutes of compression before signs and symptoms manifest. Nausea, dizziness, tachycardia, and claustrophobia are early signs of caval compression, progressing to breathing difficulty and syncopal episodes. Precipitating factors may include hypovolemia, from either blood loss or dehydration.

Management includes placing the patient in the left lateral recumbent position and treating underlying causes (ie, IV fluids, if hypovolemic). In addition, you must monitor the blood pressure and other vital signs and obtain an ECG. The cure for supine hypotensive syndrome is delivery of the fetus.

Pulmonary Embolism

One of the most common causes of maternal death during childbirth or postpartum is pulmonary embolism. An embolism may form from a number of sources, but a blood clot arising in the pelvic circulation is a frequent cause. Leakage of amniotic fluid into the maternal circulation (amniotic embolism), a clot arising from DVT (pregnancy-related venous thromboembolism), and water or air entering the vagina after a water birth (water embolism) are examples of potential embolic processes. Should the woman experience sudden dyspnea, tachycardia, atrial fibrillation, or hypotension in the postpartum state, you should suspect pulmonary embolism. The patient may complain of sudden, sharp chest pain, abdominal pain, or experience syncope. Physical examination may reveal nothing unusual except for an increased pulse rate, tachypnea, and hypotension—signs that may be mistaken for shock. Management of a postpartum embolism is the same as management of pulmonary embolism occurring in nonpregnant states (see Chapter 27).

Uterine Inversion

Uterine inversion is a potentially fatal complication of childbirth, occurring in 1 of every 2,000 pregnancies. In this condition, the placenta fails to detach properly and adheres to the uterine wall when it is expelled. As a result, the uterus literally turns inside-out. Uterine inversion usually occurs as a result of mismanaging the third stage of labour, such as placing excessive pressure on the uterus during fundal massage or by exerting strong traction on the umbilical cord in an attempt to hasten delivery of the placenta.

The severity of inversion is graded by how much the uterus has reversed itself and ranges from incomplete inversion, to complete inversion, to prolapsed inversion, and finally to total inversion. With incomplete and complete inversions, the uterus does not protrude externally. The paramedic will most likely encounter a prolapsed or a total inversion. (The other forms are not readily identifiable in the prehospital environment.) In a prolapsed inversion, the fundus of the uterus can be seen protruding from the vagina. In a total inversion, both the uterus and the vagina protrude inside-out. This is a very painful condition, and shock may develop rapidly due to hypovolemia.

Management of uterine inversion is as follows:

1. Keep the patient recumbent.
2. Administer 100% supplemental oxygen via nonrebreathing mask.
3. Start two IV lines with normal saline, and run them as rapidly as necessary to maintain blood pressure. A 250-to 500-ml initial bolus is appropriate.
4. If the placenta is still attached to the uterus, do *not* attempt to remove it.
5. Carefully monitor vital signs, and treat for shock.
6. Consider giving oxytocin (Pitocin), 10 units IM, to help control exsanguinating hemorrhage, if your local protocol permits it.

Make *one* attempt to replace the uterus. Push the uterine fundus up and through the vaginal canal by applying pressure with the fingertips and the palm of a gloved hand. If this procedure fails, cover all protruding tissues with moist sterile dressings and provide rapid transport.

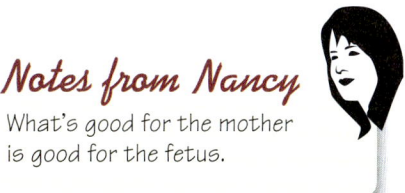

Notes from Nancy

What's good for the mother is good for the fetus.

Emergency Pharmacology in Pregnancy

There is always some concern in pregnancy of pharmacologic agents having dangerous effects on the fetus. These concerns are secondary when the life of the mother is at stake. As noted earlier, maternal physiology is altered in pregnancy, and these changes have an impact on pharmacologic therapies. Hepatic metabolism increases, as does renal excretion, which may cause IV administered medications to pass quickly through the maternal system. Volume changes may affect distribution, resulting in higher doses needed to gain appreciable systemic affects. Gastric absorption is slowed, meaning oral drugs may require a larger period than normal to achieve the desired effect.

Drugs given in the prehospital setting for pregnancy-related problems constitute a very short list.

Magnesium Sulfate

Magnesium sulfate is classified as an electrolyte. Magnesium sulfate acts as a central nervous system depressant; in pregnancy, it is principally used in the management of eclampsia. Some physicians may order a magnesium sulfate infusion with preeclampsia to prevent seizures from occurring.

Magnesium sulfate can cause respiratory depression, hypotension, and, potentially, circulatory collapse. This drug needs to be administered slowly, as rapid infusion can potentiate these effects.

Magnesium sulfate may also be considered as a slow IV push in the presence of seizures during or immediately following labour (eclampsia). (Hydralazine or labetatol can also be used to control blood pressure once seizures have stopped, if the patient is still hypertensive.) IM injection can also be used, but the total dose should be placed in two separate syringes, with an equal dose in each syringe, and administered at different sites.

Calcium Chloride

Classified as a supplement, calcium chloride is mainly used in the prehospital setting for managing cases of hypocalcemia. When magnesium sulfate has been given in cases of eclampsia and respiratory depression has developed, calcium chloride (or calcium gluconate) acts as an antidote to counter the effects of magnesium sulfate.

Side effects of calcium chloride include nausea and vomiting, syncope, bradycardia, and dysrhythmias, and the drug may precipitate cardiac arrest. This agent is typically administered as slow IV push over 10 minutes with repeat doses per provincial or regional protocol. This may be repeated in 10-minute intervals as a buffer to magnesium toxicity.

Diazepam

Diazepam (Valium) is a benzodiazepine that is classified as a sedative/anticonvulsant. It is used principally in EMS as a seizure medication. Its use is indicated in eclampsia when the patient's seizures do not respond to magnesium sulfate. Diazepam may also be ordered to treat anxiety in cases of hypertensive crisis, such as in preeclampsia.

The principal side effects of diazepam administration include nausea and vomiting, respiratory depression, and hypotension. Ancillary side effects include headache and amnesia. The dosage is 5 to 10 mg slow IV push for management of seizure states. The dosage for anxiety management is 2 to 5 mg. The anxiety dosage should be given IM if conditions permit, or IV if anxiety is high and is accompanied by significant hypertension and dependent or facial edema is present.

Diphenhydramine

Diphenhydramine (Benadryl) is an antihistamine used principally to treat allergic reactions. Due to its sedative and antiemetic properties, it is also useful in treating hyperemesis gravidarum. Side effects include drowsiness, headache, tachycardia, and hypotension. The dosage for emesis is 25 to 50 mg IV.

Oxytocin

Oxytocin (Pitocin) is a naturally occurring hormone that causes uterine contractions by acting on smooth muscle. This uterine stimulant can be used to induce labour, but is commonly used to control postpartum hemorrhage. In the prehospital setting, oxytocin should be used only to manage severe postpartum bleeding, and only after *all* products of conception have been expelled from the uterus (including additional babies).

Side effects include nausea and vomiting, tachycardia, seizures, and cardiac arrhythmias. Oxytocin can also induce coma or result in uterine rupture and hypertension if administered in excess. The dosage is 3 to 10 units IM, or 10 to 20 units in 500 or 1,000 ml normal saline, slowly titrated to effect.

Postdelivery Prehospital Care

After delivery of the baby, take the mother's vital signs. Place a sanitary napkin in front of the vagina to collect any discharge after the birth. Monitor the mother's condition closely for postpartum hemorrhage, seizure activity, or respiratory difficulty. Finally, cover the mother with blankets to prevent mild hypothermia.

Monitor the baby's vital signs as well, watching out for any signs of cardiopulmonary distress. Keep the baby warm.

You are the Paramedic Summary

1. What specific questions should you ask this patient?

There are some very important questions that you must ask any pregnant patient—especially one in labour—to determine if delivery will occur in the prehospital environment or if there is ample time to transport. The following questions will help you make this determination:

- How many weeks pregnant are you?
- When are you due?
- Is this your first baby?
- Has your bag of waters (amniotic sac) ruptured? If so, when?
- How far apart are your contractions? How long does each contraction last?
- Do you feel as though you have to push or move your bowels?

Additional questions should be asked to determine if this is a high-risk pregnancy. You must gather as much information as possible to be able to anticipate and prepare for possible resuscitation of the infant immediately following birth. Such questions include:

- Do you use drugs, drink alcohol, or take any medications?
- Have you had regular prenatal care?
- Do you have any medical problems? Inquire specifically about pregnancy-induced hypertension (eg, preeclampsia) and gestational diabetes.
- Is there any possibility that this is a multiple birth?
- If you have had prenatal care, does your obstetrician expect any complications?
- If the amniotic sac has ruptured, did it contain meconium?

2. On the basis of what the patient has told you, what do you expect to find during your physical examination?

With regular contractions that are occurring every 3 minutes and the fact that the patient feels the urge to move her bowels, you will likely see the baby's head bulging from the vaginal opening (crowning). If not, you will likely observe crowning very soon. When the patient states that she needs to push or feels the urge to move her bowels, the infant's head is pushing on the rectum; this indicates that delivery is imminent.

3. Is there adequate time to transport this patient to the hospital, or should you prepare for imminent delivery?

To not prepare for imminent delivery is not an option. Aside of the frequent and regular contractions, crowning indicates that the first stage of labour has ended and the second stage is beginning. Like it or not, this baby will *not* wait until the patient is in the controlled setting of a hospital—40-km drive!

4. What is a nuchal cord? How should you manage this situation?

A nuchal cord occurs when the umbilical cord is wrapped around the baby's neck. If a nuchal cord is present, gently attempt to slide the cord over the infant's shoulders. If this is unsuccessful, you must clamp and cut the cord at once and continue with the delivery. A cord that is tightly wrapped around the infant's neck may result in newborn asphyxia if it is not immediately treated.

5. Should the Apgar score be used to determine the need for newborn resuscitation? Why or why not?

Because the first Apgar score is not obtained until the infant is 1 minute of age, it should not be used to determine whether or not resuscitation is needed. The need for and extent of resuscitation is based on three parameters: respiratory effort, heart rate, and colour. If needed, resuscitation must commence immediately. The Apgar score can be obtained once it is determined that the infant is not in need of resuscitation.

6. Is additional treatment required for this infant other than maintaining airway patency and providing thermal management?

Although the infant is breathing adequately and has a heart rate greater than 100 beats/min, the presence of central cyanosis indicates the need for supplemental oxygen. This is most effectively provided with the blow-by method. Hold an oxygen mask or oxygen tubing near the infant's nose and mouth with the flow rate set at 5 l/min. Most infants will "pink-up" after 30 to 60 seconds of blow-by oxygen. If despite 30 seconds of blow-by oxygen, the infant remains centrally cyanotic, you must provide positive-pressure ventilations with 100% supplemental oxygen. Cyanosis of the hands and feet (acrocyanosis) is a normal finding and should be of no concern. In fact, many infants have acrocyanosis for several hours to a few days following birth.

7. How will you treat this patient's postpartum bleeding?

Up to 500 ml of blood loss can be expected following an uncomplicated delivery. To control postpartum bleeding, there are several interventions that you can perform. You can have the infant nurse on the mother; this will stimulate the mother's pituitary gland to secrete oxytocin—a hormone that promotes uterine contraction. Second, you can massage the uterine fundus, which will promote uterine vasoconstriction and decreased bleeding. Place a sanitary pad over the mother's vagina; however, never pack the vagina with gauze pads or anything else! If your interventions to control postpartum bleeding are unsuccessful, you must treat the mother for shock; administer 100% supplemental oxygen, elevate her legs 15 to 30 cm, keep her warm, and administer crystalloid fluids to maintain adequate perfusion (ie, radial pulses, adequate mental status).

8. Is a crystalloid fluid bolus indicated at this point?

Simple techniques (eg, uterine massage) have successfully controlled this patient's postpartum bleeding. She remains conscious and alert and her vital signs do not suggest shock; therefore, IV crystalloid fluid boluses are not indicated at this point. Set your IV to keep vein open, but carefully monitor the patient's condition and be prepared to treat for shock.

Prep Kit

◼ Ready for Review

- The ovaries are the beginning point for reproduction. During the menstrual cycle, one follicle releases an ovum. If the ovum becomes fertilized, it develops into an embryo, and then into a fetus.
- The fallopian tubes are the structures that transport the ovum from the ovary to the uterus (a muscular, inverted pear-shaped organ). Once an egg is fertilized, it implants in the endometrium (the inner lining of the uterus).
- The fetus is enclosed in the amniotic sac, which contains amniotic fluid, allowing the fetus to develop in a weightless environment.
- The gestational period (the time that it takes for the infant to develop in utero) normally lasts 40 weeks.
- In the first trimester of pregnancy, the placenta, umbilical cord, specialized body systems, and limbs form. In the second trimester of pregnancy, the fetus gains weight and body systems become more specialized. In the last trimester of pregnancy, the fetus primarily puts on weight.
- Pregnancy is considered at term by week 37. Babies born before 37 weeks of gestation are considered premature, and babies born after 42 weeks of gestation are considered postmature.
- Physiologic changes during pregnancy can alter a woman's normal response to trauma or exacerbate or create medical conditions that can threaten the health of woman and fetus.
- Conditions that can be exacerbated by pregnancy include heart disease, hypertension, diabetes, respiratory disorders, renal disorders, hemoglobin disorders, epilepsy, and thyroid disorders.
- Preeclampsia is the most serious hypertensive disorder, manifesting after the 20th week of pregnancy. Symptoms include edema, gradual onset of hypertension, protein in the urine, severe headache, nausea and vomiting, agitation, rapid weight gain, and visual disturbances.
- Cholestasis is a liver disease that occurs during pregnancy. In this condition, the flow of bile is altered, causing acid buildup. The acid eventually spills into the bloodstream, causing profuse and painful itching.
- Abortion is expulsion of the fetus, from any cause, before the 20th week of gestation.
- An incomplete abortion occurs when only some of the products of conception are expelled. In such cases, be alert for signs and symptoms of shock.
- The three major causes of significant antepartum hemorrhage are abruptio placenta, placenta previa, and uterine rupture.
- Assessment of third-trimester bleeding is much the same as the assessment of other vaginal bleeding. Keep the woman lying on her left side, administer supplemental oxygen, provide rapid transport, provide IV fluids and ECG monitoring, and place sanitary pads over the vagina.
- Ectopic pregnancy occurs when a fertilized ovum has implanted somewhere other than the uterus, usually in one of the fallopian tubes. The patient will be in severe pain and possibly hypovolemic shock.
- In assessing a patient with an obstetric emergency, identify the length of gestation, estimated due date, any complications with this pregnancy or others, and the presence of any vaginal bleeding.
- The major causes of injury to pregnant women are motor vehicle collisions, falls, domestic abuse, and penetrating injuries such as gunshot wounds. Treatment of trauma in a pregnant woman is the same as treatment of a nonpregnant woman, except that the pregnant patient should be transported on her left side unless spinal injury is suspected.
- Labour may begin with a bloody show, or release of mucus (sometimes with blood) from the vagina.

- The first stage of labour begins with the onset of contractions—crampy abdominal pains that may radiate into the lower back. The amniotic sac may also rupture.
- The second stage of labour begins when the baby's head enters the birth canal. The woman's contractions become more intense and more frequent. When the baby's head becomes visible at the vaginal opening (crowning), delivery is imminent.
- The third stage of labour occurs when the placenta is expelled.
- In assessing a pregnant patient, determine whether there is time to transport.
- If delivery is imminent, quickly prepare a private clean area. Behave in a calm and reassuring way. Control the delivery. Clear the baby's airway.
- Never pull on the umbilical cord to deliver the placenta. Gently massage the abdomen to aid in delivery of the placenta. Once the placenta is delivered, examine it for completeness.
- A baby born before 37 weeks' gestation or weighing less than 2.5 kg is premature. Keep a premie warm, maintain the airway, prevent umbilical cord bleeding, administer supplemental oxygen, and prevent contamination.
- Complications of labour include postpartum hemorrhage. In such cases, massage the abdomen, infuse normal saline or lactated Ringer's solution, and transport urgently.
- Meconium is the baby's first stool. A yellow or greenish-black tint to the amniotic fluid indicates the presence of meconium. Vigilantly suction the baby if meconium staining is present and the baby is not vigorous after birth.
- Pulmonary embolism can cause maternal death during childbirth or postpartum. Suspect this complication if the patient experiences sudden dyspnea, tachycardia, atrial fibrillation, or postpartum hypotension.
- Pharmacology during pregnancy may include magnesium sulfate for eclampsia; calcium chloride to reverse respiratory depression following magnesium sulfate administration; Diazepam for treating anxiety, diphenhydramine for treating hyperemesis gravidarum, and oxytocin for treatment of postpartum hemorrhage.

◼ Vital Vocabulary

abortion Expulsion of the fetus, from any cause, before the 20th week of gestation.

abruptio placenta A premature separation of the placenta from the wall of the uterus.

amniotic fluid A watery fluid that provides the fetus with a weightless environment in which to develop.

amniotic sac The fluid-filled, baglike membrane in which the fetus develops.

antepartum Before delivery.

Apgar scoring system A scoring system for assessing the status of a newborn that assigns a number value to each of five areas of assessment.

atresia The process by which an oocyte dies.

blastocyst The term for an oocyte once it has been fertilized and multiplies into cells.

bloody show A plug of mucus, sometimes mixed with blood, that is expelled from the dilating cervix and discharged from the vagina.

body In the context of the uterus, the portion below the fundus that begins to taper and narrow.

breech presentation A delivery in which the buttocks come out first.

cervical canal The interior of the cervix.

cervix The narrowest portion of the uterus that opens into the vagina.

cholestasis A common liver disease that occurs only during pregnancy, in which the flow of bile is altered resulting in acids being released into the bloodstream, causing profuse and painful itching.

chronic hypertension A blood pressure that is equal to or greater than 140/90 mm Hg, which exists prior to pregnancy, occurs before the 20th week of pregnancy, or continues to persist postpartum.

complete abortion Expulsion of all products of conception from the uterus.

corpus luteum The remains of a follicle after an oocyte has been released, and which secretes progesterone.

crowning The appearance of the infant's head at the vaginal opening during labour.

ectopic pregnancy An egg that attaches outside the uterus, typically in a fallopian tube.

embryo The fetus in the earliest stages after fertilization.

endometrium The innermost layer of tissue in the uterus.

episiotomy An incision in the perineal skin made to prevent tearing during childbirth.

external os The junction where the uterus opens into the vagina.

fallopian tubes The vehicles of transportation of the ova from the ovaries to the uterus; also called oviducts.

fetus The developing, unborn infant inside the uterus.

first stage of labour The stage of labour that begins with the onset of regular labour pains—crampy abdominal pains—during which the uterus contracts and the cervix effaces.

follicle-stimulating hormone (FSH) A hormone produced by the anterior pituitary gland which is important in the menstrual cycle.

footling breech A delivery in which one or both feet dangle through the vaginal opening.

fundus The dome-shaped top of the uterus.

gestational diabetes Diabetes that develops during pregnancy in women who did not have diabetes before pregnancy.

gestational hypertension High blood pressure that develops after the 20th week of pregnancy, in women with previously normal blood pressures, and resolves spontaneously in the postpartum period.

gestational period The time that it takes for the infant to develop in utero, normally 40 weeks.

GnRF A chemical released by the hypothalamus that stimulates the release of follicle-stimulating hormone.

gravid The number of all pregnancies a woman has had, including those not necessarily carried to term.

gravidity A term used to refer to a uterus that contains a pregnancy, whatever the outcome.

Group B streptococcus (GBS) A bacteria that lives in the genitourinary and gastrointestinal tracts of normal healthy individuals, but which can cause life-threatening infections in newborn babies.

human chorionic gonadotropin hormone A hormone that sends signals to the corpus luteum that pregnancy has initiated.

hyperemesis gravidarum A condition of persistent nausea and vomiting during pregnancy.

incomplete abortion Expulsion of the fetus which results in some products of conception remaining in the uterus.

induced abortion Intentional expulsion of the fetus.

inevitable abortion A spontaneous abortion that cannot be prevented.

internal mucosa The inner layer of tissue in the fallopian tubes.

labour The mechanism by which the baby and the placenta are expelled from the uterus.

luteinizing hormone (LH) A hormone released by the anterior pituitary gland that stimulates the process of ovulation.

meconium A dark green material in the amniotic fluid that can indicate disease in the newborn; the meconium can be aspirated into the infant's lungs during delivery; the baby's first bowel movement.

missed abortion A situation in which a fetus has died during the first 20 weeks of gestation, but has remained in utero.

molar pregnancy Pregnancy in which there is a problem at the fertilization stage, with a malfunction of the egg or sperm that results in an abnormal placenta and a fetus with an abnormal chromosome count, or which results in an empty egg.

multigravida A woman who has had two or more pregnancies, irrespective of the outcome.

multipara A woman who has had two or more deliveries.

muscularis The middle layer of tissue in the fallopian tubes.

myometrium The middle layer of tissue in the uterus.

nullipara A woman who has never delivered.

oocyte An egg produced from the female ovary.

ovulation A process in which an ovum is released from a follicle.

ovum A mature oocyte.

para The number of pregnancies a woman has carried to more than 28 weeks, regardless of whether the fetus was delivered dead or alive.

parity Number of live births a woman has had.

perimetrium The outer protective layer of tissue in the uterus.

placenta The tissue attached to the uterine wall that nourishes the fetus through the umbilical cord.

placenta previa A condition in which the placenta develops over and covers the cervix.

postpartum After birth.

preeclampsia A condition of late pregnancy that involves gradual onset of hypertension, headache, visual changes, and swelling of the hands and feet; also called pregnancy-induced hypertension or toxemia of pregnancy.

prenatal The state of the pregnant woman before birth.

primigravida A woman who is pregnant for the first time.

primipara A woman who has had one delivery only.

progesterone A hormone that influences the second phase of the menstrual cycle, when the oocyte is either fertilized or dies.

prolapsed umbilical cord A situation in which the umbilical cord comes out of the vagina before the infant.

pseudocyesis A false pregnancy that develops all the typical signs and symptoms of true pregnancy, but in which no actual pregnancy exists.

Rh factor A protein found on the red blood cells of most people; when a woman without this protein is impregnated by a man with this protein, the woman's body can create antibodies against the protein and attack future pregnancies.

second stage of labour The stage of labour in which the baby's head enters the birth canal, during which contractions become more intense and more frequent.

secretory phase The second phase of the menstrual cycle.

septic abortion A life-threatening emergency in which the uterus becomes infected following any type of abortion.

serosa The outermost layer of tissue in the fallopian tubes.

shoulder dystocia A condition in which the infant becomes trapped in between the symphysis pubis and sacrum because its shoulders are larger than its head.

spontaneous abortion Expulsion of the fetus that occurs naturally; also called miscarriage.

stratum basalis A permanent mucous membrane that makes up part of the outer endometrium.

stratum functionalis An inner mucous membrane that makes up part of the endometrium, and which is renewed following menstruation.

supine hypotensive syndrome Low blood pressure resulting from compression of the inferior vena cava by the weight of the pregnant uterus when the mother is supine.

third stage of labour The stage of labour in which the placenta is expelled.

threatened abortion Expulsion of the fetus that is attempting to take place but has not occurred yet; usually occurs in the first trimester.

tocolytics Drugs used to delay preterm labour.

transverse presentation A delivery in which the fetus lies crosswise in the uterus; one hand may protrude through the vagina.

umbilical cord The conduit connecting mother to infant via the placenta; contains two arteries and one vein.

uterine cavity The interior of the body of the uterus.

uterine inversion A potentially fatal complication of childbirth in which the placenta fails to detach properly and results in the uterus turning inside-out.

uterus A muscular inverted pear-shaped organ, that lies situated between the urinary bladder and the rectum.

vagina A tubular organ lined with mucous membranes, which is the lower portion of the birth canal.

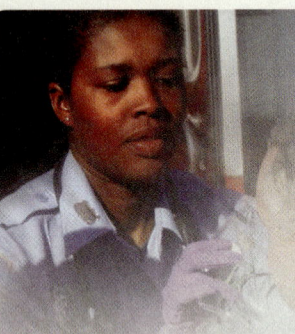

Assessment in Action

You are called to the street corner for a person who fell. When you arrive, you see an obviously pregnant woman who has fallen and sprained her ankle. As you are assessing the patient's ankle, you note that both of her ankles are swollen. You obtain a set of vital signs that include a pulse rate of 110 beats/min; blood pressure, 150/92 mm Hg; respiratory rate, 20 breaths/min; and a pulse oximetry reading of 100% on room air. When you took the patient's pulse rate, you noticed that her hands and wrists appeared swollen as well. You prepare her for transport to the hospital and while you are driving to the hospital, the patient begins to complain of abdominal cramping. The woman's eyes roll back and she has a full-body seizure.

1. **This patient's medical condition is probably related to:**
   A. preeclampsia.
   B. eclampsia.
   C. abruptio placenta.
   D. spontaneous abortion.

2. **Treatment of the above patient includes all of the following, EXCEPT:**
   A. splinting of the ankle.
   B. placing the patient in the left lateral recumbent position on a stretcher.
   C. administering IV normal saline and oxygen.
   D. placing the patient in the right lateral recumbent position on a stretcher.

3. **The criteria for the diagnosis of preeclampsia includes all of the following, EXCEPT:**
   A. hypertension.
   B. proteinuria.
   C. excessive weight gain with edema.
   D. hypotension.

4. **Which medications should you be prepared to administer?**
   A. Magnesium sulfate and diazepam
   B. Morphine and diazepam
   C. Magnesium sulfate and morphine
   D. Epinephrine and atropine

5. **When does ectopic pregnancy occur?**
   A. When a fertilized ovum implants in the uterine cavity
   B. When a fertilized ovum implants anywhere other than the uterine cavity
   C. Usually later in pregnancy
   D. When a patient becomes hypertensive

6. **The absence of abdominal pain is associated with:**
   A. spontaneous abortion.
   B. placenta previa.
   C. uterine rupture.
   D. abruptio placentae.

7. **How many stages of labour are there?**
   A. 3
   B. 5
   C. 4
   D. 6

8. **The period during which intrauterine fetal development takes place is known as:**
   A. gestation.
   B. para.
   C. uterine contractions.
   D. gravida.

9. **Pregnant patients are described by their gravid and parous states. What is the correct terminology?**
   A. Gravida and parachute
   B. Gravida and para
   C. Live and aborted
   D. Para and gravitation

10. **Uterine rupture refers to:**
    A. painless, bright red bleeding without uterine contraction.
    B. localized uterine tenderness.
    C. absent fetal heart tones.
    D. spontaneous or traumatic rupture of the uterine wall.

Challenging Question

11. **What special considerations will you need to take into account for this trauma patient?**

Points to Ponder

You respond to an obstetric emergency. On arrival you find a 23-year-old woman in the final trimester of pregnancy. She is seated in the living room on a chair. She is sobbing uncontrollably. You notice that she is sitting on a towel that has blood on it. Her chief complaint is a sudden onset of vaginal bleeding that has been occurring for 20 minutes. You ask if she is in pain, and she replies "a little." You ask if she has ever been pregnant, and she replies "once before, and I began hemorrhaging 2 weeks before delivery. I delivered a stillborn baby." She continues to sob.

How will you address this patient's emotions?

Issues: Dealing With Personal Tragedy, Determining a Pregnant Woman's History, Empathetic Response, Implementing a Treatment Plan.

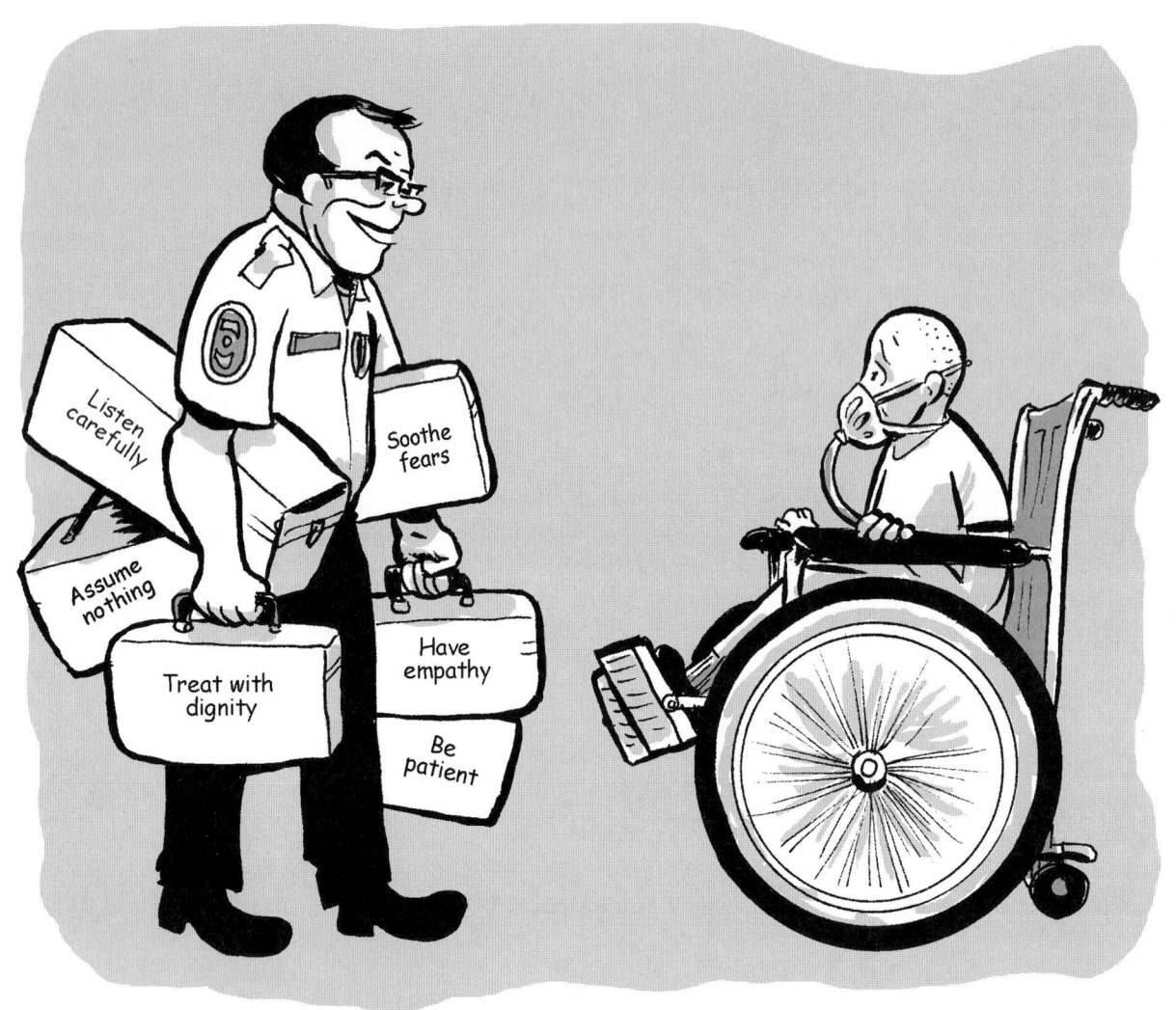

“

Special problems . . . require special approaches.”

—Nancy L. Caroline, MD

Special Considerations

Section Editor: Cory Brulotte, MD

40 Neonatology

Competency Areas

Area 1: Professional Responsibilities

1.1.b   Reflect professionalism through use of appropriate language.

Area 2: Communication

2.1.f   Speak in language appropriate to the listener.
2.1.g   Use appropriate terminology.
2.3.a   Exhibit effective non-verbal behaviour.
2.3.b   Practice active listening techniques.
2.3.c   Establish trust and rapport with patients and colleagues.
2.3.d   Recognize and react appropriately to non-verbal behaviours.
2.4.a   Treat others with respect.
2.4.b   Exhibit empathy and compassion while providing care.
2.4.c   Recognize and react appropriately to individuals and groups manifesting coping mechanisms.
2.4.d   Act in a confident manner.
2.4.f   Manage and provide support to patients, bystanders, and relatives manifesting emotional reactions.
2.4.g   Exhibit diplomacy, tact, and discretion.

Area 4: Assessment and Diagnostics

4.3.a   Conduct primary patient assessment and interpret findings.
4.3.b   Conduct secondary patient assessment and interpret findings.
4.3.f   Conduct obstetrical assessment and interpret findings.
4.3.o   Conduct neonatal assessment and interpret findings.
4.4.a   Assess pulse.
4.4.b   Assess respiration.
4.4.g   Assess skin condition.
4.4.h   Assess pupils.
4.4.i   Assess level of mentation.
4.5.b   Conduct end-tidal carbon dioxide monitoring and interpret findings.

Area 5: Therapeutics

5.1.a   Use manual maneuvers and positioning to maintain airway patency.
5.1.b   Suction oropharynx.
5.1.c   Suction beyond oropharynx.
5.1.d   Utilize oropharyngeal airway.
5.1.h   Utilize airway devices requiring visualization of vocal cords and introduced endotracheally.
5.1.i   Remove airway foreign bodies (AFB).
5.1.j   Remove foreign body by direct techniques.
5.2.a   Recognize indications for oxygen administration.
5.3.d   Administer oxygen using high concentration mask.
5.4.a   Provide oxygenation and ventilation using bag-valve-mask.
5.5.a   Conduct cardiopulmonary resuscitation (CPR).
5.5.c   Maintain peripheral intravenous (IV) access devices and infusions of crystalloid solutions without additives.

5.5.d   Conduct peripheral intravenous cannulation.
5.5.e   Conduct intraosseous needle insertion.
5.5.f   Utilize direct pressure infusion devices with intravenous infusions.
5.5.s   Conduct needle thoracostomy.
5.8.a   Recognize principles of pharmacology as applied to the medications listed in

Appendix 5.

5.8e   Administer medication via intravenous route.
5.8.f   Administer medication via intraosseous route.
5.8.g   Administer medication via endotracheal route.

Area 6: Integration

6.2.a   Provide care for neonatal patient.
6.2.b   Provide care for pediatric patient.
6.3.a   Conduct ongoing assessments based on patient presentation and interpret findings.

Appendix 4: Pathophysiology

A.   **Cardiovascular System**
Congenital Abnormalities: Transposition
B.   **Neurologic System**
Convulsive Disorders: Generalized seizures
Altered Mental Status: Metabolic
C.   **Respiratory System**
Pediatric Illness: Acute respiratory failure
Pediatric Illness: Acute sudden infant death syndrome
D.   **Female Reproductive System and Neonates**
Neonatal Complications: Cardiovascular insufficiency
Neonatal Complications: Meconium aspiration
Neonatal Complications: Respiratory insufficiency
E.   **Gastrointestinal System**
Esophagus/Stomach: Obstruction
I.   **Endocrine System**
Diabetes mellitus
J.   **Multisystem Diseases and Injuries**
Infectious Diseases: Toxic shock syndrome
Environmental Disorders: Hyperthermal injuries
Environmental Disorders: Hypothermal injuries
Shock Syndromes: Hypovolemic

Appendix 5: Medications

A.   **Medications affecting the central nervous system**
A.1   Opioid Antagonists
B.   **Medications affecting the autonomic nervous system**
B.1   Andrenergic Agonists
H.   **Medications used to treat electrolyte and substrate imbalances**
H.1   Vitamin and Electrolyte Supplements

Introduction

The prehospital care of a newborn or neonate must be tailored to meet the unique needs of this population. A newborn refers to an infant within the first day after birth; a neonate refers to an infant within the first month after birth. A healthy neonate is completely dependent on others for nourishment, warmth, and protection from the environment. Most parents recognize this need and instinctively wish to fulfill the role of nurturer and caregiver. When a neonate needs special support that necessitates intervention by trained caregivers, the parents may feel isolated and inadequate. It is important for you to support the needs of both the neonate and the parents or other caregivers by allowing them to be physically close as much as possible, explaining what is being done, and providing details of the plan for transport to the next level of care.

This chapter reviews the physiologic changes that occur in a newborn during birth, the prehospital care that should be provided during and immediately after birth, and the special needs of premature births or births complicated by other factors. It also reviews the steps involved in neonatal resuscitation and outlines the process of transporting an infant to a hospital or between hospitals.

General Pathophysiology and Assessment

Additional skilled care intervention is needed for approximately 6% to 10% of newborn deliveries, with the rate of complications increasing as the newborn's birth weight and gestational age decrease. Approximately 80% of babies born each year weighing less than 1,500 g require resuscitation. **Table 40-1** and **Table 40-2** outline risk factors for complications before and during birth. Because both short- and long-term outcomes in newborns have been linked to initial stabilization efforts, it is imperative that you anticipate problems with newborns, are knowledgeable about how to deal with them, have the appropriate resuscitation equipment readily available, and carefully consider the newborn's ultimate transport to the appropriate destination.

Table 40-1	Antepartum (Before Birth) Risk Factors
■ Multiple gestation ■ Pregnant woman's age < 16 y or > 35 y ■ Post-term (> 42 weeks') gestation ■ Premature or preterm (< 37 weeks') gestation ■ Toxemia, hypertension, diabetes ■ Polyhydramnios (excessive amount of amniotic fluid) ■ Premature rupture of the membranes	■ Inadequate prenatal care ■ Chronic maternal illness (eg, cardiac) ■ Use of drugs/medications, illicit or prescribed ■ Fetal anemia ■ Oligohydramnios (decreased volume of amniotic fluid during a pregnancy) ■ Fetal malformation

Table 40-2	Intrapartum (During Birth) Risk Factors
■ Rupture of membranes > 24 hours before delivery ■ Placenta previa, or placental abruption bleeding ■ Abnormal presentation ■ Prolapsed cord ■ Maternal fever	■ Prolonged labour or precipitous delivery ■ Meconium-stained amniotic fluid ■ Shoulder dystocia (large infant) ■ Use of narcotics within 4 hours of delivery ■ Fetal tachycardia or bradycardia

You are the Paramedic Part 1

You are called to the home of a 24-year-old woman who is 39 weeks' pregnant. She was alone when her amniotic sac ruptured. She is experiencing regular contractions that are 3 minutes apart and was afraid to drive to the hospital, so she called 9-1-1. When you and your partner arrive, you find your patient sitting on the couch. After you introduce yourselves, the patient tells you that she has already called her husband, who said he will meet her at the hospital. According to the patient, her water broke and the fluid was clear.

Initial Assessment	Recording Time: 0 Minutes
Appearance	Obviously pregnant; very nervous and in pain
Level of consciousness	A (Alert to person, place, and day)
Airway	Patent
Breathing	Respirations, increased; adequate tidal volume
Circulation	Radial pulses, increased rate and regular; no gross bleeding

1. Why is it important to determine the colour of the amniotic fluid?
2. What are some reliable indicators of imminent delivery?
3. What specific questions should you ask that will allow you to anticipate the need for resuscitation of the newborn?

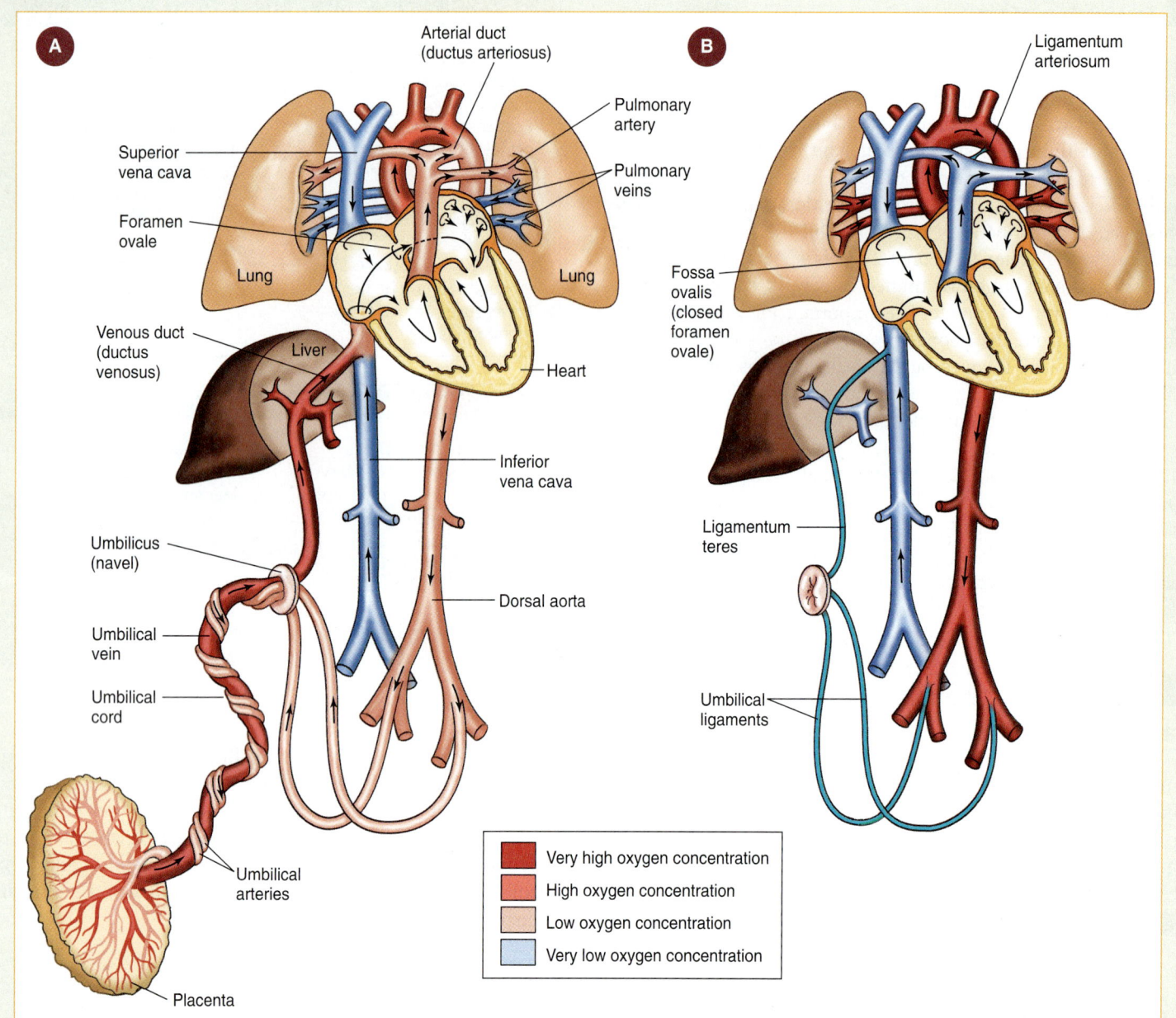

Figure 40-1 Fetal circulation. **A.** Oxygenated blood from the placenta reaches the fetus through the umbilical vein. Blood returns to the placenta via two umbilical arteries. Right-to-left shunts occur at the foramen ovale and the ductus arteriosus. **B.** Fetal circulation following transition.

Transition From Fetus to Newborn

In utero (ie, in the pregnant woman's womb), a fetus receives its oxygen from the placenta **Figure 40-1**. The fetal lung is collapsed and filled with fluid, and most (90%) of the fetal blood flow is diverted away from the lungs. As the baby is delivered, a rapid series of events needs to occur to enable the baby to breathe and use its lungs for gas exchange; this process is called fetal transition. During fetal transition, the umbilical cord is clamped, thereby removing the low-resistance placenta and increasing the systemic circulation pressure. As the newborn begins to breathe, the lungs expand with air and pulmonary vascular resistance drops. Blood flows to the lungs for gas exchange, and the fetal circulation switches to a functional adult circulation. This is characterized by the functional, then permanent, closure of the ductus venosus, the ductus arteriosus, and the foramen ovale, the three shunts that have allowed blood to bypass the fetus's lungs and use the placenta as the organ of gas exchange. Anything that delays this decline in pulmonary pressure can lead to delayed transition, with hypoxia, possible brain damage, and potentially death **Table 40-3**.

An infant delivered at less than 37 completed weeks of gestation is considered preterm; an infant born at 37 to 42 weeks of gestation is described as term; and an infant born at more than 42 weeks of gestation is described as post-term (or post-dates). Infants are also described as *small for gestational age* when the birth weight is less than the third percentile for gestational

Table 40-3	Causes of Delayed Transition in Newborns
■ Hypoxia	■ Meconium aspiration or pneumonia
■ Hypothermia	■ Delayed resorption of lung fluid (eg, cesarean section without labour)
■ Acidosis	■ Maternal narcotics or anesthesia

age (SGA) or *large for gestational age* if the birth weight is greater than the 97th percentile for the gestation (LGA). All others are *appropriate for gestational age*, or AGA.

Arrival of the Newborn

Use any time available before the infant arrives to take a patient history and prepare the environment and equipment that may be necessary. Key questions you need to ask when you are at a scene involving a pregnant woman or a recent home birth include the mother's age; has she had antenatal care; how many babies is she expecting; length of the pregnancy (preferably expressed in weeks); the onset and frequency of contractions; the presence or absence of fetal movement; whether membranes have ruptured, including its timing and the makeup of the fluid (clear, meconium stained, or bloody); whether there have been any pregnancy complications (eg, diabetes, hypertension, ultrasound-diagnosed fetal anomalies); and any medications being taken. In the excitement of the moment these questions may seem trivial, but they help determine what resuscitation and equipment may be needed.

Even if a piece of equipment is in a sealed sterile wrap, having it near at hand will expedite its use once the infant is delivered. At a minimum, you will need warm, dry blankets, a bulb syringe, two small clamps or ties, and a pair of clean scissors to cut the umbilical cord. Table 40-4 ▶ lists additional equipment that may be needed if more extensive resuscitation becomes necessary.

Notes from Nancy

Steps to Improve Fetal Circulation

■ Roll the mother onto her side, to take the weight of her uterus off the great vessels.

■ Administer 100% oxygen by mask to the mother.

Special Considerations

A delay in clamping the umbilical cord and keeping the infant below the placenta may allow blood to flow into the infant, which can in turn lead to polycythemia (an abnormally high red blood cell count). The reverse is also true, and even more concerning in the short term, because the newborn may lose half of his or her blood volume into the placenta if it is held much higher than the placenta prior to cord clamping. Never "milk" the cord before clamping.

Table 40-4	Preparation of Area for Newborn Resuscitation*

Resuscitation Equipment and Supplies
- Suction equipment
- Bulb syringe or mechanical suction and tubing, suction catheters, 5F, 6F, 8F, or 10F
- 20-ml syringe
- Meconium aspirator

Bag-Valve-Mask Equipment
- Device for delivering positive-pressure ventilation
- Face masks, newborn and premature infant size (cushioned-rim masks preferred)
- Oral airways, newborn and premature size
- Oxygen source with flow meter (flow rate up to 10 l/min)
- Oxygen blender and pulse oximeter

Intubation Equipment
- Laryngoscope with straight blades, size 0 (preterm) and 1 (term)
- Extra bulb, batteries for laryngoscope
- Endotracheal tubes size 2.5, 3.0, and 3.5
- Stylet (optional)
- Scissors and tape for securing endotracheal tube
- CO_2 detectors
- Laryngeal mask airway (optional)

Medications
- Epinephrine 1:10,000 (0.1 mg/ml), 3- or 10-ml ampules
- Isotonic crystalloid (normal saline or lactated Ringer's solution), 100- or 250-ml bag
- Sodium bicarbonate, 4.2% (5 mEq/10 ml) (optional)
- Naloxone hydrochloride, 0.4- or 1.0-mg/ml ampule (optional)
- Dextrose, 10%, 250 ml

Umbilical Cannulation Equipment
- Sterile gloves
- Scalpel or scissors
- Antiseptic solution
- Umbilical tape
- Umbilical cannulas, 3.5F, 5F (a sterile 3.5F feeding tube can be used in an emergency)
- Three-way stopcock
- Syringes, 1, 3, 5, 10, 20, and 50 ml
- Needles, 25, 21, and 18 gauge

Miscellaneous
- Gloves and appropriate PPE protection
- Radiant warmer or other heat source
- Firm, padded resuscitation surface
- Clock with second hand, timer optional
- Towels, linen
- Stethoscope, neonatal or pediatric preferred
- Cardiac monitor or saturation monitor (optional at delivery)
- Oropharyngeal airways (0, 00, and 000 sizes or 30-, 40-, and 50-mm long)
- Manometer for PPV
- Pulse oximeter

*Adapted from the American Academy of Pediatrics Neonatal Resuscitation Program

If the infant is delivered in the ambulance, the foot of the mother's bed, covered with clean, warm blankets, can be used for the initial stabilization steps. The newborn can then be placed on mother's chest after you confirm adequate patency of the airway, breathing, and pulse rate. If more extensive resuscitation is needed, the foot of the mother's bed can be used.

Optimally the newborn will be transitioned to a second ambulance equipped with a neonatal transport incubator to allow maintenance of the baby's temperature and observation of the newborn's colour, respirations, and muscle tone.

If the umbilical cord comes out ahead of the baby (which is more common with polyhydramnios, a condition characterized by extra amniotic fluid or breech presentation), the blood supply through the umbilical cord may be cut off. In this case, relieving pressure on the cord can be lifesaving. This is done by having the mother assume a knee-to-chest, or Trendelenburg position. Then, using two gloved fingers inserted into the vagina, elevate the presenting part of the baby off of the cord and maintain this position. Finally, cover the exposed cord with a moist sterile dressing.

After the infant is delivered, keep the baby at the level of the mother, with the head slightly lower than the body, to facilitate drainage of secretions **Figure 40-2** . There is evidence for delaying cord clamping for at least 1 minute in term and preterm newborns not requiring resuscitation. However, do not delay cord clamping if the newborn requires resuscitation.

Clamp the umbilical cord in two places and cut between the clamps. Suctioning of the oropharynx was once routine, but is now reserved for babies who have an obvious obstruction to spontaneous breathing or require positive-pressure ventilation.

Dry the infant well to limit body temperature loss through convection, then wrap the infant in warm blankets or place on the mother's bare skin and cover to maintain the baby's temperature via conduction from the mother.

Your initial rapid assessment of the newborn may be done simultaneously with any treatment interventions. Note the time of delivery, and monitor the ABCs. In particular, assess respiratory rate, respiratory effort, pulse rate, and pulse oximetry measures on the right upper extremity.

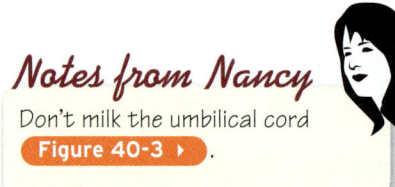

Notes from Nancy

Don't milk the umbilical cord **Figure 40-3** .

Nearly 90% of newborns are vigorous term babies. All newborns are cyanotic immediately after birth, but quickly

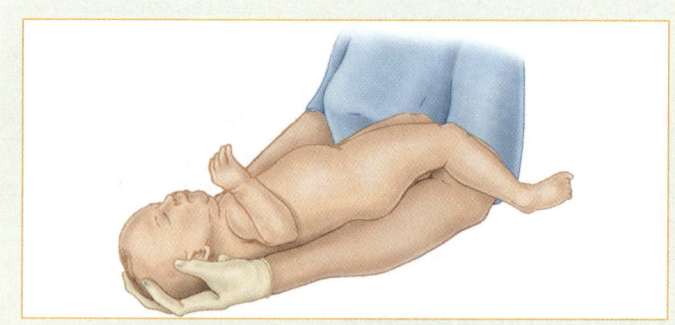

Figure 40-2 Positioning. Immediately after delivery, hold the baby with the head slightly lower than the body to facilitate drainage of secretions.

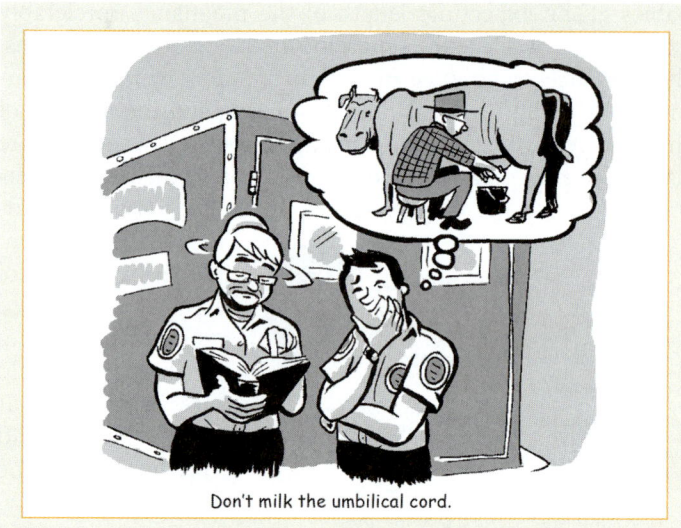

Don't milk the umbilical cord.

Figure 40-3

You are the Paramedic Part 2

Your patient tells you that this is her third pregnancy and that her first two pregnancies resulted in normal deliveries. At her last doctor's appointment, her obstetrician told her that he did not anticipate any problems and that the baby was in a head-down position in the uterus (fully engaged).

Your partner obtains baseline vital signs as you perform a visual examination of the patient's vaginal area and put on appropriate PPE attire. Your examination reveals crowning of the baby's head. You immediately position the patient appropriately and open the OB kit.

Vital Signs	Recording Time: 3 Minutes
Skin	Pink, warm, and moist
Pulse	110 beats/min, strong and regular
Blood pressure	106/60 mm Hg
Respirations	24 breaths/min; adequate tidal volume
Spo_2	98% on room air

4. What equipment and supplies should be available in case the infant requires resuscitation?

become centrally pink. The hands and feet will remain peripherally cyanosed with poor capillary refill typically for hours after delivery, so assessment of circulation should be done centrally, preferably over the sternum. If the newborn remains vigorous and pink, ongoing observation and continued thermoregulation with direct skin-to-skin contact with the mother should be maintained while on the way to a local hospital. Bonding with the mother should be encouraged in a well-appearing newborn.

The Apgar Score

The Apgar score, named after Dr. Virginia Apgar, who developed this measure in 1953, helps determine the need for and the effectiveness of resuscitation. The Apgar score is determined on the basis of the newborn's condition at 1 and 5 minutes after birth   Table 40-5 ▾ . If the 5-minute Apgar score is less than 7, the newborn's condition should be reassessed and a new score assigned every 5 minutes until 20 minutes after birth. Normal newborns have Apgar scores of 7 or 8 and 9 at 1 and 5 minutes, respectively.

Need for Resuscitation

Not all deliveries go so smoothly. Approximately 6% to 10% of newborns need additional assistance and 1% need major resuscitation to survive.

After the initial steps following delivery (bulb suctioning mouth and nose, drying, stimulating) are followed for 30 seconds, if the newborn has not responded, further intervention is indicated. Assess the newborn's respiratory rate, respiratory effort, pulse rate, and colour. Count the respiratory rate and pulse rate for 6 seconds and then multiply by 10 to quickly determine the rate per minute. The pulse rate can be determined either by auscultation or by feeling the base of the umbilical cord at the baby's abdomen, as the umbilical artery

should still have pulsatile flow   Figure 40-4 ▸ . Many newborns become centrally pink but have blue hands and feet (acrocyanosis). If the baby maintains central cyanosis of the trunk or mucous membranes, provide supplemental free-flow oxygen as well as stimulation.

If the baby is apneic (ie, has a 20-second or longer respiratory pause) or has a pulse rate less than 100 beats/min after 30 seconds of drying and stimulation and supplemental free-flow (blow-by) oxygen, begin positive-pressure ventilation (PPV) by bag-valve-mask device, being sure to use a newborn sized bag-valve-mask. You should use caution when squeezing the bag in order to avoid inadvertently delivering too much volume, potentially resulting in a pneumothorax. It is preferable to have a manometer attached to the bagging circuit to reduce the risk of barotraumas. An inspiratory pressure of 25 to 33 mm Hg is often needed to move the chest of a term newborn. After 30 seconds of adequate ventilation by PPV with 100% oxygen via a bag-valve-mask device, if the infant's pulse rate is less than 60 beats/min, begin chest compressions. Effective chest compressions should result in palpable femoral and brachial pulses.

Fewer than 1% of deliveries involve bradycardia that requires treatment with chest compressions. The most common etiology for bradycardia in a neonate is hypoxia, which is readily reversed by effective PPV. Profound hypoxia or shock is also the cause of cardiac arrest, which is almost always a secondary event in these small patients. If ventilation and chest compressions do not improve the bradycardia, administer epinephrine via the IV route, preferably an umbilical venous line. The drug may also be given via endotracheal (ET) intubation, but requires 10-fold dosing to be effective. Infants who have required active resuscitation for 20 minutes or longer rarely have positive long-term outcomes. If a spontaneous heartbeat has not been established after 10 minutes, you should consider stopping resuscitation. If spontaneous breathing has not been established after 20 minutes of resuscitation, the outcomes are likely very poor. You should seek further advice regarding

Table 40-5	The Apgar Score	
Condition	**Description**	**Score**
Appearance—skin colour	Completely pink	2
	Body pink, extremities blue	1
	Centrally blue, pale	0
Pulse rate	>100	2
	<100, >0	1
	Absent	0
Grimace—irritability	Cries	2
	Grimaces	1
	No response	0
Activity—muscle tone	Active motion	2
	Some flexion of extremities	1
	Limp	0
Respiratory—effort	Strong cry	2
	Slow and irregular	1
	Absent	0

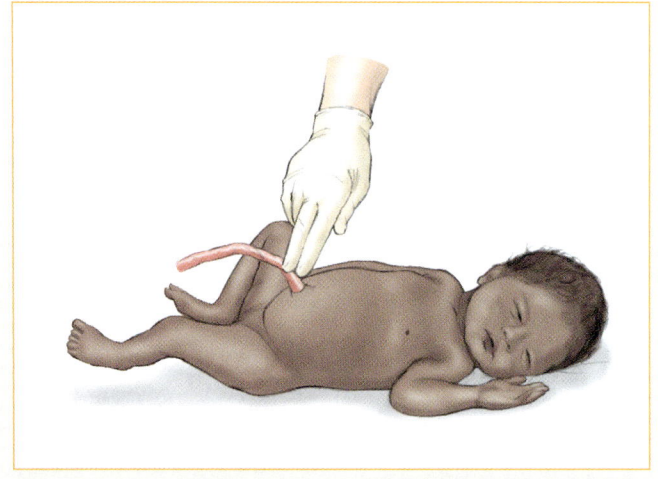

Figure 40-4 Feel for a pulse at the base of the umbilical cord.

discontinuation of life support. However, newborns are very resilient, and most respond readily to interventions.

Specific Intervention and Resuscitation Steps

Drying and Stimulation

After ensuring the patency of the airway by bulb suctioning of the newborn's mouth and nose, dry and stimulate the infant. Flick the soles of the baby's feet and gently rub the baby's back. Avoid rubbing too roughly or slapping the baby, since these actions may lead to traumatic injury.

Free-Flow Oxygen

If an infant is cyanotic or pale, provide supplemental oxygen. Given that 50 g/l of deoxygenated hemoglobin is needed before clinical cyanosis becomes apparent, a severely anemic hypoxic infant will be pale, but not cyanotic. Warm and humidify the oxygen if it will be provided for more than a few minutes. If PPV is not indicated (ie, the pulse rate is greater than 100 beats/min and the infant has adequate respiratory effort), oxygen can initially be delivered through an oxygen mask or via oxygen tubing within a hand that is cupped and held close to the infant's nose and mouth **Figure 40-5 ▼** . For babies at term, the administration of oxygen should be regulated by blending oxygen and air, and the amount delivered guided by pulse oximetry monitored from the right upper arm. Hyperoxia can be toxic to newborns, particularly the preterm baby. The oxygen flow rate should be set at 5 l/min. Do not blow oxygen directly into the newborn's eyes.

Oral Airways

Oral airways are rarely used for neonates, but they can be lifesaving if airway obstruction leads to respiratory failure. Bilateral choanal atresia (bony or membranous obstruction of the back of the nose preventing air flow) can be rapidly fatal, but usually responds to placement of an oral airway (or a gloved finger to maintain an open mouth until an adequate oral airway is

located). The Pierre Robin sequence includes a small chin, a cleft palate, and posteriorly positioned tongue that frequently leads to airway obstruction. Positioning the patient prone (chest down) may relieve the obstruction, as the tongue flops forward. If not, insert an oral airway. As with infants and small children, use a tongue blade to depress the tongue and insert the oral airway without rotating it.

Bag-Valve-Mask Ventilation

Bag-valve-mask ventilation is indicated when an infant is apneic, has inadequate respiratory effort, or has a pulse rate of less than 100 beats/min (bradycardia) after you clear the airway of secretions, relieve obstruction from the tongue, and dry and stimulate the infant. Signs of respiratory distress that suggest a need for ventilation support include periodic breathing, intercostal retractions (sucking in between the ribs), nasal flaring, and grunting on expiration. Respiratory distress occurs in approximately 8 of every 1,000 live births and accounts for approximately 15% of neonatal deaths. **Table 40-6 ▼** summarizes the most common conditions leading to respiratory distress.

Three devices may be used to deliver bag-valve-mask ventilation to a neonate. First, you may use a self-inflating bag with an oxygen reservoir (an oxygen source is not necessary to provide PPV but is necessary to provide supplementary oxygen). Second, you may use a flow-inflating bag, though it needs a gas source to provide PPV; this technique is therefore more common in the operating room. Third, you may apply a T-piece resuscitator (mostly found in neonatal intensive care units) or delivery suites.

In the prehospital setting, you will most likely use a self-inflating bag for bag-valve-mask ventilation. If available, always use the infant size (240 ml). Given that the breath size (tidal volume) of a neonate is only 5 to 8 ml/kg, less than one tenth of the bag's volume will be used for each breath—which explains why a larger bag can easily create problems.

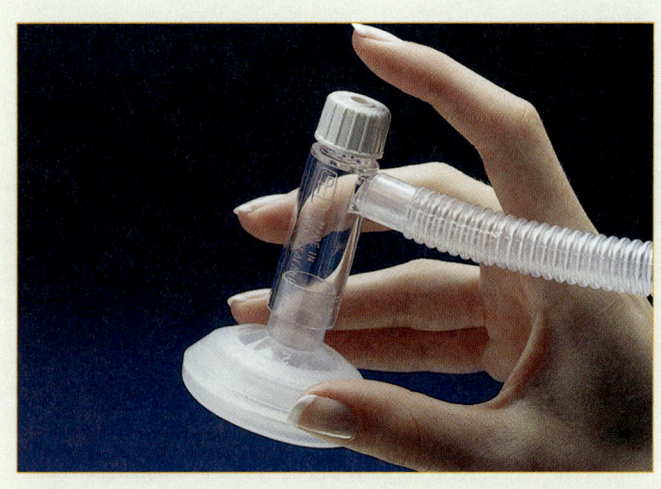

Figure 40-5 Free-flow oxygen device.

Table 40-6	Common Causes of Respiratory Distress
■ Hyaline membrane disease	■ Cardiac abnormality (eg, transposition of the great arteries, total anomalous pulmonary venous drainage, hypoplastic left heart syndrome)
■ Lung immaturity in very premature infants	■ Persistent pulmonary hypertension
■ Wet lungs, transient tachypnea of newborn	■ Choanal atresia
■ Meconium aspiration	■ Tracheo-esophageal fistula (TEF) and/or esophageal atresia (EA)
■ Congenital diaphragmatic hernia	■ Pneumonia
■ Pneumothorax	■ Metabolic derangement (eg, hypoglycemia, polycythemia)
■ Shock due to sepsis or hypovolemia	■ Central nervous system disorders (eg, vein of Galen anomaly)

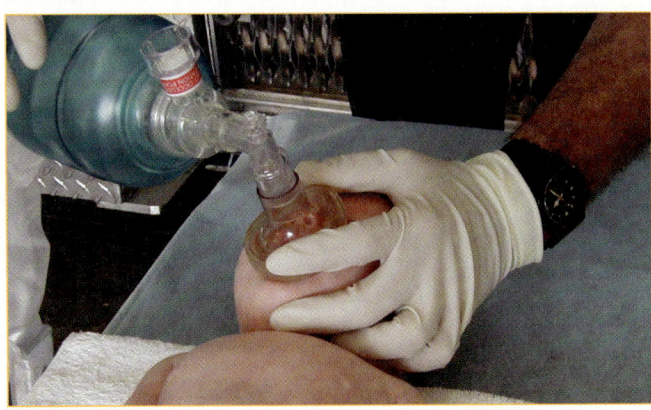

Figure 40-6 Bag-valve-mask ventilation of the newborn. Hold the mask securely to the face with your thumb and index finger. Apply countertraction under the bony part of the chin with your middle finger.

If a neonatal bag is not available and the infant is in severe respiratory distress, has apnea, or has bradycardia, you can use a bag designed for adults or older children (750 ml or greater volume) as long as you keep the delivered breath size appropriately small and monitor chest rise to avoid excessive volumes of delivered breaths. When available, a manometer connected in circuit will help to reduce the risk of barotraumas by keeping a close eye on inflating pressures.

When you are administering bag-valve-mask ventilation with 100% oxygen, the face mask needs to provide an airtight seal, fitting over the newborn's mouth and nose, and extending down to the chin but not over the eyes **Figure 40-6 ▲** . The newborn needs to have a patent airway, cleared of secretions, with his or her neck slightly extended in the sniffing position **Figure 40-7 ▼** . Because of the large occiput in neonates, placing a folded towel under the infant's shoulders will help to create the position where the airway will be most patent. The first few breaths after birth will frequently require higher pressures (perhaps 30 mm Hg or even higher) because the lungs are not yet expanded and are still full of fluid. To deliver these initial breaths, you may need to manually (cover with your finger) disable the spring-loaded pop-off valve (it is usually set by the manufacturer at 30 to 40 cm Hg). Subsequent breaths should be delivered with sufficient pressure to result in visible but not excessive chest rise.

In a newborn, the correct timing for ventilation is 40 to 60 breaths/min. In the excitement of the moment, with your adrenaline surging, it is easy to inadvertently deliver breaths at a much higher rate, which can lead to hypocapnia, air trapping, or pneumothorax. To help with the timing, count "breath–two–three, breath–two–three" as you ventilate: Give a breath on "breath," and release on "two–three." Continue PPV as long as the pulse rate remains less than 100 beats/min or respiratory effort is ineffective. If prolonged PPV is needed, hook the system to a pressure manometer to aid in monitoring and minimizing excessive pressures (target peak inspiratory pressure less than 25 mm Hg in full-term newborns, less than 20 mm Hg in preterm infants).

The most common reasons for ineffective bag-valve-mask ventilation are inadequate seal of the mask on the face and incorrect head position. Other causes such as mucous plug, pneumothorax, or equipment malfunction need to be considered as well.

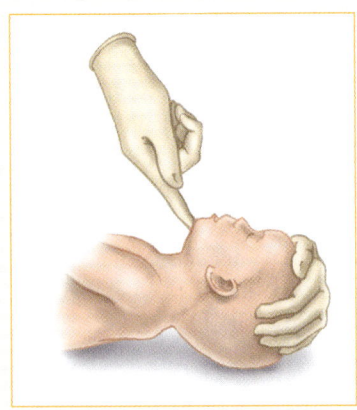

Figure 40-7 The sniffing position.

Intubation

Bag-valve-mask ventilation provides successful resuscitation of most newborns. Intubation, however, may be necessary if the newborn requires resuscitation beyond simple interventions **Figure 40-8 ▶** . Intubation is indicated in the following situations:

- Meconium-stained fluid is present and the infant is not vigorous (ie, poor muscle tone, bradycardia, inadequate ventilation), a condition for which tracheal suctioning is indicated.
- Congenital diaphragmatic hernia (a congenital defect in which abdominal organs herniate through an opening in the diaphragm into the chest cavity) is suspected and respiratory support is indicated.
- The infant does not respond to bag-valve-mask ventilation and chest compressions, necessitating endotracheal administration of epinephrine (ie, no intraosseous site has been established).

Controversies

While resuscitation with 100% oxygen is the norm, a growing body of evidence suggests that resuscitation with room air is a safe alternative. Bag-valve-mask ventilation can be initiated with room air while an oxygen source is being secured. The current recommendation includes obtaining O_2 saturations as quickly as possible and weaning the FiO_2 accordingly to maintain saturations of 90% to 95%, and no greater. Avoid hyperoxia, where possible. This of course necessitates having medical air and a blender available.

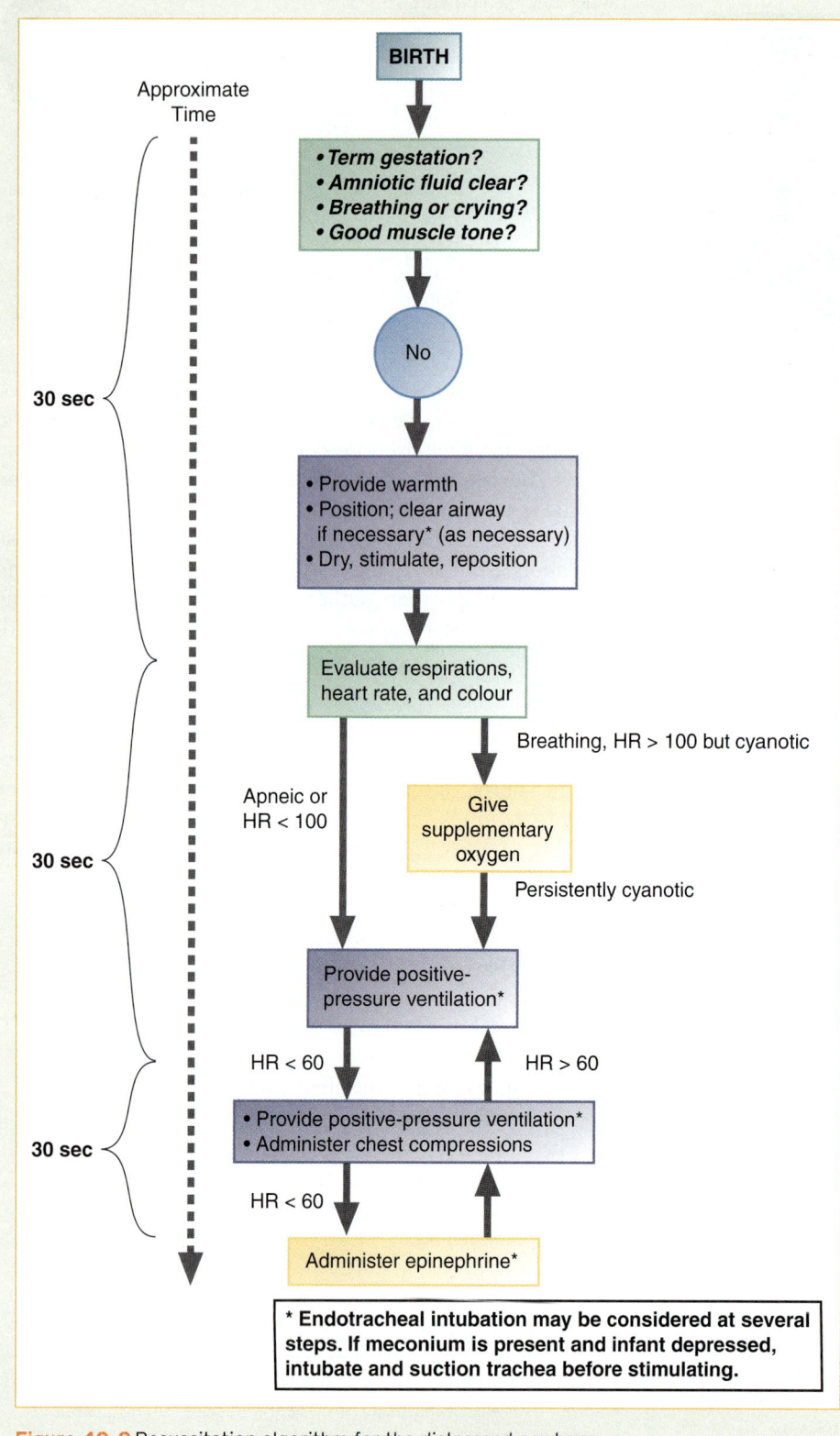

BIRTH

Approximate Time

• Term gestation?
• Amniotic fluid clear?
• Breathing or crying?
• Good muscle tone?

No

30 sec

• Provide warmth
• Position; clear airway if necessary* (as necessary)
• Dry, stimulate, reposition

Evaluate respirations, heart rate, and colour

Breathing, HR > 100 but cyanotic

Apneic or HR < 100

30 sec

Give supplementary oxygen

Persistently cyanotic

Provide positive-pressure ventilation*

HR < 60   HR > 60

• Provide positive-pressure ventilation*
• Administer chest compressions

30 sec

HR < 60

Administer epinephrine*

* Endotracheal intubation may be considered at several steps. If meconium is present and infant depressed, intubate and suction trachea before stimulating.

Figure 40-8 Resuscitation algorithm for the distressed newborn.

■ Prolonged positive-pressure ventilation is needed.

Before you begin ventilation, make sure that you have the following equipment available:

■ Suction equipment (10F tubing, with 5F to 8F being available, suction set to 100 mm Hg)
■ Laryngoscope (check the light to ensure that the bulb is bright and screwed in tightly)
■ Blades—straight: No. 1 for full-term infants, No. 0 for preterm infants
■ Shoulder roll
■ Adhesive tape, to tape the endotracheal tube
■ Endotracheal tube: 2.5 to 4.0 mm (2.5 mm if the newborn is delivered before 28 weeks of gestation, 3.0 mm if delivered before 28 to 34 weeks of gestation, 3.5 mm if delivered before 34 to 38 weeks of gestation, and 4.0 mm if delivered after 38 weeks of gestation)

Some paramedics use a stylet to provide rigidity to the ET tube. In such a case, you must secure the stylet (bending it over at the top of the ET tube so it can't advance) and make sure that it does not extend beyond the ET tube, or tracheal perforation may occur.

Intubation of the neonate is discussed in the following steps and shown in **Skill Drill 40-1 ▶** :

1. Be sure the newborn is preoxygenated by bag-valve-mask ventilation with 100% supplemental oxygen prior to making an intubation attempt, unless congenital diaphragmatic hernia is suspected, where bag-valve-mask ventilation is contraindicated, or the infant requires emergency intubation for bradycardia that is not responsive to bag-valve-mask ventilation **Step 1** .

2. Suction the oropharynx if there is an obvious obstruction to spontaneous breathing or requires positive-pressure ventilation **Step 2** . This is a vagal stimulus, so pay close attention to pulse rate and avoid deep suctioning. Bag-valve-mask ventilation may be needed if the newborn develops bradycardia at this point.

3. Place the laryngoscope blade in the oropharynx and then visualize the vocal cords **Step 3** . Avoid applying torque to the blade, as it increases the risk of trauma. Place the ET tube between the vocal cords until the black line on the tube is at

Skill Drill 40-1: Intubation of a Neonate

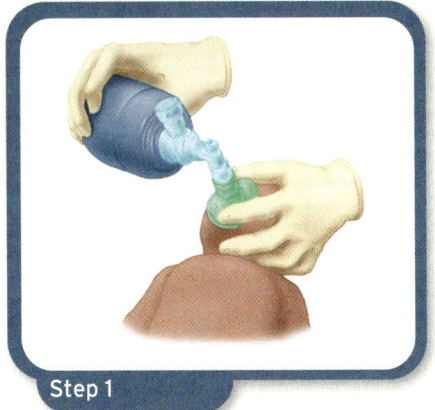

Step 1

Preoxygenate the infant by bag-valve-mask ventilation with 100% supplemental oxygen.

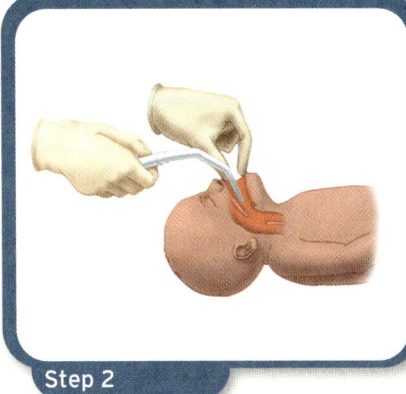

Step 2

Suction the oropharynx. Provide bag-valve-mask ventilation if bradycardia results.

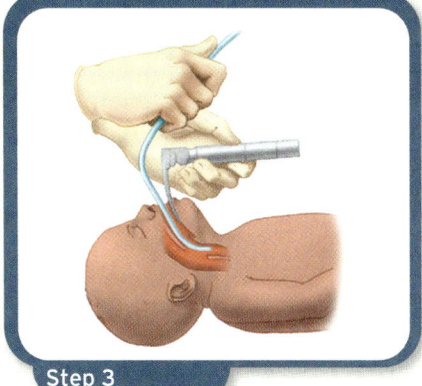

Step 3

Place the laryngoscope blade in the oropharynx. Visualize the vocal cords. Place the ET tube between the vocal cords until the black line on the ET tube is at the level of the cords.

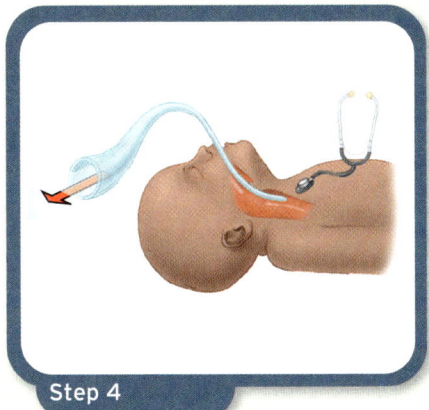

Step 4

Confirm placement. Observe chest rise, auscultate laterally and high on the chest, note the absence of significant air sounds over the stomach, and note mist in the ET tube. Note that CO_2 detector colour change is the gold standard recommendation for all ET tube placements.

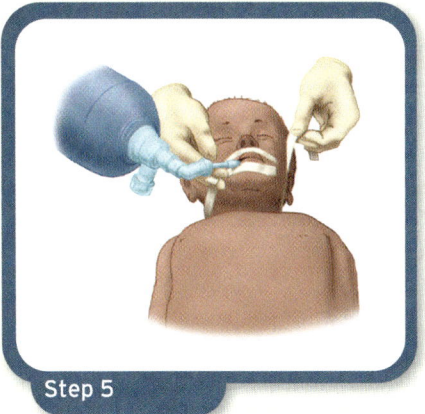

Step 5

Tape the ET tube in place. Monitor the newborn closely for complications.

the level of the cords. For full-term babies, the ET tube is usually advanced until it is at 9 cm at the lip. A premature baby may need to have the ET tube advanced to only 6.5 to 7 cm at the lip. Limit the intubation attempt to 20 seconds, and initiate bag-valve-mask ventilation if it is unsuccessful or if significant bradycardia develops.

4. Confirm placement (Step 4) by observing symmetrical chest rise when applying positive pressure through the ET tube, auscultating laterally and high on the chest to determine equal air entry on both sides, noting the absence of significant air sounds over the stomach, and observing for clinical improvement. A CO_2 detector colour change is the gold standard recommendations for all ET tube placements.

5. Tape the ET tube in place on the face to minimize the risk of the tube dislodging (Step 5). Monitor the infant closely for complications such as tube dislodgement, tube occlusion by mucous plug or meconium, or pneumothorax.

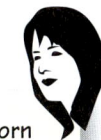

Notes from Nancy

Indications for Endotracheal Intubation of the Newborn

- Inability to ventilate effectively by bag-valve-mask device
- Necessity to perform tracheal suctioning, especially if meconium is present and infant is depressed at birth
- When prolonged ventilation will be necessary

Complications of ET tube placement include mucosal trauma causing bleeding, oropharyngeal or tracheal perforation, esophageal intubation with subsequent persistent hypoxia, and right mainstem intubation that can lead to atelectasis, persistent hypoxia, and pneumothorax. You can minimize these risks by ensuring optimal placement of the laryngoscope blade and carefully noting how far the ET tube is advanced.

Once positive-pressure ventilation or supplemental oxygen administration begins, the paramedic should reassess the patient by evaluating heart rate, respiratory rate, and oxygenation. Oxygenation is best determined by a pulse oximeter rather than simple assessment of colour, because colour is too subjective.

Gastric Decompression

Gastric decompression using an orogastric tube is indicated for prolonged bag-valve-mask ventilation (more than 5 to 10 minutes), if abdominal distension is impeding ventilation, or in the presence of diaphragmatic hernia. Many diaphragmatic hernias are diagnosed prenatally by routine ultrasound; they are suspected clinically if there are decreased breath sounds (90% of diaphragmatic hernias are on the left), a scaphoid or concave abdomen (many of the abdominal contents are in the chest), and increased work of breathing. Skill Drill 40-2 ▸ shows gastric decompression in a neonate.

1. To determine the length of tube to insert, use an 8F feeding tube and measure the length from the bottom of the earlobe to the tip of the nose to halfway between the xiphoid process (lower tip of sternum) and the umbilicus (Step 1).
2. Insert the tube through the mouth (Step 2).
3. Attach a 20-gauge syringe and suction the stomach contents (Step 3). Tape the tube to the baby's cheek. Remove the syringe from the feeding tube, leave open to free drainage, to allow venting of air from the stomach, and intermittently suction the feeding tube.

Chest Compressions

Chest compressions are indicated if the pulse rate remains less than 60 beats/min despite positioning, clearing the airway, drying and stimulation, and 30 seconds of effective PPV. Two techniques are used, depending on the number of rescuers available Figure 40-9 ▸. With the thumb (two-rescuer) technique, two thumbs are placed side by side over the sternum just below the nipples, and the hands encircle the torso. With the two-finger (one-rescuer) technique, the tips of the index and middle fingers are placed over the sternum just below the nipples and the sternum is compressed between the fingers.

The depth of compression is one third of the anteroposterior diameter of the chest. Your fingers should remain in contact with the chest at all times. In neonates, the chest compressions occur in synchrony with artificial ventilation, which you continue during chest compressions. The person delivering the chest compression counts out loud, "One and two and three and breath and. . . ." Downward strokes of chest compressions should be delivered while saying, "One and two and three." Release of the strokes should occur while saying "and." The person ventilating delivers a breath during the sequence "breath

and." This results in 90 compressions and 30 breaths/min. Pulse rate is assessed at 30-second intervals, and chest compressions stop when the pulse rate is greater than 60 beats/min. Liver laceration and rib fractures are possible risks of delivering chest compressions. Refer to Appendix A for coverage of infant CPR.

Venous Access

Emergent access becomes necessary when fluid administration is needed to support circulation, when resuscitation medications (eg, epinephrine) must be administered IV, and when therapeutic drugs (eg, IV dextrose, antibiotics) must be given IV. Establishing peripheral access in an infant can prove difficult, however.

The umbilical vein can be cannulated using an umbilical vein line in a newborn using the following steps:

1. Clean the cord with alcohol or another antiseptic. Place a sterile tie firmly, but not too tightly, around the base of the cord to control bleeding. Place a sterile drape over the site. Although the line must be placed quickly in a code situation, maintain sterile technique as much as possible.
2. Prefill a sterile 3.5F or 5F umbilical vein line cannula (a comparable-size sterile feeding tube can be used in an emergency) with normal saline using a 3-ml syringe, and three-way stopcock.
3. Cut the cord with a scalpel below the clamp placed on the cord at birth about 1 to 2 cm from the skin (between the clamp and the cord tie).
4. The umbilical vein is a large, thin-walled vessel usually found at the 12 o'clock position, as compared to the two thick-walled umbilical arteries usually found at 4 and 8 o'clock Figure 40-10 ▸. Insert the cannula into this vein for a distance of 2 to 4 cm (less in preterm infants) until blood can be aspirated. If the cannula is advanced into the liver, the infusion of hypertonic solutions may lead to irreversible damage Figure 40-11 ▸. If the cannula is advanced into the heart, arrhythmias may develop.
5. Flush the cannula with 2.0 ml of normal saline and tape it in place.

Pharmacologic Interventions

Medications are rarely needed in neonatal resuscitation, as most infants can be resuscitated with ventilatory support. Medications in neonates are based on weight, so you may need to estimate the infant's weight for dosing. A full-term infant usually weighs 3 to 4 kg; an infant born at 28 weeks of gestation, on average, weighs 1 kg.

Epinephrine

Administration of epinephrine is indicated when the infant has a pulse rate of less than 60 beats/min after 30 seconds of effective ventilation and 30 seconds of chest compressions. The recommended concentration for newborns is 1:10,000. The recommended dose is 0.1 to 0.3 ml/kg of 1:10,000 epinephrine IV, equal to 0.01 to 0.03 mg/kg, administered rapidly, followed by a 0.5- to 1-ml normal saline flush to clear the line. If IV access is not yet established, use the higher dose of 0.3 up to 1 ml/kg of 1:10,000 epinephrine given via the ET tube. Dosing may be repeated every 3 to 5 minutes in case of persistent bradycardia.

Skill Drill 40-2: Inserting an Orogastric Tube in the Newborn

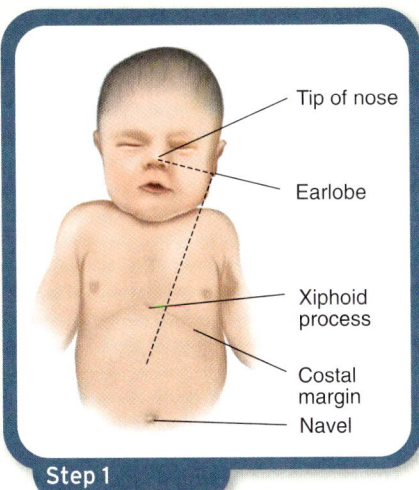

Step 1

Measure for correct depth—from the bottom of the earlobe to the tip of the nose to halfway between the xiphoid process (lower tip of sternum) and the umbilicus.

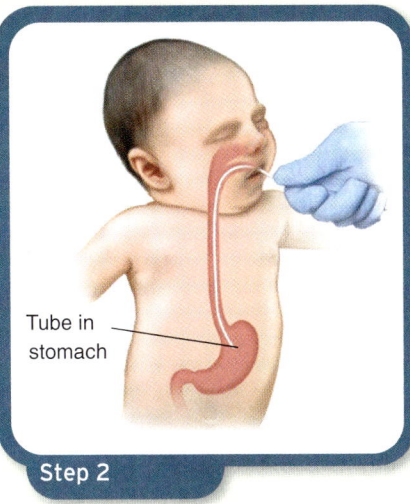

Step 2

Insert the tube to the appropriate depth. Leave the nose open to allow for ventilations.

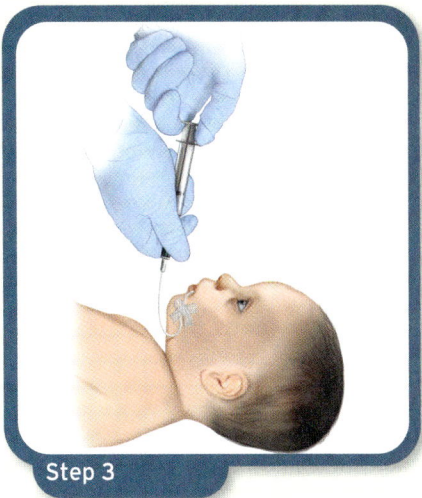

Step 3

Remove the gastric contents with a 20-ml syringe. Remove the syringe and leave the tip of the tube open to allow air to vent from the stomach. Tape the tube to the newborn's cheek.

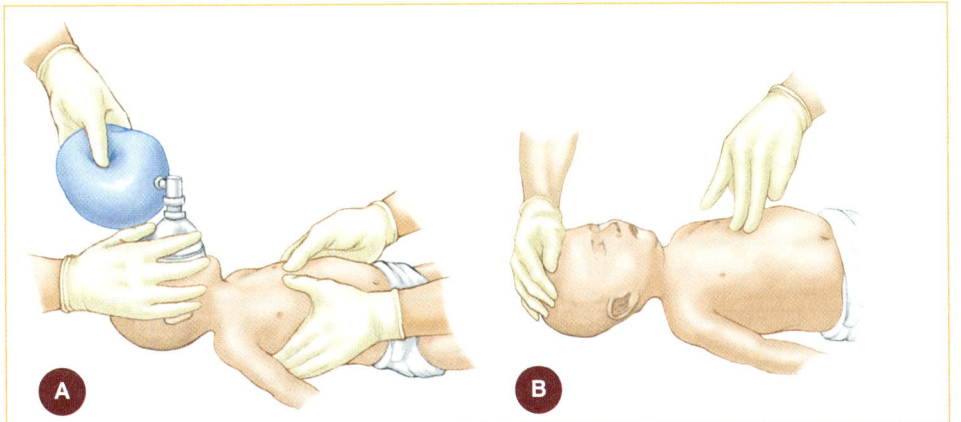

Figure 40-9 Chest compressions in the newborn. **A.** When there are two rescuers, use your thumbs side by side, placed just below an imaginary line drawn between the two nipples. **B.** When working alone, or when the baby is large, use two fingers to depress the sternum.

more than a few days old, place a peripheral IV or intraosseus (IO) line. Placement of an intraosseus line is discussed in Chapter 8. While the technique for placing an IO line is similar to that used with older children or adults, a smaller needle should be used in neonates to avoid exiting the far side of the bone. A fluid bolus in an infant consists of 10 ml/kg of normal saline IV given over 5 to 10 minutes. Multiple boluses may be administered if the patient remains clinically hypovolemic. Signs of hypovolemia include pallor, delayed capillary refill, and weak pulses despite a good pulse rate or high-quality chest compressions.

Volume Replacement

If the infant has significant intravascular volume depletion owing to conditions such as placental abruption (separation of the placenta from the uterus, which may lead to excessive bleeding) or septic shock, fluid resuscitation may be needed. In a newborn, place a low umbilical vein line as outlined earlier. In a newborn

Specific Conditions

Acidosis

If bradycardia persists after adequate ventilation, chest compressions, and volume expansion, and you suspect metabolic acidosis, sodium bicarbonate may be indicated. Direct

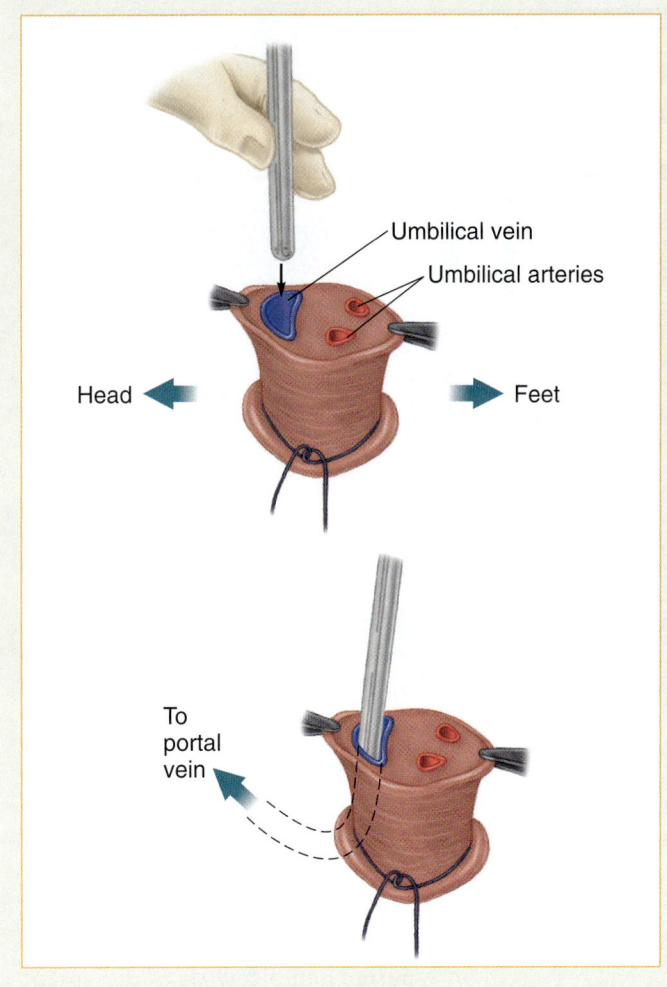

Figure 40-10 Location of the umbilical vein.

medical control may suggest an initial dose of 2 mEq/kg of 4.2% solution (0.5 mg/ml) IV to be administered over 5 to 10 minutes. Avoid rapid administration, especially in premature infants—a rapid change in pH may increase the risk of bleeding into the brain.

Respiratory Depression Secondary to Narcotic Administration

If the mother was a chronic narcotic user, administration of naloxone to the newborn to reverse the narcotic effect may precipitate life-threatening seizures. Naloxone is no longer recommended as a first-line drug in resuscitation of a newborn with an altered level of consciousness. In the case of respiratory suppression due to chronic maternal narcotic use, provide the newborn with ventilatory support and transport immediately. If, however, respiratory depression is due to the mother recently receiving narcotics and there is no chronic maternal narcotic exposure, naloxone may be administered to the newborn. A dose of 0.1 mg/kg may be carefully administered to the newborn via the IV (preferred) or IM route to reverse the narcotic-induced respiratory depression.

Pneumothorax Evacuation

If an infant has signs of a significant pneumothorax—severe respiratory distress unresponsive to PPV with unilateral decreased breath sounds and (if the pneumothorax is on the right) shift of heart sounds—a needle evacuation of the pneumothorax may be necessary. On the side of the suspected pneumothorax, clean the area around the second intercostal space, midclavicular line (usually just above the nipple), with alcohol. Prepare the equipment needed: a 22-g butterfly needle attached to extension tubing, a three-way

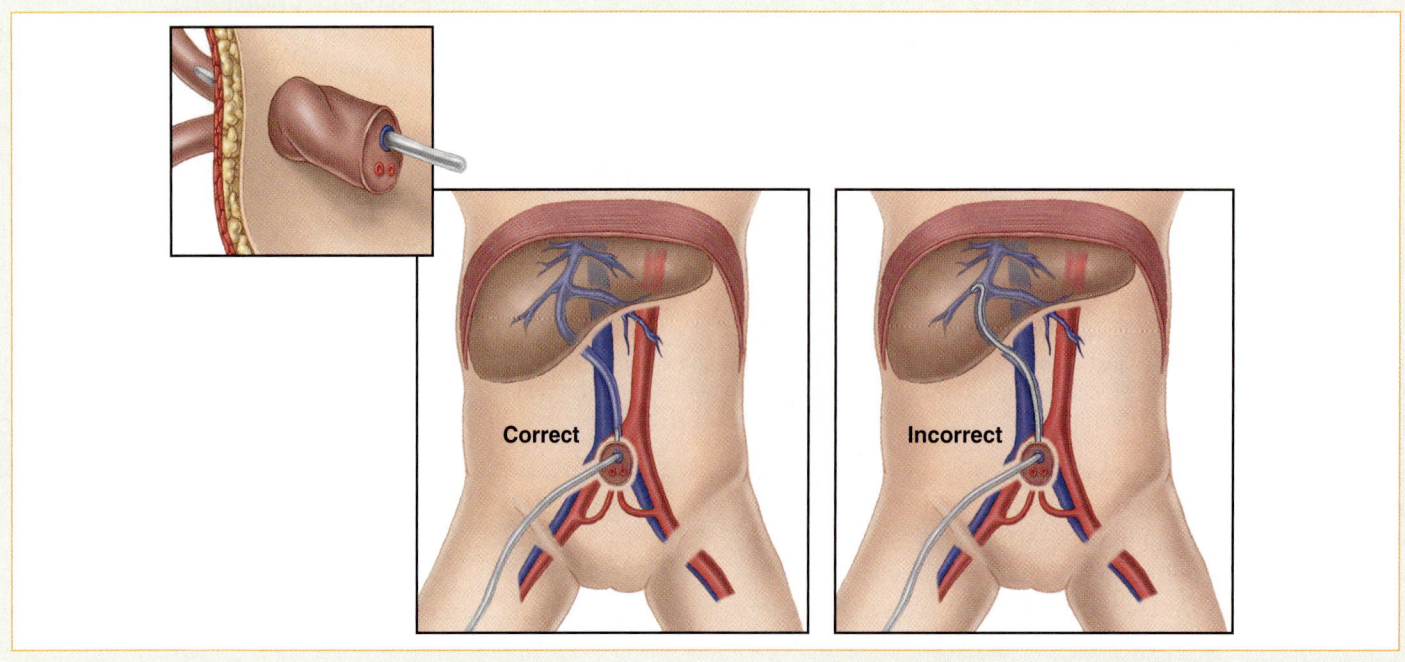

Figure 40-11 Umbilical vein cannulation.

stopcock, and a 20-ml syringe. Insert the needle above the second rib as a second paramedic pulls back on the syringe (which is open to the patient). The nerves and blood vessels run below the ribs, so avoid piercing this area. Continue to slowly advance the needle until air is recovered. The butterfly needle is rigid, so be gentle so as to avoid further tearing the lung. If the 20-ml syringe becomes filled with air, turn the stopcock off to the newborn, push out the air from the syringe, open the stopcock to the newborn, and continue withdrawing air. Once no more air can be withdrawn, remove the needle.

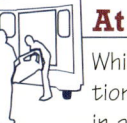

Notes from Nancy

Before you lunge for a syringe, recheck the effectiveness of artificial ventilation.

If there is a symptomatic ongoing air leak, a 22-g angio-catheter can be inserted in a similar location, the intro-ducer needle removed, and the angiocatheter attached to the exten-sion tubing. Note that the angiocatheter may further tear the lung during its initial place-ment and that it is more likely to kink than the butterfly needle.

Remove as much air as possible with the syringe. At this point, the tubing may be briefly occluded while you place the end of the tubing that had been attached to the syringe in a small bottle of sterile water and release the tubing occlusion. This can relieve the pressure buildup from the pneumothorax until the patient can be transferred to a facility for placement of a chest tube. During transport, monitor the infant very closely for signs of a reaccumulation of the pneumothorax.

While performing the pneumothorax evacuation, continue your ongoing patient assessment—use proper positioning to maintain the airway and avoid aspiration, take steps to maintain thermoregulation, and ensure adequate communication with the family and with the medical team receiving the newborn. Transport rapidly, but safely, and keep the infant warm.

Meconium-Stained Amniotic Fluid

Meconium-stained amniotic fluid, which is present in 10% to 15% of deliveries, carries a high risk of morbidity. Passage of meconium may occur either before or during delivery. It is

At the Scene

While bag-valve-mask positive-pressure ventila-tion and chest compressions can be performed in a moving emergency vehicle, you should pull the vehicle over to the side of the road while placing and secur-ing an advanced airway.

more common in post-term infants and in those who are small for their gestational age (weigh less than the 10th percentile for their age). Infants do not normally pass stool before birth, but if they do and then inhale the meconium-stained amniotic fluid either in utero or at delivery, their airways may become plugged and hypoxia may ensue. This, in turn, can lead to atelectasis, persistent pulmonary hypertension (delayed transi-tion from fetal to neonatal circulation), pneumonitis, or pneu-mothorax, which may require needle aspiration.

When a newborn is delivered through meconium-stained amniotic fluid, assess the newborn's activity level. If the baby is crying and vigorous, employ standard interventions. If the baby is depressed, it was routine to not dry or stimulate the baby and attempt intubation to clear the meconium: Intubate the tra-chea, attach a meconium aspirator and suction catheter to the end of the ET tube, and suction the ET tube until cleared of meconium-stained fluid. Continue suctioning while withdraw-ing the tube from the trachea, if the infant has a good heart rate and has begun to breathe. Be sure to cover the hole of the meco-nium aspirator with your finger in order to achieve adequate suctioning Figure 40-12 ▶ .The most current evidence does not support or refute this routine practice, so consult your local or regional protocols for the accepted practice in your service. There is no evidence, however, that an active baby benefits from airway suctioning of meconium, and there is good evidence of risk with this practice. Paramedics should not attempt to suction meconium if the baby is active and not in distress.

After tracheal suctioning, drying and stimulation may be enough to establish adequate breathing and pulse rate; in many cases where oxygen and PPV are needed, it is preferable to establish this prior to elective extubation. PPV with or without

You are the Paramedic Part 3

The baby's head delivers, and shortly thereafter the rest of the baby delivers. It is a little girl. There is no evidence of meconium on the infant's face. You dry the infant, place her in a supine position with her head slightly extended, gently suction her mouth and nose, and perform an assessment.

Newborn Assessment	Recording Time: 9 Minutes
Respiratory effort	Rapid and irregular; strong cry
Pulse rate	130 beats/min, regular
Colour	Cyanosis to the trunk and extremities

5. What prehospital treatment is indicated for this infant?

6. When is positive-pressure ventilation indicated for the newborn?

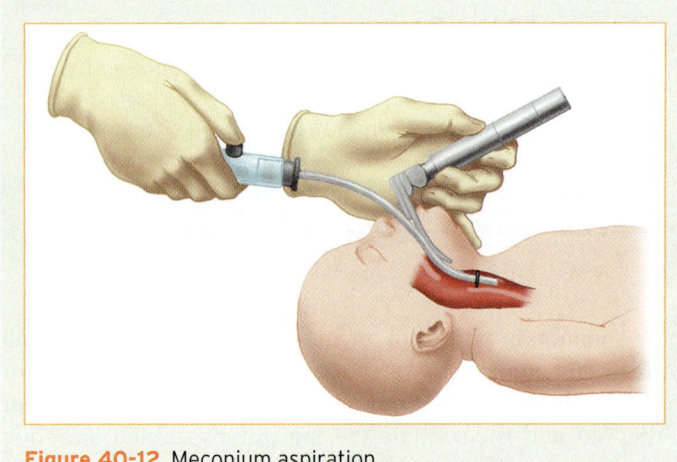

Figure 40-12 Meconium aspiration.

cardiac compression may be required. If intubation for direct tracheal suctioning is unsuccessful and the newborn has significant bradycardia, continue with standard resuscitation per NRP guidelines, including bag-valve-mask ventilation, recognizing that the newborn will be at very high risk of meconium aspiration. If the newborn has prolonged hypoxia after significantly delayed resuscitation, the outcome will likely be poor. When transporting such an infant with respiratory symptoms, stay in communication with a facility skilled at managing high-risk newborns to help with management and identification of an appropriate transport destination. To help support the family, explain what is being done for the newborn but do not discuss "chance of survival."

Diaphragmatic Hernia

Diaphragmatic hernia—that is, an abnormal opening in the diaphragm, most commonly on the left side—has an incidence of 1 in 2,200 live births. This diagnosis is often made on prenatal ultrasound before the baby's birth. The diagnosis is suspected clinically in a newborn with respiratory distress, heart sounds shifted to the right, decreased breath sounds on the left (which can also be signs of a pneumothorax), and scaphoid abdomen (ie, the abdomen, rather than being round, is sunken due to the abdominal contents being in the chest cavity). Mortality may be as high as 50% for this condition, due to the hypoplastic lungs, and associated pulmonary hypertension.

If a newborn has a diaphragmatic hernia, bag-valve-mask ventilation will introduce air that distends the intestines in the chest cavity, further compromising the newborn's ability to ventilate. If PPV is needed in such a newborn, place an ET tube and monitor peak ventilatory pressure carefully to minimize barotrauma—these babies have poorly developed lungs. Put an OG tube in place and intermittently suction the newborn to minimize intestinal distension. Ultimately, a newborn with a diaphragmatic hernia will require surgical correction, so transport him or her to a facility with a neonatal intensive care unit and a pediatric surgical team.

Apnea

Apnea is common in infants delivered before 32 weeks of gestation, but is rarely seen in the first 24 hours after delivery, even in premature infants. If prolonged (more than 20 seconds), it can lead to hypoxemia and bradycardia. Risk factors for apnea include prematurity, infection, prolonged or difficult labour and delivery, drug exposure, gastroesophageal reflux, central nervous system abnormalities including seizures, and metabolic disorders.

The pathophysiology of apnea depends on the underlying etiology. Apnea of prematurity is due to an underdeveloped central nervous system. Gastroesophageal reflux can trigger a vagal response, leading to apnea. Drug-induced apnea frequently results from direct central nervous system depression. Regardless of the cause, a newborn with apnea needs respiratory support to minimize hypoxic brain damage and other organ damage.

Assessment of an apneic infant includes a careful history to elicit possible etiologic risk factors and a physical examination that focuses on neurologic signs and symptoms or signs of infection. At birth it is important to differentiate between primary apnea and secondary apnea. If the newborn has experienced a relatively short period of hypoxia, he or she will have a period of rapid breathing, followed by apnea and bradycardia. At this point, drying and stimulation may suffice to cause a resumption of breathing and improvement in pulse rate. If hypoxia continues during primary apnea, the infant will gasp and enter secondary apnea. At this point, stimulation alone will not restart the baby's breathing. Instead, PPV by bag-valve-mask device or endotracheal intubation is required.

Additional Conditions

Additional conditions that you may encounter and your treatment response include the following:

- **Choanal atresia.** Place an oral airway.
- **Pierre Robin sequence.** Position the infant prone to maintain the airway. Use an oral airway if needed.
- **Cleft lip and/or palate.** Airway resuscitation is not needed, but you may need to apply some cricoid pressure if intubation becomes necessary. Consider delivering PPV via a bag-valve-mask device. You may need to use a little extra positive pressure in the case of a cleft palate. Owing to the risk of aspiration and regurgitation, do not feed the newborn with a cleft lip and palate in the prehospital environment.
- **Gastroschisis or omphalocoele with exposed abdominal contents.** These are developmental defects that lead to the intestines and/or other abdominal organs appearing outside the abdomen. In this situation, when providing standard resuscitation, place the newborn from the waist down into a sterile bag to keep the bowel clean and minimize heat/fluid loss. Nurse the infant on its side. Monitor the colour of the intestines (pink is good, blue/black is bad) and, if necessary, reposition the newborn so that the blood supply is not cut off due to kinking of the mesenteric blood vessels.

Premature and Low Birth Weight Infants

Infants delivered before 37 completed weeks of gestation are considered premature **Figure 40-13** . Infants born weighing less than 2,500 g are considered low birth weight. The most common etiology for low birth weight is prematurity. A number of factors can predispose a woman to deliver prematurely, including genetic factors, infection, cervical incompetence (early opening of cervix), uterine abnormalities (bicornuate uterus), abruption (placenta separation from uterine wall), multiple gestations (eg, twins, triplets), drug use, and trauma. Other factors that may contribute to low birth weight include chronic maternal hypertension, smoking, placental anomalies, and chromosomal abnormalities. If an infant is delivered prior to 24 weeks of gestation or weighs less than 500 g, the baby is unlikely to survive. The degree of immaturity can be estimated by physical characteristics such as skin appearance (more thin and translucent in more premature infants). If you observe signs of life, it is advisable to attempt resuscitation and maintain body heat until the newborn can be transported to an appropriate facility. A very preterm baby (< 28 weeks) may be slipped directly (without drying) into a plastic bag, exposing only the head, following delivery to minimize heat loss. Resuscitation should continue in the usual way.

Approximately 12% of births are preterm (< 37 weeks of gestation). Morbidity and mortality in this population are, in large part, related to the degree of prematurity. Most preterm infants delivered after 28 weeks of gestation who receive the necessary cardiorespiratory support after birth survive and do well over the long term. Infants delivered at 22 to 26 weeks of gestation have a high mortality and morbidity. Approximately one third die and one third experience significant long-term problems—typically respiratory issues, related to the need for long-term oxygen and ventilation, and neurologic issues, related to bleeding into the brain or insufficient blood supply to the brain parenchyma.

If an infant is delivered prematurely in the prehospital setting, providing cardiorespiratory support and a thermoneutral environment will optimize his or her survival and long-term outcome. Thermoregulation can be improved with careful environmental control (eg, warm blankets, plastic wrap). Premature infants are at higher risk for respiratory distress due to surfactant deficiency. The lungs of a premature infant are weak, so use only the minimum pressure necessary when you are providing PPV. The lungs and other organs are susceptible to oxygen toxicity, so attempt to reduce the amount of inspired oxygen as quickly as possible using an oxygen saturation probe as a guide. Assuming adequate perfusion, and thus accuracy of the probe, maintain saturation levels at 90% to 95%. For very premature infants, maintaining saturation levels in the region of 88% to 92% throughout their NICU course promotes a better outcome. Infants are also at risk of retinopathy of prematurity (abnormal vascular development of the retina), which may be worsened by high

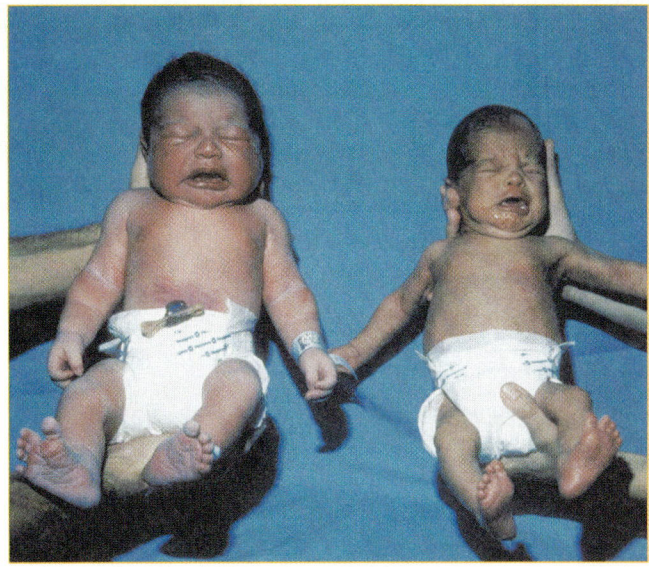

Figure 40-13 Premature infants (right) are smaller and thinner than full-term infants (left).

or long-term oxygen exposure. This may lead to severe visual deficits or blindness. Because hypoxia causes irreparable brain damage, however, do not withhold oxygen from a cyanotic premature infant. Brain injury can result from hypoxemia, rapid changes in blood pressure, hyperosmolarity leading to intraventricular hemorrhage, or periventricular leukomalacia (with inadequate brain perfusion). These brain insults may cause permanent injury with associated long-term disabilities.

Seizures in the Neonate

Seizures are the most distinctive sign of neurologic disease in the newborn. A seizure is defined clinically as a paroxysmal alteration in neurologic function (ie, behavioural and/or autonomic function). Seizures are common in premature infants, but difficult to diagnose as they are most often subtle in nature. The incidence in this population can be as high as 57.5 per 1,000 infants who weigh less than 1,500 g at birth, compared with 2.8 per 1,000 infants who weigh between 2,500 g and 3,999 g at birth.

Newborns may exhibit normal motor activity that can sometimes be mistaken for seizures. These myoclonic, dysconjugate eye movements or sucking movements are often seen when the newborn is drowsy or asleep. In addition, jitteriness is often confused with a seizure **Table 40-7** . Jitteriness is characteristically a disorder of the newborn and is rarely seen at a later age. Jitteriness is most commonly seen with hypoxic-ischemic encephalopathy, hypocalcemia, hypoglycemia, and drug withdrawal.

Table 40-7	Jitteriness Versus Seizures in the Newborn	
Characteristic	**Jitteriness**	**Seizures**
Ocular phenomenon (deviation or fixation of the eyes)	Not seen	Commonly associated
Stimulus sensitive (may be triggered by a stimulus)	Yes	No
Dominant movement	Tremor	Clonic jerking
Application of gentle pressure to limb	Stops jitteriness	Does not stop seizures
Autonomic phenomenon	Not associated	Common association

Seizures, by contrast, represent a relative medical emergency. They are usually related to a significant underlying abnormality—one that often requires specific therapy. Seizures may also interfere with cardiopulmonary function, feeding, and metabolic function. Finally, prolonged seizures may even cause brain injury.

Types of Seizures

Four major types of seizures are distinguished as follows:

- **Subtle seizure.** A seizure characterized by eye deviation, blinking, sucking, and pedaling movements of the legs and apnea.
- **Tonic seizure.** A seizure characterized by tonic extension of the limbs. Less commonly, flexion of the arms and extension of the legs may also occur. This type of seizure is more common in premature infants, especially in those with intraventricular hemorrhage.
- **Focal clonic seizure.** A seizure characterized by clonic localized jerking. This type of seizure can occur in both full-term and premature infants.
- **Myoclonic seizure.** A seizure characterized by flexion jerks of the upper or lower extremities. This type of seizure may occur singly or in a series of repetitive jerks.

When describing seizures, *multifocal* refers to clinical activity that involves more than one site, is asynchronous, and is usually migratory. *Generalized* refers to activity that is bilateral, synchronous, and nonmigratory.

Causes of Seizures

Table 40-8 ▶ lists the most common (and important) causes of neonatal seizures. The time of onset for hypoxic ischemic encephalopathy, hypoglycemia, and other metabolic disturbances is up to 3 days after delivery. With all other causes listed in Table 40-8, seizures may begin 3 days or longer after birth.

Hypoxic ischemic encephalopathy, usually secondary to perinatal asphyxia (lack of oxygen to tissues) is the single most common cause of seizures in both term and preterm infants. Seizures characteristically occur in the first 24 hours and usually become severe. Metabolic abnormalities include

Table 40-8	Causes of Neonatal Seizures
- Hypoxic ischemic encephalopathy - Intracranial infections (meningitis) - Hypoglycemia - Other metabolic disturbances - Epileptic syndromes	- Intracranial hemorrhage - Development defects - Hypocalcemia

disturbances in the levels of glucose, calcium, magnesium, or electrolytes. Other metabolic disturbances include abnormalities of amino acids, organic acids, blood ammonia, and certain toxins.

Hypoglycemia is most frequently seen in infants who are small for their gestational age, those who are large for their gestational age, and those whose mothers were diabetic during pregnancy. Neurologic symptoms consist of jitteriness, stupor, hypotonia (floppy), apnea, poor feeding, and seizures. A blood sugar level of 2.6 mmol/l or below is considered a medical emergency and immediate intervention is required, even in the absence of symptoms.

Hypocalcemia has two major peaks of incidence. The first peak occurs at 2 to 3 days after delivery and is most commonly seen in low birth weight infants and in infants of diabetic mothers. Late-onset hypocalcemia is rare but may be seen in infants who consume cow's milk or synthetic formulas high in phosphorous.

Other metabolic disturbances are uncommon in neonates, although hyponatremia, hyperammonemia, other amino acid and organic acid abnormalities, or seizures from drug withdrawal (eg, narcotic analgesics, sedative hypnotics, tricyclic antidepressants, cocaine, or alcohol) may be seen.

Assessment and Management of Seizures

Evaluation of a newborn with seizures must include a quick evaluation of prenatal and birth history and a careful physical examination. You may observe a quiet, often hypotonic infant. The newborn may be lethargic or apneic. Hypoglycemia must be recognized quickly and treated promptly. In these cases, blood glucose measurement and administration of dextrose may be lifesaving in the prehospital environment. Obtain the newborn's baseline vital signs and oxygen saturation readings and provide additional oxygen, assisted ventilation, blood pressure evaluation, and IV access as necessary. A 10% dextrose solution may be given as an IV bolus (2 ml/kg) if the newborn's blood glucose level is less than 2.6 mmol/l, with a recheck of the blood glucose level in about 30 minutes. IV bolus administration of dextrose often needs to be followed by a 10% dextrose infusion. When an IV cannot be readily established, an IM injection of glucagon is recommended until vascular access is achieved.

Consult with direct medical control if you are considering giving the newborn anticonvulsant medication. Phenobarbitol and phenytoin—the drugs most commonly used in such cases—require care in administration and may interfere with respiratory and cardiac function. Benzodiazepines, such as lorazepam, diazepam, or midazolam may also be administered IV.

Monitor the newborn's respiratory status and saturations carefully. Maintain the newborn's normal body temperature and keep the family informed about what you are doing for their infant as transport gets under way.

Thermoregulation

Thermoregulation is the body's ability to balance heat production and heat loss so as to maintain normal body temperature. This ability is very limited in the newborn. The average normal temperature of a newborn is 37.5°C. For the neonate, the thermoneutral temperature range is 36.6 to 37.2°C.

Nonshivering thermogenesis, the production of heat by metabolism, is the primary source of heat production in the neonate. Brown fat (deposited in the fetus after 28 weeks of gestation, and principally stored around the scapula, kidneys, adrenal glands, neck, and axilla) is a thermogenic tissue unique to the newborn.

Heat loss occurs when heat is lost to the environment, through any of the following four mechanisms. In evapouration, heat is lost when water evapourates from the skin and respiratory tract. In convection, heat is lost to cooler surrounding air; the extent of heat loss depends on the air temperature and air movement. In conduction, heat is lost to cooler solid objects in direct contact with the body. In radiation, heat is lost to cooler surrounding objects not in direct contact with the body.

Fever

Fever is defined as a rectal temperature greater than 38°C. Oral and axillary temperatures are, respectively, 0.6°C and 1.1°C lower than the rectal temperature on average. However, in infants younger than 2 years of age, the only reliable measurement is the rectal temperature.

A newborn's temperature regulation system is relatively immature, so fever may not always be a presenting feature with infection or illness. In fact, neonates may become hypothermic with infection. No matter what the presenting symptoms are, it is important to identify newborns with serious bacterial infection (eg, bacteremia, urinary tract infection, meningitis, bacterial gastroenteritis, and pneumonia) or serious viral infection (eg, herpes simplex) for which treatment is available. Approximately 13% of infants younger than 28 days with a temperature of more than 38.1°C will have a serious bacterial infection.

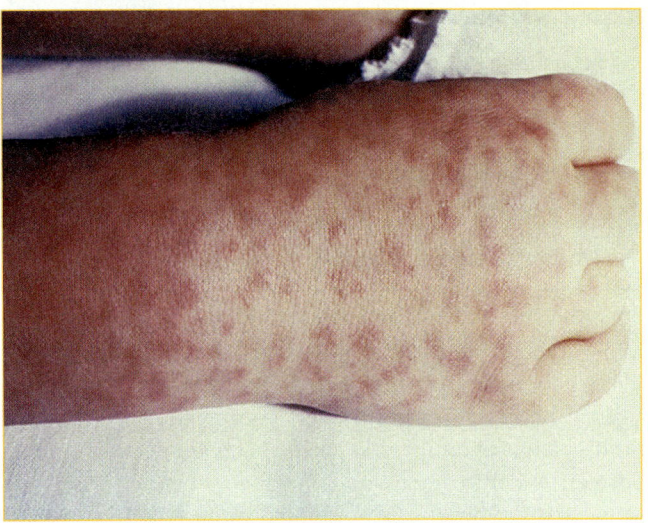

Figure 40-14 A newborn with a fever may also have petechiae (as shown here) or pinpoint pink or red skin lesions, blisters, or vesicles.

Fever may also be caused by overheating. Babies can easily become too hot when dressed in many layers of clothing, over-bundled in a heated car, or placed in direct sunlight, even through a window, or near heating vents at home. Fever related to dehydration is an important consideration in breastfeeding babies, especially in the first week after birth. These infants have often lost more than 10% of their weight and may have a history of difficulty in initiating breastfeeding.

Newborns have limited ability to control their temperature. They do not sweat to allow cooling when they are hot, and they do not shiver to raise their temperature when they are cold. Term infants may produce sweat over their brow but not the rest of their body. Premature infants do not produce sweat. Moreover, many newborns with serious life-threatening infections may actually see their core temperature drop; these infants are at a higher risk for hypoglycemia and metabolic acidosis. A careful examination will reveal irritability, somnolence, and decreased feeding. The infant may feel warm to touch. Some infants with fever, however, may be initially asymptomatic.

When fever is suspected, observe the newborn for the presence of rashes, especially petechiae or pinpoint pink or red skin lesions, blisters, or vesicles Figure 40-14 . Obtain a careful history regarding general activity, feeding, voiding, and

You are the Paramedic Part 4

After delivery of blow-by oxygen, the baby's trunk is now pink; her hands and feet, however, remain cyanotic. You take appropriate actions to keep her warm. Further assessment reveals that her respirations are rapid and her pulse rate is 120 beats/min. She resists your attempts to straighten her hips and knees and moves her foot away when you snap your finger against it.

7. What is the infant's Apgar score?

8. Is it safe to clamp and cut the umbilical cord?

Table 40-9	Risk Factors for Hypothermia

- All neonates in the first 8 to 12 hours after birth
- Home delivery
- Prolonged resuscitation
- Small for gestational age infant
- Infant with central nervous system problems
- Prematurity
- Sepsis
- Inadequate measures to keep the infant warm during transport

stooling. Obtain the newborn's vital signs and ensure adequate oxygenation and ventilation, providing free-flow supplemental oxygen if necessary. Perform chest compressions, if indicated. Administration of antipyretic agents such as acetaminophen or ibuprofen is controversial and not recommended in the prehospital setting; never give ibuprofen to an infant. To cool the newborn, remove additional layers of clothing and improve ventilation in the environment.

Hypothermia

Hypothermia is a drop in body temperature to less than 36°C. Hypothermia in the newborn occurs in all climates, but is more common during the winter months. It has been linked to impaired growth and may make the newborn vulnerable to infections. Moderate hypothermia is associated with an increased risk of death in low birth weight infants. Sick or low birth weight infants admitted to hospital with hypothermia are more likely to die than those admitted with normal temperature. Infants may die of cold exposure at temperatures adults find comfortable. Table 40-9 ▲ lists risk factors for hypothermia.

Newborn infants have increased surface area-to-volume ratio, making the newborn extremely sensitive to environmental conditions, especially when wet after delivery. An increase in metabolic function in an attempt to overcome the heat loss can cause hypoglycemia, metabolic acidosis, pulmonary hypertension, and hypoxemia. Every hypothermic newborn should also be investigated for infection.

Hypothermic neonates are cool to the touch, initially in the extremities; as their temperature drops, however, the skin becomes cool all over. The infant may also be pale and have acrocyanosis. The hypothermic newborn may present with apnea, bradycardia, cyanosis, irritability, and a weak cry. As a newborn's temperature drops, he or she may become lethargic and obtunded. In severely hypothermic babies, the face and extremities may appear bright red. Sclerema—hardening of the skin associated with reddening and edema—may be seen on the back, limbs, or all over the body. Thermal shock, disseminated intravascular coagulopathy, and death may occur in more serious cases.

Preventive measures include warming your hands before touching the baby. Dry the newborn thoroughly after birth and remove any wet blankets. Place a cap on the newborn's head, as the head is the largest source of heat loss. Place the infant

"skin to skin" with the mother, if possible. This serves two purposes: The mother keeps the baby warm, and mother and baby can more readily bond. Ensure adequate oxygenation and ventilation. If the infant is hypoglycemic, you may administer D$_{10}$W. Warm IV fluids can assist in rewarming the newborn. Current recommendations for very preterm infants (< 28 weeks) are to deliver them into a plastic bag or wrap in plastic wrap immediately to prevent heat loss, exposing only their heads, which are dried and covered with a hat. The critically ill newborn, once stabilized, should be placed in a prewarmed incubator or, if none is available, covered with warm blankets and kept on the mother's chest.

At home, skin-to-skin contact is the best method to rewarm a baby with mild hypothermia. Ideally, the room should be warm (24°C to 26.5°C), and the baby should be covered with a warm blanket and wear a prewarmed cap. Continue the rewarming process until the baby's temperature reaches the normal range or his or her feet are no longer cold. Do not use hot water bottles—they may cause burns because blood circulation is poor in the cold skin of babies.

Recent studies in neonates with hypoxic-ischemic injury indicate improved outcomes when the infant is provided mild therapeutic hypothermia within 6 hours of birth. This approach is not recommended in the out-of-hospital setting, although it is prudent to prevent hyperthermia. Maintain the infant at the lower margin of normal temperature (axillary temperature of no higher than 36.5°C).

Hypoglycemia

In full-term or preterm infants, hypoglycemia is a blood glucose level of less than 2.6 mmol/l. This condition represents an imbalance between glucose supply and utilization. Glucose levels may be low due to inadequate intake or storage or increased utilization of glucose. Most infants remain asymptomatic until the glucose falls below 2.2 mmol/l for a significant period of time. Because the brain relies on glucose as its primary fuel, hypoglycemia may result in seizures and severe, permanent brain damage. Table 40-10 ▶ lists risk factors for hypoglycemia in the newborn.

The fetus receives glucose from the mother and deposits glycogen in the liver, lung, heart, and skeletal muscle in utero. The infant then begins to utilize those glycogen stores to meet glucose needs after birth; most full-term infants will have sufficient glycogen stores to meet their glucose needs for 8 to 12 hours. Disorders related to decreased glycogen stores (small for gestational age, prematurity, postmaturity) or to increased utilization of glucose (infant of a diabetic mother, large for gestational age, hypoxia, hypothermia, sepsis) place the infant at increased risk for hypoglycemia. Metabolic adaptations to maintain normal glucose levels are regulated by counterregulatory hormones such as glucagon, epinephrine, cortisol, and growth hormone. Frequently, stressed infants will become hypoglycemic.

Table 40-10	Risk Factors for Hypoglycemia in the Newborn	
Risk Factor	**Specific Indicators**
Disorders of fetal growth and maturity	Small for gestational age
	Smaller of discordant twins (weight difference > 25%)
	Large for gestational age
	Low birth weight infant (birth weight < 2,500 g)
Prematurity	Less than 37 weeks of gestation or less than 2,500 g
Disorders of maternal glucose regulation	Insulin-dependent diabetic mother
	Gestational diabetic mother
	Morbid obesity in mother
Neonatal conditions with disturbed oxidative metabolism	Perinatal distress (eg, 5-minute Apgar score < 5)
	Hypoxemia due to cardiac or lung disease
	Shock, hypoperfusion, sepsis, cold stress
Severe anemia	Pallor (in the absence of hypovolemia)
Congenital anomalies and genetic disorders	Visible anatomical deformities/abnormalities

Symptoms of hypoglycemia may include cyanosis, apnea, irritability, poor sucking or feeding, and hypothermia. These symptoms may also be associated with lethargy, tremors, twitching or seizures, and coma. They may also have tachycardia, tachypnea, or vomiting.

Check the blood glucose level in all sick newborns (by heel stick) and evaluate the newborn's vital signs. After you establish good oxygenation, ventilation, and circulation (ABCs), manage the hypoglycemia. Direct medical control personnel may order the administration of a 10% dextrose solution as a bolus at 2 ml/kg via IV access if the newborn's blood glucose level is less than 2.6 mmol/l. This intervention may be followed by an IV infusion of 10% dextrose based on the infant's gestational age (60 ml/kg/d for a full-term infant; adjust upward based on the recommendations of the referring hospital for premature infants). As always, maintain normal body temperature—hypothermia places additional stress on glucose demand.

Vomiting

Vomiting is very common in newborns. Approximately 85% of infants vomit during the first week of life, and another 10% have vomited by 6 weeks of age. Vomiting ranges from "spitting up" to severe, bloody or bilious, projectile vomiting. Most episodes of vomiting are benign and do not result in weight loss, dehydration, or other ill effects. Bilious and/or bloody emesis (vomiting) indicates a pathologic condition that needs urgent medical attention. Persistent vomiting is a warning sign for underlying pathology and can cause excessive loss of fluid, dehydration, and changes in electrolyte levels (ie, sodium, potassium, and glucose).

Vomiting mucus, occasionally blood streaked, in the first few hours of life is not uncommon. Persistent vomiting in the first 24 hours of life suggests obstruction in the upper digestive tract such as esophageal or small intestinal atresia. Vomitus containing blood is often a sign of a life-threatening illness; it indicates bleeding in the gut due to mucosal ulceration or ectopic gastric mucosa in an intestinal duplication. Occasionally, swallowed maternal blood from an antepartum hemorrhage will cause blood-stained vomit or melena stools. Maternal blood can be easily recognized by carrying out an APT test, a test for adult hemoglobin. Sometimes bloody or tarry stools are associated with intestinal hemorrhage and thus should be considered pathological until proven otherwise. Aspiration of vomitus can cause respiratory insufficiency or obstruction of the airway.

Causes of Vomiting

A newborn's presenting symptoms may give a clue to the site of obstruction or other problem that is causing the vomiting.

Esophageal Atresia

Esophageal atresia may occur with or without a tracheoesophageal fistula. Its incidence is 1 case per 3,000 to 4,500 births. Infants are excessively mucousy soon after birth and may choke when attempting to feed, because the swallowed milk is returned promptly. If accompanied by a fistula between the esophagus and trachea, air will fill the intestines rapidly when the infant cries, and this may lead to compromised ventilation due to abdominal distension. This necessitates an urgent decompression of the stomach, typically by gastrostomy tube. The fistula also causes gastric contents to enter the lungs, which can cause severe aspiration pneumonitis. The fistula is ligated at the time of the definitive surgery for the esophageal atresia.

Gastroesophageal Reflux

Another possible cause of vomiting, pathogenic gastroesophageal reflux (GER), is common in infants, with a reported prevalence of 2% to 10%. GER is most commonly seen in infancy, with its incidence peaking in the 1- to 4-month age group. The infant may vomit either immediately or a few hours after a feeding. The vomiting may not be forceful. In uncomplicated GER, the vomitus is not bile stained or bloody. GER in infants and young children can present as typical or atypical crying and/or irritability, apnea and/or bradycardia, poor appetite, an apparent life-threatening event, vomiting, wheezing, stridor, weight loss or poor growth (failure to thrive), hoarseness, and/or laryngitis.

Pyloric Stenosis

In infantile hypertrophic pyloric stenosis (IHPS), marked hypertrophy and hyperplasia of the two (circular and longitudinal) muscular layers of the pylorus occur. As a consequence, the pylorus becomes thickened and obstructs the outlet of the stomach. The incidence of IHPS is 2 to 4 cases per 1,000 live births, with a male-to-female predominance of 4:1; 30% of patients with IHPS are first-born males. The usual age of presentation is approximately 3 weeks of life (range, 1 to 18 weeks). In IHPS, the stomach muscles contract forcibly to overcome the obstruction. Affected infants usually present with projectile vomiting, dehydration, malnutrition, and electrolyte changes. The vomitus in this case is not bile stained, but it can be brown or coffee coloured due to blood, resulting from gastritis or to a Mallory-Weiss tear at the gastroesophageal junction.

Malrotation

Malrotation is a congenital anomaly of rotation of the midgut. In this condition, the small bowel is found predominantly on the right side of the abdomen; the cecum is found in the epigastrium–right hypochondrium. In cases of malrotation, volvulus, or twisting of the gut around its mesentery, causes symptoms of vomiting and abdominal distension. The vomitus is bile stained and may be feculent (like feces/stool) if the obstruction is distal in the intestines. This is a surgical emergency because the blood supply in the mesenteric vessels may become interrupted and compromise circulation to the gut, leading to ischemia and loss of bowel integrity. Patients may die from perforation, peritonitis, or short gut syndrome when a large amount of the ischemic bowel has been surgically removed. Malrotation is estimated to occur in 1 of every 500 live births. Approximately 40% of patients are diagnosed within the first week of life; 75% are diagnosed by 1 year of age; and the remaining 25% are diagnosed later in life. With symptomatic malrotation, 75% to 90% of cases occur in infants younger than 1 year, 50% to 64% of cases occur in infants younger than 1 month, and 25% to 40% of cases occur in the first week of life. During the first week of life, the ratio of male-to-female presentation is 2:1. Early mortality rates ranged from 23% to 33%. Since the advent of corrective surgical procedures, morbidity and mortality have decreased significantly. However, bile-stained vomitus is always a red flag and should be assumed to be due to volvulus with malrotation until proven otherwise. Contrast studies must be carried out immediately to diagnose the condition, followed by immediate surgery. This is called a Ladd's procedure.

Hirschsprung Disease

Another cause of vomiting, meconium-plug syndrome, whereby the passage of meconium is delayed, is seen in Hirschsprung disease. The last segment of colon fails to relax due to lack of innervation in the wall of the intestine and causes mechanical obstruction. The infant usually has a history of not passing meconium in the first 24 hours of life. Delayed passage of meconium is also associated with microcolon seen in infants of diabetic mothers or in true meconium ileus, a common presentation of cystic fibrosis in the newborn.

Vomiting may also happen in conjunction with asphyxia, meningitis (infection of the membranes covering the brain and spine), and hydrocephalus (large head size is a clue). It is often sudden, unexpected, and forceful in such cases, and it may be accompanied by persistent irritability associated with increased intracranial pressure (ICP).

Use of drugs during pregnancy can lead to several withdrawal symptoms in infants, including vomiting. The drugs that most commonly cause vomiting in newborns are barbiturates.

Assessment and Management of Vomiting

On physical examination, you may note a distended stomach that has been caused by vomiting. Suspect an infection if the newborn has a fever or a history of contact with sick people.

Initial management steps for a newborn with vomiting start with the ABCs. Maintain a patent airway. A vomiting infant can aspirate the vomitus and compromise the airway. Keep the infant's face turned to one side to prevent aspiration. Suction or clear the vomitus from the airway with the help of a suction catheter or suction bulb. Ensure adequate oxygenation, providing either free-flow supplemental oxygen or bag-valve-mask ventilation or endotracheal intubation as necessary. Bradycardia may be caused by vagal stimulus and is usually transient; it may resolve with stimulation and free-flow oxygen.

Antiemetics should not be administered in the prehospital environment. The infant may be dehydrated, however, and need fluid resuscitation. Dry mucous membranes, tachycardia, or a sunken fontanelle are clues that the patient needs hydration. Normal saline (10 ml/kg per bolus) may be required in that case, followed by a dextrose/saline infusion.

On transport, place the newborn on his or her side, identify a facility capable of managing a high-risk infant, and explain what is being done for the infant to the family.

▎ Diarrhea

A normal number of stools per day for an infant is five to six, especially if the infant is breastfeeding, when infants often stool after every feeding. Diarrhea is an excessive loss of electrolytes and fluid in the stool. It is uncommon in newborn infants, although infants younger than 3 years have 1.3 to 2.3 episodes of diarrhea each year. The prevalence is higher in infants attending daycare centres. Nine percent of all hospitalizations of children younger than 5 years of age are for diarrhea.

The most common cause of acute diarrhea in children is viral infection (especially rotavirus infection during the winter months). More serious conditions such as intussusception, malrotation, increased ICP, and metabolic acidosis need to be ruled out. In neonates, causes of diarrhea include gastroenteritis, lactose intolerance, neonatal abstinence syndrome, thyrotoxicosis, and cystic fibrosis.

Severe cases of diarrhea can cause dehydration and subsequent electrolyte imbalance. Combinations of physical signs—such as ill general appearance, poor vital signs, capillary refill of greater than 2 seconds, dry mucous membranes, absent tears, weight loss, and low urine output—are good objective predictors of the degree of dehydration.

Assessment and Management of Diarrhea

Assessment includes estimating the number and volume of loose stools, decreased urinary output, and degree of dehydration based on skin turgor, mucous membranes, presence of sunken eyes, and other signs. Patient management, as always, begins with the ABCs. The newborn's airway and ventilation may be compromised if he or she is severely dehydrated and is obtunded, so ensure adequate oxygenation and ventilation. Perform chest compressions in addition to PPV in a newborn if the pulse rate is less than 60 beats/min.

Fluid therapy may be indicated when a newborn has diarrhea. Normal saline (10-ml/kg boluses) may be needed immediately to fluid resuscitate the infant.

Common Birth Injuries in the Newborn

Birth trauma includes both avoidable and unavoidable injuries to the infant resulting from mechanical forces (ie, compression, traction) during the delivery process. Such trauma is estimated to occur in 2 to 7 of every 1,000 live births. Most birth injuries are self-limiting and have a favourable outcome. Nearly half are potentially avoidable with recognition and anticipation of obstetric risk factors.

Birth injuries account for 2% to 3% of all infant deaths, with 5 to 8 of every 100,000 newborns dying of birth trauma and 25 of every 100,000 newborns dying of anoxic injury. Separating the effects of a hypoxic ischemic insult from the effects of a traumatic birth injury may prove difficult.

A difficult birth or injury to the baby can occur because of the infant's size or position during labour and delivery. Conditions associated with a difficult birth include primigravida (first pregnancy), cephalopelvic disproportion (the size and shape of the maternal pelvis are not adequate for the vaginal delivery of the infant or the infant's head is relatively large), prolonged or rapid labour, abnormal presentation (eg, breech or brow), large size (birth weight exceeding 4,000 g), prematurity, or low birth weight.

Birth trauma includes a variety of injuries. For example, abrasions, lacerations, bruises, and subcutaneous fat necrosis can occur with deliveries that involve instruments (eg, a vacuum or forceps). Moulding of the head and overriding parietal bones are part of the normal process of labour, but occasionally excessive moulding may be seen.

Caput succedaneum is swelling of the soft tissue of the baby's scalp as it presses against the dilating cervix. This type of cranial injury is very common. The swelling usually disappears in the first day or two after birth. It is important to distinguish this from a subaponeurotic or subgaleal hemorrhage, where bleeding occurs under the scalp as a result of shearing forces (especially common in vacuum delivery). The newborn may lose a great deal of blood into this tissue space and go into shock.

A cephalhematoma is an area of bleeding between the parietal bone and its covering periosteum. It often appears several hours after birth as a raised lump on the newborn's head, is limited by the boundaries of the bone, and may take 2 weeks to 3 months to resolve. Babies born by instrumental vaginal

You are the Paramedic Part 5

You prepare both the infant and mother for transport, load them into the ambulance, and begin transport to a hospital located 32 km away. En route, the mother experiences mild vaginal bleeding, which you control with fundal massage. As the infant is nursing, you establish an IV of normal saline on the mother and administer supplemental oxygen at 4 l/min via nasal cannula. After delivery of the placenta, you reassess the mother.

Reassessment	Recording Time: 19 Minutes
Skin	Pink, warm, and moist
Pulse	84 beats/min, strong and regular
Blood pressure	104/58 mm Hg
Respirations	20 breaths/min; adequate tidal volume
Spo$_2$	99% on oxygen via nasal cannula

When you arrive at the emergency department, you are met by a neonatologist and an emergency physician. Both the mother and baby are hemodynamically stable and are admitted to the hospital.

9. When are chest compressions indicated for the newborn?

10. When is epinephrine indicated during newborn resuscitation?

delivery are more likely to have a cephalhematoma. Do not try to drain a rapidly expanding scalp hematoma, as this may worsen or prolong the bleeding. When a large amount of blood collects, jaundice may ensue in the week after delivery as the red blood cells break down.

Linear skull fractures are occasionally seen with difficult births (spontaneous vaginal deliveries or deliveries using instruments).

The clavicle is the most frequently fractured bone in the newborn; such a bone injury is most often an unpredictable, unavoidable complication of normal birth. Risk factors may include large size, mid-forceps delivery, and shoulder dystocia (ie, the baby's shoulders get stuck in the birth canal). The infant may present with pseudoparalysis as he or she tries not to move the affected extremity to minimize pain. Examination will show crepitus and palpable bony irregularity.

Loss of spontaneous arm or leg movement is an early sign of long bone fracture. The femur and humerus are the most commonly affected long bones. The fractures are treated by splinting. Look for signs of radial nerve injury with a humerus fracture.

Brachial plexus injuries typically occur in large babies and have an incidence of 0.5 to 2.0 cases per 1,000 live births. The most common brachial plexus injury is Erb palsy (involvement of C5, C6). Klumpke paralysis (C7–C8, T1) is rare and results in the weakness of the intrinsic muscles of the hand.

Although branches of the facial nerve may be injured in forceps delivery, most facial nerve palsy is unrelated to trauma. Physical findings include asymmetric facies with crying (lack of movement on the affected side makes the face appear to be "pulled" to the opposite side). Full resolution of cranial nerve injuries may take several weeks.

Diaphragmatic paralysis may occur as an isolated finding when the cervical roots supplying the phrenic nerve are injured or in association with brachial plexus injury. The newborn may experience respiratory distress with hypoxemia, hypercapnea, and acidosis. Approximately 80% of the lesions are on the right side, and 10% are bilateral.

Laryngeal nerve injury appears to result from an intrauterine posture in which the head is rotated and flexed laterally. The infant presents with stridor or a hoarse cry. Bilateral injury may be associated with severe respiratory distress needing respiratory support. The paralysis often resolves in 4 to 6 weeks, but may occasionally take as long as 6 to 12 months to clear up.

Spinal cord injury may result from excessive traction (in a breech delivery) or rotation and torsion (in a vertex delivery). The clinical presentation is stillbirth or rapid neonatal death with failure to establish an adequate airway.

Intra-abdominal injury is uncommon and may be overlooked as a cause of death in a newborn. Hemorrhage is the most serious complication, and the liver is the organ most commonly injured. The bleeding may be catastrophic or insidious, and the patient presents with circulatory collapse. Consider intra-abdominal bleeding in every infant presenting with shock, or unexplained pallor, plus abdominal distension.

Family and Transport Considerations

Once the infant is stabilized as much as possible in the prehospital setting, transport the patient to the nearest facility that can provide the appropriate level of care. This facility will not necessarily be a tertiary hospital. A nearby community hospital, if it is located much closer, may be able to perform additional stabilization procedures for a very ill baby, such as placement of a chest tube for a clinically significant pneumothorax. Ideally, someone will contact this facility ahead to discuss the situation and obtain advice regarding care and disposition. Sometimes the infant will require immediate specialized attention, such as surgical intervention or work-up, thus you may need to discuss transfer to the most appropriate facility with direct medical control. Throughout the process, ongoing communication with the family regarding what is being done for the infant and what care is planned will help allay fears. Do not be specific about survival statistics. Many factors play into mortality and morbidity, and you don't want to be misleading. If family members have questions you can't answer, be straightforward. Tell them that you don't have a definite answer, but you will help put them in touch with the people who do (ie, the centre to which the infant is being transferred) **Figure 40-15 ▾**.

During transport, ongoing observation and frequent reassessment will ensure timely intervention should the newborn's status change. Attention to thermoregulation, respiratory effort, patency of airway, skin colour, and pulse rate is vital. A measurement of oxygen saturation and blood glucose level estimate are very helpful. If the infant is being transferred between facilities after the initial stabilization, continue to provide close observation and assessment of these factors to facilitate initiation of interventions should the infant's condition change.

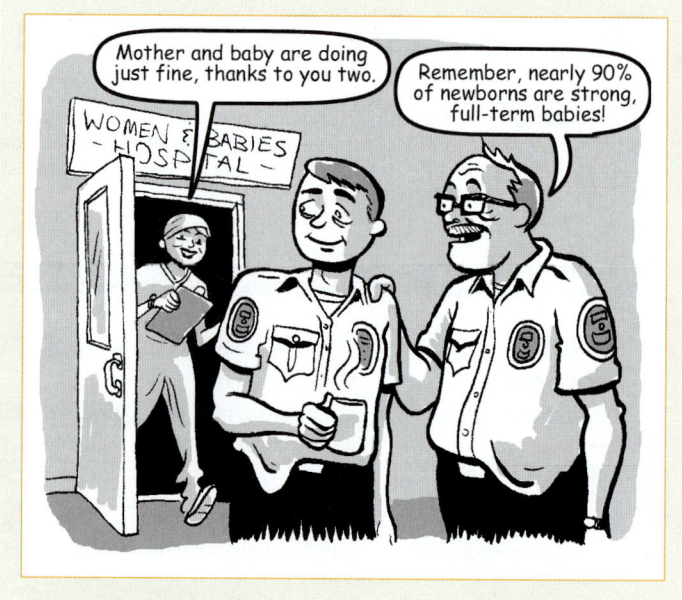

Figure 40-15

The development of new and more sophisticated techniques for the care of newborn infants, especially premature infants, together with round-the-clock care by expert medical personnel, has significantly reduced the mortality among high-risk newborns in hospitals where such capabilities are available. Because the average community hospital cannot provide the specially trained doctors and nurses or the expensive equipment needed for such care, it sometimes becomes necessary to transfer the critically ill infant to a regional centre, where the infant may benefit from highly skilled personnel and sophisticated equipment. In the well-organized regional referral system, transport of a high-risk newborn proceeds through the following several steps:

1. A physician at the referring hospital initiates a request for transport. A physician in the regional control centre decides which intensive care nursery can accommodate the patient and gives the referring physician advice on management of the infant until the transport team arrives.

2. A mode of transportation is chosen—ground transportation, helicopter, or fixed-wing aircraft, depending on the distance, availability of services, and weather conditions.

3. The transport team is mobilized, and equipment is assembled. The ideal team consists of a nurse with special training in neonatal intensive care, a respiratory therapist with similar special training, and a paramedic who has spent a period of apprenticeship in a neonatal intensive care unit. For particularly critical patients, a physician may also attend. The equipment is highly specialized, requiring appropriately designed ventilation and oxygenation units and an incubator meeting stringent criteria.

4. On arriving at the referring hospital, the transport team continues to stabilize the infant before embarking on transport. Conditions such as hypoxemia, acidosis, hypoglycemia, and hypovolemia must be treated before leaving the referring hospital.

5. While stabilizing the infant, the team collects information and materials including a copy of the mother's and infant's charts, including blood work results, and any x-rays taken of the infant. A vial of the mother's blood (clotted for group and cross-match if needed) and the placenta for pathological examination are helpful, if they can be retrieved.

You are the Paramedic Summary

1. Why is it important to determine the colour of the amniotic fluid?

A crucial part of your predelivery evaluation is to determine the colour of the amniotic fluid. Normally, it should be clear. Amniotic fluid that is brown or contains thick, particulate meconium—the baby's first bowel movement—indicates that the newborn may have aspirated the meconium. In such a case, the newborn may be severely hypoxic and may require aggressive resuscitation. Blood-stained fluid may indicate an abruption in which the mother's blood is usually lost and the infant is not anemic or hypovolemic. If there is a velamentous insertion of the umbilical cord, the abruption may interrupt fetal vessels entering the placenta along its margin, causing profound loss of blood in the infant with anemia and hypovolemia.

2. What are some reliable indicators of imminent delivery?

When determining whether you have time to transport the mother to the hospital or must prepare for imminent delivery, there are some key questions to ask and some key observations to make. Regular contractions that are less than 5 minutes apart—even if the amniotic sac has not ruptured—should be considered a sign of impending delivery. If the woman says that she feels the urge to move her bowels, the baby is pressing on her rectum and is in the birth canal. Clearly, crowning of the baby's head indicates that delivery is in progress. Perhaps one of the most reliable indicators of impending delivery is when the mother states that she is going to have her baby "now!" If she tells you this, believe her—even if it is her first baby.

3. What specific questions should you ask that will allow you to anticipate the need for resuscitation of the newborn?

Although it's impossible to predict all of the complications that might potentially occur following delivery, a thorough maternal assessment—if time permits—will enable you to identify risk factors that should increase your suspicion for a distressed newborn who will require resuscitation. Establishing how far along a woman is into her pregnancy is a key consideration. If a fetus is less than 37 weeks of gestation—in which case the woman would be in premature labour—the risk for a distressed newborn increases. You should also ask if the patient is carrying more than one baby. Of course, if she has had regular prenatal care—which typically includes an ultrasound—she will know the answer. Inquire about the use of drugs (legal and illicit), alcohol, or cigarettes during the mother's pregnancy; these factors clearly increase the risk of newborn distress. Finally, ask about her medical history, focusing specifically on conditions that can complicate pregnancy (ie, pregnancy-induced hypertension [preeclampsia] or gestational diabetes).

4. What equipment and supplies should be available in case the infant requires resuscitation?

Although approximately 90% of babies are born normal and require little more than drying, warming, and suctioning, you should be adequately prepared in the event that the infant requires more aggressive resuscitative measures. In addition to the sterile OB kit, you should have a neonatal-size bag-valve-mask device, equipment and supplies required to perform tracheal suctioning of meconium (ie, newborn-size ET tubes, meconium aspirator, suction, laryngoscope and blades), small IV cannulas, neonatal intraosseous needle, umbilical or small feeding tubes for vascular access, and epinephrine (1:10,000 only) for refractory cardiac depression. Consider carrying this equipment and supplies in a special newborn resuscitation kit, which should be checked daily, along with the other equipment and supplies on the ambulance.

5. What prehospital treatment is indicated for this infant?

Although the infant is breathing adequately and has a pulse rate of greater than 100 beats/min, the presence of central cyanosis indicates the need for free-flow supplemental oxygen. It can be delivered using an oxygen mask or oxygen tubing held near the baby's nose and mouth. Set the oxygen flow rate at 5 l/min and observe the infant for improving colour. Avoid blowing oxygen directly into the baby's eyes.

6. When is positive-pressure ventilation indicated for the newborn?

PPV is indicated in the newborn if the infant is apneic or has gasping respirations, if the infant's pulse rate is less than 100 beats/min, or if central cyanosis persists despite the delivery of free-flow supplemental oxygen. The proper ventilation rate for the newborn is 40 to 60 breaths/min.

7. What is the infant's Apgar score?

On the basis of your evaluation of the infant, her Apgar score is 9:

1. Appearance: pink body; cyanotic hands and feet (1)
2. Pulse: greater than 100 beats/min (2)
3. Grimace/irritability: infant moves her foot away when you snap your finger against her (2)
4. Activity/muscle tone: infant resists attempts to straighten hips and knees (2)
5. Respirations: rapid (2)

8. Is it safe to clamp and cut the umbilical cord?

The umbilical cord should not be clamped and cut until the baby is breathing adequately on its own and the cord has stopped pulsating. If neither of these has occurred, do not clamp and cut the cord. Instead, keep the baby at the level of the perineum, wrap the cord with sterile, moist dressings, and transport immediately with continued resuscitation en route to the hospital. The infant in this case has adequate breathing and a pulse rate greater than 100 beats/min; therefore, it is hemodynamically stable, and it is safe to clamp and cut the umbilical cord.

9. When are chest compressions indicated for the newborn?

Chest compressions are rarely needed during newborn resuscitation. However, if there is no pulse or if the pulse rate falls below 60 beats/min despite 30 seconds of *adequate* oxygenation and ventilation, begin chest compressions immediately. In the newborn, chest compressions are delivered using the two-finger technique (one rescuer) or the two-thumb encircling-hands technique (two rescuers). Compress the chest one third to one half the anteroposterior depth of the chest at a rate of 120 compressions/min. After 30 seconds of chest compressions, reassess the infant.

10. When is epinephrine indicated during newborn resuscitation?

As with chest compressions, medication therapy is rarely needed during newborn resuscitation. However, if the pulse is absent *or* less than 60 beats/min despite 30 seconds of *adequate* oxygenation and ventilation *plus* an additional 30 seconds of chest compressions (1 minute total), you should administer epinephrine. The proper newborn dose for epinephrine is 0.1 to 0.3 ml/kg of a 1:10,000 solution via rapid administration. *Never use epinephrine 1:1,000 during newborn resuscitation; it is too concentrated and may result in a spontaneous intracranial hemorrhage!* Epinephrine is recommended by IV route. It can be administered via a peripheral IV line or through the umbilical vein (if you are able to cannulate the umbilical vein) or intraosseous. If epinephrine is administered via the ET tube, consider giving a higher dose—0.3 to 1 ml/kg.

Prep Kit

Ready for Review

- The prehospital care of a newborn or neonate must be tailored to meet the unique needs of this population.
- Nearly 90% of newborns are vigorous full-term babies.
- Your initial rapid assessment of the infant may be done simultaneously with any treatment interventions.
- Not all deliveries go smoothly. Approximately 10% of newborns need additional assistance, and 1% need major resuscitation to survive.
- Additional skilled care intervention is needed for approximately 6% of newborn deliveries, with the rate of complications increasing as birth weight and gestational age decrease.
- Both short- and long-term outcomes have been linked to initial stabilization efforts.
- Infants born before 37 weeks of gestation are considered premature.
- Seizures are the most distinctive sign of neurologic disease in the newborn.
- Thermoregulation is very limited in the newborn, so the paramedic must take an active role in keeping the newborn's body temperature in the normal range.
- In full-term or preterm neonates, hypoglycemia is a blood glucose level of less than 2.6 mmol/l.
- Birth trauma includes both avoidable and unavoidable injuries to the infant resulting from mechanical forces during the delivery process. A difficult birth or injury to the baby can occur because of the infant's size or position during labour or delivery.
- Once the infant is stabilized as much as possible in the prehospital environment he or she needs to be transported to the nearest facility that can provide the appropriate level of care.

Vital Vocabulary

acrocyanosis A decrease in the amount of oxygen delivered to the extremities. The hands and feet turn blue because of narrowing (constriction) of small arterioles (tiny arteries) toward the end of the arms and legs.

amniotic fluid A clear, slightly yellowish liquid that surrounds the unborn baby (fetus) during pregnancy; contained in the amniotic sac.

Apgar score Scale used to assess newborn infant status (range, 0 to 10).

apnea Respiratory pause greater than or equal to 20 seconds.

asphyxia Condition of severely deficient supply of oxygen to the body leading to end organ damage.

bradycardia A pulse rate of less than 100 beats/min in the newborn.

central cyanosis Bluish colouration of the skin over head, neck, and trunk due to the presence of deoxygenated hemoglobin in blood vessels near the skin surface, best assessed centrally in the mucous membranes of the lips and mouth.

choanal atresia A narrowing or blockage of the nasal airway by membranous or bony tissue; a congenital condition, meaning it is present at birth. Often bilateral, and because neonates are obligatory nasal breathers, it is life-threatening.

cleft lip An abnormal defect or fissure in the upper lip that failed to close during development. It is often associated with cleft palate.

cleft palate A fissure or hole in the palate (roof of the mouth) that forms a communicating pathway between the mouth and nasal cavities.

diaphragmatic hernia A defect in the muscle of the diaphragm more common on the left side which results in passage of loops of bowel with or without other abdominal organs, through the diaphragm muscle into the chest (thoracic) cavity.

Erb palsy Lack of movement at the shoulder due to nerve injury resulting from the stretching of the cervical nerve roots (C5 and C6 most commonly) during delivery of the baby's head during birth. The effect is usually transient, but can be permanent.

free-flow oxygen Oxygen administered via oxygen tube and a cupped hand on patient's face.

gestation Period of time from conception to birth. For humans, the full period is normally 9 months (or 40 weeks).

grunting Noises heard when a baby is having difficulty breathing; short inarticulate guttural sounds as effort is expended.

hypoglycemia A deficiency of glucose in the blood caused by too much insulin or too little glucose; in the newborn it is a level less than 2.6 mmol/l.

hypotonia Low or poor muscle tone (floppy).

hypovolemia An abnormal decrease in blood volume or, strictly speaking, an abnormal decrease in the volume of blood plasma.

hypoxic ischemic encephalopathy Damage to cells in the central nervous system (the brain and spinal cord) from inadequate oxygen resulting in abnormal neurologic examination.

intercostal retractions Skin sucking in between the ribs, seen when a patient creates increased negative intrathoracic pressure to breathe.

intussusception An event where one part of the intestine telescopes into another part of the intestines and leads to a blockage in the intestine and potential for bowel ischemia.

Klumpke paralysis An injury of childbirth affecting the spinal nerves C7, C8, and T1 of the brachial plexus. It can be contrasted to Erb palsy, which affects C5 and C6.

malrotation A congenital anomaly of rotation of the midgut, the small bowel is found predominantly on the right side of the abdomen.

meconium A dark green fecal material that accumulates in the fetal intestines and is discharged around the time of birth.

nasal flaring Intermittent outward movements of the nostrils with each inspiration; indicates an increase in the work needed to breathe.

neonate Infant during the first month after birth.

newborn Infant within the first day after birth.

oligohydramnios Decreased volume of amniotic fluid during a pregnancy; a risk factor associated with abnormalities of the urinary tract, postmaturity (birth after a prolonged pregnancy), and intrauterine growth retardation.

persistent pulmonary hypertension Delayed transition from fetal to adult circulation from high pulmonary vascular resistance.

Pierre Robin sequence A condition present at birth marked by a very small lower jaw (micrognathia). The tongue tends to fall back and downward (glossoptosis), and there is a cleft soft palate.

placenta previa Abnormal location of the placenta in the lower part of the uterus partially or completely covering the cervical opening.

polycythemia Abnormally high red blood cell count.

polyhydramnios An excessive amount of amniotic fluid that can cause preterm labour. It may be associated with disorders of swallowing or intestinal blockage.

positive-pressure ventilation (PPV) Method for assisting ventilation (bag-valve-mask or intubated) with high-flow air or supplemental oxygen.

post-term Any pregnancy that lasts more than 42 weeks.

premature Underdeveloped; the condition of an infant born too soon. Refers to infants delivered before 37 weeks from the first day of the last menstrual period.

preterm Used to describe an infant delivered at less than 37 completed weeks.

primary apnea Apnea caused by oxygen deprivation; usually corrected with stimulation, such as drying or gently slapping the newborn's feet. Primary apnea is typically preceded by an initial period of rapid breathing.

primigravida First pregnancy.

prolapsed cord When the umbilical cord protrudes outside of the uterus before the baby is born. It is an obstetric emergency during pregnancy or labour that acutely endangers the life of the baby because of cord compression cutting off the blood supply. It can happen when the water breaks and often with malpresentation (eg, breech).

pulmonary hypertension Elevated blood pressure in the pulmonary arteries from constriction; causes problems with the blood flow to the lungs.

retinopathy of prematurity A disease of the eye that affects prematurely born babies, thought to be caused by disorganized growth of retinal blood vessels resulting in scarring and retinal detachment; can lead to blindness in serious cases.

secondary apnea When asphyxia continues after primary apnea, infant responds with a period of gasping respirations, falling pulse rate, and falling blood pressure.

seizure A paroxysmal alteration in neurologic function, ie, behavioural and/or autonomic function.

small for gestational age An infant whose weight is considerably less than 90% of babies of the same age.

surfactant A substance formed in the lungs that helps keep the small air sacs or alveoli from collapsing and sticking together; a low level in a premature baby contributes to respiratory distress syndrome.

term Used to describe an infant delivered at 37 to 42 weeks of gestation.

umbilical vein Blood vessel in umbilical cord may be used to administer emergency medications.

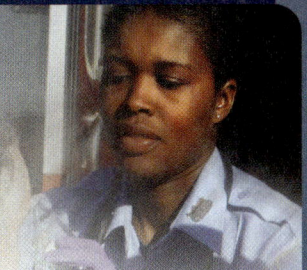

Assessment in Action

A 21-year-old woman who is 41 weeks' pregnant felt a few contractions and had the urge to go the bathroom. Her membranes ruptured (her "water broke") during this process, and she noticed it looked like "pea soup." She remembered from her prenatal visits that this wasn't a good sign and called 9-1-1. You arrive at the scene and find the infant's head presenting at the perineum.

1. **What does the "pea soup" appearance of the amniotic fluid indicate?**
   A. Dehydration of the newborn
   B. Meconium staining
   C. Cardiac arrest of the newborn
   D. Normal delivery

2. **How are delivery and resuscitation of a meconium-stained infant different from other full-term deliveries?**
   A. Higher rate of morbidity
   B. Lower rate of morbidity
   C. Higher rate of breech presentation
   D. Lower rate of breech presentation

3. **What is the most essential piece of equipment you need to prepare for this delivery?**
   A. Items to warm and dry the newborn
   B. Bulb syringe
   C. Cardiac monitor
   D. ET tube and meconium aspirator

4. **What is the primary use of the ET tube once you have it placed in the meconium-stained newborn?**
   A. It supplies positive-pressure ventilation.
   B. It serves as a suction device.
   C. It holds the airway open.
   D. It provides standard ventilation.

5. **What scale will you use to assess the newborn?**
   A. AVPU
   B. GCS
   C. Apgar
   D. SAMPLE

Challenging Question

6. **What measures will you take to provide prehospital care for the mother of this child?**

Points to Ponder

For the infant born through meconium-stained amniotic fluid discussed previously, the infant is depressed and you intubated and suctioned the trachea using a meconium aspirator while providing free-flow oxygen. You've dried and stimulated the newborn without causing injury. It is almost 2 minutes past delivery. The infant's pulse rate is 85 beats/min.

What is the next step in managing the airway—PPV or intubation?

Issues: Infant Airway Intubation, Neonatal Resuscitation.

41 Pediatrics

Competency Areas

Area 4: Assessment and Diagnostics

4.2.a	Obtain list of patient's allergies.
4.2.b	Obtain list of patient's medications.
4.2.c	Obtain chief complaint and/or incident history from patient, family members, and/or bystanders.
4.2.d	Obtain information regarding patient's past medical history.
4.2.e	Obtain information about patient's last oral intake.
4.2.f	Obtain information regarding incident through accurate and complete scene assessment.
4.3.a	Conduct primary patient assessment and interpret findings.
4.3.b	Conduct secondary patient assessment and interpret findings.
4.3.o	Conduct neonatal assessment and interpret findings.
4.4.a	Assess pulse.
4.4.b	Assess respiration.
4.4.g	Assess skin condition.
4.4.h	Assess pupils.
4.4.i	Assess level of mentation.

Area 5: Therapeutics

5.1.a	Use manual maneuvers and positioning to maintain airway patency.
5.1.b	Suction oropharynx.
5.1.c	Suction beyond oropharynx.
5.1.d	Utilize oropharyngeal airway.
5.1.e	Utilize nasopharyngeal airway.
5.1.g	Utilize airway devices not requiring visualization of vocal cords and introduced endotracheally.
5.1.h	Utilize airway devices requiring visualization of vocal cords and introduced endotracheally.
5.1.i	Remove airway foreign bodies (AFB).
5.1.j	Remove foreign body by direct techniques.
5.2.a	Recognize indications for oxygen administration.
5.3.b	Administer oxygen using low concentration mask.
5.3.d	Administer oxygen using high concentration mask.
5.4.a	Provide oxygenation and ventilation using bag-valve-mask.
5.4.b	Recognize indications for mechanical ventilation.
5.5.a	Conduct cardiopulmonary resuscitation (CPR).
5.5.c	Maintain peripheral intravenous (IV) access devices and infusions of crystalloid solutions without additives.
5.5.d	Conduct peripheral intravenous cannulation.
5.5.e	Conduct intraosseous needle insertion.
5.5.i	Conduct automated external defibrillation.
5.5.j	Conduct manual defibrillation.
5.5.q	Provide routine care for patient with non-catheter urinary drainage system.
5.5.s	Conduct needle thoracostomy.
5.5.t	Conduct oral and nasal gastric tube insertion.
5.8.a	Recognize principles of pharmacology as applied to the medications listed in Appendix 5.
5.8.c	Administer medication via subcutaneous route.
5.8.d	Administer medication via intramuscular route.
5.8.e	Administer medication via intravenous route.
5.8.f	Administer medication via intraosseous route.
5.8.g	Administer medication via endotracheal route.
5.8.k	Administer medication via rectal route.

Area 6: Integration

6.2.b	Provide care for pediatric patient.
6.3.a	Conduct ongoing assessments based on patient presentation and interpret findings.
6.3.b	Re-direct priorities based on assessment findings.

Appendix 4: Pathophysiology

A.	**Cardiovascular System**
	Cardiac Conduction Disorder: Benign arrhythmias
	Cardiac Conduction Disorder: Lethal arrhythmias
	Cardiac Conduction Disorder: Life-threatening arrhythmias
B.	**Neurologic System**
	Convulsive Disorders: Febrile Seizures
	Convulsive Disorders: Generalized seizures
	Convulsive Disorders: Partial seizures (focal)
	Altered Mental Status: Metabolic; Structural
	Infectious Disorders: Meningitis
	Pediatric: Down syndrome
	Pediatric: Hydrocephalus
	Pediatric: Spina bifida
C.	**Respiratory System**
	Pediatric Illness: Acute respiratory failure
	Pediatric Illness: Bronchiolitis
	Pediatric Illness: Croup
	Pediatric Illness: Cystic fibrosis
	Pediatric Illness: Epiglottitis
	Pediatric Illness: Sudden infant death syndrome
D.	**Female Reproductive System and Neonates**
	Neonatal Complications: Cardiovascular insufficiency
	Neonatal Complications: Meconium aspiration
	Neonatal Complications: Respiratory insufficiency
G.	**Integumentary System**
	Traumatic Injuries: Burns
J.	**Multisystem Diseases and Injuries**
	Environmental Disorders: Anaphylaxis/anaphylactoid reactions
	Shock Syndromes: Anaphylactic
	Shock Syndromes: Cardiogenic
	Shock Syndromes: Hypovolemic
	Shock Syndromes: Septic
	Trauma: Falls; Rapid deceleration injuries
L.	**Ears, Eyes, Nose, and Throat**
	Neck and Upper Airway Disorders: Epiglottitis
	External, Middle, and Inner Ear Disorders: Otitis externa
	External, Middle, and Inner Ear Disorders: Otitis media

Appendix 5: Medications

A.	**Medications affecting the central nervous system.**
A.3	Anticonvulsants
A.7	Non-narcotic analgesics
A.8	Opioid Analgesics
B.	**Medications affecting the autonomic nervous system.**
B.1	Andrenergic agonists
H.	**Medications used to treat electrolyte and substrate imbalances.**
H.1	Vitamin and electrolyte supplements
J.	**Medications used to treat poisoning and overdose.**
J.1	Antidotes or neutralizing agents.

Introduction

Children differ anatomically, physiologically, and emotionally from adults. In addition, the types of illnesses and injuries they sustain and their responses to them vary across the pediatric age span. For these reasons, you must tailor your approach to accommodate for the developmental and social issues unique to pediatrics. Some children may be afraid of the EMS crew. Depending on the child, he or she may not be able to tell you what is wrong. Also, each pediatric call involves one or more caregivers who may be stressed or frightened themselves.

This chapter addresses some of the special considerations that will enhance your effectiveness in caring for an ill or injured child. It begins by discussing the approach to pediatric patients, with a focus on their developmental level and the anatomical or physiologic differences unique to the age group. This information is used to outline an approach to pediatric assessment, review specific pediatric emergencies, and address their prehospital management. Finally, the chapter details the skills needed to care efficiently and effectively for pediatric patients, regardless of the diagnosis.

Approach to Pediatric Patients

Sick or injured children present unique challenges in evaluation and management. Their perceptions of their illness or injury, their world, and you differ from the perceptions of adults. Depending on their age, they may not be able to report what is bothering them. Fear or pain may make children difficult to assess as well. In addition, you will have to work with

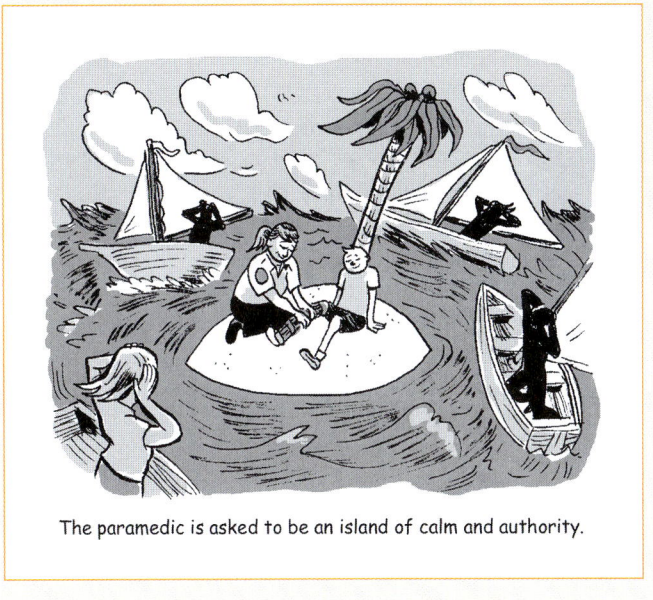

The paramedic is asked to be an island of calm and authority.

Figure 41-1

concerned parents and caregivers who may themselves be acting irrationally. In the midst of this chaos, you are expected to be an island of calm and authority, carrying out your job systematically, carefully, and confidently **Figure 41-1 ▲**.

The manner in which you approach a sick or injured child will depend on the child's age and developmental level. Childhood extends from the neonatal period, just after birth, until age 18 years. An enormous amount of physical and psychological development occurs in these 18 years. A child's anatomy, physiology, and psychosocial development will all influence your assessment and treatment.

You are the Paramedic Part 1

You and your partner are completing morning chores at the station when you are dispatched to treat a child who fell from a third-storey balcony. When you arrive in the quiet subdivision, you are flagged down by a frantic mother who points toward her 2-year-old son. You then see a toddler lying face up on the driveway approximately 1 m from the house. The mother tells you that she turned her son over but did not move him any further.

The toddler is lying motionless. His eyes are open, but he does not focus on you or his mother as she stands crying beside him. You observe an adequate respiratory rate with good bilateral chest expansion. The boy appears pale and has cool, dry skin.

Initial Assessment	Recording Time: 0 Minutes
Appearance	Pale toddler, lying motionless, making no eye contact
Level of consciousness	V (Responsive to verbal stimuli)
Airway	Open
Breathing	Adequate rate and volume; no retractions or audible sounds
Circulation	Weak radial pulses with pale, cool, dry skin

1. What assessment tool will you use to form your general impression of your patient?
2. What can you do to assist the panicked mother?

Special Considerations

Children have more head injuries than adults because of their large heads.

Pediatric Anatomy and Physiology

Head

You may have seen an infant or young child and noted the size of the child's head: Little children have very big heads. In fact, an infant's head is already two thirds the size it will be in adulthood. The large head means more surface area for heat loss. It also means more mass relative to the rest of the body—an important factor in the incidence of head injuries in young patients, who tend to lead with the head in a fall. During the school-age years, the head and body develop adult proportions.

Neck and Airway

Children have short, stubby necks, which can make it difficult to feel a carotid pulse or see jugular veins. Not surprisingly, the airway of a young child is also much smaller than an adult airway. That smaller diameter makes the airway more prone to obstruction, either by foreign body inhalation, inflammation with infection, or the child's disproportionately large tongue. During the first 4 to 6 months of life, infants are obligate nose breathers, and nasal obstruction with mucus can result in significant respiratory distress. Their epiglottis is floppy and U-shaped, which can make it difficult to visualize the cords during intubation. Finally, the narrowest part of a young child's airway occurs at the level of the cricoid cartilage, rather than at the vocal cords as in adults; these differences must influence your choice of endotracheal (ET) tubes.

Chest and Lungs

A child's chest wall is quite thin, with less musculature and less subcutaneous fat than in an adult. The thin chest wall makes it easy to hear heart and lungs sounds but also means that sounds are readily transmitted throughout the chest. Sounds originating from the nose or throat can be heard quite clearly on auscultation. The rib cage is more compliant, making retractions easy to see. Use of the diaphragm as a muscle of respiration is pronounced in infants, leading to belly breathing at baseline.

Heart

Circulation in the fetus is much different from that in the newborn, and large right-sided forces on the electrocardiogram (ECG) are normal in young infants. During the first year of life, the ECG axis and voltages shift to reflect left ventricular dominance. Cardiac output is rate-dependent in infants and young children. They have relatively poor ability to increase stroke volume, which is reflected in their normal heart rates (higher in newborns than in older children and adults) and in rate response to physiologic stress and hypovolemia.

Abdomen

The appearance of abdominal distension in a healthy infant is due to two factors: the weak abdominal wall muscles and the size of the solid organs. The liver extends below the ribcage in infants, making it more vulnerable to injury. As the child grows, the liver becomes smaller proportionately and is better protected by the bony ribcage.

Special Considerations

Because of children's shorter ribcages and less developed abdominal musculature, expect more intra-abdominal injuries in pediatric patients than in adults.

Musculoskeletal System

Reaching adult height requires active bone growth. The growth plates (ossification centres) of a child's bones are made of cartilage, are relatively weak, and are easily fractured. Overall, the bones of growing children are weaker than their ligaments, making fractures more common than sprains. Bones finish growing at differing times, but most growth plates will be closed by late adolescence.

Brain and Nervous System

The brain and nervous system continue to develop once the baby is born. As the brain matures, the infant's responses to the environment, outside stimuli, and even pain become more organized and purposeful. The rapidity of brain development can be appreciated by comparing the abilities and interactions of a 4-day-old baby, whose repertoire is limited to eating, sleeping, and defecating, with those of a 4-month-old, who smiles socially, rolls over, and plays with a rattle, and with those of a 12-month-old, who walks, is beginning to talk, and expresses preferences for individuals and activities.

Developmental Stages

Neonate and Infant

The first month of life is called the neonatal period, whereas infancy refers to the first 12 months of life. A lot of development occurs in this interval. Neonates do little else, other than eat, sleep, and cry. During the first months of life, a baby will have longer awake periods and interact more with the environment. Infants between 2 and 6 months of age are more active and social and can recognize their caregivers. By 4 months of age, infants are able to hold their heads up. Infants between 6 and 12 months of age babble, can sit unsupported, reach for objects, and are becoming more mobile—crawling and even walking. At 6 to 9 months of age, most infants develop stranger anxiety, with a strong preference for known caregivers.

Because infants cannot communicate their feelings or needs verbally, it is especially important to respect a caregiver's perception that "something is wrong." Nonspecific concerns about a young infant's behaviour, feeding, or sleep pattern may be tip-offs to a serious underlying illness or injury.

Consider the best location for performing your initial assessment. Although separating a 2-week-old from a parent will not cause distress, an older infant in stable condition will be calmest in a parent's arms. Make sure that your hands and stethoscope are warm—a startled, crying infant will be difficult to examine. Be opportunistic with your examination. If the child is quiet, listen to the heart and lungs first, perhaps listening over the clothes before you expose the chest and disturb the infant. If a young infant starts crying, letting the baby suck on a pacifier or gloved finger may quiet the child enough to allow you to complete your assessment. Jingling keys or shining a penlight may distract an older infant for long enough for you to finish an examination.

Toddler

The toddler period extends from ages 1 to 3 years. It includes the "terrible twos," a behavioural manifestation of the child's struggle between continued dependence on caregivers for food, shelter, and love and his or her emerging drive for independence. Children in this age group have limited reasoning, and a poorly developed sense of cause and effect. Language development is occurring rapidly, as is the ability to explore the world by crawling, walking, running, and climbing. Many toddlers will begin to have associations—possibly negative—with health care providers.

Your assessment of a toddler begins with observation of the child's interactions with the caregiver, vocalisations, and mobility, measured through the Pediatric Assessment Triangle (PAT), which is described in detail later. Examine a toddler in stable condition on the parent's lap. Get down to the child's level, sitting or squatting for the examination. You may need to be creative to get a good examination on a toddler with stranger anxiety: Use a parent to lift the shirt so that you can count respiratory rate, or have the parent press on the abdomen to see if that appears painful. Use play and distraction techniques whenever possible—listening to the doll's chest first may buy you a few minutes of cooperation. Offer toddlers limited choices when possible because they like to be in control. If you ask yes or no questions, the answer is likely to be "No!" Consider doing the more upsetting parts of the examination, such as palpating a tender abdomen or examining an injured extremity last. Be flexible in your approach—some toddlers will not let you complete an orderly head-to-toe examination.

Preschool-Age Child

During the preschool years (3 to 6 years), the child is becoming much more verbal and interactive. He or she can understand directions and be engaged with an activity or set of goals.

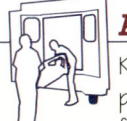

At the Scene

Keep infants and young children close to their parents during your assessment to help them feel safe and to improve your ability to perform the assessment.

Generally, a preschooler will be able to tell you what hurts and may have a story to share about the illness or injury. Preschoolers will understand as you explain what you are going to do, but choose your words carefully because preschoolers are very literal. Saying "I'm going take your pulse" may lead preschoolers to believe that you are taking something from them and wonder if you plan to give it back! Speak to them in very plain language about what you are going to do and provide lots of reassurance—this is the stage of monsters under the bed and many other fears.

As you perform your assessment, take advantage of the child's curiosity and desire to cooperate. If the patient is in medically stable condition, offer to take turns with the child in listening to the heart and lungs. Let the preschooler play with or hold equipment that is safe. To help give the child some sense of control, offer simple choices. Avoid yes or no questions. Set limits on behaviour if the child acts out. For the most part, you should be able to talk a preschooler through an orderly head-to-toe examination.

School-Age Child

As a child enters the school-age period (6 to 12 years), he or she becomes much more analytic and capable of abstract thought. At this age, the child can understand cause and effect. School-age children will have their own stories to tell about the illness or injury and may have their own ideas about the care to be given. By 8 years, the child's anatomy and physiology are similar to those of adults.

Ask the child about the history leading to calling 9-1-1 and let the child describe the symptoms, rather than focusing on the caregiver. Explain what you plan to do in simple language, and answer the child's questions. Give the child appropriate choices and control whenever possible, and provide ongoing reassurance and encouragement.

Adolescent

The adolescent years, from 13 to 18 years, can be difficult. Adolescents are struggling with issues of independence, body image, sexuality, and peer pressure. Friends are key support figures, and this is a time of experimentation and risk-taking behaviours.

With respect to CPR and foreign body airway obstruction procedures, once secondary sexual characteristics have developed (breasts or facial/axillary hair), the child should be treated as an adult. During the assessment, you must address the patient. Failure to do so can result in the adolescent feeling left out of his or her own care, which can alienate the patient, making it difficult to get an accurate assessment or give appropriate treatment. Encourage the patient's questions and involvement. Also, provide accurate information—a teen may become alienated and uncooperative if you are suspected of being misleading. When you perform the physical examination, respect the patient's privacy. If possible, address the adolescent without a caregiver present, especially about sensitive topics such as sexuality or drug use. If the adolescent's friends are on the scene, he or she may want them to remain during the assessment. Let the patient have as much control over the situation as appropriate.

Of course, do not let down your guard regarding scene safety: In a gang situation, members may have weapons and a reputation to earn.

Parents of Ill or Injured Children

The majority of children you will treat will come with at least one parent or caregiver. Thus, in many pediatric calls, you will be dealing with more than one patient—even if only the child is ill or injured. Serious illness or injury to a child is one of the most stressful situations caregivers can face. Some may react to this stress by becoming angry—at the fact that their child is sick, at the person or situation that caused the injury, or at you simply because they need someone to blame! Other parents will be frightened or guilty about the circumstances that led to the illness or injury. Establishing rapport with caregivers is vital, however, because they will be a source of important information and assistance. Children look to their parents when they are frightened and often mimic their response, so helping calm a parent may also help the patient cope.

Approach stressed caregivers in a calm, quiet, and professional manner. Enlist their help in caring for the child. Along the way, explain what you are doing and provide honest reassurance and support. Above all, don't blame the parent for what has happened. Finally, transport at least one caregiver with the child.

If the parent is extremely emotional, provide support, but remember that your first priority is the child. Don't let a distraught or aggressive parent interfere with your care. If necessary, enlist the help of other family members or law enforcement personnel.

Pediatric Assessment

Just as your general approach to a pediatric patient differs somewhat from your approach to an adult patient, so, too, will your assessment. In particular, you may need to adapt your assessment skills.

General Impression Using the Pediatric Assessment Triangle

After ensuring scene safety, the first step in an initial assessment of any patient begins with your general assessment of how the patient looks (the "sick–not sick" classification). An assessment tool called the Pediatric Assessment Triangle (PAT) **Figure 41-2 ▶** has been developed to help paramedics form a "from-the-doorway" general impression of pediatric patients. Paramedics with experience in treating ill and injured children intuitively use some version of the PAT to make the important distinction between sick and not-sick patients. The PAT standardizes this approach by including three elements—the child's appearance, work of breathing, and circulation—that

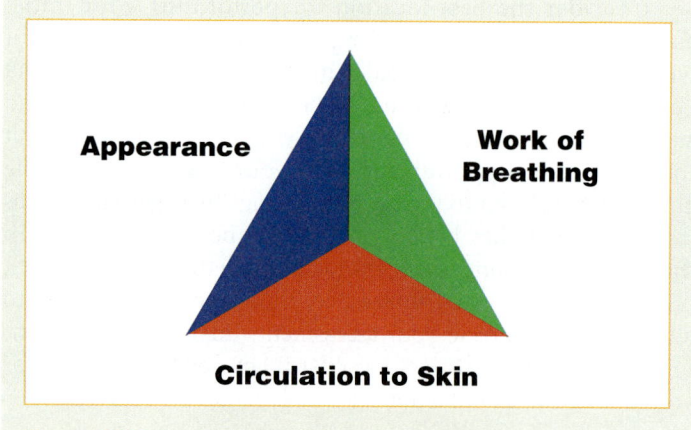

Figure 41-2 The Pediatric Assessment Triangle.

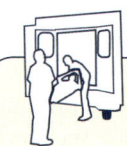

At the Scene

Use the PAT to help with your hands-off, from-the-doorway general impression of pediatric patients.

collectively paint an accurate clinical picture of the patient's cardiopulmonary status and level of consciousness. It applies a rapid, hands-off systematic approach to observing an ill or injured child and helps answer three questions:

- Is this patient sick or not sick?
- What is the most likely physiologic abnormality?
- Does this child require emergency treatment?

Appearance

The first element of the PAT is the child's appearance. In many cases, this is the most important factor in determining the severity of illness, the need for treatment, and the response to therapy. Appearance reflects the adequacy of ventilation, oxygenation, brain perfusion, body homeostasis, and central nervous system (CNS) function. The TICLS (tickles) mnemonic highlights the most important features of a child's appearance: Tone, Interactiveness, Consolability, Look or gaze, and Speech or cry **Table 41-1 ▶**.

To assess appearance, observe the child from a distance, allowing the child to interact with the caregiver as he or she chooses. Walk through the characteristics of the TICLS mnemonic while observing the child from the doorway. Delay touching the patient until you have developed your general impression because the child may become agitated by your touch. Unless a child is unconscious or critically ill, take your time in assessing his or her general appearance by observation before you begin the hands-on assessment and take vital signs. **Figure 41-3 ▶** and **Figure 41-4 ▶** demonstrate examples of an infant with a normal appearance and one with a worrisome appearance.

Table 41-1	Characteristics of Appearance: The TICLS Mnemonic
Characteristic	**Features to Look For**
Tone	Is the child moving or resisting examination vigorously? Does the child have good muscle tone? Or is the child limp, listless, or flaccid?
Interactiveness	How alert is the child? How readily does a person, object, or sound distract the child or draw the child's attention? Will the child reach for, grasp, and play with a toy or examination instrument, like a penlight or tongue blade? Or is the child uninterested in playing or interacting with the caregiver or prehospital professional?
Consolability	Can the child be consoled or comforted by the caregiver or by the prehospital professional? Or is the child's crying or agitation unrelieved by gentle reassurance?
Look or gaze	Does the child fix his or her gaze on a face, or is there a "nobody home," glassy-eyed stare?
Speech or cry	Is the child's cry strong and spontaneous or weak or high-pitched? Is the content of speech age-appropriate or confused or garbled?

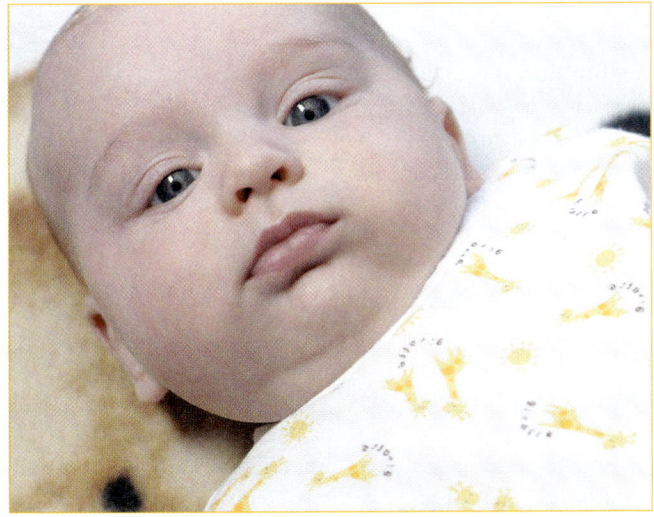

Figure 41-3 A child with a normal appearance. An infant or child who is not very sick will make good eye contact.

An abnormal appearance may result from numerous underlying physiologic abnormalities. A child may show evidence of inadequate oxygenation or ventilation, as in respiratory emergencies; inadequate brain perfusion, as from cardiovascular emergencies; systemic abnormalities or metabolic derangements, such as with poisoning, infection, or hypoglycemia; or

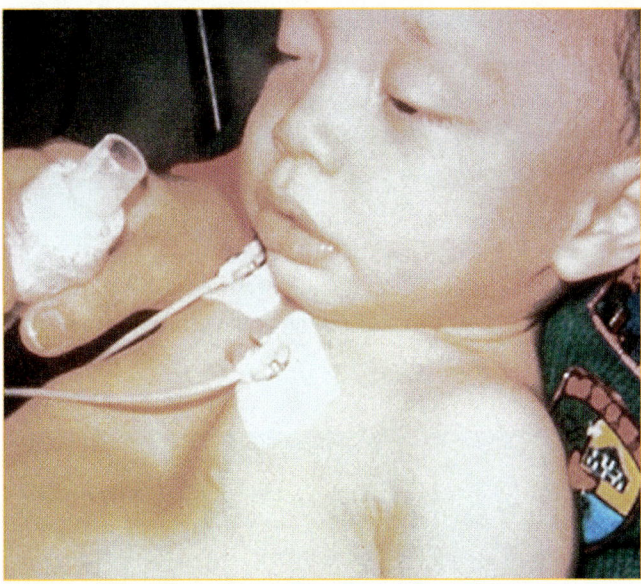

Figure 41-4 A child with an abnormal appearance. A limp child unable to maintain eye contact may be critically ill or injured.

acute or chronic brain injury. In any event, a child with a grossly abnormal appearance is seriously ill and requires immediate life-support interventions and transportation. The remainder of the PAT—work of breathing and circulation—plus the initial assessment may help identify the cause of the abnormal appearance and determine the severity of a child's illness and the need for treatment and transportation.

Work of Breathing

A child's work of breathing is often a better assessment of his or her oxygenation and ventilation status than the auscultation or respiratory rate. The work of breathing reflects the child's attempt to compensate for abnormalities in oxygenation and ventilation and, therefore, it is a proxy for effectiveness of gas exchange. The hands-off assessment of work of breathing includes listening for abnormal airway sounds and looking for signs of increased breathing effort   Table 41-2 ▸ .

Some abnormal airway sounds can be heard without a stethoscope and can indicate the likely physiology and anatomical location of the breathing problem. For example, snoring, muffled or hoarse voice, or stridor can indicate obstruction at the level of the oropharynx, glottis or supraglottic structures, or glottis or subglottic structures, respectively. Such an upper airway obstruction may result from croup, bacterial upper airway infections, or bleeding or edema.

Lower airway obstruction is suggested by abnormal grunting or wheezing. Grunting is a form of auto-PEEP (positive end-expiratory pressure), a way to distend the lower respiratory air sacs or alveoli to promote maximum gas exchange. Grunting involves exhaling against a partially closed glottis. This short, low-pitched sound is best heard at the end of exhalation and is often mistaken for whimpering. Grunting suggests moderate to severe hypoxia and is seen with lower airway conditions such as

Table 41-2	Characteristics of Work of Breathing
Characteristic	**Features to Look For**
Abnormal airway sounds	Snoring, muffled or hoarse speech, stridor, grunting or wheezing
Abnormal posturing	Sniffing position, tripod position, refusing to lie down
Retractions	Supraclavicular, intercostal, or substernal retractions of the chest wall; head bobbing in infants
Flaring	Flaring of the nares on inspiration

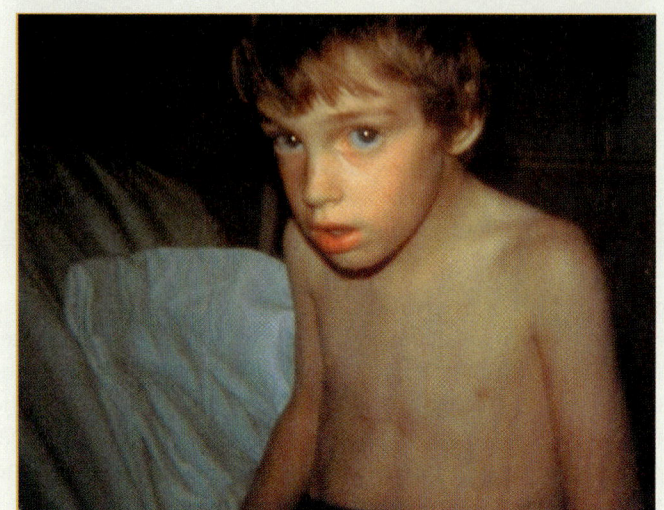

Figure 41-5 A child in a sniffing position is trying to align the airway to increase patency and improve airflow.

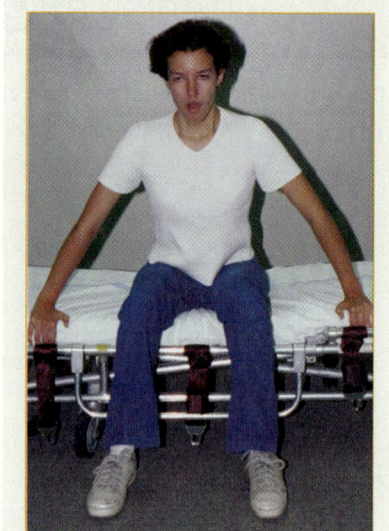

Figure 41-6 A child in a tripod position is maximizing his or her accessory muscles of respiration.

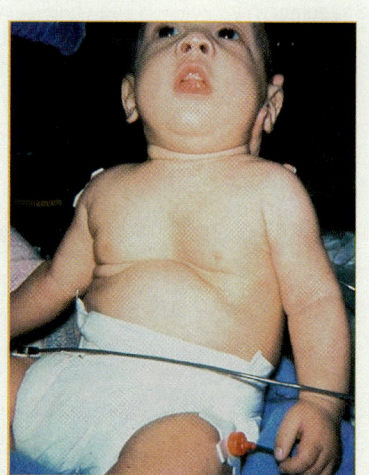

Figure 41-7 Retractions can occur in the suprasternal, intercostal, and substernal areas and indicate increased work of breathing.

pneumonia and pulmonary edema. It reflects poor gas exchange because of fluid in the lower airways and air sacs. Wheezing is a musical tone caused by air being forced through constricted or partially blocked small airways. It often occurs during exhalation only but can occur during inspiration and expiration during severe asthma attacks. Although this sound is often heard only by auscultation, severe obstruction may result in wheezing that is audible even without a stethoscope.

Abnormal positioning and retractions are physical signs of increased work of breathing that can easily be assessed without touching the patient. A child who is in the sniffing position is trying to align the axes of the airways to improve patency and increase air flow (Figure 41-5); such a position often reflects a severe upper airway obstruction. The child who refuses to lie down or who leans forward on outstretched arms (tripoding) is creating the optimal mechanical advantage to use accessory muscles of respiration (Figure 41-6).

Retractions represent the recruitment of accessory muscles of respiration to provide more "muscle power" to move air into the lungs in the face of airway or lung disease or injury. To optimally observe retractions, expose the child's chest. Retractions are a more useful measure of work of breathing in children than in

adults because a child's chest wall is less muscular, so the inward excursion of skin and soft tissue between the ribs is more apparent. Retractions may be evident in the supraclavicular area (above the clavicle), the intercostal area (between the ribs), or the substernal area (under the sternum) (Figure 41-7). Another form of retractions that is seen only in infants is head bobbing, the use of neck muscles to help breathing during severe hypoxia. The infant extends the neck as he or she inhales, then allows the head to fall forward during exhalation. Nasal flaring is the exaggerated opening of the nostrils during laboured inspiration and indicates moderate to severe hypoxia.

Combine the characteristics of work of breathing—abnormal airway sounds, abnormal positioning, retractions, and nasal flaring—to make your general assessment of the child's oxygenation and ventilation status. Together with the child's appearance, the child's work of breathing suggests the severity of the illness and the likelihood that the cause is in the airway or is respiratory.

Circulation

The goal of rapid circulatory assessment is to determine the adequacy of cardiac output and core perfusion. When cardiac output diminishes, the body responds by shunting circulation from nonessential areas (eg, skin) toward vital organs. Therefore, circulation to the skin reflects the overall status of core circulation. The three characteristics considered when assessing the circulation are pallor, mottling, and cyanosis (Table 41-3).

Pallor may be the initial sign of poor circulation or even the only visual sign in a child with compensated shock. It indicates

Table 41-3	Characteristics of Circulation to Skin
Characteristic	**Features to Look For**
Pallor	White or pale skin or mucous membranes from inadequate blood flow
Mottling	Patchy skin discolouration due to vasoconstriction or vasodilation
Cyanosis	Bluish discolouration of skin and mucous membranes

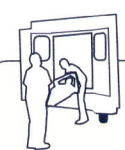

At the Scene

Note the line of demarcation of any mottling or pallor on the child's limbs during your initial assessment. An increase in mottling or pallor with movement toward the core of the body indicates a worsening "shell to core" shunt from peripheral vasoconstriction.

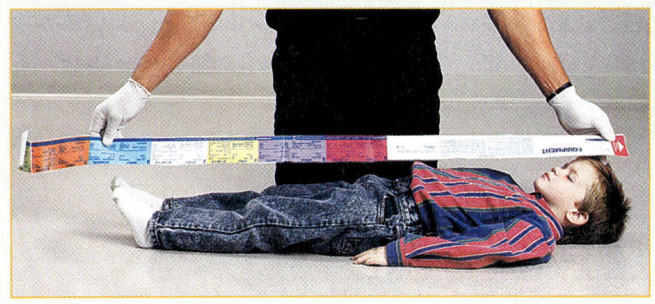

Figure 41-8 Use of a length-based resuscitation tape is one way to estimate a child's weight and identify the correct size for pediatric equipment and medication doses.

reflex peripheral vasoconstriction that is shunting blood toward the core. Pallor may also indicate anemia or hypoxia.

Mottling reflects vasomotor instability in the capillary beds demonstrated by patchy areas of vasoconstriction and vasodilation. It may also be a child's normal physiologic response to a cold environment.

Cyanosis, a bluish discolouration of the skin and mucous membranes, is the most extreme visual indicator of poor perfusion or poor oxygenation. Acrocyanosis, blue hands or feet in an infant younger than 2 months, is distinct from cyanosis; it is a normal finding when a young infant is cold. True cyanosis is seen in the skin and mucous membranes and is a late finding of respiratory failure or shock.

After assessing the child's appearance and work of breathing, visually scan the child's skin and mucous membranes looking for pallor, mottling, and cyanosis. You can then combine the three pieces of the PAT to estimate the severity of illness and the likely underlying pathologic cause. For example, a child with an abnormal appearance with poor circulation may be in shock from a cardiovascular cause.

Initial Assessment

After using the PAT to form a general impression of the patient, you will need to complete the rest of the initial assessment—that is, you must assess the child's mental status and ABCs and prioritize the care and need for transport. Threats to the ABCs are managed as they are found, providing a prioritized sequence of life-support interventions to reverse critical physiologic abnormalities. The steps are the same as with adults, albeit with differences related to the child's anatomy, physiology, and signs of distress.

Early in your assessment of a young child, you will need to estimate the child's weight, because much of your care will depend on the child's size. Ask a caregiver how much the child

weighs or make your own estimate, using a tool such as a length-based resuscitation tape **Figure 41-8 ▲**.

1. Measure the child's length, from head to heel, with the tape (with the red portion at the head).
2. Note the weight in kilograms that corresponds to the child's measured length at the heel.
3. If the child is longer than the tape, use adult equipment and medication doses.
4. From the tape, identify appropriate equipment sizes.
5. From the tape, identify appropriate medication doses.

Airway

The PAT may suggest the presence of an airway obstruction based on abnormal airway sounds and increased work of breathing. As with adults, determine if the airway is open and the patient has adequate chest rise with breathing. Check for mucus, blood, or a foreign body in the mouth or airway. If there is potential obstruction from the tongue or soft tissues, position the airway and suction as necessary. Determine whether the airway is open and patent, partially obstructed, or totally obstructed. Do not keep the suction tip or catheter in the back of a child's throat too long because young patients are extremely sensitive to vagal stimuli and the heart rate may plummet.

Breathing

The breathing component of the initial assessment involves calculating the respiratory rate, auscultating breath sounds, and checking pulse oximetry for oxygen saturation. Verify the respiratory rate per minute by counting the number of chest rises in 30 seconds and then doubling that number. Healthy infants may show periodic breathing, or variable respiratory rates with short periods of apnea greater than 20 seconds. As a consequence, counting for only 10 to 15 seconds may give a falsely low respiratory rate. Interpreting the respiratory rate requires knowing the normal values for the child's age **Table 41-4 ▶** and putting the respiratory rate in context with the rest of the PAT and initial assessment. Rapid respiratory rates may simply reflect high fever, anxiety, pain, or excitement. Normal rates, by contrast, may occur in a child who has been breathing rapidly with increased work of breathing and is becoming fatigued.

Table 41-4	Normal Respiratory Rate by Age
Age	**Respiratory Rate (breaths/min)**
Infant	25–50
Toddler	20–30
Preschool-age child	20–25
School-age child	15–20
Adolescent	12–16

Table 41-5	Normal Pulse Rates for Age
Age	**Pulse Rate (beats/min)**
Infant	100–160
Toddler	90–150
Preschool-age child	80–140
School-age child	70–120
Adolescent	60–100

At the Scene

Consider pulse oximetry readings in terms of the environmental context and the physiologic status of the child. Peripheral vasoconstriction from hypothermia or poor perfusion may alter these readings. Always correlate the pulse oximetry waveform with the patient's pulse rate and ECG reading.

Serial assessment of respiratory rates may be especially useful because the trend may be more accurate than any single value.

Auscultate the breath sounds with a stethoscope over the midaxillary line to hear abnormal lung sounds during inhalation and exhalation. Listen for extra breath sounds such as inspiratory crackles, wheezes, or rhonchi; rhonchi often indicate harsh breath sounds or sounds that may be transmitted from the upper airways. If you cannot determine whether the sounds are being generated in the lungs or the upper airway, hold the stethoscope over the nose or trachea and listen. Also, listen to the breath sounds for adequacy of air movement. Diminished breath sounds may signal severe respiratory distress. Auscultation over the trachea may also help distinguish stridor from other sounds.

Check the pulse oximetry reading to determine the oxygen saturation while the child breathes ambient air. You can place the pulse oximetry probe on a young child's finger just as you would with an adult. In infants or young children who try to remove the probe, it may be helpful to place the probe on a toe, possibly with a sock covering it. A pulse oximetry reading of greater than 94% saturation while breathing room air indicates good oxygenation.

As with the respiratory rate, evaluate the pulse oximetry reading in the context of the PAT and remainder of the initial assessment. A child with a normal pulse oximetry reading, for example, may be expending increasing amounts of energy and increasing the work of breathing to maintain his or her oxygen saturation. The PAT and initial assessment would identify the respiratory distress and point to the need for immediate intervention despite the normal oxygen saturation.

Circulation

The information obtained from the PAT about circulation to the skin directs the next step of the initial assessment. Integrate this assessment of circulation with the pulse rate and quality,

skin CTC (colour, temperature, and condition plus capillary refill time), and blood pressure to obtain an overall assessment of the child's circulatory status.

Obtain the child's pulse rate by listening to the heart or feeling the pulse for 30 seconds and doubling the number. As with respiratory rates in pediatric patients, it is important to know normal pulse rates based on age **Table 41-5 ▲**. Interpret the pulse rate within the context of the overall history, PAT, and initial assessment. Tachycardia may indicate early hypoxia or shock or a less serious condition such as fever, anxiety, pain, or excitement.

Feel for the pulse to ascertain the rate and quality of pulsations. If you cannot find a peripheral (distal) pulse (that is, radial or brachial), feel for a central pulse (that is, femoral or carotid). Check the femoral pulse in infants and young children and the carotid pulse in older children and adolescents. As with adults, if there is no pulse, start CPR.

After checking the pulse rate, do a hands-on evaluation of skin CTC. Check whether the hands and feet are warm or cool to the touch. Check capillary refill time in the fingertip, toe, heel, or pads of the fingertips; a normal refill time is less than 2 seconds. These two pieces of information need to be placed in context with the PAT and remainder of initial assessment because cool extremities and delayed capillary refill are commonly seen in a child in a cool environment.

The last step in the circulation assessment is to measure the blood pressure. It may be difficult to obtain an accurate measurement in a young child or infant because of a lack of cooperation and need for proper cuff size. Nevertheless, you should attempt to measure the blood pressure on the upper arm or thigh, making sure the cuff has a width two thirds the length of the upper arm or thigh. One formula for determining the lower limit of acceptable blood pressure in children ages 1 to 10 years is this: minimum systolic blood pressure = 70 + (2 × age in years).

At the Scene

Blood pressure is just one component of the overall assessment of pediatric patients. Determination of physiologic stability should be based on all data collected from the PAT, physical examination, and initial vital signs. Remember that compensated shock can exist in the face of adequate blood pressure.

Table 41-6	Normal Blood Pressure for Age
Age	**Minimum Systolic Blood Pressure (mm Hg)**
Infant	> 60
Toddler	> 70
Preschool-age child	> 75
School-age child	> 80
Adolescent	> 90

Table 41-7	AVPU Scale		
Category	**Stimulus**	**Response Type**	**Reaction**
Alert	Normal environment	Appropriate	Normal interactiveness for age
Verbal	Simple command or sound stimulus	Appropriate	Responds to name
		Inappropriate	Nonspecific or confused
Painful	Pain	Appropriate	Withdraws from pain
		Inappropriate	Makes sound or moves without purpose or localization of pain
		Pathologic	Posturing
Unresponsive			No perceptible response to any stimulus

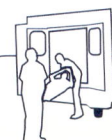

At the Scene

For children 1 to 10 years, calculate the lower limit of acceptable blood pressure for age with the following formula:

Minimum systolic blood pressure = 70 + (2 × age in years)

For example, a 2-year-old toddler should have a minimum systolic blood pressure of 74; a lower reading indicates decompensated shock. (Table 41-6 ▲ shows normal minimal systolic blood pressure values for different ages.) Given the technical difficulty of trying to measure a blood pressure, make one attempt in the prehospital setting; if unsuccessful, move on to the rest of the assessment.

Mental Status

Your general impression of the patient should provide the first clues about the child's neurologic status. As you begin the initial assessment, use the AVPU scale (Table 41-7 ▲) to evaluate the

cerebral cortex. The AVPU scale is a conventional way of assessing any patient's level of consciousness (LOC) or mental status. It categorizes motor response based on simple response to stimuli, classifying the patient as alert, responsive to verbal stimuli, responsive to painful stimuli, or unresponsive.

After evaluating the patient's response with the AVPU scale, assess the pupillary response to a beam of light to assess brain stem response. Next, evaluate motor activity, looking for symmetric movement of the extremities, seizures, posturing, or flaccidity. Combine this information with the PAT results to determine the child's neurologic status.

Exposure Considerations

Proper exposure of the child is necessary to complete the initial assessment. During the PAT, the child will have been at least partially undressed to assess the work of breathing and circulation. It is also important to evaluate the child from head to toe and to look at the child's back during the initial assessment. Be careful to avoid heat loss, especially in infants, by covering the child up as soon as possible. Keep the temperature in the ambulance high, and use blankets when necessary.

Assessment of Pain

Numerous studies have found that children are much less likely than adults to receive effective pain medications. Inadequate treatment of pain has many adverse effects on the child and family. Pain causes morbidity and misery for the child and caregivers, and it interferes with your ability to accurately assess physiologic abnormalities. Children who do not receive appropriate analgesia may be more likely to have exaggerated pain responses to subsequent painful procedures. Also, posttraumatic stress may be more common among children who experience pain during an illness or injury.

Assessment of pain must consider developmental age. The ability to identify pain improves with the age of the child. In infants and preverbal children, it may be difficult to distinguish crying and agitation due to hypoxia, hunger, or pain. Further assessment and discussion with caregivers about their perceptions of the child's pain are essential to identify pain in this age group. For verbal children, pain scales using pictures of facial expressions, such as the Wong-Baker FACES scale, may prove helpful Figure 41-9 ▶ .

Remaining calm and providing quiet, professional reassurance to parents and child is critical for managing pediatric pain and anxiety. A calm parent will help keep the child calm and more at ease. Distraction techniques with toys or stories may prove helpful in reducing pain, as may visual imagery techniques and music. Sucrose pacifiers may reduce pain in neonates. Pharmacologic methods for reducing pain—such as acetaminophen, opiates, benzodiazepines, and nitrous oxide—are available to paramedics in a number of EMS systems. The benefit of such analgesic or anxiolytic medication must be weighed against the risks of its administration (respiratory depression, bradycardia, hypoxemia, and hypotension are potential side effects of sedatives), including the potential route of administration. Medications that are given intravenously are

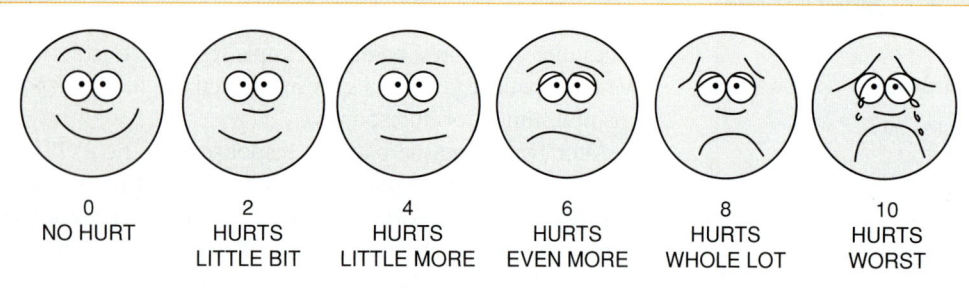

Figure 41-9 Pictures such as the Wong-Baker FACES Pain Rating Scale allow for self-assessment of pain in young children.

From Hockenberry MJ, Wilson D: *Wong's essentials of pediatric nursing, ed. 8*, St. Louis, 2009, Mosby. Used with permission. Copyright, Mosby.

Special Considerations

Consider pain to be a vital sign in pediatric patients. Assess and reassess pain along with the other vital signs. Treat pain accordingly.

often most effective at reducing pain, but they require establishing intravenous (IV) access, which itself is a painful procedure.

Today, assessment of pain is recognized as part of vital sign assessment, and management of pediatric pain and anxiety should be a routine part of prehospital care. This effort requires a thorough understanding of nonpharmacologic techniques, drugs, potential drug contraindications and complications, and management of the complications.

Transport Decision

After completing the initial assessment and beginning resuscitation when necessary, you must make a crucial decision: whether to immediately transport the child to the emergency department (ED) or continue the additional assessment and treatment on scene. Immediate transport is imperative if the emergency call is for trauma and the child has a serious mechanism of injury (MOI), a physiologic abnormality, or a potentially significant anatomical abnormality or if the scene is unsafe. In these cases, stabilize the spine, manage the airway and breathing, stop external bleeding, and begin transport. Attempt vascular access on the way to the ED. If the emergency call is for an illness, the decision to stay or go is less clear-cut and depends on the following factors: expected benefits of treatment, EMS system regulations, comfort level, and transport time.

Additional Assessment
Focused History and Physical Examination

The focused history and physical examination, which is performed on medical and trauma patients, has four objectives:

- To obtain a complete description of the chief complaint (for example, OPQRST and SAMPLE)
- To determine the MOI or nature of an illness

You are the Paramedic Part 2

You use the PAT to form a general impression of the patient. Based on his abnormal appearance and circulation, you determine that the child is sick and requires rapid treatment. The combination of your knowledge that children are more prone to head injuries than adults because of the larger size and weight of their heads compared with the rest of their bodies, the MOI, and your general impression of the patient leads you to suspect that the child may have a closed head injury.

You immediately assign one of the fire fighters the task of maintaining manual cervical spine immobilization. You ask your partner to apply 100% supplemental oxygen via a nonrebreathing mask as you expose the child to complete a rapid trauma assessment. This examination reveals a mildly distended abdomen and an obviously deformed right thigh. You ask the lieutenant to issue a trauma alert, citing the combination of your physical assessment findings and the MOI.

Vital Signs	Recording Time: 5 Minutes
Skin	Pale, cool, and dry
Pulse	170 beats/min, regular; weak distally but strong centrally
Blood pressure	86/48 mm Hg
Respirations	40 breaths/min; unlaboured, clear breath sounds
Spo$_2$	99% on nonrebreathing mask at 12 l/min of oxygen
Capillary refill	2–3 seconds

3. What do you need to carefully monitor the patient for?
4. Which interventions should you consider at this point, if any?

Table 41-8	Pediatric SAMPLE Components
Component	**Explanation**
Signs and symptoms	Onset and nature of symptoms of pain or fever
	Age-appropriate signs of distress
Allergies	Known drug reactions or other allergies
Medications	Exact names and doses of ongoing drugs (including over-the-counter, prescribed, herbal, and recreational drugs)
	Timing and amount of last dose
	Time and dose of analgesics or antipyretics
Past medical history	Previous illnesses or injuries
	Immunizations
	History of pregnancy, labour, delivery (infants and toddlers)
Last oral intake	Timing of the child's last food or drink, including bottle or breastfeeding
Events leading to illness or injury	Key events leading to the current incident
	Fever history

- To perform a rapid trauma or medical assessment or a focused or vectored physical examination of a specific body part or body system
- To obtain baseline vital signs

If the child seems to be in physiologically unstable condition based on the initial assessment, you may decide to begin transport immediately and conduct the focused history and physical examination in the ambulance. If the child is in stable condition and the scene is safe, perform the focused history and physical examination on the scene, before transport. The detailed physical examination is conducted en route to the hospital for trauma patients with a significant MOI. It can be done on the scene if you are waiting for the ambulance to arrive or if patient removal is delayed because of entrapment. As opposed to the initial assessment, which addresses immediately life-threatening pathologic problems, the focused history and physical examination narrows the focus to assessing the body part or body system specifically involved, obtaining a complete set of baseline vital signs, elaborating on the chief complaint (ie, OPQRST), and obtaining a patient history (ie, SAMPLE).

To obtain the focused history, use the SAMPLE mnemonic Table 41-8 ▲ . Tailor the physical examination to the child's age and developmental stage. In trauma patients, after the detailed physical examination is complete, reconsider the need for immediate transport.

Ongoing Assessment

The elements in the ongoing assessment include the PAT, reassessment of patient priority, vital signs (every 5 minutes if unstable condition and every 15 minutes if stable), assessment of the effectiveness of interventions (eg, medications administered,

Documentation and Communication

Perform frequent reassessment of serial vital signs, and record them on your documentation form. By recording each set of vital signs, you can visualize trends and transfer important information to the accepting physicians.

splints applied, bleeding controlled), and reassessment of the focused examination areas. Perform this kind of ongoing assessment on all patients to observe their response to treatment, to guide ongoing treatments, and to track the progression of identified pathologic and anatomical problems. New problems may also be identified on reassessment. The elements in the ongoing assessment also guide the choice of an appropriate transport destination and your radio or telephone communications with medical oversight or ED staff.

Respiratory Emergencies

Respiratory problems are among the medical emergencies that you will most frequently encounter in children. Pediatric patients with a respiratory chief complaint will span the spectrum from mildly ill to near death. In pediatrics, respiratory failure and arrest precede the majority of cardiopulmonary arrests; by contrast, a primary cardiac event is the usual cause of sudden death in adults. Early identification and intervention can stop the progression from respiratory distress to cardiopulmonary failure and help to avert much pediatric morbidity and mortality.

General Assessment and Management

When faced with a respiratory emergency, the first step is to determine the severity of the disease: Is the patient in respiratory distress, respiratory failure, or respiratory arrest?

Respiratory distress entails increased work of breathing to maintain oxygenation and/or ventilation; that is, it is a compensated state in which increased work of breathing results in adequate pulmonary gas exchange. The hallmarks of respiratory distress—which is classified as mild, moderate, or severe—are retractions (suprasternal, intercostal, subcostal), abdominal breathing, nasal flaring, and grunting.

A patient in respiratory failure can no longer compensate for the underlying pathologic or anatomical problem by increased work of breathing, so hypoxia and/or carbon dioxide retention occur. Signs of respiratory failure may include decreased or absent retractions owing to fatigue of the chest wall muscles, altered mental status owing to inadequate oxygenation and ventilation of the brain, and an abnormally low respiratory rate Table 41-9 ▶ . Respiratory failure is a decompensated state, requiring urgent intervention to ensure adequate oxygenation and ventilation and prevent respiratory arrest. Do not be afraid to assist ventilations at this point if you judge the tidal volume or respiratory effort to be inadequate.

Table 41-9	Signs of Impending Respiratory Failure
Assess	**Sign**
Mental status	Agitation, restlessness, confusion, lethargy (VPU of AVPU)
Skin colour	Cyanosis, pallor
Respiratory rate	Tachypnea → bradypnea → apnea
Respiratory effort	Severe retractions, nasal flaring, grunting, paradoxical abdominal motion, tripod positioning
Auscultation	Stridor, wheezing, rales, or diminished air movement
Blood oxygen saturation	< 90% with supplemental oxygen
Pulse rate	Tachycardia, bradycardia, or cardiac arrest

Table 41-10	Key Questions in Respiratory Emergencies
Component	**Key Questions**
Signs and symptoms	Shortness of breath? Hoarseness? Stridor? Wheezing? Cough? Chest pain? Choking? Rash/Hives? Cyanosis?
Allergies	Known drug or food allergies; smoke exposure
Medications	Names and doses of ongoing medications; recent use of corticosteroids
Past medical history	History of asthma, chronic lung disease, heart problems, prematurity; prior hospitalizations and intubation for breathing problems; history of choking or anaphylaxis; immunizations
Last oral intake	Timing of last food, including bottle or breastfeeding
Events leading to illness or injury	Fever history or recent illness; history of injury to chest; history of choking on food or object

At the Scene

Initiate aggressive airway management and ventilatory support with a bag-valve-mask device and supplemental oxygen as soon as possible for a child with respiratory failure.

Respiratory arrest implies that the patient is not breathing spontaneously. Administer immediate bag-valve-mask ventilation with supplemental oxygen to prevent progression to cardiopulmonary arrest. Resuscitation of a child from respiratory arrest is often successful, whereas resuscitation of a child in cardiopulmonary arrest usually fails.

By combining the three components of the PAT, you can determine the severity of disease before you even touch the patient. The child's appearance will give you clues about the adequacy of CNS oxygenation and ventilation. If a child with trouble breathing is sleepy, assume the child is hypoxic. Assess the work of breathing by noting the patient's position of comfort, presence or absence of retractions, and grunting or flaring. A patient who prefers to sit upright, in the sniffing position, or to use his or her arms for support is trying to optimize breathing mechanics. Deep retractions herald the use of accessory muscles of respiration to move air. Assessment of circulation for the presence of pallor or cyanosis will give further information on the adequacy of oxygenation.

After forming a general impression using the PAT, move on to the hands-on initial assessment. For respiratory emergencies, focus on the child's airway and breathing. Assess the airway by listening for stridor in awake patients or checking for obstruction in obtunded patients. Assess breathing by determining the child's respiratory rate, listening to the lungs for adequacy of air entry and abnormal breath sounds, and checking pulse oximetry readings. A rate that is too low may be more worrisome than a rate that is too high for the child's age. The presence of abnormal breath sounds may identify the anatomical or pathologic abnormality and suggest a likely diagnosis. For example, symmetric, diffuse wheezing implies bronchospasm and possibly asthma, whereas diffuse rhonchi, rales, and wheezing in an infant or toddler are typical signs of lower airway inflammation associated with bronchiolitis. The presence of stridor in the context of clear lung fields is consistent with upper airway obstruction, often due to croup. Poor air entry with decreased breath sounds is an ominous sign that must be addressed immediately. Determine oxygen saturation by assessing pulse oximetry via a finger or toe or, in a small infant, around the foot.

Your determination of whether the patient is in respiratory distress, respiratory failure, or respiratory arrest will drive your next steps, by indicating the urgency for treatment and transport. You can obtain the SAMPLE history at the scene or during transport, depending on the patient's stability. Table 41-10 ▲ lists key questions to ask during a respiratory emergency.

Most pediatric patients with a primary respiratory complaint will have respiratory distress and require only generic treatment. Allow the child to assume a position of comfort, and provide supplemental oxygen. The choice of oxygen delivery method will depend on the severity of illness and the child's developmental level. Young children may become agitated by a nasal cannula or face mask. Because crying and thrashing increase metabolic demands and oxygen consumption, you must weigh the benefits of this therapy against the potential cost. Allowing a caregiver to deliver blow-by oxygen to a calm toddler may be your best choice, if the child does not show signs of respiratory failure.

As a child becomes fatigued, respiratory distress may progress to respiratory failure. As part of your ongoing assessment, electronically monitor the patient's pulse rate, respiratory rate, and oxygen saturation. A significant change or trend in any of these variables requires prompt patient reassessment. You should also perform frequent reassessment to evaluate the effects of your treatment.

Upper Airway Emergencies
Foreign Body Aspiration or Obstruction

Infants and toddlers explore their environment by putting everything and anything into their mouths, resulting in a high risk of foreign body aspiration. Any small object or food item has the potential to obstruct a young child's narrow trachea. Peanuts, hot dogs, grapes, balloons, and small toys or pieces of toys are frequent offenders. Swallowed foreign bodies can also cause respiratory distress in infants and young children because a rigid esophageal foreign body can compress the relative pliable trachea. In addition, the tongue, owing to its large size relative to the upper airway, frequently causes upper airway obstruction in a child with a decreased LOC and diminished muscle tone.

Suspect foreign body aspiration when you encounter signs of mild or severe airway obstruction on the PAT or initial assessment. An awake patient with stridor, increased work of breathing, and good colour on the PAT has mild upper airway obstruction. Auscultation may reveal fair to good air entry, and the presence of unilateral wheezing may tip you off to a foreign body lodged in a mainstem bronchus. In contrast, a patient with severe airway obstruction is likely to be cyanotic and unconscious when you arrive, owing to profound hypoxia. If the child has spontaneous respiratory effort, you will hear poor air entry. You may *not* hear stridor owing to minimal air flow through the trachea. A typical SAMPLE history for foreign body aspiration reveals a previously healthy child with sudden onset of coughing, choking, or gagging while eating or playing.

Initial management of mild airway obstruction involves allowing the patient to assume a position of comfort, providing supplemental oxygen as tolerated, and transporting the child to an appropriate treating facility. Avoid agitating the child as this stimulus could worsen the situation. Continuous monitoring and frequent reassessments are needed to ensure that the problem does not progress to severe airway obstruction.

In severe airway obstruction, the initial management steps follow BLS guidelines for attempted removal. For a conscious infant, deliver five back slaps and five chest thrusts **Figure 41-10 ▶**:

1. Hold the infant face down, with the body resting on your forearm. Support the infant's head and face with your hand, and keep the head lower than the rest of the body.

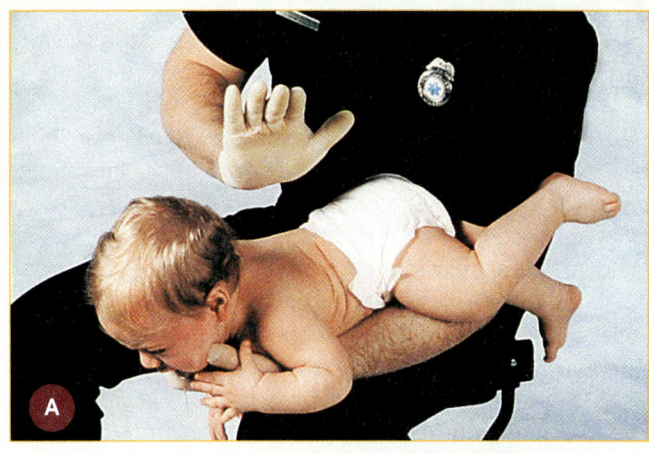

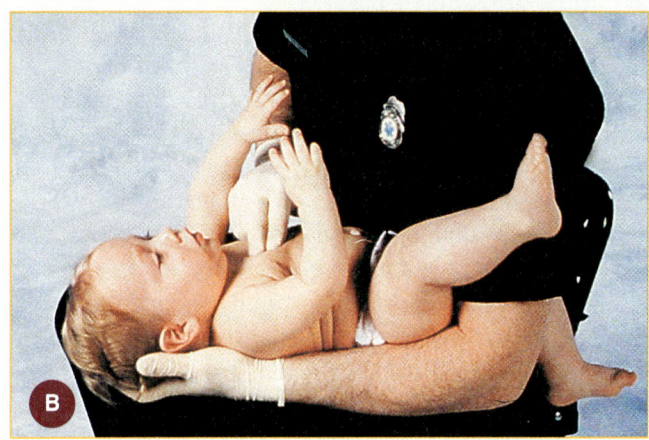

Figure 41-10 Perform back slaps and chest thrusts to clear a foreign body airway obstruction in an infant. **A.** Hold the infant face down with the body resting on your forearm. Support the jaw and face with your hand, and keep the head lower than the rest of the body. Give the infant five back slaps between the shoulder blades, using the heel of your hand. **B.** Give the infant five quick chest thrusts, using two fingers placed on the lower half of the sternum.

2. Deliver five back slaps between the shoulder blades using the heel of your hand.

3. Place your free hand behind the infant's head and back, and bring the infant upright on your thigh, sandwiching the infant's body between your two hands and arms. The infant's head should remain below the level of the body.

4. Give five quick chest thrusts in the same location and manner as for chest compressions, using two fingers placed on the lower half of the sternum. For larger infants, or if you have small hands, you can place the infant in your lap and turn the infant's whole body as a unit between back slaps and chest thrusts.

5. Repeat the sequence of back slaps and chest thrusts until the object is expelled or the infant becomes unresponsive.

6. If the infant with a severe airway obstruction becomes unresponsive, begin CPR.

If the infant regains consciousness, place him or her in the recovery position, administer 100% supplemental oxygen, and transport immediately. If you are unable to relieve the obstruction after several attempts, begin immediate transport.

If you have reason to believe that an unresponsive child has a foreign body obstruction, check the upper airway to see whether an object is visible. If so, try to remove it using a finger sweep motion. Never perform blind finger sweeps; doing so may push the object farther into the airway.

Abdominal thrusts (Heimlich maneuver) are recommended to relieve a severe airway obstruction in a conscious child. They increase the pressure in the chest, creating an artificial cough that may force a foreign body from the airway. Follow these steps to remove a foreign body obstruction from a conscious child who is in a standing position **Figure 41-11 ▼** :

1. Kneel on one knee behind the child, and circle his or her body by placing both arms around the child's chest. Prepare to give abdominal thrusts by placing your fist just above the patient's umbilicus and well below the xiphoid process. Place your other hand over that fist.
2. Give the child rapid, distinct abdominal thrusts in an upward direction. Be careful to avoid applying force to the lower ribcage or sternum.
3. Repeat this standing technique until the child expels the foreign body or becomes unresponsive.
4. If the child becomes unresponsive, place him or her supine on a firm, flat surface and inspect the airway using the head tilt–chin lift. If you can see the foreign body, try to remove it. Do not perform blind finger sweeps.
5. Attempt rescue breathing. If the first attempt fails, reposition the head and try again.
6. If the airway remains obstructed, begin CPR with chest compressions at the 30:2 compression/ventilation ratio and prepare for immediate transport.

If you manage to clear the airway obstruction in an unresponsive child (older than 1 year), but he or she remains apneic and pulseless, begin CPR and attach the automated external defibrillator (AED) as soon as possible, using appropriately sized AED pads. If you are unable to relieve the obstruction after several attempts, transport immediately.

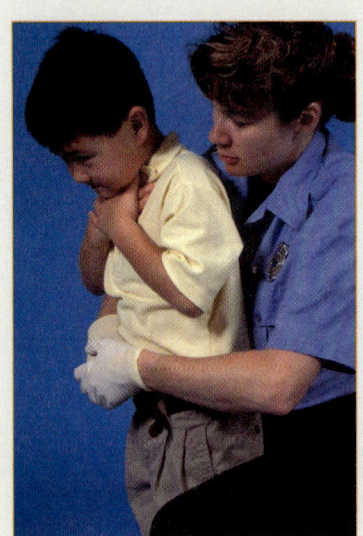

Figure 41-11 To relieve a foreign body obstruction in a responsive child who is standing, kneel behind the child, wrap your arms around his or her body, and place your fist just above the umbilicus and well below the xiphoid process.

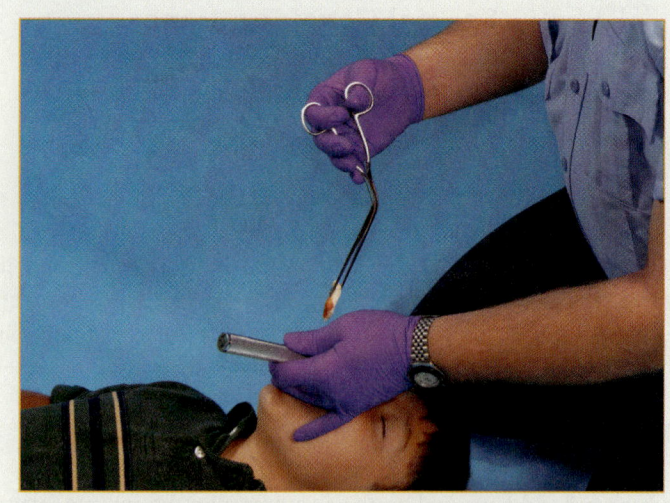

Figure 41-12 Using Magill forceps and direct laryngoscopy to remove foreign body airway obstruction.

If the BLS procedures do not dislodge the obstruction and severe airway obstruction remains, advanced airway procedures may be required. If the obstruction is more proximal, direct laryngoscopy with removal of the foreign body with Magill forceps may be successful **Figure 41-12 ▲** :

1. Hold the laryngoscope handle with your left hand.
2. Open the mouth by exerting thumb pressure on the chin.
3. Insert a pediatric straight blade into the mouth, and lift the tongue with the blade.
4. Exert gentle traction upward along the axis of the laryngoscope handle at a 45° angle, and advance the blade. Do not use the teeth or gums for leverage.
5. Watch the tip until the foreign body is visible. Do not go past the vocal cords.
6. Use suction to improve visibility if secretions are present.
7. Insert the Magill forceps into the mouth with the tips closed.
8. Grasp the foreign object and remove while looking directly at it.
9. Look at the airway to ensure that it is clear of debris. Remove the laryngoscope blade.

If you manage to remove the object, recheck the patient's breathing and circulation. Begin rescue breathing and CPR as needed and arrange for immediate transport. If direct laryngoscopy does not reveal the foreign body, use bag-valve-mask ventilation. If bag-valve-mask ventilation does not provide adequate ventilatory support, attempt to insert an advanced airway (such as ET tube, laryngeal mask airway, or Combitube). Immediate transportation to an appropriate facility is required.

Anaphylaxis

Anaphylaxis is a potentially life-threatening allergic reaction, triggered by exposure to an antigen (foreign protein). Food—especially nuts, shellfish, eggs, and milk—and bee stings are among the most common causes, although anaphylaxis to antibiotics and other medications can occur as well. Exposure to the antigen stimulates the release of histamine and other vasoactive chemical mediators from white blood cells, leading to multiple organ system involvement. Onset of symptoms generally occurs immediately after the exposure and may include hives, respiratory distress, circulatory compromise, and gastrointestinal symptoms (vomiting, diarrhea, abdominal pain).

Although a child with mild anaphylaxis may experience only hives and some wheezing, a child with severe anaphylaxis may be in respiratory failure and shock when you arrive. The PAT may reveal an anxious child (many adults describe a sense of impending doom at the onset of anaphylaxis). With severe anaphylaxis, the child may be unresponsive due to respiratory failure and shock. He or she may have increased work of breathing due to upper airway edema or bronchospasm and poor circulation. The initial assessment will usually reveal hives, with other findings potentially including swelling of the lips and oral mucosa, stridor and/or wheezing, and diminished pulses. If the child has a known allergy, the SAMPLE history may reveal recent contact with or ingestion of the potentially offending agent (including consumption of prepared foods containing traces of eggs, nuts, and milk at daycare or school).

The "gold standard" treatment for anaphylaxis is epinephrine. Epinephrine's alpha-agonist effect decreases airway edema by vasoconstriction and improves circulation by increasing peripheral vascular resistance. Its beta-agonist effect causes bronchodilation, resulting in improved oxygenation and ventilation. Epinephrine should be given by the subcutaneous (SQ) or intramuscular (IM) route at a dose of 0.01 mg/kg of the 1:1,000 solution, to a maximum dose of 0.3 mg. This dose may be repeated as necessary every 5 minutes. If several doses are needed, the child may require a continuous IV epinephrine drip. In addition to epinephrine, treatment of anaphylaxis should include supplemental oxygen, fluid resuscitation for shock, diphenhydramine for its antihistamine effect (dose: 1 to 2 mg/kg IV to a maximum of 50 mg), and bronchodilators for wheezing.

Many children with a history of anaphylaxis will have been treated with IM epinephrine by a caregiver before EMS activation. Given the short half-life of this drug, the child should be transported, even if asymptomatic on your arrival.

Croup

Croup (laryngotracheobronchitis) is a viral infection of the upper airway and the most common cause of upper airway emergencies in young children. The parainfluenza virus is the pathogen most commonly responsible for croup, but respiratory syncytial virus (RSV), influenza, and adenovirus have also been implicated. The virus is transmitted by respiratory secretions. Croup most commonly affects children 6 months to 6 years, with most cases occurring in the fall and winter months. The virus has an affinity for the subglottic space—the narrowest part of the pediatric airway—and causes edema and progressive airway obstruction. Turbulent air flow through the narrowed subglottic airway causes the hallmark sign of croup—stridor.

Most cases of croup are mild. EMS may be called when the symptoms come on abruptly or cause moderate to severe respiratory distress. The PAT for a child with croup will typically reveal an alert infant or toddler who has audible stridor with activity or agitation, a barky cough, some increased work of breathing, and normal skin colour. If a child with a history compatible with croup is sleepy or obtunded or has significant respiratory distress or cyanosis, be concerned about critical airway obstruction. On your initial assessment, breath sounds will likely be clear over the lung fields, although you may hear stridor (originating at the level of the subglottic space). Because the pathophysiology of croup largely involves the upper airway, hypoxia is uncommon, and its presence should alert you to critical obstruction and the need for immediate treatment. The SAMPLE history usually reveals several days of cold symptoms and low-grade fever, followed by onset of a barky cough, stridor, and trouble breathing. The cough and respiratory distress are often worse at night.

The initial management of croup is the same as for most respiratory emergencies. Allow the child to assume a position of comfort, and avoid agitating him or her. The use of cool mist or nebulized saline is controversial. For patients with stridor at rest, moderate to severe respiratory distress, poor air exchange, hypoxia, or altered appearance, nebulized epinephrine is the treatment of choice. The alpha-adrenergic effect results in vasoconstriction and decreased upper airway edema. Nebulized epinephrine is available as L-epinephrine. The dose for L-epinephrine is 0.25 to 0.5 mg/kg of the 1:1,000 solution (maximum, 5 mg per dose); this form can be diluted with normal saline to bring the volume to 3 ml. Although only a small amount of epinephrine is absorbed via the nebulized route, side effects may include tachycardia, agitation, tremor, and vomiting.

Special Considerations

The presence of hypoxia in a child with croup is a potentially ominous finding, indicating significant subglottic edema. Assess and transport quickly.

In the case of croup and respiratory failure, nebulized epinephrine alone may not be adequate and assisted ventilation may be necessary. Assisted ventilation with bag-valve-mask ventilation will often succeed in overcoming the upper airway obstruction. Advanced airway placement is rarely needed in croup. If performed, choose an ET tube one-half to one size smaller than normal for age or size to accommodate the subglottic edema. Children requiring nebulized epinephrine or assisted ventilation need to be transported immediately to an appropriate treatment facility.

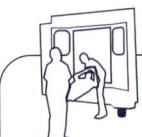

At the Scene

Bag-valve-mask ventilation is the mainstay of treatment for most upper airway emergencies.

Epiglottitis and Bacterial Infections

Epiglottitis, a once-dreaded inflammation of the supraglottic structures, usually due to bacterial infection, is now rare in children. Since the introduction of a childhood vaccine against *Haemophilus influenzae,* type B, the incidence of this life-threatening condition has decreased dramatically. Nevertheless, sporadic cases have been reported among adolescents, adults, and unimmunized children.

The classic presentation of epiglottitis is easily distinguishable using the PAT and the initial assessment. A child with epiglottitis looks sick and will be anxious, will sit upright in the sniffing position with the chin thrust forward to allow for maximal air entry, and may be drooling because of an inability to swallow secretions. The work of breathing is increased, and pallor or cyanosis may be evident. The initial assessment may reveal stridor on auscultation over the neck, a muffled voice, decreased or absent breath sounds, and hypoxia—all signs of a significant airway obstruction. The SAMPLE history will reveal a sudden onset of high fever and sore throat in preschool- or school-age children. Because symptoms progress rapidly, children with epiglottitis are generally sick for only a few hours before they come to medical attention. Remember to ask about immunizations as part of the pertinent medical history for patients suspected of having epiglottitis.

Your goal is to get the child with epiglottitis to an appropriate hospital with a maintainable airway. Because rapidly progressive disease carries a risk for acute airway obstruction and respiratory arrest, you should minimize your scene time and not attempt procedures that might agitate the child. Allow the patient to assume a position of comfort, and give supplemental oxygen only if tolerated by the patient. Do not attempt to look in the mouth because this can precipitate complete airway obstruction, and do not insert an IV line. Be prepared with a bag-valve-mask device and an ET tube one to two sizes smaller than anticipated for the child's age and length in case of complete obstruction during transport and the need for assisted ventilation. Endotracheal intubation of a child with epiglottitis is notoriously difficult owing to the extreme distortion of the airway anatomy. Alert personnel at the receiving facility to the suspected diagnosis and patient's condition because they will need to mobilize a team for the management of this difficult airway.

Some uncommon conditions can also cause upper airway obstruction, including retropharyngeal abscess, peritonsillar abscess, tracheitis, and diphtheria. Presentation may include fever, stridor, difficulty handling secretions, and respiratory distress. Regardless of the underlying diagnosis, initial assessment and management will be the same as for croup.

Lower Airway Emergencies

The underlying pathophysiology in upper airway emergencies involves restriction of air flow *into* the lungs (inhalation). By contrast, the pathophysiology of lower airway respiratory emergencies involves restriction of air flow *out* of the lungs (exhalation).

Asthma

Asthma is the most common chronic illness of childhood and the most common respiratory complaint encountered by paramedics. An estimated 5% to 10% of children are affected by asthma, many of whom will be treated in the ED. Recent studies indicate that the incidence and mortality of this disease are increasing.

There are three main components that lead to obstruction and poor gas exchange: bronchospasm, mucus production, and airway inflammation. Lower airway inflammation in asthma results in hypoxia because of ventilation-perfusion mismatch, a situation in which blood flowing to parts of the lung is poorly oxygenated. Triggers for asthma attacks include upper respiratory infections, environmental allergies, exposure to cold, changes in the weather, and secondhand smoke. Clinical signs include frequent cough, wheezing, and more general signs of respiratory distress.

The initial assessment of a child with an acute exacerbation of asthma will vary based on the degree of obstruction and the presence or absence of respiratory fatigue. A child with mild to moderate respiratory distress will be awake and alert, sometimes preferring a seated posture. Although increased work of breathing may be evident by retractions and nasal flaring, circulation will seem normal. Expiratory wheezing alone may be heard in patients with mild to moderate asthma attacks. Decreasing alertness, assumption of the tripod position, deep retractions, and cyanosis are signs of severe respiratory distress and impending respiratory failure. The initial assessment will reveal shortness of breath as evidenced by inability to speak in full sentences, increased respiratory rate, prolonged expiration phase, and wheezes noted on auscultation. The wheezing may be heard on inspiration and expiration. Decreased air movement and the absence of wheezes in a person with asthma who has activated the EMS system suggest severe lower airway obstruction and respiratory fatigue and signal the need for immediate treatment to prevent respiratory arrest.

The SAMPLE history for a patient suspected of having asthma should reveal the frequency and severity of previous asthma attacks, as reflected by ED visits and hospitalizations. A patient who has previously been admitted to an intensive care unit or intubated for asthma is at increased risk for severe—even possibly fatal—attacks. The medication history should identify any preventive treatment (controller medications) and any rescue medications administered by the caregiver before your arrival. Inhaled steroids are the most common controller medications used in pediatrics, whereas inhaled salbutamol is the most common beta-2 agonist drug used as a rescue medication.

The initial management of an asthma exacerbation remains basic respiratory care: Allow the patient to remain in a position of comfort, and start supplemental oxygen. The gold standard treatment consists of bronchodilators, beta-agonists that relax smooth muscles in the bronchioles, thereby decreasing bronchospasm and improving air movement and oxygenation.

Bronchodilators may be delivered by nebulizer or metered-dose inhaler (MDI) with a spacer-mask device. Unit doses of 2.5 mg of salbutamol premixed with 3 ml of normal saline are often used for nebulization and represent an acceptable starting dose for most young children. For a larger child or a child of any age who is in severe distress, consider administering 5 mg of salbutamol as the initial dose. If nebulized salbutamol is used, four puffs is equivalent to 2.5 mg administered by nebulizer. Children with moderate to severe respiratory distress can be given treatments every 20 minutes during transport, including back-to-back nebulizer treatments.

Although salbutamol is a relatively safe medication, its potential side effects include tachycardia, tremor, and mild hyperactivity. An isomer of salbutamol, levalbuterol, reportedly has fewer side effects. It has not been studied in the prehospital setting but is likely an acceptable alternative to salbutamol. In Canada, it is only approved for use in children older than 6 years of age.

Children with moderate to severe respiratory distress may also benefit from treatment with inhaled ipratropium, an anticholinergic bronchodilator. Studies have shown that the combination of salbutamol and ipratropium (which may be mixed and delivered together by nebulizer) is more effective than salbutamol given alone. The dose of ipratropium given is based on the patient's weight: a 0.25-mg unit dose nebulized or one puff by MDI for children weighing less than 10 kg; a 0.5-mg unit dose nebulized or two puffs by MDI for children weighing more than 10 kg.

If a child is in severe respiratory distress, is obtunded, or has markedly diminished air movement on auscultation, a dose of SQ or IM epinephrine may be required. Epinephrine will cause immediate relaxation of bronchial smooth muscles, opening the airways to allow bronchodilators to work. The dose is 0.01 mg/kg of 1:1,000 epinephrine injected SQ or IM; single doses should not exceed 0.3 mg. Initiate bronchodilator therapy immediately after administering the epinephrine.

Assisted ventilation is problematic for patients with an asthma exacerbation. High inspiratory pressures force air into the lungs, but exhalation is compromised by bronchospasm, mucus production, and inflammation, leading to air trapping and a high risk of pneumothorax and pneumomediastinum. Assisted ventilation should be undertaken only if the patient has respiratory failure and has failed to respond to SQ or IM epinephrine and high-dose bronchodilators. If this therapy is performed, use very slow rates to allow time for adequate exhalation: Your goal is adequate oxygenation.

Bronchiolitis

Bronchiolitis is an inflammation of the small airways (bronchioles) in the lower respiratory tract due to viral infection. The most common source of this disease is respiratory syncytial virus (RSV). A newly identified virus, metapneumovirus, has also been found to cause bronchiolitis. These viruses occur with highest frequency during the late fall and winter months, and they primarily affect infants and children younger than 2 years. Severity ranges from mild to moderate respiratory distress with hypoxia and respiratory failure. Younger infants are at particularly high risk for episodes of apnea associated with RSV infection, which may not be associated with severe respiratory distress.

The signs and symptoms of bronchiolitis can be difficult to distinguish from those of asthma. One clue is the child's age: Asthma is rare in children younger than 1 year. An infant with a first-time wheezing episode occurring in late fall or winter likely has bronchiolitis. Mild to moderate retractions, tachypnea, diffuse wheezing, diffuse crackles, and mild hypoxia are characteristic findings on the PAT and initial assessment. As with asthma, a sleepy or obtunded patient or one with severe retractions, diminished breath sounds, or moderate to severe hypoxia (oxygen saturation < 90%) is in danger of respiratory failure and requires immediate transport. Infants in the first months of life or who have a history of prematurity, underlying lung disease, congenital heart disease, or immunodeficiency are at greatest risk for respiratory failure and arrest.

The management of infants and young children with bronchiolitis is entirely supportive. Leave the patient in a position of comfort (eg, in the caregiver's arms, if the child does not seem to be in respiratory failure), and provide supplemental oxygen. Although bronchodilator therapy has not proved effective in the majority of cases, inhaled salbutamol or nebulized L-epinephrine (0.25 to 0.5 mg/kg of the 1:1,000 solution, maximum 5 mg per dose) may be given as a therapeutic trial in children with moderate to severe respiratory distress. Be prepared to assist ventilation with bag-valve-mask ventilation or endotracheal intubation if needed.

Management of Respiratory Emergencies

Infants and young children with severe tachypnea and retractions, in association with hypoxia, bradycardia, or altered mental status, are in respiratory failure and need immediate intervention to prevent respiratory arrest. A respiratory rate too slow for age in a child with a history of respiratory distress should also raise concerns for respiratory fatigue and failure.

Airway Management

The first step in managing any respiratory emergency is to start with the airway. Check for obstruction, and position the airway using the head tilt–chin lift or jaw-thrust maneuver Figure 41-13 ▸ . In a young infant, place a small roll under the shoulders to align the airway Figure 41-14 ▸ .

An airway adjunct may be helpful if the patient is unresponsive and cannot maintain a patent airway. The use of a nasal or oral airway will help to maintain an open airway, improve bag-valve-mask ventilation, and may avert the need for an advanced airway (such as an ET tube, laryngeal mask airway, or Combitube). When placing the adjunct, make sure to start by choosing the appropriately sized equipment.

Oropharyngeal Airway

An oropharyngeal (oral) airway is designed to keep the tongue from blocking the airway, and it makes suctioning the airway easier. This kind of airway should be used for pediatric patients who are unresponsive and cannot maintain their own airway

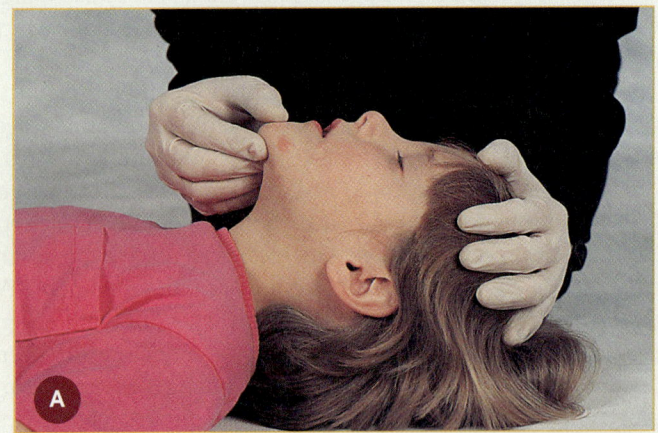

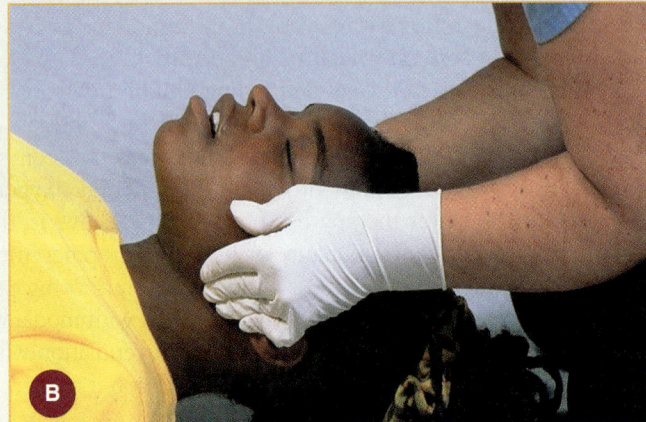

Figure 41-13 A. Use the head tilt–chin lift maneuver to open the airway of a child without trauma. **B.** For a child with suspected spinal injury, use the jaw-thrust maneuver to open the airway.

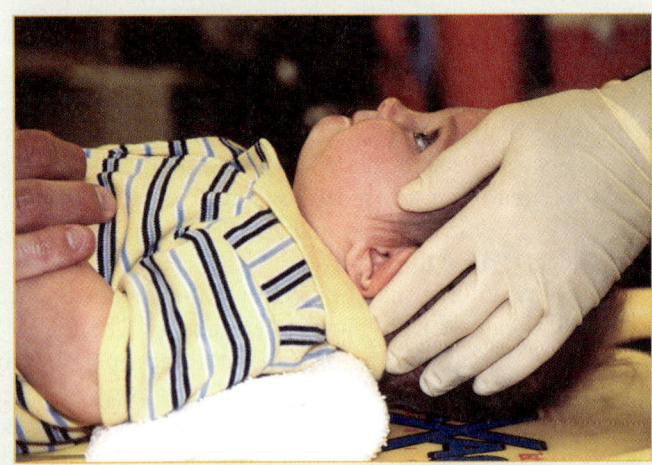

Figure 41-14 Use a shoulder roll in an infant without trauma to position the airway in a neutral position.

spontaneously. It should *not* be used for conscious patients or patients with a gag reflex—an oropharyngeal airway may stimulate vomiting, thereby increasing the risk of aspiration. In addition, this adjunct should *not* be used for children who have ingested a caustic (corrosive) or petroleum-based product.

Skill Drill 41-1 ▶ shows the preferred technique for inserting an oropharyngeal airway in a child.

1. Determine the appropriately sized airway by measuring from the corner of the mouth to the earlobe or by using the length-based resuscitation tape to measure the patient.

2. Place the airway next to the face, with the flange at the level of the central incisors and the bite block segment parallel to the hard palate. The tip of the airway should reach the angle of the jaw **Step 1**.

3. Position the patient's airway. For medical patients, use the head tilt–chin lift maneuver, avoiding hyperextension; you may place a towel under the patient's shoulders. If the patient has a traumatic injury, use the jaw-thrust maneuver and provide in-line spinal stabilization **Step 2**.

4. Open the mouth by applying pressure on the chin with your thumb.

5. Insert the airway by depressing the tongue with a tongue blade on the base of the tongue and inserting the airway directly over the tongue blade.

6. Reassess the airway after insertion **Step 3**.

Take care to avoid injuring the hard palate as you insert the airway. Rough insertion can cause bleeding, which may aggravate airway problems and cause vomiting. If the oropharyngeal airway is too small, the tongue may be pushed back into the pharynx, obstructing the airway. If it is too large, it may obstruct the larynx.

Nasopharyngeal Airway

A nasopharyngeal (nasal) airway is usually well tolerated and is not as likely as the oropharyngeal airway to cause vomiting. The nasopharyngeal airway is used for conscious patients and patients with altered levels of consciousness. In pediatric patients, it is typically used in association with respiratory failure. It is also a good choice for patients having a seizure or in a postictal state as a way of maintaining an airway. This type of airway is rarely used for children younger than 1 year because of the small diameter of their nares, which tend to become easily obstructed by secretions.

Follow the steps in **Skill Drill 41-2 ▶** to insert a nasopharyngeal airway in a child.

1. Determine the appropriately sized airway. The external diameter of the airway should not be larger than the diameter of one of the external openings of the nose (nares), and there should be no blanching (turning white) of the nare after insertion.

2. Place the airway next to the patient's face to make sure the length is correct. The airway should extend from the tip of the nose to the tragus of the ear (that is, the small cartilaginous projection in front of the opening of the ear).

3. Position the patient's airway, using the techniques described for the oropharyngeal airway **Step 1**.

Skill Drill 41-1: Inserting an Oropharyngeal Airway in a Child

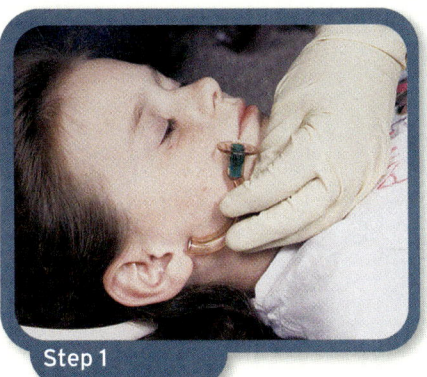

Step 1

Determine the appropriately sized airway by visualizing the device next to the patient's face.

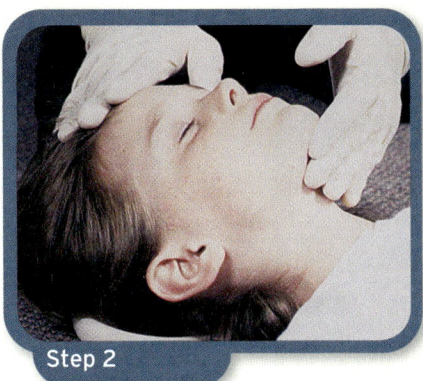

Step 2

Position the child's airway with the appropriate method.

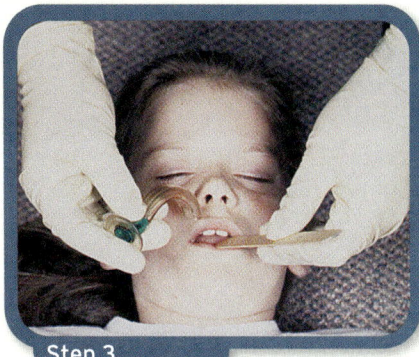

Step 3

Open the mouth.
   Insert the airway until the flange rests against the lips.
   Reassess the airway.

Skill Drill 41-2: Inserting a Nasopharyngeal Airway in a Child

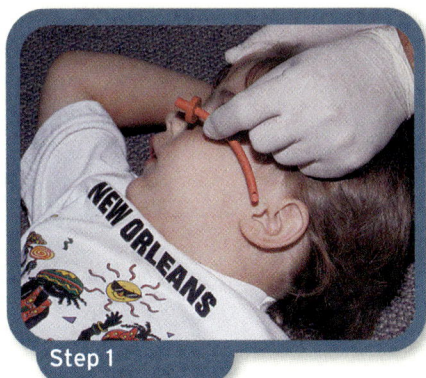

Step 1

Determine the correct airway size by comparing its diameter with the opening of the nostril (nare).
   Place the airway next to the patient's face to confirm correct length.
   Position the airway appropriately.

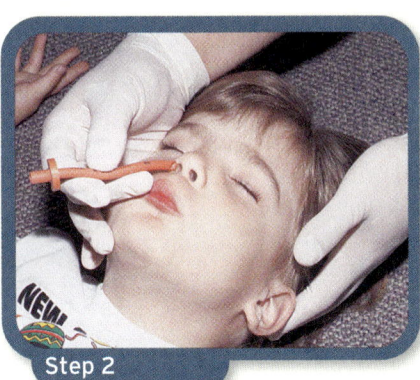

Step 2

Lubricate the airway.
   Insert the tip into the right nare with the bevel pointing toward the septum.

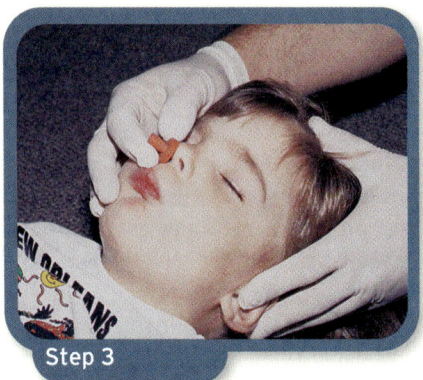

Step 3

Carefully move the tip forward until the flange rests against the outside of the nostril.
   Reassess the airway.

4. Lubricate the airway with a water-soluble lubricant.

5. Insert the tip into the right nare with the bevel pointing toward the septum, or central divider in the nose (**Step 2**).

6. Carefully move the tip forward, following the curvature of the nose, until the flange rests against the outside of the nostril. If you are inserting the airway on the left side, insert the tip into the left nare upside down, with the bevel pointing toward the septum. Move the airway forward slowly until you feel a slight resistance, and then rotate the airway 180°.

7. Reassess the airway after insertion (**Step 3**).

Several problems are possible with the nasopharyngeal airway. A diameter that is too small may become obstructed by mucus, blood, vomitus, or the soft tissues of the pharynx. If the airway is too long, it may stimulate the vagus nerve and slow the heart rate; it may also enter the esophagus, causing gastric distension. Inserting the airway in responsive patients may cause spasm of the larynx and result in vomiting. A nasopharyngeal airway should not be used when the patient has facial trauma because the airway may tear soft tissues and cause bleeding into the airway. Similarly, a nasopharyngeal airway should not be used for a patient with moderate to

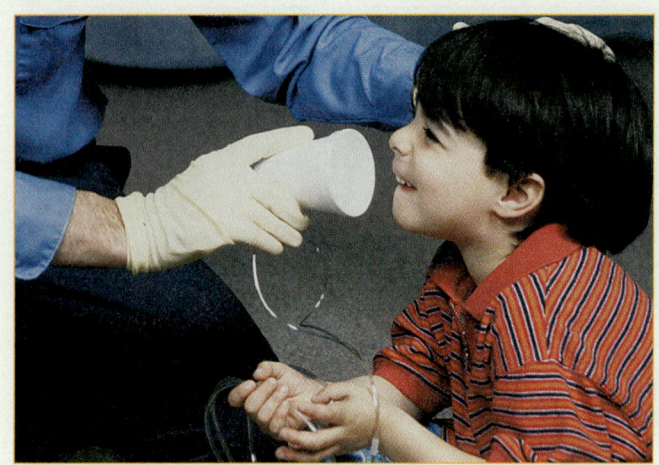

Figure 41-15 Blow-by oxygen technique can be used for a child with mild respiratory distress who won't tolerate a facial mask.

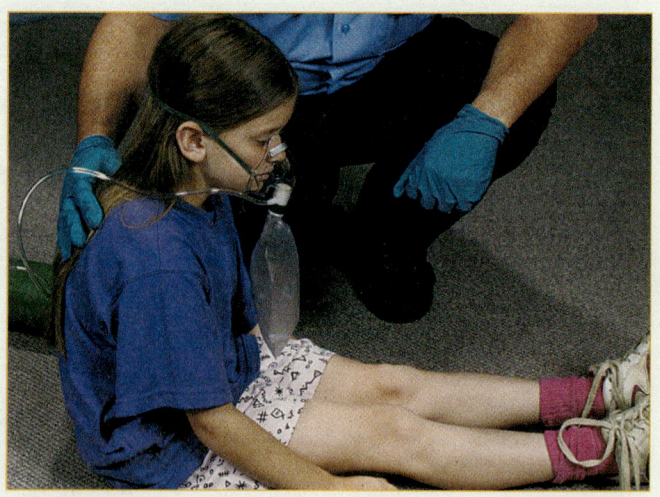

Figure 41-16 A pediatric nonrebreathing mask is the oxygen delivery method of choice for children who can tolerate it.

severe head trauma because it could increase intracranial pressure (ICP).

Oxygenation

As part of your breathing assessment, you will assess the patient's ventilatory and oxygenation status. All patients with respiratory emergencies should receive supplemental oxygen. The two most common ways to deliver oxygen to pediatric patients are the blow-by technique and the nonrebreathing mask.

The blow-by technique does not deliver high concentrations of oxygen to the patient, so it is best used when only a small amount of supplemental oxygen is needed or when the patient cannot tolerate wearing the mask needed for higher oxygen delivery. You can use oxygen tubing, a mask, a Styrofoam cup, or a similar device to deliver blow-by oxygen **Figure 41-15 ▲**. The child or caregiver can hold the device near the patient's face. The idea is to increase the oxygen concentration immediately around the patient's mouth and nose.

For children in significant respiratory distress or respiratory failure or for older children, a nonrebreathing mask is the preferred method of oxygen delivery. With this technique, the patient does not "rebreathe" exhaled air (which has a lower oxygen concentration); as a result, a nonrebreathing mask can deliver up to 90% oxygen to the patient. You must fit the mask appropriately onto the patient's face and use high flow rates (10 to 15 l/min) to achieve the maximum oxygen concentration **Figure 41-16 ▶**.

Bag-Valve-Mask Ventilation

If the patient's respiratory effort is not improved with airway positioning or insertion of an airway adjunct, start assisted ventilation with a bag-valve-mask device. Bag-valve-mask ventilation is always the first step in assisted ventilation, and it represents definitive airway management for many patients. Proficiency in bag-valve-mask ventilation is a critical skill for all paramedics and may avert the need for endotracheal intubation, a procedure with a much

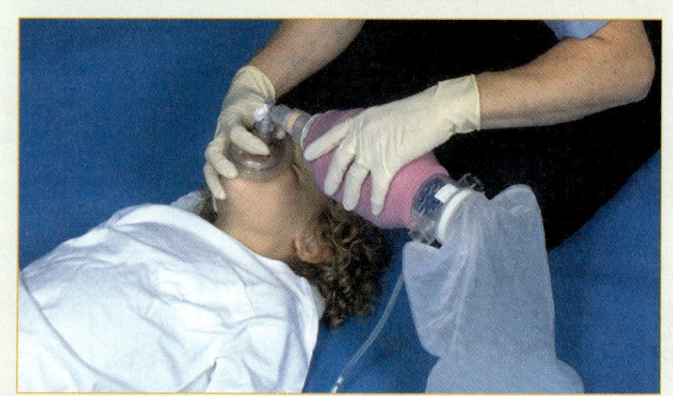

Figure 41-17 Proper mask size for bag-valve-mask ventilation.

higher complication rate. You may need to try a variety of mask sizes to find the one that gives the optimal seal. Do not hesitate to change providers, hand position, or technique if difficulty with ventilation continues.

Notes from Nancy

Limit ventilation volume to just that necessary to cause the chest to rise.

Avoid excessive tidal volumes and rate to minimize gastric distension, vomiting, and aspiration. Deliver breaths at a rate of 12 to 20 breaths/min for infants and children, squeezing the bag only until you see chest rise. Do not overdistend the chest.

Assist the ventilation of an infant or child using a bag-valve-mask device in the following way:

1. Ensure that you have the appropriate equipment in the right size. The mask should extend from the bridge of the nose to the cleft of the chin, avoiding compression of the eyes **Figure 41-17 ▲**. The mask is transparent, so

you can observe for cyanosis and vomiting. The mask volume should be small to decrease dead space and avoid rebreathing; however, the bag should contain at least 450 ml of air. Older children and adolescents may need an adult-size bag. Make sure that there is no pop-off valve on the bag or, if there is one, make sure that you can hold it shut as necessary to achieve adequate chest rise.

2. Maintain a good seal with the mask on the face. An inadequate mask-to-face seal will result in inadequate tidal volume delivery and a decreased concentration of delivered oxygen. Consider the use of airway adjuncts (nasal and oral pharyngeal airways) in tandem with bag-valve-mask ventilation.

3. Ventilate at the appropriate rate and volume (1 second per breath) until the chest visibly rises. Do not hyperventilate.

Errors in technique, including providing too much volume with each breath, squeezing the bag too forcefully, and ventilating at too fast a rate, can result in gastric distension or a pneumothorax. An inadequate mask-to-face seal or improper head position can lead to inadequately delivered tidal volume and hypoxia. Even with the best technique, however, the patient may regurgitate and aspirate the stomach contents.

One-Rescuer Bag-Valve-Mask Ventilation

Perform one-rescuer bag-valve-mask ventilation for an infant or child by following the steps in **Skill Drill 41-3 ▶**.

1. Open the airway, and insert the appropriate airway adjunct **Step 1**.

2. Hold the mask on the patient's face by using the E-C clamp method: Form a C with the thumb and index finger along the mask, while the other three fingers form an E along the mandible. With infants and toddlers, support the jaw with only your third finger. Do not compress the area under the chin because you may push the tongue into the back of the mouth and block the airway. Keep your fingers on the mandible.

3. Make sure the mask forms an airtight seal on the face. Maintain the seal while checking that the airway is open **Step 2**.

4. Squeeze the bag, using the correct ventilation rate: 12-20 breaths/min for infants and children.

5. Allow 1 second per ventilation, providing adequate time for exhalation by using the phrase "squeeze, release, release" **Step 3**.

6. Assess the effectiveness of ventilation by watching for adequate bilateral rise and fall of the chest **Step 4**.

Skill Drill 41-3: One-Rescuer Bag-Valve-Mask Ventilation for a Child

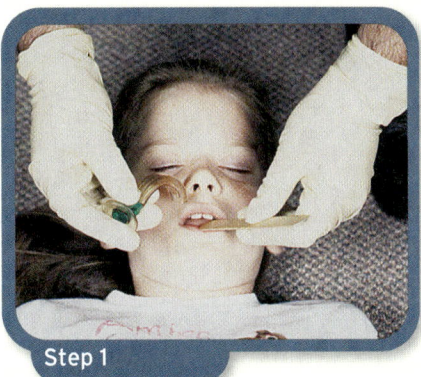

Step 1

Open the airway, and insert the appropriate airway adjunct.

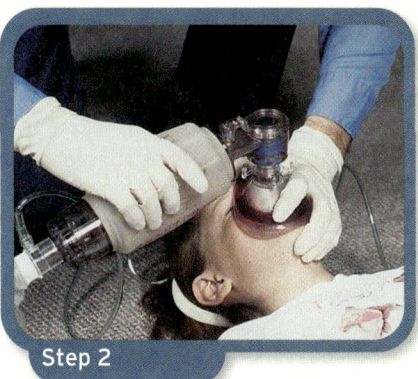

Step 2

Hold the mask on the patient's face with a one-handed head tilt–chin lift technique (E-C clamp).
Ensure a good mask-to-face seal while maintaining the airway.

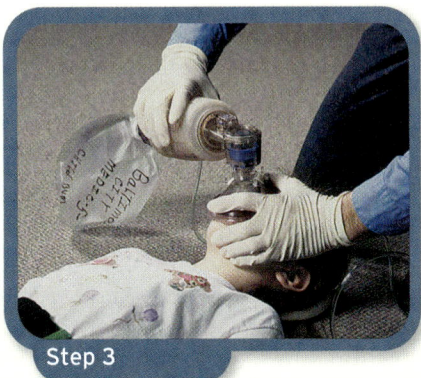

Step 3

Ventilate at a rate of 30 breaths/min for infants and 20 breaths/min for children. Allow adequate time for exhalation.

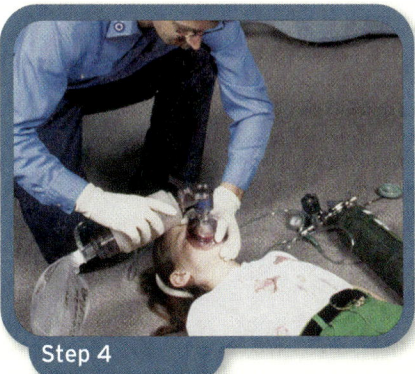

Step 4

Assess effectiveness of ventilation by watching bilateral rise and fall of the chest.

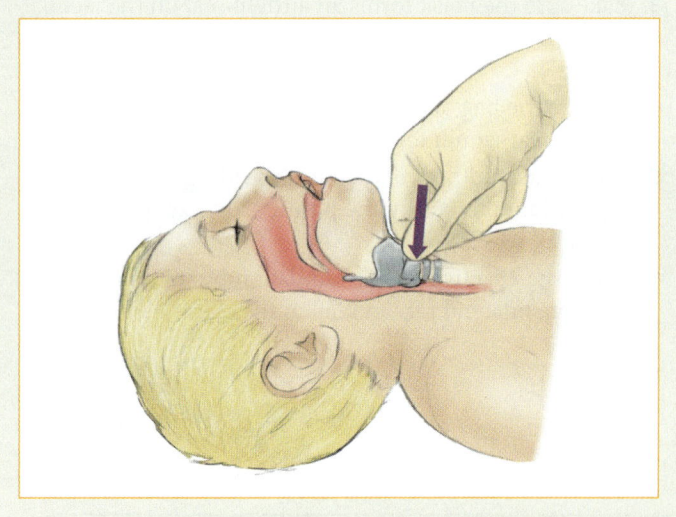

Figure 41-18 Applying cricoid pressure in an infant or child.

Two-Rescuer Bag-Valve-Mask Ventilation

This procedure requires two rescuers—one to maintain an adequate mask-to-face seal and maintain the patient's head position and one to ventilate the patient. Although this technique is more effective at delivering adequate tidal volume, you may not always be able to dedicate two providers to the patient's airway.

If a second provider is available, apply cricoid pressure using the Sellick maneuver to decrease risk of gastric distension, regurgitation, and aspiration during positive-pressure ventilation **Figure 41-18 ▲**. Only minimal pressure is needed; too much cricoid pressure can cause tracheal compression and airway obstruction. The key to successful use of the Sellick maneuver is direct posterior pressure on the cricoid ring, the complete cartilaginous ring that is caudal to the cricothyroid membrane.

Endotracheal Intubation

Consider endotracheal intubation if adequate oxygenation and ventilation cannot be achieved with good bag-valve-mask technique or if transport times are long. Intubation has the advantage of providing a definitive airway and carrying a decreased risk of aspiration, but studies have shown significant failure and complication rates when using this technique in the prehospital setting. Potential complications include damage to teeth and oral structures, aspiration of gastric contents, bradycardia due to a vagal response, bradycardia due to hypoxemia from prolonged attempts, increased ICP, and incorrect placement. Incorrect placement of the ET tube into the right mainstem bronchus may result in hypoxia and inadequate ventilation. A potentially catastrophic complication is an unrecognized esophageal intubation.

When preparing to intubate an infant or a young child, remember the differences between the adult and pediatric airways. Children have a relatively large tongue, an airway that is positioned more anteriorly, and a flexible trachea that can be easily compressed. Young infants also have a large occiput.

Equipment for Endotracheal Intubation

Access to pediatric-specific equipment is mandatory, including a range of laryngoscope blades in sizes 0 to 3 and ET tubes in sizes 2.5 (for prehospital deliveries of premature infants) to 6.0. Any size of laryngoscope handle can be used, although many paramedics prefer the thinner pediatric handles. Straight (Miller or Wis-Hipple) blades make it easy to lift the floppy epiglottis. If a curved (Macintosh) blade is used, the tip of the blade is positioned in the vallecula to lift the jaw and epiglottis to visualize the vocal cords.

The appropriately sized blade extends from the patient's mouth to the tragus of the ear. Acceptable means of measuring include using the length-based resuscitation tape and following these general guidelines:

- Premature newborn: size 0 straight blade
- Full-term newborn to 1 year: size 1 straight blade
- 2 years to adolescent: size 2 straight blade
- Adolescent or older: size 3 straight or curved blade

Use a length-based tape to choose the appropriate ET tube size or, for children older than 1 year, use this formula: (Age ÷ 4) + 4 = Size of Tube (in mm). For example, a 4-year-old child would need a 5.0-mm ET tube ((4 ÷ 4) + 4 = 5.0). Always have a tube that is one size smaller and one that is one size larger than expected available for situations in which there is variability in upper airway diameter.

Uncuffed ET tubes were long considered necessary until the child reached 8 to 10 years of age because the narrowest part of the airway was below the cords and would provide a suitable seal against a properly sized ET tube. Uncuffed tubes were also considered necessary to prevent ischemia and damage to the tracheal mucosa. With newer tube and cuff designs, it is no longer necessary to use an uncuffed tube in patients age 1 year or greater. New guidelines permit the use of a cuffed tube in these children. The advantage of using a cuffed tube is prevention of a large air leak and prevention of aspiration of stomach contents. You must always be cautious to avoid excessive cuff inflation and to prevent ischemia and damage to the tracheal mucosa at the level of the cricoid ring. You must remember that a cuffed tube is necessary in a pediatric patient once they reach adolescence, typically beyond 8 to 10 years of age.

The appropriate depth for insertion is 2 to 3 cm beyond the vocal cords. This depth should be recorded as the mark at the corner of the child's mouth. For uncuffed tubes, there is often a black glottic marker at the tube's distal end to use as a guide. When you see this line go through the vocal cord, stop. For cuffed tubes, when the cuff is just below the vocal cords, stop. Another guideline is to insert the tube to a depth that is equal to three times the inside diameter of the ET tube.

Pediatric stylets will fit into tubes sized 3.0 to 6.0 mm, whereas adult stylets are used for tubes 6.0 mm or larger. The use of a stylet is based on personal preference. If you use a stylet, insert it into the ET tube, stopping at least 1 cm from the end of the tube; a stylet that protrudes beyond the end of the tube can damage the oral mucosa and vocal cords. With the stylet in place, bend the ET tube into a gentle upward curve. In some cases, bending the tube into the shape of a hockey stick is beneficial.

Preparing for and Performing Endotracheal Intubation

Pediatric patients should be preoxygenated (but not hyperventilated) with a bag-valve-mask device and 100% supplemental oxygen for at least 30 seconds before you attempt intubation using the "squeeze, release, release" technique. Adequate preoxygenation cannot be overemphasized because respiratory failure or arrest is the most common cause of cardiopulmonary arrest in the pediatric population. During this time, you must also ensure that the child's head is in the proper position—the neutral position for patients with suspected spinal trauma or the sniffing position for patients without trauma. Insert an airway adjunct if one is needed to ensure adequate ventilation. Apply cricoid pressure once positive-pressure ventilation is initiated, and maintain it until the ET tube is correctly placed, verified, and secured.

Because stimulation of the parasympathetic nervous system and bradycardia can occur during intubation, you should apply a cardiac monitor if one is available. Use a pulse oximeter before, during, and after the intubation attempt to monitor the patient's pulse rate and oxygen saturation.

To perform endotracheal intubation in an infant or a child, follow the steps listed in **Skill Drill 41-4 ▾** :

1. Wear PPE (gloves and face shield at a minimum)　**Step 1** .
2. Check, prepare, and assemble your equipment　**Step 2** .
3. Manually open the patient's airway, and insert an adjunct if needed **Step 3** .
4. Preoxygenate the child with a bag-valve-mask device and 100% supplemental oxygen for at least 30 seconds **Step 4** .

Skill Drill 41-4: Performing Pediatric Endotracheal Intubation

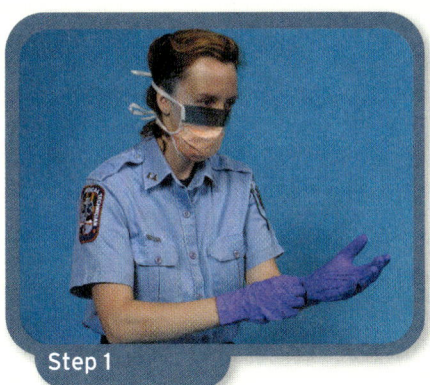

Step 1

Wear PPE (gloves and face shield at a minimum).

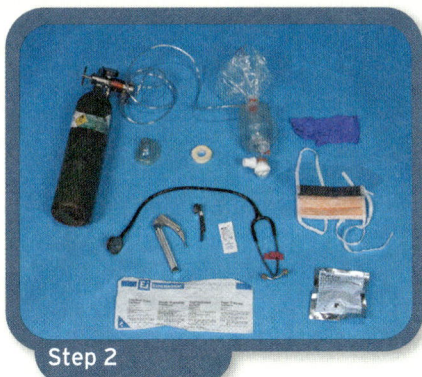

Step 2

Check, prepare, and assemble your equipment.

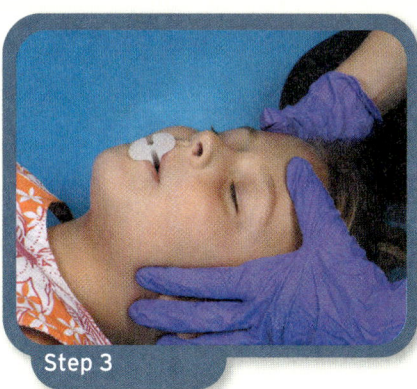

Step 3

Manually open the patient's airway and insert an adjunct if needed.

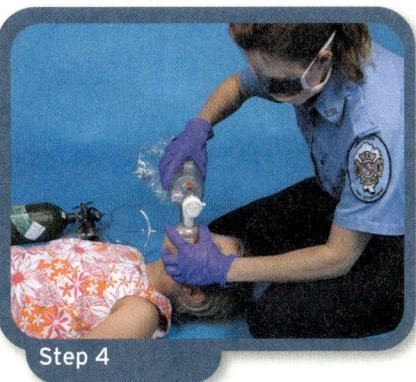

Step 4

Preoxygenate the child with a bag-valve-mask device and 100% oxygen for at least 30 seconds.

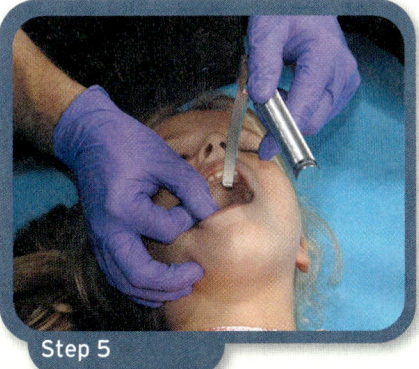

Step 5

Insert the laryngoscope blade in the right side of the mouth, and sweep the tongue to the left. Lift the tongue with firm, gentle pressure. Avoid using the teeth or gums as a fulcrum.

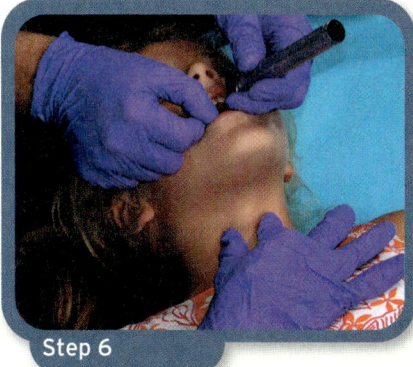

Step 6

Identify the vocal cords. If the cords are not visible, instruct your partner to apply cricoid pressure.

Skill Drill 41-4: Performing Pediatric Endotracheal Intubation (*continued*)

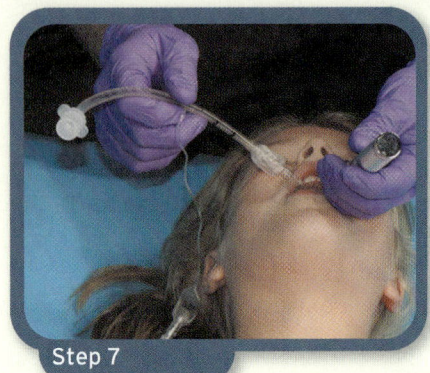

Step 7

Introduce the ET tube in the right corner of the patient's mouth.

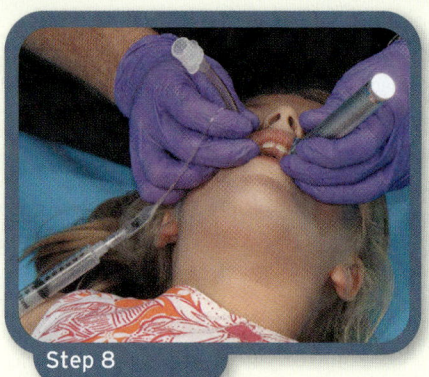

Step 8

Pass the ET tube through the vocal cords to approximately 2 to 3 cm below the vocal cords. Inflate the cuff if you are using a cuffed tube.

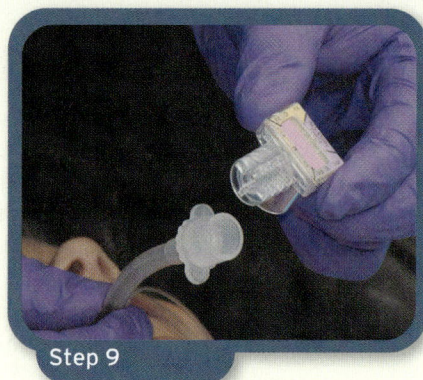

Step 9

Attach an Etco₂ detector.

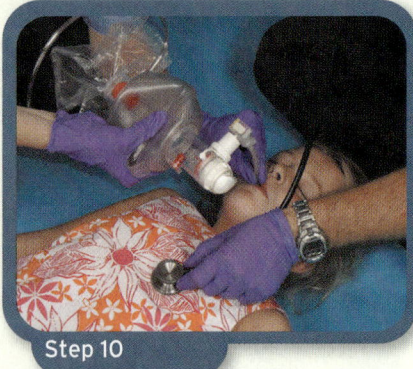

Step 10

Attach the bag-valve-mask device, ventilate, and auscultate for equal breath sounds.

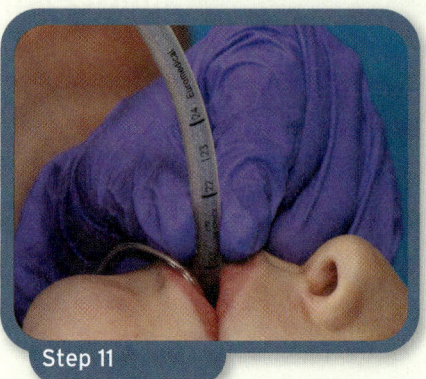

Step 11

Secure the ET tube. Reconfirm tube placement.

5. Insert the laryngoscope blade in the right side of the mouth, and sweep the tongue to the left. Lift the tongue with firm, gentle pressure. Avoid using the teeth or gums as a fulcrum (Step 5).

6. Identify the vocal cords. If they are not visible, instruct your partner to apply cricoid pressure (Step 6).

7. Introduce the ET tube in the right corner of the patient's mouth (Step 7).

8. Pass the ET tube through the vocal cords to approximately 2 to 3 cm below the vocal cords. Inflate the cuff if you are using a cuffed tube (Step 8).

9. Attach an end-tidal carbon dioxide (Etco₂) detector (Step 9).

10. Attach the bag-valve-mask device, ventilate, and auscultate for equal breath sounds over each lateral chest wall high in the axillae. Ensure absence of breath sounds over the abdomen (Step 10).

11. Secure the ET tube, noting the placement of the distance marker at the patient's teeth or gums, and reconfirm tube placement (Step 11).

Although tape may be applied in several ways to secure ET tubes, no single method is failsafe. One person should always hold the tube in place while another secures the device. Consider the use of a commercially manufactured tube-securing device for adults and children, when possible.

A critical step in endotracheal intubation is confirmation of correct placement of the tube. Watch the ET tube pass through the vocal cords, listen for breath sounds, and document the presence of Etco₂. The Etco₂ can be detected by using a colorimetric monitor or can be measured by capnometry. Most paramedic units use capnometry, whereas colorimetric Etco₂ detectors are used most commonly in the hospital setting. The colorimetric devices, which should be selected based on the weight of the child, are very accurate, even in infants and small

Table 41-11	DOPE: Troubleshooting the ET Tube	
Problem	**Assessment**	**Intervention**
Dislodgment		
Esophageal intubation	No Etco$_2$ reading or colour change Oxygen saturation < 90% Bradycardia Lack of chest rise with ventilation Auscultation of bubbling over stomach	Extubate Bag-valve-mask ventilation Reintubate
Mainstem bronchus intubation	Asymmetric chest rise Asymmetric breath sounds	Pull tube back until breath sounds and chest rise are symmetric
Accidental extubation	Same as esophageal intubation Poor or absent air movement on auscultation	Bag-valve-mask ventilation Reintubate
Obstruction		
Tube blocked with blood, secretions, or kink	Decreased chest rise Decreased breath sounds bilaterally Oxygen saturation < 90% Increased resistance to bagging	Suction Extubate Bag-valve-mask ventilation Reintubate
Pneumothorax		
Tension pneumothorax, spontaneous or induced	Asymmetric chest rise Asymmetric breath sounds Shock Oxygen saturation < 90% Jugular venous distension* Tracheal deviation*	Needle thoracostomy
Equipment		
Big air leak around tube Activated pop-off valve on resuscitator Oxygen tubing disconnected Oxygen tank empty		Check equipment "patient to tank"

*Not easily accessed or frequently seen in young children.

children. The exception is in cardiac arrest, a situation in which poor perfusion may result in levels of exhaled carbon dioxide too low to be detected by these devices.

Complications of Endotracheal Intubation

Frequent monitoring of proper tube placement, especially during any move of the patient (such as from the ground to the stretcher) is essential. The following clinical findings indicate immediate removal of the ET tube:

- No chest rise with ventilation
- Absence of breath sounds during auscultation
- Presence of epigastric gurgling sounds or vomitus in the ET tube

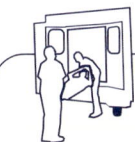

At the Scene

Calculate the endotracheal tube size for a child older than 1 year as follows:

$$(Age \div 4) + 4 = Size \ of \ ET \ tube \ (in \ mm)$$

Documentation and Communication

Vital signs, especially pulse rate and oxygen saturation, should be recorded before and after each intubation attempt. Record the size of the ET tube and the depth of insertion as measured at the patient's lip.

- Failure to confirm proper tube position with detection devices

In a patient with spontaneous circulation, lack of a colour on a colorimetric device indicates esophageal intubation. In such a case, the ET tube should be removed, bag-valve-mask ventilation resumed for 2 minutes, and endotracheal intubation reattempted.

If an intubated patient experiences a sudden decline in respiratory status, use the DOPE mnemonic (Dislodgment, Obstruction, Pneumothorax, Equipment) to identify the potential problem, and institute an appropriate intervention Table 41-11 ▲.

Special Considerations

A single intubation attempt should be limited to 20 seconds. If the attempt is not successful after 20 seconds, resume bag-valve-mask ventilation and preoxygenate the child for the next attempt.

Orogastric and Nasogastric Tube Insertion

During positive-pressure ventilation, it is common to inflate the stomach, as well as the lungs, with air. Gastric distension slows downward movement of the diaphragm and decreases tidal volume, making ventilation more difficult and necessitating higher inspiratory pressures. It also increases the risk that the patient will vomit and aspirate stomach contents into the lungs. Placement of a nasogastric (NG) tube or an orogastric (OG) tube decompresses the stomach and makes assisted ventilation easier.

Gastric decompression with an NG or OG tube is contraindicated in unresponsive children with a poor or absent gag reflex and an unsecured airway. Instead, you should perform endotracheal intubation first to decrease the risk of vomiting and aspiration.

Preparation of Equipment

To perform NG or OG tube insertion, you will need an appropriately sized NG or OG tube; a 30- to 60-ml syringe with a funnel-tipped adapter for manual removal of stomach contents through the tube; mechanical suction; adhesive tape; and a water-soluble lubricant. To prepare the patient and the equipment for NG or OG tube placement:

1. Select the proper size of tube. Use a length-based resuscitation tape to determine the proper size, or use a tube size twice the ET tube size that the child would need. For example, a child who needs a 5.0-mm ET tube requires a 10F OG or NG tube.

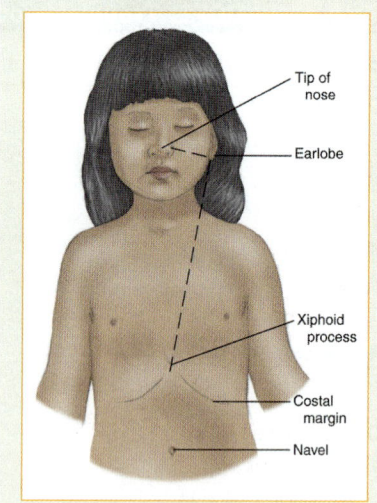

Figure 41-19 Technique for measuring the distance to insert an NG or OG tube.

2. Measure the tube on the patient. The length of the tube should be the same as the distance from the lips or tip of the nose (depending on whether the OG or NG route is used) to the earlobe *plus* the distance from the earlobe to the xiphoid process **Figure 41-19 ▲**.

3. Mark this length on the tube with a piece of tape. When the tip of the tube is in the stomach, the tape should be at the lips or nostril.

4. Place the patient in a supine position.

5. Assess the gag reflex. If the patient is unresponsive and has a poor or absent gag reflex, perform endotracheal intubation before gastric tube placement.

You are the Paramedic Part 3

As you prepare to immobilize the patient for transport, he begins to vomit. You, your partner, and the firefighter maintaining manual cervical spine stabilization log roll the child using a coordinated movement directed by the firefighter. You suction what appear to be chunks of French toast from the child's mouth and back of his throat. After suctioning, the child's oxygen saturation falls to 90%, his respiratory rate decreases to 16 breaths/min, and work of breathing increases. Your partner immediately begins bag-valve-mask ventilation using 100% oxygen, while you quickly measure the child using a length-based resuscitation tape and gather the appropriate intubation equipment.

The child is successfully intubated with a 4.5 uncuffed ET tube using in-line cervical spine stabilization for potential cervical spine injury. You confirm ET tube placement by direct visualization of the vocal cords, bilateral breath sounds, and a positive colour change on the colorimetric $Etco_2$ detector. You then secure the ET tube at the 14-cm mark at the child's lip. Your partner continues to provide bag-valve-mask ventilation at a rate of 20 breaths/min with 100% supplemental oxygen while you reassess the patient.

Reassessment	Recording Time: 10 Minutes
Skin	Pale, cool, and dry
Pulse	190 beats/min, regular; weak distally but strong centrally
ECG	Narrow complex tachycardia
Blood pressure	78/46 mm Hg
Respirations	20 breaths/min via bag-valve-mask ventilation
Spo_2	97% on bag-valve-mask ventilation at 100% oxygen
Pupils	Equal and reactive to light
Capillary refill	4 seconds

5. Is this child in shock? If so, is it compensated or decompensated?
6. How should your patient management progress?

6. In a trauma patient, maintain in-line stabilization of the cervical spine if a neck injury is possible. Choose the OG route of insertion if the patient has a severe head or midfacial injury.

7. Lubricate the end of the tube.

OG Tube Insertion

Follow these steps to insert an OG tube in an infant or child:

1. Insert the tube over the tongue, using a tongue blade if necessary to facilitate insertion.

2. Advance the tube into the hypopharynx, then insert it rapidly into the stomach.

3. If the child begins coughing or choking or has a change in voice, immediately remove the tube; it may be in the trachea.

NG Tube Insertion

Follow these steps to insert an NG tube in an infant or child:

1. Insert the tube gently through the nostril, directing the tube straight back. Do not angle the tube superiorly.

2. If the tube does not pass easily, try the opposite nostril or a smaller tube. Never force the tube.

3. If NG passage is unsuccessful, use the OG approach.

Assessing Placement of OG and NG Tubes

Follow these steps to confirm successful placement of an NG or OG tube:

1. Check tube placement by aspirating stomach contents. Use a syringe with an appropriate adapter to quickly instill 10 to 20 ml of air through the tube while auscultating over the left upper quadrant. If you hear a rush of air (or gurgling) over the stomach, the placement is correct.

2. If correct placement cannot be confirmed, remove the tube.

3. Secure the tube to the bridge of the nose or to the cheek, using adhesive tape.

4. Aspirate air from the stomach, using a 30- to 60-ml cannula-tipped syringe, or connect the tube to mechanical suction at a low, continuous suction of 20 to 40 mm Hg or to the intermittent setting.

Complications of OG or NG Tube Insertion

As with endotracheal intubation, you must be aware of the potential complications associated with the placement of an NG or OG tube—namely, placement of the tube into the trachea, resulting in hypoxia; vomiting and aspiration of stomach contents; airway bleeding or obstruction; and passage of the tube into the cranium. The last complication can occur if you insert an NG tube into a patient with severe head or midfacial trauma because the tube may be passed through the fracture and into the brain.

▌Cardiovascular Emergencies

Cardiovascular emergencies are relatively rare in children. When such problems arise, they are often related to volume or infection rather than a primary cardiac cause, unless the child has congenital heart disease. Through the PAT and initial assessment, you can quickly identify a cardiovascular emergency, understand the likely cause, and institute potentially lifesaving treatment.

General Assessment and Management

As with all pediatric emergencies, when called to a scene for a suspected cardiac complaint, begin the hands-off assessment by using the PAT and then move on to the initial assessment using the ABCs. The child's appearance gives an overview of perfusion, oxygenation, ventilation, and neurologic status. For a suspected cardiovascular problem, an abnormal appearance may indicate inadequate brain perfusion and the need for rapid intervention. Tachypnea, without retractions or abnormal airway sounds, is common in an infant or child with a primary cardiac problem; it is a mechanism for blowing off carbon dioxide to compensate for metabolic acidosis related to poor perfusion. In contrast, when cardiac compromise progresses to congestive heart failure, pulmonary edema leads to increased work of breathing and a fast respiratory rate. The presence of pallor, cyanosis, or mottling may tip you off to this problem.

For suspected cardiovascular compromise, start with airway and breathing, and provide supportive care as needed. Ensure adequate oxygenation and ventilation, and then assess the circulation by checking heart rate, pulse quality, skin CTC, and blood pressure when possible. Combine information from the PAT and initial assessment to make an initial decision about the likely underlying cause, the patient's priority, and the need for immediate treatment or transport.

If you determine that the patient's condition is stable enough for you to continue the assessment on site, continue with the SAMPLE history and the focused physical examination. (**Table 41-12 ▶** reviews key elements of a cardiovascular SAMPLE history.) Repeat the PAT and ABCs after each intervention, and monitor trends over time.

Shock

Shock is defined as inadequate delivery of oxygen and nutrients to tissues to meet metabolic demand. The types of shock that you may encounter are the same in adults and children: hypovolemic, distributive, and cardiogenic.

Besides determining the cause of shock, you must quickly determine whether the child is in a compensated or decompensated state. In compensated shock, although the child has critical abnormalities of perfusion, his or her body is (for the moment) able to mount a physiologic response to maintain adequate perfusion to vital organs by shunting blood from the periphery, increasing the heart rate, and increasing the vascular tone. A child in compensated shock will have a normal appearance, tachycardia, and signs of decreased peripheral perfusion, such as cool extremities with prolonged capillary refill. Timely intervention is needed to prevent a child in compensated shock from decompensating.

Decompensated shock is a state of inadequate perfusion in which the body's own mechanisms to improve perfusion are no longer sufficient to maintain a normal blood pressure. By definition, a child in decompensated shock will be hypotensive for his or her age **Table 41-13 ▶** . In addition to being profoundly tachycardic and showing signs of poor peripheral perfusion, a child in decompensated shock may have an altered appearance, reflecting inadequate perfusion of the brain. Because children typically

Table 41-12	SAMPLE Components for a Child With Cardiovascular Problems
Components	**Features**
Signs and symptoms	Presence of vomiting or diarrhea Number of episodes of vomiting or diarrhea Vomiting blood or bile; blood in stool External hemorrhage Presence or absence of fever Rash Respiratory distress or shortness of breath
Allergies	Known allergies History of anaphylaxis
Medications	Exact names and dosages of ongoing medications Use of laxative or antidiarrheal medications Long-term diuretic therapy Potential exposure to other medications or drugs Timing and dosages of analgesics or antipyretics
Past medical problems	History of heart problems History of prematurity Prior hospitalizations for cardiovascular problems
Last oral intake	Timing of the child's last food or drink, including bottle or breastfeeding
Events leading to injury or illness	Travel Trauma Fever history Symptoms in family members Potential toxic exposure

Table 41-13	Lower Limits of Normal Systolic Blood Pressure by Age
Age	**Minimum Systolic Blood Pressure**
Infant (1 month to 1 year)	>70 mm Hg
1-year-old child	>80 mm Hg
Child (1–10 years)	70 + (2 × age in years)
Child or adolescent >10 years	>90 mm Hg

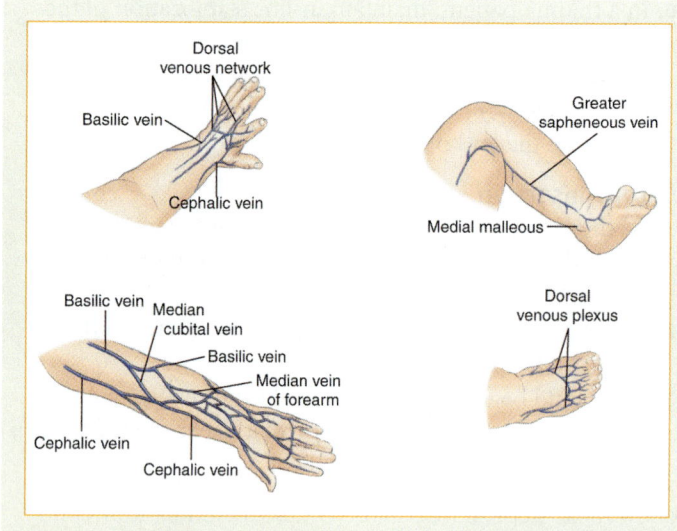

Figure 41-20 Sites for IV access in infants and children include the hands, antecubital fossa, saphenous veins at the ankle, and feet.

have strong cardiovascular systems, they are able to compensate for inadequate perfusion by increasing heart rate and peripheral vascular resistance more efficiently than adults. Hypotension is, therefore, a late and ominous sign in an infant or a young child, and urgent intervention is needed to prevent cardiac arrest.

Initial management involves allowing the child to assume a position of comfort and starting supplemental oxygen. After completing the initial assessment, make a transport decision based on the severity of the problem. Start resuscitation on scene for any child who shows signs of decompensated shock. While rapid transport is imperative, the risk of deterioration to cardiac arrest is too high to permit a "load-and-go" approach.

Hypovolemic Shock

Hypovolemia is the most common cause of shock in infants and young children, with loss of volume occurring due to illness or trauma. Because of their small blood volume (80 ml/kg body weight), a combination of excessive fluid losses and poor intake in an infant or a young child with gastroenteritis ("stomach flu") can result in shock relatively quickly. The same vulnerability exists with hemorrhage from trauma.

A patient with hypovolemic shock will often appear listless or lethargic and may have compensatory tachypnea. The child may appear pale, mottled, or cyanotic. In medical shock, further assessment may identify signs of dehydration such as sunken eyes, dry mucous membranes, poor skin turgor, or delayed capillary refill with cool extremities. In an injured child, the site of bleeding may be identified on the initial assessment or detailed physical examination.

Allow the child to remain in a position of comfort, administer supplemental oxygen, and keep the child warm. Apply direct pressure to stop any external bleeding. Volume replacement is the mainstay of treatment for hypovolemic shock, whether medical or traumatic in origin.

If the child is in compensated shock, you can attempt to establish IV or intraosseous (IO) access en route to the hospital. As with all procedures, gather all the equipment necessary before beginning this step. Cannulas—preferably an over-the-needle cannula—are available in pediatric sizes of 20, 22, and 24 gauge. A butterfly needle is a temporary alternative if an over-the-needle cannula is unavailable; this stainless steel needle stays in the vein, predisposing it to infiltration.

Many of the sites used for IV access in adults are the same for children. The most commonly used sites are the dorsum of the hand and the antecubital fossa. In children, veins in the foot may also be used **Figure 41-20 ▲** . Scalp veins and the external jugular veins are used less commonly.

The procedure for establishing IV access is as follows:

1. Check the IV fluid for proper fluid, clarity, and expiry date. Look for any discolouration or particles floating in the fluid. If any are found, discard and choose another bag of fluid.

2. Select the appropriate equipment, including an IO needle, syringe, saline, and extension set. A three-way stopcock may also be used to facilitate easier fluid administration.

3. Select the proper administration set. Connect the administration set to the bag. Prepare the administration set. Fill the drip chamber, and flush the tubing. Make sure no air bubbles remain in the tubing.

4. Prepare the syringe and extension tubing.

5. Cut or tear the tape. This can be done at any time before the IV puncture.

6. Use appropriate PPE. This must be done before the IV puncture.

7. Select the vein that you will use.

8. Secure the appropriate limb to minimize movement during the procedure.

9. Apply a tourniquet proximal to the selected site.

10. Clean the site with alcohol.

11. Insert the cannula through the skin with the bevel facing upward. Be sure to enter the skin at a shallow angle parallel to the vein.

12. Advance the cannula until you see blood return into the hub.

13. Continue to gently advance the cannula over the needle into the vein until the hub of the cannula is flush with the skin.

14. Completely remove the needle and attach IV tubing.

15. Flush the cannula with saline. Note if the line is easily flushed or if there is resistance. Resistance may mean that the cannula has infiltrated the vein. Carefully look at the surrounding skin for infiltration of fluids. If the line is infiltrated, remove it.

16. Secure the cannula with tape or a clear plastic dressing. Wrap the IV tubing with extra gauze to prevent the child from pulling out the IV cannula.

Once IV access is established, fluid resuscitation should begin with isotonic fluids *only*, such as normal saline or lactated Ringer's. Begin with 20 ml/kg of isotonic fluid, and then reassess the patient's status. The use of warm IV fluids (when possible) can counteract the effects of systemic hypothermia from environmental exposure, blood loss, or open wounds. Multiple fluid boluses may be necessary during transport.

Volume resuscitation should be addressed separately from treatment of hypoglycemia. In a child with shock due to medical illness, perform a bedside glucose check; treat with dextrose-containing fluid only for a documented low blood glucose level. Hypoglycemia is unlikely in shock due to acute injury.

Notes from Nancy

Be alert for signs of shock or respiratory insufficiency in any child who has sustained blunt chest trauma.

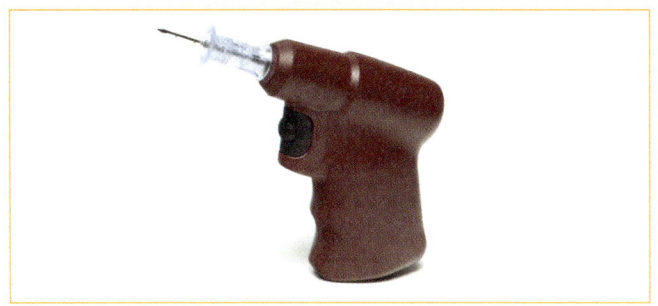

Figure 41-21 Standard pediatric size EZ-IO needle.

If a child is in decompensated shock with hypotension, begin initial fluid resuscitation at the scene. Make one attempt at IV access. If it is unsuccessful, begin IO infusion. When an IO needle is placed correctly, it will rest in the medullary canal, the space within the bone that contains bone marrow. An IO infusion is contraindicated if a secure IV line is available or if a fracture (or possible fracture) exists in the same bone in which you plan to insert the IO needle. Anything that can be administered IV can be administered through an IO line (such as isotonic fluids, medications).

The IO needles are usually double needles, consisting of a solid-bore needle inside a sharpened hollow needle. This double needle is pushed into the bone (usually the proximal tibia) with a screwing, twisting action. Once the needle pops through the bone, the solid needle is removed, leaving the hollow steel needle in place. Standard IV tubing is attached to this cannula. Newer devices, such as the EZ-IO can be used in place of traditional IO needles, making intraosseous access possible in the prehospital setting **Figure 41-21 ▲**. The EZ-IO features a sealed, hand held, lithium battery powered medical drill to which a special IO needle is attached. This device is used to insert an IO needle into the proximal humerus, proximal tibia, or distal tibia of adults and children when immediate vascular access is needed in acute situations. The EZ-IO driver (medical drill) is universal, but three different weight based, single use needle sets are available for adults, children, and patients with excessive tissue over the insertion site.

The IO lines require full and careful immobilization because they rest at a 90° angle to the bone and are easily dislodged. Stabilize the IO needle, thereby ensuring adequate flow, in the same manner that you would any impaled object. As with any invasive procedure, several complications may be associated with IO infusion: compartment syndrome, failed infusion, growth plate injury, bone inflammation caused by infection (osteomyelitis), skin infection, and bony fracture. Proper technique will help to minimize these complications.

Follow the steps in **Skill Drill 41-5 ▶** to establish an IO infusion in pediatric patients:

1. Check the IV bag for proper fluid, clarity, and expiry date. Look for any discolouration or particles floating in the fluid. If any are found, discard and choose another bag of fluid.

2. Select the appropriate equipment, including an IO needle, syringe, saline, and extension set ⟨Step 1⟩. A three-way stopcock may also be used to facilitate easier fluid administration.

3. Select the proper administration set. Connect the administration set to the bag. Prepare the administration set. Fill the drip chamber, and flush the tubing. Make sure no air bubbles remain in the tubing.

4. Prepare the syringe and extension tubing ⟨Step 2⟩.

5. Cut or tear the tape. This can be done at any time before the IO puncture.

6. Use appropriate PPE. This must be done before the IO puncture.

7. Identify the proper anatomical site for IO puncture ⟨Step 3⟩. To miss the epiphyseal (growth) plate, you should measure two fingerbreadths below the knee on the medial side of the leg.

8. Cleanse the site using aseptic technique (that is, in a circular manner from the inside out).

9. Stabilize the tibia. Place a folded towel under the knee, and hold it so that you keep your fingers away from the puncture site.

10. Insert the needle at a 90° angle to the leg. Advance the needle with a twisting motion until you feel a "pop" ⟨Step 4⟩. Unscrew the cap, and remove the stylet from the needle ⟨Step 5⟩.

11. Attach the syringe and extension set to the IO needle. Pull back on the syringe to aspirate blood and particles of bone marrow to ensure placement. If you are not able to aspirate marrow but the IO flushes easily with no signs of infiltration (swelling around insertion site), then continue to flush.

12. Slowly inject saline to ensure proper placement of the needle. Watch for infiltration, and stop the infusion immediately if any is noted.

13. It is possible to fracture the bone during insertion of the IO. If this happens, you should remove the IO needle and switch to the other leg.

14. Connect the administration set, and adjust the flow rate. Fluid does not flow well through an IO needle, and boluses are given by administering the fluid using the syringe and a three-way stopcock ⟨Step 6⟩.

15. Secure the needle with tape, and support it with a bulky dressing. Be careful not to tape around the entire circumference of the leg, which could impair circulation and create compartment syndrome.

16. Dispose of the needle in the proper container ⟨Step 7⟩. If using an EZ-IO or similar device, follow the manufacturer's instructions to ensure correct insertion.

As with IV administration, give 20-ml/kg boluses of isotonic fluid via IO infusion to treat hypovolemia, reassessing after each bolus and repeating as needed based on physiologic response. As much as 60 ml/kg may be needed during transport to improve the child's blood pressure, pulse rate, mental status, and peripheral perfusion. Rapidly transport the patient to an appropriate treatment facility.

Distributive Shock

In distributive shock, decreased vascular tone develops, resulting in vasodilation and third spacing of fluids due to increased vascular permeability (leakage of plasma out of the blood vessels and into the surrounding tissues). This results in a drop in effective blood volume and functional hypovolemia. Distributive shock may be due to sepsis, anaphylaxis, and spinal cord injury; sepsis accounts for the bulk of pediatric cases.

Early in distributive shock, the child may have warm, flushed skin and bounding pulses as a result of peripheral vasodilation. In contrast, the symptoms and signs of *late* distributive shock will look much like hypovolemic shock on initial assessment. Fever is a key finding in septic shock, whereas urticarial rash and wheezing may be noted in anaphylaxis, and neurologic deficits are apparent in shock due to spinal cord injury.

Front-line treatment of distributive shock is volume resuscitation because the child is in a state of relative hypovolemia. In a child with apparent sepsis who remains persistently hypotensive despite a total of 60 ml/kg of isotonic fluid, vasopressor support to improve vascular tone may be considered.

Anaphylactic shock should be treated immediately with SQ or IM epinephrine, 0.01 mg/kg of 1:1,000 solution (maximum dose, 0.3 mg). This dose should be repeated as necessary every 5 minutes. If several doses are needed, the child may require a low-dose, continuous epinephrine IV drip. The decision about timing of IV access and transport for distributive shock considers the same factors as for hypovolemic shock.

Cardiogenic Shock

Cardiogenic shock is the result of pump failure: Intravascular volume is normal, but myocardial function is poor. This type of shock is uncommon in the pediatric population but may be present in children with underlying congenital heart disease,

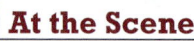

> **Special Considerations**
>
> Shock in children is most likely due to hypovolemia. Fluid resuscitation with isotonic fluid is the mainstay of treatment.

myocarditis, or rhythm disturbances. It is important to recognize cardiogenic shock by the child's history or from the initial assessment because the treatment for this type of shock is very different from that for hypovolemic or distributive shock.

A child in cardiogenic shock will appear listless or lethargic (like children in hypovolemic or distributive shock) but is likely to show signs of increased work of breathing owing to congestive heart failure and pulmonary edema. Circulation will be impaired, and skin will look pale, mottled, or cyanotic. Your initial assessment may reveal an abnormal heart rate or rhythm or a murmur or gallop. The child's skin may feel clammy, and you may palpate an enlarged liver. The caregiver may describe

> **At the Scene**
>
> A child with decompensated shock from hypovolemia needs fluid resuscitation. Do not waste time with multiple IV insertion attempts. Insert an IO needle, and begin fluid therapy.

Skill Drill 41-5: Pediatric IO Infusion

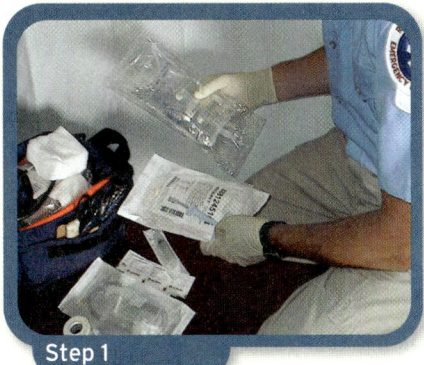

Step 1

Check selected IV bag for proper fluid, clarity, and expiry date.
   Select the appropriate equipment, including an IO needle, syringe, saline, and extension.

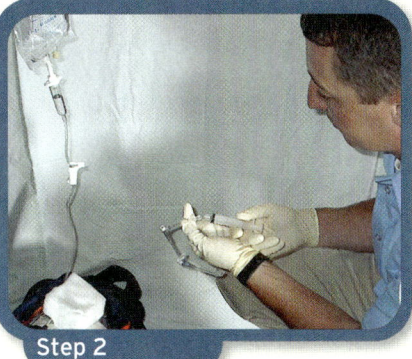

Step 2

Select the proper administration set. Connect the administration set to the bag. Prepare the administration set. Prepare the syringe and extension tubing.

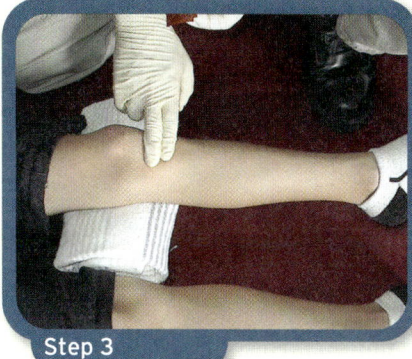

Step 3

Cut or tear the tape. Wear PPE.
   Identify the proper anatomical site for IO puncture.

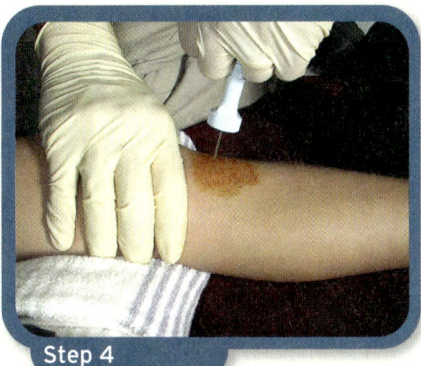

Step 4

Cleanse the site appropriately.
   Stabilize the tibia.
   Insert the needle at the proper angle.
   Advance the needle with a twisting motion until a "pop" is felt.

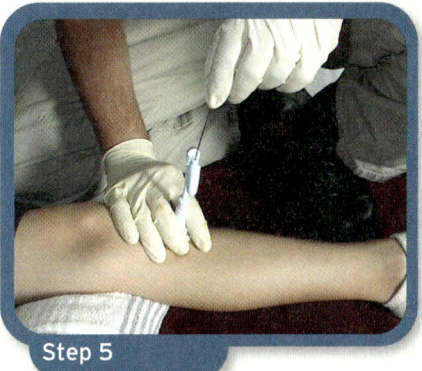

Step 5

Unscrew the cap, and remove the stylet from the needle.

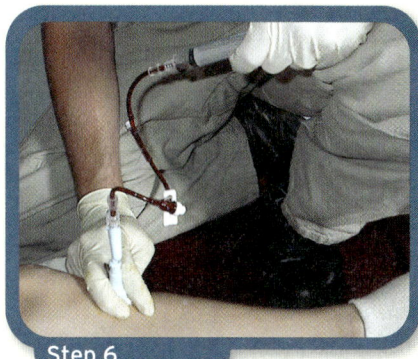

Step 6

Attach the syringe and extension set to the IO needle.
   Pull back on the syringe to aspirate blood and particles of bone marrow to ensure placement.
   Slowly inject saline to assure proper placement of the needle.
   Watch for infiltration, and stop the infusion immediately if noted.
   Connect the administration set, and adjust the flow rate as appropriate.

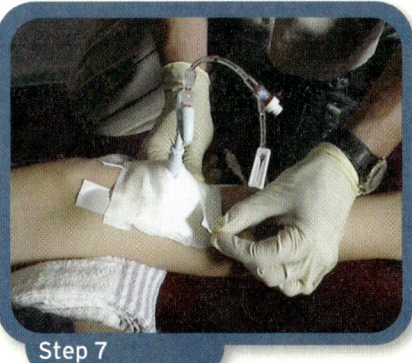

Step 7

Secure the needle with tape, and support it with a bulky dressing.
   Dispose of the needle in the proper container.

the infant sweating with feeding and, in many cases, will recount a history of congenital heart disease.

If you suspect cardiogenic shock, allow the child to remain in a position of comfort (often sitting upright), administer supplemental oxygen, and transport. The transport destination is a critical decision because the ultimate management requires pediatric critical care capability. Supplemental oxygen may not increase the SpO_2 in children with particular types of congenital heart disease, and parents will often alert you to this fact. Consider establishing IV access en route to the receiving facility. Unless you are sure of the diagnosis of cardiogenic shock (the child has a history of congenital heart disease, is afebrile, and has no history of volume loss), err on the side of fluid resuscitation. If you suspect cardiac dysfunction, administer a single isotonic fluid bolus slowly, and monitor carefully to assess its effect. Increased work of breathing, a drop in oxygen saturation, or worsening perfusion after a fluid bolus will confirm your suspicion of cardiogenic shock. Although inotropic agents may be needed to improve cardiac contractility and improve perfusion, they are rarely administered in the prehospital environment.

Arrhythmias

Rhythm disturbances can be classified based on whether the heart beat is too slow (bradyarrhythmias), too fast (tachyarrhythmias), or absent (pulseless). The signs and symptoms associated with a rhythm disturbance are often nonspecific—for example, the patient or caregiver may report fatigue, irritability, vomiting, chest or abdominal pain, palpitations, and shortness of breath. If you suspect a rhythm disturbance, quickly move through the PAT and initial assessment, supporting the airway and breathing as necessary. An ECG or rhythm strip will help to identify the underlying rhythm and suggest which specific management steps should be initiated. Address reversible causes of arrhythmias such as hypoxemia. The decision to stay on scene to obtain additional history and perform a focused physical examination will be dictated by the child's overall physiologic status.

Bradyarrhythmias

Bradyarrhythmias in children most often occur secondary to hypoxia, rather than as a result of a primary cardiac problem (such as heart block). Airway management, supplemental oxygen, and assisted ventilation as needed are always first-line treatment. Also, treat any underlying respiratory problem. Less common causes of bradycardia include congenital or acquired heart block and toxic ingestion of beta blockers, calcium channel blockers, or digoxin. Elevated ICP can also cause bradycardia and should be considered in children with ventricular shunts, a history of head injury, or suspected child maltreatment without a consistent injury history.

Initiate electronic cardiac monitoring as part of your initial assessment. If the child is asymptomatic, no further treatment is indicated in the prehospital setting. Healthy, athletic adolescents may have bradycardia as an incidental finding and should be transported to a hospital for further evaluation.

If the child's pulse rate is lower than normal for age despite oxygenation and ventilation and perfusion is poor, begin chest compressions and attempt IV or IO access. For chest compressions to be effective, the patient should be placed on a firm, flat surface with the head at the same level as the body. If you need to carry an infant while providing CPR, your forearm and hand can serve as the flat surface.

Follow the steps in **Skill Drill 41-6 ▾** to perform infant chest compressions:

1. Place the infant on a firm surface, using one hand to keep the head in an open airway position. You can also use a pad or wedge under the shoulders and upper body to keep the head from tilting forward.

Skill Drill 41-6: Performing Infant Chest Compressions

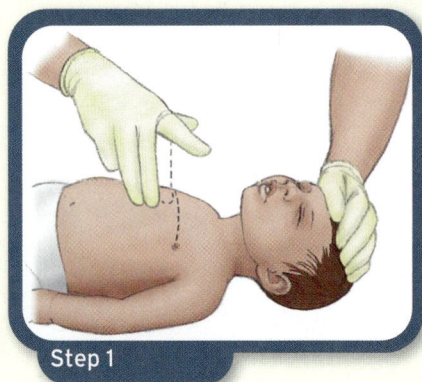

Step 1

Position the infant on a firm surface while maintaining the airway. Place two fingers in the middle of the sternum, one fingerbreadth below the imaginary intermammary line.

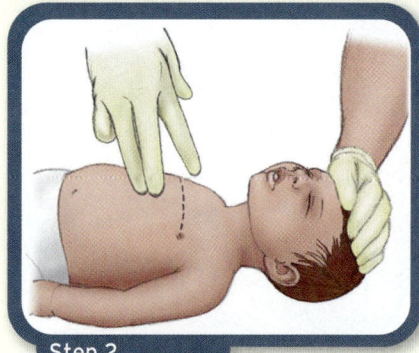

Step 2

Using two fingers, compress the sternum about one third to one half the depth of the chest. Push hard and fast, at a rate of 100 compressions/min. Allow the sternum to return briefly to its normal position between compressions.

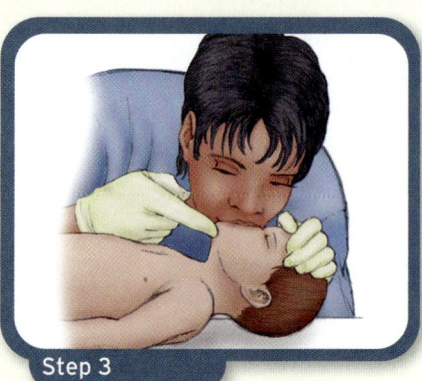

Step 3

Coordinate rapid compression and ventilation in a 30:2 ratio. Check for return of breathing and pulse after 2-minute intervals.

2. Imagine a line drawn between the nipples. Place two fingers in the middle of the sternum, one fingerbreadth below the imaginary intermammary line (Step 1).

3. Using two fingers, compress the sternum one third to one half the depth of the chest. This corresponds to approximately 4 cm (1½ inches) in most infants and about 5 cm (2 inches) in most children. Push hard and fast (at least 100 compressions/min), and allow full chest recoil. Minimize interruptions in chest compressions.

4. After each compression, allow the sternum to return briefly to its normal position. Allow equal time for compression and relaxation of the chest. Avoid jerky movements of your compressing fingers (Step 2).

5. Coordinate rapid compression and ventilation in a 30:2 ratio, making sure the infant's chest rises with each ventilation. You will find this easier to do if you use your free hand to keep the head in the open airway position. If the chest does not rise or rises only a little, use a chin lift to open the airway. The compression/ventilation ratio can be 15:2 if there are two rescuers doing CPR.

6. Reassess the infant for signs of spontaneous breathing or pulses after 2 minutes (5 cycles) and again at each 2-minute interval (Step 3).

(Skill Drill 41-7 ▶) shows the steps for performing chest compressions in children between 1 year and puberty (approximately 12 years):

1. Place the child on a firm surface, and use one hand to maintain the head tilt–chin lift (Step 1).

2. Place the heel of your hand over the middle of the sternum (between the nipples). Avoid compression over the lower tip of the sternum, which is called the xiphoid process (Step 2).

3. Compress the chest about one third to one half its total depth. Push hard and fast (100 compressions/min), and allow full chest recoil. Minimize interruptions in chest compressions. Compression and relaxation should be about the same duration. Use smooth movements, and hold your fingers off the child's ribs.

4. Coordinate rapid compression and ventilation in a 30:2 ratio, making sure that you see a visible chest rise with each ventilation (Step 3).

5. Reassess the child for signs of spontaneous breathing and pulses after 2 minutes (5 cycles of 30:2) and at 2-minute intervals.

6. If the child resumes effective breathing, place him or her in the recovery position (Step 4).

Quickly transport the patient to an appropriate receiving facility, while performing ongoing reassessments. If the child still has symptomatic bradycardia, medications are indicated. Epinephrine 0.01 mg/kg IV/IO (1:10000 dilution) is the initial medication of choice; the dose should be repeated every 3 to 5 minutes as needed for symptomatic bradycardia. If you identify heart block, give atropine as the second medication, under the direction of direct medical control. If the child continues to have symptomatic bradycardia, cardiac pacing may be indicated. If the child's rhythm deteriorates, switch to the appropriate treatment algorithm.

Tachyarrhythmias

Sinus tachycardia, a pulse rate higher than normal for age, is common in children. Although it may be a sign of serious

Skill Drill 41-7: Performing Chest Compressions on a Child

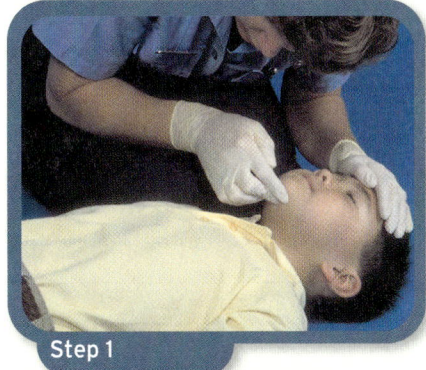

Step 1

Place the child on a firm surface, and use one hand to maintain the head tilt-chin lift.

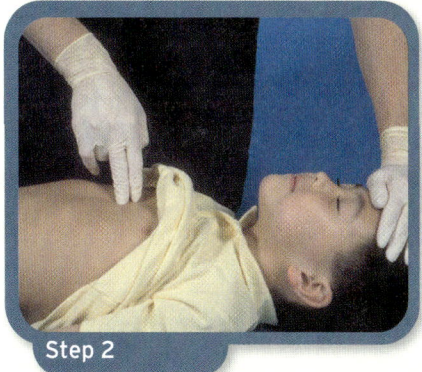

Step 2

Place the heel of your hand over the middle of the sternum (between the nipples); avoid compression of the xiphoid process.

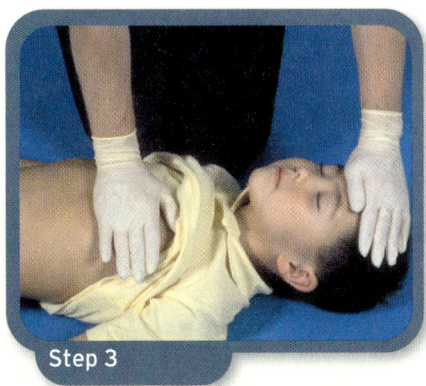

Step 3

Coordinate compression with ventilation in a 30:2 ratio, pausing for ventilation.

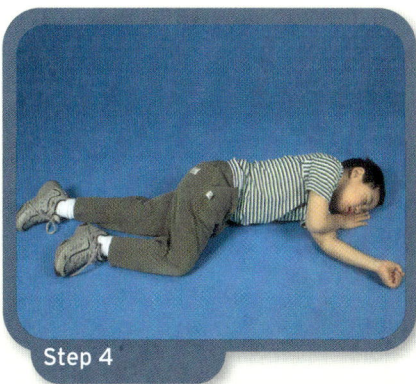

Step 4

Reassess breathing and pulse after 2 minutes and at 2-minute intervals thereafter. If the child resumes effective breathing, place him or her in the recovery position.

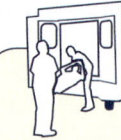

underlying illness or injury, it may also be due to fever, pain, or anxiety. Interpret the presence of tachycardia in the context of the remainder of the PAT and initial assessment. For example, if a child appears well but has a fever, sinus tachycardia is likely and treatment with antipyretics is all that is necessary. If a tachycardic child has a history of copious vomiting or diarrhea, fluid resuscitation is the appropriate treatment.

If a tachycardic child appears ill and has poor perfusion with no history of fever, trauma, or excessive volume loss, continue your assessment for a primary cardiac cause while initiating resuscitation. Your assessment should include determination of pulse rate along with interpretation of an ECG or rhythm strip.

Tachyarrhythmias are subdivided into two types based on the width of the QRS complex. A narrow complex tachycardia exists when the QRS complex is 0.09 second or less (about two or less standard boxes on the rhythm strip); a wide complex tachycardia exists when the QRS complex is greater than 0.09 second (a little more than two standard boxes on the rhythm strip).

Narrow Complex Tachycardia

Although sinus tachycardia is the most common arrhythmia in children, supraventricular tachycardia (SVT) is the most frequent tachyarrhythmia requiring antiarrhythmic treatment. **Table 41-14 ▾** compares sinus tachycardia, reentry SVT, and ventricular tachycardia (VT). You may identify sinus tachycardia based on the presence or absence of P waves, pulse rate, and history of preceding illness or injury. Its treatment is geared toward the underlying cause and may include oxygen, fluids, splinting, and analgesia.

SVT, which involves abnormal conduction pathways, can be identified by a narrow QRS complex, absence of P waves, and an unvarying pulse rate of more than 220 beats/min in an infant or more than 180 beats/min in a child. The child may have a history of SVT or exhibit nonspecific signs and symptoms, including irritability, vomiting, and chest or abdominal pain. Parents of young infants may report poor feeding for several days. The treatment of SVT depends on the patient's perfusion and overall stability. If the child is in stable condition, consider attempting vagal maneuvers while obtaining IV access: Have an older child hold his or her breath, blow into a straw with the end crimped over, or bear down as if having a bowel movement; in a younger child, place an examination glove filled with ice firmly over the midface, being careful not to obstruct the nose and mouth. Attempt these techniques only once, while continually monitoring the child's rhythm.

If the child has adequate perfusion and vagal maneuvers do not succeed in converting SVT to a sinus rhythm, consider administering adenosine (0.1 mg/kg). Adenosine has a short half-life and must be injected quickly into a vein near the heart, usually an antecubital vein. Its administration will be followed by a brief run of bradycardia, ventricular tachycardia, ventricular fibrillation, or asystole, which will convert spontaneously to sinus rhythm. Persistence of any of these rhythms is rare, but be prepared to switch arrhythmia algorithms if necessary.

For a child with SVT who has poor perfusion, synchronized cardioversion is recommended. Synchronized cardioversion is the timed administration of electrical energy to the heart to correct an arrhythmia. If the child is generating a regular but ineffective rhythm, it's important to time the jolt of electricity with the appropriate phase of the electrical activity (corresponds

Table 41-14	Features of Sinus Tachycardia, SVT, and VT					
	History	Pulse Rate	Respiratory Rate	QRS Interval	Assessment	Treatment
Sinus tachycardia	Fever Volume loss Hypoxia Pain Increased activity or exercise	< 220 beats/min (infant) < 180 beats/min (child)	Variable	Narrow: < 0.09 s	Hypovolemia Hypoxia Painful injury	Fluids Oxygen Splinting Analgesia or sedation
Supraventricular tachycardia	Congenital heart disease Known SVT Nonspecific symptoms (such as poor feeding, fussiness)	> 220 beats/min (infants) > 180 beats/min (child)	Constant	Narrow: < 0.09 s	CHF* may be present	Vagal maneuvers (ice to face) Adenosine (0.1 mg/kg) Synchronized electrical cardioversion
Ventricular tachycardia	Serious systemic illness	> 150 beats/min	Variable	Wide: > 0.09 s	CHF* may be present	Synchronized electrical cardioversion Amiodarone Procainamide

*CHF indicates congestive heart failure.

with the R wave on an ECG). A burst of electricity to the myocardium during the relative refractory period (the downward slope of the T wave) can precipitate ventricular fibrillation (VF)—a potentially lethal effect. Follow the same steps with synchronized cardioversion as with defibrillation, except that you must press the "sync" button on the defibrillator to alert the machine to time the electrical jolt. The dose of the initial synchronized cardioversion attempt is 0.5 to 1.0 joules per kilogram of body weight (J/kg). If the first dose is unsuccessful, a repeated dose of 2 J/kg can be given. In the hospital setting, sedation is provided before cardioversion, but its administration must not delay the procedure in a child in unstable condition.

An alternative approach to treating the child in SVT with poor perfusion is to give a dose of IV adenosine if vascular access is readily available. Do not delay synchronized cardioversion if vascular access is not already established, however. If the child remains in SVT and is in unstable condition or shock or is unconscious, you may give additional antiarrhythmic medications in conjunction with cardiology consultation.

Wide Complex Tachycardia

A child with a wide QRS complex tachycardia with a palpable pulse is likely in VT, a rare, but potentially life-threatening rhythm in children. Its presence may reflect underlying cardiac pathology. SVT may sometimes manifest as a wide complex rhythm, and distinguishing between the two can be challenging.

If a child with suspected VT is in hemodynamically stable condition and IV access is available, consider giving antiarrhythmic medication. Amiodarone is the drug of choice for VT with a pulse, although procainamide is an acceptable alternative. Do not give amiodarone *and* procainamide because both prolong the QT interval. If a child with VT is in unstable condition or shock or is unconscious, the treatment is synchronized cardioversion. Prior sedation is ideal, but do not delay cardioversion for this reason. The same dose of synchronized cardioversion is used for SVT and VT.

Special Considerations

The most common cause of tachycardia in an infant or a young child is sinus tachycardia from fever, dehydration, or pain.

If a child with a tachyarrhythmia is or becomes pulseless, begin CPR and follow the pulseless arrest treatment guidelines. Prepare to immediately transport any child with an arrhythmia to an appropriate receiving facility. Copies of rhythm strips or ECG tracings will be helpful to hospital personnel for diagnostic and therapeutic purposes.

Pulseless Arrest

Cardiopulmonary arrest exists when the child is unresponsive, apneic, and pulseless. In children, this type of arrhythmia is usually a secondary event—that is, the end result of profound hypoxemia and acidosis owing to respiratory failure. Asystole is the most common arrest rhythm. Pulseless electrical activity (PEA), VT, and VF are seen with lower frequency in children than

Table 41-15	Pediatric Defibrillation Paddle Size	
Age/Weight	**Paddle Size**
Older than 12 mo or > 10 kg	8-cm (adult) paddles
Up to 12 mo or < 10 kg	4.5-cm (pediatric) paddles

in adults. The survival rate for children with asystolic arrest in the prehospital setting is poor, and few survivors have good neurologic outcomes. The survival rate for children with VF arrest is slightly better and, as in adults, depends on early defibrillation.

When confronted with a pediatric patient in cardiopulmonary arrest, the most important consideration is to provide high-quality BLS skills. This starts with immediate CPR. Begin chest compressions immediately and call for a defibrillator. A second rescuer can open the airway and start rescue breathing. Attempt IV or IO access. When it becomes available, attach a monitor or defibrillator to determine the underlying cardiac rhythm. If it is asystole or PEA, defibrillation is not indicated, and additional treatment is limited to epinephrine (0.01 mg/kg IV/IO, 1:10000 dilution). After administering the medication, perform five cycles of CPR (approximately 2 minutes) before rechecking the rhythm and assessing for the presence of a pulse. If asystole or PEA persists, continue with CPR and epinephrine. High-dose epinephrine is not routinely recommended, however. Consider the "Hs" as the potential causes—for example, Hypoxia, Hypothermia, Hypovolemia, Hydrogen ions, or Hyper-/Hypokalemia. Also consider the "Ts"—Tablets (poisoning), Tamponade (cardiac), Tension pneumothorax, Thrombosis (coronary), or Thrombosis (pulmonary).

Defibrillation is performed before administration of medication in the treatment of VF or pulseless VT. Follow these steps to perform manual defibrillation in an infant or a child:

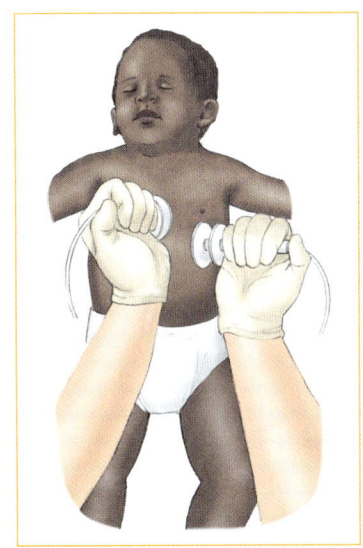

Figure 41-22 Site for defibrillation paddles or pads on anterior chest wall in small infants.

1. Confirm unresponsiveness, pulselessness, and apnea.
2. Begin CPR if a defibrillator is not immediately available.
3. Select the proper paddle or pad size **Table 41-15 ▲**.
4. Apply conductive gel to the paddles. Place one paddle on the anterior chest wall to the right of the sternum, inferior to the clavicle; place the other paddle on the left midclavicular line at the level of the xiphoid process **Figure 41-22 ▲**. Apply firm pressure to the paddles. For children who are younger than 12 months or who weigh less than 10 kg, you may use anterior-posterior paddle placement **Figure 41-23 ▶**.

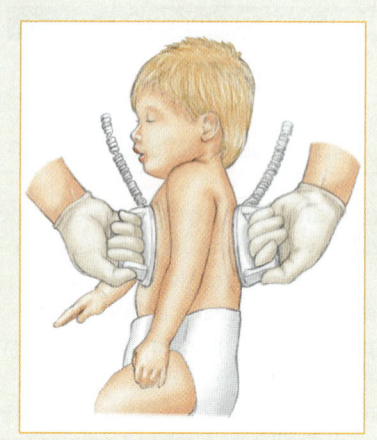

Figure 41-23 Site for defibrillation paddles or pads placed in anterior-posterior position for larger infants and children.

5. Assess the cardiac rhythm to confirm the presence of VF or pulseless VT.

6. Select the appropriate energy setting, and charge the defibrillator.

7. Verbally and visually ensure that no one is in contact with the patient; stop CPR if it is in progress.

8. Deliver the shock at the appropriate energy setting.

9. Give 5 cycles of CPR (approximately 2 minutes).

10. Reassess the rhythm.

11. If a shockable rhythm persists, give an additional shock at an increased or the same energy, and immediately resume CPR.

12. Insert an advanced airway, establish IV access, and begin medication therapy if indicated. Repeat the defibrillation after 5 cycles of CPR (approximately 2 minutes) if refractory VF or pulseless VT persists.

Many EMS systems use pregelled defibrillator pads instead of paddles. If your system uses defibrillator pads, place them in the same location as you would when using an AED. When applying the pads, ensure that there are no air pockets in the pad-skin interface because they may result in skin burns and decreased defibrillation effectiveness.

The initial energy setting for defibrillation of pediatric patients is 2 J/kg. If this level does not succeed, repeat the defibrillation at 4 J/kg. Further defibrillation should occur at 4 J/kg after cycles of CPR, as needed. There is some evidence that energy levels above 4 J/kg may be effective and safe, especially if delivered with a biphasic defibrillator. Energy levels, however, should never exceed 10 J/kg. With ongoing CPR, remember to search for and treat any underlying reversible causes. Give epinephrine only after you have delivered two shocks, doubling the dose for the second attempt.

For infants, a manual defibrillator is preferred to an AED for defibrillation. If a manual defibrillator is not available, an AED equipped with a pediatric setting or dose attenuator is preferred. If neither is available, an AED without a pediatric setting or dose attenuator may be used. Survival requires defibrillation when a shockable rhythm is present, and a high-dose shock is preferred to no shock at all.

As soon as possible, transport patients in cardiopulmonary arrest to an appropriate receiving facility. Early return of spontaneous circulation (< 5 min) and VF or VT as a presenting rhythm are associated with improved neurologic outcome for survivors of pediatric cardiopulmonary arrest.

Many EMS systems permit declaration of death in the pre-hospital setting if a child in cardiac arrest does not respond to resuscitation. In some cases, you may elect to transport the patient to an ED, even when resuscitation efforts are not successful, so as to provide social service support to the family. A child's death is a devastating event for the family and the EMS crew, and this may be one of your most difficult calls.

Medical Emergencies

Approximately half of all prehospital calls for pediatric patients are trauma-related; the other half are medical. Medical calls may include respiratory complaints (as previously discussed in this chapter), fever, seizures, and altered LOC.

Fever

Fever is a common pediatric complaint but often not a true medical emergency. A symptom of an underlying infectious or inflammatory process, fever can have multiple causes. Most pediatric fevers are caused by viral infections, which are often mild and self-limiting. In other cases, fever is a symptom of a more serious bacterial infection.

Your general impression and initial assessment will help you determine the severity of illness. Remember that young children with a fever can look quite ill—even if they only have a "bug"—because increased body temperature causes increased metabolism, tachycardia, and tachypnea. Record temperature as part of the vital signs, but recognize that the height of the fever does not reflect the severity of the illness. If the patient is a young infant, a rectal temperature is most accurate, but recognition that fever is present is more important than the exact temperature. As you move through the initial assessment, look for signs of respiratory distress, shock, seizures, stiff neck, petechial or purpuric rash, or a bulging fontanelle in an infant. These signs may tip you off to the presence of pneumonia, sepsis, or meningitis, all of which can be life threatening and require prompt transport to an appropriate facility. Ear infections (otitis externa and media) are common childhood maladies that most caregivers are experienced at managing. Occasionally, they can also lead to high fevers.

Very young infants (younger than 2 months) should always be considered at risk for serious infection. Young infants have few ways of interacting with the world, and a fever (defined as body temperature > 38°C) may be the only sign of a potentially life-threatening illness. Regardless of how well a child in this age group looks, he or she should be assessed and transported quickly to a hospital for a full sepsis workup, including blood, urine, and cerebrospinal fluid (CSF) analysis.

The focused history and physical examination will help to determine the underlying cause of the fever and the

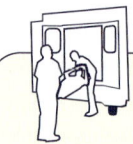

In the Field

Keep a laminated copy of the pediatric algorithms with you at all times for your reference during a cardiovascular emergency.

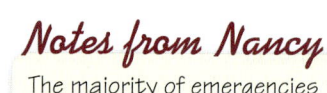

Notes from Nancy

The majority of emergencies requiring CPR in children are preventable.

Special Considerations
Fever itself is generally not an emergency, but rather a symptom of an underlying process. Use your assessment skills to determine the child's severity of illness.

severity of illness. Perform this assessment on scene if the child is in stable condition or en route to the hospital if the child appears seriously ill. Ask about the presence of vomiting, diarrhea, poor feeding, headache, neck pain or stiffness, and rash. A history of infectious exposure may provide clues to the likely cause of the child's current illness. The focused medical history may also identify a child at high risk for serious bacterial illness. For example, sickle cell disease, human immunodeficiency virus infection, and childhood cancers may all lead to an immunocompromised state.

A child with a fever may require little intervention in the prehospital environment. Simply support the ABCs as needed. Although fever by itself is not dangerous, temperature control will make the child with a minor acute illness look and feel better. Consider treating with acetaminophen or ibuprofen, but avoid aspirin in children. Use of aspirin in children has been linked with a rare illness called Reye syndrome, which can result in cerebral edema and liver failure. Other cooling measures should be limited to undressing the child. Transport the patient to an appropriate medical facility with ongoing reassessment for clinical deterioration.

Meningitis

Meningitis entails inflammation or infection of the meninges, the covering of the brain and spinal cord. It is most often caused by a viral or bacterial infection. Although children may look and feel quite ill, viral meningitis is rarely a life-threatening infection. By contrast, bacterial meningitis is potentially fatal. Children with bacterial meningitis can progress rapidly from mildly ill-appearing to coma and even death. In the early stages of illness, it is difficult to tell which type of infection is present, so take the safe route: Always proceed as if the child may have bacterial meningitis.

The symptoms of meningitis vary depending on the age of the child and the agent causing the infection. In general, the younger the child, the more vague the symptoms. A newborn with early bacterial meningitis may have fever as the only symptom. Young infants will often have fever and perhaps localizing signs such as lethargy, irritability, poor feeding, and a bulging fontanelle. Young children rarely show typical "meningeal signs" such as nuchal rigidity (neck stiffness with movement of the neck). Verbal children will often complain of headaches and neck pain. An altered LOC and seizures are ominous symptoms at any age.

Neonates most often contract meningitis-causing bacteria during the birthing process: The bacteria that may be present in the mother's vaginal tract—*Escherichia coli,* group B *Streptococcus,* and *Listeria monocytogenes*—can produce serious infections in newborns. Older infants and young children are at risk for contracting viral meningitis from enteroviruses, which are widespread during the summer and fall. Bacterial meningitis in older age groups most often involves *Streptococcus pneumoniae* (also known as pneumococcus) and *Neisseria meningitidis* (also known as meningococcus). Pneumococcus infection is becoming less

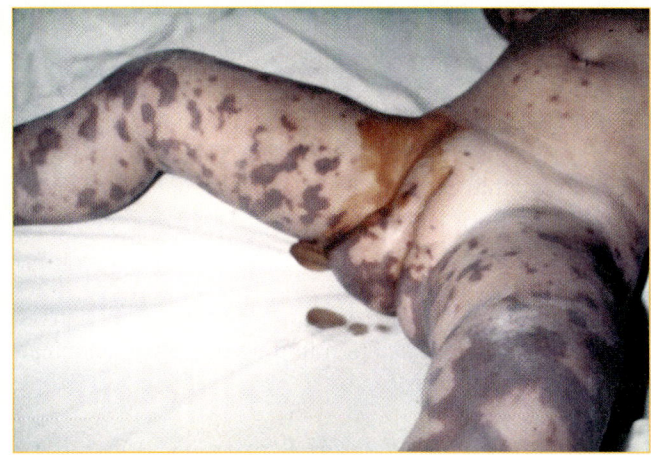

Figure 41-24 Purpura in a child with meningococcal sepsis.

Table 41-16	Pediatric SAMPLE History for Suspected Meningitis
Component	**Explanation**
Signs and symptoms	Onset and duration of illness, including "cold symptoms"–runny nose, cough Onset and duration of fever Rash? Headache? Neck pain? Photophobia? Irritability?
Allergies	Known drug reactions or other allergies
Medications	Exact names and doses of ongoing drugs Timing and amount of last dose Time and dose of analgesics and antipyretics
Past medical history	Previous illnesses or injuries Immunizations Perinatal history for young infants
Last oral intake	Timing of the child's last food or drink, including bottle or breastfeeding
Events leading to illness or injury	Any known exposures to children with illnesses and what kind of illnesses

frequent as more young children are vaccinated against this bacterium. Meningitis from *H influenzae* is rare because a vaccine against this pathogen was introduced several years ago.

Neisseria meningitidis may also cause sepsis (an overwhelming bacterial infection in the bloodstream). Meningococcal meningitis with sepsis is typically characterized by a petechial (small, pinpoint red spots) or purpuric (larger purple or black spots) rash in addition to the other symptoms of meningitis **Figure 41-24 ▶**.

Infection control is an important part of managing a child who may have meningitis. Meningococcus, in particular, is quite contagious. Protect yourself and others from contracting this illness by being vigilant about using standard and respiratory precautions. Wear a gown, gloves, and a mask if meningitis is a possibility.

Children with meningococcal sepsis and meningitis get very sick, very fast, so move quickly through your assessment. Form your general impression, and perform the initial assessment as usual, while recognizing that the initial presentation of a child with meningitis can be highly variable. Look for fever, altered mental status, bulging fontanelle, photophobia, nuchal rigidity, irritability, petechiae, purpura, and signs of shock. Perform a bedside glucose check because hypoglycemia may result from the hypermetabolic state. Helpful components of a SAMPLE history are shown in **Table 41-16 ▲** .

For children in physiologically unstable condition, provide lifesaving interventions as needed and transport them quickly, ideally to a facility with a pediatric intensive care unit. En route, perform frequent reassessments—one of the hallmarks of this disease is rapid deterioration. Monitor vital signs and changes in physical examination findings closely to anticipate a child's needs and intervene early.

Altered LOC and Mental Status

An altered LOC or mental status is an abnormal neurologic state in which a child is less alert and interactive with the environment than normal. **Table 41-17 ▼** uses the mnemonic AEIOU-TIPPS to highlight some common causes of altered LOC. Without a good history, it may be difficult to determine the underlying cause, and you may find yourself simply identifying and treating concerning symptoms.

Run through the PAT and ABCs quickly to determine possible points of intervention. Pay special attention to possible disability and dextrose issues. Use the AVPU scale (Alert, responsive to Voice, responsive to Pain, Unresponsive) to identify the level of disability. In addition, check the patient's glucose level because hypoglycemia (defined as a serum glucose

concentration < 2.2 mmol/l in a newborn and < 3.3 mmol/l in all other infants and children) is easily treatable.

The focused history and physical examination, whether performed at the scene or en route to the hospital, may also provide clues about the underlying cause. For example, a child with a history of epilepsy may be in a postictal state after an unwitnessed seizure; a child with diabetes may be hypoglycemic or in diabetic ketoacidosis. A history of toxic ingestion, recent illness, or injury may also reveal the cause of the altered mental status.

Regardless of the cause, the initial management of altered mental status is the same. Support the ABCs by carefully assessing the patient's airway and breathing. Provide assisted ventilation or airway support as needed. If the child is hypoglycemic, give glucose intravenously using 2 ml/kg of a 25% dextrose solution ($D_{25}W$) for infants and young children. Use 5 ml/kg of a 10% dextrose solution ($D_{10}W$) for neonates. Neonates do not tolerate hypertonic solutions and should not receive a dextrose solution greater than 10%. Always recheck the blood glucose level after giving IV glucose. The goal is to maintain a *normal* glucose level: Hyperglycemia is associated with worse neurologic outcomes in patients with cerebral ischemia. For children with altered mental status and signs or symptoms suggestive of an opiate toxidrome **Table 41-18 ▼** , consider giving naloxone. All patients with altered mental status should be transported expeditiously to an appropriate medical facility.

Seizures

Seizures result from abnormal electrical discharges in the brain. Although many types of seizures exist, generalized seizures manifest as abnormal motor activity and an altered LOC. Some children are predisposed to seizures because of underlying brain abnormalities, whereas others experience seizures as a result of trauma, metabolic disturbances, ingestion, or infection. Seizures associated with fever (febrile seizures) are unique to young children.

The physical manifestation of a seizure will depend on the area of the brain firing the electrical discharges and the age of

Table 41-17	AEIOU-TIPPS: Possible Causes of Altered LOC and Mental Status
A	Alcohol
E	Epilepsy, endocrine, electrolytes
I	Insulin
O	Opiates and other drugs
U	Uremia
T	Trauma, temperature
I	Infection
P	Psychogenic
P	Poison
S	Shock, stroke, space-occupying lesion, subarachnoid hemorrhage

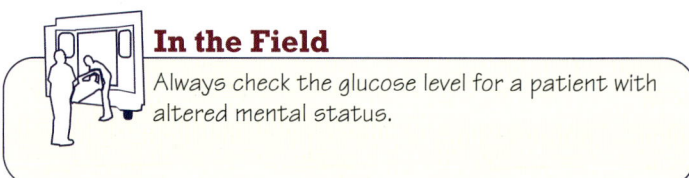

In the Field

Always check the glucose level for a patient with altered mental status.

Table 41-18	Common Toxidromes	
Toxidrome	**Agent**	**Signs and Symptoms**
Anticholinergic	Antihistamines, cyclic antidepressants	"Hot as a hare, red as a beet (hot, dry skin; hyperthermia), blind as a bat (dilated pupils), mad as a hatter (delirium, hallucinations)"
Cholinergic	Organophosphates	DUMBELS: Diarrhea/diaphoresis, Urination, Miosis, Bradycardia/bronchoconstriction, Emesis, Lacrimation, Salivation
Narcotic	Morphine, methadone	Bradycardia, hypoventilation, miosis, hypotension
Sympathomimetic	Cocaine, amphetamines	Tachycardia, hypertension, hyperthermia, mydriasis (dilated pupils), diaphoresis (sweating)

the child. Infants have immature brains, so seizures in this age group may be subtle. Repetitive movements such as lip smacking, chewing, and "bicycling" suggest seizure activity. Apnea and cyanosis can also be signs of underlying seizure activity.

The prognosis following a seizure is closely linked to the underlying cause. For example, a child with a febrile seizure will not have brain damage as a consequence of the event, whereas a child who has a seizure as a complication of a head injury or meningitis may have long-term neurologic abnormalities. All types of seizures (but especially first-time seizures) are frightening to caregivers, and they often result in 9-1-1 calls.

Types of Seizures

The classification system for seizures is the same for children and adults (see Chapter 28 for an in-depth discussion of seizures). Briefly, seizures that involve the entire brain are considered generalized seizures, whereas those that involve only one part of the brain are called partial seizures. The most common type of seizures are generalized tonic–clonic seizures (grand mal), which involve jerking of both arms and/or legs. Absence seizures are generalized seizures that involve brief loss of attention without abnormal body movements. Partial seizures can be further subclassified into simple partial seizures, which involve focal motor jerking without loss of consciousness, and complex partial seizures, which feature focal motor jerking with loss of consciousness.

Febrile Seizures

Febrile seizures occur in about 2% to 5% of young children. To make this diagnosis, the child must be between 6 months and 6 years old, have a fever, and have no identifiable precipitating cause (such as head injury, ingestion, or meningitis). Most febrile seizures occur in children between the ages of 6 months and 3 years. The strongest predictor for having a febrile seizure is a history of this diagnosis in a first-degree relative.

Simple febrile seizures are brief, generalized tonic–clonic seizures (lasting < 15 minutes) that occur in a child without underlying neurologic abnormalities. Complex febrile seizures are longer (lasting > 15 minutes), are focal, or occur in a child with baseline developmental or neurologic abnormality. They may also be associated with serious illness.

The majority of your calls for fever and seizures will involve simple febrile seizures. The postictal phase after a brief seizure tends to be short, so the child will often be waking up or back to baseline by the time you arrive at the scene. Depending on your agency's policy, a well-appearing child who has a history consistent with a simple febrile seizure may be transported by EMS or by parents but always needs urgent physician evaluation.

Special Considerations

Febrile seizures are unique to children. Reassure the parents of a child with a simple febrile seizure that the child has an excellent prognosis.

The prognosis for children with simple febrile seizures is excellent. Although one third of children who have one simple febrile seizure will have another such seizure, their prognosis does not change. There is no relationship between simple febrile seizures and brain damage or future developmental or learning disabilities, and children with this diagnosis have only a slightly increased risk for subsequent development of epilepsy.

Assessment of Seizures

The general impression and initial assessment of a child with a history of seizures should give special attention to compromised oxygenation and ventilation and signs of ongoing seizure activity. Seizures place a child at risk for respiratory distress or failure because of airway obstruction (often from the tongue), aspiration, or depressed respiratory drive. Given the typical EMS response time, any child who is still having a seizure when you arrive has likely been having seizure activity for at least 10 minutes and should be considered to be in status epilepticus; initiate treatment to stop the seizure in such cases. Status epilepticus has historically been defined as any seizure lasting more than 20 minutes or two or more seizures without return to neurologic baseline between seizures. In recent years, however, neurologists have begun urging treatment for any seizure lasting more than 5 minutes. As part of your SAMPLE history, ask about prior seizures; anticonvulsant medications; recent illness, injury, or suspected ingestion; duration of the seizure activity; and the character of the seizure.

Treatment of Seizures

Treatment at the scene will be limited to supportive care if the seizure has stopped by your arrival, but status epilepticus requires more extensive intervention. For a child with ongoing seizure activity, open the airway using the chin-lift or jaw-thrust maneuver. Very proximal airway obstruction is common during a seizure or postictal state because the tongue and jaw fall backward owing to the decreased muscle tone associated with altered mental status. If the airway is not maintainable with positioning, consider inserting a nasopharyngeal airway. Suction for secretions or vomitus, and consider the lateral decubitus position in case of ongoing vomiting. Do not attempt to intubate during an active seizure because endotracheal intubation in this setting is associated with serious complications and is rarely successful. You are better off using BLS airway management, stopping the seizure, and then considering the child's need for ALS airway support.

Provide 100% supplemental oxygen to the patient, and start bag-valve-mask ventilation as indicated for hypoventilation. Consider placing an NG tube to decompress the stomach if the patient requires assisted ventilation.

Assess the child for IV sites. Measure the serum glucose level, and treat any documented hypoglycemia.

Consider your options for anticonvulsant administration. Insertion of an IV line can be difficult in a child having a seizure, and alternative routes for medication delivery may be needed. The goal of medical therapy is to stop the seizure while minimizing anticonvulsant side effects.

First-line anticonvulsant treatment consists of a benzodiazepine—lorazepam, diazepam, or midazolam. All benzodiazepines can cause respiratory depression, so monitor oxygenation and ventilation carefully, especially when you give repeated doses or combinations of anticonvulsants. Lorazepam is an excellent choice for seizure management because of its rapid onset, lower risk of respiratory depression, and relatively long half-life. Its usefulness in the prehospital environment is limited because it must be refrigerated. Diazepam is frequently used in the prehospital setting, given by the IV or rectal route. The advantages of rectal administration include ease of access and a lower rate of respiratory depression, although onset of action is longer (approximately 5 minutes). The half-life of diazepam is relatively short, however, and breakthrough seizures may occur with longer transport times. Midazolam may be administered by the IV, IO, IM, and intranasal (using an atomizer) routes. Although it has excellent anticonvulsant effects, it has the shortest duration of action of the three benzodiazepines mentioned. Be prepared to repeat dosing for recurrent seizures.

If the seizures do not stop after two or three doses of a benzodiazepine, a second-line agent is necessary. Phenobarbital is the second-line agent of choice for neonates. Phenobarbital, phenytoin, and fosphenytoin are acceptable second-line agents for infants and children outside of the neonatal age group. Phenobarbital has sedative effects and causes respiratory depression, so be vigilant if you give it after a benzodiazepine. Although phenytoin has the advantage of not compromising the respiratory system or causing sedation, it is difficult to administer and can cause hypotension and bradycardia. Fosphenytoin, a drug that is metabolized to phenytoin, allows for more rapid infusion with fewer side effects; it may be administered by the IV or IM route.

Any child with a history suggestive of seizures requires physician evaluation to look for the cause. Although treatment at the scene is appropriate for a child in status epilepticus, detailed assessment should be performed during transport. Monitor cardiorespiratory status in any postictal child, and reassess frequently for recurrent seizure activity.

■ Toxicology Emergencies

Toxic exposures account for a significant number of pediatric emergencies. More than half of these toxic exposures occurred in children younger than 6 years, and 65% (> 1.5 million cases) occurred in patients younger than 20 years.

Toxic exposures can take the form of ingestion, inhalation, injection, or application of a substance (see Chapter 33 for more on specific exposures). A toddler or preschool-age child is most likely to have an unintentional exposure, the result of developmentally normal exploration. In this age group, ingestion tends to involve small quantities of a single cleaning product, cosmetic, or plant or a few pills. In contrast, toxic exposures in adolescents are typically the result of recreational drug use or suicide attempts and often involve multiple agents. Although intentional exposures among adolescents lead to greater morbidity and mortality, in small children, the toxic effects of some medications are such that "one pill can kill" **Table 41-19 ▶** .

You are the Paramedic Part 4

Based on the patient's vital signs and condition, you determine that he is in compensated shock. You insert a 20-gauge peripheral IV cannula in both antecubital fossae, and initiate a normal saline bolus. When you used the length-based resuscitation tape earlier, you estimated the child's weight to be approximately 12 kg, so you plan to administer a total of 240 ml (20 ml/kg). While the fluid is being delivered, you and your crew apply a cervical collar, secure the child to a pediatric backboard, and pad the voids with a blanket. You then load the patient in the ambulance, making sure to keep him warm, and contact the receiving facility. The physician agrees with your assessment and treatment and advises no further orders at this time.

Reassessment	Recording Time: 18 Minutes
Skin	Pale, cool, and dry
Pulse	165 beats/min, regular; weak distal pulses but strong central pulses
ECG	Narrow complex tachycardia
Blood pressure	84/56 mm Hg
Respirations	20 breaths/min via bag-valve-mask ventilation
Spo2	98% on bag-valve-mask ventilation with 100% supplemental oxygen
Pupils	Equal and reactive to light

7. What do you think is the cause for shock in this patient?
8. What criteria were used to determine that this patient was a "trauma alert"?

Table 41-19	One Pill Can Kill: Potentially Lethal Toddler Ingestion
Medicine	**Lethal Dose**
Camphor	5 ml of oil
Chloroquine	One 500-mg tablet
Clonidine	One 0.3-mg tablet
Glyburide	Two 5-mg tablets
Imipramine	One 150-mg tablet
Lindane	10 ml of 1% lotion
Diphenoxylate/atropine	Two 2.5-mg tablets
Propranolol	One or two 160-mg tablets
Theophylline	One 500-mg tablet
Verapamil	One or two 240-mg tablets

Table 41-20	The Pediatric SAMPLE for Toxic Exposures	
Components	**Features**	
Signs and symptoms	Time of suspected exposure Behaviour changes in child Emesis and content of vomit	
Allergies	Known drug reactions or other allergies	
Medications	Identity of suspected toxin Amount of toxin exposure (count pills or measure volume) Pill or chemical containers on scene Exact names and doses of prescribed medications	
Past medical problems	Previous illnesses or injuries	
Last oral intake	Timing of the child's last food or drink Type and time of home treatment (such as ipecac)	
Events leading to injury or illness	Key events leading to the exposure Type of exposure (inhaled, injected, ingested, or absorbed through the skin) Poison Centre contact	

Assessment

The evaluation of a child who has experienced a potentially toxic exposure follows the standard assessment sequence. Take a focused history to identify the agents to which the child was exposed, the quantity, and the route and time of exposure. Findings of physical assessment will vary widely based on these factors. Make special note of vital signs, pupillary changes, skin temperature and moisture, and any unusual odours. Putting together these pieces of the puzzle may allow you to identify a toxidrome—a pattern of symptoms and signs typical of a particular poisoning.

When performing the initial assessment, attend to airway, breathing, and circulatory support as indicated. A dextrose (glucose) check is an important test because ingestion of some common substances can lead to hypoglycemia—namely, ethanol and other alcohols, insulin, oral hypoglycemic agents, and beta blockers. Treat documented hypoglycemia as part of your resuscitation.

If the child is in stable condition without physiologic abnormalities and without a serious toxic exposure, stay on scene to obtain additional history and perform an expanded physical examination. See Table 41-20 for the SAMPLE history for a pediatric patient with a potential toxic exposure. During the expanded physical examination, look for toxidromes by assessing the patient's mental status, pupillary changes, skin CTC, gastrointestinal activity (bowel sounds, emesis, or diarrhea), and abnormal odours. Perform frequent reassessments because the child's condition may change.

Children with potentially life-threatening toxic exposures may be asymptomatic on your arrival, and the dose of drug in an accidental toddler ingestion may be high. Always attempt to collect any pill containers or bottles and transport them with the patient to the hospital to assist the ED staff in making treatment decisions.

Management

The management of any potential toxic exposure begins with supportive care and attention to the ABCs. Other management options include reducing the absorption of the substance by decontamination, enhancing elimination of the substance, and/or providing an antidote. Give special attention to the risks of environmental exposures for the paramedics, who may also require decontamination measures.

Decontamination

If the substance has been applied to the skin, reducing absorption involves removal of all clothing and a thorough washing of the skin. With ocular exposure, immediately wash out the eyes. For ingested toxins, options to reduce gastric absorption include dilution, gastric lavage, and activated charcoal.

Depending on the substance ingested, it may be useful to dilute the substance by having the child drink a glass of milk or water. This decision should be made in conjunction with a poison centre consultant or your direct medical control physician or nurse. If the child has any airway or breathing concerns, do not to allow the child to drink.

Although parents were once encouraged to keep syrup of ipecac available to induce vomiting in young children, this treatment is no longer recommended. Ipecac does not remove significant amounts of ingested toxins and can cause prolonged emesis, and it should not be used in the prehospital management of pediatric toxic ingestion.

The most common method currently used for gastrointestinal decontamination in the ED setting is the administration of activated charcoal. Activated charcoal absorbs many ingested toxins in the gut, making less drug available for systemic absorption. If it is administered within the first hour after

Table 41-21	Common Antidotes
Poison	**Antidote**
Carbon monoxide	Oxygen
Organophosphate	Atropine/pralidoxime
Tricyclic antidepressants	Bicarbonate
Opiates	Naloxone
Beta blockers	Glucagon
Calcium channel blockers	Calcium
Benzodiazepine	Flumazenil

exposure, however, some common toxins do not bind to charcoal—for example, heavy metals, alcohols, hydrocarbons, acids, and alkalis. Activated charcoal is messy to administer and is rarely readily accepted by pediatric patients. For these reasons, as well as the risk of severe chemical pneumonia if a child with altered mental status or vomiting aspirates the charcoal, this treatment may be best given in the hospital setting. If activated charcoal is given in the prehospital environment, the ideal dose is 10 times the mass of the ingested substance. The amount of drug ingested is often not known, so the typical dose is 1 to 2 g/kg.

Enhanced Elimination

Cathartics such as sorbitol are sometimes combined with activated charcoal. They work by speeding up elimination. In general, cathartics are not recommended for young children because they have been known to cause significant diarrhea with serious—sometimes life-threatening—electrolyte abnormalities. Hospital providers have additional options for enhancing elimination, such as whole bowel irrigation, urinary alkalinization for salicylate overdoses, dialysis, and hemoperfusion.

Antidotes

Antidotes can be lifesaving but are available for only a few poisonings. They work by reversing or blocking the effects of the ingested toxin. **Table 41-21 ▲** lists some of the more commonly available antidotes; indications for their use are the same for young children as for adults. The dose depends on the weight of the child.

Notes from Nancy
Any child with unexplained hyperpnea should be suspected to have salicylate poisoning.

Sudden Infant Death Syndrome

Sudden infant death syndrome (SIDS), formerly known as crib death, is the sudden and unexpected death of an infant younger than 1 year for whom a thorough postmortem examination (autopsy) fails to demonstrate an adequate cause of death. Whatever the cause, the sudden death of an apparently healthy baby is devastating to families and to the paramedics who respond to the call. Risk factors associated with SIDS include male sex; prematurity; low birth weight; young maternal age; sleeping in the prone position; sleeping with soft, bulky blankets or soft objects; sleeping on soft surfaces; and exposure to tobacco smoke.

SIDS is the leading cause of death in infants aged 1 month to 1 year, with a peak incidence between 2 and 4 months. Each week three babies in Canada die of SIDS.

Assessment and Management

The typical scenario for a SIDS call is that of a healthy infant who was put down for a nap and later found dead in bed. On arrival of EMS, the baby will be lifeless and, depending on discovery time, may have rigor mortis and dependent lividity (pooling of blood on the underside of the body). The presence of frothy or blood-tinged fluid in the mouth or nose or on the bedding is typical of SIDS. Be alert for clues to other potential causes of death, such as trauma, suffocation, or maltreatment.

Your decision to start resuscitative efforts, or to stop CPR that was started by first responders or family members, can be difficult in cases of suspected SIDS. Your actions will be guided by local protocols on declaring death in the prehospital environment and by your assessment of the patient and the needs of the family. Although a victim of SIDS cannot be resuscitated, failure to initiate care may not be acceptable to the shocked family. Likewise, ED care will not change the outcome for the infant, but hospital-based social services for the family may be an important resource. In cases that meet the criteria for declaring death at the scene and nontransport, notify the coroner, medical examiner, or law enforcement personnel, as dictated by local protocol, so that appropriate scene investigation can be undertaken. You also have an important role in mobilizing support for the survivors—for example, a chaplain or minister, SIDS team, social worker, or other family members.

Despite the emotionally charged atmosphere, doing a thorough scene assessment and obtaining the pertinent history is important. A history of recent illnesses, chronic conditions, medications, or trauma may decrease the likelihood of SIDS as the cause of death. The presence of pillows, stuffed toys, window blind cords, or sheepskin in the baby's crib may make suffocation a possibility.

Death of a Child

Whatever you suspect as the cause of death, be compassionate and nonjudgmental in dealing with caregivers. Find out the infant's name, and use it. Don't hesitate to tell the family how sorry you are. Families in this situation will often look to you for answers. Even when there is nothing to do medically, you can make a big impact by providing emotional support and care to the surviving family members.

Apparent Life-Threatening Event

An apparent life-threatening event (ALTE) is an episode during which an infant becomes pale or cyanotic; chokes, gags, or has an apneic spell; or loses muscle tone. These changes are sufficiently dramatic that the caregiver becomes frightened and may think that the baby is dying. ALTEs frequently prompt 9-1-1 calls. Their causes may include benign diagnoses, such as a brief episode of laryngospasm during feedings or gastroesophageal reflux, and serious diagnoses, such as sepsis, congenital heart disease, and seizures.

ALTEs were once thought of as existing along a spectrum with SIDS; hence they were called near-miss or aborted SIDS. More recent evidence demonstrates that although both events occur in early infancy, the two are not related.

It is common to find a distraught caregiver and a well-appearing baby on arrival at the scene of an ALTE call. Provide life support if the infant shows signs of cardiorespiratory compromise or altered mental status, and transport all infants with a history of an ALTE to an appropriate medical facility for evaluation. This is a challenging age group to assess, and overtriage is the safest path.

Child Maltreatment and Neglect

Sadly, child maltreatment is prevalent in our society. In 2003, an estimated 235,315 child maltreatment investigations were conducted in Canada (38.33 investigations per 1,000 children aged 0 to 16 years). In approximately half of these investigations (40%, or an estimated 114,607 of investigations), the child protection worker examining the case found maltreatment claims to be substantiated.

Child abuse or maltreatment comes in many forms: physical abuse, sexual abuse, emotional abuse, and child neglect. Physical abuse involves the infliction of injury to a child. Sexual abuse occurs when an adult engages in sexual activity with a child; it can range from inappropriate touching to intercourse. Emotional abuse and child neglect are often difficult to identify and may go unreported.

Keep the possibility of child maltreatment and neglect in mind when you are called to assist with an injured child. The information you gather from the initial scene assessment and interviews may prove invaluable. If you suspect child maltreatment, you should act on your suspicions because child maltreatment involves a pattern of behaviour. A child who is abused once is likely to be abused again—and next time, it may be more serious or even fatal.

Risk Factors for Maltreatment

No child asks to be abused, but certain risk factors make maltreatment more likely. Younger children are more often abused than older children, perhaps a function of their helplessness

Table 41-22	CHILD ABUSE Mnemonic for Suspicion of Child Maltreatment
C	Consistency of the injury with the child's developmental age
H	History inconsistent with injury
I	Inappropriate parental concerns
L	Lack of supervision
D	Delay in seeking care
A	Affect (of the parent or caregiver and the child in relation to the caregiver)
B	Bruises of varying ages
U	Unusual injury patterns
S	Suspicious circumstances
E	Environmental clues

and limited ability to communicate their needs. Children who require a lot of extra attention, such as children with physical or mental challenges, chronic illnesses, or other developmental problems, are also more likely to be abused.

Child maltreatment occurs across all socioeconomic levels, although it is more prevalent in lower-socioeconomic families. Divorce, financial problems, and illness can contribute to the overall stress level of parents, placing them at higher risk to abuse their children. Drug and alcohol abuse can also interfere with a caregiver's ability to parent, and both are associated with higher rates of abusive behaviour. Domestic violence in the home places a child at a much higher risk for child maltreatment.

Suspecting Maltreatment

When you are called to the home of an injured child and suspect maltreatment or neglect, trust your instincts. Use your scene assessment, focused history, and physical examination to gather additional information. Look for "red flags" that could suggest child maltreatment (summarized in the mnemonic CHILD ABUSE Table 41-22):

- A history inconsistent with the type of injury sustained—for example, a child who fell from a tree but whose bruises are only on the buttocks
- An account of the injury that is inconsistent with the developmental abilities of the child—for example, a 2-month-old child rolling off a bed
- An old injury that went unreported
- Inappropriate actions or language from the caregiver

Assessment and Management
Scene Assessment

To recognize maltreatment, you first have to suspect it. Once you begin to question whether abuse or neglect is involved, it becomes important to carefully document what you see. Although it may be difficult to remain impartial when child abuse or neglect is suspected, it is an important part of

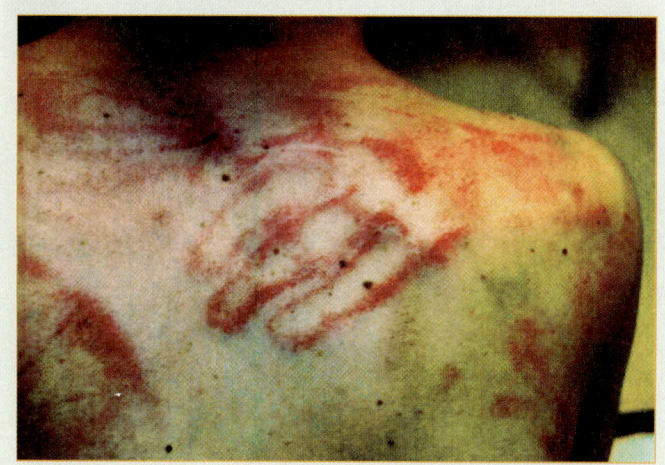

Figure 41-25 Bruises from child maltreatment. Look for bruises that look like finger or hand marks.

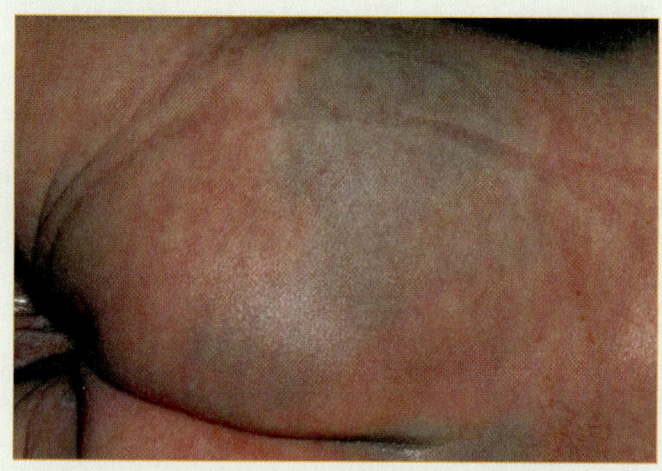

Figure 41-27 A Mongolian spot is a birthmark that can mimic a bruise. It may be on the back, buttocks, or extremities.

Documentation and Communication

If you suspect child maltreatment, take extra care with your documentation. Record conversations verbatim (in quotes) and document on your patient care report what you see and hear.

General and Initial Assessments

Although child maltreatment can generate a big emotional response from the EMS crew, remember that your primary focus should be on trauma assessment and management and on ensuring the safety of the child. Base your general impression on the PAT, which may range from normal in a child with minor inflicted injuries to grossly abnormal in a child with severe internal or CNS injuries. In shaken baby syndrome you may encounter a child with a very abnormal appearance but no external signs of injury. In such a case, the child receives a severe brain injury when a caregiver violently shakes the infant, often when the child is crying inconsolably. Given that few caregivers will admit to having hurt the child, be alert for a history that is inconsistent with the clinical picture.

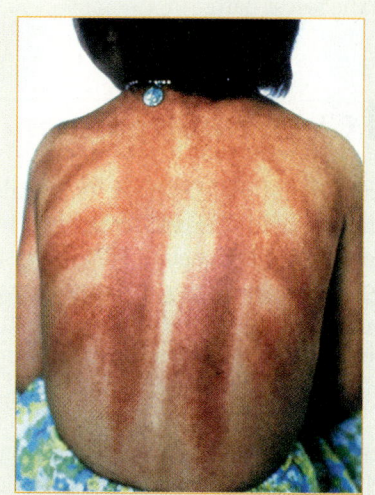

Figure 41-28 Coining, the practice of rubbing hot coins on the back as a treatment of medical illnesses, can leave impressive markings that can mimic child maltreatment.

professionalism. Record what you see and hear, but do not editorialize. Be detailed in your incident report about the child's environment, noting the condition of the home and the interactions among the caregivers, the child, and the paramedics. Record concerning comments verbatim.

Do not approach the caregiver with your concerns, but make sure that you pass them on to staff at the receiving hospital. In many provinces, paramedics are mandatory reporters of suspected child maltreatment. Be aware of local regulations; you may have a legal—and an ethical—obligation to ensure that a report is made to the local child protection services.

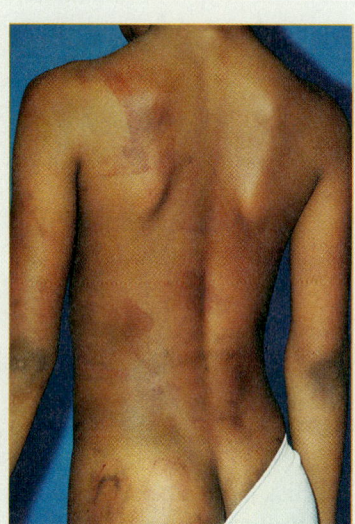

Figure 41-26 Bruises from child maltreatment. Multiple bruises or injuries that are in different stages of healing are concerns for maltreatment.

Give special attention to the child's skin while looking for bruises, especially of different ages or in concerning locations. Active toddlers often have bruises on their shins from falls and active playing but rarely on their backs or buttocks. Bruises in identifiable patterns such as belt buckles, looped cords, or straight lines are rarely incurred accidentally. **Figure 41-25** and **Figure 41-26** are examples of bruises that are suggestive of maltreatment.

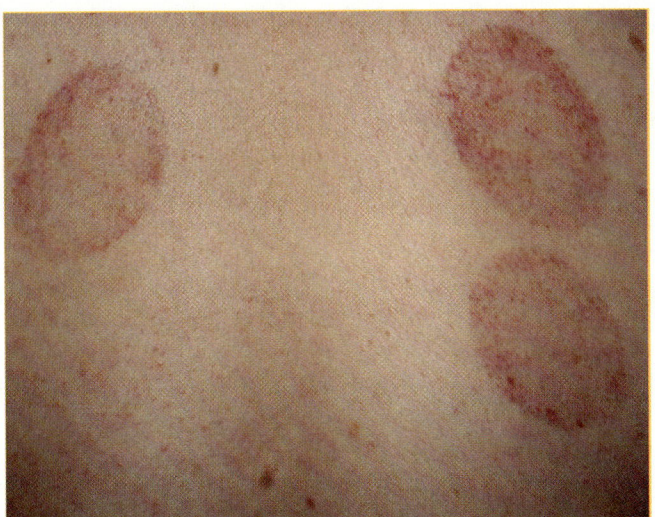

Figure 41-29 Round, flat, red circles on a child's back may be from the practice of cupping—placing warm cups on the skin to draw out illness from the body.

Use the CHILD ABUSE mnemonic when you obtain additional history. Ask yourself, "Does the caregiver's explanation make sense? Could this child produce this bruise or injury through his or her normal activities?"

Mimics of Maltreatment

It can be difficult to distinguish some normal skin findings from inflicted injuries. For example, Mongolian spots **Figure 41-27 ◂** can mimic bruises. These birthmarks are generally found on the lower back and buttocks of children of Asian or African descent; they may be mistaken for bruises because of their unique bluish colouring.

Certain cultural customs also produce skin markings that can mimic child maltreatment. Coining and cupping **Figure 41-28 ◂** and **Figure 41-29 ▴** are traditional Asian healing practices, often used in the treatment of fever. Although the skin markings can be impressive, the practice is not harmful and does not represent maltreatment.

◼ Trauma

Pediatric trauma is the leading cause of death among children older than 1 year. Motor vehicle collisions cause the most deaths in this age group, followed by falls and submersions. Among adolescents, homicide and suicide are major causes of death.

Children's age-related anatomy and physiology make their injury patterns and responses to trauma different from those seen in adults. In addition, a child's developmental stage will affect his or her response to injury. For a young child, being strapped to a backboard may be as traumatic as the injury leading to the EMS call!

Anatomical and Physiologic Differences

Head

Recall that infants and young children have heads that are large relative to the rest of their bodies. The head also has a larger mass compared with adults. The head's larger size and weight make it more prone to injury. A young child falling from a height, for example, is more likely to fall on his or her head. Traumatic brain injury is the leading cause of death and significant disability in pediatric trauma patients.

Spinal Column

The vertebral column continues to develop along with the child. When the child is younger, the cervical spine fulcrum (or bending point) is higher because the head is heavier. As the child grows, the fulcrum descends to "adult level," around C5 through C7. An infant who sustains blunt head trauma involving acceleration-deceleration forces is at high risk for a fatal, high cervical spinal injury. By comparison, a school-age child who experiences the same injury will likely sustain a lower cervical spinal injury and be paralyzed.

Fortunately, vertebral fractures and spinal cord injuries in young children are uncommon. Spinal ligaments are more lax in children than in adults, leading to increased mobility and the phenomenon of cord injury in the absence of identifiable vertebral bony fracture or dislocation.

Thoracic and lumbar spinal injuries are also encountered relatively infrequently until a child is pursuing adult activities, such as driving and diving. Nevertheless, these injuries are seen in children in association with specific mechanisms—for example, seatbelt-associated lumbar spine injuries (often associated with abdominal injury) and compression fracture due to axial loading in a fall. When confronted with a significant MOI, the safest course is to assume that the child has a bony injury and transport with spinal immobilization precautions.

Chest

Chest trauma is the third leading cause of serious injury in pediatric trauma. A child's chest wall is more pliable and flexible than that of an adult. As a result, children have fewer rib fractures and flail chest events, but injuries to the thoracic organs may be more severe because the pliable ribcage is more easily compressed during blunt trauma. As a consequence, children are more vulnerable than adults to pulmonary contusions, pericardial tamponade, and diaphragmatic rupture. Be sure to look for signs of these injuries in a child with suspected chest trauma, but note that the signs of pneumothorax or hemothorax in children are often subtle. You may not see signs such as neck vein distension, and it may be difficult to determine tracheal deviation.

Abdomen and Pelvis

Abdominal injuries are the second leading cause of serious trauma in children (after head injuries). In pediatric patients, the intra-abdominal organs are relatively large, making them vulnerable to blunt trauma. For example, the abdomen in an infant or toddler often seems protuberant because of the large liver. The liver and the spleen extend below the ribcage in young children and, therefore, do not have as much bony protection as they do in an adult. These organs have a rich blood supply, so injuries to them can result in large blood losses. The kidneys are also more vulnerable to injury in children because they are more mobile and less well supported than in adults. Finally, the duodenum and pancreas are likely to be damaged in handlebar injuries.

Pelvic fractures are relatively rare in young children and are generally seen only with high-energy MOIs. The risk for pelvic fracture increases in adolescence, when the skeleton and MOIs become more like those of adults.

Extremities

The bones of young children continue growing until well into adolescence, resulting in a higher rate of fractures than in adults. This susceptibility to fractures is a function of bone density and the presence of cartilaginous growth plates. Growth plate fractures can be seen with low-energy MOIs, and they may not present with the degree of tenderness, swelling, and bruising usually associated with a broken bone. Because a young child's ligaments are sturdier than the long bones, sprains are relatively uncommon, and joint dislocations without associated fractures are not often encountered.

Injury Patterns

Blunt trauma is the MOI in more than 90% of pediatric injury cases. Because they have less muscle and fat mass than adults, children have less protection against the forces transmitted in blunt trauma.

Falls are common in pediatric patients, and the injuries sustained will reflect the anatomy of the child and the height of the fall. For example, a 6-year-old playing on the monkey bars is most likely to sustain an upper extremity fracture when falling onto an outstretched arm. Internal or head injuries would be uncommon with this mechanism. Conversely, an infant, with a big head and no protective reflexes, who pitches out of a backpack or shopping cart will commonly have a skull fracture and could have an intracranial hemorrhage. Falls from a standing position usually result in isolated long bone injuries, whereas high-energy falls (such as from a window, ejection from a motor vehicle, car-versus-pedestrian collision) may result in multiple trauma.

Injuries from bicycle handlebars typically produce compression injuries to the intra-abdominal organs. Duodenal hematomas and/or pancreatic injuries are common with this MOI, as are upper extremity injuries. You must also consider a head injury if the patient went over the handlebars, especially if the child was not wearing a helmet.

Motor vehicle collisions can result in a variety of injury patterns depending on whether the child was properly restrained and where the child was seated in the car. For unrestrained passengers, assume multiple trauma. Restrained passengers may sustain chest and abdominal injuries associated with seatbelt use. If you see chest or abdominal bruising in a seatbelt pattern, have a high suspicion for spinal fractures. Air

Special Considerations

Always consider multiple trauma in pediatric patients. Consider head or abdominal injuries, even if they are not readily apparent.

bags pose a particular threat for head and neck injuries in young children.

A child who is the victim of a car-versus-pedestrian collision is likely to sustain multisystem trauma. Depending on the child's height and the height of the vehicle's bumper, a child may receive chest, abdominal, and lower extremity injuries at impact. Head and neck injuries may result from the fall when the child is thrown.

Assessment and Management

The first steps in managing pediatric trauma are the same as for medical emergencies. Use your hands-off assessment to establish a general impression. If the PAT findings are grossly abnormal, quickly move to initial assessment and management to prevent death or disability. Abnormal appearance should make you think immediately of a head injury. With an isolated closed head injury, the child's breathing and circulation may be normal. Of course, abnormal appearance may also reflect inadequate oxygenation of the brain owing to shock or respiratory failure. Abnormalities in work of breathing will tip you off to chest or airway injury and abnormal circulation to a hemorrhage problem. If multisystem injuries are present, all three sides of the PAT may be abnormal.

Begin the initial assessment, initiating life support interventions as you identify problems. Assess the airway for obstruction with teeth, blood, vomit, or edema. Suction as needed. For cervical spinal injury, open the airway using the jaw-thrust maneuver. If the child cannot maintain the airway, consider placement of a nasopharyngeal or oropharyngeal airway. If you attempt endotracheal intubation, maintain cervical spinal precautions. Establishment of an emergency surgical airway in a child is fraught with complications, and the failure rate is high; for these reasons, tracheotomy should be reserved for the most expert surgeons in a controlled setting. The chances of needing to perform a needle cricothyrotomy in a child are remote. In younger children, identification of the cricothyroid membrane is difficult. Appropriate needle cricothyrotomy is described in Chapter 11.

Breathing assessment includes evaluation for symmetric chest rise and equal breath sounds. Provide 100% supplemental oxygen, give bag-valve-mask ventilation as needed, and place an NG or OG tube for stomach decompression.

Pneumothorax is not common in pediatric blunt chest injury, but it may be present with penetrating trauma of the chest or upper abdomen. Remember that you are less likely to see jugular venous distension and tracheal deviation in a child. If the mechanism suggests a possible tension pneumothorax and the patient is in significant respiratory distress, perform needle decompression **Skill Drill 41-8 ▶**:

1. Assess the patient to ensure that the presentation is due to a tension pneumothorax.

2. Prepare and assemble the necessary equipment: large-bore IV cannula, preferably 14 to 16 gauge, alcohol or povidone iodine preps, and adhesive tape.

3. Locate the appropriate site. Find the second or third intercostal space in the midclavicular line on the affected side.

4. Cleanse the appropriate area using aseptic technique.

5. Insert the needle at a 90° angle, just superior to the third rib (nerves, arteries, and veins run along the inferior borders of each rib), and listen for the release of air (Step 1).

6. Advance the cannula over the needle, and place the needle in the sharps container.

7. Secure the cannula in place the same way you would secure an impaled object.

8. Monitor the patient closely for recurrence of the tension pneumothorax.

Any trauma patient should be considered to be at risk for developing shock from visible external bleeding or internal bleeding. Assess the child's circulation by checking the heart rate and quality, capillary refill, skin temperature, and blood pressure. In pediatric patients, the only sign of compensated shock might be an elevated heart rate—children have a remarkable capacity for peripheral vasoconstriction and can maintain their blood pressure despite significant blood loss. If the MOI is concerning and the child is tachycardic, assume the presence of compensated shock and initiate volume resuscitation with 20 ml/kg of isotonic fluid (normal saline or lactated Ringer's). Ideally, you will insert two peripheral IV lines, but an IO line may be best in a child with hemorrhagic shock. Control external bleeding as you would in any trauma patient. Once the ABCs are stabilized, continue your assessment of disability with the AVPU scale. Your assessment of appearance in the PAT will already have identified an altered LOC. Check the child's pupils and motor function. Place a cervical collar, and immobilize the child on a backboard as indicated.

If increased ICP is a concern, keep the head midline to facilitate jugular venous return to the heart. If the patient is not in shock, elevate the backboard or head of the stretcher to 30°. Perform shock resuscitation with IV fluids—brain hypoperfusion will make matters worse. If the child has acute signs of herniation such as a "blown" pupil or the Cushing's triad (elevated blood pressure, bradycardia, abnormal respiratory pattern), consider mild hyperventilation guided to an EtCO$_2$ of 32 to 35 mm Hg and giving mannitol.

The last piece of the initial assessment will be "exposure"—that is, a head-to-toe examination to identify all injuries. Log roll the child, and examine the back and buttocks. Once you have completed this examination, cover the child in blankets. Don't

Skill Drill 41-8: Decompression of a Tension Pneumothorax

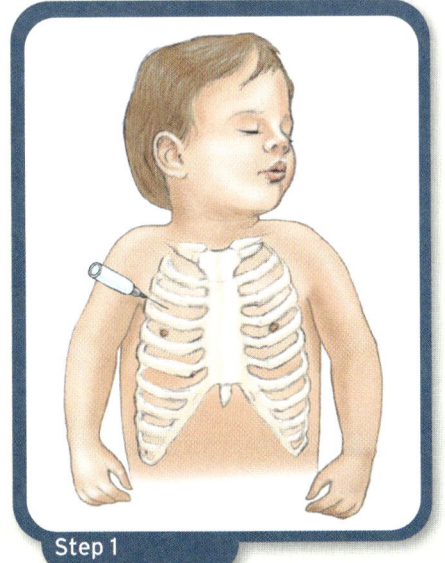

Step 1

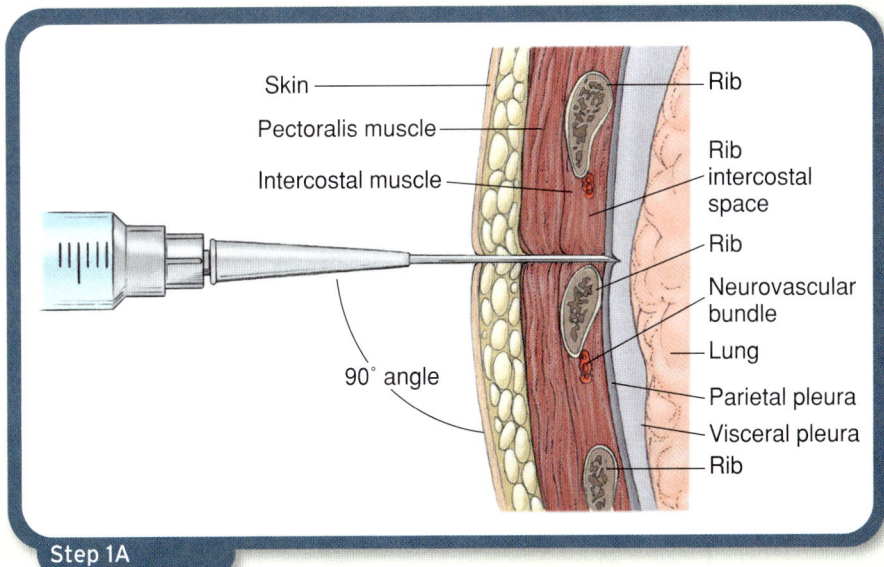

Step 1A

Locate the appropriate site. Find the second or third intercostal space in the midclavicular line on the affected side.

Cleanse the appropriate area using aseptic technique. Insert the needle at a 90° angle and listen for the release of air.

forget to cover the head, especially in infants and young children, and avoid drafts from heating or air-conditioning units. Children have a relatively large skin surface area–body mass ratio, increasing their risk for heat loss and hypothermia. Consider the use of warm IV fluids, warm oxygen, and a warm patient transport environment and keeping the patient covered. Also be sure to remove any wet clothing that could conduct heat away from the patient.

Treat any fractures—open or closed—as you would in an adult. Check out your equipment ahead of time to ensure that you have splints appropriate for smaller children.

Transport Considerations

After initial assessment and stabilization, you are faced with the transport decision. Some traumas are load-and-go situations because of the severity of injuries and the patient's unstable condition. Examples include trauma involving an ominous MOI regardless of how the patient looks on scene, a child with an unstable or compromised airway, a child in shock, a child with difficulty breathing, and a child with a severe neurologic disability. For these patients, perform lifesaving procedures on scene or en route, and quickly transfer them to an appropriate trauma centre according to local trauma triage protocols.

All trauma victims for whom spinal injury is suspected require appropriate spinal stabilization. The indications are the same for children and adults. You may have difficulty finding an appropriately sized cervical collar for infants or very young children. Do not attempt to place a collar that is too big on a small child—use towel rolls and tape to immobilize the head. Apply the tape across the temples and forehead, but avoid tape over the chin or throat because it may impair ventilation. Choose a pediatric immobilizer with a recess for the child's large occiput, or place a towel or small blanket under the shoulders and back to prevent neck flexion in infants and toddlers Figure 41-30 ▾.

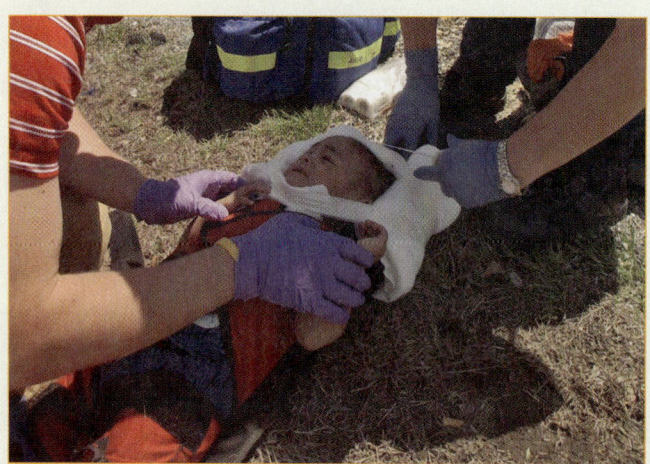

Figure 41-30 Cervical spinal stabilization with towels and tape for a young infant.

Immobilize a child with the following steps Skill Drill 41-9 ▸ :

1. Maintain a small child's head in a neutral position by placing a towel under the shoulders Step 1 .
2. Place an appropriately sized cervical collar on the patient Step 2 .
3. Carefully log roll the child onto the immobilization device Step 3 .
4. Secure the patient's torso to the immobilization device first Step 4 .
5. Secure the child's head to the immobilization device Step 5 .
6. Complete immobilization by ensuring that the child is strapped in properly Step 6 .

Secure the child firmly onto the backboard but leave room for adequate chest expansion. Being immobilized is a frightening experience, especially for a young child who cannot understand your intent. Use developmentally appropriate language to explain what you are doing and why, and keep a parent close by when possible.

Follow the steps in Skill Drill 41-10 ▸ to immobilize an infant:

1. Carefully stabilize the infant's head in a neutral position and lay the seat down into a reclined position on a hard surface Step 1 .
2. Position a pediatric board or other similar device between the patient and the surface on which the infant is resting Step 2 .
3. Carefully slide the infant into position on the board Step 3 .
4. Make sure the infant's head is in a neutral position by placing a towel under the infant's shoulders Step 4 .
5. Secure the torso first, and place padding to fill any voids Step 3 .
6. Secure the infant's head to the backboard Step 6 .

The identification of the nearest appropriate facility depends on local protocols and the capabilities of local hospitals. In some areas of the country, you may be directed to take the patient directly to a pediatric trauma centre or to arrange for air transport to a pediatric trauma centre. In other areas of the country, children are evaluated primarily at local hospitals and then transferred to a pediatric trauma centre.

Expanded History and Examination

If the patient is in stable condition and does not meet the load-and-go criteria, obtain additional history as outlined in Table 41-23 ▸ and perform a more thorough physical examination. A head-to-toe, back-to-front detailed physical examination should be performed on all trauma patients with significant MOI en route to the ED. For infants, this will

Skill Drill 41-9: Immobilizing a Child

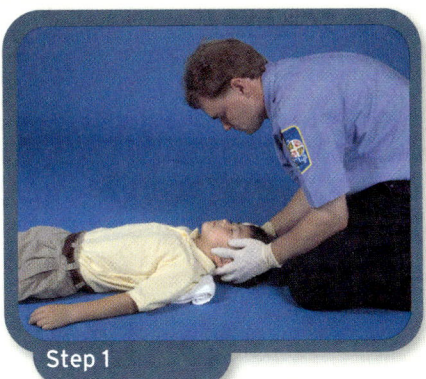

Step 1

Use a towel under the shoulders of a small child to maintain the head in a neutral position.

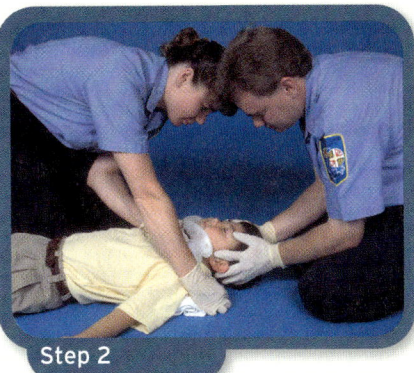

Step 2

Apply an appropriately sized cervical collar.

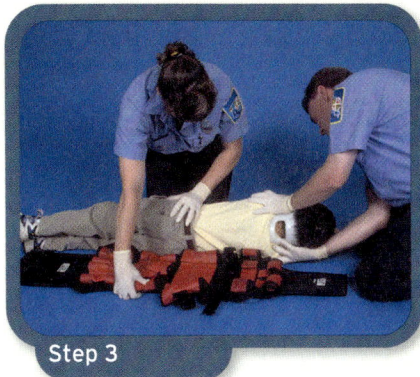

Step 3

Log roll the child onto the immobilization device.

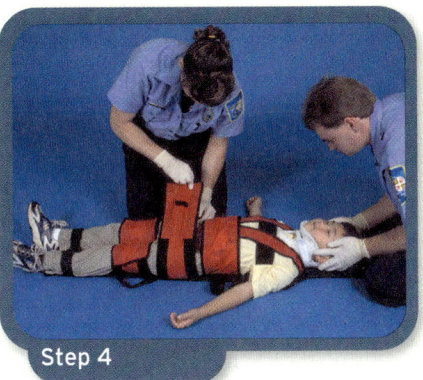

Step 4

Secure the torso first.

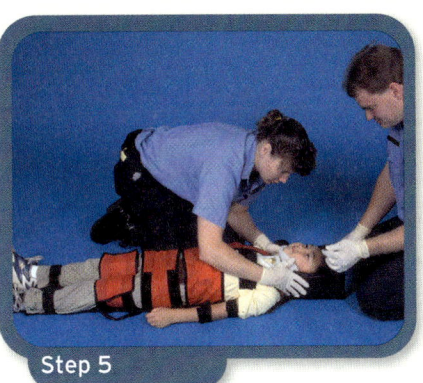

Step 5

Secure the head next.

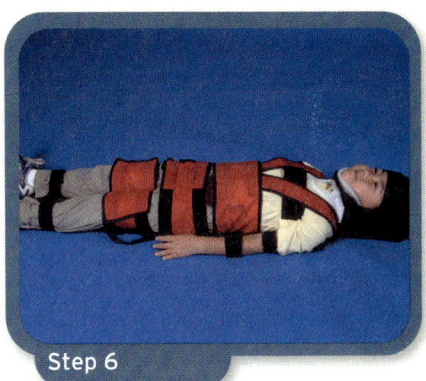

Step 6

Ensure that the child is strapped in properly.

Table 41-23	SAMPLE History in Pediatric Trauma
Component	**Explanation**
Signs and symptoms	Time of event Nature of symptoms or pain Age-appropriate signs of distress
Allergies	Known drug reactions or other allergies
Medications	Timing and last dose of long-term medications Timing and dose of analgesics or antipyretics
Past medical history	Prior surgeries Immunizations, especially last tetanus
Last oral intake	Time of child's last food and drink, including bottle or breastfeeding
Events leading to the injury	Key events leading to the current incident MOI Hazards at the scene

include checking the anterior fontanelle for bulging (a sign of increased ICP). Look for bruises, abrasions, or other subtle signs of injury that may have been missed during the initial assessment. Be sure to revisit the initial assessment during your ongoing assessment on the way to the hospital because the patient's condition can change quickly.

Pain Management

Pain is often undertreated in young children. Regardless of whether a child can communicate with you verbally, do not overlook signs of pain in pediatric trauma patients. Consider pain assessment as important as the vital signs, and use one of the many tools available to elicit the child's self-report of pain level. Tachycardia and inconsolability may be the only way a child has to express pain, and findings may be similar to those of early shock or plain old fear.

Pain treatment includes use of a calm, reassuring voice, distraction techniques, and, when appropriate, medications.

Skill Drill 41-10: Immobilizing an Infant

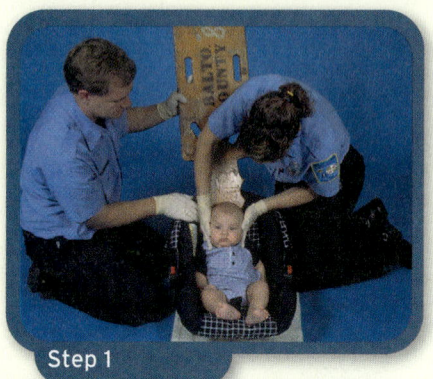

Step 1

Stabilize the head in a neutral position.

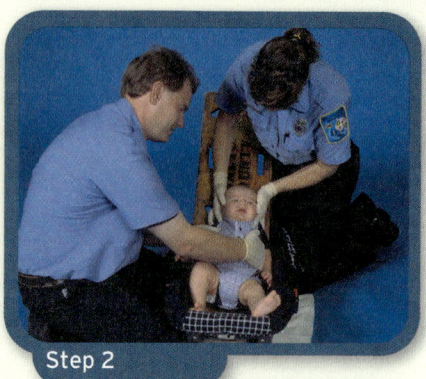

Step 2

Place an immobilization device between the infant and the surface on which he or she is resting.

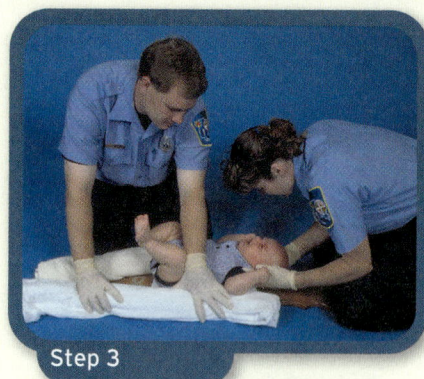

Step 3

Slide the infant onto the board.

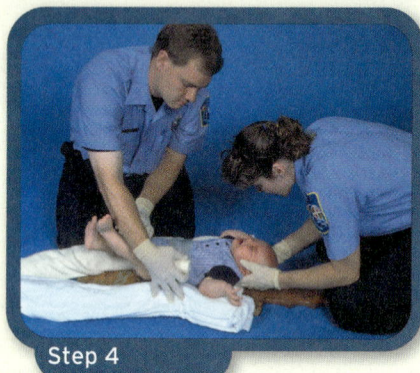

Step 4

Place a towel under the shoulders to ensure neutral head position.

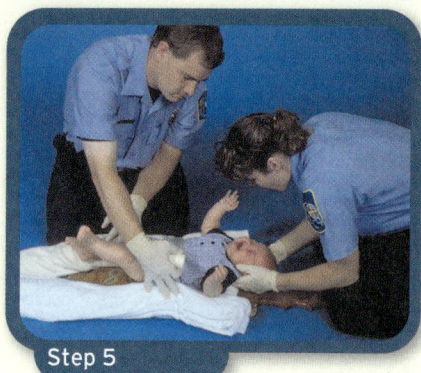

Step 5

Secure the torso first; pad any voids.

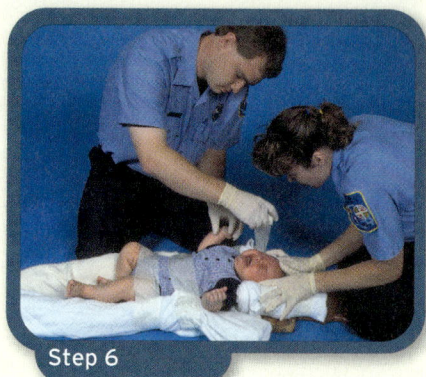

Step 6

Secure the head.

Commonly used pain medications include morphine and fentanyl. Patients who are intubated should receive pain medication and sedation (such as diazepam and midazolam) if they are in hemodynamically stable condition. These medications, which may need to be redosed depending on transport time, can also be used in conjunction with narcotics for patients in stable condition. Side effects of narcotics and benzodiazepines include respiratory depression, hypoxemia, bradycardia, and hypotension.

You must weigh the risks and benefits when deciding to administer these medications. Children who are in shock and hemodynamically unstable condition are not good candidates for narcotics or sedatives; these medications may worsen their already precarious status. All children receiving such medications should be carefully monitored in terms of their pulse rate, respiratory rate, pulse oximetry, and blood pressure.

Burns

The initial assessment and management of pediatric burn victims is similar to that of adults, with a few key differences. The larger skin surface–body mass ratio of children makes them more susceptible to heat and fluid loss. Worrisome patterns of injury or suspicious circumstances should also raise concerns of child abuse.

Assessment

The assessment of scene safety is an important element in a burn call. Check for ongoing dangers such as fire, chemicals, or other hazardous materials. Your from-the-doorway assessment may identify signs of smoke inhalation, such as abnormal airway sounds and respiratory distress, or soot around the nose. Quickly move the patient and crew to a well-ventilated area.

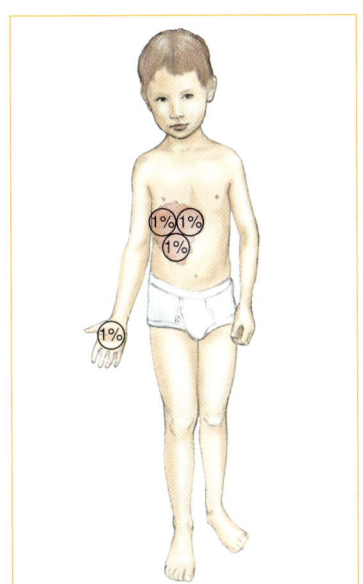

Figure 41-31 Using the child's palm to estimate burned body surface area.

An estimation of the percentage of body surface area burned may affect your decision to start fluid resuscitation in the prehospital environment and influence the transport destination. For adolescents, use the same rule of nines that you use for adult burn victims. For younger children, this rule of nines is modified to account for a child's disproportionately larger head size. For infants, the head and trunk each account for 18% of body surface area, the arms each count as 9%, and the legs each count as 14%. The size of a child's palm (not including fingers) represents about 1% total body surface area. You can also use this rule of palm to assess the extent of the burn **Figure 41-31 ▲**.

Burns suggestive of maltreatment include those in which the mechanism or pattern observed does not match the history or the child's developmental capabilities. For example, a child who cannot stand independently is unlikely to pull a hot cup of coffee off a table. Splash burns—as from tipping over a pot of boiling water—should have an irregular configuration because the hot liquid runs down the child's body. Be suspicious if a burn has clear demarcation lines or is on the buttocks.

Management

Initial management begins with removal of burning clothing and support of the ABCs. If you observe signs of smoke inhalation, consider early intubation. Make sure that you have a range of tubes available because airway edema and sloughing may mandate use of a smaller tube than originally estimated.

All burn victims should be provided 100% supplemental oxygen, regardless of the presence or absence of signs of respiratory distress. Smoke inhalation may cause bronchospasm resulting in wheezing and mild respiratory distress. Consider using a bronchodilator such as salbutamol or epinephrine (SQ or IM).

If possible, insert an IV line and initiate fluid resuscitation in transport for patients with more than 5% of burned body surface area. Start with 20 ml/kg of isotonic fluid, and reassess the need for additional boluses—as large burns can lead to huge fluid shifts.

Clean burned areas minimally to avoid hypothermia, and cover them with clean, dry cloth. Avoid putting lotions or ointments on burned skin because they can trap heat and bacteria. Avoid heat loss by covering the burn and the patient as needed.

Analgesia is a critical part of the early management of burns; these injuries can be incredibly painful. Assess and treat pain and anxiety as discussed previously. Carefully monitor any child given narcotics or benzodiazepines for signs of respiratory or hemodynamic compromise.

Once the patient's condition is stabilized, begin transport to an appropriate medical facility. Larger burns, full-thickness burns, and burns involving the face and neck are best treated at a regional burn centre.

Children With Special Health Care Needs

Children with special health care needs include those with physical, developmental, and learning disabilities. The disabilities have a broad range of causes, including premature birth, traumatic brain injury, congenital anatomical anomalies, and acquired illnesses. Advances in technology and drugs have enabled an increasing number of children with disabilities to receive care in the community, leading to a corresponding increase in the number of EMS calls for this medically complex population.

Technology-Assisted Children
Technology-assisted children constitute a subset of children with special health care needs that may require your assistance. It is important to familiarize yourself with the various types of medical technology that you may encounter and have to troubleshoot.

Tracheostomy Tubes and Artificial Ventilators
Tracheostomy is surgical procedure, involving creation of a stoma—in this case, a permanent connection between the skin of the throat and trachea—through which a tracheostomy tube can be placed for long-term ventilatory needs **Figure 41-32 ▶**. A child might need a tracheostomy for a variety of reasons, including long-term ventilator support for chronic lung disease, inability to protect the airway because of neurologic impairment, and a congenital airway anomaly leading to airway obstruction. Caregivers have been trained in the use and care of their child's tracheostomy and are a source of valuable information. In general, they will have a spare tracheostomy tube available.

At the Scene

Use the rule of palm to estimate the percentage of body surface area burned in a young child or infant: A child's palm is equal to 1% of body surface area.

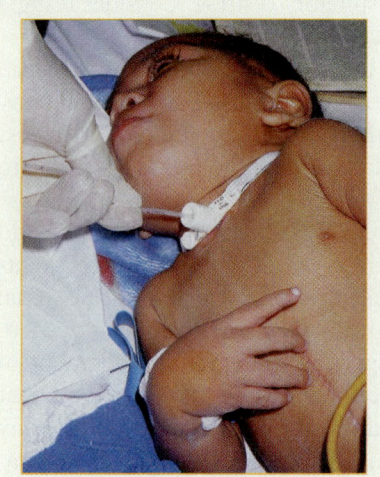

Figure 41-32 A tracheostomy is a surgical opening in the neck into the trachea, creating an artificial airway.

A child with a tracheostomy tube may breathe spontaneously with room air, if the function of the tube is simply to bypass mechanical upper airway obstruction. Alternatively, the child may be dependent on a home ventilator and supplemental oxygen if he or she has severe lung disease or problems with respiratory drive.

Although a tracheostomy tube is intended to provide a secure, permanent airway, problems can arise, as with any mechanical device. The most common problem is obstruction of the tracheostomy tube with secretions, resulting in respiratory distress or respiratory failure. Displacement of the tube is another potential problem. If you are faced with a child with a tracheostomy tube and respiratory distress, start by assessing tube position and suctioning the tube. If the child is using a home ventilator, disconnect the circuit and provide bag-valve-mask ventilation. If these measures fail to lead to improvement or if the child is cyanotic or in severe distress, you may need to remove and replace the tracheostomy tube, preferably using a tube of the same diameter and length. Confirmation of tube position is done in the same manner as for an ET tube.

Gastrostomy Tubes

Gastrostomy tubes (G-tubes) are surgically placed directly into the patient's stomach through the skin Figure 41-33 ▶ . They provide nutrition or medications directly into the stomach, bypassing the oropharynx and esophagus. Some children are unable to take food or medication by mouth and depend on a G-tube for all of their nutrition; for other patients, the tube is used to supplement intake and ensure adequate nutrition.

Problems such as obstruction, dislodgment, or leakage of a G-tube are not uncommon but rarely represent an emergency. Most such calls can be managed by supportive care and transport. Urgent physician evaluation is needed if a G-tube has been pulled out because the opening on the abdominal wall tends to constrict quickly, making replacement difficult.

Central Venous Cannulas

A central venous cannula may be inserted when a child needs long-term IV access for medications or nutrition. Such a device is placed surgically or by interventional radiologists into large central veins, such as the subclavian. Completely implanted central lines, with a port or reservoir accessible under the skin,

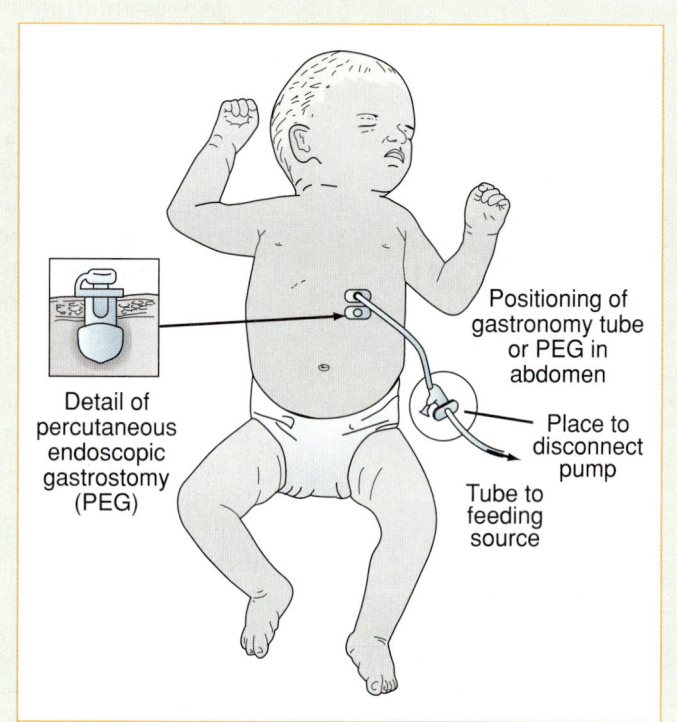

Detail of percutaneous endoscopic gastrostomy (PEG)

Positioning of gastronomy tube or PEG in abdomen

Place to disconnect pump

Tube to feeding source

Figure 41-33 A G-tube is an opening through the skin directly into the stomach.

may be left in place for months to years. For example, they are commonly placed in children with cancer who are undergoing long courses of chemotherapy. Partially implanted central lines have tubing external to the skin.

Complications associated with central venous cannulas include infections, obstruction, and dislodged or broken cannulas. Children with an infection of the central line may have redness, swelling, tenderness, or pus at the skin site of insertion; they may also have systemic signs of infection (such as fever) or signs of septic shock. Central line obstruction may be a medical emergency, depending on what is infusing through the line. If the child is not in urgent need of the infusion, simply assess the patient and transport to a hospital. Dislodged or broken cannulas may result in leakage of fluid or blood. In such a case, use sterile technique to clamp off the broken line to minimize risk of infection or air embolus.

On rare occasions, you will be confronted with a child who has a functioning central line but requires emergency IV access for prehospital treatment. Because these permanent lines carry a high risk for infection, look for peripheral access and avoid using the central line whenever possible.

CSF Shunts

Hydrocephalus is a condition resulting from impaired circulation and absorption of CSF, leading to increased size of the ventricles (fluid-filled spaces in the brain) and increased ICP. Hydrocephalus may be congenital or acquired; it is most commonly seen in children born with brain malformations as a complication of prematurity or following surgery for a brain tumour.

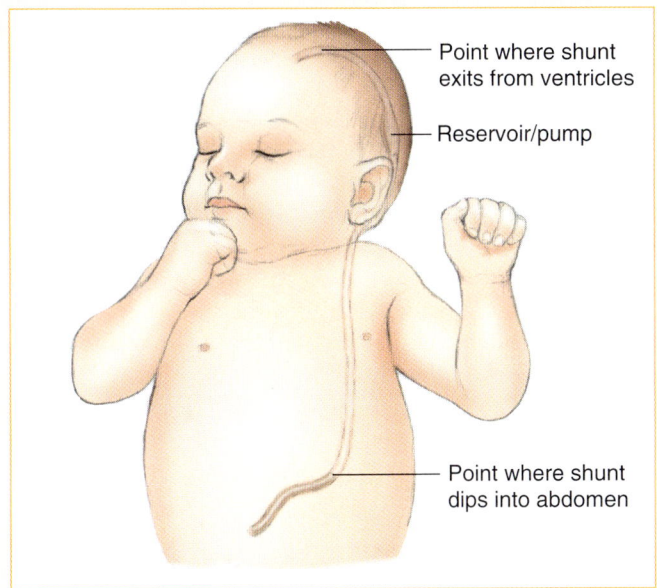

Point where shunt exits from ventricles

Reservoir/pump

Point where shunt dips into abdomen

Figure 41-34 A CSF shunt directs CSF away from the ventricles in the brain to the abdomen to relieve pressure.

Cerebrospinal fluid shunts are inserted to drain excessive fluid from the brain, thereby normalizing ICP Figure 41-34 ▲ . A neurosurgeon places the tube and connects it to a one-way, pressure-sensitive valve that runs from the enlarged ventricle subcutaneously into the abdominal peritoneal space. When pressure builds up in the ventricle, the one-way valve opens, and CSF drains into the peritoneum, where it is reabsorbed.

A CSF shunt obstruction occurs when the drainage of fluid from the brain through the shunt tubing becomes blocked—perhaps due to a break in the tubing, problems with the valve, or buildup of debris in the tubing. Without adequate fluid drainage, the CSF fluid continues to accumulate, resulting in hydrocephalus. A child with a shunt obstruction will show signs of increased ICP, which may range from subtle changes in behaviour to impending brain herniation. Typical symptoms include headache, fatigue, vomiting, and even coma. Late signs include the Cushing's triad (hypertension, bradycardia, respiratory compromise).

A CSF shunt infection results from bacterial contamination during the surgery to place the shunt or from bacteria in the blood adhering to and infecting the hardware. Infections are encountered most frequently within months of shunt surgery. Children with shunt infections are generally very sick and have fever and signs of shunt obstruction.

Shunt obstructions and shunt infections are true medical emergencies. The patient should be transported to appropriate treatment facilities where neurosurgical evaluation is available. The child's condition can deteriorate rapidly, so maintain continuous cardiopulmonary monitoring during transport.

Assessment and Management

Follow the standard pediatric assessment sequence when approaching children with special health care needs. Ask questions of the parent or caregiver to establish the child's baseline level of neurologic function and baseline physiologic status. Meet every child at his or her unique developmental level. An otherwise healthy 10-year-old with a perinatal brain injury may have the developmental skills of a toddler. Conversely, a 6-year-old with severe cardiopulmonary compromise may be ventilator-dependent and have oxygen saturation in the 80s but be cognitively intact.

Your treatment goal is to restore a child to his or her own physiologic baseline, which will require collaboration with caregivers to determine what is normal for the child and management strategies that have been successful in the past.

Special Considerations

Caregivers will be key resources when managing a child with special health care needs. Draw on their expertise to assist you in assessing and managing the child.

Transport

Most children with special health care needs will have a medical home—that is, a hospital, clinic, or private practice where they receive their care. Transporting to a facility where the clinical team is familiar with the patient's history and needs will streamline their care. If this is not possible, take along any medical records available to assist the team at the receiving facility to sort out the potentially complex issues faced by the patient. Take any assistive devices as well, including home ventilators and feeding pumps. Most important, take the parent or caregiver of the child! Children with special health care needs rely on their caregivers for much—if not all—of their care-taking needs, so it can be emotionally difficult for the child to be separated from the caretaker.

Pediatric Mental Health

During your career as a paramedic, you will undoubtedly encounter children with behavioural and psychiatric problems. The call may be for out-of-control behaviour or for a suicide attempt. Unfortunately, EMS calls for behavioural emergencies are increasing, reflecting in part the limited community resources available for children with mental health problems. A recent study of one pediatric ED found that 5% of all pediatric ED visits were for mental health concerns.

Safety

When you are called to a home for a behavioural or psychiatric emergency, safety should be your first priority. Assess the scene for your own safety and for the safety of your patient. If weapons are involved or you cannot determine the degree of risk, call for law enforcement backup.

Approach the child calmly, letting him or her know you are there to help. Address the patient directly when obtaining the history, and explain clearly what you are doing and why. Some children are flight risks, so determine how best to deploy your squad so that they do not leave the scene. As always, answer questions as honestly as possible.

A small percentage of children cannot be safely talked down for transport and must be mechanically restrained for their own protection and the protection of the paramedics. Applying these restraints may be a task for paramedics or for law enforcement personnel. If you decide to apply restraints, carefully document the reason and keep the restraints in place until arrival at the ED. An out-of-control, 27-kg 8-year-old can make a transport dangerous! Try to avoid using chemical restraint (that is, tranquilizing drugs) in the prehospital setting.

Assessment and Management

The PAT will give you a general impression of the child's mental status and cardiovascular stability. A child who has attempted suicide by ingestion may have life-threatening medical complications that trump his or her psychiatric concerns. In the absence of acute medical issues, the bulk of your assessment will be based on observation and history. In cases involving a very agitated child, your hands-on examination may be limited. **Table 41-24 ▼** lists specific SAMPLE questions for

behavioural emergencies. As always, treat any existing medical problems or injuries by using standard protocols.

An Ounce of Prevention

Emergency care for children involves a team approach by health care professionals in the community and in the hospital. Paramedics are a critical part of the community responsible for caring for sick and injured children, but their role in prevention is not always highlighted, even though this is an area where they can have a greater public health impact than possible by running a code or controlling an airway **Figure 41-35 ▼**. To be an effective child safety advocate, you must be knowledgeable about local and national prevention programs.

Prevention of Injuries

Most injuries are not accidents, but rather are predictable and preventable events. Knowledge of injury patterns helps target potential areas for intervention and prevention. For example, childhood poisonings can be prevented by effective storage of medications and chemicals. Toddler drowning and submersion can be virtually eliminated by installation of four-sided pool fencing. The risk of serious injury from a bike collision is lessened

Table 41-24	SAMPLE History for Behavioural Problems in Children	
Component	**Features**
Signs and symptoms	Out-of-control behaviour? Suicidal or homicidal thoughts or actions? Harm to self, others, or pets? Recent change in behaviour? Recent change in medication? Auditory or visual hallucinations?
Allergies	Known food or drug allergies and their reactions
Medications	List of all patient's medications and vitamins, prescribed and over-the-counter
Past medical history	History of any behaviour or psychiatric problems? Therapist, counselor, or psychiatrist contact information? Prior psychiatric or behavioural hospitalizations? Any medical illnesses?
Last oral intake	Timing and identification of last food and drink
Events leading to behavioural problems	Ongoing or new stressors? Argument or fight with boyfriend, girlfriend, or family members?

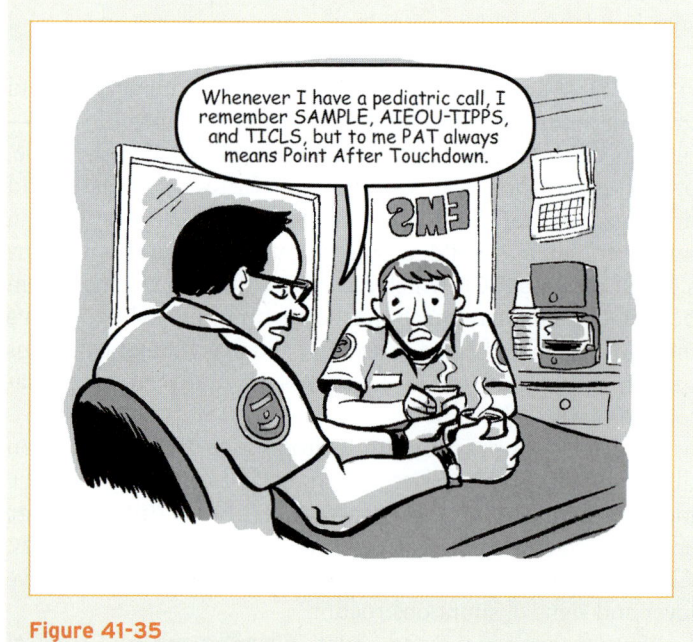

Figure 41-35

by use of a helmet. The morbidity and mortality from motor vehicle collisions is dramatically decreased by the appropriate use of child restraint devices.

As you care for children, you may be frustrated by the illnesses and injuries that you encounter, especially when they are preventable. Take this frustration as a call to action. Get involved in your community. Participate in existing prevention programs or start your own program. Numerous types of pediatric injury can be targeted Table 41-25 ; choose something that interests you, and take a leadership role.

Notes from Nancy

In the seriously injured child, all organ systems must be assumed to be injured until proved otherwise.

Table 41-25	Examples of Common Injuries and Possible Prevention Strategies
Injury	**Preventive Measures**
Vehicle trauma	Infant and child restraint seats Seatbelts and air bags Pedestrian safety programs Motorcycle helmets
Cycling	Bicycle helmets Bicycle paths separate from vehicle traffic
Recreation	Appropriate safety padding and apparel Cyclist, skateboard, and skater safety programs Soft, energy-absorbent playground surfaces
Drowning and submersion	Four-sided locked pool enclosures Pool alarms Immediate adult supervision Caretaker CPR training Swimming lessons Pool and beach safety instruction Personal flotation devices
Poisoning and household injuries	Proper storage of chemicals and medications Child safety packaging
Burns	Proper maintenance and monitoring of electrical appliances and cords Fire and smoke detectors Proper placement of cookware on stove top
Other	Discouragement of infant walker use Gated stairways Babysitter first-aid training Child care worker first-aid training

You are the Paramedic Summary

1. What assessment tool will you use to form your general impression of your patient?

The PAT provides paramedics with a quick hands-off approach to patient assessment. It can provide you with information about your patient in less than 30 seconds and without touching the patient. The three legs of the PAT—appearance, breathing, and circulation—will aid you in determining whether the child is sick or not sick. The PAT will also assist you in figuring out the physiologic status of your patient: Is he or she in respiratory distress or failure; in shock; or experiencing a neurologic problem?

2. What can you do to assist the panicked mother?

If you are a parent, you can probably relate to the fear and panic the mother is experiencing. Your best approach is to let the mother know everything that you are doing as you are doing it. Reassure her that you are doing everything possible to take care of her child, but be careful not to offer false hope by saying "Everything will be okay." Above all, remain calm and in charge of the scene. The mother needs to see that you are confident and secure with what you are doing. If possible, ask the mother to help care for the child and allow her to accompany her child to the hospital.

3. What do you need to carefully monitor your patient for?

Although the patient seems to be in stable condition at this time, he can begin to decompensate at any time without warning. The physical examination revealed a potential head injury, abdominal injury with bleeding, and a fractured femur. Any of these injuries can cause rapid deterioration of the patient's condition. Be alert for further changes in mental status, decline in respiratory status, and signs of shock.

4. Which interventions should you consider at this point, if any?

You have delegated the role of cervical spine immobilization, and the patient is receiving supplemental oxygen. At this time, you can consider establishing IV access, applying a cardiac monitor, applying a cervical collar, and immobilizing the child on a backboard.

5. Is this child in shock? If so, is it compensated or decompensated?

Yes, the child is in shock. Your patient assessment reveals an increased pulse rate, decreased respiratory status, decreased blood pressure, and increased capillary refill. Currently, he is in compensated shock based on the blood pressure, which remains higher than the minimal acceptable blood pressure. The formula for calculating minimal acceptable blood pressure for children younger than 10 years is 70 + (2 × age in years); this patient is 2 years old, so the minimal acceptable blood pressure would be 74 mm Hg.

6. How should your patient management progress?

Once the airway has been secured, you should focus on correcting the problems with circulation. Establish vascular access so you can administer fluids. Time is of the essence, meaning you should not spend a great deal of time trying to secure peripheral IV access. If you experience difficulty trying to find a vein, obtain vascular access using an IO needle. After securing vascular access, administer a fluid bolus at 20 ml/kg.

7. What do you think is the cause for shock in this patient?

This child has two potential causes for shock: abdominal injury with bleeding and a fractured femur. Both injuries could lead to a significant blood loss. Head injury will cause the blood pressure to increase as the pressure within the skull rises.

8. What criteria were used to determine that this patient was a "trauma alert"?

A trauma alert was called for this patient owing to the MOI, potential for a closed head injury, possible abdominal bleeding, and a femoral fracture.

Prep Kit

Ready for Review

- Children differ anatomically, physiologically, and emotionally from adults.
- Sick or injured children present unique challenges in evaluation and management. Their perceptions of their illness or injury, their world, and of paramedics differ from the perceptions of adults.
- The majority of children you treat will come with at least one parent or caregiver. Thus, in many pediatric calls, you will be dealing with more than one patient—even if only the child is ill or injured.
- Serious illness or injury to a child is one of the most stressful situations caregivers can face.
- An assessment tool called the Pediatric Assessment Triangle (PAT) has been developed to help paramedics form a from-the-doorway general impression of pediatric patients.
- Respiratory problems are among the medical emergencies that you will most frequently encounter in children. Pediatric patients with a respiratory chief complaint will span the spectrum from mildly ill to near death.
- In pediatrics, respiratory failure and arrest precede the majority of cardiopulmonary arrests; by contrast, a primary cardiac event is the usual cause of sudden death in adults.
- Cardiovascular emergencies are relatively rare in children. When such problems arise, they are often related to volume or infection rather than to a primary cardiac cause, unless the child has congenital heart disease.
- Through the PAT and initial assessment, you can quickly identify a cardiovascular emergency, understand the likely pathologic cause, and institute potentially lifesaving treatment.
- Pediatric medical calls may include respiratory complaints, fever, seizures, and altered LOC.
- Toxic exposures account for a significant number of pediatric emergencies.
- The sudden death of an apparently healthy baby is devastating to families and the paramedics who respond to the call.
- An apparent life-threatening event (ALTE) is an episode during which an infant becomes pale or cyanotic; chokes, gags, or has an apneic spell; or loses muscle tone.
- Child maltreatment comes in many forms: physical abuse, sexual abuse, emotional abuse, child neglect.
- Pediatric trauma is the leading cause of death among children older than 1 year.
  - Motor vehicle collisions cause the most deaths in this age group, followed by falls and submersions.
  - Among adolescents, homicide and suicide are major causes of death.
- The initial assessment and management of pediatric burn victims is similar to that of adults, with a few key differences.
  - The larger skin surface–body mass ratio of children makes them more susceptible to heat and fluid loss.
  - Worrisome patterns of injury or suspicious circumstances should raise concerns of child maltreatment.
- Children with special health care needs include children with physical, developmental, and learning disabilities.
  - These disabilities have a broad range of causes, including premature birth, traumatic brain injury, congenital anatomical anomalies, and acquired illnesses.
  - Advances in technology and drugs have enabled an increasing number of children with disabilities to receive care in the community, leading to a corresponding increase in the number of EMS calls for this medically complex population.
- During your time as a paramedic, you will undoubtedly encounter children with behavioural and psychiatric problems.
  - The call may be for out-of-control behaviour or for a suicide attempt.
  - EMS calls for behavioural emergencies are increasing, reflecting in part the limited community resources available for children with mental health problems.

Vital Vocabulary

absence seizures The type of seizures characterized by a brief lapse of attention in which the patient may stare and not respond.

acrocyanosis Cyanosis of the extremities.

apparent life-threatening event (ALTE) An unexpected sudden episode of colour change, tone change, or apnea that requires mouth-to-mouth resuscitation or vigorous stimulation.

blow-by technique A method of delivering oxygen by holding a face mask or similar device near an infant's or a child's face; used when a nonrebreathing mask is not tolerated.

bronchiolitis A condition seen in children younger than 2 years, characterized by dyspnea and wheezing.

central venous cannula A cannula inserted into the vena cava to permit intermittent or continuous monitoring of central venous pressure and to facilitate obtaining blood samples for chemical analysis.

cerebrospinal fluid shunts Tubes that drain fluid manufactured in the ventricles of the brain from the subarachnoid space to another part of the body outside of the brain, such as the peritoneum; lowers pressure in the brain.

complex febrile seizures An unusual form of seizures that occurs in association with a rapid increase in body temperature.

complex partial seizures Seizures characterized by alteration of consciousness with or without complex focal motor activity.

cricoid pressure The application of posterior pressure to the cricoid cartilage; minimizes gastric distension and the risk of vomiting and aspiration during ventilation; also referred to as the Sellick maneuver.

croup A childhood viral disease characterized by edema of the upper airways with barking cough, difficult breathing, and stridor.

cyanosis Slightly bluish, greyish, slatelike, or dark purple discolouration of the skin due to hypoxia.

epiglottitis Inflammation of the epiglottis.

generalized seizures The seizures characterized by manifestations that indicate involvement of both cerebral hemispheres.

grunting A short, low-pitched sound at the end of exhalation, present in children with moderate to severe hypoxia; reflects poor gas exchange because of fluid in the lower airways and air sacs.

head bobbing A sign of increased work of breathing in which the head lifts and tilts back during inspiration, then moves forward during expiration.

hydrocephalus The increased accumulation of cerebrospinal fluid within the ventricles of the brain.

meningitis Inflammation of the membranes of the spinal cord or brain.

Mongolian spots Blue-grey areas of discolouration of the skin caused by abnormal pigment, not by trauma or bruising.

mottling A condition of abnormal skin circulation, caused by vasoconstriction or inadequate circulation.

nasal flaring The flaring out of the nostrils, indicating increased work of breathing and hypoxia.

neonatal period The first month of life.

nuchal rigidity A stiff or painful neck; commonly associated with meningitis.

obtunded A condition when the patient is dulled to pain and sensation.

ossification centres Areas where cartilage is transformed through calcification into a new area of bone.

osteomyelitis Inflammation of the bone due to infection; a potential complication of intraosseous infusion.

pallor Lack of colour; paleness.

Pediatric Assessment Triangle (PAT) An assessment tool that allows rapid formation of a general impression of the type and level of illness or injury in an infant or child without touching him or her; consists of assessing appearance, work of breathing, and circulation to the skin.

petechial Characterized by small purplish, nonblanching spots on the skin.

purpuric Pertaining to bruising of the skin.

respiratory arrest The absence of respirations with detectable cardiac activity.

respiratory distress A clinical state characterized by increased respiratory rate, effort, and work of breathing.

respiratory failure A clinical state of inadequate oxygenation, ventilation, or both.

respiratory syncytial virus (RSV) A virus that commonly causes bronchiolitis; usually results in lifelong immunity following exposure.

retractions Physical drawing in of the chest wall between the ribs that occurs with increased work of breathing.

rhonchi Rattling respiratory sounds; also called crackles.

sepsis A pathologic state, usually in a febrile patient, resulting from the presence of invading microorganisms or their poisonous products in the bloodstream.

shaken baby syndrome A syndrome seen in abused infants and children; the patient has been subjected to violent, whiplash-type shaking injuries inflicted by the abusing individual that may cause coma, seizures, and increased intracranial pressure due to tearing of the cerebral veins with consequent bleeding into the brain.

simple febrile seizures A brief, self-limited, generalized seizure in a previously healthy child between the ages of 6 months and 6 years that is associated with the onset of or sudden increase in fever.

simple partial seizures Focal seizures that involve a motor or sensory abnormality in a patient who remains conscious.

sinus tachycardia Rapid heart rate in a child with normal conduction.

sniffing position An upright position in which the patient's head and chin are thrust slightly forward to keep the airway open; appears to be sniffing.

status epilepticus A state of continuous seizures or multiple seizures without a return to consciousness for 20 minutes.

stoma A small opening, especially an artificially created opening, such as that made by tracheostomy.

stridor A harsh sound during inspiration, high-pitched due to partial upper airway obstruction.

subglottic space The narrowest part of the pediatric airway.

sudden infant death syndrome (SIDS) The abrupt and unexplained death of an apparently healthy child younger than 1 year.

supraventricular tachycardia (SVT) An abnormal heart rhythm with a rapid, narrow QRS complex.

synchronized cardioversion The timed delivery of energy into the myocardium to correct rapid, regular cardiac rhythms in patients who are in unstable condition.

tonic–clonic seizures Seizures that feature rhythmic back-and-forth motion of an extremity and body stiffness.

tripoding An abnormal position to keep the airway open; involves leaning forward onto two arms stretched forward.

vasoconstriction A decrease in the calibre of blood vessels.

ventilation-perfusion mismatch A pathologic state in which the oxygen entering the lungs is not mixing properly with the blood circulating through the lungs.

wheezing The production of whistling sounds during expiration such as occurs in asthma and bronchiolitis.

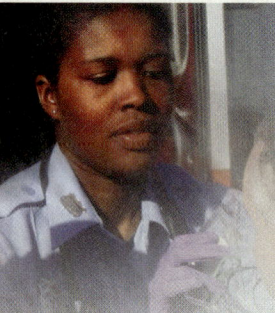

Assessment in Action

You arrive on the scene of a 6-year-old girl having difficulty breathing. Your assessment reveals that she is breathing about 40 times per minute. Her chest muscles seem to be tight and sunken between her ribs. She appears to be working very hard to breathe, and you hear grunting sounds, but the patient's skin colour and mentation seem within normal limits.

1. **Which phase of physiologic response is this patient in?**
   A. Respiratory distress
   B. Respiratory failure
   C. Respiratory arrest
   D. Cardiac arrest

2. **A child who appears to be sleepy or drowsy in addition to having difficulty breathing is called:**
   A. obtuse.
   B. obstructed.
   C. obtunded.
   D. objective.

3. **A child who uses chest muscles to help breathe is said to be using:**
   A. excessive muscles.
   B. accessory muscles.
   C. retractive muscles.
   D. tripod muscles.

4. **When counting the respiratory rate in a pediatric patient, count chest rise for:**
   A. 10 seconds and multiply by 6.
   B. 15 seconds and multiply by 4.
   C. 30 seconds and multiply by 2.
   D. a full 60 seconds.

5. **Which phase of physiologic response represents the point at which the patient will decompensate?**
   A. Respiratory distress
   B. Respiratory failure
   C. Respiratory arrest
   D. Cardiac arrest

6. **What is the best way to manage a pediatric patient in respiratory arrest?**
   A. Face mask with oxygen at 15 l/min
   B. Bag-valve-mask ventilation with oxygen at 15 l/min
   C. ET tube with bag-valve-mask ventilation
   D. Chest compressions, ET tube with bag-valve-mask ventilation

Challenging Question

7. **Why are pediatric patients more likely to have respiratory arrest before cardiac arrest?**

Points to Ponder

You have been dispatched to provide prehospital care for a pediatric patient who has a low oxygen saturation level. During your response, you wonder how this call came in for a specific problem like "low oxygen saturation level," so you ask your dispatcher to find out more about the call. The dispatcher reports that the call came from the child's mother. When you arrive at the scene, you find a child lying on a bed. The patient is connected to a number of tubes, and you notice a tracheostomy tube in place. The mother states that his saturation level is lower than normal and she is concerned that one of the drains is not working. When you look around the room, you realize that you are not familiar with any of the equipment present.

What is the best way to proceed with your assessment and treatment of this child?

Issues: Technology-Assisted Children, Work of Breathing, Airway Obstruction.

42 Geriatrics

Competency Areas

Area 2: Communication

2.1.f   Speak in language appropriate to the listener.
2.3.c   Establish trust and rapport with patients and colleagues.
2.3.d   Recognize and react appropriately to non-verbal behaviours.
2.4.g   Exhibit diplomacy, tact, and discretion.

Area 5: Therapeutics

5.1.a   Use manual maneuvers and positioning to maintain airway patency.
5.7.a   Immobilize suspected fractures involving appendicular skeleton.
5.7.b   Immobilize suspected fractures involving axial skeleton.

Area 6: Integration

6.2.c   Provide care for geriatric patient.
6.3.a   Conduct ongoing assessments based on patient presentation and interpret findings.
6.3.b   Re-direct priorities based on assessment findings.

Appendix 4: Pathophysiology

A.   **Cardiovascular System**
Cardiac Conduction Disorder: Benign arrhythmias
Cardiac Conduction Disorder: Lethal arrhythmias
Cardiac Conduction Disorder: Life-threatening arrhythmias

B.   **Neurologic System**
Altered Mental Status: Metabolic
Altered Mental Status: Structural
Chronic Neurologic Disorders: Alzheimer's
Chronic Neurologic Disorders: Parkinson's disease

C.   **Respiratory System**
Medical Illness: Chronic obstructive pulmonary disorder
Medical Illness: Pneumonia/bronchitis
Medical Illness: Pulmonary embolism

E.   **Gastrointestinal System**
Esophagus/Stomach: Obstruction
Esophagus/Stomach: Peptic ulcer disease
Esophagus/Stomach: Upper gastrointestinal bleed
Small/Large Bowel: Lower gastrointestinal bleed

G.   **Integumentary System**
Infectious and Inflammatory Illness: Infections

H.   **Musculoskeletal System**
Inflammatory Disorders: Arthritis
Inflammatory Disorders: Osteoporosis

I.   **Endocrine System**
Diabetes mellitus
Electrolyte imbalances
Thyroid disease

J.   **Multisystem Diseases and Injuries**
Toxicologic Illness: Prescription medication
Toxicologic Illness: Non-prescription medication
Toxicologic Illness: Alcohols
Environmental Disorders: Hyperthermal injuries
Environmental Disorders: Hypothermal injuries
Trauma: Falls

K.   **Psychiatric Disorders**
Affective Disorders: Depressive disorders
Affective Disorders: Suicidal ideation
Psychosocial Disorders: Antisocial disorder

Appendix 5: Medications

A.   **Medications affecting the central nervous system.**
A.5   Anxiolytics, hypnotics, and antagonists
A.8   Opioid analgesics
B.   **Medications affecting the autonomic nervous system.**
B.4   Cholinergic antagonists
B.5   Antihistamines
D.   **Medications affecting the cardiovascular system.**
D.2   Cardiac Glycosides
D.5   Class 2 Antidysrhythmics
E.   **Medications affecting blood clotting mechanisms.**
E.1   Anticoagulants
H.   **Medications used to treat electrolyte and substrate imbalances.**
H.2   Antihypoglycemic agents
I.   **Medications used to treat/prevent inflammatory responses and infections.**
I.1   Corticosteroids
I.2   NSAID
I.3   Antibiotics
J.   **Medications used to treat poisoning and overdose.**
J.1   Antidotes or neutralizing agents
K.   **Psychiatric Disorders**
Cognitive Disorders: Delirium
L.   **Ears, Eyes, Nose, and Throat**
Eyes—Medical Illness: Cataracts
Eyes—Medical Illness: Glaucoma

Introduction

Geriatrics is the assessment and treatment of disease in someone 65 years or older. In 2003, elderly Canadians accounted for 13% of the population; this percentage is expected to grow to 22%, largely driven by aging of the "baby boomers" (born in the period 1946–1964). Furthermore, the elderly population is itself growing older. The most rapidly growing segment of the Canadian population is people 85 years and older.

Elderly people constitute an ever-increasing proportion of patients in the health care system, particularly the emergency care sector. Individuals 65 years of age and older account for one third of all hospitalizations, and more than one half of all hospital stays. People are receiving more of their care out of hospital, and with insurance issues, this trend will continue in the future. This population also has more contacts with doctors than those under 65 years of age.

The old-age dependency ratio depicts the dependency individuals place upon society as they age. It is defined as the number of older people for every 100 adults (potential caregivers) between the ages of 18 and 64. In 1990, there were 20 older people for every 100 "caregivers." By 2025, it is projected that there will be 32 older people for every 100 "caregivers." The supply of caregivers is not keeping pace with the growth of the older population. The need for caregivers is going to increase, and society is going to have difficulty keeping up with the demand for services as the population continues to age. As the older population grows, paramedics will be required to offer services that are cost effective and efficient. Insurance regulations, costs associated with providing care, and facility issues will make cost a continuing concern.

Most of your geriatric patients will not reside in nursing homes. Although nursing home admissions are increasing owing to the larger number of older persons in Canada, a countertrend is for elderly people to maintain independent lives. Many older adults continue to live at home with support from a spouse or family member and a visiting nurse; others live in a more dependent care environment such as a senior centre facility. Still others may seek an assisted-living facility or a total care nursing home.

Determining how and where older adults will spend their retirement years is a difficult and complex process involving numerous social and economic issues such as the person's marital status, financial resources, religious beliefs, ethnicity, sex, and general health. Because such decisions may place a burden on family members, their wishes must be considered by health care providers. When making these decisions, older adults and their families can seek advice from medical social workers, professional care managers, discharge planners at health care facilities, and a large number of private and public resources. The range of services available includes delivered meals, personal care, housekeeping, adult day care, transportation, caregiver support, respite care, and emergency response systems, including EMS services and lifelines **Figure 42-1 ▶**.

Psychosocial factors may influence successful aging. For example, at retirement, a person may no longer feel useful or productive in society and may experience diminished self-esteem. Age also brings bereavement—sadness over the loss of friends and loved ones. Notably, the likelihood of death increases during the year following the death of one's spouse. As friends and family die, elderly persons tend to experience increasing loneliness and isolation—factors shown to have negative effects on health.

Finally, the health problems of older people are quantitatively and qualitatively different from the problems of younger people. One cannot simply transfer the principles of caring for

You are the Paramedic Part 1

You have been assigned to orient a newly hired paramedic, Mike, who graduated paramedic school 7 months ago. Your focus for the day has been on geriatric emergencies because your territory provides service to six nursing homes and assisted-living facilities. As luck would have it, your unit is dispatched to one of the smaller community nursing homes for a sick person.

Upon arrival you are escorted to the day room where the residents spend most of their time. A nurse sitting next to a patient seated in a wheelchair by the window waves you over. She introduces you to Mrs. Howard, a frail-appearing 86-year-old widow. The nurse explains that Mrs. Howard has been running a low-grade fever since last evening and is "not acting like her normal self." The physician has requested that she be transferred to the hospital to be evaluated. When asked how she is feeling, Mrs. Howard slowly turns her head away from the window toward you and replies "not well."

Initial Assessment	Recording Time: 0 Minutes
Appearance	Frail, weak, elderly woman
Level of consciousness	A (Alert to person, place, and day)
Airway	Open and clear
Breathing	Adequate chest rise and volume
Circulation	Strong, rapid radial pulse, slightly irregular

1. Why is it important to review common medical problems of elderly people?
2. Which organ systems are greatly affected by age-related changes?

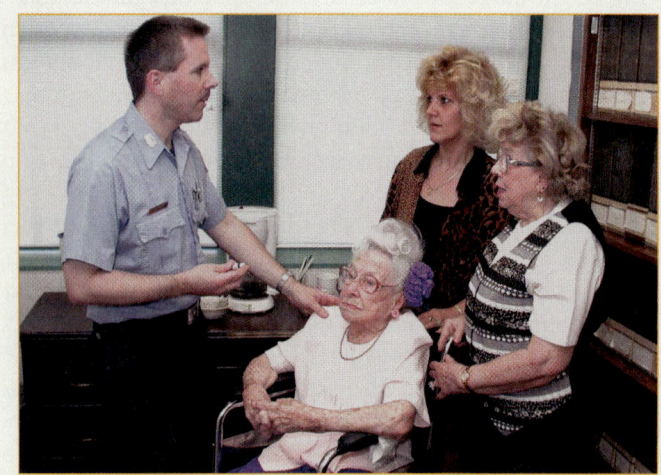

Figure 42-1 EMS professionals should be familiar with available resources.

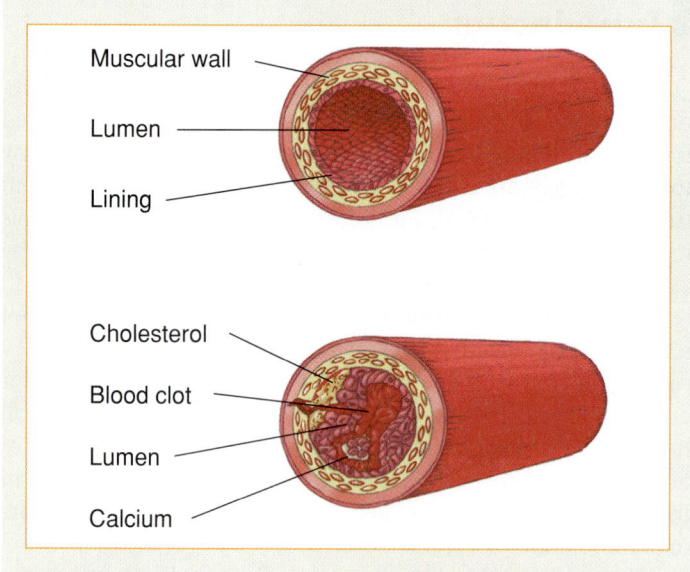

Figure 42-3 Atherosclerosis, the buildup of fatty plaque on arterial walls.

the younger population without modification. The special problems of older people require special approaches.

Anatomy and Physiology

Human growth and development peaks in the late 20s and early 30s, at which point the aging process sets in. Aging is a *linear* process; that is, the rate at which we lose functions does not increase with age. A 35-year-old is aging just as fast as an 85-year-old, but the older person exhibits the cumulative results of a longer process. Of course, the aging process can vary dramatically from one person to another. Most of us can report having seen 60-year-olds who look frail and elderly and 80-year-olds who run marathons **Figure 42-2 ◄** .

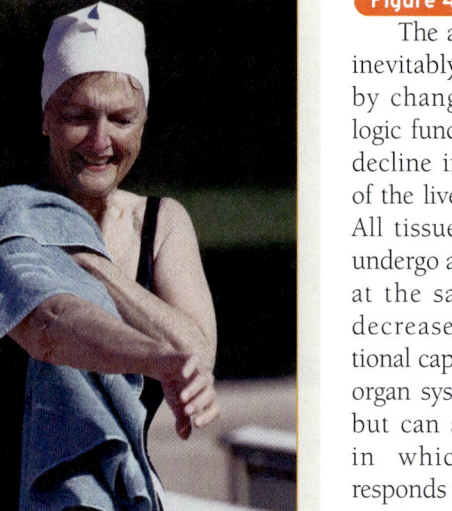

Figure 42-2 Many older people, especially those who have hobbies and activities, are healthy and vital.

The aging process is inevitably accompanied by changes in physiologic function, such as a decline in the function of the liver and kidneys. All tissues in the body undergo aging, albeit not at the same rate. The decrease in the functional capacity of various organ systems is normal but can affect the way in which a patient responds to illness.

It can also affect the way health professionals respond to a patient's illness. For example, a health care provider who is unaware of the normal changes of aging may mistake the changes for signs of illness and be tempted to give treatment when none is necessary. At the other end of the spectrum, there is a widespread—and unfortunate—tendency to attribute genuine disease symptoms to "just getting old" and to neglect their treatment.

Changes in the Cardiovascular System

A variety of changes occur in the cardiovascular system as a person grows older, with their net effect being to decrease the efficiency of this system. Specifically, the heart hypertrophies (enlarges) with age, probably in response to the chronically increased afterload imposed by stiffened blood vessels. Bigger is not better, however. Over time, cardiac output declines, mostly as a result of a decreasing stroke volume. Arteriosclerosis—the stiffening of vessel walls—contributes to systolic hypertension in many older patients, which places an extra burden on the heart. This phenomenon may be a consequence of disease states such as diabetes, atherosclerosis **Figure 42-3 ▲** , and renal compromise, and it is associated with an increased risk of cardiovascular disease, dementia, and death. Compliance of vascular walls depends on the production of collagen and elastin, proteins that are the primary components of muscle and connective tissue. An increase in pressure (normal hypertension seen in aging) leads to overproduction of abnormal collagen and decreased quantities of elastin, both of which contribute to vascular stiffening. The result is a widening pulse pressure, decreased coronary artery perfusion, and changes in cardiac ejection efficiency.

At the same time, the electric conduction system of the heart deteriorates over time. For example, the number of pacemaker cells in the sinoatrial node decreases dramatically as a person ages. In many cases, the changes in the conduction system lead to bradycardia, which can in turn contribute to the decline in cardiac output.

Some changes in cardiovascular performance are probably not a direct consequence of aging, but rather reflect the deconditioning effect of a sedentary lifestyle. Whether because of other disabilities (such as arthritis) or for psychological reasons, many people tend to limit physical activity as they grow older. The bodybuilder's slogan, "Use it or lose it," applies just as much to the cardiac muscle as to the biceps.

Changes in the Respiratory System

A person's respiratory capacity also undergoes significant reductions with age, largely due to decreases in the elasticity of the lungs and in the size and strength of the respiratory muscles. In addition, calcification of costochondral cartilage tends to make the chest wall stiffer. As a result of these changes, the vital capacity (the amount of air that can be exhaled following a maximal inhalation) decreases, and the residual volume (the amount of air left in the lungs at the end of a maximal exhalation) increases. Thus, although the total amount of air in the lungs does not change with age, the proportion of that air usefully used in gas exchange progressively declines. Air flow, which depends largely on airway size and resistance, also deteriorates somewhat with age.

Meanwhile, changes in the distribution of blood flow within the lungs result in declining Pa_{O_2}. At age 30, the Pa_{O_2} of a healthy person breathing ambient air is usually around 90 mm Hg; at 80 years, the Pa_{O_2} under the same conditions is around 75 mm Hg (Pa_{O_2} = 100 − age/3). Furthermore, the respiratory drive becomes dulled as a person ages because of decreased sensitivity to changes in arterial blood gases or decreased central nervous system (CNS) response to such changes. As a consequence, elderly people have a slower reaction to hypoxemia and hypercarbia.

Musculoskeletal changes, such as kyphosis (outward curvature of the thoracic spine; also called hunchback), may also affect pulmonary function by limiting lung volume and maximal inspiratory pressure. In addition, the lung's defence mechanisms become less effective as a natural consequence of aging. The cough and gag reflexes decrease with age, increasing the risk of aspiration. Furthermore, the ciliary mechanisms that normally help remove bronchial secretions are markedly slowed.

Changes in the Renal System

Age brings changes in the kidneys as well. The kidneys are responsible for maintaining the body's fluid and electrolyte balance and have important roles in maintaining the body's long-term acid-base balance and eliminating drugs from the body. In a young adult, the kidneys weigh 250 to 270 g; in a healthy 70-year-old, they weigh 180 to 200 g. This decline in weight results from a loss of functioning nephron units, which translates into a smaller effective filtering surface. At the same time, renal blood flow decreases by as much as 50% as a person ages.

Although the kidneys of an elderly person may be capable of dealing with day-to-day demands, they may not be able to meet unusual challenges, such as those imposed by illness. For that reason, acute illness in elderly patients is often accompanied by derangements in fluid and electrolyte balance. Aging kidneys, for example, respond sluggishly to sodium deficiency. An elderly patient may lose a great deal of sodium before the

You are the Paramedic Part 2

Recognizing an opportunity to complement your earlier review of elderly emergencies with hands-on experience, you ask Mike to begin a physical examination while your partner obtains a set of vital signs. The nurse caring for your patient is new to the facility and is not very familiar with her. She is able to tell you that your patient has a history of atrial fibrillation, congestive heart failure, diabetes, and hypertension. She is currently prescribed digoxin, pioglitazone (Actos), enalapril (Vasotec), and simvastatin (Zocor).

While you are speaking with the nurse, another patient approaches you and sets her hand on your patient's shoulder. She introduces herself as Mrs. Jessup, a good friend of Mrs. Howard. She tells you that it is normal for them to go for a walk every night after dinner; however, they have not walked for the past couple of evenings because Mrs. Howard has been feeling weak. She also volunteers that Mrs. Howard has not been eating much the past few days. Mrs. Howard brushes off her friend's concerns. You are able to ascertain from Mrs. Howard that the last meal she had was a bowl of soup yesterday at lunch.

Vital Signs	Recording Time: 5 Minutes
Level of consciousness	Alert
Pulse	110 beats/min, strong and irregular
Blood pressure	168/94 mm Hg
Respirations	22 breaths/min, regular
Skin	Hot, pink, and dry
Sp_{O_2}	93% on room air

3. Why might obtaining an accurate medical history and history of the present illness be challenging when interviewing an elderly patient?

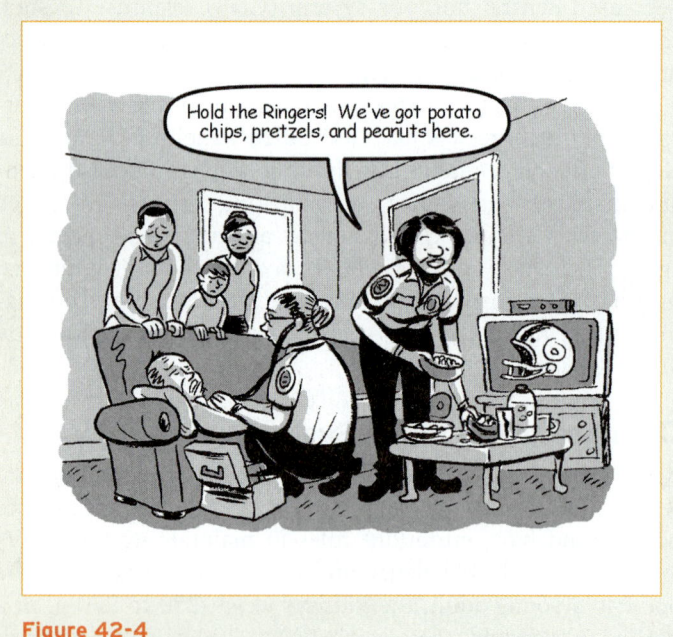

Figure 42-4

kidneys halt urinary sodium excretion, a problem that is exacerbated by the markedly decreased thirst mechanism in elderly people. The net result may be a rapid development of severe dehydration.

Conversely, elderly patients are at considerable risk of overhydration if they are exposed to large sodium loads (such as from intravenous [IV] saline solutions or heavily salted foods) **Figure 42-4 ▲** . Because of its lower glomerular filtration rate, the aging kidney is less able than its younger counterpart to excrete a large sodium load, making the patient vulnerable to acute volume overload.

The same factors that reduce an older person's ability to handle sodium also affect the body's ability to handle potassium. Thus, elderly patients are prone to hyperkalemia, which can reach serious—even lethal—levels if the patient becomes acidotic or if the potassium load is increased from any source.

Bowel and bladder continence require anatomically correct gastrointestinal (GI) and genitourinary tracts, functioning and intact sphincters, and properly working cognitive and physical functions. Urinary incontinence (involuntary loss of urine) can have significant social and emotional impact, but relatively few people admit to the problem and even fewer seek treatment. Incontinence is not a normal part of aging and can lead to skin irritation, skin breakdown, and urinary tract infections. As people age, the capacity of the bladder decreases. As a consequence, an older person may find it difficult to postpone voiding or may have involuntary bladder contractions. Two major types of incontinence are distinguished: stress and urge. Stress incontinence occurs during activities such as coughing, laughing, sneezing, lifting, and exercise. Urge incontinence is triggered by hot or cold fluids, running water, and even thinking about going to the bathroom. Treatment of incontinence consists of medications, physical therapy, and, possibly, surgery.

The opposite of incontinence is urinary retention or difficulty urinating. Patients may have difficulty voiding or absence of voiding as a result of many medical causes. In men, enlargement of the prostate can place pressure on the urethra, making voiding difficult. Bladder and urinary tract infections can also cause inflammation. In severe cases of urinary retention, patients may have acute or chronic renal failure.

Changes in the Digestive System

The process of digestion begins in the mouth, which is also where aging-related changes in the digestive system may first be noted. A decrease in the number of taste buds and changes in olfactory receptors may diminish an older person's senses of taste and smell, which may in turn interfere with the enjoyment of food. The consequent decrease in appetite may lead to malnutrition. Other changes in the mouth include a reduction in the volume of saliva, with a resulting dryness of the mouth. Dental loss is *not* a normal result of the aging process, but rather the result of disease of the teeth and gums; nevertheless, dental loss is widespread in the elderly population and contributes to nutritional and digestive problems.

Like oral secretions, gastric secretions are reduced as a person ages—although enough acid is still present to produce ulcers under certain conditions. Changes in gastric motility also occur, which may lead to slower gastric emptying—a factor of some importance when assessing the risk of aspiration.

Function of the small and large bowel changes little as a consequence of aging, although the incidence of certain diseases involving the bowel (such as diverticulosis) increases as a person grows older.

In the liver, there are changes in hepatic enzyme systems, with some systems declining in activity and others increasing. Notably, the activity of the enzyme systems concerned with the detoxification of drugs *declines* as a person ages.

Changes in the Musculoskeletal System

Aging brings a widespread decrease in bone mass in men and women, but especially among postmenopausal women. Bones become more brittle and tend to break more easily. Narrowing of the intervertebral disks and compression fractures of the vertebrae contribute to a decrease in height as a person ages, along with changes in posture. Joints lose their flexibility and may be further immobilized by arthritic changes. In fact, more than half of all elderly people have some form of arthritis. Muscle mass decreases throughout the body, with an accompanying decrease in muscle strength. From your perspective, the

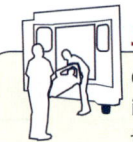

At the Scene

Growing old does not naturally or normally include confusion, dementia, delirium, depression, falls, weakness, syncope, and other conditions related to disease processes.

changes in the musculoskeletal system most often translate into fractures incurred as the result of falls.

Changes in the Nervous System

Aging produces changes in the nervous system that are reflected in the neurologic examination. Changes in thinking (cognitive) speed, memory, and postural stability are the most common normal findings in older people. Studies have documented age-associated declines in mental function, especially slower central processing of sensory stimuli and language, and longer retrieval times for short- and long-term memory. Collectively, these changes affect performance on the mental status portion of the neurologic examination, with common findings including slow responses to questioning or requests to repeat a question.

The brain decreases in terms of weight (5% to 10%) and volume as a person ages. The functional significance of these changes is not clear, however. The human brain has an enormous reserve capacity, and having a smaller and lighter brain does not interfere with the mental capabilities of productive elderly people.

Undeniably, though, the performance of most of the sense organs suffers with increasing age. The senses of taste and smell become diminished as a person ages.

Visual changes may begin as early as 40 years, such that as many as 50% of patients older than 65 years have vision problems. Causes of visual impairment in elderly people may include diabetic retinopathy and age-related macular degeneration.

The two most common causes of visual disturbances in elderly people, however, are cataracts and glaucoma. Cataracts are a result of hardening of the lenses over time. The lenses eventually become opaque, which prevents light and images from being transmitted to the rear of the eye. Patients with cataracts may complain of blurred vision, double vision, spots, and/or ghost images. Surgical repair may be required to gain vision. By contrast, glaucoma is caused by an increase in intraocular pressure severe enough to damage the optic nerve, potentially resulting in permanent loss of peripheral and central vision. Treatment of glaucoma consists of oral medications and eye drops.

Decreases in visual acuity are common in older people, even without disease processes such as cataracts. Night vision becomes impaired, as does the ability to adjust to rapid changes in lighting conditions, depth perception, and perception of colour. Changes in a patient's vision can affect independence, ability to read, and ability to drive a vehicle.

The possibility of hearing loss increases with age. A common cause of hearing impairment in geriatric patients is presbycusis, a progressive hearing loss, particularly in the high frequencies, along with lessened ability to discriminate between a particular sound and background noise. Patients who lose the ability to interpret most speech experience a decreased ability to communicate, which may lead to isolation and depression.

Another hearing-related impairment noted in the elderly population is Meniere disease (prevalence, 2 people per 1,000 population). Onset of symptoms usually occurs in early

Special Considerations
With patients who have some degree of hearing loss, don't yell! Lean closer and speak into the patient's ear using a somewhat low pitch. Remember that patients with limited vision are not necessarily hard of hearing.

middle age, with symptoms presenting in cycles that last several months at a time. The typical symptoms include vertigo (a sudden loss of normal balance or equilibrium), hearing loss, tinnitus, and pressure in the ear.

For many older people, physiologic changes make it difficult to produce speech that is loud enough, clear, and well spaced. Weakness, paralysis, poor hearing, or brain damage can damage the delicate functions that make these abilities possible.

Sense of body position (proprioception) also becomes impaired with age. Proprioception enables us to maintain postural stability by using a variety of receptors in the joints and information provided by the eyes. As these mechanisms fail with age, people become less steady on their feet, and the tendency to fall increases markedly.

Changes in the Integumentary System

Wrinkling and loss of resiliency of the skin are the most visible signs of aging. Wrinkling occurs because the skin becomes thinner, drier, less elastic, and more fragile. Subcutaneous fat becomes thinner, making for a loosened outer cover for the body. Elastin (the substance that makes the skin pliable) and collagen (the substance that makes the skin strong) decrease with age. Thinner skin tears much more easily, and the loss of elasticity allows for more bleeding before tamponade occurs.

As a person ages, the sebaceous glands produce less oil, making dryer skin. Sweat gland activity also decreases, hindering the ability to sweat and to regulate heat. Hair follicles produce thinner hair or may stop producing hair. Follicles produce less melanin (the pigment that gives hair colour), making the hair colour revert to grey or white.

The blood vessels that supply the skin also are affected by atherosclerosis and provide less oxygenated blood at the cellular level. As a consequence of the skin's lower metabolism, epidermal cells develop more slowly and do not replace outgoing cells as quickly as with younger skin. Elderly patients, therefore, are at higher risk for secondary infection after the skin breaks, for skin tumours, and for fungal or viral infections of the skin.

Homeostatic and Other Changes

Homeostasis is the process by which the body maintains a constant internal environment. Many homeostatic mechanisms work on a feedback principle, much like the thermostat in a house—that is, a change in the internal environment feeds back to the control system to induce a corrective response. For example, when the body temperature starts to rise, temperature sensors are activated, which in turn activate compensatory responses: Cutaneous blood vessels dilate, and excess heat is transferred from the body to the environment. Similarly, when the concentration of glucose in the blood rises, the pancreas is stimulated to secrete insulin, which leads to uptake of glucose by cells and reduction of the blood glucose level back toward normal.

Across the board, aging is accompanied by a progressive loss of these homeostatic capabilities. For that reason, a specific illness or injury in elderly people is more likely to result in generalized deterioration. For example, the thirst mechanism, which ordinarily protects a person from dehydration, becomes depressed in elderly patients. Likewise, temperature-regulating mechanisms tend to become disordered, which makes elderly patients much more vulnerable to environmental stresses such as heat exhaustion and accidental hypothermia after relatively minor exposures. A defect in temperature regulation also may account for the absence of a febrile response to illness in many elderly people. Infections that would ordinarily produce high fever, such as pneumococcal pneumonia, may produce only a low-grade or no fever in elderly people.

Notes from Nancy

A specific illness or injury in the elderly is more likely to result in generalized deterioration.

The regulatory system that manages the blood glucose level similarly becomes impaired with increasing age, such that an elevated blood glucose level occurs quite commonly in older patients. Ordinarily, moderate hyperglycemia does no harm, but overly aggressive treatment of this problem may produce damaging hypoglycemia.

Pathophysiology

Cardiovascular System

Diseases of the heart remain the leading cause of death among older adults in Canada, and coronary artery disease (CAD) is the number one culprit. Heart attack is the major cause of morbidity and mortality in people older than 65 years, and its potential for mortality increases significantly after a person reaches 70 years **Figure 42-5 ▶**.

Myocardial infarction (MI) is the death of part of the heart muscle due to the blockage of one of the coronary arteries. Although chest pain is a common presentation for acute myocardial infarction in older patients, it may be decreased in intensity or atypical. In fact, it may even be absent, with the patient complaining primarily of dyspnea or fatigue. Major risk factors for MI include tobacco use, hypertension, diabetes, obesity, psychosocial factors, physical activity, and alcohol consumption. Preventive strategies include measures to prevent the first MI, avoidance of recurring MIs, and lifestyle interventions. Lifestyle changes include the cessation of tobacco use, eating a healthy diet, good control of blood glucose (in diabet-

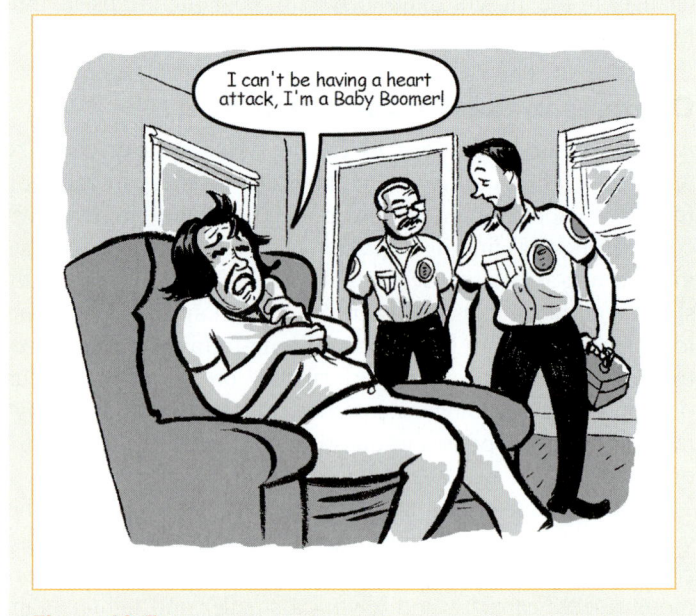

Figure 42-5

ics), exercise, weight control, and control of hypertension. A physician may also order aspirin to help reduce the risk of heart attack.

People 65 years and older are a high-risk group for heart failure. In fact, this problem is the most common reason for hospitalization in the geriatric population. Heart failure is on the rise in this cohort for two paradoxical reasons: better care of the diseases that might otherwise result in failure (such as CAD and hypertension), which enables patients to live long enough to develop heart failure, and more effective management of heart failure once it develops. Risk factors include sex, ethnicity, family history and genetics, long-term alcohol maltreatment, and multiple medical conditions—CAD, emphysema, hyperthyroidism, thiamine (vitamin B) deficiency, and human immunodeficiency virus infection, among others. As with MI, prevention is aimed at lifestyle changes: cessation of tobacco use, eating a healthy diet, good control of blood glucose (in diabetics), exercise, weight control, and control of hypertension.

Rhythm disturbances (arrhythmias) of the heart occur when the electrical system controlling the heartbeat experiences an interruption or malfunction. These irregularities cause heartbeats that are too fast, too slow, irregular, or absent. Many people experience an occasional or harmless arrhythmia, which they may describe as a skipping, fluttering, or fast heartbeat. Arrhythmias in older people are generally a result of age-related changes in the heart, existing cardiac disease, adverse drug effects, or a combination of these factors.

Cardiac arrhythmias are classified by the part of the heart from which they originate. Unlike tachyarrhythmias or bradyarrhythmias, which speed up or slow down the heart, premature beats signify no change in speed but rather alter the regularity of the heartbeat. In contrast, atrial fibrillation (coming from the atria), which is the most common arrhythmia among elderly people, increases the risk of stroke and heart failure. The fibrillating atria allow stasis of the blood, thereby encouraging clot formation and increasing the chances that a clot fragment might travel to the brain and cause a stroke. Most of the blood in the atria enters the ventricles when the valves open, with about 20% being kicked in by contraction of the atria. The aging heart may function adequately when preload provided by the atria ends up in the ventricles; however, when that 20% remains in the atria, new signs or symptoms of heart failure may develop or stable heart failure may decompensate.

Bradycardias are also more common in elderly people. The aging conduction system may produce sinus abnormalities such as sick sinus syndrome. CAD may produce high-degree blocks, whereas medications such as beta blockers or calcium channel blockers can slow the heart too much.

The human heart beats 2.5 billion times and moves 200 million litres of blood in an average lifetime. Not surprisingly, this workload affects the cardiovascular system throughout the entire body over the lifespan. For example, the incidence of aneurysm increases with age. An aneurysm is a weakness in any artery that produces a balloon defect, weakening the arterial wall. This weakness may be congenital (present at birth) or acquired. In the latter case, hypertension, atherosclerotic disease, and obesity are contributing factors to development of such a defect. For example, blood pressure greater than 160/95 mm Hg doubles the mortality risk in men and can lead to kidney loss and blindness by damaging the blood vessels that supply the kidney and eyes. Life-threatening aneurysms can develop in the brain, chest, or abdomen. A new headache or a change in chronic headache patterns, for example, may signal early cerebral bleeding from an aneurysm; all too often, the first manifestation is a sudden and devastating stroke. Preventive measures—proper diet, exercise, smoking cessation, and cholesterol control—aim to control the risk factors associated with hypertension and atherosclerotic diseases.

Aortic dissection occurs when the inside wall of the artery becomes torn and allows blood to collect between the arterial wall layers. It may occur with trauma or sustained hypertension. Dissection weakens the arterial wall, making it prone to rupture. A thoracic dissection, for example, can produce chest pain that is difficult to differentiate from cardiac ischemia. Therefore, it is helpful to take blood pressure readings in both arms in all patients with chest pain. A systolic blood pressure difference of 15 mm Hg or higher suggests a thoracic dissection.

More than half of all older persons are hypertensive. The majority have isolated systolic hypertension resulting from a loss of arterial elasticity. Controlling systolic and/or diastolic hypertension in elderly people helps prevent strokes and MIs. Geriatric hypertensive emergencies require a controlled decline in blood pressure that often cannot be achieved in the prehospital environment.

Stroke is a significant cause of death and disability in elderly people. More than 80% of all stroke deaths occur in persons older than 65 years, and stroke is the leading cause of long-term disability at any age. Strokes, which are mainly caused by atherosclerosis, are responsible for 14,000 deaths (7%) anually in Canada, making stroke the third leading cause of death. The risk of stroke doubles each decade after 35 years, mirroring the increase in risk factors such as hypertension and atrial fibrillation. Hypertension is the primary risk for stroke, but age, family history, smoking, diabetes, high cholesterol, and heart disease also contribute. Prevention is aimed at reduction of risk factors, improving diet and exercise, and lowering cholesterol.

Transient ischemic attacks (also called TIAs and mini-strokes) entail a temporary disturbance of blood supply to the brain that results in a sudden, temporary decrease in brain function. The symptoms are the same as those for a stroke but last less than 24 hours, and most will last less than 60 minutes. They are warning signs of a future stroke.

Respiratory System

Although tobacco maltreatment seems to be decreasing among elderly people, chronic lower respiratory disease, influenza, and pneumonia remain in the top five causes of geriatric deaths. In fact, one of the most common causes of death in older patients is infection with *Pneumococcus* bacteria.

Pneumonia involves an inflammation of the lung, secondary to infection by bacteria, viruses, or other organisms. Although it can affect people at any age, this disease has its biggest impact on very young and elderly people, typically during the colder seasons (winter and early spring). People considered at risk include elderly people; people with underlying health problems such as chronic obstructive pulmonary disease (COPD), diabetes mellitus, and vascular diseases; and any person with a depressed immune system because of acquired immunodeficiency syndrome, cancer therapy, or organ transplantation. Treatment is primarily supportive, consisting of bed rest, fluids, oxygen therapy via nasal cannula or mask to relieve dyspnea, analgesics to reduce fever, and antibiotics. Preventive measures include a vaccine given once and boosters after 3 to 5 years.

COPD includes chronic asthma, chronic bronchitis, and emphysema, all of which are characterized by the presence of bronchial obstruction and airway inflammation. Distinguishing these diseases can be difficult, so the problem may not be diagnosed or treated correctly. COPD affects approximately 10% of the older population, mostly owing to tobacco use. Its effects reflect the age-related loss of elastic tissue in the lungs (*senile emphysema*) and a decreased ability to defend against infection. These factors may increase the baseline disability of COPD and set up older patients for an increased risk of acute exacerbation, often caused by infection.

Preventive measures for COPD-related complications include immunization for influenza and pneumococcal pneumonia. Long-term oxygen therapy has proven helpful in hypoxemic patients. In addition, pulmonary rehabilitation may improve functional status and the quality of life for some patients.

Approximately 1 in 20 elderly people has a history of asthma or is affected by it. Onset can occur in old age with presenting symptoms of shortness of breath (especially with effort), chronic or nocturnal cough, and wheezing.

A pulmonary embolus arises when a blood vessel supplying the lung becomes blocked by a clot. Any obstruction in blood flow to the lung can result in irreversible damage or infarction. An embolus is often released from a vein in a lower extremity, the pelvis, or the abdomen but could also result from a damaged heart. The risk of pulmonary embolus increases with age because of increasing immobility. Older patients may also be bedridden after recent surgery (such as abdominal procedures). Finally, elderly patients have an increased incidence of diseases associated with a higher risk of pulmonary embolus, such as cancer, heart attack, cardiac arrhythmias, and clotting disorders.

Prevention of thromboembolism is based on the patient's risk level—high, moderate, or low. Surgical patients are in the highest-risk category for potential emboli, and prophylaxis is recommended, including warfarin (Coumadin) and/or heparin and compression stockings.

Endocrine System

Diabetes arises when the body cannot oxidize complex carbohydrates (sugars) due to impaired pancreatic activity—namely, production of insulin. Insulin moves carbohydrates out of the bloodstream, through the cellular walls, and into the cells to be metabolized. With diabetes, more glucose is present in the blood than the body can handle. Geriatric patients with diabetes are at increased risk for hypoglycemia for several reasons: medications, inadequate or irregular dietary intake, inability to recognize the warning signs due to cognitive problems, and/or blunted warning signs. Delirium may be the only indication of hypoglycemia in an elderly patient.

Over 2.25 million Canadians are estimated to have diabetes, 10% of these are over 65 years of age, primarily type 2 diabetes (adult-onset, or non–insulin-dependent diabetes). The most common risk factor for this disease is having more than one chronic disease, and many elderly people with diabetes also have hypertension, heart disease, and stroke. Other risk factors for diabetes include a family history of diabetes, genetics, age, diet, obesity, and a sedentary lifestyle. Symptoms of an elevated blood glucose level (that is, hyperglycemia) include fatigue, poor wound healing, blurred vision, and frequent infections. Other symptoms of diabetes include the three Ps: Polyuria, Polydipsia, and Polyphagia. Prevention of type 2 diabetes is aimed at changes in lifestyle that include dietary restrictions, exercise, and controlling obesity.

Older diabetics whose blood glucose levels tend to be high are more prone to hyperosmolar hyperglycemic nonketotic (HHNK) coma than diabetic ketoacidosis. The most frequent cause for HHNK coma is infection. Presentation is likely to be acute confusion with dehydration, although signs of dehydration may be altered in elderly patients (Table 42-1 ▶). Prehospital treatment remains the same as for younger patients, albeit with a cautious approach to fluid resuscitation.

Thyroid abnormalities also increase with aging. Many older patients remain asymptomatic, and the disease is diagnosed only when a routine blood test reveals a thyroid problem. With

Table 42-1	Signs of Dehydration in Elderly People

- Dry tongue
- Longitudinal furrows in the tongue
- Dry mucous membranes
- Weak upper body musculature
- Confusion
- Difficulty in speech
- Sunken eyes

hypothyroidism, for example, the signs and symptoms may match those seen with normal aging: cold intolerance, constipation, dry skin, weakness, and so on. For acute-onset hyperthyroidism (thyrotoxicosis), the presentation can be blunted; although tachycardia is generally present, older patients may experience less tremor, anxiety, or hyperactive reflexes than their younger counterparts. Atrial fibrillation is more likely to be induced by an overactive thyroid gland in a geriatric patient. A smaller percentage of elderly hyperthyroid patients present with symptoms opposite those expected: weakness, lethargy, and depression. Care in the prehospital setting is supportive.

Gastrointestinal System

Constipation is a frequent and significant problem in elderly people. Although it can cause acute abdominal pain, it should not be the initial suspect when a patient experiences such discomfort. Instead, causes with high mortality, such as bleeding from an acute abdominal aneurysm or dead bowel from mesenteric ischemia, should be investigated first. Many elderly people have diverticulosis (small outward pouches in the colon wall) and are at risk for diverticulitis and/or perforation. Appendicitis can be difficult to diagnose in older people, which probably accounts for the high perforation rate (50%) seen with this condition. The incidence of peptic ulcer disease is also increased among the older population, likely because of their relatively high use of nonsteroidal anti-inflammatory drugs (NSAIDs) for pain management.

Large bowel obstructions in elderly people are likely to be caused by cancer, impacted stool, or sigmoid volvulus. In addition, small bowel obstruction secondary to gallstones increases significantly with age. One third to one half of all elderly people have cholelithiasis (gallstones), although most remain asymptomatic for life. With one or more episodes of cholecystitis (inflammation of the gallbladder), the gallbladder adheres to the small bowel and, over time, creates an opening or fistula. The stone(s) drop into the bowel and produce the obstruction. Such a gallstone ileus may account for as many as 25% of geriatric small bowel obstructions. The large and small intestines are at risk for obstruction from adhesions due to previous surgery or infection or when a segment of bowel is forced into a fascial defect (hernia) in the abdominal wall.

Older patients are more likely than younger ones to have stomach or duodenal ulcers (peptic ulcer disease). The main risk factors for peptic ulcers are regular use of NSAIDs and infection with *Helicobacter pylori* (an ulcer-associated bacteria of the stomach), both of which are more common in older patients. Other medications have also been implicated in ulcer formation. The main symptom of peptic ulcer disease is dyspepsia (gnawing, burning pain in the upper abdomen), which usually improves immediately after eating but returns several hours later. Other causes of dyspepsia include acid reflux, gastritis, and gastric cancer.

Musculoskeletal System

Changes in physical abilities can affect older adults' confidence in their mobility. The muscle system atrophies and weakens with age. Muscle fibres become smaller and fewer, motor neurons decline in number, and strength declines. The ligaments and cartilage of the joints lose their elasticity. Cartilage also goes through degenerative changes with aging, contributing to arthritis.

The stooped posture of older people comes from atrophy of the supporting structures of the body. Two of every three older patients will show some degree of kyphosis (also called humpback, hunchback, and Pott curvature). Lost height in older adults generally results from compression in the spinal column, first in the disks and then from the process of osteoporosis in the vertebral bodies.

Osteoporosis, a condition that affects men and women, is characterized by a decrease in bone mass leading to reduction in bone strength and greater susceptibility to fracture. The extent of bone loss that a person undergoes is influenced by numerous factors, including genetics, smoking, level of activity, diet, alcohol consumption, hormonal factors, and body weight. The most rapid loss of bone occurs in women during the years following menopause, and many postmenopausal women use hormone replacement therapy as a means to reduce the loss of bone. Calcium and vitamin D supplementation is another treatment for the condition, and many other medications are available to improve bone strength. Older people should remain active and perform low-impact exercises to maintain bone and muscle strength.

Osteoarthritis is a progressive disease of the joints that destroys cartilage, promotes the formation of bone spurs in joints, and leads to joint stiffness. This type of arthritis is thought to result from "wear and tear" and, in some cases, from repetitive trauma to the joints. It affects 35% to 45% of the population older than 65 years. Typically, osteoarthritis affects several joints of the body, most commonly those in the hands, knees, hips, and spine. Patients complain of pain and stiffness that gets worse with exertion. The end result is often substantial disability and disfigurement. Patients are typically treated with anti-inflammatory medications and physical therapy to improve the range of motion.

Nervous System

Normal age-related cognitive changes have two major features: (1) They are relatively isolated (that is, they are not associated with multiple abnormal neurologic findings that suggest specific disease states), and (2) the onset and progression of these findings are "in time" with the person's aging process (that is, the findings are not sudden or extreme, and they do not extend to other abnormalities).

Delirium (also known as acute brain syndrome or acute confusional state) is a symptom, not a disease. A reflection of an underlying disturbance to a person's well-being (usually a treatable physical or mental illness), this temporary, usually reversible condition results in rapid changes in brain function. In elderly people, delirium often replaces or confounds the typical presentation caused by a medical problem, an adverse medication effect, or drug withdrawal. Disorders that cause delirium may also include poisons, electrolyte imbalances, nutritional deficiencies, and infections such as urinary tract infections and pneumonia. Onset of confusion or disorientation is abrupt (occurring during hours to days) but generally resolves with treatment of the underlying problem. The confusion and disorientation fluctuate with time, and hallucinations may occur. The patient experiences a rapid alteration between mental states, such as lethargy and agitation, serious attention disruption, disorganized thinking, and changes in perception and sensation.

Unlike delirium, dementia is a disease that produces irreversible brain failure. Disorders that cause dementia include conditions that impair vascular and neurologic structures within the brain, such as infections, strokes, head injuries, poor nutrition, and medications. The two most common degenerative types of dementia in older people are Alzheimer's disease and multi-infarct or vascular dementia, both of which cause structural damage to the brain. An estimated 6% to 10% of elderly people will eventually have dementia, although this percentage increases with advancing age. Dementia may be diagnosed when two or more brain functions are impaired. These cognitive and psychomotor functions consist of language, memory, visual perception, emotional behaviour and/or personality, and cognitive skills. Other risk factors that may predispose a patient to dementia include lower level of education, female sex, and African ethnicity. Although most cases of dementia cannot be prevented, some experts suggest that low-fat diets and exercise may help ward off vascular dementia.

Experts have not identified a single cause for Alzheimer's disease, but most believe it is not a normal part of the aging process. Although age is a significant risk factor for this disease (Alzheimer's disease typically affects patients older than 60 years), but age alone is not the cause. This progressive disease cannot be cured or reversed by any known treatment or intervention. Symptoms are subtle at onset. Over time, patients lose their ability to think, reason clearly, solve problems, and concentrate; they may present with altered behaviour that includes paranoia, delusions, and social inappropriateness. In the later stages of Alzheimer's disease, patients cannot take care of themselves and may lose the ability to speak. People with severe Alzheimer's disease become completely debilitated and totally dependent on others.

Patients with Parkinson's disease—another age-related neurologic disorder—have two or more of the following symptoms: resting tremor of an extremity, slowness of movement (bradykinesia), rigidity or stiffness of the extremities or trunk, and poor balance. Parkinson's disease is caused by degeneration of the substantia nigra, an area of the brain that controls voluntary movement by producing the neurotransmitter dopamine. Cells use dopamine to transmit impulses, so a loss of dopamine results in the loss of muscle function. Parkinson's disease can affect one or both sides of the body and produces a wide range of functional loss.

The incidence of seizures (including status epilepticus) is also increased in elderly people, partly because of the increase in risk factors such as stroke, dementia, primary or metastatic brain tumours, and acute metabolic disorders (such as hyperglycemia, hyponatremia, alcohol withdrawal). Prehospital treatment for seizures is the same for younger and older patients.

Toxicology

As the number of uses for medications increases, there is a proportional increase in the likelihood of adverse drug reactions and interactions. Elderly people are particularly prone to adverse reactions, even when they take drugs at doses that would be safe in younger people. This increased incidence of adverse drug reactions among elderly people seems to reflect changes in drug metabolism because of diminished hepatic function; in drug elimination because of diminished renal function; in body composition, including increased body fat and decreased body water, altering the distribution of drugs through the various body compartments; and in the responsiveness to drugs that affect the CNS. A change in any one of these processes can lead to toxic effects in elderly people.

Other body changes may affect medication use by geriatric patients in a more general way. As vision declines with age, reading small print becomes more difficult. Night vision becomes less acute, so reading labels in dim light can lead to errors. Short-term memory loss may lead to forgetfulness about whether medications have been taken. An inability to distinguish flavors may cause patients to take multiple doses of medications before they detect problems.

Elderly people consume more than 20% of all prescribed and over-the-counter drugs sold in Canada. Community-dwelling older persons take an average of three to five medications per day. Nursing home patients take an average of six to seven routinely scheduled medications daily (polymedicine) and two to three additional medications on an as-needed basis. This kind of polypharmacy may be therapeutic when multiple drugs are needed to manage different medical problems, but it may prove harmful when these medications interact. Elderly patients are particularly prone to having multiple chronic diseases, which may lead to a vicious circle: The presence of multiple disease states leads to the use of multiple medications, which increases the likelihood of adverse reactions, which in turn leads to treatment with more medications. In turn, a person's chance of ending up in the hospital because of an adverse reaction to a medication increases with the number of drugs taken. Ultimately, the best dosage of a drug for an elderly patient is the lowest dosage that will achieve a therapeutic effect.

Medication noncompliance in older patients is also associated with negative effects on health. Many patients—not just older patients—do not follow instructions or advice on the use of their medications. Because elderly people use more medications than the rest of the population, noncompliance issues are more likely. Noncompliance issues include failure to fill a prescription (for example, the patient doesn't have the money to pay for the drug or doesn't see the benefits of it), improper administration of medication (for example, the patient decreases the dosage to make the prescription last longer), discontinuation of medication (for example, the patient feels better and decides not to take the medication), and taking inappropriate medications (for example, the patient had medication left over from a previous prescription or shares the medicine with family or friends).

Geriatric patients are predisposed to medicine-related reactions owing to the previously mentioned age-related physiologic changes that occur in body systems and body composition. For example, an increase in the proportion of adipose tissue can prolong the half-life of a drug. In particular, medications that affect the CNS are the most common source of adverse or unexpected reactions, and barbiturates and benzodiazepines are the drugs most often associated with toxic effects. A reduction in the nervous system response—especially the decrease in parasympathetic activity typically seen with the aging process—increases the risk that adverse anticholinergic effects will occur. Reduced beta-adrenergic receptor sensitivity (which is responsible for bronchodilation) makes most bronchodilator medications less effective. The use of diuretics and antihypertensive medications by geriatric patients can cause hypotension and orthostatic changes due to reduced cardiac output and a decrease in total body water. Finally, decreased glucose tolerance may cause medications such as diuretics and corticosteroids to have hyperglycemic effects.

Notes from Nancy

The best dosage of a drug for an elderly patient is the lowest dosage that will achieve a therapeutic effect.

Drug and Alcohol Maltreatment

Alcohol is the preferred substance of maltreatment among older persons, in whom its use is on the rise. A much smaller but increasing segment of the geriatric population uses illicit drugs. Most users are men, and more than half carry their addiction into old age. About one third develop an maltreatment problem after reaching 65 years, often in response to a life-changing event such as the loss of a spouse, declining health, or low self-esteem.

The prevalence of alcohol and drug misuse among older people is also attributable to the multiplicity of medications that are prescribed for them and their heightened vulnerability to maltreatment owing to the effects of aging. Decreased body mass and total body water means higher concentrations of blood alcohol; at the same time, the combination of digestive, renal, and hepatic system changes means slower elimination of alcohol from the body.

As the geriatric population continues to grow and experiences even more chronic disabilities, the likelihood of substance maltreatment–related problems in this group will increase. Recognizing substance maltreatment in older people can be difficult. If they have engaged in this behaviour for a long time, it may be well hidden from—or even accepted by—family and friends. Because substance maltreatment can complicate your initial assessment and treatment, it is important to ask about this issue.

Psychiatric Conditions

Depression is not part of normal aging, but rather a medical disease that occurs in about 6% of the population older than 65 years. The good news is that it is treatable with medication and therapy. The bad news is that if depression goes unrecognized or untreated, it is associated with a higher suicide rate in the elderly population than in any other age group. Depression in elderly patients can mimic the effects of many other medical problems (such as dementia). Risk factors for depression in older people include a history of depression, chronic disease, and loss (function, independence, or significant others). This condition may be difficult to recognize in older people because many don't want to complain about feeling sad, worthless, or unwanted.

Disturbingly, the majority of elder suicides occur in people who have recently been diagnosed with depression. In addition, the majority of suicide victims have seen their primary care physician within the month before the event. Unlike younger people, geriatric patients typically do not make suicidal gestures or attempt to get help. Instead, the rate of completed suicide is disproportionately high in the geriatric population. Many geriatric patients see no other way out when they have a terminal illness or debilitating cardiac or neurologic condition (such as severe heart disease or stroke). At highest risk are white men 85 years and older who use firearms as their suicide method of choice.

Injury in Elderly People
Environmental Injury

Internal temperature regulation is slowed in elderly people and gets slower with increasing age. The body's ability to recognize fluctuations in temperature becomes delayed owing to a slowed endocrine system. Heat gain or loss in response to environmental changes is delayed by atherosclerotic vessels, slowed circulation, and decreased sweat production in the skin. In addition, thermoregulation can be adversely affected by chronic disease, medications, and alcohol use, all of which are more frequent in elderly people.

Not surprisingly, about half of all deaths of hypothermia occur in elderly people, and most *indoor* hypothermia deaths involve geriatric patients. Although living where harsh winters occur is a risk factor, hypothermia can develop at temperatures above freezing when an older person is exposed for a prolonged period.

The death rates from hyperthermia are more than doubled in elderly people compared with younger persons; people older than 85 years are at highest risk.

Trauma in Elderly People

Trauma is one of the top 10 causes of death among elderly people. The mortality rate for trauma in patients older than 65 years is 623 per 100,000, versus 148 per 100,000 for all other age groups. Deaths from injury in people older than 65 years account for 39% of all trauma deaths in Canada.

Several factors place an elderly person at higher risk of trauma than a younger person—namely, slower reflexes, visual and hearing deficits, equilibrium disorders, and an overall reduction in agility. In particular, changes in the body's homeostatic compensatory mechanisms combined with the effects of aging on body systems and any preexisting conditions usually add up to less-than-favourable outcomes in trauma situations. Compensation in trauma is successful when increased heart rate, increased respiration, and adequate vasoconstriction make up for trauma-related deficits. Reduced cardiac reserve, decreased respiratory function, impaired renal activity, and ineffective vasoconstriction, by contrast, may lead to unsuccessful recovery from traumatic situations. Furthermore, an elderly person is more likely to sustain serious injury in case of trauma because stiffened blood vessels and fragile tissues tear more readily, and brittle, demineralized bone is more vulnerable to fracture.

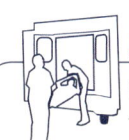

At the Scene

Compensatory mechanism changes + aging systems + preexisting conditions = bad outcomes.

Most geriatric trauma cases involve falls or motor vehicle collisions. The incidence of falls, for example, increases with increasing age. Although most falls do *not* produce serious injury, elderly people account for 75% of all fall-related deaths. This increased mortality in geriatric patients is directly related to the patient's age, preexisting disease processes, and complications related to the trauma. Falls are associated with a higher incidence of anxiety and depression, a loss of confidence, and postfall syndrome. With this syndrome, geriatric patients develop a lack of confidence and anxiety about potential falls. Ultimately, they may become immobile, risk incontinence, and develop pneumonia or pressure ulcers from lack of movement.

Falls among elderly people are evenly divided between those resulting from extrinsic (external) causes, such as

Table 42-2 Causes of Falls in the Elderly

Cause	Clues to Suggest This Cause
Extrinsic (accidental)	Obvious environmental hazard at the scene, such as poor lighting, scatter rugs, uneven sidewalk, ice or other slippery surface
Intrinsic drop attacks	Sudden fall; patient found on the ground somewhat confused, often temporarily paralyzed and unable to get up; no premonitory symptoms
Postural hypotension	Fall when getting up from a recumbent or sitting position (Check medications the patient is taking, and ask about occult blood loss, such as presence of black stools. Measure blood pressure in recumbent and sitting positions.)
Dizziness or syncope	Marked bradycardia or tachyarrhythmias
Stroke	Other characteristic signs of stroke, such as hemiparesis, hemiplegia, or aphasia
Fracture	Patient felt something snap before falling.

tripping on a loose rug or slipping on ice, and those resulting from intrinsic (internal) causes, such as a dizzy spell or a syncopal attack (**Table 42-2** ▲). The risk of falls increases in people with preexisting gait abnormalities (such as from neurologic or musculoskeletal impairment) and cognitive impairment. Older patients with osteoporosis have lower-density bones, so even a sudden, awkward turn may fracture a bone. When treating a patient who has fallen, you need to take a careful history. Although the patient often attributes the fall to an accidental cause ("I must have tripped over the rug"), meticulous questioning often reveals a period of dizziness or palpitations just before the fall, suggesting a different cause. Home safety assessments by EMS—during a routine visit or as part of an outreach program—may reduce fall incidence.

After falls, motor vehicle accidents are the second leading cause of accidental death among elderly people. Of licensed drivers, 10% are elderly people. They account for 10% of all traffic deaths, 11% of all vehicle occupant deaths, and 16% of all pedestrian deaths. Impaired vision, errors in judgment, and underlying medical conditions contribute to the higher risk. Impairments in vision and hearing, along with diminished agility, also contribute to pedestrian deaths involving elderly people.

Types of Injuries Commonly Seen in Elderly People

Changes associated with normal aging and with diseases of aging make elderly people particularly vulnerable to certain types of injuries. In particular, head trauma or injury is a serious problem. The increased fragility of cerebral blood vessels, enlargement of the subdural space, and a decrease in the supportive tissue of the meninges all contribute to make an elderly person more vulnerable than a younger person to intracranial bleeding, particularly subdural hematoma. In many cases, the hematoma develops slowly, during days or weeks. By the time the patient becomes symptomatic, the person or his or her caretakers may not remember the incident, or the family or caretakers may feel guilty about their own negligence in the incident. As a result, it may be difficult to obtain an accurate history of the initial trauma. The most important early symptom of a subdural hematoma is headache, which may be worse at night.

Sometimes the headache occurs on the same side of the head as the blood clot. With increasing intracranial pressure, the state of consciousness becomes depressed, and the patient becomes increasingly drowsy.

Elderly people are also more vulnerable than their younger counterparts to cervical spinal cord injury and cord compression, even after apparently minor trauma. Degenerative changes in the cervical spine (cervical spondylosis) cause arthritic "spurs" and narrowing of the vertebral canal; the nerve roots exiting from the cervical spine gradually become compressed, and pressure on the spinal cord increases. Any injury to the cervical spine, therefore, is much more likely to injure the already compromised spinal cord. Even a sudden movement of the neck may result in spinal cord injury.

Injuries to the chest in elderly people are much more likely to produce rib fracture and flail chest, owing to the brittleness of the ribs and overall stiffening of the chest wall as the costochondral cartilage becomes calcified. Abdominal trauma often produces liver injury, perhaps because the liver is less protected by abdominal musculature.

Orthopedic injuries are a common result of falls in geriatric patients, with hip fractures the most common acute orthopedic injury, followed, in severity and frequency, by fractures of the femur, pelvis, tibia, and upper extremities. Hip fracture may also occur without trauma, simply because of vigorous contracture of the hip musculature. The most important risk factor for hip fracture is osteoporosis: Approximately half of older women and one of eight older men will have an osteoporosis-related fracture (hip or other). An estimated 1.4 million Canadians suffer from osteoporosis. Treatment of osteoporosis-related fractures costs the Canadian health care system about $1.3 billion per year and is estimated to increase to at least $32.5 billion by 2018.

Burns are a significant risk of morbidity and mortality in elderly people because of physiologic and pathophysiologic changes. The risk of mortality is increased when preexisting medical conditions exist, defence mechanisms to protect against infection are weakened, and fluid replacement is complicated by renal compromise. In the assessment of a burn patient, paramedics need to monitor the patient's hydration status by assessing current vital signs, mucous membranes, and urine output, which is typically 50 to 60 ml/h or 1 to 2 ml/kg/h.

▌Assessment of Geriatric Patients

Although illness is common among elderly people, it is *not* an inevitable part of aging. Complaints of elderly people cannot be ascribed simply to "getting old." Aging is a continuous process and a normal development sequence that affects people in multiple ways. The normal wear-and-tear concept and genetic makeup are two theories that have been suggested to explain the biological effects of aging.

Along the same lines, there is a widespread misconception that elderly people tend to be hypochondriacs, with dozens of imaginary or minor complaints. In reality, hypochondria is far less common among elderly than among younger patients. Indeed, older patients tend *not* to complain, even when they have legitimate symptoms. When an elderly person calls for an ambulance, he or she usually has a very real problem.

Knowing what is and what is not part of the aging process constitutes the first challenge in assessing elderly people. A second challenge is that signs and symptoms of disease may be altered from their presentation in younger patients as a consequence of the aging process. An MI may present without chest pain; fever may be minimal in pneumonia; uncontrolled diabetes is more likely to present as HHNK coma than as ketoacidosis. A variety of acute illnesses—from congestive heart failure to an acute abdomen—may present simply as delirium.

Another challenge relates to the fact that the older the patient, the more likely are multiple problems—medical, psychological, and social. Interestingly, the proportion of older people with a disability has decreased; however, the total number of older people with a chronic disability has increased simply because there are more elderly people. Debilitating health conditions often found in this population include hypertension, arthritic symptoms, heart disease, cancer, diabetes, stroke, and COPD. The incidence of depression also increases with age, with 15% to 20% of people older than 85 years having some form of depression.

The co-occurrence of multiple pathologic conditions has several consequences for patients and health care providers alike. The symptoms of one disease or disability may alter or hide the symptoms of another condition. The patient with severe leg pain from arthritis, for example, may not pay much attention to new pain caused by thrombophlebitis. In addition, when several organ systems are in borderline condition, a disturbance in function in only one of the systems may have repercussions throughout the body, leading to failure of multiple organs in a dominolike manner. The presence of multiple underlying illnesses also makes it much more difficult for health professionals to sort out which problem is causing which symptom. Furthermore, chronic comorbidities may make it much more difficult to treat the patient's acute problem. For example, the medication a patient needs for a cardiac problem may be contraindicated because of a renal or hepatic problem or, at the least, may require major modification in dosage.

Notes from Nancy

Getting old is not a disease, and it does not by itself produce symptoms of disease.

Notes from Nancy

When an elderly person calls for an ambulance, there is usually a very good reason, even if it is not the reason the patient tells you.

You are the Paramedic Part 3

After gathering the information from the nurse and Mrs. Jessup, you ask Mike what he found during his physical examination. He tells you that he found the patient to have signs of dehydration as demonstrated by tenting of the skin and dry mucous membranes, diminished breath sounds bilaterally with rales at the right base, a slightly elevated irregular heartbeat, and an oral temperature of 39°C. He asks what treatment you would like him to give.

At this point you ask your partner to establish IV access so that you can administer fluids to help with the dehydration and fever. He is able to successfully insert a 20-gauge needle in the left hand. Supplemental oxygen is administered via nasal cannula at 3 l/min, and the cardiac monitor is applied.

Reassessment	Recording Time: 11 Minutes
Skin	Pink, hot, and dry
Pulse	106 beats/min, weak
Blood pressure	164/92 mm Hg
Respirations	22 breaths/min, regular
Spo$_2$	98% with supplemental oxygen at 3 l/min by nasal cannula
ECG	Atrial fibrillation with no ectopy
Pupils	PERLA
Blood glucose level	14 mmol/l

4. What are some specific respiratory illnesses commonly seen in elderly people?

5. What are the risk factors for pneumonia in elderly people? Are any present here?

The GEMS Diamond

There are many acronyms in the prehospital setting to help you remember steps in your assessment and treatment. The GEMS diamond was created to help paramedics recall key themes when dealing with geriatric patients 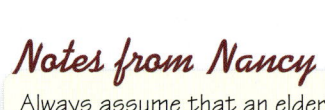. It was designed to assist the prehospital professional in the assessment and treatment of elderly patients.

"G" of the GEMS diamond is to recognize that the patient is a *geriatric* patient. The paramedic's thought process needs to be geared to the possible problems of an aging patient. When responding to an emergency involving an older patient, you should consider that older patients are different from younger patients and may present atypically.

"E" of the GEMS diamond stands for an *environmental* assessment. Assessment of the environment can help give clues to the patient's condition or the cause of the emergency. Is the home too hot or cold? Is the home well kept and secure? Are there hazardous conditions? Preventive care is also very important for a geriatric patient, who may not carefully study the environment or may not realize where risks exist.

"M" of the GEMS diamond stands for *medical* assessment. Older patients tend to have a variety of medical problems and may be taking numerous prescription, over-the-counter, and herbal medications. Obtaining a thorough history is very important in older patients.

"S" stands for *social* assessment. Older people may have less of a social network, because of the death of a spouse, family members, or friends. Older people may also need assistance with activities of daily living, such as dressing and eating. There are numerous social agencies that are readily available to help geriatric patients. Consider obtaining information pamphlets about some of the agencies for older people in your area. If you have these brochures with you and encounter a person in need, you can provide this valuable information. Social agencies that deal with the older population will be more than happy to share a listing of the services they provide.

The GEMS diamond provides a concise way to remember the important issues for older patient. Using this concept will help you make appropriate referrals, and as a result, you will help older patients maintain their quality of life.

Scene Assessment and Initial Assessment

As you move from scene assessment to the initial assessment of a patient, gather information that may prove relevant to the case. Look for potential clues from the patient's social history;

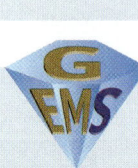

Notes from Nancy

Always assume that an elderly patient's mental status is normal until you have evidence to the contrary.

Table 42-3	The GEMS Diamond

G—Geriatric Patients

- Present atypically.
- Deserve respect.
- Experience normal changes with age.

E—Environmental Assessment

- Check the physical condition of the patient's home: Is the exterior of the home in need of repair? Is the home secure?
- Check for hazardous conditions that may be present (for example, poor wiring, rotted floors, unventilated gas heaters, broken window glass, clutter that prevents adequate egress).
- Are smoke detectors present and working?
- Is the home too hot or too cold?
- Is there an odour of feces or urine in the home? Is bedding soiled or urine-soaked?
- Is food present in the home? Is it adequate and unspoiled?
- Are liquor bottles present? If so, are they lying empty?
- If the patient has a disability, are appropriate assistive devices (for example, a wheelchair or walker) present?
- Does the patient have access to a telephone?
- Are medications out of date or unmarked, or are prescriptions for the same or similar medications from many physicians?
- If living with others, is the patient confined to one part of the home?
- If the patient is residing in a nursing facility, does the care appear to be adequate to meet the patient's needs?

M—Medical Assessment

- Older patients tend to have a variety of medical problems, making assessment more complex. Keep this in mind in all cases—both trauma and medical. A trauma patient may have an underlying medical condition that could have caused or may be exacerbated by the injury.
- Obtaining a medical history is important in older patients, regardless of the chief complaint.
- Initial assessment
- Ongoing assessment

S—Social Assessment

- Assess activities of daily living (eating, dressing, bathing, toileting).
- Are these activities being provided for the patient? If so, by whom?
- Are there delays in obtaining food, medication, or other necessary items? The patient may complain of this, or the environment may suggest this.
- If in an institutional setting, is the patient able to feed himself or herself? If not, is food still sitting on the food tray? Has the patient been lying in his or her own urine or feces for prolonged periods?
- Does the patient have a social network? Does the patient have a mechanism to interact socially with others on a daily basis?

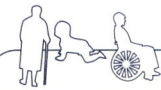

Special Considerations

Be patient when interviewing older people, recognizing that physical, intellectual, and psychological barriers may slow or interfere with effective communication.

Special Considerations

Interviewing Techniques

- Introduce yourself.
- Speak to the patient first rather than family or bystanders.
- Be aware of your body language.
- Look directly at the patient.
- Speak slowly and distinctly.
- Explain what you are doing.
- Allow time for the patient to answer.
- Show the patient respect, and preserve dignity.
- Do not talk *about* the patient with others in front of the patient.
- Be patient.
- Locate hearing aids or eyeglasses if needed.
- Turn on lights.

general living conditions; availability of social and family support; activity level; medications; overall appearance with respect to nutrition, general health, cleanliness, personal hygiene; and attitude and mental well-being. Paramedics also need to be aware of the numerous factors that affect the assessment process in geriatric patients: sensory alterations, verbal communication skills, mental and physical capabilities, and the ability of health care providers to accommodate and comprehend these conditions.

Patient History

Explain everything you plan to do, especially if the patient seems confused. Is this confused state normal, a new manifestation of a preexisting medical problem, or a patient's lack of understanding? A comprehensive patient history includes many elements—the patient's chief complaint, present illness or injury, pertinent medical history, and current health care status and needs. Pertinent medical history would *not* include information about the removal of a patient's appendix more than 50 years ago but would consider current cardiovascular health (such as palpitations or flutters), exercise tolerance, diet history, medications, smoking and drinking habits, sleep patterns, and other intrinsic and extrinsic factors.

The ability to elicit a good patient history comes from education and experience. The object is to reduce anxiety, not increase it—and if you simply whip out a lot of strange equipment and start, for example, sticking electrodes onto the patient's chest, the patient may well become frightened and wonder what is going to happen.

Communication

The ability to elicit a thorough patient history reflects education and experience. Good communication skills will help you gather the information you need during your assessment. Without good communication skills, you could frighten, alienate, insult, anger, or even harm your patients. Your first words should focus on gaining the patient's trust. Introduce yourself. Use respect when addressing the patient; use his or her name, if you know it; and avoid terms such as "honey," "dear," and "grandma" when addressing an older patient. Speak slowly, distinctly, and respectfully. Attempt to get the patient history from the patient, rather than family and bystanders, whenever possible.

Communication is not just talking; it is also listening. When asking questions of older patients, wait for their answers. Older people may need more time to process your questions, and they may speak slowly when responding. Active listening also involves paying attention to the patient's tone, especially if it conveys fear or confusion.

Nonverbal communication is just as important as verbal communication. Eye contact, hand gestures, body position, facial expressions, and touch communicate a message. When speaking with patients, get face to face with them and make sure there is plenty of light. Have patients put in hearing aids or wear glasses to facilitate better communication, and be sure to take these aids with the patients to the hospital so other health care providers can communicate as well.

Part of your task in the assessment is to determine whether this confused state is normal, a new manifestation of a preexisting medical problem, or a result of the patient's lack of understanding. Preserve the patient's dignity during exposure and when discussing his or her history around others.

Chief Complaint

Obtaining the chief complaint would seem to be a straightforward procedure, but it may not be simple with some elderly patients. Older patients tend not to report significant symptoms for several reasons. Many share the misconception that illness and assorted aches and pains are simply part of aging. Other older people may not mention even legitimate symptoms to avoid being identified as old and a hypochondriac. Some patients fear that mentioning a symptom will lead to a diagnosis or treatment that will jeopardize their independence. "If I mention those pains in my stomach," the old person may reason, "they'll put me in the hospital, and I may never come out of that place again."

Whereas elderly patients tend to underreport serious symptoms, the symptoms they *do* report are often vague and apparently trivial. Furthermore, elderly patients are likely to have several chief complaints, each of which may have a different source.

When a patient's chief complaint seems trivial, it may be necessary to go through a standard list of screening questions to confirm that you are not missing important pieces of information. In such a review of systems, questions are designed to evaluate the functions of the body's major organ systems. In the prehospital setting, there is not sufficient time to conduct a complete review of systems, but a few well-chosen questions can provide a great deal of information about the function of the patient's more important systems:

Cardiovascular
- Have you had any pain or discomfort in your chest? When?
- Have you noticed any fluttering in your chest or fast heartbeats?

Respiratory
- Do you ever get short of breath? When?
- Have you had a cough lately?

Neurologic
- Have you had any dizzy spells? Have you fainted?
- Have you had any trouble speaking?
- Have you had headaches recently?
- Have you noticed any unusual weakness or funny sensations in your arms or legs?

Gastrointestinal
- Have there been any changes in your appetite lately?
- Have you gained or lost any weight?
- Have there been any changes in your bowel movements?

Genitourinary
- Do you have any pain or difficulty urinating?
- Have you noticed any change in the colour of your urine?

If any of these screening questions yields a positive answer, follow up with further questions. For example, if the patient states that he has been coughing lately, find out whether he is bringing up sputum and, if so, what the sputum looks like (for example, Is there blood in the sputum?).

Once you have elicited what you believe to be the chief complaint, go through the usual process of assembling the history of the present illness. This history may be complicated if other chronic problems are affecting the acute problem. To sort out which symptoms relate to the current chief complaint and which are chronic difficulties, try asking questions such as "How does this problem differ from what it was like last week?" or "What happened today to make you decide to get help?"

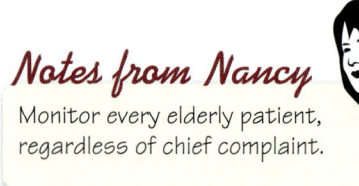

Notes from Nancy

Monitor every elderly patient, regardless of chief complaint.

Obtaining a history from an elderly patient requires patience. You must be prepared to listen, often for an extended period. But your listening will be rewarded—not only by helping you discover the patient's problem, but also by allowing you to provide part of the solution to the problem. Listening is a demonstration of caring, and your caring can mean a great deal to a lonely or frightened older person.

Other Medical History
Just as it is not practical to go through a comprehensive review of systems in the prehospital setting, it is not usually feasible to obtain a complete medical history in the prehospital setting. Nevertheless, you should inquire about recent hospitalizations and allergies.

Most important, you should obtain the most detailed history possible of the patient's medications, because medications account for a significant percentage of medical problems in elderly people. A medication history should include *all* medications, not just prescription drugs, because many people do not think to mention common over-the-counter preparations such as aspirin, antacid tablets, and herbal medicines. Ask the patient to list the medications by name, and determine the dosing and frequency for each one. Also, inquire about medications that are prescribed but not taken (such as because of cost issues or side effects) and medications that may have been provided by other sources (such as a spouse's medication). Obtain the patient's permission to take medications to the hospital, and then collect them all—prescription and nonprescription drugs. If the patient cannot tell you where the medicines are stored, check the bathroom medicine cabinet, the bedside table, the kitchen table and counters, and the refrigerator.

Physical Examination
The physical examination of an elderly patient may be fraught with difficulties. Poor cooperation and easy fatigability may require that you keep manipulations of the patient to a minimum. You may have to peel many layers of clothing off an elderly patient to perform an adequate examination. Despite these obstacles, an ill or injured geriatric patient deserves as thorough an evaluation as a younger counterpart.

Begin by observing the patient's general appearance, including dress and grooming. In some cases, inattention to appearance may be one of the first signs of depression or a serious medical condition. Evaluate the level of consciousness as you would for any patient. In a critically ill or injured patient, use the AVPU scale. If you have more time, try to perform a more detailed assessment of the patient's cognitive function. Is the patient fully alert? Is he or she oriented to place and time? Does the patient's affect seem appropriate to the situation? Are there obvious disorders in thinking, such as delusions (false beliefs)?

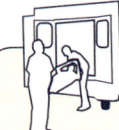

At the Scene

Cover the patient with a blanket to protect privacy and keep the patient warm. This action shows respect for the patient and will improve your examination.

Note the patient's position and degree of distress. Check the colour, moisture, and temperature of the skin, bearing in mind that the loss of elasticity in the skin of elderly patients may produce apparent signs of dehydration (such as tenting) when hydration is normal.

If you are examining the patient in his or her home, take a good look at the patient's surroundings, as well as at the patient. Try to assess the patient's self-care capability. Is everything neat and well maintained? Or is the home a mess, with dishes piled in the sink and rubbish accumulating? Do you see evidence of alcohol consumption (such as empty bottles)? Are there signs of violence, such as broken glassware, that might provide clues to elder maltreatment? Are the patient's quarters adequately heated or cooled? Is the patient living alone? Does the patient have pets? (If so, you should make arrangements for someone, such as a neighbour, to assume their care until the patient returns.) Record these observations on the patient care report to enable social service personnel to make appropriate arrangements for follow-up care.

Measure the patient's vital signs carefully. Postural changes in blood pressure vary among elderly people, but changes increase with increasing frailty and heighten the person's risk for falls. Marked postural changes in blood pressure and pulse may indicate hypovolemia or overmedication. As you measure the vital signs, bear in mind that normal blood pressure for a young person may represent significant hypotension in an elderly patient. If possible, determine the patient's baseline blood pressure. When obtaining a patient's blood pressure, be aware of the possibility of significant hypertension and orthostatic changes. Consider taking vital signs in both arms and checking pulses proximally and distally in all extremities. This process will allow you to gather information and observe for signs of dependent edema, dehydration, and the patient's circulatory status without raising his or her anxiety level.

Pay attention to the respiratory rate. Tachypnea can be a very sensitive indicator of acute illness in elderly people—especially pulmonary infection—even when patients show few, if any, other signs. When assessing the patient's respirations, listen to lung sounds in all fields, noting adventitious sounds that might aid in development of a treatment plan. You can also use the stethoscope to listen for carotid bruits; note jugular vein distension.

> ### Notes from Nancy
> Consider the possibility of hypovolemia in any elderly person whose systolic blood pressure is less than 120 mm Hg.

Detailed Physical Examination

Conduct the detailed physical examination as you would for any other patient. When examining the mouth, make a note of any upper or lower dentures. In the chest examination, keep in mind that elderly people may have pulmonary crackles without apparent pathology—so don't lunge for the nitroglycerin and furosemide at the first crackle you hear in the chest. Similarly, edema in the legs may be the result of chronic venous insufficiency and not right-sided heart failure.

Assessment and Management of Medical Complaints in Elderly People

Cardiovascular Complaints

Prehospital treatment for chest pain remains essentially unchanged in elderly patients, albeit with extra cautions because of the increased potential for medication side effects.

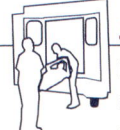

At the Scene

If the patient is hypotensive and is wearing a nitroglycerin patch, remove it. The patient's complaint could be caused by too much or too little of this medication.

As in all prehospital emergencies, paramedics must prioritize the patient's airway, breathing, and circulatory status. Nitroglycerin and morphine may produce more hypotension or respiratory compromise than in younger patients or may react adversely with long-term medications. Aspirin may increase bleeding in a patient who is already taking anticoagulants. For patients 75 years or older with ST-segment elevation infarcts, angioplasty offers a better outcome than peripheral fibrinolysis.

The presentation of heart failure in an older person can be confused by symptoms and signs symbolic of old age and shared by a number of chronic diseases—for example, dyspnea on exertion, easy fatigability (especially with left-sided heart failure), confusion, crackles on lung examination, orthopnea, dry cough progressing to productive cough, and dependent peripheral edema in right-sided heart failure. Acute exacerbations of heart failure are often related to poor diet, medication noncompliance, onset of arrhythmias such as atrial fibrillation, or acute myocardial ischemia.

Prehospital treatment is unchanged from that of younger patients, although greater consideration is given to becoming familiar with the patient's medications and their implications for your proposed treatment. For example, the patient taking long-term furosemide (Lasix) may not respond to the usual dose of the same drug that you administer as an acute therapy. Additional treatments by paramedics should include close monitoring of fluids and avoidance of excessive fluid overload, use of beta blockers in patients with systolic dysfunction (low ejection fraction), use of digoxin or diltiazem (Cardizem) in patients with atrial fibrillation or atrial flutter, and, possibly, use of anticoagulation therapy in patients with atrial arrhythmias to prevent thromboembolism.

Nonperfusing rhythms receive the same treatment as given to younger adults. Survival depends on the prearrest health of the patient and the usual factors: early recognition, prompt and effective CPR, and early defibrillation.

Thoracic aneurysms generally remain asymptomatic until they become large or rupture. Early symptoms may be related to compression by the aneurysm, such as difficulty swallowing or hoarseness from laryngeal nerve pressure. Abdominal aortic aneurysms present typically with abdominal pain or possibly only with back pain. Asymptomatic thoracic and abdominal aneurysms that do not exceed a certain size and are not expanding are generally treated without surgery but are reassessed on a regular schedule. In an older patient with back pain, examine the chest and abdomen carefully. The treatment of abdominal emergencies is surgical, so early recognition, assessment, stabilization, and rapid transport to an appropriate medical facility are essential.

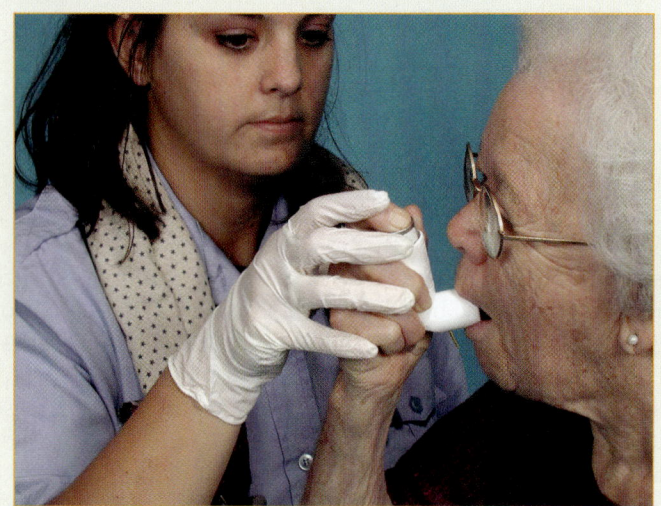

Figure 42-6 A patient having an asthma attack may have a bronchodilator medication in a metered-dose inhaler. Older patients often do not use an inhaler correctly, so you may need to help with its use if your protocols allow it.

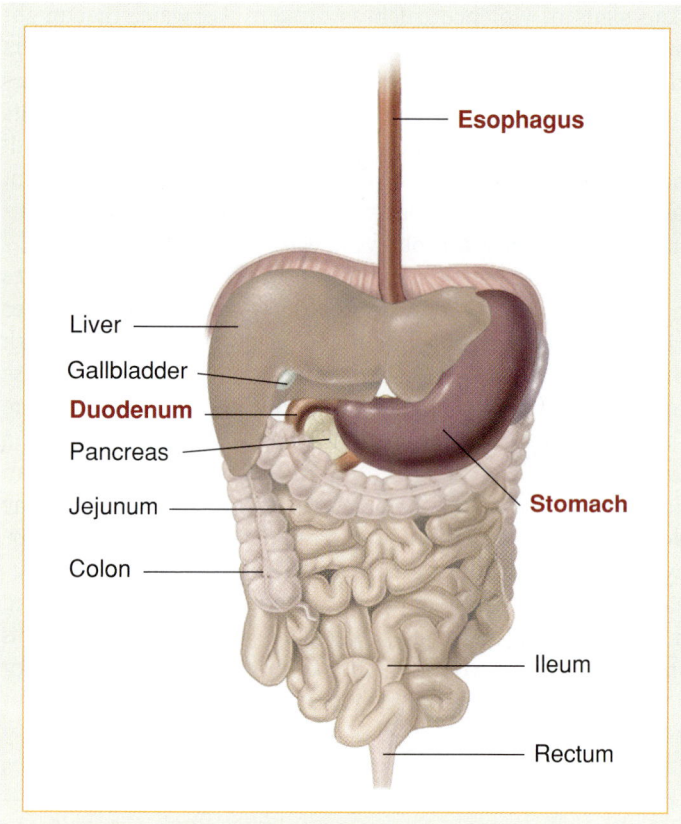

Figure 42-7 Upper GI bleeding occurs in the stomach, esophagus, and duodenum.

The usual treatments for systolic hypertension usually prove safe and effective in geriatric patients. In case of rapid onset of symptomatic systolic hypertension, treatment aims to reduce the systolic pressure with antihypertensive therapy, which can minimize cardiovascular and cerebrovascular morbidity and mortality.

Respiratory Complaints

An older patient with pneumonia often does not have the classic presentation of chills, fever, and productive cough. Instead, these symptoms are often supplanted by acute confusion (delirium), normal temperature, and a minimal to absent cough. Prehospital treatment is supportive and includes oxygen and IV access as indicated. At the receiving facility, providers will determine whether antibiotics or admission is appropriate.

Asthma clinical practice guidelines are the same for younger and older patients (**Figure 42-6 ▲**). On rare occasions, epinephrine may be indicated for a life-threatening asthma exacerbation.

In a patient of any age, treatment goals for COPD are to reduce the symptoms and complications. Along with shortness of breath, presenting symptoms may include fatigue and a decreased activity level. Treatment consists of immediate assessment and correction of respiratory difficulties with the application of supplemental oxygen. The patient may also receive bronchodilators to decrease the shortness of breath, inhaled or oral steroids to decrease inflammation, and antibiotics to treat infection.

Many pulmonary emboli are silent or present with tachypnea alone—that is, the classic triad of dyspnea, chest pain, and hemoptysis is often altered or absent. If you suspect a pulmonary embolus, check for swelling, erythema, and warmth or tenderness of the lower leg; all of these are signs of a deep venous thrombosis, which is a common cause of pulmonary embolus. If deep venous thrombosis might be present, handle the leg gently and monitor the patient for respiratory changes. Prehospital treatment is largely supportive after ensuring that airway and ventilation are adequate. Lysing the thrombus and use of anticoagulation therapies may be considered after a risk assessment is performed, with these measures being followed by rapid transport.

GI Complaints

Many causes are possible for gastric complaints. Constipation and its accompanying abdominal pain, for example, are some of the more common complaints of geriatric patients. In your assessment of a gastric emergency, ask the patient about food and fluid intake, history of abdominal complaints, current bowel and bladder habits, and medications and supplements before proceeding with a physical examination. Symptoms are often vague and manifest only as diffuse abdominal pain with no particular point of origin. Abdominal and gastric complaints often require surgical treatment, so early recognition and rapid transport for definitive hospital care are the best practice.

Upper GI hemorrhage occurs when there is bleeding from the esophagus, stomach, or duodenum (**Figure 42-7 ▲**). When severe, this condition is a true medical emergency that must be recognized and assessed quickly. Not only are older people more prone to upper GI bleeding, they are also at a greater risk of complications, the need for urgent surgery, and death.

It is not possible to determine the cause of upper GI bleeding without an endoscopic examination (inspection of the inside of a hollow organ or body cavity) of the esophagus, stomach, and duodenum. However, the history can offer clues to the cause. Regular use of NSAIDs or alcohol may result in bleeding from irritation of the lining of the stomach or from ulcers (a hollowing out or disintegration of tissue) in the stomach or duodenum. Forceful vomiting can cause tears in the esophagus that may bleed. Cirrhosis of the liver from long-term alcohol use or chronic infectious hepatitis may cause enlargement of the veins (varices) in the esophagus. These varices can rupture and result in massive bleeding. Stomach cancer or esophageal cancer can also produce upper GI bleeding. Recent weight loss or difficulty swallowing would raise the suspicion of cancer as the source of bleeding.

On arrival at the scene, even more important than knowing the cause of bleeding is being able to assess its severity. Slower bleeding is characterized by emesis with coffee-grounds appearance. With minor bleeding, the heart rate and systolic blood pressure are normal. Brisk bleeding presents with hematemesis (vomiting red blood) or melena (black, tarlike stools). It is important to note that melena, not pain, is the most common presenting symptom of GI bleeding. Prehospital treatment is supportive, including adequate pain control.

Lower GI hemorrhage primarily describes bleeding from the colon and rectum **Figure 42-8 ▶** and should never simply be attributed to hemorrhoids. Colon polyps and colon cancer are also possible causes, among others. Minor lower GI bleeding is characterized by small amounts of red blood covering formed brown stools or scant amounts of red blood noticed on the toilet paper. Severe lower GI bleeding is characterized by passing significant amounts of red blood or maroon-coloured stools.

Assessment should begin with identifying risk factors such as a history of previous lower GI bleeding, symptoms or signs suggestive of colon cancer, recent constipation or diarrhea, and use of medications such as blood thinners. Treat for shock. Severe lower GI bleeding requires immediate transportation to the nearest emergency department.

Neurologic and Endocrine Complaints

Effective prehospital acute stroke care includes early recognition, discovery of stroke-mimics such as hypoglycemia or hypoxia, and timely transport to the most appropriate facility. Use a stroke assessment tool as appropriate, taking the patient's history into account when assessing the components of the scale. An older person with severe arthritis may not move as well on one side, or damage from a previous stroke may make his or her speech difficult to assess. Always ask family or caregivers for information that may help you identify deviations from the patient's normal pattern of behaviour or activity. Assess for new weakness, fatigue, syncope, and near

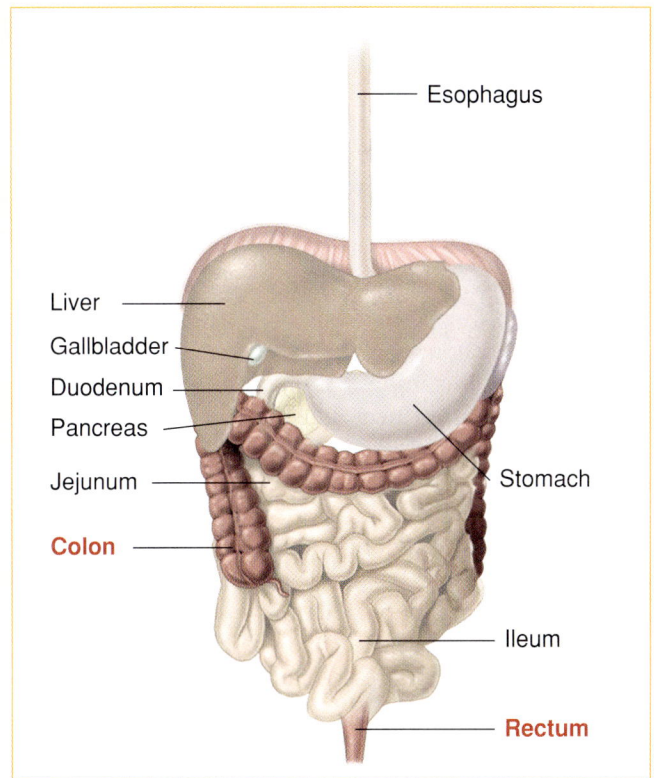

Figure 42-8 Lower GI bleeding takes place primarily in the colon and rectum.

Documentation and Communication

A stroke is a traumatic and emotional event for the patient, and a sensitive and compassionate approach is essential. Even though the patients may not be able to communicate with you, they can often understand. Communicate with them as you would any other patient—in a calm and reassuring manner.

syncope and for changes in these symptoms and in mood and sleep patterns.

Dementia signs and symptoms take months to years to become apparent and may include short-term memory loss or shortened attention span, jargon aphasia (talking nonsense), hallucinations, confusion, disorientation, difficulty in learning and retaining new information, and personality changes such as social withdrawal or inappropriate behaviour. Dementia is not synonymous with delirium, however, and a patient with dementia can also have delirium. In delirium, assess for recent changes in the patient's level of consciousness or orientation. Specifically, look for an acute onset of anxiety, an inability to think logically or maintain attention, and an inability to focus. Also assess for changes in vital signs, temperature (indicating infection), glucose level, and medications—all frequent causes of delirium. Use the mnemonic "DELIRIUMS" to identify other causes of delirium:

D Drugs or toxins
E Emotional (psychiatric)
L Low PaO_2 (carbon monoxide poisoning, COPD, congestive heart failure, acute myocardial infarction, pneumonia)
I Infection (pneumonia, urinary tract infection, sepsis)
R Retention of stool or urine
I Ictal (seizures)
U Undernutrition or underhydration
M Metabolism (thyroid or endocrine, electrolytes, kidneys)
S Subdural hematoma

Altered mental status is a symptom, not a disease. As a consequence, the assessment and subsequent management of its numerous causes is complicated. Always consider head injury (medical or traumatic), heart rhythm disturbances, dementia, medications, fluid balance changes (such as blood loss), respiratory disorders (such as hypoxia), endocrine changes (such as blood glucose level fluctuations), hyperthermia or hypothermia, and infection. Most important, paramedics need to consider neurologic causes (such as Alzheimer's disease and Parkinson's disease) and endocrine changes (such as diabetes).

In Alzheimer's disease, symptoms may present as confusion (lack of familiarity with surroundings), changes in personality or judgment, and extreme difficulty with daily activities, such as feeding, bathing, and bowel and bladder control. Parkinson's disease may present as dyskinesia (involuntary movements or tremors affecting one or both sides of the body), dementia, depression, autonomic dysfunction (bladder and GI problems), and postural instability (loss of reflexes or inability to "right oneself").

Many endocrine changes may have occurred earlier in life and been diagnosed before intervention by paramedics became necessary. Geriatric patients may have diseases such as Grave's disease (hyperthyroidism), Addison's disease (hypoadrenalism), Cushing's syndrome (hyperadrenalism), osteoporosis, or diabetes. In the assessment of geriatric patients with diagnosed diabetes, look for signs of dehydration or hyperglycemia (the three Ps: Polyuria, Polydipsia, and Polyphagia).

Notes from Nancy

Delirium in the elderly is always a sign of physical illness or drug intoxication and is always an emergency.

New-onset diabetes in geriatric patients is often a mild progression that produces no symptoms.

Toxicologic Complaints

The most common therapeutic error in cases of reported poison exposure is "inadvertently took/given medication twice" or "double dosing." In essence, medications are poisons with beneficial side effects. This definition emphasizes the need for obtaining a careful history and collecting and transporting all medications with the patient.

As mentioned earlier, many elderly people take a variety of drugs. Patients may be taking medications prescribed by more than one physician, each dispensing prescriptions without knowledge of the others' orders. Patients may also take over-the-counter medications or medications prescribed for a family member or friend.

Another factor contributing to the toxic effects of drugs in elderly people is aging-related alterations in pharmacokinetics (that is, the absorption, distribution, metabolism, and excretion of drugs). Pharmacokinetics may also be influenced by diet, smoking, alcohol consumption, and use of other drugs. Drugs such as digoxin that depend on the liver and kidney for metabolism and excretion are particularly likely to accumulate to toxic levels in older patients. With most drugs, we know little about the optimal dosage for elderly people because nearly all clinical trials to establish the safe dosages of drugs are performed in young populations. For the most part, dosages for elderly people need to be *reduced* compared with those for younger patients ("Start low, go slow").

Although almost any drug can produce toxic effects in an older person, certain drugs and classes of drugs are implicated more often than others; **Table 42-4 ▶** lists the "dirty dozen." Typically toxic effects present with psychiatric symptoms (such as hallucinations, paranoia, delusions, agitation, and psychosis) and cognitive impairment (such as delirium, confusion, disorientation, amnesia, stupor, and coma) **Figure 42-9 ▾** .

Notes from Nancy

Bring all of the patient's medications—prescription and nonprescription—to the hospital.

Sepsis

Infections in older persons can be severe and dangerous. Sepsis is the disease state that results from the presence of microorganisms or their toxic products in the bloodstream. This is a serious

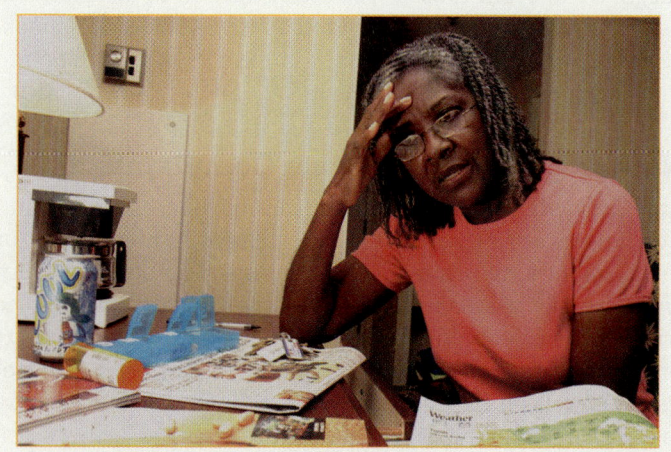

Figure 42-9 The toxic effects of drugs may initially manifest in the form of confusion.

Table 42-4	Drugs Most Commonly Causing Toxic Reactions in Elderly People	
Medication	**Symptoms**
Anti-inflammatory agents (NSAIDs, steroids)	Drowsiness, dizziness, confusion, anxiety, bradypnea, tachypnea, GI bleeding
Antibiotics	GI signs, altered mental status, seizures, coma
Anticholinergics and antihistamines	Urination difficulty, constipation, drowsiness, restlessness, irritability, hypertension
Anticoagulants (warfarin)	Ecchymosis, epistaxis, hematuria, abdominal pain, vomiting, fecal blood
Antiarrhythmics (amiodarone, lidocaine)	Restlessness, hypotension, bradycardia, tachycardia, palpitations, angina
Antidepressants (tricyclics, long-acting selective serotonin reuptake inhibitors)	Confusion, delirium, disorientation, memory impairment
Antihypertensives (diuretics, alpha blockers, beta blockers; angiotensin-converting enzyme inhibitors)	Hypotension, palpitations, angina, fluid retention, headache
Antipsychotics (phenothiazines, atypicals)	Drowsiness, tachycardia, dizziness, restlessness
Digoxin	Headache, fatigue, malaise, drowsiness, depression
Insulin and oral antidiabetic medications	Hypoglycemia presenting as confusion
Narcotics	Delirium, respiratory depression, apnea, involuntary muscle movements
Sedative-hypnotics (benzodiazepines, barbiturates)	Incoordination, dizziness, disturbances in cognitive function

problem that every paramedic should know how to recognize and treat. Think of sepsis whenever you see a hot, flushed patient who is also tachycardic and tachypneic. Other signs of sepsis include an oral temperature greater than 38°C or less than 36°C, a respiratory rate of more than 20 breaths/min or $Paco_2$ less than 32 mm Hg, and pulse rate of greater than 90 beats/min. Sepsis can be caused by bacteria, fungi, and viruses.

Skin Complaints

Herpes zoster (shingles) is caused by the reactivation of varicella virus on nerve roots. This condition is more common in the older population. Most people with herpes zoster are in good health, but people with cancer or immunosuppression are at higher risk. This condition affects any nerve in the body, but the thoracic nerves and the ophthalmic division of the trigeminal nerve are most common. The disease usually starts with pain in the affected area. Subsequently, a cluster of tiny blisters (vesicles) erupts on reddened skin in the same area. The rash is typically unilateral; it rarely crosses the midline.

One of the most common complications of herpes zoster is pain, or postherpetic neuralgia. During the acute phase of the infection, the person may have severe pain and require narcotic pain relievers. Antiviral medications such as acyclovir and famciclovir can be used, preferably within 48 hours of the activation of the disease. These medications decrease healing time, new lesion formation, and pain.

Cellulitis is an acute inflammation in the skin caused by a bacterial infection Figure 42-10 ▶ . This condition usually affects the lower extremities. Symptoms include fever, chills,

and general malaise. Cellulitis can cause warmth, swelling, redness, tenderness, and enlarged nodes in the affected area. Blood tests may show elevation of the white blood cell count and the presence of bacteria. Treatments include antibiotic therapy, ensuring adequate fluid intake, and local dressings if there is an open sore.

Psychological Complaints

Depression can be a normal, short-term reaction to a particular event. When sadness, restlessness, fatigue, and hopelessness persist for weeks, however, it becomes a larger concern. Depression in the geriatric population is a major health problem with an incidence growing in tandem with the progressive aging of the population. This trend can be attributed to increases in polypathology, psychosocial stress, and aging-related changes in the brain that collectively lead to greater cognitive impairment, increased medical illness, dependency on health care services, and more suicide attempts Figure 42-11 ▶ . Depression may also occur when a patient takes a variety of medications; such polypharmacy is more likely when the person has multiple medical conditions that result in more vulnerability to toxic effects.

When dealing with psychological emergencies with geriatric patients, paramedics need to determine whether the situation is a true behavioural emergency or a behavioural crisis. A behavioural emergency implies a significant risk of serious

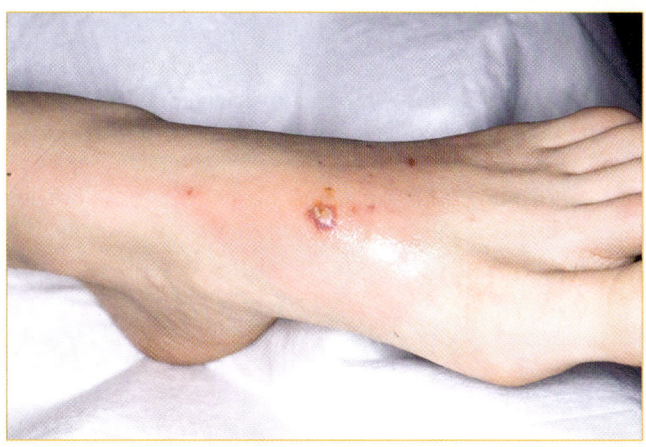

Figure 42-10 Cellulitis is a diffuse, acute inflammation in the skin caused by bacterial infection.

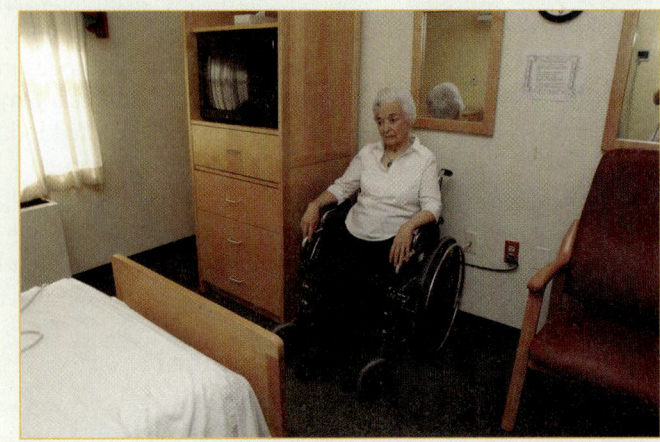

Figure 42-11 Isolation and chronic medical problems are among the factors that contribute to depression in older adults.

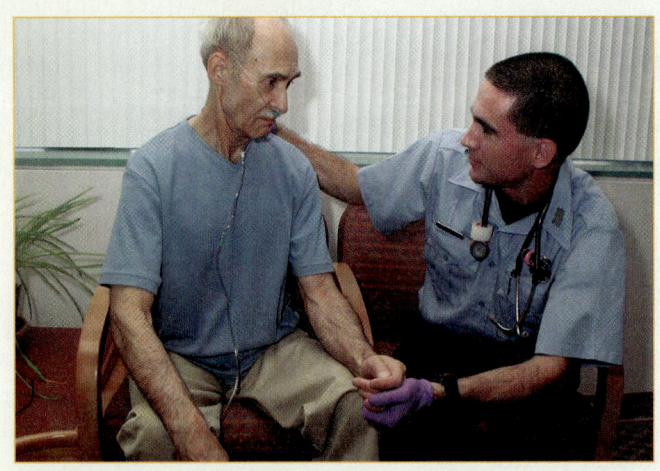

Figure 42-12 A patient in a behavioural crisis may be searching for alternative methods of coping.

harm to self or others unless intervention is undertaken immediately. Examples include serious suicidal states, potential violence, and impaired judgment that could leave a person at risk of injury or death. In a behavioural crisis, the patient's ability to cope is insufficient and becomes overwhelmed, sending the patient in search of alternative methods of coping **Figure 42-12 ▲**.

When dealing with a patient's mental illness or psychotic episodes, always remember that a person who is psychotic is out of touch with reality. Many forms of psychotic behaviour are possible, including schizophrenic and paranoid behaviours. All symptoms associated with psychotic conditions may not be present when a patient is having an episode, however. Clues to psychotic behaviour might include the patient becoming excited or angry for no apparent reason, engaging in antisocial activity or being a loner, and sleeping during the day and staying awake at night. Information about changes in the patient's normal routine may be obtained from family, friends, or caregivers.

Management of Medical Emergencies in Elderly People

The assessment and management of medical emergencies in geriatric patients can be complex. If you are well prepared to deal with these complex situations, you will not feel quite so overwhelmed and helpless.

In every emergency, you should first complete a scene size-up to confirm the scene safety, determine the nature of the call, identify the number of potential patients, and ascertain the need for additional resources. Next, you should perform an initial assessment, which consists of several quick, yet complex observations. First, formulate a general impression based on the patient's mental status and the status of his or her airway, breathing, and circulatory systems. Then, determine transportation priorities.

With the exception of patients who require immediate interventions to maintain a patent airway, adequate and supportive breathing, or circulatory status, most prehospital care is supportive and focuses on pain relief and palliative interventions. Additional steps in the patient treatment plan will depend on the patient's specific medical emergency and chief complaint.

Table 42-5 ▶ reviews common medical complications encountered with geriatric patients and their management strategies.

Assessment and Management of Trauma in Elderly Patients

Begin the assessment by looking at the mechanism of injury. Falls account for the largest number of injuries in elderly people, followed by injuries related to motor vehicles (including passenger and pedestrian trauma) and then burns and other injuries. Always look for signs or symptoms that the patient may have experienced a medical problem before the trauma. A syncopal event while driving, for example, may result in a collision.

The initial management of an injured elderly patient follows the basic ABC pattern of trauma care with some special concerns.

While securing the airway, check for dentures. If they are intact and in place, leave them where they are; if the dentures are broken or loose in the mouth, remove them and place them in a safe container. Aggressive suctioning of blood or secretions is required because of the older patient's lessened airway and gag reflexes **Figure 42-13 ▶**.

When assessing breathing, check for rib fracture. If assisted ventilation is required, use a bag-valve-mask gently, exerting just enough pressure to inflate the lungs so as to lessen the chance of creating a pneumothorax. Administer supplemental oxygen early to assist the body in compensating for early states of trauma.

| Table 42-5 | Common Medical Complications in Elderly People and Their Management |

Medical Complication	Management
Incontinence	Some cases are managed surgically. Other considerations include absorptive devices for fecal and urinary incontinence, placement of catheters, and awareness of the patient's self-esteem and social issues.
COPD	Nebulizer treatment with a bronchial dilator could include metaproterenol (Alupent), racemic epinephrine, isoetharine (Bronkosol), ipratropium (Atrovent), and salbutamol (Ventolin) or an IV dose of methylprednisolone (Solu-Medrol).
Pulmonary emboli	Lysing the thrombus and anticoagulation therapies are indicated. Once all risk factors for bleeding have been reviewed, anticoagulants such as heparin or enoxaparin (Lovenox) can be considered.
Heart failure	Heart failure that produces signs and symptoms of pulmonary edema can be managed with sublingual nitroglycerin, IV furosemide (Lasix), and IV morphine. Paramedics can also consider a vasoactive medication such as dopamine (Intropin) for patients with hemodynamically unstable hypotension.
Arrhythmias	Unless a patient is in unstable condition, arrhythmias are handled with supportive care only. Unstable arrhythmias are treated following current CPR and electrocardiographic guidelines.
Aneurysm	Treatment is handled surgically, and prehospital interventions focus on supportive care.
Hypertension	Hypertensive emergencies require a controlled decline in blood pressure, which is not often feasible in prehospital care. A hypertensive crisis or urgency may be addressed by using labetalol (Trandite) or sodium nitroprusside (Nipride).
Cerebral vascular disease	Prehospital management targets recognition and support. Definitive treatment is surgery.
Delirium	Recognize and treat the underlying cause, and provide supportive interventions.
Dementia, Alzheimer's disease, Parkinson's disease	Provide supportive care.
Diabetes	In hypoglycemia, treatments address the elevation of the blood glucose level with intramuscular or IV injections when not contraindicated. In hyperglycemia, treatment aims to eliminate additional glucose by using fluid boluses for patients with adequate renal function.
GI problems	Few treatments using medications for GI problems are possible in the prehospital environment, other than antiemetics. For nausea and vomiting, consider promethazine (Phenergan), dimenhydrinate, or prochlorperazine (Gravol) (Stemitil).
Drug toxic effects	• Lidocaine: CNS depression may occur, so be alert for respiratory changes. No antidote is used in prehospital care to reverse its effects. • Beta blockers: Provide supportive care; give activated charcoal; and consider the use of atropine, epinephrine, and glucagon in symptomatic patients. • Antihypertensives: Provide supportive care. No antidote is used in prehospital care to reverse the drugs' effects. • Diuretics: Provide supportive care. Consider treatments aimed at restoring volume depletion and electrolyte imbalance. No antidote is used in prehospital care to reverse the drugs' effects. • Digitalis: Provide supportive care. Consider fluid replacement, vasoactive medications such as dopamine, and activated charcoal. • Psychotropics: Provide supportive care. Consider aggressive fluid replacement. • Antidepressants: Provide supportive care. Give fluid therapy for hypotension and sodium bicarbonate.
Alcohol maltreatment	Provide supportive care. Later care includes identification of maltreatment potential and referral to an appropriate treatment facility.
Behavioural disorders	Use psychological support and communication strategies. Consider haloperidol (Haldol), droperidol (Inapsine), or chlorpromazine (Largactil).
Depression, suicide	Provide supportive care. Later care includes identification of the potential condition and referral to an appropriate treatment facility.

When evaluating circulation, remember that what is a normal blood pressure in a younger person may mean hypotension in an older person. If possible, try to determine the patient's normal baseline blood pressure and circulatory status.

The initial assessment of disability (neurologic status) should include an evaluation of the pupils and the level of consciousness, according to the AVPU scale. Finally, be sure to expose the entire injured area, even if it means peeling away many layers of clothing.

Once the initial assessment is complete, try to obtain a complete history of the trauma event from the patient and from anyone who may have witnessed the event Figure 42-14 ▶. If the patient fell, from what height? Did the patient have any symptoms beforehand, such as dizziness? If the patient was

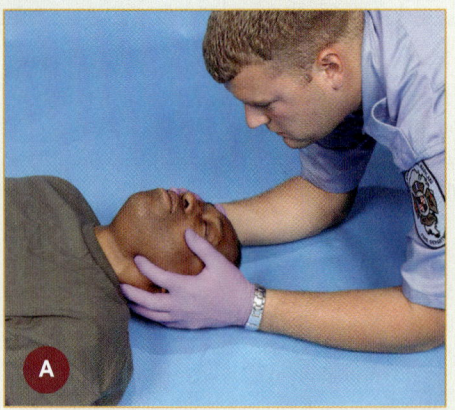 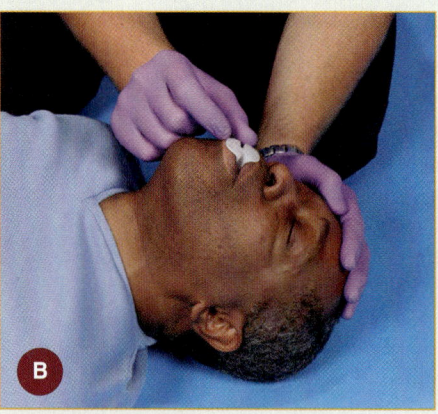 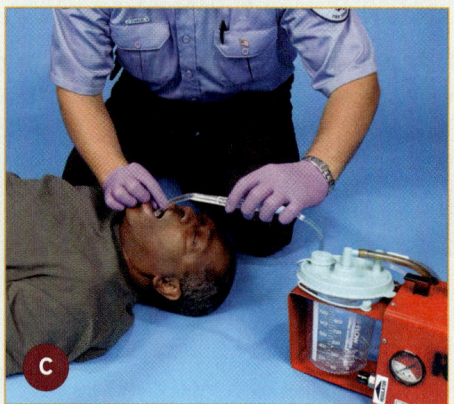

Figure 42-13 The airway should initially be addressed using simple techniques, such as (**A**) the modified jaw-thrust, (**B**) placement of an oropharyngeal or nasopharyngeal airway, and (**C**) suctioning.

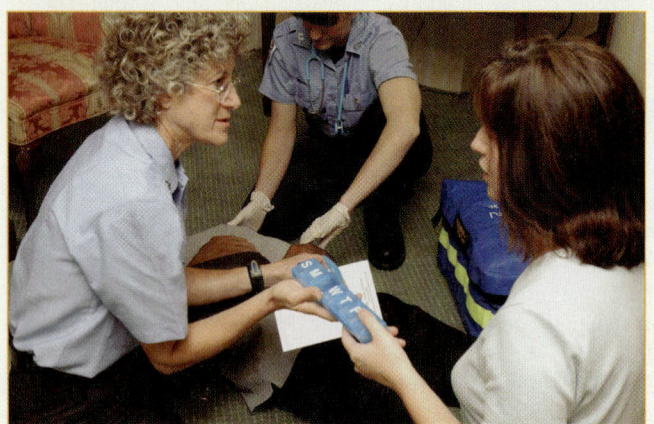

Figure 42-14 History is especially important in older patients who have lost consciousness.

struck by a car, how fast was the car moving? If the patient was the driver of a car involved in an accident, did he or she feel dizzy or black out before the collision? Did the patient have chest pain? Did witnesses notice the car moving erratically before it collided?

Obtain a complete list of all medications the patient takes regularly. Inquire in particular about beta blockers, antihypertensives, and medications for diabetes because they may affect the patient's response to resuscitation measures and to anesthesia.

Conduct the focused physical examination as usual, staying particularly alert for signs of injuries to the head, cervical spine, ribs, abdomen, and long bones. Pain from fractures or peripheral injury may be difficult to assess if the patient has decreased pain perception.

You are the Paramedic Part 4

You place your patient on a stretcher in a semi-Fowler's position and move her to the ambulance. While en route to the hospital, she begins to complain of being "a little winded." A reassessment reveals no changes in her status. Your partner suggests administering a nebulizer treatment with salbutamol. You agree, and the patient receives a nebulizer treatment with 2.5 mg of salbutamol with 2.5 ml of normal saline. Report is called en route to the emergency department, and no further orders are given.

As you arrive at the emergency department your patient says that she is breathing easier and thanks you for being so caring. She is observed in the emergency department for a few hours, and right lower lobe pneumonia is diagnosed by chest radiograph. She is admitted to the hospital for treatment with IV antibiotics and is discharged to the nursing home on the fifth day.

Reassessment	Recording Time: 20 Minutes
Skin	Pink, hot, and dry
Pulse	113 beats/min, strong and irregular
Blood pressure	158/96 mm Hg
Respirations	22 breaths/min regular
Spo₂	95% with supplemental oxygen at 3 l/min by nasal cannula
ECG	Atrial fibrillation

6. Does pneumonia present the same in elderly people as in younger people?
7. How is pneumonia managed in the prehospital setting?

Additional treatment will depend on the patient's specific injuries, although there are a few general principles to keep in mind:

- Insert an IV cannula and give an isotonic solution, but use caution. It is very easy to overload an elderly person with sodium, and you must balance that with the need to maintain adequate perfusion pressure. Use small boluses, and reassess the patient frequently, especially for signs of pulmonary edema.
- Monitor cardiac rhythm throughout prehospital care of the patient, and be alert for changes. Previous or continuing cardiac disease predisposes a person to ECG changes.
- Take steps to preserve temperature in elderly trauma patients. Regulation of temperature is slowed in elderly people, and the blood in cold patients does not clot as well.
- Frail elderly patients may not do very well with a traction splint for a femoral fracture. If possible, place the patient on a well-padded backboard and buttress him or her well with pillows secured firmly in place.
- Immobilize the cervical spine before transporting the patient. Pad the backboard generously, because the skin of an older person may be damaged by the direct trauma of the pressure and the decrease in blood flow. Target areas where the bone is near the surface, from top to bottom: occiput, scapula, spinous processes, elbows, sacrum, and heels. A pressure ulcer can develop in as little as 45 minutes and can complicate the original injury.

Elder Maltreatment

One category of geriatric trauma that deserves special mention is elder maltreatment—that is, any form of mistreatment that results in harm or loss to an older person. Five types of maltreatment are distinguished: physical, sexual, emotional, neglect, and financial. The first four are similar to the forms found in child maltreatment. Financial maltreatment involves improper use of an older person's funds, property, or assets. The average victim of elder maltreatment is 80 years old, is female, and has multiple chronic conditions. These conditions make patients unable to function on their own, leaving them dependent on others for at least part of their care. The maltreater is almost always known to the victim and is often a family member (such as adult children or a spouse).

One clue to elder maltreatment is unexplained injuries that do not fit the stated cause. Assessment of elder maltreatment must include not only the physical examination, but also the environmental and social clues. Look at the patient's overall hygiene, and review how he or she interacts with caregivers. Take adequate time to listen patiently to any concerns expressed by older patients about their care (or lack of it) **Figure 42-15 ▶**. If the patient's condition is stable but the situation is unsafe, see if the patient will accept transportation to the hospital. If the patient refuses transport, see if he or she will accept help from the local adult protective services. If the situation is immediately unsafe, notify law enforcement

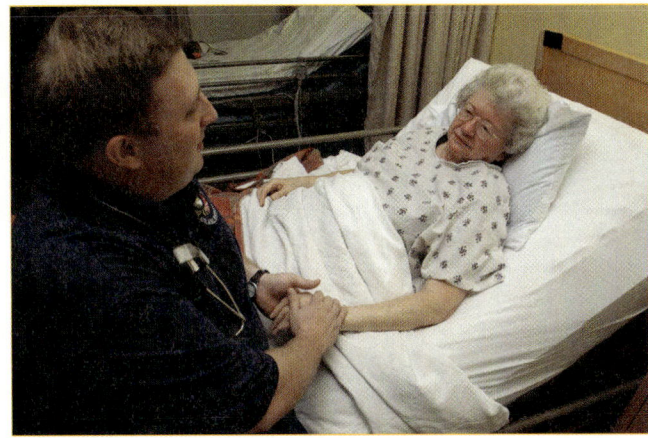

Figure 42-15 Take time to listen patiently to older patients.

personnel and remain with the patient only if the scene remains safe to do so.

Across Canada, different laws apply in different types of maltreatment situations. Four main types of laws help to protect older adults from maltreatment and neglect. Nevertheless, most elder maltreatment cases are never reported. In Canada, certain categories of maltreatment are crimes under the Criminal Code of Canada, and some types of maltreatment are also offences under provincial jurisdiction. You should become familiar with the legislation that applies to your area. However, regardless of the legislation, if you have any reason to suspect elder maltreatment in a given case of geriatric injury—for example, if you found evidence of gross patient neglect in the patient's residence—carefully document your observations and report your findings and suspicions to the receiving facility. For more information on this topic, see Chapter 43.

End-of-Life Care

You will inevitably be involved with end-of-life care for many patients. Of course, "do not resuscitate" (DNR) does *not* mean "do not respond to the needs of a terminal patient." There is much you can do, beginning with demonstrating a caring and concerned attitude and approach. Many of your visits may be "no transport" decisions and may not be perceived as valuable by those who decide on reimbursement, but they prove no less

Controversies

Many jurisdictions have implemented advance directives and "do not resuscitate" (DNR) orders in the community setting. These are similar to those used in the hospital setting. You should be aware of what policies are in place in your region and adhere to them, because they are the patient's expressed wishes in the setting of a catastrophic or terminal event.

valuable to the patient than more aggressive measures. Many communities have a local hospice, an organization that provides terminal care for patients and support for their families. If one exists in your community, consider how you or your service might collaborate on providing quality care for a person at the end of life **Figure 42-16 ▶**.

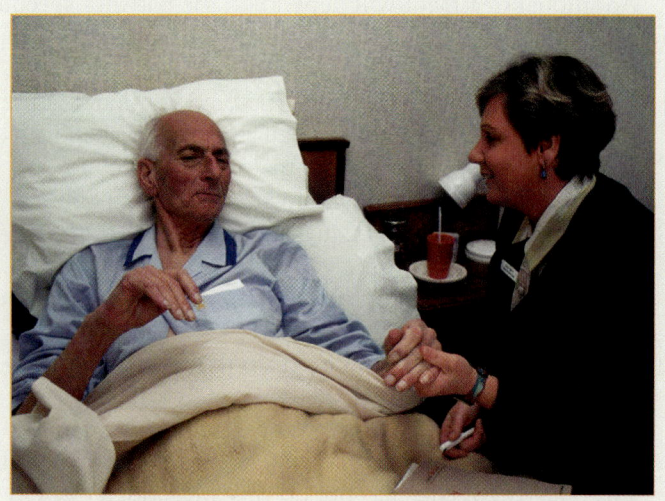

Figure 42-16 Hospice care allows people with terminal illnesses to receive palliative care in their own homes.

You are the Paramedic Summary

1. Why is it important to review common medical problems of elderly people?

Well, like it or not, we are not getting any younger. As a matter of fact, more than 4.3 million Canadians are older than 65 years; that is 13% of the population! It is predicted that by the year 2026, the older population will have increased from 4.3 million to 8 million. As we age, our bodies undergo numerous physical changes that affect the way we respond to illness and disease. Keeping up-to-date with medical problems of elderly people is just as important as staying current on other kinds of emergencies.

2. Which organ systems are greatly affected by age-related changes?

Although the aging process affects all body systems, the organ systems most relevant to older patients are the respiratory, cardiovascular, renal, nervous, and musculoskeletal.

3. Why might obtaining an accurate medical history and history of the present illness be challenging when interviewing an elderly patient?

The elderly patient can present with numerous challenges that might make patient assessment tricky. These include having more than one chronic illness, not feeling pain the same way a younger person might, difficulty distinguishing acute from chronic problems, fear of being hospitalized, and fear of losing control over their ability to care for themselves. It is important to be patient and look for subtle clues when assessing an older person.

4. What are some specific respiratory illnesses commonly seen in elderly people?

Respiratory illnesses commonly seen in elderly people include pneumonia, COPD, and pulmonary embolism.

5. What are the risk factors for pneumonia in elderly people? Are any present here?

Residing in an institutional environment, chronic illness, and a compromised immune system are all risk factors for contracting pneumonia. In our case, Mrs. Howard resides in a nursing home and has diabetes, which increases her chances of getting pneumonia.

6. Does pneumonia present the same in elderly people as it does in younger people?

If you are expecting to find a patient presenting with fever, productive cough, chest discomfort, and chest congestion, keep looking! The clinical presentation of pneumonia in elderly people will fool you. Rather than presenting with the "classic clinical picture" described above, an elderly person with pneumonia might present with altered mental status, cough, fever, shortness of breath, tachycardia, and tachypnea.

7. How is pneumonia managed in the prehospital setting?

Prehospital management of pneumonia is aimed at supportive care. Ensuring an adequate airway and oxygenation and a little tender loving care will go a long way for most of your patients. Definitive treatment for pneumonia is the administration of antibiotics.

Prep Kit

Ready for Review

- Elderly people constitute an ever-increasing proportion of patients presenting to the health care system, particularly to the emergency care sector.
- The health problems of older people are quantitatively and qualitatively different from those of younger people. The special problems of older people require special approaches.
- The aging process is accompanied by changes in physiologic function. The decrease in the functional capacity of various organ systems can affect the way in which the patient responds to illness.
- A variety of changes occur in the cardiovascular system as a person ages. The heart hypertrophies (enlarges), arteriosclerosis (the stiffening of vessel walls) develops, and the electric conduction system of the heart deteriorates.
- A person's respiratory capacity also undergoes significant reductions with age due to decreases in the elasticity of the lungs and in the size and strength of the respiratory muscles, calcification of costochrondral cartilage in the chest wall, and musculoskeletal changes.
- Geriatric patients may experience renal system changes. Although the kidneys of an elderly person may be capable of dealing with day-to-day demands, they may not be able to meet unusual challenges, such as those imposed by illness. Therefore, acute illness in elderly patients is often accompanied by derangements in fluid and electrolyte balance.
- Changes in the endocrine system may lead to diabetes and thyroid abnormalities in older patients.
- Aging brings a widespread decrease in bone mass in men and women, but especially among postmenopausal women. Bones become more brittle and tend to break more easily.
- Changes in the nervous system lead to a decrease in the performance of sense organs, as evidenced by visual changes (glaucoma and cataracts are common) and hearing loss.
- Diseases of the heart remain the leading cause of death among older adults in Canada. Heart attack is the major cause of morbidity and mortality in people older than 65 years, and its potential for mortality increases significantly after 70 years.
- Stroke is a significant cause of death and disability in elderly people. More than 80% of all stroke deaths occur in persons older than 65 years, and stroke is the leading cause of long-term disability at any age.
- Chronic lower respiratory disease, influenza, and pneumonia remain in the top five causes for geriatric deaths.
- A geriatric patient with diabetes is at increased risk for hypoglycemia for several reasons: medications, inadequate or irregular dietary intake, inability to recognize the warning signs due to cognitive problems, and/or blunted warning signs. Delirium may be the only indication of hypoglycemia in an elderly patient.
- Older diabetics whose blood glucose levels tend to be high are prone to hyperosmolar hyperglycemic nonketotic (HHNK) coma. The most frequent cause for HHNK is infection. Presentation is likely to be acute confusion with dehydration.
- Gastrointestinal problems in elderly people include peptic ulcer disease, small bowel obstruction due to gallstones, and stomach or duodenal ulcers (peptic ulcer disease).
- Osteoporosis is characterized by a decrease in bone mass leading to reduction in bone strength and greater susceptibility to fracture. Osteoarthritis is a progressive disease process of the joints that destroys cartilage, promotes the formation of bone spurs in joints, and leads to joint stiffness.
- In elderly people, delirium often replaces or confounds the typical presentation caused by a medical problem, an adverse medication effect, or drug withdrawal. Disorders that cause delirium may also include poisons, electrolyte imbalances, nutritional deficiencies, and infections such as urinary tract infections and pneumonia.
- Unlike delirium, dementia is a disease that produces irreversible brain failure. Disorders that cause dementia include conditions that impair vascular and neurologic structures within the brain, such as infections, stroke, head injuries, poor nutrition, and medications.
- The two most common degenerative types of dementia in older people are Alzheimer's disease and multi-infarct or vascular dementia, both of which cause structural damage to the brain.
- Elderly people are particularly prone to adverse drug reactions because of changes in the following: drug metabolism because of diminished hepatic function; drug elimination because of diminished renal function; body composition, including increased body fat and decreased body water, altering the distribution of drugs through the various body compartments; and the responsiveness to drugs of the central nervous system.
- Alcohol is the preferred substance of maltreatment among older persons, in whom its use is on the rise. A much smaller but increasing segment of the geriatric population uses illicit drugs.
- Depression in elderly patients can mimic the effects of many other medical problems (such as dementia). Risk factors for depression in an older person include a history of depression, chronic disease, and loss (function, independence, or significant others).
- Several factors place an elderly person at higher risk of trauma than a younger person: slower reflexes, visual and hearing deficits, equilibrium disorders, and an overall reduction in agility.
- Most geriatric trauma cases involve falls or motor vehicle collisions. Falls among elderly people are evenly divided between those resulting from extrinsic (external) causes, such as tripping on a loose rug or slipping on ice, and those resulting from intrinsic (internal) causes, such as a dizzy spell or a syncopal attack.
- Knowing what is and what is not part of the aging process constitutes the first challenge in assessing elderly patients. A second challenge is that signs and symptoms of disease may be altered from their presentation in younger patients as a consequence of aging.
- When a patient's chief complaint seems trivial, it may be necessary to go through a review of systems to confirm that you are not missing important pieces of information. If any of the screening questions yields a positive answer, follow up with further questions.
- The physical examination of older patients can be difficult. Poor cooperation and easy fatigability may require that you keep manipulations of the patient to a minimum. You may have to peel many layers of clothing off elderly patients to perform an adequate examination.
- Infections in older persons can be severe and dangerous. Consider sepsis whenever you see a hot, flushed patient who is also tachycardic and tachypneic.
- Elder maltreatment is any form of mistreatment that results in harm or loss to an older person. Five types of maltreatment are distinguished: physical, sexual, emotional, neglect, and financial.

Vital Vocabulary

bereavement Sadness from loss; grieving.

delirium An acute confusional state characterized by global impairment of thinking, perception, judgment, and memory.

dementia A chronic deterioration of mental functions.

geriatrics The assessment and treatment of disease in someone 65 years or older.

homeostasis A tendency to constancy or stability in the body's internal milieu.

hospice An organization that provides end-of-life care to patients with terminal illnesses and their families.

osteoporosis A decrease in bone mass and density.

polypharmacy The use of multiple medications.

presbycusis Progressive hearing loss, particularly in the high frequencies, along with lessened ability to discriminate between a particular sound and background noise.

proprioception The ability to perceive the position and movement of one's body or limbs.

review of systems A systematic survey of the patient's symptoms according to the major organ systems.

sepsis A disease state that results from the presence of microorganisms or their toxic products in the bloodstream.

spondylosis Immobility and consolidation of a vertebral joint.

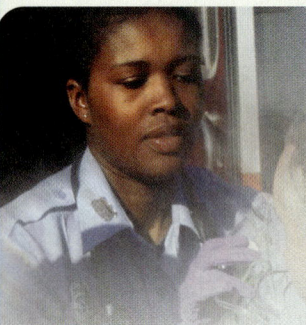

Assessment in Action

You are dispatched to a private residence for a fall. When you arrive on scene, you find an elderly man lying on his back. A large pool of blood is around his head. The patient is conscious, alert, and oriented to person, place, and day. He denies experiencing any loss of consciousness. He states that he was trying to get around the corner and tripped over his feet. His wife tells you that he has neuropathy to both his lower legs, bilateral knee replacements, and a hip replacement. He also has a history of blood clots and hypertension. His medications include lisinopril (Zestril) and warfarin (Coumadin). He has a large laceration to the back of his head. His vital signs are stable.

1. **A common change seen in the cardiovascular system of the elderly patient is:**
   A. neuropathy.
   B. hypertrophy.
   C. increased inotropy.
   D. increased automaticity.

2. **Changes in thinking, speed, memory, and postural stability are effects of the:**
   A. cardiovascular system.
   B. nervous system.
   C. pulmonary system.
   D. renal system.

3. **What is homeostasis?**
   A. Maintaining the constancy of the external environment
   B. An acute confusional state
   C. A decrease in bone mass and density
   D. Maintaining the constancy of the internal environment

4. **What is osteoarthritis?**
   A. A progressive disease process of the joints resulting in the destruction of cartilage
   B. A condition that affects only women and is characterized by a decrease in bone mass
   C. Atrophy of the supporting structures of the body
   D. A condition in which muscle fibres are smaller and fewer in numbers

5. **For what reasons are elderly persons particularly prone to adverse drug reactions?**
   A. Changes in drug metabolism because of diminished hepatic function
   B. Changes in drug elimination because of diminished renal function
   C. Changes in body composition, increased body fat, and decreased body water
   D. Changes in responsiveness to drugs that affect the central nervous system
   E. All of the above

6. **The underlying causes of falls among the elderly are classified as being:**
   A. extrinsic and intrinsic.
   B. medical illness and trauma.
   C. extrinsic and external.
   D. intrinsic and internal.

7. **In the elderly, _____ are MOST common after a fall.**
   A. epidural hematomas
   B. subdural hematomas
   C. intracerebral aneurysms
   D. ruptured cerebral arteries

Challenging Question

8. **Why do many geriatric patients present atypically when they experience an injury or illness that causes shock?**

Points to Ponder

It's 19:00 hr and your shift has just begun. You are dispatched to the assisted-living facility across town for an 86-year-old woman with chest pain. You recognize the address and apartment number as one that you have been to on several occasions. When you arrive, the patient's condition appears stable, but she has chest pain on palpation, inspiration, and movement. Her vital signs are as follows: pulse rate, 58 beats/min with sinus bradycardia on the cardiac monitor; blood pressure, 110/72 mm Hg; respiratory rate, 16 breaths/min; and pulse oximetry, 95% on room air. The patient tells you that this pain began after she received a phone call from her daughter, who was supposed to come and visit her and is now unable to do so.

Does this patient need to be transported immediately? How will you manage this patient?

Issues: Being an Advocate for the Elderly, Recognizing the Need for Independence in the Elderly.

43 Maltreatment, Neglect, and Assault

Competency Areas

Area 1: Professional Responsibilities

1.1.b   Reflect professionalism through use of appropriate language.

1.1.e   Maintain patient confidentiality.

1.1.j   Behave ethically.

1.1.k   Function as patient advocate.

1.3.b   Recognize "patient rights" and the implications on the role of the provider.

1.6.a   Exhibit reasonable and prudent judgement.

1.6.b   Practice effective problem-solving.

Area 2: Communication

2.1.e   Interact effectively with the patient, relatives, and bystanders who are in stressful situations.

2.1.g   Use appropriate terminology.

2.2.a   Record organized, accurate, and relevant patient information.

2.2.b   Prepare professional correspondence.

2.3.a   Exhibit effective non-verbal behaviour.

2.3.b   Practice active listening techniques.

2.3.c   Establish trust and rapport with patients and colleagues.

2.3.d   Recognize and react appropriately to non-verbal behaviours.

2.4.a   Treat others with respect.

2.4.b   Exhibit empathy and compassion while providing care.

2.4.c   Recognize and react appropriately to individuals and groups manifesting coping mechanisms.

2.4.d   Act in a confident manner.

2.4.e   Act assertively as required.

2.4.f   Manage and provide support to patients, bystanders, and relatives manifesting emotional reactions.

2.4.g   Exhibit diplomacy, tact, and discretion.

2.4.h   Exhibit conflict resolution skills.

Appendix 4: Pathophysiology

K.   **Psychiatric Disorders**
Anxiety Disorder: Acute stress disorder
Anxiety Disorder: Situational disturbances
Affective Disorders: Depressive disorders

Introduction

Maltreatment, neglect, and assault of children, women, and the elderly are, unfortunately, all too common Table 43-1 ▾. Because these issues are frequently encountered reasons for calls to EMS, it is important for you to recognize the signs and symptoms. You must know not only how to recognize and differentiate among maltreatment, neglect, and assault, but also how to protect yourself from injury while maintaining optimal prehospital care for the patient. Victims who survive maltreatment or neglect often have permanent disabilities, mental and physical. Although prevention strategies have improved in recent years, paramedics may be on the front lines for getting help to victims of maltreatment Figure 43-1 ▸ .

Table 43-1	Substantial Incidence of Maltreatment in Canada 2003*
Type of Maltreatment	**Percentage**
Neglect	30
Exposure to domestic violence	28
Physical abuse	24
Emotional abuse	15
Sexual abuse	3

*Excluding Quebec.

Source: Canadian Incidence Study of Reported Child Abuse and Neglect–2003. Available at: www.phac-aspc.gc.ca/cm-vee/csca-ecve/pdf/childabuse_final_e.pdf. Accessed January 16, 2009.

Child Maltreatment

Child maltreatment includes any improper or excessive action that injures or otherwise harms a child or infant or puts a child or infant at serious risk of harm, including physical abuse, sexual abuse, neglect, and emotional abuse. In Canada in

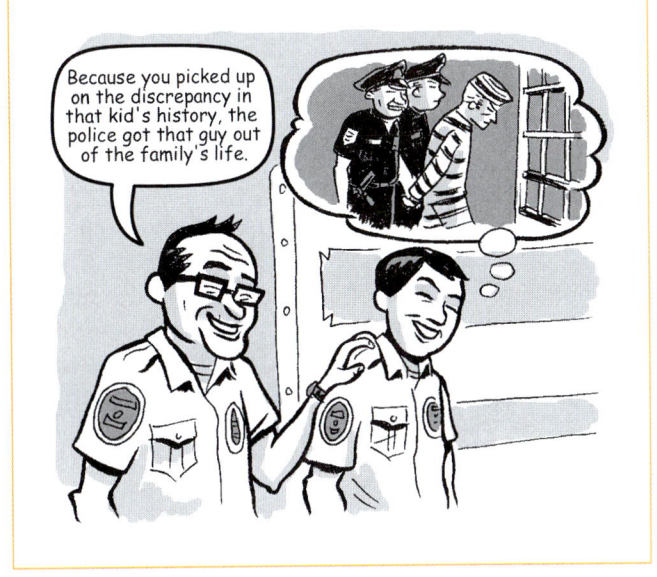

Figure 43-1

You are the Paramedic Part 1

You respond to a call for a "child who fell." On arrival, you find an unconscious 5-month-old boy. The mother just came home from work; her boyfriend had been watching the baby. The boyfriend states that the baby "fell off the couch" approximately 30 cm from the carpeted floor. The child is comatose and has ataxic breathing.

The boyfriend appears nervous. He tries to answer all questions asked of the mother and to control the scene. In the same apartment, you find a 7-year-old girl with wheezing in all fields. The mother states that the child has a puffer, but it is empty and the mother has no insurance to obtain a refill. Five other children are in the cramped apartment, all under 10 years of age. The one-bedroom apartment is clean but very small, and children must sleep on a bare mattress in the living room. The mother sleeps in the bedroom with the baby (in the same bed).

Initial Assessment	Recording Time: 0 Minutes	
	5-month-old patient	**7-year-old patient**
Appearance	Comatose	Agitated, pensive
Level of consciousness	U (Unresponsive)	A (Alert to person, place, and day)
Airway	Mildly obstructed	Mildly obstructed
Breathing	22 breaths/min; irregular	> 40 breaths/min; shallow
Circulation	78 beats/min; irregular	> 140 beats/min; regular
Skin	Acrocyanotic	Flushed

1. What are your first priorities after assessing scene safety?
2. What should raise your index of suspicion?
3. What is the 5-month-old patient's transport and treatment status, in your judgment?

Table 43-2	Potential Complications of Maltreatment

- Low self-esteem and underachievement
- Abnormal growth and development
- Poor school performance
- Social withdrawal
- Substance abuse
- Criminal behaviour beginning in young adulthood
- Suicidal tendencies
- Death
- Psychological disorders or psychiatric symptoms
- Permanent physical or neurologic damage
- Teen promiscuity and pregnancy
- Eating disorders
- Negative learned behaviour
- Vulnerability to further abuse
- Increased survivor health care costs to family and society

Source: American Academy of Pediatrics. *Pediatric Education for Prehospital Professionals*, 2nd ed. Table 12-1, p. 244. Sudbury, MA: Jones and Bartlett Publishers, Inc, 2006.

Table 43-3	Risk Factors for Child Maltreatment

Parent or Caregiver
- Parental history of maltreatment as a child
- Substance abuse by parents
- Insufficient or inaccurate parental knowledge about child development

Family
- Disorganized and disruptive family structure
- Marital or partner discord
- Financial or outside stressors present
- Inappropriate or dysfunctional parent–child interaction

Child
- Disability of the child
- Attention deficits or difficult temperament of child

Environment
- Home life affected by poverty or unemployment
- Isolation of caregivers; lack of social support
- Violent, crime-filled community

Source: Child Welfare Information Gateway. Available at: http://www.childwelfare.gov/pubs/usermanuals/foundation/foundatione.cfm. Accessed July 24, 2008.

1998, approximately 2.1% of all children were the subject of investigation by child welfare authorities. Many survivors are negatively affected by such maltreatment for the rest of their lives. Owing to the physical and psychological injuries they experience, survivors may themselves become abusive or neglectful caregivers, perpetuating the cycle of maltreatment. The number of children with long-term effects from neglect has not been well documented but is believed to be substantial. **Table 43-2 ▲** lists some of these potential long-term complications.

Child neglect occurs when a child's physical, mental, or emotional condition is harmed or endangered because the caregiver fails to supply basic necessities or engages in inadequate or dangerous child-rearing practices. Neglect includes failure to provide adequate food, clothing, or shelter; the caregiver's misuse of drugs or alcohol; failure to provide support or affection necessary to the child's psychological and social development; or child abandonment. Children who are neglected are often dirty or too thin or appear developmentally delayed because of a lack of stimulation.

As a paramedic, you will often be called to scenes because of a reported injury to a child. Many maltreated children have permanent or life-threatening injuries, and some die. If suspected child maltreatment is not reported, the child is likely to be victimized repeatedly. Therefore, you must be aware of the signs of child abuse and neglect and cognizant of your responsibility to report suspected maltreatment to law enforcement or child protection agencies. When in doubt as to whether it is an abuse or neglect situation, it is always better to err on the side of caution to protect the victim.

Profile of an At-Risk Child

Child abuse and neglect occurs in all communities and among all socioeconomic strata. Younger children are at higher risk for fatal abuse and neglect than are older children. Approximately 85% of abused or neglected children who die are younger than 6 years; more than 40% are younger than 1 year. Although no

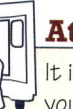

At the Scene

It is a good idea to establish a "code" between you and your partner indicating that the paramedic should discreetly call for police. This signal can be as simple as "Could you go to the ambulance and get the extra set of latex-free gloves?" This way, you will not aggravate or "tip off" the caregiver to your request for police, further riling the abuser.

geographic, ethnic, or economic setting is free of child maltreatment or neglect, children from low-income or single-parent families have more *reported* occurrences of abuse and neglect than children from higher-income families. **Table 43-3 ▲** lists other factors that put a child at risk of maltreatment.

When assessing a potential child maltreatment case, be attuned to suspicious behavioural traits. A child who does not become agitated when a parent leaves the room or who does not look to a parent for reassurance may be maltreated. Children who are maltreated may also cry excessively or not at all, may be wary of physical contact, or may appear apprehensive.

People Who Maltreat Children

Child maltreatment can be done by any person who has care, custody, or control of the child, including parents, stepparents, foster parents, babysitters, and relatives. Parents who maltreat their children frequently receive little enjoyment from parenting and are more isolated from the community than those parents who do not maltreat their children. They have unrealistic expectations of their child and try to control the

Table 43-4	"Red Flag" Caregiver Behaviours

- Apathy
- Bizarre or strange conduct
- Little or no concern about the child
- Overreaction to child misbehaviour
- Not forthcoming with events surrounding injury
- Intoxication
- Overreaction to child's condition

Source: American Academy of Pediatrics. *Pediatric Education for Prehospital Professionals*, 2nd ed. Table 12-7, p. 250. Sudbury, MA: Jones and Bartlett Publishers, Inc, 2006.

child through negative and authoritarian means. Parents who maltreat their children are often afraid of, or emotionally unable to ask for help from, sources of support in their community. Most were themselves maltreated or neglected as children. Many view themselves as victims in life generally or in the parent–child relationship in particular. They feel that they have lost control of their children and their own lives. When their children behave in a manner that parents perceive as disrespectful, they lash out in an effort to establish control. Caregivers may prefer to discipline using other means but are pushed to violence by stress.

Characteristics shared by caregivers of maltreated children include drug use, poor self-concept, immaturity, lack of parenting knowledge, and lack of interpersonal skills. **Table 43-4 ▲** lists additional "red flag" caregiver behaviours.

Assessment and Management of Child Maltreatment

One of the most important indicators of possible maltreatment is repeated calls to the same home or family for a child injury or medical problem. Nevertheless, the best indicator by far is the physical examination of the child, conducted with a keen ear for inconsistencies in the history. The physical examination must take into consideration the mental and emotional age of the child. Examining the child from toe to head may work best on toddlers and preschoolers, whereas an infant may be best examined in a parent's arms. Preadolescents and teenagers have modesty and body awareness concerns, which should be respected.

If possible, do the examination with another colleague. This approach will verify your findings and help prevent false accusations of impropriety. Also, make certain that you are very objective on your documentation. Do not include opinions or draw nonmedical conclusions; list only the objective information, and stick to the facts.

When assessing for possible child maltreatment, you may find the CHILD ABUSE mnemonic helpful:

C *Consistency* of the injury with the child's developmental age
H *History* inconsistent with injury
I *Inappropriate* parental concerns
L *Lack* of supervision
D *Delay* in seeking care
A *Affect*
B *Bruises* of varying ages
U *Unusual* injury patterns
S *Suspicious* circumstances
E *Environmental* clues

Soft-tissue injuries are the most common findings in the physical examination of an abused child. Multiple bruises in various stages of healing are another red flag **Figure 43-2 ▶**. Be alert for bruises on areas of the body where they would not be expected, such as the buttocks **Figure 43-3 ▶**, back, face, and upper legs. Bites and burns may also be noted.

You are the Paramedic Part 2

You decide to call the police to the scene, owing to the injuries and current history of the 5-month-old patient. The boyfriend becomes visibly agitated when he hears you on the radio. "What do we need cops for? Just take care of the kid," he states. After making sure you have a visible escape route, you continue caring for the child and tell the man, "It's just routine." You then ask the mother for the medical history of the child, hoping to deflect the man's attention. At this time, the 5-month-old boy is having difficulty in breathing, his extremities are becoming cyanotic, and he does not respond to external stimuli. The 7-year-old girl with asthma is in moderate distress as your partner sets up the nebulizer with the pediatric dose of salbutamol.

Vital Signs	Recording Time: 5 Minutes	
	5-month-old patient	7-year-old patient
Skin	Cool and dry, cyanotic extremities	Warm, wet
Pulse	62 beats/min	120 beats/min
Blood pressure	Unobtainable	96/50 mm Hg
Respirations	20 breaths/min; irregular	32 breaths/min
Spo2	89 mm Hg on room air	97 mm Hg on room air

4. Do you think you will have to intubate the 5-month-old boy? Why or why not?

5. Do you think you will have to intubate the 7-year-old girl? Why or why not?

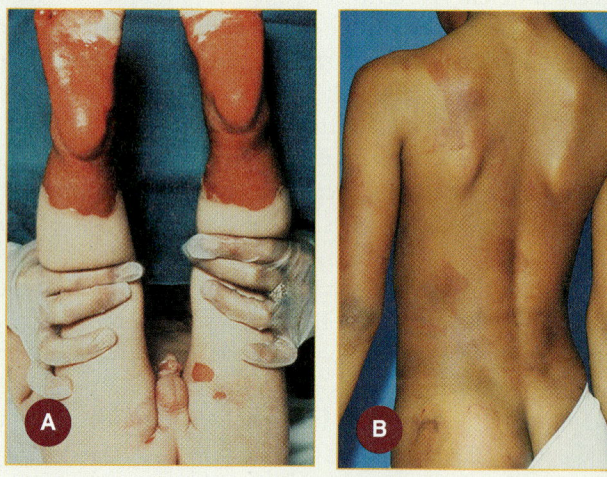

Figure 43-2 Signs of child maltreatment. **A.** Scald. **B.** Multiple injuries at different stages of healing.

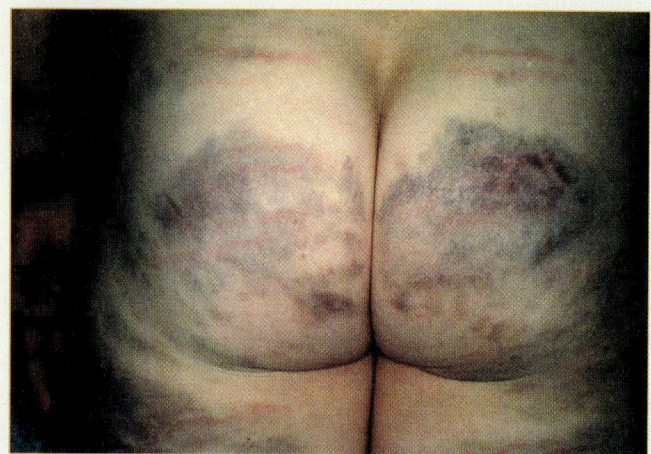

Figure 43-3 Bruises on the buttocks are usually inflicted injuries.

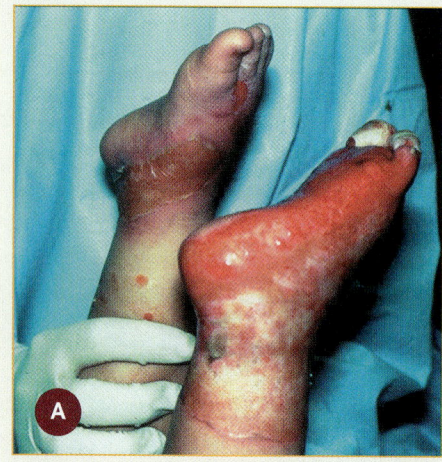
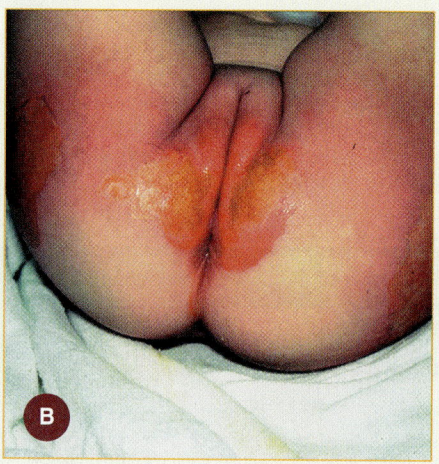

Figure 43-4 A. Stocking/glove burns of the feet or hands in an infant or a toddler are almost always inflicted injuries. **B.** A doughnut burn occurs when a child is held in a hot bath and the area in contact with the cooler porcelain is spared.

Stocking/glove burns and doughnut burns occur when a child is immersed in hot water Figure 43-4 ◂ .

Fractures can result from falls, twisting, or jerking injuries. Multiple fractures or fractures in various stages of healing are indicators of maltreatment, as are "self-healing" fractures. Head injuries are the most deadly for children; even if not fatal, they can easily produce permanent disability. Look for scalp wounds, signs and symptoms of hematoma, and concussion Figure 43-5 ▴ .

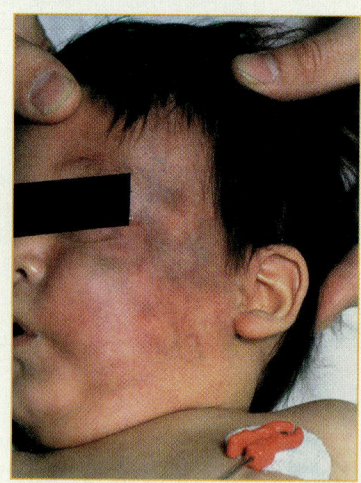

Figure 43-5 The face is a common target for physical maltreatment.

Although abdominal injuries are rare in child maltreatment cases, they are usually serious. Remember, small children have thin and underdeveloped abdominal muscles. Note the colour and rigidity of the abdomen and tenderness to palpation. Injuries to the abdomen may result in injuries to the intestines or rupture of the liver.

Sometimes, normal physical findings may suggest an inflicted injury. Other benign skin findings can also suggest maltreatment, although the lesions are actually produced by cultural rituals intended to treat illness. Some medical or folk remedies may be foreign to you or inconsistent with your training. For example, cupping Figure 43-6 ▸ and coin rubbing Figure 43-7 ▸ are alarming to most paramedics, but a reasonable explanation of the practice, which is common in some Asian cultures, should allay your suspicions.

It is important to observe the scene, including the household dynamics, as you provide prehospital care for the patient. In the "You are the Paramedic" scenario in this chapter, the first responders discovered two patients; be aware that more than one victim may be encountered. It is important to keep the scene as safe and calm as possible while still providing life support for any critical and moderately distressed patients.

In a case involving child abuse or neglect, the patient care reports (PCRs), with objective observations, will be very important to the police and child protective services (CPS). In most provinces and territories, the paramedic is a mandated reporter in child abuse or neglect cases.

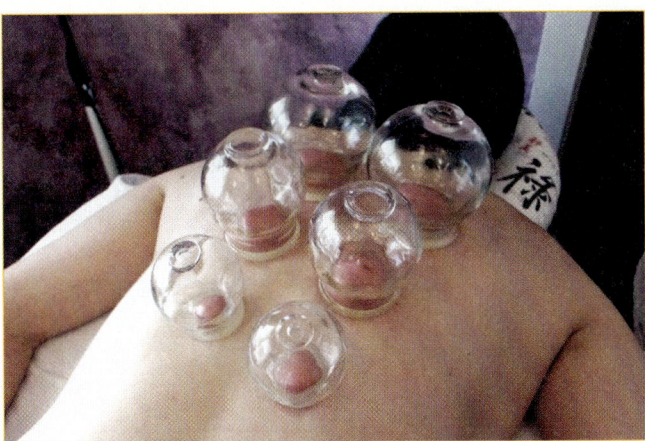

Figure 43-6 Cupping is the cultural practice of placing warm cups on the skin to pull out illness from the body. The red, flat, rounded skin lesions are often more intensely red at the borders.

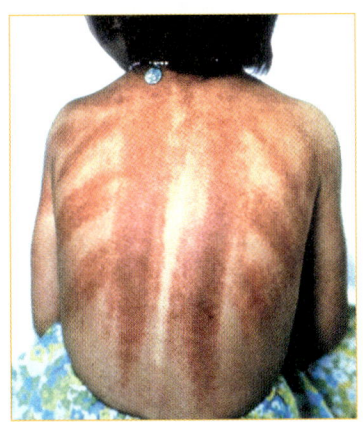

Figure 43-7 Rubbing hot coins, often on the back, produces rounded and oblong red, patchy, flat skin lesions.

Most provinces and territories have also established toll-free numbers for reporting suspected child abuse or neglect. Don't assume that someone else has already called or that the emergency department will call! It is better to have more than one person call the hotline for the same case than to see the case "fall through the cracks." Most communities also have parenting classes available through county social services.

Elder Maltreatment

The incidence of older patient maltreatment and neglect is growing. The aging of the population and the strains placed on caregivers and the nursing home systems contribute to this problem. You must use sound judgment and learn to develop good observational skills. Because geriatric patients present much differently than children and younger adults, you must be especially attuned to the possibility of maltreatment in this population. Consider the following scenario:

You respond to a call for "man down." On arrival, you find an 86-year-old man lying on his side in the living room, bleeding from the mouth and nose. He appears confused, and you cannot understand what he is trying to say. His 56-year-old daughter states that her father tripped and fell. His vital signs are as follows:

pulse, 68 beats/min; respirations, 14 breaths/min; and blood pressure, 100/68 mm Hg. The patient's skin is warm and wet. You see a walker device in the kitchen approximately 8 m away. The daughter states that the patient doesn't really need it, stating, "He just uses it to get sympathy." The daughter is very upset that the police have just pulled up. Your partner tells you that she has been to this home several times before for falls, that the patient has Alzheimer's disease, and that the daughter seems to lose patience with him, sometimes refusing to cooperate with the paramedics. The daughter then states, "Would you people hurry up and get him out of here? He's getting blood all over the rug."

In this scenario, the elderly patient clearly needs assistance, but his caregiver also seems to be overwhelmed. This situation is not unusual: Because people are living longer than ever before, their children (often baby boomers) must assume responsibility for their care. The stress on these caregivers is real—physical, emotional, and financial burdens can wear them down. Your crews should be familiar with local resources to assist caregivers and patients. This assistance can be as simple as a visiting nurse or a handy-van agency to take the patient to his or her doctor's appointments.

As with child maltreatment, elder maltreatment involves a direct action causing harm to the victim. Maltreatment of older patients includes sexual abuse, psychological or emotional abuse, neglect, and abandonment. Neglect can be active or passive. Active neglect refers to the deliberate withholding of companionship, medicine, food, exercise, or assistance with mobility; passive neglect occurs when an older person is ignored, left alone, isolated, or forgotten. Abandonment is the desertion of an older person by a person who has physical custody of the older person or by a person who has assumed responsibility for providing care. Table 43-5 ▾ lists the characteristics of older maltreated patients. In domestic maltreatment cases, the perpetrators are quite often the children of the maltreated person Table 43-6 ▾ .

Table 43-5	Profile of Maltreated Older Patients

- Women
- Persons older than 75 years
- Persons with one or more chronic physical or mental impairments placing them in a care-dependent position
- Persons who live with their abusers
- Socially isolated people
- Persons who exhibit problematic behaviour (such as incontinence or shouting)

Table 43-6	Profile of a Person Who Maltreats Elders

- Lives with the victim
- Has drug or alcohol dependency problems
- Is older than 50 years
- Depends on the victim for financial support
- Has poor impulse control
- Is ill prepared or reluctant to provide care
- Has a history of domestic violence

Factors Contributing to Elder Maltreatment

Although paramedics are concerned with treating and managing the results of abuse and neglect, an understanding of why these problems occur can be beneficial in the prehospital setting. In some cases, the violence may be a learned response. Children who were maltreated may ultimately be in a position to maltreat their elderly parents. The stress of caring for an older person may push some caregivers into abuse or neglect. Factors such as a diminishing social network, frailty, and medical illness also put older people at risk for maltreatment. Older people are at an increased risk for maltreatment in nursing facilities that have a history of providing inadequate care, are understaffed, and provide poor training for their employees.

Signs of Elder Maltreatment

The signs and symptoms of elder abuse and neglect can be subtle and, in the emergency setting, can often be overlooked. Evaluate each situation involving an older person with a critical eye toward potential abuse and neglect.

Be on the lookout for a fearful patient with unexplained bruises or sores that have not been tended to. Of course, the patient may naturally be fearful of the whole emergency situation, and there may well be a reasonable explanation for the marks on the body. Be alert for a situation in which you find an unkempt, dirty patient while the caregiver is clean. Generally speaking, a solicitous caregiver will keep the patient and the patient's surroundings tidy. Watch for a patient who allows the caregiver to answer all of your questions, while appearing mentally competent to do so; this person may look to the caregiver for approval when you ask the patient a direct question. If a patient tells you that items are being taken or money confiscated, such a complaint may be an indication of paranoia or a symptom of dementia—but it could very well be true. Don't investigate these claims; simply document them thoroughly. Be wary if a patient states that he or she is not allowed to socialize with peers and is kept in isolation.

Generally speaking, maltreated elders do not seek help. This reluctance may be due to fear of being institutionalized, fear of getting the person performing the maltreatment into "trouble," polypharmacy, confusion, or brain disorders such as Alzheimer's disease. In such cases, the physical examination, history, and observation of scene surroundings and patient interaction with caregivers are of paramount concern. The physical examination and history should address the following issues:

- Is the patient capable of answering your questions in an appropriate way?
- Is the patient fearful?
- Does the patient look clean?
- Are the pill bottles marked appropriately and consistent with purchase dates and use?
- Does the patient have bruises or sores?
- Is the patient's current history consistent with the report given by the caregiver?

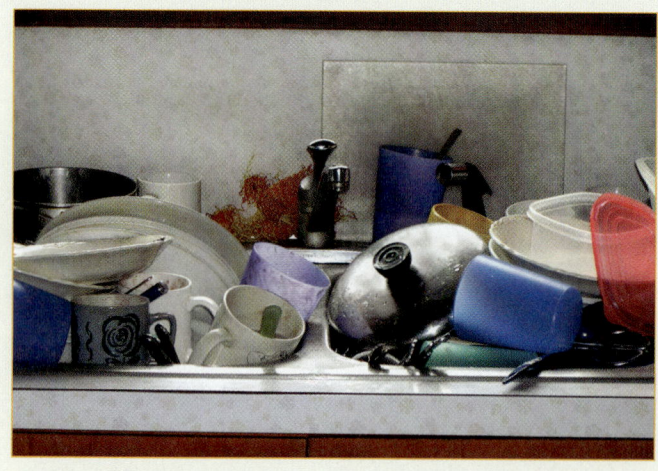

Figure 43-8 The patient's environment can provide clues to maltreatment.

Objectively record your observations on the PCR, avoiding drawing conclusions and giving opinions. Adult protective services (APS) could use these observations as an indicator of whether assistance is required.

As far as the scene goes, ask these questions **Figure 43-8 ▲** :

- Is the home tidy, and are the surroundings orderly?
- Is there food in the refrigerator?
- What is the heating or cooling situation, and is it appropriate to the weather?
- Does the patient use a walking or wheelchair device?

For patients who reside in nursing homes, signs of maltreatment include undocumented decubitus ulcers, tied-off catheters, and dangerous use of restraints. Some nursing home residents who are victims of maltreatment may not have a way to report the maltreatment, may not know how to report the maltreatment, may not be physically able to report it, or may fear retaliation for reporting it. Others may be victims of maltreatment by visiting family members.

Although the aging of the population has placed increased demands on the system, institutional caregivers have a legal obligation to meet accepted standards of care. Most communities have health departments that provide care and even transportation for elderly citizens. If the patient is institutionalized and maltreatment or neglect is suspected, you may notify the regulatory commission responsible for overseeing the facility. You should thoroughly familiarize yourself with all local assistance and keep an up-to-date directory with 24-hour phone numbers.

Domestic Maltreatment

Violence within the family has a long history. In ancient Rome, for example, husbands had the legal right to administer physical punishment to their wives within their own homes and in public. Today, paramedics are frequently called for assault and battery in the home. The statistics on intimate-partner maltreatment are sobering: Millions of women are maltreated by an intimate partner each year.

Calls of this nature challenge the skills of paramedics. Scene safety is a paramount concern, and preservation of evidence is a necessity. Consider the following scenario:

> You are called for a "woman bleeding." When you arrive, a man opens the door and tells you that his wife fell down the stairs. You find a 42-year-old woman crying and bleeding from her mouth. She has obvious contusions and abrasions on her face. Vital signs are a pulse of 124 beats/min, respirations of 28 breaths/min, and blood pressure of 132/84 mm Hg. The patient is alert and oriented to person, place, and day; her skin is warm and dry. Her husband tries to answer all of the questions you pose to her. The stairwell is carpeted and has only seven risers, but there is no blood on the stairs. Two children, ages 6 and 12, are crying in an adjacent bedroom. The father tells them to stay in the bedroom. Police have not been dispatched to this call yet.

At the Scene

If you and your partner can safely get the patient and the person suspected of maltreatment away from each other, by all means do so. This separation will help make the scene safer; it also gives you a chance to compare current histories.

Is there significance to the husband dominating the patient interview? Should the crying children raise any red flags? The children's concern and the husband's control of the scene could be perfectly normal behaviour. You must look at all the pieces of the puzzle. Document what you have observed, not what you think.

As a paramedic, you must be able to recognize the scope of domestic maltreatment and understand its various forms:

- **Physical**—hitting, kicking, pushing, shoving, choking, beating
- **Emotional**—making negative comments, calling names, playing mind games
- **Economic**—trying to keep a person from getting a job and gaining his or her own economic independence
- **Sexual**—making a person perform sexual activities against his or her will

Even though the awareness of domestic maltreatment has been raised in recent years, dealing with these cases in the prehospital environment presents a challenge to the paramedic. Battered patients may not give accurate details about their injuries, and they may avoid seeking help. Indeed, victims typically report their maltreatment only as a last resort, for many reasons—for example, shame, embarrassment, financial considerations, and low self-esteem. Moreover, many victims do not want the person responsible for the maltreatment to be charged or removed from the home, nor do they want to leave for a shelter. Many times they believe the behaviour will change, as is often promised by the abuser. Sometimes the victim believes that he or she is the reason for the maltreatment and somehow deserved it.

Finally, some victims may fear even greater maltreatment should they disclose the truth about their injuries.

Profile of a Maltreated Spouse

Physical injuries from maltreatment include broken bones, cuts, head injuries, bruises, burns, scars from old injuries, and internal injuries. A maltreated spouse may have feelings of anxiety, distress, or hopelessness and may show signs of depression, make suicide attempts, or engage in substance abuse.

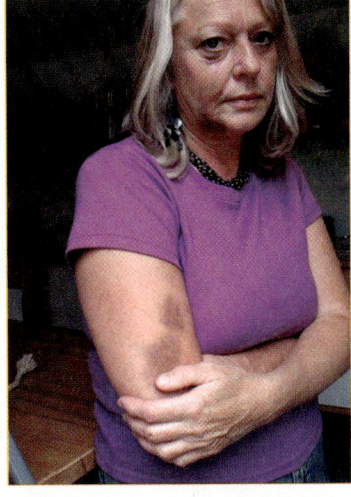

Figure 43-9 Injuries associated with intimate-partner maltreatment.

Although in the overwhelming majority of cases the victim is a woman, men also are maltreated. Men who are battered may be too humiliated to report the incident as it happened but still feel the same emotions as their female counterparts: guilt, loss of control, and shame. Because society tends to be less empathetic toward maltreated men and because fewer resources exist for them, the situation can be all the more difficult.

Same-sex relationships can be as fraught with peril as heterosexual unions. A common misconception is that participants in same-sex relationships are "on an equal playing field," so that the maltreatment cannot be as serious as that found in heterosexual relationships. In reality, concerns about "coming out" may prevent these victims from seeking help. You must be aware of and sensitive to their concerns.

Battered patients may appear fearful, apprehensive, or nonverbal. They may avoid eye contact, and their answers may be incorrect or inconsistent. Be alert for verbal clues such as "It was my fault—I really shouldn't push him" or "He's a good person—it's just that when he drinks . . ." In many provinces and territories, there are guidelines and policies that direct the police to lay a charge, as defined in the criminal code, when they suspect that an assault has occurred **Figure 43-9 ▲** .

People Who Maltreat Their Partners

Research confirms that they are a diverse population. Approximately half show no psychological deficits or difficulties, whereas others may be overly sensitive, obsessive, paranoid, or threatening. They often abuse alcohol or drugs and may have access to weapons or they may exhibit none of these characteristics. **Table 43-7 ▶** lists other characteristics of abusers.

Table 43-7	Characteristics of a Person Who Maltreats a Partner

- Was maltreated as a child
- May become more violent with each ensuing attack
- Usually comes from a family where maltreatment was common
- Very low self-esteem
- Remorseful after the attack; promises it will never happen again (but it does)
- May direct violence at children, especially children from a partner's previous relationship(s)

People who maltreat partners or spouses may use intimidation and threats to maintain their control over the person. They may throw objects in a rage or threaten regarding what he or she will do if the spouse leaves or reports the abusive behaviour. A spouse who maltreats his or her partner may also use isolation as a means to dominate the partner, not allowing the spouse to visit friends or talk openly with others, and may feel that he or she is providing discipline or is justified in these actions. Many times, the spouse who maltreats his or her partner is immediately remorseful and promises never to let the problem happen again. Historically, this is rarely true; the maltreatment usually continues and becomes even more violent.

Never forget that domestic violence calls can be dangerous. You may be dealing with a potentially violent person, and emotions on the scene will be highly charged. If the person appears to be hostile or violent, remove all unnecessary people (such as family, friends, and bystanders) from the scene. It is imperative that you put your safety and the safety of your partner first. If there is any doubt about scene safety, call for law enforcement assistance (see Chapter 51) **Figure 43-10 ▶**.

Assessment and Management of Domestic Maltreatment

Identifying a battered patient can be difficult because the victim may be protective of the attacker, frightened, or honestly unable to recall details. Patients may avoid eye contact or be

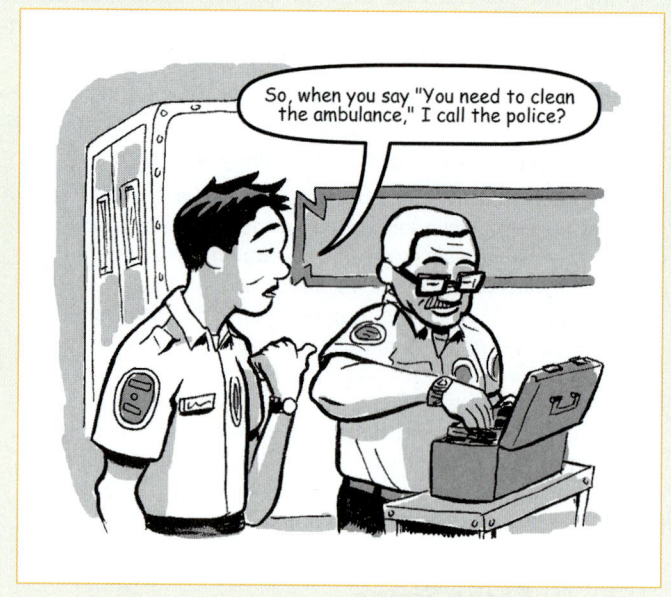

Figure 43-10

otherwise evasive about their injuries. Listen for verbal clues regarding the incident, such as "We've been having some problems." On approach to the patient, use direct questioning to ascertain the physical harm. Try to empathize and reassure the patient; this caring attitude alone may instill confidence. Be as objective and nonjudgmental as possible. Listen attentively, and be supportive. Give the patient a sense of control as much as possible. You may be the last or only chance a victim has to escape this situation, so encourage the patient to consider where he or she can go or whom he or she can call for help.

In cases involving domestic maltreatment, the PCR is more than just documentation of the transfer of care; it is a permanent record of treatment and disposition. More important, from a legal viewpoint, it represents hard evidence for the prosecution and the defence. Your statements and assessments must be objective, nonjudgmental, exact (when

You are the Paramedic Part 3

Vital Signs	Recording Time: 10 Minutes	
	5-month-old patient	7-year-old patient
Skin	Good colour; cool and dry	Warm, wet
Pulse	98 beats/min	110 beats/min
Blood pressure	60/P	96/50 mm Hg
Respirations	Intubated	Nebulizer treatment; normal breaths/min
Spo₂	98 mm Hg	100 mm Hg

6. What further treatment do you need for the 5-month-old boy? How can you check for level of consciousness at this point?

7. Is the small-volume nebulizer treatment working for the 7-year-old girl? Does this patient need to go to the hospital? Why or why not?

quoting a statement from the scene), and as neat as possible. If you make an error and want to change it, draw a line through the error and initial the lined-out statement. Usually, before testifying in court, you are allowed to review your PCR, but remember that your testimony may come many years and many patients later.

Intimate-partner maltreatment is not simply a "family issue;" it is a crime to assault another person, regardless of the relationship. The presence of law enforcement personnel is always helpful in these cases. If the patient refuses to be transported, ask if it is safe to leave information on services and resources such as victim-witness assistance programs or domestic maltreatment shelters that the patient may reference later. Learn what services are available in your area.

Sexual Assault

Sexual assault is another call that EMS receives all too often. Although most victims are women, men and children may also be attacked sexually. There are no typical characteristics of sexual offenders and unfortunately, they are very difficult to detect. Often, you can do little beyond providing compassion and transportation to the emergency department. On some occasions, patients may have multiple-system trauma and need treatment for shock. Your actions will go a long way toward providing relief. From arrival on scene to possible judicial system involvement, your professionalism is the key to proper prehospital care.

At the Scene

It is usually preferable to have a same-gender caregiver assist with the victim of sexual assault. If you have this capability and there is no unreasonable time lag for that type of response (including rape crisis teams), you should consider this option as a treatment modality.

Consider the following scenario:

You are sent to an "assist police" call. On arrival at the scene, you find a 20-year-old woman covered in a blanket and bleeding from several abrasions on her face. The police officer pulls you aside and states that the patient may have been assaulted in the alleyway on her way home from night class. Vital signs include a pulse of 134 beats/min, respirations of 32 breaths/min and irregular, and blood pressure of 122/80 mm Hg. The patient is alert and oriented to person, place, and day; her skin is warm and wet. She is very quiet, appears confused, and tells you she doesn't remember what happened. She wants to go home and shower.

The victim of sexual assault is often found in a state of denial or disbelief. Likewise, the desire to shower or douche is common. The patient should be encouraged to go to the hospital, where evidence can be collected and where access to professional services is more readily available.

Sexual assault and rape are crimes of power, force, and violence. The legal definitions of these crimes differ from jurisdiction to jurisdiction, but essentially *sexual assault* refers to any unwanted sexual contact and *rape* means penile penetration of the genitalia without the victim's consent. When the victim is underage, it is called statutory rape. Rape is an indictable offense, and you have a responsibility to preserve the crime scene in addition to treating the patient (see Chapter 51).

Treatment and Documentation

A victim of sexual assault may be hysterical, embarrassed, and/or frightened, or she may be silent and appear emotionally contained. You must be vigilant, but above all you must be professional and compassionate. If you do not observe life-threatening signs and symptoms on arrival, avoid any aggressive treatment behaviour. Leave evidence as untouched as possible, and take care to establish a chain of custody as required. The police should be notified as per protocol. Encourage the patient not to bathe, douche, urinate, or defecate, if possible. If oral penetration has occurred, advise the patient not to eat, drink, brush the teeth, or use mouthwash until he or she has been examined.

Treat all other injuries according to appropriate procedures and protocols for your EMS system. Observe routine precautions. Take the patient's history, perform a limited physical examination, and provide treatment as quickly, quietly, and calmly as possible. Take care to shield the patient from onlookers. Help the patient regain a sense of control by posing open-ended questions and allowing him or her to make decisions.

The patient may refuse assistance or transport, often because he or she wants to maintain privacy and avoid public exposure. Adult patients have the right to decline care. In these cases, you should follow your system's refusal of treatment policy or procedure for sexual assault victims without being judgmental or condescending to the patient. Your compassion is the best tool to win the patient's confidence to get further help.

Because you may need to appear in court as much as 2 or 3 years later, you should document the patient's history, assessment, treatment, and response to treatment in detail. Record only the objective facts. Subjective statements made by those on the scene or the patient should be in quotes on the PCR. Thoroughly document all patient statements pertaining to the crime, as well as statements, names, addresses, and contact information of any witnesses.

Like a battered partner, a victim of sexual assault must be treated and protected by the EMS and police. Conscientious caregivers will make a huge difference in the recovery of patients through their professional conduct. Many provinces and territories offer rape crisis teams or sexual assault treatment centres to assist patients. Your EMS system should keep an up-to-date directory of all sexual assault hotlines and assistance available, with 24-hour telephone numbers.

Child Victims

In most cases of child sexual maltreatment, the person who maltreated the child is an adult who knows the child and may be living under the same roof. Children of any age and either sex can be victims of sexual maltreatment. Although most victims of rape are older than 10 years, younger children may also be victims.

Child sexual maltreatment usually does not occur as a single incident. It does not always involve violence and physical force, and it commonly leaves no visible signs. The power of authority or the parent–child bond may be used to victimize the child instead of force or violence. The child may be manipulated into thinking that the acts are acceptable and normal behaviour. The child may also be made to feel deeply ashamed and powerless or even be kept silent by threats. The insidious nature of this maltreatment makes it difficult to detect unless the child discloses the information to a confidant or a prehospital professional.

Your assessment of a child who has been sexually maltreated should be limited to determining the type of dressing any injuries require. Sometimes, a sexually abused child is also beaten. In such cases, you should treat bruises and fractures as well. Do not examine the genitalia of a young child unless you see evidence of bleeding or an injury to this region that must be treated. In some cases, the child may present with behavioural or physical problems, such as hostility or restlessness.

You are the Paramedic Summary

1. What are your first priorities after assessing scene safety?

Your first priority in the scenario should be to open the airway of the 5-month-old boy. Your next priority is to call for a second paramedic unit to help care for the second patient you identified. Additional patient prehospital care resources such as a supervisor and engine company may also be helpful, if available in your local area.

2. What should raise your index of suspicion?

Your index of suspicion should be raised by the nervousness of the boyfriend and his attempts to control the scene.

3. What is the 5-month-old patient's transport and treatment status, in your judgment?

The 5-month-old boy should be considered in unstable condition, and treatment and transport should occur as rapidly as possible after airway maneuvering.

4. Do you think that you will have to intubate the 5-month-old boy? Why or why not?

You will have to intubate this patient on the scene because you can control his airway better than the boy can himself.

5. Do you think you will have to intubate the 7-year-old girl? Why or why not?

This patient does not have to be intubated at this point; give the salbutamol and/or ipratropium (Atrovent) treatment a chance to work before you take this step.

6. What further treatment do you need for the 5-month-old boy? How can you check for level of consciousness at this point?

This patient needs to be evaluated for brain damage due to the "fall" or to hypoxia. At this point, it is a good idea to check for painful stimuli and watch the boy's reaction, if any. A pinch of the foot may provide a response.

7. Is the nebulizer treatment working for the 7-year-old girl? Does this patient need to go to the hospital? Why or why not?

The nebulizer seems to be working for the 7-year-old girl; however, she should still be transported to the hospital. There the patient can be interviewed by professionals and, at the very least, receive another prescription for her metered-dose inhaler.

Prep Kit

■ Ready for Review

- Abuse, neglect, and assault occur at all levels of society. Because maltreatment and assault are common reasons for calls to EMS, you must recognize the signs and symptoms of these problems.
- Child maltreatment includes any improper or excessive action that injures or otherwise harms a child or infant, including physical abuse, sexual abuse, neglect, and emotional abuse. Many survivors are negatively affected for the rest of their lives.
- Reporting of child abuse or neglect is mandatory in most provinces and territories.
- Watch for the telltale signs of maltreated children and people who maltreat children.
- Maltreatment and neglect of elderly people are on the rise. Because geriatric patients present much differently than child and adult patients do, you must be especially attuned to the possibility of maltreatment in the elderly population.
- Elder maltreatment can be domestic or institutional. Adult children are often the ones who maltreat their elderly parents.
- Adult protective services exist for caregivers and victims alike.
- Domestic maltreatment happens in heterosexual and homosexual relationships.
- Victims of sexual assault may not be inclined to report the crime.

■ Vital Vocabulary

active neglect The refusal or failure to fulfill a caregiving obligation; a conscious or intentional attempt to inflict physical or emotional stress. Examples include abandonment and denial of food or health-related services.

adult protective services (APS) Organizations that investigate cases involving maltreatment and provide case management services in some cases.

assault Unlawfully placing a person in fear of immediate bodily harm.

battery Unlawfully touching a person; this includes providing emergency care without consent.

child protective services (CPS) An agency that is the community legal organization responsible for protection, rehabilitation, and prevention of child maltreatment and neglect; it has the legal authority to temporarily remove from home children who are at risk for injury or neglect and to secure foster placement.

coin rubbing A cultural ritual intended to treat an illness by rubbing hot coins, often on the back, which produces rounded and oblong red, patchy, flat skin lesions.

cupping The cultural practice of placing warm cups on the skin to pull out illness from the body. The red, flat, rounded skin lesions are often more intensely red at the borders.

maltreatment Any form of abuse that results in harm or loss. Maltreatment may be physical, sexual, psychological, or financial/material.

mandated reporter A category of professional required by some provinces and territories to report suspicions of child maltreatment. Prehospital professionals may be included.

neglect Refusal or failure on the part of the caregiver to provide life necessities, such as food, water, clothing, shelter, personal hygiene, medicine, comfort, and personal safety.

passive neglect An unintentional refusal or failure to fulfill a caregiving obligation, which results in physical or emotional distress. Examples include forgetting or isolating the person.

polypharmacy Simultaneous use of many medications.

rape Sexual intercourse inflicted forcibly on another person, against that person's will.

sexual assault An attack against a person that is sexual in nature, the most common of which is rape.

Assessment in Action

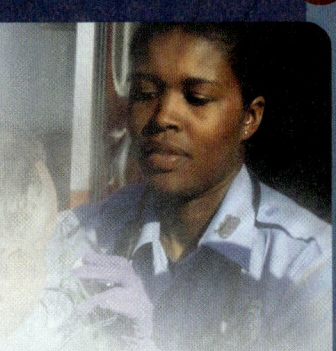

You have responded to a report of a female patient in her 40s with a possible fractured arm. As you enter the residence, you notice it is immaculately clean. Your patient is sitting on a sofa holding her left forearm, which is bruised and appears to be very tender. You ask the woman what happened, and she says that she fell on a wet floor that she had just finished mopping. As you begin your assessment, you notice a man has walked into the room. He tells you that his wife is very clumsy and "runs into everything." He states that he is sure it is not as bad as she is making it sound. As the husband is speaking, you notice the patient looks down at the floor and will not make eye contact with you.

1. **What is your primary concern in this situation?**
   A. Gathering more information about the patient
   B. Crew safety
   C. Splinting the patient's arm
   D. Questioning the husband further

2. **When you begin your assessment of the patient, you notice some bruising on her right arm. When you ask the patient how that happened, she states that she must have obtained the bruising when she fell today. How can you tell if bruising is new or old?**
   A. The bruise is larger if it is a new injury.
   B. The bruise is smaller if it is a new injury.
   C. The bruise will be a different colour or appearance.
   D. The bruise will be the same colour or appearance.

3. **As you ask the patient further about her medical history, she states that she is very clumsy and has broken that arm before. When you ask her when this occurred and what hospital treated her injuries, she states she cannot remember. The husband states that the injury was years ago and it does not matter in this case. What action should you take at this point?**
   A. If it is safe to do so, have your partner interview the husband away from the wife or interview them yourself.
   B. Immediately remove the patient to the safety of your ambulance.
   C. Ask the patient if there are any children in the home.
   D. You and your partner should leave the scene and call law enforcement.

4. **When you and your partner come back together, you find that the history of events does not match between husband and wife. You choose to splint the patient's arm and transport her to the facility of her choice. When you advise her of your intentions, she states that she does not want to go to the hospital. What is your next course of action?**
   A. Have the patient sign a refusal, and leave the scene.
   B. Have your partner go outside and contact law enforcement.
   C. Have a neighbour come over to take the patient to the hospital.
   D. Contact your supervisor.

5. **After law enforcement personnel arrive, you are able to treat and transport the patient to the hospital of her choice. Once inside your ambulance, what is a recommended way to obtain more information on how the injury occurred?**
   A. Have a law enforcement officer ride in with you and the patient.
   B. Do not ask direct questions because they will upset the patient.
   C. Ask direct questions about the potential that the injury was caused by maltreatment.
   D. Wait until you arrive at the hospital, and let the physician obtain the information.

Challenging Question

6. **You and your partner begin to write your PCR concerning this call for service. What should you be cognizant of during your documentation?**

Points to Ponder

You and your partner are called to a local kindergarten for an ill child. When you arrive at the school office, you find a 5-year-old Asian child who appears to have a common cold. You notice the child is coughing and is tugging at his ears. The school administrator pulls you aside and says that she suspects child maltreatment. When you ask why, she directs the child to come into her office and asks him to raise up his shirt. You notice large, red marks extending from the shoulders to the lumbar region of the child's back. You ask the child what happened to make these marks and the child states, "my grandmother is trying to make me better." The school administrator insists that law enforcement personnel be contacted to arrest the grandmother.

What is your opinion?

Issues: Abuse, Cultural Differences, Child Maltreatment, Physical Maltreatment.

44 Patients With Special Needs

Competency Areas

Area 2: Communication

2.1.d   Provide information to patient about their situation and how they will be treated.

2.1.g   Use appropriate terminology.

2.3.a   Exhibit effective non-verbal behaviour.

2.3.b   Practice active listening techniques.

2.3.c   Establish trust and rapport with patients and colleagues.

2.3.d   Recognize and react appropriately to non-verbal behaviours.

2.4.a   Treat others with respect.

2.4.b   Exhibit empathy and compassion while providing care.

2.4.c   Recognize and react appropriately to individuals and groups manifesting coping mechanisms.

2.4.f   Manage and provide support to patients, bystanders, and relatives manifesting emotional reactions.

2.4.g   Exhibit diplomacy, tact, and discretion.

Area 4: Assessment and Diagnostics

4.3.p   Conduct psychiatric assessment and interpret findings.

Area 6: Integration

6.1.m   Provide care to patient experiencing terminal illness.

6.2.e   Provide care for mentally-challenged patient.

Appendix 4: Pathophysiology

B.   **Neurologic System**
Chronic Neurologic Disorders: Cerebral palsy
Chronic Neurologic Disorders: Multiple sclerosis
Chronic Neurologic Disorders: Muscular dystrophy
Traumatic Injuries: Head injury
Traumatic In juries: Spinal cord injury
Pediatric: Down syndrome
Pediatric: Spina bifida

H.   **Musculoskeletal System**
Soft-Tissue Disorders: Muscular dystrophies
Soft-Tissue Disorders: Myopathies

J.   **Multisystem Diseases and Injuries**
Cancer: Malignancy

K.   **Psychiatric Disorders**
Anxiety Disorders: Generalized anxiety disorder
Anxiety Disorders: Panic disorder
Anxiety Disorders: Situational disturbances
Childhood Psychiatric Disorders: Autistic disorder

Introduction

Throughout the ages, humans have learned to adapt to the challenges they encounter. In the prehospital environment, you will encounter patients who face a variety of special challenges. Some conditions or anomalies are congenital; others have developed during the patient's lifetime or occurred as the result of a sudden event (eg, the transection of the spinal cord during a diving accident). Whatever the source of the challenge, these patients will require you to adapt your assessment and management to accommodate their needs.

Although you can still use the standard assessment plan with these patients, sometimes you may find it necessary to adapt to best meet a patient's unique needs. Can the patient see you? Can the patient hear you? Can the patient normally move all extremities? You will need to formulate a plan to care for these patients in a short amount of time. Be willing to incorporate "the experts" (ie, the patient, family members, or caregivers) as essential teammates. Learn to solve problems as part of a group, and remember your ultimate goal: to give the patient the best care possible, in the most efficient way, and still accommodate for his or her individual needs. Your confidence and caring attitude will promote trust between you, your patient, and the other members of your team.

Physical Challenges

Humans use all five senses to gather information, but we often take that sensory feedback for granted. Imagine what it would be like to go bowling while blindfolded. You hear the pins dropping—but did you knock down a couple of pins, get a strike, or just leave a 7–10 split? Imagine how frustrating it might be to see that you need to tie your shoe but to be unable to do so because an injury resulted in the loss of motor function in your hand.

Hearing Impairments

Hearing challenges are classified into two types: conductive and sensorineural deafness. Conductive deafness is a usually curable temporary condition caused by an injury to the eardrum, an infection, or simply a buildup of earwax in the external auditory canal. Sensorineural deafness, which is permanent, may be caused by a lesion or damage of the inner ear, or damage to the eighth cranial nerve. This type of hearing impairment may be congenital or secondary to a birth injury, but it may also have occurred over time from disease, medication complications, viral infections, or tumours. People may also lose their hearing due to aging (called *presbycusis*) or from prolonged exposure to loud noise.

Hearing impairment may range from a slight hearing loss to total deafness. Some patients may have difficulty with pitch, volume, and distinguishing speech. Some have learned to speak even though they have never heard speech. Others may have heard speech and learned to talk, but have since lost some or all of their hearing, leading them to speak too loudly. Parkinson's disease or other disease processes may cause the patient to slur words, speak very slowly, or speak in a monotone voice.

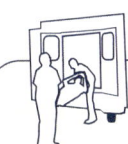

At the Scene

Consider the effect of sirens and protect your hearing . . . before it's too late.

You are the Paramedic Part 1

You and your partner are dispatched to a park for a child in respiratory distress. When you arrive at the entrance you are guided by a park officer to pavilion 4, where you find a group of active 8-year-olds enjoying a class picnic. The scene appears ordinary until you get closer to the pavilion and realize that all the children in this group have Down syndrome.

Seated on one of the picnic benches is a girl in obvious respiratory distress. You observe that she is in a tripod position and is using accessory muscles to breathe. As you get closer, you are able to hear audible expiratory wheezes. Her teacher is next to her trying to provide reassurance.

Initial Assessment	Recording Time: 0 Minutes
Appearance	Anxious; child seated in a tripod position
Level of consciousness	A (Alert to person, place, and day)
Airway	Open
Breathing	Increased work of breathing with accessory muscle use
Circulation	Strong radial pulse, slightly elevated

1. What is Down syndrome?
2. What are the characteristic physical features of Down syndrome?

Interaction With a Hearing-Impaired Patient

Clues that a person could be hearing impaired include the presence of hearing aids, poor pronunciation of words, or failure to respond to your presence or verbal questions. While communicating, face the patient so that he or she can see your mouth; don't exaggerate your lip movements or look away. Position yourself approximately 50 cm directly in front of the patient. Most people who are hearing impaired have learned to use body language, such as hand gestures and lipreading. Because hearing-impaired patients typically have more difficulty hearing higher-frequency sounds, if the patient seems to have difficulty hearing you, don't just speak louder—try lowering the pitch of your voice.

Ask the patient, "How would you like to communicate with me?" American Sign Language (ASL) may be his or her preferred method of communication 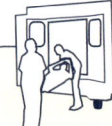 **Figure 44-1** . An interpreter, family member, or friend may prove to be a valuable teammate. If an interpreter is not readily available, call your receiving facility early on to request one. Ideally, an interpreter will arrive before you begin your assessment. Other patients may prefer written communication or communication of concepts or procedures with gestures or pictures. Simply asking a team member to retrieve the patient's hearing aid or auditory electronic enhancement device may help a great deal.

Here are some helpful hints for working with patients with hearing impairments:

- Speak slowly and distinctly into a less impaired ear, or position yourself on that side.
- Change speakers. Given that 80% of hearing loss is related to the inability to hear high-pitched sounds, look for a team

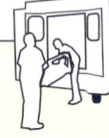
At the Scene
Some hearing-impaired patients' ears are overly sensitive to very loud noises close to their ears. Remember to use a normal tone of voice when speaking to them.

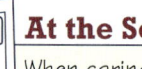
At the Scene
When caring for a hearing-impaired patient, one easy solution is to place the ear pieces of your stethoscope into the patient's ears while you speak into the bell of the stethoscope. Remember to speak softly into the bell.

member with a low-pitched voice if you think this may be the issue.

- Provide paper and pencil so that you may write your questions and the patient may write his or her responses.
- Only one person should ask interview questions, to avoid confusing the patient.
- Try the "reverse stethoscope" technique: put the earpieces of your stethoscope in the patient's ear and speak softly into the diaphragm of the stethoscope. This will amplify your voice.

At the Scene
Many patients with borderline hearing impairments may not be aware of the extent of their problem. The distracting and noisy EMS environment may worsen the situation. If a patient frequently asks you to repeat things, suspect a hearing impairment.

Hearing Aids

A hearing aid is essentially a device that makes sound louder. Hearing aids cannot restore hearing to normal, but they do improve hearing and listening ability. Several types of hearing aids are available **Figure 44-2** ▶ :

- *In-the-canal* and *completely in-the-canal*. These hearing aids are contained in a tiny case that fits partly or completely into the ear canal.
- *In-the-ear*. All parts are contained in a shell that fits in the outer part of the ear.

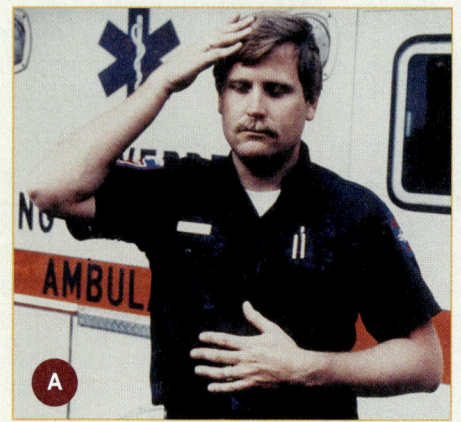
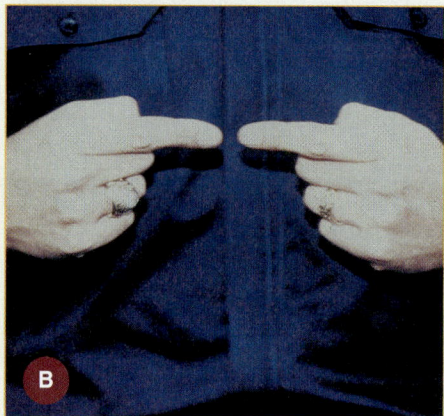
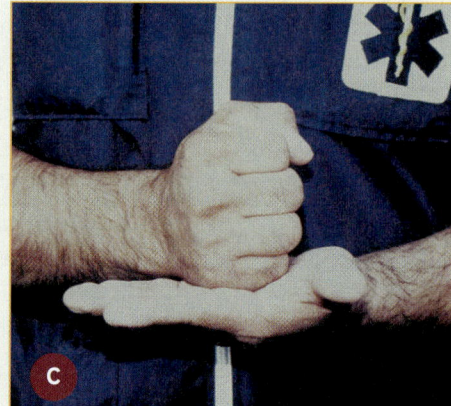

Figure 44-1 Consider learning the ASL signs for common terms related to illness and injury. **A.** Sick. **B.** Hurt. **C.** Help.

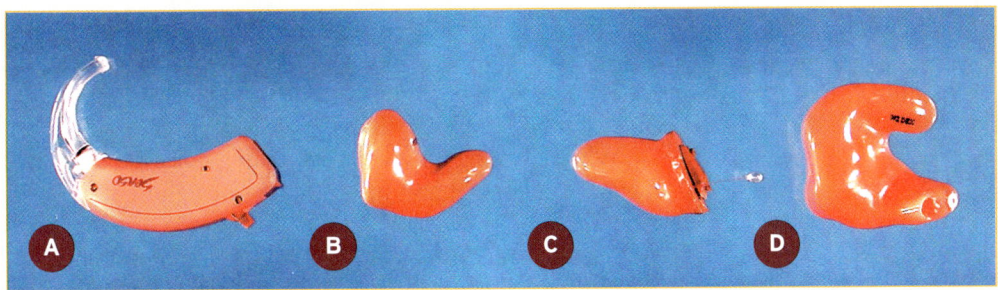

Figure 44-2 Different types of hearing aids. **A.** Behind-the-ear type. **B.** Conventional body type. **C.** In-the-canal type. **D.** In-the-ear type.

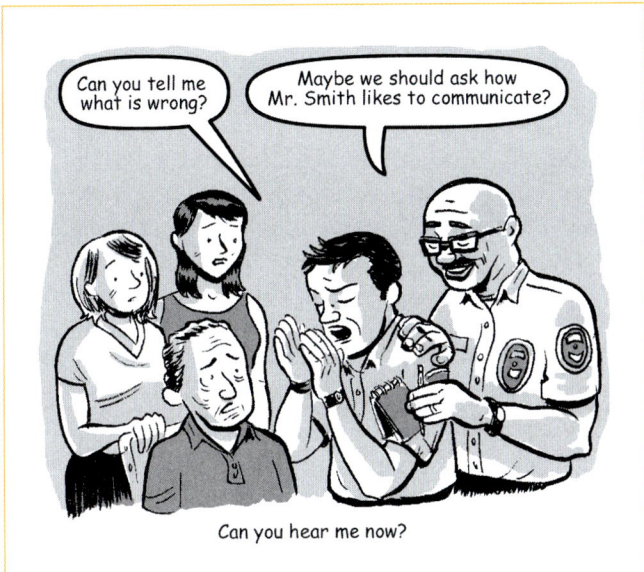

Figure 44-3

- *Behind-the-ear.* All parts are contained in a plastic case that rests behind the ear.
- *Conventional body type.* This older style is generally used by people with profound hearing loss.

Implantable hearing aids are also an option for patients with less profound hearing loss.

To insert a hearing aid, follow the natural shape of the ear. The device needs to fit snugly without forcing. If you hear a whistling sound, the hearing aid may not be in far enough to create a seal, or the volume may be too loud. Try repositioning the hearing aid, or remove it and turn down the volume. If you can't insert the hearing aid after two tries, put it in the box, take it with you, and document the transport and transfer of hearing aids to hospital personnel. Never try to clean hearing aids, and never get them wet.

If a patient's hearing aid is not working, try troubleshooting the problem. First, make sure the hearing aid is turned on Figure 44-3 ▲. Try a fresh battery, and check the tubing to make sure it isn't twisted or bent. Check the switch to make sure

it's set on M (microphone), not T (telephone). For a body aid, try a spare cord, as the old one may be broken or shorted. Finally, check the ear mould to make sure it isn't plugged with wax.

Speech Impairments

For most people, the spoken word is the primary mechanism for communicating thoughts and ideas. For some, speech may be delayed by psychological or psychosocial factors. For others, it may be altered by injury, illness, or hearing impairment.

Articulation Disorders

Articulation disorders cause the majority of speech difficulties. Dysarthria—the inability to make speech sounds correctly—results from a lack of muscle control and coordination of the larynx, tongue, mouth, and lips. Speech can be slurred, indistinct, slow, or nasal. Commonly, articulation disorders result from damage to nerve pathways passing from the brain to muscles in the larynx, mouth, or lips; delayed development from hearing problems; or slow maturation of the nervous system due to brain damage or motor disability. Articulation disorders affect both children and adults.

Language Disorders

Stroke, traumatic head/brain injury, brain tumour, delayed development, hearing loss, lack of stimulation, or emotional disturbance may cause damage to the language centre of the brain and lead to aphasia. Aphasia is the loss of ability to communicate in speech, writing, or signs. It can range from being very mild to making communication with the patient almost impossible. Aphasia may affect primarily a single aspect of language use, such as the ability to recall the names of objects, to put words into sentences, or to read.

When communicating with an aphasic patient, remember to talk to the patient as an adult, not as a child. Use focused questions rather than open-ended questions, and minimize background noise.

Fluency Disorders

In fluency disorders, the person's speech pattern is broken, interrupted, or repetitious. An example of this type of disorder is stuttering. Stuttering may be noticed only when the person attempts certain words or sounds, and it may become worse when the individual is under stress. Stuttering is normal for young children and will disappear gradually over time. The specific causes of stuttering are unknown.

When dealing with a person who has a fluency disorder, patience is the key. Impatience with or interruption of a patient who stutters may frustrate the patient more and cause the stuttering to get worse, making assessment and history-taking difficult.

Voice Production Disorders

Voice production disorders refer to the way the voice sounds and may be slightly easier to understand than other speech impairments. Signs of these disorders include hoarseness, harshness, inappropriate pitch, or abnormal nasal resonance. Causes include the closure of vocal cords, hormonal or psychiatric disturbance, or severe hearing loss.

Hypernasality may be a complication of a cleft palate, a deformity in which the two sides of the palate fail to fuse in the midline during in utero development Figure 44-4 ◂ , or it may accompany enlarged adenoids.

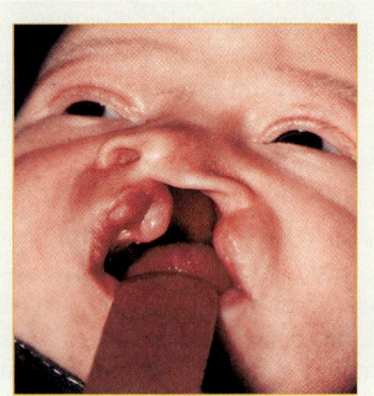

Figure 44-4 Cleft palate.

Inflammation of the larynx may produce laryngitis. Laryngitis is a common occurrence in cases involving overuse of the voice, throat infections, heavy smoking, smoke inhalation, allergic reaction, or exposure to fumes. The cause of the laryngitis may provide clues about the patient's reason for calling for your services and the severity of the situation.

Chronic laryngitis may point to long-term exposure to laryngeal irritants, which may cause polyps to develop in the larynx. Occurring more commonly in men, progressive hoarseness is usually the chief complaint in such cases. Long-term exposure to toxins such as chemicals, smoking, or weakened vocal cords from continuous strain are other risk factors.

The most ominous cause of chronic laryngitis is carcinoma of the larynx. A laryngectomy—either partial or total removal of the larynx—may be performed to battle the cancer. In case of a total laryngectomy, the patient would have *aphonia*, which is the inability to produce normal speech sounds. The patient would receive a stoma, and might communicate by burping sounds or by using an electronic or mechanical device.

Interaction With a Speech-Impaired Patient

When establishing communication, ask the speech-impaired patient how he or she would be most comfortable communicating with you. Allow an appropriate amount of time for a response, and listen carefully to establish an understanding or

At the Scene

As with all barriers to communication, remember to document whenever you enlist the help of an interpreter or a person who signs. Also remember that conclusions reached based on the information from interpreters may not be valid.

enlist someone who knows the patient to interpret. For instance, small children often have speech difficulties that spontaneously resolve, but may be difficult for a stranger to understand. If the patient prefers to speak, your ability to understand the patient will likely be affected.

When working with a patient with a voice production disorder, offer a pencil and paper or listen carefully if the patient prefers to speak. Repeat what the patient said to allow for correction or further clarification. Avoid speaking for the patient or finishing sentences for him or her. Above all, be patient!

Visual Impairments

Visual impairments may result from a multitude of causes—congenital defect, disease, injury, infection (eg, cytomegalovirus), or degeneration of the eyeball, optic nerve, or nerve pathway (eg, with aging). The degree of blindness may range from partial to total. Some patients lose peripheral or central vision; while others can only distinguish light from dark or discern general shapes.

Visual impairments may be difficult to recognize. During your scene assessment, look for signs that indicate the person is visually impaired, such as the presence of eyeglasses, a white cane, or a service dog. Make yourself known when you enter the room, and introduce yourself and others in the room or have them introduce themselves so that the patient can identify their placement and voice. In addition, retrieve any visual aids to make the interaction more comfortable for your patient Figure 44-5 ▾ .

A visually impaired person may feel vulnerable, especially during the chaos of an accident scene. He or she may have learned to use other senses such as hearing, touch, and smell to compensate for the loss of sight, and the sounds and smells of an accident may be disorienting. Remember to tell the patient what is happening, identify noises, and describe the situation and surroundings, especially if you must move the patient.

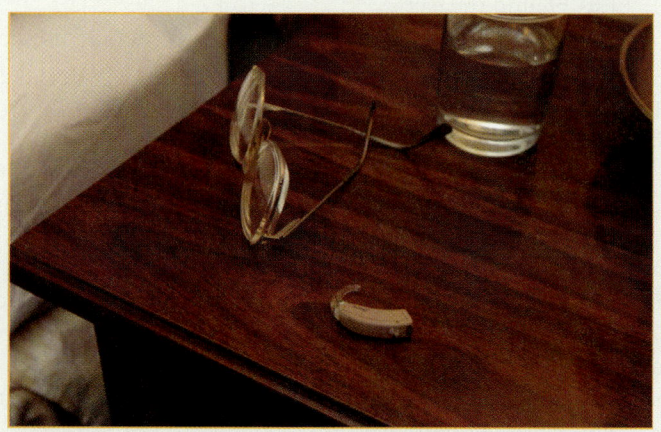

Figure 44-5 Ensuring that a patient with eyeglasses or a hearing aid is using it may reduce the patient's disorientation and stress, and will likely improve your communication with the patient during assessment.

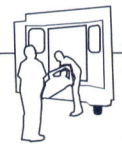

At the Scene

Remember that service dogs are "working dogs." Don't allow your crew or bystanders to play with the animal or distract it unless the patient gives permission to do so.

To ambulate safely, the patient may use a cane or walker. Even if the individual will be carried out on your stretcher, don't forget to take the patient's cane, walker, or eyeglasses. Unless the patient is critical, the service dog can remain in the room and will provide reassurance for the patient and prevent delays in transport. In some provinces, service animals are allowed in the ambulance with the patient. However, if you need to arrange for the care or accompaniment of the dog, a friend or animal control officer can be helpful in this situation.

An ambulatory patient may be led by a light touch on the arm or elbow. You may also allow the patient to rest his or her hand on your shoulder, as this may enhance the patient's sense of balance and security while moving. You may also ask the patient which method he or she prefers to use while travelling to the ambulance. Patients should be gently guided but never pushed. Obstacles need to be communicated in advance. Statements such as "You're approaching the stairs," and instructions about how many stairs to expect, will allow the patient to anticipate and navigate the obstacles safely. They will also appreciate your consideration and concern.

Paralysis

Paralysis is the inability to voluntarily move one or more body parts. It may be caused by a stroke, trauma, or birth defects, among other things. Paralysis does not always entail a loss of sensation, however. In some cases, the patient will have normal sensation or hyperesthesia (increased sensitivity), which may cause the individual to interpret touch as pain in the affected area. Paralysis of one side of the face may cause subsequent communication challenges as well.

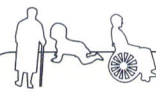

Special Considerations

- **Hemiplegia**. Paralysis of one side of the body, possibly from stroke or head injury
- **Paraplegia**. Paralysis of the lower part of the body, possibly from thoracic or lumbar spinal injury or spina bifida
- **Quadriplegia**. Paralysis of all four extremities and the trunk, possibly from a cervical spine injury

Paralyzed patients may have diaphragmatic involvement requiring the use of a ventilator. They may also rely on specialized equipment such as halo traction, Foley catheters, tracheotomies, colostomies, or feeding tubes. Each spinal cord procedure requires its own equipment and may have its own complications (see Chapter 45).

Dysphagia, caused by a partial paralysis of the esophagus, is the inability to swallow. Patients with dysphagia may choke or aspirate food and drink very easily, leading to the need for emergency airway interventions.

If patients have lost some or all of the sensation in the affected limbs, they cannot tell you when you are hurting them. Always take great care when lifting or moving a paralyzed patient. Because paralyzed limbs lack muscle tone, provide intravenous access and medication administration on the nonaffected side whenever possible. Check intravenous sites frequently for infiltration, especially after medication administration.

Special Considerations

Moving the patient without dislodging or compromising his or her extra equipment takes planning and coordination. You may need to recruit more team members so that you can efficiently move the patient without causing further complication. Strategically placed padding or pillows may also keep the patient more comfortable during transport.

Obesity

Obesity is the result of an imbalance between food eaten and calories used. The solution to the obesity problem may sound relatively simple—reestablish the balance and cure the problem. Unfortunately, obesity can be a much more complex situation. Causes of obesity are not fully understood and, in many cases, are unknown. Often, this problem may be attributed to low basal metabolic rate or genetic predisposition. Bariatrics is the branch of medicine that studies and treats obese patients.

The term obese is used when someone is 20% to 30% over his or her ideal weight. In severe or morbid obesity, the person is 20 to 40 kg over the ideal weight. Obesity afflicts about one quarter of all Canadians. These individuals may be ridiculed publicly and sometimes are victims of discrimination. Mobility and the patients' general quality of life are often negatively affected by their oversized status, and the extra weight can cause a myriad of health problems.

Interaction With the Bariatric Patient

Bariatric patients may be embarrassed by their condition or fearful of ridicule as a result of past experiences. Some of those negative interactions may have occurred at the hands of an insensitive health care professional. As with any patient, work hard to put these individuals at ease early. Establish the patient's chief complaint and then communicate your plan to help. Many have a complex and extensive past medical history, so mastering the art of conducting a patient interview will serve you well in your interactions with these individuals.

If transport is necessary, plan early for extra help and don't be afraid to call for more help if necessary. In particular, send a member of your team to find the easiest and safest exit. Remember, everyone's safety is at stake! You don't want to risk dropping the patient or injuring a team member by trying to lift too much weight. Moves, no matter how simple they may seem, become far more complex with an oversized patient.

Bariatric patients may overcome mobility difficulties by pulling, rocking, or rolling into a position. The constant strain on their body's structures may leave them with chronic joint injuries or osteoarthritis.

Some patients suffer from a condition called obesity hypoventilation syndrome, also known as Pickwickian syndrome. Patients with Pickwickian syndrome are usually *extremely* obese. They experience hypoxemia (deficient oxygenation of the blood), hypercapnia (excess carbon dioxide in the blood), and polycythemia (overabundance or overproduction of red blood cells). Physical findings may include headache, apnea (especially during sleep), sleepiness, red face, muscle twitching, and signs of right-sided heart failure. Some of these symptoms may necessitate emergency intervention in the prehospital environment.

Weight reduction is the ultimate remedy for Pickwickian syndrome. Some patients may be on a carefully monitored diet and others may benefit from surgical intervention, such as gastric bypass surgery. Surgery carries a high risk of complications, however, and not all patients are suitable candidates.

When you are moving a bariatric patient, follow these helpful tips:

- Treat the patient with dignity and respect.
- Ask your patient how best to move him or her before attempting to do so.
- Avoid trying to lift the patient by only one limb, which would risk injury to overtaxed joints.

At the Scene

When transporting an obese or bariatric patient, know the weight limits of your equipment. Use special bariatric equipment and vehicles if available and appropriate. Be sure to alert the receiving facility in advance if special accommodations, equipment, or other resources may be needed.

- Coordinate and communicate all moves to all team members *prior* to starting.
- If the move becomes uncontrolled at any point, stop, reposition, and resume.
- Look for pinch or pressure points from equipment, as they could cause a deep venous thrombosis.
- Very large patients may have difficulty breathing if you lay them flat. Keep this possibility in mind when you position these individuals.
- Many manufacturers now make specialized equipment for bariatric patients, and some areas have specially equipped bariatric ambulances for such patients. Become familiar with the resources available in your area.
- Plan egress routes to accommodate for a large patient, equipment, *and* the lifting crew members. Remember: Do no harm!
- Notify the receiving facility early to allow special arrangements to be made prior to your arrival to accommodate the patient's needs.

You are the Paramedic Part 2

You kneel down in front of the young girl, introduce yourself, and ask her name. She tells you that her name is Allison. You note that she has to take a breath after two words. She tells you that she is having a hard time "catching air," points to her bracelet, and starts to cry. You hold her hand and reassure her that you are going to help her feel better very soon. While you are doing this you look at a medical identification bracelet on her right wrist, which reveals that Allison has asthma and is allergic to penicillin. You ask the teacher if she can provide any additional information. She relates that Allison was playing kickball with her classmates when she sat down on the field. One of the aides went over to Allison and found her to be having a hard time breathing. She was brought over to the pavilion and 9-1-1 was called. Allison normally has a rescue inhaler of salbutamol (Ventolin), but it was accidentally left at the school. She has no other medical history or drug allergies. She has the emotional and developmental skills of a 4-year-old. A call was placed to her mother who authorized treatment. She will meet you at the hospital.

Vital Signs	Recording Time: 5 Minutes
Level of consciousness	Alert
Pulse	116 beats/min, regular
Blood pressure	106/72 mm Hg
Respirations	28 breaths/min, laboured
Skin	Pale, warm, and dry
SpO_2	95% on room air

3. What medical conditions are commonly seen in patients with Down syndrome?

4. Why is it important to physically be at the patient's level to speak with her?

Mental Challenges

Mental Illness

Mental illness is a generic term for a variety of illnesses that result in emotional, cognitive, or behavioural dysfunction. These conditions include bipolar disorder, depression, schizophrenia, and drug or alcohol abuse. See Chapter 37 for more detail.

Developmental Disabilities

The current terminology in Canada is "persons with disabilities," with emphasis on the person rather than the disability, be it intellectual, behavioural, developmental, or emotional. Developmental disability is a permanent condition that means a person develops slower and differently than others do. Individuals with a developmental disability may have difficulty learning and processing information with abstract ideas and changing to meet the needs of normal daily life. It may be caused by genetic factors, congenital infections, complications at birth, malnutrition, or environmental factors. Prenatal drug or alcohol use may also cause disability, as in fetal alcohol syndrome. Postnatal causes may include traumatic brain injury or poisoning (eg, with lead or other toxins).

Although IQ testing can identify the extent of the person's ability to learn and reason, just speaking to the patient and family members will give you a good idea of how well the patient can understand and interact with you. A person with a slight impairment may appear slow to understand or have a limited vocabulary. Such an individual will often act "immature" in comparison to "normal" peers. Because the individual may also have difficulty adjusting to change or a break in routine, an emergency call that generates a roomful of strangers can be overwhelming. The patient may become more difficult to interact with as his or her anxiety level increases. A severely disabled person may not have the ability to care for himself or herself, communicate, understand, or respond to the surroundings.

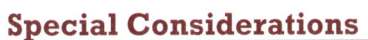

Special Considerations

Mild intellectual disability: IQ = 52–68
Moderate intellectual disability: IQ = 36–51
Severe intellectual disability: IQ = 20–35
Profound intellectual disability: IQ ≤ 19

Treatment of these patients should be based on the chief complaint, unless the illness is related to the mental disability. Patients with developmental disabilities are prone to the same disease processes as any other patients, including diabetes, heart disease, and respiratory difficulties. Transport should be accomplished without causing any more stress than necessary. In most cases, supportive care is all that is needed.

Down Syndrome

Down syndrome is characterized by a genetic chromosomal defect that can occur during fetal development, resulting in

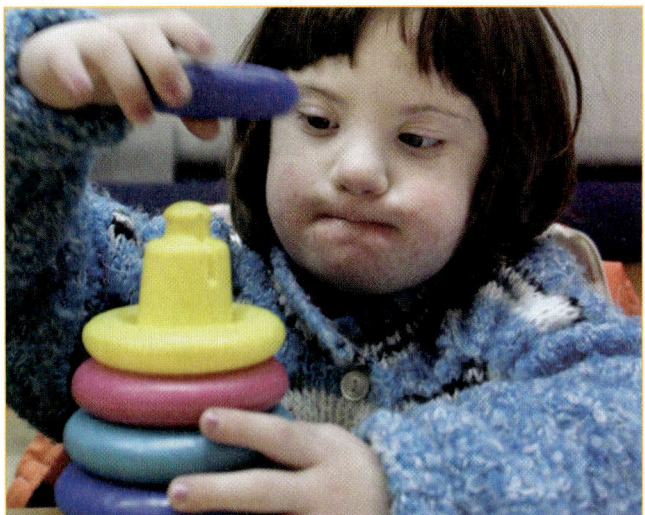

Figure 44-6 A child with Down syndrome.

a developmental disability, including mild to severe intellectual impairment **Figure 44-6 ▲**. The normal human somatic cell contains 23 chromosomes. Down syndrome, which is also known as trisomy 21, occurs when chromosome 21 fails to separate, so that the ovum contains 24 chromosomes. When the ovum is fertilized by a normal sperm with 23 chromosomes, a triplication ("trisomy") of chromosome 21 occurs.

Increased maternal age (more than 35 years old) and a family history of Down syndrome are known risk factors for this condition. A variety of abnormalities are associated with Down syndrome: a round head with a flat occiput; an enlarged, protruding tongue; slanted, wide-set eyes and folded skin on either side of the nose, covering the inner corners of the eye; short, wide hands; a small face and features; congenital heart defects; thyroid problems; and hearing and vision problems. Patients do not usually have all of these symptoms, but will have a combination of them to such a degree that the diagnosis is rapidly made at birth.

Patients with Down syndrome are at increased risk for medical complications, including those that affect the cardiovascular, sensory, endocrine, orthopaedic, dental, gastrointestinal, neurologic development, and hematologic systems. As many as 40% may suffer from heart conditions and hearing and vision problems. In particular, two thirds of children born with Down syndrome have congenital heart disease (eg, endocardial cushion defects, or ventricular or atrial septal defects). Emergency treatment should therefore include airway management, supplemental oxygen, and IV access. In patients with heart failure, administer diuretics with judicious fluid resuscitation only if necessary.

Because people with Down syndrome often have large tongues and small oral and nasal cavities, intubation of these patients may be difficult. These individuals may also have malocclusions and other dental anomalies (eg, abnormal contact of the upper and lower teeth). The enlarged tongue and dental anomalies can lead to speech abnormalities as well. In an emergency situation, if airway management is necessary, mask ventilation and intubation can be challenging. In the case of airway obstruction, a simple jaw-thrust maneuver may be all that is needed to clear the airway. In an unconscious patient, either the jaw-thrust maneuver or a nasopharyngeal airway may be necessary.

Many people with Down syndrome have epilepsy. Most of the seizures are of the tonic–clonic type. Management is the same as with other patients with seizures.

Interaction With Patients With Developmental Disabilities

When caring for a patient with any developmental disability, specifically intellectual or behavioural, obtain a complete history, treat the presenting illness, and provide supportive care. It is normal to feel somewhat uncomfortable when initiating contact with this kind of patient, especially if you've encountered such situations infrequently. Simply treating the patient as you would anyone else is the best plan.

Approach the patient in a calm and friendly manner, watching him or her for signs of increased anxiety or fear. Remember, you are a "stranger" and are approaching with a group of people. The patient may not understand your uniform or realize that you and your crew are there to help. It may be helpful to have the members of your team hold back slightly until you can establish a rapport with the patient. You can then introduce the team members and explain what they are going to do. This method will slowly bring forward the other paramedics, instead of "mobbing" the patient all at once.

You might interact with a patient as follows: "Hello Mr. Pemberton. My name is Jerry Booker." (Shake Mr. Pemberton's hand if he will allow it.) "We're here to help you. Your sister called us. She says you're not feeling well today, and we're here to help you feel better. My friend Tim is going to take your blood pressure. Do you remember having that done before?" (Allow Mr. Pemberton to see and touch the blood pressure cuff as Tim moves forward. Move slowly but deliberately, explaining beforehand what you are going to do, just as you would with any other patient. Watch carefully for signs of fear or reluctance from the patient.)

Do your best to soothe the patient's anxiety and/or discomfort as you work through your assessment and treatment. By initially establishing trust and communication, you'll have much better luck successfully executing your treatment plan, even if you eventually need to do something painful such as starting an IV.

Emotional/Disability

In the Victorian era, an emotional stress condition associated with chronic fatigue, anxiety, depression, sleep disturbances, headache, and sexual dysfunction might be lumped into the category known as *neurasthenia*—in modern terms, a "nervous breakdown." Today, physicians diagnose specific disorders such as anxiety, neurosis, compulsion, or hysteria.

Mental illness can occur in persons with mental or emotional disability just as it can arise in normal people. (The care of patients with specific mental illness is discussed in depth in Chapter 37.) In the broader sense, a person's mental status can influence his or her physical well-being, and vice versa. Emotionally or intellectually disabled individuals may be difficult to assess due to the body's normal stress response, which may alter their respiratory rate, heart rate, or perception of physical illness. Gathering a detailed history will be useful in the assessment and development of a treatment plan for these patients. Calmly ascertain the chief complaint and treat the patient accordingly, with care and understanding.

You are the Paramedic Part 3

Your partner prepares a nebulizer containing 2.5 mg of salbutamol and 3 ml of normal saline and you begin your assessment, taking care to let your patient know everything that you are doing. Your physical examination is significant for diminished air movement bilaterally with faint expiratory wheezes. You ask your partner to prepare an IV and the cardiac monitor. You load the patient onto the stretcher and into the truck to continue your treatment prior to leaving for the hospital.

In the back of the truck you give the patient a teddy bear and tell her how brave she is being. She responds with a weak smile. A 20-gauge IV is started in the left antecubital and an infusion of normal saline is started. As the ambulance departs you refill the nebulizer with 2.5 mg of salbutamol and 0.5 mg of ipratropium (Atrovent) inhalation solution.

Reassessment	Recording Time: 12 Minutes
Skin	Pale, warm, and dry
Pulse	120 beats/min, regular
Blood pressure	110/72 mm Hg
Respirations	28 breaths/min, laboured
Spo$_2$	98% on nebulizer treatment
ECG	Sinus tachycardia with no ectopy
Pupils	Reactive to light

5. What anatomical features of Down syndrome can make airway management challenging?

One of the key components of effective communication—with any type of patient—is to be a good listener. Always "listen" carefully to your patient—not just the words spoken, but also heeding the patient's tone, facial expressions, and body language. Watch for signs of aggression, clenched fists, or aggressive agitated movements or speech; they may be your only warning of an impending dangerous confrontation. Implementing active listening skills by repeating what you heard will reassure the patient that you understand and are there to help. Although these patients may present an assessment challenge, they are still patients and are prone to the same illnesses and disease processes as anyone else. Consequently, treatment and transport of such patients should focus on the chief complaint and supportive care.

When treating patients with emotional or intellectual disabilities, take care in establishing communication with the patient and/or the caregiver. Establish a baseline for the patient's emotional/mental ability so that you will be able to identify any changes. Speak in a calm voice, even if the patient does not have the ability to understand, and explain what you're going to do before doing it.

Pathologic Challenges

Pathologic challenges require special consideration when you formulate your treatment plan. Pathologies you may encounter during your career may include arthritis, cancer, cerebral palsy, cystic fibrosis, multiple sclerosis, muscular dystrophy, poliomyelitis, previous head injury, spina bifida, and myasthenia gravis. Many of these patients will be well versed in the progression, treatment, and unique nuances of their current health status.

Cancer

Simply stated, cancer is the uncontrolled overgrowth of normal tissue cells. If this growth is left unchecked, these cells have the ability to spread, destroy body systems, and kill. More than 200 different kinds of cancer are believed to exist. The type of cancer is determined by where it originates. (Cancer is discussed in greater detail in Chapters 6 and 45.)

Numerous types of treatment regimens are available for cancer—surgery, medications, radiation, and chemotherapy, to name a few. Cancer treatment may follow a single pathway, or be orchestrated into a complex combination of therapies and medications. Surgical removal has long been one of the primary methods of controlling or terminating cancer's progression; it is often used in tandem with other therapies.

Arthritis

Arthritis is a joint inflammation that causes pain, swelling, stiffness, and decreased range of motion, all of which leave patients more vulnerable to falls. Many types of arthritis exist, with symptoms ranging from mild to debilitating. For example, osteoarthritis is a degenerative joint disease associated with aging

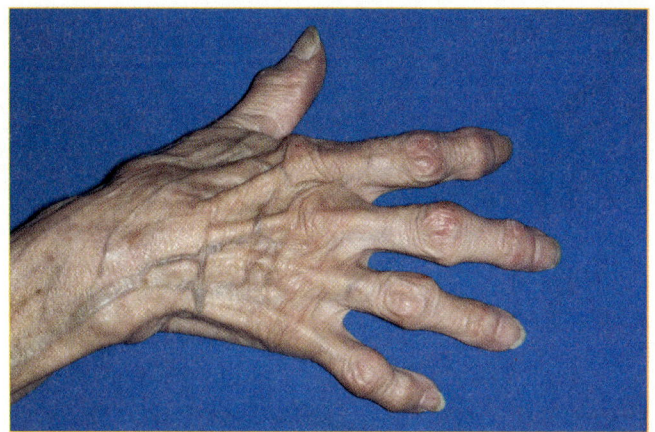

Figure 44-7 Osteoarthritis may cause substantial disfigurement.

Figure 44-7 ▲ . It initially targets the joints of the lower extremities. The pain of osteoarthritis usually grows throughout the day, with stiffness increasing following prolonged rest. In contrast, rheumatoid arthritis is an autoimmune disorder that causes inflammation and destruction of the joints and connective tissues. Some patients may experience periods of remission while others may have rapid progression of the disease.

Be sure to ask the patient with arthritis about his or her current medications before administering additional ones. Take special care when moving such a patient to incur the least amount of discomfort. Make sure the patient is as comfortable as possible and remember to use equipment that fits the patient properly.

Cerebral Palsy

Cerebral palsy is a nonprogressive, bilateral neuromuscular disorder in which voluntary muscles are poorly controlled. It results from developmental brain insults in utero (eg, cerebral hypoxia, maternal infection, or kernicterus), brain trauma at birth or in early childhood, or postpartum infections (eg, encephalitis or meningitis). Patients often have spastic movements of their limbs and display poor posture **Figure 44-8** ▶ , which impairs their ability to move in a controlled manner.

Symptoms of cerebral palsy can range from mild to severe. As children grow, these symptoms may either become exaggerated or stay the same. Related complications include visual impairments, hearing and language difficulties, seizures, and developmental disability.

Some children with severe cases of cerebral palsy are able to learn to walk with assistive devices, whereas others need support even to sit and cannot stand, walk, or speak. If the patient is able to speak, grimacing and uncontrolled movement may make speech difficult and hard to understand. To cope with ordinary tasks, many patients use computerized household controls and speaking aids. Mechanized wheelchairs may be controlled with a joystick or mouth control. Specially shaped chairs and pillows

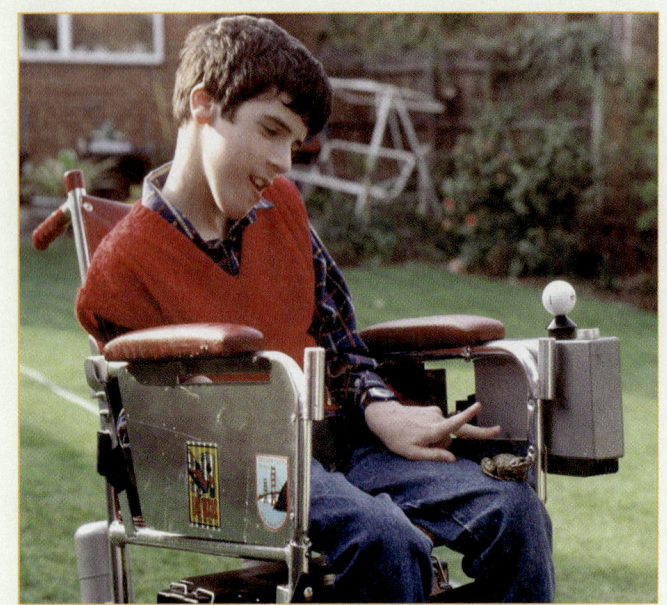

Figure 44-8 A person with cerebral palsy.

may be custom-built to facilitate the patient's comfort and ease movement. Toys may also be adapted to allow for learning and play. In addition, computers may be specially configured to aid the patient with speech simulation and provide the ability to perform household tasks, such as temperature control and lighting. Thanks to these technologies, many patients with cerebral palsy lead near-normal lives and live independently.

When caring for a patient with cerebral palsy, note the following:

- Do not assume that patients with cerebral palsy are always intellectually disabled. Although 75% of patients have some intellectual disability, many people with cerebral palsy have a normal IQ or only slight intellectual disability.
- Patients' limbs are often underdeveloped and are prone to injury (eg, from a fall from a wheelchair).
- Patients who have the ability to walk may have an ataxic or unsteady gait and are prone to falls.
- If the patient has a specially made pillow or chair (pediatric patients), the patient may prefer to use it during transport. Remember to pad the patient to ensure his or her comfort, and never force a patient's extremities into any position.
- Whenever possible, take walkers or wheelchairs along during transport.
- Approximately 25% of patients with cerebral palsy also have seizures. Be prepared to care for a seizure if one occurs, and keep suctioning available.

Cystic Fibrosis

Cystic fibrosis (CF-mucoviscidosis) is a chronic dysfunction of the endocrine system that targets multiple body systems, but primarily the respiratory and digestive systems. It is estimated that one in every 3,600 children born in Canada has CF. Although it is found in all races and ethnic groups, it most commonly occurs in Caucasian individuals of Northern European descent. The disease is usually fatal, with most children not living past their teens. With aggressive management and careful monitoring, some patients may live well into their thirties.

Cystic fibrosis is caused by a defective gene, which makes it difficult for chloride to move through cells. This causes unusually high sodium loss (resulting in salty skin) and abnormally thick mucus secretions. The secretions in the lungs cause breathing difficulties and provide an ideal growing medium for bacteria, leaving the patient highly susceptible to infection. Ultimately, the lung damage from the condition leads to lung disease, which is the primary cause of death in affected individuals.

Respiratory difficulties associated with cystic fibrosis include tachypnea, productive cough, shortness of breath, barrel chest, clubbed fingers, and cyanosis. The thick mucus may also collect in the intestines. Malnutrition and poor growth rate are common, as are intestinal blockages. Physicians strive to reduce the progression of the disease with physical therapy, exercise, vitamin supplements, and medications. Some patients may also benefit from a lung transplant.

Care of these patients should primarily focus on treating the individual's chief complaint. Keep a keen eye out for respiratory insufficiency, signs of a respiratory infection, intestinal blockage, or cardiac dysrhythmias (as a result of the electrolyte imbalance). Suctioning, high-flow supplemental oxygen, and breathing therapies may also be required during transport.

Multiple Sclerosis

Multiple sclerosis (MS) is a chronic disease of the central nervous system characterized by destruction of the myelin and nerve axons within the brain and spinal cord. It has no known cause, but is an autoimmune disorder or in some cases is genetically inherited. This disease strikes women in their 20s to 40s at a rate two to three times more often than men. Canadians have one of the highest rates of MS in the world. Every day, three new cases of MS are diagnosed. It is the most common neurologic disease affecting adults in Canada.

Myelin is a fatty covering that shields the axons. Axons are responsible for electrical conduction from neurons to muscles, leading to muscle response and communication from the body to the brain. Multiple sclerosis causes areas of myelin in random places to become inflamed, detach from the axon, and ultimately self-destruct. The area of destruction becomes scarred over—hence the name multiple (many) sclerosis (to harden) **Figure 44-9 ▶** .

Two types of multiple sclerosis are distinguished: relapsing/remitting and progressive. The relapsing/remitting form affects 90% of patients, presenting with bouts of worsening symptoms. Signs and symptoms of multiple sclerosis can be divided into those associated with the brain and those associated with the spinal cord **Table 44-1 ▶** and include numbness or tingling in parts of the body, unexplained weakness, dizziness, fatigue, double or blurry vision, and vision impairment. Periods of

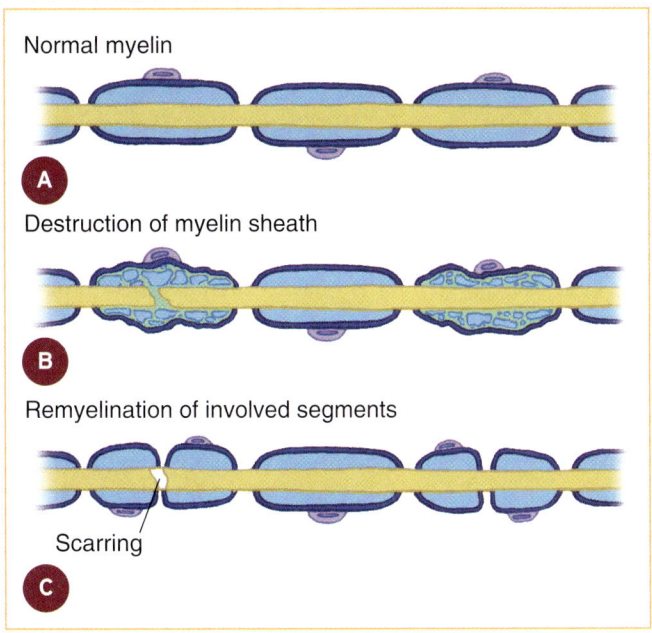

Figure 44-9 Progression of multiple sclerosis. **A.** Normal myelin. **B.** Destruction of myelin sheath. **C.** Scarring.

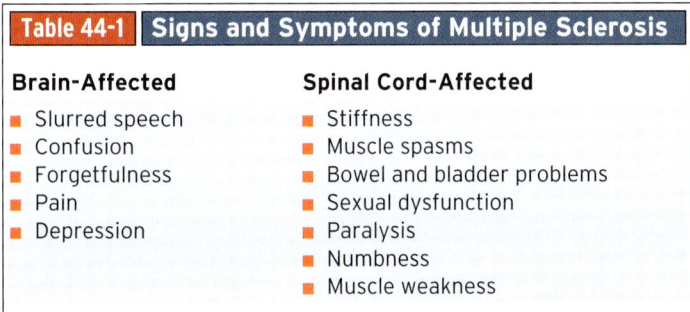

Table 44-1	Signs and Symptoms of Multiple Sclerosis
Brain-Affected	**Spinal Cord-Affected**
■ Slurred speech	■ Stiffness
■ Confusion	■ Muscle spasms
■ Forgetfulness	■ Bowel and bladder problems
■ Pain	■ Sexual dysfunction
■ Depression	■ Paralysis
	■ Numbness
	■ Muscle weakness

relapse leave the patient feeling marked improvement, with stiffness and weakness lingering for some. The other 10% of patients have the progressive form, in which symptoms get progressively worse with no periods of improvement or relief. Half of all people who have the relapsing/remitting form of the disease will develop the progressive form within 15 years if they remain untreated.

There is no cure for multiple sclerosis, although many treatments can significantly reduce the frequency of attacks and lessen symptoms when they occur. As with other illnesses, your treatment may be limited to supportive care. You may also be called to the patient's side due to tertiary complications of multiple sclerosis, such as a fall. Because of the disease process, the patient may lack feeling, so the physical examination may be difficult. A detailed medical history will help elucidate the diagnosis.

As with paralyzed patients, you must take special care when lifting and moving patients with multiple sclerosis. When these individuals are in crisis, they may not be able to walk even with their assistive devices.

Muscular Dystrophy

Muscular dystrophy is an inherited muscular disease that causes degeneration of the muscle fibres. In many cases, the destroyed fibres are replaced by fat or connective tissue. The result is a gradual weakening of muscles, slowing of motor development, and loss of muscle contractility. More than 30 types of muscular dystrophy have been identified. Some strike in early childhood and progress rapidly. Others don't strike until the late teens into the forties and progress much more slowly. Duchenne muscular dystrophy, the most common type, chiefly affects boys (1 of every 3,500 male births).

Muscular dystrophy may not be apparent in infancy, but rather appears as the child grows, presenting as muscle weakness during childhood or early adulthood. Parents or physicians may notice a delay in the normal developmental landmarks such as sitting, walking, or climbing stairs. The wasting of skeletal muscles ultimately leads to increasing disability and deformity. Kyphoscoliosis—an outward hump of the upper spine accompanied by curvature of the lower spine—may compromise pulmonary function. Cardiac involvement may also be present in as many as 95% of patients. Unfortunately, only 25% of those affected live to age 21 years, with pulmonary or cardiac complications usually being the cause of death.

Poliomyelitis

Poliomyelitis (commonly known as polio) is a highly contagious viral infection. First identified in 1789, it was once a worldwide plague, with its incidence growing to epidemic proportions from late spring through fall. Canada was declared polio-free in 1994. The last major Canadian epidemic of wild polio virus occurred in 1959, with 1,887 paralytic cases reported. Following the release of the Salk and Sabin polio vaccines in 1955, the number of cases of polio declined rapidly and the disease is now rare in Canada. Most cases involve vaccine-associated paralytic polio (VAPP), which is caused by contact between an unvaccinated individual and a person who has recently been inoculated with the live vaccine. Although live vaccines have not been used in Canada since 1996, they are still administered in many other parts of the world. Thanks to worldwide vaccination programs, promoted by the World Health Organization, the goal was to eradicate polio worldwide by 2008. However, outbreaks of polio still occur in countries where immunization programs have lapsed or where migration brings new polio cases from areas where polio is still present.

Humans are the only known hosts for the poliomyelitis virus. This pathogen enters the body by direct contact through the mouth, replicating in the pharynx, gastrointestinal system, and local lymphatic system. The virus then enters the bloodstream and spreads to the central nervous system. The spinal cord and brain are affected, which may cause paralysis or death.

In 80% to 90% of cases (usually involving young children), the illness is mild, presenting with malaise, sore throat, headache, vomiting, and slight fever. The initial symptoms are followed by a period of apparent wellness. Symptoms of major illness—fever, severe headache, stiff neck and back, deep muscle pain, or paralysis—then appear after a few days. In nonparalytic forms of polio, recovery is complete. In paralytic forms, muscle function returns gradually and completely. Any weakness or paralysis lasting longer than 12 months after the infection is a sign of permanent damage and disability.

Patients with paralysis will need special attention in order to safely lift, move, and position them. They may also need special equipment such as ventilatory assistance via an endotracheal tube or tracheotomy if they experience respiratory paralysis. They also may have an indwelling catheter in place if the lower extremities are paralyzed.

Spina Bifida

Spina bifida is the most common permanently disabling birth defect. In Canada, approximately 4 out of every 10,000 children are born with spina bifida. In this disorder, during the first month of pregnancy, the fetus' spinal column does not close properly or completely and vertebrae do not develop, leaving a portion of the spinal cord exposed **Figure 44-10 ▾**. Faithfully taking the B vitamin folic acid prior to becoming pregnant reduces the risk of spinal defects. Other maternal risk factors for spina bifida include previous neural tube defect pregnancy (increases risk by 20%), diabetes, medically diagnosed obesity, some antiseizure medications, exposure to increased temperature in early pregnancy (ie, hot baths or hot tubs, infection resulting in fever), Caucasian or Hispanic ethnicity, and lower socioeconomic status.

Symptoms of spina bifida may include partial or full paralysis (usually of the lower extremities), bladder or bowel control difficulties, learning disabilities, and latex allergy. In addition, as many as 70% to 90% of individuals with the most severe form of spina bifida also have hydrocephalus. In hydrocephalus, an increase in the amount of cerebral spinal fluid results in increased pressure on the brain. A shunt is inserted to relieve this pressure on the brain by draining excess cerebral

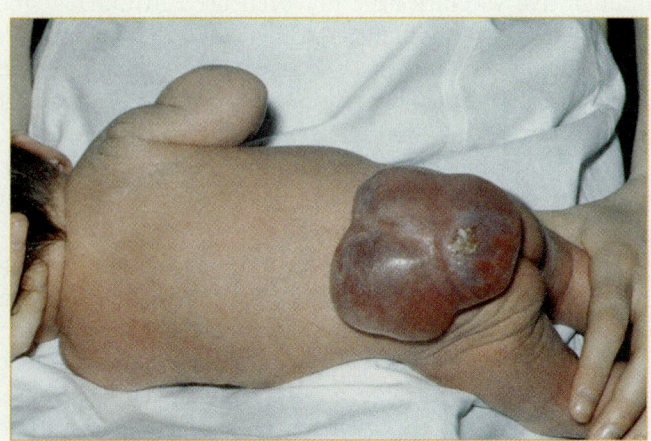

Figure 44-10 Spina bifida is characterized by exposure of part of the spinal cord.

spinal fluid. The shunt will stay in place throughout the patient's lifetime.

Spina bifida patients will likely benefit from the same considerations that you offer when treating a patient with paralysis or difficulty moving. When you are caring for these patients, ask how best to move them if possible. Remember to rule out a fall or other event that may have caused an injury. Check carefully for injuries, as patients may not be able to feel them—or the pain of an infiltrated IV, for that matter. Also, be aware that these patients may have urinary catheters or other aids in place.

Patients With Previous Head Injuries

Patients who previously experienced head injuries may be difficult to assess and treat. Brain-injured patients may face a complex array of challenges related to their injury. In such cases, gathering a complete medical history from the patient, family, and friends will assist you in the formation of a treatment plan. (Treatment will primarily be supportive care.) Your interaction with the patient will need to be tailored to his or her specific abilities. Take the time to speak with the patient and the family to establish what is normal for the patient—for example, whether the patient has cognitive, sensory, communication, motor, behavioural, or psychological deficits.

When you are caring for a patient with a previous head injury, talk to him or her in a calm and soothing tone, and watch the patient closely for signs of anxiety or aggression. In some cases, the patient may need to be specially positioned or restrained to ensure the safety of both you and the patient. Do not expect such an individual to walk to the ambulance or stretcher. As always, treat the patient with respect, use his or her name, explain procedures, and reassure the patient throughout your care.

Myasthenia Gravis

Myasthenia gravis is an abnormal condition characterized by chronic fatigability and weakness of muscles, especially in the face and throat. It is the result of a defect in the conduction of nerve impulses at the nerve junction, caused by a lack of acetylcholine. In myasthenia gravis, antibodies keep acetylcholine from reaching the muscles by blocking or damaging the receptor sites. This interruption in communication results in sudden bouts of muscle weakness, usually during activity, although the condition improves with rest. Although it affects all ethnic groups and sexes, myasthenia gravis is most commonly found in women younger than age 40 and men older than age 60.

The first symptoms usually present as weakness in eye or eyelid movement. Myasthenia gravis may also affect facial muscle control, changing the person's facial expression. In many cases, the disease is noticed initially as a sudden difficulty swallowing or chewing, or as slurred speech. Other symptoms may include blurry vision, weakness or difficulty moving the neck, shortness of breath, and weakness or difficulty moving limbs. Myasthenia gravis may be difficult to diagnosis because these symptoms can be attributed to many illnesses and disease processes.

A crisis may occur if the patient's respiratory muscles are damaged by infection, stress, or side effects of medications. These muscles could become so weak that the patient suffers an acute onset of respiratory failure. In such a case, you need to intervene immediately with airway management, ventilatory support, and possibly intubation.

Terminally Ill Patients

Unfortunately, some illnesses cannot be cured. As health care providers, you and your team will often be called upon to assist a patient who is facing imminent death, or terminal illness Figure 44-11 ▶ . Signs of impending death include decreased intake of food and drink, decreased orientation, irregular breathing patterns, and bradycardia or tachycardia. If you recognize these signs, you should help to reassure the family.

Although the goal of end-of-life care is to provide patients with a meaningful, dignified, and comfortable death, there is a surprising lack of data describing what patients and their families believe constitutes a "good death." While some patients with terminal illness choose to have the most aggressive care possible, others have a goal of comfort rather than cure or prolongation of life. In general, seriously ill patients identify pain and symptom management, preparation for death, and achieving a sense of completion as important factors in a good death.

If you are called to a scene in which death is imminent, the actions you take will have a lasting impact on the family. This is a time when compassion, understanding, and sensitivity are most needed. Some scenes may be chaotic. The family may be having a difficult time coping with the situation, and they may act out with anger and hostility. Treat everyone with compassion and understanding. The other members of your team may be

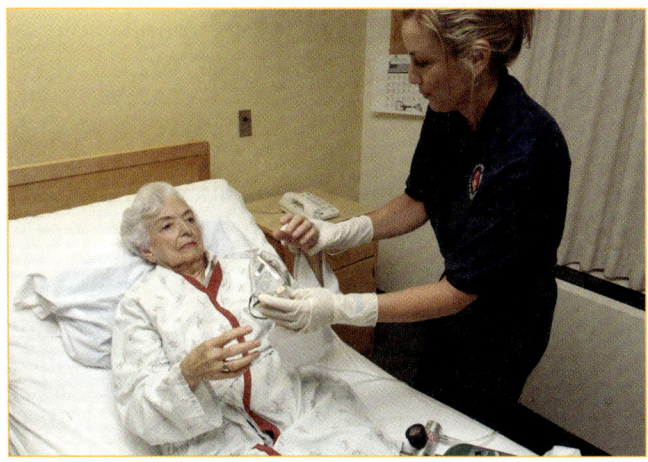

Figure 44-11 You will sometimes encounter patients with a terminal illness.

able to separate individuals and speak with them individually to diffuse intense emotions and restore order to the situation.

Terminally ill patients usually need only supportive care. Therapy is usually aimed at making the patient as comfortable as possible. The individual may have a displaced urinary catheter, need assistance in returning to bed, or need intervention in a pain crisis. Some patients may also be receiving care from hospice or a home health nurse. You may have been called because of a delay in the arrival of the regular care provider or for transport to take care of an immediate need in a clinical setting. Because terminally ill patients may use a complex array of pain medications, transdermal patches, or self-administered pain management devices, you may need to consult medical direction for guidance in their care.

You are the Paramedic Part 4

En route to the hospital you contact medical control for orders. You explain your patient's condition and her failure to improve. Your estimated time of arrival is approximately 20 minutes. Medical control asks you to administer another nebulizer treatment of 2.5 mg of salbutamol and 3 ml of normal saline, and a 20-mg methylprednisolone (Solumedrol) IV.

Upon your arrival to the emergency department you are met by Allison's mother, who is anxious to be with her daughter. A respiratory therapist is waiting at the patient's bedside to begin a continuous breathing treatment with salbutamol and Atrovent. The patient is admitted into pediatric intensive care for observation and possible intubation.

Reassessment	Recording Time: 17 Minutes
Skin	Pale, warm, and dry
Pulse	120 beats/min, strong and regular
Blood pressure	114/70 mm Hg
Respirations	24 breaths/min, laboured
Breath sounds	Diminshed bilaterally with faint expiratory wheezes
SpO_2	99% on nebulizer treatment
ECG	Sinus tachycardia without ectopy

6. Are patients with Down syndrome capable of taking an active role in their care?

If the patient has a valid do not resuscitate (DNR) order, CPR is not indicated or appropriate if the patient's heart stops and/or he or she stops breathing. If you have any question regarding the validity of a DNR or the level of interventions the patient wants, you should start resuscitation while contacting direct medical control for further instructions. When no resuscitative measures are attempted, aggressive comfort measures are required. These include oxygen administration, salbutamol-based breathing treatments, and morphine for pain and respiratory distress, as per local protocol. Place the patient in a comfortable position. Although the decision for a DNR order had already been made, family members may not understand what to do, and they may not be ready to face the death of a loved one. In such a case, take a thorough history and compassionately discuss the patient's wishes. Ask to review the DNR and keep it with the patient during transport.

Ascertain the family's wishes about having the patient remain in the home versus transport to the hospital **Figure 44-12 ▶** . During transport, contact direct medical control and advise the receiving hospital of the situation. If a family member requests to accompany the patient, he or she should be allowed to do so. If the family wishes the patient to remain at home, this request should be honoured provided it is in accordance with your local or regional protocol.

Protocols for handling the death of a patient vary, so you must learn your local or regional regulations. Your protocol will identify whether the coroner needs to be called to report

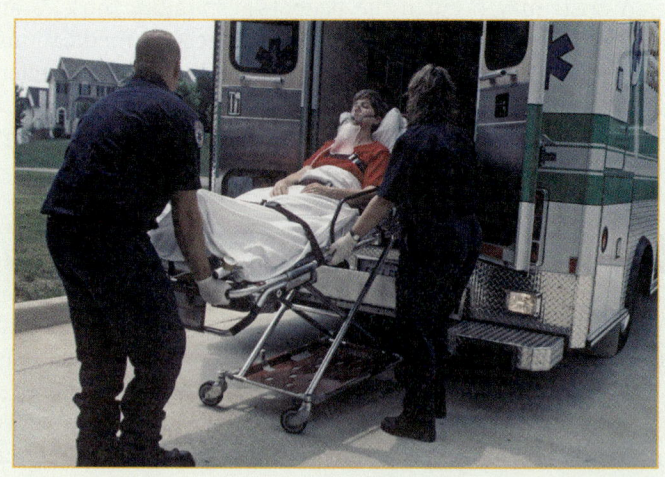

Figure 44-12 Some families may call for transport of a patient with a terminal illness.

the death and, if so, who is responsible for contacting the coroner. Also determine whether a pronouncement of death is required and, if so, who makes it.

Patients With Communicable Diseases

Some patients may have communicable diseases, which explains why appropriate PPE and routine precautions need to be followed with every patient, every time **Figure 44-13 ▼** . Gloves and eye protection should be considered basic attire. Gowns, masks, and other protective measures should be deployed if the situation warrants. Safety for yourself, your crew, and your patient is paramount. At the same time, you should treat patients with communicable diseases with the same compassion you would give to any other patient.

Clues that a patient has a communicable disease include rashes, coughing, ill appearance, health history, and medications. Offer patients with AIDS or other immuno-compromised conditions a mask prior to their arrival at a hospital to safeguard them from further exposure to illness. Masking a patient early during your assessment may be the quickest and easiest method of preventing disease transmission (see Chapters 2 and 36 for more details).

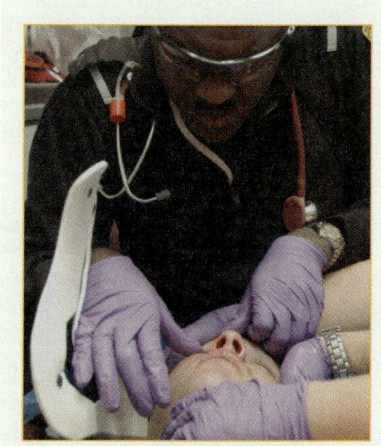

Figure 44-13 Always wear gloves and eye protection as a bare minimum.

Controversies

On some occasions, the family may disagree with the DNR order but the patient is unable to speak for himself or herself. The patient's wishes should be respected with regard to resuscitation when those wishes are clear and no reasonable doubt exists with regard to those specific wishes. If a family wants CPR started, but a DNR order states otherwise, make certain that the family is aware of the existence of the DNR order. Once aware, if they maintain their desire to initiate resuscitative efforts, you should do so.

When the family indicates a desire to start CPR in the face of a DNR order, reasonable doubt about the validity of that order is present. In such a situation, you simply cannot be certain whether the patient or another relative with medical authority for the patient initiated the DNR order or whether an individual with legal authority to make medical decisions for the patient is present. Sorting out those issues is best left for the physicians in the emergency department where more information can be obtained and more thorough discussions with the family about the gravity of the medical condition are possible.

You should thoroughly understand your local or provincial laws and protocols with regard to DNR orders and carefully consider how you would handle difficult situations with regard to DNR controversies before you face them.

Culturally Diverse Patients

Canada is a tremendously culturally diverse country, and as discussed in Chapter 10, acceptance of and awareness of the cultural backgrounds and customs of others will allow you to be a more effective paramedic and a valuable member of your community. Chapter 10 also discusses how to recognize a culturally diverse patient. Cultural diversity requires respect for all cultures, languages, and communities. In many areas, particularly large urban centres, major segments of the population do not speak English. Your job will be much easier if you learn some common words and phrases (especially medical terms) in their language.

As part of the focused history and physical examination, you must obtain a medical history. You cannot skip this step simply because the patient doesn't speak English. Most patients who don't speak English fluently will still know important words or phrases. First, find out how much English the patient can speak. Then, use short, simple questions and simple words whenever possible. Avoid difficult medical terms, and point to specific parts of the body as you ask questions.

Financial Challenges

Many patients, particularly the elderly, may be concerned about the financial aspect of the ambulance ride to the hospital. Remember, they have experienced the times before the institution of universal health care in Canada.

"I can't go to the hospital. I don't have the money!" These statements are heard from many patients who do not understand the concept of universal health care. Many of these individuals do not have private health insurance that covers ambulance services. By engaging in careful, compassionate communication with your patient, you should try to determine the source of his or her anxiety. Share with the patient your concerns about his or her current health.

You are the Paramedic Summary

1. What is Down syndrome?

Down syndrome, also known as trisomy 21, is a congenital abnormality that occurs from a failure of the number 21 chromosome to divide properly during the first stage of sperm or egg cell development. Consequently, there are three number 21 chromosomes instead of the normal pair. This extra chromosome is then passed onto the fetus and causes the abnormality.

2. What are the characteristic physical features of Down syndrome?

Classic physical features of Down syndrome include:

- Eyes that slope upward at the outer corners
- Folds of skin on either side of the nose that cover the inside corners of the eyes
- A small face and small facial features
- A large protruding tongue
- Flattening of the back of the head
- Short and broad hands

3. What medical conditions are commonly seen in patients with Down syndrome?

Children with Down syndrome may also have congenital heart defects, intestinal disorders, epilepsy, and hearing defects. They also have an increased risk of having respiratory infections.

4. Why is it important to physically be at the patient's level to speak with her?

How would you feel if you couldn't breathe, were scared, and were approached by a stranger carrying strange machines? Remember with any child it is important to make contact at eye level so you can earn his or her trust.

5. What anatomical features of Down syndrome can make airway management challenging?

Keep in mind that individuals with Down syndrome have smaller faces and facial features, a large protruding tongue, and a flattened back portion of the head. These differences may make the use of airway adjuncts a bit tricky. Be prepared to use smaller size equipment than normal, provide padding under the head, and be patient when airway management is required.

6. Are patients with Down syndrome capable of taking an active role in their care?

Many individuals with Down syndrome are capable of being functional members of society. Others may only need the assistance provided by a group home or assisted-living facility. These people would be able to take an active role in their health care and assist you in the case of an emergency.

Prep Kit

Ready for Review

- In the prehospital environment, you will encounter patients who face a variety of special challenges.
- Humans use all five senses to gather information, but we often take that sensory feedback for granted.
- Mental illness is a generic term for a variety of illnesses that result in emotional, cognitive, or behavioural dysfunction.
- A developmental disability is a permanent condition that means a person develops more slowly and differently than others. Individuals with a developmental disability may have difficulty learning and processing information with abstract ideas and changing to meet the needs of normal daily life.
- Pathologic challenges require special consideration when you formulate your treatment plan. Pathologies you may encounter during your career may include arthritis, cancer, cerebral palsy, cystic fibrosis, multiple sclerosis, muscular dystrophy, poliomyelitis, previous head injury, spina bifida, and myasthenia gravis.
- Unfortunately, some illnesses cannot be cured. As health care providers, you and your team will often be called upon to assist a patient who is facing imminent death from terminal illness.
- Some patients may have communicable diseases, which explains why appropriate PPE and routine procedures need to be followed with every patient, every time.
- Fears about payment for emergency medical services should not keep any patient from seeking help. By engaging in careful, compassionate communication with your patient, you should try to determine the source of his or her anxiety. Share with the patient your concerns about his or her current health.

Vital Vocabulary

aphasia The loss of the ability to communicate in speech, writing, or signs.

arthritis Joint inflammation that causes pain, swelling, stiffness, and decreased range of motion.

bariatrics The branch of medicine that studies and treats obese patients.

cerebral palsy A nonprogressive bilateral neuromuscular disorder in which voluntary muscles are poorly controlled.

conductive deafness A curable temporary condition, caused by an injury to the eardrum.

cystic fibrosis Chronic dysfunction of the endocrine system that affects multiple body systems, primarily the respiratory and digestive systems.

developmental disability A permanent condition that means a person develops move slowly and differently than others.

Down syndrome A genetic chromosomal defect that can occur during fetal development and that results in intellectual impairment as well as certain physical characteristics, such as a round head with a flat occiput and slanted, wide-set eyes.

emotional or intellectual disabilities Illnesses that cause a person's emotions to become out of control.

hemiplegia Paralysis of one side of the body.

mental illness A generic term for a variety of illnesses that result in emotional, cognitive, or behavioural dysfunction.

multiple sclerosis A chronic disease of the central nervous system in which there is destruction of the myelin and nerve axons within several regions of the brain and spinal cord.

muscular dystrophy An inherited muscular disease causing degeneration of the muscle fibres.

myasthenia gravis An abnormal condition characterized by the chronic fatigability and weakness of muscles, especially in the face and throat. It is the result of a defect in the conduction of nerve impulses at the nerve junction. This deficit is caused by a lack of acetylcholine.

obesity A term generally used when someone is 20% to 30% over his or her ideal weight.

osteoarthritis A degenerative joint disease associated with aging.

paraplegia Paralysis of one side of the body.

poliomyelitis A highly contagious viral infection that can cause paralysis and death, and created a serious epidemic in the past but is now prevented in Canada through a vaccine.

quadriplegia Paralysis of all four extremities and the trunk.

sensorineural deafness A permanent lack of hearing caused by a lesion or damage of the inner ear.

spina bifida The most common permanently disabling birth defect in which, during the first month of pregnancy, the spinal column of the fetus does not close properly or completely and vertebrae do not develop, leaving a portion of the spinal cord exposed.

terminal illness A sickness that the patient cannot be cured of; death is imminent.

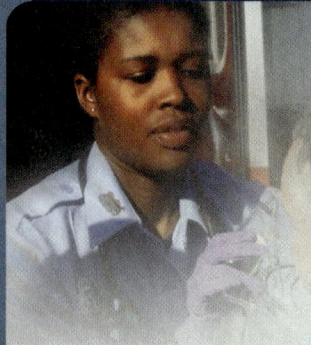

Assessment in Action

You are dispatched to a private residence for a 32-year-old patient with shortness of breath. When you arrive on scene, you find a male patient supine in his bed. You observed multiple handicapped equipment devices while walking to the patient. His family tells you that he had a spinal cord injury a year ago and is paralyzed from the neck down. They inform you that the patient is prone to pneumonia and they believe he has it now. His blood pressure is 140/70 mm Hg; pulse rate, 120 beats/min; respiratory rate, 26 breaths/min; pulse oximetry reading on room air, 95%; and the ECG shows sinus tachycardia.

1. _____ is paralysis of all four extremities and the trunk, possibly from a cervical spine injury.
   A. Hemiplegia
   B. Paraplegia
   C. Quadriplegia
   D. Hyperesthesia

2. True or false? Paralyzed patients always have diaphragmatic involvement.
   A. True
   B. False

3. A paralyzed patient may have normal sensation or:
   A. hyperesthesia.
   B. hypoesthesia.
   C. diaphragmatic involvement.
   D. hemiparesis.

4. _____ is paralysis of one side of the body.
   A. Hemiplegia
   B. Hyperesthesia
   C. Hemiparesis
   D. Paraplegia

5. _____ is defined as a nonprogressive bilateral neuromuscular disorder in which voluntary muscles are poorly controlled.
   A. Arthritis
   B. Osteoarthritis
   C. Cerebral palsy
   D. Cystic fibrosis

6. _____ is a chronic dysfunction of the endocrine system that affects multiple body systems.
   A. Arthritis
   B. Cerebral palsy
   C. Pleurisy
   D. Cystic fibrosis

7. _____ is a chronic disease of the central nervous system in which destruction of the myelin and nerve axons occur within several regions of the brain and spinal cord.
   A. Cerebral palsy
   B. Multiple sclerosis
   C. Cystic fibrosis
   D. Arthritis

Challenging Questions

You are dispatched to a private home for an unresponsive patient. When you arrive on scene, you are greeted by the patient's daughter, who tells you she believes her mother is dead, or is dying. After speaking to the daughter, you find out the patient is home with terminal liver cancer. The patient is taking agonal respirations at a rate of 2 to 4 breaths/min. She has weak, slow pulses and an unpalpable blood pressure.

8. What should you do for this patient?

9. What should you do for the family?

Points to Ponder

You and your partner are dispatched to a local residential facility for a seizure. You are familiar with this facility, as it is known as the home of severely developmentally disabled individuals. When you arrive, you find a female patient who appears postical. The patient is normally nonverbal, and her body is severely contracted. She has a history of a severe intellectual disability, seizures, diabetes, and stroke. The patient's vital signs are as follows: blood pressure, 180/90 mm Hg; respiratory rate, 24 breaths/min; pulse rate, 110 beats/min; pulse oximetry reading on room air, 96%; and the ECG shows sinus tachycardia.

How do you assess her mental status?

Issues: Understanding the Challenges of Caring for Patients With Special Needs.

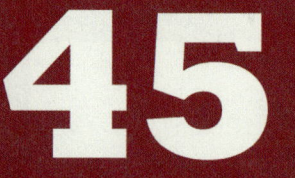

45 Acute Interventions for the Chronic Care Patient

Competency Areas

Area 3: Health and Safety

3.3.f Practice infection control techniques.
3.3.g Clean and disinfect equipment.

Area 4: Assessment and Diagnostics

4.2.c Obtain chief complaint and/or incident history from patient, family members, and/or bystanders.
4.2.d Obtain information regarding patient's past medical history.
4.2.f Obtain information regarding incident through accurate and complete scene assessment.

Area 5: Therapeutics

5.1.a Use manual maneuvers and positioning to maintain airway patency.
5.1.i Remove airway foreign bodies (AFB).
5.1.j Remove foreign body by direct techniques.
5.2.a Recognize indications for oxygen administration.
5.2.b Take appropriate safety precautions.
5.2.c Ensure adequacy of oxygen sypply.
5.2.d Recognize different types of oxygen delivery systems.
5.2.e Utilize portable oxygen delivery systems.
5.3.a Administer oxygen using nasal cannula.
5.3.b Administer oxygen using low concentration mask.
5.4.b Recognize indications for mechanical ventilation.
5.4.c Prepare mechanical ventilation equipment.
5.4.d Provide mechanical ventilation.
5.5.b Control external hemorrhage through the use of direct pressure and patient positioning.
5.5.c Maintain peripheral intravenous (IV) access devices and infusions of crystalloid solutions without additives.
5.5.o Provide routing care for patient with urinary catheter.
5.5.p Provide routing care for patient with ostomy drainage system.
5.5.u Conduct urinary catheterization.

Area 6: Integration

6.2.d Provide care for physically-challenged patient.

Appendix 4: Pathophysiology

B. **Neurologic System**
Chronic Neurologic Disorders: Amyotrophic lateral sclerosis (ALS)
Chronic Neurologic Disorders: Muscular dystrophy
Chronic Neurologic Disorders: Poliomyelitis
Infectious Disorders: Guillian Barre syndrome
J. **Multisystem Diseases and Injuries**
Cancer: Malignancy

Introduction

Breakthrough technologies, newer drugs, and research have combined to increase the average life expectancy. Thanks to these advances, persons who might have died from injuries or illnesses 50 years ago may now continue to lead satisfying and productive lives. Many of these persons, however, require physical support and care of chronic illnesses—care that may take place in the home setting. As a result of this trend, paramedics are being called upon more frequently to interact with chronic care providers and patients who are receiving home care Table 45-1 ▾ .

Quality prehospital care is the ultimate goal for paramedics, but the aims for specific patient populations are often quite different. In the acute care setting (hospital), objectives include stabilization, diagnosis, and treatment. In the prehospital setting, emergency care has historically been associated with these objectives.

In rehabilitation care, the objective is to restore a person with disabilities to his or her maximum potential in several areas: physical, social, spiritual, psychological, and vocational. Formerly, this kind of healing, exercise, and development of skills took place in hospitals. In recent years, however, rehabilitation programs have shifted from the hospital to specialized rehabilitation centres and expanded home health care programs. Rehabilitation centres are designed to promote healing and the gradual return of the patient to the community.

In patients who are unable to return to their homes, the long-term care objectives include maintenance of a safe, stimulating environment for the patient. Although paramedics often equate long-term care with nursing homes for the elderly, facilities also exist for children and patients with specific health care needs. Some long-term care facilities offer custodial care; others provide life enhancement. Clearly, long-term care covers a broad range of services.

The philosophy of hospice care began in England in the 1960s. This multidisciplinary approach seeks to improve the quality of a person's life at the end through pain and symptom management. Because many patients feel more comfortable in their own homes, surrounded by familiar people and objects, and living on their own schedule, ensuring this comfort is the primary part of the palliative plan of care.

Originally, patients resided in *hospices* (from the same Latin root as *hospitality*) to receive end-of-life care that included pain management without cure management. Over time, hospice care grew to include home and in-hospital care designed to support the dying patient and his or her family during the terminal illness and afterward through the bereavement process. Patients admitted to hospice care have a life-threatening or terminal illness that is expected to result in death within 6 months.

Table 45-1	Home Care Patients in Canada, 2000		
Year	Number of Persons Receiving Home Care	> 65 Years Old	< 65 Years Old
2000	305,538	191,645	113,893

Source: http://cansim2.statcan.ca (retrieved January 20, 2009).

You are the Paramedic Part 1

You and your partner are dispatched to a private residence for a severe headache. As your partner approaches the address, you both make mention of the wheelchair access ramp leading up to the side entrance. The door is opened by a young woman as you make your way up the walkway. She leads you into the home, explaining that her 36-year-old husband, Michael, has been experiencing a severe headache for the past 2 hours and has not experienced any relief from his normal medication.

You enter the living room and find the patient sitting in a wheelchair. He is awake, alert, and in obvious distress. You observe that he has a tracheostomy tube in place although he is not receiving supplemental oxygen. His wife tells you that he is able to breathe on his own during the day without additional oxygen, but needs a ventilator for support at night. He does not require any other special equipment or treatment.

Initial Assessment	Recording Time: 0 Minutes
Appearance	Seated upright in an electric wheelchair, face wet with sweat, grimacing
Level of consciousness	A (Alert to person, place, and day)
Airway	Open and clear
Breathing	Adequate chest rise and volume
Circulation	Slow, strong radial pulse

1. Does treating a patient with chronic health problems affect the way you deliver emergency care?
2. What types of patients are likely to benefit from home care?

Special Considerations

Chronic conditions necessitating home care occur across all ages. Different conditions are more prevalent in certain age groups. In addition, the age of the person affects his or her response to the chronic condition.

In childhood, chronic conditions may impede the attainment of normal developmental milestones and affect trust and autonomy. In adolescence, body image and peer acceptance become primary concerns, and normal teenage rebellion may interfere with treatment plans. The development of intimate relationships and achievement of vocational goals may be impaired when chronic illness strikes in early adulthood. Chronic illness in middle age may hinder professional or career growth, resulting in early retirement and the need to use retirement income for medical expenses. Spouses of older patients may become the primary caregiver even though they are experiencing a similar decline in health.

Home care used to be the norm for terminally ill patients because few patients could afford expensive hospital care and, therefore, were cared for at home. To assist some families with care of the sick, certain religious groups provided home health care, while public health nurses and visiting nurse societies provided education to home health care providers on cleanliness and prevention of disease in addition to care. Over the years, visiting nursing has evolved into a multidisciplinary specialty. Today, home health care providers are usually referred by a physician and associated with a hospital or agency.

Previously, patients receiving home health care often relied on expensive emergency department visits for management of acute incidents even when the incident could be managed at home. As a paramedic, your role in the care of these patients has expanded as more advanced technology emerges.

Home health care has become an increasingly attractive alternative both to patients, who often want to maintain control over their health care decision making, and to the provinces, which want to control acute care costs. During the 1990s, however, changes in reimbursement rules severely restricted home health care agencies in terms of who they could serve, which services could be provided, and how many visits could occur each year. Unfortunately, these informal caregivers may become overwhelmed by the care requirements and experience stress-related illnesses themselves.

The provincial and territorial governments pay for the majority of home services that are reimbursed. They regulate home health care agencies to ensure they meet the quality standards established by the federal government. Many types of agencies care for patients at home, including those reimbursed by provincial and territorial health plans, local funds, private insurance, out-of-pocket, and combinations of payers. In addition, each public program has its own method of determining reimbursement (ie, through reimbursement guidelines and ceilings).

Costs for similar home care services vary substantially. Nevertheless, studies show that home-based health care costs less than institutional health care, gives more satisfaction to those who receive it because they can remain in familiar surroundings, and often results in fewer and shorter hospital stays.

Measurement of the quality of health care is difficult in any setting but is particularly complex when care is delivered in the home. Consumers of home health care are vulnerable, are frequently too sick to advocate for themselves, and may lack advocates. Paramedics have a unique opportunity to listen to these patients and their families, observe the home care situation, and assist in securing additional resources or reporting to protective agencies. In addition, you can offer guidance for in-home injury prevention as you observe the patient at home.

The Role of the Paramedic in Injury Prevention in the Home Care Setting

The role of the paramedic is ideal for identifying and preventing illness and injury in the home care setting. You may be able to help identify causes of illness or injury, or prevention of either, in the future. For example, you may be called to the home of a patient who has fallen while trying to walk to the bathroom unassisted. As you arrive, you observe that the patient has tripped over a bath rug which caught under her walker leg. Your teachable moment comes in assisting the patient and family to recognize the need to remove scatter rugs and other hazards that might add to the cause of falls. Injuries include unintentional injuries, such as those caused by motor vehicle collisions, drowning, falls, and fires, and intentional injuries, such as suicide and violence.

An injury is defined by the US Centers for Disease Control (CDC) as "unintentional or intentional damage to the body resulting from acute exposure to thermal, mechanical, electrical or chemical energy, or from the absence of such essentials as heat or oxygen." Injuries and illness may be preventable by changing the environment or individual behaviour. One useful framework for injury prevention is the Haddon matrix.

The Haddon matrix, developed by Dr. William Haddon, who was the first administrator of what is now the National Highway Traffic Safety Administration in the United States, can be a useful tool for identifying injury prevention opportunities. According to the Haddon matrix framework, injuries occur in a certain time sequence: the pre-event phase, the event phase, and the post-event phase. Each event has a host (the person who is involved in the injury) and the equipment that is involved in the injury. There are also different environmental situations in which an injury might occur. Prevention can be focused in any "cell" of the matrix. For example, teaching the patient and family about the hazards of having scatter rugs is an intervention that addresses the host/pre-event cell; removing the rugs may address the pre-event/equipment cell.

Assessment of the Chronic Care Patient

Scene Assessment

Scene safety follows the same guidelines as for any call. Pets that live in homes with chronically ill persons may be agitated because the household has changed from a living quarters to a care facility—full of strange noises, new faces, and smells. Remember, however, that you are entering someone's home, not a health care facility. Families may keep a variety of weapons (or equipment that can function as a weapon) on hand. Caregiver stress, exhaustion, and pressure may cause some family members to react negatively to your presence or rely on you to help relieve stress **Figure 45-1 ▾**. The house may have been renovated to accommodate large equipment that may make entrances unsafe (eg, ramps intended to accommodate a wheelchair).

In addition to the usual scene assessment, perform a quick assessment of the supporting equipment. How can it be moved safely? Are backup batteries for the equipment available? Is the equipment compatible with the ambulance electrical system? Will the equipment fit?

When you assess the patient's environment, note whether nutritional support is adequate. Moreover, basic needs such as a reliable, safe heat source, good ventilation, electricity, and available water are important.

Personal Protective Equipment and Routine Precautions

PPE and routine precautions in the home care scenario are the same as in any setting. Keep contaminated supplies and equipment together and off the floor and furniture. Bring two disposable bags for supplies: Contaminated but disposable supplies can go in one bag, while contaminated but reusable supplies go in the other. Follow your agency's plan for cleaning supplies and returning them to use.

The most effective means of preventing transmission of microorganisms is handwashing. Use a waterless gel with at least 60% alcohol content before applying your gloves and after removing them. Use running water and soap to clean your hands if they are visibly soiled or if your patient has a diagnosed infection or is taking immunosuppression drugs. Use a mask, goggles, and gown if you will be exposed to respiratory secretions or if your patient is immunosuppressed and should be protected from the paramedic. Most chronically ill patients have had multiple exposures to latex, so avoid wearing latex gloves when caring for these patients. This consideration is especially critical in the pediatric population, particularly for children with spina bifida.

Basic principles of infection control should be applied to the home care setting. As a paramedic you should adhere to standard and droplet precautions for home care patients to protect your health as well as the health of others you will come in contact with.

Initial Assessment

To conduct the initial assessment of patients with chronic illness, first gather a general impression. Does the patient appear to be on the point of death? If so, do not try to troubleshoot any home care devices. Instead, remove the patient as quickly as possible from the equipment and transfer him or her to your EMS equipment. Apply portable oxygen while you assess the situation, but troubleshoot any malfunctioning devices later if you cannot fix the malfunction or failure.

Assess the patient's airway. Many patients receiving home care have artificial or altered airways such as tracheostomies or laryngectomies. Your evaluation of patients receiving home oxygen or support ventilation is no different than for any other patient. Assess the work of breathing. Look for accessory muscle use, posture, grunting, or pursed lip breathing to keep the alveoli open. Listen to the patient's breath sounds and compare them on a side-to-side basis. Finally, assess pulse oximetry.

Assess the patient's level of consciousness (LOC) or mental status. In the chronic care patient, a common alteration in LOC is dementia. Document the patient's behaviour, including accusations, but remain nonjudgmental toward caregivers. Another possible change in LOC is delirium, an often acute, reversible

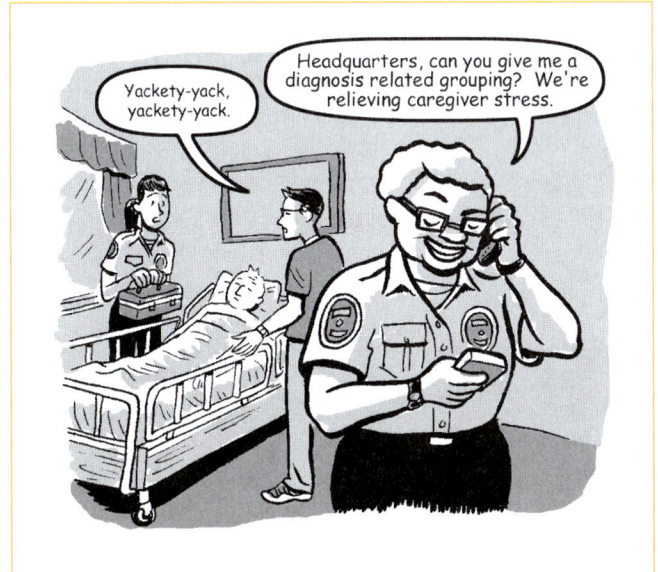

Speech bubbles: "Yackety-yack, yackety-yack." / "Headquarters, can you give me a diagnosis related grouping? We're relieving caregiver stress."

Figure 45-1

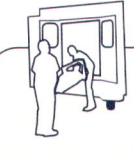

At the Scene

Pulse oximetry varies according to patient age and gender. Compare your result to the usual patient results and intervene based on your overall assessment.

change in behaviour that may be caused by glucose or electrolyte imbalances, nutritional deficiencies, hypothermia, or hyperthermia.

Focused History and Physical Examination

In a trauma patient, stabilize the patient's cervical spine, perform a rapid physical examination, provide comfort, and assess for other injuries. In a medical patient, gather a SAMPLE history, perform an assessment of the chief complaint, and take the patient's vital signs before you develop the plan of prehospital care. Once you have obtained the history, you may complete a physical examination. Treatment is based on both history and examination.

Medication Interactions in Home Care

Each patient may react differently to a particular medication. You are expected to treat any possible medication interactions by maintaining the patient's airway, breathing, and circulation.

Untoward reactions to medication interactions may be accidental. Observe the scene for signs of unsafe medication administration practices (eg, Does the patient understand his or her dosing requirements? Could similar-sounding medications cause confusion?). Is there inadequate lighting, or problematic equipment (eg, faulty infusion pumps or failing power systems)? Not all medications are meant to be crushed, yet some patients or caregivers may crush tablets before placing them in a gastric tube. Crushed extended-release medications may enter the patient's bloodstream too rapidly, causing an accidental overdose. Be suspicious for potential, accidental, or deliberate overdosing by the patient or caregiver. Report any suspicion of abuse to the proper social service agency.

Using the Home Health History

Home care providers may range from licensed personnel to friends, family, or members of fraternal or church groups. Informal caregiving networks often keep few records about the patient's care. In contrast, when home care is more formal—for example, occurring through hospitals or home care agencies—providers may be required to keep detailed records similar to those in hospitals or nursing homes. In particular, medical insurance agencies expect detailed records to support a claim for benefits.

Compliance Issues

Calls to patients receiving home care sometimes result from inoperative or damaged equipment such as IVs, tubes, artificial airways, and ventilators. Always consider that a call to a chronically ill patient may result from equipment failure rather than a worsening of the patient's condition. In such a case, care should be directed toward maintaining the patient on EMS equipment while the patient's own equipment is repaired or the patient can be transferred to new equipment. Inability to easily or expeditiously repair or replace the equipment should result in a transfer to the hospital.

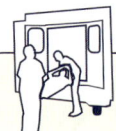

Special Considerations

Culture plays a significant role in determining what the patient and family consider adequate care. Assess the adequacy of care by speaking with the patient and family—not by making assumptions about what would be adequate in your own home. Learn the customs and cultural needs of persons in your area.

Assessing Dementia

When you are assessing a patient with dementia (or any patient, for that matter), ask two critical questions: What is the patient's usual baseline functioning? How does function today vary from baseline? Once you have identified a change from baseline behaviour, either from caregivers or from a health record, determine whether a reversible condition needs to be treated—for example, hypoglycemia, hypoxia, or hypothermia.

If no reversible conditions exist, transport the patient to the emergency department for further evaluation. Dementia

Documentation and Communication

Paramedics are often frustrated because they expect a certain level of reporting, including written transfer paperwork from a patient's home care provider. Respectfully ask the home care provider about his or her involvement with the patient. Treat this provider in the same manner as you would a close family member if he or she is unable to answer all of your questions. Whenever possible, explain the rationale for your treatment plan. Remember—you have been called because the home care treatment is not working or the situation has changed. In addition, explain that once you arrive on the scene, the law requires you to assume responsibility of the patient since you are now the primary care provider. You can have the home care provider speak with your medical control only if time permits.

At the Scene

Use the mnemonic AEIOU-TIPS to determine possible causes of altered mental status:

A Alcohol or acidosis
E Epilepsy, environment, electricity
I   Insulin
O Overdose
U Uremia
T Trauma
I   Infection
P Poisoning or psychosis
S Seizure, stroke, or shock

alone does not render a patient incompetent. In many provinces, patients cannot be transported against their will unless they are a hazard to themselves or others. Call direct medical control for assistance if the patient is unwilling to be transported. Document all assessments and interventions on your PCR.

Detailed Physical Examination

The detailed physical examination assesses a specific region or body system in the case of trauma with significant mechanism of injury (MOI). Most calls to the chronic care home will be medical in nature. The chief complaint may clue you into the mechanism or cause of the illness. The level of detail required for a physical examination in the home care setting is similar to any other physical examination encountered in paramedic practice. The need for a comprehensive examination depends on the acuity of the patient and the risk factors for further injury or illness.

Ongoing Assessment

If you are unable to resolve the patient's problem, plan to transport the patient to the appropriate facility per protocol. Streamline the patient's equipment by removing components that will not be used during transport (eg, a humidification device for a home ventilator). Document your care on the PCR or call sheet.

If the patient's own equipment will be used during transport, be sure to have battery backup for electrical devices in case of ambulance mechanical difficulties. Home care equipment is either purchased (usually as an insurance benefit) or rented, and the patient may be financially liable if it is lost or damaged. Be sure that all equipment is clearly labeled with the patient's name and contact information **Figure 45-2 ▾** . Document which pieces of equipment were transported as well as the name of the person assuming responsibility for the patient and equipment at the receiving facility.

Should the patient's problem resolve before transport, call direct medical control or follow your protocol for referring the patient to his or her own physician.

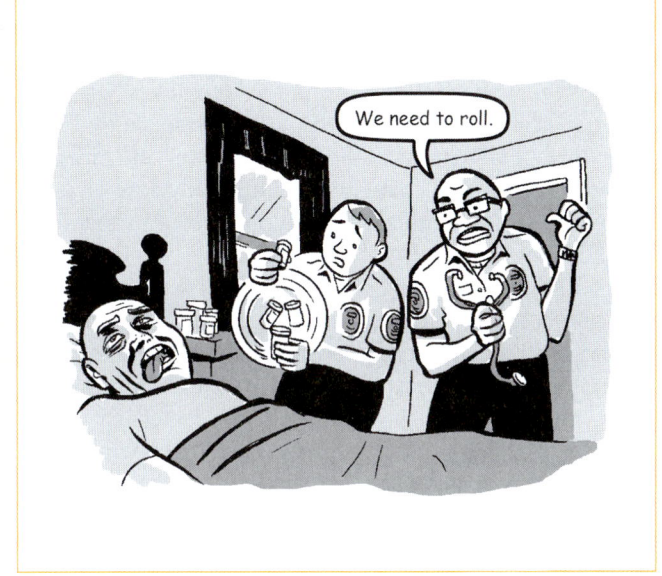

Figure 45-2

You are the Paramedic **Part 2**

You begin your assessment while your partner takes a set of vital signs. The patient was involved in a motor vehicle collision 6 months ago, resulting in a ruptured spleen, multiple rib fractures, a fractured left arm, and a C4 fracture of the neck. The spinal fracture and resulting spinal cord injury left your patient a quadriplegic. He is able to move using an electronic wheelchair. His wife was taught to straight catheterize her husband every 6 to 8 hours and assist with a bowel regimen. She is also skilled in providing tracheostomy care and setting up the ventilator at night. A home health nurse visits five times a week to provide additional assistance. He is prescribed 15 mg of baclofen three times a day to help with muscle spasms and cramping and acetaminophen (Tylenol) as needed for pain or fever.

The patient tells you that his headache began approximately 2 hours earlier while watching a football game on television. He had taken the Tylenol as prescribed with no relief. The pain has gradually gotten worse and is now a 10 on a scale of 1 to 10. He describes the pain as a relentless pounding that does not radiate. He does admit to having blurred vision. At this time he denies having experienced nausea, vomiting, chest pain, or shortness of breath.

Vital Signs	Recording Time: 5 Minutes
Level of consciousness	Alert
Pulse	56 beats/min, regular
Blood pressure	194/100 mm Hg
Respirations	16 breaths/min, regular
Skin	Flushed, warm, and diaphoretic about the face; cool, pale, and clammy elsewhere
Spo2	99% on room air

3. What type of equipment might you encounter with patients receiving home health care?

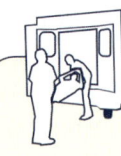

At the Scene

Transporting equipment not designed to be used during a transport may increase the risk of injury to patients and EMS professionals.

Types of Patients Who Receive Home Health Care

Chronically ill patients are cared for at home by a wide range of caregivers who may include family members, unlicensed caregivers, licensed nonprofessional caregivers, licensed professionals, or a combination of these. Many family members who care for chronically ill patients are medically knowledgeable and are often the paramedic's best source of information and care guidelines.

In addition to frail or chronically ill elderly patients in the home care setting, you may encounter individuals, for example, who have recently had a hospital stay, surgery, or a high-risk pregnancy, or a newborn with medical complications. Chronic illness or permanent injury may also necessitate home care (**Table 45-2 ▾**). Many of these patients experience similar physical problems regardless of the initial cause.

Table 45-2	Chronic Illnesses and Injuries Encountered in the Home Care Setting
Type of Disease, Injury, or Abnormality	**General Long-Term Problem**
Neuromuscular disease	Hypoventilation
Guillain-Barré syndrome	Decreased cough mechanism
Muscular dystrophy	Inability to maintain airway
Amyotrophic lateral sclerosis Multiple sclerosis Polio/postpolio syndrome Spinal cord injury Central apnea	Immobility: deep venous thrombosis, pulmonary embolus, pressure ulcers

Musculoskeletal abnormalities:
  Scoliosis or lordosis
  Pectus excavatum
  Pectus carinatum
  Pickwickian syndrome
	Hypoventilation

Pulmonary abnormalities:
  Bronchopulmonary dysplasia
  Chronic obstructive
    pulmonary disease
  Cystic fibrosis
	Decreased oxygen diffusion, infection

Cardiac abnormalities:
  Advanced-stage congestive
    heart failure
	Decreased oxygen diffusion

Patients With Abnormal Airway Conditions

Patients with respiratory compromise generally are unable to adequately ventilate themselves. In chronic obstructive pulmonary disease (COPD), loss of alveolar surface area or damage to the bronchial lining reduces the volume of air delivered to the alveoli and increases the work of breathing. Cystic fibrosis increases the amount of mucus present in the airway, limiting air flow and reducing diffusion across the pulmonary capillary membrane. Bronchopulmonary dysplasia results from early oxygen administration to (usually premature) newborns and causes permanent changes in the cells of the respiratory tract. Musculoskeletal changes such as scoliosis and chest wall abnormalities make it difficult to expand the chest adequately. Excess weight over the chest (Pickwickian syndrome) or sleep apnea may leave the patient hypoventilated during sleep. In isolated cases, ventilation would normally be adequate but the patient is experiencing an increased metabolic demand from fever or infection.

Home Oxygen-Delivery Systems

With any type of respiratory abnormality, the home care treatment plan is designed to supplement the patient's respiratory effort. Any stressor such as infection, exposure to an allergen, or psychological upset can increase the severity of signs and symptoms and render the current respiratory support inadequate.

The simplest home oxygen systems involve a nasal cannula and oxygen in various delivery systems, ranging from small portable cylinders to large oxygen-enrichment systems (**Figure 45-3 ▸**). The patient usually contracts with a respiratory home care company to purchase the cannulas, oxygen tubing, and oxygen. Patients who are anxious breathe faster, use more of the oxygen, and may run out prior to delivery; you may be called when a person's

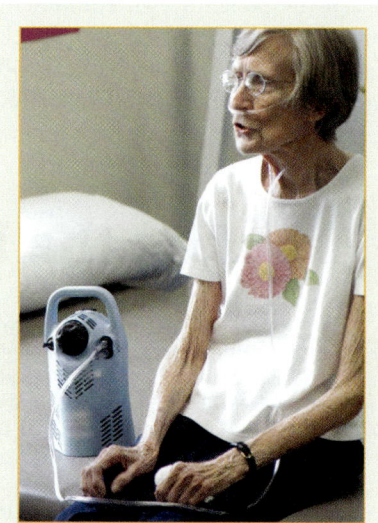

Figure 45-3 Home oxygen systems involve a nasal cannula and oxygen.

oxygen demand exceeds the current supply. If your assessment reveals that the patient needs to have more stored oxygen available, call the home care company. Meanwhile, use your cylinders to keep the patient calm and prevent decompensation. Be sure the cylinders are stored safely and within reach of the patient or caregiver.

Some patients use oxygen concentrators, which are large electrical devices that concentrate the oxygen in ambient air and eliminate other gases. Such a system eliminates frequent delivery of oxygen cylinders, is less expensive, and is easy to maintain. Its large size means that the device is not portable, however, and many concentrators are noisy and give off heat. Patients should have backup oxygen cylinders available in the event of electrical failure.

A liquid oxygen system **Figure 45-4** may also be used. With this system, more gas can be kept in a smaller container, making it an attractive option for active patients. Oxygen cannot be stored as a liquid for long as it will evapourate.

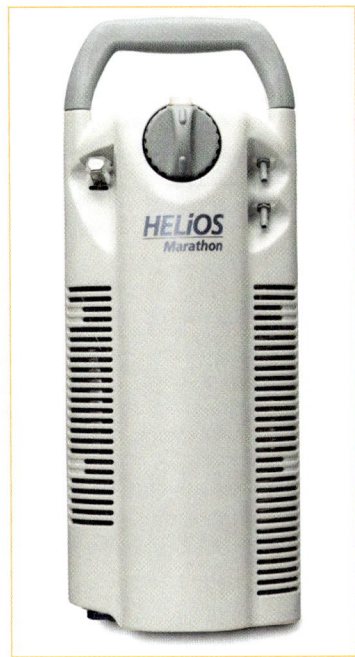

Figure 45-4 Liquid oxygen system.

To decrease the work of breathing by keeping the air passages and alveoli open during the expiratory phase, patients may use continuous positive airway pressure (CPAP) **Figure 45-5**. By keeping the airway pressure slightly higher than atmospheric pressure, CPAP keeps alveoli and airway passages stented open and decreases the work of breathing. It also increases the driving (diffusing) force of oxygen and improves overall oxygenation if a supplemental oxygen line is attached. In the home care setting, CPAP is typically used for sleep apnea. The device consists of a tight-fitting mask or nasal prongs with a thick pillow of air to decrease pressure and prevent damage to the nose and upper lip. A continuous pressure measured in centimetres of H_2O assists the patient in taking a breath and makes it difficult to completely exhale.

Bilevel airway pressure (BiPAP) exerts a different level of inspiratory pressure versus expiratory pressure. This type of support is used less often in the home care setting and does not ventilate the patient.

A ventilator, also called a respirator, mechanically delivers air to the lungs. Home ventilators are smaller than most

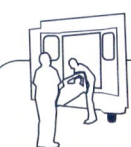

At the Scene

Both CPAP and BiPAP can be administered in the home by nasal or face mask without endotracheal intubation. This technique is referred to as "noninvasive ventilation."

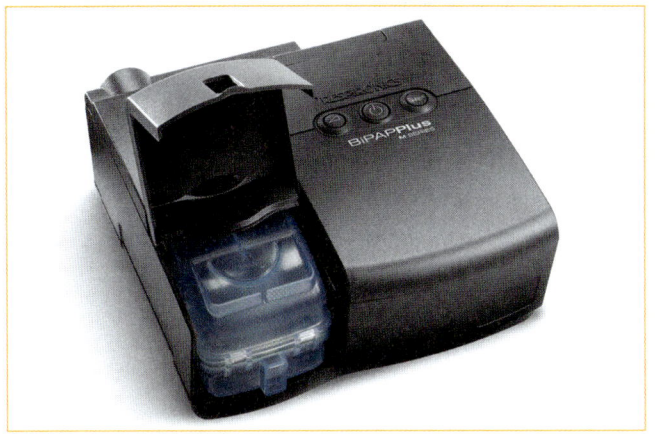

Figure 45-5 Continuous positive airway pressure machine.

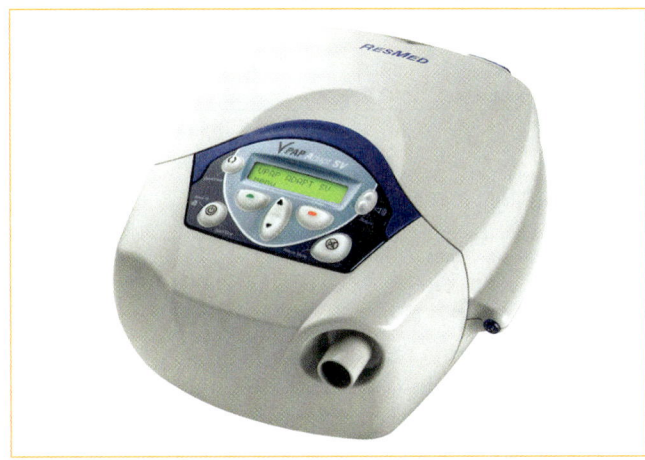

Figure 45-6 Home ventilator.

microwave ovens, use regular household electricity, and may include a battery backup **Figure 45-6**. It is important for you to become familiar with the types of units available to effectively transport your patient or assist with an equipment malfunction.

Ventilators may be set to deliver a certain volume of gas to the lungs. For example, the machine setting may specify the tidal volume (volume of air breathed in and out during a normal breath) to be delivered. This target tidal volume is based on patient-specific factors, such as resistance to flow or lung compliance (elasticity), and physician preference. Other ventilators are designed to deliver a certain pressure. Volume ventilators and pressure ventilators are used most often with an invasive airway, endotracheal intubation, or tracheostomy (discussed later in this section).

Normal breathing relies on increasing the size of the chest so that intrapulmonary and intrapleural pressures fall

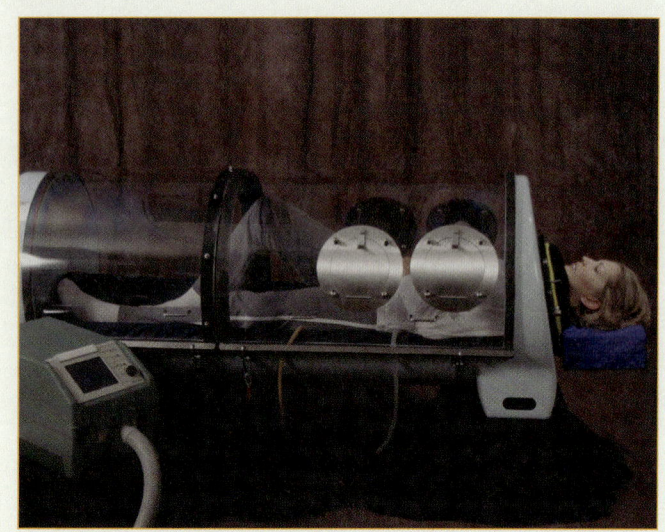

Figure 45-7 Negative-pressure ventilator.

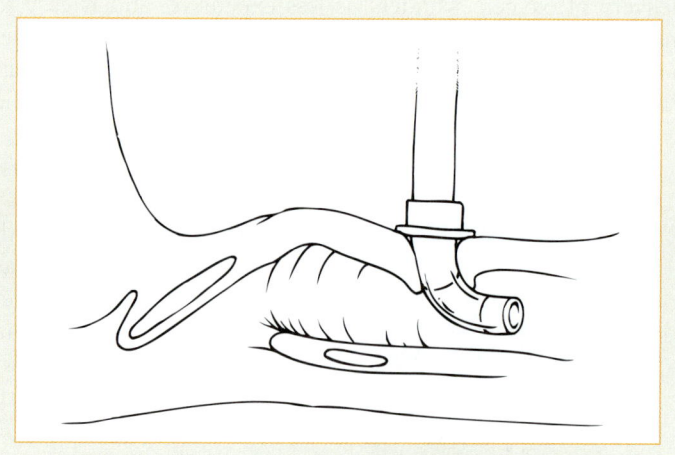

Figure 45-8 A tracheostomy is a planned surgical procedure in which an opening is placed in the trachea below the cricoid ring.

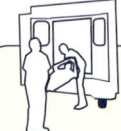 **At the Scene**

Monitor the patient's blood pressure and pulse if you are going to begin positive-pressure ventilation after a period of normal breathing.

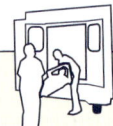 **At the Scene**

If a tracheostomy becomes plugged, the patient may be ventilated by deflating the cuff, covering the nose and mouth with a mask, and using the bag-valve-mask device. If you are unable to ventilate the patient through the tracheostomy, plug the tracheostomy stoma and attempt to ventilate the patient in the traditional manner with a bag-valve-mask device.

and air rushes in (negative-pressure ventilation). Most mechanical ventilators rely on positive-pressure ventilation—that is, air is pushed into the lungs. (You may be most familiar with positive-pressure ventilation when you are using the bag-valve-mask device.) This type of ventilation alters the hemodynamics of the body by decreasing venous return to the heart; the thoracic pump pulls blood back to the heart when the pressure within the chest is less than atmospheric pressure. During positive-pressure ventilation, the pump is not as effective and cardiac output can drop.

Negative-pressure ventilators mimic the body's normal method of breathing. These devices—which may be called ponchos, turtleshells, or belts Figure 45-7 ▲ —enlarge the chest, dropping intrapulmonary pressure below the atmospheric pressure and allowing air to rush in. Negative-pressure ventilators do not need an invasive airway and do not alter hemodynamics. They depend on a patent airway.

Invasive Airways

Improvements in artificial ventilation have transformed many homes into satellite intensive care units. As a consequence, paramedics may encounter patients who are ventilated through a tracheostomy, a surgical airway in which an opening is placed in the trachea below the cricoid ring Figure 45-8 ▶ . A tracheostomy may become necessary when prolonged use of an endotracheal (ET) tube might predispose the patient to

tracheal necrosis, tracheoesophageal fistula, ventilator-acquired pneumonia, or oral damage. (ET tubes and intubation are covered in depth in Chapter 11.)

A laryngectomy is a surgical procedure in which the larynx is removed, usually because of cancer. The trachea is then curved anteriorly and sewn to tissues of the neck. The opening that is created in the neck is called a stoma. A patient with a laryngectomy cannot be manually bagged through the nose and mouth, and you must be careful not to introduce liquids into the stoma. Most of these patients use a stoma cover to act as a filter and prevent mucus from being coughed onto others. A patient with a laryngectomy cannot produce normal speech and must learn to swallow and regurgitate air from the stomach or use an assistive device Figure 45-9 ▶ .

Tracheostomy tube designs vary, so ask the caregiver about the tube prior to beginning care. General types of tracheostomy

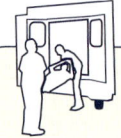 **At the Scene**

If you are transporting a child with a tracheostomy in a standard car seat, avoid using seats with a tray or shield. The tray or shield could come into contact with the tracheostomy and injure the child or block the airway.

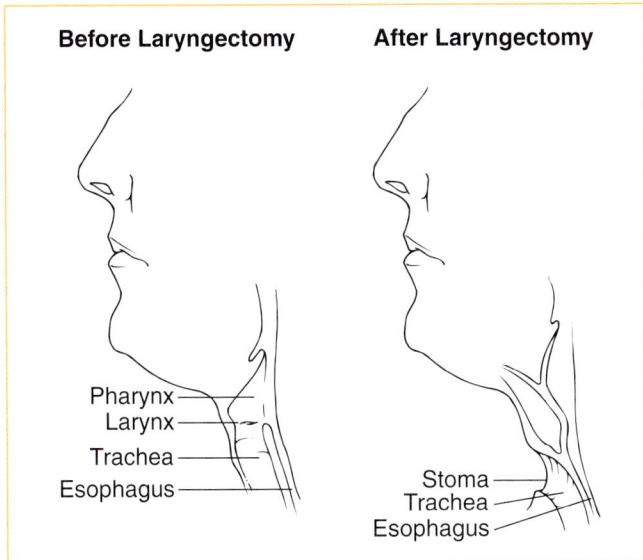

Figure 45-9 Laryngectomy.

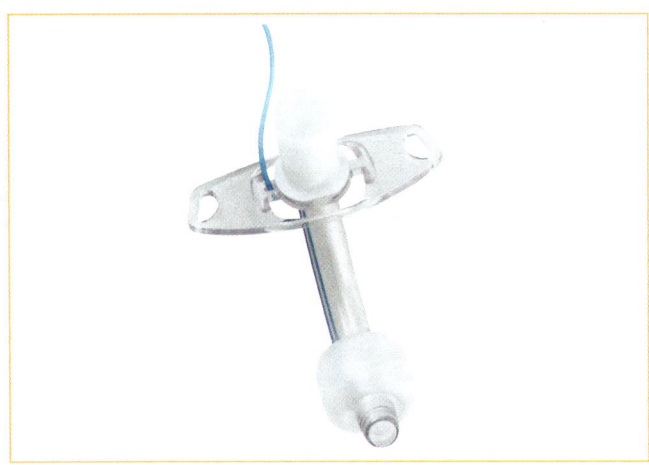

Figure 45-10 Tracheostomy tube.

tubes include a one-piece metal tube that can be plugged for speech. Such tubes are usually placed in a patient weeks to months after the tracheostomy surgery when the opening has healed well.

Airway Management

It is important to assess for airway patency in all patients, but it is especially important in patients with artificial airways. The basic airway techniques of opening, repositioning, and clearing (especially suctioning) the airway are the most critical steps in improving airway clearance and patency, thereby improving oxygenation and ventilation.

Assess the flow of oxygen and ensure that there is sufficient oxygen in the system. If you are uncertain about the oxygen flow, transfer the patient to the transport oxygen source. If a patient is on a ventilator when you arrive, assess the patient's chest for synchronous movement with the ventilator. If you have any doubt about ventilator function, do not be afraid to remove the patient from the ventilator and use manual positive-pressure ventilation. Avoid adjusting home ventilator settings unless you are specifically credentialed to work with the particular device. Soliciting the help of the patient, family, and caregivers can assist in assessment and troubleshooting of equipment.

Occasionally an artificial airway will need to be exchanged or replaced. Tracheostomy tubes are easily removed **Figure 45-10 ▶** . Untie the tracheostomy strings or device used to secure the tube, and gently slide the tube out on exhalation. When replacing this tube, have the patient take a deep breath and gently follow the contour of the tube during inhalation.

One-piece plastic tubes come either with or without cuffs. When you are working with plastic tubes, suction the patient orally with a whistle-tip catheter. Deflate the cuff and remove it

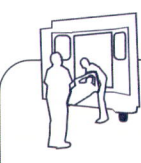

At the Scene

For infants and small children, the tracheostomy tube is usually a single-cannula plastic tube and is generally not cuffed (even if mechanical ventilation is required).

during exhalation. To replace the tracheostomy, insert an obturator (guide) into it, gently guide the tube in on inhalation, remove the obturator, and add air to the cuff.

Two-piece tracheostomies have an outer cannula that is guided into place by the obturator. When the obturator is removed, insert the inner cannula and turn the standard connector until it clicks or locks into place. Add air to the cuff, and apply the holder to secure the device around the neck. Never let go of the tube until it is secured.

On rare occasions, the paramedic will need to replace a tracheostomy with an ET tube. The easiest method is to remove the tracheostomy tube and gently guide a slightly smaller ET tube into place. (The size of the tracheostomy tube appears on its neck piece.) The ET tube will extend out from the neck, so take care to stabilize the tube. Confirm chest rise with ventilation, as it is possible—especially with new tracheostomies—to misplace the tube within the neck but outside of the trachea.

If the tracheostomy has inadvertently closed, you may intubate the patient orally or nasally. Place an occlusive dressing over the tracheostomy site to prevent air loss and observe the patient carefully for adequate chest rise.

To suction and clean a tracheostomy, follow the steps given here and in **Skill Drill 45-1 ▶** :

1. Wash your hands and apply a mask, goggles, and clean nonlatex gloves. Suctioning a home care patient is a clean procedure, not a sterile one.

2. Open supplies may be used. For cost reasons, home care patients often reuse their suction catheters. If the catheters

Skill Drill 45-1: Cleaning a Tracheostomy

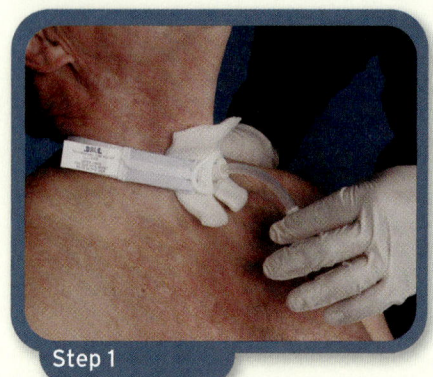

Step 1

Remove the inner cannula and place the device to soak in the proper solution.

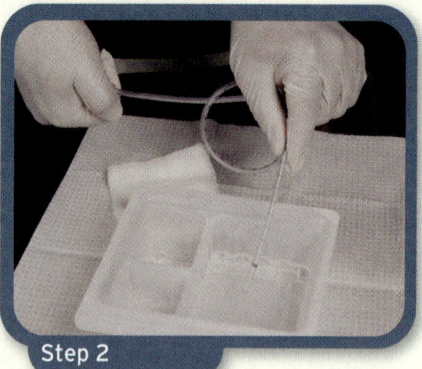

Step 2

Attach the catheter to negative pressure. Check the suction and clear the catheter by drawing up a small amount of saline.

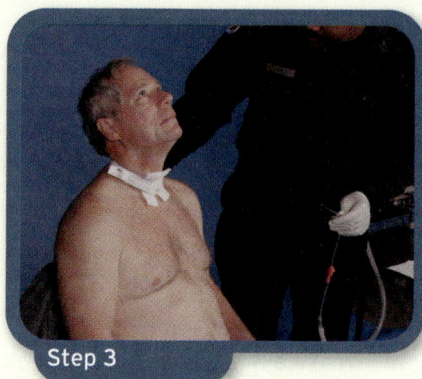

Step 3

Have the patient take a deep breath or pre-oxygenate him or her using the ventilator.

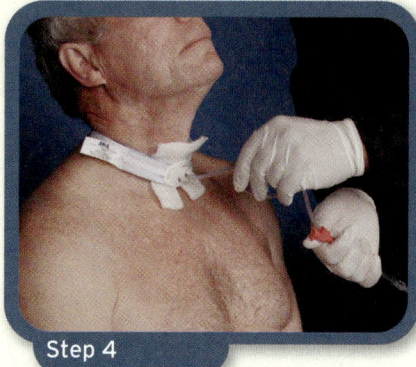

Step 4

Insert the catheter into the trachea without suction. Apply intermittent suction while removing the catheter. Repeat as necessary.

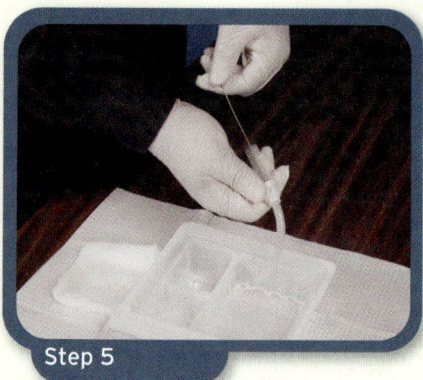

Step 5

Clean the inner cannula with the tracheostomy brush, rinse, and replace and lock into place.

do not have visible contamination and have been stored in a clean manner, they are acceptable for use.

3. Remove the inner cannula. Check with your patient's caregiver, if available, and place the device to soak in the appropriate recommended solution. If the caregiver is not available, use a mixture of hydrogen peroxide and water. Placing the cannula in plain water is acceptable in short-term situations. With one-piece tracheostomy tubes, this step is unnecessary. If the patient is dependent on a ventilator, have a replacement cannula immediately available (Step 1).

4. Attach the catheter to negative pressure. Check the suction and clear the catheter by drawing up a small amount of saline (Step 2).

5. Have the patient take a deep breath or preoxygenate him or her (Step 3).

6. Insert the catheter into the trachea without suction. Apply intermittent suction while removing the catheter. Repeat as

necessary. Keep the patient well oxygenated during the procedure (Step 4).

7. Clean the inner cannula with the tracheostomy brush, rinse, and replace and lock into place. Omit this step for a one-piece tracheostomy (Step 5).

8. Remove your gloves and wash your hands.

9. Document the procedure and assessment on your PCR.

In asthmatic patients, peak flow readings are usually obtained immediately before and after treatment for bronchospasm. A peak flow meter measures the rate of air being expired in litres per minute and gives the paramedic an indication about the condition of the larger airways. To take a peak flow reading, follow the steps in (Skill Drill 45-2 ▶):

1. Help the patient into a position of comfort, either sitting upright or standing upright, if safe to do so.

2. Place the indicator at the base of the numbered scale (Step 1).

3. Have the patient take a deep breath through the mouth.

Skill Drill 45-2: Obtaining a Peak Flow Reading

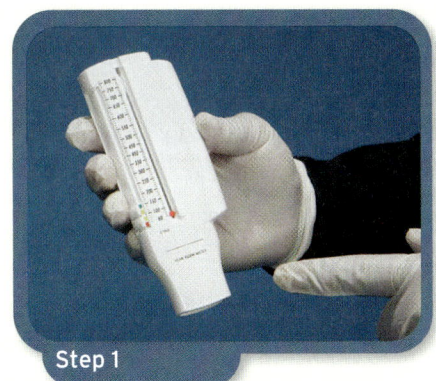

Step 1

Help the patient into a position of comfort. Place the indicator at the base of the numbered scale.

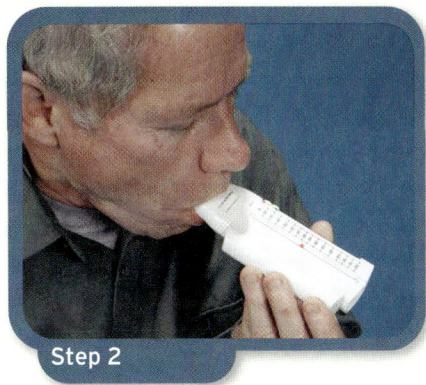

Step 2

Have the patient take a deep breath through the mouth and put the meter in the mouth. Patient blows out as hard as possible through the device for approximately 1 second. If possible, repeat two more times to obtain an average result.

4. Have the patient put the meter in the mouth and close his or her lips around the end.

5. Have the patient blow out as hard as possible through the device for approximately 1 second (Step 2).

6. If time and conditions permit, have the patient repeat steps 2 through 5 two more times to obtain an average result. Allow rest periods.

7. Document the results on the patient care record/call record.

8. Assist in cleaning the device and storing it correctly.

Patients With Chronic Cardiovascular Disease and Vascular Access

Patients who have chronic cardiovascular disease are often cared for in the home setting. Many patients have cardiac insufficiency or heart failure, an inability of the heart to keep up with the demands placed on it and failure of the heart to pump blood efficiently. The heart is then unable to provide adequate blood flow to other organs. The signs and symptoms of heart failure depend on which side of the heart is failing and include dyspnea, cardiac asthma, pooling of blood (stasis) systemically or in the liver's circulation, edema, cyanosis, and hypertrophy (enlargement) of the heart. There are many causes of congestive heart failure: coronary artery disease, leading to heart attacks and heart muscle weakness; primary heart muscle weakness from viral infections or toxins such as prolonged alcohol exposure; heart valve disease causing heart muscle weakness due to too much leaking of blood; heart muscle stiffness from a blocked valve; and hypertension. Treatment is aimed at improving the pumping function of the heart.

Some patients may have an implantable pacemaker that delivers synchronized electrical stimulation to three chambers of the heart, enabling the heart to pump blood more efficiently throughout the body.

Cardiomyopathy, a condition in which the heart muscle does not work at the optimal level, can be caused by many disease processes. Primary cardiomyopathy cannot be traced to a single cause. Hypertension, coronary artery disease, and viral infections might combine to decrease the ability of the muscle to eject blood. Secondary cardiomyopathy can be traced to a single cause, usually one that affects other body organs at the same time. All types of cardiomyopathy result in inadequate cardiac output, limiting the patient's activity. Many treatments require long-term venous access devices.

The heart never ejects 100% of the blood in the left ventricle during a heartbeat, but an ejection fraction greater than 55% is considered adequate. An ejection fraction of less than 55% may limit the patient's activity level and indicates the presence of cardiomyopathy. An ejection fraction of less than 20% can significantly alter a patient's lifestyle. In a home care patient, a change in the previous level of activity is a red flag that the heart may be temporarily or permanently deteriorating.

Vascular Access

A central venous catheter—a venous access device with the tip of the catheter in the vena cava—is used for many types of home care patients, including those receiving chemotherapy, long-term antibiotic or pain management, high-concentration glucose solutions, and hemodialysis. In contrast, a midline catheter is located in a large vessel but not the vena cava Table 45-3 ▶ .

Because the devices are used intermittently, they must be flushed to keep them open. In the past, low-concentration heparin has been the flush of choice. However, research has shown that low platelet counts develop in some patients following long-term use of heparin even at low concentrations, a condition known as heparin-induced thrombocytopenia. Flushing the device with saline eliminates the possibility of heparin-induced thrombocytopenia but means the patency of the device must be assessed frequently. Patients who are chronically ill or fragile may have devices that allow medications and fluids to be infused or body fluids to be removed and monitored. These devices place the patient at increased risk for cardiovascular complications including anticoagulation, embolus

Table 45-3	Venous Access Devices	
Type	**Use**	**Prehospital Precautions**
Midline catheters	Short-term fluids, analgesia, antibiotics	Moderate-length catheter, not good for rapid fluid resuscitation
Peripherally inserted central catheter	Long-term fluids, analgesia, chemotherapy, antibiotic therapy	Long catheter; not good for fluid resuscitation; may require direct medical direction for use
Central lines, tunneled implanted	Long-term fluids, analgesia, chemotherapy, antibiotic therapy, multiple blood draws	Have a noncutting/crush clamp available, as not all have a clamp; may require direct medical direction for use
Implanted infusion device	Long-term fluids, analgesia, chemotherapy, antibiotic therapy	Use a noncutting or nonbeveled needle for access; may require direct medical direction for use

formation, stasis, air embolus, and obstructed or malfunctioning devices.

Catheter dysfunction occurs frequently in patients receiving home infusions. Catheter-associated thrombosis can be life threatening and limit future vascular sites. Both of these complications can be minimized and treated when the paramedic is aware of preventive measures.

If a device does not seem to be working properly, ensure that it is not used for medications or any other purpose. If the patient has a gastric tube (which places him or her at increased risk for aspiration of stomach contents), position the patient in a semi-Fowler's or upright position if tolerated. Inspect and secure all external devices prior to moving the patient, especially when preparing for transport—it takes relatively little tension to inadvertently displace a tube, line, or device.

There are several things that a paramedic can do to reduce or prevent complications of vascular access devices: check the devices carefully before any treatment; keep device area clean; check that the correct medication and dose or nutrition are being infused into the device; use the device site only for what it was designed for (eg, dialysis catheters should only be used for dialysis treatment); avoid placing a blood pressure cuff on an arm that has an device port; and check pulses carefully in the device area.

Occasionally, it will be necessary to access a device for assessment, to draw blood, or to infuse medications. Proper technique is important. Patients and their caregivers will be your best resource in performing these functions. In addition, refer to your local or regional protocols and consult with direct medical control regarding accessing a venous access device when there is a need for resuscitation and you are unable to obtain any other vascular access.

Drawing Blood From a Central Venous Catheter

Central venous catheters (CVCs) offer easy access to the venous system but may present resistance to rapid fluid infusion due to their length. Because they enter the central circulation in the chest, negative pressure may draw in air (air embolus) or provide entry to microorganisms. To draw blood from a CVC, follow the steps illustrated in **Skill Drill 45-3 ▶**:

1. Wash your hands and apply a mask, goggles, and nonlatex gloves.
2. Draw the flush solution (usually normal saline but may be a heparin solution) into a syringe **Step 1**.

3. Set up the supplies, including the port access kit.
4. Swab the port with an appropriate cleansing solution (eg, Betadine) *or* clamp the catheter and remove the cap **Step 2**.
5. Attach an empty syringe or Vacutainer adapter to the hub or port **Step 3**.
6. Release the clamp (if clamped), and aspirate 5 ml of blood **Step 4**.
7. Reclamp the catheter if necessary and discard the aspirated blood **Step 5**.
8. Attach a new syringe or adapter **Step 6**.
9. Obtain the blood samples **Step 7**.
10. Reclamp the catheter if necessary and attach the syringe with the flush solution **Step 8**.
11. Release the clamp and flush the line **Step 9**.
12. Reclamp and recap the line **Step 10**.
13. Identify the tubes of blood by writing the date and time drawn and the paramedic's name on the side of the tube, and ready them for transport by securing them in a leak-proof protected container. Transport tubes to the patient's physician, hospital personnel, or usual lab. Do not shake blood collection tubes, as this may cause the blood to hemolyze.
14. Document the procedure and assessment on the PCR.
15. Dispose of contaminated equipment.

Accessing an Implantable Venous Access Device

To access an implantable venous access device, follow the steps in **Skill Drill 45-4 ▶**:

1. Wash your hands and apply a mask, goggles, and nonlatex gloves.
2. Open supplies including the port access kit.
3. Palpate the skin over the device **Step 1**.
4. Cleanse the skin over the device using a cleansing solution (eg, Betadine) **Step 2**.
5. Prime the needle tubing and needle with saline. Use a special access needle called unbeveled or noncutting to avoid slicing the silicone reservoir wall **Step 3**.
6. While stabilizing the device, insert the needle at a 90° angle to the skin until the needle tip reaches the back of the device **Step 4**.

Skill Drill 45-3: Drawing Blood From a Central Venous Catheter

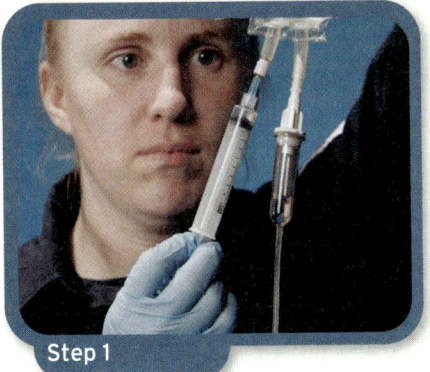

Step 1

Draw the flush solution into a syringe.

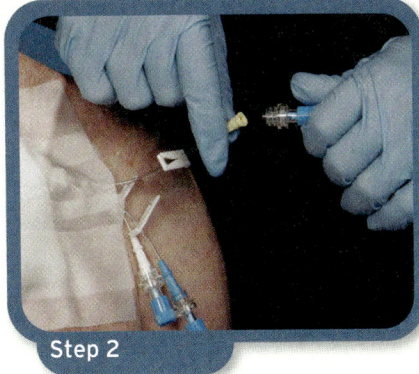

Step 2

Swab the port with an appropriate cleansing solution *or* clamp the catheter and remove the cap.

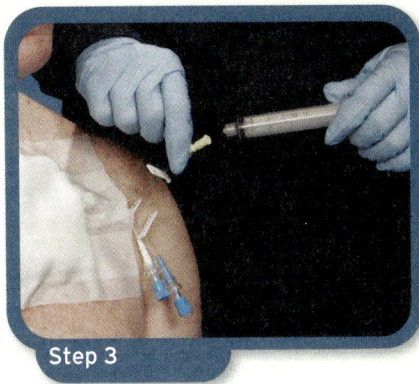

Step 3

Attach an empty syringe or Vacutainer adapter to the hub or port.

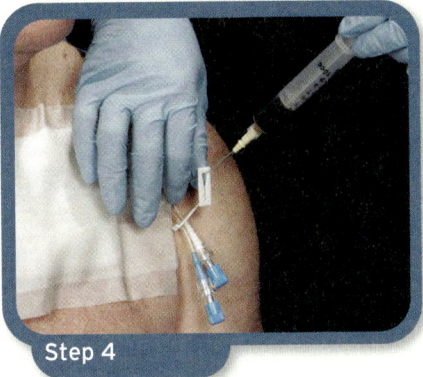

Step 4

Release the clamp (if clamped), and aspirate 5 ml of blood.

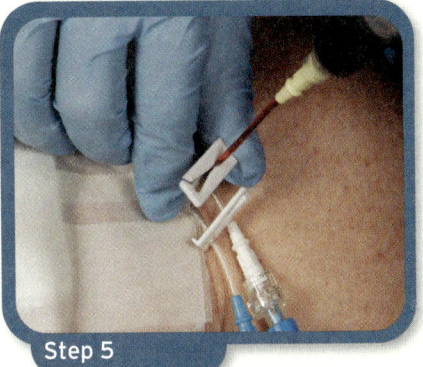

Step 5

Reclamp if necessary and discard the aspirated blood per your exposure control plan.

---

7. Aspirate 5 ml of blood (Step 5).

8. Discard the aspirate and obtain blood samples if necessary (Step 6).

9. Flush the line with normal saline (Step 7).

10. Administer medications or fluids as directed (Step 8).

11. Flush the device (Step 9).

12. Secure the needle with a sterile dressing *or* remove by pulling straight out of the device (Step 10).

13. Apply a dressing to the skin over the device if the needle was removed.

14. Identify the tubes of blood by writing the date and time drawn and the paramedic's name on the side of the tube, and ready them for transport by securing them in a leak-proof protected container. Transport tubes to the patient's physician, hospital personnel, or usual lab. Do not shake blood collection tubes, because this may cause the blood to hemolyze.

15. Document the procedure and assessment on the PCR.

16. Dispose of contaminated equipment.

Anticoagulant therapy is common in home care patients, so you should consider covert bleeding as a likely cause of hypovolemic shock in such individuals. A sudden onset of chest pain, shortness of breath, and decreased cardiac output during or immediately after opening an implanted or tunneled port may be indicators of an air embolus. Turn the patient on his or her left side to keep the embolus sequestered in the right atrium, so that air can be absorbed a little at a time, and transport the patient in that position.

Management of Vascular Access Devices

Vascular access devices relieve anxiety and the pain of frequent insertion attempts for patients. At the same time, they create potential complications. Common complications resulting from vascular access, assessment findings, and emergency interventions are shown in (Table 45-4 ▶). If a device

Skill Drill 45-3: Drawing Blood From a Central Venous Catheter (*continued*)

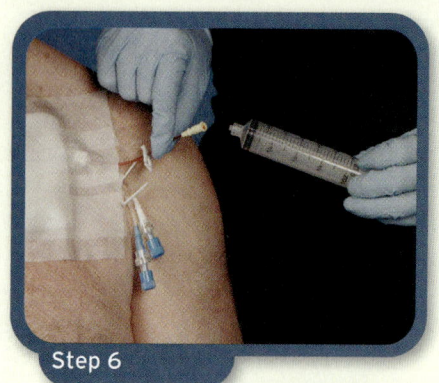

Step 6

Attach a new syringe or adapter.

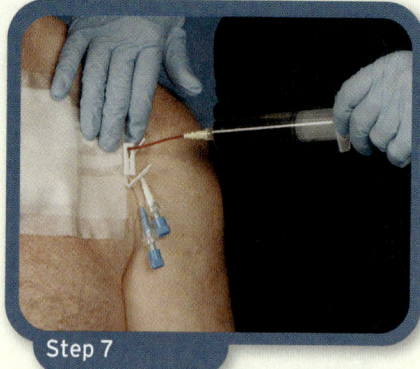

Step 7

Obtain the blood samples.

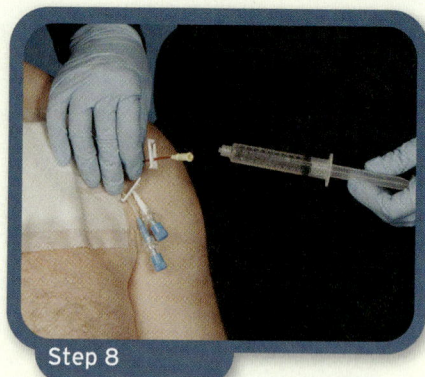

Step 8

Reclamp if necessary and attach the syringe with the flush solution.

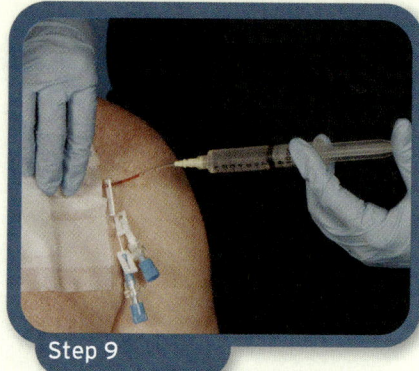

Step 9

Release the clamp and flush the line.

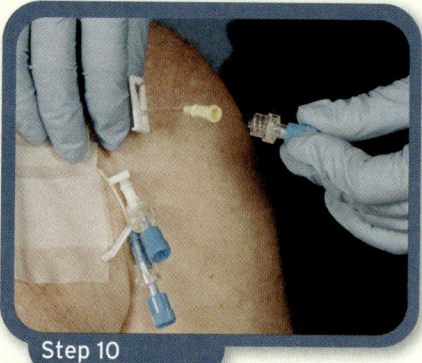

Step 10

Reclamp and recap the line.

Table 45-4	Serious Complications Associated With Vascular Access Devices
Complication	**Assessment Findings**
Occlusion	Cannot aspirate blood; infusion doesn't run
Catheter thrombosis	Swelling of arm, neck, or shoulder; pain
Sepsis	Fever, chills, malaise
Catheter migration	Change in length of exposed catheter
Catheter breakage	Leaking or bleeding from catheter
Embolism (air)	Chest pain, shortness of breath, tachycardia, hypotension, decreased level of consciousness
Embolism (PICC/midline catheter)	Inadvertent removal with distal portion of catheter missing

complication is suspected, the paramedic should not attempt to access the device. A device complication requires additional medical intervention. While not all patients will need to be transported immediately to a hospital, contact should be established and a plan made with the patient's usual health care professional. Serious complications require immediate transport of the patient to an acute care facility for further evaluation and treatment.

Patients With Gastrointestinal/Genitourinary Access

A gastric tube may be placed when the patient cannot ingest fluids, food, or medications by mouth. Tubes may be inserted through the nose or mouth into the stomach (using nasogastric or orogastric tubes). Alternatively, endoscopy procedures may be undertaken to guide the surgical entrance of the tube into the stomach, such as a percutaneous endoscopic gastric tube or placement of a percutaneous endoscopic jejunum tube into the

Skill Drill 45-4: Accessing an Implantable Venous Access Device

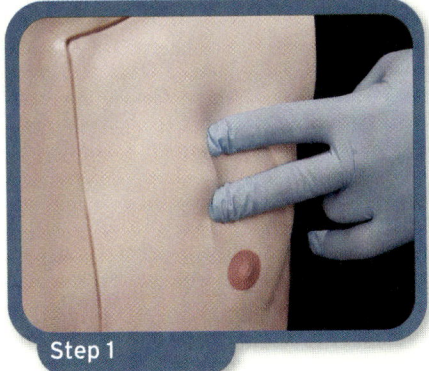

Step 1

Palpate the skin over the device.

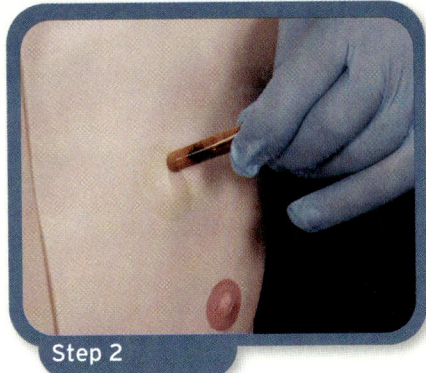

Step 2

Cleanse the skin over the device (Betadine solution).

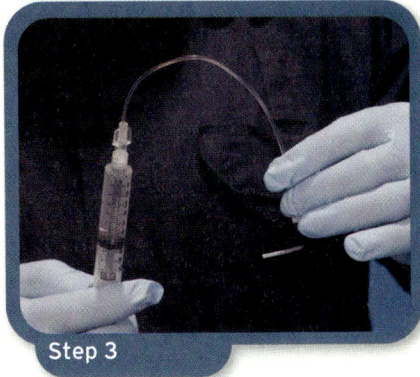

Step 3

Prime the needle tubing and needle with saline.

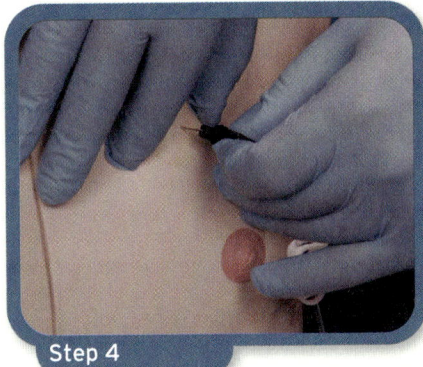

Step 4

While stabilizing the device, insert the needle at a 90° angle to the skin until the needle tip reaches the back of the device.

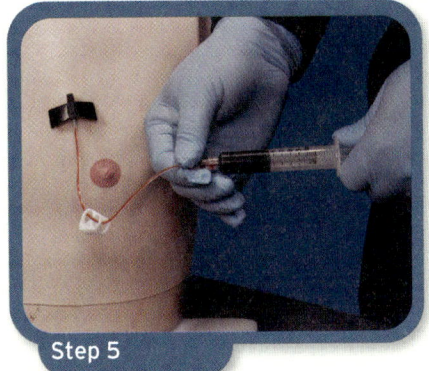

Step 5

Aspirate 5 ml of blood.

jejunum. The patient must have adequate stomach function to support use of a gastric tube. If there has been damage to the stomach, the tube may be placed into the jejunum of the small intestine.

Patients who have gastric tubes in place may still be at increased risk for aspiration. To minimize the risk of regurgitation and aspiration, the patient should be upright, at least to 30° when medications or nutrition is being infused. They should ideally be kept upright for 30 to 60 minutes after feeding. To prevent further complications such as cramping, nausea, vomiting, and diarrhea, liquids should be infused slowly. Some home care patients with gastric tubes may have their liquids delivered by an infusion pump. Occasionally a gastric tube may become nonfunctional when noncommercial foods are infused through it. This practice is highly discouraged by nutrition experts. Gastric tubes should be flushed, usually with water, after infusing medications or nutritional fluids.

Any abdominal surgery places the patient at risk for development of adhesions. Adhesions are scar tissue that may connect one loop of bowel to another or encircle a segment of bowel, constricting it and resulting in a bowel obstruction. A large-bowel obstruction (ie, obstruction in the colon) usually results from a growth within the bowel rather than adhesions. A small-bowel obstruction occurs when the small intestine becomes blocked. Improperly dissolved medications, food supplements, or the actions of certain types of medications can all lead to bowel obstruction.

Chronically ill patients who receive care at home are especially vulnerable to difficulties with normal elimination, especially normal urinary function. Such patients may require a long-term indwelling urinary catheter. Conversely, patients with neurologic damage may require intermittent urinary catheterization or placement of an indwelling catheter. The bladder is normally sterile, so introduction of any device can

Skill Drill 45-4: Accessing an Implantable Venous Access Device (continued)

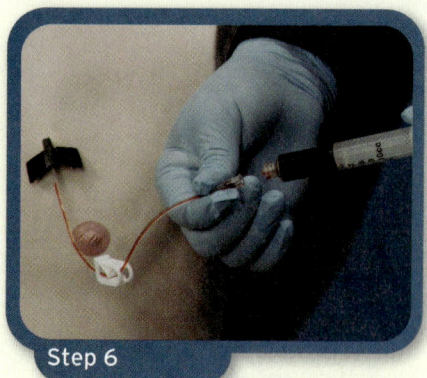

Step 6

Discard the aspirate and obtain blood samples if necessary.

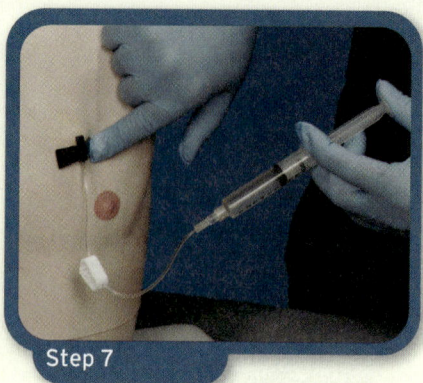

Step 7

Flush the line with normal saline.

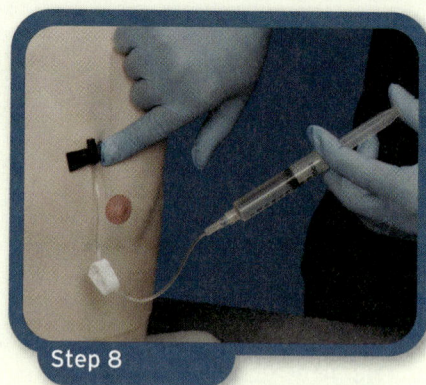

Step 8

Administer medications or fluids as directed.

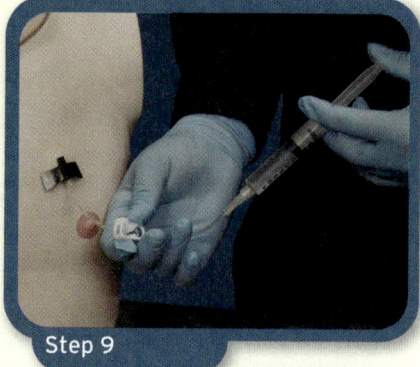

Step 9

Flush the device.

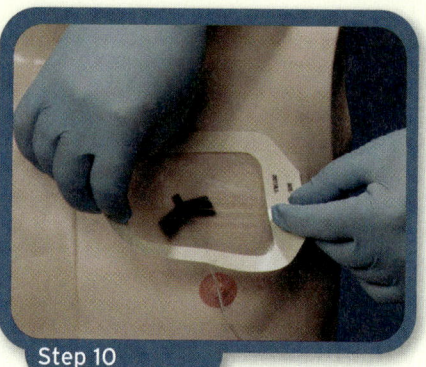

Step 10

Secure the needle with a sterile dressing.

You are the Paramedic Part 3

You perform a physical examination and find that the patient's abdomen is distended and firm upon palpation. No other significant findings are observed. Unsure of what to make of your clinical findings and the patient's clinical presentation, you decide to contact direct medical control for guidance.

The physician advises you to catheterize the patient in an attempt to relieve any pressure caused by a full bladder and to transport for further evaluation and management of the blood pressure. While you explain the doctor's recommendation for treatment and transport, the patient's wife goes to get the catheterization kit. The patient informs you that he and his wife have discussed resuscitation measures in the event that they are required and that they wish to have everything attempted.

Reassessment	Recording Time: 12 Minutes
Skin	Flushed, warm, and diaphoretic about the face; cool, pale, and clammy elsewhere
Pulse	52 beats/min, regular
Blood pressure	208/120 mm Hg
Respirations	16 breaths/min, regular
Spo₂	98% on room air
ECG	Sinus bradycardia with no ectopy
Pupils	PERLA

4. Why did the doctor recommended catheterizing the patient's bladder prior to transport?

5. Why is it important that the patient's wishes for a full resuscitation be known?

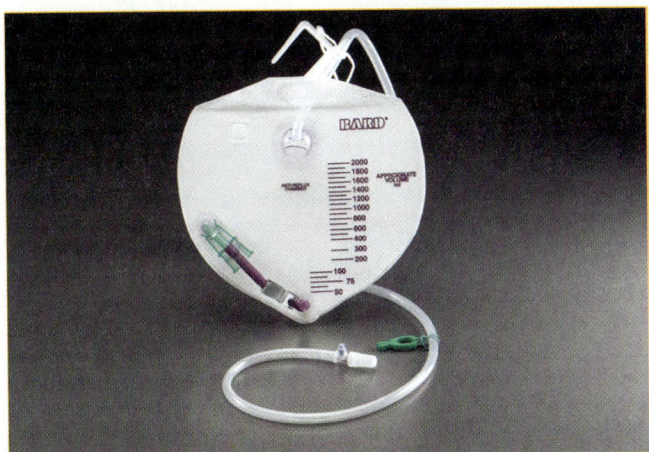

Figure 45-11 Urinary drainage bag.

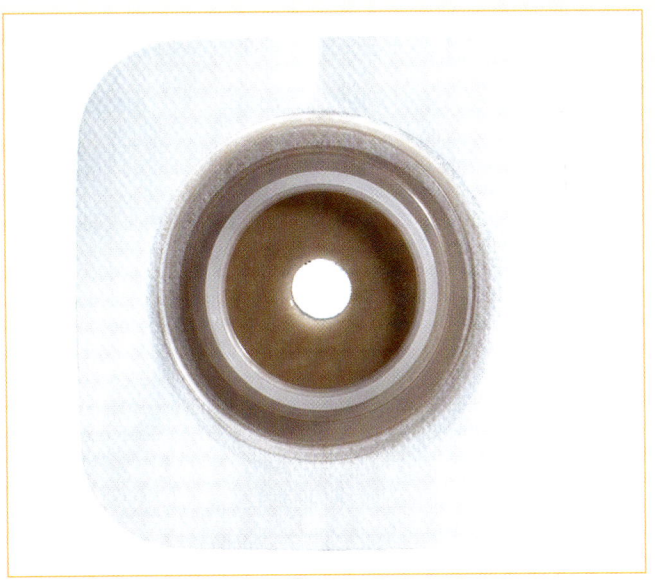

Figure 45-12 Ostomy skin wafer.

© 2009 ConvaTech Inc. Reprinted with permission.

introduce bacteria. Unless the patient is immunocompromised, however, there is low risk that clean (rather than sterile) catheterization will cause an infection **Figure 45-11 ▲** .

Indwelling catheters have a greater likelihood of contributing to urinary tract infections. The bladder is normally closed to the outside by a sphincter at the bladder-urethra junction. Indwelling catheters keep the sphincter open and provide a continuous route of entry for bacteria. Due to the short urethra in the female, women are at greater risk for urinary tract infections than men. Given the ongoing risk of an infection with an indwelling catheter, urosepsis is one of the likely causes of septic shock in such patients.

The urge to urinate occurs when the bladder fills to about 150 ml of fluid. An extreme urge to urinate occurs when approximately 400 ml of fluid fills the bladder. In susceptible individuals (eg, those with a disruption in the spinal cord), a full bladder can lead to dangerously high blood pressure, which places the patient at risk for stroke. This condition is termed autonomic dysreflexia.

Patients with small-bowel disease may need large portions of the small intestine removed (ileostomy). A stoma is constructed that connects the small intestine to the outside of the abdomen where the patient attaches a collection bag. The intestinal waste from an ileostomy is irritating to skin, as it contains some of the digestive juices. The bag must be emptied frequently.

A colostomy is a surgical opening in the large intestine that is brought to the surface of the abdomen to drain solid waste

At the Scene

Signs of potential failure of a gastrointestinal or genitourinary device in the home care setting include abdominal pain or distension, decreased or absent bowel sounds, bladder distension, dysuria, and changes in urinary output or colour.

Figure 45-12 ▲ . The drainage varies from loose (if the colostomy is along the ascending colon) to soft (if the colostomy is along the transverse or descending colon). A temporary colostomy allows the bowel to rest and heal, and is intended to be reversed at a later date. In a permanent colostomy, stool is always diverted to the stoma.

Occasionally, the ureters will be brought to the surface to a stoma, and urine will then drain directly into an appliance. Such an ureterostomy differs from a suprapubic catheter in that the catheter is surgically placed into the bladder. In the latter case, the ureters remain intact and continue to drain the kidneys into the urinary bladder.

Signs and symptoms of a large-bowel obstruction include changes in stool (may be very watery), abdominal distension, and localized pain. Signs and symptoms of a small-bowel obstruction include diffuse pain, nausea, and vomiting (often containing fecal material). Bowel sounds may vary from hypoactive to high pitched and frequent.

A bladder overfilled with urine may appear as abdominal distension. If the bladder is distended, its upper margin can usually be palpated. In abdominal distension, no upper margin will be evident. Urine production depends on factors such as fluid intake, fluid losses other than urine, and the condition of the kidneys. Urine is normally clear yellow and sterile with a slight odour. A strong ammonia smell indicates a urinary tract infection.

Inserting a Nasogastric Tube

To insert a nasogastric tube in an adult, follow the steps presented in Chapter 11. Remember to explain what you are doing to the patient and be gentle.

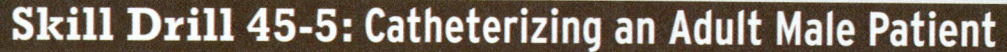

Skill Drill 45-5: Catheterizing an Adult Male Patient

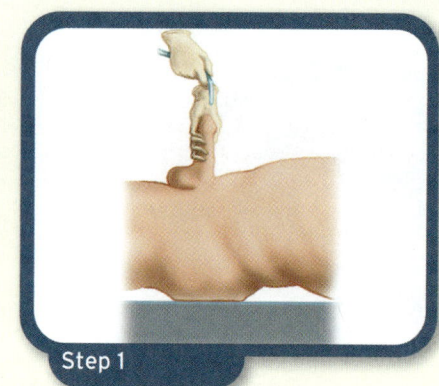

Step 1

Hold the penis at a 90° angle to the body and insert the catheter.

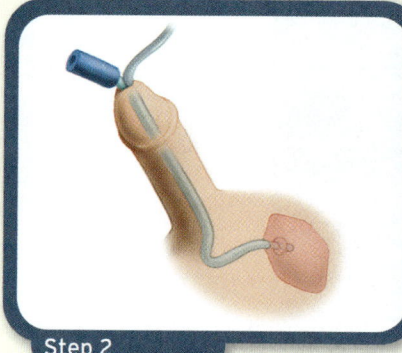

Step 2

Insert the catheter until the Y between the drainage port and the balloon port is at the tip of the penis. For a straight catheter, insert approximately 2.5 cm more.

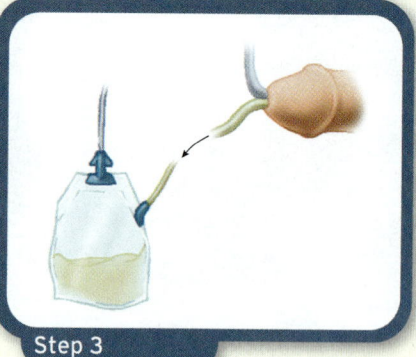

Step 3

Allow urine to drain.

At the Scene

When you are assessing bowel sounds, auscultate the abdomen to determine whether or not bowel sounds are present. Have a quiet atmosphere and auscultate *before* you palpate the abdomen.

Inserting a Catheter

Patients who are not able to void (urinate) on their own may need to be catheterized. Catheters may remain in place (ie, indwelling catheters such as Foley catheters) or may be used intermittently (straight catheters). While the principles for catheterization remain the same for either gender, anatomy differences change the process.

To catheterize adult male patients, follow these steps **Skill Drill 45-5 ▲** :

1. Help position the patient supine with legs slightly spread apart. Maintain privacy as much as possible.
2. Wash your hands and apply a mask, goggles, and clean nonlatex gloves.
3. Open supplies including the urinary catheter and placement kit. Home care patients may reuse their catheters provided that they have been stored in a clean manner. Place necessary supplies onto a clean area within reach. If you are inserting an indwelling catheter, connect a syringe filled with saline to the balloon port. Also connect the indwelling catheter to the drainage system. There are

no connecting ports for either a balloon or a drainage bag on a straight catheter.

4. Wash the penis with soap and water (or have the patient do so if he is able), making sure that the foreskin has been retracted.
5. Coat the end of the catheter with a water-soluble gel. An anesthetic gel is preferred for patients with sensation in the penile area.
6. Hold the penis at a 90° angle to the body and insert the catheter **Step 1** .
7. When urine is evident in the tubing, insert the catheter until the Y between the drainage port and the balloon port is at the tip of the penis. For a straight catheter, insert approximately 2.5 cm more **Step 2** .
8. Inflate the balloon and gently pull back on the catheter until you feel resistance, which indicates that the balloon is snug against the neck of the bladder. This step is unnecessary for a straight catheter.
9. Allow urine to drain. Note the amount and colour **Step 3** .
10. To remove a catheter, remove the saline in the balloon port and pull back gently until the catheter is free of the tip of the penis. Never remove an indwelling catheter without using a syringe to remove the saline from the balloon, as it may damage the urinary sphincter. For a straight catheter, simply pull back gently to remove the catheter. Wash according to the home care instructions.
11. Remove your gloves and wash your hands, following routine precautions.

Skill Drill 45-6: Catheterizing an Adult Female Patient

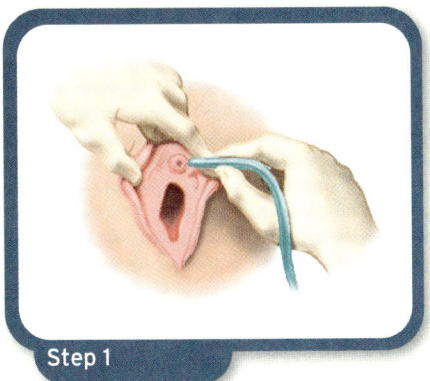

Step 1

Locate the urinary meatus anterior to the vagina and insert the catheter.

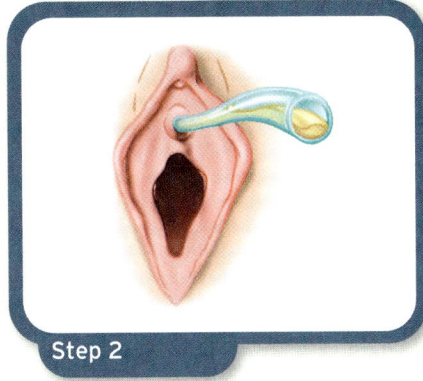

Step 2

When urine is evident in the tubing, insert the catheter another 2.5 to 7.5 cm.

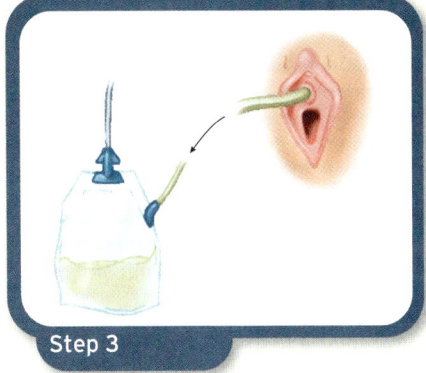

Step 3

Allow urine to drain.

12. If the catheter is to remain in place, secure it to the patient's leg according to the home care instructions.

13. Document the procedure and assessment on the PCR.

To catheterize an adult female patient, follow these steps **Skill Drill 45-6 ▲** :

1. Help position the patient supine with legs spread apart or side lying with the top knee flexed. Maintain privacy as much as possible.

2. Wash your hands and apply clean nonlatex gloves.

3. Open supplies including the urinary catheter and placement kit. Home care patients may reuse their catheters provided that they have been stored in a clean manner. Place necessary supplies onto a clean area within reach. If you are inserting an indwelling catheter, connect a syringe filled with saline to the balloon port. Also connect the indwelling catheter to the drainage system. There are no connecting ports for either a balloon or a drainage bag on a straight catheter.

4. Wash the perineal area with soap and water (or have the patient do so if she is able). First cleanse the outer area of the perineum, and then spread the labia minora and thoroughly wash the mucosa surrounding the vagina and the urinary meatus. Dry with a clean towel.

5. Coat the end of the catheter with a water-soluble gel. An anesthetic gel is preferred for patients with sensation in the perineal area.

6. Locate the urinary meatus anterior to the vagina and insert the catheter **Step 1** .

7. When urine is evident in the tubing, insert the catheter another 2.5 to 7.5 cm **Step 2** .

8. Inflate the balloon and gently pull back on the catheter until you feel resistance, which indicates that the balloon is snug against the neck of the bladder. This step is unnecessary for a straight catheter.

9. Allow urine to drain. Note the amount and colour **Step 3** .

10. To remove a catheter, remove the saline in the balloon port and pull back gently until the catheter is free of the tip of the meatus. Never remove an indwelling catheter without using a syringe to remove the saline from the balloon, as it may damage the urinary sphincter. For a straight catheter, simply pull back gently to remove the catheter. If the catheter is to be reused, it should be cleaned.

11. Remove your gloves and wash your hands.

12. If the catheter is to remain in place, secure it to the patient's leg or abdomen according to the patient's needs.

13. Document the procedure and assessment on the PCR.

Replacing an Ostomy Device

To replace an ostomy device, follow the steps in **Skill Drill 45-7 ▶** :

1. Help position the patient in a comfortable area in which to change the appliance and easily dispose of the contaminated articles.

2. Wash your hands and apply a mask, goggles, and clean nonlatex gloves.

3. Open supplies. Ostomy equipment includes a skin barrier called a wafer and one of several styles of drainage bags. Some bags can be opened along the bottom and emptied at regular intervals; others are sealed around a system similar to a urine drainage bag.

4. Empty/remove the current appliance and dispose of it appropriately **Step 1** .

5. Wash the area around the stoma with soap and water. Cleanse the stoma with water only, being careful not to rub or irritate the area **Step 2** .

6. Place a clean gauze pad over the stoma to prevent contamination of the clean skin with stool or urine (Step 3).

7. Cut the wafer to the correct size using the patient's measurement or tracing. Home care patients usually have the stoma already sized or have a tracing to cut a hole in the wafer large enough for the stoma but keeping exposed skin to a minimum (Step 4).

8. Attach the appliance to the wafer. Be sure the distal end is closed (Step 5).

9. Remove the gauze (Step 6).

10. Remove the paper backing from the wafer (Step 7).

11. Apply the appliance with the stoma centred in the wafer cutout (Step 8).

12. Remove your gloves and wash your hands.

13. Document the procedure and assessment on the PCR.

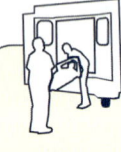

At the Scene

Be careful not to cut the ostomy appliance when using trauma shears to cut away clothing. The drainage can contaminate wounds and damage intact skin.

Patients With Wounds and Acute Infections

Wounds associated with trauma or surgery result in a break in the skin. These wounds, which may be either intentional (as with surgery) or unintentional (as during trauma), then undergo healing—that is, regeneration of living tissue.

Factors that affect wound healing include nutritional status, activity level, medications (including use of nicotine, anti-inflammatory drugs, heparin, and chemotherapy), chronic illness or immobility, diabetes, and the presence (or absence) of infection.

Immunosuppressed patients—such as early transplant recipients or individuals with human immunodeficiency virus infection—are at greater risk of acquiring infections, including wound infections. Immunocompromised patients have alterations in their immunity that increase both the risk of infection and the ability to combat infection, especially respiratory infections. Fever is often the only sign of infection in the immunocompromised patient and always requires further investigation. Special care should be taken for protection of these patients.

Drainage from a wound (called exudate) consists of fluid and cells. Serous exudate is a clear, watery drainage. Purulent exudate is pus, which consists of white blood cells, liquefied dead tissue, and bacteria. The colour of the exudate often provides a clue about the types of bacteria present. Sanguinous exudate is bloody; fresh blood is light red, while older blood is darker red.

Patients with vascular access devices are at increased risk for infections. Observe the device area for signs of infection, especially a hot to touch, reddened area that may indicate an abscess at the site. Practice good hand hygiene and site care when working with these devices.

Immobile patients with chronic illnesses are at high risk for skin breakdown, leaving them susceptible to infection. Perform a careful assessment of your patient's skin. Assess a surgical or treated wound by noting the following:

- **Appearance.** Healing appears as a pink to reddened area.
- **Size.** Measure the wound. Note any changes in size as described by the patient or caregiver.
- **Drainage.** Observe the colour, consistency, odour, and number of gauze pads soaked in a time frame to help measure the amount of drainage.
- **Swelling.** This can occur throughout the body (generalized) or in a specific area (localized). Generalized swelling or edema is a common sign in severely ill patients.
- **Pain.** Using a pain score, ask your patient to rate his or her level of pain; ask the patient or a family member for any observations of changes in level of pain. Many patients who are chronically ill may not be able to communicate their pain using a traditional 1 to 10 pain score, so be prepared to use a nonverbal scoring tool.
- **Drains or tubes.** Check the amount of drainage.
- **Temperature.** Warm to hot skin indicates a possible infection. Temperature regulation in many chronically ill or fragile patients is poor, however, so patients who have infections may not always feel warm to the touch or have a fever. Ask the patient or caregiver what is considered a normal temperature and what is different, if anything, today.

A wound with minor redness, slight warmth to the touch, and swelling may indicate a superficial infection. A painful reddened area that may have cracks or serous drainage, sometimes with red streaks extending from the area, may indicate that the patient has cellulitis. Patients with a fever and chills with an area that is hot to the touch, has purulent exudate, and is the source of pain may have a more serious infection. Cellulitis is usually treated with antibiotics, rest and elevation of the affected area, and warm compresses. Cellulitis may be more severe and require hospitalization in patients who have venous stasis, diabetes, or who are immunocompromised. If left untreated, wound infections in chronically ill patients may lead to sepsis—a serious systemic infection.

An important complication of wound healing is separation of the edges of the wound, called dehiscence. If the amount of drainage from a wound increases, especially 4 to 5 days after injury, dehiscence is likely.

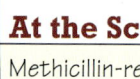

At the Scene

Methicillin-resistant Staphylococcus aureus (MRSA) is a serious problem in the community, especially among chronically ill patients. MRSA can colonize the skin and body of an individual without causing sickness and, in this way, unknowingly be passed on to other individuals.

Skill Drill 45-7: Replacing an Ostomy Device

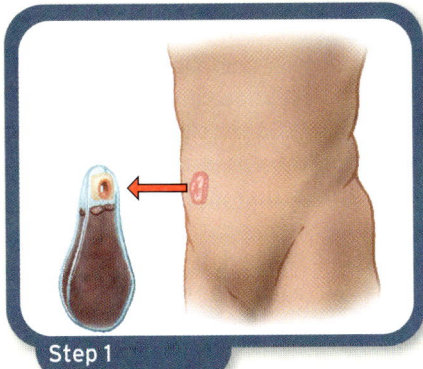

Step 1

Empty/remove the current appliance and dispose of it appropriately.

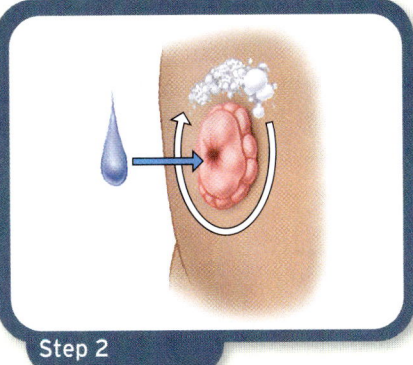

Step 2

Wash the area around the stoma with soap and water. Cleanse the stoma with water.

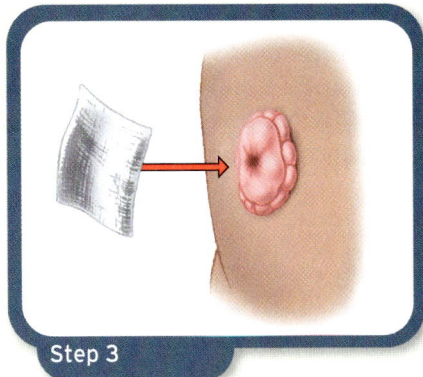

Step 3

Place a clean gauze pad over the stoma.

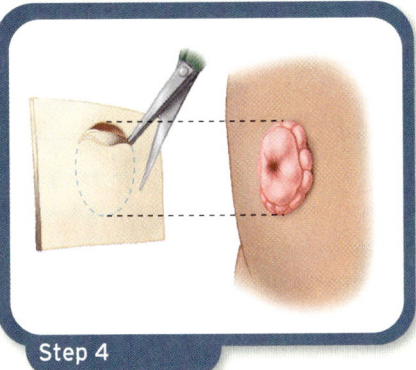

Step 4

Cut the wafer to the correct size using the patient's measurement or tracing.

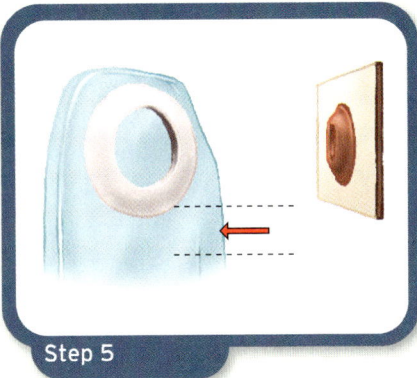

Step 5

Attach the appliance to the wafer.

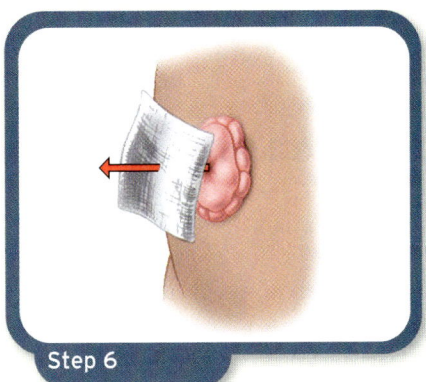

Step 6

Remove the gauze.

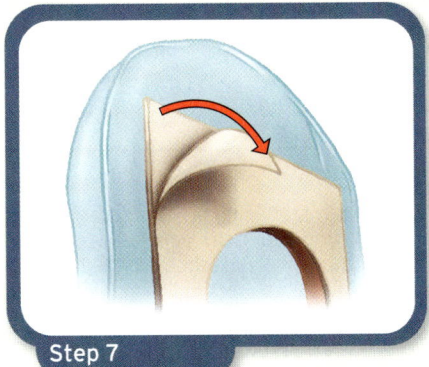

Step 7

Remove the paper backing from the wafer.

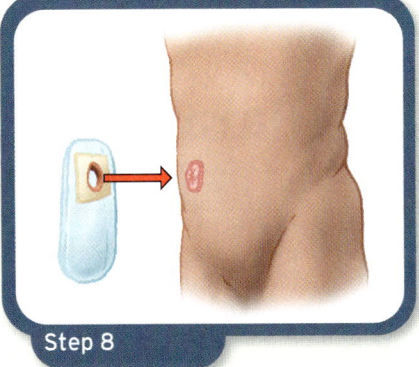

Step 8

Apply the appliance with the stoma centred in the wafer cutout.

Some wounds may be left open and unsutured to promote healing from within. In other cases, sutures or staples are used to hold the edges of a wound together; most are removed 7 to 10 days after repair. In contrast, stay sutures and retention sutures hold both skin and underlying fat or muscle together and may be left in place for 14 to 21 days.

Drains may also be sutured into place to allow liquids to escape and decrease tension on the sutures or staples. Drains are usually flat pieces of tubing that remain open on both ends. One end is placed deep within the wound; the other end lies on the skin, draining onto gauze dressing. Closed wound drainage systems rely on a tubing drain plus some type of negative pressure (suction). This kind of system prevents the entry of microorganisms into the drain and thus into the wound.

Wound Care

After exposing a wound for assessment, you should redress it to prevent further contamination. Encourage the patient to lie still while the wound is redressed. Apply a sterile dressing and secure it to the area prior to transport. This dressing should cover the surface of the wound and the surrounding area and should not be either too tight or too loose. You may need to apply a bulky dressing to a wound to help protect it during transfer and transport.

Always reassess the patient's pain level and tolerance to the dressing following the procedure. Patients with limited mobility may be uncomfortable during movement with a dressing in place. Providing reassurance, direction, and comfort to the patient and caregivers during these procedures will enhance their sense of control and comfort.

Maternal/Child Health Risks

Each year in Canada there are approximately 340,000 births. The preterm infant birth rate in Canada has been steadily rising, reaching 7.6 for every 100 live births in 2000. Infants are also more likely to be born with low birth weight (< 2,500 g). Cesarean deliveries are also at an all-time high. Women may deliver at home, or may spend anywhere from a few hours to several days in a health care setting, typically a hospital birthing centre. Each of these factors contributes to the increased need for home care for women and infants in the postpartum period.

Complications in the postpartum period include postpartum bleeding, depression, sepsis, pulmonary embolus, and infant septicemia. When you are obtaining the mother's history, asking her about postpartum bleeding in a previous pregnancy is important as a significant risk factor.

Pulmonary embolus is another complication that may occur in the postpartum period. It is the leading cause of maternal death in Canada, resulting in 6.3 deaths per 1,000,000 live births. The risk of pulmonary embolus is increased in both pregnancy and in the postpartum period. The incidence of thromboembolic disease in pregnancy has been reported to range from 1 case in 200 deliveries to 1 case in 1,400 deliveries and is caused by venous stasis, decreasing fibrinolytic activity, and increased procoagulant factors.

Depression that occurs during pregnancy or within a year after delivery is called perinatal depression, most commonly referred to as postpartum depression. During pregnancy the amount of estrogen and progesterone increases greatly. In the first 24 hours after childbirth, the amount of hormones rapidly drops back down to their normal prepregnancy levels. After pregnancy, similar hormonal changes may trigger symptoms of depression. The number of women affected with depression during this time is unknown, but some researchers suggest that depression is one of the most common complications during and after pregnancy. It is often not recognized or treated because normal changes during pregnancy such as fatigue, insomnia, strong emotional reactions, and changes in body weight may occur during pregnancy and after pregnancy. These same symptoms may also be signs of depression. The key to treatment is early recognition and referral.

Infants have immature physiology that can result in an inability to regulate temperature, adapt to respiratory problems, or respond to infection because of poorly functioning

You are the Paramedic Part 4

The patient's wife was able to catheterize her husband while he sat upright in his wheelchair. The catheter drained 800 ml of urine. An IV line was established in the right antecubital with an 18-gauge needle. During transport you note that the swelling in the patient's abdomen has almost resolved and it is now soft upon palpation. He states that his headache is almost relieved and that he no longer has blurred vision.

Upon arrival to the emergency department, the patient's symptoms have almost resolved. He is monitored in the emergency room and discharged after a short period of observation, with a diagnosis of autonomic dysreflexia syndrome.

Reassessment	Recording Time: 18 Minutes
Skin	Pale, warm, and dry
Pulse	80 beats/min
Blood pressure	144/82 mm Hg
Respirations	16 breaths/min, unlaboured
Spo$_2$	99% on room air
ECG	Sinus rhythm without ectopy

6. What is the pathophysiology of autonomic dysreflexia syndrome?

7. What are signs and symptoms of autonomic dysreflexia syndrome?

immune systems. All of these factors have an impact on sepsis, which is one of the most common causes of infant death.

In 1999, sepsis accounted for 6.7% of all infant deaths in Canada. Some pregnancy complications that can increase the risk of sepsis for a newborn include maternal bleeding, maternal fever, infection in the uterus, and premature rupture of membranes. Sepsis in newborns produces few symptoms and is difficult to determine. Frequently, these babies suddenly don't seem to be feeling well or "just don't look right" to those who care for them. Listen to the caregiver: any baby who has a change in mental status should be transported immediately for further evaluation and treatment.

Less than 1% of births occur unexpectedly at home. When an emergency home birth does occur, follow your usual paramedic practice and enjoy the experience. Once the baby has delivered, either before or on your arrival, a newborn examination should be conducted. Most newborns are healthy and need little treatment. Transport decisions should be based on local protocol and family requests. Discuss child safety restraint issues of newborns before you encounter an emergency delivery in the home. The five steps to follow in the approach to assessing a newborn are the same in any setting:

- Dry and warm the baby.
- Clear the airway.
- Assess breathing.
- Assess pulse rate.
- Assess colour.

A depressed newborn does not respond to drying, warming, and clearing the airway. These babies require resuscitation.

Pediatric Apnea

Premature newborns or those with congenital heart, lung, or neurologic problems often require home care, including an apnea monitor. Healthy infants may experience periods of apnea, especially during sleep. If the apnea is prolonged, is frequent, or occurs with a drop in pulse rate or a change in skin colour or muscle tone, it is not normal. Home monitoring of apnea may be indicated when an infant:

- Has unresolved apnea of prematurity at the time of hospital discharge.
- Has severe gastroesophageal reflux.
- Has a history of an apparent life-threatening event.
- Is the sibling of a baby who had sudden infant death syndrome.

Caregivers are taught to stimulate the infant if the low pulse rate or apnea alarm sounds; you may be called if stimulation doesn't work. Be prepared to provide positive-pressure ventila-

At the Scene

False alarms are common with apnea monitors and may be caused by movement, loose lead wires, or improperly placed electrodes. When in doubt, follow your local EMS protocols and have the family contact the manufacturer of the device.

tion and remember that newborns—especially premature babies—have difficulty in controlling their body temperatures. Keep the infant warm, including covering the infant's head.

Hospice/Comfort Care

Patients in hospice care can experience pain and discomfort from tumour growth, treatment modalities (eg, radiation and chemotherapy), immobility, inflammation, or infection. Treatment of hospice patients is based on the type and severity of pain. Patients initially receive around-the-clock anti-inflammatory medications, often coupled with antianxiety or antiemetic agents. When this regimen no longer manages the pain, the patient may receive a mild opioid. A strong opioid may be added later, along with antianxiety and antiemetic medications.

Pain may also be managed by mechanical or electrical means. Transcutaneous electrical nerve stimulators relieve pain by competing for nerve transmission pathways with the painful stimulus. Less pain stimulation reaches the brain, so the patient feels less pain. In addition, simple comfort measures are important in providing pain reduction and comfort to the patient. Turning, positioning, and supporting body parts with blanket rolls or pillows can increase comfort. Maintaining a comfortable room temperature helps. Hands-on or energy-based therapies such as massage may be used.

Many health care providers are concerned that hospice patients may overdose on pain medications. This problem, however, is not as frequent as patients being undermedicated. If you suspect that a hospice patient has received too much medication, you should begin the assessment and treatment as for any other patient. Opioids affect the respiratory drive centre, so pay close attention and care to breathing adequacy. Although naloxone can reverse the effects of opioids, the goal in these cases is to enable the patient to breathe sufficiently on his or her own. Complete reversal of the effects of the opioid will return the patient to intractable pain, initiation of the sympathetic response, and a sudden increase in blood pressure and pulse rate.

Progressive Dementia

Dementia is a progressive brain disorder with an insidious onset in which cognitive activities are lost first, followed by physical abilities. Causes of dementia may include Alzheimer's disease, Pick disease, Parkinson's disease, and stroke. Some nutritional disorders, such as Wernicke disease or Korsakoff psychosis, can also cause dementia.

Concerns regarding patients with dementia include injuries resulting from loss of judgment and insight, confusion when using medications, and becoming lost when leaving home or a familiar environment. Caregivers may also be at risk if the patient experiences paranoia. Early dementia can be managed in the home setting, but advanced dementia generally requires nursing home care.

Chronic Pain Management

Pain is a subjective term. *Nociception* is a term that more accurately describes the transmission of stimuli over specific nerve pathways. All nociceptors (ie, pain receptors) begin as free nerve endings and end in the dorsal (ascending) roots of the spinal cord. Some respond to mechanical damage, some to thermal damage, and some to chemical damage. The skin, joints, and musculature are well supplied with pain receptors, whereas the visceral organs have a limited number of pain receptors and the brain has no pain receptors. There are two major types of nociceptors: alpha (fast) fibres, which transmit a sharp, localized type of pain usually associated with an injury, and C (slow) fibres, which transmit a slow pain (often described as burning, throbbing, or achy) typically associated with long-term conditions.

Acute pain occurs immediately after an injury or surgery. Chronic pain occurs long after relief of the initiating cause is achieved. Chronic pain may also be defined as pain lasting for 6 months or longer. Some research indicates that failure to treat acute pain adequately may lead to chronic pain.

The body perceives pain as a stressor. In response, it activates the sympathetic nervous system, leading to elevated blood pressure, tachycardia, and tachypnea. Energy stores are needed to maintain this sympathetic response, even though they could be better used for healing. Effective management of pain reduces energy consumption and allows for rest and healing.

Home Chemotherapy

Chemotherapy refers to the introduction of either single cytotoxic drug or a combination of cytotoxic drugs into the body for the purpose of interrupting or eradicating malignant cellular growth. The many side effects of these treatments include alopecia (hair loss), anorexia, fatigue, leukopenia (decreased numbers of leukocytes), thrombocytopenia (decreased numbers of platelets), anemia, and increased risk of infections. During radiation therapy, painful blisters may develop at the treatment site.

Patients receiving chemotherapy routinely take multiple medications. Some of these drugs are given to battle the disease process, while others are intended to manage the symptoms of the side effects of chemotherapy. Analgesic medication patches and antiemetics are commonly prescribed. In addition, peripheral access devices may be surgically placed to aid in the delivery of these medications. Use of these devices to deliver medication requires specialized training. Follow your local protocol or direction from direct medical control when using these devices.

Patients with cancer often have seriously depressed immune systems, owing to either the treatment regimen or the disease process. To safeguard patients from infection, wash your hands after contact and wear a mask. Reverse isolation, in which the patient wears a mask, is also suggested.

Transplant Recipients

Organ transplants are considered for the treatment of a failing organ or organs. The paramedic must remember that a patient who has recently undergone a transplant is at risk of infection and take steps to protect the patient—for example, by using reverse isolation, in which the patient wears a mask.

You should encourage transplant patients and caregivers to bring all medications and any other information to the hospital with them if transport is indicated.

Psychosocial Support

Adaptation and adjustment to a chronic illness do not occur all at once. Stages of adaptation and adjustment are varied and individual, and an unexpected event can trigger readjustment needs in a patient thought to have adjusted to his or her condition. When faced with such an illness, individuals are likely to proceed through a sense of loss or mourning that is similar to that experienced by survivors of a loved one's death **Table 45-5 ▾**. The goal of adjustment is acceptance of the condition and construction of a realistic life plan incorporating the new strengths and limitations.

At the Scene

Paramedics often find it most difficult to work with patients who are in the acceptance stage of the dying process because the patient appears to have given up. In chronic illness or during injury adjustment, this stage may be the easiest. Allow the patient to do as much as possible for himself or herself. Talk with the patient or caregiver so that you are aware of what the patient expects from your treatment.

Table 45-5	Stages of Adjustment to Chronic Illness	
Stages	**Behaviours**	**Paramedic Response**
Denial	Refusal to follow plan	Treat result of refusal; stay nonjudgmental/nonargumentative; educate/reinforce plan
Anger	Verbal or physical abuse	Anger is an acceptable emotion, abuse is not; set limits; retreat if the scene is unsafe; call for assistance; provide care when the scene becomes safe; document
Bargaining	Refusal to follow plan as part of bargain	Restate options; incorporate the bargain as possible
Withdrawal with depression	Profound sadness, reduction in interaction and eye contact, listlessness	Provide reassurance
Acceptance	Adaptive behaviours	Be supportive

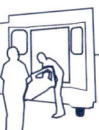

At the Scene

A terminally ill patient has the following rights:
1. The right to know the truth
2. The right to confidentiality and privacy
3. The right to consent to treatment
4. The right to choose the place to die and the time of death
5. The right to determine the disposition of his or her body

Special Considerations

Paramedics must often assume the role of health educators. At the appropriate time during a call, encourage the caregiver to prepare a list including the following items:

- Telephone list of all family and friends who should be notified of a change in the patient's condition
- Current medications, ventilator settings, tracheostomy tube type and care, tube feeding type and amount, ostomy type and appliance

Community education includes the need for an emergency information form.

Patients receiving home care are encouraged to make end-of-life decisions early in their care, if they haven't already. A durable power of attorney (DPOA; also called a health care proxy) allows a patient to appoint someone to make health care decisions in the event that he or she becomes incapacitated. The decisions covered by a DPOA include discontinuation of life support in the event of a terminal illness or injury, discontinuation and removal of life-sustaining equipment in the event of an irreversible coma, and termination of artificial nutrition and hydration. For more information, see Chapter 4.

A living will addresses the patient's wishes that life-sustaining measures be discontinued when there is no hope of recovery. A living will is not recognized in all provinces and territories.

Do not resuscitate/do not attempt resuscitation (DNR/DNAR) and do not intubate forms are physician's orders to withhold life-sustaining treatment in the event of cardiac or respiratory arrest. These orders do *not* mean that no treatment should be given. That is, patients should receive pain medication, supplemental oxygen therapy, nutrition, and hydration as needed based on assessment. Provinces and territories may require that any such order be written on approved forms with witnesses present.

You are the Paramedic Summary

1. Does treating a patient with chronic health problems affect the way you deliver emergency care?

The emergency care given to a patient with a chronic illness is no different than the care given to a person who is acutely ill. What may change is the method of delivery. For example, medications may be administered through an indwelling catheter such a PICC line or oxygen therapy may be delivered via a tracheostomy tube.

2. What groups of patients are likely to benefit from home care?

Quite a few groups of patients benefit from home health care. As technology advances, the number of illnesses that can be treated at home is on the rise. For example, you might treat patient with spinal cord injuries, chronic neuromuscular disorders such as multiple sclerosis, respiratory illnesses such as cystic fibrosis, and patients with advanced heart failure. One important thing to remember is that there is no age limit to those receiving home health care, as diseases have no age barriers.

3. What type of equipment might you encounter with patients receiving home health care?

Just as the types of disease processes you will encounter are wide and varied, so is the type of equipment you might encounter. Common examples of equipment used in the home setting include tracheostomy tubes, ventilators, CPAP machines, urinary catheters, gastrostomy tubes, and indwelling IV cannulas. A good rule of thumb to follow is: if you are unfamiliar with the equipment, do not use it! Caregivers are excellent resources for you to use. Ask for help in understanding how a specific piece of equipment works. When you are in doubt how to use a piece of equipment, call direct medical control for guidance.

4. Why did the doctor recommended catheterizing the patient's bladder prior to transport?

Spinal cord injuries can make the body work in strange ways! In some spinal cord injury patients, the pressure of a full bladder can trigger a significant rise in blood pressure and a decrease in the pulse rate. If the pressure is not relieved, the hypertension can lead to further damage or death.

5. Why is it important that the patient's wishes for a full resuscitation be known?

Knowing a person's wishes regarding resuscitation is important because the person may have a completely different view of life with a chronic illness or injury. Your patient has had time to adjust to living as a quadriplegic and may view his life as meaningful and fulfilling in a new way. You must abide by your patient's wishes and not try to impose your impressions of how a person's life must be on the patient. Remember, what you may consider as a handicap may be considered a blessing to someone who is living with the condition.

6. What is the pathophysiology of autonomic dysreflexia syndrome?

Autonomic dysreflexia syndrome is seen in patients with a spinal cord injury above the T6 level. It results from a stimulus being introduced to areas of the body below the spinal cord. Common stimuli are the pressure caused by a distended bladder or rectum. The stimulus travels up the spinal cord until it becomes blocked, preventing it from reaching the brain. As a result, the sympathetic nerve receptors below the injury site cause a rise in blood pressure. This increase in pressure is then detected by the baroreceptors, which stimulate the parasympathetic nervous system in an attempt to lower the blood pressure. Since the signals cannot travel below the injury, the blood pressure remains elevated while the pulse rate decreases. If the blood pressure remains elevated, it can become life-threatening.

7. What are signs and symptoms of autonomic dysreflexia syndrome?

The signs and symptoms include paroxysmal hypertension (systolic pressure can reach as high as 300 mm Hg), pounding headache, blurred vision, sweating above the level of injury, increased nasal congestion, nausea, bradycardia, and a distended rectum or bladder.

Prep Kit

Ready for Review

- Breakthrough technologies, newer drugs, and research have combined to increase the average life expectancy. People who might have died of injuries or illnesses 50 years ago may now continue to lead satisfying and productive lives.
- Many of these patients require physical support and care of chronic illnesses—care that may take place in the home setting.
- In rehabilitation care, the focus is on restoration of a person with disabilities to his or her maximum potential along several fronts: physical, social, spiritual, psychological, and vocational areas.
- Chronically ill patients are cared for at home by a wide range of caregivers, who may include family members, unlicensed caregivers, licensed nonprofessional caregivers, licensed professionals, or a combination of these.
- Consumers of home health care are vulnerable, are frequently too sick to advocate for themselves, and may lack advocates. Paramedics have a unique opportunity to assist in securing additional resources, reporting to protective agencies, and offering guidance for in-home injury prevention.
- Many family members who care for chronically ill patients are medically sophisticated and are often the paramedic's best source of information and care guidelines.
- In the home care setting, you may encounter patients who are chronically ill or permanently injured, as well as those who have recently had a hospital stay, surgery, or a high-risk pregnancy. You may also encounter newborns with medical complications. Many of these patients experience similar physical problems regardless of the initial cause.
- Assessment of the chronic care patient follows the standard guidelines. Ask the caregivers how the patient's condition differs today.
- It is important to assess for airway patency in all patients, but especially in patients with artificial airways.
- Patients with respiratory compromise have the inability to adequately ventilate themselves. The home care treatment plan is designed to supplement the patient's loss of respiratory effort. Any stressor can tip the balance, increase the severity of signs and symptoms, and render the current respiratory support inadequate.
- Ventilators mechanically deliver air to the lungs. Home ventilators are smaller than most microwave ovens, use regular household electricity, and may include a battery backup.
- Patients who have chronic cardiovascular disease are often cared for in the home setting. Many patients have cardiac insufficiency or heart failure, an inability of the heart to keep up with the demands placed on it and failure of the heart to pump blood efficiently.
- Central venous catheters are used for many types of home care patients, including those receiving chemotherapy, long-term antibiotic therapy or pain management, high-concentration glucose solutions, and hemodialysis.
- A gastric tube may be placed when a patient cannot ingest fluids, food, or medications by mouth.
- Chronically ill patients and patients with neurologic damage may require a long-term indwelling urinary catheter or intermittent urinary catheterization.
- A wound with minor redness, slight warmth to the touch, and swelling may indicate a superficial infection. A painful reddened area with cracks, serous drainage, or red streaks extending from the area may indicate that the patient has cellulitis. Cellulitis may be more severe and require hospitalization in patients who have venous stasis, diabetes, or who are immunocompromised.
- Complications in the postpartum period that you may see in the prehospital environment include postpartum bleeding, depression, sepsis, pulmonary embolus, and infant septicemia. You may also be called to assist with pediatric apnea monitors.
- Patients in hospice care can experience pain and discomfort from tumour growth, treatment modalities (eg, radiation and chemotherapy), immobility, inflammation, or infection. Treatment of hospice patients is based on the type and severity of pain.
- Patients receiving home care are encouraged to make end-of-life decisions early in their care. A durable power of attorney allows a patient to appoint someone to make health care decisions in the event that he or she becomes incapacitated.

Vital Vocabulary

chemotherapy The introduction of either single cytotoxic drugs or combinations of cytotoxic drugs into the body for the purpose of interrupting or eradicating malignant cellular growth.

chronic obstructive pulmonary disease (COPD) Illnesses that cause obstructive problems in the lower airways, including chronic bronchitis, emphysema, and sometimes asthma.

colostomy Establishment of an opening between the colon and the surface of the body for the purpose of providing drainage of the bowel.

dehiscence Separation of the edges of a wound.

dementia Chronic deterioration of mental functions.

Do Not Intubate Written documentation by a physician giving permission to medical personnel not to attempt intubation.

Do Not Resuscitate (DNR) Written documentation by a physician giving permission to medical personnel not to attempt resuscitation in the event of cardiac arrest.

ileostomy Surgical procedure to remove large portions of the small intestine.

laryngectomy A surgical procedure in which the larynx is removed.

negative-pressure ventilation Drawing of air into the lungs; airflow from a region of higher pressure (outside the body) to a region of lower pressure (the lungs); occurs during normal (unassisted breathing).

oxygen concentrators Large, electrical devices that concentrate the oxygen in ambient air and eliminate other gases

positive-pressure ventilation Forcing of air into the lungs.

purulent exudates Discharge that contains pus.

serous exudates Discharge that contains serum, a thin watery substance.

tidal volume Amount of air inhaled or exhaled during normal, quiet breathing; the volume of one breath.

tracheostomy Surgical opening into the trachea.

ureterostomy The formation of an opening to allow the passage of urine.

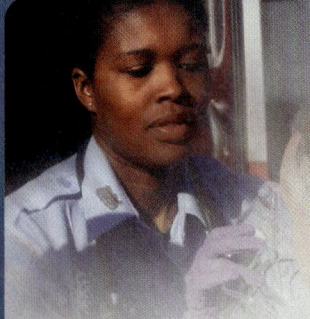

Assessment in Action

You are dispatched to the home of a 68-year-old man for an altered mental status. When you arrive on scene, you are greeted by his daughter, who tells you that the patient is an insulin-dependent diabetic whose blood sugar is 1.9 mmol/l. He is also a paraplegic from a traumatic accident 5 years before. His daughter tells you that the night before her father was experiencing upper body pain, which is typical, but it seemed to be worse yesterday. You administer IV therapy and provide dextrose. The patient becomes alert and oriented and refuses transport to the hospital. His only remaining complaint is his increased pain.

1. **Pain can be classified as _____ and _____.**
   A. acute, surgical
   B. chronic, traumatic
   C. acute, chronic
   D. subjective, stimuli

2. **Chronic pain is defined as:**
   A. pain lasting up to 3 months.
   B. pain lasting longer than 6 months.
   C. pain lasting only 2 months.
   D. pain lasting less than 3 months.

3. **The _____ nervous system is activated in the face of pain.**
   A. sympathetic
   B. parasympathetic
   C. cholinergic
   D. anticholinergic

4. **_____ is the more accurate term describing transmission of stimuli over specific nerve pathways.**
   A. Nociception
   B. Parasympathetic
   C. Sympathetic
   D. Receptor

5. **Management of pain _____, which allows for rest and healing.**
   A. increases energy consumption
   B. reduces energy consumption
   C. does nothing
   D. maintains the sympathetic response

6. **Paramedics must assume:**
   A. the patient is well cared for.
   B. the patient is being maltreated.
   C. the role of the legal guardian.
   D. the role of health educators.

7. **True or false? Conduct the initial assessment of the patient with chronic illness in the same way as for any other patient.**
   A. False
   B. True

Challenging Question

You are dispatched to the private residence of an 84-year-old man. When you arrive, the family greets you and tells you that the patient called 9-1-1 complaining of chest pain, but the patient has Alzheimer's disease. The family does not believe the patient has any complaints, and they do not want him transported to the hospital.

8. **What course of action should you take?**

Points to Ponder

You and your partner are dispatched to the home of a 72-year-old woman with a complaint of respiratory distress. When you arrive on scene, you are greeted by the patient's home health care provider. She tells you that the patient has terminal cancer. For the last 2 days, the patient has experienced an increase in shortness of breath. Her respiratory rate is 32 breaths/min; blood pressure, 100/60 mm Hg; pulse oximetry on room air, 91%; and pulse rate, 110 beats/min, sinus tachycardia on the monitor. The patient has breast cancer with metastasis to the lungs. Her family is in the process of placing the patient into hospice care, but the paperwork has not been completed yet.

Given the history of lung cancer and immunosuppression, what condition do you suspect? Should you transport the patient?

Issues: The Role of the Home Health Care Professional, Dealing With Family and Friends as Home Health Care Providers.

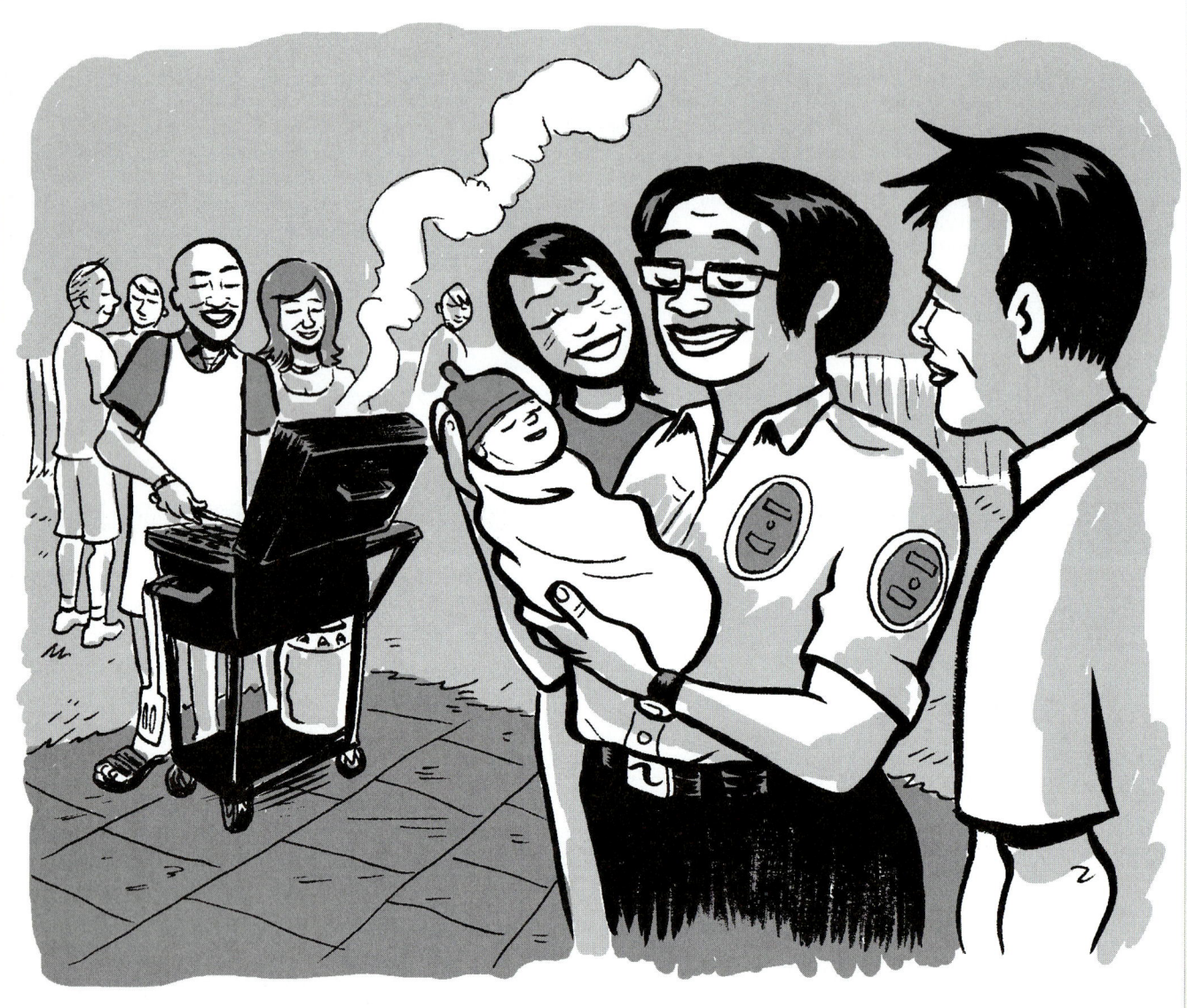

Operations

Section Editor: Steve Darling, BHSc, CCP(F)

46 Ambulance Operations

Competency Areas

Area 1: Professional Responsibilities

1.1.f Participate in quality assurance and enhancement programs.

1.4.a Function within relevant legislation, policies, and procedures.

1.5.a Work collaboratively with a partner.

Area 2: Communication

2.2.b Prepare professional correspondence.

Area 3: Health and Safety

3.2.a Practice safe biomechanics.

3.2.b Transfer patient from various positions using applicable equipment and/or techniques.

3.2.c Transfer patient using emergency evacuation techniques.

3.2.d Secure patient to applicable equipment.

3.2.e Lift patient and stretcher in and out of ambulance with partner.

Area 5: Therapeutics

5.1.a Use manual maneuvers and positioning to maintain airway patency.

5.1.i Remove airway foreign bodies (AFB).

5.1.j Remove foreign body by direct techniques.

5.2.a Recognize indications for oxygen administration.

5.2.b Take appropriate safety precautions.

5.2.c Ensure adequacy of oxygen sypply.

5.2.d Recognize different types of oxygen delivery systems.

5.2.e Utilize portable oxygen delivery systems.

5.3.a Administer oxygen using nasal cannula.

5.3.b Administer oxygen using low concentration mask.

5.4.b Recognize indications for mechanical ventilation.

5.4.c Prepare mechanical ventilation equipment.

5.4.d Provide mechanical ventilation.

5.5.b Control external hemorrhage through the use of direct pressure and patient positioning.

5.5.c Maintain peripheral intravenous (IV) access devices and infusions of crystalloid solutions without additives.

5.5.o Provide routing care for patient with urinary catheter.

5.5.p Provide routing care for patient with ostomy drainage system.

5.5.u Conduct urinary catheterization.

Area 7: Transportation

7.1.a Conduct vehicle maintenance and safety check.

7.1.b Recognize conditions requiring removal of vehicle from service.

7.1.c Utilize all vehicle equipment and vehicle devices within ambulance.

7.2.a Utilize defensive driving techniques.

7.2.b Utilize safe emergency driving techniques.

7.2.c Drive in a manner that ensures patient comfort and a safe environment for all passengers.

7.3.a Create safe landing zone for rotary-wing aircraft.

7.3.b Safely approach stationary rotary-wing aircraft.

7.3.c Safely approach stationary fixed-wing aircraft.

7.4.a Prepare patient for air medical transport.

7.4.b Recognize the stressors of flight on patient, crew, and equipment and the implications for patient care.

Introduction

Driving an emergency vehicle is a tremendous responsibility. Not only do you have to be aware of the safety of your crew and passengers, but you are also responsible for the safe passage of other vehicles you encounter on the road. Activating the lights and sirens does not ensure that you will be heard or understood by other drivers. More important, the use of lights and sirens is usually only a request for the right of way.

History of Ground Ambulances

Over the years, much has changed in the way that patients are transported to emergency care facilities. During the French Revolutionary Wars (1790s), Dr. Dominique-Jean Larrey conceived the idea of a mobile transport system for casualties. The first vehicles used for this purpose were horse-drawn wagons called flying ambulances that were part of an ambulance corps. This ambulance corps consisted of a physician, a quartermaster, a noncommissioned officer, a drummer boy to carry bandages, and 24 infantrymen to protect them. Even with such a large entourage they were able to remove victims from the battlefield within 15 minutes.

The first ambulances in Canada were commissioned in the 1880s. It is believed that the first ambulance was presented to the trustees of Toronto General Hospital in 1880. Since then, the ambulance fleet in Canada has evolved into a well-coordinated system of land, air, and communications resources.

The delivery of ambulance services is the responsibility of the provincial government. As such, current standards for ambulances are set by each province. Standards are then streamlined across the country, because all provinces and territories are represented by the EMS Chiefs of Canada. Specific vehicle standards can be referenced at provincial health ministries. These standards are updated based on operational demands and industry innovations.

The original guidelines required that all ambulances be painted Omaha orange and white, allowing them to be easily recognized by other drivers. More recently, responsibility for ambulance design schemes has been relaxed to allow for a variety of personalized paint schemes, as long as minimum illuminations and reflective standards are maintained. In North America, there are three major ambulance designs Figure 46-1 ▼ and Table 46-1 ▶ . The majority of the ambulance fleet are type II and III styles, but there are some uniquely Canadian innovations in EMS vehicles Figure 46-2 ▶ .

Improvements made to emergency vehicles over the years have not only made them safer for paramedics, but also more comfortable. Given the amount of time that paramedics spend in their vehicles, even small improvements (eg, increased headroom in the patient compartment and safety nets on the squad bench) can make it easier to perform prehospital care activities with less fear of injury. Before padded cabinet corners were used, for example, many paramedics were injured when the vehicle was in motion.

Ambulance Equipment

The patient compartment of an ambulance can seem like a complicated place to someone who is not acquainted with the prehospital profession. Every bit of space is dedicated to storing or securing the equipment it takes to do the job well. Much

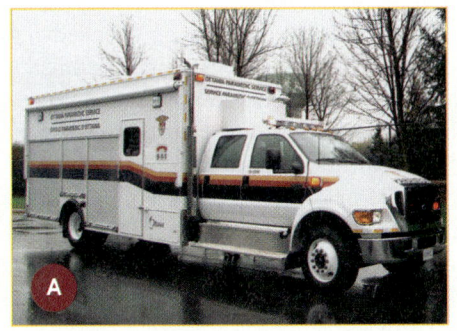 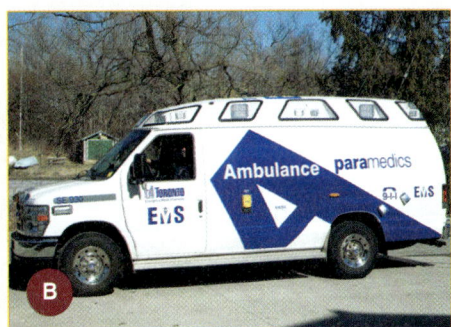 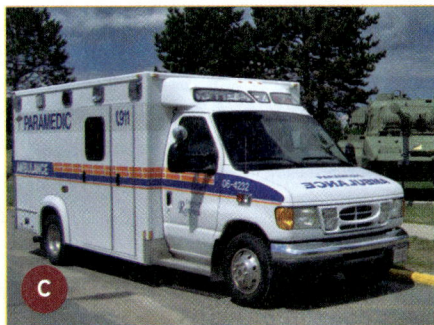

Figure 46-1 **A.** Type I (heavy duty). **B.** Type II. **C.** Type III.

You are the Paramedic Part 1

You and your partner have been dispatched to the scene of a multiple-vehicle collision on the highway. Dispatch advises you that they have received several calls regarding the crash, with the potential for multiple victims. It is 16:00 hr, and you realize that the school system in your area will be busy with traffic no matter which route you take.

1. What are some of the potential hazards you may encounter en route to the scene?
2. What dangers must be considered when approaching the scene with regard to parking and personnel protection?

Table 46-1	Basic Ambulance Designs
Type I	Conventional, truck-cab chassis with a modular ambulance body that can be transferred to a newer chassis as needed
Type II	Standard van, forward-control integral cab-body ambulance
Type III	Specialty van, forward-control integral cab-body ambulance

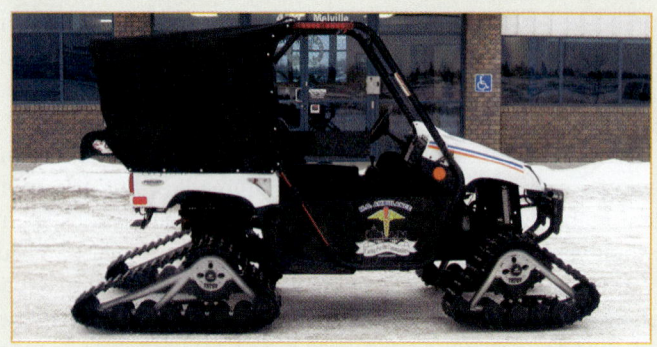

Figure 46-2 Innovative EMS response vehicle for snow-covered terrain.

like a jigsaw puzzle, everything must fit tightly together to prevent injury, yet be easily accessible.

Many organizations have influenced the development of the supplies and equipment carried on today's units. Infection control practice recommendations, including all areas of personnel protective equipment, sharps containers, and disinfecting equipment, are a provincial responsibility. Some provinces have a Medical Advisory Council (MAC) that makes recommendations based on current medical literature. Equipment standards and minimum equipment for all ambulances are written by the respective Provincial Ministries of Health. The American College of Surgeons (ACS) developed the first standardized list of equipment to be carried on an ambulance in 1970 and continues to update these lists as technological advances are made in the prehospital environment.

Checking the Ambulance

The paramedic must make sure that the ambulance carries the proper equipment. Getting ready to respond is just as important as providing prehospital care. The crew is also responsible for ensuring that the unit is capable of responding safely and efficiently to calls.

At the beginning of each shift, crew members must check the ambulance to ensure the proper equipment is available and in good working order. Each time supplies and equipment are used, they should be properly cleaned or replaced and returned to service for the next call. Consult local policy for service standards of practice. Medication expiry dates must be checked regularly to confirm that they have not expired. In addition,

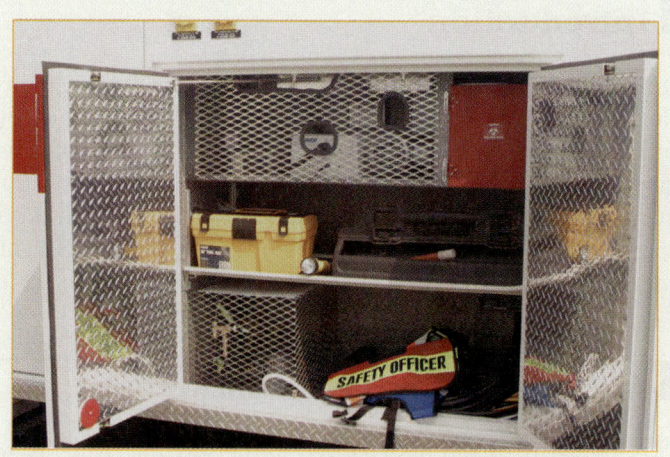

Figure 46-3 Equipment found in outside compartments.

Documentation and Communication

Because the mechanical aspects of emergency work such as driving and moving patients have an impact on your safety and the safety of others, your service should have specific procedures for daily inspections. Following these procedures protects you physically, and documenting your compliance is an important legal protection. Procedures should call for dating and either signing or initialing the check sheets. Store these sheets where they can be referenced later if needed.

diagnostic equipment, such as defibrillators, pulse oximeters, and glucometers, must be tested or calibrated regularly.

Ambulance Compartments

All compartments in the ambulance should be checked regularly, both inside and out. Most ambulances carry stabilization and splinting equipment in the outside compartments for easy access when speed may be an important factor in prehospital care **Figure 46-3 ▲**. Medications and temperature-sensitive equipment are generally stored in the patient compartment area. The following list gives some of the minimal essential equipment that should be found on all emergency ambulances:

- Airway and ventilation equipment
- Basic wound care supplies
- Monitoring devices (eg, blood pressure cuffs, pulse oximeter, electrocardiogram monitor/defibrillator)
- Selection of splints
- Childbirth supplies
- Patient transfer equipment
- Medications

Understanding Your Ambulance

An ambulance needs to be able to do four things: start, steer, stop, and stay running **Figure 46-4 ▶**. Any threat to one of the "four Ss" should prompt the operator to put the vehicle out

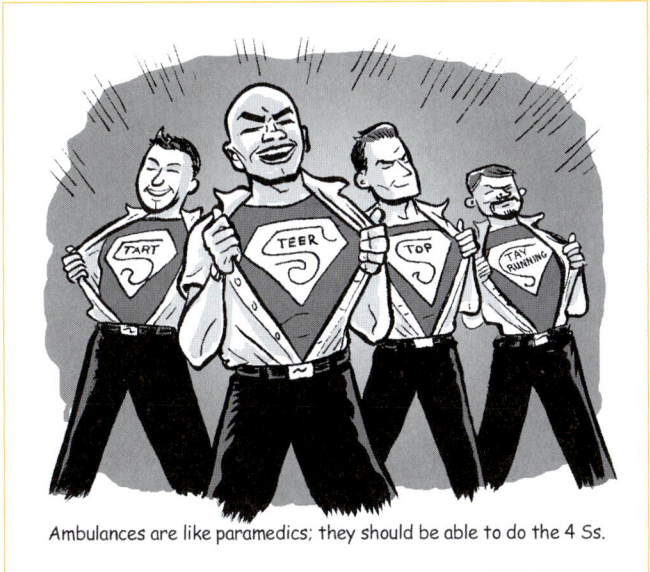

Figure 46-4

Ambulances are like paramedics; they should be able to do the 4 Ss.

of service immediately. Two other key functions that are especially important in extreme weather are adequate visibility (the wipers and lighting systems) and the internal environmental controls (heating and air conditioning).

Check It *Before* You Drive It

A standard daily checklist is essential to ensure the ambulance is in good operating order. The daily check should begin with a walk-around inspection to identify unreported body damage, major leaks, inoperative lighting, or damaged tires. A formal mechanical checklist should then guide you through a system-by-system inspection.

An operator should check the fuel levels first (some ambulances carry two fuel tanks). Next, the operator should check the motor oil prior to starting the engine. A gasoline-powered V8 motor typically contains 6 litres; a diesel motor contains more than 12 litres (all of which are critical to functioning). Make certain to consult your ambulance's owner's manual to learn the specifics of the engine. Check the oil not only to determine the level, but also for quality. Transmission fluid is often checked with the motor running and the gear selector in "park." For extra safety, be sure that the parking brake is engaged, because you will be standing in front of the running ambulance.

Lubricants of all kinds should feel slippery between the fingers, should appear clean, and should smell like fresh oil. Motor oil should be yellow or amber in a gasoline engine and may be grey or black in a diesel engine. It should never smell like fuel, which indicates that fuel is diluting the lubricant.

Transmission and steering fluids should be pink or yellow and should not smell like charcoal, which indicates that the fluids are burned. Brake fluid should be clear or yellow when fresh, but may be amber after a few years of service. Coolant may be either red or bright yellow-green. It is better to not uncap the brake fluid reservoir (because brake fluid absorbs moisture from the atmosphere) or the coolant reservoir, which

is pressurized (because hot coolant can expand rapidly and cause burns). Consult local preventive maintenance schedules for the status of your ambulance.

Look for leaks on the ground under the vehicle and inspect the inner surfaces of the tires to identify leakage of brake fluid or rear axle oil. The presence of water on the ground (eg, at the right front corner of the vehicle) is often a normal occurrence when the air conditioner has been operating.

Battery terminals should be clean, and the top surfaces of the batteries should be dry. The system voltage indicates battery condition at rest and alternator condition with the engine running. At rest, it should be between 12 and 12.5 volts; with the engine running, it should be between 13.5 and 14.5 volts. If the voltage rises to 15 volts or higher with the engine running, the alternator's voltage regulator has failed and should be replaced immediately. The ammeter measures electric current flow and indicates the condition of the battery and alternator simultaneously.

An odour like sewer gas may indicate that a battery has been boiling, perhaps because the system voltage is too high or the battery's resistance has dropped. An automotive battery is filled with concentrated sulfuric acid. When it boils, it produces sulfur dioxide (causing the odour) and pure hydrogen (odourless but highly explosive). The odour of sulfur dioxide should prompt you to take the vehicle out of service immediately, leave the hood closed, and avoid starting the engine.

Checking the brake and back-up lights requires the assistance of a second person unless the ambulance is backed up to a reflective surface like a window. Both are as essential to safe driving as the rest of the external lighting.

Check It *While* You Drive It

An ambulance has many built-in warning systems that the operator should be familiar with to avoid a critical failure that could endanger the paramedic or affect patient outcome.

Belt noise is a chirping or squealing sound, synchronous with engine speed (not road speed). It is usually related to a load on one of the appliances operated by a drive belt—the power steering pump, the water pump, the air conditioner, the vacuum pump (in a diesel), or the alternator. Belt noise is always significant and will eventually keep an ambulance from operating. It does not necessarily warrant taking a unit out of service immediately.

Brake fade is a sensation that an ambulance has lost its power brakes. Some common causes are overheating of brake surfaces, loss of vacuum, loss of brake fluid, wet or greasy brake drums, or a failed master cylinder. Even a single instance of brake fade warrants taking the vehicle out of service immediately.

Generally, you should not hear, smell, or feel a vehicle's brakes, with occasional exceptions. Cold brakes may squeak intermittently in wet weather. Some kinds of brake pads are equipped with "tell-tale tabs"—small aluminum projections that are designed to rub on the disk surfaces and squeak, warning an operator when the pads are nearing the end of their useful life. Otherwise, a consistent squeaking or grinding sound warrants immediate attention by a mechanic.

Brake pull is a sensation that, when you depress the brake pedal, someone is trying to jerk the steering wheel to the left or right. It can indicate brake fluid or grease on a brake pad, or it can result from a serious mechanical malfunction. Remove the vehicle from service immediately.

Drift is a finding that when you let go of the steering wheel, the vehicle consistently wanders left or right. A vehicle may normally drift very slightly to the right, because most roads are built with a crown in the centre (so water drains toward the gutters). A vehicle should not consistently drift to the left, however.

Steering pull is a persistent tug on the steering wheel that you can feel as the ambulance "drifts" to one side or the other. The most common cause is uneven tire pressures (possibly a flat tire). Steering pull can also be caused by one or more misaligned wheels or another mechanical problem. It can cause loss of control in the event of a sudden stop. A vehicle's steering geometry is complex. To allow for its adjustment, the entire front suspension system is held together by clamps. Misalignment can occur when a vehicle hits a curb and dislodges one or more of these clamps. The result may be control problems as well as tire and rim damage.

A pulsating brake pedal—an up-and-down motion of the brake pedal during deceleration—is an abnormal condition, especially at low speeds. A pulsing brake pedal usually indicates warped brake rotors or drums, but can also suggest a bent wheel. This motion can be severe when the brakes are hot. This condition always warrants service.

Normally, little effort should be adequate to steer an ambulance. Excessive effort to steer is therefore a serious finding and can be caused by inadequate steering fluid or a failed power steering pump or drive belt.

Steering play is a sensation of looseness or sloppiness in a vehicle's steering. This finding is important when accompanied by clunking or banging noises during steering, and it should never be noticeable in a new vehicle. This problem is typically caused by wear, but it can also result from underinflated tires. This situation warrants immediate inspection of the ambulance.

Tire squeal is a singing sound that occurs when you turn the vehicle, especially at very low speeds. Squealing is normal on very smooth concrete, but not on asphalt. The most common cause is underinflated tires, but it can also result from misaligned wheels, especially in the presence of other signs. This situation warrants a mechanic's attention as soon as possible.

Wheel bounce is a vibration, synchronous with road speed, that you can feel in the steering wheel (suggesting a front wheel) or driver's seat (rear wheel). Wheel bounce is usually detectable at freeway speeds over 72 km per hour. It suggests a defective shock absorber, a bubble in a tire, or an improperly balanced wheel.

Wheel wobble is a common finding at low speeds when a vehicle has a bent wheel. You normally detect wobble in the steering wheel if it involves a front wheel, or in the driver's seat if it is in the rear wheel. Potholes are the most common cause.

Ambulance Staffing and Deployment

Ambulance staffing has been a major source of controversy over the past decade. Escalating costs for medical care, fuel, and the financial burden of operating an ambulance service have prompted the development of alternative strategies for managing EMS systems. For example, the development of "high-performance EMS systems" represents an effort to maximize personnel productivity and minimize response times. The key factors that are analyzed in an effective, cost-efficient service are summarized below.

- **Response times.** High-performance systems typically use a fractile response time standard in which a significant fraction (usually 90%) of all responses must be achieved in an established time—for example, 8 minutes or less in an urban area. Industry standards may be adopted or standards may be established by individual provinces.
- **Productivity.** The paramedic measures how many patient transports per hour each ambulance accomplishes (known as "unit-hour utilization").
- **Unit costs.** Determined by the cost to respond to each call as well as the actual number of hours the units were actively operating, these costs include the paramedics' salaries plus the operational cost of vehicles and equipment (gas, routine maintenance, and repairs).
- **Cost for ambulance service.** The costs for ambulance service are administered by the provincial governments.

Ambulance and EMS Systems

In Canada, ambulance service is traditionally operated by municipal, hospital, or provincial agencies or run by private enterprise. Since 2001, paramedic training programs in Canada have revised their training goals and objectives to meet the National Occupational Competency Profile for Paramedicine (NOCP) developed by the Paramedic Association of Canada (PAC). The NOCP serves as the template for all training programs seeking accreditation.

Four levels of paramedic are recognized in Canada: Emergency First Responder (EMR), Primary Care Paramedic (PCP), Advanced Care Paramedic (ACP), and Critical Care Paramedic (CCP). In Canada, the majority of paramedics are certified to the PCP level. Public expectations are for ACP level of care, so availability of this level of care is increasing. CCP level of care is typically reserved for interfacility service, air ambulance operations, or other specialized services where patient complexity is very high.

The level of service varies among provinces and individual municipalities. Services consist of permanent, full-time, and part-time employees and volunteers. Some systems employ a tiered response system that attempts to assign ACP ambulances only where they are needed.

System Status Management

System Status Management (SSM) is a concept that was developed by Jack Stout in 1983. The goals of SSM are to maximize efficiency and reduce response time. SSM uses historical data to determine ambulance service demands and then tries to take fluctuations in demand into consideration when organizing service. For example, an increased demand for service may be noted during certain hours of the day or in certain geographic locations. These demands are termed peak loads. In an urban area, the demand for ambulance service may be higher during the daytime but lighter during the night. SSM attempts strategic deployment of ambulance resources in order to minimize response times. The strategic deployment of an ambulance to a location, known as posting, can take advantage of developments in satellite vehicle location and GPS technologies.

Another component of SSM is peak demand staffing. Shift schedules are designed to provide a sufficient number of ambulances during peak load hours. For example, more ambulances might be staffed between 12:00 and 18:00 hours than between midnight and 06:00 hours. One potentially negative aspect of SSM is the toll that it can take on personnel, who have less time to get out of the vehicle and relax in the ambulance station between calls.

Ambulance Stationing

The goals for establishing ambulance stations are to maximize efficiency and to minimize response times. In most urban and suburban areas, the distance factor may not be as important as the call volume. In a rural setting, both availability of first responders and distance may be equally important. Also, the district may have special facilities that create increased ambulance demand—long-term care facilities, for example. Other considerations in the design of ambulance stations include the need for maintenance of vehicles and equipment, storage, classrooms for training and meetings, and sleeping quarters for personnel who spend the night.

The Paramedic as an Emergency Health Care Professional

Paramedics working on an ambulance have a responsibility to conduct themselves as professionals. Even in times of severe stress or fatigue, the paramedic should act as an advocate for the patient. He or she should always seek to deliver high-quality prehospital care without regard to time of day, the location of the call, or the appearance or conduct of the patient. Remember, you represent your service to the public, to your colleagues, and, most importantly, to patients and their families in their time of need.

Notes from Nancy

Even in times of severe stress or fatigue, you should act as an advocate for the patient.

Emergency Vehicle Operation

All the advances made in prehospital care mean nothing if you never arrive. Driving an emergency vehicle requires you to be aware of *all* dangers on the roadway, including some that are not factors when you drive your private vehicle. Knowing where to look for these dangers is your responsibility whenever you get behind the wheel of an ambulance.

Collision Prevention

The most common causes for collisions are that the ambulance is not travelling in the proper lane or the operator is driving too fast **Figure 46-5 ▾** .

A troubling fact is that nearly half of paramedics involved in a collision had an earlier collision or moving violation in the 3 years prior to the incident. It is the responsibility of every ambulance service to ensure that personnel are not only safe drivers *before* they begin employment, but are given emergency vehicle operation courses *after* they are hired. Even if you are given specific exemptions to some traffic laws in an emergency, this privilege must be used sparingly.

Due Regard

Every province has laws regarding the use of lights and sirens when operating an emergency vehicle. The concept of due regard is an important part of those laws. Due regard means that you may use lights and sirens as a means to alert other drivers that you are in an emergency mode, but it does not exempt you from operating your vehicle with due regard for the safety of others.

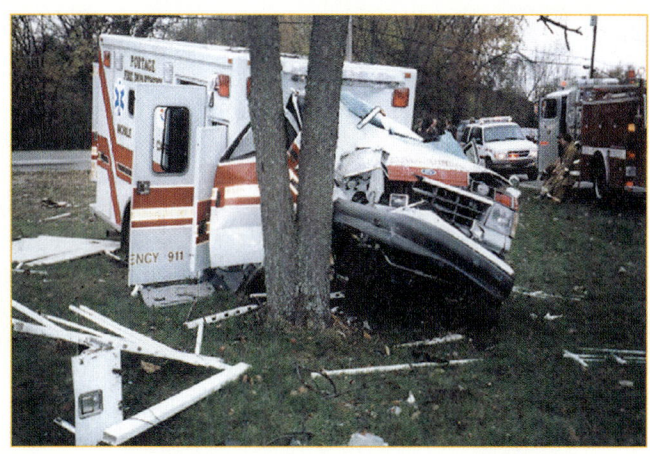

Figure 46-5 A wrecked ambulance.

You are the Paramedic Part 2

En route to the call you have received information from dispatch that the first responders are on the scene and report that you have a total of six vehicles involved with at least four pediatric patients with various degrees of injury.

3. How will knowing there are multiple patients, including children, affect your driving?

4. Where should the ambulance be positioned at the scene of a highway incident if you are the *first* to arrive?

5. Where should the ambulance be positioned at the scene of a highway incident if you are *not* the first to arrive?

Use of Escorts

It is typically *not* a good idea to follow another emergency vehicle, such as a police vehicle, through traffic as an escort. Many drivers will see only the first set of lights and sirens and assume that the way is clear once that vehicle has passed. If you are following another emergency vehicle, leave enough space between the vehicles so that other drivers (and you) have enough time to react and safely stop should someone pull in front of you unexpectedly.

Another potential danger occurs when family members follow closely behind you on the way to the hospital. Both the ambulance and other drivers may have difficulty seeing the vehicles that are following. If you need to stop suddenly, there may be no time to react and the vehicle could collide with the ambulance. Instruct family members before you leave the scene that they cannot drive closely behind you.

Use of Lights and Sirens

Despite improvements in the sophistication of 9-1-1 answering systems and in the accuracy of telephone triage protocols, EMS ambulances use their lights and sirens most of the time when responding to calls. In contrast, the decision to use lights and sirens when transporting patients to the hospital calls for judgment on the part of the paramedic. Only when transporting critical patients is the added hazard warranted. Even then, you must proceed with due regard for everyone's safety.

Driving to the Scene

When dispatched to an emergency, the paramedic must decide which route will be used to arrive at the scene safely. Avoid areas of heavy traffic if possible. School zones are especially dangerous at the beginning or ending of classes and should be avoided if possible. Be aware of construction zones in your area as well as railroad crossings. Know the best routes in your district before you head out.

The type of call can sometimes affect how you respond to it. When you hear that the call involves children or a severe trauma potential, you may want to drive with less caution, feeling that speed is more important than safety. Nothing will speed up a driver's adrenalin more than hearing that the call involves a colleague. As a professional, you must not let the nature of the call affect your judgment—always drive with caution.

When operating an emergency vehicle, the driver is responsible for his or her actions, despite the mode of dispatch. The driver must modify his or her actions, use of lights and sirens, and emergency vehicle maneuvers in traffic based on awareness and interpretation of the road and traffic conditions at each part of the route to the scene. The driver must also take into account the patient's condition and whether this mode of vehicle operation is warranted. The literature demonstrates that emergency vehicle operation with lights and sirens does not save a significant amount of time and increases the risk of having an accident.

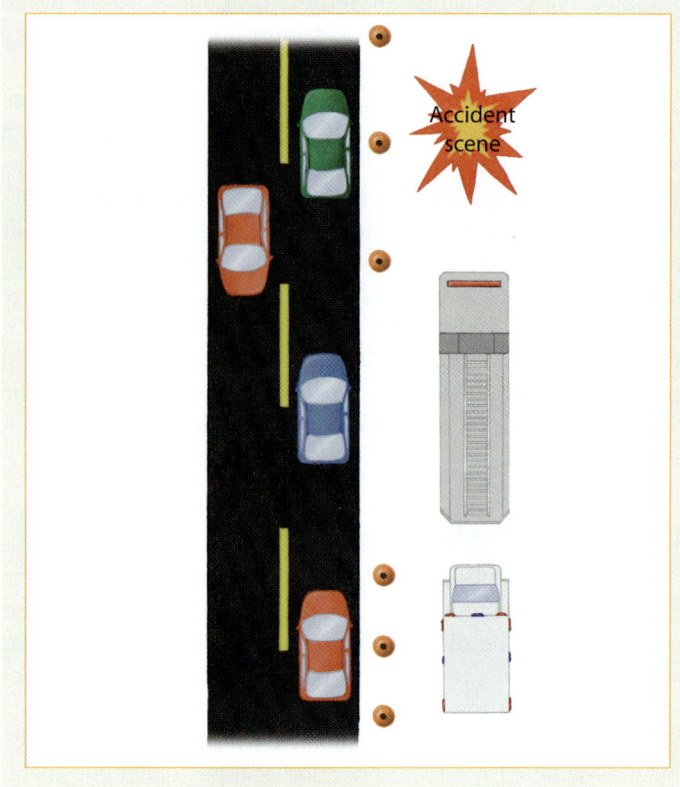

Figure 46-6 Position the vehicle to maximize your safety.

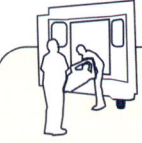 **At the Scene**

Always brake in a straight line!

Parking at an Emergency Scene

Sometimes the general public complains about the way EMS inconveniences other drivers. It may be difficult to understand why people object to blocked roads when paramedics are working diligently to save people's lives. However, sometimes the ambulance *is* parked in such a way that it unnecessarily impedes traffic flow. If you need to park an ambulance in such a way to block a traffic lane for scene and your safety, park in such a way as to protect yourself and minimize traffic flow obstruction. At the same time, however, maintain concern for others who are not involved in the incident. For example, if you are parking in an apartment complex, be aware that other people may need to leave while you are inside and try not to block parked vehicles **Figure 46-6 ▲**.

When parking off the side of the road, you must be aware of the terrain **Figure 46-7 ▶**. In dry weather, the heat from underneath the vehicle could start a grass fire. In wet weather, the weight of the ambulance makes it susceptible to sinking into mud and getting stuck.

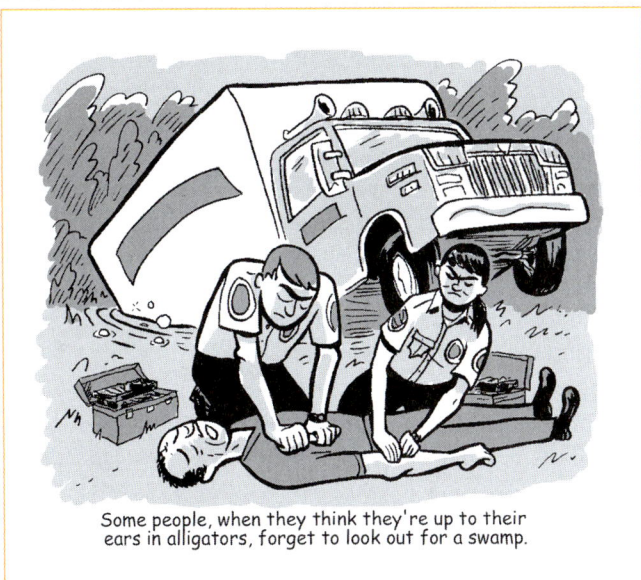

Some people, when they think they're up to their ears in alligators, forget to look out for a swamp.

Figure 46-7

some can be allowed to enter the patient compartment with assistance from the paramedic if it is appropriate for their medical condition. Always secure the patient, either on a stretcher or in a seat, with shoulder and lap belts.

A person who is accompanying the patient should usually ride in the front passenger seat with the seatbelt secured. There are reasonable exceptions to this rule, of course—for example, if the paramedic wants to keep the parent of a young child in the child's view or if the patient needs someone to translate what you say. When police presence is required, as when transporting a prisoner, the officer may need to ride in close proximity to the patient. In all cases, the riders should be secured into restraint devices, if possible. When transporting multiple patients in one ambulance, it is generally wise to load the most seriously injured last so that they will be unloaded first.

Depending on how the ambulance is equipped, follow the steps in **Skill Drill 46-1** to load a patient into an ambulance.

1. Tilt the head end of the main frame upward and place it into the patient compartment with the wheels on the floor.

Parking on a roadway at night is especially dangerous. Some drivers may have their attention distracted by the scene, and they may drift toward and collide with a parked emergency vehicle. Sometimes it may be safer to use your emergency flashers instead of all the overhead flashers; however, refer to local service policy for specific practice. Likewise, to avoid blinding oncoming traffic, it may be better to turn off the emergency vehicle's headlights when parked, especially if you are on a two-lane road.

Always wear visible protective clothing when you get out of the vehicle on roadways. Reflective vests are lightweight and have the added benefit of increasing visibility during the day as well as at night. Heavy protective clothing should also be considered when responding to collisions where extrication is being performed.

Loading and Unloading the Patient

When you are loading or unloading the ambulance, care must be taken to ensure that the patient is moved safely and quickly. Most patients will be loaded into the ambulance while on the stretcher. However,

Skill Drill 46-1: Loading the Patient

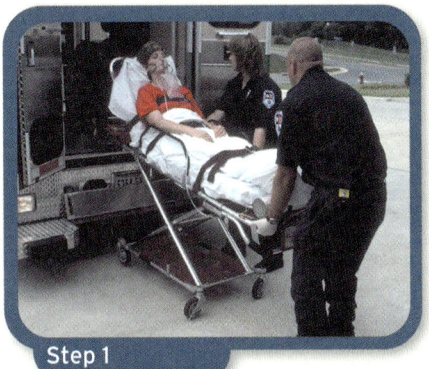

Step 1

Tilt the head of the stretcher upward, and place it into the patient compartment with the wheels on the floor.

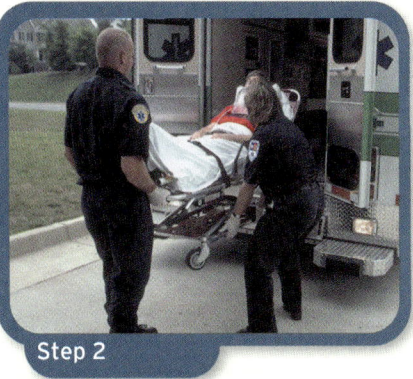

Step 2

The paramedic at the foot of the stretcher releases the undercarriage lock and lifts the undercarriage.

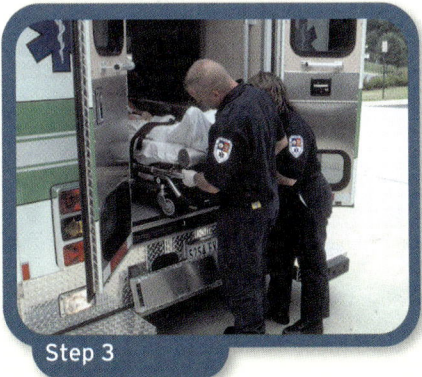

Step 3

Roll the stretcher into the back of the ambulance.

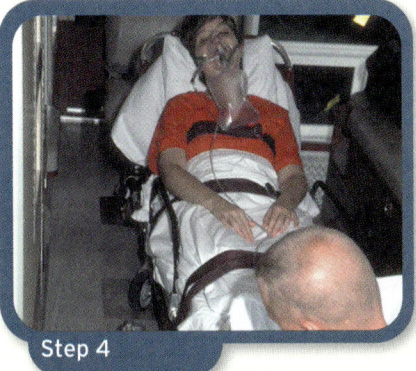

Step 4

Secure the stretcher to the brackets mounted in the ambulance.

The two additional wheels that extend just below the head end are attached to the main frame and will enable this movement (Step 1).

2. With the patient's weight supported by the two head-end wheels and the paramedic at the foot end of the stretcher, release the undercarriage lock, and your partner will lift the undercarriage up to its fully retracted position. The wheels of the undercarriage and the two head-end wheels of the main frame will now be on the same level (Step 2).

3. Roll the stretcher the rest of the way into the back of the ambulance, where it will rest on all six wheels (Step 3).

4. Secure the stretcher in the ambulance with the clamping mechanism that fastens around the undercarriage when the stretcher is pushed into them. The clamps are located in a rack on the floor or side of the patient compartment (Step 4).

Some ambulances may have a system whereby one person can load the stretcher onto the ambulance. If this is the case, the stretcher is placed in the raised "load" position at the rear of the ambulance. Place the wheels on the head of the stretcher into the ambulance, and push forward while the undercarriage collapses and retracts. Although these stretchers are designed for single-person operation, it is good practice to have both paramedics present in case uneven ground is encountered and the stretcher becomes difficult to handle. Visually check to make sure all locks are engaged. Be sure to follow your district's protocols.

To unload a patient, follow the steps in (**Skill Drill 46-2** ◄):
1. Ensure that the patient is secured to the stretcher (Step 1).
2. Unlock the head and foot locks (Step 2).
3. Lifting with your legs, carefully roll the stretcher forward until the undercarriage engages (Step 3).
4. With your partner steadying the stretcher from the side, gently bring the stretcher forward out of the ambulance (Step 4).

Skill Drill 46-2: Unloading a Patient

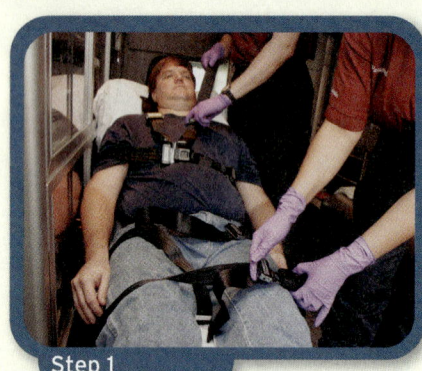

Step 1

Ensure that the patient is secured to the stretcher.

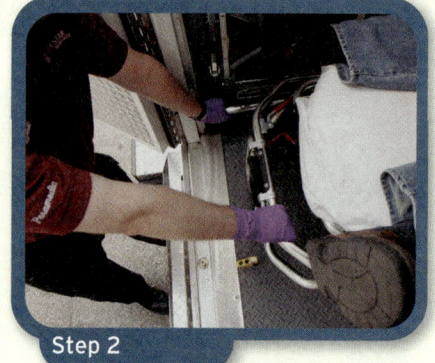

Step 2

Unlock the head and foot locks.

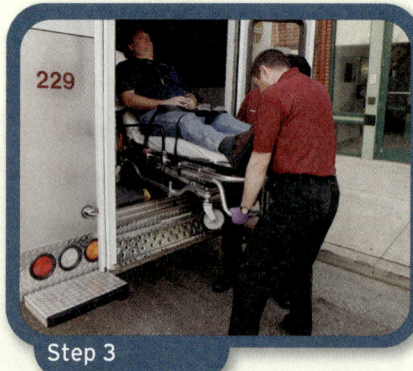

Step 3

Lifting with your legs, carefully roll the stretcher forward until the undercarriage engages.

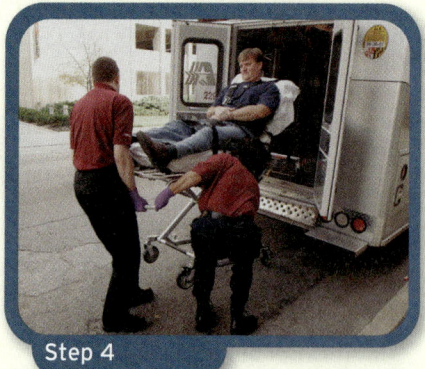

Step 4

With your partner steadying the stretcher from the side, gently bring the stretcher forward out of the ambulance.

Backing Up the Emergency Vehicle

Most EMS services have an established policy about emergency vehicle backing up procedures. Backing up a vehicle is the most common source of vehicle damage and may result in costly repairs or injuries. If possible, plan your egress strategy to avoid situations in which the ambulance will have to be backed up. If it must be done, follow these rules:

- Use a spotter to guide you (**Figure 46-8** ►).
- Talk to your partner or the spotter *before* you place the vehicle in reverse. You may be attempting to back to the left while your spotter is trying to direct you to the right.
- Keep your spotter in view at all times. If you lose sight of the spotter, stop until they are back in your line of sight.
- Agree on hand signals with your spotter before moving. Ensure that you both understand the signal for stop.
- Keep your window cracked or rolled down when in motion. This will allow you to hear people warning you of unseen dangers.

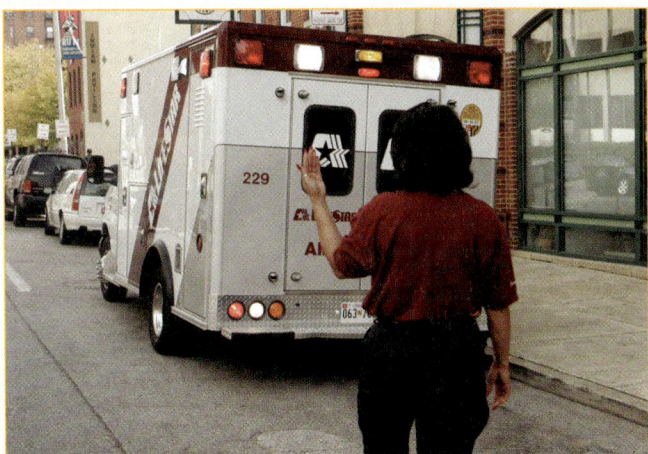

Figure 46-8 Always use a spotter when backing up the ambulance.

- Do a walk-around before getting behind the wheel and look up as well as down. Objects in the ground may not be visible once you start backing up.
- Use audible warning devices whenever the ambulance is in motion.

Use of Safety Restraints

Standard operating procedures should mandate that everyone in the ambulance use seatbelts, not just the patient. Children should not be transported on the stretcher unless properly restrained. It is not advisable to use adult seatbelts for children. Many pediatric transport devices are available, and they should be used when appropriate. Of course, when you are driving the ambulance you should always use a seatbelt. Likewise, when you are providing treatment in the patient compartment you should use the restraints whenever possible.

▌Air Medical Transports

Air medical transport—especially the use of helicopters—has done much to speed up the transfer of patients from the trauma scene to definitive care. This mode of transport provides many benefits; however, there are risks with landing a helicopter at a scene. With planning, the risk to personnel on the scene can be minimized. Several factors must be considered before calling for an air ambulance: Does the patient's condition warrant using air medical transport? Will use of the air ambulance truly save the patient time in getting to definitive care once all other factors are considered?

Fixed-Wing Air Ambulances

In 1917, a British soldier in the Camel Corps was shot in the ankle during a battle in Turkey. The soldier was evacuated from the battlefield in a deHavilland DHH. This 45-minute flight to the hospital replaced what was a 3-day trip by land. So began the transition of ground transport to the use of air ambulance. One of the first civilian air ambulance services began in Queensland, Australia, when an airplane leased from Qantas was used to treat 225 patients and make 50 emergency flights in 1928. This service, which used a pilot, nurse, and physician, evolved to become the Royal Flying Doctor Service. The first civilian air ambulance operation in North America was established in Regina by the Saskatchewan government in 1946. It is still in operation today.

The first use of a rotary-winged ambulance occurred in 1943 during the Burma Hump Airlift Operation in Southeast Asia. Flight nurses trained to care for patients in flight provided care to casualties during military operations. Civilian use of rotary-winged aircraft as an air ambulance began in 1972, with St. Anthony's Hospital in Denver, Colorado, sponsoring the Flight for Life program. In 1977, Ontario was the first Canadian province to provide helicopter-based air ambulance services to transport critically ill patients to the hospital.

Fixed-winged aircraft are used mainly for the transportation of patients over long distances **Figure 46-9 ▸** . EMS personnel are typically involved in both land and air ambulance operations. The air ambulance crew configuration may include paramedics, in addition to flight nurses, respiratory therapists, and flight physicians.

Rotary-winged aircraft are typically used for shorter distances and responses directly to the scene of accidents, where they have become essential for the transportation of critically injured patients directly to a regional trauma centre **Figure 46-10 ▸** .

You are the Paramedic Part 3

After a quick triage and assessment, you determine that air medical transportation is needed for the most critical patient. Dispatch advises you that a unit is en route and communication with you is being requested.

6. What information must you provide for the incoming helicopter?

7. How should paramedics approach the helicopter that has landed?

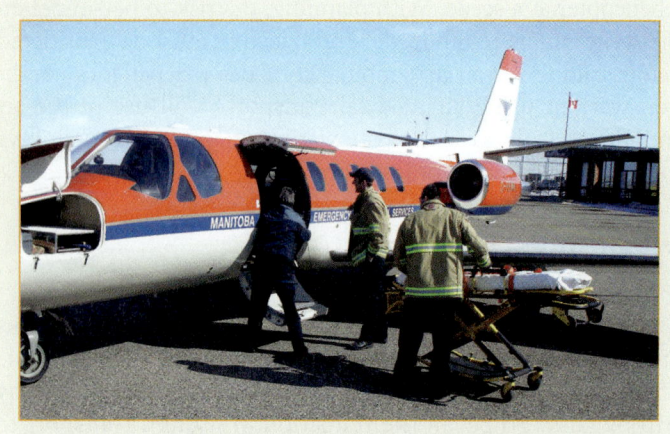

Figure 46-9 Fixed-winged aircraft.

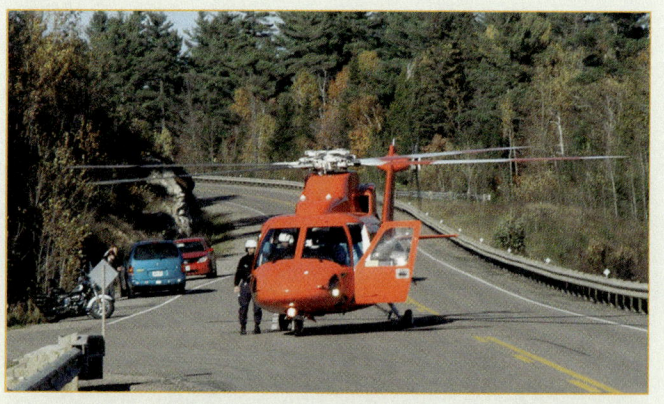

Figure 46-10 Rotary-wing air ambulance.

Advantages of Using Air Ambulances

Air ambulances have an advantage over ground transport because they can reduce transport time and may help the patient receive definitive treatment within the golden hour. In many cases, the air medical crew can provide a higher level of medical care to the patient before they even reach the hospital. The decision to use rotary-winged transport (helicopter) should be made as early in the call as possible. Most regions with rotary-winged aircraft have established policies and procedures on how and when to request the aircraft. Every paramedic should be familiar with how to activate the local or regional air medical program.

You should weigh all the factors that involve time when deciding whether the helicopter is appropriate. It takes time to get the helicopter from its base to the scene. The helicopter must be started, get clearance from air traffic controllers to take off, sometimes cover great distances, and then find a safe place to land. Once the helicopter is at the scene, time must be allotted to land the aircraft and transfer the patient to the air crew. Packaging the patient for air transport and loading the patient into the helicopter also require time. In metropolitan areas with good road access, it can be difficult to justify use of the helicopter. Severe traffic congestion or prolonged extrication times may sometimes make the use of a helicopter appropriate in urban areas.

Helicopter use may also be warranted if the patient has a spinal injury and the terrain over which the patient must be carried is very rough. When in doubt, the paramedic should refer to local or regional policies or contact the land dispatcher or direct medical control to determine if a helicopter response is indicated. (Table 46-2 ▾) summarizes the advantages of using an air ambulance.

Table 46-2	Advantages of Using an Air Ambulance
■ Specialized skills or equipment is needed
■ Rapid transport is possible
■ Can provide access to remote areas
■ Helipads available at hospital for helicopters

Disadvantages of Using Air Ambulances

Patients in cardiac arrest or those who appear to be in a pre-arrest state should be transported by ground to the nearest hospital. Treating a patient in cardiac arrest in the helicopter is difficult due to space limitations. It is also likely faster to transport this type of patient to the closest hospital by ground rather than to wait for a helicopter to arrive at the scene. The helicopter can rendezvous at the local hospital and transport the patient to a referral centre for higher level of care, if necessary, once the patient is stabilized.

In addition, helicopters must have suitable visibility and weather conditions to fly. Poor weather or anything that interferes with visibility can make it too dangerous to fly. The terrain also may make it difficult to land the helicopter safely. Uneven ground and loose objects such as rocks or debris should be taken into account before attempting to land the aircraft. (Table 46-3 ▾) lists disadvantages of using the air ambulance.

Setting Up the Landing Zone

The landing zone should be large enough to accommodate a rotary-winged aircraft of any size; standard dimensions are 30 × 30 m. The landing zone must also be firm and level, with no loose objects or debris that might be pulled up into the rotors and engine, including clothing worn by emergency workers, such as caps and scarves, and IV poles. Remove the sheet from the stretcher before putting the backboard on it so that the sheet is not pulled up into the rotor blades when the

Table 46-3	Disadvantages of Using an Air Ambulance
■ Weather/environment
■ Availability of safe landing site
■ Altitude limitations
■ Airspeed limitations
■ Aircraft cabin size
■ Terrain
■ Cost
■ Patient's condition

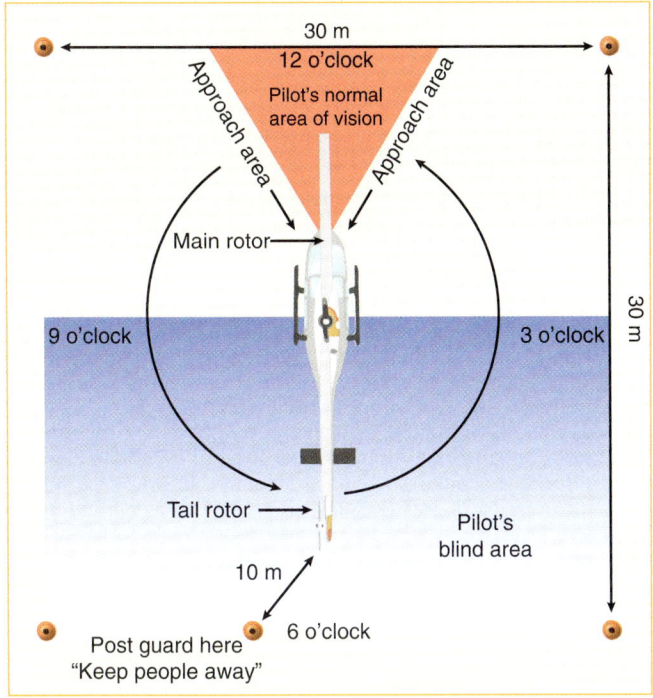

Figure 46-11 Landing zone with cones/warning devices in place.

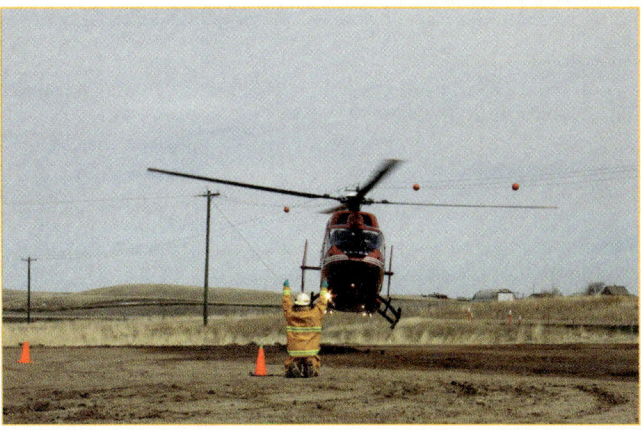

Figure 46-12 Personnel directing a helicopter for landing.

patient-loaded backboard is removed. Be aware of wires overhead that might not be visible from the air, and remove all unnecessary vehicles and people from the landing site. It is ultimately the pilot's decision to land the aircraft. Paramedics must respect the pilot's decision and not influence it in any way. Landing zone safety is essential to prevent accident or injury to personnel.

Mark the landing site with one visible light at each of the four corners **Figure 46-11 ▲**. Helicopters take off and land best into any existing wind, so it may be helpful to mark the side of prevailing winds. During a night landing, do not shine flashlights or spotlights up at the aircraft while it is descending; they may blind the pilot. Likewise, turn off headlights. Consider placing emergency vehicles under any overhead wires to signify the hazard. Some helicopter services will only land at designated helipads at night. This prevents taking unnecessary risks in landing in an unfamiliar location at night and ensures that the landing site is secure and safe.

Procedures for Landing

The most important function of the ground guide is to be aware of all hazards the pilot may not be able to see. Agree on communication channels before responding to an incident, and use standard "continue" and "abort" arm signals while at the scene **Figure 46-12 ▲**. Wear eye protection against flying debris. No matter what the situation, if a helicopter is landing at the scene, personnel on the ground should establish direct communication with the helicopter crew to advise them of the landing site, any obstacles, and any other information necessary to ensure a safe landing.

After the helicopter has landed, the paramedic should not approach the helicopter until signaled to do so by the pilot. If possible, all rotors should be stopped before you approach the aircraft. If the aircraft continues to operate in a "hot" mode (with rotor blades active), the tail rotor is the most dangerous part of the aircraft and should be avoided at all times. Always approach a helicopter from the front or side allowing the pilot to keep you in view at all times. Always follow the air crew's instructions when approaching or leaving the helicopter.

You are the Paramedic Summary

1. What are some of the potential hazards you may encounter en route to the scene?

Whenever an ambulance is en route to an emergency call, you must approach every intersection cautiously and with the thought that you could be meeting heavy traffic. In multiple-vehicle responses, always approach every intersection with caution and with the thought that you could be meeting another emergency vehicle at that intersection (police or fire).

2. What dangers must be considered upon approaching the scene with regard to parking and personnel protection?

Always approach the scene cautiously and with the thought that you could be meeting another emergency vehicle at the scene. If the scene has already been secured, park beyond the wreckage to prevent your ambulance from being exposed to the traffic. You may also receive arrival instructions if a first arriving EMS unit at the scene has already declared medical command. The arrival instructions may specify where the medical commander would like you to park your ambulance and to whom you should report. All paramedics should wear appropriate PPE such as gloves and possibly bunker gear, plus helmets when approaching the scene of a multiple-vehicle collision.

3. How will knowing there are children involved affect your driving?

It should not affect your driving at all. Whenever the ambulance is on the road, day or night, turn on the headlights to increase visibility and drive defensively.

4. Where should the ambulance be positioned at the scene of a highway incident if you are the *first* to arrive?

If you are the first to arrive at the scene of a highway incident, take time to perform a scene assessment for potential hazards to you, your crew, and the patients. Consider establishing a danger zone, parking at least 30 m from the accident, upwind and uphill (if possible) to avoid fire or any escaping hazardous liquids or fumes, and deal with the traffic until the police arrive to relieve you of that task. If there is no fire or escaping liquids or fumes, park at least 15 m from the accident. Park your vehicle between the scene and the approaching traffic to provide a collision buffer if your ambulance is the first emergency vehicle on the scene so your warning lights can warn approaching motorists before flares can be set up.

5. Where should the ambulance be positioned at the scene of a highway incident if you are *not* the first to arrive?

If the scene has already been secured, park beyond the accident to prevent your ambulance from being exposed to the traffic. You may also receive arrival instructions if the EMS unit first at the scene has already declared scene command. The arrival instructions may have specific instructions as to where the medical commander would like you to park your ambulance and to whom you should report.

6. What information must you provide for the incoming helicopter?

Once the decision has been made that a patient will be transported by helicopter, keep in mind any special considerations or limitations that will be necessary prior to loading the patient. The patient may need to be immobilized on a specific type of backboard that fits into the helicopter. Smaller helicopters only accept a specific size board. Larger helicopters may actually be able to take an entire stretcher. Some helicopter services have limitations on the length of the patient when supine, which could alter your method of immobilizing a fractured femur because a standard bipolar splint may extend the leg too long to fit in the helicopter. Methods of infection control and intubations will also be affected by air transport. Some flight crews may also need to intubate the patient prior to flight due to the limited area around the airway once the patient is on board the aircraft.

7. How should paramedics approach the helicopter that has landed?

First, wait for the approval of the pilot. Use extreme caution and follow the instructions that were discussed in your orientation with the flight crew prior to any actual calls involving patients. Some general rules to follow are listed below.

- Make sure all loose objects are secured, such as pillows and linens on your stretcher.
- Allow the flight crew to direct the loading of the patient.
- Approach in a crouched down position, as a sudden gust of wind can cause the main rotor of a helicopter to dip to a point as close as 1.5 m from the ground.
- If the helicopter is parked on a slight incline, approach it from the downhill side.
- Keep all traffic and vehicles 30 m or more away from the helicopter.
- Do not allow anyone to smoke within 100 m of the aircraft.

Prep Kit

Ready for Review

- Provincial regulations set the standards for ambulance design and manufacturing specifications.
- Three body style types are identified:
  - Type I: Conventional, truck-cab chassis with a modular ambulance body that can be transferred to a new chassis as needed
  - Type II: Standard van, forward-control integral cab-body ambulance
  - Type III: Specialty van, forward-control integral cab-body ambulance
- Check the ambulance at the beginning of every shift to ensure that all equipment is available and in good working order.
- Every ambulance needs to be able to do four things: start, steer, stop, and stay running.
- Preventive maintenance is just as important as operating skills. Looking for problems before the unit is in motion may prevent breakdowns and accidents while en route to calls.
- Any specific exemption from traffic laws does not negate the paramedic's responsibility to proceed with due regard to prevent ambulance collisions.
- Escorts should not be used due to the danger of motorists not seeing both the ambulance and the escort.
- Lights and sirens should be used when responding to emergencies but used sparingly when transporting a patient to the hospital.
- Avoid backing up the vehicle if possible. If it is necessary, use a spotter to assist in the procedure. Make sure everyone is clear on where the unit is to be placed and that hand signals used are agreed upon.
- All drivers and passengers should use safety restraints while a vehicle is in motion.
- Air transport should be considered whenever time is of the essence for the best patient outcome.

Vital Vocabulary

belt noise A chirping or squealing sound, synchronous with engine speed.

brake fade A sensation that an ambulance has lost its power brakes.

brake pull A sensation that, when an operator depresses the brake pedal, the steering wheel is being pulled to the left or the right.

calibrated The diagnostic checking and synchronizing of digital or electronic equipment to ensure that is in good working order and will measure accurately.

drift A finding that when the operator lets go of the steering wheel, a vehicle consistently wanders left or right.

due regard Driving with awareness and responsibility for other drivers on the roadways when operating an ambulance in the emergency mode.

fractile response time A fraction (not average) of all emergency responses for the purpose of setting standards in response times.

landing zone Designated location for the landing of air ambulances.

peak loads A time of day or day of week in which the call volume is at its highest.

posting The placement of an ambulance at a specific geographic location in order to cover larger areas of territory and reduce response times.

specific exemptions Limited circumstances when an emergency vehicle operator can exceed the posted signage or speed limit.

steering play A sensation of looseness or sloppiness in a vehicle's steering.

steering pull A drift that is persistent enough so an operator can feel a tug on the steering wheel.

strategic deployment The staging of ambulances to strategic locations within a service area to allow for coverage of emergency calls.

Type I Ambulance Conventional, truck-cab chassis with a modular ambulance body that can be transferred to a new chassis as needed.

Type II Ambulance Standard van, forward-control integral cab-body ambulance.

Type III Ambulance Specialty van, forward-control integral cab-body ambulance.

wheel bounce A vibration, synchronous with road speed that can be felt in the steering wheel.

wheel wobble A common finding at low speeds when a vehicle has a bent wheel.

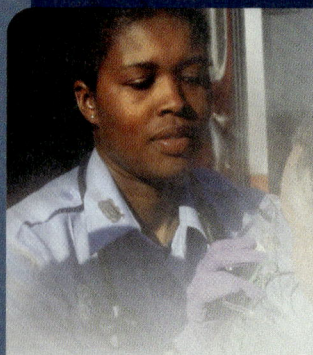

Assessment in Action

At the end of your shift you are dispatched to the scene of a vehicle that has crashed into a tree. When you arrive, you are approached by a firefighter who tells you that the patient "is in there pretty good" and there will be a delay in accessing the patient due to extrication. You see that there is heavy damage to the driver's side of the vehicle. A post is crushed to the ground and the steering wheel and dashboard are crushing the patient in the vehicle. The patient appears unresponsive and copious amounts of blood are coming from his head. You notice a compound fracture of his left femur with extensive bleeding. You and your partner decide to request a helicopter response due to the patient's condition and extended extrication time. After 15 minutes of extrication, you are able to free the patient from the vehicle. You secure the patient properly to a backboard and transfer him to the ambulance. While en route to the landing zone, you intubate him and start two large-bore IVs. When you arrive at the landing zone, the helicopter personnel are waiting for you.

1. **What is the advantage to using the helicopter for this patient?**
   A. Reduced transport time; it helps the patient receive definitive treatment within the golden hour.
   B. It is the end of your shift and you and your partner will be able to leave on time.
   C. You don't have to deal with an unstable patient for the next 20 minutes while driving the patient to the hospital.
   D. The fire department and other personnel want to practice their helicopter landing skills.

2. **A landing zone should be large enough to accommodate a rotary-winged aircraft of any size; standard dimensions are:**
   A. 30 × 15 m
   B. 45 × 30 m
   C. 30 × 30 m
   D. 15 × 30 m

3. **While intubating this patient, you need to suction blood out of the airway. You are unable to find your suction unit. At the beginning of every shift you should:**
   A. check the ambulance to ensure the proper equipment is both available and in good working order.
   B. make sure that there is enough fuel and then go get coffee.
   C. document what the previous crew has to say about supplies and equipment.
   D. start your personal work that needs to get done before anything else.

4. **Which of the following safety measures should be used when approaching the helicopter to load the patient?**
   A. Approach the helicopter as soon as it lands.
   B. At least eight people should help load the aircraft.
   C. The aircraft should be approached from the front.
   D. The aircraft should be approached from the rear.

5. **While you were driving your vehicle to the call, your steering wheel was jerking to the left. What could this be?**
   A. Brake pull
   B. Brake fade
   C. Drift
   D. Steering pull

6. **The four things that every ambulance needs to be able to do are:**
   A. start, steer, stall, and stop.
   B. start, steer, stop, and stay running.
   C. steer, stop, start, and stage.
   D. start, stop, steer, and speed.

7. **Routine ambulance equipment checks are essential so that:**
   A. accurate patient billing and reimbursement can occur in a timely manner.
   B. essential equipment is available and in working order when required for prehospital care.
   C. provincial laws and regulations can be met and licensure can be maintained.
   D. disciplinary action will not be necessary if equipment failure occurs.

Challenging Question

You are the newly appointed director of your paramedic unit. Your first course of action is to begin replacing your fleet with new ambulances. You've never done this before and are not sure what needs to be done.

8. **What do you refer to that will provide you with the essential information you need to know?**

Points to Ponder

You are dispatched to a department store for a seizure. You are responding with lights and sirens. You make a right-hand turn onto a busy roadway. As you are approaching an intersection that has a blinking yellow-red light, you notice that you have the blinking yellow. There is a vehicle on your left at a corner that has the red blinking light as well as a stop sign. The driver of the vehicle begins to drive, then stops. You are aware of what he is doing and slow down. As he stops, you begin to accelerate through the intersection. At the last moment, the vehicle at the stop sign accelerates, trying to turn in front of you. You realize that a collision is unavoidable. You see another car approaching on the opposite side of the road so you cannot maneuver into the other lane.

You turn your wheels slightly to the right and strike the vehicle in the passenger's side corner panel. Why?

Issues: Assessing Personal Safety Practices While Operating Your Emergency Vehicle, Serving as a Role Model for Others in the Operation of Emergency Vehicles.

Competency Areas

Area 1: Professional Responsibilities

1.3.c Include all pertinent and required information on ambulance call report forms.

1.5.a Work collaboratively with a partner.

1.5.c Work collaboratively with other emergency response agencies.

1.5.d Work collaboratively with other members of the health care team.

1.6.a Exhibit reasonable and prudent judgement.

1.6.b Practice effective problem-solving.

1.6.c Delegate tasks appropriately.

Area 2: Communication

2.2.a Record organized, accurate, and relevant patient information.

Area 3: Health and Safety

3.3.b Address potential occupational hazards.

3.3.e Conduct procedures and operations consistent with Workplace Hazardous Materials Information System (WHMIS) and hazardous materials management requirements.

Area 4: Assessment and Diagnostics

4.1.a Rapidly assess a scene based on the principles of a triage system.

4.1.b Assume different roles in a mass casualty incident.

4.1.c Manage a mass casualty incident.

Introduction

The most challenging situations you can be called to are disasters and mass-casualty incidents (MCIs). These incidents can be overwhelming because you will find a large number of patients and a lack of specialized equipment and/or adequate help. When you respond to an event with a large number of patients, you must use a systematic approach to manage the incident most efficiently. By learning to use the principles of the incident command system (ICS), you will be able to do the greatest good for the greatest number. As a paramedic, you will typically be assigned to work within the EMS/medical branch or group under an ICS, but you may be asked to function in other areas (which will be elabourated later in this chapter).

Disasters

Disasters overwhelm EMS and community resources because critical infrastructure has been damaged or destroyed **Figure 47-1 ▸**. Critical infrastructure includes the electrical power grid, communication systems, fuel for vehicles, water, sewage removal, food, hospitals, and transportation systems. Disaster management requires planners to take a broad look at preparedness, planning, training, response, and after-action review.

Mass-Casualty Incidents

A mass-casualty incident (MCI) is an event in which the number of patients exceeds the resources available to the initial responders **Figure 47-2 ▸**. Remember: a motor vehicle collision with several critical patients may be an MCI for a one-ambulance town. Although some EMS systems differentiate between MCIs and multiple-casualty incidents, in this chapter, either of these terms is considered an incident in which using the ICS will help paramedics work efficiently and effectively.

Your response to MCIs will differ depending on the area of land covered by the incident and the location and how spread out your patients are. You should be able to recognize an MCI as an open (uncontained) incident or a closed (contained) incident. An open incident has a number of casualties not yet located when you answer the initial call. Rescuers may have to

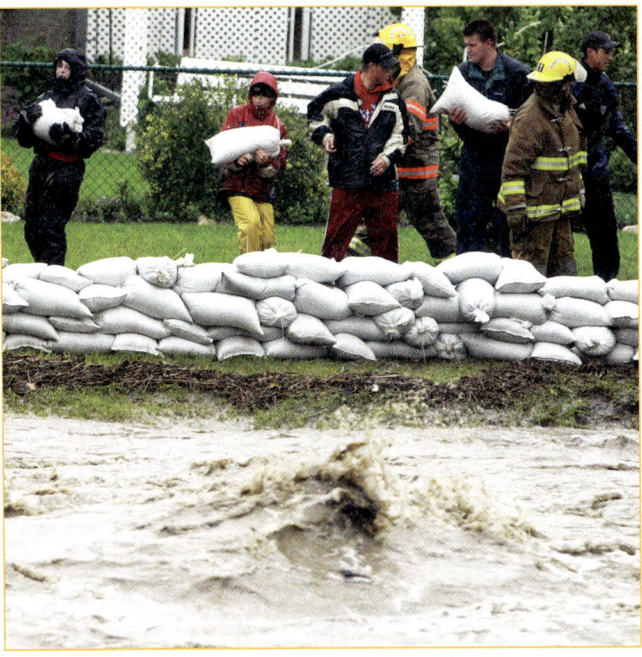

Figure 47-1 Disasters can overwhelm EMS resources and can damage critical infrastructure.

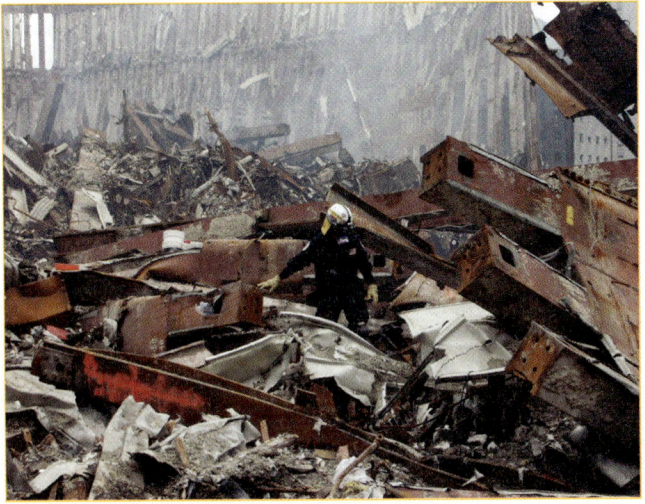

Figure 47-2 Mass-casualty incidents can be large, such as the attack on September 11, 2001, or can be much smaller in scope.

You are the Paramedic Part 1

You have been dispatched to the scene of a commercial plane down. You are the first responding rescue/EMS unit to arrive on the scene. There is no fire or other hazard noted initially. From inside the ambulance, you see approximately 30 to 40 victims walking or lying about the scene. As you arrive, 10 to 15 people approach your ambulance with cuts, bruises, and abrasions.

1. What is your plan of action?
2. Why is an incident command system (ICS) needed for handling major EMS incidents?
3. What is an "open" incident? What is a "closed" incident?

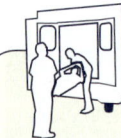

At the Scene

Table-top MCI exercises are a helpful way for paramedics to learn their roles at an MCI.

search for patients and then triage or treat them in multiple locations. There also may be an ongoing situation that produces more patients while you are at the scene, for example, school shootings, tornadoes, a hazardous materials release, or rising floodwaters.

A closed incident is a situation that is not expected to produce more patients than initially present. The patients can be triaged and treated as they are removed. Although a closed incident is often easier to handle, a closed incident may suddenly become an open incident.

Communities may establish different standards for what constitutes an MCI or for when to implement the ICS, but experience with previous MCIs is helpful in making the determination as well. Agencies and jurisdictions that regularly use the ICS will gain valuable experience and will be better prepared to respond to an MCI or a disaster. You can make significant contributions to the safety of your community by participating in disaster planning drills, table-top MCI exercises, and other ICS training opportunities.

At the Scene

The terminology used to describe an incident with multiple patients varies in different communities. Many communities use the term multiple-casualty incident to describe an emergency that involves more than one patient and the term mass-casualty incident to describe larger scale events, such as those with more than 20 patients. In this text, the term mass-casualty incident is used to describe any call that involves more than one patient or a situation that overwhelms your available resources.

The Incident Command System

It is important for you to be familiar with the terminology and concepts of the incident command system (ICS). As you know, communication is the building block of good prehospital care. Common terminology and the use of "clear text" communications (plain English as opposed to 10-codes) help responders from multiple agencies work efficiently together.

Using the ICS gives you a modular organizational structure that is built on the size and complexity of the incident. The goal of the ICS is to make the best use of your resources to manage the environment around the incident and to treat patients during an emergency. Make certain to follow your local standard operating procedures for establishing the ICS. The ICS is designed to control duplication of effort and

freelancing, in which individual units or different organizations make independent and often inefficient decisions about the next appropriate action.

One of the organizing principles of the ICS is limiting the span of control of any one individual, keeping the supervisor/worker ratio at one supervisor for three to seven workers. A supervisor who finds that his or her effective span of control is exceeded, that is, has more than seven people reporting to him or her—needs to divide tasks and delegate supervision of some tasks to another person.

Organizational divisions may include sections, branches, divisions and groups, and resources **Figure 47-3 ▸** . In some regions, emergency operations centres may exist. The centres are usually operated by city, province, or federal governments. These centres will usually only be activated in a large catastrophic event that may go on for days, that has hundreds of patients, and that taxes the whole system.

The individuals who will participate in the many tasks in an MCI or a disaster should use the ICS. You should find out from your service if one exists, who is in charge, how it is activated, and what your expected role will be.

ICS Roles and Responsibilities

There are many roles defined in the ICS. The general staff includes command, finance, logistics, operations, and planning. It is important for you to understand the specific duties of each and how they work in coordinating the response. Command functions include the public information officer (PIO), safety officer, and liaison officer.

Command

The incident commander (IC) is the person in charge of the overall incident. The IC will assess the incident, establish the strategic objectives and priorities, and develop a plan to manage the incident **Figure 47-4 ▸** . The number of command duties (public information, safety, and liaison) the IC takes on often varies by the size of the incident. Small incidents often mean the IC will do it all. In an incident of medium size or complexity, the IC may delegate some functions but retain others. For example, at a motor vehicle collision with multiple patients, the IC may designate a safety officer or assign a PIO but maintain responsibility for the other command functions. In a complex situation, the IC may appoint team members to all of the command roles.

Large MCIs, such as a hazardous materials incident, require a multiagency or multijurisdiction response and need to use a unified command system. In this case, plans are drawn up in advance by all cooperating agencies that assume a shared responsibility for decision making and cooperation. The response plan should designate the lead and support agencies in several kinds of MCIs. (The hazardous materials team will take the lead in a chemical leak, for example. However, the medical team might take the lead in a multivehicle car collision.) Agencies bordering each other should practice often with each other to ensure that a unified command system will

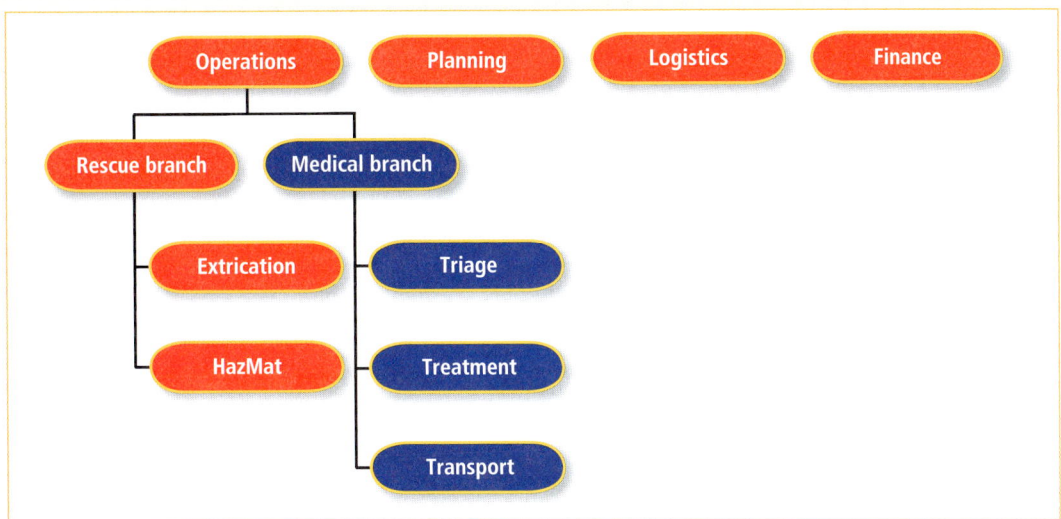

Figure 47-3 Incident command structure. Not all positions will be filled in every incident. However, the incident commander is ultimately responsible for all activity. Subordinates may be appointed to assist in managing the incident.

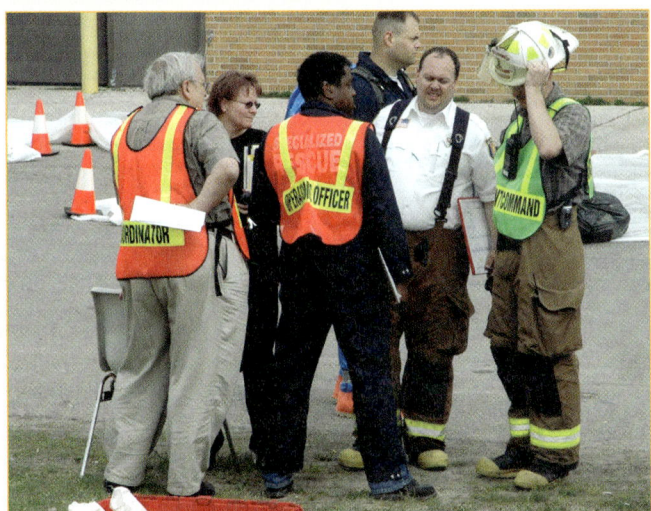

Figure 47-4 The person in command at an MCI oversees the incident and develops a plan for response.

will be reporting to a supervisor working under the IC. (Remember the rule of span of control? The number of people who can be effectively supervised is between three and seven.) To make the IC easily identifiable, some type of garment can be worn, such as a brightly coloured vest emblazoned with the word COMMAND. If the command post is set up in a vehicle, it should be well marked, and you should know its location. Make sure that your supervisor or the IC knows of any plans or operations before they are initiated.

This communication is particularly important if a transfer of command takes place. Because an MCI can be ever changing and ever increasing in scope, an IC may turn over command to someone with more experience in a critical area. This change, or transfer of command, must take place in an orderly manner and, if possible, face to face. In extreme situations, it could be done by phone, radio, or e-mail. Your agency should have standard operating procedures (SOPs) that govern the transfer of command. Make certain to follow those standard operating procedures. When an incident draws to a close, there should be a termination of command. Your agency should have demobilization procedures to implement as the situation de-escalates or comes to an end.

Finance

The finance officer is responsible for documenting all expenditures at an incident for tracking and reimbursement. A financial person is not usually needed at smaller incidents, but larger incidents or incidents that are longer in duration demand keeping track of personnel hours and expenditures for materials and supplies and reporting at meetings of the general staff. Responding agencies and organizations may be eligible for some types of reimbursement after the incident, and an efficient finance officer will help your agency to succeed in the reimbursement process. The finance officer should be trained in the process of assessing expenditures with an eye to reimbursement long before an actual event.

Logistics

The logistics section or section chief has responsibility for communications equipment, facilities, food and water, fuel, lighting, and medical equipment and supplies for patients and emergency responders. Local standard operating procedures will list the medical equipment needed for the incident,

function well and that communication among the people involved is well established before a real incident occurs.

A single command system is one in which one person is in charge, even if multiple agencies respond. It is generally used with incidents in which one agency has the majority of responsibility for incident management. Ideally, it is used for short duration, limited incidents that require the services of a single agency.

Your IC should be on or near the scene, where he or she can easily communicate with all emergency responders operating at the scene. It is important that you know who the IC is, where the command post is located, and how to communicate with your supervisor. If the incident is very large, you

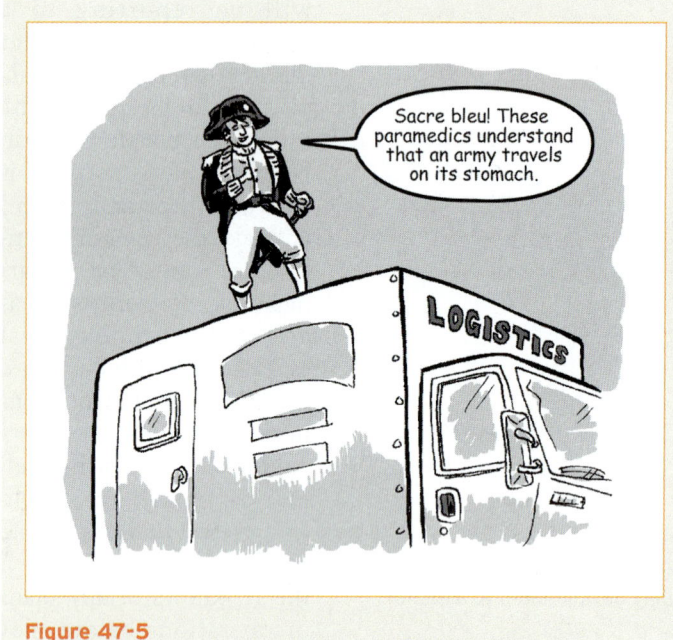

Figure 47-5

Table 47-1	MCI Equipment and Supplies*
Airway control	PPE (gloves, face shield, HEPA or N95 respirator) Oral airways, nasal airways Suction units (manual units) Rigid tip Yankauer and flexible suction catheters LMA, Combitube, ET tubes* Laryngoscope and blades* Tube check, tube restraint, tape, syringes, stylet* End-tidal CO_2 device
Breathing	Pocket mask and one-way valve Bag-valve-mask device(s) (adult and child), spare masks Oxygen delivery devices (nonrebreathing mask, cannula, extension tubing) Oxygen tank, regulator Occlusive dressings Large-bore IV cannula for thoracic decompression*
Circulation	Dressings, bandages, tape Sphygmomanometer, stethoscope Burn dressings, burn sheets, sterile water for irrigation One-handed tourniquets 1,000 ml bags of normal saline, IV start kits, cannulas*
Disability	Rigid collars (one size fits all) Head beds, wide tape, backboard straps Flashlights, spare batteries
Exposure	Space blanket to cover patients Scissors
Logistic/Command	Sector vests (triage, treatment, transport, staging, command, rescue) Pads of paper, pencils, pens, markers Triage tags or kits used by your regional system Assessment cards

Note: The items denoted by * could be packaged in an ALS kit.

depending on the type of incident. **Table 47-1 ▸** lists common MCI equipment and supplies. Logistics personnel are trained to find food, shelter, and health care for you and the other responders at the scene of an MCI **Figure 47-5 ▲**. In a large incident, it is often necessary for many people to handle logistics, even though only one person will report to the IC.

Operations

At a very large incident, the operations section is responsible for managing the tactical operations job usually handled by the IC on routine EMS calls. In a complex incident, however, the IC must coordinate with other agencies and the media, engage in strategic planning, and ensure that logistics are functioning effectively. In these cases, the IC should appoint an operations section chief. The operations section chief will supervise the

You are the Paramedic Part 2

As more units arrive on scene, you take on the role of triage officer. Patient 1 is bleeding from the nose.

Initial Assessment	Recording Time
Appearance	Pale, cool, dry skin
Level of consciousness	A (Alert to person, place, and day)
Airway	Open
Breathing	Adequate
Circulation	Pulse rapid, full, and regular

4. How should you triage this patient?
5. What is the difference between single and unified command?
6. What is "span of control"?

people working at the scene of the incident, who will be assigned to branches, divisions, and groups. Operations personnel often have experience in management within EMS.

Planning

The planning section solves problems as they arise during the MCI. Planners obtain data about the problem, analyze the previous incident plan, and predict what or who is needed to make the new plan work. Planners need to work closely with the operations, finance, and, especially logistics sections. Planners can and should call on technical experts to help with the planning process. Planners will also set out a course for demobilizing the response when needed.

Command Staff

Three important positions that help the general staff (all staff described previously) and the IC are the safety officer, the PIO, and the liaison officer. The safety officer monitors the scene for conditions that may present a hazard to responders and patients. The safety officer may need to work with environmental health and hazardous materials specialists. The importance of the safety officer cannot be underestimated—he or she has the authority to stop an emergency operation whenever a rescuer is in danger. A safety officer should remove hazards that could affect paramedics and patients before the hazards cause injury.

The public information officer (PIO) provides the public and media with clear and understandable information. A wise PIO will be positioned well away from the incident command post and, most important, away from the incident, to minimize distractions. Also, the PIO must keep the media safe and from becoming part of the incident. The designated PIO may work in cooperation with PIOs from other agencies in a joint information centre (JIC). In some circumstances, the PIO/JIC may be responsible for disseminating a message designed to help a situation, prevent panic, and provide evacuation directions.

The liaison officer (LNO) relays information and concerns among command, the general staff, and other agencies. If an agency is not represented in the command structure, questions and input should be given through the LNO.

▌EMS Response Within the ICS

Preparedness

Preparedness involves the decisions made and basic planning done before an incident occurs. Some parts of every country are prone to natural disasters, such as hurricanes, tornadoes, earthquakes, or wildfires. Therefore, preparedness in a given area would involve decisions and planning about the most likely natural disasters for the area, among other disasters.

Your EMS agency should have written disaster plans that you are regularly trained to carry out. A copy of the disaster plan should be kept in each EMS vehicle. EMS facilities should have disaster supplies so they are self-sufficient for at least the

first 72 hours. Your EMS service should have mutual aid agreements with surrounding organizations so that requests for help can be expedited in an emergency. All groups with mutual aid agreements should practice using the plans frequently. Organizations should share a list of resources with each other so they will know early on what they can access. Also, your local EMS organizations should develop an assistance program for the families of EMS responders. If EMS responders have concerns about their families during a disaster, their effectiveness on the job could be diminished.

Of course, you should have a personal disaster plan for your family. Families need to be prepared and know what to expect should you be required to be a disaster responder. You *are* up-to-date on immunizations for influenza, hepatitis A and B, and tetanus, aren't you?

Scene Assessment

You remember that assessing a scene starts with dispatch. If dispatch information indicates a possible unsafe scene, you should stay away from the scene or get only close enough to make an assessment without putting yourself in harm's way. When you arrive first on the scene of an MCI, you will make an initial assessment and some preliminary decisions. The assessment will be driven by three basic questions that responders must ask themselves:

- *What do I have?*
- *What do I need to do?*
- *What resources do I need?*

These questions have a symbiotic relationship. The answer from one helps answer the others, and each represents a piece to the puzzle. Work as team when you answer these questions because missing just one safety issue early on can start a chain of problems.

What Do I Have?

Any call starts with scene safety, and you need to assess for hazards. Warn all other responders about hazardous materials, fuel spills, electrical hazards, or other safety concerns as soon as possible. Confirm the incident location. Establish whether the incident is open or closed. Estimate the number of casualties. Your immediate report to dispatch would be "Paramedic unit number one arriving on scene, multiple vehicles involved, full road blockage, no apparent hazards at this time, paramedic unit number one is assuming command."

What Do I Need to Do?

You should keep the following priorities in mind:

- Safety
- Incident stabilization
- Preservation of property and the environment

You need to consider these priorities in the order they are given. Safety is paramount. Safety includes your life, your partner's life, and other rescuers' lives. Then, consider the safety of the patient and any bystanders. This will be difficult for anyone dedicated to saving lives, but it is important to put yourself and your partner first—you have the skills, and bystanders usually don't;

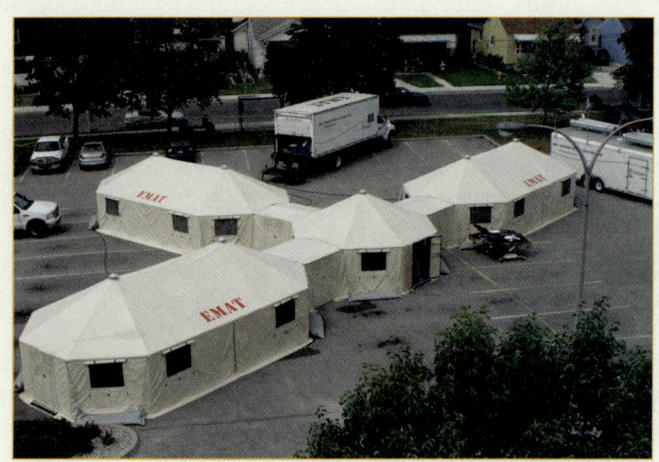

Figure 47-6 This mobile health care facility is staffed by paramedics, nurses, physicians, and other allied health care providers who are able to provide surge capacity and advanced life support.

Communications

Communications is often the key problem at an MCI or a disaster. The infrastructure can be damaged, or communications capabilities can be overwhelmed. If possible, use face-to-face communications to limit radio traffic. Some organizations responding to a disaster might not know how to use a radio, and if you do use it, don't use codes or signals. Most communications problems should be worked out before a disaster happens by designating channels strictly for command during a disaster. Whatever form of communications equipment is used, it is imperative that it is reliable, durable, field-tested, and that there are backups in place if the primary communications system does not work. Some regions have mobile self-contained communications centres, whereas others use local radio groups such as HAM radio operators to assist with communications. Most important, your plan should include a "Plan B" in case of communications failure.

the situation can be far worse if you do not put yourself first. Often, if a responder is injured, other responders will focus on "their own," removing more available resources. You may have to initially work to isolate or stabilize the incident before providing prehospital care to injured persons, another difficult concept.

What Do I Need?

Decide what resources are needed. You may need more paramedics, ambulances, or other forms of transportation. If extrication is required, a rescue unit and fire department response may be needed. If there are hazardous materials, get a hazardous materials team immediately. Many large EMS systems deploy specialized MCI units or mobile emergency room vehicles that are able to treat dozens of patients on the scene **Figure 47-6 ▲** .

Establishing Command

Once you have performed a good scene assessment and answered the three basic questions, command should be established, notification to other responders should go out, and necessary resources should be requested. A command system ensures that resources are effectively and efficiently coordinated. Command must be established early, preferably by the first-arriving, most experienced public safety official. These officials may include police, fire, or paramedics and local government officials.

At the Scene

Participating in a simulated table-top mass-casualty incident can help the paramedic better understand how command is established, how the scene is assessed, how scene objectives are determined, how an incident plan is created, how resources are requested, when ICS needs to expand, how communication is coordinated, and how EMS works with other agencies during a large emergency.

■ Medical Incident Command

What has traditionally been referred to as medical incident command is also known as the medical (or EMS) branch of the ICS **Figure 47-7 ▸** . At incidents that have a significant medical factor, the IC should appoint someone as the medical group or branch leader. This person will supervise the primary roles of the medical group—triage, treatment, and transport of the injured. The medical group leader should help ensure that EMS units responding to the scene are working within the ICS, each medical unit receives a clear assignment before beginning work at the scene, and personnel remain with their vehicle in the staging area until they are assigned their duties. **Figure 47-8 ▸** shows a diagram of an MCI with these areas.

Triage Unit

The triage officer is ultimately in charge of counting and prioritizing patients. During large incidents, a number of triage personnel may be needed. The primary duty of the triage unit is to ensure that every patient receives initial assessment of his or her condition. Paramedics doing triage will help move patients to the appropriate treatment sector. One of the most difficult parts of being a triage officer is that you must not begin treatment until all patients are triaged, or you will compromise your triage efforts.

Treatment Officer

The treatment officer will locate and set up the treatment area with a tier for each priority of patient. Treatment officers ensure that secondary triage of patients is performed and that adequate prehospital care is given as resources allow. Treatment

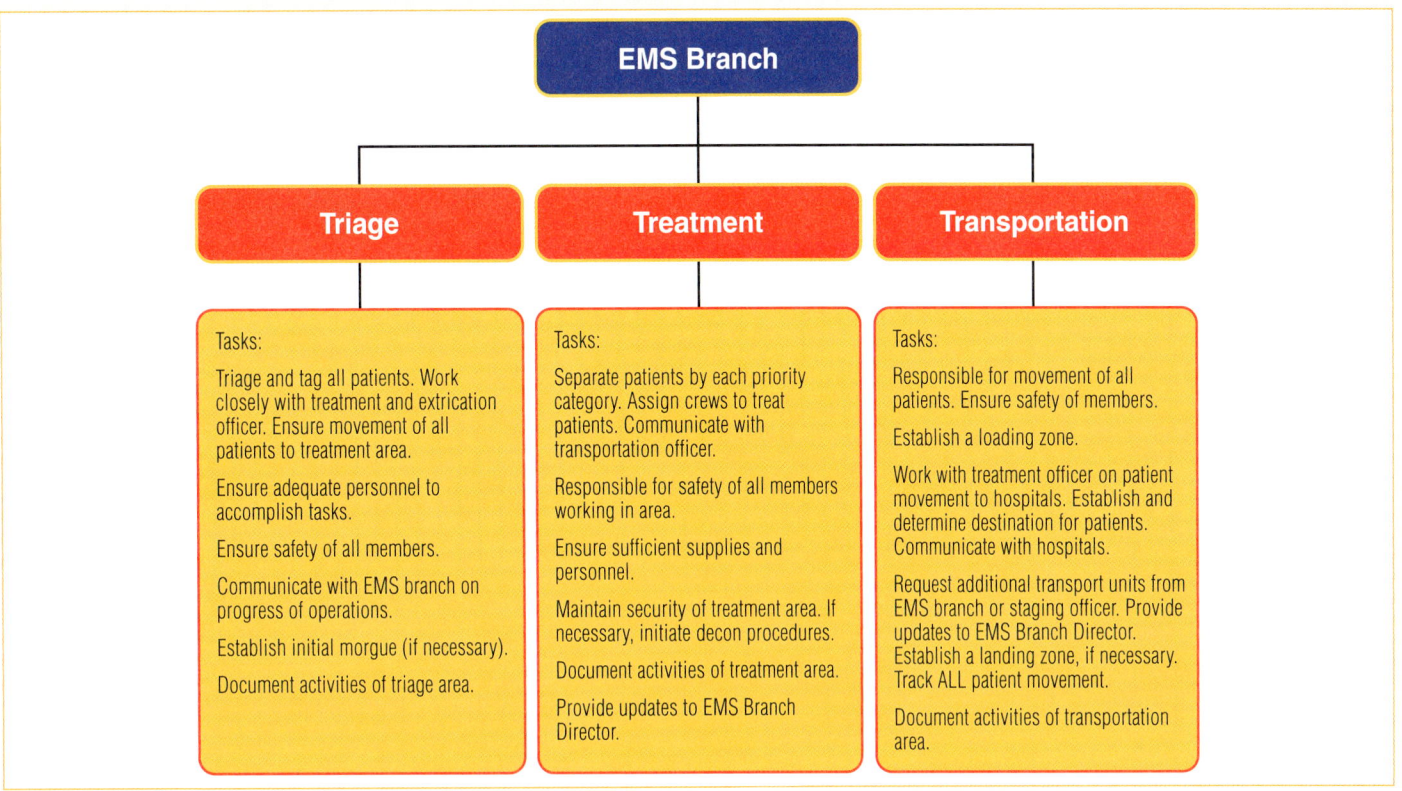

Figure 47-7 Components of the EMS branch within the incident command system.

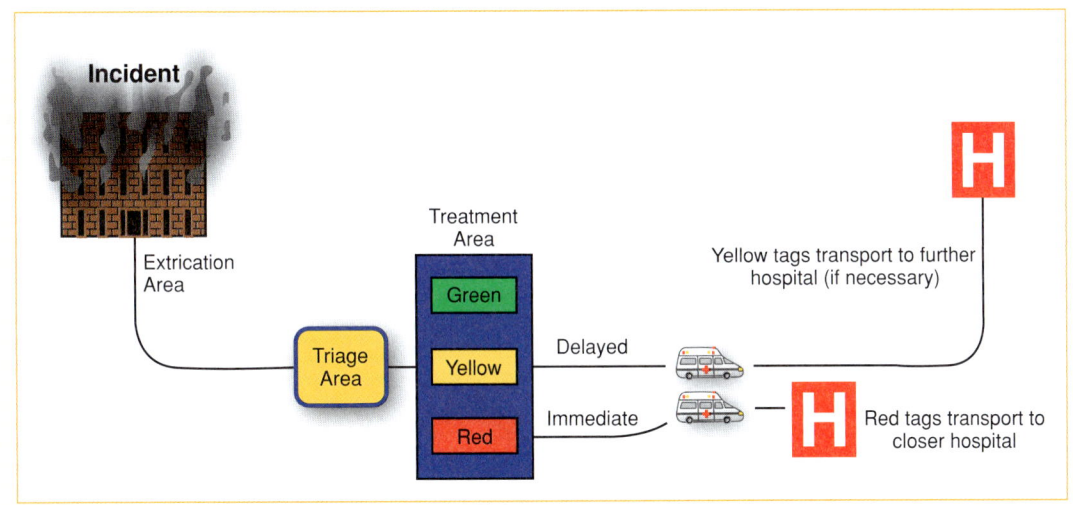

Figure 47-8 Diagram of an MCI. The ICS established at the scene of a building fire may look similar to this diagram.

Transportation Officer

The transportation officer coordinates the transportation and distribution of patients to appropriate receiving hospitals. Transportation requires coordination with incident command to help ensure that enough personnel and ambulances are in the staging area or have been requested. A key role of the transportation officer is to communicate with the area hospitals to help determine where to transport the patients. Some regions may have planned for a designated hospital within a region to perform the coordination between hospitals on destination decisions. An MCI typically disrupts the everyday functioning of the region's trauma system, so good coordination is needed. The transportation officer documents and tracks the number of vehicles transporting, patients transported, and the facility destination of each vehicle and patient.

officers also have a responsibility to assist with moving patients to the transportation area. As treatment officers supervise the responders, they must communicate with the medical group leaders to request sufficient quantities of supplies, including bandages, burn supplies, airway and respiratory supplies, and patient packaging equipment.

Staging Officer

A staging officer should be assigned when MCIs or scenes require response by numerous emergency vehicles or agencies. The vehicles cannot and should not drive into the scene of the MCI without direction from the staging officer. The staging area should be established away from the scene because the parked vehicles can be in the way. The staging officer locates an area to stage equipment and responders, tracks unit arrivals, and sends out vehicles as needed. This position plans for efficient access and exit from the disaster site and prevents traffic congestion among responding vehicles. The staging officer releases vehicles and supplies when ordered by command.

Physicians On Scene

In an MCI, some areas have plans in place for physicians on scene. Sometimes, even without a plan, the enormity of the situation may require that physicians be sent to the scene. Emergency physicians, especially, will have the ability to make difficult triage decisions. They also provide secondary triage decisions in the treatment sector, deciding which priority patients are to be transported first. Physicians can provide on-scene medical direction for paramedics, and they can provide care in the treatment sector as appropriate. Physicians who are deployed to any emergency event *must* have incident command, scene management, and scene safety training.

Rehabilitation Officer

In disasters or situations that will last for extended periods, a rehabilitation section for the responders should be established. The rehabilitation officer should establish an area that provides protection for responders from the elements and the situation. The rehabilitation area should be located away from exhaust fumes and crowds (especially members of the media) and out of view of the scene itself. Rehabilitation is where a responder's needs for rest, fluids, food, and protection from the elements are met **Figure 47-9 ▶**. The rehabilitation officer must also monitor responders for signs of stress. These signs may include

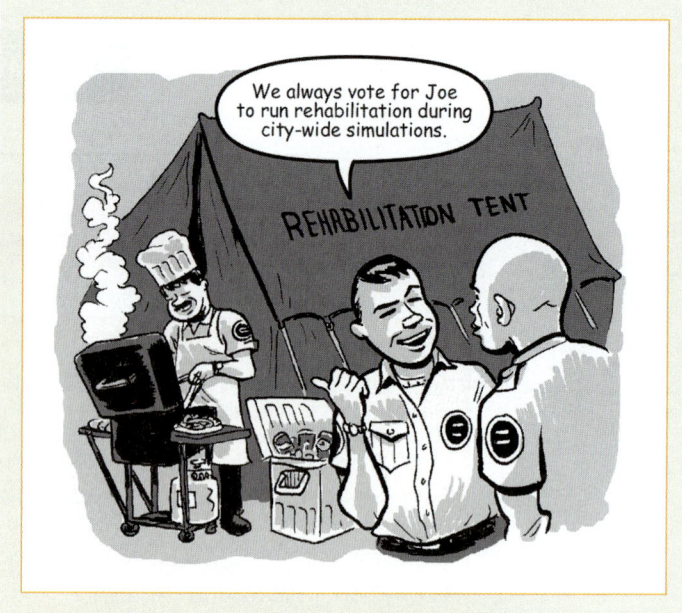

Figure 47-9

fatigue, altered thinking patterns, and complete collapse. You should remember that all EMS personnel should be responsible to be aware of signs of stress. Your service might consider having a defusing or debriefing team in this area. Responders should be encouraged to take advantage of these services but should never be forced to participate.

Extrication and Special Rescue

Some disasters require search and rescue or extrication of patients **Figure 47-10 ▶**. An extrication officer or rescue officer may need to be appointed. These officers determine the type of equipment and resources needed for the situation. In some incidents, victims may need to be extricated or rescued before they can be triaged and treated. Because extrication and rescue are medically complex, the officers will usually function under the EMS branch of the ICS. The extrication and rescue

You are the Paramedic Part 3

A teenage boy is supine and unconscious. You find a nonsucking puncture wound in his chest.

Initial Assessment	Recording Time
Appearance	Pale, cool, moist skin
Level of consciousness	P (Responsive to painful stimuli)
Airway	Open
Breathing	Rapid, shallow, laboured
Circulation	Radial pulse is rapid, weak, and regular

7. How should you triage this patient?
8. Why is there an essential need for common terminology in an ICS?

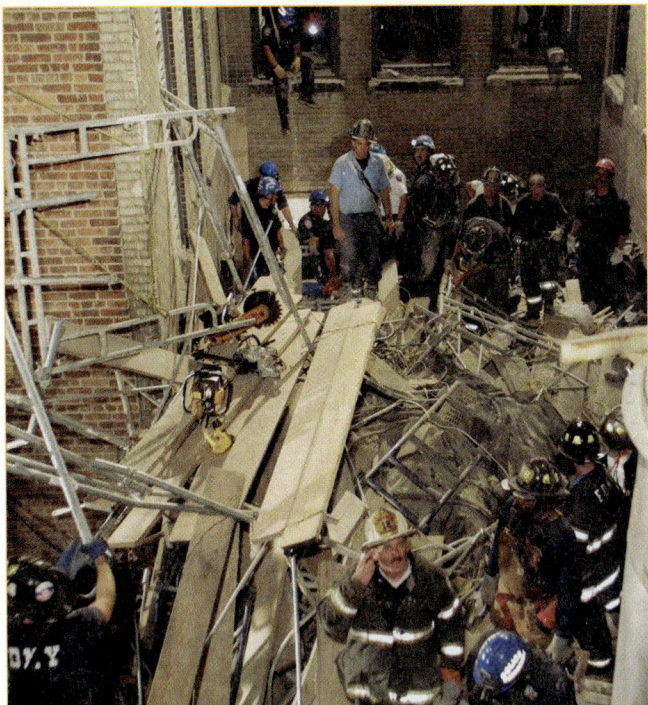

Figure 47-10 Some disasters will involve search and rescue or extrication.

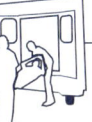

At the Scene

MCIs and disasters take a physical and emotional toll on emergency responders. Make certain that you are medically evaluated if you have been injured, come into contact with any hazardous substance, or inhale any dust, fumes, or smoke. Often, the health effects of such exposures do not manifest for years and are difficult to link to a particular event. Also, be aware of signs of stress in yourself and in your colleagues. Take full advantage of the opportunity for stress debriefing after an incident.

officers identify the special equipment and personnel needed for the rescue. Extrication and rescue can be dangerous, so crew safety is of utmost importance.

Morgue Officer

In some disasters, there will be many dead patients. The morgue officer will work with local medical examiners, coroners, disaster mortuary assistance teams, and law enforcement agencies to coordinate removal of the bodies and even, possibly, body parts. The morgue officer should attempt to leave the dead victims in the location found, if possible, until a removal and storage plan can be determined. The location of victims may help in the identification of the dead victims in mass-fatality situations, or there may be crime scene considerations. If it is determined that a morgue area is needed,

the morgue officer should ensure that the morgue is out of view of the living patients and other responders because the psychological impact could worsen the situation and that the morgue is secure from the public to prevent theft of any personal effects of the dead victims.

Triage

Triage simply means "to sort" your patients based on the severity of their injuries Figure 47-11 ▼ . The goal of doing the greatest good for the greatest number means that the triage assessment is brief and the patient condition categories are basic. Primary triage is the initial triage done in the prehospital environment, whereas secondary triage is done as patients are brought to the treatment area. During primary triage, patients are briefly assessed and then identified in some way, such as by attaching a triage tag. The main information needed on the tag is a unique number and a triage category. Rapid and accurate triage will help bring order to the chaos of the MCI scene. After the primary triage, the team leader should communicate the following information to the medical group leader.

- The total number of patients
- The number of patients in each of the triage categories
- Recommendations for extrication and movement of patients to the treatment area
- Resources needed to complete triage and begin movement of patients

Triage Categories

There are four common triage categories. They can be remembered using the mnemonic IDME, which stands for Immediate (red), Delayed (yellow), Minimal (green; hold), and Expectant (black; likely to die or dead) Table 47-2 ▶ . This is the order of priority for treatment and transport of the patients at an MCI.

Immediate (red-tag) patients are your first priority. They will need immediate prehospital care and transport.

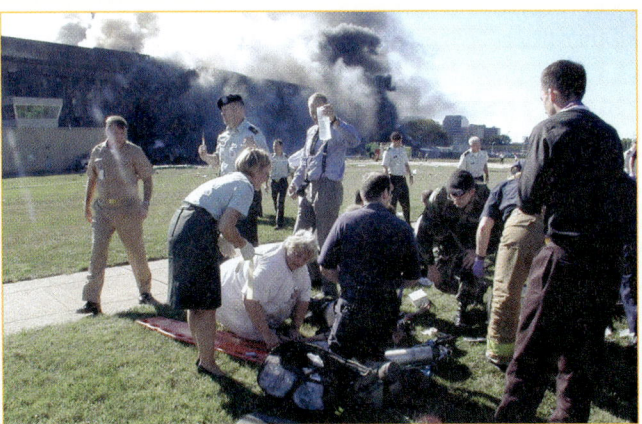

Figure 47-11 Triage is the process of sorting and prioritizing patients based on severity of conditions.

Table 47-2	Triage Priorities	
Triage Category	**Typical Injuries**

Red Tag: First Priority (immediate)
   Patients who need immediate prehospital care and transport.
   Treat these patients first, and transport as soon as possible.
	• Airway and breathing difficulties
	• Uncontrolled or severe bleeding
	• Severe medical problems
	• Signs of shock (hypoperfusion)
	• Severe burns
	• Open chest or abdominal injuries

Yellow Tag: Second Priority (delayed)
   Patients whose treatment and transport can
   be temporarily delayed.
	• Burns without airway problems
	• Major or multiple bone or joint injuries
	• Back injuries with or without spinal cord damage

Green Tag: Third Priority (walking wounded)
   Patients who require minimal or no treatment and
   transportation can be delayed until last.
	• Minor fractures
	• Minor soft-tissue injuries

Black Tag: Fourth Priority (expectant)
   Patients who are already dead or have little chance
   for survival. Treat salvageable patients before
   treating these patients.
	• Obvious death
	• Obviously nonsurvivable injury, such as major open brain trauma
	• Respiratory arrest (if limited resources)
	• Cardiac arrest

They usually have problems with the ABCs, head trauma, or signs and symptoms of shock.

Delayed (yellow-tag) patients are the second priority and will need treatment and transport, but it can be delayed. Patients usually have multiple injuries to bones or joints, including back injuries with or without spinal cord injury.

Minimal (green-tag) patients are the third priority. Patients may require no prehospital or only "minimal" treatment. In some parts of the world, this is the hold category. These patients are the "walking wounded" at the scene. If they have any apparent injuries, they are usually soft-tissue injuries such as contusions, abrasions, and lacerations.

The last priority is the expectant (black-tag) patients who are dead or whose injuries are so severe that they have, at best, a minimal chance of survival. This category may include patients who are in cardiac arrest or who have an open head injury, for example. If you have limited resources, this category may also include patients in respiratory arrest. Patients in this category receive treatment and transport only after patients in the other three categories have received prehospital care.

Triage Tags

Whatever triage system is used, it is vital that a patient has a tag or some type of label. Tagging patients early assists in tracking them and can help keep an accurate record of their condition. Triage tags should be weatherproof and easily read **Figure 47-12** ▸ . The patient tags or tape should be colour-coded and should clearly show the category of the patients. The use of symbols and colours to indicate the triage categories is important in case some rescuers are colour blind.

The tags will become part of the patient's medical record. Most have a tear-off receipt with a number correlating with the number on the tag. When torn off by the transportation officer, it will assist him or her in tracking a patient. If the patient is unconscious and cannot be identified at the scene, the tag will be an identifier for tracking purposes. Some areas use digital photography of patients to assist in later identification. The photo is catalogued with the patient's tag number, and the patient's location is tracked with this. When family members are brought to crisis centres to help locate loved ones, the pictures may be of assistance. This technique has been used quite effectively in Europe and Israel with Polaroid and digital pictures. Another way of tracking and accounting for patients is to only issue 20 to 25 cards or tags at a time with a score card to mark how patients are triaged and their priority. When the medic returns for more tags, the scorecard will assist command to count the number of patients and assist command and the staff in developing a plan to respond and ensuring that appropriate resources are available

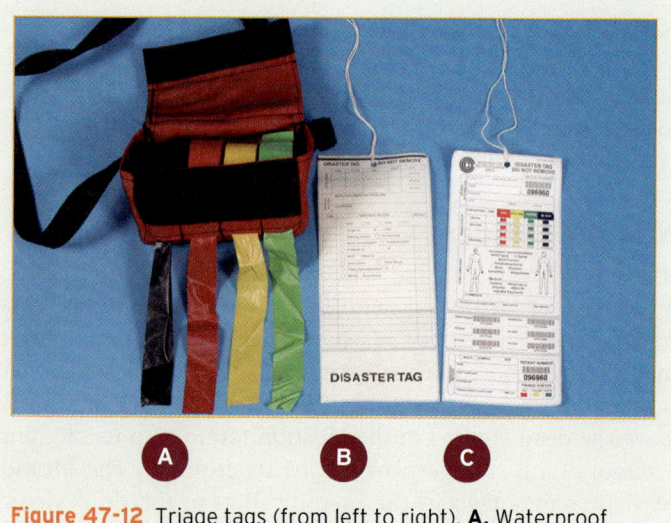

Figure 47-12 Triage tags (from left to right). **A.** Waterproof coloured tape. **B.** Back of triage tag. **C.** Front of triage tag.

or summoned. Whatever labeling system is used, it is imperative for the transportation officer to be able to identify which patient went by which unit and to which destination, as well as the priority of the patient's condition.

START Triage

START triage is one of the easiest methods of triage. START stands for Simple Triage And Rapid Treatment. The staff members at Hoag Memorial Hospital, Newport Beach, California, are responsible for developing this method of triage. It is easily mastered with practice and will give you the ability to rapidly categorize patients at an MCI. START triage uses a limited assessment of the patient's ability to walk, respiratory status, hemodynamic status, and neurologic status.

The first step of the START triage system is performed on arrival at the scene by calling out to the disaster site, "If you can hear my voice and are able to walk . . ." and then directing patients to an easily identifiable landmark. The injured persons in this group are the "walking wounded" and are considered minimal priority, or third-priority patients.

The second step in the START process is directed toward nonwalking patients. You move to the first nonambulatory patient and assess the respiratory status. If the patient is not breathing, you should open the airway by using a simple manual maneuver. A patient who still does not begin to breathe is triaged as expectant (black). If the patient begins to breathe, tag him or her as immediate (red) and place in the recovery position and move on to the next patient.

If the patient is breathing, a quick estimation of the respiratory rate should be made. A patient who is breathing faster than 30 breaths per minute is triaged as an immediate priority (red). If the patient is breathing fewer than 30 breaths/min, move to the next step of the assessment.

The next step is to assess the hemodynamic status of the patient by checking for a radial pulse. An absent radial pulse implies the patient is hypotensive and should be triaged as an immediate priority. If the radial pulse is present, go to the next assessment.

The final assessment in START triage is to assess the patient's neurologic status, which simply means to assess the patient's ability to follow simple commands such as, "show me three fingers." This assessment establishes that the patient can understand and follow commands. A patient who is unconscious or cannot follow simple commands is an immediate priority patient. A patient who complies with a simple command should be triaged in the delayed category. The START system is shown in **Figure 47-13 ▶**.

JumpSTART Triage for Pediatric Patients

Lou Romig, MD, recognized that the START triage system does not take into account the physiologic and developmental differences of pediatric patients. She developed the JumpSTART triage system for pediatric patients. JumpSTART is intended for use in children younger than 8 years or who appear to weigh less than 45 kg. As in START, the JumpSTART system begins by identifying the walking wounded. Infants or children not developed enough to walk or follow commands (including children with special needs) should be taken as soon as possible to the treatment sector for immediate secondary triage. This action assists in getting children who cannot take care of their own basic needs into a caregiver's hands. There are several differences within the respiratory status assessment compared with that in START. First, if you find that a pediatric patient is not breathing, immediately check the pulse. If there is no pulse, label the patient as expectant. If the patient is not breathing but has a pulse, open the airway with a manual maneuver. If the patient does not begin to breathe, give five rescue breaths and check respirations again. A child who does not begin to breathe should be labeled expectant. The primary reason for this difference is that the most common cause of cardiac arrest in children is respiratory arrest.

You are the Paramedic Part 4

A man has a 50-cm long steel rod from the aircraft impaled in his thigh. There is minor bleeding from the wound; however, there is no apparent fracture.

Initial Assessment	Recording Time
Appearance	Pale, cool, dry skin
Level of consciousness	A (Alert to person, place, and day); feels pain
Airway	Open
Breathing	Rapid and deep
Circulation	Radial pulses are fast and regular

9. How should you triage this patient?

10. What is START?

11. What is the value of using triage tags?

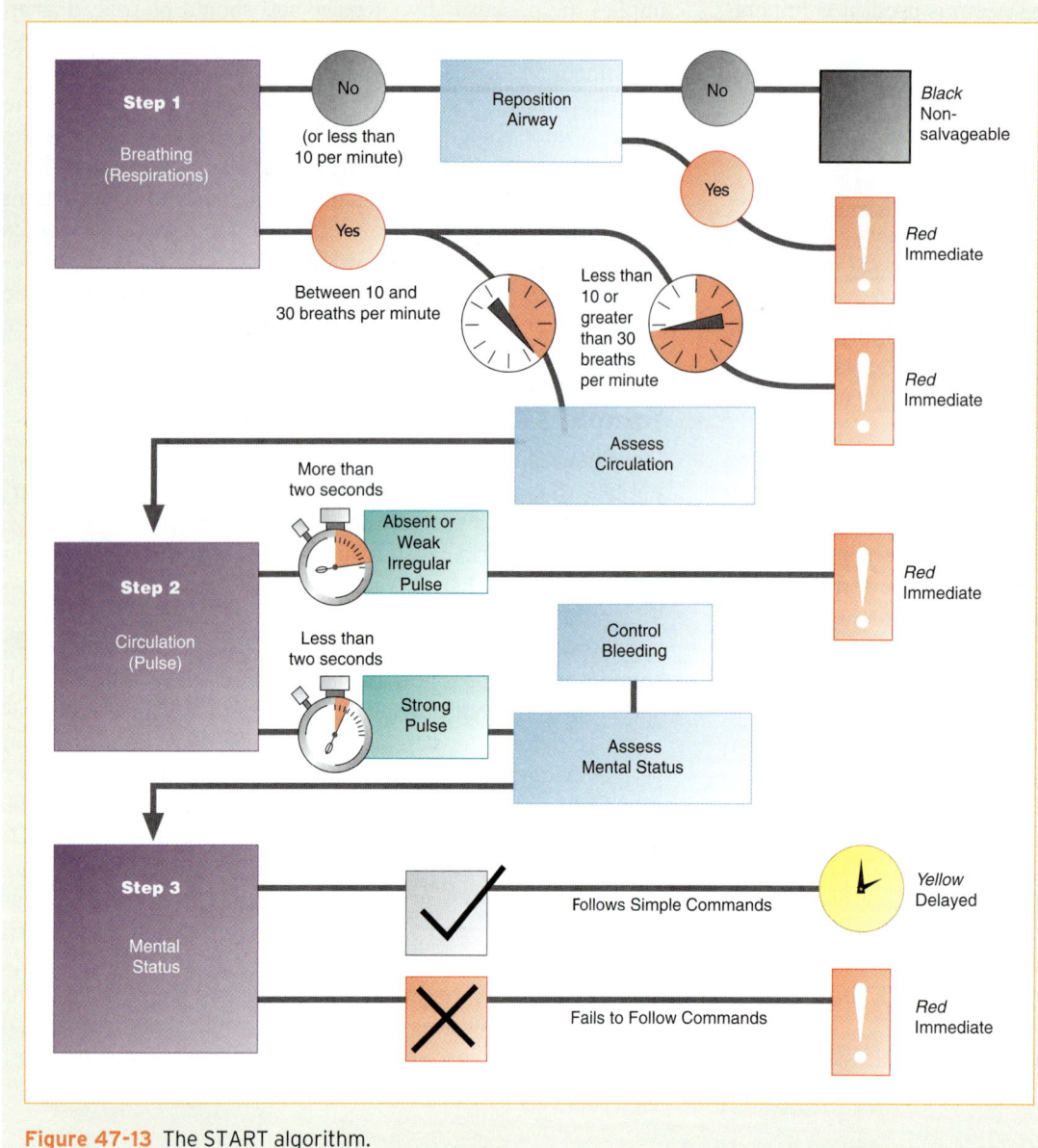

Figure 47-13 The START algorithm.

will vary. For JumpSTART, a modified AVPU score is used. A child who is unresponsive or responds to pain by posturing or with incomprehensible sounds or is unable to localize pain is considered an immediate priority and tagged as such. A child who responds to pain by localizing it or withdrawing from it or is alert is considered a delayed priority patient. The JumpSTART system is shown in **Figure 47-14 ▶**.

Triage Special Considerations

There are a few special situations in triage. Patients who are hysterical and disruptive to rescue efforts may need to be made an immediate priority and transported out of the disaster site, even if they are not seriously injured. Panic breeds panic, and this type of behaviour could have a detrimental impact on other patients and on the rescuers.

A rescuer who becomes sick or injured during the rescue effort should be handled as an immediate priority and be transported off the site as soon as possible to avoid negative impact to the morale of remaining rescuers.

Hazardous materials and weapons of mass destruction incidents force the hazardous materials team to identify patients as contaminated or noncontaminated before the regular triage process. Contamination by chemicals or biological weapons in a treatment area, a hospital, or trauma centre could obstruct all systems and organizations coping with the MCI. Bear in mind that some incidents may require multiple triage areas or teams because the victims are located far apart.

Transportation of Patients

All patients triaged as immediate (red) or delayed (yellow) should preferably be transported by ambulance. In extremely large situations, a bus may transport the walking wounded. If a bus is used for walking wounded patients, it is strongly

The next step of the JumpSTART process is to assess the approximate rate of respirations. A patient who is breathing less than 15 breaths/min or more than 45 breaths/min is tagged as immediate priority, and you move on to the next patient. If the respirations are within the range of 15 to 45 breaths/min, the patient is assessed further.

The next assessment in JumpSTART triage is also the hemodynamic status of the patient. Just like in START, you are simply checking for a distal pulse. This does not need to be the brachial pulse; assess the pulse that you feel the most competent and comfortable checking. If there is an absence of a distal pulse, label the child as an immediate priority and move to the next patient. If the child has a distal pulse, move on to the next assessment.

The final assessment is for neurologic status. Because of the developmental differences in children, their responses

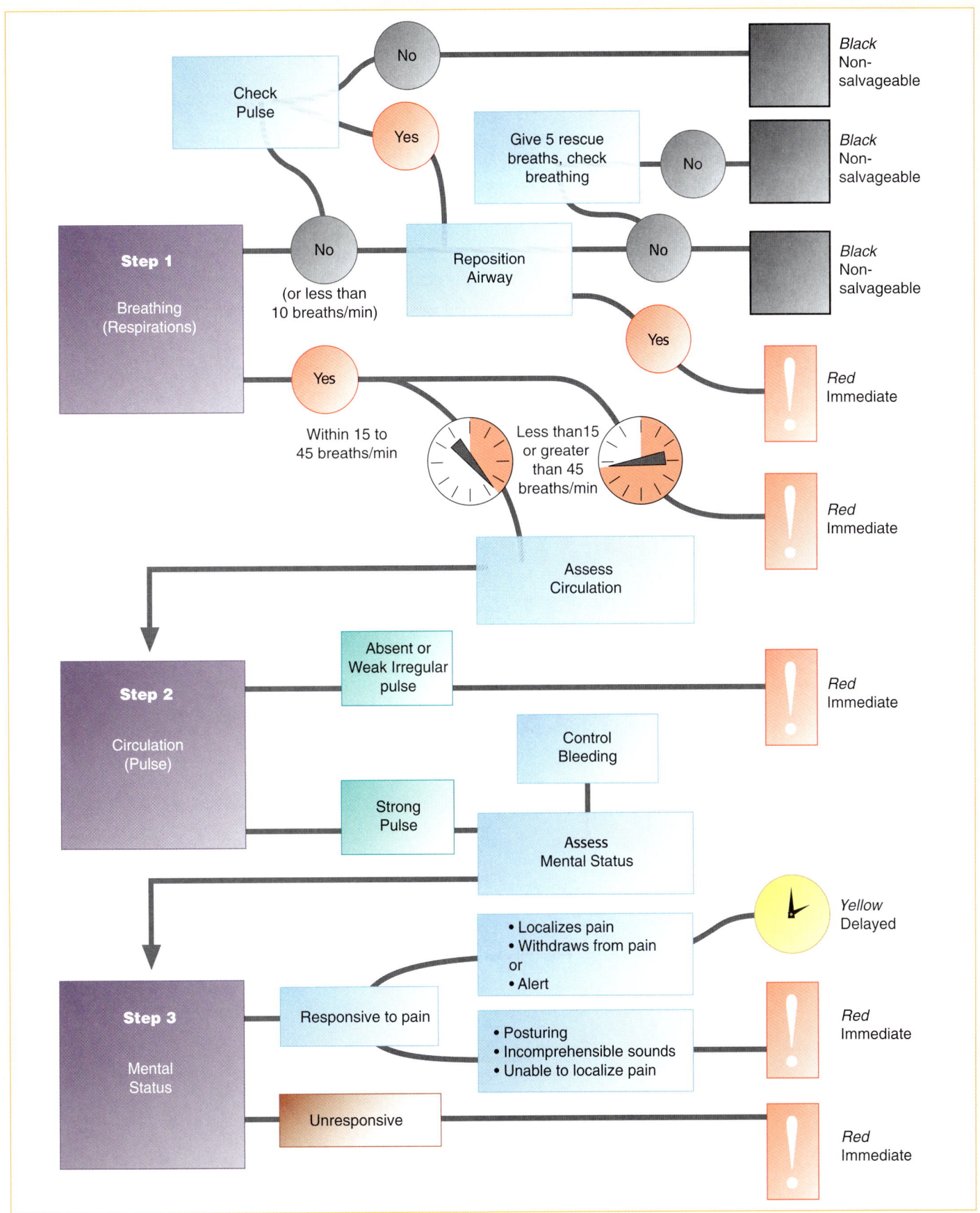

Figure 47-14 The JumpSTART algorithm.

suggested that they be transported to a hospital or clinic distant from the MCI or disaster site to avoid overwhelming the local area hospital resources. It is advisable when using a bus to plan for at least one first responder (FR) or paramedic to ride on the bus and to have an ambulance follow the bus. If a walking wounded patient's condition worsens, the patient could be moved to the ambulance and transported to a closer facility. The paramedic can stay with the patients triaged as needing minimal prehospital care until their arrival at the designated hospital. Any worsening of a patient's condition must be relayed to the receiving hospital as soon as possible in whatever manner the incident dictates.

Immediate priority patients should be transported two at a time until all are transported from the site. Then patients in the delayed category can be transported two or three at a time until all are at a hospital. Finally, the walking wounded are transported. Expectant patients who are still alive would receive treatment and transport at this time. Dead victims are handled or transported according to the standing operating procedure for the area.

Critical Incident Stress Management

Responders at a disaster or an MCI may become overwhelmed. Critical incident stress management should be available and spoken about to all responders and should start within the rehabilitation sector. All responders are encouraged to participate, but stress management should not be imposed or forced. Forcing stress management can do more harm than good to the psychological well-being of rescuers. Some rescuers have a preference for and personal support to recover from these situations alone.

After-Action Reviews

After any incident, an after-action review should be done. All agencies involved in the response should participate in the effort to improve future reactions to disasters. If something worked well in the plan, keep it. If something did not work at all, remove it or fix it.

No response is ever perfect, but it is up to all participants to keep perfecting their training, equipment, plans, and skills. Leaders in EMS suggest that all observations should be noted, in writing if possible, to allow future review. Discourage all finger pointing, which is not problem solving. All MCIs are different, and the way you react to each of them will be different, too.

Conclusion

No paramedic ever wants the "Big One" to happen. These events can happen anywhere and at anytime. They can overwhelm EMS systems with huge demands on materials and people, and people can be affected physically and psychologically. By keeping the basic goal of "doing the most good for the most patients" in the forefront, developing plans, using the ICS, and applying a systematic approach to triage, even an MCI can be handled effectively. By practicing plans often or on everyday smaller-scale incidents, they will become instinctive, which will help you use them in larger incidents.

You are the Paramedic Summary

1. What is your plan of action?

Tag them green, and designate an area for them to be placed.

2. Why is an incident command system (ICS) needed for handling major EMS incidents?

Any incident that involves multiple units responding to an incident requires management of the resources and personnel for a timely and efficient operation. When multiple agencies, especially from different jurisdictions, are involved, it is even more urgent that a system be in place to manage the incident and coordinate the response. Paramedics are trained to manage a single patient with multiple priorities. This is practiced on a daily basis. When a situation arises in which multiple patients must be managed and multiple units are responding (not a daily practice), there must be an ICS that is simple and well understood by all providers. Each community needs to have an ICS that has been practiced and is understood by all of the providers in each of the agencies that may be asked to respond to any major incident.

3. What is an "open" incident? What is a "closed" incident?

An open incident has a number of casualties not yet located when you answer the initial call. Rescuers may have to search for patients and then triage or treat them in multiple locations. There may also be an ongoing situation that produces more patients while you are at the scene, for example, school shootings, tornadoes, a hazardous materials release, or rising floodwaters. A closed incident is a situation that is not expected to produce more patients than initially present. The patients can be triaged and treated as they are removed.

4. How should you triage this patient?

Yellow

5. What is the difference between single and unified command?

Single command usually only works well when there is one emergency service agency responsible for the entire operation and no need for other disciplines to be involved. A unified command structure is more common and a key component of an ICS. This means that all involved agencies contribute to the command process by determining the overall goals and objectives, joint planning for tactical activities, and maximizing the use of all assigned resources at the incident.

6. What is "span of control?"

Another key component of an ICS is the span of control. A manageable span of control is the number of subordinates that one supervisor can manage effectively. The desired range is from three to seven. It can be very easy to lose track of workers at an incident if they are not assigned to small units.

7. How should you triage this patient?

Red

8. Why is there an essential need for common terminology in an ICS?

Common terminology is needed because there may be units from many different jurisdictions. It is easier to use simple sector titles indicating the function they serve (that is, staging, command, operations, triage, treatment, transportation, extrication). An MCI is not the time to begin figuring out another agency's "code system." Plain English works best in these situations. It is much easier for responding units to report to the IC instead of trying to remember that the medic on unit 620 is the person commanding the EMS unit at the scene.

9. How should you triage this patient?

Yellow

10. What is START?

START is an acronym for Simple Triage And Rapid Treatment. This is a method of triaging developed in Newport Beach, CA, in the early 1980s. Under START, the first concept is to clear an area and tell all walking wounded to walk to that location. After clearing walking wounded patients from the scene, the next step is to triage each remaining patient, assessing their respiratory status, hemodynamic status, and mental status. Basically, patients who have adequate respiratory status and hemodynamic status and are alert are classified as "delayed." If they do not have an adequate respiratory status or hemodynamic status or are not alert, they are usually classified as "immediate." The START process permits a few rescuers to triage large numbers of patients very rapidly. If this is the system used in your region, check with your medical director for more specifics on how to use the system.

11. What is the value of triage tags?

Triage tags can be very useful tools. The hardest part is getting crews to start using them! Some EMS agencies have tag days in which all patients are tagged to give the crews practice using the tags. Typically, there are a few different types of triage tags commercially available for services to purchase. Some provinces have designed their own tags and issued supplies to all EMS agencies. One very useful aspect to triage tags is that they help to eliminate the need to reassess each patient over and over again. Once the patient is tagged, it is clear that a paramedic has assessed the patient at least once.

Prep Kit

Ready for Review

- Disaster management requires planners to take a broad look at preparedness, planning, training, response, and after-action review.
- A mass-casualty incident (MCI) is an event in which the number of patients exceeds the resources available to the initial responders.
- Using the incident command system (ICS) gives you a modular organizational structure that is built on the size and complexity of the incident.
- Major incidents require the involvement and coordination of multiple jurisdictions, functional agencies, and emergency response disciplines.
- Your EMS agency should have written disaster plans that you are regularly trained to carry out.
- What has traditionally been referred to as medical incident command is also known as the medical (or EMS) branch of the incident command system. At incidents that have a significant medical factor, the incident commander should appoint someone as the medical group or branch leader who will supervise triage, treatment, and transport of injured patients.
- The goal of triage is to do the greatest good for the greatest number. This means that the triage assessment is brief and patient condition categories are basic.

Vital Vocabulary

closed incident A contained incident in which patients are found in one focal location and the situation is not expected to produce more patients than initially present.

command In incident command, the position that oversees the incident, establishes the objectives and priorities, and from there develops a response plan.

critical infrastructure The external foundation in communities made up of structures and services critical in the day-to-day living activities of humans: energy sources, fuel, water, sewage removal, food, hospitals, and transportation systems.

demobilization The process of directing responders to return to their facilities when work at a disaster or mass-casualty incident has finished, at least for the particular responders.

disaster management A planned, coordinated response to a disaster that involves cooperation of multiple responders and agencies and enables effective triage and provision of care according to triage decisions.

disasters Widespread events that disrupt community resources and functions, in turn threatening public safety, lives, and property.

extrication officer In incident command, the person appointed to determine the type of equipment and resources needed for a situation involving extrication or special rescue; also called the rescue officer.

finance officer In incident command, the position in an incident responsible for accounting of all expenditures and authorizing the release of emergency funds. This person is usually responsible for negotiating *just in time* contracts with suppliers to ensure adequate supplies.

freelancing When individual units or different organizations make independent and often inefficient decisions about the next appropriate action.

incident commander (IC) The overall leader of the incident command system to whom commanders or leaders of incident command system divisions report.

incident command system (ICS) A system implemented to manage disasters and mass- and multiple-casualty incidents in which section chiefs, including finance, logistics, operations, and planning, report to the incident commander.

joint information centre (JIC) An area designated by the incident commander, or a designee, in which public information officers from multiple agencies disseminate information about the incident.

JumpSTART triage A sorting system for pediatric patients less than 8 years old or weighing less than 45 kg. There is a minor adaptation for infants since they cannot ambulate on their own.

liaison officer (LNO) In incident command, the person who relays information, concerns, and requests among responding agencies.

logistics In incident command, the position that helps procure and stockpile equipment and supplies during an incident.

mass-casualty incident (MCI) An emergency situation that can place great demand on the equipment or personnel of the EMS system or has the potential to overwhelm your available resources.

medical incident command A branch of operations in a unified command system, whose three designated sector positions are triage, treatment, and transport.

morgue officer In incident command, the person who works with area medical examiners, coroners, and law enforcement agencies to coordinate the disposition of dead victims.

open incident An ongoing or uncontained incident in which rescuers will have to search for patients and then triage or treat them. The situation may produce more patients. Examples include school shootings, tornadoes, a hazardous materials release, and rising floodwaters.

operations In incident command, the position that carries out the orders of the commander to help resolve the incident.

planning In incident command, the position that ultimately produces a plan to resolve any incident.

primary triage A type of patient sorting used to rapidly categorize patients; the focus is on speed in locating all patients and determining an initial priority as their condition warrants.

public information officer (PIO) In incident command, the person who keeps the public informed and relates any information to the press.

rehabilitation officer In incident command, the person who establishes an area that provides protection for responders from the elements and the situation.

rescue officer In incident command, the person appointed to determine the type of equipment and resources needed for a situation involving extrication or special rescue; also called the extrication officer.

safety officer In incident command, the person who gives the "go ahead" to a plan or who may stop an operation when rescuer safety is an issue.

secondary triage A type of patient sorting used in the treatment sector that involves retriage of patients.

single command system A command system in which one person is in charge, generally used with small incidents that involve only one responding agency or one jurisdiction.

span of control In incident command, the subordinate positions under the commander's direction to which the workload is distributed; the supervisor/worker ratio.

staging officer In incident command, the person who locates an area to stage equipment and personnel and tracks unit arrival and deployment from the staging area.

START triage A patient sorting process that stands for Simple Triage And Rapid Treatment and uses a limited assessment of the patient's ability to walk, respiratory status, hemodynamic status, and neurologic status.

termination of command The end of the incident command structure when an incident draws to a close.

transfer of command In incident command, when an incident commander turns over command to someone with more experience in a critical area.

transportation officer In incident command, the person who coordinates transportation and distribution of patients to appropriate receiving hospitals.

treatment officer In incident command, the person responsible for locating, setting up, and supervising the treatment area.

triage To sort patients based on the severity of their conditions and prioritize them for care accordingly.

triage officer The person in charge of prioritizing patients, whose primary duty is to ensure that every patient receives initial triage.

unified command system A command system used in larger incidents in which there is a multiagency response or multiple jurisdictions are involved.

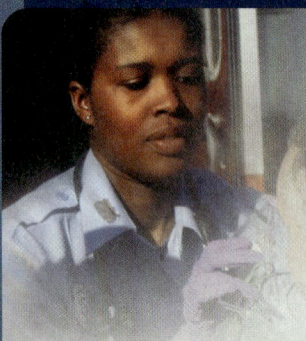

Assessment in Action

You are dispatched to a motor vehicle collision involving a commuter bus on the highway. You are the first unit on scene. When you exit your vehicle, you immediately begin your initial scene assessment. There are several walking wounded, and you are informed that the bus was full, was cut off by another vehicle, and swerved to the right. It travelled down an embankment, rolled over, and landed on its wheels. There are no other vehicles involved, but many people are exiting their vehicles to try to help.

1. **The first assessment radio report to your dispatcher is very important and should include all of the following, EXCEPT:**
   A. location of the triage sector.
   B. specific location of the incident.
   C. extent of the incident.
   D. approximate number of patients involved.

2. **As the first responder arriving at the scenario, you should ask yourself all of the following questions, EXCEPT:**
   A. What do I have?
   B. What do I need?
   C. What do I need to do it?
   D. When do shifts change?

3. **A mass-casualty incident is defined as:**
   A. the greatest challenge facing a paramedic because the resources are severely limited initially.
   B. those things that are critical in the day-to-day living activities of humans, such as energy sources, fuel, water, sewage removal, food, hospitals, and transportation systems.
   C. an event in which the number of patients exceeds the number of patient care providers or the resources available to responders.
   D. the result of a natural or human-made disaster, subcategorized as open or closed.

4. **Regardless of the cause of this MCI, how would this scenario be subcategorized?**
   A. Closed incident
   B. Open incident
   C. Open-ended incident
   D. Human-made disaster

5. **What are the two types of incident command systems?**
   A. Single command and unified command systems
   B. Span of control and consolidated action systems
   C. Unified command and dual command systems
   D. Single command and multiple command systems

6. **What are the designated sector positions within medical incident command?**
   A. Triage
   B. Treatment
   C. Transportation
   D. All of the above

7. **What is span of control?**
   A. Individual units or different organizations making independent and often inefficient decisions about the next appropriate action
   B. Establishing the objectives and priorities by the person overseeing the incident
   C. The subordinate positions under a commander's direction to which the workload is distributed; the supervisor/worker ratio
   D. Assistance in procuring and stockpiling equipment

8. **The commander's support staff can be remembered by using the mnemonic:**
   A. C-LAP.
   B. C-ICS.
   C. C-ICE.
   D. C-FLOP.

9. **There are several positions that fall under the incident commander to assist him or her. They are:**
   A. safety officer.
   B. public information officer.
   C. liaison officer.
   D. all of the above.

Challenging Questions

You arrive to work your night shift. You learn the day crew has been at a structure fire all afternoon. Your supervisor tells you to go and relieve your colleagues. You arrive on scene and are asked to take over the triage sector. The off-going triage officer informs you that they have already triaged approximately 22 patients and that they are expecting another 15 to 20 victims. You've never done this before and are a little nervous. After taking in a few deep breaths, you begin your role.

10. **What is your role?**

Points to Ponder

You are dispatched to your local high school at 13:00 hr because of the smell of smoke. When you arrive, the local fire department is there assessing the situation. The cooking class left something burning on the stove and it caught fire. There are approximately 10 to 15 students who were in the classroom who are experiencing possible smoke inhalation symptoms.

What should you do first? Who should you contact?

Issues: Initiating Incident Command at Smaller Events, Knowing Your Department's Standard Operating Procedures for an MCI.

48 Terrorism and Weapons of Mass Destruction

Competency Areas

Area 2: Communication

2.4.f Manage and provide support to patients, bystanders, and relatives manifesting emotional reactions.

Area 3: Health and Safety

3.3.a Assess scene for safety.
3.3.b Address potential occupational hazards.
3.3.c Conduct basic extrication.
3.3.e Conduct procedures and operations consistent with Workplace Hazardous Materials Information System (WHMIS) and hazardous materials management requirements.
3.3.f Practice infection control techniques.
3.3.g Clean and disinfect equipment.
3.3.h Clean and disinfect an emergency vehicle.

Area 4: Assessment and Diagnostics

4.1.a Rapidly assess a scene based on the principles of a triage system
4.1.b Assume different roles in a mass casualty incident.
4.1.c Manage a mass casualty incident.

Appendix 4: Pathophysiology

C. **Respiratory System**
Traumatic Injuries: Burns
Traumatic Injuries: Toxic inhalation
G. **Integumentary System**
Traumatic Injuries: Burns
Infectious and Inflammatory Illness: Infections
J. **Multisystem Diseases and Injuries**
Toxicologic Illness: Poisons (absorption, inhalation, ingestion)
Toxicologic Illness: Asphyxiants
Toxicologic Illness: Cyanide
Environmental Disorders: Radiation exposure

Appendix 5: Medications

A. **Medications affecting the central nervous system.**
A.3 Anticonvulsants
A.6 Neuroleptics
A.9 Paralytics
B. **Medications affecting the autonomic nervous system.**
B.4 Cholinergic Antagonists
J. **Medications used to treat poisoning and overdose.**
J.1 Antidotes or Neutralizing Agents

Introduction

According to the Canadian Security Intelligence Service (CSIS), with the exception of the United States, more terrorist groups are active in Canada today than in any other country. The presence of these organizations probably can be attributed to the fact that we live and work next door to the world's largest terrorist target—the United States.

Although the most visible aspect of terrorism is physical violence, the CSIS and the Royal Canadian Mounted Police (RCMP) track a number of different activities, such as fundraising, bases of operations, and attempts to procure weapons and materials.

Canada has had experience with violent acts of terrorism. In the 1970s, domestic terrorism unfolded in Quebec with the Front de liberation du Québec (FLQ). In 1985, 280 Canadians were killed in the bombing of Air India flight 182. Twenty-five Canadians were killed in the 2001 bombing of the World Trade Center in New York City. Because Canada plays a significant military role in combating terrorism overseas, Canadians and Canada are potential targets for future terrorist activity.

The CSIS has identified other contributing factors to the threat of terrorism:

- Persons trained in terrorist training camps, as well as veterans of campaigns in Afghanistan, Bosnia, Chechnya, and elsewhere, are known to reside in Canada.
- Canadian citizens have travelled to Iraq to fight in the insurgency, and they may return to Canada with new skills and motivations.
- Terrorist groups continue to intimidate and exploit Canada's immigrant and expatriate communities, sometimes through front organizations.
- Terrorists in Canada have conducted preliminary reconnaissance against potential Canadian targets.

Trends in Transnational Terrorism

A growing number of countries have experienced attacks by terrorist groups affiliated with Al Qaeda. Many of these groups have similar goals and motivations to Al Qaeda. These goals include the elimination of Western influences and secular forms of government in Muslim countries. Because these groups are borderless and terrorist incidents are not specifically contained within defined borders of established nations, these groups are often referred to as transnational terrorist groups.

Many of these groups are becoming increasingly sophisticated. Many members are well-educated and multilingual, with skills in modern technology, such as communicating via encrypted messages. Members may display a willingness to die for their cause. These groups display the following characteristics:

- Launch attacks globally, including in countries not previously targeted.
- Target soft (nonmilitary) targets, with the aim of killing as many people as possible.
- Attempt to acquire more lethal weapons, including chemical, biological, radiological, and nuclear devices.
- Use the Internet, particularly the Internet news media, as a propaganda and recruitment tool.

You are the Paramedic Part 1

You and your partner are dispatched to the Northside Regional Shopping Centre for a patient having a seizure. While en route, dispatch informs you that they have received numerous 9-1-1 calls from within the shopping centre. Callers are stating that a large number of people are vomiting and having seizures. Many appear to be unconscious.

Additional information received from dispatch states that shopping centre security is reporting a high-pitched whistling sound, much like a gas leak. The HazMat team has been dispatched and has an established time of arrival (ETA) of 4 minutes. All units are given the order to not enter the shopping centre until HazMat has evaluated the scene.

On arrival in the parking lot, you note that your supervisor is on the scene and has donned the "EMS Command" vest. Your supervisor, as well as numerous other responders from law enforcement, fire, and shopping centre security, meets you at the front entrance. Your unit is assigned to report to the temporary hospital that has been set up in a fast food restaurant across the street. As part of the START system, the "walking wounded" who have already exited the building were told to go to the fast food restaurant to be medically evaluated. There are a number of higher priority patients who are being evaluated or are yet to be evaluated pending authorization that the site is actually safe to enter, but they are clearly not your responsibility at this time.

Initial Assessment	Recording Time: 0 Minutes
Appearance	Female in her 30s who is pacing and appears to be crying
Level of consciousness	A (Alert to person, place, and day)
Airway	Open and clear
Breathing	Rapid and shallow
Circulation	Weak, slow radial pulse

1. What is your first priority at a call in this situation?
2. What does the dispatch information indicate as far as the need for additional resources?

- Recruit a growing number of young, second-generation immigrants with little or no previous links to terrorism.

Espionage in Canada

Transnational terrorist organizations are taking advantage of globalization and are involved in such criminal activities as drug trafficking, migrant smuggling, government corruption, arms dealing, and money laundering, all in an effort to fund their organizations.

Today, most espionage activities directed against Canada involve economic espionage. This is illegal, clandestine, or coercive activity by either a foreign government or terrorist organization to gain unauthorized access to economic intelligence, such as proprietary information or technology. Canada is a world leader in the following fields:

- Aerospace
- Biotechnology
- Chemicals
- Communications
- Information technology
- Mining
- Metallurgy
- Nuclear energy
- Oil
- Natural gas

All of this makes Canada a potential target, not only for information theft, but for violent activities, such as blowing up a refinery in a densely populated area.

As a result of the increase in terrorist activity, it is possible that you may respond to a terrorist event during your career. International terrorists as well as domestic groups have increased their targeting of civilian populations with acts of terror. The question is not will terrorists strike again, but rather when and where they will strike. The paramedic must be mentally and physically prepared for the possibility of a terrorist event.

The use of weapons of mass destruction, or weapons of mass casualty, further complicates the management of the terrorist incident and places the paramedic in greater danger. Although it is difficult to anticipate and plan a response to many terrorist events, there are several key principles that apply to every response. This chapter describes how you can prepare to respond to these events by discussing types of terrorist events, personal safety, and patient management. You will learn the signs, symptoms, and treatment of patients who have been exposed to nuclear, chemical, or biological agents or an explosive attack. At the end of this chapter, you will be able to answer the following key questions:

- What are your initial actions?
- Who should you notify, and what should you tell them?
- What type of additional resources might you require?
- How should you proceed to address the needs of the victims?
- How do you ensure your own and your partner's safety, as well as the safety of the victims?
- What is the clinical presentation of a patient exposed to a WMD?
- How are WMD patients to be assessed and treated?
- How do you avoid becoming contaminated or cross-contaminated with a WMD agent?

What Is Terrorism?

The Canadian Department of Justice defines terrorism through its Anti-terrorism Act, which makes it a crime to:

- Knowingly participate in or contribute to any activity of a terrorist group.
- Knowingly facilitate a terrorist activity.
- Knowingly instruct anyone to carry out a terrorist activity or a terrorist activity in connection with a terrorist group.
- Knowingly harbor or conceal a person who has carried out or is likely to carry out a terrorist activity.

Today, terrorists pose a threat to nations and cultures everywhere. International terrorism has brought a new fear into the lives of many Canadian citizens Figure 48-1 ▾ .

Modern-day terrorism is common in the Middle East, where terrorist groups have frequently attacked civilian populations. In Ireland terrorist groups have attacked the civilian population for decades under the guise of religious freedom. In

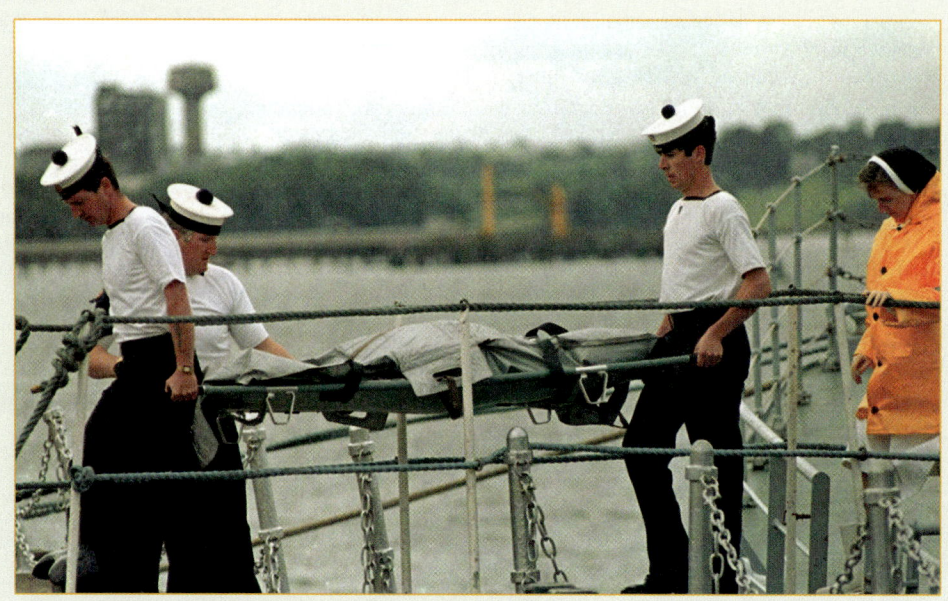

Figure 48-1 The effects of terrorism, such as the Air India bombing, are broad and unimaginable. Paramedics must be prepared to work in the most austere environments.

Colombia, political terrorist groups target oil resources as a means to instill fear.

In the United States, domestic terrorists have struck multiple times within the last decade. The Centennial Park bombing during the 1996 Summer Olympics and the destruction of the Alfred P. Murrah Federal Building in Oklahoma City in 1995 are examples. Terrorist organizations are generally categorized. Only a small percentage of groups, such as the following, actually turn toward terrorism as a means to achieve their goals:

1. **Violent religious groups/doomsday cults.** These include groups such as Aum Shinrikyo, who carried out chemical and biological attacks in Tokyo between 1994 and 1995. Some of these groups may participate in apocalyptic violence.

2. **Extremist political groups.** They may include violent separatist groups and those who seek political, religious, economic, and social freedom.

3. **Technology terrorists.** Those who attack a population's technological infrastructure as a means to draw attention to their cause, such as cyberterrorists.

4. **Single-issue groups.** These include anti-abortion groups, animal rights groups, anarchists, racists, or even ecoterrorists who threaten or use violence as a means to protect the environment.

Canada has not experienced any major mass-casualty incidents involving chemical, biological, radiological, or nuclear terrorism. However, there have been a range of incidents:

- **1993:** 130 grams of ricin, a known biological warfare agent, were seized by Canadian customs at an Alaska–Yukon border crossing.
- **1996:** Various news media outlets received envelopes containing razor blades purportedly coated with rat poison from an extremist animal group.
- **1996:** Gas masks and chemical protection suits were among the items seized from the cache in British Columbia of a US-based militia group.
- **1999:** A sports bag containing a pipe bomb, potassium cyanide, and procaine was found in a luggage locker in Edmonton.
- **2000:** A booby-trap consisting of a pipe bomb with a flask of liquid cyanide attached was found in the home of a hydroponic marijuana grower in British Columbia.
- **2001:** Hoax letters threatening exposure to anthrax were received in Victoria, Ottawa, and Toronto.
- **2006:** 12 Ontario men were arrested in Toronto in a homegrown terror cell. RCMP recovered 3 tons of ammonium nitrate fertilizer, three times the amount used by Timothy McVeigh to destroy the federal building in Oklahoma City in 1995.

Most terrorist attacks require the coordination of multiple terrorists or "actors" working together. Nineteen hijackers worked together to commit the worst act of terrorism in United States history on September 11, 2001. At least four terrorists worked together to commit the London Subway bombings on July 7, 2005. However, in a few instances there has been a single terrorist who struck with devastating results. Terrorists who acted alone carried out all of the Atlanta abortion clinic attacks, the 1996 Summer Olympics attack, and the Oklahoma City bombing.

Weapons of Mass Destruction

What Are Weapons of Mass Destruction?

A weapon of mass destruction (WMD), or weapon of mass casualty (WMC), is any agent designed to bring about mass death, casualties, and/or massive damage to property and infrastructure (bridges, tunnels, airports, and seaports). These instruments of death and destruction include biological, nuclear, chemical, and explosives/incendiary weapons. To date, the preferred WMD for terrorists has been explosive devices. Terrorist groups have favoured tactics that use truck bombs or car or pedestrian suicide bombers. Many previous terrorist attempts to use either chemical or biological weapons to their full capacity have been unsuccessful. Nonetheless, as a paramedic you should understand the destructive potential of these weapons.

As discussed earlier, the motives and tactics of the new-age terrorist groups have begun to change. As with the doomsday cults, many terrorist groups participate in apocalyptic, indiscriminate killing. This doctrine of total carnage would make the use of WMDs highly desirable. WMDs are easy to obtain or create and are specifically geared toward killing large numbers of people. Had the proper techniques been used during the 1995 attack on the Tokyo subway, there may have been tens of thousands of casualties. With the fall of the former Soviet Union, the technology and expertise to produce WMDs may be available to terrorist groups with sufficient funding. Moreover, the technical recipes for making nuclear, biological, and chemical (NBC) weapons and explosive devices can be found readily on the Internet; in fact, they have even been published on terrorist group websites.

There are five categories of terrorist incidents that first responder agencies may confront in the prehospital environment. They are easily remembered with the mnemonic: BNICE as shown in Table 48-1 ▾.

Biological Terrorism/Warfare

Biological agents are organisms that cause disease or death. They are generally found in nature; for terrorist use, however, they are cultivated, synthesized, and mutated in a laboratory. The weaponization of biological agents is performed to artificially maximize the target population's exposure to the germ, thereby exposing the greatest number of people and achieving the desired result.

Table 48-1	The Categories of Terrorist Incidents
B	Biological
N	Nuclear
I	Incendiary
C	Chemical
E	Explosives

The primary types of biological agents that you may come into contact with during a biological event include:

- Viruses
- Bacteria
- Toxins

Nuclear/Radiological Terrorism

There have been only two publicly known incidents involving the use of a nuclear device. During World War II, Hiroshima and Nagasaki were devastated when they were targeted with nuclear bombs. It has been estimated that a death toll of 214,000 occurred due to the two bombs and their associated effects. The awesome destructive power demonstrated by the attack ended World War II and has served as a deterrent to nuclear war.

There are also nations that hold close ties with terrorist groups (known as state-sponsored terrorism) and have obtained some degree of nuclear capability. It is also possible for a terrorist to secure radioactive materials or waste to perpetrate an act of terror. Such materials are far easier for the determined terrorist to acquire and would require less expertise to use. The difficulties in developing a nuclear weapon are well documented. Radioactive materials, however, such as those in Radiological Dispersal Devices (RDDs), also known as "dirty bombs," can cause widespread panic and civil disturbances. More on these devices will be covered later in this chapter.

Chemical Terrorism/Warfare

Chemical agents are manmade substances that can have devastating effects on living organisms. They can be produced in liquid, powder, or vapour form depending on the desired route of exposure and dissemination technique. Developed during World War I, these agents have been implicated in thousands of deaths since being introduced on the battlefield, and since

then have been used to terrorize civilian populations. These agents consist of the following five categories:

- Vesicants or blister agents (ie, mustard gas and Lewisite)
- Respiratory or choking agents (ie, phosgene or chlorine)
- Nerve agents (ie, sarin, soman, tabun, or V agent)
- Metabolic or blood agents (ie, hydrogen cyanide, cyanogens chloride)
- Irritating agents (ie, mace, chloropicrin, tear gas, capsicum/pepper spray, and dibenzoxazepine)

Explosives/Incendiary Weapons

Explosives are the most likely method used by terrorists **Figure 48-2 ▸** . Incendiary weapons involve agents and chemicals used to start fires. Incendiary agents, such as acetone, can be combined with chemicals to produce explosives capable of massive destruction. Ranging from suicide bombings on public buses to trucks loaded with explosives set to go off in underground parking

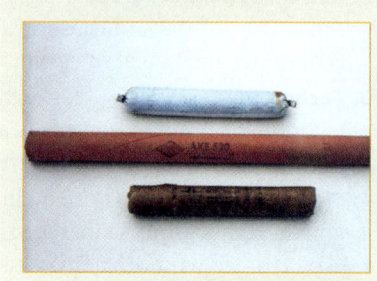

Figure 48-2 Every year, thousands of pounds of explosives are stolen.

garages of government buildings, these explosions can be very destructive. Explosives are substances that fit into one of the following two categories:

- A substance or article, including a device designed to function by explosion
- A substance or article, including a device, which by chemical reaction within itself can function in a similar manner even if not designated to function by explosion, unless the substance or article is otherwise classified

You are the Paramedic Part 2

The HazMat team is on the scene and has entered the shopping centre. The word is coming back through EMS Command that they believe a small canister of a nerve gas was released in the sporting goods store. The actual number of patients still inside the shopping centre who are unconscious or may have had seizures is approximately eight patients. The HazMat team is attempting a rapid decontamination on these patients so they can be removed to the cold zone and lifesaving treatment begun. EMS Command has already been in contact with the Poison Centre and they have advised that all patients, even those who are alert like your patient, be evaluated for nerve agent symptoms (DUMBELS) and if necessary managed with a MARK 1 kit. You begin to evaluate your patient further and note she is still tearing and has vomited.

Vital Signs	Recording Time: 10 Minutes
Level of consciousness	Alert, with a Glasgow Coma Scale score of 15
Skin	Pale, warm, and dry
Pulse	Weak radial at 52 beats/min
Respirations	12 breaths/min
SpO_2	97% with oxygen at 10 l/min via nonrebreathing mask

3. What precautions can you take to ensure your own safety?

4. What does your index of suspicion tell you about this scene?

Paramedic Response to Terrorism and WMD Incidents

EMS Planning for a WMD Incident

The ability of an EMS organization to respond effectively begins with the development of plans, procedures, and training. Does your organization have plans to respond to a WMD incident, or does it rely on existing policy and procedures? It is important to note that a WMD incident is different from a hazardous materials incident in that the incident is deliberate in nature, so the EMS organization is responding to a crime scene where criminal activity has occurred and may be continuing to occur. The WMD incident may produce a large number of casualties and even fatalities. Many of these casualties will seek immediate medical attention, with the potential of plugging up your existing medical infrastructure. Instead of a few individuals requiring decontamination, as typically occurs in a hazardous materials incident, responding organizations may be required to decontaminate large numbers of people. Some of these people will require dry decontamination, whereas others may require wet decontamination.

Note that any response to a WMD incident will generally require a multi-agency coordinated response, which is a challenge in itself. Numerous after-action reports to various incidents mention communication, information sharing, and equipment compatibility as challenges to such a response. For example, does your EMS organization have the ability to directly communicate with the police and fire services? If this is the case, do you know what communication tools and procedures are available to you to assist in a multi-agency response? A proper response to a WMD incident takes planning, equipment allocation, and training. In order to respond effectively to these incidents, your organization needs the experience of training in multi-agency coordinated drills and/or exercises.

EMS Terrorist Response Plan

EMS organizations should have a terrorist response plan, and every paramedic should know his or her role in such a plan. Such roles may require the paramedic to take on additional responsibilities or work in a nontraditional manner. For example, it may be necessary to utilize paramedics in alternative treatment facilities or have paramedics fill various positions within the Incident Command System. These plans should include specific information on responding to WMD incidents. EMS organizations should have knowledge of their community's vulnerabilities, and this information should be passed along to the paramedic. EMS organizations should participate in risk assessments that identify key community areas or events that present targets for terrorists. For example, important community dates such as national holidays, large public gatherings, and meetings of political and social groups with either domestic or international agendas.

Recalling Paramedics During Times of Disaster

Many EMS organizations have part-time staff who hold part- or full-time positions in other organizations. During a disaster, many of these individuals will be recalled to their full-time positions or to what they consider to be their primary job. EMS organizations should have an accurate count of how many actual paramedics they are able to recall during an emergency. From a planning standpoint, EMS organizations should know if individual paramedics work for other response organizations. As a point of reflection, do you know any paramedics who work for multiple emergency response organizations? In a WMD incident, how would you choose which organization to work for? Is there the potential that you or your colleagues could be called by several organizations?

Paramedic WMD Training

The reality is that responding to a mass-casualty incident caused by a WMD will place the average paramedic into a much riskier position than normal. There will be the possibility of potentially being exposed to a situation that a HazMat team or joint CBRN team would normally be trained to handle. All paramedics should be trained at least an awareness level with respect to WMD incidents. In addition, all paramedics should be fit tested and trained in respiratory protection, as well as the basic elements of PPE and decontamination.

Alternative Health Care Facilities

A WMD incident can produce an enormous amount of casualties that can overload any health care system. It is recognized that most hospitals will not be able to handle the number of patients who may seek medical attention after a WMD incident. To effectively manage this situation, paramedics may be involved in working in temporary off-site treatment centres. Such treatment centres may be pre-identified community buildings, such as arenas, sports complexes, or schools, that can be quickly converted to treat patients. In addition, paramedics may be part of specialized Provincial Emergency Response Teams. As an example, Ontario has the Emergency Medical Assistance Team comprised of physicians, nurses, paramedics, and other allied health care professionals. This team is equipped and designed to use existing community facilities and its own infrastructure to lessen the impact of a WMD incident.

The facility that is chosen should be able to house and care for a large number of patients. It needs to have water, restrooms, food provisions, furniture, electricity, and heating. High schools generally can maintain and sustain patients because they have amenities such as chairs, desks, cafeterias, water fountains, auditoriums, and public address systems.

Patient Tracking During a WMD Incident

Patient identification and tracking should begin immediately. Because EMS is the first medical provider to respond, it should have an established patient-tracking mechanism that can be deployed. Paramedics may be involved in tracking patients as they are triaged, decontaminated, treated, and transported from the scene. Patients may be separated from family members as well as from personal belongings. Relatives from across the country will seek information on family members whom they believe were involved in the attack.

In a WMD incident, patient belongings become part of the criminal investigation, and need to be tracked along with medical treatment, specimen results, and patient outcomes. In addition, it is important for the paramedic to recognize that suspects may be among the patients treated by EMS. This emphasizes the importance of maintaining patient tracking information on everyone from the incident.

In the interest of time, basic information, such as name, date of birth, chief complaint, and destination, should be recorded on a colour-coded triage tag. The tag itself should be waterproof, because patients may require decontamination. The tag should have several barcode stickers that can be placed on bags of patient belongings, destination rosters, and ambulance call reports. Alternative treatment centres and hospitals should use the same system.

Paramedics Situational Awareness

Paramedics are often involved in providing medical coverage for special events or areas of mass gatherings that are potential targets for terrorist activities. It is important for paramedics to recognize potential signs of a potential terrorist incident, because almost all successful terrorist attacks involve reconnaissance, intelligence gathering, and even dry runs. Therefore, the first line of defence against terrorism is being cognizant of potential precursor activities for a terrorist attack and then reporting such activities when they occur. In Canada, reports of suspicious activity should be reported to the National Security Hotline at 1-800-425-5805. Also contact local law enforcement. For more information, visit the RCMP website.

Table 48-2 ▶ lists situations that should trigger your suspicions of a potential terrorist attack.

Recognizing a Terrorist Event (Indicators)

Most acts of terror are covert, which means that the public safety community generally has no prior knowledge of the time, location, or nature of the attack. This element of surprise makes responding to an event more complex. You must constantly be aware of your surroundings and understand the possible risks for terrorism associated with certain locations, at certain times.

Understanding and being aware of the current threat is only the beginning of responding safely to calls. Once you are on duty, you must be able to make appropriate decisions regarding the potential for a terrorist event. In determining the potential for a terrorist attack, on every call you should observe the following:

- **Type of location.** Is the location a monument, infrastructure, government building, or a specific type of location such as a temple? Is there a large gathering? Is there a special event taking place?

- **Type of call.** Is there a report of an explosion or suspicious device nearby? Does the call come into dispatch as someone having unexplained coughing and difficulty breathing? Are there reports of people fleeing the scene?
- **Number of patients.** Are there multiple patients with similar signs and symptoms? This is probably the single most important clue that a terrorist attack or an incident involving a WMD has occurred.

At the Scene

One of the easiest ways to distinguish between a nonterrorist mass-casualty event and a terrorist event is that the intentional use of WMD affects multiple persons. These casualties will generally exhibit the same signs and symptoms. It is highly unlikely for more than one person to experience a seizure at any given time. It is not uncommon to find multiple patients complaining of difficulty breathing at the scene of a fire. However, the same report in the subway at rush hour, when no smell of smoke has been reported, is certainly cause for suspicion. In these situations, you must use good judgment and resist the urge to "rush in and help," especially when there are multiple victims from an unknown cause.

- **Victims' statements.** This is probably the second best indication of a terrorist or WMD event. Are the patients fleeing the scene giving statements such as, "Everyone is passing out," "There was a loud explosion," or "There are a lot of people shaking on the ground." If so, something is occurring that you do not want to rush into, even if it is determined not to be a terrorist event.
- **Pre-incident indicators.** Has there been a recent increase in violent political activism? Are you aware of any credible threats made against the location, gathering, or occasion?

Response Actions

Once you suspect that a terrorist event has occurred or WMD have been used, there are certain actions to take to ensure that you will be safe and be in the proper position to help the community.

Scene Safety

Ensure that the scene is safe. If you have any doubt that it may not be safe, do not enter. When dealing with a WMD scene, it is safe to assume that you will not be able to enter where the event has occurred—nor do you want to. The best location for staging is upwind and uphill from the incident. Wait for assistance from those who are trained in assessing and managing WMD scenes Figure 48-3 ▶ . Also remember:
- Failure to park your vehicle at a safe location can place you and your partner in danger Figure 48-4 ▶ .
- If your vehicle is blocked in by other emergency vehicles or damaged by a secondary device (or event), you will be unable to provide patients with transportation, or escape yourself Figure 48-5 ▶ .

Table 48-2 | Situational Awareness for Potential Terrorist Activity

Situational Awareness of Suspicious Situations

- The theft or loss of badges, credentials, ID cards, or uniforms.
- The creation of false IDs.
- Photographing, sketching, or surveillance of buildings and facilities.
- Trespassing near key facilities or in supposedly secure areas, particularly by multiple persons.
- The presence of uncommon or abandoned vehicles, packages, or containers.
- Persons who seem to be making careful note of the presence of security cameras, antivehicle bollards, and similar security measures around potential targets.
- Observing people who are searching trash containers or placing unusual items in them (particularly around transit systems or the lobbies of crowded buildings).
- Purchases at government surplus sales of military, police, fire, or paramedic vehicles and equipment, particularly if there is an indication to refurbish them.
- The attempted purchase of supplies necessary for the manufacture of explosive devices, which include the unusual frequent purchase of fertilizer or cleaning supplies. Acetone and peroxide are key components in a particularly devastating homemade explosive.
- An increase in the number of threats or false alarms to facilities that require evacuation. If a false alarm is rung, watch for onlookers who are observing your reaction.
- Attempts to gain information from janitors, receptionists, and other entry-level employees.

Situational Awareness of Mail Bombs

- Mail that has no return address.
- Mail addressed only to the title of the prospective recipient or that uses an incorrect title.
- Misspelled words or defective addresses.
- Restrictive markings such as "personal for" or "to be opened only by."
- Stains, discolourations, oiliness, crystallization, or a strange odour.
- Abnormal size or excessive wrapping, particularly if the package is heavily taped or wrapped with twine.
- Wires, metal, foil, string, or cell phone antenna protruding from the package.
- A very rigid envelope.
- An unusually heavy or unbalanced feel to the package.
- Lopsided or uneven envelope.

Situational Awareness of Suicide Attackers

- Suspects have been seen praying fervently, giving the appearance of whispering to someone. Others have been described as agitated or very nervous.
- Suspects may be hugging a package or routinely checking the contents of a backpack or heavy shopping bag.
- Suspect may look furtive and may be having a hard time fitting in with the normal street scene.
- Loose or bulky clothing, often inappropriate for the weather and circumstances, can conceal a vest bomb.
- Look for someone maneuvering to get close to a VIP or a large cluster of people.
- Suicide bombers often try to avoid coming near security or into contact with any authority figure until it is time to launch the attack.

Situational Awareness of Vehicle Bombs

- Vehicle that has a strong chemical smell or the scent of something burning.
- Signs of recent body work, especially of poor quality, or with patches welded to the cab or body of the vehicle.
- Extra fuel tanks, extra antennas, or recent signs of reinforced suspension.
- Inappropriate license plates or misspelled artwork.
- Heavily tinted windows, particularly if used in an unusual manner.
- Be wary of signs of large boxes, fuel canisters, extra batteries, and similar objects that can be seen inside the vehicle.
- Signs that the vehicle is heavily overloaded on its suspension.
- Drivers whose behaviour is suspicious or who insist on parking close to a crowded or hardened target.

Source: Mackenzie Institute.

Paramedics arriving at an incident should stop their vehicle at a distance and do an initial visual assessment of the area. The *North American Emergency Response Guidebook* may be helpful in determining initial hazard distances. This assessment should include any new information obtained from bystanders, victims, or witnesses to the incident. The fire department's HazMat team is usually responsible for determining safety zones, which are marked as hot, warm, and cold. These zones not only mark the site where hazardous materials and joint CBRN personnel work, but it also establishes the crime scene perimeter. Only authorized personnel with specialized training and equipment should enter either the warm zone or the hot zone. The cold zone is normally where the paramedics perform triage and patient treatment.

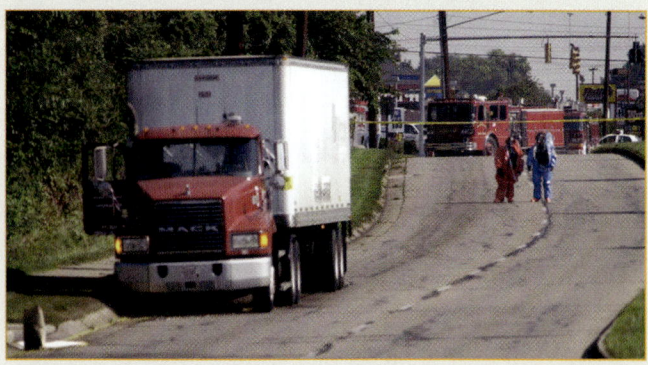

Figure 48-3 Improper staging of a mass-casualty scene could lead to injury or even death of paramedics. Wait for assistance from persons who are trained in assessing and managing such scenes.

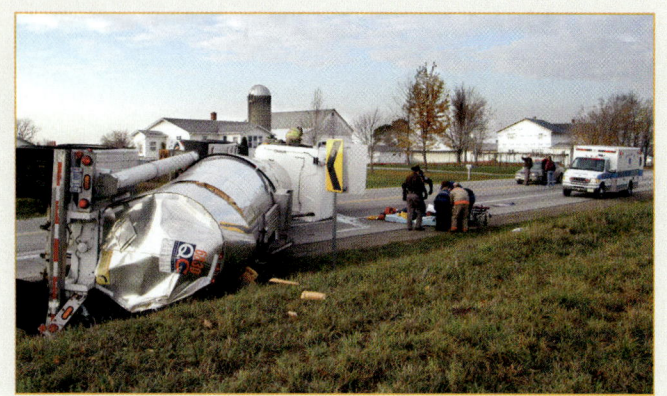

Figure 48-4 Park your vehicle at a safe location and distance.

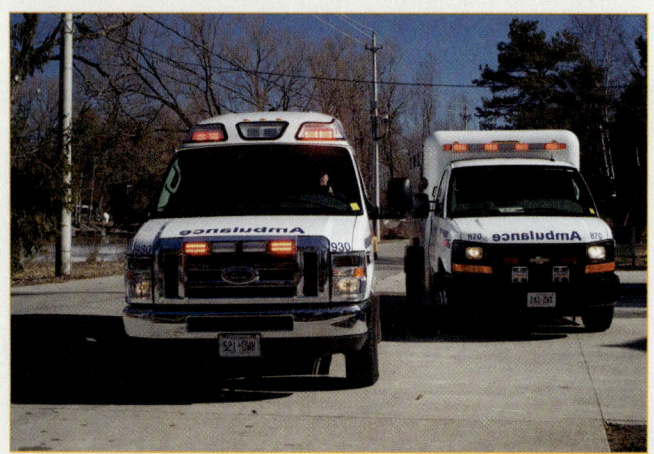

Figure 48-5 Make sure that your vehicle is not blocked in by other emergency vehicles.

EMS Scene Safety Officer

The safety of paramedics and other EMS responders is a priority during a WMD response. These incidents are complex, involving a multitude of potential risks that could cause injury or harm to individual paramedics. This not only affects the paramedic's well-being, but it also decreases his or her ability to effectively respond to those patients who need care the most. An EMS safety officer should be appointed who is responsible for identifying all potential risks and placing control measures in place to mitigate them. The safety officer monitors EMS activities at the scene to ensure that the paramedics are working within established safety guidelines that are included in the incident action plan.

Responder Safety (Personnel Protection)

The best form of protection from a WMD agent is preventing yourself from coming into contact with the agent. The greatest threats facing a paramedic in a WMD attack are contamination and cross-contamination. Contamination with an agent occurs when you have direct contact with the WMD or are exposed to it. Cross-contamination occurs when you come into contact with a contaminated person who has not yet been decontaminated.

Day-to-day emergency calls typically require paramedics to face risks for short periods of time. Most of the personal protective equipment (PPE) issued to paramedics is designed to work for short periods of time. Response to a WMD attack may require days or weeks of constant work in PPE. The PPE used should reflect the complexity and duration of the incident.

Notification Procedures

When you suspect a terrorist or WMD event has taken place, notify the dispatch centre, provided that communication is functioning properly. Vital information needs to be communicated effectively if you are to receive the appropriate assistance (see Chapter 16 for information on effective communication). Inform dispatch of the nature of the event, any additional resources that may be required, the estimated number of patients, and the upwind route of approach or optimal route of approach. If there is the presence of a plume, that information should be communicated, along with the wind direction and the potential areas to avoid.

It is extremely important to establish a staging area, where other units will converge. Be mindful of access and egress routes when you direct units to respond to a location. It is unwise to have units respond to the front entrance of a hotel or apartment building that has had an explosion. Last, trained responders in the proper protective equipment are the only persons equipped to handle the WMD incident. These specialized units, traditionally hazardous materials (HazMat) teams, must be requested as early as possible due to the time required to assemble and dispatch the team and their equipment. Many jurisdictions share HazMat teams, and the team may have to travel a long distance to reach the location of the event. It is always better to be safe than sorry; call the team early and the outcome of the call will be more favourable. Keep in mind that there may be more than one type of device or agent present.

Establishing Command

The first arriving provider on the scene must begin to sort out the chaos and define his or her responsibilities under the

Incident Command System (ICS). As the first person on scene, the paramedic may need to establish "EMS or Medical Command" until additional personnel arrive. Depending on the circumstances, you and other paramedics may function as medical branch officers, triage officers, treatment officers, transportation or logistic officers, or staff. If the ICS is already in place, then you should immediately seek out the medical staging officer to receive your assignment. The incident command system and its components are discussed in further detail in Chapter 47.

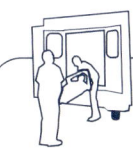

At the Scene

Secondary devices may include various types of electronic equipment such as cell phones or pagers that are detonated when "answered."

Secondary Device or Event (Reassessing Scene Safety)

Terrorists have been known to plant additional explosives that are set to explode after the initial bomb. This type of secondary device is intended primarily to injure responders and to secure media coverage, because the media generally arrives on scene just after the initial response. Do not rely on others to secure your safety. It is every paramedic's responsibility to constantly assess and reassess the scene for safety. It is easy to overlook a suspicious package lying on the floor while you are treating casualties. Stay alert. Something as subtle as a change in the wind direction during a gas attack or an increase in the number of contaminated patients can place you in danger. Never become so involved with the tasks that you are performing that you do not look around and make sure that the scene remains safe.

At the Scene

You are of no help to the public if you become a patient. More importantly, once you become a victim of the event, you place an additional burden on your fellow responders, who must treat you. Assess the scene and resist the urge to run in and help (do not develop tunnel vision). You may place your life and your partner in danger. Remember . . . do not become a victim.

Chemical Agents

Chemical agents are liquids or gases that are dispersed to kill or injure. Modern-day chemicals were first developed during the two World Wars. During the Cold War, many of these agents were perfected and stockpiled. While Canada has long renounced the use of chemical weapons, many nations still develop and stockpile them. These agents are deadly and pose a threat if acquired by terrorists. Note that injury from chemical agents can also occur from industrial accidents or incidents, whether intentional or not. Industrial accidents continue to be a significant potential source of exposure to the agents used in chemical weapons. In Canada, common chemicals such as phosgene, cyanide, ammonia, and chlorine are transported on highways. This means that chemical facilities and the transportation industry are potential targets for terrorism.

Chemical weapons have several classifications. The properties or characteristics of an agent can be described as liquid, gas, or solid material. Persistency and volatility are terms used to describe how long the agent will stay on a surface before it evapourates. Persistent or nonvolatile agents can remain on a surface for long periods of time, usually longer than 24 hours. Nonpersistent or volatile agents evapourate relatively fast when left on a surface in the optimal temperature range. An agent that is described as highly persistent (such as VX, a nerve agent) can remain in the environment for weeks to months, whereas an agent that is highly volatile (such as sarin, also a nerve agent) will turn from liquid to gas (evapourate) within minutes to seconds. Generally speaking, volatile liquids pose a dual risk of dermal and inhalation exposure, whereas liquids that are persistent are more likely to be absorbed through the skin.

Route of exposure is a term used to describe how the agent most effectively enters the body. Chemical agents can have either a vapour or contact hazard. Agents with a vapour hazard enter the body through the respiratory tract in the form of vapours. Agents with a contact hazard (or skin hazard) give off very little vapour or no vapours and enter the body through the skin. The effects of vapours are largely influenced by ambient wind conditions and whether the release was in an enclosed space.

The paramedic should take an all-hazard approach to managing patients exposed to chemical agents. This may include:

- Using appropriate PPE.
- Ensuring that patients are appropriately decontaminated.
- Providing supportive prehospital care to patients.
- Providing specific antidotes to patients when indicated.

Personal Protective Equipment

The paramedic is generally expected to operate primarily on the outer perimeter of a contaminated area and should encounter minimal contamination. However, cross-contamination from patients, wind shifts, and secondary agent releases could put the paramedic at an increased risk for contamination. Also, properly trained paramedics may be called upon to perform limited duties in support of decontamination operations within the outer limits of the warm zone.

As with any other call, paramedics need to ensure that they have adequate PPE for the zone of operation they may be working in Figure 48-6 ▶. Usually it will only be members of joint CBRN teams or HazMat teams who will be working in the hot or warm zones. However, all paramedics need to ensure that they are protected from direct or cross-contamination and that they understand what zone they are in. Generally speaking, EMS will stage and operate in the cold zone. Properly trained paramedics may also be assigned to joint CBRN

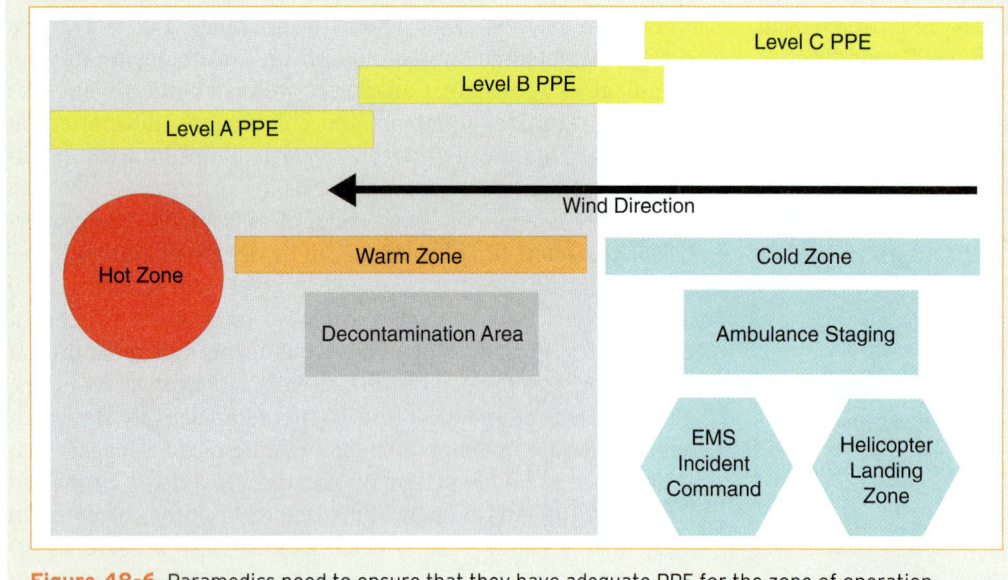

Figure 48-6 Paramedics need to ensure that they have adequate PPE for the zone of operation.

teams and tasked with medical management and decontamination in the warm or hot zones.

Anyone entering either the warm or hot zones is considered dirty and must wear the appropriate PPE, as established by incident command. All personnel and patients are to be decontaminated before entering the cold zone to decrease the risk of potential secondary contamination.

Decontamination is a special aspect in the response to primarily chemical agents, but it can be applied to radiological and biological incidents to remove agents that may pose harm to an individual's health. Chapter 50 discusses decontamination and the levels of proper PPE in full detail.

Vesicants (Blister Agents)

The primary route of exposure of blister agents, or vesicants, is the skin (contact); however, if vesicants are left on the skin or clothing long enough, they produce vapours that can enter the respiratory tract. Vesicants cause burn-like blisters to form on the patient's skin as well as in the respiratory tract. The vesicant agents consist of sulfur mustard (H), Lewisite (L), and phosgene oxime (CX) (the symbols H, L, and CX are military designations for these chemicals). The vesicants usually cause the most damage to damp or moist areas of the body, such as the armpits, groin, and the respiratory tract. Signs of vesicant exposure on the skin include:

- Skin irritation, burning, and reddening
- Immediate intense skin pain (with L and CX)
- Formation of large blisters
- Grey discolouration of skin (a sign of permanent damage seen with L and CX)
- Swollen and closed or irritated eyes
- Permanent eye injury (including blindness)

If vapours were inhaled, the patient may experience the following:

- Hoarseness and stridor
- Severe cough
- Hemoptysis (coughing up of blood)
- Severe dyspnea

Sulfur mustard (agent H) is a brownish, yellowish oily substance that is generally considered very persistent. When released, mustard has the distinct smell of garlic or mustard and is quickly absorbed into the skin and/or mucous membranes. As the agent is absorbed into the skin, it begins an irreversible process of damage to the cells. Absorption through the skin or mucous membranes usually occurs within seconds, and damage to the underlying cells takes place within 1 to 2 minutes.

Mustard is considered a mutagen, which means that it mutates, damages, and changes the structures of cells. Eventually, cellular death will occur. On the surface, the patient will generally not produce any signs or symptoms until 4 to 6 hours after exposure (depending on concentration and amount of exposure) Figure 48-7 ▾.

The patient will experience a progressive reddening of the affected area, which will gradually develop into large blisters. These blisters are very similar in shape and appearance to those associated with thermal second-degree burns. The fluid within the blisters does not contain any of the agent; however, the skin covering the area is considered to be contaminated until decontamination by trained personnel has been performed.

Mustard also attacks vulnerable cells within the bone marrow and depletes the body's ability to reproduce white blood cells. As with burns, the primary complication associated with vesicant blisters is secondary infection. If the patient does survive the

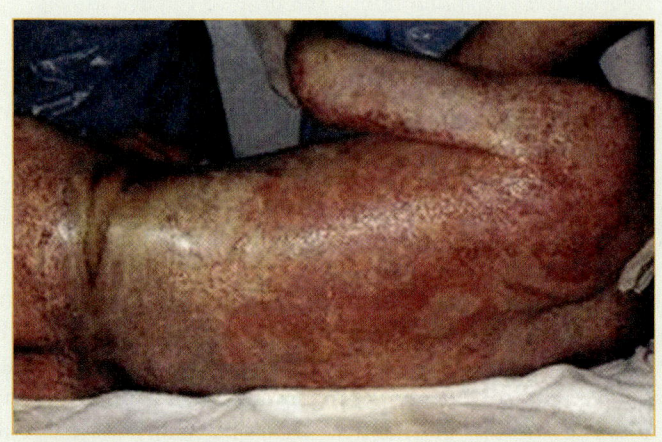

Figure 48-7 Skin damage resulting from exposure to sulfur mustard (agent H).

initial direct injury from the agent, the depletion of the white blood cells leaves the patient with a decreased resistance to infections. Although sulfur mustard is regarded as persistent, it does release enough vapours when dispersed to be inhaled. This creates upper and lower airway compromise. The result is damage and swelling of the airways. The airway compromise makes the patient's condition far more serious.

Lewisite (L) and phosgene oxime (CX) produce blister wounds very similar to mustard. They are highly volatile and have a rapid onset of symptoms, as opposed to the delayed onset seen with mustard. These agents produce immediate intense pain and discomfort when contact is made. The patient may have a greyish discolouration at the contaminated site. While tissue damage also occurs with exposure to these agents, they do not cause the secondary cellular injury that is associated with mustard.

Vesicant Agent Treatment

There are no antidotes for mustard or CX exposure. BAL (British Anti-Lewisite) is the antidote for agent L; however, it is not carried by civilian EMS. The paramedic must ensure that the patient has been decontaminated before ABCs are initiated. The patient may require prompt airway support if any agent has been inhaled, but this should not occur until after decontamination. Initiate transport and gain IV access as soon as possible. Generally, burn centres are best equipped to handle the wounds and subsequent infections produced by vesicants. Follow your local protocols when deciding what facility to transport the patient to.

Pulmonary Agents (Choking Agents)

The pulmonary agents are gases that cause immediate harm to persons exposed to them. The primary route of exposure for these agents is through the respiratory tract, which makes them

an inhalation or vapour hazard. Once inside the lungs, they damage the lung tissue and fluid leaks into the lungs. Pulmonary edema develops in the patient, resulting in difficulty breathing due to the inability for air exchange. These agents produce respiratory-related symptoms such as dyspnea, tachypnea, and pulmonary edema. This class of chemical agents consists of chlorine (CL) and phosgene.

Chlorine (CL) was the first chemical agent ever used in warfare. It has a distinct odour of bleach and creates a green haze when released as a gas. Initially it produces upper airway irritation and a choking sensation. The patient may later experience:

- Shortness of breath
- Chest tightness
- Hoarseness and stridor due to upper airway constriction
- Gasping and coughing

With serious exposures, patients may experience pulmonary edema, complete airway constriction, and death. The fumes from a mixture of household bleach (CL) and ammonia create an acid gas that produces similar effects. Each year, such mixtures overcome hundreds of people when they try to mix household cleaners.

Phosgene should not be confused with phosgene oxime, a blistering agent, or vesicant. Not only has phosgene been produced for chemical warfare, but it is a product of combustion such as might be produced in a fire at a textile factory or house, or from metalwork or burning Freon (a liquid chemical used in refrigeration). Therefore, you may encounter a patient who was exposed to this gas during the course of a normal call or at a fire scene. Phosgene is a very potent agent that has a delayed onset of symptoms, usually hours. Unlike CL, when phosgene enters the body, it generally does not produce severe irritation, which would possibly cause the patient to leave the area or hold his or her breath. In fact, the odour produced by the chemical is similar to that of freshly mown grass or hay. The result is that much

You are the Paramedic Part 3

Your patient receives a rapid decontamination and she is now the first patient who is ready to be transported to the nearest facility. You are notified that the patient has been administered a nerve agent antidote, or MARK 1 kit, which involved auto-injectors of atropine and 2-PAM chloride. Your patient, who is a 30-year-old woman who was working in the shopping centre when the incident took place, is still conscious, alert, and oriented. She is complaining of nausea and vomiting. She is experiencing excessive lacrimation and has already urinated twice while in the treatment area. She also has pinpoint pupils and denies any pertinent medical history.

Reassessment	Recording Time: 20 Minutes
Skin	Pale, warm, and dry
Pulse	110 beats/min (after atropine), bounding, regular radial pulse
Blood pressure	150/92 mm Hg
Respirations	12 breaths/min
Spo₂	97% with supplemental oxygen at 12 l/min via nonrebreathing mask
ECG	Sinus tachycardia without ectopy

5. What could your patient's signs and symptoms represent?
6. What are your treatment options for this patient?

more of the gas is allowed to enter the body unnoticed. The initial symptoms of a mild exposure may include:

- Nausea
- Chest tightness
- Severe cough
- Dyspnea upon exertion

The patient with a severe exposure may present with dyspnea at rest and excessive pulmonary edema (the patient will actually expel large amounts of pulmonary edema from their lungs). The pulmonary edema that is seen with a severe exposure produces such large amounts of fluid from the lungs that the patient may actually become hypovolemic and subsequently hypotensive.

Pulmonary Agent Treatment

The best initial treatment for any pulmonary agent is to remove the patient from the contaminated atmosphere. This should be done by trained personnel in the proper PPE. Aggressive management of the ABCs should be initiated, paying particular attention to oxygenation, ventilation, and suctioning if required. Do not allow the patient to be active, as this will worsen the condition much faster. There are no antidotes to counteract the pulmonary agents. Performing the ABCs, gaining IV access, allowing the patient to rest in a position of comfort with the head elevated, and initiating rapid transport are the primary goals for care provided in the prehospital setting. Pharmacotherapy of this patient may include the standard treatment for bronchospasm, pulmonary edema, potential steroid use (per local medical direction) and positive-pressure ventilation with supplementary oxygen. The use of positive end-expiratory pressure (PEEP) valves attached to a bag-valve-mask may improve oxygenation.

Nerve Agents

The nerve agents are among the most deadly chemicals developed. Designed to kill large numbers of people with small quantities, nerve agents can cause cardiac arrest within seconds to minutes of exposure. Nerve agents, discovered while in search of a superior pesticide, are a class of chemical called organophosphates, which are found in household bug sprays, agricultural pesticides, and some industrial chemicals, at far lower strengths than in nerve agents.

Almost 900 different pesticides are available for use in Canada. Approximately 37 of these belong to a class of insecticides known as organophosphates. The chemicals in this class kill insects by disrupting their brains and nervous systems. Unfortunately, these chemicals or nerve agents (at greater strengths) also can harm the brains and nervous systems of animals and humans. These chemicals block the essential enzyme in the nervous system called cholinesterase from working, causing the body's organs to become overstimulated and burn out.

G agents came from the early nerve agents, the G series, which were developed by German scientists (hence the G) in the period after WWI and into WWII. There are three G series agents, which are all designed with the same basic chemical

structure with slight variations to produce different properties. The two variations of these agents are lethality and volatility. The following G agents are listed from high volatility to low volatility:

- **Sarin (GB).** Highly volatile colourless and odourless liquid. Turns from liquid to gas within seconds to minutes at room temperature. Highly lethal, with an LD_{50} of 1,700 mg/70 kg (about 1 drop, depending on the purity). The LD_{50} is the amount that will kill 50% of people who are exposed to this level. Sarin is primarily a vapour hazard, with the respiratory tract as the main route of entry. This agent is especially dangerous in enclosed environments such as office buildings, shopping centres, or subway cars. When this agent comes into contact with skin, it is quickly absorbed and evapourates. When sarin is on clothing, it has the effect of off-gassing, which means that the vapours are continuously released over a period of time (like perfume). This renders the patient as well as the patient's clothing contaminated.

- **Soman (GD).** Twice as persistent as sarin and five times as lethal. It has a fruity odour as a result of the type of alcohol used in the agent and generally has no colour. This agent is both a contact and inhalation hazard that can enter the body through skin absorption and through the respiratory tract. A unique additive in GD causes it to bind to the cells that it attacks faster than any other agent. This irreversible binding is called aging, which makes it more difficult to treat patients who have been exposed.

- **Tabun (GA).** Approximately half as lethal as sarin and 36 times more persistent; under the proper conditions it will remain for several days. It also has a fruity smell and an appearance similar to sarin. The components used to manufacture GA are easy to acquire and the agent is easy to manufacture, which make it unique. GA is both a contact and inhalation hazard that can enter the body through skin absorption as well as through the respiratory tract.

- **V agent (VX).** Clear oily agent that has no odour and looks like baby oil. V agent was developed by the British after World War II and has similar chemical properties to the G series agents. The difference is that VX is over 100 times more lethal than sarin and is extremely persistent **Figure 48-8 ▶**. In fact, VX is so persistent that given the proper conditions it will remain relatively unchanged for weeks to months.

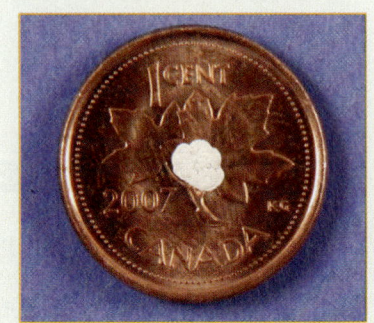

Figure 48-8 VX is the most toxic chemical ever produced. The dot on the penny demonstrates the amount needed to achieve the lethal dose.

These properties make VX primarily a contact hazard, because it lets off very little vapour. It is easily absorbed into the skin, and the oily residue that remains on the skin's surface is extremely difficult to decontaminate.

Nerve agents all produce similar symptoms but have varying routes of entry. Nerve agents differ slightly in lethal concentration or dose and also differ in their volatility. Some agents are designed to become a gas quickly (nonpersistent or highly volatile), while others remain liquid for a period of time (persistent or nonvolatile). These agents have been used successfully in warfare and to date represent the only type of chemical agent that has been used successfully in a terrorist act. Once the agent has entered the body through skin contact or through the respiratory system, the patient will begin to exhibit a pattern of predictable symptoms. Like all chemical agents, the severity of the symptoms will depend on the route of exposure and the amount of agent to which the patient was exposed. The resulting symptoms are described below using the military mnemonic SLUDGEM and the medical mnemonic DUMBELS. These two mnemonics are used to describe the symptoms of nerve agent exposure and are shown in ◖ **Table 48-3 ▼** ◗. The medical mnemonic is more useful to you because it lists the more dangerous symptoms associated with exposure to nerve agents.

There are only a handful of medical conditions that are associated with the bilateral pinpoint constricted pupils (miosis) seen with nerve agent exposure. Conditions such as a suspected stroke, direct light to both eyes, and a drug overdose all can cause bilateral constricted pupils. You should therefore assess the patient for all of the SLUDGEM/DUMBELS signs and symptoms to determine whether the patient has been exposed to a nerve agent.

Table 48-3	Symptoms of Persons Exposed to Nerve Agents
Military Mnemonic: SLUDGEM	
S	Salivation
L	Lacrimation
U	Urination
D	Defecation
G	GI distress
E	Emesis
M	Miosis
Medical Mnemonic: DUMBELS	
D	Defecation
U	Urination
M	Miosis
B	Bradycardia, Bronchorrhea
E	Emesis
L	Lacrimation
S	Salivation

Miosis is the most common symptom of nerve agent exposure and can remain for days to weeks. This symptom, along with the others listed in Table 48-3, will help you recognize exposure to a nerve agent early. The seizures that are associated with nerve agent exposure are unlike those found in patients with a history of seizure. The patient will continue to seize until death or until treatment is given with a nerve agent antidote (MARK 1 or NAAK).

Nerve Agent Treatment (MARK 1/NAAK)

Fatalities from severe exposure occur as a result of respiratory complications, which lead to respiratory arrest. Once the patient has been decontaminated, the paramedic should be prepared to treat these patients aggressively, if they are to be saved. You can greatly increase the patient's chances of survival simply by providing airway and ventilatory support. As with all emergencies, managing the ABCs is the best and most important treatment that you can provide. Often patients exposed to these agents will begin seizing and will not stop. These patients will require administration of nerve agent antidote kits in addition to support of the ABCs.

Fortunately, there is an antidote for nerve agent exposure. MARK 1 kits, also known as Nerve Agent Antidote Kits (NAAK), contain two auto-injector medications: atropine and 2-PAM chloride (pralidoxime chloride). In some regions, the paramedic may carry MARK 1 kits on the unit and will be called upon to administer one or both of the antidotes. These medications are delivered using the same technique as the EpiPen auto-injector; however, multiple doses may need to be administered.

Atropine is used to block the nerve agent's overstimulation of the body. However, because the nerve agent may remain in the body for long periods of time, 2-PAM chloride is used to eliminate the agent from the body. The 2-PAM antidote is effective at relieving the respiratory muscle paralysis and twitching caused by the nerve agent. Many of the symptoms described in the DUMBELS mnemonic will be reversed with the use of atropine; however, many doses may need to be administered to see these results. If your service carries a nerve agent antidote, please refer to your medical director and local protocols for dose and usage information.

◖ **Table 48-4 ▶** ◗ has been provided for quick reference and comparison of the nerve agents.

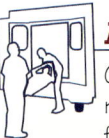

At the Scene

On March 20, 1995, members of a Japanese cult released sarin (GB) in the Tokyo subway. The first arriving medical responders were met with chaos as hundreds and then thousands of people fled the subway system. Many were contaminated and showing signs and systems of nerve agent exposure. In the end more than 5,000 people sought medical care for exposure to sarin, and 12 people died. None of the paramedics wore protective clothing and most became cross-contaminated. Remember, you can avoid becoming exposed. Don't become a victim yourself!

Table 48-4	Nerve Agents					
Name	Code Name	Odour	Special Features	Onset of Symptoms	Volatility	Route of Exposure
Tabun	GA	Fruity	Easy to manufacture	Immediate	Low	Both contact and vapour hazard
Sarin	GB	None (if pure) or strong	Will off-gas while on victim's clothing	Immediate	High	Primarily respiratory vapour hazard; extremely lethal if skin contact is made
Soman	GD	Fruity	Ages rapidly, making it difficult to treat	Immediate	Moderate	Contact with skin; minimal vapour hazard
V agent	VX	None	Most lethal chemical agent; difficult to decontaminate	Immediate	Very low	Contact with skin; no vapour hazard (unless aerosolized)

Industrial Chemicals/Insecticides

As previously mentioned, the basic chemical ingredient in nerve agents is organophosphate. This is a common chemical that is used in lesser concentrations for insecticides. While industrial chemicals do not possess sufficient lethality to be effective WMDs, they are easy to acquire, inexpensive, and would have similar effects as the nerve agents. Crop-duster planes could be used to disseminate these chemicals. You should be cautious when responding to calls where insecticide equipment is stored and used, such as a farm or supply store that sells these products. The symptoms and medical management of patients poisoned by organophosphate insecticide are identical to those of the nerve agents.

Metabolic Agents (Cyanides)

Hydrogen cyanide (AC) and cyanogens chloride (CK) are both agents that affect the body's ability to use oxygen. Cyanide is a colourless gas that has an odour similar to almonds. The effects of the cyanides begin on the cellular level and are very rapidly seen at the organ system level. Beside the nerve agents, metabolic agents are the only chemical weapons known to kill within seconds to minutes. Unlike nerve agents, however, these deadly gases are commonly found in many industrial settings. Cyanides are produced in massive quantities for industrial uses such as gold and silver mining, photography, lethal injections, and plastics processing. They are often present in fires associated with textile or plastic factories. In fact, cyanide is naturally found in the pits of many fruits in very low doses. There is very little difference in the symptoms found between AC and CK. In low doses, these chemicals are associated with dizziness, light-headedness, headache, and vomiting. Higher doses will produce symptoms that include:

- Shortness of breath and gasping respirations
- Tachypnea
- Flushed skin colour
- Tachycardia
- Altered mental status
- Seizures
- Coma
- Apnea
- Cardiac arrest

At the Scene

Always make sure that your patients have been thoroughly decontaminated by trained personnel before you come into contact with them. Chemical agents are primarily a vapour hazard, and all of the patient's clothing must be removed to prevent off-gassing. Finally, never perform mouth-to-mouth or mouth-to-mask ventilation on a victim of a chemical agent. Many of the vapours may linger in the patient's airway and cross-contamination may occur.

The symptoms associated with the inhalation of a large amount of cyanide will all appear within several minutes. Death is likely unless the patient is treated promptly.

Cyanide Agent Treatment

Cyanide binds with the body's cells, preventing oxygen from being used. Several medications act as antidotes, but many services do not carry them. Once trained personnel wearing the proper PPE have removed the patient from the source of exposure, even if there is no liquid contamination, all of the patient's clothes must be removed to prevent off-gassing in the ambulance. Trained and protected personnel must decontaminate any patients who may have been exposed to liquid contamination before a paramedic can initiate treatment. Then you should support the patient's ABCs and gain IV access. Mild effects of cyanide exposure will generally resolve by simply removing the victim from the source of contamination and administering supplementary oxygen. Severe exposure, however, will require aggressive oxygenation and perhaps ventilation with supplementary oxygen. Always use a bag-valve-mask device or oxygen-powered ventilator device to ventilate a patient exposed to a metabolic agent. The agent can easily be passed on from the patient to the paramedic through mouth-to-mouth or mouth-to-mask ventilations. If no antidote is available, initiate transport immediately.

Table 48-5 ▶ summarizes the chemical agents. The odours of the particular chemicals are provided for informational purposes only. The sense of smell is a poor tool to use to determine whether there is a chemical agent present. Many

Table 48-5	Chemical Agents					
Class	**Military Designations**	**Odour**	**Lethality**	**Onset of Symptoms**	**Volatility**	**Primary Route of Exposure**
Nerve agents	Tabun (GA) Sarin (GB) Soman (GD) VX	Fruity or none	Most lethal chemical agents can kill within minutes; effects are reversible with antidotes	Immediate	Moderate (GA, GD) Very high (GB) Low (VX)	Vapour hazard (GB) Both vapour and contact hazard (GA, GD) Contact hazard (VX)
Vesicants	Mustard (H) Lewisite (L) Phosgene oxime (CX)	Garlic (H) Geranium (L)	Causes large blisters to form on victims; may severely damage upper airway if vapours are inhaled; severe intense pain and greyish skin discolouration (L, CX)	Delayed (H) Immediate (L, CX)	Very low (H, L) Moderate (CX)	Primarily contact; with some vapour hazard
Pulmonary agents	Chlorine (CL) Phosgene (CG)	Bleach (CL) Cut grass (CG)	Causes irritation; choking (CL); severe pulmonary edema (CG)	Immediate (CL) Delayed (CG)	Very high	Vapour hazard
Cyanide agents	Hydrogen cyanide (AC) Cyanogens chloride (CK)	Almonds (AC) Irritating (CK)	Highly lethal chemical gases; can kill within minutes; effects are reversible with antidotes	Immediate	Very high	Vapour hazard

persons are unable to smell the agents, and the odour could be derived from another source. This information is useful to you if you receive reports from victims claiming to smell bleach or garlic, for example. You should never enter a potentially hazardous area and "smell" to determine whether a chemical agent is present.

Biological Agents

Biological agents pose many difficult issues when used as a WMD. Biological agents can be almost completely undetectable. Also, most of the diseases caused by these agents will be similar to other minor illnesses commonly seen by paramedics.

Biological agents are grouped as viruses, bacteria, or neurotoxins and may be spread in various ways. Dissemination is the means by which a terrorist will spread the agent—for example, poisoning the water supply or aerosolizing the agent into the air or ventilation system of a building. A disease vector is an animal that spreads disease, once infected, to another animal. For example, the plague can be spread by infected rats, smallpox by infected persons, and West Nile virus by infected mosquitoes. How easily the disease is able to spread from one human to another human is called communicability. Some diseases, such as those caused by human immunodeficiency virus, are difficult to spread by routine contact. Therefore communicability is considered low. In other instances when communicability is high, such as with smallpox, the person is considered contagious. Typically, routine precautions are enough to prevent contamination from contagious biological organisms.

Incubation describes the period of time between the person becoming exposed to the agent and when symptoms begin. The incubation period is especially important for the

paramedic to understand. Although your patient may not exhibit signs or symptoms, he or she may be contagious.

Paramedics need to be aware of when they should suspect the use of biological agents. If the agent is in the form of a powder, such as in the October 2001 incidents in the United States involving anthrax powder mailed in letters, the call must be handled by HazMat specialists. Patients who have come into direct contact with the agent need to be decontaminated before any EMS contact or treatment is initiated.

Viruses

Viruses are germs that require a living host to multiply and survive. A virus is a simple organism and cannot thrive outside of a host (living body). Once in the body, the virus will invade healthy cells and replicate itself to spread through the host. As the virus spreads, so does the disease that it carries. Viruses survive by moving from one host to another by using its transport system-vectors.

Viral agents that may be used during a biological terrorist release pose an extraordinary problem for health care providers, especially those in EMS. Although some viral agents do have vaccines, there is no treatment for a viral infection other than antivirals for some agents. Because of this characteristic, the following viruses have been used as terrorist agents.

Smallpox

Smallpox is a highly contagious disease. All forms of routine precautions and PPE must be used to prevent cross-contamination to health care providers. Simply by wearing examination gloves, a HEPA-filtered respirator, and eye protection, you will greatly reduce your risk of contamination. The last natural case of smallpox in the world was seen in 1977. Before the rash and blisters show, the illness will start with a high fever and body aches and headaches. The patient's temperature is usually in the range of 38°C to 40°C.

An easy, quick way to differentiate the smallpox rash from other skin disorders is to observe the size, shape, and location of the lesions. In smallpox, all the lesions are identical in their development. In other skin disorders, the lesions will be in various stages of healing and development. Smallpox blisters also begin on the face and extremities and eventually move toward the chest and abdomen. The disease is in its most contagious phase when the blisters begin to form Figure 48-9 ▾ . Unprotected contact with these blisters will promote transmission of the disease. There is a vaccine to prevent smallpox; however, it has been linked to medical complications and in very rare cases death Table 48-6 ▾ . Vaccination against the disease is part of a national strategy to respond to a terrorist threat. Because the vaccine does have some risk, only first responders have been offered the vaccine. Should an outbreak occur, vaccine would be offered to people at risk.

Viral Hemorrhagic Fevers

Viral hemorrhagic fevers (VHF) consist of a group of diseases that include the Ebola, Rift Valley, and yellow fever viruses, among others. This group of viruses causes the blood in the body to seep out from the tissues and blood vessels Figure 48-10 ▾ . Initially, the patient will have flu-like symptoms, progressing to more serious symptoms such as internal and external hemorrhaging. Outbreaks are not uncommon in Africa and South America. Outbreaks in Canada, however, are extremely rare. All PPE and routine precautions must be taken when treating these illnesses. Mortality rates can range from 5% to 90%, depending on the strain of virus, the patient's age and health condition, and the availability of a modern health care system Table 48-7 ▸ .

Bacteria

Unlike viruses, bacteria do not require a host to multiply and live. Bacteria are much more complex and larger than viruses and can grow up to 100 times larger than the largest virus. Bacteria contain all the cellular structures of a normal cell and are completely self-sufficient. Most importantly, bacterial infections can be fought with antibiotics.

Most bacterial infections will generally begin with flu-like symptoms, which make it quite difficult to identify whether the cause is a biological attack or a natural epidemic. Biological agents have been developed and used for centuries during times of war.

Inhalation and Cutaneous Anthrax (*Bacillus anthracis*)

Anthrax is a deadly bacteria that lays dormant in a spore (protective shell). When exposed to the optimal temperature and

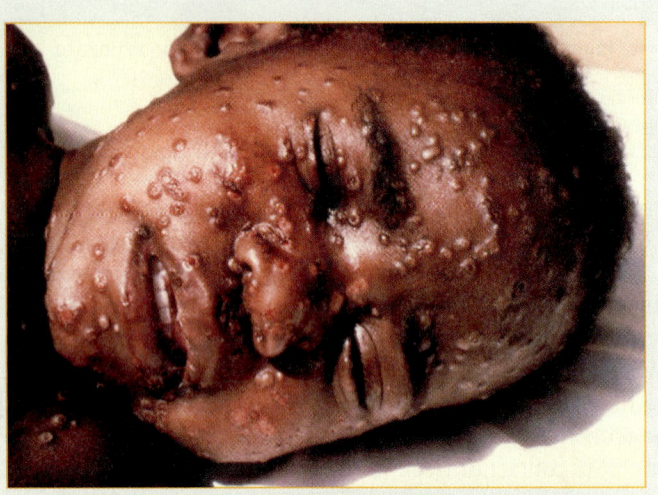

Figure 48-9 In smallpox, all the lesions are identical in their development. In other skin disorders, the lesions will be in various stages of healing and development.

Table 48-6	Characteristics of Smallpox
Dissemination	Aerosolized for warfare or terrorist uses
Communicability	High from infected individuals or items (such as blankets used by infected patients). Person-to-person transmission is possible.
Route of entry	Through inhalation of coughed droplets or direct skin contact with blisters
Signs and symptoms	Severe fever, malaise, body aches, headaches, small blisters on the skin, bleeding of the skin and mucous membranes. Incubation period is 10 to 12 days and the duration of the illness is approximately 4 weeks.
Medical management	BSI precautions. There is no specific treatment for smallpox victims. Patients should be provided with supportive prehospital care (ABCs).

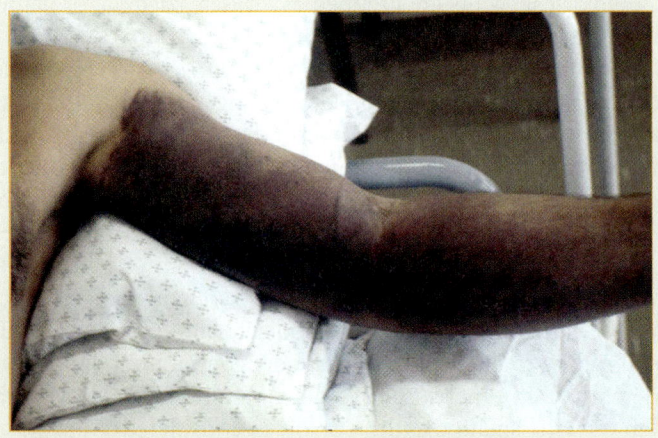

Figure 48-10 Viral hemorrhagic fevers cause the blood vessels and tissues to seep blood. The end result is ecchymosis, hemoptysis, and blood in the patient's stool. Notice the severe discolouration in this patient with Crimean Congo hemorrhagic fever, indicating internal bleeding.

moisture, the germ will be released from the spore. The routes of entry for anthrax are inhalation, cutaneous, or gastrointestinal (from consuming food that contain spores) **Figure 48-11 ▾** . The inhalational form or pulmonary anthrax is the most deadly and often presents as a severe cold. Pulmonary anthrax infections are associated with a 90% death rate if untreated. Antibiotics can be used to treat anthrax successfully. There is also a vaccine to prevent anthrax infections **Table 48-8 ▸** .

Plague—Bubonic/Pneumonic

Of all the infectious diseases known to humans, none has killed as many as the plague. The 14th century plague that ravaged Asia, the Middle East, and finally Europe (the Black Death) killed an estimated 33 to 42 million people. Later on, in the early 19th century, almost 20 million people in India and China

Table 48-7	Characteristics of Viral Hemorrhagic Fevers
Dissemination	Direct contact with an infected person's body fluids. It can also be aerosolized for use in an attack.
Communicability	Moderate from person to person or from contaminated items.
Route of entry	Direct contact with an infected person's body fluids.
Signs and symptoms	Sudden onset of fever, weakness, muscle pain, headache, and sore throat. All of these symptoms are followed by vomiting and as the virus runs it course, internal and external bleeding.
Medical management	Routine precautions and PPE. There is no specific treatment for viral hemorrhagic fever. Patients should be provided supportive prehospital care (ABCs) and treatment for shock and hypotension, if present.

Table 48-8	Characteristics of Anthrax
Dissemination	Aerosol
Communicability	Only in the cutaneous form (rare)
Route of entry	Through inhalation of spore or skin contact with spore or direct contact with skin wound (cutaneous)
Signs and symptoms	Flu-like symptoms, fever, respiratory distress with tachycardia, shock, pulmonary edema and respiratory failure after 3 to 5 days of flu-like symptoms
Medical management	Pulmonary/inhalation: PPE and routine precautions, supplemental oxygen, ventilatory support for pulmonary edema or respiratory failure and transport. Cutaneous: BSI precautions, apply dry sterile dressing to prevent accidental contact with wound and fluids.

perished due to plague. The plague's natural vectors are infected rodents and fleas. When a person is either bit by an infected flea or comes into contact with an infected rodent (or the waste of the rodent), the person can contract bubonic plague.

Bubonic plague infects the lymphatic system (a passive circulatory system in the body that bathes the tissues in lymph and works with the immune system). When this occurs, the patient's lymph nodes (area of the lymphatic system where infection-fighting cells are housed) become infected and grow. The glands of the nodes will grow large (up to the size of a tennis ball) and round, forming buboes **Figure 48-12 ▸** . If left untreated, the infection may spread through the body, leading to sepsis and possibly death. This form of plague is not contagious and is not likely to be seen in a bioterrorist incident.

Pneumonic plague is a lung infection, also known as plague pneumonia, that results from inhalation of plague bacteria. This form of the disease is contagious and has a much higher death rate than the bubonic form. This form of plague therefore would be easier to disseminate (aerosolized), has a higher mortality, and is contagious **Table 48-9 ▸** .

Neurotoxins

Neurotoxins are the most deadly substances known to humans. The strongest neurotoxin is 15,000 times more lethal than VX and 100,000 times more lethal than sarin. These toxins are produced from plants, marine animals, moulds, and bacteria. The route of entry for these toxins is through ingestion, inhalation from aerosols, or injection. Unlike viruses and bacteria, neurotoxins are not contagious and have a faster onset of symptoms. Although these biological toxins have immense destructive potential, they have not been used successfully as a WMD.

Botulinum Toxin

The most potent neurotoxin is botulinum, which is produced by bacteria. When introduced into the body, this neurotoxin

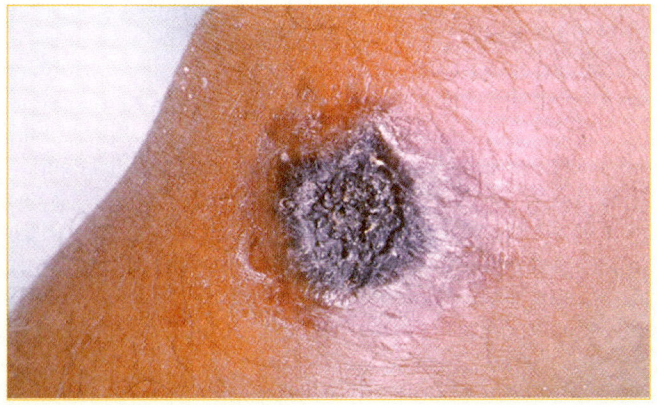

Figure 48-11 Cutaneous anthrax.

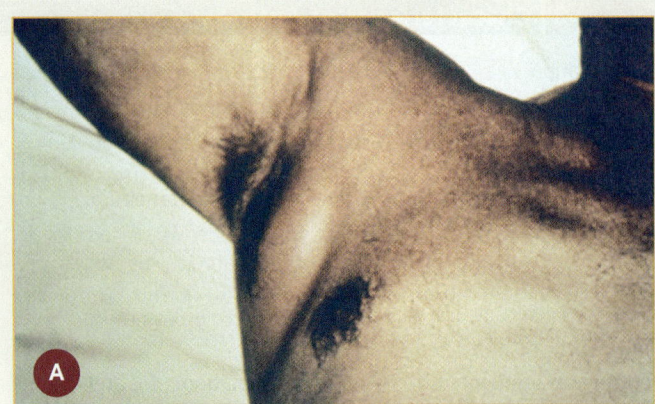

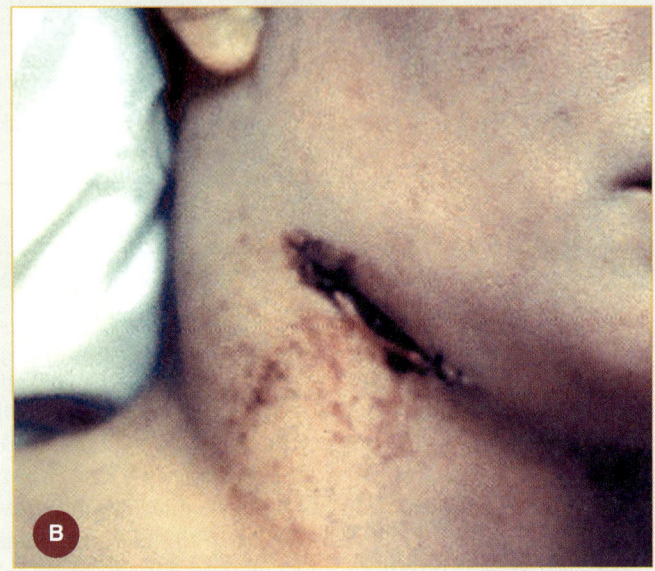

Figure 48-12 A. Plague buboe at lymph node under arm. **B.** Plague buboe at lymph node on neck.

Table 48-10	Characteristics of Botulinum Toxin
Dissemination	Aerosol or food supply sabotage or injection
Communicability	None
Route of entry	Ingestion or gastrointestinal
Signs and symptoms	Dry mouth, intestinal obstruction, urinary retention, constipation, nausea and vomiting, abnormal pupil dilation, blurred vision, double vision, drooping eyelids, difficulty swallowing, difficulty speaking, and respiratory failure due to paralysis
Medical management	ABCs, provide supplemental oxygen and transport. Ventilatory support may be needed due to paralysis of the respiratory muscles. A vaccine is available.

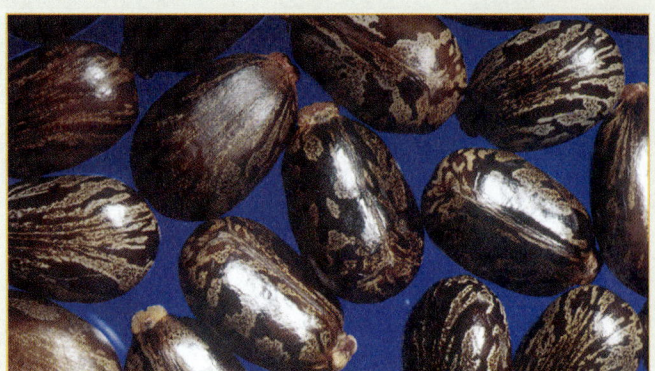

Figure 48-13 These seemingly harmless castor beans contain the key ingredient for ricin, one of the most potent toxins known to humans.

Table 48-9	Characteristics of Plague
Dissemination	Aerosol
Communicability	Bubonic: low, only from contact with fluid in buboe Pneumonic: high, from person to person
Route of entry	Ingestion, inhalation, or cutaneous
Signs and symptoms	Fever, headache, muscle pain and tenderness, pneumonia, shortness of breath, extreme lymph node pain and enlargement (bubonic)
Medical management	PPE and routine precautions, ABCs, provide supplemental oxygen, and transport

Ricin

While not as deadly as botulinum, ricin is still five times more lethal than VX. This toxin is derived from mash that is left from the castor bean Figure 48-13 ▲ . When introduced into the body, ricin causes pulmonary edema and respiratory and circulatory failure leading to death Table 48-11 ▶ .

The clinical picture depends on the route of exposure. The toxin is quite stable and extremely toxic by many routes of exposure, including inhalation. Perhaps 1 to 3 mg of ricin can kill an adult, and the ingestion of one seed can probably kill a child.

Although all parts of the castor bean are actually poisonous, it is the seeds that are the most toxic. Castor bean ingestion causes a rapid onset of nausea, vomiting, abdominal cramps, and severe diarrhea, followed by vascular collapse. Death usually occurs on the third day in the absence of appropriate medical intervention.

Ricin is least toxic by the oral route. This is probably a result of poor absorption in the gastrointestinal tract, some digestion in the gut, and, possibly, some expulsion of the agent

affects the nervous system's ability to function. Voluntary muscle control will diminish as the toxin spreads. Eventually the toxin will cause muscle paralysis that begins at the head and face and travels downward throughout the body. The patient's accessory muscles and diaphragm will become paralyzed, and the patient will go into respiratory arrest Table 48-10 ▶ .

Table 48-11	Characteristics of Ricin
Dissemination	Aerosol or contamination of a food or water supply by sabotage
Communicability	None
Route of entry	Inhalation, ingestion, injection
Signs and symptoms	Inhaled: Cough, difficulty breathing, chest tightness, nausea, muscle aches, pulmonary edema, and hypoxia Ingested: Nausea and vomiting, internal bleeding, and death Injection: No signs except swelling at the injection site and death
Medical management	ABCs. No treatment or vaccine exists.

as caused by the rapid onset of vomiting. Ingestion causes local hemorrhage and necrosis of the liver, spleen, kidney, and gastrointestinal tract. Signs and symptoms appear 4 to 8 hours after exposure.

Signs and symptoms of ricin ingestion are as follows:

- Fever
- Chills
- Headache
- Muscle aches
- Nausea
- Vomiting
- Diarrhea
- Severe abdominal cramping
- Dehydration
- Gastrointestinal bleeding
- Necrosis of liver, spleen, kidneys, and gastrointestinal tract

Inhalation of ricin causes nonspecific weakness, cough, fever, hypothermia, and hypotension. Symptoms occur about 4 to 8 hours after inhalation, depending on the inhaled dose. The onset of profuse sweating some hours later signifies the termination of the symptoms.

Signs and symptoms of ricin inhalation are as follows:

- Fever
- Chills
- Nausea

- Local irritation of eyes, nose, and throat
- Profuse sweating
- Headache
- Muscle aches
- Nonproductive cough
- Chest pain
- Dyspnea
- Pulmonary edema
- Severe lung inflammation
- Cyanosis
- Convulsions
- Respiratory failure

Treatment is supportive and includes both respiratory support and cardiovascular support as needed. Early intubation, ventilation, and positive end expiratory pressure, combined with treatment of pulmonary edema, are appropriate. Intravenous fluids and electrolyte replacement are useful for treating the dehydration caused by profound vomiting and diarrhea. **Table 48-12** ▾ summarizes the biological agents.

Other Paramedic Roles During a Biological Event

Syndromic Surveillance

Syndromic surveillance is the monitoring, usually by local or provincial health departments, of patients presenting to emergency departments and alternative care facilities, and the recording of EMS call volume and the use of over-the-counter medications. Patients with signs and symptoms that resemble influenza are particularly important. Local and provincial health departments monitor for an unusual influx of patients with these symptoms in hopes of catching an outbreak early. The EMS role in syndromic surveillance is a small one, yet valuable in the overall tracking of a biological terrorist event or infectious disease outbreak. Quality assurance and dispatch operations need to be aware of an unusual number of calls from patients with "unexplainable flu" coming from a particular region or community.

Points of Distribution

The federal and provincial governments have developed and distributed regional stockpiles of key antibiotics, antidotes, and

Table 48-12	Biological Agents			
Disease	**Transmission Person to Person**	**Incubation Period**	**Duration of Illness**	**Lethality (approximate case fatality rates)**
Inhalation anthrax	No	1 to 6 d	3 to 5 d (usually fatal if untreated)	High
Pneumonic plague	High	2 to 3 d	1 to 6 d (usually fatal)	High unless treated within 12 to 24 h
Smallpox	High	7 to 17 d (average 12 d)	4 wk	High to moderate
Viral hemorrhagic fevers	Moderate	4 to 21 d	Death between 7 to 16 d	High to moderate, depending on type of fever
Botulinum	No	1 to 5 d	Death in 24 to 72 h; lasts months if patient does not die	High without respiratory support
Ricin	No	18 to 24 h	Days; death within 10 to 12 d for ingestion	High

other supplies for rapid deployment in the event that immediate treatment of large numbers of people is required. Each province has established its own warehousing and distribution system as part of their respective disaster or contingency plans Figure 48-14 ▾ . EMS agencies are integral to this system. As a paramedic, it is your responsibility to know how you fit into this plan.

Paramedics may be called on to assist in the delivery of the medications to the public (depending on local emergency management planning). The paramedic's role may include triage, treatment of seriously ill patients, and patient transport to the hospital. Most plans for PODs include at least one

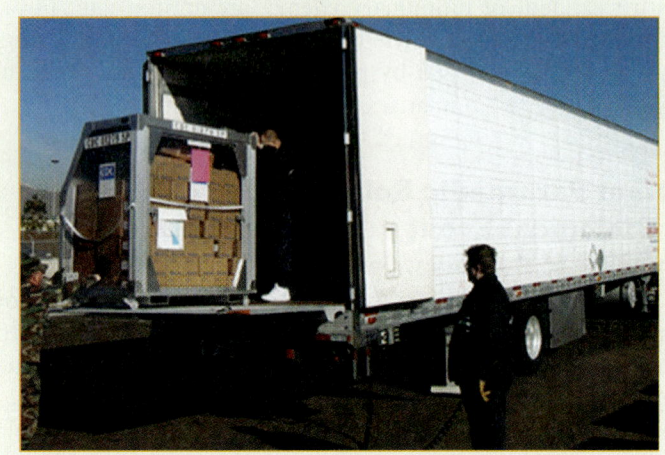

Figure 48-14 The federal and provincial governments have a plan in place to deliver supplies in the event of an emergency.

ambulance on standby for the transport of seriously ill patients.

Radiological/Nuclear Devices

What Is Radiation?

Ionizing radiation is energy that is emitted in the form of rays, or particles. This energy can be found in radioactive material, such as rocks and metals. Radioactive material is any material that emits radiation. This material is unstable, and attempts to stabilize itself by changing its structure is a natural process called decay. As the substance decays, it gives off radiation until it stabilizes. The process of radioactive decay can take from as little as minutes to billions of years; meanwhile, the substance remains radioactive.

The energy that is emitted from a strong radiological source is either alpha, beta, gamma (x-rays), or neutron radiation Figure 48-15 ▸ . Alpha is the least harmful penetrating type of radiation and cannot travel fast or through most objects. In fact, a sheet of paper or the body's skin easily stops it. Beta radiation is slightly more penetrating than alpha and requires a layer of clothing to stop it. Gamma or x-rays are far faster and stronger than alpha and beta rays. These rays easily penetrate through the human body and

Notes from Nancy

Before you enter the "hot" zone, remember: Your best allies are time, distance, and shielding.

You are the Paramedic Part 4

Your patient has a patent airway. You immediately apply high-flow oxygen via a nonrebreathing mask. Lung sounds are raspy and moist sounding. Her oxygen saturation is at 97% on 15 l/min of oxygen. Because the patient report that you received from the HazMat team indicates that a nerve agent antidote kit was used on the patient, you will need to closely monitor her vital signs and watch to see if symptoms develop. Take along another MARK 1 kit and contact direct medical control once en route to the ED.

While en route, your patient states that she does not feel right. She is becoming disoriented. She suddenly begins to have a seizure. You quickly place padding around the patient to keep her from injuring herself. She becomes incontinent.

Reassessment	Recording Time: 30 Minutes
Skin	Pale, warm, and dry
Pulse	120 beats/min
Blood pressure	148/94 mm Hg
Respirations	12 breaths/min
Spo_2	96% with supplemental oxygen
ECG	Sinus tachycardia with an occasional PVC

7. What does the nerve agent antidote kit include?

8. Is this kit part of your local protocol in dealing with patients exposed to a nerve agent?

9. What is your next step in treatment?

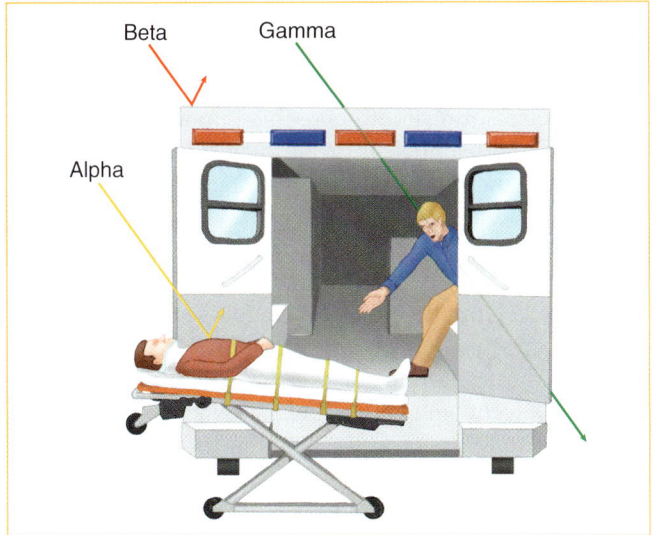

Figure 48-15 Alpha, beta, and gamma radiation.

require either several centimetres of lead or concrete to prevent penetration. Neutron energy is the fastest moving and most powerful form of radiation. Neutrons easily penetrate through lead and require several feet of concrete to stop them.

Sources of Radiological Material

There are thousands of radioactive materials found on the earth. These materials are generally used for purposes that benefit humankind, such as medicine, killing germs in food (irradiating), and construction work. Once radiological material has been used for its purpose, the material remaining is called radiological waste. Radiological waste remains radioactive but has no more usefulness. These materials can be found at:

- Hospitals
- Colleges and universities
- Chemical and industrial sites
- Power plants

Not all radioactive material is tightly guarded, and the waste is often not guarded. This makes use of radioactive material and substances appealing to terrorists.

Radiological Dispersal Devices

A radiological dispersal device (RDD) is any container that is designed to disperse radioactive material. This would generally require the use of a bomb, hence the nickname dirty bomb. A dirty bomb would carry the potential to injure victims with not only the radioactive material but also the explosive material used to deliver it. Just the thought of an RDD creates fear in a population, and so the ultimate goal of the terrorist—fear—is accomplished. In reality, however, the destructive capability of a dirty bomb is limited to the explosives that are attached to it. Therefore, if the explosive is sufficient to kill 10 persons without

radioactive material, it will also kill 10 persons with the radioactive material added. There may be long-term injuries and illness associated with the use of an RDD, yet not much more than the bomb by itself would create. In short, the dirty bomb is an ineffective WMD.

Nuclear Energy

Nuclear energy is artificially made by altering (splitting) radioactive atoms. The result is an immense amount of energy that usually takes the form of heat. Nuclear material is used in medicine, weapons, naval vessels, and power plants. Nuclear material gives off all forms of radiation including neutrons (the most deadly type). Like radioactive material, when nuclear material is no longer useful it becomes waste that is still radioactive.

Nuclear Weapons

The destructive energy of a nuclear explosion is unlike any other weapon in the world. That is why nuclear weapons are kept only in secure facilities throughout the world. There are nations that have ties to terrorists and that have actively attempted to build nuclear weapons. However, the ability of these nations to deliver a nuclear weapon, such as a missile or bomb, is as of yet, incomplete. There is also the deterrent of complete mutual annihilation. Therefore, the likelihood of a nuclear attack is extremely remote.

Unfortunately, due to the collapse of the former Soviet Union, the whereabouts of many small nuclear devices is unknown. These small suitcase-sized nuclear weapons are called Special Atomic Demolition Munitions (SADM). The SADM, or "suit-case nuke," was designed to destroy individual targets, such as important buildings, bridges, tunnels, or large ships. The estimate is that perhaps as many as 80 are missing as of 1998. No other information or updates on the whereabouts of these devices have been made public.

How Radiation Affects the Body

The effects of radiation exposure will vary depending on the amount of radiation that a person receives and the route of entry. Radiation can be introduced into the body by all routes of entry as well as through the body (irradiation). The patient can inhale radioactive dust from nuclear fallout or from a dirty bomb, or have radioactive liquid absorbed into the body through the skin. Once in the body, the radiation source will irradiate the person from within rather than from an external source (such as x-ray equipment). Some common signs of acute radiation sickness are nausea, vomiting, and diarrhea. Additional injuries will occur with a nuclear blast such as thermal and blast trauma, trauma from flying objects, and eye injuries.

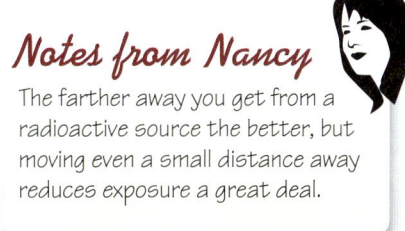

Notes from Nancy
The farther away you get from a radioactive source the better, but moving even a small distance away reduces exposure a great deal.

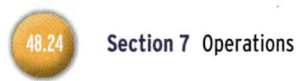

Medical Management

Being exposed to a radiation source does not make a patient contaminated or radioactive. However, when patients have a radioactive source on their body (such as debris from a dirty bomb), they are contaminated and must be initially cared for by a HazMat responder. Once the patient is decontaminated and there is no threat to you, you may begin treatment with the ABCs and treat the patient for any burns or trauma.

Protective Measures

There are no suits or protective gear designed to completely shield from radiation. Those who work in high-risk areas do wear some protection (lead-lined suits); however, this equipment is not available to the paramedic. The best ways to protect yourself from the effects of radiation are to use time and distance, and shield yourself in Level C protection from the source.

- **Time.** Radiation has a cumulative effect on the body. The less time that you are exposed to the source, the less the effects will be. If you realize that the patient is near a radiation source, leave the area immediately.

- **Distance.** Radiation is limited as to how far it can travel. Depending on the type of radiation, often moving only a few feet is enough to remove you from immediate danger. Alpha radiation cannot travel more than a few centimetres. You should take this into account when responding to a nuclear or radiological incident and make certain that responders are stationed far enough from the incident.

- **Shielding.** As discussed earlier, the path of all radiation can be stopped by a specific object. It will be impossible for you to recognize the type of radiation being emitted, or even from which direction it is coming. Therefore, you should always assume that you are dealing with the strongest form of radiation and use concrete shielding (such as buildings or walls) between yourself and the incident. The importance of shielding cannot be overemphasized. In one atomic test, a car was parked on the side of a house, opposite the direction of the oncoming blast. The house was completely destroyed, yet the car that was directly next to it sustained almost no damage.

You are the Paramedic Summary

1. What is your first priority at a call in this situation?

Because there are multiple patients and a potential hazard to the rescuers, the first priority is your personal safety and that of your crew. That is why it was smart to stage the units until more information was determined about the cause of the incident.

2. What does the dispatch information indicate as far as the need for additional resources?

The dispatch information paints a picture of multiple patients with medical complaints. While it is not uncommon to get multiple patients with traumatic complaints at a typical motor vehicle collision, we rarely get multiple patients with medical complaints unless there is something they all were exposed to causing the symptoms.

3. What precautions can you take to ensure your own safety?

Immediately make sure help is on the way with self-contained breathing apparatus (SCBA) and the appropriate level of Haz-Mat training. Each community has a plan and the best thing you can do at this point is don't just rush in, rather activate the plan.

4. What does your index of suspicion tell you about this scene?

The specifics are slowly being identified as the HazMat team identifies the product that the patients were exposed to. However, the slow pulse rate, vomiting, and tearing lead you in the direction of a nerve agent even before the actual substance is identified.

5. What could your patient's signs and symptoms represent?

As you have learned, patients who have been exposed to a nerve agent are likely to have the symptoms paramedics remember using the mnemonic DUMBELS. That stands for:

Defecation, Urination, Miosis, Bradycardia/bronchorrhea, Emesis, Lacrimation, and Salivation.

6. What are your treatment options for this patient?

Always manage the ABCs and symptoms. In a case of suspected nerve gas exposure, contact medical direction or the Poison Centre for authorization to administer the MARK 1 kit, which usually consists of two auto-injectors: one with a high dose of atropine and the other with 2-PAM chloride (pralidoxime chloride). Then transport the patient with ongoing assessment and support of her ABCs.

7. What does the nerve agent antidote kit include?

The MARK 1 kit includes two auto-injectors, which contain a high dose of atropine and the other with 2-PAM chloride (pralidoxime chloride).

8. Is this kit part of your local protocol in dealing with patients exposed to a nerve agent?

If it is not, you should ask your medical director what the plan is for treating large numbers of patients who have been exposed to a nerve agent.

9. What are your next steps in treatment?

Ongoing assessment, manage the ABCs, and transport the patient. Depending on how fast she comes out of the seizure and how well she can ventilate, it may be necessary to consider intubation and the need to support or assist her ventilations with a bag-valve-mask device and supplementary oxygen. Consult with direct medical control to consider the need to potentially medicate the patient for (1) nausea and vomiting, (2) developing fluid in the lungs, and (3) seizure activity if lengthy.

Prep Kit

■ Ready for Review

- As a result of the increase in terrorist activity, it is possible that you could witness a terrorist event. You must be mentally and physically prepared for the possibility of a terrorist event.
- The use of weapons of mass destruction or mass casualty further complicates the management of the terrorist incident. Be aware of your surroundings at all times. The best form of protection from a WMD agent is to avoid contact with the agent.
- A WMD is any agent designed to bring about mass death, casualties, and/or massive damage to property and infrastructure (bridges, tunnels, airports, and seaports). These can be nuclear, chemical, biological, and explosive weapons.
- Indicators that may give you clues as to whether the emergency is the result of an attack include the type of location, type of call, number of patients, patients' statements, and preincident indicators.
- If you suspect that a terrorist or WMD event has occurred, ensure that the scene is safe. If you have any doubt that it may not be safe, do not enter. Wait for assistance.
- Notification of the dispatcher is essential. Inform dispatch of the nature of the event, any additional resources that may be required, the estimated number of patients, and the upwind route of approach or optimal route of approach.
- Establish a staging area, where other units will converge. Be mindful of access and exit routes.
- Terrorists may set secondary devices to explode after the initial bomb, to injure responders and secure media coverage. Constantly assess and reassess the scene for safety.
- Paramedics may be called upon to assist in the delivery of the medications to the public. The paramedic's role may include triage, treatment of seriously ill patients, and patient transport to the hospital.

■ Vital Vocabulary

alpha Type of energy that is emitted from a strong radiological source; it is the least harmful penetrating type of radiation and cannot travel fast or through most objects.

anthrax A deadly bacteria (*Bacillus anthracis*) that lays dormant in a spore (protective shell); the germ is released from the spore when exposed to the optimal temperature and moisture. The route of entry is inhalation, cutaneous, or gastrointestinal (from consuming food that contains spores).

bacteria Microorganisms that reproduce by binary fission. These single-cell creatures reproduce rapidly. Some can form spores (encysted variants) when environmental conditions are harsh.

beta Type of energy that is emitted from a strong radiological source; is slightly more penetrating than alpha, and requires a layer of clothing to stop it.

BNICE A mnemonic for the five types of terrorist incidents that first responder agencies may be confronted with in the prehospital environment.

botulinum Produced by bacteria, this is a very potent neurotoxin. When introduced into the body, this neurotoxin affects the nervous system's ability to function and causes muscle paralysis.

buboes Enlarged lymph nodes (up to the size of tennis balls) that were characteristic of people infected with the bubonic plague.

bubonic plague An epidemic that spread throughout Europe in the Middle Ages, also called the Black Death, transmitted by infected fleas and characterized by acute malaise, fever, and the formation of tender, enlarged, inflamed lymph nodes that appear as lesions, called buboes.

chlorine (CL) The first chemical agent ever used in warfare. It has a distinct odour of bleach, and creates a green haze when released as a gas. Initially it produces upper airway irritation and a choking sensation.

communicability Describes how easily a disease spreads from one human to another human.

contact hazard A hazardous agent that gives off very little or no vapours; the skin is the primary route for this type of chemical to enter the body; also called a skin hazard.

contagious A person infected with a disease that is highly communicable.

covert Act in which the public safety community generally has no prior knowledge of the time, location, or nature of the attack.

cross-contamination Occurs when a person is contaminated by an agent as a result of coming into contact with another contaminated person.

cyanide Agent that affects the body's ability to use oxygen. It is a colourless gas that has an odour similar to almonds. The effects begin on the cellular level and are very rapidly seen at the organ system level.

decay A natural process in which a material that is unstable attempts to stabilize itself by changing its structure.

dirty bomb Name given to a bomb that is used as a radiological dispersal device (RDD).

disease vector An animal that once infected, spreads a disease to another animal.

dissemination The means with which a terrorist will spread a disease, for example, by poisoning of the water supply, or aerosolizing the agent into the air or ventilation system of a building.

domestic terrorists Native citizens who carry out terrorist acts against their own country.

G agents Early nerve agents that were developed by German scientists in the period after WWI and into WWII. There are three such agents: sarin, soman, and tabun.

gamma (x-rays) Type of energy that is emitted from a strong radiological source that is far faster and stronger than alpha and beta rays. These rays easily penetrate through the human body and require either several centimetres of lead or concrete to prevent penetration.

incubation Describes the period of time from a person being exposed to a disease to the time when symptoms begin.

international terrorism Terrorism that is carried out by those not of the host's country; also known as cross-border terrorism.

ionizing radiation Energy that is emitted in the form of rays, or particles.

LD$_{50}$ The amount of an agent or substance that will kill 50% of people who are exposed to this level.

Lewisite (L) A blistering agent that has a rapid onset of symptoms and produces immediate intense pain and discomfort on contact.

lymphatic system A passive circulatory system that transports a plasma-like liquid called lymph, a thin fluid that bathes the tissues of the body.

lymph nodes Area of the lymphatic system where infection-fighting cells are housed.

MARK 1 A nerve agent antidote kit containing two auto-injector medications, atropine and 2-PAM chloride (pralidoxime chloride); also known as a Nerve Agent Antidote Kit (NAAK).

miosis Bilateral pinpoint constricted pupils.

mutagen Substance that mutates, damages, and changes the structures of DNA in the body's cells.

NAAK A nerve agent antidote kit containing two auto-injector medications, atropine and 2-PAM chloride (pralidoxime chloride); also known as a MARK 1 kit.

nerve agents A class of chemicals called organophosphates; they function by blocking an essential enzyme in the nervous system, which causes the body's organs to become overstimulated and burn out.

neurotoxins Biological agents that are the most deadly substances known to humans; they include botulinum toxin and ricin.

neutron radiation Type of energy that is emitted from a strong radiological source; neutron energy is the fastest moving and most powerful form of radiation. Neutrons easily penetrate through lead, and require several feet of concrete to stop them.

off-gassing The emitting of an agent after exposure, for example from a person's clothes that have been exposed to the agent.

persistency Term used to describe how long a chemical agent will stay on a surface before it evapourates.

phosgene A pulmonary agent that is a product of combustion, such as might be produced in a fire at a textile factory or house, or from metalwork or burning Freon. Phosgene is a very potent agent that has a delayed onset of symptoms, usually hours.

phosgene oxime (CX) A blistering agent that has a rapid onset of symptoms and produces immediate intense pain and discomfort on contact.

pneumonic plague A lung infection, also known as plague pneumonia, that is the result of inhalation of plague bacteria.

radioactive material Any material that emits radiation.

radiological dispersal device (RDD) Any container that is designed to disperse radioactive material.

ricin Neurotoxin derived from mash that is left from pressing oil from the castor bean; causes pulmonary edema and respiratory and circulatory failure, leading to death.

route of exposure Manner by which a toxic substance enters the body.

sarin (GB) A nerve agent that is one of the G agents; a highly volatile colourless and odourless liquid that turns from liquid to gas within seconds to minutes at room temperature.

secondary device Additional explosives used by terrorists, which are set to explode after the initial bomb.

smallpox A highly contagious disease; it is most contagious when blisters begin to form.

soman (GD) A nerve agent that is one of the G agents; twice as persistent as sarin and five times as lethal; it has a fruity odour as a result of the type of alcohol used in the agent, and is both a contact and inhalation hazard that can enter the body through skin absorption and through the respiratory tract.

Special Atomic Demolition Munitions (SADM) Small suitcase-sized nuclear weapons that were designed to destroy individual targets, such as important buildings, bridges, tunnels, or large ships.

state-sponsored terrorism Terrorism that is funded and/or supported by nations that hold close ties with terrorist groups.

sulfur mustard (H) A vesicant; it is a brownish-yellowish oily substance that is generally considered very persistent; has the distinct smell of garlic or mustard and, when released, it is quickly absorbed into the skin and/or mucous membranes and begins an irreversible process of damaging the cells.

syndromic surveillance The monitoring, usually by local or provincial health departments, of patients presenting to emergency departments and alternative care facilities, the recording of EMS call volume, and the use of over-the-counter medications.

tabun (GA) A nerve agent that is one of the G agents; is 36 times more persistent than sarin and approximately half as lethal; has a fruity smell and is unique because the components used to manufacture the agent are easy to acquire and the agent is easy to manufacture.

terrorism A violent act dangerous to human life, to intimidate or coerce a government, the civilian population or any segment there of, in furtherance of political or social objectives.

V agent (VX) One of the G agents; it is a clear, oily agent that has no odour and looks like baby oil; over 100 times more lethal than sarin and is extremely persistent.

vapour hazard An agent that enters the body through the respiratory tract.

vesicants Blister agents; the primary route of entry for vesicants is through the skin.

viral hemorrhagic fevers (VHF) A group of diseases that include the Ebola, Rift Valley, and yellow fever viruses among others. This group of viruses causes the blood in the body to seep out from the tissues and blood vessels.

viruses Germs that require a living host to multiply and survive.

volatility Term used to describe how long a chemical agent will stay on a surface before it evapourates.

weapon of mass casualty (WMC) Any agent designed to bring about mass death, casualties, and/or massive damage to property and infrastructure (bridges, tunnels, airports, and seaports); also known as a weapon of mass destruction (WMD).

weapon of mass destruction (WMD) Any agent designed to bring about mass death, casualties, and/or massive damage to property and infrastructure (bridges, tunnels, airports, and seaports); also known as a weapon of mass casualty (WMC).

weaponization The creation of a weapon from a biological agent generally found in nature and that causes disease; the agent is cultivated, synthesized, and/or mutated to maximize the target population's exposure to the germ.

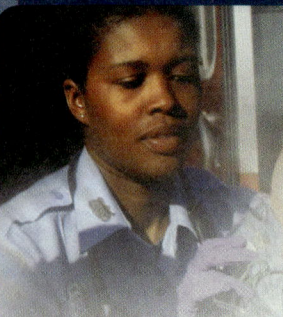

Assessment in Action

Events over the past decade have shown that terrorists, foreign and domestic, are willing to attack. Terrorists now have access to a broad array of lethal materials worldwide and can strike a specific target at any given time. Terrorists are no longer limited to conventional weapons.

1. **As a paramedic you must be familiar with the nonconventional agents that may be used in a WMD attack. All of the following are nonconventional weapons, EXCEPT:**
   A. chemical.
   B. nuclear.
   C. biological.
   D. explosives.

2. **A weapon of mass destruction is any agent that will bring about:**
   A. mass casualty.
   B. mass death.
   C. massive damage to infrastructure.
   D. all of the above.

3. **Terrorism carried out by individuals or groups who are not from the host country is known as:**
   A. domestic terrorism.
   B. doomsday terrorism.
   C. international terrorism.
   D. Al Qaeda.

4. **Chemical agents are manmade substances that can have devastating effects on living organisms. All of the following are agents that can be used for chemical warfare, EXCEPT:**
   A. nerve agents.
   B. pulmonary agents.
   C. bacterial agents.
   D. blood agents.

5. **Time, distance, and shielding are the three most important factors in staying safe when dealing with what type of WMD?**
   A. Chemical weapon
   B. Radiological weapon
   C. Biological weapon
   D. Bacterial weapon

6. **A chemical agent that is described as highly persistent can:**
   A. evapourate relatively fast.
   B. remain in the environment for weeks to months.
   C. cause extensive blistering within minutes.
   D. all of the above.

Challenging Questions

You are responding to a train station where there was a reported small explosion. Dispatch reports there are now a number of patients complaining of difficulty breathing and nausea. As you walk into the station you observe that two patients are unconscious and seizing, while numerous others are pleading with you to help them.

7. **What type of event do you suspect?**

8. **What concerns do you have for your safety?**

www.Paramedic.EMSzone.com/Canada

Points to Ponder

You are responding to a WMD incident where a primary explosion has disseminated chemical agents at the National Bank. You are told by the Incident Commander (IC) to stage about two blocks from the incident location while they wait for the HazMat team to evaluate the situation. The staging area is near a park and the IC wants triage to be set up in the park. There are about 40 patients confirmed by the IC. A total of six ambulances within the city are responding.

What are your concerns with both the location of the triage area and the number of ambulances that are responding? What do you want to know about the chemical agent?

Issues: Scene Safety, Staging Location, Incident Commander, Need for Decontamination, Secondary Devices.

www.Paramedic.EMSzone.com/Canada

49 Rescue Awareness and Operations

Competency Areas

Area 2: Communication

2.2.a Record organized, accurate, and relevant patient information.

2.2.b Prepare professional correspondence.

Area 3: Health and Safety

3.2.a Practice safe biomechanics.

3.2.b Transfer patient from various positions using applicable equipment and/or techniques.

3.2.c Transfer patient using emergency evacuation techniques.

3.2.d Secure patient to applicable equipment.

3.2.e Lift patient and stretcher in and out of ambulance with partner.

3.3.a Assess scene for safety.

3.3.b Address potential occupational hazards.

3.3.c Conduct basic extrication.

Area 4: Assessment and Diagnostics

4.1.a Rapidly assess a scene based on the principles of a triage system.

4.1.b Assume different roles in a mass casualty incident.

4.1.c Manage a mass casualty incident.

Appendix 4: Pathophysiology

J. **Multisystem Diseases and Injuries**
Toxicologic Illness: Poisons (absorption, inhalation, ingestion)
Toxicologic Illness: Acids and alkalis
Toxicologic Illness: Hydrocarbons
Toxicologic Illness: Asphyxiants
Toxicologic Illness: Cyanide
Environmental Disorders: Local cold injuries
Environmental Disorders: Near drowning and drowning

Appendix 5: Medications

A. **Medications affecting the central nervous system.**

A.7 Non-narcotic analgesics

A.8 Opioid Analgesics

Introduction

"Rescue" means to deliver from danger or imprisonment. As paramedics, we must remove from peril or confinement every patient we encounter. Paramedics cannot simply push a button and magically transport patients to an emergency department—which means technically that every emergency scene is a rescue situation. Patients are found in every imaginable situation. Imagine you have a patient on the second floor of a three-storey brick structure. This bariatric patient is lying on the floor of a half-bathroom in the back of the structure. Your assessment shows the patient is experiencing a myocardial infarction and acute exacerbation of chronic obstructive pulmonary disease (COPD). The treatment is easy, but the rescue is difficult. You must extricate this patient to your waiting squad with a monitor, two IVs, a nitro drip, and a continuous positive airway pressure machine attached **Figure 49-1 ▶**.

Rescue and removal of patients involves several steps. You must access the patient and then quickly assess him or her for medical/trauma complications to determine which treatments should be started. Treatment must begin at the site, but this is often difficult because of the circumstances surrounding the event. The patient must be released or removed from the entrapment, and medical care must continue throughout the incident. The most difficult process in any rescue is neither the rescue nor the treatment process, but rather the coordination and balance of both.

A technical rescue incident (TRI) is a complex rescue incident involving vehicles, water, trench collapse, confined spaces, or wilderness search and rescue that requires specially trained personnel and special equipment. In many settings,

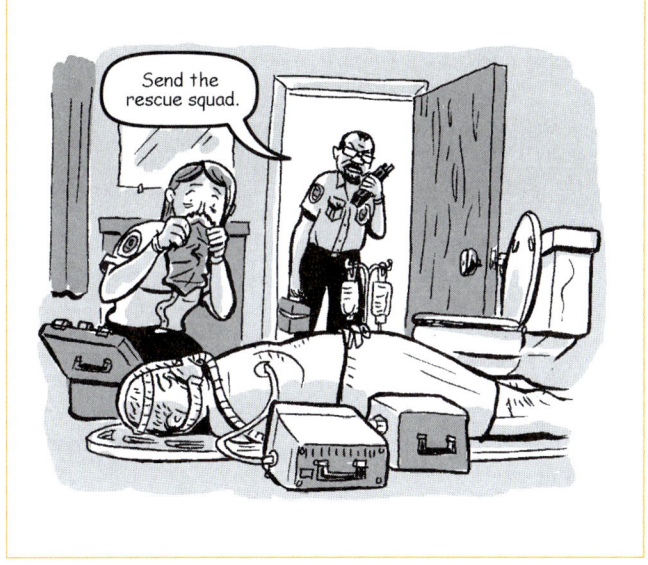

Figure 49-1

rescues are conducted by specially trained personnel from services other than EMS. Nevertheless, all paramedics must understand basic rescue techniques in order to function effectively as part of a team at a TRI. This chapter describes how to assist specially trained rescue personnel in carrying out the tasks, but it will not make you an expert in the skills that require specialized training.

Training in technical rescue areas is conducted at three levels:

- **Awareness.** This training level is an introduction to the topic, with an emphasis on recognizing the hazards,

You are the Paramedic **Part 1**

It is a blistering hot summer day in July. The meteorologist has warned people to stay indoors. The current temperature is 35°C with a heat index of 40.5°C. You and your partner make your way back to the station from the hospital after treating the third heat-related illness of the day. The two of you chuckle as a call is dispatched for the local police department regarding chickens in the road. Five minutes later your laughter is replaced by surprise as your unit is dispatched to the same location for a truck in a ditch.

Upon arrival, you and your partner are stunned as you navigate the unit through what appears to be at least 100 chickens wandering aimlessly across a two-lane paved road. Beyond the chickens, buried in a ditch, is a flatbed truck turned on its side. Wire mesh cages, feathers, and dead chickens are strewn about. The cab of the truck has landed on the driver's side with major intrusion into the driver's compartment and spidering of the windshield. Inside you find a middle-age man with active bleeding from a forehead laceration. He is screaming that he has severe abdominal pain and cannot move his legs, which are pinned beneath the dashboard. You let him know that help is there and advise him to keep as still as possible and not to move his neck. You decide to wait until fire department personnel advise you that the scene is safe prior to proceeding with prehospital care.

Initial Assessment	Recording Time: 0 Minutes
Appearance	Middle-aged man in obvious pain
Level of consciousness	A (Alert to person, place, and day)
Airway	Open
Breathing	Chest rise appears adequate
Circulation	Unable to assess

1. What are some examples of situations requiring special rescue teams?
2. Identify the ten steps of a special rescue sequence.

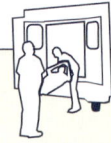

At the Scene

One of the benefits of rescue awareness and operations education is that it helps you avoid rescue situations that you are not trained to handle.

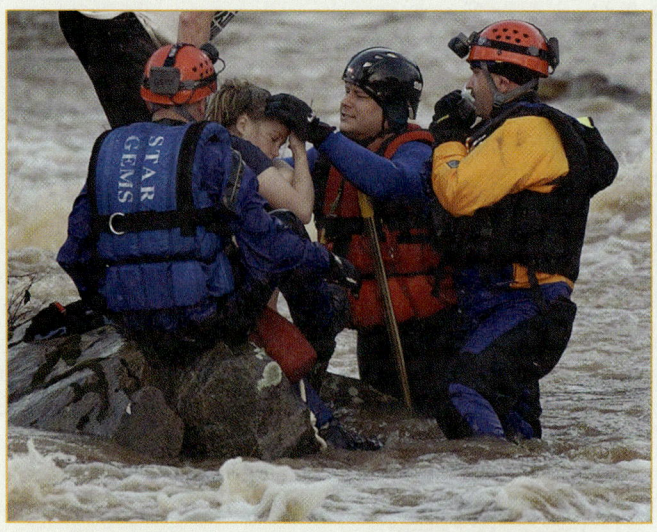

Figure 49-2 EMS agencies may respond to a variety of special rescue situations.

securing the scene, and calling for appropriate assistance. There is no actual use of rescue skills at the awareness level.

- **Operations.** Geared toward working in the "warm zone" of an incident (the area directly around the hazard area), this kind of training will allow you to directly assist those conducting the rescue operation.
- **Technician.** At this level, you are directly involved in the rescue operation itself. Training includes the use of specialized equipment, care of patients during the rescue, and management of the incident and of all personnel at the scene.

Most of the training and education paramedics receive is aimed at the awareness level, enabling them to identify the hazards and secure the scene to prevent additional people from becoming patients. Your function as a paramedic in rescue operations depends on the type of services you provide and the level of expertise your company has attained.

Notes from Nancy

The paramedic's job at the scene of an accident is to provide prehospital care to the patients.

All paramedics must wear proper personal protective equipment (PPE) to allow them to access patients and safely administer treatment that will continue throughout the incident. Once the scene is safe, and the technical aspects of the patient rescue or extrication are understood, patient access and prehospital care can begin.

Types of Rescues

EMS agencies may respond to a variety of special rescue situations **Figure 49-2 ▶**, including vehicle, confined space, trench, water, and wilderness rescue. It is important for awareness-level responders to have an understanding of these types of rescues. Often, the first emergency unit to arrive at a rescue incident is an ambulance with paramedics who may not be trained in special rescue techniques. The initial actions taken by paramedics may determine the safety of both patients and paramedics. They may also determine how efficiently the rescue is completed.

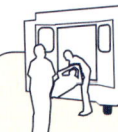

At the Scene

Just as in prehospital care, the first priority in rescue is "rescuer safety."

Guidelines for Operations

When assisting rescue team members, the following guidelines will prove useful:

- Be safe.
- Follow orders.
- Work as a team.
- Think.
- Follow the golden rule of public service.

Be Safe

Rescue situations have many hidden hazards, including oxygen-deficient atmospheres and strong water currents. Knowledge, education, and training are required to recognize the signs that indicate a hazardous rescue situation exists. Once the hazards are identified, determine what actions are necessary to ensure your own safety as well as the safety of your partner, the patients, and any bystanders. It requires experience and skill to determine that a rescue scene is not safe to enter, and that determination could save lives.

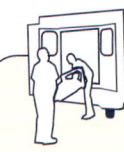

At the Scene

All rescue teams should have written safety procedures or SOPs that are familiar to every team member.

Follow Orders

The officers and the rescue teams you'll work with on special rescue incidents have received extensive specialized training. They've been chosen for those duties because they have experience and skills in a particular area of rescue. It is critical to follow the orders of personnel who understand exactly what needs to be done to ensure everyone's safety and to mitigate the dangers involved in the rescue situation. Follow their orders exactly as given. If you do not understand what's expected of you, *ask*. Have the orders clarified so you'll be able to complete your assigned task safely.

Work as a Team

Rescue efforts often require many people to complete a wide variety of tasks. Some personnel may be trained in specific tasks, such as rope rescue or swift water rescue. However, they cannot do their jobs without the support and assistance of others. Rescue is a team effort, and you play an essential role on this team.

Think

As you're working on a rescue situation, you must constantly assess and reassess the scene. You may see something that the incident commander (IC) doesn't see. If you think your assigned task may be unsafe, bring it to the attention of the IC or safety officer. Do not try to reorganize the total rescue effort, because it is being directed by people who are highly trained and experienced, but do not ignore what's happening around you either. Observations that you should bring to the IC's attention include changing weather conditions that might affect the rescue scene operations, suspicious packages or items on the scene, and broken equipment.

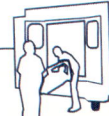

At the Scene

F-A-I-L-U-R-E

The reasons for rescue failures can be referred to by the mnemonic "FAILURE":

F Failure to understand the environment, or underestimating it
A Additional medical problems not considered
I Inadequate rescue skills
L Lack of teamwork or experience
U Underestimating the logistics of the incident
R Rescue versus recovery mode not considered
E Equipment not mastered

Follow the Golden Rule of Public Service

When you're involved in carrying out a rescue effort, it is all too easy to concentrate on the technical aspects of the rescue and forget to focus on the scared person who needs your emotional support and encouragement. It is helpful to have a rescuer stay with the patient whenever possible, keeping the patient updated on which actions will be performed during the rescue process.

Steps of Special Rescue

The role of the paramedic in special rescue operations is often vague and can change as the rescue operation progresses. All paramedics must have some formalized education or training in rescue techniques. This educational process is aimed at preparing responders to understand and identify potential

You are the Paramedic Part 2

You are slightly relieved by the sound of the engine company sirens in the distance, but you know that you will require additional resources for extrication and transport. The closest rescue squad with extrication capabilities is 30 minutes away, and transport time to the trauma centre is approximately 1 hour by ground. Your partner contacts dispatch and asks them to dispatch the rescue assignment for extrication assistance and a helicopter for transport.

After fire personnel stabilize the vehicle with cribbing and advise you that it is safe to gain access to the patient, you ask for assistance from one of the police officers to hold the patient's c-spine by leaning through the window on the driver's side of the cab. You are able to open the door on the passenger's side and carefully climb into the cab positioning yourself next to the patient. You introduce yourself to the patient, who tells you that he was driving down the road when he became "blinded by the sunlight" and ran off the road and landed in the ditch. The patient denies having any loss of consciousness, headache, dizziness, or visual disturbances. He has a medical history of panic attacks, for which he takes 40 mg of Prozac every day. He has no known drug allergies.

Vital Signs	Recording Time: 5 Minutes
Level of consciousness	Alert
Pulse	122 beats/min, strong and regular
Blood pressure	134/72 mm Hg
Respirations	22 breaths/min, nonlaboured
Skin	Pink, warm, and slightly diaphoretic
Spo$_2$	95% on room air

3. Why is it important to maintain good communication with the patient during a special rescue incident?

4. What is the patient at risk of experiencing as a result of being pinned underneath the dashboard from the pelvis down?

hazards and to determine when it is safe or potentially unsafe to access and rescue patients. All paramedics will be involved with a rescue at some point in their careers, so they must be skilled in specialized patient packaging techniques to allow for safe extrication and prehospital medical care.

Although special rescue situations may take many different forms, all rescuers should follow ten steps to perform these rescues in a safe, effective, and efficient manner:

1. Preparation
2. Response
3. Arrival and assessment
4. Stabilization
5. Access
6. Disentanglement
7. Removal
8. Transport
9. Security of the scene and preparation for the next call
10. Postincident analysis

Preparation

You can prepare for responses to emergency rescue incidents by training with fire departments and special rescue teams in your area. This educational process will prepare you to respond to a mutual aid call and teach you about the type of rescue equipment other departments have access to and the training levels of their personnel. Knowing the terminology used in the prehospital setting will also make communicating with other rescuers easier and more effective.

Prior to any technical rescue call, your department must consider the following issues:

- Does the department have the personnel and equipment needed to handle a TRI from start to finish?
- What equipment and which personnel will the department send on a technical rescue call?
- Do members of the department know the potential hazard areas in their response area? Have they visited those areas with local representatives?

Response

A dispatch protocol should be established for a TRI. If your department has its own technical rescue team, it will usually respond with a rescue squad, an ambulance, fire engine company, and fire chief. Otherwise, it will respond with a medic unit, engine company, and chief. In many EMS departments, the rescue squad will come from an outside agency. Often, it is necessary to notify utility companies during a TRI and seek their assistance. Many technical rescues involve electricity, sewer pipes, or factors that may create the need for heavy equipment, to which utility companies have ready access.

Arrival and Assessment

Immediately upon arrival, the IC will assume command. A rapid and accurate scene assessment is needed to avoid placing rescuers

in danger and to determine what additional resources may be needed. Paramedics must assess the extent of injuries and the number of patients; this information will then help to determine how many medic units and other resources are needed.

Do *not* rush into the incident scene until an assessment of the situation is complete. A paramedic approaching a trench collapse may cause further collapse. A paramedic entering a swiftly flowing river might be quickly knocked off his or her feet and carried downstream. A paramedic climbing into a well to evaluate an unconscious patient may be overcome by an oxygen-deficient atmosphere. Paramedics need to *stop and think about the dangers that may be present.* Do not make yourself part of the problem.

Stabilization

Once the resources are on the way and the scene is safe to enter, it is time to stabilize the incident. Look around you, identifying and evaluating the hazards at the scene, observing the geographical area, noting the routes of access and exit, observing weather and wind conditions, and considering evacuation problems and transport distances. Establish an outer perimetre to keep the public and media out of the staging area and maintain a smaller perimetre directly around the rescue. The rescue area is the area that surrounds the incident site (eg, collapsed structure, collapsed trench, hazardous spill area). The size of the rescue area is proportional to the hazards that exist.

As part of the stabilization effort, you should establish three controlled zones:

- **Hot zone.** For entry teams and rescue teams only. This zone immediately surrounds the dangers of the site (eg, hazardous materials releases) to protect personnel outside the zone.
- **Warm zone.** For properly trained and equipped personnel only. This zone is where personnel and equipment decontamination and hot zone support take place.
- **Cold zone.** For staging vehicles and equipment. This zone contains the command post. The public and the media should be kept clear of the cold zone at all times.

Police or fire line tape is often used to demarcate these controlled zones. Red tape is typically used for the hot zone, orange tape for the warm zone, and yellow tape for the cold zone. Of course, someone must ensure that the zones of the emergency scene are enforced. Scene control activities are sometimes assigned to law enforcement personnel.

During stabilization, atmospheric monitoring should be started to identify any immediately dangerous to life and health (IDLH) environments for rescuers and patients. After considering the type of incident, you may begin planning how to safely rescue patients. In a trench rescue, for example, you might set up ventilation fans for air flow, set up lights for visibility, and protect the trench from further collapse.

Access

With the scene stabilized, now you must gain access to the patient. How is he or she trapped? In a trench situation, the culprit may be a dirt pile. In a rope rescue, scaffolding may have fallen. In a confined space, a hazardous atmosphere may have caused the patient to collapse. To reach a patient who is buried or trapped beneath debris, it is sometimes necessary to dig a tunnel as a means of rescue and escape. Identify the actual reason for the rescue and work toward freeing the patient safely.

Communicate with patients at all times during the rescue to make sure they are not injured further by the rescue operation. Even if they're not injured, they need to be reassured that the team is working as quickly as possible to free them.

Emergency medical care should be initiated as soon as access to the patient is achieved. Technical rescue paramedics are crucial resources at TRIs; not only can these responders start IVs and treat medical conditions, but they also know how to deal with the special equipment being used and the procedures taking place around them. It is vitally important that the actions of paramedics be effectively coordinated into ongoing operations during rescue incidents. Their main functions are to treat patients and to stand by in case a rescue team member needs medical assistance. As soon as a rescue area is secured and stabilized, paramedics must be allowed access to the patients for medical assessment and stabilization. Some fire departments have trained paramedics to the technical rescue level so that they can enter hazardous areas and provide direct assistance to patients there. Throughout the course of the rescue operation, which may span many hours, paramedics must continually monitor and ensure the stability of all patients.

Gaining access to the patient depends on the type of incident. For example, in an incident involving a motor vehicle, its location and position, the damage to the vehicle, and the position of the patient are important considerations. The means of gaining access to the patient must also take into account the nature and severity of the patient's injuries. The chosen means of access may change during the course of the rescue as the nature or severity of the patient's injuries becomes apparent.

Disentanglement

Once precautions have been taken and the reason for entrapment has been identified, the patient needs to be freed as safely as possible. A team member should remain with the patient to direct the rescuers who are performing the disentanglement. In a trench incident, this would include digging either with a shovel or by hand to free the patient.

In a motor vehicle collision, the vehicle should be removed from around the patient rather than trying to remove the patient through the wreckage. Parts of the vehicle—for example, the steering wheel, seats, pedals, and dashboard—may trap the occupants. Disentanglement is the cutting of a vehicle (or machinery) away from trapped or injured patients, using extrication and rescue tools along with various extrication methods.

Removal

Once the patient has been disentangled, efforts shift to removing the patient ⬤ **Figure 49-3 ▸** . In some instances, this may simply amount to having someone assist the patient up a

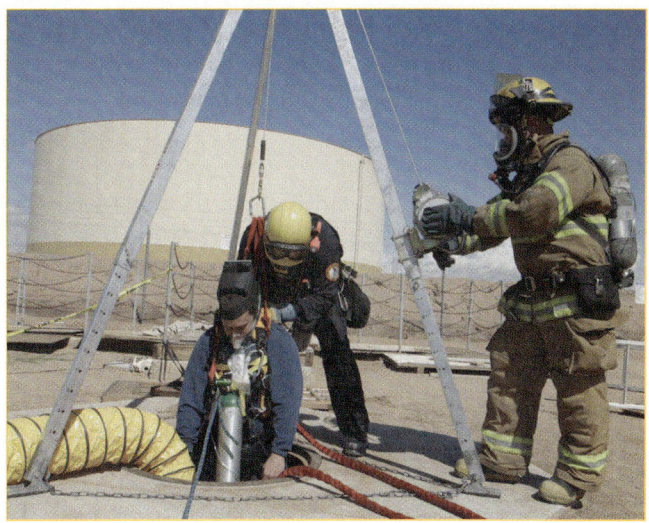

Figure 49-3 Patient removal.

ladder; in other situations, it may require removal with spinal immobilization due to possible injuries. A wide variety of equipment, including Stokes baskets, backboards, stretchers, and other immobilization devices, is used to remove injured patients from trenches, confined spaces, and elevated points.

Preparing the patient for removal involves maintaining continued control of all life-threatening problems, dressing all wounds, and immobilizing all suspected fractures and spinal injuries. The use of standard splints in confined areas is difficult and frequently impossible, but stabilization of the arms to the patient's trunk and of the legs to each other will often suffice until the patient is positioned on a long backboard, which may serve as the ultimate splint for the whole body. The Kendrick extrication device (KED) is typically used for stabilization of a sitting patient.

Sometimes a patient must be removed quickly (rapid extrication; covered in Chapter 25) because his or her general condition is deteriorating and time does not permit meticulous splinting and dressing procedures. Quick removal may also occur if hazards are present, such as spilled gas or other materials that could endanger the patient or rescue personnel. The only time the patient should be moved prior to completion of initial prehospital care, assessment, stabilization, and treatment is when the patient's or emergency responder's life is in immediate danger.

Packaging is preparing the patient for movement as a unit. It is often accomplished by means of a long backboard, scoop stretcher, or similar device. These boards are essential for moving patients with potential or actual spine injuries.

Rough-terrain rescues may require passing a multiple-person stretcher across rough terrain, fording streams, or climbing over rocks. These operations require at least one person to take each corner of the litter or backboard if possible. In extreme cases, a four-person team may have to hand a litter around or over obstacles to another team ("leapfrogging"). Rescues in rough terrain often require ingenuity to suspend or pad a stretcher so that the patient is provided with a reasonably comfortable ride. Padding may consist of inflated inner tubes, 10 to 15 cm foam padding, or loosely rolled blankets. This technique is superior to "slinging" the stretcher on straps, which may lead to excessive swaying and bouncing.

Transport

Once the patient has been removed from the hazard area, EMS will undertake transport to an appropriate medical facility. Depending on the severity of the patient's injuries and the distance to the medical facility, the type of transport will vary. For example, if a patient is critically injured or if the rescue is taking place some distance from the hospital, air transportation may be more appropriate than a ground ambulance.

In rough-terrain rescues, four-wheel drive, high-clearance vehicles may be required to transport patients on stretchers to an awaiting ambulance. Snowmobiles with attached sleds can be used to transport patients down snow-covered mountains. Helicopters are increasingly used for quick evacuation from remote areas, but they have their limitations in bad weather conditions.

▌General Rescue Scene Procedures

As a paramedic, you know that your own safety as well as the safety of your partner and the public is paramount. At a TRI, while you may be tempted to approach the patient or the accident area, it is critically important to slow down and properly evaluate the situation. Consider the potential general hazards and risks of utilities, confined spaces, and environmental conditions, as well as hazards that are IDLH. In confined-space rescue incidents, potential hazards may include deep or isolated spaces, multiple complicating hazards (eg, water or chemicals), failure of essential equipment or service, and environmental conditions (eg, snow or rain).

Approaching the Scene

Beginning with the initial dispatch of the rescue call, you should be compiling facts and impressions about the call. Scene assessment begins with the information gained from the person reporting the incident and then from the bystanders at the scene upon arrival.

The information gathered when an emergency call is received is important to the success of the rescue operation. Information collected should include the following:

- Location of the incident
- Nature of the incident (kinds and number of vehicles)
- Condition and position of patients
- Condition and position of vehicles
- Number of people trapped or injured and types of injuries
- Any specific or special hazard information (confined space concerns)
- Name of person calling and a number where the person can be reached

As you approach the scene of a TRI, however, you may not always know what kind of scene you are entering. Is it a construction scene? Do you see piles of dirt that would indicate a

trench? What actions are the civilians taking? Are they attempting to rescue trapped people, possibly placing themselves at considerable danger? Identify any life-threatening hazards, and take corrective measures to mitigate them. Determine whether the situation is a search, rescue, or recovery. If additional resources are needed, they should be ordered by the IC.

A scene assessment should include the initial and ongoing evaluation of the following issues:

- Scope and magnitude of the incident
- Risk and benefit analysis
- Number of known and potential patients
- Hazards
- Access to the scene
- Environmental factors
- Available and necessary resources
- Establishment of a control perimetre

Utility Hazards

In case of utility hazards, your goal is to control as many of the hazards as possible. Minimize all risks and ensure that all paramedics are using appropriate PPE. Are there any downed electrical wires near the scene **Figure 49-4 ▼** ? Is equipment or machinery electrically charged so as to present a danger to the patient or the rescuers? The IC should ensure that the proper procedures are taken to shut off the utilities in the rescue area. Remember—utility hazards can be above or below ground, and the rescue situation will dictate which ones need to be addressed first.

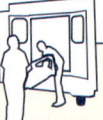

At the Scene

Treat all downed wires as if they are charged (live) until you receive specific clearance from the electric company. Even if the lights are out along the street where the wires are down, never assume that the wires are dead. Be especially alert for downed wires after a storm that has blown down trees or tree limbs.

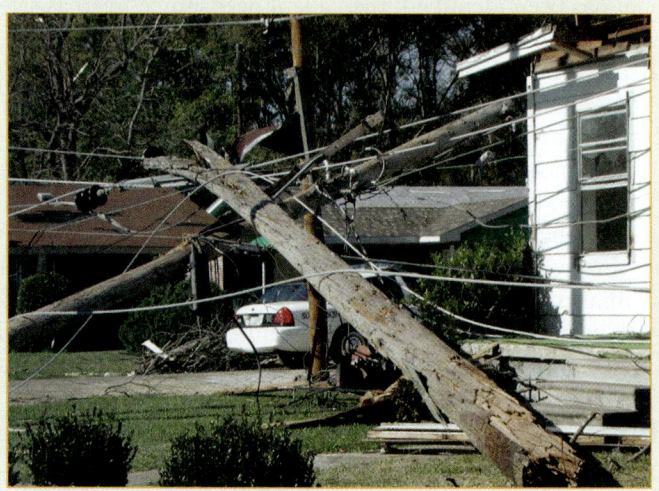

Figure 49-4 Downed electrical wires present a hazard.

Utility hazards require the assistance of trained personnel. For electrical hazards, such as downed lines, park at least one truck span away. Watch for falling utility poles; a damaged pole may bring other poles down with it. Do not touch any wires, power lines, or other electrical sources until they have been deenergized by a power company representative. It isn't just the wires that are hazardous; any metal that they touch is also energized. Metal fences or guardrails may become energized along their entire unbroken length. Be careful around running or standing water, as water is an excellent conductor of electricity.

Natural gas and liquefied petroleum gas are nontoxic but are classified as asphyxiates because they displace breathing air. In addition, both are explosive. If a call involves leaking gas, call the gas company immediately. If a patient has been overcome by leaking gas, wear positive-pressure self-contained breathing apparatus and remove the patient from the hazardous atmosphere before beginning treatment.

Scene Security

Has the area been secured to prevent people from entering? Colleagues, family members, and even other rescuers may unwittingly enter an unsafe scene and become patients themselves. The IC should coordinate with law enforcement to help secure the scene and control access. In addition, the fire department should implement a strict accountability system to control access to the rescue scene.

Protective Equipment

Most specialized teams carry items such as harnesses; smaller, lighter helmets; and jumpsuits that are easier to move in than turnout gear. For personnel who perform water rescues, the minimum PPE includes a personal flotation device (PFD), thermal protection, a helmet appropriate for water rescue, a cutting device, a whistle, and contamination protection (if necessary). Rescuers should use a properly sized PFD that is designed and certified for their specific mission. They must be familiar with the manufacturer's procedures for donning and removing (doffing) their PFD. All straps should be tightened with loose straps secured to prevent entanglement Figure 49-5 ◂ .

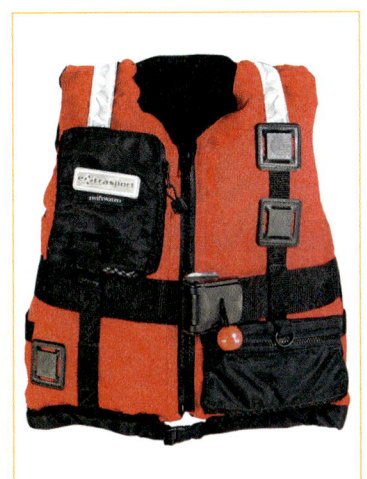

Figure 49-5 A PFD.

A handheld strobe light may help paramedics keep track of each other in a crowd or in rural or wilderness locations. When working along highways, they can hook these lights onto their belts or attach them to their upper arms to provide additional visibility to oncoming vehicles. Strobe lights are lightweight, quite durable, and readily visible at night at a distance of approximately 1.6 km.

When considering the use of protective head gear, paramedics must use approved devices that meet certain standards and are appropriate for the rescue environment (eg, climbing helmets, firefighter helmets). Footwear must be designed and certified for a specific rescue environment. The environment may require thermal protection (hot or cold), chemical protection, insole puncture barriers, and ankle support. Water rescue operations require specialized foot protection such as wetsuit-type booties. Paramedics must also consider the use of Canadian Standards Association (CSA)-approved safety glasses or goggles, puncture- or cut-resistant gloves, flame- or flash-protective clothing that is highly visible, and appropriate footwear to support ankles and provide traction. Other useful items that are easily carried by paramedics include binoculars, chalk or spray paint for marking searched areas, a compass for wilderness rescues, first aid kits, a whistle, a handheld global positioning system, and cyalume-type light sticks. The IC and the technical rescue team will help to determine what protective equipment you will need to wear while assisting.

Incident Command System

The first arriving officer immediately assumes command and starts using the incident command system (ICS). This step is critically important because many TRIs will eventually become very complex and require a large number of assisting units. Without the ICS in place, it will be difficult—if not impossible—to ensure the rescuers' safety.

Accountability

Accountability should be practiced at all emergencies, no matter how small. The accountability system is the single most important process to ensure rescuers' safety. It tracks the personnel on the scene, including their identities, assignments, and locations. This system ensures that only rescuers who have been given specific assignments are operating within the area where the rescue is taking place. By using an accountability system and working within the ICS, an IC can track the resources at the scene, task out assignments, and ensure that every person at the scene operates safely.

Patient Contact

At any rescue scene, you must try to communicate with the patient. Technical rescue situations often last for hours, with the patient being left alone for long periods of time. If at all possible, you should attempt to communicate via a radio, cell phone, or yelling. Reassure the patient that everything is being done to ensure his or her safety.

If you succeed in making contact, it is important to stay in communication with the patient. Ideally, someone should be assigned to talk to the patient, while others focus on making the rescue. Realize that the patient could be sick or injured and is probably frightened. If you are calm, your demeanour will in turn calm the patient:

- Make and keep eye contact with the patient.
- Tell the truth. Lying destroys trust and confidence. You may not always tell the patient everything, but if the patient asks a specific question, answer truthfully.
- Communicate at a level that the patient can understand.
- Be aware of your own body language.
- Always speak slowly, clearly, and distinctly.
- Use a patient's proper name. Use the patient's surname, preceded by the proper qualifier (ie, Mr. or Ms.).
- If a patient is hard of hearing, speak clearly and directly at the person, so that he or she can read your lips.
- Allow time for the patient to answer or respond to your questions.
- Try to make the patient comfortable and relaxed whenever possible.

▌Assisting Rescue Crews

If you will be assisting a technical rescue team, training with the team is probably the most important step you can take so that you can work together effectively during a TRI. Training allows you to get a feel for how the team members operate; likewise, they can get an idea of which duties they can trust you with. The more knowledge you have, the more you'll be able to do.

At any TRI, follow the IC's orders. Your ultimate goal is to protect the team and patients. No matter what type of rescue scene you enter, keep these three guidelines in mind:

- Approach the scene cautiously.
- Position apparatus properly.
- Assist specialized team members as needed.

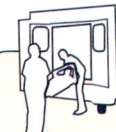

At the Scene

Always assume that oncoming traffic cannot see you, and act appropriately.

Vehicles

Determine where to locate your emergency vehicle, taking into account the safety of emergency workers, patients, and other motorists. Whenever possible, park emergency vehicles in a manner that will ensure safety and not disrupt traffic any more than necessary. Traffic flow is the largest single hazard associated with any operation that takes place on a highway. Provide a safe ambulance loading zone. On limited-access highways, keep vehicles and apparatus not directly involved in the rescue off the roadway. Have staging areas away from the scene. Do not hesitate to request that the road be closed if necessary.

Use large emergency vehicles to provide a barrier against motorists who fail to heed emergency warning lights. Many departments place apparatus at an angle to the collision. This position ensures that the apparatus is pushed to the side of a collision in the event that it is struck from behind. You can also place traffic cones or flares to direct motorists away from the

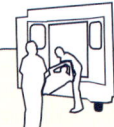

At the Scene

Most newer cars and pickup trucks have driver-side and passenger-side airbags. Some newer vehicles have supplemental airbags in other places as well. Airbags that do not activate during a collision present a danger to rescuers until they're deactivated.

You are the Paramedic Part 3

A rapid trauma survey yields an actively bleeding 10-cm laceration across the patient's forehead and diffuse abdominal tenderness. Assessment below the abdomen is not possible because the patient is pinned beneath the dashboard from the pelvis down. The patient is anxious about not being able to feel his legs. You do your best to reassure him that additional help is on its way and encourage him to focus on taking slow, deep breaths.

You place the patient on a nonrebreathing mask at 12 l/min of oxygen. Your partner applies a c-collar and manual c-spine continues to be held by the police officer. Bleeding from the forehead laceration is controlled with direct pressure and bandaging by one of the firefighters. You are able to initiate a 16-gauge IV cannula in the right antecubital vein and begin a normal saline infusion to keep vein open. Dispatch advises that the ETA for an additional unit is approximately 20 minutes and the ETA for the helicopter is approximately 10 minutes. Two of the firefighters leave to establish a landing zone.

Reassessment	Recording Time: 13 Minutes
Skin	Pink, warm, and slightly diaphoretic
Pulse	130 breaths/min, strong and regular
Blood pressure	128/70 mm Hg
Respirations	22 breaths/min, regular
Spo$_2$	98% via nonrebreathing mask on 100% supplemental oxygen
ECG	Sinus tachycardia with no ectopy
Pupils	PERLA

5. What needs to be monitored on this patient?

collision. If using flares, be aware of flammable material and liquids that could be ignited.

You need to be visible at a collision scene. Use only essential warning lights, because too many lights tend to distract or confuse other drivers. Turn off headlights and consider the use of amber lighting at the scene. Your PPE should be bright to help ensure your visibility during daylight hours. Any PPE that is used at night needs to be equipped with reflective material to increase your visibility in the darkness. PPE must be worn at all motor vehicle collisions. Before exiting the ambulance at an emergency scene, be alert for any vehicles that might cause you injury. Do not assume that motorists will heed your warning lights, and let law enforcement personnel coordinate traffic control.

Paramedics must be aware of all potential hazards at rescue scenes—both obvious (eg, sharp metal and broken glass) and less obvious or hidden dangers. Downed power lines may fall from above, and underground electrical feeds may become exposed. Energy-absorbing bumpers can explode when subjected to heat and can spring out when loaded. Airbags or supplemental restraint systems (SRS) can deploy at any time after an accident and must be deactivated even if the power supply to the vehicle has been disconnected. Conventional fuel systems with highly flammable vapours may ignite if they come in contact with hot catalytic converters or heated engine components. New vehicles that use alternative fuel sources (eg, electric or propane-fueled vehicles) can also pose problems for rescuers. For example, paramedics must be aware of the electrical power, any storage cells, and high-pressure cylinders used in natural-gas–powered vehicles.

Vehicle-Related Terminology

To reduce confusion and mistakes at extrication scenes, it is important to use standardized terminology when referring to specific parts of vehicles. The front of a vehicle normally travels down the road first. The hood is located on the front of the vehicle. The rear of a vehicle is where the trunk is usually located.

The left side of a vehicle is on your left as you sit in the vehicle. In Canada, the driver's seat is on the left side of the vehicle. The right side of a vehicle is where the passenger's seat is located. Always refer to left and right as they relate to *the vehicle*—not as they refer to *your* left and right.

Vehicles contain A, B, C, and D posts, which are the vertical supports that hold up the roof and form the upright columns of the occupant cage. The A posts are located closest to the front of the vehicle; they form the sides of the windshield. In four-door vehicles, the B posts are located between the front and rear doors of a vehicle; in some vehicles, they do not reach all of the way to the roof. In four-door vehicles, the C posts are located behind the rear doors, if present. D posts can be found on larger vehicles such as sport utility vehicles and vans that have a passenger window on the side behind the rear doors. The D post is located behind the rear passenger windows.

The hood covers the engine compartment. The bulkhead divides the engine compartment from the passenger compartment.

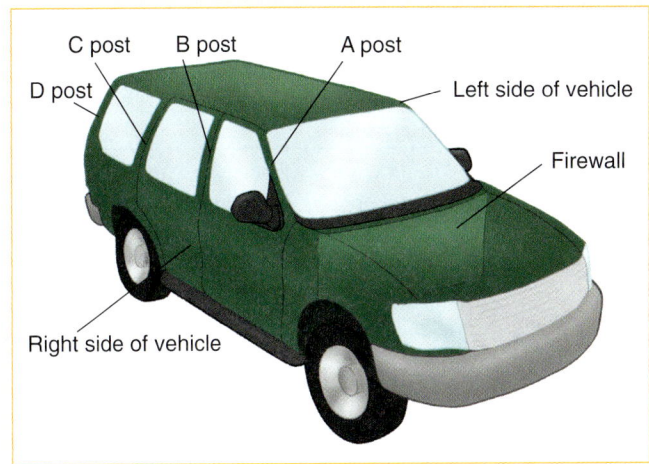

Figure 49-6 The anatomy of a vehicle.

An insulating metal piece known as the firewall protects the passengers in the event of an engine fire. The passenger compartment includes the front and back seats. This part of a vehicle is sometimes called the occupant cage or occupant compartment **Figure 49-6 ▲** .

There are two common types of vehicle frames: *platform frame* construction and *unibody* construction.

Platform frame construction uses beams to fabricate the load-bearing frame of a vehicle. The engine, transmission, and body components are then attached to this basic platform frame. This type of frame construction is found primarily in trucks and sport utility vehicles; it is rare in smaller passenger cars. Platform frame construction provides a structurally sound base for stabilizing the vehicle and an anchor point for attaching cables or extrication tools.

Unibody construction, which is used for most modern cars, combines the vehicle body and the frame into a single component. By folding multiple thicknesses of metal together, a column can be formed that is strong enough to serve as the frame for a lightweight vehicle. Unibody construction allows auto manufacturers to produce lighter weight vehicles. When extricating a person from such a vehicle, remember that unibody vehicles do not have the frame rails that are present with platform frame–constructed vehicles.

Vehicle Stabilization

Unstable objects pose a threat to both rescuers and victims of the collision. These objects—most often, the damaged vehicles—need to be stabilized before your approach.

Vehicles that end up on their wheels need to be stabilized with cribbing in the front and back of the wheels **Figure 49-7 ▲** . Cribbing is

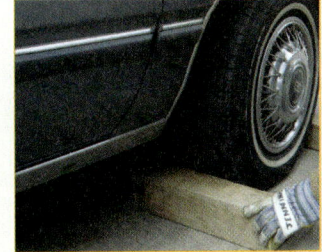

Figure 49-7 Cribbing.

short lengths of robust timber (10 × 10 cm) used to stabilize a vehicle. It prevents the vehicle from rolling backward or forward.

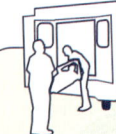

At the Scene

Even vehicles that are positioned upright on all four wheels should be stabilized.

After the cribbing has been placed, a vehicle can still move because of the give and motion generated by the suspension system. This motion may occur as rescuers enter the vehicle and the patients are extricated from the vehicle, and it can cause further injuries to the patients of the collision. The suspension system of most vehicles can be stabilized with step blocks, which are stairstep-shaped blocks that are placed under the side of the vehicle. Place one step block toward the front of the vehicle and a second step block toward the rear of the vehicle **Figure 49-8 ▾**. Once the step blocks are in place, the tires can be deflated by pulling out the valve stem with a pair of pliers or puncturing the tires. This creates a stable vehicle. If step blocks are not available or are not the right size, you can build a box crib by placing cribbing at right angles to the first layer of cribbing **Figure 49-9 ▸**.

After a collision, some vehicles will come to rest on their roof or sides. These vehicles are very unstable, and the slightest weight on them can cause them to move. To stabilize these vehicles, use box cribs or step blocks on each end of the vehicle.

Wedges are used to snug loose cribbing under the load or when using lift airbags to fill the void between the crib and the object as it is raised. Wedges should be the same width as the cribbing, with the tapered end no less than 6 mm thick. When the ends are less than 6 mm, the end will commonly fracture under a load.

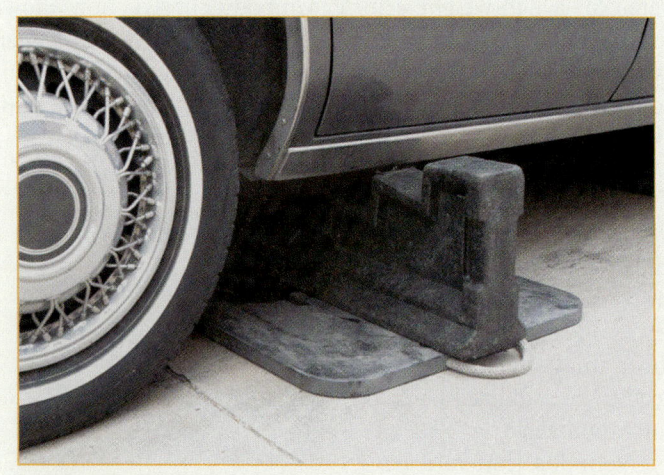

Figure 49-8 Step blocks can be used to stabilize a vehicle.

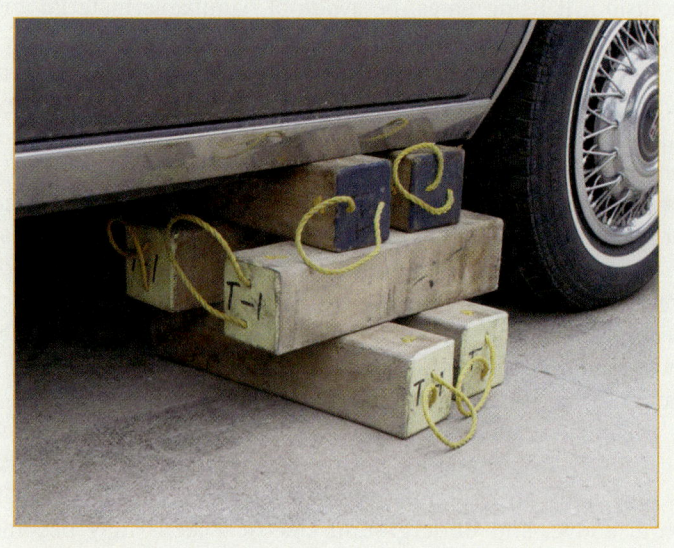

Figure 49-9 Box crib.

Gain Access to the Patient
Open the Door

After stabilizing the vehicle, the simplest way to access a crash victim is to open a door. Try all of the doors first—even if they appear to be badly damaged. It is an embarrassing waste of time and energy to open a jammed door with heavy rescue equipment when another door can be opened easily and without any special equipment.

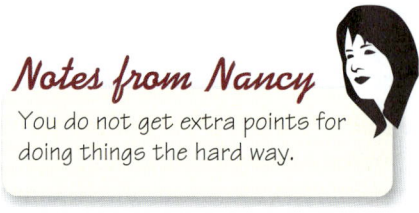

Notes from Nancy

You do not get extra points for doing things the hard way.

Attempt to unlock and open the least damaged door first. Make sure the locking mechanism is released. Try the outside and inside handles at the same time if possible.

If you have an open door but still need more room, have two rescuers lean against the door and push; most vehicle doors will easily bend open, creating a much wider opening for patient removal.

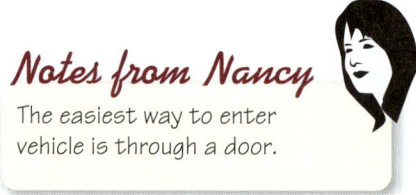

Notes from Nancy

The easiest way to enter vehicle is through a door.

Break Tempered Glass

If a patient's condition is serious enough to require immediate prehospital care and you cannot enter the vehicle through a door, consider breaking a window. Do not try to break and enter through the windshield because it is made of laminated windshield glass, which is difficult to break. The side and rear windows are made of tempered glass, also known as safety glass, and will break easily into small pieces when hit with a sharp, pointed object such as a spring-loaded centre punch or

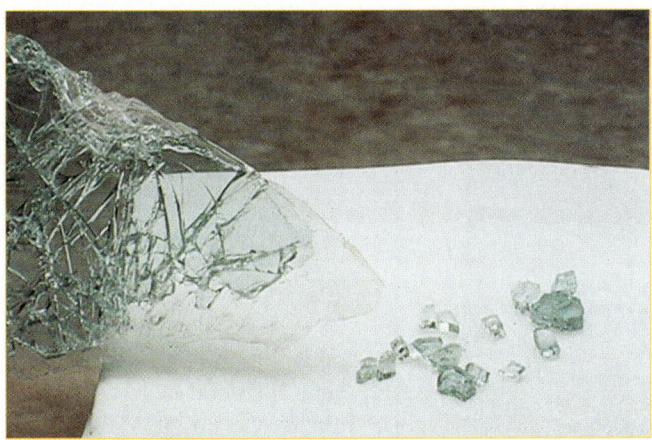

Figure 49-10 The two types of glass in vehicles: laminated glass (left) and tempered glass (right).

At the Scene

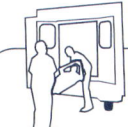

Always warn trapped car passengers that you're going to break the glass!

the point of an axe Figure 49-10 ▲ . Because these windows do not pose as great a safety threat, they can be your primary access route.

If you must break a window to unlock a door or gain access, try to break one that is far away from the patient. If the patient's condition warrants your immediate entry, however, do not hesitate to break the closest window. Small pieces of tempered glass do not usually pose a danger to people trapped in cars.

During this step of the rescue, all rescuers should be in proper PPE, including dust mask, safety glasses, or goggles.

Notes from Nancy

Do not use a sledgehammer to crack a walnut.

Attempt to lower windows as far as possible before breaking glass, and then select a spring-loaded centre punch. If you're using something other than a spring-loaded centre punch, always aim for a low corner. The window frame will help prevent the tool (such as an axe or screwdriver) from sailing into the vehicle and hitting the person inside. Personnel are given a verbal warning "Breaking glass," unless a stop/freeze call is made. After breaking the window, use your gloved hands to pull the remaining glass out of the window frame so it doesn't fall onto any passengers or injure any rescuers.

To break tempered glass, follow the steps in Skill Drill 49-1 ▶ .

1. Ensure that the patient and rescuers are properly protected.
2. Place the centre punch in the lower corner of the window and apply pressure until the spring is activated Step 1 .
3. Press on the centre punch to break the window Step 2 .
4. Remove any loose glass around the window opening Step 3 .
5. Follow this procedure until all glass has been removed Step 4 .

Once you have removed the pieces of glass from the frame, try to unlock the door again. Release the locking mechanism, and then use both the inside and outside door handles at the same time. This action may force a jammed locking mechanism, even in a door that appears to be badly damaged.

Breaking the rear window will sometimes provide an opening large enough to enable a rescuer to reach a patient if there is no other rapid means for gaining access. Using the simple techniques of opening a door or breaking the rear window will enable you to gain access to most patients in motor vehicle collisions, even those in upside-down vehicles.

Force the Door

If you cannot gain access to the vehicle by the methods already described, heavier extrication tools must be used to gain access to the patient. The most common technique is door displacement Figure 49-11 ▼ . The opening and displacement of vehicle doors may be difficult and somewhat unpredictable, however.

At the Scene

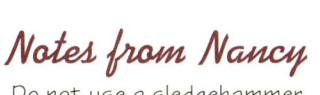

To reduce the risk of tempered glass pieces falling on patients, cover the window with duct tape or shelf paper prior to breaking it. Most of the glass can be removed as a unit.

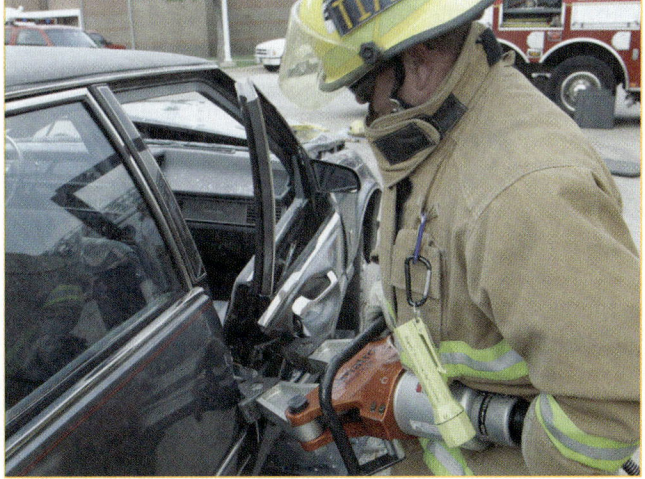

Figure 49-11 The most common technique for gaining access is door displacement.

Skill Drill 49-1: Breaking Tempered Glass

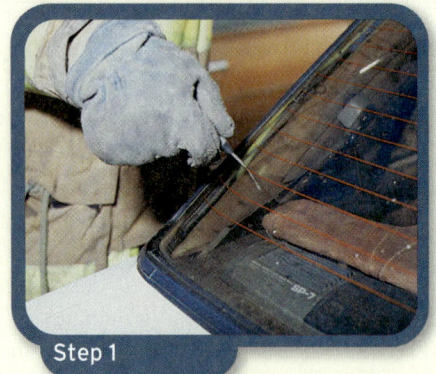

Step 1

Place the spring-loaded centre punch at the lower corner of the window.

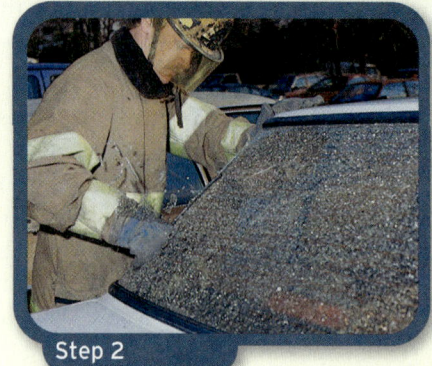

Step 2

Press on the centre punch.

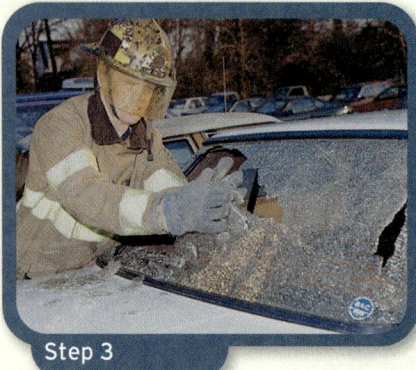

Step 3

Remove glass to the outside.

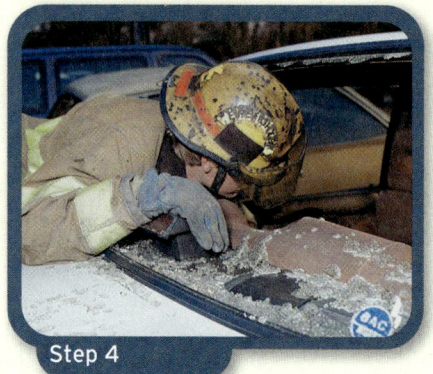

Step 4

Follow this procedure until all glass has been removed.

When it is necessary to force a door to gain access to the patient, choose a door that will not endanger the safety of the patient. For example, do not try to force a door open if the patient is leaning against it.

Powered hydraulic tools are the most efficient and widely used tools for opening a jammed door that can be opened by releasing the door from the latch side or the hinge side of the door. The decision regarding which method to use will depend on the structure of the vehicle and the type of damage the door has sustained.

First, use a pry tool to bend the sheet metal away from the edge of the door where the spreader of the hydraulic tool is to be inserted. Next, place the spreader in a position so that it is not in the pathway that the door will take when the hinges or latch break. Do not stand in a position that might put you in danger. Activate the hydraulic tool to push apart the outer sheet metal skin of the vehicle to expose the hinges or door latch. Once the outer sheet metal has been exposed, close the tips of the spreader and remove them.

If the side bar is crushed onto the patient and the compartment is still intact, you should consider the "vertical crush" technique: Peel the door down and away from the patient with the jaws on the roof and the top of the door.

At this point, insert the closed tips onto the inner skin of the door and the door jamb just above the latch or hinges. Activate the spreader to extend the tips until the latch or hinge separates. When separating a door at the latch side, you can place 10×10 cm cribbing under the bottom of the door to hold it up and then start to separate the hinges of the door. When separating a door from the hinge side, place the spreader on the top of the bottom hinge. Use the hydraulic spreader to separate the door from the hinge. Once the hinges have separated, place 10×10 cm cribbing underneath the door to hold it in place while you work on the latch side of the door. Note that some hydraulic tools are capable of cutting door hinges.

Once the door has been removed, move it away from the vehicle, where it will not be a safety hazard to other rescuers.

Provide Initial Medical Care

As soon as you've secured access to the patient, a paramedic should begin to provide emergency medical care. Being trapped in a damaged vehicle is a frightening experience, so it is important that one caregiver remain with the patient and provide both emotional comfort and physical care. Prehospital care should occur simultaneously with extrication **Figure 49-12 ▶**. Although it may be necessary to delay some elements of these processes for a short period, it is important to work toward the goal of stabilizing the patient and removing him or her from the vehicle as quickly and safely as possible.

Notes from Nancy

Try before you pry.

Notes from Nancy

A good extrication is a safe extrication.

Disentangle the Patient

The next step in the extrication sequence is disentangling the patient, a measure that seeks to remove those parts of the vehicle

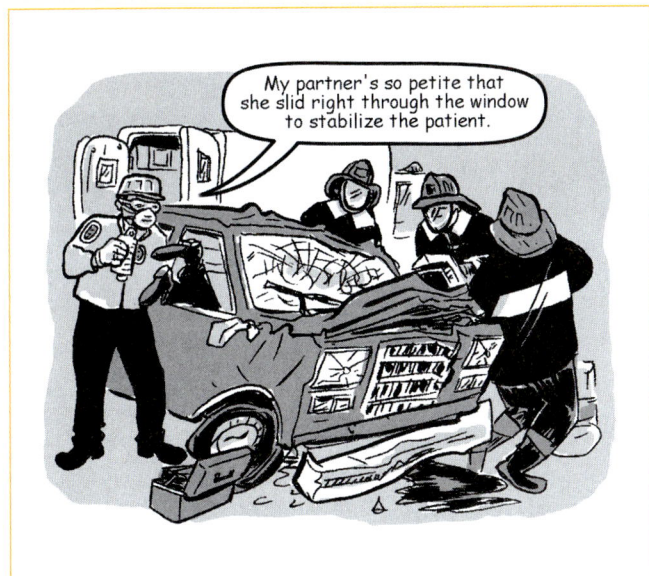

My partner's so petite that she slid right through the window to stabilize the patient.

Figure 49-12

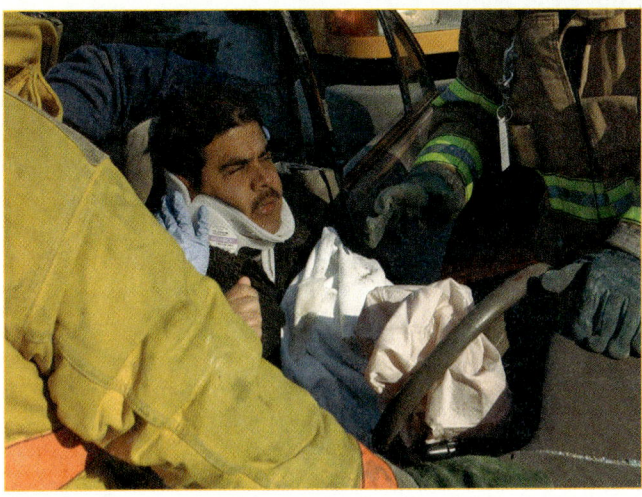

Figure 49-13 The driver may be trapped between the steering wheel and the back of the front seat.

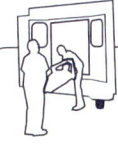

At the Scene

If you're wearing a heavy coat for protection from the weather during a rescue operation, then the patient will also be cold if not covered with blankets.

that are trapping the patient. The goal here is to remove the sheet metal and plastic from around the patient—not to "cut the patient out of the vehicle."

Before attempting disentanglement, study the situation. What is trapping the patient in the vehicle? Perform only those disentanglement procedures that are necessary to remove the patient safely from the vehicle. The order in which these procedures are performed will be dictated by the specific conditions at the incident. Many times it will be necessary to perform one procedure before you can access the parts of the vehicle needed to perform another procedure.

As you work to disentangle the patient from the wrecked vehicle, protect the patient by covering him or her with a blanket or by using a backboard. Be sure that the patient understands what's being done—the sounds made by extrication procedures can be quite frightening for patients.

To learn all of the methods of disentangling a patient, you need to take an approved extrication course. The five procedures presented below are the ones that are most commonly performed.

Displace the Seat

In frontal and rear-end collisions, the vehicle may become compressed. As the front of the vehicle is pushed back, the space between the steering wheel and the seat becomes smaller. In some cases, the driver may be trapped between the steering

wheel and the back of the front seat 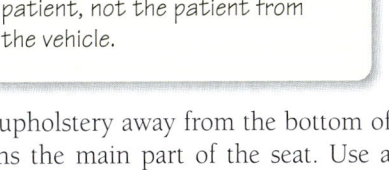 **Figure 49-13 ▲** . Displacing the seat can relieve pressure on the driver and give rescuers more space for removal.

If it is necessary to displace a seat backward, start with the simplest steps. Many times you can gain some room by moving the seat backward on its track, especially with short drivers who have the seat forward. To move a seat back, first be sure that the patient is supported. With manually operated seats, you need to release the seat-adjusting lever and carefully slide the seat back as far as it will go. If the seat is electrically operated, check that the car has power, and engage the lever to electrically move the seat backward. With seats that have adjustable backs and adjustable heights, you can use these features to give the patient more room or lower the seat to help disentangle the patient.

If these methods are unsuccessful, perform a dash displacement. As a last resort, you can use a manual hydraulic spreader or a powered hydraulic tool to move the seat back. Place one tip of the hydraulic tool on the bottom of the seat. Avoid pushing on the seat channel that is attached to the floor of the vehicle. Place the other tip of the spreader at the bottom of the A-post door jamb. Support the patient carefully. Engage the seat adjustment lever on manually operated seats, and open the spreader in a careful and controlled fashion. The seat should move backward smoothly in a controlled manner.

In some cases, it may be helpful to remove the back of

Notes from Nancy

Remove the vehicle from the patient, not the patient from the vehicle.

the seat. To do so, cut the upholstery away from the bottom of the seat back where it joins the main part of the seat. Use a reciprocating saw or a hydraulic cutter to cut the supports for the seat back. Be certain that the patient is supported and protected during this procedure.

Remove the Windshield

A second technique that's often part of disentanglement is the removal of glass. Removing the rear window, side glass, or windshield improves communication between rescue personnel inside the vehicle and personnel outside the vehicle. Sometimes all you need to do is to roll a window down. Open windows provide a good route for passing medical care supplies to the inside caregiver. When the roof of a vehicle must be removed, all of the glass must first be removed from the vehicle.

On most vehicles, the side windows and rear window are tempered glass that can be removed by striking the glass in a lower corner with a sharp object, such as a spring-loaded centre punch. In contrast, windshields cannot be broken with a spring-loaded centre punch. They consist of plastic laminated glass—a type of "sandwich," in which the two pieces of bread are thin sheets of specially constructed glass and the filling is a thin layer of a special flexible plastic. When laminated glass is struck by a sharp stone or by a spring-loaded centre punch, a small mark is formed, but the structure of the glass remains intact. For this reason, the windshield must be removed in one large piece. The windshields of most passenger vehicles are glued in place with a strong, plastic-type adhesive.

Removing a windshield is an essential step before removing the roof of a vehicle. It will also provide added space when administering emergency medical care to an injured patient. The windshield of a damaged vehicle may be removed using either an axe or a saw.

To remove a windshield using an axe **Figure 49-14 ▸**, first be certain that the patient is protected from flying glass. One rescuer then begins to cut the top of the windshield at the centre of the windshield, using short strokes of the axe. He or she continues cutting along the top of the windshield with the next cut down the side of the windshield close to the A post. Finally, the first rescuer cuts along the bottom of the windshield. At this point, the first rescuer stabilizes the half of the windshield that has been cut free. Next, a second rescuer starts

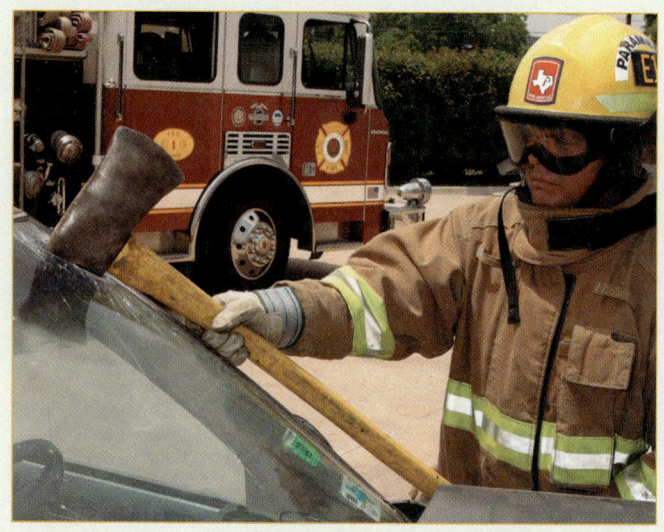

Figure 49-14 Removing the windshield with an axe.

at the top of the windshield where the initial cuts were made by the first rescuer. He or she cuts the second half of the windshield following the same sequence of cuts used by the first rescuer. The windshield is then lifted out of its frame and removed to a place where it will not present a safety hazard.

When using a saw, the windshield is removed by making the cuts in the same order as those made with an axe.

Displace the Dash

During a frontal collision, the vehicle's dash may be pushed down or backward. When a patient is trapped by the dash, you must remove it using a technique called the dash displacement or dash roll-up. The objective of the dash displacement is to lift the dash up and move it forward.

Dash displacement requires a cutting tool such as a hacksaw, reciprocating saw, air chisel, or hydraulic cutter. This cutting tool is used to make a cut on the A post. A mechanical

You are the Paramedic **Part 4**

About 10 minutes later the patient becomes extremely anxious and complains about excruciating abdominal pain. A reassessment of the abdomen shows marked distension and rigidity. The patient is becoming pale and increasingly diaphoretic. His radial pulses are weakening. He begs you to do something for the pain, although you have explained that you are not able to do so. Despite your best efforts to be reassuring, the patient's anxiety continues to escalate and he keeps repeating "I'm dying." You increase the flow of the IV and silently hope that additional help arrives soon. Off in the distance the whir of helicopter blades can be heard.

Reassessment	Recording Time: 23 Minutes
Skin	Pale, cool, and diaphoretic
Pulse	140 beats/min, carotid
Blood pressure	92/68 mm Hg
Respirations	20 breaths/min
Spo$_2$	97% on 100% supplemental oxygen
ECG	Sinus rhythm without ectopy

At the Scene

Airbag Safety

- Steering wheels on most recently manufactured vehicles contain a driver's side airbag, which is a lifesaving safety feature for the occupants of the vehicle.
- If the airbag has deployed during the collision, it does not present a safety hazard for rescuers.
- If not deployed during the collision, an airbag presents a hazard for the passenger of the vehicle and for rescue personnel. It could potentially deploy if wires are cut or if it becomes activated during the rescue operation.
- If the airbag did not deploy, disconnect the battery and allow the airbag capacitor to discharge. The time required to discharge the capacitor varies from one model of airbag to another.
- Some newer-model vehicles have a switch mounted on or under the dash that allows drivers to disconnect or shut off the SRS.
- Do not place a hard object such as a backboard between the patient and an undeployed airbag.
- Do not attempt to cut a steering wheel if the airbag hasn't deployed.
- There are times when you will be attending to a patient sitting next to or in front of an undeployed airbag. You must try to maintain a safe distance between you and the airbag when doing so. You could suffer serious injury if it is unexpectedly activated.
- Some vehicles contain side-mounted airbags or curtains that provide lateral protection for passengers. Check vehicles for the presence of these devices.

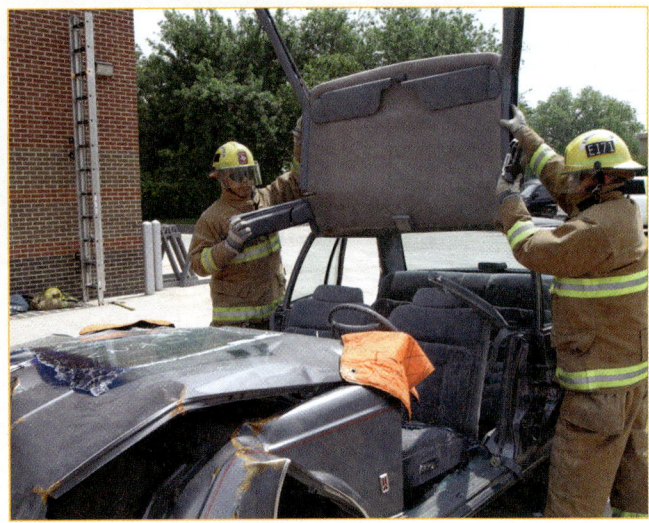

Figure 49-15 Removing the roof provides a large exit route for the patient.

high-lift jack or a hydraulic ram then pushes the dash forward, and cribbing maintains the opening made with these tools.

The first step of the dash displacement is to open both front doors. Tie them in the open position so they won't move as the dash is being displaced. Alternatively, you can remove the doors.

Next, place a backboard or other protective device between the patient and the bottom part of the A post, where the relief cut will be made. Cut the bottom of the A post where it meets the sill or floor of the vehicle. It is critical to make the cut perpendicular to the A post; failure to do so may cut the fuel or power line located in the rocker panels.

Place the base of a high-lift mechanical jack or a hydraulically powered ram at the base of the B post where the sill and the B post meet. Place the tip of the jack or ram at the bend in the A post, which is located toward the top of the A post. In a controlled manner, extend the jack or ram to push the dash up and off of the patient.

Once the dash has been removed, build a crib to hold the sill in the proper position and to prevent the dash from moving. You can then remove the jack or ram.

Performing dash displacement requires careful monitoring of the movement of the dash to be certain that it is moving away from the patient and that it isn't causing additional harm to the patient. Be sure that the patient is protected and have someone keep the patient updated on what is being done.

Displace the Roof

Removing the roof of a vehicle allows equipment to be more easily passed in to the paramedic. It also increases the amount of space available to perform medical care and increases the visibility and space for performing disentanglement. Both paramedic and patient will benefit from the fresh air supply, too. The increased space helps to reduce the feeling of panic caused by the confined space of the wrecked vehicle. Removing the roof also provides a large exit route for the patient **Figure 49-15 ▲**.

One method of displacing the roof is to cut the A posts and fold the roof back toward the rear of the vehicle. This method provides limited space and takes about the same time as removing the entire roof. Accordingly, in most cases, it is preferable to remove the entire roof.

Roof displacement can be accomplished with hand tools such as hacksaws, air chisels, or manual hydraulic cutters. Appropriate power tools include reciprocating saws and powered hydraulic cutters.

A key consideration in displacing the roof is to ensure the safety of rescuers and the patient inside the vehicle. In particular, as you cut the posts that support the roof, rescuers must support the roof to keep it from falling on the patient.

To displace the roof, first remove the glass to prevent it from falling on the patients. Cut the vehicle posts farthest away from the patient. Cut the posts at a level to ensure that the least amount of post will remain after roof removal. It is very important to cut the shoulder harness on seatbelts because they're attached to the roof in many vehicles and will be the only thing preventing roof removal. When cutting the wider rear posts, cut them at the narrowest point of the post. As each post is cut, a rescuer needs to support that post. Cut the post closest to the patient last. Working together, remove the roof and place it away from the vehicle, where it doesn't

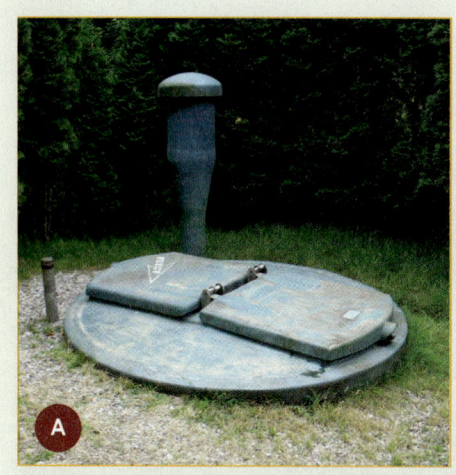 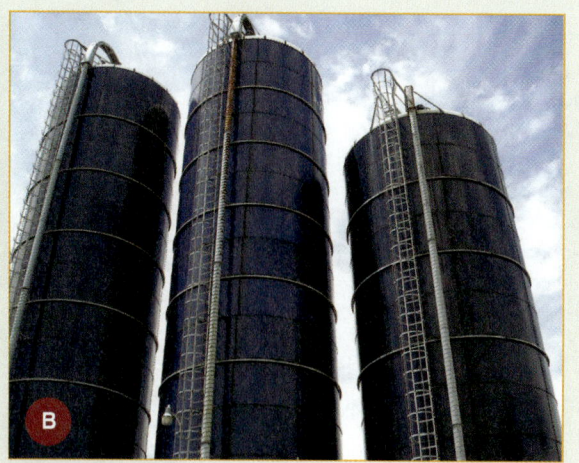

Figure 49-16 Confined spaces **A.** Below ground. **B.** Silo.

pose a safety hazard. Cover the sharp ends of the cut posts with a protective device.

Confined Spaces

A confined space is a location surrounded by a structure that isn't designed for continuous occupancy. Confined spaces have limited openings for entrance and exit. Confined spaces can occur in farm, commercial, and industrial settings. Structures such as grain silos, industrial pits, tanks, and below-ground structures are all considered confined spaces. Automobile trunks are also considered confined spaces. Cisterns, well casings, and septic tanks are also confined spaces that are found in many residential settings **Figure 49-16 ▲**.

Confined spaces present a special hazard because they may have limited ventilation to provide for air circulation and exchange, which can make them an oxygen-deficient atmosphere, or they may contain poisonous gases. Entering a confined space without testing the atmosphere for safety and without the proper breathing apparatus can result in death. Additionally, there is a risk of fire and explosion in confined spaces because inadequate ventilation may trap flammable mixtures. Grain silos and trenches can suddenly become "quicksand" and lead to engulfment. Machinery may often have confined spaces containing augers or screws that can be hazardous to rescue workers. All rescue personnel must consider the potential for stored electrical energy in any machinery and should never attempt any rescue without being properly trained.

Do not be overwhelmed by the urgency to start treating patients; scene safety must always be considered first.

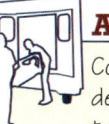 **At the Scene**

Confined spaces such as manholes can be deceiving. They may look habitable but can contain minimal oxygen or deadly invisible toxins.

A confined-space call is sometimes dispatched as a heart attack or medical illness call, because the caller assumes the person who entered a confined space and became unresponsive suffered a heart attack or medical illness.

Examples of Oxygen Deficiency/Poisonous Gases in Confined Spaces

Hydrogen sulfide (H_2S) is a colourless, toxic, flammable gas that is released when bacteria break down organic matter in the absence of oxygen. It can be found in swamps, standing water, sewers, volcanic gases, natural gas, and in some wells. Hydrogen sulfide is heavier than air and has a very pungent odour at first but deadens the sense of smell very quickly.

At the Scene

More rescuers die in confined spaces than victims! Of all deaths in confined-space rescue incidents, 60% are rescuers. Do not enter a confined space without proper breathing apparatus and special training.

Carbon monoxide (CO) is a colourless, odourless, tasteless gas that cannot be detected by your normal senses. Inhaling relatively small quantities of CO gas can result in severe poisoning because it binds to red blood cells about 200 to 250 times more readily than oxygen. Therefore, a small quantity of CO can "monopolize" the red blood cells and prevent them from transporting oxygen to all parts of the body. The signs and symptoms of CO poisoning include headache, nausea, disorientation, and unconsciousness.

Carbon dioxide (CO_2) is a colourless gas associated with asphyxiation risks. It is actually the end product of a metabolism process in which sugar and fats combine with oxygen. Carbon dioxide is used to make dry ice and is found in fire extinguishers. It produces a sour taste in the mouth and a stinging sensation in the nose and mouth.

Methane (CH_4)—the principal component of natural gas— isn't toxic but will cause burns if ignited. Flammable or explosive mixtures form at much lower concentrations than the concentrations at which asphyxiation risks arise. Methane is used as a fuel from natural gas fields but can also be generated from fermentation of organic matter (eg, manure, waste water, sludge, and municipal solid waste).

Ammonia (NH_3) is a toxic and corrosive chemical with a characteristic pungent odour. Because ammonia is lighter than air, it rises to the upper atmospheric level in confined spaces. It is typically found in rural areas and is used extensively for fertilizing agricultural crops.

Nitrogen dioxide (NO_2) is a reddish-brown gas that has a characteristic sharp, biting odour. It is most prominent in air pollution and is considered toxic by inhalation.

Safe Approach

As you approach a confined-space rescue scene, look for a bystander who might have witnessed the emergency. Information gathered prior to the technical rescue team's arrival will save valuable time during the actual rescue. Do not automatically assume that a person in a pit has simply suffered a heart attack; instead, assume that there is an IDLH atmosphere at any confined-space call. An IDLH atmosphere can immediately incapacitate anyone who enters the confined space without breathing protection. Toxic gases may be present, or oxygen levels may be insufficient to support life. Inevitably, it will take some time for qualified rescuers to arrive on the scene and prepare for a safe entry into the confined space. The victim of the original incident may have died before your arrival—do not put your life in danger for a dead patient.

Assisting Other Rescuers

You and your partner can prevent a confined-space incident from becoming worse by recognizing it, securing the scene, and ensuring that no one enters the space until additional rescue resources arrive. As highly trained personnel arrive, you may provide help by giving these rescuers a situation report.

The first responding rescuers must share whatever information is discovered at the rescue scene with the arriving crew. Anything that may be important to the response should be noted by the first arriving unit. Observed conditions should be compared to reported conditions, and a determination should be made as to the relative change over the time period. Whether an incident appears to be stable or has changed significantly since the first report will affect the operation strategy for the rescue. An assessment should be quickly completed immediately upon arrival, and this information should be relayed to the specialized rescue team members when they arrive at the scene. Other items of importance that should be included in a situation report are a description of any rescue attempts that have been made, exposures, hazards, extinguishment of fires, the facts and probabilities of the scene, the situation and resources of the fire company, the identity of any hazardous materials present, and a progress evaluation.

Confined-space rescues can be complex and can take a long time to complete. You may be asked to assist by bringing rescue equipment to the scene, maintaining a charged hose line, or providing crowd control. By understanding the hazards of confined spaces, you will be better prepared to assist a specialized team that's dealing with an emergency involving a confined space.

Trenches

Trench rescues may become necessary when earth is removed for placement of a utility line or for other construction and the sides of the excavation collapse, trapping a worker **Figure 49-17 ▾** . Entrapments may also occur when children play around a pile of sand or earth that collapses. Unfortunately, many entrapments occur because the required safety precautions were not taken.

Whenever a collapse occurs, you need to understand that the collapsed product is unstable and prone to further collapse. Earth and sand are very heavy, and a person who's partly entrapped cannot simply be pulled out. Instead, the patient must be carefully dug out after shoring has stabilized the sides of the excavation.

Vibration or additional weight on top of displaced earth will increase the probability of a secondary collapse. A secondary collapse occurs after the initial collapse; it can be caused by equipment vibration, personnel standing at the edge of the trench, or water eroding away the soil. Safe removal of trapped

At the Scene

Most trench collapses occur in trenches less than 4 m deep and 2 m wide. Patients are suddenly covered with heavy soil, resulting in asphyxia. Specially trained rescuers should make safe access only after shoring is in place.

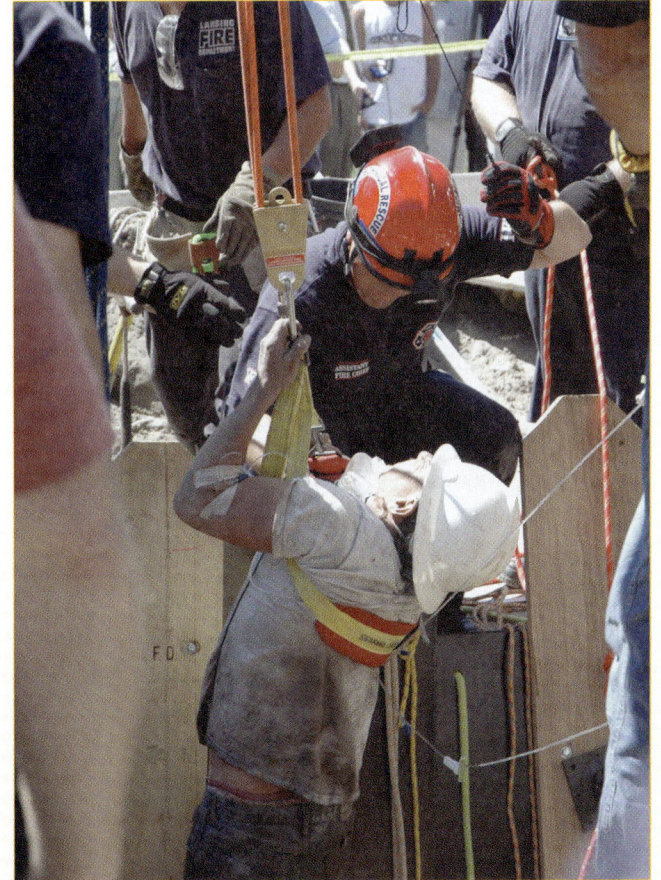

Figure 49-17 Trench rescue.

persons requires a special rescue team that is trained and equipped to erect shoring that will protect the rescuers and the entrapped person from secondary collapse.

Safety is of paramount importance when approaching a trench or excavation collapse. Walking close to the edge of a collapse can trigger a secondary collapse. Stay away from the edge of the site, and keep all workers and bystanders away. Vibration from equipment and machinery can cause secondary collapses, so shut off all heavy equipment. Vibrations caused by nearby traffic can also cause collapse, so it may be necessary to stop or divert traffic.

Soil that has been removed from the excavation and placed in a pile is called the spoil pile. This material is very unstable and may collapse if placed too close to the excavation. Avoid disturbing the spoil pile.

Make verbal contact with the trapped person if possible, but do *not* place yourself in danger while doing so. If you approach the trench, do so from the narrow end, where the soil will be more stable. However, it is best *not* to approach the trench unless absolutely necessary; paramedics should stay out of a trench unless properly trained.

Provide reassurance by letting the trapped person know that a trained rescue team is on the way. By removing people from the edges of the excavation, shutting down machinery, and establishing contact with the patient, you start the rescue process.

You can also assess the scene, looking for evidence that would indicate where the trapped workers may be located. Hand tools and hard hats are one indicator of their presence. By questioning the workers, paramedics may also determine where the patients were last seen.

Water

Almost all EMS departments may be called to perform a water rescue—whether from a small stream, a large river, a lake, the ocean, a reservoir, or a swimming pool. A static source such as a lake may have no current and is considered flat water or slow moving. In contrast, a whitewater stream or flooded river may have a very swift current. During a flood, a dry wash in the desert can quickly become a raging monster.

Rescuers may suddenly find themselves immersed in moving water during a water rescue, so they should be aware of self-rescue techniques. A PFD is essential. In addition, if suddenly immersed in fast-moving water, rescuers should adopt the self-rescue position. The first step is to roll into a face-up arched position with the lower back higher than the feet to avoid subsurface objects. Keep the feet together and facing in the direction of travel (feet first) with arms to the side. Use the hands for changing direction to avoid objects and for diversion to a safe area. Keep the head down, with the chin tucked in.

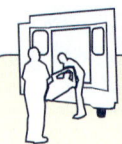
At the Scene
Do not attempt a water rescue unless you are specially trained.

This position protects the rescuer's head, face, and lower back from striking objects and provides a means for controlling direction.

Cold Water Rescue

Water temperature varies widely by season and by geographical area. Even on warm days, water temperatures can be very low. Water causes heat loss 25 times greater than ambient air temperature. Indeed, any water temperature less than 37°C will cause hypothermia; patients who become hypothermic lose the ability to self-rescue. Maintaining body heat is critical because hypothermia becomes an immediate problem that progresses to unconsciousness and death. In extremely cold water (4°C), a submersion time of 15 to 20 minutes will rapidly lead to death.

If you find yourself in cold water, make every effort to keep your face above water, protect your head, and assume the heat-escape-lessening position (HELP) **Figure 49-18 ▾** , which helps keep heat in the core of your body. Immersion victims should minimize movement and assume the HELP position. In a group, victims should huddle together to share body warmth.

At the Scene
Humans cannot maintain body heat in water that is less than 32°C. The colder the water, the faster the loss of heat. Compared with air, water causes a heat loss at a rate 25 times faster. Immersion for 15 to 20 minutes in 4°C water is likely to be fatal.

In water colder than 21°C, immersion victims may actually benefit from a phenomenon known as the cold protective response. Essentially, when a person is submerged in cold water, heat is conducted from the body to the water. The resulting hypothermia can protect vital organs from the lack of oxygen. In addition, exposure to cold water will occasionally activate certain primitive reflexes, which may preserve body functions for prolonged periods. In one case, a 2½-year-old girl recovered after

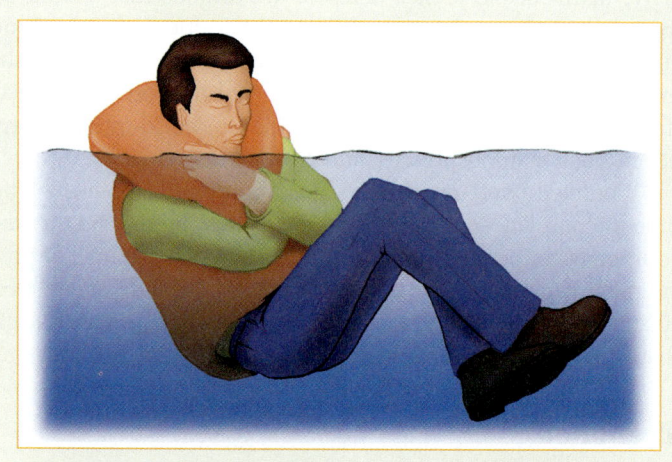
Figure 49-18 The heat-escape-lessening position (HELP).

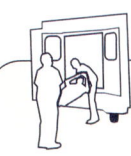

At the Scene

The HELP position can decrease heat loss by 60% compared with treading water.

being submerged in cold water for at least 66 minutes. For this reason, you should continue to provide full resuscitative efforts for a victim of cold water submersion until the patient recovers or is pronounced dead by a physician (see Chapter 35 for a more detailed discussion of hypothermia).

Whenever a person dives or jumps into very cold water, the diving reflex (also known as the mammalian diving reflex)—the slowing of the heart rate caused by submersion in cold water—may cause immediate bradycardia. Although loss of consciousness may follow, the person may be able to survive for an extended time under water because of a lowering of the metabolic rate and decreased oxygen demand and consumption associated with hypothermia.

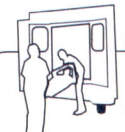

At the Scene

Remember that hypothermic patients are dehydrated due to "cold diuresis," and should be removed from the water in a horizontal position to avoid orthostatic changes.

Other Water Rescue Situations

In North America, the most common swift water rescue scenario involves people who have attempted to drive vehicles through a pool of water created by a flooded stream. The vehicle stalls because of the depth of the water, leaving the vehicle occupants stranded in a rising stream with a swift current. If the water is high enough, the vehicle can be swept away. These incidents are especially dangerous for rescue personnel, because it is difficult to determine the depth of the water around the vehicle.

In surface water rescues, rescuers must consider hazards such as the dangerous hydraulics created by moving water as well as "strainers" (objects in the water such as trees, branches, debris, or wire mesh that can pose a serious pinning risk for rescuers). Dams and hydroelectric sites are also treacherous for even the most skilled rescuers. It is important to remember that the height of a dam does not indicate the degree of hazard to rescuers. Intakes at the base of a dam can act like strainers. Low-head dams are often associated with recirculating currents (sometimes referred to as a "boil") **Figure 49-19 ▶** . These currents can trap victims and unwary rescuers alike, forcing them underwater, away from the dam, and back to the surface again, where the cycle repeats itself. For this reason, low-head dams are often referred to as "drowning machines." Never underestimate the power or intensity of moving water.

Safe Approach

When responding to water rescue incidents, your safety and the safety of other rescuers are your primary concerns. Your

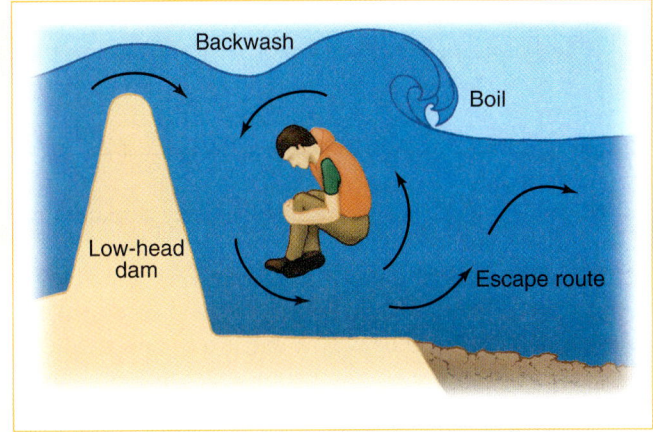

Figure 49-19 Recirculating current at a low-head dam.

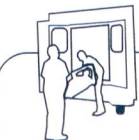

At the Scene

The hydraulics of moving water change with variables such as depth, velocity, and obstruction to flow.

gear is not designed for water rescue activities. When working at a water rescue scene, you should use personal protective gear designed for water rescue. Whenever you are within 3 metres of the water, you should wear an approved PFD. Shoes that provide solid traction are preferable to boots.

If you are part of the first arriving ambulance's crew, and the endangered people are in a vehicle or holding on to a tree or other solid object, try to communicate with them. Let them know that more help is on the way.

Do not exceed your level of training. If you cannot swim, operating around or near water is not recommended. A person who is trained as a lifeguard for still water is not prepared to enter flowing water with a strong current, such as in a river, stream, or ocean. Make sure that bystanders do not try to rescue the patient and place themselves in a situation where they need to be rescued, too.

When you see a person struggling in the water, your first impulse may be to jump in to assist. However, that action may not result in a successful rescue and can endanger your life. The model most commonly used in water rescue is *reach-throw-row-go*:

- Attempt to *reach* out to the threatened person first, using any readily available object. If the person is close to shore, a branch, pole, oar, or paddle may be long enough.
- If you cannot reach the person, *throw* something—for example, a life buoy or a throw bag (a small sack containing two ropes and a piece of foam). In an emergency situation, a rescuer opens the bag, pulls out enough rope to grasp firmly (some rescuers prefer to wrap the rope around their backs), and then throws the bag to the victim. The victim should be instructed to grab the

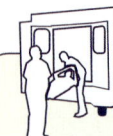

rope and not the bag, because the bag may contain more rope that can uncoil.

- If you cannot reach the person by throwing something that floats, you may be able to *row* out to the drowning person if a small boat or canoe is available. Do so only if you know how to operate or propel the craft properly. Protect yourself by wearing an approved PFD.
- As a last resort, *go* into the water to save the victim. Enter the water only if you are a capable swimmer trained in lifesaving and water rescue techniques. Remove encumbering clothing before doing so, and take a flotation device with you if one is available.

Many departments in colder regions have developed specialized equipment to assist in ice rescues. Throwing a rope or flotation device may be helpful initially. Ladders can be used to distribute the weight of the rescuer on ice-covered water. Specially designed hose lines have been used with end-caps and an air line to create a flotation buoy. Special rescue suits are available to prevent hypothermia and provide flotation for the rescuer. If your department is involved in ice rescues, you should receive training in these specialized procedures.

Recovery Situations

On occasion, you may be called to the scene of a drowning and find that the patient is not floating or visible in the water. An organized rescue effort in these circumstances calls for personnel who are experienced with recovery techniques and equipment, including snorkels, masks, and scuba gear. As a last resort, when standard procedures for recovery are unsuccessful, you may have to use a grappling hook or large hook to drag the bottom for the victim. Although the hook could seriously wound the patient, it may be the only effective way to bring him or her to the surface for resuscitative efforts.

Spinal Incidents in Submersion Incidents

Submersion incidents may be complicated by spinal fractures and spinal cord injuries. You must assume that spinal injury exists with the following conditions:

- The submersion has resulted from a diving mishap or fall.
- The patient is unconscious, and no information is available to rule out the possibility of a mechanism causing neck injury.
- The patient is conscious but complains of weakness, paralysis, or numbness in the arms or legs.
- You suspect the possibility of spinal injury despite what witnesses say.

Most spinal injuries in diving incidents affect the cervical spine. When spinal injury is suspected, the neck must be protected from further injury. This means that you will have to

stabilize the suspected injury while the patient is still in the water. Follow the steps in **Skill Drill 49-2 ▶**:

1. Turn the patient supine. Two rescuers are usually required to turn the patient safely, although in some cases one rescuer will suffice. Always rotate the entire upper half of the patient's body as a single unit. Twisting only the head, for example, may aggravate any injury to the cervical spine **Step 1**.
2. Restore the airway and begin ventilation. Immediate ventilation is the primary treatment of all submersion patients as soon as the patient is face up in the water. Use a pocket mask if it is available. Have the other rescuer support the head and trunk as a unit while you open the airway and begin artificial ventilation **Step 2**.
3. Float a buoyant backboard under the patient as you continue ventilation **Step 3**.
4. Secure the trunk and head to the backboard to eliminate motion of the cervical spine. Do not remove the patient from the water until this is done **Step 4**.
5. Remove the patient from the water, on the backboard **Step 5**.
6. Cover the patient with a blanket. Give supplemental oxygen if the patient is breathing spontaneously. Begin CPR if there is no pulse. Effective cardiac compression or CPR is extremely difficult to perform when the patient is still in the water **Step 6**.

Rope Rescue

Rope rescue skills are the most versatile and widely used technical rescue skills. Sometimes a rope rescue is performed to remove a person from a position of peril; at other times, rope rescues are needed to remove ill or injured persons—for example, from inside a tank.

Types of Rope Rescues

Rope rescue incidents are divided into low-angle and high-angle operations. Low-angle operations are situations where the slope of the ground over which the rescuers are working is less than 45°. In these cases, rescuers depend on the ground for their primary support, and the rope system serves as a secondary means of support. An example of a low-angle system is a rope stretched from the top of an embankment and used for support by rescuers who are carrying a patient up an incline.

Low-angle operations are used when the scene requires ropes to be used only as assistance to pull or haul up a patient or rescuer. They are usually necessary when adequate footing is not present, in areas such as a dirt or rock embankment. In

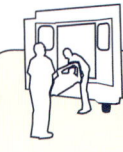

Skill Drill 49-2: Stabilizing a Suspected Spinal Injury in the Water

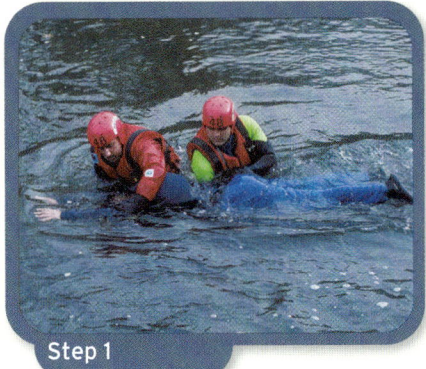

Step 1

Turn the patient to a supine position in the water by rotating the entire upper half of the body as a single unit.

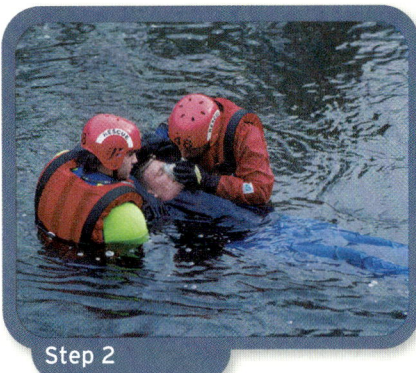

Step 2

As soon as the patient is turned, begin artificial ventilation using the mouth-to-mouth method or a pocket mask.

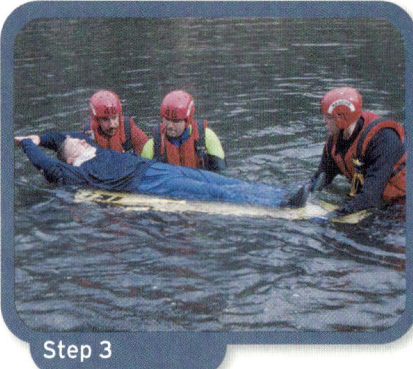

Step 3

Float a buoyant backboard under the patient.

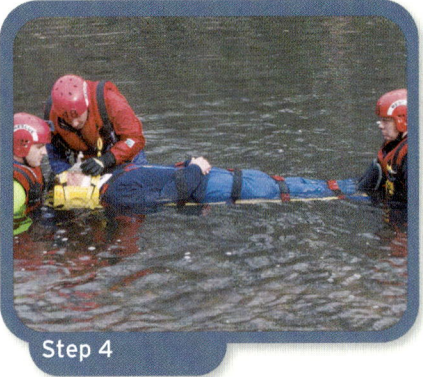

Step 4

Secure the patient to the backboard.

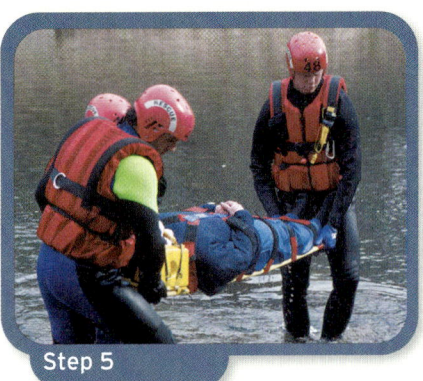

Step 5

Remove the patient from the water.

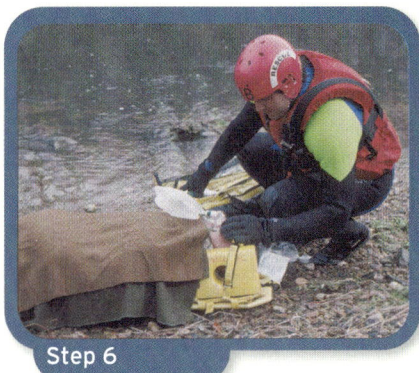

Step 6

Cover the patient with a blanket and apply oxygen if breathing. Begin CPR if breathing and a pulse are still absent.

---

such an incident, a rope will be tied to the rescuer's harness and the rescuer will climb the embankment by himself/herself, using the rope to keep from falling. Low-angle operations also include lifelines placed during ice or water rescues.

Ropes can also be used to assist in raising or lowering a Stokes basket. This technique frees the rescuers from having to carry all of the weight over rough terrain. Rescuers at the top of the embankment can help to pull up or lower the basket using a rope system.

When using any rope system to assist in rescue operations, a safety feature is to belay the rope. Belay in climbing is a technique of controlling the rope as it is fed out to the climbers. A critical part of the climbing system, it can be accomplished with a self-belay or a secondary lifeline. The use of belay systems has become a controversial issue in rescue, and their benefits are being researched. One potential complication is that belays depend on the angle of operations; as a consequence, the entire load may be transferred to the belay line. This could prove dangerous depending on the load and the length of rope.

Another aspect of climbing or rescue situations is the act of descending. In some descents, the angle is so severe that a technique known as rappelling is performed. To rappel is to descend on a fixed rope. Scrambling is a method used to ascend rocky faces and ridges and can be considered a cross between hill climbing (where an individual walks up a steep incline using both hands and feet) and rock climbing.

A hasty rope slide is a self-escape procedure when there is no other means of egress. This kind of semicontrolled fall without a descent device should not be attempted without proper training. The rope is wrapped around the back and under the arms or placed between the feet to provide resistance for slowing the rate of descent. Gloved hands are also effective for slowing the descent rate.

High-angle operations are situations where the slope of the ground is greater than 45°, and rescuers or patients are dependent on a life safety rope and not a fixed surface of support such as the ground. High-angle rescue techniques are used to raise or lower a person when other means of raising or lowering are not readily available. These rescues are extremely demanding and dangerous, and they should be attempted only by personnel who are thoroughly trained in proper procedure.

Safe Approach

If you respond to an incident that may require a rope rescue operation, consider both your safety and the safety of those around you. Rope rescues are among the most time-consuming calls that you will encounter. Extensive setup is necessary, and a considerable amount of equipment needs to be assembled prior to initiating any rescue. Protect your safety by remaining away from the area under the patient and away from any loose materials that might potentially fall. Work to control the scene so that bystanders move to an area where they will not be injured.

Wilderness Search and Rescue

Wilderness search and rescue (SAR) is an activity that is conducted by a limited number of departments. SAR missions consist of two parts: search (looking for a lost or overdue person) and rescue (removing a patient from a hostile environment).

Several types of situations may result in the initiation of SAR missions. Small children may wander off and be unable to find their way back to a known place. Older adults who are suffering from Alzheimer's disease may fail to remember where they're going and become lost. People who are hiking, hunting, or participating in other wilderness activities may become lost because they lack the proper training or equipment, because the weather changes unexpectedly, or if they become sick or injured.

Safe Approach

"Wilderness" can include many different environments, such as forests, mountains, deserts, natural parks, animal refuges, and rain forests. Depending on the terrain and environmental factors, the wilderness can be as little as a few minutes into the backcountry or a few feet off the roadway. Despite the short access time, the scene could require an extended evacuation and thus qualify as a wilderness incident. Examples of wilderness terrains include cliffs, steep slopes, rivers, streams, valleys, mountainsides, and beaches. Terrain hazards include cliffs, caves, wells, mines, avalanches, and rock slides.

When you participate in SAR missions, prepare for the weather conditions by bringing suitable clothing. Make sure that you do not exceed your physical limitations, and do not get in situations that are beyond your ability to handle in the wilderness. Call for a special wilderness rescue team, depending on the situation and your local protocols.

Using a Litter

Litters facilitate moving patients to a place of safety and can be used in a variety of situations. The manner in which a patient is packaged in a litter depends on his or her medical condition, the environment, and the manner in which the patient will be evacuated. Litters can be lifted by rope, carried by vehicles, or, most commonly, hand-carried by rescuers. In case of vertical evacuation, pack excess gear around the patient to prevent undue movement. While handling the patient, be sure to communicate and keep him or her apprised of the situation and your progress.

The standard litter carry involves a team of six to eight rescuers distributed around the litter, three or four to a side. Normally, the person at the front of the left side is in charge and directs the activities of the others. This method has the advantages of being fast, as little teamwork is required, and it usually gives the patient a comfortable ride. Its disadvantages include the fact that this carrying method is very tiring for the handlers, because it puts constant strain on certain muscles, and ground vision is difficult, especially at night; a handler can easily trip over a rock and drop the litter.

More than one team will be needed if the litter must be carried over a distance further than the team can cover in about 15 to 20 minutes. Team *leapfrogging* is a good method to use on long evacuations, ie, one team takes the litter for a given distance while the other team goes ahead to rest and preplan the next stretch. At the pass-off point, the first team advances to the next point for rest and planning.

When footing is highly unstable, an obstacle prevents the litter team from progressing, or falling becomes a possible hazard, the caterpillar or lap pass is a useful option. When the

You are the Paramedic **Part 5**

The engine company has been on scene for 45 minutes and just finished widening access to the cab of the truck when the rescue company arrives. They are now ready to begin the process of removing the dashboard. Earplugs are provided for both you and the patient to protect your hearing from the hydraulic tools that will be used. A yellow blanket is placed over the two of you to prevent injury from debris. The helicopter crew is waiting, ready to assist in extrication and packaging.

Prior to the start of the dashboard removal you were able to increase the patient's blood pressure to 114/66 mm Hg. Your main concerns are keeping him calm and being prepared for the potential decline in his status once the dashboard is lifted off of his pelvis. It requires an additional 35 minutes to remove the dashboard. As feared, once the pressure of the dashboard is relieved from your patient's pelvis, he becomes pale and loses consciousness. One of the helicopter medics is able to palpate a weak carotid pulse. The patient is quickly but carefully moved over to the stretcher for resuscitative care by the flight crew. He is immediately intubated and has a second large-bore IV line placed.

Upon arrival to the trauma centre, the patient is found to have a shattered pelvis, bilateral femur fractures, and a small subdural hematoma. He is evaluated in the emergency department and then taken promptly to the operating room for stabilization of his pelvis and lower extremities, and evacuation of the subdural hematoma.

litter reaches the obstacle, the team pauses while every extra person lines up on the route ahead of the difficult terrain or obstacles. The rescuers form two lines facing each other about the width of the litter apart and alternate (in other words, they aren't all opposite each other). They usually sit down and try to make themselves as stable as possible. When everyone is set, rescuers pass the litter down between the two lines. As the litter passes a person, he or she gets up and carefully but quickly moves around the line in the direction of travel, and gets set to pass the litter again. Done correctly, this technique provides a very stable and secure passage.

Table 49-1	Medications for Pain Management in Rescue Situations
Medication	**Characteristics**
Morphine sulfate	Narcotic analgesic and central nervous system depressant often used in the treatment of myocardial infarction, kidney stones, and pulmonary edema. It should be used with caution in patients who are volume-depleted or suffering from severe hypotension.
Nitrous oxide (Nitronox, Entonox)	Narcotic analgesic and central nervous system depressant primarily used for the treatment of moderate to severe pain. It should be used with caution in patients who are volume depleted or who suffer from severe hypotension.
Fentanyl citrate (Sublimaze)	This central nervous system depressant with analgesic properties is used for musculoskeletal pain, fractures, and burns. It should not be used in patients who cannot follow verbal instructions, those with head injuries, COPD patients, and patients with thoracic injuries or possible pneumothorax. Use caution in environments less than −6°C, which could make administration difficult to impossible.
Ketorolac (Toradol)	Classified as a nonsteroidal anti-inflammatory drug (NSAID), ketorolac has analgesic, anti-inflammatory, and antipyretic effects. It is considered in controlling moderate to severe pain. Its only true contraindication is in patients with a known hypersensitivity to the drug and patients with reported allergies to aspirin or NSAIDs.

Prehospital Care

Many medical and trauma conditions can and will be assessed during the rescue process. In confined-space rescues, especially with cave-ins and trench rescues, paramedics need to consider the potential for crush injuries—in particular, the possibility of compartment syndrome. When human tissue goes without an adequate supply of oxygen-enriched blood, tissue (cells) continues to metabolize (produce energy) without oxygen (anaerobic metabolism), producing lactic acid as a by-product. When entrapped or compressed areas of the body are eventually reperfused, these metabolic by-products are released into the circulation. Treatment with high-flow oxygen therapy or positive-pressure ventilations, along with administration of sodium bicarbonate, can help to reverse the effects of respiratory and metabolic acidosis.

Pain Management

Patients involved in many rescue situations will be experiencing pain from injuries received during the incident. Pain control should take the form of nonpharmacologic methods such as splinting to minimize movement, gentle handling, or talking with patients to create a distraction during assessment and movement. Paramedics must also keep patients warm, as a shivering patient will aggravate pain with his or her every movement.

Pharmacologic treatment in the prehospital setting remains controversial, and paramedics should consult with their medical directors on issues related to pain management. All medications are contraindicated in patients with a known hypersensitivity to the drug. Table 49-1 ▶ lists some of the medications that can be considered in the pain management of patients during rescue efforts. Because most analgesics have the potential to induce nausea and vomiting, all medications must be administered slowly and use of antiemetics should be considered.

Medical Supplies

Table 49-2 ▶ lists the basic medical supplies that you should carry in an off-road medical pack.

Patient Packaging

A number of special patient packaging tools are available to help you extricate patients out of their situation and up, down, or out to your ambulance. The Stokes basket, for example, is a rigid framed structure that the patient is set into and then secured. It comes in two general types. The most common is the wire Stokes basket, which consists of a rigid metal (aluminum, steel, or titanium) frame and ribs with a chicken-wire mesh attached to the frame. The other style is the plastic or fibreglass Stokes basket, which consists of a steel or aluminum frame with a rigid plastic or fibreglass basket. Both types of Stokes baskets are available as one- or two-piece units that can be latched or joined together for easier packing into the rescue scene.

The wire Stokes basket is more suitable for water rescue and helicopter hoist situations, as the wire mesh allows water or air to easily pass through it. Given that water weighs 1 kg per litre, this is a significant weight reduction. In the case of moving air (eg, a helicopter's rotor downwash) or moving water, such a basket allows the fluid to pass through it rather than spinning or dragging in response to the air or hydraulic forces being exerted on it.

Table 49-2	**Supplies for an Off-Road Medical Pack**
■ Vinyl or latex gloves	■ 2 glucose or energy gel packets
■ Face masks	■ Heat packs
■ Hand sanitizer	■ Abdominal dressing
■ Mouth-to-mask resuscitation device	■ Survival blanket
■ 1 triangular bandage (cravat)	■ Scissors
■ Universal trauma dressings	■ Irrigation fluid or wound cleansing soap
■ 10 × 10 cm and 13 × 23 cm sterile dressings	■ Goggles
■ Roller gauze bandage	■ SAM splint
■ Gauze-adhesive strips	■ Steri-strips
■ Occlusive dressing for sealing chest wounds	■ Cervical collars
■ Adhesive tape	■ Blood pressure cuff
■ Blankets	■ Rapid immobilization straps
■ Cold packs	■ Pocket flashlight
■ Alcohol pads	■ Batteries
■ 1 12-ml or larger syringe for irrigation of wounds	

Unfortunately, a wire Stokes basket catches every bit of debris and hooks on most any obstruction or obstacle. Thus for most other types of evacuations, a plastic or fibreglass Stokes basket is the superior choice as it more easily slides over the top of surfaces such as snow or debris, or down ladders.

Both types of Stokes baskets have a litter wheel device that can be attached to the bottom to facilitate movement over trails and low-level debris/screen. Also, both devices have minimal (or no) belts or straps to secure the patient into the basket. Instead, a number of patient packaging systems may be used, including those featuring 5- to 6-mm cord or 2.5-cm tubular webbing. Each packaging system relies on the same basic principle: securing the patient's pelvis, which is the fulcrum of the body, into the Stokes basket. Separate securing techniques are then deployed to secure the patient's legs and/or chest, or to lash/lace the patient's entire body into the Stokes basket.

One difficulty that may arise is packaging the patient with a fractured pelvis, as these techniques will cause such a patient an incredible amount of pain. Indeed, any sort of patient packaging that involves first anchoring the pelvis will result in a significant amount of patient "discomfort."

One highly effective solution to this problem is to secure the patient in a full-body vacuum mattress. Once the patient is adequately splinted and secured in this device, then the mattress is placed and secured inside the Stokes basket. Now the main attachment/focal point is the entire vacuum splint and not the patient's broken pelvis.

Another difficulty frequently encountered is the need to transport a spine-immobilized patient in a Stokes basket. Some devices have a leg divider portion for the lower extremities that prohibits use of a backboard. Also, most backboards are too wide and their rectangular shape will not readily fit inside a Stokes basket.

There are two solutions to this problem. The first is to place the patient in a Kendrick Extrication Device (KED) rather than a backboard and then secure them into the Stokes basket. The second is to hold the cervical spine, surround the patient with enough rescuers to lift/levitate the patient up while maintaining spinal immobilization, slide the Stokes basket underneath the patient, and then lower the patient back down into the Stokes basket. The patient may then be secured, with the Stokes basket serving as the spinal immobilization device.

Once the patient has been safely extricated or evacuated, you can reverse the process and lower/secure the patient to a backboard in preparation for transportation. This consideration is especially important in a multiple-patient rescue scenario, as most rescue services possess only one or, at best, several Stokes baskets but have multiple backboards. Do not let the ambulance crew drive off with your Stokes basket unless you have a replacement for it. The loss of a specialized litter can put a rescue team out of service or necessitate having to improvise with alternative patient packaging.

When packaging a patient into a Stokes basket, you need to consider all of his or her needs. If you have placed the patient on supplemental oxygen, then the portable oxygen tank (preferably an aluminum one) must be secured in the litter as well. Likewise, the oxygen tubing to the mask or cannula must be secured, as it might potentially catch on a piece of debris or inadvertently become entangled in the raising or lowering system.

The same holds true for IVs. You do not want to rely on a gravity-fed system if possible: The IV tubing is just waiting for an opportunity to hang up on something at best, or to hang up on something and rip your hard-earned IV out of the patient at worst. If the patient requires an IV, use a pressure infuser and secure the IV and tubing along with the patient prior to extrication/transportation.

Stokes baskets are poor insulators. Thus, when packaging the patient into the Stokes basket, you must also protect him or her from the elements. Keep the patient (and any IV lines) warm.

If you will be transporting a patient through or out of an area where falling debris such as rocks, ice, or building material is a factor, you'll want to package your patient with head and eye protection. This may be as simple as placing a rock helmet and goggles or other protective glasses on the patient, or as comprehensive as using a litter shield to protect the patient's head and neck.

Some tight or confined spaces are so narrow that they cannot accommodate the passage of a Stokes basket. Your patient, however, may require spinal immobilization. In such a case, the solution is a KED or KED/SKED combination.

A KED is an excellent spinal immobilization device that captures the three planes of the spinal column (ie, the head, shoulders, and pelvis). This narrow-profile device was originally designed by an EMT for extrication of Formula One racecar drivers. You apply the KED to the patient and then rig it for raising or lowering as you would an uninjured patient—namely, by using a seat harness and applying a chest harness around the patient and the KED.

Another option is to place the patient in a KED and then secure both into a SKED device. A SKED litter is the classic example of a flexible, wrap-around litter. It is essentially a drag sheet made from heavy-duty polyethylene plastic that wraps around (cocoons) the patient with prerigged securing and attachment points. It is a great tool for sliding patients through narrow passageways and over rough surfaces.

Adaptability and improvisation are an essential part of prehospital care practices. In rescue and extrication situations, the patient's needs, your resources, and the techniques used can change as the rescue process develops. Should you find yourself at a rescue situation without all the necessary equipment, you may have to use your ingenuity to improvise the tools needed to get the patient to safety. If necessary, you can always rely on the technique of splinting one body part to another, by attaching upper extremities to the torso and lower legs to each other. This is a very effective means of splinting when no other devices are available.

You are the Paramedic Summary

1. What are some examples of situations requiring special rescue teams?

Special rescue teams are trained in specific areas such as cave rescue, dive rescue, confined space rescue, trench rescue, swift water rescue, rope rescue, and wilderness rescue. Being a member of a special rescue team requires personal dedication to maintaining personal fitness as well as to numerous hours of rigorous training.

2. Identify the ten steps of a special rescue sequence.

The ten steps of a special rescue sequence are as follows: (1) preparation, (2) response, (3) arrival and assessment, (4) stabilization, (5) access, (6) disentanglement, (7) removal, (8) transport, (9) security of the scene and preparation for the next call, and (10) postincident analysis.

3. Why is it important to maintain good communication with the patient during a special rescue incident?

Patients need to know that you are there and that everything possible is being done to remove them from the situation and provide the necessary prehospital care. In our case, communication is easily maintained because you are able to be in the vehicle with the patient. This is not possible in all special rescue incidents. Occasionally the patient or patients must remain alone for several hours while the scene is made safe and access can be made. This is a traumatic time for the patient. A reassuring voice can go a long way to helping keep the patient calm and maintain his or her level of confidence.

4. What is the patient at risk of experiencing as a result of being pinned underneath the dashboard from the pelvis down?

The patient is at risk for experiencing crush syndrome. While his inability to feel his legs may be the result of a spinal cord injury, lack of perfusion can also produce loss of sensation to the areas distal to the source of obstruction, which in this case is the dashboard.

5. What needs to be monitored on this patient?

In a word, SHOCK! Currently he is compensating for the injuries we suspect; at the very minimum you can suspect an abdominal bleed and fractured pelvis. There is no way of knowing how long his body can compensate for the blood loss. Also keep in mind that the dashboard is acting as a tourniquet. You need to anticipate that once the dashboard is removed from the pelvis and blood flow is restored to the lower extremities, the blood pressure might change significantly.

Prep Kit

◼ Ready for Review

- "Rescue" means to deliver from danger or imprisonment.
- The most difficult process in any rescue is neither the rescue nor the treatment process, but rather the coordination and balance of both.
- A technical rescue incident (TRI) is a complex rescue incident involving vehicles, water, trench collapse, confined spaces, or wilderness search and rescue that requires specially trained personnel and special equipment.
- Technical rescue training occurs on three levels: awareness, operations, and technician. Most of the training and education paramedics receive is aimed at the awareness level, enabling them to identify the hazards and secure the scene to prevent additional people from becoming patients.
- When assisting rescue team members, the following guidelines will prove useful:
  - Be safe.
  - Follow orders.
  - Work as a team.
  - Think.
  - Follow the golden rule of public service.
- Although special rescue situations may take many different forms, all rescuers should follow ten steps to perform these rescues in a safe, effective, and efficient manner:
  - Preparation
  - Response
  - Arrival and assessment
  - Stabilization
  - Access
  - Disentanglement
  - Removal
  - Transport
  - Security of the scene and preparation for the next call
  - Postincident analysis
- At a TRI, it is critically important to slow down and properly evaluate the situation. Consider the potential general hazards and risks of utilities, confined spaces, and environmental conditions, as well as hazards that are immediately dangerous to life and health (IDLH).
- The first arriving officer at a rescue scene should immediately assume command and start using the incident command system (ICS). This step is critically important because many TRIs will eventually become very complex and require a large number of assisting units.
- Accountability should be practiced at all emergencies, no matter how small.
- Whenever possible, park emergency vehicles in a manner that will ensure safety and not disrupt traffic any more than necessary. Traffic flow is the largest single hazard associated with any operation that takes place on a highway.
- A confined space is a location surrounded by a structure that isn't designed for continuous occupancy. Confined spaces have limited openings for entrance and exit.
- Confined spaces present a special hazard because they may have limited ventilation to provide for air circulation and exchange, which can make them an oxygen-deficient atmosphere, or they may contain poisonous gases.
- Trench rescues may become necessary when earth is removed for placement of a utility line or for other construction and the sides of the excavation collapse, trapping a worker.
- Because almost all paramedics have the potential to be called to a water rescue situation, you should know how to properly don a personal flotation device as well as how to use the self-rescue position.

- Rope rescue incidents are divided into low-angle and high-angle operations.
  - Low-angle operations are situations where the slope of the ground over which the rescuers are working is less than 45°. Low-angle operations are used when the scene requires ropes to be used only as assistance to pull or haul up a patient or rescuer.
  - High-angle operations are situations where the slope of the ground is greater than 45°, and rescuers or patients are dependent on a life safety rope and not a fixed surface of support such as the ground.
- Wilderness search and rescue (SAR) missions consist of two parts: search (looking for a lost or overdue person) and rescue (removing a patient from a hostile environment).
- Litters facilitate moving patients to a place of safety and can be used in a variety of situations. The manner in which a patient is packaged in a litter depends on his or her medical condition, the environment, and the manner in which the patient will be evacuated.
- Pain control in rescue situations should take the form of nonpharmacologic methods such as splinting to minimize movement, and gentle handling. Pharmacologic treatment in the prehospital setting remains controversial, and paramedics should consult with their medical directors on issues related to pain management.
- A number of special patient packaging tools are available to help extricate patients out of their situation and up, down, or out to the ambulance. The Stokes basket is an example of a packaging tool.

◼ Vital Vocabulary

accountability system A method of accounting for all personnel at an emergency incident and ensuring that only personnel with specific assignments are permitted to work within the various zones.

awareness The first level of rescue training provided to all responders, with an emphasis on recognizing the hazards, securing the scene, and calling for appropriate assistance. There is no actual use of rescue skills.

belay Technique of controlling the rope as it is fed out to climbers.

cold protective response Phenomenon associated with cold water immersion in which reflexes in the body and a lowered metabolic rate help preserve basic body functions.

cold zone A safe area for those agencies involved in the operations; the incident commander (IC), command post, paramedics, and other support functions necessary to control the incident should be located in the cold zone.

confined space A space with limited or restricted access that is not meant for continuous occupancy, such as a manhole, well, or tank.

cribbing Short lengths of wood that are used to stabilize vehicles.

entrapment A condition in which a patient is trapped by debris, soil, or other material and is unable to extricate himself or herself.

hasty rope slide Self-escape procedure when there is no other means of egress.

high-angle operations A rope rescue operation where the angle of the slope is greater than 45°; rescuers depend on life safety rope rather than a fixed support surface such as the ground.

hot zone The area immediately surrounding an incident site that is directly dangerous to life and health. All personnel working in the hot zone must wear complete and appropriate protective clothing and equipment. Entry requires approval by the IC or a designated sector officer. Complete backup, rescue, and decontamination teams must be in place at the perimetre before operations begin.

immediately dangerous to life and health (IDLH) An atmospheric concentration of any toxic, corrosive, or asphyxiant substance that poses an immediate threat to life or could cause irreversible or delayed adverse health effects. There are three general IDLH atmospheres: toxic, flammable, and oxygen-deficient.

laminated windshield glass Type of window glazing that incorporates a sheeting material that stops the glass from breaking into shards.

low-angle operations A rope rescue operation on a mildly sloping surface (less than 45°) or flat land where rescuers are dependent on the ground for their primary support, and the rope system is a secondary means of support.

operations The technical rescue training level geared toward working in the warm zone of an incident. Training at this level allows responders to directly assist those conducting the rescue operation and to use certain rescue skills and procedures.

personal flotation device (PFD) Also commonly known as a life vest, a PFD allows the body to float in water.

rappelling To descend on a fixed rope.

scrambling A method used to ascend rocky faces and ridges and can be considered a cross between hill climbing and rock climbing.

search and rescue (SAR) The process of locating and removing a patient from the wilderness.

secondary collapse A collapse that occurs following the primary collapse. This can occur in trench, excavation, and structural collapses.

self-rescue position Position used in fast-moving water rescue situations. The rescuer rolls into a face-up arched position with the lower back higher than the feet to avoid objects below the surface. The feet should be together and facing in the direction of travel (feet first), with arms at the sides.

shoring A method of supporting a trench wall or building components such as walls, floors, or ceilings using either hydraulic, pneumatic, or wood shoring systems. Shoring is used to prevent collapse.

spoil pile The pile of dirt that has been removed from an excavation. The pile may be unstable and prone to collapse.

step blocks Specialized cribbing assemblies made out of wood or plastic blocks in a step configuration.

technician The training level that provides a high level of competency in the various disciplines of technical or hazardous materials rescue for rescuers who will be directly involved in the rescue operation itself.

technical rescue incident (TRI) A complex rescue incident involving vehicles or machinery, water or ice, rope techniques, a trench or excavation collapse, confined spaces, a structural collapse, wilderness search and rescue, or hazardous materials, and which requires specially trained personnel and special equipment.

technical rescue team A group of rescuers specially trained in the various disciplines of technical rescue.

tempered glass A type of safety glass that is heat-treated so that it will break into small pieces.

warm zone The area located between the hot zone and the cold zone at an incident. Decontamination stations are located in the warm zone.

wedges Used to snug loose cribbing.

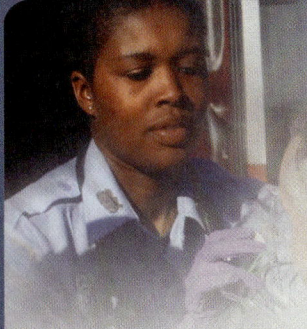

Assessment in Action

You are dispatched to the scene of a motor vehicle collision. Upon your arrival, you find a single-car motor vehicle collision involving one patient. You immediately notice parts of the vehicle that lie approximately 30 m away from the vehicle body. You safely and cautiously approach the vehicle, performing your mental scene assessment. The patient is heavily entrapped in the driver's seat of the vehicle. The truck company is preparing their jaws and other rescue equipment to extricate the patient from the vehicle. You notice the patient is gurgling and unconscious; you ask the incident commander approximately how long the extrication will take. They inform you that it will be at least 20 minutes due to the type of entrapment.

1. **At which three levels is training in technical rescue areas conducted?**
   A. Awareness, operations, training
   B. Awareness, technician, basic
   C. Awareness, operations, technician
   D. Awareness, basic level, advanced level

2. **Most of the training and education paramedics receive is aimed at the _____ level.**
   A. basic
   B. operations
   C. technician
   D. awareness

3. **In a motor vehicle collision, what is the most important thing to remember?**
   A. The vehicle is to be removed from around the patient rather than trying to remove the patient through the wreckage.
   B. The patient is to be removed through the wreckage rather than trying to remove the vehicle from around the patient.
   C. You need to remove the patient immediately without any securing of the vehicle or scene assessment.
   D. Allow the family of the patient to climb into the car and be with the patient to calm him or her.

4. **The rescue operations commander informs you that the vehicle's A post has been crushed onto the patient's upper torso. You understand the A post to be:**
   A. between the front and rear doors of a vehicle.
   B. between the rear doors of the vehicle and the trunk.
   C. near the front bumper.
   D. closest to the front of the vehicle—it forms the sides of the windshield.

5. **You notice that the vehicle remains unstable and could pose a threat to the rescuers. What type of objects can be used to help support this vehicle?**
   A. Cribbing, wedges, or step blocks
   B. Cutting the battery cable
   C. Deflating the tires
   D. Removing the key from the ignition

6. **The next step after the extrication is completed is to:**
   A. perform prehospital care.
   B. disentangle the patient.
   C. displace the seat.
   D. remove the windshield.

Challenging Question

You are dispatched to the scene of a 25-year-old man who fell into a lake. The patient had been drinking alcohol heavily throughout the course of the day. The water is extremely cold, and the patient begins to panic.

7. **What should you do?**

Points to Ponder

Toward the end of your shift, you're dispatched to a residential area for a construction worker who fell into a pit. When you arrive on scene, you find a 30-year-old man lying in a prone position at the bottom of a dirt hole, which is about 3 m deep and 2.5 m wide. The fire department is shoring up the hole to allow you access to the patient.

You are told by his supervisors that the patient was climbing up a ladder while carrying a bucket; he slipped on the ladder and fell. His supervisor tells you that the patient initially was not responsive and stayed that way for approximately 2 minutes. The patient is verbally responsive now, and complains of back and head pain.

What PPE should you don?

Issues: Understanding What Your Needs Are at the Scene of a Technical Rescue Incident; Knowing What Information You Should Have at Initial Dispatch, En Route, and Arriving on Scene; Understanding the Importance of Scene Assessment.

50

Hazardous Materials Incidents

Competency Areas

Area 3: Health and Safety

3.3.a   Assess scene for safety.
3.3.b   Address potential occupational hazards.
3.3.c   Conduct basic extrication.
3.3.e   Conduct procedures and operations consistent with Workplace Hazardous Materials Information System (WHMIS) and hazardous materials management requirements.
3.3.g   Clean and disinfect equipment.
3.3.h   Clean and disinfect an emergency vehicle.

Area 4: Assessment and Diagnostics

4.1.a   Rapidly assess a scene based on the principles of a triage system
4.1.b   Assume different roles in a mass casualty incident.
4.1.c   Manage a mass casualty incident.

Appendix 4: Pathophysiology

C.   **Respiratory System**
     Traumatic Injuries: Burns
     Traumatic Injuries: Toxic inhalation
G.   **Integumentary System**
     Traumatic Injuries: Burns
J.   **Multisystem Diseases and Injuries**
     Toxicologic Illness: Poisons (absorption, inhalation, ingestion)
     Toxicologic Illness: Acids and alkalis
     Toxicologic Illness: Hydrocarbons
     Toxicologic Illness: Asphyxiants
     Toxicologic Illness: Cyanide
     Toxicologic Illness: Organophosphates

Appendix 5: Medications

B.   **Medications affecting the autonomic nervous system**.
B.4   Cholinergic Antagonists
D.   **Medications affecting the cardiovascular system**.
D.3   Diuretics

Introduction

One of the inevitable consequences of living in an industrialized world is the proliferation of hazardous materials. The products of our civilization require the manufacture, transport, storage, use, and disposal of thousands of potentially toxic substances. Approximately 10,000 hazardous materials releases occur in Canada each year, 10% of these are related to transportation incidents.

This chapter will take a broad look at some of the special considerations involved in responding to incidents that may involve hazardous materials. It is not intended to be a comprehensive coverage of hazardous materials. The general rule for paramedics responding to industrial, highway, and many other types of incidents is to maintain a high index of suspicion and to stay away from the hazardous materials incident.

Laws and Regulations

Training requirements and standards are put forth by the 2002 edition of *NFPA 473: Standard for Competencies for EMS Personnel Responding to Hazardous Materials Incidents* published by the National Fire Protection Association (NFPA). All paramedics should receive training to the basic Awareness Level and those more involved (working on medical monitoring or decontamination of the team) will need to be trained to the Operations or Technician Level.

With Awareness Level training, you may be the first to discover a hazardous materials release. Topics covered in the course include recognizing potential hazards, initiating protective measures for yourself and your community, and requesting additional response resources.

The Operations Level (EMS/HM Level I Responder) of training will allow you to perform defensive actions against the hazardous material. You can perform patient prehospital care activities in the cold zone (the command and support centre) at an incident for patients who no longer present a significant risk of secondary contamination.

The Technician Level (EMS/HM Level II Responder) of training will allow you to perform patient prehospital care activities in the warm zone at a hazardous materials incident, working with patients who may still present a significant risk of secondary contamination. At this level, you should be able to coordinate activities at a hazardous materials incident and provide medical support for hazardous materials teams.

Federal, provincial, and local rules govern the use, storage, and transportation of hazardous materials. These regulations are designed to improve the public's right to know and to help protect workers and emergency responders as they try to protect the public. Paramedics should become familiar with the laws of the provinces and localities in which they serve.

You are the Paramedic Part 1

You and a member of ABC Ambulance Service are responding to a chemical spill at a semiconductor manufacturing plant. The dispatch centre reports that there is one patient who has been removed from the structure by the HazMat entry team. When you arrive, you notice that the zones have been set up and the patient is just entering the cold zone from the decontamination corridor. The patient is conscious, well oriented, and answering all questions appropriately, although she is in pain. The HazMat officer reports that a forklift inside the building collided with some shelving, causing it to fall. The shelving stored several different chemicals.

You are handed a stack of MSDS that were provided by the manufacturing facility. Among the chemicals you notice a variety of acids (including 70% hydrofluoric, 10% sulfuric, and 20% acetic acid), 50% sodium hydroxide, a solvent, and methylene chloride.

The patient was the driver of the forklift. She is a 35-year-old woman who is conscious and experiencing minor pain. Fire department personnel on-scene currently are assisting ventilations with high-flow supplemental oxygen by nonrebreathing mask at 15 l/min.

Initial Assessment	Recording Time: 0 Minutes
Appearance	Entering the "cold zone" by fire personnel on-scene
Level of consciousness	A (Alert to person, place, and day)
Airway	Patent
Breathing	Rapid, shallow
Circulation	Slow, regular pulse: flushed skin

1. What is a hazardous material?
2. What is your role during a HazMat incident?
3. How would you manage this patient?

Paramedics and Hazardous Materials Incidents

Paramedics must use their street smarts to identify potential hazardous materials scenes and determine how to handle the scene if they are the first responders. You also need to know how and when to request medical backup (consult with direct medical control or Poison Centre) and a hazardous materials team. You should understand how a hazardous materials scene should be organized, including how you fit into the scheme. Paramedics also need to know the principles of personal protection equipment used at a hazardous materials scene, how the hazardous materials team will decontaminate patients, what immediate actions should be taken, and how to treat exposures. In addition, paramedics may be called upon to support hazardous materials teams through medical monitoring.

Hazardous materials incidents may include:

- A truck or train collision in which a substance is leaking from a tank truck or railroad tank car
- A leak, fire, or other emergency at an industrial plant, refinery, or other complex where chemicals or explosives are produced, used, or stored
- A leak or rupture of an underground natural gas pipe
- Deterioration of underground fuel tanks and seepage of oil or gasoline into the surrounding ground
- Buildup of methane or other by-products of waste decomposition in sewers or sewage processing plants
- A motor vehicle collision in which a gas tank has ruptured

Often, the presence of hazardous materials is easily recognized from warning signs, placards, or labels found in the following locations:

- On buildings or in areas where hazardous materials are produced, used, or stored
- On trucks and railroad cars that carry any hazardous material
- On barrels or boxes that contain hazardous material

When you first arrive at a call and recognize a hazardous material incident, your most important job will be to identify the hazardous material. Unfortunately, identifying materials can be difficult. Little consistency is used on labels and placards, and sometimes transporters won't label containers or vessels appropriately. The labeling of packages and transport vehicles can also be misleading.

In most cases, the package or tank must contain a certain amount of a hazardous material before a placard is required. A truck carrying 100 kg of Hazardous Material #1 and 100 kg of both Hazardous Material #2 and Hazardous Material #3 may not be required by law to display any labels or placards; because the quantities are so "small," there is no law governing these materials. The truck may show only "Please drive carefully" on its flip placard. Although a collision involving this truck might not seem serious, the wise paramedic will keep a high index of suspicion when approaching the scene of any truck or train tanker collision.

Maintain that high index of suspicion as you follow up on your first assessment of the scene. Some substances are not hazardous until mixed with another substance. The Hazardous Material #1 and the Hazardous Material #3 in the truck collision may become highly toxic if they combine. As a paramedic with a high index of suspicion, you need to remember that there may be no regulations against carrying such substances together on one truck or railroad car (or adjacent tank cars). The driver of a commercial truck and the conductor of a train, however, must carry papers that identify what is being transported in their care. If you can, without sacrificing your own safety or prehospital care, look for these papers. These papers may be your first clue that you are in a hazardous materials incident.

You can often identify leaks or spills of hazardous materials by the following:

- A visible cloud or strange-looking smoke resulting from the escaping substance
- A leak or spill from a tank, container, truck, or railroad car with or without hazardous material placards or labels
- An unusual, strong, noxious, acrid odour in the area

Manufacturers may add substances that produce a strong noxious odour to indicate the presence of normally odourless toxic gases or fluids during a leak or spill. However, a large number of hazardous gases and fluids don't smell at all, or don't smell bad, even when a substantial leak or spill has occurred. A large number of people can be exposed and injured or killed before the presence of a hazardous material incident is identified.

If you approach a scene where more than one person has collapsed or is unconscious or in respiratory distress, you should assume that there has been a hazardous material leak or spill and that it is unsafe to enter the area.

If you don't follow the proper safety measures when faced with a hazardous materials incident, you and many others could end up needlessly injured or dead. The safety of you and your team, the other responders, and the public must be your most important concern. Just because you can't see or smell the hazard doesn't mean you can't still be affected by it. *Dead heroes can't save lives.*

There will be times when the ambulance is the first vehicle to arrive at the scene. If, as you approach, any signs suggest that a hazardous materials incident has occurred, you should stop at a safe distance, upwind from the scene. After rapidly sizing up the scene, call for a hazardous materials team. If you don't recognize the danger until you're too close, immediately leave the danger zone. Once you've reached a safe place, try to rapidly assess the situation and provide as

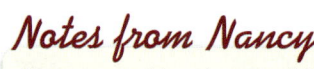

Notes from Nancy

Always consider the possibility of hazardous materials when responding to a road or rail accident. Every cargo should be considered dangerous until proven otherwise.

much information as possible when calling for the hazardous materials team, including your specific location, the size and shape of the containers of the hazardous material, what you've observed, and what you've been told has occurred. Don't re-enter the scene and don't leave the area until you've been cleared by the hazardous material team, or you may contribute to the situation by spreading hazardous materials. Finally, if possible, don't allow civilians to enter the scene.

Hazardous Material Assessment

If the dispatch centre says there could be a hazardous material involved in the call you're going on, assume that you have a hazardous materials incident. If you're responding to an incident that involves a commercial vehicle or a noncommercial vehicle and a train, maintain your high index of suspicion. Tractor trailers, tanker trucks, alternative fuel vehicles, and pesticide control vehicles should be high on your list. Be suspicious if you're called to industrial facilities, warehouses, tank farms, pipeline facilities, manufacturing operations, and chemical plants. Agricultural operations and supply stores use many different chemicals that, in spite of the benign nature of the business, demand utmost care and alertness. Consider the possibility of terrorist incidents in places such as large offices, government buildings, and shopping centres.

Notes from Nancy

Do not rush into a hazardous materials scene. Stop and assess the situation first.

Remember, hazardous materials may be solids, liquids, or gases. When you approach any scene as a paramedic, be alert for evidence of spilled liquids or

powders, vapour clouds, or odours. If your EMS dispatcher or fire and law enforcement dispatchers give you reports that there are many people who seem to be ill or people with symptoms that raise your index of suspicion about exposure to a toxic material, you should stop far away from the scene to think through your approach, assessing the risks of the scene.

Use binoculars to get a clearer picture of what's going on. The standard rule of thumb for hazardous materials scene assessment says that if the entire scene cannot be covered by your thumb held out at arm's length, you are too close! You should use every piece of technology at your disposal to get information about what has happened, who is involved, how many patients there are, what their injuries or symptoms are, and if possible what hazardous materials may be involved.

Identification of Hazardous Materials

One of the most valuable pieces of information at a hazardous materials scene is the identification of the specific material involved. This information will be of tremendous value to the responding hazardous materials team. Particularly if there are a number of casualties, this knowledge is critical to prepare for the possible health effects on patients and to alert the EMS teams that will be dispatched to help you. Take no risks, but try to read the marking and placards required at hazardous materials storage sites and on vehicles. If you are at a permanent manufacturing or storage facility, you should ask anyone you can for the Material Safety Data Sheets (MSDS) for in-depth information about the hazardous materials **Figure 50-1 ▶**. What you do at this point—even though you might rather be using your patient skills—could save lives later.

You are the Paramedic **Part 2**

As you assume prehospital care, you begin with assessment of the patient's airway by continuing high-flow oxygen by nonrebreathing mask at 15 l/min. Her mental status remains conscious and well oriented. You place the patient on the monitor and the ECG indicates a first-degree block with a sinus bradycardia. There are no signs of trauma but you notice a garlicky, almond smell about the patient. You start an IV to administer normal saline to keep vein open.

Vital Signs	Recording Time: 10 Minutes
Level of consciousness	Alert, with a Glasgow Coma Scale score of 15
Skin	Warm, dry, and flushed
Pulse	Radial pulse, 54 beats/min, regular
Respirations	36 breaths/min via nonrebreathing mask
SpO_2	100%

4. Evaluating the symptoms presented by this patient, what do you expect to be the primary offending chemical?
5. You have confirmed your diagnosis. Now how would you treat the patient? What supportive prehospital care would you use (include any drugs and dosages)?
6. What resources can the paramedic use to identify hazardous materials during the scene assessment?

---

syngenta

MATERIAL SAFETY DATA SHEET

Syngenta Crop Protection Canada, Inc. 140 Research Lane, Research Park Guelph, ON N1G 4Z3	**In Case of Emergency, Call** **1-800-327-8633 (FAST MED)**
Date of MSDS Preparation (Y/M/D): 2006-12-31	**Supersedes date (Y/M/D): 2005-09-01**
MSDS prepared by: Department of Regulatory & Biology Development Syngenta Crop Protection Canada, Inc.	**For further information contact:** 1-87-SYNGENTA (1-877-964-3682)

SECTION – 1: PRODUCT IDENTIFICATION

Product Identifier: RIDOMIL® GOLD 1G   Formulation No.: A9603A

Registration Number: 26612 (Pest Control Products Act)
Chemical Classes: Phenylamide Fungicide
Synonym: None.

Active Ingredient(%): Metalaxyl-M (1.0 %)   CAS No.: 70630-17-0
{Metalaxyl-M is the active isomer of metalaxyl.}
Chemical Name: (R)-2-[(2,6-dimethylphenyl)-methoxyacetylamino]-propionic acid methyl ester

Product Use: RIDOMIL GOLD 1G is a systemic fungicide for the control of cavity spot in carrots, damping-off or stunt in head lettuce and the control of *Phytophthora* root rot in ginseng. For further details please refer to product label.

SECTION – 2 : COMPOSITION/INFORMATION ON INGREDIENTS

Material	OSHA PEL	ACGIH TLV	Other	NTP/IARC/OSHA Carcinogen	WHMIS†
Attapulgite Clay	Not Established	Not Established	Not Established	IARC Group 3	Not Established
Crystalline Silica, Quartz	10 mg/m³/ (%SiO₂+2) (respirable dust)	0.05 mg/m³ (respirable silica)	0.05 mg/m³ (respirable dust)**	IARC Group 2A	Yes
n- Methylpyrrolidone (≥ 4%)	Not Established	Not Established	10 ppm TWA****	No	Not Established
Metalaxyl-M (1.0%)	Not Established	Not Established	10 mg/m³ TWA***	No	Not Established

**	Recommended by NIOSH
***	Syngenta Occupational Exposure Limit (OEL)
****	Recommended by AIHA (American Industrial Hygiene Association)
†	Material listed in Ingredient Disclosure List under Hazardous Products Act.

Ingredients not precisely identified are proprietary or non-hazardous. Values are not product specifications.

SECTION – 3: HAZARDS IDENTIFICATION

<u>Symptoms of Acute Exposure</u>
May cause eye, skin and respiratory irritation.

Figure 50-1 Material Safety Data Sheets (MSDS). The MSDS contains a great deal of critical safety information including product identification, accidental release measures, exposure control/personal protection, and toxicological information on multiple pages. Be certain to read the entire MSDS.

gases, flammable liquids and solids, oxidizers and organic peroxides, radioactive materials, and corrosives. The four-digit numbers on the placards correspond with information guides in the Transport Canada's Emergency Response Guidebook (ERG). You can download a free copy of the ERG by visiting the CANUTEC website. The most recent edition of the *Emergency Response Guidebook* should be carried on every emergency response vehicle. The ERG provides information on specific properties and hazards of substances, what's shown on placards, and recommended isolation distances. See **Figure 50-2 ▸** for examples of hazardous materials placards, and **Figure 50-3 ▸** for samples of hazardous materials warning labels.

Other good sources of information for identifying hazardous materials to relay through dispatch to other responders include the bill of lading, which should be carried by the truck driver in the cab, and the waybill or "consist" that is carried by the conductor of a train. The dispatch centre may assist in collecting further information from organizations such as CANUTEC, which operates a 24-hour telephone line (call collect at 613-996-6666 or *666 from a mobile phone) and has an extensive database to assist emergency responders. To be of assistance, CANUTEC needs to know the product involved, the shipper, and the transporter. CANUTEC has a website listing many educational events and activities for all hazardous materials responders, including paramedics.

Hazardous Materials Placarding System

Different systems of placards are used at fixed facilities and on transportation vehicles, and it's important for you to recognize them. The most common is the four-digit numbers that are part of the United Nations/North American coding system for identification of hazardous materials. In addition to the numbers, different symbols are used to help identify different classes of hazardous materials including explosives, poisonous

Initial Isolation and Protection Distance

Until the hazardous materials technical team arrives to determine the hazard zone, you should be aware of the safety perimeters that are necessary for hazardous materials that are toxic (poisonous) and those that pose danger of fire or explosion. In general, the safe distance is a lot further away than most people would believe. Remember the "rule of thumb" described above. Also, the *Emergency Response Guidebook* can help determine appropriate

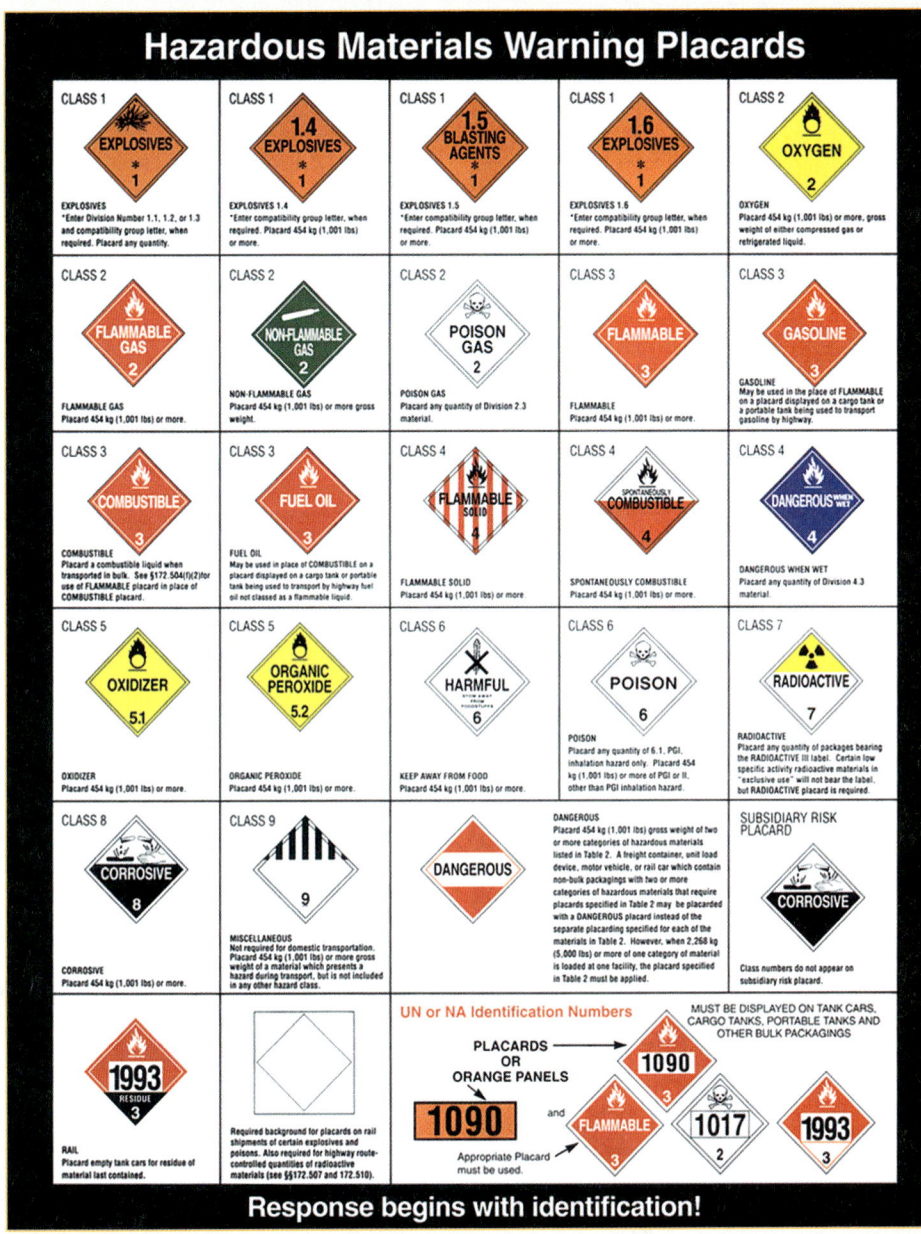

Figure 50-2 Hazardous materials warning placards.

oxygen levels, and the concentration of hydrogen sulfide and carbon monoxide. They will also be able to determine the pH of spills and may have capability for specific agent testing using colourimetric devices. They may also use tools such as Computer-Aided Management of Emergency Operations (CAMEO) to help predict downwind concentrations of hazardous materials based on the input of environmental factors into a computer model.

Classification of Hazardous Materials

The National Fire Protection Association (NFPA) 704 Hazardous Materials Classification ranks hazardous materials according to health hazard or toxicity levels, fire hazard, chemical reactive hazard, and special hazards (such as radiation or acids) for permanent facilities that store hazardous materials. Levels of personal protection gear are rated according to the toxicity of the material. Before you enter any potential hazardous materials area, you must know the type and degree of health, fire, and reactive hazard protection needed to operate safely near these substances. Much of this specialized personal protective equipment is not carried on the ambulance on a daily basis and needs to be acquired through a hazardous materials team. **Figure 50-4 ▶** shows hazardous materials classifications from the NFPA.

Toxicity Level

Toxicity levels are measures of the health risk that a substance poses to someone who comes into contact with it. There are five toxicity levels: 0, 1, 2, 3, and 4. The higher the number, the greater the toxicity. Most ambulances are unlikely to have the specialized protective gear that would be required for dealing with any hazardous materials over Level 0.

- **Level 0** includes materials that would cause little, if any, health hazard if you came into contact with them. This is the only level that does not require special PPE.
- **Level 1** includes materials that would cause irritation on contact but only mild residual injury, even without treatment.
- **Level 2** includes materials that could cause temporary damage or residual injury unless prompt medical treatment is provided. Both levels 1 and 2 are considered slightly hazardous but require use of self-contained

safe distances for isolation of the incident. However, if you are able to read placards with the naked eye, you may already be too close and should consider moving farther away. In general, you should stay uphill and upwind from any hazardous materials scene. To help determine wind direction, a piece of narrow roller bandage approximately 1 m long can be tied to the top of your antenna. Be sure to check the wind direction periodically, and relocate if a change in wind direction dictates.

Once on the scene, hazardous materials teams have many sophisticated tools to help identify hazardous materials and to establish safe scene perimeters. Hazardous materials teams use air monitoring equipment to help determine explosive limits,

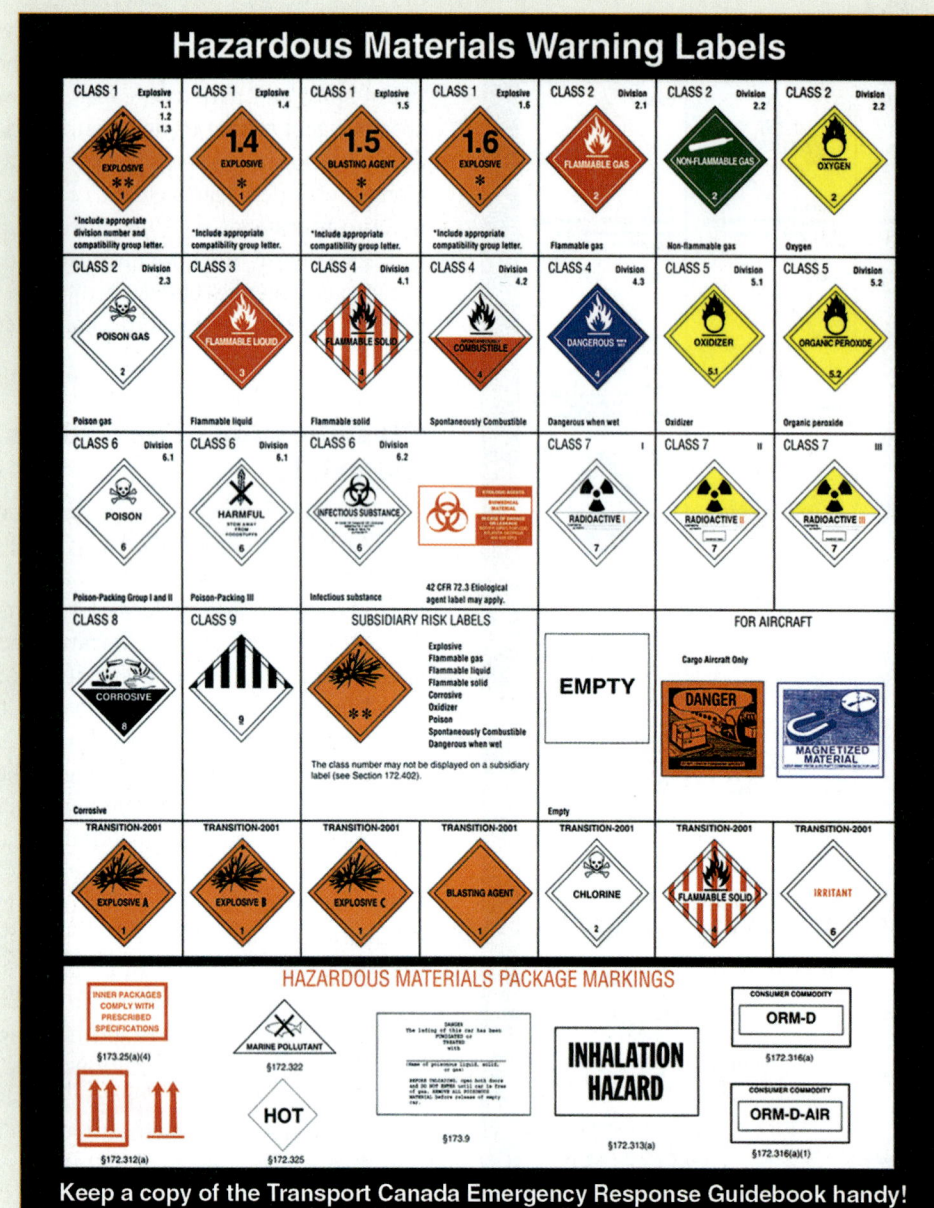

Figure 50-3 Hazardous materials warning labels.

breathing apparatus (SCBA) if you are going to come into contact with them. You would need training in using SCBA in a hazardous materials incident.

- **Level 3** includes materials that are extremely hazardous to health. Contact with these materials requires full protective gear so that none of your skin surface is exposed.
- **Level 4** includes materials that are so hazardous that minimal contact will cause death. For level 4 substances, you need specialized gear that is designed for protection against that particular hazard.

Table 50-1 ▾ further describes the four hazard classes.

Hazardous Materials Scene Management

To ensure efficiency and safety when responding to a potential hazardous materials incident, you should learn the concepts and principles of the National Incident Management System (NIMS) and the Incident Command System (ICS) discussed in Chapter 47. Hazardous materials incident management may seem labourious, slow, or cumbersome to you, but the potentially extreme hazards and the need to protect rescuers, other health care personnel, and the public from harm mandate a cautious approach.

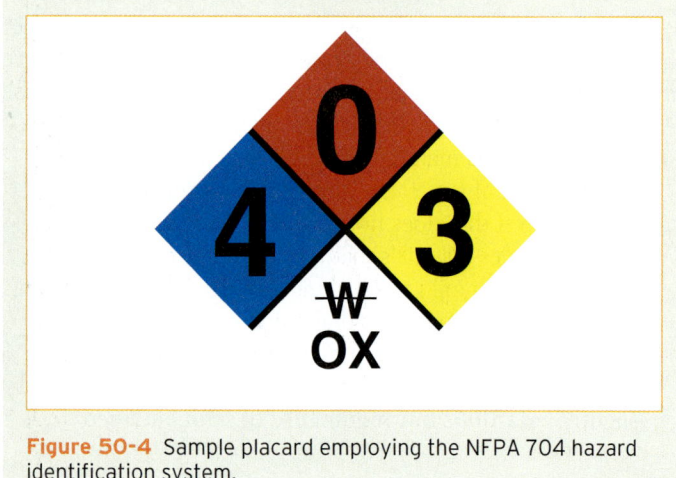

Figure 50-4 Sample placard employing the NFPA 704 hazard identification system.

Table 50-1	Toxicity Levels of Hazardous Materials	
Level	Health Hazard	Protection Needed
0	Little or no hazard	None
1	Slightly hazardous	SCBA (level C suit) only
2	Slightly hazardous	SCBA (level C suit) only
3	Extremely hazardous	Full protection, with no exposed skin (level A or B suit)
4	Minimal exposure causes death	Special hazardous materials gear (level A suit)

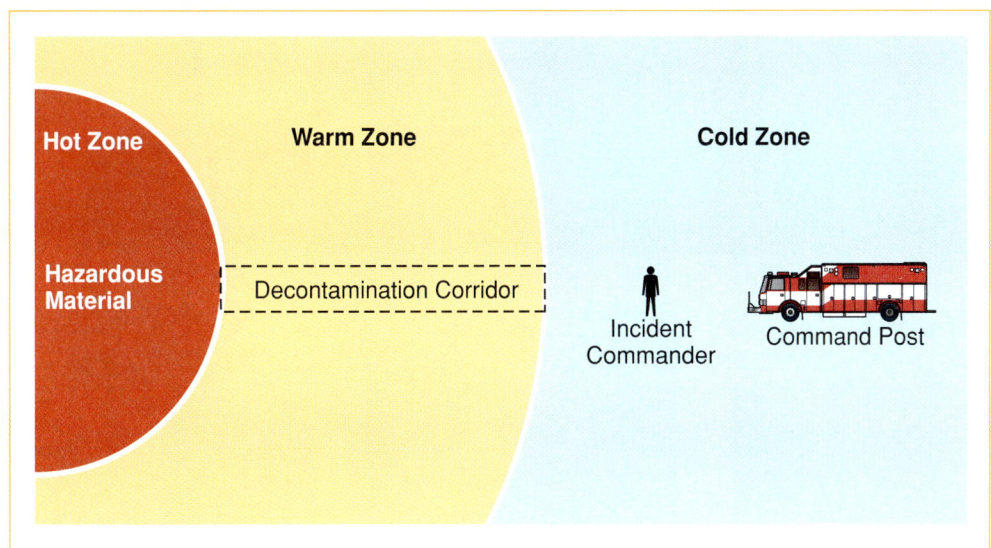

Figure 50-5 Hot, warm, and cold zones.

Establishing Safety Zones

If you discover that an ordinary ambulance call is really a hazardous materials incident, you must take the following steps:

- Notify your dispatcher and any other EMS, fire, or law enforcement responders that you can.
- Identify and tell the others what you observe about wind direction and terrain features.
- Approach and position yourself upwind and uphill from the scene.
- Keep in mind the rule of thumb (if you can't cover the scene with your thumb held at arm's length, you are too close to the hazardous material).
- Isolate the incident as much as possible to avoid the risk of further harm to other people—laypeople, paramedics, firefighters, and law enforcement. No one should risk life or health at a hazardous materials incident. The *Emergency Response Guidebook*, which you should carry in your vehicle, can help determine initial isolation distances.

As the hazardous materials incident progresses, hazardous materials specialists will establish several zones. Easy to remember, they're called the hot, warm, and cold zones. The hot zone is the contamination zone where only properly trained rescuers wearing appropriate personal protective equipment (PPE) are allowed. The warm zone surrounds the hot zone. Typically the decontamination corridor is located in the warm zone. This zone should only be entered by trained hazardous materials specialists wearing appropriate PPE. Trained hazardous materials paramedics may provide urgent lifesaving prehospital care in the warm zone before patients are fully decontaminated. The cold zone provides a further buffer from the hazards present in the hot and warm zones. Paramedics normally perform triage and patient treatment in the cold zone **Figure 50-5 ▲**.

Personal Safety

You should be familiar with the PPE used at hazardous materials scenes even if you are not trained to use it. Hazardous materials technicians call this PPE Level A through Level D, and the equipment is used depending on what and how much of the hazardous material is at the site **Figure 50-6 ▶**. Most paramedic ambulances do not carry this equipment.

Level A provides the greatest protection from exposure to hazardous substances. These suits look like an astronaut's suit because they are "fully encapsulating" **Figure 50-7 ▶**. Some hazardous materials technicians refer to Level A protection as fully encapsulating protection. These suits fully cover and protect the SCBA worn by hazardous materials technicians. The suits are rigorously tested by the manufacturers to determine resistance and permeability to many chemicals. Because they are so gas- and liquid-tight, you may be asked to monitor the technicians for heat stress.

Level B is called for when the technician needs protection from splashes and inhaled toxins. It is not fully encapsulating like Level A, and it is worn with SCBA. B suits are typically worn by the hazardous materials decontamination team in the warm zone.

Level C is designed to protect against a known agent. The equipment provides splash protection and is worn with an air-purifying respirator that must have filters specifically chosen to provide protection against the known agent. Offering eye and hand protection and foot coverings, Level C protection could be used during transport of patients with the potential of secondary contamination.

Level D is the level of PPE offered by firefighters' turnout gear. It is typically not worn in hazardous materials incidents but may be used by some personnel in the cold zone.

The hazardous materials team should determine the appropriate PPE needed for a specific hazardous material. After identifying any hazardous material, the hazardous materials team will consult a permeability chart to determine breakthrough time for the fabrics the Level A suits are made of. The hazardous materials team will also determine which type of gloves and boots will be worn. The team might decide that a double- or triple-glove system is necessary for the incident.

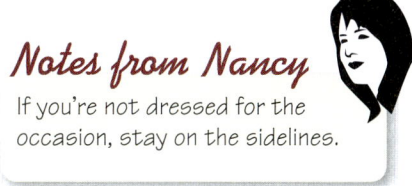

Notes from Nancy
If you're not dressed for the occasion, stay on the sidelines.

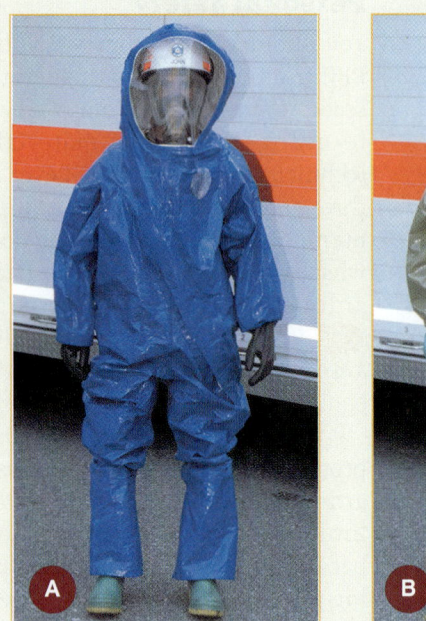
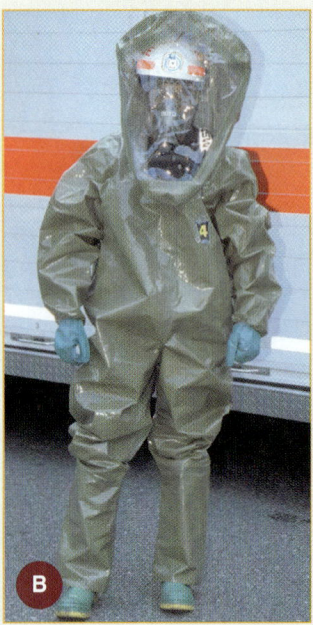
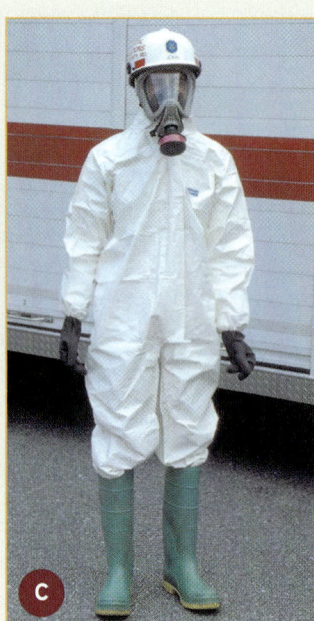
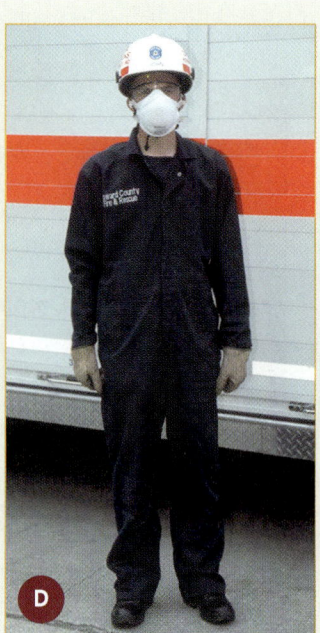

Figure 50-6 Four levels of protection. **A.** Level A protection. **B.** Level B protection. **C.** Level C protection. **D.** Level D protection.

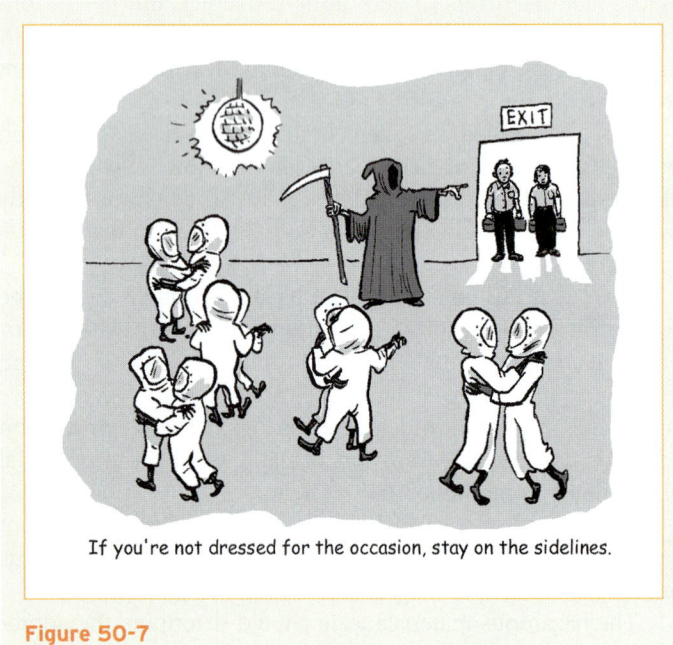

If you're not dressed for the occasion, stay on the sidelines.

Figure 50-7

■ Contamination and Toxicology

The dangers that hazardous materials present to the human body depend on the ability of the hazardous material to interfere with the body's processes. The bodily harm caused by a hazardous material is affected by the route of exposure, the dose and concentration, how long the toxin was in contact with the body, and whether it exhibits acute or delayed toxicity. If a patient has a chronic preexisting condition, like a respiratory ailment, then a minor chlorine spill in an enclosed warehouse could prove to be more dangerous than would be expected.

Primary and Secondary Contamination

There are two basic types of contamination, primary and secondary. Primary contamination is the direct exposure of a patient to a hazardous material. Secondary contamination takes place when a hazardous material is transferred to a person from another person or from contaminated objects. Secondary contamination occurs when solids or liquids accumulate on a person, clothes, or an object, but doesn't normally occur with the diffusion of a toxic gas.

Routes of Exposure

The physical properties of hazardous materials and the physical surroundings at the hazardous materials spill can expose your patient in different ways. Air temperature, the concentration of the hazardous materials, and the amount of time that a patient is exposed will help you determine what your primary concern in treating your patient should be. If a material is not volatile and does not give off vapour but touches your patient's skin, it is called a dermal exposure. Many hazardous materials can be taken into other body systems through the skin. Skin conditions like abrasions may accelerate the absorption. Dermal exposure, also known as topical exposure, may result in only a local effect, such as reddening of the skin or the formation of blisters.

However, if the hazardous material is absorbed through the skin, a systemic effect may occur. Hazardous materials, when absorbed through the skin, can have a toxic effect on the neurologic, renal, or hepatic systems. These toxic effects may be seen immediately in the prehospital environment, or may be delayed for hours or even years later with the appearance of a cancer. When the reaction shows up hours after your initial treatment, your careful medical records become invaluable to patients, who might not be able to speak for themselves. Your records should include a description of the scene, anything the hazardous materials team told you about what the toxin was, and how your patient looked initially.

Regardless of the route of exposure, the dose effect principle applies—the greater the length of time or the greater the concentration of the material, the greater the effect probably will be on the human body. For example, people who have a toxin briefly splashed on their skin will be exposed to a much lower dose of toxin than if they were lying in a puddle of that same toxin for 30 minutes. The cycle of poison action includes absorption into the body, delivery to target organs, and binding to the organs. The cycle continues with biotransformation and elimination of the toxin through the gastrointestinal, kidney, or respiratory systems. These concepts should be considered as decontamination decisions are made with the hazardous materials team.

In addition, paramedics should be aware that a synergistic effect may occur when two hazardous materials interact, producing a much greater impact than either substance alone. If your extrication patient is lying in a puddle of gasoline, his or her level of consciousness will be compounded if also exposed to carbon monoxide.

Respiratory exposure can be efficient, rapid, and lethal. Many hazardous gases, the gases formed when some liquids spill, or even dustlike powders can harm the respiratory membranes or be absorbed into the body by passing through the bronchial tree or alveoli directly into the bloodstream.

When hazardous materials are injected into the body or are absorbed through an open wound, this is known as parenteral exposure. Parenteral exposure could occur at a vehicle collision if your patient has an open wound that is exposed to a toxin leaking from a container.

Gastrointestinal exposure occurs when your patient swallows a hazardous material like an organophosphate pesticide. You will need all your patient communication skills when assessing such a patient, because often the ingestion is deliberate.

Chemical and Toxicology Terminology

Learning some of the terms that describe the properties of hazardous materials and the toxicologic effects on people will help you as you work with others in handling a hazardous materials event.

Chemical Terms

When you are working at the scene of a hazardous materials event, you can often assess the scope of the problem by considering the physical properties of the toxin in relation to environmental factors. For example, if the liquid leaking from a tank has a high boiling point and the air temperature is low, then the paramedic will have less concern that the vapours of the liquid will be a respiratory hazard.

If vapours arise as a liquid turns to gas, it's important to know that as the air temperature becomes hotter, the vapour pressure of a hazardous material will also increase (as should your concern for more toxin being released to affect you and your patients).

Vapour density is another concept for figuring out where a gas or vapour might go. Vapour density compares the hazardous material gas to air (air has a vapour density of 1). If the toxic gas is heavier than air, the toxin will sink into little valleys

You are the Paramedic Part 3

You monitor your patient's vital signs on the way to the hospital and note no further deterioration. You administer IV fluids at a TKVO rate and monitor the ECG for further changes en route to the local trauma centre.

On arrival at the trauma centre, you and your partner provide a concise, complete report to the team, including the HazMat incident, your initial physical assessment, interventions, and the patient's response to your treatment. Patient care is assumed by the trauma team.

The patient is evaluated in the emergency department and found to have exposure to hydrofluoric acid and phenol.

Reassessment	Recording Time: 20 Minutes
Skin	Pink, warm, and dry
Pulse	100 beats/min, regular
Blood pressure	160/86 mm Hg
Respirations	30 breaths/min via nonrebreathing mask
SpO_2	100%
ECG	Sinus bradycardia with a first-degree heart block

7. What information about HazMat medical monitoring and rehabilitation operation must be documented?

and ditches. But if the vapour rises and dissipates as it travels with the wind, then the vapour density is less than that of the air. This is why you are taught to approach a scene from upwind and uphill!

Of course, all bets are off if a fire is involved. If a hazardous material reaches a temperature at which its vapours can be ignited by a spark, then it has reached its flash point. If it gets warmer than the flash point, the vapours will burst into sustained burning; it has reached its ignition temperature. If the percentage concentration of the hazardous material as it mixes with air reaches its lower explosive limit (LEL), also known as lower flammable limit, then it can burn in the air (or explode). If the concentration of the hazardous material gets too high (or too "rich"), there will not be enough oxygen to support the combustion in air and the mixture has exceeded its upper explosive limit (UEL).

Hazardous materials teams can, in many cases, cool down the heat or dissipate the concentration of vapours by pouring on streams of cool water. However, before any water is applied, the hazardous materials team will make critical decisions about whether or not the material may be water reactive or water soluble. If they are going to use water, they will also determine the hazardous material's specific gravity—whether or not the hazardous material will sink or float in water.

Toxicology Terms

Chemistry experts and medical providers should communicate with each other using agreed-upon terms to describe the health hazards any incident might present. You will be a better reporter if you can master these terms for all the health care providers who will care for your patient in the hospital.

Safe and unsafe concentrations of various substances are often expressed in parts per billion (ppb) or parts per million (ppm). The threshold limit value (TLV) is the maximum concentration of a toxin that someone can be exposed to for a 40-hour work week. If you look up a chemical in a reference text and find that it has a very low ppb number for its TLV, this means it is more dangerous than if it had a high TLV. The threshold limit value short-term exposure limit (TLV-STEL) is the concentration that a person can be exposed to for a limited number of brief time periods (eg, four 15-minute exposures per day). The threshold limit value ceiling level (TLV-CL) is the concentration that a person should never be exposed to. A permissible exposure limit (PEL) is the maximum concentration of a chemical that a person may be exposed to. In Canada, occupational exposure limits are set by provincial or territorial regulations. Sometimes you will hear the experts refer to the lethal dose or LD, which is the amount of the substance sure to cause death. You might hear the hazardous materials team refer to immediately dangerous to life and health (IDLH), which indicates that a respirator is mandatory. This means that the atmospheric concentration of any toxic, corrosive, or asphyxiant substance will pose an immediate threat to life, irreversible or delayed adverse effects, or serious interference for a team member's attempt to escape from the dangerous atmosphere.

Decontamination and Treatment

Treating hazardous materials patients can be a difficult and emotionally challenging experience. Remember, your safety comes first. *If you are first on the scene, you cannot immediately begin prehospital care.* Even when a patient is visible and in need of rescue, you must not rush in. Staying safe is a tough decision that requires discipline and emotional coolness. You must work as part of the team to prevent more casualties. Use the incident command system, which permits only properly trained and equipped hazardous materials personnel to enter the hot zone. Wait until your patients have been decontaminated. Then you can apply your knowledge and skills to actually treat the patient safely in a hands-on fashion.

Because hazardous materials can cause harmful effects, protecting the environment should be one of your considerations. If your patient's injuries are treated and not life-threatening, environmental issues should be a major consideration. You should take steps to prevent runoff during decontamination. If your patient is suffering, environmental considerations are still important but a lower priority than patient prehospital care.

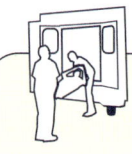

At the Scene

No patient is ever completely decontaminated, even if he or she has been decontaminated by the hazardous materials team on-site. Always protect yourself first!

Decontamination

The team's approach to decontamination will depend on the type of hazardous material involved; the stability of the scene; and the number, condition, and location of patients. Decontamination is undertaken to reduce the dose of hazardous material in contact with the patient and decrease the risk of secondary contamination to others (including rescuers and hospital personnel). Protection of the environment during decontamination is important; plans should be made for containment of runoff.

There are four types of decontamination methods—dilution, absorption, neutralization, and disposal. Dilution uses copious amounts of water to flush the contaminant from the skin or eyes. This decreases the dose effect of the hazardous material on the patient. Sometimes a simple soap, such as tincture of green soap, is used in the decontamination process. Other decontamination agents are rarely used, however, isopropyl alcohol might be used to help with removal of isocyanates and vegetable oil is sometimes used if the contaminant is a water-reactive substance. Be cautious if you or any team member is using brushes; abrasion of a patient's skin increases the potential for hazardous material absorption.

Absorption is accomplished with large pads that the hazardous materials team carry to soak up liquid and remove it from the patient. Towels can also be used in the same way.

Neutralization involves the use of a chemical to change the hazardous material into less harmful substances. Neutralization is almost never used by hazardous materials teams because of the dangers of uncontrolled exothermic reactions. Disposal of as much clothing and equipment as possible to reduce the magnitude of the problem is another method of decontamination.

Emergency Decontamination in "Fast-Breaking" Situations

In some of the most difficult situations, you may be faced with the need to make an immediate decision about ambulatory patients who are approaching the ambulance, or who attempt to leave the scene to seek transportation despite being contaminated. In this case, you should provide patient assessment information to the incident commander, who is responsible for deciding whether to proceed with a rapid, emergency decontamination.

In such situations, you must still don appropriate PPE. Even if no respirator is available, the paramedic should take maximum barrier precautions. Put on turnouts or a splash-resistant (Tyvek) jumpsuit, eye protection, mask (such as a HEPA mask), and at least two layers of gloves. In addition, booties should be worn over footwear if possible. In general, nitrile gloves offer superior protection against many hazardous materials. Leather materials should be removed because these often absorb hazardous materials.

Once protected as much as possible, the paramedic should instruct patients to disrobe and remove as much of the hazardous materials from their bodies as they can. If you can, give the patients plastic bags in which they can place their personal belongings and clothing. If the hazardous material is a powder, then it should be brushed away first. If the hazardous material is water reactive, then no water should be used during decontamination. Most often, however, water is considered to be the universal decontamination solution. In any emergency decontamination method, you need to minimize the risk to yourself. This type of decontamination is also referred to as the two-step approach to decontamination. Unmanned hose streams can be set up by the fire department to douse patients with large amounts of water.

An example of such a set-up is the creation of an emergency decontamination corridor made by parking two fire engines parallel to each other and approximately 3 to 6 metres apart **Figure 50-8 ▶**. Nozzles can be attached to the side discharge ports of the engines and set to create a fine-particle fog-stream decontamination shower. Patients should disrobe on one end and enter the shower in single file. From a remote location, patients could be advised how to decontaminate and directed to pay special attention to the areas of the body that are difficult to rinse such as the axillae, between fingers and toes, around the groin, the scalp, and between the buttocks. Soap and soft brushes should be made available. At the other end of the shower corridor, towels, blankets, and temporary garments should be available. It is at the *end* of this corridor that you, the paramedic, would make initial contact with the

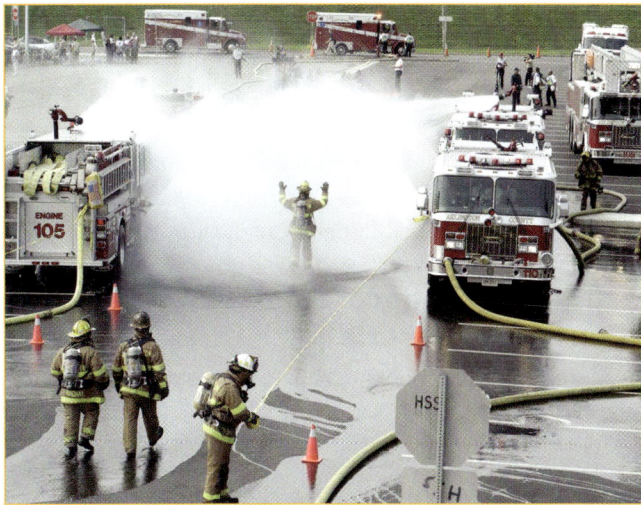

Figure 50-8 Emergency decontamination corridor.

patients and begin the triage process. Ideally, the runoff water from decontamination should be contained. At a minimum, the runoff should not be allowed to become a source of secondary contamination.

Technical Decontamination

You will hear the hazardous materials team refer to an "eight-step" process, which is only carried out by trained personnel.

1. Rescuers access the patients in the hot zone and remove as much of the contamination as possible as they move patients to the decontamination corridor.

2. Contaminated tools, equipment, and clothing should be left behind at the hot zone end of the decontamination corridor.

3. Patients and hazardous materials personnel are showered and washed using water, brushes, soap, or other appropriate decontamination agents to remove all surface contaminants. This is done with the assistance of other hazardous materials personnel who should wear not less than one step lower PPE than the entry team. This decontamination is done in a manner that will contain runoff. Often this is accomplished inside a small wading pool or other disposable basin. Any remaining clothing or jewelry is removed from the patients. At this point, the patients may be handed off to a separate decontamination team who should again wash the patients before they are handed off to medical personnel. Even at this point, the patients should not be considered fully decontaminated and paramedics should continue to wear PPE as they assess and treat the patients. Paramedics should stay alert for signs of an ongoing primary or potential secondary contamination problem.

4. Rescuers continue to decontaminate themselves. In this step, they remove their possibly contaminated SCBA.

5. Rescuers remove their contaminated protective clothing and equipment, placing these items into a bag or receptacle for later decontamination or disposal.

6. Depending on the potential of the situation, the rescuers may need to take off their clothing as well.

7. Personnel shower to further reduce the potential for contamination.

8. Entry team personnel undergo medical evaluation.

Treatment of Patients Exposed to Hazardous Materials

In general, the treatment of hazardous materials patients is straightforward. You can use many of the concepts learned in the chapters on burns and toxicology. There are some special considerations for hazardous materials patients, however. One of these is that invasive procedures should be minimized if possible. If you know from the hazardous materials team that your patient is contaminated, the process of endotracheal intubation may expose the patient to airway contamination. Placement of an IV may help contamination bypass the skin barrier. You will need to weigh the risks of invasive procedures against their benefits.

You should be familiar with references and how to access technical expertise when deciding how to treat patients from a hazardous materials incident. Some assistance may be obtained from the *Emergency Response Guidebook* and CANUTEC. In addition, paramedics may consult with Poison Centres, the Agency for Toxic Substance Registry, and their local direct medical control. The hazardous materials team may have comprehensive reference textbooks that can guide the paramedic in treatment decisions and also be of assistance to emergency department physicians. Never forget that you are the eyes and ears of the physician in the prehospital environment. Share the knowledge you've gained from the hazardous materials team for your patient's sake.

Corrosives: Acids and Bases

Corrosives are chemicals that include both acids and bases. Some examples are toilet bowl cleaner, lye, and hydrochloric acids. Acids have a low pH, while bases have a high pH. Agents with both high and low pH can cause severe burns. Signs and symptoms include skin irritation, reddening or other discolouration, and blistering. Exposure of fumes to mucous membranes can also cause burns, including severe life-threatening airway burns.

Decontamination of materials with a high pH will require considerably more time to flush from the skin. High pH materials have a soap-like resistance to being flushed from the skin as compared to low pH acids. Once the patient is decontaminated appropriately, treatment is symptomatic. Treat burns appropriately and consider transport to a burn centre. Patients showing signs of pulmonary edema may need to be treated for this based on local or regional protocols.

Hydrocarbon Solvents

Many of these solvents give off potent vapours that can be inhaled and can also be absorbed through the skin. Respiratory exposure in particular can cause immediate pulmonary symptoms such as pulmonary edema. Prolonged dermal exposure can cause symptoms as well, including cardiac dysrhythmias and seizures.

Pulmonary Irritants

Many gases react with the moisture of mucous membranes to cause irritation ranging from minor to severe or choking. Examples of such gases are chlorine gas and ammonia. The first thing to do for your patients is to make sure they (and you as well) are away from the contamination and in fresh air. Removal of clothing may help dissipate trapped gases. Pulmonary edema should be treated according to protocols.

Pesticides

Exposure to organophosphate and carbamate pesticides can produce severe signs and symptoms. These hazardous materials interfere with the enzyme cholinesterase, which promotes uptake of the neurotransmitter acetylcholine. Runaway nerve stimulation produces a syndrome that is known by the mnemonic, SLUDGE (Salivation, Lacrimation, Urination, Defecation, Gastrointestinal distress, and Emesis). Also look for excess pulmonary secretions. As always, paramedics should protect themselves from secondary contamination, including that from emesis when the exposure has been gastrointestinal. Treatment of organophosphate poisoning includes protection of the airway with possibly frequent suctioning, and the use of atropine to block the overstimulation of muscarinic receptors of the parasympathetic nervous system. The use of pralidoxime is recommended for organophosphate exposures but not for carbamates.

Chemical Asphyxiants

Any gas that displaces oxygen from the atmosphere is termed an asphyxiant. Colourless, odourless gases (eg, carbon monoxide and hydrogen sulfide) confined to an area may represent a deadly trap for would-be rescuers who rush in to help a collapsed victim. Substances known as chemical asphyxiants interfere with the utilization of oxygen at the cellular level; cyanide is a common example of such an agent. Hydrogen cyanide is used in many industrial processes. The release of cyanide in Bhopal, India, was a major hazardous materials incident that caused thousands of fatalities. Cyanide poisoning can also occur during exposure to the by-products of combustion at structure fires. Two commercially available kits are available for treatment of cyanide poisoning. One treatment kit consists of hydroxocobalamin, which binds to cyanide and forms a nontoxic by-product. Alternatively, cyanide exposure can be treated with amyl nitrate ampules that the patient should inhale for 15 seconds of every minute. This is followed by the IV administration of 300 mg of sodium nitrite, followed by 12.5 g of sodium thiosulfate. Another common exposure that results in a cellular respiratory failure is carbon monoxide. This gas ties up hemoglobin to the extent that oxygen in the blood becomes inaccessible to the cells. Treatment includes removal of the patient from the source and administration of 100% supplemental oxygen.

Transportation Considerations

The ideal transportation scenario at a hazardous materials incident would be to have a team of paramedics who were not involved with decontamination or cold zone patient treatment standing by to transport patients to the hospital emergency department. However, if the incident is a large one, the cold zone paramedics may well need to both treat and transport.

Paramedics should remember that patients received after decontamination should not be assumed to be completely decontaminated. Accordingly, paramedics should take certain precautions to prepare themselves and their equipment for assuming prehospital care of the patient from the hazardous materials team and for getting the patient to the hospital. First, the paramedic should wear appropriate PPE. The hazardous materials team may be able to supply some of the PPE if the transporting paramedic does not have access to a splash-proof Tyvek jumpsuit, for example. The transporting paramedic should be given a complete report on what hazardous materials have been involved, what the patient's exposure has been, and what has been done to decontaminate and treat the patient. In no event should a transporting paramedic have to transport a patient if decontamination has not been sufficient for the driver to operate the ambulance. An example of insufficient decontamination would be when hazardous material on the patient continues to produce toxic gases.

Before receiving and transporting a patient exposed to hazardous material, the paramedic can do several things in preparation. One principle is to reduce the amount of supplies and equipment that the patient will come in contact with. You could remove the mattress from the stretcher because the patient will probably be carried on a backboard; removing the mattress will make later decontamination easier. In general, use as much disposal equipment as possible. Supplies and equipment inside the ambulance should be removed and set aside in a clean, safe place for later retrieval.

It is impractical and time-consuming to line the inside of the ambulance with plastic. Instead, plan to isolate the patient by wrapping him or her in a plastic barrier to reduce the potential for secondary contamination. A double-wrap procedure is preferable. In this procedure, the patient is first wrapped in a plastic blanket, preferably one that helps protect the patient from hypothermia. Then the patient is placed on a backboard and the backboard placed on the stretcher. Paramedics should know which hospitals in their area have facilities for receiving patients with possible hazardous materials contamination. The hospital should be given plenty of notice prior to the transport so that they can assemble the appropriately trained personnel and prepare equipment. Often hospitals will have a separate or dedicated treatment and decontamination room for these situations.

Medical Monitoring and Rehabilitation

You may be asked to assist with medical monitoring of the hazardous materials team. Rehabilitation (or "rehab") refers to the process through which hazardous materials entry teams are rested, rehydrated, and evaluated before being sent back into the hot zone. The PPE the team wears often causes heat stress, and of course the toxins the team is working with can cause serious health effects. Factors that influence hazardous materials team members' health include level of physical fitness, activity, level of PPE, and environment factors such as temperature.

Medical monitoring should include documentation of the incident factors including the hazardous materials involved, their toxic effects, what PPE was worn, its resistance to permeability with the hazardous materials, and what type of decontamination was used. You should have a plan for treatment, transport, and potential availability of antidotes in case a hazardous materials team member needs medical assistance.

You might be asked to assess hazardous materials team members before they suit up for entry into the hot zone and then again after they come out. Your assessment should include complete vital signs, as well as the ECG, temperature, and body weight. Team members should be encouraged to prehydrate with water or a sports drink. Working inside a Level A suit is like being inside a sauna, with no way to lose heat through evapouration, conduction, convection, or radiation. A useful fact that can help you with your assessment is that some hazardous materials teams keep a file of their members' baseline medical status. Be sure to ask for this information.

Before being allowed to re-enter the hot zone, the hazardous materials team should be evaluated by the paramedic in the rehab sector (located in the cold zone) for hydration status, vital signs, and any potential symptoms of exposure to the toxic agent the incident involves **Figure 50-9 ▼** . Team members should take off their protective clothing and be given a chance to rest. Complete vital signs are again taken as well as other assessments, including neurologic assessment

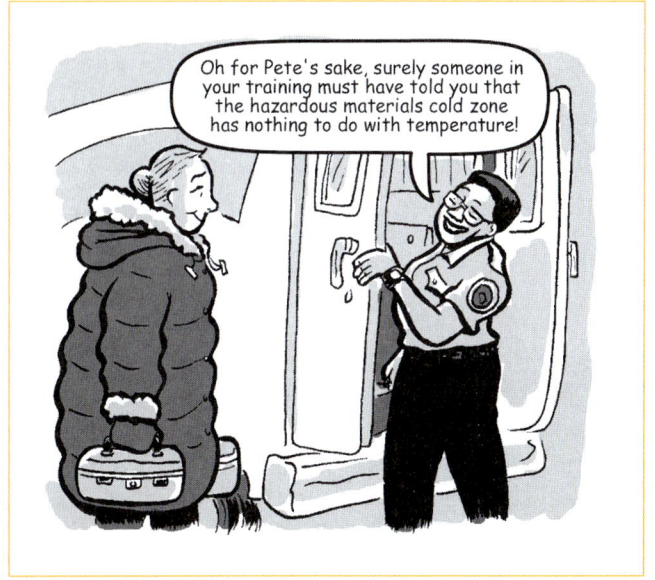

Figure 50-9

(eg, orientation to time, place, and events) as well as fine motor skills. Team members with elevated temperatures should be monitored closely for possible heat stroke. The loss of body weight is a direct correlation to the loss of fluids and the risk of dehydration and hypovolemia. Members should be encouraged to rehydrate by drinking water or other appropriate fluids. If there are abnormalities in vital signs or if the team member has signs or symptoms, they should not be allowed to return to work until their physical status returns to normal. An example of a hazardous materials team rehabilitation log that can assist paramedics in the hazardous materials rehab sector is shown in **Figure 50-10 ▶**.

HazMat Medical Monitoring Worksheet

Date:_____ Entry Person:_____

Incident #_____ Medical Monitor:_____

Important: HazMat team members shall not be allowed to don PPE if any of the following conditions are present: systolic BP < 100 or > 160, diastolic BP > 100, pulse rate > 120, temperature > 37.8°C, Respirations > 24. Medical monitors must read and be familiar with the "Medical Monitoring Guidelines" before beginning medical evaluations.

Pre-entry Evaluation
Before donning PPE, take and record baseline vital signs.

Time_____ BP_____ Pulse Rate_____ Resp._____ Temp._____°C

Post-entry Evaluation
Immediately after doffing PPE, take vital signs and assess for hyperthermia.

Time_____ BP_____ Pulse Rate_____ Resp._____ Temp._____°C

Re-entry Evaluation
Before redonning PPE, take vital signs and reassess for hyperthermia.
Entry person must remain in rehab for a minimum of 30 minutes between entries.

Time_____ BP_____ Pulse Rate_____ Resp._____ Temp._____°C

HazMat Exposure Suspected?
Immediately contact HazMat Team Leader and see "HazMat Exposure Protocols."

Figure 50-10 Rehabilitation log.

You are the Paramedic Summary

1. What is a hazardous material?

The National Fire Protection Association (NFPA) 704 Hazardous Materials Classification defines a hazardous material (substance or waste) as: "Any substance that causes or may cause adverse effects on the health or safety of employees, the general public, or the environment; any biological agent and other disease-causing agent, or a waste or combination of wastes."

2. What is your role during a HazMat incident?

The role of paramedics is to first keep themselves from being exposed or injured. Then a scene assessment is performed to assess for risks of primary or secondary contamination of the patient and the responders, determine the need for additional resources, and decide what safety parameters must be immediately established. Depending on the role your agency plays in local HazMat response plans and the level of training provided, you may also assess the level of decontamination, treatment, and transportation considerations.

3. How would you manage this patient?

Don the appropriate level PPE for the specific type of substance exposure. Then an initial assessment can be performed. If ambulatory, the patient should be instructed to remove all clothing and move to a predetermined decontamination centre. Copious amounts of water are the decontamination solution of choice.

4. Evaluating the symptoms presented by this patient, what do you expect to be the primary offending chemical?

Phenol and hydrofluoric as well as sulfuric acids.

5. You have confirmed your diagnosis. Now how would you treat the patient? What supportive prehospital care would you use (include any drugs and dosages)?

- **Phenol.** Decontaminate initially with large volumes of water. Support respirations, control seizures, and manage ventricular ectopy with recognized means of treatment.
- **Bronchospasms secondary to toxic inhalation.** Immediately give 100% humidified oxygen. Provide salbutamol by nebulizer or metered dose inhaler with aerochamber. If wheezing continues, repeat the dose. For severe respiratory distress, consider administration of 0.01 mg/kg epinephrine subcutaneously while assisting ventilations.
- **Supraventricular tachydysrhythmias.** Administer a 6-mg rapid IV push of adenosine (Adenocard) followed by a saline bolus.
- **Hydrofluoric acid.** Once the affected areas are decontaminated, the burned areas should be covered with calcium gluconate gel. If calcium gluconate is not available, Epsom salt (magnesium sulfate), magnesium-containing antacids such as Maalox or Mylanta, or Tums can be used as a topical agent.

    In the case of hydrofluoric acid burns, pain is an excellent indicator that the injury is continuing. If pain continues after calcium gluconate gel is applied, then calcium gluconate infiltration is needed. Calcium gluconate in a 5% solution is injected SQ in a volume of 0.5 ml every ½ to 1 cm into the burned area.

- **Cardiac symptoms of hypocalcemia.** Provide continuous monitoring of the ECG, watching for prolongation of the QT interval. Muscle contractions or cardiac arrest should be treated with an IV bolus of 5 ml 10% calcium chloride or 10 ml of 10% calcium gluconate. IV calcium should be considered for any patient with exposure to hydrofluoric acid in a concentration of greater than 10% over 5% or more of body surface area.

6. What resources can the paramedic use to identify hazardous materials during the scene assessment?

There are several methods for identifying hazardous materials. Many EMS agencies are required to carry some form of reference to identify hazardous materials.

- *Emergency Response Guidebook:* Provides the names of substances, UN (United Nations) numbers, placard facsimiles, an emergency action guide, and evacuation and isolation information.
- NFPA 704 placard system: This is a fixed placard system used in many fixed facilities. The placards are coloured and indicate specific hazards (red = fire hazard, blue = health hazard, and yellow = reactivity hazard).
- UN numbers and Transport Canada placards: Placarding vehicles is required by law, but many owners do not comply.
- MSDS: Material Safety Data Sheets (MSDS) provide detailed information about a substance and are used when exposure occurs with that product. MSDS are used throughout the industry as a means of identifying chemicals and complying with employees' right to know. These must be readily available for employees to review.
- Packaging labels.
- Shipping papers: Carried by the shipper when transporting substances and contain the name of the product.
- Textbooks, handbooks.
- Dispatcher: When resources are not immediately available to the paramedic, the dispatcher may be able to obtain information for you.
- Assistance from CANUTEC (an information resource available through a collect call to 613-966-6666 with detailed information on the chemicals involved and their manufacturers).

7. What information about HazMat medical monitoring and rehabilitation operation must be documented?

The type of substance involved, its toxicity, and the danger of secondary contamination must be documented. Additional information to record includes appropriate PPE and suit breakthrough time, appropriate antidotes, medical treatment, and transportation method.

Prep Kit

■ Ready for Review

- Approximately 10,000 hazardous materials incidents occur in Canada each year.
- Handling hazardous materials emergencies requires specialized extra training and equipment.
- You should never enter a hazardous materials scene because specialized training and PPE are required.
- The three levels of hazardous materials training are: awareness, operations, and technician.
- Specific laws dictate that all paramedics should receive awareness level hazardous materials training.
- The great majority of hazardous materials emergencies are transportation incidents.
- When you are approaching transport incidents, especially those involving commercial vehicles, you should be alert for signs of hazardous materials.
- Signs of hazardous materials include vapour clouds, strange odours, spilled liquids, and multiple victims.
- Hazardous materials incident management follows NIMS and ICS principles.
- Hazardous material incidents have hot, warm, and cold zones.
- Without proper PPE, you should not enter the hot and warm zones.
- The four levels of hazardous materials PPE are level A, level B, level C, and level D.
- Sources of information about hazardous materials include placards, transport documents, and MSDS.
- Primary hazardous materials contamination comes from direct contact with the toxin.
- Secondary contamination is spread by people (patients, the hazardous materials team, or paramedics), clothing, or objects.
- Effects from hazardous materials exposure may be local on the body or systemic.
- Routes of exposure include dermal, respiratory, parenteral, and gastrointestinal.
- Rescue and decontamination of victims is secondary to rescuer and public protection.
- Decontamination should be undertaken as a methodical eight-step process.
- In some situations, decontamination may have to be done rapidly in a two-step process.
- Treatment of hazardous materials victims is usually symptomatic and supportive of the ABCs.
- Invasive procedures should be minimized to avoid the risk of introducing contamination.
- Paramedics may be directed to support a hazardous materials operation with medical monitoring of the hazardous materials personnel.

■ Vital Vocabulary

absorption A type of decontamination that is done with large pads that the hazardous materials team carry to soak up liquid and remove it from the patient.

Agency for Toxic Substance Registry An information source for toxicologic effects of hazardous materials.

asphyxiant Any gas that displaces oxygen from the atmosphere; can be deadly if exposure occurs in a confined space.

Awareness Level The training level to which all paramedics should be trained; topics include recognizing potential hazards, initiating protective measures for yourself and your community, and requesting additional response resources.

bill of lading A document carried by drivers of commercial vehicles that should provide specific information about what is carried on the vehicle.

CAMEO Computer-Aided Management of Emergency Operations; a tool to help predict downwind concentrations of hazardous materials based on the input of environmental factors into a computer model.

CANUTEC A resource available to emergency responders via telephone on a 24-hour basis.

carbon monoxide A chemical asphyxiant that results in a cellular respiratory failure; this gas ties up hemoglobin to the extent that oxygen in the blood becomes inaccessible to the cells.

chemical asphyxiants Substances that interfere with the utilization of oxygen at the cellular level.

cold zone The outermost zone of management at a hazardous materials scene; the area where paramedics typically first encounter the patient.

corrosives A class of chemicals with either high or low pH levels. Exposure can cause severe soft-tissue damage.

cyanide A chemical asphyxiant used in many industrial processes; exposure can occur from by-products of combustion at structure fires.

decontamination The process of removing hazardous materials from the body or clothing of victims or rescuers. Includes the methods of dilution, absorption, disposal, and (in rare cases only) neutralization.

dermal exposure Skin exposure, also known as topical exposure. Some hazardous materials may be absorbed through the skin to produce a systemic effect.

dilution A type of decontamination method that uses copious amounts of water to flush the contaminant from the skin or eyes.

disposal A type of decontamination in which as much clothing and equipment as possible is disposed of to reduce the magnitude of the problem.

dose effect The principle that the longer a hazardous material is in contact with the body or the greater the concentration, the greater the effect will probably be.

Emergency Response Guidebook (ERG) A hazardous materials reference that provides valuable information about hazardous materials, isolation distances, etc; should be carried on every emergency response unit, and every paramedic should know how to use it.

flash point The temperature at which a vapour can be ignited by a spark.

gastrointestinal exposure Exposure to a hazardous material through intentional or unintentional swallowing of the substance.

hazardous material Any substance that is toxic, poisonous, radioactive, flammable, or explosive and causes injury or death with exposure.

hot zone The central area of a hazardous materials scene and the location of the greatest hazard.

ignition temperature The temperature at which a vapour will burst into sustained burning.

immediately dangerous to life and health (IDLH) A phrase that means the atmospheric concentration of any toxic, corrosive, or asphyxiant substance will pose an immediate threat to life, irreversible or delayed adverse effects, or serious interference for a team member attempting to escape from the dangerous atmosphere; a respirator is mandatory.

lethal dose (LD) Amount of a hazardous substance sure to cause death.

Level A The highest level of protective suit worn by hazardous materials personnel. Also referred to as fully encapsulating, because the suit covers everything, including the breathing apparatus.

Level B PPE that is one step less protective than level A.

Level C A level of PPE that provides splash protection.

Level D The level of protection that firefighter turnout gear provides.

local effect An effect of a hazardous material on the body that is limited to the area of contact.

lower explosive limit (LEL) The concentration of the hazardous material that can burn or explode in the air when it mixes with air.

Material Safety Data Sheets (MSDS) Information documents that are supposed to be kept on site at workplaces for every potentially hazardous chemical at the workplace.

medical monitoring The process of assessing the health status of hazardous materials team members before and after entry to a hazardous materials incident site.

neutralization A type of decontamination that uses one chemical to change the hazardous material into two less harmful substances; rarely used by hazardous materials teams.

Operations Level This training level, also called EMS/HM Level I Responder, allows paramedics to perform prehospital care activities in the cold zone (the command and support centre) at an incident for patients who no longer present a significant risk of secondary contamination.

parenteral exposure Entry of a hazardous material into the bloodstream, either through force of injection or through an open wound.

permissible exposure limit (PEL) The maximum concentration of a chemical that a person may be exposed to.

ppb Parts per billion; an expression of concentration.

ppm Parts per million; an expression of concentration.

primary contamination An exposure that occurs with direct contact with the hazardous material.

respiratory exposure Exposure of the airways and lungs to a gas or vapour.

rule of thumb A reminder of the proper distance from a hazardous materials scene; the entire scene should be hidden by a thumb held at arm's length.

secondary contamination Exposure to a hazardous material by contact with a contaminated person or object.

SLUDGE An mnemonic that stands for salivation, lacrimation, urination, defecation, gastrointestinal distress, and emesis, which are the signs and symptoms that can be produced by exposure to organophosphate and carbamate pesticides or other nerve-stimulating agents.

specific gravity The measure that indicates whether or not a hazardous material will sink or float in water.

synergistic effect When two substances interact to produce an overall greater effect than either alone or combined.

systemic effect A physiologic effect on the entire body or one of the body's systems.

Technician Level This training level, also called EMS/HM Level II Responder, allows paramedics to perform prehospital care activities in the warm zone at a hazardous materials incident, working with patients who may still present a significant risk of secondary contamination.

threshold limit value (TLV) The concentration of a substance that is supposed to be safe for exposure no more than 8 hours per day and 40 hours per week.

threshold limit value ceiling level (TLV-CL) The concentration that a person should never be exposed to.

threshold limit value short-term exposure limit (TLV-STEL) The concentration of a substance that a worker can be exposed to for up to 15 minutes but no more than 4 times per day with at least an hour between each exposure.

toxicity levels Measures of the risk that a hazardous material poses to the health of an individual who comes into contact with it.

upper explosive limit (UEL) The concentration of a hazardous material at which there is not enough oxygen to support the combustion in air.

vapour density A measure that compares the hazardous material gas to air; toxic gases that are heavier than air will sink, while vapours that are lighter than air will dissipate and travel with the wind.

vapour pressure The pressure exerted by a vapour when the liquid and vapour states of a material are in equilibrium; this measure changes as a material is heated.

warm zone The division of the HazMat scene that surrounds the hot zone and is inside the cold zone.

water reactive A property that indicates that a material will undergo a chemical reaction (for example, explosion) when mixed with water.

water soluble A property that indicates that a material can be dissolved in water.

waybill A cargo document kept by the conductor of a train.

www.Paramedic.EMSzone.com/Canada

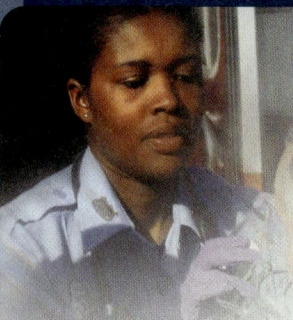

Assessment in Action

You are dispatched to an overturned tractor trailer on a busy highway. When you arrive, you notice the truck is leaking something. You're not sure what it is. You immediately call for additional resources.

1. **On arrival, you see a placard with white and red stripes. This truck is most likely carrying:**
   A. oxidizers.
   B. flammable liquids.
   C. flammable solids.
   D. explosives.

2. **All paramedics should be trained to:**
   A. Technician Level.
   B. Operations Level.
   C. Hazard Level.
   D. Awareness Level.

3. **All of the following are responsibilities of hazardous material awareness-trained personnel, EXCEPT:**
   A. having knowledge of hazardous materials and risks involved in case of an accident.
   B. recognizing the need for additional resources.
   C. understanding the potential outcomes of a hazardous material incident.
   D. entering the hot zone and mitigating the incident.

4. **The standard rule of thumb for hazardous materials scene assessment is:**
   A. if the entire scene cannot be covered by your thumb held out at arm's length, then you are too close.
   B. approach should include stopping at a distance away.
   C. the identification of the hazardous material on scene.
   D. preparing the paramedic for the possible health risks.

5. **The guidebook that paramedics should have in their vehicle to help identify a hazardous material is the:**
   A. *Emergency Response Guidebook.*
   B. *Hazardous Material Textbook.*
   C. Material Safety Data Sheets.
   D. Truck placard chart.

6. **You should stay _____ from any hazardous material scene.**
   A. uphill and upwind
   B. downhill and downwind
   C. uphill and downwind
   D. upwind and downhill

7. **While on scene, to help get additional information regarding a specific chemical product, you may call:**
   A. CANUTEC.
   B. FEMA.
   C. CDC.
   D. Poison Centre.

8. **The measure of health risk that a substance poses to someone who comes into contact with it is called the:**
   A. health hazard.
   B. bill of lading.
   C. toxicity level.
   D. primary contamination.

9. **The type of personal protective equipment that provides the highest level of protection at a hazardous materials incident is known as:**
   A. Level A.
   B. Level B.
   C. Level C.
   D. Level D.

Challenging Questions

You are dispatched to a warehouse for three patients who are complaining of nausea, vomiting, diarrhea, and sweating. When you arrive on scene, you find the patients located outside on a bench. During your assessment, you note that the patients are also hypotensive and have constricted pupils. You begin to ask questions and you find out that this "warehouse" manufactures pesticides.

10. **What should you immediately begin to suspect?**

11. **What treatment should you provide for these patients?**

Points to Ponder

You are dispatched to an explosion at an apartment complex. While you are en route, you see red balls of flames high in the air in the distance. When you arrive, several fire engines are already on scene. They are keeping you at a staging area until they figure out what happened and if any hazardous materials were involved.

What can you do while waiting for clearance? Once you can enter the scene, what precautions should you take?

Issues: Understanding What to Do at a Hazardous Materials Incident.

Crime Scene Awareness

Competency Areas

Area 1: Professional Responsibilities

1.3.a   Comply with scope of practice.
1.3.b   Recognize "patient rights" and the implications on the role of the provider.
1.5.a   Work collaboratively with a partner.
1.5.c   Work collaboratively with other emergency response agencies.
1.5.d   Work collaboratively with other members of the health care team.
1.6.a   Exhibit reasonable and prudent judgement.
1.6.b   Practice effective problem-solving.

Area 2: Communication

2.4.a   Treat others with respect.
2.4.b   Exhibit empathy and compassion while providing care.
2.4.c   Recognize and react appropriately to individuals and groups manifesting coping mechanisms.
2.4.d   Act in a confident manner.
2.4.e   Act assertively as required.
2.4.f   Manage and provide support to patients, bystanders, and relatives manifesting emotional reactions.
2.4.g   Exhibit diplomacy, tact, and discretion.
2.4.h   Exhibit conflict resolution skills.

Area 3: Health and Safety

3.3.a   Assess scene for safety.
3.3.b   Address potential occupational hazards.
3.3.d   Exhibit defusing and self-protection behaviours appropriate for use with patients and bystanders.

Appendix 4: Pathophysiology

K.   **Psychiatric Disorders**
Psychotic Disorders: Homicidal ideation

Introduction

Thousands of times each year, paramedics face potentially violent situations. With any call, you may find yourself in the middle of a physical domestic argument when responding to an injured patient **Figure 51-1 ▾** . You might realize that another room in the house where you are treating an unconscious patient is a methamphetamine lab. As you read the many cautions in this textbook about questionable scenes, remember that paramedics have been severely injured or killed in violent incidents while attempting to reach and treat sick and injured people.

As an educated and effective health care provider, you need to know how to avoid violence when possible and how to protect yourself when violence erupts. Because all emergency services agencies respond to potentially life-threatening situations daily, you should make time for every self-protection course that you can. Sound survival skills training will help you identify potentially dangerous situations. Once you recognize a violent situation, you will be able to retreat to a safe location and await the assistance of law enforcement. *Your main mission is to return home safely at the end of each shift.*

Awareness

Some paramedics-in-training are surprised to hear how serious and widespread attacks against emergency responders have become. Violence is not only an urban event; a call in a rural area can be just as deadly as a call in a large city. In many rural areas, paramedics may arrive at the scene of an emergency long before law enforcement personnel. You should never be complacent about the possibility of encountering violence. Problems can occur at every social and economic level and in every size of community.

En route to the scene, you need to prepare yourself mentally for what could occur once you get there. Discussing the options with your fellow paramedics is a good way to anticipate reactions. Before you begin prehospital care, you need to perform a scene assessment with an eye to your safety. If you feel the scene is not safe, contact law enforcement personnel and wait for them to secure the scene. Remember: If you rush in to a scene and are injured by violence, you will complicate the scene for your partner and other responders.

Being Confused With Law Enforcement Personnel

Many patients and bystanders mistake paramedics for police officers. The uniform you wear may be adorned with a badge, patch, collar insignias, and a name plate. The uniform worn by most police officers is strikingly similar. Aggressive behaviour intended for the police may be unintentionally directed at you. Your options for defending yourself may be severely limited. To counteract this, many agencies have adopted a more casual uniform for paramedics, such as golf shirts with only the service's logo printed on the shirt. You might want to request low-key uniforms if you see a need as you become more experienced.

Body Armour

Most police officers routinely wear soft body armour. Should this protective garment be mandated for your personal safety? Your agency will have guidelines. Some agencies provide all paramedics with soft body armour, and some fire services provide it for firefighters.

Body armour is not bulletproof; there are six levels of protection. Body armour does not shield your neck or head, so whatever your level of protection, you will still be vulnerable to injury. Consult with your service and local law enforcement officials to decide if you need protection and at what level. Remember that using sound survival skills to avoid dangerous situations gives you more protection than body armour.

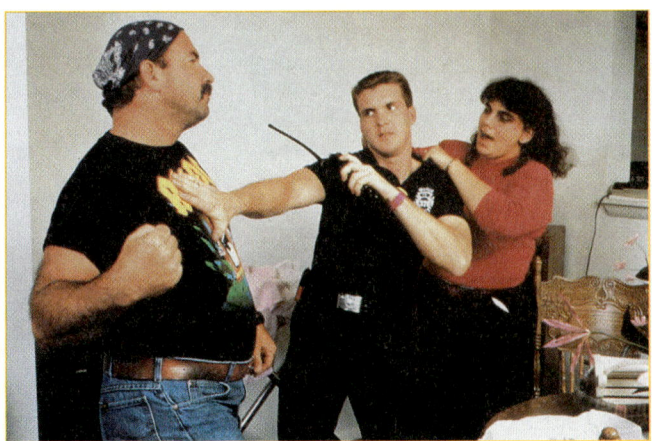

Figure 51-1 The most routine call can quickly turn violent.

You are the Paramedic Part 1

You and your partner have just finished a light dinner on a warm summer evening. In your community, you mostly respond to cardiac incidents and occasional motor vehicle collisions. You see very few incidents involving violence, especially domestic violence. In fact, you have never responded to a domestic violence incident.

Shortly after dinner, you and your partner are dispatched to a residence to care for an injured person. Information about the injury is unavailable. You and your partner head over to the residence.

1. Does the lack of violent incidents in your response district ensure your safety?
2. What measures will you take to stay safe on this call?

Indicators of Violence

Violence can often be predicted, as most experienced paramedics already know. If you are dispatched to a shooting, stabbing, or attempted suicide, the potential for violence can be obvious. You may not expect aggressive behaviour when you arrive at the scene of an injured person. But if you are met by an agitated family member pacing the room with fists clenched and using profane language, your antenna should go up. The potential for such behaviour to escalate to physically violent behaviour should not be discounted. You must quickly identify potentially dangerous situations and act to remove yourself, your team, and, if possible the patient, to a safe place. You must not become so completely involved with patient care that you fail to see the possibility of physical harm to the patient or other care providers. Experts call this tunnel vision **Figure 51-2 ▾** .

Standard Operating Procedures

Some agencies have developed standard operating procedures (SOPs) for dealing with potentially violent incidents. Specific procedures for response to methamphetamine labs, civil disturbances, and hostage or barricade incidents provide paramedics with specific steps to be taken at such scenes. If your agency has an SOP manual, consult it as soon as you take the job for direction on handling specific situations.

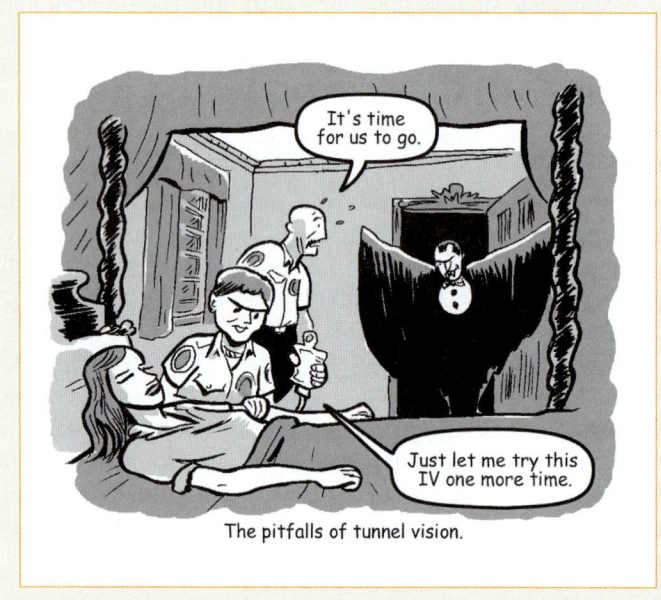

The pitfalls of tunnel vision.

Figure 51-2

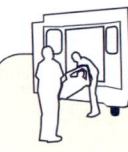

At the Scene

Violence can often be predicted. If your unit is dispatched to a shooting, stabbing, or attempted suicide, the potential for violence should be obvious.

▌Highway Incidents

Law enforcement dashboard cameras mounted in vehicles have provided the public a rare view of the dangers routinely faced by law enforcement officers when approaching vehicles. You face similar dangers whenever you walk to the door of a motor vehicle. Calls to a "man slumped over the steering wheel" or an "unconscious person in a vehicle" can be disastrous for an unsuspecting paramedic. Remember, your uniform can lead to you being mistaken for a police officer as you approach a vehicle—especially if the occupant's level of consciousness has been altered by alcohol or illegal drugs.

Approach and Vehicle Positioning

For maximum safety when arriving at incidents with a single vehicle in which the potential for danger is high, your vehicle should be positioned a minimum of 5 m behind the stopped vehicle at a 10° angle to the driver's side facing the shoulder **Figure 51-3 ▸** . The wheels should be turned all the way to the left. In this position, the wheels and the motor block will provide limited protection in the event of gunfire.

After dark, use your vehicle's high beams and spotlights to illuminate the interior and exterior of the patient's vehicle. Bright light will also conceal you as you approach the vehicle. Do not walk between the spotlight and the vehicle because you will provide a silhouette in the patient's rearview mirror and alert any conscious occupants to your position.

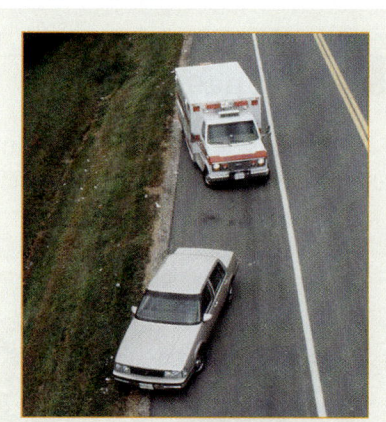

Figure 51-3 Position the unit a minimum of 5 m behind the stopped vehicle at a 10° angle to the left if you are the only emergency vehicle on the scene.

Before leaving your vehicle, the license number of the motor vehicle should be recorded and left by the radio. Include the name of the province or territory where the license tag was issued. If something happens to you and your partner, a written record of the motor vehicle will exist. It is even more effective to notify your dispatcher of the situation, location of the emergency, and the number and province or territory of the license plate because that information will allow your agency to react quickly, instead of searching your vehicle for paper. In some services and in certain situation, paramedics are not permitted to approach a vehicle until police are on the scene. This is to ensure the safety of those responding to the incident. Consult and follow local or regional policies and protocols to deal with the incident.

Approaching the Motor Vehicle

A systematic approach to a motor vehicle with people inside is not usually needed in cases of personal injury accidents at a busy intersection, accidents where the motor vehicle is found torn wide open, or situations with bystanders already around the motor vehicle. When you have an uncomfortable feeling about *this* motor vehicle, a system is vital to protect everyone on your team. Here are some procedures that you can use.

When there are two or more paramedics in the unit, the person riding in the right front seat, the incident commander (IC) of the emergency vehicle, makes the approach. All other members of the emergency response team remain with the ambulance or medical unit in case something goes wrong.

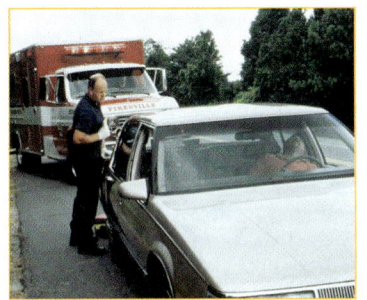

Figure 51-4 The IC moves from the right front of the unit directly to the right rear-trunk area of the vehicle.

Proceed to the rear passenger-side trunk area and place the response bag or jump kit at the rear of the motor vehicle out of the path of travel **Figure 51-4 ◂**. Look out for people hiding in the trunk of a motor vehicle, and check the trunk lid to ensure that it is properly closed. Use only a light touch on the trunk seam to detect motion or an unsecured trunk lid. If the trunk is open, retreat to your vehicle. Using a belly-in movement, proceed to the "C" column on the passenger side of the motor vehicle **Figure 51-5 ▾**. Moving belly-in toward the motor vehicle creates as small an image as possible for the occupants of the motor vehicle to see.

Stop at the left C column and look in the rear and side windows **Figure 51-6 ▸**. Notice the number of people in the vehicle. Pay particular attention to the location of their hands. Any attempt to stab, strike, or shoot will be accomplished using the hands. Try to see if there are items lying on the seat or on the floor. Look for weapons. These might include the obvious guns or knives, but may also include baseball bats, beer bottles, or pieces of pipe. If you see a deadly weapon, a gun, or a knife, retreat to a safe location, and call for law enforcement assistance. Wait for law enforcement—officers are trained to extricate and secure weapons; paramedics are not. *Never* attempt to unload a weapon. And although you cannot retreat every time you see a weapon, your awareness that the object is within reach of the people in the car gives you time to react if that object becomes a weapon.

If the back seat is occupied, do not pass the C column. If you pass the C column, the back-seat passengers will be behind you. You will have to divide your attention between the front and rear seats.

If there are no passengers in the back seat, move forward to the B column with the same belly-in movement **Figure 51-7 ▾**. As with the C column, the B column will conceal you from the

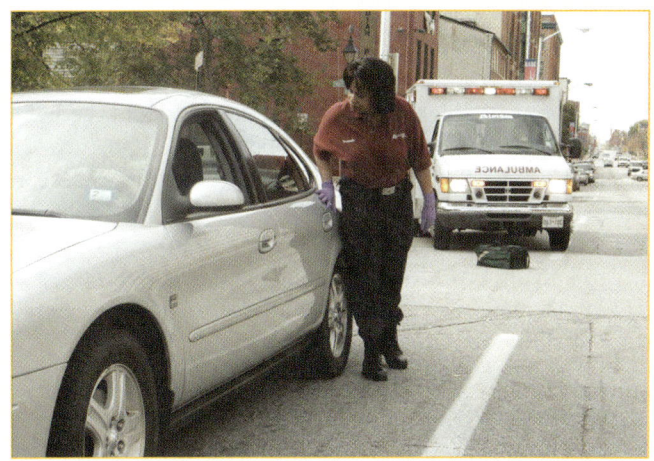

Figure 51-6 Stop at the right C column and look in the rear and side windows. Until the IC declares the vehicle safe, the medical kit remains on the ground at the rear of the vehicle.

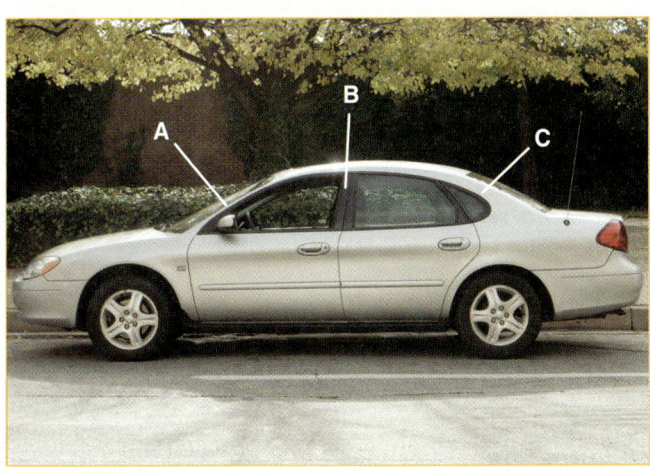

Figure 51-5 "A," "B," and "C" columns of a vehicle.

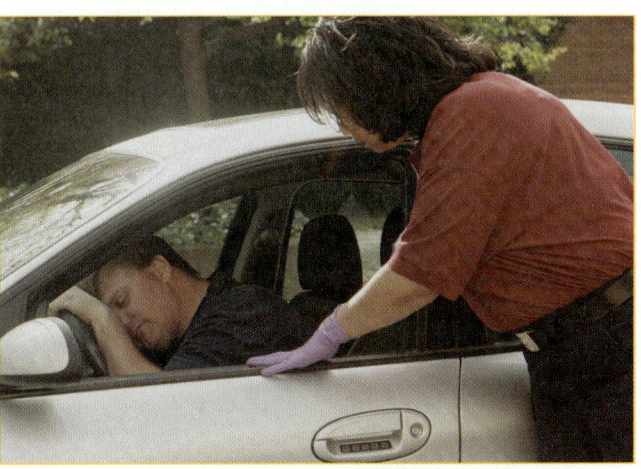

Figure 51-7 At this stage of the approach, do not move past the B column for any reason.

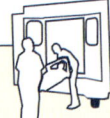

At the Scene

Weapon Locations
- Glove box
- On top of the sun visor
- Arm rest
- Under either side of the seat
- In the centre console
- In side-door pockets
- Next to driver's right thigh

passengers of the vehicle. Examine the front-seat area. Where are the occupants' hands? What are the occupants doing? Are any weapons visible? When you are ready to let the driver know that you are there, do so without moving past the B column into the driver's door area. Law enforcement personnel refer to this area as the kill zone. Tap lightly on the window of the vehicle to get the driver's attention and announce yourself: "Paramedic. Do you need help?"

After the IC declares that the incident scene is safe and determines that the occupants of the motor vehicle need medical or other assistance, you should follow the SOPs for your service.

Keep your flashlight off until you need it. Hold the light at arms-length and away from your body before you turn it on Figure 51-8 ▾ . Illuminate the scene for only a few seconds during each use.

Take special precautions when you approach vans. Vans can carry many types of cargo, and your inability to see that cargo is a danger. A van can carry a large number of people or a large quantity of weapons.

A safe approach to a van is modified from the approach made to the passenger side of a standard motor vehicle. When you exit the unit with the jump kit, move 5 m away from the passenger side of the van. If you are belly-in to the van, an occupant may suddenly open the side door and grab you. Instead, remain clear of the side door of the van throughout the approach Figure 51-9 ▾ . From this distance, walk parallel to the van until you are approximately 45° forward of the A column. This position gives you the greatest visibility inside of the van but keeps you at a safe distance until you can determine that the situation is secure Figure 51-10 ▾ .

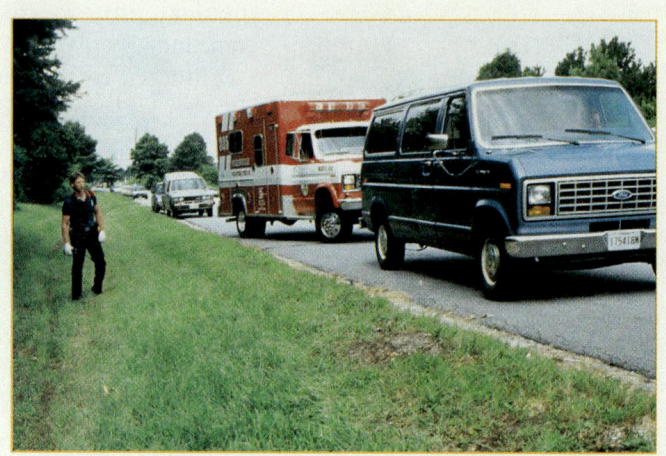

Figure 51-9 Until you are 45° forward of the A column, maintain 5 m between yourself and the passenger side of the van.

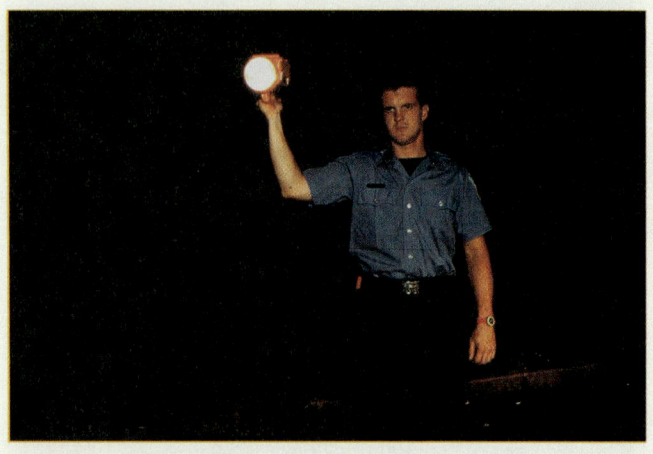

Figure 51-8 Because a light makes a good target, hold a flashlight away from your body when illuminating an area.

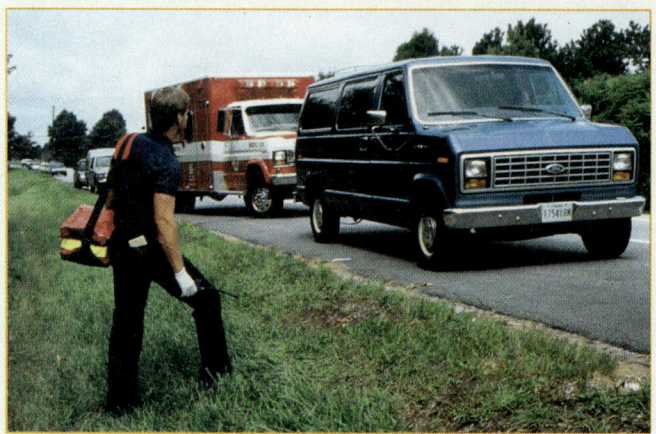

Figure 51-10 Position yourself 45° forward of the A column before making contact with the occupants of a van.

You are the Paramedic Part 2

You arrive at a single-family residence. You gather your equipment and prepare to approach the house. While walking toward the house, you can hear a female screaming. A male voice is yelling profanities over the woman's screaming. Your partner pauses on the walkway and looks over at you, eyebrows raised.

3. What information can be obtained as you walk toward the house?

4. What actions should you take in response to the hostilities heard from within the residence?

Retreating From Danger

You will be in situations in which unsafe circumstances dictate your retreat to a safe area. The safest means of retreat is to back away and call for law enforcement assistance. If your partner is injured while approaching a motor vehicle, the best way to ensure help will arrive quickly is to back away and call for assistance yourself. Back away from the danger zone, remain in your vehicle, and provide the dispatcher with all the needed information. This would include:

- The number of aggressors involved
- The number and type of injuries
- The number and type of weapons involved
- The make, colour, body style, and license number of the vehicle involved
- The direction of travel if the vehicle leaves the scene before the law enforcement personnel arrive

In addition, make certain to document in detail why you had to leave the scene.

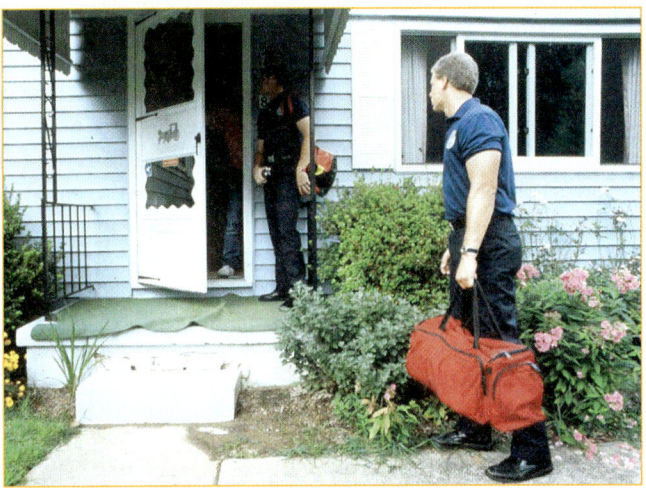

Figure 51-11 Stand on the doorknob side of the entrance when announcing your arrival.

Residential Incidents

Warning Signs

Emergency response personnel are frequently called to residential areas to assist someone injured in an assault, domestic dispute, shooting, or stabbing. These calls require an obvious level of caution. But many routine calls have the potential for violent outcomes. An attempted suicide may turn into a homicide, with you as the victim. The response to an "injured person" may have been an intentional attack by a person who remains on the scene as you arrive.

Your standard procedure for responding to any call involving violence should be to allow law enforcement personnel to arrive and secure the scene before your entry. Securing a scene demands more than the simple presence of a law enforcement officer at the scene. Responding paramedics must ensure that the scene is safe before going in to provide prehospital care.

Approaching a Residence

Information provided to dispatchers may be limited, and a complete picture of the circumstances at the scene may not be available to paramedics. Keep in mind that all calls have a potential for violence. When arriving at a residence, listen for loud, threatening voices. Glance through available windows for signs of a struggle. In addition, look for visible weapons. By obtaining such information, you can make a decision about the relative safety of the scene. Anytime you perceive danger, abort the approach and back away to your vehicle. Call for law enforcement assistance, and wait for the officers to arrive.

Entering a Residence

Law enforcement officers consider entry doors to residences extremely dangerous. Many law enforcement officers have been shot and killed while standing in front of a door after knocking to gain entry. Most bullets pass easily through all but the heaviest doors. You should stand to the doorknob side of the door when preparing to knock **Figure 51-11 ▲**. If you stand on the hinged side of the door, any person in the room can observe you by opening the door only slightly, and you would have a limited view of conditions inside the room. Knock on the door and announce: "Paramedics," "Fire service," or "Rescue squad." In doing so, you will reduce the chance of being mistaken for a law enforcement officer. Ask whoever answers the door to lead you to the patient. If you do this, you will not only get to the patient quickly, but the person who leads you acts as a shield for you and gives you a few extra moments to react if the situation deteriorates.

When entering any type of structure you should pick a primary exit and a secondary exit. Your primary exit is usually the door that was used to enter the building. A secondary exit might be a rear door or, in an emergency, a window. Whenever you are in a building, try to keep at least one means of escape accessible at all times.

As you arrive at the patient's location, scan the room for weapons. If there is a gun or knife, back your way out of the residence and call for law enforcement assistance. Today, many people keep loaded firearms in the house for personal protection. Be aware that objects like ashtrays, scissors, bottles, fireplace pokers, and knitting needles can be used as weapons. Move any potential weapon out of the patient's reach.

Domestic Violence

Domestic disturbances are among the most dangerous situations faced by law enforcement officers and paramedics. In Canada, one in four females seen in the emergency department has a complaint related to domestic violence. For an in-depth discussion on domestic violence, refer to Chapter 43.

As a paramedic, you must be aware of the dangers involved and handle these incidents with extreme caution.

If a violent or physical dispute is in progress when you arrive at a residence, wait for law enforcement assistance before you enter. Tempers may flare while you are treating a patient. Using good communication skills in conjunction with eye contact and appropriate body language can defuse the situation. Your voice is the most effective tool you can use to keep out of trouble in a dispute. Knowing what words to use or not to use in a situation is only part of your goal. You must also be aware of the tone, pacing, pitch, and rhythm of your voice. Talk to people with the same respect that you expect from them, regardless of your personal opinion of them. A good paramedic is always respectful because it puts patients at ease and can suppress the anger of a violent person who is not the patient. That person may turn on you, and the situation can quickly deteriorate to a dangerous level if you do not use respectful language and tone.

You may also use a technique known as contact and cover, which will be described in greater depth later in the chapter. One aspect of the technique involves one paramedic making contact with the patient to provide prehospital care. The second paramedic obtains patient information, and more important, gauges the level of tension and warns his or her partner at the first sign of trouble.

Your most important mandate is to conduct yourself as a professional in a patient-care environment. Your duty is to act in a professional manner, no matter how unpleasant or difficult the situation.

Most paramedics are not trained as marriage counselors, psychologists, psychiatrists, or clergy. Crisis intervention is not part of your job and should be left to the professionals. You may be required by law to report certain conditions such as domestic violence or child maltreatment to local authorities. Be sure to check your community's laws to learn your mandatory reporting duties. Seven provinces and territories have introduced civil legislation to better protect women in situations of domestic violence. Be sure to check legislation in your jurisdiction to learn your mandatory reporting duties.

Violence on the Streets

The increase in gang activity and the prevalence of clandestine drug laboratories pose unique challenges to paramedics. Mass-casualty shootings, resulting from what law enforcement characterizes as an active shooter, have struck fear in many communities. In addition, you may be responding to an assault or robbery scene before law enforcement personnel arrive.

Clandestine Drug Laboratories

Clandestine drug laboratories are a growing problem. The most popular substance manufactured in clandestine labs is methamphetamine, known on the street as meth, speed, and crank. With a small investment of a few hundred dollars, a drug producer, or "cooker," can begin producing methamphetamine   Figure 51-12 ▼ .

Everything associated with a clandestine lab is hazardous! Because of the highly flammable properties of some chemicals associated with cooking methamphetamine and the toxic nature of others, extreme caution must be exercised when a lab is found. Although some methamphetamine "cooking" operations may look like a typical high school chemistry laboratory, others are much harder to recognize. Large quantities of over-the-counter cold remedies containing ephedrine or pseudoephedrine, gallon containers of camping fuel, and sulfuric acid in the form of lye may be the only signs of methamphetamine production. Almost every chemical involved is a hazardous material   Figure 51-13 ▶ .

In addition to the chemical hazards found at clandestine labs, some cookers use booby traps to safeguard their operations. These may include fragmentation and incendiary devices, animal traps, and impaling stakes.

Once a clandestine laboratory is identified, it is your job to remain clear of the area until the scene is secured by trained law enforcement personnel and hazardous materials specialists. If possible, take any patients with you if you can do so without exposing yourself and your team to additional hazardous materials.

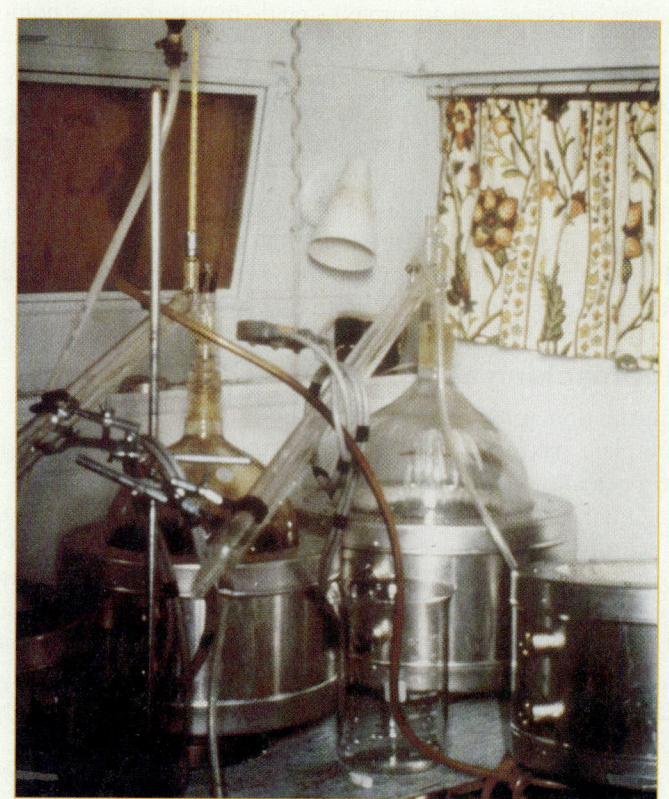

Figure 51-12 Some methamphetamine labs may resemble a high school chemistry laboratory. Do not touch anything!

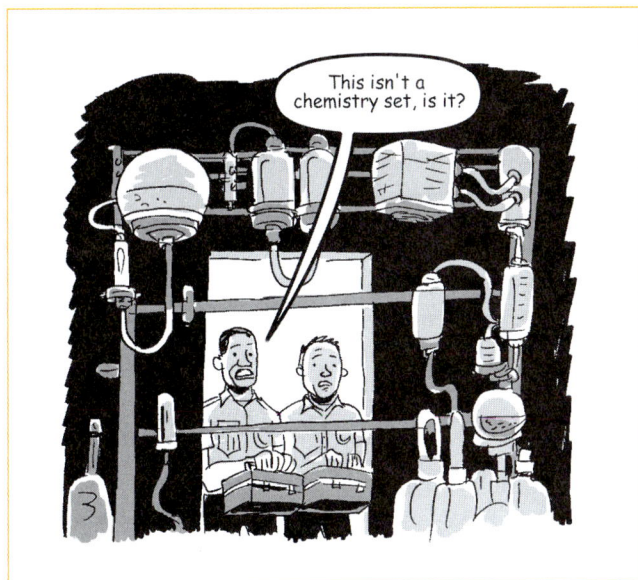

Figure 51-13

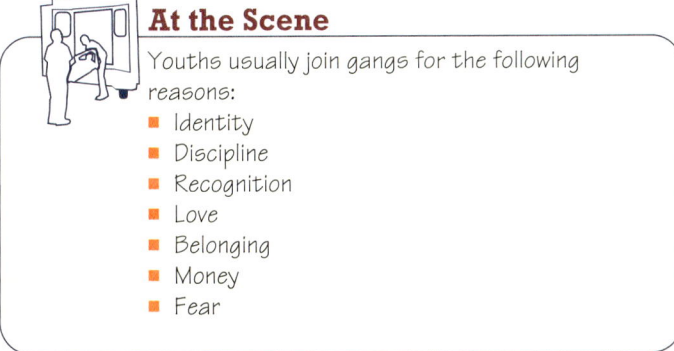

At the Scene

Youths usually join gangs for the following reasons:
- Identity
- Discipline
- Recognition
- Love
- Belonging
- Money
- Fear

Gangs

Gangs pose an increasing threat in communities across the nation. What was once a problem only in major cities is now a problem in smaller suburban and rural communities. Data about the extent of gang activity in Canada are very limited. Gang-related homicides, which stem from the activities of organized crime groups and street gangs, gained steadily from 4% of all homicides in 1994 to 16% in 2005.

Gang members often operate on what might be considered their own "three Rs": Reputation, Respect, and Retaliation. Reputation provides status for individual members and the gang itself and is gained by committing crimes. Closely associated with reputation is respect, which may actually be fear. The thought of gaining respect from peers is a common force that drives adolescents to gangs. To maintain their respect and reputation, a gang or an individual gang member must retaliate whenever disrespected or "dissed." For example, the simple act of cutting a motorcycle gang member's jacket or "colours" may be viewed as a sign of disrespect. Such disrespect will usually lead to the third R, retaliation.

Always use common sense when dealing with gangs. Even if you know gang hand signs or slang, it would be dangerous for you to use them around gang members—you are not a member of the group. In many gang strongholds, you may be advised to obtain police escorts into the area for all emergency medical incidents. When treating a patient wounded in a drive-by shooting, limit the amount of prehospital care provided out in the open. The wisest move is to get your prehospital patient into the ambulance to avoid being seen, and possibly targeted, for a second round of gunfire.

Multiple-Casualty Shootings and Snipers

Well-publicized mass shootings gave all emergency services a mandate to focus on responses to such catastrophes. You, as the paramedic, are an integral part of emergency operations at these scenes. Paramedics must prepare, plan, and train for these complex and difficult violent incidents.

As with any other shooting or stabbing incident, responding paramedic units should remain in the staging area until the scene is secured by law enforcement personnel. Staging, treatment, and triage areas may need to be up to 1 kilometre away from the actual scene. Line-of-sight and, thus, line-of-fire from windows must be avoided when establishing these sites. Although parking lots or playing fields at schools may seem to be ideal locations, an assailant could have a wide field of fire, causing a chaotic situation to deteriorate even further.

Paramedics in mass or serial shootings need to know how to use cover and concealment. You need to know the difference between objects that provide cover and those that offer concealment only. Cover objects, such as trees, utility poles, mail-collection boxes, dumpsters, curbs, vehicles, and depressions in the ground, are usually impenetrable to bullets. Tall grass, shrubbery, and dark shadows are areas of concealment. When cover is not readily available, use concealment to provide some protection while you assess your position. Your job at that point is to find cover.

Many services are using tactical paramedics in mass-casualty shootings. In addition, these specially trained medics provide prehospital care for barricaded patients, patients being held hostage, and other special operations in which a paramedic without special training might not be able to work. These specially trained responders are a critical link in providing medical care in hostile situations, including multiple-casualty shootings.

Hostage Situations

EMS personnel sometimes arrive on a scene before it is secure. Remember, hostage situations are law enforcement problems until the scene is secure. Have you considered what you would do if you met an armed adversary? Because no hard and fast rules apply, you should take all the additional training you can in handling armed people in the prehospital environment. Anything can happen, depending on the assailant, your position, and your reactions. The possibility of being taken hostage is extremely remote, but it exists. If you are taken hostage, remember that most hostage incidents in Canada last between

4½ and 5 hours. Your behaviour can greatly enhance your chances of surviving the ordeal.

Hostages are usually held as a form of human collateral to ensure compliance with a promise. If you are taken hostage, you can increase your chances of survival if you can anticipate the feelings and actions of the hostage taker and the negotiators.

The psychological results of being held hostage are of greater concern than physical problems. Even if you are physically unharmed, you may experience strong psychological reactions during the incident. The aftereffects of being held hostage can become posttraumatic stress disorder (PTSD). It is often wise to seek professional counseling after your release, even if you do not think you need it, to prevent long-term problems later. Knowing what to expect if you are held hostage can help you keep your psychological equilibrium during the situation and help you deal with the psychological stress that often accompanies your release.

Stages of a Hostage Situation

The six stages involved in taking and maintaining hostages are surveillance, capture, transport, holding, move, and resolution. Paramedics who are taken hostage are most affected by the capture, transport, and holding stages.

When a paramedic is taken hostage, the hostage taker is usually as surprised as the captured paramedic. Mentally disturbed people and criminals rarely plan to capture a paramedic, but if it happens, they may use the hostage as a medium of exchange or as a safety shield when they attempt to escape.

During the capture, the hostage taker will probably be extremely nervous and try to gain control of what has unexpectedly become an unsettled situation. At this stage, you are in grave personal danger. You must assume that the person on the other end of the gun will use violence if you do not follow instructions.

Do not attempt to escape. Consider the safety of any other hostages. If your escape attempt fails, what will your new position be with your abductor? If your actions antagonize your captor, your chances of being hurt increase. You must avoid personal injury, remain calm, and control the instinctive anger that occurs when you are physically attacked.

At the moment of capture, you may feel that it is all a bad dream because your mind cannot adjust quickly to such a radical change. This almost-automatic psychological denial can help you as you make the transition from being in control of your surroundings to acknowledging your inability to defend yourself.

The hostage taker may order you to move to a more secure location. This move may be only to the other side of the room or to another part of the same building. If you are transported soon after capture, the aggressor will still be agitated. During this stage, expect to receive harsh commands from your captor. If the captor feels you are moving too slowly, expect physical maltreatment such as pushing, dragging, or kicking.

If your abductor has time, you may be tied, gagged, and blindfolded before being transported. Your body's reflexes may slow down, and if you have been slow in following instructions, your captors might use physical pain to speed you up. You might find yourself feeling a loss of emotional equilibrium. Your perceptions may be distorted, especially if you are blindfolded.

If you are prepared and have planned ahead, you can reduce the shock of this experience, recover your senses quickly, and regain your composure. Obtain as much information as possible about your location by using all your senses, especially if you are blindfolded during the move. What do you hear? Do you smell animals, chemicals, or food? If you used stairs, try to remember the number of floors. Did you leave the original building? Note the number of captors involved. The more you can remember about the transport stage of your captivity, the more help you will be to law enforcement agencies after your release.

During the holding stage, many hostages may begin to develop psychological and emotional problems. The situation has calmed slightly, law enforcement personnel are at the scene, and release negotiations are ongoing. The holding stage is tedious; you sit, wait, and hope for a safe release. Hostage negotiators count on time to bring an incident to a safe and successful conclusion. Your chances of survival increase proportionally from the time of your capture to the time of your release. In the beginning stages, the hostage taker may threaten to kill you. But as time goes on, you are kept alive so that the hostage taker's demands will be met.

Even if negotiations have started, do not try predict an exact time or date of release, even to yourself. If you set an unrealistic goal (such as 4 hours) and are wrong, you will feel demoralized. Only your abductors will decide when or whether you will be released. If you have been captured by terrorists, plan for a much longer time in captivity than if your captors were criminals or mentally disturbed people. Accept the fact that you have no control over when you will be freed.

During the holding stage, your mental state is a greater danger to you than your captors are. After you reach the holding area, your captors will try to break your spirit. You may be forced to ask for food and permission to sleep or to use the toilet.

Manage yourself and your personal environment. Do not do anything that will attract unwanted attention, and do not stare at your captors. If you convincingly fake a heart attack or sickness, you become less valuable and more expendable to your captors. If the hostage takers believe you are in their way or on their nerves, they may kill you. Remember that any one of your captors can walk in and kill you at any time. Your only chance for survival is to maintain your role as a bargaining chip.

Because you are wearing a uniform, other hostages may look to you for guidance and strength. Your captors may consider this image of authority as a threat. Anything that draws attention to you increases the possibility of violence. Make every effort to be inconspicuous. Develop a nonthreatening image by removing the badge, collar pins, and patches from your uniform, or turn your uniform shirt inside out so these items are not visible.

Contact and Cover

In any violent situation, you must never assume that you will not be harmed because you are clearly identified as a paramedic. Always assume that the person with a gun will shoot anyone in sight. If you see law enforcement personnel seeking cover, you must not remain in the immediate vicinity.

Remember the difference between objects that provide cover and those that offer concealment only. You should make your body conform to the shape of the object as much as possible Figure 51-14 ▼.

People shooting from a higher position than you (such as in an upper floor window or on a roof) can usually see the upper part of your torso or head over the top of your cover, especially if you are using a wall or motor vehicle as cover Figure 51-15 ▼. If this occurs, use the engine block and wheel area of a motor vehicle as cover. Avoid the area near the fuel tank, and do not use the area between the wheels as cover. Even though the aggressor cannot see you if you are between

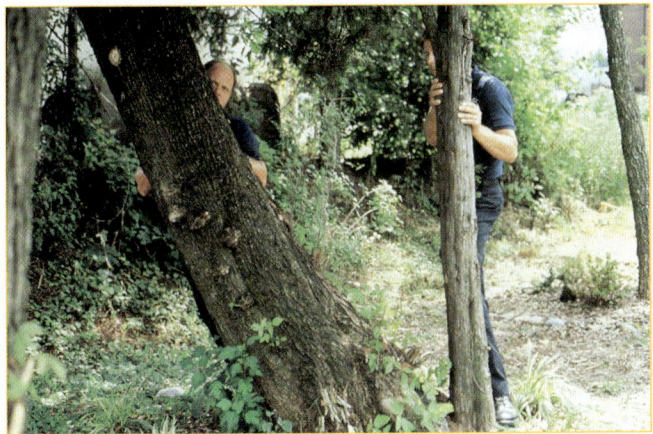

Figure 51-14 Choose a tree that is large enough to conceal all of your body.

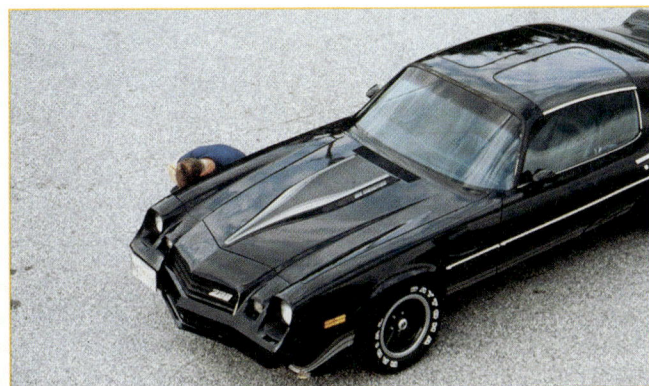

Figure 51-15 A sniper can see part of your body from above your position of cover.

the wheels, a skilled shooter can hit you by ricocheting bullets off the pavement in front of you.

Select a fire hydrant as cover only if you cannot immediately find larger objects. You will soon become uncomfortable trying to match your body to the small hydrant. There is a very real possibility in such a situation that you could be shot in the arm, knee, or shoulder. However, your central body mass vital organs will be protected. If this is the only cover available, it is better than remaining in the open.

If you are not outdoors, items inside a structure and the structure itself can provide cover or concealment, depending on their construction. Furniture and appliances, such as a solid oak desk or a refrigerator, can be used for cover because they can stop a bullet. If you dive behind the sofa or a stuffed chair, you have concealed yourself but are not protected by cover.

Using Walls as Cover

You cannot assume that a wall will provide safe cover—many provide only concealment. For your safety and survival, you must determine whether the type of wall you have chosen gives you cover or concealment only. For example, brick and concrete-block walls are much safer than cinder-block walls. The porous nature of cinder blocks will not absorb the bullet's energy and stop it. However, most interior walls are constructed with wood or aluminum studs and covered with drywall or siding. They may conceal you but are not good cover because they are not impenetrable. If your only protection is behind a frame wall, try to stand near the door or window frames. These areas are usually constructed with extra framing materials and contain more wood than other areas of the wall.

Evasive Tactics

Change locations only if the new location is better cover, farther from the hostile atmosphere, and can be reached without your revealing yourself to the attacker. Do not change your position of cover just for the sake of changing. Before changing locations, quickly look out from your cover several times Figure 51-16 ▶. Look from a different height and angle each time. Use this "quick-peek" technique to evaluate the advisability of changing locations. Always return to cover as quickly as possible.

If you decide that you would be safer in another location, do not run directly away from the assailant's position; run in a zigzag pattern. You have less chance of being hit if your movement takes you across the assailant's field of view.

Concealment Techniques

Tall grass, shrubbery, and dark shadows are considered areas of concealment. When cover is not readily available, use concealment to provide some protection while you assess your position and seek cover.

Areas of concealment are more common after dark than during daylight hours. If you are involved in a violent situation at night, move into the darkness or shadows and stand still. The assailant cannot see you and may not shoot. If the assailant fires shots at random, chances are you will not be hit.

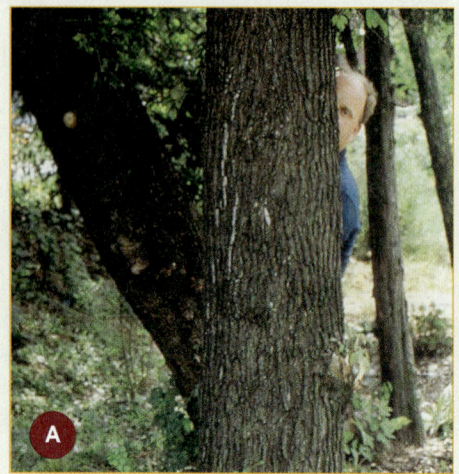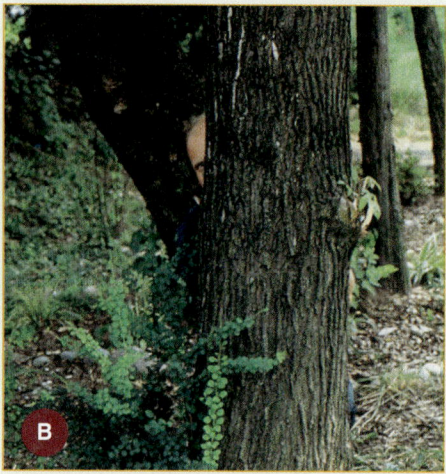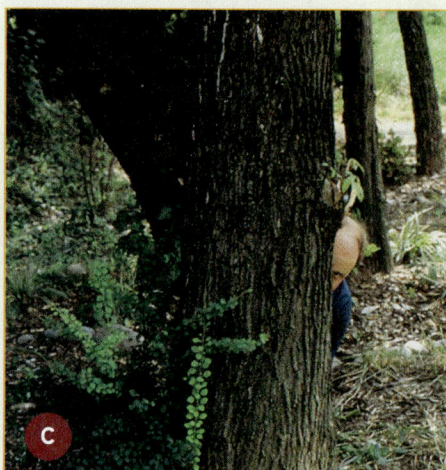

Figure 51-16 If you must analyze your position, look from a different height and angle each time.

In rural areas, tall grass or a cornfield can conceal you whether it is day or night. Remain motionless so that the foliage does not move. After you finish analyzing the situation, move toward cover.

Self-defence

Recognizing the potential for violence when you arrive on the scene gives you time to request support and protection from law enforcement officers. With their protection, you should be able to treat your patient safely after the scene is secure. However, you must also consider what to do if the violence is ongoing or breaks out while you are providing prehospital care. If you know some effective defensive moves, you may be able to resolve the situation without getting hurt yourself.

If someone prevents you from reaching your patient, identify yourself and say, "Move back! That person may die if you don't let me help!" If the person blocking your way moves, you have attained your goal, and no additional force is required. If the person does not move, take a side step and repeat the verbal challenge. Inform the person, "If you don't get out of my way, I'm calling the police!" This threat

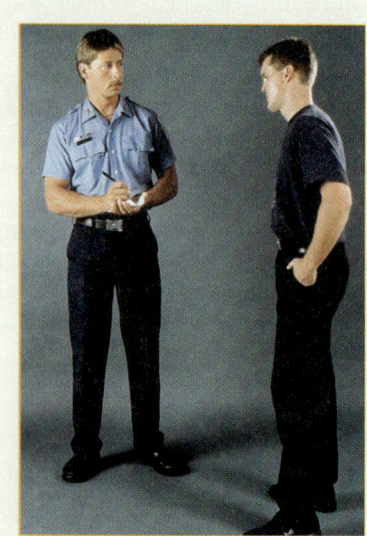

Figure 51-17 The interview stance.

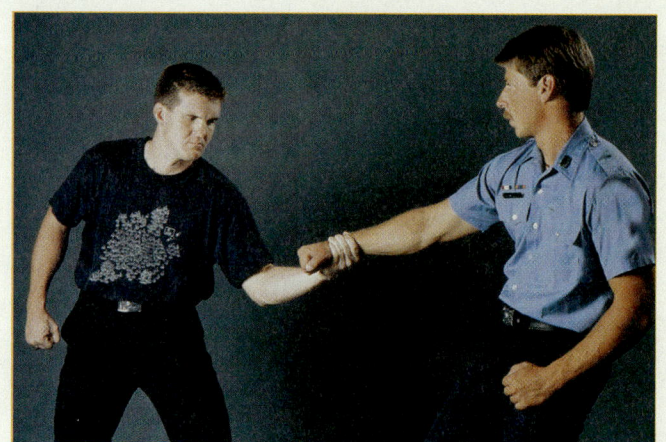

Figure 51-18 When someone grabs you, the normal reaction is to pull away.

usually makes the person move, but not always in the direction you wanted. There are some techniques that you can learn to physically defend yourself.

You can control an unexpected attack. Always use the interview stance so you will be in a defensive position if violence suddenly erupts. This stance is especially helpful in domestic encounters.

To assume the interview stance, stand approximately an arm's length from the person with your body at a 45° angle to the person. Your feet should be shoulder-width apart, your knees slightly bent, and your hands relaxed **Figure 51-17** .

If someone unexpectedly grabs your wrists, your normal reaction is to pull away or jerk back from the attacker. Fight against your natural tendencies. Do not jerk back; think through your moves. First, figure out where your attacker's thumbs are. If you try to break the grip by pulling against the assailant's fingers, you will have difficulty in breaking the hold **Figure 51-18** .

But if you jerk your forearm against the assailant's thumb (**Figure 51-19** ▾), you can easily break free. Usually this means you will pull toward your body instead of away from it. This move is more effective because the thumb is weaker than the combined strength of the fingers. Once you are free of the assailant's grip, retreat to a safe area.

If an assailant grabs the front of your shirt, seize the hand of the attacker and twist it toward the thumb. At the same time, flash your free hand through your attacker's field of vision. This unexpected action should break the person's

concentration long enough for you to break the hold and escape (**Figure 51-20** ▾).

Self-defence in Armed Encounters

Distraction techniques are very useful in breaking the chain of events (turn, locate, focus, and fire) in a shooting incident and in preventing attacks with knives or other sharp objects. Again, the purpose of the distraction is to increase your chances of survival by giving you time to escape. The distraction does not have to be elabourate.

When something is coming at you, your initial instinct is to blink or flinch. Consider what happens when you are driving during a heavy rain and a passing vehicle throws water on your car's windshield. Even though you know the water is not going to hit you, you still blink or flinch when the water strikes the windshield. This is the reaction you want to provoke.

Throwing your patient care report pad at the person provides the same distraction as the water hitting the windshield. It interrupts the chain of

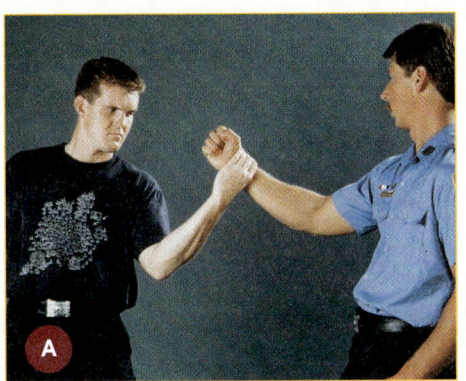
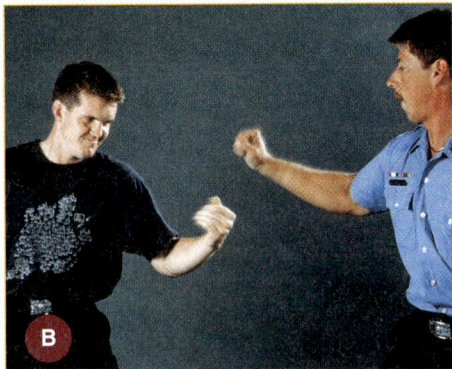

Figure 51-19 To break a hold, pull toward the thumb (**A**) and break the hold (**B**), turn, and run.

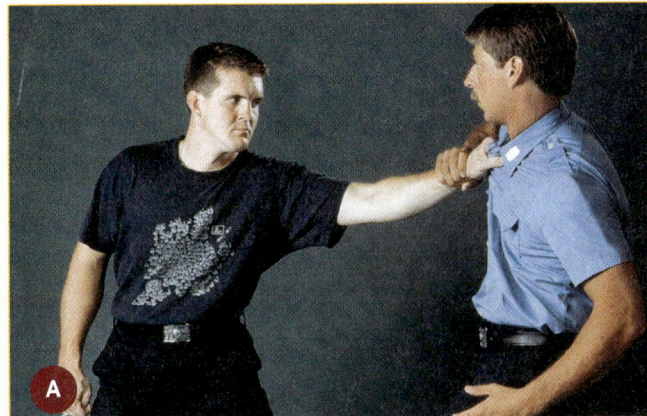

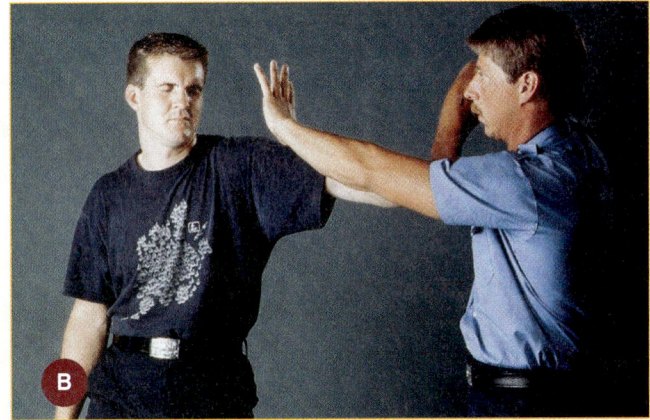

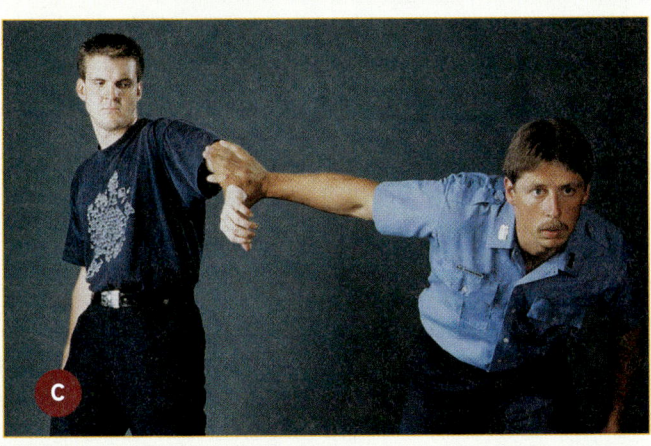

Figure 51-20 To break away from a person who has grabbed your shirt, do the following: **A.** Seize your attacker's hand and twist toward the thumb. **B.** Flash your free hand in the attacker's face, which will break the concentration long enough for you to escape. **C.** After you feel the grip relaxing on your shirt, twist your body away from your assailant and run to a safer area.

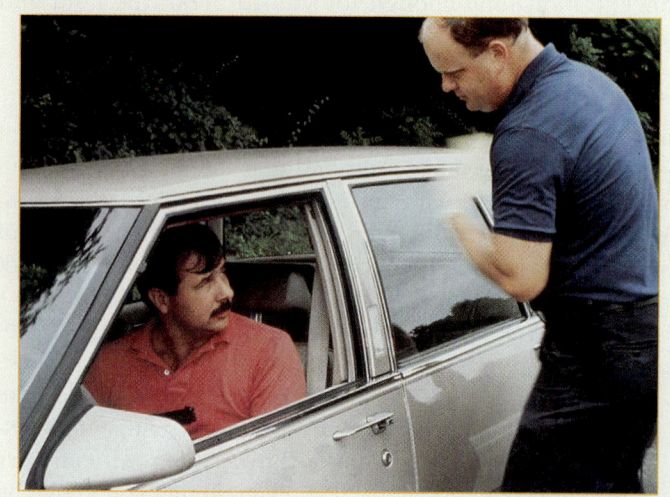

Figure 51-21 If aggressive action occurs, throw the pad directly at the nose of the aggressor.

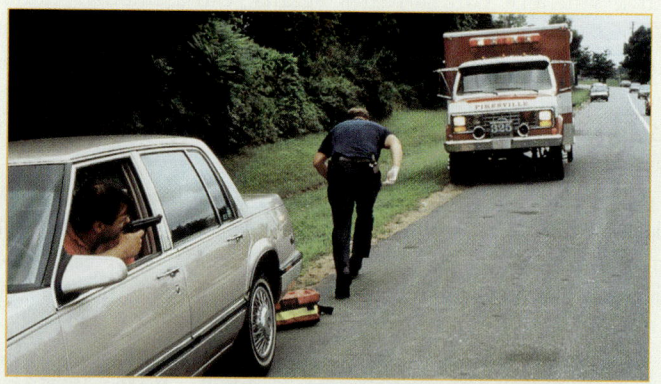

Figure 51-22 While the aggressor flinches and attempts to refocus, run toward the unit.

events long enough to permit you to get out of the line of fire and run to safety.

Carry the clipboard in your nondominant hand when you make an approach. Raise the pad to your nondominant shoulder. If the patient takes aggressive action during your initial interview, be prepared to throw the pad directly at the aggressor's nose Figure 51-21 ▲ . Use only a soft pad of paper for this technique. A hard object such as an aluminum report book or clipboard may cause needless injuries. The soft pad will not cause undue harm. If the person is reaching for a lighter instead of a weapon and you react by throwing the pad, you only have to apologize and explain. Explain that you have had calls during which the patient took aggressive action toward you, and you thought it was going to happen again.

After you throw the pad, do not wait for a reaction. As soon as it is out of your hand, turn toward your vehicle, get out of the possible line of fire, and run to safety.

Put as much distance as possible between you and the aggressor. If possible, run to your vehicle Figure 51-22 ▶ . You can call for help or drive to a safer location. If you are cut off from the ambulance, evaluate the surrounding area for the best possible cover and concealment.

Use physical force as a defensive technique, not an aggressive motion. Properly executed defensive motions can be as effective as physical strikes and are easier to defend if you face civil liability charges.

The amount of defensive force needed to protect yourself varies with each incident. If you believe that your life is in imminent danger, any action that gets you out of the situation is a reasonable level of force.

Crime Scenes

As a paramedic, you will respond to assist the victims of violent crime. Clearly, your first responsibility, beyond that of personal safety, is to the patient. However, you also have a responsibility to the community at large. By assisting law enforcement personnel to maintain the integrity of the crime scene, you increase the probability that a suspect will be captured and convicted.

Preserving Evidence

It is best to remember what is known as Locard's principle, "Every contact leaves a trace." Generally, there are two types of evidence: testimonial and real or physical. Testimonial evidence is the oral documentation by a witness of the facts. Real or physical evidence ties a suspect or a victim to a crime and includes body materials, objects, and impressions.

You are the Paramedic Part 3

You retreat and stage a safe distance from the house. When law enforcement officers arrive, you brief them on the situation and wait until they have the scene secured. Once the law enforcement officers feel they have the scene secured, they have you enter the house and treat a badly beaten female patient. The officers tell you they have arrested a man with a handgun in his waistband, who had been beating the woman. You and your partner look at each other realizing the danger you would have placed yourself in had you elected to enter the house alone.

5. How can your approach to the scene be an important part of the scene assessment?

6. What would you or your partner have done if you elected to enter the house alone and found the gun in the patient's waist?

Follow law enforcement direction when you are asked to park in a specific area or to avoid a certain location. Officers may be attempting to safeguard tire imprints, bullet casings, or blood. Once you are at your patient's side, try to alter the scene as little as possible. Be mindful of bullet casings, weapons, blood spatter, and puddles. Whenever possible, walk around such evidence **Figure 51-23 ▾**. This is best referred to as "the path of contamination," which is the area where emergency personnel should walk in order to avoid interfering with potential evidence. It is usually away from a path that a victim and/or suspect may have used. This path can be determined by your own personal observations (ie, bloodstained areas, areas where footwear impressions can be seen, areas where weapons can be seen). The path might be determined already by other on-scene personnel, such as the fire department, other paramedics, or law enforcement. If you are the first agency on the scene, walk along the wall into the room to the patient. Generally, criminals will exit the scene quickly, which is usually the shortest path. Walking along the wall will not contaminate the exit path. Be prepared to tell law enforcement officers where you have walked to differentiate it from the victim or suspect's footwear.

Do not pick up expended cartridge casings to determine the calibre. Do not use telephones, flush toilets, or turn on water in a sink. In each case, valuable evidence can be lost. When you remove clothes to expose a wound, do not cut through bullet holes, knife cuts, or tears. Once the clothes are removed, do not shake them because valuables, including valuable trace evidence, may fall from the pockets to the floor. Always inform law enforcement personnel of any change in the crime scene that resulted during patient treatment.

You can be called to provide testimonial evidence in court regarding what you saw or heard at the scene of a crime. Because a criminal case might not go to trial for a year or more, it is imperative the incident be properly documented. Writing a complete report is the mark of a professional paramedic. Incomplete reports seldom keep anyone out of court.

Three elements require proper documentation: what you saw, what you heard, and the chain of custody. Documentation should include a description of the scene. How many patients? Was the victim supine or prone? Where was the weapon? Were any characteristics of the scene noteworthy? Do not draw conclusions or overstate facts. Any statements made by the patient during transfer to a medical facility should be documented.

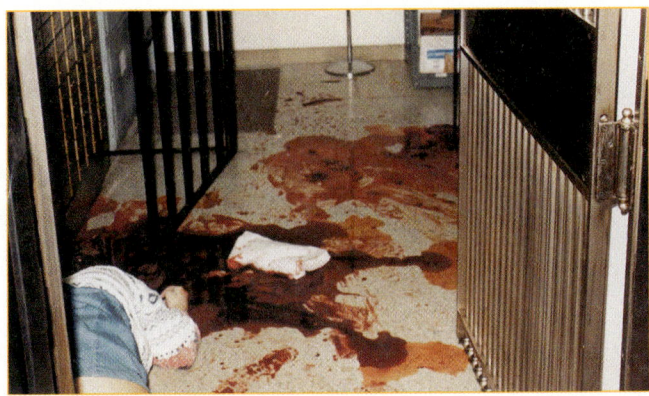

Figure 51-23 Do not disturb bullet casings, and avoid stepping in blood spatter and puddles.

Documentation and Communication

Your report should answer the following questions.
- What did you see?
  - Overturned or damaged furniture
  - Weapons
  - Position of victim and other persons at the scene
- What did you hear?
  - Arguing or screams
  - Weapons being chambered or talk of the use of a weapon
  - Incriminating statements by persons on the scene
- What was done with evidence taken from the victim?
  - Clothing
  - Weapons (Law enforcement personnel should secure weapons whenever possible.)

As always, clearly note your actions on the scene.

Documentation and Communication

Document as much as you can at the crime scene, but know that your notes can be your best friend or worst enemy when it comes time to testify. Your documentation may become evidence in a court case. It is best to document what you are sure of. If you are called to testify, your documentation will help you remember the specifics of the call.

You are the Paramedic Summary

1. Does the lack of violent incidents in your response district ensure your safety?

Absolutely not! Violence knows no geographic boundaries; it can happen anywhere and at any time. A statistically low rate of violence—although good—simply means that it's a matter of time before you are faced with such a call. It is crucial to remember that all calls you respond to pose a potential threat to your safety. It is your responsibility to carefully size up every scene—regardless of how docile it may appear—to ensure that you are not walking into a volatile situation.

2. What measures will you take to stay safe on this call?

First, you should request law enforcement response to the scene. You should exercise caution on every call; however, you should be especially cautious of calls in which the details are sketchy or unknown. A call for an "injured person" is very generic; it could range from a minor injury sustained during a family picnic to an intoxicated man with an assault rifle. You should also ask the dispatcher to attempt to gather more information about the call while you are en route; forewarned is forearmed. If this is not possible, err on the side of caution and stage in a safe place until law enforcement personnel arrive at the scene and ensure that it's safe.

3. What information can be obtained as you walk toward the house?

Screaming and profanity should immediately indicate that this is not a safe scene. Other signs of a violent situation include the sound of breaking glass, loud music, other unusual sounds, or an obvious struggle that you can see through a window. Keep your ears and eyes open at all times and never let your guard down.

4. What actions should you take in response to the hostilities heard from within the residence?

Unless you and your partner wish to become part of a situation that may result in your own deaths, it would be extremely wise to immediately withdraw from the scene and move to a place of safety. However, when doing so, you should back away from the residence. If you turn your back, and the person inside knows that you are there, you will never see an attack coming. Stage in a safe area and wait for law enforcement personnel to arrive.

5. How can your approach to the scene be an important part of the scene assessment?

Remember this: the life you save (or attempt to save) may take your own! Never hastily enter a scene without making a deliberate and concerted effort to look for safety hazards and taking appropriate action to buffer any hazards. This may include requesting law enforcement, fire personnel, the power company, or the animal warden. The scene assessment—with emphasis on remaining cognizant of threats to your safety—is not a one-time assessment; it is an ongoing process until the call has ended. Many scenes are safe initially, only to deteriorate with alarming speed and unpredictability.

6. What would you or your partner have done if you elected to enter the house alone and found the gun in the patient's waistband?

The obvious must be pointed out: if you recognize that a scene is clearly unsafe (screaming and profane language should raise a red flag), then you should never place yourself in such a situation. The answer to this question is "it depends." Can you egress before the person has a chance to draw the gun? Is there an escape route? If so, where is it in proximity to the person with the gun? Is there an object that you can use as cover if the person opens fire? Although you have no way of predicting how a person who is carrying a weapon is going to react or behave, you can safely assume that it will not be pleasant. If egression is not an option (ie, you are trapped in between the assailant and the door), try to remain calm and use your skills of diplomacy to assure the person that you are there to help.

Prep Kit

Ready for Review

- No community, socioeconomic group, race, or religion is immune to violence. The use of sound survival skills will reduce the potential for you to fall victim to an act of violence while on an emergency call.
- Allow law enforcement personnel to secure the scene of violent incidents before you enter.
- Should violence erupt while you are on scene, retreat to a safe place and summon the police.

Vital Vocabulary

clandestine drug laboratories Locations where illegal drugs such as methamphetamine, lysergic acid diethylamide (LSD), ecstasy, and phencyclidine hydrochloride (PCP) are manufactured.

concealment Protection from being seen.

contact and cover Technique that involves one paramedic making contact with the patient to provide prehospital care, while the second paramedic obtains patient information, gauges the level of tension, and warns his or her partner at the first sign of trouble.

cover Obstacles that are difficult or impossible for bullets to penetrate.

physical evidence The evidence that ties a suspect or victim to a crime. It may include body materials, objects, and impressions.

primary exit The main means of escape should violence erupt. This is usually the door you used to enter the building.

secondary exit Any other means of egress, including windows and rear doors.

tactical paramedics Specially trained medics who provide prehospital care for barricaded patients, patients being held hostage, and other special operations.

testimonial evidence The oral documentation by a witness of the facts of a criminal act.

tunnel vision Dangerous situation when a paramedic becomes so completely involved with prehospital care that he or she fails to see the possibility of physical harm to the patient or other care providers.

Points to Ponder

You are dispatched to an assault on a corner in your local town. The local police department asks you to stage approximately two blocks away. After approximately 10 minutes, you are notified that the scene is safe. When you approach the patient, you see that he has two stab wounds to his chest. You and your partner provide spinal precautions and provide immediate lifesaving prehospital care to him. You transport him to the nearest trauma centre.

What would you have done if you arrived at the scene before the police? If the perpetrator were on the scene, what would you do?

Issues: Potential Exposure to Scene Violence, How to Approach the Scene.

Assessment in Action

You and your partner are dispatched to the highway for an unconscious patient in a car. You are informed by your dispatch centre that the scene appears to be safe. The person who called 9-1-1 was travelling in the opposite direction and noticed the motor vehicle pulled over on the shoulder of the highway.

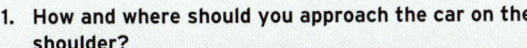

1. **How and where should you approach the car on the shoulder?**
   A. At a minimum of 5 m to the rear of the car and on a 20° angle
   B. At a minimum of 5 m in front of the car on a 1° angle
   C. At a minimum of 5 m to the rear of the car and on a 10° angle
   D. At a minimum of 5 m to the rear of the car and on a 15° angle

2. **If you are the person riding in the passenger seat, how should you approach the vehicle?**
   A. Proceed to the rear passenger side trunk area.
   B. Proceed to the rear driver's side trunk area.
   C. Proceed directly to the driver's side door.
   D. Proceed directly to the passenger side door.

3. **Special attention should be taken when approaching:**
   A. cars.
   B. motorcycles.
   C. SUVs.
   D. vans.

4. **What should you do if the situation turns unsafe?**
   A. Stay and deal with it.
   B. Adapt and overcome.
   C. Retreat from the scene.
   D. Try to talk to the patient.

5. **Information that you need to give to your dispatcher if there is an unsafe condition includes all of the following, EXCEPT:**
   A. the number of aggressors involved.
   B. the patient's name and estimated transport time to the hospital.
   C. the number and type of weapons involved, if any.
   D. the make, colour, body style, and license number of the car.

6. **True or false? Once on the scene, and there do not appear to be any threats to the paramedics, you can move on to other things, such as treating the patient.**
   A. True
   B. False

7. **True or false? Only certain calls require a scene assessment for violence hazards.**
   A. True
   B. False

Challenging Question

You are dispatched to the scene of a pediatric pedestrian struck outside of an apartment complex. When you arrive on scene, you see an ambulance and a fire truck on scene already. You look for them and notice a crowd of approximately 100 angry individuals. You find a police officer and you ask her to lead you to where the patient is. When you arrive at the patient's side, you find the ambulance and fire crew. You immediately direct BLS to secure the patient, who appears to be stable, and transfer him to the ambulance.

8. **What dangers do large crowds pose to the paramedics?**

Appendix A: Cardiac Life Support Fundamentals

Competency Areas

Area 1: Professional Responsibilities

1.5.a   Work collaboratively with a partner.

1.5.b   Accept and deliver constructive feedback.

1.5.c   Work collaboratively with other emergency response agencies.

1.5.d   Work collaboratively with other members of the health care team.

1.6.c   Delegate tasks appropriately.

Area 5: Therapeutics

5.1.a   Use manual maneuvers and positioning to maintain airway patency.

5.1.b   Suction oropharynx.

5.1.c   Suction beyond oropharynx.

5.1.d   Utilize oropharyngeal airway.

5.1.g   Utilize airway devices not requiring visualization of vocal cords and introduced endotracheally.

5.1.h   Utilize airway devices requiring visualization of vocal cords and introduced endotracheally.

5.5.i   Conduct automated external defibrillation.

5.5.j   Conduct manual defibrillation.

Appendix 4: Pathophysiology

A.   **Cardiovascular System**

Cardiac Conduction Disorder: Benign arrhythmias

Cardiac Conduction Disorder: Lethal arrhythmias

Cardiac Conduction Disorder: Life-threatening arrhythmias

Introduction

Paramedics and first responders are frequently dispatched to calls involving a cardiac arrest. An estimated 60% to 70% of all prehospital cardiac arrests occur in the home; the remainder occur in public places. Having a bystander who has initiated the proper prehospital care at the scene is definitely a plus—indeed, it often means the difference between life and death. Some paramedics might even find it difficult to remember successfully resuscitating a patient from cardiac arrest who did not either have citizen CPR or for whom the arrest was a witnessed event and an AED was immediately available.

This appendix explores planning for the resuscitation or "code," the roles of the code team leader and code team members, and ways that practice and planning can help increase your resuscitation success. The International Liaison Committee on Resuscitation and the American Heart Association, in conjunction with national agencies, such as the Canadian Heart and Stroke Foundation, revises the guidelines for emergency cardiovascular care and CPR every 5 years. This appendix describes how your agency can incorporate the latest guidelines into your codes.

Managing Cardiac Arrest

Although survival rates from prehospital cardiac arrest vary greatly, survival averages 6.4% based on reports from Canada and the United States. The "Chain of Survival" includes four essential links: early access, early CPR, early defibrillation, and early definitive care **Figure A-1 ▸** . Those communities that have made survival of a prehospital cardiac arrest a benchmark for measurable improvements in their health care systems have worked hard on each of these links.

Improving the Response to Cardiac Arrest: The SMART Way

When you are undertaking a community-based program to improve survival of prehospital cardiac arrest, consider adopting the management acronym SMART to describe the program's objectives: Specific, Measurable, Attainable and Achievable, Realistic and Relevant, and Timely. Here are a few questions that progressive communities should ask:

- Is there a universal access number (ie, 9-1-1), and do all members of the public know how and when to use it?
- Are all the dispatchers/communicators trained in CPR telephone instruction?
- Is a community CPR training program readily available at all times of the day and days of the week at little to no cost for the citizens? If so, does the public know it is available? Have 10% to 20% of the population been trained? (Part of attaining this objective can be addressed by convincing the public to take the self-help approach to CPR training as provided by the 30-minute CPR Anytime program.)
- Is CPR a requirement to graduate high school?

You are the Paramedic Part 1

Jim, a 54-year-old man, is playing basketball in an adult league on a Saturday afternoon at the local elementary school. He leaves the game to get a drink and starts to feel dizzy as he returns to the court. He suddenly drops to his knees and then to the floor. Fortunately, one of his teammates, Tom, took a cardiopulmonary resuscitation (CPR) course about 2 months ago, so he takes charge of the situation. Tom orders a teammate, "Go call 9-1-1 and tell them we have a cardiac arrest." Next, he tells someone else, "Go search for an AED."

About 2 minutes pass as the nearest first responder agency, which was located only a few blocks away, arrives on the scene. Your paramedics are still responding from a few kilometres away.

Upon arrival of your paramedic unit, you are led into the court by a teammate. You hear over the radio that a supervisor is en route as a back-up. As you approach the patient's side, you do a quick assessment of the scene for safety and potential hazards and then begin an initial assessment. Your general impression indicates a middle-aged, overweight male who is receiving good-quality CPR as judged by the counting you hear and the compressions. A first responder is attaching the pads and cables to their AED. These cables can easily be switched to your monitor, but this can wait until after the first shock.

You note the following findings while getting an initial report.

Initial Assessment	Recording Time: 2 Minutes
Appearance	CPR is in progress, patient is not vomiting, and the belly is not distended
Level of consciousness	U (Unresponsive)
Airway	Open with a head tilt–chin lift
Breathing	Being ventilated with a bag-valve-mask device with high-flow supplemental oxygen
Circulation	Receiving compressions at the two-rescuer rate/ratio

1. Arriving on the scene of an apparent cardiac arrest with bystanders who have initiated prehospital care, how should you evaluate the quality of the CPR?
2. Many elementary schools and public places have an AED available. How might that have helped in this situation?

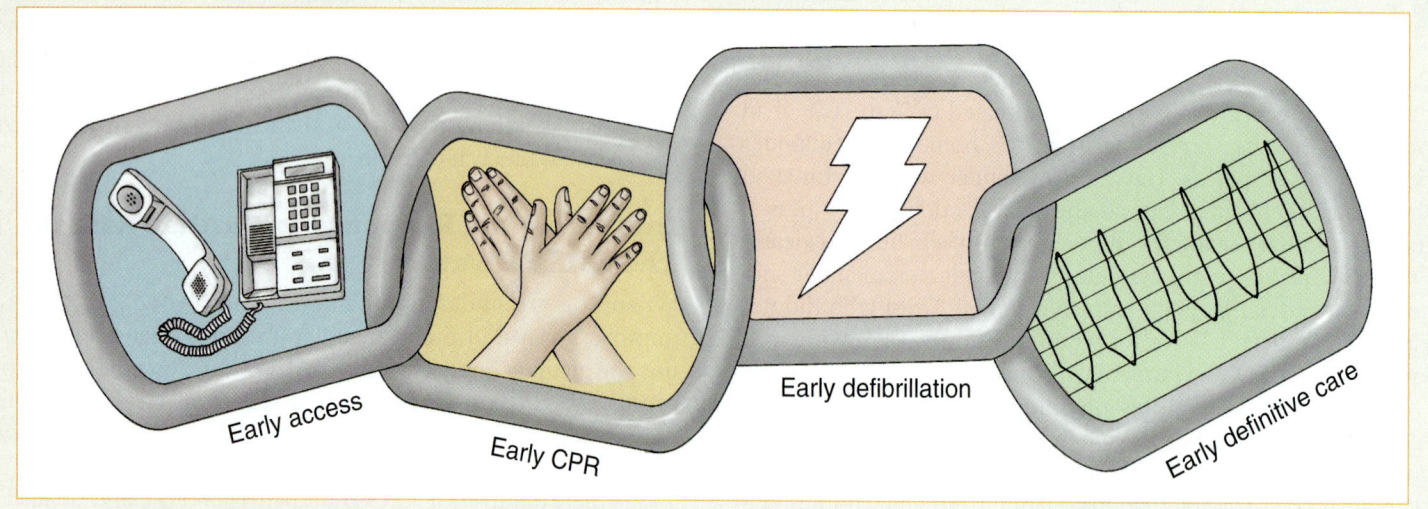

Figure A-1 The four links of the Chain of Survival.

- Are 100% of the responders to emergencies (police, fire, EMS) currently trained in CPR and the AED? Do all response vehicles have an AED?
- Are AEDs and qualified personnel who are trained in their use available in all locations of public assembly for more than 500 people or in high-risk locations?
- How long does it take for the first emergency responder to arrive on the scene? How long does it take for the paramedics to arrive?
- Is the EMS agency's medical director actively involved in reviewing all cardiac arrests and making quality improvements to the EMS system's response on a regular basis?
- Are the cardiac arrest events reported using the Recommended Guidelines for Uniform Reporting of Data from Out-of-Hospital Cardiac Arrest (The Utstein Style) so your community's data can be compared to the data of other progressive communities?

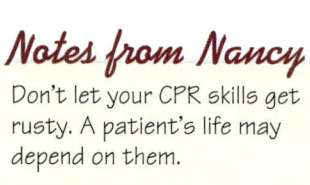

Notes from Nancy

Don't let your CPR skills get rusty. A patient's life may depend on them.

- How often does the code team practice its response and its teamwork in an effort to improve the success of future codes?

Guidelines 2005: A Reemphasis on Quality CPR

During the past 15 years the emphasis on quality CPR has seemed to slip as paramedics became more focused on intubation, drug administration, defibrillation, and other aspects of code management. Recent studies have shown that the quality of CPR is poor in both in-hospital and prehospital settings: The depth of compressions is inadequate, the rate of compressions is too slow, almost half the time no compressions are provided, the ventilations are too fast, and the chest is rarely allowed to

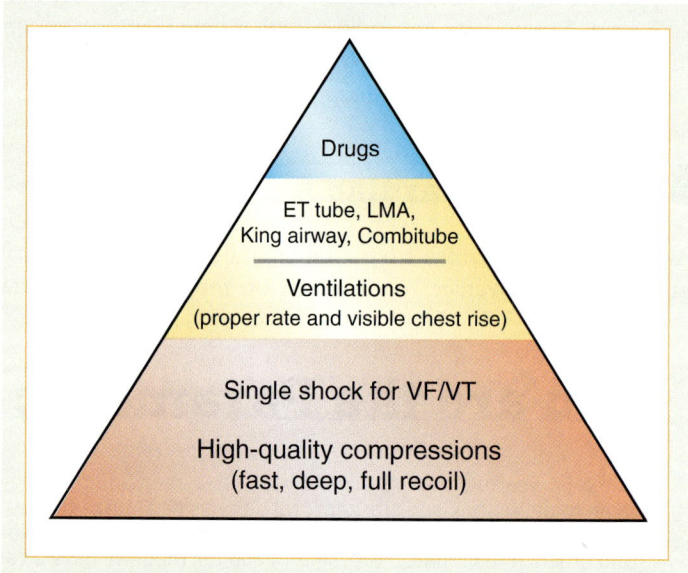

Figure A-2 The resuscitation pyramid. The success of a code relies on high-quality CPR.

fully recoil. Studies investigating the value of intubation and resuscitation drugs are inconclusive at best, but CPR is clearly important both before and after defibrillation. In addition, immediate CPR can double or triple the rate of survival from ventricular fibrillation (VF) sudden cardiac arrest.

The 2005 CPR guidelines reemphasize the importance of providing high-quality CPR (push hard and fast, and allow full chest recoil). In fact, the "resuscitation pyramid" is built on a strong base of high-quality CPR, as illustrated in **Figure A-2 ▲** . The recognition that a paramedic's best chance of succeeding at resuscitation hinges on continuous, uninterrupted high-quality CPR changes the focus of prehospital care. Today, given the renewed attention to high-quality CPR, the focus is on how to treat the patient without any interruptions in manual CPR.

As you arrive on the scene of the code, you need to clearly understand that the success of the code relies on high-quality compressions and not on an IV, an ET tube, or any drug in your box. Work together with the BLS providers, assist them, compliment their efforts, and relieve them as they tire but do not interrupt or disrupt their efforts!

The Steps of CPR

The basic life support steps of CPR for the adult patient follow the algorithm shown in **Figure A-3 ▼**. They presume that an AED is not immediately available at the patient's side. Integration of the AED will be discussed later in this appendix. Prehospital providers (first responders and paramedics) must be trained and prepared to provide either one-rescuer CPR or two-rescuer CPR as available personnel dictate.

In some instances, single-rescuer CPR may have been started before EMS personnel arrive. To help make CPR easier to learn, remember, and perform, the general public or "lay rescuers" are taught a universal compression–ventilation ratio of 30:2. They are not taught to take a pulse, to perform rescue breathing, or to perform two-rescuer CPR. Paramedics should be thrilled and thankful to arrive on the scene and find a bystander who is both properly trained and willing to provide CPR. Unfortunately, studies have shown that bystander CPR is performed in only one third or fewer of witnessed cardiac arrests and that when performed, even by health care providers, it is not done well. Bystanders who have been trained previously in CPR are often reluctant to begin this procedure for the following reasons:

- CPR steps may have been too complicated and included too many steps to remember. The 2005 guidelines made a significant effort to simplify the steps taught to the public.
  - Training methods may have been inadequate, and skill retention typically declines very rapidly after a course. This issue is being studied to try to determine which methods of training will produce the greatest skill retention. A video-based watch-and-do method, as opposed to watch-then-do, has been incorporated into many course revisions.
  - Some members of the public may be afraid of transmitted diseases and therefore may be reluctant to perform mouth-to-mouth resuscitation. Although the 2005 guidelines strongly emphasize that the risk of transmission of infection is very low, those who are still concerned are encouraged to use barrier devices. In addition, the technique of compression-only CPR is encouraged for those who are reluctant to do ventilations and for dispatcher-assisted CPR instruction.

Single-Rescuer CPR

Tom immediately began single-rescuer CPR when his teammate Jim dropped suddenly on the basketball court. The steps are shown in **Skill Drill A-1 ▶**.

1. Establish unresponsiveness. If there is no movement or response to shouting and shaking the adult patient, then the patient is considered "unresponsive."
   - If you are by yourself, phone 9-1-1 (or the emergency number) and make sure the AED is immediately available.
   - If there is a second rescuer, send him or her to call 9-1-1 (or the emergency number) and get the AED.
2. Open the airway **Step 1**. Use the head tilt–chin lift method unless trauma to the neck is suspected, in which case the jaw-thrust maneuver may be more appropriate.

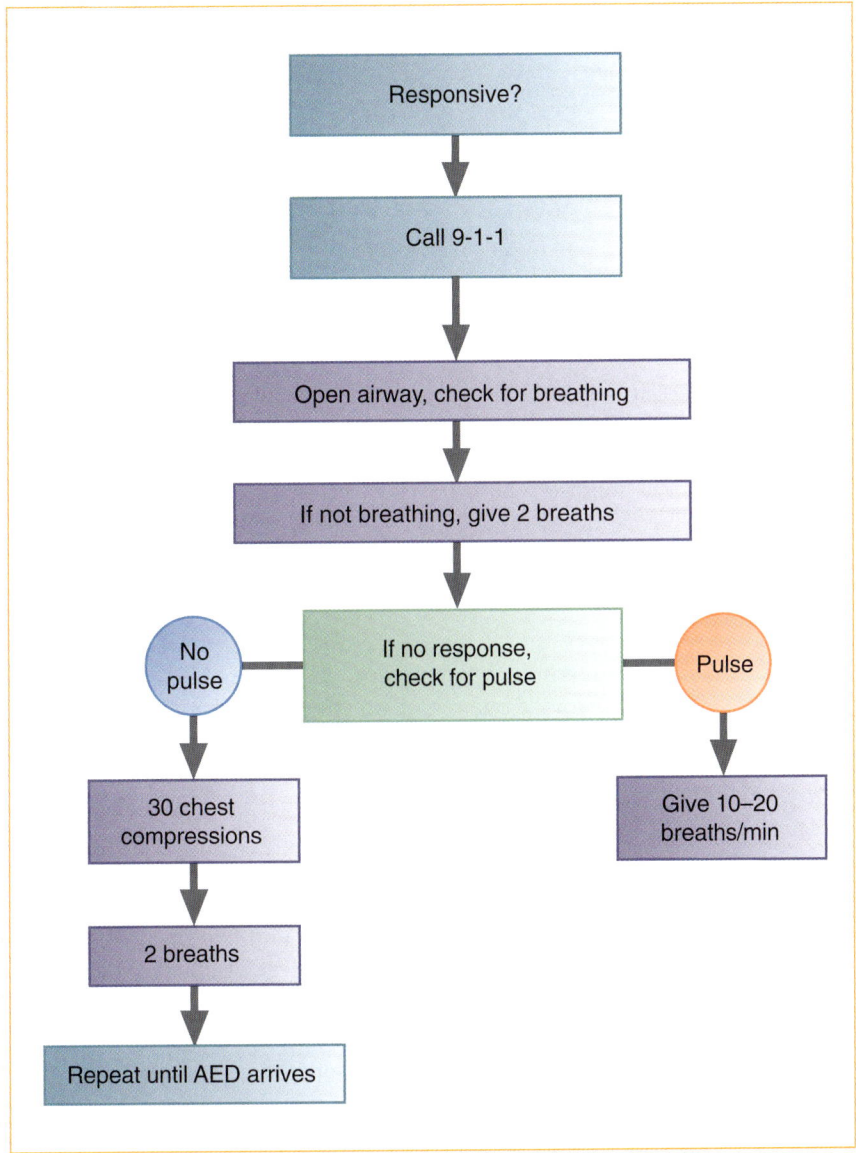

Figure A-3 The BLS adult health care provider algorithm.

Skill Drill A-1: Single-Rescuer Adult CPR

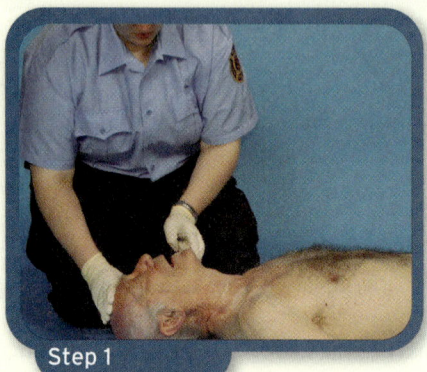

Step 1

Establish unresponsiveness. Open the airway.

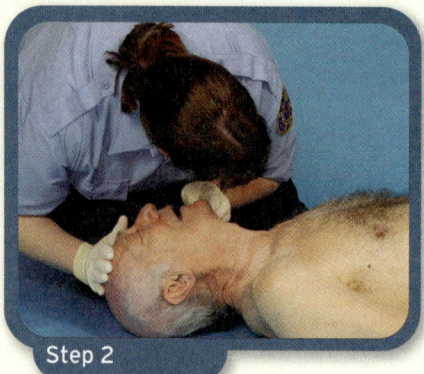

Step 2

Check for breathing (look, listen, and feel). If no breaths, administer two breaths, each 1 second, achieving visible chest rise.

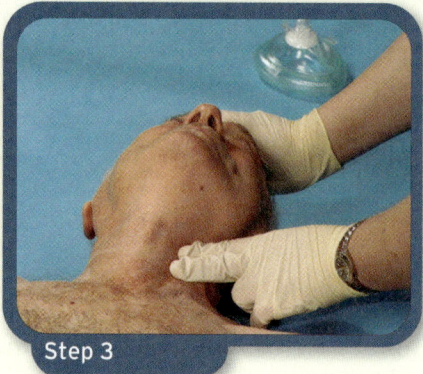

Step 3

Perform a carotid pulse check (maximum of 10 seconds).

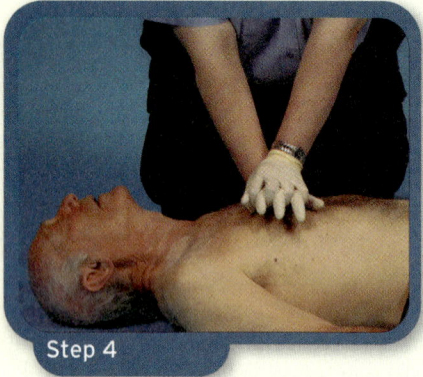

Step 4

Begin 30 compressions—centre of the chest, push hard and fast (rate of 100/min), and allow full chest recoil.

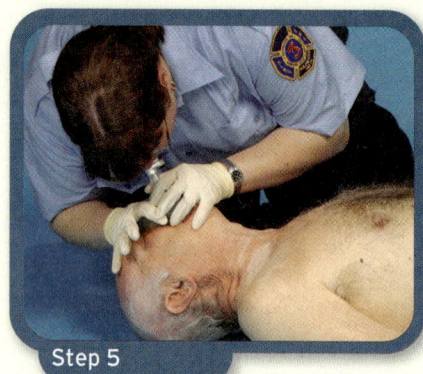

Step 5

Ventilate two times for 1 second each to achieve visible chest rise. Complete five cycles (approximately 2 minutes) and reassess the patient for a maximum of 10 seconds. If AED has arrived, attach it without interrupting compressions.

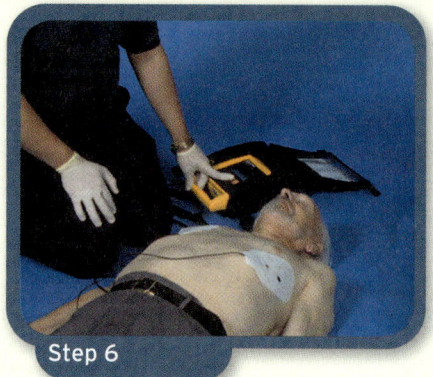

Step 6

Check the patient's rhythm.
If it is shockable, administer a single shock and then resume CPR immediately for five cycles. Reanalyze the rhythm.
If it is not shockable, resume CPR immediately for five cycles.

---

3. Check for breathing (**Step 2**). Look, listen, and feel for 5 seconds to a maximum of 10 seconds.

- If there is no breathing, give two rescue breaths over 1 second each to achieve a visible chest rise. Do not over-ventilate the patient, as it can cause gastric distention and regurgitation.
- If the patient is breathing or resumes effective breathing, place him or her in the recovery position and monitor closely.

4. Health care providers are taught to check for a carotid pulse in the adult for at least 5 seconds but to spend no more than 10 seconds trying to locate the pulse (**Step 3**). Compressions are delivered in the centre of the chest between the nipples with the heel of the hand and with the second hand on top of the first. Compressions on an adult should be provided at a rate of 100/min, pressing 4 to 5 cm and ensuring full chest recoil after each compression.

- If a pulse were present, the health care provider would provide one rescue breath every 5 to 6 seconds.
- If no pulse were present, the health care provider would begin chest compressions (**Step 4**). All compressors will eventually get tired. As help becomes available, be prepared to change compressors without interrupting compressions every 2 minutes.

5. Continue the cycles of 30 compressions (push hard and fast, and allow full chest recoil) and two breaths (**Step 5**) (1-second duration each to achieve visible chest rise) until the AED or defibrillator arrives.

6. Check the patient's rhythm (**Step 6**) once the AED arrives, with the least amount of interruption in chest compressions as possible.

- If it is a shockable rhythm, administer a single shock, resume CPR immediately for five cycles (approximately 2 minutes), and then reanalyze the rhythm.

■ If it is not a shockable rhythm, resume CPR immediately for five cycles (approximately 2 minutes). Continue until ALS providers take over or the patient starts to move. The health care provider would determine whether the patient has a pulse at this point.

Two-Rescuer CPR

Two-rescuer adult CPR provides the same cycle of 30 compressions to every two breaths as in the single-rescuer technique. Because the work is split between the two rescuers, it is more efficient and there is less interruption in the chest compressions to provide the ventilations. If an advanced airway has been inserted, asynchronous compressions and ventilations are possible. That is, the compressor simply presses hard, fast, and with full chest recoil at the rate of 100/min while the ventilator provides one breath (over 1 second's time, while observing for visible chest rise) every 6 to 8 seconds.

When you are using the two-rescuer technique, rotate the compressor every 2 minutes. To do so, ask the bystander to continue to assist and kneel on the other side of the patient. Now you can have an "active compressor" and an "on-deck compressor" who is ready to take over after the five cycles or 2-minute interval. Studies of rescuer fatigue show that the compressor tires after 2 to 5 minutes and that the quality of compressions will suffer if the compressor is not replaced. The steps in two-rescuer CPR are outlined here and in **Skill Drill A-2 ▾** :

1. Establish unresponsiveness. Send a helper to phone 9-1-1 and get the AED.

Skill Drill A-2: Two-Rescuer Adult CPR

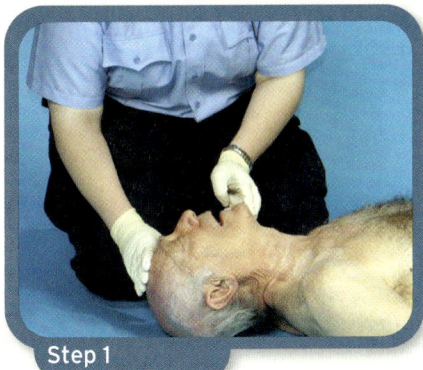

Step 1

Establish unresponsiveness. Open the airway.

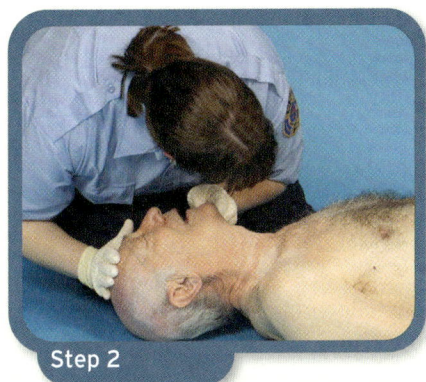

Step 2

Check for breathing. If there are no breaths, administer two breaths, each 1 second, achieving visible chest rise.

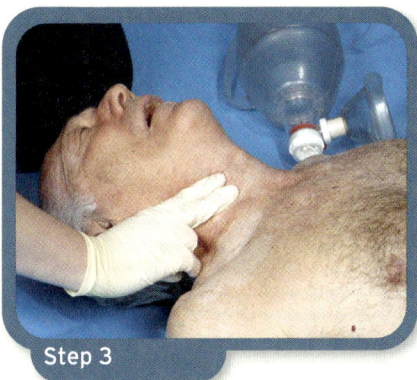

Step 3

Perform a carotid pulse check (maximum of 10 seconds).

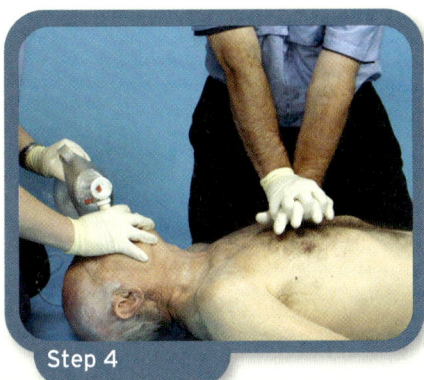

Step 4

One rescuer begins 30 compressions, counting out loud.

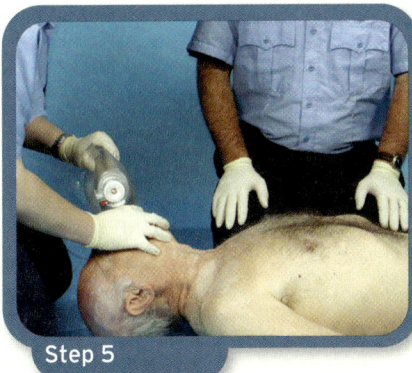

Step 5

Second rescuer ventilates two times and applies the AED pads while waiting. Complete five cycles and reassess the patient for a maximum of 10 seconds.

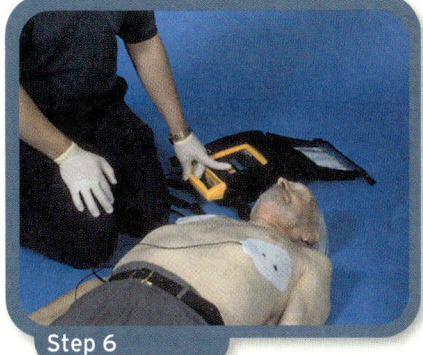

Step 6

Analyze the patient's ECG rhythm.

If it is shockable, administer a single shock at the device-specific dose. If it is nonshockable or immediately following the shock (unless the patient wakes up), begin five cycles of 30 compressions to two ventilations.

Repeat cycles of compressions/ventilations and AED shocks.

2. Open the airway using the head tilt–chin lift maneuver (Step 1).

3. Check for breathing (look, listen, and feel) (Step 2). If there are no breaths, administer two breaths, each 1 second in duration and achieving visible chest rise.

4. The health care provider should perform a carotid pulse check for 5 seconds (maximum of 10 seconds) (Step 3).

5. One rescuer begins 30 compressions—centre of the chest, push hard and fast (rate of 100/min), and allow full chest recoil (Step 4). Count out loud so the second rescuer is prepared to ventilate as you get to "28 and 29 and 30."

6. The second rescuer ventilates two times, each 1 second in duration and achieving visible chest rise (Step 5). The ventilator should use a bag-valve-mask device with supplementary oxygen and an OPA. Position yourself approximately 45 cm above the head of the supine patient to allow for the proper "E-C" or "OK" hand position and mask seal. During the waiting time, the second rescuer could apply the AED pads so it is ready to analyze at the 2-minute point.

7. Complete five cycles (approximately 2 minutes) and reassess the patient for a maximum of 10 seconds. If the AED has arrived and is attached, analyze the patient's ECG rhythm to determine whether it is shockable or nonshockable (Step 6).

8. If it is a shockable rhythm, administer a single shock at the device-specific dose. Ensure that all parties are clear prior to administering the shock. ("I'm clear, you're clear, we're all clear.")

9. If it is a nonshockable rhythm or immediately following the shock (unless the patient wakes up), begin five cycles (approximately 2 minutes) of 30 compressions to two ventilations.

10. Repeat Steps 7, 8, and 9 until ALS arrives and takes over or the medical director orders otherwise. As additional help arrives, prepare for transport or contact direct medical control.

Note: Once an advanced airway has been inserted, the compressions and ventilations are no longer in cycles. Instead, they are asynchronous, with the compressor providing 100/min without pauses for breaths and the ventilator giving 8 to 10 breaths/min (every 6 to 8 seconds). The compressor will get tired so be prepared to switch compressors every 2 minutes with no more than 10-second pauses, if any.

Modification in Technique for Children

Definitions

The age-old question raised to the pediatricians has been "For the purposes of resuscitation, what age defines a child?" Many pediatricians would simply say, "If the patient looks like a child, then he or she is a child; if the patient looks like an adult, then he or she is an adult." This vagueness is further complicated by the epidemic of childhood obesity. The 2005 guidelines use the following definitions of age groups for the purposes of resuscitation:

- **Newly born**—the infant at time of birth
- **Neonate**—the infant until discharge from the initial hospitalization
- **Infant**—younger than 1 year
- **Child**
  - health care providers: age 1 year to adolescence (signs of puberty or secondary sexual characteristic development)
  - lay rescuers: ages 1 to 8
- **Adult**—adolescent and older

This appendix concentrates on infant, child, and adult patients. The care of newly born and neonatal patients is discussed in Chapter 40.

Child CPR

The technique of CPR has a few slight variations for children, as shown below in italics. (**Skill Drill A-3 ▶**) shows the steps of one-rescuer child CPR.

1. Establish unresponsiveness. If there is no movement or response to *tapping and asking loudly "Are you okay?"* the child is unresponsive.
   - Send someone to phone 9-1-1 (or the emergency number) and get the AED.
   - If you are a lone rescuer *for a sudden collapse,* phone 9-1-1 (or the emergency number) and get the AED.
   - If you are a lone rescuer and it was not a sudden collapse, proceed to the next step.

2. Open the airway (Step 1). Use the head tilt–chin lift method unless trauma to the neck is suspected, in which case the jaw-thrust maneuver may be more appropriate.

3. Check for breathing (Step 2). Look, listen, and feel for a maximum of 10 seconds.
   - If there is no breathing, give two *effective* rescue breaths over 1 second each to achieve a visible chest rise. Do not over-ventilate the patient, as it can cause gastric distension and regurgitation. *Use a child-sized bag-valve-mask* device with supplementary oxygen, implement an oropharyngeal airway, and position the second rescuer or ventilator approximately 45 cm above the supine child's head. Use the "E-C" or "OK" method to ensure proper mask seal.
   - If the patient is breathing or resumes effective breathing, place him or her in the recovery position and monitor closely.

4. At this point the lay rescuer begins compressions. Health care providers are taught to check for a carotid pulse in the child (as long as they do not exceed 10 seconds) (Step 3).

Compressions are delivered in the centre of the chest between the nipples with the heel of *either one hand or both hands as in the adult technique.* They should be provided at a rate of 100/min, pressing *one third to one half the depth of the chest* and ensuring full chest recoil after each compression Step 4 .

- If a pulse is present, the health care provider gives one rescue breath *every 3 to 5 seconds* Step 5 .
- If no pulse is present, the health care provider begins chest compressions. Be prepared to change compressors every 2 minutes.

5. *If not already done, phone 9-1-1 (or the emergency number) and get the AED.*

6. Continue the cycles of 30 compressions (push hard and fast, and allow full chest recoil) and two breaths (1-second duration each to achieve visible chest rise) until the AED or defibrillator arrives. *If there are two rescuers, health care providers are taught to give cycles of 15 compressions to two ventilations.*

7. Check the patient's rhythm once the AED arrives, with the least amount of interruption in chest compressions as possible Step 6 . *If the child is between 1 and 8 years old, use child pads if available. If the AED has a key or switch to deliver a child shock dose, activate it to decrease the energy level. If no child pads are available, use adult pads.*

- If there is a shockable rhythm, administer a single shock. Resume CPR immediately for five cycles (approximately 2 minutes), and then reanalyze the rhythm.
- If there is not a shockable rhythm, resume CPR immediately for five cycles (approximately 2 minutes). The public is trained to continue until ALS paramedics take over or the child starts to move. The health care provider would determine whether the patient has a pulse at this point.

Skill Drill A-4 ▶ shows the steps of two-rescuer child CPR, also summarized here.

1. Establish unresponsiveness, and send a helper to phone 9-1-1 and get the AED. If there is no helper, continue with the steps of CPR and then phone and look for an AED at the 2-minute point.

2. Open the airway using the head tilt–chin lift maneuver Step 1 .

3. Check for breathing (look, listen, and feel) Step 2 . If there are no breaths, administer two effective breaths, each lasting 1 second and achieving visible chest rise.

4. Perform a carotid pulse check (maximum of 10 seconds) Step 3 .

5. One rescuer begins 15 compressions—centre of the chest, push hard and fast (rate of 100/min), and allow full chest

You are the Paramedic Part 2

During the first 2 minutes of CPR with Tom and the first responders, a lot of teamwork has been going on. Tom is beginning to tire yet still wants to stay involved, so he becomes the "on-deck compressor." Another first responder has placed the AED next to Jim and relieved Tom; he becomes the compressor. Because Tom has been shown how to apply the AED electrodes, he is able to work around the compressor.

After approximately 2 minutes (five cycles) of CPR, a brief pause in care allows the team to analyze Jim's ECG. The AED begins to charge up, displaying a shockable rhythm such as ventricular fibrillation. In the meantime, Tom administers a few more compressions, and the ventilator removes the bag-valve-mask so oxygen does not flow near the patient. The first responder at the AED states, "I'm clear, you're clear, we're all clear," and proceeds to deliver a single shock. Jim's heavy body bounces on the hardwood floor but he does not awaken. The code team immediately begins the next five cycles of 30 compressions and two ventilations.

Vital Signs	Recording Time: 3 Minutes
Skin	Pale and clammy
Pulse	None palpable at carotid
Blood pressure	None
Respirations	Being ventilated with a bag-valve-mask device

Previously, the duration of time from stopping compressions to analyzing to charging and providing the traditional three-shock series would have been almost 2 minutes of no chest compressions. No perfusion of the brain and vital organs occurs when there is no circulation from rescuers compressing the chest properly. Every pause in compressions, even when it lasts for as little as a few seconds, requires the next few compressions to reprime the pump. For this reason, a pause to analyze the rhythm should last no longer than 10 seconds without chest compressions.

When a patient has a shockable rhythm and does respond appropriately to a shock, it often takes a minute or so for return of spontaneous circulation (ROSC). Unless the patient actually wakes up, immediately after the shock the rescuers should begin CPR with chest compressions.

3. What should you do next as the paramedic on the scene?
4. What is the advantage to perfusion and chest compressions from inserting an advanced airway during two-rescuer CPR?

Skill Drill A-3: Single-Rescuer Child CPR

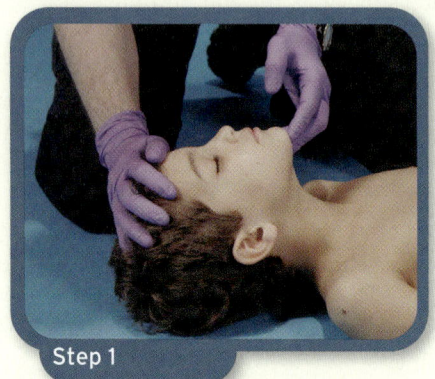

Step 1

Establish unresponsiveness. Open the airway.

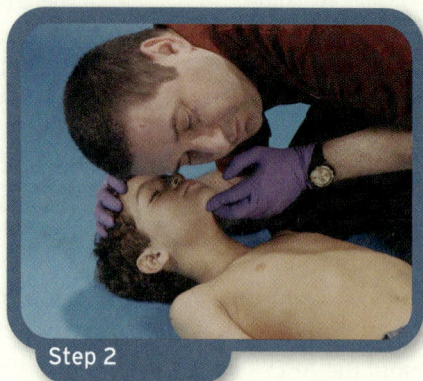

Step 2

Check for breathing (look, listen, and feel). If no breaths, administer two effective breaths.

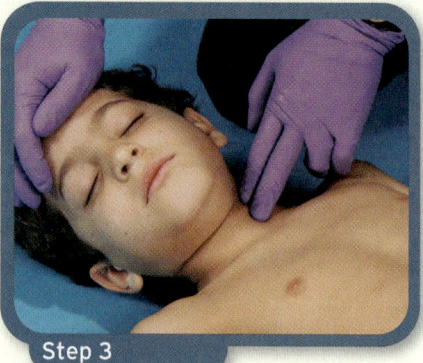

Step 3

Perform a carotid pulse check for 5 seconds (maximum of 10 seconds).

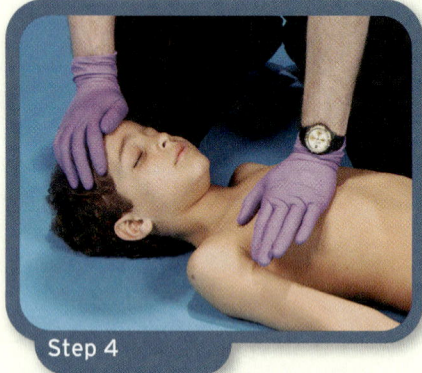

Step 4

Begin 30 compressions—centre of the chest, push hard and fast (rate of 100/min), and allow full chest recoil—using either one or two hands depending on the child's size. Compress one third to one half the depth of the chest.

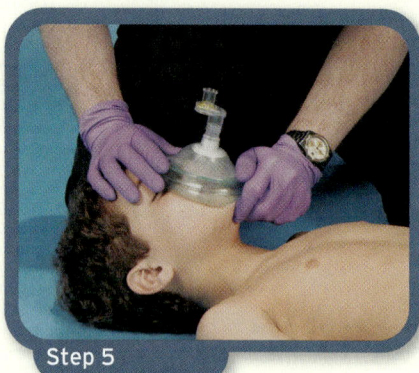

Step 5

Ventilate two times for 1 second each to achieve visible chest rise. Use a child-sized pocket mask with a one-way valve.

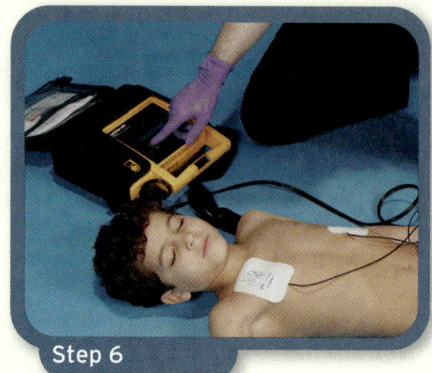

Step 6

Complete five cycles (approximately 2 minutes) and reassess the patient for a maximum of 10 seconds. If the AED has arrived, attach it, using child pads if the child is between 1 and 8 years old. Decrease the AED energy level. Analyze the rhythm.

If the rhythm is shockable, administer a single shock and then resume CPR immediately for five cycles. Reanalyze the rhythm.

If the rhythm is not shockable, resume CPR immediately for five cycles.

recoil (**Step 4**). Count out loud so the second rescuer is prepared to ventilate as you get to "13 and 14 and 15."

6. The second rescuer ventilates two times, each lasting 1 second and achieving visible chest rise (**Step 5**). The ventilator should use a child-sized bag-valve-mask device with supplementary oxygen and an OPA. Position yourself approximately 45 cm above the head of the supine patient to allow for the proper "E-C" or "OK" hand position and mask seal. During the waiting time, the second rescuer could apply the AED pads so the AED is ready to analyze at the 2-minute point.

7. Complete five cycles (approximately 2 minutes) and reassess the patient for a maximum of 10 seconds. If the

AED has arrived and is attached, analyze the patient's ECG rhythm to determine whether it is shockable or nonshockable (**Step 6**). If the child is between 1 and 8 years old, use child pads if available. If the AED has a key or switch to deliver a child shock dose, activate it to decrease the energy level.

8. If there is a shockable rhythm, administer a single shock at the device-specific dose (200 J is the default). Ensure that all parties are clear prior to administering the shock. ("I'm clear, you're clear, we're all clear.")

9. If there is a nonshockable rhythm or immediately following the shock (unless the patient wakes up), begin

Skill Drill A-4: Two-Rescuer Child CPR

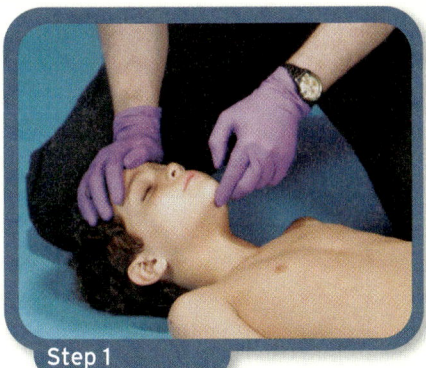

Step 1

Establish unresponsiveness. Open the airway.

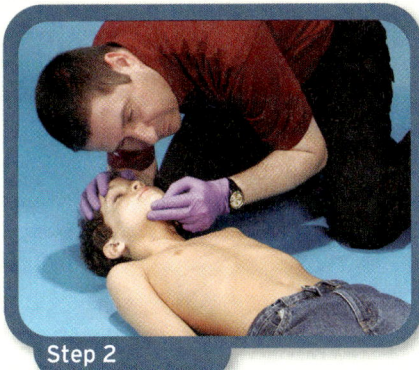

Step 2

Check for breathing (look, listen, and feel). If no breaths, administer two effective breaths.

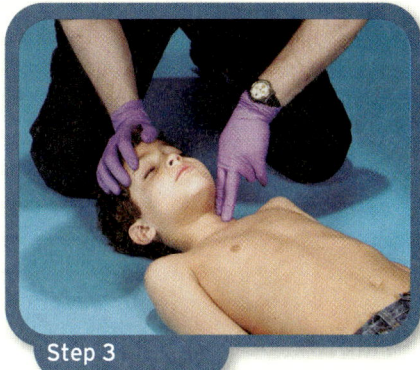

Step 3

Perform a carotid pulse check (maximum of 10 seconds).

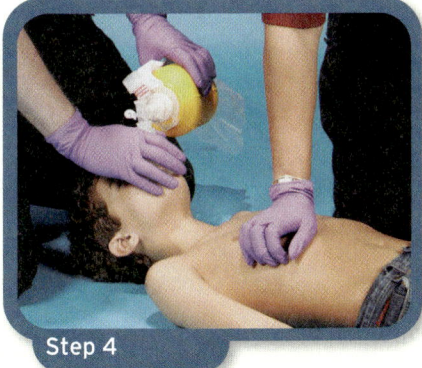

Step 4

One rescuer begins 15 compressions—centre of the chest, push hard and fast (rate of 100/min) and allow full chest recoil.

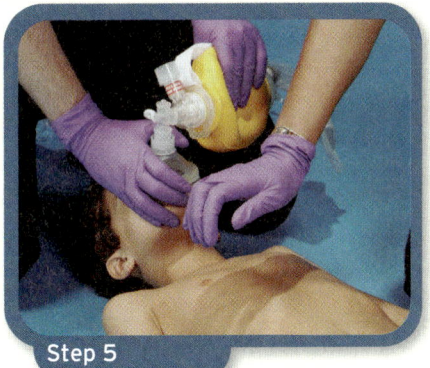

Step 5

The second rescuer ventilates two times for 1 second each to achieve visible chest rise. The ventilator should use a child-sized bag-valve-mask device with supplementary oxygen and an oropharyngeal airway. Position yourself approximately 45 cm above the head of the supine patient to allow for the proper hand position/mask seal.

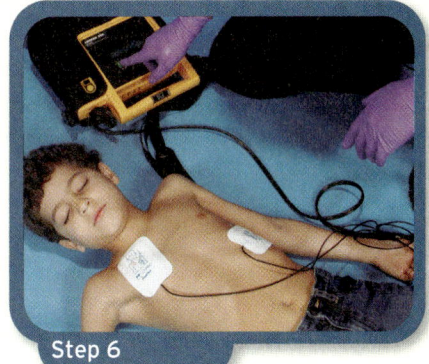

Step 6

Complete five cycles (approximately 2 minutes) and reassess the patient for a maximum of 10 seconds. If an AED has arrived and is attached, analyze the patient's ECG rhythm. Use child pads if the child is between 1 and 8 years old. Decrease the AED energy level.

If the rhythm is shockable, administer a single shock.

If the rhythm is not shockable or immediately following the shock, begin five cycles of 15 compressions to two ventilations.

five cycles (approximately 2 minutes) of 15 compressions to two ventilations.

10. Repeat Steps 7, 8, and 9 until ALS arrives and takes over or the medical director orders otherwise. As additional help arrives, prepare for transport or contact direct medical control.

Note: Once an advanced airway has been inserted, the compressions and ventilations are no longer in cycles. Instead, they are asynchronous with the compressor providing 100/min without pauses for breaths and the ventilator giving 8 to 10 breaths/min (every 6 to 8 seconds). Because the compressor will inevitably get tired, switch compressors every 2 minutes with no more than 10-second pauses, if any.

Infant CPR

The technique of CPR for an infant has a few slight variations (shown in italics below), as described in **Skill Drill A-5 ▶** .

1. Establish unresponsiveness. If there is no movement or response to *tapping and asking loudly "Are you okay?"* you *may consider flicking the infant's heels with your fingertips.* If there is no response, the infant is then considered unresponsive.

   ■ Send someone to phone 9-1-1 (or the emergency number).

   ■ If you are a lone rescuer, proceed to the next step.

2. Open the airway Step 1 . Use the head tilt–chin lift method (*do not hyperextend the neck*) unless trauma to the

Skill Drill A-5: Infant CPR

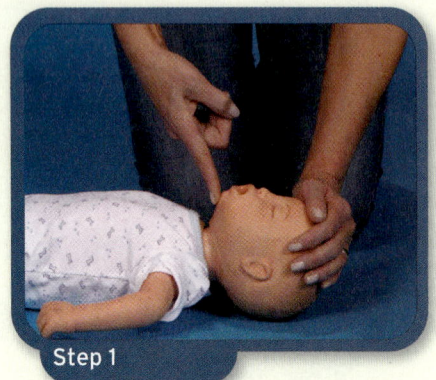

Step 1

Establish unresponsiveness. Open the airway.

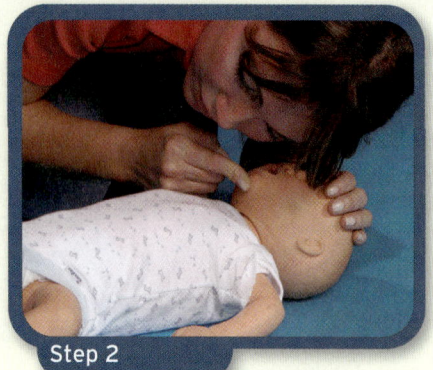

Step 2

Check for breathing.

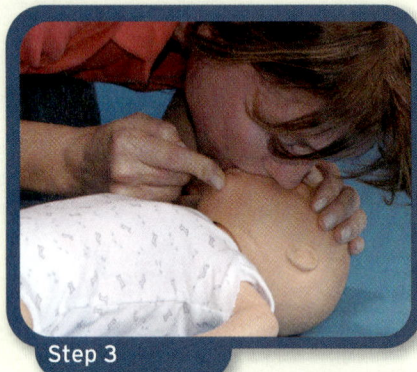

Step 3

If there is no breathing, give two *effective* rescue breaths over 1 second each to achieve a visible chest rise.
    Check for a *brachial or femoral pulse in the infant* (do not exceed 10 seconds).

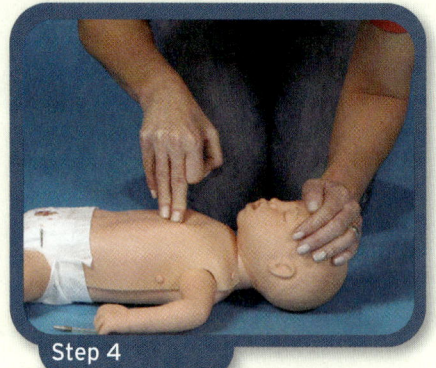

Step 4

Give compressions at a rate of 100 per minute to a depth of one third to one half the depth of the chest, allowing full chest recoil.

one half the depth of the chest and ensuring full chest recoil after each compression (Step 4).

- If a pulse is present, the health care provider provides one rescue breath *every 3 to 5 seconds.*
- If no pulse is present, the health care provider begins chest compressions. All compressors will inevitably get tired, so be prepared to change compressors without interrupting compressions every 2 minutes.

5. *If not already done, phone 9-1-1 (or the emergency number).*

6. Continue the cycles of 30 compressions (push hard and fast, and allow full chest recoil) and two breaths (1-second duration each to achieve visible chest rise) until the ALS unit arrives. If there are two rescuers, health care providers are taught to provide cycles of 15 compressions to two ventilations. The compressions can be done using the two-hands encircling method (Figure A-4 ▶). Use of an AED is not recommended with an infant.

neck is suspected, in which case the jaw-thrust maneuver may be more appropriate.

3. Check for breathing (Step 2). Look, listen, and feel for a maximum of 10 seconds.
   - If there is no breathing, give two *effective* rescue breaths with a barrier device or appropriate-size pocket mask over 1 second each to achieve a visible chest rise. Do not over-ventilate the patient, as it can cause gastric distention and regurgitation.

4. At this point, the lay rescuer begins compressions. Health care providers check for a *brachial or femoral pulse in the infant* as long as they do not spend more than 10 seconds trying to locate the pulse (Step 3). Compressions are delivered in the centre of the chest just below the nipple line. *Use two fingers to compress.* Compressions on an infant should be provided at a rate of 100/min, pressing *one third to*

▌ Defibrillation

Early in the steps of CPR, a rescuer or helper is sent to fetch the AED. Many communities have placed AEDs in public places such as health clubs, public pools, concert halls, sports venues, airports, schools, and government buildings.

The AED has been shown to be an effective lifesaving treatment for adults and children older than 1 year. The AEDs used on children from 1 to 8 years of age usually will have a pediatric-sized electrode and some type of switch or attenuator device designed to reduce the amount of electricity delivered to the smaller-sized patient. The AEDs used on patients older than 8 years do not require attenuator devices and the adult electrodes are acceptable to use. These units are preprogrammed so that the user does not have to select a dose. Manual defibrillator units require the operator to select the appropriate dose.

Shockable Rhythms

The two shockable ECG rhythms are ventricular fibrillation (VF) and pulseless ventricular tachycardia (VT). When a patient is in a shockable rhythm, the heart is quivering but blood is not pumping. Defibrillation stuns the heart muscle momentarily and allows the patient's normal conduction system to resume control. If the patient is not defibrillated, the VF will ultimately deteriorate to asystole or flatline.

In the first moments of a cardiac arrest, when the patient is in VF or VT, the heart is oxygenated and "ready" to receive a shock. This explains why the rescuer should begin the steps of CPR and get the AED attached as quickly as possible. If a shock is recommended in this circumstance, administer it immediately—the chances of a successful defibrillation drop 7% to 10% for every minute that passes.

When the VF or VT is not "fresh," however, a rapid shock is not always the best initial treatment. When a patient is in cardiac arrest for an interval of 4 to 5 minutes or longer, even if the initial ECG showed a shockable rhythm, the success rate is poor because the heart is no longer "ready" for a shock. Instead, perfusion and oxygenation are needed first. The 2005 guidelines state that it would be more appropriate to begin the steps of CPR, proceeding with five cycles or approximately 2 minutes of 30 compressions to two ventilations, and then analyze the patient's ECG. If the patient is still in VF or VT at this point, he or she would be ready for a dose of electricity.

Shock First or Compressions First?

The decision to deliver a shock first versus provide CPR compressions first is a local direct medical control policy decision. Many medical directors implement a policy similar to the following:

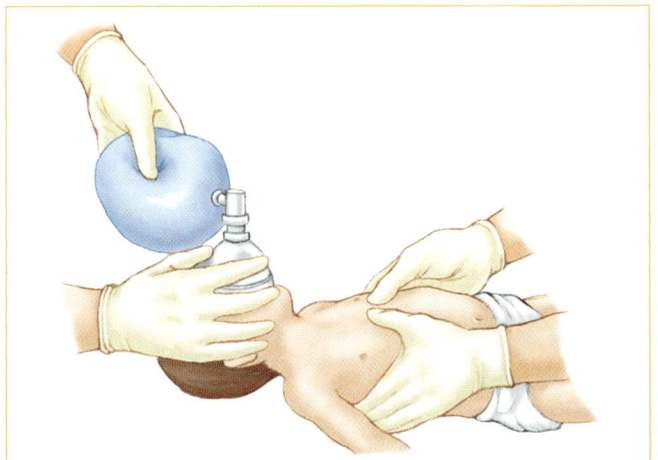

Figure A-4 The primary method of providing chest compressions to the infant when there are two rescuers is to use the two-hands chest encircling method. Compress one third to one half the depth of the chest just below the imaginary line between the nipples.

Controversies

What Happened to the Gold Standard of Airway Care?

The use of advanced airway devices seems to be deemphasized in the 2005 guidelines—particularly the use of the endotracheal (ET) tube, which previously was considered the "gold standard." When used by skilled BLS paramedics, bag-valve-mask ventilation with supplementary oxygen can be as effective as an ET tube in terms of oxygenation, ventilation, and protection from aspiration for short transportation times.

Many service medical directors have been reluctant to train their first responders in the optional endotracheal intubation skill because of the marginal results when the skill is not practiced frequently. In the past, unrecognized, uncorrected esophageal intubations or tube dislodgements occurred with unacceptable frequency. One study of paramedics providing pediatric intubations in the prehospital environment revealed that 8% of patients arriving at the emergency department had a tube in their esophagus. Another study in a large adult group of cardiac arrests found that 25% of the tubes were in the esophagus or pharynx. As a consequence, airway options now favour good bag-valve-mask ventilation technique and use of easier-to-insert devices such as the laryngeal mask airway (LMA), King airway, Combitube, or similar airways.

- If the paramedic witnesses the cardiac arrest and has the AED in hand, he or she should analyze the rhythm first and, if it is a shockable rhythm, proceed with a shock.
- If the cardiac arrest is not witnessed by the paramedic, then five cycles (2 minutes) of CPR should be performed prior to analyzing and then shocking the patient if the AED recommends it.
- The decision of whether to count bystander CPR as the first 2 minutes is a judgment call. If you enter the room and observe high-quality compressions being performed (at the proper rate and depth, and with full chest recoil), it probably makes the most sense to allow the bystander to finish out the 2 minutes, unless he or she is tiring, and apply the electrodes around the compressor. Then, at the 2-minute point, you will be ready to analyze and shock, if recommended.

The success rate for a biphasic dose is excellent (better than 93%) if the heart is ready to receive the shock. The three-shock series of defibrillation that was taught prior to 2005 no longer makes sense because it would mean delaying compressions for the sake of two additional shocks that will probably not work at this point. If the shock does not work, the patient needs 2 minutes of high-quality CPR. The health care provider can then quickly reanalyze the rhythm and shock as recommended by the device.

Effective Shocks and Special Circumstances

When a shock is effective, occasionally the patient wakes up. That result is dramatic, of course, but the majority of the effective defibrillations will take a minute or so to produce an effective return of circulation. For this reason, as soon as the patient is defibrillated, you should immediately begin compressions. Don't be surprised if the patient does begin to move after a minute or so; you can then cease the compressions and check for a pulse, respirations, and blood pressure.

Because defibrillator pads or electrodes are safer, paddles are rarely used today. Instead, the patient's ECG is monitored and displayed throughout the arrest—not just when taking a "quick look" or when asking the AED to analyze the rhythm. Thus it is possible to observe VF or VT while compressions are being done and begin to charge up the unit. Once the AED is fully charged, the operator should clear all rescuers and deliver the shock. With this approach, compressions can be delivered while the unit is charging, which minimizes the interruption.

The code team member who delivers the shock *must* always first clear the patient! It is also recommended that the ventilation device be removed from the patient mask or detached from the advanced airway to prevent oxygen from flowing across the patient's chest while a shock is being delivered, as the simultaneous delivery poses a fire hazard.

You should review the following special circumstances for defibrillation and understand the solutions or modifications to the procedure should they arise:

- **The patient is an infant.** Use a manual defibrillator with the proper paddles or pads and appropriate dose per your pediatric protocols.
- **The patient has a hairy chest and the electrodes will not stick.** Quickly shave the patient just as you would to do a 12-lead ECG.
- **The patient is submersed in water or soaking wet.** Get out of the rain, quickly move the patient to your office (the ambulance), or remove the patient from the pool and dry him or her off prior to applying the electrodes or shocking.
- **The patient has an AICD or pacemaker.** Avoid these devices by a few centimetres when placing the electrodes.
- **The patient has a transdermal medication patch on the chest.** Quickly remove the patch and wipe the chest dry. Be aware that you can absorb nitroglycerin into your own skin if you do not use disposable gloves.

The Adult Pulseless Arrest Algorithm

The algorithm used to manage an adult in cardiac arrest builds on the BLS adult health care provider algorithm discussed earlier in this appendix. After making sure the patient has been placed on supplementary oxygen, the monitor or defibrillator is used to determine whether the patient is still in a shockable rhythm. The algorithm **Figure A-5 ▶** separates the treatment

Controversies

Advanced Airways

In some settings, the LMA, King airway, and Combitube are superior to bag-valve-mask ventilation and oxygenation. Surprisingly, research shows that these devices are equivalent to the ET tube in the adult patient. In addition, the Combitube and King airway offer protection from aspiration of the stomach contents into the lungs. The LMA, King airway, and Combitube are similar in several ways:

- They are advanced airway techniques that are inserted blindly.
- They are placed orally and inserted past the hypopharyngeal space.
- They are easy to use and do not require extensive training in laryngoscopy.

Training selected paramedics on the use of these devices may expand the number of patients who are afforded an advanced airway when one is needed.

approach into two basic pathways: shockable rhythms (VF or VT) or nonshockable rhythms (asystole or pulseless electrical activity).

The key difference in management from the past approaches is that some preplanning is done so that the medications are drawn up and ready to administer prior to the rhythm checks. The medications are administered during CPR and compressions need not stop for this treatment.

As long as the patient has an effective BLS airway and is being adequately ventilated, placement of an advanced airway (ET tube, LMA, King airway, or Combitube)—although helpful—should never take priority over delivery of high-quality compressions or a shock when needed. Practice your intubation techniques so you are able to insert the advanced airway device with no more than a 10-second interruption in chest compressions.

At the Scene

IV or IO?

The 2005 guidelines expanded the use of intraosseous (IO) access beyond children to adults. The algorithm for the adult pulseless arrest patient clearly states that IO is an acceptable type of access to the patient's circulation. Due to the hollow nature of the long bones, infused fluids or medications administered by the IO route will reach the central circulation as fast as those injected into a central venous line (eg, internal jugular or subclavian vein). With the introduction of newer, easier-to-use IO devices such as the FAST1 for the sternum site and the bone injection gun (BIG) and EZ-IO bone drill for the leg, use of IO cannulation is becoming more common in the cardiac arrest patient.

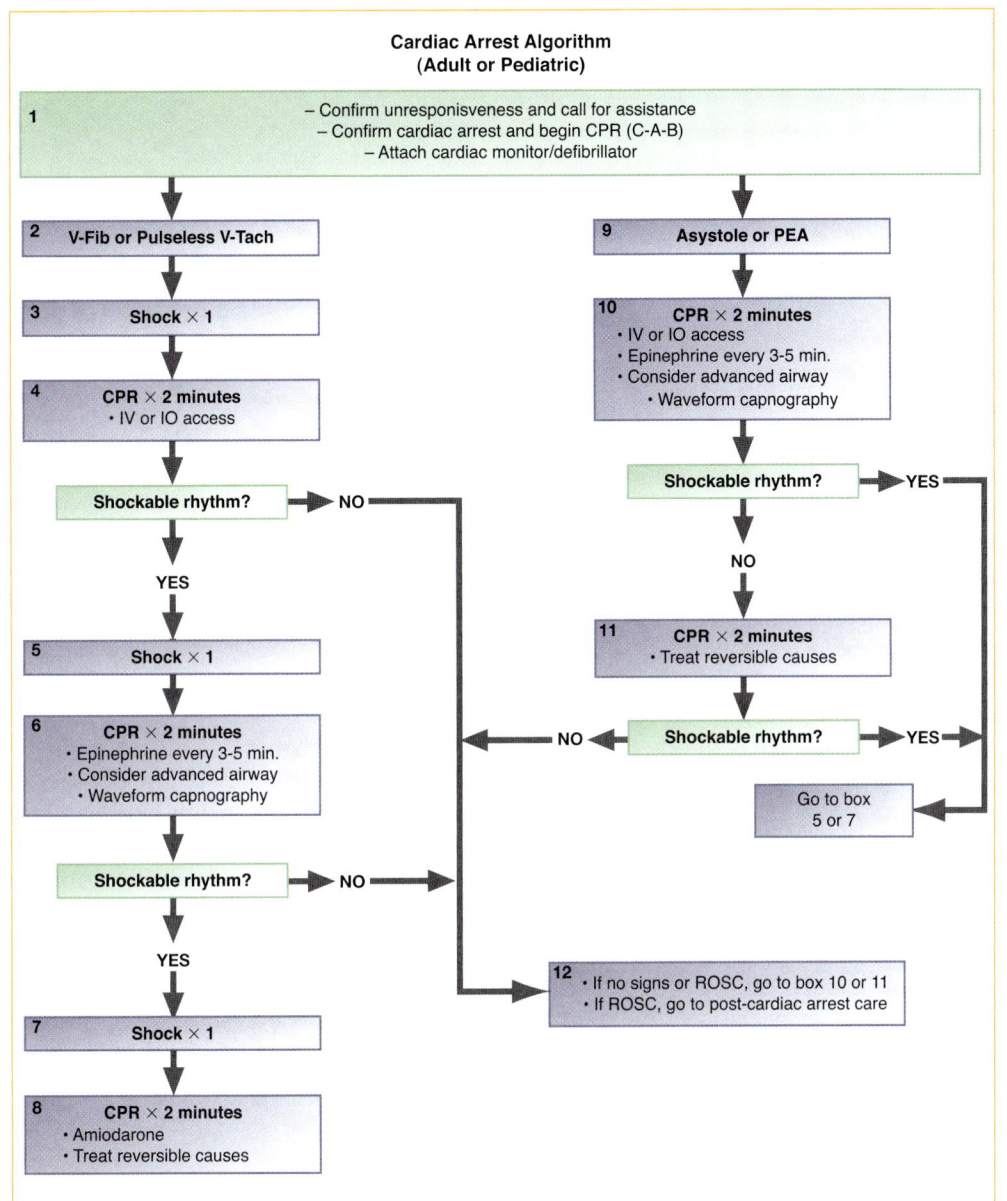

Figure A-5 The pulseless arrest algorithm from the 2010 guidelines.

been administered, allow it to circulate and then reanalyze the patient at the next 2-minute point. If the patient remains in a shockable rhythm, administer another shock.

Managing Patients in Asystole or Pulseless Electrical Activity

This arm of the algorithm calls for the paramedic to provide CPR and do a rhythm check at each 2-minute point. If the patient is in a nonshockable rhythm, such as asystole or pulseless electrical activity (PEA), the potential cause must be taken into consideration. The "Hs and Ts" listed in **Table A-1 ▸** are a good way to remember the causes of asystole or PEA. Some of these issues can be managed in the prehospital environment; others will require intervention in the emergency department.

If three rescuers are doing CPR (ventilator, active compressor, and on-deck compressor) and an advanced airway has been placed, the compressions and ventilations can be asynchronous. Medications should be prepared and administered while doing CPR. A timekeeper can remind the code team leader what should be coming up in the next 30 seconds, in the next 15 seconds, and so on.

team leader what should be coming up in the next 30 seconds, in the next 15 seconds, and so on.

Drug therapy for VF or VT includes a vasopressor given every 3 to 5 minutes. The vasopressor of choice is 1 mg of epinephrine administered either IV or IO. A single dose of vasopressin 40 U IV or IO may be substituted for the first and/or second dose of epinephrine.

After the third shock, you may decide to administer an antiarrhythmic such as amiodarone (300 mg IV or IO once) or lidocaine (1 to 1.5 mg/kg first dose, then 0.5 to 0.75 mg/kg IV or IO, up to a maximum of 3 doses, or 3 mg/kg). If the patient has torsade de pointes, consider giving magnesium (loading dose 1 to 2 g IV or IO). After each drug has

Drug therapy for asystole and PEA includes a vasopressor every 3 to 5 minutes. The vasopressor of choice is 1 mg of epinephrine administered either IV or IO. A single dose of vasopressin 40 U IV or IO may be substituted for either the first or second epinephrine dose (but not both).

Consider administering atropine, 1 mg IV/IO, for asystole or a slow PEA rate of less than 60. This dose can be repeated every 3 to 5 minutes up to a maximum of three doses. If the patient changes to VF or VT at any point or when the rhythm is checked every five cycles of CPR (approximately 2 minutes), move back to the shockable side of the algorithm. After each drug has been administered, allow it to circulate and then reanalyze the patient at the next 2-minute point.

Table A-1	The "Hs and Ts": Factors Contributing to Cardiac Arrest	
▪ Hypovolemia	▪ Toxins	
▪ Hypoxia	▪ Tamponade, cardiac	
▪ Hydrogen ion (acidosis)	▪ Tension pneumothorax	
▪ Hypokalemia/hyperkalemia	▪ Thrombosis (coronary or pulmonary)	
▪ Hypoglycemia		
▪ Hypothermia	▪ Trauma	

leader what should be coming up in the next 30 seconds, in the next 15 seconds, and so on.

Drug therapy for asystole and PEA includes a vasopressor every 3 to 5 minutes. The vasopressor of choice is 1 mg of epinephrine administered either IV or IO. A single dose of vasopressin 40 U IV or IO may be substituted for either the first or second epinephrine dose (but not both).

Consider administering atropine, 1 mg IV/IO, for asystole or a slow PEA rate of less than 60. This dose can be repeated every 3 to 5 minutes up to a maximum of three doses. If the patient changes to VF or VT at any point or when the rhythm is checked every five cycles of CPR (approximately 2 minutes), move back to the shockable side of the algorithm. After each drug has been administered, allow it to circulate and then reanalyze the patient at the next 2-minute point.

Useful Adjuncts to Assist in the Return of Spontaneous Circulation

Several devices are available to provide feedback to rescuers on the quality of their compressions (rate, depth, and chest recoil). In addition, three devices hold considerable promise in improving the quality and consistency of the compressions as well as improving the blood flow during CPR: the impedance threshold device (ITD) and two mechanical compression adjuncts.

Impedance Threshold Device

The impedance threshold device (ITD) has been shown to enhance the vacuum in the chest, which forms during the chest recoil phase of CPR. Imagine a bellows fanning a fireplace. As the bellows opens to its full size, it sucks in air. A similar process occurs when the chest wall re-expands—the vacuum that results pulls air into the lungs and blood back into the heart. An ITD selectively prevents that unnecessary air from rushing into the chest, maximizing the vacuum during the recoil phase of the compression. This results in enhanced return of blood that increases cardiac output, blood pressure, and perfusion to vital organs. In theory, this may improve survival rates. Use of the ITD may improve circulation during CPR and may increase the return of spontaneous circulation in cardiac arrest patients. This device was considered acceptable and useful (a Class IIa rating) in the 2005 guidelines, but not yet considered definitive. It is currently the subject of an ongoing

large, multicentre prehospital trial to determine its true role in the management of a patient in cardiac arrest. Paramedics and first responders must remember that when the patient's pulse returns, the ITD should be removed from the ventilation system because it is designed to be used in conjunction with compressions and may impair blood flow, if not removed, when there is a return of spontaneous circulation **Figure A-6 ▸**.

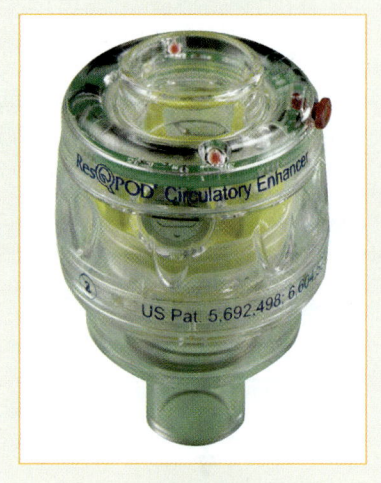

Figure A-6 The ResQPOD®, an impedance threshold device.

Load-Distributing Band CPR Device

The AutoPulse device is a mechanical device designed to deliver consistent, uninterrupted chest compressions and potentially improve hemodynamics during cardiac arrest. This automated, portable device squeezes the entire chest, thereby improving blood flow to the heart and brain during cardiac arrest **Figure A-7 ▾**. Its use can also free up rescuers to focus on other lifesaving interventions and eliminate fatigue from the performance of CPR chest compressions.

The AutoPulse can be integrated into a code as follows:

1. Ensure that CPR is in progress and that effective, high-quality compressions are being provided.
2. Align the patient on the AutoPulse platform.
3. Close the band over the patient's chest.
4. Press the start button (AutoPulse performs the compressions automatically).
5. Provide bag-valve-mask ventilation at a rate of two ventilations for every 30 compressions. Each ventilation should be given over 1 second to provide visible chest rise.

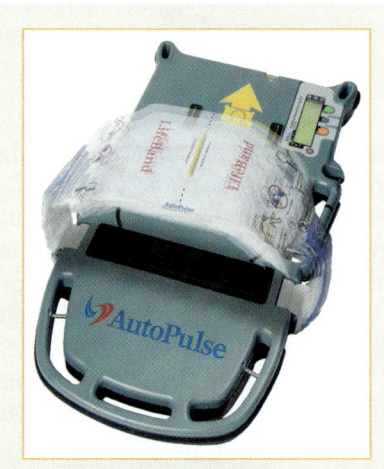

Figure A-7 The AutoPulse® noninvasive cardiac support pump.

6. If an advanced airway is in place (ET tube, LMA, King airway, or Combitube), there are no longer cycles of compressions to ventilations. The compression rate is a continuous 100/min; the ventilation rate is 8 to 10/min.

7. After 2 minutes of CPR, reassess for pulse and/or shockable rhythm (maximum of 10 seconds).

Thumper CPR Device

The Thumper Figure A-8 ▾ is an adjunct to CPR that provides both continuous chest compressions (100/min) and ventilations. It can be used with a pocket mask or an advanced airway. Because this device is powered by oxygen and delivers oxygen when it ventilates, it does go through a large volume of oxygen. If you use the Thumper, plan to carry additional portable oxygen tanks equipped with high-pressure hose adapters to facilitate rapid transfer of the gas. Use these high-pressure adapters in the ambulance and keep them available for use in the emergency department if the Thumper is used to transport the patient to the emergency department. The Thumper has been particularly helpful in prolonged resuscitation attempts.

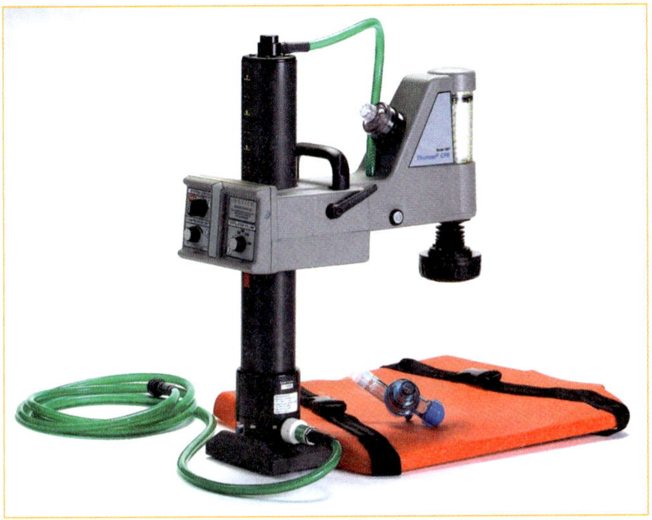

Figure A-8 The Thumper CPR system.

At the Scene

Beware the Misplaced Tube!

The 2005 guidelines include recommendations on tube placement confirmation and continuous monitoring of the tube's position to avoid its dislodgment. To ensure that the tube is inserted in the correct location, after the tube is seen to pass through the vocal cords and the tube position is verified by chest expansion and auscultation during positive-pressure ventilation, the rescuer should obtain additional confirmation of placement using an end-tidal CO_2 or esophageal detection device. No single confirmation technique including clinical signs or the presence of water vapour in the tube, is completely reliable.

You are the Paramedic Part 3

After providing CPR, two shocks with the AED, BLS airway management, an IV, a vasopressor, and then a third shock, the patient has a return of spontaneous circulation. He is being closely monitored and assisted with ventilation at 12 times/min because he is beginning to take some breaths on his own.

Reassessment	Recording Time: 10 Minutes
Level of consciousness	P (Responsive to painful stimuli)
Pulse	96 beats/min, regular
Blood pressure	110/70 mm Hg
Respirations	8 breaths/min, assisted to 12
Spo₂	96% being ventilated with supplemental oxygen
ECG	12-lead shows acute myocardial infarction

5. Because this patient has experienced a return of spontaneous circulation prior to an advanced airway being placed, should one now be inserted?

6. If so, which device would be appropriate if experienced paramedics are present?

7. If you were using an impedance threshold device on the bag-valve-mask device, should it be continued?

Scene Choreography and Teamwork

During resuscitation, plenty of tasks need to be performed. This is where teamwork comes in. Teamwork divides the task while multiplying the chances for a successful resuscitation. There is a role for each health care provider who is committed to fulfilling his or her part. Experience tells us that teams who practice together regularly are more successful in their resuscitation attempts.

Hockey is a team sport that requires every team member to play a specific role. The coach determines who will be on the bench and selects the lines for a particular game. The team captain and assistant captains have a leadership role on and off the ice, using their skill and experience to mentor newer players. The job of the centre and wing men is to forecheck and try to put the puck in the opponent's net, while defensemen and goalie protect the net from the other team's attempts to score. Hockey is a team sport. Each member of the team has a specific role, whether it is scoring, defense, or penalty killing. All team members must be totally committed to the success of the team rather than their own personal achievements **Figure A-9** .

The intense preparation and teamwork that characterize any type of high-level sports team hold a few pertinent lessons for code team members:

- Athletes do not only excel on their own. They need the support of their team and coach.
- The coach helps the team members understand the rules of the game and prepare for its challenges.
- The coach drills the athletes with routines or plays and provides constant feedback and plenty of practice opportunities to measure their progress.
- The team trains with the best equipment, eats nutritious meals, develops a positive mental attitude about winning, and gets plenty of rest after enduring rigorous demanding physical and mental exercise.
- When it is time to compete, team members are well prepared, on time, and ready to go. The coach can support them from the sidelines and may offer signals and guidance or "plays" in some sports, but he or she can't compete for the team.

Code team members who are rested, fit, and well nourished, and who bring a positive attitude to their work, practice their skills, know the "plays," and work together as a team are on top of their game. They are ready to resuscitate patients. To be successful, your team needs to take the following steps:

- Know the plays expertly and automatically. This takes a lot of practice. When there are questions, use posters and pocket cards to explain and prepare.
- Listen to your "coaches." They have the best interests of the patients in mind—and your best interests, too.
- Have a "practice ethic." Pull out the manikins and run mock codes or simulations frequently. Collect data on the cumulative time of interruptions of compressions so that the team has feedback and can work to improve its performance.

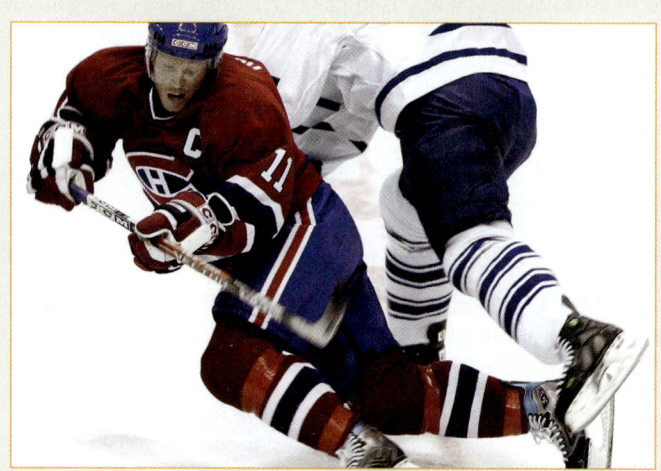

Figure A-9 Even though Saku Koivo is an individual, hockey is a team sport.

- Remember that success equals practice, a positive mental attitude, well-designed plays (ie, algorithms), and excellent coaching.
- Recognize that the effectiveness of the team is not about you. It's about succeeding as a group. Patients are counting on you to get this right!

Code Team Member and Code Team Leader Roles

Whether you are a code team member or a code team leader, you should know both your own role and the roles of the other members of your code team during the resuscitation attempt. This will help you anticipate what steps are coming next and see how your role is an essential part of the resuscitation attempt. Whatever skills you are trained and appropriately authorized to perform, it is essential to the success of the resuscitation that you are prepared, have practiced regularly, have mastered the algorithms, and are committed to success.

Code Team Member Roles

A code team member may be called on to perform all of the following roles (and more):

- **Ventilator**—managing the airway. This team member's duties include suctioning the patient, applying cricoid pressure, ventilating the patient with a bag-valve-mask device, inserting an advanced airway device (ie, LMA, ET tube, King airway, or Combitube), and maintaining manual in-line immobilization of the head and neck.
- **Active compressor**—providing high-quality chest compressions. The only responsibility of this team member is to compress for 2 minutes and be the on-deck compressor for 2 minutes.

- **On-deck compressor.** At the 2-minute point, this team member needs to be ready to relieve the compressor without any interruption in compressions. Other functions include assisting with application of mechanical CPR adjunct device (if available), checking on vital signs, and preparing the patient for transport.
- **Other support personnel**—responsible for analyzing the ECG and delivering shocks, gaining venous (IV or IO) access, providing documentation for the patient care report, and supporting family members.

Code Team Leader Roles

Every resuscitation team needs a leader to organize the efforts of the group in a manner similar to that of a conductor leading the individual musicians in an orchestra. Clearly the code team leader must know all of the specific skills and be able to perform each skill expertly—occasionally the code team leader will serve as the backup for a team member who may be having a tough time inserting a tube or gaining IV access. The code team leader is often responsible for making sure everything gets done at the right time in the right way, however.

The roles of the code team leader may include all of the following:

- Taking the patient's history and performing the physical examination.
- Interpreting the ECG.
- Keeping track of the time.
- Making a medication decision following the algorithm.
- Clearly delegating tasks to code team members.
- Completing documentation after the resuscitation attempt.
- Talking with direct medical control.
- Controlling the resuscitation scene.

Code team leaders must also model excellent behaviour and leadership skills for their team and all others who may be involved in the resuscitation. The code team leader should help train future team leaders, seek to improve the effectiveness of the entire team through continuous quality improvement, and practice after the resuscitation to help prepare for the next code.

The 2005 guidelines say the following about lengthy resuscitative efforts and transporting cardiac arrest patients:

- There are very few instances that require transporting a nontraumatic cardiac arrest patient who has failed a successfully executed prehospital ACLS resuscitation effort to an emergency department to continue the resuscitation attempt.
- In the absence of mitigating factors, prolonged resuscitative efforts are unlikely to be successful. If ROSC

Controversies

To Terminate or Not to Terminate in the Prehospital Environment

Rescuers who begin BLS are taught to continue until one of the following events occurs:

- Effective spontaneous circulation and ventilation are restored.
- Care is transferred to a higher level of care provider, who in turn may determine whether the patient is not responsive to the resuscitative attempt.
- Reliable criteria indicating irreversible death are present.
- The rescuer is unable to continue because of exhaustion or the presence of dangerous environmental hazards or because continuation of the resuscitation effort places other lives in jeopardy.
- A valid DNR order is presented to the rescuers.
- The resuscitation reaches a point where termination of resuscitation is appropriate based on local or regional protocols, where available.

of any duration occurs, however, it may be appropriate to consider extending the resuscitative effort.

- Rare exceptions may include severe prehospital hypothermia (eg, submersion in icy water) and drug overdose. A successfully executed prehospital resuscitation includes an "adequate trial" of BLS and ALS.

Transporting a deceased patient who is refractory to proper BLS and ACLS is considered unethical. Protocols for pronouncement of death and appropriate transport of the body by non-EMS vehicles should be established. Many jurisdictions have developed or adopted termination of resuscitation protocols that permit paramedics to discontinue a resuscitation effort after a predetermined endpoint is reached. Although paramedics may terminate a resuscitation, pronouncement of death may require a physician. Many services access direct medical control for this pronouncement. Every paramedic should be aware of termination of resuscitation protocols that exist in their jurisdiction, be knowledgeable in their regional protocols, and know how to obtain pronouncement of death, if required.

■ A Plan for a Code

The following plan is merely an example and is not the "only way"; obviously, different communities have different resources

You are the Paramedic **Part 4**

Your patient experienced an acute myocardial infarction, causing his heart to go into VF. Fortunately, his teammate responded quickly and initiated the links in the Chain of Survival. After a week in the hospital, the patient went home to his family with a supervised weight loss and exercise program.

that arrive at different times in different ways. The point is that you need a plan and you need to practice this plan diligently.

This example focuses on a prehospital EMS agency response to a cardiac arrest in a private home, assuming a five-person team that could arrive on different units (eg, first responder, paramedic, supervisor) at different times in the first few minutes. Roles for the adult scenario include Compressor 1, Compressor 2, Ventilator, Code Team Leader, and the paramedic supervisor:

- **Compressor 1.** Responsible for doing high-quality chest compressions (100/min, press hard and fast, and full chest recoil), stays in position and compresses for 2 minutes and then rests for 2 minutes (for the duration of the time the patient is pulseless), may assist with application of the Thumper (provided Compressor 2 is continuing uninterrupted compressions).

- **Compressor 2.** Responsible for doing high-quality chest compressions (100/min, press hard and fast, and full chest recoil), stays in position and compresses for 2 minutes and then rests for 2 minutes (for the duration of the time the patient is pulseless), may assist with application of the Thumper (provided Compressor 1 is continuing uninterrupted compressions).

- **Ventilator.** Responsible for providing ventilations (bag-valve-mask, oropharyngeal airway, oxygen) at a ratio of 30:2 ensuring visible chest rise with each ventilation (1 second in duration). May need to briefly suction the patient as necessary. Will assist with the transition from BLS airway to advanced airway (not a high priority). Once an advanced airway is placed, ventilate 8 to 10 times/min to achieve visible chest rise over a 1-second duration for each ventilation.

- **Code team leader.** Responsible for initial ECG analysis and defibrillation with a single shock. Responsible for overall timing of the code and reassessment after 2 minutes of cycles of CPR with the interruption not to exceed 10 seconds. After the initial shock (or ascertaining "no shock" rhythm), proceed to establish IV or IO access (no medications down the tube), then begin a vasopressor every 3 to 5 minutes (1 mg epinephrine, with vasopressin as an acceptable substitute for the first or second—but not both—doses of epinephrine), help to transition the airway from BLS to an advanced airway (ET tube, Combitube, King airway, or LMA), and continue with single shocks every 2 minutes if patient is still in VT or VF. Make the decision with input from the code team and direct medical control that the resuscitation should be terminated if there is no ROSC in the first 15 minutes. If there is ROSC, administer the appropriate antidysrrhythmic (eg, amiodarone, lidocaine), ensure appropriate ventilations, and assist the team in preparing for transport.

- **Paramedic supervisor.** Bring in the Thumper and work with one of the compressors to transition the patient to mechanical CPR compressions with minimal interruption. Assist the medic with IV or IO, advanced airway placement, and preparation of medications, and contact direct medical control, per local protocols.

Vital Vocabulary

asynchronous In CPR, when two rescuers do ventilations and compressions individually and not timed or waiting for the other rescuer to pause.

code team leader The code team member who has the responsibility for managing the rescuers or team members during a cardiac arrest, as well as choreographing the effort of the group.

code team member A member of the resuscitation team trying to revive the patient.

You are the Paramedic Summary

1. **Arriving on the scene of an apparent cardiac arrest with bystanders who have initiated prehospital care, how should you evaluate the quality of CPR?**

Look at the depth of compressions, listen to hear if the compressor is counting to 30, and observe for full chest recoil.

2. **Many elementary schools and public places have an AED available. How might that have helped in this situation?**

The teammates could have quickly obtained the AED, and Tom could have used it within the first 4 minutes or the electrical phase of the arrest.

3. **What should you do next as the paramedic on the scene?**

Take over the role of the code team leader and focus on perfusion and choreographing the arrest.

4. **What is the advantage to perfusion and chest compressions from inserting an advanced airway during two-rescuer CPR?**

With an advanced airway inserted, the two rescuers can switch over to asynchronous CPR with compressions at 100/min and ventilations every 6 to 8 seconds.

5. **Because this patient experienced a return of spontaneous circulation prior to an advanced airway being placed, should one be inserted?**

As time is available. As long as the patient will tolerate an ET tube and you have an experienced paramedic, it would be appropriate to insert one.

6. **If so, which device would be appropriate if an experienced paramedic is present?**

For the patient with ROSC and no gag reflex, the ET tube makes the most sense.

7. **If you were using an impedance threshold device on the bag-valve-mask device, should it be continued?**

No. This device is designed for use with the patient in cardiac arrest during CPR. It should not be used after resuscitation.

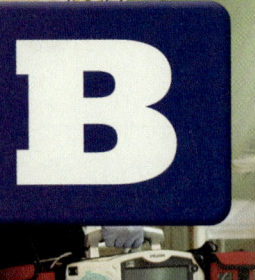

Appendix B: Assessment-Based Management

Competency Areas

Area 1: Professional Responsibilities

1.5.a   Work collaboratively with a partner.

1.5.b   Accept and deliver constructive feedback.

1.5.c   Work collaboratively with other emergency response agencies.

1.5.d   Work collaboratively with other members of the health care team.

Area 2: Communication

2.1.a   Deliver an organized, accurate, and relevant report utilizing telecommunication devices.

2.1.b   Deliver an organized, accurate, and relevant verbal report.

2.1.c   Deliver an organized, accurate, and relevant patient history.

2.1.f   Speak in language appropriate to the listener.

2.3.c   Establish trust and rapport with patients and colleagues.

Area 4: Assessment and Diagnostics

4.3.a   Conduct primary patient assessment and interpret findings.

4.3.b   Conduct secondary patient assessment and interpret findings.

Area 6: Integration

6.3.a   Conduct ongoing assessments based on patient presentation and interpret findings.

6.3.b   Re-direct priorities based on assessment findings.

Area 7: Transportation

7.1.c   Utilize all vehicle equipment and vehicle devices within ambulance.

Introduction

This appendix reviews the standardized approach to patient assessment, which is the format used and reinforced throughout each chapter of this text. Mastery of the standardized approach to patient assessment is a key clinical skill that helps characterize the best paramedics. Only after you have developed a strong foundation in patient assessment and broad clinical experience can you confidently make clinical judgments and adapt the standardized format to meet each patient's immediate needs.

This appendix also covers some of the finer points about assessment, dealing with people, and the importance of working as a team. Many of these strategies are presented throughout the text in the cases and will be used in the laboratory exercises in your paramedic training program.

Effective Assessment

The prehospital care that you provide is built on a strong base consisting of quality assessment of the patient. For this reason, much of your training program emphasizes assessment, and the scenarios or simulations you participate in during your classroom activities involve constant practice assessing patients. You simply cannot properly treat a patient without taking the time and effort to assess his or her situation. Likewise, you cannot obtain medical orders for patient treatment interventions or medication orders without first assessing the patient so you can report your findings.

Paramedics follow a uniform format to gather, evaluate, and synthesize the information. This consistency helps you make the right prehospital care management decisions and take the corresponding appropriate actions. Conversely, not doing an effective assessment can lead you down a bumpy road where the decision making can have disastrous results for the patient. In any situation where the medical directives and standing orders do not address the patient's problem or situation, paramedics should access direct medical control to ensure the situation is managed appropriately.

Accurate information is critical to your decision making. If a first responder is too embarrassed to admit he or she could not really hear the patient's blood pressure and makes up data, this can lead to inappropriate decision making, poor prehospital care, or a lack of confidence in the paramedic's abilities. If you cannot feel, hear, or interpret essential information, such

You are the Paramedic Part 1

After you check out the ambulance and grab a quick cup of coffee, it is 19:00 hours already. The pager tones go off, and the dispatcher alerts you to an incoming call. A head-on collision has just occurred in a suburban neighbourhood not far from your station. The police, the fire department, a second ambulance, and a supervisor are all en route because they have received multiple calls on the collision that may involve a fire and entrapment.

The police arrive first and begin to control the flow of traffic. They report that the smoke was from an airbag, not a vehicle fire. They notify the dispatcher to continue the response because there are two older patients, one in each vehicle, and it is not clear whether either is trapped. The fire department arrives next, and the incident command system is set up. The incident commander (IC) reports that there is no fire but a rescue company is needed to open the car doors. Both patients are conscious, elderly women. One patient may have her legs trapped; the other is very confused.

Your ambulance arrives next, and you assess the scene as you approach it. The mechanism of injury (MOI) is significant: There is a considerable amount of damage to the front ends of both vehicles, and the rear of the second vehicle has been pushed into a telephone pole. There are also some cracks in the windshield, which may explain the bleeding from the driver's head.

The IC fills you in on the details as you quickly don your personal protective gear—standard operating procedure at all collisions involving a rescue. The police officer said that one woman is acting as if she is highly intoxicated but he has not yet gotten a breathalyzer reading on her. The second ambulance and the supervisor are just arriving, so you are assigned to deal with the confused woman who, according to the police, "may have been the one to cause the collision."

Initial Assessment	Recording Time: 1 Minute
Appearance	A woman in her late 50s. She is bleeding from a head laceration, nervous, scared, and very confused.
Level of consciousness	V (Responsive to verbal stimuli); knows name, not sure of day or where she is
Airway	Open and clear
Breathing	Rapid, but no obvious life threats at this time
Circulation	She has a weak radial pulse and no life-threatening bleeding.

1. What are some of the potential causes of a head-on collision in which the driver never hit the brakes?
2. What is the significance of the MOI in this collision for your patient?
3. If it is clear that your patient was not wearing a seatbelt, how could this fact change things?

as vital signs, the best course is to immediately say you are having some difficulty obtaining the information and get some help. Perhaps the blood pressure is so low that it is not easy to hear or feel, or perhaps you are just having a bad day. It isn't always important that you make a mistake—it is what you do with your mistakes when they occur that is very important!

In patient assessment, the history is critically important. Some experts believe that 80% of a medical diagnosis is based solely on the history and not on objective data, such as vital signs, laboratory test results, and ECGs. If you have gained a broad knowledge of diseases and medical conditions through your training, reading, and experience, you will have many profiles with which you can compare the objective and subjective findings of the history. This "pattern recognition," helps you develop an "initial differential diagnosis." With excellent history gathering and interviewing skills, you can focus the physical examination and assessment to arrive at the most accurate initial diagnosis and assist emergency department (ED) staff in arriving at the admission diagnosis.

The Importance of the Physical Examination

The physical examination should be "vectored"—that is, focused on the body system that the chief complaint and history suggest is the source of the problem. (Table B-1 ▾) summarizes the types of physical examinations that you have encountered in this text.

You will practice these physical examinations as part of your training program numerous times until you master them. The examinations will then be incorporated into classroom lab simulations of patient scenarios to help prepare you for their application in the prehospital environment.

Observational studies show that paramedics who have clearly demonstrated in practical skills testing that they know the steps and sequences of the examinations and know when they are supposed to use them nevertheless overlook the physical examinations or apply them in only a cursory manner in the prehospital environment. Ideally, your paramedic instructors and partners will model and instill excellent work habits and a practice ethic so that you will conduct the physical examinations appropriately when your patient's condition warrants their use.

Developing an Action Plan

After you obtain subjective information from the patient through your interviewing skills (that is, OPQRST and SAMPLE) and then obtain objective findings by obtaining vital signs and other parameters (such as ECG, SpO_2, $EtCO_2$ blood glucose level, and other clinical findings), the next step is assessment and developing a treatment plan. The more extensive the knowledge base of clinical profiles (that is, typical clinical pictures) you have, the better your chances of making an accurate assessment. Pattern recognition and "gut instinct" based on lots of hands-on experience have key roles in this decision process. Once the assessment has been completed, a treatment or action plan must be developed. Some of the treatment will have already begun if the initial assessment revealed life threats based on the patient's mental status or ABCs.

Your action plan for treatment of the patient must consider the priority and severity of the patient's condition, the environmental conditions, and the BLS and ALS treatment protocols used in your region. In Canada, paramedics may operate under local, regional, or provincial protocols. Typically, these protocols are developed by EMS medical directors or medical advisory committees of the respective service. In addition, these protocols usually address the prehospital care of trauma patients following the standards and the appropriate prehospital management requested by their trauma and burn centres.

Some protocols are written in an assessment-based format in which the topics are typical assessment findings such as breathing difficulty, chest pain, and altered mental status. Most protocols—including the asthma, allergic reaction, head trauma, and suspected stroke protocols—involve a combination of assessment findings and presumptive clinical assessments (an "initial diagnosis"). You would need to arrive at the right clinical impression to know which protocol to use. In most protocols, a statement in the preface discusses the issue of clinical judgment. Sometimes it takes this kind of clinical judgment to realize which specific protocol is the best to follow, especially when a patient has multiple presenting problems. Good judgment is developed over time and is based on supervised clinical experience plus common sense. Protocols have been described as "cookbooks for a thinking cook." Paramedics with good judgment know when and how to consult with medical direction to consider deviating from their cookbook.

Table B-1	Types of Physical Examinations
Examination	**Description**
Rapid trauma examination/ assessment	Provided for a trauma patient with significant MOI
Rapid physical examination/ assessment	Provided for a medical patient who is not responsive
Detailed physical examination	Provided en route to the ED for a trauma patient with a significant MOI
Neurologic examination	Assesses the Cincinnati Stroke Scale, cranial nerves, and sensory and motor function in each extremity
Cardiopulmonary (heart/lungs) examination	Includes an assessment of the lung sounds, heart sounds, JVD (jugular venous distension), pedal edema, and ECG
Obstetric examination	Includes checking for crowning in a woman in labour
Other examinations	For specific patient complaints

Factors Affecting the Ability to Assess Patients and Make Decisions

Your attitude can significantly influence your assessment and decision-making abilities. We all have spent a good part of our lives developing attitudes, values, and biases—some helpful and some destructive. When you become a paramedic, you must leave your attitude and your ego at the door! Not everyone keeps their home the way you do, nor does every person look the same, act the same, or have the same values. Your patients' choices are not good or bad, just as yours are not good or bad. They just might be different from what you have become accustomed to. Steer clear of assigning "labels" to or stereotyping patients and their families. Referring to patients by derogatory names or slurs is disrespectful and distracting and often leads to a biased and incomplete assessment. Remember, patients call us to provide medical care—not to judge them or their families or their homes. Don't try to judge your patients, but rather treat their conditions as you would expect prehospital care to be provided to one of your loved ones.

Attempting to prejudge the situation or the patient leads to a form of myopia (tunnel vision), as if you have blinders on and miss everything in the periphery. This behaviour can hamper your information gathering and cause you not to collect enough information for a thorough assessment. It is distracting and leads you to "lock on" to an initial impression too early before you have analyzed all the facts. Such an inappropriate gut instinct can cause you to make poor judgments about a patient's medical condition based on past experiences. If you have collected insufficient information to recognize the patterns of injury or a medical condition, you may not be able to make an accurate assessment, or if you do, it will often take longer. Quality management of the patient depends on an accurate medical assessment, not whether you like the patient.

Uncooperative patients can be difficult to assess. When a patient is nasty, your first reaction may be to pack up and leave. Nevertheless, it is important to remember that this person may be "under the influence"—not necessarily of alcohol or drugs. Many patients who are acting out, belligerent, or restless may be reacting to a medical or traumatic situation such as hypoxia, hypovolemia, hypoglycemia, hypothermia, head injury, or concussion. Always rule out medical or traumatic causes for irritability and lack of cooperation before assuming the behaviour is due to intoxication or a behavioural problem.

Sometimes patients have a very distracting injury, such as the fracture shown in **Figure B-1** ▸. Always follow the plan you have been taught: scene assessment, initial assessment (mental status, ABCs, priority decision), determination of the significance of the MOI, and then appropriate focused history and physical examination. Do not allow a distracting injury to divert your attention from the assessment plan. If necessary, temporarily cover the injury with a towel and con-

tinue your assessment! You will ultimately get to it at the proper point in the assessment. You do not want to treat the leg and lose the life because the patient was not breathing adequately.

The number of responders is a factor that definitely needs to be worked into the team's approach to patient assessment and management. Regardless of the various ways in which your local EMS system responds (one, two, or multiple tiers), once at the scene, the team can consist of two to four or more paramedics with varying levels of training. How the scene is managed, who the team leader is, and how assessment information is gathered (sequential versus simultaneous) needs to be practiced in advance. Patients dislike assessment by committee, in which two or more paramedics grill the patient at the same time. This practice can be confusing, often no one gets the entire story, and the patient may repeatedly be asked the same questions.

Sometimes the prehospital environment can prove a major distraction to your assessment. If you are prepared for the possibilities, you can consider strategies to deal with them proactively rather than reacting to them. Examples of environmental distracters include crowds, unruly bystanders, potentially violent or dangerous situations, high noise levels, and an excessive number of paramedics at the scene. If the presence of too many people makes it difficult for you to do your job, politely ask them to wait elsewhere or release the extra responders from the scene. You might also move the patient into your "office" (the back of the ambulance). If an unruly crowd obstructs your assessment or rocks the ambulance, drive around the block!

Finally, patient compliance issues may sometimes present obstacles to assessment and management. If the patient has difficulty confiding in you or any of the other rescuers, it can limit the information you have to make accurate decisions.

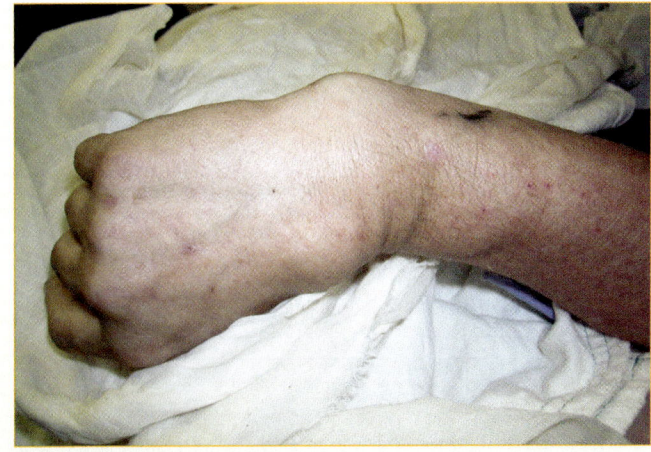

Figure B-1 This fracture is distracting but not an immediate life threat. Don't let it interfere with your initial assessment to locate the real life threats.

Some patients simply will not tell you their medical history. Be careful not to spark this "problem" by displaying an attitude or body language that says you are disinterested or not really someone the patient can trust. Sensitivity to cultural, ethnic, and religious factors is also important and should be included in your training and classroom lab simulations.

Scene Choreography

The importance of a team leader choreographing the activities of the team at the scene of an emergency cannot be overstated. As described in Appendix A, the code team leader and code team members have specific roles that must be constantly practiced and carried out correctly to increase the success of prehospital resuscitations. Indeed, the role of the team leader is key to the coordinated effort of the entire team. Achieving this kind of coordination can be challenging when there are too few or too many responders at the scene. Clearly, the team gives its best response when a single leader manages and monitors the team's efforts with a clear understanding of the strategies, goals, and plans for the particular situation.

The team concept should be practiced not just for a cardiac arrest call. Instead, the team concept needs to be reinforced in the classroom lab setting with practice in numerous simulated responses. The team members and team leader will then be better prepared to respond quickly and effectively in the prehospital setting with real emergencies.

Practice is critically important, including practice in rotating roles and cross-training to assume various roles should the need arise. Some two-paramedic ambulance teams rotate responsibilities or roles by the call, with one partner being the driver/skills paramedic and the other the patient contact/assessment paramedic (team leader) who will ride in the patient compartment en route to the ED. If the call involves more team members, they are added to this basic response and one paramedic assumes the team leader role. If only two paramedics are on the scene, one establishes rapport and conducts the assessment of the patient, while the other handles the on-scene skills such as obtaining vital signs, applying oxygen, and inserting an IV. Because one paramedic will drive to the ED, he or she will most likely clean the stretcher and the back of the ambulance and prepare for the next call while the paramedic who rode with the patient to the ED gives the radio report, gives the face-to-face verbal report on arrival, and completes the patient care report (PCR).

Is this approach the perfect strategy for all EMS units? No, it is just one good way. Other strategies might work equally well. What is essential is that the roles have been practiced and worked out before arriving at the patient's side. If the team has a plan and the situation is complex, the responders have a basic starting point to adapt the response or actions to meet the challenges of the environment or situation.

Pull out the equipment, break into teams, and practice simulated responses with experienced educator/evaluators to document your actions for a post-simulation analysis. Discuss what went right and what did not, and figure out how improvements can be made to the equipment, the team members' performance, and their communication within the team, with patients and families, and with leadership. The next simulation—which could be the real thing—can flow smoothly and look as if it had been practiced a hundred times.

You are the Paramedic Part 2

From your initial patient assessment, it was clear that the patient is confused, yet the rest of the initial assessment seems unremarkable. Her chief complaint seems to be medical (altered mental status), so you proceed down the patient assessment algorithm and conduct a focused history and physical examination of a responsive medical patient—that is, you interview the patient and obtain a history before conducting the physical examination. Your partner obtains the baseline vital signs while you interview the patient.

Vital Signs	Recording Time: 4 Minutes
Skin	Pale, warm, and clammy
Pulse	118 beats/min; weak, regular rate
Blood pressure	110/70 mm Hg
Respirations	24 breaths/min and normal

4. What is the value of using mnemonics such as OPQRST and SAMPLE in your assessment?
5. If the patient had been "not responsive," which steps would your focused history and physical examination involve?

EMS Equipment

When Tom Wolfe wrote *The Right Stuff* in 1979, he was describing what it took to be one of the first seven astronauts selected by NASA for the space program. Similarly, a paramedic responding to emergency calls must carry the "right stuff"—that is, equipment that is packaged and at the patient's side when you need it. As paramedics, we always need to be prepared for the worst-case scenarios, which are threats to the patient's ABCs.

Not having equipment readily available compromises prehospital care. Consider a patient who has struck his head and has altered mental status. If he started vomiting and you did not have PPE (personal protective equipment) and a suction unit, the patient could easily aspirate.

Planning which EMS equipment to carry is a bit like travelling on a plane with only a carry-on bag that will fit in the overhead bin. You need to carry the essential items, downsize to facilitate rapid movement throughout the airport, and minimize the bulk and weight of the baggage. The essential equipment needs to be carried on every call to every patient's side. It includes the equipment to conduct the initial assessment and treat life threats you may find, as well as the cardiac monitor and defibrillator. **Table B-2 ◄** summarizes this set of equipment.

The specific equipment, bags, and boxes depend on your local protocols, standing order flexibility, the typical number of paramedics and first responders, and the difficulty in accessing the patient. Many EMS services continue to use the same plastic "fishing tackle" boxes that have long served as paramedic drug boxes.

Table B-2	Essential Equipment
Function	**Essential Items**
Airway control	PPE (gloves, face shield, and HEPA or N-95 mask)
	Oral airways, nasal airways
	Suction unit (electric or manual)
	Rigid tip Yankauer and flexible suction catheters
	LMA, Combitube, ET tubes
	Laryngoscope and blades
	Tube check, tube restraint, tape, syringes, stylet
	Cricothyrotomy supplies, end-tidal carbon dioxide device
Breathing	Pocket mask and one-way valve
	Bag-valve-mask ventilation device(s) (adult and child), spare masks
	Oxygen-delivery devices (nonrebreathing mask, nasal cannula, extension tubing)
	Oxygen tank, regulator, transport ventilator
	Occlusive dressings
	Large-bore IV cannula for thoracic decompression
	Pulse oximeter
Circulation	Dressings, bandages, and tape
	Sphygmomanometer, stethoscope
	Assessment card and pen
	Impedance threshold device (ITD) and CPR prompt
	AED or manual defibrillator
	Drug box
	Glucometer
	Venous access supplies (IV and IO)
Disability and dysrhythmia	Rigid collars
	Flashlight
	ECG monitor
Exposure	Space blanket to cover the patient
	Scissors

General Approach to the Patient

Your general approach to the patient entails more than simply following the standardized assessment plan. You must have a calm demeanour, look the part, act the part, and have a kind manner. For some paramedics, these details come naturally; for others, they take practice. Practicing your approach is essential for ensuring that you can communicate effectively and provide the level of service patients expect to receive. Most patients are not in a position to rate your ability to conduct an accurate assessment, intubate, or insert an IV line (aside from how much it hurt or how big a mess you made), but they do gauge the quality of prehospital care in terms of the "people skills" provided and the level of compassion you showed.

Your approach to the patient should be planned in advance, in terms of which team member will do most of the talking and questioning and establish the rapport with the patient while the other team members focus on the necessary skills and equipment issues. Make sure you take in the right stuff and are ready to provide resuscitative care because confusion about equipment can unnecessarily add to the level of chaos. As the paramedic doing the assessment, you must carry on an active, concerned dialogue. Take notes—and listen to what the patient tells you!

Review of the Standardized Approach to Assessment

Throughout this book, we have emphasized using the same basic approach to the assessment of the patient. In summary, every scene is assessed to locate the hazards, recognize the MOI, and ensure you have the appropriate PPE and adequate help. The first assessment for every patient is the initial assessment, which is designed to find and deal with life threats. It includes the MS-ABC-priority elements: a check of the patient's mental status using AVPU; assessment and management of the airway, breathing, and circulation; and setting the priority as high or low for this specific patient. Next, the patient is classified as medical or trauma. Although there are some crossovers (such as a geriatric patient with a broken hip who had a syncopal episode), usually a patient will have one overwhelming problem type.

Trauma patients are further subclassified into one of two groups: those with a significant MOI and those without a significant MOI. A patient with a significant MOI will get a rapid trauma examination, with baseline vital signs and SAMPLE history being taken as you prepare the patient for transport. He or she will then get a detailed physical examination and ongoing assessment en route to the regional trauma centre. For patients with a nonsignificant MOI, the examination focuses on the injured body part and then baseline vital signs, a SAMPLE history, and transport. These patients do not routinely receive a detailed physical examination, rather they receive an ongoing assessment en route to the ED.

Patients are likewise subclassified into two groups: those who are responsive and those who are not responsive. The focus in these cases is on the chief complaint, because your line of questioning will depend on how the patient presents. In all cases, you can use the OPQRST mnemonic to remember how to elaborate on the patient's chief complaint. The patient who does not respond appropriately (is not responsive) receives the same rapid examination that the trauma patient with significant MOI would receive, but it is termed the rapid physical examination in medical cases (rather than the rapid trauma examination, as in trauma cases). Next, baseline vital signs and a SAMPLE history are obtained; for a patient who is not responsive, this history may come from bystanders and family members. All patients receive an ongoing assessment en route to the ED.

A medical patient who is responsive will provide you with most of the information needed to arrive at an initial diagnosis if you ask the right questions. In a responsive patient, you should elaborate on the chief complaint, obtain baseline vital signs and a SAMPLE history, and conduct a physical examination that focuses on the body system involved in the chief complaint (such as a neurologic examination, a cardiopulmonary examination, or an obstetric examination). You can then conduct the ongoing assessment en route to the ED.

From a priority or sense of urgency perspective, some trauma patients have a significant MOI and some medical patients are not responsive; with these patients, you should take an urgent, rapid resuscitative approach. Conversely, with trauma patients without a significant MOI and medical patients who are responsive, you can take a slightly more contemplative and less rushed approach. Of course, we are still cognizant of the time with some responsive medical patients (such as for a possible MI or stroke)!

This approach to the patient assessment is the same for all levels of paramedics. The only difference between assessment provided by emergency responders, primary care paramedics, advanced care paramedics, and critical care paramedics is the addition of specific lab tests (such as blood glucose or ECG) and the clinical treatment prerogatives in your "toolbox."

You are the Paramedic Part 3

From your focused history and physical examination of the patient, you have learned that she is confused about the motor vehicle collision and does not remember what happened. She is not sure if she passed out, although a bystander who heard the collision states that the patient was sleepy just after the accident.

The patient denies having any pain but thinks she is going to miss her morning meeting with her friends. By using the SAMPLE history, you find out that the patient has medication in her pocketbook, which is a clue that she has type 2 diabetes. The patient is not sure whether she had any breakfast this morning because she was running very late for her appointment.

You decide to obtain an ECG and a finger stick to check her blood glucose level. Your partner starts an IV. Her blood glucose level is very low, which is one of many possible explanations for her altered mental state.

After receiving 50 ml/25 mg of dextrose IV, the patient seems like a different person. She is alert and very apologetic about causing so much trouble. She says she must have forgotten to eat this morning because she was in a big rush to meet her friends. She asks you to contact her daughter who lives nearby and laughs as the police officer has her take a breathalyzer test, which is found to be negative. As you prepare to leave the scene, your patient inquires about the other woman whose vehicle she hit. You are able to tell her that fortunately, after she was disentangled, the injuries were minor because she was wearing her seatbelt.

Vital Signs	Recording Time: 10 Minutes
Skin	Pale, warm, and clammy
Pulse	118 beats/min; weak, regular rate
Blood pressure	110/p mm Hg
Respirations	24 breaths/min; normal
Blood glucose	2 mmol/l

6. Why might you suspect that the patient has type 2 diabetes?

7. As long as she has a gag reflex, which medication options do you have?

Presenting the Patient

Your ability to present your patient to the next link in the chain of medical care can be a key element in ensuring continuity of care. Effective communication and transfer of the patient's assessment and management data are vital to prehospital caregivers and in-hospital providers who will ultimately be responsible for the patient. Refining this skill is important so that the right amount of the right information is presented to the right person at the right time.

An Essential Skill

The number of calls involving other typical paramedic skills (such as IV insertion or drug administration) may be minimal compared with the number of times you must present the patient to another health care provider face-to-face, over the telephone, over the radio, or in writing on the PCR. Effective presentation and communications skills are essential for continuity of care and to establish trust and credibility with the direct medical control physician.

Good assessment and excellent presentation skills go hand in hand. After all, you can't report or treat anything that you haven't found! A good presentation suggests effective patient assessment; a poor presentation suggests poor assessment and prehospital care. The format that we use minimizes rambling and disjointed presentations that cover inconsequential information but omit vital information. Most health care providers are also programmed to mentally receive a patient presentation in a specific format. The format we recommend follows the SOAP mnemonic: Subjective information, Objective information, Assessment, and Plan for treatment.

A poor presentation can compromise the prehospital care because the paramedic often relies on physician orders to administer specific medications and procedures. If the report was inaccurate or so disjointed that it was "not listened to" or understood by the physician, essential care may not be ordered when needed.

An effective patient presentation is concise, usually lasting about a minute. It should be free of medical jargon and follow the same basic information pattern (that is, the SOAP format). It should also include pertinent positives (such as dyspnea with clear lung sounds) and pertinent negatives (such as head injury with no loss of consciousness).

Components of an Effective Patient Presentation

The format for a radio report to direct medical control typically includes the following key components:

- Your unit identifier, level of training, and appropriate medical channel authorized for transmission
- Patient identification information, such as age, sex, and degree of distress
- The chief complaint or reason the ambulance was called
- The present illness or injury, which includes the MOI and an elaboration of the chief complaint using OPQRST
- The medical history obtained using the SAMPLE protocol
- Physical examination findings—pertinent positives and pertinent negatives
- Your assessment or initial diagnosis
- The treatment plan, including what has been done so far, what you will be doing, and any medical orders you are requesting
- Your estimated time of arrival (ETA) at the facility

Radio reports that do not involve direct medical control (BLS reports for notification) are usually briefer. Face-to-face reports are usually slightly more detailed, bringing the ED nurse or physician up-to-date on what has transpired during your prehospital care of the patient.

An example of a direct medical control radio report using this format follows:

Telemetry Dispatcher: *Go ahead, Medic 785. You are clear to transmit with MD 802 from Saint Peter's Hospital on Med Channel 2.*

Medic 785: *MD 802, this is Medic 785 on Med 2. How do you read?*

MD 802: *Medic 785, this is MD 802. You are loud and clear. Proceed with your transmission.*

Medic 785: *I am treating a 58-year-old male in moderate distress with a chief complaint of chest pain. He states it came on suddenly while shoveling snow. He describes the pain as "a crushing sensation under his breastbone" and states it radiates down his left arm. The pain is a 7 on 10, and he has had the pain for about 20 minutes. The patient states he has no relevant history and denies shortness of breath. He has an allergy to Novocain and takes 325 mg of aspirin daily and 10 mg of Lipitor (atorvastatin). He has a history of hypertension and high cholesterol with CAD (coronary artery disease) in his family. His last oral intake was lunch 3 hours ago and the 162 mg of chewable aspirin the dispatcher advised him to take before our arrival. The events leading up to the incident involved shoveling heavy snow.*

Physical examination reveals some crackles at the bases of both lungs, but no JVD or pedal edema. His vital signs are respirations of 20 and regular; pulse of 110, strong and regular; and a BP of 146/82 mm Hg. His pulse ox is 96 on a nonrebreathing mask. His ECG is sinus tach with no ectopy, but the 12-lead shows ST-segment elevation in V_3 and V_4 (a possible anterior wall MI). We are treating him as a rule-out MI and have administered morphine, oxygen, and nitro; aspirin was self-administered. We are currently transporting, and our plan is to continue monitoring him and go through the rest of the fibrinolytic checklist. We are requesting an order for 5 mg of metoprolol.

MD 802: *Medic 785, go ahead and administer 5 mg metoprolol and I will alert the cath lab staff right away.*

Medic 785: *Received. Be advised our ETA is 20 minutes.*

The keys to developing proficiency with a radio report or a face-to-face report are repetition and understanding the format. We suggest you use an assessment card that highlights the key areas of the radio report. Many pocket guides include this sample format for reference. Eventually, after much practice, you will no longer need the form or pocket guide to refer to because the communication format will be second nature. It is also helpful to practice giving radio reports for simulated patients into a cassette recorder. Soon you will notice that reports on real patients in the prehospital environment come easily and flow off your tongue.

Simulations Using Common Complaints Found in the Prehospital Setting

Your paramedic program will offer scenario-based practice in the lab setting designed to help prepare you for the internship experience. In fact, there are many simulations that you must be examined on in order to practice. These simulations take place after you have learned core paramedic skills (that is, ECG, IV, drug administration) and the treatment algorithms for complaints commonly encountered in the prehospital environment. You will have the opportunity to work with the typical equipment and team members just as interactions would occur in the prehospital setting.

The goals of these simulations include practicing the teamwork, team leadership, and scene choreography discussed in this appendix. You will have many opportunities to work with the equipment and practice the assessment format and skills of paramedics. Likewise, you will have a chance to work on your leadership and decision-making abilities so you can provide interventions that are based on assessment and the treatment modalities in the regional treatment protocols and the ACLS algorithms. In addition, you will have ample opportunities to practice your verbal presentation skills and documentation using the PCR for review by your paramedic faculty.

Most simulations in the lab setting can be done on pre-programmed "patients" or manikins designed to allow you to use your core skills. Some paramedic programs use highly sophisticated training simulators and labs that provide realistic feedback to students on a real-time basis **Figure B-2 ▾** . Video has also been incorporated as a means of reviewing the simulations.

Ideally, simulations will include scenarios that allow you to practice each of the situations in **Table B-3 ▸** and **Table B-4 ▸** . Paramedic students will encounter simulations covering any manner of patient presentations. In fact, the Paramedic Association of Canada has recognized this in their National Occupational Competency Profile document and recognizes simulation as a minimum requirement for exhibiting competence in specific areas. It may be helpful to associate these scenarios with the treatment protocols and algorithms used in your EMS system.

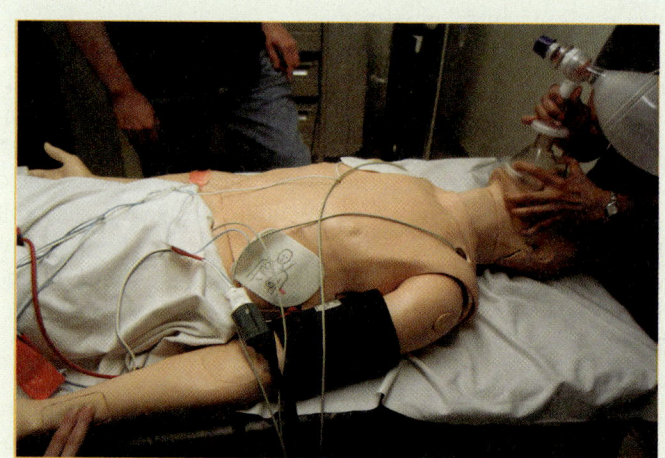

Figure B-2 This is an example of a simulations lab used in a number of paramedic training programs. The manikins and video can provide real-time feedback on changes in the "patient's" vital signs and reactions to your interventions.

Table B-3	General Competency 6.1: Utilize Differential Diagnosis Skills, Decision-Making Skills, and Psychomotor Skills in Providing Care to Patients		
Specific Competency	**Simulated**	**Clinical**	**Precepted**
Provide care to patient experiencing illness or injury primarily involving cardiovascular system.	❏	❏	❏
Provide care to patient experiencing illness or injury primarily involving neurologic system.	❏	❏	❏
Provide care to patient experiencing illness or injury primarily involving respiratory system.	❏	❏	❏
Provide care to patient experiencing illness or injury primarily involving genitourinary/reproductive systems.	❏	❏	❏
Provide care to patient experiencing illness or injury primarily involving gastrointestinal system.	❏	❏	❏
Provide care to patient experiencing illness or injury primarily involving integumentary system.	❏	❏	❏
Provide care to patient experiencing illness or injury primarily involving musculoskeletal system.	❏	❏	❏
Provide care to patient experiencing illness primarily involving immune system.	❏	❏	❏
Provide care to patient experiencing illness primarily involving endocrine system.	❏	❏	❏
Provide care to patient experiencing illness or injury primarily involving eyes, ears, nose, or throat.	❏	❏	❏
Provide care to patient experiencing illness or injury due to poisoning or overdose.	❏	❏	❏
Provide care to patient experiencing non-urgent medical problem.	❏	❏	❏
Provide care to patient experiencing terminal illness.	❏	❏	❏
Provide care to patient experiencing illness or injury due to extremes of temperature or adverse environments.	❏	❏	❏
Provide care to patient based on understanding of common physiologic, anatomical, incident, and patient-specific trauma criteria that determine appropriate decisions for triage, transport, and destination.	❏	❏	❏
Provide care for patient experiencing psychiatric crisis.	❏	❏	❏
Provide care for patient in labour.	❏	❏	❏
Provide care for neonatal patient.	❏	❏	❏
Provide care for pediatric patient.	❏	❏	❏
Provide care for geriatric patient.	❏	❏	❏
Provide care for mentally challenged patient.	❏	❏	❏
Conduct ongoing assessments based on patient presentation and interpret findings.	❏	❏	❏
Redirect priorities based on assessment findings.	❏	❏	❏

Table B-4	Basic Knowledge of Cardiovascular System Illnesses, Conditions, and Injuries Required in Order for Practitioners to Achieve the Competencies Defined in Area 4 of the National Occupational Competency Profile	

Cardiovascular System	Primary Care Paramedic	Advanced Care Paramedic and Critical Care Paramedic
Vascular disease	■ Aneurysm ■ Arteriosclerosis ■ Deep vein thrombosis ■ Hypertension ■ Peripheral vascular disease	■ Aneurysm (intracranial, abdominal aortic) ■ Arteriosclerosis ■ Deep vein thrombosis ■ Hypertension ■ Peripheral vascular disease ■ Thoracic aortic dissection
Inflammatory disorders	■ Endocarditis ■ Myocarditis ■ Pericarditis	■ Endocarditis ■ Myocarditis ■ Pericarditis
Valvular disease		■ Prolasped mitral valve ■ Regurgitation ■ Stenosis
Acute coronary syndromes	■ Infarction ■ Ischemia/angina	■ Infarction ■ Ischemia/angina
Heart failure	■ Cardiomyopathies ■ Left sided ■ Pericardial tamponade ■ Right sided	■ Cardiomyopathies ■ Left sided ■ Pericardial tamponade ■ Right sided
Cardiac conduction disorder	■ Benign arrhythmias ■ Lethal arrhythmias ■ Life-threatening arrhythmias	■ Benign arrhythmias ■ Lethal arrhythmias ■ Life-threatening arrhythmias
Congenital abnormalities		■ Atrial septal defect ■ Patent ductus arteriosus ■ Transposition ■ Ventricular septal defect
Traumatic injuries		■ Aortic disruption ■ Myocardial contusion ■ Peripheral vascular disruption

You are the Paramedic Summary

1. **What are some of the potential causes of a head-on collision in which the driver never hit the brakes?**

Patients who suddenly lose consciousness, fall asleep at the wheel, commit suicide, or are highly intoxicated often veer off the road without hitting their brakes.

2. **What is the significance of the MOI in this collision for your patient?**

There was significant damage to the front of both vehicles, which means the patient's body may have absorbed significant energy in the form of blunt trauma. This possibility sets the tone of and priority for the assessment.

3. **If it is clear that your patient was not wearing a seatbelt, how could this fact change things?**

Without a seatbelt, the focus in a frontal collision is whether the patient took the up-and-over or down-and-under pathway in relationship to the dashboard and steering wheel. The up-and-over pathway is associated with head, neck, and chest injuries. The down-and-under pathway is associated with knee, leg, hip, and lower spine injuries.

4. **What is the value of using mnemonics like the OPQRST and SAMPLE in your assessment?**

The mnemonics help you remember key assessment questions during the focused history and physical examination. OPQRST is used to elaborate on the chief complaint. It stands for Onset; Provocation; Quality; Region, referral, or radiation; Severity; and Time. The SAMPLE history helps you obtain the patient's medical history. It stands for Signs/symptoms, Allergies, Medications, Pertinent past medical history (such as recent hospitalizations, diseases or conditions such as epilepsy, a heart condition, or diabetes), Last oral intake, and Events leading up to today's incident.

5. **If the patient had been "not responsive," which steps would your focused history and physical examination have involved?**

If your patient was not responsive, the focused history and physical examination would take a fast track that involves the rapid medical examination and the baseline vital signs. The SAMPLE history would be obtained from bystanders or family members because the patient was unable to talk. The rapid medical examination would be basically the same as the rapid trauma assessment which involves a quick hands-on examination of the head, neck, chest, abdomen, back, buttocks, and four extremities.

6. **Why might you suspect that your patient has type 2 diabetes?**

Because she has no obvious trauma and altered mental status, hypoglycemia is one of several differential diagnoses you might consider. The blood glucose test is a quick way to see exactly what her blood glucose level is. In this case, with a blood glucose level of less than 4 mmol/l and her oral diabetic medications, you suspect type 2 diabetes. As a general rule, people with type 1 diabetes take insulin because their pancreas does not make insulin. People with type 2 diabetes usually regulate their blood glucose level with diet, exercise, and oral medications.

7. **As long as she has a gag reflex, which medication options do you have?**

When a person with diabetes has a gag reflex and altered mental status and the glucometer reads 2 mmol/l, you can administer glucose onto the gums with a tongue depressor or a small glass of juice with extra sugar added. If you have a good IV site that will not infiltrate, give 25 g $D_{50}W$ IV. Glucagon is another option.

Appendix C: National Occupational Competency Profiles for Paramedic Practitioners Correlation Guide

Area 1: Professional Responsibilities

Competency		Chapter Reference
1.1	**Function as a professional.**	
1.1.a	Maintain patient dignity.	1, 2, 5, 16, 39
1.1.b	Reflect professionalism through use of appropriate language.	1, 2, 5, 10, 12, 16, 40, 43
1.1.c	Dress appropriately and maintain personal hygiene.	1, 2, 12, 16, 35, 36
1.1.d	Maintain appropriate personal interaction with patients.	1, 2, 10, 12, 16
1.1.e	Maintain patient confidentiality.	1, 2, 4, 5, 10, 16, 39, 43
1.1.f	Participate in quality assurance and enhancement programs.	1, 16, 46
1.1.g	Utilize community support agencies as appropriate.	2, 3, 16, 35
1.1.h	Promote awareness of emergency medical system and profession.	1, 3, 16
1.1.i	Participate in professional association.	1, 16
1.1.j	Behave ethically.	1, 2, 4, 5, 10, 43
1.1.k	Function as patient advocate.	1, 2, 3, 5, 10, 20, 39, 43
1.2	**Participate in continuing education.**	
1.2.a	Develop personal plan for continuing professional development.	1
1.2.b	Self-evaluate and set goals for improvement, as related to professional practice.	1, 2, 3
1.2.c	Interpret evidence in medical literature and assess relevance to practice.	1, 5
1.3	**Possess an understanding of the medicolegal aspects of the profession.**	
1.3.a	Comply with scope of practice.	1, 4, 11, 20, 51
1.3.b	Recognize "patient rights" and the implications on the role of the provider.	1, 4, 5, 10, 39, 43, 51
1.3.c	Include all pertinent and required information on ambulance call report forms.	4, 47
1.4	**Recognize and comply with relevant provincial and federal legislation.**	
1.4.a	Function within relevant legislation, policies, and procedures.	1, 4, 5, 17, 46

Competency		Chapter Reference
1.5	**Function effectively in a team environment.**	
1.5.a	Work collaboratively with a partner.	1, 11, 12, 46, 47, 51, Appendix A, Appendix B
1.5.b	Accept and deliver constructive feedback.	1, Appendix A, Appendix B
1.5.c	Work collaboratively with other emergency response agencies.	1, 14, 35, 47, 51, Appendix A, Appendix B
1.5.d	Work collaboratively with other members of the health care team.	1, 47, 51, Appendix A, Appendix B
1.6	**Make decisions effectively.**	
1.6.a	Exhibit reasonable and prudent judgement.	1, 5, 11, 15, 43, 47, 51
1.6.b	Practice effective problem-solving.	1, 5, 15, 43, 47, 51
1.6.c	Delegate tasks appropriately.	1, 11, 15, 47, Appendix A

Area 2: Communication

Competency		Chapter Reference
2.1	**Practice effective oral communication skills.**	
2.1.a	Deliver an organized, accurate, and relevant report utilizing telecommunication devices.	16, Appendix B
2.1.b	Deliver an organized, accurate, and relevant verbal report.	1, 16, Appendix B
2.1.c	Deliver an organized, accurate, and relevant patient history.	1, 12, 16, Appendix B
2.1.d	Provide information to patient about their situation and how they will be treated.	1, 2, 5, 9, 10, 12, 16, 20, 38, 44
2.1.e	Interact effectively with the patient, relatives, and bystanders who are in stressful situations.	1, 2, 5, 10, 12, 16, 37, 39, 43
2.1.f	Speak in language appropriate to the listener.	1, 9, 10, 12, 16, 38, 39, 40, 42, Appendix B
2.1.g	Use appropriate terminology.	1, 5, 9, 10, 12, 16, 20, 38, 39, 40, 43, 44

Competency	Chapter Reference
2.2	**Practice effective written communication skills.**
2.2.a Record organized, accurate, and relevant patient information.	14, 16, 26, 43, 47, 49
2.2.b Prepare professional correspondence.	16, 43, 46, 49
2.3	**Practice effective non-verbal communication skills.**
2.3.a Exhibit effective non-verbal behaviour.	2, 9, 10, 12, 14, 15, 16, 38, 40, 43, 44
2.3.b Practice active listening techniques.	1, 2, 9, 10, 12, 14, 15, 16, 37, 38, 40, 43, 44
2.3.c Establish trust and rapport with patients and colleagues.	2, 5, 9, 10, 12, 14, 15, 16, 38, 39, 40, 42, 43, 44, Appendix B
2.3.d Recognize and react appropriately to non-verbal behaviours.	2, 9, 10, 12, 14, 15, 16, 38, 40, 42, 43, 44
2.4	**Practice effective interpersonal relations.**
2.4.a Treat others with respect.	1, 2, 5, 10, 15, 38, 39, 40, 43, 44, 51
2.4.b Exhibit empathy and compassion while providing care.	1, 2, 5, 10, 15, 32, 37, 38, 40, 43, 44, 51
2.4.c Recognize and react appropriately to individuals and groups manifesting coping mechanisms.	2, 10, 12, 38, 39, 40, 43, 44, 51
2.4.d Act in a confident manner.	1, 2, 10, 11, 15, 38, 40, 43, 51
2.4.e Act assertively as required.	1, 2, 10, 11, 38, 43, 51
2.4.f Manage and provide support to patients, bystanders, and relatives manifesting emotional reactions.	2, 10, 37, 38, 40, 43, 44, 48, 51
2.4.g Exhibit diplomacy, tact, and discretion.	1, 2, 5, 10, 12, 15, 38, 39, 40, 42, 43, 44, 51
2.4.h Exhibit conflict resolution skills.	2, 10, 37, 38, 43, 51

Area 3: Health and Safety

Competency	Chapter Reference
3.1	**Maintain good physical and mental health.**
3.1.a Maintain balance in personal lifestyle.	2
3.1.b Develop and maintain an appropriate support system.	2
3.1.c Manage personal stress.	2
3.1.d Practice effective strategies to improve physical and mental health related to shift work.	2
3.1.e Exhibit physical strength and fitness consistent with the requirements of professional practice.	2

Competency	Chapter Reference
3.2	**Practice safe lifting and moving techniques.**
3.2.a Practice safe biomechanics.	46, 49
3.2.b Transfer patient from various positions using applicable equipment and/or techniques.	14, 46, 49
3.2.c Transfer patient using emergency evacuation techniques.	14, 46, 49
3.2.d Secure patient to applicable equipment.	46, 49
3.2.e Lift patient and stretcher in and out of ambulance with partner.	46, 49
3.3	**Create and maintain a safe work environment.**
3.3.a Assess scene for safety.	1, 2, 11, 14, 20, 31, 35, 48, 49, 50, 51
3.3.b Address potential occupational hazards.	1, 2, 11, 14, 20, 35, 36, 47, 48, 49, 50, 51
3.3.c Conduct basic extrication.	48, 49, 50
3.3.d Exhibit defusing and self-protection behaviours appropriate for use with patients and bystanders.	2, 51
3.3.e Conduct procedures and operations consistent with Workplace Hazardous Materials Information System (WHMIS) and hazardous materials management requirements.	2, 14, 20, 47, 48, 50
3.3.f Practice infection control techniques.	2, 11, 14, 20, 31, 36, 45, 48
3.3.g Clean and disinfect equipment.	2, 11, 31, 36, 45, 48, 50
3.3.h Clean and disinfect an emergency vehicle.	2, 31, 36, 48, 50

Area 4: Assessment and Diagnostics

Competency	Chapter Reference
4.1	**Conduct triage.**
4.1.a Rapidly assess a scene based on the principles of a triage system.	14, 47, 48, 49, 50
4.1.b Assume different roles in a mass casualty incident.	14, 47, 48, 49, 50
4.1.c Manage a mass casualty incident.	14, 47, 48, 49, 50
4.2	**Obtain patient history.**
4.2.a Obtain list of patient's allergies.	7, 11, 12, 14, 26, 27, 29, 30, 31, 33, 38, 41
4.2.b Obtain list of patient's medications.	7, 11, 12, 14, 26, 27, 29, 30, 31, 33, 37, 38, 41

Competency		Chapter Reference
4.2.c	Obtain chief complaint and/or incident history from patient, family members, and/or bystanders.	11, 12, 14, 26, 27, 29, 30, 31, 33, 35, 37, 38, 39, 41, 45
4.2.d	Obtain information regarding patient's past medical history.	11, 12, 14, 26, 27, 29, 30, 31, 33, 37, 38, 39, 41, 45
4.2.e	Obtain information about patient's last oral intake.	12, 14, 30, 31, 33, 39, 41
4.2.f	Obtain information regarding incident through accurate and complete scene assessment.	11, 14, 17, 20, 26, 27, 29, 31, 33, 35, 37, 41, 45

4.3   Conduct complete physical assessment demonstrating appropriate use of inspection, palpation, percussion, and auscultation and interpret findings.

4.3.a	Conduct primary patient assessment and interpret findings.	11, 13, 14, 17, 18, 19, 20, 26, 27, 28, 29, 30, 31, 32, 33, 38, 39, 40, 41, Appendix B
4.3.b	Conduct secondary patient assessment and interpret findings.	11, 13, 14, 17, 18, 19, 20, 26, 27, 28, 30, 31, 32, 33, 38, 39, 40, 41, Appendix B
4.3.c	Conduct cardiovascular system assessment and interpret findings.	13, 14, 18, 27, 30
4.3.d	Conduct neurological system assessment and interpret findings.	13, 14, 18, 21, 22, 28
4.3.e	Conduct respiratory system assessment and interpret findings.	11, 13, 14, 18, 21, 26, 30
4.3.f	Conduct obstetrical assessment and interpret findings.	18, 39, 40
4.3.g	Conduct gastrointestinal system assessment and interpret findings.	13, 14, 18, 24, 31
4.3.h	Conduct genitourinary system assessment and interpret findings.	13, 14, 18, 24, 32, 38
4.3.i	Conduct integumentary system assessment and interpret findings.	13, 14, 18, 19, 20, 30
4.3.j	Conduct musculoskeletal assessment and interpret findings.	13, 14, 18, 23, 25
4.3.k	Conduct assessment of the immune system and interpret findings.	18, 30
4.3.l	Conduct assessment of the endocrine system and interpret findings.	18, 29
4.3.m	Conduct assessment of the ears, eyes, nose, and throat and interpret findings.	13, 14, 18
4.3.n	Conduct multisystem assessment and interpret findings.	14, 17, 18, 21, 27, 34, 36
4.3.o	Conduct neonatal assessment and interpret findings.	9, 14, 39, 40, 41
4.3.p	Conduct psychiatric assessment and interpret findings.	14, 33, 37, 44

4.4   Assess vital signs.

4.4.a	Assess pulse.	11, 13, 14, 18, 20, 26, 27, 28, 30, 31, 38, 39, 40, 41
4.4.b	Assess respiration.	11, 13, 14, 18, 20, 26, 27, 28, 30, 31, 38, 39, 40, 41
4.4.c	Conduct non-invasive temperature monitoring.	13, 14, 18, 20, 35
4.4.d	Measure blood pressure by auscultation.	11, 13, 14, 18, 20, 26, 27, 28, 30, 31, 38
4.4.e	Measure blood pressure by palpation.	13, 14, 18, 20, 27, 28, 31
4.4.f	Measure blood pressure with non-invasive blood pressure monitor.	18, 20
4.4.g	Assess skin condition.	11, 13, 14, 18, 20, 26, 27, 28, 30, 38, 40, 41
4.4.h	Assess pupils.	13, 14, 18, 20, 21, 26, 27, 28, 30, 40, 41
4.4.i	Assess level of mentation.	11, 13, 14, 18, 20, 21, 26, 27, 28, 30, 31, 38, 40, 41

4.5   Utilize diagnostic tests.

4.5.a	Conduct oximetry testing and interpret findings.	14, 18, 31, 33
4.5.b	Conduct end-tidal carbon dioxide monitoring and interpret findings.	18, 40
4.5.c	Conduct glucometric testing and interpret findings.	18, 28, 29, 33
4.5.d	Conduct peripheral venipuncture.	8, 18, 20, 27, 28
4.5.e	Obtain arterial blood samples via radial artery puncture.	18
4.5.f	Obtain arterial blood samples via arterial line access.	18
4.5.g	Conduct invasive core temperature monitoring and interpret findings.	18
4.5.h	Conduct pulmonary artery catheter monitoring and interpret findings.	18
4.5.i	Conduct central venous pressure monitoring and interpret findings.	18
4.5.j	Conduct arterial line monitoring and interpret findings.	18
4.5.k	Interpret laboratory and radiological data.	18
4.5.l	Conduct 3-lead electrocardiogram (ECG) and interpret findings.	18, 27
4.5.m	Obtain 12-lead electrocardiogram and interpret findings.	18, 27

Area 5: Therapeutics

Competency	Chapter Reference
5.1	**Maintain patency of upper airway and trachea.**
5.1.a	Use manual maneuvers and positioning to maintain airway patency.	11, 20, 26, 30, 33, 40, 41, 42, 45, 46, Appendix A
5.1.b	Suction oropharynx.	11, 33, 40, 41, Appendix A
5.1.c	Suction beyond oropharynx.	11, 33, 40, 41, Appendix A
5.1.d	Utilize oropharyngeal airway.	11, 40, 41, Appendix A
5.1.e	Utilize nasopharyngeal airway.	11, 41
5.1.f	Utilize airway devices not requiring visualization of vocal cords and not introduced endotracheally.	11
5.1.g	Utilize airway devices not requiring visualization of vocal cords and introduced endotracheally.	11, 27, 41, Appendix A
5.1.h	Utilize airway devices requiring visualization of vocal cords and introduced endotracheally.	11, 20, 27, 33, 39, 40, 41, Appendix A
5.1.i	Remove airway foreign bodies (AFB).	11, 40, 41, 45, 46
5.1.j	Remove foreign body by direct techniques.	11, 40, 41, 45, 46
5.1.k	Conduct percutaneous cricothyroidotomy.	11
5.1.l	Conduct surgical cricothyroidotomy.	11
5.2	**Prepare oxygen delivery devices.**
5.2.a	Recognize indications for oxygen administration.	11, 26, 27, 28, 30, 31, 33, 39, 40, 41, 45, 46
5.2.b	Take appropriate safety precautions.	11, 45, 46
5.2.c	Ensure adequacy of oxygen supply.	11, 45, 46
5.2.d	Recognize different types of oxygen delivery systems.	11, 45, 46
5.2.e	Utilize portable oxygen delivery systems.	11, 45, 46
5.3	
5.3.a	Administer oxygen using nasal cannula.	11, 27, 32, 45, 46
5.3.b	Administer oxygen using low concentration mask.	11, 26, 41, 45, 46
5.3.c	Administer oxygen using controlled concentration mask.	11, 39
5.3.d	Administer oxygen using high concentration mask.	11, 26, 27, 28, 32, 33, 40, 41
5.3.e	Administer oxygen using pocket mask.	11, 27
5.4	**Utilize ventilation equipment.**
5.4.a	Provide oxygenation and ventilation using bag-valve-mask.	9, 11, 26, 27, 28, 33, 40, 41
5.4.b	Recognize indications for mechanical ventilation.	11, 20, 26, 41, 45, 46

Competency	Chapter Reference
5.4.c	Prepare mechanical ventilation equipment.	11, 26, 45, 46
5.4.d	Provide mechanical ventilation.	11, 26, 45, 46
5.5	**Implement measures to maintain hemodynamic stability.**
5.5.a	Conduct cardiopulmonary resuscitation (CPR).	27, 40, 41
5.5.b	Control external hemorrhage through the use of direct pressure and patient positioning.	21, 25, 31, 45, 46
5.5.c	Maintain peripheral intravenous (IV) access devices and infusions of crystalloid solutions without additives.	8, 20, 27, 28, 29, 30, 31, 32, 33, 38, 39, 40, 41, 45, 46
5.5.d	Conduct peripheral intravenous cannulation.	8, 20, 27, 28, 30, 31, 32, 33, 38, 40, 41
5.5.e	Conduct intraosseous needle insertion.	8, 40, 41
5.5.f	Utilize direct pressure infusion devices with intravenous infusions.	40
5.5.g	Administer volume expanders (colloid and non-crystalloid).	8
5.5.h	Administer blood and/or blood products.	NA
5.5.i	Conduct automated external defibrillation.	27, 41, Appendix A
5.5.j	Conduct manual defibrillation.	27, 41, Appendix A
5.5.k	Conduct cardioversion.	27
5.5.l	Conduct transcutaneous pacing.	27
5.5.m	Maintain transvenous pacing.	NA
5.5.n	Maintain intra-aortic balloon pumps.	NA
5.5.o	Provide routine care for patient with urinary catheter.	32, 45, 46
5.5.p	Provide routine care for patient with ostomy drainage system.	45, 46
5.5.q	Provide routine care for patient with non-catheter urinary drainage system.	32, 41
5.5.r	Monitor chest tubes.	NA
5.5.s	Conduct needle thoracostomy.	23, 40, 41
5.5.t	Conduct oral and nasal gastric tube insertion.	41
5.5.u	Conduct urinary catheterization.	45, 46
5.6	**Provide basic care for soft tissue injuries.**
5.6.a	Treat soft tissue injuries.	25
5.6.b	Treat burn.	20
5.6.c	Treat eye injury.	21
5.6.d	Treat penetration wound.	19
5.6.e	Treat local cold injury.	35

Competency		Chapter Reference
5.7	**Immobilize actual and suspected fractures.**	
5.7.a	Immobilize suspected fractures involving appendicular skeleton.	25, 42
5.7.b	Immobilize suspected fractures involving axial skeleton.	22, 42
5.8	**Administer medications.**	
5.8.a	Recognize principles of pharmacology as applied to the medications listed in Appendix 5.	7, 11, 26, 27, 31, 32, 33, 40, 41
5.8.b	Follow safe process for responsible medication administration.	7, 8, 27, 31, 32, 33
5.8.c	Administer medication via subcutaneous route.	8, 26, 41
5.8.d	Administer medication via intramuscular route.	8, 26, 30, 41
5.8e	Administer medication via intravenous route.	8, 11, 26, 27, 30, 40, 41
5.8.f	Administer medication via intraosseous route.	8, 40, 41
5.8.g	Administer medication via endotracheal route.	8, 26, 40, 41
5.8.h	Administer medication via sublingual route.	8, 27
5.8.i	Administer medication via topical route.	8
5.8.j	Administer medication via oral route.	8
5.8.k	Administer medication via rectal route.	8, 41
5.8.l	Administer medication via inhalation.	8

Area 6: Integration

Competency		Chapter Reference
6.1	**Utilize differential diagnosis skills, decision-making skills, and psychomotor skills in providing care to patients.**	
6.1.a	Provide care to patient experiencing illness or injury primarily involving cardiovascular system.	15, 19, 23, 27
6.1.b	Provide care to patient experiencing illness or injury primarily involving neurological system.	15, 21, 22, 28
6.1.c	Provide care to patient experiencing illness or injury primarily involving respiratory system.	11, 15, 19, 23, 26
6.1.d	Provide care to patient experiencing illness or injury primarily involving genitourinary/reproductive systems.	15, 24, 32, 38, 39
6.1.e	Provide care to patient experiencing illness or injury primarily involving gastrointestinal system.	15, 24

Competency		Chapter Reference
6.1.f	Provide care to patient experiencing illness or injury primarily involving integumentary system.	15, 19, 20, 25
6.1.g	Provide care to patient experiencing illness or injury primarily involving musculoskeletal system.	15, 17, 19, 25
6.1.h	Provide care to patient experiencing illness primarily involving immune system.	15, 30
6.1.i	Provide care to patient experiencing illness primarily involving endocrine system.	15, 29
6.1.j	Provide care to patient experiencing illness or injury primarily involving eyes, ears, nose, or throat.	11, 15, 19, 21
6.1.k	Provide care to patient experiencing illness or injury due to poisoning or overdose.	15, 33, 37, 38
6.1.l	Provide care to patient experiencing non-urgent medical problem.	15, 32
6.1.m	Provide care to patient experiencing terminal illness.	2, 15, 44
6.1.n	Provide care to patient experiencing illness or injury due to extremes of temperature or adverse environments.	15, 19, 20, 35
6.1.o	Provide care to patient based on understanding of common physiological, anatomical, incident, and patient-specific field trauma criteria that determine appropriate decisions for triage, transport, and destination.	15, 17, 19, 20
6.1.p	Provide care for patient experiencing psychiatric crisis.	15, 37
6.1.q	Provide care for patient in labour.	39
6.2	**Provide care to meet the needs to unique patient groups.**	
6.2.a	Provide care for neonatal patient.	9, 39, 40
6.2.b	Provide care for pediatric patient.	9, 15, 20, 40, 41
6.2.c	Provide care for geriatric patient.	9, 15, 20, 42
6.2.d	Provide care for physically-challenged patient.	15, 45
6.2.e	Provide care for mentally-challenged patient.	15, 44
6.3	**Conduct ongoing assessments and provide care.**	
6.3.a	Conduct ongoing assessments based on patient presentation and interpret findings.	14, 15, 17, 20, 27, 32, 33, 38, 39, 40, 41, 42, Appendix B
6.3.b	Re-direct priorities based on assessment findings.	14, 15, 17, 20, 27, 32, 41, 42, Appendix B

Area 7: Transportation

Competency	Chapter Reference
7.1 **Prepare ambulance for service.**	
7.1.a Conduct vehicle maintenance and safety check.	46
7.1.b Recognize conditions requiring removal of vehicle from service.	46
7.1.c Utilize all vehicle equipment and vehicle devices within ambulance.	46, Appendix B
7.2 **Drive ambulance or similar type vehicle.**	
7.2.a Utilize defensive driving techniques.	2, 46
7.2.b Utilize safe emergency driving techniques.	2, 46
7.2.c Drive in a manner that ensures patient comfort and a safe environment for all passengers.	2, 46
7.3 **Transfer patient to air ambulance.**	
7.3.a Create safe landing zone for rotary-wing aircraft.	46
7.3.b Safely approach stationary rotary-wing aircraft.	46
7.3.c Safely approach stationary fixed-wing aircraft.	46
7.4 **Transport patient in air ambulance.**	
7.4.a Prepare patient for air medical transport.	46
7.4.b Recognize the stressors of flight on patient, crew, and equipment and the implications for patient care.	17, 46

Appendix 4: Pathophysiology

System and Illness, Condition, Injury	Chapter
A. Cardiovascular System	
Vascular Disease	
Aneurysm	27
Arteriosclerosis	6, 27
Deep vein thrombosis	27
Hypertension	6, 27, 39
Peripheral vascular disease	27
Thoracic aortic dissection	6, 27
Inflammatory Disorders	
Endocarditis	27, 36
Myocarditis	27
Pericarditis	6
Valvular Disease	
Prolapsed mitral valve	6
Regurgitation	6
Stenosis	6

System and Illness, Condition, Injury	Chapter
Acute Coronary Syndromes	
Infarction	6, 27
Ischemia/angina	27
Heart Failure	
Cardiomyopathies	6
Left-sided	6, 27
Pericardial tamponade	6, 27
Right-sided	6, 27
Cardiac Conduction Disorder	
Benign arrhythmias	6, 27, 41, 42, Appendix A
Lethal arrhythmias	6, 27, 32, 41, 42, Appendix A
Life-threatening arrhythmias	6, 26, 27, 41, 42, Appendix A
Congenital Abnormalities	
Atrial septal defect	9
Patent ductus arteriosus	9
Transposition	9, 40
Ventricular septal defect	6, 9
Traumatic Injuries	
Aortic disruption	27
Myocardial contusion	6
Peripheral vascular disruption	27
B. Neurologic System	
Convulsive Disorders	
Febrile Seizures	28, 41
Generalized seizures	28, 33, 39, 40, 41
Partial seizures (focal)	28, 41
Headache and Facial Pain	
Infection	6, 28
Intracranial hemorrhage	28
Migraine	28
Tension	28
Cerebrovascular Disorders	
Ischemic/hemorrhagic stroke	28
Transient ischemic attack	28
Altered Mental Status	
Metabolic	6, 28, 32, 40, 41, 42
Structural	6, 28, 41, 42
Chronic Neurologic Disorders	
Alzheimers	6, 28, 42
Amyotrophic lateral sclerosis (ALS)	28, 45
Bell's palsy	28
Cerebral palsy	28, 44
Multiple sclerosis	6, 28, 44
Muscular dystrophy	6, 28, 44, 45
Parkinson's disease	6, 28, 42
Poliomyelitis	28, 45
Infectious Disorders	
Encephalitis	28, 36
Guillian Barre syndrome	26, 28, 45
Meningitis	28, 36, 41

System and Illness, Condition, Injury	Chapter
Tumors	
Structural	28
Vascular	28
Traumatic Injuries	
Head injury	14, 26, 44
Hematoma (epidural, subdural, subarachnoid)	19, 21
Spinal cord injury	44
Pediatric	
Downs syndrome	41, 44
Hydrocephalus	41
Spina bifida	28, 41, 44

C. Respiratory System

System and Illness, Condition, Injury	Chapter
Medical Illness	
Acute respiratory failure	26, 27
Adult respiratory disease syndrome	26
Aspiration	11, 26
Chronic obstructive pulmonary disorder	6, 26, 42
Hyperventilation syndrome	26
Pleural effusion	26
Pneumonia/bronchitis	6, 26, 36, 42
Pulmonary edema	6, 26, 27
Pulmonary embolism	6, 26, 32, 39, 42
Reactive airways disease/asthma	6, 26, 27, 39
Traumatic Injuries	
Aspirated foreign body	11, 26
Burns	20, 48, 50
Diaphragmatic injuries	23, 24
Flail chest	17, 23
Hemothorax	23
Penetrating injury	17
Pneumothorax (simple, tension)	14, 26
Pulmonary contusion	23
Toxic inhalation	20, 48, 50
Tracheobronchial disruption	11
Pediatric Illness	
Acute respiratory failure	40, 41
Bronchiolitis	36, 41
Croup	26, 36, 41
Cystic fibrosis	6, 41
Epiglottitis	36, 41
Sudden infant death syndrome	40, 41

D. Female Reproductive System and Neonates

System and Illness, Condition, Injury	Chapter
Pregnancy Complications	
Abruptio placenta	39
Eclampsia	39
Ectopic pregnancy	14, 38, 39
First trimester bleeding	39
Placenta previa	39
Pre-eclampsia	39
Third trimester bleeding	39
Uterine rupture	39
Childbirth Complications	
Abnormal presentations	39
Postpartum complications	39
Postpartum hemorrhage	39
Prolapsed cord	39
Uterine inversion	39

System and Illness, Condition, Injury	Chapter
Neonatal Complications	
Cardiovascular insufficiency	40, 41
Meconium aspiration	40, 41
Respiratory insufficiency	40, 41

E. Gastrointestinal System

System and Illness, Condition, Injury	Chapter
Esophagus/Stomach	
Esophageal varices	31
Esophagitis	31
Gastritis	31
Gastroesophageal reflux	31
Obstruction	40, 42
Peptic ulcer disease	6, 42
Upper gastrointestinal bleed	31, 42
Liver/Gall Bladder	
Cholecystitis/biliary colic	6, 31
Cirrhosis	31, 33
Hepatitis	6, 31
Pancreas	
Pancreatitis	31
Small/Large Bowel	
Appendicitis	14, 31
Diverticulitis	31
Gastroenteritis	31, 36
Inflammatory bowel disease	31
Lower gastrointestinal bleed	31, 42
Obstruction	31
Traumatic Injuries	
Abdominal injury—penetrating/blunt	24
Esophageal disruption	24, 31
Evisceration	24

F. Genitourinary System

System and Illness, Condition, Injury	Chapter
Reproductive Disorders	
Bleeding/discharge	38
Infection	38
Ovarian cyst	38
Testicular torsion	32
Renal/Bladder	
Colic/calculi	32
Infection	32
Obstruction	32, 38, 39
Renal failure	32
Traumatic injuries	32

G. Integumentary System

System and Illness, Condition, Injury	Chapter
Traumatic Injuries	
Burns	20, 41, 48, 50
Lacerations/avulsions/abrasions	17, 19
Infectious and Inflammatory Illness	
Allergy/urticaria	6, 30
Infections	20, 42, 48
Infestations	36

H. Musculoskeletal System

System and Illness, Condition, Injury	Chapter
Soft Tissue Disorders	
Amputations	19, 25
Compartment syndrome	19, 25

System and Illness, Condition, Injury	Chapter
Contusions	19, 21
Dislocations	25
Muscular dystrophies	28, 44
Myopathies	28, 44
Neocrotizing fasciitis	19
Sprains	25
Strains	25
Subluxations	25

Skeletal Fractures

Appendicular	17
Axial	17
Open, closed	25

Inflammatory Disorders

Arthritis	6, 42
Gout	6
Osteomyelitis	8, 19, 36
Osteoporosis	42

I. Endocrine System

Acid-base disturbances	6
Addison's disease	29
Cushing's disease	29
Diabetes mellitus	6, 29, 39, 40, 42
Electrolyte imbalances	6, 42
Thyroid disease	6, 29, 31, 32, 39, 42

J. Multisystem Diseases and Injuries

Cancer

Malignancy	6, 26, 28, 44, 45

Hematologic Disorders

Anemia	6, 34
Bleeding disorders	34
Leukemia	34
Lymphomas (Hodgkins, non-Hodgkins)	34
Multiple myeloma	34
Sickle cell disease	6, 34, 39

Infectious Diseases

Acquired immune deficiency syndrome	6, 36
Antibiotic resistant infection	36
Influenza virus	6, 36
Malaria	36
Meningococcemia/bacteremia	6
Tetanus	6, 36
Toxic shock syndrome	38, 40

Toxicologic Illness

Prescription medication	6, 33, 42
Non-prescription medication	6, 33, 38, 42
Recreational	6, 33, 38
Poisons (absorption, inhalation, ingestion)	6, 33, 48, 49, 50
Acids and alkalis	33, 49, 50
Hydrocarbons	33, 49, 50
Asphyxiants	33, 48, 49, 50
Cyanide	33, 48, 49, 50
Organophosphates	33, 50
Alcohols	33, 42
Food poisoning	31, 33, 36

Alcohol Related

Chronic alcoholism	33
Delerium tremens	33

System and Illness, Condition, Injury	Chapter
Korsakov's psychosis	33
Wernicke's encephalopathy	33

Environmental Disorders

Barotrauma	35
Hyperthermal injuries	20, 40, 42
Hypothermal injuries	40, 42
Air embolism	35
Anaphylaxis/anaphylactoid reactions	30, 41
Decompression sickness	35
Descent, ascent barotrauma	35
Heat cramps	35
Heat exhaustion	35
Heat stroke	35
High altitude cerebral edema	35
High altitude pulmonary edema	35
Local cold injuries	35, 49
Near drowning and drowning	6, 35, 49
Radiation exposure	20, 48
Stings and bites	30, 33
Systemic hypothermia	25

Immunologic Disorders

Autoimmune disorders	6, 31

Shock Syndromes

Anaphylactic	6, 18, 30, 41
Cardiogenic	6, 14, 18, 27, 41
Hypovolemic	6, 18, 20, 27, 31, 32, 38, 40, 41
Neurogenic	6, 18, 28
Obstructive	6, 18
Septic	6, 18, 38, 41

Trauma

Assault	14, 17
Blast injuries	17
Crush injuries	17, 19
Falls	14, 17, 41, 42
Rapid deceleration injuries	14, 17, 41

K. Psychiatric Disorders

Anxiety Disorders

Acute stress disorder	2, 43
Generalized anxiety disorder	2, 37, 44
Panic disorder	2, 37, 44
Post-traumatic stress disorder	2, 37
Situational disturbances	2, 43, 44

Childhood Psychiatric Disorders

Attention-deficit disorder	37
Autistic disorder	44

Cognitive Disorders

Delirium	33, 37, 42

Eating Disorders

Anorexia nervosa	37
Bulimia nervosa	37

Affective Disorders

Bipolar disorder	6, 37
Depressive disorders	6, 37, 42, 43
Suicidal ideation	37, 42

System and Illness, Condition, Injury	Chapter
Psychotic Disorders	
Delusional disorder	37
Homicidal ideation	37, 51
Schizophrenia	37
Psychosocial Disorders	
Antisocial disorder	42

L. Ears, Eyes, Nose, and Throat

Eyes–Traumatic Injuries	
Burns/chemical exposure	20
Corneal injuries	21
Hyphema	21
Penetrating injury	21
Eyes–Medical Illness	
Cataracts	13, 21, 42
Central retinal artery occlusion	NA
Glaucoma	21, 42
Infection	21
Retinal detachment	21
External, Middle, and Inner Ear Disorders	
Otitis externa	41
Otitis media	41
Traumatic ear injuries	17, 19, 21
Vertigo	28
Face and Jaw Disorders	
Dental abscess	21
Trauma injury	21
Trismus	11, 21, 28
Nasal and Sinus Disorders	
Epistaxis	21
Sinusitis	6
Trauma injury	21
Oral and Dental Disorders	
Dental fractures	21
Penetrating injury	21
Neck and Upper Airway Disorders	
Epiglottitis	11, 41
Obstruction	11, 26
Peritonsillar abscess	26
Retropharyngeal abscess	26
Tonsillitis	6, 26
Tracheostomies	11
Trauma injury—blunt/penetrating	11

Appendix 5: Medications

Medication	Chapter
A. Medications affecting the central nervous system.	
A.1	Opioid Antagonists	7, 20, 33
A.2	Anaesthetics	7
A.3	Anticonvulsants	7, 28, 33, 39, 41, 48
A.4	Antiparkinsonism Agents	28

Medication		Chapter
A.5	Anxiolytics, Hypnotics, and Antagonists	7, 11, 28, 33, 42
A.6	Neuroleptics	48
A.7	Non-narcotic analgesics	7, 31, 32, 41, 49
A.8	Opioid Analgesics	7, 11, 26, 27, 31, 32, 33, 38, 41, 42, 49
A.9	Paralytics	7, 11, 48
B. Medications affecting the autonomic nervous system.		
B.1	Adrenergic Agonists	7, 27, 30, 41
B.2	Adrenergic Antagonists	7, 27
B.3	Cholinergic Agonists	7, 27
B.4	Cholinergic Antagonists	7, 26, 27, 42, 48, 50
B.5	Antihistamines	27, 30, 33, 42
C. Medications affecting the respiratory system.		
C.1	Bronchodilators	7, 26
D. Medications affecting the cardiovascular system.		
D.1	Antihypertensive Agents	7, 27
D.2	Cardiac Glycosides	7, 27, 42
D.3	Diuretics	7, 26, 27, 50
D.4	Class 1 Antidysrhythmics	7, 11, 27
D.5	Class 2 Antidysrhythmics	7, 27, 42
D.6	Class 3 Antidysrhythmics	7, 27
D.7	Class 4 Antidysrhythmics	7, 27
D.8	Antianginal Agents	7, 27
E. Medications affecting blood clotting mechanisms.		
E.1	Anticoagulants	7, 27, 42
E.2	Thrombolytics	7, 27
E.3	Platelet Inhibitors	7, 27
F. Medications affecting the gastrointestinal system.		
F.1	Antiemetics	7
G. Medications affecting labour, delivery, and postpartum hemorrhage.		
G.1	Uterotonics	7, 39
G.2	Tocolytics	7, 39
H. Medications used to treat electrolyte and substrate imbalances.		
H.1	Vitamin and Electrolyte Supplements	7, 33, 39, 41
H.2	Antihypoglycemic Agents	7, 29, 39, 42
H.3	Insulin	29, 39

Medication		Chapter
I. Medications used to treat/prevent inflammatory responses and infections.		
I.1	Corticosteroids	7, 26, 30, 42
I.2	NSAID	7, 42
I.3	Antibiotics	7, 42
I.4	Immunizations	7

Medication		Chapter
J. Medications used to treat poisoning and overdose.		
J.1	Antidotes or Neutralizing Agents	7, 11, 28, 33, 41, 42, 48

Medication Formulary

Medication References

American Heart Association (AHA) Classification of Recommendations and Level of Evidence

A system of classifying recommendations based on strength of the supporting scientific evidence was used.

Class I   This indicates that a treatment should be administered.

Class IIa   This indicates that it is reasonable to administer treatment.

Class IIb   This indicates that treatment may be considered.

Class III   This indicates that treatment should NOT be administered. It is not helpful and may be harmful.

Class Indeterminate   This indicates that either research is beginning on the treatment or that research is continuing on this treatment. There are no recommendations until further research is performed (eg, cannot recommend for or against).

Pregnancy Category Ratings for Drugs

Drugs have been categorized by the US Food and Drug Administration (FDA) according to the level of risk to the fetus and are routinely used by health care providers in Canada. Categories are listed for each herein under "Pregnancy Safety" and are interpreted as follows:

Category A   Controlled studies in women fail to demonstrate a risk to the fetus in the first trimester, and there is no evidence of risk in later trimesters; the possibility of fetal harm appears to be remote.

Category B   Either; (1) animal reproductive studies have not demonstrated a fetal risk but there are no controlled studies in women or, (2) animal reproductive studies have shown an adverse effect (other than decreased fertility) that was not confirmed in controlled studies on women in the first trimester and there is no evidence of risk in later trimesters.

Category C   Either; (1) studies in animals have revealed adverse effects on the fetus and there are no controlled studies in women or, (2) studies in women and animals are not available. Drugs in this category should be given only if the potential benefit justifies the risk to the fetus.

Category D   There is positive evidence of human fetal risk, but the benefits for pregnant women may be acceptable despite the risk, as in life-threatening diseases for which safer drugs cannot be used or are ineffective. An appropriate statement must appear in the "Warnings" section of the labelling of drugs in this category.

Category X   Studies in animals and humans have demonstrated fetal abnormalities, there is evidence of fetal risk based on human experience, or both; the risk of using the drug in pregnant women clearly outweighs any possible benefit. The drug is contraindicated in women who are or may become pregnant. An appropriate statement must appear in the "Contraindications" section of the labelling of drugs in this category.

Canadian Food and Drug Act

The Food and Drug Act, first passed in 1920, and most recently revised in 1985, aims to protect the public from mislabelled, poisonous, or otherwise harmful foods and medications. It applies to all food, drugs, natural health products, and medical devices sold in Canada and governs the sale, advertisement, and labelling of products to ensure consumer safety and prevent deception.

The Controlled Drugs and Substances Act (1996) replaced the Narcotic Control Act, which was passed in 1961. It governs the production, registration, distribution, and possession of narcotics and controlled substances. The drugs are organized into eight schedules, each associated with varying control measures, depending on their dependence and abuse potential and their usefulness in medical therapy. Schedules I through V list different controlled substances, schedule VI lists precursors to "designer drugs" or other controlled substances, and schedules VII and VIII specify amounts of substances in schedule II associated with lesser penalties. It is illegal to import, export, traffic, or possess substances in schedules I, II, and III. The offences in schedule IV are similar to those for I, II, and III, except that there is no offence for simple possession. It is illegal to import, export, or possess for trafficking substances in schedules V and VI.

- **Schedule I** includes narcotics, such as opium, heroin, morphine, and cocaine.
- **Schedule II** includes cannabis and cannabis resin.
- **Schedule III** includes stimulants, such as amphetamines, and hallucinogens, such as LSD.
- **Schedule IV** includes substances such as anabolic steroids, barbiturates, and benzodiazepines.
- **Schedule V** includes phenylpropanolamine.
- **Schedule VI** includes precursors that can be converted into or used to produce "designer drugs" or other controlled substances.
- **Schedule VII** defines limits associated with application of cannabis-related penalties: cannabis (3 kg) and cannabis resin (3 kg).
- **Schedule VIII** defines limits associated with application of cannabis-related penalties: cannabis (30 g) and cannabis resin (1 g).

Weights and Measures

Commonly Used Prefixes		
Prefix Name	**Prefix Symbol**	**Prefix Value**
micro	μ	1/1,000,000 or 0.000001
milli	m	1/1,000 or 0.001
centi	c	1/100 or 0.01
kilo	k	1,000
mega	M	1 million or 1,000,000

Common Metric Conversions

Weight

1 kilogram (kg)	2.2 pounds (lb)
1 kilogram (kg)	1,000 grams (g or gm)
1 gram (g or gr)	1,000 milligrams (mg)
1 milligram (mg)	1,000 micrograms (µg or mcg)

Volume

1 litre (l)	1,000 millilitres or cubic centimetres (ml or cc)

Temperature

37° Celsius (°C)	98.6° Fahrenheit (°F)

Length

1 centimetre (cm)	10 millimetres (mm)
100 centimetres (cm)	1 metre (m)

Common Medical Abbreviations Related to Pharmacology

Common Medical Abbreviations Related to Pharmacology

Abbreviation	Meaning	Abbreviation	Meaning
ā	before	NKA	no known allergies
α	alpha	NKDA	no known diagnosed allergies
amp.	ampule	NTG	nitroglycerin
APAP	acetaminophen	ø	null or none
ASA	aspirin	p̄	after
β	beta	pc	post cibos (after eating)
bid	Bis in die (twice a day)	pedi	pediatric
c̄	with	po	per os (by mouth)
caps	capsules	pr	per rectus (by rectum)
cc	cubic centimetre	prn	per re nata (when necessary)
D/C	discontinue	q̄	quisque (every)
dig	digoxin	qd	quisque die (every day)
elix	elixir	qh	quisque hora (every hour)
ET	endotracheal	qid	quarter in die (four times a day)
ETOH	ethyl alcohol	qod	every other day
g or gr	gram	RL	Ringer's lactate
gtt	gutta (drop)	s̄	sine (without)
gtts	guttae (drops)	SC	subcutaneous
HHN	handheld nebulizer	sol	solution
Hs	hora somni (at bedtime)	SQ	subcutaneous
IC	intracardiac	stat	statim (now or immediately)
IM	intramuscular	SVN	small volume nebulizer
IO	intraosseous	tid	ter in die (three times a day)
IV	intravenous	TKO	to keep open
IVP	intravenous push	TKVO	to keep vein open
IVPB	intravenous piggyback	u	unit
kg	kilogram	ut dict	ut dictum (as directed)
L or l	litre	®	registered trademark
lb	pound	♀	female
LR	lactated Ringer's	♂	male
MAX	maximum	>	greater than
MDI	metered dose inhaler	<	less than
µ	micro	≥	greater than or equal to
µgtt	microdrop	≤	less than or equal to
µg or mcg	microgram	≈	approximately
mEq	milliequivalent	=	equal
mg	milligram	≠	not equal
min	minute	Δ	change(s)
ml	millilitre	±	plus or minus
MS or MSO4	morphine sulfate	°	degree(s)
nitro	nitroglycerin	™	trademark

Drug Dosage Calculations

Terminology

Desired dose   The quantity of a medication that is to be administered to a patient. This is usually expressed in milligrams, grams, or units.

Concentration (of the medication on hand)   The amount of a medication that is present in the ampule or vial. This is usually expressed in milligrams, grams, or units.

Volume   (of the medication on hand) The amount of a fluid that is present in the ampule or vial in which the medication is dissolved. This is usually expressed in millilitres or litres.

Formulas

$$\text{Concentration on hand} = \frac{\text{concentration on hand (mg)}}{\text{volume on hand (ml)}}$$

EXAMPLE

How many milligrams of medication "Q" are in each ml/cc? Medication "Q" is packaged 500 mg in 10 ml of saline.

$$\text{Concentration on hand} = \frac{\text{concentration on hand (500 mg)}}{\text{volume on hand (10 ml)}}$$

$$\text{Concentration on hand} = \frac{500 \text{ mg}}{10 \text{ ml}}$$

$$\text{Concentration on hand} = 50 \text{ mg/ml}$$

EXAMPLE

You are ordered to administer 70 mg of medication "Y" to a patient. The medication is prepared as follows, 100 mg in 5 ml of saline.

$$\text{Volume to be administered} = \frac{\text{volume on hand} \times \text{desired dose}}{\text{concentration on hand}}$$

$$\text{Volume to be administered} = \frac{\text{volume on hand (5 ml)} \times \text{desired dose (70 mg)}}{\text{concentration on hand (100 mg)}}$$

$$\text{Volume to be administered} = \frac{(5 \text{ ml}) \times (70 \text{ mg})}{(100 \text{ mg})}$$

Note: (mg) can be crossed out leaving the final units notation (ml).

$$\text{Volume to be administered} = \frac{350 \text{ ml}}{100}$$

$$\text{Volume to be administered} = 3.5 \text{ ml}$$

Intravenous Infusion Drip Rate Calculation

$$\text{Formula: Drops per minute (gtt/min)} = \frac{\text{total amount of fluid to be administered in ml} \times \text{drop factor*}}{\text{total time in minutes}}$$

*The drop factor for the IV tubing will be indicated on the package for the tubing. Standard values are as follows: 10, 15, and 20 gtt lines (macrodrip) and 50 or 60 gtt/ml lines (microdrip).

EXAMPLE

You are ordered to administer 1,000 ml of normal saline every 8 hours using a 10 gtt IV tubing set. Calculate the number of drops per minute.

Total volume: 1,000 ml

Drop factor: 10 gtt/ml

Total time: 8 hours × 60 = 480 minutes

$$\text{Drops per minute (gtt/min)} = \frac{\begin{array}{c}\text{Total amount of fluid to be}\\ \text{administered (1,000 ml)} \times\\ \text{drop factor (10 gtt/ml)}\end{array}}{\text{Total time in minutes (480)}}$$

$$\text{Drops per minute (gtt/min)} = \frac{(1,000 \text{ ml}) \times (10 \text{ gtt/ml})}{480 \text{ min}}$$

$$\text{Drops per minute (gtt/min)} = \frac{10,000}{480}$$

$$\text{Drops per minute (gtt/min)} = 20.83 \qquad \text{Note: Round to the nearest drop}$$

$$\text{Drops per minute (gtt/min)} = 21 \text{ gtt(s)/min}$$

Medications

Reference for Medication Listings

Name of Medication (Other Common Names)

Class How the medication is categorized as compared to other medications. This is usually done by grouping those medications with similar characteristics, traits, or primary components.

Mechanism of action The manner of combination of parts, processes, etc., which form a common function.

Indications A circumstance that points to or shows the cause, pathology, treatment, or issue of an attack of disease; that which points out; that which serves as a guide or warning.

Contraindications Any condition, especially any condition of disease, which renders some particular line of treatment improper or undesirable.

Adverse reactions This is an abnormal or harmful effect to an organism caused by exposure to a chemical. It is indicated by some result such as death, a change in food or water consumption, altered body and organ weights, altered enzyme levels, or visible illness. An effect may be classed as adverse if it causes functional or anatomic damage, causes irreversible change in the homeostasis of the organism, or increases the susceptibility of the organism to other chemical or biologic stress. A nonadverse effect will usually be reversed when the organism is no longer being exposed to the chemical.

Drug interactions This refers to any potential effects that a medication may have when administered in conjunction or in the presence of another medication already in the patient's system, a medication delivery device, or fluid.

How supplied This is how the manufacturer packages the medication for distribution and sale. Typical methods of packaging are prefilled syringes, vials, or ampules.

Dosage and administration This is the typical or average volume of the medication that is to be administered to the patient and the route of introduction of the medication to the patient.

Duration of action Three values are given; (1) Onset: the estimated amount of time it will take for the medication to enter the body/system and begin to take effect, (2) Peak effect: the estimated amount of time it will take for the medication to have its greatest effect on the patient/system and (3) Duration: the estimated amount of time that the medication will have any effect on the patient/system.

Special considerations Additional pertinent information concerning a medication.

Acetylcysteine Sodium (Mucomyst)

Class Mucolytic, glutathione donor.

Mechanism of action Protects liver by maintaining or restoring glutathione levels or by acting as an alternate substrate for conjugation with and thus detoxification of reactive metabolites.

Indications Antidote to prevent or lessen hepatic injury following ingestion of potentially toxic quantities of acetaminophen.

Contraindications Known hypersensitivity to the drug.

Adverse reactions Nausea, vomiting, hypersensitivity reactions.

Drug interactions Should not be mixed with or run in same IV site as antibiotics.

How supplied 30- and 50-ml vials of a 20% solution.

Dosage and Administration												
	10-15 kg	15-20 kg	20-25 kg	25-30 kg	30-40 kg	40-50 kg	50-60 kg	60-70 kg	70-80 kg	80-90 kg	90-100 kg	100-110 kg
Initial infusion of acetylcysteine (in D_5W over 15 min)	11.25 ml	15 ml	18.75 ml	22.5 ml	30 ml	37.5 ml	45 ml	52.5 ml	60 ml	67.5 ml	75 ml	82.5 ml
Volume of 5% Dextrose for initial infusion	40 ml	50 ml	75 ml	75 ml	100 ml	200 ml	200 ml	200 ml	200 ml	200 ml	200 ml	200 ml
Second infusion of acetylcysteine (500 ml D_5W over 4 hrs)	3.75 ml	5 ml	6.25 ml	7.5 ml	10 ml	12.5 ml	15 ml	17.5 ml	20 ml	22.5 ml	25 ml	27.5 ml
Third infusion of acetylcysteine (in 1 l D_5W over 16 hrs)	7.5 ml	10 ml	12.5 ml	15 ml	20 ml	25 ml	30 ml	35 ml	40 ml	45 ml	50 ml	55 ml

Special considerations Anaphylactoid reactions.

Activated Charcoal

Class   Adsorbent.

Mechanism of action   Adsorbs toxic substances from the gastrointestinal tract; onset of action is immediate.

Indications   Most oral poisonings and medication overdoses; can be used after evacuation of poisons.

Contraindications   Oral administration to comatose patient; after ingestion of corrosives, caustics, or petroleum distillates (ineffective and may induce vomiting); simultaneous administration with other oral drugs.

Adverse reactions   May induce nausea and vomiting; may cause constipation; may cause black stools.

Drug interactions   Bonds with and generally inactivates whatever it is mixed with, eg, syrup of ipecac.

How supplied   25 g (black powder)/125-ml bottles (200 mg/ml); 50 g (black powder)/250-ml bottles (200 mg/ml).

Dosage and administration   *Note:* if not in premixed slurry, dilute with 1 part charcoal/4 parts water. *Adult:* 1–2 g/kg PO or via NGT. *Pediatric:* 1–2 g/kg PO or via NGT.

Duration of action   Depends on gastrointestinal function; will act until excreted.

Special considerations   Often used in conjunction with magnesium citrate. Must be stored in a closed container. Does not adsorb cyanide, lithium, iron, lead, arsenic, or alcohols.

Adenosine (Adenocard)

Class   Endogenous nucleotide.

Mechanism of action   Slows conduction time through the AV node; can interrupt re-entrant pathways; slows heart rate; acts directly on sinus pacemaker cells. Is drug of choice for reentry SVT. Can be used diagnostically for stable, wide-complex tachycardias of unknown type.

Indications   Conversion of PSVT to sinus rhythm. May convert reentry SVT due to Wolff-Parkinson-White syndrome. Not effective in converting atrial fibrillation/flutter or VT.

Contraindications   Second- or third-degree block or sick sinus syndrome, atrial flutter/atrial fibrillation, ventricular tachycardia, hypersensitivity to adenosine, poison-induced tachycardia.

Adverse reactions   Facial flushing, shortness of breath, chest pain, headache, paresthesia, diaphoresis, palpitations, hypotension, nausea, metallic taste.

Drug interactions   Methylxanthines (theophylline-like drugs) antagonize the effects of adenosine. Dipyridamole (Persantine) potentiates the effects of adenosine. Carbamazepine (Tegretol) may potentiate the AV node, blocking the effects of adenosine. May cause bronchoconstriction in asthmatic patients.

How supplied   3 mg/ml in 2-ml flip-top vials for IV injection.

Dosage and administration   *Adult:* 6 mg over 1–3 seconds, followed by a 20-ml saline flush and elevate extremity; if no response after 1–2 minutes, administer 12 mg over 1–3 seconds; maximum total dose, 30 mg; *Pediatric:* 0.1–0.2 mg/kg rapid IV; maximum single dose, 12 mg.

Duration of action   Onset and peak effect: within seconds. Duration: 12 seconds.

Special considerations   Short half-life limits side effects in most patients. Pregnancy safety: Category C.

Amiodarone (Cordarone)

Class   Antiarrhythmic.

Mechanism of action   Blocks sodium channels and myocardial potassium channels.

Indications   VF/pulseless VT and unstable VT in patients refractory to other therapy.

Contraindications   Known hypersensitivity, cardiogenic shock, sinus bradycardia, and second- or third-degree AV block (unless a functional pacemaker is available).

Adverse reactions   Hypotension, bradycardia, prolongation of the PR, QRS, and QT intervals.

Drug interactions   Use with digoxin may cause digoxin toxicity. Antiarrhythmics may cause increased serum levels. Beta blockers and calcium channel blockers may potentiate bradycardia, sinus arrest, and AV heart blocks.

How supplied   Ampules containing 150 mg/3 ml (50 mg/ml) and prefilled syringes containing 150 mg/3 ml (50 mg/ml).

Dosage and administration   *Adult: VF/pulseless VT unresponsive to CPR, defibrillation, and vasopressors:* 300 mg IV/IO push (recommend dilution in 20–30 ml D₅W). Initial dose can be followed **one time** in 3–5 minutes at 150 mg IV/IO push. *Recurrent life-threatening ventricular arrhythmias:* Maximum cumulative dose is 2.2 g/24 hours, administered as follows: *Rapid infusion:* 150 mg IV/IO over 10 minutes (15 mg/min). May repeat rapid infusion (150 mg IV/IO) every 10 minutes as needed. *Slow infusion:* 360 mg IV/IO over 6 hours (1 mg/min). *Maintenance infusion:* 540 mg IV/IO over 18 hours (0.5 mg/min). *Pediatric: Refractory VF/pulseless VT:* 5 mg/kg IV/IO bolus. Can repeat the 5 mg/kg IV/IO bolus up to a total dose of 15 mg/kg per 24 hours. Maximum single dose is 300 mg. *Perfusing supraventricular and ventricular tachycardias:* Loading dose of 5 mg/kg IV/IO over 20–60 minutes (maximum single dose of 300 mg). Can repeat to maximum of 15 mg/kg per day.

Duration of action   Onset: immediate with peak effect in 10–15 minutes. Duration: 30–45 minutes.

Special considerations   Pregnancy safety: Category D. Monitor patient for hypotension. May worsen arrhythmias or precipitate new arrhythmias.

Amyl Nitrite, Sodium Nitrite, Sodium Thiosulfate (Cyanide Antidote Kit)

Class   Antidote.

Mechanism of action   Amyl nitrite: affinity for cyanide ions; reacts with hemoglobin to form methemoglobin (low toxicity); sodium nitrite: same as amyl nitrite; sodium thiosulfate: produces thiocyanate, which is then excreted.

Indications   Cyanide or hydrocyanic acid poisoning.

Contraindications   Not applicable.

Adverse reactions   Excessive doses of amyl nitrite and sodium nitrite can produce severe, life-threatening methemoglobinemia. Use only recommended doses.

Drug interactions   None.

How supplied   Amyl nitrite: in capsules similar to ammonia capsules.

Dosage and administration *Adult:* Amyl nitrite: breathe 30 seconds out of every minute. Sodium thiosulfate and sodium nitrite: IV per antidote kit directions. *Pediatric:* Same as adult.

Duration of action variable.

Special considerations Cyanide poisoning must be recognized quickly and treated quickly; if pulse persists, even in presence of apnea, prognosis is good with treatment. The antidote kit must be used in conjunction with administration of oxygen.

Aspirin

Class Platelet inhibitor, anti-inflammatory agent.

Mechanism of action Prostaglandin inhibition.

Indications New onset chest pain suggestive of acute myocardial infarction. Signs and symptoms suggestive of recent cerebrovascular accident.

Contraindications Hypersensitivity. Relatively contraindicated in patients with active ulcer disease or asthma.

Adverse reactions Heartburn, GI bleeding, prolonged bleeding, nausea, and vomiting. Wheezing in allergic patients.

Drug interactions Use with caution in patients allergic to NSAIDs.

How supplied 81-mg, 160-mg, or 325-mg tablets (chewable and standard).

Dosage and administration *Adult:* 160 mg to 325 mg PO (chewed if possible). *Pediatric:* Not recommended.

Duration of action Onset: 30–45 minutes. Peak effect: variable. Duration: variable.

Special considerations Pregnancy safety: Category D. Not recommended in pediatric population.

Atropine Sulfate

Class Anticholinergic agent.

Mechanism of action Parasympatholytic: inhibits action of acetylcholine at postganglionic parasympathetic neuroeffector sites. Increases heart rate in life-threatening bradyarrhythmias.

Indications Hemodynamically unstable bradycardia, asystole, bradycardic (< 60 beats/min) pulseless electrical activity (PEA), organophosphate poisoning, bronchospastic pulmonary disorders.

Contraindications Tachycardia, hypersensitivity, unstable cardiovascular status in acute hemorrhage and myocardial ischemia, narrow-angle glaucoma.

Adverse reactions Headache; dizziness; palpitations; nausea and vomiting; tachycardia; arrhythmias; anticholinergic effects (blurred vision, dry mouth, urinary retention); paradoxical bradycardia when pushed slowly or at low doses; flushed, hot, dry skin.

Drug interactions Potential adverse effects when administered with digoxin, cholinergics, and physostigmine. Effects enhanced by antihistamines, procainamide, quinidine, antipsychotics, benzodiazepines, and antidepressants.

How supplied Prefilled syringes: 1 mg in 10 ml (0.1 mg/ml). Nebulizer: 0.2% (1 mg in 0.5 ml) and 0.5% (2.5 mg in 0.5 ml). Ampules: 0.4 or 0.6 mg/ml.

Dosage and administration *Adult: Asystole or bradycardic PEA:* 1 mg IV/IO push. May repeat every 3–5 minutes (if asystole or PEA persists) to a maximum of 3 doses (3 mg). *Unstable bradycardia:* 0.5 mg IV/IO every 3–5 minutes as needed, not to exceed total dose of 3 mg. Use shorter dosing interval (3 minutes) and higher doses in severe clinical conditions. *Organophosphate poisoning:* Extremely large doses (2–4 mg or higher) may be needed. *Pediatric:* 0.02 mg/kg via IV/IO push; may double this dose for second IV/IO dose. *Minimum single dose:* 0.1 mg. *Maximum doses:* child single dose: 0.5 mg, child total dose: 1 mg, adolescent single dose: 1 mg, adolescent total dose: 2 mg.

Duration of action Onset: immediate. Peak effect: rapid to 1–2 minutes. Duration: 2–6 hours.

Special considerations Pregnancy safety: Category C. Moderate doses may cause pupillary dilation.

Calcium Chloride

Class Electrolyte.

Mechanism of action Increases cardiac contractile state (positive inotropic effect). May enhance ventricular automaticity.

Indications Hypocalcemia, hyperkalemia, magnesium sulfate overdose, calcium channel blocker overdose, adjunctive therapy in treatment of insect bites and stings.

Contraindications Hypercalcemia, VF, digoxin toxicity.

Adverse reactions Bradycardia, asystole, hypotension, peripheral vasodilation, metallic taste, local necrosis, coronary and cerebral artery spasm, nausea and vomiting.

Drug interactions May worsen arrhythmias secondary to digoxin toxicity. May antagonize the effects of verapamil. Do not mix with or infuse immediately before or after sodium bicarbonate without intervening flush.

How supplied Prefilled syringes containing a 10% solution in 10 ml (100 mg/ml).

Dosage and administration *Adult:* 500 mg to 1,000 mg (5–10 ml of a 10% solution) IV/IO push for hyperkalemia and calcium channel blocker overdose. May be repeated as needed. *Pediatric:* 20 mg/kg (0.2 ml/kg) slow IV/IO push. Maximum 1 g dose; may repeat in 10 minutes.

Duration of action Onset: 5–15 minutes. Peak effect: 3–5 minutes. Duration: 15–30 minutes, but may persist for 4 hours (dose dependent).

Special considerations Pregnancy safety: Category C. Do not use routinely in cardiac arrest.

Dexamethasone Sodium Phosphate (Decadron)

Class Corticosteroid.

Mechanism of action Suppresses acute and chronic inflammation; immunosuppressive effects.

Indications Anaphylaxis, asthma, spinal cord injury, croup, elevated intracranial pressure due to edema from space occupying lesion (prevention and treatment), as an adjunct to treatment of shock.

Contraindications Hypersensitivity to product.

Adverse reactions Hypertension, sodium and water retention, gastrointestinal bleeding, TB. None from single dose.

Drug interactions Calcium.

How supplied 100 mg/5-ml vials or 20 mg/1-ml vials.

Dosage and administration   *Adult:* 10–100 mg IV (1 mg/kg slow IV bolus) (considerable variance through medical control). *Pediatric:* 0.25–1.0 mg/kg/dose IV, IO, IM.

Duration of action   Onset: Hours. Peak effect: 8–12 hours. Duration: 24–72 hours.

Special considerations   Pregnancy safety: unknown. Protect medication from heat. Toxicity and side effects with long-term use.

Dextrose (25% or 50%)

Class   Carbohydrate, hypertonic solution.

Mechanism of action   Rapidly increases serum glucose levels. Short-term osmotic diuresis.

Indications   Hypoglycemia, altered level of consciousness, coma of unknown etiology, seizure of unknown etiology, status epilepticus.

Contraindications   Intracranial hemorrhage.

Adverse reactions   Extravasation leads to tissue necrosis. Warmth, pain, burning, thrombophlebitis, rhabdomyolysis, hyperglycemia.

Drug interactions   Sodium bicarbonate, Coumadin.

How supplied   25 g/50-ml prefilled syringes (500 mg/ml) or 12.5 g/50-ml prefilled syringes (2.50 mg/ml).

Dosage and administration   *Adult:* 12.5–25 g slow IV; may be repeated as necessary. *Pediatric:* 0.5–1 g/kg/dose slow IV; may be repeated as necessary.

Duration of action   Onset: less than 1 minute. Peak effect: variable. Duration: variable.

Special considerations   Administer thiamine prior to dextrose in known alcoholic patients. Draw blood to determine glucose level before administering. Do not administer to patients with known CVA unless hypoglycemia documented.

Diazepam (Valium)

Class   Benzodiazepine, sedative-hypnotic, anticonvulsant.

Mechanism of action   Potentiates effects of inhibitory neurotransmitters. Raises seizure threshold. Induces amnesia and sedation.

Indications   Acute anxiety states, acute alcohol withdrawal (delirium tremens), muscle relaxant, seizure activity, agitation. Analgesia for elective medical procedures (fracture reduction, cardioversion).

Contraindications   Hypersensitivity, glaucoma, coma, shock, substance abuse, head injury.

Adverse reactions   Respiratory depression, hypotension, drowsiness, ataxia, reflex tachycardia, nausea, confusion, thrombosis, and phlebitis.

Drug interactions   Incompatible with most drugs, fluids.

How supplied   10 mg/5-ml prefilled syringes, ampules, and vials.

Dosage and administration   Seizure activity: *Adult:* 5–10 mg IV q 10–15 minutes prn (5 mg over 5 min)(maximum dose, 30 mg). Seizure activity: *Pediatric:* 0.2–0.5 mg slowly q 2–5 minutes up to 5 mg (maximum dose, 10 mg/kg). Rectal diazepam: 0.5 mg/kg via 5-cm rectal catheter and flush with 2–3 ml air after administration. Sedation for nonemergent cardioversion: 5–15 mg IV over 5–10 minutes prior to cardioversion.

Duration of action   Onset: 1–5 minutes. Peak effect: minutes. Duration: 20–50 minutes.

Special considerations   Pregnancy safety: Category D. Short duration of anticonvulsant effect. Reduce dose 50% in elderly patient.

Digoxin (Lanoxin)

Class   Inotropic agent.

Mechanism of action   Rapid-acting cardiac glycoside with direct and indirect effects that increase force of myocardial contraction, increase refractory period of AV node, and increase total peripheral resistance.

Indications   Congestive heart failure, reentry SVT, especially atrial flutter and atrial fibrillation.

Contraindications   Ventricular fibrillation, ventricular tachycardia, digoxin toxicity, hypersensitivity to digoxin.

Adverse reactions   Headache, weakness, blurred yellow or green vision, confusion, seizures, arrhythmias, nausea, vomiting, and skin rash.

Drug interactions   Amiodarone, verapamil, and quinidine may increase serum digoxin concentrations by 50%–70%. Concurrent use of digoxin and verapamil may lead to severe heart block. Diuretics may potentiate cardiac toxicity.

How supplied   2-ml ampules of 0.5 mg digoxin; also as tablets, capsules, and elixirs.

Dosage and administration   *Adult:* Loading dose of 10 to 15 µg/kg. *Pediatric:* not recommended in the prehospital setting.

Duration of action   Onset: IV: 5–30 minutes; Peak effect: 30–120 minutes. Duration: several days.

Special considerations   Pregnancy safety: Category A. Patients receiving IV digoxin must be on a monitor. Patients with known renal failure are prone to digoxin toxicity. Hypokalemia, hypomagnesemia, and hypercalcemia potentiate digoxin toxicity. Use carefully in patients with Wolff-Parkinson-White Syndrome (ventricular arrhythmias).

Diltiazem Hydrochloride (Cardizem)

Class   Calcium channel blocker.

Mechanism of action   Block influx of calcium ions into cardiac muscle; prevents spasm of coronary arteries. Arterial and venous vasodilator. Reduces preload and afterload. Reduces myocardial oxygen demand.

Indications   Control of rapid ventricular rates due to atrial flutter, atrial fibrillation, and reentry SVT; angina pectoris.

Contraindications   Hypotension, sick sinus syndrome, second- or third-degree AV block, cardiogenic shock, wide-complex tachycardias, poison/drug-induced tachycardia.

Adverse reactions   Bradycardia, second- or third-degree AV blocks, chest pain, CHF, syncope. VF, VT, nausea, vomiting, dizziness, dry mouth, dyspnea, headache.

Drug interactions   Caution in patients using medications that affect cardiac contractility. In general, should not be used in patients on beta blockers.

How supplied   25 mg/5-ml vial; 50 mg/10-ml vial.

Dosage and administration   *Adult:* Initial bolus: 0.25 mg/kg (average dose 15–20 mg) IV over 2 minutes. If inadequate response, may re-bolus in 15 minutes: 0.35 mg/kg (average dose 20–25 mg) IV over 2 minutes. Maintenance infusion of 5–15 mg/h. *Pediatric:* Not recommended.

Duration of action   Onset: 2–5 minutes. Peak effect: variable. Duration: 1–3 hours.

Special considerations   Pregnancy safety: Category C. Use with caution in patients with renal or hepatic dysfunction. PVCs may be noted at time of conversion of PSVT to sinus rhythm.

Diphenhydramine (Benadryl)

Class Antihistamine; anticholinergic.

Mechanism of action Blocks cellular histamine receptors; decreases vasodilation; decreases motion sickness. Reverses extrapyramidal reactions.

Indications Symptomatic relief of allergies, allergic reactions, anaphylaxis, acute dystonic reactions (phenothiazines). Blood administration reactions; used for motion sickness, hay fever.

Contraindications Asthma, glaucoma, pregnancy, hypertension, narrow-angle glaucoma, infants, patients taking monoamine oxidase inhibitors (MAOIs).

Adverse reactions Sedation, hypotension, seizures, visual disturbances, vomiting, urinary retention, palpitations, arrhythmias, dry mouth and throat, and paradoxical CNS excitation in children.

Drug interactions Potentiates effects of alcohol and other anticholinergics, may inhibit corticosteroid activity; MAOIs prolong anticholinergic effects of diphenhydramine.

How supplied Tablets: 25, 50 mg; Capsules: 25, 50 mg; Prefilled syringes: 50- or 100-mg; vials (IV or IM); elixir, 12.5 mg/5 ml.

Dosage and administration *Adult:* 25–50 mg IM or IV or PO. *Pediatric:* 1–2 mg/kg IV, IO slowly or IM. If given PO: 5 mg/kg/24 hours.

Duration of action Onset: 15–30 minutes. Peak effect: 1 hour. Duration: 3–12 hours.

Special considerations Not used in infants or in pregnancy: Category B. If used in anaphylaxis, will be in conjunction with epinephrine and corticosteroids.

Dobutamine (Dobutrex)

Class Sympathomimetic, inotropic agent.

Mechanism of action Synthetic catecholamine. Increased myocardial contractility and stroke volume, increased cardiac output. Minimal chronotropic activity. Increases renal blood flow.

Indications Cardiogenic shock, CHF, left ventricular dysfunction. Often used in conjunction with other drugs.

Contraindications Tachyarrhythmias, Idiopathic Hypertrophic Subaortic Stenosis (IHSS), severe hypotension.

Adverse reactions May increase infarct size in patient with MI, headache, arrhythmias, hypertension, PVCs.

Drug interactions Incompatible with sodium bicarbonate and furosemide. Beta blockers may blunt inotropic effects.

How supplied 250 mg/20-ml vials.

Dosage and administration *Adult:* IV infusion at 2–20 µg/kg/min titrated to desired effect. *Pediatric:* 2–20 µg/kg/min titrated to desired effect.

Duration of action Onset: 2 minutes. Peak effect: 10 minutes. Duration: 1–2 minutes after infusion discontinued.

Special considerations Pregnancy safety: not well established. Monitor blood pressure closely. Always monitor drip rate. Avoid extravasation injury.

Dopamine (Intropin)

Class Sympathomimetic, inotropic agent.

Mechanism of action Immediate metabolic precursor to norepinephrine. Increases systemic vascular resistance, dilates renal and splanchnic vasculature. Increases myocardial contractility and stroke volume.

Indications Cardiogenic, septic, or spinal shock, hypotension with low cardiac output states, distributive shock.

Contraindications Hypovolemic shock, pheochromocytoma, tachyarrhythmias, VF.

Adverse reactions Cardiac arrhythmias, hypertension, increased myocardial oxygen demand; extravasation may cause tissue necrosis.

Drug interactions Incompatible in alkaline solutions. MAOIs will enhance effects of dopamine. Bretylium may potentiate effect of dopamine. Beta blockers may antagonize effects of dopamine. When administered with phenytoin: may cause hypotension, bradycardia, and seizures.

How supplied 200 mg/5 ml–400 mg/5 ml prefilled syringes, ampules for IV infusion; 400 mg in 250-ml D₅W premixed solutions.

Dosage and administration *Adult:* 2–20 µg/kg/min titrated to patient response; *Pediatric:* 2–20 µg/kg/min titrated to patient response.

Duration of action Onset: 1–4 minutes. Peak effect: 5–10 minutes. Duration: Effects cease almost immediately after infusion is shut off.

Special considerations Pregnancy safety not established. Effects are dose-dependent. Dopaminergic response: 2–4 µg/kg/min: dilates vessels in kidneys; increased urine output. Beta-adrenergic response: 4–10 µg/kg/min: positive chronotropic and inotropic adrenergic response: 10–20 µg/kg/min: primarily alpha stimulant/vasoconstriction. Greater than 20 µg/kg/min: reversal of renal effects/override alpha effects. Always monitor drip rate. Avoid extravasation injury.

Epinephrine (Adrenalin)

Class Sympathomimetic.

Mechanism of action Direct-acting alpha- and beta-agonist. Alpha: vasoconstriction. Beta-1: positive inotropic, chronotropic, and dromotropic effects. Beta-2: bronchial smooth muscle relaxation and dilation of skeletal vasculature.

Indications Cardiac arrest (VF/pulseless VT, asystole, PEA), symptomatic bradycardia as an alternative infusion to dopamine, severe hypotension secondary to bradycardia when atropine and transcutaneous pacing are unsuccessful, allergic reactions, anaphylaxis, asthma.

Contraindications Hypertension, hypothermia, pulmonary edema, myocardial ischemia, hypovolemic shock.

Adverse reactions Hypertension, tachycardia, arrhythmias, pulmonary edema, anxiety, restlessness, psychomotor agitation, nausea, headache, angina.

Drug interactions Potentiates other sympathomimetics, deactivated by alkaline solutions (ie, sodium bicarbonate), monamine oxidase inhibitors (MAOIs) may potentiate effects, beta blockers may blunt effects.

How supplied 1:1,000 solution: ampules and vials containing 1 mg/ml. 1:10,000 solution: prefilled syringes containing 1 mg in 10 ml (0.1 mg/ml). Auto-injector (EpiPen): 0.5 mg/ml (1:2,000).

Dosage and administration *Adult: Mild allergic reactions and asthma:* 0.3–0.5 mg (0.3–0.5 ml of 1:1,000) SC. *Anaphylaxis:* 0.1 mg (1 ml of 1:10,000) IV/IO over 5 minutes. *Cardiac arrest:* IV/IO dose: 1 mg (10 ml of 1:10,000 solution) every 3–5 minutes during resuscitation. Follow each dose with 20-ml flush and elevate arm for 10 to 20 seconds after dose. Higher dose: Higher doses (up to 0.2 mg/kg) may be used for specific indications (beta blocker or calcium channel blocker overdose). Continuous infusion: Add 1 mg (1 ml of 1:1,000 solution) to 500 ml of normal saline or D$_5$W. Initial infusion rate of 1 μg/min titrated to effect (typical dose: 2–10 μg/min). *Profound bradycardia or hypotension:* 2–10 μg/min; titrate to patient response. *Pediatric: Mild allergic reactions and asthma:* 0.01 mg/kg (0.01 ml/kg) of 1:1,000 solution SC (maximum of 0.3 ml). *Cardiac arrest:* IV/IO dose: 0.01 mg/kg (0.1 ml/kg) of 1:10,000 solution every 3–5 minutes during arrest. *Symptomatic bradycardia:* IV/IO dose: 0.01 mg/kg (0.1 ml/kg) of 1:10,000 solution. *Continuous*

IV/IO infusion: Begin with rapid infusion, then titrate to response. Typical initial infusion: 0.1–1 μg/min. Higher doses may be effective.

Duration of action   Onset: immediate. Peak effect: minutes. Duration: several minutes.

Special considerations   Pregnancy safety: Category C. May cause syncope in asthmatic children. May increase myocardial oxygen demand.

Epinephrine Racemic (Vaponefrin)

Class   Sympathomimetic.

Mechanism of action   Stimulates beta-2 receptors in lungs: bronchodilation with relaxation of bronchial smooth muscles. Reduces airway resistance. Useful in treating laryngeal edema; inhibits histamine release.

Indications   Bronchial asthma, prevention of bronchospasm. Croup, laryngotracheobronchitis, laryngeal edema.

Contraindications   Hypertension, underlying cardiovascular disease, epiglottitis.

Adverse reactions   Tachycardia, arrhythmias.

Drug interactions   MAOIs and bretylium may potentiate effects. Beta blockers may blunt effects.

How supplied   MDI: 0.16–0.25 mg/spray. Solution: 7.5, 15, 30 ml in 1%, 2.25% solutions.

Dosage and administration   *Adult:* MDI: 2–3 inhalations, repeated every 5 minutes PRN. Solution: dilute 5 ml (1%) in 5.0 ml NS, administer over 15 minutes. *Pediatric:* Solution: dilute 0.25 ml (0.1%) in 2.5 ml NS (if less than 20 kg); dilute 0.5 ml in 2.5 ml NS (if 20–40 kg); dilute 0.75 ml in 2.5 ml NS (if greater than 40 kg). Administer by aerosolization.

Duration of action   Onset: within 5 minutes. Peak effect: 5–15 minutes. Duration: 1–3 hours.

Special considerations   May cause tachycardia and other arrhythmias. Monitor vital signs. Excessive use may cause bronchospasm.

Etomidate (Amidate)

Class   Anesthetic.

Mechanism of action   Produces hypnosis rapidly, causing CNS depression and anesthesis. Offers no analgesic effect.

Indications   Induction of anesthesia for rapid sequence intubation (RSI).

Contraindications   Hypersensitivity.

Adverse reactions   Apnea, transient muscle movements, myoclonus, suppression of cortisol levels, nausea, vomiting.

Drug interactions   Synergistic with benzodiazepines, may decrease analgesic effects of opiates, antagonizes aminophylline.

How supplied   2 mg/ml; 10-ml vial.

Dosage and administration   0.3 mg/kg IV over 30–60 seconds, to a maximum dose of 20 mg.

Duration of action   Onset: within 60 seconds (may be as rapid as 5–15 seconds). Duration of 3–15 minutes.

Special considerations   Other medications should be used if prolonged sedation is required; this drug is not intended for administration by infusion.

Fentanyl Citrate (Sublimaze)

Class   Opioid analgesic.

Mechanism of action   Alleviates pain through CNS action, suppresses fear and anxiety centres in brain; depresses brainstem respiratory centres, increases peripheral venous capacitance and decreases venous return, decreases preload and afterload, which decreases myocardial oxygen demand.

Indications   Induction of anesthesia for rapid sequence intubation (RSI), analgesia for moderate to severe acute and chronic pain.

Contraindications   Patients who have taken MAOIs within the past 14 days.

Adverse reactions   Respiratory depression, may trigger laryngospasm or muscle rigidity if administered rapidly; hypotension.

Drug interactions   Not compatible with barbiturates, MAOIs may cause paradoxical excitation.

How supplied   25 mcg/ml (2- or 5-ml vials).

Dosage and administration   *Anesthesia (induction):* 1–2 mcg/kg IV. *Adult analgesia:* 25–50 mcg IV every 5–15 minutes. *Pediatric analgesia:* 0.5–1.0 mcg/kg IV every 5 to 15 minutes.

Duration of action   Onset: immediate. Peak effect: 3–15 minutes. Duration: 30–90 minutes.

Special considerations   Pregnancy safety: Category C. Naloxone should be readily available as an antidote.

Flumazenil (Romazicon)

Class   Benzodiazepine receptor antagonist.

Mechanism of action   Antagonizes the actions of benzodiazepines on the CNS.

Indications   Reversal of respiratory depression and sedative effects from pure benzodiazepine overdose.

Contraindications   Hypersensitivity, tricyclic antidepressant overdose, seizure-prone patients, coma of unknown etiology, benzodiazepine dependence.

Adverse reactions   Nausea, vomiting, agitation, injection site pain, visual disturbances, seizures, cutaneous vasodilation.

Drug interactions   Toxic effects of mixed-drug overdose (especially tricyclics and antidepressants).

How supplied   5- and 10-ml vials (0.1 mg/ml).

Dosage and administration   *Adult: First dose:* 0.2 mg IV/IO over 15 seconds. *Second dose:* 0.3 mg IV/IO over 30 seconds. If no response, give third dose. *Third dose:* 0.5 mg IV/IO over 30 seconds. If no response, repeat once every minute until adequate response or a total of 3 mg is given. *Pediatric:* Not recommended.

Duration of action   Onset: 1–2 minutes. Peak effect and duration: related to plasma concentration of benzodiazepines.

Special considerations Pregnancy safety: Category C. Romazicon may precipitate withdrawal syndromes in patients dependent on benzodiazepines. Be prepared to manage seizures in patients who are physically dependent on benzodiazepines or who have ingested large doses of other drugs or consider not administering the drug to this patient population. Monitor patients for resedation and respiratory depression. Be prepared to assist ventilations.

Furosemide (Lasix)

Class Loop diuretic.

Mechanism of action Inhibits electrolyte reabsorption and promotes excretion of sodium, potassium, chloride.

Indications CHF, pulmonary edema, hypertensive crisis.

Contraindications Hypovolemia, anuria, hypotension (relative contraindication); hypersensitivity, hepatic coma.

Adverse reactions May exacerbate hypovolemia, hypokalemia, ECG changes, dry mouth, hypochloremia, hyponatremia, hyperglycemia (due to hemoconcentration).

Drug interactions Lithium toxicity may be potentiated by sodium depletion. Digoxin toxicity may be potentiated by potassium depletion.

How supplied 100 mg/5-ml, 20-mg/2-ml, 40 mg/4-ml vials.

Dosage and administration *Adult:* 0.5–1.0 mg/kg injected IV over 1 to 2 minutes. If no response, double the dose to 2 mg/kg over 1 to 2 minutes. *Pediatric:* 1 mg/kg/dose IV, IO.

Duration of action Onset: 5 minutes. Peak effect: 20–60 minutes. Duration: 4–6 hours.

Special considerations Pregnancy safety: Category C. Ototoxicity and deafness can occur with rapid administration. Should be protected from light.

Glucagon

Class Hyperglycemic agent, pancreatic hormone, insulin antagonist.

Mechanism of action Increases blood glucose level by stimulating glycogenolysis. Unknown mechanism of stabilizing cardiac rhythm in beta blocker overdose. Minimal positive inotropic and chronotropic response. Decreases gastrointestinal motility and secretions.

Indications Altered level of consciousness when hypoglycemia is suspected. May be used as inotropic agent in beta blocker overdose or assist with the passage of esophageal food boluses.

Contraindications Hyperglycemia, hypersensitivity.

Adverse reactions Nausea, vomiting, tachycardia, hypertension.

Drug interactions Incompatible in solution with most other substances. No significant drug interactions with other emergency medications.

How supplied 1-mg ampules (requires reconstitution with diluent provided).

Dosage and administration *Adult: Hypoglycemia:* 0.5–1 mg IM; may repeat in 7–10 minutes. *Calcium channel blocker or beta blocker overdose:* 3 mg initially, followed by infusion at 3 mg/h as necessary. *Pediatric: Hypoglycemia:* 0.5–1 mg IM (for children < 20 kg). *Calcium channel blocker or beta blocker overdose:* not recommended.

Duration of action Onset: 1 minute. Peak effect: 30 minutes. Duration: variable (generally 9–17 minutes).

Special considerations Pregnancy safety: Category C. Ineffective if glycogen stores depleted. Should always be used in conjunction with 50% dextrose whenever possible. If patient does not respond to second dose glucagon, 50% dextrose must be administered.

Haloperidol (Haldol)

Class Tranquilizer, antipsychotic.

Mechanism of action Inhibits central nervous system (CNS) catecholamine receptors: strong antidopaminergic and weak anticholinergic. Acts on CNS to depress subcortical areas, mid-brain, and ascending reticular activating system in the brain.

Indications Acute psychotic episodes.

Contraindications Agitation secondary to shock or hypoxia. Hypersensitivity.

Adverse reactions Extrapyramidal signs and symptoms, restlessness, spasms, Parkinson-like symptoms, drooling, dystonia, hypotension, orthostatic, hypotension, nausea, vomiting, blurred vision.

Drug interactions Enhanced CNS depression and hypotension in combination with alcohol. Antagonized amphetamines and epinephrine. Other CNS depressants may potentiate effects.

How supplied 5 mg/ml ampule.

Dosage and administration *Adult:* 2–5 mg IM every 30–60 minutes until sedation achieved. *Pediatric:* Not recommended.

Duration of action Onset: 10 minutes. Peak effect: 30–45 minutes. Duration: variable (generally 12–24 hours).

Special considerations Pregnancy safety: not established. Treat hypotension secondary to haloperidol with fluids and norepinephrine, not epinephrine. Patient may also be taking benztropine mesylate (Cogentin) if on long-term therapy with haloperidol.

Hydrocortisone Sodium Succinate (Solu-Cortef)

Class Corticosteroid.

Mechanism of action Anti-inflammatory and immunosuppressive with salt-retaining actions.

Indications Shock due to acute adrenocortical insufficiency.

Contraindications None if given as single dose.

Adverse reactions Only for long-term use.

Drug interactions Incompatible with heparin.

How supplied 100-mg, 250-mg, or 500-mg vials.

Dosage and administration *Adult:* 1–4 mg/kg slow IV bolus. *Pediatric:* 0.16–1.0 mg/kg slow IV bolus.

Duration of action Onset: 1 hour. Peak effect: variable. Duration: 8–12 hours.

Special considerations May be used in status asthmaticus as a second-line drug.

Hydroxyzine (Atarax)

Class   Antihistamine, antiemetic, antianxiety agent.

Mechanism of action   Potentiates effects of analgesics; calming effect without impairing mental alertness.

Indications   To potentiate the effects of analgesics; to control nausea and vomiting, anxiety reactions, and motion sickness; preoperative and postoperative sedation.

Contraindications   Hypersensitivity.

Adverse reactions   Dry mouth and drowsiness.

Drug interactions   Potentiates the effects of CNS depressants such as narcotics, barbiturates, and alcohol.

How supplied   25 mg/ml or 50 mg/ml in 1-ml vials.

Dosage and administration   *Adult:* 25–100 mg IM. *Pediatric:* 0.5–1.0 mg/kg/dose IM.

Duration of action   Onset: IM: 15–30 minutes. Peak effect: 45 minutes to 1.5 hours. Duration: 4–6 hours.

Special considerations   Should be given by IM injection only. Localized burning at injection site is common complaint.

Ketamine

Class   Anesthetic.

Mechanism of action   Dissociative anesthetic, producing analgesia.

Indications   Sole anesthetic agent for diagnostic and minor surgical procedures; induction agent in special circumstances (status asthmaticus).

Contraindications   Hypersensitivity to the medication, hypertension, elevated intracranial pressure, thyrotoxicosis, psychosis, congestive heart failure.

Adverse reactions   Laryngospasm, respiratory depression, increased intracranial pressure, hypotension, bradycardia, delirium, hypersalivation, fasciculations.

Drug interactions   Inhaled anesthetics may prolong duration of action of ketamine.

How supplied   10 mg in 20-ml vial; 50 mg in 10-ml vial.

Dosage and administration   *Induction:* 0.5–2 mg/kg IV or 4–6 mg/kg IM.

Duration of action   Onset: rapid. Peak effect: 5 minutes. Duration: 20–60 minutes.

Special considerations   Pregnancy safety: Category C.

Ketorolac Tromethamine (Toradol IM)

Class   Nonsteroidal anti-inflammatory (NSAID) analgesic.

Mechanism of action   NSAID that also exhibits peripherally acting nonnarcotic analgesic activity by inhibiting prostaglandin synthesis.

Indications   Short-term management of moderate to severe pain.

Contraindications   Allergy to salicylates or other NSAIDs; patients with history of asthma; bleeding disorders, especially gastrointestinal (GI) related (peptic ulcer disease); renal failure.

Adverse reactions   Anaphylaxis due to hypersensitivity, nausea, GI bleeding, sedation, hypotension or hypertension, rash, headache, edema.

Drug interactions   May increase bleeding time in patients taking anticoagulants.

How supplied   15 or 30 mg in 1-ml vial or 60 mg in 2-ml vials.

Dosage and administration   *Adult:* 30–60 mg IM. *Pediatric:* Not recommended.

Duration of action   Onset: 10 minutes. Peak effect: 1–2 hours. Duration: 2–6 hours.

Special considerations   Pregnancy safety: Category C. Use with caution in elderly patient. May be given IV in lower dosage (15–30 mg).

Labetolol (Normodyne, Trandate)

Class   Selective alpha and nonselective beta-adrenergic blocker.

Mechanism of action   Blood pressure reduced without reflex tachycardia; total peripheral resistance reduced without significant alteration in cardiac output.

Indications   Moderate to severe hypertension.

Contraindications   Bronchial asthma, CHF, cardiogenic shock, second- and third-degree heart block, bradycardia.

Adverse reactions   Headache, dizziness, ventricular arrhythmias, hypotension, dyspnea, facial flushing, postural hypotension, diaphoresis, allergic reaction.

Drug interactions   Trandate may block bronchodilator effects of beta-adrenergic agonists. Nitroglycerine may augment hypotensive effects of Labetolol.

How supplied   Trandate injection 5 mg/ml, 20-ml (100 mg) and 40-ml (200 mg) vials.

Dosage and administration   *Adult:* 5–20 mg slow IV over 2 minutes (additional injections of 10–40 mg can be given at 10-minute intervals). Infusion: 2 mg/min titrated to acceptable supine blood pressure. *Pediatric:* safety not established.

Duration of action   Onset: less than 5 minutes. Peak effect: variable. Duration: 3–6 hours.

Special considerations   Pregnancy safety: Category C. Continuous monitoring of BP, pulse rate, and ECG. Observe for signs of CHF, bradycardia, bronchospasm. Should only be administered with patient in supine position.

Lidocaine Hydrochloride (Xylocaine)

Class   Antiarrhythmic.

Mechanism of action   Decreases automaticity by slowing the rate of phase 4 depolarization.

Indications   Alternative to amiodarone in cardiac arrest from VF/pulseless VT, stable monomorphic VT, stable polymorphic VT with normal baseline QT interval.

Contraindications   Hypersensitivity, second- and third-degree AV blocks in the absence of artificial pacemaker, Stokes-Adams syndrome, prophylactic use in AMI, wide-complex ventricular escape beats with bradycardia.

Adverse reactions   Slurred speech, seizures (with high doses), altered mental status, confusion, lightheadedness, blurred vision, bradycardia.

Drug interactions   Apnea induced with succinylcholine may be prolonged with high doses of lidocaine. Cardiac depression may occur in conjunction with IV phenytoin (Dilantin). Procainamide may exacerbate CNS effects. Metabolic clearance is decreased in patients with liver disease or in patients taking beta blockers.

How supplied   100 mg in 5-ml prefilled syringes and ampules (20 mg/ml), 1-g and 2-g additive syringes, 1-g and 2-g vials in 30 ml of solution.

Dosage and administration   *Adult: Cardiac arrest from VF/pulseless VT:* Initial dose: 1–1.5 mg/kg IV/IO. Repeat dose: 0.5–0.75 mg/kg, repeated in 5–10 minutes to maximum dose of 3 mg/kg. *Stable VT, wide-complex tachycardia of uncertain type, significant ectopy:* Doses ranging from 0.5–0.75 mg/kg and up to 1–1.5 mg/kg may be used. Repeat 0.5–0.75 mg/kg every 5–10 minutes. Maximum total dose is 3 mg/kg. *Maintenance infusion:* 1–4 mg/min (30–50 µg/kg/min); can dilute in D_5W or normal saline. *Pediatric:* IV/IO dose: 1 mg/kg rapid IV/IO push.

Maximum dose: 100 mg. *Continuous IV/IO infusion:* 20–50 µg/kg/min. Administer bolus dose (1 mg/kg) when infusion is initiated if bolus has not been given within previous 15 minutes.

Duration of action   Onset: 1–3 minutes. Peak effect: 5–10 minutes. Duration: variable (15 minutes–2 hours).

Special considerations   Pregnancy safety: Category B. Reduce maintenance infusions by 50% if patient is over 70 years of age, has liver or renal disease, or is in CHF or shock. A 75–100 mg bolus maintains blood levels for only 20 minutes (if not in shock). Exceedingly high doses of lidocaine can result in coma or death. Avoid lidocaine for reperfusion arrhythmias after fibrinolytic therapy. Cross-reactivity with other forms of local anesthetics.

Lidocaine Spray

Class   Topical anesthetic.

Mechanism of action   Stabilizes neuronal membrane.

Indications   Used as a lubricant and topical anesthetic to facilitate passage of diagnostic and treatment devices. Suppresses the pharyngeal and tracheal gag reflex.

Contraindications   Patients with a known hypersensitivity to lidocaine

Adverse reactions   Methemoglobinemia has been reported following the use of lidocaine on extremely rare occasions.

Drug interactions   No significant interactions found or known.

How supplied   Multidose aerosol can, 20% lidocaine.

Dosage and administration   *Adult:* 0.5–1.0 second spray, repeat as needed. *Pediatric:* 0.25–0.5 second spray, repeat as needed.

Duration of action   Onset: Immediate. Peak effect: 30 seconds. Duration: 15 minutes.

Special considerations   Pregnancy safety: Category A. Topical use only, not for ocular use or injection.

Lorazepam (Ativan)

Class   Benzodiazepine; sedative; anticonvulsant.

Mechanism of action   Anxiolytic, anticonvulsant, and sedative effects; suppresses propagation of seizure activity produced by foci in cortex, thalamus, and limbic areas.

Indications   Initial control of status epilepticus or severe recurrent seizures, severe anxiety, sedation.

Contraindications   Acute narrow-angle glaucoma. Coma, shock, or suspected drug abuse.

Adverse reactions   Respiratory depression, apnea, drowsiness, sedation, ataxia, psychomotor impairment, confusion, restlessness, delirium, hypotension, bradycardia.

Drug interactions   May precipitate CNS depression if patient is already taking CNS depressant medications.

How supplied   2 and 4 mg/ml concentrations in 1-ml vials.

Dosage and administration   *Note:* When given IV or IO, must dilute with equal volume of sterile water or sterile saline; when given IM, lorazepam is not to be diluted. *Adult:* 2–4 mg slow IV at 2 mg/min or IM; may repeat in 15–20 minutes to maximum dose of 8 mg. For sedation: 0.05 mg/kg up to 4 mg IM. *Pediatric:* 0.05–0.20 mg/kg slow IV, IO slowly over 2 minutes or IM; may repeat in 15–20 minutes to maximum dose of 0.2 mg/kg.

Duration of action   Onset: 1–5 minutes. Peak effect: variable. Duration: 6–8 hours.

Special considerations   Pregnancy safety: Category D. Monitor BP and respiratory rate during administration. Have advanced airway equipment readily available. Inadvertent arterial injection may result in vasospasm and gangrene. Lorazepam expires in 6 weeks if not refrigerated.

Magnesium Sulfate

Class   Electrolyte.

Mechanism of action   Reduces striated muscle contractions and blocks peripheral neuromuscular transmission by reducing acetylcholine release at the myoneural junction, manages seizures in toxemia of pregnancy, induces uterine relaxation, can cause bronchodilation after beta-agonists and anticholinergics have been used.

Indications   Seizures of eclampsia (toxemia of pregnancy), torsade de pointes, hypomagnesemia, Class IIa agent for VF/pulseless VT that is refractory to lidocaine.

Contraindications   Heart blocks, myocardial damage.

Adverse reactions   CNS depression, facial flushing, diaphoresis, depressed reflexes, circulatory collapse, hypotension.

Drug interactions   May enhance effects of other CNS depressants, serious changes in overall cardiac function may occur with cardiac glycosides.

How supplied   10%, 12.5%, 50% solution in 40, 80, 100, and 125 mg/ml.

Dosage and administration   *Adult: Seizure activity associated with pregnancy:* 1–4 g IV/IO over 3 minutes; maximum dose of 30–40 g/day. *Cardiac arrest due to hypomagnesemia or torsade de pointes:* 1–2 g diluted in 10 ml of D_5W IV/IO over 5–20 minutes. *Torsade de pointes with a pulse or AMI with hypomagnesemia:* Loading dose of 1–2 g mixed in 50–100 ml of D_5W over 5–60 minutes IV. Follow with 0.5–1 g/h IV (titrate to control torsade de pointes). *Pediatric: IV/IO infusion:* 25–50 mg/kg (maximum dose: 2 g) over 10–20 minutes; faster for torsade de pointes. *For asthma:* 25–50 mg/kg (maximum dose: 2 g) over 10–20 minutes.

Duration of action   Onset: IV/IO: immediate, IM: 3–4 hours, Duration: 30 minutes (IV/IO), 3–4 hours (IM).

Special considerations   Pregnancy safety: Category B. Recommended that the drug not be given in the 2 hours before delivery, if possible. IV calcium chloride or calcium gluconate should be available as a magnesium antagonist if needed. Use with caution in patients with renal failure.

Mannitol (Osmitrol)

Class Osmotic diuretic.

Mechanism of action Induces osmotic diuresis; decreases cerebral edema, thus reducing intracranial pressure.

Indications Temporizing measure to decrease intracranial pressure in patient with signs of acute herniation.

Contraindications Pulmonary edema, hypovolemia, hypotension, hypersensitivity.

Adverse reactions Thrombophlebitis, hypotension, acute pulmonary edema, congestive heart failure and circulatory overload; seizures, hyponatremia.

Drug interactions Incompatible with alkaline solutions and other commonly used IV solutions; must be run in dedicated IV line; do not use if crystals appear in bag.

How supplied 100 g/250-ml bag (20% solution).

Dosage and administration 0.25–5 g/kg over 15 minutes; repeat after 30 minutes, if necessary; must be administered through a 40-micron filter.

Duration of action Onset: 15 minutes. Peak effect: 60–90 minutes. Duration: 3–8 hours.

Meperidine (Demerol)

Class Opioid analgesic.

Mechanism of action Synthetic opioid agonist that acts on opioid receptors to produce analgesia, euphoria, respiratory and physical depression; a schedule II drug with potential for physical dependency and abuse.

Indications Analgesia for moderate to severe pain.

Contraindications Hypersensitivity to narcotic agents, diarrhea caused by poisoning, patients taking MAOIs, during labour or delivery of a premature infant, undiagnosed abdominal pain or head injury.

Adverse reactions Respiratory depression, sedation, apnea, circulatory depression, arrhythmias, shock, euphoria, delirium, agitation, hallucinations, visual disturbances, coma, seizures, headache, facial flushing, increased ICP, nausea, vomiting.

Drug interactions Do not give concurrently with MAOIs (even with a dose in the last 14 days!). Exacerbates CNS depression when given with these medications.

How supplied 50/ml in 1-ml prefilled syringes.

Dosage and administration *Adult:* 50–100 mg IM, SC or 25–50 mg slowly IV. *Pediatric:* 1–2 mg/kg/dose IV, IO, IM, SC.

Duration of action Onset: IM: 10–45 minutes; IV: immediate. Peak effect: 30–60 minutes. Duration: 2–4 hours.

Special considerations Pregnancy safety: Category C. Use with caution in patients with asthma and COPD. May aggravate seizures in patients with known convulsive disorders. Naloxone should be readily available as antagonist.

Methylprednisolone (Solu-Medrol)

Class Anti-inflammatory glucocorticoid.

Mechanism of action Synthetic corticosteroid that suppresses acute and chronic inflammation; potentiates vascular smooth muscle relaxation by beta-adrenergic agonists.

Indications Anaphylaxis, bronchodilator for unresponsive asthma.

Contraindications Premature infants, systemic fungal infections; use with caution in patients with gastrointestinal bleeding.

Adverse reactions Headache, hypertension, sodium and water retention, CHF, hypokalemia, alkalosis, peptic ulcer disease, nausea, vomiting.

Drug interactions Hypoglycemic responses to insulin and hypoglycemic agents may be blunted. Potassium-depleting agents may exacerbate hypokalemic effects.

How supplied 40-, 125-, 500- and 1,000-mg vials.

Dosage and administration 1–2 mg/kg IV.

Duration of action Onset of action: 1–2 hours. Peak effect: variable. Duration: 8–24 hours.

Special considerations Pregnancy safety: not established. Crosses the placenta and may cause fetal harm.

Midazolam (Versed)

Class Short-acting benzodiazepine CNS depressant.

Mechanism of action Anxiolytic and sedative properties similar to other benzodiazepines, memory impairment.

Indications Sedation, anxiolytic prior to endotracheal or nasotracheal intubation; administer for conscious sedation.

Contraindications Glaucoma, shock, coma, alcohol intoxication, overdose, depressed vital signs, concomitant use with other CNS depressants, barbiturates, alcohol, narcotics.

Adverse reactions Hiccough, cough, oversedation, nausea, vomiting, injection site pain, headache, blurred vision, hypotension, respiratory depression, and arrest.

Drug interactions Should not be used in patients who have taken a CNS depressant.

How supplied 2-, 5-, 10-ml vials (1 mg/ml); 1-, 2- , 5-, 10-ml vials (5 mg/ml).

Dosage and administration *Adult:* 2.0–2.5 mg slow IV over 2–3 minutes; may be repeated to total maximum: 0.1 mg/kg. *Pediatric:* Not recommended.

Duration of action Onset: 1–3 minutes, IV and dose dependent. Peak effect: variable. Duration: 2–6 hours, dose dependent.

Special considerations Pregnancy safety: Category D. Administer immediately prior to intubation procedure. Requires continuous monitoring of respiratory and cardiac function. Never administer as IV bolus.

Morphine Sulfate

Class Opioid analgesic.

Mechanism of action Alleviates pain through CNS action, suppresses fear and anxiety centres in brain; depresses brain stem respiratory centres, increases peripheral venous capacitance and decreases venous return, decreases preload and afterload, which decreases myocardial oxygen demand.

Indications Severe CHF, pulmonary edema, chest pain associated with acute MI, analgesia for moderate to severe acute and chronic pain (use with caution).

Contraindications Head injury, exacerbated COPD, depressed respiratory drive, hypotension, undiagnosed abdominal pain, decreased level of consciousness, suspected hypovolemia, patients who have taken MAOIs within the past 14 days.

Adverse reactions   Respiratory depression, hypotension, decreased level of consciousness, nausea, vomiting, bradycardia, tachycardia, syncope, facial flushing, euphoria, bronchospasm, dry mouth.

Drug interactions   Potentiates sedative effects of phenothiazines. CNS depressant may potentiate effects of morphine. MAOIs may cause paradoxical excitation.

How supplied   10 mg in 1 ml of solution, ampules, and preloaded syringes.

Dosage and administration   *Adult: Initial dose:* 2–4 mg IV (over 1–5 minutes) every 5–30 minutes. *Repeat dose:* 2–8 mg at 5- to 15-minute intervals. *Pediatric:* 0.1–0.2 mg/kg per dose via IV, IO, IM, or SC; maximum dose of 5 mg.

Duration of action   Onset: immediate. Peak effect: 20 minutes. Duration: 2–7 hours.

Special considerations   Pregnancy safety: Category C. Morphine rapidly crosses the placenta. Safety in neonate not established. Use with caution in geriatric population and those with COPD, asthma. Vagotonic effect in patient with acute inferior MI (bradycardia, heart block). Naloxone should be readily available as an antidote.

Naloxone Hydrochloride (Narcan)

Class   Narcotic antagonist.

Mechanism of action   Competitive inhibition at narcotic receptor sites, reverse respiratory depression secondary to opiate drugs, completely inhibits the effect of morphine.

Indications   Opiate overdose, coma; complete or partial reversal of CNS and respiratory depression induced by opioids; decreased level of consciousness; coma of unknown origin; narcotic agonist for the following: morphine, heroin, hydromorphone (Dilaudid), methadone, meperidine (Demerol), paregoric, fentanyl (Sublimase), oxycodone (Percodan), codeine, propoxyphene (Darvon); narcotic agonist and antagonist for the following: butorphanol (Stadol), pentazocine (Talwin), nalbuphine (Nubain).

Contraindications   Use with caution in narcotic-dependent patients; use with caution in neonates of narcotic-addicted mothers.

Adverse reactions   Withdrawal symptoms in the addicted patient, tachycardia, hypertension, arrhythmias, nausea, vomiting, diaphoresis.

Drug interactions   Incompatible with bisulfite and alkaline solutions.

How supplied   0.02 mg/ml (neonate); 0.4 mg/ml, 1 mg/ml; 2.0 mg/5-ml ampules; 2 mg/5-ml prefilled syringe.

Dosage and administration   *Adult:* 0.4–2.0 mg IV, IM, or SC; minimum recommended dose, 2.0 mg; repeat at 5-minute intervals to a maximum dose of 10 mg (medical control may request higher amounts). Infusion: 2 mg in 500 ml of D_5W (4 µg/ml), infuse at 0.4 mg/h (100 ml/h). *Pediatric:* 0.1 mg/kg/dose IV, IM, or SC; maximum dose of 0.8 mg; if no response in 10 minutes, administer an additional 0.1 mg/kg/dose.

Duration of action   Onset: within 2 minutes. Peak effect: variable. Duration: 30–60 minutes.

Special considerations   Pregnancy safety: Category B. Seizures without causal relationship have been reported. May not reverse hypotension. Morphine may precipitate withdrawal syndromes in patients dependant on morphine or other opiates. Be prepared to manage seizures in patients who are physically dependant on opiates or who have ingested large doses of other drugs, or consider not administering the drug to this patient population. Monitor patients for resedation and respiratory depression. Be prepared to assist ventilations.

Nifedipine (Procardia)

Class   Calcium channel blocker.

Mechanism of action   Inhibits movement of calcium ions across cell membranes; calcium channel blocker, arterial and venous vasodilator; reduces preload and afterload; prevents coronary artery spasm and decreases total peripheral resistance; reduces myocardial oxygen demand; does not prolong AV nodal conduction.

Indications   Hypertensive crisis, angina pectoris, premature labour pulmonary edema (investigational).

Contraindications   Compensatory hypertension, hypotension, hypersensitivity.

Adverse reactions   Hypotension, CHF, headache, dizziness, lightheadedness, facial flushing, heat sensation, weakness, nausea, muscle cramps, mood changes, peripheral edema, myocardial infarction.

Drug interactions   Beta blockers may potentiate effects. Effects of theophylline may be increased. Antihypertensives may potentiate hypotensive effects.

How supplied   Soft gelatin capsules, 10–20 mg. Extended-release tablets, 30, 60, 90 mg.

Dosage and administration   *Adult:* 10 mg SL or buccal (puncture end of capsule with needle and squeeze; may administer SL or buccally or may have patient bite and swallow); may repeat in 30 minutes. *Pediatric:* Not recommended.

Duration of action   Onset: 15–30 minutes. Peak effect: 1–3 hours. Duration: 6–8 hours.

Special considerations   Pregnancy safety: Category C. Does not slow AV nodal activity. Have beta blocker available for control of reflex tachycardia. Use with caution in geriatric population; hypotension and angina pectoris may occur.

Nitroglycerin (Nitrostat, Tridil, and others)

Class   Vasodilator.

Mechanism of action   Smooth muscle relaxant acting on vascular, bronchial, uterine, and intestinal smooth muscle; dilation of arterioles and veins in the periphery; reduces preload and afterload; decreases the workload of the heart and, thereby, myocardial oxygen demand.

Indications   Acute angina pectoris, ischemic chest pain, hypertension, CHF, pulmonary edema.

Contraindications   Hypotension, hypovolemia; intracranial bleeding or head injury; previous administration of Viagra, Revatio, Levitra, Cialis, or other erectile dysfunction agents within past 24 hours.

Adverse reactions   Headache, hypotension, syncope, reflex tachycardia, flushing, nausea, vomiting, diaphoresis, muscle twitching.

Drug interactions   Additive effects with other vasodilators; incompatible with other drugs IV.

How supplied   Tablets: 0.3 mg; 0.4 mg; 0.6 mg. NTG spray: 0.4 mg–0.8 mg under the tongue. NTG IV (Tridil).

Dosage and administration   *Adult:* Tablets: 0.3–0.4 mg SL; may repeat in 3–5 minutes to maximum of 3 doses. NTG spray: 0.4 mg under the tongue; 1–2 sprays, may repeat in 3–5 minutes to maximum of 3 doses. NTG IV infusion: begin at 10 to 20 µg/min; increase by 5–10 µg/min every 5 minutes until desired effect. *Pediatric:* Not recommended.

Duration of action   Onset: 1–3 minutes. Peak effect: 5–10 minutes. Duration: 20–30 minutes or if IV, 1–10 minutes after discontinuation of infusion.

Special considerations   Pregnancy safety: Category C. Hypotension more common in geriatric population. NTG decomposes if exposed to light or heat. Must be kept in airtight containers. Active ingredient may have a stinging effect when administered.

Nitrous Oxide:Oxygen (50:50) (Entenox, Nitronox)

Class   Gaseous analgesic and anesthetic.

Mechanism of action   Exact mechanism unknown; affects central nervous system phospholipids.

Indications   Moderate to severe pain, anxiety, apprehension.

Contraindications   Impaired level of consciousness, head injury, inability to comply with instructions; decompression sickness (nitrogen narcosis, air embolism, air transport); undiagnosed abdominal pain or marked distension, bowel obstruction; hypotension, shock, COPD (with history/suspicion of carbon dioxide retention); cyanosis; chest trauma with pneumothorax.

Adverse reactions   Dizziness, apnea, expansion of gas-filled pockets, cyanosis, nausea, vomiting, malignant hyperthermia, drowsiness, euphoria.

Drug interactions   None of significance.

How supplied   D and E cylinders (blue and green); of 50% nitrous oxide and 50% oxygen compressed gas.

Dosage and administration   *Adult:* (*Note:* Invert cylinder several times before use) Instruct the patient to inhale deeply through demand valve and mask or mouthpiece. *Pediatric:* Same as adult.

Duration of action   Onset: 2–5 minutes. Peak effect: variable. Duration: 2–5 minutes.

Special considerations   Pregnancy safety: Nitrous oxide increases the incidence of spontaneous abortion. Ventilate patient area during use. Nitrous oxide is a nonflammable and nonexplosive gas. Nitrous oxide is ineffective in 20% of the population.

Norepinephrine (Levophed)

Class   Sympathomimetic.

Mechanism of action   Potent alpha-agonist resulting in intense vasoconstriction; positive chronotropic and increased inotropic effect (from 10% beta effects) with increased cardiac output.

Indications   Cardiogenic shock, significant hypotensive (< 70 mm Hg) states.

Contraindications   Hypotensive patients with hypovolemia, pregnancy (relative contraindication).

Adverse reactions   Headache, arrhythmias, tachycardia, reflex bradycardia; angina pectoris, hypertension; decreased blood flow to gastrointestinal tract, kidneys, skeletal muscle, and skin.

Drug interactions   Can be deactivated by alkaline solutions. Sympathomimetics and phosphodiesterase inhibitors may exacerbate arrhythmias.

How supplied   1 mg/ml, 4-ml ampules.

Dosage and administration   *Adult:* Dilute 8 mg in 500 ml of D_5W or 4 mg in 250 ml of D_5W (16 mg/ml); infuse by IV piggyback at 0.5–1.0 µg/min, titrated to improve blood pressure (up to 30 µg/min). *Pediatric:* 0.1–1.0 µg/min IV infusion, titrated to patient response.

Duration of action   Onset: 1–3 minutes. Peak effect: variable. Duration: 5–10 minutes and lasts only 1 minute after infusion discontinued.

Special considerations   Pregnancy safety: not established. May cause fetal anoxia when used in pregnancy. Must be infused through large stable vein to avoid tissue necrosis (antidote: local phentolamine injection). Often used with low-dose dopamine to spare renal and mesenteric blood flow.

Oral Glucose

Class   Hyperglycemic.

Mechanism of action   Provides quickly absorbed glucose to increase blood glucose levels.

Indications   Conscious patients with suspected hypoglycemia.

Contraindications   Decreased level of consciousness, nausea, vomiting.

Adverse reactions   Nausea, vomiting.

Drug interactions   None.

How supplied   Glucola: 300-ml bottles. Glucose pastes and gels in various forms.

Dosage and administration   *Adult:* Should be sipped slowly by patient until clinical improvement noted. *Pediatric:* Same as adult.

Duration of action   Onset: immediate. Peak effect: variable. Duration: variable.

Special considerations   As noted in indications section.

Oxygen

Class   Naturally occurring atmospheric gas.

Mechanism of action   Reverses hypoxemia.

Indications   Confirmed or expected hypoxemia, ischemic chest pain, respiratory insufficiency, prophylactically during air transport, confirmed or suspected carbon monoxide poisoning, all other causes of decreased tissue oxygenation, decreased level of consciousness.

Contraindications   Flammable environment where oxygen may support combustion.

Adverse reactions   Decreased level of consciousness and respiratory depression in patients with chronic carbon dioxide retention. Retrolental fibroplasia if high concentrations given to premature infants (maintain 30%–40% oxygen).

Drug interactions   None.

How supplied   Oxygen cylinders (usually green and white) of 100% compressed oxygen gas.

Dosage and administration *Adult:* Cardiac arrest and carbon monoxide poisoning: 100%. Hypoxemia: 10–15 l/min via nonrebreathing mask. COPD: 1–6 l/min via nasal catheter or 28%–35% Venturi mask. Be prepared to provide ventilatory support if higher concentrations of oxygen needed. *Pediatric:* Same as for adult with exception of premature infant.

Duration of action Onset: immediate. Peak effect: not applicable. Duration: Less than 2 minutes.

Special considerations Certain patients with COPD or emphysema depend on their hypoxic drive for ventilation. Supplemental oxygen suppresses this drive and may result in respiratory arrest. Do not withhold supplemental oxygen from hypoxic patients, but titrate the amount of supplemental oxygen and be prepared to provide respiratory support. Be familiar with litre flow and each type of delivery device used. Supports possibility of combustion.

Oxytocin (Pitocin)

Class Hormone.

Mechanism of action Increases uterine contractions.

Indications Postpartum hemorrhage after infant and placental delivery.

Contraindications Presence of second fetus, unfavourable fetal position, hypersensitivity.

Adverse reactions Hypotension, hypertension, tachycardia, arrhythmias, angina pectoris; anxiety, seizures, nausea, vomiting, uterine rupture; anaphylaxis.

Drug interactions Other vasopressors may potentiate hypertension.

How supplied 10 USP units/1-ml ampule (10 U/ml) and prefilled syringe. 5 USP units/1-ml ampule (5 U/ml) and prefilled syringe.

Dosage and administration IM administration: 3–10 units after delivery of placenta. IV administration: Mix 10–40 units in 1,000 ml of a nonhydrating diluent: Infused at 20–40 milliunits/min, titrated to severity of bleeding and uterine response.

Duration of action Onset: IM: 3–5 minutes; IV: immediate. Peak effect: variable. Duration: IM; 30–60 minutes; IV: 20 minutes after infusion discontinued.

Special considerations Pregnancy safety: not applicable. Monitor vital signs, including fetal heart rate and uterine tone closely.

Pancuronium (Pavulon)

Class Nondepolarizing neuromuscular blocker/paralytic.

Mechanism of action Binds to the receptor for acetylcholine at the neuromuscular junction.

Indications Induction or maintenance of paralysis after intubation to assist ventilations.

Contraindications Hypersensitivity, inability to control airway and support ventilations with oxygen and positive pressure, neuromuscular disease (myasthenia gravis), hepatic or renal failure.

Adverse reactions Apnea, weakness, salivation, premature ventricular contractions, tachycardia; transient hypotension, increased blood pressure; pain, burning at injection site.

Drug interactions Positive chronotropic drugs may potentiate tachycardia.

How supplied 4 mg/2-ml ampule.

Dosage and administration *Adult:* 0.1 mg/kg slow IV; repeat every 30–60 minutes PRN. *Pediatric:* 0.1 mg/kg slow IV, IO.

Duration of action Onset: 30 seconds. Peak effect: paralysis in 3–5 minutes. Duration: 45–60 minutes.

Special considerations Pregnancy safety: not established. If patient is conscious, explain the effect of the medication before administration and always sedate the patient before using pancuronium. Intubation and ventilatory support must be readily available. Monitor the patient carefully. Effects may be reversed with neostigmine (Prostigmin) 0.05 mg/kg and should be accompanied by atropine (0.5–1.2 mg IV). Pancuronium has no effect on consciousness or pain and will not stop neuronal seizure activity. Pulse rate and cardiac output are increased. Decrease doses for patients with renal disease.

Phenobarbital

Class Barbiturate, anticonvulsant.

Mechanism of action Generally unknown but believed to reduce neuronal excitability by increasing the motor cortex threshold to electrical stimulation.

Indications Prevention and treatment of seizure activity; prophylaxis for febrile seizures; anxiety, apprehension; status epilepticus.

Contraindications Patients with porphyria, hypersensitivity, severe liver or respiratory diseases.

Adverse reactions Respiratory depression, hypotension, coma, bradycardia, nausea, vomiting; central nervous system (CNS) depression, ataxia, nystagmus, pupillary constriction; burning at injection site.

Drug interactions Effects potentiated by other CNS depressants, anticonvulsants, and MAOIs; incompatible with all other drugs; flush line before and after use.

How supplied Elixir: 20 mg/5 ml. Tablets: 8, 15, 30, 60, 90, 100 mg. Parenteral: 30, 60, 65 mg, 130-mg/ml ampule; dose may be diluted with D_5W prior of administration.

Dosage and administration *Adult:* 100–250 mg slow IV, or IM; may repeat as needed in 20–30 minutes. *Pediatric:* 10–20 mg/kg IV, IO (less than 1 mg/kg/min) or IM; repeat as needed in 20–30 minutes.

Duration of action Onset: 3–30 minutes. Peak effect: 30 minutes. Duration: 4–6 hours.

Special considerations Pregnancy safety: Category B. Potential for abuse. Carefully monitor vital signs. Use with caution in patients with pulmonary, cardiovascular, hepatic, or renal insufficiency. Use a large, stable vein for injection.

Phenytoin (Dilantin)

Class Anticonvulsant, antiarrhythmic.

Mechanism of action Promotes sodium efflux from neurons, thereby stabilizing the neuron's threshold against excitability caused by excess stimulation; in similar fashion, decreases abnormal ventricular automaticity and decreases the refractory period in the myocardial conduction system.

Indications Prophylaxis and treatment of major motor seizures, digoxin-induced arrhythmias.

Contraindications Hypersensitivity, bradycardia, second- and third-degree heart block.

Adverse reactions Hypotension with too rapid IV push, heart block, arrhythmias, cardiovascular collapse, nausea, vomiting, ataxia, central nervous system depression, nystagmus, pain at injection site, respiratory depression.

Drug interactions   Serum dilantin levels increased by: anticoagulants, tagamet, sulfonamides, salicylates. Metabolism increased by chronic alcohol use. Cardiac depressant effects increased by lidocaine, propranolol, and other beta blockers. Precipitation may occur when mixed with D_5W. Incompatible with many solutions and medications.

How supplied   50 mg/ml in 2- and 5-ml ampules, 2-ml prefilled syringes. May be diluted in normal saline (NS) (1–10 mg/ml); use in-line filter. *Note:* IV line should be flushed with 0.9% NS before and after drug administration.

Dosage and administration   *Adult:* Seizures: 15–20 mg/kg slow IV, not to exceed 1 g or rate of 50 mg/min). Arrhythmias: 50–100 mg (diluted) slow IV every 5–15 min PRN. *Pediatric:* Seizures: 15–20 mg/kg slow IV (1–3 mg/kg/min). Arrhythmias: 5 mg/kg slow IV; maximum, 1 g.

Duration of action   Onset: 20–30 minutes for seizure disorder. Peak effect: 1–3 hours. Duration: 18–24 hours but as long as 15 days reported.

Special considerations   Pregnancy safety: not established. Carefully monitor vital signs. Venous irritation may occur (use large stable vein).

Pralidoxime Chloride (2-PAM Chloride, Protopam)

Class   Cholinesterase reactivator.

Mechanism of action   Reactivation of cholinesterase to effectively act as an antidote to organophosphate pesticide poisoning. This action allows for destruction of accumulated acetylcholine at the neuromuscular junction.

Indications   As an antidote in the treatment of poisoning by organophosphate pesticides and chemicals. In the prehospital arena, is used when atropine is or has become ineffective in management of organophosphate poisoning.

Contraindications   Use with caution in patients with reduced renal function; patients with myasthenia gravis and organophosphate poisoning.

Adverse reactions   Dizziness, blurred vision, diplopia, headache, drowsiness, nausea, tachycardia, hyperventilation, muscular weakness, excitement, and manic behaviour.

Drug interactions   No direct drug interactions; however, patients with organophosphate poisoning should not be given barbiturates, morphine, theophylline, aminophylline, succinylcholine, reserpine, and phenothiazines.

How supplied   Emergency Single Dose Kit containing: One 20-ml vial of 1 g sterile protopam chloride. One 20-ml ampule of sterile diluent. Sterile, disposable 20-ml syringe. Needle and alcohol swab.

Dosage and administration   *Note:* If Protopam is to be used, it should be administered almost simultaneously with atropine. *Adult:* Initial dose of 1–2 g as an IV infusion with 100 ml of saline over 15–30 minutes. *Pediatric:* 20–40 mg/kg as IV infusion over 15–30 minutes. Doses may be repeated every 1 hour if muscle weakness persists. If IV administration is not feasible, IM or SC injection may be utilized.

Duration of action   Onset: minutes. Peak effect: variable. Duration: variable.

Special considerations   Pregnancy safety: unknown. Treatment will be most effective if given within a few hours after poisoning. Cardiac monitoring should be considered in all cases of severe organophosphate poisoning.

Procainamide (Pronestyl)

Class   Antiarrhythmic.

Mechanism of action   Suppresses phase 4 depolarization in normal ventricular muscle and Purkinje fibres, reducing ectopic pacemaker automaticity; suppresses intraventricular conduction.

Indications   Stable monomorphic VT with normal QT interval, reentry SVT uncontrolled by vagal maneuvers and adenosine, stable wide-complex tachycardia of unknown origin, atrial fibrillation with rapid ventricular rate in patients with Wolff-Parkinson-White syndrome.

Contraindications   Torsade de pointes, second- and third-degree AV block (without functional artificial pacemaker), digoxin toxicity, tricyclic antidepressant overdose.

Adverse reactions   Widening of the PR, QRS, and QT intervals, AV heart block, hypotension, reflex tachycardia, bradycardia, nausea and vomiting.

Drug interactions   May increase plasma levels of amiodarone and quinidine.

How supplied   1 g in 10-ml vials (100 mg/ml); 1 g in 2-ml vials (500 mg/ml) for infusion.

Dosage and administration   *Adult: Recurrent VF/pulseless VT:* 20 mg/min IV infusion (maximum dose: 17 mg/kg). In urgent situations, up to 50 mg/min may be administered (maximum dose of 17 mg/kg). *Other indications:* 20 mg/min IV infusion until any **one** of the following occurs: arrhythmia suppression, hypotension, QRS widens by > 50% of its pretreatment width, or total dose of 17 mg/kg has been given. *Maintenance infusion:* 1–4 mg/min (dilute in D_5W or normal saline). *Pediatric:* Loading dose of 15 mg/kg IV/IO over 30–60 minutes.

Duration of action   Onset: 10–30 minutes. Peak effect: variable. Duration: 3–6 hours.

Special considerations   Pregnancy safety: Category C. Potent vasodilating and negative inotropic effects. Hypotension may occur with rapid infusion. Administer cautiously to patients with renal, hepatic, or cardiac insufficiency. Administer cautiously to patients with asthma or digoxin-induced arrhythmias.

Propofol (Diprivan)

Class   Anesthetic.

Mechanism of action   Dose-dependent CNS depression similar to benzodiazipines and barbiturates; involves a positive modulation of the inhibitory function of the neurotransmitter gamma-aminobutyrate (GABA) through GABA-A receptors.

Indications   Induction and maintenance of sedation in intubated and mechanically ventilated patients.

Contraindications   Disorders of lipid metabolism; patients younger than 12 years old or less than 40 kg in weight; sensitivity to drug or components of emulsion, including soybean oil, egg lecithin, and glycerol.

Adverse reactions Hypotension, apnea, bradycardia, airway obstruction following rapid infusion.

Drug interactions Extreme caution when given with opiate analgesics or sedatives; must be administered in a separate IV line—do not mix with other drugs or blood products.

How supplied Lipid emulsion of (check concentration).

Dosage and administration Induction as part of rapid sequence intubation: 1–2 mg/kg IV administered at a rate of 40 mg every 10 seconds until induction onset. Maintenance of ICU sedation: 0.3 mg/kg/h, increased by increments of 0.3–5 mg/kg/h every 5 min

until desired level of sedation. Maximum dose of 5 mg/kg/h (0.5 ml/kg/h) (higher doses have been associated with heart failure when administered to neurologic patients). May administer boluses of 10–20 mg to rapidly increase sedation in patients not prone to hypotension; may need to decrease dose by 20%–30% in elderly, debilitated, or hypovolemic patients.

Duration of action Onset: 20–40 seconds. Duration: 30–60 seconds.

Special considerations Pregnancy safety: Category C. Closely monitor patient during administration.

Propranolol (Inderal)

Class Beta-adrenergic blocker, antiarrhythmic (Class II).

Mechanism of action Nonselective beta-adrenergic blocker that inhibits chronotropic, inotropic, and vasodilator response to beta-adrenergic stimulation.

Indications Hypertension, angina pectoris, VT and VF refractory to lidocaine; selected supraventricular tachycardias.

Contraindications Sinus bradycardia, second- or third-degree AV block, asthma, CHF, COPD.

Adverse reactions Bradycardia, heart blocks, angina pectoris, palpitations, syncope. Bronchospasm, dyspnea, hallucinations, anxiety, nausea, vomiting, visual disturbances.

Drug interactions Verapamil may worsen AV conduction abnormalities. Succinylcholine effects may be enhanced. Effects may be reversed by isoproterenol (Isuprel), norepinephrine, dopamine.

How supplied Solution of 1-mg/ml vials.

Dosage and administration *Adult:* Dilute 1–3 mg in 10–30 ml of D$_5$W; administer slowly IV at rate of 1 mg/min; maximum, 5 mg. *Pediatric:* 0.01–0.05 mg/kg/dose slow IV over 10 minutes; maximum, 3 mg.

Duration of action Onset: 15–60 minutes. Peak effect: variable. Duration: 6–12 hours.

Special considerations Pregnancy safety: Category C. Closely monitor patient during administration. Use cautiously in geriatric population. Atropine should be readily available.

Rocuronium (Zemuron)

Class Paralytic agent.

Mechanism of action Nondepolarizing neuromuscular blocking agent, paralytic.

Indications To facilitate intubation, to terminate laryngospasm, to promote muscle relaxation, to facilitate electroconvulsive shock therapy.

Contraindications Acute narrow-angle glaucoma, penetrating eye injuries, inability to control airway or support ventilations with oxygen and positive pressure, newborns, myasthenia gravis, hepatic or renal failure.

Adverse reactions Apnea, weakness, tachycardia, hypotension, hypetension, bronchospasm, edema at injection site.

Drug interactions Use of inhalational anesthetics will enhance neuromuscular blockade.

How supplied 10 mg/10-ml (5-ml) rocuronium vials.

Dosage and administration *Adult:* initial dose 0.6 mg/kg IV push; maintenance dose of 0.3 mg/kg IV push every 20 to 30 minutes. *Pediatric:* 0.6 mg/kg IV.

Duration of action Onset: 30–60 seconds. Peak effect: 3 minutes. Duration: 20–30 minutes.

Special considerations Pregnancy safety: Category C. Intubation and ventilatory support must be readily available. Monitor the patient carefully. Rocuronium has no effect on consciousness or pain. Will not stop neuronal seizure activity.

Salbutamol (Ventolin)

Class Sympathomimetic, bronchodilator.

Mechanism of action Selective beta-2 agonist that stimulates adrenergic receptors of the sympathomimetic nervous system resulting in smooth muscle relaxation in the bronchial tree and peripheral vasculature.

Indications Treatment of bronchospasm in patients with reversible obstructive airway disease (COPD/asthma). Prevention of exercise-induced bronchospasm.

Contraindications Known prior hypersensitivity reactions to salbutamol. Tachycardia arrhythmias, especially those caused by digoxin. Synergistic with other sympathomimetics.

Adverse reactions Often dose-related and include restlessness, tremors, dizziness, palpitations, tachycardia, nervousness, peripheral vasodilation, nausea, vomiting, hyperglycemia, increased blood pressure, and paradoxical bronchospasm.

Drug interactions Tricyclic antidepressants may potentiate vasculature effects. Beta blockers are antagonistic. May potentiate hypokalemia caused by diuretics.

How supplied *Solution for aerosolization:* 0.5% (5 mg/ml). Metered dose inhaler: 100 µg/metered spray (canister with 200–600 inhalations). Also available in premixed nebules of 2.5 mg/2.5 ml.

Dosage and administration *Adult:* Administer 2.5–5.0 mg. Dilute 0.5–1.0 ml of 0.5% solution for inhalation with 2–3 ml normal saline in nebulizer and administer over 10–15 minutes. *MDI:* 1–2 inhalations; 5 minutes between inhalations. *Pediatric:* Administer solution of 0.01–0.03 ml (0.05–0.15 mg/kg/dose diluted in 2 ml of 0.9% normal saline. May repeat every 20 minutes three times.

Duration of action Onset: 5-15 minutes. Peak effect: 30 minutes–2 hours. Duration: 3-4 hours.

Special considerations Pregnancy safety: Category C. Antagonized by beta blockers (eg, Inderal, Lopressor). May precipitate angina pectoris and arrhythmias. Solution designed for inhalation should only be administered by the inhalation route.

Succinylcholine (Anectine)

Class   Depolarizing neuromuscular blocker, paralyzing agent.

Mechanism of action   Bind to the receptors for acetylcholine.

Indications   To facilitate intubation, to terminate laryngospasm, to promote muscle relaxation, to facilitate electroconvulsive shock therapy.

Contraindications   Acute narrow-angle glaucoma, penetrating eye injuries, inability to control airway or support ventilations with oxygen and positive pressure.

Adverse reactions   Apnea, malignant hyperthermia, arrhythmias, bradycardia, hypertension, hypotension, cardiac arrest, hyperkalemia, increased intraocular pressure, fasciculations, exacerbation of hyperkalemia in trauma patients.

Drug interactions   Effects potentiated by oxytocin, beta blockers, and organophosphates. Diazepam may reduce duration of action.

How supplied   40 mg in 2-ml ampule (20 mg/ml). 100 mg in 5-ml ampule (20 mg/ml). Multidose vial.

Dosage and administration   *Adult:* 1–1.5 mg/kg rapid IV; repeat once if needed. *Pediatric:* 1.5–2 mg/kg dose rapid IV, IO; repeat once if needed.

Duration of action   Onset: 1 minute. Peak effect: 1–3 minutes. Duration: 5 minutes.

Special considerations   Pregnancy safety: Category C. Paramedics use primarily to facilitate endotracheal intubation. If the patient is conscious, explain the effects of the drug before administration. Consider premedication with atropine, particularly in pediatric age group. Premedication with lidocaine may blunt any increase in intracranial pressure during intubation. Diazepam or midazolam should be used in any conscious patient undergoing neuromuscular blockade.

Tenectaplase (TNK)

Class   Fibrinolytic agent.

Mechanism of action   Modified form of TPA that binds to fibrin and converts plasminogen to plasmin.

Indications   Lysis of suspected occlusive coronary artery thrombi associated with evolving transmural myocardial infarction.

Contraindications   Recent surgery (within 3 weeks), active bleeding, recent hemorrhagic CVA, prolonged CPR, intracranial or intraspinal surgery; recent significant trauma, especially head trauma; uncontrolled hypertension (generally BP over 200 mm Hg).

Adverse reactions   GI, GU, intracranial, and other site bleeding; hypotension, allergic reactions, chest pain, abdominal pain, hemorrhagic CVA, reperfusion arrhythmias.

Drug interactions   Do not mix with dextrose-containing solutions.

How supplied   50-mg vial.

Dosage and administration   0.5 mg/kg to a maximum dose of 50 mg.

Special considerations   Pregnancy safety: contraindicated. Closely monitor vital signs. Observe for bleeding. Do not give IM injection to patient receiving tenectaplase.

Thiamine

Class   Vitamin (B1).

Mechanism of action   Combines with ATP to form thiamine pyrophosphate coenzyme, a necessary component for carbohydrate metabolism. The brain is extremely sensitive to thiamine deficiency.

Indications   Coma of unknown origin, delirium tremens, beriberi, Wernicke's encephalopathy.

Contraindications   None.

Adverse reactions   Hypotension from too rapid of an injection or too high a dose, anxiety, diaphoresis, nausea, vomiting, allergy (rare).

Drug interactions   Give thiamine before glucose under all circumstances.

How supplied   1,000 mg in 10-ml vial (100 mg/ml).

Dosage and administration   *Adult:* 100 mg slow IV or IM. *Pediatric:* 10–25 mg slow IV or IM.

Duration of action   Onset: rapid. Peak effect: variable. Duration: dependent upon degree of deficiency.

Special considerations   Pregnancy safety: Category A. Large IV doses may cause respiratory difficulties. Anaphylaxis reactions reported.

Tissue Plasminogen Activator (TPA)

Class   Thrombolytic agent.

Mechanism of action   Binds to fibrin-bound plasminogen at the clot site, converting plasminogen to plasmin; plasmin digests the fibrin strands of the clot, restoring perfusion.

Indications   Acute evolving myocardial infarction, massive pulmonary emboli, arterial thrombosis and embolism, to clear arteriovenous cannulas, acute ischemic stroke.

Contraindications   Recent surgery (within 3 weeks), active bleeding, recent hemorrhagic CVA, prolonged CPR, intracranial or intraspinal surgery; recent significant trauma, especially head trauma; uncontrolled hypertension (generally BP over 200 mm Hg).

Adverse reactions   GI, GU, intracranial, and other site bleeding; hypotension, allergic reactions, chest pain, abdominal pain, hemorrhagic CVA, reperfusion arrhythmias.

Drug interactions   Acetylsalicylic acid may increase risk of hemorrhage. Heparin and other anticoagulants may be required and can increase risk of hemorrhage.

How supplied   20 mg with 20-ml diluent vial. 50 mg with 50-ml diluent vial.

Dosage and administration Acute MI   *Adult:* 10-mg bolus IV over 2 minutes; then 50 mg over 1 hour, then 20 mg over the second hour and 20 mg over the third hour, for a total dose of 100 mg (other dosing schedules are also used and may be prescribed through direct medical control). *Pediatric:* safety not established. Acute ischemic stroke: 0.9 mg/kg IV, 10% given as bolus over 1 minute, with remaining 90% given over 1 hour.

Duration of action   Onset: clot lysis most often within 60–90 minutes. Peak effect: variable. Duration: 30 minutes with 80% cleared within 10 minutes.

Special considerations   Pregnancy safety: contraindicated. Closely monitor vital signs. Observe for bleeding. Do not give IM injection to patient receiving tissue plasminogen activator.

Vasopressin (Pitressin synthetic)

Class   Antidiuretic hormone.

Mechanism of action   Stimulation of V_1 smooth muscle receptors, potent vasoconstrictor when given in high doses.

Indications   Alternate vasopressor to the first or second dose of epinephrine in cardiac arrest, may be useful in cases of vasodilatory shock (ie, septic shock).

Contraindications　Responsive patients with coronary artery disease.

Adverse reactions　Bronchoconstriction, ischemic chest pain, nausea and vomiting, abdominal pain.

Drug interactions　None reported.

How supplied　1-ml vials containing 20 units (20 U/ml).

Dosage and administration　*Adult:* 40-unit one-time dose IV/IO to replace the first or second dose of epinephrine in cardiac arrest. *Pediatric:* Not recommended.

Duration of action　Onset: immediate. Duration: variable.

Special considerations　Pregnancy safety: Category C. May increase peripheral vascular resistance and provoke cardiac ischemia and angina.

Vecuronium (Norcuron)

Class　Paralytic agent.

Mechanism of action　Nondepolarizing neuromuscular blocking agent, paralytic.

Indications　To facilitate intubation, to terminate laryngospasm, to promote muscle relaxation, to facilitate electroconvulsive shock therapy.

Contraindications　Acute narrow-angle glaucoma, penetrating eye injuries, inability to control airway or support ventilations with oxygen and positive pressure, newborns, myasthenia gravis, hepatic or renal failure.

Adverse reactions　Apnea, weakness, salivation, premature ventricular contractions, tachycardia, transient hypotension, increased blood pressure.

Drug interactions　Use of inhalational anesthetics will enhance neuromuscular blockade.

How supplied　10 mg/10-ml vecuronium bromide vials with diluent. 20-ml vials (20 mg vecuronium) without diluent.

Dosage and administration　*Adult:* 0.1 mg/kg IV push; maintenance dose within 25–40 minutes: 0.01–0.05 mg/kg IV push. *Pediatric:* 0.1 mg/kg IV, IO; maintenance dose within 20–35 minutes: 0.01–0.05 mg/kg IV push.

Duration of action　Onset: 30 seconds. Peak effect: 2.5–3 minutes. Duration: 25–30 minutes.

Special considerations　Pregnancy safety: Category C. Intubation and ventilatory support must be readily available. Monitor the patient carefully. Vecuronium has no effect on consciousness or pain. Will not stop neuronal seizure activity. Pulse rate, cardiac output are increased. Decrease doses for patients with renal disease.

Verapamil (Isoptin)

Class　Antiarrhythmic.

Mechanism of action　Calcium channel blocker, Class IV antiarrhythmic, prolongs AV nodal refractory period, dilates coronary arteries and arterioles.

Indications　PSVT, PAT, atrial fibrillation and atrial flutter with rapid ventricular response.

Contraindications　Wolff-Parkinson-White syndrome, second-degree or third-degree AV block, sick sinus syndrome (unless patient has functioning pacemaker), hypotension, cardiogenic shock, severe CHF, pulmonary edema, patients receiving IV beta blockers, wide-complex tachycardias, children younger than 12 months of age.

Adverse reactions　Hypotension, AV block, bradycardia, asystole, dizziness, headache, nausea, vomiting, complete AV block, peripheral edema.

Drug interactions　Increases serum concentration of digoxin. Beta-adrenergic blockers may have additive negative inotropic and chronotropic effects. Antihypertensives may potentiate hypotensive effects.

How supplied　5 mg/2 ml in 2-, 4-, 5-ml vials or 2-, 4-ml ampules.

Dosage and administration　*Adult:* 2.5–5.0 mg IV bolus over 2 minutes (over 3 minutes in older patients). Repeat doses of 5–10 mg may be given every 15–30 minutes to a maximum of 20 mg. *Pediatric:* 0.1–0.2 mg/kg/dose IV, IO push over 2 minutes. Repeat dose in 30 minutes if not effective. (*Note:* not to be used in children younger than 12 months of age.).

Duration of action　Onset: 2–5 minutes. Peak effect: variable. Duration: 30–60 minutes.

Special considerations　Pregnancy safety: Category C. Closely monitor patient's vital signs. Be prepared to resuscitate. AV block or asystole may occur as result of slowed AV conduction.

IV Solutions (Colloids and Crystalloids)

Colloids expand plasma volume by colloidal osmotic pressure. Colloids are most often used in hypovolemic shock states. Crystalloids are substances in solution that can diffuse through the intravascular compartment. Crystalloid solutions are used for electrolyte replacement, a route for medication, and short-term intravascular volume expansion.

Dextran

Class   Artificial colloid.

Mechanism of action   Dextran is a sugar-containing colloid used as an intravascular volume expander. It remains in the intravascular compartment for approximately 12 hours. It increases intravascular volume by attracting water from other fluid compartments by virtue of its colloid osmotic pressure.

Indications   Hypovolemic shock.

Contraindications   Dextran should not be administered to patients who have a known hypersensitivity to the drug. It should not be administered to patients suffering congestive heart failure, renal failure, or known bleeding disorders.

Adverse reactions   Rash, itching, dyspnea, chest tightness, and mild hypotension have all been reported with dextran use. The incidence of these side effects is, however, very low, and reactions are generally mild. Increased bleeding time has also been reported with dextran use due to its interference with platelet function.

Drug interactions   Dextran should not be administered to patients who are receiving anticoagulants as it significantly retards blood clotting.

How supplied   Dextran 40 and Dextran 70 are supplied in 250- and 500-ml bottles.

Dosage and administration   The dosage of dextran is titrated according to the patient's physiologic response.

Duration of action   8–12 hours.

Special considerations   In the management of burn shock, it is especially important to follow standard fluid resuscitation regimens to prevent possible circulatory overload.

Lactated Ringer's (Hartman's Solution)

Class   Isotonic crystalloid solution.

Mechanism of action   Lactated Ringer's replaces water and electrolytes.

Indications   Hypovolemic shock; to keep open IV.

Contraindications   Lactated Ringer's should not be used in patients with congestive heart failure or renal failure.

Adverse reactions   Rare in therapeutic dosages.

Drug interactions   Few in the emergency setting.

How supplied   Lactated Ringer's is supplied in 250-, 500-, and 1,000-ml bags, IV infusion.

Dosage and administration   Hypovolemic shock; titrate according to patient's physiologic response.

Duration of action   Short-term therapy.

Special considerations   None.

Pentaspan (Pentastarch, Hespan)

Class   Artificial colloid.

Mechanism of action   Starch-containing colloid used as an intravascular volume expander. Following administration, the plasma volume is expanded slightly in excess of the volume administered. This effect has been observed for up to 24 to 36 hours. It increases intravascular volume by virtue of its colloid osmotic pressure.

Indications   Hypovolemic shock, especially burn shock; septic shock.

Contraindications   There are no major contraindications when used in the management of life-threatening hypovolemic states.

Adverse reactions   Nausea, vomiting, mild febrile reactions, chills, itching, and urticaria (hives) have been reported with hetastarch administration. Severe anaphylactic reactions have been rarely reported.

Drug interactions   Should not be administered to patients who are receiving anticoagulants.

How supplied   250- and 500-ml bags; each 100 ml contains 10 g pentastarch.

Dosage and administration   500 to 2,000 ml/24 hours, depending on volume lost; typical adult dose is 500-ml bolus.

Duration of action   18–24 hours.

Special considerations   Pregnancy safety: Category C. Patients allergic to corn may be allergic to pentaspan. Not recommended for use in pediatric population.

5% Dextrose in Water (D$_5$W)

Class   Hypotonic dextrose-containing solution.

Mechanism of action   D$_5$W provides nutrients in the form of dextrose as well as free water.

Indications   IV access for emergency drugs; for dilution of concentrated drugs for intravenous infusion.

Contraindications   D$_5$W should not be used as a fluid replacement for hypovolemic states.

Adverse reactions   Rare in therapeutic dosages.

Drug interactions   D$_5$W should not be used with phenytoin (Dilantin) or amrinone (Inocor).

How supplied   D$_5$W is supplied in bags of 50, 100, 150, 250, 500, and 1,000 ml.

Dosage and administration   D$_5$W is usually administered through a minidrip (60 drops/ml) set at a rate of "to keep open" (TKO).

Duration of action   Short-term therapy.

Special considerations   None.

10% Dextrose in Water (D$_{10}$W)

Class Hypertonic dextrose-containing solution.

Mechanism of action D$_{10}$W provides nutrients in the form of dextrose as well as free water.

Indications Neonatal resuscitation, hypoglycemia.

Contraindications D$_{10}$W should not be used as a fluid replacement for hypovolemic states.

Adverse reactions Rare in therapeutic dosages.

Drug interactions Should not be used with phenytoin (Dilantin) or amrinone (Inocor).

How supplied D$_{10}$W is supplied in bags of 50, 100, 150, 250, 500, and 1,000 ml.

Dosage and administration The administration rate of D$_{10}$W will usually be dependent on the patient's condition.

Duration of action Short-term therapy.

Special considerations None.

0.9% Sodium Chloride (Normal Saline)

Class Isotonic crystalloid solution.

Mechanism of action Normal saline replaces water and electrolytes.

Indications Heat-related problems (heat exhaustion, heat stroke), freshwater drowning, hypovolemia, diabetic ketoacidosis, to keep open IV.

Contraindications The use of 0.9% sodium chloride should not be considered in patients with congestive heart failure, because circulatory overload can be easily induced.

Adverse reactions Rare in therapeutic dosages.

Drug interactions Few in the emergency setting.

How supplied Normal saline is supplied in 250-, 500-, and 1,000-ml bags. Sterile normal saline for irrigation should not be confused with that designed for intravenous administration.

Dosage and administration The specific situation being treated will dictate the rate in which normal saline will be administered. In severe heat stroke, diabetic ketoacidosis, and freshwater drowning, it is likely that you will be called on to administer the fluid quite rapidly. In other cases, it is advisable to administer the fluid at a moderate rate (for example, 100 ml/h).

Duration of action Short-term therapy.

Special considerations None.

0.45% Sodium Chloride (½ Normal Saline)

Class Hypotonic crystalloid solution.

Mechanism of action One-half normal saline replaces free water and electrolytes.

Indications Patients with diminished renal or cardiovascular function for which rapid rehydration is not indicated.

Contraindications Cases in which rapid rehydration is indicated.

Adverse reactions Rare in therapeutic dosages.

Drug interactions Few in the emergency setting.

How supplied One-half normal saline is supplied in 250-, 500-, and 1,000-ml bags.

Dosage and administration The specific situation and patient condition will dictate the rate at which one-half normal saline will be administered.

Duration of action Short-term therapy.

Special considerations None.

5% Dextrose in 0.45% Sodium Chloride (D$_5$½NS)

Class Hypertonic dextrose-containing crystalloid solution.

Mechanism of action D$_5$½NS replaces free water and electrolytes and provides nutrients in the form of dextrose.

Indications Heat exhaustion, diabetic disorders; for use as a way to keep open solution in patients with impaired renal or cardiovascular function.

Contraindications D$_5$½NS should not be used when rapid fluid resuscitation is indicated.

Adverse reactions Rare in therapeutic dosages.

Drug interactions D$_5$½NS should not be used with phenytoin (Dilantin) or amrinone (Inocor).

How supplied D$_5$½NS is supplied in bags containing 250, 500, and 1,000 ml of the fluid.

Dosage and administration The specific situation and patient condition will dictate the rate at which D$_5$½NS should be administered.

Duration of action Short-term therapy.

Special considerations None.

5% Dextrose in 0.9% Sodium Chloride (D$_5$NS)

Class Hypertonic dextrose-containing crystalloid solution.

Mechanism of action D$_5$NS replaces free water and electrolytes and provides nutrients in the form of dextrose.

Indications Heat-related disorders, freshwater drowning, hypovolemia, peritonitis.

Contraindications D$_5$NS should not be administered to patients with impaired cardiac or renal function.

Adverse reactions Rare in therapeutic dosages.

Drug interactions D$_5$NS should not be used with phenytoin (Dilantin) or amrinone (Inocor).

How supplied D$_5$NS is supplied in bags containing 250, 500, and 1,000 ml of the solution.

Dosage and administration The specific situation and patient condition will dictate the rate at which D$_5$NS is given.

Duration of action Short-term therapy.

Special considerations None.

5% Dextrose in Lactated Ringer's (D₅LR)

Class   Hypertonic dextrose-containing crystalloid solution.

Mechanism of action D_5LR replaces water and electrolytes and provides nutrients in the form of dextrose.

Indications   Hypovolemic shock, hemorrhagic shock, certain cases of acidosis.

Contraindications D_5LR should not be administered to patients with decreased renal or cardiovascular function.

Adverse reactions   Rare in therapeutic dosages.

Drug interactions D_5LR should not be used with phenytoin (Dilantin) or amrinone (Inocor).

How supplied D_5LR is supplied in bags containing 250, 500, and 1,000 ml of the fluid.

Dosage and administration   In severe hypovolemic shock D_5LR should be infused through a large-bore cannula (14 or 16 gauge). This infusion should be administered "wide open" until a blood pressure of 100 mm Hg is achieved. When the blood pressure is attained, the infusions should be reduced to 100 ml/h. In other cases, the specific situation and patient condition will dictate the rate of administration.

Duration of action   Short-term therapy.

Special considerations   None.

Glossary

6 Ps of musculoskeletal assessment Pain, Paralysis, Parasthesias, Pulselessness, Pallor, and Pressure.

abandonment Abrupt termination of contact with the patient without giving the patient sufficient opportunity to find another suitable health care professional to take over his or her medical treatment.

abduction Movement *away* from the midline of the body.

aberrant conduction The abnormal conduction of the electrical impulse through the heart.

ABO system The antigen classification given to blood.

abortion Expulsion of the fetus, from any cause, before the 20th week of gestation.

abrasion An injury in which a portion of the body is denuded of epidermis by scraping or rubbing.

abruptio placenta A premature separation of the placenta from the wall of the uterus.

abscess A collection of pus in a sac, formed by necrotic tissues and an accumulation of white blood cells.

absence seizures The type of seizures characterized by a brief lapse of attention in which the patient may stare and not respond; formerly known as petit mal seizures.

absolute refractory period The early phase of cardiac repolarization, wherein the heart muscle cannot be stimulated to depolarize.

absorption The process by which a substance's molecules are moved from the site of entry or administration into the body and into systemic circulation.

absorption (hazardous materials) A type of decontamination that is done with large pads that the hazardous materials team carry to soak up liquid and remove it from the patient.

abuse Any form of maltreatment that results in harm or loss. Maltreatment may be physical, sexual, psychological, or financial/material.

acceleration The rate of change in velocity.

access port A sealed hub on an administration set designed for sterile access to the IV fluid.

accessory muscles Muscles not normally used during normal breathing; includes the sternocleidomastoid muscles of the neck.

accountability system A method of accounting for all personnel at an emergency incident and ensuring that only personnel with specific assignments are permitted to work within the various zones.

acetabulum The cup-shaped cavity in which the rounded head of the femur rotates.

acetylcholine (ACh) Chemical neurotransmitter of the parasympathetic nervous system.

acholic stools Light, clay-coloured stools caused by liver failure.

acidosis A blood pH of less than 7.35. A pathologic condition resulting from the accumulation of acids in the body.

acquired immunity The immunity the body develops as part of exposure to an antigen.

acquired immunodeficiency syndrome (AIDS) The end-stage disease process caused by the human immunodeficiency virus (HIV). A person with this is extremely vulnerable to numerous bacterial, viral, and fungal infections that would not affect a person with an intact immune system.

acrocyanosis A decrease in the amount of oxygen delivered to the extremities. The hands and feet turn blue because of narrowing (constriction) of small arterioles (tiny arteries) toward the end of the arms and legs.

acromion Lateral extension of the scapula that forms the highest point of the shoulder.

activation Mediators of inflammation trigger the appearance of molecules known as selectins and integrins on the surfaces of endothelial cells and PMNs, respectively.

active hyperemia The dilation of arterioles after transient arteriolar constriction, which allows influx of blood under increased pressure.

active neglect The refusal or failure to fulfill a caregiving obligation; a conscious or intentional attempt to inflict physical or emotional stress. Examples include abandonment and denial of food or health-related services.

activities of daily living (ADLs) Normal everyday activities such as getting dressed, brushing teeth, taking out the garbage, etc.

acute coronary syndrome Term used to describe any group of clinical symptoms consistent with acute myocardial ischemia.

acute dystonic reaction A syndrome that may occur in patients taking typical antipsychotic agents. The patient develops muscle spasms of the neck, face, and back within a few days of starting treatment with the drug.

acute mountain sickness (AMS) An altitude illness characterized by headache plus at least one of the following: fatigue or weakness, gastrointestinal symptoms (nausea, vomiting or anorexia), dizziness or lightheadedness, or difficulty sleeping.

acute myocardial infarction (AMI) A condition present when a period of cardiac ischemia caused by sudden narrowing or complete occlusion of a coronary artery leads to death (necrosis) of myocardial tissue.

acute radiation syndrome The clinical course that usually begins within hours of exposure to a radiation source. Symptoms include nausea, vomiting, diarrhea, fatigue, fever, and headache. The long-term symptoms are dose-related and are hematopoietic and gastrointestinal.

acute renal failure (ARF) A sudden decrease in filtration through the glomeruli.

acute respiratory distress syndrome (ARDS) A respiratory syndrome characterized by respiratory insufficiency and hypoxemia.

adduction Movement *toward* the midline of the body.

adenoids Lymphatic tissues located on the posterior nasopharyngeal wall that filter bacteria.

adhesion The attachment of PMNs to endothelial cells, mediated by selectins and integrins.

adipose tissue A connective tissue containing large amounts of lipids. Also referred to as fat tissue.

administration set Tubing that connects to the IV bag access port and the cannula to deliver IV fluid.

adolescents Persons who are 12 to 18 years of age.

adrenal cortex The outer part of the adrenal glands that produces corticosteroids.

adrenal glands Endocrine glands located on top of the kidneys that release adrenaline when stimulated by the sympathetic nervous system.

adrenal medulla The inner portion of the adrenal glands that synthesizes, stores, and eventually releases epinephrine and norepinephrine.

adrenaline The hormone produced by the adrenal gland with alpha and beta sympathomimetic properties.

adrenergic Pertaining to nerves that release the neurotransmitter norepinephrine or noradrenaline (such as adrenergic nerves, adrenergic response). The term also pertains to the receptors acted on by norepinephrine, that is, the adrenergic receptors.

adrenocorticotropic hormone (ACTH) Hormone that targets the adrenal cortex to secrete cortisol (a glucocorticoid).

adult protective services (APS) Organizations that investigate cases involving maltreatment and provide case management services in some cases.

advance care planning Expression of oral and/or written advance directives by capable patients in anticipation of their wishes regarding future health care choices and expected quality of life.

advance directive A written document that expresses the wants, needs, and desires of a patient in reference to future medical care; examples include living wills, do not resuscitate (DNR) orders, and organ donation.

adventitious A type of breath sound that occurs in addition to the normal breath sounds; examples are crackles and wheezes.

aerobic metabolism Metabolism that can proceed only in the presence of oxygen.

affect The outward expression of a person's mood.

afferent arteriole The structure in the kidney that supplies blood to the glomerulus.

afferent nerves The nerves that carry sensory impulses from all parts of the body to the brain.

affinity The force attraction between medications and receptors causing them to bind together.

afterdrop Continued fall in core temperature after a victim of hypothermia has been removed from a cold environment, due at least in part to the return of cold blood from the body surface to the body core.

afterload The pressure in the aorta against which the left ventricle must pump blood.

Agency for Toxic Substance Registry An information source for toxicologic effects of hazardous materials.

agitation Extreme restlessness and anxiety.

agnosia Inability to connect an object with its correct name.

agonal Pertaining to the period of dying.

agonal respirations Slow, shallow, irregular respirations or occasional gasping breaths; results from cerebral anoxia.

agonal rhythm A cardiac dysrhythmia seen just before the heart stops altogether; essentially asystole with occasional QRS complexes that are not associated with cardiac output.

agonist A substance that mimics the actions of a specific neurotransmitter or hormone by binding to the specific receptor of the naturally occurring substance.

agoraphobia Literally, "fear of the market-place"; fear of entering a public place from which escape may be impeded.

alarm reaction The body's first, "startle" response to a stressor.

alcoholism A state of physical and psychological addiction to ethanol.

aldosterone One of the two main hormones responsible for adjustments to the final composition of urine, aldosterone increases the rate of active resorption of sodium and chloride ions into the blood and decreases resorption of potassium.

alert and oriented (A x O) A determination made when assessing mental status by looking at whether the patient is oriented to four elements: person, place, time, and the event itself. Each element provides information about different aspects of the patient's memory.

alert response The first reaction in the alarm reaction, in which you immediately stop whatever you are doing and focus on the source of the stimulus.

alkalosis A pathologic condition resulting from the accumulation of bases in the body. A blood pH of greater than 7.45.

allergen Any substance that causes a hypersensitivity reaction.

allergic reaction An abnormal immune response the body develops when reexposed to a substance or allergen.

allergy Hypersensitivity reaction to the presence of an agent (allergen) that is intrinsically harmless.

alpha Type of energy that is emitted from a strong radiological source; it is the least harmful penetrating type of radiation and cannot travel fast or through most objects.

alternative time sampling Time parameters that are set during a research project.

altitude illnesses Conditions caused by the effects from hypobaric (low atmospheric pressure) hypoxia on the CNS and pulmonary systems as result of unacclimatized people ascending to altitude; range from acute mountain sickness to high altitude cerebral edema (HACE) and high altitude pulmonary edema (HAPE).

alveolar ridges The ridges between the teeth, which are covered with thickened connective tissue and epithelium.

alveolar volume Volume of inhaled air that reaches the alveoli and participates in gas exchange; equal to tidal volume minus dead space volume and is approximately 350 ml in the average adult.

alveoli Saclike units at the end of the bronchioles where gas exchange takes place (singular: alveolus).

Alzheimer's disease A progressive organic condition in which neurons die, causing dementia.

amenorrhea Absence of menstruation.

amnesia Loss of memory.

amniotic fluid A clear, slightly yellowish liquid that surrounds the unborn baby (fetus) during pregnancy; contained in the amniotic sac.

amniotic sac The fluid-filled, baglike membrane in which the fetus develops.

amphetamines A class of drugs that increase alertness and excitation (that is, stimulants); includes methamphetamine (crank or ice), methylenedioxyamphetamine (MDA, Adam), and methylenedioxymethamphetamine (MDMA, Eve, ecstasy).

ampules Small glass containers that are sealed and the contents sterilized.

amputation An injury in which part of the body is completely severed.

amyotrophic lateral sclerosis (ALS) Also known as Lou Gehrig's disease, this disease strikes the voluntary motor neurons, causing their death. It is characterized by fatigue and general weakness of muscle groups; eventually, the patient will not be able to walk, eat, or speak.

anaerobic metabolism The metabolism that takes place in the absence of oxygen; the principal product is lactic acid.

analgesia The absence of the sensation of pain.

analgesics A classification for medications that relieve pain, or induce analgesia.

anaphylactic shock A severe hypersensitivity reaction that involves bronchoconstriction and cardiovascular collapse.

anaphylaxis An extreme systemic form of an allergic reaction involving two or more body systems.

anatomical dead space Includes the trachea and larger bronchi. The air remaining in these areas is the result of residual gas in the upper airway at the end of inhalation.

androgens Male sex hormones that regulate body changes associated with sexual development (puberty), including growth spurts, deepening of the voice, growth of facial and pubic hair, and muscle growth and strength.

anemia A lower than normal hemoglobin or erythrocyte level.

anesthesia Lack of feeling within a body part.

anesthetic A type of medication intended to induce a loss of sensation to touch or pain.

aneurysm A swelling or enlargement of part of a blood vessel, resulting from weakening of the vessel wall.

anger A strong, negative emotion that may be a response to illness, and which could result in aggressive behaviour on the part of the patient.

angina pectoris The sudden pain from myocardial ischemia, caused by diminished circulation to the cardiac muscle. The pain is usually substernal and often radiates to the arms, jaw, or abdomen and usually lasts 3 to 5 minutes and disappears with rest.

angioedema An allergic reaction that may cause profound swelling of the tongue and lips.

angiogenesis The growth of new blood vessels.

angiotensin converting enzyme (ACE) inhibitors Medications that suppress the conversion of angiotensin I to angiotensin II.

angiotensin II receptor antagonists Medications that are similar to ACE inhibitors but work by selectively blocking angiotensin II at their receptor sites.

angle of impact The angle at which an object hits another; this characterizes the force vectors involved and has a bearing on patterns of energy dissipation.

angle of Louis Prominence on the sternum that lies opposite the second intercostal space.

angulation The presence of an abnormal angle or bend in an extremity.

anion An ion that contains an overall negative charge.

anisocoria A condition in which the pupils are not of equal size.

anorexia nervosa An eating disorder in which a person diets by exerting extraordinary control over his or her eating, and loses weight to the point of jeopardizing his or her health and life.

anoxia An absence of oxygen.

antagonist A molecule that blocks the ability of a given chemical to bind to its receptor, preventing a biologic response.

antecubital The anterior aspect of the elbow.

antegrade amnesia Inability to remember from this point in time forward.

antepartum Before delivery.

anterior chamber The anterior area of the globe between the lens and the cornea that is filled with aqueous humour.

anterior cord syndrome A condition that occurs with flexion injuries or fractures resulting in the displacement of bony fragments into the anterior portion of the spinal cord; findings include paralysis below the level of the insult and loss of pain, temperature, and touch sensation.

anterior tibial artery The artery that travels through the anterior muscles of the leg and continues to the foot as the dorsalis pedis.

anterograde (posttraumatic) amnesia Loss of memory relating to events that occurred after the injury.

anthrax A deadly bacteria (*Bacillus anthracis*) that lays dormant in a spore (protective shell); the germ is released from the spore when exposed to the optimal temperature and moisture. The route of entry is inhalation, cutaneous, or gastrointestinal (from consuming food that contains spores).

antiarrhythmic medications The medications used to treat and prevent cardiac rhythm disorders.

antibiotic medications The medications that fight bacterial infection by killing the bacteria or by preventing multiplication of the bacteria to allow the body's immune system to overcome them.

antibodies Proteins secreted by certain immune cells that bind antigens to make them more visible to the immune system.

anticholinergic Of or pertaining to the blocking of acetylcholine receptors, resulting in inhibition of transmission of parasympathetic nerve impulses.

anticoagulant A substance that prevents blood from clotting.

anticoagulant drugs The medications used to prevent intravascular thrombosis by preventing blood coagulation in the vascular system.

anticonvulsant medications The medications used to treat seizures, which are believed to work by inhibiting the influx of sodium into cells.

antidiuretic hormone (ADH) One of the two main hormones responsible for adjustments to the final composition of urine, ADH causes ducts in the kidney to become more permeable to water.

antigen An agent that, when taken into the body, stimulates the formation of specific protective proteins called antibodies.

antihypertensives The medications used to control blood pressure.

antineoplastic medications The medications designed to combat cancer.

antiplatelet agents The medications that interfere with the collection of platelets.

antipsychotic drugs Medications used to control psychosis.

antiseptics Chemicals used to cleanse an area before performing an invasive procedure, such as starting an IV; not toxic to living tissues; examples include isopropyl alcohol and iodine.

anuria A complete stop in the production of urine.

anxiety disorder A mental disorder in which the dominant mood is fear and apprehension.

anxiolysis Relief of anxiety.

anxious avoidant attachment A bond between an infant and his or her parent or caregiver in which the infant is repeatedly rejected and develops an isolated lifestyle that does not depend upon the support and care of others.

aorta The largest artery in the body, originating from the left ventricle.

aortic valve The valve between the left ventricle and the aorta.

Apgar scoring system A scoring system for assessing the status of a newborn that assigns a number value to each of five areas of assessment.

aphasia The impairment of language that affects the production or understanding of speech and the ability to read or write.

aphonia Inability to speak.

apnea Respiratory pause greater than or equal to 20 seconds.

apneustic centre Portion of the brain stem that influences the respiratory rate by increasing the number of inspirations per minute.

apoptosis Normal, genetically programmed cell death.

apparent life-threatening event (ALTE) An unexpected sudden episode of colour change, tone change, or apnea that requires mouth-to-mouth resuscitation or vigorous stimulation.

appendicular skeleton The part of the skeleton comprising the upper and lower extremities.

apraxia Inability to connect an object with its proper use.

aqueous humour The clear, watery fluid in the anterior chamber of the globe.

arachnoid The middle membrane of the three meninges that enclose the brain and spinal cord.

arrhythmias Disturbances in cardiac rhythm.

arterial air embolism Air bubbles in the arterial blood vessels.

arterial gas embolism (AGE) The resultant gaseous emboli from the forcing of gas into the pulmonary vasculature from barotrauma.

arteries The muscular, thick-walled blood vessels that carry blood away from the heart.

arteriole A small blood vessel that carries oxygenated blood, branching into yet smaller vessels called capillaries.

arteriosclerosis A pathologic condition in which the arterial walls become thickened and inelastic.

arthritis Joint inflammation that causes pain, swelling, stiffness, and decreased range of motion.

Arthus reaction A localized reaction involving vascular inflammation in response to an IgG-mediated allergic response.

articulations The locations where two or more bones meet; joints.

artifact An artificial product; in cardiology, is used to refer to noise or interference in an ECG tracing.

arytenoid cartilages Pyramid-like cartilaginous structures that form the posterior attachment of the vocal cords.

ascites Abnormal accumulation of fluid in the peritoneal cavity.

aseptic technique A method of cleansing used to prevent contamination of a site when performing an invasive procedure, such as starting an IV.

asphyxia Condition of severely deficient supply of oxygen to the body leading to end organ damage.

asphyxiant Any gas that displaces oxygen from the atmosphere; can be deadly if exposure occurs in a confined space.

aspiration Entry of fluids or solids into the trachea, bronchi, and lungs.

assault To create in another person a fear of immediate bodily harm or invasion of bodily security.

asthma A chronic inflammatory lower airway condition resulting in intermittent wheezing and excess mucus production.

asymmetric chest wall movement When one side of the chest moves less than the other; indicates decreased airflow into one lung.

asynchronous In CPR, when two rescuers do ventilations and compressions individually and not timed or waiting for the other rescuer to pause.

asystole The absence of ventricular contractions; a "straight-line ECG."

ataxia Inability to coordinate the muscles properly; often used to describe a staggering gait.

atelectasis Alveolar collapse that prevents use of that portion of the lung for ventilation and oxygenation.

atherosclerosis A disorder in which cholesterol and calcium build up inside the walls of the blood vessels, forming plaque, which eventually leads to partial or complete blockage of blood flow.

atlanto-occipital joint Joint formed at the articulation of the atlas of the vertebral column and the occipital bone of the skull.

atmosphere absolute (ATA) A measurement of ambient pressure; the weight of air at sea level.

atopic The medical term for having an allergic tendency.

atresia The process by which an oocyte dies.

atrial kick The addition to ventricular volume contributed by contraction of the atria.

atrioventricular (AV) node A specialized structure located in the AV junction that slows conduction through the AV junction.

atrioventricular (AV) valves The mitral and tricuspid valves.

atrophy Wasting away of a tissue.

atropine A parasympathetic blocker; opposes the action of acetylcholine on the heart and elsewhere, thereby allowing the body's natural sympathetic system to speed up the heart rate.

atropine-like effects Results of some antipsychotic medications that include side effects similar to atropine, resulting in dry mouth, blurred vision, urinary retention, and cardiac arrhythmias.

auditory ossicles The bones that function in hearing and are located deep within cavities of the temporal bone.

aura Sensations experienced before an attack occurs. Common in seizures and migraine headaches.

aural Pertaining to the ear.

auricle The large outside portion of the ear through which sound waves enter the ear; also called the pinna.

auscultation The method of listening to sounds within the body with a stethoscope.

autoantibodies Antibodies directed against the patient.

autocrine hormone A hormone that acts on the cell that has secreted it.

autoimmune disorders Disorders in which the body identifies its own antigen as a foreign body and activates the inflammatory system.

autoimmunity The production of antibodies or T cells that work against the tissues of a person's own body, producing autoimmune disease or a hypersensitivity reaction.

automaticity Spontaneous initiation of depolarizing electric impulses by pacemaker sites within the electric conduction system of the heart.

autonomic dysreflexia A potentially life-threatening late complication of spinal cord injury in which massive, uninhibited uncompensated cardiovascular response occurs due to stimulation of the sympathetic nervous system below the level of injury. Also known as autonomic hyperreflexia.

autonomic nervous system (ANS) A subdivision of the nervous system that controls primarily involuntary body functions. It comprises the sympathetic and parasympathetic nervous systems.

autoregulation An increase in mean arterial pressure to compensate for decreased cerebral perfusion pressure; compensatory response of the body to shunt blood to the brain; manifests clinically as hypertension.

autosomal dominant A pattern of inheritance that involves genes that are located on autosomes or the nonsex chromosomes. You only need to inherit a single copy of a particular form of a gene to show the trait.

autosomal recessive A pattern of inheritance that involves genes located on autosomes or the nonsex chromosomes. You must inherit two copies of a particular form of a gene to show the trait.

AV junction The atrioventricular junction; the portion of the electric conduction system of the heart located in the upper part of the interventricular septum that conducts the excitation impulse from the atria to the bundle of His.

avascular necrosis Tissue death resulting from the loss of blood supply.

avian (bird) flu A disease caused by a virus that occurs naturally in the bird population. Signs and symptoms include fever, sore throat, cough, and muscle aches.

AVPU A method of assessing mental status by determining whether a patient is Awake and alert, responsive to Verbal stimuli or Pain, or Unresponsive; used principally in the initial assessment.

avulsing A tearing away or forcible separation.

avulsion An injury that leaves a piece of skin or other tissue partially or completely torn away from the body.

avulsion fracture A fracture that occurs when a piece of bone is torn free at the site of attachment of a tendon or ligament.

Awareness Level The training level to which all EMS personnel should be trained; topics include recognizing potential hazards, initiating protective measures for yourself and your community, and requesting additional response resources.

axial skeleton The part of the skeleton comprising the skull, spinal column, and rib cage.

axilla The armpit.

axillary artery The artery that runs through the axilla, connecting the subclavian artery to the brachial artery.

axon Long, slender extension of a neuron (nerve cell) that conducts electrical impulses away from the neuronal soma.

azotemia Increased nitrogenous wastes in the blood.

Babinski reflex When the toe(s) moves upward in response to stimulation to the sole of the foot. Under normal circumstances, the toe(s) moves downward.

bacteria Small organisms that can grow and reproduce outside the human cell in the presence of the temperature and nutrients, and cause disease by invading and multiplying in the tissues of the host.

bacterial vaginosis An overgrowth of bacteria in the vagina, characterized by itching, burning, or pain, and possibly a "fishy" smelling discharge.

bag-valve-mask device Manual ventilation device that consists of a bag, mask, reservoir, and oxygen inlet; capable of delivering up to 100% oxygen.

bandage Material used to secure a dressing in place.

barbiturates Any medications of a group of barbituric acid derivatives that act as central nervous system depressants and are used as sedatives or hypnotics.

bariatrics The branch of medicine that studies and treats obese patients.

barometric energy The energy that results from sudden changes in pressure as may occur in a diving accident or sudden decompression in an airplane.

barotrauma Injury resulting from pressure disequilibrium across body surfaces.

Bartholin glands The glands that secrete mucus for sexual lubrication.

basal ganglia Structures located deep within the cerebrum, diencephalon, and midbrain that have an important role in coordination of motor movements and posture.

basal metabolic rate (BMR) The heat energy produced at rest from normal body metabolic reactions, determined mostly by the liver and skeletal muscles.

base station Assembly of radio equipment consisting of at least a transmitter, receiver, and antenna connection at a fixed location.

basilar skull fractures Usually occur following diffuse impact to the head (such as falls, motor vehicle collisions); generally result from extension of a linear fracture to the base of the skull and can be difficult to diagnose with a radiograph (x-ray).

basophils White blood cells that work to produce chemical mediators during an immune response.

battery Unlawfully touching a person; this includes providing emergency care without consent.

Battle's sign Bruising over the mastoid bone behind the ear commonly seen following a basilar skull fracture; also called retroauricular ecchymosis.

Beck's triad The combination of a narrowed pulse pressure, muffled heart tones, and JVD associated with cardiac tamponade; usually resulting from penetrating chest trauma.

behaviour The way people act or perform, for example how they react/respond to a situation.

behavioural disorder An emergency in which the patient's presenting problem is some disorder of mood, thought, or behaviour that interferes with their activities of daily living (ADLs).

behavioural emergency A situation in which abnormal behaviour threatens an individual's health and safety or the health and safety of another.

belay Technique of controlling the rope as it is fed out to climbers.

Bell's palsy A temporary paralysis of the facial nerve (7th cranial nerve), which controls the muscles on each side of the face.

belt noise A chirping or squealing sound, synchronous with engine speed.

benzodiazepines Sedative-hypnotic drugs that provide muscle relaxation and mild sedation; includes drugs such as diazepam (Valium) and midazolam (Versed).

bereavement Sadness from loss; grieving.

beta Type of energy that is emitted from a strong radiological source; is slightly more penetrating than alpha, and requires a layer of clothing to stop it.

beta-2 agonists Pharmacologic agents that stimulate the beta-2 receptor sites found in smooth muscle; include common bronchodilators like salbutamol.

bigeminy An arrhythmia in which every other heartbeat is a premature contraction.

bill of lading A document carried by drivers of commercial vehicles that should provide specific information about what is carried on the vehicle.

bioavailability The amount of a medication that is still active once it reaches its target tissue.

biologic half-life The time it takes the body to eliminate half of the drug.

biomechanics The study of the physiology and mechanics of a living organism using the tools of mechanical engineering.

Biot respirations Characterized by an irregular rate, pattern, and volume of breathing with intermittent periods of apnea; results from increased intracranial pressure. Also called ataxic respirations.

biotelemetry Transmission of physiologic data, such as an ECG, from the patient to a distant point of reception (commonly referred to in EMS as "telemetry").

biotransformation A process by which a medication is chemically converted to a different compound or metabolite.

bipolar mood disorder A disorder in which a person alternates between mania and depression.

bivalent An ion that contains two charges.

blast front The leading edge of the shock wave.

blastocyst The term for an oocyte once it has been fertilized and multiplies into cells.

blind panic A fear reaction in which a person's judgment seems to disappear entirely; it is particularly dangerous because it may precipitate mass panic among others.

blinding The method of not giving the specifics of a project to the individuals participating in a research or study.

blood The fluid tissue that is pumped by the heart through the arteries, veins, and capillaries and consists of plasma and formed elements or cells, such as red blood cells, white blood cells, and platelets.

bloodborne pathogens Pathogenic microorganisms that are present in human blood and can cause disease in humans. These pathogens include, but are not limited to, hepatitis B virus (HBV) and human immunodeficiency virus (HIV).

blood pressure The pressure exerted by the pulsatile flow of blood against the arterial walls.

blood tubing A special type of macrodrip administration set designed to facilitate rapid fluid replacement by manual infusion of multiple IV bags or IV-blood replacement combinations.

bloody show A plug of mucus, sometimes mixed with blood, that is expelled from the dilating cervix and discharged from the vagina.

blow-by technique A method of delivering oxygen by holding a face mask or similar device near an infant's or a child's face; used when a nonrebreathing mask is not tolerated.

blowout fracture A fracture to the floor of the orbit usually caused by a blow to the eye.

blunt cardiac injury Contusion as the heart is compressed between the sternum and the spine.

blunt trauma Injury resulting from compression or deceleration forces, potentially crushing an organ or causing it to rupture.

BNICE A mnemonic for the five types of terrorist incidents that first responder agencies may be confronted with in the prehospital setting.

body In the context of the uterus, the portion below the fundus that begins to taper and narrow.

bolus A term used to describe "in one mass"; in medication administration, a single dose given by the IV or IO route; may be a small or large quantity of the drug.

bonding The formation of a close, personal relationship.

Bone Injection Gun (BIG) A spring-loaded device that is used for inserting an IO needle into the proximal tibia in adult and pediatric patients.

bone marrow Specialized tissue found within bone.

borborygmi A bowel sound characterized by increased activity within the bowel.

borderline personality disorder A disorder characterized by disordered images of self, impulsive and unpredictable behaviour, marked shifts in mood, and instability in relationships with others.

botulinum Produced by bacteria, this is a very potent neurotoxin. When introduced into the body, this neurotoxin affects the nervous system's ability to function and causes muscle paralysis.

botulism Poisoning from eating food containing botulinum toxin.

Bourdon-gauge flowmeter An oxygen flowmeter that is commonly used because it is not affected by gravity and can be placed in any position.

bowing fracture An incomplete fracture typically occurring in children in which the bone becomes bent as the result of a compressive force.

boxer's fracture A fracture of the head of the fifth metacarpal that usually results from striking an object with a clenched fist.

Boyle's law At a constant temperature, the volume of a gas is inversely proportional to its pressure (if you double the pressure on a gas, you halve its volume); written as $PV = K$, where P = pressure, V = volume, and K = a constant.

brachial artery The artery that runs through the arm and branches into the radial and ulnar arteries.

bradycardia A slow heart rate, less than 60 beats/min; a pulse rate of less than 100 beats/min in the newborn.

bradykinesia The slowing down of voluntary body movements. Found in Parkinson's disease.

brain Part of the central nervous system, located within the cranium and containing billions of neurons that serve a variety of vital functions.

brain stem The area of the brain between the spinal cord and cerebrum, surrounded by the cerebellum; controls functions that are necessary for life, such as respirations.

brake fade A sensation that an ambulance has lost its power brakes.

brake pull A sensation that, when an operator depresses the brake pedal, the steering wheel is being pulled to the left or the right.

breath-hold diving Also called free diving, this type of diving does not require any equipment, except sometimes a snorkel.

breech presentation A delivery in which the buttocks come out first.

brisance The shattering effect of a shock wave and its ability to cause disruption of tissues and structures.

bronchioles Subdivision of the smaller bronchi in the lungs; made of smooth muscle and dilate or constrict in response to various stimuli.

bronchiolitis A condition seen in children younger than 2 years, characterized by dyspnea and wheezing.

bronchoconstriction Narrowing of the bronchial tubes.

bronchodilation Widening of the bronchial tubes.

bronchospasm Severe constriction of the bronchial tree.

Brown-Sequard syndrome A condition associated with penetrating trauma with hemisection of the spinal cord and complete damage to all spinal tracts on the involved side.

bruit An abnormal "whoosh"-like sound of turbulent blood flow moving through a narrowed artery.

buboes Enlarged lymph nodes (up to the size of tennis balls) that were characteristic of people infected with the bubonic plague.

bubonic plague An epidemic that spread throughout Europe in the Middle Ages, also called the Black Death, transmitted by infected fleas and characterized by acute malaise, fever, and the formation of tender, enlarged, inflamed lymph nodes that appear as lesions, called buboes.

buccal route A medication route in which medication is administered between the cheeks and gums.

buckle fracture A common incomplete fracture in children in which the cortex of the bone fractures from an excessive compression force.

buddy splinting Securing an injured digit to an adjacent uninjured one to allow the intact digit to act as a splint.

buffers Molecules that modulate changes in pH to keep it in the physiologic range.

bulimia nervosa An eating disorder characterized by consumption of large amounts of food, and for which the patient then sometimes compensates by using purging techniques.

bundle branch block A disturbance in electric conduction through the right or left bundle branch from the bundle of His.

bundle of His The portion of the electric conduction system in the interventricular septum that conducts the depolarizing impulse from the atrioventricular junction to the right and left bundle branches.

burn shock The shock or hypoperfusion caused by a burn injury and the tremendous loss of fluids.

burnout The exhaustion of physical or emotional strength.

BURP maneuver Acronym for Backward, Upward, Rightward Pressure.

bursa A fluid-filled sac located adjacent to joints that reduces the amount of friction between moving structures.

bursitis Inflammation of a bursa.

butterfly cannula A rigid, hollow, venous cannulation device identified by its plastic "wings" that act as anchoring points for securing the cannula.

butyrophenones Potent, effective sedatives; includes drugs such as haloperidol (Haldol) and droperidol (Inapsine).

caladium A common houseplant that contains caladium oxalate crystals; ingestion leads to nausea, vomiting, and diarrhea.

calcaneous The heel bone; the largest of the tarsal bones.

calcitonin The hormone secreted by the thyroid gland that helps maintain normal calcium levels in the blood.

calcium channel blockers The medications that suppress arrhythmias, provide more oxygen to the heart via coronary artery dilation, and reduce peripheral vascular resistance.

calibrated The diagnostic checking and synchronizing of digital or electronic equipment to ensure that is in good working order and will measure accurately.

calyces (singular: calyx) Large urinary tubes that branch off the renal pelvis and connect with the renal pyramids to collect the urine draining from the collecting tubules.

CAMEO Computer-Aided Management of Emergency Operations; a tool to help predict downwind concentrations of hazardous materials based on the input of environmental factors into a computer model.

cancellous bone Trabecular or spongy bone.

cannula shear Occurs when a needle is reinserted into the cannula, and it slices through the cannula, creating a free-floating segment.

cannulation The insertion of a cannula, such as into a vein to allow for fluid flow.

CANUTEC A resource available to emergency responders via telephone on a 24-hour basis.

capacitance vessels The smallest venules.

cape cyanosis Deep cyanosis of the face and neck and across the chest and back; associated with little or no blood flow; it is particularly ominous.

capillaries Extremely narrow blood vessels composed of a single layer of cells through which oxygen and nutrients pass to the tissues. Capillaries form a network between arterioles and venules.

capillary refill time A test done on the fingers or toes by briefly squeezing the toe or finger, then evaluating the time it takes for the pink colour to return.

capnographer Device that attaches in between the endotracheal tube and bag-valve-mask device; contains colourimetric paper, which should turn yellow during exhalation, indicating proper tube placement.

capnometer Device that attaches in the same way as a capnographer, but provides a light-emitting diode (LED) readout of the patient's exhaled carbon dioxide.

capsule A cylindrical gelatin container enclosing a dose of medication.

carbon monoxide A chemical asphyxiant that results in a cellular respiratory failure; this gas ties up hemoglobin to the extent that oxygen in the blood becomes inaccessible to the cells.

carboxyhemoglobin Abnormal hemoglobin that is formed by the attachment of carbon monoxide to the hemoglobin molecule.

cardiac cycle The period from one cardiac contraction to the next. Each cardiac cycle consists of ventricular contraction (systole) and relaxation (diastole).

cardiac glycosides A classification of medications that naturally occur in plant substances and that block certain ionic pumps in the heart cells' membranes, which indirectly increases calcium concentrations; an example is digoxin.

cardiac output (CO) Amount of blood pumped by the heart per minute, calculated by multiplying the stroke volume by the heart rate per minute.

cardiac tamponade A condition in which the atria and right ventricle are collapsed by a collection of blood or other fluid within the pericardial sac, resulting in a diminished cardiac output.

cardiogenic shock A condition caused by loss of 40% or more of the functioning myocardium; the heart is no longer able to circulate sufficient blood to maintain adequate oxygen delivery.

cardiopulmonary arrest The sudden and often unexpected cessation of adequate cardiac output.

cardiovascular collapse Failure of the heart and blood vessels; shock.

cardioversion The use of a synchronized direct current (DC) electric shock to convert tachyarrhythmias (such as atrial flutter) to normal sinus rhythm.

carina Point at which the trachea bifurcates (divides) into the left and right mainstem bronchi.

carpals The eight small bones of the wrist.

carpopedal spasm Contorted position of the hand in which the fingers flex in a clawlike attitude and the thumb curls toward the palm.

carrier An individual who harbors an infectious agent and, although not personally ill, can transmit the infection to another person.

cartilage Tough, elastic substance that covers opposable surfaces of moveable joints and forms part of the skeleton.

cartilaginous joints Joints that are spanned completely by cartilage and allow for minimal motion.

castor bean A seed that contains the poison ricin; causes a variety of toxic effects: burning of the mouth and throat; nausea, vomiting, diarrhea, and severe stomach pains; prostration; failing vision and kidney failure, which is the usual cause of death.

catatonic Lacking expression or movement, or appearing rigid.

catatonic type A type of schizophrenia in which the person displays odd motor activity, such as strange facial expression or rigidity.

catecholamines Hormones produced by the adrenal medulla (epinephrine and norepinephrine) that assist the body in coping with physical and emotional stress by increasing the heart and respiratory rates and the blood pressure.

cation An ion that contains an overall positive charge.

cauda equina The location where the spinal cord separates, composed of nerve roots.

caustics Chemicals that are acids or alkalis; cause direct chemical injury to the tissues they contact.

cavitation Cavity formation; shock waves that push tissues in front of and lateral to the projectile and may not necessarily increase the wound size or cause permanent injury but can result in cavitation.

cell-mediated immunity Immune process by which T-cell lymphocytes recognize antigens and then secrete cytokines (specifically lymphokines) that attract other cells or stimulate the production of cytotoxic cells that kill the infected cells.

cell signaling The process by which cells communicate with one another.

cellular immunity The immunity provided by special white blood cells called T cells that attack and destroy invaders.

cellular telephones Low-power portable radios that communicate through an interconnected series of repeater stations called "cells."

Celsius scale A scale for measuring temperature in which water freezes at 0° and boils at 100°.

central cord syndrome A condition resulting from hyperextension injuries to the cervical area that cause damage with hemorrhage or edema to the central cervical segments; findings include greater loss of function in the upper extremities with variable sensory loss of pain and temperature.

central cyanosis Bluish colouration of the skin due to the presence of deoxygenated hemoglobin in blood vessels near the skin surface.

central nervous system (CNS) The system containing the brain and spinal cord.

central neurogenic hyperventilation Deep, rapid respirations; similar to Kussmaul, but without an acetone breath odour; commonly seen following brain stem injury.

central shock A term that describes shock secondary to central pump failure; it includes both cardiogenic shock and obstructive shock.

central venous cannula A cannula inserted into the vena cava to permit intermittent or continuous monitoring of central venous pressure and to facilitate obtaining blood samples for chemical analysis.

central vision The visualization of objects directly in front of you.

cerebellum The region of the brain essential in coordinating muscle movements in the body; also called the athlete's brain.

cerebral concussion Occurs when the brain is jarred around in the skull; a mild diffuse brain injury that does not result in structural damage or permanent neurologic impairment.

cerebral contusion A focal brain injury in which brain tissue is bruised and damaged in a defined area.

cerebral cortex The largest portion of the cerebrum; regulates voluntary skeletal movement and one's level of awareness—a part of consciousness.

cerebral edema Cerebral water; causes or contributes to swelling of the brain.

cerebral palsy (CP) A developmental condition in which damage is done to the brain. It presents during infancy as delays in walking or crawling, and can take on a spastic form in which muscles are in a near constant state of contraction.

cerebral perfusion pressure (CPP) The pressure of blood flow through the brain; the difference between the mean arterial pressure (MAP) and intracranial pressure (ICP).

cerebrospinal fluid (CSF) Fluid produced in the ventricles of the brain that flows in the subarachnoid space and bathes the meninges.

cerebrospinal fluid shunts Tubes that drain fluid manufactured in the ventricles of the brain from the subarachnoid space to another part of the body outside of the brain, such as the peritoneum; lowers pressure in the brain.

cerebrospinal otorrhea Cerebrospinal fluid drainage from the ears.

cerebrospinal rhinorrhea Cerebrospinal fluid drainage from the nose.

cerebrovascular accident (CVA) An interruption of blood flow to the brain that results in the loss of brain function.

cerebrum The largest portion of the brain; responsible for higher functions, such as reasoning; divided into right and left hemispheres, or halves.

certification Evidence of a certain level of training, such as a certificate of completion from a course or school.

certified A title given when a person has shown that he or she has met requirements based on knowledge of certain facts.

cervical canal The interior of the cervix.

cervix The narrowest portion of the uterus that opens into the vagina.

chancre The primary hard lesion or ulcer of syphilis that occurs at the entry site of the infection.

chancroid A highly contagious sexually transmitted disease caused by the bacteria Haemophilus ducreyi, which causes painful sores (ulcers), usually of the genitals.

chemical asphyxiants Substances that interfere with the utilization of oxygen at the cellular level.

chemical energy The energy released as a result of a chemical reaction.

chemical mediators Chemicals that work to cause the immune or allergic response, for example, histamine.

chemical name A description of the drug's chemical composition and molecular structure.

chemoreceptors Monitor the levels of O_2, CO_2, and the pH of the CSF and then provide feedback to the respiratory centres to modify the rate and depth of breathing based on the body's needs at any given time.

chemotactic factors The factors that cause cells to migrate into an area.

chemotaxins Components of the activated complement system that attract leukocytes from the circulation to help fight infections.

chemotaxis The movement of additional white blood cells to an area of inflammation in response to the release of chemical mediators, such as neutrophils, injured tissue, and monocytes.

chemotherapy The introduction of either single cytotoxic drugs or combinations of cytotoxic drugs into the body for the purpose of interrupting or eradicating malignant cellular growth.

CHEMTREC (Chemical Emergency Transportation Center) A resource available to emergency responders via telephone on a 24-hour basis.

Cheyne-Stokes respirations Respirations that are fast and then become slow, with intervening periods of apnea; commonly seen following brain stem injury.

chickenpox A very contagious disease caused by varicella zoster virus, which is part of the herpes virus family, occurring most often in the winter and early spring.

chief complaint The problem for which the patient is seeking help.

child protective services (CPS) An agency that is the community legal organization responsible for protection, rehabilitation, and prevention of child maltreatment and neglect; it has the legal authority to temporarily remove from home children who are at risk for injury or neglect and to secure foster placement.

chlamydia A sexually transmitted disease caused by the bacterium Chlamydia trachomatis.

chlorine (CL) The first chemical agent ever used in warfare. It has a distinct odour of bleach, and creates a green haze when released as a gas. Initially it produces upper airway irritation and a choking sensation.

choanal atresia A narrowing or blockage of the nasal airway by membranous or bony tissue; a congenital condition, meaning it is present at birth.

cholestasis A common liver disease that occurs only during pregnancy, in which the flow of bile is altered resulting in acids being released into the bloodstream, causing profuse and painful itching.

cholinergic Fibres in the parasympathetic nervous system that release a chemical called acetylcholine.

chordae tendineae Fibrous strands shaped like umbrella stays that attach the free edges of the leaflets, or cusps, of the atrioventricular valves to the papillary muscles.

choroid plexus Specialized cells within the hollow areas in the ventricles of the brain that produce CSF.

chronic bronchitis Chronic inflammatory condition affecting the bronchi that is associated with excess mucous production that results from overgrowth of the mucous glands in the airways.

chronic hypertension A blood pressure that is equal to or greater than 140/90 mm Hg, which exists prior to pregnancy, occurs before the 20th week of pregnancy, or continues to persist postpartum.

chronic obstructive pulmonary disease (COPD) Illnesses that cause obstructive problems in the lower airways, including chronic bronchitis, emphysema, and sometimes asthma.

chronic renal failure (CRF) Progressive and irreversible inadequate kidney function due to permanent loss of nephrons.

chronotropic effect The rate of contraction of the heart.

chyme The partially digested food that exits the stomach, entering the duodenum.

cilia Hairlike microtubule projections on the surface of a cell that can move materials over the cell surface.

circumferential burns Burns on the neck or chest that may compress the airway or on an extremity that might act like a tourniquet.

circumflex coronary artery One of the two branches of the left main coronary artery.

circumstantial thinking Situation in which a patient includes many irrelevant details in his or her account of things.

civil suit An action instituted by a private individual or corporation against another private individual or corporation.

clandestine drug laboratories Locations where illegal drugs such as methamphetamine, lysergic acid diethylamide (LSD), ecstasy, and phencyclidine hydrochloride (PCP) are manufactured.

classic heat stroke Also called passive heat stroke, this is a serious heat illness that usually occurs during heat waves and is most likely to strike very old, very young, or bedridden people.

clavicle An S-shaped bone, also called the collarbone, that articulates medially with the sternum and laterally with the shoulder.

cleft lip An abnormal defect or fissure in the upper lip that failed to close during development. It is often associated with cleft palate.

cleft palate A fissure or hole in the palate (roof of the mouth) that forms a communicating pathway between the mouth and nasal cavities.

climacteric End phase of a woman's life menstrual cycle.

clitoris A small, cylindrical mass of erectile tissue and nerves located at the anterior junction of the labia minora, homologous to the glans penis of the male.

clonic activity Type of seizure movement involving the contraction and relaxation of muscle groups.

closed abdominal injury An injury in which there is soft-tissue damage inside the body, but the skin remains intact.

closed-ended question A question that is specific and focused, either demanding a yes or no answer, or an answer chosen from specific options.

closed fracture A fracture in which the skin is not broken.

closed incident A contained incident in which patients are found in one focal location and the situation is not expected to produce more patients than initially present.

closed wound An injury in which damage occurs beneath the skin or mucous membrane but the surface remains intact.

clotting factors Substances in the blood that are necessary for clotting; also called coagulation factors.

CNS stimulants Any medications or agents that increase brain activity.

coagulation Clotting.

coagulation system The system that forms blood clots in the body and facilitates repairs to the vascular tree.

cochlea The shell-shaped structure within the inner ear that contains the organ of Corti.

cochlear duct A canal within the cochlea that receives vibrations from the ossicles.

code team leader The code team member who has the responsibility for managing the rescuers or team members during a cardiac arrest, as well as choreographing the effort of the group.

code team member A member of the resuscitation team trying to revive the patient.

coin rubbing A cultural ritual intended to treat an illness by rubbing hot coins, often on the back, which produces rounded and oblong red, patchy, flat skin lesions.

cold diuresis Secretion of large amounts of urine in response to cold exposure and the consequent shunting of blood volume to the body core.

cold protective response Phenomenon associated with cold water immersion in which reflexes in the body and a lowered metabolic rate help preserve basic body functions.

cold zone A safe area for those agencies involved in the operations; the incident commander (IC), command post, paramedics, and other support functions necessary to control the incident should be located in the cold zone.

collagen A protein that gives tensile strength to the connective tissues of the body.

collateral circulation The mesh of arteries and capillaries that furnishes blood to a segment of tissue whose original arterial supply has been obstructed.

colloid solutions Solutions that contain molecules (usually proteins) that are too large to pass out of the capillary membranes and, therefore, remain in the vascular compartment.

colostomy Establishment of an opening between the colon and the surface of the body for the purpose of providing drainage of the bowel.

coma A state in which one does not respond to verbal or painful stimuli.

Combitube Multilumen airway device that consists of a single tube with two lumens, two balloons, and two ventilation ports; an alternative device if endotracheal intubation is not possible or has failed.

comedo A noninflammatory acne lesion.

command In incident command, the position that oversees the incident, establishes the objectives and priorities, and from there develops a response plan.

comminuted fracture A fracture in which the bone is broken into three or more pieces.

commotio cordis An event in which an often fatal cardiac dysrhythmia is produced by a sudden blow to the thoracic cavity.

communicability Describes how easily a disease spreads from one human to another human.

communicable disease A disease that can be transmitted from one person to another under certain conditions.

communicable period The period during which an infected person is capable of transmitting illness to someone else.

communication The transmission of information to another person—whether it be verbal or through body language.

compartment syndrome A condition that develops when edema and swelling result in increased pressure within soft tissues,

causing circulation to be compromised, possibly resulting in tissue necrosis.

compensated shock The early stage of shock, in which the body can still compensate for blood loss.

complement system A group of plasma proteins whose function is to do one of three things: attract leukocytes to sites of inflammation, activate leukocytes, and directly destroy cells.

complete abortion Expulsion of all products of conception from the uterus.

complete fracture A fracture in which the bone is broken into two or more completely separate pieces.

complete spinal cord injury Total disruption of all tracts of the spinal cord, with all cord-mediated functions below the level of transection lost permanently.

complex febrile seizures An unusual form of seizures that occurs in association with a rapid increase in body temperature.

complex partial seizures Seizures characterized by alteration of consciousness with or without complex focal motor activity.

compound fracture An open fracture; a fracture beneath an open wound.

compulsion A repetitive action carried out to relieve the anxiety of obsessive thoughts.

computer-aided dispatch An automated computer system that processes the information received and assists the dispatcher with multiple functions and tasks.

concealment Protection from being seen.

concentration The total weight of a drug contained in a specific volume of liquid.

concentration gradient The natural tendency for substances to flow from an area of higher concentration to an area of lower concentration, within or outside the cell.

concept formation Pattern of understanding based on initially obtained information.

conduction Transfer of heat to a solid object or a liquid by direct contact.

conductive deafness A curable temporary condition, caused by an injury to the eardrum.

confabulation The invention of experiences to cover gaps in memory, seen in patients with certain organic brain syndromes.

confined space A space with limited or restricted access that is not meant for continuous occupancy, such as a manhole, well, or tank.

confrontation Interviewing technique in which the interviewer points out to the patient something of interest in his/her conversation or behaviour.

confusion An impaired understanding of one's surroundings.

conjunctiva A thin, transparent membrane that covers the sclera and internal surfaces of the eyelids.

conjunctivitis An inflammation of the conjunctivae that usually is caused by bacteria, viruses, allergies, or foreign bodies; should be considered highly contagious; also called pink eye.

connective tissue   Tissue that serves to bind various tissue types together.

consent   Agreement by the patient to accept a medical intervention.

contact and cover   Technique that involves one paramedic making contact with the patient to provide care, while the second paramedic obtains patient information, gauges the level of tension, and warns his or her partner at the first sign of trouble.

contact burn   A burn produced by touching a hot object.

contact hazard   A hazardous agent that gives off very little or no vapours; the skin is the primary route for this type of chemical to enter the body; also called a skin hazard.

contagious   A person infected with a disease that is highly communicable.

contaminated   The presence or the reasonably anticipated presence of blood or other potentially infectious materials on an item or surface.

contaminated stick   The puncturing of an emergency care provider's skin with a needle or cannula that was used on a patient.

continuous positive airway pressure (CPAP)   A form of noninvasive ventilation in which the patient exhales against positive-pressure via a tight-fitting face mask; used to treat patients with cardiogenic pulmonary edema.

contraceptive device   A device used to prevent pregnancy.

contractility   The strength of heart muscle contractions.

contraindications   In health care, conditions or factors that increase the risk involved in using a particular drug, carrying out a medical procedure, or engaging in a particular activity.

contusion   A bruise; an injury that causes bleeding beneath the skin but does not break the skin.

convection   Mechanism by which body heat is picked up and carried away by moving air currents.

convenience sampling   A type of research in which subjects are manually assigned to a specific person or crew, rather than being randomly assigned; the least-preferred component of research.

conventional reasoning   A type of reasoning in which a child looks for approval from peers and society.

conversion hysteria   A reaction in which a person subconsciously transforms his or her anxiety into a bodily dysfunction; the person may be unable to see or hear or may become partially paralyzed.

cookbook medicine   Treatment based on a protocol or algorithm without adequate knowledge of the patient being treated.

cor pulmonale   Heart disease that develops secondary to a chronic lung disease, usually affecting primarily the right side of the heart.

core body temperature (CBT)   The temperature in the part of the body comprising the heart, lungs, brain, and abdominal viscera.

cornea   The transparent anterior portion of the eye that overlies the iris and pupil.

coronal suture   The point where the parietal bones join with the frontal bone.

coronary arteries   The blood vessels of the heart that supply blood to its walls.

coronary artery disease (CAD)   A pathologic process caused by atherosclerosis that leads to progressive narrowing and eventual obstruction of the coronary arteries.

coronary sinus   A large vessel in the posterior part of the coronary sulcus into which the coronary veins empty.

coronary sulcus   The groove along the exterior surface of the heart that separates the atria from the ventricles.

corpus luteum   The remains of a follicle after an oocyte has been released, and which secretes progesterone.

corrosives   A class of chemicals with either high or low pH levels. Exposure can cause severe soft-tissue damage.

cortex   Part of the internal anatomy of the kidney; the lighter-coloured outer region closest to the capsule.

corticosteroids   Hormones that regulate the body's metabolism, the balance of salt and water in the body, the immune system, and sexual function.

cortisol   Hormone that stimulates most body cells to increase their energy production.

countercurrent multiplier   The process in which the body produces either concentrated or diluted urine, depending on the body's needs.

coup–contrecoup injury   Dual impacting of the brain into the skull; coup injury occurs at the point of impact; contrecoup injury occurs on the opposite side of impact, as the brain rebounds.

couplet   Two premature ventricular contractions occurring sequentially.

cover   Obstacles that are difficult or impossible for bullets to penetrate.

covert   Act in which the public safety community generally has no prior knowledge of the time, location, or nature of the attack.

crackles   Abnormal breath sounds that have a fine, crackling quality; previously called rales.

cranial vault   The bones that encase and protect the brain, including the parietal, temporal, frontal, occipital, sphenoid, and ethmoid bones; also called the cranium or skull.

craniofacial disjunction   A Le Fort III fracture; involves a fracture of all of the midfacial bones, thus separating the entire midface from the cranium.

crepitus   A grating sensation made when two pieces of broken bone are rubbed together or subcutaneous emphysema is palpated.

cribbing   Short lengths of wood that are used to stabilize vehicles.

cribriform plate   A horizontal bone perforated with numerous foramina for the passage of the olfactory nerve filaments from the nasal cavity.

cricoid cartilage   Forms the lowest portion of the larynx; also referred to as the cricoid ring;

the first ring of the trachea and is the only upper airway structure that forms a complete ring.

cricoid pressure   The application of posterior pressure to the cricoid cartilage; minimizes gastric distension and the risk of vomiting and aspiration during ventilation; also referred to as the Sellick maneuver.

cricothyroid membrane   A thin, superficial membrane located between the thyroid and cricoid cartilages that is relatively avascular and contains few nerves; the site for emergency surgical and nonsurgical access to the airway.

criminal prosecution   An action instituted by the government against a private individual for violation of criminal law.

crista galli   A prominent bony ridge in the centre of the anterior fossa and the point of attachment of the meninges.

critical incident   An event that overwhelms the ability to cope with the experience, either at the scene or later.

critical incident stress debriefings (CISDs)   A confidential peer group discussion in which specially trained teams work with emergency personnel who have been involved in traumatic calls or other painful incidents; CISDs usually occur within 24 to 72 hours of the incident.

critical infrastructure   The external foundation in communities made up of structures and services critical in the day-to-day living activities of humans: energy sources, fuel, water, sewage removal, food, hospitals, and transportation systems.

critical minimum threshold   Minimum cerebral perfusion pressure required to adequately perfuse the brain; 60 mm Hg in the adult.

cross-contamination   Occurs when a person is contaminated by an agent as a result of coming into contact with another contaminated person.

cross-sectional research   A type of research in which information is gathered from a group of individuals over a specific time frame.

cross-tolerance   A form of drug tolerance in which patients who take a particular medication for an extended period can build up a tolerance to other medications in the same class.

croup   A childhood viral disease characterized by edema of the upper airways with barking cough, difficult breathing, and stridor.

crown   The part of the tooth that is external to the gum.

crowning   The appearance of the infant's head at the vaginal opening during labour.

crush injury   An injury in which the body or part of the body is crushed, preventing tissue function and, possibly, resulting in permanent tissue damage.

crush syndrome   Significant metabolic derangement that can lead to renal failure and death. It develops when crushed extremities or other body parts remain trapped for prolonged periods.

crystalloid solutions   Solutions of dissolved crystals (for example, salts or sugars) in water; contain compounds that quickly dissociate in solution.

cumulative effect An effect that occurs when several successive doses of a medication are administered or when absorption of a medication occurs faster than excretion or metabolism.

cupping The cultural practice of placing warm cups on the skin to pull out illness from the body. The red, flat, rounded skin lesions are often more intensely red at the borders.

current health status A composite picture of a number of factors in a patient's life, such as dietary habits, current medications, allergies, exercise, alcohol or tobacco use, recreational drug use, sleep patterns and disorders, and immunizations.

curved laryngoscope blade Also called the Macintosh blade; designed to fit into the vallecula, indirectly lifting the epiglottis and exposing the vocal cords.

Cushing's reflex The combination of a slowing pulse, rising blood pressure, and erratic respiratory patterns; a grave sign for patients with head trauma.

Cushing's syndrome A condition caused by an excess of cortisol production by the adrenal glands or by excessive use of cortisol or other similar steroid (glucocorticoid) hormones.

Cushing's triad Hypertension (with a widening pulse pressure), bradycardia, and irregular respirations; classic trio of findings associated with increased ICP.

cusps Points at the top of a tooth.

cutaneous Pertaining to the skin.

cyanide Agent that affects the body's ability to use oxygen. It is a colourless gas that has an odour similar to almonds. The effects begin on the cellular level and are very rapidly seen at the organ system level.

cyanosis A bluish-grey skin colour that is caused by reduced levels of oxygen in the blood.

cystadenomas Fluid-filled cysts that form on the outer ovarian surface.

cystic fibrosis Chronic dysfunction of the endocrine system that affects multiple body systems, primarily the respiratory and digestive systems.

cytokines Products of cells that affect the function of other cells.

cytomegalovirus (CMV) A herpesvirus that can produce the symptoms of prolonged high fever, chills, headache, malaise, extreme fatigue, and an enlarged spleen.

D5W An intravenous solution made up of 5% dextrose in water.

Dalton's law Each gas in mixture exerts the same partial pressure that it would exert if it were alone in the same volume, and the total pressure of a mixture of gases is the sum of the partial pressures of all the gases in the mixture.

damages Compensation for injury awarded by a court.

data interpretation The process of formulating a conclusion based on comparing the

patient's condition with information from your training, education, and past experiences.

dead space The portion of the tidal volume that does not reach the alveoli and thus does not participate in gas exchange.

decay A natural process in which a material that is unstable attempts to stabilize itself by changing its structure.

deceleration A negative acceleration, that is, slowing down.

decerebrate (extensor) posturing Abnormal posture characterized by extension of the arms and legs; indicates pressure on the brain stem.

decision-making capacity The patient's ability to understand and process the information you give him or her about your proposed plan of care.

decompensated shock The late stage of shock, when blood pressure is falling.

decompression sickness (DCS) A broad range of signs and symptoms caused by nitrogen bubbles in blood and tissues coming out of solution on ascent.

decontamination The process of removing hazardous materials from the body or clothing of victims or rescuers. Includes the methods of dilution, absorption, disposal, and (in rare cases only) neutralization.

decorticate (flexor) posturing Abnormal posture characterized by flexion of the arms and extension of the legs; indicates pressure on the brain stem.

decussation Movement of nerves from one side of the brain to the opposite side of the body.

deep fascia A dense layer of fibrous tissue below the subcutaneous tissue; composed of tough bands of tissue that ensheath muscles and other internal structures.

deep frostbite A type of frostbite in which the affected part looks white, yellow-white, or mottled blue-white and is hard, cold, and without sensation.

deep vein thrombosis (DVT) The formation of a blood clot within the larger veins of an extremity, typically following a period of prolonged immobilization.

defamation Intentionally making a false statement, through written or verbal communication, which injures a person's good name or reputation.

defence mechanisms Psychological ways to relieve stress; they are usually automatic or subconscious. Defence mechanisms include denial, regression, projection, and displacement.

defendant In a civil suit, the individual against whom a legal action is brought.

defibrillation The use of an unsynchronized direct current (DC) electric shock to terminate ventricular fibrillation.

degloving A traumatic injury that results in the soft tissue of the hand being drawn downward like a glove being removed.

degranulate To release granules into the surrounding tissue.

dehiscence Separation of the edges of a wound.

dehydration Depletion of the body's systemic fluid volume.

delirium An acute confessional state characterized by global impairment of thinking, perception, judgment, and memory.

delirium tremens (DTs) A severe withdrawal syndrome seen in people with alcoholism who are deprived of ethyl alcohol; characterized by restlessness, fever, sweating, disorientation, agitation, and seizures; can be fatal if untreated.

delta wave The slurring of the upstroke of the first part of the QRS complex that occurs in Wolff-Parkinson-White syndrome.

delusion A fixed belief that is not shared by others of a person's culture or background and that can't be changed by reasonable argument; a false belief.

delusions of grandeur A state in which a person believes oneself to be someone of great importance.

delusions of persecution A state in which a person believes that others are plotting against him or her.

dementia The slow onset of progressive disorientation, shortened attention span, and loss of cognitive function.

demobilization The process of directing responders to return to their facilities when work at a disaster or mass-casualty incident has finished, at least for the particular responders.

dendrites Part of the neuron that receives impulses from the axon and contains vesicles for release of neurotransmitters.

denial An early response to a serious medical emergency, in which the severity of the emergency is diminished or minimized. Denial is the first coping mechanism for people who believe they are going to die.

dentin The principal mass of the tooth, which is made up of a material that is much more dense and stronger than bone.

depersonalization A type of dissociative disorder in which a person loses his or her sense of reality, and may experience events as being "dream-like."

depolarization The process of discharging resting cardiac muscle fibres by an electric impulse that causes them to contract.

depolarizing neuromuscular blocking agents Medications designed to keep muscles in a contracted state.

depressed skull fractures Result from high-energy direct trauma to a small surface area of the head with a blunt object (such as a baseball bat to the head); commonly result in bony fragments being driven into the brain, causing injury.

depression A persistent mood of sadness, despair, and discouragement; may be a symptom of many different mental and physical disorders, or it may be a disorder on its own.

depression fracture A fracture in which the broken region of the bone is pushed deeper into the body than the remaining intact bone.

derealization A symptom of a dissociative disorder in which objects seem to change size or shape; people may seem dead or behave like robots when viewed during a moment of acute stress.

dermal exposure Skin exposure, also known as topical exposure. Some hazardous materials may be absorbed through the skin to produce a systemic effect.

dermatomes Distinct areas of skin that correspond to specific spinal or cranial nerve levels where sensory nerves enter the CNS.

dermis The inner layer of skin, containing hair follicle roots, glands, blood vessels, and nerves.

dermoid cysts Ovarian cysts containing formational tissue, such as hair and teeth.

descriptive research A type of research in which an observation of an event is made, but without attempts to alter or change it.

designated infection control officer (DICO) An individual trained to ensure that proper postexposure medical treatment and counseling is provided to an exposed employee or volunteer.

desired dose The amount of a drug that the physician orders for a patient; the drug order.

desquamation The continuous shedding of the dead cells on the surface of the skin.

detailed physical examination The part of the assessment process in which a detailed area-by-area examination is performed on patients whose problems cannot be readily identified or when more specific information is needed about problems identified in the focused history and physical examination.

devascularization The loss of blood to a part of the body.

developmental disability Insufficient development of the brain, resulting in some level of dysfunction or impairment.

diabetes mellitus Disease characterized by the body's inability to sufficiently metabolize glucose. The condition occurs either because the pancreas doesn't produce enough insulin or the cells don't respond to the effects of the insulin that's produced.

diabetic ketoacidosis (DKA) A form of acidosis in uncontrolled diabetes in which certain acids accumulate when insulin is not available.

diaphragm Large skeletal muscle that plays a major role in breathing and separates the chest cavity from the abdominal cavity.

diaphragmatic hernia Passage of loops of bowel with or without other abdominal organs, through the diaphragm muscle; occurs as the bowel from the abdomen "herniates" upward through the diaphragm into the chest (thoracic) cavity.

diaphysis The shaft of a long bone.

diarrhea Liquid stool.

diastasis An increase in the distance between the two sides of a joint.

diastole The period of ventricular relaxation during which the ventricles passively fill with blood.

dieffenbachia A common houseplant that resembles "elephant ears"; ingestion leads to burns of the mouth and tongue and, possibly, paralysis of the vocal cords and nausea and vomiting; in severe cases, may be edema of the tongue and larynx, leading to airway compromise.

diencephalon The part of the brain between the brain stem and the cerebrum that includes the thalamus, the subthalamus, hypothalamus, and epithalamus.

diffuse axonal injury (DAI) Diffuse brain injury that is caused by stretching, shearing, or tearing of nerve fibres with subsequent axonal damage.

diffuse brain injury Any injury that affects the entire brain.

diffusion A process in which molecules move from an area of higher concentration to an area of lower concentration.

digital arteries The arteries that supply blood to the fingers and toes.

digital intubation Method of intubation that involves directly palpating the glottic structures and elevating the epiglottis with your middle finger while guiding the ET tube into the trachea by feel.

digoxin preparations Medications prescribed for the treatment of chronic CHF or for certain rapid atrial arrhythmias.

diluent A solution (usually water or normal saline) used for diluting a medication.

dilution A type of decontamination method that uses copious amounts of water to flush the contaminant from the skin or eyes.

diplopia Double vision.

direct laryngoscopy Visualization of the airway with a laryngoscope.

direct medical control Type of medical control in which the paramedic is in direct contact with a physician, usually via two-way radio or telephone.

dirty bomb Name given to a bomb that is used as a radiological dispersal device (RDD).

disaster management A planned, coordinated response to a disaster that involves cooperation of multiple responders and agencies and enables effective triage and provision of care according to triage decisions.

disasters Widespread events that disrupt community resources and functions, in turn threatening public safety, lives, and property.

disease vector An animal that once infected, spreads a disease to another animal.

disinfectants Chemicals used on nonliving objects to kill organisms; toxic to living tissues; examples include Virex, Cidex, and Microcide.

dislocation The displacement of a bone from its normal position within a joint.

disorganization A condition in which a person is characterized by uncontrolled and disconnected thought, is usually incoherent or rambling in speech, and may or may not be oriented to person and place.

disorganized symptoms Refers to erratic speech, emotional responses, and motor behaviour.

disorganized type A type of schizophrenia in which the person usually displays the wrong emotion for a particular situation, often self-absorbed.

disorientation Confusion regarding a person's sense of who one is (person), where one is (place), and at what point in time one finds oneself (time).

dispatch To send to a specific destination or to send on a task.

displacement Redirection of an emotion from yourself to another person.

disposal A type of decontamination in which as much clothing and equipment as possible is disposed of to reduce the magnitude of the problem.

dissection In references to blood vessels, an aneurysm, or bulge, formed by the separation of the layers of an arterial wall.

disseminated intravascular coagulopathy (DIC) A life-threatening condition commonly found in severe trauma.

dissemination The means with which a terrorist will spread a disease, for example, by poisoning of the water supply, or aerosolizing the agent into the air or ventilation system of a building.

dissociation Feelings of being detached from yourself, as if you were dreaming.

distal convoluted tubule (DCT) Connects with the kidney's collecting tubules.

distractibility The patient's attention is easily diverted.

distraction injury An injury that results from a force that tries to increase the length of a body part or separate one body part from another.

distress A type of stress that a person finds overwhelming and debilitating.

distribution The movement and transportation of a medication throughout the bloodstream to tissues and cells of the body and, ultimately, to its target receptor.

distributive shock A condition that occurs when there is widespread dilation of the resistance vessels (small arterioles), the capacitance vessels (small venules), or both.

diuresis Secretion of large amounts of urine by the kidney.

diuretic medications The medications designed to promote elimination of excess salt and water by the kidneys.

diuretics Chemicals that increase urinary output.

Do Not Intubate forms Written documentation by a physician giving permission to medical personnel not to attempt intubation.

do not resuscitate (DNR) forms Written documentation by a physician giving permission to medical personnel not to attempt resuscitation in the event of cardiac arrest.

do not resuscitate (DNR) order A type of advance directive that describes which life-sustaining procedures should be performed in the event of a sudden deterioration in a patient's medical condition.

domestic terrorists Native citizens who carry out terrorist acts against their own country.

dopaminergic receptors The receptors believed to cause dilation of the renal, coronary, and cerebral arteries.

dorsal Referring to the back or posterior side of the body or an organ.

dorsiflex To bend the foot or hand backward.

dose effect The principle that the longer a hazardous material is in contact with the body or the greater the concentration, the greater the effect will probably be.

Down syndrome A genetic chromosomal defect that can occur during fetal development and that results in mental retardation as well as certain physical characteristics, such as a round head with a flat occiput and slanted, wide-set eyes.

dressing Material used to directly cover a wound.

drift A finding that when the operator lets go of the steering wheel, a vehicle consistently wanders left or right.

drip chamber The area of the administration set where fluid accumulates so that the tubing remains filled with fluid.

dromotropic Relating to or influencing the conductivity of nerve fibres or cardiac muscle fibres.

dromotropic effect The effect on the velocity of conduction.

drowning The process of experiencing respiratory impairment from submersion or immersion in liquid.

drug Substance that has some therapeutic effect (such as reducing inflammation, fighting bacteria, or producing euphoria) when given in the appropriate circumstances and in the appropriate dose.

drug abuse Any use of drugs that causes physical, psychological, economic, legal, or social harm to the user or others affected by the user's behaviour.

drug addiction A chronic disorder characterized by the compulsive use of a substance that results in physical, psychological, or social harm to the user who continues to use the substance despite the harm.

drug reconstitution Injecting sterile water or saline from one vial into another vial containing a powdered form of the drug.

ductus arteriosus A duct that is present before birth that connects the pulmonary artery to the aorta in order to move unoxygenated blood back to the placenta.

ductus venosus A duct that is present before birth that connects the placenta to the heart in order to move oxygenated blood to the fetus.

due process A right to a fair procedure for a legal action against a person or agency; has two components: *Notice* and *Opportunity to be Heard*.

due regard Driving with awareness and responsibility for other drivers on the roadways when operating an ambulance in the emergency mode.

duodenum The first part of the small intestine.

duplex Radio system using more than one frequency to permit simultaneous transmission and reception.

dura mater The outermost layer of the three meninges that enclose the brain and spinal cord; it is the toughest meningeal layer.

duration of action How long the medication concentration can be expected to remain above the minimum level needed to provide the intended action.

duty Legal obligation of public and certain other ambulance services to respond to a call for help in their jurisdiction.

dysconjugate gaze Paralysis of gaze or lack of coordination between the movements of the two eyes.

dysmenorrhea Painful menstruation.

dysphagia Difficulty in swallowing.

dysphonia Difficulty speaking.

dysplasia An alteration in the size, shape, and organization of cells.

dyspnea Any difficulty in respiratory rate, regularity, or effort.

dystonia Contractions of the body into a bizarre position.

early adults Persons who are 19 to 40 years of age.

ecchymosis Localized bruising or blood collection within or under the skin.

echolalia Meaningless echoing of the interviewer's words by the patient.

ecstasy A drug officially named methylenedioxymethamphetamine (MDMA) that is sometimes used to facilitate date rape; a methamphetamine derivative with hallucinogenic properties; street names include XTC, Adam, X, lover's speed, and clarity.

ectopic pregnancy A pregnancy in which the ovum implants somewhere other than the uterine endometrium.

edema A condition in which excess fluid accumulates in tissues, manifested by swelling.

efferent arteriole The structure in the kidney where blood drains from the glomerulus.

efferent nerves The nerves that carry messages from the brain to the muscles and all other organs of the body.

ejection fraction The portion of the blood ejected from the ventricle during systole.

elastin A protein that gives the skin its elasticity.

electrical alternans An ECG pattern in which the QRS vector changes with each heart beat. This pattern is pathognomonic for cardiac tamponade.

electrical conduction system In the heart, the specialized cardiac tissue that initiates and conducts electric impulses. The system includes the SA node, internodal atrial conduction pathways, atrioventricular junction, atrioventricular node, bundle of His, and the Purkinje network.

electrical energy The energy delivered in the form of high voltage.

electrolytes Charged atoms or compounds that result from the loss or gain of an electron. These are ions that the body uses to perform certain critical metabolic functions.

elixir A syrup with alcohol and flavouring added.

embryo The fetus in the earliest stages after fertilization.

emergence phenomenon Nightmares associated with the use of ketamine.

emergency medical dispatch First aid instructions given by specially trained dispatchers to callers over the telephone while an ambulance is en route to the call.

emergency medical dispatcher (EMD) A person who receives information and relays that information in an organized manner during the emergency.

emergency medical services (EMS) A health care system designed to bring immediate on-scene prehospital care to those in need along with transport to a definitive medical care facility.

Emergency Response Guidebook (ERG) A hazardous materials reference that provides valuable information about hazardous materials, isolation distances, etc; should be carried on every emergency response unit, and every paramedic should know how to use it.

emotional or intellectual impairment Illnesses that cause a person's emotions to become out of control.

emphysema Infiltration of any tissue by air or gas; a chronic obstructive pulmonary disease characterized by distension of the alveoli and destructive changes in the lung parenchyma.

emulsion A preparation of one liquid (usually an oil) distributed in small globules in another liquid (usually water).

encoded A message is put into a code before it is transmitted.

endocardium The thin membrane lining the inside of the heart.

endocrine glands Glands that secrete or release chemicals that are used inside the body. Endocrine glands lack ducts and release hormones directly into the surrounding tissue and blood.

endocrine hormones Hormones that are carried to their target or cell group in the bloodstream.

endometriomas Ovarian cysts formed from endometrial tissue.

endometriosis A condition in which endometrial tissue grows outside the uterus.

endometritis An inflammation of the endometrium that often is associated with a bacterial infection.

endometrium The innermost layer of tissue in the uterus.

endoscopy The insertion of a flexible tube into the esophagus with the intent of visualizing and repairing damage or disease.

endosteum The inner lining of a hollow bone.

endothelial cells Specific types of epithelial cells that serve the function of lining the blood vessels.

endotoxin A toxin released by some bacteria when they die.

endotracheal (ET) tube Tube that is inserted into the trachea; equipped with a distal cuff, proximal inflation port, a 15/22-mm adapter, and cm markings on the side.

endotracheal intubation Passing an endotracheal (ET) tube through the glottic opening and sealing the tube with a cuff inflated against the tracheal wall.

end-tidal carbon dioxide The numeric percentage of carbon dioxide contained in the last few millilitres of the patient's exhaled air.

end-tidal carbon dioxide (ETCO₂) detectors Device that detects the presence of carbon dioxide in exhaled air.

enhanced 9-1-1 system An emergency call-in system in which additional information such as the phone number and location of the caller is recorded automatically through sophisticated telephone technology and the dispatcher need only confirm the information on the screen.

enteral route A route of medication administration that involves the medication passing through a portion of the gastrointestinal tract.

enterococcus A common, normal organism of the GI tract, urinary tract, and genitourinary tract, and which may become resistant to vancomycin.

entrapment A condition in which a patient is trapped by debris, soil, or other material and is unable to extricate himself or herself.

entry wound The point at which a penetrating object enters the body.

environmental emergencies Medical conditions caused or exacerbated by the weather, terrain, or unique atmospheric conditions such as high altitude or underwater.

eosinophils Cells that make up approximately 1% to 3% of the leukocytes, which play a major role in allergic reactions and bronchoconstriction in an asthma attack.

epicardium The thin membrane lining the outside of the heart.

epidermis The outermost layer of the skin.

epidural hematoma An accumulation of blood between the skull and dura.

epigastric The right upper region of the abdomen directly inferior to the xyphoid process and superior to the umbilicus.

epiglottis Leaf-shaped cartilaginous structure that closes over the trachea during swallowing.

epiglottitis Inflammation of the epiglottis.

epinephrine Hormone produced by the adrenal medulla that plays a vital role in the function of the sympathetic nervous system.

epiphyseal plate The growth plate of a bone; a major site of bone development during childhood.

epiphyses The ends of a long bone.

episiotomy An incision in the perineal skin made to prevent tearing during childbirth.

epithelialization The formation of fresh epithelial tissue to heal a wound.

epithelium Type of tissue that covers all external surfaces of the body.

Erb palsy Lack of movement at the shoulder due to nerve injury resulting from the stretching of the cervical nerve roots (C5 and C6 most commonly) during delivery of the baby's head during birth. The effect is usually transient, but can be permanent.

erythema Reddening of the skin.

erythrocytes Red blood cells.

escharotomy A surgical cut through the eschar or leathery covering of a burn injury to allow for swelling and minimize the potential for development of compartment syndrome in a circumferentially burned limb or the thorax.

esophageal detector device (EDD) Bulb or syringe that is attached to the proximal end of the ET tube; a device used to confirm proper ET tube placement.

estrogen One of the three major female hormones. At puberty, estrogen brings about the secondary sex characteristics.

ethical A behaviour expected by an individual or group following a set of rules.

ethics A set of values in society that differentiates right from wrong.

etiology The cause of a disease process.

etomidate A nonnarcotic, nonbarbiturate hypnotic-sedative drug; also called Amidate.

eustress A type of stress that motivates an individual to achieve.

evaluation Collection of the methods, skills, and activities necessary to determine whether a service or program is needed, likely to be used, conducted as planned, and actually helps people.

evapouration The conversion of a liquid to a gas.

evisceration Displacement of an organ outside the body.

excretion The elimination of toxic or inactive metabolites from the body. This is primarily done by the kidneys, intestines, lungs, and assorted glands.

exertional heat stroke A serious type of heat stroke usually affecting young and fit people exercising in hot and humid conditions.

exertional hyponatremia A condition due to prolonged exertion in hot environments coupled with excessive hypotonic fluid intake that leads to nausea, vomiting, and, in severe cases, mental status changes and seizures.

exhalation Passive movement of air out of the lungs; also called expiration.

exit wound The point at which a penetrating object leaves the body, which may or may not be in a straight line from the entry wound.

exocrine glands Glands that excrete chemicals for elimination.

exocrine hormones Hormones that are secreted through ducts into an organ or onto epithelial surfaces.

exopthalmos Protrusion of the eyes from the normal position within the socket.

exotoxin A toxin that is secreted by living cells to aid in the death and digestion of other cells.

experimental research Describes a new product, skill, or idea that is undergoing research and will be trialed, with the effects evaluated.

expiration Passive movement of air out of the lungs; also called exhalation.

expiratory reserve volume The amount of air that you can exhale following a normal exhalation; average volume is about 1,200 ml.

expressed consent A type of informed consent that occurs when the patient does something, either through words or by taking some sort of action, that demonstrates permission to provide care.

expressive aphasia Damage to or loss of the ability to speak.

external auditory canal The area in which sound waves are received from the auricle (pinna) before they travel to the eardrum; also called the ear canal.

external ear One of three anatomical parts of the ear; it contains the pinna, the ear canal, and the external portion of the tympanic membrane.

external jugular (EJ) vein Large neck vein that is lateral to the carotid artery.

external os The junction where the uterus opens into the vagina.

external respiration The exchange of gases between the lungs and the blood cells in the pulmonary capillaries; also called pulmonary respiration.

extracellular fluid (ECF) The water outside the cells; accounts for 15% of body weight.

extract A concentrated preparation of a drug made by putting the drug into solution (in alcohol or water) and evaporating off the excess solvent to a prescribed standard.

extrication officer In incident command, the person appointed to determine the type of equipment and resources needed for a situation involving extrication or special rescue; also called the rescue officer.

extubation The process of removing the tube from an intubated patient.

eyelash reflex Contraction of the patient's lower eyelid when it is gently stroked; fairly reliable indicator of the presence or absence of an intact gag reflex.

EZ-IO A hand-held, battery-powered driver to which a special IO needle is attached; used for insertion of the IO needle into the proximal tibia of children and adults.

facet joint The joint on which each vertebra articulates with adjacent vertebrae.

facial nerve The seventh cranial nerve; supplies motor activity to all muscles of facial expression, the sense of taste, and anterior two thirds of the tongue and cutaneous sensation to the external ear, tongue, and palate.

facilitation An interviewing technique in which the interviewer uses noncommittal words and gestures to encourage the patient to proceed.

Fahrenheit scale A scale for measuring temperature in which water freezes at 32° and boils at 212°.

fallopian tubes The vehicles of transportation of the ova from the ovaries to the uterus; also called oviducts.

false imprisonment The intentional and unjustified detention of a person against his or her will.

fascia The fibrelike connective tissue that covers arteries, veins, tendons, and ligaments.

fasciculations Characterized by brief, uncoordinated twitching of small muscle groups in the face, neck, trunk, and extremities; caused by the administration of depolarizing neuromuscular blocking agents (eg, succinylcholine).

fasciotomy A surgical procedure that cuts away fascia to relieve pressure.

FAST1® A sternal IO device used in adults; stands for First Access for Shock and Trauma.

fatigue fractures Fractures that result from multiple compressive loads.

fear Also sometimes referred to as a phobia, this is an anxious feeling, usually about specific things or situations.

feculent Smelling of feces.

feedback inhibition Negative feedback resulting in the decrease of an action in the body.

femoral artery The main artery supplying the thigh and leg.

femoral shaft fractures A break in the diaphysis of the femur.

femur The proximal bone of the leg that extends from the pelvis to the knee.

fetus The developing, unborn infant inside the uterus.

fibrin A whitish, filamentous protein formed by the action of thrombin on fibrinogen. Fibrin is the protein that polymerizes (bonds) to form the fibrous component of a blood clot.

fibrinolysis cascade The breakdown of fibrin in blood clots, and the prevention of the polymerization of fibrin into new clots.

fibrinolytic agents The only medications available to dissolve blood clots after they have already formed; the drugs promote the digestion of fibrin.

fibrinolytic system The mechanism by which fibrin undergoes dissolution owing to the action of enzymes; clots are destroyed.

fibrinolytic therapy The therapy that uses medications that act to dissolve blood clots.

fibrous joints The joints that contain dense fibrous tissue and allow for no motion.

fibula The smaller of the two bones of the lower leg.

fight-or-flight syndrome A physiologic response to a profound stressor that helps one deal with the situation at hand; features increased sympathetic tone and resulting in dilation of the pupils, increased heart rate, dilation of the bronchi, mobilization of glucose, shunting of blood away from the gastrointestinal tract and cerebrum, and increased blood flow to the skeletal muscles.

finance officer In incident command, the position in an incident responsible for accounting of all expenditures.

first-degree heart block A partial disruption of the conduction of the depolarizing impulse from the atria to the ventricles, causing prolongation of the P-R interval.

first stage of labour The stage of labour that begins with the onset of regular labour pains—crampy abdominal pains—during which the uterus contracts and the cervix effaces.

flail chest An injury that involves two or more adjacent ribs fractured in two or more places, allowing the segment between the fractures to move independently of the rest of the thoracic cage.

flame burn A thermal burn caused by flames touching the skin.

flash burn An electrothermal injury caused by arcing of electric current.

flash chamber The area of an IV cannula that fills with blood to help indicate when a vein is cannulated.

flash point The temperature at which a vapour can be ignited by a spark.

flat Used to describe behaviour in which the patient doesn't seem to feel much of anything at all.

flat bones Bones that are thin and broad, such as the scapula.

flexion injury A type of injury that results from forward movement of the head, typically as the result of rapid deceleration, such as in a car crash, or with a direct blow to the occiput.

flight of ideas Accelerated thinking in which the mind skips very rapidly from one thought to the next.

flow-restricted, oxygen-powered ventilation device (FROPVD) Also referred to as a manually triggered ventilator or demand valve. Can be used to ventilate apneic or to administer supplemental oxygen to spontaneously breathing patients.

fluid extract A concentrated form of a drug prepared by dissolving the crude drug in the fluid in which it is most readily soluble.

focal brain injury A specific, grossly observable brain injury.

focused history and physical examination The part of the assessment process in which the patient's major complaints or any problems that are immediately evident are further and more specifically evaluated.

focused physical examination The examination done on a responsive medical patient, driven by the information gathered during the initial assessment and the history-taking phase.

follicle-stimulating hormone (FSH) A hormone produced by the anterior pituitary gland which is important in the menstrual cycle.

fomite An inanimate object contaminated with microorganisms that serves as a means of transmitting an illness.

fontanelles The soft spots in the skull of a newborn and infant where the sutures of the skull have not yet grown together.

footling breech A delivery in which one or both feet dangle through the vaginal opening.

foramen magnum A large opening at the base of the skull through which the spinal cord exits the brain.

foramen ovale An opening in the septum of the heart before birth, and which closes after birth.

foramina Small natural openings, perforations, or orifices, such as in the bones of the cranial vault; plural of foramen.

Fowler's position A sitting position with the head elevated to 90° (sitting straight upright).

foxglove A plant that contains cardiac glycosides used in making digoxin; ingestion of leaves causes nausea, vomiting, diarrhea, abdominal cramps, hyperkalemia, and a variety of arrhythmias.

fractile response time A fraction (not average) of all emergency responses for the purpose of setting standards in response times.

fraction of inspired oxygen (F_{IO_2}) The percentage of oxygen in inhaled air.

fracture A break or rupture in the bone.

free-flow oxygen Oxygen administered via oxygen tube and a cupped hand on patient's face.

freelancing When individual units or different organizations make independent and often inefficient decisions about the next appropriate action.

free radicals Molecules that are missing one electron in their outer shell.

frequency In radio communications, the number of cycles per second of a signal, inversely related to the wavelength.

frontal lobe The portion of the brain that is important in voluntary motor actions and personality traits.

frostbite Localized damage to tissues resulting from prolonged exposure to extreme cold.

frostnip   Early frostbite, characterized by numbness and pallor without significant tissue damage.

fsw   Abbreviation for feet of seawater, an indirect measure of pressure under water.

full-thickness burn   A burn that extends through the epidermis and dermis into the subcutaneous tissues beneath; previously called a third-degree burn.

functional residual capacity   The amount of air that can be forced from the lungs in a single exhalation.

fundus   The dome-shaped top of the uterus.

fungus (plural: fungi)   A small organism that can grow rapidly in the presence of nutrients and organic material, and can cause infection related to contact with decaying organic matter or from airborne spores in the environment such as moulds.

futile intervention   A medical intervention that will not work or will not benefit the patient in any way.

G agents   Early nerve agents that were developed by German scientists in the period after WWI and into WWII. There are three such agents: sarin, soman, and tabun.

gag reflex   Automatic reaction when something touches an area deep in the oral cavity; helps protect the lower airway from aspiration.

gait   Walking pattern.

galea aponeurotica   Tough, tendinous layer of the scalp.

gamma (x-rays)   Type of energy that is emitted from a strong radiological source that is far faster and stronger than alpha and beta rays. These rays easily penetrate through the human body and require either several centimetres of lead or concrete to prevent penetration.

gamma-hydroxybutrate (GHB)   A drug used to facilitate date rape; is colourless with a salty taste disguised when mixed with a drink; street names include Georgia home boy, grievous bodily harm, easy lay, G, scoop, liquid X, soap, and salty water.

ganglia   Groupings of nerve cell bodies located in the peripheral nervous system.

gangrene   An infection commonly caused by *C perfringens*. The result is tissue destruction and gas production that may lead to death.

gastric distension   Inflation of the patient's stomach with air.

gastric tubes   Tubes that are commonly inserted in patients in the prehospital setting to decompress the stomach; can also be used to administer certain enteral medications.

gastroenteritis   A term that comprises many types of infections and irritations of the gastrointestinal tract; symptoms include nausea and vomiting, fever, abdominal cramps, and diarrhea.

gastrointestinal exposure   Exposure to a hazardous material through intentional or unintentional swallowing of the substance.

gauge   The internal diameter of an IV cannula or needle.

general adaptation syndrome   A three-stage description of the body's short-term and long-term reactions to stress.

general impression   The overall initial impression that determines the priority for patient care; based on the patient's surroundings, the mechanism of injury, signs and symptoms, and the chief complaint.

generalized anxiety disorder (GAD)   A disorder in which a person worries about everything for no particular reason, or their worrying is unproductive and they can't decide what to do about an upcoming situation.

generalized seizures   The seizures characterized by manifestations that indicate involvement of both cerebral hemispheres.

generic drug   A medication that is not patented.

generic name   A general name for a drug that is not manufacturer-specific; usually the name given to the drug by the company that first manufactures it.

genital herpes   An infection of the genitals, buttocks, or anal area caused by herpes simplex virus (HSV), which may cause sores of the genitals, mouth, or lips.

genital warts   Warts caused by the human papillomavirus (HPV), a sexually transmitted disease; also called condylomata acuminata or venereal warts.

geriatrics   The assessment and treatment of disease in someone 65 years or older.

gestation   Period of time from conception to birth. For humans, the full period is normally 9 months.

gestational diabetes   Diabetes that develops during pregnancy in women who did not have diabetes before pregnancy.

gestational hypertension   High blood pressure that develops after the 20th week of pregnancy, in women with previously normal blood pressures, and resolves spontaneously in the postpartum period.

gestational period   The time that it takes for the infant to develop in utero, normally 40 weeks.

glands   Cells or organs that selectively remove, concentrate, or alter materials in the blood and then secrete them back into the body.

Glasgow Coma Scale (GCS)   An evaluation tool used to determine level of consciousness, which evaluates and assigns point values (scores) for eye opening, verbal response, and motor response, which are then totaled; effective in helping predict patient outcomes.

glenoid fossa   Socket in the scapula in which the head of the humerus rotates.

global aphasia   Damage to or loss of both the ability to speak and the ability to understand speech.

globe   The eyeball.

glomerular (Bowman's) capsule   A double-layered cup with the inner layer infiltrating and surrounding the capillaries of the glomerulus.

glomerular filtration   The first step in the formation of urine; calculated to determine renal function.

glomerular filtration rate (GFR)   The rate at which blood is filtered through the glomerula.

glomerulus   A tuft of capillaries located in the kidney that serve as the main filter for the blood in the kidney.

glossopharyngeal nerve   Ninth cranial nerve; supplies motor fibres to the pharyngeal muscle, providing taste sensation to the posterior portion of the tongue, and carrying parasympathetic fibres to the parotid gland.

glottis   The space in between the vocal cords that is the narrowest portion of the adult's airway; also called the glottic opening.

glucagon   Hormone produced by the pancreas that is vital to the control of the body's metabolism and blood sugar level. Glucagon stimulates the breakdown of glycogen to glucose.

GnRF   A chemical released by the hypothalamus that stimulates the release of follicle-stimulating hormone.

goals   The end points toward which intervention efforts are directed. A statement of changes sought in an injury problem, stated in broad terms.

goblet cells   Cells that produce a protective mucous lining.

gonads   The reproductive glands; the main source of sex hormones.

gonorrhea   A sexually transmitted disease which results in infection caused by the gonococcal bacteria, *Neisseria gonorrhea*. Signs and symptoms include pus-containing discharge from the urethra and painful urination in males, and signs and symptoms of an acute abdomen in females.

Good Samaritan law   A statute providing limited immunity from liability to persons responding voluntarily and in good faith to the aid of an injured person outside the hospital.

gout   A painful disorder characterized by the crystallization of uric acid within a joint.

granulocytes   Cells that contain granules.

gravid   The number of all pregnancies a woman has had, including those not necessarily carried to term.

gravidity   A term used to refer to a uterus that contains a pregnancy, whatever the outcome.

gravity   The acceleration of a body by the attraction of the earth's gravitational force, normally 9.8 m/sec^2.

Greenfield filter   A mesh filter placed in the inferior vena cava to catch blood clots in patients who are at high risk of pulmonary embolus.

greenstick fracture   A type of fracture occurring most frequently in children in which there is incomplete breakage of the bone.

gross negligence   Negligence that is willful, wanton, intentional, or reckless; a serious departure from the accepted standards.

ground substance   Material between cells.

group B streptococcus (GBS) A bacteria that lives in the genitourinary and gastrointestinal tracts of normal healthy individuals, but which can cause life-threatening infections in newborn babies.

growth plates Structures located on either end of an infant's bone, which aid in lengthening bones as the child grows.

grunting A short, low-pitched sound at the end of exhalation, present in children with moderate to severe hypoxia; reflects poor gas exchange because of fluid in the lower airways and air sacs.

gtt A unit of measure that indicates drops.

guarding Contraction of the abdominal muscles in patients.

Guillain-Barré syndrome A disease of unknown etiology that causes paralysis that progresses from the feet to the head (ascending paralysis). If the paralysis reaches the diaphragm, the patient may require respiratory support.

gum elastic bougie Also called the Eschmann stylet; a flexible device that is inserted in between the glottis under direct laryngoscopy. The ET tube is then threaded over the device, facilitating its entry into the trachea.

gut-associated lymphoid tissue (GALT) The lymphoid tissue that lies under the inner lining of the esophagus and intestines.

habituation The situation in which there is a physical tolerance and psychological dependence on a drug or drugs.

Haddon matrix A framework developed by William Haddon, Jr, MD as a method to generate ideas about injury prevention that address the host, agent, and environment and their impact in the pre-event, event, and post-event phases of the injury process.

hallucination A sense perception not founded on objective reality; a false perception.

hallucinogen An agent that produces false perceptions in any one of the five senses.

hantavirus Also known as hemorrhagic fever with renal syndrome, this is a type of virus found in wild rodents, which can also cause disease in humans, characterized by fever, headache, abdominal pain, loss of appetite, and vomiting.

hapten A substance that normally does not stimulate an immune response but can be combined with an antigen and at a later point initiate an antibody response.

hard palate The bony anterior part of the palate, which forms the roof of the mouth.

hasty rope slide Self-escape procedure when there is no other means of egress.

hazardous material Any substance that is toxic, poisonous, radioactive, flammable, or explosive and causes injury or death with exposure.

head bobbing A sign of increased work of breathing in which the head lifts and tilts back during inspiration, then moves forward during expiration.

head injury A traumatic insult to the head that may result in injury to soft tissue, bony structures, or the brain.

head tilt–chin lift maneuver Manual airway maneuver that involves tilting the head back while lifting up on the chin; used to open the airway of a semiconscious or unconscious nontrauma patient.

health care professional A person who follows specific professional attributes that are outlined in this profession.

heart rate (HR) The number of heart contractions per minute.

heat cramps Acute and involuntary muscle pains, usually in the lower extremities, the abdomen, or both, that occur because of profuse sweating and subsequent sodium losses in sweat.

heat exhaustion A clinical syndrome characterized by volume depletion and heat stress that is thought to be a milder form of heat illness and on a continuum leading to heat stroke.

heat illness The increase in core body temperature due to inadequate thermolysis.

heat stroke The least common and most deadly heat illness, caused by a severe disturbance in thermoregulation, usually characterized by a core temperature of more than 40°C and altered mental status.

heat syncope An orthostatic or near-syncopal episode that typically occurs in nonacclimated individuals who may be under heat stress.

Heimlich maneuver Abdominal thrusts performed to relieve a foreign body airway obstruction.

helminths Invertebrates with long, flexible, rounded, or flattened bodies, commonly called worms; a type of parasite.

helper T cells A type of T lymphocyte that is involved in both cell-mediated and antibody-mediated immune responses. It secretes cytokines that stimulate the B cells and other T cells.

hematemesis Vomit with blood. Can either be like coffee grounds in appearance, indicating partially digested blood, or bright red blood indicating current active bleeding.

hematochezia Blood with the stool that is separate. Caused by lower GI bleeds.

hematocrit The percentage of RBCs in total blood volume.

hematoma A localized collection of blood in the soft tissues as a result of injury or a broken blood vessel.

hematopoiesis The generation of blood cells.

hematopoietic system The system that includes all blood components and the organs involved in their development and production.

hematuria The presence of blood in the urine.

hemiparesis Weakness of one side of the body.

hemiplegia Paralysis of one side of the body.

hemochromatosis An inherited disease in which the body absorbs more iron than it needs and stores it in the liver, kidneys, and pancreas.

hemoglobin An iron-containing protein within red blood cells that has the ability to combine with oxygen.

hemolytic anemia A disease characterized by increased destruction of the red blood cells. It can occur from an Rh factor reaction, exposure to chemicals, or a disorder of the immune system.

hemolytic disorder A disorder relating to the breakdown of RBCs.

hemoperitoneum The presence of extravasated blood in the peritoneal cavity.

hemophilia A bleeding disorder that is primarily hereditary, in which clotting does not occur or occurs insufficiently.

hemopneumothorax A collection of blood and air in the pleural cavity.

hemoptysis Coughing up blood.

hemorrhage Profuse bleeding.

hemorrhagic One of the two main types of stroke; occurs as a result of bleeding inside the brain.

hemorrhagic cyst A blood-filled sac that forms when a blood vessel bursts in a cyst wall and the blood fills the sac.

hemostasis The body's natural blood-clotting mechanism.

hemothorax The collection of blood within the normally closed pleural space.

Henry's law The amount of gas dissolved in a liquid is directly proportional to the partial pressure of the gas above the liquid.

Hering-Breuer reflex The nervous system mechanism that terminates inhalation and prevents lung overexpansion.

hernia Protrusion of any organ through an opening into a body cavity where it does not belong.

herniation Process in which tissue is forced out of its normal position, such as when the brain is forced from the cranial vault, either through the foramen magnum or over the tentorium.

hertz (Hz) Unit of frequency equal to 1 cycle per second.

Hi-Ox mask A mask that allows the patient to inhale oxygen from a reservoir bag via a one-way valve and exhale breath through another one-way valve through a high-efficiency filter before exiting the mask.

high-altitude cerebral edema (HACE) An altitude illness in which there is a change in mental status and/or ataxia in a person with AMS or the presence of mental status changes and ataxia in a person without AMS.

high-altitude pulmonary edema (HAPE) An altitude illness characterized by dyspnea at rest, cough, severe weakness, and drowsiness that may eventually lead to central cyanosis, audible rales or wheezing, tachypnea, and tachycardia.

high-angle operations A rope rescue operation where the angle of the slope is greater than 45°; rescuers depend on life safety rope rather than a fixed support surface such as the ground.

hilum Point of entry of all of the blood vessels and the bronchi into each lung.

hilum A cleft where the ureters, renal blood vessels, lymphatic vessels, and nerves enter and leave the kidney.

histamine A chemical found in mast cells that, when released, causes vasodilation, capillary leaking, and bronchiole constriction.

history of the present illness Information about the chief complaint, obtained using the OPQRST mnemonic.

homeostasis A tendency to constancy or stability in the body's internal environment.

hormones Proteins formed in specialized organs or glands and carried to another organ or group of cells in the same organism. Hormones regulate many body functions, including metabolism, growth, and temperature.

hospice An organization that provides end-of-life care to patients with terminal illnesses and their families.

host resistance One's ability to fight off infection.

hot zone The area immediately surrounding an incident site that is directly dangerous to life and health. All personnel working in the hot zone must wear complete and appropriate protective clothing and equipment. Entry requires approval by the IC or a designated sector officer. Complete backup, rescue, and decontamination teams must be in place at the perimetre before operations begin.

human chorionic gonadotropin hormone A hormone that sends signals to the corpus luteum that pregnancy has initiated.

human immunodeficiency virus (HIV) AIDS (acquired immunodeficiency syndrome) is caused by HIV, which kills or damages the cells in the body's immune system so that the body is unable to fight infections and certain cancers.

humerus The bone of the upper arm.

humoural immunity The use of antibodies dissolved in the plasma and lymph to destroy foreign substances.

hydrocarbons Compounds made up principally of hydrogen and carbon atoms mostly obtained from the distillation of petroleum.

hydrocephalus The increased accumulation of cerebrospinal fluid within the ventricles of the brain.

hymen A membrane that protects the vaginal orifice before first intercourse.

hyoid bone A small, horseshoe-shaped bone to which the jaw, tongue, epiglottis, and thyroid cartilage attach.

hypercalcemia A condition in which calcium levels are elevated.

hypercarbia Increased carbon dioxide levels in the bloodstream.

hypercholesterolemia An elevated blood cholesterol level.

hyperemesis gravidarum A condition of persistent nausea and vomiting during pregnancy.

hyperesthesia Hyperacute pain to touch.

hyperextension Extension of a limb of other body part beyond its usual range of motion.

hyperglycemia Abnormally high blood glucose level.

hyperkalemia An increased level of potassium in the blood.

hypermagnesemia An increased serum magnesium level.

hypernatremia A blood serum sodium level greater than 148 mmol/l and a serum osmolarity greater than 295 mOsm/kg.

hyperosmolar hyperglycemic nonketotic coma (HHNC), also known as hyperosmolar nonketotic coma (HONK), is a metabolic derangement that occurs principally in patients with type 2 diabetes. The condition is characterized by hyperglycemia, hyperosmolarity, and an absence of significant ketosis.

hyperosmolar nonketotic coma (HONK), also known as hyperosmolar hyperglycemic nonketotic coma (HHNC), is a metabolic derangement that occurs principally in patients with type 2 diabetes. The condition is characterized by hyperglycemia, hyperosmolarity, and an absence of significant ketosis.

hyperperistalsis Increased movement within the bowel.

hyperphosphatemia An increased level of phosphate in the blood.

hyperplasia An increase in the actual number of cells in an organ or tissue, usually resulting in an increase in size of the organ or tissue.

hyperpyrexia A very high body temperature.

hypersensitivity Occurs when a patient reacts with exaggerated or inappropriate allergic symptoms after coming into contact with a substance the body perceives as harmful.

hypertension High blood pressure, usually a diastolic pressure greater than 90 mm Hg.

hyperthermia Unusually elevated body temperature.

hypertonic solution A solution that has a greater concentration of sodium than does the cell; the increased osmotic pressure can draw water out of the cell and cause it to collapse.

hypertrophic scar An abnormal scar with excess collagen that does not extend over the wound margins.

hypertrophy An increase in the size of the cells due to synthesis of more subcellular components, leading to an increase in tissue and organ size.

hyperventilation Occurs when CO_2 elimination exceeds CO_2 production.

hyphema Bleeding into the anterior chamber of the eye; results from direct ocular trauma.

hypnosis Altered consciousness often caused by hypnotic drugs, which are used to induce sleep.

hypocalcemia A low level of calcium in the blood.

hypocarbia Decreased CO_2 content in arterial blood.

hypoglossal nerve Twelfth cranial nerve; provides motor function to the muscles of the tongue and throat.

hypoglycemia A deficiency of glucose in the blood caused by too much insulin or too little glucose.

hypokalemia A low blood serum potassium level.

hypomagnesemia A decreased serum magnesium level.

hyponatremia A blood serum sodium level that is below 135 mmol/l and a serum osmolarity that is less than 280 mOsm/kg.

hypoperfusion A condition that occurs when the level of tissue perfusion decreases below that needed to maintain normal cellular functions.

hypoperistalsis Decreased bowel movement.

hypophosphatemia A decreased blood serum phosphate level.

hypothalamic-pituitary-adrenal (HPA) axis A major part of the neuroendocrine system that controls reactions to stress. It is the mechanism for a set of interactions among glands, hormones, and parts of the midbrain that mediate the general adaptation syndrome.

hypothalamus The most inferior portion of the diencephalon; responsible for control of many body functions, including heart rate, digestion, sexual development, temperature regulation, emotion, hunger, thirst, and regulation of the sleep cycle.

hypothermia Condition in which the core body temperature is significantly below normal.

hypotonia Low or poor muscle tone (floppy).

hypotonic solution A solution that has a lower concentration of sodium than does the cell; the increased osmotic pressure lets water flow into the cell, causing it to swell and possibly burst.

hypoventilate To not move adequate volumes of gas; underventilate.

hypoventilation Occurs when CO_2 production exceeds the body's ability to eliminate it by ventilation.

hypovolemia An abnormal decrease in blood volume or, strictly speaking, an abnormal decrease in the volume of blood plasma.

hypovolemic shock A condition that occurs when the circulating blood volume is inadequate to deliver adequate oxygen and nutrients to the body.

hypoxemia A decrease in arterial oxygen levels.

hypoxia A lack of oxygen to the body's cells and tissues.

hypoxic drive Secondary control of breathing that stimulates breathing based on decreased PaO_2 levels.

hypoxic ischemic encephalopathy Damage to cells in the central nervous system (the brain and spinal cord) from inadequate oxygen.

iatrogenic response An adverse condition inadvertently induced in a patient by the treatment given.

icterus Jaundice; the yellow appearance of the skin and other tissues caused by an accumulation of bile pigments.

ideas of reference The belief that external forms of communication (television, radio, and newspaper) are directed specifically at the individual.

idiopathic Of no known cause.

idiosyncrasy An abnormal (and usually unexplained) reaction by a person to a medication, to which most other people do not react.

ignition temperature The temperature at which a vapour will burst into sustained burning.

ileostomy Surgical procedure to remove large portions of the small intestine.

ilium The broad, uppermost bone of the pelvis.

illicit In relation to drugs, illegal drugs such as marijuana, cocaine, and LSD.

illusion A misinterpretation of sensory stimuli.

immediately dangerous to life and health (IDLH) A phrase that means the atmospheric concentration of any toxic, corrosive, or asphyxiant substance will pose an immediate threat to life, irreversible or delayed adverse effects, or serious interference for a team member attempting to escape from the dangerous atmosphere; a respirator is mandatory. There are three general IDLH atmospheres: toxic, flammable, and oxygen-deficient.

immune response The body's defence reaction to any substance that is recognized as foreign.

immune system The body system that includes all of the structures and processes designed to mount a defence against foreign substances and disease-causing agents.

immunity The body's ability to protect itself from acquiring a disease.

immunity (legal) Legal protection from penalties that could normally be incurred under the law.

immunobiologic medications The medications that include serums, vaccines, and other immunizing agents.

immunodeficiency An abnormal condition in which some part of the body's immune system is inadequate, and consequently resistance to infectious disease is decreased.

immunogen An antigen that activates immune cells to generate an immune response against itself.

immunoglobulins Antibodies secreted by the B cells.

immunosuppressant medications The medications intended to inhibit the body's ability to attack the "foreign" organ or, in the case of autoimmune diseases, the medications that inhibit the body's attack on itself.

impacted fracture A broken bone in which the end of one bone becomes wedged into another bone, as could be the case in a fall from a significant height.

impaled object An object that has caused a puncture wound and remains embedded in the wound.

imperforate hymen A situation in which the hymen completely covers the vaginal orifice.

implementation plan A strategy for carrying out an intervention. Includes goals, objectives, activities, evaluation measures, resource assessment, and time line.

implied consent Assumption on behalf of a person unable to give consent that he or she would have done so.

implosion A bursting inward.

impulse control disorders A condition in which an individual lacks the ability to resist a temptation or can't stop acting on a drive.

inattention Used to describe patients with whom it is difficult to gain their attention or focus.

incidence The frequency with which a disease occurs.

incident command system (ICS) A system implemented to manage disasters and mass- and multiple-casualty incidents in which section chiefs, including finance, logistics, operations, and planning, report to the incident commander.

incident commander (IC) The overall leader of the incident command system to whom commanders or leaders of incident command system divisions report.

incision A wound usually made deliberately, as in surgery; a clean cut, as opposed to a laceration.

incomplete abortion Expulsion of the fetus which results in some products of conception remaining in the uterus.

incomplete fracture A fracture in which the bone does not fully break.

incomplete spinal cord injury Spinal cord injury in which there is some degree of cord-mediated function; initial dysfunction may be temporary and there may be potential for recovery.

incubation Describes the period of time from a person being exposed to a disease to the time when symptoms begin.

incubation period The time period between exposure to an organism and the first symptoms of illness, during which the organism multiplies within the body and starts to produce symptoms.

indications The reasons or conditions for which the medication is given.

indirect injury An injury that results from a force that is applied to one region of the body but leads to an injury in another area.

indirect medical control Medical direction given through a set of protocols, policies, and/or standards.

induced abortion Intentional expulsion of the fetus.

inevitable abortion A spontaneous abortion that cannot be prevented.

infants Persons who are from 1 month to 1 year of age.

infarction Death (necrosis) of a localized area of tissue caused by the cutting off of its blood supply.

infection The abnormal invasion of a host or host tissue by organisms such as bacteria, viruses, or parasites, with or without signs or symptoms of disease.

infectious hepatitis Another name for hepatitis A, an inflammation from a virus that causes mild fatigue, loss of appetite, fever, nausea, abdominal pain, and eventually, jaundice, dark-coloured urine, and whitish stools.

inferential A research format that uses a hypothesis to prove one finding from another.

infiltration The escape of fluid into the surrounding tissue; the result of vein perforation during IV cannulation.

inflammatory response A reaction by tissues of the body to irritation or injury, characterized by pain, swelling, redness, and heat.

influenza The flu, a respiratory infection caused by a variety of viruses. It differs from the common cold in that the flu involves a fever, headache, and extreme exhaustion.

informed consent A patient's voluntary agreement to be treated after being told about the nature of the disease, the risks and benefits of the proposed treatment, alternative treatments, or the choice of no treatment at all.

ingestion Eating or drinking materials for absorption through the gastrointestinal tract.

inhalation Breathing into the lungs; a medication delivery route.

initial assessment The part of the assessment process that helps you identify immediately or potentially life-threatening conditions so that you can initiate lifesaving prehospital care.

initial diagnosis A determination of what a paramedic thinks is the patient's current problem, usually based on the patient history and the chief complaint.

injection When the skin is pierced, and foreign material is deposited into the skin.

injuries Any unintentional or intentional damage to the body resulting from acute exposure to thermal, mechanical, electrical, or chemical energy or from the absence of such essentials as heat or oxygen.

injury risk A potentially hazardous situation that puts people in a position in which they could be harmed.

injury surveillance The ongoing systematic collection, analysis, and interpretation of injury data essential to the planning, implementation, and evaluation of public health practice.

inner ear One of three anatomical parts of the ear; it consists of the cochlea and semicircular canals.

inotropic Affecting the contractility of muscle tissue, especially cardiac muscle.

inspection Looking at the patient, either in general or at a specific area (ie, a patient's overall appearance from the doorway, versus looking specifically at the chest wall for abnormalities/deformities).

inspiration The active process of moving air into the lungs; also called inhalation.

inspiratory reserve volume The amount of air that can be inhaled after a normal inhalation; the amount of air that can be inhaled in addition to the normal tidal volume.

institutional review board (IRB) A group or institution that follows a set of requirements for review that were devised by the US Public Health Service.

insulin Hormone produced by the pancreas that's vital to the control of the body's metabolism and blood sugar level. Insulin causes sugar, fatty acids, and amino acids to be taken up and metabolized by cells.

insulin resistance Condition in which the pancreas produces enough insulin but the body can't effectively utilize it.

integument The skin.

intension tremors Tremors that occur when trying to accomplish a task.

intentional injuries Injuries that are purposefully inflicted by a person on himself or herself or on another person. Examples include suicide or attempted suicide, homicide, rape, assault, domestic maltreatment, elder maltreatment, and child maltreatment.

intercostal nerves Nerves that innervate the external intercostal muscles, the muscles between the ribs.

intercostal retractions Skin sucking in between the ribs, seen when a patient creates increased negative intrathoracic pressure to breathe.

intercostal space The space between two ribs, named according to the number of the rib above it, that contains the intercostal muscles and neurovascular bundle.

interference A direct biochemical interaction between two drugs.

interferon Protein produced by cells in response to viral invasion. Interferon is released into the bloodstream or intercellular fluid to induce healthy cells to manufacture an enzyme that counters the infection.

interleukins Chemical substances that attract white blood cells to the sites of injury and bacterial invasion.

internal mucosa The inner layer of tissue in the fallopian tubes.

internal respiration The exchange of gases between the blood cells and the tissues; also called cellular respiration.

internal shunt Also called an arteriovenous (AV) fistula, this device is an artificial connection between a vein and an artery, usually in the forearm or upper arm.

international terrorism Terrorism that is carried out by those not of the host's country; also known as cross-border terrorism.

internodal pathways The three pathways of the electrical conduction system found in the atria that transmit the impulse from the SA node to the AV node.

interstitial fluid The water bathing the cells; accounts for about 10.5% of body weight;

includes special fluid collections, such as cerebrospinal fluid and intraocular fluid.

interstitial nephritis A chronic inflammation of the interstitial cells surrounding the nephrons.

intertrochanteric fractures Fractures that occur in the region between the lesser and greater trochanters.

interventions Specific prevention measures or activities designed to meet a program objective. Categories include education/behaviour change, enforcement/legislation, engineering/technology, and economic incentives.

interventricular septum A thick wall that separates the right and left ventricles.

intracellular fluid (ICF) The water contained inside the cells; normally accounts for 45% of body weight.

intracerebral hematoma Bleeding within the brain tissue (parenchyma) itself; also referred to as an intraparenchymal hematoma.

intracranial pressure (ICP) The pressure within the cranial vault; normally 0 to 15 mm Hg in adults.

intradermal the layer of the dermis, just beneath the epidermis; a medication delivery route.

intramuscular (IM) route A method of delivering a medication into the muscle of the body. This is accomplished by placing a needle into a muscle space and injecting the medication into the tissue.

intranasal Within the nose.

intraosseous Within the bone.

intraosseous (IO) infusion A technique of administering fluids, blood and blood products, and medications into the intraosseous space of a long bone, usually the proximal tibia.

intraosseous (IO) route A method of delivering a medication into the marrow cavity of a bone. This is accomplished by placing a rigid needle into the marrow cavity and flushing a medication into the space.

intraosseous (IO) space The spongy cancellous bone of the epiphyses and the medullary cavity of the diaphysis, collectively.

intrapulmonary shunting Bypassing of oxygen-poor blood past nonfunctional alveoli.

intrarenal acute renal failure (IARF) A type of acute renal failure due to damage in the kidney itself, often caused by immune-mediated diseases, prerenal ARF, toxins, heavy metals, some medications, or some organic compounds.

intravascular fluid Plasma; the water within the blood vessels, which carries red blood cells, white blood cells, and vital nutrients; normally accounts for about 4.5% of body weight.

intravenous Within a vein.

intravenous (IV) therapy Cannulation of a vein with an IV cannula to access the patient's vascular system.

intussusception An event where one part of the intestine folds into another part of the intestines leads to a blockage.

iodine An essential element in the diet and an important component of thyroxine. Without the proper level of iodine intake, thyroxine can't be produced, and physical and mental growth are diminished.

ionic concentration The amount of charged particles found in a particular area.

ionizing radiation Energy that is emitted in the form of rays, or particles.

ions Charged atoms or compounds that result from the loss or gain of an electron.

iris The coloured portion of the eye.

iron deficiency anemia The most common type of anemia in which iron stores are low or lacking and the serum iron concentration is low.

irregular bones Bones with unique shapes that allow them to perform a specific function and that do not fit into the other categories based on shape.

irreversible shock The final stage of shock, resulting in death.

ischemia Tissue anoxia from diminished blood flow to tissue, usually caused by narrowing or occlusion of the artery.

ischemic One of the two main types of stroke; occurs when blood flow to a particular part of the brain is cut off by a blockage (eg, a clot) inside a blood vessel.

ischium The lowermost dorsal bone of the pelvis.

islets of Langerhans A specialized group of cells in the pancreas where insulin and glucagon are produced.

isoelectric When referring to a wave, the wave is neither positive nor negative.

isoelectric line The baseline of the ECG.

isoimmunity Formation of antibodies or T cells that are directed against antigens or another person's cells.

isotonic crystalloids Intravenous solutions that do not cause a fluid shift into or out of the cell; examples include normal saline and lactated Ringer's solutions.

isotonic solution A solution that has the same concentration of sodium as does the cell. In this case, water does not shift, and no change in cell shape occurs.

Jacksonian March The wave-like movement of a seizure from a point of focus to other areas of the brain.

jaundice The presence of excessive bile pigments in the bloodstream that give the skin, mucous membranes, and eyes a distinct yellow colour; jaundice is often associated with liver disease.

jaw-thrust maneuver Manual airway maneuver that involves stabilizing the patient's head and thrusting the jaw forward; the preferred method of opening the airway of a semiconscious or unconscious trauma patient.

jaw-thrust maneuver with head tilt Manual airway maneuver that involves thrusting the jaw forward while tilting back on the head.

joint The point at which two or more bones articulate, or come together.

joint capsule   A saclike envelope that encloses the cavity of a synovial joint.

joint information centre (JIC)   An area designated by the incident commander, or a designee, in which public information officers from multiple agencies disseminate information about the incident.

jugular vein distension (JVD)   A prominence of the jugular veins due to increased volume or increased pressure within the central venous system or the thoracic cavity.

JumpSTART triage   A sorting system for pediatric patients less than 8 years old or weighing less than 45 kg. There is a minor adaptation for infants since they cannot ambulate on their own.

junctional rhythm   An arrhythmia arising from ectopic foci in the area of the atrioventricular junction; often shows an absence of the P wave, a short P-R interval, or a P wave appearing after the QRS complex.

juxtaglomerular apparatus   A structure formed at the site where the efferent arteriole and distal convoluted tubule meet.

Kehr's sign   Left shoulder pain that may indicate a ruptured spleen.

keloid scar   An abnormal scar commonly found in people with darkly pigmented skin. It extends over the wound margins.

ketamine   A drug with sedative, analgesic, and hypnotic properties; created in the laboratory from phencyclidine (PCP).

ketamine hydrochloride   A drug used to facilitate date rape but that is predominantly marketed in Canada as a veterinary anesthetic and is a phencyclidine hydrochloride derivative; street names include special K, vitamin K, cat Valium, and Fort Dodge.

kidneys   Solid, bean-shaped organs located in the retroperitoneal space that filter blood and excrete body wastes in the form of urine.

kidney stones   Solid crystalline masses formed in the kidney, resulting from an excess of insoluble salts or uric acid crystallizing in the urine; may become trapped anywhere along the urinary tract.

kinetic energy   The energy associated with bodies in motion, expressed mathematically as half the mass times the square of the velocity.

kinetics   The study of the relationship among speed, mass, vector direction, and physical injury.

King airway   A single-lumen airway device that serves as an alternative to ventilation with a bag-valve-mask or for procedures where tracheal intubation is not possible.

kinin system   A general term for a group of polypeptides that mediate inflammatory responses by stimulating visceral smooth muscle and relaxing vascular smooth muscle to produce vasodilation.

Klumpke paralysis   An injury of childbirth affecting the spinal nerves C7, C8, and T1 of the brachial plexus. It can be contrasted to Erb palsy, which affects C5 and C6.

Korotkoff sounds   Sounds related to blood pressure that are heard by stethoscope.

Kussmaul respirations   Deep, gasping respirations; common in diabetic coma (ketoacidosis).

kyphosis   Outward curve of the thoracic spine.

labia majora   Outer fleshy "lips" covered with pubic hair that protect the vagina.

labia minora   Inner fleshy "lips" devoid of pubic hair that protect the vagina.

labile   Used to describe a rapid shift in mood.

labour   The mechanism by which the baby and the placenta are expelled from the uterus.

laceration   A wound made by tearing or cutting tissues.

lacrimal apparatus   The structures in which tears are secreted and drained from the eye.

lactated Ringer's (LR) solution   A sterile isotonic crystalloid IV solution of specified amounts of calcium chloride, potassium chloride, sodium chloride, and sodium lactate in water.

lactic acid   A metabolic end product of the breakdown of glucose that accumulates when metabolism proceeds in the absence of oxygen.

lambdoid suture   The point where the occipital bones attach to the parietal bones.

lamina   Arise from the posterior pedicles and fuse to form the posterior spinous processes.

laminated windshield glass   Type of window glazing that incorporates a sheeting material that stops the glass from breaking into shards.

landing zone   Designated location for the landing of air ambulances.

landline   Communications system linked by wires, usually in reference to a conventional telephone system.

lantana   A perennial flowering shrub with clusters of red berries that can lead to serious and even fatal poisoning; Also known as red sage or wild sage; ingestion causes stomach upsets, muscle weakness, shock, and, sometimes, death.

laryngeal mask airway (LMA)   Device that surrounds the opening of the larynx with an inflatable silicone cuff positioned in the hypopharynx; an alternative device to bag-valve-mask ventilation.

laryngectomy   A surgical procedure in which the larynx is removed.

laryngoscope   Device that is used in conjunction with a laryngoscope blade in order to perform direct laryngoscopy.

laryngospasm   Severe constriction of the larynx in response to allergy, noxious stimuli, or illness.

larynx   A complex structure formed by many independent cartilaginous structures that all work together; where the upper airway ends and the lower airway begins.

lassitude   Condition of listlessness and fatigue.

late adults   Persons who are 61 years old or older.

lateral compression   A force that is directed from the side toward the midline of the body.

law of conservation of energy   The principle that energy can be neither created nor destroyed, it can only change form.

LD₅₀   The amount of an agent or substance that will kill 50% of people who are exposed to this level.

Le Fort fractures   Maxillary fractures that are classified into three categories based on their anatomical location.

lead   Any one of the conductors, composed of two or more electrodes, in the ECG that shows the electrical conduction in the heart.

left atrium   The upper left chamber of the heart; receives blood from the pulmonary veins.

left ventricle   The thick-walled, muscular, lower left chamber of the heart; receives blood from the left atrium and pumps it out through the aorta into the systemic arteries.

lens   A transparent body within the globe that focuses light rays.

lethal dose (LD)   Amount of a hazardous substance sure to cause death.

leukemia   Cancer or malignancy of the blood-forming organs, particularly affecting the white blood cells that develop abnormally and/or excessively at the expense of normal blood cells.

leukocytes   The white blood cells responsible for fighting off infection.

leukopenia   Reduction in the number of white blood cells.

leukotrienes   Arachidonic acid metabolites that function as chemical mediators of inflammation. Also known as slow-reacting substances of anaphylaxis (SRS-A).

Level A   The highest level of protective suit worn by hazardous materials personnel. Also referred to as fully encapsulating because the suit covers everything, including the breathing apparatus.

Level B   Personal protective equipment that is one step less protective than level A.

Level C   A level of personal protective equipment that provides splash protection.

Level D   The level of protection that fire fighter turnout gear provides.

Lewisite (L)   A blistering agent that has a rapid onset of symptoms and produces immediate intense pain and discomfort on contact.

liability   A finding in civil cases that the preponderance of the evidence shows the defendant was responsible for the plaintiff's injuries.

liaison officer (LNO)   In incident command, the person who relays information, concerns, and requests among responding agencies.

libel   Making a false statement in written form that injures a person's good name.

lice   Tiny, wingless, parasitic insects that feed on the patient's blood. This infestation is easily spread through close personal contact. Several types exist: head, body, and pubic lice.

licensed Similar to certified, a person who has shown a degree of competency in a specific occupation and is granted ability to function through a governmental body.

licensure The privilege to practice at a carefully defined level, usually granted by a provincial government agency or self-governing professional body.

licit In relation to drugs, legalized drugs such as coffee, alcohol, and tobacco.

life expectancy The average amount of years a person can be expected to live.

ligaments Tough bands of tissue that connect bone to bone around a joint or support internal organs within the body.

ligand Any molecule that binds a receptor leading to a reaction.

limb leads The ECG leads attached to the limbs and that form the hexaxial system, dividing the heart along a coronal plane into the anterior and posterior segments.

limbic system Structures within the cerebrum and diencephalon that influence emotions, motivation, mood, and sensations of pain and pleasure.

linear fracture A fracture that runs parallel to the long axis of a bone.

linear skull fractures Account for 80% of skull fractures; also referred to as nondisplaced skull fractures; commonly occur in the temporal-parietal region of the skull; not associated with deformities to the skull.

liniments Liquid preparations of drugs for external use, usually to relieve some discomfort (such as pain, itching) or to protect the skin.

lithium The cornerstone drug for the treatment of bipolar disorder.

living will A type of advance directive, generally requiring a precondition for withholding resuscitation when the patient is incapacitated.

local anesthesia A type of anesthesia that causes a loss of sensation to touch or pain at a specific isolated spot on the body where a procedure is to take place.

local effect (hazardous material) An effect of a hazardous material on the body that is limited to the area of contact.

local effects The effects that result from the direct application of a drug to a tissue, for example when lotions are applied to the skin to relieve itching.

local reaction When the body limits a response to a specific area after being exposed to a foreign substance.

logistics In incident command, the position that helps procure and stockpile equipment and supplies during an incident.

long bones Bones that are longer than they are wide.

loop diuretics Medications that inhibit the reabsorption of sodium and calcium ions and that can cause an excessive loss of potassium.

loop of Henle The U-shaped portion of the renal tubule that extends from the proximal to the distal convoluted tubule; concentrates the filtrate and converts it to urine.

loosening of associations A situation in which the logical connection between one idea and the next becomes obscure, at least to the listener.

lordosis Inward curve of the lumbar spine just above the buttocks. An exaggerated form of lordosis results in the condition known as swayback.

low-angle operations A rope rescue operation on a mildly sloping surface (less than 45°) or flat land where rescuers are dependent on the ground for their primary support, and the rope system is a secondary means of support.

lower explosive limit (LEL) The concentration of the hazardous material that can burn or explode in the air when it mixes with air.

lumen The inside diameter of an artery or other hollow structure.

Lund and Browder chart A detailed version of the rule of nines chart that takes into consideration the changes in body surface area brought on by growth.

lung compliance The ability of the alveoli to expand when air is drawn into the lungs, either during negative-pressure ventilation or positive-pressure ventilation.

luteinizing hormone (LH) Hormone that regulates the production of both eggs and sperm, as well as production of reproductive hormones.

Lyme disease A tick-borne disease which primarily affects the skin, heart, joints, and nervous system, and characterized by a round, red lesion or bull's-eye rash.

lymph A thin, watery fluid that bathes the tissues of the body.

lymphangitis Inflammation of a lymph channel.

lymphatic system A network of capillaries, vessels, ducts, nodes, and organs that helps to maintain the fluid environment of the body by producing lymph and transporting it through the body.

lymph nodes Area of the lymphatic system where infection-fighting cells are housed.

lymphoblasts Lymphocytes transformed because of stimulation by an antigen.

lymphocytes The white blood cells responsible for a large part of the body's immune protection.

lymphoid system The system primarily made up of the bone marrow, lymph nodes, and spleen that participates in formation of lymphocytes and immune responses.

lymphokines Cytokines released by lymphocytes, including many of the interleukins, gamma interferon, tumour necrosis factor beta, and chemokines.

lymphomas Malignant diseases that arise within the lymphoid system; includes non-Hodgkin and Hodgkin lymphomas.

macrodrip sets Administration sets named for the large orifice between the piercing spike and the drip chamber; allow for rapid fluid flow into the vascular system; allow 10 or 15 gtt/ml, depending on the manufacturer.

macrophages Cells that developed from the monocytes that provide the body's first line of defence in the inflammatory process.

Magill forceps A special type of forcep that is curved, thus allowing the paramedic to maneuver it in the airway.

malignant hyperthermia A condition that can result from common anesthesia medications (notably succinylcholine) and present with hyperthermia, muscular rigidity, altered mental status, and a hyperdynamic state.

malleolus The large, rounded bony protuberance on either side of the ankle joint.

mallet finger An avulsion fracture of the extensor tendon of the distal phalynx caused by jamming a finger into an object.

malocclusion Misalignment of the teeth.

malrotation A congenital anomaly of rotation of the midgut, the small bowel is found predominantly on the right side of the abdomen.

maltreatment Any form of abuse that results in harm or loss. Maltreatment may be physical, sexual, psychological, or financial/material.

mandated reporter A category of professional required by some provinces and territories to report suspicions of child maltreatment. Prehospital professionals may be included.

mandible The movable lower jaw bone.

mandibular nerve A sensory and motor nerve that supplies the muscles of chewing and skin of the lower lip, chin, temporal region, and part of the external ear.

mania A mental disorder characterized by abnormally exaggerated happiness, joy, or euphoria with hyperactivity, insomnia, and grandiose ideas.

manic-depressive illness A bipolar disorder in which mood fluctuates between depression and mania. The alterations in mood are usually episodic and recurrent.

manubrium The superior segment of the sternum; its lower border defines the angle of Louis.

march fractures *See* fatigue fractures.

margination Loss of fluid from the blood vessels into the tissue, causing the blood left in the vessels to have an increased viscosity, which in turn slows the flow of blood and produces stasis.

marijuana The dried leaves and flower buds of the *Cannabis sativa* plant that are smoked to achieve a high.

MARK 1 A nerve agent antidote kit containing two auto-injector medications, atropine and 2-PAM chloride (pralidoxime chloride); also known as a Nerve Agent Antidote Kit (NAAK).

mass-casualty incident (MCI) An emergency situation that can place great demand on the equipment or personnel of the EMS system or has the potential to overwhelm your available resources.

mast cells The cells that resemble basophils but do not circulate in the blood. Mast cells play a role in allergic reactions, immunity, and wound healing.

mastication The process of chewing with the teeth.

mastoid process A cone-shaped section of bone at the base of the temporal bone.

Material Safety Data Sheets (MSDS) Information documents that are supposed to be kept on site at workplaces for every potentially hazardous chemical at the workplace.

maxillary nerve A sensory nerve; supplies the skin on the posterior part of the side of the nose, lower eyelid, cheek, and upper lip.

mean The average number in a given research project.

mean arterial pressure (MAP) The average (or mean) pressure against the arterial wall during a cardiac cycle.

measles An infectious viral disease that occurs most often in late winter and spring. It begins with a fever followed by a cough, running nose, and pink eye. Then a rash spreads from the face and neck down the back and trunk.

mechanical energy The energy that results from motion (kinetic energy) or that is stored in an object (potential energy).

mechanism of action The way in which a medication produces the intended response.

mechanism of injury (MOI) The way in which traumatic injuries occur; the forces that act on the body to cause damage.

meconium A dark green material in the amniotic fluid that can indicate disease in the newborn; the meconium can be aspirated into the infant's lungs during delivery; the baby's first bowel movement.

median The midpoint number in a given research project.

mediastinitis Inflammation of the mediastinum, often a result of the gastric contents leaking into the thoracic cavity after esophageal perforation.

mediastinum Space within the chest that contains the heart, major blood vessels, vagus nerve, trachea, and esophagus; located between the two lungs.

medical ambiguity Uncertainty regarding the specific cause of the patient's condition.

medical asepsis A term applied to the practice of preventing contamination of the patient by using aseptic technique.

medical direction Direction given to an EMS service or paramedic by a physician.

medical incident command A branch of operations in a unified command system, whose three designated sector positions are triage, treatment, and transport.

medical monitoring The process of assessing the health status of hazardous materials team members before and after entry to a hazardous materials incident site.

Medical Practice Act An act that usually defines the minimum qualifications of those who may perform various health services, defines the skills that each type of practitioner is legally permitted to use, and

establishes a means of certification for different categories of health care professionals.

medication A licensed drug taken to cure or reduce symptoms of an illness or medical condition or as an aid in the diagnosis, treatment, or prevention of a disease or other abnormal condition.

medulla Continuous inferiorly with the spinal cord; serves as a conduction pathway for ascending and descending nerve tracts; coordinates heart rate, blood vessel diameter, breathing, swallowing, vomiting, coughing, and sneezing. Also refers to part of the internal anatomy of the kidney; the middle layer.

medulla oblongata The inferior portion of the midbrain, which serves as a conduction pathway for both ascending and descending nerve tracts.

medullary canal The hollow centre portion of a long bone.

melanin The pigment that gives skin its colour.

melena Dark, tarry, very odorous stools caused by upper gastrointestinal bleeds.

membrane attack complex (MAC) Molecules that insert themselves into the bacterial membrane, leading to weakened areas in the membrane.

menarche The beginning phase of a woman's life cycle of menstruation.

meninges A set of three tough membranes, the dura mater, arachnoid, and pia mater, that encloses the entire brain and spinal cord.

meningitis An inflammation of the meningeal coverings of the brain and spinal cord; it is usually caused by a virus or bacterium.

meningococcal meningitis An infection of the fluid of a person's spinal cord and the fluid that surrounds the brain. Sometimes referred to as spinal meningitis, it is caused by bacteria or virus. The viral type is less severe than the bacterial; the bacterial type can result in brain damage, hearing loss, learning disability, or death.

menopause The ending phase of a woman's life cycle of menstruation.

menorrhagia Menstrual blood flow that lasts several days longer than it should or flow that is abnormally excessive.

menstrual cycle The entire monthly cycle of menstruation from start to finish.

menstruation Monthly flow of blood.

mental illness A generic term for a variety of illnesses that result in emotional, cognitive, or behavioural dysfunction.

mental status examination (MSE) A way of measuring the "mental vital signs" in a disturbed patient. The mnemonic COASTMAP can be used to conduct this examination, assessing consciousness, orientation, activity, speech, thought, memory, affect and mood, and perception.

mesentery A membranous double fold of tissue in the abdomen that attaches various organs to the body wall.

metabolic Pertaining to the breakdown of ingested foodstuffs into smaller and smaller

molecules and atoms that are used as energy sources for cellular function.

metacarpals The five bones that form the palm and back of the hand.

metaphysis The region of the long bone between the epiphysis and diaphysis.

metaplasia A reversible, cellular adaptation in which one adult cell type is replaced by another adult cell type.

metastasis Change in location of a disease from one organ or part of the body to another. Often used to describe a cancer that has migrated to other parts of the body.

metatarsals The five long bones extending from the tarsus to the phalanges of the foot.

metered-dose inhaler (MDI) A pressurized canister that delivers a specific dose of a medication; commonly used for beta-agonist bronchodilators.

methamphetamine A highly addictive drug in the amphetamine family.

metric system A decimal system based on tens for the measurement of length, weight, and volume.

metrorrhagia Irregular but frequent vaginal bleeding.

microdrip sets Administration sets named for the small needlelike orifice between the piercing spike and the drip chamber; allow for carefully controlled fluid flow and are ideally suited for medication administration; allow for 60 gtt/ml.

micturition reflex A spinal reflex that causes contraction of the bladder's smooth muscles, producing the urge to void as pressure is exerted on the internal urinary sphincter.

midbrain The part of the brain that is responsible for helping to regulate level of consciousness.

middle adults Persons who are 41 to 60 years of age.

middle ear One of three anatomical parts of the ear; it consists of the inner portion of the tympanic membrane and the ossicles.

milk In the context of pharmacology, an aqueous suspension of an insoluble drug.

mineralocorticoids Any of a group of steroid hormones, such as aldosterone, that are secreted by the adrenal cortex and regulate the balance of water and electrolytes in the body.

minute alveolar volume The amount of air that actually reaches the alveoli per minute and participates in gas exchange.

minute volume The amount of air that moves in and out of the respiratory tract per minute.

miosis Bilateral pinpoint constricted pupils.

missed abortion A situation in which a fetus has died during the first 20 weeks of gestation, but has remained in utero.

missile fragmentation A primary mechanism of tissue disruption from certain rifles in which pieces of the projectile break apart, allowing the pieces to create their own separate paths through tissues.

mitochondria The metabolic centre or powerhouse of the cell. They are small and rod-shaped organelles.

mitral valve The valve located between the left atrium and the left ventricle of the heart.

Mix-o-Vial A single vial divided into two compartments by a rubber stopper; Solu-Medrol is stored this way.

mobile In radio communications, a radio that is affixed to an EMS vehicle, but the vehicle can move around.

mobile intensive care units (MICUs) An early title given to an ambulance-style unit.

mode The most common number in any given research project.

molar pregnancy Pregnancy in which there is a problem at the fertilization stage, with a malfunction of the egg or sperm that results in an abnormal placenta and a fetus with an abnormal chromosome count, or which results in an empty egg.

Mongolian spots Blue-grey areas of discolouration of the skin caused by abnormal pigment, not by trauma or bruising.

monoamine oxidase inhibitors (MAOIs) Psychiatric medication used primarily to treat atypical depression by increasing norepinephrine and serotonin levels in the central nervous system.

monocytes Mononuclear phagocytic white blood cells derived from myeloid stem cells. They circulate in the bloodstream for about 24 hours and then move into tissues to mature into macrophages.

monomorphic Having only one common shape.

mononucleosis Infectious mononucleosis or mono (glandular fever), caused by the Epstein-Barr virus, is often called the kissing disease. It is also spread by coughing or sneezing.

monophonic The sound of one note during wheezing, caused by the vibration of a single bronchus.

monovalent An ion that contains one charge.

mons veneris Also called the mons pubis, this is a rounded pad of fatty tissue that overlies the symphysis pubis and is anterior to the urethral and vaginal openings.

mood A person's sustained and pervasive emotional state.

mood disorder A group of disorders in which the disturbance of mood is accompanied by full or partial manic or depressive syndrome.

morality Code of conduct defined by society, religion, culture, or another person that affects one's character, conduct, and conscience.

morbidity Number of nonfatally injured or disabled people. Usually expressed as a rate, meaning the number of nonfatal injuries in a certain population in a given time period divided by the size of the population.

morgue officer In incident command, the person who works with area medical examiners, coroners, and law enforcement agencies to coordinate the disposition of dead victims.

moro reflex An infant reflex in which, when an infant is caught off guard, the infant opens his or her arms wide, spreads the fingers, and seems to grab at things.

mortality Deaths caused by injury and disease. Usually expressed as a rate, meaning the number of deaths in a certain population in a given time period divided by the size of the population.

mottling A condition of abnormal skin circulation, caused by vasoconstriction or inadequate circulation.

mucopolysaccharide gel One of the complex materials found, along with the collagen fibres and elastin fibres, in the dermis of the skin.

mucosal atomizer device (MAD) A device that attaches to the end of a syringe that is used to spray (atomize) certain medications via the intranasal route.

mucosal-associated lymphoid tissue (MALT) The lymphoid tissue associated with the skin and the respiratory, urinary, and reproductive traits as well as the tonsils.

multifocal Arising from or pertaining to many foci or locations.

multigravida A woman who has had two or more pregnancies, irrespective of the outcome.

multipara A woman who has had two or more deliveries.

multiple myeloma A disease in which an abnormal plasma cell infiltrates the bone marrow with a cancerous (neoplastic) cell, causing tumours to form inside the bones.

multiple-organ dysfunction syndrome (MODS) A progressive condition usually characterized by combined failure of several organs, such as the lungs, liver, and kidney, along with some clotting mechanisms, which occurs after severe illness or injury.

multiple sclerosis (MS) An autoimmune condition in which the body attacks the myelin of the brain and spinal cord, leading to gaps in the insulation normally provided by the myelin, causing scarring.

multiplex Method by which simultaneous transmission of voice and ECG signals can be achieved over a single radio frequency.

mumps A viral infection that primarily affects the parotid glands, which are one of the three pairs of salivary glands, causing swelling in front of the ears.

murmur An abnormal "whoosh"-like sound heard over the heart that indicates turbulent blood flow around a cardiac valve.

Murphy's eye An opening on the side of an endotracheal tube at its distal tip that enables ventilation to occur even if the tip becomes occluded by blood, mucus, or the tracheal wall.

Murphy's sign Pain when pressure is applied to the right upper quadrant of the abdomen in a specific manner; helps detect gallbladder problems.

muscarinic cholinergic antagonists Medications that block acetylcholine exclusively at the muscarinic receptors; an example is atropine.

muscle fatigue The condition that arises when a muscle depletes its supply of energy.

muscular dystrophy (MD) A nonneurologic condition of genetic origin in which defective DNA causes an error in the creation of muscle tissue, resulting in the degeneration of muscular tissue. This presents with progressive muscle weakness, delayed development of muscle motor skills, ptosis, drooling, and poor muscle tone.

muscularis The middle layer of tissue in the fallopian tubes.

mutagen Substance that mutates, damages, and changes the structures of DNA in the body's cells.

mutism The absence of speech.

myasthenia gravis An abnormal condition characterized by the chronic fatigability and weakness of muscles, especially in the face and throat. It is the result of a defect in the conduction of nerve impulses at the nerve junction. This deficit is caused by a lack of acetylcholine.

myelin An insulating-type substance present in some neurons that allows the cell to consistently send its signal along the axon without "shorting out" or losing electricity to surrounding fluids and tissues.

myocardial contusion Blunt force injury to the heart that results in capillary damage, interstitial bleeding, and cellular damage in the area.

myocardial rupture An acute traumatic perforation of the ventricles, atria, intraventricular septum, intra-atrial septum, chordae, papillary muscles, or valves.

myocardium The cardiac muscle.

myoclonus Jerking motions of the body.

myoglobin A protein found in muscle that is released into the circulation after crush injury or other muscle damage and whose presence in the circulation may produce kidney damage.

myometrium The middle layer of tissue in the uterus.

myotomes Regions of the body innervated by the motor components of spinal nerves.

myxedema coma A rare condition that can occur in patients who have severe, untreated hypothyroidism.

NAAK A nerve agent antidote kit containing two auto-injector medications, atropine and 2-PAM chloride (pralidoxime chloride); also known as a MARK 1 kit.

narcotic The generic term for opiates and opioids, drugs that act as a CNS depressant and produce insensibility or stupor.

nasal cannula Delivers oxygen via two small prongs that fit into the patient's nostrils. With an oxygen flow rate of 1 to 6 l/min, the nasal cannula can deliver an oxygen concentration of 24% to 44%.

nasal cavity The chamber inside the nose that lies between the floor of the cranium and the roof of the mouth.

nasal flaring Intermittent outward movements of the nostrils with each inspiration; indicates an increase in the work needed to breathe.

nasal septum A rigid partition composed of bone and cartilage; divides the nasopharynx into two passages.

nasogastric (NG) tube Gastric tube is inserted into the stomach through the nose.

nasolacrimal duct The passage through which tears drain from the lacrimal sacs into the nasal cavity.

nasopharyngeal (nasal) airway A soft rubber tube about 15 cm long that is inserted through the nose into the posterior pharynx behind the tongue, thereby allowing passage of air from the nose to the lower airway.

nasopharynx The nasal cavity; formed by the union of the facial bones.

nasotracheal intubation Insertion of an endotracheal tube into the trachea through the nose.

native immunity A nonspecific cellular and humoural response that operates as the body's first line of defence against pathogens.

natural immunity The immunity the body develops as part of being exposed to an antigen and developing antibodies, for example, exposure to measles, having the measles, and developing immunity to the measles.

nature of illness (NOI) The general type of illness a patient is experiencing.

nebulizer A device for producing a fine spray or mist that is used to deliver inhaled medications.

necrosis The death of tissue, usually caused by a cessation of its blood supply.

needle cricothyrotomy Insertion of a 14- to 16-gauge over-the-needle IV cannula (angiocath) through the cricothyroid membrane and into the trachea.

needle decompression Also referred to as a needle thoracentesis, this procedure introduces a needle or angiocath into the pleural space in an attempt to relieve a tension pneumothorax.

needleless systems A device that does not use needles for: (1) collection of body fluids or withdrawal of body fluids after initial venous or arterial access is established; (2) administration of medication or fluids; or (3) any other procedure involving the potential for occupational exposure to bloodborne pathogens due to percutaneous injuries from contaminated sharps.

negative feedback The concept that once the desired effect of a process has been achieved, further action is inhibited until it is needed again; also called feedback inhibition.

negative-pressure ventilation Drawing of air into the lungs; airflow from a region of higher pressure (outside the body) to a region of lower pressure (the lungs); occurs during normal (unassisted breathing).

negative symptoms Evidence of a disease or condition, noted by lack of normal circumstances, rather than the presence of new physical evidence or a physical change; with regard to schizophrenia, refers to a lack of normal behaviour, and apathy, mutism, a flat affect, and a lack of interest in pleasure.

negative wave pulse The phase of an explosion in which pressure from the blast is less than atmospheric pressure.

neglect Refusal or failure on the part of the caregiver to provide life necessities, such as food, water, clothing, shelter, personal hygiene, medicine, comfort, and personal safety.

negligence Professional action or inaction on the part of the health care worker that does not meet the standard of ordinary care expected of similarly trained and prudent health care practitioners and that results in injury to the patient.

neologism An invented word that has meaning only to its inventor.

neonatal period The first month of life.

neonate Infant during the first month after birth.

neoplasms Tumours.

neovascularization Development of vessels to aid in healing an injured soft tissue.

nephrons The structural and functional units of the kidney that form urine; composed of the glomerulus, the glomerular (Bowman's) capsule, the proximal convoluted tubule (PCT), loop of Henle, and the distal convoluted tubule (DCT).

nerve agents A class of chemicals called organophosphates; they function by blocking an essential enzyme in the nervous system, which causes the body's organs to become overstimulated and burn out.

neurogenic shock Circulatory failure caused by paralysis of the nerves that control the size of the blood vessels, leading to widespread dilation; seen in spinal cord injuries.

neuroleptic malignant syndrome (NMS) A condition caused by antipsychotic and even common antiemetic medications that presents with hyperthermia, muscular rigidity, altered mental status, and a hyperdynamic state.

neuromuscular blocking agents Medications that affect the parasympathetic nervous system by inducing paralysis.

neuronal soma The body of a neuron (nerve cell).

neurotoxins Biological agents that are the most deadly substances known to humans; they include botulinum toxin and ricin.

neurotransmission The process of chemical signaling between cells.

neurotransmitters Proteins that transmit signals between cells of the nervous system.

neurovascular bundle A closely placed grouping of an artery, vein, and nerve that lies beneath the inferior edge of a rib.

neurovascular compromise The loss of the nerve supply, blood supply, or both to a region of the body, typically distal to a site of injury; characterized by alterations in sensation, including numbness and tingling, or by a loss or decrease of motor function; vascular compromise is indicated by weak or absent pulses, poor skin colour, and cool skin.

neutralization A type of decontamination that uses one chemical to change the hazardous material into two less harmful substances; rarely used by hazardous materials teams.

neutron radiation Type of energy that is emitted from a strong radiological source; neutron energy is the fastest moving and most powerful form of radiation. Neutrons easily penetrate through lead, and require several feet of concrete to stop them.

neutrophils Cells that make up approximately 55% to 70% of the leukocytes responsible in large part for the body's protection against infection. They are readily attracted by foreign antigens and destroy them by phagocytosis.

newborn Infant within the first few hours after birth.

Newton's first law of motion The principle that a body at rest will remain at rest unless acted on by an outside force.

Newton's second law of motion The principle that the force that an object can exert is the product of its mass times its acceleration.

nicotinic cholinergic antagonists Medications that block the acetylcholine only at nicotinic receptors.

nitrogen narcosis A state resembling alcohol intoxication produced by nitrogen gas dissolved in the blood at high ambient pressure; also called rapture of the deep.

noise In radio communications, interference in a radio signal.

nonbarbiturate hypnotics Medications designed to sedate without the side effects of a barbiturate.

nondepolarizing neuromuscular blocking agents Medications designed to cause temporary paralysis by binding in a competitive but nonstimulatory manner to part of the ACh receptor. Do not cause fasciculations.

nondisplaced fracture A break in which the bone remains aligned in its normal position.

nonelectrolytes Solutes that have no electrical charge; include glucose and urea; measured in milligrams (mg).

nonopioid analgesics Medications designed to relieve pain without the side effects of opioids.

nonrebreathing mask A combination mask and reservoir bag system. Oxygen fills a reservoir bag that is attached to the mask by a one-way valve. This permits the patient to inhale from the reservoir bag but not to exhale back into it. With a good mask-to-face seal and a flow rate of 15 l/min, it is capable of delivering up to 90% inspired oxygen.

nonspecific agents Medications that produce effects on different cells through a variety of mechanisms. Generally classified by the focus of action or specific therapeutic use.

nonsteroidal anti-inflammatory drugs (NSAIDs) Medications with analgesic and fever reducing properties.

norepinephrine A neurotransmitter and drug sometimes used in the treatment of shock; produces vasoconstriction through its alpha stimulator properties.

normal saline A solution of 0.9% sodium chloride; an isotonic crystalloid.

normal sinus rhythm The normal rhythm of the heart, wherein the excitation impulse arises in the SA node, travels through the internodal pathways to the atrioventricular junction, down the bundle of His, through the bundle branches, and into the Purkinje network without interference.

nosocomial infection An infection acquired from a health care setting.

nuchal rigidity A stiff or painful neck; commonly associated with meningitis.

nucleus A cellular organelle that contains the genetic information. The nucleus controls the function and structure of a cell.

nullipara A woman who has never delivered.

nursemaid's elbow The subluxation of the radial head that often results from pulling on an outstretched arm.

nystagmus The rhythmic shaking of the eyes.

obesity A term generally used when someone is 20% to 30% over his or her ideal weight.

objectives Specific, time-limited, and quantifiable statements that summarize an expected result of an intervention.

oblique fracture A fracture that travels diagonally from one side of the bone to the other.

obsession A persistent idea that a person cannot dismiss from his or her thoughts.

obstructive shock Shock that occurs when there is a block to blood flow in the heart or great vessels, causing an insufficient blood supply to the body's tissues.

obtunded A condition when the patient is dulled to pain and sensation.

occipital condyles Articular surfaces on the occipital bone where the skull articulates with the atlas on the vertebral column.

occipital lobe The portion of the brain that is responsible for the processing of visual information.

occiput The most posterior portion of the cranium.

occlusion Blockage, usually of a tubular structure such as a blood vessel or IV cannula.

ocular Pertaining to the eye.

oculomotor nerve Third cranial nerve; innervates the muscles that cause motion of the eyeballs and upper eyelid.

off-gassing The emitting of an agent after exposure, for example from a person's clothes that have been exposed to the agent.

official name The name listed in the United States Pharmacopeia (USP) once the generic name has been approved by the United States Adopted Name Council and the drug has been approved by the US Food and Drug Administration.

ointment A semisolid preparation for external application to the body, usually containing a medicinal substance.

olecranon The proximal bony projection of the ulna at the elbow; the part of the ulna that constitutes the "funny bone."

olfactory nerves Participates in the transmission of scent impulses.

oligohydramnios Decreased volume of amniotic fluid during a pregnancy; a risk factor associated with abnormalities of the urinary tract, postmaturity (birth after a prolonged pregnancy), and intrauterine growth retardation.

oliguria A decrease in urine output to the extent that total urine output drops below 500 ml/day.

ongoing assessment The part of the assessment process in which problems are reevaluated and responses to treatment are assessed.

ongoing cyanosis Deep cyanosis of the face and neck and across the chest and back; associated with little or no blood flow; it is particularly ominous.

online (direct) medical control Type of medical control in which the paramedic is in direct contact with a physician, usually via two-way radio or telephone.

onset of action The time needed for the concentration of the medication at the target tissue to reach the minimum effective level.

oocyte An egg produced from the female ovary.

open abdominal injury An injury in which there is a break in the surface of the skin or mucous membrane, exposing deeper tissue to potential contamination.

open book pelvic fracture A life-threatening fracture of the pelvis caused by a force that displaces one or both sides of the pelvis laterally and posteriorly.

open cricothyrotomy Also referred to as a surgical cricothyrotomy; an emergent procedure that involves incising the cricothyroid membrane with a scalpel and inserting an endotracheal or tracheostomy tube directly into the subglottic area of the trachea.

open-ended question A question that does not have a yes or no answer, and which does not give the patient specific options to choose from.

open fracture Any break in a bone in which the overlying skin has been damaged.

open incident An ongoing or uncontained incident in which rescuers will have to search for patients and then triage or treat them. The situation may produce more patients. Examples include school shootings, tornadoes, a hazardous materials release, and rising floodwaters.

open pneumothorax The result of a defect in the chest wall that allows air to enter the thoracic space.

open wound An injury in which there is a break in the surface of the skin or the mucous membrane, exposing deeper tissue to potential contamination.

operations The technical rescue training level geared toward working in the warm zone of an incident. Training at this level allows responders to directly assist those conducting the rescue operation and to use certain rescue skills and procedures.

Operations Level This training level, also called EMS/HM Level I Responder, allows paramedics to perform patient care activities in the cold zone (the command and support centre) at an incident for patients who no longer present a significant risk of secondary contamination.

operations (incident command) The position that carries out the orders of the commander to help resolve the incident.

ophthalmic nerve A sensory nerve that supplies the skin of the forehead, the upper eyelid, and conjunctiva.

opiate Various alkaloids derived from the opium or poppy plant.

OPIM An acronym that stands for other potentially infectious materials. These include CSF, pericardial fluid, synovial fluid, pleural fluid, amniotic fluid, peritoneal fluid, and any fluid containing gross visible blood.

opioid A synthetic narcotic not derived from opium; potent analgesics with sedative properties, including drugs such as fentanyl (Sublimaze) and alfentanil (Alfenta).

opioid agonist-antagonists Medications designed to relieve pain without the side effects of opioids.

opioid agonists Chemicals that are similar to or derived from the opium plant.

opioid antagonists A classification of medications that reverses the effects of opioid drugs.

opsoninization Occurs when an antibody coats an antigen to facilitate its recognition by immune cells.

opthalmoscope An instrument used to look into a patient's eyes and view the retina and aqueous fluid; consists of a concave mirror and a battery-powered light that is usually contained in the handle.

optic nerve Either of the second cranial nerves that enter the eyeball posteriorly, through the optic foramen.

orbits Bony cavities in the frontal part of the skull that enclose and protect the eyes.

ordinary negligence Negligence that is a failure to act, or a simple mistake that causes harm to a patient.

organ of Corti A structure located in the cochlea that contains hairs that are stimulated by vibrations to form nerve impulses that travel to the brain and are perceived as sound.

organelles Internal cellular structures that carry out specific functions for the cell.

organic brain syndrome Temporary or permanent dysfunction of the brain, caused by a disturbance in the physical or physiologic functioning of brain tissue.

organophosphates A class of chemical found in many insecticides used in agriculture and in the home.

orientation A person's sense of who one is (person), where one is (place), and at what day of the week one finds oneself (day), and an understanding of events leading up to where one finds oneself (events).

orogastric (OG) tube Gastric tube inserted into the stomach through the mouth.

oropharyngeal (oral) airway A hard plastic device that is curved in such a way that it fits over the back of the tongue with the tip in the posterior pharynx.

oropharynx Forms the posterior portion of the oral cavity, which is bordered superiorly by the hard and soft palates, laterally by the cheeks, and inferiorly by the tongue.

orotracheal intubation Insertion of an endotracheal tube into the trachea through the mouth.

orthopnea Severe dyspnea experienced when lying down and relieved by sitting or standing up.

orthostatic hypotension A drop in systolic blood pressure when moving from a sitting to a standing position.

orthostatic vital signs Assessing vital signs in two different patient positions to determine the degree of hypovolemia.

osmolarity The ability to influence the movement of water across a semipermeable membrane.

osmosis The movement of water across a semipermeable membrane (for example, the cell wall) from an area of lower to higher concentration of solute molecules.

ossicles The three small bones in the inner ear that transmit vibrations to the cochlear duct at the oval window.

ossification centres Areas where cartilage is transformed through calcification into a new area of bone.

osteoarthritis (OA) The degeneration of a joint surface caused by wear and tear that leads to pain and stiffness.

osteogenesis imperfecta A congenital bone disease that results in fragile bones.

osteomyelitis Inflammation of the bone due to infection; a potential complication of intraosseous infusion.

osteoporosis A condition characterized by decreased bone mass and density and increased susceptibility to fractures.

otoscope A tool used to examine the ears of a patient; consists of a head and a handle. The head contains an electric light source and a low-power magnifying lens.

outcome (impact) objectives State the intended effect of the program on participants or on the community in such terms as the participants' increased knowledge, changed behaviours or attitudes, or decreased injury rates.

oval window An oval opening between the middle ear and the vestibule.

ovaries Female gonads; ovaries release eggs and secrete the female hormones.

overhydration An increase in the body's systemic fluid volume.

overriding The overlap of a bone that occurs from the muscle spasm that follows a fracture, leading to a decrease in the length of the bone.

over-the-needle cannula A Teflon (plastic) cannula inserted over a hollow needle.

ovulation A process in which an ovum is released from a follicle.

ovum A mature oocyte.

oxygen concentrators Large, electrical devices that concentrate the oxygen in ambient air and eliminate other gases.

oxygen humidifier Small bottle of water through which the oxygen leaving the cylinder is moisturized before it reaches the patient.

oxygenation The process of delivering oxygen to the blood by diffusion from the alveoli following inhalation into the lungs.

oxyhemoglobin Hemoglobin that is occupied by oxygen.

P waves The first wave of the ECG complex, representing depolarization of the atria.

pacemaker The specialized tissue within the heart that initiates excitation impulses; an electronic device used to stimulate cardiac contraction when the electric conduction system of the heart is malfunctioning, especially in complete heart block. An electronic pacemaker consists of a battery-powered pulse generator and a wire that transmits the electric impulse to the ventricles.

palate Forms the roof of the mouth and separates the oropharynx and nasopharynx.

palatine bone An irregularly shaped bone found in the posterior part of the nasal cavity.

palatine tonsils One of three sets of lymphatic organs that comprise the tonsils; located in the back of the throat, on each side of the posterior opening of the oral cavity; help protect the body from bacteria introduced into the mouth and nose.

pallor Lack of colour; paleness.

palmar grasp An infant reflex that occurs when something is placed in the infant's palm; the infant grasps the object.

palpation Physical touching for the purpose of obtaining information.

palpitations A sensation felt under the left breast of the heart "skipping a beat," usually caused by a premature ventricular contraction.

pancreas The digestive gland that secretes digestive enzymes into the duodenum through the pancreatic duct. The pancreas is considered both an endocrine gland and an exocrine gland.

pancuronium A nondepolarizing neuromuscular blocking agent; used to maintain paralysis following succinylcholine-facilitated intubation; also called Pavulon.

papillary muscles Protrusions of the myocardium into the ventricular cavities to which the chordae tendineae are attached.

para The number of pregnancies a woman has carried to more than 28 weeks, regardless of whether the fetus was delivered dead or alive.

para-aminophenol derivatives Medications designed to reduce fevers and relieve pain.

paracrine hormones Hormones that diffuse through intracellular spaces to their target.

paralytics Also called neuromuscular blocking agents; paralyzes skeletal muscles; used in an emergency situation to facilitate intubation.

parameters Outlined measures that may be difficult to obtain in a research project.

paranasal sinuses The sinuses, or hollowed sections of bone in the front of the head, that are lined with mucous membrane and drain into the nasal cavity.

paranoid type A type of schizophrenia in which the person experiences delusions or hallucinations usually centred around a specific theme, where their cognitive functions remain intact.

paraplegia Paralysis of the lower part of the body.

parasite Any living organism in or on any other living creature; takes advantage of the host by feeding off cells and tissues.

parasympathetic nervous system A subdivision of the autonomic nervous system that is involved in control of involuntary, vegetative functions, mediated largely by the vagus nerve through the chemical acetylcholine.

parathyroid hormone (PTH) A hormone secreted by the parathyroids that acts as an antagonist to calcitonin. PTH is secreted when calcium blood levels are low.

parenchyma The substance of a gland or solid organ.

parenteral exposure Entry of a hazardous material into the bloodstream, either through force of injection or through an open wound.

parenteral routes Medication routes in which medications are administered via any route other than the alimentary canal (digestive tract), skin, or mucous membranes.

paresthesias Abnormal sensations such as burning, numbness, or tingling.

parietal lobe The portion of the brain that is the site for reception and evaluation of most sensory information, except smell, hearing, and vision.

parietal pain Pain caused by inflammation of the parietal peritoneum that is generally described as steady, aching, and aggravated by movement.

parietal pleura Thin membrane that lines the chest cavity.

parity Number of live births a woman has had.

Parkinson's disease A neurologic condition in which the portion of the brain responsible for production of dopamine is damaged or overused, resulting in tremors.

Parkland formula A formula that recommends giving 4 ml of normal saline for each kilogram of body weight, multiplied by the percentage of body surface area burned; sometimes used to calculate fluid needs during lengthy transport times.

paroxysmal nocturnal dyspnea (PND) Severe shortness of breath occurring at night after several hours of recumbency, during which fluid pools in the lungs; the person is forced to sit up to breathe. PND is caused by left heart failure or decompensation of chronic obstructive pulmonary disease.

partial laryngectomy   Surgical removal of a portion of the larynx.

partial pressure   The amount of the total pressure contributed by various gases in solution.

partial rebreathing mask   Similar to the nonrebreathing mask except that there is no one-way valve between the mask and the reservoir. Room air is not entrained with inspiration; however, residual expired air is mixed in the mask and rebreathed.

partial-thickness burn   A burn that involves the epidermis and part of the dermis, characterized by pain and blistering; previously called a second-degree burn.

passive interventions   Something that offers automatic protection from injury, often without requiring any conscious change of behaviour by the individual; child-resistant bottles and air bags are some examples.

passive neglect   An unintentional refusal or failure to fulfill a caregiving obligation, which results in physical or emotional distress. Examples include forgetting or isolating the person.

past medical history   Information obtained during the patient history, such as the patient's general state of health, childhood and adult diseases, surgeries and hospitalizations, psychiatric and mental illnesses, or traumatic injuries, which may relate to the patient's current problem.

patch   A connection between a telephone line and a radio communications system enabling a caller to get "on the air" by dialing into a special telephone.

patch (medication)   A solid medication impregnated into a membrane or adhesive that is applied to the surface of the skin.

patella   The kneecap.

patent   Open.

pathologic fracture   A fracture that occurs in an area of abnormally weakened bone.

pathophysiology   The study of how normal physiologic processes are affected by disease.

pathway expansion   The tissue displacement that occurs as a result of low-displacement shock waves that travel at the speed of sound in tissue.

patient autonomy   The right to direct one's own care, and to decide how you want your end-of-life medical care provided.

patient history   Information about the patient's chief complaint, present symptoms, and previous illnesses.

peak expiratory flow   An approximation of the extent of bronchoconstriction; used to determine whether patients are

improving with therapy (eg, inhaled bronchodilators).

peak loads   A time of day or day of week in which the call volume is at its highest.

pectoral girdle   The shoulder girdle.

Pediatric Assessment Triangle (PAT)   An assessment tool that allows rapid formation of a general impression of the type and level of illness or injury in an infant or child without touching him or her; consists of assessing appearance, work of breathing, and circulation to the skin.

pedicles   Thick lateral bony struts that connect the vertebral body with spinous and transverse processes and make up the lateral and posterior portions of the spinal foramen; also, a narrow strip of tissue by which an avulsed piece of tissue remains connected to the body.

pelvic girdle   The large bone that arises in the area of the last nine vertebrae and sweeps around to form a complete ring.

pelvic inflammatory disease (PID)   An infection of the female upper organs of reproduction, specifically the uterus, ovaries, and fallopian tubes.

penetrating trauma   Injury caused by objects that pierce the surface of the body, such as knives and bullets, and damage internal tissues and organs.

Penrose drain   A type of surgical drain; often used as a tourniquet.

peptic ulcer disease (PUD)   Abrasion of the stomach or small intestine.

perception   The way a person processes the data supplied by the five senses.

percussion   Gently striking the surface of the body, typically overlying various body cavities to detect changes in the densities of the underlying structures.

percutaneous   Through the skin or mucous membrane.

percutaneous routes   The medication routes of any medication absorbed through the skin or a mucous membrane.

perfusion   The circulation of blood within an organ or tissue in adequate amounts to meet the cells' needs.

pericardial sac   The potential space between the layers of the pericardium.

pericardial tamponade   Impairment of diastolic filling of the right ventricle due to significant amounts of fluid in the pericardial sac surrounding the heart, leading to a decrease in the cardiac output.

pericardiocentesis   A procedure in which a needle or angiocath is introduced into the pericardial sac to relieve cardiac tamponade.

pericardium   The double-layered sac containing the heart and the origins of the superior vena cava, inferior vena cava, and pulmonary artery.

perimetrium   The outer protective layer of tissue in the uterus.

perineum   The area between the vaginal opening and the anus.

periorbital ecchymosis   Bruising under or around the orbits that is commonly seen following a basilar skull fracture; also called raccoon eyes.

periosteum   The fibrous tissue that covers bone.

peripheral nerves   All of the nerves of the body extending from the brain and spinal cord.

peripheral nervous system (PNS)   Consists of all nervous tissue outside of the brain and spinal cord and is subdivided into two divisions, the somatic and autonomic nervous systems. Consists of 31 pairs of spinal nerves and 12 pairs of cranial nerves, which may be sensory, motor, or connecting nerves.

peripheral neuropathy   A group of conditions in which the nerves leaving the spinal cord are damaged, resulting in distortion of signals to or from the brain. One type is diabetic, in which the peripheral nerves are damaged as blood glucose levels rise, causing loss of sensation, numbness, burning, pain, paresthesia, and muscle weakness.

peripheral shock   A term that describes shock secondary to peripheral circulatory abnormalities—includes both hypovolemic shock and distributive shock.

peripheral vein cannulation   Cannulating veins of the periphery, that is, those that can be seen and/or palpated. Examples of peripheral veins include those of the hand, arm, and lower extremity and the external jugular vein.

peripheral vision   Visualization of lateral objects while looking forward.

peristalsis   The rhythmic contractions of the intestines and esophagus that allow material to move.

peritoneum   A membrane in the abdomen encasing the liver, spleen, diaphragm, stomach, and transverse colon.

peritonitis   Inflammation of the peritoneum (the lining around the abdominal cavity) that results from either blood or hollow organ contents spilling into the abdominal cavity.

peritubular capillaries   A set of capillaries unique to the kidney that branch off from the efferent arteriole; the site of tubular resorption.

periumbilical   Pertaining to the area around the umbilicus (the navel).

permanent cavity   The path of crushed tissue produced by a missile traversing part of the body.

permissible exposure limit (PEL)   The maximum concentration of a chemical that a person may be exposed to.

perseveration   Repeating the same idea over and over again.

persistency   Term used to describe how long a chemical agent will stay on a surface before it evapourates.

persistent pulmonary hypertension Delayed transition from fetal to neonatal circulation.

personal flotation device (PFD) Also commonly known as a life vest, a PFD allows the body to float in water.

personality disorder The term used to describe a condition a person has when he or she behaves or thinks in a way that is dysfunctional or causes distress to other people.

pertussis An acute infectious disease characterized by a catarrhal stage, followed by a paroxysmal cough that ends in a whooping inspiration. Also called whooping cough.

petechiae Tiny purple or red spots that appear on the skin due to bleeding within the skin or under mucous membranes.

petechial Characterized by small purplish, nonblanching spots on the skin.

pH The measure of acidity or alkalinity of a solution.

phagocyte A kind of cell that engulfs and consumes foreign material such as microorganisms and debris.

phagocytosis Process in which one cell eats or engulfs a foreign substance to destroy it.

phalanges The bones of the fingers or toes.

pharmacodynamics The branch of pharmacology that studies reactions between medications and living structures, including the processes of body responses to pharmacologic, biochemical, physiologic, and therapeutic effects.

pharmacokinetics The study of the metabolism and action of medications with particular emphasis on the time required for absorption, duration of action, distribution in the body, and method of excretion.

pharmacology The branch of medicine dealing with the actions of drugs in the body—therapeutic and toxic effects—and development and testing of new drugs and new uses of existing ones.

pharyngeotracheal lumen airway (PtL) Multi-lumen airway device that consists of two tubes and two cuffs; an alternative device if endotracheal intubation is not possible or has failed.

pharynx Throat.

phlebitis Inflammation of the wall of a vein, sometimes caused by an IV line, manifested by tenderness, redness, and slight edema along part of the length of the vein.

phlebotomy The withdrawal of blood from a vein.

phobia An abnormal and persistent dread of a specific object or situation.

phosgene A pulmonary agent that is a product of combustion, such as might be produced in a fire at a textile factory or house, or from metalwork or burning Freon. Phosgene is a very potent agent that has a delayed onset of symptoms, usually hours.

phosgene oxime (CX) A blistering agent that has a rapid onset of symptoms and produces immediate intense pain and discomfort on contact.

phrenic nerves Nerves that innervate the diaphragm.

physical dependence A physiologic state of adaptation to a drug, usually characterized by tolerance to the drug's effects and a withdrawal syndrome if use of the drug is stopped, especially abruptly.

physical evidence The evidence that ties a suspect or victim to a crime. It may include body materials, objects, and impressions.

physical examination The process by which quantifiable, objective information is obtained from a patient about his or her overall state of health.

physiologic dead space Additional dead space created by intrapulmonary obstructions or atelectasis.

physiologic fracture A fracture that occurs when abnormal forces are applied to normal bone structures.

physis The growth plate in long bones.

pia mater The innermost of the three meninges that enclose the brain and spinal cord, it rests directly on the brain and spinal cord.

piercing spike The hard, sharpened plastic spike on the end of the administration set designed to pierce the sterile membrane of the IV bag.

Pierre Robin sequence A condition present at birth marked by a very small lower jaw (micrognathia). The tongue tends to fall back and downward (glossoptosis), and there is a cleft soft palate.

pill A drug shaped into a ball or oval to be swallowed; often coated to disguise an unpleasant taste.

pinna The large outside portion of the ear through which sound waves enter the ear; also called the auricle.

piriform fossa Hollow pockets on the lateral sides of the glottic opening.

pituitary gland Gland whose secretions control, or regulate, the secretions of other endocrine glands. Often called the "master gland."

placenta The tissue attached to the uterine wall that nourishes the fetus through the umbilical cord.

placenta previa A condition in which the placenta develops over and covers the cervix.

plaintiff In a civil suit, the individual who brings a legal action against another individual.

planning In incident command, the position that ultimately produces a plan to resolve any incident.

plantar Referring to the sole of the foot.

plantar flexion Bending of the foot toward the ground.

plaque In cardiology, the white to yellow lesion found in atherosclerosis that is made up of lipids, cell debris, and smooth muscles cells; in older people, may also include calcium.

plasma A component of blood, made of 92% water, 6% to 7% proteins, and electrolytes, clotting factors, and glucose; this makes up 55% of the total blood volume.

plasmin A naturally occurring clot-dissolving enzyme, usually present in the body in its inactive form, plasminogen.

platelets Small cells in the blood that are essential for clot formation.

pleura Membrane lining the outer surface of the lungs (visceral pleura), the inner surface of the chest wall, and the thoracic surface of the diaphragm (parietal pleura).

pleural effusion Excessive accumulation of fluid in the pleural space.

plexus A cluster of nerve roots that permits peripheral nerve roots to rejoin and function as a group.

pneumonia An inflammation of the lungs caused by bacteria, viruses, fungi, or other organisms.

pneumonic plague A lung infection, also known as plague pneumonia, that is the result of inhalation of plague bacteria.

pneumonitis Inflammation of the lung. Implies lung inflammation from an irritant such as a chemical, dust, or radiation, or from aspiration. When lung inflammation is caused by an infectious agent, it would typically be called pneumonia.

pneumotaxic centre Area of the brain stem that has an inhibitory influence on inspiration.

pneumothorax The collection of air within the normally closed pleural space.

podocytes Special cells in the inner membrane of the glomerulus that wrap around the capillaries in the glomerulus, forming filtration slits.

point of maximal impulse (PMI) The palpable beat of the apex of the heart against the chest wall during ventricular contraction; normally palpated in the fifth left intercostal space in the midclavicular line.

point tenderness The tenderness that is sharply localized at the site of the injury, found by gently palpating along the bone with the tip of one finger.

poison A substance whose chemical action could damage structures or impair function when introduced into the body.

poliomyelitis A viral infection that attacks the axons, especially motor axons, and destroys them, causing weakness, paralysis, and respiratory arrest. An effective vaccine has been developed and this disease is now rare.

polycythemia An overabundance or production of RBCs, WBCs, and platelets, which makes the blood thick.

polyhydramnios An excessive amount of amniotic fluid. May cause preterm labour.

polymenorrhea Menstrual blood flow that occurs more often than a 24-day interval.

polymorphonuclear neutrophils (PMNs) A type of white blood cell formed by bone marrow tissue that possesses a nucleus consisting of several parts or lobes connected by fine strands; a variety of leukocyte.

polypharmacy Simultaneous use of many medications.

polyphonic The sound of multiple notes during wheezing, caused by the vibrations of many bronchi.

polyuria Frequent and plentiful urination.

pons The portion of the brain stem that lies below the midbrain and contains nerve fibres that affect sleep and respiration.

popliteal artery The artery in the area or space behind the knee joint.

portable A hand-held radio that can be carried on a person and used for communications away from a vehicle.

portal vein A large vessel created by the intersection of blood vessels from the GI system. The portal vein empties into the liver.

positive symptoms Evidence of or physical change due to a disease or condition, which can be physically noted by the patient or health care provider; with regard to schizophrenia, refers to delusions and hallucinations.

positive wave pulse The phase of the explosion in which there is a pressure front with a pressure higher than atmospheric pressure.

positive-pressure ventilation (PPV) Method for assisting ventilation (bag-valve-mask or intubated) with high-flow air or oxygen.

postconventional reasoning A type of reasoning in which a child bases decisions upon his or her conscience.

posterior chamber The posterior area of the globe between the lens and the iris.

posterior cord syndrome A condition associated with extension injuries with isolated injury to the dorsal column; presents as decreased sensation to light touch, proprioception, and vibration while leaving most other motor and sensory functions intact.

posterior spinous process Formed by the fusion of the posterior lamina, this is an attachment site for muscles and ligaments.

posterior tibial artery The artery that travels through the calf muscles to the plantar aspect of the foot.

postictal The period of time after a seizure during which the brain is reorganizing activity.

posting The placement of an ambulance at a specific geographic location in order to cover larger areas of territory and reduce response times.

postpartum After birth.

postpolio syndrome A result of polio in which neurons break down and die, resulting in difficulty swallowing, weakness, fatigue, or breathing problems even after the patient has healed.

post-term Any pregnancy that lasts more than 42 weeks.

postrenal ARF A type of acute renal failure caused by obstruction of urine flow from the kidneys, commonly caused by a blockage of the urethra by prostate enlargement, renal calculi, or strictures.

posttraumatic stress disorder (PTSD) A severe form of anxiety that stems from a traumatic experience. PTSD is characterized by the reliving of the stress and nightmares of the original situation.

postural hypotension Symptomatic drop in blood pressure related to the patient's body position; detected by measuring pulse and blood pressure while the patient is lying supine, sitting up, and standing. An increase in pulse rate and a decrease in blood pressure in any one of these positions is considered a positive sign for this condition.

postural tremors Tremors that occur as the person holds a body part still.

posture The position of one's body.

potential energy The amount of energy stored in an object, the product of mass, gravity, and height, that is converted into kinetic energy and results in injury, such as from a fall.

potentiation In health care, the effect of increasing the potency or effectiveness of a drug or other treatment; may occur by administering two medications concurrently, and one increases the effect of the other.

powder A drug that has been ground into pulverized form.

power of attorney for personal care A legal document that contains advance directives and appoints another person to make health care decisions, including withdrawal or withholding of care, for the patient in the event that he or she becomes incapable of making such decisions.

ppb Parts per billion; an expression of concentration.

ppm Parts per million; an expression of concentration.

P-R interval The period between the beginning of the P wave (atrial depolarization) and the onset of the QRS complex (ventricular depolarization), signifying the time required for atrial depolarization and passage of the excitation impulse through the atrioventricular junction.

preconventional reasoning A type of reasoning in which a child acts almost purely to avoid punishment or to get what he or she wants.

precordial leads Another term used to describe the chest leads in an ECG.

preeclampsia A condition of late pregnancy that involves gradual onset of hypertension, headache, visual changes, and swelling of the hands and feet; also called pregnancy-induced hypertension or toxemia of pregnancy.

prefilled syringes Medication syringes that are prepackaged and prepared with a specific concentration.

preload The pressure under which the ventricle fills.

premature Underdeveloped; the condition of an infant born too soon. Refers to infants delivered before 37 weeks from the first day of the last menstrual period.

premenstrual syndrome (PMS) A cluster of all or some of the troubling symptoms that occur during a woman's menstrual phase that can include fluid retention, breast pain and tenderness, headache, severe cramping, and emotional changes, including agitation, irritability, depression, and anger.

prenatal The state of the pregnant woman before birth.

prepuce In the anatomy of the female genitalia, a layer of skin directly above the clitoris.

prerenal ARF A type of acute renal failure that is caused by hypoperfusion of the kidneys, resulting from hypovolemia (hemorrhage, dehydration), trauma, shock, sepsis, and heart failure (congestive heart failure, myocardial infarction); often reversible if the underlying condition can be found and perfusion restored to the kidney.

presbycusis Progressive hearing loss, particularly in the high frequencies, along with lessened ability to discriminate between a particular sound and background noise.

preschoolers Persons who are 3 to 6 years of age.

pressure infuser device A sleeve that is placed around the IV bag and inflated to force fluid to flow from the IV bag and into the tubing.

pressure of speech Speech in which words seem to tumble out under immense emotional pressure.

pressure-compensated flowmeter An oxygen flowmeter that incorporates a float ball within a tapered calibrated tube. The float rises or falls according to the gas flow within the tube. Because this type of flowmeter is affected by gravity, it must remain in an upright position to obtain an accurate flow reading.

preterm Used to describe an infant delivered at less than 37 completed weeks.

prevalence The number of cases of a disease in a specific population over time.

priapism A sustained, painful erection of the penis.

primary adrenal insufficiency Also known as Addison's disease. A rare condition in which the adrenal glands produce an insufficient amount of adrenal hormones.

primary apnea Apnea caused by oxygen deprivation; usually corrected with stimulation, such as drying or slapping the newborn's feet. Primary apnea is typically preceded by an initial period of rapid breathing.

primary brain injury An injury to the brain and its associated structures that is a direct result of impact to the head.

primary contamination An exposure that occurs with direct contact with the hazardous material.

primary exit The main means of escape should violence erupt. This is usually the door you used to enter the building.

primary injury prevention Keeping an injury from occurring.

primary respiratory drive Normal stimulus to breathe; based on fluctuations in $PaCO_2$ and pH of the CSF.

primary response The first encounter with the foreign substance to begin the immune response.

primary spinal cord injury Injury to the spinal cord that is a direct result of trauma, for example transection of the spinal cord from penetrating trauma or displacement of ligaments and bone fragments, resulting in compression of the spinal cord.

primary triage A type of patient sorting used to rapidly categorize patients; the focus is on speed in locating all patients and determining an initial priority as their condition warrants.

primigravida First pregnancy.

primipara A woman who has had one delivery only.

primitive reflexes Reflex reactions such as Babinski, grasping, and sucking signs normally found in very young patients.

process objectives State how a program will be implemented, describing the service to be provided, the nature of the service, and to whom it will be directed.

prodrome The early signs and symptoms that occur before a disease or condition fully appears, eg, dizziness before fainting.

profession A specialized set of knowledge, skills, and/or expertise.

professional A person who follows expected standards and performance parameters in a specific profession.

progesterone One of the three major female hormones.

projection Blaming unacceptable feelings, motives, or desires on others.

prolapsed umbilical cord When the umbilical cord presents itself outside of the uterus while the fetus is still inside; an obstetric emergency during pregnancy or labour that acutely endangers the life of the baby; can happen when the water breaks and with the gush of water the cord comes along.

pronation The act of turning the palm of the hand backward or downward, performed by internal rotation of the forearm.

proprioception The ability to perceive the position and movement of one's body or limbs.

prospective research Specific reason a task or research will be performed before it is started.

prostaglandins A group of lipids that act as chemical messengers.

protocol A treatment plan developed for a specific illness or injury.

protozoans Single-celled, usually microscopic, eukaryotic organisms such as amoebas, ciliates, flagellates, and sporozoans; a type of parasite.

protuberant A convex or distended shape of the abdomen. This can be caused by edema.

proximal convoluted tubule (PCT) One of two complex sections of the nephron, the PCT includes an enlargement at the end called the glomerular capsule.

proximate cause The specific reason that an injury occurred; one of the items that must be proven in order for a paramedic to be held liable for negligence.

pruritus Unspecified itching.

pseudocyesis A false pregnancy that develops all the typical signs and symptoms of true pregnancy, but in which no actual pregnancy exists.

pseudomembrane A false membrane formed by a dead tissue layer. Seen in the posterior pharynx of patients with diphtheria.

psychiatric emergency An emergency in which abnormal behaviour threatens an individual's health and safety or the health and safety of another person, for example when a person becomes suicidal, homicidal, or has a psychotic episode.

psychological dependence The emotional state of craving a drug to maintain a feeling of well-being.

psychosis A mental disorder characterized by loss of contact with reality.

psychotropic drugs Drugs that affect mood, thought, or behaviour.

ptosis Drooping of an eyelid.

pubic symphysis The midline articulation of the pubic bones.

pubis One of two bones that form the anterior portion of the pelvic ring.

public information officer (PIO) In incident command, the person who keeps the public informed and relates any information to the press.

pudendum The female external genitalia.

pulmonary artery One of two arteries that carry deoxygenated blood from the right ventricle to the lungs.

pulmonary blast injuries Pulmonary trauma resulting from short-range exposure to the detonation of high explosives.

pulmonary circulation The flow of blood from the right ventricle through the pulmonary arteries and all of their branches and capillaries in the lungs and back to the left atrium through the venules and pulmonary veins; also called the lesser circulation.

pulmonary contusion Injury to the lung parenchyma that results in capillary hemorrhage into the tissue.

pulmonary edema Congestion of the pulmonary air spaces with exudate and foam, often secondary to left heart failure.

pulmonary embolism Obstruction of a pulmonary artery or arteries by solid, liquid, or gaseous material swept through the right side of the heart into the lungs.

pulmonary hypertension Elevated blood pressure in the pulmonary arteries from constriction; causes problems with the blood flow in the lungs, and makes the heart work harder.

pulmonary overpressurization syndrome Also called "POPS" or "burst lung," this diving emergency can occur during ascent and can cause pneumothorax, mediastinal and subcutaneous emphysema, alveolar hemorrhage, and the lethal arterial gas embolism (AGE).

pulmonary route A medication route in which medication is administered directly to the pulmonary system through inhalation or injection.

pulmonary veins The vessels that carry oxygenated blood from the lungs to the left atrium.

pulmonic valve The valve between the right ventricle and the pulmonary artery.

pulp Specialized connective tissue within the pulp cavity of a tooth.

pulse oximeter Device that measures oxygen saturation.

pulse oximetry An assessment tool that measures oxygen saturation of hemoglobin in the capillary beds.

pulse pressure The difference between the systolic and diastolic pressures.

pulsus paradoxus A drop in the systolic BP of 10 mm Hg or more; commonly seen in patients with pericardial tamponade or severe asthma.

pulvule A solid medication form that resembles a capsule but it is not made of gelatin and does not separate.

puncture wound A stab injury from a pointed object, such as a nail or a knife.

pupil The circular opening in the centre of the eye through which light passes to the lens.

Purkinje fibres A system of fibres in the ventricles that conducts the excitation impulse from the bundle branches to the myocardium.

purpuric Pertaining to bruising of the skin.

purulent Full of pus; having the character of pus.

purulent exudates Discharge that contains pus.

push-to-talk Commonly abbreviated as PTT, a method for communicating on a half-duplex communications system by pushing a button on the communication device to send and releasing the button to receive.

pyelonephritis Inflammation of the kidney linings.

pylorus A circumferential muscle at the end of the stomach that acts as a valve between the stomach and duodenum.

pyriform fossae Two pockets of tissue on the lateral borders of the larynx.

pyrogenic reaction A reaction characterized by an abrupt temperature elevation (as high as 41°C) with severe chills, backache, headache, weakness, nausea, and vomiting; a potential complication of IV or IO therapy.

pyrogens Chemicals or proteins that travel to the brain and affect the hypothalamus, and stimulate a rise in the body's core temperature.

QRS complex Deflections of the ECG produced by ventricular depolarization.

quadriplegia Paralysis of all four extremities and the trunk.

qualitative   A type of descriptive statistic in research that does not use numerical information.

quantitative   A type of measurement in research that uses a mean, median, and mode.

rabies   A fatal infection of the central nervous system caused by a bite from an animal that has been infected with the rabies virus.

raccoon or panda eyes   Bruising under or around the orbits that is commonly seen following a basilar skull fracture; also called periorbital ecchymosis.

radial artery   The artery pertaining to the wrist.

radiation   Emission of heat from an object into surrounding, colder air.

radioactive material   Any material that emits radiation.

radiological dispersal device (RDD)   Any container that is designed to disperse radioactive material.

radiopaque   Feature of an IV cannula (or any other object) that allows it to appear on an x-ray.

radius   The bone on the thumb side of the forearm.

rales   Old terminology for abnormal breath sounds that have a fine, crackling quality; now called crackles.

randomly   A way of choosing subjects for a research project without specific reasons.

range of motion (ROM)   The arc of movement of an extremity at a joint in a particular direction.

rape   Sexual intercourse inflicted forcibly on another person, against that person's will.

rapid trauma assessment   A unique and specialized assessment performed between the initial assessment and the focused physical examination of a trauma patient, usually on patients with a significant mechanism of injury, assessing specific parts of the entire body.

rapid-sequence intubation (RSI)   A specific set of procedures, combined in rapid succession, to induce sedation and paralysis and intubate a patient quickly.

rappelling   To descend on a fixed rope.

reactive airway disease   A term used to describe any condition that causes hyperreactive bronchioles and bronchospasm.

recall   The ability to retrieve a specific piece of stored information on demand.

recanalization   The opening up of new channels through a blocked artery.

receptive aphasia   Damage to or loss of the ability to understand speech.

receptors   Specialized areas in tissues that initiate certain actions after specific stimulation.

reciprocity   The process of granting licensing or certification to a provider from another province or agency.

recognition   The ability to identify information that one has encountered before.

recovery position   Left-lateral recumbent position; used in all semiconscious and unconscious nontrauma patients, who are able to maintain their own airway spontaneously and are breathing adequately.

recruitment   The process of signaling additional muscle fibres to contract to create a more forceful contraction.

referred pain   Pain that originates in one area of the body but is interpreted as coming from a different area of the body.

reflexes   Involuntary motor responses to specific sensory stimuli, such as a tap on the knee or stroking the eyelash.

refractory period   A short period immediately after depolarization in which the myocytes are not yet repolarized and are unable to fire or conduct an impulse.

regional anesthesia   A type of anesthesia that focuses on a particular portion of the body, such as the legs or the arms.

registration   Giving information that will be stored in some form of record book or the ability to add new items to the cerebral data bank.

regression   A return to more childish behaviour while under stress.

rehabilitation officer   In incident command, the person who establishes an area that provides protection for responders from the elements and the situation.

relative refractory period   That period in the cell-firing cycle at which it is possible but difficult to restimulate the cell to fire another impulse.

renal columns   Inward extensions of cortical tissue that surround the renal pyramids.

renal dialysis   A technique for "filtering" the blood of its toxic wastes, removing excess fluids, and restoring the normal balance of electrolytes.

renal fascia   Dense, fibrous connective tissue that anchors the kidney to the abdominal wall.

renal pelvis   Part of the internal anatomy of the kidney; a flat, funnel-shaped tube filling the sinus at the level of the hilus.

renal pyramids   Parallel cone-shaped bundles of urine-collecting tubules that are located in the medulla of the kidneys.

renin   A hormone produced by cells in the juxtaglomerular apparatus when the blood pressure is low.

renin-angiotensin-aldosterone system (RAAS)   A complex feedback mechanism responsible for the kidney's regulation of sodium in the body.

repeater   Miniature transmitter that picks up a radio signal and rebroadcasts it, extending the range of a radio communications system.

reperfusion   The resumption of blood flow through an artery.

rescue officer   In incident command, the person appointed to determine the type of equipment and resources needed for a situation involving extrication or special rescue; also called the extrication officer.

research ethics board (REB)   A group or institution that follows a set of requirements for ethical review of a research protocol or project, initially devised by the Medical Research Council of Canada.

reservoir   In the context of communicable disease, a place where organisms may live and multiply.

residual volume   The air that remains in the lungs after maximal expiration.

resistance vessels   The smallest arterioles.

respiration   The exchange of gases between a living organism and its environment.

respiratory arrest   The absence of respirations with detectable cardiac activity.

respiratory distress   A clinical state characterized by increased respiratory rate, effort, and work of breathing.

respiratory exposure   Exposure of the airways and lungs to a gas or vapour.

respiratory failure   A clinical state of inadequate oxygenation, ventilation, or both.

respiratory syncytial virus (RSV)   A labile paramyxovirus that produces its characteristic fusion of human cells in a tissue culture known as the syncytial effect. Two subtypes, A and B, have been identified. RSV can affect both the upper and lower respiratory tracts but is more prevalent with the lower, causing pneumonias and bronchiolitis.

restlessness   A situation in which the patient can't sit still.

rest tremors   Tremors that occur when the body part is not in motion.

retardation of thought   The patient seems to take a very long time to get from one thought to the next.

retention   The ability to store items in an accessible place in the mind.

reticular activating system (RAS)   Located in the upper brain stem; responsible for maintenance of consciousness, specifically one's level of arousal.

reticuloendothelial system   The system in the body that is primarily used to defend against infection.

retina   A delicate 10-layered structure of nervous tissue located in the rear of the interior of the globe that receives light and generates nerve signals that are transmitted to the brain through the optic nerve.

retinal detachment   Separation of the inner layers of the retina from the underlying choroid, the vascular membrane that nourishes the retina.

retinopathy of prematurity   A disease of the eye that affects prematurely born babies, thought to be caused by disorganized growth of retinal blood vessels resulting in scarring and retinal detachment; can lead to blindness in serious cases.

retractions   Physical drawing in of the chest wall between the ribs that occurs with increased work of breathing.

retrograde amnesia   Loss of memory relating to events that occurred before the injury.

retroperitoneal space   The area in the abdomen containing the aorta, vena cava, pancreas, kidneys, ureters, and portions of the duodenum and large intestine.

retrospective research Research performed from current available information.

retrosternal Situated or occurring behind the sternum.

review of systems A systematic survey of the patient's symptoms according to the major organ systems.

Rh factor A protein found on the red blood cells of most people; when a woman without this protein is impregnated by a man with this protein, the woman's body can create antibodies against the protein and attack future pregnancies.

rhabdomyolysis The destruction of muscle tissue leading to a release of potassium and myoglobin.

rheumatoid arthritis (RA) An inflammatory disorder that affects the entire body and leads to degeneration and deformation of joints.

rhonchi Rattling respiratory sounds that may resemble snoring; also called crackles.

rhonchus A coarse, low-pitched breath sound heard in patients who have chronic mucus in the airways (plural: rhonchi).

ribonucleic acid (RNA) Nucleic acid associated with controlling cellular activities.

ricin Neurotoxin derived from mash that is left from pressing oil from the castor bean; causes pulmonary edema and respiratory and circulatory failure, leading to death.

right atrium The upper right chamber of the heart; receives blood from the venae cavae and supplies blood to the right ventricle.

right ventricle The lower right chamber of the heart; receives blood from the right atrium and pumps blood out through the pulmonic valve into the pulmonary artery.

risk factors Characteristics of people, behaviours, or environments that increase the chances of disease or injury. Some examples are alcohol use, poverty, or gender.

rocuronium A nondepolarizing neuromuscular blocking agent; used to maintain paralysis following succinylcholine-facilitated intubation; also called Zemuron.

Rohypnol A benzodiazepine used to facilitate date rape and that can create memory loss; street names include roofies, roof, roachies, rocha, and Mexican Valium.

rooting reflex An infant reflex that occurs when something touches an infant's cheek, and the infant instinctively turns his or her head toward the touch.

rotation-flexion injury A type of injury typically resulting from high acceleration forces; can result in a stable unilateral facet dislocation in the cervical spine.

round bones The small bones that are found adjacent to joints that assist with motion.

route of exposure Manner by which a toxic substance enters the body.

routine practices Term used to describe infection control practices that merge aspects of universal precautions and body substance isolation and that relies on knowledge of signs and symptoms and communicable disease modes of transmission rather than diagnosis.

R-R interval The period between the onset of one QRS complex and the onset of the next QRS complex.

rubella A viral disease similar to measles, best known by the distinctive red rash on the skin. It is not nearly as infectious or severe as measles.

rubor Redness; one of the classic signs of inflammation.

rubs Lung sound produced by a partial loss of intrapleural integrity, when an abnormal collection of fluid has accumulated between a portion of the visceral and parietal pleura, resulting in "pleuritic" pain and a perceived rub on auscultation.

rule of nines A system that assigns percentages to sections of the body, allowing calculation of the amount of skin surface involved in the burn area.

rule of palm A system that estimates total body surface area burned by comparing the affected area with the size of the patient's palm, which is roughly equal to 1% of the patient's total body surface area.

rule of thumb A reminder of the proper distance from a hazardous materials scene; the entire scene should be hidden by a thumb held at arm's length.

ruptured ovarian cyst A fluid-filled sac within the ovary that bursts from internal pressure.

ST segment The interval between the end of the QRS complex and the beginning of the T wave; often elevated or depressed with respect to the isoelectric line when there is significant myocardial ischemia.

sacroiliac joints The points of attachment of the *ilium* to the sacrum.

safe residual pressure A term that implies that it is *unsafe* to continue using an oxygen cylinder with a pressure of less than 200 psi.

safety officer In incident command, the person who gives the "go ahead" to a plan or who may stop an operation when rescuer safety is an issue.

sagittal suture The point of the skull where the parietal bones join.

saline locks Special types of IV devices that eliminate the need to hang a bag of IV fluid; also called a buff cap or INT (intermittent); commonly used for patients who do not require fluid boluses but may require medication therapy.

sampling errors Expected errors that occur in the sampling phase of research.

sarin (GB) A nerve agent that is one of the G agents; a highly volatile colourless and odourless liquid that turns from liquid to gas within seconds to minutes at room temperature.

saturation diving A type of diving in which the diver remains at depth for prolonged periods.

scabies An infestation of the skin with the mite *Sarcoptes scabei*. It spreads rapidly when there is skin-to-skin contact.

scald burn A burn produced by hot liquids.

scaphoid A concave shape of the abdomen. This can be caused by evisceration.

scaphoid (bone) The wrist bone that is found just beyond that most distal portion of the radius.

scapula A large, flat, triangular bone along the posterior thorax that articulates with the clavicle and humerus.

scar revision A surgical procedure to improve the appearance of a scar, reestablish function, or correct disfigurement from soft-tissue damage, surgical incision, or lesion.

scene assessment A quick assessment of the scene and its surroundings made to provide information about scene safety and the mechanism of injury or nature of illness, before you enter and begin patient care.

school age A person who is 6 to 12 years of age.

sclera The white part of the eye.

scoliosis Sideways curvature of the spine.

scope of practice What a province permits a paramedic practicing under its license or certification to do.

scrambling A method used to ascend rocky faces and ridges and can be considered a cross between hill climbing and rock climbing.

search and rescue (SAR) The process of locating and removing a patient from the wilderness.

sebaceous gland A gland located in the dermis that secretes sebum.

sebum An oily substance secreted by sebaceous glands.

second stage of labour The stage of labour in which the baby's head enters the birth canal, during which contractions become more intense and more frequent.

secondary apnea When asphyxia continues after primary apnea, infant responds with a period of gasping respirations, falling pulse rate, and falling blood pressure.

secondary brain injury The "after effects" of the primary injury; includes abnormal processes such as cerebral edema, increased intracranial pressure, cerebral ischemia and hypoxia, and infection; onset is often delayed following the primary brain injury.

secondary collapse A collapse that occurs following the primary collapse. This can occur in trench, excavation, and structural collapses.

secondary contamination Exposure to a hazardous material by contact with a contaminated person or object.

secondary device Additional explosives used by terrorists, which are set to explode after the initial bomb.

secondary exit Any other means of egress, including windows and rear doors.

secondary injury prevention Reducing the effects of an injury that has already happened.

secondary response The body's reaction when it is exposed to an antigen for which it already has antibodies, in which it responds by killing the invading substance.

secondary spinal cord injury Injury to the spinal cord, thought to be the result of multiple factors that result in a progression of inflammatory responses from primary spinal cord injury.

secondary triage A type of patient sorting used in the treatment sector that involves retriage of patients.

secretory phase The second phase of the menstrual cycle.

secure attachment A bond between an infant and his or her parent or caregiver, in which the infant understands that his or her parents or caregivers will be responsive to his or her needs and take care of him or her when help is needed.

sedation Reduction of a patient's anxiety, induction of amnesia, and suppression of the gag reflex.

sedative-hypnotic A drug used to reduce anxiety, calm agitated patients, and help produce drowsiness and sleep (CNS depressants).

segmental fracture A bone that is broken in more than one place.

seizure A paroxysmal alteration in neurologic function, ie, behavioural and/or autonomic function.

selective serotonin reuptake inhibitors (SSRIs) A class of antidepressants that inhibit the reuptake of serotonin.

self-contained underwater breathing apparatus The expansion of the acronym (SCUBA) for specialized underwater breathing equipment.

self-rescue position Position used in fast-moving water rescue situations. The rescuer rolls into a face-up arched position with the lower back higher than the feet to avoid objects below the surface. The feet should be together and facing in the direction of travel (feet first), with arms at the sides.

self-sealing blood tubes Glass tubes with self-sealing rubber caps; used to obtain blood samples for laboratory analysis.

Sellick maneuver The application of posterior pressure to the cricoid cartilage to minimize the risk of regurgitation during positive-pressure ventilation; also referred to as cricoid pressure.

semilunar valves The two valves, the aortic and pulmonic, that divide the heart from the aorta and pulmonary arteries.

sensitivity The ability to recognize a foreign substance the next time it is encountered.

sensitization Developing sensitivity to a substance that initially caused no allergic reaction.

sensorineural deafness A permanent lack of hearing caused by a lesion or damage of the inner ear.

sepsis A pathologic state, usually in a febrile patient, resulting from the presence of invading microorganisms or their toxic products in the bloodstream.

septic abortion A life-threatening emergency in which the uterus becomes infected following any type of abortion.

septic shock Shock that occurs as a result of widespread infection, usually bacterial. Untreated, the result is multiple organ dysfunction syndrome (MODS) and often death.

seropositive Having a positive blood test for an infectious agent, such as HIV or hepatitis B or C virus.

serosa The outermost layer of tissue in the fallopian tubes.

serotonin A vasoactive amine that increases vascular permeability to cause vasodilation.

serotonin syndrome An idiosyncratic complication that occurs with antidepressant therapy in which patients have lower extremity muscle rigidity, confusion or disorientation, and/or agitation.

serous exudates Discharge that contains serum, a thin watery substance.

serum sickness A condition in which antigen antibody complexes formed in the bloodstream deposit in sites around the body, most notably in the kidney, with resultant inflammatory reactions.

severe acute respiratory syndrome (SARS) Potentially life-threatening viral infection that usually starts with flu-like symptoms.

sexual assault An attack against a person that is sexual in nature, the most common of which is rape.

sexually transmitted diseases (STDs) A group of diseases usually acquired by sexual contact, and which include gonorrhea, syphilis, chlamydia, scabies, pubic lice, herpes, hepatitis, and HIV infection.

shaken baby syndrome A syndrome seen in maltreated infants and children; the patient has been subjected to violent, whiplash-type shaking injuries inflicted by the abusing individual that may cause coma, seizures, and increased intracranial pressure due to tearing of the cerebral veins with consequent bleeding into the brain.

shallow water blackout A diving emergency that occurs when a person hyperventilates just before submerging underwater and loses consciousness before resurfacing due to hypoxemia and cerebral vasoconstriction.

sharps Any contaminated item that can cause injury; includes IV needles and cannulas, broken ampules or vials, or anything else that can penetrate or lacerate the skin.

shearing An applied force or pressure exerted against the surface and layers of the skin as tissues slide in opposite but parallel planes.

Shiley A type of tracheostomy tube.

shock An abnormal state associated with inadequate oxygen and nutrient delivery to the metabolic apparatus of the cell.

shoring A method of supporting a trench wall or building components such as walls, floors, or ceilings using either hydraulic, pneumatic, or wood shoring systems. Shoring is used to prevent collapse.

short bones The bones that are nearly as wide as they are long.

shoulder dystocia A condition in which the infant becomes trapped in between the symphysis pubis and sacrum because its shoulders are larger than its head.

shunt Situation in which a portion of the output of the right side of the heart reaches the left side of the heart without being oxygenated in the lungs; may be caused by atelectasis, pulmonary edema, or a variety of other conditions. In hemodialysis, an anastomosis between a peripheral artery and vein.

sickle cell disease A disease that causes red blood cells to be misshapen, resulting in poor oxygen-carrying capability and potentially resulting in lodging of the red blood cells in blood vessels or the spleen.

side effects Reactions that can manifest as signs or symptoms that are not desired but are expected based on how the medication works.

signs Indications of illness or injury that the examiner can see, hear, feel, smell, and so on.

silver fork deformity The dorsal deformity of the forearm that results from a Colles fracture.

simple face mask A full mask enclosure with open side ports. Room air is drawn in through the side ports on inhalation, diluting the concentration of inspired oxygen. Exhaled air is vented through holes on each side of the mask. The simple face mask will deliver between 40% and 60% oxygen at 10 l/min.

simple febrile seizures A brief, self-limited, generalized seizure in a previously healthy child between the ages of 6 months and 6 years that is associated with the onset of or sudden increase in fever.

simple partial seizures Focal seizures that involve a motor or sensory abnormality in a patient who remains conscious.

simple phobia A fear that is focused on one class of objects (eg, mice, spiders, dogs) or situations (eg, high places, darkness, flying).

simplex Method of radio communication using a single frequency that enables transmission or reception of voice or an ECG signal but is incapable of simultaneous transmission and reception.

single command system A command system in which one person is in charge, generally used with small incidents that involve only one responding agency or one jurisdiction.

sinoatrial (SA) node The dominant pacemaker of the heart, located at the junction of the superior vena cava and the right atrium.

sinus arrhythmia A slight irregularity of the heart rate caused by changes in parasympathetic tone during breathing.

sinus bradycardia A sinus rhythm with a heart rate less than 60 beats/min.

sinus tachycardia A sinus rhythm with a heart rate greater than 100 beats/min.

sinuses Cavities formed by the cranial bones that trap contaminants from entering the respiratory tract and act as tributaries for fluid to and from the eustachian tubes and tear ducts.

skeletal muscle Muscle that is attached to bones and usually crosses at least one joint; striated or voluntary muscle.

skeletal muscle relaxants Medications that provide relief of skeletal muscle spasms.

skull The structure at the top of the axial skeleton that houses the brain and consists of 28 bones that comprise the auditory ossicles, the cranium, and the face.

slander Verbally making a false statement that injures a person's good name.

slow-reacting substances of anaphylaxis (SRS-A) Biologically active compounds derived from arachidonic acid called leukotrienes.

SLUDGE An mnemonic that stands for salivation, lacrimation, urination, defecation, gastrointestinal distress, and emesis, which are the signs and symptoms that can be produced by exposure to organophosphate and carbamate pesticides or other nerve-stimulating agents.

small for gestational age An infant whose size and weight are considerably less than the average for babies of the same age.

smallpox A highly contagious disease; it is most contagious when blisters begin to form.

smooth muscle Nonstriated involuntary muscle found in vessel walls, glands, and the gastrointestinal tract.

sniffing position An upright position in which the patient's head and chin are thrust slightly forward to keep the airway open; appears to be sniffing.

snoring Noise made on inhalation when the upper airway is partially obstructed by the tongue.

snuffbox The region at the base of the thumb where the scaphoid may be palpated.

sodium channel blockers Antiarrhythmic medications that slow conduction through the heart.

sodium-potassium (Na+-K+) pump The mechanism by which the cell brings in two potassium (K+) ions and releases three sodium (Na+) ions.

solute The dissolved particles contained in the solvent.

solution A liquid containing one or more chemical substances entirely dissolved, usually in water.

solvent The fluid that does the dissolving, or the solution that contains the dissolved components.

soman (GD) A nerve agent that is one of the G agents; twice as persistent as sarin and five times as lethal; it has a fruity odour as a result of the type of alcohol used in the agent, and is both a contact and inhalation hazard that can enter the body through skin absorption and through the respiratory tract.

somatic motor neurons The nerve fibres that transmit impulses to a muscle.

somatoform disorder A condition in which a person is overly concerned with physical health and appearance to the point that it dominates his or her life; an example is hypochondria.

source individual Any individual, living or dead, whose blood or other potentially infectious materials may be a source of occupational exposure to the member/volunteer. Examples include, but are not limited to, hospital and clinic patients; clients in institutions for the developmentally disabled; trauma victims; clients of drug and alcohol treatment facilities; residents of hospices and nursing homes; human remains; and individuals who donate or sell blood or blood components.

spacer A device that collects medication as it is released from the canister of a metered-dose inhaler, allowing more to be delivered to the lungs and less to be lost to the environment.

spalling Delaminating or breaking off into chips and pieces.

span of control In incident command, the subordinate positions under the commander's direction to which the workload is distributed; the supervisor/worker ratio.

Special Atomic Demolition Munitions (SADM) Small suitcase-sized nuclear weapons that were designed to destroy individual targets, such as important buildings, bridges, tunnels, or large ships.

specific agents Medications that bring about an identifiable mechanism with unique receptors for the agent.

specific exemptions Limited circumstances when an emergency vehicle operator can exceed the posted signage or speed limit.

specific gravity The measure that indicates whether or not a material will sink or float in water.

spina bifida The most common permanently disabling birth defect in which, during the first month of pregnancy, the spinal column of the fetus does not close properly or completely and vertebrae do not develop, leaving a portion of the spinal cord exposed.

spinal cord The part of the central nervous system that extends downward from the brain through the foramen magnum and is protected by the spine.

spinal shock The temporary local neurologic condition that occurs immediately after spinal trauma; swelling and edema of the spinal cord begin immediately after injury, with severe pain and potential paralysis.

spiral fracture A break in a bone that appears like a spring on a radiograph.

spirits A preparation of a volatile substance dissolved in alcohol.

spoil pile The pile of dirt that has been removed from an excavation. The pile may be unstable and prone to collapse.

spondylosis Immobility and consolidation of a vertebral joint.

spontaneous abortion Expulsion of the fetus that occurs naturally; also called miscarriage.

sprains Injuries, including a stretch or a tear, to the ligaments of a joint that commonly lead to pain and swelling.

stable angina Angina pectoris characterized by periodic pain with a predictable pattern.

staging officer In incident command, the person who locates an area to stage equipment and personnel and tracks unit arrival and deployment from the staging area.

standard deviation In research this outlines how much change from the mean is expected.

standard of care What a reasonable paramedic with training would do in the same or a similar situation.

standard precautions The new term used to describe the infection control practices that will reduce the opportunity for exposure of providers in the daily care of patients.

standing order A form of off-line or indirect medical control; a written document signed by the EMS system's medical director that outlines specific directions, permissions, and sometimes prohibitions regarding patient care that is rendered prior to contacting direct medical control.

Staphylococcus aureus A strain of bacteria that became resistant to the drug methicillin, creating a new strain called methicillin-resistant *Staphylococcus aureus*; symptoms include infection and possibly localized skin abscesses and cellulites, empyemas, and endocarditis.

START triage A patient sorting process that stands for Simple Triage And Rapid Treatment and uses a limited assessment of the patient's ability to walk, respiratory status, hemodynamic status, and neurologic status.

state-sponsored terrorism Terrorism that is funded and/or supported by nations that hold close ties with terrorist groups.

status asthmaticus A severe, prolonged asthma attack that cannot be broken with epinephrine.

status epilepticus A state of continuous seizures or multiple seizures without a return to consciousness for 20 minutes.

steam burn A burn that has been caused by direct exposure to hot steam exhaust, as from a broken pipe.

steatorrhea Foamy, fatty stools caused by liver failure or gallbladder problems.

steering play A sensation of looseness or sloppiness in a vehicle's steering.

steering pull A drift that is persistent enough so an operator can feel a tug on the steering wheel.

stem cells Cells that can develop into other types of cells in the body.

stenosis Narrowing.

step blocks Specialized cribbing assemblies made out of wood or plastic blocks in a step configuration.

stereotyped activity Repetitive movements that don't appear to serve any purpose.

sterile The destruction of all living organisms; achieved by using heat, gas, or chemicals.

sternum Also known as the breastbone, this bony structure along the midline of the thorax provides a point of anterior attachment for the thoracic cage.

stimulants An agent that increases the level of body activity.

stoma A small opening, especially an artificially created opening, such as that made by tracheostomy.

straddle fracture A fracture of the pelvis that results from landing on the perineal region.

straight laryngoscope blade Also called the Miller blade; designed to lift the epiglottis and expose the vocal cords.

strain Stretching or tearing of a muscle by excessive stretching or overuse.

strategic deployment The staging of ambulances to strategic locations within a service area to allow for coverage of emergency calls.

stratum basalis A permanent mucous membrane that makes up part of the outer endometrium.

stratum functionalis An inner mucous membrane that makes up part of the endometrium, and which is renewed following menstruation.

stress A nonspecific response of the body to any demand made upon it.

stress fracture A fracture that results from exaggerated stress on the bone caused by unusually rapid muscle development.

stressor Any agent or situation that causes stress.

striae Stretch marks on the abdomen caused by size changes.

striated muscle Skeletal muscle that is under voluntary control.

stridor A harsh, high-pitched, crowing inspiratory sound, such as the sound often heard in acute laryngeal obstruction.

stroke volume (SV) The volume of blood pumped forward with each ventricular contraction.

stylet A semirigid wire that is inserted into the ET tube to mould and maintain the shape of the tube.

subarachnoid hemorrhage Bleeding into the subarachnoid space, where the cerebrospinal fluid (CSF) circulates.

subarachnoid space The space located between the pia mater and the arachnoid mater.

subclavian artery The artery that travels from the aorta to each upper extremity.

subconjunctival hematoma The collection of blood within the sclera of the eye, presenting as a bright red patch of blood over the sclera but not involving the cornea.

subcutaneous (SC) Beneath the skin.

subcutaneous emphysema A physical finding of air within the subcutaneous tissue.

subcutaneous (SC or SQ) route A medication route in which injections are given beneath the skin into the fat or connective tissue immediately underlying it.

subdural hematoma An accumulation of blood beneath the dura but outside the brain.

subglottic space The narrowest part of the pediatric airway.

sublingual (SL) A medication route in which medication is administered under the tongue.

subluxation A partial or incomplete dislocation.

substance abuse Use of a substance that disrupts activities of daily living.

substance dependence Use of a substance that results in addiction and physiologic dependence on the substance.

substance intoxication Use of a substance that results in impaired thinking and motor function.

substance use Use of moderate amounts of a substance without seriously affecting activities of daily living.

substitute decision maker A person designated by a patient (or by default depending on law in a given practice jurisdiction) to make health care decisions for that person when he or she is unable to do so.

subthalamus The part of the diencephalon that is involved in controlling motor functions.

succinylcholine chloride A depolarizing neuromuscular blocker frequently used as the initial paralytic during rapid-sequence intubation; causes muscle fasciculations; also referred to as Anectine.

sucking reflex An infant reflex in which the infant starts sucking when his or her lips are stroked.

sudden infant death syndrome (SIDS) The abrupt and unexplained death of an apparently healthy child younger than 1 year.

suicide Any willful act designed to bring an end to one's own life.

sulfur mustard (H) A vesicant; it is a brownish-yellowish oily substance that is generally considered very persistent; has the distinct smell of garlic or mustard and, when released, it is quickly absorbed into the skin and/or mucous membranes and begins an irreversible process of damaging the cells.

summation effect The process whereby multiple medications can produce a response that the individual medications alone do not produce.

superficial burn A burn involving only the epidermis, producing very red, painful skin; previously called a first-degree burn.

superficial frostbite A type of frostbite characterized by altered sensation (numbness, tingling, or burning) and white, waxy skin that is firm to palpation, but the underlying tissues remain soft.

supination To turn the forearm laterally so that the palm faces forward (if standing) or upward (if lying supine).

supine hypotensive syndrome Low blood pressure resulting from compression of the inferior vena cava by the weight of the pregnant uterus when the mother is supine.

suppository A drug mixed in a firm base that melts at body temperature and is shaped to fit the rectum, urethra, or vagina.

supracondylar fractures Fractures of the distal humerus that occur just proximal to the elbow.

supraglottic Located above the glottic opening, as in the upper airway structures.

suprapubic The region of the abdomen superior to the pubic bone and inferior to the umbilicus.

suprasternal notch The indentation formed by the superior border of the manubrium and the clavicles, often used as a landmark for procedures such as subclavian vein access.

supraventricular tachycardia (SVT) An abnormal heart rhythm with a rapid, narrow QRS complex.

surface-tended diving A type of diving in which air is piped to the diver through a tube from the surface.

surfactant A liquid protein substance that coats the alveoli in the lungs, decreases alveolar surface tension, and keeps the alveoli expanded; a low level in a premature baby contributes to respiratory distress syndrome.

surrogate decision maker A person designated by a patient to make health care decisions for them when they are unable to make decisions for themselves.

suspension A preparation of a finely divided drug intended to be (or already) incorporated in a suitable liquid.

sympathetic blocking agent An antihypertensive medication that decreases cardiac output and rennin secretions.

sympathetic eye movement The movement of both eyes in unison.

sympathetic nervous system Subdivision of the autonomic nervous system that governs the body's fight-or-flight reactions by inducing smooth muscle contraction or relaxation of the blood vessels and bronchioles.

sympathomimetics The medications administered to stimulate the sympathetic nervous system.

symptoms The pain, discomfort, or other abnormality that the patient feels.

synapses Gaps between nerve cells across which nervous stimuli are transmitted.

synchronized cardioversion The timed delivery of energy into the myocardium to correct rapid, regular cardiac rhythms in patients who are in unstable condition.

syncopal episodes Fainting; brief losses of consciousness caused by transiently inadequate blood flow to the brain.

syncope Fainting; brief loss of consciousness caused by transiently inadequate blood flow to the brain.

syndromic surveillance The monitoring, usually by local or provincial health departments, of patients presenting to emergency departments and alternative care facilities, the recording of EMS call volume, and the use of over-the-counter medications.

synergism An interaction of two or more medications that results in an effect that is greater than the sum of their effects if taken independently.

synovial joints Joints that permit movement of the component bones.

synovial membrane The lining of a joint that secretes synovial fluid into the joint space.

syphilis A sexually transmitted disease caused by the spiral-shaped bacteria *Treponema pallidum* and whose signs and symptoms include an ulcerative lesion or chancre of the skin or mucous membrane at the site of infection, commonly in the genital region.

syrup A drug suspended in sugar and water to improve its taste.

systematic sampling A computer-generated list of subjects or groups for research.

systemic anesthesia A type of anesthesia often done through the inhalation of volatile vapourized liquids and predominantly reserved for operating room use; also called general anesthesia.

systemic circulation The flow of blood from the left ventricle through the aorta, to all of its branches and capillaries in the tissues, and back to the right atrium through the venules, veins, and venae cavae; also called the greater circulation.

systemic complications Reactions that affect systems of the body.

systemic effect A physiologic effect on the entire body or one of the body's systems.

systemic inflammatory response syndrome (SIRS) The systemic inflammatory response to a variety of severe clinical insults.

systemic reaction A reaction that occurs throughout the body, possibly affecting multiple body systems.

systole The period during which the ventricles contract.

T killer cells Cells released during a type IV allergic reaction that kill antigen-bearing target cells.

T wave The upright, flat, or inverted wave following the QRS complex of the ECG, representing ventricular repolarization.

tablet A powdered drug that has been moulded or compressed into a small disk.

tabun (GA) A nerve agent that is one of the G agents; is 36 times more persistent than sarin and approximately half as lethal; has a fruity smell and is unique because the components used to manufacture the agent are easy to acquire and the agent is easy to manufacture.

tachycardia A rapid heart rate, more than 100 beats/min.

tachyphylaxis A condition in which the patient rapidly becomes tolerant to a medication.

tactical paramedics Specially trained medics who provide prehospital care of barricaded patients, patients being held hostage, and other special operations.

tactile fremitus Vibrations in the chest as the patient breathes.

talus The bone of the foot that articulates with the tibia.

tangential thinking Leaving the current topic midconversation to talk about something else, inhibiting interpersonal communication.

target tissues Tissues to which hormones are directed to act on.

tarsals The ankle bones.

technical rescue incident (TRI) A complex rescue incident involving vehicles or machinery, water or ice, rope techniques, a trench or excavation collapse, confined spaces, a structural collapse, wilderness search and rescue, or hazardous materials, and which requires specially trained personnel and special equipment.

technical rescue team A group of rescuers specially trained in the various disciplines of technical rescue.

Technician Level This training level, also called EMS/HM Level II Responder, allows paramedics to perform prehospital care activities in the warm zone at a hazardous materials incident, working with patients who may still present a significant risk of secondary contamination.

tempered glass A type of safety glass that is heat-treated so that it will break into small pieces.

temporal lobe The portion of the brain that has an important role in hearing and memory.

temporomandibular joint (TMJ) The joint between the temporal bone and the posterior condyle that allows for movements of the mandible.

ten-code A radio code system using the number 10 plus another number.

tendinitis Inflammation of a tendon that most commonly results from overuse.

tendons The fibrous portions of muscle that attach to bone.

tension lines The pattern of tautness of the skin, which is arranged over body structures and affects how well wounds heal.

tension pneumothorax A life-threatening collection of air within the pleural space; the volume and pressure have both collapsed the involved lung and caused a shift of the mediastinal structures to the opposite side.

tenting A condition in which the skin slowly retracts after being pinched and pulled away slightly from the body; a sign of dehydration.

tentorium A structure that separates the cerebral hemispheres from the cerebellum and brain stem.

term Used to describe an infant delivered at 37 to 42 weeks of gestation.

terminal drop hypothesis The theory that a person's mental function declines in the last 5 years of life.

terminal illness A sickness that the patient cannot be cured of; death is imminent.

termination of action The amount of time after the medication's concentration falls below the minimum effective level until it is eliminated from the body.

termination of command The end of the incident command structure when an incident draws to a close.

terrorism A violent act dangerous to human life, to intimidate or coerce a government, the civilian population or any segment thereof, in furtherance of political or social objectives.

testes Male gonads located in the scrotum that produce hormones called androgens.

testimonial evidence The oral documentation by a witness of the facts of a criminal act.

testosterone The most important androgen in men.

tetanus A disease caused by spores that enter the body through a puncture wound contaminated with animal feces, street dust, or soil, or which can enter through contaminated street drugs, and whose signs and symptoms include pain at the wound site and painful muscle contractions in the neck and trunk muscles.

thalamus The part of the diencephalon that processes most sensory input and influences mood and general body movements, especially those associated with fear or rage.

thalassemia A type of anemia in which not enough hemoglobin is produced, or the hemoglobin is defective.

theophylline A naturally occurring alkaloid found in a variety of plants (such as tea leaves).

therapeutic The desired or intended action of a medication.

therapeutic index The ratio of a drug's lethal dose for 50% (LD_{50}) of the population to its effective dose for 50% (ED_{50}) of the population; a medication's margin of safety.

therapy regulator Attaches to the stem of the oxygen cylinder, and reduces the high pressure of gas to a safe range (about 50 psi).

thermal burn An injury caused by radiation or direct contact with a heat source on the skin.

thermogenesis The production of heat in the body.

thermolysis The liberation of heat from the body.

thermoregulation The process by which the body maintains temperature through a combination of heat gain by metabolic processes and muscular movement and heat loss through respiration, evaporation, conduction, convection, and perspiration.

thiazides A type of diuretic medication that specifically controls the sodium and water quantities excreted by the kidneys.

third spacing The shifting of fluid into the tissues, creating edema.

third stage of labour The stage of labour in which the placenta is expelled.

Thompson test Squeezing of the calf muscle to evaluate for plantar flexion of the foot to determine whether the Achilles tendon is intact.

thoracic inlet The superior aspect of the thoracic cavity, this ring-like opening is created by the first vertebral vertebra, the first rib, the clavicles, and the manubrium.

thorax The part of the body between the neck and the diaphragm, encased by the ribs.

thought broadcasting The belief that others can hear one's thoughts.

thought control The belief that outside forces are controlling one's thoughts.

thought insertion The belief that thoughts are being thrust into one's mind by another person.

thought withdrawal The belief that thoughts are being removed from one's mind.

threatened abortion Expulsion of the fetus that is attempting to take place but has not occurred yet; usually occurs in the first trimester.

threshold limit value (TLV) The concentration of a substance that is supposed to be safe for exposure no more than 8 hours per day and 40 hours per week.

threshold limit value ceiling level (TLV-CL) The concentration that a person should never be exposed to.

threshold limit value short-term exposure limit (TLV-STEL) The concentration of a substance that a worker can be exposed to for up to 15 minutes but no more than four times per day with at least an hour between each exposure.

thrombin An enzyme that causes the conversion of fibrinogen to fibrin, which binds to the platelet plugs, forming the final mature blood clot.

thrombocytes Platelets.

thrombocytopenia Reduction in the number of platelets.

thromboembolic disease The condition in which a patient has a DVT or pulmonary embolism.

thrombophlebitis Inflammation of a vein.

through-the-needle cannulas Plastic cannulas inserted through a hollow needle; referred to as Intracaths.

thyroid Large gland located at the base of the neck that produces and excretes hormones that influence growth, development, and metabolism.

thyroid cartilage The main supporting cartilage of the larynx; a shield-shaped structure formed by two plates that join in a "V" shape anteriorly to form the laryngeal prominence known as the Adam's apple.

thyroid-stimulating hormone (TSH) Hormone that controls the release of thyroid hormone from the thyroid gland.

thyroid storm A rare, life-threatening condition that may occur in patients with thyrotoxicosis. The condition is usually triggered by a stressful event or increased volume of thyroid hormones in the circulation.

thyrotoxicosis A toxic condition caused by excessive levels of circulating thyroid hormone.

thyroxine The body's major metabolic hormone. Thyroxine stimulates energy production in cells, which increases the rate at which the cells consume oxygen and use carbohydrates, fats, and proteins.

tibia The shin bone.

tidal volume A measure of the depth of breathing; the volume of air that is inhaled or exhaled during a single respiratory cycle.

tincture A dilute alcoholic extract of a drug.

toddlers Persons who are 1 to 3 years of age.

tokolytics Drugs used to delay preterm labour.

tolerance Physiologic adaptation to the effects of a drug such that increasingly larger doses of the drug are required to achieve the same effect.

tongue-jaw lift maneuver A manual maneuver that involves grasping the tongue and jaw and lifting; commonly used to suction the airway and to place certain airway devices.

tonic activity Type of seizure movement involving the constant contraction and trembling of muscle groups.

tonic–clonic seizures Seizures that feature rhythmic back-and-forth motion of an extremity and body stiffness.

tonicity The osmotic pressure of a solution, based on the relationship between sodium and water inside and outside the cell, that takes advantage of their chemical and osmotic properties to move water to areas of higher sodium concentration.

tonsils Lymphatic tissues that are located in the posterior pharynx; they help to trap bacteria.

tonsil-tip catheter A hard or rigid suction catheter; also called a Yankauer catheter.

tort A wrongful act that gives rise to a civil suit.

torus fracture *See* buckle fracture.

total body surface area (TBSA) Used in the calculation of a burn injury to determine the percentage of the surface of the patient's body that has been injured. This is commonly estimated by using the rule of palm or the rule of nines.

total body water (TBW) Total amount of water in the human body; accounts for approximately 60% of the weight of an average man; divided into various compartments.

total laryngectomy Surgical removal of the entire larynx.

total lung capacity The total volume of air that the lungs can hold; approximately 6 l in the average adult male.

toxic shock syndrome (TSS) A form of septic shock caused by *Streptococcus pyogenes* (group A strep) or *Staphylococcus aureus;* initial symptoms include syncope, myalgia, diarrhea, vomiting, headache, fever, and sore throat.

toxicity levels Measures of the risk that a hazardous material poses to the health of an individual who comes into contact with it.

toxicologic emergencies Medical emergencies caused by toxic agents such as poison.

toxidrome The syndrome-like symptoms of a poisonous agent.

toxoid A modified bacterial toxin that has been made nontoxic but retains the ability to stimulate the formation of antibodies.

trachea The conduit for all entry into the lungs; a tubular structure that is approximately 10 to 12 cm in length and is composed of a series of C-shaped cartilaginous rings; also called the windpipe.

tracheal transection Traumatic separation of the trachea from the larynx.

tracheobronchial suctioning Passing a suction catheter into the endotracheal tube to remove pulmonary secretions.

tracheostomy Surgical opening into the trachea.

tracheostomy tube Plastic tube placed within the tracheostomy site (stoma).

track marks The visible scars from repeated cannulation of a vein; commonly associated with illicit drug use.

trade name The brand name registered to a specific manufacturer or owner; also called proprietary name.

transceiver A radio transmitter and receiver housed in a single unit; a two-way radio.

transdermal Across the skin; a medication delivery route.

transdermal route A medication route generally performed by placing medication directly onto the patient's skin.

transfer of command In incident command, when an incident commander turns over command to someone with more experience in a critical area.

transient ischemic attack (TIA) A disorder of the brain in which brain cells temporarily stop working because of insufficient oxygen, causing stroke-like symptoms that resolve completely within 24 hours of onset.

transillumination intubation Method of intubation that uses a lighted stylet to guide the endotracheal tube into the trachea.

translaryngeal cannula ventilation Used in conjunction with needle cricothyrotomy to ventilate a patient; requires a high-pressure jet ventilator.

transmission—airborne The spread of infection by droplet nuclei or dust through the air. Without the intervention of winds or drafts the distance over which airborne infection takes place is short (< 5 m).

transmission—droplet The direct dissemination of a pathogen from a reservoir to a susceptible host's conjunctiva, nose, or mouth by spray with relatively large, short-ranged (±1 m) aerosols produced by sneezing, coughing, or talking.

transmigration (diapedesis) The PMNs permeate through the vessel wall, moving into the interstitial space.

transportation officer In incident command, the person who coordinates transportation and distribution of patients to appropriate receiving hospitals.

transposition Congenital abnormality where the aorta and pulmonary artery positions on the heart are reversed.

transverse fracture A fracture that runs in a straight line from one edge of the bone to the other and that is perpendicular to each edge.

transverse presentation A delivery in which the fetus lies crosswise in the uterus; one hand may protrude through the vagina.

transverse spinous process The junction of each pedicle and lamina on each side of a vertebra; these project laterally and posteriorly and form points of attachment for muscles and ligaments.

trauma Acute physiologic and structural change that occurs in a victim as a result of the rapid dissipation of energy delivered by an external force.

traumatic asphyxia A pattern of injuries seen after a severe force is applied to the thorax, forcing blood from the great vessels and back into the head and neck.

traumatic brain injury (TBI) A traumatic insult to the brain capable of producing physical, intellectual, emotional, social, and vocational changes.

treatment officer In incident command, the person responsible for locating, setting up, and supervising the treatment area.

trench foot A process similar to frostbite but caused by prolonged exposure to cool, wet conditions.

triage To sort patients based on the severity of their conditions and prioritize them for care accordingly.

triage officer The person in charge of prioritizing patients, whose primary duty is to ensure that every patient receives initial triage.

trichomoniasis A parasitic infection.

tricuspid valve The valve between the right atrium and right ventricle of the heart.

tricyclic antidepressants (TCAs) A group of drugs used to treat severe depression and manage pain; minimal dosing errors can cause toxic results.

trigeminal nerve Fifth cranial nerve; supplies sensation to the scalp, forehead, face, and lower jaw and innervates the muscles of mastication, the throat, and the inner ear.

trigeminy A premature complex in every third heartbeat.

tripoding An abnormal position to keep the airway open; involves leaning forward onto two arms stretched forward.

trismus Clenched teeth caused by spasms of the jaw muscles; occurs during seizures and head injuries.

trunking Sharing of radio frequencies by multiple agencies or systems.

trust and mistrust A phrase that refers to a stage of development from birth to approximately 18 months of age, during which infants gain trust of their parents or caregivers if their world is planned, organized, and routine.

tuberculin skin test A test to determine if a person has ever been infected with tuberculosis.

tuberculosis (TB) A chronic bacterial disease caused by *Mycobacterium tuberculosis* that usually affects the lungs but can also affect other organs such as the brain or kidneys; may be characterized by a persistent cough, night sweats, headache, weight loss, hemoptysis, or chest pain.

tubo-ovarian abscess An infectious mass growing within the ovaries and fallopian tubes.

tubules Sections of the kidney where the filtration of wastes, electrolytes, and water is controlled.

tunica adventitia The outer layer of tissue of a blood vessel wall, composed of elastic and fibrous connective tissue.

tunica intima The smooth, thin, inner lining of a blood vessel.

tunica media The middle and thickest layer of tissue of a blood vessel wall, composed of elastic tissue and smooth muscle cells that allow the vessel to expand or contract in response to changes in blood pressure and tissue demand.

tunnel vision Dangerous situation when a paramedic becomes so completely involved with prehospital care that he or she fails to see the possibility of physical harm to the patient or other care providers.

turbinates Three bony shelves that protrude from the lateral walls of the nasal cavity and extend into the nasal passageway, parallel to the nasal floor; serve to increase the surface area of the nasal mucosa, thereby improving the processes of warming, filtering, and humidification of inhaled air.

turgor Loss of elasticity in the skin.

twisting injuries Injuries that commonly occur during athletic activities in which an extremity rotates around a planted foot or hand.

tympanic membrane The eardrum; a thin, semitransparent membrane in the middle ear that transmits sound vibrations to the internal ear by means of the auditory ossicles.

type 1 diabetes The type of diabetic disease that usually starts in childhood and requires daily injections of supplemental synthetic insulin to control blood glucose. Sometimes called juvenile or juvenile-onset diabetes.

type 2 diabetes The type of diabetic disease that usually starts in later life and often can be controlled through diet and oral medications. Sometimes called adult-onset diabetes.

Type I Ambulance Conventional, truck-cab chassis with a modular ambulance body that can be transferred to a new chassis as needed.

Type II Ambulance Standard van, forward-control integral cab-body ambulance.

Type III Ambulance Specialty van, forward-control integral cab-body ambulance.

U wave A small flat wave sometimes seen after the T wave and before the next P wave.

ulna The larger bone of the forearm, on the side opposite the thumb.

ulnar artery The artery of the forearm that travels along its medial aspect.

ultrahigh frequency (UHF) band The portion of the radio frequency spectrum between 300 and 3,000 mHz.

umbilical The region of the abdomen surrounding the umbilicus.

umbilical cord The conduit connecting mother to infant via the placenta; contains two arteries and one vein.

umbilical vein Blood vessel in umbilical cord used to administer emergency medications.

unblinded study A type of study in which the subjects are advised of all aspects of the study.

undifferentiated type Schizophrenia that does not fit neatly into another category.

unified command system A command system used in larger incidents in which there is a multiagency response or multiple jurisdictions are involved.

unifocal Arising from a single site.

unintentional injuries Injuries that occur without intent to harm (commonly called accidents). Some examples are motor vehicle collisions, poisonings, drownings, falls, and most burns.

unstable angina Angina pectoris characterized by a changing, unpredictable pattern of pain, which may signal an impending acute myocardial infarction.

upper airway Consists of all anatomical airway structures above the level of the vocal cords.

upper explosive limit (UEL) The concentration of a hazardous material at which there is not enough oxygen to support the combustion in air.

uremia Severe kidney failure resulting in the buildup of waste products within the blood. Eventually brain functions will be impaired.

uremic frost A powdery buildup of uric acid, especially around the face.

ureterostomy The formation of an opening to allow the passage of urine.

ureters A pair of thick-walled, hollow tubes that transport urine from the kidneys to the bladder.

urethra A hollow, tubular structure that drains urine from the bladder, passing it outside of the body.

uricosuric medications The medications designed to lower the uric acid level in the blood by increasing the excretion by the kidneys into the urine.

urinary bladder A hollow, muscular sac in the midline of the lower abdominal area that stores urine until it is released from the body.

urinary tract infections (UTIs) Infections, usually of the lower urinary tract (urethra and bladder), which occur when normal flora bacteria enter the urethra and grow.

urine Liquid waste products filtered out of the body by the urinary system.

urticaria Multiple small, raised areas on the skin that may be one of the warning signs of impending anaphylaxis. Also known as hives.

uterine cavity The interior of the body of the uterus.

uterine inversion A potentially fatal complication of childbirth in which the placenta fails to detach properly and results in the uterus turning inside-out.

uterus A muscular inverted pear-shaped organ, that lies situated between the urinary bladder and the rectum.

uvula A soft-tissue structure that resembles a punching bag; located in the posterior aspect of the oral cavity, at the base of the tongue.

V agent (VX) One of the G agents; it is a clear, oily agent that has no odour and looks like baby oil; it is over 100 times more lethal than sarin and is extremely persistent.

vaccine A suspension of whole (live or inactivated) or fractionated bacteria or viruses that have been made nonpathogenic; given to induce an immune response and prevent disease.

Vacutainer A cylindrical device that attaches to an 18- or 20-gauge sampling needle; accommodates self-sealing blood tubes when obtaining blood samples.

vagina The lower portion of the birth canal, which also serves as a passage for menstrual bleeding and as a receptacle of the penis during sexual intercourse.

vaginal bleeding Bleeding from the vagina.

vaginal yeast infection An infection caused by the fungus *Candida albicans*, in which fungi overpopulate the vagina.

vagus nerve The 10th cranial nerve, the chief mediator of the parasympathetic nervous system.

vallecula An anatomical space, or "pocket," located between the base of the tongue and the epiglottis; an important anatomical landmark for endotracheal intubation.

Valsalva maneuver Forced exhalation against a closed glottis, the effect of which is to stimulate the vagus nerve and, thereby, slow the heart rate.

vapour A gaseous medication form primarily used in operating room anesthesia.

vapour density A measure that compares the hazardous material gas to air; toxic gases that are heavier than air will sink, while vapours that are lighter than air will dissipate and travel with the wind.

vapour hazard An agent that enters the body through the respiratory tract.

vapour pressure The pressure exerted by a vapour when the liquid and vapour states of a material are in equilibrium; this measure changes as a material is heated.

vasa recta A series of peritubular capillaries that surround the loop of Henle, into which water moves after passing through the descending and ascending limbs of the loop of Henle.

vasculitis An inflammation of the blood vessels.

vasoactive amines Substances such as histamine and serotonin that increase vascular permeability.

vasoconstriction Narrowing of a blood vessel, such as with hypoperfusion or cold extremities.

vasodilation Widening of a blood vessel.

vasodilator medications The medications that work on the smooth muscles of the arterioles and/or the veins.

vecuronium A nondepolarizing neuromuscular blocking agent; used to maintain paralysis following succinylcholine-facilitated intubation; also called Norcuron.

veins The blood vessels that carry blood to the heart.

velocity The speed of an object in a given direction.

venae cavae The largest veins of the body; they return blood to the right atrium.

venous thrombosis The development of a stationary blood clot in the venous circulation.

ventilation The process of eliminating carbon dioxide from the blood by diffusion into the alveoli and exhalation from the lungs.

ventilation-perfusion mismatch A pathologic state in which the oxygen entering the lungs is not mixing properly with the blood circulating through the lungs.

ventricles Specialized hollow areas in the brain.

Venturi mask A mask that has a number of interchangeable adapters that draws room air into the mask along with the oxygen flow; allows for the administration of highly specific oxygen concentrations.

venules Very small veins.

vertebral body Anterior weight-bearing structure in the spine made of cancellous bone and surrounded by a layer of hard, compact bone that provides support and stability.

vertical compression A type of injury typically resulting from a direct blow to the crown of the skull or rapid deceleration from a fall through the feet, legs, and pelvis, possibly causing a burst fracture or disk herniation.

vertical shear The type of pelvic fracture that occurs when a massive force displaces the pelvis superiorly.

very high frequency (VHF) band The portion of the radio frequency spectrum between 30 and 150 mHz.

vesicants Blister agents; the primary route of entry for vesicants is through the skin.

vesicle A tiny fluid-filled sac; a small blister.

vestibule A cleft between the labia minora, where the urethral opening (orifice), the vaginal opening (orifice), and the hymen are located.

vials Small glass or plastic bottles that contain medication; may contain single or multiple doses.

vicarious liability Protection whereby the employer is held liable to compensate persons for the harm caused by their employees in the course of their employment.

viral hemorrhagic fevers (VHF) A group of diseases that include the Ebola, Rift Valley, and yellow fever viruses among others. This group of viruses causes the blood in the body to seep out from the tissues and blood vessels.

viral hepatitis An inflammation of the liver produced by one of five distinct forms of the virus—A, B, C, D, and E. The five types differ in transmission but present with the same signs and symptoms.

virulence A measure of the disease-causing ability of a microorganism. Also refers to the ability of an organism to survive outside the living host.

virus A small organism that can only multiply inside a host, such as a human, and cause disease.

visceral pain Crampy, aching pain deep within the body, the source of which is usually hard to pinpoint; common with urologic problems.

visceral pleura Thin membrane that lines the lungs.

visual acuity (VA) The ability or inability to see, and how well one can see.

visual cortex The area in the brain where signals from the optic nerve are converted into visual images.

vitreous humour A jellylike substance found in the posterior compartment of the eye between the lens and the retina.

vocal cords White bands of tough tissue that are the lateral borders of the glottis.

volar Pertaining to the palm or sole; referring to the flexor surfaces of the forearm, wrist, or hand.

volatility Term used to describe how long a chemical agent will stay on a surface before it evapourates.

Volkmann ischemic contracture Deformity of the hand, fingers, and wrist resulting from damage to forearm muscles; develops from muscle ischemia and is associated with compartment syndrome.

voluntary muscle Muscle that can be controlled by a person.

Volutrol A special type of microdrip set that features a 100- or 200-ml calibrated drip chamber; used for fluid regulation in patients prone to circulatory overload, such as pediatric and elderly patients; also called a Buretrol.

Waddell triad A pattern of vehicle-pedestrian injuries in children and people of short stature in which (1) the bumper hits pelvis and femur, (2) the chest and abdomen hit the grille or low hood, and (3) the head strikes the ground.

warm zone The area located between the hot zone and the cold zone at an incident.

Decontamination stations are located in the warm zone.

water reactive A property that indicates that a material will undergo a chemical reaction (for example, explosion) when mixed with water.

water soluble A property that indicates that a material can be dissolved in water.

wavelength The distance in a propagating wave from one point to the corresponding point on the next wave.

waybill A cargo document kept by the conductor of a train.

weapon of mass casualty (WMC) Any agent designed to bring about mass death, casualties, and/or massive damage to property and infrastructure (bridges, tunnels, airports, and seaports); also known as a weapon of mass destruction (WMD).

weapon of mass destruction (WMD) Any agent designed to bring about mass death, casualties, and/or massive damage to property and infrastructure (bridges, tunnels, airports, and seaports); also known as a weapon of mass casualty (WMC).

weaponization The creation of a weapon from a biological agent generally found in nature and that causes disease; the agent is cultivated, synthesized, and/or mutated to maximize the target population's exposure to the germ.

wedges Used to snug loose cribbing.

West Nile virus (WNV) A type of virus that is transmitted by mosquitos, and which usually only causes mild disease in humans, but can cause encephalitis, meningitis, or death. Symptoms, if exhibited, include fever, headache, body rash, and swollen lymph glands.

wheel bounce A vibration, synchronous with road speed that can be felt in the steering wheel.

wheel wobble A common finding at low speeds when a vehicle has a bent wheel.

wheezing The production of whistling sounds during expiration such as occurs in asthma and bronchiolitis.

whiplash An injury to the cervical vertebrae or their supporting ligaments and muscles, usually resulting from sudden acceleration or deceleration.

whistle-tip catheters Soft plastic, nonrigid catheters; also called French catheters.

windchill factor The factor that takes into account the temperature and wind velocity in calculating the effect of a given ambient temperature on living organisms.

withdrawal syndrome A predictable set of signs and symptoms, usually involving altered central nervous system activity, that occurs after the abrupt cessation of a drug or after rapidly decreasing the usual dosage of a drug.

Wolff-Parkinson-White (WPW) syndrome A syndrome characterized by short P-R intervals, delta waves, nonspecific ST-T wave changes, and paroxysmal episodes of tachycardia caused by the presence of an accessory pathway.

working diagnosis The overall initial impression that determines the priority for patient prehospital care; based on the patient's surroundings, the mechanism or injury, signs and symptoms, and the chief complaint.

xanthines A classification of medications that affect the respiratory smooth muscle and that relax bronchiole smooth muscles, stimulate cardiac muscle, and stimulate the central nervous system.

xyphoid process An inferior segment of the sternum often used as a landmark for CPR.

years of potential life lost A way of measuring and comparing the overall impact of deaths resulting from different causes. It is calculated based on a fixed age minus the age at death. Usually the fixed age is 65 or 70 or the life expectancy of the group in question.

zone of coagulation The reddened area surrounding the leathery and sometimes charred tissue that has sustained a full-thickness burn.

zone of hyperemia In a thermal burn, the area that is least affected by the burn injury.

zone of stasis The peripheral area surrounding the zone of coagulation that has decreased blood flow and inflammation. This area can undergo necrosis within 24 to 48 hours after the injury, particularly if perfusion is compromised due to burn shock.

zygomatic arch The bone that extends along the front of the skull below the orbit.

Index

References to figures and tables are denoted by f and t following page numbers.

Credits

Chapter 1
Opener Courtesy of Multimedia Group/Toronto EMS; 1-3 © National Library of Medicine; 1-4 Courtesy of Eugene L. Nagel and the Miami Fire Department; 1-7 © Glen E. Ellman; 1-8 © Michael Ledray/ShutterStock, Inc; 1-10 (inset) © Dan Myers; 1-11 Courtesy of Captain David Jackson, Saginaw Township Fire Department; 1-14 © Design Pics Inc/Alamy Images.

Chapter 2
Opener © Mark C. Ide; 2-2A Source: Eating Well with Canada's Food Guide (2007), http://www.hc-sc.gc.ca/fn-an/food-guide-aliment/index-eng.php, Health Canada. Reproduced with the permission of the Minister of Public Works and Government Services Canada, 2009; 2-2B © Monika Adamczyk/ShutterStock, Inc; 2-4 © LiquidLibrary; 2-9 Courtesy of Island Photography/US Air Force; 2-11 © David Buffington/Photodisc/Getty Images; 2-13 © Eddie M. Sperling; 2-15 © Mike Schrengohst/ShutterStock, Inc; 2-18 © Glen E. Ellman; 2-21 © Peter Jones/Reuters; 2-24 Courtesy of Moldex-Metric, Inc (www.moldex.com); 2-26 © LM Otero/AP Photos; 2-27 © Steven Townsend/Code 3 Images.

Chapter 3
Opener Courtesy of Captain David Jackson, Saginaw Township Fire Department; 3-1 © Alison Grippo/ShutterStock, Inc; 3-2 © Steven Townsend/Code 3 Images; 3-3 (left) © Ryan McVay/Photodisc/Getty Images; 3-3 (right) © Carolyn Brule/ShutterStock, Inc; 3-5 © Steven Pepple/ShutterStock, Inc; 3-6A Courtesy of Henry Pollak; 3-6B © Vladimir Korostyshevskiy/ShutterStock, Inc; 3-6C Courtesy of Captain David Jackson, Saginaw Township Fire Department; 3-7 (top left) © Cristina Fumi/ShutterStock, Inc; 3-7 (top right) © Photos.com; 3-7 (bottom) © Andreas Nilsson/ShutterStock, Inc; 3-9 © Craig Jackson/Inthe DarkPhotography.com; 3-10 © SuperStock/age footstock; 3-11 © Steven Townsend/Code 3 Images; 3-12 © Mark Humphrey/AP Photos; Table 3-1 Source: 'Leading Causes of Death and Hospitalization in Canada', Table 1: Leading causes of death, males and females combined, http://www.phac-aspc.gc.ca/publicat/lcd-pcd97/index-eng.php, Public Health Agency of Canada, 2004. Reproduced with the permission of the Minister of Public Works and Government Services Canada, 2009.

Chapter 4
Opener © AioK/ShutterStock, Inc; 4-1 © Brand X Pictures/Creatas; 4-3 © Dan Myers; 4-4 © Photodisc; 4-10 Courtesy of LifeScan, Inc; 4-14 © Brian Snyder/Reuters/Landov.

Chapter 5
5-2 Courtesy of Dr. Russell D. MacDonald; 5-6 Do Not Resuscitate Confirmation Form © Queen's Printer for Ontario, 2008. Reproduced with permission; 5-8 © UPI/HO/Landov; 5-9 © The Express Times/AP Photos.

Chapter 6
Opener © National Cancer Institute/Photodisc/Getty Images; 6-11A&B Courtesy of Leonard V. Crowley, MD, Century College; 6-13B Courtesy of Rocky Mountain Laboratory, NIAID, NIH; 6-16A&B, 6-19, 6-20A&B, 6-22A&B Courtesy of Leonard V. Crowley, MD, Century College.

Chapter 7
7-2A © Stephen Aaron Rees/ShutterStock, Inc; 7-2B © Photos.com; 7-2C Courtesy of Yellowstone National Park; 7-2D Courtesy of Linda Bartlett/National Cancer Institute; 7-7 Courtesy of Schwarz Pharma AG. Used with permission.

Chapter 8
8-31 Courtesy of Pyng Medical Corporation; 8-32 Courtesy of Vidacare Corporation; 8-33&34 Used with permission of PerSys Medical and Bound Tree Medical; 8-38 © ajt/ShutterStock, Inc; 8-56&57 Courtesy of Baxter International, Inc; 8-59 Courtesy of Wolfe Tory Medical, Inc; Skill Drill 8-13 Courtesy of Dr. Russell D. MacDonald.

Chapter 9
Opener © Photodisc; 9-1 © Johanna Goodyear/ShutterStock, Inc; 9-5 © Scott Milless/ShutterStock, Inc; 9-6 © EML/ShutterStock, Inc; 9-7 © Maxim Bolotnikov/ShutterStock, Inc; 9-8 © GeoTrac/Alamy Images; 9-9 © Trout55/ShutterStock, Inc; 9-10 © Jamie Wilson/ShutterStock, Inc; 9-11 © SW Productions/Jupiterimages; 9-13 © Rubberball Productions; 9-14 © Photodisc; 9-15 © Blend Images/Alamy Images; 9-16, 9-20 © Photodisc.

Chapter 10
10-3 © Keith Cullom; 10-5 © Glen E. Ellman; 10-6 © Eddie M. Sperling; 10-8 © Craig Jackson/Inthe DarkPhotography.com.

Chapter 11
11-24 HELiOS® Marathon™ portable oxygen unit. Courtesy of Nellcor Puritan Bennett in affiliation with Tyco Healthcare; 11-56, 11-59, 11-60–62, 11-69A&B Courtesy of Marianne Gausche-Hill, MD, FACEP, FAAP; 11-73 Courtesy of King Systems. Used with permission; 11-79–82 Courtesy of Dr. Russell D. MacDonald; 11-92 © Eddie M. Sperling.

Chapter 12
12-1 © Mark C. Ide; 12-5 © Glen E. Ellman; 12-11 © Jack Dagley Photography/ShutterStock, Inc.

Chapter 13
13-7 © Denis Pepin/ShutterStock, Inc; 13-8 © WizData, Inc/ShutterStock, Inc; 13-9 © Kenneth Chelette/ShutterStock, Inc; 13-12 Courtesy of Ronald Dieckmann, MD; 13-14 © Germán Ariel Berra/ShutterStock, Inc; 13-31 © Dr. P. Marazzi/Photo Researchers, Inc.

Chapter 14
Opener © VStock/Alamy Images; 14-2 © Adam Alberti, NJFirePictures.com; 14-3 Courtesy of Tempe Fire Department; 14-4 © Paul Chiasson, CP/AP Photos; 14-5 Courtesy of James Tourtellotte/U.S. Customs and Border Protection; 14-8A © Mark C. Ide; 14-8B © Corbis; 14-8D © Dan Myers; 14-8E © Jack Dagley Photography/ShutterStock, Inc; 14-8F © Larry St. Pierre/ShutterStock, Inc; 14-8G © micheal ledray/ShutterStock, Inc; 14-10 © Thinkstock/Getty Images; 14-12 © E.M. Singletary, MD. Used with permission.

Chapter 15
Opener © Mike Meadows/AP Photos; 15-1 © Mark C. Ide; 15-4 © Peter Willott, The St. Augustine Record/AP Photos; 15-6, 15-8 © Craig Jackson/IntheDark Photography.com; 15-12 © Mark C. Ide.

Chapter 16
16-12 Courtesy of ZOLL Data Systems, Inc.

Chapter 17
17-1 © Shout Pictures/Custom Medical Stock Photo; 17-2 © Dan Myers; 17-3 Courtesy of Mr. Ron Tracey; 17-5 © Terry Dickson, Florida Times-Union/AP Photos; 17-6 © Dan Myers; 17-8 Courtesy of Captain David Jackson, Saginaw Township Fire Department; 17-12 © Dan Myers; 17-13 © Dennis Wetherhold, Jr; 17-14 © Dan Myers; 17-16 © Michael Ledray/ShutterStock, Inc; 17-20A © Charles Stewart & Associates; 17-20B © D. Willoughby/Custom Medical Stock Photography.

Chapter 18
Opener © Glen E. Ellman; 18-4 © Mark C. Ide; 18-5 Courtesy of David Clark Company Incorporated; 18-7 © SPL/Photo Researchers, Inc.

Chapter 19
Opener Courtesy of Moose Jaw Police Service; 19-3 Courtesy of Rhonda Beck; 19-5 (left) © English/Custom Medical Stock Photo; 19-6 (left) © E.M. Singletary, MD. Used with permission; 19-7 © Custom Medical Stock Photo; 19-9 © E.M. Singletary, MD. Used with permission; 19-10 © Mark C. Ide; 19-11 Courtesy of FEMA; 19-12 © Zoom 77/AP Photos; 19-14 Courtesy of Matthew J. Belan, MD; 19-17 Combat Application Tourniquet® (C-A-T®) photo courtesy of North American Rescue Products, Inc; 19-19 © E.M. Singletary, MD. Used with permission.

Chapter 20
Opener © Glen E. Ellman; 20-1 © Dale A. Stock/ShutterStock, Inc; 20-2 © Dr. P. Marazzi/Photo Researchers, Inc; 20-6 © J. Yakwichuk/Custom Medical Stock Photo; 20-7 Courtesy of Health Resources and Services Administration, Maternal and Child Health Bureau, Emergency Medical Services for Children Program; 20-8 © Kevin Frayer/AP Photos; 20-11A&B © Charles Stewart & Associates; 20-13A © Amy Walters/ShutterStock, Inc; 20-13B © E.M. Singletary, MD. Used with permission; 20-16 Courtesy of Water-Jel® Technologies; 20-20 © Charles Stewart & Associates.

Chapter 21
Opener © E.M. Singletary, MD. Used with permission; 21-25 © Eddie M. Sperling; 21-29 Courtesy of John T. Halgren, MD, University of Nebraska Medical Center; 21-41 © E.M. Singletary, MD. Used with permission; 21-54 © Joe Gough/ShutterStock, Inc.

Chapter 22
22-10 Courtesy of Thomas EMS; 22-14 © Reuters Photographer/Reuters.

Chapter 23
Opener © PHT/Photo Researchers, Inc; 23-1 © Shout Pictures/Custom Medical Stock Photo; 23-13 © Charles Stewart & Associates; 23-18 © SIU Bio Med Comm./Custom Medical Stock Photo.

Chapter 24
Opener © Charles Stewart & Associates; 24-9 © Dr. P. Marazzi/Photo Researchers, Inc; 24-11 © Custom Medical Stock Photo.

Chapter 25
Opener © Charles Stewart & Associates; 25-9A&B Courtesy of International Osteoporosis Foundation; 25-19 © Charles Stewart & Associates; 25-34 © Custom Medical Stock Photo; 25-35 Courtesy of Anand M. Murthi, MD.

Chapter 26
26-3 © E.M. Singletary, MD. Used with permission; 26-6 Courtesy of The Milton J. Dance, Jr. Head and Neck Rehabilitation Center (www.gbmc.org/voice); 26-7 © Eddie M. Sperling; 26-8 (inset) © David M. Martin, MD/Photo Researchers, Inc; 26-9 (inset) © Dr. Kessel & Dr. Kardon/Tissue & Organs/Visuals Unlimited; 26-17 Courtesy of Health Resources and Services Administration, Maternal and Child Health Bureau, Emergency Medical Services for Children Program; 26-18 © Logical Images/Custom Medical Stock Photo; 26-19 © Uschi Hering/ShutterStock, Inc; 26-20B Courtesy of Stuart Mirvis, MD; 26-22 © Mediscan/Visuals Unlimited; 26-23 © Jones and Bartlett Publishers. Sprague-Rappaport Stethoscope courtesy of MDF Instruments USA, Inc; 26-27A Courtesy of Nonin Medical, Inc; 26-28 Image of Masimo Rad-57® Pulse CO-Oximeter™ is © 2009 Masimo Corporation. All rights reserved. Masimo, Rad-57, and Pulse CO-Oximeter are trademarks of Masimo Corporation; 26-30 Courtesy of Marianne Gausche-Hill, MD, FACEP, FAAP; 26-31A LIFEPAK® defibrillator/monitor. Courtesy of